Get everything in this book

PLUS PHOTOS at

www.IdentADrug.com

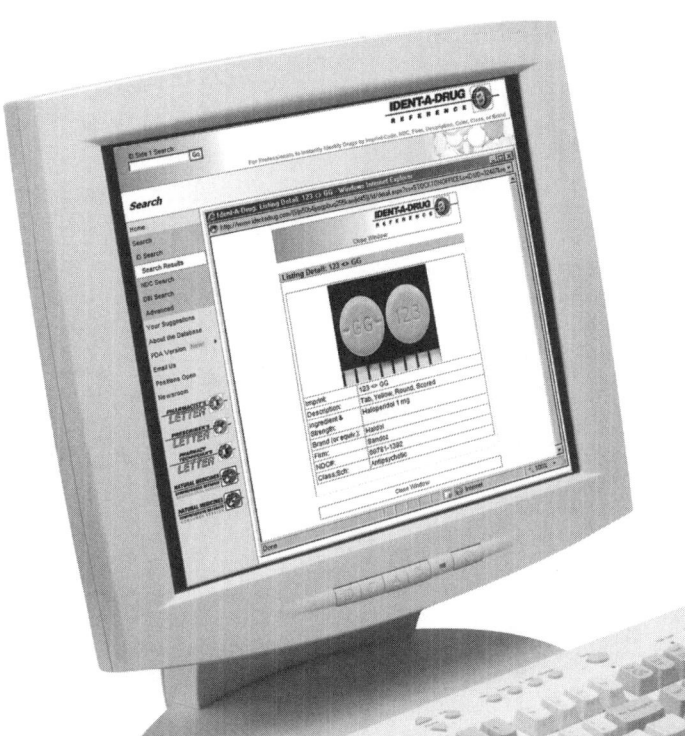

Get individual access for only $39 per year...

or ask about a multi-user license for your whole organization.

Further details and order forms are located on the last pages of this book.

- **Updated Daily**
  New products added immediately.

- **Most comprehensive database of its kind**

- **Easy, Fast Searching**
  Advanced search features give you instant answers.

- **NDC Numbers and DEA Classifications**

- **Drug Identification Numbers (DIN)**
  For identifying Canadian drugs

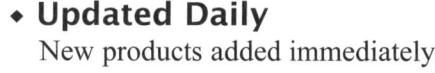

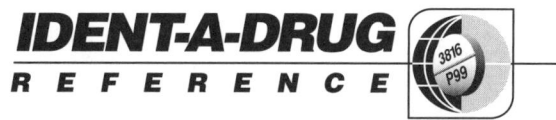

For instant access, order online at IdentADrug.com
Call: (209) 472-2240 ◆ Fax: (209) 472-2249
Email: mail@IdentADrug.com
3120 W. March Lane, PO Box 8190, Stockton, CA 95208

For Tablet and Capsule Identification

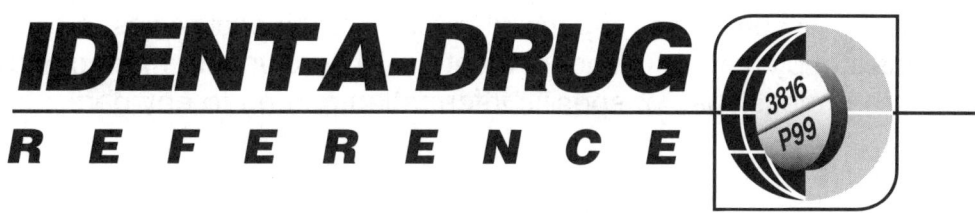

2011 Edition

Published by Therapeutic Research Center

3120 W. March Lane • PO Box 8190 • Stockton CA 95208
Phone (209) 472-2240 • Fax (209) 472-2249
mail@IdentADrug.com • IdentADrug.com

Compiled by the Editors of:

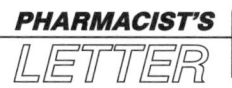   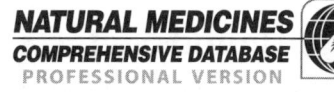 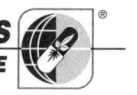   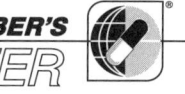

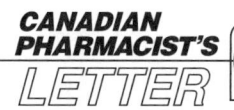   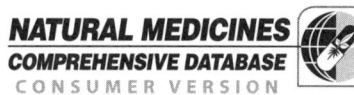   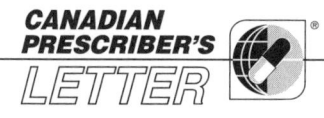

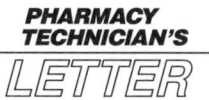   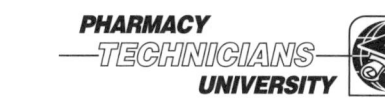   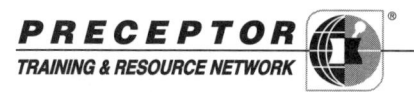

Copyright © 2010 by Therapeutic Research Center
All rights reserved. No part of this book may be reproduced or transmitted in any form or by any means electronic or mechanical, including photocopying, recording, scanning, or by any information storage or retrieval system without written permission from the publisher.

The authors have attempted to compile a comprehensive and accurate reference. The publisher assumes no responsibility for errors, inaccuracies, omissions, or any inconsistency herein. Readers must use their own judgment or consult an appropriate professional for specific information related to any particular medical situation.

For information on additional copies of this edition, or access to the Web version, mobile version, or the PDA version of *Ident-A-Drug Reference,* use the order form in the back of the book or contact:

Therapeutic Research Center, PO Box 8190, Stockton, CA 95208
TEL: 209-472-2240 • FAX: 209-472-2249
E-MAIL: mail@IdentADrug.com • IdentADrug.com

We wish to recognize some of the people who created this reference:

Stephanie Feilzer, Database Coordinator
Alicia Calvillo, Product Coordinator
Adam Kaye, Pharm.D., FASCP
Sean D. Tomlinson, Pharm.D.
Linda Hneitina, Editorial Quality Manager
Henry Gardiner, Marketing Associate

Printed in the United States of America
ISBN-13: 978-0-9788205-8-9

Preface

Over 100,000 patients die annually in North America due to medical errors, and over 7,000 die due to medication errors. Some medication errors result from a patient taking the wrong drug.

All pharmaceutical capsules and tablets are imprinted with identification codes. The *Ident-A-Drug Reference* is organized by these codes so that drug products can be correctly identified.

The *Ident-A-Drug Reference* includes brand name and generic products from the United States and Canada. It lists the code imprinted on the front and the back of the tablet or capsule. It describes each product's color, shape, graphics, imprint codes, etc., and gives the product's ingredients and the strength of each ingredient. For U.S. products, *Ident-A-Drug Reference* also lists the National Drug Code (NDC) and drug class. If the drug is a narcotic or in one of the schedules determined by the Drug Enforcement Administration (DEA), the schedule is also given. For Canadian products, all relevant information is provided, including the Health Canada Drug Identification Number (DIN).

The web and PDA versions are even more powerful than this printed version. IdentADrug.com contains everything in this book plus photos of the tablets and capsules. It's updated constantly as new drugs are introduced.

Pharmacists, physicians, and nurses use the *Reference* to identify tablets and capsules when a patient is admitted to a hospital, long-term care facility, or intermediate-care facility. It is especially important to identify the medication in the patient's possession when they are admitted.

Pharmacists use the *Reference* to help patients refill prescriptions, or to communicate with physician offices about refills. It can also be used to put identification information on prescription labels.

Emergency medical personnel often use this information. The medication found on a patient is sometimes the only clue to that person's medical history or disease states.

Law enforcement officers find the *Reference* extremely useful as a quick and easy way to identify drugs found on a person.

Parents and school officials also use *Ident-A-Drug* to identify medications when needed.

One of the fastest growing groups of *Ident-A-Drug Reference* users is consumers who need to check their own medications or medications of loved ones. Medication identifications frequently change as patients obtain medications from different manufacturers, or as insurance companies and managed care companies require patients to switch medications or pharmacies.

The *Ident-A-Drug Reference* is a unique resource dedicated to promoting health and well-being by accurately identifying thousands of drug products. Stephanie Feilzer and her Editorial Team have done society a tremendous service by providing this easy-to-use and constantly updated *Reference*. The publisher encourages any user of the *Reference* who is not a health professional to seek advice from an appropriate professional regarding drug or medical questions.

If you ever have difficulty locating a product in this book or on IdentADrug.com, feel free to contact us. We always look forward to helping you and making this *Reference* even more useful.

Jeff M. Jellin, Pharm.D.
Editor-in-Chief
Pharmacist's Letter, Prescriber's Letter, and *Natural Medicines Comprehensive Database*
IdentADrug.com

How to Use *IDENT-A-DRUG Reference*

Guidelines for Use:
To use *Ident-A-Drug Reference*, start with the code that's imprinted on either side of the oral medication. Use the following rules:
- First look up the number or letter that is farthest to the left, then the number or letter next to it, etc.
- The entries are listed in typical dictionary or phonebook order. For example, 469 is followed by 47, followed by 471, followed by 4711, followed by 48, etc.
- Letters follow numbers. For example, 469 would be followed by 46A. 999999 would be followed by A.
- Only letters and numbers are listed in the imprint column. When looking up a medication, ignore any spaces, dashes, slashes, periods, or other symbols. Logos are also not included in the imprint column. For example, if you're trying to find information on a tablet that's imprinted 345 33, look up 34533. For 0.5 look up 05. For 45/GG look up 45GG. For a Logo 25, look up 25. For imprints that do contain symbols other than numbers and letters, a more detailed description will be given in the Description column.
- Oral medications that have an imprint on the front and back are listed as two separate listings. In *Ident-A-Drug*, a symbol that looks like <> separates the code that is imprinted on the front of the tablet, and the code that is imprinted on the back of the tablet. You should be able to find the medication by looking up either side and then verifying the alternate side's information.

Description of Columns:

Imprint: This column contains the numerical and alphabetical imprints on oral medications. Other symbols are omitted, i.e. dashes, periods, slashes, logos, etc. If a tablet has imprints on both sides, the information is listed, separated by a <>. Entries that include the front-back symbol (<>) are listed twice in the *Reference*; one listing for the imprint on the front and one listing for the imprint on the back.

Description: This column contains a physical description of the oral medication. The information occurs in the following order: Tab (for Tablet) or Cap (for Capsule), Color, Shape (if a tablet), and other information which may include scoring, embossing, debossing, etc. Clarification of the imprint information by including dashes, slashes, decimals, spaces, and logo information is also included in the Description column.

Ingredient & Strength: This column contains a listing of the active ingredients and their amounts.

Brand (Or Equiv.) by Firm: This column lists the brand name and/or manufacturer or distributor of a product. For generic drugs, the equivalent brand name is given in this column.

NDC#: The NDC number is given in the following format: 00000-0000. The third segment of the NDC number, the packaging information, is omitted because it is not necessary for the identification of an oral medication by imprint. Some older drugs or drugs no longer manufactured may not have an NDC# listed. Canadian drugs are listed in this column. If Canadian drugs have an accompanying DIN, it is listed in this column.

Class; Schedule: This column contains the class of drug and the schedule assigned by the Drug Enforcement Agency (DEA) if the medication is a controlled substance. This schedule is shown in the following format: Schedule 2 is listed as C II, Schedule 3 as C III, and so forth. Canadian products do not utilize a controlled substance rating, even if they are a controlled substance in the United States.

If you find a tablet or capsule that is not listed in *Ident-A-Drug Reference*, or if you find anything that you think should be changed, please alert the publisher. It's possible that a new drug has come on the market after the current print version of the book. This information may be available on our website, **IdentADrug.com**, which is updated daily.

ID FRONT <> BACK	DESCRIPTION FRONT <> BACK	INGREDIENT & STRENGTH	BRAND (or Generic Equiv.) by FIRM	NDC#	CLASS; SCH.
0014 <> 20	Tab, Yellow, Rectangular	Pravastatin Sodium 20 mg	Pravachol by Watson	00591-0014	Antihyperlipidemic
0016 <> 40	Tab, Green, Rounded Rectangle	Pravastatin Sodium 40 mg	Pravachol by Watson	00591-0016	Antihyperlipidemic
002 <> A	Tab, Blue, Round, Scored	Dextromethorphan 60 mg, Guaifenesin 1200 mg	Aquatab DM by Adams	63824-0002	Cold Remedy
002 <> AMIDE	Tab, Orange, Pink & Purple, Pillow Shaped, Chewable	Ascorbic Acid 30 mg, Sodium Ascorbate 33 mg, Sodium Fluoride, Vitamin A Acetate, Vitamin D 400 Units	Tri Vitamin Fluoride by Schein	00364-0846	Vitamin
002 <> AMIDE	Tab, Orange, Pink & Purple, Pillow Shaped, Chewable	Ascorbic Acid 30 mg, Sodium Ascorbate 33 mg, Sodium Fluoride, Vitamin A Acetate, Vitamin D 400 Units	Tri Vitamin Fluoride by Major	00904-7810	Vitamin
0025 <> PHARMICS	Tab, 00 over 25	Acetaminophen 500 mg, Hydrocodone Bitartrate 5 mg	Vicodin by Quality Care	60346-0442	Analgesic; C III
0027V	Tab, White, Round	Acetaminophen 325 mg	Tylenol by Qualitest	00603-0263	Analgesic
0029V	Tab, White, Oblong	Acetaminophen 500 mg	Tylenol Ex Strength by Qualitest	00603-0265	Analgesic
003 <> RPC25	Tab, White, Round, Scored, RPC over 2.5	Midodrine HCl 2.5 mg	Amatine by Shire	Canadian DIN 01934392	Antihypotensive
003 <> RPC25	Tab, White, Round, Scored, RPC over 2.5	Midodrine HCl 2.5 mg	ProAmatine by Roberts	54092-0003	Antihypotensive
003 <> RPC25	Tab, White, Round, Scored, RPC over 2.5	Midodrine HCl 2.5 mg	ProAmatine by Nycomed	57585-0103	Antihypotensive
0030 <> G	Tab, White to Off-White, Round, Film Coated, G <> 00 / 30	Ranitidine HCl 150 mg	Zantac by Genpharm	15330-0030	Gastrointestinal
0030 <> G	Tab, Off-White, Film Coated, 00 over 30	Ranitidine HCl 168 mg	Zantac by Genpharm	55567-0030	Gastrointestinal
0031 <> G	Tab, Off-White, Film Coated, 00 over 31	Ranitidine HCl 336 mg	Zantac by Genpharm	55567-0031	Gastrointestinal
0031 <> G	Tab, White to Off-White, Cap Shaped, Film Coated	Ranitidine HCl 300 mg	Zantac by Genpharm	15330-0031	Gastrointestinal
0031V	Tab, White, Round	Acetaminophen 500 mg		00603-0268	Analgesic
0034	Tab	Acetaminophen 300 mg, Codeine Phosphate 60 mg	Tylenol Ex Strength by Qualitest	55289-0916	Analgesic; C III
0037 <> G	Tab, Blue, Oval	Acyclovir 800 mg	Tylenol w/ Codeine by PDRX	55567-0037	Antiviral
0037 <> G	Tab, Blue, Oval	Acyclovir 800 mg	Zovirax by Genpharm	49884-0567	Antiviral
0037 <> G	Tab, Blue, Oval	Acyclovir 800 mg	Zovirax by Par		
0370681	Tab, Mauve, Cap Shaped, Scored	Carbetapentane Tannate 60 mg, Chlorpheniramine Tannate 5 mg	Tussi-12 S by Mallinckrodt	00406-8867	Cold Remedy
004 <> ACF	Tab, White to Off-White, Round, A over CF	Candesartan Cilexetil 4 mg	Atacand by AstraZeneca	Canadian DIN 02239090	Antihypertensive
004 <> ACF	Tab, White to Off-White, Round, A over CF	Candesartan Cilexetil 4 mg	Atacand by AstraZeneca	17228-0018	Antihypertensive
004 <> ACF	Tab, White to Off-White, Round, A over CF	Candesartan Cilexetil 4 mg	Atacand by AstraZeneca	00186-0004	Antihypertensive
004 <> RPC5	Tab, Orange, Round, Scored, RPC over 5	Midodrine HCl 5 mg	Amatine by Shire	Canadian DIN 01934406	Antihypotensive
004 <> RPC5	Tab, Orange, Round, Scored, RPC over 5	Midodrine HCl 5 mg	ProAmatine by Roberts	54092-0004	Antihypotensive
004 <> RPC5	Tab, Orange, Round, Scored, RPC over 5	Midodrine HCl 5 mg	ProAmatine by Nycomed	57585-0104	Antihypotensive
004 <> RPC50	Tab, Orange, Round, Scored, RPC over 5.0 <> 004	Midodrine HCl 5 mg	ProAmatine by Shire	54092-0004	Antihypotensive
0048V	Tab, Maroon, Round	Phenazopyridine HCl 95 mg	AZO-Standard by Qualitest	00603-0048	Urinary Analgesic
0053	Tab, White, Round	Niacin 500 mg	Nicolar by Moore		Vitamin
0053 <> G	Tab, White, Oval, Scored, Film Coated	Oxaprozin 600 mg	Daypro by Par	49884-0723	NSAID
0057	Cap, Maroon, Oval, Soft Gel	Docusate Sodium 100 mg, Casanthranol 30 mg	Peri-Colace by UDL	51079-0039 Discontinued	Laxative
0057	Cap, Maroon, Oval, Soft Gel	Docusate Sodium 100 mg, Casanthranol 30 mg	Peri-Colace by Sandoz by Sovereign	00781-2653	Laxative
0058MAJOR	Cap	Chlorpheniramine Maleate 8 mg, Pseudoephedrine HCl 120 mg		58716-0014	Cold Remedy
005R	Tab, Coated	Acetaminophen 650 mg, Propoxyphene Napsylate 100 mg	Darvocet-N 100 by Med Pro	53978-5013	Analgesic; C IV
006 <> ADAMS	Tab, Yellow, Oblong, Scored	Pseudoephedrine HCl 120 mg, Methscopolamine Nitrate 2.5 mg	Allerx-D by Adams	63824-0006	Cold Remedy
006 <> COP	Tab, Pink, Round	Sodium Fluoride 1 mg	Luride by Colgate	00126-0006	Element
006 <> HOYT	Tab, Pink, Chewable	Sodium Fluoride 2.2 mg	Luride Cherry by Colgate	00126-0006	Element
00631390	Tab, Peach, Round, 0063 / 1390	Hydralazine 25 mg, Hydrochlorothiazide 15 mg, Reserpine 0.1 mg	Ser-Ap-Es by Reid-Rowell		Antihypertensive; Diuretic
007 <> ADAMS	Tab, Blue, Oval, Scored	Chlorpheniramine Maleate 8 mg, Methscopolamine Nitrate 2.5 mg	Allerx by Adams	63824-0067	Cold Remedy
007 <> RPC10	Tab, Blue, Round, Scored, RPC over 10	Midodrine HCl 10 mg	ProAmatine by Roberts	54092-0007	Antihypotensive
008 <> ACG	Tab, Light Pink, Round, A over CG	Candesartan Cilexetil 8 mg	Atacand by AstraZeneca	Canadian DIN 02239091	Antihypertensive
008 <> ACG	Tab, Light Pink, Round, A over CG	Candesartan Cilexetil 8 mg	Atacand by AstraZeneca	00186-0008	Antihypertensive

ID FRONT <> BACK	DESCRIPTION FRONT <> BACK	INGREDIENT & STRENGTH	BRAND (or Generic Equiv.) by FIRM	NDC#	CLASS; SCH.
008 <> ACG	Tab, Light Pink, Round, A over CG	Candesartan Cilexetil 8 mg	Atacand by AstraZeneca	17228-0017	Antihypertensive
0088 <> 018	Tab, Peach, Oblong, Film Coated	Fexofenadine HCl 180 mg	Allegra by Aventis	00088-1109	Antihistamine
0088 <> 03	Tab, Peach, Oblong, Film Coated	Fexofenadine HCl 30 mg	Allegra by Aventis	00088-1106	Antihistamine
0088 <> 06	Tab, Peach, Oblong, Film Coated	Fexofenadine HCl 60 mg	Allegra by Aventis	00088-1107	Antihistamine
009 <> AP	Tab, Orange, Round, Scored, Chewable, p inside A	Aspirin 81 mg	Bayer Aspirin-Children by Qualitest	00603-0024	Analgesic
009 <> AP	Tab, Orange, Round, Scored, Chewable, p inside A	Aspirin 81 mg	Bayer Aspirin-Children by Rugby	00536-3297	Analgesic
009 <> DURA	Tab, Light Blue	Guaifenesin 600 mg	Robitussin by Anabolic	00722-6139	Expectorant
00951674	Cap, Green	Acetaminophen 325 mg, Butalbital 50 mg, Caffeine 40 mg	Fioricet by Blansett	51674-0009	Analgesic
01	Tab, White, Round, 0.1	Desmopressin Acetate 0.1 mg	DDAVP by Ferring	Canadian	Antidiuretic
01	Tab, White, Oval, Uncoated	Desmopressin Acetate 0.1 mg.	Minirin by Ferring	Canadian DIN 02246500	Antidiuretic
01 <> 36AV	Tab, White, Oval, Scored, 0.1 <> 36 over AV	Desmopressin Acetate 0.1 mg	DDAVP by Aventis	00075-0016	Antidiuretic
01 <> A	Tab, Light Pink, Round, Film Coated	Simvastatin 10 mg	Zocor by Aurobindo	65862-0051	Antihyperlipidemic
01 <> CBP	Tab, Yellow, Oblong, Scored, CBP <> / 01	Pseudoephedrine HCl 120 mg, Methscopolamine 2.5 mg	RhinaClear by Amneal	65162-0550	Cold Remedy
01 <> DAN5609	Tab, White, Pentagonal, Scored, 0.1 <> Dan over 5609	Clonidine HCl 0.1 mg	Catapres by Watson	00591-5609	Antihypertensive
01 <> E	Tab, White to Off-White, Oval, Film Coated	Carvedilol 3.125 mg	Coreg by Aurobindo	65862-0142	Antihypertensive
01 <> NOVO	Tab, White, Round, No/Vo/0.1	Clonidine HCl 0.1 mg	Catapres by Novopharm	Canadian DIN 02046121	Antihypertensive
010	Cap, Barr Logo	Tetracycline HCl 500 mg	Sumycin by Apotheca	12634-0162	Antibiotic
010	Cap, Barr Logo	Tetracycline HCl 500 mg	Sumycin by Major	00904-2407	Antibiotic
010	Tab, Orange, Diamond Shaped, Scored	Estropipate 0.75 mg	by Duramed	51285-0010	Hormone
0100	Cap, Red	Amantadine HCl 100 mg	Symmetrel by Pharmascience	Canadian	Antiviral
0100	Tab, White	Fluoride 3.75 mg, Calcium 145 mg	by Mericon	00394-0100	Mineral
0100	Cap, Yellow	Vitamin A Palmitate 25,000 Units	by Richlyn		Vitamin
0101	Cap, Yellow	Vitamin A Natural 25,000 Units	by Richlyn		Vitamin
0102	Cap, Red	Vitamin A Palmitate 50,000 Units	by Richlyn		Vitamin
0104	Cap, Yellow	Vitamin A Solubilized 25,000 Units	by Richlyn		Vitamin
0105	Cap, Red	Fluoride 3 mg, Calcium 250 mg	Monocal by Mericon		Mineral
0105	Tab, White, 0105/Mericon Logo				
0109	Cap, Yellow	Vitamin A Solubilized 50,000 Units	by Richlyn		Vitamin
011	Tab, Pink, Round, Schering Logo 011	Betamethasone 0.6 mg	Celestone by Schering	00085-0011	Steroid
0111	Tab, White, Round	Acetaminophen 325 mg, Butalbital 50 mg, Caffeine 40 mg	Fioricet by D M Graham		Analgesic
0111V	Tab, White, Round	Dimenhydrinate 50 mg	Dramamine by Qualitest	00603-3327	Antiemetic
0115 <> 7025	Tab, Light Orange, Compressed	Hyoscyamine Sulfate 0.375 mg	Levsin by Global	00115-7025	Gastrointestinal
0115 <> 7026	Tab, White, Round	Oxycodone HCl 5 mg	OxyContin by Global	00115-7026	Analgesic; C II
0115 <> 7029	Tab, Tan, Round	Pancrelipase 8000 Units	Creon 8 by Global	00115-7029	Gastrointestinal
01151111	Cap	Diphenhydramine HCl 50 mg	by Ivax	00182-0135	Antihistamine
01151142	Cap, Pink	Ephedrine Sulfate 0.75 g	by Richlyn		Antiasthmatic
01151300	Cap, Yellow	Oxytetracycline 250 mg	Terramycin by Richlyn		Antibiotic
01151398	Cap, Orange & Yellow	Tetracycline HCl 100 mg	Achromycin V by Richlyn		Antibiotic
01151400	Cap, Orange & Yellow	Tetracycline HCl 250 mg	Achromycin V by Richlyn		Antibiotic
01151402	Cap, Black & Yellow	Tetracycline HCl 500 mg	Achromycin V by Richlyn		Antibiotic
01151405	Cap, Black & Yellow	Tetracycline HCl 250 mg	Achromycin V by Richlyn		Antibiotic
01152150	Tab, White, Round	Aminophylline 100 mg	Aminophylline by Richlyn		Antiasthmatic
01152151	Tab, Beige, Round	Aminophylline 100 mg	Aminophylline by Richlyn		Antiasthmatic
01152158	Tab, White, Round	Aminophylline 200 mg	Aminophylline by Richlyn		Antiasthmatic

ID FRONT <> BACK	DESCRIPTION FRONT <> BACK	INGREDIENT & STRENGTH	BRAND (or Generic Equiv.) by FIRM	NDC#	CLASS; SCH.
01152162	Tab, White, Round	Aminophylline 200 mg	Aminophylline by Richlyn		Antiasthmatic
01152390	Tab, Maroon, Round	Sulfisoxazole 500 mg, Phenazopyridine HCl 50 mg	Azo-Gantrisin by Richlyn		Antibiotic; Urinary Analgesic
01152400	Tab, Green, Round	Phenobarbital 16.2 mg, Belladonna 10.8 mg	Bellophen by Richlyn		Gastrointestinal; C IV
01152758	Cap, Green & Yellow	Chlordiazepoxide 5 mg	Librium by Richlyn		Antianxiety; C IV
01152760	Cap, Black & Green	Chlordiazepoxide 10 mg	Librium by Richlyn		Antianxiety; C IV
01152762	Cap, Green & White	Chlordiazepoxide 25 mg	Librium by Richlyn		Antianxiety; C IV
01152790	Tab, White, Round, Scored, 0015 over 2790	Chloroquine Phosphate 250 mg	Aralen Phosphate by Global	00115-2790	Antimalarial
01152810	Tab, Yellow, Round	Chlorpheniramine Maleate 4 mg	Chlor-Trimeton by Richlyn		Antihistamine
01152920	Tab, White, Round	Cortisone Acetate 25 mg	Cortone by Richlyn		Steroid
01153030	Tab, White, Round	Dehydrocholic Acid 250 mg	Decholin by Richlyn		Gastrointestinal
01153100	Tab, Blue, Pentagonal	Dexamethasone 0.75 mg	Decadron by Richlyn		Steroid
01153200	Cap, Blue	Dicyclomine HCl 10 mg	Bentyl by Richlyn		Gastrointestinal
01153210	Cap, Blue & Clear	Dicyclomine HCl 10 mg, Phenobarbital 15 mg	Bentyl w/ Pb by Richlyn		Gastrointestinal; C IV
01153220	Tab, Blue	Dicyclomine HCl 20 mg	Bentyl by Richlyn		Gastrointestinal
01153225	Tab, White	Dicyclomine HCl 20 mg, Phenobarbital 15 mg	Bentyl w/ Pb by Richlyn		Gastrointestinal; C IV
01153250	Tab, White, Round	Pepsin 250 mg, Pancreatin 300 mg, Dehydrocholic Acid 150 mg	Entozyme by Richlyn		Gastrointestinal
01153585	Tab, Yellow, Round	Folic Acid 1 mg	Folvite by Richlyn		Vitamin
01153660	Tab, Blue, Round	Hydralazine HCl 25 mg	Apresoline by Richlyn		Antihypertensive
01153662	Tab, Blue, Round	Hydralazine HCl 50 mg	Apresoline by Richlyn		Antihypertensive
01153670	Tab, Peach, Round	Hydrochlorothiazide 25 mg	Hydrodiuril by Richlyn		Diuretic; Antihypertensive
01153675	Tab, Peach, Round	Hydrochlorothiazide 50 mg	Hydrodiuril by Richlyn		Diuretic; Antihypertensive
01153677	Tab, Peach, Round	Hydrochlorothiazide 100 mg	Hydrodiuril by Richlyn		Diuretic; Antihypertensive
01153685	Tab, White, Round	Hydrocortisone 20 mg	Hydrocortone by Richlyn		Steroid
01153706	Tab, White, Round	Isoniazid 100 mg	Laniazid by Richlyn		Antimycobacterial
01153888	Tab, White, Round	Meprobamate 200 mg	Equanil by Richlyn		Sedative/Hypnotic; C IV
01153890	Tab, White, Round	Meprobamate 400 mg	Equanil by Richlyn		Sedative/Hypnotic; C IV
01153900	Tab, White, Round	Methocarbamol 500 mg	Robaxin by Richlyn		Muscle Relaxant
01153902	Tab, White, Oblong	Methocarbamol 750 mg	Robaxin by Richlyn		Muscle Relaxant
01153975	Tab, Brown, Round	Methenamine Mandelate 250 mg	Mandelamine by Richlyn		Antibiotic; Urinary Tract
01153976	Tab, Brown, Oblong	Methenamine Mandelate 500 mg	Mandelamine by Richlyn		Antibiotic; Urinary Tract
01153977	Tab, Lavender, Oval	Methenamine Mandelate 1000 mg	Mandelamine by Richlyn		Antibiotic; Urinary Tract
01153982	Tab, Yellow, Oblong	Methyltestosterone 10 mg	Metandren by Richlyn		Hormone; C III
01153986	Tab, Yellow, Round	Methyltestosterone 25 mg	Metandren by Richlyn		Hormone; C III
01154086	Tab, White, Round	Nicotinic Acid 500 mg	Niacin by Richlyn		Vitamin
01154214	Tab, Green, Round	Phenobarbital 15 mg	Phenobarbital by Richlyn		Sedative/Hypnotic; C IV
01154214	Tab, White, Round	Phenobarbital 15 mg	Phenobarbital by Richlyn		Sedative/Hypnotic; C IV
01154214	Tab, Pink, Round	Phenobarbital 15 mg	Phenobarbital by Richlyn		Sedative/Hypnotic; C IV
01154233	Tab, White, Round	Phenobarbital 30 mg	by Richlyn		Sedative/Hypnotic; C IV
01154233	Tab, Green, Round	Phenobarbital 30 mg	by Richlyn		Sedative/Hypnotic; C IV
01154233	Tab, Pink, Round	Phenobarbital 30 mg	by Richlyn		Sedative/Hypnotic; C IV

ID FRONT <> BACK	DESCRIPTION FRONT <> BACK	INGREDIENT & STRENGTH	BRAND (or Generic Equiv.) by FIRM	NDC#	CLASS; SCH.
01154252	Tab, White, Round	Piperazine Citrate 250 mg	by Richlyn		Antihelmintic
01154280	Tab, Orange, Round	Prednisolone 5 mg	by Richlyn		Steroid
01154294	Tab, White, Round	Prednisone 5 mg	by Richlyn		Steroid
01154302	Tab, White, Oblong	Colchicine 0.5 mg, Probenecid 500 mg	ColBenemid by Richlyn		Antigout
01154308	Tab, Peach, Round	Propantheline Bromide 15 mg	Pro-Banthine by Richlyn		Gastrointestinal
01154322	Tab, White, Round	Propylthiouracil 50 mg	Propylthiouracil by Richlyn		Antithyroid
01154331	Tab, White, Round	Triprolidine 2.5 mg, Pseudoephedrine 60 mg	Actifed by Richlyn		Cold Remedy
01154332	Tab, White, Round	Pseudoephedrine 60 mg	Sudafed by Richlyn		Decongestant
01154334	Tab, Dark Red, Round	Phenazopyridine HCl 100 mg	Pyridium by Richlyn		Urinary Analgesic
01154336	Tab, Dark Red, Round	Phenazopyridine HCl 200 mg	Pyridium by Richlyn		Urinary Analgesic
01154360	Tab, Yellow, Round	Pyrilamine Maleate 25 mg	by Richlyn		Antihistamine
01154380	Tab, White, Round	Quinidine Sulfate 200 mg	by Richlyn		Antiarrhythmic
01154400	Tab, Orange, Round	Rauwolfia Serpentina 50 mg	Raudixin by Richlyn		Antihypertensive
01154404	Tab, Orange, Round	Rauwolfia Serpentina 100 mg	Raudixin by Richlyn		Antihypertensive
01154423	Tab, White, Round	Reserpine 0.25 mg	Serpasil by Qualitest		Antihypertensive
01154426	Tab, White, Round	Reserpine 0.1 mg	Serpasil by Richlyn		Antihypertensive
01154428	Tab, White, Round	Reserpine 0.25 mg	Serpasil by Richlyn		Antihypertensive
01154631	Tab, Pink, Round	Sodium Fluoride 2.2 mg	Luride by Richlyn		Element
01154711	Tab, White, Round	Sulfadiazine 2.5 g, Sulfamerazine 2.5 g, Sulfamethazine 2.5 g	Terfonyl by Richlyn		Antibiotic
01154714	Tab, White, Round	Sulfadiazine 500 mg	by Richlyn		Antibiotic
01154747	Tab, White, Round	Sulfisoxazole 500 mg	Gantrisin by Richlyn		Antibiotic
01154812	Tab, Beige, Round	Thyroglobulin 1 g	Proloid by Richlyn		Thyroid Hormone
01154824	Tab, Beige, Round	Thyroid 1 g	by Richlyn		Thyroid Hormone
01154825	Tab, Red, Round	Thyroid 1 g	by Richlyn		Thyroid Hormone
01154826	Tab, Beige, Round	Thyroid 2 g	by Richlyn		Thyroid Hormone
01154827	Tab, Red, Round	Thyroid 2 g	by Richlyn		Thyroid Hormone
01154840	Tab, White, Round	Triamcinolone 4 mg	Aristocort by Richlyn		Steroid
01154860	Tab, Light Blue	Trichlormethiazide 4 mg	Aq 4B Aquazide by Jones	52604-9780	Diuretic; Antihypertensive
01154871	Tab, Blue, Round	Tripelennamine HCl 50 mg	PBZ by Richlyn		Antihistamine
01154895	Tab, Purple, Round	Atropine Sulfate, Benzoic Acid, Hyoscyamine Sulfate, Methenamine, Phenyl Salicylate	Urised by Richlyn		Urinary Tract
01154900	Tab, Blue, Round	Atropine Sulfate, Benzoic Acid, Hyoscyamine Sulfate, Methenamine, Phenyl Salicylate	Urised by Richlyn		Urinary Tract
01154902	Tab, Purple, Round	Atropine Sulfate, Benzoic Acid, Hyoscyamine Sulfate, Methenamine, Phenyl Salicylate	Urised by Richlyn		Urinary Tract
01157001	Cap, White, 0115-7001	Pancrelipase 4500 Units	Pancrease by Major	00904-5413	Gastrointestinal
01157003	Cap, Brown & Flesh	Amylase 33,200 Units, Lipase 10,000 Units, Protease 37,500 Units	Lipram 10000 by Global	00115-7003	Gastrointestinal
01157017	Cap, Brown & Olive	Minocycline HCl 50 mg	Minocin by Global	00115-7017	Antibiotic
01157017	Cap, Brown & Olive	Minocycline HCl 50 mg	Minocin by Neuman	64579-0305	Antibiotic
01157018	Cap, Olive & White	Minocycline HCl 100 mg	Minocin by Global	00115-7018	Antibiotic
01157023	Cap, Flesh	Pancrelipase 16,000 Units	Pancrease MT16 by Global	00115-7023	Gastrointestinal
01157024	Cap, Brown & White	Pancrelipase 20,000 Units	Creon 20 by Global	00115-7024	Gastrointestinal
01157035	Cap, White	Pancrelipase 4500 Units	Pancrease by Global	00115-7035	Gastrointestinal

ID FRONT <> BACK	DESCRIPTION FRONT <> BACK	INGREDIENT & STRENGTH	BRAND (or Generic Equiv.) by FIRM	NDC#	CLASS; SCH.
01157036	Cap, Brown and Flesh	Pancrelipase 10,000 Units	Creon 10 by Global	00115-7036	Gastrointestinal
01157040	Cap, Brown & Clear	Pancrelipase 10,000 Units	Pancrease MT10 by Global	00115-7040	Gastrointestinal
01157041	Cap, Flesh & White	Pancrelipase 18,000 Units	Ultrase MT 18 by Global	00115-7041	Gastrointestinal
01157042	Cap, Clear & White	Pancrelipase 12,000 Units	Ultrase MT 12 by Global	00115-7042	Gastrointestinal
01157043	Cap, Brown	Pancrelipase 20,000 Units	Ultrase MT 20 by Global	00115-7043	Gastrointestinal
01157054	Cap, Olive	Minocycline HCl 75 mg	Minocin by Global	00115-7054	Antibiotic
01157055	Cap, Clear and Natural	Pancrelipase 20,000 Units	Pancrease MT20 by Global	00115-7055	Gastrointestinal
01157057	Cap, Natural and White, Opaque	Pancrelipase 5000 Units	Creon 5 by Global	00115-7057	Gastrointestinal
01159743	Cap, White Print	Acetaminophen 500 mg, Hydrocodone Bitartrate 5 mg	Vicodin by Alphagen	59743-0011	Analgesic; C III
0117 <> BVF	Tab, White, Oblong, Ex Release	Pentoxifylline 400 mg	Trental by Pharmafab	62542-0725	Anticoagulant
0117 <> BVF	Tab, White, Oblong, Ex Release	Pentoxifylline 400 mg	Trental by Teva	00093-5116	Anticoagulant
0117 <> BVF	Tab, White, Oblong, Ex Release	Pentoxifylline 400 mg	Trental by Vangard	00615-4523	Anticoagulant
01170 <> C	Cap, Yellow, Oval, Scored, C <> 01 70	Oxaprozin 600 mg	Daypro by Dr. Reddy's	55111-0170	NSAID
0119 <> 25	Tab, White, Round	Topiramate 25 mg	Topamax by Dava	67253-0751	Anticonvulsant
012	Tab, Peach, Oblong, 012 is underlined	Fexofenadine HCl 120 mg	Allegra 24 hr by Aventis	Canadian DIN 02242819	Antihistamine
012	Tab, White, Round	Acetaminophen 325 mg	Tylenol by Rugby	00536-3222	Analgesic
012	Tab, Green, Round	Chlorzoxazone 250 mg, Acetaminophen 300 mg	Parafon Forte by Amide		Muscle Relaxant
012 <> ADAMS	Tab	Guaifenesin 600 mg	Robitussin by Nat Pharmpak	55154-5903	Expectorant
012 <> MEDEVA	Tab, Light Green, Scored	Guaifenesin 600 mg	Robitussin by Medeva	53014-0012	Expectorant
012 <> PAR	Tab, Coated	Hydroxyzine HCl 10 mg	by Par	49884-0012	Antianxiety; Antihistamine
0120 <> 50	Tab, Light Orange, Round	Topiramate 50 mg	Topamax by Dava	67253-0752	Anticonvulsant
0121	Tab, Ross Logo 0121	Prenatal, Folic Acid	Pramilet by Ross		Vitamin
0121 <> 100	Tab, Orange, Round	Topiramate 100 mg	Topamax by Dava	67253-0753	Anticonvulsant
0122 <> 200	Tab, Pink, Capsule Shaped	Topiramate 200 mg	Topamax by Dava	67253-0754	Anticonvulsant
0127 <> LUNSCO	Tab, Film Coated	Acetaminophen 500 mg, Chlorpheniramine Maleate 8 mg, Phenylephrine HCl 40 mg	Protid by Lunsco	10892-0127	Cold Remedy
0127 <> LUNSCO	Tab, Film Coated	Acetaminophen 500 mg, Chlorpheniramine Maleate 8 mg, Phenylephrine HCl 40 mg	Protid by Mikart	46672-0161	Cold Remedy
013	Cap, Black & Clear	Niacin TD 125 mg	Nicobid by Time Caps		Vitamin
013 <> PAR	Tab, Coated	Hydroxyzine HCl 25 mg	by Par	49884-0013	Antianxiety; Antihistamine
0131 2008	Tab, Peach, Oblong	Chlorpheniramine Maleate 2 mg, Pseudoephedrine HCl 30 mg, Acetaminophen 325 mg	Codimal by Schwarz		Cold Remedy
0131 2008	Cap, Red & White	Chlorpheniramine Maleate 8 mg, Pseudoephedrine HCl 120 mg	Codimal LA by Schwarz		Cold Remedy
014	Cap, Clear & Green	Niacin TD 250 mg	Nicobid by Time Caps		Vitamin
014	Tab, Yellow, Oval	Dexchlorpheniramine Maleate 4 mg	Polaramine by Ivax	00182-1014	Antihistamine
014 <> COP	Tab, Chewable	Sodium Fluoride 1.1 mg	Luride Half Strength by Colgate	00126-0014	Element
014 <> PAR	Tab, Coated	Hydroxyzine HCl 50 mg	Atarax by Par	49884-0014	Antianxiety; Antihistamine
014 <> THERRX	Tab, Yellow, Diamond Shaped, Film Coated	Ascorbic Acid 60 mg, Calcium Carbonate 200 mg, Iron 30 mg, Vitamin E 30 IU, Thiamine Mononitrate 3 mg, Riboflavin 3.4 mg, Niacinamide 20 mg, Pyridoxine HCl 50 mg, Folic Acid 1 mg, Magnesium Oxide 100 mg, Cyanocobalamin 12 mcg, Zinc Oxide 15 mg, Cupric Oxide 2 mg, Folic Acid 1 mg	Precare Conceive by Ther Rx	64011-0014	Vitamin
0140	Cap, Green, Clear Gel, Coated, Graphic enclosed in an Inverted Triangle	Ergocalciferol 1.25 mg	Ergo D by Optimum	61298-0020	Vitamin
0140P	Cap, Gelatin, P in a Triangle	Ergocalciferol 1.25 mg	Vitamin D by Banner Pharma	10888-0140	Vitamin
0140P	Cap, Gelatin, P in a Triangle	Ergocalciferol 1.25 mg	Vitamin D by URL Mutual	00677-0765	Vitamin
0140P	Cap, Gelatin, P in a Triangle	Ergocalciferol 1.25 mg	Vitamin D by URL Mutual	00144-0639	Vitamin
0140P	Cap, Gelatin, P in a Triangle	Ergocalciferol 1.25 mg	Vitamin D by URL Mutual	00904-0291	Vitamin

ID FRONT <> BACK	DESCRIPTION FRONT <> BACK	INGREDIENT & STRENGTH	BRAND (or Generic Equiv.) by FIRM	NDC#	CLASS; SCH.
0140P	Cap, Gelatin, P in a Triangle	Ergocalciferol 1.25 mg	Vitamin D by URL Mutual	00223-1971	Vitamin
01425MG	Cap, Light Green Cap, Light Green Body	Zaleplon 5 mg	Sonata by Dava	67253-0950	Sedative/Hypnotic
014310MG	Cap, Green Cap, Green Body	Zaleplon 10 mg	Sonata by Dava	67253-0951	Sedative/Hypnotic
0144125MG	Cap, Yellow Opaque Cap, White Opaque Body	Ramipril 1.25 mg	Altace by Dava	67253-0671	Antihypertensive
0145	Cap, Orange, Soft Gel	Docusate Sodium 100 mg	Colace by Qualitest	00603-0145	Laxative
0145 <> P400	Tab, Light Yellow, Oval, Scored	Amiodarone 400 mg	Cordarone by Upsher Smith	00245-0145	Antiarrhythmic
014525MG	Cap, Orange Opaque Cap, White Opaque Body	Ramipril 2.5 mg	Altace by Dava	67253-0672	Antihypertensive
01465MG	Cap, Red Opaque Cap, White Opaque Body	Ramipril 5 mg	Altace by Dava	67253-0673	Antihypertensive
014710MG	Cap, Aqua Blue Opaque Cap, Aqua Blue Opaque Body	Ramipril 10 mg	Altace by Dava	67253-0674	Antihypertensive
0147CC	Cap, C-C in a box	Phentermine HCl 30 mg	T Diet by Jones	52604-0010	Anorexiant; C IV
0149 0436 <> ENTEXLA	Tab	Guaifenesin 400 mg, Phenylpropanolamine HCl 75 mg	Entex LA by Amerisource	62584-0436	Cold Remedy
0149 0436 <> ENTEXLA	Tab	Guaifenesin 400 mg, Phenylpropanolamine HCl 75 mg	Entex LA by Leiner	59606-0641	Cold Remedy
0149 0436 <> ENTEXLA	Tab	Guaifenesin 400 mg, Phenylpropanolamine HCl 75 mg	Entex LA by Caremark	00339-5128	Cold Remedy
0149 0436 <> ENTEXLA	Tab	Guaifenesin 400 mg, Phenylpropanolamine HCl 75 mg	Entex LA by Urgent Care Center	50716-0436	Cold Remedy
0149 0436 <> ENTEXLA	Tab	Guaifenesin 400 mg, Phenylpropanolamine HCl 75 mg	Entex LA by Nat Pharmpak	55154-2303	Cold Remedy
015	Cap, Maroon & Pink	Niacin TD 400 mg	Nicobid by Time Caps		Vitamin
015 <> MEDEVA	Tab, Light Blue, Scored	Guaifenesin 400 mg, Pseudoephedrine HCl 120 mg	Sudafed Sinus by Medeva	53014-0015	Cold Remedy
015 <> PAR	Tab	Meclizine HCl 50 mg	by Par	49884-0015	Antiemetic
0158	Tab, Blue, Round, Scored, Duramed Logo-Diamond	Estradiol 1.5 mg	Gyndiol by Medicis	99207-0499	Hormone
0158	Tab, Blue, Round, Scored, Duramed Logo-Diamond	Estradiol 1.5 mg	Gyndiol by Heartland	61392-0042	Hormone
0158	Tab, Blue, Round, Scored, Duramed Logo-Diamond	Estradiol 1.5 mg	Gyndiol by Fielding	00421-0158	Hormone
015AMIDE	Tab, White, Oval, Ex Release	Dexchlorpheniramine Maleate 6 mg	Polaramine by Watson	00591-4009	Antihistamine
016 <> ACH	Tab, Pink, Round, A over CH	Candesartan Cilexetil 16 mg	Atacand by AstraZeneca	Canadian DIN 02239092	Antihypertensive
016 <> ACH	Tab, Pink, Round, A over CH	Candesartan Cilexetil 16 mg	Atacand by AstraZeneca	00186-0016	Antihypertensive
016 <> DP	Tab, Orange, Round	Levonorgestrel 0.10 mg, Ethinyl Estradiol 0.02 mg	Aviane by Barr	00555-9045	Oral Contraceptive
016 <> DP	Tab, Orange, Round	Levonorgestrel 0.10 mg, Ethinyl Estradiol 0.02 mg	Aviane by Duramed	51285-0017	Oral Contraceptive
016 <> DP	Tab, Orange, Round	Levonorgestrel 0.10 mg, Ethinyl Estradiol 0.02 mg	Aviane by Apotex	Canadian DIN 02298538	Oral Contraceptive
016 <> DP	Tab, Orange, Round	Levonorgestrel 0.10 mg, Ethinyl Estradiol 0.02 mg	Aviane by Apotex	Canadian DIN 02298546	Oral Contraceptive
016 <> PAR	Tab	Chlorzoxazone 250 mg	by Par	49884-0016	Muscle Relaxant
016 <> US	Tab, Yellow, Oval, Film Coated	Folic Acid 2.2 mg, Vitamin B-6 25 mg, Vitamin B-12 500 mcg	Folgard Rx by Upsher Smith	00245-0183	Vitamin
016 <> US	Tab, Yellow, Oval, Film Coated	Folic Acid 2.2 mg, Vitamin B-6 25 mg, Vitamin B-12 500 mcg	Folgard Rx by Upsher Smith	00245-0016	Vitamin
017 <> DECII	Tab, Dark Blue, Scored	Guaifenesin 600 mg, Pseudoephedrine HCl 60 mg	Deconsal II by Celltech	53014-0017	Cold Remedy
017 <> MEDEVA	Tab, Dark Blue, Scored	Guaifenesin 600 mg, Pseudoephedrine HCl 60 mg	Deconsal II by Medeva	53014-0017	Cold Remedy
017 <> US	Tab, Green, Round, Film Coated	Folic Acid 800 mcg, Vitamin B 115 mcg, Vitamin B-6 10 mg	Folgard by Upsher Smith	00245-0017	Vitamin
018	Tab, Oblong, Peach	Fexofenadine HCl 180 mg	Allegra by Prasco	66993-0109	Antihistamine
018	Tab, Greek Letter Alpha	Guaifenesin 600 mg	Robitussin by Sovereign	58716-0600	Expectorant
018	Tab, Greek Letter Alpha	Guaifenesin 600 mg	Robitussin by Pharmafab	62542-0700	Expectorant
018 <> 0088	Tab, Peach, Oblong, Film Coated	Fexofenadine HCl 180 mg	Allegra by Aventis	00088-1109	Antihistamine
018 <> E	Tab, Peach, Oblong, Film Coated, Scripted E	Fexofenadine HCl 180 mg	Allegra by Aventis	00088-1109	Antihistamine
018A	Cap, Green, Opaque	Chlordiazepoxide 5 mg, Clidinium Bromide 2.5 mg	Librax by Schein	00364-0559	Gastrointestinal
019 <> A	Tab, Pink, Round	Guaifenesin 200 mg	Aquabid by Ivax	00182-2614 Discontinued	Expectorant
019 <> THERRX	Tab, Blue, Oval, Film Coated	Calcium 200 mg, Folic Acid 1 mg, Vitamin B6 75 mg, Vitamin B12 12 mcg	PremesisRx by KV Pharma	64011-0019	Vitamin; Mineral
0198	Cap, Gray, Savage Logo 0198	Butalbital 50 mg, Acetaminophen 650 mg	Axocet by Savage	00281-0198	Analgesic
019TCL	Cap	Papaverine HCl 150 mg	by Schein	00364-0181	Vasodilator
01A	Cap, Ivory & Red, Gelatin, BI Logo	Dipyridamole 200 mg, Aspirin 25 mg	Aggrenox by Boehringer Ingelheim Canada	Canadian DIN 02242119	Antiplatelet

ID FRONT <> BACK	DESCRIPTION FRONT <> BACK	INGREDIENT & STRENGTH	BRAND (or Generic Equiv.) by FIRM	NDC#	CLASS; SCH.
01A	Cap, Ivory & Red, Gelatin, BI Logo	Dipyridamole 200 mg, Aspirin 25 mg	Aggrenox by Boehringer Ingelheim	00597-0001	Antiplatelet
01A	Cap, Ivory & Red, Gelatin, BI Logo	Dipyridamole 200 mg, Aspirin 25 mg	Aggrenox by Boehringer Ingelheim	12714-0125	Antiplatelet
01B	Tab, White, Round, 0.2	Fenoterol 2.5 mg	by Boehringer Ingelheim	Canadian	Antiasthmatic
02	Tab, White, Round, 0.2	Desmopressin Acetate 0.2 mg	DDAVP by Ferring	Canadian	Antidiuretic
02 <> 37AV	Tab, White, Round, Scored, 0.2 <> 37 over AV	Desmopressin Acetate 0.2 mg	DDAVP by Aventis	00075-0026	Antidiuretic
02 <> A	Tab, Light Pink, Round, Film Coated	Simvastatin 20 mg	Zocor by Aurobindo	65862-0052	Antihyperlipidemic
02 <> CBP	Tab, Blue, Oblong, Scored, CBP <> / 02	Chlorpheniramine Maleate 8 mg, Methscopolamine 2.5 mg	RhinaClear by Amneal	65162-0550	Cold Remedy
02 <> DAN5612	Tab, Yellow, Pentagonal, Scored, 0.2 <> Dan over 5612	Clonidine HCl 0.2 mg	by Schein	00364-0821	Antihypertensive
02 <> DAN5612	Tab, Yellow, Pentagonal, Scored, 0.2 <> Dan over 5612	Clonidine HCl 0.2 mg	by Watson	00591-5612	Antihypertensive
02 <> E	Tab, White to Off-White, Oval, Film Coated	Carvedilol 6.25 mg	Coreg by Aurobindo	65862-0143	Antihypertensive
02 <> NOVO	Tab, Orange, Round, No/Vo <> 0.2	Clonidine HCl 0.2 mg	Catapres by Novopharm	Canadian DIN 02046148	Antihypertensive
020	Cap	Loperamide 2 mg	Imodium by URL Mutual	00677-1422	Antidiarrheal
020 <> CL	Tab, White, Round	Colchicine 0.6 mg	Colchicine by Concord	20254-0020	Antigout
020N2	Cap	Loperamide 2 mg	Imodium by Schein	00364-2481	Antidiarrheal
021	Tab, Tan, Round	Thyroid 32.5 mg	Thyroid by Major	00904-7865	Thyroid Hormone
021	Tab, Tan, Round	Thyroid 32.5 mg	Thyroid by Time Caps	49483-0021	Thyroid Hormone
021 <> DP	Tab, White, Round	Desogestrel 0.15 mg, Ethinyl Estradiol 0.02 mg	Kariva by Barr	00555-9050	Oral Contraceptive
021 <> KOS	Tab, Blue, Extended Release	Niacin 500 mg, Simvastatin 20mg	Simcor by Abbott	00074-3312	Antihyperlipidemic
021MJ	Tab, White, Round, Scored	Estradiol 0.5 mg	Estrace by Warner Chilcott	00430-0021	Hormone
021MJ	Tab, White, Round, Scored	Estradiol 0.5 mg	Estrace by Caremark	00339-5464	Hormone
022 <> DP	Tab, Light Blue, Round	Ethinyl Estradiol 0.01 mg	Kariva by Barr	00555-9050	Oral Contraceptive
022 <> KOS	Tab, Blue, Extended Release	Niacin 750 mg, Simvastatin 20mg	Simcor by Abbott	00074-3315	Antihyperlipidemic
0221	Tab, Circa Logo	Glipizide 5 mg	by Moore	00839-7939	Antidiabetic
0221	Tab, Circa Logo	Glipizide 5 mg	by URL Mutual	00677-1544	Antidiabetic
0221	Tab, Circa Logo	Glipizide 5 mg	by Circa	71114-0221	Antidiabetic
0222	Tab, Circa Logo	Glipizide 10 mg	by Circa	71114-0222	Antidiabetic
0222	Tab, Circa Logo	Glipizide 10 mg	by URL Mutual	00677-1545	Antidiabetic
0222	Tab, Circa Logo	Glipizide 10 mg	by Schein	00364-2605	Antidiabetic
0222	Tab, Circa Logo	Glipizide 10 mg	by Moore	00839-7940	Antidiabetic
023 <> KOS	Tab, Blue, Extended Release	Niacin 1000 mg, Simvastatin 20mg	Simcor by Abbott	00074-3316	Antihyperlipidemic
023 <> PH	Tab, Yellow, Round	Aspirin 81 mg	Aspirin by Pharbest	16103-0356	Analgesic
023 <> R	Tab, White, Round	Aspirin 325 mg, Butalbital 50 mg, Caffeine 40 mg	Fiorinal by Actavis	00228-2023	Analgesic; C III
023R	Tab	Aspirin 325 mg, Butalbital 50 mg, Caffeine 40 mg	Fiorinal by Allscripts		Analgesic; C III
024 <> ADAMS	Tab, Yellow	Atropine Sulfate 0.04 mg, Chlorpheniramine Maleate 8 mg, Hyoscyamine Sulfate 0.19 mg, Phenylephrine 25 mg, Phenylpropanolamine 50 mg, Scopolamine 0.01 mg	Atrohist Plus by Drug Distr	52985-0227	Cold Remedy
024 <> ADAMS	Tab, Yellow	Atropine Sulfate 0.04 mg, Chlorpheniramine Maleate 8 mg, Hyoscyamine Sulfate 0.19 mg, Phenylephrine 25 mg, Phenylpropanolamine 50 mg, Scopolamine 0.01 mg	Atrohist Plus by Medeva	53014-0024	Cold Remedy
024 <> THX	Tab, Orange, Oval, Film Coated, Chewable	Calcium 250 mg, Copper 2 mg, Folic Acid 1 mg, Iron 40 mg, Magnesium 50 mg, Vitamin B6 2 mg, Vitamin C 50 mg, Vitamin D3 6 mcg, Vitamin E 3.5 mg, Zinc 15 mg	Precare Prenatal by Ther Rx	64011-0024	Vitamin; Mineral
025	Cap	Amylase 20,000 Units, Lipase 4000 Units, Protease 25,000 Units	Pancreatic Enzyme by Ivax	00182-1554	Gastrointestinal
025	Tab, White, Round	Calcium Carbonate 648 mg	Os-Cal by Watson	00536-3414	Vitamin; Mineral
025 <> APO	Tab, Blue, Round	Clonidine 0.025 mg	Dixarit by Apotex	Canadian DIN 02248732	Antihypertensive
025 <> N126	Tab, White, Round, Scored, 0.25 <> N over 126	Alprazolam 0.25 mg	Xanax by Teva	55953-8131	Antianxiety; C IV
025 <> N126	Tab, White, Round, Scored, 0.25 <> N over 126	Alprazolam 0.25 mg	Xanax by Medirex	57480-0520	Antianxiety; C IV
025 <> N126	Tab, White, Round, Scored, 0.25 <> N over 126	Alprazolam 0.25 mg	Xanax by PDRX	55289-0962	Antianxiety; C IV

ID FRONT <> BACK	DESCRIPTION FRONT <> BACK	INGREDIENT & STRENGTH	BRAND (or Generic Equiv.) by FIRM	NDC#	CLASS; SCH.
025 <> NOVO	Tab, White, Oval, no\vo <> 0.25	Alprazolam 0.25 mg	Xanax by Novopharm	Canadian DIN 01913484	Antianxiety; C IV
025 <> R	Tab, Tan, Oblong	Risperidone 0.25 mg	Risperdal by Pharmascience	Canadian DIN 02252007	Antipsychotic
025 <> SP321	Tab, Yellow, Round, Scored, Orally Disintegrating, 0.25	Alprazolam 0.25 mg	Niravam by Schwarz	00091-3321	Antianxiety; C IV
025 <> THERRX	Tab, Peach, Cap Shaped, Scored, Film Coated	Ascorbic Acid 50 mg, Calcium Carbonate 250 mg, Cyanocobalamin 12 mcg, Cholecalciferol 6 mcg, Thiamine Mononitrate 3 mg, Riboflavin 3.4 mg, Niacinamide 20 mg, Pyridoxine HCl 20 mg, Folic Acid 1 mg, Magnesium Oxide 50 mg, Zinc Sulfate 15 mg, Cupric Sulfate 2 mg	Precare Prenatal by Ther Rx	64011-0025	Vitamin; Mineral
0252240MG	Cap, Black Bands, RPR Logo over 240 mg	Diltiazem HCl 240 mg	Dilacor by Watson	00075-0252	Antihypertensive
0258	Cap, Maroon & Brown, Savage Logo 0258	Vitamin, Iron	Chromagen FA by Savage	00281-0259	Vitamin
025ALG	Tab, Light Yellow, 0.25/ALG	Alprazolam 0.25 mg	Xanax by Schein	00364-2582	Antianxiety; C IV
025AP	Tab	Estradiol 0.5 mg	by BMS	15548-0025	Hormone
026 <> R	Tab, White, Round	Phenobarbital 15 mg	Phenobarbital by Heartland	61392-0382	Sedative/Hypnotic; C IV
026 <> R	Tab, White, Round	Phenobarbital 15 mg	Phenobarbital by Actavis	00228-2026	Sedative/Hypnotic; C IV
026 <> R	Tab, White, Round	Phenobarbital 15 mg	Phenobarbital by Vangard	00615-0420	Sedative/Hypnotic; C IV
026 <> R	Tab, White, Round	Phenobarbital 15 mg	Phenobarbital by UDL	51079-0094 Discontinued	Sedative/Hypnotic; C IV
0262	Cap, Brown, Savage Logo 0262	Vitamin, Iron	Chromagen Forte by Savage	00281-0262	Vitamin
026AP	Tab	Estradiol 1 mg	Estrace by BMS	15548-0026	Hormone
026G	Cap, Powder Blue	Piroxicam 10 mg	Feldene by Genpharm	Canadian	NSAID
026G	Cap, Dark Green & Olive	Piroxicam 10 mg	Feldene by Genpharm	55567-0026	NSAID
027 <> R	Tab, White, Round, Scored	Alprazolam 0.25 mg	Xanax by Ivax	00182-0027	Antianxiety; C IV
027 <> R	Tab, White, Round, Scored	Alprazolam 0.25 mg	Xanax by Actavis	00228-2027	Antianxiety; C IV
027 <> R	Tab, White, Round, Scored	Alprazolam 0.25 mg	Xanax by Heartland	61392-0034	Antianxiety; C IV
027AP	Tab	Estradiol 2 mg	by BMS	15548-0027	Hormone
028 <> R	Tab, White, Round, Scored	Phenobarbital 30 mg	by Actavis	00228-2028	Sedative/Hypnotic; C IV
028 <> R	Tab, White, Round, Scored	Phenobarbital 30 mg	by Vangard	00615-0421	Sedative/Hypnotic; C IV
0282V	Cap, Clear	Quinine Sulfate 325 mg	Quinamm by Qualitest	00603-5622	Antimalarial
029 <> R	Tab, Peach, Round, Scored	Alprazolam 0.5 mg	Xanax by Ivax	00182-0028	Antianxiety; C IV
029 <> R	Tab, Peach, Round, Scored	Alprazolam 0.5 mg	Xanax by Heartland	61392-0035	Antianxiety; C IV
029 <> R	Tab, Peach, Round, Scored	Alprazolam 0.5 mg	Xanax by Actavis	00228-2029	Antianxiety; C IV
029 <> TENCON	Tab, White, Cap Shaped	Acetaminophen 650 mg, Butalbital 50 mg	Tencon by Int'l Ethical Labs	11584-0029	Analgesic
02C <> SEPTRADS	Tab	Sulfamethoxazole 800 mg, Trimethoprim 160 mg	by Nat Pharmpak	55154-0703	Antibiotic
03	Tab, Round, Peach	Fexofenadine HCl 30 mg	Allegra by Prasco	66993-0106	Antihistamine
03 <> 0088	Tab, Peach, Oblong, Film Coated	Fexofenadine HCl 30 mg	Allegra by Aventis	00088-1106	Antihistamine
03 <> A	Tab, Pink, Round, Film Coated	Simvastatin 40 mg	Zocor by Aurobindo	65862-0053	Antihyperlipidemic
03 <> DAN5613	Tab	Clonidine HCl 0.3 mg	Catapres by Watson	00591-5613	Antihypertensive
03 <> E	Tab, Peach, Round, Film Coated, Scripted E	Fexofenadine HCl 30 mg	Allegra by Aventis	00088-1106	Antihistamine
03 <> E	Tab, White to Off-White, Oval, Film Coated	Carvedilol 12.5 mg	Coreg by Aurobindo	65862-0144	Antihypertensive
03 <> SP	Tab, Yellow, Round	Aspirin 81 mg	Aspirin by Amneal	65162-0241	Analgesic
030 <> HUMDM	Tab, Dark Green, Cap Shaped, Scored	Dextromethorphan 30 mg, Guaifenesin 600 mg	Humibid-DM by Celltech	53014-0030	Cold Remedy
030 <> MEDEVA	Tab, Dark Green, Scored	Dextromethorphan 30 mg, Guaifenesin 600 mg	Humibid-DM by Medeva	53014-0030	Cold Remedy
031 <> A	Tab, Chewable	Ascorbic Acid 34.5 mg, Cyanocobalamin 4.9 mcg, Folic Acid 0.35 mg, Niacinamide 14.16 mg, Pyridoxine HCl 1.1 mg, Riboflavin 1.2 mg, Sodium Ascorbate 32.2 mg, Sodium Fluoride 1.1 mg, Thiamine Mononitrate 1.15 mg, Vitamin A Acetate 5.5 mg, Vitamin D 0.194 mg	Poly Vitamins by Ivax	00182-1819	Vitamin
031 <> R	Tab, Blue, Round, Scored	Alprazolam 1 mg	Xanax by Actavis	00228-2031	Antianxiety; C IV
031 <> R	Tab, Blue, Round, Scored	Alprazolam 1 mg	Xanax by Ivax	00182-0029	Antianxiety; C IV
0310	Tab, White, Cap Shaped, Scored	Magnesium Salicylate 600 mg	Mobidin by B F Ascher	00225-0310	Analgesic
0319	Cap, Purple, Savage Logo 0319	Folic Acid 1 mg	Chromagen OB by Savage	00281-0319	Vitamin

ID FRONT <> BACK	DESCRIPTION FRONT <> BACK	INGREDIENT & STRENGTH	BRAND (or Generic Equiv.) by FIRM	NDC#	CLASS; SCH.
032 <> ACL	Tab, Pink, Round, A over CL	Candesartan Cilexetil 32 mg	Atacand by AstraZeneca	17228-0032	Antihypertensive
032 <> ACL	Tab, Pink, Round, A over CL	Candesartan Cilexetil 32 mg	Atacand by AstraZeneca	00186-0032	Antihypertensive
032 <> PAL	Tab, Purple, Oval, Scored	Acetaminophen 712.8 mg, Caffeine 60 mg, Dihydrocodeine Bitartrate 32 mg	Panlor SS by Mikart	46672-0141	Analgesic; C III
032 <> PAL	Tab, Purple, Oval, Scored	Acetaminophen 712.8 mg, Caffeine 60 mg, Dihydrocodeine Bitartrate 32 mg	Panlor SS by Pamlab	00525-0032	Analgesic; C III
032032 <> ENTEXPSE	Tab, Yellow, Scored, Film Coated, 032 over 032 <> Entex PSE	Guaifenesin 600 mg, Pseudoephedrine HCl 120 mg	Entex PSE by Dura	51479-0032	Cold Remedy
032032 <> ENTEXPSE	Tab, Yellow, Scored, Film Coated, 032 over 032 <> Entex PSE	Guaifenesin 600 mg, Pseudoephedrine HCl 120 mg	Entex PSE by Welpharm	63375-6376	Cold Remedy
0321US	Tab, Green, Oblong	Magnesium Salicylate 600 mg, Phenyltoloxamine Citrate 25 mg	Magsal by Nat Pharmpak	55154-5238	Analgesic
0321US	Tab, Green, Oblong	Magnesium Salicylate 600 mg, Phenyltoloxamine Citrate 25 mg	Magsal by US Pharma	52747-0321	Analgesic
033 <> 57344	Tab, White, Oblong	Diphenhydramine HCl 50 mg	by AAA		Antihistamine
033033 <> ENTEXLA	Tab, Orange, Oblong, Scored	Guaifenesin 400 mg, Phenylpropanolamine HCl 75 mg	Entex LA by Dura	51479-0033	Cold Remedy
033033 <> ENTEXLA	Tab, Orange, Oblong, Scored	Guaifenesin 400 mg, Phenylpropanolamine HCl 75 mg	Entex LA by Martec		Cold Remedy
033033 <> ENTEXLA	Tab, Orange, Oblong, Scored	Guaifenesin 400 mg, Phenylpropanolamine HCl 75 mg	Entex LA by Welpharm	63375-6377	Cold Remedy
0331 <> MP	Tab, Dark Red, Cap Shaped, Film Coated	Calcium Carbonate 312 mg, Cyanocobalamin 3 mcg, Ferric Polysaccharide Complex, Folic Acid 1 mg, Niacinamide 10 mg, Pyridoxine HCl 2 mg, Riboflavin 3 mg, Sodium Ascorbate, Thiamine Mononitrate 3 mg, Vitamin A 4000 Units, Vitamin D 400 Units	Nu Iron V by Merz	00259-0331	Vitamin; Mineral
033BARR	Cap, Black & Green	Chlordiazepoxide 10 mg	Librium by UDL	51079-0375	Antianxiety; C IV
033BARR	Cap, Black & Green	Chlordiazepoxide 10 mg	Librium by Sandoz	00781-2082	Antianxiety; C IV
033BARR	Cap, Black & Green	Chlordiazepoxide 10 mg	Librium by Med Pro	53978-3175	Antianxiety; C IV
034 <> PAR	Tab, Blue & White, Oval	Meclizine HCl 12.5 mg	Antivert by UDL	51079-0089	Antiemetic
034 <> PAR	Tab, Blue & White, Oval	Meclizine HCl 12.5 mg	Antivert by Schein	00364-0411	Antiemetic
034 <> PAR	Tab, Blue & White, Oval	Meclizine HCl 12.5 mg	Antivert by Vangard	00615-1553	Antiemetic
034 <> PAR	Tab, Blue & White, Oval	Meclizine HCl 12.5 mg	Antivert by Qualitest	00603-4319	Antiemetic
034 <> PAR	Tab, Blue & White, Oval	Meclizine HCl 12.5 mg	Antivert by Major	00904-2384	Antiemetic
034 <> PAR	Tab, Blue & White, Oval	Meclizine HCl 12.5 mg	Antivert by URL Mutual	00677-0418	Antiemetic
034 <> PAR	Tab, Blue & White, Oval	Meclizine HCl 12.5 mg	Antivert by Amerisource	62584-0772	Antiemetic
034 <> PAR	Tab, Blue & White, Oval	Meclizine HCl 12.5 mg	Antivert by PDRX	55289-0982	Antiemetic
034 <> PAR	Tab, Blue & White, Oval	Meclizine HCl 12.5 mg	Antivert by Ivax	00182-0871	Antiemetic
034 <> PAR	Tab, Blue & White, Oval	Meclizine HCl 12.5 mg	Antivert by Par	49884-0034	Antiemetic
03451032	Cap, Gray & Red	Aspirin 389 mg, Caffeine 32.4 mg, Propoxyphene 65 mg	Darvon Compound by Lemmon		Analgesic; C IV
035 <> PAR	Tab, Yellow & White, Oval, Scored	Meclizine HCl 25 mg	Antivert by Qualitest	00603-4320	Antiemetic
035 <> PAR	Tab, Yellow & White, Oval, Scored	Meclizine HCl 25 mg	Antivert by Amerisource	62584-0774	Antiemetic
035 <> PAR	Tab, Yellow & White, Oval, Scored	Meclizine HCl 25 mg	Antivert by Par	49884-0035	Antiemetic
035 <> PAR	Tab, Yellow & White, Oval, Scored	Meclizine HCl 25 mg	Antivert by Pharmedix	53002-0351	Antiemetic
035 <> PAR	Tab, Yellow & White, Oval, Scored	Meclizine HCl 25 mg	Antivert by Ivax	00182-0872	Antiemetic
035 <> PAR	Tab, Yellow & White, Oval, Scored	Meclizine HCl 25 mg	Antivert by URL Mutual	00677-0419	Antiemetic
035 <> PAR	Tab, Yellow & White, Oval, Scored	Meclizine HCl 25 mg	Antivert by Vangard	00615-1554	Antiemetic
035 <> PAR	Tab, Yellow & White, Oval, Scored	Meclizine HCl 25 mg	Antivert by UDL	51079-0090	Antiemetic
035 <> PAR	Tab, Yellow & White, Oval, Scored	Meclizine HCl 25 mg	Antivert by Schein	00364-0412	Antiemetic
0375 <> ER	Tab, White to Off White, Round, Ex Release, "0.375" <> ER	Pramipexole DiHCl 0.375 mg	Mirapex ER by Boehringer Ingelheim	00597-0109	Antiparkinson
0379 <> MR	Tab, Off-White, Film Coated	Guaifenesin 400 mg, Pseudoephedrine HCl 120 mg	Sudafed Sinus by Merz	00259-0379	Cold Remedy
03Z3636	Tab, White, Round, 0.3/Z 3636	Conjugated Estrogens 0.3 mg	Premarin by Ivax		Hormone
04	Tab, Yellow, Round	Tamsulosin HCl 0.4 mg	Flomax CR by Boehringer Ingelheim	Canadian DIN 02270102	Antiadrenergic
04 <> A	Tab, Pink, Cap Shaped, Film Coated	Simvastatin 80 mg	Zocor by Aurobindo	65862-0054	Antihyperlipidemic
04 <> E	Tab, White to Off-White, Oval, Film Coated	Carvedilol 25 mg	Coreg by Aurobindo	65862-0145	Antihypertensive
042	Tab, Pink, Oval	Diphenhydramine HCl 25 mg	Benadryl by Watson	00536-3597	Antihistamine

ID FRONT <> BACK	DESCRIPTION FRONT <> BACK	INGREDIENT & STRENGTH	BRAND (or Generic Equiv.) by FIRM	NDC#	CLASS; SCH.
043	Tab, White, Round	Vitamin B-1, Thiamin	B-Vitamin by Watson	00536-4680	Vitamin
0430 <> WALLACE	Tab, Yellow, Cap Shaped, Scored	Felbamate 400 mg	Felbatol by Wallace	00037-0430	Anticonvulsant
0431 <> WALLACE	Tab, Peach, Oblong, Scored	Felbamate 600 mg	Felbatol by Wallace	00037-0431	Anticonvulsant
0431 <> WALLACE	Tab, Peach, Oblong, Scored	Felbamate 600 mg	Felbatol by Hoffmann La Roche	00004-6200	Anticonvulsant
044	Tab, White, Round	Colchicine 0.6 mg	Colchicine by Alphagen	59743-0085	Antigout
044HD	Tab, White, Round	Meprobamate 400 mg	Neuramate by Halsey	Discontinued	Sedative/Hypnotic; C IV
04785477	Tab, White, Round, Scored	Atropine Sulfate 0.0194 mg, Hyoscyamine Sulfate 0.1037 mg, Phenobarbital 16.2 mg, Scopolamine 0.0065 mg	Donnatal by Shire	58521-0754	Gastrointestinal; C IV
04785477	Tab	Phenobarbital 16.2 mg	by Physician Total Care	54868-3720	Sedative/Hypnotic; C IV
048	Tab, Red, Cap Shaped	Calcium Pantothenate 10 mg, Cyanocobalamin 25 mcg, Ferrous Sulfate 525 mg, Folic Acid 800 mcg, Niacinamide 30 mg, Pyridoxine HCl 5 mg, Riboflavin 6 mg, Sodium Ascorbate 500 mg, Thiamine Mononitrate 6 mg	Multiret Folic 500 by Amide	52152-0048	Vitamin; Mineral
048	Tab, Pink, Oblong, 048 <> I) logo	Diphenhydramine HCl 25 mg	Benadryl by A & Z Pharma	58716-0026	Antihistamine
04WE	Cap	Brompheniramine Maleate 6 mg, Pseudoephedrine HCl 60 mg	Ultrabrom PD by Sovereign	00182-1806	Cold Remedy
05 <> 18060524O	Tab, 0.05 <> 1806.05-240	Lorazepam 0.5 mg	Ativan by Ivax	00677-1056	Antianxiety; C IV
05 <> 240	Tab, White, Round, Film Coated, 0.5 <> Royce Logo 240	Lorazepam 0.5 mg	Ativan by URL Mutual	00603-4243	Antianxiety; C IV
05 <> 240	Tab, White, Round, Film Coated, 0.5 <> Royce Logo 240	Lorazepam 0.5 mg	Ativan by Qualitest	44514-0098	Antianxiety; C IV
05 <> 240	Tab, White, Round, Film Coated, 0.5 <> Royce Logo 240	Lorazepam 0.5 mg	Ativan by Talbert	51875-0240	Antianxiety; C IV
05 <> 240	Tab, White, Round, Film Coated, 0.5 <> Royce Logo 240	Lorazepam 0.5 mg	Ativan by Royce	00093-5420	Antianxiety; C IV
05 <> 5420	Tab, White, Oval, Scored, Hourglass Logo 0.5	Cabergoline 0.5 mg	Dostinex by Teva	65862-0005	Antiparkinson
05 <> A	Tab, Peach, Round, Film Coated	Citalopram HBr 10 mg	Celexa by Aurobindo	13107-0005	Antidepressant
05 <> A	Tab, Peach, Round, Film Coated	Citalopram HBr 10 mg	Celexa by Aurobindo	Canadian DIN 00655740	Antidepressant
05 <> APO	Tab, White, Round, APO/0.5	Lorazepam 0.5 mg	Ativan by Apotex	00555-0491	Antianxiety; C IV
05 <> B491	Tab, White, Round, b over 491 <> 0.5, Ex Release	Alprazolam 0.5 mg	Xanax XR by Barr	59762-0057	Antianxiety; C IV
05 <> G	Tab, White, Pentagonal, G <> 0.5, Ex Release	Alprazolam 0.5 mg	Xanax XR by Greenstone	00093-1057	Antianxiety; C IV
05 <> G	Tab, White, Oval, Scored, 0.5 <> G	Estradiol 0.5 mg	by Teva	Discontinued	Hormone
05 <> G	Tab, White, Oval, Scored, 0.5 <> G	Estradiol 0.5 mg	by AAI Pharma	27280-0004	Hormone
05 <> N	Tab, White, Round, N <> 0.5	Lorazepam 0.5 mg	Ativan by Novopharm	Canadian DIN 00711101	Antianxiety; C IV
05 <> N127	Tab, Orange, Round, Scored, 0.5 <> N over 127	Alprazolam 0.5 mg	Xanax by Medirex	57480-0521	Antianxiety; C IV
05 <> N127	Tab, Orange, Round, Scored, 0.5 <> N over 127	Alprazolam 0.5 mg	Xanax by Teva	55953-8127	Antianxiety; C IV
05 <> N127	Tab, Orange, Round, Scored, 0.5 <> N over 127	Alprazolam 0.5 mg	Xanax by Moore	00839-7852	Antianxiety; C IV
05 <> NN	Tab, Orange, Round, Scored, N / N <> 0.5	Clonazepam 0.5 mg	Rivotril by Novopharm	Canadian DIN 02239024	Anticonvulsant
05 <> NOVO	Tab, Peach, Oval, no/vo <> 0.5	Alprazolam 0.5 mg	Xanax by Novopharm	Canadian DIN 01913492	Antianxiety; C IV
05 <> NU	Tab, White, Round, 0.5 <> NU	Lorazepam 0.5 mg	Ativan by Nu Pharm	Canadian DIN 00865672	Antianxiety; C IV
05 <> P	Tab, White, Round	Lorazepam 0.5 mg	Ativan by Pharmascience	Canadian DIN 00728187	Antianxiety; C IV
05 <> R	Tab, Brownish Red, Oblong, Scored	Risperidone 0.5 mg	Risperdal by Pharmascience	Canadian DIN 02252015	Antipsychotic
05 <> SP322	Tab, Yellow, Round, Scored, Orally Disintegrating, 05	Alprazolam 0.5 mg	Niravam by Schwarz	00091-3322	Antianxiety; C IV
05 <> W	Tab, White, Round, W/0.5	Lorazepam 0.5 mg	Ativan by Wyeth	Canadian DIN 02041413	Antianxiety; C IV
05 <> W	Tab, Pale Green, Round, W <> 0.5, Sublingual	Lorazepam 0.5 mg	Ativan by Wyeth	Canadian DIN 02041456	Antianxiety; C IV
05 <> X	Tab, White, Pentagonal, Ex Release, 0.5 <> X	Alprazolam 0.5 mg	Xanax XR by Pharmacia	00009-0057	Antianxiety; C IV

ID FRONT <> BACK	DESCRIPTION FRONT <> BACK	INGREDIENT & STRENGTH	BRAND (or Generic Equiv.) by FIRM	NDC#	CLASS; SCH.
05 <> Z4232	Tab, Green, Round, Scored, Z over 4232 <> 0.5	Bumetanide 0.5 mg	Bumex by Teva	00093-4232	Diuretic
05 <> Z4232	Tab, Green, Round, Scored, 0.5 <> Z over 4232	Bumetanide 0.5 mg	Bumex by Vangard	00615-4541	Diuretic
05 <> Z4232	Tab, Green, Round, Scored, 0.5 <> Z over 4232	Bumetanide 0.5 mg	Bumex by Caraco		Diuretic
05 <> Z4232	Tab, Green, Round, Scored, 0.5 <> Z over 4232	Bumetanide 0.5 mg	Bumex by Ivax	00172-4232 Discontinued	Diuretic
05 <> Z4232	Tab, Green, Round, Scored, 0.5 <> Z over 4232	Bumetanide 0.5 mg	Bumex by Sandoz	00781-1821	Diuretic
05 <> Z4232	Tab, Green, Round, Scored, 0.5 <> Z over 4232	Bumetanide 0.5 mg	Bumex by Ivax	00182-2615	Diuretic
05 <> Z4232	Tab, Green, Round, Scored, 0.5 <> Z over 4232	Bumetanide 0.5 mg	Bumex by Moore	00839-8011	Diuretic
05 <> Z4232	Tab, Green, Round, Scored, 0.5 <> Z over 4232	Bumetanide 0.5 mg	Bumex by Major	00904-5102	Diuretic
05OHISTEXIE	Cap, Green and White	Carbinoxamine Maleate Immediate Release 2 mg, Carbinoxamine Maleate Extended Release 8 mg	Histex I/E by Teamm	67336-0050 Discontinued	Cold Remedy
051 <> R	Tab, White, Round, Scored	Diazepam 2 mg	Valium by Actavis	00228-2051	Antianxiety; C IV
051 <> R	Tab, White, Round, Scored	Diazepam 2 mg	Valium by Heartland	61392-0726	Antianxiety; C IV
052 <> R	Tab, Yellow, Round, Scored	Diazepam 5 mg	Valium by Heartland	61392-0831	Antianxiety; C IV
052 <> R	Tab, Yellow, Round, Scored	Diazepam 5 mg	Valium by Actavis	00228-2052	Antianxiety; C IV
052 <> R	Tab, Yellow, Round, Scored	Diazepam 5 mg	Valium by Urgent Care Center	50716-0132	Antianxiety; C IV
052 <> R	Tab, Yellow, Round, Scored	Diazepam 5 mg	Valium by Physician Total Care	54868-0059	Antianxiety; C IV
052 <> R	Tab, Yellow, Round, Scored	Diazepam 5 mg	Valium by Talbert	44514-0955	Antianxiety; C IV
05240405	Tab, White, Round, Scored, 0524 over 0405	Allopurinol 100 mg	Zyloprim by Vangard	00615-1592	Antigout
05240405	Tab, White, Round, Scored, 0524 over 0405	Allopurinol 100 mg	Zyloprim by H J Harkins Co	52959-0473	Antigout
05240405	Tab, White, Round, Scored, 0524 over 0405	Allopurinol 100 mg	Zyloprim by Apotheca	12634-0491	Antigout
05240405	Tab, White, Round, Scored, 0524 over 0405	Allopurinol 100 mg	Zyloprim by BASF	10117-0602	Antigout
05240405	Tab, White, Round, Scored, 0524 over 0405	Allopurinol 100 mg	Zyloprim by Par	49884-0602	Antigout
05240405	Tab, White, Round, Scored, 0524 over 0405	Allopurinol 100 mg	Zyloprim by Vangard	49884-0104	Antigout
05240410	Tab, Peach, Round, Scored, 0524 over 0410	Allopurinol 300 mg	Zyloprim by Par	49884-0105	Antigout
05240410	Tab, Peach, Round, Scored, 0524 over 0410	Allopurinol 300 mg	Zyloprim by BASF	10117-0603	Antigout
05240410	Tab, Peach, Round, Scored, 0524 over 0410	Allopurinol 300 mg	Zyloprim by IDE Inter	00814-0511	Antigout
05240410	Tab, Orange, Round, Scored, 0524 over 0410	Allopurinol 300 mg	Zyloprim by Par	49884-0603	Antigout
05271552	Cap, Dark Green & Light Green	Aspirin 325 mg, Butalbital 50 mg, Caffeine 40 mg	Fiorinal by Major	00904-3934	Analgesic; C III
05271552LANNETT	Cap, Dark Green & Light Green	Aspirin 325 mg, Butalbital 50 mg, Caffeine 40 mg	Fiorinal by Ivax	00182-0140	Analgesic; C III
05271552LANNETT	Cap, Dark Green & Light Green	Aspirin 325 mg, Butalbital 50 mg, Caffeine 40 mg	Fiorinal by Teva	55953-0633	Analgesic; C III
05271552LANNETT	Cap, Dark Green & Light Green	Aspirin 325 mg, Butalbital 50 mg, Caffeine 40 mg	Fiorinal by URL Mutual	00677-1439 Discontinued	Analgesic; C III
053 <> R	Tab, Blue, Round, Scored	Diazepam 10 mg	Valium by URL Mutual	00677-1050	Antianxiety; C IV
053 <> R	Tab, Blue, Round, Scored	Diazepam 10 mg	Valium by Actavis	00228-2053	Antianxiety; C IV
053 <> R	Tab, Blue, Round, Scored	Diazepam 10 mg	Valium by H J Harkins Co	52959-0306	Antianxiety; C IV
0546 <> BARR	Tab, Dark Orange, Cap Shaped, Film Coated	Cephalexin 500 mg	by Barr	00555-0546 Discontinued	Antibiotic
05510123	Tab, Pink, Round, Scored	Dyphylline 200 mg, Guaifenesin 200 mg	Dyline GG by Seatrace	00551-0123	Antiasthmatic; Expectorant
0552 <> M	Tab, White, Round, Scored, M in square	Oxycodone HCl 5 mg	Roxicodone by Mallinckrodt	00406-0552	Analgesic; C II
0554M5MG	Cap, Brown & Light Brown, Black Print, Opaque, 0554/M over 5 mg	Oxycodone HCl 5 mg	Roxicodone by Mallinckrodt	00406-0554	Analgesic; C II
058	Tab, Cream & Orange, Round, Chewable	Vitamin 1 mg, Fluoride 1 mg	PolyVi-Flor by Amide		Vitamin
05915238	Tab, White, Round	Meprobamate 400 mg	Miltown by Schein		Sedative/Hypnotic; C IV
05915239	Tab, White, Round	Meprobamate 200 mg	Miltown by Schein		Sedative/Hypnotic; C IV
059BARR	Cap, Pink	Diphenhydramine HCl 50 mg	Benadryl by UDL	51079-0066 Discontinued	Antihistamine
05ALG	Tab, Dark Yellow, 0.5/ALG	Alprazolam 0.5 mg	Xanax by Schein	00364-2583	Antianxiety; C IV

ID FRONT <> BACK	DESCRIPTION FRONT <> BACK	INGREDIENT & STRENGTH	BRAND (or Generic Equiv.) by FIRM	NDC#	CLASS; SCH.
05MG05MG	Cap, White, Opaque	Anagrelide HCl 0.5 mg	Agrylin by Pharmascience	Canadian DIN 02274949	Antiplatelet
05MG607	Cap, Light Yellow, 0.5 mg 607	Tacrolimus 0.5 mg	Prograf by Astellas	00469-0607	Immunosuppressant
05MG607	Cap, Light Yellow, 0.5 mg 607	Tacrolimus 0.5 mg	Prograf by St. Mary's Med	60760-0457	Immunosuppressant
05MG607	Cap, Light Yellow, 0.5 mg 607	Tacrolimus 0.5 mg	Prograf by Astellas	Canadian DIN 02243144	Immunosuppressant
05MGF607	Cap, Light Yellow, 0.5 mg "f" in square, 607	Tacrolimus 0.5 mg	Prograf by Astellas	Canadian DIN 02243144	Immunosuppressant
06	Tab, Oval, Peach	Fexofenadine HCl 60 mg	Allegra by Prasco	66993-0102	Antihistamine
06	Tab, Oval, Peach	Fexofenadine HCl 60 mg	Allegra by Prasco	66993-0107	Antihistamine
06 <> 0088	Tab, Peach, Oblong, Film Coated	Fexofenadine HCl 60 mg	Allegra by Aventis	00088-1107	Antihistamine
06 <> A	Tab, Light Pink, Cap Shaped, Scored, A <> 0 / 6	Citalopram HBr 20 mg	Celexa by Aurobindo	65862-0006	Antidepressant
06 <> A	Tab, Light Pink, Cap Shaped, Scored, A <> 0 / 6	Citalopram HBr 20 mg	Celexa by Aurolife	13107-0006	Antidepressant
06 <> A1	Tab, Light Green, Oblong, Ex Release	Guaifenesin 600 mg	Robitussin by Ivax	00182-1188	Expectorant
06 <> E	Tab, Peach, Oblong, Film Coated, Scripted E	Fexofenadine HCl 60 mg	Allegra by Aventis	00088-1107	Antihistamine
06 <> E	Tab, Peach, Oblong, Film Coated, Scripted E, 06 is underlined	Fexofenadine HCl 60 mg	Allegra 12 hr by Aventis	Canadian DIN 02231462	Antihistamine
06012D	Tab, Tan & White, Film Coated	Fexofenadine HCl 60 mg, Pseudoephedrine HCl 120 mg	Allegra-D 12 hr by Aventis	00088-1090	Antihistamine
061 <> PAR	Tab, Film Coated	Fluphenazine HCl 1 mg	Prolixin by Qualitest	00603-3666	Antipsychotic
061 <> PAR	Tab, Film Coated	Fluphenazine HCl 1 mg	Prolixin by Schein	00364-2265	Antipsychotic
061 <> T	Tab, Pink, Oblong, Line under 061	Diphenhydramine HCl 25 mg	Benadryl by Time Caps	49483-0061	Antihistamine
0610	Tab, Yellow, Scored	Oxycodone HCl 5 mg, Aspirin 325 mg	Endodan by BMS	Canadian DIN 01916483	Analgesic
0617	Cap, Red and White	Acetaminophen 500 mg	Tylenol Ex Strength by Major	00904-1987	Analgesic
062 <> PAR	Tab, Coated	Fluphenazine HCl 2.5 mg	Prolixin by Qualitest	00603-3667	Antipsychotic
062 <> PAR	Tab, Coated	Fluphenazine HCl 2.5 mg	Prolixin by Schein	00364-2266	Antipsychotic
0625Z2042	Tab, White, Round, 0.625 Z/2042	Conjugated Estrogens 0.625 mg	Premarin by Ivax		Hormone
063 <> ADAMS	Tab, Yellow, Oval, Scored	Dextromethorphan 60 mg, Guaifenesin 1200 mg, Pseudoephedrine 60 mg	Aquatab C by Adams	63824-0063	Cold Remedy
063 <> R	Tab, White, Round, Scored	Lorazepam 2 mg	Ativan by Actavis	00228-2063	Antianxiety; C IV
063 <> R	Tab, White, Round, Scored	Lorazepam 2 mg	Ativan by Nat Pharmpak	55154-0552	Antianxiety; C IV
063 <> R	Tab, White, Round, Scored	Lorazepam 2 mg	Ativan by Compumed	00403-0012	Antianxiety; C IV
063 <> R	Tab, White, Round, Scored	Lorazepam 2 mg	Ativan by Talbert	44514-0100	Antianxiety; C IV
0636	Tab, White to Off-White, Scored	Oxycodone HCl 5 mg, Acetaminophen 325 mg	Endocet by BMS	Canadian DIN 01916548	Analgesic
064 <> PAR	Tab, Film Coated	Fluphenazine HCl 10 mg	Prolixin by Qualitest	00603-3669	Antipsychotic
064 <> PAR	Tab, Film Coated	Fluphenazine HCl 10 mg	Prolixin by Schein	00364-2268	Antipsychotic
6654160	Cap	Lithium Carbonate 300 mg	Eskalith by Major	00904-2912	Antipsychotic
0659 <> ULTRAM	Tab, White, Oblong	Tramadol HCl 50 mg	Ultram by Ortho-McNeil	00045-0659	Analgesic
066100 <> B	Tab, White to Off-White, Round, Scored, 066 over 100	Isoniazid 100 mg	Laniazid by Barr	00555-0066	Antimycobacterial
066100 <> B	Tab, White to Off-White, Round, Scored, 066 over 100	Isoniazid 100 mg	Laniazid by UDL	51079-0082	Antimycobacterial
0665 <> 4001	Tab	Medroxyprogesterone Acetate 10 mg	by Int'l Lab	00665-4001	Hormone
06654001	Tab	Medroxyprogesterone Acetate 10 mg	by Talbert	44514-0542	Hormone
06654120	Cap, Orange, Black Print	Valproic Acid 250 mg	Depakene by Int'l Lab	00665-4120	Anticonvulsant
06654120	Cap, Orange, Black Print	Valproic Acid 250 mg	Depakene by Major	00904-2101	Anticonvulsant
06654120	Cap, Orange, Black Print	Valproic Acid 250 mg	Depakene by URL Mutual	00677-1079	Anticonvulsant
06654120	Cap, Orange, Black Print	Valproic Acid 250 mg	Depakene by Sandoz	00781-2203	Anticonvulsant
06654120	Cap, Orange, Black Print	Valproic Acid 250 mg	Depakene by RP Scherer	11014-0790	Anticonvulsant
06654140	Cap, Green	Hydralazine 25 mg, Hydrochlorothiazide 25 mg	Apresazide by Solvay	Discontinued	Antihypertensive; Diuretic
06654160	Cap, White, Red Print, 0665 over 4160	Lithium Carbonate 300 mg	Eskalith by URL Mutual	00677-1092	Antipsychotic

ID FRONT <> BACK	DESCRIPTION FRONT <> BACK	INGREDIENT & STRENGTH	BRAND (or Generic Equiv.) by FIRM	NDC#	CLASS; SCH.
06654160	Cap, White, Red Print, 0665 over 4160	Lithium Carbonate 300 mg	Eskalith by Qualitest	00603-4220	Antipsychotic
06654160	Cap, White, Red Print, 0665 over 4160	Lithium Carbonate 300 mg	Eskalith by Moore	00839-7149	Antipsychotic
06654160	Cap, White, Red Print, 0665 over 4160	Lithium Carbonate 300 mg	Eskalith by DRX	55045-2324	Antipsychotic
06654160	Cap, White, Red Print, 0665 over 4160	Lithium Carbonate 300 mg	Eskalith by Sandoz	00781-2100	Antipsychotic
06654160	Cap, White, Red Print, 0665 over 4160	Lithium Carbonate 300 mg	Eskalith by Int'l Lab	00665-4160	Antipsychotic
06654160	Cap, White, Red Print, 0665 over 4160	Lithium Carbonate 300 mg	Eskalith by Mylan		Antipsychotic
06654160	Cap, White, Red Print, 0665 over 4160	Lithium Carbonate 300 mg	Eskalith by Schein	00364-0855	Antipsychotic
06654160	Cap, White, Red Print, 0665 over 4160	Lithium Carbonate 300 mg	Eskalith by Solvay	00032-7512	Antipsychotic
0675AP	Cap, White	Quinine Sulfate 325 mg	Quinine by Allan	13279-0675 Discontinued	Antimalarial
068 <> ADAMS	Tab, Green, Oval, Scored	Guaifenesin 1200 mg, Pseudoephedrine 75 mg	Aquatab D by Adams	63824-0068	Cold Remedy
0698	Cap, Yellow, Round	Benzonatate 200 mg	Tessalon by Forest	00456-0698	Antitussive
0699	Cap, Red, Soft Gel	Amantadine HCl 100 mg	Endantadine by BMS	Canadian DIN 02034468	Antiviral
06WE	Cap	Brompheniramine Maleate 12 mg, Pseudoephedrine HCl 120 mg	Ultrabrom by Sovereign	58716-0025	Cold Remedy
07 <> A	Tab, White, Cap Shaped, Film Coated, Scored, A <> 0/7	Citalopram HBr 40 mg	Celexa by Aurobindo	65862-0007	Antidepressant
07 <> A	Tab, White, Cap Shaped, Film Coated, Scored, A <> 0/7	Citalopram HBr 40 mg	Celexa by Aurolife	13107-0007	Antidepressant
07 <> SL	Tab, White, Round, Sugar Coated	Hydroxyzine HCl 10 mg	Atarax by Talbert	44514-0418	Antianxiety; Antihistamine
07 <> SL	Tab, White, Round, Sugar Coated	Hydroxyzine HCl 10 mg	Atarax by Qualitest	00603-3970	Antianxiety; Antihistamine
07 <> SL	Tab, White, Round, Sugar Coated	Hydroxyzine HCl 10 mg	Atarax by Kaiser	00179-0294	Antianxiety; Antihistamine
07 <> SL	Tab, White, Round, Sugar Coated	Hydroxyzine HCl 10 mg	Atarax by Sidmak	Discontinued	Antianxiety; Antihistamine
07 <> SL	Tab, White, Round, Film Coated	Hydroxyzine HCl 10 mg	Atarax by Mutual	53489-0126	Antianxiety; Antihistamine
070	Tab, RP Logo	Theophylline Anhydrous 300 mg	Quibron T Sr Accudose by Monarch	61570-0019	Antiasthmatic
070 <> USL	Tab, Yellow, Round	Potassium Citrate 5 mEq	Potassium Citrate by Upsher-Smith	00245-0070	Electrolytes
0700US	Tab, Light Red, Oval	Phenyltoloxamine 30 mg, Magnesium Salicylate 600 mg	Novasal by US Pharma	52747-0700	Analgesic
071 <> USL	Tab, Yellow, Oval	Potassium Citrate 10 mEq	Potassium Citrate by Upsher-Smith	00245-0071	Electrolytes
071300 <> B	Tab, White to Off-White, Round, Scored, 071 over 300	Isoniazid 300 mg	Laniazid by Barr	00555-0071	Antimycobacterial
071300 <> B	Tab, White to Off-White, Round, Scored, 071 over 300	Isoniazid 300 mg	Laniazid by UDL	51079-0083	Antimycobacterial
073 <> RPC	Tab, Sugar Coated	Propantheline Bromide 7.5 mg	Pro Banthine by Roberts	54092-0073	Gastrointestinal
074 <> RPC	Tab, Sugar Coated	Propantheline Bromide 15 mg	Pro Banthine by Roberts	54092-0074	Gastrointestinal
0748	Tab, Blue, Round, Scored	Estradiol 2 mg	Gynodiol by Fielding	00421-0748	Hormone
0748 <> 0748	Tab, Blue, Scored	Estradiol 2 mg	by Heartland		Hormone
075 <> ER	Tab, White to Off White, Round, Ex Release, "0.75" <> ER	Pramipexole DiHCl 0.75 mg	Mirapex ER by Boehringer Ingelheim	00597-0285	Antiparkinson
0754 <> PAL	Tab, Green, Oblong, Scored	Pseudoephedrine HCl 45 mg, Guaifenesin 600 mg, Dextromethorphan HBr 30 mg	Panmist DM by Pamlab	00525-0754 Discontinued	Cold Remedy
0754 <> PAL	Tab, Green, Oblong, Scored	Pseudoephedrine HCl 45 mg, Guaifenesin 600 mg, Dextromethorphan HBr 30 mg	Panmist DM by Sovereign	58716-0687	Cold Remedy
0759 <> PAL	Tab, Green, Oblong, Scored	Pseudoephedrine HCl 48 mg, Guaifenesin 595 mg, Dextromethorphan HBr 32 mg	Panmist DM by Pamlab	00525-0759 Discontinued	Cold Remedy
076	Tab, Green, Oval, Film Coated	Ascorbic Acid 500 mg, Calcium Pantothenate 18 mg, Cyanocobalamin 5 mcg, Folic Acid 0.5 mg, Niacinamide 100 mg, Pyridoxine HCl 4 mg, Riboflavin 15 mg, Thiamine Mononitrate 15 mg	Formula B by Major	00904-2630	Vitamin
076	Tab, Green, Oval, Film Coated	Ascorbic Acid 500 mg, Calcium Pantothenate 18 mg, Cyanocobalamin 5 mcg, Folic Acid 0.5 mg, Niacinamide 100 mg, Pyridoxine HCl 4 mg, Riboflavin 15 mg, Thiamine Mononitrate 15 mg	Vitaplex by Amide	52152-0076	Vitamin
0768	Tab, Purple, Round, Scored	Estradiol 0.5 mg	Gynodiol by Fielding	00421-0768	Hormone
0768	Tab, Purple, Round, Scored	Estradiol 0.5 mg	Gynodiol by Heartland		Hormone
0768 <> PAL	Tab, White, Cap Shaped	Pseudoephedrine HCl 48 mg, Guaifenesin 595 mg	Panmist JR by Pamlab	00525-0768 Discontinued	Cold Remedy
077	Tab, Gray, Round, Schering Logo 077	Perphenazine 16 mg	Trilafon by Schering		Antipsychotic

ID FRONT <> BACK	DESCRIPTION FRONT <> BACK	INGREDIENT & STRENGTH	BRAND (or Generic Equiv.) by FIRM	NDC#	CLASS; SCH.
077	Tab, Yellow, Oval	Ascorbic Acid 500 mg, Biotin 0.15 mg, Chromic Nitrate 0.1 mg, Cupric Oxide, Cyanocobalamin 50 mcg, Ferrous Fumarate 27 mg, Folic Acid 0.8 mg, Magnesium Oxide 50 mg, Manganese Dioxide 5 mg, Niacin 100 mg, Pantothenic Acid 25 mg, Pyridoxine HCl 25 mg, Riboflavin 20 mg, Thiamine Mononitrate 20 mg, Vitamin A Acetate 5000 Units, Vitamin E Acetate 30 Units	Vitaplex Plus by Amide	52152-0077	Vitamin
077 <> ADAMS	Tab, Blue, Oblong, Scored	Chlorpheniramine 8 mg, Methscopolamine 2.5 mg	AllerRx PM by Adams	63824-0077	Antihistamine
0775 <> PAL	Tab	Guaifenesin 600 mg, Pseudoephedrine HCl 90 mg	Panmist LA by Sovereign	58716-0658 Discontinued	Cold Remedy
0775 <> PAL	Tab	Guaifenesin 600 mg, Pseudoephedrine HCl 90 mg	Panmist LA by Pamlab	00525-0775 Discontinued	Cold Remedy
078 <> OHM	Tab, Orange, Round	Acetaminophen 325 mg, Phenyltoloxamine Citrate 30 mg	Percogesic by Ivax	00182-1413 Discontinued	Analgesic
0780 <> PAL	Tab, White w/ Green Specks	Chlorpheniramine Maleate 8 mg, Methscopolamine Nitrate 2.5 mg, Phenylpropanolamine HCl 75 mg	Pannaz by Murfreesboro	51129-1429 Discontinued	Cold Remedy
0780 <> PAL	Tab, White w/ Green Specks	Chlorpheniramine Maleate 8 mg, Methscopolamine Nitrate 2.5 mg, Phenylpropanolamine HCl 75 mg	Pannaz by Pamlab	00525-0780	Cold Remedy
0780 <> PAL	Tab, White w/ Green Specks	Chlorpheniramine Maleate 8 mg, Methscopolamine Nitrate 2.5 mg, Phenylpropanolamine HCl 75 mg	Pannaz by Anabolic	00722-6337 Discontinued	Cold Remedy
0788 <> PAL	Tab, White w/ Green Specks, Scored	Pseudoephedrine HCl 90 mg, Chlorpheniramine 8 mg, Methscopolamine 2.5 mg	Durahist by Pamlab	00525-0788 Discontinued	Cold Remedy
079	Tab, White, Oblong	Aspirin 800 mg	Aspirin by Amide		Analgesic
0792 <> PAL	Tab, White with Red Spots, Cap Shaped, 07/92 <> PAL	Pseudoephedrine HCl 85 mg, Guaifenesin 795 mg	Panmist LA by Pamlab	00525-0792 Discontinued	Cold Remedy
08 <> A	Tab, Yellow, Cap Shaped, Film Coated, Scored, A <> 0 / 8	Mirtazapine 15 mg	Remeron by Aurobindo	65862-0031	Antidepressant
08 <> A	Tab, Yellow, Cap Shaped, Film Coated, Scored, A <> 0 / 8	Mirtazapine 15 mg	Remeron by Aurolife	13107-0031	Antidepressant
08 <> SL	Tab, White, Black Print, Round, Sugar Coated	Hydroxyzine HCl 25 mg	Atarax by Murfreesboro	51129-1481	Antianxiety; Antihistamine
08 <> SL	Tab, White, Black Print, Round, Sugar Coated	Hydroxyzine HCl 25 mg	Atarax by Moore	00839-7438	Antianxiety; Antihistamine
08 <> SL	Tab, White, Black Print, Round, Sugar Coated	Hydroxyzine HCl 25 mg	Atarax by Baker Cummins	63171-1493	Antianxiety; Antihistamine
08 <> SL	Tab, White, Black Print, Round, Sugar Coated	Hydroxyzine HCl 25 mg	Atarax by Apotheca	12634-0474	Antianxiety; Antihistamine
08 <> SL	Tab, White, Black Print, Round, Sugar Coated	Hydroxyzine HCl 25 mg	Atarax by Darby Group	66467-4568	Antianxiety; Antihistamine
08 <> SL	Tab, White, Black Print, Round, Sugar Coated	Hydroxyzine HCl 25 mg	Atarax by Sandoz	00781-1334	Antianxiety; Antihistamine
08 <> SL	Tab, White, Black Print, Round, Sugar Coated	Hydroxyzine HCl 25 mg	Atarax by Rx Dispensing	61807-0032	Antianxiety; Antihistamine
08 <> SL	Tab, White, Black Print, Round, Sugar Coated	Hydroxyzine HCl 25 mg	Atarax by Amerisource	62584-0743	Antianxiety; Antihistamine
08 <> SL	Tab, White, Black Print, Round, Sugar Coated	Hydroxyzine HCl 25 mg	Atarax by H J Harkins Co	52959-0074	Antianxiety; Antihistamine
08 <> SL	Tab, White, Black Print, Round, Sugar Coated	Hydroxyzine HCl 25 mg	Atarax by Pharmedix	53002-0320	Antianxiety; Antihistamine
08 <> SL	Tab, White, Black Print, Round, Sugar Coated	Hydroxyzine HCl 25 mg	Atarax by Richmond	54738-0308	Antianxiety; Antihistamine
08 <> SL	Tab, White, Black Print, Round, Sugar Coated	Hydroxyzine HCl 25 mg	Atarax by Physician Total Care	54868-0063	Antianxiety; Antihistamine
08 <> SL	Tab, White, Black Print, Round, Sugar Coated	Hydroxyzine HCl 25 mg	Atarax by Ivax	00182-1493	Antianxiety; Antihistamine
08 <> SL	Tab, White, Black Print, Round, Sugar Coated	Hydroxyzine HCl 25 mg	Atarax by Med Pro	53978-3066	Antianxiety; Antihistamine
08 <> SL	Tab, White, Black Print, Round, Sugar Coated	Hydroxyzine HCl 25 mg	Atarax by Major	00904-0358	Antianxiety; Antihistamine
08 <> SL	Tab, White, Black Print, Round, Sugar Coated	Hydroxyzine HCl 25 mg	Atarax by Caremark	00339-6009	Antianxiety; Antihistamine
08 <> SL	Tab, White, Black Print, Round, Sugar Coated	Hydroxyzine HCl 25 mg	Atarax by Kaiser	00179-0295	Antianxiety; Antihistamine
08 <> SL	Tab, White, Black Print, Round, Sugar Coated	Hydroxyzine HCl 25 mg	Atarax by Qualitest	00603-3971	Antianxiety; Antihistamine
08 <> SL	Tab, White, Black Print, Round, Sugar Coated	Hydroxyzine HCl 25 mg	Atarax by Talbert	44514-0419	Antianxiety; Antihistamine
080 <> SCHERING	Tab, Yellow, Round, Scored, "Schering" over a Logo <> / 080	Chlorpheniramine 4 mg	Chlor-Trimeton by Schering-Plough	00085-0080	Antihistamine
0812	Cap, Purple, Opaque, Soft Gel, White Ink	Calcium Citrate 100 mg, Iron 27 mg, Vitamin D3 400 IU, Vitamin E 30 IU, Vitamin B6 25 mg, Folic Acid 1 mg, Docusate Sodium 50 mg, Docosahexaenoic Acid 250 mg	CitraNatal Harmony by Mission	00178-0812	Prenatal Vitamin
081IMPAX10	Cap, Light Brown and Lavender, Opaque, Hard Gelatin, IMPAX/10, Delayed Release	Omeprazole 10 mg	Prilosec by Teva Pharmaceuticals	00093-5210 Discontinued	Gastrointestinal

ID FRONT <> BACK	DESCRIPTION FRONT <> BACK	INGREDIENT & STRENGTH	BRAND (or Generic Equiv.) by FIRM	NDC#	CLASS; SCH.
0822	Tab, Pink, Round, Chewable	Sodium Fluoride 2.2 mg	Luride by Pharmafair		Element
08220405	Tab, White, Round	Allopurinol 100 mg	Zyloprim by Boots		Antigout
08220410	Tab, Peach, Round	Allopurinol 300 mg	Zyloprim by Boots		Antigout
08220430	Tab, White, Round	Butalbital 50 mg, Aspirin 325 mg, Caffeine 40 mg	Fiorinal by Halsey		Analgesic; C III
08220576	Tab, Pink, Round, Chewable	Meclazine 25 mg	Bonine by Boots		Antiemetic
08220841	Tab, Pink, Round, Chewable	Sodium Fluoride 2.2 mg	Luride Lozi-tabs by Boots		Element
08221530	Tab, Pink, Round	Levothyroxine Sodium 300 mcg	Synthroid by Boots		Thyroid Hormone
08221531	Tab, Green, Round	Levothyroxine Sodium 300 mcg	Synthroid by Boots		Thyroid Hormone
08225	Tab, White, Round	Atropine Sulfate 0.025 mg, Diphenoxylate HCl 2.5 mg	Lomotil by Pharmafair		Antidiarrheal; C V
0829 <> CN90	Tab, White, Oval, Scored, 08 / 29	Vitamin C 120 mg, Calcium 160 mg, Iron 90 mg, Vitamin D3 400 IU, Vitamin E 30 IU, Thiamin 3 mg, Riboflavin 3.4 mg, Niacinamide 20 mg, Vitamin B6 20 mg, Folic Acid 1 mg, Iodine 150 mcg, Zinc 25 mg, Copper 2 mg, Docusate Sodium 50 mg	CitraNatal 90 DHA by Mission	00178-0829	Vitamin
082IMPAX20	Cap, Lavender, Opaque, Hard Gelatin, IMPAX/20, Delayed Release	Omeprazole 20 mg	Prilosec by Teva Pharmaceuticals	00093-5211 Discontinued	Gastrointestinal
083	Tab, Reddish Brown, Cap Shaped	Ibuprofen 200 mg, Pseudoephedrine 30 mg	Dristan by Perrigo	00113-0083	Cold Remedy
083	Tab, Reddish Brown, Cap Shaped	Ibuprofen 200 mg, Pseudoephedrine 30 mg	Advil Cold and Sinus by Ivax	00182-1195	Cold Remedy
083 <> APO	Tab, White to Off-White, Oval, Film Coated	Paroxetine HCl 20 mg	Paxil by Apotex	60505-0083	Antidepressant
083 <> KALI	Tab, Reddish Orange, Round	Acetaminophen 325 mg, Tramadol 37.5 mg	Ultracet by Kali	66893-	Analgesic
083 <> KALI	Tab, Orange, Capsule Shaped, Film Coated	Tramadol HCl 37.5 mg, Acetaminophen 325 mg	Ultracet by Par	49884-0946	Analgesic
0832G536C	Cap, Yellow	Phentermine HCl 30 mg	by Forest	00456-0766	Anorexiant; C IV
0832G536C	Cap, Black	Phentermine HCl 30 mg	by Forest	00456-0606	Anorexiant; C IV
0835	Cap, Pink and White	Diphenhydramine HCl 25 mg	Benadryl by Major	00904-5306	Antihistamine
0835	Cap, Pink	Diphenhydramine HCl 25 mg	Benadryl by Major	00904-2035	Antihistamine
0836	Cap, Pink	Diphenhydramine HCl 50 mg	Benadryl by Major	00904-5306	Antihistamine
083IMPAX40	Cap, Brown and Lavender, Opaque, Hard Gel, IMPAX/40, Delayed Release	Omeprazole 40 mg	Prilosec by Teva Pharmaceuticals	00093-5212 Discontinued	Gastrointestinal
084 <> AMIDE	Tab, Peach, Oblong	Choline Magnesium Trisalicylate 500 mg	Trilisate by Ivax	00182-1899 Discontinued	NSAID
084 <> APO	Tab, White to Off-White, Oval, Film Coated	Paroxetine HCl 30 mg	Paxil by Apotex	60505-0084	Antidepressant
084 <> WC	Tab, White, Blue Print, Oval, Partially Scored, Film Coated	Gemfibrozil 600 mg	by Moore	00839-7787	Antihyperlipidemic
084 <> WC	Tab, White, Blue Print, Oval, Partially Scored, Film Coated	Gemfibrozil 600 mg	by Sidmak	Discontinued	Antihyperlipidemic
084 <> WC	Tab, White, Blue Print, Oval, Partially Scored, Film Coated	Gemfibrozil 600 mg	by Kaiser	62224-1226	Antihyperlipidemic
084 <> WC	Tab, White, Blue Print, Oval, Partially Scored, Film Coated	Gemfibrozil 600 mg	by Med Pro	53978-2033	Antihyperlipidemic
084 <> WC	Tab, White, Blue Print, Oval, Partially Scored, Film Coated	Gemfibrozil 600 mg	by Allscripts		Antihyperlipidemic
084 <> WC	Tab, White, Blue Print, Oval, Partially Scored, Film Coated	Gemfibrozil 600 mg	by Warner Chilcott	00047-0084	Antihyperlipidemic
084 <> WC	Tab, White, Blue Print, Oval, Partially Scored, Film Coated	Gemfibrozil 600 mg	by Kaiser	00179-1171	Antihyperlipidemic
085 <> AMIDE	Tab, White, Oblong	Choline Magnesium Trisalicylate 750 mg	Trilisate by Ivax	00182-1895 Discontinued	NSAID
085 <> R	Tab, Pink, Cap Shaped, Film Coated	Acetaminophen 650 mg, Propoxyphene Napsylate 100 mg	Darvocet-N 100 by Urgent Care Center	50716-0364	Analgesic; C IV
085 <> R	Tab, Pink, Cap Shaped, Film Coated	Acetaminophen 650 mg, Propoxyphene Napsylate 100 mg	Darvocet-N 100 by Rugby	00536-4361	Analgesic; C IV
085 <> R	Tab, Pink, Cap Shaped, Film Coated	Acetaminophen 650 mg, Propoxyphene Napsylate 100 mg	Darvocet-N 100 by Heartland	61392-0446	Analgesic; C IV
085 <> R	Tab, Pink, Cap Shaped, Film Coated	Acetaminophen 650 mg, Propoxyphene Napsylate 100 mg	Darvocet-N 100 by Golden State	60429-0518	Analgesic; C IV
085 <> R	Tab, Pink, Cap Shaped, Film Coated	Acetaminophen 650 mg, Propoxyphene Napsylate 100 mg	Darvocet-N 100 by Actavis	00228-2085	Analgesic; C IV
086	Tab, Brownish Orange, Round	Bisacodyl 5 mg	Dulcolax by Perrigo	00113-0086	Gastrointestinal
0863 <> 93	Tab, White to Off-White, Round, Film Coated	Ciprofloxacin 250 mg	Cipro by Teva	00093-0863 Discontinued	Antibiotic

ID FRONT <> BACK	DESCRIPTION FRONT <> BACK	INGREDIENT & STRENGTH	BRAND (or Generic Equiv.) by FIRM	NDC#	CLASS; SCH.
0864 <> 93	Tab, White to Off-White, Cap Shaped, Film Coated	Ciprofloxacin 500 mg	Cipro by Teva	00093-0864 Discontinued	Antibiotic
0865 <> 93	Tab, White to Off-White, Cap Shaped, Film Coated	Ciprofloxacin 750 mg	Cipro by Teva	00093-0865	Antibiotic
0866	Cap, Red, Oblong, Soft Gel	Docusate Calcium 240 mg	Surfak by RP Scherer		Laxative
0866	Tab, White, Oval, Coated	Vitamin C 120 mg, Calcium 125 mg, Iron 20 mg, Vitamin D3 400 IU, Vitamin B6 25 mg, Folic Acid 1 mg	CitraNatal B-Calm by Mission	00178-0866	Vitamin; Supplement
0893	Tab, White, Oval, Coated	Vitamin C 120 mg, Calcium 125 mg, Iron 35 mg, Vitamin D3 400 IU, Vitamin E 30 IU, Thiamin 3 mg, Riboflavin 3.4 mg, Niacinamide 20 mg, Vitamin B6 25 mg, Folic Acid 1 mg, Iodine 150 mcg, Zinc 25 mg, Copper 2 mg, Docusate Sodium 50 mg	CitraNatal Assure by Mission	00178-0893	Vitamin; Supplement
0894	Tab, Light Brown, Scored	Hydrocodone Bitartrate 5 mg	by RPR	Canadian	Analgesic; C III
0897	Cap, Orange, Oval, Soft Gel	Docusate Sodium 100 mg	Colace by UDL	Discontinued	Laxative
0898	Cap, Orange, White Print, Soft Gel	Docusate Sodium 250 mg	Colace by Sandoz	00781-2795	Laxative
0898	Cap, Orange, White Print, Soft Gel	Docusate Sodium 250 mg	Colace by UDL	51079-0048 Discontinued	Laxative
09 <> A	Tab, Reddish Brown, Cap Shaped, Film Coated, Scored, A <> 0 / 9	Mirtazapine 30 mg	Remeron by Aurobindo	65862-0003	Antidepressant
09 <> A	Tab, Reddish Brown, Cap Shaped, Film Coated, Scored, A <> 0 / 9	Mirtazapine 30 mg	Remeron by Aurobindo	13107-0003	Antidepressant
091 <> PAR	Tab, Yellow, Round, Film Coated	Doxycycline 50 mg	Monoclox by Par	49884-0091	Antibiotic
092 <> PAR	Tab, Light Orange, Round, Film Coated	Doxycycline 75 mg	Monoclox by Par	49884-0092	Antibiotic
0920	Cap, Pink & Clear, Royce Logo	Isosorbide Dinitrate 40 mg	Isordil by Eon		Antianginal
0924 <> 93	Tab, White to Off-White, Cap Shaped, Scored, 9 over 3	Oxaprozin 600 mg	Daypro by Teva	00093-0924	NSAID
093 <> APO	Tab, White, Round	Doxazosin Mesylate 1 mg	Cardura by Major	00904-5522	Antihypertensive
093 <> APO	Tab, White, Round	Doxazosin Mesylate 1 mg	Cardura by Apotex	60505-0093	Antihypertensive
093 <> MIA	Tab	Chlorpheniramine 8 mg, Phenylephrine 25 mg, Pyrilamine 25 mg	Histatan by Ivax	00182-1912	Cold Remedy
093 <> MIA	Tab	Chlorpheniramine 8 mg, Phenylephrine 25 mg, Pyrilamine 25 mg	Histatan by Ivax	00172-4376	Cold Remedy
093 <> MIA	Tab	Chlorpheniramine 8 mg, Phenylephrine 25 mg, Pyrilamine 25 mg	Rhinatate by Major	00904-1669	Cold Remedy
093 <> PAR	Tab, Yellow, Round, Film Coated	Doxycycline 100 mg	Monoclox by Par	49884-0093	Antibiotic
094 <> APO	Tab, White, Cap Shaped	Doxazosin Mesylate 2 mg	Cardura by Apotex	60505-0094	Antihypertensive
094 <> APO	Tab, White, Cap Shaped	Doxazosin Mesylate 2 mg	Cardura by Major	00904-5523	Antihypertensive
095	Tab, Red, Oval, Ex Release, Schering Logo 095	Dexchlorpheniramine Maleate 4 mg	Polaramine by Schering		Antihistamine
095 <> APO	Tab, White, Cap Shaped	Doxazosin Mesylate 4 mg	Cardura by Apotex	60505-0095	Antihypertensive
095 <> APO	Tab, White, Cap Shaped	Doxazosin Mesylate 4 mg	Cardura by Major	00904-5524	Antihypertensive
096 <> APO	Tab, White, Cap Shaped	Doxazosin Mesylate 8 mg	Cardura by Major	00904-5525	Antihypertensive
096 <> APO	Tab, White, Cap Shaped	Doxazosin Mesylate 8 mg	Cardura by Apotex	60505-0096	Antihypertensive
097 <> APO	Tab, White to Off-White, Oval, Film Coated	Paroxetine HCl 10 mg	Paxil by Apotex	60505-0097	Antidepressant
0993	Cap, Orange	Acetaminophen 250 mg, Dextromethorphan HBr 10 mg, Guaifenesin 100 mg, Pseudoephedrine HCl 30 mg	Tylenol Cold by PFI		Cold Remedy
1	Tab, Orange, Oval	Dextrothyroxine Sodium 1 mg	Choloxin by Boots		Thyroid Hormone
1	Tab, White, Round	Clonazepam 1 mg	Klonopin Wafers by Hoffmann La Roche	00004-0282	Sedative; C IV
1	Tab, White, Round, Film Coated	Metoprolol Tartrate 25 mg	Lopressor by Caraco	57664-0506	Antihypertensive
1	Tab, Blue, Buccal	Fentanyl 100 mcg	Fentora by Cephalon	63459-0541	Opioid Agonist; C II
1	Tab, White, Round	Nitroglycerin 0.3 mg (1/200 gr)	Nitrostat by Able	53265-0249 Discontinued	Vasodilator
1	Tab, Ex Release	Nitroglycerin 1 mg	Sustachron by Forest		Vasodilator
1	Tab, White, Round	Nitroglycerin CR Buccal 1 mg	Nitrogard by Forest	10418-0136	Vasodilator
1	Tab, Off-White to White, Round, Ex Release	Nitroglycerin 1 mg	Nitrogard 1 by Forest	00456-0686	Vasodilator
1	Tab, Blue, Round	Trifluoperazine HCl 1 mg	Apo Trifluoperazine by Apotex	Canadian DIN 00345539	Antipsychotic

ID FRONT <> BACK	DESCRIPTION FRONT <> BACK	INGREDIENT & STRENGTH	BRAND (or Generic Equiv.) by FIRM	NDC#	CLASS; SCH.
1	Tab, Bright Pink, Round	Fluphenazine HCl 1 mg	Fluphenazine by Apotex	Canadian DIN 00405345	Antipsychotic
1	Tab, White, Round, Vanda Logo <> 1	Iloperidone 1 mg	Fanapt by Vanda	43068-0101	Antipsychotic
1 <> 113	Tab, White, Barrel Shaped	Granisetron HCl 1 mg	Kytril by Dava	67253-0417	Antiemetic
1 <> 241	Tab	Lorazepam 1 mg	Ativan by URL Mutual	00677-1057	Antianxiety; C IV
1 <> 241	Tab	Lorazepam 1 mg	Ativan by Qualitest	00603-4244	Antianxiety; C IV
1 <> 274	Tab, Blue, Round, Scored	Clonazepam 1 mg	Klonopin by Caraco	57664-0274	Sedative; C IV
1 <> 3685	Tab, White, Round, Scored, Hourglass Logo 1	Doxazosin Mesylate 1 mg	Cardura by Ivax	00172-3685	Antihypertensive
1 <> 4036	Tab, White, Square, Hourglass Logo 1	Estazolam 1 mg	Prosom by Ivax	00172-4036	Sedative/Hypnotic; C IV
1 <> 54050	Tab, White, Hexagonal, Scored, 54 over 050	Haloperidol 1 mg	Haldol by Merck Sharp & Dohme	60312-0072	Antipsychotic
1 <> 54050	Tab, White, Hexagonal, Scored, 54 over 050	Haloperidol 1 mg	Haldol by Roxane	00054-8343 Discontinued	Antipsychotic
1 <> 54050	Tab, White, Hexagonal, Scored, 54 over 050	Haloperidol 1 mg	Haldol by Nat Pharmpak	55154-4924	Antipsychotic
1 <> 54050	Tab, White, Hexagonal, Scored, 54 over 050	Haloperidol 1 mg	Haldol by Amerisource	62584-0725	Antipsychotic
1 <> 5624DAN	Tab	Lorazepam 1 mg	Ativan by Quality Care	60346-0047	Antianxiety; C IV
1 <> A	Tab, Light Yellow	Dextromethorphan HBr 30 mg, Guaifenesin 600 mg, Phenylephrine HCl 15 mg	Albatussin Sr by Anabolic	00722-6211	Cold Remedy
1 <> ALVA	Tab, White, Oval	Acetaminophen 250 mg, Caffeine 32.5 mg, Magnesium Salicylate Tetrahydrate 310 mg	Arthriten by Alva		Analgesic
1 <> ALVA	Tab, Light Blue, Oval	Pamabrom 50 mg	Diurex Maximum Relief by Alva		Diuretic
1 <> ATIVAN	Tab, White, Oblong, l/Ativan	Lorazepam 1 mg	Ativan by Wyeth	Canadian DIN 02041421	Antianxiety; C IV
1 <> B492	Tab, Yellow, Round, b over 492, Ex Release	Alprazolam 1 mg	Xanax XR by Barr	00555-0492	Antianxiety; C IV
1 <> B97	Tab, White, Round, Orally Disintegrating	Clonazepam 1 mg	Klonopin Wafers by Barr	00555-0097	Sedative; C IV
1 <> DAN5604	Tab, Peach, Round, Scored, DAN over 5604	Haloperidol 1 mg	Haldol by Schein	00364-2205	Antipsychotic
1 <> DRL50	Tab, White, Oval	Nefazodone HCl 50 mg	Serzone by Dr. Reddy's	55111-0138	Antidepressant
1 <> DRL50	Tab, White, Oval	Nefazodone HCl 50 mg	Serzone by Par	49884-0916	Antidepressant
1 <> EP905	Tab, White, Round	Lorazepam 1 mg	Ativan by Excellium	64125-0905	Antianxiety; C IV
1 <> G	Tab, Yellow, Square, Ex Release	Alprazolam 1 mg	Xanax XR by Greenstone	59762-0059	Antianxiety; C IV
1 <> G	Tab, White, Hexagonal, Scored	Estradiol 1 mg	by AAI Pharma	27280-0005	Hormone
1 <> G	Tab, White, Hexagonal, Scored	Estradiol 1 mg	by Teva	00093-1058 Discontinued	Hormone
1 <> GG51	Tab, Lavender, Round, GG over 51	Trifluoperazine HCl 1 mg	by Apotheca	12634-0678	Antipsychotic
1 <> GG51	Tab, Lavender, Round, GG over 51	Trifluoperazine HCl 1 mg	by Sandoz	00781-1030	Antipsychotic
1 <> INV309	Tab, Pink, Square, Scored, 1 <> INV over 309	Warfarin Sodium 1 mg	Coumadin by Apothecon	59772-0352	Anticoagulant
1 <> KC	Tab, White, Round, Film Coated	Pitavastatin 1 mg	Livalo by Kowa Pharmaceuticals	00002-4770	Antihyperlipidemic
1 <> N	Tab, Yellow, Round, Scored, Large N	Haloperidol 1 mg	Haldol by Novopharm	Canadian DIN 00363677	Antipsychotic
1 <> N	Tab, White, Round	Terazosin HCl 1 mg	Hytrin by Novopharm	Canadian DIN 02230805	Antihypertensive
1 <> N590	Tab, White to Off-White, Round, Scored, N over 590	Doxazosin Mesylate 1 mg	Cardura by Teva	00093-8120	Antihypertensive
1 <> NN	Tab, Yellow, Oval, Scored, N / N <> 1	Cilazapril 1 mg	Inhibace by Novopharm	Canadian DIN 02266350	Antihypertensive
1 <> NN	Tab, White, Round, Scored, N/N	Ketotifen Fumarate 1 mg	Zaditen by Novopharm	Canadian DIN 02230730	Antiasthmatic
1 <> NN	Tab, White, Round, Scored, N / N	Doxazosin Mesylate 1 mg	Cardura by Novopharm	Canadian DIN 02247728	Antihypertensive
1 <> NOVO	Tab, Peach, Oblong, NO/VO <> 1	Prazosin HCl 1 mg	Minipress by Novopharm	Canadian DIN 01934198	Antihypertensive
1 <> P	Tab, White, Round	Terazosin HCl 1 mg	Hytrin by Pharmascience	Canadian DIN 02243518	Antihypertensive

ID FRONT <> BACK	DESCRIPTION FRONT <> BACK	INGREDIENT & STRENGTH	BRAND (or Generic Equiv.) by FIRM	NDC#	CLASS; SCH.
1 <> P	Tab, Blue, Round, Scored	Methadone Hydrochloride 1 mg	Metadol by Pharmascience	Canadian DIN 02247698	Analgesic
1 <> PMS	Tab, Pale Green, Round, Scored	Hydromorphone HCl 1 mg	by Pharmascience	Canadian DIN 00885444	Analgesic; C II
1 <> SEARLE	Tab	Mestranol 0.05 mg, Norethindrone 1 mg	Norinyl by Searle	00025-0263	Oral Contraceptive
1 <> SP323	Tab, White, Round, Scored, Orally Disintegrating	Alprazolam 1 mg	Niravam by Schwarz	00091-3323	Antianxiety; C IV
1 <> W	Tab, White, Round, Sublingual	Lorazepam 1 mg	Ativan by Wyeth	Canadian DIN 02041464	Antianxiety; C IV
1 <> WARFARINTARO	Tab, Light Pink, Cap Shaped	Warfarin Sodium 1 mg	Coumadin by Taro	51672-4027	Anticoagulant
1 <> X	Tab, Yellow, Square, Ex Release	Alprazolam 1 mg	Xanax XR by Pharmacia	00009-0059	Antianxiety; C IV
1 <> Z	Tab, White to Off-White, Round, Film Coated	Carvedilol 3.125 mg	Coreg by Zydus	68382-0092	Antihypertensive
1 <> Z4233	Tab, Yellow, Round, Scored, Z over 4233	Bumetanide 1 mg	Bumex by Teva	00093-4233	Diuretic
1 <> Z4233	Tab, Yellow, Round, Scored, Z over 4233	Bumetanide 1 mg	Bumex by Ivax	00172-4233 Discontinued	Diuretic
1 <> Z4233	Tab, Yellow, Round, Scored, Z over 4233	Bumetanide 1 mg	Bumex by Sandoz	00781-1822	Diuretic
1 <> Z4233	Tab, Yellow, Round, Scored, Z over 4233	Bumetanide 1 mg	Bumex by Moore	00839-8012	Diuretic
1 <> Z4233	Tab, Yellow, Round, Scored, Z over 4233	Bumetanide 1 mg	Bumex by Murfreesboro	51129-1337	Diuretic
1 <> Z4233	Tab, Yellow, Round, Scored, Z over 4233	Bumetanide 1 mg	Bumex by Major	00904-5103	Diuretic
1 <> Z4233	Tab, Yellow, Round, Scored, Z over 4233	Bumetanide 1 mg	Bumex by Ivax	00182-2616	Diuretic
1 <> Z4233	Tab, Yellow, Round, Scored, Z over 4233	Bumetanide 1 mg	Bumex by Nat Pharmpak	55154-5819	Diuretic
10	Tab, Orange, Round	Bethanechol Chloride 10 mg	Urecholine by Roberts	Canadian	Urinary Tract
10	Tab, Blue, Round	Amitriptyline HCl 10 mg	Elavil by Apotex	Canadian DIN 00335053	Antidepressant
10	Tab, White, Cap Shaped, Film Coated, four point star <> 10	Valdecoxib 10 mg	Bextra by Searle	00025-1975 Discontinued	COX 2 Inhibitor
10	Tab, Red, Round, Scored	Chlorpheniramine Maleate 5 mg, Phenylephrine HCl 10 mg, Carbetapentane Tannate 60 mg	Ricotuss by Rico Pharma	62453-0103	Cold Remedy
10	Tab, Red, Round, Scored	Chlorpheniramine Maleate 5 mg, Phenylephrine HCl 10 mg, Carbetapentane Tannate 60 mg	Ricotuss by Pegasus	55246-0055	Cold Remedy
10	Tab, Yellow, Oval, Dish Logo/10	Loratadine 10 mg	Claritin by Schering	Canadian DIN 00782696	Antihistamine
10	Tab, Dark Orange, Round, Ex Release, Andrx Logo 10	Lovastatin 10 mg	Altoprev by Andrx	62022-0627	Antihyperlipidemic
10	Tab, Dark Orange, Round, Ex Release, Andrx Logo 10	Lovastatin 10 mg	Altocor by Andrx	62022-0760	Antihyperlipidemic
10	Tab, White, Round	Buspirone HCl 10 mg	Buspar by Amide	52152-0223	Antianxiety
10	Tab, Yellow, Round, Hourglass Logo <> 10	Prochlorperazine 10 mg	Compazine by Ivax	00172-3691	Antiemetic
10	Tab, Yellow, Round, Orally Disintegrating	Olanzapine 10 mg	Zyprexa Zydis by Eli Lilly	00002-4454	Antipsychotic
10	Tab, White, Round	Buspirone HCl 10 mg	Buspar by Major	00904-5588	Antianxiety
10	Tab	Yohimbine HCl	by Jerome Stevens	50564-0509	Impotence Agent
10	Tab, Light Green, Round	Thioridazine HCl 10 mg	by Apotex	Canadian	Antipsychotic
10	Tab, Rose, Round	Nifedipine 10 mg	Adalat 10 by Bayer	Canadian	Antihypertensive
10	Tab, Blue, Round	Trifluoperazine HCl 10 mg	by Apotex	Canadian DIN 00326836	Antipsychotic
10	Cap, Orange, Oval	Hydroxyzine HCl 10 mg	Atarax by Novopharm	Canadian DIN 00738824	Antianxiety; Antihistamine
10	Tab, Light Orange, Octagonal, Film Coated, E674 over 10, Extended Release	Oxymorphone HCl 10 mg	Opana ER by Endo	63481-0674	Analgesic; C II
10	Tab, Light Brown, Round	Imipramine HCl 10 mg	Tofranil by Apotex	Canadian DIN 00360201	Antidepressant
10	Tab, Pink, Square	Famotidine 10 mg	Famotidine by Apotex	Canadian DIN 02231119	Gastrointestinal

ID FRONT <> BACK	DESCRIPTION FRONT <> BACK	INGREDIENT & STRENGTH	BRAND (or Generic Equiv.) by FIRM	NDC#	CLASS; SCH.
10	Cap, Orange, Oval	Hydroxyzine HCl 10 mg	by Apotex	Canadian DIN 00646059	Antianxiety; Antihistamine
10	Tab, Pale Yellow, Triangular	Clomipramine HCl 10 mg	Anafranil by Apotex	Canadian DIN 02040786	OCD
10	Tab, Blue, Round	Desipramine HCl 10 mg	Apo Desipramine by Apotex	Canadian DIN 02216248	Antidepressant
10	Tab, Tan, Round, Film Coated	Citalopram 10 mg	Celexa by Torrent	13668-0009	Antidepressant
10	Tab, White, Oval	Citalopram HBr 10 mg	Celexa by Pharmascience	Canadian DIN 02270609	Antidepressant
10	Tab, White, Round, Vanda Logo <> 10	Iloperidone 10 mg	Fanapt by Vangard	43068-0110	Antipsychotic
10	Tab, White to Off-White, Round, Sublingual	Asenapine 10 mg	Saphris by Organon	00052-0119	Antipsychotic
10	Tab, White, Round	Metoclopramide HCl 10 mg	Metozolv ODT by Salix	65649-0432	Gastrointestinal
10 <> 0013	Tab, Pink to Peach, Rounded Rectangle	Pravastatin Sodium 10 mg	Pravachol by Watson	00591-0013	Antihyperlipidemic
10 <> 103	Tab, White, Oval, Scored, Boehringer Logo 103 <> 10	Torsemide 10 mg	Demadex by Nat Pharmpak	55154-0406	Diuretic
10 <> 103	Tab, White, Oval, Scored, Boehringer Logo 103 <> 10	Torsemide 10 mg	Demadex by Boehringer Mannheim	Canadian	Diuretic
10 <> 103	Tab, White, Oval, Scored, Boehringer Logo 103 <> 10	Torsemide 10 mg	Demadex by Hoffmann La Roche	00004-0263	Diuretic
10 <> 255	Tab, Coated, 10/Royce Logo	Baclofen 10 mg	Lioresal by Qualitest	00603-2408	Muscle Relaxant
10 <> 257	Tab, Coated, 10/Royce Logo <> 257	Cyclobenzaprine HCl 10 mg	by Qualitest	00603-3077	Muscle Relaxant
10 <> 2662	Tab, Peach, Round, Hourglass logo 10 <> 2662	Famotidine 10 mg	Pepcid AC by Ivax	00172-2662	Gastrointestinal
10 <> 2737	Tab, Off-White, Diamond Shaped	Fosinopril Sodium 10 mg	Monopril by Sandoz	00781-5083	Antihypertensive
10 <> 335	Tab, Coated, 10/Royce Logo	Piroxicam 10 mg	Feldene by Qualitest	00603-5222	NSAID
10 <> 341	Tab, Coated, 10/Royce Logo	Pindolol 10 mg	by Qualitest	00603-5221	Antihypertensive
10 <> 3691	Tab, Gold, Round	Prochlorperazine 10 mg	Compazine by Ivax	00182-8211	Antiemetic
10 <> 4197	Tab, Pink, Round	Enalapril Maleate 10 mg	Vasotec by Ivax	00172-4197	Antihypertensive
10 <> 4197	Tab, Pink, Round, Hourglass Logo over 4197	Enalapril Maleate 10 mg	Vasotec by Ivax	Discontinued	Antihypertensive
10 <> 4740	Tab, Light Beige, Cap Shaped	Citalopram HBr 10 mg	Celexa by Ivax	00172-4740 Discontinued	Antidepressant
10 <> 5351	Tab, Dark Yellow, Oblong, Hourglass Logo 5351	Benazepril HCl 10 mg	Lotensin by Ivax	00172-5351 Discontinued	Antihypertensive
10 <> 54382	Tab, White, Hexagonal, Scored, 54 over 382	Haloperidol 10 mg	Haldol by Roxane	00054-4346 Discontinued	Antipsychotic
10 <> 5656	Tab, White, Round	Tamoxifen Citrate 10 mg	Nolvadex by Ivax	00172-5656 Discontinued	Antiestrogen
10 <> 5664	Tab, White, Oval, Scored, Hourglass Logo over 10	Buspirone HCl 10 mg	BuSpar by Ivax	00172-5664	Antianxiety
10 <> 5664	Tab, White, Oval	Buspirone HCl 10 mg	BuSpar by Teva	00172-5664	Anxiolytic
10 <> 5732	Tab, White, Round, Hourglass Logo 10 <> 5732	Bisoprolol 10 mg, Hydrochlorothiazide 6.25 mg	Ziac by Ivax	00172-5732	Antihypertensive; Diuretic
10 <> 7815	Tab, White, Cap Shaped, Film Coated	Valdecoxib 10 mg	Bextra by Pfizer	Canadian DIN 02246621 Discontinued	COX 2 Inhibitor
10 <> 832	Tab, Butterscotch Yellow, Sugar Coated	Chlorpromazine HCl 10 mg	by Schein	00364-0380	Antipsychotic
10 <> 832	Tab, Butterscotch Yellow, Sugar Coated	Chlorpromazine HCl 10 mg	by Qualitest	00603-2808	Antipsychotic
10 <> A	Tab, White, Cap Shaped, Film Coated	Mirtazapine 45 mg	Remeron by Aurobindo	65862-0032	Antidepressant
10 <> A	Tab, White, Cap Shaped, Film Coated	Mirtazapine 45 mg	Remeron by Aurolife	13107-0032	Antidepressant
10 <> ABG	Tab, White, Round, Controlled Release	Oxycodone HCl 10 mg	OxyContin by Ivax	00172-6354	Analgesic; C II
10 <> AD	Tab, Blue, Round, Scored	Mixed Amphetamine Salts 10 mg: Amphetamine Aspartate 2.5 mg, Amphetamine Sulfate 2.5 mg, Dextroamphetamine Saccharate 2.5 mg, Dextroamphetamine Sulfate 2.5 mg	Adderall by DRX	55045-2607	Stimulant; C II
10 <> AD	Tab, Blue, Round, Scored	Mixed Amphetamine Salts 10 mg: Amphetamine Aspartate 2.5 mg, Amphetamine Sulfate 2.5 mg, Dextroamphetamine Saccharate 2.5 mg, Dextroamphetamine Sulfate 2.5 mg	Adderall by Physician Total Care	54868-3674	Stimulant; C II

ID FRONT <> BACK	DESCRIPTION FRONT <> BACK	INGREDIENT & STRENGTH	BRAND (or Generic Equiv.) by FIRM	NDC#	CLASS; SCH.
10 <> AD	Tab, Blue, Round, Scored	Mixed Amphetamine Salts 10 mg: Amphetamine Aspartate 2.5 mg, Amphetamine Sulfate 2.5 mg, Dextroamphetamine Saccharate 2.5 mg, Dextroamphetamine Sulfate 2.5 mg	Adderall by Shire	58521-0032	Stimulant; C II
10 <> AFE	Tab, Reddish Brown, Round, Film Coated, Extended Release	Felodipine 10 mg	Plendil by AstraZeneca	Canadian DIN 00851787	Antihypertensive
10 <> AMIDE009	Tab, White, Round, Amide 009	Isoxsuprine HCl 10 mg	Vasodilan by Ivax	00182-1055	Vasodilator
10 <> AMIDE009	Tab, White, Round, Amide 009	Isoxsuprine HCl 10 mg	Vasodilan by Amide	52152-0009	Vasodilator
10 <> AMIDE009	Tab, White, Round, Amide 009	Isoxsuprine HCl 10 mg	Vasodilan by Qualitest	00603-4146	Vasodilator
10 <> APO	Tab, Grayish Pink, Round	Nifedipine 10 mg	Nifed PA by Apotex	Canadian DIN 02197448	Antihypertensive
10 <> APO	Tab, White, Round, Biconvex	Domperidone 10 mg	Apo Domperidone by Apotex	Canadian DIN 02103613	Gastrointestinal
10 <> APO	Tab, Yellow, Round, APO/10	Oxazepam 10 mg	Apo Oxazepam by Apotex	Canadian DIN 00402680	Sedative/Hypnotic; C IV
10 <> APO	Tab, White, Cap Shaped, Film Coated	Zolpidem Tartrate 10 mg	Ambien by Apotex	60505-2605	Sedative/Hypnotic; C IV
10 <> APO	Tab, Pink, Shield-Shaped	Simvastatin 10 mg	Zocor by Apotex	Canadian DIN 02247012	Antihyperlipidemic
10 <> APO	Tab, Yellow, Oblong	Paroxetine HCl 10 mg	Paxil by Apotex	Canadian DIN 02240907	Antidepressant
10 <> ARICEPT	Tab, Yellow, Round, Orally Disintegrating	Donepezil HCl 10 mg	Aricept RDT by Pfizer	Canadian DIN 02269465	Antialzheimers
10 <> ARICEPT	Tab, Yellow, Round, Orally Disintegrating	Donepezil HCl 10 mg	Aricept ODT by Eisai	62856-0832	Antialzheimers
10 <> ARICEPT	Tab, Yellow, Round, Film Coated	Donepezil HCl 10 mg	Aricept by Eisai	62856-0246	Antialzheimers
10 <> ARICEPT	Tab, Yellow, Round, Film Coated	Donepezil HCl 10 mg	Aricept by Pfizer	Canadian DIN 02232044	Antialzheimers
10 <> B351	Tab, White, Round, Film Coated, b over 351	Leflunomide 10 mg	Arava by Barr	00555-0351	Antiarthritic
10 <> B972	Tab, Blue, Oval, Scored, b over 972	Mixed Amphetamine Salts 10 mg: Dextroamphetamine Saccharate 2.5 mg, Amphetamine Aspartate 2.5 mg, Amphetamine Sulfate 2.5 mg, Dextroamphetamine Sulfate 2.5 mg	Adderall by Barr	00555-0972	Stimulant; C II
10 <> BAYER	Tab, Orange, Round, Film-Coated, BAYER BAYER in cross	Vardenafil HCl 10 mg	Levitra by Bayer	Canadian DIN 02250470	Impotence Agent
10 <> BAYER	Tab, Orange, Round, Film-Coated, BAYER BAYER in cross	Vardenafil HCl 10 mg	Levitra by Bayer	00026-8730	Impotence Agent
10 <> BTG	Tab, White, Cap Shaped	Oxandrolone 10 mg	Oxandrin by BTG	54396-0110	Steroid; C III
10 <> D	Tab, White, D-Shaped	Dexmethylphenidate HCl 10 mg	Focalin by Novartis	00078-0382	Stimulant; C II
10 <> DAN5554	Tab, Orange, Round, Scored, DAN over 5554	Propranolol HCl 10 mg	Inderal by Med Pro	53978-0034	Antihypertensive
10 <> DAN5554	Tab, Orange, Round, Scored, DAN over 5554	Propranolol HCl 10 mg	Inderal by Schein	00364-0756	Antihypertensive
10 <> DAN5554	Tab, Orange, Round, Scored, DAN over 5554	Propranolol HCl 10 mg	Inderal by Watson	00591-5554	Antihypertensive
10 <> DAN5620	Tab, Light Blue, Round, Scored	Diazepam 10 mg	Valium by St. Mary's Med	60760-0776	Antianxiety; C IV
10 <> DAN5620	Tab, Light Blue, Round, Scored	Diazepam 10 mg	Valium by Watson	00591-5620	Antianxiety; C IV
10 <> DAN5643	Tab, White, Round, Scored, DAN over 5643	Minoxidil 10 mg	Rogaine by Watson	00591-5643	Antihypertensive
10 <> DAN5643	Tab, White, Round, Scored, DAN over 5643	Minoxidil 10 mg	Rogaine by Schein	00364-2173	Antihypertensive
10 <> DAN5730	Tab, White, Round, Scored	Baclofen 10 mg	Lioresal by Watson	00591-5730	Muscle Relaxant
10 <> DAN5730	Tab, White, Round, Scored	Baclofen 10 mg	Lioresal by Amerisource	62584-0623	Muscle Relaxant
10 <> DAN5730	Tab, White, Round, Scored	Baclofen 10 mg	Lioresal by Schein	00364-2312	Muscle Relaxant
10 <> DAN5730	Tab, White, Round, Scored	Baclofen 10 mg	Lioresal by Heartland	61392-0706	Muscle Relaxant
10 <> DAN5730	Tab, White, Round, Scored	Baclofen 10 mg	Lioresal by Heartland	61392-0090	Muscle Relaxant
10 <> E	Tab, Red, Octagonal	Acetaminophen 400 mg, Hydrocodone Bitartrate 10 mg	Zydone by Endo	63481-0698	Analgesic; C III
10 <> E	Tab, Red, Octagonal	Acetaminophen 400 mg, Hydrocodone Bitartrate 10 mg	Zydone by West Pharm	52967-0275	Analgesic; C III
10 <> E530	Tab, White, Round	Isoxsuprine HCl 10 mg	Vasodilan by Eon	00185-0530	Vasodilator
10 <> E702	Tab, White, Round, Coated, Extended Release	Oxycodone HCl 10 mg	OxyContin by Endo	60951-0702	Analgesic; C II
10 <> E797	Tab, Yellow, Oval	Oxycodone HCl 10 mg, Acetaminophen 650 mg	Endocet by Endo	60951-0797	Analgesic; C II

ID FRONT <> BACK	DESCRIPTION FRONT <> BACK	INGREDIENT & STRENGTH	BRAND (or Generic Equiv.) by FIRM	NDC#	CLASS; SCH.
10 <> F	Tab, White	Medroxyprogesterone Acetate 10 mg	Proclim by Fournier	Canadian	Hormone
10 <> FL	Tab, White to Off-White, Round, Scored, Film Coated, F over L <> 10	Escitalopram Oxalate 10 mg	Lexapro by Forest	00456-2010	Antidepressant
10 <> FL	Tab, Gray, Cap Shaped, Film Coated	Memantine HCl 10 mg	Namenda Titration Pak by Forest	00456-3200	Antialzheimers
10 <> FL	Tab, Gray, Cap Shaped, Film Coated	Memantine HCl 10 mg	Namenda by Forest	00456-3210	Antialzheimers
10 <> FL	Tab, Pinkish-Purple, Triangular	Nebivolol HCl 10 mg	Bystolic by Forest	00456-1410	Antihypertensive
10 <> G019	Tab, Brown, Triangular, Film Coated	Quinapril HCl 10 mg	Accupril by Greenstone	59762-5020	Antihypertensive
10 <> G1540	Tab, White, Round	Amlodipine Besylate 10 mg	Norvasc by Greenstone	59762-1540	Antihypertensive
10 <> G5	Tab, Yellow, Circular	Pravastatin Sodium 10 mg	Pravachol by Glenmark	68462-0195	Antihyperlipidemic
10 <> G58	Tab, White to Off White, Round	Amlodipine Besylate 10 mg	Norvasc by Glenmark	68462-0212	Antihypertensive
10 <> GG455	Tab, Yellow, Round, Film Coated, GG over 455	Chlorpromazine HCl 10 mg	Thorazine by Sandoz	00781-1715	Antipsychotic
10 <> GG58	Tab, Lavender, Round, Film Coated, GG over 58	Trifluoperazine HCl 10 mg	Stelazine by Sandoz	00781-1036	Antipsychotic
10 <> GG953	Tab, Pale Yellow, Round	Prochlorperazine 10 mg	Compazine by Sandoz	00781-5021	Antiemetic
10 <> INV276	Tab, Pale Yellow, Round, Film Coated, 10 <> INV over 276	Prochlorperazine 10 mg	Compazine by Apothecon	62269-0276	Antiemetic
10 <> INV276	Tab, Pale Yellow, Round, Film Coated, 10 <> INV over 276	Prochlorperazine 10 mg	Compazine by Invamed	52189-0276	Antiemetic
10 <> INV276	Tab, Pale Yellow, Round, Film Coated, 10 <> INV over 276	Prochlorperazine 10 mg	Compazine by Apotheca	12634-0676	Antiemetic
10 <> INV281	Tab, Purple, Round, Film Coated	Trifluoperazine HCl 10 mg	by Invamed	52189-0281	Antipsychotic
10 <> INV315	Tab, White, Square, Scored, INV over 315	Warfarin Sodium 10 mg	Coumadin by Sandoz	00781-0387	Anticoagulant
10 <> INV315	Tab, White, Square, Scored, INV over 315	Warfarin Sodium 10 mg	Coumadin by Apothecon	59772-0387	Anticoagulant
10 <> JANSSENP	Tab, 10 <> Janssen/P	Cisapride 10 mg	Propulsid by Janssen	50458-0430	Gastrointestinal
10 <> KU106	Tab, White, Round, Scored	Isosorbide Mononitrate 10 mg	Ismo by Kremers Urban	62175-0106	Antianginal
10 <> L093	Tab, Peach, Oval, Film-Coated	Simvastatin 10 mg	Zocor by Perrigo	45802-0384	Antihyperlipidemic
10 <> LOTENSIN	Tab, Dark Yellow, Round, Film Coated	Benazepril HCl 10 mg	Lotensin by Southwood	58016-0420	Antihypertensive
10 <> LOTENSIN	Tab, Dark Yellow, Round, Film Coated	Benazepril HCl 10 mg	Lotensin by Novartis	00078-0448	Antihypertensive
10 <> LOTENSIN	Tab, Dark Yellow, Round, Film Coated	Benazepril HCl 10 mg	Lotensin by PDRX	55289-0109	Antihypertensive
10 <> LOTENSIN	Tab, Dark Yellow, Round, Film Coated	Benazepril HCl 10 mg	Lotensin by DRX	55045-2374	Antihypertensive
10 <> LOTENSIN	Tab, Dark Yellow, Round, Film Coated	Benazepril HCl 10 mg	Lotensin by Amerisource	62584-0063	Antihypertensive
10 <> LOTENSIN	Tab, Dark Yellow, Round, Film Coated	Benazepril HCl 10 mg	Lotensin by Pharm Util	60491-0383	Antihypertensive
10 <> LUPIN	Tab, Pink, Round	Lisinopril 10 mg	Zestril by Lupin	68180-0514	Antihypertensive
10 <> M	Tab, White, Round, M in a double circle <> 10	Dicyclomine HCl 10 mg	Bentylol by Axcan	Canadian DIN 02103087	Gastrointestinal
10 <> M	Tab, White, Diamond Shaped, Scored, M inside square <> 10	Dextroamphetamine Sulfate 10 mg	Dexedrine by Mallinckrodt	00406-8959	Stimulant; C II
10 <> M	Tab, Coral, Triangular, Film Coated, M inside a Box	Imipramine HCl 10 mg	Tofranil by Mallinckrodt	00406-9920	Antidepressant
10 <> M	Tab, White to Cream Colored, Pillow-Shaped, M inside square	Mixed Amphetamine Salts 10 mg; Dextroamphetamine Saccharate 2.5 mg, Amphetamine Aspartate 2.5 mg, Dextroamphetamine Sulfate 2.5 mg, Amphetamine Sulfate 2.5 mg	Adderall by Mallinckrodt	00406-8892	Stimulant; C II
10 <> M	Tab, White, Round, Scored	Methylphenidate HCl 10 mg	Ritalin by D M Graham	00756-0284	Stimulant; C II
10 <> M	Tab, White, Round, Scored	Methylphenidate HCl 10 mg	Ritalin by Mallinckrodt	00406-1122	Stimulant; C II
10 <> M54	Tab, Orange, Round, Film Coated, M over 54	Thioridazine 10 mg	Mellaril by Mylan	00378-0612	Antipsychotic
10 <> M54	Tab, Orange, Round, Film Coated, M over 54	Thioridazine 10 mg	Mellaril by UDL	51079-0565	Antipsychotic
10 <> M54	Tab, Orange, Round, Film Coated, M over 54	Thioridazine 10 mg	Mellaril by Dixon Shane	17236-0318	Antipsychotic
10 <> M54	Tab, Orange, Round, Film Coated, M over 54	Thioridazine 10 mg	Mellaril by Qualitest	00603-5992	Antipsychotic
10 <> M54	Tab, Orange, Round, Film Coated, M over 54	Thioridazine 10 mg	Mellaril by Vangard	00615-2504	Antipsychotic
10 <> MJ543	Tab, White, Round	Isoxsuprine HCl 10 mg	Vasodilan by BMS	00087-0543	Vasodilator
10 <> MYLAN182	Tab, Orange, Round, Scored, Mylan over 182	Propranolol HCl 10 mg	Inderal by UDL	51079-0277 Discontinued	Antihypertensive
10 <> MYLAN182	Tab, Orange, Round, Scored, Mylan over 182	Propranolol HCl 10 mg	Inderal by Mylan	00378-0182	Antihypertensive
10 <> N	Tab, Pink, Shield Shaped	Simvastatin 10 mg	Zocor by Novopharm	Canadian DIN 02250152	Antihyperlipidemic

ID FRONT <> BACK	DESCRIPTION FRONT <> BACK	INGREDIENT & STRENGTH	BRAND (or Generic Equiv.) by FIRM	NDC#	CLASS; SCH.
10 <> N	Tab, Light Blue, Round, Scored, Large N	Haloperidol 10 mg	Haldol by Novopharm	Canadian DIN 00713449	Antipsychotic
10 <> N	Tab, Yellow, Cap Shaped	Paroxetine HCl 10 mg	Paxil by Novopharm	Canadian DIN 02248556	Antidepressant
10 <> N	Tab, Dark Orange, Round, Large N	Imipramine 10 mg	Tofranil by Novopharm	Canadian DIN 00021504	Antidepressant
10 <> N	Tab, Pink, Rounded Square	Pravastatin Sodium 10 mg	Pravachol by Novopharm	Canadian DIN 02247008	Antihyperlipidemic
10 <> N	Tab, Green, Round	Terazosin HCl 10 mg	Hytrin by Novopharm	Canadian DIN 02230808	Antihypertensive
10 <> N	Tab, Blue, Round	Amitriptyline HCl 10 mg	Elavil by Novopharm	Canadian DIN 00037400	Antidepressant
10 <> N	Tab, White, Diamond Shaped, Scored, 1 / 0	Fosinopril Sodium 10 mg	Monopril by Novopharm	Canadian DIN 02247802	Antihypertensive
10 <> N	Tab, White, Round, Black Ink	Ketorolac Tromethamine 10 mg	Toradol by Novopharm	Canadian DIN 02230201	NSAID
10 <> N	Tab, White, Round	Leflunomide 10 mg	Arava by Novopharm	Canadian DIN 02261251	Antiarthritic
10 <> N	Tab, White, Round, Scored, 1|0	Medroxyprogesterone Acetate 10 mg	Provera by Novopharm	Canadian DIN 02221306	Hormone
10 <> N	Tab, White, Oval, Squared Ends, Scored, N <> 1/0	Buspirone HCl	Buspar by Novopharm	Canadian DIN 02231492	Antianxiety
10 <> N	Tab, White, Oval	Alendronate Sodium 10 mg	Fosamax by Novopharm	Canadian DIN 02247373	Antiosteoporosis
10 <> N093	Tab, White, Round, Scored, N over 093 <> 10	Pindolol 10 mg	by Med Pro	53978-2025	Antihypertensive
10 <> N131	Tab, Blue, Round, Scored, 1,0 <> N over 131	Alprazolam 1 mg	Xanax by Teva	55953-0131	Antianxiety; C IV
10 <> N131	Tab, Blue, Round, Scored, 1,0 <> N over 131	Alprazolam 1 mg	Xanax by Medirex	57480-0522	Antianxiety; C IV
10 <> N525	Tab, White, Oval, Scored	Glipizide 10 mg	by Novopharm	43806-0525	Antidiabetic
10 <> NOVO	Tab, Yellow, Shield-Shaped	Cyclobenzaprine HCl 10 mg	Flexeril by Novopharm	Canadian DIN 02080052	Muscle Relaxant
10 <> NOVO	Tab, Light Blue, Round, NO/VO <> 10	Timolol Maleate 10 mg	Blocadren by Novopharm	Canadian DIN 01947818	Antihypertensive
10 <> NU	Tab, Grayish-Pink, Round, Film Coated	Nifedipine 10 mg	by Nu Pharm	Canadian DIN 02212102	Antihypertensive
10 <> OC	Tab, White, Round, Film Coated	Oxycodone HCl 10 mg	OxyContin by Purdue	59011-0100	Analgesic; C II
10 <> OX	Tab, White, Oval, Scored	Oxandrolone 10 mg	Oxandrin by Watson	00591-3545	Steroid; C III
10 <> P	Tab, White, Round	Bisoprolol Fumarate 10 mg	Monocor by Pharmascience	Canadian DIN 02302640	Antihypertensive
10 <> P	Tab, Peach, Round, Scored	Bethanechol Chloride 10 mg	Urecholine by Pharmascience	Canadian DIN 00759171	Urinary Tract
10 <> P	Tab, White, Round	Leflunomide 10 mg	ARAVA by Pharmascience	Canadian DIN 02288265	Antiarthritic
10 <> P	Tab, Light Pink, Shield Shaped	Simvastatin 10 mg	Zocor by Pharmascience	Canadian DIN 02269260	Antihyperlipidemic
10 <> P	Tab, Yellow, Oval, Scored, P Logo <> 1 / 0	Paroxetine HCl 10 mg	Paxil by Pharmascience	Canadian DIN 02247750	Antidepressant
10 <> P	Tab, Pale Green, Round, Scored	Methadone Hydrochloride 10 mg	Metadol by Pharmascience	Canadian DIN 02247700	Analgesic
10 <> P	Tab, White, Round, Film Coated	Bisoprolol Fumarate 10 mg	Zym-Bisoprolol by Zymcan Pharm	Canadian DIN 02321572	Antihypertensive
10 <> P	Tab, Blue, Round	Terazosin HCl 10 mg	Hytrin by Pharmascience	Canadian DIN 02243521	Antihypertensive

ID FRONT <> BACK	DESCRIPTION FRONT <> BACK	INGREDIENT & STRENGTH	BRAND (or Generic Equiv.) by FIRM	NDC#	CLASS; SCH.
10 <> PAL	Tab, Light Yellow, Round, Coated, PAL <> 1.0	L-methylfolate (Metafolin) 1.0 mg	Zervalx by PAMLAB	00525-1010	Supplement
10 <> PAR652	Tab, White, Round, Scored	Torsemide 10 mg	Demadex by Par	49884-0652	Diuretic
10 <> PAR708	Tab, Peach, Oval, Scored	Buspirone HCl 10 mg	Buspar by Par	49884-0708	Antianxiety
10 <> PAXIL	Tab, Yellow, Oblong, Film Coated	Paroxetine HCl 10 mg	Paxil by Med Pro	53978-2059	Antidepressant
10 <> PAXIL	Tab, Yellow, Oblong, Film Coated	Paroxetine HCl 10 mg	Paxil by SB	59742-3210	Antidepressant
10 <> PAXIL	Tab, Yellow, Oblong, Film Coated	Paroxetine HCl 10 mg	Paxil by Pharmacy Care	65070-0144	Antidepressant
10 <> PAXIL	Tab, Yellow, Oblong, Film Coated	Paroxetine HCl 10 mg	Paxil by SKB	00029-3210	Antidepressant
10 <> PAXIL	Tab, Yellow, Oblong, Film Coated	Paroxetine HCl 10 mg	Paxil by GSK	Canadian DIN 02027887	Antidepressant
10 <> PD155	Tab, White, Oval, Film Coated	Atorvastatin Calcium 10 mg	Lipitor by Parke Davis	Canadian DIN 02230711	Antihyperlipidemic
10 <> PD155	Tab, White, Oval, Film Coated	Atorvastatin Calcium 10 mg	Lipitor by Pharm Util	60491-0803	Antihyperlipidemic
10 <> PD155	Tab, White, Oval, Film Coated	Atorvastatin Calcium 10 mg	Lipitor by Goedecke	53869-0155	Antihyperlipidemic
10 <> PD155	Tab, White, Oval, Film Coated	Atorvastatin Calcium 10 mg	Lipitor by Parke Davis	00071-0155	Antihyperlipidemic
10 <> PD530	Tab, Brown, Triangular, Film Coated	Quinapril HCl 10 mg	Accupril by Parke Davis	00071-0530	Antihypertensive
10 <> PD530	Tab, Brown, Triangular, Film Coated	Quinapril HCl 10 mg	Accupril by Parke Davis	Canadian DIN 01947672	Antihypertensive
10 <> PD530	Tab, Brown, Triangular, Film Coated	Quinapril HCl 10 mg	Accupril by PDRX	55289-0553	Antihypertensive
10 <> PD530	Tab, Brown, Triangular, Film Coated	Quinapril HCl 10 mg	Accupril by Direct Dispensing	57866-4420	Antihypertensive
10 <> PD530	Tab, Brown, Triangular, Film Coated	Quinapril HCl 10 mg	Accupril by RX Pak	65084-0124	Antihypertensive
10 <> PERCOCET	Tab, Yellow, Oval	Acetaminophen 650 mg, Oxycodone HCl 10 mg	Percocet by Endo	63481-0622	Analgesic; C II
10 <> PERCOCET	Tab, Yellow, Oval	Acetaminophen 650 mg, Oxycodone HCl 10 mg	Percocet by BMS	00056-0622	Analgesic; C II
10 <> PERCOCET	Tab, Yellow, Oval	Acetaminophen 650 mg, Oxycodone HCl 10 mg	Percocet by West Pharm	52967-0280	Analgesic; C II
10 <> PF	Tab, White, Round	Morphine Sulfate 10 mg	MS Contin by Purdue	Canadian	Analgesic; C II
10 <> SCHWARZ610	Tab, White, Round, Scored	Isosorbide Mononitrate 10 mg	Monoket by Schwarz	00091-3610	Antianginal
10 <> SP2309	Tab, White, Cap Shaped, Scored, Film Coated	Ascorbic Acid, Calcium Carbonate, Cupric Oxide, Cyanocobalamin 12 mcg, Vitamin D, Polysaccharide Iron Complex, Folic Acid 1 mg, Magnesium Oxide, Niacinamide 20 mg, Potassium Iodide, Pyridoxine HCl, Riboflavin 3.4 mg, Thiamine Mononitrate, Vitamin A, Vitamin E Acetate, Zinc Sulfate	Niferex PN Forte by Schwarz	00131-2309	Vitamin
10 <> SP351	Tab, White, Round, Orally Disintegrating, SP above Score, 351 below	Baclofen 10 mg	Kemstro by Schwarz	00091-3351	Muscle Relaxant
10 <> TARO	Tab, Peach, Shield-Shaped, Film-Coated	Simvastatin 10 mg	Zocor by Taro	Canadian DIN 02265885	Antihyperlipidemic
10 <> U137	Tab, White, Round, Scored	Minoxidil 10 mg	by Pharmacia	Canadian DIN 00514500	Antihypertensive
10 <> WARFARINTARO	Tab, White, Cap Shaped	Warfarin Sodium 10 mg	Coumadin by Taro	51672-4035	Anticoagulant
10 <> WYETH	Tab, White, Round	Isosorbide Dinitrate 10 mg	Isordil by Wyeth	00008-4161	Antianginal
10 <> Z3927	Tab, Light Blue, Round, Scored, Z over 3927	Diazepam 10 mg	Valium by PDRX	55289-0091	Antianxiety; C IV
10 <> Z3927	Tab, Light Blue, Round, Scored, Z over 3927	Diazepam 10 mg	Valium by Ivax	00172-3927	Antianxiety; C IV
10 <> Z3927	Tab, Light Blue, Round, Scored, Z over 3927	Diazepam 10 mg	Valium by Ivax	00182-1757	Antianxiety; C IV
10 <> Z4096	Tab, White, Round, Scored, Z over 4096	Baclofen 10 mg	Lioresal by Baker Cummins	63171-1295	Muscle Relaxant
10 <> Z4096	Tab, White, Round, Scored, Z over 4096	Baclofen 10 mg	Lioresal by Caremark	00339-5834	Muscle Relaxant
10 <> Z4096	Tab, White, Round, Scored, Z over 4096	Baclofen 10 mg	Lioresal by Ivax	00172-4096	Muscle Relaxant
10 <> Z4096	Tab, White, Round, Scored, Z over 4096	Baclofen 10 mg	Lioresal by Major	00904-3365	Muscle Relaxant
10 <> Z4096	Tab, White, Round, Scored, Z over 4096	Baclofen 10 mg	Lioresal by Ivax	00182-1295	Muscle Relaxant
10 <> Z4218	Tab, White, Round, Z over 4218	Pindolol 10 mg	Visken by Ivax	00172-4218 Discontinued	Antihypertensive
10 <> ZAROXOLYN	Tab, Yellow	Metolazone 10 mg	Zaroxolyn by Medeva	53014-0835	Diuretic
10 <> ZLP	Tab, Yellow, Round, Film Coated	Zolpidem Tartrate 10 mg	Ambien by Sandoz	00781-5318	Sedative/Hypnotic; C IV
10 <> ZM	Tab, White, Round, Film Coated	Zolpidem Tartrate 10 mg	Ambien by Genpharm	15330-0265	Sedative/Hypnotic; C IV
10 <> ZT	Tab, Blue, Round, White Specks, Orally Disintegrating	Zolpidem Tartrate 10 mg	Tovalt ODT by Biovail	64455-0159	Sedative/Hypnotic; C IV

ID FRONT <> BACK	DESCRIPTION FRONT <> BACK	INGREDIENT & STRENGTH	BRAND (or Generic Equiv.) by FIRM	NDC#	CLASS; SCH.
10 <> ZYRTEC	Tab, White, Rectangular, Film Coated	Cetirizine HCl 10 mg	Zyrtec by Southwood	58016-0367	Antihistamine
10 <> ZYRTEC	Tab, White, Rectangular, Film Coated	Cetirizine HCl 10 mg	Zyrtec by Murfreesboro	51129-1379	Antihistamine
10 <> ZYRTEC	Tab, White, Rectangular, Film Coated	Cetirizine HCl 10 mg	Zyrtec by Pfizer	00069-5510	Antihistamine
100	Tab, White	Atenolol 100 mg	Tenormin by Schein	Canadian	Antihypertensive
100	Tab, Yellow, Round	Ketoprofen 100 mg	Orudis by Rhodiapharm	Canadian	NSAID
100	Tab, Yellow, Round, Scored, 100 <> Forest Logo	Levothyroxine Sodium 100 mcg	Levothroid by Nat Pharmpak	55154-4007	Thyroid Hormone
100	Tab, White, Oblong, Film Coated, Fournier Logo <> 100	Fenofibrate 100 mg	Lipidil Supra by Fournier	Canadian DIN 02241601	Antihyperlipidemic
100	Cap, White, Red Print	Theophylline Anhydrous 100 mg	Slo-Bid by RPR	00801-0100	Antiasthmatic
100	Cap, Red Print, Ex Release	Theophylline Anhydrous 100 mg	by Nat Pharmpak	55154-4025	Antiasthmatic
100	Tab, Green, Round	Thioridazine HCl 100 mg	Apo Thioridazine by Apotex	Canadian	Antipsychotic
100	Tab, Pink, Round	Trimipramine 100 mg	Rhotrimine by Rhodiapharm	Canadian	Antidepressant
100	Tab, Yellow, Round, Scored	Levothyroxine Sodium 100 mcg	Eltroxin by GSK	Canadian DIN 02213206	Thyroid Hormone
100	Tab, White, Round	Modafinil 100 mg	Alertec by Shire	Canadian DIN 02239665	Stimulant; C IV
100	Tab, Blue, Cap Shaped, Scored, Film Coated	Metoprolol Tartrate 100 mg	Lopressor by Nu Pharm	Canadian DIN 00865613	Antihypertensive
100	Tab, Blue, Cap Shaped, Scored, Film Coated	Metoprolol Tartrate 100 mg	Lopressor by Apotex	Canadian DIN 00751170	Antihypertensive
100	Tab, Peach, Round	Desipramine HCl 100 mg	Apo Desipramine by Apotex	Canadian DIN 02216280	Antidepressant
100	Tab, Pink, Trapezoid-Shaped	Fluconazole 100 mg	Diflucan by Glenmark	68462-0102	Antifungal
100	Tab, Pink, Trapezoid-Shaped	Fluconazole 100 mg	Diflucan by Cobalt	Canadian DIN 02281279	Antifungal
100	Tab, Yellow, Round, 100 <> Cobalt Logo	Topiramate 100 mg	Topamax by Cobalt	Canadian DIN 02287773	Antimigraine
100 <> 1021	Tab, Orange, Round	Topiramate 100 mg	Topamax by Dava	67253-0753	Anticonvulsant
100 <> 105	Tab, White, Cap Shaped, Scored, Boehringer Logo/105 <> 100	Torsemide 100 mg	Demadex by Boehringer Mannheim	Canadian	Diuretic
100 <> 105	Tab, White, Cap Shaped, Scored, Boehringer Logo/105 <> 100	Torsemide 100 mg	Demadex by Hoffmann La Roche	00004-0265	Diuretic
100 <> 274INV	Tab, 274/INV	Captopril 100 mg	Capoten by Schein	00364-2631	Antihypertensive
100 <> 350	Tab, 100/Royce Logo <> 350	Captopril 100 mg	Capoten by Qualitest	00603-2558	Antihypertensive
100 <> 4332	Tab, Peach, Oval, Scored, Logo 4332 <> 100	Nefazodone 100 mg	Serzone by Ivax	00172-4332	Antidepressant
100 <> 4360	Tab, Pale Yellow, Round, Hourglass Logo over 4360	Clozapine 100 mg	Clozaril by Dixon Shane	17236-0356	Antipsychotic
100 <> 4360	Tab, Pale Yellow, Round, Hourglass Logo over 4360	Clozapine 100 mg	Clozaril by Ivax	00172-4360 Discontinued	Antipsychotic
100 <> 4364	Tab, Yellow, Round, Hourglass Logo 4364	Labetalol HCl 100 mg	Trandate by Ivax	00172-4364	Antihypertensive
100 <> 4364	Tab, Yellow, Round, Hourglass Logo 4364	Labetalol HCl 100 mg	Trandate by Ivax	00182-8202 Discontinued	Antihypertensive
100 <> 4430	Tab, White, Round, Ivax Hourglass Logo 100 <> 4430	Misoprostol 100 mcg	Cytotec by Ivax	00172-4430	Gastrointestinal
100 <> 4440	Tab, White, Round, Hourglass Logo 4440 <> 100	Gabapentin 100 mg	Neurontin by Ivax	00172-4440 Discontinued	Anticonvulsant
100 <> 5411	Tab, Pink, Oval, Ivax Logo 100	Fluconazole 100 mg	Diflucan by Ivax	00054-5411	Antifungal
100 <> 54862	Tab, White, Round	Morphine Sulfate SR 100 mg	Oramorph by Roxane	00054-8793 00054-4793	Analgesic; C II
100 <> 5674	Tab, Light Blue, Oblong, Scored, Ivax Logo 100	Sertraline HCl 100 mg	Zoloft by Ivax	00172-5674 Discontinued	Antidepressant
100 <> 5841	Tab, White, Round, Ivax Logo 100 <> 5841	Cilostazol 100 mg	Pletal by Ivax	00172-5841 Discontinued	Antiplatelet

ID FRONT <> BACK	DESCRIPTION FRONT <> BACK	INGREDIENT & STRENGTH	BRAND (or Generic Equiv.) by FIRM	NDC#	CLASS; SCH.
100 <> 734N	Tab, Film Coated, 734/N	Metoprolol Tartrate 100 mg	Lopressor by Schein	00364-2561	Antihypertensive
100 <> 7772	Tab, Pale Yellow, Round, Hourglass Logo over 4360	Clozapine 100 mg	Clozaril by Teva Pharmaceuticals	00093-7772	Antipsychotic
100 <> 832	Tab, Butterscotch Yellow, Sugar Coated	Chlorpromazine HCl 100 mg	Thorazine by URL Mutual	00677-0456	Antipsychotic
100 <> 832	Tab, Butterscotch Yellow, Sugar Coated	Chlorpromazine HCl 100 mg	Thorazine by Qualitest	00603-2811	Antipsychotic
100 <> 832	Tab, Butterscotch Yellow, Sugar Coated	Chlorpromazine HCl 100 mg	Thorazine by Schein	00364-0383	Antipsychotic
100 <> ABG	Tab, Green, Capsule-Shaped, Film-Coated, Controlled Release	Morphine Sulfate 100 mg	MS Contin by Ivax	00172-2165	Analgesic; C II
100 <> ANZEMET	Tab, Pink, Oval, Film Coated	Dolasetron 100 mg	Anzemet by Merrell	00068-1203	Antiemetic
100 <> ANZEMET	Tab, Pink, Oval, Film Coated	Dolasetron 100 mg	Anzemet by Aventis	00088-1203	Antiemetic
100 <> ANZEMET	Tab, Pink, Oval, Film Coated	Dolasetron 100 mg	Anzemet by Aventis	Canadian DIN 02231379	Antiemetic
100 <> CIPRO	Tab, Yellow, Round, Film Coated	Ciprofloxacin HCl 100 mg	Ciprobay by Bayer	00026-8511	Antibiotic
100 <> CLOZARIL	Tab, Pale Yellow, Round, Scored	Clozapine 100 mg	Clozaril by Novartis	00078-0127	Antipsychotic
100 <> CLOZARIL	Tab, Pale Yellow, Round, Scored	Clozapine 100 mg	Clozaril by Physician Total Care	54868-3576	Antipsychotic
100 <> CLOZARIL	Tab, Pale Yellow, Round, Scored	Clozapine 100 mg	Clozaril by Novartis	Canadian DIN 00894745	Antipsychotic
100 <> CLOZARIL	Tab, Yellow, Round, Scored	Clozapine 100 mg	Clozaril by Dixon Shane	17236-0303	Antipsychotic
100 <> COBALT LOGO	Tab, Pink, Trapezoidal, Cobalt Logo	Fluconazole 100 mg	Co Fluconazole by Cobalt	Canadian DIN 02281279	Antifungal
100 <> DEPADE	Tab, Beige, Cap Shaped, Film Coated	Naltrexone HCl 100 mg	Depade by Mallinckrodt	00406-0119	Opioid Antagonist
100 <> E	Tab, Grey, Oval, Extended Release	Morphine Sulfate 100 mg	MS Contin by Ethex	58177-0340	Analgesic; C II
100 <> E658	Tab, Blue, Cap Shaped, Ex Release	Morphine Sulfate 100 mg	MS Contin by Endo	60951-0658	Analgesic; C II
100 <> FL	Tab, Blue, Oval, Film Coated	Milnacipran HCl 100 mg	Savella by Forest	00456-1510	Antidepressant; Antifibromyalgia
100 <> FLINT	Tab, Yellow, Round, Scored	Levothyroxine Sodium 100 mcg	Synthroid by Abbott	Canadian DIN 02172100	Thyroid Hormone
100 <> FLINT	Tab, Yellow, Round, Scored	Levothyroxine Sodium 100 mcg	Synthroid by Med Pro	53978-1038	Thyroid Hormone
100 <> FLINT	Tab, Yellow, Round, Scored	Levothyroxine Sodium 100 mcg	Synthroid by Pharmedix	53002-1056	Thyroid Hormone
100 <> FLINT	Tab, Yellow, Round, Scored	Levothyroxine Sodium 100 mcg	Synthroid by Giant Food	11146-0305	Thyroid Hormone
100 <> FLINT	Tab, Yellow, Round, Scored	Levothyroxine Sodium 100 mcg	Synthroid by Rite Aid	11822-5193	Thyroid Hormone
100 <> FLINT	Tab, Yellow, Round, Scored	Levothyroxine Sodium 100 mcg	Synthroid by Amerisource	62584-0014	Thyroid Hormone
100 <> FLINT	Tab, Yellow, Round, Scored	Levothyroxine Sodium 100 mcg	Synthroid by Murfreesboro	51129-1665	Thyroid Hormone
100 <> FLINT	Tab, Yellow, Round, Scored	Levothyroxine Sodium 100 mcg	Synthroid by Nat Pharmpak	55154-0906	Thyroid Hormone
100 <> FLINT	Tab, Yellow, Round, Scored	Levothyroxine Sodium 100 mcg	Synthroid by Abbott	00048-1070	Thyroid Hormone
100 <> FLINT	Tab, Yellow, Round, Scored	Levothyroxine Sodium 100 mcg	Synthroid by Forest	00456-0323	Thyroid Hormone
100 <> FLINT	Tab, Yellow, Round, Scored	Levothyroxine Sodium 100 mcg	Synthroid by Kaiser	00179-0458	Thyroid Hormone
100 <> GG	Tab, White, Cap Shaped, Scored	Cabergoline 0.5 mg	Dostinex by Greenstone	59762-0100	Antiparkinson
100 <> GG335	Tab, Yellow, Cap Shaped, Scored, 100 <> GG over 335	Levothyroxine 100 mcg	Levo-T by Alara	64909-0126	Thyroid Hormone
100 <> GG335	Tab, Yellow, Cap Shaped, Scored, 100 <> GG over 335	Levothyroxine 100 mcg	Levo-T by Sandoz	00781-5184	Thyroid Hormone
100 <> GG34	Tab, Orange, Round, Film Coated, GG over 34	Thioridazine 100 mg	Mellaril by Sandoz	00781-1644	Antipsychotic
100 <> GG437	Tab, Yellow, Round, GG over 437	Chlorpromazine HCl 100 mg	Thorazine by Sandoz	00781-1718	Antipsychotic
100 <> GLYSET	Tab, White, Round	Miglitol 100 mg	Glyset by Pharmacia	00009-5014	Antidiabetic
100 <> IMITREX	Tab, Pink, Triangular Shaped, Film Coated	Sumatriptan Succinate 100 mg	Imitrex by GSK	00173-0450	Antimigraine
100 <> INV274	Tab, Scored	Captopril 100 mg	Capoten by Invamed	52189-0274	Antihypertensive
100 <> LAMICTAL	Tab, White, Round, Orally Disintegrating	Lamotrigine 100 mg	Lamictal ODT by GSK	00173-0776	Anticonvulsant
100 <> M	Tab, Gray, Round, M inside square <> 100	Morphine Sulfate 100 mg	MS Contin by Mallinckrodt	00406-8390	Analgesic; C II
100 <> M61	Tab, Orange, Round, Film Coated, M over 61	Thioridazine 100 mg	Mellaril by Dixon Shane	17236-0305	Antipsychotic
100 <> M61	Tab, Orange, Round, Film Coated, M over 61	Thioridazine 100 mg	Mellaril by Qualitest	00603-5995	Antipsychotic
100 <> M61	Tab, Orange, Round, Film Coated, M over 61	Thioridazine 100 mg	Mellaril by Mylan	00378-0618	Antipsychotic
100 <> M61	Tab, Orange, Round, Film Coated, M over 61	Thioridazine 100 mg	Mellaril by Vangard	00615-2508	Antipsychotic
100 <> M61	Tab, Orange, Round, Film Coated, M over 61	Thioridazine 100 mg	Mellaril by UDL	51079-0580	Antipsychotic

ID FRONT <> BACK	DESCRIPTION FRONT <> BACK	INGREDIENT & STRENGTH	BRAND (or Generic Equiv.) by FIRM	NDC#	CLASS; SCH.
100 <> MYLAN167	Tab, Beige, Round, Film Coated, 100 <> Mylan over 167	Doxycycline Hyclate 100 mg	Vibra-Tabs by UDL	51079-0554	Antibiotic
100 <> MYLAN167	Tab, Beige, Round, Film Coated, 100 <> Mylan over 167	Doxycycline Hyclate 100 mg	Vibra-Tabs by Mylan	00378-0167	Antibiotic
100 <> MYLAN197	Tab, Green, Round, Scored, Mylan over 197	Chlorpropamide 100 mg	Diabinese by Mylan	00378-0197	Antidiabetic
100 <> MYLAN197	Tab, Green, Round, Scored, Mylan over 197	Chlorpropamide 100 mg	Diabinese by UDL	51079-0202 Discontinued	Antidiabetic
100 <> N	Tab, White, Round, Scored	Chlorpromazine HCl 100 mg	Largactil by Novopharm	Canadian DIN 00232831	Antipsychotic; Antiemetic
100 <> N	Tab, White, Round	Misoprostol 100 mcg	Cytotec by Novopharm	Canadian DIN 02240754	Gastrointestinal
100 <> N	Tab, Pink, Shield Shaped	Fluconazole 100 mg	Diflucan by Novopharm	Canadian DIN 02236979	Antifungal
100 <> N	Tab, Pink, Triangle Shaped	Sumatriptan 100 mg	Imitrex by Novopharm	Canadian DIN 02239367	Antimigraine
100 <> N	Tab, Orange, Round	Topiramate 100 mg	Topamax by Novopharm	Canadian DIN 02248861	Anticonvulsant
100 <> N	Tab, Grey, Round	Morphine Sulfate 100 mg	MS Contin by Novopharm	Canadian DIN 02302799	Analgesic; N
100 <> N135	Tab, White, Oblong, Scored, N over 135 <> 100	Captopril 100 mg	Capoten by Teva	00093-8135	Antihypertensive
100 <> N135	Tab, White, Oblong, Scored, 100 <> N over 135	Captopril 100 mg	Capoten by Teva	55953-0135 Discontinued	Antihypertensive
100 <> N135	Tab, White, Oblong, Scored, 100 <> N over 135	Captopril 100 mg	Capoten by Medirex	57480-0841	Antihypertensive
100 <> N135	Tab, White, Oblong, Scored, 100 <> N over 135	Captopril 100 mg	Capoten by Major	00904-5048	Antihypertensive
100 <> N401	Tab, White, Round, 100 <> N over 401	Atenolol 100 mg	Tenormin by Allscripts		Antihypertensive
100 <> N401	Tab, White, Round, 100 <> N over 401	Atenolol 100 mg	Tenormin by Novopharm	62528-0401	Antihypertensive
100 <> N401	Tab, White, Round, 100 <> N over 401	Atenolol 100 mg	Tenormin by Medirex	57480-0447	Antihypertensive
100 <> N401	Tab, White, Round, 100 <> N over 401	Atenolol 100 mg	Tenormin by Teva	55953-0401	Antihypertensive
100 <> N551	Tab, Peach, Round, N over 551	Fluconazole 100 mg	Diflucan by Teva	00093-7203 Discontinued	Antifungal
100 <> N577	Tab, Dark Blue, Round, Film Coated	Flurbiprofen 100 mg	Ansaid by Allscripts		NSAID
100 <> N577	Tab, Dark Blue, Round, Film Coated	Flurbiprofen 100 mg	Ansaid by Warrick	59930-1772	NSAID
100 <> N577	Tab, Dark Blue, Round, Film Coated	Flurbiprofen 100 mg	Ansaid by Qualitest	00603-3700	NSAID
100 <> N577	Tab, Dark Blue, Round, Film Coated	Flurbiprofen 100 mg	Ansaid by Moore	00839-8004	NSAID
100 <> N734	Tab, White, Cap Shaped, Film Coated	Metoprolol Tartrate 100 mg	Lopressor by Brightstone	62939-2221	Antihypertensive
100 <> N734	Tab, White, Cap Shaped, Film Coated	Metoprolol Tartrate 100 mg	Lopressor by Direct Dispensing	57866-6579	Antihypertensive
100 <> N734	Tab, White, Cap Shaped, Film Coated	Metoprolol Tartrate 100 mg	Lopressor by Medirex	57480-0803	Antihypertensive
100 <> N734	Tab, White, Cap Shaped, Film Coated	Metoprolol Tartrate 100 mg	Lopressor by Teva	55953-0734 Discontinued	Antihypertensive
100 <> N969	Tab, Pale Yellow, Oval, Scored, N/969	Clozapine 100 mg	Clozaril by Teva	00093-0276 Discontinued	Antipsychotic
100 <> N969	Tab, Pale Yellow, Oval, Scored, N/969	Clozapine 100 mg	Clozaril by Par	49884-0089	Antipsychotic
100 <> NN	Tab, Light Yellow, Round, Scored, N/N <> 100	Spironolactone 100 mg	Aldactone by Novopharm	Canadian DIN 00613223	Diuretic
100 <> NN	Tab, White, Round, Scored, N/N <> 100	Theophylline Anhydrous 100 mg	Theo-Dur by Novopharm	Canadian DIN 02230085	Antiasthmatic
100 <> NN	Tab, White, Oval, Scored, N / N <> 100	Fluvoxamine Maleate 100 mg	Luvox by Novopharm	Canadian DIN 02239954	OCD
100 <> NN	Tab, Orange, Oval, Scored, N/N	Moclobemide 100 mg	Manerix by Novopharm	Canadian DIN 02239746	Antidepressant
100 <> NN	Tab, Peach, Shield Shaped, Scored, N/N <> 100	Lamotrigine 100 mg	Lamictal by Novopharm	Canadian DIN 02248233	Antiepileptic

ID FRONT <> BACK	DESCRIPTION FRONT <> BACK	INGREDIENT & STRENGTH	BRAND (or Generic Equiv.) by FIRM	NDC#	CLASS; SCH.
100 <> NOVO	Tab, White, Oval, novo/100	Captopril 100 mg	Capoten by Novopharm	Canadian DIN 01942999	Antihypertensive
100 <> NOVO	Tab, White, Round, Scored no/vo <> 100	Atenolol 100 mg	Tenormin by Novopharm	Canadian DIN 01912054	Antihypertensive
100 <> NOVO	Tab, White, Round, Scored	Trazodone HCl 100 mg	Desyrel by Novopharm	Canadian DIN 02144271	Antidepressant
100 <> NU	Tab, White, Oval, Film Coated	Fluvoxamine Maleate 100 mg	Luvox by Nu Pharm	Canadian DIN 02231193	OCD
100 <> OM	Tab, Orange, Round	Tapentadol Hydrochloride 100 mg	Tapentadol Hydrochloride by Janssen-Ortho	50458-0840	Analgesic; C II
100 <> P	Tab, Yellow, Round	Topiramate 100 mg	Topamax by Pharmascience	Canadian DIN 02263009	Anticonvulsant
100 <> P	Tab, Light Pink, Trapezoidal	Fluconazole 100 mg	Diflucan by Pharmascience	Canadian DIN 02245644	Antifungal
100 <> P	Tab, Pink, Round, Pharmascience Logo	Amiodarone 100 mg	Cordarone by Pharmascience	Canadian DIN 02292173	Antiarrhythmic
100 <> PAR654	Tab, White, Round, Scored	Torsemide 100 mg	Demadex by Par	49884-0654	Diuretic
100 <> PF	Tab, Gray, Round	Morphine Sulfate 100 mg	MS Contin by Purdue	59011-0263	Analgesic; C II
100 <> S	Tab, Orange, Round, Film Coated	Pinaverium Bromide 100 mg	Dicetel by Solvay	Canadian DIN 02230684	Gastrointestinal
100 <> S	Tab, White, Triangle Shaped	Sumatriptan 100 mg	Imitrex by Dr. Reddy's	55111-0737	Antimigraine
100 <> SCHERING244	Tab, Brown, Round, Scored	Labetalol HCl 100 mg	Normodyne by Rightpak	65240-0705	Antihypertensive
100 <> SP	Tab, Dark Yellow, Oval, Film Coated	Lacosamide 100 mg	Vimpat by Schwarz	00091-2478	Antiepileptic
100 <> SYNTHROID	Tab, Yellow, Round, Scored	Levothyroxine Sodium 100 mcg	Synthroid by Abbott	00074-6624	Thyroid Hormone
100 <> T4	Tab, Yellow, Cap Shaped, Scored	Levothyroxine Sodium 100 mcg	Levothroid by Forest	00456-1323	Thyroid Hormone
100 <> TMC125	Tab, White to Off-White, Oval	Etravirine 100 mg	Intelence by Tibotec	59676-0570	Antiviral
100 <> TOP	Tab, Yellow, Round, Film Coated	Topiramate 100 mg	Topamax by Janssen-Ortho	Canadian DIN 02230894	Anticonvulsant
100 <> TOPAMAX	Tab, Yellow, Round, Film Coated	Topiramate 100 mg	Topamax by McNeil	00045-0641	Anticonvulsant
100 <> TOPAMAX	Tab, Yellow, Round, Film Coated	Topiramate 100 mg	Topamax by Ortho-McNeil	00062-0641	Anticonvulsant
100 <> TOPAMAX	Tab, Yellow, Round, Film Coated	Topiramate 100 mg	Topamax by McNeil	52021-0641	Anticonvulsant
100 <> VIDEX	Tab, Off-White to Light Orange/Yellow, Round, Chewable	Didanosine 100 mg	Videx by BMS	Canadian DIN 01940546	Antiviral
100 <> VIDEX	Tab, Off-White to Light Orange/Yellow, Round, Chewable	Didanosine 100 mg	Videx by BMS	00087-6652	Antiviral
100 <> VOLTARENSR	Tab, Light Pink, Round, Film Coated, Voltaren-XR	Diclofenac Sodium 100 mg	Voltaren XR by Novartis	Canadian DIN 00590827	NSAID
100 <> VOLTARENXR	Tab, Light Pink, Round, Film Coated, Voltaren-XR	Diclofenac Sodium 100 mg	Voltaren XR by H J Harkins Co	52959-0472	NSAID
100 <> VOLTARENXR	Tab, Light Pink, Round, Film Coated, Voltaren-XR	Diclofenac Sodium 100 mg	Voltaren XR by Caremark	00339-6091	NSAID
100 <> VOLTARENXR	Tab, Light Pink, Round, Film Coated, Voltaren-XR	Diclofenac Sodium 100 mg	Voltaren XR by Novartis	00028-0205	NSAID
100 <> VOLTARENXR	Tab, Light Pink, Round, Film Coated, Voltaren-XR	Diclofenac Sodium 100 mg	Voltaren XR by Novartis	17088-0205	NSAID
100 <> WELLBUTRIN	Tab	Bupropion HCl 100 mg	Wellbutrin by GSK	00173-0178	Antidepressant
100 <> Z4362	Tab, Green, Oval	Flurbiprofen 100 mg	Ansaid by Ivax	00182-2621	NSAID
100 <> ZOLOFT	Tab, Yellow, Oblong	Sertraline HCl 100 mg	Zoloft by PDRX	55289-0550	Antidepressant
1000	Tab, Off White, Capsule Shaped	Nicotinic Acid 1000 mg	Niaspan FCT by Sepracor	Canadian DIN 02262339	Antihyperlipidemic
1000 <> 4432	Tab, White, Oval, Scored, Hourglass Logo 4432	Metformin HCl 1000 mg	Glucophage by Ivax	00172-4432 Discontinued	Antidiabetic
1000 <> ANDRX676	Tab, White, Round, Film Coated	Metformin HCl 1000 mg	Glucophage by Andrx	62037-0676	Antidiabetic
1000 <> B387	Tab, White to Off-White, Oval, Scored, Film Coated	Metformin HCl 1000 mg	Glucophage by Barr	00555-0387	Antidiabetic
1000 <> BMS6071	Tab, White, Cap Shaped, Scored, Film Coated	Metformin HCl 1000 mg	Glucophage by Direct Dispensing	57866-9057	Antidiabetic
1000 <> BMS6071	Tab, White, Cap Shaped, Scored, Film Coated	Metformin HCl 1000 mg	Glucophage by BMS	00087-6071	Antidiabetic

ID FRONT <> BACK	DESCRIPTION FRONT <> BACK	INGREDIENT & STRENGTH	BRAND (or Generic Equiv.) by FIRM	NDC#	CLASS; SCH.
1000 <> BMS6071	Tab, White, Cap Shaped, Scored, Film Coated	Metformin HCl 1000 mg	Glucophage by Caremark	00339-6173	Antidiabetic
1000 <> G45	Tab, White, Round	Metformin 1000 mg	Glucophage by Glenmark	68462-0161	Antihyperglycemic
1000 <> IP177	Tab, White to Off White, Oval, Scored	Metformin HCl 1000 mg	Glucophage by Amneal	65162-0177	Antihyperglycemic
1000 <> KOS	Tab, White, Cap Shaped	Niacin 1000 mg	Niaspan by KOS	60598-0003	Antihyperlipidemic
1000 <> KOS	Tab, Orange, Cap Shaped, Film Coated, Extended Release	Niacin 1000 mg	Niaspan by KOS	60958-0142	Antihyperlipidemic
1000 <> PROCANBID	Tab, Gray, Black Print, Oval, Film Coated, Ex Release	Procainamide HCl 1000 mg	Procanbid by King	61570-0071	Antiarrhythmic
1000 <> PROCANBID	Tab, Gray, Black Print, Oval, Film Coated, Ex Release	Procainamide HCl 1000 mg	Procanbid by Parke Davis	00071-0564	Antiarrhythmic
1000A	Tab, Orange, Oval, Film Coated, Extended Release, 1000 "Abbott Logo"	Niacin 1000 mg	Niaspan by Abbott	00074-3080	Antihyperlipidemic
1001	Tab, White, Round	Aminophylline 100 mg	Aminophylline by Vortech		Antiasthmatic
10010 <> NOVO	Tab, Blue, Oval, Scored	Levodopa 100 mg, Carbidopa 10 mg	Sinemet by Novopharm	Canadian DIN 02244494	Antiparkinson
10010 <> NU	Tab, Blue, Oval, Scored, 100 over 10 <> NU	Carbidopa 10 mg, Levodopa 100 mg	by Nu Pharm	Canadian DIN 02182831	Antiparkinson
100100	Tab, White, Oblong, SR	Guaifenesin 900 mg, Phenylephrine 25 mg	by Brighton	10914-0100	Cold Remedy
100100100 <> BARR733	Tab, White, Oval, Scored	Trazodone HCl 300 mg	Desyrel by Teva	00480-0292	Antidepressant
100100100 <> BARR733	Tab, White, Oval, Scored	Trazodone HCl 300 mg	Desyrel by Barr	00555-0733	Antidepressant
100100100 <> MJ796	Tab, Yellow, Scored	Trazodone HCl 300 mg	Desyrel by BMS	00087-0796	Antidepressant
100101 <> JACOBUS	Tab, Scored, Jacobus <> 100/101	Dapsone 100 mg	Dapsone by Jacobus	49938-0101	Antimycobacterial
100101 <> JACOBUS	Tab, Scored, Jacobus <> 100/101	Dapsone 100 mg	Dapsone by Physician Total Care	54868-3801	Antimycobacterial
10010ENDO	Tab, Red & Blue, Oval, 100/10/Endo	Levodopa 100 mg, Carbidopa 10 mg	Sinemet by AltiMed	Canadian	Antiparkinson
1002 <> KOS	Tab, Dark Pink and Light Purple, Cap Shaped	Lovastatin 20 mg, Niacin 1000 mg	Advicor by KOS	60598-0008	Antihyperlipidemic
10025 <> APO	Tab, White, Round, Scored, Film Coated	Atenolol 100 mg, Chlorthalidone 25 mg	Tenoretic by Apotex	Canadian DIN 02248764	Antihypertensive; Diuretic
10025 <> N	Tab, White, Round, Scored	Atenolol 100 mg, Chlorthalidone 25 mg	Tenoretic by Novopharm	Canadian DIN 02302926	Antihypertensive
10025 <> NOVO	Tab, Yellow, Oval, Scored	Levodopa 100 mg, Carbidopa 25 mg	Sinemet by Novopharm	Canadian DIN 02244495	Antiparkinson
10025ENDO	Tab, Yellow, Oval, 100/25/Endo	Levodopa 100 mg, Carbidopa 25 mg	Sinemet by AltiMed	Canadian	Antiparkinson
10025MG	Tab, White, Round, 100/25 mg	Atenolol 100 mg, Chlorthalidone 25 mg	Tenoretic by Zeneca	Canadian	Antihypertensive; Diuretic
1008	Tab, Round	Dextroamphetamine Sulfate 5 mg	Dexedrine by Vortech		Stimulant; C II
1009	Tab, Round	Digitoxin 0.2 mg	by Vortech	00182-0559	Cardiac Agent
100BARR066	Tab	Isoniazid 100 mg	Laniazid by Ivax		Antimycobacterial
100ER	Tab, White, Round, Black Ink, ER	Tramadol HCl 100 mg	Ultram ER by Ortho-McNeil	00062-0653	Analgesic
100LLT28	Tab, Orange, Round	Thioridazine 100 mg	Mellaril by Lederle		Antipsychotic
100M	Tab	Levothyroxine Sodium 100 mcg	Levo-T by Mova	55370-0129	Thyroid Hormone
100M <> Z	Tab, Yellow, Round, Scored	Levothyroxine Sodium 100 mcg	Levo-T by Zoetica	64909-0109	Thyroid Hormone
100M10 <> MOVA	Tab, White, Cap Shaped	Captopril 100 mg	Capoten by Mova	55370-0145	Antihypertensive
100MCG <> FLINT	Tab, Yellow, Round, Scored	Levothyroxine Sodium 0.1 mg	Synthroid by Amerisource	62584-0070	Thyroid Hormone
100MCG <> FLINT	Tab, Yellow, Round, Scored	Levothyroxine Sodium 0.1 mg	Synthroid by Wal Mart	49035-0194	Thyroid Hormone
100MCG <> FLINT	Tab, Yellow, Round, Scored	Levothyroxine Sodium 0.1 mg	Synthroid by Rightpac	65240-0742	Thyroid Hormone
100MG	Cap, Yellowish-Brown, Ivax Logo 100 mg	Cyclosporine 100 mg	Neoral by Ivax	00172-7312	Immunosuppressant
100MG <> CLOZARIL	Tab, Pale Yellow, Round, Scored	Clozapine 100 mg	Clozaril by Novartis	Canadian DIN 00894745	Antipsychotic
100MG <> G4910	Tab, Light Yellow, Cap Shaped, Scored	Sertraline HCl 100 mg	Zoloft by Greenstone	59762-4910	Antidepressant
100MG <> N	Tab, Diamond-Shaped, Yellow, Scored	Azathioprine 100 mg	Azasan by Salix	65649-0241	Immunosuppressant
100MG <> N	Tab, Light Yellow, Diamond Shaped	Azathioprine 100 mg	Azasan by AAI Pharma	66591-0241	Immunosuppressant
100MG <> PF	Tab, Grey, Round, Sustained-Release, Film-Coated, Biconvex	Morphine Sulfate 100 mg	MS Contin by Purdue	Canadian DIN 02014319	Analgesic; C II

ID FRONT <> BACK	DESCRIPTION FRONT <> BACK	INGREDIENT & STRENGTH	BRAND (or Generic Equiv.) by FIRM	NDC#	CLASS; SCH.
100MG <> PF	Tab, Grey, Round, Sustained-Release, Film-Coated, Biconvex	Morphine Sulfate 100 mg	MS Contin by Pharmascience	Canadian DIN 02245287	Analgesic
100MG <> PROVIGIL	Tab, White, Cap Shaped	Modafinil 100 mg	Provigil by Neuman	64579-0319	Stimulant; C IV
100MG <> PROVIGIL	Tab, White, Cap Shaped	Modafinil 100 mg	Provigil by Cephalon	63459-0101	Stimulant; C IV
100MG <> T	Tab, White, Yellow Imprint, Round, Film Coated, Ex Release	Carbamazepine 100 mg	Tegretol by Caremark	00339-6131	Anticonvulsant
100MG <> T	Tab, White, Yellow Imprint, Round, Film Coated, Ex Release	Carbamazepine 100 mg	Tegretol by Novartis	00083-0061	Anticonvulsant
100MG <> ZOLOFT	Tab, Light Yellow, Cap Shaped, Scored, Film Coated	Sertraline HCl 100 mg	Zoloft by Roerig	00049-4910	Antidepressant
100MG <> ZOLOFT	Tab, Light Yellow, Cap Shaped, Scored, Film Coated	Sertraline HCl 100 mg	Zoloft by Va Cmop	65243-0063	Antidepressant
100MG <> ZOLOFT	Tab, Light Yellow, Cap Shaped, Scored, Film Coated	Sertraline HCl 100 mg	Zoloft by Heartland	61392-0939	Antidepressant
100MG <> ZOLOFT	Tab, Light Yellow, Cap Shaped, Scored, Film Coated	Sertraline HCl 100 mg	Zoloft by PDRX	55289-0550	Antidepressant
100MG <> ZOLOFT	Tab, Light Yellow, Cap Shaped, Scored, Film Coated	Sertraline HCl 100 mg	Zoloft by DRX	55045-2208	Antidepressant
100MG <> ZOLOFT	Tab, Light Yellow, Cap Shaped, Scored, Film Coated	Sertraline HCl 100 mg	Zoloft by Nat Pharmpak	55154-2712	Antidepressant
100MG <> ZOLOFT	Tab, Light Yellow, Cap Shaped, Scored, Film Coated	Sertraline HCl 100 mg	Zoloft by Physician Total Care	54868-2637	Antidepressant
100MG <> ZOLOFT	Tab, Light Yellow, Cap Shaped, Scored, Film Coated	Sertraline HCl 100 mg	Zoloft by Allscripts		Antidepressant
100MG <> ZOLOFT	Tab, Light Yellow, Cap Shaped, Scored, Film Coated	Sertraline HCl 100 mg	Zoloft by Amerisource	62584-0910	Antidepressant
100MG <> ZOLOFT	Tab, Light Yellow, Cap Shaped, Scored, Film Coated	Sertraline HCl 100 mg	Zoloft by Direct Dispensing	57866-6305	Antidepressant
100MG2131	Cap, Pink & White	Nitrofurantoin 100 mg	by Direct Dispensing	57866-6590	Antibiotic
100MGFLUVOX	Tab, White, Oval, 100 mg Fluvox	Fluvoxamine Maleate 100 mg	Luvox by AltiMed	Canadian DIN 02218461	OCD
100MGLEDERLEM4	Tab, Orange & Purple	Minocycline HCl 100 mg	Minocin by Lederle		Antibiotic
100MGWATSON498	Cap, Blue, 100MG on Cap and WATSON498 on body	Doxycycline Hyclate 100 mg	Vibramycin by Watson	52544-0498	Antibiotic
100P	Cap, Orange and Lavender	Minocycline HCl 100 mg	Minocin by Pharmascience	Canadian DIN 02294427	Antibiotic
100P <> DAN	Tab, White, Round, Scored	Phenobarbital 100 mg	Phenobarbital by Schein	00364-0206	Sedative/Hypnotic; C IV
100TRP2SL44150	Tab, White, Trapezoidal, Scored	Trazodone HCl 150 mg	Desyrel by Sandoz	00781-1826	Antidepressant
100WYETH	Tab, White, Round	Acebutolol HCl 100 mg	Sectral by Wyeth	Canadian	Antihypertensive
101 <> APO	Tab, White to Off-White, Oval, Film Coated	Paroxetine HCl 40 mg	Paxil by Apotex	60505-0101	Antidepressant
101 <> GG	Tab, White, Scored	Methocarbamol 750 mg	Robaxin by Sandoz	00781-1750	Muscle Relaxant
101 <> KP	Tab, Yellowish Orange, Round, Scored	Sulfasalazine 500 mg	Azulfidine by Pharmacia		Gastrointestinal
101 <> KPH	Tab, Gold, Round, Scored	Sulfasalazine 500 mg	Azulfidine by Pharmacia	59632-0101	Gastrointestinal
101 <> KPH	Tab, Gold, Round, Scored	Sulfasalazine 500 mg	Azulfidine by Thrift Drug	59198-0010	Gastrointestinal
101 <> KPH	Tab, Gold, Round, Scored	Sulfasalazine 500 mg	Azulfidine by Amerisource	62584-0005	Gastrointestinal
101 <> KPH	Tab, Gold, Round, Scored	Sulfasalazine 500 mg	Azulfidine by Pharmacia	Canadian DIN 02064480	Gastrointestinal
101 <> KPH	Tab, Gold, Round, Scored	Sulfasalazine 500 mg	Azulfidine by Pharmacia	00013-0101	Gastrointestinal
101 <> KU	Tab, White, Round, Scored	Hyoscyamine Sulfate 0.125 mg	Levsin by Kremers Urban	62175-0101	Gastrointestinal
101 <> TENORMIN	Tab, White, Round	Atenolol 100 mg	Tenormin by Pharm Util	60491-0629	Antihypertensive
101 <> TENORMIN	Tab, White, Round	Atenolol 100 mg	Tenormin by AstraZeneca	00310-0101	Antihypertensive
1010 <> 20	Tab, Tan, Oval, Film Coated	Citalopram 20 mg	Celexa by Torrent	13668-0010	Antidepressant
10100 <> SP341	Tab, Blue, Round, Scored, 10/100 <> SP over 341, Orally Disintegrating	Carbidopa 10 mg, Levodopa 100 mg	Parcopa by Schwarz	00091-3341	Antiparkinson
101010 <> 935200	Tab, White to Off-White, Rectangular, Trisect Scored	Buspirone HCl 30 mg	BuSpar by Teva	00093-5200	Antianxiety
101010 <> MB4	Tab, White, Cap Shaped, Scored	Buspirone HCl 30 mg	BuSpar by Mylan	00378-1175	Antianxiety
101010 <> MB4	Tab, White, Cap Shaped, Scored	Buspirone HCl 30 mg	BuSpar by UDL	51079-0994	Antianxiety
101010 <> MJ824	Tab, Pink, Scored, MJ Logo	Buspirone HCl 30 mg	BuSpar by BMS	00087-0824	Antianxiety
1011 <> 40	Tab, Tan, Oval, Film Coated, 4 / 0	Citalopram 40 mg	Celexa by Torrent	13668-0011	Antidepressant
1011 <> STASON	Tab, White, Diamond Shaped	Captopril 12.5 mg	Capoten by Stason	60763-1011	Antihypertensive
1011 <> STASON	Tab, White, Diamond Shaped	Captopril 12.5 mg	Capoten by Duramed	51285-0955	Antihypertensive
1012 <> STASON	Tab, Off-White, Diamond Shaped, Scored	Captopril 25 mg	Capoten by Stason	60763-1012	Antihypertensive

ID FRONT <> BACK	DESCRIPTION FRONT <> BACK	INGREDIENT & STRENGTH	BRAND (or Generic Equiv.) by FIRM	NDC#	CLASS; SCH.
10125 <> 5033	Tab, Blue, Round, Ivax Hourglass Logo 5033 <> 10/12.5	Lisinopril 10 mg, HCTZ 12.5 mg	Prinzide by Ivax	00172-5033	Antihypertensive; Diuretic
10125 <> APO	Tab, Pink, Oval, APO <> 10 over 12.5	Lisinopril 10 mg, HCTZ 12.5 mg	Prinzide by Apotex	60505-0205	Antihypertensive; Diuretic
10125 <> APO	Tab, Pink, Round	Hydrochlorothiazide 12.5 mg, Lisinopril 10 mg	Zestoretic by Apotex	Canadian DIN 02261979	Diuretic; Antihypertensive
1013 <> STASON	Tab, White, Diamond Shaped, Scored	Captopril 50 mg	Capoten by Stason	60763-1013	Antihypertensive
101362	Cap, Yellow, 10-1362	Ephedrine 25 mg	by PDK		Cold Remedy
1014 <> STASON	Tab, White, Cap Shaped, Scored	Captopril 100 mg	Capoten by Stason	60763-1014	Antihypertensive
1014 <> STASON	Tab, White, Cap Shaped, Scored	Captopril 100 mg	Capoten by Duramed	51285-0958	Antihypertensive
102 <> 5	Tab, White, Oval, Scored, Boehringer Logo and 102 <> 5	Torsemide 5 mg	Demadex by Hoffmann La Roche	00004-0262	Diuretic
102 <> 5	Tab, White, Oval, Scored	Torsemide 5 mg	Demadex by Boehringer Mannheim	12871-6477	Diuretic
102 <> K	Tab, Orange, Round, K with Arrow Logo	Bisacodyl 5 mg	Dulcolax Laxative by Qualitest	00603-0054	Gastrointestinal
102 <> K	Tab, Orange, Round, K with Arrow Logo	Bisacodyl 5 mg	Dulcolax by Watson	00536-3381	Gastrointestinal
102 <> KPH	Tab, Gold, Oval, Film Coated	Sulfasalazine 500 mg	Azulfidine EN Tabs by Thrift Drug	59198-0230	Gastrointestinal
102 <> KPH	Tab, Gold, Oval, Film Coated	Sulfasalazine 500 mg	Azulfidine EN Tabs by Pharmacia	Canadian DIN 02064472	Gastrointestinal
102 <> KPH	Tab, Gold, Oval, Film Coated	Sulfasalazine 500 mg	Azulfidine EN Tabs by Pharmacia	59632-0102	Gastrointestinal
102 <> KPH	Tab, Gold, Oval, Film Coated	Sulfasalazine 500 mg	Azulfidine EN Tabs by Pharmacia	00013-0102	Gastrointestinal
102 <> KPH	Tab, Gold, Oval, Film Coated	Sulfasalazine 500 mg	Azulfidine EN Tabs by Wal Mart	49035-0167	Gastrointestinal
102 <> KPH	Tab, Gold, Oval, Film Coated	Sulfasalazine 500 mg	Azulfidine EN Tabs by Nat Pharmpak	55154-2801	Gastrointestinal
102 <> KPH	Tab, Gold, Oval, Film Coated	Sulfasalazine 500 mg	Azulfidine EN Tabs by Rx Pak	65084-0171	Gastrointestinal
102 <> KU	Tab, White, Round, Scored, Sublingual	Hyoscyamine Sulfate 0.125 mg	Levsin by Murfreesboro	51129-1503	Gastrointestinal
102 <> KU	Tab, White, Round, Scored, Sublingual	Hyoscyamine Sulfate 0.125 mg	Levsin by Kremers Urban	62175-0102	Gastrointestinal
102 <> SLX	Tab, White to Off-White, Oval, Scored	Sodium phosphate (Monobasic, monohydrate) 1.102 g, Sodium Phosphate (Dibasic, Anhydrous) 0.398 g	OsmoPrep by Salix	65649-0701	Gastrointestinal
1022 <> SOLVAY	Tab, Sugar Coated	Esterified Estrogens 0.625 mg	by Apotheca	12634-0509	Hormone
1024 <> 93	Tab, White to Off-White, Oblong, Scored, 93 to left of Score <> 1024	Nefazodone HCl 100 mg	Serzone by Teva	00093-1024	Antidepressant
1025	Tab, White, Oval, 102/5	Torsemide 5 mg	Demadex by Boehringer Mannheim	Canadian	Diuretic
1025 <> 93	Tab, Light Yellow to Yellow, Oblong	Nefazodone HCl 200 mg	Serzone by Teva	00093-1025	Antidepressant
10251025 <> VISKAZIDES	Tab, Peach, Round, Scored, 10/25 10/25 <> Viskazide S in a Triangle	Hydrochlorothiazide 25 mg, Pindolol 10 mg	Viskazide by Novartis	Canadian DIN 00566827	Diuretic; Antihypertensive
1026 <> 93	Tab, White to Off-White, Oblong	Nefazodone HCl 250 mg	Serzone by Teva	00093-1026	Antidepressant
103	Tab, White, Round	Simethicone 80 mg	Mylanta by Ivax	00182-1460 Discontinued	Antiflatulent
103	Tab, White, Round	Simethicone 80 mg	Mylicon by Ivax	00182-8643 Discontinued	Antiflatulent
103 <> 10	Tab, White, Oval, Scored, Boehringer Logo 103 <> 10	Torsemide 10 mg	Demadex by Boehringer Mannheim	Canadian	Diuretic
103 <> 10	Tab, White, Oval, Scored, Boehringer Logo 103 <> 10	Torsemide 10 mg	Demadex by Hoffmann La Roche	00004-0263	Diuretic
103 <> 10	Tab, White, Oval, Scored, Boehringer Logo 103 <> 10	Torsemide 10 mg	Demadex by Nat Pharmpak	55154-0406	Diuretic
10300 <> TP	Tab, White, Oblong, Scored, TP <> 10 / 300	Hydrocodone 10 mg, Acetaminophen 300 mg	Xodol by Teamm	67336-0911	Analgesic; C III
1031	Tab	Carbetapentane Tannate 60 mg, Chlorpheniramine Tannate 5 mg, Ephedrine Tannate 10 mg, Phenylephrine Tannate 10 mg	Tri Tannate Plus by Rugby	00536-4394	Cold Remedy
103103 <> C	Tab, Blue, Round, 103 over 103 <> Caraco Logo	Salsalate 500 mg	Disalcid by Caraco	57664-0103	NSAID
1032	Tab, White, Round	Reserpine 0.25 mg	Serpasil by Vortech		Antihypertensive
10325 <> E712	Tab, Yellow, Oval	Oxycodone 10 mg, Acetaminophen 325 mg	Endocet by Endo	60951-0712	Analgesic; C II
10325 <> M523	Tab, White to Off-White, Cap Shaped, M523 <> 10/325	Oxycodone 10 mg, Acetaminophen 325 mg	Percocet by Mallinckrodt	00406-0523	Analgesic; C II
10325 <> PERCOCET	Tab, Yellow, Oval, 10-325 <> PERCOCET	Acetaminophen 325 mg, Oxycodone HCl 10 mg	Percocet by Endo	63481-0629	Analgesic; C II
1033	Tab, Round	Rauwolfia Serpentina 100 mg	Raudixin by Vortech		Antihypertensive
1035 <> 93	Tab, Peach, Round	Lisinopril 10 mg, HCTZ 12.5 mg	Prinzide by Teva	00093-1035	Antihypertensive; Diuretic

ID FRONT <> BACK	DESCRIPTION FRONT <> BACK	INGREDIENT & STRENGTH	BRAND (or Generic Equiv.) by FIRM	NDC#	CLASS; SCH.
10MG	Tab, Light Pink, Oblong, Film-Coated, Delayed Release, Logo <> 10MG	Omeprazole 10 mg	Losec MUPS by AstraZeneca	Canadian DIN 02242461	Gastrointestinal
10MG <> 4759	Tab, Beige, Hexagonal, Film-Coated,	Prasugrel 10 mg	Effient by Eli Lilly	00002-4759	Antiplatelet
10MG <> 4759	Tab, Beige, Double Arrow Shaped, Film-Coated	Prasugrel 10 mg	Effient by Eli Lilly	Canadian DIN 02349124	Antiplatelet
10MG <> APO	Tab, White, Ovoid, Scored	Cetirizine HCl 10 mg	Reactine by Apotex	Canadian DIN 02231603	Antihistamine
10MG <> BUSPAR	Tab, MJ Logo	Buspirone HCl 10 mg	Buspar by Med Pro	53978-3024	Antianxiety
10MG <> ETHEX265	Tab, Yellow, Oval, Scored	Buspirone HCl 10 mg	BuSpar by Ethex	58177-0265	Antianxiety
10MG <> FP	Tab, Beige, Oval, Scored, Film Coated	Citalopram 10 mg	Celexa by Forest	00456-4010	Antidepressant
10MG <> IL	Tab, Beige, Oval, Film Coated	Citalopram HBr 10 mg	Celexa by Inwood	00258-3695	Antidepressant
10MG334410MGSB	Cap, Ivory & Natural with White & Yellow Pellets	Prochlorperazine 10 mg	Compazine by Int'l Processing	59885-3344	Antiemetic
10MG351310MGSB	Cap, Brown & Clear	Dextroamphetamine Sulfate 10 mg	Dexedrine by DRX	55045-2616	Stimulant; C II
10MG351310MGSB	Cap, Brown & Clear	Dextroamphetamine Sulfate 10 mg	Dexedrine by Physician Total Care	54868-3811	Stimulant; C II
10MG709TRADE DRESSLICD	Cap, Yellow & White, Hard Gel, Trade Dress Lic'd	Nortriptyline HCl 10 mg	by Pharmascience	Canadian DIN 5760676924	Antidepressant
10MGLEDERLE12	Cap, Green & Yellow	Loxapine 10 mg	Loxitane by Lederle		Antipsychotic
10MGSARAFEM	Cap, Lavender, Opaque	Fluoxetine HCl 10 mg	Sarafem by Warner Chilcott	00430-0435	Antidepressant
10MGSB10MG3344	Cap, Ivory & Natural with White & Yellow Pellets	Prochlorperazine 10 mg	Compazine by Int'l Processing	59885-3344	Antiemetic
10MGSB10MG3513	Cap, Brown & Clear	Dextroamphetamine Sulfate 10 mg	Dexedrine by Physician Total Care	54868-3811	Stimulant; C II
10MGSONATA	Cap, Green & Opaque	Zaleplon 10 mg	Sonata by Wyeth	00008-0926	Sedative/Hypnotic; C IV
10MGSONATA	Cap, Green & Opaque	Zaleplon 10 mg	Sonata by King	60793-0146	Sedative/Hypnotic; C IV
10MGWPC001	Cap, Red, White Ink	Phenoxybenzamine HCl 10 mg	Dibenzyline by Wellspring	65197-0001	Antihypertensive
10MGZAR	Tab, Yellow, Round, 10 mg/Zar	Metolazone 10 mg	Zaroxolyn by Medeva		Diuretic
10MJ <> BUSPAR	Tab, 10 over MJ <> Buspar	Buspirone HCl 10 mg	Buspar by Nat Pharmpak	55154-2010	Antianxiety
10NOVO	Tab, Yellow, D-Shaped, 10/Novo	Cyclobenzaprine HCl 10 mg	Novo Cycloprine by Novopharm	Canadian	Muscle Relaxant
10TRIANGLE <> BAYERCROSS	Tab, Light Red, Round, Film Coated	Rivaroxaban 10 mg	Xarelto by Bayer	Canadian DIN 02316986	Anticoagulant
10VALIUM <> ROCHE	Tab, Blue, Round, Scored	Diazepam 10 mg	Valium by Roche	00140-0006	Antianxiety; C IV
10XL	Tab, Pink, Round	Oxybutynin Chloride 10 mg	Ditropan XL by Janssen-Ortho	Canadian DIN 02243961	Urinary Tract
10XL	Tab, Pink, Round	Oxybutynin Chloride 10 mg	Ditropan XL by Alza	17314-8501	Urinary Tract
10ZESTRIL	Tab, Pink, Round, 10ZESTRIL inside Heart Logo	Lisinopril 10 mg	Zestril by AstraZeneca	Canadian DIN 02049376	Diuretic; Antihypertensive
11	Tab, White, Round, Scored, 11 <> Triangle	Biperiden HCl 2 mg	Akineton by Par	49884-0693	Antiparkinson
11	Tab, White, Round, Scored, 11 <> Triangle	Biperiden HCl 2 mg	Akineton by Physician Total Care	54868-2432	Antiparkinson
11	Tab, White, Round, Scored, 11 <> Triangle	Biperiden HCl 2 mg	Akineton by Abbott	Canadian DIN 00124982	Antiparkinson
11 <> A	Tab, White, Cap Shaped, Film Coated	Mirtazapine 7.5 mg	Remeron by Aurobindo	65862-0001	Antidepressant
11 <> A	Tab, White, Cap Shaped, Film Coated	Mirtazapine 7.5 mg	Remeron by Aurolife	13107-0001	Antidepressant
11 <> B	Tab, Light Green, Round, Film Coated	Inert	Tri-Levlen 28 by Berlex	50419-0111	Oral Contraceptive; Placebo
11 <> D	Tab, White, Round, Film Coated	Zidovudine 300 mg	Retrovir by Aurobindo	65862-0024	Antiviral
11 <> DUPONT	Tab, Pale Yellow, Cap Shaped, Scored, Film Coated	Naltrexone HCl 50 mg	Revia by Dupont	Canadian	Opioid Antagonist
11 <> P	Tab, Dye Free, Round, Chewable, 1.1	Sodium Fluoride 1.1 mg	Pharmaflur 1.1 by Pharmics	00813-0065	Element
11 <> RX	Tab, White, Oblong, Scored, R / X <> 1 / 1	Fosinopril 10 mg	Monopril by Ranbaxy	63304-0775	Antihypertensive
11 <> SL	Tab, Sugar Coated	Dipyridamole 25 mg	by Pliva	50111-0311	Antiplatelet
11 <> VP	Tab, White, Round, Scored, Film Coated	Ethambutol HCl 100 mg	Myambutol by Versapharm	61748-0011	Antituberculosis
11 <> VP	Tab, White, Round, Film Coated	Ethambutol HCl 100 mg	by West-Ward	00143-9100	Antituberculosis

ID FRONT <> BACK	DESCRIPTION FRONT <> BACK	INGREDIENT & STRENGTH	BRAND (or Generic Equiv.) by FIRM	NDC#	CLASS; SCH.
110	Tab, White, Scored, 110 Prasco Logo	Phenylephrine HCl 20 mg, Chlorpheniramine Maleate 8 mg, Methscopolamine Nitrate 2.5 mg	DriHist SR by Prasco	66993-0110	Cold Remedy
110	Tab, Light Beige, Round, Film Coated, Scored	Moexipril HCl 7.5 mg	Univasc by Paddock	00574-0110	Antihypertensive
110	Tab, White to Off White, Round, Scored, Orally Disintegrating	Alprazolam ODT .25 mg	Niravam by Par	49884-0110	Antianxiety
110 <> AP	Tab, Light Blue, Cap Shaped, Scored	Acetaminophen 650 mg, Butalbital 50 mg	Promacet by Atley	59702-0650	Analgesic
110 <> CIBA	Tab, Orange, Oval, Scored	Maprotiline HCl 25 mg	Ludiomil by Novartis	00083-0110	Antidepressant
110 <> CSCOTT	Tab, Sugar Coated, C Scott	Thyroid 1 g	by JMI Canton	00252-7007	Thyroid Hormone
110 <> PMS10	Tab, Blue, Round, Scored	Methylphenidate HCl 10 mg	Ritalin by Pharmascience	Canadian DIN 00584991	Stimulant; C II
110260MG	Cap, Pink & White	Fexofenadine HCl 60 mg	Allegra by Allscripts		Antihistamine
1105	Cap, Red, Soft Gel	Docusate Sodium 50 mg	Colace by UDL	51079-0521 Discontinued	Laxative
1105	Cap, Red, Soft Gel	Docusate Sodium 50 mg	Colace by RP Scherer		Laxative
111	Tab, White to Off White, Round, Scored, Orally Disintegrating	Alprazolam ODT .5 mg	Niravam by Par	49884-0111	Antianxiety
111 <> 93	Tab, White, Round, Film Coated	Cimetidine HCl 200 mg	Tagamet by Teva	00093-0111	Gastrointestinal
111 <> A	Tab, Brown, Oval, Film Coated, Scored	Methenamine Mandelate 500 mg	Mandelamine by Murfreesboro	51129-1430	Antibiotic; Urinary Tract
111 <> COPLEY	Tab, Yellowish Tan, Coated	Ascorbic Acid 120 mg, Beta-Carotene 4.2 mg, Calcium Carbonate 490.76 mg, Cholecalciferol 0.49 mg, Cupric Oxide 2.5 mg, Cyanocobalamin 12 mcg, Ferrous Fumarate 197.75 mg, Folic Acid 1 mg, Niacinamide 21 mg, Pyridoxine HCl 10.5 mg, Riboflavin 3.15 mg, Thiamine Mononitrate 1.575 mg, Vitamin A Acetate 8.4 mg, Vitamin E Acetate 44 mg, Zinc Oxide 31.12 mg	by Teva	38245-0111 Discontinued	Vitamin
111 <> COR	Tab, Orange, Round, Film Coated	Rimantadine HCl 100 mg	Flumadine by Sandoz	00781-5029	Antiviral
111 <> GDC	Tab, White, Round	Calcium Carbonate, Magnesium Hydroxide	Mi-Acid by Major	00904-5115	Gastrointestinal
111 <> PMS	Tab, Yellow, D Shaped, Film Coated	Cyclobenzaprine HCl 10 mg	Flexeril by Pharmascience	Canadian DIN 02212048	Muscle Relaxant
1111 <> 93	Tab, White, Round	Lisinopril 2.5 mg	Prinivil by Teva	00093-1111 Discontinued	Antihypertensive
1111 <> BTG	Tab, White, Oval	Oxandrolone 2.5 mg	Oxandrin by BTG	54396-0111	Steroid; C III
1111 <> E	Tab, Light Pink, Round, Sustained Release	Bupropion HCl 200 mg	Wellbutrin SR by Eon	00185-1111	Antidepressant
1111 <> OX	Tab, White, Oval, Scored	Oxandrolone 2.5 mg	Oxandrin by Watson	00591-3544	Steroid; C III
1113 <> 93	Tab, Red, Round	Lisinopril 10 mg	Prinivil by Teva	00093-1113 Discontinued	Antihypertensive
1114 <> 93	Tab, Red, Cap Shaped	Lisinopril 20 mg	Prinivil by Teva	00093-1114 Discontinued	Antihypertensive
1114 <> BEACH	Tab, Yellow, Oblong, Film Coated	Methenamine Mandelate 500 mg, Sodium Phosphate, Monobasic 500 mg	Uroqid Acid No. 2 by Neogen	59051-0090	Antibiotic; Urinary Tract
1114 <> BEACH	Tab, Yellow, Oblong, Film Coated	Methenamine Mandelate 500 mg, Sodium Phosphate, Monobasic, Monohydrate 500 mg	Uroqid Acid No. 2 by Pharmaceutical Assoc	00121-0352	Antibiotic; Urinary Tract
1114 <> BEACH	Tab, Yellow, Oblong, Film Coated	Methenamine Mandelate 500 mg, Sodium Phosphate, Monobasic, Monohydrate 500 mg	Uroqid Acid No. 2 by Beach	00486-1114	Antibiotic; Urinary Tract
1114 <> BEACH	Tab, Yellow, Oblong, Film Coated	Methenamine Mandelate 500 mg, Sodium Phosphate, Monobasic 500 mg	Uroqid Acid No. 2 by West-Ward	00143-9023	Antibiotic; Urinary Tract
1115	Tab, Blue, Round, Savage Logo 1115	Dyphylline 200 mg	Dilor by Savage	00281-1115	Antiasthmatic
1115 <> 93	Tab, Yellow, Cap Shaped	Lisinopril 40 mg	Prinivil by Teva	00093-1115 Discontinued	Antihypertensive
1116	Tab, White, Round, Large Triangle over Small Triangle	Dyphylline 400 mg	Dilor-400 by Savage	00281-1116	Antiasthmatic
1117 <> W	Tab, Yellow, Round, Film-Coated	Levonorgestrel 90 mcg, Ethinyl Estradiol 20 mcg	Lybrel by Wyeth	00008-1117	Oral Contraceptive
1117 <> WPI	Tab, White, Oblong, Film Coated	Mirtazapine 15 mg	Remeron by Watson	00591-1117	Antidepressant
1118 <> 93	Tab, Light Blue, Oval, Ex Release	Etodolac 600 mg	Lodine XL by Teva	00093-1118	NSAID
112	Tab, Light Beige, Round, Film Coated	Sitagliptin 50 mg	Januvia by Merck	00006-0112	Antidiabetic

42

Copyright © 2010 Ident-A-Drug (209) 472-2240 • May not be reproduced without permission • For updated data, go to www.IdentADrug.com

ID FRONT <> BACK	DESCRIPTION FRONT <> BACK	INGREDIENT & STRENGTH	BRAND (or Generic Equiv.) by FIRM	NDC#	CLASS; SCH.
112	Tab, Ex Release, 1 1/2	Nitroglycerin 1.5 mg	Nitrobid by Forest	10418-0143	Vasodilator
112	Tab, White to Off-White, Cap Shaped, Film Coated	Acetaminophen 500 mg	Tylenol Ex Strength by UDL	51079-0396 Discontinued	Analgesic
112 <> 93	Tab, White, Round, Film Coated	Cimetidine HCl 300 mg	Tagamet by PDRX	55289-0799	Gastrointestinal
112 <> 93	Tab, White, Round, Film Coated	Cimetidine HCl 300 mg	Tagamet by Teva	00093-0112	Gastrointestinal
112 <> AP	Tab, Blue, Round	Hyoscyamine Sulfate 0.125 mg	Levsin by Alaven Pharmaceutical	68220-0112	Gastrointestinal
112 <> FLINT	Tab, Rose, Round, Scored	Levothyroxine Sodium 112 mcg	Synthroid by Abbott	00048-1080	Thyroid Hormone
112 <> FLINT	Tab, Rose, Round, Scored	Levothyroxine Sodium 112 mcg	Synthroid by Nat Pharmpak	55154-0911	Thyroid Hormone
112 <> FLINT	Tab, Rose, Round, Scored	Levothyroxine Sodium 112 mcg	Synthroid by CVS	51316-0201	Thyroid Hormone
112 <> FLINT	Tab, Rose, Round, Scored	Levothyroxine Sodium 112 mcg	Synthroid by Forest	00456-0330	Thyroid Hormone
112 <> FLINT	Tab, Rose, Round, Scored	Levothyroxine Sodium 112 mcg	Synthroid by Abbott	Canadian DIN 02171228	Thyroid Hormone
112 <> GG336	Tab, Rose, Cap Shaped, Scored, 112 <> GG over 336	Levothyroxine 112 mcg	Levo-T by Alara	64909-0127	Thyroid Hormone
112 <> GG336	Tab, Rose, Cap Shaped, Scored, 112 <> GG over 336	Levothyroxine 112 mcg	Levo-T by Sandoz	00781-5185	Thyroid Hormone
112 <> SYNTHROID	Tab, Pink, Round, Scored	Levothyroxine Sodium 112 mcg	Synthroid by Abbott	00074-9296	Thyroid Hormone
112 <> T4	Tab, Rose, Cap Shaped	Levothyroxine Sodium 112 mcg	Levothroid by Forest	00456-1330	Thyroid Hormone
1120UAD	Cap, Maroon, Opaque	Acetaminophen 500 mg, Hydrocodone Bitartrate 5 mg	Vicodin by Forest	00785-1120	Analgesic; C III
1122	Tab, Brown, Round	Sennosides 8.6 mg	Senokot by Cypress	60258-0950	Laxative
1122 <> 93	Tab, Orange, Oval, Ex Release	Etodolac 400 mg	Lodine XL by Teva	00093-1122	NSAID
1125	Tab, White, Cap Shaped, Film Coated	Potassium Phosphate (Dibasic, Anhydrous 852 mg), Sodium Phosphate (Monobasic, Monohydrate 130 mg)	K-Phos Neutral by Pharmaceutical Assoc	00121-0349	Electrolytes
1125	Tab	Potassium Phosphate (Monobasic 155 mg), Sodium Phosphate (Dibasic, Anhydrous 852 mg), Sodium Phosphate (Monobasic, Monohydrate 130 mg)	K-Phos Neutral by Beach	00486-1125	Electrolytes
1127 <> BRL	Tab, White, Oblong, Scored	Sucralfate 1 g	Carafate by Blue Ridge	59273-0001	Gastrointestinal
1127 <> BRL	Tab, White, Oblong, Scored	Sucralfate 1 g	Carafate by SKB	00135-0176	Gastrointestinal
112M	Tab	Levothyroxine Sodium 112 mcg	Synthroid by Em Pharma	63254-0440	Thyroid Hormone
112M	Tab	Levothyroxine Sodium 112 mcg	Synthroid by Mova	55370-0161	Thyroid Hormone
112M <> Z	Tab, Pink, Round, Scored	Levothyroxine Sodium 112 mcg	Synthroid by Zoetica	64909-0116	Thyroid Hormone
112MCG	Tab, Rose, Round, Scored	Levothyroxine Sodium 112 mcg	Synthroid by Amerisource	62584-0080	Thyroid Hormone
112MCG	Tab, Rose, Round, Scored	Levothyroxine Sodium 112 mcg	Synthroid by Rightpac	65240-0743	Thyroid Hormone
112MCG	Tab, Rose, Round, Scored	Levothyroxine Sodium 112 mcg	Synthroid by GSK	53873-0118	Thyroid Hormone
112MCG	Tab, Rose, Round, Scored	Levothyroxine Sodium 112 mcg	Synthroid by Physician Total Care	54868-3849	Thyroid Hormone
113 <> 1	Tab, White, Barrel Shaped	Granisetron HCl 1 mg	Kytril by Dava	67253-0417	Antiemetic
113 <> 93	Tab, Film Coated	Cimetidine HCl 400 mg	Tagamet by Vangard	00615-3566	Gastrointestinal
113 <> AP	Tab, Blue, Round, Sublingual	Hyoscyamine Sulfate 0.125 mg	Levsin by Alaven Pharmaceutical	68220-0113	Gastrointestinal
113 <> COPLEY	Tab, Buff	Chlorpheniramine Tannate 8 mg, Phenylephrine Tannate 25 mg, Pyrilamine Tannate 25 mg	R-Tannate by Schein	00364-2196	Cold Remedy
1134 <> BEACH	Tab, White, Oblong, Scored, Film Coated	Potassium Phosphate (Monobasic 305 mg), Sodium Phosphate (Monobasic 700 mg)	K-Phos No 2 by West-Ward	00143-9024	Electrolytes
1134 <> BEACH	Tab, White, Oblong, Scored, Film Coated	Potassium Phosphate (Monobasic 305 mg), Sodium Phosphate (Monobasic 700 mg)	K-Phos No 2 by Pharmaceutical Assoc	00121-0386	Electrolytes
1134 <> BEACH	Tab, White, Oblong, Scored, Film Coated	Potassium Phosphate (Monobasic 305 mg), Sodium Phosphate (Monobasic 700 mg)	K-Phos No 2 by Beach	00486-1134	Electrolytes
1136 <> BEACH	Tab, White, Cap Shaped	Potassium Citrate Anhydrous 50 mg, Sodium Citrate, Anhydrous 950 mg	Citrolith by Beach	00486-1136	Electrolytes
1136 <> BEACH	Tab, White, Cap Shaped	Potassium Citrate Anhydrous 50 mg, Sodium Citrate, Anhydrous 950 mg	Citrolith by Pharmaceutical Assoc	00121-0374	Electrolytes
113BIOCRAFT	Cap, Light Green	Cephradine 500 mg	by Schein	00364-2142	Antibiotic
114	Cap, Black, Oval, Softgel	Vitamin C 100 mg, Folic Acid 1 mg, Niacinamide 20 mg, Thiamine Mononitrate 1.5 mg, Riboflavin 1.7 mg, Vitamin B6 10 mg, Vitamin B12 6 mcg, Calcium Pantothenate 5 mg, Biotin 150 mcg	Renaphro by Rising	64980-0114	Vitamin; Supplement

ID FRONT <> BACK	DESCRIPTION FRONT <> BACK	INGREDIENT & STRENGTH	BRAND (or Generic Equiv.) by FIRM	NDC#	CLASS; SCH.
114 <> COPLEY	Tab, Light Orange, Cap Shaped, Scored, Film Coated, Ex Release	Procainamide HCl 750 mg	Procan SR by Murfreesboro	51129-1174	Antiarrhythmic
114 <> COPLEY	Tab, Light Orange, Cap Shaped, Scored, Film Coated, Ex Release	Procainamide HCl 750 mg	Procan SR by Moore	00839-7029	Antiarrhythmic
114 <> COPLEY	Tab, Light Orange, Cap Shaped, Scored, Film Coated, Ex Release	Procainamide HCl 750 mg	Procan SR by Teva	00093-9114 Discontinued	Antiarrhythmic
114 <> COPLEY	Tab, Light Orange, Cap Shaped, Scored, Film Coated, Ex Release	Procainamide HCl 750 mg	Procan SR by Ivax	00182-1709	Antiarrhythmic
115	Cap, Maroon, Oval, Softgel	Ferrous Fumarate 200 mg, Ascorbic Acid 250 mg, Desiccated Stomach Powder 100 mg, Cyanocobalamin 10 mcg	FeoGen by Rising	64980-0115	Vitamin; Supplement
115 <>AP	Tab, White, Cap Shaped, Extended Release	Hyoscyamine Sulfate 0.375 mg	Levbid by Alaven Pharmaceutical	68220-0115	Gastrointestinal
115 <> KPI	Tab, Round, Light Gray	Liothyronine Sodium 5 mcg	Cytomel by King	52604-3414	Thyroid Hormone
115 <> TENORETIC	Tab, White, Round	Atenolol 50 mg, Chlorthalidone 25 mg	Tenoretic by AstraZeneca	00310-0115	Antihypertensive; Diuretic
1155 <> MYLAN	Tab, White, Cap Shaped, Film Coated	Acetaminophen 650 mg, Propoxyphene Napsylate 100 mg	Darvocet-N 100 by Mylan	51079-0934 Discontinued	Analgesic; C IV
1155 <> MYLAN	Tab, White, Cap Shaped, Film Coated	Acetaminophen 650 mg, Propoxyphene Napsylate 100 mg	Darvocet-N 100 by UDL	49884-0644	Analgesic; C IV
1157018	Cap, Green & White	Minocycline HCl 100 mg	Minocin by Par	64980-0116	Antibiotic
116	Cap, Maroon and Brown, Softgel	Ferrous Fumarate 200 mg, Vitamin C 250 mg, Vitamin B12 0.01 mg, FA 1 mg	FeoGen FA by Rising	46672-0147	Vitamin
116 <> MIA	Tab, Orange, Cap Shaped, Scored	Acetaminophen 325 mg, Hydrocodone 7.5 mg	Vicodin by Mikart	00781-5223	Analgesic; C III
116 <> SZ	Tab, White, Oblong	Carvedilol 12.5 mg	Coreg by Sandoz	53978-5032	Antihypertensive
1161	Tab	Furosemide 40 mg	by Med Pro	00364-1075	Diuretic
1166 <> COPLEY	Tab, Orange, Pink & Purple, Chewable	Ascorbic Acid 34.5 mg, Cyanocobalamin 4.9 mcg, Folic Acid 0.35 mg, Niacinamide 14.17 mg, Pyridoxine HCl 1.1 mg, Riboflavin 1.26 mg, Sodium Ascorbate 32.2 mg, Sodium Fluoride 2.21 mg, Thiamine Mononitrate 1.15 mg, Vitamin A Palmitate 5.5 mg, Vitamin D 0.194 mg, Vitamin E Acetate 15.75 mg	Polyvitamin by Schein		Vitamin
117	Cap, Green & Yellow	Vitamin B Complex, C	Allbee with C by Fresh		Vitamin
117 <> SZ	Tab, White, Oval	Carvedilol 25 mg	Coreg by Sandoz	00781-5224	Antihypertensive
117 <> TENORETIC	Tab, White, Round	Atenolol 100 mg, Chlorthalidone 25 mg	Tenoretic by AstraZeneca	00310-0117	Antihypertensive; Diuretic
1170 <> 50	Tab, Pale Yellow, Cap Shaped, Scored, Film Coated	Naltrexone HCl 50 mg	Revia by Mallinckrodt	00406-1170	Opioid Antagonist
1171 <> 75	Tab, Pink, Round, Film Coated	Clopidogrel 75 mg	Plavix by Nat Pharmpak	55154-2016	Antiplatelet
1171 <> 75	Tab, Pink, Round, Film Coated	Clopidogrel 75 mg	Plavix by Sanofi-Aventis	Canadian DIN 02238682	Antiplatelet
1171 <> 75	Tab, Pink, Round, Film Coated	Clopidogrel 75 mg	Plavix by BMS	63653-1171	Antiplatelet
1172 <> 93	Tab, White to Off-White, Oval	Penicillin V Potassium 250 mg	by Teva Pharmaceuticals	00093-1172	Antibiotic
1174 <> 93	Tab, White to Off-White, Oval, Scored	Penicillin V Potassium 500 mg	V-Cillin K by Teva Pharmaceuticals	00093-1174	Antibiotic
1177 <> 93	Tab, Off-White, Round	Neomycin Sulfate 500 mg	Mycifradin by UDL	51079-0015	Antibiotic
1177 <> 93	Tab, Off-White, Round	Neomycin Sulfate 500 mg	Mycifradin by Teva	00093-1177	Antibiotic
117COPLEY	Tab, Red, Oblong, Ex Release	Procainamide HCl 1000 mg	PROCAN by Copley		Antiarrhythmic
118 <> THERRX	Tab, Peach, Cap Shaped, Film Coated	Folic Acid 1 mg, Vitamin B1 3 mg, Vitamin B2 3.4 mg, Vitamin B3 20 mg, Vitamin B6 50 mg, Vitamin B12 12 mg, Vitamin C 50 mg, Vitamin D3 6 mcg, Vitamin E 3.5 IU, Calcium Carbonate 250 mg, Copper 2 mg, Iron 40 mg, Magnesium 50 mg, Zinc 15 mg	PreCare by KV Pharma	64011-0118	Vitamin; Mineral
1189500 <> G	Tab	Chlorzoxazone 500 mg	by Royce	51875-0239	Muscle Relaxant
119	Tab, Orange, Round, Schering Logo 119	Perphenazine 4 mg, Amitriptyline HCl 10 mg	Etrafon-A by Schering		Antipsychotic; Antidepressant

ID FRONT <> BACK	DESCRIPTION FRONT <> BACK	INGREDIENT & STRENGTH	BRAND (or Generic Equiv.) by FIRM	NDC#	CLASS; SCH.
119 <> THERRX	Tab, White, Pink Print, Oval, Film Coated	Biotin 35 mcg, Folic Acid 1 mg, Vitamin B1 3 mg, Vitamin B2 3.4 mg, Vitamin B3 20 mg, Vitamin B6 10 mg, Vitamin B12 12 mcg, Vitamin C 100 mg, Vitamin D3 230 IU, Vitamin K 90 mcg, Pantothenic Acid 7 mg, Calcium Carbonate 250 mg, Chromium 45 mcg, Copper 1.3 mg, Iron 30 mg, Molybdenum 50 mcg, Selenium 75 mcg, Zinc 11 mg	PrimaCare by KV Pharma	64011-0015	Vitamin; Mineral
1191	Cap, Green, Soft Gel	Simethicone 125 mg	Mylicon by Perrigo	00113-0428	Antiflatulent
12	Tab, White, Round, 1/2	Clonazepam 0.5 mg	Klonopin Wafers by Hoffmann La Roche	00004-0281	Sedative; C IV
12	Cap	Oxacillin Sodium Monohydrate	by DRX	55045-2277	Antibiotic
12	Tab, White, Round, Vanda Logo <> 12	Iloperidone 12 mg	Fanapt by Vanda	43068-0112	Antipsychotic
12 <> 54169	Tab, White, Hexagonal, 1 over 2	Haloperidol 0.5 mg	Haldol by Nat Pharmpak	55154-4923	Antipsychotic
12 <> 54169	Tab, White, Hexagonal, 1 over 2	Haloperidol 0.5 mg	Haldol by Murfreesboro	51129-1130	Antipsychotic
12 <> 54169	Tab, White, Hexagonal, 1 over 2	Haloperidol 0.5 mg	Haldol by Roxane	00054-8342	Antipsychotic
12 <> A	Tab, White, Round, Film Coated	Metformin HCl 500 mg	Glucophage by Aurobindo	65862-0008	Antidiabetic
12 <> B96	Tab, White, Round, Orally Disintegrating, 1/2	Clonazepam 0.5 mg	Klonopin Wafers by Barr	00555-0096	Sedative; C IV
12 <> F	Tab, Blue, Cap Shaped, Film Coated	Paroxetine HCl 30 mg	Paxil by Aurobindo	65862-0156	Antidepressant
12 <> G	Tab, Purple, Round	Dipyridamole 25 mg	Persantine by Glenmark	68462-0116	Antiplatelet
12 <> MEDEVA	Tab, Green, Oblong, Scored	Guaifenesin 600 mg	Robitussin by Physician Total Care	54868-1777	Expectorant
12 <> MEDEVA	Tab, Green, Oblong, Scored	Guaifenesin 600 mg	Robitussin by Adams	63824-0012	Expectorant
12 <> MEDEVA	Tab, Green, Oblong, Scored	Guaifenesin 600 mg	Robitussin by Compumed	00403-1009	Expectorant
12 <> MEDEVA	Tab, Green, Oblong, Scored	Guaifenesin 600 mg, Pseudoephedrine 60 mg	Syn Rx by Adams	63824-0308	Cold Remedy
12 <> MYKROX	Tab, White, Round, 1/2 <> Mykrox	Metolazone 0.5 mg	Mykrox by Medeva	53014-0847	Diuretic
12 <> OV	Tab, White	Methamphetamine HCl 5 mg	Desoxyn by Ovation	67386-0102	Stimulant; C II
12 <> WW	Tab, White, Oblong	Ondansetron HCl 8 mg	Zofran by West-Ward	00143-2423	Antiemetic
120	Tab, White, Scored, 120 Prasco Logo	Pseudoephedrine HCl 120 mg, Methscopolamine Nitrate 2.5 mg	Amdry-D by Prasco	66993-0120	Cold Remedy
120	Tab, Ivory, Round, Ex Release, Hourglass Logo <> 120	Verapamil HCl 120 mg	Isoptin SR by Ivax	00172-4285	Antihypertensive
120	Tab, Ivory, Round, Ex Release, Hourglass Logo <> 120	Verapamil HCl 120 mg	Isoptin SR by Southwood	58016-0509	Antihypertensive
120	Tab, Ivory, Round, Ex Release, Hourglass Logo <> 120	Verapamil HCl 120 mg	Isoptin SR by Caremark	00339-5812	Antihypertensive
120 <> B	Tab, White, Cap Shaped, Ex Release	Diltiazem HCl 120 mg	Cardizem LA by Biovail	64455-0100	Antihypertensive
120 <> B	Tab, White, Cap Shaped, Ex Release	Diltiazem HCl 120 mg	Tiazac XC by Biovail	Canadian DIN 02256738	Antihypertensive
120 <> IMDUR	Tab, White, Oval	Isosorbide Mononitrate 120 mg	Imdur by Murfreesboro	51129-1574	Antianginal
120 <> IMDUR	Tab, White, Oval	Isosorbide Mononitrate 120 mg	Imdur by Schering	00085-1153	Antianginal
120 <> IMDUR	Tab, White, Oval	Isosorbide Mononitrate 120 mg	Imdur by Pharm Util	60491-0314	Antianginal
120 <> STARLIX	Tab, Yellow, Oval	Nateglinide 120 mg	Starlix by Novartis	00078-0352	Antidiabetic
120 <> STARLIX	Tab, Yellow, Oval	Nateglinide 120 mg	Starlix by Novartis	Canadian DIN 02245439	Antidiabetic
120 <> US13	Tab, White, Cap Shaped	Sotalol HCl 120 mg	Sorine by Upsher Smith	00245-0013	Antiarrhythmic
120 <> W587	Tab, White, Oval, Scored	Isosorbide Mononitrate 120 mg	Imdur by Warrick	59930-1587	Antianginal
120 <> Z4238	Tab, White, Cap Shaped	Nadolol 120 mg	Corgard by Ivax	00172-4238 Discontinued	Antihypertensive
1200	Tab, Light Green, Cap Shaped, Film Coated, Scored, SR, Star Logo 1200	Guaifenesin 1200 mg, Phenylephrine HCl 40 mg	Liquibid-D 1200 by Capellon	64543-0140	Cold Remedy
1200 <> ADAMS	Tab, Green & White, Oval, Ex Release	Guaifenesin 1200 mg	Robitussin by Adams	63824-0052	Expectorant
1202MJ <> M	Tab	Fosinopril Sodium 40 mg	Monopril by BMS	15548-0202	Antihypertensive
12059911	Cap, White & Dark Blue	Propranolol HCl 120 mg	Inderal LA by ESI Lederle	59911-5473	Antihypertensive
120ANDRX687	Cap, White	Diltiazem HCl 120 mg	Cardizem LA by Heartland	61392-0957	Antihypertensive
120INNOPRANXL	Cap, Gray & Off-White, Ex Release, 120, 3 Bands InnoPranXL Reliant Logo	Propranolol HCl 120 mg	InnoPran XL by Reliant	65726-0251	Antihypertensive
120MG <> BERLEX	Tab, White, Cap Shaped, Scored	Sotalol 120 mg	Betapace AF by Berlex	50419-0119	Antiarrhythmic
120MG <> BETAPACE	Tab, Light Blue, Cap Shaped, Scored	Sotalol 120 mg	Betapace by Berlex	50419-0109	Antiarrhythmic

ID FRONT <> BACK	DESCRIPTION FRONT <> BACK	INGREDIENT & STRENGTH	BRAND (or Generic Equiv.) by FIRM	NDC#	CLASS; SCH.
120MGANDRX597	Cap, Orange & White, Ex Release	Diltiazem HCl 120 mg	Cartia XT by Andrx	62037-0597	Antihypertensive
120SR <> KNOLL	Tab, Light Violet, Oval, Film Coated	Verapamil HCl 120 mg	Isoptin SR by Abbott	00044-1827	Antihypertensive
120SR <> KNOLL	Tab, Light Violet, Oval, Film Coated	Verapamil HCl 120 mg	Isoptin SR by Abbott	Canadian DIN 01907123	Antihypertensive
120WATSON662	Cap, Pink & White, 120/Watson/662	Diltiazem HCl 120 mg	Dilacor XR by Watson		Antihypertensive
121	Tab, White, Cap Shaped	Acetaminophen 500 mg	Tylenol Ex Strength by Marlex	10135-0144	Analgesic
121	Tab, White, Cap Shaped	Acetaminophen 500 mg	Tylenol Ex Strength by Amneal	65162-0607	Analgesic
121 <> BOCA	Tab, White, Ex Release	Guaifenesin 600 mg, Pseudoephedrine HCl 45 mg	by Boca	64376-0030	Cold Remedy
121 <> H	Tab, White, Round, Film Coated	Ropinirole HCl 0.25 mg	Requip by Heritage	23155-0121	Antiparkinson
121 <> PMS	Tab, Orange, Round, Scored	Procyclidine HCl 2.5 mg	Kemadrin by Pharmascience	Canadian DIN 00649392	Antiparkinson
1212 <> B776	Tab, Peach, Oval, Scored, 12 over 1/2	Mixed Amphetamine Salts 12.5 mg: Dextroamphetamine Saccharate 3.125 mg, Amphetamine Aspartate 3.125 mg, Dextroamphetamine Sulfate 3.125 mg, Amphetamine Sulfate 3.125 mg	Adderall by Barr	00555-0776	Stimulant; C II
1215 <> 93	Tab, Dark Blue, Oval, Ex Release	Cefaclor 375 mg	Ceclor CD by Teva	00093-1215 Discontinued	Antibiotic
122	Tab, Light Green, Cap Shaped	Loperamide 2 mg	Imodium by Rugby	00536-3966	Antidiarrheal
122	Tab, Light Green, Cap Shaped	Loperamide 2 mg	Imodium by Qualitest	00603-0208	Antidiarrheal
122	Tab, Light Green, Cap Shaped	Loperamide 2 mg	Imodium by OHM		Antidiarrheal
122	Tab, Light Green, Cap Shaped	Loperamide 2 mg	Imodium by Ivax	00182-1082 Discontinued	Antidiarrheal
122 <> BOCA	Tab, White, Oblong, Scored	Dextromethorphan HBr 60 mg, Guaifenesin 1000 mg	Dex GG by Boca	64376-0031	Cold Remedy
122 <> GDC	Tab, Pink, Round	Bismuth 262 mg	Pepto-Bismol by Ivax	00182-1091 Discontinued	Gastrointestinal
122 <> H	Tab, Yellow, Round, Film Coated	Ropinirole HCl 0.5 mg	Requip by Heritage	23155-0122	Antiparkinson
12210	Cap, Yellow	D-Alpha Tocopheryl Acetate 100 Units	Epsilan-M by Adria		Vitamin
123	Tab, Pink, Cap Shaped	Efavirenz 600 mg, Emtricitabine 200 mg, Tenofovir 300 mg	Atripla by BMS	15584-0101	Antiviral
123	Tab, Pink, Cap Shaped	Efavirenz 600 mg, Emtricitabine 200 mg, Tenofovir 300 mg	Atripla by Pfizer	Canadian DIN 02300699	Antiviral
123 <> BOCA	Tab, White, Ex Release	Pseudoephedrine HCl 120 mg, Chlorpheniramine Maleate 8 mg, Methscopolamine Nitrate 2.5 mg	by Boca	64376-0032	Cold Remedy
123 <> GG	Tab, Yellow, Round, Scored	Haloperidol 1 mg	Haldol by Sandoz	00781-1392	Antipsychotic
123 <> H	Tab, Green, Round, Film Coated	Ropinirole HCl 1 mg	Requip by Heritage	23155-0123	Antiparkinson
123 <> MH	Tab, Beige, Round, Film Coated	Ergotamine Tartrate 1 mg, Caffeine 100 mg	Cafergot by Mikart	46672-0198	Antimigraine
123 <> PMS20	Tab, Yellow, Round, Scored	Methylphenidate HCl 20 mg	by Pharmascience	Canadian DIN 00588009	Stimulant; C II
1237	Tab, Round	Pentaerythritol Tetranitrate 20 mg	Peritrate by Vortech		Antianginal
124	Tab, White, Scored, 124 Prasco Logo	Chlorpheniramine Maleate 8 mg, Pseudoephedrine HCl 120 mg, Methscopolamine Nitrate 2.5 mg	Amdry-C by Prasco	66993-0124	Cold Remedy
124	Tab, Yellow, Round, Delayed Release	Pantoprazole Sodium 40 mg	Protonix by Caraco	41616-0580	Gastrointestinal
124 <> BOCA	Tab, White, Cap Shaped, Extended Release	Guaifenesin 595 mg, Pseudoephedrine HCl 48 mg	Pseudo GG TR by Boca	64376-0033	Cold Remedy
124 <> COR	Tab, Light Yellow, Round, Scored	Glyburide 2.5 mg	Micronase by Ivax	00182-2646	Antidiabetic
124 <> H	Tab, Peach, Round, Film Coated	Ropinirole HCl 2 mg	Requip by Heritage	23155-0124	Antiparkinson
1242	Tab, Round	Prednisolone 5 mg	by Vortech		Steroid
125	Tab, White & Orange, Oval, Film Coated	Anhydrous Bosentan 125 mg	Tracleer by Actelion	66215-0102	Antihypertensive
125	Cap, White, Red Print	Theophylline Anhydrous 125 mg	Slo-Bid by RPR	00801-1125	Antiasthmatic
125	Tab, White & Orange, Oval, Film Coated	Anhydrous Bosentan 125 mg	Tracleer by Actelion	Canadian DIN 02244982	Antihypertensive
125	Tab, Oval, Red, Enteric Coated	Divalproex Sodium 125 mg	Depakote by Nu Pharm	Canadian DIN 02239517	Anticonvulsant

ID FRONT <> BACK	DESCRIPTION FRONT <> BACK	INGREDIENT & STRENGTH	BRAND (or Generic Equiv.) by FIRM	NDC#	CLASS; SCH.
125 <> 355	Tab, 12.5/Royce Logo <> 355	Captopril 12.5 mg	Capoten by Qualitest	00603-2555	Antihypertensive
125 <> AD	Tab, Orange, Round, Scored, 12.5 <> AD	Mixed Amphetamine Salts 12.5 mg: Amphetamine Aspartate 3.125 mg, Amphetamine Sulfate 3.125 mg, Dextroamphetamine Saccharate 3.125 mg, Dextroamphetamine Sulfate 3.125 mg	Adderall by Shire	58521-0125	Stimulant; C II
125 <> AMOXIL	Tab, Chewable	Amoxicillin 125 mg	Amoxil by Quality Care	60346-0100	Antibiotic
125 <> APO	Tab, Red, Oval, Biconvex	Divalproex Sodium 125 mg	Depakote by Apotex	Canadian DIN 02239698	Anticonvulsant
125 <> APO	Tab, White, Oblong, APO <> 12.5	Captopril 12.5 mg	Capoten by Apotex	Canadian DIN 00893595	Antihypertensive
125 <> APO	Tab, Orange, Round, APO <> 1.25	Indapamide 1.25 mg	Lozol by Apotex	Canadian DIN 02245246	Diuretic
125 <> APO	Tab, White, Oval, Film Coated, APO <> 12.5	Carvedilol 12.5 mg	Apo Carvedilol by Apotex	Canadian DIN 02247935	Antihypertensive
125 <> APO046	Tab, White to Off-White, Oval	Divalproex Sodium 125 mg	Depakote by Apotex	60505-3065	Anticonvulsant
125 <> BOCA	Tab, White, Round, SR	Chlorpheniramine Maleate 12 mg, Pseudoephedrine HCl 20 mg, Methscopolamine Nitrate 2.5 mg	PCM Allergy by Boca	64376-0036	Cold Remedy
125 <> CAPOTEN	Tab, White, Cap Shaped, Capoten <> 12.5	Captopril 12.5 mg	Capoten by Par	49884-0793	Antihypertensive
125 <> CAPOTEN	Tab, White, Cap Shaped, Capoten <> 12.5	Captopril 12.5 mg	Capoten by BMS	Canadian DIN 00695661	Antihypertensive
125 <> CAPOTEN	Tab, White, Cap Shaped, 12.5	Captopril 12.5 mg	Capoten by Med Pro	53978-0939	Antihypertensive
125 <> CAPOTEN	Tab, White, Cap Shaped, 12.5	Captopril 12.5 mg	Capoten by Par	00003-0450	Antihypertensive
125 <> CAPOTEN	Tab, White, Cap Shaped, 12.5	Captopril 12.5 mg	Capoten by Nat Pharmpak	55154-3706	Antihypertensive
125 <> COR	Tab, Light Green, Round, Scored	Glyburide 5 mg	Micronase by Ivax	00182-2647 Discontinued	Antidiabetic
125 <> FAMVIR	Tab, White, Round, Film Coated	Famciclovir 125 mg	Famvir by Apotheca	12634-0508	Antiviral
125 <> FAMVIR	Tab, White, Round, Film Coated	Famciclovir 125 mg	Famvir by SKB	60351-4115	Antiviral
125 <> FAMVIR	Tab, White, Round, Film Coated	Famciclovir 125 mg	Famvir by Physician Total Care	54868-3882	Antiviral
125 <> FAMVIR	Tab, White, Round, Film Coated	Famciclovir 125 mg	Famvir by SKB	00007-4115	Antiviral
125 <> FAMVIR	Tab, White, Round, Film Coated	Famciclovir 125 mg	Famvir by Allscripts	00078-0366	Antiviral
125 <> FAMVIR	Tab, White, Round, Film Coated	Famciclovir 125 mg	Famvir by Novartis	Canadian DIN 02229110	Antiviral
125 <> FLINT	Tab, Light Brown, Round, Scored	Levothyroxine Sodium 125 mcg	Synthroid by Abbott	00048-1130	Thyroid Hormone
125 <> FLINT	Tab, Light Brown, Round, Scored	Levothyroxine Sodium 125 mcg	Synthroid by Forest	00456-0324	Thyroid Hormone
125 <> FLINT	Tab, Light Brown, Round, Scored	Levothyroxine Sodium 125 mcg	Synthroid by Murfreesboro	51129-1653	Thyroid Hormone
125 <> FLINT	Tab, Light Brown, Round, Scored	Levothyroxine Sodium 125 mcg	Synthroid by Giant Food	11146-0303	Thyroid Hormone
125 <> FLINT	Tab, Light Brown, Round, Scored	Levothyroxine Sodium 125 mcg	Synthroid by Rite Aid	11822-5285	Thyroid Hormone
125 <> FLINT	Tab, Light Brown, Round, Scored	Levothyroxine Sodium 125 mcg	Synthroid by Nat Pharmpak	55154-0909	Thyroid Hormone
125 <> FLINT	Tab, Light Brown, Round, Scored	Levothyroxine Sodium 125 mcg	Synthroid by Kaiser	00179-1210	Thyroid Hormone
125 <> FLINT	Tab, Light Brown, Round, Scored	Levothyroxine Sodium 125 mcg	Synthroid by Abbott	Canadian DIN 02172119	Thyroid Hormone
125 <> GG330	Tab, Turquoise, Cap Shaped, Scored, 125 <> GG over 330	Levothyroxine 137 mcg	Levo-T by Alara	64909-0140	Thyroid Hormone
125 <> GG337	Tab, Brown, Cap Shaped, Scored, 125 <> GG over 337	Levothyroxine 125 mcg	Levo-T by Alara	64909-0129	Thyroid Hormone
125 <> GG337	Tab, Brown, Cap Shaped, Scored, 125 <> GG over 337	Levothyroxine 125 mcg	Levo-T by Sandoz	00781-5186	Thyroid Hormone
125 <> GRISPEG	Tab, White, Elliptical, Film Coated, Scored, 125 <> GRIS-PEG	Griseofulvin 125 mg	Gris-PEG by Allergan	00023-0763	Antifungal
125 <> GRISPEG	Tab, White, Elliptical, Film Coated, Scored, 125 <> GRIS-PEG	Griseofulvin 125 mg	Fulvicin P/G by Novartis	00043-0800	Antifungal
125 <> H	Tab, Purple, Round, Film Coated	Ropinirole HCl 3 mg	Requip by Heritage	23155-0125	Antiparkinson

ID FRONT <> BACK	DESCRIPTION FRONT <> BACK	INGREDIENT & STRENGTH	BRAND (or Generic Equiv.) by FIRM	NDC#	CLASS; SCH.
125 <> M	Tab, White to Cream Colored, Octagon, M inside square <> 12.5	Mixed Amphetamine Salts 12.5 mg: Dextroamphetamine Saccharate 3.125 mg, Amphetamine Aspartate 3.125 mg, Dextroamphetamine Sulfate 3.125 mg, Amphetamine Sulfate 3.125 mg	Adderall by Mallinckrodt	00406-8886	Stimulant; C II
125 <> N	Tab, White, Oval, N <> 12.5	Carvedilol 12.5 mg	Coreg by Novopharm	Canadian DIN 02246531	Antihypertensive
125 <> N132	Tab, White, Oval, Scored, N score 132 <> 12.5	Captopril 12.5 mg	Capoten by Teva	00093-8132 Discontinued	Antihypertensive
125 <> N132	Tab, White, Oval, Scored, N score 132 <> 12.5	Captopril 12.5 mg	Capoten by Major	57480-0838	Antihypertensive
125 <> N132	Tab, White, Oval, Scored, N score 132 <> 12.5	Captopril 12.5 mg	Capoten by Medirex	55953-0132	Antihypertensive
125 <> N132	Tab, White, Oval, Scored, N score 132 <> 12.5	Captopril 12.5 mg	Capoten by Teva	55953-0132 Discontinued	Antihypertensive
125 <> N342	Tab, White, Round, Scored, N over 342 <> 1.25	Glyburide 1.25 mg	Micronase by Teva	55953-0342	Antidiabetic
125 <> N342	Tab, White, Round, Scored, N over 342 <> 1.25	Glyburide 1.25 mg	Micronase by Warrick	59930-1592	Antidiabetic
125 <> N342	Tab, White, Round, Scored, N over 342 <> 1.25	Glyburide 1.25 mg	Micronase by Brightstone	62939-3211	Antidiabetic
125 <> N342	Tab, White, Round, Scored, N over 342 <> 1.25	Glyburide 1.25 mg	Micronase by Qualitest	00603-3762	Antidiabetic
125 <> N342	Tab, White, Round, Scored, N over 342 <> 1.25	Glyburide 1.25 mg	Micronase by Moore	00839-8039	Antidiabetic
125 <> N342	Tab, White, Round, Scored, N over 342 <> 1.25	Glyburide 1.25 mg	Micronase by Ivax	00182-2645	Antidiabetic
125 <> N342	Tab, White, Round, Scored, N over 342 <> 1.25	Glyburide 1.25 mg	Micronase by Major	00904-5075	Antidiabetic
125 <> N342	Tab, White, Round, Scored, N over 342 <> 1.25	Glyburide 1.25 mg	Micronase by Teva	00093-8342	Antidiabetic
125 <> N747	Tab, Cherry & Rose, Chewable, 25 <> N over 747	Amoxicillin 155 mg	Amoxil by Teva	55953-0747	Antibiotic
125 <> N747	Tab, Cherry & Rose, Chewable, 25 <> N over 747	Amoxicillin 155 mg	Amoxil by Warrick	59930-1573	Antibiotic
125 <> N853	Tab, Light Yellow, Film Coated, 1.25 <> N853	Indapamide 1.25 mg	Lozol by Teva	55953-0853	Diuretic
125 <> N853	Tab, Light Yellow, Film Coated, 1.25 <> N853	Indapamide 1.25 mg	Lozol by Novopharm	43806-0853	Diuretic
125 <> NN	Tab, White, Cap Shaped, Scored, N/N <> 12.5	Captopril 12.5 mg	Capoten by Novopharm	Canadian DIN 01942964	Antihypertensive
125 <> NOVO	Tab, Pink, Oval, Scored, NO / VO, Chewable	Amoxicillin 125 mg	Amoxil by Novopharm	Canadian DIN 02036347	Antibiotic
125 <> NU	Tab, White, Cap Shaped, Scored, 12.5 <> NU	Captopril 12.5 mg	Capoten by Nu Pharm	Canadian DIN 01913824	Antihypertensive
125 <> P	Tab, White, Oval, Film Coated, P <> 12.5	Carvedilol 12.5 mg	Coreg by Pharmascience	Canadian DIN 02245916	Antihypertensive
125 <> P	Tab, White, Round	Famciclovir 125 mg	Famvir by Pharmascience	Canadian DIN 02278081	Antiviral
125 <>PAXILCR	Tab, Yellow, Round, Film Coated, Paxil over CR <> 12.5	Paroxetine HCl 12.5 mg	Paxil CR by GSK	Canadian DIN 02248503	Antidepressant
125 <>PAXILCR	Tab, Yellow, Round, Film Coated, Paxil over CR <> 12.5	Paroxetine HCl 12.5 mg	Paxil CR by SKB	00029-3206	Antidepressant
125 <> R	Tab, White, Oval, Film Coated	Ciprofloxacin 100 mg	Cipro by Dr. Reddy's	55111-0125	Antibiotic
125 <> SYNTHROID	Tab, Brown, Round, Scored	Levothyroxine Sodium 125 mcg	Synthroid by Abbott	00074-7068	Thyroid Hormone
125 <> T4	Tab, Brown, Cap Shaped	Levothyroxine Sodium 125 mcg	Levothroid by Forest	00456-1324	Thyroid Hormone
125 <> Z4262	Tab, Orange, Round, 1.25 <> Z over 4262	Indapamide 1.25 mg	Lozol by Ivax	00172-4262 Discontinued	Diuretic
125 <> Z4262	Tab, Orange, Round, 1.25 <> Z over 4262	Indapamide 1.25 mg	Lozol by Ivax	00182-8201	Diuretic
125250 <> 5710	Tab, Light Yellow, Oval, Ivax Logo 5710 <> 1.25'250	Glyburide 1.25 mg, Metformin 250 mg	Glucovance by Ivax	00172-5710 Discontinued	Antidiabetic
125250 <> 5710	Tab, Light Yellow, Oval, Ivax Logo 5710 <> 1.25/250	Glyburide 1.25 mg, Metformin 250 mg	Glucovance by Teva	00093-5710 Discontinued	Antidiabetic
1253	Tab, Pink, Oblong	Hematinic Vitamin	Theragran by Moore		Vitamin
12530 <>WATSON	Tab, Pink, Round	Ethinyl Estradiol 0.03 mg, Levonorgestrel 0.125 mg	Trivora-28 by Watson	52544-0291	Oral Contraceptive
12530 <>WATSON	Tab, Pink, Round	Levonorgestrel 0.03 mg, Ethinyl Estradiol 0.125 mg	Trivora-28 by Murfreesboro	51129-1632	Oral Contraceptive
1259	Tab, Pink, Round, Scored, 1259 over Score <> Diamond	Estradiol 1 mg	Gynodiol by Fielding	00421-1259	Hormone

ID FRONT <> BACK	DESCRIPTION FRONT <> BACK	INGREDIENT & STRENGTH	BRAND (or Generic Equiv.) by FIRM	NDC#	CLASS; SCH.
1259	Tab, Pink, Round, Scored, 1259 over Score <> Diamond	Estradiol 1 mg	Gynodiol by Novavax	66500-0259	Hormone
125ALTACE	Cap, Yellow and White, Opaque, Hard Gel, 1.25 ALTACE	Ramipril 1.25 mg	Altace by Aventis	Canadian DIN 02221829	Antihypertensive
125DPI	Tab, 125/DPI	Estropipate 1.5 mg	by Schein	00364-2601	Hormone
125M	Tab	Levothyroxine Sodium 0.125 mg	Euthyrox by Em Pharma	63254-0441	Thyroid Hormone
125M	Tab	Levothyroxine Sodium 0.125 mg	Levo-T by Mova	55370-0130	Thyroid Hormone
125M <> Z	Tab, Brown, Round, Scored	Levothyroxine Sodium 125 mcg	Levo-T by Zoetica	64909-0110	Thyroid Hormone
125MCG <> FLINT	Tab, Brown, Round, Scored	Levothyroxine Sodium 0.125 mg	by Amerisource	62584-0130	Thyroid Hormone
125MCG <> FLINT	Tab, Brown, Round, Scored	Levothyroxine Sodium 0.125 mg	Synthroid by Rightpac	65240-0744	Thyroid Hormone
125N	Cap, Pink	Amoxicillin 250 mg	Amoxil by Southwood	58016-0103	Antibiotic
125NAXEN	Tab, Green, Oval, 125/Naxen	Naproxen 125 mg	Navalbine by BW Inc	Canadian	NSAID
125Z2045	Tab, White, Round, 1.25 Z/2045	Conjugated Estrogens 1.25 mg	Premarin by Ivax		Hormone
126	Tab, White, Round	Calcium Carbonate 500 mg	Tums by Guardian		Vitamin; Mineral
126	Tab, White to Off-White, Cap Shaped	Hydrocodone Bitartrate 5 mg, Acetaminophen 325 mg	Norco by Caraco	57664-0126	Analgesic; C III
126 <> H	Tab, Pale Brown, Round, Film Coated	Ropinirole HCl 4 mg	Requip by Heritage	23155-0126	Antiparkinson
126 <> R	Tab, White, Oval, Film Coated	Ciprofloxacin 250 mg	Cipro by Pharmascience	Canadian DIN 02248437	Antibiotic
126 <> R	Tab, White, Oval, Film Coated	Ciprofloxacin 250 mg	Cipro by Dr. Reddy's	55111-0126	Antibiotic
126FLINT	Tab	Levothyroxine Sodium 0.125 mg	by Med Pro	53978-1120	Thyroid Hormone
127 <> H	Tab, Blue, Round, Film Coated	Ropinirole HCl 5 mg	Requip by Heritage	23155-0127	Antiparkinson
127 <> R	Tab, Orange, Round, Scored	Clonidine HCl 0.1 mg	Catapres by Qualitest	00603-2954	Antihypertensive
127 <> R	Tab, Orange, Round, Scored	Clonidine HCl 0.1 mg	Catapres by Med Pro	53978-0936	Antihypertensive
127 <> R	Tab, Orange, Round, Scored	Clonidine HCl 0.1 mg	Catapres by Ivax	00182-1250	Antihypertensive
127 <> R	Tab, Orange, Round, Scored	Clonidine HCl 0.1 mg	Catapres by Apotheca	12634-0465	Antihypertensive
127 <> R	Tab, Orange, Round, Scored	Clonidine HCl 0.1 mg	Catapres by Heartland	61392-0513	Antihypertensive
127 <> R	Tab, Orange, Round, Scored	Clonidine HCl 0.1 mg	Catapres by PDRX	55289-0073	Antihypertensive
127 <> R	Tab, Orange, Round, Scored	Clonidine HCl 0.1 mg	Catapres by Golden State	60429-0050	Antihypertensive
127 <> R	Tab, Orange, Round, Scored	Clonidine HCl 0.1 mg	Catapres by Vangard	00615-2572	Antihypertensive
127 <> R	Tab, White, Oval, Film Coated	Ciprofloxacin 500 mg	Cipro by Pharmascience	Canadian DIN 02248438	Antibiotic
127 <> R	Tab, White, Oval, Film Coated	Ciprofloxacin 500 mg	Cipro by Dr. Reddy's	55111-0127	Antibiotic
1276	Tab, Tan, Round	Thyroid 0.5 g	by Vortech		Thyroid Hormone
128	Tab, White, Ovoid, 128 <> Assyrian Lion	Pivampicillin 500 mg	Pondocillin by Leo Pharma	Canadian DIN 0058224	Antibiotic
128 <> R	Tab, Orange, Round, Scored	Clonidine HCl 0.2 mg	Catapres by Major	00904-5657	Antihypertensive
128 <> R	Tab, White, Cap Shaped, Film Coated	Ciprofloxacin 750 mg	Cipro by Pharmascience	Canadian DIN 02248439	Antibiotic
128 <> R	Tab, White, Cap Shaped, Film Coated	Ciprofloxacin 750 mg	Cipro by Dr. Reddy's	55111-0128	Antibiotic
128 <> R	Tab, Orange, Round, Scored	Clonidine HCl 0.2 mg	Catapres by Heartland	61392-0516	Antihypertensive
128 <> R	Tab, Orange, Round, Scored	Clonidine HCl 0.2 mg	Catapres by Golden State	60429-0051	Antihypertensive
128 <> R	Tab, Orange, Round, Scored	Clonidine HCl 0.2 mg	Catapres by Qualitest	00603-2955	Antihypertensive
128 <> R	Tab, Orange, Round, Scored	Clonidine HCl 0.2 mg	Catapres by Actavis	00228-2128	Antihypertensive
128 <> R	Tab, Orange, Round, Scored	Clonidine HCl 0.2 mg	Catapres by Ivax	00182-1251	Antihypertensive
129 <> R	Tab, Orange, Round, Scored	Clonidine HCl 0.3 mg	Catapres by Actavis	00228-2129	Antihypertensive
129 <> R	Tab, Orange, Round, Scored	Clonidine HCl 0.3 mg	Catapres by Qualitest	00603-2956	Antihypertensive
129 <> R	Tab, Orange, Round, Scored	Clonidine HCl 0.3 mg	Catapres by Ivax	00182-1252	Antihypertensive
129 <> R	Tab, Orange, Round, Scored	Clonidine HCl 0.3 mg	Catapres by Heartland	61392-0519	Antihypertensive
129 <> R	Tab, Orange, Round, Scored	Clonidine HCl 0.3 mg	Catapres by Major	00904-5658	Antihypertensive
12H <> DALLERGY	Tab, White, Cap Shaped, Scored, Ex Release	Chlorpheniramine Maleate 12 mg, Methscopolamine Nitrate 2.5 mg, Phenylephrine HCl 20 mg	Dallergy ER by Laser	00277-0182	Cold Remedy

ID FRONT <> BACK	DESCRIPTION FRONT <> BACK	INGREDIENT & STRENGTH	BRAND (or Generic Equiv.) by FIRM	NDC#	CLASS; SCH.
12H <> DALLERGY	Tab, White, Cap Shaped, Scored	Chlorpheniramine Maleate 8 mg, Methscopolamine Nitrate 2.5 mg, Phenylephrine HCl 20 mg	Dallergy ER by Laser	00277-0180 Discontinued	Cold Remedy
12KLONOPIN <> ROCHE	Tab, Orange, Round, Scored, 1/2 Klonopin, K perforation	Clonazepam 0.5 mg	Klonopin by Roche	59643-0068	Sedative; C IV
12KLONOPIN <> ROCHE	Tab, Orange, Round, Scored, 1/2 Klonopin, K perforation	Clonazepam 0.5 mg	Klonopin by Hoffmann La Roche	00004-0068	Sedative; C IV
13 <> A	Tab, White, Round, Film Coated	Metformin HCl 850 mg	Glucophage by Aurobindo	65862-0009	Antidiabetic
13 <> G	Tab, White, Oval	Gabapentin 800 mg	Neurontin by Glenmark	68462-0127	Anticonvulsant
13 <> GG220	Tab	Acetaminophen 300 mg, Codeine Phosphate 30 mg	Tylenol w/ Codeine by Med Pro	53978-2086	Analgesic; C III
13 <> KPI	Tab	Guaifenesin 600 mg	Robitussin by Monarch	61570-0026	Expectorant
130	Tab, White	Methoxide 13 mg	Robaxin by Chemaide	36678-5533	Muscle Relaxant
130	Tab, White, Oval	Ondansetron HCl 4 mg	Zofran by Caraco	62756-0130	Antiemetic
130 <> BL	Tab, White, Round, Scored	Albuterol Sulfate 2 mg	Proventil by Teva	00093-2226	Antiasthmatic
130 <> EL	Tab	Hyoscyamine Sulfate 0.125 mg	Levsin by Anabolic	00722-6294	Gastrointestinal
130 <> MYLAN	Tab, Orange, Cap Shaped, Film Coated	Acetaminophen 650 mg, Propoxyphene HCl 65 mg	Wygesic by Mylan	00378-0130	Analgesic; C IV
130 <> MYLAN	Tab, Orange, Cap Shaped, Film Coated	Acetaminophen 650 mg, Propoxyphene HCl 65 mg	Wygesic by Qualitest	00603-5463	Analgesic; C IV
130 <> MYLAN	Tab, Orange, Cap Shaped, Film Coated	Acetaminophen 650 mg, Propoxyphene HCl 65 mg	Wygesic by UDL	51079-0741	Analgesic; C IV
130 <> PMS5	Tab, Orange, Round, Scored	Methylphenidate HCl 5 mg	by Pharmascience	Canadian DIN 02234749	Stimulant; C II
130 <> ZESTRIL	Tab, Pink, Cap Shaped, Scored	Lisinopril 5 mg	Zestril by AstraZeneca	00310-0130	Antihypertensive
130 <> ZESTRIL	Tab, Pink, Cap Shaped, Scored	Lisinopril 5 mg	Zestril by Kaiser	00179-1168	Antihypertensive
130 <> ZESTRIL	Tab, Pink, Cap Shaped, Scored	Lisinopril 5 mg	Zestril by Med Pro	53978-3063	Antihypertensive
130RH405RELIANT	Cap, Dark Green and White, Segmented Band, Reliant Logo	Fenofibrate 130 mg	Antara by Reliant	65726-0403	Antihyperlipidemic
131 <> BL	Tab, White, Round, Scored	Albuterol Sulfate 4 mg	Proventil by Teva	00093-2228	Antiasthmatic
131 <> BOCA	Tab, Purple, Oval, Chewable	Phenylephrine HCl 10 mg, Methscopolamine Nitrate 1.25 mg, Chlorpheniramine Maleate 2 mg	PCM Chewable by Boca	64376-0530	Cold Remedy
131 <> ZESTRIL10	Tab, Pink, Round	Lisinopril 10 mg	Prinivil by Kaiser	00179-1157	Antihypertensive
131 <> ZESTRIL10	Tab, Pink, Round	Lisinopril 10 mg	Zestril by AstraZeneca	00310-0131	Antihypertensive
131 <> ZESTRIL10	Tab, Pink, Round	Lisinopril 10 mg	Prinivil by Med Pro	53978-1000	Antihypertensive
13105 <> SP2209	Tab, Blue, Oval, Film Coated	Calcium Carbonate 125 mg, Cyanocobalamin 3 mcg, Vitamin D 400 Units, Polysaccharide Iron Complex 60 mg, Folic Acid 1 mg, Niacinamide 10 mg, Pyridoxine HCl 1.64 mg, Riboflavin 3 mg, Sodium Ascorbate 50 mg, Thiamine Mononitrate 2.43 mg, Vitamin A 4000 Units, Zinc Sulfate 18 mg	Niferex PN by Ther-Rx	00131-2209	Vitamin; Mineral
13120	Tab, Orange, Round	Aspirin 250 mg, Phenacetin 120 mg, Phenobarbital 15 mg	Axotal by Adria		Analgesic; C IV
1313 <> LAN	Tab, White, Round	Pilocarpine HCl 5 mg	Salagen by Lannett	00527-1313	Cholinergic Agonist
132 <> 93	Tab, White to Off-White, Oval, Chewable	Lamotrigine 25 mg	Lamictal by Teva	00093-0132	Anticonvulsant
132 <> BL	Tab, White, Round, Scored	Metaproterenol Sulfate 10 mg	Alupent by Nat Pharmpak	55154-5586	Antiasthmatic
132 <> BOCA	Tab, White, Cap Shaped	Pseudoephedrine HCl 50 mg, Guaifenesin 1200 mg	Sudal SR by Boca	64376-0531	Cold Remedy
132 <> BP	Tab, Yellow, Round	Magnesium 600 mg, Vitamin B-6 25 mg	Beelith by Beach	00486-1132	Mineral; Vitamin
132 <> ZESTRIL20	Tab, Red, Round	Lisinopril 20 mg	Prinivil by Kaiser	00179-1169	Antihypertensive
132 <> ZESTRIL20	Tab, Red, Round	Lisinopril 20 mg	Zestril by AstraZeneca	00310-0132	Antihypertensive
132 <> ZESTRIL20	Tab, Red, Round	Lisinopril 20 mg	Prinivil by Med Pro	53978-1017	Antihypertensive
132GG	Tab, White, Round, Scored, Film Coated, GG/132	Verapamil HCl 80 mg	Isoptin by Sandoz	00781-1016	Antihypertensive
133	Tab, White, Circular, Scored	Bumetanide 1 mg	Burinex by Leo Pharma	Canadian DIN 00728284	Diuretic
133	Tab, Tan, Round, Chewable	Chlorpheniramine Maleate 2 mg, Methscopolamine Nitrate 1.25 mg, Phenylephrine HCl 10 mg	Extendryl Chews by Fleming	00256-0133	Cold Remedy
133 <> AP	Tab, Blue, Oblong, AP logo (Upside down V over p) <> 133	Acetaminophen 500 mg, Diphenhydramine HCl 25 mg	Tylenol PM by Advance	00093-2232 Discontinued	Cold Remedy
133 <> BL	Tab, Buff, Round, Scored	Metaproterenol Sulfate 20 mg	by Teva		Antiasthmatic
133 <> BOCA	Tab, Purple, Oval	Chlorpheniramine Maleate 2 mg, Pseudoephedrine HCl 15 mg	Pediox by Boca	64376-0532	Cold Remedy
133 <> ZESTRIL30	Tab, Red, Round	Lisinopril 30 mg	Zestril by AstraZeneca	00310-0133	Antihypertensive

For updated data, go to www.IdentADrug.com

ID FRONT <> BACK	DESCRIPTION FRONT <> BACK	INGREDIENT & STRENGTH	BRAND (or Generic Equiv.) by FIRM	NDC#	CLASS; SCH.
13308	Cap, Green, 13/308	Potassium Chloride 10 mEq	K-Lease by Adria		Electrolytes
1332	Tab, Round	Chlorpheniramine Maleate 4 mg	Chlor-Trimeton by Vortech		Antihistamine
1332 <> MP53	Tab, Peach, Scored	Prednisone 20 mg	by Southwood	58016-0217	Steroid
1335 <> LCI	Tab, Yellow, Round	Doxycycline 50 mg	Adoxa by Lannett	00527-1335	Antibiotic
1339	Tab, Round	Phenylpropanolamine HCl 40 mg, Phenylephrine HCl 10 mg, Phentoloxamine 15 mg, Chlorpheniramine 5 mg	Amaril by Vortech		Cold Remedy
134 <> BOCA	Tab, White, Cap Shaped	Pseudoephedrine HCl 80 mg, Dextromethorphan HBr 40 mg, Guaifenesin 700 mg	Maxifed DMX by Boca	64376-0533	Cold Remedy
134 <> E	Tab	Reserpine 0.25 mg	by Allscripts		Antihypertensive
134 <> ZESTRIL40	Tab, Yellow, Round	Lisinopril 40 mg	Prinivil by Kaiser	00179-1203	Antihypertensive
134 <> ZESTRIL40	Tab, Yellow, Round	Lisinopril 40 mg	Zestril by AstraZeneca	00310-0134	Antihypertensive
13411	Tab, Pink, Oblong	Magnesium Salicylate 650 mg	Magan by Adria		Analgesic
1342	Tab, Round	Penicillin G 400,000 Units	Pentids by Vortech		Antibiotic
135	Cap, Light Yellow, Opaque	Nimodipine 30 mg	Nimotop by Caraco	57664-0135	Antihypertensive
135 <> 93	Tab, White, Oval, Film Coated	Carvedilol 6.25 mg	Coreg by Teva	00093-0135	Antihypertensive
135 <> A	Cap, Blue Cap, Yellow Body, Hard Gelatin Cap Contains White Mini Tabs	Choline Fenofibrate 135 mg	Trilipix by Abbott	00074-9189	Treats Cholesterol
135 <> BOCA	Tab, Green, Cap Shaped	Pseudoephedrine HCl 80 mg, Guaifenesin 700 mg	Maxifed by Boca	64376-0538	Cold Remedy
135 <> ORTHO	Tab	Ethinyl Estradiol 0.035 mg, Norethindrone 1 mg	Ortho Novum 1 Plus 35 by Dept Health	53808-0031	Oral Contraceptive
135 <> ZESTRIL212	Tab, White, Round	Lisinopril 2.5 mg	Zestril by AstraZeneca	00310-0135	Antihypertensive
13511	Cap, Green, Oval	Docusate Sodium 100 mg	Modane Soft by Adria		Laxative
135COPLEY	Tab, White, Oval, 135/Copley	Doxylamine Succinate 25 mg	Unisom by Copley		Sleep Aid
136 <> BL	Tab, White, Cap Shaped, Scored	Cephalexin 250 mg	Keflex by Teva	00093-2238	Antibiotic
136 <> COPLEY	Tab	Metoprolol Tartrate 50 mg	Lopressor by Teva	38245-0136	Antihypertensive
1367 <> LCI	Tab, Yellow, Cap Shaped	Probenecid 500 mg	Benemid by Lannett	00527-1367	Antigout
137	Tab, White, 137 <> Assyrian Lion	Pivmecillinam HCl 200 mg	Selexid by Leo Pharma	Canadian	Antibiotic
137	Tab, White, Round	Aspirin 325 mg	Aspirin by Granutec		Analgesic
137 <> BL	Tab, White, Cap Shaped, Scored	Cephalexin 500 mg	Keflex by Teva	00093-2240	Antibiotic
137 <> FLINT	Tab, Blue, Round, Scored	Levothyroxine Sodium 137 mcg	Synthroid by Forest	00456-0331	Thyroid Hormone
137 <> FLINT	Tab, Blue, Round, Scored	Levothyroxine Sodium 137 mcg	Synthroid by Abbott	Canadian DIN 02233852	Thyroid Hormone
137 <> G	Tab, Yellow, Oval, Scored	Oxcarbazepine 150 mg	Trileptal by Glenmark	68462-0137	Anticonvulsant
137 <> GG330	Tab, White, Cap Shaped, Scored, 137 <> GG over 330	Levothyroxine 137 mcg	Levo-T by Sandoz	00781-5191	Thyroid Hormone
137 <> SYNTHROID	Tab, Turquoise-Blue, Round, Scored	Levothyroxine Sodium 137 mcg	Synthroid by Abbott	00074-3727	Thyroid Hormone
137 <> T4	Tab, Cap Shaped, Dark Blue, Scored	Levothyroxine Sodium 137 mcg	Levothroid by Forest	00456-1331	Thyroid Hormone
1375 <> DITROPAN	Tab, 13/75	Oxybutynin Chloride 5 mg	Ditropan by Ortho-McNeil	00088-1375	Urinary Tract
1375 <> DITROPAN	Tab, 13/75	Oxybutynin Chloride 5 mg	Ditropan by Nat Pharmpak	55154-2209	Urinary Tract
137BL	Tab, Coated, 137/BL	Cephalexin	by Schein	00364-2293	Antibiotic
137MCG	Tab, Debossed	Levothyroxine Sodium 137 mcg	Eltroxin by GSK	53873-0119	Thyroid Hormone
138 <> SQUIBB	Tab, White, Round, Scored	Sulfamethoxazole 400 mg, Trimethoprim 80 mg	by Mutual	53489-0145	Antibiotic
138 <> SQUIBB	Tab, White, Round, Scored	Sulfamethoxazole 400 mg, Trimethoprim 80 mg	SMZ TMP 400/80 by Apothecon	59772-0139	Antibiotic
1381 <> DAYPRO	Tab, White, Cap Shaped, Scored, Film Coated	Oxaprozin 600 mg	Daypro by PF	48692-0013	NSAID
1381 <> DAYPRO	Tab, White, Cap Shaped, Scored, Film Coated	Oxaprozin 600 mg	Daypro by Searle	00025-1381	NSAID
1381 <> DAYPRO	Tab, White, Cap Shaped, Scored, Film Coated	Oxaprozin 600 mg	Daypro by Searle	00014-1381	NSAID
1381 <> DAYPRO	Tab, White, Cap Shaped, Scored, Film Coated	Oxaprozin 600 mg	Daypro by Caremark	00339-5881	NSAID
1381 <> DAYPRO	Tab, White, Cap Shaped, Scored, Film Coated	Oxaprozin 600 mg	Daypro by H J Harkins Co	52959-0252	NSAID
1381 <> DAYPRO	Tab, White, Cap Shaped, Scored, Film Coated	Oxaprozin 600 mg	Daypro by DRX	55045-2120	NSAID
1381 <> DAYPRO	Tab, White, Cap Shaped, Scored, Film Coated	Oxaprozin 600 mg	Daypro by Allscripts		NSAID

ID FRONT <> BACK	DESCRIPTION FRONT <> BACK	INGREDIENT & STRENGTH	BRAND (or Generic Equiv.) by FIRM	NDC#	CLASS; SCH.
1381 <> DAYPRO	Tab, White, Cap Shaped, Scored, Film Coated	Oxaprozin 600 mg	Daypro by Rx Dispensing	61807-0079	NSAID
1381 <> DAYPRO	Tab, White, Cap Shaped, Scored, Film Coated	Oxaprozin 600 mg	Daypro by St. Mary's Med	60760-0381	NSAID
1381 <> DAYPRO	Tab, White, Cap Shaped, Scored, Film Coated	Oxaprozin 600 mg	Daypro by Amerisource	62584-0381	NSAID
1381 <> DAYPRO	Tab, White, Cap Shaped, Scored, Film Coated	Oxaprozin 600 mg	Daypro by Pharmacia	Canadian DIN 02027860	NSAID
1388	Tab, Blue, Round	Atropine, Methylene Blue, Benzoic Acid, Hyoscyamine, Methenamine, Phenyl Salicylate	Uritabs by Vortech		Urinary Tract
139 <> G	Tab, Yellow, Oval, Scored	Oxcarbazepine 600 mg	Trileptal by Glenmark	68462-0139	Anticonvulsant
1390	Tab, Round	Levothyroxine Sodium 0.2 mg	Synthroid by Vortech		Hormone
14	Tab, White, Round, 1/4	Clonazepam 0.25 mg	Klonopin Wafers by Hoffmann La Roche	00004-0280	Sedative; C IV
14	Tab, White, Round, Triangle Logo	Ephedrine 24 mg, Phenobarbital 24 mg, Theophylline 65 mg, Potassium Iodide 320 mg	Quadrinal by Knoll		Antiasthmatic; C IV
14 <> A	Tab, White, Oblong, Film Coated, Scored, A <> 1/4	Metformin HCl 1000 mg	Glucophage by Aurobindo	65862-0010	Antidiabetic
14 <> A	Tab, White, Oblong, Film Coated, Scored, A <> 1/4	Metformin HCl 1000 mg	Glucophage by Eon	00185-0221	Antidiabetic
14 <> B	Tab, Light Yellow, Round, b <> 14	Ethinyl Estradiol 35 mcg, Ethynodiol Diacetate 1 mg	Demulen by Barr	00555-9064	Oral Contraceptive
14 <> B95	Tab, White, Round, Orally Disintegrating, 1/4	Clonazepam 0.25 mg	Klonopin Wafers by Barr	00555-0095	Sedative; C IV
14 <> VP	Tab, White, Round, Scored	Ethambutol HCl 400 mg	Myambutol by Versapharm	61748-0014	Antituberculosis
14 <> VP	Tab, White, Round, Film Coated, Scored	Ethambutol HCl 400 mg	by West-Ward	00143-9101	Antituberculosis
1400015	Cap, Orange & Yellow	Tetracycline HCl 250 mg	by Global	00115-1400	Antibiotic
1402015	Cap, Black & Yellow	Tetracycline HCl 500 mg	by Global	00115-1402	Antibiotic
140KLX	Cap, Green and White, Opaque	Cephalexin 250 mg	Keflex by Karalex	42043-0140	Antibiotic
141	Tab, Off White, Round, Film Coated, Ex Release	Bupropion HCl 150 mg	Wellbutrin XL by Actavis	67767-0141	Antidepressant
141 <> ZESTORETIC	Tab, Peach, Round	Hydrochlorothiazide 12.5 mg, Lisinopril 10 mg	Zestoretic by IPR	54921-0141	Diuretic; Antihypertensive
141 <> ZESTORETIC	Tab, Peach, Round	Hydrochlorothiazide 12.5 mg, Lisinopril 10 mg	Zestoretic by AstraZeneca	00310-0141	Diuretic; Antihypertensive
141KLX	Cap, Light Green and Dark Green, Opaque	Cephalexin 500 mg	Keflex by Karalex	42043-0141	Antibiotic
142	Tab, White, Round	Acetaminophen 325 mg	Tylenol by Granutec		Analgesic
142	Tab, White to Off-White, Cap Shaped, Extended Release	Metformin HCl 500 mg	Glucophage XR by Caraco	62756-0142	Antidiabetic
142 <> ZESTORETIC	Tab, White, Round	Hydrochlorothiazide 12.5 mg, Lisinopril 20 mg	Zestoretic by AstraZeneca	00310-0142	Diuretic; Antihypertensive
142 <> ZESTORETIC	Tab, White, Round	Hydrochlorothiazide 12.5 mg, Lisinopril 20 mg	Zestoretic by IPR	54921-0142	Diuretic; Antihypertensive
1423 <> M	Tab, White, Round, Ex Release, M inside square, Extended Release	Methylphenidate HCl 10 mg	Ritalin by Mallinckrodt	00406-1423	Stimulant; C II
1423 <> M	Tab, White, Round, Ex Release, M inside square, Extended Release	Methylphenidate HCl 10 mg	Ritalin by D M Graham	00756-0285	Stimulant; C II
143	Tab	Carbenicillin Indanyl Sodium	Geocillin by Pharm Util	60491-0277	Antibiotic
143	Tab, Red, Cap Shaped, Extended Release	Metformin HCl 750 mg	Glucophage XR by Caraco	62756-0143	Antidiabetic
143	Tab, Green, Orange, Pink or Yellow	Sodium Fluoride 2.21 mg	Luride T by Colgate	00126-0143	Element
143 <> B	Tab, White, Round	Inert	Demulen by Barr	00555-9064	Oral Contraceptive; Placebo
143 <> B	Tab, White, Round	Inert	Tri-Sprintec by Barr	00555-9018	Oral Contraceptive; Placebo
143 <> B	Tab, White, Round	Inert	Sprintec by Barr	00555-9016	Oral Contraceptive; Placebo
143 <> R	Tab, Peach, Oval	Fluconazole 50 mg	Diflucan by Dr. Reddy's	55111-0143	Antifungal
143 <> R	Tab, White, Round, Scored	Carbamazepine 200 mg	Tegretol by Actavis	00228-2143	Anticonvulsant
143 <> R	Tab, White, Round, Scored	Carbamazepine 200 mg	Tegretol by Vangard	00615-3505	Anticonvulsant
143 <> R	Tab, White, Round, Scored	Carbamazepine 200 mg	Tegretol by Heartland	61392-0038	Anticonvulsant
143 <> R	Tab, White, Round, Scored	Carbamazepine 200 mg	Tegretol by PDRX	55289-0210	Anticonvulsant
143 <> ROERIG	Tab, Yellow, Cap Shaped, Film Coated	Carbenicillin Indanyl Sodium 382 mg	Geocillin by Roerig	00049-1430	Antibiotic
144 <> M	Tab, White, Round	Tamoxifen Citrate 10 mg	Nolvadex by Mylan	00378-0144	Antiestrogen

ID FRONT <> BACK	DESCRIPTION FRONT <> BACK	INGREDIENT & STRENGTH	BRAND (or Generic Equiv.) by FIRM	NDC#	CLASS; SCH.
144 <> PD	Tab, White, D-Shaped	Norethindrone Acetate 1 mg, Ethinyl Estradiol 5 mcg	Femhrt by Pfizer	Canadian DIN 02244531	Oral Contraceptive
144 <> PD	Tab, White, D-Shaped	Norethindrone Acetate 1 mg, Ethinyl Estradiol 5 mcg	Femhrt by Parke Davis	00071-0144	Oral Contraceptive
144 <> R	Tab, Peach, Oval	Fluconazole 100 mg	Diflucan by Dr. Reddy's	55111-0144	Antifungal
1445 <> LCI	Tab, Blue, Speckled, Cap Shaped, Scored	Phentermine HCl 37.5 mg	Adipex-P by Lannett	00527-1445	Anorexiant; C IV
145	Tab, White, Oblong, Film-Coated, Fournier logo <> 145	Fenofibrate 145 mg	Lipidil EZ by Fournier	Canadian DIN 02269082	Antihyperlipidemic
145	Tab	Digoxin 0.125 mg	Lanoxin by Physician Total Care	54868-2134	Cardiac Agent
145	Tab, Blue, Hexagon-Shaped	Lisinopril 10 mg, Hydrochlorothiazide 12.5 mg	Prinzide by Merck Frosst	Canadian DIN 02108194	Antihypertensive; Diuretic
145 <> R	Tab, Peach, Oval	Fluconazole 150 mg	Diflucan by Dr. Reddy's	55111-0145	Antifungal
145 <> ZESTORETIC	Tab, Peach, Round	Hydrochlorothiazide 25 mg, Lisinopril 20 mg	Zestoretic by AstraZeneca	00310-0145	Diuretic; Antihypertensive
145 <> ZESTORETIC	Tab, Peach, Round	Hydrochlorothiazide 25 mg, Lisinopril 20 mg	Zestoretic by IPR	54921-0145	Diuretic; Antihypertensive
1451 <> M	Tab, White, Round, M inside Box, Ex Release	Methylphenidate HCl 20 mg	Ritalin SR by Mallinckrodt	00406-1451	Stimulant; C II
1451 <> SEARLE	Tab, White, Round	Misoprostol 100 mcg	Cytotec by Searle	00025-1451	Gastrointestinal
1451 <> SEARLE	Tab, White, Round	Misoprostol 100 mcg	Cytotec by H J Harkins Co	52959-0353	Gastrointestinal
146 <> R	Tab, Peach, Oval	Fluconazole 200 mg	Diflucan by Dr. Reddy's	55111-0146	Antifungal
146 <> R	Tab, Peach, Oval	Fluconazole 200 mg	Diflucan by Dr. Reddy's	55111-0146	Antifungal
14611461	Tab, 1461 Debossed Above Line and Below Line	Misoprostol 200 mcg	by PDRX	55289-0698	Gastrointestinal
1463	Tab, Round	Conjugated Estrogens 0.625 mg	Premarin by Vortech		Hormone
1468	Cap, Red	Ferrous Sulfate 325 mg	Feosol by Nutro Labs		Mineral
147 <> 93	Tab, Light Red, Round	Naproxen 250 mg	Naprosyn by Brightstone	62939-8311	NSAID
147 <> 93	Tab, Light Red, Round	Naproxen 250 mg	Naprosyn by Heartland	61392-0289	NSAID
147 <> 93	Tab, Light Red, Round	Naproxen 250 mg	Naprosyn by Teva	00093-0147	NSAID
147 <> 93	Tab, Light Red, Round	Naproxen 250 mg	Naprosyn by Ivax	00182-8240 Discontinued	NSAID
147 <> THERRX	Tab, Oval, Light Pink, Film-Coated, Scored	Calcium 400 mg, Vitamin D3 200 IU, Vitamin C 25 mg, Folic Acid 2 mg, Vitamin B6 25 mg	Encora AM by Ther-Rx	64011-0166	Supplement
1472 <> SOLVAY	Tab, Coated	Ascorbic Acid 70 mg, Calcium 200 mg, Cyanocobalamin 2.2 mcg, Folic Acid 1 mg, Iodine 175 mcg, Iron 65 mg, Magnesium 100 mg, Niacin 17 mg, Pyridoxine HCl 2.2 mg, Riboflavin 1.6 mg, Thiamine Mononitrate 1.5 mg, Vitamin A 3000 Units, Vitamin D 400 Units, Vitamin E 10 Units, Zinc 15 mg	Zenate by Leiner	59606-0497	Vitamin
1472 <> SOLVAY	Tab, Coated	Ascorbic Acid 70 mg, Calcium 200 mg, Cyanocobalamin 2.2 mcg, Folic Acid 1 mg, Iodine 175 mcg, Iron 65 mg, Magnesium 100 mg, Niacin 17 mg, Pyridoxine HCl 2.2 mg, Riboflavin 1.6 mg, Thiamine Mononitrate 1.5 mg, Vitamin A 3000 Units, Vitamin D 400 Units, Vitamin E 10 Units, Zinc 15 mg	Zenate by Solvay	00032-1472	Vitamin
148	Tab, Red, Oval, Ex Release, Schering Logo 148	Dexchlorpheniramine Maleate 6 mg	Polaramine by Schering		Antihistamine
148 <> 93	Tab, Peach, Oval	Naproxen 375 mg	Naprosyn by Teva	00093-0148 Discontinued	NSAID
148 <> 93	Tab, Peach, Oval	Naproxen 375 mg	Naprosyn by Brightstone	62939-8321	NSAID
148 <> 93	Tab, Peach, Oval	Naproxen 375 mg	Naprosyn by Heartland	61392-0292	NSAID
148 <> 93	Tab, Peach, Oval	Naproxen 375 mg	Naprosyn by Otsuka	46602-0004	NSAID
1481	Tab, Peach, Oval	Prenatal Vitamins	Precare by Pecos		Vitamin
149 <> 93	Tab, Light Red, Oval	Naproxen 500 mg	Naprosyn by Ivax	00182-8241 Discontinued	NSAID
149 <> 93	Tab, Light Red, Oval	Naproxen 500 mg	Naprosyn by Teva	00093-0149	NSAID
149 <> 93	Tab, Light Red, Oval	Naproxen 500 mg	Naprosyn by Heartland	61392-0295	NSAID
149 <> 93	Tab, Light Red, Oval	Naproxen 500 mg	Naprosyn by Brightstone	62939-8331	NSAID

ID FRONT <> BACK	DESCRIPTION FRONT <> BACK	INGREDIENT & STRENGTH	BRAND (or Generic Equiv.) by FIRM	NDC#	CLASS; SCH.
149 <> 93	Tab, Light Red, Oval	Naproxen 500 mg	Naprosyn by Vangard	0615-3563	NSAID
1492	Tab, Peach, Round	Fosinopril Sodium 10 mg, Hydrochlorothiazide 12.5 mg	Monopril HCT by BMS	00087-1492	Antihypertensive; Diuretic
1492	Tab, Peach, Round	Fosinopril Sodium 10 mg, Hydrochlorothiazide 12.5 mg	Monopril HCT by BMS	12698-1492	Antihypertensive; Diuretic
1493	Tab, Peach, Round, Scored	Fosinopril Sodium 20 mg, Hydrochlorothiazide 12.5 mg	Monopril HCT by BMS	00087-1493	Antihypertensive; Diuretic
1493	Tab, Peach, Round, Scored	Fosinopril Sodium 20 mg, Hydrochlorothiazide 12.5 mg	Monopril HCT by BMS	12698-1493	Antihypertensive; Diuretic
149BIOCRAFT	Cap	Clindamycin HCl 150 mg	Cleocin HCl by Biocraft		Antibiotic
15	Tab, Light Yellow, Oval	Meloxicam 15 mg	Mobic by Lupin	68180-0502	NSAID
15	Tab, Yellow, Round, Orally Disintegrating	Olanzapine 15 mg	Zyprexa Zydis by Eli Lilly	00002-4455	Antipsychotic
15	Tab, White to Yellowish White, Orange to Dark Brown Specks	Lansoprazole 15 mg	Prevacid by Tap	00300-1543	Gastrointestinal
15	Tab, White, Octagonal, Film-Coated	Oxymorphone HCl 15 mg	Opana ER by Endo	63481-0553	Analgesic; C II
15	Tab, White to Yellowish White, Orange to Dark Brown Specks	Lansoprazole 15 mg	Prevacid FasTab by Tap	Canadian DIN 02249464	Gastrointestinal
15	Tab, White, Round	Pioglitazone 15 mg	Actos by Cobalt	Canadian DIN 02302861	Antidiabetic
15 <> 25	Tab, White, Round, 15 <> Hourglass Logo 25	Captopril 25 mg, HCTZ 15 mg	Capozide by Ivax	00172-2515	Antihypertensive; Diuretic
15 <> 50	Tab, White, Oval, 15 <> Hourglass Logo 50	Captopril 50 mg, HCTZ 15 mg	Capozide by Ivax	00172-5015	Antihypertensive; Diuretic
15 <> 5675	Tab, Yellow, Round, Hourglass Logo 5675 <> 15	Mirtazapine 15 mg	Remeron by Ivax	00172-5675 Discontinued	Antidepressant
15 <> 93	Tab, White, Oval, Film Coated	Nabumetone 500 mg	Relafen by UDL	51079-0989	NSAID
15 <> 93	Tab, White, Oval, Film Coated	Nabumetone 500 mg	Relafen by Teva	00093-1015	NSAID
15 <> A	Tab, Yellow, Round, Film Coated	Simvastatin 5 mg	Zocor by Aurobindo	65862-0050	Antihyperlipidemic
15 <> ABG	Tab, Blue, Round, Film-Coated, Controlled Release	Morphine Sulfate 15 mg	MS Contin by Neuman	64579-0349	Analgesic; C II
15 <> ABG	Tab, Blue, Round, Film-Coated, Controlled Release	Morphine Sulfate 15 mg	MS Contin by Ivax	00172-2162	Analgesic; C II
15 <> ACTOS	Tab, White to Off-White, Round	Pioglitazone HCl 15 mg	Actos by Eli Lilly	Canadian DIN 02242572	Antidiabetic
15 <> ACTOS	Tab, White, Round, Convex	Pioglitazone HCl 15 mg	Actos by Prestige	58056-0337	Antidiabetic
15 <> ACTOS	Tab, White, Round	Pioglitazone HCl 15 mg	Actos by Takeda	64764-0151	Antidiabetic
15 <> AD	Tab, Orange, Oval, Scored	Mixed Amphetamine Salts 15 mg: Amphetamine Aspartate 3.75 mg, Amphetamine Sulfate 3.75 mg, Dextroamphetamine Saccharate 3.75 mg, Dextroamphetamine Sulfate 3.75 mg	Adderall by Shire	58521-0150	Stimulant; C II
15 <> B1	Tab, White, Round, B1 <> 1 over 5	Penicillin V Potassium 250 mg	V-Cillin K by Teva	00093-1171	Antibiotic
15 <> B777	Tab, Peach, Round, Scored, 1 over 5	Mixed Amphetamine Salts 15 mg: Dextroamphetamine Saccharate 3.75 mg, Amphetamine Aspartate 3.75 mg, Dextroamphetamine Sulfate 3.75 mg, Amphetamine Sulfate 3.75 mg	Adderall by Barr	00555-0777	Stimulant; C II
15 <> BL	Tab, White, Round, Scored	Penicillin V Potassium 250 mg	Pen*Vee K by UDL	51079-0615	Antibiotic
15 <> BL	Tab, White, Round, Scored	Penicillin V Potassium 250 mg	by Teva	00093-1171 Discontinued	Antibiotic
15 <> BL	Tab, White, Round, Scored	Penicillin V Potassium 250 mg	by PDRX	55289-0206	Antibiotic
15 <> BL	Tab, White, Round, Scored	Penicillin V Potassium 250 mg	by Pharmedix	53002-0201	Antibiotic
15 <> BL	Tab, White, Round, Scored	Penicillin V Potassium 250 mg	by Diversified Healthcare	55887-0980	Antibiotic
15 <> BL	Tab, White, Round, Scored	Penicillin V Potassium 250 mg	by Southwood	58016-0146	Antibiotic
15 <> DF	Tab, Light Peach, Round, Extended Release	Darifenacin 15 mg	Enablex by Novartis	00078-0420	Urinary Tract
15 <> DF	Tab, Light Peach, Round, Extended Release	Darifenacin 15 mg	Enablex by Novartis	Canadian DIN 02273225	Urinary Tract
15 <> DORAL	Tab, Light Orange w/ White Speckles, Capsule-shaped, 15 <> Doral	Quazepam 15 mg	Doral by Wallace	00037-9002	Sedative/Hypnotic; C IV
15 <> DURA	Tab, White, Oblong, Scored	Guaifenesin 600 mg, Pseudoephedrine HCl 120 mg	by DJ Pharma	64455-0015	Cold Remedy
15 <> DURA	Tab, White, Oblong, Scored	Guaifenesin 600 mg, Pseudoephedrine 120 mg	Guai Vent PSE by Anabolic	00722-6310	Cold Remedy
15 <> E	Tab, Green, Oval, Extended Release	Morphine Sulfate 15 mg	MS Contin by Ethex	58177-0310	Analgesic; C II
15 <> E	Tab, Dark Yellow, Round	Benazepril HCl 10 mg	Lotensin by Aurobindo	65862-0116	Antihypertensive
15 <> E652	Tab, Blue, Round	Morphine Sulfate 15 mg	MS Contin by Endo	60951-0652	Analgesic; C II

ID FRONT <> BACK	DESCRIPTION FRONT <> BACK	INGREDIENT & STRENGTH	BRAND (or Generic Equiv.) by FIRM	NDC#	CLASS; SCH.
15 <> ER	Tab, White to Off-White, Oval, Ex Release, "1.5" <> ER	Pramipexole DiHCl 1.5 mg	Mirapex ER by Boehringer Ingelheim	00597-0113	Antiparkinson
15 <> ETH	Tab, Brown, Round, Scored, Immediate Release	Morphine Sulfate 15 mg	MSIR by Ethex	58177-0313	Analgesic; C II
15 <> FL	Tab, Purple, Cap Shaped, Film Coated	Memantine 15 mg	Namenda by Forest	00456-3215	Antialzheimers
15 <> G	Tab, Peach, Round	Meloxicam 15 mg	Mobic by Genpharm	15330-0219	NSAID
15 <> G14	Tab, Light Yellow, Oval	Meloxicam 15 mg	Mobic by Glenmark	68462-0141	NSAID
15 <> GG31	Tab, Orange, Round, Film Coated, GG over 31	Thioridazine 15 mg	Mellaril by Sandoz	00781-1614	Antipsychotic
15 <> M	Tab, White to Cream Colored, Octagon, M inside square	Mixed Amphetamine Salts 15 mg: Dextroamphetamine Saccharate 3.75 mg, Amphetamine Aspartate 3.75 mg, Dextroamphetamine Sulfate 3.75 mg, Amphetamine Sulfate 3.75 mg	Adderall by Mallinckrodt	00406-8885	Stimulant; C II
15 <> M	Tab, Light Green, Round, Convex, Scored, M inside square	Oxycodone HCl 15 mg	Roxicodone by Mallinckrodt	00406-8515	Analgesic; C II
15 <> M	Tab, Blue, Round, M inside square <> 15	Morphine Sulfate 15 mg	MS Contin by Mallinckrodt	00406-8315	Analgesic; C II
15 <> M	Tab, Yellow, Oblong	Meloxicam 15 mg	Mobic by Boehringer Ingelheim	00597-0030	NSAID
15 <> MSD	Tab, White, Round	Lisinopril 2.5 mg	Prinivil by Merck	00006-0015	Antihypertensive
15 <> N	Tab, Off-White, Round, Scored, N <> 1/5	Meloxicam 15 mg	Mobicox by Novopharm	Canadian DIN 02258323	NSAID
15 <> N	Tab, White, Round	Codeine Phosphate 15 mg	by AltiMed	Canadian DIN 00779458	Analgesic; C II
15 <> OC	Tab, Grey, Round, CR	Oxycodone HCl 15 mg	OxyContin by Purdue	59011-0815	Analgesic; C II
15 <> P	Tab, Yellow, Oval, Scored	Mirtazapine 15 mg	Remeron by Pharmascience	Canadian DIN 02273942	Antidepressant
15 <> P	Tab, White, Round	Pioglitazone HCl 15 mg	Actos by Pharmascience	Canadian DIN 02303124	Antihyperglycemic
15 <> TC	Tab, Green, Oval	Morphine Sulfate 15 mg ER	Ratio-Morphine by Ratiopharm	Canadian DIN 02244790	Analgesic; C II
15 <> WATSON365	Tab, Pink, Round, Scored	Clorazepate Dipotassium 15 mg	Tranxene by Ivax	00182-0014	Antianxiety; C IV
15 <> WATSON365	Tab, Pink, Round, Scored	Clorazepate Dipotassium 15 mg	Tranxene by Major	00904-5159	Antianxiety; C IV
15 <> WATSON365	Tab, Pink, Round, Scored	Clorazepate Dipotassium 15 mg	Tranxene by Watson	00591-0365	Antianxiety; C IV
150	Tab, Peach, Round, Schering Logo 150	Ethinyl Estradiol 0.5 mg	Estinyl by Schering		Hormone
150	Tab, Light Yellow, Round, Film Coated, a Logo 150	Solifenacin Succinate 5 mg	VESIcare by Astellas	Canadian DIN 02277263	Urinary Tract
150	Tab, Light Blue, Round, Scored	Levothyroxine Sodium 150 mcg	Eltroxin by GSK	Canadian DIN 02213214	Thyroid Hormone
150	Tab, Light Yellow, Round, Film Coated, a Logo 150	Solifenacin Succinate 5 mg	VESIcare by Astellas	51248-0150	Urinary Tract
150	Tab, White, Round, Scored, Film Coated, 150 over Triangle	Propafenone HCl 150 mg	Rythmol by Abbott	00044-5022	Antiarrhythmic
150	Tab, White, Round, Scored, Film Coated, 150 over Triangle	Propafenone HCl 150 mg	Rythmol by Caremark	00339-6050	Antiarrhythmic
150	Tab, White, Round, Scored, Film Coated, 150 over Triangle	Propafenone HCl 150 mg	Rythmol by Nat Pharmpak	55154-1606	Antiarrhythmic
150	Tab, White, Round, Scored, Film Coated, 150 over Triangle	Propafenone HCl 150 mg	Rythmol by Abbott	00603708	Antiarrhythmic
150	Tab, White to Off-White, Round, Film Coated, Cobalt Logo <> 150	Ranitidine HCl 150 mg	Zantac by Cobalt	Canadian DIN 02248570	Gastrointestinal
150	Tab, White, Round, Scored, Film Coated, 150 over Triangle	Propafenone HCl 150 mg	Rythmol by Pharmascience	Canadian DIN 02294559	Antiarrhythmic
150	Tab, Pink, Oval	Fluconazole 150 mg	Diflucan by Glenmark	68462-0103	Antifungal
150 <> 4333	Tab, Peach, Round, Scored, Logo 4333 <> 150	Nefazodone 150 mg	Serzone by Ivax	00172-4333	Antidepressant
150 <> 4357	Tab, Beige, Round	Ranitidine HCl 150 mg	Zantac by Ivax	00172-4357 Discontinued	Gastrointestinal
150 <> 5412	Tab, Pink, Oval	Fluconazole 150 mg	Diflucan by Ivax	00172-5412	Antifungal
150 <> B701	Tab, Pink, Round, Film Coated, b over 701	Demeclocycline HCl 150 mg	Declomycin by Barr	00555-0701	Antibiotic
150 <> BNVA	Tab, White, Oblong, Film-Coated	Ibandronate Sodium 150 mg	Boniva by Hoffmann La Roche	00004-0186	Bisphosphonate
150 <> COPLEY	Tab, Off-White, Cap Shaped	Naproxen 550 mg	Naprosyn by Rx Dispensing	61807-0021	NSAID
150 <> COPLEY	Tab, Off-White, Cap Shaped	Naproxen 500 mg	Naprosyn by Teva	38245-0150	NSAID

ID FRONT <> BACK	DESCRIPTION FRONT <> BACK	INGREDIENT & STRENGTH	BRAND (or Generic Equiv.) by FIRM	NDC#	CLASS; SCH.
150 <> COPLEY	Tab, Off-White, Cap Shaped	Naproxen 500 mg	Naprosyn by Qualitest	00603-4732	NSAID
150 <> COPLEY	Tab, Off-White, Cap Shaped	Naproxen 500 mg	Naprosyn by Southwood	58016-0289	NSAID
150 <> FLINT	Tab, Light Blue, Round, Scored	Levothyroxine Sodium 150 mcg	Synthroid by Abbott	00048-1090	Thyroid Hormone
150 <> FLINT	Tab, Light Blue, Round, Scored	Levothyroxine Sodium 150 mcg	Synthroid by Kaiser	00179-0459	Thyroid Hormone
150 <> FLINT	Tab, Light Blue, Round, Scored	Levothyroxine Sodium 150 mcg	Synthroid by Forest	00456-0325	Thyroid Hormone
150 <> FLINT	Tab, Light Blue, Round, Scored	Levothyroxine Sodium 150 mcg	Synthroid by Amerisource	62584-0015	Thyroid Hormone
150 <> FLINT	Tab, Light Blue, Round, Scored	Levothyroxine Sodium 150 mcg	Synthroid by Nat Pharmpak	55154-0905	Thyroid Hormone
150 <> FLINT	Tab, Light Blue, Round, Scored	Levothyroxine Sodium 150 mcg	Synthroid by Giant Food	11146-0304	Thyroid Hormone
150 <> FLINT	Tab, Light Blue, Round, Scored	Levothyroxine Sodium 150 mcg	Synthroid by Rite Aid	11822-5210	Thyroid Hormone
150 <> FLINT	Tab, Light Blue, Round, Scored	Levothyroxine Sodium 150 mcg	Synthroid by Rx Pak	65084-0182	Thyroid Hormone
150 <> FLINT	Tab, Light Blue, Round, Scored	Levothyroxine Sodium 150 mcg	Synthroid by Abbott	Canadian DIN 02172127	Thyroid Hormone
150 <> FLINT	Tab, Light Blue, Round, Scored	Levothyroxine Sodium 150 mcg	Synthroid by Med Pro	53978-0999	Thyroid Hormone
150 <> GG338	Tab, Blue, Cap Shaped, Scored, 150 <> GG over 338	Levothyroxine 150 mcg	Levo-T by Sandoz	00781-5187	Thyroid Hormone
150 <> GG338	Tab, Blue, Cap Shaped, Scored, 150 <> GG over 338	Levothyroxine 150 mcg	Levo-T by Alara	64909-0141	Thyroid Hormone
150 <> N	Tab, Lavender, Round Sustained Release	Bupropion HCl 150 mg	Wellbutrin SR by Novopharm	Canadian DIN 02260239	Antidepressant
150 <> N	Tab, Yellow, Hexagonal	Sulindac 150 mg	Clinoril by Novopharm	Canadian DIN 00745588	NSAID
150 <> N	Tab, White, Round	Ranitidine HCl 150 mg	Zantac by Novopharm	Canadian DIN 00828564	Gastrointestinal
150 <> N544	Tab, White, Round, Film Coated, N over 544	Ranitidine HCl 150 mg	Zantac by Teva	00093-8544 Discontinued	Gastrointestinal
150 <> N544	Tab, White, Round, Film Coated, N over 544	Ranitidine HCl 150 mg	Zantac by UDL	51079-0879	Gastrointestinal
150 <> N544	Tab, White, Round, Film Coated, N over 544	Ranitidine HCl 150 mg	Zantac by Murfreesboro	51129-1197	Gastrointestinal
150 <> N544	Tab, White, Round, Film Coated, N over 544	Ranitidine HCl 150 mg	Zantac by Pharmacy Care	65070-0053	Gastrointestinal
150 <> N544	Tab, White, Round, Film Coated, N over 544	Ranitidine HCl 150 mg	Zantac by Med Pro	53978-2075	Gastrointestinal
150 <> N544	Tab, White, Round, Film Coated, N over 544	Ranitidine HCl 150 mg	Zantac by Nat Pharmpak	55154-5581	Gastrointestinal
150 <> N548	Tab, Peach, Round, N over 548	Fluconazole 150 mg	Diflucan by Teva	00093-7204 Discontinued	Antifungal
150 <> NN	Tab, Tan, Oval, Scored, N/N	Moclobemide 150 mg	Manerix by Novopharm	Canadian DIN 02239747	Antidepressant
150 <> NN	Tab, White, Shield Shaped, Scored, N/N <> 150	Lamotrigine 150 mg	Lamictal by Novopharm	Canadian DIN 02248234	Antiepileptic
150 <> ORTHO	Tab	Mestranol 0.05 mg, Norethindrone 1 mg	Ortho Novum 1 Plus 50 by Dept Health	53808-0030	Oral Contraceptive
150 <> ORTHO	Tab	Ethinyl Estradiol 0.035 mg, Norgestimate 0.215 mg, Norgestimate 0.18 mg, Norgestimate 0.25 mg	Ortho Tri-Cyclen 28 by Dept Health	53808-0043	Oral Contraceptive
150 <> PRIFTIN	Tab, Dark Pink, Round, Film Coated	Rifapentine 150 mg	Priftin by Aventis	00088-2100	Antibiotic
150 <> PRIFTIN	Tab, Dark Pink, Round, Film Coated	Rifapentine 150 mg	Priftin by Gruppo Lepetit	12522-8598	Antibiotic
150 <> SP	Tab, Salmon, Oval, Film Coated	Lacosamide 150 mg	Vimpat by Schwarz	00091-2479	Antiepileptic
150 <> SYNTHROID	Tab, Blue, Round, Scored	Levothyroxine Sodium 150 mcg	Synthroid by Abbott	00074-7069	Thyroid Hormone
150 <> T4	Tab, Blue, Cap Shaped, Scored	Levothyroxine Sodium 150 mcg	Levothroid by Forest	00456-1325	Thyroid Hormone
150 <> TMC	Tab, White, Oval, Film Coated	Darunavir 150 mg	Prezista by Tibotec	59676-0564	Antiviral
150 <> VIDEX	Tab, Off-White to Light Orange/Yellow, Round, Chewable	Didanosine 150 mg	Videx by BMS	Canadian DIN 01940554	Antiviral
150 <> VIDEX	Tab, Off-White to Light Orange/Yellow, Round, Chewable	Didanosine 150 mg	Videx by BMS	00087-6653	Antiviral
150 <> XELODA	Tab, Light Peach, Oblong, Film Coated	Capecitabine 150 mg	Xeloda by Hoffmann La Roche	00004-1101	Antineoplastic
150 <> XELODA	Tab, Light Peach, Oblong, Film Coated	Capecitabine 150 mg	Xeloda by Roche	Canadian DIN 02238453	Antineoplastic
150 <> Z	Tab, Rust Colored, Five-Sided	Ranitidine 150 mg	Zantac OTC by Pfizer		Gastrointestinal

ID FRONT <> BACK	DESCRIPTION FRONT <> BACK	INGREDIENT & STRENGTH	BRAND (or Generic Equiv.) by FIRM	NDC#	CLASS; SCH.
1500 <> GSK	Tab, Yellow, Oval, Film Coated, 1/500	Metformin HCl 500 mg, Rosiglitazone 1 mg	Avandamet by GSK	Canadian DIN 02247085	Antidiabetic
1500 <> GSK	Tab, Yellow, Oval, Film Coated, 1/500	Metformin HCl 500 mg, Rosiglitazone 1 mg	Avandamet by SKB	00007-3166	Antidiabetic
15034 <> N	Tab, White, Oval, Scored, 1.5 034	Glyburide 1.5 mg	Glynase by Teva	00093-8034	Antidiabetic
150AXIDRELIANT	Cap, Dark and Pale Yellow, Opaque, Black Ink	Nizatidine 150 mg	Axid by Reliant	65726-0144	Gastrointestinal
150LLA18	Tab, Peach, Heptagonal	Amoxapine 150 mg	Asendin by Lederle		Antidepressant
150M	Tab	Levothyroxine Sodium 150 mcg	Levo-T by Mova	55370-0131	Thyroid Hormone
150M	Tab	Levothyroxine Sodium 150 mcg	Euthyrox by Em Pharma	63254-0442	Thyroid Hormone
150M <> Z	Tab, Blue, Round, Scored	Levothyroxine Sodium 150 mcg	Levo-T by Zoetica	64909-0117	Thyroid Hormone
150MCG <> FLINT	Tab, Blue, Round, Scored	Levothyroxine Sodium 150 mcg	Synthroid by Wal Mart	49035-0193	Thyroid Hormone
150MCG <> FLINT	Tab, Blue, Round, Scored	Levothyroxine Sodium 150 mcg	Synthroid by Amerisource	62584-0090	Thyroid Hormone
150MG <> RSN	Tab, Blue, Oval, Film Coated	Risedronate Sodium 150 mg	Actonel by Procter and Gamble	00149-0478	Bisphosphonate
150P	Cap, Scarlet and Purple	Clindamycin HCl 150 mg	Dalacin C by Pharmascience	Canadian DIN 02294826	Antibiotic
150PT	Cap, Clear, 150 <> P/T	Chlorpheniramine Maleate 12 mg, Phenylpropanolamine 75 mg	Ornade by Kaiser	00179-1136	Cold Remedy
150PT	Cap, Clear, 150 <> P/T	Chlorpheniramine Maleate 12 mg, Phenylpropanolamine 75 mg	Ornade by Jones	52604-0405	Cold Remedy
150WALLACE374001	Cap, Blue & White, 150 Wallace 37-4001	Methacycline HCl 150 mg	Rondomycin by Wallace		Antibiotic
151	Tab, Light Pink, Round, Film Coated, a Logo 151	Solifenacin Succinate 10 mg	VESIcare by Astellas	Canadian DIN 02277271	Urinary Tract
151	Tab, Light Pink, Round, Film Coated, a Logo 151	Solifenacin Succinate 10 mg	VESIcare by Astellas	51248-0151	Urinary Tract
151 <> GXCJ7	Tab, White, Diamond, Film	Lamivudine 150 mg	Epivir by Murfreesboro	51129-1620	Antiviral
151 <> M	Tab, White, Round	Finasteride 5 mg	Proscar by Mylan	00378-3151	Antiandrogen
151 <> M	Tab, White, Round	Finasteride 5 mg	Proscar by UDL	51079-0520	Antiandrogen
151 <> SEARLE	Tab, White, Round	Ethinyl Estradiol 35 mcg, Ethynodiol Diacetate 1 mg	Demulen 1/35 by Pharm Util	60491-0181	Oral Contraceptive
151 <> SEARLE	Tab, White, Round	Ethinyl Estradiol 35 mcg, Ethynodiol Diacetate 1 mg	Demulen 1/35 by Searle	00025-0151	Oral Contraceptive
151 <> SEARLE	Tab, White, Round	Ethinyl Estradiol 35 mcg, Ethynodiol Diacetate 1 mg	Demulen 1/35 by Nat Pharmpak	55154-3612	Oral Contraceptive
151 <> SEARLE	Tab, White, Round	Ethinyl Estradiol 35 mcg, Ethynodiol Diacetate 1 mg	Demulen 1/35 by Physician Total Care	54868-0404	Oral Contraceptive
151 <> SEARLE	Tab, White, Round	Ethinyl Estradiol 35 mcg, Ethynodiol Diacetate 1 mg	Demulen 1/35 by Rx Pak	65084-0219	Oral Contraceptive
151LUNSCO	Cap	Acetaminophen 300 mg, Phenyltoloxamine Citrate 20 mg, Salicylamide 200 mg	Durabac by Seatrace	00551-0151	Analgesic
152	Tab, Coated	Ascorbic Acid 500 mg, Biotin 0.15 mg, Chromic Nitrate 0.1 mg, Cupric Oxide, Cyanocobalamin 50 mcg, Ferrous Fumarate 27 mg, Folic Acid 0.8 mg, Magnesium Oxide 50 mg, Manganese Dioxide 5 mg, Niacin 100 mg, Pantothenic Acid 25 mg, Pyridoxine HCl 25 mg, Riboflavin 20 mg, Thiamine Mononitrate 20 mg, Vitamin A Acetate 5000 Units, Vitamin E Acetate 30 Units	B C w Folic Acid Plus by Sandoz	00781-1102	Vitamin
152	Tab, Green, Round, Film Coated, White Print	Dexbrompheniramine 6 mg, Pseudoephedrine 120 mg	by Sovereign	58716-0659	Cold Remedy
152	Tab, White, Round, Scored, A logo (a letter "C" with a dash in the middle) 152	Buspirone HCl 10 mg	BuSpar by Ranbaxy	63304-0501	Antianxiety
152 <> AP	Tab, Purple, Cap Shaped, Scored, Chewable	Pseudoephedrine HCl 15 mg, Chlorpheniramine Maleate 2 mg	Pediox by Atley	59702-0152	Cold Remedy
152 <> CARACO	Tab	Guaifenesin 600 mg	Robitussin by Caraco	57664-0152	Expectorant
152 <> COPLEY	Tab, Golden Yellow, Film Coated	Ascorbic Acid 200 mg, Biotin 0.15 mg, Calcium Pantothenate 27.17 mg, Chromic Chloride 0.51 mg, Cupric Oxide 3.75 mg, Cyanocobalamin 50 mcg, Ferrous Fumarate 82.2 mg, Folic Acid 0.8 mg, Magnesium Oxide 82.89 mg, Manganese 50 mg, Manganese Sulfate 15.5 mg, Niacinamide Ascorbate 400 mg, Pyridoxine HCl 30.25 mg, Riboflavin 20 mg, Thiamine Mononitrate 20 mg, Vitamin A Acetate 10.75 mg, Vitamin E Acetate 30 mg, Zinc Oxide 27.99 mg	Berplex Plus by Schein	00364-0814	Vitamin

ID FRONT <> BACK	DESCRIPTION FRONT <> BACK	INGREDIENT & STRENGTH	BRAND (or Generic Equiv.) by FIRM	NDC#	CLASS; SCH.
152 <> COPLEY	Tab, Golden Yellow, Film Coated	Ascorbic Acid 200 mg, Biotin 0.15 mg, Calcium Pantothenate 27.17 mg, Chromic Chloride 0.51 mg, Cupric Oxide 3.75 mg, Cyanocobalamin 50 mcg, Ferrous Fumarate 82.2 mg, Folic Acid 0.8 mg, Magnesium Oxide 82.89 mg, Manganese 50 mg, Manganese Sulfate 15.5 mg, Niacinamide Ascorbate 400 mg, Pyridoxine HCl 30.25 mg, Riboflavin 20 mg, Thiamine Mononitrate 20 mg, Vitamin A Acetate 10.75 mg, Vitamin E Acetate 30 mg, Zinc Oxide 27.99 mg	by Teva	38245-0152 Discontinued	Vitamin
152 <> COPLEY	Tab, Yellow, Oval, Film Coated	Ascorbic Acid 200 mg, Biotin 0.15 mg, Calcium Pantothenate 27.17 mg, Chromic Chloride 0.51 mg, Cupric Oxide 3.75 mg, Cyanocobalamin 50 mcg, Ferrous Fumarate 82.2 mg, Folic Acid 0.8 mg, Magnesium Oxide 82.89 mg, Manganese 50 mg, Manganese Sulfate 15.5 mg, Niacinamide Ascorbate 400 mg, Pyridoxine HCl 30.25 mg, Riboflavin 20 mg, Thiamine Mononitrate 20 mg, Vitamin A Acetate 10.75 mg, Vitamin E Acetate 30 mg, Zinc Oxide 27.99 mg	B Complex Vit Plus by Teva	00093-9152	Vitamin
152 <> GXCJ7	Tab, White, Diamond, Film Coated	Lamivudine 150 mg	Epivir by Murfreesboro	51129-1622	Antiviral
152 <> WPPH	Tab, Yellow, Round, Film Coated	Methyldopa 250 mg	by Endo	60951-0776	Antihypertensive
1520 <> WARRICK	Tab, White, Round, Scored	Albuterol Sulfate 2 mg	Proventil by Allscripts		Antiasthmatic
1520 <> WARRICK	Tab, White, Round, Scored	Albuterol Sulfate 2 mg	Proventil by Southwood	58016-0473	Antiasthmatic
153 <> R	Tab, White, Round, Film Coated	Ondansetron HCl 4 mg	Zofran by Dr. Reddy's	55111-0153	Antiemetic
153 <> WPPH	Tab, White, Round, Film Coated	Hydrochlorothiazide 25 mg, Methyldopa 250 mg	by Merck	00006-0153	Diuretic; Antihypertensive
153 <> WPPH	Tab, White, Round, Film Coated	Hydrochlorothiazide 25 mg, Methyldopa 250 mg	by West Point	59591-0153	Diuretic; Antihypertensive
153 <> WPPH	Tab, White, Round, Film Coated	Hydrochlorothiazide 25 mg, Methyldopa 250 mg	by Endo	60951-0779	Diuretic; Antihypertensive
1530 <> SCS	Tab, White, Round	Ethinyl Estradiol 0.03 mg, Levonorgestrel 0.15 mg	Levora by Patheon	63285-0100	Oral Contraceptive
1530 <> SCS	Tab, White, Round	Ethinyl Estradiol 0.03 mg, Levonorgestrel 0.15 mg	by SCS Pharms	00905-0279	Oral Contraceptive
1530 <> WATSON	Tab, White, Round	Ethinyl Estradiol 0.03 mg, Levonorgestrel 0.15 mg	Levora by Watson	52544-0279	Oral Contraceptive
1531	Tab, Round	Sulfisoxazole 500 mg	Gantrisin by Vortech		Antibiotic
1533	Tab, Round	Digoxin 0.25 mg	Lanoxin by Vortech		Cardiac Agent
154	Tab, Yellow, Scored	Sulindac 200 mg	by Kaiser	00179-1334	NSAID
154 <> 93	Tab, White, Oval, Film Coated	Ticlopidine HCl 250 mg	Ticlid by Pharmascience	Canadian DIN 02243327	Anticoagulant
154 <> 93	Tab, White, Oval, Film Coated	Ticlopidine HCl 250 mg	Ticlid by UDL	51079-0920	Anticoagulant
154 <> 93	Tab, White, Oval, Film Coated	Ticlopidine HCl 250 mg	Ticlid by Teva	00093-0154	Anticoagulant
154 <> R	Tab, Yellow, Round, Film Coated	Ondansetron HCl 8 mg	Zofran by Dr. Reddy's	55111-0154	Antiemetic
154 <> WPPH	Tab, Bright Yellow, Hexagonal, Scored	Sulindac 200 mg	by Endo	60951-0781	NSAID
154 <> WPPH	Tab, Bright Yellow, Hexagonal, Scored	Sulindac 200 mg	by Merck Sharp & Dohme	62904-0154	NSAID
154 <> WPPH	Tab, Bright Yellow, Hexagonal, Scored	Sulindac 200 mg	by West Point	59591-0154	NSAID
155	Tab, White, Circular, Assyrian Lion Logo	Bumetanide 2 mg	Bumex by Leo Pharma	Canadian	Diuretic
155 <> 93	Tab, White to Off-White, Cap Shaped	Topiramate 25 mg	Topamax by Teva	00093-0155	Anticonvulsant
155 <> MYLAN	Tab, Pink, Oblong, Film Coated	Acetaminophen 650 mg, Propoxyphene Napsylate 100 mg	Darvocet-N 100 by Med Pro	53978-5013	Analgesic; C IV
155 <> MYLAN	Tab, Pink, Oblong, Film Coated	Acetaminophen 650 mg, Propoxyphene Napsylate 100 mg	Darvocet-N 100 by UDL	51079-0322 Discontinued	Analgesic; C IV
155 <> MYLAN	Tab, Pink, Oblong, Film Coated	Acetaminophen 650 mg, Propoxyphene Napsylate 100 mg	Darvocet-N 100 by Qualitest	00603-5466	Analgesic; C IV
155 <> MYLAN	Tab, Pink, Oblong, Film Coated	Acetaminophen 650 mg, Propoxyphene Napsylate 100 mg	Darvocet-N 100 by Vangard	00615-0455	Analgesic; C IV
155 <> MYLAN	Tab, Pink, Oblong, Film Coated	Acetaminophen 650 mg, Propoxyphene Napsylate 100 mg	Darvocet-N 100 by Mylan	00378-0155	Analgesic; C IV
155 <> MYLAN	Tab, Pink, Oblong, Film Coated	Acetaminophen 650 mg, Propoxyphene Napsylate 100 mg	Darvocet-N 100 by Allscripts		Analgesic; C IV
155 <> R	Tab, White, Round, Film Coated	Ondansetron HCl 16 mg	Zofran by Dr. Reddy's	55111-0155	Antiemetic
15500 <> 4833M	Tab, White to Off-White, Oblong, Film Coated, '15/500	Pioglitazone HCl 15 mg, Metformin HCl 500 mg	Actoplus Met by Takeda	64764-0155	Antidiabetic
15520527	Cap	Aspirin 325 mg, Butalbital 50 mg, Caffeine 40 mg	Fiorinal by URL Mutual	00677-1439	Analgesic; C III
1554	Tab, Round	Dextroamphetamine Sulfate 10 mg	Dexedrine by Vortech		Stimulant; C II
156 <> A	Tab	Hyoscyamine Sulfate 0.375 mg	Levsin by Ivax	00182-2657	Gastrointestinal

For updated data, go to www.IdentADrug.com

ID FRONT <> BACK	DESCRIPTION FRONT <> BACK	INGREDIENT & STRENGTH	BRAND (or Generic Equiv.) by FIRM	NDC#	CLASS; SCH.
156 <> R	Tab, Pink, Round, Film Coated	Ondansetron HCl 24 mg	Zofran by Dr. Reddy's	55111-0156	Antiemetic
156 <> WPPH	Tab, Butterscotch Yellow, D-Shaped, Film Coated	Cyclobenzaprine HCl 10 mg	by Med Pro	53978-1035	Muscle Relaxant
156 <> WPPH	Tab, Butterscotch Yellow, D-Shaped, Film Coated	Cyclobenzaprine HCl 10 mg	by West Point	59591-0156	Muscle Relaxant
156 <> WPPH	Tab, Butterscotch Yellow, D-Shaped, Film Coated	Cyclobenzaprine HCl 10 mg	by Endo	60951-0767	Muscle Relaxant
156 <> WPPH	Tab, Butterscotch Yellow, D-Shaped, Film Coated	Cyclobenzaprine HCl 10 mg	by PDRX	55289-0567	Muscle Relaxant
157 <> CARACO	Tab	Guaifenesin 400 mg, Phenylpropanolamine HCl 75 mg	Entex LA by Caraco	57664-0157	Cold Remedy
1571 <> 252	Tab	Phenobarbital 64.8 mg	by URL Mutual	00677-0762	Sedative/Hypnotic; C IV
157WPPH	Cap, Blue & White Beads	Indomethacin 75 mg	Indocin SR by Endo	60951-0774	NSAID
157WPPH	Cap, Blue & White Beads	Indomethacin 75 mg	Indocin SR by West Point	59591-0157	NSAID
158 <> COPLEY	Tab, Chewable	Ascorbic Acid 34.5 mg, Cyanocobalamin 4.9 mcg, Folic Acid 0.35 mg, Niacinamide 14.16 mg, Pyridoxine HCl 1.1 mg, Riboflavin 1.2 mg, Sodium Ascorbate 32.2 mg, Sodium Fluoride 1.1 mg, Thiamine Mononitrate 1.15 mg, Vitamin A Acetate 5.5 mg, Vitamin D 0.194 mg, Vitamin E Acetate 15.75 mg	Polyvitamin by Schein	00364-1157	Vitamin
15850 <> 4833M	Tab, White to Off-White, Oblong, Film Coated, 15/850	Pioglitazone HCl 15 mg, Metformin HCl 850 mg	Actoplus Met by Takeda	64764-0158	Antidiabetic
159 <> COPLEY	Tab, Chewable	Cholecalciferol 0.194 mg, Cupric Oxide 1.25 mg, Cyanocobalamin 4.9 mcg, Ferrous Fumarate 36.5 mg, Folic Acid 0.35 mg, Niacinamide 14.17 mg, Pyridoxine HCl 1.1 mg, Riboflavin 1.26 mg, Sodium Ascorbate 32.2 mg, Sodium Fluoride 2.21 mg, Thiamine Mononitrate 1.15 mg, Vitamin A Acetate 5.5 mg, Vitamin E 15.75 mg, Zinc Oxide 12.5 mg	Polyvitamin by Schein	00364-0770	Vitamin
159879	Cap	Tetracycline HCl 500 mg	by Qualitest	00603-5920	Antibiotic
159BARR	Cap, Green & White	Chlordiazepoxide 25 mg	Librium by UDL	51079-0141	Antianxiety; C IV
159BARR	Cap, Green & White	Chlordiazepoxide 25 mg	Librium by PDRX	55289-0126	Antianxiety; C IV
159WPPH	Cap, Blue	Indomethacin 50 mg	Indocin by Endo	60951-0773	NSAID
159WPPH	Cap, Blue	Indomethacin 50 mg	Indocin by West Point	59591-0159	NSAID
159WPPH	Cap, Blue	Indomethacin 50 mg	Indocin by Southwood	58016-0236	NSAID
15BL	Tab	Penicillin V Potassium 250 mg	by Med Pro	53978-5042	Antibiotic
15M <> P	Tab, White, Round, Scored	Meloxicam 15 mg	Mobicox by Pharmascience	Canadian DIN 02248268	NSAID
15MG <> DEPLIN	Tab, Orange, Oval, Coated	L-methylfolate (Metafolin) 15 mg	Deplin by PAMLAB, LLC.	00525-0450	Supplement
15MG <> P	Tab, Green, Round, Sustained Release	Morphine Sulfate 15 mg	MS Contin by Pharmascience	Canadian DIN 02245284	Analgesic
15MG <> PF	Tab, Green, Round	Morphine Sulfate 15 mg	MS Contin by Purdue	Canadian	Analgesic; C II
15MG334615MGSB	Cap, White & Yellow Pellets, 15 MG/3346 in White Print	Prochlorperazine 24.3 mg	Compazine by SKB	00007-3346	Antiemetic
15MG334615MGSB	Cap, White & Yellow Pellets	Prochlorperazine 15 mg	Compazine by Int'l Processing	59885-3346	Antiemetic
15MG351415MGSB	Cap, Brown & Natural	Dextroamphetamine Sulfate 15 mg	Dexedrine by Int'l Processing	59885-3514	Stimulant; C II
15MGSB15MG3346	Cap, White & Yellow Pellets	Prochlorperazine 15 mg	Compazine by Int'l Processing	59885-3346	Antiemetic
15MGSB15MG3346	Cap, White & Yellow Pellets	Prochlorperazine 15 mg	Compazine by SKB	00007-3346	Antiemetic
15MGSB15MG3514	Cap, Brown & Natural	Dextroamphetamine Sulfate 15 mg	Dexedrine by Int'l Processing	59885-3514	Stimulant; C II
15P <> DAN	Tab, White, Round, Scored	Phenobarbital 15 mg	Phenobarbital by Schein	00364-2444	Sedative/Hypnotic; C IV
15SYCBMZ	Tab, White, Round, 1.5/Syc-BMZ	Bromazepam 1.5 mg	Lectopam by AltiMed	Canadian DIN 02167808 Discontinued	Sedative; C IV
15WESTWARDFLURAZE	Cap	Flurazepam HCl 15 mg	by West-Ward		Hypnotic; C IV
15XL	Tab, Gray, Oval	Oxybutynin Chloride 15 mg	Ditropan XL by Alza	17314-8502	Urinary Tract
16	Tab, White, Round	Perphenazine 16 mg	Apo Perphenazine by Apotex	Canadian DIN 00335096	Antipsychotic
16 <> 93	Tab, Beige, Oval	Nabumetone 750 mg	by Teva	00093-1016	NSAID
16 <> A	Tab, Green, Cap Shaped, Film Coated, A <> 1 / 6	Sertraline HCl 25 mg	Zoloft by Aurobindo	65862-0011	Antidepressant
16 <> ACH	Tab, White, Oval	Candesartan Cilexetil 16 mg	by AstraZeneca	17228-0016	Antihypertensive
16 <> BIOCRAFT	Tab, White, Oval	Penicillin V Potassium 250 mg	by Qualitest	00603-5067	Antibiotic

ID FRONT <> BACK	DESCRIPTION FRONT <> BACK	INGREDIENT & STRENGTH	BRAND (or Generic Equiv.) by FIRM	NDC#	CLASS; SCH.
16 <> BIOCRAFT	Tab, White, Oval	Penicillin V Potassium 250 mg	by Apotheca	12634-0468	Antibiotic
16 <> BIOCRAFT	Tab, White, Oval	Penicillin V Potassium 250 mg	by Major	00904-2450	Antibiotic
16 <> BIOCRAFT	Tab, White, Oval	Penicillin V Potassium 250 mg	by Moore	00839-5188	Antibiotic
16 <> BIOCRAFT	Tab, White, Oval	Penicillin V Potassium 250 mg	by Southwood	58016-0146	Antibiotic
16 <> BIOCRAFT	Tab, White, Oval	Penicillin V Potassium 250 mg	by Teva	Discontinued	Antibiotic
16 <> CIBA	Tab, White, Round, Film Coated	Methylphenidate HCl 20 mg	Ritalin by Caremark	00339-4084	Stimulant; C II
16 <> CIBA	Tab, White, Round, Film Coated	Methylphenidate HCl 20 mg	Ritalin SR by Novartis	00083-0016	Stimulant; C II
16 <> CIBA	Tab, White, Round, Film Coated	Methylphenidate HCl 20 mg	Ritalin by Novartis	Canadian DIN 00632775	Stimulant; C II
16 <> E	Tab, Pink, Round	Benazepril HCl 20 mg	Lotensin by Aurobindo	65862-0117	Antihypertensive
16 <> N	Tab, White, Round, Biconvex, Bevelled-Edge, Scored	Betahistine Dihydrochloride 16 mg	Novo-Betahistine by Novopharm	Canadian DIN 02280191	Antivertigo
160	Tab, White, Oval, Scored	Megestrol acetate 160 mg	Megace by BMS	Canadian DIN 00731323	Antineoplastic
160	Tab, White, Oblong, Film Coated, Fournier Logo <> 160	Fenofibrate 160 mg	Lipidil Supra by Fournier	Canadian DIN 02241602	Antihyperlipidemic
160	Tab	Acetaminophen 160 mg	Children's Tylenol by Mead Johnson	Canadian DIN 00876038	Analgesic
160	Tab	Acetaminophen 160 mg	Children's Tylenol by Mead Johnson	Canadian DIN 02231805	Analgesic
160	Tab, Pink, Round, Schering Logo 160	Carisoprodol 350 mg	Rela by Schering		Muscle Relaxant
160	Tab, White, Round	Triprolidine 2.5 mg, Pseudoephedrine 60 mg	Actifed by Ivax	00182-1605 Discontinued	Cold Remedy
160 <> COR	Tab, White, Round	Levocarnitine 330 mg	Carnitor by Rising	64980-0130	Supplement
160 <> NN	Tab, Light Blue, Cap Shaped, Scored, N/N <> 160	Sotalol HCl 160 mg	Sotacor by Novopharm	Canadian DIN 02231182	Antiarrhythmic
160 <> OC	Tab, Blue, Cap Shaped, Film Coated	Oxycodone HCl 160 mg	OxyContin by Purdue	59011-0109	Analgesic; C II
160 <> R	Tab, Yellow, Cap Shaped	Ofloxacin 200 mg	Floxin by Dr. Reddy's	55111-0160	Antibiotic
160 <> TY	Tab, Pink, Round, Scored, Chewable	Acetaminophen 160 mg	Junior Tylenol Meltaways by McNeil	50580-0513	Analgesic
160 <> TY	Tab, Purple, Round, Scored, Chewable	Acetaminophen 160 mg	Junior Tylenol Meltaways by McNeil	50580-0514	Analgesic
160 <> TY	Tab, Pink or Purple, Round, Scored, Chewable	Acetaminophen 160 mg	Children's Tylenol by McNeil	Canadian DIN 02241361	Analgesic
160 <> US14	Tab, White, Cap Shaped	Sotalol HCl 160 mg	Sorine by Upsher Smith	00245-0014	Antiarrhythmic
160 <> Z4239	Tab, White, Cap Shaped	Nadolol 160 mg	Corgard by Ivax	00172-4239 Discontinued	Antihypertensive
1605 <> W	Tab, Sugar-Coated	Perphenazine 8 mg	by Schein	00364-2625	Antipsychotic
160MG <> BERLEX	Tab, White, Cap Shaped, Scored	Sotalol 160 mg	Betapace AF by Berlex	50419-0116	Antiarrhythmic
160MG <> BETAPACE	Tab, Light Blue, Cap Shaped, Scored	Sotalol 160 mg	Betapace by Berlex	50419-0106	Antiarrhythmic
161 <> R	Tab, White, Cap Shaped	Ofloxacin 300 mg	Floxin by Dr. Reddy's	55111-0161	Antibiotic
161 <> THERRX	Tab, Oval, Purple, Film-Coated, Scored	Calcium 600 mg, Vitamin D3 600 IU, Vitamin C 25 mg, Folic Acid 0.5 mg, Vitamin B6 12.5 mg	Encora PM by Ther-Rx	64011-0166	Supplement
1611 <> BMS	Tab, White to Off-White, Triangular	Entecavir 0.5 mg	Baraclude by BMS	Canadian DIN 02282224	Antiviral
1611 <> BMS	Tab, White to Off-White, Triangular	Entecavir 0.5 mg	Baraclude by BMS	00003-1611	Antiviral
1612 <> BMS	Tab, Pink, Triangular	Entecavir 1 mg	Baraclude by BMS	00003-1612	Antiviral
162	Tab, White & Yellow, Round	Aluminum Hydroxide 200 mg, Magnesium Hydroxide 200 mg	Maalox by Guardian		Gastrointestinal
162 <> ACS	Tab, Peach, Oval, A over CS	Candesartan Cilexetil 16 mg, Hydrochlorothiazide 12.5 mg	Atacand HCT by AstraZeneca	00186-0162	Antihypertensive; Diuretic
162 <> ACS	Tab, Peach, Oval, A over CS	Candesartan Cilexetil 16 mg, Hydrochlorothiazide 12.5 mg	Atacand HCT by AstraZeneca	17228-0162	Antihypertensive; Diuretic
162 <> R	Tab, Yellow, Cap Shaped	Ofloxacin 400 mg	Floxin by Dr. Reddy's	55111-0162	Antibiotic
162 <> WPPH	Tab, Peach, Diamond Shaped, Scored	Amiloride HCl 5 mg, Hydrochlorothiazide 50 mg	Moduretic by West Point	59591-0162	Antihypertensive; Diuretic

ID FRONT <> BACK	DESCRIPTION FRONT <> BACK	INGREDIENT & STRENGTH	BRAND (or Generic Equiv.) by FIRM	NDC#	CLASS; SCH.
162 <> WPPH	Tab, Peach, Diamond Shaped, Scored	Amiloride HCl 5 mg, Hydrochlorothiazide 50 mg	Moduretic by Endo	60951-0764	Antihypertensive; Diuretic
164	Tab, Beige, Round, Film Coated	Flurbiprofen 50 mg	Ansaid by Caraco	57664-0164	NSAID
164 <> G	Tab, White, Oblong	Carvedilol 12.5 mg	Coreg by Glenmark	68462-0164	Antihypertensive
164PAR	Tab	Benztropine Mesylate 0.5 mg	Cogentin by Schein	00364-0834	Antiparkinson
165	Tab, Beige, Round, Film Coated	Flurbiprofen 100 mg	Ansaid by Caraco	57664-0165	NSAID
165 <> COPLEY	Tab, Oval, White	Ascorbic Acid 17.53 mg, Beta-Carotene 0.56 mg, Calcium Carbonate 249.41 mg, Calcium Pantothenate 4.18 mg, Cholecalciferol 0.25 mg, Cupric Oxide 2.02 mg, Ferrous Fumarate 82.15 mg, Magnesium Oxide 82.93 mg, Niacinamide Ascorbate 8.54 mg, Pyridoxine HCl 2.43 mg, Riboflavin 0.84 mg, Thiamine Mononitrate 1 mg, Vitamin A Acetate 2680 Units, Zinc Oxide 15.56 mg	Enfamil Natalins by Teva	00093-9165 Discontinued	Vitamin
165 <> COPLEY	Tab, Oval, White	Ascorbic Acid 17.53 mg, Beta-Carotene 0.56 mg, Calcium Carbonate 249.41 mg, Calcium Pantothenate 4.18 mg, Cholecalciferol 0.25 mg, Cupric Oxide 2.02 mg, Ferrous Fumarate 82.15 mg, Magnesium Oxide 82.93 mg, Niacinamide Ascorbate 8.54 mg, Pyridoxine HCl 2.43 mg, Riboflavin 0.84 mg, Thiamine Mononitrate 1 mg, Vitamin A Acetate 2680 Units, Zinc Oxide 15.56 mg	Enfamil Natalins by Teva	38245-0165 Discontinued	Vitamin
165PAR	Tab	Benztropine Mesylate 1 mg	Cogentin by Schein	00364-0703	Antiparkinson
166	Tab, White, Cap Shaped, Scored, Film Coated	Metoprolol Tartrate 50 mg	Lopressor by Caraco	57664-0166	Antihypertensive
166	Tab, White, Oblong, Scored	Metoprolol Tartrate 50 mg	Lopressor by Neuman	64579-0071	Antihypertensive
166	Tab, Brown, Oblong	Methenamine Mandelate 0.5 g	Mandelamine by Warner Chilcott	00430-0166	Antibiotic; Urinary Tract
166	Tab, Brown, Oblong	Methenamine Mandelate 0.5 g	Mandelamine by Parke Davis	00430-0166	Antibiotic; Urinary Tract
167	Tab, Purple, Oblong, Film Coated	Methenamine Mandelate 1 g	Mandelamine by Warner Chilcott	00430-0167	Antibiotic; Urinary Tract
167	Tab, White, Cap Shaped, Convex, Scored	Metoprolol Tartrate 100 mg	Lopressor by Caraco	57664-0167	Antihypertensive
167	Tab, White, Oblong, Convex, Scored	Metoprolol Tartrate 100 mg	Lopressor by Neuman	64579-0076	Antihypertensive
167	Tab, White, Oblong, Convex, Scored	Metoprolol Tartrate 100 mg	Lopressor by Qualitest	00603-4628	Antihypertensive
167	Tab, White, Oblong, Convex, Scored	Metoprolol Tartrate 100 mg	Lopressor by Qualitest	00603-4628	Antihypertensive
167	Tab, Purple, Oblong, Film Coated	Methenamine Mandelate 1 g	Mandelamine by Parke Davis	00071-0167	Antibiotic; Urinary Tract
168	Tab, White, Round, Triangular Logo	Nilutamide 50 mg	Nilandron by Aventis	00088-1110 Discontinued	Antiandrogen
168	Tab, White, Round, Triangular Logo	Nilutamide 50 mg	Nilandron by Aventis	12579-0808	Antiandrogen
168D	Tab, White, Round, Triangular Logo <> 168D	Nilutamide 150 mg	Nilandron by Aventis	00088-1111	Antiandrogen
17	Tab, Pink, Oval, Scored	Moexipril 7.5 mg	Univasc by Teva	00093-0017	Antihypertensive
17 <> A	Tab, Blue, Cap Shaped, Film Coated, A <> 1/7	Sertraline HCl 50 mg	Zoloft by Aurobindo	65862-0012	Antidepressant
17 <> ADAMS	Tab	Guaifenesin 600 mg, Pseudoephedrine HCl 60 mg	by Nat Pharmpak	55154-5901	Cold Remedy
17 <> B1	Tab, White, Round, B1 <> 1 over 7	Penicillin V Potassium 500 mg	V-Cillin K by Teva	00093-1173	Antibiotic
17 <> BL	Tab, White, Round, Scored	Penicillin V Potassium 500 mg	Pen*Vee K by UDL	51079-0616	Antibiotic
17 <> BL	Tab, White, Round, Scored	Penicillin V Potassium 500 mg	Pen*Vee K by Talbert	44514-0645	Antibiotic
17 <> BL	Tab, White, Round, Scored	Penicillin V Potassium 500 mg	Pen*Vee K by Teva	00093-1173	Antibiotic
17 <> BL	Tab, White, Round, Scored	Penicillin V Potassium 500 mg	Pen*Vee K by Pharmafab	62542-0724	Antibiotic
17 <> BL	Tab, White, Round, Scored	Penicillin V Potassium 500 mg	Pen*Vee K by St. Mary's Med	60760-0174	Antibiotic
17 <> BL	Tab, White, Round, Scored	Penicillin V Potassium 500 mg	Pen*Vee K by Pharmedix	53002-0202	Antibiotic
17 <> BL	Tab, White, Round, Scored	Penicillin V Potassium 500 mg	Pen*Vee K by Qualitest	00603-5068	Antibiotic
17 <> BL	Tab, White, Round, Scored	Penicillin V Potassium 500 mg	Pen*Vee K by Moore	00839-1766	Antibiotic
17 <> E	Tab, Dark Pink, Round	Benazepril HCl 40 mg	Lotensin by Aurobindo	65862-0118	Antihypertensive
17 <> E	Tab, Dark Pink, Round	Benazepril HCl 40 mg	Lotensin by Aurobindo	65862-0118	Antihypertensive
17 <> M	Tab, Orange, Round, Scored, M <> 1/7	Quinapril HCl 5 mg	Accupril by Mylan	00378-1117	Antihypertensive
17 <> MEDEVA	Tab, Blue, Oblong, Scored	Guaifenesin 600 mg, Pseudoephedrine HCl 60 mg	Deconsal LA by Adams	63824-0017	Cold Remedy
17 <> MEDEVA	Tab, Blue, Oblong, Scored	Guaifenesin 600 mg, Pseudoephedrine 60 mg	Syn Rx by Adams	63824-0308	Cold Remedy
170 <> WPHH	Tab, Bright Yellow, Round	Sulindac 150 mg	by Merck Sharp & Dohme	62904-0170	NSAID

ID FRONT <> BACK	DESCRIPTION FRONT <> BACK	INGREDIENT & STRENGTH	BRAND (or Generic Equiv.) by FIRM	NDC#	CLASS; SCH.
170 <> WPHH	Tab, Bright Yellow, Round	Sulindac 150 mg	by Kaiser	00179-1333	NSAID
170 <> WPPH	Tab, Bright Yellow, Round	Sulindac 150 mg	by West Point	59591-0170	NSAID
170 <> WPPH	Tab, Bright Yellow, Round	Sulindac 150 mg	by Endo	60951-0780	NSAID
1705	Tab, White, Round	Atropine Sulfate 0.025 mg, Diphenoxylate HCl 2.5 mg	Lomotil by Vortech		Antidiarrheal; C V
171 <> SQUIBB	Tab, White, Oval Shaped, Scored	Sulfamethoxazole 800 mg, Trimethoprim 160 mg	by Mutual	53489-0146	Antibiotic
171 <> SQUIBB	Tab, White, Oval Shaped, Scored	Sulfamethoxazole 800 mg, Trimethoprim 160 mg	SMZ TMP 800/160 by Apothecon	59772-0174	Antibiotic
171 <> W	Tab, Green, Hexagon Shaped	Ropinirole HCl 1 mg	Requip by Wockhardt	64679-0171	Antiparkinson
1710 <> PHA	Tab, Yellow, Diamond Shaped, Film Coated	Eplerenone 25 mg	Inspra by Pharmacia		Antihypertensive
1712 <> CARAFATE	Tab, Light Pink, Oblong, Scored	Sucralfate 1 g	Carafate by Giant Food	11146-0041	Gastrointestinal
1712 <> CARAFATE	Tab, Light Pink, Oblong, Scored	Sucralfate 1 g	Carafate by Amerisource	62584-0712	Gastrointestinal
1712 <> CARAFATE	Tab, Light Pink, Oblong, Scored	Sucralfate 1 g	Carafate by Murfreesboro	51129-1166	Gastrointestinal
1712 <> CARAFATE	Tab, Light Pink, Oblong, Scored	Sucralfate 1 g	Carafate by Aventis	00088-1712	Gastrointestinal
1712 <> CARAFATE	Tab, Light Pink, Oblong, Scored	Sucralfate 1 g	Carafate by H J Harkins Co	52959-0052	Gastrointestinal
1712 <> CARAFATE	Tab, Light Pink, Oblong, Scored	Sucralfate 1 g	Carafate by Med Pro	53978-0305	Gastrointestinal
1712 <> CARAFATE	Tab, Light Pink, Oblong, Scored	Sucralfate 1 g	Carafate by Nat Pharmpak	55154-2207	Gastrointestinal
1712 <> CARAFATE	Tab, Light Pink, Oblong, Scored	Sucralfate 1 g	Carafate by Heartland	61392-0606	Gastrointestinal
1712 <> CARAFATE	Tab, Light Pink, Oblong, Scored	Sucralfate 1 g	Carafate by SKB		Gastrointestinal
172 <> M	Tab, White, Round	Metolazone 2.5 mg	Zaroxolyn by UDL	51079-0023	Diuretic
172 <> M	Tab, White, Round	Metolazone 2.5 mg	Zaroxolyn by Mylan	00378-6172	Diuretic
172 <> R	Tab, Green, Oval	Finasteride 5 mg	Proscar by Dr. Reddy's	55111-0172	Antiandrogen
1720 <> PHA	Tab, Pink, Diamond Shaped, Film Coated	Eplerenone 50 mg	Inspra by Pharmacia		Antihypertensive
1721 <> M	Tab, White, Oval, M inside square <> 1721	Acetaminophen 650 mg, Propoxyphene Napsylate 100 mg	Darvocet-N 100 by Mallinckrodt	00406-1721	Analgesic; C IV
172172	Tab, Orange, Oblong	Magnesium 500 mg	Magonate by Fleming	00256-	Supplement
173 <> 93	Tab, White, Round, Film Coated	Leflunomide 10 mg	Arava by Teva	00093-0173	Antiarthritic
173 <> M	Tab, Orange, Round	Metolazone 5 mg	Zaroxolyn by Mylan	00378-6173	Diuretic
173 <> M	Tab, Orange, Round	Metolazone 5 mg	Zaroxolyn by UDL	51079-0024	Diuretic
173 <> MSD	Tab, Green, Squared Cap Shape	Enalapril Maleate 5 mg, Hydrochlorothiazide 12.5 mg	Vaseretic by Biovail	64455-0145	Antihypertensive; Diuretic
173 <> MSD	Tab, Green, Squared Cap Shape	Enalapril Maleate 5 mg, Hydrochlorothiazide 12.5 mg	Vaseretic by Merck-Frosst	Canadian DIN 02242826	Antihypertensive; Diuretic
173 <> MSD	Tab, Green, Squared Cap Shape	Enalapril Maleate 5 mg, Hydrochlorothiazide 12.5 mg	Vaseretic by Merck	00006-0173	Antihypertensive; Diuretic
1730 <> PHA	Tab, Red, Diamond Shaped, Film Coated	Eplerenone 100 mg	Inspra by Searle	00025-1730	Antihypertensive
1739	Tab, Round	Butabarbital 30 mg	Butisol Sodium by Vortech		Sedative/Hypnotic; C III
174	Tab, Pink, Round	Bisacodyl 5 mg	Dulcolax by Perrigo	00113-0174	Gastrointestinal
174	Tab, White, Round	Magnesium Oxide 400 mg	Mag-Ox by Qualitest	00603-0209	Mineral
174 <> 93	Tab, Yellow, Round, Film-Coated	Leflunomide 20 mg	Arava by Teva	00093-0174	Antiarthritic
174 <> M	Tab, Light Green, Round	Metolazone 10 mg	Zaroxolyn by Mylan	00378-6174	Diuretic
174 <> WPPH	Tab, Yellow, Round, Film Coated	Methyldopa 125 mg	by Endo	60951-0775	Antihypertensive
174040MG	Cap, Dark Pink and Salmon	Omeprazole 40 mg	Prilosec by Ranbaxy	63304-0445	Gastrointestinal
175	Cap, Red	Hexavitamin	by West-Ward		Vitamin
175	Cap, Green and Yellow, Black Ink	Paromomycin Sulfate 250 mg	Humatin by Caraco	57664-0175	Antibiotic
175 <> FLINT	Tab, Lilac, Round, Scored	Levothyroxine Sodium 175 mcg	Synthroid by Abbott	Canadian DIN 02172135	Thyroid Hormone
175 <> FLINT	Tab, Lilac, Round, Scored	Levothyroxine Sodium 175 mcg	Synthroid by Abbott	00048-1100	Thyroid Hormone
175 <> FLINT	Tab, Lilac, Round, Scored	Levothyroxine Sodium 175 mcg	Synthroid by Forest	00456-0326	Thyroid Hormone
175 <> FLINT	Tab, Lilac, Round, Scored	Levothyroxine Sodium 175 mcg	Synthroid by Murfreesboro	51129-1643	Thyroid Hormone
175 <> GG339	Tab, Lilac, Cap Shaped, Scored, 175 <> GG over 339	Levothyroxine 175 mcg	Levo-T by Alara	64909-0142	Thyroid Hormone
175 <> GG339	Tab, Lilac, Cap Shaped, Scored, 175 <> GG over 339	Levothyroxine 175 mcg	Levo-T by Sandoz	00781-5188	Thyroid Hormone
175 <> ID	Tab, White, Cap Shaped, Scored	Guaifenesin 600 mg	Robitussin by Iopharm	61646-0125	Expectorant
175 <> SYNTHROID	Tab, Purple, Round, Scored	Levothyroxine Sodium 175 mcg	Synthroid by Abbott	00074-7070	Thyroid Hormone

ID FRONT <> BACK	DESCRIPTION FRONT <> BACK	INGREDIENT & STRENGTH	BRAND (or Generic Equiv.) by FIRM	NDC#	CLASS; SCH.
175 <> T4	Tab, Lilac, Cap Shaped	Levothyroxine Sodium 175 mcg	Levothroid by Forest	00456-1326	Thyroid Hormone
1757	Tab, Pink, Round	Phenobarbital 15 mg	Phenobarbital by Vortech		Sedative/Hypnotic; C IV
1758	Tab, White, Round	Phenobarbital 15 mg	Phenobarbital by Vortech		Sedative/Hypnotic; C IV
1759	Tab, Pink, Round	Phenobarbital 30 mg	by Vortech		Sedative/Hypnotic; C IV
175M	Tab	Levothyroxine Sodium 175 mcg	Levo-T by Mova	55370-0162	Thyroid Hormone
175M	Tab	Levothyroxine Sodium 175 mcg	Euthyrox by Em Pharma	63254-0443	Thyroid Hormone
175M <> Z	Tab, Purple, Round, Scored	Levothyroxine Sodium 175 mcg	Levo-T by Zoetica	64909-0111	Thyroid Hormone
175MCG	Tab, Debossed	Levothyroxine Sodium 175 mcg	Eltroxin by GSK	53873-0120	Thyroid Hormone
175MCG <> FLINT	Tab, Purple, Round, Scored	Levothyroxine Sodium 0.175 mg	Synthroid by Rightpac	65240-0758	Thyroid Hormone
176	Tab, White to Off White, Cap Shaped	Hydrocodone Bitartrate 10 mg, Acetaminophen 325 mg	Norco by Caraco	57664-0176	Analgesic; C III
176 <> WC	Tab, White, Cap Shaped, Scored, Ex Release	Isosorbide Mononitrate 60 mg	Imdur by Warner Chilcott	00047-0176	Antianginal
176 <> WPPH	Tab, Yellow, Round, Film Coated	Methyldopa 500 mg	by Merck	00006-0176	Antihypertensive
176 <> WPPH	Tab, Yellow, Round, Film Coated	Methyldopa 500 mg	by Endo	60951-0777	Antihypertensive
1761	Tab, White, Round	Phenobarbital 30 mg	by Vortech		Sedative/Hypnotic; C IV
177	Tab, Off-White to Light Yellow, Mottled, Round	Sapropterin Dihydrochloride 100 mg	Kuvan by BioMarin	68135-0300	Phenylketonuria Treatment
177	Tab, Off-White to Light Yellow, Mottled, Round	Sapropterin Dihydrochloride 100 mg	Kuvan by BioMarin	Canadian DIN 02350580	Phenylketonuria Treatment
177 <> REVIA	Tab, Pale Yellow, Cap Shaped, Scored	Naltrexone 50 mg	Revia by Apotex	Canadian DIN 02213826	Opioid Antagonist
1772	Tab, White, Round	Phenobarbital 16 mg	by Vortech		Sedative/Hypnotic; C IV
1772 <> M	Tab, Pink, Oval, M inside square	Acetaminophen 650 mg, Propoxyphene Napsylate 100 mg	Darvocet-N 100 by Mallinckrodt	00406-1772	Analgesic; C IV
1772 <> MARION	Tab, Coated	Diltiazem HCl 60 mg	Cardizem by Drug Distr	52985-0191	Antihypertensive
1778	Tab, Round	Phenobarbital, Hyoscyamine, Atropine	Hypnaldyne by Vortech		Gastrointestinal; C IV
1779	Tab, Round	Colchicine 0.6 mg	Colsalide Improved by Vortech		Antigout
179 <> WPPH	Tab, Salmon, Round, Film Coated	Hydrochlorothiazide 15 mg, Methyldopa 250 mg	by Merck	00006-0179	Diuretic; Antihypertensive
179 <> WPPH	Tab, Salmon, Round, Film Coated	Hydrochlorothiazide 15 mg, Methyldopa 250 mg	by Endo	60951-0778	Diuretic; Antihypertensive
1796180MG	Cap, Blue & Light Blue	Diltiazem HCl 180 mg	Cardizem CD by Marion		Antihypertensive
1797240MG	Cap, Blue	Diltiazem HCl 240 mg	Cardizem CD by Marion		Antihypertensive
1798300MG	Cap, 1798/300 mg	Diltiazem HCl 300 mg	Cardizem by Murfreesboro	51129-9732	Antihypertensive
17BL	Tab, Film Coated	Penicillin V Potassium 500 mg	by Med Pro	53978-5055	Antibiotic
18	Tab, White, Round, 1/8	Clonazepam 0.125 mg	Klonopin Wafers by Hoffmann La Roche	00004-0279	Sedative; C IV
18	Tab, White to Off-White, Round, Film Coated, Scored	Quinapril HCl 5 mg	Accupril by Teva	00093-5456 Discontinued	Antihypertensive
18 <> A	Tab, Yellow, Cap Shaped, Film Coated, A <> 1 / 8	Sertraline HCl 100 mg	Zoloft by Aurobindo	65862-0013	Antidepressant
18 <> B94	Tab, White to Off-White, Round, 1/8, b over 94, Orally Disintegrating	Clonazepam 0.125 mg	Klonopin Wafers by Barr	00555-0094	Sedative; C IV
18 <> BI	Tab, Reddish Orange, Sugar Coated	Dipyridamole 50 mg	by Nat Pharmpak	55154-0402	Antiplatelet
18 <> BI	Tab, Reddish Orange, Sugar Coated	Dipyridamole 50 mg	Persantine-50 by Boehringer Ingelheim	00597-0018	Antiplatelet
18 <> BL	Tab, Off-White, Round	Neomycin Sulfate 500 mg	by Teva	00093-1177 Discontinued	Antibiotic
18 <> D	Tab, Pink, Oval, Scored	Hydrochlorothiazide 12.5 mg, Quinapril 10 mg	Accuretic by Aurobindo	65862-0161	Diuretic; Antihypertensive
18 <> F	Tab, White to Off-White, Round	Alendronate Sodium 10 mg	Fosamax by Aurobindo	65862-0327	Antiosteoporosis
180	Tab, White, Round	Norgestimate 0.180 mg, Ethinyl Estradiol 0.025 mg	Tri-Cyclen LO 21 by Janssen-Ortho	Canadian DIN 02258560	Oral Contraceptive
180	Tab, White, Round	Norgestimate 0.180 mg, Ethinyl Estradiol 0.025 mg	Tri-Cyclen LO 28 by Janssen-Ortho	Canadian DIN 02258587	Oral Contraceptive
180	Cap, Green and White	Diltiazem HCl 180 mg	Tiazac by Inwood	00258-3688	Antihypertensive

ID FRONT <> BACK	DESCRIPTION FRONT <> BACK	INGREDIENT & STRENGTH	BRAND (or Generic Equiv.) by FIRM	NDC#	CLASS; SCH.
180 <> B	Tab, White, Cap Shaped, Ex Release	Diltiazem HCl 180 mg	Cardizem LA by Biovail	64455-0101	Antihypertensive
180 <> B	Tab, White, Cap Shaped, Ex Release	Diltiazem HCl 180 mg	Tiazac XC by Biovail	Canadian DIN 02256746	Antihypertensive
180 <> OM	Tab, White, Round, O-M 180	Ethinyl Estradiol 0.025 mg, Norgestimate 0.180 mg	Ortho Tri-Cyclen Lo by Ortho-McNeil	00062-1251	Oral Contraceptive
180 <> STARLIX	Tab, Red, Oval, Film-Coated	Nateglinide 180 mg	Starlix by Novartis	Canadian DIN 02245440	Antidiabetic
180010	Cap, Clear, 18-0010	Potassium Chloride 750 mg	K-Norm by Penwalt		Electrolytes
180605 <> G	Tab, 1806, 1806 0.5 <> G	Lorazepam 0.5 mg	Ativan by Royce	51875-0240	Antianxiety; C IV
18060 5240 <> 005	Tab, 1806.05-240 <> 0.05	Lorazepam 0.5 mg	Ativan by Ivax	00182-1806	Antianxiety; C IV
18060 5G	Tab	Lorazepam 1 mg	Ativan by Ivax	00182-1807	Antianxiety; C IV
18071 <> G	Tab	Lorazepam 1 mg	Ativan by Royce	51875-0241	Antianxiety; C IV
18082 <> G	Tab	Lorazepam 2 mg	Ativan by Royce	51875-0242	Antianxiety; C IV
180MG <> ISOPTINSR	Tab, Light Pink, Oval, Scored, Film Coated	Verapamil HCl 180 mg	Isoptin SR by Abbott	00044-1825	Antihypertensive
180MGANDRX549	Cap, Gray & White	Diltiazem HCl 180 mg	Cardizem by Kaiser	00179-1375	Antihypertensive
180MGANDRX598	Cap, Orange & Yellow, Ex Release	Diltiazem HCl 180 mg	Cartia XT by Heartland	61392-0958	Antihypertensive
180MGANDRX598	Cap, Orange & Yellow, Ex Release	Diltiazem HCl 180 mg	Cartia XT by Andrx	62037-0598	Antihypertensive
180MGDILACORXR	Cap	Diltiazem HCl 180 mg	Dilacor by Kaiser		Antihypertensive
180WATSON663	Cap, Pink & White, 180/Watson/663	Diltiazem HCl 180 mg	Dilacor XR by Watson	62224-9339	Antihypertensive
181	Tab, Yellow, Oval, Film Coated	Trandolapril 1 mg, Verapamil HCl 180 mg	Tarka by Abbott	Canadian	Antihypertensive
181 <> G	Tab, White, Round	Flavoxate HCl 100 mg	Urispas by Global	00115-1811	Antispasmodic
181 <> RDY	Tab, Beige, Cap Shaped, Scored	Levetiracetam 250 mg	Keppra by Dr. Reddy's	55111-0181	Anticonvulsant
1812	Tab, Round	Benzthiazide 50 mg	Aquatag by Vortech	Discontinued	Diuretic; Antihypertensive
182	Tab, Pink, Oval, Film Coated, Ex Release, Triangle 182	Trandolapril 2 mg, Verapamil 180 mg	Tarka by Abbott	00074-3287	Antihypertensive
182	Tab, Pink, Oval, Film Coated, Ex Release, Triangle 182	Trandolapril 2 mg, Verapamil 180 mg	Tarka by Abbott	00048-5921	Antihypertensive
182	Tab, Pink, Oval, Film Coated, Ex Release, Triangle 182	Trandolapril 2 mg, Verapamil 180 mg	Tarka by Knoll	00048-5921	Antihypertensive
182	Tab, Pink, Oval, Film Coated, Ex Release, Triangle 182	Trandolapril 2 mg, Verapamil 180 mg	Tarka by Abbott	Canadian DIN 02238096	Antihypertensive
182 <> RDY	Tab, Beige, Cap Shaped, Scored, 1 / 82 <> RDY	Levetiracetam 500 mg	Keppra by Dr. Reddy's	55111-0182	Anticonvulsant
182 <> TARKA	Tab, Pink, Oval, Film Coated	Trandolapril 2 mg, Verapamil 180 mg	Tarka by Abbott	00044-5921	Antihypertensive
183	Tab, Yellow, Cap Shaped, Scored, Film Coated	Oxcarbazepine 150 mg	Trileptal by Caraco	62756-0183	Anticonvulsant
183 <> 44	Tab, White, Round	Aspirin 325 mg	Aspirin by Ivax	00182-1909 Discontinued	Analgesic
183 <> R	Tab, Coated	Dipyridamole 50 mg	by Vangard	00615-1573	Antiplatelet
183 <> RDY	Tab, Beige, Cap Shaped, Scored	Levetiracetam 750 mg	Keppra by Dr. Reddy's	55111-0183	Anticonvulsant
184	Tab, Yellow, Cap Shaped, Scored, Film Coated	Oxcarbazepine 300 mg	Trileptal by Caraco	62756-0184	Anticonvulsant
1840	Tab, Round	Nitrofurantoin 50 mg	Furatoin by Vortech		Antibiotic
184Q	Cap, Buff, 184/Q	Doxepin HCl 10 mg	Sinequan by Quantum		Antidepressant
185	Tab, Yellow, Cap Shaped, Scored, Film Coated	Oxcarbazepine 600 mg	Trileptal by Caraco	62756-0185	Anticonvulsant
185 <> BEECHAM	Tab	Penicillin V Potassium	by SKB		Antibiotic
185Q	Ivory & White, 185/Q	Doxepin HCl 25 mg	Sinequan by Quantum		Antidepressant
186 <> COP	Tab, Chewable	Fluoride Ion .25 mg	Luride by Colgate	00126-0186	Mineral
186QPL	Cap, Ivory, 186/QPL	Doxepin HCl 50 mg	Sinequan by Quantum		Antidepressant
187 <> PAR	Tab, Film Coated	Hydrochlorothiazide 25 mg, Methyldopa 250 mg	by Par	49884-0187	Diuretic; Antihypertensive
1876	Tab, Round	Phentermine HCl 8 mg	Phentrol by Vortech		Anorexiant; C IV
1879	Tab, Yellow, Round	Phendimetrazine 35 mg	Weightrol by Vortech		Anorexiant; C III
187Q	Cap, Green, 187/Q	Doxepin HCl 75 mg	Sinequan by Quantum		Antidepressant
188 <> COPLEY	Tab, Pink, Cap Shaped, Scored, Film Coated, Ex Release	Procainamide HCl 500 mg	Procan SR by Ivax	00182-1708	Antiarrhythmic
188 <> COPLEY	Tab, Pink, Cap Shaped, Scored, Film Coated, Ex Release	Procainamide HCl 500 mg	Procan SR by Qualitest	00603-5411	Antiarrhythmic

ID FRONT <> BACK	DESCRIPTION FRONT <> BACK	INGREDIENT & STRENGTH	BRAND (or Generic Equiv.) by FIRM	NDC#	CLASS; SCH.
188 <> COPLEY	Tab, Pink, Cap Shaped, Scored, Film Coated, Ex Release	Procainamide HCl 500 mg	Procan SR by Moore	00839-7028	Antiarrhythmic
188 <> COPLEY	Tab, Pink, Cap Shaped, Scored, Film Coated, Ex Release	Procainamide HCl 500 mg	Procan SR by Teva	00093-9188 Discontinued	Antiarrhythmic
188 <> COPLEY	Tab, Pink, Cap Shaped, Scored, Film Coated, Ex Release	Procainamide HCl 500 mg	Procan SR by URL Mutual	00677-0987	Antiarrhythmic
188 <> PAR	Tab, Coated	Hydrochlorothiazide 30 mg, Methyldopa 500 mg	by Par	49884-0188	Diuretic; Antihypertensive
1886	Tab, Round	Propantheline Bromide 15 mg	Pro-Banthine by Vortech		Gastrointestinal
1893 <> 93	Tab, Blue, Oval, Film Coated	Etodolac 500 mg	Lodine by Teva	00093-1893	NSAID
19 <> BI	Tab, Sugar Coated	Dipyridamole 75 mg	Persantine-75 by Boehringer Ingelheim	00597-0019	Antiplatelet
19 <> BL	Tab, Yellow, Round	Imipramine HCl 10 mg	Tofranil by Teva	00093-2111	Antidepressant
19 <> D	Tab, Pink, Round, Film Coated	Hydrochlorothiazide 12.5 mg, Quinapril 20 mg	Accuretic by Aurobindo	65862-0162	Diuretic; Antihypertensive
19 <> F	Tab, White to Off-White, Oval	Alendronate Sodium 35 mg	Fosamax by Aurobindo	65862-0328	Antiosteoporosis
19 <> RE	Tab, White, Round	Atenolol 25 mg	Tenormin by Ranbaxy	63304-0621	Antihypertensive
19 <> WYETH	Tab, Orange, Round, Scored	Promethazine 12.5 mg	Phenergan by Wyeth	00008-0019	Antiemetic; Antihistamine
190 <> GG	Tab, White, Round, Scored	Methocarbamol 500 mg	Robaxin by Sandoz	00781-1760	Muscle Relaxant
1908	Tab, White, Round	Orphenadrine Citrate 100 mg	Norflex by Vortech		Muscle Relaxant
190JC <> E2NOM	Tab, White, Round, 1/90 J-C <> E2/N O-M	Estradiol 1 mg, Norgestimate 0.09 mg	Ortho-Prefest by Ortho-McNeil	00062-1840	Hormone
191 <> GG	Tab, Blue, Round	Amoxapine 100 mg	Asendin by Sandoz	00781-1846	Antidepressant
1911 <> G	Tab, Orange, Oval, Film Coated	Rimantadine HCl 10 mg	Flumadine by Global	00115-1911	Antiviral
1915	Tab, Round	Hydrochlorothiazide 50 mg	Hydrodiuril by Vortech		Diuretic; Antihypertensive
1919PRINIVIL	Tab, White, Shield Shaped	Lisinopril 20 mg	Prinivil by MSD	Canadian	Antihypertensive
192 <> R	Tab, Pink, Oval	Fexofenadine 30 mg	Allegra by Dr. Reddy's	55111-0192	Antihistamine
192 <> WPPH	Tab, Light Blue, Round	Timolol Maleate 5 mg	Blocadren by West Point	59591-0192	Antihypertensive
192 <> WPPH	Tab, Light Blue, Round	Timolol Maleate 5 mg	Blocadren by Endo	60951-0782	Antihypertensive
1922	Tab, Round	Brompheniramine Maleate 12 mg, Phenylephrine HCl 15 mg, Phenylpropanolamine HCl 15 mg	Normatane TD by Vortech		Cold Remedy
192Q	Cap, Green & White, 192-Q	Temazepam 15 mg	Restoril by Quantum		Sedative/Hypnotic; C IV
193 <> R	Tab, Pink, Oval	Fexofenadine HCl 60 mg	Allegra by Dr. Reddy's	55111-0193	Antihistamine
1934	Cap, Red & Clear, Savage Logo 1934	Chlorpheniramine Maleate 8 mg, Pseudoephedrine HCl 120 mg	Brexin LA by Savage	00281-1934	Cold Remedy
193PAR	Cap	Flurazepam HCl 15 mg	by Qualitest		Hypnotic; C IV
193Q	Cap, White, 193-Q	Temazepam 30 mg	Restoril by Quantum	00603-3691	Sedative/Hypnotic; C IV
194 <> R	Tab, Pink, Oval	Fexofenadine HCl 180 mg	Allegra by Dr. Reddy's	55111-0194	Antihistamine
194 <> WPPH	Tab, Light Blue, Round	Timolol Maleate 10 mg	Blocadren by Endo	60951-0783	Antihypertensive
194 <> WPPH	Tab, Light Blue, Round	Timolol Maleate 10 mg	by West Point	59591-0194	Antihypertensive
1945	Tab, Round	Trichlormethiazide 4 mg	Marazide II by Vortech		Diuretic; Antihypertensive
194PAR	Cap	Flurazepam HCl 30 mg	by Qualitest	00603-3692	Hypnotic; C IV
195 <> THERRX	Tab, Peach, Cap Shaped, Film Coated	Vitamin C 50 mg, Vitamin D3 6 mcg, Vitamin E 3.5 IU, Vitamin B1 3 mg, Vitamin B2 3.4 mg, Vitamin B3 20 mg, Vitamin B6 50 mg, Folic Acid 1 mg, Vitamin B12 12 mcg, Calcium 250 mg, Iron 30 mg, Magnesium 25 mg, Zinc 15 mg, Copper 2 mg, Docusate Sodium 50 mg, Succinic Acid 35 mg	PreCare Premier by Ther-Rx	64011-0195	Supplement
195 <> WPPH	Tab, Peach, Cap Shaped, Film Coated	Diflunisal 250 mg	by Endo	60951-0768	NSAID
196 <> WPPH	Tab, Orange, Cap Shaped, Film Coated	Diflunisal 500 mg	by Quality Care	60346-0053	NSAID
196 <> WPPH	Tab, Orange, Cap Shaped, Film Coated	Diflunisal 500 mg	by Endo	60951-0769	NSAID
196 <> WPPH	Tab, Orange, Cap Shaped, Film Coated	Diflunisal 500 mg	by H J Harkins Co	52959-0379	NSAID
197 <> COPLEY	Tab, Dark Red, Chewable	Ascorbic Acid 34.47 mg, Cholecalciferol 0.194 mg, Cupric Oxide 1.25 mg, Cyanocobalamin 4.9 mcg, Ferrous Fumarate 36.48 mg, Folic Acid 0.35 mg, Niacinamide 14.16 mg, Pyridoxine HCl 1.1 mg, Riboflavin 1.258 mg, Sodium Fluoride 1.1 mg, Thiamine Mononitrate 1.15 mg, Vitamin A Acetate 5.5 mg, Vitamin E Acetate 15.75 mg, Zinc Oxide 12.5 mg	Polyvitamin by Schein	00364-2506	Vitamin
197 <> RDY	Tab, Brown, Round, Film Coated	Simvastatin 5 mg	Zocor by Dr. Reddy's	55111-0197	Antihyperlipidemic

ID FRONT <> BACK	DESCRIPTION FRONT <> BACK	INGREDIENT & STRENGTH	BRAND (or Generic Equiv.) by FIRM	NDC#	CLASS; SCH.
197 <> S	Tab, White Round	Inert	Seasonale by Duramed	51285-0058	Oral Contraceptive; Placebo
197 <> THERRX	Tab, Maroon, Cap Shaped, Film Coated, Ther-Rx <> 197	Iron 151 mg (Iron Sumalate 50 mg) (Iron Fumarate 101 mg), Succinic Acid 50 mg, Vitamin C 60.8 mg (Ascorbic Acid 60 mg) (Threonic Acid 0.8 mg), Folic Acid 1 mg, Vitamin B12 10 mcg	Chromagen Forte by Ther-Rx	64011-0197	Supplement
1975	Tab, Round	Triprolidine 2.5 mg, Pseudoephedrine 60 mg	Actifed by Vortech		Cold Remedy
198 <> RDY	Tab, Brown, Round, Film Coated	Simvastatin 10 mg	Zocor by Dr. Reddy's	55111-0198	Antihyperlipidemic
198 <> THERRX	Tab, Maroon, Cap Shaped, Film Coated, Ther-Rx <> 198	Iron 70 mg, Succinic Acid 75 mg, Vitamin C 152 mg (Ascorbic Acid 150 mg) (Threonic Acid 2 mg), Vitamin B12 10 mcg, Desiccated Stomach Substance 50 mg	Chromagen by Ther-Rx	64011-0198	Supplement
199 <> 93	Tab, Peach, Round, Scored, Mottled	Venlafaxine HCl 25 mg	Effexor by Teva	00093-0199	Antidepressant
199 <> RDY	Tab, Brown, Round, Film Coated	Simvastatin 20 mg	Zocor by Dr. Reddy's	55111-0199	Antihyperlipidemic
199 <> THERRX	Tab, Green, Cap Shaped, Film Coated, Ther-Rx <> 199	Iron 70 mg, Succinic Acid 75 mg, Vitamin C 152 mg (Ascorbic Acid 150 mg) (Threonic Acid 2 mg), Folic Acid 1 mg, Vitamin B12 10 mcg	Chromagen FA by Ther-Rx	64011-0199	Supplement
1998	Tab, Oblong	Methocarbamol 750 mg	Robaxin by Vortech		Muscle Relaxant
19WYETH	Tab	Promethazine HCl 12.5 mg	by Wyeth		Antiemetic; Antihistamine
1AHR <> TENEX	Tab, Light Pink, Diamond Shaped, AHR imprinted inside 1	Guanfacine HCl 1 mg	Tenex by A H Robins	00031-8901	Antihypertensive
1AHR <> TENEX	Tab, Light Pink, Diamond Shaped, AHR imprinted inside 1	Guanfacine HCl 1 mg	Tenex by Nat Pharmpak	55154-3008	Antihypertensive
1AHR <> TENEX	Tab, Light Pink, Diamond Shaped, AHR imprinted inside 1	Guanfacine HCl 1 mg	Tenex by Rightpac	65240-0748	Antihypertensive
1AHR <> TENEX	Tab, Light Pink, Diamond Shaped, AHR imprinted inside 1	Guanfacine HCl 1 mg	Tenex by Amerisource	62584-0901	Antihypertensive
1AHR <> TENEX	Tab, Light Pink, Diamond Shaped, AHR imprinted inside 1	Guanfacine HCl 1 mg	Tenex by Leiner	59606-0748	Antihypertensive
1AHR <> TENEX	Tab, Light Pink, Diamond Shaped, AHR imprinted inside 1	Guanfacine HCl 1 mg	Tenex by Pharmedix	53002-1045	Antihypertensive
1D300	Cap, Blue and Clear	Chlorpheniramine Maleate 8 mg, Pseudoephedrine HCl 120 mg	De Congestine by Qualitest	00603-3143	Cold Remedy
1JC <> E2OM	Tab, Pink, Round, 1 J-C <> E2 O-M	Estradiol 1 mg	Ortho-Prefest by Ortho-McNeil	00062-1840	Hormone
1KLONOPIN <> ROCHE	Tab, Blue, Round, K perforation	Clonazepam 1 mg	Klonopin by Hoffmann La Roche	00004-0058	Sedative; C IV
1LLL11	Tab, Yellow, Round	Levothyroxine Sodium 0.1 mg	Synthroid by Lederle		Thyroid Hormone
1MG <> 503	Tab, White to Off-White, Round	Guanfacine 1 mg	Intuniv by Shire	54092-0513	Non-Stimulant Anti-ADHD
1MG <> 511	Tab, White, Pentagon	Lorazepam 1 mg	Ativan by Wyeth	52903-5812	Antianxiety; C IV
1MG <> CARDURA	Tab, White, Oblong, Scored	Doxazosin Mesylate 1 mg	Cardura by Roerig	00049-2750	Antihypertensive
1MG <> ETH266	Tab, Gray, Oblong	Doxazosin Mesylate 1 mg	Cardura by Ethex	58177-0266	Antihypertensive
1MG <> MLP16	Tab, Gray, Oblong, Scored	Doxazosin Mesylate 1 mg	Cardura by Dava	67253-0380	Antihypertensive
1MGF617	Cap, White, Red Ink	Anhydrous Tacrolimus 1 mg	Prograf by Astellas	Canadian DIN 02175991	Immunosuppressant
1P96	Tab	Guaifenesin 400 mg, Phenylpropanolamine HCl 75 mg	Entex LA by Major	00904-3264	Cold Remedy
1R	Cap, Beige, Oval, Opaque, Soft Gel	Terazosin HCl 1 mg	Hytrin by Ranbaxy	63304-0662	Antihypertensive
1W	Tab, White, Round, 1/W	Lorazepam 1 mg	Ativan by Wyeth	Canadian	Antianxiety; C IV
2	Cap, Blue-Green, White Print, Ex Release	Tolterodine 2 mg	Detrol LA by Pharmacia	00009-5190	Urinary Tract
2	Tab, Yellow, Oval	Dextrothyroxine Sodium 2 mg	Choloxin by Boots		Thyroid Hormone
2	Tab, White, Round	Clonazepam 2 mg	Klonopin Wafers by Hoffmann La Roche	00004-0283	Sedative; C IV
2	Cap, Blue-Green, White Print, Ex Release	Tolterodine 2 mg	Detrol LA by Pfizer	Canadian DIN 02244612	Urinary Tract
2	Tab, Orange, Buccal	Fentanyl 200 mcg	Fentora by Cephalon	63459-0542	Opioid Agonist; C II
2	Tab, Round, Peach, Coated	Folic (Folic Acid) 2.5 mg, Pyridoxine (B6) 25 mg, Cyanocobalamin (B12) 1 mg	Folbalin by Red River Pharma	12593-0040 Discontinued	Vitamin; Supplement
2	Tab, White, Round	Nitro Tab 0.4 mg	by Teva	55953-0295 Discontinued	Vasodilator
2	Tab, Off-White to White, Round, Ex Release	Nitroglycerin 2 mg	Nitrogard 2 by Forest	00456-0687	Vasodilator
2	Tab	Nitroglycerin 2 mg	Sustachron ER Buccal by Forest	10418-0137	Vasodilator
2	Tab, White, Round	Nitroglycerin 0.4 mg (1/150 gr)	Nitrostat by Able	53265-0250 Discontinued	Vasodilator

ID FRONT <> BACK	DESCRIPTION FRONT <> BACK	INGREDIENT & STRENGTH	BRAND (or Generic Equiv.) by FIRM	NDC#	CLASS; SCH.
2	Tab, Gray, Round, Schering Logo/2	Perphenazine 2 mg	Trilafon by Schering	Canadian	Antipsychotic
2	Tab, White, Round	Perphenazine 2 mg	Apo Perphenazine by Apotex	Canadian DIN 00335134	Antipsychotic
2	Tab, Blue, Round	Trifluoperazine HCl 2 mg	Apo Trifluoperazine by Apotex	Canadian DIN 00312754	Antipsychotic
2	Tab, Blue and White, Triangular, Bilayered, Scored, Star Logo 2	Guaifenesin 120 mg IR, Phenylephrine HCl 5 mg IR, Guaifenesin 195 mg SR, Phenylephrine HCl 15 mg SR	Liquibid-PD by Capellon	64543-0246	Cold Remedy
2	Tab, Yellow, Round	Methotrimeprazine Maleate 2 mg	Methoprazine by Apotex	Canadian DIN 02238403	Antipsychotic
2	Tab, Pink, Round	Fluphenazine HCl 2 mg	Fluphenazine by Apotex	Canadian DIN 00410632	Antipsychotic
2	Tab, White, Round, Vanda Logo <> 2	Iloperidone 2 mg	Fanapt by Vanda	43068-0102	Antipsychotic
2 <> 107	Tab, Pale Yellow, Round	Trandolapril 2 mg	Mavik by Dava	67253-0107	Antihypertensive
2 <> 2063V	Tab	Acetaminophen 300 mg, Codeine Phosphate 15 mg	Tylenol w/ Codeine by PDRX	55289-0449	Analgesic; C III
2 <> 242	Tab	Lorazepam 2 mg	Ativan by Qualitest	00603-4245	Antianxiety; C IV
2 <> 256	Tab, White, Round	Betahistine DiHCl 8 mg	Serc by Solvay	Canadian DIN 02240601	Antivertigo
2 <> 275	Tab, White, Round, Scored	Clonazepam 2 mg	Klonopin by Caraco	57664-0275	Sedative; C IV
2 <> 3686	Tab, White, Round, Scored, Hourglass Logo 2	Doxazosin Mesylate 2 mg	Cardura by Ivax	00172-3686	Antihypertensive
2 <> 4037	Tab, Pink, Square, Hourglass Logo 2	Estazolam 2 mg	Prosom by Ivax	00172-4037	Sedative/Hypnotic; C IV
2 <> 521	Tab, White, Round, AstraZeneca Logo 521 <> 2	Acetaminophen 300 mg, Codeine Phosphate 15 mg	Tylenol w/ Codeine by AstraZeneca	62037-0521	Analgesic; C III
2 <> 54570	Tab, White, Hexagonal, Scored, 54 over 570	Haloperidol 2 mg	Haldol by Roxane	00054-8344	Antipsychotic
2 <> 54743	Tab, White, Round, Scored, 54 over 743	Hydromorphone HCl 2 mg	Dilaudid by Roxane	00054-8392	Analgesic; C II
2 <> 9350	Tab, White, Round, 93 over 50	Acetaminophen 300 mg, Codeine Phosphate 15 mg	Tylenol w/ Codeine by Teva	00093-0050	Analgesic; C III
2 <> A	Tab, Orange, Round, Abbott Logo (a)	Hydromorphone HCl 2 mg	Dilaudid by Abbott	00074-2415	Analgesic; C II
2 <> ALVA	Tab, Dark Red, Round	Magnesium Salicylate 162.5 mg, Pamabrom 25 mg	Diurex Caffeine Free by Alva		Analgesic; Diuretic
2 <> ATIVAN	Tab, White, Oval	Lorazepam 2 mg	Ativan by Wyeth	Canadian DIN 02041448	Antianxiety; C IV
2 <> B305	Tab, White, Round, Scored	Acetaminophen 300 mg, Codeine Phosphate 15 mg	Tylenol w/ Codeine by Barr	00555-0305	Analgesic; C III
2 <> B493	Tab, Blue, Round, b over 493, Ex Release	Alprazolam 2 mg	Xanax XR by Barr	00555-0493	Antianxiety; C IV
2 <> CPI	Tab, CPI Logo	Phenobarbital 30 mg	Phenobarbital by Century	00436-0870	Sedative/Hypnotic; C IV
2 <> CPI	Tab, CPI Logo	Phenobarbital 30 mg	Phenobarbital by Century	00436-0129	Sedative/Hypnotic; C IV
2 <> CPI	Tab, CPI Logo	Phenobarbital 30 mg	Phenobarbital by Century	00436-0869	Sedative/Hypnotic; C IV
2 <> DAN5621	Tab, White, Round, Scored	Diazepam 2 mg	Valium by DRX	55045-2652	Antianxiety; C IV
2 <> DAN5621	Tab, White, Round, Scored	Diazepam 2 mg	Valium by Murfreesboro	51129-1302	Antianxiety; C IV
2 <> DAN5621	Tab, White, Round, Scored	Diazepam 2 mg	Valium by Vangard	00615-1532	Antianxiety; C IV
2 <> DAN5621	Tab, White, Round, Scored	Diazepam 2 mg	Valium by Watson	00591-5621	Antianxiety; C IV
2 <> DRL100	Tab, White, Oval	Nefazodone HCl 100 mg	Serzone by Par	49884-0917	Antidepressant
2 <> DRL100	Tab, White, Oval	Nefazodone HCl 100 mg	Serzone by Dr. Reddy's	55111-0139	Antidepressant
2 <> E	Tab, Blue, Round, Film Coated	Hydromorphone HCl 2 mg	Dilaudid by Ethex	58177-0298	Analgesic; C II
2 <> G	Tab, Blue, Round, Ex Release	Alprazolam 2 mg	Xanax XR by Greenstone	59762-0066	Antianxiety; C IV
2 <> G	Tab, White, Round, Scored	Estradiol 2 mg	by AAI Pharma	27280-0006	Hormone
2 <> G	Tab, White, Round, Scored	Estradiol 2 mg	by Teva	00093-1059 Discontinued	Hormone
2 <> GG53	Tab, Lavender, Round, Film Coated, GG over 53	Trifluoperazine HCl 2 mg	Stelazine by Sandoz	00781-1032	Antipsychotic
2 <> INV279	Tab, Purple, Round, Film Coated	Trifluoperazine HCl 2 mg	by Invamed	52189-0279	Antipsychotic
2 <> INV310	Tab, Lavender, Square, Scored, INV over 310	Warfarin Sodium 2 mg	Coumadin by Sandoz	00781-0363	Anticoagulant
2 <> INV310	Tab, Lavender, Square, Scored, INV over 310	Warfarin Sodium 2 mg	Coumadin by Apothecon	59772-0363	Anticoagulant
2 <> KC	Tab, White, Round, Film Coated	Pitavastatin 2 mg	Livalo by Kowa Pharmaceuticals	00002-4771	Antihyperlipidemic

ID FRONT <> BACK	DESCRIPTION FRONT <> BACK	INGREDIENT & STRENGTH	BRAND (or Generic Equiv.) by FIRM	NDC#	CLASS; SCH.
2 <> M	Tab, White, Round	Hydromorphone HCl 2 mg	Dilaudid by Murfreesboro	51129-1465	Analgesic; C II
2 <> M	Tab, White, Round, M inside a square <> 2	Acetaminophen 300 mg, Codeine Phosphate 15 mg	Tylenol w/ Codeine by Mallinckrodt	00406-0483	Analgesic; C III
2 <> M	Tab, White, Round	Hydromorphone HCl 2 mg	Dilaudid by Mallinckrodt	00406-3243	Analgesic; C II
2 <> MCNEIL	Tab, White, Round, McNeil	Acetaminophen 300 mg, Caffeine 15 mg, Codeine Phosphate 15 mg	Tylenol w/ Codeine by Janssen-Ortho	Canadian DIN 02163934	Analgesic; C III
2 <> MP111	Tab	Acetaminophen 300 mg, Codeine Phosphate 15 mg	Tylenol w/ Codeine by Pharmedix	53002-0122	Analgesic; C III
2 <> MP111	Tab	Acetaminophen 300 mg, Codeine Phosphate 15 mg	Tylenol w/ Codeine by URL Mutual	00677-0611	Analgesic; C III
2 <> N	Tab, Peach, Round	Terazosin HCl 2 mg	Hytrin by Novopharm	Canadian DIN 02230806	Antihypertensive
2 <> N	Tab, Pink, Round, Scored, Large N	Haloperidol 2 mg	Haldol by Novopharm	Canadian DIN 00363669	Antipsychotic
2 <> N125	Tab, White, 2 <> N over 125	Alprazolam 2 mg	Xanax by Teva	55953-8125	Antianxiety; C IV
2 <> N480	Tab, White, Round, Scored, N over 480 <> 2	Albuterol Sulfate 2 mg	Proventil by Heartland	61392-0567	Antiasthmatic
2 <> N480	Tab, White, Round, Scored, N over 480 <> 2	Albuterol Sulfate 2 mg	Proventil by Teva	55953-0480	Antiasthmatic
2 <> N480	Tab, White, Round, Scored, N over 480 <> 2	Albuterol Sulfate 2 mg	Proventil by Amerisource	62584-0821	Antiasthmatic
2 <> N480	Tab, White, Round, Scored, N over 480 <> 2	Albuterol Sulfate 2 mg	Proventil by Anabolic	00722-6436	Antiasthmatic
2 <> N480	Tab, White, Round, Scored, N over 480 <> 2	Albuterol Sulfate 2 mg	Proventil by Apotheca	12634-0090	Antiasthmatic
2 <> N480	Tab, White, Round, Scored, N over 480 <> 2	Albuterol Sulfate 2 mg	Proventil by Warner Chilcott	00047-0956	Antiasthmatic
2 <> N593	Tab, White to Off-White, Cap Shaped, Scored	Doxazosin Mesylate 2 mg	Cardura by Teva	00093-8121	Antihypertensive
2 <> NN	Tab, White, Oblong, Scored, N / N	Doxazosin Mesylate 2 mg	Cardura by Novopharm	Canadian DIN 02242729	Antihypertensive
2 <> NN	Tab, White, Round, Scored, N / N <> 2	Clonazepam 2 mg	Rivotril by Novopharm	Canadian DIN 02239025	Anticonvulsant
2 <> NOVO	Tab, White, Round, Scored	Prazosin HCl 2 mg	Minipress by Novopharm	Canadian DIN 01934201	Antihypertensive
2 <> P	Tab, Orange, Round	Terazosin HCl 2 mg	Hytrin by Pharmascience	Canadian DIN 02243519	Antihypertensive
2 <> PAL	Tab, Peach, Round	Folic Acid 2.5 mg, Pyridoxine HCl 25 mg, Cyanocobalamin 1 mg	Foltx by Pamlab	00525-0855 Discontinued	Vitamin
2 <> PMS	Tab, Pale Orange, Round, Scored	Hydromorphone HCl 2 mg	by Pharmascience	Canadian DIN 00885436	Analgesic; C II
2 <> SB	Tab, Pink, Pentagonal	Rosiglitazone Maleate 2 mg	Avandia by SKB	00029-3158	Antidiabetic
2 <> SB	Tab, Pink, Pentagonal, Film Coated	Rosiglitazone Maleate 2 mg	Avandia by GSK	Canadian DIN 02241112	Antidiabetic
2 <> SP324	Tab, White, Round, Scored, Orally Disintegrating	Alprazolam 2 mg	Niravam by Schwarz	00091-3324	Antianxiety; C IV
2 <> U	Tab, White, Round	Pramipexole DiHCl 0.125 mg	Mirapex by Boehringer Ingelheim	00597-0083	Antiparkinson
2 <> U	Tab, White, Round	Pramipexole DiHCl 0.125 mg	Mirapex by Pharmacia	00009-0002	Antiparkinson
2 <> U	Tab, White, Round	Pramipexole DiHCl 0.125 mg	Mirapex by Promex Med	62301-0026	Antiparkinson
2 <> V2063	Tab, White, V-Scored, Round	Acetaminophen 300 mg, Codeine Phosphate 15 mg	Tylenol w/ Codeine by Vintage	00254-2063	Analgesic; C III
2 <> W	Tab, Blue, Round, Sublingual	Lorazepam 2 mg	Ativan by Wyeth	Canadian DIN 02041472	Antianxiety; C IV
2 <> WARFARINTARO	Tab, Lavender, Cap Shaped	Warfarin Sodium 2 mg	Coumadin by Taro	51672-4028	Anticoagulant
2 <> X	Tab, Blue, Round, Ex Release	Alprazolam 2 mg	Xanax XR by Pharmacia	00009-0066	Antianxiety; C IV
2 <> XANAX	Tab, White, Cap Shaped, Scored, Film Coated	Alprazolam 2 mg	Xanax by Pharmacia	Canadian	Antianxiety; C IV
2 <> XANAX	Tab, White, Cap Shaped, Scored, Film Coated	Alprazolam 2 mg	Xanax by Pharmacia	00009-0094	Antianxiety; C IV
2 <> Z3925	Tab, White, Round, Scored, Z over 3925	Diazepam 2 mg	Valium by Ivax	00172-3925	Antianxiety; C IV
2 <> Z3925	Tab, White, Round, Scored, Z over 3925	Diazepam 2 mg	Valium by Kaiser	00179-1085	Antianxiety; C IV
2 <> Z3925	Tab, White, Round, Scored, Z over 3925	Diazepam 2 mg	Valium by Ivax	00182-1755	Antianxiety; C IV
2 <> Z4234	Tab, Peach, Round, Scored, Z over 4234	Bumetanide 2 mg	Bumex by Teva	00093-4234	Diuretic
2 <> Z4234	Tab, Peach, Round, Scored, Z over 4234	Bumetanide 2 mg	Bumex by Ivax	00182-2617	Diuretic
2 <> Z4234	Tab, Peach, Round, Scored, Z over 4234	Bumetanide 2 mg	Bumex by Major	00904-5104	Diuretic

ID FRONT <> BACK	DESCRIPTION FRONT <> BACK	INGREDIENT & STRENGTH	BRAND (or Generic Equiv.) by FIRM	NDC#	CLASS; SCH.
2 <> Z4234	Tab, Peach, Round, Scored, Z over 4234	Bumetanide 2 mg	Bumex by Murfreesboro	51129-1383	Diuretic
2 <> Z4234	Tab, Peach, Round, Scored, Z over 4234	Bumetanide 2 mg	Bumex by Ivax	00172-4234 Discontinued	Diuretic
2 <> Z4234	Tab, Peach, Round, Scored, Z over 4234	Bumetanide 2 mg	Bumex by Sandoz	00781-1823	Diuretic
2 <> Z4234	Tab, Peach, Round, Scored, Z over 4234	Bumetanide 2 mg	Bumex by Caraco		Diuretic
20	Tab, White, Cap Shaped, Film Coated, four point star <> 20	Valdecoxib 20 mg	Bextra by Searle	00025-1980 Discontinued	COX 2 Inhibitor
20	Tab, Orange, Round, Ex Release, Andrx Logo 20	Lovastatin 20 mg	Altoprev by Andrx	62022-0628	Antihyperlipidemic
20	Tab, Yellow, Round, Orally Disintegrating	Olanzapine 20 mg	Zyprexa Zydis by Eli Lilly	00002-4456	Antipsychotic
20	Tab, Rose	Nifedipine 20 mg	Adalat 20 by Bayer	Canadian	Antihypertensive
20	Cap, Opaque & Pink	Omeprazole 20 mg	Prilosec by AstraZeneca	Canadian	Gastrointestinal
20	Tab, Light Green, Octagonal, Film Coated, Extended Release	Oxymorphone HCl 20 mg	Opana ER by Endo	63481-0617	Analgesic; C II
20	Tab, White, Oval, Film-Coated, Scored	Citalopram HBr 20 mg	Celexa by Pharmascience	Canadian DIN 02248010	Antidepressant
20	Cap, White, Opaque, Santarus Triangle logo 20	Omeprazole 20 mg, Sodium Bicarbonate 1100 mg	Zegerid by Santarus	68012-0102	Gastrointestinal
20 <> 0014	Tab, Yellow, Rectangular	Pravastatin Sodium 20 mg	Pravachol by Watson	00591-0014	Antihyperlipidemic
20 <> 1010	Tab, Tan, Oval, Film Coated	Citalopram 20 mg	Celexa by Torrent	13668-0010	Antidepressant
20 <> 104	Tab, White, Oval, Scored, Boehringer Logo 104 <> 20	Torsemide 20 mg	Demadex by Teva	00480-0147	Diuretic
20 <> 104	Tab, White, Oval, Scored, Boehringer Logo 104 <> 20	Torsemide 20 mg	Demadex by Compumed	00403-0715	Diuretic
20 <> 104	Tab, White, Oval, Scored, Boehringer Logo 104 <> 20	Torsemide 20 mg	Demadex by Hoffmann La Roche	00004-0264	Diuretic
20 <> 104	Tab, White, Oval, Scored, Boehringer Logo 104 <> 20	Torsemide 20 mg	Demadex by Nat Pharmpak	55154-0405	Diuretic
20 <> 104	Tab, White, Oval, Scored, Boehringer Logo 104 <> 20	Torsemide 20 mg	Demadex by Caremark	00339-6012	Diuretic
20 <> 256	Tab	Baclofen 20 mg	Lioresal by Qualitest	00603-2409	Muscle Relaxant
20 <> 2729	Tab, Off-White, Oval	Fosinopril Sodium 20 mg	Monopril by Sandoz	00781-5084	Antihypertensive
20 <> 4198	Tab, Peach, Round	Enalapril Maleate 20 mg	Vasotec by Ivax	00172-4198 Discontinued	Antihypertensive
20 <> 4198	Tab, Peach, Round, Hourglass Logo over 4198	Enalapril Maleate 20 mg	Vasotec by Ivax		Antihypertensive
20 <> 4626	Tab, White, Round, Film Coated, Ivax Logo 20	Doxycycline Hyclate 20 mg	Periostat by Ivax	00172-4626	Antibiotic
20 <> 4741	Tab, Light Pink, Cap Shaped, Scored	Citalopram HBr 20 mg	Celexa by Ivax	00172-4741 Discontinued	Antidepressant
20 <> 5352	Tab, Pink, Oblong, Hourglass Logo 5352	Benazepril HCl 20 mg	Lotensin by Ivax	00172-5352 Discontinued	Antihypertensive
20 <> 54690	Tab, White, Hexagonal, Scored, 54 over 690	Haloperidol 20 mg	Haldol by Roxane	00054-8347	Antipsychotic
20 <> 5657	Tab, White, Round	Tamoxifen Citrate 20 mg	Nolvadex by Ivax	00172-5657 Discontinued	Antiestrogen
20 <> 5728	Tab, Beige, Round, Hourglass Logo 20	Famotidine 20 mg	Pepcid by Ivax	00172-5728	Gastrointestinal
20 <> 5728	Tab, Beige, Round	Famotidine 20 mg	Pepcid by Teva	00172-5728	Histamine H2 Antagonist
20 <> 7815	Tab, White, Cap Shaped, Film Coated	Valdecoxib 20 mg	Bextra by Pfizer	Canadian DIN 02246622 Discontinued	COX 2 Inhibitor
20 <> A	Tab, White to Off-White, Round	Lisinopril 2.5 mg	Zestril by Aurobindo	65862-0037	Antihypertensive
20 <> ABG	Tab, Pink, Round, Controlled Release	Oxycodone HCl 20 mg	OxyContin by Ivax	00172-6355	Analgesic; C II
20 <> AD	Tab, Orange, Round, Scored	Mixed Amphetamine Salts 20 mg: Amphetamine Aspartate 5 mg, Amphetamine Sulfate 5 mg, Dextroamphetamine Saccharate 5 mg, Dextroamphetamine Sulfate 5 mg	Adderall by DRX	55045-2608	Stimulant; C II
20 <> AD	Tab, Orange, Round, Scored	Mixed Amphetamine Salts 20 mg: Amphetamine Aspartate 5 mg, Amphetamine Sulfate 5 mg, Dextroamphetamine Saccharate 5 mg, Dextroamphetamine Sulfate 5 mg	Adderall by Shire	58521-0033	Stimulant; C II
20 <> AMIDE010	Tab, White, Round	Isoxsuprine HCl 20 mg	Vasodilan by Ivax	00182-1056	Vasodilator
20 <> AMIDE010	Tab, White, Round	Isoxsuprine HCl 20 mg	Vasodilan by Amide	52152-0010	Vasodilator

ID FRONT <> BACK	DESCRIPTION FRONT <> BACK	INGREDIENT & STRENGTH	BRAND (or Generic Equiv.) by FIRM	NDC#	CLASS; SCH.
20 <> AMIDE010	Tab, Amide 010	Isoxsuprine HCl 20 mg	Vasodilan by Qualitest	00603-4147	Vasodilator
20 <> AO	Tab, Coated	Salsalate 750 mg	by Quality Care	60346-0034	NSAID
20 <> APO	Tab, White, Oval, Film Coated	Citalopram 20 mg	Celexa by Apotex	Canadian DIN 02246056	Antidepressant
20 <> APO	Tab, Grayish Pink, Round	Nifedipine 20 mg	Nifed PA by Apotex	Canadian DIN 02181525	Antihypertensive
20 <> APO	Tab, Peach, Shield-Shaped	Simvastatin 20 mg	Zocor by Apotex	Canadian DIN 02247013	Antihyperlipidemic
20 <> APO	Tab, Yellow, Oval, Film Coated	Tenoxicam 20 mg	Mobiflex by Apotex	Canadian DIN 02230661	NSAID
20 <> APO	Tab, Pink, Oblong, Scored	Paroxetine HCl 20 mg	Paxil by Apotex	Canadian DIN 02240908	Antidepressant
20 <> B352	Tab, Yellow, Round, Film Coated	Leflunomide 20 mg	Arava by Barr	005555-0352	Antiarthritic
20 <> B973	Tab, Peach, Oval, Scored, b over 973, 2 over 0	Mixed Amphetamine Salts 20 mg: Amphetamine Aspartene 5 mg, Amphetamine Sulfate 5 mg, Dextroamphetamine Saccharate 5 mg, Dextroamphetamine Sulfate 5 mg	Adderall by Barr	005555-0973	Stimulant; C II
20 <> BAYER	Tab, Orange, Round, Film-Coated, BAYER BAYER in cross	Vardenafil HCl 20 mg	Levitra by Bayer	Canadian DIN 02250489	Impotence Agent
20 <> BAYER	Tab, Orange, Round, Film-Coated, BAYER BAYER in cross	Vardenafil HCl 20 mg	Levitra by Bayer	00026-8740	Impotence Agent
20 <> BL	Tab, Salmon, Round, Coated	Imipramine HCl 25 mg	Tofranil by Teva	00093-2113	Antidepressant
20 <> BL	Tab, Salmon, Round, Coated	Imipramine HCl 25 mg	Tofranil by Schein	00364-0406	Antidepressant
20 <> BL	Tab, Salmon, Round, Coated	Imipramine HCl 25 mg	Tofranil by UDL	51079-0080	Antidepressant
20 <> D	Tab, Pink, Round, Film Coated	Hydrochlorothiazide 25 mg, Quinapril 20 mg	Accuretic by Aurobindo	65862-0163	Diuretic; Antihypertensive
20 <> DAN5555	Tab, Blue, Round, Scored, DAN over 5555	Propranolol HCl 20 mg	Inderal by Rx Pak	65084-0101	Antihypertensive
20 <> DAN5555	Tab, Blue, Round, Scored, DAN over 5555	Propranolol HCl 20 mg	Inderal by Schein	00364-0757	Antihypertensive
20 <> DAN5555	Tab, Blue, Round, Scored, DAN over 5555	Propranolol HCl 20 mg	Inderal by Watson	00591-5555	Antihypertensive
20 <> DAN5555	Tab, Blue, Round, Scored, DAN over 5555	Propranolol HCl 20 mg	Inderal by Vangard	00615-2562	Antihypertensive
20 <> DAN5731	Tab, White, Round, Scored	Baclofen 20 mg	Lioresal by Watson	00591-5731	Muscle Relaxant
20 <> DAN5731	Tab, White, Round, Scored	Baclofen 20 mg	Lioresal by Schein	00364-2313	Muscle Relaxant
20 <> DAN5731	Tab, White, Round, Scored	Baclofen 20 mg	Lioresal by Amerisource	62584-0624	Muscle Relaxant
20 <> E531	Tab, White, Round	Isoxsuprine HCl 20 mg	Vasodilan by Eon	00185-0531	Vasodilator
20 <> E703	Tab, Pink, Round, Coated, Extended Release	Oxycodone HCl 20 mg	OxyContin by Endo	60951-0703	Analgesic; C II
20 <> EFF	Tab	Methazolamide 50 mg	Neptazane by Mikart	46672-0109	Antiglaucoma Agent
20 <> ETH	Tab, White, Cap Shaped, Scored, Ex Release	Potassium Chloride 20 mEq	by Ethex	58177-0202	Electrolytes
20 <> FL	Tab, White to Off-White, Round, Scored, Film Coated	Escitalopram Oxalate 20 mg	Lexapro by Forest	00456-2020	Antidepressant
20 <> G020	Tab, Brown, Round, Film Coated	Quinapril HCl 20 mg	Accupril by Greenstone	59762-5021	Antihypertensive
20 <> G5	Tab, Yellow, Rounded Rectangular	Pravastatin Sodium 20 mg	Pravachol by Glenmark	68462-0196	Antihyperlipidemic
20 <> INV236	Tab, White, Round, Scored, INV over 236	Nadolol 20 mg	Corgard by Ivax	00182-2632	Antihypertensive
20 <> INV236	Tab, White, Round, Scored, INV over 236	Nadolol 20 mg	Nadolol by Schein	00364-2652	Antihypertensive
20 <> INV236	Tab, White, Round, Scored, INV over 236	Nadolol 20 mg	Nadolol by Invamed	52189-0236	Antihypertensive
20 <> INV236	Tab, White, Round, Scored, INV over 236	Nadolol 20 mg	Nadolol by Sandoz	00781-1181	Antihypertensive
20 <> INV236	Tab, White, Round, Scored, INV over 236	Nadolol 20 mg	Nadolol by Moore	00839-7869	Antihypertensive
20 <> INV236	Tab, White, Round, Scored	Nadolol 20 mg	Nadolol by Major	00904-5069	Antihypertensive
20 <> KU107	Tab, White, Round, Scored	Isosorbide Mononitrate 20 mg	Ismo by Physician Total Care	54868-3822	Antianginal
20 <> KU107	Tab, White, Round, Scored	Isosorbide Mononitrate 20 mg	Ismo by Kremers Urban	62175-0107	Antianginal
20 <> L540	Tab, Orange, Oval, Film-Coated	Simvastatin 20 mg	Zocor by Perrigo	45802-0384	Antihyperlipidemic
20 <> LOTENSIN	Tab, Beige, Round, Film Coated	Benazepril HCl 20 mg	Lotensin by PDRX	55289-0086	Antihypertensive
20 <> LOTENSIN	Tab, Beige, Round, Film Coated	Benazepril HCl 20 mg	Lotensin by Amerisource	62584-0079	Antihypertensive
20 <> LOTENSIN	Tab, Beige, Round, Film Coated	Benazepril HCl 20 mg	Lotensin by Novartis	00078-0449	Antihypertensive
20 <> LUPIN	Tab, Dark Pink, Round	Lisinopril 20 mg	Zestril by Lupin	68180-0515	Antihypertensive

For updated data, go to www.IdentADrug.com

ID FRONT <> BACK	DESCRIPTION FRONT <> BACK	INGREDIENT & STRENGTH	BRAND (or Generic Equiv.) by FIRM	NDC#	CLASS; SCH.
20 <> M	Tab, White, Round, Scored, M in a double circle <> 20	Dicyclomine HCl 20 mg	Bentylol by Axcan	Canadian DIN 02103095	Gastrointestinal
20 <> M	Tab, White to Cream Colored, Octagon, M inside square	Mixed Amphetamine Salts 20 mg: Dextroamphetamine Saccharate 5 mg, Amphetamine Aspartate 5 mg, Dextroamphetamine Sulfate 5 mg, Amphetamine Sulfate 5 mg	Adderall by Mallinckrodt	00406-8893	Stimulant; C II
20 <> M	Tab, White, Round, Scored, M inside square <> 20 above Score	Methylphenidate HCl 20 mg	Ritalin by Mallinckrodt	00406-1124	Stimulant; C II
20 <> M	Tab, White, Round, Scored, M inside square <> 20 above Score	Methylphenidate HCl 20 mg	Ritalin by Neuman		Stimulant; C II
20 <> MC	Tab, M/C	Isoxsuprine HCl 20 mg	Vasodilan by Shire	58521-0576	Vasodilator
20 <> MJ544	Tab, White, Round, Scored	Isoxsuprine HCl 20 mg	Vasodilan by BMS	00087-0544	Vasodilator
20 <> MYLAN183	Tab, Blue, Round, Scored, Mylan over 183	Propranolol HCl 20 mg	Inderal by Mylan	00378-0183	Antihypertensive
20 <> MYLAN183	Tab, Blue, Round, Scored, Mylan over 183	Propranolol HCl 20 mg	Inderal by UDL	51079-0278	Antihypertensive
20 <> N	Tab, Light Orange, Shield Shaped	Simvastatin 20 mg	Zocor by Novopharm	Canadian DIN 02250160	Antihyperlipidemic
20 <> N	Tab, Cream, Rounded Square	Pravastatin Sodium 20 mg	Pravachol by Novopharm	Canadian DIN 02247009	Antihyperlipidemic
20 <> N	Tab, Blue, Hexagonal, Scored, N <> 2/0	Propranolol HCl 20 mg	Inderal by Novopharm	Canadian DIN 00740675	Antihypertensive
20 <> N	Tab, Pink, Oval, Scored, N <> 2/0	Paroxetine HCl 20 mg	Paxil by Novopharm	Canadian DIN 02248557	Antidepressant
20 <> N	Tab, Dark Pink, Round, Scored, Large N	Haloperidol 20 mg	Haldol by Novopharm	Canadian DIN 00768820	Antipsychotic
20 <> N	Tab, Orange, Round, Scored, Film Coated	Isosorbide Dinitrate 20 mg, Hydralazine HCl 37.5 mg	BiDil by NitroMed	12948-0001	Antianginal; Antihypertensive
20 <> N	Tab, White, Oblong	Fosinopril Sodium 20 mg	Monopril by Novopharm	Canadian DIN 02247803	Antihypertensive
20 <> N	Tab, White, Shield Shaped	Leflunomide 20 mg	Arava by Novopharm	Canadian DIN 02261278	Antiarthritic
20 <> NN	Tab, Blue, Octagonal, 20 <> N/N	Lovastatin 20 mg	Mevacor by Novopharm	Canadian DIN 02246542	Antihyperlipidemic
20 <> NN	Tab, White, Oval, Scored, N / N <> 20	Citalopram 20 mg	Celexa by Novopharm	Canadian DIN 02251558	Antidepressant
20 <> NOVO	Tab, Beige, D-Shaped, Novo/20	Famotidine 20 mg	Pepcid by Novopharm	Canadian DIN 02022133	Gastrointestinal
20 <> NOVO	Tab, Light Blue, Oblong, NO/VO <> 20	Timolol Maleate 20 mg	Blocadren by Novopharm	Canadian DIN 01947826	Antihypertensive
20 <> NU	Tab, Grayish-Pink, Round, Film Coated	Nifedipine 20 mg	by Nu Pharm	Canadian DIN 02200937	Antihypertensive
20 <> OC	Tab, Pink, Round, Film Coated	Oxycodone HCl 20 mg	OxyContin by Purdue	59011-0103	Analgesic; C II
20 <> P	Tab, Pink, Oval, Scored, P Logo <> 2 / 0	Paroxetine HCl 20 mg	Paxil by Pharmascience	Canadian DIN 02247751	Antidepressant
20 <> P	Tab, Beige, Shield Shaped	Simvastatin 20 mg	Zocor by Pharmascience	Canadian DIN 02269279	Antihyperlipidemic
20 <> P	Tab, White, Triangle Shaped	Leflunomide 20 mg	ARAVA by Pharmascience	Canadian DIN 02288273	Antiarthritic
20 <> PAR653	Tab, White, Round, Scored	Torsemide 20 mg	Demadex by Par	49884-0653	Diuretic
20 <> PAXIL	Tab, Pink, Oblong, Film Coated	Paroxetine HCl 20 mg	Paxil by GSK	Canadian DIN 01940481	Antidepressant
20 <> PAXIL	Tab, Pink, Oblong, Film Coated	Paroxetine HCl 20 mg	Paxil by Kaiser	00179-1182	Antidepressant
20 <> PAXIL	Tab, Pink, Oblong, Film Coated	Paroxetine HCl 20 mg	Paxil by Allscripts		Antidepressant

ID FRONT <> BACK	DESCRIPTION FRONT <> BACK	INGREDIENT & STRENGTH	BRAND (or Generic Equiv.) by FIRM	NDC#	CLASS; SCH.
20 <> PAXIL	Tab, Pink, Oblong, Film Coated	Paroxetine HCl 20 mg	Paxil by Nat Pharmpak	55154-4504	Antidepressant
20 <> PAXIL	Tab, Pink, Oblong, Film Coated	Paroxetine HCl 20 mg	Paxil by H J Harkins Co	52959-0360	Antidepressant
20 <> PAXIL	Tab, Pink, Oblong, Film Coated	Paroxetine HCl 20 mg	Paxil by Amerisource	62584-0211	Antidepressant
20 <> PAXIL	Tab, Pink, Oblong, Film Coated	Paroxetine HCl 20 mg	Paxil by SB	59742-3211	Antidepressant
20 <> PAXIL	Tab, Pink, Oblong, Film Coated	Paroxetine HCl 20 mg	Paxil by Kaiser	62224-2340	Antidepressant
20 <> PAXIL	Tab, Pink, Oblong, Film Coated	Paroxetine HCl 20 mg	Paxil by SKB	00029-3211	Antidepressant
20 <> PD156	Tab, White, Oval, Film Coated	Atorvastatin Calcium 20 mg	Lipitor by Pharm Util	60491-0804	Antihyperlipidemic
20 <> PD156	Tab, White, Oval, Film Coated	Atorvastatin Calcium 20 mg	Lipitor by Parke Davis	Canadian DIN 02230713	Antihyperlipidemic
20 <> PD156	Tab, White, Oval, Film Coated	Atorvastatin Calcium 20 mg	Lipitor by Parke Davis	00071-0156	Antihyperlipidemic
20 <> PD156	Tab, White, Oval, Film Coated	Atorvastatin Calcium 20 mg	Lipitor by Goedecke	53869-0156	Antihyperlipidemic
20 <> PD156	Tab, White, Oval, Film Coated	Atorvastatin Calcium 20 mg	Lipitor by Physician Total Care	54868-3946	Antihyperlipidemic
20 <> PD532	Tab, Brown, Round, Film Coated, PD over 532	Quinapril HCl 20 mg	Accupril by PDRX	55289-0554	Antihypertensive
20 <> PD532	Tab, Brown, Round, Film Coated, PD over 532	Quinapril HCl 20 mg	Accupril by Parke Davis	00071-0532	Antihypertensive
20 <> PD532	Tab, Brown, Round, Film Coated, PD over 532	Quinapril HCl 20 mg	Accupril by Parke Davis	Canadian DIN 01947680	Antihypertensive
20 <> PF	Tab, White, Cap Shaped	Morphine Sulfate 20 mg	MS Contin by Purdue	Canadian	Analgesic; C II
20 <> SCHWAR2620	Tab, White, Round, Scored	Isosorbide Mononitrate 20 mg	Monoket by Schwarz	00091-3620	Antianginal
20 <> SCHWAR2620	Tab, White, Round, Scored	Isosorbide Mononitrate 20 mg	Monoket by Heartland	61392-0630	Antianginal
20 <> SP352	Tab, White, Round, Orally Disintegrating, SP above Score, 352 below	Baclofen 20 mg	Kemstro by Schwarz	00091-3352	Muscle Relaxant
20 <> TARO	Tab, Tan, Shield-Shaped, Film-Coated	Simvastatin 20 mg	Zocor by Taro	Canadian DIN 02265893	Antihyperlipidemic
20 <> VISTA065	Tab, White, Round, Scored	Isoxsuprine HCl 20 mg	Vasodilan by Vista	61970-0066	Vasodilator
20 <> VISTA065	Tab, White, Round, Convex, Scored	Isoxsuprine HCl 20 mg	Vasodilan by Murfreesboro	51129-1587	Vasodilator
20 <> VISTA065	Tab, Coated, Embossed	Isoxsuprine HCl 20 mg	Vasodilan by Vista	61970-0065	Vasodilator
20 <> WATSON334	Tab, 2.0, <> Watson 334	Lorazepam 2 mg	Ativan by Watson	00781-1403	Antianxiety; C IV
20 <> Z4097	Tab, White, Round, Scored, Z over 4097	Baclofen 20 mg	Lioresal by Ivax	00172-4097	Muscle Relaxant
20 <> Z4097	Tab, White, Round, Scored, Z over 4097	Baclofen 20 mg	Lioresal by Med Pro	53978-3167	Muscle Relaxant
20 <> Z4097	Tab, White, Round, Scored, Z over 4097	Baclofen 20 mg	Lioresal by UDL	51079-0284	Muscle Relaxant
20 <> Z4097	Tab, White, Round, Scored, Z over 4097	Baclofen 20 mg	Lioresal by Baker Cummins	63171-1296	Muscle Relaxant
20 <> Z4097	Tab, White, Round, Scored, Z over 4097	Baclofen 20 mg	Lioresal by Rx Dispensing	61807-0131	Muscle Relaxant
20 <> Z4097	Tab, White, Round, Scored, Z over 4097	Baclofen 20 mg	Lioresal by Major	00904-5222	Muscle Relaxant
20 <> Z4097	Tab, White, Round, Scored, Z over 4097	Baclofen 20 mg	Lioresal by Ivax	00182-1296	Muscle Relaxant
20 <> Z4235	Tab, White, Round, Z over 4235	Nadolol 20 mg	Corgard by Ivax	00093-4235	Antihypertensive
20 <> Z4235	Tab, White, Round, Z over 4235	Nadolol 20 mg	Corgard by Ivax	00182-2632	Antihypertensive
200	Cap, White	Etodolac 200 mg	by ESI Lederle		NSAID
200	Tab, Yellow, Cap Shaped	Ibuprofen 200 mg	Motrin by Apotex	Canadian	NSAID
200	Cap, White, Ex Release, Printed in Red	Theophylline Anhydrous 200 mg	Slo-Bid by RPR	00801-0200	Antiasthmatic
200	Tab, Buff, Round, Savage Logo 200	Pancrelipase 400 mg, Lipase 400 mg, Protease NLT 400 mg, Amylase NLT 400 mg	Ilozyme by Savage	00281-2001	Gastrointestinal
200	Tab, White, Diamond Shaped	Cimetidine HCl 200 mg	Tagamet HB 200 by SKB		Gastrointestinal
200	Tab, Pink, Round, Scored	Levothyroxine Sodium 200 mcg	Eltroxin by GSK	Canadian DIN 02213222	Thyroid Hormone
200	Tab, White, Round, Hourglass Logo <> 200	Cimetidine HCl 200 mg	Tagamet by Ivax	00182-2660 Discontinued	Gastrointestinal
200	Tab, Pink, Trapezoid-Shaped	Fluconazole 200 mg	Diflucan by Glenmark	68462-0104	Antifungal
200	Tab, Pink, Round, 200 <> Cobalt Logo	Topiramate 200 mg	Topamax by Cobalt	Canadian DIN 02287781	Antimigraine
200 <> 0122	Tab, Pink, Capsule Shaped	Topiramate 200 mg	Topamax by Dava	67253-0754	Anticonvulsant

ID FRONT <> BACK	DESCRIPTION FRONT <> BACK	INGREDIENT & STRENGTH	BRAND (or Generic Equiv.) by FIRM	NDC#	CLASS; SCH.
200 <> 3RP	Tab, Light Blue, Cap-Shaped, Film-Coated	Ribavirin 200 mg	Copegus by Three Rivers	66435-0102	Antiviral
200 <> 4334	Tab, Peach, Oval, Logo 4334 <> 200	Nefazodone 200 mg	Serzone by Ivax	00172-4334	Antidepressant
200 <> 4365	Tab, White, Round, Hourglass Logo 4365	Labetalol HCl 200 mg	Trandate by Ivax	00182-8203 Discontinued	Antihypertensive
200 <> 4365	Tab, White, Round, Hourglass Logo 4365	Labetalol HCl 200 mg	Trandate by Ivax	00172-4365	Antihypertensive
200 <> 4405	Tab, Pale Yellow, Oval, Hourglass Logo over 4405, Scored	Clozapine 200 mg	Clozaril by Teva	00093-4405	Antipsychotic
200 <> 4431	Tab, White, Round, Ivax Hourglass Logo 200 mcg	Misoprostol 200 mcg	Cytotec by Ivax	00172-4431	Gastrointestinal
200 <> 5413	Tab, Pink, Oval, Ival Logo 200	Fluconazole 200 mg	Diflucan by Ivax	00172-5413	Antifungal
200 <> 832	Tab, Butterscotch Yellow, Sugar Coated	Chlorpromazine HCl 200 mg	by Qualitest	00603-2812	Antipsychotic
200 <> 832	Tab, Butterscotch Yellow, Sugar Coated	Chlorpromazine HCl 200 mg	by Schein	00364-0384	Antipsychotic
200 <> 832	Tab, Coated	Chlorpromazine HCl 200 mg	by URL Mutual	00677-0787	Antipsychotic
200 <> ABG	Tab, Green, Oblong, Convex, Film Coated	Morphine Sulfate 200 mg	MS Contin by Novartis	00043-0148	Analgesic; C II
200 <> ALTI200	Tab, Pink, Round, Scored	Amiodarone 200 mg	Cordarone by AltiMed	Canadian DIN 02240071	Antiarrhythmic
200 <> APO	Tab, Light Yellow, Oval	Ofloxacin 200 mg	Apo Ofloxacin by Apotex	Canadian DIN 02231529	Antibiotic
200 <> APO	Tab, White, Round, Biconvex, SR	Ketoprofen 200 mg	Orudis by Apotex	Canadian DIN 02172577	NSAID
200 <> APO	Tab, Pink, Round	Amiodarone HCl 200 mg	Pacerone by Apotex	Canadian	Antiarrhythmic
200 <> BAYER	Tab, Red, Round, Film Coated, Bayer Cross <> 200	Sorafenib 200 mg	Nexavar by Bayer	Canadian DIN 02284227	Cancer Treatment
200 <> BAYER	Tab, Red, Round, Film Coated, Bayer Cross <> 200	Sorafenib 200 mg	Nexavar by Bayer	00026-8488	Cancer Treatment
200 <> C	Tab, Pink, Round	Amiodarone 200 mg	Cordarone by Wyeth	52903-4188	Antiarrhythmic
200 <> CP	Tab, Light Green, Oblong, Scored	Guaifenesin 600 mg, Potassium Guaiacolsulfonate 300 mg	Humibid LA by Carolina	68249-0200	Cold Remedy
200 <> CTD	Tab, White, Oblong	Cimetidine HCl 200 mg	QC Heartburn by Chain Drug	63868-0519	Gastrointestinal
200 <> DP	Tab	Levothyroxine Sodium 200 mcg	Levoxyl by Jones	52604-1112	Thyroid Hormone
200 <> E	Tab, Brown, Oval, Extended Release	Morphine Sulfate 200 mg	MS Contin by Ethex	58177-0380	Analgesic; C II
200 <> E659	Tab, Green, Oval, Ex Release	Morphine Sulfate 200 mg	MS Contin by Endo	60951-0659	Analgesic; C II
200 <> FLINT	Tab, Pink, Round, Scored	Levothyroxine Sodium 200 mcg	Synthroid by Abbott	Canadian DIN 02172143	Thyroid Hormone
200 <> FLINT	Tab, Pink, Round, Scored	Levothyroxine Sodium 200 mcg	Synthroid by Med Pro	53978-0856	Thyroid Hormone
200 <> FLINT	Tab, Pink, Round, Scored	Levothyroxine Sodium 200 mcg	Synthroid by Murfreesboro	51129-1654	Thyroid Hormone
200 <> FLINT	Tab, Pink, Round, Scored	Levothyroxine Sodium 200 mcg	Synthroid by Abbott	00048-1140	Thyroid Hormone
200 <> FLINT	Tab, Pink, Round, Scored	Levothyroxine Sodium 200 mcg	Synthroid by Forest	00456-0327	Thyroid Hormone
200 <> FLINT	Tab, Pink, Round, Scored	Levothyroxine Sodium 200 mcg	Synthroid by Kaiser	00179-0460	Thyroid Hormone
200 <> FLINT	Tab, Pink, Round, Scored	Levothyroxine Sodium 200 mcg	Synthroid by Rx Pak	65084-0160	Thyroid Hormone
200 <> FLINT	Tab, Pink, Round, Scored	Levothyroxine Sodium 200 mcg	Synthroid by Wal Mart	49035-0172	Thyroid Hormone
200 <> FLINT	Tab, Pink, Round, Scored	Levothyroxine Sodium 200 mcg	Synthroid by Nat Pharmpak	55154-0907	Thyroid Hormone
200 <> FLINT	Tab, Pink, Round, Scored	Levothyroxine Sodium 200 mcg	Synthroid by Rite Aid	11822-5194	Thyroid Hormone
200 <> FLINT	Tab, Pink, Round, Scored	Levothyroxine Sodium 200 mcg	Synthroid by Giant Food	11146-0306	Thyroid Hormone
200 <> GG340	Tab, Pink, Cap Shaped, Scored, 200 <> GG over 340	Levothyroxine 200 mcg	Levo-T by Alara	64909-0144	Thyroid Hormone
200 <> GG340	Tab, Pink, Cap Shaped, Scored, 200 <> GG over 340	Levothyroxine 200 mcg	Levo-T by Sandoz	00781-5189	Thyroid Hormone
200 <> GG457	Tab, Yellow, Round, GG over 457	Chlorpromazine HCl 200 mg	Thorazine by Sandoz	00781-1719	Antipsychotic
200 <> IBU	Tab, Yellow, Cap Shaped, Biconvex	Ibuprofen 200 mg	Motrin by Apotex	Canadian DIN 00441643	NSAID
200 <> IG	Tab, White, Round, Scored	Fosinopril Sodium 10 mg	Monopril by Deca	68552-0221	Antihypertensive
200 <> IG	Tab, White, Round, Scored	Fosinopril Sodium 10 mg	Monopril by Zydus	24658-0100	Antihypertensive
200 <> IP138	Tab, White, Oblong, Film Coated	Ibuprofen 200 mg	Advil by Interpharm	53746-0138	NSAID
200 <> K	Tab, White, Round	Oxandrolone 2.5 mg	Oxandrin by Par	49884-0301	Steroid; CIII
200 <> L124	Tab, White, Oval	Cimetidine HCl 200 mg	Tagamet by Perrigo	00113-0124	Gastrointestinal

ID FRONT <> BACK	DESCRIPTION FRONT <> BACK	INGREDIENT & STRENGTH	BRAND (or Generic Equiv.) by FIRM	NDC#	CLASS; SCH.
200 <> LAMICTAL	Tab, White, Round, Orally Disintegrating	Lamotrigine 200 mg	Lamictal ODT by GSK	00173-0777	Anticonvulsant
200 <> M	Tab, Green, Oblong, M inside square <> 200	Morphine Sulfate 200 mg	MS Contin by Mallinckrodt	00406-8320	Analgesic; C II
200 <> N	Tab, Yellow, Hexagonal	Sulindac 200 mg	Clinoril by Novopharm	Canadian DIN 00745596	NSAID
200 <> N	Tab, Pink, Round	Topiramate 200 mg	Topamax by Novopharm	Canadian DIN 02248862	Anticonvulsant
200 <> N	Tab, Off-White, Oval	Ofloxacin 200 mg	Floxin by Novopharm	Canadian DIN 02243474	Antibiotic
200 <> N	Tab, Yellow, Cap Shaped	Ibuprofen 200 mg	Motrin by Novopharm	Canadian DIN 00629324	NSAID
200 <> N	Tab, Blue, Shield-Shaped, Compressed	Acyclovir 200 mg	Zovirax by Novopharm	Canadian DIN 02285959	Antiviral
200 <> N181	Tab, Green, Oval, Film Coated	Cimetidine HCl 200 mg	Tagamet by Darby Group	66467-3480	Gastrointestinal
200 <> N181	Tab, Green, Oval, Film Coated	Cimetidine HCl 200 mg	Tagamet by Teva	00093-8181 Discontinued	Gastrointestinal
200 <> N181	Tab, Green, Oval, Film Coated	Cimetidine HCl 200 mg	Tagamet by Brightstone	62939-2111	Gastrointestinal
200 <> N181	Tab, Green, Oval, Film Coated	Cimetidine HCl 200 mg	Tagamet by URL Mutual	00677-1527	Gastrointestinal
200 <> N214	Tab, Pink, Oval, Scored	Amiodarone 200 mg	Cordarone by Teva	55953-0214 Discontinued	Antiarrhythmic
200 <> N214	Tab, Pink, Oval, N 214/200	Amiodarone 200 mg	Cordarone by Novopharm	43806-0214	Antiarrhythmic
200 <> N552	Tab, Peach, Round, N over 552	Fluconazole 200 mg	Diflucan by Teva	00093-7205 Discontinued	Antifungal
200 <> NN	Tab, Red, Cap Shaped, N/N	Morphine Sulfate 200 mg	MS Contin by Novopharm	Canadian DIN 02302802	Analgesic; N
200 <> NN	Tab, Pink, Round, Scored, N / N <> 200	Amiodarone HCl 200 mg	Cordarone by Novopharm	Canadian DIN 02239835	Antiarrhythmic
200 <> NN	Tab, White, Round, Scored, N/N <> 200	Ketoconazole 200 mg	Nizoral by Novopharm	Canadian DIN 02231061	Antifungal
200 <> NOVO	Tab, White, Oval	Acebutolol HCl 200 mg	Monitan by Novopharm	Canadian DIN 02204525	Antihypertensive
200 <> P	Tab, Salmon, Round	Topiramate 200 mg	Topamax by Pharmascience	Canadian DIN 02263017	Anticonvulsant
200 <> P	Tab, White, Round, Pharmascience Logo	Bezafibrate 200 mg	Bezalip by Pharmascience	Canadian DIN 02240331	Antihyperlipidemic
200 <> PD352	Tab, Light Yellow, Oval, Film Coated	Troglitazone 200 mg	Rezulin by Murfreesboro	51129-1286	Antidiabetic
200 <> PD352	Tab, Light Yellow, Oval, Film Coated	Troglitazone 200 mg	Rezulin by Parke Davis	00071-0352	Antidiabetic
200 <> RDY	Tab, Brown, Round, Film Coated	Simvastatin 40 mg	Zocor by Dr. Reddy's	55111-0200	Antihyperlipidemic
200 <> SCHERING752	Tab, White, Round, Scored	Labetalol HCl 200 mg	Normodyne by Rightpak	65240-0706	Antihypertensive
200 <> SP	Tab, Blue, Oval, Film Coated	Lacosamide 200 mg	Vimpat by Schwarz	00091-2480	Antiepileptic
200 <> SW	Tab	Tiludronate Disodium 240 mg	Skelid by Sanofi	00024-1800	Bisphosphonate
200 <> SW	Tab	Tiludronate Disodium 240 mg	Skelid by Sanofi Winthrop	53360-1800	Bisphosphonate
200 <> SYNTHROID	Tab, Pink, Round, Scored	Levothyroxine Sodium 200 mcg	Synthroid by Abbott	00074-7148	Thyroid Hormone
200 <> T4	Tab, Pink, Cap Shaped	Levothyroxine Sodium 200 mcg	Levothroid by Forest	00456-1327	Thyroid Hormone
200 <> TOP	Tab, Salmon, Round, Film Coated	Topiramate 200 mg	Topamax by Janssen-Ortho	Canadian DIN 02230896	Anticonvulsant
200 <> TOPAMAX	Tab, Salmon, Round, Film Coated	Topiramate 200 mg	Topamax by Ortho-McNeil	00062-0642	Anticonvulsant
200 <> TOPAMAX	Tab, Salmon, Round, Film Coated	Topiramate 200 mg	Topamax by McNeil	00045-0642	Anticonvulsant
200 <> TOPAMAX	Tab, Salmon, Round, Film Coated	Topiramate 200 mg	Topamax by McNeil	52021-0642	Anticonvulsant
200 <> VIDEX	Tab, Off-White to Light Orange/Yellow, Round, Chewable	Didanosine 200 mg	Videx by BMS	00087-6665	Antiviral
200 <> WYETH4188	Tab, Pink, Round, Scored, 200 inside C <> Wyeth over 4188	Amiodarone 200 mg	Cordarone by Wyeth	00008-4188	Antiarrhythmic
2002PP	Cap, Clear & White	Phenylpropanolamine HCl 75 mg, Caraminephen Edisylate 40 mg	Tuss Ornade by Pioneer		Antitussive

ID FRONT <> BACK	DESCRIPTION FRONT <> BACK	INGREDIENT & STRENGTH	BRAND (or Generic Equiv.) by FIRM	NDC#	CLASS; SCH.
20050 <> APO	Tab, Peach, Oval, Scored	Carbidopa 50 mg Levodopa 200 mg	Sinemet by Apotex	Canadian DIN 0245211	Antiparkinson
200A05	Cap, Blue	Acyclovir 200 mg	Zovirax by Mova	55370-0557	Antiviral
200ER	Tab, White, Round, Black Ink, ER	Tramadol HCl 200 mg	Ultram ER by Ortho-McNeil	00062-0655	Analgesic
200G60	Tab, White, Oval	Cimetidine HCl 200 mg	Tagamet by Novopharm		Gastrointestinal
200M	Tab	Levothyroxine Sodium 200 mcg	Levo-T by Mova	55370-0132	Thyroid Hormone
200M <> Z	Tab, Pink, Round, Scored	Levothyroxine Sodium 200 mcg	Levo-T by Zoetica	64909-0119	Thyroid Hormone
200MCG <> 283	Tab, Coated	Cerivastatin Sodium 0.2 mg	Baycol by Bayer	00026-2883	Antihyperlipidemic
200MCG <> FLINT	Tab, Debossed	Levothyroxine Sodium 200 mcg	by Amerisource	62584-0140	Thyroid Hormone
200MG <> PF	Tab, Red, Cap-Shaped, Scored, Film-Coated, Sustained-Release	Morphine Sulfate 200 mg	MS Contin by Purdue	Canadian DIN 02014327	Analgesic
200MG <> PF	Tab, Red, Cap-Shaped, Scored, Film-Coated, Sustained-Release	Morphine Sulfate 200 mg	MS Contin by Pharmascience	Canadian DIN 02245288	Analgesic
200MG <> PROVIGIL	Tab, White, Cap Shaped	Modafinil 200 mg	Provigil by Neuman	64579-0324	Stimulant; C IV
200MG <> PROVIGIL	Tab, White, Cap Shaped	Modafinil 200 mg	Provigil by Cephalon	63459-0201	Stimulant; C IV
200MG <> T	Tab, White, Pink Imprint, Round, Film Coated, Ex Release	Carbamazepine 200 mg	Tegretol by Novartis	00083-0062	Anticonvulsant
200MG4176	Cap, Light Gray, Red Print	Etodolac 200 mg	by Ivax	00172-4176	NSAID
200MG4176	Cap, Light Gray, Red Print	Etodolac 200 mg	by Ivax	00182-2664	NSAID
200MGGILEAD	Cap, Blue and White, Hard Gel	Emtricitabine 200 mg	Emtriva by Gilead	61958-0601	Antiviral
200NORMODYNE <> SCHERING752	Tab, Film Coated	Labetalol HCl 200 mg	Normodyne by Schering	53922-0752	Antihypertensive
200NORMODYNE <> SCHERING752	Tab, Film Coated, 200 Normodyne <> Schering 752	Labetalol HCl 200 mg	Normodyne by Thrift Drug	59198-0081	Antihypertensive
200WYETH	Tab, White, Oval	Acebutolol HCl 200 mg	Sectral by Wyeth	Canadian	Antihypertensive
201	Tab, Film Coated	Naproxen 375 mg	Naprelan by Elan	56125-0201	NSAID
201 <> COR	Tab, White, Round, Coated	Ropinirole HCl 0.25 mg	Requip by CorePharma	64720-0201	Antiparkinson
201 <> IG	Tab, White, Round	Fosinopril Sodium 20 mg	Monopril by Blu	24658-0101	Antihypertensive
201 <> IG	Tab, White, Round	Fosinopril Sodium 20 mg	Monopril by Deca	68552-0222	Antihypertensive
201 <> K	Tab, White, Round	Oxandrin 10 mg	by Par	49884-0302	Steroid; CIII
201 <> RDY	Tab, Yellow, Round	Risperidone 0.25 mg	Risperdal by Dr. Reddy's	55111-0201	Antipsychotic
201 <> THERRX	Tab, Red, Scored, Film-Coated	Iron Sumalate 70 mg, Iron Ferrous Fumarate 81 mg, Succinic Acid 150 mg, Vitamin C 140 mg, Vitamin C (Ascorbic Acid 60 mg) (Threonic Acid 0.8 mg), Folic Acid 1 mg, Vitamin B12 10 mg	Repliva 21/7 by Ther-Rx	64011-0207	Supplement
201 <> UU	Tab, White, Cap Shaped, Scored	Acetaminophen 650 mg, Hydrocodone Bitartrate 7.5 mg	Lorcet Plus by Amerisource	62584-0028	Analgesic; C III
201 <> UU	Tab, White, Cap Shaped, Scored	Acetaminophen 650 mg, Hydrocodone Bitartrate 7.5 mg	Lorcet Plus by Nat Pharmpak	55154-7302	Analgesic; C III
201 <> UU	Tab, White, Cap Shaped, Scored	Acetaminophen 650 mg, Hydrocodone Bitartrate 7.5 mg	Lorcet Plus by Murfreesboro	51129-0053	Analgesic; C III
201 <> UU	Tab, White, Cap Shaped, Scored	Acetaminophen 650 mg, Hydrocodone Bitartrate 7.5 mg	Lorcet Plus by Med Pro	53978-2071	Analgesic; C III
201 <> UU	Tab, White, Cap Shaped, Scored	Acetaminophen 650 mg, Hydrocodone Bitartrate 7.5 mg	Lorcet Plus by Forest	00785-1122	Analgesic; C III
201 <> UU	Tab, White, Cap Shaped, Scored	Acetaminophen 650 mg, Hydrocodone Bitartrate 7.5 mg	Lorcet Plus by Mikart	46672-0025	Analgesic; C III
2011 <> G	Tab, White, Round, Extended Release	Orphenadrine Citrate 100 mg	Norflex by Global	00115-2011	Muscle Relaxant
20110 <> B	Tab, Beige, Oval, Scored, Film Coated	Fluoxetine HCl 10 mg	Prozac by Barr	00555-0201	Antidepressant
20125 <> 5034	Tab, Yellow, Round, Ivax Hourglass Logo 5034 <> 20/12.5	Lisinopril 20 mg, HCTZ 12.5 mg	Prinzide by Ivax	00172-5034	Antihypertensive; Diuretic
20125 <> APO	Tab, White to Off-White, Oval, APO <> 20 over 12.5	Lisinopril 20 mg, HCTZ 12.5 mg	Prinzide by Apotex	60505-0206	Antihypertensive; Diuretic
20125 <> APO	Tab, White, Round	Lisinopril 20 mg, HCTZ 12.5 mg	Zestoretic by Apotex	Canadian DIN 02261987	Antihypertensive; Diuretic
2013	Tab, Yellow, Round	Chlorpheniramine Maleate 4 mg	Chlor-Trimeton by Circa		Antihistamine
201SEARLE	Tab, White to Off-White, Round, 201/Searle	Hydrochlorothiazide 25 mg, Spironolactone 25 mg	Aldactazide by Searle	Canadian DIN 00180408	Diuretic; Antihypertensive
202	Tab, White to Off-White, Oval, Scored, Coated	Gabapentin 600 mg	Neurontin by Caraco	62756-0202	Anticonvulsant
202	Tab, Film Coated, Logo	Naproxen 550 mg	Naprelan by Elan	56125-0202	NSAID

ID FRONT <> BACK	DESCRIPTION FRONT <> BACK	INGREDIENT & STRENGTH	BRAND (or Generic Equiv.) by FIRM	NDC#	CLASS; SCH.
202 <> IG	Tab, White, Round	Fosinopril Sodium 40 mg	Monopril by Deca	68552-0223	Antihypertensive
202 <> IG	Tab, White, Round	Fosinopril Sodium 40 mg	Monopril by Blu	24658-0102	Antihypertensive
202 <> RDY	Tab, Pink, Round	Risperidone 0.5 mg	Risperdal by Dr. Reddy's	55111-0202	Antipsychotic
2020	Tab, White with Specks, Oblong	Caffeine 175 mg	Caffeine by B & M Labs		Stimulant
2020MYLAN	Cap, Green	Piroxicam 20 mg	Feldene by Va Cmop	65243-0057	NSAID
2025 <> 5032	Tab, Peach, Round, Ivax Hourglass Logo 5032 <> 20/25	Lisinopril 20 mg, HCTZ 25 mg	Prinzide by Ivax	00172-5032	Antihypertensive; Diuretic
2025 <> APO	Tab, Pink, Oval, APO <> 20 over 25	Lisinopril 20 mg, HCTZ 25 mg	Prinzide by Apotex	60505-0207	Antihypertensive; Diuretic
2025 <> APO	Tab, Pink, Round, APO <> 20 over 25	Lisinopril 20 mg, HCTZ 25 mg	Zestoretic by Apotex	Canadian DIN 02261995	Antihypertensive; Diuretic
202NORMODYNE <> SCHERING752	Tab, Film Coated	Labetalol HCl 200 mg	Normodyne by Amerisource	62584-0752	Antihypertensive
203 <> IG	Tab, Pink, Round, I / G	Glimepiride 1 mg	Amaryl by Perrigo	10768-7150	Antidiabetic
203 <> RDY	Tab, White, Round	Risperidone 1 mg	Risperdal by Dr. Reddy's	55111-0203	Antipsychotic
20336	Cap, Off-White to Light Yellow Powder	Piroxicam 20 mg	Feldene by Qualitest	00603-5223	NSAID
2035	Cap	Chlordiazepoxide 10 mg	Librium by Vortech		Antianxiety; C IV
203A <> TEC	Tab, White to Off-White, Rectangular, Scored	Doxazosin Mesylate 2 mg	Cardura by AltiMed	Canadian DIN 02243216 Discontinued	Antihypertensive
203A <> TEC	Tab, White to Off-White, Round, Scored	Doxazosin Mesylate 1 mg	Cardura by Ratiopharm	Canadian DIN 02243215 Discontinued	Antihypertensive
203B	Tab, Green, Round	Amitriptyline HCl 25 mg	Elavil by Barr		Antidepressant
204	Tab, White to Off-White, Oval, Scored, Coated	Gabapentin 800 mg	Neurontin by Caraco	62756-0204	Anticonvulsant
204	Tab, White, Oblong	Pseudoephedrine 120 mg	Sudafed by OHM Labs		Cold Remedy
204 <> 400N	Tab, Light Green, Coated, 400/N	Cimetidine HCl 400 mg	Tagamet by Schein	00364-2593	Gastrointestinal
204 <> IG	Tab, Green, Round, I / G	Glimepiride 2 mg	Amaryl by Perrigo	10768-7475	Antidiabetic
204 <> M	Tab, White, Round	Diclofenac Sodium 50 mg	by Martec	65413-0001	NSAID
204 <> RDY	Tab, White, Round	Risperidone 2 mg	Risperdal by Dr. Reddy's	55111-0204	Antipsychotic
204 <> UAD	Tab, White, Oblong	Guaifenesin 300 mg, Phenylephrine HCl 20 mg	Endal by Mikart	46672-0145	Cold Remedy
204 <> UAD	Tab, White, Oblong	Guaifenesin 300 mg, Phenylephrine HCl 20 mg	Endal by Forest	00785-2204	Cold Remedy
204 <> UAD	Tab, White, Oblong	Guaifenesin 300 mg, Phenylephrine HCl 20 mg	Endal by Physician Total Care	54868-4094	Cold Remedy
205	Tab, Pink, Oval	Diphenhydramine HCl 25 mg	Benadryl by Granutec		Antihistamine
205 <> C	Tab, White, Round	Armodafinil 50 mg	Nuvigil by Cephalon	63459-0205	Stimulant; C IV
205 <> ETHEX	Tab, White, Oblong, Ex Release	Guaifenesin 600 mg	Guaifenex LA by Ethex	58177-0205 Discontinued	Expectorant
205 <> IG	Tab, Blue, Round, I / G	Glimepiride 4 mg	Amaryl by Perrigo	10768-7700	Antidiabetic
205 <> INV	Tab, Film Coated	Hydrochlorothiazide 15 mg, Methyldopa 250 mg	by Qualitest	00603-4543	Diuretic; Antihypertensive
205 <> M	Tab, White, Round	Diclofenac Sodium 75 mg	by Martec	65413-0002	NSAID
205 <> RDY	Tab, White, Round	Risperidone 3 mg	Risperdal by Dr. Reddy's	55111-0205	Antipsychotic
206 <> IG	Tab, Beige, Round, Coated	Citalopram HBr 10 mg	Celexa by Blu	24658-0140	Antidepressant
206 <> INV	Tab, Film Coated	Hydrochlorothiazide 25 mg, Methyldopa 250 mg	by Qualitest	00603-4544	Diuretic; Antihypertensive
206 <> RDY	Tab, White, Round	Risperidone 4 mg	Risperdal by Dr. Reddy's	55111-0206	Antipsychotic
206 <> THERRX	Tab, Purple, Scored, Film-Coated	Succinic Acid 150 mg	Repliva 21/7 by Ther-Rx	64011-0207	Supplement
2063V <> 2	Tab	Acetaminophen 300 mg, Codeine Phosphate 15 mg	Tylenol w/ Codeine by PDRX	55289-0449	Analgesic; C III
2064V <> 3	Tab, White, Round	Acetaminophen 300 mg, Codeine Phosphate 30 mg	Tylenol w/ Codeine by Vintage	00254-2064	Analgesic; C III
2064V <> 3	Tab, White, Round	Acetaminophen 300 mg, Codeine Phosphate 30 mg	Tylenol w/ Codeine by Qualitest	00603-2338	Analgesic; C III
2065V <> 4	Tab, 2065 over V <> 4	Acetaminophen 300 mg, Codeine Phosphate 60 mg	Tylenol w/ Codeine by Quality Care	60346-0632 Discontinued	Analgesic; C III
207	Tab, Scored	Nadolol 40 mg	Corgard by King	61570-0201	Antihypertensive

ID FRONT <> BACK	DESCRIPTION FRONT <> BACK	INGREDIENT & STRENGTH	BRAND (or Generic Equiv.) by FIRM	NDC#	CLASS; SCH.
207 <> IG	Tab, Pink, Round, Scored, Coated	Citalopram HBr 20 mg	Celexa by Blu	24658-0141	Antidepressant
207 <> TT	Tab	Guaifenesin 600 mg, Pseudoephedrine HCl 60 mg	by URL Mutual	00677-1487	Cold Remedy
2078213	Tab, White, Round, 20 78-213	Metaproterenol 20 mg	Metaprel by Sandoz		Antiasthmatic
208	Tab, Scored	Nadolol 120 mg	Corgard by King	61570-0203	Antihypertensive
208 <> B	Tab, White, Round	Inert	Portia by Barr	00555-9020	Oral Contraceptive; Placebo
208 <> B	Tab, White, Round	Inert	Jolessa by Barr	00555-9123	Oral Contraceptive; Placebo
208 <> B	Tab, White, Round	Inert	Levlite by Barr	00555-9014	Oral Contraceptive; Placebo
208 <> B	Tab, White, Round	Inert	Tri-Lo-Sprintec by Barr	00555-9065	Oral Contraceptive; Placebo
208 <> B	Tab, White, Round, Stylized b	Inert	Gianvi by Teva Pharmaceuticals	00093-5661	Oral Contraceptive; Placebo
208 <> ETHEX	Tab, White, Cap Shaped, Ex Release	Guaifenesin 600 mg, Pseudoephedrine HCl 120 mg	Duratuss by Ethex	58177-0208	Cold Remedy
208 <> ETHEX	Tab, White, Cap Shaped, Ex Release	Guaifenesin 600 mg, Pseudoephedrine 120 mg	Duratuss by Murfreesboro	51129-1390	Cold Remedy
208 <> IG	Tab, White, Round, Scored, Coated	Citalopram HBr 40 mg	Celexa by Blu	24658-0142	Antidepressant
2080	Tab, White, Round, Red Print	Almotriptan Maleate 6.25 mg	Axert by Janssen-Ortho	Canadian DIN 02248128	Antimigraine
2080	Tab, White, Round, Red Print	Almotriptan Maleate 6.25 mg	Axert by Ortho-McNeil	00062-2080	Antimigraine
2080	Tab, White, Round, Red Print	Almotriptan Maleate 6.25 mg	Axert by Searle	00025-2080	Antimigraine
2083	Tab, Orange, Round, Scored	Hydrochlorothiazide 25 mg	Hydrodiuril by Va Cmop	65243-0039	Diuretic; Antihypertensive
2083	Tab, Orange, Round, Scored	Hydrochlorothiazide 25 mg	Hydrodiuril by Vangard	00615-1561	Diuretic; Antihypertensive
2083V	Tab, White, Round, Scored	Allopurinol 100 mg	Zyloprim by Vintage	00603-2115	Antigout
2084V	Tab, Peach, Round, Scored	Allopurinol 300 mg	Zyloprim by Vintage	00603-2116	Antigout
2087V	Tab, White, Oval	Alprazolam 0.25 mg	Xanax by Qualitest	00603-2127	Antianxiety; C IV
2088V	Tab, Orange, Oval	Alprazolam 0.5 mg	Xanax by Qualitest	00603-2128	Antianxiety; C IV
2089	Tab, Orange, Round, Scored	Hydrochlorothiazide 50 mg	by Va Cmop	65243-0040	Diuretic; Antihypertensive
2089V	Tab, Blue, Oval	Alprazolam 1 mg	Xanax by Qualitest	00603-2129	Antianxiety; C IV
209	Tab, White to Off White, Round	Amlodipine Besylate 10 mg	Norvasc by Breckenridge	51991-0668	Antihypertensive
209 <> IG	Tab, White, Round	Terbinafine HCl 250 mg	Lamisil by Glenmark	68462-0136	Antifungal
209 <> IG	Tab, White, Round	Terbinafine HCl 250 mg	Lamisil by Blu	24658-0180	Antifungal
209 <> IG	Tab, White, Round	Terbinafine 250 mg	Lamisil by Interpharm	68462-0136	Antifungal
2090 <> V	Tab, White, Oblong	Alprazolam 2 mg	Xanax by Qualitest	00603-2130	Antianxiety; C IV
2095	Cap	Docusate Sodium 100 mg	Dio-Sul by Vortech		Laxative
209B	Tab, Pink, Round	Amitriptyline HCl 10 mg	Elavil by Barr		Antidepressant
20A	Tab, White, Round, 20A/Tower Symbol	Metaproterenol Sulfate 20 mg	Alupent by Boehringer Ingelheim	Canadian Discontinued	Antiasthmatic
20BAYER	Tab, Round, Orange	Vardenafil 20 mg	Levitra by Bayer	00085-1934	Impotence Agent
20F	Tab, White, Round	Tamoxifen Citrate 20 mg	Nolvadex by Pharmacia	Canadian	Antiestrogen
20M	Tab, White	Benzoyl Peroxide 20 mg	Benoxyl by Stiefel	Canadian	Antiacne
20M	Tab, White	Dicyclomine HCl 20 mg	by Aventis	Canadian	Gastrointestinal
20MG	Cap, Blue	Pericyazine 20 mg	by RPR	Canadian	Psychotropic Agent
20MG	Tab, Pink, Oblong, Film-Coated, Delayed Release, Logo <> 20MG	Omeprazole 20 mg	Losec MUPS by AstraZeneca	Canadian DIN 02242462	Gastrointestinal
20MG <> AEH	Tab, Light Pink, Oblong, Delayed-Release	Esomeprazole 20 mg	Nexium by AstraZeneca	Canadian DIN 02244521	Proton Pump Inhibitor
20MG <> FP	Tab, Pink, Oval, Scored, Film Coated	Citalopram 20 mg	Celexa by Compumed	00403-4894	Antidepressant
20MG <> FP	Tab, Pink, Oval, Scored, Film Coated	Citalopram 20 mg	Celexa by Forest	00456-4020	Antidepressant
20MG <> FP	Tab, Pink, Oval, Scored, Film Coated	Citalopram 20 mg	Celexa by Forest	63711-0120	Antidepressant

ID FRONT <> BACK	DESCRIPTION FRONT <> BACK	INGREDIENT & STRENGTH	BRAND (or Generic Equiv.) by FIRM	NDC#	CLASS; SCH.
20MG <> IL	Tab, Pink, Oval, Scored, Film Coated, I / L	Citalopram HBr 20 mg	Celexa by Inwood	00258-3696	Antidepressant
20MGSARAFEM	Cap, Pink and Lavender, Opaque	Fluoxetine HCl 20 mg	Sarafem by Warner Chilcott	00430-0436	Antidepressant
20N640	Cap, Dark Green	Piroxicam 20 mg	Feldene by Heartland	61392-0401	NSAID
20N640	Cap, Dark Green	Piroxicam 20 mg	Feldene by Moore	00839-7774	NSAID
20P	Tab, White, Round, Scored, 20 over P	Furosemide 20 mg	Lasix by Pharmascience	Canadian DIN 02247493	Diuretic
20R <> RPR	Tab	Chlorthalidone 50 mg	Hygroton by RPR	00801-0020	Diuretic
20R <> RPR	Tab	Chlorthalidone 50 mg	Hygroton by RPR	00075-0020 Discontinued	Diuretic
20ZESTRIL	Tab, Pink, Round, 20ZESTRIL inside Heart Logo	Lisinopril 20 mg	Zestril by AstraZeneca	Canadian DIN 02049384	Diuretic; Antihypertensive
21 <> A	Tab, Light Red, Round, Scored, A <> 2 / 1	Lisinopril 5 mg	Zestril by Aurobindo	65862-0038	Antihypertensive
21 <> B	Tab, Light Orange, Round	Ethinyl Estradiol 0.03 mg, Levonorgestrel 0.15 mg	Levlen 28 by Berlex	50419-0411	Oral Contraceptive
21 <> B	Tab, Light Orange, Round	Ethinyl Estradiol 0.03 mg, Levonorgestrel 0.15 mg	Levlen 21 by Berlex	50419-0410	Oral Contraceptive
21 <> BL	Tab, Green, Round	Imipramine HCl 50 mg	Tofranil by Teva	00093-2117	Antidepressant
21 <> BL	Tab, Green, Round	Imipramine HCl 50 mg	Tofranil by UDL	51079-0081	Antidepressant
21 <> D	Tab, White to Off White, Round	Atenolol 25 mg	Tenormin by Aurobindo	65862-0168	Antihypertensive
21 <> EFF	Tab, White, Round, Debossed	Methazolamide 25 mg	Neptazane by Lederle	55806-0021	Antiglaucoma Agent
21 <> EFF	Tab, White, Round, Debossed	Methazolamide 25 mg	Neptazane by Duramed	51285-0968	Antiglaucoma Agent
21 <> F	Tab, White to Off-White, Oval	Alendronate Sodium 70 mg	Fosamax by Aurobindo	65862-0329	Antiosteoporosis
21 <> I	Tab, White, Round, Scored	Glycopyrrolate 1 mg	Robinul by Dr. Reddy's	55111-0648	Anticholinergic Agent
21 <> M	Tab, White, Round, Scored, M inside square	Methylphenidate HCl 20 mg	Methylin by Neuman	64579-0034	Stimulant; C II
210	Tab, Yellow	Perphenazine 2 mg, Amitriptyline 10 mg	by Schering	Canadian	Antipsychotic; Antidepressant
210	Tab, White to Off White, Round	Amlodipine Besylate 5 mg	Norvasc by Breckenridge	51991-0667	Antihypertensive
210 <> ANTIVERT	Tab, Blue & White, Oblong	Meclizine HCl 12.5 mg	Antivert by Roerig	00662-2100	Antiemetic
210 <> ANTIVERT	Tab, Blue & White, Oblong	Meclizine HCl 12.5 mg	Antivert by Roerig	00049-2100	Antiemetic
21000 <> GSK	Tab, Yellow, Oval, Film Coated, 2/1000	Metformin HCl 1000 mg, Rosiglitazone 2 mg	Avandamet by SKB	00007-3163	Antidiabetic
21000 <> GSK	Tab, Yellow, Oval, Film Coated, 2/1000	Metformin HCl 1000 mg, Rosiglitazone 2 mg	Avandamet by GSK	Canadian DIN 02248440	Antidiabetic
2101V	Tab, Blue, Round, Film Coated	Amitriptyline HCl 10 mg	Elavil by Vintage	00254-2101	Antidepressant
2102 <> V	Tab, Yellow, Round	Amitriptyline HCl 25 mg	Elavil by Vintage	00603-2213	Antidepressant
2102V	Tab, Yellow, Round, Film Coated	Arritriptyline HCl 25 mg	Elavil by Vintage	00254-2102	Antidepressant
2103V	Tab, Beige, Round, Film Coated	Amitriptyline HCl 50 mg	Elavil by Caremark	00339-6137	Antidepressant
2103V	Tab, Beige, Round, Film Coated	Amitriptyline HCl 50 mg	Elavil by Vintage	00254-2103	Antidepressant
21040	Tab, White, Round	Furosemide 40 mg	Lasix by Martec		Diuretic
2104V	Tab, Orange, Round, 2104 over V	Amitriptyline HCl 75 mg	Elavil by Vintage	00254-2104	Antidepressant
2104V	Tab, Orange, Round, 2104 over V	Amitriptyline HCl 75 mg	Elavil by Qualitest	00603-2215	Antidepressant
2105V	Tab, Pink, Round, Film Coated, 2105 over V	Amitriptyline HCl 100 mg	Elavil by Vintage	00254-2105	Antidepressant
2106 <> V	Tab, Blue, Oblong	Amitriptyline HCl 150 mg	Elavil by Vintage		Antidepressant
211	Tab, Coated	Amitriptyline 12.5 mg, Chlordiazepoxide 5 mg	Limbitrol by Qualitest	00603-2690	Antianxiety; C IV
211	Tab, White, Round	Amlodipine Besylate 2.5 mg	Norvasc by Breckenridge	51991-0666	Antihypertensive
211 <> ANTIVERT	Tab, White & Yellow, Oblong	Meclizine HCl 25 mg	Antivert by Roerig	00049-2110	Antiemetic
211 <> ANTIVERT	Tab, White & Yellow, Oblong	Meclizine HCl 25 mg	Antivert by Rightpak	65240-0605	Antiemetic
211 <> ANTIVERT	Tab, White & Yellow, Oblong	Meclizine HCl 25 mg	Antivert by Roerig	00662-2110	Antiemetic
211 <> MYLAN	Tab, Green, Coated	Amitriptyline 12.5 mg, Chlordiazepoxide 5 mg	Limbitrol by Mylan	00378-0211	Antianxiety; C IV
211 <> US25	Tab, White, Round, Scored, US over 2.5 <> 211	Midodrine HCl 2.5 mg	Orvaten by Upsher Smith	00245-0211	Antihypotensive
2111 <> G	Tab, Red, Round, Film Coated	Demeclocycline HCl 150 mg	Declomycin by Global	00115-2111	Antibiotic
2115 <> B	Tab, White, Oval, Scored	Norethindrone Acetate 5 mg	Aygestin by Barr	00555-0211	Hormone
212	Tab, Blue, Round, Savage Logo 212	Potassium Chloride 600 mg	Kaon-CL 8 by Savage		Electrolytes

ID FRONT <> BACK	DESCRIPTION FRONT <> BACK	INGREDIENT & STRENGTH	BRAND (or Generic Equiv.) by FIRM	NDC#	CLASS; SCH.
212	Tab, 2 1/2	Nitroglycerin 2.5 mg	Sustachron ER Buccal by Forest	10418-0138	Vasodilator
212 <> 643	Tab, Pink, Round, 643 <> 2 1/2	Metolazone 2.5 mg	Zaroxolyn by Upstate Pharma	65580-0643	Diuretic
212 <> ETHEX	Tab, Pink, Oval, Film Coated	Ascorbic Acid 120 mg, Calcium 250 mg, Copper 2 mg, Cyanocobalamin 12 mcg, Docusate Sodium 50 mg, Folic Acid 1 mg, Iodine 0.15 mg, Iron 90 mg, Niacinamide 20 mg, Pyridoxine HCl 20 mg, Riboflavin 3.4 mg, Thiamine Mononitrate 3 mg, Vitamin A 4000 Units, Vitamin D 400 Units, Vitamin E 30 Units, Zinc 25 mg	Prenatal MR 90 by Ethex	58177-0212	Vitamin
212 <> FL	Tab, Light Blue, Triangular, FL <> 2 1/2	Nebivolol HCl 2.5 mg	Bystolic by Forest	00456-1402	Antihypertensive
212 <> U121	Tab, White, Half Oval, Scored, U/121 <> 2 1/2	Minoxidil 2.5 mg	Loniten by Pharmacia	Canadian DIN 00514497	Antihypertensive
212 <> U121	Tab, White, Half Oval, Scored, U/121 <> 2 1/2	Minoxidil 2.5 mg	Loniten by Pharmacia	00009-0121	Antihypertensive
212 <> US5	Tab, Pink, Round, Scored, US over 5 <> 212	Midodrine HCl 5 mg	Orvaten by Upsher Smith	00245-0212	Antihypotensive
212 <> WARFARINTARO	Tab, Green, Cap Shaped, 2 1/2	Warfarin Sodium 2.5 mg	Coumadin by Taro	51672-4029	Anticoagulant
212 <> ZAROXOLYN	Tab, Pink, Round, 2 1/2 <> Zaroxolyn	Metolazone 2.5 mg	Zaroxolyn by Medeva	53014-0975	Diuretic
212 <> ZAROXOLYN	Tab, Pink, Round, 2 1/2 <> Zaroxolyn	Metolazone 2.5 mg	Zaroxolyn by Amerisource		Diuretic
212 <> ZAROXOLYN	Tab, Pink, Round, 2 1/2 <> Zaroxolyn	Metolazone 2.5 mg	Zaroxolyn by Prestige	58056-0355	Diuretic
212 <> ZAROXOLYN	Tab, Pink, Round, 2 1/2 <> Zaroxolyn	Metolazone 2.5 mg	Zaroxolyn by Compumed	00403-1597	Diuretic
212 <> ZAROXOLYN	Tab, Pink, Round, 2 1/2 <> Zaroxolyn	Metolazone 2.5 mg	Zaroxolyn by Caremark	00339-5426	Diuretic
212 <> ZAROXOLYN	Tab, Pink, Round, 2 1/2 <> Zaroxolyn	Metolazone 2.5 mg	Zaroxolyn by Nat Pharmpak	55154-2504	Diuretic
2120V <> 3	Tab, White, Round, Scored	Aspirin 325 mg, Codeine Phosphate 30 mg	Aspirin w/ Codeine by Vintage	00254-2120	Analgesic; C III
2120V <> 3	Tab, White, Round, Scored	Aspirin 325 mg, Codeine Phosphate 30 mg	Aspirin w/ Codeine by URL Mutual	00677-0647	Analgesic; C III
2120V <> 3	Tab, White, Round, Scored	Aspirin 325 mg, Codeine Phosphate 30 mg	Aspirin w/ Codeine by Qualitest	00603-2361	Analgesic; C III
2121V <> 4	Tab	Aspirin 325 mg, Codeine Phosphate 60 mg	Aspirin w/ Codeine by Vintage	00254-2121	Analgesic; C III
2121V <> 4	Tab, White	Aspirin 325 mg, Codeine Phosphate 60 mg	Aspirin w/ Codeine by Qualitest	00603-2362	Analgesic; C III
2122 <> G	Tab, Red, Round, Film Coated	Demeclocycline HCl 300 mg	Declomycin by Global	00115-2122	Antibiotic
2125 <> IMO	Tab, White, Cap Shaped, 2 over 125	Loperamide HCl 2 mg, Simethicone 125 mg	Imodium by McNeil Consumer		Antidiarrheal; Antiflatulent
212COUMADIN <> DUPONT	Tab, Green, Round, Scored, 2 1/2 Coumadin <> Dupont	Warfarin Sodium 2.5 mg	by Thrift Drug	59198-0349	Anticoagulant
213	Tab, White, Round	Acetaminophen 500 mg	Tylenol Ex Strength by Ivax		Analgesic
213	Tab, White to Off White, Round, Scored, Orally Disintegrating	Alprazolam ODT 1 mg	Niravam by Par	49884-0213	Antianxiety
213 <> ETHEX	Tab, Green, Cap Shaped, Ex Release	Dextromethorphan 30 mg, Guaifenesin 600 mg	Humibid-DM by DRX	55045-2623	Cold Remedy
213 <> ETHEX	Tab, Green, Cap Shaped, Ex Release	Dextromethorphan 30 mg, Guaifenesin 600 mg	Humibid-DM by Ethex	58177-0213	Cold Remedy
213 <> US10	Tab, Purple, Round, Scored, US over 10 <> 213	Midodrine HCl 10 mg	Orvaten by Upsher Smith	00245-0213	Antihypotensive
2130V	Tab, Light Brown, Round	Amitriptyline HCl 50 mg	Elavil by Vintage		Antidepressant
214	Tab, White to Off White, Round, Scored, Orally Disintegrating	Alprazolam ODT 2 mg	Niravam by Par	49884-0214	Antianxiety
214 <> ANTIVERT	Tab, Blue & Yellow, Oblong	Meclizine HCl 50 mg	Antivert by Roerig	00049-2140	Antiemetic
214 <> ETHEX	Tab, Blue, Cap Shaped, Scored	Guaifenesin 600 mg, Pseudoephedrine HCl 60 mg	Guaifenex AM by Ethex	58177-0214 Discontinued	Cold Remedy
215	Tab, Light Blue, Round	Norgestimate 0.215 mg, Ethinyl Estradiol 0.025 mg	Tri-Cyclen LO 28 by Janssen-Ortho	Canadian DIN 02258587	Oral Contraceptive
215	Tab, Light Blue, Round	Norgestimate 0.215 mg, Ethinyl Estradiol 0.025 mg	Tri-Cyclen LO 21 by Janssen-Ortho	Canadian DIN 02258560	Oral Contraceptive
215 <> C	Tab, White, Oval	Armodafinil 150 mg	Nuvigil by Cephalon	63459-0215	Stimulant; C IV
215 <> OM	Tab, Light Blue, Round, O-M 215	Ethinyl Estradiol 0.025 mg, Norgestimate 0.215 mg	Ortho Tri-Cyclen Lo by Ortho-McNeil	00062-1251	Oral Contraceptive
2158 <> 93	Tab, White, Round, Scored, 9 over 3 <> 2158	Trimethoprim 100 mg	Proloprim by Teva	00093-2158	Antibiotic
215Q	Cap, Ivory, 215/Q	Meclofenamate Sodium 50 mg	Meclomen by Quantum		NSAID

ID FRONT <> BACK	DESCRIPTION FRONT <> BACK	INGREDIENT & STRENGTH	BRAND (or Generic Equiv.) by FIRM	NDC#	CLASS; SCH.
216 <> ETHEX	Tab, White, Oval	Ascorbic Acid 80 mg, Beta-Carotene 0.4 mg, Biotin 30 mcg, Calcium 200 mg, Copper 3 mg, Cyanocobalamin 2.5 mcg, Folic Acid 1 mg, Iron 60 mg, Magnesium 100 mg, Niacinamide 17 mg, Pantothenic Acid 7 mg, Pyridoxine HCl 4.86 mg, Riboflavin 1.6 mg, Thiamine 1.5 mg, Vitamin A 0.8 mcg, Vitamin D 10 mcg, Vitamin E 10 mg, Zinc 25 mg	Natalins Rx by Ethex	58177-0216	Vitamin
216Q	Cap, Yellow, 216/Q	Meclofenamate Sodium 100 mg	Meclomen by Quantum		NSAID
217	Tab, White	Aspirin 325 mg, Caffeine 30 mg	Anacin by Frosst	Canadian	Analgesic
217 <> COPLEY	Tab, White, Oval	Prenatal Vitamins	Prenatal Optima Tablet by Teva	00093-9217	Vitamin; Mineral
217ABANA	Cap, White & Green Beads	Phentermine HCl 37.5 mg	Obenix by Elge	58298-0952	Anorexiant; C IV
217FORT	Tab, White	Aspirin 500 mg, Caffeine 30 mg	Anacin by Frosst	Canadian	Analgesic
218BARR	Tab, White, Round	Ergoloid Mesylate 0.5 mg	Hydergine by Barr		Ergot Alkaloids
219	Tab, Yellow, Oblong, Scored, Film Coated	Choline Magnesium Trisalicylate 500 mg	by Compumed	00403-0544	NSAID
219	Tab, Yellow, Cap Shaped, Scored, Film Coated	Choline Magnesium Trisalicylate 500 mg	Trilisate by Caraco	57664-0219	NSAID
219 <> BARR	Tab, Pink, Cap Shaped, Film Coated	Erythromycin Stearate 500 mg	by Barr	00555-0219 Discontinued	Antibiotic
22 <> A	Tab, Light Yellow, Round	Lisinopril 10 mg	Zestril by Aurobindo	65862-0039	Antihypertensive
22 <> B	Tab, Pink, Round, Sugar Coated	Ethinyl Estradiol 0.02 mg, Levonorgestrel 0.1 mg	Levlite by Schering	64259-1165	Oral Contraceptive
22 <> B	Tab, Pink, Round, Sugar Coated	Ethinyl Estradiol 0.02 mg, Levonorgestrel 0.1 mg	Levlite by Schering	12866-1163	Oral Contraceptive
22 <> B	Tab, Pink, Round, Coated	Ethinyl Estradiol 0.02 mg, Levonorgestrel 0.1 mg	Levlite 28 by Berlex	50419-0022	Oral Contraceptive
22 <> BL	Tab, Pink, Round, Coated	Amitriptyline HCl 10 mg	Elavil by Teva	00093-2120	Antidepressant
22 <> D	Tab, White to Off White, Round, Scored	Atenolol 50 mg	Tenormin by Aurobindo	65862-0169	Antihypertensive
22 <> E	Tab, 25, White, Round, Film Coated	Topiramate 25 mg	Topiramate by Aurobindo	65862-0171	Anticonvulsant
22 <> I	Tab, White, Round, Scored	Glycopyrrolate 2 mg	Robinul by Dr. Reddy's	55111-0649	Anticholinergic Agent
22 <> M	Tab, White, Round	Albuterol Sulfate 4 mg	VoSpire ER by Mylan	00378-4122	Antiasthmatic
22 <> P	Tab, White, Round, Chewable, 2.2	Sodium Fluoride 2.21 mg	Pharmaflur by Pharmics	00813-0066	Element
220	Tab, Blue, Oblong, Scored, Film Coated	Choline Magnesium Trisalicylate 750 mg	Trilisate by Caraco	57664-0220	NSAID
220	Tab, Blue, Oblong, Scored, Film Coated	Choline Magnesium Trisalicylate 750 mg	by Compumed	00403-0561	NSAID
220 <> 93	Tab, White, Round, Film-Coated	Bicalutamide 50 mg	Casodex by Novopharm	Canadian DIN 02270226	Antiandrogen
220 <> 93	Tab, White to Off White, Round	Bicalutamide 50 mg	Casodex by Teva	00093-0220	Antiandrogen
220 <> RDY	Tab, Light Yellow, Round	Lamotrigine 25 mg	Lamictal by Dr. Reddy's	55111-0220	Anticonvulsant
2205	Tab, Green, Round	Ferrous Sulfate 325 mg	Feosol by Ivax	00182-4028 Discontinued	Mineral
221	Tab, Pink, Round, Film Coated	Sitagliptin 25 mg	Januvia by Merck	00006-0221	Antidiabetic
221	Tab, Pink, Cap Shaped, Scored, Film Coated	Choline Magnesium Trisalicylate 1000 mg	Trilisate by Caraco	57664-0221	NSAID
221	Tab, Pink, Oblong, Scored, Film Coated	Choline Magnesium Trisalicylate 1000 mg	by Compumed	00403-0694	NSAID
221 <> 3M	Tab, White, Round, Ex Release	Orphenadrine Citrate 100 mg	by Perrigo	00113-0381	Muscle Relaxant
221 <> 3M	Tab, White, Round, Ex Release	Orphenadrine Citrate 100 mg	Norflex by Rightpak	65240-0703	Muscle Relaxant
221 <> 3M	Tab, White, Round, Ex Release	Orphenadrine Citrate 100 mg	Norflex ER by 3M	00089-0221	Muscle Relaxant
221 <> 3M	Tab, White, Round, Ex Release	Orphenadrine Citrate 100 mg	by Allscripts	Discontinued	Muscle Relaxant
221 <> 3M	Tab, White, Round, Ex Release	Orphenadrine Citrate 100 mg	by Nat Pharmpak	55154-2907	Muscle Relaxant
221 <> 3M	Tab, White, Round, Ex Release	Orphenadrine Citrate 100 mg	Norflex by H J Harkins Co	52959-0178	Muscle Relaxant
221 <> 3M	Tab, White, Round, Ex Release	Orphenadrine Citrate 100 mg	Norflex by Rx Pak	65084-0229	Muscle Relaxant
221 <> 3M	Tab, White, Round, Ex Release	Orphenadrine Citrate 100 mg	by PDRX	55289-0646	Muscle Relaxant
221 <> 3M	Tab, White, Round, Ex Release	Orphenadrine Citrate 100 mg	by Amerisource	62584-0221	Muscle Relaxant
221 <> 93	Tab, Dark Yellow, Round, Film Coated	Risperidone 0.25 mg	Risperdal by Teva	00093-0221	Antipsychotic
221 <> BL	Tab, White to Off-White, Cap Shaped, Chewable	Amoxicillin 125 mg	Amoxil by Teva	00093-2267	Antibiotic
221 <> BL	Tab, White to Off-White, Cap Shaped, Chewable	Amoxicillin 125 mg	Amoxil by Moore	00839-7776 Discontinued	Antibiotic

ID FRONT <> BACK	DESCRIPTION FRONT <> BACK	INGREDIENT & STRENGTH	BRAND (or Generic Equiv.) by FIRM	NDC#	CLASS; SCH.
221 <> R	Tab, Peach, Round, Scored	Hydrochlorothiazide 25 mg	Hydrodiuril by Apotheca	12634-0445	Diuretic; Antihypertensive
221 <> R	Tab, Peach, Round, Scored	Hydrochlorothiazide 25 mg	Hydrodiuril by H J Harkins Co	52959-0132	Diuretic; Antihypertensive
221 <> R	Tab, Peach, Round, Scored	Hydrochlorothiazide 25 mg	Hydrodiuril by Actavis	00228-2221	Diuretic; Antihypertensive
221 <> RDY	Tab, Light Yellow, Round	Lamotrigine 100 mg	Lamictal by Dr. Reddy's	55111-0221	Anticonvulsant
22190	Tab, Coated, Debossed	Probenecid 500 mg	by PDRX	55289-0715	Antigout
222	Tab, White, Round, Scored	Aspirin 375 mg, Caffeine 30 mg, Codeine Phosphate 8 mg	Atasol-8 by Johnson & Johnson	Canadian DIN 00108162	Analgesic; C III
222 <> 93	Tab, White to Off-White, Cap Shaped, Film Coated	Sumatriptan Succinate 25 mg	Imitrex by Teva	00093-0222	Antimigraine
222 <> BL	Tab, White to Off-White, Oblong, Scored, Chewable	Amoxicillin 250 mg	Amoxil by Teva	00093-2268	Antibiotic
222 <> BL	Tab, White to Off-White, Oblong, Scored, Chewable	Amoxicillin 250 mg	Amoxil by Casa DeAmigos	62138-6005	Antibiotic
222 <> BL	Tab, White to Off-White, Oblong, Scored, Chewable	Amoxicillin 250 mg	Amoxil by DRX	55045-2004	Antibiotic
222 <> BL	Tab, White to Off-White, Oblong, Scored, Chewable	Amoxicillin 250 mg	Amoxil by St. Mary's Med	60760-0268 Discontinued	Antibiotic
222 <> CARACO	Tab, Mottled Yellow, Round, Scored	Guaifenesin 600 mg, Pseudoephedrine HCl 120 mg	by Med Pro	53978-3330	Cold Remedy
222 <> CARACO	Tab, Mottled Yellow, Cap Shaped, Scored	Guaifenesin 600 mg, Pseudoephedrine HCl 120 mg	Miraphen by Caraco	57664-0222	Cold Remedy
222 <> R	Tab, Peach, Round, Scored	Hydrochlorothiazide 50 mg	Hydrodiuril by Actavis	00228-2222	Diuretic; Antihypertensive
222 <> RDY	Tab, Light Yellow, Round	Lamotrigine 150 mg	Lamictal by Dr. Reddy's	55111-0222	Anticonvulsant
223 <> 93	Tab, White to Off-White, Cap Shaped, Film Coated	Sumatriptan Succinate 50 mg	Imitrex by Teva	00093-0223	Antimigraine
223 <> ETHEX	Tab, Red, Oval	Codeine Phosphate 10 mg, Guaifenesin 300 mg	Brontex by Ethex	58177-0223	Cold Remedy; C III
223 <> RDY	Tab, Light Yellow, Round	Lamotrigine 200 mg	Lamictal by Dr. Reddy's	55111-0223	Anticonvulsant
2238 <> 93	Tab, White, Cap Shaped, Scored	Cephalexin 250 mg	Keflex by Teva	00093-2238	Antibiotic
224 <> 93	Tab, Light Pink, Cap Shaped, Film Coated	Sumatriptan Succinate 100 mg	Imitrex by Teva	00093-0224	Antimigraine
2240 <> 93	Tab, White, Cap Shaped, Scored	Cephalexin 500 mg	Keflex by Teva	00093-2240	Antibiotic
22425	Tab, White, Round, 224 / 2.5	Minoxidil 2.5 mg	Loniten by Royce		Antihypertensive
225	Tab	Baclofen 10 mg	Lioresal by Sandoz	00781-1641	Muscle Relaxant
225	Tab, White, Round, Scored, Film Coated, 225 over Triangle	Propafenone HCl 225 mg	Rythmol by Abbott	00044-5024	Antiarrhythmic
225	Cap, Maroon, Logo/225	Clindamycin HCl 150 mg	Dalacin C by Upjohn	Canadian	Antibiotic
225	Tab, White, Round, Scored, Film Coated, 225 over Triangle	Propafenone HCl 225 mg	by Murfreesboro	51129-1362	Antiarrhythmic
225 <> 93	Tab, Reddish Brown, Round, Film Coated	Risperidone 0.5 mg	Risperdal by Teva	00093-0225	Antipsychotic
225 <> C	Tab, White, Oval	Armodafinil 250 mg	Nuvigil by Cephalon	63459-0225	Stimulant; C IV
225 <> COPLEY	Tab, Film Coated	Potassium Chloride 600 mg	by Schein	00364-0861	Electrolytes
225 <> ETHEX	Tab, Pink, Oval, Scored	Ascorbic Acid 120 mg, Calcium 200 mg, Copper 2 mg, Cyanocobalamin 12 mcg, Folic Acid 1 mg, Iron 27 mg, Niacinamide 20 mg, Pyridoxine HCl 10 mg, Riboflavin 3 mg, Thiamine HCl 1.84 mg, Vitamin A 4000 Units, Vitamin D 400 Units, Vitamin E 22 mg, Zinc 25 mg	NatalCare Plus by Ethex	58177-0225	Vitamin
225 <> IG	Tab, White, Cap Shaped, Film Coated, Scored	Gemfibrozil 600 mg	Lopid by Zydus	68382-0100	Antihyperlipidemic
225 <> IG	Tab, White, Capsule Shaped	Gemfibrozil 600 mg	Lopid by Blu	24658-130	Antihyperlipidemic
225 <> PAR	Tab	Haloperidol 2 mg	Haldol by Ivax	00182-1264	Antipsychotic
225 <> RDY	Tab, White, Round	Lamotrigine 5 mg	Lamictal by Dr. Reddy's	55111-0225	Anticonvulsant
22510	Tab, White, Round	Minoxidil 10 mg	Loniten by Royce		Antihypertensive
225105	Tab, Coated	Ascorbic Acid 100 mg, Cyanocobalamin 25 mcg, Ferrous Fumarate 600 mg	Tolfrinic by B F Ascher	00225-0105	Vitamin
225245	Tab, 225/245 <> Ascher Logo	Hyoscyamine Sulfate 0.125 mg	Levsin by Sovereign	58716-0612	Gastrointestinal
225250	Tab, White	Ethaverine HCl 100 mg	by B F Ascher		Vasodilator
225295	Tab, Pale Yellow, Round, Scored, 225/295 <> Ascher Logo	Hyoscyamine Sulfate 0.125 mg	Levsin by DRX	55045-2362	Gastrointestinal
225295	Tab, Pale Yellow, Round, Scored, 225/295 <> Ascher Logo	Hyoscyamine Sulfate 0.125 mg	Levsin by B F Ascher	00225-0295	Gastrointestinal
225356	Tab, White, Round, Scored, Ascher Logo <> 225/356	Magnesium Salicylate 325 mg, Phenyltoloxamine Citrate 30 mg	Mobigesic by B F Ascher	00225-0356	Analgesic
225405	Cap, 225/405	Chlorpheniramine Maleate 12 mg, Phenylpropanolamine 75 mg	Ornade by B F Ascher		Cold Remedy
225450	Tab, 225-450 <> 2 Ascher Logos	Acetaminophen 500 mg, Hydrocodone Bitartrate 5 mg	Vicodin by B F Ascher	00225-0450	Analgesic; C III
225470	Cap, Clear & White, 225/470	Phendimetrazine Tartrate 105 mg	by B F Ascher		Anorexiant; C III

ID FRONT <> BACK	DESCRIPTION FRONT <> BACK	INGREDIENT & STRENGTH	BRAND (or Generic Equiv.) by FIRM	NDC#	CLASS; SCH.
225480	Cap, 225 over 480	Brompheniramine Maleate 12 mg, Pseudoephedrine HCl 120 mg	Allent by Pharmafab	62542-0154	Cold Remedy
225480	Cap, 225 over 480	Brompheniramine Maleate 12 mg, Pseudoephedrine HCl 120 mg	Allent by B F Ascher	00225-0480	Cold Remedy
226	Tab, Orange, Round, Enteric Coated	Aspirin 325 mg	Aspirin by Granutec	54499-0226	Analgesic
226	Tab	Baclofen 20 mg	Lioresal by Sandoz	00781-1642	Muscle Relaxant
226 <> M	Tab, Orange, Round, Scored	Quinapril HCl 10 mg	Accupril by Mylan	00378-0226	Antihypertensive
226 <> RDY	Tab, White, Cap Shaped	Lamotrigine 25 mg	Lamictal by Dr. Reddy's	55111-0226	Anticonvulsant
2263 <> 93	Tab, Off-White, Cap Shaped, Film Coated	Amoxicillin 500 mg	Amoxil by Novopharm	00093-2263	Antibiotic
2263 <> 93	Tab, Off-White, Cap Shaped, Film Coated	Amoxicillin 500 mg	Amoxil by Teva	55953-2263	Antibiotic
2265 <> V	Tab, Off-White, Oval, Scored	Baclofen 10 mg	Lioresal by Vintage	00254-2265	Muscle Relaxant
2265 <> V	Tab, Off-White, Oval, Scored	Baclofen 10 mg	Lioresal by Qualitest	00603-2406	Muscle Relaxant
2266 <> V	Tab, Off-White, Cap Shaped, Scored	Baclofen 20 mg	Lioresal by Qualitest	00603-2407	Muscle Relaxant
2266 <> V	Tab, Off-White, Cap Shaped, Scored	Baclofen 20 mg	Lioresal by Vintage	00254-2266	Muscle Relaxant
2267 <> 93	Tab, White to Off-White, Cap Shaped	Amoxicillin 125 mg	Amoxil by Teva	00093-2267	Antibiotic
2268 <> 93	Tab, White to Off-White, Oblong	Amoxicillin 250 mg	Amoxil by Teva	00093-2268	Antibiotic
227	Tab, Invamed Logo	Metoclopramide 5 mg	Reglan by Med Pro	53978-2094	Gastrointestinal
227	Tab, Pink, Oval, Film-Coated	Raltegravir 400 mg	Isentress by Merck	00006-0227	Antiviral
227	Tab, Pink, Round	Raltegravir 400 mg	Isentress by Merck Frosst	Canadian DIN 02301881	Antiviral
227 <> WC	Tab, Light Buff, Round	Vitamin A 1000 Units, Cholecalciferol 400 Units, Vitamin E 11 Units, Ascorbic Acid 120 mg, Folic Acid 1 mg, Thiamine Mononitrate 2 mg, Riboflavin 3 mg, Niacinamide 20 mg, Cyanocobalamin 12 mcg, Pyridoxine HCl 10 mg, Iron 29 mg	Natachew by Warner Chilcott	00430-0227	Vitamin
227 <> WC	Tab, Light Buff, Round	Vitamin A 1000 Units, Cholecalciferol 400 Units, Vitamin E 11 Units, Ascorbic Acid 120 mg, Folic Acid 1 mg, Thiamine Mononitrate 2 mg, Riboflavin 3 mg, Niacinamide 20 mg, Cyanocobalamin 12 mcg, Pyridoxine HCl 10 mg, Iron 29 mg	Natachew by Amide	52152-0210	Vitamin
227 <> WYETH	Tab, Pink, Scored	Promethazine HCl 50 mg	Phenergan by Wyeth	52903-0227	Antiemetic; Antihistamine
227 <> WYETH	Tab, Pink, Round	Promethazine HCl 50 mg	Phenergan by Wyeth	00008-0227	Antiemetic; Antihistamine
2270 <> 93	Tab, Mottled Pink, Oval, Chewable	Amoxicillin 200 mg, Clavulanate Potassium 28.5 mg	Augmentin by Teva	00093-2270	Antibiotic
2272 <> 93	Tab, Mottled Pink, Oval, Chewable	Amoxicillin 400 mg, Clavulanate Potassium 57 mg	Augmentin by Teva	00093-2272	Antibiotic
2274 <> 93	Tab, White, Oblong	Amoxicillin 500 mg, Clavulanate Potassium 125 mg	Augmentin by Teva	00093-2274	Antibiotic
2275 <> 93	Tab, White, Oblong, Scored	Amoxicillin 875 mg, Clavulanate Potassium 125 mg	Augmentin by Teva	00093-2275	Antibiotic
227555	Tab, White, Oval	Ergoloid Mesylate 1 mg	Hydergine by Barr		Ergot Alkaloids
228	Tab, Yellow, Round, Enteric Coated	Aspirin 81 mg	Aspirin by Granutec		Analgesic
228 <> SCHERING	Tab, White, Round, Score, Schering Logo	Griseofulvin, Ultramicrosize 125 mg	Fulvicin P/G by Schering	00085-0228	Antifungal
228QPL10	Tab, White, Round	Minoxidil 10 mg	Loniten by Quantum		Antihypertensive
229 <> RDY	Tab, White, Round	Pravastatin Sodium 10 mg	Pravachol by Dr. Reddy's	55111-0229	Antihyperlipidemic
22905	Tab, White, Round, 229/0.5	Haloperidol 0.5 mg	Haldol by Royce		Antipsychotic
2293	Cap	Diltiazem HCl 90 mg	Cardizem by Allscripts		Antihypertensive
22R <> RPR	Tab	Chlorthalidone 25 mg	Hygroton by RPR	00801-0022	Diuretic
22R <> RPR	Tab	Chlorthalidone 25 mg	Hygroton by RPR	00075-0022 Discontinued	Diuretic
23 <> A	Tab, Light Yellow, Cap Shaped	Lisinopril 20 mg	Zestril by Aurobindo	65862-0040	Antihypertensive
23 <> BL	Tab, Light Green, Round, Coated	Amitriptyline HCl 25 mg	Elavil by Teva	00093-2122	Antidepressant
23 <> D	Tab, White to Off White, Round, Scored	Atenolol 100 mg	Tenormin by Aurobindo	65862-0170	Antihypertensive
23 <> E	Tab, Dark Yellow, Round, Film Coated	Topiramate 100 mg	Topiramate by Aurobindo	65862-0173	Anticonvulsant
230	Tab, Yellow, Round	Bisacodyl 5 mg	Dulcolax by UDL	51079-0907	Gastrointestinal
230	Tab, Yellow, Round	Bisacodyl 5 mg	Dulcolax by Major	00904-7927	Gastrointestinal
230 <> RDY	Tab, White, Round	Pravastatin Sodium 20 mg	Pravachol by Dr. Reddy's	55111-0230	Antihyperlipidemic

ID FRONT <> BACK	DESCRIPTION FRONT <> BACK	INGREDIENT & STRENGTH	BRAND (or Generic Equiv.) by FIRM	NDC#	CLASS; SCH.
230 <> SYNTHO	Tab, Light Blue, Cap Shaped, Film Coated	Esterified Estrogens 0.625 mg, Methyltestosterone 1.25 mg	Syntest H.S. by Breckenridge	51991-0078	Hormone
230 <> SYNTHO	Tab, Light Blue, Cap Shaped, Film Coated	Esterified Estrogens 0.625 mg, Methyltestosterone 1.25 mg	Syntest H.S. by Breckenridge	66756-0230	Hormone
2301	Tab, Yellow, Round	Haloperidol 1 mg	Haldol by Royce		Antipsychotic
231	Tab, Red, Round, Schering Logo 231	Dexbrompheniramine Maleate 6 mg, Pseudoephedrine Sulfate 120 mg	Disophrol by Schering		Cold Remedy
231	Tab, White, Round, Savage Logo 231	Choline Bitartrate 25 mg, Dexpanthenol 50 mg	Ilopan-Choline by Savage	00281-2311	Antiflatulent
231 <> M	Tab, White, Round, Scored	Atenolol 50 mg	Tenormin by Mylan	00378-0231	Antihypertensive
231 <> M	Tab, White, Round, Scored	Atenolol 50 mg	Tenormin by UDL	51079-0684	Antihypertensive
231 <> M	Tab, White, Round, Scored	Atenolol 50 mg	Tenormin by Heartland	61392-0543	Antihypertensive
231 <> RDY	Tab, White, Round	Pravastatin Sodium 40 mg	Pravachol by Dr. Reddy's	55111-0231	Antihyperlipidemic
231 <> SYNTHO	Tab, Light Green, Cap Shaped, Film Coated	Esterified Estrogens 1.25 mg, Methyltestosterone 2.5 mg	Syntest D.S. by Breckenridge	66756-0231	Hormone
231 <> SYNTHO	Tab, Light Green, Cap Shaped, Film Coated	Esterified Estrogens 1.25 mg, Methyltestosterone 2.5 mg	Syntest D.S. by Breckenridge	51991-0079	Hormone
2312	Tab, Purple, Round	Haloperidol 2 mg	Haldol by Royce		Antipsychotic
232	Tab, Scored	Nadolol 20 mg	Corgard by King	61570-0200	Antihypertensive
232 <> ETHEX	Tab, Peach, Film Coated	Ascorbic Acid 50 mg, Calcium 250 mg, Copper 2 mg, Folic Acid 1 mg, Iron 40 mg, Magnesium 50 mg, Pyridoxine HCl 2 mg, Vitamin D 6 mcg, Vitamin E 3.5 mg, Zinc 15 mg	Natalcare X by Ethex	58177-0232 Discontinued	Vitamin
23201 <> BARR	Tab, White, Oval, Scored, barr <> 232/0.1	Desmopressin Acetate 0.1 mg	DDAVP by Barr	00555-0232	Antidiuretic
2320V	Tab, White, Round, 2320 over V	Belladonna, Phenobarbital 16.2 mg	Donnatal by Qualitest	00603-2418	Gastrointestinal; C IV
232232	Tab, Pink, Oval, Scored, Chewable, 232 over 232 <> Mova Logo	Amoxicillin 250 mg	Amoxil by Bayer	00280-0036	Antibiotic
232232	Tab, Pink, Oval, Scored, Chewable, 232 over 232 <> Mova Logo	Amoxicillin 250 mg	Amoxil by Mova	55370-0892	Antibiotic
232232	Tab, Pink, Oval, Scored, Chewable, 232 over 232 <> Mova Logo	Amoxicillin 250 mg	Amoxil by Clonmell	55190-0232	Antibiotic
2325	Tab, Green, Round, 232/5	Haloperidol 5 mg	Haldol by Royce		Antipsychotic
2325 <> V	Tab, White, Round, Scored	Benztropine Mesylate 0.5 mg	Cogentin by UDL	51079-0404	Antiparkinson
2325 <> V	Tab, White, Oval, Scored	Benztropine Mesylate 0.5 mg	Cogentin by Qualitest	00603-2433	Antiparkinson
2326 <> V	Tab, White, Round, Scored	Benztropine Mesylate 1 mg	Cogentin by Qualitest	00603-2434	Antiparkinson
2326 <> V	Tab, White, Oval, Scored	Benztropine Mesylate 1 mg	Cogentin by UDL	51079-0406	Antiparkinson
2327 <> V	Tab, White, Round, Scored	Benztropine Mesylate 2 mg	Cogentin by UDL	51079-0407	Antiparkinson
2327 <> V	Tab, White, Oval, Scored	Benztropine Mesylate 2 mg	Cogentin by Qualitest	00603-2435	Antiparkinson
23280	Tab, White, Round, 232/80	Furosemide 80 mg	Lasix by Martec		Diuretic
233 <> 93	Tab, White, Round, Film Coated	Ondansetron HCl 4 mg	Zofran by Teva	00093-0233	Antiemetic
233 <> RDY	Tab, Yellow, Oval	Meloxicam 7.5 mg	Mobic by Dr. Reddy's	55111-0233	NSAID
23302 <> BARR	Tab, White, Oval, Scored, barr <> 233/0.2	Desmopressin Acetate 0.2 mg	DDAVP by Barr	00555-0233	Antidiuretic
23310	Tab, Bluish Green, Round, 233/10	Haloperidol 10 mg	Haldol by Royce		Antipsychotic
234 <> M	Tab, White, Round, Film Coated	Metformin HCl 500 mg	Glucophage by UDL	51079-0972 Discontinued	Antidiabetic
234 <> M	Tab, White, Round, Film Coated	Metformin HCl 500 mg	Glucophage by Mylan	00378-0234	Antidiabetic
234 <> RDY	Tab, Yellow, Round	Meloxicam 15 mg	Mobic by Dr. Reddy's	55111-0234	NSAID
23420	Tab, Salmon, Round, 234/20	Haloperidol 20 mg	Haldol by Royce		Antipsychotic
235 <> 800N	Tab, Light Green, Coated, 800/N	Cimetidine HCl 800 mg	Tagamet by Schein	00364-2594	Gastrointestinal
235 <> WATSON	Tab, Yellow	Norethindrone 0.35 mg	Aygestin by Watson	52544-0235	Hormone
2355 <> V	Tab, White, Round, Scripted V	Acetaminophen 325 mg, Butalbital 50 mg, Caffeine 40 mg	Fioricet by Qualitest	00603-2546	Analgesic
2357 <> V	Tab, White, Oblong	Acetaminophen 500, Butalbital 50 mg, Caffeine 40 mg	Esgic Plus by Vintage	00254-2357	Analgesic
2357 <> V	Tab, White, Oblong	Acetaminophen 500, Butalbital 50 mg, Caffeine 40 mg	Esgic Plus by Qualitest	00603-2545	Analgesic
236 <> PAR	Tab, Peach, Round, Scored, Film Coated	Doxycycline 150 mg	Monoclox by Par	49884-0236	Antibiotic
237 <> A	Tab, White to Off-White, Round	Atropine Sulfate 0.025 mg, Diphenoxylate HCl 2.5 mg	Lomotil by Able	53265-0237 Discontinued	Antidiarrheal; C V

ID FRONT <> BACK	DESCRIPTION FRONT <> BACK	INGREDIENT & STRENGTH	BRAND (or Generic Equiv.) by FIRM	NDC#	CLASS; SCH.
237 <> ETHEX	Tab, White, Ex Release	Hyoscyamine Sulfate 0.375 mg	Levbid by Ethex	58177-0237	Gastrointestinal
237 <> IG	Tab, White, Round	Amlodipine Besylate 2.5 mg	Norvasc by Blu	24658-0190	Antihypertensive
237 <> MYLAN	Tab, White, Oval, Film Coated	Etodolac 400 mg	Lodine by Aventis	64734-0002	NSAID
237 <> MYLAN	Tab, White, Oval, Film Coated	Etodolac 400 mg	Lodine by Mylan	00378-0237	NSAID
237 <> MYLAN	Tab, White, Oval, Film Coated	Etodolac 400 mg	Lodine by Allscripts		NSAID
238 <> IG	Tab, White, Round	Amlodipine Besylate 5 mg	Norvasc by Blu	24658-0191	Antihypertensive
2384	Cap	Hematinic Combination	Tri-Tinic by Vortech		Vitamin
239 <> IG	Tab, White, Round	Amlodipine Besylate 10 mg	Norvasc by Blu	24658-0192	Antihypertensive
239500	Tab, Green, Oblong, Royce Logo 239 500	Chlorzoxazone 500 mg	Parafon DSC by Royce		Muscle Relaxant
239500	Tab, Green, Oblong, Royce Logo 239 500	Chlorzoxazone 500 mg	by Royce	51875-0239	Muscle Relaxant
24 <> 93	Tab, White, Oval, Film Coated, Extended Release	Oxycodone HCl 10 mg	OxyContin by Teva	00093-0024 Discontinued	Analgesic; C II
24 <> A	Tab, Light Yellow, Round	Lisinopril 30 mg	Zestril by Aurobindo	65862-0041	Antihypertensive
24 <> BL	Tab, Brown, Round, Coated	Amitriptyline HCl 50 mg	Elavil by Teva	00093-2124	Antidepressant
24 <> E	Tab, Pink, Round, Film Coated	Topiramate 200 mg	Topiramate by Aurobindo	65862-0174	Anticonvulsant
24 <> GXCF7	Tab, Pink, Oval	Ondansetron HCl 24 mg	Zofran by GSK	00173-0680	Antiemetic
24 <> M	Tab, Blue, Round	Albuterol Sulfate 8 mg	VoSpire ER by Mylan	00378-4124	Antiasthmatic
24 <> N	Tab, White, Round, Biconvex, Bevelled-Edge, Scored	Betahistine Dihydrochloride 24 mg	Novo-Betahistine by Novopharm	Canadian DIN 02280205	Antivertigo
24 <> WW	Tab, White, Cap Shaped	Ondansetron HCl 24 mg	Zofran by West-Ward	00143-2424	Antiemetic
240	Cap, Blue-Green and Purple	Diltiazem 240 mg	Tiazac by Inwood	00258-3689	Antihypertensive
240 <> 05	Tab, White, Round, Film Coated, 0.5 <> Royce Logo 240	Lorazepam 0.5 mg	Ativan by Royce	51875-0240	Antianxiety; C IV
240 <> 05	Tab, White, Round, Film Coated, 0.5 <> Royce Logo 240	Lorazepam 0.5 mg	Ativan by Qualitest	00603-4243	Antianxiety; C IV
240 <> 05	Tab, White, Round, Film Coated, 0.5 <> Royce Logo 240	Lorazepam 0.5 mg	Ativan by URL Mutual	00677-1056	Antianxiety; C IV
240 <> 05	Tab, White, Round, Film Coated, 0.5 <> Royce Logo 240	Lorazepam 0.5 mg	Ativan by Talbert	44514-0098	Antianxiety; C IV
240 <> 05	Tab, White, Round, Film Coated, 0.5 <> Royce Logo 240	Lorazepam 0.5 mg	Ativan by Royce		Antianxiety; C IV
240 <> B	Tab, White, Cap Shaped, Ex Release	Diltiazem HCl 240 mg	Tiazac XC by Biovail	Canadian DIN 02256754	Antihypertensive
240 <> B	Tab, White, Cap Shaped, Ex Release	Diltiazem HCl 240 mg	Cardizem LA by Biovail	64455-0102	Antihypertensive
240 <> M	Tab, White, Round, Film Coated	Metformin HCl 850 mg	Glucophage by Mylan	00378-0240	Antidiabetic
240 <> M	Tab, White, Round, Film Coated	Metformin HCl 850 mg	Glucophage by UDL	51079-0973	Antidiabetic
240 <> NOVO	Tab, Off White, Cap Shaped, Scored, NO/VO <> 2/40, Sustained Release	Verapamil HCl 240 mg	Isoptin SR by Novopharm	Canadian DIN 002211920	Antihypertensive
240 <> US15	Tab, White, Cap Shaped	Sotalol HCl 240 mg	Sorine by Upsher Smith	00245-0015	Antiarrhythmic
240 <> WPPH	Tab, White, Round, Scored	Chlorothiazide 250 mg	Diuril by Endo	60951-0765	Diuretic; Antihypertensive
240 <> WPPH	Tab, White, Round, Scored	Chlorothiazide 250 mg	Diuril by Circa	71114-4207	Diuretic; Antihypertensive
240 <> WPPH	Tab, White, Round, Scored	Chlorothiazide 250 mg	Diuril by Merck	00006-0240	Diuretic; Antihypertensive
24005 <> WATSON	Tab, White, Round, Scored, 240 over 0.5	Lorazepam 0.5 mg	Ativan by Watson	52544-0240	Antianxiety; C IV
24005 <> WATSON	Tab, White, Round, Scored, 240 over 0.5	Lorazepam 0.5 mg	Ativan by Watson	00591-0240	Antianxiety; C IV
240Z	Cap, in White Ink	Tetracycline HCl 500 mg	by Kaiser	00179-1021	Antibiotic
240MG <> BETAPACE	Tab, Light Blue, Cap Shaped, Scored	Sotalol 240 mg	Betapace by Berlex	50419-0107	Antiarrhythmic
240MGANDRX599	Cap, Brown & Orange, Ex Release	Diltiazem HCl 240 mg	Cartia XT by Andrx	62037-0599	Antihypertensive
240WATSON664	Cap, Red & White, 240/Watson/664	Diltiazem HCl 240 mg	Dilacor XR by Watson		Antihypertensive
241	Tab, White, Oval, Film Coated, Ex Release, Triangle 241	Trandolapril 1 mg, Verapamil 240 mg	Tarka by Abbott	00074-3288	Antihypertensive
241	Tab, White, Oval, Film Coated, Ex Release, Triangle 241	Trandolapril 1 mg, Verapamil 240 mg	Tarka by Knoll	00048-5912	Antihypertensive
241	Tab, Scored	Nadolol 80 mg	Corgard by King	61570-0202	Antihypertensive
241	Tab, White, Oval, Film Coated, Ex Release, Triangle 241	Trandolapril 1 mg, Verapamil 240 mg	Tarka by Abbott	00048-5912	Antihypertensive
241	Tab, Blue, T-Shaped, Scored	Clorazepate Dipotassium 3.75 mg	Tranxene by Actavis	00228-3067	Antianxiety; C IV
241	Tab, Yellow, Round, Scored	Clozapine 50 mg	Clozaril by Caraco	57664-0241	Antipsychotic

ID FRONT <> BACK	DESCRIPTION FRONT <> BACK	INGREDIENT & STRENGTH	BRAND (or Generic Equiv.) by FIRM	NDC#	CLASS; SCH.
241	Tab, Blue, T-Shaped, Scored	Clorazepate Dipotassium 3.75 mg	Tranxene by Pliva	50111-0986	Antianxiety; C IV
241	Tab, White, Oval, Film Coated, Ex Release, Triangle 241	Trandolapril 1 mg, Verapamil 240 mg	Tarka by Abbott	Canadian DIN 02240945	Antihypertensive
241 <> 1	Tab, 1/Royce Logo	Lorazepam 1 mg	Ativan by Qualitest	00603-4244	Antianxiety; C IV
241 <> 1	Tab, 1/Royce Logo	Lorazepam 1 mg	Ativan by URL Mutual	00677-1057	Antianxiety; C IV
241 <> TARKA	Tab, White, Oval, Film Coated	Trandolapril 1 mg, Verapamil 240 mg	Tarka by Abbott	00044-5912	Antihypertensive
241 <> WPPH	Tab, Peach, Round	Hydrochlorothiazide 25 mg	Hydrodiuril by Endo	60951-0770	Diuretic; Antihypertensive
241 <> WPPH	Tab, Peach, Round	Hydrochlorothiazide 25 mg	Hydrodiuril by Merck	00006-0241	Diuretic; Antihypertensive
2410V	Tab, White, Round, Straight or Stylized "V"	Carisoprodol 350 mg	Soma by Qualitest	00603-2582	Muscle Relaxant
2410V	Tab, White, Round, Straight or Stylized "V"	Carisoprodol 350 mg	Soma by Vintage	00254-2410	Muscle Relaxant
2411	Tab, White, Round, Scored, Royce Logo 241/1	Lorazepam 1 mg	Ativan by Royce	00591-0241	Antianxiety; C IV
2411	Tab, White, Round, Scored, Royce Logo 241/1	Lorazepam 1 mg	Ativan by St. Mary's Med	60760-0241	Antianxiety; C IV
2411	Tab, White, Round, Scored, Royce Logo 241/1	Lorazepam 1 mg	Ativan by Talbert	44514-0099	Antianxiety; C IV
2411	Tab, White, Round, Scored, Royce Logo 241/1	Lorazepam 1 mg	Ativan by Royce	51875-0241	Antianxiety; C IV
2411 <> WATSON	Tab, White, Round, Scored, 241 over 1	Lorazepam 1 mg	Ativan by Watson	52544-0241	Antianxiety; C IV
2411 <> WATSON	Tab, White, Round, Scored, 241 over 1	Lorazepam 1 mg	Ativan by Watson	00591-0241	Antianxiety; C IV
242	Tab, Gold, Oval, Film Coated, Ex Release, Triangle 242	Trandolapril 2 mg, Verapamil 240 mg	Tarka by Abbott	00048-5922	Antihypertensive
242	Tab, Peach, T-Shaped, Scored	Clorazepate Dipotassium 7.5 mg	Tranxene by Actavis	00228-3068	Antianxiety; C IV
242	Tab, Peach, T-Shaped, Scored	Clorazepate Dipotassium 7.5 mg	Tranxene by Pliva	50111-0987	Antianxiety; C IV
242	Tab, Gold, Oval, Film Coated, Ex Release, Triangle 242	Trandolapril 2 mg, Verapamil 240 mg	Tarka by Knoll	00048-5922	Antihypertensive
242	Tab, Gold, Oval, Film Coated, Ex Release, Triangle 242	Trandolapril 2 mg, Verapamil 240 mg	Tarka by Abbott	00074-3289	Antihypertensive
242	Tab, Gold, Oval, Film Coated	Carvedilol 3.125 mg	Coreg by Caraco	57664-0242	Antihypertensive
242	Tab, Gold, Oval, Film Coated, Ex Release, Triangle 242	Trandolapril 2 mg, Verapamil 240 mg	Tarka by Abbott	Canadian DIN 02240946	Antihypertensive
242 <> MYLAN	Tab, Pink, Oval, Film Coated	Etodolac 500 mg	Lodine by Mylan	00378-1242	NSAID
242 <> TARKA	Tab, Gold, Oval, Film Coated	Trandolapril 2 mg, Verapamil 240 mg	Tarka by Abbott	00044-5922	Antihypertensive
2422	Tab, White, Round, Scored, 242 over 2 <> Royce Logo	Lorazepam 2 mg	Ativan by Compumed	00403-0012	Antianxiety; C IV
2422	Tab, White, Round, Scored, 242 over 2 <> Royce Logo	Lorazepam 2 mg	Ativan by Royce	51875-0242	Antianxiety; C IV
2422	Tab, White, Round, Scored, 242 over 2 <> Royce Logo	Lorazepam 2 mg	Ativan by Royce	60760-0242	Antianxiety; C IV
2422	Tab, White, Round, Scored, 242 over 2 <> Royce Logo	Lorazepam 2 mg	Ativan by St. Mary's Med	00603-4245	Antianxiety; C IV
2422	Tab, White, Round, Scored, 242 over 2 <> Royce Logo	Lorazepam 2 mg	Ativan by Qualitest	55154-0651	Antianxiety; C IV
2422 <> WATSON	Tab, White, Round, Scored, 242 over 2	Lorazepam 2 mg	Ativan by Nat Pharmpak	52544-0242	Antianxiety; C IV
2422 <> WATSON	Tab, White, Round, Scored, 242 over 2	Lorazepam 2 mg	Ativan by Watson	00591-0242	Antianxiety; C IV
2428	Cap	Phenytoin 100 mg	Di-Phen by Vortech		Anticonvulsant
243	Tab, Lavender, T-Shaped, Scored	Clorazepate Dipotassium 15 mg	Tranxene by Actavis	00228-3069	Antianxiety; C IV
243	Tab, Lavender, T-Shaped, Scored	Clorazepate Dipotassium 15 mg	Tranxene by Pliva	50111-0988	Antianxiety; C IV
243 <> WATSON	Tab, Light Blue, Round	Norethindrone 0.5 mg, Ethinyl Estradiol 0.035 mg	Leena by Watson	52544-0219	Oral Contraceptive
243 <> WPPH	Tab, Peach, Round	Hydrochlorothiazide 50 mg	by Merck	00006-0243	Diuretic; Antihypertensive
243 <> WPPH	Tab, Peach, Round	Hydrochlorothiazide 50 mg	by Endo	60951-0771	Diuretic; Antihypertensive
244	Tab, Reddish Brown, Oval, Film Coated, Ex Release, Triangle 244	Trandolapril 4 mg, Verapamil 240 mg	Tarka by Abbott	00074-3290	Antihypertensive
244	Tab, Reddish Brown, Oval, Film Coated, Ex Release, Triangle 244	Trandolapril 4 mg, Verapamil 240 mg	Tarka by Abbott	00048-5942	Antihypertensive
244	Tab, Reddish Brown, Oval, Film Coated, Ex Release, Triangle 244	Trandolapril 4 mg, Verapamil 240 mg	Tarka by Knoll	00048-5942	Antihypertensive
244	Tab, Reddish Brown, Oval, Film Coated, Ex Release, Triangle 244	Trandolapril 4 mg, Verapamil 240 mg	Tarka by Abbott	Canadian DIN 02238097	Antihypertensive
244	Tab, White, Oval, Film Coated	Carvedilol 6.25 mg	Coreg by Caraco	57664-0244	Antihypertensive
244 <> MYLAN	Tab, Blue, Oval, Film Coated, Ex Release	Verapamil HCl 120 mg	Isoptin SR by UDL	51079-0894	Antihypertensive
244 <> MYLAN	Tab, Blue, Oval, Film Coated, Ex Release	Verapamil HCl 120 mg	Isoptin SR by Mylan	00378-1120	Antihypertensive

ID FRONT <> BACK	DESCRIPTION FRONT <> BACK	INGREDIENT & STRENGTH	BRAND (or Generic Equiv.) by FIRM	NDC#	CLASS; SCH.
244 <> MYLAN	Tab, Blue, Oval, Film Coated, Ex Release	Verapamil HCl 120 mg	Isoptin SR by Murfreesboro	51129-1298	Antihypertensive
244 <> TARKA	Tab, Reddish Brown, Oval, Film Coated	Trandolapril 4 mg, Verapamil 240 mg	Tarka by Abbott	00044-5942	Antihypertensive
244 <> WATSON	Tab, Yellowish Green, Round	Norethindrone 1 mg, Ethinyl Estradiol 0.035 mg	Leena by Watson	52544-0219	Oral Contraceptive
2442 <> G	Tab, Yellow, Round, Film Coated	Bupropion HCl 100 mg	Wellbutrin SR by Teva	00093-3501	Antidepressant
2444 <> G	Tab, Light Yellow, Round, Film Coated, Sustained Release	Bupropion HCl 150 mg	Wellbutrin SR by Teva	00093-3502	Antidepressant
2444 <> G	Tab, Light Yellow, Round, Film Coated, Sustained Release	Bupropion HCl 150 mg	Zyban by Teva	00093-5703	Antidepressant
244SEARLE	Tab, White to Off-White, Round, 244/Searle	Hydrochlorothiazide 50 mg, Spironolactone 50 mg	Aldactazide by Searle	Canadian DIN 00594377	Diuretic; Antihypertensive
245	Tab, White, Oval, Film Coated	Carvedilol 12.5 mg	Coreg by Caraco	57664-0245	Antihypertensive
245 <> MYLAN	Tab, Green, Oval, Scored	Bumetanide 0.5 mg	Bumex by Caraco	57664-0317	Diuretic
245 <> MYLAN	Tab, Green, Oval, Scored	Bumetanide 0.5 mg	Bumex by Heartland	61392-0048	Diuretic
245 <> MYLAN	Tab, Green, Oval, Scored	Bumetanide 0.5 mg	Bumex by Mylan	00378-0245	Diuretic
245 <> MYLAN	Tab, Green, Oval, Scored	Bumetanide 0.5 mg	Bumex by Hoffmann La Roche	00004-0290	Diuretic
245 <> WPPH	Tab, White, Round, Scored	Chlorothiazide 500 mg	Diuril by Endo	60951-0766	Diuretic; Antihypertensive
2455 <> WPIWPI	Tab, Light Peach, Cap Shaped, Scored, Film Coated	Metformin HCl 1000 mg	Glucophage by Watson	00591-2455	Antidiabetic
246	Tab, Scored	Nadolol 160 mg	Corgard by King	61570-0204	Antihypertensive
246 <> IG	Tab, Blue, Cap Shaped, Scored, I / G <> 246	Levetiracetam 250 mg	Keppra by Glenmark	68462-0545	Antiepileptic
246 <> PAR	Tab, Lavender	Aspirin 325 mg, Carisoprodol 200 mg	Soma Compound by Schein	00364-2524	Analgesic; Muscle Relaxant
247	Tab, White, Oval, Film Coated	Carvedilol 25 mg	Coreg by Caraco	57664-0247	Antihypertensive
247 <> B	Tab, Brown, Round	Ferrous Fumarate	Junel 1/20 Fe by Barr	00555-9026	Oral Contraceptive; Placebo
247 <> B	Tab, Brown, Round	Ferrous Fumarate	Junel 1.5/30 Fe by Barr	00555-9028	Oral Contraceptive; Placebo
247 <> IG	Tab, Yellow, Cap Shaped, Scored, I / G	Levetiracetam 500 mg	Keppra by Glenmark	68462-0546	Antiepileptic
2472	Cap	Diphenhydramine HCl 25 mg	Benadryl by Vortech		Antihistamine
247210	Tab	Amitriptyline 25 mg, Perphenazine 2 mg	Triavil by Qualitest	00603-5115	Antidepressant; Antipsychotic
247210	Tab	Amitriptyline 10 mg, Perphenazine 2 mg	Triavil by Ivax	00182-1235	Antidepressant; Antipsychotic
247210	Tab	Amitriptyline 10 mg, Perphenazine 2 mg	Triavil by Royce	51875-0247	Antidepressant; Antipsychotic
2473	Cap	Diphenhydramine HCl 50 mg	Benadryl by Vortech		Antihistamine
248 <> IG	Tab, Pink, Cap Shaped, Scored	Levetiracetam 750 mg	Keppra by Glenmark	68462-0547	Antiepileptic
248 <> RDY	Tab, Beige, Oval, Scored	Levetiracetam 1000 mg	Keppra by Dr. Reddy's	55111-0248	Anticonvulsant
248225	Tab, Orange, Round, Royce Logo 248/2-25	Amitriptyline 25 mg, Perphenazine 2 mg	Triavil by Royce	51875-0248	Antidepressant; Antipsychotic
248225	Tab, Orange, Round, Royce Logo 248/2-25	Amitriptyline 25 mg, Perphenazine 2 mg	Triavil by Ivax	00182-1236	Antidepressant; Antipsychotic
249410	Tab, Salmon	Amitriptyline 10 mg, Perphenazine 4 mg	Triavil by Ivax	00182-1237	Antidepressant; Antipsychotic
249410	Tab, Salmon	Amitriptyline 10 mg, Perphenazine 4 mg	Triavil by Royce	51875-0249	Antidepressant; Antipsychotic
25	Tab, Yellow, Round	Amitriptyline HCl 25 mg	Elavil by Apotex	Canadian DIN 00335061	Antidepressant
25	Tab, White, Round	Bethanechol Chloride 25 mg	Urecholine by Roberts	Canadian	Urinary Tract
25	Tab, Pale Yellow, Round	Clomipramine HCl 25 mg	Apo Clomipramine by Apotex	Canadian DIN 02040778	OCD
25	Tab, Pink, Round, Film Coated	Trimipramine Maleate 25 mg	by Nu Pharm	Canadian DIN 02020602	Antidepressant

ID FRONT <> BACK	DESCRIPTION FRONT <> BACK	INGREDIENT & STRENGTH	BRAND (or Generic Equiv.) by FIRM	NDC#	CLASS; SCH.
25	Tab, Brown, Round	Thioridazine HCl 25 mg	Apo Thioridazine by Apotex	Canadian	Antipsychotic
25	Tab, White, Round	Terbutaline Sulfate 2.5 mg	Bricanyl by AstraZeneca	Canadian	Antiasthmatic
25	Tab, Pink, Round, Film Coated	Trimipramine 25 mg	Rhotrimine by Rhodiapharm	Canadian	Antidepressant
25	Tab, Red, Round	Phenazopyridine HCl 100 mg	Pyridium by Breckenridge	51991-0520	Urinary Analgesic
25	Cap, White	Amylase 20,000 Units, Lipase 4500 Units, Protease 25,000 Units	Pancrease by Eurand		Gastrointestinal
25	Tab, Pink, Round, Film Coated	Trimipramine Maleate 25 mg	Trimip by Apotex	Canadian DIN 00740802	Antidepressant
25	Cap, Green, Oval	Hydroxyzine HCl 25 mg	Atarax by Novopharm	Canadian DIN 00738832	Antianxiety; Antihistamine
25	Tab, Orangish Yellow, Round, Film Coated	Desipramine HCl 25 mg	Apo Desipramine by Apotex	Canadian DIN 02216256	Antidepressant
25	Tab, Orange, Round	Dipyridamole 25 mg	Dipyridamole by Apotex	Canadian DIN 00895644	Antiplatelet
25	Tab, Yellow, Round, Coated	Diclofenac Sodium 25 mg	Apo Diclo by Apotex	Canadian DIN 00839175	NSAID
25	Cap, Green	Hydroxyzine HCl 25 mg	Apo Hydroxyzine by Apotex	Canadian DIN 00646024	Antianxiety; Antihistamine
25	Tab, Blue, Round, Film Coated	Hydralazine HCl 25 mg	Hydralazine by Apotex	Canadian DIN 00441627	Antihypertensive
25	Tab, Light Brown, Round	Imipramine HCl 25 mg	Tofranil by Apotex	Canadian DIN 00312797	Antidepressant
25	Tab, White, Round, 25 <> Cobalt Logo	Topiramate 25 mg	Topamax by Cobalt	Canadian DIN 02287765	Antimigraine
25 <> 0119	Tab, White, Round	Topiramate 25 mg	Topamax by Dava	67253-0751	Anticonvulsant
25 <> 15	Tab, White, Round, Hourglass Logo 25 <> 15	Captopril 25 mg, HCTZ 15 mg	Capozide by Ivax	00172-2515	Antihypertensive; Diuretic
25 <> 25	Tab, Peach, Round, Hourglass Logo 25 <> 25	Captopril 25 mg, HCTZ 25 mg	Capozide by Ivax	00172-2525	Antihypertensive; Diuretic
25 <> 348	Tab, 25/Royce Logo <> 348	Captopril 25 mg	Capoten by Qualitest	00603-2556	Antihypertensive
25 <> 4195	Tab, Yellow, Round, Scored, 2.5 <> Hourglass Logo over 4195	Enalapril Maleate 2.5 mg	Vasotec by Ivax	00172-4195	Antihypertensive
25 <> 4214	Tab, Light Yellow, Round, Film Coated, Blue Ink, 2.5 <> 4214	Saxagliptin 2.5 mg	Onglyza by BMS	00003-4214	Antidiabetic
25 <> 4359	Tab, Pale Yellow, Round, Hourglass Logo over 4359	Clozapine 25 mg	Clozaril by Ivax	00093-4359	Antipsychotic
25 <> 4359	Tab, Pale Yellow, Round, Hourglass Logo over 4359	Clozapine 25 mg	Clozaril by Dixon Shane	17236-0357	Antipsychotic
25 <> 50	Tab, Off-White, Oval, 25 <> Hourglass Logo 50	Captopril 50 mg, HCTZ 25 mg	Capozide by Ivax	00172-5025	Antihypertensive; Diuretic
25 <> 5672	Tab, Blue, Round, Scored, Ivax Logo 25	Sertraline HCl 25 mg	Zoloft by Ivax	00172-5672 Discontinued	Antidepressant
25 <> 5732	Tab, Yellow, Round, Hourglass Logo 2.5 <> 5732	Bisoprolol 2.5 mg, Hydrochlorothiazide 6.25 mg	Ziac by Ivax	00172-5730	Antihypertensive; Diuretic
25 <> 832	Tab, Butterscotch Yellow, Sugar Coated	Chlorpromazine HCl 25 mg	by Qualitest	00603-2809	Antipsychotic
25 <> A	Tab, Light Yellow, Cap Shaped	Lisinopril 40 mg	Zestril by Aurobindo	65862-0042	Antihypertensive
25 <> AFL	Tab, Yellow, Round, Film Coated, Extended Release, AFL <> 2.5	Felodipine 2.5 mg	Plendil by AstraZeneca	00172-5672	Antihypertensive
25 <> APO	Tab, Pink, Round, Film Coated, 2.5	Indapamide 2.5 mg	Lozol by Apotex	Canadian DIN 02057778	Diuretic
25 <> APO	Tab, White to Off-White, Round, APO <> 2.5	Lisinopril 2.5 mg	Zestril by Apotex	Canadian DIN 02223678	Antihypertensive
25 <> APO	Tab, White, Shield Shaped	Lamotrigine 25 mg	Lamictal by Apotex	60505-0184	Anticonvulsant
25 <> B	Tab, Bright Pink, Cap Shaped	Diphenhydramine HCl 25 mg	Benadryl by Warner Lambert	Canadian DIN 02245208	Antihistamine
25 <> BAYER	Tab, Orange, Round, Film-Coated, 2.5	Vardenafil HCl 2.5 mg	Levitra by Bayer	00501-2002	Impotence Agent
25 <> BL	Tab, Lavender, Round, Coated	Amitriptyline HCl 75 mg	Elavil by Teva	00026-8710	Antidepressant
25 <> CLOZARIL	Tab, Pale Yellow, Round, Scored	Clozapine 25 mg	Clozaril by Novartis	00093-2126	Antipsychotic
25 <> CLOZARIL	Tab, Pale Yellow, Round, Scored	Clozapine 25 mg	Clozaril by Nat Pharmpak	55154-3412	Antipsychotic

ID FRONT <> BACK	DESCRIPTION FRONT <> BACK	INGREDIENT & STRENGTH	BRAND (or Generic Equiv.) by FIRM	NDC#	CLASS; SCH.
25 <> CLOZARIL	Tab, Yellow, Round, Scored	Clozapine 25 mg	Clozaril by Novartis	Canadian DIN 00894737	Antipsychotic
25 <> CLOZARIL	Tab, Yellow, Round, Scored	Clozapine 25 mg	Clozaril by Direct Dispensing	57866-4421	Antipsychotic
25 <> D	Tab, Blue, D-Shaped, D <> 2.5	Dexmethylphenidate HCl 2.5 mg	Focalin by Novartis	00078-0380	Stimulant; C II
25 <> DAN5642	Tab, White, Round, Scored, 2.5 <> Dan over 5642	Minoxidil 2.5 mg	Rogaine by Schein	00364-2172	Antihypertensive
25 <> DAN5642	Tab, White, Round, Scored, 2.5 <> Dan over 5642	Minoxidil 2.5 mg	Rogaine by Watson	00591-5642	Antihypertensive
25 <> DEPADE	Tab, Pink, Cap Shaped, Film Coated	Naltrexone HCl 25 mg	Depade by Mallinckrodt	00406-0089	Opioid Antagonist
25 <> E	Tab, White, Round, Film Coated, 2.5 <> Elan Logo	Frovatriptan 2.5 mg	Frova by Endo	63481-0025	Antimigraine
25 <> F	Tab, Pink, 2.5 <> F	Medroxyprogesterone Acetate 2.5 mg	Provim by Fournier	Canadian	Hormone
25 <> FL	Tab, White, Round, Film Coated	Milnacipran HCl 25 mg	Savella by Forest	00456-1525	Antidepressant; Antifibromyalgia
25 <> FLINT	Tab, Orange, Round, Scored	Levothyroxine Sodium 25 mcg	Synthroid by Abbott	00048-1020	Thyroid Hormone
25 <> FLINT	Tab, Orange, Round, Scored	Levothyroxine Sodium 25 mcg	Synthroid by Forest	00456-0320	Thyroid Hormone
25 <> FLINT	Tab, Orange, Round, Scored	Levothyroxine Sodium 25 mcg	Synthroid by Nat Pharmpak	55154-0910	Thyroid Hormone
25 <> FLINT	Tab, Orange, Round, Scored	Levothyroxine Sodium 25 mcg	Synthroid by Rite Aid	11822-5287	Thyroid Hormone
25 <> FLINT	Tab, Orange, Round, Scored	Levothyroxine Sodium 25 mcg	Synthroid by Abbott	Canadian DIN 02172062	Thyroid Hormone
25 <> FLINT	Tab, Orange, Round, Scored	Levothyroxine Sodium 25 mcg	Synthroid by Rx Pak	65084-0174	Thyroid Hormone
25 <> FLINT	Tab, Orange, Round, Scored	Levothyroxine Sodium 25 mcg	Synthroid by Haines	59564-0115	Thyroid Hormone
25 <> G1520	Tab, White, Diamond-Shaped	Amlodipine Besylate 2.5 mg	Norvasc by Greenstone	59762-1520	Antihypertensive
25 <> G41	Tab, White, Round	Carvedilol 25 mg	Coreg by Glenmark	68462-0165	Antihypertensive
25 <> GG32	Tab, Orange, Round, Film Coated, GG over 32	Thioridazine 25 mg	Mellaril by Sandoz	00781-1624	Antipsychotic
25 <> GG331	Tab, Orange, Cap Shaped, Scored, 25 <> GG over 331	Levothyroxine 25 mcg	Levo-T by Sandoz	00781-5180	Thyroid Hormone
25 <> GG331	Tab, Orange, Cap Shaped, Scored, 25 <> GG over 331	Levothyroxine 25 mcg	Levo-T by Alara	64909-0121	Thyroid Hormone
25 <> GG476	Tab, Yellow, Round, GG over 476	Chlorpromazine HCl 25 mg	Thorazine by Sandoz	00781-1716	Antipsychotic
25 <> GG476	Tab, Yellow, Round, GG over 476	Chlorpromazine HCl 25 mg	Thorazine by Heartland	61392-0040	Antipsychotic
25 <> GLYSET	Tab, White, Round	Miglitol 25 mg	Glyset by Pharmacia	00009-5012	Antidiabetic
25 <> I	Tab, White, Triangular, Film Coated	Sumatriptan Succinate 25 mg	Imitrex by GSK	Canadian DIN 0223938	Antimigraine
25 <> I	Tab, White, Triangular, Film Coated	Sumatriptan Succinate 25 mg	Imitrex by GSK	00173-0735	Antimigraine
25 <> I	Tab, White, Triangular, Film Coated	Sumatriptan Succinate 25 mg	Imitrex by GSK	00173-0460	Antimigraine
25 <> I	Tab, White, Triangular, Film Coated	Sumatriptan Succinate 25 mg	Imitrex by Physician Total Care	54868-3777	Antimigraine
25 <> INV272	Tab, Scored, INV over 272	Captopril 25 mg	Capoten by Invamed	52189-0272	Antihypertensive
25 <> INV272	Tab, Scored, INV over 272	Captopril 25 mg	Capoten by Schein	00364-2629	Antihypertensive
25 <> INV277	Tab, Yellow, Round, Film Coated	Prochlorperazine Maleate 25 mg	by Invamed	52189-0277	Antiemetic
25 <> INV311	Tab, Green, Square, Scored, 2.5 <> INV over 311	Warfarin Sodium 2.5 mg	Coumadin by Sandoz	00781-0364	Anticoagulant
25 <> INV311	Tab, Green, Square, Scored, 2.5 <> INV over 311	Warfarin Sodium 2.5 mg	Coumadin by Apothecon	59772-0364	Anticoagulant
25 <> L479	Tab, Pink, Cap Shaped	Diphenhydramine HCl 25 mg	Benadryl by Perrigo	00113-0479	Antihistamine
25 <> LMT	Tab, White, Round, Orally Disintegrating	Lamotrigine 25 mg	Lamictal ODT by GSK	00173-0772	Anticonvulsant
25 <> LUPIN	Tab, White to Off-White, Round, LUPIN <> 2.5	Lisinopril 2.5 mg	Zestril by Lupin	68180-0512	Antihypertensive
25 <> M	Tab, Coral, Round, Biconvex, Film Coated, M inside Box	Imipramine HCl 25 mg	Tofranil by Mallinckrodt	00406-9921	Antidepressant
25 <> M1	Tab, Yellow, Round, Scored	Methotrexate Sodium 2.5 mg	Methotrexate by Wyeth Canada	Canadian DIN 02170698	Antineoplastic
25 <> M58	Tab, Orange, Round, Film Coated, M over 58	Thioridazine 25 mg	Mellaril by Mylan	00378-0614	Antipsychotic
25 <> M58	Tab, Orange, Round, Film Coated, M over 58	Thioridazine 25 mg	Mellaril by Dixon Shane	17236-0301	Antipsychotic
25 <> M58	Tab, Orange, Round, Film Coated, M over 58	Thioridazine 25 mg	Mellaril by Vangard	00615-2506	Antipsychotic
25 <> M58	Tab, Orange, Round, Film Coated, M over 58	Thioridazine 25 mg	Mellaril by UDL	51079-0566	Antipsychotic
25 <> MJ504	Tab, White w/ Blue Flecks, Round, MJ over 504	Cyclophosphamide 25 mg	Cytoxan by BMS	Canadian DIN 00344877	Antineoplastic
25 <> MJ504	Tab, White w/ Blue Flecks, Round, MJ over 504	Cyclophosphamide 25 mg	Cytoxan by Mead Johnson	00015-0504	Antineoplastic
25 <> MYLAN146	Tab, White, Round, Scored, Mylan over 146	Spironolactone 25 mg	Aldactone by Mylan	00378-2146	Diuretic

ID FRONT <> BACK	DESCRIPTION FRONT <> BACK	INGREDIENT & STRENGTH	BRAND (or Generic Equiv.) by FIRM	NDC#	CLASS; SCH.
25 <> MYLAN146	Tab, White, Round, Scored, Mylan over 146	Spironolactone 25 mg	Aldactone by Vangard	00615-1535	Diuretic
25 <> MYLAN146	Tab, White, Round, Scored, Mylan over 146	Spironolactone 25 mg	Aldactone by UDL	51079-0103	Diuretic
25 <> MYLAN146	Tab, White, Round, Scored, Mylan over 146	Spironolactone 25 mg	Aldactone by Qualitest	00603-5766	Diuretic
25 <> MYLAN146	Tab, White, Round, Scored, Mylan over 146	Spironolactone 25 mg	Aldactone by Heartland	61392-0083	Diuretic
25 <> MYLAN146	Tab, White, Round, Scored, Mylan over 146	Spironolactone 25 mg	Aldactone by Nat Pharmpak	55154-5517	Diuretic
25 <> MYLAN146	Tab, White, Round, Scored, Mylan over 146	Spironolactone 25 mg	Aldactone by Pharmedix	53002-0472	Diuretic
25 <> MYLAN146	Tab, White, Round, Scored, Mylan over 146	Spironolactone 25 mg	Aldactone by Vangard	00615-1535	Diuretic
25 <> N	Tab, White, Round	Topiramate 25 mg	Topamax by Novopharm	Canadian DIN 02248860	Anticonvulsant
25 <> N	Tab, Yellow, Round	Amitriptyline HCl 25 mg	Elavil by Novopharm	Canadian DIN 00037419	Antidepressant
25 <> N	Tab, Yellow, Round, Scored, N <> 2/5	Spironolactone 25 mg	Aldactone by Novopharm	Canadian DIN 00613215	Diuretic
25 <> N	Tab, Dark Orange, Round, Large N	Imipramine 25 mg	Tofranil by Novopharm	Canadian DIN 00021512	Antidepressant
25 <> N	Tab, Blue, Round, N/25	Hydralazine HCl 25 mg	Apresoline by Novopharm	Canadian DIN 00759473	Antihypertensive
25 <> N	Tab, Dark Pink, Round, N <> 2.5	Indapamide 2.5 mg	Lozide by Novopharm	Canadian DIN 02231184	Diuretic
25 <> N	Tab, White, Oval	Carvedilol 25 mg	Coreg by Novopharm	Canadian DIN 02246532	Antihypertensive
25 <> N	Tab, White, Round, Scored, N <> 2 / 5	Chlorpromazine HCl 25 mg	Largactil by Novopharm	Canadian DIN 00232823	Antipsychotic; Antiemetic
25 <> N343	Tab, Peach, Round, Scored, 2.5 <> N over 343	Glyburide 2.5 mg	Micronase by Teva	00093-8343	Antidiabetic
25 <> N343	Tab, Peach, Round, Scored, 2.5 <> N over 343	Glyburide 2.5 mg	Micronase by Moore	00839-8040	Antidiabetic
25 <> N343	Tab, Peach, Round, Scored, 2.5 <> N over 343	Glyburide 2.5 mg	Micronase by Brightstone	62939-3221	Antidiabetic
25 <> N343	Tab, Peach, Round, Scored, 2.5 <> N over 343	Glyburide 2.5 mg	Micronase by Heartland	61392-0709	Antidiabetic
25 <> N343	Tab, Peach, Round, Scored, 2.5 <> N over 343	Glyburide 2.5 mg	Micronase by Teva	55953-0343	Antidiabetic
25 <> N343	Tab, Peach, Round, Scored, 2.5 <> N over 343	Glyburide 2.5 mg	Micronase by Medirex	57480-0408	Antidiabetic
25 <> N343	Tab, Peach, Round, Scored, 2.5 <> N over 343	Glyburide 2.5 mg	Micronase by Murfreesboro	51129-1405	Antidiabetic
25 <> N343	Tab, Peach, Round, Scored, 2.5 <> N over 343	Glyburide 2.5 mg	Micronase by UDL	51079-0872 Discontinued	Antidiabetic
25 <> N343	Tab, Peach, Round, Scored, 2.5 <> N over 343	Glyburide 2.5 mg	Micronase by Major	00904-5076	Antidiabetic
25 <> N343	Tab, Peach, Round, Scored, 2.5 <> N over 343	Glyburide 2.5 mg	Micronase by Kaiser	62224-1331	Antidiabetic
25 <> N343	Tab, Peach, Round, Scored, 2.5 <> N over 343	Glyburide 2.5 mg	Micronase by Warrick	59930-1622	Antidiabetic
25 <> N837	Tab, Film Coated, 2.5	Indapamide 2.5 mg	Lozol by Teva	55953-0837	Diuretic
25 <> N958	Tab, Pale Yellow, Oval, Scored, N/958	Clozapine 25 mg	Clozaril by Par	49884-0088	Antipsychotic
25 <> N958	Tab, Pale Yellow, Oval, Scored, N/958	Clozapine 25 mg	Clozaril by Teva	00093-0275 Discontinued	Antipsychotic
25 <> NN	Tab, Pink, Oval, Scored, N / N <> 2.5	Cilazapril 2.5 mg	Inhibace by Novopharm	Canadian DIN 02266369	Antihypertensive
25 <> NN	Tab, White, Round, N/N <> 25	Atenolol 25 mg	Tenormin by Novopharm	Canadian DIN 02266660	Antihypertensive
25 <> NN	Tab, White, Shield Shaped, Scored, N/N <> 25	Lamotrigine 25 mg	Lamictal by Novopharm	Canadian DIN 02248232	Antiepileptic
25 <> NN	Tab, Peach, Round, Scored, N/N	Medroxyprogesterone Acetate 2.5 mg	Provera by Novopharm	Canadian DIN 02221284	Hormone
25 <> NORVASC	Tab, White, Diamond Shaped, 2.5 <> Norvasc	Amlodipine Besylate 2.5 mg	Norvasc by Pfizer	00069-1520	Antihypertensive
25 <> NORVASC	Tab, White, Diamond Shaped, 2.5 <> Norvasc	Amlodipine Besylate 2.5 mg	Norvasc by Murfreesboro	51129-1260	Antihypertensive
25 <> NORVASC	Tab, White, Diamond Shaped, 2.5 <> Norvasc	Amlodipine Besylate 2.5 mg	Norvasc by Physician Total Care	54868-3853	Antihypertensive
25 <> NORVASC	Tab, White, Diamond Shaped, 2.5 <> Norvasc	Amlodipine Besylate 2.5 mg	Norvasc by DRX	55045-2377	Antihypertensive

ID FRONT <> BACK	DESCRIPTION FRONT <> BACK	INGREDIENT & STRENGTH	BRAND (or Generic Equiv.) by FIRM	NDC#	CLASS; SCH.
25 <> NOVO	Tab, White, Round, Scored, no/vo <> 2.5	Glyburide 2.5 mg	DiaBeta by Novopharm	Canadian DIN 01913670	Antidiabetic
25 <> P	Tab, White, Round, Oval, Film Coated	Carvedilol 25 mg	Coreg by Pharmascience	Canadian DIN 02245917	Antihypertensive
25 <> P	Tab, White, Round	Topiramate 25 mg	Topamax by Pharmascience	Canadian DIN 02262991	Anticonvulsant
25 <> P	Tab, White, Round, P logo <> 2.5	Oxybutynin Chloride 2.5 mg	Ditropan by Pharmascience	Canadian DIN 02240549	Urinary Tract
25 <> P	Tab, Yellow, Round	Diclofenac Sodium 25 mg	Voltaren by Pharmascience	Canadian DIN 02231502	NSAID
25 <> P	Tab, Pink, Round, Scored	Loxapine Succinate 25 mg	Loxapac by Pharmascience	Canadian DIN 02230839	Antipsychotic
25 <> P	Tab, Yellow, Round	Methotrimeprazine Maleate 25 mg	Nozinan by Pharmascience	Canadian DIN 02232904	Antipsychotic
25 <> P	Tab, White to Off White, Caplet Shaped, Scored	Methadone HCl 25 mg	Metadol by Pharmascience	Canadian DIN 02247701	Analgesic
25 <> PAXILCR	Tab, Pink, Round, Film Coated, Paxil CR 25	Paroxetine HCl 25 mg	Paxil CR by GSK	Canadian DIN 02248504	Antidepressant
25 <> PAXILCR	Tab, Pink, Round, Film Coated, Paxil CR 25	Paroxetine HCl 25 mg	Paxil CR by SKB	00029-3207	Antidepressant
25 <> PERCOCET	Tab, Pink, Oval, 2.5 <> Percocet	Oxycodone HCl 2.5 mg, Acetaminophen 325 mg	Percocet by Endo	63481-0627	Analgesic; C II
25 <> PERCOCET	Tab, Pink, Oval, 2.5 <> Percocet	Oxycodone HCl 2.5 mg, Acetaminophen 325 mg	Percocet by West Pharm	52967-0278	Analgesic; C II
25 <> PRECOSE	Tab, White, Round	Acarbose 25 mg	Precose by Bayer	00026-2863	Antidiabetic
25 <> S	Tab, White, Triangle Shaped	Sumatriptan 25 mg	Imitrex by Dr. Reddy's	55111-0738	Antimigraine
25 <> SANDOZ	Tab, Red, Round, Sugar Coated	Mesoridazine Besylate 25 mg	Serentil by Novartis	Canadian DIN 00027456	Antipsychotic
25 <> SYNTHROID	Tab, Orange, Round, Scored	Levothyroxine Sodium 25 mcg	Synthroid by Abbott	00074-4341	Thyroid Hormone
25 <> T4	Tab, Orange, Cap Shaped	Levothyroxine Sodium 25 mcg	Levothroid by Forest	00456-1320	Thyroid Hormone
25 <> TOP	Tab, White, Round, Film Coated	Topiramate 25 mg	Topamax by Janssen-Ortho	Canadian DIN 02230893	Anticonvulsant
25 <> TOP	Tab, White, Round, Film Coated	Topiramate 25 mg	Topamax by McNeil	00045-0639	Anticonvulsant
25 <> TOP	Tab, White, Round, Film Coated	Topiramate 25 mg	Topamax by Ortho-McNeil	00062-0639	Anticonvulsant
25 <> TOP	Tab, White, Round, Film Coated	Topiramate 25 mg	Topamax by McNeil	52021-0639	Anticonvulsant
25 <> VIDEX	Tab, Off-White to Light Orange/Yellow, Round, Chewable	Didanosine 25 mg	Videx by BMS	Canadian DIN 01940511	Antiviral
25 <> VIDEX	Tab, Off-White to Light Orange/Yellow, Round, Chewable	Didanosine 25 mg	Videx by BMS	00087-6650	Antiviral
25 <> VOLTAREN	Tab, Yellow, Round, Enteric Coated	Diclofenac Sodium 25 mg	Voltaren by Novartis	Canadian DIN 00514004	NSAID
25 <> W	Tab, Yellow, Round	Isosorbide Dinitrate 2.5 mg	Isordil by Wyeth	00008-4139	Antianginal
25 <> ZAROXOLYN	Tab, Debossed, 2.5 <> Zaroxolyn	Metolazone 2.5 mg	Zaroxolyn by Drug Distr	52985-0218	Diuretic
250	Tab, Orange, Oval, Enteric Coated	Divalproex Sodium 250 mg	by Nu Pharm	Canadian DIN 02239518	Anticonvulsant
250	Tab, Blue, Round	Norgestimate 0.250 mg, Ethinyl Estradiol 0.025 mg	Tri-Cyclen LO 21 by Janssen-Ortho	Canadian DIN 02258560	Oral Contraceptive
250	Tab, Blue, Round	Norgestimate 0.250 mg, Ethinyl Estradiol 0.025 mg	Tri-Cyclen LO 28 by Janssen-Ortho	Canadian DIN 02258587	Oral Contraceptive
250	Tab, Pink, Cap Shaped, Scored	Niacin 250 mg	Slo-Niacin by Upsher Smith	00245-0062	Vitamin
250 <> 347	Tab, White to Cream, Oval, Film Coated	Cefprozil 250 mg	Cefzil by Sandoz	00781-5043	Antibiotic
250 <> 400	Tab, Red, Oblong	Amoxicillin 400 mg	Amoxil by Allscripts		Antibiotic
250 <> 4335	Tab, Peach, Round, Logo 4335 <> 250	Nefazodone 250 mg	Serzone by Ivax	00172-4335	Antidepressant
250 <> 5311	Tab, White to Off White, Oval, Ivax Logo 5311 <> 250	Ciprofloxacin 250 mg	Cipro by Ivax	00172-5311	Antibiotic

ID FRONT <> BACK	DESCRIPTION FRONT <> BACK	INGREDIENT & STRENGTH	BRAND (or Generic Equiv.) by FIRM	NDC#	CLASS; SCH.
250 <> 7720	Tab, Light Orange, Film Coated	Cefprozil 250 mg	Cefzil by BMS	Canadian DIN 02163659	Antibiotic
250 <> 7720	Tab, Light Orange, Film Coated	Cefprozil 250 mg	Cefzil by BMS	00087-7720	Antibiotic
250 <> AMOXIL	Tab, Pink, Oval, Chewable	Amoxicillin 250 mg	Amoxil by Allscripts		Antibiotic
250 <> AMOXIL	Tab, Pink, Oval, Chewable	Amoxicillin 250 mg	Amoxil by SKB	00029-6005	Antibiotic
250 <> APO	Tab, White, Round, Biconvex, Enteric Coated	Naproxen 250 mg	Naprosyn by Apotex	Canadian DIN 02246699	NSAID
250 <> APO	Tab, White, Oval	Ticlopidine HCl 250 mg	Ticlopidine by Apotex	Canadian DIN 02237701	Anticoagulant
250 <> APO	Tab, Peach, Oval, Biconvex	Divalproex Sodium 250 mg	Depakote by Apotex	Canadian DIN 02239699	Anticonvulsant
250 <> APO047	Tab, White to Off-White, Oval	Divalproex Sodium 250 mg	Depakote by Apotex	60505-3066	Anticonvulsant
250 <> B814	Tab, Round, Film Coated, Biconvex	Ciprofloxacin HCl 250 mg	Cipro by Barr	00555-0814	Antibiotic
250 <> CIPRO	Tab, White to Light Yellow, Round, Film Coated	Ciprofloxacin HCl 250 mg	Cipro by Bayer	00085-1758	Antibiotic
250 <> CIPRO	Tab, White to Light Yellow, Round, Film Coated	Ciprofloxacin HCl 250 mg	Cipro by Compumed	00403-4258	Antibiotic
250 <> CIPRO	Tab, White to Light Yellow, Round, Film Coated	Ciprofloxacin HCl 250 mg	Cipro by Pharmedix	53002-0279	Antibiotic
250 <> CIPRO	Tab, White to Light Yellow, Round, Film Coated	Ciprofloxacin HCl 250 mg	Cipro by Bayer	Canadian DIN 02155958	Antibiotic
250 <> CIPRO	Tab, White to Light Yellow, Round, Film Coated	Ciprofloxacin HCl 250 mg	Cipro by Direct Dispensing	57866-6250	Antibiotic
250 <> CIPRO	Tab, White to Light Yellow, Round, Film Coated	Ciprofloxacin HCl 250 mg	Cipro by Amerisource	62584-0335	Antibiotic
250 <> CIPRO	Tab, White to Light Yellow, Round, Film Coated	Ciprofloxacin HCl 250 mg	Cipro by Bayer	00026-8512	Antibiotic
250 <> CIPRO	Tab, White to Light Yellow, Round, Film Coated	Ciprofloxacin HCl 250 mg	Cipro by Nat Pharmpak	55154-4806	Antibiotic
250 <> CIPRO	Tab, White to Light Yellow, Round, Film Coated	Ciprofloxacin HCl 250 mg	Cipro by Apotheca	12634-0423	Antibiotic
250 <> CIPRO	Tab, White to Light Yellow, Round, Film Coated	Ciprofloxacin HCl 250 mg	Cipro by H J Harkins Co	52959-0171	Antibiotic
250 <> CITRACAL	Tab, White, Modified Rectangle, Film Coated	Calcium Citrate 250 mg, Vitamin D 62.5 IU	Citracal 250 mg + D by Mission	00178-0837	Vitamin; Supplement
250 <> FAMVIR	Tab, White, Round, Film Coated	Famciclovir 250 mg	Famvir by SKB	60351-4116	Antiviral
250 <> FAMVIR	Tab, White, Round, Film Coated	Famciclovir 250 mg	Famvir by SKB	00007-4116	Antiviral
250 <> FAMVIR	Tab, White, Round, Film Coated	Famciclovir 250 mg	Famvir by Novartis	00078-0367	Antiviral
250 <> FAMVIR	Tab, White, Round, Film Coated	Famciclovir 250 mg	Famvir by Physician Total Care	54868-3969	Antiviral
250 <> FAMVIR	Tab, White, Round, Film Coated	Famciclovir 250 mg	Famvir by Novartis	Canadian DIN 02229129	Antiviral
250 <> G	Tab, Dark Pink, Cap Shaped, Film Coated	Azithromycin 250 mg	Zithromax by Genpharm	Canadian DIN 02278359	Antibiotic
250 <> G2	Tab, White, Round	Terbinafine HCl 250 mg	Lamisil by Glenmark	68462-0136	Antifungal
250 <> G32	Tab, Pink, Round, G-32 <> 250	Naproxen 250 mg	Naprosyn by Glenmark	68462-0188	NSAID
250 <> GLAXO	Tab, White, Oblong	Cefuroxime Axetil 250 mg	Ceftin by GSK	00173-7004	Antibiotic
250 <> GRISPEG	Tab, White, Cap Shaped, Film Coated, Gris-Peg <> 250, Scored	Griseofulvin 250 mg	Fulvicin P/G by Leiner	59606-0654	Antifungal
250 <> GRISPEG	Tab, White, Cap Shaped, Film Coated, Gris-Peg <> 250, Scored	Griseofulvin 250 mg	Fulvicin P/G by Amerisource	62584-0773	Antifungal
250 <> GRISPEG	Tab, White, Cap Shaped, Film Coated, Gris-Peg <> 250, Scored	Griseofulvin 250 mg	Fulvicin P/G by Novartis	00043-0801	Antifungal
250 <> GRISPEG	Tab, White, Cap Shaped, Film Coated, Gris-Peg <> 250, Scored	Griseofulvin 250 mg	Fulvicin P/G by Allergan	00023-0773	Antifungal
250 <> INV	Tab, White, Oblong, Film Coated	Hydroxychloroquine Sulfate 200 mg	by Murfreesboro	51129-1426	Antimalarial
250 <> INV	Tab, White, Oblong, Film Coated	Hydroxychloroquine Sulfate 200 mg	by DRX	55045-2766	Antimalarial
250 <> INV	Tab, White, Oblong, Film Coated	Hydroxychloroquine Sulfate 200 mg	by Invamed	52189-0250	Antimalarial
250 <> IP188	Tab, White, Round	Naproxen 250 mg	Naprosyn by Amneal	65162-0076 Discontinued	NSAID
250 <> IP188	Tab, White, Round	Naproxen 250 mg	Naprosyn by Dr. Reddy's	55111-0366	NSAID
250 <> IP188	Tab, White, Round	Naproxen 250 mg	Naprosyn by Interpharm	53746-0188	NSAID

ID FRONT <> BACK	DESCRIPTION FRONT <> BACK	INGREDIENT & STRENGTH	BRAND (or Generic Equiv.) by FIRM	NDC#	CLASS; SCH.
250 <> K	Tab, Dark Pink, Round, Film Coated	Tranylcypromine Sulfate 10 mg	Parnate by Par	49884-0032	Antidepressant
250 <> LAMISIL	Tab, White, Round	Terbinafine HCl 250 mg	by Allscripts		Antifungal
250 <> LAMISIL	Tab, White, Round	Terbinafine HCl 250 mg	Lamisil by Novartis	00078-0179	Antifungal
250 <> LEVAQUIN	Tab, Pink, Oblong, Film Coated	Levofloxacin 250 mg	Levaquin by Physician Total Care	54868-4175	Antibiotic
250 <> LEVAQUIN	Tab, Pink, Rectangular, Film Coated	Levofloxacin 250 mg	Levaquin by Janssen-Ortho	Canadian DIN 02236841	Antibiotic
250 <> LEVAQUIN	Tab, Pink, Rectangular, Film Coated	Levofloxacin 250 mg	Levaquin by McNeil	00045-1520	Antibiotic
250 <> LUPIN	Tab, Light Orange, Oval, Film Coated	Cefprozil 250 mg	Cefzil by Lupin	68180-0403	Antibiotic
250 <> MCNEIL1520	Tab, Pink, Rectangle, Film Coated	Levofloxacin 250 mg	Levaquin by Johnson & Johnson	59604-0520	Antibiotic
250 <> MCNEIL1520	Tab, Pink, Rectangle, Film Coated	Levofloxacin 250 mg	Levaquin by Ortho-McNeil	00062-1520	Antibiotic
250 <> MCNEIL1520	Tab, Pink, Rectangle, Film Coated	Levofloxacin 250 mg	Levaquin by McNeil	00045-1520	Antibiotic
250 <> MYLAN106	Tab, Film Coated, 250 <> Mylan over 106	Erythromycin Stearate 250 mg	by Diversified Healthcare	55887-0994	Antibiotic
250 <> MYLAN106	Tab, Film Coated, 250 <> Mylan over 106	Erythromycin Stearate 250 mg	by Rx Dispensing	61807-0013	Antibiotic
250 <> MYLAN106	Tab, Film Coated, 250 <> Mylan over 106	Erythromycin Stearate 250 mg	by Mylan	00378-0106	Antibiotic
250 <> MYLAN210	Tab, Green, Round, Scored, Mylan over 210	Chlorpropamide 250 mg	Diabinese by Physician Total Care	54868-0036	Antidiabetic
250 <> MYLAN210	Tab, Green, Round, Scored, Mylan over 210	Chlorpropamide 250 mg	Diabinese by Mylan	00378-0210	Antidiabetic
250 <> MYLAN210	Tab, Green, Round, Scored, Mylan over 210	Chlorpropamide 250 mg	Diabinese by UDL	51079-0203 Discontinued	Antidiabetic
250 <> MYLAN217	Tab, White, Scored, 250 <> Mylan over 217	Tolazamide 250 mg	Tolinase by Mylan	00378-0217	Antidiabetic
250 <> N	Tab, Peach, Oblong	Diflunisal 250 mg	Dolobid by Novopharm	Canadian DIN 02048493	NSAID
250 <> N	Tab, Pink, Oblong	Levofloxacin 250 mg	Levaquin by Novopharm	Canadian DIN 02248262	Antibiotic
250 <> N	Tab, Dark Pink, Oval	Azithromycin 250 mg	Zithromax by Novopharm	Canadian DIN 02267845	Antibiotic
250 <> N517	Tab, Peach & Yellow, Oval, N over 517	Naproxen 250 mg	by Teva	55953-0517 Discontinued	NSAID
250 <> N751	Tab, Pink, Round, Scored, Chewable, 250 <> N over 751	Amoxicillin 250 mg	Amoxil by Teva	55953-0751 Discontinued	Antibiotic
250 <> N751	Tab, Pink, Round, Scored, Chewable, 250 <> N over 751	Amoxicillin 250 mg	Amoxil by Warrick	59930-1611	Antibiotic
250 <> NAPROSYN	Tab	Naproxen 250 mg	Naprosyn by H J Harkins Co	52959-0110	NSAID
250 <> NN	Tab, Off-White, Round, Scored, N / N	Flutamide 250 mg	Euflex by Novopharm	Canadian DIN 02230089	Antiandrogen
250 <> NN	Tab, White, Round, Scored, N/N <> 250	Terbinafine HCl 250 mg	Lamisil by Novopharm	Canadian DIN 02240346	Antifungal
250 <> NOVO	Tab, Pink, Oval, Scored, NO / VO, Chewable	Amoxicillin 250 mg	Amoxil by Novopharm	Canadian DIN 02036355	Antibiotic
250 <> NOVO	Tab, White, Round, Film-Coated	Ciprofloxacin Hydrochloride 250 mg	Novo-Ciprofloxacin by Novopharm	Canadian DIN 02161737	Antibiotic
250 <> OM	Tab, Dark Blue, Round, O-M 250	Ethinyl Estradiol 0.025 mg, Norgestimate 0.250 mg	Ortho Tri-Cyclen Lo by Ortho-McNeil	00062-1251	Oral Contraceptive
250 <> P	Tab, White, Round	Famciclovir 250 mg	Famvir by Pharmascience	Canadian DIN 02278103	Antiviral
250 <> P	Tab, Red, Oblong	Azithromycin 250 mg	Zithromax by Pharmascience	Canadian DIN 02261634	Antibiotic
250 <> P	Tab, White, Oval	Ursodiol 250 mg	Urso by Pharmascience	Canadian DIN 02273497	Gastrointestinal
250 <> PL	Tab, Pink, Round, Film Coated, Scored	Tinidazole 250 mg	Tindamax by Presutti Labs	66378-0250 Discontinued	Antibiotic
250 <> R	Tab, White, Round	Terbinafine 250 mg	Lamisil by Dr. Reddy's	Lamisil	Antifungal
250 <> SYCTCP	Tab, White, Oval, Film Coated, 250 <> Syc-TCP	Ticlopidine HCl 250 mg	Ticlid by AltiMed	Canadian DIN 02194422	Anticoagulant

ID FRONT <> BACK	DESCRIPTION FRONT <> BACK	INGREDIENT & STRENGTH	BRAND (or Generic Equiv.) by FIRM	NDC#	CLASS; SCH.
250 <> T	Tab, Pink, Round, Scored	Tinidazole 250 mg	Tindamax by Teva	44523-0042	Antibiotic
250 <> TICLID	Tab, White, Blue Print, Oval, Film Coated	Ticlopidine HCl 250 mg	Ticlid by Wal Mart	49035-0165	Anticoagulant
250 <> TICLID	Tab, White, Blue Print, Oval, Film Coated	Ticlopidine HCl 250 mg	Ticlid by Med Pro	53978-3027	Anticoagulant
250 <> TICLID	Tab, White, Blue Print, Oval, Film Coated	Ticlopidine HCl 250 mg	Ticlid by Physician Total Care	54868-3783	Anticoagulant
250 <> TICLID	Tab, White, Blue Print, Oval, Film Coated	Ticlopidine HCl 250 mg	Ticlid by Syntex	18393-0431	Anticoagulant
250 <> TICLID	Tab, White, Blue Print, Oval, Film Coated	Ticlopidine HCl 250 mg	Ticlid by Hoffmann La Roche	00004-0018	Anticoagulant
250 <> TICLID	Tab, White, Blue Print, Oval, Film Coated	Ticlopidine HCl 250 mg	Ticlid by Roche	Canadian DIN 02162776 Discontinued	Anticoagulant
250 <> TM	Tab, Pink, Round, Film Coated	Tinidazole 250 mg	Tindamax by Mission	00178-8250	Antibiotic
250 <> UCB	Tab, Blue, Oblong, Scored, Film Coated	Levetiracetam 250 mg	Keppra by UCB	50474-0591	Anticonvulsant
2500 <> GSK	Tab, Pink, Oval, Film Coated, 2/500	Metformin HCl 500 mg, Rosiglitazone 2 mg	Avandamet by GSK	Canadian DIN 02247086	Antidiabetic
2500 <> GSK	Tab, Pink, Oval, Film Coated, 2/500	Metformin HCl 500 mg, Rosiglitazone 2 mg	Avandamet by SKB	00007-3167	Antidiabetic
2500V	Cap	Chlorpheniramine Maleate 8.8 mg	by Vintage	00254-2500	Antihistamine
250125 <> APO	Tab, White, Oval, Film Coated	Amoxicillin 250 mg, Clavulanate Potassium 125 mg	Clavulin by Apotex	Canadian DIN 02243350	Antibiotic
250125 <> AUGMENTIN	Tab, White, Oblong, Film Coated, 250/125	Amoxicillin 250 mg, Clavulanate Potassium 125 mg	Augmentin by Southwood	58016-0107	Antibiotic
250125 <> AUGMENTIN	Tab, White, Oblong, Film Coated, 250/125	Amoxicillin 250 mg, Clavulanate Potassium 125 mg	Augmentin by Casa DeAmigos	62138-6075	Antibiotic
250125 <> AUGMENTIN	Tab, White, Oblong, Film Coated, 250/125	Amoxicillin 250 mg, Clavulanate Potassium 125 mg	Augmentin by Pharmedix	53002-0250	Antibiotic
250125 <> AUGMENTIN	Tab, White, Oblong, Film Coated, 250/125	Amoxicillin 250 mg, Clavulanate Potassium 125 mg	Augmentin by Bayer	00280-1001	Antibiotic
250125 <> AUGMENTIN	Tab, White, Oblong, Film Coated, 250/125	Amoxicillin 250 mg, Clavulanate Potassium 125 mg	Augmentin by SKB	00029-6075	Antibiotic
2501V	Cap	Chlorpheniramine Maleate 12 mg	Chlor-Trimeton by Vintage	00254-2501	Antihistamine
25025 <> NOVO	Tab, Light Blue, Oval, Scored	Levodopa 250 mg, Carbidopa 25 mg	Sinemet by Novopharm	Canadian DIN 02244496	Antiparkinson
25025 <> NU	Tab, Blue, Oval, Scored, 250 over 25 <> NU	Carbidopa 25 mg, Levodopa 250 mg	by Nu Pharm	Canadian DIN 02182831	Antiparkinson
25025ENDO	Tab, Red & Blue, Oval, 250/25/Endo	Levodopa 250 mg, Carbidopa 25 mg	Sinemet by AltiMed	Canadian	Antiparkinson
250425	Tab	Amitriptyline 25 mg, Perphenazine 4 mg	Triavil by Ivax	00182-1238	Antidepressant; Antipsychotic
250425	Tab	Amitriptyline 25 mg, Perphenazine 4 mg	Triavil by Royce	51875-0250	Antidepressant; Antipsychotic
250AP7491	Cap	Cefaclor 250 mg	Ceclor by Golden State	60429-0701	Antibiotic
250AP7491	Cap	Cefaclor 250 mg	Ceclor by Apothecon	59772-7491	Antibiotic
250BRISTOL7375	Cap, Blue & Purple, 250/Bristol 7375	Cephalexin 250 mg	Keflex by BMS		Antibiotic
250CP	Cap, Branded Nortriptyline	Nortriptyline 10 mg	by Moore	00839-7798	Antidepressant
250GLAXO	Tab, White, Oblong, 250/Glaxo	Cefuroxime Axetil 250 mg	by GSK	Canadian	Antibiotic
250LUPIN	Cap, Dark Green and White	Cephalexin 250 mg	Keflex by Lupin	68180-0121	Antibiotic
250M25	Tab, Rose, Round, Scored, 250 / M25	Naproxen 250 mg	Naprosyn by Dava	67253-0620	NSAID
250M25	Tab, Rose, Round, Scored, 250 / M25	Naproxen 250 mg	Naprosyn by Major	00904-5535	NSAID
250M25 <> MOVA	Tab, Rose, Round	Naproxen 250 mg	by Caremark	00339-5870	NSAID
250M25 <> MOVA	Tab, Rose, Round	Naproxen 250 mg	Naprosyn by Mova	55370-0139	NSAID
250MG <> TRYPTAN	Tab, White, Oval, Film Coated	L-Tryptophan 250 mg	Tryptan by Valeant	Canadian DIN 02239326	Supplement
250MG <> VIRACEPT	Tab, Light Blue, Oblong	Nelfinavir Mesylate 250 mg	Viracept by Mova	55370-0560	Antiviral
250MG <> VIRACEPT	Tab, Light Blue, Oblong	Nelfinavir Mesylate 250 mg	Viracept by Agouron	63010-0010	Antiviral
250MG <> VIRACEPT	Tab, Light Blue, Oblong	Nelfinavir Mesylate 250 mg	Viracept by Circa	71114-4206	Antiviral
250MG <> VIRACEPT	Tab, Light Blue, Oblong	Nelfinavir Mesylate 250 mg	Viracept by Patheon	63285-0010	Antiviral
250MG7375BRISTOL	Cap, Printed in White Ink	Cephalexin 250 mg	by Golden State	60429-0036	Antibiotic
250MLA05	Cap, Blue & White	Cefaclor 250 mg	Ceclor by Mova	55370-0894	Antibiotic

ID FRONT <> BACK	DESCRIPTION FRONT <> BACK	INGREDIENT & STRENGTH	BRAND (or Generic Equiv.) by FIRM	NDC#	CLASS; SCH.
250MLA07	Cap, Green & White	Cephalexin 250 mg	Keflex by Mova	55370-0900	Antibiotic
250MYLAN106	Tab, Film Coated	Erythromycin Stearate 250 mg	by Med Pro	53978-5029	Antibiotic
250N253	Cap, Bright Orange & White, Opaque, 250 <> N over 253	Cefaclor 250 mg	Ceclor by Teva	55953-0253 Discontinued	Antibiotic
250N253	Cap, Bright Orange & White, Opaque, 250 <> N over 253	Cefaclor 250 mg	Ceclor by Qualitest	00603-2586	Antibiotic
250N253	Cap, Bright Orange & White, Opaque, 250 <> N over 253	Cefaclor 250 mg	Ceclor by H J Harkins Co	52959-0367	Antibiotic
250N253	Cap, Bright Orange & White, Opaque, 250 <> N over 253	Cefaclor 250 mg	Ceclor by Major	00904-5204	Antibiotic
250N253	Cap, Bright Orange & White, Opaque, 250 <> N over 253	Cefaclor 250 mg	Ceclor by UDL	51079-0617	Antibiotic
250NAXEN	Tab, Yellow, Oval	Naproxen 250 mg	Navalbine by BW Inc	Canadian	NSAID
250NORTRIPTYLINE10	Cap, Green & White	Nortriptyline HCl 10 mg	by H J Harkins Co	52959-0358	Antidepressant
250SP	Cap, Green and White	Amoxicillin 250 mg	Amoxil by 4349121 Canada Inc	Canadian DIN 02241826	Antibiotic
251	Tab, Red, Round	Pseudoephedrine 30 mg	Sudafed by Granutec		Decongestant
251	Tab, Orange, Round, Schering Logo 251	Halazepam 20 mg	Paxipam by Schering		Antianxiety; C IV
25100 <> SP342	Tab, Yellow, Round, Scored, 25/100 <> SP over 342, Orally Disintegrating	Carbidopa 25 mg, Levodopa 100 mg	Parcopa by Schwarz	00091-3342	Antiparkinson
25102 <> JACOBUS	Tab, White, Round, 25 over 102	Dapsone 25 mg	Dapsone by PDRX	55289-0188	Antimycobacterial
25102 <> JACOBUS	Tab, White, Round, 25 over 102	Dapsone 25 mg	Dapsone by Jacobus	49938-0102	Antimycobacterial
251CP	Cap, Branded Nortriptyline 25MG	Nortriptyline HCl 25 mg	by Moore	00839-7799	Antidepressant
251CPNORTRIPTYLINE25	Cap, Imprinted in Black Ink <> Imprinted in White Ink	Nortriptyline HCl 25 mg	by Rx Dispensing	61807-0142	Antidepressant
251NORTRIPTYLINE25	Cap, Green & White	Nortriptyline HCl 25 mg	by H J Harkins Co	52959-0359	Antidepressant
252 <> 1571	Tab	Phenobarbital 64.8 mg	Phenobarbital by URL Mutual	00677-0762	Sedative/Hypnotic; C IV
252 <> B	Tab, White, Round, Film Coated	Dipyridamole 25 mg	Persantine by Ivax	00182-1568	Antiplatelet
252 <> B	Tab, White, Round, Film Coated	Dipyridamole 25 mg	Persantine by Qualitest	00603-3383	Antiplatelet
252 <> B	Tab, White, Round, Film Coated	Dipyridamole 25 mg	Persantine by Genpharm	55567-0088	Antiplatelet
252 <> B	Tab, White, Round	Dipyridamole 25 mg	Persantine by Major	00904-1086	Antiplatelet
252 <> B	Tab, White, Round, Film Coated	Dipyridamole 25 mg	Persantine by Heartland	61392-0549	Antiplatelet
252 <> B	Tab, White, Round, Film Coated	Dipyridamole 25 mg	Persantine by Kaiser	00179-1153	Antiplatelet
252 <> B	Tab, White, Round, Film Coated	Dipyridamole 25 mg	Persantine by Sandoz	00781-1890	Antiplatelet
252 <> B	Tab, White, Round, Film Coated	Dipyridamole 25 mg	Persantine by Schein	00364-2491	Antiplatelet
252 <> B	Tab, White, Round, Film Coated	Dipyridamole 25 mg	Persantine by Barr	00555-0252	Antiplatelet
252 <> B	Tab, White, Round, Film Coated	Dipyridamole 25 mg	Persantine by UDL	51079-0068	Antiplatelet
252 <> INV	Tab, Film Coated	Cyclobenzaprine HCl 10 mg	by Physician Total Care	54868-1110	Muscle Relaxant
252 <> R	Tab, Yellow, Round	Carvedilol 3.125 mg	Coreg by Dr. Reddy's	55111-0252	Antihypertensive
2520220	Tab, Natural, Round, 252/0220	Thyroid 130 mg	by Jones		Thyroid Hormone
2520400	Tab	Phenobarbital 15 mg	Phenobarbital by Moore	00839-1478	Sedative/Hypnotic; C IV
2520400	Tab	Phenobarbital 15 mg	Phenobarbital by JMI Canton	00252-6712	Sedative/Hypnotic; C IV
2520400	Tab	Phenobarbital 15 mg	Phenobarbital by Kaiser	00179-0602	Sedative/Hypnotic; C IV
2520400	Tab	Phenobarbital 15 mg	Phenobarbital by Jones	52604-6712	Sedative/Hypnotic; C IV
2520400	Tab	Phenobarbital 15 mg	Phenobarbital by URL Mutual	00677-0236	Sedative/Hypnotic; C IV
2520401	Tab, White, Round, Scored	Phenobarbital 30 mg	Phenobarbital by Ivax	00182-0292	Sedative/Hypnotic; C IV
2520401	Tab, White, Round, Scored	Phenobarbital 30 mg	Phenobarbital by JMI Canton	00252-6722	Sedative/Hypnotic; C IV
2520401	Tab, White, Round, Scored	Phenobarbital 30 mg	Phenobarbital by Kaiser	00179-0601	Sedative/Hypnotic; C IV
2520401	Tab, White, Round, Scored	Phenobarbital 30 mg	Phenobarbital by Jones	52604-6722	Sedative/Hypnotic; C IV
2520401	Tab, White, Round, Scored	Phenobarbital 30 mg	Phenobarbital by Physician Total Care	54868-3903	Sedative/Hypnotic; C IV
2520401	Tab, White, Round, Scored	Phenobarbital 30 mg	Phenobarbital by Moore	00839-1484	Sedative/Hypnotic; C IV
2520494	Tab, Natural, Round	Thyroid 32 mg	by Jones		Thyroid Hormone
2520495	Tab, Natural, Round	Thyroid 65 mg	by Jones		Thyroid Hormone
2521571	Tab	Phenobarbital 60 mg	Phenobarbital by Moore	00839-6257	Sedative/Hypnotic; C IV

ID FRONT <> BACK	DESCRIPTION FRONT <> BACK	INGREDIENT & STRENGTH	BRAND (or Generic Equiv.) by FIRM	NDC#	CLASS; SCH.
2521571	Tab	Phenobarbital 60 mg	Phenobarbital by Ivax	00182-0590	Sedative/Hypnotic; C IV
2521571	Tab	Phenobarbital 60 mg	Phenobarbital by JMI Canton	00252-6731	Sedative/Hypnotic; C IV
2521571	Tab	Phenobarbital 60 mg	Phenobarbital by Kaiser	00179-1019	Sedative/Hypnotic; C IV
2521571	Tab	Phenobarbital 60 mg	Phenobarbital by Jones	52604-6731	Sedative/Hypnotic; C IV
25222	Tab, White to Off White, Round, Flat	Liothyronine Sodium 25 mcg	Cytomel by Paddock	00574-0222	Thyroid Hormone
252252 <> PROVENTIL2	Tab, Off-White, Round, 252 over 252 <> Proventil 2	Albuterol Sulfate 2 mg	Proventil by Schering	00085-0252	Antiasthmatic
2523089	Tab	Phenobarbital 90 mg	Phenobarbital by JMI Canton	00252-6740	Sedative/Hypnotic; C IV
2523089	Tab	Phenobarbital 90 mg	Phenobarbital by Jones	52604-6740	Sedative/Hypnotic; C IV
2523089	Tab	Phenobarbital 90 mg	Phenobarbital by URL Mutual	00677-0238	Sedative/Hypnotic; C IV
2523089	Tab	Phenobarbital 90 mg	Phenobarbital by URL Mutual	00677-0237	Sedative/Hypnotic; C IV
25237	Tab, Chewable	Sodium Fluoride 2.2 mg	by JMI Canton	00252-7928	Element
25237	Tab, Chewable	Sodium Fluoride 2.2 mg	by URL Mutual	00677-0132	Element
252389	Tab, White, Round	Phenobarbital 100 mg	Phenobarbital by JMI Canton		Sedative/Hypnotic; C IV
2525	Cap	Butalbital 50 mg, Aspirin 200 mg, Phenacetin 130 mg, Caffeine 40 mg	Marnal by Vortech		Analgesic; C III
2525	Tab, Ivory, Round, 25/25	Hydrochlorothiazide 25 mg, Spironolactone 25 mg	Novo Spirozine by Novopharm	Canadian	Diuretic; Antihypertensive
2525 <> NOVO	Tab, Light Peach, Round, Scored, NOVO <> 25/25	Hydrochlorothiazide 25 mg, Spironolactone 25 mg	Aldactazide by Novopharm	Canadian DIN 00613231	Diuretic; Antihypertensive
25250 <> SP343	Tab, Blue, Round, Scored, 25/250 <> SP over 343, Orally Disintegrating	Carbidopa 25 mg, Levodopa 250 mg	Parcopa by Schwarz	00091-3343	Antiparkinson
25255050 <> MP168	Tab, White, Round, Scored, 2525 over 5050	Trazodone HCl 150 mg	Desyrel by Mutual	53489-0517	Antidepressant
25255050 <> MP168	Tab, White, Round, Scored	Trazodone HCl 150 mg	Desyrel by Watson	00591-2300	Antidepressant
25255050 <> MP168	Tab, White, Round, Scored, 2525 over 5050	Trazodone HCl 150 mg	Desyrel by Schein	00364-2300	Antidepressant
25255050 <> MP168	Tab, White, Round, Scored, 2525 over 5050	Trazodone HCl 150 mg	Desyrel by Teva	00480-0319	Antidepressant
25255050 <> MP168	Tab, White, Round, Scored, 2525 over 5050	Trazodone HCl 150 mg	Desyrel by Major	00904-5221	Antidepressant
253 <> A	Tab, Yellow, Round	Methylphenidate HCl 5 mg	Ritalin by Able	53265-0253 Discontinued	Stimulant; C II
253 <> R	Tab, White, Round	Carvedilol 6.25 mg	Coreg by Dr. Reddy's	55111-0253	Antihypertensive
2530 <> V	Tab, Yellow, Round, Scored	Clonazepam 0.5 mg	Klonopin by Vintage	00254-2530	Sedative; C IV
2531 <> V	Tab, Light Blue, Round	Clonazepam 1 mg	Klonopin by Vintage	00254-2531	Sedative; C IV
25310	Cap, Royce Logo	Doxepin HCl 25 mg	by Quality Care	60346-0553	Antidepressant
2532 <> V	Tab, White, Round	Clonazepam 2 mg	Klonopin by Vintage	00254-2532	Sedative; C IV
253MIA	Cap, White Print	Acetaminophen 325 mg, Dichloralantipyrine 100 mg, Isomeheptene Mucate (1:1) 65 mg	Migratine by Major		Analgesic; C IV
253MIA	Cap, White Print	Acetaminophen 325 mg, Dichloralantipyrine 100 mg, Isomeheptene Mucate (2:1) 65 mg	Midrin by Carnrick	00086-0120	Analgesic; C IV
254	Tab, White, Round	Triprolidine 2.5 mg, Pseudoephedrine 60 mg	Actifed by Granutec		Cold Remedy
254 <> A	Tab, White to Off-White, Round, Scored	Methylphenidate HCl 10 mg	Ritalin by Able	53265-0254 Discontinued	Stimulant; C II
254 <> M	Tab, Orange, Round, Scored	Quinapril HCl 20 mg	Accupril by Mylan	00378-0254	Antihypertensive
254 <> R	Tab, White, Round, Film-Coated	Carvedilol 12.5 mg	Coreg by Dr. Reddy's	55111-0254	Antihypertensive
254 <> WATSON	Tab, Blue, Round	Norethindrone 0.5 mg, Ethinyl Estradiol 0.035 mg	Tri-Norinyl by Watson	52544-0274	Oral Contraceptive
254 <> WATSON	Tab, Blue, Round	Norethindrone 0.5 mg, Ethinyl Estradiol 0.035 mg	Brevicon by Watson	52544-0254	Oral Contraceptive
25400 <> ADG	Tab, White, Cap Shaped, 2.5/400	Acetaminophen 400 mg, Oxycodone 2.5 mg	Percocet by Mikart	46672-0828	Analgesic; C II
2541 <> V	Tab, Light Tan, Oval, Scored	Clonidine HCl 0.1 mg	Catapres by Vintage	00254-2541	Antihypertensive
2542 <> V	Tab, Orange, Oval, Scored	Clonidine HCl 0.2 mg	Catapres by Vintage	00254-2542	Antihypertensive
2543 <> V	Tab, Peach, Oval, Scored	Clonidine HCl 0.3 mg	Catapres by Vintage	00254-2543	Antihypertensive
255	Tab, Yellow, Round	Chlorpheniramine Maleate 4 mg	Chlor-Trimeton by Granutec		Antihistamine
255 <> 10	Tab, 10/Royce Logo	Baclofen 10 mg	Lioresal by Qualitest	00603-2408	Muscle Relaxant
255 <> A	Tab, Orange, Round, Scored	Methylphenidate HCl 20 mg	Ritalin by Able	53265-0255 Discontinued	Stimulant; C II

ID FRONT <> BACK	DESCRIPTION FRONT <> BACK	INGREDIENT & STRENGTH	BRAND (or Generic Equiv.) by FIRM	NDC#	CLASS; SCH.
255 <> R	Tab, White, Round	Carvedilol 25 mg	Coreg by Dr. Reddy's	55111-0255	Antihypertensive
2550	Tab, Peach, Round, 25/50	Triamterene 25 mg, Hydrochlorothiazide 50 mg	Novo Triazide by Novopharm	Canadian	Antihypertensive; Diuretic
2550 <> NOVO	Tab, Light Orange, Round, Scored, 25/50	Hydrochlorothiazide 25 mg, Triamterene 50 mg	Dyazide by Novopharm	Canadian DIN 00532657	Diuretic; Antihypertensive
25500 <> 5711	Tab, Light Orange, Oval, Ivax Logo 5711 <> 2.5/500	Glyburide 2.5 mg, Metformin 500 mg	Glucovance by Teva	00093-5711	Antidiabetic
25510	Tab, White, Oval, Royce Logo 255/10	Baclofen 10 mg	Lioresal by Royce	51875-0255	Muscle Relaxant
256 <> 2	Tab, White, Round	Betahistine DiHCl 8 mg	SERC by Solvay	Canadian DIN 02240601	Antivertigo
256 <> 20	Tab, 20/Royce Logo	Baclofen 20 mg	Lioresal by Qualitest	00603-2409	Muscle Relaxant
256 <> S	Tab, White to Off-White, Round	Betahistine DiHCl 8 mg	by Solvay	Canadian DIN 02240601	Antivertigo
25620	Tab, White, Round, Royce Logo 256/20	Baclofen 20 mg	Lioresal by Royce	51875-0256	Muscle Relaxant
25650 <> WATSON	Tab, Light Aqua, Cap Shaped, 25/650 <> Watson	Pentazocine HCl 25 mg, Acetaminophen 650 mg	Talacen by Watson	52544-0396	Analgesic; C IV
257	Tab, White, Coated	Pseudoephedrine HCl 60 mg, Triprolidine HCl 2.5 mg	Actifed by Granutec		Cold Remedy
257 <> 10	Tab, Coated, 257 <> 10/Royce Logo	Cyclobenzaprine HCl 10 mg	by Qualitest	00603-3077	Muscle Relaxant
257 <> B	Tab, Pink, Round, Film Coated, Stylized b	Drospirenone 3 mg, Ethinyl Estradiol 0.02 mg	Gianvi by Teva Pharmaceuticals	00093-5661	Oral Contraceptive
257 <> ETHEX	Tab, Blue, Oval, Film Coated	Ascorbic Acid 50 mg, Calcium 125 mg, Cyanocobalamin 3 mcg, Folic Acid 1 mg, Iron 60 mg, Niacinamide 10 mg, Pyridoxine HCl 2 mg, Riboflavin 3 mg, Thiamine Mononitrate 3 mg, Vitamin A 4000 Units, Vitamin D 400 Units, Zinc 18 mg	Niferex PN by Ethex	58177-0257	Vitamin
257 <> IG	Tab, White, Oval	Nabumetone 500 mg	Relafen by Glenmark	68462-0358	NSAID
25710	Tab, Dark Yellow, Film Coated, 257/10 <> Royce Logo	Cyclobenzaprine HCl 10 mg	by Royce	51875-0257	Muscle Relaxant
2577 <> V	Tab, Yellow, Round	Colchicine 0.6 mg	by Vintage	00254-2577	Antigout
258	Tab, Blue, Round, Schering Logo 258	Pseudoephedrine Sulfate 120 mg	Afrinol by Schering		Decongestant
258	Tab, Blue, Round, Scored, Film Coated	Carbinoxamine Maleate 8 mg	Histex CT by Teamm	67336-0258 Discontinued	Cold Remedy
258	Tab, Blue, Round, Schering Logo 258	Diphenhydramine HCl 25 mg	by Granutec		Antihistamine
258 <> ETHEX	Tab, White, Oval, Film Coated	Ascorbic Acid 80 mg, Calcium 250 mg, Copper 2 mg, Cyanocobalamin 12 mcg, Folic Acid 1 mg, Iodine 0.2 mg, Iron 60 mg, Magnesium 10 mg, Niacinamide 20 mg, Pyridoxine HCl 4 mg, Riboflavin 3.4 mg, Thiamine 3 mg, Vitamin A Acetate 5000 Units, Vitamin D 400 Units, Vitamin E 30 Units, Zinc 25 mg	Niferex PN Forte by Ethex	58177-0258	Vitamin
258 <> IG	Tab, White to Light Pink, Oval	Nabumetone 750 mg	Relafen by Glenmark	68462-0359	NSAID
258258	Cap, White, Opaque, Black Ink	Zonisamide 25 mg	Zonegran by Caraco	62756-0258	Anticonvulsant
258A	Cap, Yellow, Opaque	Phentermine HCl 30 mg	by Able	53265-0258 Discontinued	Anorexiant; C IV
259 <> BARR	Tab, Beige, Oval, Film Coated	Erythromycin Ethylsuccinate 400 mg	by Barr	00555-0259 Discontinued	Antibiotic
259 <> IG	Tab, Pink, Oval	Zolpidem Tartrate 5 mg	Ambien by Glenmark	68462-0279	Sedative/Hypnotic; C IV
259 <> INV	Tab	Atenolol 25 mg	Tenormin by Invamed	52189-0259	Antihypertensive
259 <> INV	Tab	Atenolol 25 mg	Tenormin by Apothecon	62269-0259	Antihypertensive
259 <> WATSON	Tab, Yellowish Green, Round	Norethindrone 1 mg, Ethinyl Estradiol 0.035 mg	Tri-Norinyl by Watson	52544-0274	Oral Contraceptive
259 <> WATSON	Tab, Yellow-Green, Round	Norethindrone 1 mg, Ethinyl Estradiol 0.035 mg	Noriyl 1+35 28 by Watson	52544-0259	Oral Contraceptive
259259	Cap, Light Gray, White, Opaque, Black Ink	Zonisamide 50 mg	Zonegran by Caraco	62756-0259	Anticonvulsant
25ALTACE	Cap, Orange and White, Opaque, Hard Gel, 2.5 ALTACE	Ramipril 2.5 mg	Altace by Aventis	Canadian DIN 02221837	Antihypertensive
25BARR323	Cap, Black Print	Hydroxyzine Pamoate 42.61 mg	by Qualitest	00603-3994	Antianxiety; Antihistamine
25C <> GS	Tab, White to Pale Yellow, Round, Effervescent	Ranitidine HCl 25 mg	Zantac Efferdose by GSK	00173-0734	Gastrointestinal
25DAN5542	Tab, Beige, Triangular, 25/Dan 5542	Thioridazine 25 mg	Mellaril by Danbury		Antipsychotic
25FLINT	Tab	Levothyroxine Sodium 0.025 mg	Synthroid by Med Pro	53978-1221	Thyroid Hormone

For updated data, go to www.IdentADrug.com

ID FRONT <> BACK	DESCRIPTION FRONT <> BACK	INGREDIENT & STRENGTH	BRAND (or Generic Equiv.) by FIRM	NDC#	CLASS; SCH.
25LLA13	Tab, White, Heptagonal	Amoxapine 25 mg	Asendin by Lederle		Antidepressant
25M	Tab	Levothyroxine Sodium 25 mcg	Levo-T by Mova	55370-0125	Thyroid Hormone
25M	Tab	Levothyroxine Sodium 25 mcg	Euthyrox by Em Pharma	63254-0435	Thyroid Hormone
25M <> Z	Tab, Orange, Round, Scored	Levothyroxine Sodium 25 mcg	Levo-T by Zoetica	64909-0106	Thyroid Hormone
25MCG	Tab	Levothyroxine Sodium 25 mcg	Eltroxin by GSK	53873-0104	Thyroid Hormone
25MCG <> FLINT	Tab, Orange, Round, Scored	Levothyroxine Sodium 25 mcg	by Amerisource	62584-0020	Thyroid Hormone
25MCG <> FLINT	Tab, Orange, Round, Scored	Levothyroxine Sodium 25 mcg	Synthroid by Rightpac	65240-0739	Thyroid Hormone
25MG	Cap, Yellowish-Brown, Ivax Logo 25 mg	Cyclosporine 25 mg	Neoral by Ivax	00172-7310	Immunosuppressant
25MG <> CLOZARIL	Tab, Pale Yellow, Round, Scored	Clozapine 25 mg	Clozaril by Novartis	Canadian DIN 00894737	Antipsychotic
25MG <> G4960	Tab, Light Green, Cap Shaped, Scored	Sertraline HCl 25 mg	Zoloft by Greenstone	59762-4960	Antidepressant
25MG <> N	Tab, Light Yellow, Oval	Azathioprine 25 mg	Azasan by AAI Pharma	66591-0211	Immunosuppressant
25MG <> ZOLOFT	Tab, Light Green, Cap Shaped, Scored, Film Coated	Sertraline HCl 25 mg	Zoloft by Pharmacy Care	65070-0210	Antidepressant
25MG <> ZOLOFT	Tab, Light Green, Cap Shaped, Scored, Film Coated	Sertraline HCl 25 mg	Zoloft by Direct Dispensing	57866-1057	Antidepressant
25MG <> ZOLOFT	Tab, Light Green, Cap Shaped, Scored, Film Coated	Sertraline HCl 25 mg	Zoloft by Roerig	00049-4960	Antidepressant
25MG <> ZOLOFT	Tab, Light Green, Cap Shaped, Scored, Film Coated	Sertraline HCl 25 mg	Zoloft by Murfreesboro	51129-1333	Antidepressant
25N031	Cap, Bright Yellow & Deep Orange, 25 <> N over 031	Clomipramine HCl 25 mg	by Teva	55953-0031 Discontinued	OCD
25N420	Cap, Light Green	Indomethacin 25 mg	Indocin by Allscripts		NSAID
25N420	Cap, Light Green	Indomethacin 25 mg	Indocin by Apotheca	12634-0455	NSAID
25NOVO	Tab, Beige, Round, 25/Novo	Clomipramine HCl 25 mg	Novo Clopamine by Novopharm	Canadian	OCD
25P	Tab, Peach	Hydrochlorothiazide 25 mg	Urozide by Pharmascience	Canadian DIN 02247386	Diuretic; Antihypertensive
25Z2160	Tab, White, Round, 2.5 Z/2160	Conjugated Estrogens 2.5 mg	Premarin by Ivax		Hormone
26 <> A	Tab, Light Pink, Round	Lisinopril 10 mg, HCTZ 12.5 mg	Prinzide by Aurobindo	65862-0043	Antihypertensive; Diuretic
26 <> BL	Tab, Orange, Round, Coated, Scored	Amitriptyline HCl 100 mg	Elavil by Teva	00093-2128	Antidepressant
26 <> CIBA	Tab, Orange, Round, Scored	Maprotiline HCl 50 mg	by Novartis	00083-0026	Antidepressant
26 <> EFF	Tab, White, Round	Isoniazid 100 mg	Laniazid by Mikart	46672-0158	Antimycobacterial
260 <> 715	Tab, White, Round	Quinine Sulfate 260 mg	Quinamm by Ivax	00182-8615 Discontinued	Antimalarial
260 <> DBETHEX	Tab, Coated, Scored	Ascorbic Acid 100 mg, Biotin 30 mcg, Calcium Carbonate, Precipitated 250 mg, Chromic Chloride 25 mcg, Cupric Oxide 2 mg, Cyanocobalamin 12 mcg, Ferrous Fumarate 60 mg, Folic Acid 1 mg, Magnesium Oxide 25 mg, Manganese Sulfate 5 mg, Niacinamide 20 mg, Pantothenic Acid 10 mg, Potassium Iodide 150 mcg, Pyridoxine HCl 10 mg, Riboflavin 3.4 mg, Sodium Molybdate 25 mcg, Thiamine HCl 3 mg, Vitamin A 5000 Units, Vitamin D 400 Units, Vitamin E 30 Units, Zinc Oxide 25 mg	Prenatal MTR by Ethex	58177-0260 Discontinued	Vitamin
260 <> IG	Tab, White, Oval	Zolpidem Tartrate 10 mg	Ambien by Glenmark	68462-0280	Sedative/Hypnotic; C IV
260 <> WESTWARD	Tab, White, Round, Scored	Isoniazid 100 mg	Laniazid by Amneal	65162-0180	Antimycobacterial
260 <> WESTWARD	Tab, White, Round, Scored	Isoniazid 100 mg	Laniazid by Versapharm	61748-0016	Antimycobacterial
260 <> WESTWARD	Tab, White, Round, Scored	Isoniazid 100 mg	Laniazid by West-Ward	00143-1260	Antimycobacterial
260 <> WESTWARD	Tab, White, Round, Scored	Isoniazid 100 mg	Laniazid by Amerisource	62584-0759	Antimycobacterial
260260	Cap, Light Orange, White, Opaque, Black Ink	Zonisamide 100 mg	Zonegran by Caraco	62756-0260	Anticonvulsant
261 <> INV	Tab, White, Round	Methazolamide 25 mg	Neptazane by Invamed	52189-0261	Antiglaucoma Agent
261 <> INV	Tab, White, Round	Methazolamide 25 mg	Neptazane by Apothecon	62269-0261	Antiglaucoma Agent
2611 <> G	Tab, White, Football Shaped	Terbutaline Sulfate 2.5 mg	Brethine by Global	00115-2611	Antiasthmatic
2614SCHEINCE-FACLOR250MG	Cap, Purple	Cefaclor 250 mg	Ceclor by Schein	00364-2614	Antibiotic

Copyright © 2010 Ident-A-Drug (209) 472-2240 • May not be reproduced without permission •

ID FRONT <> BACK	DESCRIPTION FRONT <> BACK	INGREDIENT & STRENGTH	BRAND (or Generic Equiv.) by FIRM	NDC#	CLASS; SCH.
2615SCHEINCE-FACLOR500MG	Cap, Purple & Yellow	Cefaclor 500 mg	by Schein	00364-2615	Antibiotic
262	Tab, White, Round	Dimenhydrinate 50 mg	Dramamine by Granutec		Antiemetic
262 <> BARR	Tab, Coated	Thioridazine HCl 50 mg	by Barr	00555-0262	Antipsychotic
2622 <> G	Tab, White, Round	Terbutaline Sulfate 5.0 mg	Brethine by Global	00115-2622	Antiasthmatic
263 <> BARR	Tab, Coated	Thioridazine HCl 100 mg	by Barr	00555-0263	Antipsychotic
2631 <> V	Tab, Orange, Round	Cyclobenzaprine HCl 5 mg	Flexeril by Qualitest	00603-3078	Muscle Relaxant
2632 <> V	Tab, Yellow, Round	Cyclobenzaprine HCl 10 mg	Flexeril by Qualitest	00603-3079	Muscle Relaxant
265 <> PAR	Tab, Coated	Amitriptyline 12.5 mg, Chlordiazepoxide 5 mg	Limbitrol by Par	49884-0265	Antianxiety; C IV
265 <> WATSON	Tab, White, Round	Norethindrone 1 mg, Mestranol 0.05 mg	Norinyl 1+50 28 by Watson	52544-0265	Oral Contraceptive
266 <> CP	Tab, Coated, Imprinted in Black Ink	Thioridazine HCl 25 mg	by Heartland	61392-0463	Antipsychotic
266 <> MRK	Tab, Light Pink, Cap Shaped	Rizatriptan Benzoate 5 mg	Maxalt by Merck	00006-0266	Antimigraine
266 <> MSD	Tab, Pale Pink, Cap-Shaped	Rizatriptan 5 mg	Maxalt by Merck Frosst	Canadian DIN 02240520	Antimigraine
266 <> PAR	Tab, Coated	Amitriptyline 25 mg, Chlordiazepoxide 10 mg	Limbitrol DS by Par	49884-0266	Antianxiety; C IV
2662 <> 10	Tab, Peach, Round, Hourglass logo 10 <> 2662	Famotidine 10 mg	Pepcid AC by Ivax	00172-2662	Gastrointestinal
267 <> IG	Tab, Brown, Round	Quinapril 5 mg	Accupril by Dr. Reddy's	55111-0621	Antihypertensive
267 <> WW	Tab, Pink, Round	Lisinopril 10 mg	Zestril by West-Ward	00143-1267	Antihypertensive
267267 <> S	Tab, White to Off-White, Round, Scored	Betahistine Dihydrochloride 16 mg	Serc by Solvay	Canadian DIN 02243878	Antivertigo
268 <> IG	Tab, Brown, Round	Quinapril 10 mg	Accupril by Dr. Reddy's	55111-0622	Antihypertensive
268 <> RDY	Tab, Brown, Round, Film Coated	Simvastatin 80 mg	Zocor by Dr. Reddy's	55111-0268	Antihyperlipidemic
2682 <> V	Tab, White, Round, Scored	Diazepam 2 mg	Valium by Vintage	00254-2682	Antianxiety; C IV
2683 <> V	Tab, Yellow, Round, Scored	Diazepam 5 mg	Valium by Vintage	00254-2683	Antianxiety; C IV
2684 <> V	Tab, Blue, Round, Scored	Diazepam 10 mg	Valium by Vintage	00254-2684	Antianxiety; C IV
269 <> IG	Tab, Brown, Round	Quinapril 20 mg	Accupril by Dr. Reddy's	55111-0623	Antihypertensive
269 <> R	Tab, White, Round, Scored	Metoclopramide HCl 10 mg	Reglan by Actavis	00228-2269	Gastrointestinal
269 <> R	Tab, White, Round, Scored	Metoclopramide HCl 10 mg	Reglan by UDL	Discontinued	Gastrointestinal
269 <> R	Tab, White, Round, Scored	Metoclopramide HCl 10 mg	Reglan by Nat Pharmpak	55154-5510	Gastrointestinal
269 <> RDY	Tab, White, Oval	Amlodipine Besylate 2.5 mg	Norvasc by Dr. Reddy's	55111-0269	Antihypertensive
2690V	Tab, White, Oval, 2960 over V	Diethylpropion HCl 75 mg	Durad by 3M	00089-0212	Anorexiant; C IV
2690V	Tab, White, Oval, 2960 over V	Diethylpropion HCl 75 mg	Durad by URL Mutual	00677-0436	Anorexiant; C IV
2690V	Tab, White, Oval, 2960 over V	Diethylpropion HCl 75 mg	Durad by Qualitest	00603-3290	Anorexiant; C IV
2690V	Tab, White, Oval, 2960 over V	Diethylpropion HCl 75 mg	Durad by Macnary	55982-0008	Anorexiant; C IV
2690V	Tab, White, Oval, 2960 over V	Diethylpropion HCl 75 mg	Durad by PDRX	55289-0368	Anorexiant; C IV
27 <> A	Tab, Light Pink, Round	Lisinopril 20 mg, HCTZ 25 mg	Prinzide by Aurobindo	65862-0045	Antihypertensive; Diuretic
27 <> EFF	Tab, White, Round	Isoniazid 300 mg	Laniazid by Mikart	46672-0159	Antimycobacterial
27 <> R	Tab, Orange, Round	Propranolol HCl 10 mg	Inderal by Actavis	00228-2327	Antihypertensive
270	Tab, White to Off-White, Rectangle-Shaped, 270 <> Bone Image	Alendronate Sodium 70 mg, Cholecalciferol 5600 IU	Fosamax Plus D by Merck	68263-0270	Antiosteoporosis
270 <> CP	Tab, Coated	Thioridazine HCl 200 mg	by Creighton	50752-0270	Antipsychotic
270 <> IG	Tab, Brown, Oval	Quinapril 40 mg	Accupril by Dr. Reddy's	55111-0624	Antihypertensive
270 <> RDY	Tab, White, Oval	Amlodipine Besylate 5 mg	Norvasc by Dr. Reddy's	55111-0270	Antihypertensive
271 <> INV	Tab, Scored	Captopril 12.5 mg	Capoten by Invamed	52189-0271	Antihypertensive
271 <> INV	Tab, Scored	Captopril 12.5 mg	Capoten by Schein	00364-2628	Antihypertensive
271 <> RDY	Tab, White, Oval	Amlodipine Besylate 10 mg	Norvasc by Dr. Reddy's	55111-0271	Antihypertensive
2711 <> G	Tab, Light Blue, Cap Shaped	Sotalol 80 mg	Betapace by Global	00115-2711	Antiarrhythmic
2713 <> WPI	Tab, Light Peach, Cap Shaped, Film Coated	Metformin HCl 500 mg	Glucophage by Watson	00591-2713	Antidiabetic
2715	Cap	Nitroglycerine SA 6.5 mg	Nitrobid by Vortech		Vasodilator
2718	Cap	Nitroglycerine SA 2.5 mg	Nitrobid by Vortech		Vasodilator

ID FRONT <> BACK	DESCRIPTION FRONT <> BACK	INGREDIENT & STRENGTH	BRAND (or Generic Equiv.) by FIRM	NDC#	CLASS; SCH.
272 <> DMSP	Tab	Carbidopa 25 mg, Levodopa 100 mg	by Murfreesboro	51129-1127	Antiparkinson
272 <> M	Tab, Orange, Round, Scored	Quinapril HCl 40 mg	Accupril by Mylan	00378-0272	Antihypertensive
2722 <> G	Tab, Light Blue, Cap Shaped	Sotalol 120 mg	Betapace by Global	00115-2722	Antiarrhythmic
2722 <> V	Tab, White, Oblong	Guaifenesin 1200 mg, Pseudoephedrine 120 mg	Entex PSE by Qualitest	00603-3504	Cold Remedy
2727 <> TEGRETOL	Tab, Pink, Cap Shaped, Scored	Carbamazepine 200 mg	Tegretol by Novartis	00083-0027	Anticonvulsant
2727 <> TEGRETOL	Tab, Pink, Cap Shaped, Scored	Carbamazepine 200 mg	Tegretol by Nat Pharmpak	55154-1012	Anticonvulsant
2729 <> 20	Tab, Off-White, Oval	Fosinopril Sodium 20 mg	Monopril by Sandoz	00781-5084	Antihypertensive
272CPTEMAZEPAM15MG	Cap, Red Print	Temazepam 15 mg	Restoril by Creighton	50752-0272	Sedative/Hypnotic; C IV
272TEMAZEPAM15MG	Cap, 272 and Creighton's Logo <> Imprint in Red Ink	Temazepam 15 mg	Restoril by Kaiser	00179-1106	Sedative/Hypnotic; C IV
273 <> 5	Tab, Yellow, Round, 5 <> 273	Clonazepam 0.5 mg	Klonopin by Caraco	57664-0273	Sedative; C IV
2732 <> 40	Tab, Off-White, Hexagonal	Fosinopril Sodium 40 mg	Monopril by Sandoz	00781-5085	Antihypertensive
2732V	Cap	Chlordiazepoxide 5 mg, Clidinium Bromide 2.5 mg	Librax by Vintage	00254-2732	Gastrointestinal
2733 <> G	Tab, Light Blue, Cap Shaped	Sotalol 160 mg	Betapace by Global	00115-2733	Antiarrhythmic
2734	Tab, Orange, Round	Enalapril Maleate 20 mg	Vastoec by Schein		Antihypertensive
2737 <> 10	Tab, Off-White, Diamond Shaped	Fosinopril Sodium 10 mg	Monopril by Sandoz	00781-5083	Antihypertensive
273CPTEMAZEPAM30MG	Cap, Red Print	Temazepam 30 mg	Restoril by Creighton	50752-0273	Sedative/Hypnotic; C IV
273INV <> 50	Tab	Captopril 50 mg	Capoten by Schein	00364-2630	Antihypertensive
274 <> 1	Tab, Blue, Round, Scored	Clonazepam 1 mg	Klonopin by Caraco	57664-0274	Sedative; C IV
274 <> ETH	Tab, White, Oval, Partially Scored, Film Coated	Hyoscyamine Sulfate 0.125 mg	Levsin by Ethex	58177-0274	Gastrointestinal
274 <> M	Tab, White to Off-White, Round	Tamoxifen Citrate 20 mg	Nolvadex by Mylan	00378-0274	Antiestrogen
274 <> RDY	Tab, White, Oval	Pravastatin 80 mg	Pravachol by Dr. Reddy's	55111-0274	Antihyperlipidemic
274 <> ROCHE	Tab, Light Blue, Oval, Film Coated	Naproxen 275 mg	Naprosyn by Syntex	18393-0274	NSAID
2744 <> G	Tab, Light Blue, Cap Shaped	Sotalol 240 mg	Betapace by Global	00115-2744	Antiarrhythmic
274INV <> 100	Tab	Captopril 100 mg	Capoten by Schein	00364-2631	Antihypertensive
275 <> 2	Tab, White, Round, Scored	Clonazepam 2 mg	Klonopin by Caraco	57664-0275	Sedative; C IV
275 <> CP	Tab	Acetaminophen 325 mg, Butalbital 50 mg, Caffeine 40 mg	Fioricet by Creighton	50752-0275	Analgesic
275 <> ETHEX	Tab, White, Film Coated	Ascorbic Acid 1 mg, Calcium 200 mg, Cyanocobalamin 2.2 mcg, Folic Acid 1 mg, Iodine 175 mcg, Iron 65 mg, Magnesium 100 mg, Niacin 17 mg, Pyridoxine HCl 2.2 mg, Riboflavin 1.6 mg, Thiamine HCl 1.5 mg, Vitamin A 3000 Units, Vitamin D 400 Units, Vitamin E 10 Units, Zinc 15 mg	Prenatal Z by Ethex	58177-0275	Vitamin
275 <> G0	Tab, Blue, Oval	Naproxen 275 mg	Anaprox by Glenmark	68462-0178	NSAID
275 <> IG	Tab, White, Round	Hydroxyzine 10 mg	Atarax by Glenmark	68462-0360	Antianxiety; Antihistamine
275 <> N531	Tab, White, Round, Film Coated, N over 531	Naproxen 275 mg	Naprosyn by Moore	00839-7889	NSAID
275 <> N531	Tab, White, Round, Film Coated, N over 531	Naproxen 275 mg	Naprosyn by Teva	55953-0531 Discontinued	NSAID
275 <> N531	Tab, White, Round, Film Coated, N over 531	Naproxen 275 mg	Naprosyn by Major	00904-5040	NSAID
276 <> IG	Tab, White, Round	Hydroxyzine 25 mg	Atarax by Glenmark	68462-0361	Antianxiety; Antihistamine
2768	Cap	Tetracycline HCl 250 mg	Nor-Tet by Vortech		Antibiotic
277	Tab, Beige, Round, Film Coated	Sitagliptin 100 mg	Januvia by Merck	00006-0277	Antidiabetic
277	Tab, Logo 277	Isoniazid 300 mg	Laniazid by Quality Care	60346-0483	Antimycobacterial
277	Tab, Coated	Amitriptyline 25 mg, Chlordiazepoxide 10 mg	Limbitrol DS by Qualitest	00603-2691	Antianxiety; C IV
277 <> IG	Tab, White, Round	Hydroxyzine 50 mg	Atarax by Glenmark	68462-0362	Antianxiety; Antihistamine
277 <> MYLAN	Tab, White, Coated	Amitriptyline 25 mg, Chlordiazepoxide 10 mg	Limbitrol DS by Mylan	00378-0277	Antianxiety; C IV
2771	Tab, White to Off-White, Oval, 2771 <> Heart	Irbesartan 75 mg	Avapro by Sanofi	Canadian DIN 02237923	Antihypertensive
2771	Tab, White to Off-White, Oval, 2771 <> Heart	Irbesartan 75 mg	Avapro by BMS	00087-2771	Antihypertensive
2772	Tab, White to Off-White, Oval, 2772 <> Heart	Irbesartan 150 mg	Avapro by Sanofi	Canadian DIN 02237924	Antihypertensive
2772	Tab, White to Off-White, Oval, 2772 <> Heart	Irbesartan 150 mg	Avapro by BMS	00087-2772	Antihypertensive

ID FRONT <> BACK	DESCRIPTION FRONT <> BACK	INGREDIENT & STRENGTH	BRAND (or Generic Equiv.) by FIRM	NDC#	CLASS; SCH.
2772	Tab, White to Off-White, Oval, 2772 <> Heart	Irbesartan 150 mg	Avapro by Murfreesboro	51129-1339	Antihypertensive
2773	Tab, White to Off-White, Oval, 2773 <> Heart	Irbesartan 300 mg	Avapro by Sanofi	Canadian DIN 02237925	Antihypertensive
2773	Tab, White to Off-White, Oval, 2773 <> Heart	Irbesartan 300 mg	Avapro by BMS	00087-2773	Antihypertensive
2775	Tab, Peach, Oval, 2775 <> Heart	Irbesartan 150 mg, HCTZ 12.5 mg	Avalide by BMS	00087-2775	Antihypertensive; Diuretic
2775	Tab, Peach, Oval, 2775 <> Heart	Irbesartan 150 mg, HCTZ 12.5 mg	Avalide by Sanofi	Canadian DIN 02241818	Antihypertensive; Diuretic
2775 <> WPI	Tab, Light Peach, Cap Shaped, Film Coated	Metformin HCl 850 mg	Glucophage by Watson	00591-2775	Antidiabetic
2776	Tab, Peach, Oval, 2776 <> Heart	Irbesartan 300 mg, HCTZ 12.5 mg	Avalide by Sanofi	Canadian DIN 02241819	Antihypertensive; Diuretic
2776	Tab, Peach, Oval, 2776 <> Heart	Irbesartan 300 mg, HCTZ 12.5 mg	Avalide by BMS	00087-2776	Antihypertensive; Diuretic
278 <> IG	Tab, White, Round	Topiramate 25 mg	Topamax by Invagen	31722-0278	Anticonvulsant
278 <> INV	Tab, Purple, Round, Film Coated	Trifluoperazine HCl 1 mg	Stelazine by Invamed	52189-0278	Antipsychotic
278 <> INV	Tab, Purple, Round, Film Coated	Trifluoperazine HCl 1 mg	by Apothecon	62269-0278	Antipsychotic
2788	Tab, Pink, Oval, 2788 <> Heart	Irbesartan 300 mg, HCTZ 25 mg	Avalide by BMS	00087-2788	Antihypertensive; Diuretic
2788	Tab, Pink, Oval, 2788 <> Heart	Irbesartan 300 mg, HCTZ 25 mg	Avalide by Sanofi	Canadian DIN 02280213	Antihypertensive; Diuretic
279 <> IG	Tab, Yellow, Round	Topiramate 50 mg	Topamax by Invagen	31722-0279	Anticonvulsant
2790 <> 0115	Tab, White, Round	Chloroquine Phosphate 250 mg	Aralen Phosphate by Global	00115-2790	Antimalarial
27TEGRETAL27	Tab	Carbamazepine 200 mg	Tegretol by Med Pro	53978-1070	Anticonvulsant
28 <> A	Tab, Light Yellow, Round	Lisinopril 20 mg, HCTZ 12.5 mg	Prinzide by Aurobindo	65862-0044	Antihypertensive; Diuretic
28 <> B	Tab, Light Pink, Round	Inert	Levlen 28 by Berlex	50419-0411	Oral Contraceptive; Placebo
28 <> B	Tab, Pink, Round	Inert	Levlen 28 by Berlex	50419-0028	Oral Contraceptive; Placebo
28 <> B	Tab, Orange, Round	Levonorgestrel 0.10 mg, Ethinyl Estradiol 0.02 mg	Lo Seasonique by Duramed	51285-0092	Oral Contraceptive
28 <> M	Tab	Nadolol 20 mg	Nadolol by Qualitest	00603-4740	Antihypertensive
280 <> IG	Tab, Light Yellow, Round	Topiramate 100 mg	Topamax by Invagen	31722-0280	Anticonvulsant
280 <> KALI	Tab, Beige, Round	Citalopram HBr 10 mg	Celexa by Perrigo	10768-7060	Antidepressant
281	Tab, White, Oblong	Acetaminophen 500 mg	Tylenol Ex Strength by Ivax		Analgesic
281 <> IG	Tab, Pink, Round	Topiramate 200 mg	Topamax by Invagen	31722-0281	Anticonvulsant
281 <> KALI	Tab, Pink, Round	Citalopram HBr 20 mg	Celexa by Perrigo	10768-7191	Antidepressant
282	Tab, White, Round, Schering Logo 282	Azatadine Maleate 1 mg	Optimine by Schering	00085-0282	Antihistamine
282 <> KALI	Tab, White, Round	Citalopram HBr 40 mg	Celexa by Perrigo	10768-7616	Antidepressant
282MEP	Tab, White	Acetaminophen 350 mg, Caffeine 30 mg, Codeine Phosphate 15 mg	by Frosst	Canadian	Analgesic; C III
283	Tab, White & Blue, Round, Scored	Bendroflumethiazide 5 mg, Nadolol 40 mg	Corzide by King	61570-0175	Diuretic; Antihypertensive
283200MCG	Tab, Light Yellow-Brown, Round	Cerivastatin Sodium 0.2 mg	Baycol by Bayer	00026-2883	Antihyperlipidemic
284	Tab, White & Blue, Round, Scored	Bendroflumethiazide 5 mg, Nadolol 80 mg	Corzide by King	61570-0176	Diuretic; Antihypertensive
284300MCG	Tab, Yellow-Brown	Cerivastatin Sodium 0.3 mg	Baycol by Bayer	00026-2884	Antihyperlipidemic
285 <> 400MCG	Tab, Gold, Round, 400 over mcg	Cerivastatin Sodium 0.4 mg	Baycol by Bayer	00026-2885	Antihyperlipidemic
285 <> 400MCG	Tab, Gold, Round, 400 over mcg	Cerivastatin Sodium 0.4 mg	Baycol by DSM	63552-0031	Antihyperlipidemic
285 <> B	Tab, White, Round, Film Coated	Dipyridamole 50 mg	Persantine by Barr	00555-0285	Antiplatelet
285 <> B	Tab, White, Round, Film Coated	Dipyridamole 50 mg	Persantine by UDL	51079-0069	Antiplatelet
285 <> B	Tab, White, Round	Dipyridamole 50 mg	Persantine by Major	00904-1087	Antiplatelet
285 <> B	Tab, White, Round, Film Coated	Dipyridamole 50 mg	Persantine by Ivax	00182-1569	Antiplatelet
286 <> 800MCG	Tab, Brown	Cerivastatin Sodium 0.8 mg	Baycol by Bayer	00026-2886	Antihyperlipidemic
286 <> BARR	Tab, White, Round, Film Coated	Dipyridamole 75 mg	Persantine by Ivax	00182-1570	Antiplatelet
286 <> BARR	Tab, White, Round, Film Coated	Dipyridamole 75 mg	Persantine by UDL	51079-0070	Antiplatelet

ID FRONT <> BACK	DESCRIPTION FRONT <> BACK	INGREDIENT & STRENGTH	BRAND (or Generic Equiv.) by FIRM	NDC#	CLASS; SCH.
286 <> BARR	Tab, White, Round, Film Coated	Dipyridamole 75 mg	Persantine by Barr	00555-0286	Antiplatelet
286 <> BARR	Tab, White, Round	Dipyridamole 75 mg	Persantine by Major	00904-1088	Antiplatelet
2867	Cap	Tetracycline HCl 500 mg	Nor-Tet by Vortech		Antibiotic
2869	Cap	Propoxyphene HCl 65 mg	Margesic by Vortech		Analgesic; C IV
287	Tab, Yellow, Round, Schering Logo 287	Perphenazine 2 mg, Amitriptyline HCl 10 mg	Etrafon by Schering		Antipsychotic; Antidepressant
287	Tab, Pink, Round	Acetaminophen 325 mg, Pseudoephedrine HCl 30 mg	Sinutab by Granutec		Cold Remedy
2874	Cap	Dicyclomine HCl 10 mg	Bentyl by Vortech		Gastrointestinal
289288 <> S	Tab, White to Off-White, Round, Scored	Betahistine Dihydrochloride 24 mg	Serc by Solvay	Canadian DIN 02247998	Antivertigo
29	Tab, Purepac Logo 29	Propranolol HCl 20 mg	Inderal by Quality Care	60346-0598	Antihypertensive
29 <> B	Tab, White, Round, Coated	Inert	Levlite 28 by Berlex	50419-0029	Oral Contraceptive; Placebo
2907	Tab, White, Round	Furosemide 40 mg	Lasix by Teva	00172-2907	Antihypertensive/Diuretic
2908	Tab, White, Round, Hourglass Logo 2908	Furosemide 20 mg	Lasix by Kaiser	00179-1373	Diuretic
2908	Tab, White, Round, Hourglass Logo 2908	Furosemide 20 mg	Lasix by Ivax	00172-2908	Diuretic
2908	Tab, White, Round, Hourglass Logo 2908	Furosemide 20 mg	Lasix by Ivax	00182-1170 Discontinued	Diuretic
2908	Tab, White, Round, Hourglass Logo 2908	Furosemide 20 mg	Lasix by Quality Care	60346-0761	Diuretic
2908	Tab, White, Round, Hourglass Logo 2908	Furosemide 20 mg	Lasix by Baker Cummins	63171-1170	Diuretic
291	Tab, White, Round, Scored	Baclofen 10 mg	Lioresal by Caraco	57664-0291	Muscle Relaxant
291291 <> S	Tab, White, Round, Scored, Film Coated	Fluvoxamine Maleate 50 mg	Luvox by Solvay	Canadian DIN 01919342	OCD
291BARR	Tab, Off-White, Round	Metronidazole 250 mg	Flagyl by Barr		Antibiotic
292	Tab, White, Round, Scored	Baclofen 20 mg	Lioresal by Caraco	57664-0292	Muscle Relaxant
292 <> ETHEX	Tab, Beige, Oval, Scored, Film Coated	Ascorbic Acid 120 mg, Calcium 200 mg, Cholecalciferol 400 Units, Copper 2 mg, Cyanocobalamin 12 mcg, Docusate Sodium 50 mg, Folic Acid 1 mg, Iodine 150 mcg, Iron 90 mg, Niacinamide 20 mg, Pyridoxine HCl 20 mg, Riboflavin 3.4 mg, Thiamine HCl 3 mg, Vitamin A 2700 Units, Vitamin E 30 Units, Zinc 25 mg	Ultra Natalcare by Ethex	58177-0292	Vitamin
292BARR	Tab, Off-White, Oblong	Metronidazole 500 mg	Flagyl by Barr		Antibiotic
293	Tab, White, Round, Scored, Film Coated	Metoprolol Succinate 25 mg	Toprol XL by Apotex	51877-0293	Antihypertensive
293	Tab, White, Round, Scored, Film Coated	Metoprolol Succinate 25 mg	Toprol XL by Ethex	58177-0293	Antihypertensive
294	Tab, Red, Round	Pseudoephedrine 30 mg	Pseudoval Plus by Granutec		Decongestant
295DP	Tab, Duramed Logo	Guaifenesin 400 mg, Phenylpropanolamine HCl 75 mg	Entex LA by Schein	00364-2138	Cold Remedy
2975	Cap	Propoxyphene HCl 65 mg, Aspirin 227 mg, Phenacetin 162 mg, Caffeine 32 mg	Margesic Comp. 65 by Vortech		Analgesic; C IV
298	Tab, Brown, Black Print, Round, Schering Logo over 298	Ethinyl Estradiol 0.02 mg	by Amerisource	62584-0298	Hormone
298	Tab, Brown, Black Print, Round, Schering Logo over 298	Ethinyl Estradiol 0.02 mg	Estinyl by Schering	00085-0298	Hormone
298 <> 44	Tab, Greenish Brown, Round	Sennosides 8.6 mg	Senna by LNK	50844-0298	Gastrointestinal
2985Z	Cap, Light Blue	Doxycycline Hyclate 100 mg	by H J Harkins Co	52959-0463	Antibiotic
298B	Tab, Orange, Round	Hydroxyzine HCl 25 mg	Atarax by Barr		Antianxiety; Antihistamine
298ER	Tab, Beige, Oblong	Ethinyl Estradiol 0.02 mg	by Heartland	61392-0799	Hormone
299BARR	Tab, Orange, Round	Hydroxyzine HCl 50 mg	Atarax by Barr		Antianxiety; Antihistamine
2AHR <> TENEX	Tab, Yellow, Diamond Shaped, 2 over AHR	Guanfacine HCl 2 mg	Tenex by Rightpac	65240-0748	Antihypertensive
2AHRTENEX	Tab	Guanfacine HCl 2.3 mg	Tenex by Pharmedix	53002-1052	Antihypertensive
2AMPMVERSACAP	Cap, 2-AM over PM <> Versacap	Guaifenesin 300 mg, Pseudoephedrine HCl 60 mg	Sudafed Sinus by Pharmafab	62542-0403	Cold Remedy
2C	Tab, Pink, Oval	Clonidine HCl 0.1 mg, Chlorthalidone 15 mg	Combipres by Boehringer Ingelheim	Canadian	Antihypertensive; Diuretic

ID FRONT <> BACK	DESCRIPTION FRONT <> BACK	INGREDIENT & STRENGTH	BRAND (or Generic Equiv.) by FIRM	NDC#	CLASS; SCH.
2KLONOPIN <> ROCHE	Tab, White, Round, K perforation	Clonazepam 2 mg	Klonopin by Hoffmann La Roche	00004-0098	Sedative; C IV
2LLL12	Tab, Pink, Round	Levothyroxine Sodium 0.2 mg	Synthroid by Lederle		Thyroid Hormone
2MG	Cap, Blue, Opaque	Tizanidine HCl 2 mg	Zanaflex by Acorda	10144-0602	Muscle Relaxant
2MG <> 503	Tab, White to Off-White, Cap Shaped	Guanfacine 2 mg	Intuniv by Shire	54092-0515	Non-Stimulant Anti-ADHD
2MG <> 511	Tab, White, Pentagon	Lorazepam 2 mg	Ativan by Wyeth	52903-5813	Antianxiety; C IV
2MG <> CARDURA	Tab, Yellow, Oblong, Scored	Doxazosin Mesylate 2 mg	Cardura by Roerig	00049-2760	Antihypertensive
2MG <> CARDURA	Tab, Yellow, Oblong, Scored	Doxazosin Mesylate 2 mg	Cardura by H J Harkins Co	52959-0003	Antihypertensive
2MG <> ETH267	Tab, Yellow, Oblong	Doxazosin Mesylate 2 mg	Cardura by Ethex	58177-0267	Antihypertensive
2MG <> IODIUMAD	Tab, Light Green, Cap Shaped, Scored, 2 mg <> Imodium A-D	Loperamide 2 mg	Imodium by McNeil	Canadian DIN 02183862	Antidiarrheal
2MG <> LOP	Tab, Light Green, Cap Shaped	Loperamide 2 mg	Imodium by Novopharm	Canadian DIN 02132591	Antidiarrheal
2MG <> MLP17	Tab, Yellow, Oval, Scored	Doxazosin Mesylate 2 mg	Cardura by Dava	67253-0381	Antihypertensive
2MG500MG <> BULLSYMBOL	Tab, Pink	Repaglinide 2 mg, Metformin 500 mg	PrandiMet by Novo Nordisk	00169-0092	Diabetic Glycemic Control
2N	Cap, White	Loperamide 2 mg	Imodium by Mova	55370-0169	Antidiarrheal
2N	Cap, White	Loperamide 2 mg	Imodium by Teva	55953-0020 Discontinued	Antidiarrheal
2N	Cap, White	Loperamide 2 mg	Imodium by Moore	00839-7623	Antidiarrheal
2N020	Cap, White, Opaque, N over 020	Loperamide 2 mg	Imodium by Heartland	61392-0336	Antidiarrheal
2N020	Cap, White, Opaque, N over 020	Loperamide 2 mg	Imodium by Amerisource	62584-0768	Antidiarrheal
2N020	Cap, White, Opaque, N over 020	Loperamide 2 mg	Imodium by Medirex	57480-0830	Antidiarrheal
2N020	Cap, White, Opaque, N over 020	Loperamide 2 mg	Imodium by Major	00904-7617	Antidiarrheal
2N020	Cap, White, Opaque, N over 020	Loperamide 2 mg	Imodium by DHHS Prog	11819-0036	Antidiarrheal
2NS	Tab, Purple, Oblong	Divalproex Sodium 500 mg	by Heartland	61392-0610	Anticonvulsant
2R	Cap, Yellow, Oval, Opaque, Soft Gel	Terazosin HCl 2 mg	Hytrin by Ranbaxy	63304-0663	Antihypertensive
2RORER142	Tab, White, Round	Aspirin 325 mg, Codeine Phosphate 15 mg, Maalox 150 mg	Ascriptin Codeine #2 by Rorer		Analgesic; C III
2VALIUM <> ROCHE	Tab, White, Round, Scored	Diazepam 2 mg	Valium by Roche	00140-0004	Antianxiety; C IV
2W	Tab, Blue, Round, 2/W	Lorazepam 2 mg	Ativan by Wyeth	Canadian	Antianxiety; C IV
3	Tab, White, Round, # and 3	Nitroglycerin 0.3 mg	Nitrostat by Endo	60951-0692	Vasodilator
3	Tab, Off-White to White, Round, Ex Release	Nitroglycerin 3 mg	Nitrogard 3 by Forest	00456-0683	Vasodilator
3	Tab	Nitroglycerin 3 mg	Sustachron ER Buccal by Forest	10418-0139	Vasodilator
3	Tab, White, Round	Nitroglycerin 0.6 mg (1/100 gr)	Nitrostat by Able	53265-0251 Discontinued	Vasodilator
3	Tab, White, Round, Sublingual	Nitroglycerin 0.3 mg	Nitrostat by Glenmark	68462-0145	Vasodilator
3 <> 2064V	Tab, White, Round	Acetaminophen 300 mg, Codeine Phosphate 30 mg	Tylenol w/ Codeine by Vintage	00254-2064	Analgesic; C III
3 <> 2064V	Tab, White, Round	Acetaminophen 300 mg, Codeine Phosphate 30 mg	Tylenol w/ Codeine by Qualitest	00603-2338	Analgesic; C III
3 <> 2120V	Tab, White, Round, Scored	Aspirin 325 mg, Codeine Phosphate 30 mg	Aspirin w/ Codeine by Allscripts		Analgesic; C III
3 <> 2120V	Tab, White, Round, Scored	Aspirin 325 mg, Codeine Phosphate 30 mg	Aspirin w/ Codeine by URL Mutual	00677-0647	Analgesic; C III
3 <> 2120V	Tab, White, Round, Scored	Aspirin 325 mg, Codeine Phosphate 30 mg	Aspirin w/ Codeine by Qualitest	00603-2361	Analgesic; C III
3 <> 2120V	Tab, White, Round, Scored	Aspirin 325 mg, Codeine Phosphate 30 mg	Aspirin w/ Codeine by Vintage	00254-2120	Analgesic; C III
3 <> 3984	Tab	Aspirin 325 mg, Codeine Phosphate 30 mg	Aspirin w/ Codeine by DRX	55045-2307	Analgesic; C III
3 <> 522	Tab, White, Round, Andrx Logo 522 <> 3	Acetaminophen 300 mg, Codeine 30 mg	Tylenol w/ Codeine by Andrx	62037-0522	Analgesic; C III
3 <> 93150	Tab, White, Round, 93 over 150	Acetaminophen 300 mg, Codeine Phosphate 30 mg	Tylenol w/ Codeine by Major	00904-0175	Analgesic; C III
3 <> 93150	Tab, White, Round, 93 over 150	Acetaminophen 300 mg, Codeine Phosphate 30 mg	Tylenol w/ Codeine by Nat Pharmpak	55154-5548	Analgesic; C III
3 <> 93150	Tab, White, Round, 93 over 150	Acetaminophen 300 mg, Codeine Phosphate 30 mg	Tylenol w/ Codeine by UDL	51079-0161 Discontinued	Analgesic; C III
3 <> 93150	Tab, White, Round, 93 over 150	Acetaminophen 300 mg, Codeine Phosphate 30 mg	Tylenol w/ Codeine by Urgent Care Center	50716-0465	Analgesic; C III
3 <> 93150	Tab, White, Round, 93 over 150	Acetaminophen 300 mg, Codeine Phosphate 30 mg	Tylenol w/ Codeine by Pharmedix	53002-0101	Analgesic; C III
3 <> 93150	Tab, White, Round, 93 over 150	Acetaminophen 300 mg, Codeine Phosphate 30 mg	Tylenol w/ Codeine by Murfreesboro	51129-0089	Analgesic; C III

ID FRONT <> BACK	DESCRIPTION FRONT <> BACK	INGREDIENT & STRENGTH	BRAND (or Generic Equiv.) by FIRM	NDC#	CLASS; SCH.
3 <> 93150	Tab, White, Round, 93 over 150	Acetaminophen 300 mg, Codeine Phosphate 30 mg	Tylenol w/ Codeine by Teva	00093-0150	Analgesic; C III
3 <> A	Tab, White, Octagonal, Film Coated	Indapamide 2.5 mg	Lozol by Arcola	00070-3000 Discontinued	Diuretic
3 <> A	Tab, Pink, Round, Film Coated, Scored	Guaifenesin 1200 mg, Phenylpropanolamine 75 mg	Aquatab D by Adams	63824-0003	Cold Remedy
3 <> A	Tab, White, Octagonal, Film Coated	Indapamide 2.5 mg	Lozol by RPR	00801-3000	Diuretic
3 <> A	Tab, White, Octagonal, Film Coated	Indapamide 2.5 mg	Lozol by Murfreesboro	51129-1537	Diuretic
3 <> A285	Tab, White to Off-White, Round	Acetaminophen 300 mg, Codeine Phosphate 30 mg	Tylenol w/ Codeine by Able	53265-0285 Discontinued	Analgesic; C III
3 <> ALVA	Tab, Olive, Cap Shaped	Riboflavin 1 mg, Green Tea Leaf 300 mg	Thinz by Alva		Supplement
3 <> B303	Tab, White, Round, B/303 <> 3	Acetaminophen 300 mg, Codeine Phosphate 30 mg	Tylenol w/ Codeine by Barr	00555-0303 Discontinued	Analgesic; C III
3 <> B303	Tab, White, Round, B/303 <> 3	Acetaminophen 300 mg, Codeine Phosphate 30 mg	Tylenol w/ Codeine by Duramed	51285-0303	Analgesic; C III
3 <> B494	Tab, Green, Round, b over 494, Ex Release	Alprazolam 3 mg	Xanax XR by Barr	00555-0494	Antianxiety; C IV
3 <> BARR198	Tab	Acetaminophen 300 mg, Codeine Phosphate 30 mg	Tylenol w/ Codeine by Barr	00555-0198	Analgesic; C III
3 <> BARR198	Tab	Acetaminophen 300 mg, Codeine Phosphate 30 mg	Tylenol w/ Codeine by Pharmedix	53002-0101	Analgesic; C III
3 <> BIOCRAFT	Tab	Sulfamethoxazole 800 mg, Trimethoprim 160 mg	by Nat Pharmpak	55154-5805	Antibiotic
3 <> BIOCRAFT	Tab	Sulfamethoxazole 800 mg, Trimethoprim 160 mg	by Ivax	00182-8844	Antibiotic
3 <> CIBA	Tab, Pale Green, Round, Scored	Methylphenidate HCl 10 mg	Ritalin by Caremark	00339-4083	Stimulant; C II
3 <> CIBA	Tab, Pale Green, Round, Scored	Methylphenidate HCl 10 mg	Ritalin by Novartis	00083-0003	Stimulant; C II
3 <> CL	Tab, White to Off-White, Rectangle, Sublingual	Nitroglycerin 0.3 mg	Nitrostat by Pliva	50111-0992	Vasodilator
3 <> DRL150	Tab, White, Oval	Nefazodone HCl 150 mg	Serzone by Dr. Reddy's	55111-0140	Antidepressant
3 <> DRL150	Tab, White, Oval	Nefazodone HCl 150 mg	Serzone by Par	49884-0918	Antidepressant
3 <> E	Tab, Pink, Oval, Film Coated	Conjugated Estrogens 0.625 mg	Enjuvia by Barr	51285-0408	Hormone
3 <> ETH	Tab, White, Oval	Nitroglycerin 0.3 mg	Nitrostat by PDRX	55289-0308	Vasodilator
3 <> ETH	Tab, White, Oval	Nitroglycerin 0.3 mg	NitroQuick by Ethex	58177-0323	Vasodilator
3 <> G	Tab, Green, Triangular, Ex Release	Alprazolam 3 mg	Xanax XR by Greenstone	59762-0068	Antianxiety; C IV
3 <> GG220	Tab	Acetaminophen 300 mg, Codeine Phosphate 30 mg	Tylenol w/ Codeine by Golden State	60429-0500	Analgesic; C III
3 <> LOGO001	Tab, Logo 001	Acetaminophen 300 mg, Codeine Phosphate 30 mg	Tylenol w/ Codeine by Quality Care	60346-0059	Analgesic; C III
3 <> M	Tab, White, Round, M inside square <> 3	Acetaminophen 300 mg, Codeine Phosphate 30 mg	Tylenol w/ Codeine by Mallinckrodt	00406-0484	Analgesic; C III
3 <> MCNEIL	Tab, White, Round, McNeil	Acetaminophen 300 mg, Caffeine 15 mg, Codeine Phosphate 30 mg	Tylenol w/ Codeine by Janssen-Ortho	Canadian DIN 02163926	Analgesic; C III
3 <> MP122	Tab, 3 <> MP over 122	Acetaminophen 300 mg, Codeine Phosphate 30 mg	Tylenol w/ Codeine by URL Mutual	00677-0612	Analgesic; C III
3 <> N	Tab, White, Round	Nitroglycerin 0.3 mg	Nitrostat by Parke Davis	00071-0417	Vasodilator
3 <> N	Tab, White, Round	Nitroglycerin 0.3 mg	Nitrostat by Parke Davis	Canadian DIN 00037613	Vasodilator
3 <> NOVO	Tab, Pink, Round	Bromazepam 3 mg	Lectopam by Novopharm	Canadian DIN 02230584	Sedative; C IV
3 <> P001	Tab	Acetaminophen 300 mg, Codeine Phosphate 30 mg	Tylenol w/ Codeine by Talbert	44514-0223	Analgesic; C III
3 <> R001	Tab	Acetaminophen 300 mg, Codeine Phosphate 30 mg	Tylenol w/ Codeine by Pharmedix	53002-0101	Analgesic; C III
3 <> R001	Tab	Acetaminophen 300 mg, Codeine Phosphate 30 mg	Tylenol w/ Codeine by Vangard	00615-0430	Analgesic; C III
3 <> R20	Tab, White, Round	Acetaminophen 300 mg, Codeine Phosphate 30 mg	Tylenol w/ Codeine by Actavis	00228-3020	Analgesic; C III
3 <> R20	Tab, White, Round	Acetaminophen 300 mg, Codeine Phosphate 30 mg	Tylenol w/ Codeine by Heartland	61392-0714	Analgesic; C III
3 <> R56	Tab, White to Off-White, Round	Acetaminophen 300 mg, Codeine Phosphate 30 mg	Tylenol w/ Codeine by Actavis	00228-3056	Analgesic; C III
3 <> RX562	Tab, White, Round	Acetaminophen 300 mg, Codeine Phosphate 30 mg	Tylenol w/ Codeine by Ranbaxy	63304-0562	Analgesic; C III
3 <> SP	Tab, Blue, Oval	Doxepin 3 mg	Silenor by Somaxon	42847-0103	Sedative/Hypnotic
3 <> WARFARINTARO	Tab, Tan, Cap Shaped	Warfarin Sodium 3 mg	Coumadin by Taro	51672-4030	Anticoagulant
3 <> X	Tab, Green, Triangular, Ex Release	Alprazolam 3 mg	Xanax XR by Pharmacia	00009-0068	Antianxiety; C IV
3 <> Z3984	Tab, White, Round, Z over 3984	Aspirin 325 mg, Codeine Phosphate 30 mg	Aspirin w/ Codeine by Ivax	00172-3984 Discontinued	Analgesic; C III

ID FRONT <> BACK	DESCRIPTION FRONT <> BACK	INGREDIENT & STRENGTH	BRAND (or Generic Equiv.) by FIRM	NDC#	CLASS; SCH.
30	Tab, White to Yellowish White, Orange to Dark Brown Specks	Lansoprazole 30 mg	Prevacid by Tap	00300-1544	Gastrointestinal
30	Tab, White to Yellowish White, Orange to Dark Brown Specks	Lansoprazole 30 mg	Prevacid FasTab by Tap	Canadian DIN 02249472	Gastrointestinal
30	Tab, Red, Octagonal, Film-Coated	Oxymorphone HCl 30 mg	Opana ER by Endo	63481-0571	Analgesic; C II
30	Tab, White, Round	Pioglitazone 30 mg	Actos by Cobalt	Canadian DIN 02302888	Antidiabetic
30 <> 54409	Tab, White, Round	Morphine Sulfate SR 30 mg	Oramorph by Roxane	00054-8805 00054-4805	Analgesic; C II
30 <> 5676	Tab, Tan, Round, Hourglass Logo 5676 <> 30	Mirtazapine 30 mg	Remeron by Ivax	00172-5676 Discontinued	Antidepressant
30 <> ABG	Tab, Orange, Round, Film-Coated, Controlled Release	Morphine Sulfate 30 mg	MS Contin by Ivax	00172-2163	Analgesic; C II
30 <> ACTOS	Tab, White to Off-White, Round	Pioglitazone HCl 30 mg	Actos by Eli Lilly	Canadian DIN 02242573	Antidiabetic
30 <> ACTOS	Tab, White, Round, Flat, Scored	Pioglitazone HCl 30 mg	Actos by Prestige	58056-0338	Antidiabetic
30 <> ACTOS	Tab, White, Round	Pioglitazone HCl 30 mg	Actos by Takeda	64764-0301	Antidiabetic
30 <> AD	Tab, Orange, Round, Scored	Mixed Amphetamine Salts 30 mg; Amphetamine Aspartate 7.5 mg, Amphetamine Sulfate 7.5 mg, Dextroamphetamine Saccharate 7.5 mg, Dextroamphetamine Sulfate 7.5 mg	Adderall by Shire	58521-0034	Stimulant; C II
30 <> ADALATCC	Tab, Reddish Pink, Round, Film Coated, Adalat over CC	Nifedipine 30 mg	Adalat CC by DRX	55045-2788	Antihypertensive
30 <> ADALATCC	Tab, Reddish Pink, Round, Film Coated, Adalat over CC	Nifedipine 30 mg	Adalat CC by Va Cmop	65243-0053	Antihypertensive
30 <> ADALATCC	Tab, Reddish Pink, Round, Film Coated, Adalat over CC	Nifedipine 30 mg	Adalat CC by Southwood	58016-0120	Antihypertensive
30 <> ADALATCC	Tab, Reddish Pink, Round, Film Coated, Adalat over CC	Nifedipine 30 mg	Adalat CC by Bayer	00026-8841	Antihypertensive
30 <> ADALATCC	Tab, Reddish Pink, Round, Film Coated, Adalat over CC	Nifedipine 30 mg	Adalat CC by Nat Pharmpak	55154-4805	Antihypertensive
30 <> ADALATCC	Tab, Reddish Pink, Round, Film Coated, Adalat over CC	Nifedipine 30 mg	Adalat CC by Wal Mart	49035-0154	Antihypertensive
30 <> ADALATCC	Tab, Reddish Pink, Round, Film Coated, Adalat over CC	Nifedipine 30 mg	Adalat CC by Med Pro	53978-3033	Antihypertensive
30 <> ADALATCC	Tab, Reddish Pink, Round, Film Coated, Adalat over CC	Nifedipine 30 mg	Adalat CC by Allscripts		Antihypertensive
30 <> ADALATCC	Tab, Reddish Pink, Round, Film Coated, Adalat over CC	Nifedipine 30 mg	Adalat CC by Smiths Food & Drug	58341-0058	Antihypertensive
30 <> ADALATCC	Tab, Reddish Pink, Round, Film Coated, Adalat over CC	Nifedipine 30 mg	Adalat CC by Amerisource	62584-0841	Antihypertensive
30 <> ADALATCC	Tab, Reddish Pink, Round, Film Coated, Adalat over CC	Nifedipine 30 mg	Adalat CC by Compumed	00403-4957	Antihypertensive
30 <> ADALATCC	Tab, Reddish Pink, Round, Film Coated, Adalat over CC	Nifedipine 30 mg	Adalat CC by Eckerd	19458-0878	Antihypertensive
30 <> ADALATCC	Tab, Reddish Pink, Round, Film Coated, Adalat over CC	Nifedipine 30 mg	Adalat CC by Talbert	44514-0701	Antihypertensive
30 <> ADAMS	Tab	Dextromethorphan HBr 30 mg, Guaifenesin 600 mg	by Nat Pharmpak	55154-5902	Cold Remedy
30 <> AMGEN	Tab, Light Green, Oval, Film Coated	Cinacalcet HCl 30 mg	Sensipar by Amgen	55513-0073	Calcimimetic
30 <> APO	Tab, Blue, Oblong	Paroxetine HCl 30 mg	Paxil by Apotex	Canadian DIN 02240909	Antidepressant
30 <> B	Tab, Yellow, Round, Extended Release	Nifedipine 30 mg	Adalat CC by Teva	00093-5272	Antihypertensive
30 <> B	Tab, Yellow, Round, Extended Release	Nifedipine 30 mg	Adalat CC by Ivax	00182-8232 Discontinued	Antihypertensive
30 <> B	Tab, Reddish Brown, Round, Film Coated, Ex Release	Nifedical 30 mg	Procardia XL by Teva	00093-0819	Antihypertensive
30 <> B974	Tab, Peach, Oval, Scored, b over 974, 3 over 0	Mixed Amphetamine Sulfate 30 mg; Amphetamine Aspartene 7.5 mg, Amphetamine Sulfate 7.5 mg, Dextroamphetamine Saccharate 7.5 mg, Dextroamphetamine Sulfate 7.5 mg	Adderall by Barr	00555-0974	Stimulant; C II
30 <> E	Tab, Pink, Oval, Extended Release	Morphine Sulfate 30 mg	MS Contin by Ethex	58177-0320	Analgesic; C II
30 <> E653	Tab, Green, Round	Morphine Sulfate 30 mg	MS Contin by Endo	60951-0653	Analgesic; C II
30 <> ER	Tab, White to Off-White, Oval, Ex Release, "3.0" <> ER	Pramipexole DiHCl 3.0 mg	Mirapex ER by Boehringer Ingelheim	00597-0115	Antiparkinson
30 <> ETHEX	Tab, Brown, Cap Shaped, Scored, Immediate Release	Morphine Sulfate 30 mg	MSIR by Ethex	58177-0314	Analgesic; C II
30 <> G	Tab, White, Round, Film Coated	Ranitidine HCl 150 mg	by Mylan	00378-3252	Gastrointestinal
30 <> GG	Tab, Reddish-Orange, Round, Film Coated	Thioridazine 10 mg	Mellaril by Sandoz	00781-1604	Antipsychotic
30 <> LUPIN	Tab, Red, Round	Lisinopril 30 mg	Zestril by Lupin	68180-0516	Antihypertensive
30 <> M	Tab, Purple, Round, M inside square <> 30	Morphine Sulfate 30 mg	MS Contin by Mallinckrodt	00406-8330	Analgesic; C II

ID FRONT <> BACK	DESCRIPTION FRONT <> BACK	INGREDIENT & STRENGTH	BRAND (or Generic Equiv.) by FIRM	NDC#	CLASS; SCH.
30 <> M	Tab, Light Blue, Round, Convex, Scored, M inside square	Oxycodone HCl 30 mg	Roxicodone by Mallinckrodt	00406-8530	Analgesic; C II
30 <> M	Tab, White to Cream Colored, Octagon, M inside square	Mixed Amphetamine Salts 30 mg: Dextroamphetamine Saccharate 7.5 mg, Amphetamine Aspartate 7.5 mg, Dextroamphetamine Sulfate 7.5 mg, Amphetamine Sulfate 7.5 mg	Adderall by Mallinckrodt	00406-8894	Stimulant; C II
30 <> MEDEVA	Tab, Green, Oblong, Scored	Dextromethorphan 30 mg, Guaifenesin 600 mg	Humibid-DM by Adams	63824-0030	Cold Remedy
30 <> MOSSR	Tab, Blue, Round, M.O.S.-SR/30	Morphine HCl 30 mg	M.O.S.-S.R. by ICN	Canadian DIN 00776181	Analgesic; C II
30 <> N	Tab, Orange, Oval, Scored, N <> 3/0	Mirtazapine 30 mg	Remeron by Novopharm	Canadian DIN 02259354	Antidepressant
30 <> N	Tab, Blue, Oval, N <> 3/0	Paroxetine HCl 30 mg	Paxil by Novopharm	Canadian DIN 02248558	Antidepressant
30 <> NOVO	Tab, Green, Round	Diltiazem HCl 30 mg	Cardizem by Novopharm	Canadian DIN 00862924	Antihypertensive
30 <> OC	Tab, Round, Brown, CR	Oxycodone HCl 30 mg	OxyContin by Purdue	59011-0830	Analgesic; C II
30 <> P	Tab, Brown, Oval, Scored	Mirtazapine 30 mg	Remeron by Pharmascience	Canadian DIN 02248762	Antidepressant
30 <> P	Tab, Blue, Oval, P Logo	Paroxetine HCl 30 mg	Paxil by Pharmascience	Canadian DIN 02247752	Antidepressant
30 <> PAXIL	Tab, Blue, Oblong, Film Coated	Paroxetine HCl 30 mg	Paxil by GSK	Canadian DIN 01940473	Antidepressant
30 <> PAXIL	Tab, Blue, Oblong, Film Coated	Paroxetine HCl 30 mg	Paxil by SB	59742-3212	Antidepressant
30 <> PAXIL	Tab, Blue, Oblong, Film Coated	Paroxetine HCl 30 mg	Paxil by Physician Total Care	54868-3526	Antidepressant
30 <> PAXIL	Tab, Blue, Oblong, Film Coated	Paroxetine HCl 30 mg	Paxil by SKB	00029-3212	Antidepressant
30 <> PF	Tab, White, Cap Shaped	Morphine Sulfate 30 mg	MS Contin by Purdue	Canadian	Analgesic; C II
30 <> PG	Tab, White, Round	Pioglitazone HCl 30 mg	Actos by Pharmascience	Canadian DIN 02303132	Antihyperglycemic
30 <> WW	Tab, Pink, Oval, Scored, Extended Release	Isosorbide Mononitrate 30 mg	Imdur by West-Ward	00143-2230	Antianginal
300	Cap, White	Etodolac 300 mg	Lodine by ESI Lederle		NSAID
300	Tab, White, Round, Scored, Film Coated, 300 over Triangle	Propafenone HCl 300 mg	Rythmol by Abbott	00044-5023	Antiarrhythmic
300	Tab, Peach, Round, Logo/300	Penicillin V Potassium 300 mg	by Nadeau	Canadian	Antibiotic
300	Cap, White, Red Print, Ex Release	Theophylline Anhydrous 300 mg	Slo-Bid by RPR	00801-0300	Antiasthmatic
300	Tab, White, Oblong	Theophylline Anhydrous 300 mg	Slo-Bid by RPR	Canadian	Antiasthmatic
300	Tab, Green, Round, Scored	Levothyroxine Sodium 300 mcg	Eltroxin by GSK	Canadian DIN 02213230	Thyroid Hormone
300	Tab, White, Round, Scored, Film Coated, 300 over Triangle	Propafenone HCl 300 mg	Rythmol by Abbott	Canadian DIN 00603716	Antiarrhythmic
300	Tab, White to Off-White, Cap-Shaped, Film Coated, Cobalt Logo <> 300	Ranitidine HCl 300 mg	Zantac by Cobalt	Canadian DIN 02248571	Gastrointestinal
300	Tab, Red, Round	Ferrous Sulfate 300 mg	Ferrous Sulfate by Apotex	Canadian DIN 01912518	Mineral
300	Tab, White, Round, Scored, Film Coated, 300 over Triangle	Propafenone HCl 300 mg	Rythmol by Pharmascience	Canadian DIN 02243728	Antiarrhythmic
300 <> 4366	Tab, Green, Round, Hourglass Logo 4366	Labetalol HCl 300 mg	Trandate by Ivax	00172-4366	Antihypertensive
300 <> 4441	Tab, White, Round, Hourglass Logo over 4441	Gabapentin 300 mg	Neurontin by Ivax	00172-4441 Discontinued	Anticonvulsant
300 <> APO	Tab, White, Oval	Ofloxacin 300 mg	Oflox by Apotex	Canadian DIN 02231531	Antibiotic
300 <> B	Tab, White, Cap Shaped, Ex Release	Diltiazem HCl 300 mg	Cardizem LA by Biovail	64455-0103	Antihypertensive
300 <> B	Tab, White, Cap Shaped, Ex Release	Diltiazem HCl 300 mg	Tiazac XC by Biovail	Canadian DIN 02256762	Antihypertensive
300 <> B702	Tab, Pink, Round, Film Coated, b over 702	Demeclocycline HCl 300 mg	Declomycin by Barr	00555-0702	Antibiotic

ID FRONT <> BACK	DESCRIPTION FRONT <> BACK	INGREDIENT & STRENGTH	BRAND (or Generic Equiv.) by FIRM	NDC#	CLASS; SCH.
300 <> BARR071	Tab, White, Round, Scored, Barr over 071	Isoniazid 300 mg	Laniazid by Schein	00364-0151	Antimycobacterial
300 <> BARR071	Tab, White, Round, Scored, Barr over 071	Isoniazid 300 mg	Laniazid by Barr	Discontinued	Antimycobacterial
300 <> FLINT	Tab, Green, Round, Scored	Levothyroxine Sodium 300 mcg	Synthroid by CVS	51316-0246	Thyroid Hormone
300 <> FLINT	Tab, Green, Round, Scored	Levothyroxine Sodium 300 mcg	Synthroid by Thrift Drug	59198-0298	Thyroid Hormone
300 <> FLINT	Tab, Green, Round, Scored	Levothyroxine Sodium 300 mcg	Synthroid by Amerisource	62584-0170	Thyroid Hormone
300 <> FLINT	Tab, Green, Round, Scored	Levothyroxine Sodium 300 mcg	Synthroid by Abbott	00048-1170	Thyroid Hormone
300 <> FLINT	Tab, Green, Round, Scored	Levothyroxine Sodium 300 mcg	Synthroid by Forest	00456-0328	Thyroid Hormone
300 <> FLINT	Tab, Green, Round, Scored	Levothyroxine Sodium 300 mcg	Synthroid by Abbott	Canadian DIN 02172151	Thyroid Hormone
300 <> GG341	Tab, Pink, Cap Shaped, Scored, 300 <> GG over 341	Levothyroxine 300 mcg	Levo-T by Alara	64909-0145	Thyroid Hormone
300 <> GG341	Tab, Green, Cap Shaped, Scored, 300 <> GG over 341	Levothyroxine 300 mcg	Levo-T by Sandoz	00781-5190	Thyroid Hormone
300 <> GILEAD4331	Tab, Light Blue, Almond Shaped, Film Coated	Tenofovir Disoproxil Fumarate 300 mg	Viread by Gilead	61958-0401	Antiviral
300 <> GILEAD4331	Tab, Light Blue, Almond Shaped, Film Coated	Tenofovir Disoproxil Fumarate 300 mg	Viread by Gilead	Canadian DIN 02247128	Antiretroviral Agent
300 <> GXCW3	Tab, White, Round, Film Coated	Zidovudine 300 mg	Retrovir by Allscripts		Antiviral
300 <> GXCW3	Tab, White, Round, Film Coated	Zidovudine 300 mg	Retrovir by DSM	63552-0501	Antiviral
300 <> GXCW3	Tab, White, Round, Film Coated	Zidovudine 300 mg	Retrovir by GSK	00173-0501	Antiviral
300 <> GXCW3	Tab, White, Round, Film Coated	Zidovudine 300 mg	Retrovir by DRX	55045-2488	Antiviral
300 <> N	Tab, White, Oval	Ofloxacin 300 mg	Floxin by Novopharm	Canadian DIN 02243475	Antibiotic
300 <> N	Tab, White, Cap Shaped	Ranitidine HCl 300 mg	Zantac by Novopharm	Canadian DIN 00828556	Gastrointestinal
300 <> N192	Tab, Dark Green, Oval, Film Coated	Cimetidine HCl 300 mg	Tagamet by Teva	00093-8192 Discontinued	Gastrointestinal
300 <> N192	Tab, Green, Oval, Film Coated	Cimetidine HCl 300 mg	Tagamet by Dixon Shane	17236-0171	Gastrointestinal
300 <> N192	Tab, Green, Oval, Film Coated	Cimetidine HCl 300 mg	Tagamet by DRX	55045-2272	Gastrointestinal
300 <> N192	Tab, Green, Oval, Film Coated	Cimetidine HCl 300 mg	Tagamet by Warrick	59930-1801	Gastrointestinal
300 <> N192	Tab, Green, Oval, Film Coated	Cimetidine HCl 300 mg	Tagamet by Medirex	57480-0813	Gastrointestinal
300 <> N192	Tab, Green, Oval, Film Coated	Cimetidine HCl 300 mg	Tagamet by URL Mutual	00677-1528	Gastrointestinal
300 <> N192	Tab, Green, Oval, Film Coated	Cimetidine HCl 300 mg	Tagamet by Teva	55953-0192	Gastrointestinal
300 <> N192	Tab, Green, Oval, Film Coated	Cimetidine HCl 300 mg	Tagamet by Nat Pharmpak	55154-9303	Gastrointestinal
300 <> N192	Tab, Green, Oval, Film Coated	Cimetidine HCl 300 mg	Tagamet by Brightstone	62939-2121	Gastrointestinal
300 <> N547	Tab, White, Cap Shaped, Film Coated, N over 547	Ranitidine HCl 300 mg	Zantac by Teva	00093-8547 Discontinued	Gastrointestinal
300 <> N547	Tab, White, Cap Shaped, Film Coated, N over 547	Ranitidine HCl 300 mg	Zantac by Teva	55953-0547	Gastrointestinal
300 <> N547	Tab, White, Cap Shaped, Film Coated, N over 547	Ranitidine HCl 300 mg	Zantac by UDL	51079-0880	Gastrointestinal
300 <> NN	Tab, White, Cap Shaped, Scored, N/N <> 300	Theophylline Anhydrous 300 mg	Theo-Dur by Novopharm	Canadian DIN 02230087	Antiasthmatic
300 <> NN	Tab, White, Oval, Scored, N/N	Moclobemide 300 mg	Manerix by Novopharm	Canadian DIN 02239748	Antidepressant
300 <> PD357	Tab, White, Oval, Film Coated	Troglitazone 300 mg	Rezulin by Murfreesboro	511129-1423	Antidiabetic
300 <> PD357	Tab, White, Oval, Film Coated	Troglitazone 300 mg	Rezulin by Parke Davis	00071-0357	Antidiabetic
300 <> PLZID	Tab, White, Round, Film-Coated	Zidovudine 300 mg	Retrovir by Teva	00093-5530 Discontinued	Antiviral
300 <> SCHERING438	Tab, Blue, Round	Labetalol HCl 300 mg	Normodyne by Rightpak	65240-0670	Antihypertensive
300 <> SEROQUEL	Tab, White, Cap Shaped, Film Coated	Quetiapine Fumarate 300 mg	Seroquel by AstraZeneca	00310-0274	Antipsychotic
300 <> SEROQUEL	Tab, White, Cap Shaped, Film Coated	Quetiapine Fumarate 300 mg	Seroquel by AstraZeneca	Canadian DIN 02244107	Antipsychotic
300 <> SYNTHROID	Tab, Green, Round, Scored	Levothyroxine Sodium 300 mcg	Synthroid by Abbott	00074-7149	Thyroid Hormone
300 <> T4	Tab, Green, Cap Shaped	Levothyroxine Sodium 300 mcg	Levothroid by Forest	00456-1328	Thyroid Hormone

ID FRONT <> BACK	DESCRIPTION FRONT <> BACK	INGREDIENT & STRENGTH	BRAND (or Generic Equiv.) by FIRM	NDC#	CLASS; SCH.
300 <> TAGAMETSB	Tab, Film Coated	Cimetidine HCl 300 mg	Tagamet by H J Harkins Co	52959-0270	Gastrointestinal
300 <> TMC114	Tab, Orange, Oval, Film-Coated	Darunavir 300 mg	Prezista by Tibotec	59676-0560 Discontinued	Antiviral
3000	Tab, White, Round	Quinidine Gluconate 324 mg	Quinaglute by Roxane		Antiarrhythmic
300599113607	Cap, White, Oblong	Etodolac 300 mg	Lodine by ESI Lederle	59911-3607	NSAID
300599223607	Cap, White	Etodolac 300 mg	Lodine by Wyeth	52903-3607	NSAID
300AXIDRELIANT	Cap, Brown and Pale Yellow, Opaque, Black Ink	Nizatidine 300 mg	Axid by Reliant	65726-0145	Gastrointestinal
300BARR	Tab, Orange, Round	Hydroxyzine HCl 100 mg	Atarax by Barr		Antianxiety; Antihistamine
300ER	Tab, White, Round, Black Ink, ER	Tramadol HCl 300 mg	Ultram ER by Ortho-McNeil	00062-0657	Analgesic
300M	Tab	Levothyroxine Sodium 300 mcg	Synthroid by Mova	55370-0134	Thyroid Hormone
300M	Tab	Levothyroxine Sodium 300 mcg	Synthroid by Em Pharma	63254-0445	Thyroid Hormone
300M <> Z	Tab, Green, Round, Scored	Levothyroxine Sodium 300 mcg	Synthroid by Zoetica	64909-0112	Thyroid Hormone
300M30	Tab, White, Round, Scored	Cimetidine 300 mg	Tagamet by Dava	67253-0340	Gastrointestinal
300M30 <> MOVA	Tab, White, Round, Film Coated	Cimetidine HCl 300 mg	Tagamet by Mova	55370-0135	Gastrointestinal
300M30 <> MOVA	Tab, White, Round, Film Coated	Cimetidine HCl 300 mg	Tagamet by Compumed	00403-1340	Gastrointestinal
300MCG <> 284	Tab, Coated	Cerivastatin Sodium 0.3 mg	Baycol by Bayer	00026-2884	Antihyperlipidemic
300MG <> TMC114	Tab, Orange, Oval, Film-Coated	Darunavir 300 mg	Prezista by Janssen-Ortho	Canadian DIN 02284057	Antiviral
300MG4177	Cap, Red Print	Etodolac 300 mg	by Ivax	00172-4177	NSAID
300MG4177	Cap, Red Print	Etodolac 300 mg	by Ivax	00182-2665	NSAID
300MGANDRX600	Cap, Orange, Ex Release	Diltiazem HCl 300 mg	Cartia XT by Andrx	62037-0600	Antihypertensive
300NORMODYNE <> SCHERING438	Tab, Blue, Round, Film, Schering 438 <> 300 Normodyne	Labetalol HCl 300 mg	Normodyne by Thrift Drug	59198-0082	Antihypertensive
300P	Cap, Light Blue	Clindamycin HCl 300 mg	Dalacin C by Pharmascience	Canadian DIN 02294834	Antibiotic
300SB <> TAGAMET	Tab, Light Green, Film Coated	Cimetidine HCl 300 mg	Tagamet by Quality Care	60346-0001	Gastrointestinal
300SKF <> TAGAMET	Tab, Film Coated	Cimetidine HCl 300 mg	Tagamet by Pharmedix	53002-0328	Gastrointestinal
300WALLACE374101	Cap, Blue & White, 300 Wallace 37-4101	Methacycline HCl 300 mg	Rondomycin by Wallace		Antibiotic
301 <> ETHEX	Tab, White, Red Print, Round, Film Coated	Ketorolac Tromethamine 10 mg	Toradol by Ethex	58177-0301	NSAID
301 <> ETHEX	Tab, White, Red Print, Round, Film Coated	Ketorolac Tromethamine 10 mg	Toradol by Compumed	00403-4136	NSAID
301 <> ETHEX	Tab, White, Red Print, Round, Film Coated	Ketorolac Tromethamine 10 mg	Toradol by Syntex	18393-0301	NSAID
301 <> ETHEX	Tab, White, Red Print, Round, Film Coated	Ketorolac Tromethamine 10 mg	Toradol by Murfreesboro	51129-1437	NSAID
301 <> HOPE	Tab, White, Round	Scopolamine Hydrobromide 0.4 mg	Scopace by Hope	60267-0301	Antiemetic
301 <> HOPE	Tab, White, Round	Scopolamine Hydrobromide 0.4 mg	Scopace by Anabolic	00722-6383	Antiemetic
301 <> RS	Tab, White, Round	Atropine Sulfate 0.025 mg, Diphenoxylate HCl 2.5 mg	Lomotil by Corepharma	64720-0301	Antidiarrheal; C V
301 <> RS	Tab, White, Round	Atropine Sulfate 0.025 mg, Diphenoxylate HCl 2.5 mg	Lomotil by Amneal	65162-0301	Antidiarrheal; C V
301 <> WATSON	Tab, White, Round	Furosemide 40 mg	Lasix by Allscripts		Diuretic
3012	Cap, Orange & White, 3 Mericon Logo/0102	Fluoride 3.74 mg, Calcium 145 mg	Florical by Mericon		Mineral
301B	Tab, Yellow, Round	Hydroxyzine HCl 10 mg	Atarax by Barr		Antianxiety, Antihistamine
302 <> 4833G	Tab, White to Off-White, Round, 30/2	Pioglitazone 30 mg, Glimepiride 2 mg	Duetact by Takeda	64764-0302	Antidiabetic
302 <> LUPIN	Tab, White, Oblong	Cefuroxime Axetil 250 mg	Ceftin by Watson	00591-3224	Antibiotic
302 <> LUPIN	Tab, White, Oblong	Cefuroxime Axetil 250 mg	Ceftin by Lupin	68180-0302	Antibiotic
302 <> MYLAN	Tab, White, Round	Acyclovir 800 mg	Zovirax by Mylan	00378-0302	Antiviral
302BARR50	Cap, Black Print	Hydroxyzine Pamoate 85.22 mg	Vistaril by Qualitest	00603-3995	Antianxiety, Antihistamine
303 <> ICN	Tab, White, Round, ICN/303	Trioxsalen 5 mg	Trisoralen by ICN	Canadian DIN 01966383	Psoralen
303 <> ICN	Tab, White, Round, ICN/303	Trioxsalen 5 mg	Trisoralen by ICN	00187-0303	Psoralen
303 <> LUPIN	Tab, White, Oblong	Cefuroxime Axetil 500 mg	Ceftin by Watson	00591-3225	Antibiotic
303 <> LUPIN	Tab, White, Oblong	Cefuroxime Axetil 500 mg	Ceftin by Lupin	68180-0303	Antibiotic

ID FRONT <> BACK	DESCRIPTION FRONT <> BACK	INGREDIENT & STRENGTH	BRAND (or Generic Equiv.) by FIRM	NDC#	CLASS; SCH.
3030	Tab, Blue, Oblong, 30/30	Caffeine 200 mg	30-30's by D&E Pharma		Stimulant
3030 <> IMDUR	Tab, Light Red, Oval, Scored	Isosorbide Mononitrate 30 mg	Imdur by Caremark	00339-6002	Antianginal
3030 <> IMDUR	Tab, Light Red, Oval, Scored	Isosorbide Mononitrate 30 mg	Imdur by Schering	00085-3306	Antianginal
3030 <> IMDUR	Tab, Light Red, Oval, Scored	Isosorbide Mononitrate 30 mg	Imdur by AstraZeneca	17228-3306	Antianginal
3030 <> IMDUR	Tab, Light Red, Oval, Scored	Isosorbide Mononitrate 30 mg	Imdur by Murfreesboro	51129-1573	Antianginal
303303 <> GILGIL	Tab, White, Oval, Scored	Guaifenesin 600 mg, Dextromethorphan HBr 30 mg, Phenylephrine HCl 20 mg	Giltuss TR by Gil Pharma	58552-0303	Cold Remedy
303303 <> GILGIL	Tab, White, Oval, Scored	Guaifenesin 600 mg, Dextromethorphan HBr 30 mg, Phenylephrine HCl 20 mg	Giltuss by Sovereign	58716-0646	Cold Remedy
303325	Cap, White, Royce Logo 303/325	Quinine Sulfate 324 mg	by Royce		Antimalarial
3035 <> N	Tab, Pale Blue, Oval, Scored	Glyburide 3 mg	Glynase by Teva	00093-8035 Discontinued	Antidiabetic
304 <> 4833G	Tab, White to Off-White, Round, 30/4	Pioglitazone 30 mg, Glimepiride 4 mg	Duetact by Takeda	64764-0304	Antidiabetic
304 <> AP	Tab, Purple, Chewable, A/P <> 30/4	Pseudoephedrine HCl 30 mg, Chlorpheniramine Maleate 4 mg	Sudal 12 by Atley	59702-0809	Cold Remedy
304304 <> GILGIL	Tab, White, Oblong, Scored	Guaifenesin 600 mg, Phenylephrine HCl 25 mg	Gilphex TR by Gil Pharma	58552-0304	Cold Remedy
305 <> PMS	Tab, White, Round, Scored	Procyclidine HCl 5 mg	Kemadrin by Pharmascience	Canadian DIN 00587354	Antiparkinson
305305 <> GILGIL	Tab, White, Cap Shaped, Scored	Chlorpheniramine 8 mg, Phenylephrine HCl 20 mg	Phenabid by Gil Pharma	58552-0305	Cold Remedy
3054090	Tab, White, 30/54/090	Morphine Sulfate 30 mg	MS Contin by Boehringer Ingelheim	Canadian	Analgesic; C II
306 <> PFIZER	Tab, Pink, Cap Shaped, Film Coated	Azithromycin 250 mg	Zithromax by Physician Total Care	54868-4183	Antibiotic
306 <> PFIZER	Tab, Pink, Cap Shaped, Film Coated	Azithromycin 250 mg	Zithromax by Pfizer	Canadian DIN 02212021	Antibiotic
306 <> PFIZER	Tab, Pink, Cap Shaped, Film Coated	Azithromycin 250 mg	Zithromax by Pfizer	00069-3060	Antibiotic
306 <> PFIZER	Tab, Pink, Cap Shaped, Film Coated	Azithromycin 250 mg	Zithromax by Allscripts		Antibiotic
3060 <> G	Tab, Pink, Cap Shaped, Film Coated	Azithromycin 250 mg	Zithromax by Greenstone	59762-3060	Antibiotic
3061	Cap	Cefaclor 250 mg	Ceclor by Eli Lilly	00110-3061	Antibiotic
3062	Cap	Cefaclor 500 mg	Ceclor by Eli Lilly	00110-3062	Antibiotic
306306 <> GILGIL	Tab, White, Cap Shaped, Scored	Chlorpheniramine 8 mg, Dextromethorphan HBr 30 mg, Phenylephrine HCl 20 mg	Phenabid DM by Gil Pharma	58552-0306	Cold Remedy
307 <> PA	Tab, White, Round, Film Coated	Hydroxyzine HCl 10 mg	Atarax by Pliva	50111-0307	Antianxiety; Antihistamine
307 <> PA	Tab, White, Round, Film Coated	Hydroxyzine HCl 10 mg	Atarax by UDL	51079-0413	Antianxiety; Antihistamine
3070 <> G	Tab, Pink, Cap Shaped, Film Coated	Azithromycin 500 mg	Zithromax by Greenstone	59762-3070	Antibiotic
308 <> 93	Tab	Clemastine Fumarate 2.68 mg	by H J Harkins Co	52959-0501	Antihistamine
308 <> ETHEX	Tab, White, Cap Shaped, Scored, Ex Release	Guaifenesin 1200 mg	Guaifenex G by Ethex	58177-0308 Discontinued	Expectorant
308 <> PA	Tab, White, Round, Sugar Coated	Hydroxyzine HCl 25 mg	Atarax by Pliva	50111-0308	Antianxiety; Antihistamine
308 <> PFIZER	Tab, White, Oval, Film Coated	Azithromycin 600 mg	Zithromax by Pfizer	00069-3080	Antibiotic
308 <> PFIZER	Tab, White, Oval, Film Coated	Azithromycin 600 mg	Zithromax by Pfizer	Canadian DIN 02231143	Antibiotic
3080 <> G	Tab, White, Oval, Film Coated	Azithromycin 600 mg	Zithromax by Greenstone	59762-3080	Antibiotic
308AV	Tab, White, Round, Film Coated, Black Ink	Fexofenadine HCl 180 mg, Pseudoephedrine HCl 240 mg	Allegra-D 24 hr by Aventis	00088-1095	Antihistamine; Decongestant
308US	Tab, Maroon, Oval	Calcium Pantothenate 10 mg, Copper Sulfate, Cu-64, Cyanocobalamin 15 mcg, Ferrous Fumarate 324 mg, Folic Acid 1 mg, Magnesium Sulfate, Manganese Sulfate, Niacinamide 30 mg, Pyridoxine HCl 5 mg, Riboflavin 6 mg, Sodium Ascorbate 200 mg, Thiamine Mononitrate 10 mg, Zinc Sulfate	Hemocyte Plus by US Pharma	52747-0308	Vitamin; Mineral

ID FRONT <> BACK	DESCRIPTION FRONT <> BACK	INGREDIENT & STRENGTH	BRAND (or Generic Equiv.) by FIRM	NDC#	CLASS; SCH.
308US	Tab, Maroon, Oval	Calcium Pantothenate 10 mg, Copper Sulfate,Cu-64, Cyanocobalamin 15 mcg, Ferrous Fumarate 324 mg, Folic Acid 1 mg, Magnesium Sulfate, Manganese Sulfate, Niacinamide 30 mg, Pyridoxine HCl 5 mg, Riboflavin 6 mg, Sodium Ascorbate 200 mg, Thiamine Mononitrate 10 mg, Zinc Sulfate	Hemocyte Plus by JLM	63369-0308	Vitamin; Mineral
309 <> MEDEVA	Tab, Yellow, Oblong, Scored	Dextromethorphan 30 mg, Guaifenesin 600 mg, Pseudoephedrine 60 mg	Syn Rx DM by Medeva	53014-0311 Discontinued	Cold Remedy
309 <> MEDEVA	Tab, Yellow, Oblong, Scored	Dextromethorphan 30 mg, Guaifenesin 600 mg, Pseudoephedrine 60 mg	Syn Rx by Adams	63824-0311	Cold Remedy
309 <> PA	Tab, White, Round, Sugar Coated	Hydroxyzine HCl 50 mg	Atarax by Pliva	50111-0309	Antianxiety; Antihistamine
309 <> SL	Tab, White, Black Print, Round, Sugar Coated	Hydroxyzine HCl 50 mg	Atarax by Ivax	00182-1494	Antianxiety; Antihistamine
309 <> SL	Tab, White, Black Print, Round, Sugar Coated	Hydroxyzine HCl 50 mg	Atarax by Direct Dispensing	57866-3876	Antianxiety; Antihistamine
309 <> SL	Tab, White, Black Print, Round, Sugar Coated	Hydroxyzine HCl 50 mg	Atarax by Richmond	54738-0309	Antianxiety; Antihistamine
309 <> SL	Tab, White, Black Print, Round, Sugar Coated	Hydroxyzine HCl 50 mg	Atarax by Darby Group	66467-4569	Antianxiety; Antihistamine
309 <> SL	Tab, White, Black Print, Round, Sugar Coated	Hydroxyzine HCl 50 mg	Atarax by Sandoz	00781-1336	Antianxiety; Antihistamine
309 <> SL	Tab, White, Black Print, Round, Sugar Coated	Hydroxyzine HCl 50 mg	Atarax by Major	00904-0359	Antianxiety; Antihistamine
309 <> SL	Tab, White, Black Print, Round, Sugar Coated	Hydroxyzine HCl 50 mg	Atarax by Baker Cummins	63171-1494	Antianxiety; Antihistamine
309 <> SL	Tab, White, Black Print, Round, Sugar Coated	Hydroxyzine HCl 50 mg	Atarax by Moore	00839-7439	Antianxiety; Antihistamine
309 <> SL	Tab, White, Black Print, Round, Sugar Coated	Hydroxyzine HCl 50 mg	Atarax by Qualitest	00603-3972	Antianxiety; Antihistamine
309 <> SL	Tab, White, Black Print, Round, Sugar Coated	Hydroxyzine HCl 50 mg	Atarax by Allscripts		Antianxiety; Antihistamine
309 <> SL	Tab, White, Black Print, Round, Sugar Coated	Hydroxyzine HCl 50 mg	Atarax by Sidmak		Antianxiety; Antihistamine
309 <> SL	Tab, White, Black Print, Round, Sugar Coated	Hydroxyzine HCl 50 mg	Atarax by Murfreesboro	51129-1477	Antianxiety; Antihistamine
309543	Cap, White Opaque Body, Blue Opaque Cap	Duloxetine 30 mg	Cymbalta by Eli Lilly	Canadian DIN 02301482	Antidepressant, Anxiolytic, Analgesic
30BLANSETT	Cap, Red Print	Guaifenesin 250 mg, Pseudoephedrine HCl 120 mg	Sudafed Sinus by Sovereign	58716-0010	Cold Remedy
30MG <> P	Tab, Violet, Round, Sustained Release	Morphine Sulfate 30 mg	MS Contin by Pharmascience	Canadian DIN 02245285	Analgesic
30MG <> PF	Tab, Violet, Round	Morphine Sulfate 30 mg	MS Contin by Purdue	Canadian	Analgesic; C II
30MG <> RSN	Tab, White, Oval, Film Coated	Risedronate Sodium 30 mg	Actonel by Proc & Gamble	Canadian DIN 02239146	Bisphosphonate
30MG <> RSN	Tab, White, Oval, Film Coated	Risedronate Sodium 30 mg	Actonel by Procter and Gamble	00149-0470	Bisphosphonate
30P <> DAN	Tab, White, Round, Scored	Phenobarbital 30 mg	by Schein	00364-0203	Sedative/Hypnotic; C IV
31	Tab, White, Oval, 31 <> Bone Image	Alendronate Sodium 70 mg	Fosamax by Merck	00006-0031	Antiosteoporosis
31	Tab, White, Oval, 31 <> Bone Image	Alendronate Sodium 70 mg	Fosamax by Merck Frosst	Canadian DIN 02245329	Antiosteoporosis
31 <> 93	Tab, Pink, Oval, Film Coated, Extended Release	Oxycodone HCl 20 mg	OxyContin by Teva	00093-0031 Discontinued	Analgesic; C II
31 <> BMS50	Tab, Light Pink, Hexagonal	Nefazodone HCl 50 mg	Serzone by Direct Dispensing	57866-0911	Antidepressant
31 <> BMS50	Tab, Light Pink, Hexagonal	Nefazodone HCl 50 mg	Serzone by BMS	00087-0031	Antidepressant
31 <> BMS50	Tab, Light Pink, Hexagonal	Nefazodone HCl 50 mg	Serzone by BMS	15548-0031	Antidepressant
31 <> BMS50	Tab, Light Pink, Hexagonal	Nefazodone HCl 50 mg	Serzone by BMS	Canadian	Antidepressant
31 <> BMS50	Tab, Light Pink, Hexagonal	Nefazodone HCl 50 mg	Serzone by Murfreesboro	51129-1106	Antidepressant
31 <> D	Tab, White, Round	Carisoprodol 350 mg	Soma by Aurobindo	65862-0158	Muscle Relaxant
31 <> DX	Tab, Yellow, Oblong	Isosorbide Mononitrate 60 mg	Imdur by Ivax	00182-2687	Antianginal
31 <> G	Tab, White, Oblong, Film Coated	Ranitidine HCl 300 mg	by Mylan	00378-3254	Gastrointestinal
31 <> G	Tab, White, Oval	Gabapentin 600 mg	Neurontin by Glenmark	68462-0126	Anticonvulsant
310	Tab, Yellow, Oblong, Ascher Logo 310	Magnesium Salicylate 600 mg	Mobidin by B F Ascher	00225-0310	Analgesic
310	Tab	Hematinic	Trihemic 600 by Marlop		Vitamin
310 <> 54	Tab, Yellow to Speckled Yellow, Oval	Nefazodone HCl 200 mg	Serzone by Roxane	00054-4674	Antidepressant
310 <> MEDEVA	Tab, Blue, Oblong, Scored	Dextromethorphan 30 mg, Guaifenesin 600 mg, Pseudoephedrine 60 mg	Syn Rx by Adams	63824-0311	Cold Remedy

ID FRONT <> BACK	DESCRIPTION FRONT <> BACK	INGREDIENT & STRENGTH	BRAND (or Generic Equiv.) by FIRM	NDC#	CLASS; SCH.
310 <> MEDEVA	Tab, Blue, Oblong, Scored	Dextromethorphan 30 mg, Guaifenesin 600 mg, Pseudoephedrine 60 mg	Syn Rx DM by Medeva	53014-0311 Discontinued	Cold Remedy
3100	Cap, Yellow	Phentermine 30 mg	Ionamin by Vortech	Canadian	Anorexiant; C IV
3101	Cap, Blue & White, Pulvule	Nabilone 1 mg	by Eli Lilly	Canadian	Antiemetic; C II
3101 <> BRL30	Tab, Light Blue, Round, BRL over 30	Diltiazem HCl 30 mg	Cardizem by Blue Ridge	59273-0002	Antihypertensive
3101 <> BRL30	Tab, Light Blue, Round, BRL over 30	Diltiazem HCl 30 mg	Cardizem by Elan Hold	60274-0884	Antihypertensive
3102 <> BRL60	Tab, White, Round, Scored, BRL over 60	Diltiazem HCl 60 mg	Cardizem by Blue Ridge	59273-0003	Antihypertensive
31025	Cap, Blue & Pink, Royce Logo 310/25	Doxepin HCl 25 mg	Sinequan by Royce		Antidepressant
31025	Cap, Royce Logo 310	Doxepin HCl 25 mg	by Quality Care	60346-0553	Antidepressant
31025	Cap, Blue & Pink, Royce Logo 310/25	Doxepin HCl 25 mg	Sinequan by Royce	51875-0310	Antidepressant
3103 <> BRL90	Tab, Light Blue, Oblong, Scored	Diltiazem HCl 90 mg	Cardizem by Blue Ridge	59273-0004	Antihypertensive
3104 <> BRL120	Tab, White, Oblong, Scored	Diltiazem HCl 120 mg	Cardizem by Blue Ridge	59273-0005	Antihypertensive
3104 <> BRL120	Tab, White, Oblong, Scored	Diltiazem HCl 120 mg	Cardizem by Watson	52544-0778	Antihypertensive
3104PROZAC10	Cap, Green	Fluoxetine HCl 10 mg	Prozac by Eli Lilly		Antidepressant
3105	Cap, Off-White, Gelatin Coated	Fluoxetine HCl 20 mg	Prozac by Nat Pharmpak	55154-0802	Antidepressant
3105PROZAC20	Cap, Green & Yellow	Fluoxetine HCl 20 mg	Prozac by Eli Lilly		Antidepressant
311	Tab, Brown	Vitamin Combination	Pronemia by Marlop		Vitamin
311	Tab, White, Round, Schering Logo 311	Methyltestosterone 10 mg	Oreton by Schering		Hormone; C III
311	Tab, White to Off-White, Cap Shaped	Ezetimibe 10 mg, Simvastatin 10 mg	Vytorin 10/10 by Schering-Plough	66582-0311	Antihyperlipidemic
311 <> WATSON	Tab	Furosemide 20 mg	Lasix by Watson	52544-0311	Diuretic
311 <> WATSON	Tab	Furosemide 20 mg	Lasix by DRX	55045-1553	Diuretic
311 <> WATSON	Tab	Furosemide 20 mg	Lasix by Major	00904-1580	Diuretic
311 <> WATSON	Tab	Furosemide 20 mg	Lasix by Macnary	55982-0010	Diuretic
311 <> WATSON	Tab	Furosemide 20 mg	Lasix by Golden State	60429-0078	Diuretic
3111 <> WPI	Tab, Mottled White to Off-White, Oval, Extended-Release	Methylphenidate HCl 20 mg	Ritalin by Watson	00591-3111	Stimulant; C II
3111DARVONCOMP65	Cap, Gray & Red, 3111/Darvon Comp 65	Aspirin 389 mg, Caffeine 32.4 mg, Propoxyphene 65 mg	Darvon Compound by Eli Lilly		Analgesic; C IV
3115	Cap, Black	Phentermine 30 mg	Phentrol #5 by Vortech		Anorexiant; C IV
31150	Cap, Flesh & Pink, Royce Logo 311/50	Doxepin HCl 50 mg	Sinequan by Royce	51875-0311	Antidepressant
31150	Cap, Flesh & Pink, Royce Logo 311/50	Doxepin HCl 50 mg	Sinequan by Royce		Antidepressant
312	Tab	Therapeutic Multivitamin	Berocca by Marlop		Vitamin
312	Tab, White to Off-White, Cap Shaped	Ezetimibe 10 mg, Simvastatin 20 mg	Vytorin 10/20 by Schering-Plough	66582-0312	Antihyperlipidemic
312	Tab, White, Scored, 312 Prasco Logo	Guaifenesin 1000 mg, Dextromethorphan HBr 60 mg	Guaifenesin DM by Prasco	66993-0312	Cold Remedy
312 <> ETHEX	Tab, Orange, Round, Scored	Dextroamphetamine Sulfate 10 mg	Dexedrine by Ethex	58177-0311	Stimulant; C II
312 <> SL	Tab, Sugar Coated	Dipyridamole 50 mg	by Pliva	50111-0312	Antiplatelet
312393	Cap, Light Green & Green, Oval	Dicloxacillin Sodium 250 mg	by Allscripts	00480-0778	Antibiotic
3125VANCOCINHCL 125MG	Cap, Blue and Brown, Opaque	Vancomycin HCl 125 mg	Vancocin HCl Pulvules by Nat Pharmpak	55154-1805	Antibiotic
3125VANCOCINHCL 125MG	Cap, Blue and Brown, Opaque	Vancomycin HCl 125 mg	Vancocin HCl Pulvules by Eli Lilly	00002-3125	Antibiotic
3126VANCOCINHCL 250MG	Cap, Blue and Brown, Opaque	Vancomycin HCl 250 mg	Vancocin HCl Pulvules by Eli Lilly	00002-3126	Antibiotic
3126VANCOCINHCL 250MG	Cap, Blue & Purple, Opaque	Vancomycin HCl 250 mg	Vancocin HCl Pulvules by Teva	00480-0778	Antibiotic
312R <> RBX	Tab, White, Round, Film Coated	Zopiclone 5 mg	Imovane by Ranbaxy	Canadian DIN 02267918	Sedative; Hypnotic
313	Tab	Therapeutic Multivitamin, Minerals	Berocca Plus by Marlop		Vitamin
313	Tab, Gray, Blue Print, Round, Schering Logo over 313	Perphenazine 8 mg	Trilafon by Schering	00085-0313	Antipsychotic

ID FRONT <> BACK	DESCRIPTION FRONT <> BACK	INGREDIENT & STRENGTH	BRAND (or Generic Equiv.) by FIRM	NDC#	CLASS; SCH.
313	Tab, White to Off-White, Cap Shaped	Ezetimibe 10 mg, Simvastatin 40 mg	Vytorin 10/40 by Schering-Plough	66582-0313	Antihyperlipidemic
313 <> SL	Tab, Sugar Coated	Dipyridamole 75 mg	by Pliva	50111-0313	Antiplatelet
3131	Tab, White, Round, Film Coated, Ex Release	Potassium Chloride 750 mg	Kaon-CL by Savage	00281-3131	Electrolytes
313313 <> S	Tab, White, Oval, Scored, Film Coated	Fluvoxamine Maleate 100 mg	Luvox by Solvay	Canadian DIN 01919369	OCD
3137WPI	Cap, Off-White	Nizatidine 150 mg	Axid by Watson	00591-3137	Gastrointestinal
3138WPI	Cap, Light Brown	Nizatidine 300 mg	Axid by Watson	00591-3138	Gastrointestinal
314 <> 93	Tab, White, Round, Film Coated	Ketorolac Tromethamine 10 mg	Toradol by Allscripts		NSAID
314 <> 93	Tab, White, Round, Film Coated	Ketorolac Tromethamine 10 mg	Toradol by Southwood	58016-0247	NSAID
314 <> 93	Tab, White, Round, Film Coated	Ketorolac Tromethamine 10 mg	Toradol by Teva	00093-0314	NSAID
3144	Cap, Yellow	Nizatidine 150 mg	Axid by Eli Lilly	Canadian	Gastrointestinal
3145	Cap, Brown & Yellow	Nizatidine 300 mg	Axid by Eli Lilly	Canadian	Gastrointestinal
315	Tab, White to Off-White, Cap Shaped	Ezetimibe 10 mg, Simvastatin 80 mg	Vytorin 10/80 by Schering-Plough	66582-0315	Antihyperlipidemic
315	Cap, Red	Vitamin Combination	Pronemia by Marlop		Vitamin
315 <> ETH	Tab, Orange, Scored	Oxycodone HCl 5 mg	Roxicodone by Ethex	58177-0315	Analgesic; C II
315 <> M	Tab, White	Ondansetron HCl 4 mg	Zofran by UDL	51079-0524	Antiemetic
315 <> M	Tab, White, Round	Ondansetron HCl 4 mg	Zofran by Mylan	00378-7732	Antiemetic
315 <> PRASCO	Tab, White, Oval	Guaifenesin 600 mg, Phenylephrine HCl 40 mg	WellBid-D by Prasco	66993-0315	Cold Remedy
315 <> PROFENFORTE	Tab, White, Oval, Scored, Ex Release	Guaifenesin 800 mg, Pseudoephedrine HCl 90 mg	Profen Forte by Ivax Labs	59310-0315	Cold Remedy
315UCB	Cap, Black & Orange	Niacinamide 25 mg, Vitamin A 8000 Units, Magnesium Sulfate 70 mg, Zinc Sulfate 80 mg, Ascorbic Acid 150 mg, Vitamin E 50 Units, Thiamine Mononitrate 10 mg, Calcium Pantothenate 10 mg, Riboflavin 5 mg, Manganese Chloride 4 mg, Pyridoxine HCl 2 mg, Folic Acid 1 mg	Vicon Forte by Rx Pak	65084-0211	Vitamin
316	Tab, Yellow, Round	Acetaminophen 325 mg, Chlorpheniramine Maleate 2 mg, Phenylephrine HCl 5 mg	Tylenol Allergy by Major	00904-2021	Cold Remedy
316	Tab, Red, Oval, Schering Logo 316	Fluphenazine HCl 10 mg	Permitil by Schering	00085-0316	Antipsychotic
316 <> ETHEX	Tab, Tan, Scored, Film Coated	Ascorbic Acid 120 mg, Biotin 30 mcg, Calcium 200 mg, Chromium 25 mcg, Copper 2 mg, Cyanocobalamin 12 mcg, Folic Acid 1 mg, Iodine 150 mcg, Iron 27 mg, Magnesium 25 mg, Manganese 5 mg, Molybdenum 25 mcg, Niacinamide 20 mg, Pantothenic Acid 10 mg, Pyridoxine HCl 10 mg, Riboflavin 3.4 mg, Selenium 20 mg, Thiamine HCl 3 mg, Vitamin A 5000 Units, Vitamin D 400 Units, Vitamin E 30 mg, Zinc 25 mg	Prenatal MTR by Ethex	58177-0316	Vitamin
316 <> PRASCO	Tab, Green, Oblong	Guaifenesin 1200 mg, Phenylephrine HCl 40 mg	WellBid-D 1200 by Prasco	66993-0316	Cold Remedy
3169 <> V	Tab, White, Oval	Furosemide 20 mg	Lasix by Vintage	00254-3169	Diuretic
316UCB	Cap	Ascorbic Acid 150 mg, Calcium Pantothenate 10 mg, Cyanocobalamin 10 mcg, Folic Acid 1 mg, Magnesium Sulfate 70 mg, Manganese Chloride 4 mg, Niacinamide 25 mg, Pyridoxine HCl 2 mg, Riboflavin 5 mg, Thiamine Mononitrate 10 mg, Vitamin A 8000 Units, Vitamin E 50 Units, Zinc Sulfate 80 mg	by Eckerd	19458-0847	Vitamin
317 <> ETHEX	Tab, White, Oval	Vitamin A 4000 IU, Vitamin C 80 mg, Calcium 200 mg, Iron 54 mg, Vitamin D 400 IU, Vitamin E 15 IU, Thiamine 1.5 mg, Riboflavin 1.6 mg, Niacin 7 mg, Vitamin B6 4 mg, Folate 1 mg, Vitamin B12 2.5 mcg, Biotin 30 mg, Pantothenic Acid 7 mg, Magnesium 100 mg, Zinc 25 mg, Copper 3 mg	Enfamil Natalins by Ethex	58177-0317	Vitamin
317 <> M	Tab, Green, Shield Shaped, Film Coated	Cimetidine HCl 300 mg	Tagamet by Qualitest	00603-2891	Gastrointestinal
317 <> M	Tab, Green, Shield Shaped, Film Coated	Cimetidine HCl 300 mg	Tagamet by Heartland	61392-0197	Gastrointestinal
317 <> M	Tab, Green, Shield Shaped, Film Coated	Cimetidine HCl 300 mg	Tagamet by Nat Pharmpak	55154-5560	Gastrointestinal
317 <> M	Tab, Green, Shield Shaped, Film Coated	Cimetidine HCl 300 mg	Tagamet by H J Harkins Co	52959-0345	Gastrointestinal
317 <> M	Tab, Green, Shield Shaped, Film Coated	Cimetidine HCl 300 mg	Tagamet by UDL	51079-0807 Discontinued	Gastrointestinal
317 <> M	Tab, Green, Shield Shaped, Film Coated	Cimetidine HCl 300 mg	Tagamet by Mylan	00378-0317	Gastrointestinal

ID FRONT <> BACK	DESCRIPTION FRONT <> BACK	INGREDIENT & STRENGTH	BRAND (or Generic Equiv.) by FIRM	NDC#	CLASS; SCH.
317 <> M	Tab, Green, Shield Shaped, Film Coated	Cimetidine HCl 300 mg	Tagamet by Murfreesboro	51129-1181	Gastrointestinal
3170V	Tab, White, Round	Furosemide 40 mg	Lasix by Vintage	00254-3170	Diuretic
3171	Cap, Coated	Loracarbef 400 mg	Lorabid by Eli Lilly	00110-3171	Antibiotic
3171	Cap, Coated	Loracarbef 400 mg	Lorabid by DRX	55045-2259	Antibiotic
3171V	Tab, White, Round, 3171/V	Furosemide 80 mg	Lasix by Vintage	00254-3171	Diuretic
3171V	Tab, White, Round, 3171/V	Furosemide 80 mg	Lasix by Qualitest	00603-3741	Diuretic
3176 <> WPI	Tab, White, Round, Film Coated	Citalopram HBr 10 mg	Celexa by Watson	00591-3176	Antidepressant
317B	Tab, White, Oblong	Acetaminophen 325 mg, Propoxyphene Napsylate 50 mg	Darvocet-N 50 by Barr		Analgesic; C IV
3180 <> V	Tab, White, Round	Glycopyrrolate 1 mg	Robinul by Heritage	51079-0700	Gastrointestinal
3186 <> V	Tab, Red, Oblong	Codeine Phosphate 10 mg, Guaifenesin 300 mg	Robitussin by Qualitest	00603-3781	Analgesic; C III
3186 <> V	Tab, Red, Oblong	Codeine Phosphate 10 mg, Guaifenesin 300 mg	Robitussin by Vintage	00254-3186	Analgesic; C III
3189 <> V	Tab, Scored, Film Coated	Guaifenesin 600 mg, Pseudoephedrine HCl 120 mg	by Vintage	00254-3189	Cold Remedy
318BARR	Tab, Orange, Oblong	Acetaminophen 650 mg, Propoxyphene Napsylate 100 mg	Darvocet-N 100 by Barr		Analgesic; C IV
3190 <> V	Tab, Yellow, Cap Shaped	Guaifenesin 600 mg, Pseudoephedrine 120 mg	Entex PSE by Qualitest	00603-3767	Cold Remedy
32 <> 93	Tab, Yellow, Oval, Film Coated, Extended Release	Oxycodone HCl 40 mg	OxyContin by Teva	00093-0032 Discontinued	Analgesic; C II
32 <> BL	Tab	Sulfamethoxazole 400 mg, Trimethoprim 80 mg	by PDRX	55289-0457	Antibiotic
32 <> BMS100	Tab, White, Hexagonal, Scored	Nefazodone HCl 100 mg	Serzone by BMS	Canadian	Antidepressant
32 <> BMS100	Tab, White, Hexagonal, Scored	Nefazodone HCl 100 mg	Serzone by Direct Dispensing	57866-0912	Antidepressant
32 <> BMS100	Tab, White, Hexagonal, Scored	Nefazodone HCl 100 mg	Serzone by BMS	00087-0032	Antidepressant
32 <> BMS100	Tab, White, Hexagonal, Scored	Nefazodone HCl 100 mg	Serzone by Kaiser	00179-1241	Antidepressant
32 <> BMS100	Tab, White, Hexagonal, Scored	Nefazodone HCl 100 mg	Serzone by BMS	15548-0032	Antidepressant
32 <> C	Tab, White to Off White, Round	Sumatriptan Succinate 25 mg	Imitrex by Aurobindo	65862-0146	Antimigraine
32 <> MSD	Tab, White, Round	Ivermectin 3 mg	Stromectol by Murfreesboro	51129-1590	Antihelmintic
32 <> MSD	Tab, White, Round	Ivermectin 3 mg	Stromectol by Merck	00006-0032	Antihelmintic
320 <> RDY	Tab, Peach, Oval, Scored, 3 / 20	Glimepiride 1 mg	Amaryl by Dr. Reddy's	55111-0320	Antidiabetic
3202 <> WATSON	Tab, White, Orange Specks, Cap Shaped, Bisected	Hydrocodone 5 mg, Acetaminophen 325 mg	Norco by Watson	00591-3202	Analgesic; C III
321 <> M	Tab, White, Round	Lorazepam 0.5 mg	Ativan by Caremark	00339-4018	Antianxiety; C IV
321 <> M	Tab, White, Round	Lorazepam 0.5 mg	Ativan by Nat Pharmpak	55154-5550	Antianxiety; C IV
321 <> M	Tab, White, Round	Lorazepam 0.5 mg	Ativan by UDL	51079-0417 Discontinued	Antianxiety; C IV
321 <> M	Tab, White, Round	Lorazepam 0.5 mg	Ativan by Vangard	00615-0450	Antianxiety; C IV
321 <> M	Tab, White, Round	Lorazepam 0.5 mg	Ativan by Murfreesboro	51129-1344	Antianxiety; C IV
321 <> M	Tab, White, Round	Lorazepam 0.5 mg	Ativan by Mylan	00378-0321	Antianxiety; C IV
321 <> R	Tab, Pink, Round	Propranolol HCl 60 mg	Inderal by Actavis	00228-2321	Antihypertensive
321 <> RDY	Tab, Green, Oval, Scored, 3 / 21	Glimepiride 2 mg	Amaryl by Dr. Reddy's	55111-0321	Antidiabetic
322 <> ACJ	Tab, Yellow, Oval, A over CJ	Candesartan Cilexetil 32 mg, Hydrochlorothiazide 12.5 mg	Atacand HCT by AstraZeneca	17228-0322	Antihypertensive; Diuretic
322 <> ACJ	Tab, Yellow, Oval, A over CJ	Candesartan Cilexetil 32 mg, Hydrochlorothiazide 12.5 mg	Atacand HCT by AstraZeneca	00186-0322	Antihypertensive; Diuretic
322 <> ETHEX	Tab, Orange, Oval, Film Coated	Vitamin A 1000 Units, Ascorbic Acid 120 mg, Iron 60 mg, Cholecalciferol, Vitamin E, Thiamine 2 mg, Riboflavin 3 mg, Niacinamide 20 mg, Pyridoxine HCl 10 mg, Folic Acid 1 mg, Cyanocobalamin 12 mcg	NatalCare by Thrift Drug	59198-0320	Vitamin
322 <> ETHEX	Tab, Orange, Oval, Film Coated	Vitamin A 1000 Units, Ascorbic Acid 120 mg, Iron 60 mg, Cholecalciferol, Vitamin E, Thiamine 2 mg, Riboflavin 3 mg, Niacinamide 20 mg, Pyridoxine HCl 10 mg, Folic Acid 1 mg, Cyanocobalamin 12 mcg	NatalCare by Ethex	58177-0322 Discontinued	Vitamin
322 <> M	Tab, Orange, Round	Ciprofloxacin 250 mg	Cipro by Mylan	00378-1322	Antibiotic
322 <> M	Tab, Orange, Round, Film Coated	Ciprofloxacin 250 mg	Cipro by UDL	51079-0402	Antibiotic
322 <> RDY	Tab, Blue, Oval, Scored, 3 / 22	Glimepiride 4 mg	Amaryl by Dr. Reddy's	55111-0322	Antidiabetic
323	Cap, Maroon	Piroxicam 20 mg	Feldene by Rx Pak	65084-0156	NSAID
323	Cap, Maroon	Piroxicam 20 mg	Feldene by Rightpak	65240-0648	NSAID
323 <> MYLAN	Tab, Orange, Cap Shaped	Ciprofloxacin 500 mg	Cipro by Mylan	00378-1323	Antibiotic

ID FRONT <> BACK	DESCRIPTION FRONT <> BACK	INGREDIENT & STRENGTH	BRAND (or Generic Equiv.) by FIRM	NDC#	CLASS; SCH.
323 <> MYLAN	Tab, Orange, Cap Shaped	Ciprofloxacin 500 mg	Cipro by Mylan	51079-0403	Antibiotic
3230WPI	Tab, Yellow, Round	Meloxicam 7.5 mg	Mobic by Watson	00591-3230	NSAID
3238 <> WPI	Tab, Green, Cap Shaped, Film Coated, Scored, 32 / 38	Sertraline HCl 25 mg	Zoloft by Watson	00591-3238	Antidepressant
3239 <> WPI	Tab, Blue, Cap Shaped, Film Coated, Scored, 32 / 39	Sertraline HCl 50 mg	Zoloft by Watson	00591-3239	Antidepressant
324 <> ML	Tab, Round, Pink, Film Coated	Folic Acid 2.2 mg, Pyridoxine 25 mg, Cyanocobalamin 500 mcg	Folcaps by Midlothian	68308-0324	Vitamin
324 <> MYLAN	Tab, Orange, Cap Shaped	Ciprofloxacin 750 mg	Cipro by Mylan	00378-1324	Antibiotic
324 <> MYLAN	Tab, Orange, Cap Shaped	Ciprofloxacin 750 mg	Cipro by UDL	51079-0234 Discontinued	Antibiotic
3240 <> WPI	Tab, Yellow, Cap Shaped, Film Coated, Scored, 32 / 40	Sertraline HCl 100 mg	Zoloft by Watson	00591-3240	Antidepressant
325	Tab, White, Round	Acetaminophen 325 mg	Tylenol by Apotex	Canadian	Analgesic
325 <> APO	Tab, White, Cap Shaped	Acetaminophen 325 mg	Tylenol by Apotex	Canadian DIN 02229873	Analgesic
325 <> NOVO	Tab, White, Oblong	Acetaminophen 325 mg	Tylenol by Novopharm	Canadian DIN 00389218	Analgesic
325 <> TYLENOL	Tab, White, Round, Scored, Film Coated	Acetaminophen 325 mg	Tylenol by McNeil	Canadian DIN 00559393	Analgesic
325 <> TYLENOL	Tab, White, Round, Scored, Film Coated	Acetaminophen 325 mg	Tylenol by McNeil	Canadian DIN 00723894	Analgesic
3256 <> WATSON	Tab, White, Round	Cyclobenzaprine HCl 5 mg	Flexeril by Watson	00591-3256	Muscle Relaxant
325MG <> L403	Tab, White, Round	Acetaminophen 325 mg	Tylenol by Perrigo	00113-0403	Analgesic
325MG <> L406	Tab, Light Blue, Round	Diphenhydramine HCl 25 mg	Benadryl by Perrigo	00113-0406	Antihistamine
326 <> ML	Tab, Round, Pink, Film-Coated	Folic Acid 2.2 mg, Vitamin B-6 25 mg, Vitamin B-12 1 mg	FaBB by Midlothian	68308-0326	Vitamin; Supplement
326 <> PRASCO	Tab, White, Oblong, Scored	Phenylephrine 25 mg, Guaifenesin 900 mg	by Prasco	66993-0326	Cold Remedy
327	Tab, Peach, Oval	Ticlopidine 250 mg	Ticlid by Caraco	57664-0327	Anticoagulant
327	Tab, Orange, Round, Enteric Coated, Black Print	Bisacodyl 5 mg	Dulcolax by Major		Gastrointestinal
327 <> SZ	Tab, Grayish Lavender, Oblong, Film Coated	Mycophenolate Mofetil 500 mg	CellCept by Sandoz	00781-5175	Immunosuppressant
328 <> ETHEX	Tab, White, Oval	Vitamin A 4,000 IU, Vitamin C 120 mg, Calcium 200 mg, Iron 50 mg, Vitamin D 400 IU, Vitamin E 30 IU, Vitamin B1 3 mg, Vitamin B2 3 mg, Niacin 20 mg, Vitamin B6 3 mg, Folic Acid 1 mg, Vitamin B12 8 mcg, Iodine 150 mcg, Zinc 15 mg	Nata Tab Cfe by Ethex	58177-0328	Vitamin
329 <> ETHEX	Tab, Purple, Oval	Vitamin A 4,000 IU, Vitamin C 120 mg, Calcium 200 mg, Iron 29 mg, Vitamin D3 400 IU, Vitamin E 30 IU, Vitamin B1 3 mg, Vitamin B2 3 mg, Niacin 20 mg, Vitamin B6 3 mg, Folic Acid 1 mg, Vitamin B12 8 mcg, Iodine 150 mcg, Zinc 15 mg	Nata Tab FA by Ethex	58177-0329	Vitamin
32BL	Tab	Sulfamethoxazole 400 mg, Trimethoprim 80 mg	by Quality Care	60346-0559	Antibiotic
33 <> 93	Tab, Green, Oval, Film Coated, Extended Release	Oxycodone HCl 80 mg	OxyContin by Teva	00093-0033 Discontinued	Analgesic; C II
33 <> BIOCRAFT	Tab	Sulfamethoxazole 800 mg, Trimethoprim 160 mg	by Vangard	00615-0170	Antibiotic
33 <> BMS200	Tab, Light Yellow, Hexagonal	Nefazodone HCl 200 mg	Serzone by BMS	Canadian	Antidepressant
33 <> BMS200	Tab, Light Yellow, Hexagonal	Nefazodone HCl 200 mg	Serzone by BMS	00087-0033	Antidepressant
33 <> BMS200	Tab, Light Yellow, Hexagonal	Nefazodone HCl 200 mg	Serzone by Kaiser	00179-1243	Antidepressant
33 <> BMS200	Tab, Light Yellow, Hexagonal	Nefazodone HCl 200 mg	Serzone by BMS	15548-0033	Antidepressant
33 <> C	Tab, White to Off White, Cap Shaped	Sumatriptan Succinate 50 mg	Imitrex by Aurobindo	65862-0147	Antimigraine
33 <> E	Tab, Light Yellow, Round, Film Coated	Topiramate 50 mg	Topiramate by Aurobindo	65862-0172	Anticonvulsant
330 <> GRISACTIN	Tab	Griseofulvin, Ultramicrosize 330 mg	Grisactin Ultra by Pharm Util	60491-0290	Antifungal
330 <> MYLAN	Tab, White, Round	Amitriptyline 10 mg, Perphenazine 2 mg	Triavil by Mylan	00378-0330	Antidepressant; Antipsychotic
330 <> MYLAN	Tab, White, Round	Amitriptyline 10 mg, Perphenazine 2 mg	Triavil by Direct Dispensing	57866-3077	Antidepressant; Antipsychotic
331	Tab, Beige, Round	Sennosides 15 mg	Senokot by OHM Labs	00113-0331	Gastrointestinal
331	Tab, Beige, Round	Sennosides 15 mg	Senokot by Perrigo	51660-0428	Laxative

For updated data, go to www.IdentADrug.com

ID FRONT <> BACK	DESCRIPTION FRONT <> BACK	INGREDIENT & STRENGTH	BRAND (or Generic Equiv.) by FIRM	NDC#	CLASS; SCH.
331 <> DP	Tab, Light Green, Round	Inert	Kariva by Barr	00555-9050	Oral Contraceptive; Placebo
331 <> DP	Tab, Light Green, Round	Inert	Lo Ovral by Barr	00555-9049	Oral Contraceptive; Placebo
331 <> ETH	Tab, White, Round, Scored, Film Coated	Propafenone HCl 150 mg	Rythmol by Ethex	58177-0331	Antiarrhythmic
33110	Tab	Lorazepam 1 mg	Ativan by Ivax	00182-1807	Antianxiety; C IV
332	Tab, White, Scored, 332 Prasco Logo	Pseudoephedrine HCl 120 mg, Guaifenesin 1200 mg	Entex PSE by Prasco	66993-0332	Cold Remedy
332 <> B	Tab, Round, Orange, Coated	Desogestrel 0.125 mg, Ethinyl Estradiol 0.025 mg	Velivet by Barr	00555-9051	Oral Contraceptive
332 <> ETH	Tab, White, Round, Scored, Film Coated	Propafenone HCl 225 mg	Rythmol by Ethex	58177-0332	Antiarrhythmic
33205 <> WATSON	Tab, White, Round, Scored	Lorazepam 0.5 mg	Ativan by Murfreesboro	51129-1410	Antianxiety; C IV
3327G <> 4	Tab, White, Oval, 3327 over G <> 4	Methylprednisolone 4 mg	Medrol by Pharmacia	00009-3327	Steroid
3327G <> 4	Tab, White, Oval, 3327 over G <> 4	Methylprednisolone 4 mg	Medrol by Greenstone	59762-3327	Steroid
3328G150MG	Cap	Clindamycin HCl 150 mg	Cleocin HCl by Quality Care	60346-0018	Antibiotic
333	Tab, White, Round, Enteric Coated	Acamprosate 333 mg	Campral by Forest	00456-3330	Antialcoholism
333	Tab, White, Round, Enteric Coated	Acamprosate 333 mg	Campral by Prempharm	Canadian DIN 02293269	Antialcoholism
333 <> B	Tab, Round, Beige, Coated	Desogestrel 0.1 mg, Ethinyl Estradiol 0.025 mg	Velivet by Barr	00555-9051	Oral Contraceptive
333 <> ETH	Tab, White, Round, Scored, Film Coated	Propafenone HCl 300 mg	Rythmol by Ethex	58177-0333	Antiarrhythmic
333 <> R	Tab, Yellow, Round	Propranolol HCl 80 mg	Inderal by Actavis	00228-2333	Antihypertensive
33310 <> WATSON	Tab	Lorazepam 1 mg	Ativan by Watson		Antianxiety; C IV
334 <> B	Tab, Round, White	Inert	Velivet by Barr	00555-9051	Oral Contraceptive; Placebo
33420	Tab	Lorazepam 2 mg	Ativan by Ivax	00182-1808	Antianxiety; C IV
334410MGSB10MG	Cap, Black & Clear w/ White & Yellow Beads, 33410MG on one end, SB10MG on the other	Prochlorperazine 10 mg	Compazine by SKB	00007-3344	Antiemetic
335 <> B	Tab, Round, Pink, Coated	Desogestrel 0.15 mg, Ethinyl Estradiol 0.025 mg	Velivet by Barr	00555-9051	Oral Contraceptive
33510	Cap, Blue & White, Royce Logo 335/10	Piroxicam 10 mg	Feldene by Royce		NSAID
33510	Cap, Blue & White, Royce Logo 335/10	Piroxicam 10 mg	Feldene by Qualitest	00603-5222	NSAID
33510	Cap, Blue & White, Royce Logo 335/10	Piroxicam 10 mg	Feldene by Mutual	53489-0441	NSAID
3354 <> M	Tab, White & Yellow, Round	Orphenadrine Citrate 25 mg, Aspirin 385 mg, Caffeine 30 mg	Norgesic by Mylan	00378-3354	Muscle Relaxant
3358 <> M	Tab, White, Round, Ex Release	Orphenadrine Citrate 100 mg	Norflex by 3M	00089-1221	Muscle Relaxant
3358 <> M	Tab, White, Round, Ex Release	Orphenadrine Citrate 100 mg	Norflex by Mylan	00378-3358	Muscle Relaxant
3358 <> M	Tab, White, Round, Ex Release	Orphenadrine Citrate 100 mg	Norflex by Physician Total Care	54868-4102	Muscle Relaxant
3620	Cap, Blue, Royce Logo 336/20	Piroxicam 20 mg	Feldene by Royce		NSAID
33620	Cap, Blue, Royce Logo 336/20	Piroxicam 20 mg	Feldene by Mutual	53489-0442	NSAID
33620	Cap, Blue, Royce Logo 336/20	Piroxicam 20 mg	Feldene by Med Pro	53978-1255	NSAID
33620	Cap, Blue, Royce Logo 336/20	Piroxicam 20 mg	Feldene by Qualitest	00603-5223	NSAID
3366 <> WPI	Tab, Pink, Cap Shaped, Film Coated	Zolpidem Tartrate 5 mg	Ambien by Watson	00591-3366	Sedative/Hypnotic; C IV
3367 <> WPI	Tab, White, Cap Shaped, Film Coated	Zolpidem Tartrate 10 mg	Ambien by Watson	00591-3367	Sedative/Hypnotic; C IV
3369 <> WATSON	Tab, White, Round, Scored	Butalbital 50 mg, Acetaminophen 325 mg, Caffeine 40 mg	Fioricet by Watson	00591-3369 Discontinued	Analgesic
337 <> R	Tab, Peach, Round	Prednisone 20 mg	Deltasone by Actavis	00228-2337	Steroid
338 <> R	Tab, White, Round	Prednisone 10 mg	Deltasone by Actavis	00228-2338	Steroid
3399	Cap	Chlorpheniramine Maleate 12 mg, Phenylpropanolamine 75 mg	Ornade by Vortech		Cold Remedy
33BIOCRAFT	Tab	Sulfamethoxazole 800 mg, Trimethoprim 160 mg	SMX TMP DS by Prepackage Specialists	58864-0478	Antibiotic
33BIOCRAFT	Tab	Sulfamethoxazole 800 mg, Trimethoprim 160 mg	SMZ TMP DS by Diversified Healthcare	55887-0983	Antibiotic
34	Tab, Med Pro Logo	Clonazepam 1 mg	by Med Pro	53978-3185	Sedative, C IV
34 <> B	Tab, White, Round, Film Coated, Stylized b	Estradiol 1 mg, Norethindrone Acetate 0.5 mg	Mimvey by Teva Pharmaceuticals	00093-5455	Hormone
34 <> BIOCRAFT	Tab, White, Round, Scored, 3 over 4 <> Biocraft	Trimethoprim 100 mg	by Teva	Discontinued	Antibiotic
34 <> BIOCRAFT	Tab, White, Round, Scored, 3 over 4 <> Biocraft	Trimethoprim 100 mg	by Murfreesboro	51129-1204	Antibiotic

ID FRONT <> BACK	DESCRIPTION FRONT <> BACK	INGREDIENT & STRENGTH	BRAND (or Generic Equiv.) by FIRM	NDC#	CLASS; SCH.
34 <> C	Tab, White to Off White, Cap Shaped	Sumatriptan Succinate 100 mg	Imitrex by Aurobindo	65862-0148	Antimigraine
34 <> CIBA	Tab, Pale Yellow, Round, Scored	Methylphenidate HCl 20 mg	Ritalin by Novartis	00083-0034	Stimulant; C II
34 <> CIBA	Tab, Pale Yellow, Round, Scored	Methylphenidate HCl 20 mg	Ritalin by Physician Total Care	54868-2762	Stimulant; C II
34 <> CIBA	Tab, Pale Yellow, Round, Scored	Methylphenidate HCl 20 mg	Ritalin by Caremark	00339-4085	Stimulant; C II
34 <> M	Tab, White	Anastrozole 1 mg	Arimidex by UDL	51079-0323	Antineoplastic
3405	Tab, 340 Above Bisect, 5 Below <> Mortar and Pestle Logo	Pindolol 5 mg	Visken by Royce	51875-0340	Antihypertensive
3405	Tab, 5/Royce Logo	Pindolol 5 mg	Visken by Qualitest	00603-5220	Antihypertensive
341 <> 44	Tab, Gray, Oval	Calcium Polycarbophil 125 mg	Fibercon by LNK	50844-	Gastrointestinal
341 <> B	Tab, Light Yellow, Round	Norethindrone 0.5 mg, Ethinyl Estradiol 0.035 mg	Aranelle by Barr	00555-9066	Oral Contraceptive
341 <> ETH	Tab, White, Round	Benazepril HCl 5 mg	Lotensin by Ethex	58177-0341	Antihypertensive
34110	Tab, White, Round, 341/10 Royce Logo	Pindolol 10 mg	Visken by Qualitest	00603-5221	Antihypertensive
3416 <> WPI	Tab, White, Cap Shaped, Scored	Butalbital 50 mg, Acetaminophen 325 mg, Caffeine 40 mg	Fioricet by Watson	00591-3416	Analgesic
342	Tab, Pink, Round, Chewable	Carbamazepine 100 mg	Tegretol by Ranbaxy	63304-0747	Anticonvulsant
342	Tab, Pink, Round, Scored, Chewable	Carbamazepine 100 mg	Tegretol by Caraco	57664-0342	Anticonvulsant
342	Tab, Greenish Brown, Round	Sennosides 8.6 mg	Senokot by Ivax	00182-1093	Gastrointestinal
342 <> 3M	Tab, White, Round, Scored	Theophylline Anhydrous 125 mg	Theolair by 3M	00089-0342	Antiasthmatic
342 <> B	Tab, White, Round	Norethindrone 1 mg, Ethinyl Estradiol 0.035 mg	Aranelle by Barr	00555-9066	Oral Contraceptive
342 <> ETH	Tab, Red, Round	Benazepril HCl 10 mg	Lotensin by Ethex	58177-0342	Antihypertensive
342 <> RDY	Tab, Brown, Round, Film Coated	Citalopram 10 mg	Celexa by Dr. Reddy's	55111-0342	Antidepressant
343 <> B	Tab, Peach, Round	Inert	Aranelle by Barr	00555-9066	Oral Contraceptive; Placebo
343 <> ETH	Tab, Grey, Round	Benazepril HCl 20 mg	Lotensin by Ethex	58177-0343	Antihypertensive
343 <> RDY	Tab, Pink, Round	Citalopram 20 mg	Celexa by Dr. Reddy's	55111-0343	Antidepressant
3436 <> WATSON	Tab, White, Oval	Furosemide 20 mg	Lasix by Watson	00591-3436	Diuretic
3438 <> A	Tab, White, Round, Apotex Logo	Selegiline 5 mg	Eldepryl by Major	00904-5266	Antiparkinson
3438 <> A	Tab, White, Round, Apotex Logo	Selegiline 5 mg	Eldepryl by Apotex	60505-3438	Antiparkinson
344	Tab, Coated	Verapamil HCl 80 mg	Verelan by Moore	00839-7267	Antihypertensive
344	Tab, Coated	Verapamil HCl 80 mg	Verelan by IDE Inter	00814-8280	Antihypertensive
344 <> B	Tab, Yellow, Round	Norethindrone 0.35 mg	Errin by Barr	00555-0344	Oral Contraceptive
344 <> ETH	Tab, Blue, Round	Benazepril HCl 40 mg	Lotensin by Ethex	58177-0344	Antihypertensive
344 <> M	Tab, Orange	Ondansetron HCl 8 mg	Zofran by UDL	51079-0525	Antiemetic
344 <> RDY	Tab, White, Round	Citalopram 40 mg	Celexa by Dr. Reddy's	55111-0344	Antidepressant
345	Tab, Yellow, Round, Scored	Clozapine 25 mg	Clozaril by Caraco	57664-0345	Antipsychotic
345 <> B	Tab, Off White, Round, Film Coated, Biconvex	Lithium Carbonate 300 mg	Lithobid by Barr	00555-0345	Antipsychotic
34510	Tab, Orange, Round, Film Coated, Royce Logo 345/10	Hydroxyzine HCl 10 mg	Atarax by Royce	51875-0345	Antianxiety; Antihistamine
346	Tab, Coated	Verapamil HCl 120 mg	Verelan by IDE Inter	00814-8281	Antihypertensive
346	Tab, Coated	Verapamil HCl 120 mg	Verelan by Moore	00839-7268	Antihypertensive
34625	Tab, Green, Round, Film Coated, Royce Logo 346/25	Hydroxyzine HCl 25 mg	Atarax by Royce	51875-0346	Antianxiety; Antihistamine
34625	Tab, Green, Round, Film Coated, Royce Logo 346/25	Hydroxyzine HCl 25 mg	Atarax by Rx Dispensing	61807-0032	Antianxiety; Antihistamine
347	Tab, Blue, Oblong	Acetaminophen 500 mg, Diphenhydramine HCl 25 mg	Tylenol PM by Granutec		Cold Remedy
347	Tab, Yellow, Round, Scored	Clozapine 100 mg	Clozaril by Caraco	57664-0347	Antipsychotic
347 <> 250	Tab, White to Cream, Oval, Film Coated	Cefprozil 250 mg	Cefzil by Sandoz	00781-5043	Antibiotic
34750	Tab, Yellow, Round, Film Coated, Royce Logo 347/50	Hydroxyzine HCl 50 mg	Atarax by Royce	51875-0347	Antianxiety; Antihistamine
347BARR	Tab, White, Round	Chlorpropamide 100 mg	Diabinese by Barr		Antidiabetic
348 <> 500	Tab, Oval, Beige, Film Coated	Cefprozil 500 mg	Cefzil by Sandoz	00781-5044	Antibiotic
348 <> R	Tab, White, Round, Scored	Propylthiouracil 50 mg	Propylthiouracil by Activas	00228-2348	Antithyroid
34825	Tab	Captopril 25 mg	Capoten by Royce	51875-0348	Antihypertensive
34825	Tab	Captopril 25 mg	Capoten by Qualitest	00603-2556	Antihypertensive
3494 <> WATSON	Tab, White, Cap Shaped, Scored, 34 / 94	Oxycodone 5 mg, Ibuprofen 400 mg	Combunox by Watson	00591-3494	Analgesic; NSAID; C II
34950	Tab, White, Oval, Royce Logo 349/50	Captopril 50 mg	Capoten by Ivax	00182-2624	Antihypertensive

ID FRONT <> BACK	DESCRIPTION FRONT <> BACK	INGREDIENT & STRENGTH	BRAND (or Generic Equiv.) by FIRM	NDC#	CLASS; SCH.
34950	Tab, White, Oval, Royce Logo 349/50	Captopril 50 mg	Capoten by Qualitest	00603-2557	Antihypertensive
34950	Tab, White, Oval, Royce Logo 349/50	Captopril 50 mg	Capoten by Royce		Antihypertensive
35	Tab, Blue, Round, Scored, Logo <> 35	Phendimetrazine Tartrate 35 mg	Bontril by Mikart	46672-0057	Anorexiant; C III
35 <> BL	Tab, White, Round, Scored	Trimethoprim 200 mg	by Teva	Discontinued	Antibiotic
35 <> E	Tab, Salmon, Round, Scored, E above score <> 35	Trandolapril 1 mg	Mavik by Aurobindo	65862-0164	Antihypertensive
35 <> ORTHO	Tab	Ethinyl Estradiol 0.035 mg, Norethindrone 0.5 mg, Norethindrone 1 mg, Norethindrone 0.75 mg	Ortho Novum 777 by Dept Health	53808-0032	Oral Contraceptive
35 <> T	Tab, Yellow, Round, Scored, 3 / 5, Stylized T	Phendimetrazine Tartrate 35 mg	Bontril by Mikart	46672-0138	Anorexiant; C III
35 <> X	Tab, White, Round, Scored	Phendimetrazine Tartrate 35 mg	Bontril by Mikart	46672-0174	Anorexiant; C III
35 <> X	Tab, White, Round	Phendimetrazine Tartrate 35 mg	by Allscripts		Anorexiant; C III
350 <> ETHEX	Tab, White, Oval	Vitamin A 2700 Units, Ascorbic Acid 120 mg, Calcium 200 mg, Iron 90 mg, Vitamin D 400 Units, Thiamine HCl 3 mg, Riboflavin 3.4 mg, Niacinamide 20 mg, Pyridoxine HCl 20 mg, Folic Acid 1 mg, Cyanocobalamin 12 mcg, Zinc 25 mg, Copper 2 mg, Magnesium 30 mg, Docusate Sodium	Prenate Advance by Ethex	58177-0350	Vitamin
350100	Tab, White, Oval, Royce Logo 350/100	Captopril 100 mg	Capoten by Qualitest	00603-2558	Antihypertensive
350100	Tab, White, Oval, Royce Logo 350/100	Captopril 100 mg	Capoten by Royce		Antihypertensive
350100	Tab, RPR Logo over 351	Theophylline Anhydrous 100 mg	Capoten by Ivax	00182-2625	Antihypertensive
351			Slo Phyllin by RPR	00075-0351 Discontinued	Antiasthmatic
351 <> ETHEX	Tab, Mottled White, Round	Vitamin A 1000 Units, Cholecalciferol 400 Units, Vitamin E 11 Units, Ascorbic Acid 120 mg, Folic Acid 1 mg, Thiamine Mononitrate 2 mg, Riboflavin 3 mg, Niacinamide 20 mg, Pyridoxine HCl 10 mg, Cyanocobalamin 12 mcg, Iron 29 mg	Nutrinate Chewable by Ethex	58177-0351	Vitamin
351 <> G	Tab, Yellow, Oval, Film Coated	Fenofibrate 54 mg	Lofibra by Global	00115-5511	Antihyperlipidemic
351 <> RPR	Tab, White, Round	Theophylline Anhydrous 100 mg	Slo Phyllin by RPR	00801-0351	Antiasthmatic
35131OMGSB10MG	Cap, Clear & Brown, 3513/10 mg	Dextroamphetamine Sulfate 10 mg	Dexedrine by GSK	Canadian DIN 01924559	Stimulant; C II
35131OMGSB10MG	Cap, Clear & Brown, 3513/10 mg	Dextroamphetamine Sulfate 10 mg	Dexedrine by SKB	00007-3513	Stimulant; C II
3514SB15MG15MG	Cap, Brown & Clear	Dextroamphetamine Sulfate 15 mg	Dexedrine by SKB	00007-3514	Stimulant; C II
3514SB15MG15MG	Cap, Brown & Clear	Dextroamphetamine Sulfate 15 mg	Dexedrine by GSK	Canadian DIN 01924567	Stimulant; C II
352	Tab, RPR Logo over 352	Theophylline Anhydrous 200 mg	Slo Phyllin by RPR	00075-0352 Discontinued	Antiasthmatic
352 <> FULVICINPG	Tab, Off-White, Fulvicin P/G	Griseofulvin, Ultramicrocrystalline 330 mg	Fulvicin P/G by Pharm Util	60491-0275	Antifungal
352 <> RPR	Tab, White, Round	Theophylline Anhydrous 200 mg	Slo Phyllin by RPR	00801-0352	Antiasthmatic
3535 <> GEIGY	Tab, White, Mottled Blue, Cap Shaped, Scored	Hydrochlorothiazide 25 mg, Metoprolol Tartrate 50 mg	Lopressor HCT by Novartis	00078-0460	Diuretic; Antihypertensive
3549IL	Tab, Peach, Round, Scored, 3549 over IL inside diamond, ER	Isosorbide Dinitrate 40 mg	Isordil by Schein	00364-0401	Antianginal
3549IL	Tab, Peach, Round, Scored, 3549 over IL inside diamond, ER	Isosorbide Dinitrate 40 mg	Isordil by Inwood	00258-3549	Antianginal
3549IL	Tab, Peach, Round, Scored, 3549 over IL inside diamond, ER	Isosorbide Dinitrate 40 mg	Isordil by Ivax	00182-0879	Antianginal
3549IL	Tab, Peach, Round, Scored, 3549 over IL inside diamond, ER	Isosorbide Dinitrate 40 mg	Isordil by Allscripts		Antianginal
3549IL	Tab, Peach, Round, Scored, 3549 over IL inside diamond, ER	Isosorbide Dinitrate 40 mg	Isordil by Murfreesboro	51129-1329	Antianginal
3549IL	Tab, Peach, Round, Scored, 3549 over IL inside diamond, ER	Isosorbide Dinitrate 40 mg	Isordil by Murfreesboro	51129-1315	Antianginal

ID FRONT <> BACK	DESCRIPTION FRONT <> BACK	INGREDIENT & STRENGTH	BRAND (or Generic Equiv.) by FIRM	NDC#	CLASS; SCH.
3549IL	Tab, Peach, Round, Scored, 3549 over IL inside diamond, ER	Isosorbide Dinitrate 40 mg	Isordil by Sandoz	00781-1417	Antianginal
3549IL	Tab, Peach, Round, Scored, 3549 over IL inside diamond, ER	Isosorbide Dinitrate 40 mg	Isordil by URL Mutual	00677-0473	Antianginal
3549IL	Tab, Peach, Round, Scored, 3549 over IL inside diamond, ER	Isosorbide Dinitrate 40 mg	Isordil by Major	00904-2149	Antianginal
355 <> C	Tab, Mottled Green, Cap Shaped	Guaifenesin 600 mg, Dextromethorphan HBr 30 mg	Humibid DM by Caraco	57664-0355	Cold Remedy
355125	Tab, White, Oblong, Royce Logo 355/12.5	Captopril 12.5 mg	Capoten by Qualitest	00603-2555	Antihypertensive
355125	Tab, White, Oblong, Royce Logo 355/12.5	Captopril 12.5 mg	Capoten by Ivax	00182-2622	Antihypertensive
355125	Tab, White, Oblong, Royce Logo 355/12.5	Captopril 12.5 mg	Capoten by Royce	00904-2149	Antihypertensive
357	Tab, Oval, Beige, Film Coated, Scored	Fluvoxamine Maleate 25 mg	Luvox by Caraco	57664-0357	OCD
357 <> MYLAN	Tab, Lavender, Cap Shaped, Film Coated, Ex Release	Pentoxifylline 400 mg	Trental by Mylan	00378-0357	Anticoagulant
357 <> MYLAN	Tab, Lavender, Cap Shaped, Film Coated, Ex Release	Pentoxifylline 400 mg	Trental by UDL	51079-0889 Discontinued	Anticoagulant
3571V	Tab, Peach, Round, Scored, 3571 over V	Hydrochlorothiazide 25 mg	Oretic by Pliva	50111-0886	Diuretic; Antihypertensive
3571V	Tab, Peach, Round, Scored	Hydrochlorothiazide 25 mg	Oretic by Qualitest	00603-3856	Diuretic; Antihypertensive
3571V	Tab, Peach, Round, Scored, 3571 over V	Hydrochlorothiazide 25 mg	Oretic by Vintage	00254-3571	Diuretic; Antihypertensive
3572V	Tab, Peach, Round, Scored, 3572 over V	Hydrochlorothiazide 50 mg	Oretic by Pliva	50111-0887	Diuretic; Antihypertensive
3572V	Tab, Peach, Round, Scored, 3572 over V	Hydrochlorothiazide 50 mg	Oretic by Qualitest	00603-3857	Diuretic; Antihypertensive
357HRMAGNUM	Cap, Pink & White, 357 HR/Magnum	Caffeine 200 mg	Caffeine by BDI		Stimulant
357MAGNUM	Tab, Pink, Bullet Shaped	Caffeine 200 mg	Caffeine by B & M Labs		Stimulant
358	Tab, White, Oval, Scored	Metoprolol Succinate 200 mg	Toprolol XL by Ethex	58177-0358	Antihypertensive
358 <> 550	Tab	Amiloride HCl 5 mg, Hydrochlorothiazide 50 mg	Moduretic by URL Mutual	00677-1223	Antihypertensive; Diuretic
3585 <> V	Tab, White, Film-Coated, Round	Hydrocodone Bitartrate 7.5 mg, Ibuprofen 200 mg	Vicoprofen by Vintage	00254-3585	Analgesic; C III
358550	Tab, Peach, Round, 358 5-50 <> Mortar and Pestle Logo (Royce)	Amiloride HCl 5 mg, Hydrochlorothiazide 50 mg	Moduretic by Royce	51875-0358	Antihypertensive; Diuretic
3586 <> V	Tab, Purple, Film-Coated, Oval, Scored	Hydrocodone Bitartrate 10 mg, Ibuprofen 200 mg	Vicoprofen by Vintage	00254-3586	Analgesic; C III
358R	Tab, 358/R	Hydrochlorothiazide 25 mg, Propranolol HCl 40 mg	by Schein	00364-0838	Diuretic; Antihypertensive
3591 <> V	Tab, White, Red Specks, Cap Shaped, Scored, 35/91 V	Acetaminophen 500 mg, Hydrocodone Bitartrate 2.5 mg	Lortab by Vintage	00254-3591	Analgesic; C III
3591V	Tab, White, Red Specks, 35/91 V	Acetaminophen 500 mg, Hydrocodone Bitartrate 2.5 mg	Lortab by Qualitest	00603-3880	Analgesic; C III
3592 <> V	Tab, White, Oblong, Scored, 35/92	Acetaminophen 500 mg, Hydrocodone Bitartrate 5 mg	Vicodin by Kaiser	00179-1026	Analgesic; C III
3592 <> V	Tab, White, Oblong, Scored, 35/92	Acetaminophen 500 mg, Hydrocodone Bitartrate 5 mg	Vicodin by Pharmedix	53002-0119	Analgesic; C III
3592 <> V	Tab, White, Oblong, Scored, 35/92	Acetaminophen 500 mg, Hydrocodone Bitartrate 5 mg	Vicodin by Vangard	00615-0400	Analgesic; C III
3592 <> V	Tab, White, Oblong, Scored, 35/92	Acetaminophen 500 mg, Hydrocodone Bitartrate 5 mg	Vicodin by UDL	51079-0780	Analgesic; C III
3592 <> V	Tab, White, Cap Shaped, Scored	Acetaminophen 500 mg, Hydrocodone Bitartrate 5 mg	Vicodin by Vintage	00254-3592	Analgesic; C III
3592 <> V	Tab, White w/ Green Specks, Cap Shaped, Scored, V <> 35 over 94	Acetaminophen 500 mg, Hydrocodone Bitartrate 7.5 mg	Lortab by UDL	51079-0781 Discontinued	Analgesic; C III
3594 <> V	Tab, White w/ Green Specks, Oblong, V <> 35 over 94	Acetaminophen 500 mg, Hydrocodone Bitartrate 7.5 mg	Lortab by Ivax	00182-0691	Analgesic; C III
3594 <> V	Tab, White w/ Green Specks, Oblong, V <> 35 over 94	Acetaminophen 500 mg, Hydrocodone Bitartrate 7.5 mg	Lortab by Qualitest	00603-3882	Analgesic; C III
3594 <> V	Tab, White w/ Green Specks, Cap Shaped, Scored, V <> 35 over 94	Acetaminophen 500 mg, Hydrocodone Bitartrate 7.5 mg	Lortab by Vintage	00254-3594	Analgesic; C III
3594V	Tab, White w/ Green Specks, Oblong, V <> 35 over 94	Acetaminophen 500 mg, Hydrocodone Bitartrate 7.5 mg	Lortab by Murfreesboro	51129-1381	Analgesic; C III
3594V	Tab, White w/ Green Specks, Oblong, V <> 35 over 94	Acetaminophen 500 mg, Hydrocodone Bitartrate 7.5 mg	Lortab by St. Mary's Med	60760-0594	Analgesic; C III
3595 <> V	Tab, White, Cap Shaped, Scored	Acetaminophen 650 mg, Hydrocodone Bitartrate 7.5 mg	Lorcet Plus by Vintage	00254-3595	Analgesic; C III
3596 <> V	Tab, White, Cap Shaped, Scored	Acetaminophen 750 mg, Hydrocodone Bitartrate 7.5 mg	Vicodin ES by Vintage	00254-3596	Analgesic; C III
3596 <> V	Tab, White, Oblong	Acetaminophen 750 mg, Hydrocodone Bitartrate 7.5 mg	Vicodin ES by Ivax	00182-0681	Analgesic; C III
3596 <> V	Tab, White, Oblong	Acetaminophen 750 mg, Hydrocodone Bitartrate 7.5 mg	Vicodin ES by Qualitest	00603-3883	Analgesic; C III
3597 <> V	Tab, Light Blue, Cap Shaped, 35/97 V	Acetaminophen 650 mg, Hydrocodone Bitartrate 10 mg	Lorcet by Vintage	00254-3597	Analgesic; C III
3597 <> V	Tab, Light Blue, 35/97 V	Acetaminophen 650 mg, Hydrocodone Bitartrate 10 mg	Lorcet by Qualitest	00603-3885	Analgesic; C III
3597V	Tab, 35/97 V	Acetaminophen 650 mg, Hydrocodone Bitartrate 10 mg	Lorcet by Vintage	00254-3597	Analgesic; C III

ID FRONT <> BACK	DESCRIPTION FRONT <> BACK	INGREDIENT & STRENGTH	BRAND (or Generic Equiv.) by FIRM	NDC#	CLASS; SCH.
3597V	Tab, Light Blue, 35/97 V	Acetaminophen 650 mg, Hydrocodone Bitartrate 10 mg	Lorcet by Qualitest	00603-3885	Analgesic; C III
3598 <> V	Tab, White, Oblong, Scored	Acetaminophen 660 mg, Hydrocodone Bitartrate 10 mg	Lorcet by Vintage	00254-3598	Analgesic; C III
35A	Cap, Green, Soft Gel	Acetaminophen 325 mg, Dextromethorphan HBr 15 mg, Doxylamine Succinate 6.25 mg	NyQuil by Walgreens	00363-0535	Cold Remedy
35MG <> RSN	Tab, Orange, Oval, Film Coated	Risedronate Sodium 35 mg	Actonel by Procter and Gamble	00149-0472	Bisphosphonate
35MG <> RSN	Tab, Orange, Oval, Film Coated	Risedronate Sodium 35 mg	Actonel by Proc & Gamble	Canadian DIN 02246896	Bisphosphonate
35MG <> RSN	Tab, Light Orange, Oval, Film-Coated	Risedronate Sodium 5 mg	Actonel Plus Calcium by Proc and Gamble	Canadian DIN 02279657	Bisphosphonate
36	Tab, Brown, Round, Inverted Triangle over 36	Herbal Blend: Valerian, Passiflora, Magnesium Carbonate	Valerian by Wonder Labs	99528-0606	Homeopathic
36 <> A	Tab, White, Round, Scored, Orally Disintegrating	Mirtazapine 15 mg	Remeron SolTab by Aurobindo	65862-0021	Antidepressant
36 <> E	Tab, Yellow, Round	Trandolapril 2 mg	Mavik by Aurobindo	65862-0165	Antihypertensive
36 <> SL	Tab, Light Yellow, Sugar Coated	Desipramine HCl 25 mg	by Schein	00364-2209	Antidepressant
36 <> SL	Tab, Light Yellow, Round, Sugar Coated	Desipramine HCl 25 mg	Norpramin by Pliva	50111-0436	Antidepressant
360 <> B	Tab, White, Cap Shaped, Ex Release	Diltiazem HCl 360 mg	Tiazac XC by Biovail	Canadian DIN 02256770	Antihypertensive
360 <> B	Tab, White, Cap Shaped, Ex Release	Diltiazem HCl 360 mg	Cardizem LA by Biovail	64455-0104	Antihypertensive
3600 <> V	Tab, Pink, Oval	Acetaminophen 500 mg, Hydrocodone Bitartrate 10 mg	Lortab by Qualitest	00603-3888	Analgesic; C III
3600 <> V	Tab, Pink, Cap Shaped	Hydrocodone Bitartrate 10 mg, Acetaminophen 500 mg	Lortab by Vintage	00254-3600	Analgesic; C III
3600 <> V	Tab, Pink, Cap Shaped	Acetaminophen 500 mg, Hydrocodone Bitartrate 10 mg	Lortab by UDL	51079-0254	Analgesic; C III
3601 <> V	Tab, Yellow, Oblong	Acetaminophen 325 mg, Hydrocodone Bitartrate 10 mg	Norco by UDL	51079-0779	Analgesic; C III
3601 <> V	Tab, Yellow, Oblong	Acetaminophen 325 mg, Hydrocodone Bitartrate 10 mg	Norco by Vintage	00254-3601	Analgesic; C III
3604 <> V	Tab, White with Orange Specks, Oblong	Hydrocodone Bitartrate 5 mg, Acetaminophen 325 mg	Norco by Vintage	51079-0777	Analgesic; C III
3604 <> V	Tab, White with Orange Specks, Oblong	Hydrocodone Bitartrate 5 mg, Acetaminophen 325 mg	Norco by Vintage	00254-3604	Analgesic; C III
3605 <> V	Tab, Light Orange, Oval, Scored	Hydrocodone Bitartrate 7.5 mg, Acetaminophen 325 mg	Norco by UDL	51079-0778	Analgesic; C III
3608 <> 59911	Tab, White, Oval, Film Coated	Etodolac 400 mg	by Wyeth	52903-3608	NSAID
3608 <> 59911	Tab, White, Oval	Etodolac 400 mg	by ESI Lederle	59911-3608	NSAID
3609IL	Cap, ER	Propranolol HCl 60 mg	Inderal by Qualitest	00603-5497	Antihypertensive
361	Tab, Oval, Yellow, Film Coated, Scored	Fluvoxamine Maleate 50 mg	Luvox by Caraco	57664-0361	OCD
361 <> M	Tab, Blue, Oblong, Scored	Acetaminophen 650 mg, Hydrocodone Bitartrate 10 mg	Lortab by Southwood	58016-0232	Analgesic; C III
3612V	Tab, Bisected V	Hydromorphone HCl 4 mg	by Vintage	00254-3612	Analgesic; C II
3613 <> IL	Tab, Peach, Round, Scored, Ex Release	Isosorbide Dinitrate 40 mg	Isochron by Forest	00456-0637	Antianginal
3613IL	Tab, Peach, Round, Scored, Ex Release	Isosorbide Dinitrate 40 mg	Isordil by Murfreesboro	51129-1566	Antianginal
3613IL	Tab, Peach, Round, Scored, Ex Release	Isosorbide Dinitrate 40 mg	Isordil by Inwood	00258-3613	Antianginal
3615 <> V	Tab, Orange, Round	Hydroxyzine HCl 10 mg	Atarax by Vintage	00254-3615	Antianxiety; Antihistamine
36154	Tab, 361, 5.4 <> Mortar and Pestle Logo	Yohimbine HCl 5.4 mg	by Royce	51875-0361	Impotence Agent
3616 <> V	Tab, Green, Round	Hydroxyzine HCl 25 mg	Atarax by Vintage	00254-3616	Antianxiety; Antihistamine
3616 <> V	Tab, Green, Round	Hydroxyzine HCl 25 mg	Atarax by Qualitest	00603-3968	Antianxiety; Antihistamine
3617 <> V	Tab, Light Orange, Round	Hydroxyzine HCl 50 mg	Atarax by Vintage	00254-3617	Antianxiety; Antihistamine
3618 <> TISH	Tab, Beige, Oblong	Polycarbophil 500 mg	Fibercon by Rugby		Laxative
362	Tab, Oval, Red, Film Coated	Fluvoxamine Maleate 100 mg	Luvox by Caraco	57664-0362	OCD
363025	Tab, White, Oval, Royce Logo 363/0.25	Alprazolam 0.25 mg	Xanax by Royce		Antianxiety; C IV
3640061	Cap, Clear & Light Green	Chloral Hydrate 500 mg	Chloral Hydrate by RP Scherer	11014-0913	Sedative/Hypnotic; C IV
36405	Tab, Peach, Oval, Royce Logo, 364/0.5	Alprazolam 0.5 mg	Xanax by Royce		Antianxiety; C IV
3642	Cap	Papaverine HCl 150 mg	Pavabid by Vortech		Vasodilator
364364 <> GLYBUR	Tab, Light Blue, Oblong, Scored	Glyburide 5 mg	DiaBeta by Copley	38245-0364	Antidiabetic
364364 <> GLYBUR	Tab, Light Blue, Oblong, Scored	Glyburide 5 mg	DiaBeta by Teva	38245-0364 Discontinued	Antidiabetic
364364 <> GLYBUR	Tab, Light Blue, Oblong, Scored	Glyburide 5 mg	DiaBeta by Merrell	00068-3202	Antidiabetic

ID FRONT <> BACK	DESCRIPTION FRONT <> BACK	INGREDIENT & STRENGTH	BRAND (or Generic Equiv.) by FIRM	NDC#	CLASS; SCH.
364364 <> GLYBUR	Tab, Light Blue, Oblong, Scored	Glyburide 5 mg	DiaBeta by Blue Ridge	59273-0015	Antidiabetic
364364 <> GLYBUR	Tab, Light Blue, Oblong, Scored	Glyburide 5 mg	DiaBeta by PDRX	55289-0892	Antidiabetic
364DPI	Cap, Scarlet, Black Print	Acetaminophen 325 mg, Dichloralantipyrine 100 mg, Isometheptene Mucate (1:1) 65 mg	Midchlor by Schein	00364-2342	Analgesic; C IV
364DPI	Cap, Scarlet, Black Print	Acetaminophen 325 mg, Dichloralantipyrine 100 mg, Isometheptene Mucate (1:1) 65 mg	by Kaiser	00179-1222	Analgesic; C IV
3651	Tab, Blue, Oval, Royce Logo 365/1	Alprazolam 1 mg	Xanax by Royce		Antianxiety; C IV
3651	Tab, Blue, Oval, Scored, 365 over 1 <> Royce Logo	Alprazolam 1 mg	Xanax by Apotheca	12634-0522	Antianxiety; C IV
367 <> C	Tab, Red, Oblong, Film Coated	Guaifenesin 300 mg, Codeine Phosphate 10 mg	Robitussin A-C by Martec	52555-0160	Analgesic; C III
3678	Cap, Clear & Yellow	Benzonatate 200 mg	Tessalon by Inwood	00258-3678	Antitussive
3678	Cap	Phentermine 30 mg	Phentrol #6 by Vortech		Anorexiant; C IV
368	Tab, White, Round, Scored, Extended-Release	Metoprolol Succinate 100 mg	Toprol XL by Ethex	58177-0368	Antihypertensive
368 <> SL	Tab, Brown, Black Print, Round	Amitriptyline HCl 50 mg	Elavil by Ivax	00182-1020	Antidepressant
368 <> SL	Tab, Brown, Black Print, Round	Amitriptyline HCl 50 mg	Elavil by Amerisource	62584-0308	Antidepressant
368 <> SL	Tab, Brown, Black Print, Round	Amitriptyline HCl 50 mg	Elavil by H J Harkins Co	52959-0514	Antidepressant
368 <> SL	Tab, Brown, Black Print, Round	Amitriptyline HCl 50 mg	Elavil by Qualitest	00603-2214	Antidepressant
368 <> SL	Tab, Brown, Black Print, Round	Amitriptyline HCl 50 mg	Elavil by Nat Pharmpak	55154-5809	Antidepressant
368 <> SL	Tab, Brown, Black Print, Round	Amitriptyline HCl 50 mg	Elavil by Apothecon	59772-8554	Antidepressant
368 <> SL	Tab, Brown, Black Print, Round	Amitriptyline HCl 50 mg	Elavil by Baker Cummins	63171-1020	Antidepressant
368 <> SL	Tab, Brown, Black Print, Round	Amitriptyline HCl 50 mg	Elavil by Pliva	50111-0368	Antidepressant
3685 <> 0115	Tab, White, Oval	Hydrocortisone 20 mg	by Global	00115-3685	Steroid
3685 <> 1	Tab, White, Round, Scored, Hourglass Logo 1	Doxazosin Mesylate 1 mg	Cardura by Ivax	00172-3685	Antihypertensive
3686 <> 2	Tab, White, Round, Scored, Hourglass Logo 2	Doxazosin Mesylate 2 mg	Cardura by Ivax	00172-3686	Antihypertensive
3687 <> 4	Tab, Orange, Round, Scored, Hourglass Logo 4	Doxazosin Mesylate 4 mg	Cardura by Ivax	00172-3687	Antihypertensive
369	Tab, White, Oval, Scored	Metoprolol Succinate 50 mg	Toprol XL by Ethex	58177-0369	Antihypertensive
3690 <> 5	Tab, Gold, Round	Prochlorperazine 5 mg	Compazine by Ivax	00182-8210	Antiemetic
3691 <> 10	Tab, Gold, Round	Prochlorperazine 10 mg	Compazine by Ivax	00182-8211	Antiemetic
36954	Cap, Green	Loperamide 2 mg	Imodium by Nat Pharmpak	55154-4912	Antidiarrheal
36954	Cap, Green	Loperamide 2 mg	Imodium by Roxane	00054-8537	Antidiarrheal
36AV <> 01	Tab, White, Oval, Scored, 36 over AV <> 0.1	Desmopressin Acetate 0.1 mg	DDAVP by Aventis	00075-0016	Antidiuretic
36SL	Tab, Sugar Coated	Desipramine HCl 25 mg	by Med Pro	53978-2076	Antidepressant
37 <> 149	Tab, Light Red, Oblong, Mottled	Naproxen 500 mg	by Allscripts		NSAID
37 <> A	Tab, White, Round, Scored, Orally Disintegrating	Mirtazapine 30 mg	Remeron SolTab by Aurobindo	65862-0022	Antidepressant
37 <> E	Tab, Rose, Round	Trandolapril 4 mg	Mavik by Aurobindo	65862-0166	Antihypertensive
370 <> MYLAN	Tab, Yellow, Scored	Bumetanide 1 mg	Bumex by Mylan	00378-0370	Diuretic
370 <> SL	Tab, Orange, Round	Amitriptyline HCl 100 mg	Elavil by Ivax	00182-1063	Antidepressant
37046 <> BUTIBEL	Tab, Red, Round, 37 over 046	Belladonna Extract 15 mg, Butabarbital Sodium 15 mg	Butibel by Wallace	00037-0046	Gastrointestinal; C IV
370B	Tab, White, Round	Lorazepam 0.5 mg	Ativan by Barr		Antianxiety; C IV
371001 <> WALLACE	Tab, White, Round, Scored, 37-1001 <> Wallace	Meprobamate 400 mg	Miltown by Wallace	00037-1001	Sedative/Hypnotic; C IV
371101 <> WALLACE	Tab, White, Round, Sugar Coated	Meprobamate 200 mg	Miltown by Wallace	00037-1101	Sedative/Hypnotic; C IV
37112 <> BUTISOLSODIUM	Tab, Lavender, Scored, 37 over 112	Butabarbital 15 mg	Butisol Sodium by Wallace	00037-0112	Sedative/Hypnotic; C III
37113 <> BUTISOLSODIUM	Tab, Blue-Green, Round, Scored, 37 over 113	Butabarbital 30 mg	Butisol Sodium by Wallace	00037-0113	Sedative/Hypnotic; C III
37114 <> BUTISOLSODIUM	Tab, Orange, Scored, 37 over 114	Butabarbital 50 mg	Butisol Sodium by Wallace	00037-0114	Sedative/Hypnotic; C III
3712 <> TISH	Tab, Green, Triangular	Ferrous Sulfate 324 mg	Feosol by ADH Health Products		Mineral
371B	Tab, White, Round	Lorazepam 1 mg	Ativan by Barr		Antianxiety; C IV
372 <> M	Tab, Green, Pentagonal, Scored, Film Coated	Cimetidine HCl 400 mg	Tagamet by Mylan	00378-0372	Gastrointestinal

ID FRONT <> BACK	DESCRIPTION FRONT <> BACK	INGREDIENT & STRENGTH	BRAND (or Generic Equiv.) by FIRM	NDC#	CLASS; SCH.
372 <> M	Tab, Green, Pentagonal, Scored, Film Coated	Cimetidine HCl 400 mg	Tagamet by H J Harkins Co	52959-0375	Gastrointestinal
372 <> M	Tab, Green, Pentagonal, Scored, Film Coated	Cimetidine HCl 400 mg	Tagamet by UDL	51079-0808 Discontinued	Gastrointestinal
372 <> M	Tab, Green, Pentagonal, Scored, Film Coated	Cimetidine HCl 400 mg	Tagamet by Murfreesboro	51129-1179	Gastrointestinal
372 <> M	Tab, Green, Pentagonal, Scored, Film Coated	Cimetidine HCl 400 mg	Tagamet by Nat Pharmpak	55154-5555	Gastrointestinal
3725 <> MYLAN	Tab, Scored	Hydrochlorothiazide 25 mg, Triamterene 37.5 mg	Maxzide 25 by Mylan	00378-3725	Diuretic; Antihypertensive
372BARR	Tab, White, Round	Lorazepam 2 mg	Ativan by Barr		Antianxiety; C IV
373 <> ETHEX	Tab, White, Oval, Film Coated, Ex Release	Guaifenesin 1200 mg, Pseudoephedrine HCl 120 mg	Aquabid D by Ethex	58177-0373	Cold Remedy
373 <> M	Tab, White, Round, Film Coated	Hydroxychloroquine Sulfate 200 mg	Plaquenil by Mylan	00378-0373	Antimalarial
3737	Tab, White, Oblong	Dyphylline 400 mg	Lufyllin by Lemmon		Antiasthmatic
3737 <> UU	Tab, White, Round, Scored	Pramipexole DiHCl 1.5 mg	Mirapex by Boehringer Ingelheim	00597-0091	Antiparkinson
3737 <> UU	Tab, White, Round, Scored	Pramipexole DiHCl 1.5 mg	Mirapex by Pharmacia	00009-0037	Antiparkinson
373BARR	Tab, Yellow, Round	Oxazepam 15 mg	Serax by Barr		Sedative/Hypnotic; C IV
373WATSON	Tab, Film Coated, Watson 373	Maprotiline HCl 25 mg	by Ivax	00182-1882	Antidepressant
373WATSON	Tab, Film Coated, Watson 373	Maprotiline HCl 25 mg	by Sandoz	00781-1631	Antidepressant
373WATSON	Tab, Film Coated, Watson 373	Maprotiline HCl 25 mg	by Medirex	57480-0493	Antidepressant
374401 <> WALLACE	Tab, White, Oval, Scored, 37 over 4401	Penicillamine 250 mg	by Horner	Canadian	Chelating Agent
374401 <> WALLACE	Tab, White, Oval, Scored, 37 over 4401	Penicillamine 250 mg	Depen Titratable by Wallace	00037-4401	Chelating Agent
375 <> APO	Tab, White, Cap Shaped, Biconvex, Enteric Coated	Naproxen 375 mg	Naprosyn by Apotex	Canadian DIN 02246700	NSAID
375 <> ECNAPROSYN	Tab, White, Cap Shaped, Enteric Coated	Naproxen 375 mg	EC-Naprosyn by Hoffmann La Roche	00004-6415	NSAID
375 <> ECNAPROSYN	Tab, White, Cap Shaped	Naproxen 375 mg	Naprosyn by Syntex	18393-0255	NSAID
375 <> ECNAPROSYN	Tab, White, Cap Shaped	Naproxen 375 mg	Naprosyn by PDRX	55289-0267	NSAID
375 <> ECNAPROSYN	Tab, White, Cap Shaped	Naproxen 375 mg	Naprosyn by DRX	55045-2425	NSAID
375 <> ETHEX	Tab, Pink & Beige, Oval	Prenatal Multivitamin	Stuartnatal Plus 3 by Ethex	58177-0375	Vitamin
375 <> G32	Tab, Pink, Cap Shaped	Naproxen 375 mg	Naprosyn by Glenmark	68462-0189	NSAID
375 <> IP189	Tab, White, Oblong	Naproxen 375 mg	Naprosyn by Interpharm	53746-0189	NSAID
375 <> IP189	Tab, White, Oblong	Naproxen 375 mg	Naprosyn by Dr. Reddy's	55111-0367	NSAID
375 <> IP189	Tab, White, Oblong	Naproxen 375 mg	Naprosyn by Amneal	65162-0077 Discontinued	NSAID
375 <> N	Tab, White, Cap Shaped	Naproxen Sodium 375 mg	Naprelan by Victory	68453-0375	NSAID
375 <> N	Tab, White, Cap Shaped	Naproxen 375 mg	Naprelan by Elan	00086-0090	NSAID
375 <> N518	Tab, Pink, Oval, N over 518	Naproxen 375 mg	Naprosyn by Medirex	57480-0834	NSAID
375 <> N518	Tab, Pink, Oval, N over 518	Naproxen 375 mg	Naprosyn by Teva	55953-0518	NSAID
375 <> NAPROSYN	Tab, Peach, Oblong	Naproxen 375 mg	Naprosyn by Nat Pharmpak	55154-3803	NSAID
375 <> NAPROSYN	Tab, Peach, Oblong	Naproxen 375 mg	Naprosyn by Amerisource	62584-0273	NSAID
375 <> NAPROSYN	Tab, Peach, Oblong	Naproxen 375 mg	Naprosyn by Syntex	18393-0273	NSAID
375 <> NAPROSYN	Tab, Peach, Oblong	Naproxen 375 mg	Naprosyn by H J Harkins Co	52959-0192	NSAID
375 <> NAPROSYN	Tab, Peach, Oblong	Naproxen 375 mg	Naprosyn by Thrift Drug		NSAID
375 <> NAPROSYN	Tab, Peach, Oblong	Naproxen 375 mg	Naprosyn by Allscripts	59198-0238	NSAID
375 <> NAPROSYN	Tab, Peach, Oblong	Naproxen 375 mg	Naprosyn by Rightpak	65240-0700	NSAID
375 <> PAXILCR	Tab, Blue, Round, Film Coated, Paxil over CR <> 37.5	Paroxetine HCl 37.5 mg	Paxil CR by SKB	00029-3208	Antidepressant
375 <> SIDMAK	Tab, Off-White, Oval	Nystatin 100,000 Units	Mycostatin by Pliva	50111-0375	Antifungal
375 <> SIDMAK	Tab, Off-White, Oval	Nystatin 100,000 Units	Mycostatin by Qualitest	00603-4831	Antifungal
375 <> TP189	Tab, White, Oval	Naproxen 375 mg	Naprosyn by Major	00904-5590	NSAID
375 <> WATSON363	Tab, Blue, Round, Scored, 3.75 <> Watson 363	Clorazepate Dipotassium 3.75 mg	Tranxene by Major	00904-3970	Antianxiety; C IV
375 <> WATSON363	Tab, Blue, Round, Scored, 3.75 <> Watson 363	Clorazepate Dipotassium 3.75 mg	Tranxene by Watson	52544-0363	Antianxiety; C IV
375 <> WATSON363	Tab, Blue, Round, Scored, 3.75 <> Watson 363	Clorazepate Dipotassium 3.75 mg	Tranxene by Ivax	00182-0009	Antianxiety; C IV
375 <> WATSON363	Tab, Blue, Round, Scored, 3.75 <> Watson 363	Clorazepate Dipotassium 3.75 mg	Tranxene by Watson	00591-0363	Antianxiety; C IV

ID FRONT <> BACK	DESCRIPTION FRONT <> BACK	INGREDIENT & STRENGTH	BRAND (or Generic Equiv.) by FIRM	NDC#	CLASS; SCH.
37520	Tab, Yellow, Oval, Film Coated, Imprint in Black Ink	Naproxen 375 mg, Esomeprazole 20 mg	Vimovo by AstraZeneca	00186-0510	Antiarthritis
3757	Tab, White, Round, 3757 <> Ivax Hourglass Logo	Lisinopril 2.5 mg	Prinivil by Ivax	00172-3757	Antihypertensive
3758	Tab, White, Square, Scored, 3758 <> Ivax Hourglass Logo	Lisinopril 5 mg	Prinivil by Ivax	00172-3758	Antihypertensive
3759 <> I	Tab, White, Oval, Scored	Lisinopril 10 mg	Prinivil by Ivax	00172-3759	Antihypertensive
375FLAGYL	Cap, Green & Gray	Metronidazole 375 mg	Flagyl by Searle	00025-1942	Antibiotic
375FLAGYL	Cap, Green & Gray	Metronidazole 375 mg	Flagyl by Physician Total Care	54868-3786	Antibiotic
375M37	Tab, White, Cap Shaped, Scored, 375 / M37	Naproxen 375 mg	Naprosyn by Major	00904-5536	NSAID
375M37	Tab, White, Cap Shaped, Scored, 375 / M37	Naproxen 375 mg	Naprosyn by Dava	67253-0621	NSAID
375M37 <> MOVA	Tab, White, Cap Shaped	Naproxen 375 mg	Naprosyn by Caremark	00339-5872	NSAID
375M37 <> MOVA	Tab, White, Cap Shaped	Naproxen 375 mg	Naprosyn by Mova	55370-0140	NSAID
375NAXEN	Tab, Peach, Oblong	Naproxen 375 mg	Naprosyn by BW Inc	Canadian	NSAID
376 <> ETHEX	Tab, Yellow, Oval	Vitamin A 4,000 IU, Vitamin D 400 IU, Vitamin E 30 IU, Vitamin C 120 mg, Folic Acid 1 mg, Vitamin B1 3 mg, Vitamin B2 3 mg, Niacin 20 mg, Vitamin B6 3 mg, Vitamin B12 8 mcg, Biotin 30 mcg, Pantothenic Acid 7 mg, Calcium 200 mg, Iodine 150 mcg, Zinc 15 mg, Magnesium 100 mg, Iron 29 mg, Copper 3 mg	NataTab by Ethex	58177-0376	Vitamin
3760	Tab, White, Pentagonal-Shaped, Scored, 3760 <> Ivax Hourglass Logo	Lisinopril 20 mg	Prinivil by Ivax	00172-3760	Antihypertensive
3761	Tab, White, Round, 3761 <> Ivax Hourglass Logo	Lisinopril 40 mg	Prinivil by Ivax	00172-3761	Antihypertensive
3762	Tab, White, Oval, Scored, 3762 <> Ivax Hourglass Logo	Lisinopril 30 mg	Prinivil by Ivax	00172-3762	Antihypertensive
377	Tab, White, Cap Shaped, Film Coated	Tramadol 50 mg	Ultram by Caraco	57664-0377	Analgesic
377 <> MYLAN	Tab, White, Round	Naproxen 250 mg	Naprosyn by Dixon Shane	17236-0076	NSAID
377 <> MYLAN	Tab, White, Round	Naproxen 250 mg	Naprosyn by UDL	510079-0793 Discontinued	NSAID
377 <> MYLAN	Tab, White, Round	Naproxen 250 mg	Naprosyn by Kaiser	00179-1186	NSAID
377 <> MYLAN	Tab, White, Round	Naproxen 250 mg	Naprosyn by Mylan	00378-0377	NSAID
377 <> MYLAN	Tab, White, Round	Naproxen 250 mg	Naprosyn by H J Harkins Co	52959-0190	NSAID
3770008	Tab, White, Round, 377-0008	Aminophylline 100 mg	Aminophylline by Vale		Antiasthmatic
3770106	Tab, Yellow, Round, 377-0106	Chlorpheniramine Maleate 1 mg, Pyrilamine 12.5 mg, Phenylephrine HCl 5 mg	Duphrene by Vale		Cold Remedy
3770109	Tab, Yellow, Round, 377-0109	Ephedrine 16.2 mg, Sodium Phenobarbital 24.3 mg	by Vale		Antiasthmatic; C IV
3770125	Tab, White, Round, 377-0125	Guaifenesin 100 mg	Robitussin by Vale		Expectorant
3770167	Tab, White, Round, 377-0167	Pyrilamine Maleate 25 mg	Nisaval by Vale		Antihistamine
3770187	Tab, Pink, Round, 377-0187	Phenobarbital 15 mg	Phenobarbital by Vale		Sedative/Hypnotic; C IV
3770188	Tab, White, Round, 377-0188	Phenobarbital 15 mg	Phenobarbital by Vale		Sedative/Hypnotic; C IV
3770189	Tab, Green, Round, 377-0189	Phenobarbital 15 mg	Phenobarbital by Vale		Sedative/Hypnotic; C IV
3770192	Tab, White, Round, 377-0192	Phenobarbital 30 mg	by Vale		Sedative/Hypnotic; C IV
3770193	Tab, Pink, Round, 377-0193	Phenobarbital 30 mg	by Vale		Sedative/Hypnotic; C IV
3770196	Tab, White, Round, 377-0196	Phenobarbital 90 mg	by Vale		Sedative/Hypnotic; C IV
3770214	Tab, Red, Round, 377-0214	Rauwolfia Serpentina 50 mg	Raudixin by Vale		Antihypertensive
3770215	Tab, Pink, Round, 377-0215	Rauwolfia Serpentina 100 mg	Raudixin by Vale		Antihypertensive
3770216	Tab, Green & White Mottled, Round, 377-0216	Phenylephrine 5 mg, Chlorpheniramine 2 mg, Salicylamide 250 mg, Acetaminophen 150 mg	Rhinogesic by Vale		Cold Remedy
3770217	Tab, Green & White Mottled, Round, 377-0217	Phenylephrine 2 mg, Chlorpheniramine 1 mg, Salicylamide 90 mg, Acetaminophen 60 mg	Rhinogesic JR by Vale		Cold Remedy
3770232	Tab, Pink, Round, 377-0232	Butabarbital 15 mg	Butisol Sodium by Vale		Sedative/Hypnotic; C III
3770233	Tab, Green, Round, 377-0233	Butabarbital 30 mg	Butisol Sodium by Vale		Sedative/Hypnotic; C III

ID FRONT <> BACK	DESCRIPTION FRONT <> BACK	INGREDIENT & STRENGTH	BRAND (or Generic Equiv.) by FIRM	NDC#	CLASS; SCH.
3770238	Tab, Pink, Round, 377-0238	Sodium Salicylate 324 mg	by Vale		Analgesic
3770240	Tab, Red, Round, 377-0240	Sodium Salicylate 324 mg	by Vale		Analgesic
3770242	Tab, Purple, Round, 377-0242	Sodium Salicylate 324 mg	by Vale		Analgesic
3770272	Tab, Tan, Round, 377-0272	Thyroid 30 mg	by Vale		Thyroid Hormone
3770277	Tab, Pink, Round, 377-0277	Sulfadiazine 167 mg, Sulfamerazine 167 mg, Sulfamethazine 167 mg	Triple Sulfoid by Vale		Antibiotic
3770290	Tab, Orange, Round, 377-0290	Diphenhydramine HCl 50 mg	Valdrene by Vale		Antihistamine
3770311	Tab, Green & White, Round, 377-0311	Phenylephrine 5 mg, Chlorpheniramine 2 mg, Salicylamide 250 mg, Acetaminophen 150 mg, Guaifenesin 100 mg	Rhinogesic GG by Vale		Cold Remedy
3770332	Tab, Tan, Round, 377-0332	Pepsin 259 mg, Pancreatin 32 mg, Diastase 2 mg	Pepsin & Pancreatin by Vale		Gastrointestinal
3770349	Tab, Yellow, Round, 377-0349	Magnesium Trisilicate 500 mg	Trioval by Vale		Antiarthritic
3770351	Tab, Yellow, Round, 377-0351	Phendimetrazine Tartrate 35 mg	Obeval by Vale		Anorexiant; C III
3770358	Tab, Green, Round, 377-0358	Pseudoephedrine 60 mg	Sudafed by Vale		Decongestant
3770359	Tab, Mottled White, Round, 377-0359	Guaifenesin 100 mg, Pseudoephedrine HCl 30 mg	Glycofed by Vale		Cold Remedy
3770365	Tab, Green, Round, 377-0365	Phenobarbital, Hyoscyamine, Scopolamine, Atropine	Barbeloid by Vale		Gastrointestinal; C IV
3770396	Tab, Green, Round, 377-0396	Thyroid 65 mg	by Vale		Thyroid Hormone
3770498	Tab, Yellow, Round, 377-0498	Phenobarbital, Hyoscyamine, Scopolamine, Atropine	Barbeloid by Vale		Gastrointestinal; C IV
3770630	Tab, Blue & White, Round, 377-0630	Dover's Pwd 24 mg, Aspirin 324 mg, Caffeine 32 mg	Dovacet by Vale		Analgesic
3770636	Tab, Red, Round, 377-0636	Dover's Pwd 15 mg, Aspirin 162 mg, Caffeine 8.1 mg	Acedoval by Vale		Analgesic
3770642	Tab, Yellow, Round, 377-0642	Phenobarbital, Hyoscyamine, Scopolamine, Camphor, Valerian, Passiflora	Nevrotose #3 by Vale		Gastrointestinal; C IV
3770650	Tab, Blue, Round, 377-0650	Barbital, Hyoscyamine Sulfate, Scopolamine, Passiflora, Valerian	Barbatose #2 by Vale		Gastrointestinal
377200	Tab, White, Oval, Scored, Film Coated, 377/200 <> Royce Logo	Hydroxychloroquine Sulfate 200 mg	Plaquenil by Royce		Antimalarial
377200	Tab, White, Oval, Scored, Film Coated, 377/200 <> Royce Logo	Hydroxychloroquine Sulfate 200 mg	by Major	00904-5107	Antimalarial
377200	Tab, White, Oval, Scored, Film Coated, 377/200 <> Royce Logo	Hydroxychloroquine Sulfate 200 mg	by Qualitest	00603-3944	Antimalarial
377200	Tab, White, Oval, Scored, Film Coated, 377/200 <> Royce Logo	Hydroxychloroquine Sulfate 200 mg	by Royce	51875-0377	Antimalarial
377200	Tab, White, Oval, Scored, Film Coated, 377/200 <> Royce Logo	Hydroxychloroquine Sulfate 200 mg	by Ivax	00182-2609	Antimalarial
377200	Tab, White, Oval, Scored, Film Coated, 377/200 <> Royce Logo	Hydroxychloroquine Sulfate 200 mg	by Schein	00364-2627	Antimalarial
3774280	Tab, Orange, Round, 377-4280	Prednisone 5 mg	Deltasone by Vale		Steroid
3774294	Tab, White, Round, 377-4294	Prednisone 5 mg	Deltasone by Vale		Steroid
378 <> PFIZER	Tab, Blue, Round, Film Coated	Trovafloxacin 100 mg	Trovan by Roerig	00049-3780	Antibiotic
378 <> PFIZER	Tab, Blue, Round, Film Coated	Trovafloxacin 100 mg	Trovan by Pfizer	Canadian DIN 02239191	Antibiotic
379 <> PFIZER	Tab, Blue, Oval, Film Coated	Trovafloxacin 200 mg	Trovan by Pfizer	Canadian DIN 02239192	Antibiotic
379 <> PFIZER	Tab, Blue, Oval, Film Coated	Trovafloxacin 200 mg	Trovan by Roerig	00049-3790	Antibiotic
3796	Cap	Dextroamphetamine Sulfate 15 mg	Dexedrine by Vortech		Stimulant; C II
37AV <> 02	Tab, White, Round, Scored, 37 over AV <> 0.2	Desmopressin Acetate 0.2 mg	DDAVP by Aventis	00075-0026	Antidiuretic
37WALLACE2001 <> SOMA	Tab, White, Round, 37-Wallace 2001 <> Soma Logo	Carisoprodol 350 mg	Soma by Wallace	00037-2001	Muscle Relaxant
37WALLACE2001 <> SOMA	Tab, White, Round, 37-Wallace 2001 <> Soma Logo	Carisoprodol 350 mg	by Thrift Drug	59198-0361	Muscle Relaxant

ID FRONT <> BACK	DESCRIPTION FRONT <> BACK	INGREDIENT & STRENGTH	BRAND (or Generic Equiv.) by FIRM	NDC#	CLASS; SCH.
37WALLACE2001 <> SOMA	Tab, White, Round, 37-Wallace 2001 <> Soma Logo	Carisoprodol 350 mg	Soma by Horner	Canadian	Muscle Relaxant
37WALLACE2001 <> SOMA	Tab, White, Round, 37-Wallace 2001 <> Soma Logo	Carisoprodol 350 mg	Soma by Rightpac	65240-0738	Muscle Relaxant
37WALLACE2001 <> SOMA	Tab, White, Round, 37-Wallace 2001 <> Soma Logo	Carisoprodol 350 mg	by Caremark	00339-6145	Muscle Relaxant
37WALLACE2001 <> SOMA	Tab, White, Round, 37-Wallace 2001 <> Soma Logo	Carisoprodol 350 mg	by Nat Pharmpak	55154-4102	Muscle Relaxant
37WALLACE4224	Tab, Dark Pink, Round, Scored, 37 over Wallace over 4224	Guaifenesin 200 mg	Aquabid by Wallace	00037-4224	Expectorant
37WALLACE4312	Tab, Rose, Round, 37 over Wallace over 4312	Guaifenesin 200 mg	Aquabid by Wallace	00037-4312	Expectorant
38 <> 832	Tab, White, Round, Scored	Oxybutynin Chloride 5 mg	Ditropan by Dixon Shane	17236-0850	Urinary Tract
38 <> 832	Tab, White, Round, Scored	Oxybutynin Chloride 5 mg	Ditropan by UDL	51079-0628	Urinary Tract
38 <> 832	Tab, White, Round, Scored	Oxybutynin Chloride 5 mg	Ditropan by Rosemont	00832-0038	Urinary Tract
38 <> GG	Tab, Lavender, Film Coated	Hydroxyzine HCl 25 mg	by Sandoz		Antianxiety; Antihistamine
381	Tab	Amoxapine 100 mg	Asendin by Watson	52544-0381	Antidepressant
381381 <> COPLEY	Tab, Green, Hexagonal, Scored	Micronized Glyburide 3 mg	by DRX	55045-2267	Antidiabetic
381381 <> COPLEY	Tab, Green, Hexagonal, Scored	Micronized Glyburide 3 mg	by Teva	38245-0381	Antidiabetic
381B	Tab, White, Round, Scored, 381 over b	Meperidine 50 mg	Demerol by Barr	00555-0381	Analgesic; C II
381B	Tab, White, Round, Scored, 381 over b	Meperidine 50 mg	Demerol by Physician Total Care	54868-1233	Analgesic; C II
382	Tab	Amoxapine 150 mg	Asendin by Watson	52544-0382	Antidepressant
382 <> BARR	Tab, White, Round	Meperidine 100 mg	Demerol by Barr	00555-0382	Analgesic; C II
383 <> ETH	Tab, Light Orange, Oval, Scored, ETH to left of Score <> 383	Carbidopa 50 mg, Levodopa 200 mg	Sinemet CR by Ethex	58177-0383	Antiparkinson
384260	Tab, 384, 260 <> Mortar and Pestle Logo	Quinine Sulfate 260 mg	by Royce	51875-0384	Antimalarial
384260R	Tab, White, Round	Quinine Sulfate 260 mg	Quinamm by Ivax	00182-1213	Antimalarial
386	Cap, Maroon	Phenylpropanolamine HCl 75 mg, Brompheniramine Sulfate 12 mg	Dimetapp Gelcaps by Granutec		Cold Remedy
38625500	Tab, Scored, 386 Left of Score, 2.5 over 500 Right of Score <> Royce Logo	Acetaminophen 500 mg, Hydrocodone Bitartrate 2.5 mg	Lortab by Royce	51875-0386	Analgesic; C III
387 <> A	Tab, White to Off White, Round, Film Coated	Hydroxyzine HCl 10 mg	Atarax by Able	53265-0387 Discontinued	Antianxiety; Antihistamine
387 <> GLAXO	Tab, Light Blue, Cap Shaped, Film Coated	Cefuroxime Axetil 250 mg	Ceftin by GSK	51947-8121	Antibiotic
387 <> GLAXO	Tab, Light Blue, Cap Shaped, Film Coated	Cefuroxime Axetil 250 mg	Ceftin by Allscripts	55154-1109	Antibiotic
387 <> GLAXO	Tab, Light Blue, Cap Shaped, Film Coated	Cefuroxime Axetil 250 mg	Ceftin by GSK	53978-2088	Antibiotic
387 <> GLAXO	Tab, Light Blue, Cap Shaped, Film Coated	Cefuroxime Axetil 250 mg	Ceftin by Nat Pharmpak	62584-0325	Antibiotic
387 <> GLAXO	Tab, Light Blue, Cap Shaped, Film Coated	Cefuroxime Axetil 250 mg	Ceftin by Med Pro		Antibiotic
387 <> GLAXO	Tab, Light Blue, Cap Shaped, Film Coated	Cefuroxime Axetil 250 mg	Ceftin by Amerisource		Antibiotic
387 <> SL	Tab, Film Coated, Debossed	Ibuprofen 400 mg	Motrin by Pliva	50111-0387	NSAID
387500	Tab, 387 5 over 500	Acetaminophen 500 mg, Hydrocodone Bitartrate 5 mg	Vicodin by Quality Care	60346-0442	Analgesic; C III
387500	Tab, Scored, 387 Left of the Score, 5 over 500 Right of the Score <> Royce Logo	Acetaminophen 500 mg, Hydrocodone Bitartrate 5 mg	Vicodin by Royce	51875-0387	Analgesic; C III
388 <> A	Tab, White to Off White, Round, Film Coated	Hydroxyzine HCl 25 mg	Atarax by Able	53265-0388 Discontinued	Antianxiety; Antihistamine
388 <> SL	Tab, Film Coated	Ibuprofen 600 mg	Motrin by Pliva	50111-0388	NSAID
38832	Tab, White, Round, Scored, 38/832	Oxybutynin Chloride 5 mg	Ditropan by Martec	52555-0685	Urinary Tract
38875500	Tab, White, Oblong, Scored, 388 7.5/500 w/ Royce Logo	Acetaminophen 500 mg, Hydrocodone Bitartrate 7.5 mg	Lortab by Royce	51875-0388	Analgesic; C III
38875500	Tab, White, Oblong, Scored, 388 7.5/500 w/ Royce Logo	Acetaminophen 500 mg, Hydrocodone Bitartrate 7.5 mg	Lortab by Royce	51875-0388	Analgesic; C III
389 <> A	Tab, White to Off White, Round, Film Coated	Hydroxyzine HCl 50 mg	Atarax by Able	53265-0389 Discontinued	Antianxiety; Antihistamine
38975650	Tab, White, Oblong, Scored, 389 7.5/650 w/ Royce Logo	Acetaminophen 650 mg, Hydrocodone Bitartrate 7.5 mg	Lorcet Plus by Royce	51875-0389	Analgesic; C III
38975650	Tab, White, Oblong, Scored, 389 7.5/650 w/ Royce Logo	Acetaminophen 650 mg, Hydrocodone Bitartrate 7.5 mg	Lorcet Plus by Qualitest	00603-3884	Analgesic; C III
38975650	Tab, White, Oblong, Scored, 389 7.5/650 w/ Royce Logo	Acetaminophen 650 mg, Hydrocodone Bitartrate 7.5 mg	Lorcet Plus by Royce		Analgesic; C III

ID FRONT <> BACK	DESCRIPTION FRONT <> BACK	INGREDIENT & STRENGTH	BRAND (or Generic Equiv.) by FIRM	NDC#	CLASS; SCH.
38G	Cap, Gray	Etodolac 200 mg	Lodine by Genpharm	55567-0038	NSAID
39	Tab, White	Naltrexone HCl 50 mg	by Drugabuse	65694-0100	Opioid Antagonist
39 <> 93	Tab, White to Off-White, Diamond Shaped, Scored, 9 / 3	Lamotrigine 25 mg	Lamictal by Teva	00093-0039	Anticonvulsant
39 <> BMS150	Tab, Peach, Hexagonal, Scored	Nefazodone HCl 150 mg	Serzone by BMS	15548-0039	Antidepressant
39 <> BMS150	Tab, Peach, Hexagonal, Scored	Nefazodone HCl 150 mg	Serzone by Kaiser	00179-1242	Antidepressant
39 <> BMS150	Tab, Peach, Hexagonal, Scored	Nefazodone HCl 150 mg	Serzone by Allscripts		Antidepressant
39 <> BMS150	Tab, Peach, Hexagonal, Scored	Nefazodone HCl 150 mg	Serzone by BMS	00087-0039	Antidepressant
39 <> BMS150	Tab, Peach, Hexagonal, Scored	Nefazodone HCl 150 mg	Serzone by Par	49884-0569	Antidepressant
39 <> BMS150	Tab, Peach, Hexagonal, Scored	Nefazodone HCl 150 mg	Serzone by BMS	Canadian	Antidepressant
39 <> SB	Tab, White, Oval, Film Coated	Carvedilol 3.125 mg	Coreg by SKB	59742-4139	Antihypertensive
39 <> SB	Tab, White, Oval, Film Coated	Carvedilol 3.125 mg	Coreg by SKB	00007-4139	Antihypertensive
39 <> SB	Tab, White, Oval, Film Coated	Carvedilol 3.125 mg	Coreg by Murfreesboro	51129-1126	Antihypertensive
390 <> WYETH	Tab, White, Round, Scored	Penicillin V Potassium 500 mg	Pen Vee K by Wyeth	00008-0390	Antibiotic
390 <> WYETH	Tab, White, Round, Scored	Penicillin V Potassium 500 mg	Pen Vee K by Casa DeAmigos	62138-0390	Antibiotic
3900P	Cap, Gelatin	Guaifenesin 90 mg, Theophylline 150 mg	Bronchial by Banner Pharma	10888-3900	Antiasthmatic
39010650	Tab, Scored, 390 Left of Score, 10 over 650 Right of Score <> Royce Logo	Acetaminophen 650 mg, Hydrocodone Bitartrate 10 mg	Lorcet by Med Tek	52349-0202	Analgesic; C III
39010650	Tab, Scored, 390 Left of Score, 10 over 650 Right of Score <> Royce Logo	Acetaminophen 650 mg, Hydrocodone Bitartrate 10 mg	Lorcet by Royce	51875-0390	Analgesic; C III
39010650	Tab, Scored, 390 Left of Score, 10 over 650 Right of Score <> Royce Logo	Acetaminophen 650 mg, Hydrocodone Bitartrate 10 mg	Lorcet by Ivax	00182-0034	Analgesic; C III
391	Tab, White, Cap Shaped, Film Coated, Scored	Oxaprozin 600 mg	Daypro by Caraco	57664-0391	NSAID
391 <> G	Tab, Purple, Oval, Convex	Carbidopa 50 mg, Levodopa 200 mg	Sinemet CR by Global	00115-3911	Antiparkinson
391V	Tab, Peach, Round, Scored	Levothyroxine Sodium 25 mcg	by URL Mutual	00677-1648	Thyroid Hormone
391V	Tab, Peach, Round, Scored	Levothyroxine Sodium 25 mcg	by Vintage	00254-3911	Thyroid Hormone
391V	Tab, Peach, Round, Scored	Levothyroxine Sodium 25 mcg	by Direct Dispensing	57866-5503	Thyroid Hormone
3912V	Tab, White, Round, Scored	Levothyroxine Sodium 50 mcg	by Vintage	00254-3912	Thyroid Hormone
3912V	Tab, White, Round, Scored	Levothyroxine Sodium 50 mcg	by URL Mutual	00677-1649	Thyroid Hormone
3913V	Tab, Purple, Round, Scored	Levothyroxine Sodium 75 mcg	by Direct Dispensing	57866-5505	Thyroid Hormone
3913V	Tab, Purple, Round, Scored	Levothyroxine Sodium 75 mcg	Synthroid by Vintage	00254-3913	Thyroid Hormone
3913V	Tab, Purple, Round, Scored	Levothyroxine Sodium 75 mcg	Synthroid by URL Mutual	00677-1650	Thyroid Hormone
3913V	Tab, Purple, Round, Scored	Levothyroxine Sodium 75 mcg	by Allscripts		Thyroid Hormone
3914V	Tab, Yellow, Round, Scored, 3914/V	Levothyroxine Sodium 25 mcg	by Direct Dispensing	57866-3953	Thyroid Hormone
3914V	Tab, Yellow, Round, Scored, 3914/V	Levothyroxine Sodium 100 mcg	by Vintage	00254-3914	Thyroid Hormone
3914V	Tab, Yellow, Round, Scored, 3914/V	Levothyroxine Sodium 100 mcg	by Heartland	61392-0201	Thyroid Hormone
3914V	Tab, Yellow, Round, Scored, 3914/V	Levothyroxine Sodium 100 mcg	by Murfreesboro	51129-1649	Thyroid Hormone
3915V	Tab	Levothyroxine Sodium 150 mcg	by PDRX	55289-0084	Thyroid Hormone
3916V	Tab, Pink, Round, Scored	Levothyroxine Sodium 200 mcg	by Vintage	00254-3916	Thyroid Hormone
3916V	Tab, Pink, Round, Scored	Levothyroxine Sodium 200 mcg	by Direct Dispensing	57866-4381	Thyroid Hormone
39175750	Tab, White, Oblong, Scored, 391 7.5/750 w/ Royce Logo	Acetaminophen 750 mg, Hydrocodone Bitartrate 7.5 mg	Vicodin ES by Royce		Analgesic; C III
39175750	Tab, White, Oblong, Scored, 391 7.5/750 w/ Royce Logo	Acetaminophen 750 mg, Hydrocodone Bitartrate 7.5 mg	Vicodin ES by Royce	51875-0391	Analgesic; C III
3917V	Tab, Green, Round, Scored	Levothyroxine Sodium 300 mcg	by Direct Dispensing	57866-3958	Thyroid Hormone
3917V	Tab, Green, Round, Scored	Levothyroxine Sodium 300 mcg	by URL Mutual	00677-0769	Thyroid Hormone
3917V	Tab, Green, Round, Scored	Levothyroxine Sodium 300 mcg	by Vintage	00254-3917	Thyroid Hormone
3919V	Tab, Brown, Round	Levothyroxine Sodium 125 mcg	by URL Mutual	00677-1637	Thyroid Hormone
3919V	Tab, Brown, Round	Levothyroxine Sodium 125 mcg	by Vintage	00254-3919	Thyroid Hormone
392 <> G	Tab, Purple, Oval, Convex	Carbidopa 25 mg, Levodopa 100 mg	Sinemet CR by Global	00115-3922	Antiparkinson
3925	Cap, Blue & Clear	Phentermine 30 mg	Phentrol #2 by Vortech		Anorexiant; C IV
3938	Cap, Blue & Pink	Phentermine 15 mg	Phentrol #3 by Vortech		Anorexiant; C IV

ID FRONT <> BACK	DESCRIPTION FRONT <> BACK	INGREDIENT & STRENGTH	BRAND (or Generic Equiv.) by FIRM	NDC#	CLASS; SCH.
394	Tab, Peach, Round, Schering Logo 394	Reserpine 0.1 mg, Trichlormethiazide 4 mg	Naquival by Schering		Antihypertensive; Diuretic
394	Tab, Scored	Chlorpropamide 250 mg	Diabinese by Rightpak	65240-0634	Antidiabetic
394 <> GLAXO	Tab, Dark Blue, Cap Shaped, Film Coated	Cefuroxime Axetil 500 mg	Ceftin by Nat Pharmpak	55154-1111	Antibiotic
394 <> GLAXO	Tab, Dark Blue, Cap Shaped, Film Coated	Cefuroxime Axetil 500 mg	Ceftin by GSK	Discontinued	Antibiotic
39465650	Tab, 394 65 over 650 <> Royce Logo	Acetaminophen 650 mg, Propoxyphene HCl 65 mg	Wygesic by Royce	51875-0394	Analgesic; C IV
395 <> GLAXO	Tab, White, Cap Shaped, Film Coated	Cefuroxime Axetil 125 mg	Ceftin by GSK	00173-0395	Antibiotic
3955005 <> WATSON	Tab, Green, Cap Shaped, Scored	Pentazocine HCl 50 mg, Naloxone HCl 0.5 mg	Talwin by Watson	52544-0395	Analgesic; C IV
3955005 <> WATSON	Tab, Green, Cap Shaped, Scored, 50 0.5	Naloxone HCl 0.5 mg, Pentazocine HCl 50 mg	Talwin NX by Watson	00591-0395	Analgesic; C IV
396 <> A	Tab, Light Peach, Mottled, Round,	Methamphetamine HCl 5 mg	Desoxyn by Able	53265-0396	Stimulant; C II
				Discontinued	
39625650 <> WATSON	Tab, Light Aqua, Cap Shaped, Scored	Pentazocine HCl 25 mg, Acetaminophen 650 mg	Talacen by Watson	00591-0396	Analgesic; C IV
3966	Tab, White, Round, Hourglass Logo over 3966	Atropine Sulfate 0.025 mg, Diphenoxylate HCl 2.5 mg	Lomotil by Ivax	00172-3966	Antidiarrheal; C V
				Discontinued	
3966	Tab, White, Round, Hourglass Logo over 3966	Atropine Sulfate 0.025 mg, Diphenoxylate HCl 2.5 mg	Lomotil by Mallinckrodt	00406-0463	Antidiarrheal; C V
397	Tab, White, Round	Metformin HCl 500 mg	Glucophage by Caraco	57664-0397	Antidiabetic
398	Tab, White to Off-White, Round, Scored	Glipizide 5 mg	Glucotrol by Caraco	57664-0398	Antidiabetic
3984 <> 0115	Tab, White, Round	Methyltestosterone 10 mg	Methitest by Global	00115-3984	Hormone; C III
3984 <> 3	Tab	Aspirin 325 mg, Codeine Phosphate 30 mg	Aspirin w/ Codeine by DRX	55045-2307	Analgesic; C III
3985 <> 4	Tab	Aspirin 325 mg, Codeine Phosphate 60 mg	Aspirin w/ Codeine by DRX	55045-2355	Analgesic; C III
3986 <> 0115	Tab, Yellow, Round	Methyltestosterone 25 mg	by Global	00115-3986	Hormone; C III
399	Tab, Yellow, Round	Caffeine 200 mg	Vivarin by Granutec		Stimulant
399	Tab, White to Off-White, Round, Scored	Glipizide 10 mg	Glucotrol by Caraco	57664-0399	Antidiabetic
39G	Cap, Gray	Etodolac 300 mg	Lodine by Genpharm	55567-0039	NSAID
3LLL13	Tab, Green, Round	Levothyroxine Sodium 0.3 mg	Synthroid by Lederle		Thyroid Hormone
3M <> 221	Tab, White, Round, Ex Release	Orphenadrine Citrate 100 mg	by Amerisource	62584-0221	Muscle Relaxant
3M <> 221	Tab, White, Round, Ex Release	Orphenadrine Citrate 100 mg	by PDRX	55289-0646	Muscle Relaxant
3M <> 221	Tab, White, Round, Ex Release	Orphenadrine Citrate 100 mg	by Perrigo	00113-0381	Muscle Relaxant
3M <> 221	Tab, White, Round, Ex Release	Orphenadrine Citrate 100 mg	Norflex ER by 3M	00089-0221	Muscle Relaxant
				Discontinued	
3M <> 221	Tab, White, Round, Ex Release	Orphenadrine Citrate 100 mg	Norflex by H J Harkins Co	52959-0178	Muscle Relaxant
3M <> 221	Tab, White, Round, Ex Release	Orphenadrine Citrate 100 mg	Norflex by Rx Pak	65084-0229	Muscle Relaxant
3M <> 221	Tab, White, Round, Ex Release	Orphenadrine Citrate 100 mg	by Nat Pharmpak	55154-2907	Muscle Relaxant
3M <> 221	Tab, White, Round, Ex Release	Orphenadrine Citrate 100 mg	by Allscripts		Muscle Relaxant
3M <> 221	Tab, White, Round, Ex Release	Orphenadrine Citrate 100 mg	Norflex by Rightpak	65240-0703	Muscle Relaxant
3M <> 342	Tab, White, Round, Scored	Theophylline Anhydrous 125 mg	Theolair by 3M	00089-0342	Antiasthmatic
3M <> DISALCID	Tab, Aqua, Round, Scored, Film Coated	Salsalate 500 mg	Disalcid by 3M	00089-0149	NSAID
3M <> DISALCID	Tab, Aqua, Round, Scored, Film Coated	Salsalate 500 mg	Disalcid by 3M	00089-0148	NSAID
3M <> DISALCID750	Tab, Aqua, Cap Shaped, Scored, Film Coated	Salsalate 750 mg	Disalcid by Rx Pak	65084-0212	NSAID
3M <> DISALCID750	Tab, Aqua, Cap Shaped, Scored, Film Coated	Salsalate 750 mg	Disalcid by 3M	00089-0151	NSAID
3M <> DISALCID750	Tab, Aqua, Cap Shaped, Scored, Film Coated	Salsalate 750 mg	by Amerisource	62584-0151	NSAID
3M <> DISALCID750	Tab, Aqua, Cap Shaped, Scored, Film Coated	Salsalate 750 mg	Disalcid by Leiner	59606-0635	NSAID
3M <> DISALCID750	Tab, Aqua, Cap Shaped, Scored, Film Coated	Salsalate 750 mg	by Nat Pharmpak	55154-2902	NSAID
3M <> DISALCID750	Tab, Aqua, Cap Shaped, Scored, Film Coated	Salsalate 750 mg	by Thrift Drug	59198-0121	NSAID
3M <> NORGESIC	Tab, White & Yellow, Round	Aspirin 385 mg, Caffeine 30 mg, Orphenadrine Citrate 25 mg	Norgesic by 3M	00089-0231	Analgesic; Muscle Relaxant
				Discontinued	
3M <> NORGESICFORTE	Tab, Green & White, Cap Shaped, Scored	Aspirin 770 mg, Caffeine 60 mg, Orphenadrine Citrate 50 mg	Norgesic Forte by Thrift Drug	59198-0158	Analgesic
3M <> NORGESICFORTE	Tab, Green & White, Cap Shaped, Scored	Aspirin 770 mg, Caffeine 60 mg, Orphenadrine Citrate 50 mg	Norgesic Forte by CVS	00894-6767	Analgesic
3M <> NORGESICFORTE	Tab, Green & White, Cap Shaped, Scored	Aspirin 770 mg, Caffeine 60 mg, Orphenadrine Citrate 50 mg	Norgesic Forte by Amerisource	62584-0233	Analgesic
3M <> NORGESICFORTE	Tab, Green & White, Cap Shaped, Scored	Aspirin 770 mg, Caffeine 60 mg, Orphenadrine Citrate 50 mg	Norgesic Forte by 3M	00089-0233	Analgesic
				Discontinued	

ID FRONT <> BACK	DESCRIPTION FRONT <> BACK	INGREDIENT & STRENGTH	BRAND (or Generic Equiv.) by FIRM	NDC#	CLASS; SCH.
3M <> NORGESICFORTE	Tab, Green & White, Cap Shaped, Scored	Aspirin 770 mg, Caffeine 60 mg, Orphenadrine Citrate 50 mg	Norgesic Forte by Nat Pharmpak	55154-2905	Analgesic
3M <> NORGESICFORTE	Tab, Green & White, Cap Shaped, Scored	Aspirin 770 mg, Caffeine 60 mg, Orphenadrine Citrate 50 mg	Norgesic Forte by CVS	51316-0050	Analgesic
3M <> NORGESICFORTE	Tab, Green & White, Cap Shaped, Scored	Aspirin 770 mg, Caffeine 60 mg, Orphenadrine Citrate 50 mg	Norgesic Forte by Allscripts	Canadian	Analgesic
3M <> NORGESICFORTE	Tab, Green & White, Cap Shaped, Scored	Aspirin 770 mg, Caffeine 60 mg, Orphenadrine Citrate 50 mg	Norgesic Forte by 3M	53978-3384	Analgesic
3M <> NORGESICFORTE	Tab, Green & White, Cap Shaped, Scored	Aspirin 770 mg, Caffeine 60 mg, Orphenadrine Citrate 50 mg	Norgesic Forte by Med Pro	00089-0341	Analgesic
3M <> SR200	Tab, White, Round, Scored	Theophylline Anhydrous 200 mg	Theolair SR by 3M	50716-0505	Antiasthmatic
3M <> SR200	Tab, White, Round, Scored	Theophylline Anhydrous 200 mg	by Urgent Care Center	Canadian	Antiasthmatic
3M <> SR250	Tab, White, Round, Scored, SR over 250	Theophylline Anhydrous 250 mg	Theolair SR by 3M	00089-0345	Antiasthmatic
3M <> SR250	Tab, White, Round, Scored, SR over 250	Theophylline Anhydrous 250 mg	Theolair by 3M	Canadian	Antiasthmatic
3M <> SR300	Tab, White, Oval, Scored	Theophylline Anhydrous 300 mg	Theolair SR by 3M	00089-0343	Antiasthmatic
3M <> SR500	Tab, White, Cap Shaped, Scored	Theophylline Anhydrous 500 mg	Theolair SR by 3M	00089-0347	Antiasthmatic
3M <> SR500	Tab, White, Oblong, Scored	Theophylline Anhydrous 500 mg	Theolair by 3M	Canadian	Antiasthmatic
3M <> THEOLAIR250	Tab, White, Cap Shaped, Scored	Theophylline Anhydrous 250 mg	Theolair by 3M	00089-0344	Antiasthmatic
3M <> TR100	Tab, White, Round, Scored, TR over 100	Flecainide Acetate 100 mg	Tambocor by 3M	00089-0307	Antiarrhythmic
3M <> TR150	Tab, White, Oval, Scored	Flecainide Acetate 150 mg	Tambocor by Integrity	64731-0945	Antiarrhythmic
3M <> TR150	Tab, White, Oval, Scored	Flecainide Acetate 150 mg	Tambocor by 3M	00089-0314	Antiarrhythmic
3M <> TR50	Tab, White, Round, TR over 50	Flecainide Acetate 50 mg	by Murfreesboro	51129-1378	Antiarrhythmic
3M <> TR50	Tab, White, Round, TR over 50	Flecainide Acetate 50 mg	Tambocor by 3M	00089-0305	Antiarrhythmic
3M <> UREX	Tab, White, Cap Shaped, Scored	Methenamine Hippurate 1 g	Urex by 3M	00089-0371	Antibiotic; Urinary Tract
3M107	Tab, Green, Oblong	Aluminum Hydroxide 600 mg	Amphojel by 3M	00089-0107	Gastrointestinal
3M161	Tab, Green, Round	Orphenadrine Citrate 50 mg	by 3M	Canadian Discontinued	Muscle Relaxant
3M221	Tab, White	Orphenadrine Citrate 100 mg	by 3M	Canadian Discontinued	Muscle Relaxant
3M342	Tab, White, Round	Theophylline Anhydrous 125 mg	Theolair by 3M	00089-0342	Antiasthmatic
3MDISALCID	Cap, Aqua & White	Salsalate 500 mg	Disalcid by 3M	00089-0148	NSAID
3MDISALCID	Tab, Aqua, Round, Scored, Film Coated	Salsalate 500 mg	by 3M	Canadian Discontinued	NSAID
3MDISALCID750	Tab, Aqua, Cap Shaped, Scored, Film Coated	Salsalate 750 mg	by 3M	Canadian Discontinued	NSAID
3MG <> 503	Tab, Green, Round	Guanfacine 3 mg	Intuniv by Shire	54092-0517	Non-Stimulant Anti-ADHD
3MSR300	Tab, White, Oval, Scored	Theophylline Anhydrous 300 mg	by 3M	Canadian	Antiasthmatic
3P1153	Tab, Purple, Round	Levothyroxine Sodium 0.175 mg	Synthroid by Wal Mart	49035-0191	Thyroid Hormone
3R	Cap, Red, Oval, Opaque, Soft Gel	Terazosin HCl 5 mg	Hytrin by Ranbaxy	63304-0664	Antihypertensive
3RORER143	Tab, White, Round	Aspirin 325 mg, Codeine Phosphate 30 mg, Maalox 150 mg	Ascriptin Codeine #3 by Rorer		Analgesic; C III
3RP <> 200	Tab, Light Blue, Cap-Shaped, Film-Coated	Ribavirin 200 mg	Copegus by Three Rivers	66435-0102	Antiviral
3RP <> 400	Tab, Medium Blue, Cap-Shaped, Film-Coated	Ribavirin 400 mg	Copegus by Three Rivers	66435-0103	Antiviral
3RP <> 600	Tab, Dark Blue, Cap-Shaped, Film-Coated	Ribavirin 600 mg	Copegus by Three Rivers	66435-0104	Antiviral
3SYCBMZ	Tab, Pink, Cylindrical, 3/Syc-BMZ	Bromazepam 3 mg	Lectopam by AltiMed	Canadian DIN 02167816	Sedative; C IV
3V2 <> GS	Tab, Pink, Cap Shaped, Film Coated	Ropinirole HCl 2 mg	Requip XL by GSK	00007-4885	Antiparkinson
4	Cap, Blue, White Print, Ex Release	Tolterodine 4 mg	Detrol LA by Pharmacia	00009-5191	Urinary Tract
4	Tab, White, Oval	Dextrothyroxine Sodium 4 mg	Choloxin by Boots		Thyroid Hormone
4	Tab, White, Round, Film Coated	Ibuprofen 400 mg	Motrin by Norton		NSAID
4	Tab, White, Round, Film Coated	Ibuprofen 400 mg	Motrin by Murfreesboro	51129-1522	NSAID
4	Tab, White, Round, Scored	Acetaminophen 300 mg, Codeine Phosphate 60 mg	Tylenol w/ Codeine by Mikart	46672-0056	Analgesic; C III
4	Cap, Blue, White Print, Ex Release	Tolterodine 4 mg	Detrol LA by Pfizer	Canadian DIN 02244613	Urinary Tract
4	Tab, Green, Buccal	Fentanyl 400 mcg	Fentora by Cephalon	63459-0544	Opioid Agonist; C II
4	Tab, White, Round, # and 4	Nitroglycerin 0.4 mg	Nitrostat by Endo	60951-0718	Vasodilator

ID FRONT <> BACK	DESCRIPTION FRONT <> BACK	INGREDIENT & STRENGTH	BRAND (or Generic Equiv.) by FIRM	NDC#	CLASS; SCH.
4	Tab, Gray, Round, Schering Logo/4	Perphenazine 4 mg	Trilafon by Schering	Canadian	Antipsychotic
4	Tab, Gray, Round	Perphenazine 4 mg	Apo Perphenazine by Apotex	Canadian DIN 00335126	Antipsychotic
4	Tab, White, Oval	Ondansetron 4 mg	Zofran by Actavis	52152-0538	Antiemetic
4	Tab, White, Round, Sublingual	Nitroglycerin 0.4 mg	Nitrostat by Glenmark	68462-0146	Vasodilator
4	Tab, White, Round, Vanda Logo <> 4	Iloperidone 4 mg	Fanapt by Vanda	43068-0104	Antipsychotic
4 <> 108	Tab, Pale Pink, Round	Trandolapril 4 mg	Mavik by Dava	67253-0108	Antihypertensive
4 <> 2065V	Tab, 2065 over V <> 4	Acetaminophen 300 mg, Codeine Phosphate 60 mg	Tylenol w/ Codeine by Quality Care	60346-0632 Discontinued	Analgesic; C III
4 <> 2121V	Tab	Aspirin 325 mg, Codeine Phosphate 60 mg	Aspirin w/ Codeine by Vintage	00254-2121	Analgesic; C III
4 <> 2121V	Tab, White	Aspirin 325 mg, Codeine Phosphate 60 mg	Aspirin w/ Codeine by Qualitest	00603-2362	Analgesic; C III
4 <> 3327G	Tab, White, Oval, 3327 over G <> 4	Methylprednisolone 4 mg	Medrol by Greenstone	59762-3327	Steroid
4 <> 3327G	Tab, White, Oval, 3327 over G <> 4	Methylprednisolone 4 mg	Medrol by Pharmacia	00009-3327	Steroid
4 <> 3687	Tab, Orange, Round, Scored, Hourglass Logo 4	Doxazosin Mesylate 4 mg	Cardura by Ivax	00172-3687	Antihypertensive
4 <> 3985	Tab	Aspirin 325 mg, Codeine Phosphate 60 mg	Aspirin w/ Codeine by DRX	55045-2355	Analgesic; C III
4 <> 4216V	Tab, White, Oval	Methylprednisolone 4 mg	Medrol by Vintage	00254-4216	Steroid
4 <> 523	Tab, White, Round, Andrx Logo 523 <> 4	Acetaminophen 300 mg, Codeine 60 mg	Tylenol w/ Codeine by Andrx	62037-0523	Analgesic; C III
4 <> 54196	Tab, White to Off-White, Round	Hydromorphone HCl 4 mg	Dilaudid by Roxane	00054-0264	Analgesic; C II
4 <> 54609	Tab, White, Round, Scored, 54 over 609	Hydromorphone HCl 4 mg	Dilaudid by Roxane	00054-4394	Analgesic; C II
4 <> 54609	Tab, White, Round, Scored, 54 over 609	Hydromorphone HCl 4 mg	Dilaudid by Roxane	00054-8394	Analgesic; C II
4 <> 93350	Tab, White, Round, 93 over 350	Acetaminophen 300 mg, Codeine Phosphate 60 mg	Tylenol w/ Codeine by Southwood	58016-0272	Analgesic; C III
4 <> 93350	Tab, White, Round, 93 over 350	Acetaminophen 300 mg, Codeine Phosphate 60 mg	Tylenol w/ Codeine by Teva	00093-0350	Analgesic; C III
4 <> 93350	Tab, White, Round, 93 over 350	Acetaminophen 300 mg, Codeine Phosphate 60 mg	Tylenol w/ Codeine by UDL	51079-0106	Analgesic; C III
4 <> 93350	Tab, White, Round, 93 over 350	Acetaminophen 300 mg, Codeine Phosphate 60 mg	Tylenol w/ Codeine by Murfreesboro	51129-6662	Analgesic; C III
4 <> 93350	Tab, White, Round, 93 over 350	Acetaminophen 300 mg, Codeine Phosphate 60 mg	Tylenol w/ Codeine by Sandoz	00781-1654	Analgesic; C III
4 <> 93350	Tab, White, Round, 93 over 350	Acetaminophen 300 mg, Codeine Phosphate 60 mg	Tylenol w/ Codeine by St. Mary's Med	60760-0350	Analgesic; C III
4 <> A	Tab, Yellow, Round, Abbott Logo (a)	Hydromorphone HCl 4 mg	Dilaudid by Abbott	00074-2416	Analgesic; C II
4 <> A	Tab, Yellow, Round, Scored	Guaifenesin 1200 mg, Phenylpropanolamine 75 mg	Aquatab D by Adams	63824-0004	Cold Remedy
4 <> A286	Tab, White to Off-White, Round	Acetaminophen 300 mg, Codeine Phosphate 60 mg	Tylenol w/ Codeine by Able	53265-0286 Discontinued	Analgesic; C III
4 <> B304	Tab, White, Round, Scored	Acetaminophen 300 mg, Codeine Phosphate 60 mg	Tylenol w/ Codeine by Barr	00555-0304	Analgesic; C III
4 <> BARR229	Tab	Acetaminophen 300 mg, Codeine Phosphate 60 mg	Tylenol w/ Codeine by Pharmedix	53002-0103	Analgesic; C III
4 <> CL	Tab, White to Off-White, Rectangle, Sublingual	Nitroglycerin 0.4 mg	Nitrostat by Pliva	50111-0989	Vasodilator
4 <> COPLEY717	Tab	Guanabenz Acetate 5.14 mg	by Teva	38245-0717 Discontinued	Antihypertensive
4 <> CPI	Tab, CPI Logo	Phenobarbital 16.2 mg	by Century	00436-0866	Sedative/Hypnotic; C IV
4 <> CPI	Tab, CPI Logo	Phenobarbital 16.2 mg	by Century	00436-0867	Sedative/Hypnotic; C IV
4 <> DPI	Tab	Acetaminophen 300 mg, Codeine Phosphate 60 mg	Tylenol w/ Codeine by Quality Care	60346-0632 Discontinued	Analgesic; C III
4 <> DRL200	Tab, White, Oval	Nefazodone HCl 200 mg	Serzone by Dr. Reddy's	55111-0141	Antidepressant
4 <> DRL200	Tab, White, Oval	Nefazodone HCl 200 mg	Serzone by Par	49884-0919	Antidepressant
4 <> E	Tab, Yellow, Oval, Film Coated	Conjugated Estrogens 1.25 mg	Enjuvia by Barr	51285-0410	Hormone
4 <> E	Tab, Tan, Film Coated	Hydromorphone HCl 4 mg	Dilaudid by Ethex	58177-0299	Analgesic; C II
4 <> ETH	Tab, White, Oval	Nitroglycerin 0.4 mg	Nitrostat by PDRX	55289-0309	Vasodilator
4 <> ETH	Tab, White, Oval	Nitroglycerin 0.4 mg	NitroQuick by Ethex	58177-0324	Vasodilator
4 <> G	Tab, White, Round	Ondansetron ODT 4 mg	Zofran ODT by Glenmark	68462-0157	Antiemetic
4 <> G1	Tab, White, Oval	Ondansetron HCl 8 mg	Zofran by Glenmark	68462-0105	Antiemetic
4 <> GG	Tab	Atropine Sulfate 0.025 mg, Diphenoxylate HCl 2.5 mg	Lomotil by Sandoz		Antidiarrheal; C V
4 <> GLAXO	Tab, White, Oval, Film Coated	Ondansetron HCl 4 mg	Zofran by GSK		Antiemetic

ID FRONT <> BACK	DESCRIPTION FRONT <> BACK	INGREDIENT & STRENGTH	BRAND (or Generic Equiv.) by FIRM	NDC#	CLASS; SCH.
4 <> GLAXO	Tab, Yellow, Oval, Film Coated	Ondansetron HCl 4 mg	Zofran by GSK	Canadian DIN 02213567	Antiemetic
4 <> H304	Tab, White, Oval, Film Coated, Scored	Acetaminophen 300 mg, Codeine Phosphate 60 mg	Tylenol w/ Codeine by Barr	51285-0304	Analgesic; C III
4 <> I	Tab, White, Round	Meprobamate 400 mg	Miltown by Dr. Reddy's	55111-0641	Tranquilizer
4 <> INV312	Tab, Blue, Square, Scored, INV over 312	Warfarin Sodium 4 mg	Coumadin by Sandoz	00781-0369	Anticoagulant
4 <> INV312	Tab, Blue, Square, Scored, INV over 312	Warfarin Sodium 4 mg	Coumadin by Apothecon	59772-0369	Anticoagulant
4 <> KC	Tab, White, Round, Film Coated	Pitavastatin 4 mg	Livalo by Kowa Pharmaceuticals	00002-4772	Antihyperlipidemic
4 <> M	Tab, White, Round	Hydromorphone HCl 4 mg	Dilaudid by Murfreesboro	51129-1466	Analgesic; C II
4 <> M	Tab, White, Round, M inside square <> 4	Acetaminophen 300 mg, Codeine Phosphate 60 mg	Tylenol w/ Codeine by Mallinckrodt	00406-0485	Analgesic; C III
4 <> M	Tab, White, Round	Hydromorphone HCl 4 mg	Dilaudid by Mallinckrodt	00406-3244	Analgesic; C II
4 <> M	Tab, White, Triangular, Film Coated	Fluphenazine HCl 1 mg	Prolixin by UDL	51079-0485	Antipsychotic
4 <> M	Tab, White, Triangular, Film Coated	Fluphenazine HCl 1 mg	Prolixin by Mylan	00378-6004	Antipsychotic
4 <> MCNEIL	Tab, White, Round, McNeil	Acetaminophen 300 mg, Codeine Phosphate 60 mg	Tylenol w/ Codeine by Janssen-Ortho	Canadian DIN 02163918	Analgesic; C III
4 <> MP127	Tab	Acetaminophen 300 mg, Codeine Phosphate 60 mg	Tylenol w/ Codeine by URL Mutual	00677-0632	Analgesic; C III
4 <> N	Tab, White, Round	Nitroglycerin 0.4 mg	Nitrostat by Parke Davis	00071-0418	Vasodilator
4 <> N499	Tab, White, Round, Scored, N over 499 <> 4	Albuterol Sulfate 4 mg	Proventil by Teva	55953-0499 Discontinued	Antiasthmatic
4 <> N499	Tab, White, Round, Scored, N over 499 <> 4	Albuterol Sulfate 4 mg	Proventil by Medirex	57480-0423	Antiasthmatic
4 <> N499	Tab, White, Round, Scored, N over 499 <> 4	Albuterol Sulfate 4 mg	Proventil by Heartland	61392-0570	Antiasthmatic
4 <> N499	Tab, White, Round, Scored, N over 499 <> 4	Albuterol Sulfate 4 mg	Proventil by DRX	55045-2283	Antiasthmatic
4 <> N499	Tab, White, Round, Scored, N over 499 <> 4	Albuterol Sulfate 4 mg	Proventil by Anabolic	00722-6437	Antiasthmatic
4 <> N596	Tab, White to Off-White, Diamond Shaped, Scored, N over 596	Doxazosin Mesylate 4 mg	Cardura by Teva	00603-2094	Antihypertensive
4 <> NN	Tab, White, Diamond-Shaped, Scored, N / N	Doxazosin Mesylate 4 mg	Cardura by Novopharm	Canadian DIN 02242730	Antihypertensive
4 <> P	Tab, Yellow, Oval, P logo <> 4	Ondansetron HCl 4 mg	Zofran by Pharmascience	Canadian DIN 02258188	Antiemetic
4 <> PAL	Tab, White, Round, Scored	Carbinoxamine Maleate 4 mg	Palgic by PamLab	00525-6748	Cold Remedy
4 <> PLOND	Tab, White, Oval	Ondansetron 4 mg	Zofran by Sandoz	00781-5257	Antiemetic
4 <> PMS	Tab, Yellow, Round, Scored	Hydromorphone HCl 4 mg	by Pharmascience	Canadian DIN 00885401	Analgesic; C II
4 <> PROVENTIL	Tab, Film Coated	Albuterol Sulfate 4 mg	Proventil by Nat Pharmpak	55154-3507	Antiasthmatic
4 <> R003	Tab	Acetaminophen 300 mg, Codeine Phosphate 60 mg	Tylenol w/ Codeine by Actavis	00228-2003	Analgesic; C III
4 <> R003	Tab, White, Round	Acetaminophen 300 mg, Codeine Phosphate 60 mg	Tylenol w/ Codeine by Ivax	00182-1338	Analgesic; C III
4 <> R21	Tab, White, Round	Acetaminophen 300 mg, Codeine Phosphate 60 mg	Tylenol w/ Codeine by Actavis	00228-3021	Analgesic; C III
4 <> R58	Tab, White to Off-White, Round	Acetaminophen 300 mg, Codeine Phosphate 60 mg	Tylenol w/ Codeine by Actavis	00228-3058	Analgesic; C III
4 <> RPC5	Tab, Orange, Round, Scored	Midodrine HCl 5 mg	Proamatine by Murfreesboro	51129-1433	Antihypotensive
4 <> RX561	Tab, White, Round	Acetaminophen 300 mg, Codeine Phosphate 60 mg	Tylenol w/ Codeine by Ranbaxy	63304-0561	Analgesic; C III
4 <> SAMPLE	Tab, Film Coated	Ondansetron HCl 4 mg	Zofran by GSK		Antiemetic
4 <> SB	Tab, Orange, Pentagonal	Rosiglitazone Maleate 4 mg	Avandia by SKB	00029-3159	Antidiabetic
4 <> SB	Tab, Orange, Pentagonal, Film Coated	Rosiglitazone Maleate 4 mg	Avandia by GSK	Canadian DIN 02241113	Antidiabetic
4 <> V	Tab, Green, Round, Ex Release	Albuterol Sulfate 4 mg	Vospire ER by Dava	68774-0600	Antiasthmatic
4 <> V	Tab, Green, Round, Ex Release	Albuterol Sulfate 4 mg	Vospire ER by Odyssey	65473-0754	Antiasthmatic
4 <> VOLMAX	Tab, Powder Blue, Dark Blue Print, Hexagonal, Ex Release	Albuterol Sulfate 4 mg	Volmax by Anabolic	00722-6429	Antiasthmatic
4 <> VOLMAX	Tab, Powder Blue, Dark Blue Print, Hexagonal, Ex Release	Albuterol Sulfate 4 mg	Volmax by McNeil	00045-1039	Antiasthmatic
4 <> VOLMAX	Tab, Powder Blue, Dark Blue Print, Hexagonal, Ex Release	Albuterol Sulfate 4 mg	Proventil by Eckerd	19458-0848	Antiasthmatic
4 <> VOLMAX	Tab, Powder Blue, Dark Blue Print, Hexagonal, Ex Release	Albuterol Sulfate 4 mg	Volmax by CVS	51316-0240	Antiasthmatic

ID FRONT <> BACK	DESCRIPTION FRONT <> BACK	INGREDIENT & STRENGTH	BRAND (or Generic Equiv.) by FIRM	NDC#	CLASS; SCH.
4 <> VOLMAX	Tab, Powder Blue, Dark Blue Print, Hexagonal, Ex Release	Albuterol Sulfate 4 mg	Volmax by Muro	00451-0398	Antiasthmatic
4 <> VOLMAX	Tab, Powder Blue, Dark Blue Print, Hexagonal, Ex Release	Albuterol Sulfate 4 mg	Volmax by Med Pro	53978-2026	Antiasthmatic
4 <> VOLMAX	Tab, Powder Blue, Dark Blue Print, Hexagonal, Ex Release	Albuterol Sulfate 4 mg	Volmax by Wal Mart	49035-0159	Antiasthmatic
4 <> VOLMAX	Tab, Powder Blue, Dark Blue Print, Hexagonal, Ex Release	Albuterol Sulfate 4 mg	Volmax by Nat Pharmpak	55154-4304	Antiasthmatic
4 <> WARFARINTARO	Tab, Blue, Cap Shaped	Warfarin Sodium 4 mg	Coumadin by Taro	51672-4031	Anticoagulant
4 <> Z	Tab, Dark Yellow, Round, Film Coated	Risperidone 25 mg	Risperdal by Zydus	68382-0112	Antipsychotic
4 <> Z3985	Tab, White, Round, Z over 3985	Aspirin 325 mg, Codeine Phosphate 60 mg	Aspirin w/ Codeine by Ivax	00172-3985 Discontinued	Analgesic; C III
4 <> ZER	Tab, White, Round, Scored	Carbinoxamine Maleate 4 mg	Palgic by Zerxis	18011-0674 Discontinued	Cold Remedy
4 <> ZOFRAN	Tab, White, Oval, Film	Ondansetron HCl 4 mg	Zofran by PDRX	55289-0480	Antiemetic
4 <> ZOFRAN	Tab, White, Oval, Film Coated	Ondansetron HCl 4 mg	Zofran by GSK	00173-0446	Antiemetic
40	Tab, Blue, Round, Film Coated, 40 inside Knoll Triangle	Verapamil HCl 40 mg	by Med Pro	53978-3076	Antihypertensive
40	Tab, Peach, Round, Ex Release, Andrx Logo 40	Lovastatin 40 mg	Altoprev by Andrx	62022-0629	Antihyperlipidemic
40	Tab, Yellow, Octagonal, Film Coated, Extended Release	Oxymorphone HCl 40 mg	Opana ER by Endo	63481-0693	Analgesic; C II
40	Tab, White, Oval, Film-Coated, Scored	Citalopram HBr 40 mg	Celexa by Pharmascience	Canadian DIN 02248011	Antidepressant
40 <> 0016	Cap, Dark Blue and White, Opaque	Omeprazole 40 mg, Sodium Bicarbonate 1100 mg	Zegerid by Santarus	68012-0104	Gastrointestinal
40 <> 0016	Tab, Green, Rounded Rectangle	Pravastatin Sodium 40 mg	Pravachol by Watson	00591-0016	Antihyperlipidemic
40 <> 1011	Tab, Tan, Oval, Film Coated, 4 / 0	Citalopram 40 mg	Celexa by Torrent	13668-0011	Antidepressant
40 <> 2732	Tab, Off-White, Hexagonal	Fosinopril Sodium 40 mg	Monopril by Sandoz	00781-5085	Antihypertensive
40 <> 4742	Tab, White, Cap Shaped, Scored	Citalopram HBr 40 mg	Celexa by Ivax	00172-4742 Discontinued	Antidepressant
40 <> 5353	Tab, Red, Oblong, Hourglass Logo 5353	Benazepril HCl 40 mg	Lotensin by Ivax	00172-5353 Discontinued	Antihypertensive
40 <> 5729	Tab, Tan, Round, Hourglass Logo 5729	Famotidine 40 mg	Pepcid by Ivax	00172-5729	Gastrointestinal
40 <> 5729	Tab, Beige, Round	Famotidine 40 mg	Pepcid by Teva	00172-5729	Histamine H2 Antagonist
40 <> ABG	Tab, Yellow, Round, Controlled Release	Oxycodone HCl 40 mg	OxyContin by Ivax	00172-6356	Analgesic; C II
40 <> APO	Tab, White, Oval, Film Coated	Citalopram HBr 40 mg	Celexa by Apotex	Canadian DIN 02246057	Antidepressant
40 <> APO	Tab, Dusty Rose, Shield-Shaped	Simvastatin 40 mg	Zocor by Apotex	Canadian DIN 02247014	Antihyperlipidemic
40 <> B	Tab, White, Round, Film Coated, Heart Outline around B	Bisoprolol 10 mg, Hydrochlorothiazide 6.25 mg	Ziac by Duramed	51285-0040	Antihypertensive; Diuretic
40 <> CALAN	Tab, Pink, Round, Coated	Verapamil HCl 40 mg	Calan by Searle	00025-1771	Antihypertensive
40 <> CRESTOR	Tab, Pink, Oval, Coated	Rosuvastatin 40 mg	Crestor by AstraZeneca	00310-0754	Antihyperlipidemic
40 <> DAN5556	Tab, Green, Round, Scored, DAN over 5556	Propranolol HCl 40 mg	Inderal by Rx Pak	65084-0102	Antihypertensive
40 <> DAN5556	Tab, Green, Round, Scored, DAN over 5556	Propranolol HCl 40 mg	Inderal by Schein	00364-0758	Antihypertensive
40 <> DAN5556	Tab, Green, Round, Scored, DAN over 5556	Propranolol HCl 40 mg	Inderal by Watson	00591-5556	Antihypertensive
40 <> DAN5556	Tab, Green, Round, Scored, DAN over 5556	Propranolol HCl 40 mg	Inderal by Vangard	00615-2563	Antihypertensive
40 <> E705	Tab, Yellow, Round, Coated, Extended Release	Oxycodone HCl 40 mg	OxyContin by Endo	60951-0705	Analgesic; C II
40 <> ELAVIL	Tab, Blue, Round, Film Coated	Amitriptyline HCl 10 mg	Elavil by H J Harkins Co	52959-0396	Antidepressant
40 <> ELAVIL	Tab, Blue, Round, Film Coated	Amitriptyline HCl 10 mg	Elavil by Zeneca	00310-0040	Antidepressant
40 <> G	Tab, Orange, Oval, Film Coated	Etodolac 400 mg	Lodine by Genpharm	55567-0040	NSAID
40 <> G021	Tab, Brown, Elliptical, Film Coated	Quinapril HCl 40 mg	Accupril by Greenstone	59762-5022	Antihypertensive
40 <> G5	Tab, Green, Rounded Rectangular	Pravastatin Sodium 40 mg	Pravachol by Glenmark	68462-0197	Antihyperlipidemic
40 <> INV237	Tab, White, Round, Scored, INV over 237	Nadolol 40 mg	Corgard by Ivax	00182-2633	Antihypertensive
40 <> INV237	Tab, White, Round, Scored, INV over 237	Nadolol 40 mg	Nadolol by Schein	00364-2653	Antihypertensive
40 <> INV237	Tab, White, Round, Scored, INV over 237	Nadolol 40 mg	Nadolol by Major	00904-5070	Antihypertensive
40 <> INV237	Tab, White, Round, Scored, INV over 237	Nadolol 40 mg	Nadolol by Invamed	52189-0237	Antihypertensive
40 <> INV237	Tab, White, Round, Scored, INV over 237	Nadolol 40 mg	Nadolol by Moore	00839-7870	Antihypertensive
40 <> INV237	Tab, White, Round, Scored, INV over 237	Nadolol 40 mg	Nadolol by Sandoz	00781-1182	Antihypertensive

ID FRONT <> BACK	DESCRIPTION FRONT <> BACK	INGREDIENT & STRENGTH	BRAND (or Generic Equiv.) by FIRM	NDC#	CLASS; SCH.
40 <> L879	Tab, Light Pink, Oval, Film-Coated	Simvastatin 40 mg	Zocor by Perrigo	45802-0879	Antihyperlipidemic
40 <> LOTENSIN	Tab, Rose, Round, Film Coated	Benazepril HCl 40 mg	Lotensin by Physician Total Care	54868-2352	Antihypertensive
40 <> LOTENSIN	Tab, Rose, Round, Film Coated	Benazepril HCl 40 mg	Lotensin by Novartis	00078-0450	Antihypertensive
40 <> LUPIN	Tab, Yellow, Round	Lisinopril 40 mg	Zestril by Lupin	68180-0517	Antihypertensive
40 <> MEGACE	Tab, Light Blue, Round, Scored	Megestrol Acetate 40 mg	Megace by Mead Johnson	00015-0596	Hormone
40 <> MYLAN184	Tab, Green, Round, Scored, Mylan over 184	Propranolol HCl 40 mg	Inderal by UDL	51079-0279	Antihypertensive
40 <> MYLAN184	Tab, Green, Round, Scored, Mylan over 184	Propranolol HCl 40 mg	Inderal by Mylan	00378-0184	Antihypertensive
40 <> MYLAN216	Tab, White, Round, Scored, Mylan over 216	Furosemide 40 mg	Lasix by Heartland	61392-0253	Diuretic
40 <> MYLAN216	Tab, White, Round, Scored, Mylan over 216	Furosemide 40 mg	Lasix by Allscripts		Diuretic
40 <> MYLAN216	Tab, White, Round, Scored, Mylan over 216	Furosemide 40 mg	Lasix by Kaiser	62224-1222	Diuretic
40 <> MYLAN216	Tab, White, Round, Scored, Mylan over 216	Furosemide 40 mg	Lasix by Murfreesboro	51129-1389	Diuretic
40 <> MYLAN216	Tab, White, Round, Scored, Mylan over 216	Furosemide 40 mg	Lasix by Mylan	00378-0216	Diuretic
40 <> MYLAN216	Tab, White, Round, Scored, Mylan over 216	Furosemide 40 mg	Lasix by UDL	51079-0073 Discontinued	Diuretic
40 <> N	Tab, Pink, Shield Shaped	Simvastatin 40 mg	Zocor by Novopharm	Canadian DIN 02250179	Antihyperlipidemic
40 <> N	Tab, Green, Rounded Square	Pravastatin Sodium 40 mg	Pravachol by Novopharm	Canadian DIN 02247010	Antihyperlipidemic
40 <> N	Tab, Green, Octagonal	Lovastatin 40 mg	Mevacor by Novopharm	Canadian DIN 02246543	Antihyperlipidemic
40 <> NN	Tab, White, Oval, Scored, N / N <> 40	Citalopram 40 mg	Celexa by Novopharm	Canadian DIN 02251566	Antidepressant
40 <> NOVO	Tab, Brown & Orange, D-Shaped, novo/40	Famotidine 40 mg	Pepcid by Novopharm	Canadian DIN 02022141	Gastrointestinal
40 <> OC	Tab, Yellow, Round, Film Coated	Oxycodone HCl 40 mg	OxyContin by Purdue	59011-0105	Analgesic; C II
40 <> P	Tab, Green, Oblong, P logo	Paroxetine HCl 40 mg	Paxil by Pharmascience	Canadian DIN 02293749	Antidepressant
40 <> P	Tab, Brick Red, Shield Shaped	Simvastatin 40 mg	Zocor by Pharmascience	Canadian DIN 02269287	Antihyperlipidemic
40 <> PAXIL	Tab, Light Green, Oblong, Film Coated	Paroxetine HCl 40 mg	Paxil by SB	59742-3213	Antidepressant
40 <> PAXIL	Tab, Light Green, Oblong, Film Coated	Paroxetine HCl 40 mg	Paxil by SKB	00029-3213	Antidepressant
40 <> PD157	Tab, White, Oval, Film Coated	Atorvastatin Calcium 40 mg	Lipitor by Parke Davis	Canadian DIN 02230714	Antihyperlipidemic
40 <> PD157	Tab, White, Oval, Film Coated	Atorvastatin Calcium 40 mg	Lipitor by Murfreesboro	51129-1424	Antihyperlipidemic
40 <> PD157	Tab, White, Oval, Film Coated	Atorvastatin Calcium 40 mg	Lipitor by Physician Total Care	54868-4229	Antihyperlipidemic
40 <> PD157	Tab, White, Oval, Film Coated	Atorvastatin Calcium 40 mg	Lipitor by Goedecke	53869-0157	Antihyperlipidemic
40 <> PD157	Tab, White, Oval, Film Coated	Atorvastatin Calcium 40 mg	Lipitor by Parke Davis	00071-0157	Antihyperlipidemic
40 <> PD535	Tab, Brown, Oval, Film Coated	Quinapril HCl 40 mg	Accupril by PDRX	55289-0555	Antihypertensive
40 <> PD535	Tab, Brown, Oval, Film Coated	Quinapril HCl 40 mg	Accupril by Parke Davis	00071-0535	Antihypertensive
40 <> PD535	Tab, Brown, Oval, Film Coated	Quinapril HCl 40 mg	Accupril by Parke Davis	Canadian DIN 01947699	Antihypertensive
40 <> PLC	Tab, Mottled Pink, Round	Amoxicillin 400 mg, Clavulanate Potassium 20 mg	Augmentin by Ivax	00172-7402	Antibiotic
40 <> TAP	Tab, Green, Round	Febuxostat 40 mg	Uloric by Takeda	64764-0918	Antigout
40 <> TARO	Tab, Brick Red, Shield-Shaped, Film-Coated	Simvastatin 40 mg	Zocor by Taro	Canadian DIN 02265907	Antihyperlipidemic
40 <> Z4236	Tab, White, Round, Z over 4236	Nadolol 40 mg	Corgard by Ivax	00093-4236	Antihypertensive
40 <> ZD4522	Tab, Pink, Oval, Coated	Rosuvastatin 40 mg	Crestor by AstraZeneca	Canadian DIN 02247164	Antihyperlipidemic
40 <> ZD4522	Tab, Pink, Oval, Coated	Rosuvastatin 40 mg	Crestor by AstraZeneca	00310-0754	Antihyperlipidemic
400	Tab, Film Coated, Upjohn Logo and 400	Ibuprofen 400 mg	Motrin by Quality Care	60346-0430	NSAID

ID FRONT <> BACK	DESCRIPTION FRONT <> BACK	INGREDIENT & STRENGTH	BRAND (or Generic Equiv.) by FIRM	NDC#	CLASS; SCH.
400 <> 250	Tab, Red, Oblong	Amoxicillin 400 mg	Amoxil by Allscripts		Antibiotic
400 <> 3RP	Tab, Medium Blue, Cap-Shaped, Film-Coated	Ribavirin 400 mg	Copegus by Three Rivers	66435-0103	Antiviral
400 <> 4175	Tab, White, Cap Shaped, Hourglass Logo 4175	Etodolac 400 mg	Lodine by Heartland	61392-0917	NSAID
400 <> 4175	Tab, White, Cap Shaped, Hourglass Logo 4175	Etodolac 400 mg	Lodine by Ivax	00172-4175	NSAID
400 <> 4175	Tab, White, Cap Shaped, Hourglass Logo 4175	Etodolac 400 mg	Lodine by Qualitest	00603-3570	NSAID
400 <> 4267	Tab, White, Round, Hourglass Logo over 4267	Acyclovir 400 mg	Zovirax by Ivax	00172-4267 Discontinued	Antiviral
400 <> 4267	Tab, White, Round, Hourglass Logo over 4267	Acyclovir 400 mg	Zovirax by Ivax	00182-8200 Discontinued	Antiviral
400 <> 4267	Tab, White, Round, Hourglass Logo over 4267	Acyclovir 400 mg	Zovirax by Amerisource	62584-0606	Antiviral
400 <> 4442	Tab, White, Oval, Hourglass Logo 4442 <> 400	Gabapentin 400 mg	Neurontin by Ivax	00172-4442 Discontinued	Anticonvulsant
400 <> A02	Tab, White, Oval	Acyclovir 400 mg	Zovirax by Mova	55370-0555	Antiviral
400 <> A04	Tab, White, Oval	Etodolac 400 mg	Lodine by Mova	55370-0552	NSAID
400 <> APO	Tab, Yellow, Oval	Ofloxacin 400 mg	Oflox by Apotex	Canadian DIN 02231532	Antibiotic
400 <> APO	Tab, Pink, Oblong	Pentoxifylline 400 mg	Trental by Apotex	Canadian DIN 02230090	Anticoagulant
400 <> APO041	Tab, White to Off-White, Oblong	Etodolac 400 mg	Lodine by Apotex	60505-0041	NSAID
400 <> C101	Tab, White, Round, Film Coated	Ibuprofen 400 mg	Motrin by Dr. Reddy's	55111-0101	NSAID
400 <> H3647	Tab, Light Orange, Oval, Film Coated	Telithromycin 400 mg	Ketek by Aventis	00088-2225	Antibiotic
400 <> IP131	Tab, White, Round, Film Coated	Ibuprofen 400 mg	Motrin by Major	00904-1748	NSAID
400 <> IP131	Tab, White, Round, Film Coated	Ibuprofen 400 mg	Motrin by Ivax	00182-1809 Discontinued	NSAID
400 <> IP131	Tab, White, Round, Film Coated	Ibuprofen 400 mg	Motrin by Amneal	65162-0568	NSAID
400 <> IP131	Tab, White, Round, Film Coated	Ibuprofen 400 mg	Motrin by Watson	00591-3464	NSAID
400 <> IP131	Tab, White, Round, Film Coated	Ibuprofen 400 mg	Motrin by Interpharm	53746-0131	NSAID
400 <> IP131	Tab, White, Round, Film Coated	Ibuprofen 400 mg	Motrin by Golden State	60429-0092	NSAID
400 <> IP131	Tab, White, Round, Film Coated	Ibuprofen 400 mg	Motrin by Rx Dispensing	61807-0027	NSAID
400 <> IP131	Tab, White, Round, Film Coated	Ibuprofen 400 mg	Motrin by Qualitest	00603-4018	NSAID
400 <> IP138	Tab, White, Round, Film Coated	Ibuprofen 400 mg	Motrin by Breckenridge	51991-0720	NSAID
400 <> N	Tab, Pink, Shield-Shaped, Compressed tablet	Acyclovir 400 mg	Zovirax by Novopharm	Canadian DIN 02285967	Antiviral
400 <> N	Tab, Gold, Oval	Ofloxacin 400 mg	Floxin by Novopharm	Canadian DIN 02243476	Antibiotic
400 <> N204	Tab, Green, Oval, Scored, Film Coated, Scored, N over 204	Cimetidine HCl 400 mg	Tagamet by Compumed	00403-1005	Gastrointestinal
400 <> N204	Tab, Green, Oval, Film Coated, Scored, N over 204	Cimetidine HCl 400 mg	Tagamet by Rx Dispensing	61807-0066	Gastrointestinal
400 <> N204	Tab, Dark Green, Oval, Scored, Film Coated, N over 204	Cimetidine HCl 400 mg	Tagamet by Teva	00093-8204 Discontinued	Gastrointestinal
400 <> N204	Tab, Green, Oval, Film Coated, Scored, N over 204	Cimetidine HCl 400 mg	Tagamet by Brightstone	62939-2131	Gastrointestinal
400 <> N204	Tab, Green, Oval, Film Coated, Scored, N over 204	Cimetidine HCl 400 mg	Tagamet by URL Mutual	00677-1529	Gastrointestinal
400 <> N204	Tab, Green, Oval, Film Coated, Scored, N over 204	Cimetidine HCl 400 mg	Tagamet by Medirex	57480-0814	Gastrointestinal
400 <> N204	Tab, Green, Oval, Film Coated, Scored, N over 204	Cimetidine HCl 400 mg	Tagamet by Warrick	59930-1802	Gastrointestinal
400 <> N943	Tab, Blue, Cap Shaped	Acyclovir 400 mg	Zovirax by UDL	51079-0877 Discontinued	Antiviral
400 <> N943	Tab, Blue, Cap Shaped	Acyclovir 400 mg	Zovirax by Major	00904-5232	Antiviral
400 <> N943	Tab, Blue, Cap Shaped	Acyclovir 400 mg	Zovirax by Warrick	59930-1576	Antiviral
400 <> N943	Tab, Blue, Cap Shaped	Acyclovir 400 mg	Zovirax by Teva	55953-0943	Antiviral
400 <> N943	Tab, Blue, Cap Shaped	Acyclovir 400 mg	Zovirax by Amerisource	62584-0437	Antiviral
400 <> N943	Tab, Blue, Cap Shaped	Acyclovir 400 mg	Zovirax by Teva	00093-8943	Antiviral

ID FRONT <> BACK	DESCRIPTION FRONT <> BACK	INGREDIENT & STRENGTH	BRAND (or Generic Equiv.) by FIRM	NDC#	CLASS; SCH.
400 <> NOVO	Tab, Green, Oval	Cimetidine 400 mg	Tagamet by Novopharm	Canadian DIN 00603678	Gastrointestinal
400 <> NOVO	Tab, White, Oval	Acebutolol HCl 400 mg	Monitan by Novopharm	Canadian DIN 02204533	Antihypertensive
400 <> NU	Tab, Pink, Cap Shaped	Pentoxifylline 400 mg	Trental by Nu Pharm	Canadian DIN 02230401	Anticoagulant
400 <> PAR162	Tab, White, Round, Film Coated, Par over 162	Ibuprofen 400 mg	Motrin by Ivax	00172-4018	NSAID
400 <> PAR162	Tab, White, Round, Film Coated, Par over 162	Ibuprofen 400 mg	Motrin by UDL	51079-0281 Discontinued	NSAID
400 <> PAR162	Tab, White, Round, Film Coated, Par over 162	Ibuprofen 400 mg	Motrin by Par	49884-0162	NSAID
400 <> PAR162	Tab, White, Round, Film Coated, Par over 162	Ibuprofen 400 mg	Motrin by Amerisource	62584-0746	NSAID
400 <> PAR162	Tab, White, Round, Film Coated, Par over 162	Ibuprofen 400 mg	Motrin by Rx Dispensing	61807-0027	NSAID
400 <> PAR162	Tab, White, Round, Film Coated, Par over 162	Ibuprofen 400 mg	Motrin by PDRX	55289-0590	NSAID
400 <> PD353	Tab, Tan, Oval, Film Coated	Troglitazone 400 mg	Rezulin by Parke Davis	00071-0353	Antidiabetic
400 <> PD353	Tab, Tan, Oval, Film Coated	Troglitazone 400 mg	Rezulin by Teva	00480-0756	Antidiabetic
400 <> SEROQUEL	Tab, Yellow, Cap Shaped. Film Coated	Quetiapine Fumarate 400 mg	Seroquel by AstraZeneca	00310-0279	Antipsychotic
400 <> SL	Tab, Dark Yellow to Brownish-Orange, Oval, Film Coated, Scored	Imatinib 400 mg	Gleevec by Novartis	00078-0438	Antineoplastic
400 <> SL	Tab, Dark Yellow to Brownish-Orange, Oval, Film Coated, Scored	Imatinib 400 mg	Gleevec by Novartis	Canadian DIN 02253283	Antineoplastic
400 <> TMC	Tab, Light Orange, Oval, Film Coated	Darunavir 400 mg	Prezista by Tibotec	59676-0561	Antiviral
400 <> UAD	Tab, White, Scored	Guaifenesin 400 mg, Pseudoephedrine HCl 120 mg	Sudafed Sinus by Forest	00785-6301	Cold Remedy
400000LLP17	Tab, White, Round	Penicillin G Potassium 400,000 Units	Pentids by Lederle		Antibiotic
4001 <> 0665	Tab	Medroxyprogesterone Acetate 10 mg	by Int'l Lab	00665-4001	Hormone
4001 <> 6666	Tab	Medroxyprogesterone Acetate 10 mg	by Apotheca	12634-0108	Hormone
4005R	Tab, 4005 and R inside Diamond	Meprobamate 200 mg	by Rugby	00536-4005	Sedative/Hypnotic; C IV
4005R	Tab, 4005 and R inside Diamond	Meprobamate 200 mg	by Chelsea	46193-0902	Sedative/Hypnotic; C IV
4006R	Tab, 4006 and R inside Diamond	Meprobamate 400 mg	by Rugby	00536-4006	Sedative/Hypnotic; C IV
4006R	Tab, 4006 and R inside Diamond	Meprobamate 400 mg	by Chelsea	46193-0901	Sedative/Hypnotic; C IV
400M40	Tab, White, Oblong, Scored	Cimetidine 400 mg	Tagamet by Dava	67253-0341	Gastrointestinal
400M40 <> MOVA	Tab, White, Oblong, Film Coated	Cimetidine HCl 400 mg	Tagamet by Compumed	00403-1067	Gastrointestinal
400M40 <> MOVA	Tab, White, Oblong, Film Coated	Cimetidine HCl 400 mg	Tagamet by Rosemont	00832-0103	Gastrointestinal
400M40 <> MOVA	Tab, White, Oblong, Film Coated	Cimetidine HCl 400 mg	Tagamet by Mova	55370-0136	Gastrointestinal
400M40 <> MOVA	Tab, White, Oblong, Film Coated	Cimetidine HCl 400 mg	Tagamet by Compumed		Gastrointestinal
400MCG <> 285	Tab, Gold, Round, 400 over mcg	Cerivastatin Sodium 0.4 mg	Baycol by Bayer	00026-2885	Antihyperlipidemic
400MCG <> 285	Tab, Gold, Round, 400 over mcg	Cerivastatin Sodium 0.4 mg	Baycol by DSM	63552-0031	Antihyperlipidemic
400MEDEVA	Cap, White & Yellow	Chlorpheniramine Maleate 4 mg, Pseudoephedrine HCl 60 mg	Atrohist by Adams	63824-0400	Cold Remedy
400MEDEVA	Cap, White & Yellow	Chlorpheniramine Maleate 4 mg, Pseudoephedrine HCl 60 mg	Atrohist Ped by Medeva	53014-0400	Cold Remedy
400MG <> T	Tab, Brown, Round, Film Coated, Ex Release	Carbamazepine XR 400 mg	Tegretol XR by Novartis	00083-0060	Anticonvulsant
400MG <> T	Tab, Brown, Round, Film Coated, Ex Release	Carbamazepine 400 mg	Tegretol by Physician Total Care	54868-3862	Anticonvulsant
400mg <> TMC	Tab, Light Orange, Oval, Film Coated	Darunavir 400 mg	Prezista by Janssen-Ortho	Canadian DIN 02324016	Antiviral
400MONITAN	Tab, White, Oblong	Acebutolol HCl 400 mg	Sectral by Wyeth	Canadian	Antihypertensive
400N <> 204	Tab, Light Green, Film Coated	Cimetidine HCl 400 mg	Tagamet by Schein	00364-2593	Gastrointestinal
401 <> MYLAN	Tab, Coated, Beveled Edge	Ibuprofen 400 mg	Motrin by Mylan	00378-0401	NSAID
402	Cap, Green & Yellow, Schering Logo 402	Theophylline Anhydrous LA 125 mg	Theovent by Schering		Antiasthmatic
402	Tab, White, Scored, 402 Prasco Logo	Hyoscyamine Sulfate 0.15 mg	Levsin by Prasco	66993-0402	Gastrointestinal
402 <> C	Tab, Peach, Round, Film Coated	Tiagabine 2 mg	Gabitril by Cephalon	63459-0402	Anticonvulsant
402 <> DP	Tab, Yellow, Cap Shaped, Scored	Pseudoephedrine HCl 120 mg, Guaifenesin 600 mg	by Duramed	51285-0402	Cold Remedy

ID FRONT <> BACK	DESCRIPTION FRONT <> BACK	INGREDIENT & STRENGTH	BRAND (or Generic Equiv.) by FIRM	NDC#	CLASS; SCH.
402 <> P&G	Tab, White, Rectangular	Etidronate Disodium 200 mg	Didronel by Proc & Gamble	Canadian DIN 01997629	Calcium Metabolism
402 <> P&G	Tab, White, Rectangular	Etidronate Disodium 200 mg	Didronel by Pharm Util	60491-0801	Calcium Metabolism
402 <> P&G	Tab, White, Rectangular	Etidronate Disodium 200 mg	Didronel by DRX	55045-2326	Calcium Metabolism
402 <> P&G	Tab, White, Rectangular	Etidronate Disodium 200 mg	Didronel by Procter and Gamble	00149-0405	Calcium Metabolism
402400	Tab, Yellow, Oblong, Royce Logo 402/400	Etodolac 400 mg	Lodine by Royce		NSAID
402402	Cap, Clear, White Powder, Ex Release	Phenytoin Sodium 100 mg	Dilantin by Caraco	62756-0402	Anticonvulsant
402MEDEVA	Cap, Clear & Green, White Beads	Guaifenesin 300 mg	Robitussin by Medeva	53014-0402	Expectorant
402MEDEVA	Cap, Clear & Green, White Beads	Guaifenesin 300 mg	Robitussin by Adams	63824-0402	Expectorant
403	Tab, Red, Round	Pseudoephedrine 30 mg	Sudafed by Ivax	00182-1459	Decongestant
403 <> PMS	Tab, Pink, Round	Sennosides 12 mg	Senokot by Pharmascience	Canadian DIN 00896403	Laxative
4036 <> 1	Tab, White, Square, Hourglass Logo 1	Estazolam 1 mg	Prosom by Ivax	00172-4036	Sedative/Hypnotic; C IV
4037 <> 2	Tab, Pink, Square, Hourglass Logo 2	Estazolam 2 mg	Prosom by Ivax	00172-4037	Sedative/Hypnotic; C IV
404 <> C	Tab, Yellow, Round, Film Coated	Tiagabine 4 mg	Gabitril by Cephalon	63459-0404	Anticonvulsant
404SEMPREXD	Cap, Dark Green & White, Yellow Band	Acrivastine 8 mg, Pseudoephedrine HCl 60 mg	Semprex D by Celltech	53014-0404	Cold Remedy
405 <> WATSON	Tab, White, Round	Lisinopril 2.5 mg	Prinivil by Watson	00591-0405	Antihypertensive
4059	Tab, White, Oval, Ivax Logo / 4059	Cefadroxil 1000 mg	Duricef by Ivax	00172-4059 Discontinued	Antibiotic
4059 <> 93	Tab, White, Oval, Scored, 9 / 3	Cefadroxil 1000 mg	Duricef by Teva	00093-4059	Antibiotic
405HD	Tab, Pink, Round	Amitriptyline HCl 10 mg	Elavil by Halsey	Discontinued	Antidepressant
406	Cap	Indomethacin 50 mg	Indocin by URL Mutual	00677-0873	NSAID
406 <> NE	Tab, White, Cap Shaped, Scored	Etidronate Disodium 400 mg	Didronel by Pharm Util	60491-0802	Calcium Metabolism
406 <> NE	Tab, White, Cap Shaped, Scored	Etidronate Disodium 400 mg	Didronel by Procter and Gamble	00149-0406	Calcium Metabolism
406 <> WATSON	Tab, White, Cap Shaped	Lisinopril 5 mg	Prinivil by Watson	00591-0406	Antihypertensive
4067	Tab, White, Round	Codeine Phosphate 30 mg, Aspirin 380 mg, Caffeine 30 mg	A.S.A. by Eli Lilly		Analgesic; C III
406HD	Tab, Green, Round	Amitriptyline HCl 25 mg	Elavil by Halsey	Discontinued	Antidepressant
407HD	Tab, Brown, Round	Amitriptyline HCl 50 mg	Elavil by Halsey	Discontinued	Antidepressant
408HD	Tab, Purple, Round	Amitriptyline HCl 75 mg	Elavil by Halsey	Discontinued	Antidepressant
4098 <> 500	Tab, Light Yellow, Oval, Film Coated, Double-Triangle Logo	Nabumetone 500 mg	Relafen by Par	49884-0649	NSAID
4099 <> 750	Tab, Dark Yellow, Oval, Film Coated, Double-Triangle Logo	Nabumetone 750 mg	Relafen by Par	49884-0650	NSAID
409HD	Tab, Orange, Round	Amitriptyline HCl 100 mg	Elavil by Halsey	Discontinued	Antidepressant
40MG <> AEI	Tab, Pink, Oblong, Delayed-Release	Esomeprazole 40 mg	Nexium by AstraZeneca	Canadian DIN 02244522	Proton Pump Inhibitor
40MG <> FP	Tab, White, Oval, Scored, Film Coated	Citalopram 40 mg	Celexa by Forest	00456-4040	Antidepressant
40MG <> IL	Tab, White, Oval, Scored, Film Coated, I / L	Citalopram HBr 40 mg	Celexa by Inwood	00258-3697	Antidepressant
41 <> BMS250	Tab, White, Hexagonal	Nefazodone HCl 250 mg	Serzone by Par	49884-0574	Antidepressant
41 <> BMS250	Tab, White, Hexagonal	Nefazodone HCl 250 mg	Serzone by BMS	00087-0041	Antidepressant
41 <> BMS250	Tab, White, Hexagonal	Nefazodone HCl 250 mg	Serzone by Kaiser	00179-1244	Antidepressant
41 <> BMS250	Tab, White, Hexagonal	Nefazodone HCl 250 mg	Serzone by BMS	15548-0041	Antidepressant
41 <> C	Tab, White to Off White, Oval, Scored	Torsemide 5 mg	Demadex by Aurobindo	65862-0125	Diuretic
41 <> DP	Tab, Green, Round, Film Coated, 41 <> dp	Conjugated Estrogens 0.3 mg	Cenestin by Barr	51285-0441	Hormone
41 <> ELAVIL	Tab, Beige, Round, Film Coated	Amitriptyline HCl 50 mg	Elavil by Zeneca	00310-0041	Antidepressant
41 <> G	Tab, White, Round	Carvediol 6.25 mg	Coreg by Glenmark	68462-0163	Antihypertensive
41 <> GG	Tab, Yellow, Round	Imipramine HCl 10 mg	Tofranil by Sandoz	00781-1762	Antidepressant
41 <> GSK	Tab, Yellow, Triangular (Rounded), GSK <> 4/1	Rosiglitazone Maleate 4 mg, Glimepiride 1 mg	Avandaryl by GSK	00007-3151	Antidiabetic
41 <> GSK	Tab, Yellow, Triangular (Rounded), GSK <> 4/1	Rosiglitazone Maleate 4 mg, Glimepiride 1 mg	Avandaryl by GSK	Canadian DIN 02258781	Antidiabetic
41000 <> GSK	Tab, Pink, Oval, Film Coated, 4/1000	Metformin HCl 1000 mg, Rosiglitazone 4 mg	Avandamet by GSK	Canadian DIN 02248441	Antidiabetic

ID FRONT <> BACK	DESCRIPTION FRONT <> BACK	INGREDIENT & STRENGTH	BRAND (or Generic Equiv.) by FIRM	NDC#	CLASS; SCH.
41000 <> GSK	Tab, Pink, Oval, Film Coated, 4/1000	Metformin HCl 1000 mg, Rosiglitazone 4 mg	Avandamet by SKB	00007-3164	Antidiabetic
4107 <> Z	Tab	Naproxen 250 mg	Naprosyn by Quality Care	60346-0816	NSAID
411 <> COPLEY	Tab, White, Square	Methazolamide 25 mg	Neptazane by Teva	3245-0411 Discontinued	Antiglaucoma Agent
411 <> PMS	Tab, White, Round	Sennosides 8.6 mg	Senokot by Pharmascience	Canadian DIN 00896411	Laxative
411 <> USE	Tab, Scored, US over E	Nitroglycerin 2.6 mg	Nitrong by RPR	00075-0221	Vasodilator
4116 <> LILLY	Tab, White, Round, Film Coated, Imprint in Blue Ink	Olanzapine 7.5 mg	Zyprexa by PDRX		Antipsychotic
4117 <> LILLY	Tab, White, Round, Film Coated, Imprint in Blue Ink	Olanzapine 10 mg	Zyprexa by PDRX		Antipsychotic
4117 <> W	Tab, Orange, Film Coated	Ethionamide 250 mg	Trecator by Wyeth	00008-4117	Antituberculosis
412	Tab, Pink, Oblong, Savage Logo 412	Magnesium Salicylate 545 mg	Magan by Adria		Analgesic
412 <> C	Tab, Green, Oval, Film Coated	Tiagabine 12 mg	Gabitril by Cephalon	63459-0412	Anticonvulsant
412 <> USE	Tab, Scored, Film Coated, US over E	Nitroglycerin 6.5 mg	Nitrong by RPR	00075-0274	Vasodilator
41200665	Cap, Black Print, Ex Release	Valproic Acid 250 mg	Depakene by Int'l Lab	00665-4120	Anticonvulsant
4125 <> WYETH	Tab, Light Green, Ex Release	Isosorbide Dinitrate 40 mg	Isordil by Wyeth	00008-4125	Antianginal
413 <> ETHEX	Tab, White, Cap Shaped, Scored	Guaifenesin 800 mg, Pseudoephedrine HCl 80 mg	Panmist LA by Ethex	58177-0413	Cold Remedy
4131	Tab, Ivory, Rectangular, 4131/Logo	Pergolide Mesylate 0.05 mg	Permax by Draxis	Canadian Discontinued	Antiparkinson
4133	Tab, Green, Rectangular, 4133/Logo	Pergolide Mesylate 0.25 mg	Permax by Draxis	Canadian Discontinued	Antiparkinson
4135	Tab, Pink, Rectangular, Draxis Logo	Pergolide Mesylate 1 mg	Permax by Draxis	Canadian Discontinued	Antiparkinson
414	Tab, White to Off-White, Cap Shaped	Ezetimibe 10 mg	Zetia by Schering	66582-0414	Antihyperlipidemic
414	Tab, White to Off-White, Cap Shaped	Ezetimibe 10 mg	Ezetrol by Merck Frosst	Canadian DIN 02247521	Antihyperlipidemic
414 <> ETHEX	Tab, White, Cap Shaped	Guaifenesin 600 mg, Pseudoephedrine HCl 45 mg, Dextromethorphan HBr 30 mg	Pseudovent DM by Ethex	58177-0414	Cold Remedy
4140 <> V	Tab	Meclizine HCl 12.5 mg	by Qualitest	00603-4319	Antiemetic
4142	Tab, White, Oblong, "Wave" Logo <> 4142	Dronedarone 400 mg	Multaq by Sanofi	00024-4142	Antiarrhythmic
415 <> ETHEX	Tab, Pink & Beige, Oval	Vitamin A 3,000 IU, Vitamin D 400 IU, Vitamin E 22 mg, Vitamin C 120 mg, Folic Acid 1 mg, Vitamin B1 1.8 mg, Vitamin B2 4 mg, Niacinamide 20 mg, Vitamin B6 25 mg, B12 12 mcg, Calcium 200 mg, Copper 2 mg, Iron 28 mg, Zinc 25 mg, Magnesium 25 mg	NatalCare 3 by Ethex	58177-0415	Vitamin
416 <> C	Tab, Blue, Oval, Film Coated	Tiagabine 16 mg	Gabitril by Cephalon	63459-0416	Anticonvulsant
416 <> ETH	Tab, Tan, Round	Lipase 8000 Units, Amylase 30,000 Units, Protease 30,000 Units	Plaretase by Ethex	58177-0416	Gastrointestinal
4160665	Cap, Red Print	Lithium Carbonate 300 mg	Eskalith by URL Mutual	00677-1092	Antipsychotic
4160665	Cap, Red Print	Lithium Carbonate 300 mg	Eskalith by Schein	00364-0855	Antipsychotic
4160665	Cap, Red Print	Lithium Carbonate 300 mg	Eskalith by Int'l Lab	00665-4160	Antipsychotic
4165	Tab, White, Blue Print, Oval	Raloxifene HCl 60 mg	Evista by Eli Lilly	Canadian DIN 02239028	Antiosteoporosis
417 <> COPLEY	Tab, Light Blue	Metoprolol Tartrate 100 mg	Lopressor by Teva	38245-0417	Antihypertensive
417 <> MYLAN	Tab, Peach, Scored	Bumetanide 2 mg	Bumex by Mylan	00378-0417	Diuretic
4171V	Tab, White, Round	Meperidine HCl 50 mg	Demerol by Qualitest	00603-4415	Analgesic; C II
4172V	Tab, White, Round	Meperidine HCl 100 mg	Demerol by Qualitest	00603-4416	Analgesic; C II
4174 <> 500	Tab, White, Cap Shaped, Hourglass Logo 4174	Etodolac 500 mg	Lodine by Ivax	00172-4174	NSAID
4175 <> 400	Tab, White, Cap Shaped, Hourglass Logo 4175	Etodolac 400 mg	Lodine by Ivax	00172-4175	NSAID
4175 <> 400	Tab, White, Cap Shaped, Hourglass Logo 4175	Etodolac 400 mg	Lodine by Qualitest	00603-3570	NSAID
4175 <> 400	Tab, White, Cap Shaped, Hourglass Logo 4175	Etodolac 400 mg	Lodine by Heartland	61392-0917	NSAID
418 <> ETHEX	Tab, Pink, Oval, Gloss Coated	Prenatal Multivitamin	Natalcare GlossTabs by Ethex	58177-0418	Vitamin
418 <> WATSON	Tab, White, Round, Film Coated	Cyclobenzaprine HCl 10 mg	Flexeril by DHHS Prog	118819-0069	Muscle Relaxant

ID FRONT <> BACK	DESCRIPTION FRONT <> BACK	INGREDIENT & STRENGTH	BRAND (or Generic Equiv.) by FIRM	NDC#	CLASS; SCH.
418 <> WATSON	Tab, White, Round, Film Coated	Cyclobenzaprine HCl 10 mg	Flexeril by Watson	52544-0418	Muscle Relaxant
418 <> WATSON	Tab, White, Round, Film Coated	Cyclobenzaprine HCl 10 mg	Flexeril by Apotheca	12634-0528	Muscle Relaxant
418 <> WATSON	Tab, White, Round, Film Coated	Cyclobenzaprine HCl 10 mg	Flexeril by Prepackage Specialists	58864-0128	Muscle Relaxant
419 <> BARR	Tab, White, Round, Film Coated	Ibuprofen 400 mg	Motrin by Barr	00555-0419 Discontinued	NSAID
4194 <> 500	Tab, Blue, Oval, Ex Release, Hourglass Logo 4194	Cefaclor 500 mg	Ceclor by Ivax	00172-4194	Antibiotic
4195 <> 25	Tab, Yellow, Round, Scored, Hourglass Logo over 4195 <> 2.5	Enalapril Maleate 2.5 mg	Vasotec by Ivax	00172-4195 Discontinued	Antihypertensive
4196 <> 5	Tab, White, Round, Scored, Hourglass Logo over 4196	Enalapril Maleate 5 mg	Vasotec by Ivax	00172-4196 Discontinued	Antihypertensive
4196 <> 5	Tab, White, Round, Scored, W over 924	Enalapril Maleate 5 mg	Vasotec by Ivax	00172-4196	Antihypertensive
4197 <> 10	Tab, Pink, Round	Enalapril Maleate 10 mg	Vasotec by Ivax	00172-4197 Discontinued	Antihypertensive
4197 <> 10	Tab, Pink, Round, Hourglass Logo over 4197	Enalapril Maleate 10 mg	Vasotec by Ivax		Antihypertensive
4198 <> 20	Tab, Peach, Round, Hourglass Logo over 4198	Enalapril Maleate 20 mg	Vasotec by Ivax		Antihypertensive
4198 <> 20	Tab, Peach, Round	Enalapril Maleate 20 mg	Vasotec by Ivax	00172-4198 Discontinued	Antihypertensive
42 <> C	Tab, White to Off White, Oval, Scored	Torsemide 10 mg	Demadex by Aurobindo	65862-0126	Diuretic
42 <> DP	Tab, Red, Round, Film Coated, 42 <> dp	Conjugated Estrogens 0.625 mg	Cenestin by Barr	51285-0442	Hormone
42 <> ELAVIL	Tab, Orange, Round, Film Coated	Amitriptyline HCl 75 mg	Elavil by Zeneca	00310-0042	Antidepressant
42 <> GG	Tab, Green, Round, Film Coated	Imipramine HCl 50 mg	Tofranil by Sandoz	00781-1766	Antidepressant
42 <> GSK	Tab, Orange, Triangular (Rounded), GSK <> 4/2	Rosiglitazone Maleate 4 mg, Glimepiride 2 mg	Avandaryl by GSK	Canadian DIN 02258803	Antidiabetic
42 <> GSK	Tab, Orange, Triangular (Rounded), GSK <> 4/2	Rosiglitazone Maleate 4 mg, Glimepiride 2 mg	Avandaryl by GSK	00007-3152	Antidiabetic
420	Tab, White, Round, Sugar-Coated, Circle around 420	Ibuprofen 200 mg	Motrin by OHM		NSAID
420	Tab, White, Round, Sugar-Coated, Circle around 420	Ibuprofen 200 mg	Motrin by UDL	51079-0731 Discontinued	NSAID
420	Tab, White, Round, Sugar-Coated, Circle around 420	Ibuprofen 200 mg	Motrin by Ivax	00182-8688 Discontinued	NSAID
420 <> B	Tab, White, Cap Shaped, Ex Release	Diltiazem HCl 420 mg	Cardizem LA by Biovail	64455-0105	Antihypertensive
420 <> BARR	Tab, White, Oval, Film Coated	Ibuprofen 600 mg	Motrin by Barr	00555-0420 Discontinued	NSAID
420 <> BARR	Tab, White, Oval, Film Coated	Ibuprofen 600 mg	Motrin by Barr		NSAID
420 <> C	Tab, Pink, Oval, Film Coated	Tiagabine 20 mg	Gabitril by Cephalon	63459-0420	Anticonvulsant
420 <> S	Tab, White, Round	Atenolol 25 mg	Tenormin by Dava	67253-0420	Antihypertensive
421	Tab, Yellow, Cap Shaped, Film Coated, Scored	Paroxetine 10 mg	Paxil by Caraco	57664-0421	Antidepressant
421 <> MYLAN	Tab, Beige, Cap Shaped, Film Coated	Methyldopa 500 mg	Aldomet by Mylan	00378-0421	Antihypertensive
421 <> MYLAN	Tab, Beige, Cap Shaped, Film Coated	Methyldopa 500 mg	Aldomet by UDL	51079-0201	Antihypertensive
4211V	Tab, White, Round	Methocarbamol 500 mg	Robaxin by Qualitest	00603-4485	Muscle Relaxant
4212 <> V	Tab, White, Oblong	Methocarbamol 750 mg	Robaxin by Qualitest	00603-4486	Muscle Relaxant
4214 <> 25	Tab, Light Yellow, Round, Film Coated, Blue Ink, 2.5 <> 4214	Saxagliptin 2.5 mg	Onglyza by BMS	00003-4214	Antidiabetic
4215 <> 5	Tab, Pink, Round, Film Coated, Blue Ink	Saxagliptin 5 mg	Onglyza by BMS	00003-4215	Antidiabetic
4216V <> 4	Tab, White, Oval	Methylprednisolone 4 mg	Medrol by Vintage	00254-4216	Steroid
422	Tab, White to Off White, Film Coated, Cap Shaped, Scored	Paroxetine 20 mg	Paxil by Caraco	57664-0422	Antidepressant
422 <> RDY	Tab, White, Oblong, Ex Release	Ciprofloxacin 500 mg	Cipro XR by Dr. Reddy's	55111-0422	Antibiotic
422 <> S	Tab, White, Round	Atenolol 100 mg	Tenormin by Dava	67253-0422	Antihypertensive
4220	Tab	Cefaclor 375 mg	Ceclor CD by Eli Lilly	00110-4220	Antibiotic
4220	Tab	Cefaclor 375 mg	Ceclor CD by Dura	51479-0036	Antibiotic
4221	Tab	Cefaclor 500 mg	Ceclor CD by Eli Lilly	00110-4221	Antibiotic

ID FRONT <> BACK	DESCRIPTION FRONT <> BACK	INGREDIENT & STRENGTH	BRAND (or Generic Equiv.) by FIRM	NDC#	CLASS; SCH.
4221	Tab	Cefaclor 500 mg	Ceclor CD by Dura	51479-0035	Antibiotic
4226 <> Z	Tab, Peach, Round	Guanabenz Acetate 4 mg	Wytensin by Ivax	00172-4226	Antihypertensive
4227 <> Z	Tab, Gray, Round	Guanabenz Acetate 8 mg	Wytensin by Ivax	00172-4227	Antihypertensive
423 <> E	Tab, White, Round	Hyoscyamine Sulfate 0.125 mg	NuLev by Ethex	58177-0423	Gastrointestinal
423 <> RDY	Tab, White, Oblong, Ex Release	Ciprofloxacin 1000 mg	Cipro XR by Dr. Reddy's	55111-0423	Antibiotic
4234 <> V	Tab, White, Oval	Metoclopramide 5 mg	Reglan by Qualitest	00603-4614	Gastrointestinal
4235 <> V	Tab, White, Oval	Metoclopramide 10 mg	Reglan by Qualitest	00603-4615	Gastrointestinal
424 <> C	Tab, Blue, Film Coated, Cap Shaped	Paroxetine 30 mg	Paxil by Caraco	57664-0424	Antidepressant
425 <> C	Tab, Green, Film Coated, Cap Shaped	Paroxetine 40 mg	Paxil by Caraco	57664-0425	Antidepressant
425 <> P	Tab, White, Round, Scored	Atropine Sulfate 0.0194 mg, Scopolamine HBr 0.0065 mg, Hyoscyamine HBr 0.1037 mg, Phenobarbital 16.2 mg	Donnatal by PBM	66213-0425	Gastrointestinal; C IV
4259 <> Z	Tab, White, Round	Indapamide 2.5 mg	Lozol by Ivax	00172-4259 Discontinued	Diuretic
4259 <> Z	Tab, White, Round	Indapamide 2.5 mg	Lozol by Ivax	00182-2610 Discontinued	Diuretic
4259 <> Z	Tab, White, Round	Indapamide 2.5 mg	Lozol by Qualitest	00603-4061	Diuretic
4259 <> Z	Tab, White, Round	Indapamide 2.5 mg	Lozol by Major	00904-5074	Diuretic
4259 <> Z	Tab, White, Round	Indapamide 2.5 mg	Lozol by Physician Total Care	54868-3106	Diuretic
4259 <> Z	Tab, White, Round	Indapamide 2.5 mg	Lozol by Sandoz	00781-1051	Diuretic
4259 <> Z	Tab, White, Round	Indapamide 2.5 mg	Lozol by Qualitest	00603-4161	Diuretic
426 <> ETHEX	Tab, White, Oblong, Scored	Chlorpheniramine Maleate 8 mg, Pseudoephedrine HCl 120 mg, Methscopolamine Nitrate 2.5 mg	Hista-Vent PSE by Ethex	58177-0426	Cold Remedy
42616	Tab, White, Round	Aspirin 325 mg	Aspirin by Pennex Labs		Analgesic
4266200	Cap, White, Opaque	Acyclovir 200 mg	Zovirax by Watson		Antiviral
4267 <> 400	Tab, White, Round, Hourglass Logo over 4267	Acyclovir 400 mg	Zovirax by Ivax	00182-8200 Discontinued	Antiviral
4267 <> 400	Tab, White, Round, Hourglass Logo over 4267	Acyclovir 400 mg	Zovirax by Ivax	00172-4267	Antiviral
4267 <> 400	Tab, White, Round, Hourglass Logo over 4267	Acyclovir 400 mg	Zovirax by Amerisource	62584-0606	Antiviral
4268 <> 800	Tab, White, Oval, Hourglass Logo 4268	Acyclovir 800 mg	Zovirax by Ivax	00172-4268 Discontinued	Antiviral
4268 <> 800	Tab, White, Oval, Hourglass Logo 4268	Acyclovir 800 mg	Zovirax by Ivax	00182-2667 Discontinued	Antiviral
427 <> ETHEX	Tab, Yellow, Cap Shaped, Scored	Pseudoephedrine HCl 120 mg, Methscopolamine Nitrate 2.5 mg	HistaClear by Ethex	58177-0427 Discontinued	Cold Remedy
427 <> MYLAN	Tab, Yellowish Orange, Round	Sulindac 150 mg	Clinoril by Mylan	00378-0427	NSAID
427 <> MYLAN	Tab, Yellowish Orange, Round	Sulindac 150 mg	Clinoril by UDL	51079-0666 Discontinued	NSAID
427 <> ZANTAC150	Tab	Ranitidine HCl 168 mg	Zantac Efferdose by GSK	60937-0427	Gastrointestinal
4270V	Cap	Acetaminophen 325 mg, Dichloralantipyrine 100 mg, Isometheptene Mucate (1:1) 65 mg	Migquin by Vintage	00254-4270	Analgesic; C IV
427COPLEY	Tab, Pink, Round, 427/Copley	Diclofenac Sodium 75 mg	Voltaren by Copley	38245-0427	NSAID
4285	Cap, Dark Red, Opaque, Gelatin, Scherer Logo 4285	Ascorbic Acid 250 mg, Cyanocobalamin 10 mcg, Ferrous Fumarate 200 mg, Stomach Extract 100 mg	Chromagen by RP Scherer	11014-0222	Vitamin
4285	Cap, Maroon, Savage Logo 4285	Vitamin, Iron	Chromagen by Savage	00281-4285	Vitamin
429	Tab, White, Round, Scored	Fludrocortisone Acetate 0.1 mg	Florinef Acetate by King	61570-0190	Steroid
429 <> RDY	Tab, White, Round, Film Coated	Metformin HCl 500 mg	Glucophage by Dr. Reddy's	55111-0429	Antidiabetic
43 <> C	Tab, White to Off White, Oval, Scored	Torsemide 20 mg	Demadex by Aurobindo	65862-0127	Diuretic
43 <> DP	Tab, White, Round, Film Coated, 43 <> dp	Conjugated Estrogens 0.9 mg	Cenestin by Barr	51285-0443	Hormone
43 <> ELAVIL	Tab, Mauve, Round, Film Coated	Amitriptyline HCl 100 mg	Elavil by Zeneca	00310-0043	Antidepressant

ID FRONT <> BACK	DESCRIPTION FRONT <> BACK	INGREDIENT & STRENGTH	BRAND (or Generic Equiv.) by FIRM	NDC#	CLASS; SCH.
43 <> ELAVIL	Tab, Reddish Purple, Round, Film Coated	Amitriptyline HCl 100 mg	Elavil by Merck	00006-0435	Antidepressant
430 <> GG	Tab, Green, Cap Shaped	Cimetidine HCl 800 mg	Tagamet by Sandoz	00781-1444	Gastrointestinal
430 <> RDY	Tab, White, Cap Shaped, Film Coated	Metformin HCl 850 mg	Glucophage by Dr. Reddy's	55111-0430	Antidiabetic
4303	Tab, Yellow, Oval, Scored, Logo 4303	Clozapine 12.5 mg	Clozaril by Ivax	00172-4303 Discontinued	Antipsychotic
4306 <> 0115	Tab	Promethazine HCl 25 mg	by Global	00115-4306	Antiemetic; Antihistamine
431	Tab, Red Print, Film Coated, Schering Logo 431	Albuterol Sulfate 4 mg	Proventil by Leiner	59606-0771	Antiasthmatic
431	Tab, Red Print, Film Coated, Schering Logo 431	Albuterol Sulfate 4 mg	Proventil by Thrift Drug	59198-0318	Antiasthmatic
431	Tab, Red Print, Film Coated, Schering Logo 431	Albuterol Sulfate 4 mg	Proventil by Med Pro	53978-0820	Antiasthmatic
431	Tab, Red Print, Film Coated, Schering Logo 431	Albuterol Sulfate 4 mg	Proventil by Allscripts		Antiasthmatic
431	Tab, Red Print, Film Coated, Schering Logo 431	Albuterol Sulfate 4 mg	Proventil by Pharmedix	53002-1036	Antiasthmatic
431 <> RDY	Tab, White, Oval, Film Coated, Scored, RD / Y <> 43 / 1	Metformin HCl 1000 mg	Glucophage by Dr. Reddy's	55111-0431	Antidiabetic
431COPLEY	Tab, Pink, Round, 431/Copley	Diclofenac Sodium 25 mg	Voltaren by Copley		NSAID
432 <> ETH	Tab, Yellow, Round, Chewable, Vanilla Flavor	Fluoride Ion 0.25 mg	Luride by Ethex	58177-0432	Mineral
4324RUGBY	Tab	Prednisone 5 mg	by Pharmedix	53002-0352	Steroid
433 <> ETH	Tab, White, Round, Chewable, Grape Flavor	Fluoride Ion 0.50 mg	EtheDent by Ethex	58177-0433	Mineral
433 <> M	Tab, Peach, Round, Film Coated	Bupropion HCl 75 mg	Wellbutrin by Mylan	00378-0433	Antidepressant
433 <> M	Tab, Peach, Round, Film Coated	Bupropion HCl 75 mg	Wellbutrin by UDL	51079-0943	Antidepressant
4330 <> 850	Tab, White, Oval, Hourglass Logo 4330	Metformin HCl 850 mg	Glucophage by Ivax	00172-4330 Discontinued	Antidiabetic
4331 <> 500	Tab, White, Oval, Hourglass Logo 4331	Metformin HCl 500 mg	Glucophage by Ivax	00172-4331 Discontinued	Antidiabetic
4332 <> 100	Tab, Peach, Oval, Scored, Logo 4332 <> 100	Nefazodone 100 mg	Serzone by Ivax	00172-4332	Antidepressant
4333 <> 150	Tab, Peach, Round, Scored, Logo 4333 <> 150	Nefazodone 150 mg	Serzone by Ivax	00172-4333	Antidepressant
4334 <> 200	Tab, Peach, Oval, Logo 4334 <> 200	Nefazodone 200 mg	Serzone by Ivax	00172-4334	Antidepressant
433433 <> GLYBUR	Tab, Pink, Oblong, Scored	Glyburide 2.5 mg	DiaBeta by Coventry	61372-0577	Antidiabetic
433433 <> GLYBUR	Tab, Pink, Oblong, Scored	Glyburide 2.5 mg	DiaBeta by Teva	38245-0433	Antidiabetic
433433 <> GLYBUR	Tab, Pink, Oblong, Scored	Glyburide 2.5 mg	DiaBeta by Blue Ridge	59273-0014	Antidiabetic
433433 <> GLYBUR	Tab, Pink, Oblong, Scored	Glyburide 2.5 mg	DiaBeta by Merrell	00068-3201	Antidiabetic
4335 <> 250	Tab, Peach, Round, Logo 4335 <> 250	Nefazodone 250 mg	Serzone by Ivax	00172-4335	Antidepressant
43385	Cap, Orange and White, Hourglass Logo 4338 / 5	Terazosin HCl 5 mg	Hytrin by Ivax	00172-4338	Antihypertensive
433COPLEY	Tab, Pink, Oblong, 433/Copley	Glyburide 2.5 mg	Micronase by Copley		Antidiabetic
434	Tab, White to Off-White, Round, Raised Hexagon <> 434	Allopurinol 100 mg	Zyloprim by Caraco	57664-0434	Antigout
434 <> ETH	Tab, Red, Round, Chewable, Cherry Flavor	Fluoride Ion 1.0 mg	Luride by Ethex	58177-0434	Mineral
4343 <> 50	Tab, Peach, Oval, Logo 4343 <> 50	Nefazodone 50 mg	Sezone by Ivax	00172-4343	Antidepressant
434640MG	Cap, Light Blue, Opaque	Fluoxetine 40 mg	Prozac by Ivax	00172-4346 Discontinued	Antidepressant
434640MG	Cap, Light Blue, Opaque	Fluoxetine 40 mg	Prozac by Teva	00093-7198	Antidepressant
4348 <> 600	Tab, White, Oval, Scored, Hourglass Logo / 4348	Oxaprozin 600 mg	Daypro by Ivax	00172-4348 Discontinued	NSAID
435	Tab, White to Off-White, Round, Film Coated	Metformin HCl 850 mg	Glucophage by Caraco	57664-0435	Antidiabetic
435 <> ETHEX	Tab, Yellow, Oval	Vitamin C 60 mg, Iron 90 mg, Vitamin D3 400 IU, Vitamin E 30 IU, Vitamin B1 2 mg, Vitamin B2 3 mg, Vitamin B6 3 mg, Folic Acid 1 mg, Magnesium 25 mg, Zinc 20 mg, Copper 2 mg, Vitamin A 3500 IU, Vitamin B12 12 mcg, Dioctylsulfosuccinate Sodium 50 mg	Care Nate 600 by Ethex	58177-0437	Vitamin; Supplement
435 <> M	Tab, Light Blue, Round, Film Coated	Bupropion HCl 100 mg	Wellbutrin by Mylan	00378-0435	Antidepressant
435 <> M	Tab, Light Blue, Round, Film Coated	Bupropion HCl 100 mg	Wellbutrin by UDL	51079-0944	Antidepressant
4354	Tab, White, Round, Scored	Isoniazid 100 mg	Laniazid by Southwood	58016-0912	Antimycobacterial
435620MG	Cap, Aqua Blue, Black Print, Opaque, Hourglass Logo 4356 over 20 mg	Fluoxetine HCl 20 mg	Prozac by Ivax	00093-4356	Antidepressant

ID FRONT <> BACK	DESCRIPTION FRONT <> BACK	INGREDIENT & STRENGTH	BRAND (or Generic Equiv.) by FIRM	NDC#	CLASS; SCH.
435620MG	Cap, Aqua Blue Opaque	Fluoxetine 20 mg	Prozac by Teva	00172-4356	Antidepressant
435620MG	Cap, White to Off White Cap, Aqua Blue Opaque Body	Fluoxetine 20 mg	Prozac by Teva	00093-4356	Antidepressant
4357 <> 150	Tab, Beige, Round	Ranitidine HCl 150 mg	Zantac by Ivax	00172-4357 Discontinued	Gastrointestinal
4359 <> 25	Tab, Pale Yellow, Round, Hourglass Logo over 4359	Clozapine 25 mg	Clozaril by Dixon Shane	17236-0357	Antipsychotic
4359 <> 25	Tab, Pale Yellow, Round, Hourglass Logo over 4359	Clozapine 25 mg	Clozaril by Ivax	00093-4359	Antipsychotic
436	Tab, White to Off-White, Round, Raised Hexagon <> 436	Allopurinol 300 mg	Zyloprim by Caraco	57664-0436	Antigout
436 <> ETHEX	Tab, Yellow, Round, Chewable	Calcium Carbonate 600 mg	Care Nate 600 by Ethex	58177-0437	Vitamin; Supplement
4360 <> 100	Tab, Pale Yellow, Round, Hourglass Logo over 4360	Clozapine 100 mg	Clozaril by Dixon Shane	17236-0356	Antipsychotic
4360 <> 100	Tab, Pale Yellow, Round, Hourglass Logo over 4360	Clozapine 100 mg	Clozaril by Ivax	00172-4360 Discontinued	Antipsychotic
436310MG	Cap, Aqua Blue & White, Black Print, Opaque, 4363 over 10 mg	Fluoxetine HCl 10 mg	Prozac by Ivax	00172-4363 Discontinued	Antidepressant
436310MG	Cap, Aqua Blue Opaque Cap, White Opaque Body	Fluoxetine 10 mg	Prozac by Teva	00172-4363	Antidepressant
4364 <> 100	Tab, Yellow, Round, Hourglass Logo 4364	Labetalol HCl 100 mg	Trandate by Ivax	00182-8202 Discontinued	Antihypertensive
4364 <> 100	Tab, Yellow, Round, Hourglass Logo 4364	Labetalol HCl 100 mg	Trandate by Ivax	00172-4364	Antihypertensive
4365 <> 200	Tab, White, Round, Hourglass Logo 4365	Labetalol HCl 200 mg	Trandate by Ivax	00172-4365	Antihypertensive
4365 <> 200	Tab, White, Round, Hourglass Logo 4365	Labetalol HCl 200 mg	Trandate by Ivax	00182-8203 Discontinued	Antihypertensive
4366 <> 300	Tab, Green, Round, Hourglass Logo 4366	Labetalol HCl 300 mg	Trandate by Ivax	00172-4366	Antihypertensive
437	Tab, Yellow, Round, Scored	Digoxin 0.125 mg	Lanoxin by Caraco	57664-0437	Cardiac Agent
437 <> SL	Tab, Light Green, Black Print, Round, Sugar Coated	Desipramine HCl 50 mg	by Qualitest	00603-3167	Antidepressant
437 <> SL	Tab, Light Green, Black Print, Round, Sugar Coated	Desipramine HCl 50 mg	by URL Mutual	00677-1199	Antidepressant
437 <> SL	Tab, Light Green, Black Print, Round, Sugar Coated	Desipramine HCl 50 mg	by Richmond	54738-0437	Antidepressant
437 <> SL	Tab, Light Green, Black Print, Round, Sugar Coated	Desipramine HCl 50 mg	by Ivax	00182-1333	Antidepressant
437 <> SL	Tab, Light Green, Black Print, Round, Sugar Coated	Desipramine HCl 50 mg	by Warner Chilcott	00047-0595	Antidepressant
437 <> SL	Tab, Light Green, Black Print, Round, Sugar Coated	Desipramine HCl 50 mg	by DRX	55045-1909	Antidepressant
437 <> SL	Tab, Light Green, Black Print, Round, Sugar Coated	Desipramine HCl 50 mg	by Moore	00839-7552	Antidepressant
437 <> SL	Tab, Light Green, Black Print, Round, Sugar Coated	Desipramine HCl 50 mg	by Med Pro	53978-2077	Antidepressant
437 <> SL	Tab, Light Green, Black Print, Round, Sugar Coated	Desipramine HCl 50 mg	by Schein	00364-2210	Antidepressant
437 <> SL	Tab, Light Green, Black Print, Round, Sugar Coated	Desipramine HCl 50 mg	Norpramin by Pliva	50111-0437	Antidepressant
43797007	Tab, Green, Hexagonal, 43797-007	Hyoscyamine Sulfate 0.125 mg	Levsin by Hauck		Gastrointestinal
438 <> ETHEX	Tab, White Cap Shaped	Guaifenesin 595 mg, Pseudoephedrine HCl 48 mg, Dextromethorphan HBr 32 mg	Pseudovent DM by Ethex	58177-0438	Cold Remedy
438 <> GG	Tab, White, Round, Scored, Compressed	Pindolol 5 mg	Visken by Sandoz	00781-1168	Antihypertensive
438 <> SL	Tab, Light Orange, Sugar Coated	Desipramine HCl 75 mg	by Schein	00364-2243	Antidepressant
438 <> SL	Tab, Light Orange, Round, Sugar Coated	Desipramine HCl 75 mg	Norpramin by Pliva	50111-0438	Antidepressant
438100MG	Cap, White, Opaque	Gabapentin 100 mg	Neurontin by Teva	00172-4381	Anticonvulsant
438300MG	Cap, Yellow Opaque Cap, White Opaque Body	Gabapentin 300 mg	Neurontin by Teva Pharmaceuticals	00172-4382 Discontinued	Anticonvulsant
438230MG	Cap, Yellow and White, Opaque, Ivax Logo 4382	Gabapentin 300 mg	Neurontin by Ivax	00172-4382	Anticonvulsant
438340MG	Cap, Orange and White, Opaque, Ivax Logo 4383	Gabapentin 400 mg	Neurontin by Ivax	00172-4383 Discontinued	Anticonvulsant
438340MG	Cap, Orange Opaque Cap, White Opaque Body	Gabapentin 400 mg	Neurontin by Teva	00172-4383	Anticonvulsant
4389	Tab, White, Round, Hourglass Logo over 4389	Fluvoxamine Maleate 25 mg	Luvox by Ivax	00172-4389 Discontinued	OCD

ID FRONT <> BACK	DESCRIPTION FRONT <> BACK	INGREDIENT & STRENGTH	BRAND (or Generic Equiv.) by FIRM	NDC#	CLASS; SCH.
439 <> ETHEX	Tab, White, Oval, Scored	Vitamin A 2700 IU, Vitamin C 120 mg, Calcium Citrate 125 mg, Iron 27 mg, Vitamin D3 400 IU, Vitamin E 30 IU, Thiamine 3 mg, Riboflavin 3.4 mg, Niacinamide 20 mg, Vitamin B6 20 mg, Folic Acid 1 mg, Iodine 150 mcg, Zinc 25 mg, Copper 2 mg, Docusate Sodium 50 mg	Cal-Nate by Ethex	58177-0439	Vitamin
439 <> GG	Tab, White, Round, Scored, Compressed	Pindolol 10 mg	Visken by Sandoz	00781-1169	Antihypertensive
439 <> R	Tab, White to Off-White, Round, Clear Film Coated	Trazodone HCl 50 mg	Desyrel by Vangard	00615-2578	Antidepressant
439 <> R	Tab, White to Off-White, Round, Clear Film Coated	Trazodone HCl 50 mg	Desyrel by Heartland	61392-0487	Antidepressant
439 <> R	Tab, White to Off-White, Round, Clear Film Coated	Trazodone HCl 50 mg	Desyrel by Med Pro	53978-0495	Antidepressant
439 <> R	Tab, White to Off-White, Round, Clear Film Coated	Trazodone HCl 50 mg	Desyrel by Nat Pharmpak	55154-1910	Antidepressant
439 <> R	Tab, White to Off-White, Round, Clear Film Coated	Trazodone HCl 50 mg	Desyrel by Actavis	00228-2439	Antidepressant
4391	Tab, Yellow, Round, Hourglass Logo over 4391	Fluvoxamine Maleate 50 mg	Luvox by Ivax	00172-4391 Discontinued	OCD
4392	Tab, Beige, Round, Hourglass Logo over 4392	Fluvoxamine Maleate 100 mg	Luvox by Ivax	00172-4392 Discontinued	OCD
43RH405RELIANT	Cap, Light Green and Off-White, Segmented Band, Reliant Logo	Fenofibrate 43 mg	Antara by Reliant	65726-0401	Antihyperlipidemic
44	Tab, Red, Round	Pseudoephedrine HCl 30 mg	Sudafed by Major	00904-5053	Decongestant
44 <> 183	Tab, White, Round	Aspirin 325 mg	Aspirin by Ivax	00182-1909 Discontinued	Analgesic
44 <> 298	Tab, Greenish Brown, Round	Sennosides 8.6 mg	Senna by LNK	50844-0298	Gastrointestinal
44 <> 341	Tab, Gray, Oval	Calcium Polycarbophil 125 mg	Fibercon by LNK	50844-	Gastrointestinal
44 <> C	Tab, White to Off White, Cap Shaped, Scored	Torsemide 100 mg	Demadex by Aurobindo	65862-0128	Diuretic
44 <> DP	Tab, Blue, Round, Film Coated	Conjugated Estrogens 1.25 mg	Cenestin by Duramed	51285-0444	Hormone
44 <> GSK	Tab, Pink, Triangular (Rounded), GSK <> 4/4	Rosiglitazone Maleate 4 mg, Glimepiride 4 mg	Avandaryl by GSK	Canadian DIN 02258811	Antidiabetic
44 <> GSK	Tab, Pink, Triangular (Rounded), GSK <> 4/4	Rosiglitazone Maleate 4 mg, Glimepiride 4 mg	Avandaryl by GSK	00007-3153	Antidiabetic
44 <> UU	Tab, White, Oval, Scored	Pramipexole DiHCl 0.25 mg	Mirapex by Boehringer Ingelheim	00597-0084	Antiparkinson
44 <> UU	Tab, White, Oval, Scored	Pramipexole DiHCl 0.25 mg	Mirapex by Pharmacia	00009-0004	Antiparkinson
440 <> ETH	Tab, Tan, Oval, Film Coated, Scored	Folic Acid 2.2 mg, Vitamin B6 25 mg, Vitamin B12 500 mcg	ComBgen by Ethex	58177-0440	Vitamin
440 <> FH10	Tab, Oyster, Round, Film Coated, Extended Release	Nisoldipine 10 mg	Sular by Horizon	59630-0440	Antihypertensive
4404 <> 50	Tab, Pale Yellow, Round, Hourglass Logo 4404 <> 50	Clozapine 50 mg	Clozaril by Ivax	00093-4404	Antipsychotic
4405 <> 200	Tab, Pale Yellow, Oval, Hourglass Logo over 4405, Scored	Clozapine 200 mg	Clozaril by Teva	00093-4405	Antipsychotic
441	Tab, White, Round, Scored	Digoxin 0.25 mg	Lanoxin by Caraco	57664-0441	Cardiac Agent
441 <> FH20	Tab, Yellow, Round, Film Coated, Extended Release	Nisoldipine 20 mg	Sular by Horizon	59630-0441	Antihypertensive
441 <> M	Tab, White, Round, Film Coated	Benazepril HCl 5 mg	Lotensin by Mylan	00378-0441	Antihypertensive
441 <> R	Tab, White, Round, Coated	Trazodone HCl 100 mg	Desyrel by Vangard	00615-2579	Antidepressant
441 <> R	Tab, White to Off-White, Round, Clear Film Coated	Trazodone HCl 100 mg	Desyrel by Actavis	00228-2441	Antidepressant
441 <> R	Tab, White, Round, Coated	Trazodone HCl 100 mg	Desyrel by Heartland	61392-0490	Antidepressant
44104	Tab, White, Round	Acetaminophen 325 mg	Tylenol by LNK	50844-0104	Analgesic
44104	Tab, White, Round, 44-104	Acetaminophen 325 mg	Tylenol by Ivax	00182-8447	Analgesic
44104	Tab, White, Round, 44-104	Acetaminophen 325 mg	Tylenol by Ivax	00182-0141 Discontinued	Analgesic
44107	Cap, Pink & Natural, Bands, 44-107, <> 44-107	Diphenhydramine HCl 25 mg	Benadryl by Wal Mart	49035-0190	Antihistamine
441074 4107	Cap, Pink & Natural, Bands, 44-107, <> 44-107	Diphenhydramine HCl 25 mg	Benadryl by Major	00904-2035	Antihistamine
441074 4107	Cap, Pink & Natural, Bands, 44-107, <> 44-107	Diphenhydramine HCl 25 mg	Benadryl by Ivax	00182-2092 Discontinued	Antihistamine
441074 4107	Cap, Pink & Natural, Bands, 44-107, <> 44-107	Diphenhydramine HCl 25 mg	Benadryl by Heartland	61392-0220	Antihistamine
441074 4107	Cap, Pink & Natural, Bands, 44-107, <> 44-107	Diphenhydramine HCl 25 mg	Benadryl by Quality Care	60346-0589	Antihistamine
44111	Tab, White, Round, 44-111	Pseudoephedrine 60 mg, Chlorpheniramine Maleate 4 mg	Sudafed Plus by LNK	50844-0111	Cold Remedy

ID FRONT <> BACK	DESCRIPTION FRONT <> BACK	INGREDIENT & STRENGTH	BRAND (or Generic Equiv.) by FIRM	NDC#	CLASS; SCH.
44111	Tab, White, Round, 44-111	Pseudoephedrine 60 mg, Chlorpheniramine Maleate 4 mg	Sudafed Plus by Ivax	00182-1471 Discontinued	Cold Remedy
44112	Tab, Red, Round, Film Coated	Pseudoephedrine 30 mg	Sudafed by LNK	50844-	Decongestant
44113	Tab, White, Round, Scored	Pseudoephedrine HCl 60 mg	Sudafed by Major	00904-5125	Decongestant
44137	Tab, White, Round, Scored	Simethicone 80 mg	Mylanta by Major	00904-5068	Antiflatulent
44137	Tab, Chewable	Simethicone 80 mg	Mylanta Gas by LNK	50844-0137	Antigas
44148	Tab, White, Round, 44-148	Acetaminophen 500 mg	Tylenol Ex Strength by Ivax	00182-8453	Analgesic
44148	Tab, White, Round, 44/148	Acetaminophen 500 mg	Tylenol Ex Strength by LNK	50844-0148	Analgesic
44148	Tab, White, Round, 44-148	Acetaminophen 500 mg	Tylenol Ex Strength by Ivax	00182-1453	Analgesic
44156	Tab, Orange, Round	Acetaminophen 325 mg, Phenyltoloxamine Citrate 30 mg	Percogesic by Major	Discontinued 00904-5141	Analgesic
44156	Tab, Orange, Round	Acetaminophen 325 mg, Phenyltoloxamine Citrate 30 mg	Percogesic by LNK	50844-0156	Analgesic
44156	Tab, Orange, Round	Acetaminophen 325 mg, Phenyltoloxamine Citrate 30 mg	Percogesic by Ivax	00182-1027 Discontinued	Analgesic
44157	Tab, White, Round, 44/157	Aspirin 325 mg	Aspirin by Major	00904-2019	Analgesic
44157	Tab, Film Coated	Aspirin 325 mg	Bayer by LNK	50844-0157	Analgesic
44157 <> ASPIRIN	Tab, White, Round, Film Coated, 44 over 157 <> Aspirin	Aspirin 325 mg	Aspirin by UDL	51079-0005	Analgesic
44159	Tab, White, Round	Acetaminophen 250 mg, Aspirin 250 mg, Caffeine 65 mg	Excedrin Migraine by LNK	50844-0159	Analgesic
44159	Tab, White, Round, 44-159	Acetaminophen 250 mg, Aspirin 250 mg, Caffeine 65 mg	Genaced by Ivax	00182-1455	Analgesic
44160	Tab, White, Round	Aspirin, Magnesium Hydroxide, Aluminum Hydroxide	Ascriptin by Ivax	00182-1058 Discontinued	Analgesic
44160	Tab, White, Round	Aspirin, Magnesium Hydroxide, Aluminum Hydroxide	Ascriptin by Major	00904-0346	Analgesic
44160	Cap, Red, Oval	Beta Carotene 25,000 IU	Beta Carotene by Watson	00536-4902	Vitamin
44160	Tab, White, Round	Aspirin, Magnesium Hydroxide, Aluminum Hydroxide	Ascriptin by LNK	50844-4902	Analgesic
44161	Tab, Yellow & White, Round	Aluminum Hydroxide 200 mg, Magnesium Hydroxide 200 mg	Maalox by Rugby	00536-3035	Gastrointestinal
44164	Tab, White, Round, Scored, 44-164	Aspirin 400 mg, Caffeine 32 mg	Anacin by Rugby	00536-3278	Analgesic
44164	Tab, White, Round, Scored, 44-164	Aspirin 400 mg, Caffeine 32 mg	Anacin by Major	00904-5101	Analgesic
44165	Tab, White, Cap Shaped	Aspirin, Magnesium Hydroxide, Aluminum Hydroxide	Ascriptin by Major	00904-0347	Analgesic
44165	Tab, White, Cap Shaped	Aspirin, Magnesium Hydroxide, Aluminum Hydroxide	Ascriptin by Ivax	00182-1060 Discontinued	Analgesic
44165	Tab, White, Cap Shaped	Aspirin, Magnesium Hydroxide, Aluminum Hydroxide	Ascriptin by LNK	50844-0165	Analgesic
44175	Cap, White	Acetaminophen 500 mg	Tylenol Ex Strength by LNK	50844-0175	Analgesic
44175	Tab, White, Cap Shaped, 44-175	Acetaminophen 500 mg	Tylenol Ex Strength by Ivax	00182-2152 Discontinued	Analgesic
44178	Tab, White, Round, Scored, 44 over 178	Triprolidine 2.5 mg, Pseudoephedrine 60 mg	Aprodine by Rugby	00536-3421	Cold Remedy
44178	Tab, White, Round, Scored, 44 over 178	Triprolidine 2.5 mg, Pseudoephedrine 60 mg	Aprodine by Major	00904-0250	Cold Remedy
44181	Tab, Sugar Coated	Suphedrine 30 mg	Sudafed by LNK	50844-0181	Decongestant
44183	Tab, White, Round	Aspirin 325 mg	Aspirin by Major	00904-2015	Analgesic
44183	Tab, White, Round	Aspirin 325 mg	Aspirin by LNK	50844-0183	Analgesic
44184	Cap, Red & White	Acetaminophen 500 mg	Tylenol Ex Strength by LNK	50844-0184	Analgesic
44185	Tab, Pink w/ white specks, Round, Chewable	Acetaminophen 80 mg	Children's Tylenol by LNK	50844-0185	Analgesic
44185	Tab, Pink, Round, 44-185, Chewable	Acetaminophen 80 mg	Children's Tylenol by Major	00904-5258	Analgesic
44185	Tab, Pink, Round, 44-185, Chewable	Acetaminophen 80 mg	Children's Tylenol by Ivax	00182-1585	Analgesic
44186	Tab, Pink, Round, Scored, Chewable	Acetaminophen 80 mg	Children's Tylenol by Major	00904-5256	Analgesic
44186	Tab, Grape, Chewable	Acetaminophen 80 mg	Children's Tylenol by LNK	50844-0186	Analgesic
44189	Tab, Blue, Round	Diphenhydramine HCl 25 mg	Sominex by Major	00904-4274	Antihistamine
44189	Tab, Blue, Round	Diphenhydramine HCl 25 mg	Sominex by LNK	50844-0189	Antihistamine
44191	Tab, Pink, Oblong	Diphenhydramine HCl 25 mg	Benadryl by LNK	50844-0191	Antihistamine
44191	Tab, Pink, Oval, Film Coated	Diphenhydramine HCl 25 mg	Benadryl by UDL	51079-0862	Antihistamine

ID FRONT <> BACK	DESCRIPTION FRONT <> BACK	INGREDIENT & STRENGTH	BRAND (or Generic Equiv.) by FIRM	NDC#	CLASS; SCH.
44191	Tab, Pink, Oval, 44-191	Genahist 25 mg	Benadryl by Ivax	00182-2091 Discontinued	Antihistamine
44194	Tab, Yellow, Round, Scored, 44 over 194	Chlorpheniramine Maleate 4 mg	Chlor-Trimeton by Major	00904-0012	Antihistamine
44194	Tab, Yellow, Round, Scored, 44 over 194	Chlorpheniramine Maleate 4 mg	Chlor-Trimeton by LNK	50844-0194	Antihistamine
44194	Tab, Yellow, Round, Scored, 44 over 194	Chlorpheniramine Maleate 4 mg	Chlor-Trimeton by Circa	71114-4208	Antihistamine
44194	Tab, Yellow, Round, Scored, 44 over 194	Chlorpheniramine Maleate 4 mg	Chlor-Trimeton by UDL	51079-0163	Antihistamine
44194	Tab, Yellow, Round	Chlorpheniramine Maleate 4 mg	Chlor-Trimeton by Ivax	00182-0471 Discontinued	Antihistamine
44197	Tab, Blue, Round	Brompheniramine Maleate 12 mg, Phenylephrine HCl 15 mg, Phenylpropanolamine HCl 15 mg	Dimetapp by LNK	50844-0197	Cold Remedy
44198	Tab, White, Round, Scored	Dimenhydrinate 50 mg	Dramamine by LNK	50844-0198	Antiemetic
44198	Tab, White, Round, Scored	Dimenhydrinate 50 mg	Dramamine by Major	00904-2051	Antiemetic
44198	Tab, White, Round, Scored	Dimenhydrinate 50 mg	Dramamine by Ivax	00182-0195 Discontinued	Antiemetic
442	Tab, Pink, Round	Phenolphthalein 65 mg, Docusate Sodium 100 mg	by Perrigo	00113-0442	Gastrointestinal
442	Tab, Orange, Oval, Schering Logo 442	Fluphenazine HCl 2.5 mg	Permitil by Schering	00085-0442	Antipsychotic
442 <> FH30	Tab, Mustard, Round, Film Coated, Extended Release	Nisoldipine 30 mg	Sular by Horizon	59630-0442	Antihypertensive
442 <> MYLAN	Tab, Purple, Round, Film Coated	Perphenazine 2 mg, Amitriptyline HCl 25 mg	Triavil by Pharmafab	62542-0914	Antipsychotic; Antidepressant
442 <> MYLAN	Tab, Purple, Round, Film Coated	Amitriptyline 25 mg, Perphenazine 2 mg	Triavil by Mylan	00378-0442	Antidepressant; Antipsychotic
44201	Tab, White, Round	Aluminum Hydroxide 200 mg, Magnesium Hydroxide 200 mg	Maalox by LNK	50844-0201	Gastrointestinal
44211	Tab, Oval, Film Coated	Aspirin 500 mg	Bufferin by LNK	50844-0211	Analgesic
44218	Tab, Orange, Round, White Specks	Aspirin 81 mg	Aspirin by LNK	50844-0218	Analgesic
44218	Tab, Orange, Round, White Specks	Aspirin 81 mg	Aspirin by Major	00904-4040	Analgesic
44222	Tab, White, Round	Aspirin 81 mg	Aspirin by LNK	50844-0222	Analgesic
44224	Tab, Multi-Flavor	Calcium Carbonate 500 mg	Tums by LNK	50844-0224	Antacid
44225	Tab, Yellow, Round	Aspirin 81 mg	Aspirin by LNK	50844-0225	Analgesic
44226	Tab, Yellow, Round	Caffeine 200 mg	Stay Awake by Major	00904-7955	Stimulant
44226	Tab	Caffeine 200 mg	Vivarin by LNK	50844-0226	Alertness Aid
44227	Tab, Orange, Black Print, Round, Enteric Coated, 44 over 227	Aspirin 325 mg	Aspirin by LNK	50844-0227	Analgesic
44235	Tab, Light Blue, Oblong	Acetaminophen 500 mg, Diphenhydramine 25 mg	Tylenol PM by LNK	50844-0235	Cold Remedy
44236	Cap, White, Oblong	Aspirin 500 mg	Aspirin by Rite Aid		Analgesic
44236	Tab, Oval, Film Coated	Aspirin 500 mg	Bayer by LNK	50844-0236	Analgesic
44237	Tab, Green, Cap Shaped, 44-237	Acetaminophen 500 mg, Pseudoephedrine 30 mg	Tylenol Sinus Ex Strength by Ivax	00182-2145 Discontinued	Analgesic
44239	Tab, Purple, Round	Acetaminophen 160 mg	Tylenol Jr by Major	00904-7589	Analgesic
44239	Tab, Grape	Acetaminophen 160 mg	Tylenol Jr. by LNK	50844-0239	Analgesic
44240	Tab, White, Oblong, Film Coated, 44-240	Acetaminophen 325 mg	Tylenol by LNK	50844-0240	Analgesic
44242	Tab, Pink, Round, Scored	Acetaminophen 325 mg, Pseudoephedrine 30 mg	Tylenol Sinus by Major	00904-0321	Cold Remedy
44243	Tab, Red, Round, Enteric Coated	Aspirin 500 mg	Aspirin by LNK	50844-0243	Analgesic
44246	Tab	Acetaminophen 500 mg	Tylenol PM by LNK	50844-0246	Analgesic
44247	Tab, Enteric Coated	Aspirin 500 mg	Ecotrin by LNK	50844-0247	Analgesic
44249	Tab, White, Round	Aspirin 325 mg	Aspirin by LNK	50844-0249	Analgesic
44255	Tab, Yellow, Round, Enteric Coated, 44/255	Aspirin 81 mg	Aspirin by LNK	50844-0255	Analgesic
44258	Tab, Yellow, Oblong	Acetaminophen 325 mg, Pseudoephedrine 30 mg, Dextromethorphan 15 mg, Chlorpheniramine Maleate 2 mg	Tylenol Cold by Major	00904-7655	Cold Remedy
44276	Tab	Doxylamine Succinate 25 mg	Unisom by LNK	50844-0276	Sleep Aid
44290	Cap, 44-290	Diphenhydramine HCl 50 mg	by Quality Care	60346-0045	Antihistamine

ID FRONT <> BACK	DESCRIPTION FRONT <> BACK	INGREDIENT & STRENGTH	BRAND (or Generic Equiv.) by FIRM	NDC#	CLASS; SCH.
44290	Cap	Diphenhydramine HCl 50 mg	Benadryl by LNK	50844-0290	Antihistamine
44291	Tab, Brown, Film Coated	Ibuprofen 200 mg	Advil by LNK	50844-0291	Analgesic
44291	Tab, Brown, Round, 44-291	Ibuprofen 200 mg	Motrin by Ivax	00182-1039 Discontinued	NSAID
44292	Tab, Brown, Oval, Film Coated	Ibuprofen 200 mg	Advil by LNK	50844-0292	Analgesic
44293	Liquigel	Doxylamine Succinate 50 mg	Unisom by LNK	50844-0293	Sleep Aid
44298	Tab	Senna 8.6 mg	Senokot by LNK	50844-0298	Laxative
443 <> COPLEY	Tab, Off-White, Cap Shaped	Naproxen 375 mg	by Teva	38245-0443	NSAID
443 <> COPLEY	Tab	Naproxen 375 mg	by Qualitest	00603-4731	NSAID
443 <> COPLEY	Tab, White, Oblong	Naproxen 375 mg	by Southwood	58016-0267	NSAID
443 <> FH40	Tab, Burnt Orange, Round, Film Coated, Extended Release	Nisoldipine 40 mg	Sular by Horizon	59630-0443	Antihypertensive
443 <> M	Tab, White, Round, Film Coated	Benazepril HCl 10 mg	Lotensin by Mylan	00378-0443	Antihypertensive
443 <> M	Tab, White, Round, Film Coated	Benazepril HCl 10 mg	Lotensin by UDL	51079-0145	Antihypertensive
4430 <> 100	Tab, White, Round, Ivax Hourglass Logo 100 <> 4430	Misoprostol 100 mcg	Cytotec by Ivax	00172-4430	Gastrointestinal
44304	Tab, Yellow, Round	Acetaminophen 500 mg, Chlorpheniramine Maleate 2 mg, Dextromethorphan HBr 15 mg, Pseudoephedrine HCl 30 mg	Tylenol Cold by Major	00904-3650	Cold Remedy
4431 <> 200	Tab, White, Round, Ivax Hourglass Logo 200 mcg	Misoprostol 200 mcg	Cytotec by Ivax	00172-4431	Gastrointestinal
44317	Tab, Mint	Calcium Carbonate 500 mg	Tums by LNK	50844-0317	Antacid
44318	Tab, Bubblegum, Chewable	Acetaminophen 80 mg	Children's Tylenol by LNK	50844-0318	Analgesic
44319	Tab, Pink, Cherry, Chewable	Bismuth 262 mg	Pepto Bismol by LNK	50844-0319	Anti-Diarrheal, Anti-Nausea
4432 <> 1000	Tab, White, Oval, Scored, Hourglass Logo 4432	Metformin HCl 1000 mg	Glucophage by Ivax	00172-4432 Discontinued	Antidiabetic
44326	Tab, Pink, Round, Coated, 44 over 326	Bisacodyl 5 mg	Correctol by LNK	50844-0326	Gastrointestinal
44327	Tab, Orange	Bisacodyl 5 mg	Dulcolax by LNK	50844-0327	Laxative
44329	Tab, Pink, Cap Shaped, Film Coated	Diphenhydramine HCl 25 mg	Benadryl by Major	00904-5551	Antihistamine
44329	Tab, Pink, Cap Shaped, Film Coated	Diphenhydramine HCl 25 mg	Benadryl by UDL	51079-0967 Discontinued	Antihistamine
44335	Tab, Multi-Fruit Flavor	Calcium Carbonate 750 mg	Tums EX by LNK	50844-0335	Antacid
44336	Tab, Multi-Fruit	Calcium Carbonate 1000 mg	Tums Ultra Strength by LNK	50844-0336	Antacid
44338	Tab, White, Oblong	Magnesium Salicylate 580 mg	by LNK	50844-0338	Analgesic
44339	Tab, Tropical Fruit Flavor	Calcium Carbonate 750 mg	Tums EX by LNK	50844-0339	Antacid
44340	Tab, Wintergreen	Calcium Carbonate 750 mg	Tums EX by LNK	50844-0340	Antacid
44341	Tab	Fiberlax 625 mg	Fibercon by LNK	50844-0341	Laxative
44344	Tab, Mint, Oval, Film Coated	Caffeine 200 mg	No-Doz by LNK	50844-0344	Alertness Aid
44345	Tab, Mint, Chewable	Magnesium Hydroxide 311 mg	Phillips Milk of Magnesia by LNK	50844-0345	Antacid
44346	Tab, Pink, Oval, Film Coated	Bismuth 262 mg	Pepto Bismol by LNK	50844-0346	Anti-Diarrheal, Anti-Nausea
44347	Tab	Senna 15 mg	Ex-Lax by LNK	50844-0347	Laxative
4435 <> 500	Tab, White, Oval, Ivax Logo 4435, ER	Metformin HCl 500 mg	Glucophage XR by Ivax	00172-4435 Discontinued	Antidiabetic
44352	Tab, White, Round	Ibuprofen 200 mg	Motrin by LNK	50844-0352	NSAID
44353	Tab, White, Cap Shaped, 44-353	Ibuprofen 200 mg	Motrin by LNK	50844-0353	NSAID
44367	Tab, Blue	Diphenhydramine 25 mg	Simply Sleep by LNK	50844-0367	Sleep Aid
44369	Tab, White, Oval	Acetaminophen 500 mg, Pamabrom 25 mg, Pyrilamine 15 mg	Midol by LNK	50844-0369	PMS Relief
44371	Gelcap	Acetaminophen 500 mg	Tylenol PM by LNK	50844-0371	Analgesic
44373	Tab, Blue, Round, 44/373	Acetaminophen 500 mg, Diphenhydramine HCl 38 mg	Tylenol PM by LNK	50844-0373	Cold Remedy
44375	Tab, Oval, Film Coated	Loperamide HCl 2 mg	Immodium AD by LNK	50844-0375	Anti-Diarrheal, Anti-Nausea
44377	Tab	Cimetidine 200 mg	Tagamet by LNK	50844-0377	Antacid
44378	Tab	Ranitidine 75 mg	Zantac by LNK	50844-0378	Antacid

ID FRONT <> BACK	DESCRIPTION FRONT <> BACK	INGREDIENT & STRENGTH	BRAND (or Generic Equiv.) by FIRM	NDC#	CLASS; SCH.
44382	Tab, Blue, Round, 44-382	Pseudoephedrine HCl 60 mg, Chlorpheniramine Maleate 4 mg	Sudogest by Major	00904-5351	Cold Remedy
44386	Tab	Doxylamine Succinate 25 mg	Unisom by LNK	50844-0386	Sleep Aid
44388	Tab, Pink, Wintergreen, Chewable	Bismuth 262 mg	Pepto Bismol by LNK	50844-0388	Anti-Diarrheal, Anti-Nausea
44389	Tab, Oval, Film Coated	Aspirin 325 mg	Bayer by LNK	50844-0389	Analgesic
44392	Tab, Orange, Round, 44 over 392	Ibuprofen 200 mg	Motrin by LNK	50844	Analgesic
44393	Tab, Bright Orange, Cap Shaped	Ibuprofen 200 mg	Advil by LNK	50844-0393	NSAID
44396	Tab, Assorted Berries	Calcium Carbonate 750 mg	Tums EX by LNK	50844-0396	Antacid
44397	Tab, Cherry, Chewable	Aspirin 81 mg	Bayer by LNK	50844-0397	Analgesic
44399	Tab, Fruit	Acetaminophen 160 mg	Tylenol Jr by LNK	50844-0399	Analgesic
444 <> ETHEX	Tab, White, Cap Shaped, Film Coated, Scored	Guaifenesin 1200 mg, Phenylephrine HCl 40 mg	PhenaVent D by Ethex	58177-0444	Cold Remedy
4440 <> 100	Tab, White, Round, Hourglass Logo 4440 <> 100	Gabapentin 100 mg	Neurontin by Ivax	00172-4440 Discontinued	Anticonvulsant
44400	Tab, Assorted Fresh Blend	Calcium Carbonate	Tums EX by LNK	50844-0400	Antacid
44402	Tab, Yellow	Senna 8.6 mg, Docusate Sodium 50 mg	Senokot S by LNK	50844-0402	Laxative
44403	Tab	Meclizine 25 mg	Dramamine II by LNK	50844-0403	Antiemetic
44404	Tab, Pink, Round, Scored, Chewable	Meclizine 25 mg	Bonine by LNK	50844-0404	Antiemetic
4441 <> 300	Tab, White, Round, Hourglass Logo over 4441	Gabapentin 300 mg	Neurontin by Ivax	00172-4441 Discontinued	Anticonvulsant
44412	Tab	Aspirin 81 mg, Calcium 300 mg	Bayer by LNK	50844-0412	Analgesic
44413	Tab	Aspirin 500 mg, Caffeine 32.5 mg	Bayer by LNK	50844-0413	Analgesic
44414	Tab, Enteric Coated	Aspirin 81 mg	St. Joseph's by LNK	50844-0414	Analgesic
4441W	Cap, Yellow	Temilian 10 mg	Restoril by LentLife	73245-5679	Cold Remedy
4442 <> 400	Tab, White, Oval, Hourglass Logo 4442 <> 400	Gabapentin 400 mg	Neurontin by Ivax	00172-4442 Discontinued	Anticonvulsant
4443 <> 600	Tab, White, Oval, Scored, Ivax Logo 4443	Gabapentin 600 mg	Neurontin by Ivax	00093-4443	Anticonvulsant
44438	Tab, White, Round, Film Coated	Ibuprofen 200 mg	Motrin by LNK	50844-0438	NSAID
44439	Tab, Enteric Coated	Aspirin 81 mg	Ecotrin by LNK	50844-0439	Analgesic
4444 <> 800	Tab, White, Oval, Scored, Ivax Logo 4444	Gabapentin 800 mg	Neurontin by Ivax	00093-4444	Anticonvulsant
44445	Tab, Oval, Film Coated	Acetaminophen 500 mg	Tylenol Ex Strength by LNK	50844-0445	Analgesic
44447	Tab, Bubblegum, Chewable	Acetaminophen 80 mg	Children's Tylenol by LNK	50844-0447	Analgesic
44448	Tab, Watermelon, Chewable	Acetaminophen 80 mg	Children's Tylenol by LNK	50844-0448	Analgesic
44449	Tab, Grape, Rapid Meltaways	Acetaminophen 160 mg	Tylenol Jr by LNK	50844-0449	Analgesic
44450	Tab, Bubblegum	Acetaminophen 160 mg	Tylenol Jr by LNK	50844-0450	Analgesic
44452	Tab, Grape, Chewable	Acetaminophen 80 mg	Children's Tylenol by LNK	50844-0452	Analgesic
44453	Tab, Red, Round, Coated, 44 / 453	Phenylephrine 10 mg	Sudafed PE by LNK	50844-	Decongestant
44456	Liquidgel	Suphedrine 60 mg	Suphedrine by LNK	50844-0456	Decongestant
44458	Tab, Blue	Guaifenesin 400 mg	Mucinex by LNK	50844-0458	Expectorant
44459	Tab, Yellow, Oval	Guaifenesin 400 mg, Dextromethorphan HBr 20 mg	by LNK	50844-0459	Cold Remedy
44464	Tab, Green, Cap Shaped	Acetaminophen 325 mg, Diphenhydramine HCl 12.5 mg, Phenylephrine HCl 5 mg	Benadryl Allergy/Sinus/Headache by LNK	50844-0464	Cold Remedy
445 <> ETH	Tab, Yellow, Round, Scored	Oxycodone HCl 15 mg	Roxicodone by Ethex	58177-0445	Analgesic; C II
44500	Tab, White & Red, Cap Shaped, Gel Coated, 44-500	Acetaminophen 500 mg	Tylenol Ex Strength by Major	00904-1989	Analgesic
44500	Tab, White & Red, Cap Shaped, Gel Coated, 44-500	Acetaminophen 500 mg	Tylenol Ex Strength by Ivax	00182-2154 Discontinued	Analgesic
44500	Press Fit Gelcap, Quick Release	Acetaminophen 500 mg	Tylenol Ex Strength by LNK	50844-0500	Analgesic
44519	Press Fit Gelcap, Quick Release	Acetaminophen 500 mg	Tylenol Rapid Release by LNK	50844-0519	Analgesic
44531	Tab	Acetaminophen 500 mg	Tylenol Ex Strength by LNK	50844-0531	Analgesic
44532	Tab, White, Round	Guaifenesin 400 mg	Robitussin by LNK	50844-0532	Cold Remedy
44533	Tab, White, Oval	Dextromethorphan 20 mg, Guaifenesin 400 mg	Mucinex DM by LNK	50844-0533	Cold Remedy
44536	Tab, Oval, Film Coated, Vanilla	Acetaminophen 500 mg	Tylenol PM by LNK	50844-0536	Analgesic

ID FRONT <> BACK	DESCRIPTION FRONT <> BACK	INGREDIENT & STRENGTH	BRAND (or Generic Equiv.) by FIRM	NDC#	CLASS; SCH.
44542	Tab, White, Oval	Guaifenesin 400 mg, Phenylephrine 10 mg	Mucinex D by LNK	50844-0547	Cold Remedy
44547	Tab	Guaifenesin 400 mg	Mucinex D by LNK	Discontinued	Expectorant
4455RUGBY	Tab, Tan, Round, 4455/Rugby	Ranitidine 150 mg	by Rugby	00069-4460	Gastrointestinal
446	Tab	Polythiazide 2 mg, Reserpine 0.25 mg	Renese R by Pfizer	00555-0446	Diuretic; Antihypertensive
446 <> BARR	Tab, White, Round	Tamoxifen Citrate 10 mg	Nolvadex by Barr	00310-0446	Antiestrogen
446 <> BARR	Tab, White, Round	Tamoxifen Citrate 10 mg	Nolvadex by Zeneca	59564-0144	Antiestrogen
446 <> BARR	Tab, White, Round	Tamoxifen Citrate 10 mg	Nolvadex by Haines	58177-0446	Antiestrogen
446 <> ETH	Tab, White, Round, Scored	Oxycodone HCl 30 mg	Roxicodone by Ethex	66302-0467	Analgesic; C II
4467	Tab, Orange, Oval	Tadalafil 20 mg	Adcirca by United	Canadian DIN 02302896	Antihypertensive
44MAG	Cap, Red	Caffeine 200 mg	Caffeine by BDI	00172-5695	Stimulant
45	Tab, White, Round	Pioglitazone 45 mg	Actos by Cobalt	Discontinued	Antidiabetic
45 <> 5695	Tab, White, Round, Hourglass Logo 5695 <> 45	Mirtazapine 45 mg	Remeron by Ivax	00074-9642	Antidepressant
45 <> A	Cap, Reddish-Brown Cap, Yellow Body, Hard Gelatin Cap Contains White Mini Tabs	Choline Fenofibrate 45 mg	Trilipix by Abbott	58056-0339	Treats Cholesterol
45 <> ACTOS	Tab, White, Round, Flat	Pioglitazone HCl 45 mg	Actos by Prestige	Canadian DIN 02242574	Antidiabetic
45 <> ACTOS	Tab, White to Off-White, Round	Pioglitazone HCl 45 mg	Actos by Eli Lilly	64764-0451	Antidiabetic
45 <> ACTOS	Tab, White, Round	Pioglitazone HCl 45 mg	Actos by Takeda	54868-0409	Antidiabetic
45 <> ELAVIL	Tab, Film Coated	Amitriptyline HCl 25 mg	Elavil by Physician Total Care	00310-0045	Antidepressant
45 <> ELAVIL	Tab, Yellow, Round, Film Coated	Amitriptyline HCl 25 mg	Elavil by Zeneca	65240-0637	Antidepressant
45 <> ELAVIL	Tab, Yellow, Round	Amitriptyline HCl 25 mg	Elavil by Rightpak	00597-0116	Antidepressant
45 <> ER	Tab, White to Off-White, Oval, Ex Release, "4.5" <> ER	Pramipexole DiHCl 4.5 mg	Mirapex ER by Boehringer Ingelheim	Canadian DIN 02303140	Antiparkinson
45 <> PG	Tab, White, Round	Pioglitazone HCl 45 mg	Actos by Pharmascience	00245-0450	Antihyperglycemic
450	Cap, Brown & Light Green	Hypericum perforatum 450 mg	Alterra by Upsher Smith by Jones	52604-9160	Supplement
450 <> MD	Tab	Diethylpropion HCl 75 mg		00186-0450	Anorexiant; C IV
450 <> PLENDIL	Tab, Sage Green, Round, Ex Release	Felodipine 2.5 mg	Plendil by AstraZeneca	00004-0038	Antihypertensive
450 <> VGC	Tab, Pink, Oval, Film Coated	Valganciclovir HCl 450 mg	Valcyte by Hoffmann La Roche	Canadian DIN 02245777	Antiviral
450 <> VGC	Tab, Pink, Oval, Film Coated	Valganciclovir HCl 450 mg	Valcyte by Roche	Canadian DIN 02247087	Antiviral
4500 <> GSK	Tab, Orange, Oval, Film Coated, 4/500	Metformin HCl 500 mg, Rosiglitazone 4 mg	Avandamet by GSK	00007-3168	Antidiabetic
4500 <> GSK	Tab, Orange, Oval, Film Coated, 4/500	Metformin HCl 500 mg, Rosiglitazone 4 mg	Avandamet by SKB		Antidiabetic
450MD <> B	Tab, White, Oval	Diethylpropion HCl 75 mg	Tenuate Dosepan by MD	00555-9065	Anorexiant; C IV
451 <> B	Tab, Gray, Round, Film Coated	Norgestimate 0.18 mg, Ethinyl Estradiol 0.025 mg	Tri-Lo-Sprintec by Barr	62224-2119	Oral Contraceptive
451 <> MYLAN	Tab, White, Cap Shaped	Naproxen 500 mg	Naprosyn by Kaiser	60760-0451	NSAID
451 <> MYLAN	Tab, White, Cap Shaped	Naproxen 500 mg	Naprosyn by St. Mary's Med	00378-0451	NSAID
451 <> MYLAN	Tab, White, Cap Shaped	Naproxen 500 mg	Naprosyn by Mylan	00179-1188	NSAID
451 <> MYLAN	Tab, White, Cap Shaped	Naproxen 500 mg	Naprosyn by Kaiser	17236-0078	NSAID
451 <> MYLAN	Tab, White, Cap Shaped	Naproxen 500 mg	Naprosyn by Dixon Shane	44514-0651	NSAID
451 <> MYLAN	Tab, White, Cap Shaped	Naproxen 500 mg	Naprosyn by Talbert	51079-0795	NSAID
451 <> MYLAN	Tab, White, Cap Shaped	Naproxen 500 mg	Naprosyn by UDL	51129-1314	NSAID
451 <> MYLAN	Tab, White, Cap Shaped	Naproxen 500 mg	Naprosyn by Murfreesboro	51660-0701	NSAID
451 <> MYLAN	Tab, White, Cap Shaped	Naproxen 500 mg	Naprosyn by OHM	00186-0451	NSAID
451 <> PLENDIL	Tab, Light Red-Brown, Round, Ex Release	Felodipine 5 mg	Plendil by AstraZeneca	50111-0451	Antihypertensive
451 <> SL	Tab, Film Coated, Debossed	Ibuprofen 800 mg	Motrin by Pliva	00172-4510	NSAID
4510	Tab, Light Green, Oval, Hourglass Logo 4510	Fluoxetine HCl 10 mg	Prozac by Ivax	Discontinued	Antidepressant

ID FRONT <> BACK	DESCRIPTION FRONT <> BACK	INGREDIENT & STRENGTH	BRAND (or Generic Equiv.) by FIRM	NDC#	CLASS; SCH.
4519	Tab, Pink, Ross Logo 4519	Multivitamin Chewable	Vi-Daylin by Ross		Vitamin
452 <> B	Tab, Light Blue, Round, Film Coated	Norgestimate 0.215 mg, Ethinyl Estradiol 0.025 mg	Tri-Lo-Sprintec by Barr	00555-9065	Oral Contraceptive
452 <> PLENDIL	Tab, Red-Brown, Round, Ex Release	Felodipine 10 mg	Plendil by AstraZeneca	00186-0452	Antihypertensive
4520	Tab, Orange, Ross Logo 4520	Multivitamin, Iron Chewable	Vi-Daylin by Ross		Vitamin
453 <> B	Tab, Blue, Round, Film Coated	Norgestimate 0.25 mg, Ethinyl Estradiol 0.025 mg	Tri-Lo-Sprintec by Barr	00555-9065	Oral Contraceptive
454 <> M	Tab, Round	Pindolol 5 mg	by Merckle	58107-0004	Antihypertensive
454 <> WATSON	Tab, Orange, Oblong	Gemfibrozil 600 mg	Lopid by Watson	00591-0454	Antihyperlipidemic
45435	Cap, Green, Oval, 45-435	Chloral Hydrate 500 mg	Chloral Hydrate by Chase		Sedative/Hypnotic; C IV
455	Cap, One-Piece Gelatin Capsule	Ipodate Sodium 500 mg	Oragrafin Sodium by Bracco	00270-0455	Diagnostic
455 <> M	Tab, Round	Pindolol 10 mg	by Merckle	58107-0005	Antihypertensive
4556	Tab, Yellow, Round	Phenylpropanolamine 50 mg, Pheniramine 25 mg, Pyrilamine 25 mg	by Eon		Cold Remedy
457	Tab, Blue, Round	Sennosides 25 mg	by Perrigo	00113-0457	Gastrointestinal
457	Tab, Blue, Round	Sennosides 25 mg	Senokot by Perrigo	51660-0429	Laxative
457 <> MYLAN	Tab	Lorazepam 1 mg	Ativan by Vangard	00615-0451	Antianxiety; C IV
458 <> CLARITIN10	Tab, White, Round, Claritin over 10	Loratadine 10 mg	Claritin by Nat Pharmpak	55154-3513	Antihistamine
458 <> CLARITIN10	Tab, White, Round, Claritin over 10	Loratadine 10 mg	Claritin by Patient First	57575-0100	Antihistamine
458 <> CLARITIN10	Tab, White, Round, Claritin over 10	Loratadine 10 mg	Claritin by Southwood	58016-0560	Antihistamine
458 <> CLARITIN10	Tab, White, Round, Claritin over 10	Loratadine 10 mg	Claritin DR by Schering	00085-0458	Antihistamine
458 <> CLARITIN10	Tab, White, Round, Claritin over 10	Loratadine 10 mg	Claritin by Urgent Care Center	50716-0267	Antihistamine
458 <> CLARITIN10	Tab, White, Round, Claritin over 10	Loratadine 10 mg	Claritin by H J Harkins Co	52959-0452	Antihistamine
458 <> CLARITIN10	Tab, White, Round, Claritin over 10	Loratadine 10 mg	Claritin by Allscripts		Antihistamine
458 <> CLARITIN10	Tab, White, Round, Claritin over 10	Loratadine 10 mg	Claritin by Direct Dispensing	57866-3500	Antihistamine
458 <> CLARITIN10	Tab, White, Round, Claritin over 10	Loratadine 10 mg	Claritin by Amerisource	62584-0458	Antihistamine
458 <> CLARITIN10	Tab, White, Round, Claritin over 10	Loratadine 10 mg	Claritin by Compumed	00403-4369	Antihistamine
458 <> CLARITIN10	Tab, White, Round, Claritin over 10	Loratadine 10 mg	Claritin by Neuman	64579-0251	Antihistamine
458 <> CLARITIN10	Tab, White, Round, Claritin over 10	Loratadine 10 mg	Claritin by Mylan	00378-3358	Antihistamine
458 <> ETHEX	Tab, White, Oval	Vitamin C 120 mg, Calcium Carbonate 200 mg, Elemental Iron 90 mg, Vitamin D3 400 IU, Vitamin E 30 IU, Vitamin B1 3 mg, Vitamin B2 3.4 mg, Niacinamide 20 mg, Vitamin B6 20 mg, Folic Acid 1 mg, Vitamin B12 12 mcg, Zinc 25 mg, Copper 2 mg, Magnesium 30 mg, Docusate Sodium 50 mg	Advanced-RF NatalCare by Ethex	58177-0458	Vitamin
458B	Tab, White, Oblong	Amitriptyline HCl 150 mg	Elavil by Barr	65862-0080	Antidepressant
46 <> A	Tab, Yellow, Cap Shaped, Film Coated	Glyburide 1.25 mg, Metformin 250 mg	Glucovance by Aurobindo	14656-0046	Antidiabetic
46 <> CIBA	Tab, Tan, Round, Scored	Hydrochlorothiazide 50 mg	Esidrix by Ciba	51285-0446	Diuretic; Antihypertensive
46 <> DP	Tab, Orange, Round, Film Coated, 46 <> dp	Conjugated Estrogens 0.45 mg	Cenestin by Barr	Discontinued	Hormone
4600	Cap, Yellow, White Print, Soft Gel	Benzonatate 100 mg	Tessalon by Sidmak	00677-1472	Antitussive
4600	Gelcap, Yellow, Soft	Benzonatate 100 mg	Tessalon Perles by URL Mutual	10888-4600	Antitussive
4600P	Cap, Gelatin, P in a Triangle	Benzonatate 100 mg	Tessalon by Banner Pharma		Antitussive
461 <> ETH	Tab, Pink, Round, Scored	Oxycodone HCl 10 mg	OxyContin by Ethex	58177-0461	Analgesic; C II
46180MG	Cap, White, Opaque, Hard Gel	Aprepitant 80 mg	Emend by Merck	00006-0461	Antiemetic
46180MG	Cap, White, Opaque, Hard Gel	Aprepitant 80 mg	Emend by Merck	00006-3862	Antiemetic
46180MG	Cap, White, Opaque, Hard Gel	Aprepitant 80 mg	Emend by Merck	Canadian DIN 02298791	Antiemetic
462 <> ETH	Tab, Grey, Round, Scored	Oxycodone HCl 20 mg	Oxycodone by Ethex	58177-0462	Analgesic; C II
46212 5MG	Cap, White, Pink, Opaque, Hard Gel	Aprepitant 125 mg	Emend by Merck	00006-3862	Antiemetic
46212 5MG	Cap, White, Pink, Opaque, Hard Gel	Aprepitant 125 mg	Emend by Merck	00006-0462	Antiemetic
46212 5MG	Cap, White, Pink, Opaque, Hard Gel	Aprepitant 125 mg	Emend by Merck	Canadian DIN 02298805	Antiemetic
4626 <> 20	Tab, White, Round, Film Coated, Ivax Logo 20	Doxycycline Hyclate 20 mg	Periostat by Ivax	00172-4626	Antibiotic
463 <> 93	Tab, Peach, Diamond Shaped, Scored, 9 / 3	Lamotrigine 100 mg	Lamictal by Teva	00093-0463	Anticonvulsant

ID FRONT <> BACK	DESCRIPTION FRONT <> BACK	INGREDIENT & STRENGTH	BRAND (or Generic Equiv.) by FIRM	NDC#	CLASS; SCH.
463 <> ETHEX	Tab, Blue, Cap Shaped	Vitamin D3 400 IU, Vitamin E 30 IU, Vitamin C 120 mg, Folic Acid 1 mg, Vitamin B1 3 mg, Vitamin B2 3 mg, Niacin 20 mg, Vitamin B6 3 mg, Vitamin B12 8 mcg, Calcium 200 mg, Iodine 150 mcg, Zinc 15 mg, Iron 29 mg	NutriSpire by Ethex	58177-0463	Vitamin
466 <> WATSON	Tab, White, Round	Tramadol HCl 50 mg	Ultram by Watson	00591-0466	Analgesic
467	Tab, White to Off-White, Round	Meperidine HCl 50 mg	Demerol by Caraco	57664-0467	Analgesic; C II
467HD	Tab, White, Round	Dipyridamole 75 mg	Persantine by Halsey	Discontinued	Antiplatelet
468 <> MJ	Tab, Chewable	Ascorbic Acid 60 mg, Cholecalciferol 400, Cyanocobalamin 4.5 mcg, Folic Acid 0.3 mg, Niacin 13.5 mg, Niacinamide, Pyridoxine HCl, Riboflavin Phosphate Sodium, Sodium Fluoride, Thiamine Mononitrate, Vitamin A Acetate, Vitamin E 15 Units	Poly Vi Flor by BMS	00087-0468	Vitamin
468 <> PAR	Tab, Elongated Shape, Film Coated	Ibuprofen 600 mg	Motrin by Par		NSAID
469 <> PAR	Tab, Film Coated	Ibuprofen 400 mg	Motrin by Quality Care	60346-0030	NSAID
47 <> A	Tab, Light Pink, Cap Shaped, Film Coated	Glyburide 2.5 mg, Metformin 500 mg	Glucovance by Aurobindo	65862-0081	Antidiabetic
47 <> ELAVIL	Tab, Blue, Cap Shaped, Film Coated	Amitriptyline HCl 150 mg	Elavil by Zeneca	00310-0047	Antidepressant
47 <> GG	Tab, Beige, Round, Film Coated	Imipramine HCl 25 mg	Tofranil by Sandoz	00781-1764	Antidepressant
470BARR	Tab, Pink, Oblong, 470/Barr	Acetaminophen 650 mg, Propoxyphene Napsylate 100 mg	Darvocet-N 100 by Barr		Analgesic; C IV
471	Tab, White to Off-White, Round	Meperidine HCl 100 mg	Demerol by Caraco	57664-0471	Analgesic; C II
471 <> SL	Tab, Yellow, Round, Scored	Propranolol HCl 80 mg	Inderal by Ivax	00182-1815	Antihypertensive
4719RUGBY	Tab	Triazolam 0.25 mg	by Chelsea	46193-0978	Sedative/Hypnotic; C IV
473 <> R	Tab, White, Round, Scored, Film Coated	Verapamil HCl 80 mg	Verelan by Actavis	00228-2473	Antihypertensive
473 <> R	Tab, White, Round, Scored, Film Coated	Verapamil HCl 80 mg	Verelan by Heartland	61392-0493	Antihypertensive
473 <> WESTWARD	Tab	Prednisone 10 mg	by West-Ward		Steroid
474 <> MJ	Tab, Orange, Pink & Purple, Pillow Shaped, Chewable	Ascorbic Acid 60 mg, Cyanocobalamin 4.5 mcg, Fluoride Ion 1 mg, Folic Acid 0.3 mg, Niacin 13.5 mg, Pyridoxine HCl 1.05 mg, Riboflavin 1.2 mg, Thiamine 1.05 mg, Vitamin A 2500 Units, Vitamin D 400 Units, Vitamin E 15 Units	Poly Vi Flor by BMS	00087-0474	Vitamin
4740 <> 10	Tab, Light Beige, Cap Shaped	Citalopram HBr 10 mg	Celexa by Ivax	00172-4740 Discontinued	Antidepressant
4740 <> 93	Tab, Light Beige, Cap-Shaped	Citalopram HBr 10 mg	Celexa by Teva	00093-4740	Antidepressant
4741 <> 20	Tab, Light Pink, Cap Shaped, Scored	Citalopram HBr 20 mg	Celexa by Ivax	00172-4741 Discontinued	Antidepressant
4741 <> 93	Tab, Light Pink, Cap-Shaped, Scored, 9 / 3	Citalopram HBr 20 mg	Celexa by Teva	00093-4741	Antidepressant
4742 <> 93	Tab, White, Cap Shaped, Scored	Citalopram HBr 40 mg	Celexa by Ivax	00172-4742 Discontinued	Antidepressant
4742 <> 93	Tab, White to Off-White, Cap-Shaped, Scored, 9 / 3	Citalopram HBr 40 mg	Celexa by Teva	00093-4742	Antidepressant
474COPLEY	Tab, Pink, Round, 474/Copley	Diclofenac Sodium 50 mg	Voltaren by Copley	38245-0474	NSAID
475	Tab, Imprint Begins West-Ward	Prednisone 5 mg	Sterapred by Merz	00259-0390	Steroid
475 <> R	Tab, White, Round, Scored, Film Coated	Verapamil HCl 120 mg	Verelan by Actavis	00228-2475	Antihypertensive
475 <> R	Tab, White, Round, Scored, Film Coated	Verapamil HCl 120 mg	Verelan by Prepackage Specialists	58864-0530	Antihypertensive
475 <> R	Tab, White, Round, Scored, Film Coated	Verapamil HCl 120 mg	Verelan by PDRX	55289-0481	Antihypertensive
475 <> R	Tab, White, Round, Scored, Film Coated	Verapamil HCl 120 mg	Verelan by Heartland	61392-0496	Antihypertensive
4759 <> 10MG	Tab, Beige, Hexagonal, Film-Coated	Prasugrel 10 mg	Effient by Eli Lilly	00002-4759	Antiplatelet
4759 <> 10MG	Tab, Beige, Double Arrow Shaped, Film-Coated	Prasugrel 10 mg	Effient by Eli Lilly	Canadian DIN 02349124	Antiplatelet
476 <> MJ	Tab, Pillow-Shaped, Chewable	Ascorbic Acid 60 mg, Copper 1 mg, Cyanocobalamin 4.5 mcg, Fluoride Ion 1 mg, Folic Acid 0.3 mg, Iron 12 mg, Niacin 13.5 mg, Pyridoxine HCl 1.05 mg, Riboflavin 1.2 mg, Thiamine 1.05 mg, Vitamin A 2500 Units, Vitamin D 400 Units, Vitamin E 15 Units, Zinc 10 mg	Poly Vi Flor Iron by BMS	00087-0476	Vitamin
4760 <> 5MG	Tab, Yellow, Hexagonal, Film-Coated	Prasugrel 5 mg	Effient by Eli Lilly	00002-4760	Antiplatelet
4761CEFACLOR500MG	Cap, Zenith Logo	Cefaclor 500 mg	Ceclor CD by DRX	55045-2337	Antibiotic

ID FRONT <> BACK	DESCRIPTION FRONT <> BACK	INGREDIENT & STRENGTH	BRAND (or Generic Equiv.) by FIRM	NDC#	CLASS; SCH.
477	Tab, Round, White, Film Coated, Scored	Metoprolol Tartrate 50 mg	Lopressor by Caraco	57664-0477	Antihypertensive
477 <> MJ	Tab, Orange, Pink & Purple, Pillow Shaped, Chewable	Ascorbic Acid 60 mg, Cholecalciferol 400 Units, Sodium Fluoride, Vitamin A Acetate 2500 Units	Tri Vi Flor by BMS	00087-0477	Vitamin
477477 <> GLYBUR	Tab, White, Oblong, Scored	Glyburide 1.25 mg	DiaBeta by Blue Ridge	59273-0015	Antidiabetic
477477 <> GLYBUR	Tab, White, Oblong, Scored	Glyburide 1.25 mg	DiaBeta by Teva	38245-0477	Antidiabetic
477477 <> GLYBUR	Tab, White, Oblong, Scored	Glyburide 1.25 mg	DiaBeta by Blue Ridge	59273-0013	Antidiabetic
477477 <> GLYBUR	Tab, White, Oblong, Scored	Glyburide 1.25 mg	DiaBeta by Merrell	00068-3200	Antidiabetic
477477 <> GLYBUR	Tab, White, Oblong, Scored	Glyburide 1.25 mg	DiaBeta by Coventry	61372-0576	Antidiabetic
477COPLEY	Tab, White, Oblong, 477/Copley	Glyburide 1.25 mg	Diabeta by Copley		Antidiabetic
478 <> RDY	Tab, Light Pink, Cap Shaped, Film Coated	Zolpidem Tartrate 5 mg	Ambien by Dr. Reddy's	55111-0478	Sedative/Hypnotic; C IV
479 <> RDY	Tab, White, Cap Shaped, Film Coated	Zolpidem Tartrate 10 mg	Ambien by Dr. Reddy's	55111-0479	Sedative/Hypnotic; C IV
479HD	Tab, White, Round	Dipyridamole 50 mg	Persantine by Halsey	Discontinued	Antiplatelet
48	Tab, Fushchia, Film Coated	Calcium Pantothenate 10 mg, Cyanocobalamin 25 mcg, Ferrous Sulfate 525 mg, Folic Acid 800 mcg, Niacinamide 30 mg, Pyridoxine HCl 5 mg, Riboflavin 6 mg, Sodium Ascorbate 500 mg, Thiamine Mononitrate 6 mg	Generet 500 Folic Acid by Ivax	00182-4333	Vitamin; Mineral
48	Tab, Yellow, Oblong, Film-Coated, Fournier logo <> 48	Fenofibrate 48 mg	Lipidil EZ by Fournier	Canadian DIN 02269074	Antihyperlipidemic
48 <> 93	Tab, White to Off-White, Oval	Metformin HCl 500 mg	Glucophage by Teva	00093-1048	Antidiabetic
48 <> A	Tab, Green, Yellow, White, Round, Scored	Phendimetrazine Tartrate 35 mg	Bontril PDM by Amarin	65234-0048	Anorexiant; C III
48 <> A	Tab, Yellow, Cap Shaped, Film Coated	Glyburide 5 mg, Metformin 500 mg	Glucovance by Aurobindo	65862-0082	Antidiabetic
480 <> R	Tab, White, Oval, Film Coated	Tolmetin Sodium 600 mg	by Physician Total Care	54868-2421	NSAID
480 <> R	Tab, White, Oval, Film Coated	Tolmetin Sodium 600 mg	by Ivax	00182-1932	NSAID
480 <> R	Tab, White, Oval, Film Coated	Tolmetin Sodium 600 mg	by Actavis	00228-2480	NSAID
480 <> R	Tab, White, Oval, Film Coated	Tolmetin Sodium 600 mg	by Qualitest	00603-6131	NSAID
4804	Cap, Blue & White	Oxazepam 10 mg	by PF	48692-0094	Sedative/Hypnotic; C IV
4804	Cap, Blue & White	Oxazepam 10 mg	by PF	48692-0030	Sedative/Hypnotic; C IV
4805	Tab, Clear, Oval, Logo	Oxazepam 15 mg	by PF	48692-0106	Sedative/Hypnotic; C IV
481 <> WC	Tab, Green, Cap Shaped, W/C	Inert	Ovcon 35 by Warner Chilcott	00430-0582	Oral Contraceptive; Placebo
4810 <> V	Tab, White, Round, Scored	Oxycodone HCl 5 mg	OxyContin by Qualitest	00603-4990	Analgesic; C II
4811 <> V	Tab, Light Green, Round, Scored	Oxycodone HCl 15 mg	OxyContin by Qualitest	00603-4991	Analgesic; C II
4811 <> V	Tab, Light Green, Round, Scored	Oxycodone HCl 15 mg	Roxicodone by Vintage	00254-4811	Analgesic; C II
4812 <> V	Tab, Light Blue, Round, Scored	Oxycodone HCl 30 mg	Roxicodone by Vintage	00254-4812	Analgesic; C II
4812 <> V	Tab, Light Blue, Round, Scored	Oxycodone HCl 30 mg	OxyContin by Qualitest	00603-4992	Analgesic; C II
481BARR	Tab, Aqua, Round	Haloperidol 10 mg	Haldol by Barr		Antipsychotic
482 <> MJ	Tab, Pillow-Shaped, Chewable	Ascorbic Acid 60 mg, Copper 1 mg, Cyanocobalamin 4.5 mcg, Fluoride Ion 0.5 mg, Folic Acid 0.3 mg, Iron 12 mg, Niacin 13.5 mg, Pyridoxine HCl 1.05 mg, Riboflavin 1.2 mg, Thiamine 1.05 mg, Vitamin A 2500 Units, Vitamin D 400 Units, Vitamin E 15 Units, Zinc 10 mg	Poly Vi Flor Iron by BMS	00087-0482	Vitamin
4821 <> I1	Tab, White, Round, Scored	Lorazepam 1 mg	Ativan by Teva	00093-4821	Antianxiety; C IV
4822 <> I2	Tab, White, Round, Scored	Lorazepam 2 mg	Ativan by Teva	00093-4822	Antianxiety; C IV
482A <> RBX	Tab, White, Oval, Film Coated	Carvedilol 3.125 mg	Coreg by Ranbaxy	Canadian DIN 02268027	Antihypertensive
482B <> RBX	Tab, White, Oval, Film Coated	Carvedilol 6.25 mg	Coreg by Ranbaxy	Canadian DIN 02268035	Antihypertensive
482BARR	Tab, Salmon, Round	Haloperidol 20 mg	Haldol by Barr		Antipsychotic
482C <> RBX	Tab, White, Oval, Film Coated	Carvedilol 12.5 mg	Coreg by Ranbaxy	Canadian DIN 02268043	Antihypertensive

ID FRONT <> BACK	DESCRIPTION FRONT <> BACK	INGREDIENT & STRENGTH	BRAND (or Generic Equiv.) by FIRM	NDC#	CLASS; SCH.
482D <> RBX	Tab, White, Oval, Film Coated	Carvedilol 25 mg	Coreg by Ranbaxy	Canadian DIN 02268051	Antihypertensive
4832V	Cap, Red, 4832V	Acetaminophen 500 mg, Oxycodone HCl 5 mg	Percocet by Vintage	00254-4832	Analgesic; C II
4832V	Cap, Red, 4832V	Acetaminophen 500 mg, Oxycodone HCl 5 mg	Percocet by Qualitest	00603-4997	Analgesic; C II
4833G <> 302	Tab, White to Off-White, Round, 30/2	Pioglitazone 30 mg, Glimepiride 2 mg	Duetact by Takeda	64764-0302	Antidiabetic
4833G <> 304	Tab, White to Off-White, Round, 30/4	Pioglitazone 30 mg, Glimepiride 4 mg	Duetact by Takeda	64764-0304	Antidiabetic
4833M <> 15500	Tab, White to Off-White, Oblong, Film Coated, 15/500	Pioglitazone HCl 15 mg, Metformin HCl 500 mg	Actoplus Met by Takeda	64764-0155	Antidiabetic
4833M <> 15850	Tab, White to Off-White, Oblong, Film Coated, 15/850	Pioglitazone HCl 15 mg, Metformin HCl 850 mg	Actoplus Met by Takeda	64764-0158	Antidiabetic
4839V	Tab, White, Round, Scored	Acetaminophen 325 mg, Oxycodone HCl 5 mg	Percocet by Ivax	00182-1465	Analgesic; C II
4839V	Tab, White, Round, Scored	Acetaminophen 325 mg, Oxycodone HCl 5 mg	Percocet by Qualitest	00603-4998	Analgesic; C II
4839V	Tab, White, Round, Scored	Acetaminophen 325 mg, Oxycodone HCl 5 mg	Percocet by Vintage	00254-4839	Analgesic; C II
484 <> B	Tab, White, Round	Leucovorin Calcium 5 mg	Wellcovorin by UDL	51079-0581	Antineoplastic
484 <> B	Tab, White, Round	Leucovorin Calcium 5 mg	Wellcovorin by Barr	00555-0484	Antineoplastic
484 <> B	Tab, White, Round	Leucovorin Calcium 5 mg	Wellcovorin by Major	00904-2315	Antineoplastic
484 <> B	Tab, White, Round	Leucovorin Calcium 5 mg	Wellcovorin by Qualitest	00603-4183	Antineoplastic
484 <> B	Tab, White, Round	Leucovorin Calcium 5 mg	Wellcovorin by Supergen		Antineoplastic
4841	Tab, White, Round	Neomycin Sulfate 500 mg	Neomycin by Eon	62701-0900	Antibiotic
485 <> B	Tab, Pale Green, Round	Leucovorin Calcium 25 mg	Wellcovorin by Supergen	62701-0901	Antineoplastic
485 <> B	Tab, Pale Green, Round	Leucovorin Calcium 25 mg	Wellcovorin by Qualitest	00603-4184	Antineoplastic
485 <> B	Tab, Pale Green, Round	Leucovorin Calcium 25 mg	Wellcovorin by Barr	00555-0485	Antineoplastic
485 <> B	Tab, Pale Green, Round	Leucovorin Calcium 25 mg	Wellcovorin by UDL	51079-0582	Antineoplastic
4853V	Tab, 4853 and V Separated by Horizontal Line	Oxybutynin Chloride 5 mg	by Qualitest	00603-4975	Urinary Tract
4853V	Tab, 4853 and V Separated by Horizontal Line	Oxybutynin Chloride 5 mg	Ditropan by Vintage	00254-4835	Urinary Tract
486 <> RDY	Tab, White, Oval	Nabumetone 500 mg	Relafen by Dr. Reddy's	55111-0486	NSAID
487 <> MJ	Tab, Orange, Pink & Purple, Chewable	Cyanocobalamin 4.5 mcg, Folic Acid 0.3 mg, Niacinamide, Pyridoxine HCl 1.05 mg, Riboflavin 1.2 mg, Sodium Ascorbate, Sodium Fluoride, Thiamine Mononitrate, Vitamin A Acetate, Vitamin D 400 Units, Vitamin E Acetate	Poly Vi Flor by BMS	00087-0487	Vitamin
487 <> RDY	Tab, White, Oval	Nabumetone 750 mg	Relafen by Dr. Reddy's	55111-0487	NSAID
4870125MG	Cap, White, Opaque, Hourglass Logo 4870 <> 12.5mg	Hydrochlorothiazide 12.5 mg	Hydrodiuril by Ivax	00172-4870	Diuretic; Antihypertensive
4870125MG	Cap, White, Opaque	Hydrochlorothiazide 12.5 mg	Microzide by Teva	00172-4870	Antihypertensive/Diuretic
488 <> MJ	Tab, Chewable	Cupric Oxide, Cyanocobalamin 4.5 mcg, Ferrous Fumarate, Folic Acid 0.3 mg, Niacinamide, Pyridoxine HCl 1.05 mg, Riboflavin 1.2 mg, Sodium Ascorbate, Sodium Fluoride, Thiamine Mononitrate, Vitamin A Acetate, Vitamin D 400 Units, Vitamin E Acetate, Zinc Oxide	Poly Vi Flor Iron by BMS	00087-0488	Vitamin
488DPI	Cap, White, Black Print, Opaque	Hydrochlorothiazide 25 mg, Triamterene 37.5 mg	Dyazide by Barr	00555-0488	Diuretic; Antihypertensive
4890 <> SB	Tab, White, Pentagonal, Film Coated	Ropinirole HCl 0.25 mg	Requip by GSK	Canadian DIN 02232565	Antiparkinson
4890 <> SB	Tab, White, Pentagonal, Film Coated	Ropinirole HCl 0.25 mg	Requip by SKB	60351-4890	Antiparkinson
4890 <> SB	Tab, White, Pentagonal, Film Coated	Ropinirole HCl 0.25 mg	Requip by RX Pak	65084-0202	Antiparkinson
4890 <> SB	Tab, White, Pentagonal, Film Coated	Ropinirole HCl 0.25 mg	Requip by SKB	00007-4890	Antiparkinson
4891 <> SB	Tab, Yellow, Pentagonal, Film Coated	Ropinirole HCl 0.5 mg	Requip by SKB	00007-4891	Antiparkinson
4891 <> SB	Tab, Yellow, Pentagonal, Film Coated	Ropinirole HCl 0.5 mg	Requip by SKB	60351-4891	Antiparkinson
4892 <> SB	Tab, Green, Pentagonal, Film Coated	Ropinirole HCl 1 mg	Requip by SKB	60351-4892	Antiparkinson
4892 <> SB	Tab, Green, Pentagonal, Film Coated	Ropinirole HCl 1 mg	Requip by SKB	00007-4892	Antiparkinson
4892 <> SB	Tab, Green, Pentagonal, Film Coated	Ropinirole HCl 1 mg	Requip by RX Pak	65084-0203	Antiparkinson
4892 <> SB	Tab, Green, Pentagonal, Film Coated	Ropinirole HCl 1 mg	Requip by GSK	Canadian DIN 02232567	Antiparkinson
4893 <> SB	Tab, Light Pink, Pentagonal, Film Coated	Ropinirole HCl 2 mg	Requip by GSK	Canadian DIN 02232568	Antiparkinson

ID FRONT <> BACK	DESCRIPTION FRONT <> BACK	INGREDIENT & STRENGTH	BRAND (or Generic Equiv.) by FIRM	NDC#	CLASS; SCH.
4893 <> SB	Tab, Light Pink, Pentagonal, Film Coated	Ropinirole HCl 2 mg	Requip by SKB	00007-4893	Antiparkinson
4893 <> SB	Tab, Light Pink, Pentagonal, Film Coated	Ropinirole HCl 2 mg	Requip by SKB	60351-4893	Antiparkinson
4894 <> SB	Tab, Blue, Pentagonal, Film Coated	Ropinirole HCl 5 mg	Requip by SKB	60351-4894	Antiparkinson
4894 <> SB	Tab, Blue, Pentagonal, Film Coated	Ropinirole HCl 5 mg	Requip by SKB	00007-4894	Antiparkinson
4894 <> SB	Tab, Blue, Pentagonal, Film Coated	Ropinirole HCl 5 mg	Requip by GSK	Canadian DIN 02232569	Antiparkinson
4895 <> SB	Tab, Purple, Pentagonal	Ropinirole HCl 3 mg	Requip by SKB	00007-4895	Antiparkinson
4896 <> SB	Tab, Brown, Pentagonal	Ropinirole HCl 4 mg	Requip by SKB	00007-4896	Antiparkinson
49 <> 93	Tab, White to Off-White, Oval	Metformin HCl 850 mg	Glucophage by Teva	00093-1049	Antidiabetic
49 <> A	Tab, Yellow, Round, Film Coated	Risperidone 0.25 mg	Risperdal by Aurobindo	65862-0119	Antipsychotic
49 <> BIOCRAFT	Tab, White, Oval, Scored	Penicillin V Potassium 500 mg	by Rx Dispensing	61807-0004	Antibiotic
49 <> BIOCRAFT	Tab, White, Oval, Scored	Penicillin V Potassium 500 mg	by Apotheca	12634-0422	Antibiotic
49 <> BIOCRAFT	Tab, White, Oval, Scored	Penicillin V Potassium 500 mg	by Ivax	00182-1537	Antibiotic
49 <> BIOCRAFT	Tab, White, Oval, Scored	Penicillin V Potassium 500 mg	by Teva	Discontinued	Antibiotic
49 <> RB	Tab, Light Blue, Oval	Glimepiride 2 mg	Amaryl by Ranbaxy	63304-0426 Discontinued	Antidiabetic
49 <> RB	Tab, White, Dumbbell-Shaped, Scored	Glimepiride 2 mg	Amaryl by Ranbaxy	63304-0426	Antidiabetic
4940V	Tab, Gray, Round, Sugar Coated	Perphenazine 2 mg	Trilafon by Qualitest	00603-5090	Antipsychotic
4941V	Tab, Gray, Round, Sugar Coated	Perphenazine 4 mg	Trilafon by Qualitest	00603-5091	Antipsychotic
4942V	Tab, Gray, Round, Sugar Coated	Perphenazine 8 mg	Trilafon by Qualitest	00603-5092	Antipsychotic
494HD	Tab, White, Round	Dipyridamole 25 mg	Persantine by Halsey	Discontinued	Antiplatelet
496 <> SCHERING	Tab, White, Round, Scored	Griseofulvin, Microsize 500 mg	Fulvicin-U/F by Schering	00085-0496	Antifungal
4960	Cap, Light Brown, Opaque, Hourglass Logo 4960	Flutamide 125 mg	Eulexin by Ivax	00172-4960	Antiandrogen
497	Cap, Yellow	Nifedipine 10 mg	Procardia by Novopharm		Antihypertensive
4971V	Tab, Maroon, Round, Scored, Coated	Phenazopyridine HCl 100 mg	by Pharmafab	62542-0917	Urinary Analgesic
4971V	Tab, Maroon, Round, Scored, Coated	Phenazopyridine HCl 100 mg	by Kaiser	00179-0542	Urinary Analgesic
4971V	Tab, Maroon, Round, Scored, Coated	Phenazopyridine HCl 100 mg	by Direct Dispensing	57866-4388	Urinary Analgesic
4972V	Tab, Burgundy, Scored, Coated	Phenazopyridine HCl 200 mg	by Direct Dispensing	57866-4392	Urinary Analgesic
4972V	Tab, Burgundy, Scored, Coated	Phenazopyridine HCl 200 mg	by Kaiser	00179-0545	Urinary Analgesic
4972V	Tab, Burgundy, Scored, Coated	Phenazopyridine HCl 200 mg	by Physician Total Care	54868-0879	Urinary Analgesic
497DYNACIN50MG	Cap, White	Minocycline HCl 50 mg	Dynacin by Nat Pharmpak	55154-9102	Antibiotic
4980	Tab, Pink, Cap Shaped, Hourglass Logo 4980	Acetaminophen 650 mg, Propoxyphene Napsylate 100 mg	Darvocet-N 100 by Ivax	00172-4980 Discontinued	Analgesic; C IV
499	Tab, Yellow, Oval, Film Coated	Mirtazapine 15 mg	Remeron by Caraco	57664-0499	Antidepressant
499	Tab, Peach, Round, Sch. Logo 499	Methyltestosterone 25 mg	Oreton by Schering		Hormone; C III
499 <> BARR	Tab, White, Oval, Film Coated	Ibuprofen 800 mg	Motrin by Barr	00555-0499 Discontinued	NSAID
4G87C879	Tab	Aspirin 325 mg, Codeine Phosphate 60 mg	Aspirin w/ Codeine by URL Mutual	00677-0676	Analgesic; C III
4H2	Tab, White, Oval	Cetirizine HCl 10 mg	Zyrtec by Perrigo	45802-0919	Antihistamine
4I	Tab, White, Oval	Ibuprofen 400 mg	Motrin by Dr. Reddy's	55111-0682	NSAID
4LLA39	Tab, White, Round	Acetaminophen 300 mg, Codeine Phosphate 60 mg	Tylenol w/ Codeine by Lederle		Analgesic; C III
4MG	Cap, White and Blue, Opaque	Tizanidine HCl 4 mg	Zanaflex by Acorda	10144-0604	Muscle Relaxant
4MG <> 503	Tab, Green, Cap Shaped	Guanfacine 4 mg	Intuniv by Shire	54092-0519	Non-Stimulant Anti-ADHD
4MG <> CARDURA	Tab, Orange, Oblong, Scored	Doxazosin Mesylate 4 mg	Cardura by Roerig	00049-2770	Antihypertensive
4MG <> CARDURA	Tab, Orange, Oblong, Scored	Doxazosin Mesylate 4 mg	Cardura by Nat Pharmpak	55154-3216	Antihypertensive
4MG <> ETH268	Tab, Pink, Oblong	Doxazosin Mesylate 4 mg	Cardura by Ethex	58177-0268	Antihypertensive
4MG <> MLP18	Tab, Orange, Oblong, Scored	Doxazosin Mesylate 4 mg	Cardura by Dava	67253-0382	Antihypertensive
4MGWATSON151	Cap, White, Opaque, Hard Gelatin	Silodosin 4 mg	Rapaflo by Watson	52544-0151	Alpha Blocker
4R	Cap, Blue, Oval, Opaque, Soft Gel	Terazosin HCl 10 mg	Hytrin by Ranbaxy	63304-0665	Antihypertensive
5	Tab, White, Round	Buspirone HCl 5 mg	Buspar by Amide	52152-0222	Antianxiety

ID FRONT <> BACK	DESCRIPTION FRONT <> BACK	INGREDIENT & STRENGTH	BRAND (or Generic Equiv.) by FIRM	NDC#	CLASS; SCH.
5	Tab, Yellow, Round, Hourglass Logo <> 5	Prochlorperazine 5 mg	Compazine by Ivax	00172-3690	Antiemetic
5	Tab, Yellow, Round, Orally Disintegrating	Olanzapine 5 mg	Zyprexa Zydis by Eli Lilly	00002-4453	Antipsychotic
5	Tab, White, Round	Buspirone HCl 5 mg	Buspar by Major	00904-5587	Antianxiety
5	Tab, Yellow, Round	Bisacodyl 5 mg	Dulcolax by Major	00904-7927	Gastrointestinal
5	Tab, Pink, Round, Scored	Lisinopril 5 mg	Zestril by Lupin	68180-0513	Antihypertensive
5	Tab, White, Round	Terbutaline Sulfate 5 mg	Bricanyl by AstraZeneca	Canadian	Antiasthmatic
5	Tab	Warfarin Sodium 5 mg	Coumadin by Pharmedix	53002-1048	Anticoagulant
5	Cap, Mustard	Nifedipine 5 mg	Apo Nifed by Apotex	Canadian DIN 00725110	Antihypertensive
5	Tab, ER	Nitroglycerin 5 mg	Sustachron ER Buccal by Forest by AltiMed	10418-0140	Vasodilator
5	Tab, White, Oblong, 5 Albert Logo	Glyburide 5 mg	Glyburide	Canadian	Antidiabetic
5	Tab, Pink, Round, 5 Inside Heart Logo	Lisinopril 5 mg	Zestril by AstraZeneca	Canadian DIN 02049333	Antihypertensive
5	Tab, Yellow, Round	Bisacodyl 5 mg	Dulcolax by Apotex	Canadian DIN 00545023	Gastrointestinal
5	Tab, Pink, Round	Isosorbide Dinitrate 5 mg	Isordil by Apotex	Canadian DIN 00670944	Antianginal
5	Tab, Yellow, Round	Methotrimeprazine Maleate 5 mg	Methoprazine by Apotex	Canadian DIN 02238404	Antipsychotic
5	Tab, White, Oblong, 5/Logo	Glyburide 5 mg	Ratio Glyburide by Ratiopharm	Canadian DIN 01900935	Antidiabetic
5	Tab, White, Round	Fluphenazine HCl 5 mg	Fluphenazine by Apotex	Canadian DIN 00405361	Antipsychotic
5	Tab, Blue, Round	Trifluoperazine HCl 5 mg	Apo Trifluoperazine by Apotex	Canadian DIN 00312746	Antipsychotic
5	Tab, Pink, Octagonal, Film Coated, E907 over 5, Extended Release	Oxymorphone HCl 5 mg	Opana ER by Endo	63481-0907	Analgesic; C II
5	Tab, Salmon, Oblong, Film Coated, Scored, 5 <> Servier Logo	Ivabradine 5 mg	Procoralan by Servier		Antianginal
5	Tab, White to Off-White, Round, Sublingual	Asenapine 5 mg	Saphris by Organon	00052-0118	Antipsychotic
5	Tab, White, Round	Metoclopramide HCl 5 mg	Metozolv ODT by Salix	65649-0431	Gastrointestinal
5 <> 102	Tab, White, Oval, Scored, Boehringer Logo and 102 <> 5	Torsemide 5 mg	Demadex by Hoffmann La Roche	00004-0262	Diuretic
5 <> 102	Tab, White, Oval, Scored	Torsemide 5 mg	Demadex by Boehringer Mannheim	12871-6477	Diuretic
5 <> 273	Tab, Yellow, Round, ,5 <> 273	Clonazepam 0.5 mg	Klonopin by Caraco by Qualitest	57664-0273	Sedative; C IV
5 <> 340	Tab, 5/Royce Logo	Pindolol 5 mg		00603-5220	Antihypertensive
5 <> 3690	Tab, Gold, Round	Prochlorperazine 5 mg	Compazine by Ivax	00182-8210	Antiemetic
5 <> 4196	Tab, White, Round, Scored, W over 924	Enalapril Maleate 5 mg	Vasotec by Ivax	00172-4196	Antihypertensive
5 <> 4196	Tab, White, Round, Scored, Hourglass Logo over 4196	Enalapril Maleate 5 mg	Vasotec by Ivax	Discontinued	Antihypertensive
5 <> 4215	Tab, Pink, Round, Film Coated, Blue Ink	Saxagliptin 5 mg	Onglyza by BMS	00003-4215	Antidiabetic
5 <> 511	Tab, White, Pentagon	Lorazepam 0.5 mg	Ativan by Wyeth	52903-5811	Antianxiety; C IV
5 <> 5350	Tab, Yellow, Oblong, Hourglass Logo 5350	Benazepril HCl 5 mg	Lotensin by Ivax	00172-5350 Discontinued	Antihypertensive
5 <> 5663	Tab, White, Oval	Buspirone HCl 5 mg	BuSpar by Teva	00172-5663	Anxiolytic
5 <> 5732	Tab, Pink, Round, Hourglass Logo 5 <> 5732	Bisoprolol 5 mg, Hydrochlorothiazide 6.25 mg	Ziac by Ivax	00172-5731	Antihypertensive; Diuretic
5 <> 644	Tab, Blue, Round	Metolazone 5 mg	Zaroxolyn by Upstate	65580-0644	Diuretic
5 <> A	Tab, White, Round, Flat-Faced, A<>5	Alendronate 5 mg	Fosamax by Apotex	Canadian DIN 02248727	Antiosteoporosis
5 <>AD	Tab, Blue, Round, Scored	Mixed Amphetamine Salts 5 mg; Amphetamine Aspartate 1.25 mg, Amphetamine Sulfate 1.25 mg, Dextroamphetamine Saccharate 1.25 mg, Dextroamphetamine Sulfate 1.25 mg	Adderall by DRX	55045-2606	Stimulant; C II

ID FRONT <> BACK	DESCRIPTION FRONT <> BACK	INGREDIENT & STRENGTH	BRAND (or Generic Equiv.) by FIRM	NDC#	CLASS; SCH.
5 <> AD	Tab, Blue, Round, Scored	Mixed Amphetamine Salts 5 mg; Amphetamine Aspartate 1.25 mg, Amphetamine Sulfate 1.25 mg, Dextroamphetamine Saccharate 1.25 mg, Dextroamphetamine Sulfate 1.25 mg	Adderall by Shire	58521-0031	Stimulant; C II
5 <> AFM	Tab, Pink, Round, Film Coated, Extended Release	Felodipine 5 mg	Plendil by AstraZeneca	Canadian DIN 00851779	Antihypertensive
5 <> APO	Tab, Yellow, Shield-Shaped	Simvastatin 5 mg	Zocor by Apotex	Canadian DIN 02247011	Antihyperlipidemic
5 <> ARICEPT	Tab, White, Round, Film Coated	Donepezil HCl 5 mg	Aricept by Eisai	62856-0245	Antialzheimers
5 <> ARICEPT	Tab, White, Round, Film Coated	Donepezil HCl 5 mg	Aricept by Pfizer	Canadian DIN 02232043	Antialzheimers
5 <> ARICEPT	Tab, White, Round, Orally Disintegrating	Donepezil HCl 5 mg	Aricept ODT by Eisai	62856-0831	Antialzheimers
5 <> ARICEPT	Tab, White, Round, Orally Disintegrating	Donepezil HCl 5 mg	Aricept RDT by Pfizer	Canadian DIN 02269457	Antialzheimers
5 <> B971	Tab, Blue, Oval, Scored, b over 971	Mixed Amphetamine Salts 5 mg; Amphetamine Aspartene 1.25 mg, Amphetamine Sulfate 1.25 mg, Dextroamphetamine Saccharate 1.25 mg, Dextroamphetamine Sulfate 1.25 mg	Adderall by Barr	00555-0971	Stimulant; C II
5 <> BAYER	Tab, Orange, Round, Film-Coated	Vardenafil HCl 5 mg	Levitra by Bayer	Canadian DIN 02250462	Impotence Agent
5 <> BAYER	Tab, Orange, Round, Film-Coated	Vardenafil HCl 5 mg	Levitra by Bayer	00026-8720	Impotence Agent
5 <> D	Tab, Yellow, D-Shaped	Dexmethylphenidate HCl 5 mg	Focalin by Novartis	00078-0381	Stimulant; C II
5 <> DAN5619	Tab, Yellow, Round, Scored, Dan over 5619	Diazepam 5 mg	Valium by DRX	55045-2656	Antianxiety; C IV
5 <> DAN5619	Tab, Yellow, Round, Scored, Dan over 5619	Diazepam 5 mg	Valium by Schein	00364-0775	Antianxiety; C IV
5 <> DAN5619	Tab, Yellow, Round, Scored, Dan over 5619	Diazepam 5 mg	Valium by Watson	00591-5619	Antianxiety; C IV
5 <> DAN5619	Tab, Yellow, Round, Scored, Dan over 5619	Diazepam 5 mg	Valium by Vangard	00615-1533	Antianxiety; C IV
5 <> DAN5619	Tab, Yellow, Round, Scored, Dan over 5619	Diazepam 5 mg	Valium by St. Mary's Med	60760-0775	Antianxiety; C IV
5 <> DRL250	Tab, White, Oval	Nefazodone HCl 250 mg	Serzone by Par	49884-0920	Antidepressant
5 <> DRL250	Tab, White, Oval	Nefazodone HCl 250 mg	Serzone by Dr. Reddy's	55111-0142	Antidepressant
5 <> E	Tab, Yellow, Octagonal	Acetaminophen 400 mg, Hydrocodone Bitartrate 5 mg	Zydone by Endo	63481-0668	Analgesic; C III
5 <> E	Tab, Yellow, Octagonal	Acetaminophen 400 mg, Hydrocodone Bitartrate 5 mg	Zydone by West Pharm	52967-0273	Analgesic; C III
5 <> EPI132	Tab, White, Round, Scored, 5 <> EPI over 132	Oxycodone HCl 5 mg	Percolone by BMS	00056-0132	Analgesic; C II
5 <> EPI132	Tab, White, Round, Scored, 5 <> EPI over 132	Oxycodone HCl 5 mg	Percolone by Endo	63481-0132	Analgesic; C II
5 <> F	Tab, Blue	Medroxyprogesterone Acetate 5 mg	Proclim by Fournier	Canadian	Hormone
5 <> FL	Tab, Beige, Triangular	Nebivolol HCl 5 mg	Bystolic by Forest	00456-1405	Antihypertensive
5 <> FL	Tab, Tan, Cap Shaped, Film Coated	Memantine HCl 5 mg	Namenda by Forest	00456-3205	Antialzheimers
5 <> FL	Tab, Tan, Cap Shaped, Film Coated	Memantine HCl 5 mg	Namenda Titration Pak by Forest	00456-3200	Antialzheimers
5 <> FL	Tab, White to Off-White, Round, Film Coated	Escitalopram Oxalate 5 mg	Lexapro by Forest	00456-2005	Antidepressant
5 <> G022	Tab, Brown, Elliptical, Scored, Film Coated	Quinapril HCl 5 mg	Accupril by Greenstone	59762-5019	Antihypertensive
5 <> G1530	Tab, White, Elongated Octagon-Shaped	Amlodipine Besylate 5 mg	Norvasc by Greenstone	59762-1530	Antihypertensive
5 <> G58	Tab, White to Off White, Round	Amlodipine Besylate 5 mg	Norvasc by Glenmark	68462-0211	Antihypertensive
5 <> GG55	Tab, Lavender, Round, Film Coated, GG over 55	Trifluoperazine HCl 5 mg	Stelazine by Sandoz	00781-1034	Antipsychotic
5 <> GG952	Tab, Pale Yellow, Round	Prochlorperazine 5 mg	Compazine by Sandoz	00781-5020	Antiemetic
5 <> GSCL2	Tab, White to Off-White, Oblong	Lamotrigine 5 mg	Lamictal by GSK	Canadian DIN 02240115	Anticonvulsant
5 <> GSI	Tab, Pale Pink, Square	Ambrisentan 5 mg	Letairis by Gilead	61958-0801	Antihypertensive
5 <> INV275	Tab, Pale Yellow, Round, Film Coated, 5 <> INV over 275	Prochlorperazine Maleate 5 mg	by Apothecon	62269-0275	Antiemetic
5 <> INV275	Tab, Yellow, Round, Film Coated	Prochlorperazine Maleate 5 mg	by Invamed	52189-0275	Antiemetic
5 <> INV275	Tab, Yellow, Round, Film Coated	Prochlorperazine Maleate 5 mg	by Murfreesboro	51129-1427	Antiemetic
5 <> INV280	Tab, Purple, Round, Film Coated	Trifluoperazine HCl 5 mg	Stelazine by Apothecon	62269-0280	Antipsychotic
5 <> INV280	Tab, Purple, Round, Film Coated	Trifluoperazine HCl 5 mg	Stelazine by Invamed	52189-0280	Antipsychotic
5 <> INV313	Tab, Peach, Square, Scored, INV over 313	Warfarin Sodium 5 mg	Coumadin by Sandoz	00781-0377	Anticoagulant

ID FRONT <> BACK	DESCRIPTION FRONT <> BACK	INGREDIENT & STRENGTH	BRAND (or Generic Equiv.) by FIRM	NDC#	CLASS; SCH.
5 <> INV313	Tab, Peach, Square, Scored, INV over 313	Warfarin Sodium 5 mg	Coumadin by Apothecon	59772-0377	Anticoagulant
5 <> L	Tab, White, Oval, Film-Coated	Simvastatin 5 mg	Zocor by Perrigo	45802-0924	Antihyperlipidemic
5 <> LL	Tab, Salmon Pink, Round, Biconvex, Film-Coated	Bisoprolol Fumarate 5 mg	Monocor by Biovail Corp.	Canadian DIN 02241148	Antihypertensive
5 <> LOTENSIN	Tab, Light Yellow, Round	Benazepril HCl 5 mg	Lotensin by Southwood	58016-0264	Antihypertensive
5 <> LOTENSIN	Tab, Light Yellow, Round	Benazepril HCl 5 mg	Lotensin by Novartis	00078-0447	Antihypertensive
5 <> M	Tab, White, Triangular, Scored, M inside square <> over 5	Dextroamphetamine Sulfate 5 mg	Dexedrine by Mallinckrodt	00406-8958	Stimulant; C II
5 <> M	Tab, White to Cream Colored, Pillow-Shaped, M inside square	Mixed Amphetamine Salts 5 mg: Dextroamphetamine Saccharate 1.25 mg, Amphetamine Aspartate 1.25 mg, Dextroamphetamine Sulfate 1.25 mg, Amphetamine Sulfate 1.25 mg	Adderall by Mallinckrodt	00406-8891	Stimulant; C II
5 <> M	Tab, White, Round, M inside square	Methylphenidate HCl 5 mg	Methylin by Mallinckrodt	00406-1121	Stimulant; C II
5 <> M	Tab, White, Round	Methylin Methylphenidate HCl 5 mg	Ritalin by Mallinckrodt	00406-1121	Stimulant; C II
5 <> MOXY	Tab, White, Round, Scored, 5 <> M-OXY	Oxycodone HCl 5 mg	Roxicodone by Mallinckrodt		Analgesic; C II
5 <> N	Tab, White, Round	Alendronate Sodium 5 mg	Fosamax by Novopharm	Canadian DIN 02248251	Antiosteoporosis
5 <> N	Tab, Brown, Round	Terazosin HCl 5 mg	Hytrin by Novopharm	Canadian DIN 02230807	Antihypertensive
5 <> N	Tab, Light Yellow, Shield Shaped	Simvastatin 5 mg	Zocor by Novopharm	Canadian DIN 02250144	Antihyperlipidemic
5 <> N179	Tab, White, Round, 5 <> N over 179	Selegiline HCl 5 mg	by Teva	55953-0179	Antiparkinson
5 <> N179	Tab, White, Round, 5 <> N over 179	Selegiline HCl 5 mg	by Major	00904-5206	Antiparkinson
5 <> N179	Tab, White, Round, 5 <> N over 179	Selegiline HCl 5 mg	by Warrick	59930-1537	Antiparkinson
5 <> N344	Tab, Light Green, Round, Scored, N over 344	Glyburide 5 mg	Micronase by Teva	00093-8344	Antidiabetic
5 <> N344	Tab, Light Green, Round, Scored, N over 344	Glyburide 5 mg	Micronase by Warrick	59930-1639	Antidiabetic
5 <> N344	Tab, Light Green, Round, Scored, N over 344	Glyburide 5 mg	Micronase by Medirex	57480-0409	Antidiabetic
5 <> N344	Tab, Light Green, Round, Scored, N over 344	Glyburide 5 mg	Micronase by PDRX	55289-0892	Antidiabetic
5 <> N344	Tab, Light Green, Round, Scored, N over 344	Glyburide 5 mg	Micronase by Brightstone	62939-3231	Antidiabetic
5 <> N344	Tab, Light Green, Round, Scored, N over 344	Glyburide 5 mg	Micronase by Murfreesboro	51129-1288	Antidiabetic
5 <> N344	Tab, Light Green, Round, Scored, N over 344	Glyburide 5 mg	Micronase by Kaiser	00179-1205	Antidiabetic
5 <> N344	Tab, Light Green, Round, Scored, N over 344	Glyburide 5 mg	Micronase by Moore	00839-8041	Antidiabetic
5 <> N344	Tab, Light Green, Round, Scored, N over 344	Glyburide 5 mg	Micronase by Qualitest	00603-3764	Antidiabetic
5 <> N344	Tab, Light Green, Round, Scored, N over 344	Glyburide 5 mg	Micronase by Talbert	44514-0385	Antidiabetic
5 <> N344	Tab, Light Green, Round, Scored, N over 344	Glyburide 5 mg	Micronase by Major	00904-5077	Antidiabetic
5 <> N344	Tab, Light Green, Round, Scored, N over 344	Glyburide 5 mg	Micronase by UDL	51079-0873	Antidiabetic
5 <> N344	Tab, Light Green, Round, Scored, N over 344	Glyburide 5 mg	Micronase by Teva	55953-0344	Antidiabetic
5 <> N344	Tab, Light Green, Round, Scored, N over 344	Glyburide 5 mg	Micronase by Novopharm	62528-0344	Antidiabetic
5 <> N524	Tab, White, Oval, Scored	Glipizide 5 mg	by Novopharm	43806-0524	Antidiabetic
5 <> NN	Tab, Blue, Round, N/N/5	Oxybutynin Chloride 5 mg	Ditropan by Novopharm	Canadian DIN 02230394	Urinary Tract
5 <> NN	Tab, Orange, Oval, Scored, N / N <> 5	Cilazapril 5 mg	Inhibace by Novopharm	Canadian DIN 02266377	Antihypertensive
5 <> NN	Tab, White, Oblong, Scored, N/N	Glyburide 5 mg	DiaBeta by Novopharm	Canadian DIN 01913689	Antidiabetic
5 <> NN	Tab, Blue, Round, Scored, N/N	Medroxyprogesterone Acetate 5 mg	Provera by Novopharm	Canadian DIN 02221292	Hormone
5 <> NOVO	Tab, White, Diamond, Scored, NO/VO <> 5	Prazosin HCl 5 mg	Minipress by Novopharm	Canadian DIN 01934228	Antihypertensive
5 <> NOVO	Tab, White, Round, Scored, NO/VO <> 5	Timolol Maleate 5 mg	Blocadren by Novopharm	Canadian DIN 01947796	Antihypertensive

ID FRONT <> BACK	DESCRIPTION FRONT <> BACK	INGREDIENT & STRENGTH	BRAND (or Generic Equiv.) by FIRM	NDC#	CLASS; SCH.
5 <> NVR	Tab, White to Light Yellow, Oblong	Everolimus 5 mg	Afinitor by Novartis	00078-0566	Cancer Therapy
5 <> P	Tab, White, Shield Shaped	Simvastatin 5 mg	Zocor by Pharmascience	Canadian DIN 02269252	Antihyperlipidemic
5 <> P	Tab, Yellow, Round	Methotrimeprazine Maleate 5 mg	Nozinan by Pharmascience	Canadian DIN 02232903	Antipsychotic
5 <> P	Tab, Peach, Round, Scored	Methadone Hydrochloride 5 mg	Metadol by Pharmascience	Canadian DIN 02247699	Analgesic
5 <> P	Tab, Brown, Round	Terazosin HCl 5 mg	Hytrin by Pharmascience	Canadian DIN 02243520	Antihypertensive
5 <> PAL	Tab, Yellow, Round	Folacin 5 mg, Niacinamide 20 mg, Cobalamin 1 mg, Pantothenic Acid 10 mg, Pyridoxine HCl 50 mg, D-Biotin 300 mcg, Thiamine HCl 1.5 mg, Vitamin C 60 mg, Riboflavin 1.5 mg,	Diatx by PamLab	00525-0316	Vitamin
5 <> PAR651	Tab, White, Round, Scored	Torsemide 5 mg	Demadex by Par	49884-0651	Diuretic
5 <> PAR707	Tab, Peach, Oval, Scored	Buspirone HCl 5 mg	Buspar by Par	49884-0707	Antianxiety
5 <> PD527	Tab, Brown, Oval, Scored, Film Coated	Quinapril HCl 5 mg	Accupril by PDRX	55289-0552	Antihypertensive
5 <> PD527	Tab, Brown, Oval, Scored, Film Coated	Quinapril HCl 5 mg	Accupril by Parke Davis	00071-0527	Antihypertensive
5 <> PD527	Tab, Brown, Oval, Scored, Film Coated	Quinapril HCl 5 mg	Accupril by Pharm Util	60491-0001	Antihypertensive
5 <> PD527	Tab, Brown, Oval, Scored, Film Coated	Quinapril HCl 5 mg	Accupril by Parke Davis	Canadian DIN 01947664	Antihypertensive
5 <> PF	Tab, White, Round	Morphine Sulfate 5 mg	MS Contin by Purdue	Canadian	Analgesic; C II
5 <> PROVERA	Tab	Medroxyprogesterone Acetate 5 mg	by Quality Care	60346-0603	Hormone
5 <> S	Tab, White, Shield Shaped	Selegiline 5 mg	Eldepryl by Watson	52544-0136	Antiparkinson
5 <> S	Tab, White, Shield Shaped	Selegiline 5 mg	Eldepryl by Mylan		Antiparkinson
5 <> SAL	Tab, White, Round, Film Coated	Pilocarpine HCl 5 mg	Salagen by MGI	58063-0705	Cholinergic Agonist
5 <> W	Tab, Pink, Round	Isosorbide Dinitrate 5 mg	Isordil by Wyeth	00008-4126	Antianginal
5 <> WARFARINTARO	Tab, Peach, Cap Shaped	Warfarin Sodium 5 mg	Coumadin by Taro	51672-4032	Anticoagulant
5 <> Z3926	Tab, Yellow, Round, Scored, Z over 3926	Diazepam 5 mg	Valium by Pharmedix	53002-0334	Antianxiety; C IV
5 <> Z3926	Tab, Yellow, Round, Scored, Z over 3926	Diazepam 5 mg	Valium by Qualitest	00603-3217	Antianxiety; C IV
5 <> Z3926	Tab, Yellow, Round, Scored, Z over 3926	Diazepam 5 mg	Valium by Ivax	00172-3926	Antianxiety; C IV
5 <> Z4217	Tab, White, Round, Z over 4217	Pindolol 5 mg	Visken by Ivax	00172-4217 Discontinued	Antihypertensive
5 <> Z4232	Tab, Green, Round, Scored	Bumetanide 0.5 mg	Bumex by Vangard	00615-4541	Diuretic
5 <> ZAROXOLYN	Tab, Blue, Round	Metolazone 5 mg	Zaroxolyn by Amerisource	62584-0850	Diuretic
5 <> ZAROXOLYN	Tab, Blue, Round	Metolazone 5 mg	Zaroxolyn by Prestige	58056-0356	Diuretic
5 <> ZAROXOLYN	Tab, Blue, Round	Metolazone 5 mg	Zaroxolyn by Nat Pharmpak	55154-2505	Diuretic
5 <> ZAROXOLYN	Tab, Blue, Round	Metolazone 5 mg	Zaroxolyn by Medeva	53014-0850	Diuretic
5 <> ZAROXOLYN	Tab, Blue, Round	Metolazone 5 mg	Zaroxolyn by Compumed	00403-1603	Diuretic
5 <> ZAROXOLYN	Tab, Blue, Round	Metolazone 5 mg	Zaroxolyn by Caremark	00339-5428	Diuretic
5 <> ZAROXOLYN	Tab, Blue, Round	Metolazone 5 mg	Zaroxolyn by Neuman	64579-0057	Diuretic
5 <> ZLP	Tab, White, Round, Film Coated	Zolpidem Tartrate 5 mg	Ambien by Sandoz	00781-5317	Sedative/Hypnotic; C IV
5 <> ZM	Tab, Pink, Round, Film Coated	Zolpidem Tartrate 5 mg	Ambien by Genpharm	15330-0264	Sedative/Hypnotic; C IV
5 <> ZT	Tab, White, Round, Off-White Specks, Orally Disintegrating	Zolpidem Tartrate 5 mg	Tovalt ODT by Biovail	64455-0158	Sedative/Hypnotic; C IV
5 <> ZYRTEC	Tab, White, Rectangular, Film Coated	Cetirizine HCl 5 mg	Zyrtec by Murfreesboro	51129-1192	Antihistamine
5 <> ZYRTEC	Tab, White, Rectangular, Film Coated	Cetirizine HCl 5 mg	Zyrtec by Pfizer	00069-5500	Antihistamine
50	Tab, White, Biconvex	Atenolol 50 mg	Tenormin by Schein	Canadian	Antihypertensive
50	Tab, Round	Bethanechol Chloride 50 mg	Urecholine by Roberts	Canadian	Urinary Tract
50	Tab, Pink, Oblong	Metoprolol Tartrate 50 mg	Lopressor by Nu Pharm	Canadian	Antihypertensive
50	Tab, Symbol	Levothyroxine Sodium 50 mcg	Synthroid by Nat Pharmpak	55154-4006	Thyroid Hormone
50	Tab	Levothyroxine Sodium 0.05 mg	Synthroid by Nat Pharmpak	55154-0903	Thyroid Hormone
50	Tab, White	Levothyroxine Sodium 50 mcg	Synthroid by Direct Dispensing	57866-5400	Thyroid Hormone

ID FRONT <> BACK	DESCRIPTION FRONT <> BACK	INGREDIENT & STRENGTH	BRAND (or Generic Equiv.) by FIRM	NDC#	CLASS; SCH.
50	Tab, Yellow, Round	Ketoprofen 50 mg	Orudis by Rhodiapharm	Canadian	NSAID
50	Tab, Pink, Round, Film Coated	Hydralazine HCl 50 mg	Apo Hydralazine by Apotex	Canadian DIN 02004836	Antihypertensive
50	Tab, White, Round, Scored	Levothyroxine Sodium 50 mcg	Eltroxin by GSK	Canadian DIN 02213192	Thyroid Hormone
50	Tab, Pink, Round, Film Coated	Trimipramine Maleate 50 mg	Surmontil by Nu Pharm	Canadian DIN 02020599	Antidepressant
50	Tab, Pink, Round	Trimipramine 50 mg	Rhotrimine by Rhodiapharm	Canadian	Antidepressant
50	Cap, White, Red Print, Ex Release	Theophylline Anhydrous 50 mg	Slo-Bid by RPR	00801-0057	Antiasthmatic
50	Tab, White, Round	Thioridazine HCl 50 mg	Apo Thioridazine by Apotex	Canadian	Antipsychotic
50	Tab, Pink, Round	Hydralazine HCl 50 mg	Apresoline by Apotex	Canadian DIN 00441635	Antihypertensive
50	Cap, Red, Oval	Hydroxyzine HCl 50 mg	Atarax by Novopharm	Canadian DIN 00738840	Antianxiety; Antihistamine
50	Cap, Red	Hydroxyzine HCl 50 mg	Apo Hydroxyzine by Apotex	Canadian DIN 00646016	Antianxiety; Antihistamine
50	Tab, Yellow, Round	Ketoprofen 50 mg	Orudis by Apotex	Canadian DIN 00790435	NSAID
50	Tab, Yellow, Round	Ketoprofen 50 mg	Orudis by Nu Pharm	Canadian DIN 02044633	NSAID
50	Tab, Light Brown, Round	Imipramine HCl 50 mg	Tofranil by Apotex	Canadian DIN 00326852	Antidepressant
50	Tab, Pink, Cap Shaped, Film Coated, Scored	Metoprolol Tartrate 50 mg	Lopressor by Apotex	Canadian DIN 00749354	Antihypertensive
50	Tab, Brown, Round	Amitriptyline HCl 50 mg	Elavil by Apotex	Canadian DIN 00335088	Antidepressant
50	Tab, Green, Round, Film Coated	Desipramine HCl 50 mg	Apo Desipramine by Apotex	Canadian DIN 02216264	Antidepressant
50	Tab, Reddish Brown, Round, Coated	Diclofenac Sodium 50 mg	Voltaren by Apotex	Canadian DIN 02243433	NSAID
50	Tab, Pink, Trapezoid-Shaped	Fluconazole 50 mg	Diflucan by Cobalt	Canadian DIN 02281260	Antifungal
50	Tab, Pink, Trapezoid-Shaped	Fluconazole 50 mg	Diflucan by Glenmark	68462-0101	Antifungal
50	Tab, Light Orange, Round	Topiramate 50 mg	Topamax by Dava	67253-0752	Anticonvulsant
50 <> 1170	Tab, Pale Yellow, Cap Shaped, Scored, Film Coated	Naltrexone HCl 50 mg	Revia by Mallinckrodt	00406-1170	Opioid Antagonist
50 <> 15	Tab, White, Oval, Hourglass Logo 50 <> 15	Captopril 50 mg, HCTZ 15 mg	Capozide by Ivax	00172-5015	Antihypertensive; Diuretic
50 <> 25	Tab, Off-White, Oval, Hourglass Logo 50 <> 25	Captopril 50 mg, HCTZ 25 mg	Capozide by Ivax	00172-5025	Antihypertensive; Diuretic
50 <> 273INV	Tab, 273/INV	Captopril 50 mg	Capoten by Schein	00364-2630	Antihypertensive
50 <> 349	Tab, 50/Royce Logo <> 349	Captopril 50 mg	Capoten by Qualitest	00603-2557	Antihypertensive
50 <> 4343	Tab, Peach, Oval, Logo 4343 <> 50	Nefazodone 50 mg	Sezone by Ivax	00172-4343	Antidepressant
50 <> 4404	Tab, Pale Yellow, Round, Hourglass Logo 4404 <> 50	Clozapine 50 mg	Clozaril by Ivax	00093-4404	Antipsychotic
50 <> 5410	Tab, Pink, Oval	Fluconazole 50 mg	Diflucan by Ivax	00172-5410	Antifungal
50 <> 5673	Tab, Light Blue, Oval, Scored, Ivax Logo 50	Sertraline HCl 50 mg	Zoloft by Ivax	00172-5673 Discontinued	Antidepressant
50 <> 727N	Tab, 727/N	Metoprolol Tartrate 50 mg	Lopressor by Schein	00364-2560	Antihypertensive
50 <> 832	Tab, Sugar Coated	Chlorpromazine HCl 50 mg	Thorazine by Schein	00364-0382	Antipsychotic
50 <> 832	Tab, Sugar Coated	Chlorpromazine HCl 50 mg	Thorazine by URL Mutual	00677-0455	Antipsychotic
50 <> 832	Tab, Butterscotch Yellow, Sugar Coated	Chlorpromazine HCl 50 mg	Thorazine by Qualitest	00603-2810	Antipsychotic
50 <> A	Tab, Light Pink, Round, Film Coated	Dolasetron 50 mg	Anzemet by Aventis	00088-1202	Antiemetic
50 <> A	Tab, Pale Violet, Scored	Acetaminophen 325 mg, Butalbital 50 mg	Phrenilin by Amarin	65234-0050	Analgesic

ID FRONT <> BACK	DESCRIPTION FRONT <> BACK	INGREDIENT & STRENGTH	BRAND (or Generic Equiv.) by FIRM	NDC#	CLASS; SCH.
50 <> ANANDRON	Tab, White, Round, Biconvex	Nilutamide 50 mg	Anandron by Aventis	Canadian DIN 02221861	Antiandrogen
50 <> ANZEMET	Tab, Light Pink, Round, Film Coated	Dolasetron 50 mg	Anzemet by Merrell	00068-1202	Antiemetic
50 <> APO	Tab, White, Round	Fluvoxamine Maleate 50 mg	Luvox by Apotex	Canadian DIN 02231329	OCD
50 <> B	Tab, White, Cap Shaped, Film Coated	Diphenhydramine HCl 50 mg	Benadryl by Pfizer	Canadian DIN 02239138	Antihistamine
50 <> B	Tab, Pink, Round, Film Coated, Heart Outline around B	Bisoprolol 5 mg, Hydrochlorothiazide 6.25 mg	Ziac by Duramed	51285-0050	Antihypertensive; Diuretic
50 <> CATAFLAM	Tab, Light Brown, Round, Sugar Coated	Diclofenac Potassium 50 mg	Cataflam by Novartis	00078-0436	NSAID
50 <> CATAFLAM	Tab, Light Brown, Round, Sugar Coated	Diclofenac Potassium 50 mg	Cataflam by PDRX	55289-0818	NSAID
50 <> CATAFLAM	Tab, Light Brown, Round, Sugar Coated	Diclofenac Potassium 50 mg	Cataflam by Direct Dispensing	57866-1182	NSAID
50 <> CATAFLAM	Tab, Light Brown, Round, Sugar Coated	Diclofenac Potassium 50 mg	Cataflam by H J Harkins Co	52959-0344	NSAID
50 <> CATAFLAM	Tab, Light Brown, Round, Sugar Coated	Diclofenac Potassium 50 mg	Cataflam by Novartis	00028-0151	NSAID
50 <> CATAFLAM	Tab, Light Brown, Round, Sugar Coated	Diclofenac Potassium 50 mg	Cataflam by Allscripts		NSAID
50 <> CATAFLAM	Tab, Light Brown, Round, Sugar Coated	Diclofenac Potassium 50 mg	Cataflam by DRX	55045-2225	NSAID
50 <> CATAFLAM	Tab, Light Brown, Round, Sugar Coated	Diclofenac Potassium 50 mg	Cataflam by Novartis	17088-0151	NSAID
50 <> COBALTLOGO	Tab, Pink, Trapezoidal	Fluconazole 50 mg	Co Fluconazole by Cobalt	Canadian DIN 02281260	Antifungal
50 <> DEPADE	Tab, Pale Yellow, Cap Shaped, Scored, Film Coated	Naltrexone HCl 50 mg	Depade by Mallinckrodt	00406-0092	Opioid Antagonist; Antialcoholism
50 <> FL	Tab, Green, Oval, Film-Coated	Milnacipran HCl 50 mg	Savella by Forest	00456-1550	Antidepressant; Antifibromyalgia
50 <> FLINT	Tab, White, Round, Scored	Levothyroxine Sodium 50 mcg	Synthroid by Abbott	Canadian DIN 02172070	Thyroid Hormone
50 <> FLINT	Tab, White, Round, Scored	Levothyroxine Sodium 50 mcg	Synthroid by Med Pro	53978-0589	Thyroid Hormone
50 <> FLINT	Tab, White, Round, Scored	Levothyroxine Sodium 50 mcg	Synthroid by Physician Total Care	54868-1011	Thyroid Hormone
50 <> FLINT	Tab, White, Round, Scored	Levothyroxine Sodium 50 mcg	Synthroid by Murfreesboro	51129-1657	Thyroid Hormone
50 <> FLINT	Tab, White, Round, Scored	Levothyroxine Sodium 50 mcg	Synthroid by Giant Food	11146-0301	Thyroid Hormone
50 <> FLINT	Tab, White, Round, Scored	Levothyroxine Sodium 50 mcg	Synthroid by Knoll	55445-0104	Thyroid Hormone
50 <> FLINT	Tab, White, Round, Scored	Levothyroxine Sodium 50 mcg	Synthroid by Amerisource	62584-0013	Thyroid Hormone
50 <> FLINT	Tab, White, Round, Scored	Levothyroxine Sodium 50 mcg	Synthroid by Forest	00456-0321	Thyroid Hormone
50 <> FLINT	Tab, White, Round, Scored	Levothyroxine Sodium 50 mcg	Synthroid by Kaiser	00179-0457	Thyroid Hormone
50 <> FLINT	Tab, White, Round, Scored	Levothyroxine Sodium 50 mcg	Synthroid by Abbott	00048-1040	Thyroid Hormone
50 <> GG33	Tab, Orange, Round, Film Coated, GG over 33	Thioridazine 50 mg	Mellaril by Sandoz	00781-1634	Antipsychotic
50 <> GG332	Tab, White, Cap Shaped, Scored, 50 <> GG over 332	Levothyroxine 50 mcg	Levo-T by Sandoz	00781-5181	Thyroid Hormone
50 <> GG332	Tab, White, Cap Shaped, Scored, 50 <> GG over 332	Levothyroxine 50 mcg	Levo-T by Alara	64909-0122	Thyroid Hormone
50 <> GG407	Tab, Yellow, Round, GG over 407	Chlorpromazine HCl 50 mg	Thorazine by Sandoz	00781-1717	Antipsychotic
50 <> GLYSET	Tab, White, Round	Miglitol 50 mg	Glyset by Pharmacia	00009-5013	Antidiabetic
50 <> IMITREX	Tab, White, Triangular, Coated	Sumatriptan Succinate 50 mg	Imitrex by Physician Total Care	54868-3852	Antimigraine
50 <> IMITREX	Tab, White, Triangular, Coated	Sumatriptan Succinate 50 mg	Imitrex by Pharm Util	60491-0318	Antimigraine
50 <> IMITREX	Tab, White, Triangular, Coated	Sumatriptan Succinate 50 mg	Imitrex by GSK	00173-0459	Antimigraine
50 <> INV273	Tab, Scored	Captopril 50 mg	Capoten by Invamed	52189-0273	Antihypertensive
50 <> LMT	Tab, White, Round, Orally Disintegrating	Lamotrigine 50 mg	Lamictal ODT by GSK	00173-0774	Anticonvulsant
50 <> M	Tab, Coral, Round, Biconvex, Film Coated, M inside Box	Imipramine HCl 50 mg	Tofranil by Mallinckrodt	00406-6922	Antidepressant
50 <> M59	Tab, Orange, Round, Film Coated, M over 59	Thioridazine 50 mg	Mellaril by UDL	51079-0567	Antipsychotic
50 <> M59	Tab, Orange, Round, Film Coated, M over 59	Thioridazine 50 mg	Mellaril by Mylan	00378-0616	Antipsychotic
50 <> M59	Tab, Orange, Round, Film Coated, M over 59	Thioridazine 50 mg	Mellaril by Dixon Shane	17236-0302	Antipsychotic
50 <> M59	Tab, Orange, Round, Film Coated, M over 59	Thioridazine 50 mg	Mellaril by Qualitest	00603-5994	Antipsychotic
50 <> M59	Tab, Orange, Round, Film Coated, M over 59	Thioridazine 50 mg	Mellaril by Vangard	00615-2507	Antipsychotic

ID FRONT <> BACK	DESCRIPTION FRONT <> BACK	INGREDIENT & STRENGTH	BRAND (or Generic Equiv.) by FIRM	NDC#	CLASS; SCH.
50 <> MJ503	Tab, White w/ Blue Flecks, Round, MJ over 503	Cyclophosphamide 50 mg	Cytoxan by BMS	Canadian DIN 00344885	Antineoplastic
50 <> MJ503	Tab, White w/ Blue Flecks, Round, MJ over 503	Cyclophosphamide 50 mg	Cytoxan by Mead Johnson	00015-0503	Antineoplastic
50 <> N	Tab, Pink, Round, N/50	Hydralazine HCl 50 mg	Apresoline by Novopharm	Canadian DIN 00759481	Antihypertensive
50 <> N	Tab, White, Round, Scored, N <> 5 / 0	Fluvoxamine Maleate 50 mg	Luvox by Novopharm	Canadian DIN 02239953	OCD
50 <> N	Tab, White, Round, Scored, N <> 5 / 0	Chlorpromazine HCl 50 mg	Largactil by Novopharm	Canadian	Antipsychotic; Antiemetic
50 <> N	Tab, White, Round, N <> 5 / 0	Cyproterone Acetate 50 mg	Androcur by Novopharm	Canadian DIN 02232872	Antiandrogen
50 <> N	Tab, Yellow, Cap Shaped, Scored, N <> 5/0	Azathioprine 50 mg	Imuran by Novopharm	Canadian DIN 02236819	Immunosuppressant
50 <> N	Tab, Light Pink, Round	Amitriptyline HCl 50 mg	Elavil by Novopharm	Canadian DIN 00037427	Antidepressant
50 <> N	Tab, Dark Orange, Round, Large N	Imipramine 50 mg	Tofranil by Novopharm	Canadian DIN 00021520	Antidepressant
50 <> N039	Tab, White, Round, Scored	Atenolol 50 mg	Tenormin by Novopharm	62528-0039	Antihypertensive
50 <> N039	Tab, White, Round, 50 <> N over 039	Atenolol 50 mg	Tenormin by Teva	55953-0039 Discontinued	Antihypertensive
50 <> N039	Tab, 50 <> N over 039	Atenolol 50 mg	Tenormin by Medirex	57480-0446	Antihypertensive
50 <> N039	Tab, 50 <> N over 039	Atenolol 50 mg	Tenormin by DRX	55045-1860	Antihypertensive
50 <> N039	Tab, 50 <> N over 039	Atenolol 50 mg	Tenormin by Apotheca	12634-0436	Antihypertensive
50 <> N134	Tab, White, Oblong, Scored, N score 134 <> 50	Captopril 50 mg	Capoten by Major		Antihypertensive
50 <> N134	Tab, White, Oblong, Scored, N score 134 <> 50	Captopril 50 mg	Capoten by Moore	00839-7996	Antihypertensive
50 <> N134	Tab, White, Oblong, Scored, N score 134 <> 50	Captopril 50 mg	Capoten by Medirex	57480-0840	Antihypertensive
50 <> N134	Tab, White, Oblong, Scored, N score 134 <> 50	Captopril 50 mg	Capoten by Teva Pharmaceuticals	00093-8134 Discontinued	Antihypertensive
50 <> N550	Tab, Peach, Round, N over 550	Fluconazole 50 mg	Diflucan by Teva	00093-0237 Discontinued	Antifungal
50 <> N573	Tab, Film Coated	Flurbiprofen 50 mg	Ansaid by Warrick	59930-1771	NSAID
50 <> N573	Tab, Film Coated	Flurbiprofen 50 mg	Ansaid by Moore	00839-8003	NSAID
50 <> N727	Tab, White, Oblong, Scored	Metoprolol Tartrate 50 mg	Lopressor by Va Cmop	65243-0048	Antihypertensive
50 <> N727	Tab, Film Coated	Metoprolol Tartrate 50 mg	Lopressor by Medirex	57480-0802	Antihypertensive
50 <> N727	Tab, White, Cap Shaped, Film Coated	Metoprolol Tartrate 50 mg	Lopressor by Teva	55953-0727 Discontinued	Antihypertensive
50 <> N727	Tab, Film Coated, N 727	Metoprolol Tartrate 50 mg	Lopressor by Brightstone	62939-2211	Antihypertensive
50 <> N735	Tab, Dark Orange, Round, Film Coated	Diclofenac Sodium 50 mg	Voltaren by Allscripts		NSAID
50 <> NOVO	Tab, Light Orange, Round, Scored	Trazodone HCl 50 mg	Desyrel by Novopharm	Canadian DIN 02114263	Antidepressant
50 <> NOVO	Tab, White, Oval, Scored	Captopril 50 mg	Capoten by Novopharm	Canadian DIN 01942980	Antihypertensive
50 <> NOVO	Tab, Peach, Round, Scored, 50 below Score	Hydrochlorothiazide 50 mg	HydroDiuril by Novopharm	Canadian DIN 00021482	Diuretic; Antihypertensive
50 <> NU	Tab, White, Round, Film Coated	Fluvoxamine Maleate 50 mg	Luvox by Nu Pharm	Canadian DIN 02231192	OCD
50 <> OM	Tab, Yellow, Round	Tapentadol Hydrochloride 50 mg	Tapentadol Hydrochloride by Janssen-Ortho	50458-0820	Analgesic; C II
50 <> P	Tab, Yellow, Round	Methotrimeprazine Maleate 50 mg	Nozinan by Pharmascience	Canadian DIN 02232905	Antipsychotic
50 <> P	Tab, Pink, Trapezoid Shaped	Fluconazole 50 mg	Diflucan by Pharmascience	Canadian DIN 02245643	Antifungal

ID FRONT <> BACK	DESCRIPTION FRONT <> BACK	INGREDIENT & STRENGTH	BRAND (or Generic Equiv.) by FIRM	NDC#	CLASS; SCH.
50 <> P	Tab, Reddish Brown, White Print, Round	Diclofenac Sodium 50 mg	Voltaren by Pharmascience	Canadian DIN 02231503	NSAID
50 <> R11	Tab, Pale Yellow, Cap Shaped, Scored, Film Coated	Naltrexone HCl 50 mg	ReVia by BMS	00056-0011	Opioid Antagonist
50 <> R11	Tab, Pale Yellow, Cap Shaped, Scored, Film Coated	Naltrexone HCl 50 mg	ReVia by Duramed	51285-0011	Opioid Antagonist
50 <> R11	Tab, Pale Yellow, Cap Shaped, Scored, Film Coated	Naltrexone HCl 50 mg	Revia by BMS	00056-0011	Opioid Antagonist
50 <> ROBERTS103	Tab	Bethanechol Chloride 50 mg	Urecholine by Pharm Util	60491-0221	Urinary Tract
50 <> S	Tab, Orange, Round, Film Coated, 50 <> S over Triangle	Pinaverium Bromide 50 mg	Dicetel by Solvay	Canadian DIN 01950592	Gastrointestinal
50 <> S	Tab, White, Triangle Shaped	Sumatriptan 50 mg	Imitrex by Dr. Reddy's	55111-0736	Antimigraine
50 <> SP	Tab, Pink, Oval, Film	Lacosamide 50 mg	Vimpat by Schwarz	00091-2477	Antiepileptic
50 <> SYNTHROID	Tab, White, Round, Scored	Levothyroxine Sodium 50 mcg	Synthroid by Abbott	00074-4552	Thyroid Hormone
50 <> T	Tab, Light Yellow, Round	Topiramate 50 mg	Topamax by Pharmascience	Canadian DIN 02312085	Anticonvulsant
50 <> T4	Tab, White, Cap Shaped	Levothyroxine Sodium 50 mcg	Levothroid by Forest	00456-1321	Thyroid Hormone
50 <> TOPAMAX	Tab, Light Yellow, Round, Coated	Topiramate 50 mg	Topamax by Ortho-McNeil	00045-0640	Anticonvulsant
50 <> VIDEX	Tab, Off-White to Light Orange/Yellow, Round, Chewable	Didanosine 50 mg	Videx by BMS	00087-6651	Antiviral
50 <> VOLTAREN	Tab, Light Brown, Round, Enteric Coated	Diclofenac Sodium 50 mg	Voltaren by Novartis	Canadian DIN 00514012	NSAID
500	Tab, Coated	Metformin HCl 500 mg	Glucophage by Lipha	64130-1010	Antidiabetic
500	Cap, Gray & Green	Metronidazole 500 mg	Flagyl by RPR	Canadian	Antibiotic
500	Tab, Oval, Pink, Enteric Coated	Divalproex Sodium 500 mg	Depakote by Nu Pharm	Canadian DIN 02239519	Anticonvulsant
500	Tab, Reddish Brown, Oval, Film Coated	Mirtazapine 30 mg	Remeron by Caraco	57664-0500	Antidepressant
500	Tab, Pink, Cap Shaped, Scored	Niacin 500 mg	Slo-Niacin by Upsher Smith	00245-0063	Vitamin
500	Tab, Off White, Capsule Shaped	Nicotinic Acid 500 mg	Niaspan FCT by Sepracor	Canadian DIN 02262347	Antihyperlipidemic
500 <> 348	Tab, Oval, Beige, Film Coated	Cefprozil 500 mg	Cefzil by Sandoz	00781-5044	Antibiotic
500 <> 4098	Tab, Light Yellow, Oval, Film Coated, Double-Triangle Logo	Nabumetone 500 mg	Relafen by Par	49884-0649	NSAID
500 <> 4174	Tab, White, Cap Shaped, Hourglass Logo 4174	Etodolac 500 mg	Lodine by Ivax	00172-4174	NSAID
500 <> 4194	Tab, Blue, Oval, Ex Release, Hourglass Logo 4194	Cefaclor 500 mg	Ceclor by Ivax	00172-4194	Antibiotic
500 <> 4331	Tab, White, Oval, Hourglass Logo 4331	Metformin HCl 500 mg	Glucophage by Ivax	00172-4331	Antidiabetic
500 <> 4435	Tab, White, Oval, Ivax Logo 4435, ER	Metformin HCl 500 mg	Glucophage XR by Ivax	00172-4435 Discontinued	Antidiabetic
500 <> 5312	Tab, White to Off White, Oval, Ivax Logo 5312 <> 500	Ciprofloxacin 500 mg	Cipro by Ivax	00172-5312	Antibiotic
500 <> 571	Tab, White to Off-White, Cap Shaped, Ex Release, Andrx Logo	Metformin HCl 500 mg	Glucophage XR by Andrx	62037-0571	Antidiabetic
500 <> 6065	Tab, White to Off-White, Cap Shaped, Extended Release	Metformin HCl 500 mg	Glucophage XR by Par	49884-0921	Antidiabetic
500 <> 7721	Tab, White, Cap Shaped, Film Coated	Cefprozil 500 mg	Cefzil by BMS	Canadian DIN 02163667	Antibiotic
500 <> 7721	Tab, White, Cap Shaped, Film Coated	Cefprozil 500 mg	Cefzil by BMS	00087-7721	Antibiotic
500 <> AMOXIL	Tab, Pink, Cap Shaped	Amoxicillin 500 mg	Amoxil by SKB	00029-6046	Antibiotic
500 <> ANDRX674	Tab, White, Round, Film Coated	Metformin HCl 500 mg	Glucophage by Andrx	62037-0674	Antidiabetic
500 <> APO	Tab, Pink, Oval, Biconvex	Divalproex Sodium 500 mg	Depakote by Apotex	Canadian DIN 02239700	Anticonvulsant
500 <> APO	Tab, White, Oval	Nabumetone 500 mg	Nabumetone by Apotex	Canadian DIN 02238639	NSAID
500 <> APO	Tab, White, Cap Shaped, Biconvex, Enteric Coated	Naproxen 500 mg	Naprosyn by Apotex	Canadian DIN 02246701	NSAID
500 <> APO	Tab, White, Cap Shaped	Acetaminophen 500 mg	Tylenol by Apotex	Canadian DIN 02229977	Analgesic

ID FRONT <> BACK	DESCRIPTION FRONT <> BACK	INGREDIENT & STRENGTH	BRAND (or Generic Equiv.) by FIRM	NDC#	CLASS; SCH.
500 <> APO048	Tab, White to Off-White, Oval	Divalproex Sodium 500 mg	Depakote by Apotex	60505-3067	Anticonvulsant
500 <> APO102	Tab, White to Off-White, Oblong	Etodolac 500 mg	Lodine by Apotex	60505-0102	NSAID
500 <> ASPIRIN	Tab, White, Round	Aspirin 500 mg	Aspirin by Perrigo	00113-0448	Analgesic
500 <> B385	Tab, White to Off-White, Oval, Film Coated	Metformin HCl 500 mg	Glucophage by Barr	00555-0385	Antidiabetic
500 <> B815	Tab, White, Cap Shaped, Film Coated, b815	Ciprofloxacin 500 mg	Cipro by Barr	00555-0815	Antibiotic
500 <> BMS6060	Tab, White to Off-White, Round, Film Coated	Metformin HCl 500 mg	Glucophage by PDRX	55289-0211	Antidiabetic
500 <> BMS6060	Tab, White to Off-White, Round, Film Coated	Metformin HCl 500 mg	Glucophage by Heartland	61392-0717	Antidiabetic
500 <> BMS6060	Tab, White to Off-White, Round, Film Coated	Metformin HCl 500 mg	Glucophage by BMS	00087-6060	Antidiabetic
500 <> BMS6063	Tab, White to Off-White, Cap Shaped, Film Coated, Ex Release	Metformin HCl 500 mg	Glucophage XR by BMS	00087-6063	Antidiabetic
500 <> CIPRO	Tab, White to Light Yellow, Oblong, Film Coated	Ciprofloxacin HCl 500 mg	Cipro by Compumed	00403-4522	Antibiotic
500 <> CIPRO	Tab, White to Light Yellow, Oblong, Film Coated	Ciprofloxacin HCl 500 mg	Cipro by St. Mary's Med	60760-0513	Antibiotic
500 <> CIPRO	Tab, White to Light Yellow, Oblong, Film Coated	Ciprofloxacin HCl 500 mg	Cipro by Bayer	Canadian DIN 02155966	Antibiotic
500 <> CIPRO	Tab, White to Light Yellow, Oblong, Film Coated	Ciprofloxacin HCl 500 mg	Cipro by Bayer	00085-1754	Antibiotic
500 <> CIPRO	Tab, White to Light Yellow, Oblong, Film Coated	Ciprofloxacin HCl 500 mg	Cipro by Nat Pharmpak	55154-4801	Antibiotic
500 <> CIPRO	Tab, White to Light Yellow, Oblong, Film Coated	Ciprofloxacin HCl 500 mg	Cipro by PDRX	55289-0371	Antibiotic
500 <> CIPRO	Tab, White to Light Yellow, Oblong, Film Coated	Ciprofloxacin HCl 500 mg	Cipro by Allscripts		Antibiotic
500 <> CIPRO	Tab, White to Light Yellow, Oblong, Film Coated	Ciprofloxacin HCl 500 mg	Cipro by Amerisource	62584-0336	Antibiotic
500 <> CIPRO	Tab, White to Light Yellow, Oblong, Film Coated	Ciprofloxacin HCl 500 mg	Cipro by Rx Dispensing	61807-0035	Antibiotic
500 <> CIPRO	Tab, White to Light Yellow, Oblong, Film Coated	Ciprofloxacin HCl 500 mg	Cipro by Bayer	00026-8513	Antibiotic
500 <> CIPRO	Tab, White to Light Yellow, Oblong, Film Coated	Ciprofloxacin HCl 500 mg	Cipro by Med Pro	53978-3075	Antibiotic
500 <> CIPRO	Tab, White to Light Yellow, Oblong, Film Coated	Ciprofloxacin HCl 500 mg	Cipro by Physician Total Care	54868-0939	Antibiotic
500 <> CIPRO	Tab, White to Light Yellow, Oblong, Film Coated	Ciprofloxacin HCl 500 mg	Cipro by H J Harkins Co	52959-0036	Antibiotic
500 <> DMI	Tab, Blue, Oval, Film Coated, Extended Release	Ciprofloxacin 500 mg	Proquin XR by Depomed	13913-0001	Antibiotic
500 <> ECNAPROSYN	Tab, White, Cap Shaped, Enteric Coated	Naproxen 500 mg	EC-Naprosyn by Hoffmann La Roche	00004-6416	NSAID
500 <> ECNAPROSYN	Tab, White, Cap Shaped	Naproxen 500 mg	Naprosyn by PDRX	55289-0693	NSAID
500 <> ECNAPROSYN	Tab, White, Cap Shaped	Naproxen 500 mg	Naprosyn by Par	49884-0568	NSAID
500 <> ECNAPROSYN	Tab, White, Cap Shaped	Naproxen 500 mg	Naprosyn by Syntex	18393-0256	NSAID
500 <> ECNAPROSYN	Tab, White, Cap Shaped	Naproxen 500 mg	Naprosyn by H J Harkins Co	52959-0456	NSAID
500 <> ECNAPROSYN	Tab, White, Cap Shaped	Naproxen 500 mg	Naprosyn by Compumed	00403-0717	NSAID
500 <> ECNAPROSYN	Tab, White, Cap Shaped	Naproxen 500 mg	Naprosyn by DRX	55045-2441	NSAID
500 <> FAMVIR	Tab, White, Oblong, Film Coated	Famciclovir 500 mg	Famvir by SKB	60351-4117	Antiviral
500 <> FAMVIR	Tab, White, Oblong, Film Coated	Famciclovir 500 mg	Famvir by SKB	00007-4117	Antiviral
500 <> FAMVIR	Tab, White, Oblong, Film Coated	Famciclovir 500 mg	Famvir by Novartis	00078-0368	Antiviral
500 <> FAMVIR	Tab, White, Oblong, Film Coated	Famciclovir 500 mg	Famvir by Novartis	Canadian DIN 02177102	Antiviral
500 <> FLAGYL	Tab, Film Coated, Debossed	Metronidazole 500 mg	by Thrift Drug	59198-0030	Antibiotic
500 <> FLAGYL	Tab, Blue, Oblong, Film Coated	Metronidazole 500 mg	Flagyl by Searle	00025-1821	Antibiotic
500 <> G32	Tab, Off White to Light Pink, Cap Shaped	Naproxen 500 mg	Naprosyn by Glenmark	68462-0190	NSAID
500 <> G45	Tab, White, Round	Metformin 500 mg	Glucophage by Glenmark	68462-0159	Antihyperglycemic
500 <> GLAXO	Tab, White, Oblong	Cefuroxime Axetil 500 mg	Ceftin by GSK	00173-7005	Antibiotic
500 <> GMZ	Tab, Blue, Oval, Film Coated	Metformin HCl 500 mg	Glumetza by Depomed	13913-0002	Antidiabetic
500 <> HAW	Tab, White, Oval, Scored	Methscopolamine Nitrate 2.5 mg, Chlorpheniramine Maleate 8 mg, Pseudoephedrine HCl 120 mg	Xiral by Hawthorn	63717-0500	Cold Remedy
500 <> IP175	Tab, White to Off White, Round	Metformin HCl 500 mg	Glucophage by Amneal	65162-0175	Antihyperglycemic
500 <> IP190	Tab, White, Oblong	Naproxen 500 mg	Naprosyn by Dr. Reddy's	55111-0368	NSAID
500 <> IP190	Tab, White, Oblong	Naproxen 500 mg	Naprosyn by Amneal	65162-0078 Discontinued	NSAID
500 <> IP190	Tab, White, Oblong	Naproxen 500 mg	Naprosyn by Interpharm	53746-0190	NSAID

ID FRONT <> BACK	DESCRIPTION FRONT <> BACK	INGREDIENT & STRENGTH	BRAND (or Generic Equiv.) by FIRM	NDC#	CLASS; SCH.
500 <> KOS	Tab, White, Cap Shaped, Extended Release	Niacin 500 mg	Niaspan by KOS	60598-0001	Antihyperlipidemic
500 <> KOS	Tab, White, Cap Shaped, Extended Release	Niacin 500 mg	Niaspan by Allscripts	54569-5267	Antihyperlipidemic
500 <> KOS	Tab, Orange, Cap Shaped, Film Coated, Extended Release	Niacin 500 mg	Niaspan by KOS	60958-0140	Antihyperlipidemic
500 <> LEVAQUIN	Tab, Peach, Rectangular, Film Coated	Levofloxacin 500 mg	Levaquin by Janssen-Ortho	Canadian DIN 02236842	Antibiotic
500 <> LEVAQUIN	Tab, Peach, Rectangular, Film Coated	Levofloxacin 500 mg	Levaquin by McNeil	00045-1525	Antibiotic
500 <> LEVAQUIN	Tab, Peach, Rectangular, Film Coated	Levofloxacin 500 mg	Levaquin by Physician Total Care	54868-3923	Antibiotic
500 <> LUPIN	Tab, White, Oval, Film Coated	Cefzil 500 mg	Cefzil by Lupin	68180-0404	Antibiotic
500 <> MCNEIL1525	Tab, Peach, Oblong, Film Coated	Levofloxacin 500 mg	Levaquin by Murfreesboro	51129-1629	Antibiotic
500 <> MCNEIL1525	Tab, Peach, Oblong, Film Coated	Levofloxacin 500 mg	Levaquin by Ortho-McNeil	00062-1525	Antibiotic
500 <> MCNEIL1525	Tab, Peach, Oblong, Film Coated	Levofloxacin 500 mg	Levaquin by Johnson & Johnson	59604-0525	Antibiotic
500 <> MPC	Tab, White, Round	Acetohydroxamic Acid 250 mg	Lithostat by Mission	00178-0500	Urinary Tract
500 <> MYLAN107	Tab, Film Coated, 500 <> Mylan over 107	Erythromycin Stearate 500 mg	by St. Mary's Med	60760-0107	Antibiotic
500 <> MYLAN107	Tab, Coated	Erythromycin Stearate 500 mg	by PDRX	55289-0705	Antibiotic
500 <> MYLAN107	Tab, Film Coated, Mylan over 107	Erythromycin Stearate 500 mg	by DRX	55045-1113	Antibiotic
500 <> MYLAN107	Tab, Film Coated, 500 <> Mylan over 107	Erythromycin Stearate 500 mg	by Mylan	00378-0107	Antibiotic
500 <> MYLAN107	Tab, Film Coated	Erythromycin Stearate 500 mg	by Med Pro	53978-0026	Antibiotic
500 <> MYLAN107	Tab, Film Coated, 500 <> Mylan over 107	Erythromycin Stearate 500 mg	by Rx Dispensing	61807-0015	Antibiotic
500 <> MYLAN107	Tab, Coated	Erythromycin Stearate 500 mg	by Direct Dispensing	57866-0265	Antibiotic
500 <> MYLAN156	Tab, Yellow, Oblong, Film Coated	Probenecid 500 mg	Benemid by Med Pro	53978-0014	Antigout
500 <> MYLAN156	Tab, Yellow, Oblong, Film Coated	Probenecid 500 mg	Benemid by Mylan	00378-0156	Antigout
500 <> N	Tab, Orange, Oblong	Diflunisal 500 mg	Dolobid by Novopharm	Canadian DIN 02048507	NSAID
500 <> N	Tab, Light Pink, Oblong	Levofloxacin 500 mg	Levaquin by Novopharm	Canadian DIN 02248263	Antibiotic
500 <> N	Tab, White, Cap Shaped	Naproxen Sodium 500 mg	Naprelan by Victory	68453-0850	NSAID
500 <> N	Tab, White, Cap Shaped	Naproxen Sodium 500 mg	Naprelan by Elan	00086-0091	NSAID
500 <> N520	Tab, Light Yellow, Oval, 500 <> N over 520	Naproxen 500 mg	by Teva	55953-0520 Discontinued	NSAID
500 <> N520	Tab, N over 520	Naproxen 500 mg	by Medirex	67480-0835	NSAID
500 <> NAPROSYN	Tab, Yellow, Round, Scored	Naproxen 500 mg	by Thrift Drug	59198-0239	NSAID
500 <> NAPROSYN	Tab, Yellow, Round, Scored	Naproxen 500 mg	by Nat Pharmpak	55154-3804	NSAID
500 <> NAPROSYN	Tab, Yellow, Round, Scored	Naproxen 500 mg	by Allscripts		NSAID
500 <> NAPROSYN	Tab, Yellow, Round, Scored	Naproxen 500 mg	by Syntex	18393-0277	NSAID
500 <> NAPROSYN	Tab, Yellow, Round, Scored	Naproxen 500 mg	Naprosyn by Rightpak	65240-0701	NSAID
500 <> NAPROSYN	Tab, Yellow, Round, Scored	Naproxen 500 mg	by H J Harkins Co	52959-0516	NSAID
500 <> NAPROSYN	Tab, Yellow, Round, Scored	Naproxen 500 mg	Naprosyn by H J Harkins Co	52959-0111	NSAID
500 <> NAPROSYN	Tab, Yellow, Round, Scored	Naproxen 500 mg	Naprosyn by Novopharm	43806-0139	NSAID
500 <> NOVO	Tab, White, Cap-Shaped, Film-Coated	Ciprofloxacin 500 mg	Novo-Ciprofloxacin by Novopharm	Canadian DIN 02161745	Antibiotic
500 <> P	Tab, White, Oval	Famciclovir 500 mg	Famvir by Pharmascience	Canadian DIN 02278111	Antiviral
500 <> PL	Tab, Pink, Cap Shaped, Film Coated, Scored	Tinidazole 500 mg	Tindamax by Presutti Labs	66378-0500 Discontinued	Antibiotic
500 <> RELAFEN	Tab, White, Oblong, Film Coated	Nabumetone 500 mg	by PDRX	55289-0015	NSAID
500 <> RELAFEN	Tab, White, Oblong, Film Coated	Nabumetone 500 mg	Relafen by Rx Dispensing	61807-0051	NSAID
500 <> RELAFEN	Tab, White, Oblong, Film Coated	Nabumetone 500 mg	Relafen by SKB	Canadian	NSAID
500 <> RELAFEN	Tab, White, Oblong, Film Coated	Nabumetone 500 mg	by Eli Lilly	Canadian	NSAID
500 <> RELAFEN	Tab, White, Oblong, Film Coated	Nabumetone 500 mg	Relafen by SKB	00029-4851	NSAID
500 <> RELAFEN	Tab, White, Oblong, Film Coated	Nabumetone 500 mg	Relafen by H J Harkins Co	52959-0227	NSAID

ID FRONT <> BACK	DESCRIPTION FRONT <> BACK	INGREDIENT & STRENGTH	BRAND (or Generic Equiv.) by FIRM	NDC#	CLASS; SCH.
500 <> RELAFEN	Tab, White, Oblong, Film Coated	Nabumetone 500 mg	by Nat Pharmpak	55154-4505	NSAID
500 <> RELAFEN	Tab, White, Oblong, Film Coated	Nabumetone 500 mg	Relafen by SB	59742-4851	NSAID
500 <> RELAFEN	Tab, White, Oblong, Film Coated	Nabumetone 500 mg	by Amerisource	62584-0851	NSAID
500 <> SP	Tab, Light Orange, Round, Scored, Film Coated	Methocarbamol 500 mg	Robaxin by Schwarz		Muscle Relaxant
500 <> TM	Tab, Pink, Oval, Film Coated	Tinidazole 500 mg	Tindamax by Mission	00178-8500	Antibiotic
500 <> TP190	Tab, White, Oval	Naproxen 500 mg	Naprosyn by Major	00904-4591	NSAID
500 <> TYLENOL	Tab, White, Round	Acetaminophen 500 mg	Tylenol Ex Strength by McNeil	Canadian DIN 00559407	Analgesic
500 <> UCB	Tab	Aspirin 500 mg, Hydrocodone Bitartrate 5 mg	Lortab ASA by UCB	50474-0500	Analgesic; C III
500 <> UCB	Tab, Yellow, Oblong, Scored, Film Coated	Levetiracetam 500 mg	Keppra by UCB	50474-0592	Anticonvulsant
500 <> US67	Tab, White, Oval, Scored, US over 67	Niacin 500 mg	Niacor by Upsher Smith	00245-0067	Vitamin
500 <> XELODA	Tab, Peach, Oblong, Film Coated	Capecitabine 500 mg	Xeloda by Roche	Canadian DIN 02238454	Antineoplastic
500 <> XELODA	Tab, Peach, Oblong, Film Coated	Capecitabine 500 mg	Xeloda by Hoffmann La Roche	00004-1100	Antineoplastic
5000	Cap, 5000 Proceeded By Eon Logo <> Blue & White Pellets	Phentermine HCl 30 mg	by Quality Care	62682-7025	Anorexiant; C IV
500125 <> AMC	Tab, White, Oblong	Amoxicillin 500 mg, Clavulanate Potassium 125 mg	Augmentin by LEK	66685-1002	Antibiotic
500125 <> APO	Tab, White, Oval, Film Coated, 500-125	Amoxicillin 500 mg, Clavulanate Potassium 125 mg	Clavulin by Apotex	Canadian DIN 02243351	Antibiotic
500125 <> AUGMENTIN	Tab, White, Oblong, Film Coated, 500/125	Amoxicillin 500 mg, Clavulanate Potassium 125 mg	Augmentin by Bayer	00280-1011	Antibiotic
500125 <> AUGMENTIN	Tab, White, Oblong, Film Coated, 500/125	Amoxicillin 500 mg, Clavulanate Potassium 125 mg	Augmentin by Casa DeAmigos	62138-6080	Antibiotic
500125 <> AUGMENTIN	Tab, White, Oblong, Film Coated, 500/125	Amoxicillin 500 mg, Clavulanate Potassium 125 mg	Augmentin by Allscripts		Antibiotic
500125 <> AUGMENTIN	Tab, White, Oblong, Film Coated, 500/125	Amoxicillin 500 mg, Clavulanate Potassium 125 mg	Augmentin by PDRX	55289-0296	Antibiotic
500125 <> AUGMENTIN	Tab, White, Oblong, Film Coated, 500/125	Amoxicillin 500 mg, Clavulanate Potassium 125 mg	Augmentin by H J Harkins Co	52959-0021	Antibiotic
500125 <> AUGMENTIN	Tab, White, Oblong, Film Coated, 500/125	Amoxicillin 500 mg, Clavulanate Potassium 125 mg	Augmentin by Pharmedix	53002-0239	Antibiotic
500125 <> AUGMENTIN	Tab, White, Oblong, Film Coated, 500/125	Amoxicillin 500 mg, Clavulanate Potassium 125 mg	Augmentin by Amerisource	62584-0312	Antibiotic
500125 <> AUGMENTIN	Tab, White, Oblong, Film Coated, 500/125	Amoxicillin 500 mg, Clavulanate Potassium 125 mg	Augmentin by SKB	00029-6080	Antibiotic
50020	Tab, Yellow, Oval, Film Coated, Imprint in Black Ink	Naproxen 500 mg, Esomeprazole 20 mg	Vimovo by AstraZeneca	00186-0520	Antiarthritis
500222AF	Cap, White, 500/222 AF	Acetaminophen 500 mg	Tylenol Ex Strength by Johnson & Johnson	Canadian	Analgesic
5002DAN	Cap, Clear & Pink	Diphenhydramine HCl 25 mg	by Schein	00364-0116	Antihistamine
5003DAN	Cap, Pink	Diphenhydramine HCl 50 mg	by Schein	00364-0117	Antihistamine
5005 <> SP2104	Tab, White, Oval, Scored	Acetaminophen 500 mg, Hydrocodone Bitartrate 5 mg	Co-Gesic by Schwarz	00131-2104	Analgesic; C III
500A	Tab, Film Coated, 500/A	Salsalate 500 mg	by Schein	00364-0832	NSAID
500A	Tab, Orange, Cap Shaped, Film Coated, Extended Release, 500 "Abbott Logo"	Niacin 500 mg	Niaspan by Abbott	00074-3074	Antihyperlipidemic
500AP7494	Cap	Cefaclor 500 mg	by Golden State	60429-0702	Antibiotic
500AP7494	Cap	Cefaclor 500 mg	by Apothecon	59772-7494	Antibiotic
500BRISTOL7376	Cap, Blue, 500 Bristol 7376	Cephalexin 500 mg	Keflex by BMS		Antibiotic
500CIPRO	Tab, Yellow, Oblong, Film Coated	Ciprofloxacin HCl 500 mg	Cipro by Pharmedix	53002-0264	Antibiotic
500ESTAC	Cap, Blue, Film Coated	Acetaminophen 500 mg	Tylenol Ex Strength by McNeil	Canadian DIN 02155214	Analgesic
500GLAXO	Tab, White, Oblong, 500/Glaxo	Cefuroxime Axetil 500 mg	Ceftin by GSK	Canadian	Antibiotic
500LUPIN	Cap, Dark Green and Light Green	Cephalexin 500 mg	Keflex by Lupin	68180-0122	Antibiotic
500M50	Tab, Rose, Cap Shaped, Scored, 500 / M50	Naproxen 500 mg	Naprosyn by Dava	67253-0622	NSAID
500M50 <> MOVA	Tab, Rose, Cap Shaped	Naproxen 500 mg	Naprosyn by Compumed	00403-1442	NSAID
500M50 <> MOVA	Tab, Rose, Cap Shaped	Naproxen 500 mg	Naprosyn by Mova	55370-0141	NSAID
500M50 <> MOVA	Tab, Rose, Cap Shaped	Naproxen 500 mg	Naprosyn by JLM	63369-0560	NSAID
500M50 <> MOVA	Tab, Rose, Cap Shaped	Naproxen 500 mg	Naprosyn by Caremark	00339-5874	NSAID
500MG	Tab, Green	Cephalexin 500 mg	Keftabs by H J Harkins Co	52959-0086	Antibiotic
500MG <> L405	Tab, White, Round	Acetaminophen 500 mg	Tylenol Ex Strength by Perrigo	00113-0405	Analgesic
500MG <> L407	Tab, Pink, Cap Shaped	Pseudoephedrine 120 mg	Sudafed 12 Hr by Perrigo	00113-0407	Decongestant

ID FRONT <> BACK	DESCRIPTION FRONT <> BACK	INGREDIENT & STRENGTH	BRAND (or Generic Equiv.) by FIRM	NDC#	CLASS; SCH.
500MG <> OV111	Tab, White, Oval, Film-Coated, Scored	Vigabatrin 500 mg	Sabril by Lundbeck	67386-0111	Anticonvulsant
500MG <> TRYPTAN	Tab, White, Oval, Film Coated	L-Tryptophan 500 mg	Tryptan by Valeant	Canadian DIN 02029456	Supplement
500MG <> TRYPTAN	Tab, White, Oval, Film Coated	L-Tryptophan 500 mg	by AltiMed	Canadian DIN 02240333	Supplement
500MG4761CEFACLOR	Cap, Zenith Logo	Cefaclor 500 mg	Ceclor CD by DRX	55045-2337	Antibiotic
500MG7376BRISTOL	Cap, Blue, White Print	Cephalexin 500 mg	by Golden State	60429-0037	Antibiotic
500MGBRISTOL/7376	Cap, 500 mg <> Bristol over 7376	Cephalexin 500 mg	by BMS		Antibiotic
500MGCALSAN	Cap, White, 500 mg/Calsan	Calcium Carbonate 500 mg	Os-Cal by Novartis	Canadian DIN 02232482	Vitamin; Mineral
500MGZ4761CEFACLOR	Cap	Cefaclor 500 mg	Ceclor CD by Ivax	00172-4761	Antibiotic
500MGZENITH	Cap, Yellowish White Powder	Cefadroxil Monohydrate 500 mg	by Physician Total Care	54868-3742	Antibiotic
500MLA06	Cap, Blue & Gray, 500ML-A06	Cefaclor 500 mg	Ceclor by Mova	55370-0895	Antibiotic
500MLA08	Cap, Light Green & Dark Green, 500ML-A08	Cephalexin 500 mg	Keflex by Mova	55370-0901	Antibiotic
500N	Cap, Brown	Amoxicillin 500 mg	Amoxil by Nat Pharmpak	55154-1750	Antibiotic
500N	Cap	Cephalexin 500 mg	by Rx Dispensing	61807-0006	Antibiotic
500N114	Cap, 500 <> N over 114	Cephalexin 500 mg	by H J Harkins Co	52959-0031	Antibiotic
500N114	Cap, 500 <> N over 114	Cephalexin 500 mg	by Apotheca	12634-0434	Antibiotic
500N114	Cap, Orange, 500 <> N over 114	Cephalexin 500 mg	by Teva	55953-0114	Antibiotic
500N251	Cap, Bright Orange & Gray, Opaque, 500 <> N over 251	Cefaclor 500 mg	Ceclor by UDL	51079-0618	Antibiotic
500N251	Cap, Bright Orange & Gray, Opaque, 500 <> N over 251	Cefaclor 500 mg	by Qualitest	00603-2587	Antibiotic
500N251	Cap, Bright Orange & Gray, Opaque, 500 <> N over 251	Cephalexin 500 mg	by Warrick	59930-1536	Antibiotic
500N251	Cap, Bright Orange & Gray, Opaque, 500 <> N over 251	Cephalexin 500 mg	Ceclor CD by Major	00904-5205	Antibiotic
500N251	Cap, Bright Orange & Gray, Opaque, 500 <> N over 251	Cefaclor 500 mg	by Teva	55953-0251 Discontinued	Antibiotic
500N716	Cap	Amoxicillin 500 mg	Amoxil by Casa DeAmigos	62138-0601	Antibiotic
500N716	Cap, Buff, Opaque, 500 <> N over 716	Amoxicillin 500 mg	Amoxil by Novopharm	43806-0716	Antibiotic
500N716	Cap, 500 <> N over 716	Amoxicillin 500 mg	Amoxil by St. Mary's Med	60760-0716	Antibiotic
500P	Cap, Purepac Logo	Prazosin HCl 1 mg	by Actavis		Antihypertensive
500POLY	Cap, Blue Print	Acetaminophen 500 mg, Hydrocodone Bitartrate 5 mg	Vicodin by Poly	50991-0005	Analgesic; C III
500SP	Cap, Green and White	Amoxicillin 500 mg	Amoxil by 4349121 Canada Inc	Canadian DIN 02241827	Antibiotic
500TAS	Cap, Yellow, Film Coated	Acetaminophen 500 mg, Chlorpheniramine Maleate 2 mg, Pseudoephedrine HCl 30 mg	Extra Strength Tylenol Allergy Sinus by McNeil	Canadian DIN 01933728	Cold Remedy
500TCMND	Cap, Yellow, Film Coated	Acetaminophen 500 mg, Pseudoephedrine HCl 30 mg, Dextromethorphan HBr 15 mg	Tylenol Flu Daytime Ex Strength by McNeil	Canadian DIN 00743267	Cold Remedy
500TYLENOL	Cap, White, Film Coated	Acetaminophen 500 mg	Tylenol Ex Strength by McNeil	Canadian DIN 00723908	Analgesic
501	Tab, Lavender, Round, Scored, Martec Logo 501	Estradiol 0.5 mg	Estrace by Martec	52555-0716	Hormone
501	Tab, Off-White, Oval, Film Coated	Mirtazapine 45 mg	Remeron by Caraco	57664-0501	Antidepressant
501 <> DP	Tab, Lavender, Round, Duramed Logo	Estradiol 0.5 mg	Estrace by Duramed	51285-0501	Hormone
501 <> M	Tab, Orange, Round, Film Coated	Bisoprolol 2.5 mg, Hydrochlorothiazide 6.25 mg	Ziac by UDL	51079-0954 Discontinued	Antihypertensive; Diuretic
501 <> M	Tab, Orange, Round, Film Coated	Bisoprolol 2.5 mg, Hydrochlorothiazide 6.25 mg	Ziac by Mylan	00378-0501	Antihypertensive; Diuretic
50100 <> SL441	Tab, White, Trapezoid, Scored, SL 441 <> 50/100	Trazodone HCl 150 mg	Desyrel by Heartland	61392-0179	Antidepressant
50100 <> SL441	Tab, White, Trapezoid, Scored, SL 441 <> 50/100	Trazodone HCl 150 mg	Desyrel by Physician Total Care	54868-1959	Antidepressant
5011 <> G	Tab, Light Yellow, Round	Spironolactone 25 mg	Aldactone by Greenstone	59762-5011	Diuretic
5011V	Tab, White, Round	Phenobarbital 15 mg	by Qualitest	00603-5165	Sedative/Hypnotic; C IV
5011V	Tab, Bisected V	Phenobarbital 15 mg	by Vintage	00254-5011	Sedative/Hypnotic; C IV
5012 <> G	Tab, Orange, Oval, Scored	Spironolactone 50 mg	Aldactone by Greenstone	59762-5012	Diuretic

For updated data, go to www.IdentADrug.com

ID FRONT <> BACK	DESCRIPTION FRONT <> BACK	INGREDIENT & STRENGTH	BRAND (or Generic Equiv.) by FIRM	NDC#	CLASS; SCH.
5012V	Tab, White, Round	Phenobarbital 32.4 mg	by Vangard	00615-0463	Sedative/Hypnotic; C IV
5012V	Tab, White, Round	Phenobarbital 32.4 mg	by Vintage	00254-5012	Sedative/Hypnotic; C IV
5012V	Tab, White, Round	Phenobarbital 32.4 mg	by PDRX	55289-0535	Sedative/Hypnotic; C IV
5012V	Tab, White, Round	Phenobarbital 32.4 mg	by Ivax	00182-0292	Sedative/Hypnotic; C IV
5012V	Tab, White, Round	Phenobarbital 32.4 mg	by Qualitest	00603-5166	Sedative/Hypnotic; C IV
5012V	Tab, White, Round	Phenobarbital 32.4 mg	by Physician Total Care		Sedative/Hypnotic; C IV
5013 <> G	Tab, Peach, Round, Scored	Spironolactone 100 mg	Aldactone by Greenstone	59762-5013	Diuretic
5013 <> V	Tab, White, Round, Convex	Phenobarbital 64.8 mg	by Physician Total Care	54868-3933	Sedative/Hypnotic; C IV
5013V	Tab, 5013/V	Phenobarbital 64.8 mg	by Heartland	61392-0392	Sedative/Hypnotic; C IV
5013VV	Tab	Phenobarbital 64.8 mg	by DRX	55045-2387	Sedative/Hypnotic; C IV
5014 <> G	Tab, Tan, Round	Hydrochlorothiazide 25 mg, Spironolactone 25 mg	Aldactazide by Greenstone	59762-5014	Diuretic; Antihypertensive
5014 <> V	Tab, White, Round, Convex	Phenobarbital 97.2 mg	by Physician Total Care	54868-3958	Sedative/Hypnotic; C IV
502	Tab, White to Off-White, Round, Scored	Tizanidine HCl 2 mg	Zanaflex by Caraco	57664-0502	Muscle Relaxant
502	Tab, Pink, Round	Estradiol 1 mg	Estrace by Duramed		Hormone
502	Tab, Rose, Round, Scored, Martec Logo 502	Estradiol 1 mg	Estrace by Martec	52555-0717	Hormone
502 <> DP	Tab, Rose, Round, Duramed Logo	Estradiol 1 mg	by Duramed	51285-0502	Hormone
502 <> DP	Tab, Pink, Round, Scored, 502 <> D over P	Estradiol 1 mg	by Heartland	61392-0178	Hormone
502 <> KOS	Tab, Light Yellow, Cap Shaped	Lovastatin 20 mg, Niacin 500 mg	Advicor by KOS	60598-0006	Antihyperlipidemic
502 <> MD	Tab, Dark Green	Dextromethorphan HBr 30 mg, Guaifenesin 600 mg	Humigen DM by MD	43567-0502	Cold Remedy
50223	Tab, White to Off White, Round, Flat	Liothyronine Sodium 50 mcg	Cytomel by Paddock	00574-0223	Thyroid Hormone
5025	Tab, White, Round, 50/25	Atenolol 50 mg, Chlorthalidone 25 mg	Tenoretic by Zeneca	Canadian	Antihypertensive; Diuretic
5025 <> APO	Tab, White, Round, Scored, Film Coated	Atenolol 50 mg, Chlorthalidone 25 mg	Tenoretic by Apotex	Canadian DIN 02248763	Antihypertensive; Diuretic
5025 <> N	Tab, White, Round, Scored	Atenolol 50 mg, Chlorthalidone 25 mg	Tenoretic by Novopharm	Canadian DIN 02302918	Antihypertensive
502502	Cap, Purepac Logo	Prazosin HCl	by Heartland	61392-0112	Antihypertensive
50252550 <> APO150	Tab, Pale Orange, Rectangular, Scored, APO-150 <> 50/25/25/50	Trazodone HCl 150 mg	Apo Trazodone by Apotex	Canadian DIN 02147653	Antidepressant
50252550 <> NU150	Tab, Pale Orange, Rectangular, Scored, 50 over 25 over 25 over 50 <> NU-150	Trazodone HCl 150 mg	Desyrel by Nu Pharm	Canadian DIN 02165406	Antidepressant
503	Tab, White to Off-White, Round, Scored	Tizanidine HCl 4 mg	Zanaflex by Caraco	57664-0503	Muscle Relaxant
503 <> 1MG	Tab, White to Off-White, Round	Guanfacine 1 mg	Intuniv by Shire	54092-0513	Non-Stimulant Anti-ADHD
503 <> 2MG	Tab, White to Off-White, Cap Shaped	Guanfacine 2 mg	Intuniv by Shire	54092-0515	Non-Stimulant Anti-ADHD
503 <> 3MG	Tab, Green, Round	Guanfacine 3 mg	Intuniv by Shire	54092-0517	Non-Stimulant Anti-ADHD
503 <> 4MG	Tab, Green, Cap Shaped	Guanfacine 4 mg	Intuniv by Shire	54092-0519	Non-Stimulant Anti-ADHD
503 <> M	Tab, Blue, Round, Film Coated	Bisoprolol 5 mg, Hydrochlorothiazide 6.25 mg	Ziac by Mylan	00378-0503	Antihypertensive; Diuretic
503 <> M	Tab, Blue, Round, Film Coated	Bisoprolol 5 mg, Hydrochlorothiazide 6.25 mg	Ziac by UDL	51079-0955	Antihypertensive; Diuretic
				Discontinued	
5030 <> V	Tab, Light Blue with Dark Blue Specks	Phentermine 37.5 mg	Adipex-P by Qualitest	00603-5192	Anorexiant; C IV
5030 <> V	Tab, Light Blue with Dark Blue Specks	Phentermine 37.5 mg	Adipex-P by Vintage	00254-5030	Anorexiant; C IV
5030 <> WATSON	Tab, Blue, Round	Levonorgestrel 0.03 mg, Ethinyl Estradiol 0.05 mg	Trivora-28 by Murfreesboro	51129-1631	Oral Contraceptive
5030 <> WATSON	Tab, Blue, Round	Ethinyl Estradiol 0.03 mg, Levonorgestrel 0.05 mg	Trivora-28 by Watson	52544-0291	Oral Contraceptive
5032 <> 2025	Tab, Peach, Round, Ivax Hourglass Logo 5032 <> 20/25	Lisinopril 20 mg, HCTZ 25 mg	Prinzide by Ivax	00172-5032	Antihypertensive; Diuretic
5033 <> 10125	Tab, Blue, Round, Ivax Hourglass Logo 5033 <> 10/12.5	Lisinopril 10 mg, HCTZ 12.5 mg	Prinzide by Ivax	00172-5033	Antihypertensive; Diuretic
5034 <> 20125	Tab, Yellow, Round, Ivax Hourglass Logo 5034 <> 20/12.5	Lisinopril 20 mg, HCTZ 12.5 mg	Prinzide by Ivax	00172-5034	Antihypertensive; Diuretic
503HD	Tab, Blue, Round	Chlorpropamide 250 mg	Diabinese by Halsey	Discontinued	Antidiabetic
504	Tab, Blue, Round, Scored, Martec Logo 504	Estradiol 2 mg	Estrace by Martec	52555-0718	Hormone
504	Tab, White, Blue Specks, Cap Shaped	Phentermine HCl 37.5 mg	Adipex-P by Caraco	57664-0504	Anorexiant; C IV
504 <> DP	Tab, Blue, Round, Duramed Logo	Estradiol 2 mg	Estrace by Duramed	51285-0504	Hormone
5044	Tab, Pink, Oval, Scored	Eprosartan 400 mg	Teveten by SKB	60351-5044	Antihypertensive

ID FRONT <> BACK	DESCRIPTION FRONT <> BACK	INGREDIENT & STRENGTH	BRAND (or Generic Equiv.) by FIRM	NDC#	CLASS; SCH.
5044	Tab, Pink, Oval, Scored	Eprosartan 400 mg	Teveten by Halsey		Antihypertensive
5044 <> SOLVAY	Tab, Pink, Oval	Eprosartan 400 mg	Teveten by Solvay	Canadian DIN 02240432	Antihypertensive
5044 <> SOLVAY	Tab, Pink, Oval	Eprosartan 400 mg	Teveten by Biovail	64455-0130	Antihypertensive
5046 <> SOLVAY	Tab, White, Cap Shaped	Eprosartan 600 mg	Teveten by Biovail	64455-0131	Antihypertensive
5046 <> SOLVAY	Tab, White, Cap Shaped	Eprosartan 600 mg	Teveten by Solvay	Canadian DIN 02243942	Antihypertensive
505 <> M	Tab, White, Round, Film Coated	Bisoprolol 10 mg, Hydrochlorothiazide 6.25 mg	Ziac by Mylan	00378-0505	Antihypertensive; Diuretic
505 <> M	Tab, White, Round, Film Coated	Bisoprolol 10 mg, Hydrochlorothiazide 6.25 mg	Ziac by UDL	51079-0956	Antihypertensive; Diuretic
5050	Tab, White, Cap Shaped, Scored	Ephedrine HCl 25 mg, Guaifenesin 400 mg	Ephedrine Formula 400 by D & E Pharma	Discontinued	Cold Remedy
5050	Tab, White, Round, 50/50	Hydrochlorothiazide 50 mg, Spironolactone 50 mg	Novo Spirozine by Novopharm	Canadian	Diuretic; Antihypertensive
5050 <> DAN	Tab, Orange, Round, Film Coated	Hydralazine HCl 25 mg	by Schein	00364-0144	Antihypertensive
5050 <> NOVO	Tab, Light Peach, Round, Scored, NOVO <> 50/50	Hydrochlorothiazide 50 mg, Spironolactone 50 mg	Aldactazide by Novopharm	Canadian DIN 00657182	Diuretic; Antihypertensive
505050 <> AP3171	Tab, Off-White, Rectangular, Scored	Trazodone HCl 150 mg	Desyrel by Apothecon	59772-3171	Antidepressant
505050 <> APOT150	Tab, White, Oval, Scored	Trazodone HCl 150 mg	Desyrel by Apotex	60505-2655	Antidepressant
505050 <> BARR732	Tab, White, Oval, Scored	Trazodone HCl 150 mg	Desyrel by Barr	00555-0732	Antidepressant
505050 <> BARR732	Tab, White, Oval, Scored	Trazodone HCl 150 mg	Desyrel by Teva	00480-0290	Antidepressant
505050 <> BLBL	Tab, Orange, Rectangular, Scored, Trisected	Trazodone HCl 150 mg	Desyrel by BMS	Canadian DIN 00702277	Antidepressant
505050 <> MJ778	Tab, Orange, Rectangular, Scored	Trazodone HCl 150 mg	Desyrel by Apothecon	59772-3171	Antidepressant
505050 <> MJ778	Tab, Orange, Rectangular, Scored	Trazodone HCl 150 mg	Desyrel by Rx Pak	65084-0221	Antidepressant
505050 <> MJ778	Tab, Orange, Rectangular, Scored	Trazodone HCl 150 mg	Desyrel by Amerisource	62584-0778	Antidepressant
505050 <> MJ778	Tab, Orange, Rectangular, Scored	Trazodone HCl 150 mg	Desyrel by Pharm Util	60491-0912	Antidepressant
505050 <> MJ778	Tab, Orange, Rectangular, Scored	Trazodone HCl 150 mg	Desyrel by Leiner	59606-0631	Antidepressant
505050 <> MJ778	Tab, Orange, Rectangular, Scored	Trazodone HCl 150 mg	Desyrel by BMS	00087-0778	Antidepressant
505050 <> MJ778	Tab, Orange, Rectangular, Scored	Trazodone HCl 150 mg	Desyrel by Nat Pharmpak	55154-2011	Antidepressant
505050 <> MJ778	Tab, Orange, Rectangular, Scored	Trazodone HCl 150 mg	Desyrel by Physician Total Care	54868-2549	Antidepressant
505050 <> NOVO	Tab, Light Orange, Rectangular, NOVO <> 50/50/50	Trazodone HCl 150 mg	Desyrel by Novopharm	Canadian DIN 02144298	Antidepressant
505050 <> PLIVA441	Tab, White, Trapezoidal, Scored	Trazodone HCl 150 mg	Desyrel by Pliva	50111-0441	Antidepressant
505050 <> SL441	Tab, White, Trapezoidal, Scored, 50 50 50 <> SL441	Trazodone HCl 150 mg	Desyrel by Parmed	00349-8824	Antidepressant
505050 <> SL441	Tab, White, Trapezoidal, Scored, 50 50 50 <> SL441	Trazodone HCl 150 mg	Desyrel by Ivax	00182-1298	Antidepressant
505050 <> SL441	Tab, White, Trapezoidal, Scored, 50 50 50 <> SL441	Trazodone HCl 150 mg	Desyrel by Qualitest	00603-6146	Antidepressant
505050 <> SL441	Tab, White, Trapezoidal, Scored, 50 50 50 <> SL441	Trazodone HCl 150 mg	Desyrel by URL Mutual	00677-1302	Antidepressant
505050 <> SL441	Tab, White, Trapezoidal, Scored, 50 50 50 <> SL441	Trazodone HCl 150 mg	Desyrel by Moore	00839-7507	Antidepressant
505050 <> SL441	Tab, White, Trapezoidal, Scored, 50 50 50 <> SL441	Trazodone HCl 150 mg	Desyrel by Sandoz	00781-1826	Antidepressant
505050 <> SL441	Tab, White, Trapezoidal, Scored, 50 50 50 <> SL441	Trazodone HCl 150 mg	Desyrel by Warner Chilcott	00047-0716	Antidepressant
505050 <> SL441	Tab, White, Trapezoidal, Scored, 50 50 50 <> SL441	Trazodone HCl 150 mg	Desyrel by Major	00904-3992	Antidepressant
5052 <> DANDAN	Tab, White, Round, Scored	Prednisone 5 mg	Deltasone by Schein	00364-0218	Steroid
5052 <> DANDAN	Tab, White, Round, Scored	Prednisone 5 mg	Deltasone by Watson	00591-5052	Steroid
5052 <> DANDAN	Tab, White, Round, Scored	Prednisone 5 mg	Deltasone by Vedco	50989-0601	Steroid
5052 <> DANDAN	Tab, White, Round, Scored	Prednisone 5 mg	Deltasone by Nat Pharmpak	55154-5208	Steroid
5052 <> DANDAN	Tab, White, Round, Scored	Prednisone 5 mg	Deltasone by Danbury	61955-0218	Steroid
5052 <> DANDAN	Tab, White, Round, Scored	Prednisone 5 mg	Deltasone by Merz	00259-0390	Steroid
5052 <> DANDAN	Tab, White, Round, Scored	Prednisone 5 mg	Deltasone by WA Butler	11695-1801	Steroid
5052 <> DANDAN	Tab, White, Round, Scored	Prednisone 5 mg	Deltasone by Southwood	58016-0216	Steroid
5052JMI	Tab, Yellow, Round	Chlorpheniramine Maleate 4 mg	by JMI Canton		Antihistamine
5052V	Tab, Film Coated, 5052/V	Guaifenesin 400 mg, Phenylpropanolamine HCl 75 mg	Entex LA by Vintage	00254-5052	Cold Remedy

For updated data, go to www.IdentADrug.com

ID FRONT <> BACK	DESCRIPTION FRONT <> BACK	INGREDIENT & STRENGTH	BRAND (or Generic Equiv.) by FIRM	NDC#	CLASS; SCH.
5053 <> V	Tab	Guaifenesin 600 mg, Phenylpropanolamine HCl 75 mg	Entex LA by Qualitest	00603-3778	Cold Remedy
5053 <> V	Tab, 50/53 <> V	Guaifenesin 600 mg, Phenylpropanolamine HCl 75 mg	Entex LA by Vintage	00254-5053	Cold Remedy
5058 <> DANDAN	Tab, Blue-Green, Round, Scored	Tripelennamine HCl 50 mg	by Schein	00364-0281	Antihistamine
5059 <> DANDAN	Tab, Peach, Round, Scored	Prednisolone 5 mg	Prednisolone by Schein	00364-0217	Steroid
5059 <> DANDAN	Tab, Peach, Round, Scored	Prednisolone 5 mg	Prednisolone by Darby Group	66467-4346	Steroid
5059 <> DANDAN	Tab, Peach, Round, Scored	Prednisolone 5 mg	Prednisolone by WA Butler	11695-1800	Steroid
5059 <> DANDAN	Tab, Peach, Round, Scored	Prednisolone 5 mg	Prednisolone by Vedco	50989-0600	Steroid
5059 <> DANDAN	Tab, Peach, Round, Scored	Prednisolone 5 mg	Prednisolone by Watson	00591-5059	Steroid
506HD	Tab, White, Round	Metronidazole 250 mg	Flagyl by Halsey	Discontinued	Antibiotic
507	Tab, White, Round, Schering Logo 507	Griseofulvin, Ultramicrosize 250 mg	Fulvicin P/G by Schering	00591-5059	Antifungal
507 <> MYLAN	Tab, Green, Coated, Beveled Edge	Hydrochlorothiazide 15 mg, Methyldopa 250 mg	Aldoril by Mylan	00378-0507	Diuretic; Antihypertensive
507 <> WATSON	Tab, Light Yellow, Round	Ethinyl Estradiol 0.035 mg, Norethindrone 0.5 mg	Necon 0.5 35 21 by Watson	52544-0507	Oral Contraceptive
507 <> WATSON	Tab, Light Yellow, Round	Ethinyl Estradiol 0.035 mg, Norethindrone 0.5 mg	Necon 1 10/11-21 by Watson	52544-0553	Oral Contraceptive
507 <> WATSON	Tab, Light Yellow, Round	Ethinyl Estradiol 0.035 mg, Norethindrone 0.5 mg	Necon 0.5 35 28 by Watson	52544-0550	Oral Contraceptive
507 <> WATSON	Tab, Light Yellow, Round	Ethinyl Estradiol 0.035 mg, Norethindrone 0.5 mg	Necon 1 10/11-28 by Watson	52544-0554	Oral Contraceptive
507HD	Cap, Green	Indomethacin 25 mg	Indocin by Halsey	Discontinued	NSAID
508	Cap, Off-White & Red	Acetaminophen 325 mg, Dichloralphenazone 100 mg, Isometheptene Mucate 65 mg	by Jerome Stevens Pharm		Analgesic; C IV
508	Tab, Pink, Oval, Film Coated	Citalopram HBr 20 mg	Celexa by Caraco	57664-0508	Antidepressant
508 <> WATSON	Tab, Light Yellow, Round	Ethinyl Estradiol 0.035 mg, Norethindrone 1 mg	Necon 1 10/11-28 by Watson	52544-0554	Oral Contraceptive
508 <> WATSON	Tab, Dark Yellow, Round	Ethinyl Estradiol 0.035 mg, Norethindrone 1 mg	Necon 1 35 21 by Watson	52544-0508	Oral Contraceptive
508 <> WATSON	Tab, Light Yellow, Round	Ethinyl Estradiol 0.035 mg, Norethindrone 1 mg	Necon 1 10/11-21 by Watson	52544-0553	Oral Contraceptive
508 <> WATSON	Tab, Dark Yellow, Round	Ethinyl Estradiol 0.035 mg, Norethindrone 1 mg	Necon 1 35 28 by Watson	52544-0552	Oral Contraceptive
5084 <> V	Tab, White, Round, Scored	Prednisone 1 mg	Deltasone by Vintage	00254-5084	Steroid
5085 <> V	Tab, White, Round, Scored	Prednisone 2.5 mg	Deltasone by Vintage	00254-5085	Steroid
508HD	Cap, Green	Indomethacin 50 mg	Indocin by Halsey	Discontinued	NSAID
509	Tab, White, Oval, Film Coated	Citalopram HBr 40 mg	Celexa by Caraco	57664-0509	Antidepressant
50902 <> B	Tab, Beige, Round, Scored, Film Coated, 50 over 902	Naltrexone HCl 50 mg	ReVia by Barr	00555-0902	Opioid Antagonist
5092 <> V	Tab, Peach, Round, Scored	Prednisone 20 mg	Deltasone by Vintage	00254-5092	Steroid
5093 <> V	Tab, White, Round, Scored	Prednisone 10 mg	Deltasone by Vintage	00254-5093	Steroid
5093 <> V	Tab, White, Round, Scored	Prednisone 10 mg	Deltasone by Qualitest	00603-5338	Steroid
5094 <> V	Tab, White, Round, Scored	Prednisone 5 mg	Deltasone by Qualitest	00603-5337	Steroid
5094 <> V	Tab, White, Round, Scored	Prednisone 5 mg	Deltasone by Vintage	00254-5094	Steroid
5097V	Tab, Coated, Scored	Ascorbic Acid 80 mg, Beta-Carotene, Biotin 0.03 mg, Calcium Carbonate, Cholecalciferol 400 Units, Cupric Oxide, Cyanocobalamin 2.5 mcg, Ferrous Fumarate, Folic Acid 1 mg, Magnesium Oxide, Niacinamide 17 mg, Pantothenic Acid 7 mg, Pyridoxine HCl 4 mg, Riboflavin 1.6 mg, Thiamine Mononitrate 1.5 mg, Vitamin A Acetate, Vitamin E Acetate 15 mg, Zinc Oxide	Prenatal Rx by Vintage	00254-5097	Vitamin
5097V	Tab, Coated, Scored	Ascorbic Acid 80 mg, Beta-Carotene, Biotin 0.03 mg, Calcium Carbonate, Cholecalciferol 400 Units, Cupric Oxide, Cyanocobalamin 2.5 mcg, Ferrous Fumarate, Folic Acid 1 mg, Magnesium Oxide, Niacinamide 17 mg, Pantothenic Acid 7 mg, Pyridoxine HCl 4 mg, Riboflavin 1.6 mg, Thiamine Mononitrate 1.5 mg, Vitamin A Acetate, Vitamin E Acetate 15 mg, Zinc Oxide	by Physician Total Care	54868-3828	Vitamin
50DAN5568	Tab, White, Triangular, 50/Dan 5568	Thioridazine 50 mg	Mellaril by Danbury		Antipsychotic
50H	Tab, White to Off-White, Round, BI Logo	Telmisartan 20 mg	Micardis by Boehringer Ingelheim	00597-0039	Antihypertensive
50K <> P	Tab, Orange, Round, White Print, Coated	Diclofenac Sodium 50 mg	Voltaren Rapide by Pharmascience	Canadian DIN 02239753	NSAID
50LLA15	Tab, Orange, Heptagonal	Amoxapine 50 mg	Asendin by Lederle		Antidepressant

For updated data, go to www.IdentADrug.com

ID FRONT <> BACK	DESCRIPTION FRONT <> BACK	INGREDIENT & STRENGTH	BRAND (or Generic Equiv.) by FIRM	NDC#	CLASS; SCH.
1036 <> 93	Tab, White, Round	Lisinopril 20 mg, HCTZ 12.5 mg	Prinzide by Teva	00093-1036 Discontinued	Antihypertensive; Diuretic
1037 <> 93	Tab, Peach, Round	Lisinopril 20 mg, HCTZ 25 mg	Prinzide by Teva	00093-1037 Discontinued	Antihypertensive; Diuretic
1039 <> NUMARK	Tab, Soluble	Chlorpheniramine Maleate 4 mg, Phenylephrine 10 mg, Phenylpropanolamine 50 mg, Pyrilamine Maleate 25 mg	Histalet Forte by Numark	55499-1039	Cold Remedy
1039 <> NUMARK	Tab, Soluble	Chlorpheniramine Maleate 4 mg, Phenylephrine HCl 10 mg, Phenylpropanolamine HCl 50 mg, Pyrilamine Maleate 25 mg	Histalet Forte by Mikart	46672-0021	Cold Remedy
104	Tab, Orange, Oval	Sulfasalazine 500 mg	by AltiMed	Canadian DIN 00685925	Gastrointestinal
104 <> 20	Tab, White, Oval, Scored, Boehringer Logo 104 <> 20	Torsemide 20 mg	Demadex by Hoffmann La Roche	00004-0264	Diuretic
104 <> 20	Tab, White, Oval, Scored, Boehringer Logo 104 <> 20	Torsemide 20 mg	Demadex by Teva	00480-0147	Diuretic
104 <> 20	Tab, White, Oval, Scored, Boehringer Logo 104 <> 20	Torsemide 20 mg	Demadex by Caremark	00339-6012	Diuretic
104 <> 20	Tab, White, Oval, Scored, Boehringer Logo 104 <> 20	Torsemide 20 mg	Demadex by Nat Pharmpak	55154-0405	Diuretic
104 <> 20	Tab, White, Oval, Scored, Boehringer Logo 104 <> 20	Torsemide 20 mg	Demadex by Compumed	00403-0715	Diuretic
104 <> SZ	Tab, Round, Peach, Chewable	Cetirizine HCl 5 mg	Zyrtec by Sandoz	00781-5283	Antihistamine
1041 <> 93	Tab, Pink, Round, Film Coated, Ex Release	Diclofenac Sodium 100 mg	Voltaren XR by Biovail	62660-0021	NSAID
1041 <> 93	Tab, Pink, Round, Film Coated, Ex Release	Diclofenac Sodium 100 mg	Voltaren XR by Teva	00093-1041	NSAID
1043	Tab, Tan, Round	Thyroid 2 g	by Vortech		Thyroid Hormone
1044	Tab, Tan, Round	Thyroid 1 g	by Vortech		Thyroid Hormone
1044 <> 93	Tab, White, Cap Shaped	Enalapril Maleate 5 mg, Hydrochlorothiazide 12.5 mg	Vaseretic by Teva	00093-1044	Antihypertensive; Diuretic
1045	Tab, Red, Round	Thyroid 1 g	by Vortech		Thyroid Hormone
1045 <> 93	Tab, Brown, Cap Shaped, Film Coated	Quinapril 20 mg	Accupril by Teva	00093-1045	Antihypertensive
105 <> 100	Tab, White, Cap Shaped, Scored, Boehringer Logo/105 <> 100	Torsemide 100 mg	Demadex by Hoffmann La Roche	00004-0265	Diuretic
105 <> 100	Tab, White, Cap Shaped, Scored, Boehringer Logo/105 <> 100	Torsemide 100 mg	Demadex by Boehringer Mannheim	Canadian	Diuretic
105 <> CC	Tab, Blue, Cap Shaped, Scored, C C on opposite sides of Score	Salsalate 750 mg	Disalcid by Caraco	57664-0105	NSAID
105 <> TENORMIN	Tab, White, Round, Scored	Atenolol 50 mg	Tenormin by Pharm Util	60491-0627	Antihypertensive
105 <> TENORMIN	Tab, White, Round, Scored	Atenolol 50 mg	Tenormin by Wal Mart	49035-0166	Antihypertensive
105 <> TENORMIN	Tab, White, Round, Scored	Atenolol 50 mg	Tenormin by AstraZeneca	00310-0105	Antihypertensive
1050 <> 93	Tab, Brown, Round, Film-Coated, Scored	Quinapril 5 mg	Accupril by Teva	00093-1050	Antihypertensive
10500 <> ADG	Tab, White, Cap Shaped, 10/500	Acetaminophen 500 mg, Oxycodone 10 mg	Percocet by Mikart	46672-0826	Analgesic; C II
10501050 <> VISKAZIDES	Tab, Orange, Round, Scored, 10/50 10/50 <> Viskazide S in a Triangle	Hydrochlorothiazide 50 mg, Pindolol 10 mg	Viskazide by Novartis	Canadian DIN 00568635	Diuretic; Antihypertensive
1051 <> 93	Tab, Brown, Oval, Film-Coated	Quinapril 10 mg	Accupril by Teva	00093-1051	Antihypertensive
105105 <> BIOCRAFT	Tab, White, Oblong, Scored	Sucralfate 1 g	Carafate by Murfreesboro	51129-1266	Gastrointestinal
105105 <> BIOCRAFT	Tab, White, Oblong, Scored	Sucralfate 1 g	Carafate by Teva	00093-2210	Gastrointestinal
105105 <> BIOCRAFT	Tab, White, Oblong, Scored	Sucralfate 1 g	Carafate by UDL	51079-0871	Gastrointestinal
105105 <> BIOCRAFT	Tab, White, Oblong, Scored	Sucralfate 1 g	Carafate by Golden State	60429-0706	Gastrointestinal
105105 <> BIOCRAFT	Tab, White, Oblong, Scored	Sucralfate 1 g	Carafate by Vangard	00615-4517	Gastrointestinal
1052 <> 93	Tab, Rust, Cap Shaped	Enalapril Maleate 10 mg, Hydrochlorothiazide 25 mg	Vaseretic by Teva	00093-1052	Antihypertensive; Diuretic
1053 <> 93	Tab, Brown, Oblong, Film-Coated	Quinapril 40 mg	Accupril by Teva	00093-1053	Antihypertensive
106	Tab, Pale Yellow, Round	Trandolapril 1 mg	Mavik by Dava	67253-0106	Antihypertensive
106 <> SZ	Tab, Round, Peach, Chewable	Cetirizine HCl 10 mg	Zyrtec by Sandoz	00781-5284	Antihistamine
107	Tab	Acetaminophen 500 mg, Chlorpheniramine Maleate 4 mg, Phenylpropanolamine 25 mg	Alumadrine by Fleming	00256-0107	Cold Remedy
107	Tab, Brown & Yellow, Round	Sulfasalazine 500 mg	Azulfidine by Ratiopharm	Canadian DIN 00685933	Gastrointestinal

ID FRONT <> BACK	DESCRIPTION FRONT <> BACK	INGREDIENT & STRENGTH	BRAND (or Generic Equiv.) by FIRM	NDC#	CLASS; SCH.
107 <> 2	Tab, Pale Yellow, Round	Trandolapril 2 mg	Mavik by Dava	67253-0107	Antihypertensive
107 <> A	Tab, Coated	Ascorbic Acid 120 mg, Calcium 200 mg, Copper 2 mg, Cyanocobalamin 12 mcg, Folic Acid 1 mg, Iron 65 mg, Niacinamide 20 mg, Pyridoxine HCl 10 mg, Riboflavin 3 mg, Thiamine Mononitrate 1.84 mg, Vitamin A 4000 Units, Vitamin D 400 Units, Vitamin E 22 mg, Zinc 25 mg	Prenatal Plus by Ivax	00182-4464	Vitamin
107 <> B	Tab, White, Oblong, b <> 107, Extended Release	Metformin HCl 750 mg	Glucophage XR by Barr	00555-0107 Discontinued	Antidiabetic
107 <> RDY	Tab, White, Capsule Shaped	Naproxen Sodium 275 mg	Anaprox by Dr. Reddy's	55111-0107	Anti-inflammatory
107 <> T	Tab, White, Round	Atenolol 25 mg	Tenormin by AstraZeneca	00310-0107	Antihypertensive
1073 <> 93	Tab, White to Off-White, Cap Shaped, Biconvex	Cefuroxime Axetil 250 mg	Ceftin by Teva	00093-1073 Discontinued	Antibiotic
1074 <> 93	Tab, White to Off-White, Cap Shaped, Biconvex	Cefuroxime Axetil 500 mg	Ceftin by Teva	00093-1074	Antibiotic
1077	Tab, Round	Chlorpheniramine Maleate 8 mg	Chlor-Trimeton by Vortech		Antihistamine
1077 <> 93	Tab, Light Orange, Round, Film Coated	Cefprozil 250 mg	Cefzil by Teva	00093-1077	Antibiotic
1078	Tab, Round	Phenobarbital 15 mg, Belladonna 10 mg	Bellophen by Vortech		Gastrointestinal; C IV
1078 <> 93	Tab, White, Cap Shaped, Film Coated	Cefprozil 500 mg	Cefzil by Teva	00093-1078	Antibiotic
1078212	Tab, White, Round, 10 78-212	Metaproterenol 10 mg	Metaprel by Sandoz		Antiasthmatic
1079	Tab, Round	Digitoxin 0.1 mg	by Vortech		Cardiac Agent
108 <> 4	Tab, Pale Pink, Round	Trandolapril 4 mg	Mavik by Dava	67253-0108	Antihypertensive
108 <> RDY	Tab, White, Capsule Shaped, Scored	Naproxen Sodium 550 mg	Anaprox by Dr. Reddy's	55111-0108	Anti-inflammatory
1087 <> 93	Tab, Dark Blue, Oval, Ex Release	Cefaclor 500 mg	Ceclor by Teva	00093-1087	Antibiotic
108MIA	Tab, 108/MIA	Acetaminophen 500 mg, Hydrocodone Bitartrate 5 mg	Vicodin by Schein	00364-0744	Analgesic; C III
109	Cap, Dark Brown, Softgel	Ferrous Fumarate 460 mg, Vitamin C 60 mg, Vitamin B12 0.01 mg, FA 1 mg	FeoGen Forte by Rising	64980-0109	Vitamin
109	Tab, Peach, Oblong	Ortho Phosphate 1 g	Uro-KP-Neutral by Star		Vitamin
109 <> T	Tab	Carbamazepine 200 mg	Tegretol by Baker Cummins	63171-1233	Anticonvulsant
1091 <> NUMARK	Tab, Orange, Oblong, Scored	Hydrocodone Bitartrate 5 mg, Pseudoephedrine HCl 60 mg	P V Tussin by Numark	55499-1091	Decongestant/Analgesic; C III
1091 <> NUMARK	Tab, Orange, Oblong, Scored	Hydrocodone Bitartrate 5 mg, Pseudoephedrine HCl 60 mg	P V Tussin by Mikart	46672-0133	Decongestant/Analgesic; C III
1093	Tab, Red, Round	Thyroid 2 g	by Vortech		Thyroid Hormone
1094	Tab, Round	Penicillin G 250,000 Units	Pentids by Vortech		Antibiotic
1098	Tab, Round	Prednisone 5 mg	by Vortech		Steroid
10ALG	Tab, 1.0/ALG	Alprazolam 1 mg	Xanax by Schein	00364-2584	Antianxiety; C IV
10ALTACE	Cap, Blue and White, Opaque, Hard Gel	Ramipril 10 mg	Altace by Aventis	Canadian DIN 02221853	Antihypertensive
10CL <> P	Tab, White, Round, Scored, P <> 10/CL	Clobazam 10 mg	Frisium by Pharmascience	Canadian DIN 02244474	Anticonvulsant
10DAN5566	Tab, Yellowish Green, Triangular, 10/Dan 5566	Thioridazine 10 mg	Mellaril by Danbury		Antipsychotic
10F	Tab, White, Round, 10/F	Tamoxifen Citrate 10 mg	Nolvadex by Pharmacia	Canadian	Antiestrogen
10GILEAD	Tab, White	Adefovir Dipivoxil 10 mg	Hepsera by Gilead	61958-0501	Antiviral
10LLC12	Tab, Yellow, Square	Leucovorin Calcium 10 mg	Wellcovorin by Lederle	Canadian	Antineoplastic
10M	Tab, White, 10/M	Benzoyl Peroxide 10 mg	Benoxyl by Stiefel	Canadian	Antiacne
10M	Tab, White, 10/M	Dicyclomine HCl 10 mg	by Aventis	Canadian	Gastrointestinal
10MG	Tab, Black Print	Glipizide 10 mg	Glucotrol XL by Direct Dispensing	57866-6303	Antidiabetic
10MG	Cap, Blue	Pericyazine 10 mg	by RPR	Canadian	Psychotropic Agent
10MG	Cap, Pamelor Logo <> Sandoz Logo 10 mg	Nortriptyline HCl 10 mg	by Allscripts		Antidepressant

ID FRONT <> BACK	DESCRIPTION FRONT <> BACK	INGREDIENT & STRENGTH	BRAND (or Generic Equiv.) by FIRM	NDC#	CLASS; SCH.
50LLT27	Tab, Orange, Round	Thioridazine 50 mg	Mellaril by Lederle	63254-0436	Antipsychotic
50M	Tab, Mova Logo	Levothyroxine Sodium 50 mcg	Euthyrox by Em Pharma	55370-0126	Thyroid Hormone
50M	Tab	Levothyroxine Sodium 50 mcg	Levo-T by Mova		Thyroid Hormone
50M <> Z	Tab, White, Round, Scored	Levothyroxine Sodium 50 mcg	Levo-T by Zoetica	64909-0114	Thyroid Hormone
50MCG	Tab, Color Coded	Levothyroxine Sodium 50 mcg	by Med Pro	53978-3022	Thyroid Hormone
50MCG <> FLINT	Tab, Debossed	Levothyroxine Sodium 0.05 mg	Synthroid by Amerisource	62584-0040	Thyroid Hormone
50MCG <> FLINT	Tab, White, Round, Scored	Levothyroxine Sodium 0.05 mg	Synthroid by Rightpac	65240-0740	Thyroid Hormone
50MG	Cap, Yellowish-Brown, Ivax Logo 50 mg	Cyclosporine 50 mg	Neoral by Ivax	00172-7311	Immunosuppressant
50MG	Tab, White to Off-White, Cap Shaped, Torrent Logo <> 50mg	Sertraline HCl 50 mg	Zoloft by Torrent	13668-0005	Antidepressant
50MG <> G4900	Tab, Light Blue, Cap Shaped, Scored	Sertraline HCl 50 mg	Zoloft by Greenstone	59762-4900	Antidepressant
50MG <> N	Tab, Light Yellow, Oblong	Azathioprine 50 mg	Azasan by AAI Pharma	66591-0221	Immunosuppressant
50MG <> ZOLOFT	Tab, Light Blue, Cap Shaped, Scored, Film Coated	Sertraline HCl 50 mg	Zoloft by Nat Pharmpak	55154-2709	Antidepressant
50MG <> ZOLOFT	Tab, Light Blue, Cap Shaped, Scored, Film Coated	Sertraline HCl 50 mg	Zoloft by Med Pro	53978-3019	Antidepressant
50MG <> ZOLOFT	Tab, Light Blue, Cap Shaped, Scored, Film Coated	Sertraline HCl 50 mg	Zoloft by Direct Dispensing	57866-6304	Antidepressant
50MG <> ZOLOFT	Tab, Light Blue, Cap Shaped, Scored, Film Coated	Sertraline HCl 50 mg	Zoloft by Amerisource	62584-0900	Antidepressant
50MG <> ZOLOFT	Tab, Light Blue, Cap Shaped, Scored, Film Coated	Sertraline HCl 50 mg	Zoloft by Heartland	61392-0629	Antidepressant
50MG <> ZOLOFT	Tab, Light Blue, Cap Shaped, Scored, Film Coated	Sertraline HCl 50 mg	Zoloft by Compumed	00403-4721	Antidepressant
50MG <> ZOLOFT	Tab, Light Blue, Cap Shaped, Scored, Film Coated	Sertraline HCl 50 mg	Zoloft by Roerig	00049-4900	Antidepressant
50MG <> ZOLOFT	Tab, Light Blue, Cap Shaped, Scored, Film Coated	Sertraline HCl 50 mg	Zoloft by Pharmacy Care	65070-0035	Antidepressant
50MG <> ZOLOFT	Tab, Light Blue, Cap Shaped, Scored, Film Coated	Sertraline HCl 50 mg	Zoloft by Southwood	58016-0366	Antidepressant
50MGFLUVOX	Tab, White, Round, 50/mg/Fluvox	Fluvoxamine Maleate 50 mg	Luvox by AltiMed	Canadian DIN 02218453	OCD
50MGLEDERLEL4	Cap, Blue & Green	Loxapine 50 mg	Loxitane by Lederle		Antipsychotic
50MGLEDERLEM2	Cap, Orange	Minocycline HCl 50 mg	Minocin by Lederle		Antibiotic
50MGWATSON500	Cap, Blue & White, 50MG on cap, WATSON500 on body	Doxycycline Hyclate 50 mg	Vibramycin by Watson	52544-0500	Antibiotic
50MO <> MOVA	Tab, Debossed	Captopril 50 mg	Capoten by Mova		Antihypertensive
50MO5 <> MOVA	Tab, White, Cap Shaped	Captopril 50 mg	Capoten by Mova	55370-0144	Antihypertensive
50MYSOLINE	Tab, White, Rounded Square, Scored, 50 over Mysoline	Primidone 50 mg	Mysoline by Wal Mart	49035-0168	Anticonvulsant
50MYSOLINE	Tab, White, Rounded Square, Scored, 50 over Mysoline	Primidone 50 mg	Mysoline by Ayerst	00046-0431	Anticonvulsant
50N <> 727	Tab, Film Coated	Metoprolol Tartrate 50 mg	Lopressor by Ivax	00182-1987	Antihypertensive
50N032	Cap, Bright Yellow & Turquoise, 50 <> N over 032	Clomipramine HCl 50 mg	Anafranil by Teva	55953-0032 Discontinued	OCD
50NOVO	Tab, White, Round, 50/Novo	Clomipramine HCl 50 mg	Novo Clopamine by Novopharm	Canadian	OCD
50P	Tab, Peach, Round	Hydrochlorothiazide 50 mg	PMS-Hydrochlorothiazide by Pharmascience	Canadian DIN 02247387	Diuretic
50P	Cap, Orange	Minocycline HCl 50 mg	Minocin by Pharmascience	Canadian DIN 02294419	Antibiotic
51 <> 93	Tab, White, Oval, Film Coated	Carvedilol 3.125 mg	Coreg by Teva	00093-0051	Antihypertensive
51 <> A	Tab, White, Round	Benazepril HCl 5 mg	Lotensin by Amneal	65162-0751	Antihypertensive
51 <> BN	Tab, White, Round	Ephedrine HCl 25 mg, Guaifenesin 200 mg	Ephedrine Plus Tabs by Neil Labs	60242-0225	Cold Remedy
51 <> C	Tab	Atenolol 50 mg, Chlorthalidone 25 mg	Tenoretic by IPR	54921-0115	Antihypertensive; Diuretic
51 <> RP	Tab, Yellow, Round, Scored	Dextroamphetamine Sulfate 5 mg	Dexedrine by Shire	58521-0451	Stimulant; C II
510 <> DP	Tab, Pink, Round, Film Coated	Levonorgestrel 0.050 mg, Ethinyl Estradiol 0.03 mg	Triphasil by Barr	51285-0514	Oral Contraceptive
510 <> DP	Tab, Pink, Round, Film Coated	Levonorgestrel 0.050 mg, Ethinyl Estradiol 0.03 mg	Triphasil by Barr	00555-9047	Oral Contraceptive
510 <> WATSON	Tab, Light Blue, Round	Norethindrone 1 mg, Mestranol 0.05 mg	Necon 1 50 28 by Watson	52544-0556	Oral Contraceptive
510 <> WATSON	Tab, Light Blue, Round	Norethindrone 1 mg, Mestranol 0.05 mg	Necon 1 50 21 by DRX	55045-2722	Oral Contraceptive
510 <> WATSON	Tab, Light Blue, Round	Norethindrone 1 mg, Mestranol 0.05 mg	Necon 1 50 21 by PDRX	55289-0379	Oral Contraceptive
510 <> WATSON	Tab, Light Blue, Round	Norethindrone 1 mg, Mestranol 0.05 mg	Necon 1 50 21 by Watson	52544-0510	Oral Contraceptive

ID FRONT <> BACK	DESCRIPTION FRONT <> BACK	INGREDIENT & STRENGTH	BRAND (or Generic Equiv.) by FIRM	NDC#	CLASS; SCH.
5100 <> RPR	Tab, Light Blue, Oblong, Film Coated	Enoxacin 200 mg	Penetrex by RPR	00801-5100	Antibiotic
5100 <> RPR	Tab, Light Blue, Oblong, Film Coated	Enoxacin 200 mg	Penetrex by RPR	00075-5100 Discontinued	Antibiotic
511	Tab, White, Oval, Film Coated, Extended Release	Divalproex Sodium 125 mg	Depakote ER by Northstar RX	16714-0511	Anticonvulsant
511 <> 05	Tab, White, Pentagonal, 511 <> 0.5	Lorazepam 0.5 mg	Ativan by ESI Lederle	59911-5811	Antianxiety; C IV
511 <> 05	Tab, White, Pentagonal, 511 <> 0.5	Lorazepam 0.5 mg	Ativan by Mylan	55160-0129	Antianxiety; C IV
511 <> 1MG	Tab, White, Pentagonal, Scored, 1 over MG	Lorazepam 1 mg	Ativan by Nat Pharmpak	55154-1914	Antianxiety; C IV
511 <> 1MG	Tab, White, Pentagonal, Scored, 1 over MG	Lorazepam 1 mg	Ativan by ESI Lederle	59911-5812	Antianxiety; C IV
511 <> 1MG	Tab, White, Pentagonal, Scored, 1 over MG	Lorazepam 1 mg	Ativan by Wyeth	52903-5812	Antianxiety; C IV
511 <> 2MG	Tab, White, Pentagonal, Scored, 2 over MG	Lorazepam 2 mg	Ativan by ESI Lederle	59911-5813	Antianxiety; C IV
511 <> 2MG	Tab, White, Pentagonal, Scored, 2 over MG	Lorazepam 2 mg	Ativan by Nat Pharmpak	55154-2002	Antianxiety; C IV
511 <> 2MG	Tab, White, Pentagonal, Scored, 2 over MG	Lorazepam 2 mg	Ativan by Wyeth	52903-5813	Antianxiety; C IV
511 <> 7065	Tab, Light Yellow, Round	Bisoprolol 2.5 mg, Hydrochlorothiazide 6.25 mg	Ziac by ESI Lederle	59911-7065	Antihypertensive; Diuretic
511 <> 7066	Tab, Light Pink, Round	Bisoprolol 5 mg, Hydrochlorothiazide 6.25 mg	Ziac by ESI Lederle	59911-7066	Antihypertensive; Diuretic
511 <> 7067	Tab, White, Round	Bisoprolol 10 mg, Hydrochlorothiazide 6.25 mg	Ziac by ESI Lederle	59911-7067	Antihypertensive; Diuretic
511 <> A75	Tab, White, Round	Acyclovir 400 mg	Zovirax by ESI Lederle	59911-3163	Antiviral
511 <> A77	Tab, White, Oval	Acyclovir 800 mg	Zovirax by ESI Lederle	59911-3164	Antiviral
511 <> B71	Tab, Orange, Round	Bupropion HCl 75 mg	Wellbutrin by ESI Lederle	59911-5861	Antidepressant
511 <> B77	Tab, Orange, Oval	Bupropion HCl 100 mg	Wellbutrin by ESI Lederle	59911-5862	Antidepressant
511 <> DP	Tab, White, Round, Film Coated	Levonorgestrel 0.075 mg, Ethinyl Estradiol 0.04 mg	Triphasil by Barr	00555-9047	Oral Contraceptive
511 <> DP	Tab, White, Round, Film Coated	Levonorgestrel 0.075 mg, Ethinyl Estradiol 0.04 mg	Triphasil by Barr	51285-0514	Oral Contraceptive
511 <> E1	Tab, Off-White, Round, Scored	Estradiol 0.5 mg	Estrace by Ayerst	00046-5879	Hormone
511 <> E1	Tab, Off-White, Round, Scored	Estradiol 0.5 mg	Estrace by ESI Lederle	59911-5879	Hormone
511 <> E7	Tab, Off-White, Round, Scored	Estradiol 1 mg	Estrace by Ayerst	00046-5880	Hormone
511 <> E7	Tab, Off-White, Round, Scored	Estradiol 1 mg	Estrace by ESI Lederle	59911-5880	Hormone
511 <> E77	Tab, Off-White, Round, Scored	Estradiol 2 mg	Estrace by Ayerst	00046-5882	Hormone
511 <> E77	Tab, Off-White, Round, Scored	Estradiol 2 mg	Estrace by ESI Lederle	59911-5882	Hormone
511 <> LODOSYN	Tab, Orange, Round, Scored	Carbidopa 25 mg	Lodosyn by BMS	00056-0511	Antiparkinson
511 <> MX	Tab, Yellow, Round, Scored	Methotrexate Sodium 2.5 mg	Rheumatrex by Lederle	00005-5874	Antineoplastic
511 <> MX	Tab, Yellow, Round, Scored	Methotrexate Sodium 2.5 mg	Rheumatrex by ESI Lederle	59911-5874	Antineoplastic
511 <> P77	Tab, White, Oblong, Ex Release	Pentoxifylline 400 mg	Trental by ESI Lederle	59911-3290	Anticoagulant
511 <> PAR	Tab, White, Cap Shaped, Coated	Minocycline 50 mg	Dynacin by Par	49884-0511	Antibiotic
51105	Tab, White, Pentagonal, 511/0.5	Lorazepam 0.5 mg	Ativan by ESI Lederle	59911-5811	Antianxiety; C IV
5111V	Tab, Orange, Oblong	Acetaminophen 325 mg, Propoxyphene 50 mg	Darvocet N-50 by Qualitest	00603-5465	Analgesic; C IV
5111V	Tab, Orange, Oblong	Acetaminophen 325 mg, Propoxyphene 50 mg	Darvocet N-50 by Vintage	00254-5111	Analgesic; C IV
5112V	Tab, Orange, Oblong	Acetaminophen 650 mg, Propoxyphene Napsylate 100 mg	Darvocet-N 100 by Direct Dispensing	57866-4361	Analgesic; C IV
5112V	Tab, Orange, Oblong	Acetaminophen 650 mg, Propoxyphene Napsylate 100 mg	Darvocet-N 100 by Vintage	00254-5112	Analgesic; C IV
5112V	Tab, Orange, Oblong	Acetaminophen 650 mg, Propoxyphene Napsylate 100 mg	Darvocet-N 100 by Qualitest	00603-5466	Analgesic; C IV
5113V	Tab, White, Oblong, Film Coated	Acetaminophen 650 mg, Propoxyphene Napsylate 100 mg	Darvocet-N 100 by Qualitest	00603-5467	Analgesic; C IV
5113V	Tab, White, Oblong, Film Coated	Acetaminophen 650 mg, Propoxyphene Napsylate 100 mg	Darvocet-N 100 by Vintage	00254-5113	Analgesic; C IV
5113V	Tab, White, Oblong, Film Coated	Acetaminophen 650 mg, Propoxyphene Napsylate 100 mg	Darvocet-N 100 by Direct Dispensing	57866-4361	Analgesic; C IV
5114V	Tab, Pink, Oblong, Film Coated	Acetaminophen 650 mg, Propoxyphene Napsylate 100 mg	Darvocet-N 100 by Direct Dispensing	00603-5468	Analgesic; C IV
5114V	Tab, Pink, Oblong, Film Coated	Acetaminophen 650 mg, Propoxyphene Napsylate 100 mg	Darvocet-N 100 by Qualitest	00254-5114	Analgesic; C IV
5114V	Tab, Pink, Oblong, Film Coated	Acetaminophen 650 mg, Propoxyphene Napsylate 100 mg	Darvocet-N 100 by Vintage	62584-0840	Analgesic; C IV
5114V	Tab, Pink, Oblong, Film Coated	Acetaminophen 650 mg, Propoxyphene Napsylate 100 mg	Darvocet-N 100 by Amerisource	27280-0007	Analgesic; C IV
5114V	Tab, Pink, Oblong, Film Coated	Acetaminophen 650 mg, Propoxyphene Napsylate 100 mg	Darvocet-N 100 by AAI Pharma		Analgesic; C IV
511ACYCLOVIR200MG	Cap, White, Black Print, 511 over ACYCLOVIR over 200 mg	Acyclovir 200 mg	Zovirax by ESI Lederle	59911-5831	Antiviral
511MX	Tab, Yellow, Round, 511/MX	Methotrexate 2.5 mg	Rheumatrex by ESI Lederle		Antineoplastic
511P77	Tab, White, Oval, 511/P77	Pentoxifylline 400 mg	Trental by ESI Lederle	59911-3290	Anticoagulant
511SELEGILINEHCL5MG	Cap, White, Red Print, 511 over Selegiline HCl over 5 mg	Selegiline 5 mg	Eldepryl by SB	59742-3158	Antiparkinson

ID FRONT <> BACK	DESCRIPTION FRONT <> BACK	INGREDIENT & STRENGTH	BRAND (or Generic Equiv.) by FIRM	NDC#	CLASS; SCH.
511SELEGILINEHCL5MG	Cap, White, Red Print, 511 over Selegiline HCl over 5 mg	Selegiline 5 mg	Eldepryl by Sanofi	00024-2775	Antiparkinson
511SELEGILINEHCL5MG	Cap, White, Red Print, 511 over Selegiline HCl over 5 mg	Selegiline 5 mg	Eldepryl by ESI Lederle	59911-5886	Antiparkinson
511SELEGILINEHCL5MG	Cap, White, Red Print, 511 over Selegiline HCl over 5 mg	Selegiline 5 mg	Eldepryl by Dava	67253-	Antiparkinson
512	Tab, Yellow, Round	Meloxicam 7.5 mg	Mobic by Caraco	57664-0512	NSAID
512	Tab, White, Round, Scored	Acetaminophen 325 mg, Oxycodone HCl 5 mg	Percocet by Mallinckrodt	00406-0512	Analgesic; C II
512	Tab, Brown, Oval, Film Coated, Extended Release	Divalproex Sodium 250 mg	Depakote ER by Northstar RX	16714-0512	Anticonvulsant
512 <> DP	Tab, Orange, Round, Film Coated	Levonorgestrel 0.125 mg, Ethinyl Estradiol 0.03 mg	Triphasil by Barr	00555-9047	Oral Contraceptive
512 <> DP	Tab, Orange, Round, Film Coated	Levonorgestrel 0.125 mg, Ethinyl Estradiol 0.03 mg	Triphasil by Barr	51285-0514	Oral Contraceptive
512 <> HD	Tab	Acetaminophen 325 mg, Oxycodone HCl 5 mg	Percocet by Schein	00364-0605 Discontinued	Analgesic; C II
512 <> MILES	Tab, Film Coated	Ciprofloxacin HCl 250 mg	Cipro by Quality Care	60346-0433	Antibiotic
512 <> PAR	Tab, White, Cap Shaped, Coated	Minocycline 75 mg	Dynacin by Par	49884-0512	Antibiotic
5123	Tab, White, Round, Scored	Captopril 50 mg	Capoten by Caremark	00339-6116	Antihypertensive
5124 <> 93	Tab, Light Yellow, Triangular, Coated	Benazepril HCl 5 mg	Lotensin by Teva	00093-5124	Antihypertensive
5124 <> V	Tab, White, Round, Scored, Film Coated	Propafenone HCl 150 mg	Rythmol by Vintage	00254-5124	Antiarrhythmic
5125 <> 93	Tab, Mustard Yellow, Triangular, Coated	Benazepril HCl 10 mg	Lotensin by Teva	00093-5125	Antihypertensive
5125 <> APO	Tab, Pink, Oval, Scored, 5 / 12.5	Cilazapril 5 mg, Hydrochlorothiazide 12.5 mg	Inhibace Plus by Apotex	Canadian DIN 02284987	Antihypertensive
5125 <> V	Tab, White, Round, Scored, Film Coated	Propafenone HCl 225 mg	Rythmol by Vintage	00254-5125	Antiarrhythmic
5126 <> 93	Tab, Pink, Triangular, Coated	Benazepril HCl 20 mg	Lotensin by Teva	00093-5126	Antihypertensive
5126 <> V	Tab, White, Round, Scored, Film Coated	Propafenone HCl 300 mg	Rythmol by Vintage	00254-5126	Antiarrhythmic
5127 <> 93	Tab, Pink to Light Red, Triangular, Coated	Benazepril HCl 40 mg	Lotensin by Teva	00093-5127	Antihypertensive
513	Tab, Yellow, Oval	Meloxicam 15 mg	Mobic by Caraco	57664-0513	NSAID
513	Tab, Red, Round, Sav. Logo 513	Phenolphthalein 130 mg	Modane by Savage	00281-0298	Gastrointestinal
513	Tab, Blue, Oval, Enteric Coated, Delayed Release	Divalproex Sodium 500 mg	Depakote ER by Northstar RX	16714-0513	Anticonvulsant
513 <> JSP	Tab, Peach, Round	Levothyroxine Sodium 25 mcg	Synthroid by Lannett	00527-1341	Thyroid Hormone
513 <> JSP	Tab, Peach, Round, Scored	Levothyroxine Sodium 0.025 mg	Synthroid by Ivax	00182-1529	Thyroid Hormone
513 <> JSP	Tab, Peach, Round, Scored	Levothyroxine Sodium 0.025 mg	Synthroid by Jerome Stevens	50564-0513	Thyroid Hormone
513 <> JSP	Tab, Peach, Round, Scored	Levothyroxine Sodium 0.025 mg	Synthroid by Watson	52544-0902	Thyroid Hormone
513 <> MILES	Tab, Yellow, Oblong, Film Coated	Ciprofloxacin HCl 500 mg	Cipro by Bayer	00026-8513	Antibiotic
513 <> MILES	Tab, Film Coated	Ciprofloxacin HCl 500 mg	Cipro by Nat Pharmpak	55154-4801	Antibiotic
513 <> PAR	Tab, White, Cap Shaped, Coated	Minocycline 100 mg	Dynacin by Par	49884-0513	Antibiotic
5130 <> V	Tab, White, Round, Scored	Primidone 50 mg	Mysoline by Vintage	00254-5130	Anticonvulsant
5136 <> V	Tab, Pink, Round	Promethazine HCl 50 mg	Phenergan by Vintage	00254-5136	Antiemetic; Antihistamine
5137 <> V	Tab, White, Round, Scored	Promethazine HCl 25 mg	Phenergan by Vintage	00254-5137	Antiemetic; Antihistamine
5138 <> V	Tab, Orange, Round, Scored	Promethazine HCl 12.5 mg	Phenergan by Vintage	00254-5138	Antiemetic; Antihistamine
514 <> JSP	Tab, White, Round	Levothyroxine Sodium 50 mcg	Synthroid by Lannett	00527-1342	Thyroid Hormone
514 <> JSP	Tab, White, Round, Scored	Levothyroxine Sodium 0.05 mg	Unithroid by Watson	52544-0903	Thyroid Hormone
514 <> JSP	Tab, White, Round, Scored	Levothyroxine Sodium 0.05 mg	Synthroid by Jerome Stevens	50564-0514	Thyroid Hormone
5140 <> 93	Tab, White to Off-White, Round	Alendronate Sodium 5 mg	Fosamax by Teva	00093-5140	Antiosteoporosis
5140 <> RPR	Tab, Dark Blue, Oblong, Film Coated	Enoxacin 400 mg	Penetrex by RPR	00801-5140	Antibiotic
5140 <> RPR	Tab, Dark Blue, Oblong, Film Coated	Enoxacin 400 mg	Penetrex by RPR	00075-5140 Discontinued	Antibiotic
5141 <> 93	Tab, White to Off-White, Round	Alendronate Sodium 10 mg	Fosamax by Teva	00093-5141	Antiosteoporosis
5142 <> 93	Tab, White to Off-White, Oval	Alendronate Sodium 40 mg	Fosamax by Teva	00093-5142	Antiosteoporosis
5147 <> SOLVAY	Tab, Butterscotch, Cap Shaped, Film Coated	Eprosartan 600 mg, Hydrochlorothiazide 12.5 mg	Teveten HCT by Solvay	Canadian DIN 02253631	Antihypertensive; Diuretic
5147 <> SOLVAY	Tab, Butterscotch, Cap Shaped, Film Coated	Eprosartan 600 mg, Hydrochlorothiazide 12.5 mg	Teveten HCT by Biovail	64455-0132	Antihypertensive; Diuretic
51479019	Cap, Gray & Red	Cycloserine 250 mg	Seromycin by Eli Lilly		Antibiotic
51479019	Cap, Gray & Red	Cycloserine 250 mg	Seromycin by Dura	51479-0019	Antibiotic

ID FRONT <> BACK	DESCRIPTION FRONT <> BACK	INGREDIENT & STRENGTH	BRAND (or Generic Equiv.) by FIRM	NDC#	CLASS; SCH.
51479DURA005GEST	Cap, 51479/Dura <> 005/Gest	Guaifenesin 200 mg, Phenylephrine HCl 5 mg, Phenylpropanolamine HCl 45 mg	Dura Gest by Anabolic	00722-6060	Cold Remedy
515	Cap, Green, Oval, Savage Logo 515	Docusate Sodium 100 mg	Modane Soft by Savage	00281-5111	Laxative
515	Tab, Pink, Cap Shaped, Film Coated	Zolpidem Tartrate 5 mg	Ambien by Caraco	57664-0515	Sedative/Hypnotic; C IV
515 <> JSP	Tab, Purple, Round	Levothyroxine Sodium 75 mcg	Synthroid by Lannett	00527-1343	Thyroid Hormone
515 <> JSP	Tab, Purple, Round, Scored	Levothyroxine Sodium 75 mcg	Synthroid by Watson	52544-0904	Thyroid Hormone
515 <> JSP	Tab, Purple, Round, Scored	Levothyroxine Sodium 75 mcg	Unithroid by Pharm Pkg Ctr	54383-0086	Thyroid Hormone
515 <> JSP	Tab, Purple, Round, Scored	Levothyroxine Sodium 75 mcg	Unithroid by Jerome Stevens	50564-0515	Thyroid Hormone
5150 <> 93	Tab, Pink, Oval, Scored	Moexipril 15 mg	Univasc by Teva	00093-5150	Antihypertensive
5150 <> SOLVAY	Tab, Brick Red, Cap Shaped, Film Coated	Eprosartan 600 mg, Hydrochlorothiazide 25 mg	Teveten HCT by Biovail	64455-0133	Antihypertensive; Diuretic
5151 <> GEIGY	Tab, Reddish Pink, Cap Shaped, Scored, Film Coated	Metoprolol Tartrate 50 mg	Lopressor by Caremark	00339-5213	Antihypertensive
5151 <> GEIGY	Tab, Reddish Pink, Cap Shaped, Scored, Film Coated	Metoprolol Tartrate 50 mg	Lopressor by Novartis	00078-0458	Antihypertensive
5151 <> GEIGY	Tab, Reddish Pink, Cap Shaped, Scored, Film Coated	Metoprolol Tartrate 50 mg	Lopressor by Nat Pharmpak	55154-1009	Antihypertensive
5151 <> GEIGY	Tab, Reddish Pink, Cap Shaped, Scored, Film Coated	Metoprolol Tartrate 50 mg	Lopressor by Novartis	Canadian DIN 00397423	Antihypertensive
5151 <> GEIGY	Tab, Reddish Pink, Cap Shaped, Scored, Film Coated	Metoprolol Tartrate 50 mg	Lopressor by Wal Mart	49035-0179	Antihypertensive
5156	Cap, ER, Logo 5156	Papaverine HCl 150 mg	by DRX	55045-1629	Vasodilator
5157 <> 93	Tab, White, Round	Lisinopril 30 mg	Prinivil by Teva	00093-5157 Discontinued	Antihypertensive
516	Tab, Light Orange, Round, Film Coated, Andrx Logo <> 516	Benazepril HCl 5 mg	Lotensin by Andrx	62037-0516	Antihypertensive
516	Tab, White to Off-White, Oval, Film Coated	Zolpidem Tartrate 10 mg	Ambien by Caraco	57664-0516	Sedative/Hypnotic; C IV
516 <> JSP	Tab, Yellow, Round, Scored	Levothyroxine Sodium 100 mcg	Unithroid by Lannett	00527-1345	Thyroid Hormone
516 <> JSP	Tab, Yellow, Round, Scored	Levothyroxine Sodium 100 mcg	Unithroid by Jerome Stevens	50564-0516	Thyroid Hormone
516 <> JSP	Tab, Yellow, Round, Scored	Levothyroxine Sodium 100 mcg	Unithroid by Watson	52544-0906	Thyroid Hormone
516 <> JSP	Tab, Yellow, Round, Scored	Levothyroxine Sodium 100 mcg	Unithroid by URL Mutual	00677-0078	Thyroid Hormone
516 <> JSP	Tab	Levothyroxine Sodium 0.1 mg	by Jones	52604-7701	Thyroid Hormone
516 <> ML	Tab, Round, Pink, Film Coated	Folic Acid 2.5 mg, Pyridoxine 25 mg, Cyanocobalamin 1 mg	Foltx by Midlothian	68308-0516	Vitamin
5161	Tab, White, Round, Film Coated	Hydrocodone Bitartrate 7.5 mg, Ibuprofen 200 mg	Vicoprofen Tablets by Teva	00093-5161	Analgesic; C III
5162 <> AP	Tab, White, Oval, Scored	Captopril 50 mg, HCTZ 15 mg	Capozide by Apothecon	59772-5162	Antihypertensive; Diuretic
5162DAN	Cap, Orange & Yellow	Tetracycline HCl 250 mg	by Schein	00364-2026	Antibiotic
5163 <> AP	Tab, Peach, Oval, Scored	Captopril 50 mg, HCTZ 25 mg	Capozide by Apothecon	59772-5163	Antihypertensive; Diuretic
51674009	Cap, Green	Acetaminophen 325 mg, Butalbital 50 mg, Caffeine 40 mg	Fioricet by Blansett	51674-0009	Analgesic
517	Tab, Orange, Round, Film Coated, Andrx Logo <> 517	Benazepril HCl 10 mg	Lotensin by Andrx	62037-0517	Antihypertensive
517 <> MYLAN	Tab, White, Film Coated, Scored	Gemfibrozil 600 mg	by Mylan	00378-0517	Antihyperlipidemic
5171 <> 93	Tab, White to Off-White, Oval	Alendronate Sodium 70 mg	Fosamax by Teva	00093-5171	Antiosteoporosis
5172 <> 93	Tab, White to Off-White, Pillow-Shaped	Alendronate Sodium 35 mg	Fosamax by Teva	00093-5172	Antiosteoporosis
517GG	Cap, Light Green	Indomethacin 25 mg	Indocin by Sandoz		NSAID
518	Tab, Peach, Round, Film Coated, Andrx Logo <> 518	Benazepril HCl 20 mg	Lotensin by Andrx	62037-0518	Antihypertensive
518MD	Tab, Blue, Round	Diethylpropion HCl 25 mg	Tenuate by MD		Anorexiant; C IV
519	Tab, Orange-Red, Round, Film Coated. Andrx Logo <> 519	Benazepril HCl 40 mg	Lotensin by Andrx	62037-0519	Antihypertensive
519 <> DP	Tab, Light Green, Round, Film Coated	Inert	Triphasil by Barr	00555-9047	Oral Contraceptive; Placebo
519 <> DP	Tab, Light Green, Round, Film Coated	Inert	Triphasil by Barr	51285-0514	Oral Contraceptive; Placebo
519 <> DP	Tab, Light Green, Round, Film Coated	Inert	Aviane by Barr	00555-9045	Oral Contraceptive; Placebo
519 <> JSP	Tab, Tan, Round	Levothyroxine Sodium 125 mcg	Unithroid by Lannett	00527-1347	Thyroid Hormone
519 <> JSP	Tab, Tan, Round, Scored	Levothyroxine Sodium 0.125 mg	Unithroid by Watson	52544-0908	Thyroid Hormone
519 <> JSP	Tab, Tan, Round, Scored	Levothyroxine Sodium 0.125 mg	Unithroid by Ivax	00182-1516	Thyroid Hormone
519 <> JSP	Tab, Tan, Round, Scored	Levothyroxine Sodium 0.125 mg	Unithroid by Jerome Stevens	50564-0519	Thyroid Hormone

ID FRONT <> BACK	DESCRIPTION FRONT <> BACK	INGREDIENT & STRENGTH	BRAND (or Generic Equiv.) by FIRM	NDC#	CLASS; SCH.
5194 <> 93	Tab, White, Oval	Penicillin V Potassium 250 mg	V-Cillin K by Teva	00093-5194 Discontinued	Antibiotic
5195 <> 93	Tab, White, Oval	Penicillin V Potassium 500 mg	V-Cillin K by Teva	00093-5195 Discontinued	Antibiotic
5196DAN	Cap, Brown & Clear	Papaverine HCl 150 mg	by Schein	00364-0181	Vasodilator
51H	Tab, White, Oblong, Scored	Telmisartan 40 mg	Micardis by Boehringer Ingelheim	12714-0109	Antihypertensive
51H	Tab, White, Oblong, Scored	Telmisartan 40 mg	Micardis by Boehringer Ingelheim Canada	Canadian DIN 02240769	Antihypertensive
51H	Tab, White to Off-White, Oblong, BI Logo	Telmisartan 40 mg	Micardis by Boehringer Ingelheim	00597-0040	Antihypertensive
52 <> A	Tab, White, Round	Benazepril HCl 10 mg	Lotensin by Amneal	65162-0752	Antihypertensive
52 <> MP	Tab, White, Round, Scored	Prednisone 10 mg	by Allscripts		Steroid
52 <> MP	Tab, White, Round, Scored	Prednisone 10 mg	by Allscripts		Steroid
52 <> RP	Tab, Yellow, Round, Scored	Dextroamphetamine Sulfate 10 mg	Dexedrine by Shire	58521-0452	Stimulant; C II
520 <> JSP	Tab, Debossed	Levothyroxine Sodium 0.15 mg	Estre by Macnary	55982-0015	Thyroid Hormone
520 <> JSP	Tab	Levothyroxine Sodium 0.15 mg	by JMI Canton	00252-7700	Thyroid Hormone
520 <> JSP	Tab, Blue, Round, Scored	Levothyroxine Sodium 150 mcg	Unithroid by Lannett	00527-1349	Thyroid Hormone
520 <> JSP	Tab, Blue, Round, Scored	Levothyroxine Sodium 150 mcg	Unithroid by Watson	52544-0909	Thyroid Hormone
520 <> JSP	Tab, Blue, Round, Scored	Levothyroxine Sodium 150 mcg	Unithroid by URL Mutual	00677-0992	Thyroid Hormone
520 <> JSP	Tab, Blue, Round, Scored	Levothyroxine Sodium 150 mcg	Unithroid by Ivax	00182-1117	Thyroid Hormone
520 <> JSP	Tab, Blue, Round, Scored	Levothyroxine Sodium 150 mcg	Unithroid by Jerome Stevens	50564-0520	Thyroid Hormone
520 <> N517	Tab, Film Coated	Naproxen 550 mg	Naprosyn by URL Mutual	00677-1514	NSAID
52001PRIMUS	Cap, Turquoise Green	Flavocoxid 250 mg	Limbrel by Primus	68040-0601	Antiosteoporosis
521 <> 2	Tab, White, Round, AstraZeneca Logo 521 <> 2	Acetaminophen 300 mg, Codeine Phosphate 15 mg	Tylenol w/ Codeine by AstraZeneca	62037-0521	Analgesic; C III
521 <> DP	Tab, Orange, Round	Prochlorperazine 5 mg	Compazine by Barr	00555-0521 Discontinued	Antiemetic
521 <> MYLAN	Tab, Coated	Acetaminophen 650 mg, Propoxyphene Napsylate 100 mg	Darvocet-N 100 by Mylan	00378-0521	Analgesic; C IV
521 <> SINEMETCR	Tab, Peach, Oval, Scored, Sustained Release, SINEMET over CR	Carbidopa 50 mg, Levodopa 200 mg	Sinemet CR by BMS	00056-0521	Antiparkinson
521 <> SINEMETCR	Tab, Peach, Oval, Scored, Sustained Release, SINEMET over CR	Carbidopa 50 mg, Levodopa 200 mg	Sinemet CR by BMS	Canadian DIN 00870935	Antiparkinson
5213 <> 93	Tab, Yellow, Cap Shaped, Film Coated, Scored, 9 / 3	Moexipril HCl 7.5 mg, Hydrochlorothiazide 12.5 mg	Uniretic by Teva	00093-5213	Antihypertensive; Diuretic
5214 <> 93	Tab, White, Cap Shaped, Film Coated, Scored, 9 / 3	Moexipril HCl 15 mg, Hydrochlorothiazide 12.5 mg	Uniretic by Teva	00093-5214	Antihypertensive; Diuretic
5215 <> 93	Tab, Yellow, Cap Shaped, Film Coated, Scored, 9 / 3	Moexipril HCl 15 mg, Hydrochlorothiazide 25 mg	Uniretic by Teva	00093-5215	Antihypertensive; Diuretic
5216 <> DANDAN	Tab, Tan, Round, Scored	Folic Acid 1 mg	Folvite by Amerisource	62584-0708	Vitamin
5216 <> DANDAN	Tab, Tan, Round, Scored	Folic Acid 1 mg	Folvite by JB	51111-0087	Vitamin
5216 <> DANDAN	Tab, Tan, Round, Scored	Folic Acid 1 mg	Folvite by Vangard	00615-0664	Vitamin
5216 <> DANDAN	Tab, Tan, Round, Scored	Folic Acid 1 mg	Folvite by Watson	00591-5216	Vitamin
5216 <> DANDAN	Tab, Tan, Round, Scored	Folic Acid 1 mg	Folvite by Schein	00364-0137	Vitamin
522 <> 3	Tab, White, Round, Andrx Logo 522 <> 3	Acetaminophen 300 mg, Codeine 30 mg	Tylenol w/ Codeine by Andrx	62037-0522	Analgesic; C III
522 <> DP	Tab, Yellow, Round	Prochlorperazine 10 mg	Compazine by Barr	00555-0522 Discontinued	Antiemetic
522 <> JSP	Tab, Pink, Round, Scored	Levothyroxine Sodium 200 mcg	Unithroid by Lannett	00527-1351	Thyroid Hormone
522 <> JSP	Tab, Pink, Round, Scored	Levothyroxine Sodium 200 mcg	Unithroid by Jerome Stevens	50564-0522	Thyroid Hormone
522 <> JSP	Tab, Pink, Round, Scored	Levothyroxine Sodium 200 mcg	Unithroid by Watson	52544-0911	Thyroid Hormone
522 <> JSP	Tab, Pink, Round, Scored	Levothyroxine Sodium 200 mcg	Unithroid by URL Mutual	00677-0079	Thyroid Hormone
5220	Tab, White to Off White, Round, Flat	Liothyronine Sodium 5 mcg	Cytomel by Paddock	00574-0220	Thyroid Hormone
52273111Q	Tab, Yellow, Diamond, 52273-111/Q	Nystatin Vaginal 100,000 Units	Mycostatin by Quantum		Antifungal
522HD	Tab, Blue, Round	Chlorpropamide 100 mg	Diabinese by Halsey	Discontinued	Antidiabetic
523 <> 4	Tab, White, Round, Andrx Logo 523 <> 4	Acetaminophen 300 mg, Codeine 60 mg	Tylenol w/ Codeine by Andrx	62037-0523	Analgesic; C III
523 <> JSP	Tab, Green, Round, Scored	Levothyroxine Sodium 300 mcg	Unithroid by Lannett	00527-1352	Thyroid Hormone

ID FRONT <> BACK	DESCRIPTION FRONT <> BACK	INGREDIENT & STRENGTH	BRAND (or Generic Equiv.) by FIRM	NDC#	CLASS; SCH.
523 <> JSP	Tab, Green, Round, Scored	Levothyroxine Sodium 300 mcg	Unithroid by Ivax	00182-1119	Thyroid Hormone
523 <> JSP	Tab, Green, Round, Scored	Levothyroxine Sodium 300 mcg	Unithroid by Watson	52544-0912	Thyroid Hormone
523 <> JSP	Tab, Green, Round, Scored	Levothyroxine Sodium 300 mcg	Unithroid by Jerome Stevens	50564-0523	Thyroid Hormone
523 <> M	Tab, Pink, Round Scored, M <> 523 to side of score	Bisoprolol Fumarate 5 mg	Zebeta by Mylan	00378-0523	Antihypertensive
52354	Cap	Mexitil 150 mg	Mexitil by Roxane	00054-2616	Antiarrhythmic
524	Tab, White, Round, Film Coated, Andrx Logo 524	Hydrocodone Bitartrate 7.5 mg, Ibuprofen 200 mg	Vicoprofen by Andrx	62037-0524	Analgesic; C III
524 <> BMS	Tab, White to Off-White, Round, Film Coated	Dasatinib 70 mg	Sprycel by BMS	Canadian DIN 02293145	Cancer Treatment
524 <> BMS	Tab, White to Off-White, Round, Film Coated	Dasatinib 70 mg	Sprycel by BMS	00003-0524	Cancer Treatment
524 <> M	Tab, White, Round	Bisoprolol Fumarate 10 mg	Zebeta by Mylan	00378-0524	Antihypertensive
524 <> WATSON	Tab, White, Round	Norgestimate 0.180 mg, Ethinyl Estradiol 0.035 mg	TriNessa by Watson	52544-0935	Oral Contraceptive
52401MG	Cap, White, Ivax logo 5240 <> 1 mg	Anagrelide HCl 1 mg	Agrylin by Ivax	00172-5240	Antiplatelet
52105MG	Cap, Light Green and White, Opaque, Ivax Logo 5241 <> 0.5 mg	Anagrelide HCl 0.5 mg	Agrylin by Ivax	00172-5241	Antiplatelet
524HD	Tab, White, Round	Cyproheptadine HCl 4 mg	Periactin by Halsey	Discontinued	Antihistamine
525 <> WATSON	Tab, Light Blue, Round	Norgestimate 0.215 mg, Ethinyl Estradiol 0.035 mg	TriNessa by Watson	52544-0935	Oral Contraceptive
5250 <> BMS	Tab, Coated, Mottled	Diltiazem HCl 30 mg	Cardizem by BMS	00003-5250 Discontinued	Antihypertensive
5252 <> TEGRETOL	Tab, White w/ Pink Specks, Round, Scored, 52 over 52, Chewable	Carbamazepine 100 mg	Tegretol by Nat Pharmpak	55154-1011	Anticonvulsant
5252 <> TEGRETOL	Tab, White w/ Pink Specks, Round, Scored, 52 over 52, Chewable	Carbamazepine 100 mg	Tegretol by Basel	58887-0052	Anticonvulsant
5252 <> TEGRETOL	Tab, White w/ Pink Specks, Round, Scored, 52 over 52, Chewable	Carbamazepine 100 mg	Tegretol by Neuman	64579-0325	Anticonvulsant
5252 <> TEGRETOL	Tab, White w/ Pink Specks, Round, Scored, 52 over 52, Chewable	Carbamazepine 100 mg	Tegretol by Allscripts		Anticonvulsant
5252 <> TEGRETOL	Tab, White w/ Pink Specks, Round, Scored, 52 over 52, Chewable	Carbamazepine 100 mg	Tegretol by Novartis	00083-0052	Anticonvulsant
525879	Cap	Doxycycline Hyclate	by URL Mutual	00677-0598	Antibiotic
526 <> DANDAN	Tab, White, Round	Isoniazid 300 mg	Laniazid by Schein	00364-0151	Antimycobacterial
526 <> WATSON	Tab, Blue, Round	Norgestimate 0.250 mg, Ethinyl Estradiol 0.035 mg	TriNessa by Watson	52544-0935	Oral Contraceptive
526 <> WATSON	Tab, Blue, Round	Norgestimate 0.250 mg, Ethinyl Estradiol 0.035 mg	Mononessa by Watson	52544-0526	Oral Contraceptive
526879	Cap, Blue	Doxycycline Hyclate 100 mg	by Dixon Shane	17236-0527	Antibiotic
527 <> BMS	Tab, White to Off-White, Round, Film Coated	Dasatinib 20 mg	Sprycel by BMS	00003-0527	Cancer Treatment
527 <> BMS	Tab, White to Off-White, Round, Film Coated	Dasatinib 20 mg	Sprycel by BMS	Canadian DIN 02293129	Cancer Treatment
527093	Tab, Pink, Round, Film Coated, Scored	Bisoprolol Fumarate 5 mg	Zebeta by Teva	00093-5270	Antihypertensive
527093	Tab, Pink, Round, Film Coated, Scored	Bisoprolol Fumarate 5 mg	Zebeta by Novopharm	Canadian DIN 02267470	Antihypertensive
5271043	Tab, Round, 527/1043	Isobutylallylbarbituric Acid 50 mg, Caffeine 40 mg, Aspirin 200 mg, Phenacetin 130 mg	Lanorinal by Lannett		Analgesic
5271060	Tab, White, Round, 527/1060	Glutethimide 500 mg	Doriden by Lannett		Hypnotic; C II
5271088	Tab, White, Round, 527/1088	Glutethimide 250 mg	Doriden by Lannett		Hypnotic; C II
5271123	Tab, Green, Round, 527/1123	Dextroamphetamine Sulfate 15 mg	Dexedrine by Lannett		Stimulant; C II
5271138	Tab, Round, 527/1138	Amphetamine Sulfate 5 mg	by Lannett		Stimulant; C II
5271139	Tab, Round, 527/1139	Amphetamine Sulfate 10 mg	by Lannett		Stimulant; C II
5271143	Tab, Yellow, Round, 527/1143	Dextroamphetamine Sulfate 5 mg	Dexedrine by Lannett		Stimulant; C II
5271170	Tab, White, Round, 527/1170	Atropine Sulfate 0.025 mg, Diphenoxylate HCl 2.5 mg	Lofene by Lannett		Antidiarrheal; C V
5271179	Tab, Lavender, Round, 527/1179	Butabarbital 0.25 g	Butisol Sodium by Lannett		Sedative/Hypnotic; C III

ID FRONT <> BACK	DESCRIPTION FRONT <> BACK	INGREDIENT & STRENGTH	BRAND (or Generic Equiv.) by FIRM	NDC#	CLASS; SCH.
5271180	Tab, Green, Round, 527/1180	Butabarbital 0.5 g	Butisol Sodium by Lannett		Sedative/Hypnotic; C III
5271184	Tab, Pink, Round, 527/1184	Butabarbital 1.5 g	Butisol Sodium by Lannett		Sedative/Hypnotic; C III
5271219	Tab, Orange, Round, 527/1219	Dextroamphetamine Sulfate 10 mg	Dexedrine by Lannett		Stimulant; C II
5271224	Tab, White, Round, 527/1224	Meprobamate 400 mg	Equanil by Lannett		Sedative/Hypnotic; C IV
5271250	Tab, White, Round, 527/1250	Meprobamate 200 mg	Equanil by Lannett		Sedative/Hypnotic; C IV
5271252	Tab, Green, Round, 527/1252	Phendimetrazine Tartrate 35 mg	Obalan by Lannett		Anorexiant; C III
5271269	Tab, Oval, Speckled, 527/1269	Phendimetrazine Tartrate 35 mg	P-D-M Ovals by Lannett		Anorexiant; C III
5271270	Tab, Pink, Round, 527/1270	Phendimetrazine Tartrate 35 mg	P-D-M by Lannett		Anorexiant; C III
5271271	Tab, Yellow, Round, 527/1271	Phendimetrazine Tartrate 35 mg	P-D-M by Lannett		Anorexiant; C III
5271272	Tab, Gray, Round, 527/1272	Phendimetrazine Tartrate 35 mg	P-D-M by Lannett		Anorexiant; C III
5271273	Tab, White, Round, 527/1273	Phendimetrazine Tartrate 35 mg	P-D-M by Lannett		Anorexiant; C III
5271274	Tab, Speckled Green & White, Round, 527/1274	Phendimetrazine Tartrate 35 mg	P-D-M by Lannett		Anorexiant; C III
527155LANNETT	Cap, Dark Green & Light Green	Aspirin 325 mg, Butalbital 50 mg, Caffeine 40 mg	Fiorinal by Duramed	51285-0908	Analgesic; C III
527193	Tab, White, Round, Film Coated, 5271 over 93	Bisoprolol Fumarate 10 mg	Zebeta by Teva	00093-5271	Antihypertensive
527193	Tab, White, Round, Film Coated, 5271 over 93	Bisoprolol Fumarate 10 mg	Zebeta by Novopharm	Canadian DIN 02267489	Antihypertensive
5275 <> 93	Tab, Blue, Round	Dexmethylphenidate HCl 2.5 mg	Focalin by Teva	00093-5275	Stimulant; C II
527508	Cap, Yellow, 527/508	Pentobarbital Sodium 1.5 g	Nembutal by Lannett		Sedative/Hypnotic; C II
527510	Cap, Black, 527/510	Phendimetrazine Tartrate 35 mg	P-D-M by Lannett		Anorexiant; C III
527511	Cap, Clear & Yellow, 527/511	Pentobarbital Sodium 0.75 g	Nembutal by Lannett		Sedative/Hypnotic; C II
527515	Cap, Blue, 527/515	Amobarbital Sodium 3 g	Amytal by Lannett		Sedative/Hypnotic; C II
527535	Cap, 527/535	Secobarbital Sodium 0.5 g, Butalbital Sodium 0.5 g, Phenobarbital 0.5 g	Tribarb by Lannett		Sedative/Hypnotic; C III
527544	Cap, Reddish-Orange, 527/544	Secobarbital Sodium 1.5 g	Seconal by Lannett		Sedative/Hypnotic; C II
527546	Cap, Reddish-Orange, 527/546	Secobarbital Sodium 0.75 g	Seconal by Lannett		Sedative/Hypnotic; C II
527549	Cap, Brown & Clear, 527/549	Phentermine HCl 30 mg	by Lannett		Anorexiant; C IV
527557	Cap, Green, 527/557	Chloral Hydrate 500 mg	Chloral Hydrate by Lannett		Sedative/Hypnotic; C IV
527558	Cap, Blue & White, 527/558	Glutethimide 500 mg	by Lannett		Hypnotic; C II
527561	Cap, Pink & White, 527/561	Dover's Powder, Phenacetin, Aspirin, Camphor, Caffeine, Atropine	Doverin by Lannett		Analgesic
527566	Cap, Blue & Orange, 527/566	Amobarbital Sodium 0.75 g, Secobarbital Sodium 0.75 g	Tuinal by Lannett		Sedative/Hypnotic; C II
527567	Cap, Blue & Orange, 527/567	Amobarbital Sodium 1.5 g, Secobarbital Sodium 1.5 g	Tuinal by Lannett		Sedative/Hypnotic; C II
527568	Cap, Blue & Gold, 527/568	Dover's Powder, Phenacetin, Aspirin, Camphor, Caffeine, Atropine	Doverin by Lannett		Analgesic
527584	Cap, Gray & Red, 527/584	Aspirin 389 mg, Caffeine 32.4 mg, Propoxyphene 65 mg	Darvon Compound 65 by Lannett		Analgesic; C IV
527591	Cap, Green & Yellow, 527/591	Chlordiazepoxide 5 mg	Librium by Lannett		Antianxiety; C IV
527592	Cap, Black & Green, 527/592	Chlordiazepoxide 10 mg	Librium by Lannett		Antianxiety; C IV
527593	Cap, Green & White, 527/593	Chlordiazepoxide 25 mg	Librium by Lannett		Antianxiety; C IV
527595	Cap, Pink, 527/595	Propoxyphene 65 mg	Darvon by Lannett		Analgesic; C IV
5276 <> 93	Tab, Yellow, Round	Dexmethylphenidate HCl 5 mg	Focalin by Teva	00093-5276	Stimulant; C II
527625	Cap, Yellow, 527/625	Phendimetrazine Tartrate 35 mg	P-D-M by Lannett		Anorexiant; C III
527626	Cap, Blue & Clear, 527/626	Phendimetrazine Tartrate 35 mg	P-D-M by Lannett		Anorexiant; C III
527627	Cap, Brown & Clear, 527/627	Phendimetrazine Tartrate 35 mg	P-D-M by Lannett		Anorexiant; C III
527628	Cap, Clear & Green, 527/628	Phendimetrazine Tartrate 35 mg	P-D-M by Lannett		Anorexiant; C III

ID FRONT <> BACK	DESCRIPTION FRONT <> BACK	INGREDIENT & STRENGTH	BRAND (or Generic Equiv.) by FIRM	NDC#	CLASS; SCH.
527637	Cap, Brown & Clear, 527/637	Phendimetrazine Tartrate 35 mg	Obalan by Lannett		Anorexiant; C III
527638	Cap, Red & Yellow, 527/638	Phendimetrazine Tartrate 35 mg	Obalan by Lannett		Anorexiant; C III
527639	Cap, Clear & Green, 527/639	Phendimetrazine Tartrate 35 mg	Obalan by Lannett		Anorexiant; C III
5277 <> 93	Tab, White to Off-White, Round	Dexmethylphenidate HCl 10 mg	Focalin by Teva	00093-5277	Stimulant; C II
527900	Tab, White, Round, 527/900	Acetaminophen 300 mg, Codeine Phosphate 30 mg	Tylenol w/ Codeine by Lannett		Analgesic; C III
527903	Tab, Orange, Round, 527/903	Codeine 8 mg, Salicylamide 230 mg, Acetaminophen 150 mg, Caffeine 30 mg	Codalan No.1 by Lannett		Analgesic; C III
527904	Tab, White, Round, 527/904	Codeine 15 mg, Salicylamide 230 mg, Acetaminophen 150 mg, Caffeine 30 mg	Codalan No.2 by Lannett		Analgesic; C III
527905	Tab, Green, Round, 527/905	Codeine 30 mg, Salicylamide 230 mg, Acetaminophen 150 mg, Caffeine 30 mg	Codalan No.3 by Lannett		Analgesic; C III
528 <> BMS	Tab, White to Off-White, Oval, Film Coated	Dasatinib 50 mg	Sprycel by BMS	Canadian DIN 02293137	Cancer Treatment
528 <> BMS	Tab, White to Off-White, Oval, Film Coated	Dasatinib 50 mg	Sprycel by BMS	00003-0528	Cancer Treatment
5282 <> 93	Tab, White, Round, Film Coated	Ropinirole HCl 0.25 mg	Requip by Teva	00093-5282	Antiparkinson
5283 <> 93	Tab, Yellow, Round, Film Coated	Ropinirole HCl 0.5 mg	Requip by Teva	00093-5283	Antiparkinson
5284 <> 93	Tab, Green, Round, Film-Coated	Ropinirole HCl 1 mg	Requip by Teva	00093-5284	Antiparkinson
5285 <> 93	Tab, Pink, Round, Film-Coated	Ropinirole HCl 2 mg	Requip by Teva	00093-5285	Antiparkinson
5286 <> 93	Tab, Purple, Round, Film-Coated	Ropinirole HCl 3 mg	Requip by Teva	00093-5286	Antiparkinson
5287 <> 93	Tab, Beige, Round, Film-Coated	Ropinirole HCl 4 mg	Requip by Teva	00093-5287	Antiparkinson
5288 <> 93	Tab, Blue, Round, Film Coated	Ropinirole HCl 5 mg	Requip by Teva	00093-5288	Antiparkinson
529 <> 54	Tab, Yellow, Black Print, Round, Film Coated	Thiethylperazine Maleate 10 mg	Torecan by Roxane	00054-8748	Antiemetic
529MD	Tab, White, Round	Glutethimide 500 mg	Doriden by MD		Hypnotic; C II
52H	Tab, White, Oblong, Scored	Telmisartan 80 mg	Micardis by Boehringer Ingelheim	12714-0110	Antihypertensive
52H	Tab, White, Oblong, Scored, BI Logo	Telmisartan 80 mg	Micardis by Boehringer Ingelheim	00597-0041	Antihypertensive
52H	Tab, White to Off-White, Oblong	Telmisartan 80 mg	Micardis by Boehringer Ingelheim Canada	Canadian DIN 02240770	Antihypertensive
53 <> A	Tab, White, Round	Benazepril HCl 20 mg	Lotensin by Amneal	65162-0753	Antihypertensive
53 <> M	Tab, Green, Pentagonal, Film Coated	Cimetidine HCl 200 mg	Tagamet by Qualitest	00603-2890	Gastrointestinal
53 <> M	Tab, Green, Pentagonal, Film Coated	Cimetidine HCl 200 mg	Tagamet by Mylan	00378-0053	Gastrointestinal
53 <> M	Tab, Green, Pentagonal, Film Coated	Cimetidine HCl 200 mg	Tagamet by H J Harkins Co	52959-0374	Gastrointestinal
53 <> M	Tab, Green, Pentagonal, Film Coated	Cimetidine HCl 200 mg	Tagamet by Murfreesboro	51129-1177	Gastrointestinal
53 <> M	Tab, Green, Pentagonal, Film Coated	Cimetidine HCl 200 mg	Tagamet by Heartland	61392-0194	Gastrointestinal
53 <> MP	Tab, Peach, Round, Scored	Prednisone 20 mg	Deltasone by Allscripts		Steroid
530 <> MD	Tab, Blue & Green, Round, Scored	Methylphenidate HCl 10 mg	Ritalin by Sandoz	00781-8841	Stimulant; C II
530 <> MD	Tab, Light Blue, Round, Scored	Methylphenidate HCl 10 mg	Ritalin by AltiMed	Canadian DIN 02230321	Stimulant; C II
530 <> MD	Tab, Light Blue, Round, Scored	Methylphenidate HCl 10 mg	Ritalin by Apothecon	59772-8841	Stimulant; C II
530 <> MD	Tab, Light Blue, Round, Scored	Methylphenidate HCl 10 mg	Ritalin by Qualitest	00603-4570	Stimulant; C II
530 <> WC	Tab, White, Round	Norethindrone Acetate 1 mg, Ethinyl Estradiol 20 mcg	Loestrin 24 Fe by Warner Chilcott	00430-0530	Oral Contraceptive
5307 <> DANDAN	Tab, White, Round, Scored	Promethazine HCl 25 mg	Phenergan by Pharmedix	53002-0402	Antiemetic; Antihistamine
5307 <> DANDAN	Tab, White, Round, Scored	Promethazine HCl 25 mg	Phenergan by Schein	00364-0222	Antiemetic; Antihistamine
5307 <> DANDAN	Tab, White, Round, Scored	Promethazine HCl 25 mg	Phenergan by Watson	00591-5307	Antiemetic; Antihistamine
530MD	Tab, Pale Blue/Green	Methylphenidate HCl 10 mg	Ritalin by MD	43567-0530	Stimulant; C II
530MD	Tab, Pale Blue/Green	Methylphenidate HCl 10 mg	Ritalin by Caremark	00339-4093	Stimulant; C II
530MD	Tab, Pale Blue Green, Round, Scored	Methylphenidate HCl 10 mg	Ritalin by Medeva	53014-0530	Stimulant; C II
530MD	Tab, Blue-Green	Methylphenidate HCl 10 mg	Ritalin by Caremark	00339-4096	Stimulant; C II
530MD	Tab, Pale Blue/Green	Methylphenidate HCl 10 mg	Ritalin by Int'l Med Systems	00548-7010	Stimulant; C II
530MD	Tab	Methylphenidate HCl 10 mg	Ritalin by Ivax	00182-1066	Stimulant; C II

ID FRONT <> BACK	DESCRIPTION FRONT <> BACK	INGREDIENT & STRENGTH	BRAND (or Generic Equiv.) by FIRM	NDC#	CLASS; SCH.
531 <> MD	Tab	Methylphenidate HCl 5 mg	Ritalin by Qualitest	00603-4569	Stimulant; C II
531 <> SCHWARZ	Tab, White, Round, Scored	Hyoscyamine Sulfate 0.125 mg	Levsin by Schwarz	00091-3531	Gastrointestinal
531 <> SCHWARZ	Tab, White, Round, Scored	Hyoscyamine Sulfate 0.125 mg	Levsin by Thrift Drug	59198-0287	Gastrointestinal
531 <> SCHWARZ	Tab, White, Round, Scored	Hyoscyamine Sulfate 0.125 mg	Levsin by Prestige	58056-0351	Gastrointestinal
5311 <> 250	Tab, White to Off White, Oval, Ivax Logo 5311 <> 250	Ciprofloxacin 250 mg	Cipro by Ivax	00172-5311	Antibiotic
5311 <> V	Tab, Green, Oblong, Scored	Dextromethorphan HBr 30 mg, Guaifenesin 600 mg	by DRX	55045-2623	Cold Remedy
5311V	Tab, Film Coated	Dextromethorphan HBr 30 mg, Guaifenesin 600 mg	by PDRX	55289-0625	Cold Remedy
5311V	Tab, Film Coated, V-Scored	Dextromethorphan HBr 30 mg, Guaifenesin 600 mg	Guaibid DM by Vintage	00254-5311	Cold Remedy
5311V	Tab, Green, Oblong, Scored, Film	Guaifenesin 600 mg, Dextromethorphan HBr 30 mg	by Med Pro	53978-3312	Cold Remedy
5312	Tab, Light Green, Delayed Release, 5312	Guaifenesin 600 mg	Robitussin by Quality Care	60346-0863	Expectorant
5312 <> 500	Tab, White to Off White, Oval, Ivax Logo 5312 <> 500	Ciprofloxacin 500 mg	Cipro by Ivax	00172-5312	Antibiotic
5312V	Tab, Green, Oblong, Scored	Guaifenesin 600 mg	Robitussin by Vangard	00615-4524	Expectorant
5312V	Tab, V-Scored	Guaifenesin 600 mg	Robitussin by Vintage	00254-5312	Expectorant
5313 <> 750	Tab, White to Off White, Oval, Ivax Logo 5313 <> 750	Ciprofloxacin 750 mg	Cipro by Ivax	00172-5313	Antibiotic
5319 <> DAN	Tab, White, Round	Promethazine HCl 50 mg	Phenergan by Watson	00591-5319	Antiemetic; Antihistamine
5319 <> DAN	Tab, White, Round	Promethazine HCl 50 mg	Phenergan by Schein	00364-0345	Antiemetic; Antihistamine
531MD	Tab	Methylphenidate HCl 5 mg	by Caremark	00339-4097	Stimulant; C II
531MD	Tab, Yellow, Round	Methylphenidate HCl 5 mg	by Medeva	53014-0531	Stimulant; C II
531MD	Tab	Methylphenidate HCl 5 mg	by Ivax	00182-1173	Stimulant; C II
531MD	Tab	Methylphenidate HCl 5 mg	by MD	43567-0531	Stimulant; C II
531MD	Tab, Yellow, Round, Scored	Methylphenidate HCl 5 mg	by Apothecon	59772-8840	Stimulant; C II
531MD	Tab	Methylphenidate HCl 5 mg	by Schein	00364-0561	Stimulant; C II
531MD	Tab, Debossed	Methylphenidate HCl 5 mg	by Int'l Med Systems	00548-7005	Stimulant; C II
532 <> MD	Tab, Orange, Round, Scored	Methylphenidate HCl 20 mg	Ritalin by AltiMed	Canadian DIN 02230322	Stimulant; C II
532 <> MD	Tab, Orange, Round, Scored	Methylphenidate HCl 20 mg	Ritalin by Apothecon	59772-8842	Stimulant; C II
532 <> SCHWARZ	Tab, White, Octagonal, Scored, Sublingual	Hyoscyamine Sulfate 0.125 mg	Levsin by Prestige	58056-0352	Gastrointestinal
532 <> SCHWARZ	Tab, White, Octagonal, Scored, Sublingual	Hyoscyamine Sulfate 0.125 mg	Levsin by Amerisource	62584-0007	Gastrointestinal
532 <> SCHWARZ	Tab, White, Octagonal, Scored, Sublingual	Hyoscyamine Sulfate 0.125 mg	Levsin by Physician Total Care	54868-1767	Gastrointestinal
532 <> SCHWARZ	Tab, White, Octagonal, Scored, Sublingual	Hyoscyamine Sulfate 0.125 mg	Levsin by Thrift Drug	59198-0173	Gastrointestinal
532 <> SCHWARZ	Tab, White, Octagonal, Scored, Sublingual	Hyoscyamine Sulfate 0.125 mg	Levsin by Schwarz	00091-3532	Gastrointestinal
532 <> SCHWARZ	Tab, White, Octagonal, Scored, Sublingual	Hyoscyamine Sulfate 0.125 mg	Levsin by Med Pro	53978-3372	Gastrointestinal
532 <> SCHWARZ	Tab, White, Octagonal, Scored, Sublingual	Hyoscyamine Sulfate 0.125 mg	Levsin by Nat Pharmpak	55154-0952	Gastrointestinal
532 <> SCHWARZ	Tab, White, Octagonal, Scored, Sublingual	Hyoscyamine Sulfate 0.125 mg	Levsin by Murfreesboro	51129-1489	Gastrointestinal
5321 <> DANDAN	Tab, White, Round, Scored	Primidone 250 mg	Mysoline by Vangard	00615-2521	Anticonvulsant
5321 <> DANDAN	Tab, White, Round, Scored	Primidone 250 mg	Mysoline by Schein	00364-0366	Anticonvulsant
5321 <> DANDAN	Tab, White, Round, Scored	Primidone 250 mg	Mysoline by Watson	00591-5321	Anticonvulsant
5325 <> DANDAN	Tab, White, Cap Shaped, Scored	Colchicine 0.5 mg, Probenecid 500 mg	ColBenemid by Schein	00364-0315	Antigout
5325 <> DANDAN	Tab, White, Cap Shaped, Scored	Colchicine 0.5 mg, Probenecid 500 mg	ColBenemid by Watson	00591-5325	Antigout
5325V	Tab, 53/25V	Atropine Sulfate 0.04 mg, Chlorpheniramine Maleate 8 mg, Hyoscyamine Sulfate 0.19 mg, Phenylephrine 25 mg, Phenylpropanolamine 50 mg, Scopolamine 0.01 mg	Atrohist Plus by Ivax	00172-4375	Cold Remedy
5325V	Tab	Atropine Sulfate 0.04 mg, Chlorpheniramine Maleate 8 mg, Hyoscyamine Sulfate 0.19 mg, Phenylephrine 25 mg, Phenylpropanolamine 50 mg, Scopolamine 0.01 mg	Atrohist Plus by Qualitest	00603-5549	Cold Remedy
532HD	Tab, Red & White	Oxycodone 5 mg, Acetaminophen 500 mg	Tylox by Halsey	Discontinued	Analgesic; C II
532MD	Tab, Orange, Round, 532/MD	Methylphenidate HCl 20 mg	Ritalin by Pharmascience	Canadian	Stimulant; C II
532MD	Tab	Methylphenidate HCl 20 mg	Ritalin by Caremark	00339-4094	Stimulant; C II
532MD	Tab	Methylphenidate HCl 20 mg	Ritalin by Int'l Med Systems	00548-7020	Stimulant; C II
532MD	Tab, Orange, Round, Scored	Methylphenidate HCl 20 mg	Ritalin by Medeva	53014-0532	Stimulant; C II

ID FRONT <> BACK	DESCRIPTION FRONT <> BACK	INGREDIENT & STRENGTH	BRAND (or Generic Equiv.) by FIRM	NDC#	CLASS; SCH.
532MD	Tab	Methylphenidate HCl 20 mg	Ritalin by Caremark	00339-4098	Stimulant; C II
532MD	Tab	Methylphenidate HCl 20 mg	Ritalin by MD	43567-0532	Stimulant; C II
533	Tab, Pink, Cap Shaped, Scored	Carbamazepine 200 mg	Tegretol by Caraco	57664-0533	Anticonvulsant
5333DAN	Cap, Orange & Yellow	Procainamide HCl 500 mg	by Schein	00364-0344	Antiarrythmic
5335 <> DANDAN	Tab, White, Round, Scored	Trihexyphenidyl HCl 2 mg	Artane by Heartland	61392-0634	Antiparkinson
5335 <> DANDAN	Tab, White, Round, Scored	Trihexyphenidyl HCl 2 mg	Artane by Schein	00364-0408	Antiparkinson
5335 <> DANDAN	Tab, White, Round, Scored	Trihexyphenidyl HCl 2 mg	Artane by Vangard	00615-0675	Antiparkinson
5335 <> DANDAN	Tab, White, Round, Scored	Trihexyphenidyl HCl 2 mg	Artane by Watson	00591-5335	Antiparkinson
5335 <> DANDAN	Tab, White, Round, Scored	Trihexyphenidyl HCl 2 mg	Artane by Amerisource	62584-0886	Antiparkinson
5335 <> DANDAN	Tab, White, Round, Scored	Trihexyphenidyl HCl 2 mg	Artane by Octofoil	63467-0301	Antiparkinson
5335 <> DANDAN	Tab, White, Round, Scored	Trihexyphenidyl HCl 2 mg	Artane by Danbury	61955-0408	Antiparkinson
5337 <> DANDAN	Tab, White, Round, Scored	Trihexyphenidyl HCl 5 mg	Artane by Schein	00364-0409	Antiparkinson
5337 <> DANDAN	Tab, White, Round, Scored	Trihexyphenidyl HCl 5 mg	Artane by Watson	00591-5337	Antiparkinson
5337 <> DANDAN	Tab, White, Round, Scored	Trihexyphenidyl HCl 5 mg	Artane by Amerisource	62584-0887	Antiparkinson
5337 <> DANDAN	Tab, White, Round, Scored	Trihexyphenidyl HCl 5 mg	Artane by Danbury	61955-0409	Antiparkinson
5337 <> DANDAN	Tab, White, Round, Scored	Trihexyphenidyl HCl 5 mg	Artane by Heartland	61392-0956	Antiparkinson
533HD	Cap, Blue	Flurazepam HCl 30 mg	Dalmane by Halsey	Discontinued	Hypnotic; C IV
534 <> SCHWARZ	Tab, Pink	Hyoscyamine Sulfate 0.125 mg, Phenobarbital 15 mg	Levsin Phenobarb by Schwarz	00091-3534	Gastrointestinal; C IV
5342 <> DANDAN	Tab, White, Round, Scored	Nylidrin 6 mg	by Schein	00364-0391	Vasodilator
5345 <> DANDAN	Tab	Hydrochlorothiazide 50 mg	Hydrodiuril by Talbert	44514-0411	Diuretic; Antihypertensive
5345 <> DANDAN	Tab, Peach, Round, Scored	Hydrochlorothiazide 50 mg	Hydrodiuril by Schein	00364-0328	Diuretic; Antihypertensive
5347 <> DANDAN	Tab, Yellow, Cap Shaped, Scored, Film Coated	Probenecid 500 mg	Benemid by Watson	00591-5347	Antigout
5347 <> DANDAN	Tab, Yellow, Cap Shaped, Scored, Film Coated	Probenecid 500 mg	Benemid by Schein	00364-0314	Antigout
5347 <> DANDAN	Tab, Yellow, Cap Shaped, Scored, Film Coated	Probenecid 500 mg	Benemid by Pharmedix	53002-0397	Antigout
534HD	Cap, Blue & White	Flurazepam HCl 15 mg	Dalmane by Halsey	Discontinued	Hypnotic; C IV
535	Tab, Pink, Cap Shaped, Scored	Carbamazepine 300 mg	Tegretol by Caraco	57664-0535	Anticonvulsant
535 <> MD	Tab	Atropine Sulfate 0.025 mg, Diphenoxylate HCl 2.5 mg	Lomotil by Quality Care	60346-0437	Antidiarrheal; C V
5350 <> 5	Tab, Yellow, Oblong, Hourglass Logo 5350	Benazepril HCl 5 mg	Lotensin by Ivax	00172-5350	Antihypertensive
				Discontinued	
5351 <> 10	Tab, Dark Yellow, Oblong, Hourglass Logo 5351	Benazepril HCl 10 mg	Lotensin by Ivax	00172-5351	Antihypertensive
				Discontinued	
53511	Tab, Debossed 535-11 <> Gilbert Logo	Acetaminophen 325 mg, Butalbital 50 mg, Caffeine 40 mg	Fioricet by Amerisource	62584-0630	Analgesic
53511	Tab, White, Oblong, Scored, Accucaps Logo 535/11	Acetaminophen 325 mg, Butalbital 50 mg, Caffeine 40 mg	Fioricet by Accucaps	61474-4073	Analgesic
53511	Tab, White, Oblong, Scored, Logo	Butalbital 50 mg, Acetaminophen 325 mg, Caffeine 40 mg	Fioricet by Nat Pharmpak	59198-0331	Analgesic
53511 <> G	Tab, Gilbert Logo	Acetaminophen 325 mg, Butalbital 50 mg, Caffeine 40 mg	Fioricet by Prestige	55154-4601	Analgesic
53511 <> GL	Tab, 535-11 <> Gilbert Logo G with overlaid L	Butalbital 50 mg, Acetaminophen 325 mg, Caffeine 40 mg	Esgic by Rx Pak	58056-0354	Analgesic
53511 <> GL	Tab, White, Oblong, Scored	Acetaminophen 325 mg, Butalbital 50 mg, Caffeine 40 mg	Fioricet by Accucaps	65084-0126	Analgesic
53512	Cap, Opaque & White, Logo and 535-12 in Kelly Green	Benazepril HCl 20 mg	Lotensin by Ivax	61474-4074	Antihypertensive
5352 <> 20	Tab, Pink, Oblong, Hourglass Logo 5352			00172-5352	
				Discontinued	
5353 <> 40	Tab, Red, Oblong, Hourglass Logo 5353	Benazepril HCl 40 mg	Lotensin by Ivax	00172-5353	Antihypertensive
				Discontinued	
5353 <> GEIGY	Tab, White, Mottled Pink, Cap Shaped, Scored	Hydrochlorothiazide 25 mg, Metoprolol Tartrate 100 mg	Lopressor HCT by Novartis	00078-0461	Diuretic; Antihypertensive
5353 <> GEIGY	Tab, White, Mottled Pink, Cap Shaped, Scored	Hydrochlorothiazide 25 mg, Metoprolol Tartrate 100 mg	Lopressor HCT by Pharm Util	60491-0371	Diuretic; Antihypertensive
535HD	Tab, Pink, Round	Hydralazine HCl 10 mg	Apresoline by Halsey	Discontinued	Antihypertensive
535ll	Tab, Gilbert Logo	Acetaminophen 325 mg, Butalbital 50 mg, Caffeine 40 mg	Fioricet by Leiner	59606-0643	Analgesic
536	Tab, Pink, Cap Shaped, Scored	Carbamazepine 400 mg	Tegretol by Caraco	57664-0536	Anticonvulsant
536 <> 93	Tab, White, Oval, Film Coated	Naproxen 275 mg	Anaprox by Ivax	00182-1974	NSAID
536 <> 93	Tab, White, Oval, Film Coated	Naproxen 275 mg	Anaprox by Brightstone	62939-8431	NSAID
536 <> 93	Tab, White, Oval, Film Coated	Naproxen 275 mg	Anaprox by Teva	00093-0536	NSAID

ID FRONT <> BACK	DESCRIPTION FRONT <> BACK	INGREDIENT & STRENGTH	BRAND (or Generic Equiv.) by FIRM	NDC#	CLASS; SCH.
536 <> 93	Tab, White, Oval, Film Coated	Naproxen 275 mg	Anaprox by Kaiser	00179-1206	NSAID
536 <> E	Tab, White, Oval	Amlodipine Besylate 2.5 mg	Norvasc by Ethex	58177-0536	Antihypertensive
5360	Tab, Pale Yellow, Oblong, Hourglass Logo 5360	Benazepril HCl 5 mg, HCTZ 6.25 mg	Lotensin HCT by Ivax	00172-5360	Antihypertensive; Diuretic
5360 <> 93	Tab, White to Off White, Oval, Film Coated	Ursodiol 250 mg	Urso by Teva	00093-5360	Gastrointestinal
5361	Tab, Pink, Oblong, Hourglass Logo 5361	Benazepril HCl 10 mg, HCTZ 12.5 mg	Lotensin HCT by Ivax	00172-5361 Discontinued	Antihypertensive; Diuretic
5361 <> 93	Tab, White to Off White, Oval, Film Coated, Scored	Ursodiol 500 mg	Urso Forte by Teva	00093-5361	Gastrointestinal
5361 <> ANEXSIA	Tab, White, Cap Shaped, Scored	Acetaminophen 500 mg, Hydrocodone Bitartrate 5 mg	Anexsia by Mallinckrodt	00406-5361	Analgesic; C III
5361 <> DAN075	Tab, Light Blue, Round, Scored, 5361 <> Dan 0.75	Dexamethasone 0.75 mg	by Schein	00364-0098	Steroid
5362	Tab, Orange, Oblong, Hourglass Logo 5362	Benazepril HCl 20 mg, HCTZ 12.5 mg	Lotensin HCT by Ivax	00172-5362 Discontinued	Antihypertensive; Diuretic
5362 <> ANEXSIA	Tab, White, Cap Shaped, Scored	Acetaminophen 650 mg, Hydrocodone Bitartrate 7.5 mg	Anexsia by Mallinckrodt	00406-5362	Analgesic; C III
5363	Tab, Dark Orange, Oblong, Hourglass Logo 5363	Benazepril HCl 20 mg, HCTZ 25 mg	Lotensin HCT by Ivax	00172-5363 Discontinued	Antihypertensive; Diuretic
5363 <> ANEXSIA	Tab	Acetaminophen 660 mg, Hydrocodone Bitartrate 10 mg	Vicodin HP by Mallinckrodt	00406-5363	Analgesic; C III
5368 <> DANDAN	Tab, Off-White, Round, Scored	Disulfiram 500 mg	Antabuse by Schein	00364-0337	Antialcoholism
5369 <> DANDAN	Tab, White, Round, Scored	Bethanechol Chloride 10 mg	Urecholine by Schein	00364-0349	Urinary Tract
5369 <> DANDAN	Tab, White, Round, Scored	Bethanechol Chloride 10 mg	Urecholine by Watson	00591-5369	Urinary Tract
5369 <> DANDAN	Tab, White, Round, Scored	Bethanechol Chloride 10 mg	Urecholine by Bryant	63629-1164	Urinary Tract
536HD	Tab, Peach, Round	Hydralazine HCl 25 mg	Apresoline by Halsey	Discontinued	Antihypertensive
537	Tab, Light Yellow, Film Coated, Cap Shaped	Tramadol HCl 37.5 mg, Acetaminophen 325 mg	Ultracet by Caraco	57664-0537	Analgesic
537 <> 93	Tab, Off-White, Oval, Film Coated	Naproxen 550 mg	Anaprox DS by Kaiser	00179-1223	NSAID
537 <> 93	Tab, Off-White, Oval, Film Coated	Naproxen 550 mg	Anaprox DS by Teva	00093-0537	NSAID
537 <> 93	Tab, Off-White, Oval, Film Coated	Naproxen 550 mg	Anaprox DS by Brightstone	62939-8441	NSAID
537 <> E	Tab, White, Oval	Amlodipine Besylate 5mg	Norvasc by Ethex	58177-0537	Antihypertensive
537 <> M	Tab, Light Blue, Film Coated, Beveled Edge	Naproxen 275 mg	Naprosyn by Mylan	00378-0537	NSAID
537 <> M	Tab, Film Coated	Naproxen 275 mg	Naprosyn by Allscripts	Discontinued	NSAID
537 <> M	Tab, Light Blue, Film Coated	Naproxen 275 mg	Naprosyn by H J Harkins Co	52959-0357	NSAID
5373 <> DAN	Tab	Isosorbide Dinitrate 10 mg	Isordil by Watson	00591-5373	Antianginal
5373 <> DANDAN	Tab, White, Round, Scored	Isosorbide Dinitrate 10 mg	Isordil by Schein	00364-0341	Antianginal
5374 <> DANDAN	Tab, White, Round, Scored	Isosorbide Dinitrate 5 mg	Isordil by Watson	00591-5374	Antianginal
5374 <> DANDAN	Tab, White, Round, Scored	Isosorbide Dinitrate 5 mg	Isordil by Schein	00364-0340	Antianginal
5375MYLAN	Cap	Doxepin HCl 75 mg	by PDRX	55289-0258	Antidepressant
537V	Tab, Grey, Round, Scored, 5377 over V	Yohimbine HCl 5.4 mg	by Ivax	00172-4368	Impotence Agent
537HD	Tab, Orange, Round	Hydralazine HCl 50 mg	Apresoline by Halsey	Discontinued	Antihypertensive
537KREMERSURBAN	Cap	Hyoscyamine Sulfate 0.375 mg	Levsin by Drug Distr	52985-0228	Gastrointestinal
537SCHWARZ	Cap, Brown & White	Hyoscyamine Sulfate 0.375 mg	Levsin by Thrift Drug	59198-0288	Gastrointestinal
538	Tab, White, Round, Schering Logo 538	Halazepam 40 mg	Paxipam by Schering		Antianxiety; C IV
538 <> E	Tab, White, Oval	Amlodipine Besylate 10 mg	Norvasc by Pfizer	58177-0538	Antihypertensive
538 <> R	Tab, Mottled Dark Blue, Round, Scored	Carbidopa 10 mg, Levodopa 100 mg	Sinemet by Heartland	61392-0177	Antiparkinson
538 <> R	Tab, Mottled Dark Blue, Round, Scored	Carbidopa 10 mg, Levodopa 100 mg	Sinemet by Murfreesboro	51129-1301	Antiparkinson
538 <> R	Tab, Mottled Dark Blue, Round, Scored	Carbidopa 10 mg, Levodopa 100 mg	Sinemet by Actavis	00228-2538	Antiparkinson
538 <> R	Tab, Mottled Dark Blue, Round, Scored	Carbidopa 10 mg, Levodopa 100 mg	Sinemet by Qualitest	00603-2568	Antiparkinson
5381 <> DANDAN	Tab, White, Round, Scored	Methocarbamol 500 mg	Robaxin by Talbert	44514-0557	Muscle Relaxant
5381 <> DANDAN	Tab, White, Round, Scored	Methocarbamol 500 mg	Robaxin by Schein	00364-0346	Muscle Relaxant
5381 <> DANDAN	Tab, White, Round, Scored	Methocarbamol 500 mg	Robaxin by Watson	00591-5381	Muscle Relaxant
5381 <> DANDAN	Tab, White, Round, Scored	Methocarbamol 500 mg	Robaxin by Kaiser	00179-0446	Muscle Relaxant
5381 <> DANDAN	Tab, White, Round, Scored	Methocarbamol 500 mg	Robaxin by Pharmedix	53002-0304	Muscle Relaxant
5382 <> DANDAN	Tab, White, Cap Shaped, Scored	Methocarbamol 750 mg	Robaxin by Watson	00591-5382	Muscle Relaxant
5382 <> DANDAN	Tab, White, Cap Shaped, Scored	Methocarbamol 750 mg	Robaxin by Talbert	44514-0558	Muscle Relaxant

ID FRONT <> BACK	DESCRIPTION FRONT <> BACK	INGREDIENT & STRENGTH	BRAND (or Generic Equiv.) by FIRM	NDC#	CLASS; SCH.
5382 <> DANDAN	Tab, White, Cap Shaped, Scored	Methocarbamol 750 mg	Robaxin by Kaiser	00179-0447	Muscle Relaxant
5382 <> DANDAN	Tab, White, Cap Shaped, Scored	Methocarbamol 750 mg	Robaxin by Schein	00364-0347	Muscle Relaxant
5385 <> DAN	Tab	Isosorbide Dinitrate 5 mg	Isordil by Watson	00591-5385	Antianginal
5385 <> DAN	Tab, White, Round	Isosorbide Dinitrate 5 mg	Isordil by Schein	00364-0368	Antianginal
5387 <> DAN	Tab, Yellow, Round	Isosorbide Dinitrate 2.5 mg	Isordil by Watson	00591-5387	Antianginal
5387 <> DAN	Tab, Yellow, Round	Isosorbide Dinitrate 2.5 mg	Isordil by Schein	00364-0367	Antianginal
5388 <> DANDAN	Tab, White, Cap Shaped, Scored	Triamcinolone 4 mg	by Schein	00364-0352	Steroid
538HD	Tab, Orange, Round	Hydralazine HCl 100 mg	Apresoline by Halsey	Discontinued	Antihypertensive
539	Tab, Pink, Cap Shaped	Carbamazepine 100 mg	Tegretol by Schein	57664-0539	Anticonvulsant
539 <> BP	Tab, Layered, Round	Guaifenesin 275 mg, Phenylephrine HCl 25 mg	Guaiphen-PD by Boca	64376-0539	Cold Remedy
539 <> R	Tab, Mottled Yellow, Round, Scored	Carbidopa 25 mg, Levodopa 100 mg	Sinemet by Actavis	00228-2539	Antiparkinson
539 <> R	Tab, Mottled Yellow, Round, Scored	Carbidopa 25 mg, Levodopa 100 mg	Sinemet by Heartland	61392-0180	Antiparkinson
539 <> R	Tab, Mottled Yellow, Round, Scored	Carbidopa 25 mg, Levodopa 100 mg	Sinemet by Med Pro	53978-2078	Antiparkinson
539 <> R	Tab, Mottled Yellow, Round, Scored	Carbidopa 25 mg, Levodopa 100 mg	Sinemet by Qualitest	00603-2569	Antiparkinson
5390 <> DANDAN	Tab, White, Round, Scored	Nylidrin 12 mg	by Schein	00364-0392	Vasodilator
54 <> 310	Tab, Yellow to Speckled Yellow, Oval	Nefazodone HCl 200 mg	Serzone by Roxane	00054-4674	Antidepressant
54 <> 529	Tab, Yellow, Black Print, Round, Film Coated	Thiethylperazine Maleate 10 mg	Torecan by Roxane	00054-8748	Antiemetic
54 <> 643	Tab, Beige, Round	Naproxen 250 mg	Naprosyn by Roxane	00054-8641	NSAID
54 <> 899	Tab	Prednisone 10 mg	Deltasone by Med Pro	53978-3037	Steroid
54 <> A	Tab, White, Round	Benazepril HCl 40 mg	Lotensin by Amneal	65162-0754	Antihypertensive
54 <> PAR	Tab, Yellow, Triangular, Sugar Coated	Imipramine HCl 10 mg	Tofranil by Allscripts		Antidepressant
540 <> BP	Tab, White, Oval	Guaifenesin 600 mg, Phenylephrine HCl 40 mg	Liquibid-D by Boca	64376-0540	Cold Remedy
540 <> C	Tab, White, Barrel Shaped	Cetirizine HCl 5 mg	Zyrtec by Caraco	57664-0540	Antihistamine
540 <> R	Tab, Mottled Light Blue, Round, Scored	Carbidopa 25 mg, Levodopa 250 mg	Sinemet by Qualitest	00603-2570	Antiparkinson
540 <> R	Tab, Mottled Light Blue, Round, Scored	Carbidopa 25 mg, Levodopa 250 mg	Sinemet by Actavis	00228-2540	Antiparkinson
540 <> R	Tab, Mottled Light Blue, Round, Scored	Carbidopa 25 mg, Levodopa 250 mg	Sinemet by Heartland	61392-0183	Antiparkinson
540 <> R	Tab, Mottled Light Blue, Round, Scored	Carbidopa 25 mg, Levodopa 250 mg	Sinemet by Murfreesboro	51129-1292	Antiparkinson
5400 <> FP	Tab, White to Off-White, Cap Shaped, Scored, F / P <> 5400	Oxycodone HCl 5 mg, Ibuprofen 400 mg	Combunox by Forest	00456-5200	Analgesic; NSAID; C II
54009	Tab, White, Round, 54-009	Propranolol HCl 20 mg	Inderal by Roxane		Antihypertensive
5401 <> AMB5	Tab, Pink, Cap Shaped, Film Coated	Zolpidem Tartrate 5 mg	Ambien by Caremark	00339-4064	Sedative/Hypnotic; C IV
5401 <> AMB5	Tab, Pink, Cap Shaped, Film Coated	Zolpidem Tartrate 5 mg	Ambien by Nat Pharmpak	55154-3617	Sedative/Hypnotic; C IV
5401 <> AMB5	Tab, Pink, Cap Shaped, Film Coated	Zolpidem Tartrate 5 mg	Ambien by H J Harkins Co	52959-0362	Sedative/Hypnotic; C IV
5401 <> AMB5	Tab, Pink, Cap Shaped, Film Coated	Zolpidem Tartrate 5 mg	Ambien by Searle	00025-5401	Sedative/Hypnotic; C IV
5401 <> AMB5	Tab, Pink, Cap Shaped, Film Coated	Zolpidem Tartrate 5 mg	Ambien by Sanofi	00024-5401	Sedative/Hypnotic; C IV
5401 <> V	Tab, White, Round, Scored	Quinine Sulfate 260 mg	Quinamm by Qualitest	00603-5618	Antimalarial
54010	Tab, Orange, Oblong	Diflunisal 250 mg	Dolobid by Roxane	00054-8210	NSAID
54012	Tab, White, Round, 54-012	Amitriptyline HCl 25 mg	Elavil by Roxane		Antidepressant
54013	Tab, Yellow, Round, Scored	Leucovorin Calcium 25 mg	Wellcovorin by Schein	00054-8499	Antineoplastic
54013	Tab, Yellow, Round, Scored	Leucovorin Calcium 25 mg	Wellcovorin by Roxane	00054-4499	Antineoplastic
54015	Tab, White to Off-White, Round, Scored	Torsemide 5 mg	Demadex by Roxane	00054-0075	Diuretic
54016	Tab, White to Off-White, Round, Scored	Torsemide 10 mg	Demadex by Roxane	00054-0076	Diuretic
54017	Tab, White to Off-White, Round, Scored	Torsemide 20 mg	Demadex by Roxane	00054-0077	Diuretic
54019	Tab, Yellow, Round, 54-019	Chlorpheniramine Maleate 4 mg	Chlor-Trimeton by Roxane		Antihistamine
5402 <> DANDAN	Tab, Tan, Round, Scored	Bethanechol Chloride 25 mg	Urecholine by Schein	00364-0410	Urinary Tract
5402 <> DANDAN	Tab, Tan, Round, Scored	Bethanechol Chloride 25 mg	Urecholine by Watson	00591-5402	Urinary Tract
54024	Tab, White, Round, 54 over 024	Flecainide Acetate 50 mg	Tambocor by Roxane	00054-0010	Antiarrhythmic
54039	Tab, Beige, Oblong, 54-039	Naproxn 500 mg	Naprosyn by Roxane	00054-8643	NSAID
54042	Tab, White, Oval, Scored	Nefazodone HCl 100 mg	Serzone by Roxane	00054-4672	Antidepressant
54043	Tab, Yellow, Round, Scored	Azathioprine 50 mg	Imuran by Roxane	00054-8084	Immunosuppressant

ID FRONT <> BACK	DESCRIPTION FRONT <> BACK	INGREDIENT & STRENGTH	BRAND (or Generic Equiv.) by FIRM	NDC#	CLASS; SCH.
54043	Tab, Yellow, Round, Scored	Azathioprine 50 mg	Imuran by Roxane	00054-4084	Immunosuppressant
54050 <> 1	Tab, White, Hexagonal, Scored, 54 over 050	Haloperidol 1 mg	Haldol by Roxane	00054-8343 Discontinued	Antipsychotic
54050 <> 1	Tab, White, Hexagonal, Scored, 54 over 050	Haloperidol 1 mg	Haldol by Nat Pharmpak	55154-4924	Antipsychotic
54050 <> 1	Tab, White, Hexagonal, Scored, 54 over 050	Haloperidol 1 mg	Haldol by Merck Sharp & Dohme	60312-0072	Antipsychotic
54050 <> 1	Tab, White, Hexagonal, Scored, 54 over 050	Haloperidol 1 mg	Haldol by Amerisource	62584-0725	Antipsychotic
54053300	Tab, White, Round, 54-053 300	Quinidine Sulfate 300 mg	Lin-Qin, Quinova by Roxane	00054-8735	Antiarrhythmic
5406 <> DANDAN	Tab, Green, Round, Scored	Reserpine 0.125 mg, Hydrochlorothiazide 25 mg	by Schein	00364-0354	Antihypertensive; Diuretic
54062	Tab, Round, 54-062	Propranolol HCl 60 mg	Inderal by Roxane		Antihypertensive
54063	Tab, White, Round, 54-063	Acetaminophen 325 mg	Tylenol by Roxane	00054-8014	Analgesic
5407 <> DANDAN	Tab, Green, Round, Scored	Reserpine 0.125 mg, Hydrochlorothiazide 50 mg	by Schein	00364-0355	Antihypertensive; Diuretic
54070	Tab, White, Round, Scored, 54 over 070	Flecainide Acetate 100 mg	Tambocor by Roxane	00054-0011	Antiarrhythmic
54072	Cap, Flesh & Green, White Print, Hard Gel	Hydroxyurea 500 mg	Hydrea by Roxane	00054-2247	Antineoplastic
54072	Cap, Flesh & Green, White Print, Hard Gel	Hydroxyurea 500 mg	Hydrea by Nat Pharmpak	55154-4930	Antineoplastic
54072	Cap, Flesh & Green, White Print, Hard Gel	Hydroxyurea 500 mg	Hydrea by Roxane	00054-8247	Antineoplastic
54076	Tab, Round, White, Scored	Sertraline HCl 25 mg	Zoloft by Roxane	00054-0022	Antidepressant
54080	Tab, White, Round	Prednisone 25 mg	Deltasone by Roxane		Steroid
54092	Tab, White, Round, Scored, 54 over 092	Prednisone 1 mg	Deltasone by Allscripts		Steroid
54092	Tab, White, Round, Scored, 54 over 092	Prednisone 1 mg	Deltasone by Roxane	00054-8739	Steroid
54092	Tab, White, Round, Scored, 54 over 092	Prednisone 1 mg	Deltasone by Pharmedix	53002-0483	Steroid
54092	Tab, White, Round, Scored, 54 over 092	Prednisone 1 mg	Deltasone by Nat Pharmpak	55154-4926	Steroid
54092	Tab, White, Round, Scored, 54 over 092	Prednisone 1 mg	Deltasone by Roxane	00054-8247	Steroid
54093	Tab, Orange, Oblong	Diflunisal 500 mg	Dolobid by Roxane	00054-4741	NSAID
54099	Tab, White, Round, 54-099	Amitriptyline HCl 50 mg	Elavil by Roxane	00054-8220	Antidepressant
540HD	Tab, White, Round	Metronidazole 500 mg	Flagyl by Halsey	Discontinued	Antibiotic
541 <> BP	Tab, Cap Shaped, Coated, Scored	Guaifenesin 1200 mg, Phenylephrine HCl 40 mg	Guaiphen-PD by Boca	64376-0541	Cold Remedy
541 <> C	Tab, White, Barrel Shaped	Cetirizine HCl 10 mg	Zyrtec by Caraco	57664-0541	Antihistamine
5410 <> 50	Tab, Pink, Oval	Fluconazole 50 mg	Diflucan by Ivax	00172-5410	Antifungal
54103	Tab, Round, 54-103	Bisacodyl 5 mg	Dulcolax by Roxane		Gastrointestinal
54104	Tab, Pink, Round, Speckled, 54/104	Fluconazole 100 mg	Diflucan by Roxane		Antifungal
54107	Tab, Beige, Round, Film Coated	Lithium Carbonate 300 mg	Lithobid by Roxane	00054-4288 00054-8288	Antipsychotic
5411 <> 100	Tab, Pink, Oval, Ivax Logo 100	Fluconazole 100 mg	Diflucan by Ivax	00172-5411	Antifungal
5411 <> ZM5	Tab, Pink, Cap-Shaped, Film-Coated	Zolpidem Tartrate 5 mg	Ambien by Prasco	66993-0715	Sedative/Hypnotic; C IV
54111	Tab, Off White, Round	Mefloquine HCl 200 mg	Lariam by Roxane	00054-0025	Antimalarial
5412 <> 150	Tab, Pink, Oval	Fluconazole 150 mg	Diflucan by Ivax	00172-5412	Antifungal
5413 <> 200	Tab, Pink, Oval, Ival Logo 200	Fluconazole 200 mg	Diflucan by Ivax	00172-5413	Antifungal
54140	Tab, White, Black Print, Round, Film Coated, 54 over 140	Diclofenac Sodium 25 mg	Voltaren by Roxane	00054-8223	NSAID
54142	Tab, White, Round, Scored, 54 over 142	Methadone HCl 10 mg	Dolophine by Roxane	00054-4571	Analgesic; C II
54142	Tab, White, Round, Scored	Methadone HCl 10 mg	Dolophine by Roxane	00054-8854	Analgesic; C II
54143	Tab, White, Round, 54-143	Amitriptyline HCl 100 mg	Elavil by Roxane		Antidepressant
54145	Cap, Red, Opaque	Ramipril	Altace by Roxane	00054-0108	Antihypertensive
54149	Tab, Round, White, Scored	Sertraline HCl 50 mg	Zoloft by Roxane	00054-0023	Antidepressant
54150	Tab, White, Cap Shaped	Flecainide Acetate 150 mg	Tambocor by Roxane	00054-0012	Antiarrhythmic
54162	Tab, White, Round, 54 over 162	Methadone HCl 5 mg	Dolophine by Roxane	00054-4218	Analgesic; C II
54163	Tab, White, Round, Scored, 54 over 163	Meperidine 100 mg	Demerol by Roxane	00054-8596	Analgesic; C II
54163	Tab, White, Round, Scored, 54 over 163	Meperidine 100 mg	Demerol by Roxane	00054-4596	Analgesic; C II
54169 <> 12	Tab, White, Hexagonal, 1 over 2	Haloperidol 0.5 mg	Haldol by Nat Pharmpak	55154-4923	Antipsychotic
54169 <> 12	Tab, White, Hexagonal, 1 over 2	Haloperidol 0.5 mg	Haldol by Murfreesboro	51129-1130	Antipsychotic

ID FRONT <> BACK	DESCRIPTION FRONT <> BACK	INGREDIENT & STRENGTH	BRAND (or Generic Equiv.) by FIRM	NDC#	CLASS; SCH.
54169 <> 12	Tab, White, Hexagonal, 1 over 2	Haloperidol 0.5 mg	Haldol by Roxane	00054-8342	Antipsychotic
54171	Tab, Peach, Oblong, Scored	Oxcarbazepine 600 mg	Trileptal by Roxane	00054-0099	Anticonvulsant
54179	Cap, Reddish Orange, 54-179	Chloral Hydrate 500 mg	Chloral Hydrate by Roxane	00054-8140	Sedative/Hypnotic; C IV
54180	Tab, Blue, Oval, 54-180	Naproxen 275 mg	Anaprox by Roxane	00054-8638	NSAID
54183	Tab, White, Round, 54-183	Prednisolone 5 mg	by Roxane		Steroid
54193	Tab, White, Oblong, Scored	Nevirapine 200 mg	Viramune by Roxane	00054-8647	Antiviral
54193	Tab, White, Oblong, Scored	Nevirapine 200 mg	Viramune by Roxane	00054-4647	Antiviral
54193	Tab, White, Oblong, Scored	Nevirapine 200 mg	Viramune by Boehringer Ingelheim	00597-0046	Antiviral
54193	Tab, White, Oblong, Scored	Nevirapine 200 mg	Viramune by Physician Total Care	54868-3844	Antiviral
54193	Tab, White, Oblong, Scored	Nevirapine 200 mg	Viramune by Boehringer Ingelheim Canada	Canadian DIN 02238748	Antiviral
54196; <> 4	Tab, White to Off-White, Round	Hydromorphone HCl 4 mg	Dilaudid by Roxane	00054-0264	Analgesic; C II
54199	Tab, Light Blue, Round, Scored	Oxycodone HCl 30 mg	Roxicodone by Roxane	00054-4665	Analgesic; C II
				00054-8665	
542 <> BP	Tab, Red Speckled, Cap Shaped	Guaifenesin 1200 mg, Dextromethorphan HBr 60 mg	Tussi-Bid by Boca	64376-0542	Cold Remedy
5420 <> 05	Tab, White, Oval, Scored, Hourglass Logo 0.5	Cabergoline 0.5 mg	Dostinex by Teva	00093-5420	Antiparkinson
54200	Tab, Pink, Round, Speckled, 54/200	Fluconazole 150 mg	Diflucan by Roxane	00054-8289	Antifungal
54201	Tab, Yellow, Round, Scored, Film Coated	Mirtazapine 15 mg	Remeron by Roxane	00054-4676	Antidepressant
54201	Tab, Yellow, Round, Scored, Film Coated	Mirtazapine 15 mg	Remeron by Roxane	00054-8676	Antidepressant
5421 <> AMB10	Tab, White, Cap Shaped, Film Coated	Zolpidem Tartrate 10 mg	Ambien by Sanofi	00024-5421	Sedative/Hypnotic; C IV
5421 <> AMB10	Tab, White, Cap Shaped, Film Coated	Zolpidem Tartrate 10 mg	Ambien by Searle	00025-5421	Sedative/Hypnotic; C IV
5421 <> AMB10	Tab, White, Cap Shaped, Film Coated	Zolpidem Tartrate 10 mg	Ambien by Caremark	00339-4065	Sedative/Hypnotic; C IV
5421 <> AMB10	Tab, White, Cap Shaped, Film Coated	Zolpidem Tartrate 10 mg	Ambien by H J Harkins Co	52959-0363	Sedative/Hypnotic; C IV
5421 <> AMB10	Tab, White, Cap Shaped, Film Coated	Zolpidem Tartrate 10 mg	Ambien by PDRX	55289-0792	Sedative/Hypnotic; C IV
54210	Tab, White, Round, Scored, 54 over 210	Methadone HCl 5 mg	Dolophine by Roxane	00054-4570	Analgesic; C II
54210	Tab, White, Round, Scored	Methadone HCl 5 mg	Dolophine by Roxane	00054-8554	Analgesic; C II
54212	Tab, White, Round, 54-212	Neomycin Sulfate 500 mg	by Roxane	00054-8600	Antibiotic
54213	Cap, White, Black Print, Opaque, Hard Gel	Lithium Carbonate 150 mg	Eskalith by Roxane	00054-8526	Antipsychotic
54213	Cap, White, Black Print, Opaque, Hard Gel	Lithium Carbonate 150 mg	Eskalith by Roxane	00054-2526	Antipsychotic
5422 <> ZM10	Tab, White, Cap-Shaped, Film-Coated	Zolpidem Tartrate 10 mg	Ambien by Prasco	66993-0716	Sedative/Hypnotic; C IV
54223	Cap, Pink, 54-223	Diphenhydramine HCl 50 mg	Benadryl by Roxane		Antihistamine
54231	Tab, Orange to Speckled Orange, Round	Ropinirole HCl 2 mg	Requip by Roxane	00054-0119	Antiparkinson
54233	Tab, White, Round	Amlodipine Besylate 10 mg	Norvasc by Roxane	00054-0102	Antihypertensive
54249	Tab, White, Round, 54-249	Propranolol HCl 80 mg	Inderal by Roxane		Antihypertensive
54251	Tab, White, Round	Acarbose 100 mg	Precose by Roxane	00054-0142	Antidiabetic
54252	Tab, White, Round, 54-252	Acetaminophen 500 mg	Tylenol Ex Strength by Roxane	00054-8016	Analgesic
54253	Tab, White, Oblong	Sulfamethoxazole 400 mg, Trimethoprim 80 mg	Septra by Roxane		Antibiotic
54259	Tab, Red, Round, 54/259	Ferrous Sulfate 300 mg	by Roxane	00054-8284	Mineral
54262	Tab, White, Round, Scored, 54 over 262	Morphine Sulfate 30 mg	MSIR by Roxane	00054-8583	Analgesic; C II
54262	Tab, White, Round, Scored	Morphine Sulfate 30 mg	MSIR by Roxane	00054-4583	Analgesic; C II
54263	Tab, White, Round, 54-263	Phenobarbital 100 mg	Phenobarbital by Roxane	00054-8707	Sedative/Hypnotic; C IV
54271	Tab, White, Round, Film Coated	Clarithromycin 250 mg	Biaxin by Roxane	00054-0037	Antibiotic
54273	Tab, Brown to Speckled Brown, Round	Ropinirole 4 mg	Requip by Roxane	00054-0121	Antiparkinson
5428 <> DAN	Tab, Light Yellow, Round	Reserpine 0.1 mg, Hydralazine HCl 25 mg, Hydrochlorothiazide 15 mg	by Schein	00364-0361	Antihypertensive; Diuretic
54280	Tab, White, Round, 54 over 280	Dihydrotachysterol 0.125 mg	DHT by Roxane	00054-4190	Vitamin
54284	Tab, Yellow, Capsule Shaped, Film Coated	Levetiracetam 500 mg	Keppra by Roxane	00054-0151	Anticonvulsant
54293	Tab, Off-White, Round, Scored, 54 over 293	Leucovorin Calcium 5 mg	Wellcovorin by Roxane	00054-8496	Antineoplastic
54293	Tab, Off-White, Round, Scored, 54 over 293	Leucovorin Calcium 5 mg	Wellcovorin by Roxane	00054-4496	Antineoplastic

ID FRONT <> BACK	DESCRIPTION FRONT <> BACK	INGREDIENT & STRENGTH	BRAND (or Generic Equiv.) by FIRM	NDC#	CLASS; SCH.
54299	Tab, Light Yellow, Round, Scored, 54 over 299	Dexamethasone 0.5 mg	Decadron by Roxane	00054-4179	Steroid
54299	Tab, Light Yellow, Round, Scored, 54 over 299	Dexamethasone 0.5 mg	Decadron by Roxane	00054-8179	Steroid
543 <> 80	Tab, Brick Red, Cap Shaped, Film Coated	Simvastatin 80 mg	Zocor by Merck-Frosst	Canadian DIN 02240332	Antihyperlipidemic
543 <> 80	Tab, Brick Red, Cap Shaped, Film Coated	Simvastatin 80 mg	Zocor by Merck	00006-0543	Antihyperlipidemic
543 <> DP	Tab, White, Round, Film Coated	Ethinyl Estradiol 0.03 mg, Norgestrel 0.3 mg	Lo Ovral by Barr	51285-0546	Oral Contraceptive
543 <> DP	Tab, White, Round, Film Coated	Ethinyl Estradiol 0.03 mg, Norgestrel 0.3 mg	Lo Ovral by Barr	00555-9049	Oral Contraceptive
5430 <> DANDAN	Tab, White, Round, Scored	Acetazolamide 250 mg	Diamox by Compumed	00403-0058	Antiglaucoma Agent
5430 <> DANDAN	Tab, White, Round, Scored	Acetazolamide 250 mg	Diamox by Amerisource	62584-0043	Antiglaucoma Agent
5430 <> DANDAN	Tab, White, Round, Scored	Acetazolamide 250 mg	Diamox by Schein	00364-0400	Antiglaucoma Agent
5430 <> DANDAN	Tab, White, Round, Scored	Acetazolamide 250 mg	Diamox by Watson	00591-5430	Antiglaucoma Agent
54302	Tab, White, Cap Shaped, Scored, Film Coated	Calcium Carbonate 1250 mg	Os-Cal by Roxane	00054-8120	Vitamin; Mineral
54302	Tab, White, Cap Shaped, Scored	Calcium Carbonate 1250 mg	Os-Cal by Roxane	00054-4120	Vitamin; Mineral
54303	Tab, White, Black Print, Round, Film Coated, 54 over 303	Propantheline Bromide 15 mg	Pro-Banthine by Roxane	00054-8737	Gastrointestinal
54303	Tab, White, Black Print, Round, Film Coated, 54 over 303	Propantheline Bromide 15 mg	Pro-Banthine by Kaiser	00179-0627	Gastrointestinal
54303	Tab, White, Black Print, Round, Film Coated, 54 over 303	Propantheline Bromide 15 mg	Pro-Banthine by Roxane	00054-4721	Gastrointestinal
54306	Tab, White, Round	Protriptyline HCl 5 mg	Vivactil by Roxane	00054-0210	Antidepressant
54311	Tab, White, Round	Acarbose 25 mg	Precose by Roxane	00054-0140	Antidiabetic
54312	Tab, White, Capsule Shaped, Film Coated	Clarithromycin 500 mg	Biaxin by Roxane	00054-0037	Antibiotic
54323	Tab, Yellow, Round, Scored, 54 over 323	Methotrexate 2.5 mg	Rheumatrex by Roxane	00054-4550	Antineoplastic
54323	Tab, Yellow, Round, Scored, 54 over 323	Methotrexate 2.5 mg	Rheumatrex by Roxane	00054-8550	Antineoplastic
54328	Cap, Yellow, Opaque	Ramipril 1.25 mg	Altace by Roxane	00054-0106	Antihypertensive
54329	Cap, Green, 54-329	Indomethacin 50 mg	Indocin by Roxane		NSAID
54331	Tab, Peach, Round, Scored	Oxcarbazepine 150 mg	Trileptal by Roxane	00054-0097	Anticonvulsant
54333	Tab, White, Round, 54-333	Propranolol HCl 40 mg	Inderal by Roxane		Antihypertensive
54334	Tab, Pink, Round, Speckled, 54/334	Fluconazole 200 mg	Diflucan by Roxane	00054-4290 00054-8290	Antifungal
54337	Tab, Yellow, Round	Ropinirole 0.5 mg	Requip by Roxane	00054-0117	Antiparkinson
54339	Tab, White, Round, Scored, 54 over 339	Prednisone 2.5 mg	Deltasone by Roxane	00054-4742	Steroid
54339	Tab, White, Round, Scored, 54 over 339	Prednisone 2.5 mg	Deltasone by Roxane	00054-8740	Steroid
54339	Tab, White, Round, Scored, 54 over 339	Prednisone 2.5 mg	Deltasone by Nat Pharmpak	55154-4918	Steroid
54343	Tab, White, Round, Scored, 54 over 343	Prednisone 50 mg	Deltasone by DRX	55045-1928	Steroid
54343	Tab, White, Round, Scored, 54 over 343	Prednisone 50 mg	Deltasone by Qualitest	00603-5022	Steroid
54343	Tab, White, Round, Scored, 54 over 343	Prednisone 50 mg	Deltasone by Roxane	00054-4733	Steroid
54343	Tab, White, Round, Scored	Prednisone 50 mg	Deltasone by Roxane	00054-8729	Steroid
54343	Tab, White, Round, Scored	Prednisone 50 mg	Deltasone by Roxane	00054-0019	Steroid
54346	Tab, White, Round, Scored, Extended Release	Lithium Carbonate 450 mg	Eskalith CR by Roxane	00054-0020	Antipsychotic
54352	Tab, White, Round, Scored, 54 over 352	Megestrol Acetate 40 mg	Megace by Roxane	00054-4604	Hormone
54352	Tab, White, Round, Scored, 54 over 352	Megestrol Acetate 40 mg	Megace by Roxane	00054-8604	Hormone
54353	Tab, Round, Beige, Film Coated	Mirtazapine 30 mg	Remeron by Roxane	00054-4677	Antidepressant
54353	Tab, Round, Beige, Film Coated	Mirtazapine 30 mg	Remeron by Roxane	00054-8677	Antidepressant
54360	Tab, White, Round, 54-360	Amitriptyline HCl 75 mg	Elavil by Roxane		Antidepressant
54369	Cap	Loperamide 2 mg	Imodium by Nat Pharmpak	55154-4912	Antidiarrheal
54369	Cap	Loperamide 2 mg	Imodium by Roxane	00054-8537	Antidiarrheal
54371	Tab, Pink, Round, Film Coated	Zolpidem Tartrate 5 mg	Ambien by Roxane	00054-0086	Sedative/Hypnotic; C IV
54372	Tab, White, Cap Shaped	Calcium Gluconate 500 mg	Caltrate by Roxane	00054-8121	Vitamin; Mineral
54372	Tab, White to Off White, Capsule Shaped	Calcium Gluconate 500 mg	Caltrate by Roxane	00054-0262	Vitamin; Mineral
54372	Tab, White, Cap Shaped	Calcium Gluconate 500 mg	Caltrate by Roxane	00054-4121	Vitamin; Mineral
5438 <> DANDAN	Tab, White, Round, Scored	Quinidine Sulfate 200 mg	Quinidine Sulfate by Schein	00364-0229	Antiarrhythmic
5438 <> DANDAN	Tab, White, Round, Scored	Quinidine Sulfate 200 mg	Quinidine Sulfate by Watson	00591-5438	Antiarrhythmic

ID FRONT <> BACK	DESCRIPTION FRONT <> BACK	INGREDIENT & STRENGTH	BRAND (or Generic Equiv.) by FIRM	NDC#	CLASS; SCH.
5438 <> DANDAN	Tab, White, Round, Scored	Quinidine Sulfate 200 mg	Quinidine Sulfate by Heartland	61392-0953	Antiarrhythmic
54382 <> 10	Tab, White, Hexagonal, Scored, 54 over 382	Haloperidol 10 mg	Haldol by Roxane	00054-4346	Antipsychotic
				Discontinued	
54383	Tab, Beige, Round, 54-383	Methyldopa 500 mg	Aldomet by Roxane		Antihypertensive
54392	Cap, Red & White, Black Print, Opaque	Oxycodone 5 mg, Acetaminophen 500 mg	Tylox by Roxane	00054-2795	Analgesic; C II
543HD	Tab, White, Round	Acetaminophen 325 mg, Butalbital 50 mg, Caffeine 40 mg	Fioricet by Halsey	Discontinued	Analgesic
54403	Tab, Off-White, Round, Scored, 54 over 403	Hydromorphone HCl 8 mg	Dilaudid by Roxane	00054-4370	Analgesic; C II
54409 <> 30	Tab, White, Round	Morphine Sulfate SR 30 mg	Oramorph by Roxane	00054-8805	Analgesic; C II
				00054-4805	
54410	Tab, White, Round, Scored	Levorphanol Tartrate 2 mg	Levo-Dromoran by Roxane	00054-8494	Analgesic; C II
54410	Tab, White, Round, Scored	Levorphanol Tartrate 2 mg	Levo-Dromoran by Roxane	00054-4494	Analgesic; CII
54412	Tab, White, Round, Scored	Codeine Sulfate 60 mg	by Roxane	00054-4157	Analgesic; CII
54412	Tab, White, Round, Scored	Codeine Sulfate 60 mg	by Roxane	00054-8157	Analgesic; C II
54413	Tab, White, Oblong, 54-413	Aluminum Hydroxide 500 mg	Amphojel by Roxane		Gastrointestinal
5442 <> DANDAN	Tab, White, Round, Scored	Prednisone 10 mg	Deltasone by Med Pro	53978-3037	Steroid
5442 <> DANDAN	Tab, White, Round, Scored	Prednisone 10 mg	Deltasone by Nat Pharmpak	55154-5215	Steroid
5442 <> DANDAN	Tab, White, Round, Scored	Prednisone 10 mg	Deltasone by Watson	00591-5442	Steroid
5442 <> DANDAN	Tab, White, Round, Scored	Prednisone 10 mg	Deltasone by Schein	00364-0461	Steroid
5442 <> DANDAN	Tab, White, Round, Scored	Prednisone 10 mg	Deltasone by Danbury	61955-0461	Steroid
5442 <> DANDAN	Tab, White, Round, Scored	Prednisone 10 mg	Deltasone by Heartland	61392-0417	Steroid
5442 <> DANDAN	Tab, White, Round, Scored	Prednisone 10 mg	Deltasone by Merz	00259-0364	Steroid
5442 <> DANDAN	Tab, White, Round, Scored	Prednisone 10 mg	Deltasone by Amerisource	62584-0833	Steroid
54420	Tab, Light Yellow	Mercaptopurine 50 mg	Purinethol by Roxane	00054-4581	Antineoplastic
54422	Cap, 54-422	Indomethacin 25 mg	Indocin by Roxane		NSAID
54425	Tab, White to Off-White, Round	Hydromorphone HCl 8 mg	Dilaudid by Roxane	00054-0265	Analgesic; C II
5443 <> DANDAN	Tab, Peach, Round, Scored	Prednisone 20 mg	Deltasone by Qualitest	00603-2551	Steroid
5443 <> DANDAN	Tab, Peach, Round, Scored	Prednisone 20 mg	Deltasone by Vangard	00615-1542	Steroid
5443 <> DANDAN	Tab, Peach, Round, Scored	Prednisone 20 mg	Deltasone by H J Harkins Co	52959-0127	Steroid
5443 <> DANDAN	Tab, Peach, Round, Scored	Prednisone 20 mg	Deltasone by Watson	00591-5443	Steroid
5443 <> DANDAN	Tab, Peach, Round, Scored	Prednisone 20 mg	Deltasone by Schein	00364-0442	Steroid
5443 <> DANDAN	Tab, Peach, Round, Scored	Prednisone 20 mg	Deltasone by WA Butler	11695-1802	Steroid
5443 <> DANDAN	Tab, Peach, Round, Scored	Prednisone 20 mg	Deltasone by Vedco	50989-0602	Steroid
5443 <> DANDAN	Tab, Peach, Round, Scored	Prednisone 20 mg	Deltasone by Danbury	61955-0442	Steroid
5444 <> DAN	Tab, White, Round, Scored	Chlorothiazide 250 mg	Diuril by Schein	00364-0389	Diuretic; Antihypertensive
54452	Tab, White, Round, Scored, 54 over 452	Lithium Carbonate 300 mg	Eskalith by Roxane	00054-8528	Antipsychotic
54452	Tab, White, Round, Scored, 54 over 452	Lithium Carbonate 300 mg	Eskalith by Roxane	00054-4527	Antipsychotic
54460	Tab, Green, Oval	Cimetidine HCl 800 mg	Tagamet by Roxane	00054-8226	Gastrointestinal
54463	Cap, Flesh, Black Print, Opaque, Hard Gel	Lithium Carbonate 300 mg	Eskalith by Roxane	00054-8527	Antipsychotic
54463	Cap, Flesh, Black Print, Opaque, Hard Gel	Lithium Carbonate 300 mg	Eskalith by Direct Dispensing	57866-6523	Antipsychotic
54463	Cap, Flesh, Black Print, Opaque, Hard Gel	Lithium Carbonate 300 mg	Eskalith by Heartland	61392-0131	Antipsychotic
54463	Cap, Flesh, Black Print, Opaque, Hard Gel	Lithium Carbonate 300 mg	Eskalith by Med Pro	53978-0523	Antipsychotic
54463	Cap, Flesh, Black Print, Opaque, Hard Gel	Lithium Carbonate 300 mg	Eskalith by Nat Pharmpak	55154-4920	Antipsychotic
54463	Cap, Flesh, Black Print, Opaque, Hard Gel	Lithium Carbonate 300 mg	Eskalith by Mylan	00378-1912	Antipsychotic
54463	Cap, Flesh, Black Print, Opaque, Hard Gel	Lithium Carbonate 300 mg	Eskalith by Roxane	00054-2527	Antipsychotic
54470	Tab, White, Capsule Shaped, Film Coated	Levetiracetam 1000 mg	Keppra by Roxane	00054-0257	Anticonvulsant
54472	Cap, Blue, 54-472	Piroxicam 10 mg	Feldene by Roxane	00054-8660	NSAID
54479	Cap, Blue, 54-479	Piroxicam 20 mg	Feldene by Roxane	00054-8661	NSAID
54482	Tab, White, Round, 54 over 482	Tamoxifen Citrate 20 mg	Nolvadex by Roxane	00054-4834	Antiestrogen
54482	Tab, White, Round, 54 over 482	Tamoxifen Citrate 20 mg	Nolvadex by Roxane	00054-8834	Antiestrogen
54486	Tab, Round, White, Scored	Sertraline HCl 100 mg	Zoloft by Roxane	00054-0024	Antidepressant

ID FRONT <> BACK	DESCRIPTION FRONT <> BACK	INGREDIENT & STRENGTH	BRAND (or Generic Equiv.) by FIRM	NDC#	CLASS; SCH.
54489	Tab, Yellow, Round, Scored	Dexamethasone 1 mg	Decadron by Roxane	00054-8174	Steroid
54489	Tab, Yellow, Round	Dexamethasone 1 mg	by Roxane	00054-4181	Steroid
5449 <> DAN025	Tab, Orange, Pentagonal, Scored, 5449 <> Dan 0.25	Dexamethasone 0.25 mg	Decadron by Schein	00364-0397	Steroid
54492	Tab, White, Round, 54-492	Amitriptyline HCl 150 mg	Elavil by Roxane		Antidepressant
54499	Tab, Peach, Round, 54-499	Hydrochlorothiazide 50 mg	Hydrodiuril by Roxane		Diuretic; Antihypertensive
544HD5	Tab, Yellow, Round	Diazepam 5 mg	Valium by Halsey	Discontinued	Antianxiety; C IV
545 <> BARR	Tab, Light Orange, Cap Shaped, Film Coated	Cephalexin 250 mg	by Barr	00555-0545	Antibiotic
				Discontinued	
545 <> R	Tab, Purepac Logo 545 <> R	Diflunisal 250 mg	by Actavis	00228-2545	NSAID
545 <> RDY	Tab, Peach, Round, Biconvex	Venlafaxine 25 mg	Effexor by Dr. Reddy's	55111-0545	Antidepressant
5450 <> 93	Tab, White, Round, Ex Release	Alprazolam 0.5 mg	Xanax XR by Teva	00093-5450	Antianxiety; C IV
5450 <> DAN050	Tab, Yellow, Pentagonal, Scored, Dan over 0.50	Dexamethasone 0.5 mg	by Schein	00364-0398	Steroid
54503	Tab, White, Round, 54-503	Phenobarbital 15 mg	Phenobarbital by Roxane	00054-8703	Sedative/Hypnotic; C IV
54511	Tab, Yellow, Round	Dextroamphetamine Sulfate 10 mg	Dexedrine by Richwood		Stimulant; C II
5451 <> 93	Tab, Yellow, Round, Ex Release	Alprazolam 1 mg	Xanax XR by Teva	00093-5451	Antianxiety; C IV
5451 <> DAN15	Tab, White, Pentagonal, Scored, 5451 <> Dan 1.5	Dexamethasone 1.5 mg	by Schein	00364-0399	Steroid
54511	Tab, White to Off White, Round	Ropinirole HCl .25 mg	Requip by Roxane	00054-0116	Antiparkinson
54512	Tab, White, Oval, 54/512	Alprazolam 1 mg	Xanax by Roxane	00054-8104	Antianxiety; C IV
54513	Tab, White, Round	Amlodipine Besylate 2.5 mg	Norvasc by Roxane	00054-0100	Antihypertensive
54515	Tab, Peach, Speckled, Round	Oxcarbazepine 300 mg	Trileptal by Roxane	00054-0098	Anticonvulsant
54519	Tab, White, Oval	Triazolam 0.125 mg	Halcion by Roxane	00054-4858	Sedative/Hypnotic; C IV
54519	Tab, White, Oval	Triazolam 0.125 mg	Halcion by Roxane	00054-8858	Sedative/Hypnotic; C IV
54522	Tab, Yellow, Round	Dextroamphetamine Sulfate 5 mg	Dexedrine by Richwood		Stimulant; C II
5452 <> 93	Tab, Blue, Oval, Ex Release	Alprazolam 2 mg	Xanax XR by Teva	00093-5452	Antianxiety; C IV
54521	Tab, White, Round	Cilostazol 50 mg	Pletal by Roxane	00054-0028	Antiplatelet
54523	Cap, Brown & Red, White Print, Hard Gel	Mexiletine 150 mg	Mexitil by Roxane	00054-2616	Antiarrhythmic
54523	Cap, Brown & Red, White Print, Hard Gel	Mexiletine 150 mg	Mexitil by Ridgebury	60921-0066	Antiarrhythmic
5453 <> 93	Tab, Green, Round, Ex Release	Alprazolam 3 mg	Xanax XR by Teva	00093-5453	Antianxiety; C IV
54532	Tab, White, Round, Scored, 54 over 532	Pseudoephedrine 60 mg	Sudafed by Roxane	00054-4744	Decongestant
54532	Tab, White, Round, Scored, 54 over 532	Pseudoephedrine 60 mg	Sudafed by Roxane	00054-8744	Decongestant
54533	Tab, White, Round, Scored, 54 over 533	Furosemide 80 mg	Lasix by Roxane	00054-4301	Diuretic
54533	Tab, White, Round, Scored, 54 over 533	Furosemide 80 mg	Lasix by Med Pro	53978-0927	Diuretic
54533	Tab, White, Round, Scored, 54 over 533	Furosemide 80 mg	Lasix by Nat Pharmpak	55154-4909	Diuretic
54533	Tab, White, Round, Scored, 54 over 533	Furosemide 80 mg	Lasix by Roxane	00054-8301	Diuretic
5454 <> DANDAN	Tab, White, Round, Scored	Quinidine Sulfate 300 mg	Quinidine Sulfate by Watson	00591-5454	Antiarrhythmic
5454 <> DANDAN	Tab, White, Round, Scored	Quinidine Sulfate 300 mg	Quinidine Sulfate by Schein	00364-0582	Antiarrhythmic
54543	Tab, White, Round, Scored, 54 over 543	Oxycodone HCl 5 mg, Acetaminophen 325 mg	Percocet by Boehringer Ingelheim	Canadian	Analgesic; C II
54543	Tab, White, Round, Scored, 54 over 543	Oxycodone HCl 5 mg, Acetaminophen 325 mg	Percocet by Roxane	00054-4650	Analgesic; C II
54543	Tab, White, Round, Scored, 54 over 543	Oxycodone HCl 5 mg, Acetaminophen 325 mg	Percocet by Roxane	00054-8650	Analgesic; C II
54549	Tab, White, Round, Scored, 54 over 549	Methadone HCl 10 mg	Dolophine by Roxane	00054-4219	Analgesic; C II
54555	Tab, Pink, Round	Methamphetamine HCl 5 mg	Desoxyn by Richwood		Stimulant; C II
5455 <> DANDAN	Tab, Blue, Tab, Blue, Round, Scored	Chlorpropamide 250 mg	by Schein	00364-0510	Antidiabetic
54552	Tab, White, Round	Clotrimazole Troche 10 mg	Mycelex by Roxane	00054-4146	Antifungal
54553	Tab, White, Round, Film Coated	Zolpidem Tartrate 10 mg	Ambien by Roxane	00054-0087	Sedative/Hypnotic; C IV
54566	Tab, Pink, Round	Methamphetamine HCl 10 mg	Desoxyn by Richwood		Stimulant; C II
54577	Tab, Green, Round	Phendimetrazine Tartrate 35 mg	X-Trozine by Richwood		Anorexiant; C III
54570 <> 2	Tab, White, Hexagonal, Scored, 54 over 570	Haloperidol 2 mg	Haldol by Roxane	00054-8344	Antipsychotic
54572	Tab, White, Round, 54-572	Phenobarbital 30 mg	by Roxane	00054-8705	Sedative/Hypnotic; C IV

ID FRONT <> BACK	DESCRIPTION FRONT <> BACK	INGREDIENT & STRENGTH	BRAND (or Generic Equiv.) by FIRM	NDC#	CLASS; SCH.
54575	Tab, Red to Speckled Red, Round	Ropinirole HCl 3 mg	Requip by Roxane	00054-0120	Antiparkinson
54582	Tab, White, Round, Scored	Oxycodone HCl 5 mg	Roxicodone by Roxane	00054-8657	Analgesic; C II
				00054-4657	
54583	Tab, White, Round, Scored, 54 over 583	Furosemide 40 mg	Lasix by Roxane	00054-8299	Diuretic
54583	Tab, White, Round, Scored, 54 over 583	Furosemide 40 mg	Lasix by Nat Pharmpak	55154-4908	Diuretic
54583	Tab, White, Round, Scored, 54 over 583	Furosemide 40 mg	Lasix by Med Pro	53978-5032	Diuretic
54583	Tab, White, Round, Scored, 54 over 583	Furosemide 40 mg	Lasix by Roxane	00054-4299	Diuretic
54583	Tab, White, Round, Scored, 54 over 583	Furosemide 40 mg	Lasix by JB	51111-0481	Diuretic
54592	Tab, White, Black Print, Round, Film Coated, 54 over 592	Diclofenac Sodium 50 mg	Voltaren by Roxane	00054-8221	NSAID
54592	Tab, White, Black Print, Round, Film Coated, 54 over 592	Diclofenac Sodium 50 mg	Voltaren by Roxane	00054-4221	NSAID
54599	Tab, White, Oval, 54-599	Alprazolam 0.5 mg	Xanax by Roxane	00054-8105	Antianxiety; C IV
545BARR	Cap	Cephalexin	by Warner Chilcott	00047-0938	Antibiotic
546 <> PA	Tab, White, Round, Enteric Coated	Diclofenac Sodium 50 mg	Voltaren by Pliva	50111-0546	NSAID
546 <> RDY	Tab, Peach, Round, Biconvex	Venlafaxine 37.5 mg	Effexor by Dr. Reddy's		Antidepressant
54601	Tab, Yellow, Round	Phendimetrazine Tartrate 35 mg	Plegine by Richwood	55111-0546	Anorexiant; C III
54602	Cap, Blue, Opaque	Ramipril 10 mg	Altace by Roxane	00054-0109	Antihypertensive
54603	Tab, Blue, Oblong, 54-603	Naproxen 550 mg	Anaprox by Roxane	00054-8639	NSAID
54609 <> 4	Tab, White, Round, Scored, 54 over 609	Hydromorphone HCl 4 mg	Dilaudid by Roxane	00054-8394	Analgesic; C II
54609 <> 4	Tab, White, Round, Scored, 54 over 609	Hydromorphone HCl 4 mg	Dilaudid by Roxane	00054-4394	Analgesic; C II
54612	Tab, White, Round, Scored, 54 over 612	Prednisone 5 mg	Deltasone by Roxane	00054-4728	Steroid
54612	Tab, White, Round, Scored, 54 over 612	Prednisone 5 mg	Deltasone by Southwood	58016-0218	Steroid
54612	Tab, White, Round, Scored, 54 over 612	Prednisone 5 mg	Deltasone by Roxane	00054-8724	Steroid
54612	Tab, White, Round, Scored, 54 over 612	Prednisone 5 mg	Deltasone by Kaiser	00179-0610	Steroid
54612	Tab, White, Round, Scored, 54 over 612	Prednisone 5 mg	Deltasone by Caremark	00339-5292	Steroid
54612	Tab, White, Round, Scored, 54 over 612	Prednisone 5 mg	Deltasone by Med Pro	53978-0060	Steroid
54612	Tab, White, Round, Scored, 54 over 612	Prednisone 5 mg	Deltasone by Murfreesboro	51129-1307	Steroid
54613	Tab, White, Round, Scored	Codeine Sulfate 15 mg	by Roxane	00054-8155	Analgesic; C II
54462	Cap, Brown & Clear	Phendimetrazine Tartrate 105 mg	X-Trozine LA-105 by Richwood		Anorexiant; C III
54620	Tab, Light Blue, Oval, Scored, 54 over 620	Triazolam 0.25 mg	Halcion by Roxane	00054-4859	Sedative/Hypnotic; C IV
54620	Tab, Light Blue, Oval, Scored, 54 over 620	Triazolam 0.25 mg	Halcion by Roxane	00054-8859	Sedative/Hypnotic; C IV
54622	Tab, Beige, Round	Methyldopa 250 mg	Aldomet by Roxane		Antihypertensive
546233	Tab, White, Round, Scored, 54/623 3	Acetaminophen 300 mg, Codeine Phosphate 30 mg	Tylenol w/ Codeine by Roxane	00054-8022	Analgesic; C III
54623	Cap, Blue	Phendimetrazine Tartrate 35 mg	X-Trozine by Richwood		Anorexiant; C III
54632	Cap, Red, White Print, Hard Gel	Mexiletine 200 mg	Mexitil by Ridgebury	60921-0067	Antiarrhythmic
54632	Cap, Red, White Print, Hard Gel	Mexiletine 200 mg	Mexitil by Roxane	00054-2617	Antiarrhythmic
54636	Tab, Light Beige, Capsule Shaped, Film Coated	Levetiracetam 750 mg	Keppra by Roxane	00054-0152	Anticonvulsant
54639	Tab, Light Blue, Round, 54 over 639	Cyclophosphamide 25 mg	Cytoxan by Roxane	00054-8089	Antineoplastic
54639	Tab, Light Blue, Round, 54 over 639	Cyclophosphamide 25 mg	Cytoxan by Roxane	00054-4129	Antineoplastic
54643	Tab	Naprosyn 250 mg	Naprosyn by Nat Pharmpak	55154-5907	NSAID
54647	Tab, White, Round, Film Coated	Pilocarpine HCl 5 mg	Salagen by Roxane	00054-0056	Cholinergic Agonist
54650	Tab, Yellow, Round, Scored	Leucovorin Calcium 15 mg	Wellcovorin by Roxane	00054-4498	Antineoplastic
54650	Tab, Yellow, Round, Scored	Leucovorin Calcium 15 mg	Wellcovorin by Roxane	00054-8498	Antineoplastic
54656	Cap, Light Green, Opaque	Zaleplon 5 mg	Sonata by Roxane	00054-0084	Hypnotic
54662	Tab, White, Round, Scored, 54 over 662	Dexamethasone 2 mg	Decadron by Nat Pharmpak	55154-4914	Steroid
54662	Tab, White, Round, Scored, 54 over 662	Dexamethasone 2 mg	Decadron by DRX	55045-2605	Steroid
54662	Tab, White, Round, Scored	Dexamethasone 2 mg	Decadron by Roxane	00054-8176	Steroid
54662	Tab, White, Round, Scored	Dexamethasone 2 mg	Decadron by Roxane	00054-4183	Steroid
5468	Cap, Black	Phentermine HCl 30 mg	Oby-Trim 30 by Richwood		Anorexiant; C IV

ID FRONT <> BACK	DESCRIPTION FRONT <> BACK	INGREDIENT & STRENGTH	BRAND (or Generic Equiv.) by FIRM	NDC#	CLASS; SCH.
54680	Tab, White, Round	Vitamin C 500 mg	by Roxane		Vitamin
54690 <> 20	Tab, White, Hexagonal, Scored, 54 over 690	Haloperidol 20 mg	Haldol by Roxane	00054-8347	Antipsychotic
54694	Tab, White, Round	Protriptyline HCl 10 mg	Vivactil by Roxane	00054-0211	Antidepressant
546HD2	Tab, White, Round	Diazepam 2 mg	Valium by Halsey	Discontinued	Antianxiety; C IV
547	Cap, Yellow, Oval	Calcitriol 0.25 mcg	by Roxane	00054-0007	Vitamin; Mineral
547 <> PA	Tab, White, Round, Enteric Coated	Diclofenac Sodium 75 mg	Voltaren by Pliva	50111-0547	NSAID
547 <> RDY	Tab, Peach, Round, Biconvex	Venlafaxine 50 mg	Effexor by Dr. Reddy's	55111-0547	Antidepressant
54702	Cap, Flesh & White, Black Print, Opaque, Hard Gel	Lithium Carbonate 600 mg	Eskalith by Roxane	00054-8531	Antipsychotic
54702	Cap, Flesh & White, Black Print, Opaque, Hard Gel	Lithium Carbonate 600 mg	Eskalith by Roxane	00054-2531	Antipsychotic
54703	Tab, Coral, Round, 54-703	Imipramine HCl 50 mg	Tofranil by Roxane		Antidepressant
54710	Tab, Green, Round, Scored	Oxycodone HCl 15 mg	Roxicodone by Roxane	00054-4658 00054-8658	Analgesic; C II
54715	Tab, White, Round, Scored	Perindopril Erbumine 8 mg	ACEON by Roxane	00054-0112	Antihypertensive
54722	Tab, Blue to Speckled Blue, Round	Ropinirole 5 mg	Requip by Roxane	00054-0122	Antiparkinson
54730	Tab, White, Cap Shaped, Scored, 54 730	Oxycodone HCl 5 mg, Acetaminophen 500 mg	Roxicet by Roxane	00054-4784	Analgesic; C II
54732	Tab, White, Round, 54-732	Atropine Sulfate 0.025 mg, Diphenoxylate HCl 2.5 mg	Lomotil by Roxane		Antidiarrheal; C V
54733	Tab, White, Round, Scored, 54 over 733	Morphine Sulfate 15 mg	MSIR by Physician Total Care	54868-3191	Analgesic; C II
54733	Tab, White, Round, Scored, 54 over 733	Morphine Sulfate 15 mg	MSIR by Roxane	00054-4582	Analgesic; C II
54733	Tab, White, Round, Scored	Morphine Sulfate 15 mg	MSIR by Roxane	00054-8582	Analgesic; C II
54733	Tab, White, Round	Morphine Sulfate 15 mg	by Roxane	00054-0235	Analgesic; CII
54737	Tab, White, Round	Acarbose 50 mg	Precose by Roxane	00054-0141	Antidiabetic
54743 <> 2	Tab, White, Round, Scored, 54 over 743	Hydromorphone HCl 2 mg	Dilaudid by Roxane	00054-8392 00054-4392	Analgesic; C II
54744	Tab, White, Round	Terbinafine HCl 250 mg	Lamisil by Roxane	00054-0065	Antifungal
54749	Tab, Speckled Peach, Oval	Nefazodone HCl 150 mg	Serzone by Roxane	00054-4673	Antidepressant
54751	Tab, Green, Round	Ropinirole HCl 1 mg	Requip by Roxane	00054-0118	Antiparkinson
54757	Tab, White, Round	Cilostazol 100 mg	Pletal by Roxane	00054-0044	Antiplatelet
54760	Tab, White, Round, Scored, 54 over 760	Prednisone 20 mg	Deltasone by Roxane	00054-4729	Steroid
54760	Tab, White, Round, Scored, 54 over 760	Prednisone 20 mg	Deltasone by PDRX	55289-0352	Steroid
54760	Tab, White, Round, Scored, 54 over 760	Prednisone 20 mg	Deltasone by Med Pro	53978-0084	Steroid
54760	Tab, White, Round, Scored, 54 over 760	Prednisone 20 mg	Deltasone by Nat Pharmpak	55154-4905	Steroid
54760	Tab, White, Round, Scored	Prednisone 20 mg	Deltasone by Roxane	00054-8726	Steroid
54763	Tab, White, Round, Scored, 54 over 763	Megestrol Acetate 20 mg	Megace by Roxane	00054-4603	Hormone
54763	Tab, White, Round, Scored, 54 over 763	Megestrol Acetate 20 mg	Megace by Roxane	00054-8603	Hormone
54769	Tab, Aqua, Round, Scored	Dexamethasone 6 mg	Decadron by Roxane	00054-4186	Steroid
54769	Tab, Aqua, Round, Scored	Dexamethasone 6 mg	Decadron by Roxane	00054-4186	Steroid
54771	Tab, White, Round	Amlodipine Besylate 5 mg	Norvasc by Roxane	00054-0101	Antihypertensive
54772	Tab, White, Round, 54 over 772	Dihydrotachysterol 0.4 mg	DHT by Roxane	00054-4191	Vitamin
547735	Tab, White, Hexagonal, 54-773 5	Haloperidol 5 mg	Haldol by Roxane	00054-8345	Antipsychotic
54777	Tab, White, Round, Film Coated	Zidovudine 300 mg	Retrovir by Roxane	00054-0052	Antiviral
54779	Tab, White, Round, 54-779	Phenobarbital 60 mg	by Roxane	00054-8708	Sedative/Hypnotic; C IV
54780	Tab, White, Round, 54 over 780	Tamoxifen Citrate 10 mg	Nolvadex by Roxane	00054-8831	Antiestrogen
54780	Tab, White, Round, 54 over 780	Tamoxifen Citrate 10 mg	Nolvadex by Roxane	00054-4831	Antiestrogen
5478215	Tab, White, Round, Ex Release, 54/782 15	Morphine Sulfate 15 mg	Oramorph SR by Roxane	00054-4790 00054-8790	Analgesic; C II
54783	Tab, White, Round, Scored	Codeine Sulfate 30 mg	by Roxane	00054-8156	Analgesic; C II
54783	Tab, White, Round, Scored	Codeine Sulfate 30 mg	by Roxane	00054-4156	Analgesic; C II
54794	Cap, Orange, Opaque	Ramipril 2.5 mg	Altace by Roxane	00054-0107	Antihypertensive
54795	Cap, Light Orange, Opaque	Balsalazide Disodium 750 mg	Colazal by Roxane	00054-0079	Gastrointestinal

ID FRONT <> BACK	DESCRIPTION FRONT <> BACK	INGREDIENT & STRENGTH	BRAND (or Generic Equiv.) by FIRM	NDC#	CLASS; SCH.
54799	Tab	Cimetidine HCl 400 mg	Tagamet by Roxane	00054-8225	Gastrointestinal
5479DAN	Cap, Red & Ivory	Erythromycin Estolate 250 mg	by Schein	00364-0530	Antibiotic
548	Cap, Green & Tan	Hydroxyurea 500 mg	by Murfreesboro	51129-1469	Antineoplastic
548	Cap, Green & Tan	Hydroxyurea 500 mg	by URL Mutual	00677-1680	Antineoplastic
548	Cap, Green & Tan	Hydroxyurea 500 mg	by Qualitest	00603-3946	Antineoplastic
548 <> RDY	Tab, Peach, Round, Biconvex	Venlafaxine 75 mg	Effexor by Dr. Reddy's	55111-0548	Antidepressant
54810	Tab, White, Round, 54-810	Propranolol HCl 90 mg	Inderal by Roxane		Antihypertensive
54819	Tab, White, Oblong, 54-819	Acetaminophen 650 mg	Tylenol by Roxane	00054-8015	Analgesic
54820	Tab, 54 over 820	Ranitidine HCl 300 mg	Zantac by Eon	00185-0136	Gastrointestinal
54820	Tab, 54 over 820	Ranitidine HCl 336 mg	Zantac by Ridgebury	60921-0098	Gastrointestinal
54820	Tab, 54 over 820	Ranitidine HCl 336 mg	Zantac by Roxane	00054-4854	Gastrointestinal
54822	Tab, White, Oblong	Sulfamethoxazole 800 mg, Trimethoprim 160 mg	Septra DS by Roxane		Antibiotic
54823	Tab, White, Round, 54 over 823	Pseudoephedrine 30 mg	Sudafed by Roxane	00054-8743	Decongestant
54823	Tab, White, Round, 54 over 823	Pseudoephedrine 30 mg	Sudafed by Roxane	00054-4743	Decongestant
54839	Tab, White, Black Print, Round, Film Coated, 54 over 839	Diclofenac Sodium 75 mg	Voltaren by Roxane	00054-4222	NSAID
54839	Tab, White, Black Print, Round, Film Coated, 54 over 839	Diclofenac Sodium 75 mg	Voltaren by Roxane	00054-8222	NSAID
54839	Tab, White, Black Print, Round, Film Coated, 54 over 839	Diclofenac Sodium 75 mg	Voltaren by Murfreesboro	51129-1348	NSAID
54840	Tab, White, Round, 54 over 840	Furosemide 20 mg	Lasix by PDRX	55289-0593	Diuretic
54840	Tab, White, Round, 54 over 840	Furosemide 20 mg	Lasix by JB	51111-0484	Diuretic
54840	Tab, White, Round, 54 over 840	Furosemide 20 mg	Lasix by Murfreesboro	51129-1275	Diuretic
54840	Tab, White, Round, 54 over 840	Furosemide 20 mg	Lasix by Nat Pharmpak	55154-4906	Diuretic
54840	Tab, White, Round, 54 over 840	Furosemide 20 mg	Lasix by Med Pro	53978-5031	Diuretic
54840	Tab, White, Round, 54 over 840	Furosemide 20 mg	Lasix by Roxane	00054-8297	Diuretic
54840	Tab, White, Round, 54 over 840	Furosemide 20 mg	Lasix by Roxane	00054-4297	Diuretic
54843	Tab, White, Square with Rounded Corners, Scored, 54/843	Methadone HCl 40 mg	Dolophine by Roxane	00054-4547	Analgesic; C II
54853	Tab, Beige, Round, 54-853	Methyldopa 125 mg	Aldomet by Roxane		Antihypertensive
54859	Tab, White, Round, 54-859	Aminophylline 100 mg	Aminophylline by Roxane	00054-8025	Antiasthmatic
54860	Tab, White, Oval, 54-860	Alprazolam 1 mg	Xanax by Roxane	00054-8107	Antianxiety; C IV
54862 <> 100	Tab, White, Round	Morphine Sulfate SR 100 mg	Oramorph by Roxane	00054-8793	Analgesic; C II
				00054-4793	
54875	Tab, Blue, Round, Film Coated	Levetiracetam 250 mg	Keppra by Roxane	00054-0150	Anticonvulsant
54878	Tab, Blue, Round, Film Coated	Pilocarpine HCl 7.5 mg	Salagen by Roxane	00054-0144	Cholinergic Agonist
54879	Tab, White, Round, Scored, 54 over 879	Meperidine 50 mg	Demerol by Roxane	00054-8595	Analgesic; C II
54879	Tab, White, Round, Scored, 54 over 879	Meperidine 50 mg	Demerol by Roxane	00054-4595	Analgesic; C II
54880	Tab, Coral, Round, 54-880	Imipramine HCl 25 mg	Tofranil by Roxane		Antidepressant
54883	Tab, Light Pinkish-Orange, Pillow-Shaped, 54-883	Methadone HCl 40 mg	Diskets by Roxane	00054-4538	Analgesic; C II
54883	Tab, Light Pinkish-Orange, Pillow-Shaped, 54-883	Methadone HCl 40 mg	Diskets by Eli Lilly	00002-2153	Analgesic; C II
54883	Tab, Light Pinkish-Orange, Pillow-Shaped, 54-883	Methadone HCl 40 mg	Diskets by Cebert	64019-0538	Analgesic; C II
54888	Cap, Green, Opaque	Zaleplon 10 mg	Sonata by Roxane	00054-0085	Hypnotic
54892	Tab, Green, Round, Scored, 54 over 892	Dexamethasone 4 mg	Decadron by Nat Pharmpak	55154-4901	Steroid
54892	Tab, Green, Round, Scored, 54 over 892	Dexamethasone 4 mg	Decadron by Med Pro	53978-2057	Steroid
54892	Tab, Green, Round, Scored	Dexamethasone 4 mg	Decadron by Roxane	00054-4184	Steroid
54892	Tab, Green, Round, Scored	Dexamethasone 4 mg	Decadron by Roxane	00054-4184	Steroid
54899	Tab, White, Round, Scored, 54 over 899	Prednisone 10 mg	Deltasone by Roxane	00054-4730	Steroid
54899	Tab, White, Round, Scored, 54 over 899	Prednisone 10 mg	Deltasone by Nat Pharmpak	55154-4919	Steroid
54899	Tab, White, Round, Scored, 54 over 899	Prednisone 10 mg	Deltasone by Kaiser	00179-1154	Steroid
54899	Tab, White, Round, Scored	Prednisone 10 mg	Deltasone by Roxane	00054-0017	Steroid
54899	Tab, White, Round, Scored	Prednisone 10 mg	Deltasone by Roxane	00054-8725	Steroid
549 <> RDY	Tab, Peach, Round, Flat	Venlafaxine 100 mg	Effexor by Dr. Reddy's	55111-0549	Antidepressant

ID FRONT <> BACK	DESCRIPTION FRONT <> BACK	INGREDIENT & STRENGTH	BRAND (or Generic Equiv.) by FIRM	NDC#	CLASS; SCH.
54902	Tab, White, Round, 54-902	Oxycodone HCl 4.5 mg, Oxycodone Terephthalate 0.38 mg, Aspirin 325 mg	Roxiprin by Roxane	00054-8653 Discontinued	Analgesic; C II
54903	Tab, Pink, Round, 54 over 903	Dihydrotachysterol 0.2 mg	DHT by Roxane	00054-4189	Vitamin
54903	Tab, Pink, Round, 54 over 903	Dihydrotachysterol 0.2 mg	DHT by Roxane	00054-8182	Vitamin
				00054-4182	
54912	Tab, Light Green, Round	Cimetidine HCl 300 mg	Tagamet by Roxane	00054-8224	Gastrointestinal
54919	Tab, 54 over 919	Ranitidine HCl 168 mg	Zantac by Ridgebury	60921-0097	Gastrointestinal
54919	Tab, Orange, Round, 54 over 919	Ranitidine HCl 168 mg	Zantac by Roxane	00054-4853	Gastrointestinal
54922	Tab, White, Round	Granisetron HCl 1 mg	Kytril by Roxane	00054-0143	Antiemetic
54923	Cap, Blue, 54/923	Acyclovir 200 mg	Zovirax by Roxane	00054-2080	Antiviral
54930	Tab, White, Round, 54-930	Aminophylline 200 mg	Aminophylline by Roxane	00054-8026	Antiasthmatic
54932	Tab, White, Round, 54-932	Acetaminophen 300 mg, Codeine Phosphate 60 mg	Tylenol w/ Codeine by Roxane		Analgesic; C III
54933 <> 60	Tab, White, Round, Sustained Release	Morphine Sulfate 60 mg	Oramorph SR by Xanodyne	66479-0542	Analgesic; C II
5493360	Tab, White, Round, Sustained Release	Morphine Sulfate 60 mg	Oramorph SR by Roxane	00054-8792	Analgesic; C II
				00054-4792	
54939	Tab, Coral, Round, 54-939	Imipramine HCl 10 mg	Tofranil by Roxane		Antidepressant
54942	Tab, Off-White, Round, Scored	Leucovorin Calcium 10 mg	Wellcovorin by Roxane	00054-8497	Antineoplastic
54942	Tab, Off White, Round, Scored	Leucovorin Calcium 10 mg	Wellcovorin by Roxane	00054-4497	Antineoplastic
54943	Tab, Pink, Round, Scored, 54 over 943	Dexamethasone 1.5 mg	Decadron by DRX	55045-2591	Steroid
54943	Tab, Pink, Round, Scored	Dexamethasone 1.5 mg	Decadron by Roxane	00054-8181	Steroid
54943	Tab, Pink, Round, Scored	Dexamethasone 1.5 mg	Decadron by Roxane	00054-4182	Steroid
54949	Tab, 54 over 949	Ranitidine HCl 150 mg	Zantac by Eon	00185-0135	Gastrointestinal
54959	Cap, Green & Red, White Print	Mexiletine 250 mg	Mexitil by Roxane	00054-2618	Antiarrhythmic
54959	Cap, Green & Red, White Print	Mexiletine 250 mg	Mexitil by Ridgebury	60921-0068	Antiarrhythmic
5496 <> DANDAN	Tab, Buff, Round, Scored	Hydrochlorothiazide 25 mg, Spironolactone 25 mg	Aldactazide by Schein	00364-0513	Diuretic; Antihypertensive
54960	Tab, Pale Blue, Round, Scored	Dexamethasone 0.75 mg	Decadron by Roxane	00054-8180	Steroid
54960	Tab, Pale Blue, Round, Scored	Dexamethasone .75 mg	Decadron by Roxane	00054-4180	Steroid
54969	Tab, Round, 54-969	Diazepam 2 mg	Valium by Roxane		Antianxiety; C IV
54970	Tab, White, Round, 54-970	Propranolol HCl 10 mg	Inderal by Roxane		Antihypertensive
54972	Cap, Pink, 54-972	Propoxyphene 65 mg	Darvon by Roxane		Analgesic; C IV
549735	Tab, Peach, Round, 54-973 5	Diazepam 5 mg	Valium by Roxane		Antianxiety; C IV
54979	Tab	Quinidine Sulfate 200 mg	by PDRX	55289-0222	Antiarrhythmic
54979200	Tab, White, Round, 54-979 200	Quinidine Sulfate 200 mg	Lin-Qin, Quinova by Roxane	00054-8733	Antiarrhythmic
54980	Tab, Blue, Round, Scored, 54 over 980	Cyclophosphamide 50 mg	Cytoxan by Roxane	00054-4130	Antineoplastic
54980	Tab, Blue, Round, Scored, 54 over 980	Cyclophosphamide 50 mg	Cytoxan by Roxane	00054-8130	Antineoplastic
549821 0	Tab, Peach, Round	Diazepam 10 mg	Valium by Roxane		Antianxiety; C IV
54983	Tab, White, Round, 54-983	Amitriptyline HCl 10 mg	Elavil by Roxane		Antidepressant
54989	Cap, Celery & Green, 54/989	Phendimetrazine Tartrate 105 mg	Prelu-2 by Roxane	00054-2719	Anorexiant; C III
54992	Tab, Pink, Oblong, 54-992	Naproxen 375 mg	Naproxyn by Roxane	00054-8642	NSAID
54997	Tab, White, Round, Film Coated	Mirtazapine 45 mg	Remeron by Roxane	00054-4678	Antidepressant
549HD10	Tab, Blue, Round	Diazepam 10 mg	Valium by Halsey	Discontinued	Antianxiety; C IV
55 <> N	Tab, White to Off-White, Round, Film-Coated	Fluvoxamine Maleate 50 mg	Novo-Fluvoxamine by Novopharm	Canadian DIN 02239953	OCD
55 <> P	Tab, Salmon Pink, Round, Film Coated	Bisoprolol Fumarate 5 mg	Zym-Bisoprolol by Zymcan Pharm	Canadian DIN 02321556	Antihypertensive
55 <> P	Tab, Pink, Round, Scored, P <> 5 / 5	Bisoprolol Fumarate 5 mg	Monocor by Pharmascience	Canadian DIN 02247573	Antihypertensive
55 <> PAR	Tab, Brown, Black Print, Round, Sugar Coated	Imipramine HCl 25 mg	Tofranil by Ivax	00182-0827	Antidepressant
55 <> PAR	Tab, Brown, Black Print, Round, Sugar Coated	Imipramine HCl 25 mg	Tofranil by URL Mutual	00677-0422	Antidepressant

ID FRONT <> BACK	DESCRIPTION FRONT <> BACK	INGREDIENT & STRENGTH	BRAND (or Generic Equiv.) by FIRM	NDC#	CLASS; SCH.
55 <> PAR	Tab, Brown, Black Print, Round, Sugar Coated	Imipramine HCl 25 mg	Tofranil by Amerisource	62584-0750	Antidepressant
55 <> PAR	Tab, Brown, Black Print, Round, Sugar Coated	Imipramine HCl 25 mg	Tofranil by Par	49884-0055	Antidepressant
550	Tab, Pinkish Purple, Oval, Schering Logo 550	Fluphenazine HCl 5 mg	Permitil by Schering	00085-0550	Antipsychotic
550	Tab, Peach, Diamond Shaped, Scored, 5 / 50	Amiloride HCl 5 mg, Hydrochlorothiazide 50 mg	Moduret by Genpharm	Canadian DIN 02257378	Antihypertensive; Diuretic
550 <> 358	Tab	Amiloride HCl 5 mg, Hydrochlorothiazide 50 mg	Moduretic by URL Mutual	00677-1223	Antihypertensive; Diuretic
550 <> N533	Tab, Film Coated	Naproxen 550 mg	Naprosyn by Major	00904-5041	NSAID
550 <> N533	Tab, Light Blue, Coated	Naproxen 550 mg	Naprosyn by Moore	00839-7890	NSAID
550 <> N533	Tab, White, Oval, Film Coated, 550 <> N over 533	Naproxen 550 mg	Naprosyn by Teva	55953-0533	NSAID
550 <> N|N	Tab, Peach, Diamond-Shaped, Compressed, 5 over 50	Amiloride 5 mg, Hydrochlorothiazide 50 mg	Novamilor by Novopharm	Canadian DIN 01937219	Antihypertensive; Diuretic
550 <> NN	Tab, Pink, Diamond Shaped, N/N <> 5 over 50	Amiloride HCl 5 mg, Hydrochlorothiazide 50 mg	Moduret by Novopharm	Canadian DIN 01937219	Antihypertensive; Diuretic
550 <> R	Tab, White, Round, Enteric Coated, Delayed Release	Diclofenac Sodium 50 mg	Voltaren by PDRX	55289-0166	NSAID
550 <> R	Tab, White, Round, Enteric Coated, Delayed Release	Diclofenac Sodium 50 mg	Voltaren by Actavis	00228-2550	NSAID
550 <> R	Tab, White, Round, Enteric Coated, Delayed Release	Diclofenac Sodium 50 mg	Voltaren by CVS	00894-5841	NSAID
550 <> R	Tab, White, Round, Enteric Coated, Delayed Release	Diclofenac Sodium 50 mg	Voltaren by Ivax	00182-2618	NSAID
5500 <> 5712	Tab, Yellow, Oval, Ivax Logo 5712 <> 5/500	Glyburide 5 mg, Metformin 500 mg	Glucovance by Teva	00093-5712	Antidiabetic
5500 <> 5712	Tab, Yellow, Oval, Ivax Logo 5712 <> 5/500	Glyburide 5 mg, Metformin 500 mg	Glucovance by Ivax	00172-5712 Discontinued	Antidiabetic
5501 <> DAN	Tab, White, Oval, Sublingual	Ergoloid Mesylate 1 mg	by Schein	00364-0446	Ergot Alkaloids
5502 <> DAN	Tab, White, Round, Sublingual	Ergoloid Mesylate 0.5 mg	by Schein	00364-0415	Ergot Alkaloids
5503 <> DAN	Tab, Amber-Yellow, Round	Sulfasalazine 500 mg	by Schein	00364-0444	Gastrointestinal
5504 <> DAN	Tab, White, Round	Ergoloid Mesylate 1 mg	by Schein	00364-0622	Ergot Alkaloids
5507 <> DAN	Tab, Yellow, Round	Chlorthalidone 25 mg	by Schein	00364-0564	Diuretic
5507 <> DAN	Tab, Yellow, Round	Chlorthalidone 25 mg	by Schein	00364-0592	Diuretic
5508 <> DANDAN	Tab, White, Round, Scored	Tolbutamide 500 mg	by Schein	00364-0477	Antidiabetic
550HD	Tab, White, Round	Glutethimide 500 mg	Doriden by Halsey	Discontinued	Hypnotic; C II
551 <> PFIZER	Tab, Rounded Rectangle, Film Coated	Cetirizine HCl 10 mg	by Physician Total Care	54868-3876	Antihistamine
551 <> PFIZER	Tab, Rounded Rectangle, Film Coated	Cetirizine HCl 10 mg	by PDRX	55289-0108	Antihistamine
551 <> PFIZER	Tab, Rounded Rectangle, Film Coated	Cetirizine HCl 10 mg	by Caremark	00339-6097	Antihistamine
551 <> PFIZER	Tab, Rounded Rectangle, Film Coated	Cetirizine HCl 10 mg	by Allscripts		Antihistamine
551 <> R	Tab, White, Round, Enteric Coated, Delayed Release	Diclofenac Sodium 75 mg	Voltaren by Actavis	00228-2551	NSAID
551 <> R	Tab, White, Round, Enteric Coated, Delayed Release	Diclofenac Sodium 75 mg	Voltaren by DRX	55045-2247	NSAID
551 <> R	Tab, White, Round, Enteric Coated, Delayed Release	Diclofenac Sodium 75 mg	Voltaren by Rugby	00536-5738	NSAID
551 <> R	Tab, White, Round, Enteric Coated, Delayed Release	Diclofenac Sodium 75 mg	Voltaren by PDRX	55289-0150	NSAID
551 <> R	Tab, White, Round, Enteric Coated, Delayed Release	Diclofenac Sodium 75 mg	Voltaren by Ivax	00182-2619	NSAID
551 <> R	Tab, White, Round, Enteric Coated, Delayed Release	Diclofenac Sodium 75 mg	Voltaren by CVS	00894-5846	NSAID
5510 <> 93	Tab, Round, Pale Yellow to Buff, Scored	Mercaptopurine 50 mg	Purinethol by Teva	00093-5510	Antineoplastic
5513 <> DAN	Tab, White, Round	Carisoprodol 350 mg	Soma by Heartland	61392-0949	Muscle Relaxant
5513 <> DAN	Tab, White, Round	Carisoprodol 350 mg	Soma by Pharmedix	53002-0356	Muscle Relaxant
5513 <> DAN	Tab, White, Round	Carisoprodol 350 mg	Soma by Watson	00591-5513	Muscle Relaxant
5513 <> DAN	Tab, White, Round	Carisoprodol 350 mg	Soma by Schein	00364-0475	Muscle Relaxant
5513 <> DAN	Tab, White, Round	Carisoprodol 350 mg	Soma by Urgent Care Center	50716-0202	Muscle Relaxant
5513 <> DAN	Tab, White, Round	Carisoprodol 350 mg	Soma by Kaiser	00179-1349	Muscle Relaxant
5515 <> DANDAN	Tab, Yellow, Round, Scored	Bethanechol Chloride 50 mg	Urecholine by Watson	00591-5515	Urinary Tract
5515 <> DANDAN	Tab, Yellow, Round, Scored	Bethanechol Chloride 50 mg	Urecholine by Schein	00364-0590	Urinary Tract
5516 <> DAN	Tab, White, Round	Quinine Sulfate 260 mg	by Schein	00364-0560	Antimalarial
5518 <> DAN	Tab, Light Green, Round	Chlorthalidone 50 mg	by Schein	00364-0593	Diuretic
5518 <> DAN	Tab, Light Green, Round	Chlorthalidone 50 mg	by Schein	00364-0528	Diuretic

ID FRONT <> BACK	DESCRIPTION FRONT <> BACK	INGREDIENT & STRENGTH	BRAND (or Generic Equiv.) by FIRM	NDC#	CLASS; SCH.
5520DAN	Cap, Black & Yellow	Tetracycline HCl 500 mg	by Schein	00364-2029	Antibiotic
5522 <> DAN	Tab, Orange, Round, Film Coated	Hydroxyzine HCl 10 mg	Atarax by Heartland	61392-0012	Antianxiety; Antihistamine
5522 <> DAN	Tab, Orange, Round, Film Coated	Hydroxyzine HCl 10 mg	Atarax by Schein	00364-0494	Antianxiety; Antihistamine
5522 <> DAN	Tab, Orange, Round, Film Coated	Hydroxyzine HCl 10 mg	Atarax by Watson	00591-5522	Antianxiety; Antihistamine
5523 <> DAN	Tab, Green, Round, Film Coated	Hydroxyzine HCl 25 mg	Atarax by Vangard	00615-1526	Antianxiety; Antihistamine
5523 <> DAN	Tab, Green, Round, Film Coated	Hydroxyzine HCl 25 mg	Atarax by Watson	00591-5523	Antianxiety; Antihistamine
5523 <> DAN	Tab, Green, Round, Film Coated	Hydroxyzine HCl 25 mg	Atarax by Heartland	61392-0013	Antianxiety; Antihistamine
5523 <> DAN	Tab, Green, Round, Film Coated	Hydroxyzine HCl 25 mg	Atarax by Schein	00364-0495	Antianxiety; Antihistamine
5523 <> DAN	Tab, Green, Round, Film Coated	Hydroxyzine HCl 25 mg	Atarax by Med Pro	53978-3066	Antianxiety; Antihistamine
5523 <> DAN	Tab, Green, Round, Film Coated	Hydroxyzine HCl 25 mg	Atarax by Nat Pharmpak	55154-5203	Antianxiety; Antihistamine
5538 <> DAN	Tab, Off-White, Round, Ex Release	Quinidine Gluconate 324 mg	Quinaglute by Watson	00591-5538	Antiarrhythmic
5538 <> DAN	Tab, Off-White, Round	Quinidine Gluconate 324 mg	Quinaglute by Schein	00364-0604	Antiarrhythmic
554 <> R	Tab, Film Coated	Metoprolol Tartrate 50 mg	Lopressor by Vangard	00615-3552	Antihypertensive
5540 <> DAN	Tab, Off-White to White, Round	Metronidazole 250 mg	Flagyl by Watson	00591-5540	Antibiotic
5540 <> DAN	Tab, Off-White to White, Round	Metronidazole 250 mg	Flagyl by Schein	00364-0595	Antibiotic
5540 <> DAN	Tab, Off-White to White, Round	Metronidazole 250 mg	Flagyl by Nat Pharmpak	55154-5212	Antibiotic
5540 <> DAN	Tab, Off-White to White, Round	Metronidazole 250 mg	Flagyl by Allscripts		Antibiotic
5540 <> DAN	Tab, Off-White to White, Round	Metronidazole 250 mg	Flagyl by Med Pro	53978-0215	Antibiotic
5542 <> DAN25	Tab, Beige, Triangular, Film Coated	Thioridazine HCl 25 mg	by Schein	00364-0662	Antipsychotic
5543 <> DANDAN	Tab, White, Round, Scored	Allopurinol 100 mg	Zyloprim by Danbury	61955-0632	Antigout
5543 <> DANDAN	Tab, White, Round, Scored	Allopurinol 100 mg	Zyloprim by Nat Pharmpak	55154-5239	Antigout
5543 <> DANDAN	Tab, White, Round, Scored	Allopurinol 100 mg	Zyloprim by Schein	00364-0632	Antigout
5543 <> DANDAN	Tab, White, Round, Scored	Allopurinol 100 mg	Zyloprim by Watson	00591-5543	Antigout
5544 <> DANDAN	Tab, Orange, Round, Scored	Allopurinol 300 mg	Zyloprim by Danbury	61955-0633	Antigout
5544 <> DANDAN	Tab, Orange, Round, Scored	Allopurinol 300 mg	Zyloprim by Watson	00591-5544	Antigout
5544 <> DANDAN	Tab, Orange, Round, Scored	Allopurinol 300 mg	Zyloprim by Nat Pharmpak	55154-5216	Antigout
5544 <> DANDAN	Tab, Orange, Round, Scored	Allopurinol 300 mg	Zyloprim by Med Pro	53978-5001	Antigout
5544 <> DANDAN	Tab, Orange, Round, Scored	Allopurinol 300 mg	Zyloprim by Schein	00364-0633	Antigout
5546 <> DANDAN	Tab, White, Round, Scored	Sulfamethoxazole 400 mg, Trimethoprim 80 mg	Septra by Schein	00364-2068	Antibiotic
5546 <> DANDAN	Tab, White, Round, Scored	Sulfamethoxazole 400 mg, Trimethoprim 80 mg	Septra by Watson	00591-5546	Antibiotic
5546 <> DANDAN	Tab, White, Round, Scored	Sulfamethoxazole 400 mg, Trimethoprim 80 mg	Septra by St. Mary's Med	60760-0004	Antibiotic
5547 <> DANDAN	Tab, White, Oval, Scored	Sulfamethoxazole 800 mg, Trimethoprim 160 mg	Septra by Southwood	58016-0109	Antibiotic
5547 <> DANDAN	Tab, White, Oval, Scored	Sulfamethoxazole 800 mg, Trimethoprim 160 mg	Septra by Nat Pharmpak	55154-5205	Antibiotic
5547 <> DANDAN	Tab, White, Oval, Scored	Sulfamethoxazole 800 mg, Trimethoprim 160 mg	Septra by Amerisource	62584-0399	Antibiotic
5547 <> DANDAN	Tab, White, Oval, Scored	Sulfamethoxazole 800 mg, Trimethoprim 160 mg	Septra by Va Cmop	65243-0067	Antibiotic
5547 <> DANDAN	Tab, White, Oval, Scored	Sulfamethoxazole 800 mg, Trimethoprim 160 mg	Septra by Watson	00591-5547	Antibiotic
5547 <> DANDAN	Tab, White, Oval, Scored	Sulfamethoxazole 800 mg, Trimethoprim 160 mg	Septra by Schein	00364-2069	Antibiotic
5547 <> DANDAN	Tab, White, Oval, Scored	Sulfamethoxazole 800 mg, Trimethoprim 160 mg	Septra by Pharmedix	53002-0210	Antibiotic
5548 <> DANDAN	Tab, White, Round, Film Coated	Chloroquine Phosphate 250 mg	Aralen Phosphate by Schein	00364-0470	Antimalarial
5549 <> DAN	Tab, White, Round, Film Coated	Chloroquine Phosphate 500 mg	Aralen Phosphate by Schein	00364-2431	Antimalarial
555	Tab, Pale Orange, Round, Extended Release	Bupropion HCl 200 mg	Wellbutrin SR by Global	00115-5445	Antidepressant
555 <> 5665	Tab, White, Cap Shaped, Scored, Hourglass Logo 5665	Buspirone HCl 15 mg	BuSpar by Ivax	00172-5665	Antianxiety
555 <> 5665	Tab, White, Capsule Shaped, Scored	Buspirone HCl 15 mg	BuSpar by Teva	00172-5665	Anxiolytic
555 <> 931003	Tab, White to Off-White, Rectangular, Scored	Buspirone HCl 15 mg	BuSpar by Teva Pharmaceuticals	00093-1003	Antianxiety
555 <> B	Tab, Light Blue-Green, Round, Film Coated	Levonorgestrel 0.15 mg, Ethinyl Estradiol 0.03 mg	Seasonique by Duramed	51285-0087	Oral Contraceptive
555 <> ETH309	Tab, Yellow, Cap Shaped, Scored	Buspirone HCl 15 mg	BuSpar by Ethex	58177-0309	Antianxiety
555 <> MB3	Tab, White, Cap Shaped, Scored	Buspirone HCl 15 mg	BuSpar by Mylan	00378-1165	Antianxiety
555 <> MB3	Tab, White, Cap Shaped, Scored	Buspirone HCl 15 mg	BuSpar by UDL	51079-0960	Antianxiety
555 <> MJ822	Tab, White, Rectangular, Scored	Buspirone HCl 15 mg	BuSpar by Murfreesboro	51129-1375	Antianxiety
555 <> MJ822	Tab, White, Rectangular, Scored	Buspirone HCl 15 mg	BuSpar by Wal Mart	49035-0188	Antianxiety

ID FRONT <> BACK	DESCRIPTION FRONT <> BACK	INGREDIENT & STRENGTH	BRAND (or Generic Equiv.) by FIRM	NDC#	CLASS; SCH.
555 <> MJ822	Tab, White, Rectangular, Scored	Buspirone HCl 15 mg	BuSpar by Direct Dispensing	57866-0904	Antianxiety
555 <> MJ822	Tab, White, Rectangular, Scored	Buspirone HCl 15 mg	BuSpar by BMS	00087-0822	Antianxiety
555 <> MJ822	Tab, White, Rectangular, Scored	Buspirone HCl 15 mg	BuSpar by BMS	15548-0822	Antianxiety
555 <> MJ822	Tab, White, Rectangular, Scored	Buspirone HCl 15 mg	BuSpar by Caremark	00339-4105	Antianxiety
555 <> MYLAN	Tab, White, Cap Shaped	Naproxen 375 mg	Naprosyn by Novartis	61615-0016	NSAID
555 <> MYLAN	Tab, White, Cap Shaped	Naproxen 375 mg	Naprosyn by Dixon Shane	17236-0077	NSAID
555 <> MYLAN	Tab, White, Cap Shaped	Naproxen 375 mg	Naprosyn by Kaiser	62224-4552	NSAID
555 <> MYLAN	Tab, White, Cap Shaped	Naproxen 375 mg	Naprosyn by Mylan	00378-0555	NSAID
555 <> MYLAN	Tab, White, Cap Shaped	Naproxen 375 mg	Naprosyn by Kaiser	00179-1187	NSAID
555 <> MYLAN	Tab, White, Cap Shaped	Naproxen 375 mg	Naprosyn by UDL	51079-0794	NSAID
555 <> MYLAN	Tab, White, Cap Shaped	Naproxen 375 mg	Naprosyn by H J Harkins Co	52959-0191	NSAID
555 <> PAR721	Tab, Peach, Rectangular, Scored, 5-5-5	Buspirone HCl 15 mg	Buspar by Par	49884-0721	Antianxiety
555 <> BMS	Tab, Mottled Clear, Film Coated, Scored	Diltiazem HCl 60 mg	Cardizem by BMS	00003-5550 Discontinued	Antihypertensive
5550 <> BMS	Tab, Mottled Clear, Film Coated, Scored	Diltiazem HCl 60 mg	Cardizem by Med Pro	53978-1235 Discontinued	Antihypertensive
555013 <> BARR	Tab, Pink, Round, Film Coated	Erythromycin Stearate 250 mg	by Barr	00555-0013 Discontinued	Antibiotic
555013BARR	Tab, Red, Round, 555/013 Barr	Erythromycin Stearate 250 mg	Erythrocin by Barr		Antibiotic
555064	Tab, Orange, Round, 555/064	Hydralazine HCl 25 mg	Apresoline by Barr		Antihypertensive
555065	Tab, Orange, Round, 555/065	Hydralazine HCl 50 mg	Apresoline by Barr		Antihypertensive
555089	Tab, White, Round, 555/089	Propylthiouracil 50 mg	by Barr		Antithyroid
555126	Tab, Blue, Round, 555/126	Dicyclomine HCl 20 mg	Bentyl by Barr		Gastrointestinal
555153LLP21	Tab, White, Round, 555/153 LL P21	Phenobarbital 30 mg	by Lederle		Sedative/Hypnotic; C IV
555157BARR	Tab, Peach, Round, 555/157 Barr	Prednisone 20 mg	Deltasone by Barr		Steroid
555163 <> BARR	Tab, White, Round, Scored, 555 over 163	Diazepam 2 mg	Valium by Southwood	58016-0274	Antianxiety; C IV
555163 <> BARR	Tab, White, Round, Scored, 555 over 163	Diazepam 2 mg	Valium by Barr	00555-0163 Discontinued	Antianxiety; C IV
555164 <> BARR	Tab, Blue, Round, Scored, 555 over 164	Diazepam 10 mg	Valium by Southwood	58016-0273	Antianxiety; C IV
555164 <> BARR	Tab, Blue, Round, Scored, 555 over 164	Diazepam 10 mg	Valium by Barr	00555-0164	Antianxiety; C IV
555169BARR	Tab, White, Round, 555/169 Barr	Furosemide 40 mg	Lasix by Barr		Diuretic
555174	Tab, Pink, Round, 555/174	Isosorbide Dinitrate 5 mg	Isordil by Barr		Antianginal
555175	Tab, White, Round, 555/175	Isosorbide Dinitrate 10 mg	Isordil by Barr		Antianginal
555186	Tab, Green, Round, 555/186	Isosorbide Dinitrate 20 mg	Isordil by Barr		Antianginal
555188BARR	Tab, White, Round, 555/188 Barr	Quinidine Sulfate 200 mg	by Barr		Antiarrhythmic
55519 <> DANDAN	Tab, Flat-faced, Bevel-edged, 555/19	Hydrochlorothiazide 25 mg	Hydrodiuril by Watson	00591-5552	Diuretic; Antihypertensive
555192BARR	Tab, Peach, Round, 555/192 Barr	Hydrochlorothiazide 100 mg	Hydrodiuril by Barr		Diuretic; Antihypertensive
5552 <> DANDAN	Tab, White to Off-White, Round, Scored	Metronidazole 500 mg	Flagyl by Watson	00555-5552	Antibiotic
5552 <> DANDAN	Tab, White to Off-White, Round, Scored	Metronidazole 500 mg	Flagyl by Nat Pharmpak	55154-5234	Antibiotic
5552 <> DANDAN	Tab, White to Off-White, Round, Scored	Metronidazole 500 mg	Flagyl by Schein	00364-0687	Antibiotic
555520	Tab, 555/20	Hydrochlorothiazide 50 mg	by Barr	00555-0020	Diuretic; Antihypertensive
555200	Tab, White, Round, 555/200	Atropine Sulfate 0.025 mg, Diphenoxylate HCl 2.5 mg	Lomotil by Barr		Antidiarrheal; C V
555210	Tab, Brown, Round, 555/210	Amitriptyline HCl 50 mg	Elavil by Barr		Antidepressant
555211	Tab, Purple, Round, 555/211	Amitriptyline HCl 75 mg	Elavil by Barr		Antidepressant
555212	Tab, Orange & Red, Round	Amitriptyline HCl 100 mg	Elavil by Barr		Antidepressant
555233	Tab, 555/233	Prednisone 10 mg	by Barr		Steroid

ID FRONT <> BACK	DESCRIPTION FRONT <> BACK	INGREDIENT & STRENGTH	BRAND (or Generic Equiv.) by FIRM	NDC#	CLASS; SCH.
555241BARR	Tab, White, Round, 555/241 Barr	Allopurinol 100 mg	Zyloprim by Barr		Antigout
555242	Tab, Peach, Round, 555/242	Allopurinol 300 mg	Zyloprim by Barr		Antigout
555251	Tab, White, Round, 555/251	Tolbutamide 500 mg	Orinase by Barr		Antidiabetic
555255	Tab, Green, Round, 555/255	Chlorzoxazone 250 mg, Acetaminophen 300 mg	Parafon Forte by Barr		Muscle Relaxant
55526	Tab, White, Round, 555/26	Prednisone 5 mg	Deltasone by Barr		Steroid
555265	Tab, 555/265	Hydrochlorothiazide 25 mg, Spironolactone 25 mg	by Barr	00555-0265	Diuretic; Antihypertensive
555266	Tab, 555/266	Spironolactone 25 mg	by Barr	00555-0266	Diuretic
555271 <> BARR	Tab, White, Round, Scored, 555 over 271	Sulfinpyrazone 100 mg	Anturane by Barr	00555-0271	Uricosuric
555278	Tab, White, Round, Scored, 555 over 278	Acetaminophen 325 mg, Oxycodone HCl 5 mg	Percocet by Barr	00555-0278	Analgesic; C II
555279	Tab, Blue, Round, 555/279	Isosorbide Dinitrate 30 mg	Isordil by Barr		Antianginal
555288	Tab, Green, Round, 555/288	Isosorbide Dinitrate Oral 40 mg	Isordil by Barr		Antianginal
555293BARR	Tab, Yellow, Round, 555/293 Barr	Oxycodone HCl 4.5 mg, Oxycodone Terephthalate 0.38 mg, Aspirin 325 mg	Percodan by Barr		Analgesic; C II
5553 <> DAN	Tab, Light Orange, Round, Film Coated	Doxycycline Hyclate 100 mg	Vibramycin by Pharmedix	53002-0271	Antibiotic
5553 <> DAN	Tab, Light Orange, Round, Film Coated	Doxycycline Hyclate 100 mg	Vibramycin by Med Pro	53978-3028	Antibiotic
5553 <> DAN	Tab, Light Orange, Round, Film Coated	Doxycycline Hyclate 100 mg	Vibramycin by Schein	00364-2063	Antibiotic
5553 <> DAN	Tab, Light Orange, Round, Film Coated	Doxycycline Hyclate 100 mg	Vibramycin by Watson	00591-5553	Antibiotic
5553 <> DAN	Tab, Light Orange, Round, Film Coated	Doxycycline Hyclate 100 mg	Vibramycin by Murfreesboro	51129-1357	Antibiotic
55535	Tab, White, Round, 555/35	Meprobamate 200 mg	Miltown by Barr		Sedative/Hypnotic; C IV
55536	Tab, 555/36 Debossed	Meprobamate 400 mg	by Barr	00555-0036	Sedative/Hypnotic; C IV
555363 <> BARR	Tab, Yellow, Round, Scored, 555/363 <> Barr	Diazepam 5 mg	Valium by Barr	00555-0363 Discontinued	Antianxiety; C IV
555363 <> BARR	Tab, Yellow, Round, Scored	Diazepam 5 mg	by Southwood	58016-0275	Antianxiety; C IV
555365	Tab, Peach, Round, 555/365	Propranolol HCl 10 mg	Inderal by Barr		Antihypertensive
555366	Tab, Blue, Round, 555/366	Propranolol HCl 20 mg	Inderal by Barr		Antihypertensive
555367	Tab, Green, Round, 555/367	Propranolol HCl 40 mg	Inderal by Barr		Antihypertensive
555368	Tab, Pink, Round, 555/368	Propranolol HCl 60 mg	Inderal by Barr		Antihypertensive
555369	Tab, Yellow, Round, 555/369	Propranolol HCl 80 mg	Inderal by Barr		Antihypertensive
5553DAN	Tab, Film Coated	Doxycycline Hyclate 100 mg	Vibramycin by Allscripts		Antibiotic
555424B	Tab, White, Round, 555/424 B	Metoclopramide 10 mg	Reglan by Barr		Gastrointestinal
555427 <> BARR	Tab, White, Round, Scored, 555/427 <> Barr	Hydrochlorothiazide 25 mg, Propranolol HCl 40 mg	by Barr	00555-0427	Diuretic; Antihypertensive
555428 <> BARR	Tab, White, Round, Scored, 555/428 <> Barr	Hydrochlorothiazide 25 mg, Propranolol HCl 80 mg	by Barr	00555-0428	Diuretic; Antihypertensive
555429	Tab, White, Round, 555/429	Trimethoprim 100 mg	Trimpex by Barr		Antibiotic
555430	Tab, White, Round, 555/430	Trimethoprim 200 mg	Trimpex by Barr		Antibiotic
555444 <> BARR	Tab, Yellow, Oval, Scored, 555/444 <> barr	Hydrochlorothiazide 50 mg, Triamterene 75 mg	Maxzide by Barr	00555-0444	Diuretic; Antihypertensive
555444 <> BARR	Tab, Yellow, Oval, Scored, 555/444 <> barr	Hydrochlorothiazide 50 mg, Triamterene 75 mg	Maxzide by PDRX	55289-0488	Diuretic; Antihypertensive
555444 <> BARR	Tab, Yellow, Oval, Scored, 555/444 <> barr	Hydrochlorothiazide 50 mg, Triamterene 75 mg	Maxzide by Major	00904-1965	Diuretic; Antihypertensive
555483 <> BARR	Tab, Light Yellow, Round, Scored, 555 over 483 <> barr	Amiloride HCl 5 mg, Hydrochlorothiazide 50 mg	Moduretic by Barr	00555-0483	Antihypertensive; Diuretic
555489 <> BARR	Tab, White, Round, Scored, 555 over 489 <> barr	Trazodone HCl 50 mg	Desyrel by Nat Pharmpak	55154-1406	Antidepressant
555489 <> BARR	Tab, White, Round, Scored, 555 over 489 <> barr	Trazodone HCl 50 mg	Desyrel by UDL	51079-0427 Discontinued	Antidepressant
555489 <> BARR	Tab, White, Round, Scored, 555 over 489 <> barr	Trazodone HCl 50 mg	Desyrel by Barr	00555-0489	Antidepressant
555490 <> BARR	Tab, White, Round, Scored, 555 over 490 <> barr	Trazodone HCl 100 mg	Desyrel by UDL	51079-0428 Discontinued	Antidepressant
555490 <> BARR	Tab, White, Round, Scored, 555 over 490 <> barr	Trazodone HCl 100 mg	Desyrel by Murfreesboro	51129-1131	Antidepressant
555490 <> BARR	Tab, White, Round, Scored, 555 over 490 <> barr	Trazodone HCl 100 mg	Desyrel by Barr	00555-0490	Antidepressant
555585 <> BARR	Tab, Light Green, Round, Scored, 555 over 585 <> barr	Chlorzoxazone 500 mg	Parafon Forte by Barr	00555-0585	Muscle Relaxant

ID FRONT <> BACK	DESCRIPTION FRONT <> BACK	INGREDIENT & STRENGTH	BRAND (or Generic Equiv.) by FIRM	NDC#	CLASS; SCH.
555585 <> BARR	Tab, Light Green, Round, Scored, 555 over 585 <> barr	Chlorzoxazone 500 mg	Parafon Forte by PDRX	55289-0633	Muscle Relaxant
555585 <> BARR	Tab, Light Green, Round, Scored, 555 over 585 <> barr	Chlorzoxazone 500 mg	Parafon Forte by UDL	51079-0476	Muscle Relaxant
555585 <> BARR	Tab, Light Green, Round, Scored, 555 over 585 <> barr	Chlorzoxazone 500 mg	Parafon Forte by Direct Dispensing	57866-3444	Muscle Relaxant
555606 <> B	Tab, White, Round, Scored, 555 over 606	Megestrol Acetate 20 mg	Megace by UDL	51079-0434	Hormone
555606 <> B	Tab, White, Round, Scored, 555 over 606	Megestrol Acetate 20 mg	Megace by Barr	00555-0606	Hormone
555606 <> B	Tab, White, Round, Scored, 555 over 606	Megestrol Acetate 20 mg	Megace by Major	00904-3570	Hormone
555607 <> B	Tab, White, Round, Scored, 555 over 607	Megestrol Acetate 40 mg	Megace by UDL	51079-0435 Discontinued	Hormone
555607 <> BARR	Tab, White, Round, Scored, 555 over 607	Megestrol Acetate 40 mg	Megace by Supergen	62701-0920	Hormone
555607 <> BARR	Tab, White, Round, Scored, 555 over 607	Megestrol Acetate 40 mg	Megace by Barr	00555-0607	Hormone
555607 <> BARR	Tab, White, Round, Scored, 555 over 607	Megestrol Acetate 40 mg	Megace by CVS	51316-0239	Hormone
555607 <> BARR	Tab, White, Round, Scored, 555 over 607	Megestrol Acetate 40 mg	Megace by CVS	00894-6651	Hormone
555607 <> BARR	Tab, White, Round, Scored, 555 over 607	Megestrol Acetate 40 mg	Megace by URL Mutual	00677-1206	Hormone
555607 <> BARR	Tab, White, Round, Scored, 555 over 607	Megestrol Acetate 40 mg	Megace by Warner Chilcott	00047-0108	Hormone
555607 <> BARR	Tab, White, Round, Scored, 555 over 607	Megestrol Acetate 40 mg	Megace by Qualitest	00603-4392	Hormone
555607 <> BARR	Tab, White, Round, Scored, 555 over 607	Megestrol Acetate 40 mg	Megace by Major		Hormone
555643 <> BARR	Tab, Green, Oval, Scored, 555/643 <> barr	Hydrochlorothiazide 25 mg, Triamterene 37.5 mg	Maxzide by Barr	00555-0643	Diuretic; Antihypertensive
555727 <> BARR	Tab, Yellow, Round, Scored, 555 over 727	Estropipate 0.75 mg	Ogen by Barr	00555-0727	Hormone
555727 <> BARR	Tab, Yellow, Round, Scored, 555 over 727	Estropipate 0.75 mg	Ogen by Heartland	61392-0617	Hormone
555728 <> BARR	Tab, Peach, Round, Scored, 555 over 728	Estropipate 1.5 mg	Ogen by Heartland	61392-0707	Hormone
555728 <> BARR	Tab, Peach, Round, Scored, 555 over 728	Estropipate 1.5 mg	Ogen by Barr	00555-0728 Discontinued	Hormone
555729 <> BARR	Tab, Blue, Round, Scored, 555 over 729	Estropipate 3 mg	Ogen by Barr	00555-0729	Hormone
555729 <> BARR	Tab, Blue, Round, Scored, 555 over 729	Estropipate 3 mg	Ogen by Heartland	61392-0715	Hormone
555779 <> B	Tab, White, Round, Scored, 555 over 779	Medroxyprogesterone Acetate 10 mg	Provera by Barr	00555-0779	Hormone
555779 <> B	Tab, White, Round, Scored, 555 over 779	Medroxyprogesterone Acetate 10 mg	Provera by URL Mutual	00677-1619	Hormone
555779 <> B	Tab, White, Round, Scored, 555 over 779	Medroxyprogesterone Acetate 10 mg	Provera by Major	00904-2690	Hormone
555779 <> B	Tab, White, Round, Scored, 555 over 779	Medroxyprogesterone Acetate 10 mg	Provera by Qualitest	00603-4367	Hormone
555779 <> B	Tab, White, Round, Scored, 555 over 779	Medroxyprogesterone Acetate 10 mg	Provera by Nat Pharmpak	55154-5575	Hormone
555831 <> BARR	Tab, Pink, Oval, Scored	Warfarin Sodium 1 mg	Coumadin by Barr	00555-0831 Discontinued	Anticoagulant
555832 <> BARR	Tab, Green, Oval, Scored, 555/832 <> Barr	Warfarin Sodium 2.5 mg	Coumadin by Barr	00555-0832 Discontinued	Anticoagulant
555833 <> BARR	Tab, Peach, Oval, Scored, 555/833 <> Barr	Warfarin Sodium 5 mg	by Barr	Discontinued	Anticoagulant
555834 <> BARR	Tab, Yellow, Oval, Scored, 555/834 <> Barr	Warfarin Sodium 7.5 mg	by Barr	Discontinued	Anticoagulant
555835 <> BARR	Tab, White, Oval, Scored, 555/835 <> Barr	Warfarin Sodium 10 mg	by Barr	Discontinued	Anticoagulant
555869 <> BARR	Tab, Lavender, Oval, Scored, 555/869 <> Barr	Warfarin Sodium 2 mg	by Barr	Discontinued	Anticoagulant
555872 <> B	Tab, White, Round, Scored, 555 over 872	Medroxyprogesterone Acetate 2.5 mg	Provera by Major	00904-5227	Hormone
555872 <> B	Tab, White, Round, Scored, 555 over 872	Medroxyprogesterone Acetate 2.5 mg	Provera by Southwood	58016-0374	Hormone
555872 <> B	Tab, White, Round, Scored, 555 over 872	Medroxyprogesterone Acetate 2.5 mg	Provera by Murfreesboro	51129-1373	Hormone
555872 <> B	Tab, White, Round, Scored, 555 over 872	Medroxyprogesterone Acetate 2.5 mg	Provera by Barr	00555-0872	Hormone
555872 <> B	Tab, White, Round, Scored, 555 over 872	Medroxyprogesterone Acetate 2.5 mg	Provera by URL Mutual	00677-1617	Hormone
555872 <> B	Tab, White, Round, Scored, 555 over 872	Medroxyprogesterone Acetate 2.5 mg	Provera by Qualitest	00603-4365	Hormone
555872 <> B	Tab, White, Round, Scored, 555 over 872	Medroxyprogesterone Acetate 2.5 mg	Provera by Nat Pharmpak	55154-5569	Hormone
555873 <> B	Tab, White, Round, Scored, 555 over 873	Medroxyprogesterone Acetate 5 mg	Provera by Nat Pharmpak	55154-5571	Hormone
555873 <> B	Tab, White, Round, Scored, 555 over 873	Medroxyprogesterone Acetate 5 mg	Provera by Major	00904-5228	Hormone
555873 <> B	Tab, White, Round, Scored, 555 over 873	Medroxyprogesterone Acetate 5 mg	Provera by Qualitest	00603-4366	Hormone
555873 <> B	Tab, White, Round, Scored, 555 over 873	Medroxyprogesterone Acetate 5 mg	Provera by URL Mutual	00677-1618	Hormone
555873 <> B	Tab, White, Round, Scored, 555 over 873	Medroxyprogesterone Acetate 5 mg	Provera by Barr	00555-0873	Hormone

ID FRONT <> BACK	DESCRIPTION FRONT <> BACK	INGREDIENT & STRENGTH	BRAND (or Generic Equiv.) by FIRM	NDC#	CLASS; SCH.
555874 <> BARR	Tab, Blue, Oval, Scored, 555/874 <> Barr	Warfarin Sodium 4 mg	by Barr	Discontinued	Anticoagulant
556 <> B	Tab, Yellow, Round, Film Coated	Ethinyl Estradiol 0.01 mg	Seasonique by Duramed	51285-0087	Oral Contraceptive
556 <> B	Tab, Yellow, Round	Ethinyl Estradiol 0.01 mg	Lo Seasonique by Duramed	51285-0092	Oral Contraceptive
556 <> PAR	Tab, White, Oval	Lisinopril 2.5 mg	Zestril by Par	49884-0556	Antihypertensive
5561DAN	Cap, Brown, Opaque	Disopyramide Phosphate 150 mg	Norpace by Schein	00364-0740	Antiarrhythmic
5562 <> DAN	Tab, White, Oval, Film Coated, Ex Release	Procainamide HCl 250 mg	Procan by Schein	00364-0715	Antiarrhythmic
5562 <> DAN	Tab, White, Oval, Film Coated, Ex Release	Procainamide HCl 250 mg	Procan by Watson	00591-5562	Antiarrhythmic
5563 <> DANDAN	Tab, White, Oval, Scored, Film Coated, Ex Release	Procainamide HCl 500 mg	Procan by Schein	00364-0716	Antiarrhythmic
5564 <> DANDAN	Tab, White, Oval, Film Coated, Scored, Ex Release	Procainamide HCl 750 mg	Procan by Schein	00364-0717	Antiarrhythmic
5565 <> DAN	Tab, Yellow, Round, Film Coated	Hydroxyzine HCl 50 mg	Atarax by Watson	00591-5565	Antianxiety; Antihistamine
5565 <> DAN	Tab, Coated	Hydroxyzine HCl 50 mg	Atarax by Med Pro	53978-3186	Antianxiety; Antihistamine
5565 <> DAN	Tab, Yellow, Round, Film Coated	Hydroxyzine HCl 50 mg	Atarax by Schein	00364-0496	Antianxiety; Antihistamine
5566 <> DAN10	Tab, Yellow-Green, Triangular	Thioridazine 10 mg	Mellaril by Schein	00364-2317	Antipsychotic
5568 <> DAN50	Tab, White, Triangular, Film Coated	Thioridazine 50 mg	Mellaril by Schein	00364-2318	Antipsychotic
5569 <> DAN	Tab, Orange, Round, Film Coated	Thioridazine 100 mg	Mellaril by Schein	00364-0670	Antipsychotic
557 <> PAR	Tab, White, Cap Shaped	Lisinopril 5 mg	Zestril by Par	49884-0557	Antihypertensive
557 <> SL	Tab, Debossed	Naproxen 500 mg	Naprosyn by Pliva	50111-0557	NSAID
5571 <> DANDAN	Tab, White, Oval, Scored	Trimethoprim 100 mg	Trimpex by Watson	00591-5571	Antibiotic
5571 <> DANDAN	Tab, White, Oval, Scored	Trimethoprim 100 mg	Trimpex by Schein	00364-0649	Antibiotic
5572 <> DAN	Tab, White, Round, Film Coated	Thioridazine HCl 15 mg	by Schein	00364-0669	Antipsychotic
5575 <> DANDAN	Tab, White, Round, Scored	Furosemide 40 mg	by Schein	00364-0514	Diuretic
5579 <> B	Tab, White, Round, Convex, Scored	Medroxyprogesterone Acetate 10 mg	by Nat Pharmpak	55154-5579	Hormone
5579 <> DANDAN	Tab, Blue, Round, Scored	Chlorpropamide 100 mg	by Schein	00364-0699	Antidiabetic
557HD	Tab, White, Round	Ibuprofen 200 mg	Motrin by Halsey	Discontinued	NSAID
558 <> PAR	Tab, White, Round	Lisinopril 10 mg	Zestril by Par	49884-0558	Antihypertensive
5580 <> DAN	Tab, Orange, Round, Film Coated	Thioridazine HCl 150 mg	by Schein	00364-0723	Antipsychotic
5581 <> DAN	Tab, Reddish Pink, Round, Film Coated	Thioridazine HCl 200 mg	by Schein	00364-0724	Antipsychotic
5582 <> DANDAN	Tab, White, Round, Scored	Tolazamide 250 mg	by Schein	00364-0720	Antidiabetic
5584 <> DAN	Tab, White, Round, Film Coated	Ibuprofen 400 mg	Motrin by Schein	00364-0765	NSAID
5585 <> DAN	Tab, White, Round, Film Coated	Ibuprofen 200 mg	Motrin by Schein	00364-2145	NSAID
5587 <> DAN	Tab, White, Round, Scored, Film Coated	Methyldopa 500 mg	by Schein	00364-0708	Antihypertensive
5588 <> DAN	Tab, White, Round, Scored, Film Coated	Methyldopa 250 mg	by Schein	00364-0707	Antihypertensive
5589 <> DANDAN	Tab, White, Round, Scored	Metoclopramide HCl 10 mg	Reglan by Watson	00591-5589	Gastrointestinal
5589 <> DANDAN	Tab, White, Round, Scored	Metoclopramide HCl 10 mg	Reglan by Schein	00364-0769	Gastrointestinal
5589 <> DANDAN	Tab, White, Round, Scored	Metoclopramide HCl 10 mg	Reglan by Med Pro	53978-5011	Gastrointestinal
5589 <> DANDAN	Tab, White, Round, Scored	Metoclopramide HCl 10 mg	Reglan by Nat Pharmpak	55154-5202	Gastrointestinal
559 <> PAR	Tab, White, Round	Lisinopril 20 mg	Zestril by Par	49884-0559	Antihypertensive
5590 <> DANDAN	Tab, White, Round, Scored	Tolazamide 500 mg	by Schein	00364-0722	Antidiabetic
5591 <> DANDAN	Tab, White, Round, Scored	Tolazamide 100 mg	by Schein	00364-0721	Antidiabetic
5597 <> DANDAN	Tab, White, Cap Shaped, Scored	Acetohexamide 500 mg	Dymelor by Schein	00364-2233	Antidiabetic
5597 <> DANDAN	Tab, White, Cap Shaped, Scored	Acetohexamide 500 mg	Dymelor by Watson	00591-5597	Antidiabetic
5598 <> DANDAN	Tab, White, Cap Shaped, Scored	Acetohexamide 250 mg	Dymelor by Schein	00364-2232	Antidiabetic
5598 <> DANDAN	Tab, White, Cap Shaped, Scored	Acetohexamide 250 mg	Dymelor by Watson	00591-5598	Antidiabetic
5599 <> DANDAN	Tab, White, Round, Scored, Film Coated	Trazodone HCl 100 mg	Desyrel by Schein	00364-2110	Antidepressant
5599 <> DANDAN	Tab, White, Round, Scored, Film Coated	Trazodone HCl 100 mg	Desyrel by Watson	00591-5599	Antidepressant
559HD	Tab, White, Round	Ibuprofen 400 mg	Motrin by Halsey	Discontinued	NSAID
56 <> 93	Tab, Yellow, Cap Shaped, Film Coated, Scored, 9 / 3	Fluvoxamine Maleate 50 mg	Luvox by Teva	00093-0056	OCD
56 <> C	Tab, Pink, Cap-Shaped, Film-Coated, Biconvex	Paroxetine 20mg	Paroxetine by Aurobindo	65862-0155	Antidepressant
56 <> PAR	Tab, Green, Round, Sugar Coated	Imipramine HCl 50 mg	Tofranil by Par	49884-0056	Antidepressant
56 <> PAR	Tab, Sugar Coated, Printed in Black	Imipramine HCl 50 mg	Tofranil by Amerisource	62584-0751	Antidepressant

ID FRONT <> BACK	DESCRIPTION FRONT <> BACK	INGREDIENT & STRENGTH	BRAND (or Generic Equiv.) by FIRM	NDC#	CLASS; SCH.
56 <> W	Tab, Yellow, Oval	Sertraline HCl 100 mg	Zolot by West-Ward	00143-9580	Antidepressant
56 <> WYETH	Tab, White, Round	Ethinyl Estradiol 0.05 mg, Norgestrel 0.5 mg	Ovral by PDRX	55289-0245	Oral Contraceptive
56 <> WYETH	Tab, White, Round	Ethinyl Estradiol 0.05 mg, Norgestrel 0.5 mg	Ovral by Wyeth	00008-0056	Oral Contraceptive
560	Tab, White, Cap Shaped, Ascher Logo <> 560	Acetaminophen 500 mg, Melatonin 1.5 mg	Melagesic by B F Ascher	00225-0560	Analgesic; Supplement
560 <> PAR	Tab, White to Off-White, Round	Lisinopril 40 mg	Zestril by Par	49884-0560	Antihypertensive
5600 <> DANDAN	Tab, White, Round, Scored, Film Coated	Trazodone HCl 50 mg	Desyrel by Schein	00364-2109	Antidepressant
5600 <> DANDAN	Tab, White, Round, Scored, Film Coated	Trazodone HCl 50 mg	Desyrel by Watson	00591-5600	Antidepressant
5601 <> DAN	Tab, Film Coated	Verapamil HCl 80 mg	by Nat Pharmpak	55154-5227	Antihypertensive
5601 <> DANDAN	Tab, Film Coated	Verapamil HCl 80 mg	Verelan by Watson	00591-5601	Antihypertensive
5601 <> DANDAN	Tab, Film Coated	Verapamil HCl 80 mg	Verelan by Amerisource	62584-0888	Antihypertensive
5601 <> DANDAN	Tab, White, Round, Film Coated, Scored	Verapamil HCl 80 mg	by Schein	00364-2111	Antihypertensive
5602 <> DANDAN	Tab, Coated	Verelan by Amerisource		62584-0889	Antihypertensive
5602 <> DANDAN	Tab, Coated	Verapamil HCl 120 mg	by Watson	00591-5602	Antihypertensive
5602 <> DANDAN	Tab, White, Round, Coated, Scored	Verapamil HCl 120 mg	by Schein	00364-2112	Antihypertensive
5602 <> DANDAN	Tab, 5602 <> Dan/Dan	Verapamil HCl 120 mg	by Nat Pharmpak	55154-5229	Antihypertensive
5603 <> DAN2	Tab, Yellow, Round, Scored	Haloperidol 2 mg	Haldol by Schein	00364-2206	Antipsychotic
5605 <> DAN05	Tab, White, Round, Scored, 5605 <> Dan 0.5	Haloperidol 0.5 mg	Haldol by Schein	00364-2204	Antipsychotic
5606 <> DAN5	Tab, Blue, Round, Scored	Haloperidol 5 mg		00364-2207	Antipsychotic
5607 <> DAN15	Tab, White, Round, Film Coated	Methyldopa 250 mg, Hydrochlorothiazide 15 mg	by Schein	00364-0827	Antihypertensive; Diuretic
5608 <> DAN25	Tab, White, Round, Film Coated	Methyldopa 250 mg, Hydrochlorothiazide 25 mg	by Schein	00364-0828	Antihypertensive; Diuretic
560HD	Tab, White, Oval	Ibuprofen 600 mg	Motrin by Halsey	Discontinued	NSAID
561 <> JSP	Tab, Green, Round, Scored	Levothyroxine Sodium 88 mcg	Synthroid by Lannett	00527-1344	Thyroid Hormone
561 <> JSP	Tab, Green, Round, Scored	Levothyroxine Sodium 88 mcg	Synthroid by Watson	52544-0905	Thyroid Hormone
5610 <> DAN50	Tab, White, Round, Film Coated, Scored	Methyldopa 500 mg, Hydrochlorothiazide 50 mg	by Schein	00364-2401	Antihypertensive; Diuretic
5611 <> DAN30	Tab, White, Round, Film Coated	Methyldopa 500 mg, Hydrochlorothiazide 30 mg	by Schein	00364-2400	Antihypertensive; Diuretic
5613 <> DAN03	Tab, Light Blue, Pentagonal, Scored, 5613 <> Dan 0.3	Clonidine HCl 0.3 mg	by Schein	00364-0824	Antihypertensive
5614DAN	Cap, Blue & White	Flurazepam HCl 15 mg	by Schein	00364-0801	Hypnotic; C IV
5615DAN	Cap, Blue	Flurazepam HCl 30 mg	by Schein	00364-0802	Hypnotic; C IV
5616DAN	Cap, Red	Oxazepam 15 mg	by Schein	00364-2152	Sedative/Hypnotic; C IV
5617DAN	Cap, White	Oxazepam 10 mg	by Schein	00364-2154	Sedative/Hypnotic; C IV
5618DAN	Cap, Maroon	Oxazepam 30 mg	by Schein	00364-2153	Sedative/Hypnotic; C IV
561HD	Tab, White, Oblong	Metoclopramide HCl 10 mg	Reglan by Halsey	Discontinued	Gastrointestinal
562 <> JSP	Tab, Pink, Round, Scored	Levothyroxine Sodium 112 mcg	Unithroid by Lannett	00527-1346	Thyroid Hormone
562 <> JSP	Tab, Pink, Round, Scored	Levothyroxine Sodium 112 mcg	Unithroid by Watson	52544-0907	Thyroid Hormone
5620 <> DAN10	Tab, Light Blue, Round, Scored	Diazepam 10 mg	by Schein	00364-0776	Antianxiety; C IV
5621 <> DAN2	Tab, White, Round, Scored	Diazepam 2 mg	by Schein	00364-0774	Antianxiety; C IV
5622 <> DAN2	Tab, White, Round, Scored	Lorazepam 2 mg	Ativan by Schein	00364-0795	Antianxiety; C IV
5623150MG	Cap, Yellow & White, Ivax Hourglass Logo 5623 on the cap and 150 mg on the body	Nizatidine 150 mg	Axid by Ivax	00172-5623	Gastrointestinal
				Discontinued	
5624 <> DAN1	Tab, White, Round, Scored	Lorazepam 1 mg	Ativan by Schein	00364-0794	Antianxiety; C IV
5624300MG	Cap, Brown & White, Ivax Hourglass Logo 5624 on the cap 300 mg on the body	Nizatidine 300 mg	Axid by Ivax	00172-5624	Gastrointestinal
				Discontinued	
5624DAN <> 1	Tab	Lorazepam 1 mg	Ativan by Quality Care	60346-0047	Antianxiety; C IV
5625 <> DAN05	Tab, White, Round, Scored, 5625 <> Dan 0.5	Lorazepam 0.5 mg	Ativan by Schein	00364-0793	Antianxiety; C IV
562HD	Tab, Peach, Round	Brompheniramine Maleate 4 mg	Dimetane by Halsey	Discontinued	Antihistamine
562MD	Tab, White, Round, Ex Release	Methylphenidate HCl 20 mg	Metadate ER by Medeva	53014-0594	Stimulant; C II
562MD	Tab, White, Round, Ex Release	Methylphenidate HCl 20 mg	Ritalin by MD	43667-0562	Stimulant; C II
562MD	Tab, White, Round, Ex Release	Methylphenidate HCl 20 mg	Ritalin by Caremark	00339-4099	Stimulant; C II
562MD	Tab, White, Round, Ex Release	Methylphenidate HCl 20 mg	Ritalin by Int'l Med Systems	00548-7029	Stimulant; C II
563 <> JSP	Tab, Purple, Round, Scored	Levothyroxine Sodium 175 mcg	Unithroid by Lannett	00527-1350	Thyroid Hormone

ID FRONT <> BACK	DESCRIPTION FRONT <> BACK	INGREDIENT & STRENGTH	BRAND (or Generic Equiv.) by FIRM	NDC#	CLASS; SCH.
563 <> JSP	Tab, Purple, Round, Scored	Levothyroxine Sodium 175 mcg	Unithroid by Watson	52544-0910	Thyroid Hormone
563 <> PLIVA	Tab, Yellow, Round, Film Coated	Cyclobenzaprine HCl 10 mg	Flexeril by Teva	00093-1919	Muscle Relaxant
563 <> PLIVA	Tab, Yellow, Round, Film Coated	Cyclobenzaprine HCl 10 mg	Flexeril by Pliva	50111-0563	Muscle Relaxant
563 <> SL	Tab, Yellow, Round, Film Coated	Cyclobenzaprine HCl 10 mg	Flexeril by URL Mutual	00677-1429	Muscle Relaxant
563 <> SL	Tab, Yellow, Round, Film Coated	Cyclobenzaprine HCl 10 mg	Flexeril by Warner Chilcott	00047-0057	Muscle Relaxant
563 <> SL	Tab, Yellow, Round, Film Coated	Cyclobenzaprine HCl 10 mg	Flexeril by Qualitest	00603-3077	Muscle Relaxant
563 <> SL	Tab, Yellow, Round, Film Coated	Cyclobenzaprine HCl 10 mg	Flexeril by Sidmak		Muscle Relaxant
5644 <> DAN	Tab, White, Oval, Film Coated	Ibuprofen 800 mg	Motrin by Schein	00364-2137	NSAID
5656 <> 10	Tab, White, Round	Tamoxifen Citrate 10 mg	Nolvadex by Ivax	00172-5656 Discontinued	Antiestrogen
5657 <> 20	Tab, White, Round	Tamoxifen Citrate 20 mg	Nolvadex by Ivax	00172-5657 Discontinued	Antiestrogen
5658 <> DAN	Tab, White, Round, Film Coated	Cyclobenzaprine HCl 10 mg	Flexeril by DJ Pharma	64455-0013	Muscle Relaxant
5658 <> DAN	Tab, White, Round, Film Coated	Cyclobenzaprine HCl 10 mg	Flexeril by Danbury	61955-2348	Muscle Relaxant
5658 <> DAN	Tab, White, Round, Film Coated	Cyclobenzaprine HCl 10 mg	Flexeril by Pharmedix	53002-0308	Muscle Relaxant
5658 <> DAN	Tab, White, Round, Film Coated	Cyclobenzaprine HCl 10 mg	Flexeril by Heartland	61392-0098	Muscle Relaxant
5658 <> DAN	Tab, White, Round, Film Coated	Cyclobenzaprine HCl 10 mg	Flexeril by Nat Pharmpak	55154-5217	Muscle Relaxant
5658 <> DAN	Tab, White, Round, Film Coated	Cyclobenzaprine HCl 10 mg	Flexeril by Schein	00364-2348	Muscle Relaxant
5658 <> DAN	Tab, White, Round, Film Coated	Cyclobenzaprine HCl 10 mg	Flexeril by Vangard	00615-3520	Muscle Relaxant
5658 <> DAN	Tab, White, Round, Film Coated	Cyclobenzaprine HCl 10 mg	Flexeril by Watson	00591-5658	Muscle Relaxant
5658 <> DAN	Tab, White, Round, Film Coated	Cyclobenzaprine HCl 10 mg	Flexeril by Southwood	58016-0234	Muscle Relaxant
5658 <> DAN	Tab, White, Round, Film Coated	Cyclobenzaprine HCl 10 mg	Flexeril by PDRX	55289-0567	Muscle Relaxant
5658 <> DAN	Tab, White, Round, Film Coated	Cyclobenzaprine HCl 10 mg	Flexeril by Amerisource	62584-0354	Muscle Relaxant
5658 <> DAN	Tab, White, Round, Film Coated	Cyclobenzaprine HCl 10 mg	Flexeril by Heartland	61392-0830	Muscle Relaxant
5659 <> DANDAN	Tab, White, Round, Scored	Furosemide 80 mg	by Schein	00364-0700	Diuretic
565HD05	Tab, White, Round, 565 HD 0.5	Lorazepam 0.5 mg	Ativan by Halsey	Discontinued	Antianxiety; C IV
5660 <> 60	Tab, Yellow, Round, Scored	Isosorbide Mononitrate 60 mg	Imdur by Ivax	00172-5660	Antianginal
5660 <> DANDAN	Tab, Yellow, Round, Scored	Sulindac 200 mg	Clinoril by Pharmedix	53002-0388	NSAID
5660 <> DANDAN	Tab, Yellow, Round, Scored	Sulindac 200 mg	Clinoril by Heartland	61392-0955	NSAID
5660 <> DANDAN	Tab, Yellow, Round, Scored	Sulindac 200 mg	Clinoril by H J Harkins Co	52959-0195	NSAID
5660 <> DANDAN	Tab, Yellow, Round, Scored	Sulindac 200 mg	Clinoril by Watson	00591-5660	NSAID
5660 <> DANDAN	Tab, Yellow, Round, Scored	Sulindac 200 mg	Clinoril by Schein	00364-2442	NSAID
5660 <> DANDAN	Tab, Yellow, Round, Scored	Sulindac 200 mg	Clinoril by PDRX	55289-0930	NSAID
5660 <> DANDAN	Tab, Yellow, Round, Scored	Sulindac 200 mg	Clinoril by St. Mary's Med	60760-0424	NSAID
5660 <> DANDAN	Tab, Yellow, Round, Scored	Sulindac 200 mg	Clinoril by St. Mary's Med	60760-0330	NSAID
5661 <> DAN	Tab, Yellow, Round	Sulindac 150 mg	Clinoril by Watson	00591-5661	NSAID
5661 <> DAN	Tab, Yellow, Round	Sulindac 150 mg	Clinoril by Schein	00364-2441	NSAID
5661 <> DAN	Tab, Yellow, Round	Sulindac 150 mg	Clinoril by Direct Dispensing	57866-4621	NSAID
5661 <> DAN	Tab, Yellow, Round	Sulindac 150 mg	Clinoril by St. Mary's Med	60760-0290	NSAID
5661 <> DAN	Tab, Yellow, Round	Sulindac 150 mg	Clinoril by Heartland	61392-0954	NSAID
5662 <> DAN	Tab, Off-White, Oval, Scored	Nalidixic Acid 1 g	by Schein	00364-2325	Antibiotic
5663 <> 5	Tab, White, Oval	Buspirone HCl 5 mg	BuSpar by Teva	00172-5663	Anxiolytic
5664 <> 10	Tab, White, Oval, Scored, Hourglass Logo over 10	Buspirone HCl 10 mg	BuSpar by Ivax	00172-5664	Antianxiety
5664 <> 5	Tab, White, Oval	Buspirone HCl 10 mg	BuSpar by Teva	00172-5664	Anxiolytic
5665 <> 555	Tab, White, Capsule Shaped, Scored	Buspirone HCl 15 mg	BuSpar by Teva	00172-5665	Anxiolytic
5665 <> 555	Tab, White, Cap Shaped, Scored, Hourglass Logo 5665	Buspirone HCl 15 mg	BuSpar by Ivax	00172-5665	Antianxiety
566HD	Tab, White, Round	Butalbital 50 mg, Aspirin 325 mg, Caffeine 40 mg	Fiorinal by Halsey	Discontinued	Analgesic; C III
567	Tab, White, Cap Shaped, Scored, Andrx Logo 567	Hydrocodone Bitartrate 10 mg, Acetaminophen 660 mg	Vicodin HP by Andrx	62037-0567	Analgesic; C III
567 <> HD	Tab	Acetaminophen 325 mg, Butalbital 50 mg, Caffeine 40 mg	Fioricet by Schein	00364-2297	Analgesic

ID FRONT <> BACK	DESCRIPTION FRONT <> BACK	INGREDIENT & STRENGTH	BRAND (or Generic Equiv.) by FIRM	NDC#	CLASS; SCH.
5672 <> 25	Tab, Blue, Round, Scored, Ivax Logo 25	Sertraline HCl 25 mg	Zoloft by Ivax	00172-5672 Discontinued	Antidepressant
5673 <> 50	Tab, Light Blue, Oval, Scored, Ivax Logo 50	Sertraline HCl 50 mg	Zoloft by Ivax	00172-5673 Discontinued	Antidepressant
5674 <> 100	Tab, Light Blue, Oblong, Scored, Ivax Logo 100	Sertraline HCl 100 mg	Zoloft by Ivax	00172-5674 Discontinued	Antidepressant
5675 <> 15	Tab, Yellow, Round, Hourglass Logo 5675 <> 15	Mirtazapine 15 mg	Remeron by Ivax	00172-5675 Discontinued	Antidepressant
5676 <> 30	Tab, Tan, Round, Hourglass Logo 5676 <> 30	Mirtazapine 30 mg	Remeron by Ivax	00172-5676 Discontinued	Antidepressant
5677 <> DANDAN	Tab, Off-White, Round, Scored	Nalidixic Acid 500 mg	by Schein	00364-2324	Antibiotic
5678 <> DAN	Tab, White, Round, Film Coated	Amitriptyline 25 mg, Chlordiazepoxide 10 mg	Limbitrol by Schein	00364-2158	Antianxiety; C IV
5679 <> DAN	Tab, Light Green, Round, Film Coated	Amitriptyline 12.5 mg, Chlordiazepoxide 5 mg	Limbitrol by Schein	00364-2157	Antianxiety; C IV
568100MG	Cap, White, Opaque, Black Ink	Vorinostat 100 mg	Zolinza by Merck	00006-0568	Cancer Treatment
5695 <> 45	Tab, White, Round, Hourglass Logo 5695 <> 45	Mirtazapine 45 mg	Remeron by Ivax	00172-5695 Discontinued	Antidepressant
5696DANPRAZOSIN	Cap, Dark Gray, Opaque	Prazosin HCl 2 mg	by Schein	00364-2390	Antihypertensive
5697DANPRAZOSIN	Cap, Yellow, Opaque	Prazosin HCl 1 mg	by Schein	00364-2389	Antihypertensive
57	Cap, Maroon, Oval, Soft Gel	Docusate Sodium 100 mg, Casanthranol 30 mg	Peri-Colace by Ivax	00182-0150	Laxative
57	Tab, White, Oblong, Boots Logo	Aspirin 800 mg	ZORprin by Par	49884-0657	Analgesic
57 <> 93	Tab, Light Pink to Brick, Cap Shaped, Film Coated, Scored, 9/3	Fluvoxamine Maleate 100 mg	Luvox by Teva	00093-0057	OCD
57 <> C	Tab, White to Off-White, Round	Amlodipine Besylate 2.5 mg	Norvasc by Aurobindo	65862-0101	Antihypertensive
57 <> D	Tab, White to Off White, Round, Scored	Perindopril Erbumine 2 mg	Aceon by Aurobindo	65862-0286	Antihypertensive
57 <> LOTENSINHCT	Tab, White, Oblong, Coated	Benazepril HCl 5 mg, Hydrochlorothiazide 6.25 mg	Lotensin HCT by Novartis	00078-0451	Antihypertensive; Diuretic
57 <> LOTENSINHCT	Tab, White, Oblong, Scored	Benazepril HCl 5 mg, Hydrochlorothiazide 6.25 mg	Lotensin HCT by Novartis	00083-0057	Antihypertensive; Diuretic
57 <> M	Tab, White, Oblong, Scored	Sucralfate 1000 mg	by Warrick	59930-1532	Gastrointestinal
57 <> M	Tab, Round	Sucralfate 1000 mg	by Merckle	58107-0001	Gastrointestinal
57 <> R	Tab, White, Round, Scored, Coated	Lorazepam 0.5 mg	Ativan by Mylan	55160-0130	Antianxiety; C IV
57 <> R	Tab, White, Round, Scored, Coated	Lorazepam 0.5 mg	Ativan by Actavis	00228-2057	Antianxiety; C IV
57 <> R	Tab, White, Round, Scored, Coated	Lorazepam 0.5 mg	Ativan by Nat Pharmpak	55154-1116	Antianxiety; C IV
57 <> R	Tab, White, Round, Scored, Coated	Lorazepam 0.5 mg	Ativan by Kaiser	00179-1174	Antianxiety; C IV
570 <> DP	Tab, White, Round	Inert	Ortho-Cept by Barr	00555-9043	Oral Contraceptive; Placebo
570 <> DP	Tab, White, Round	Inert	Apri 28 Day by Duramed	51285-0576	Oral Contraceptive; Placebo
5704 <> DANDAN	Tab, White, Cap Shaped, Film Coated, Scored	Fenoprofen Calcium 600 mg	by Schein	00364-2316	NSAID
5706 <> DAN500	Tab, Light Green, Round, Scored	Chlorzoxazone 500 mg	by Schein	00364-2255	Muscle Relaxant
571 <> 500	Tab, White to Off-White, Cap Shaped, Ex Release, Andrx Logo	Metformin HCl 500 mg	Glucophage XR by Andrx	62037-0571	Antidiabetic
571 <> R	Tab, White, Round, Coated	Indapamide 2.5 mg	Lozol by Caremark	00339-6183	Diuretic
571 <> R	Tab, White, Round, Film Coated	Indapamide 2.5 mg	Lozol by Actavis	00228-2571	Diuretic
5710 <> 125250	Tab, Light Yellow, Oval, Ivax Logo 5710 <> 1.25/250	Glyburide 1.25 mg, Metformin 250 mg	Glucovance by Ivax	00172-5710 Discontinued	Antidiabetic
5710 <> 125250	Tab, Light Yellow, Oval, Ivax Logo 5710 <> 1.25/250	Glyburide 1.25 mg, Metformin 250 mg	Glucovance by Teva	00093-5710 Discontinued	Antidiabetic
5710 <> DAN2	Tab, White, Round, Scored	Albuterol Sulfate 2 mg	Proventil by Schein	00364-2438	Antiasthmatic
5711 <> 25500	Tab, Light Orange, Oval, Ivax Logo 5711 <> 2.5/500	Glyburide 2.5 mg, Metformin 500 mg	Glucovance by Teva	00093-5711	Antiasthmatic
5711 <> DAN4	Tab, White, Round, Scored	Albuterol Sulfate 4 mg	Proventil by Schein	00364-2439	Antiasthmatic
5712 <> 5500	Tab, Yellow, Oval, Ivax Logo 5712 <> 5/500	Glyburide 5 mg, Metformin 500 mg	Glucovance by Ivax	00172-5712 Discontinued	Antidiabetic

ID FRONT <> BACK	DESCRIPTION FRONT <> BACK	INGREDIENT & STRENGTH	BRAND (or Generic Equiv.) by FIRM	NDC#	CLASS; SCH.
5712 <> 5500	Tab, Yellow, Oval, Ivax Logo 5712 <> 5/500	Glyburide 5 mg, Metformin 500 mg	Glucovance by Teva	00093-5712	Antidiabetic
5713 <> DAN25	Tab, White, Round, Scored	Amoxapine 25 mg	Asendin by Schein	00364-2432	Antidepressant
5713 <> DAN25	Tab, White, Round, Scored	Amoxapine 25 mg	Asendin by Watson	00591-5713	Antidepressant
5714 <> DAN50	Tab, Red, Round, Scored, DAN over 50	Amoxapine 50 mg	Asendin by Schein	00364-2433	Antidepressant
5714 <> DAN50	Tab, Red, Round, Scored, DAN over 50	Amoxapine 50 mg	Asendin by Watson	00591-5714	Antidepressant
5715 <> DAN100	Tab, Blue, Round, Scored, DAN over 100	Amoxapine 100 mg	Asendin by Watson	00591-5715	Antidepressant
5715 <> DAN100	Tab, Blue, Round, Scored, DAN over 100	Amoxapine 100 mg	Asendin by Schein	00364-2434	Antidepressant
5715 <> TEVA	Tab, White to Off-White, Cap Shaped, Chewable	Lamotrigine 5 mg	Lamictal by Teva	00093-5715 Discontinued	Anticonvulsant
5716 <> DAN150	Tab, Orange, Round, Scored	Amoxapine 150 mg	Asendin by Schein	00364-2435	Antidepressant
5716 <> DAN150	Tab, Orange, Round, Scored	Amoxapine 150 mg	Asendin by Watson	00591-5716	Antidepressant
5716 <> TEVA	Tab, White, Elliptical, Chewable, 57 over 16	Lamotrigine 25 mg	Lamictal by Teva	00093-5716 Discontinued	Anticonvulsant
572	Tab, 572 <> Barr Logo	Methotrexate 2.5 mg	Rheumatrex by Qualitest	00603-4499	Antineoplastic
572	Tab, 572 <> Barr Logo	Methotrexate 2.5 mg	Rheumatrex by URL Mutual	00677-1610	Antineoplastic
5721DAN	Cap, Flesh & Pink	Fenoprofen Calcium 300 mg	by Schein	00364-2315	NSAID
5724 <> DAN10	Tab, White, Round, Scored	Metaproterenol Sulfate 10 mg	by Schein	00364-2283	Antiasthmatic
5725 <> DAN20	Tab, White, Round, Scored	Metaproterenol Sulfate 20 mg	by Schein	00364-2284	Antiasthmatic
5725RUGBY	Cap, White and Light Blue, Opaque	Acyclovir 200 mg	Zovirax by Rugby	00536-5725 Discontinued	Antiviral
5728 <> 20	Tab, Beige, Round, Hourglass Logo 20	Famotidine 20 mg	Pepcid by Ivax	00172-5728	Gastrointestinal
5728 <> 20	Tab, Beige, Round	Famotidine 20 mg	Pepcid by Teva	00172-5728	Histamine H2 Antagonist
5729 <> 40	Tab, Beige, Round	Famotidine 40 mg	Pepcid by Teva	00172-5729	Histamine H2 Antagonist
5729 <> 40	Tab, Tan, Round, Hourglass 40	Famotidine 40 mg	Pepcid by Ivax	00172-5729	Gastrointestinal
572HD1	Tab, White, Round	Lorazepam 1 mg	Ativan by Halsey	Discontinued	Antianxiety; C IV
573 <> PROVENTIL4	Tab, White, Film Coated	Albuterol Sulfate 4 mg	Proventil by PDRX	55289-0634	Antiasthmatic
573 <> PROVENTIL4	Tab, White, Film Coated	Albuterol Sulfate 4 mg	Proventil by Amerisource	62584-0463	Antiasthmatic
5731	Tab, Pink, Round	Bisoprolol 5 mg, Hydrochlorothiazide 6.25 mg	Ziac by Zenith	00172-5731	Antihypertensive; Diuretic
5732 <> 10	Tab, White, Round, 5732 <> Hourglass Logo 10	Bisoprolol 10 mg, Hydrochlorothiazide 6.25 mg	Ziac by Ivax	00172-5732	Antihypertensive; Diuretic
5732 <> 25	Tab, Yellow, Round, 5732 <> Hourglass Logo 2.5	Bisoprolol 2.5 mg, Hydrochlorothiazide 6.25 mg	Ziac by Ivax	00172-5730	Antihypertensive; Diuretic
5732 <> 5	Tab, Pink, Round, 5732 <> Hourglass Logo 5	Bisoprolol 5 mg, Hydrochlorothiazide 6.25 mg	Ziac by Ivax	00172-5731	Antihypertensive; Diuretic
57344 <> 033	Tab, White, Oblong	Diphenhydramine HCl 50 mg	by AAA		Antihistamine
573573 <> PROVENTIL4	Tab, Off-White, Round, 573/573 <> Proventil 4	Albuterol Sulfate 4 mg	Proventil by Schering	00085-0573	Antiasthmatic
5736 <> DAN5	Tab, White, Round	Timolol Maleate 5 mg	by Schein	00364-2357	Antihypertensive
5737 <> DAN10	Tab, White, Round, Scored	Timolol Maleate 10 mg	Blocadren by Schein	00364-2358	Antihypertensive
5738 <> DAN20	Tab, White, Cap Shaped, Scored	Timolol Maleate 20 mg	Blocadren by Schein	00364-2359	Antihypertensive
573HD2	Tab, White, Round	Lorazepam 2 mg	Ativan by Halsey	Discontinued	Antianxiety; C IV
574	Tab, White, Biconvex, Film Coated, Extended Release, Andrx Logo 574	Metformin HCl 500 mg	Fortamet by Andrx	62022-0574	Antidiabetic
574 <> MYLAN	Tab, Orange, Round, Film Coated	Amitriptyline 25 mg, Perphenazine 4 mg	Triavil by Mylan	00378-0574	Antidepressant; Antipsychotic
574HD	Tab, White, Oblong	Acetaminophen 500 mg, Hydrocodone Bitartrate 5 mg	Vicodin by Halsey	Discontinued	Analgesic; C III
575	Tab, White, Biconvex, Film Coated, Extended Release, Andrx Logo 575	Metformin HCl 1000 mg	Fortamet by Andrx	62022-0575	Antidiabetic
575	Tab, Light Pink, Cap Shaped, Film Coated	Sitagliptin 50 mg, Metformin HCl 500 mg	Janumet by Merck	00006-0575	Antidiabetic
575 <> DP	Tab, Rose, Round	Desogestrel 0.15 mg, Ethinyl Estradiol 0.03 mg	Ortho-Cept by Barr	00555-9043	Oral Contraceptive
575 <> DP	Tab, Rose, Round	Desogestrel 0.15 mg, Ethinyl Estradiol 0.03 mg	Ortho-Cept by Allscripts		Oral Contraceptive
5751V	Tab, Tan, Oval	Chlorpheniramine Tannate 8 mg, Phenylephrine Tannate 25 mg, Pyrilamine Tannate 25 mg	by Vintage		Cold Remedy
5755 <> M	Tab, White, Rectangle Shaped, Scored, M inside of Box	Methadone HCl 5 mg	Dolophine by Mallinckrodt	00406-5755	Analgesic; C II

ID FRONT <> BACK	DESCRIPTION FRONT <> BACK	INGREDIENT & STRENGTH	BRAND (or Generic Equiv.) by FIRM	NDC#	CLASS; SCH.
576 <> 93	Tab, Blue, Round	Lovastatin 20 mg	Mevacor by Teva	00093-0576	Antihyperlipidemic
57693	Tab, Light Blue, Round	Lovastatin 20 mg	Mevacor by Teva	00093-0576	Antihyperlipidemic
577	Tab, Red, Cap Shaped, Film Coated	Sitagliptin 50 mg, Metformin HCl 1000 mg	Janumet by Merck	00006-0577	Antidiabetic
577 <> 750	Tab, Light Yellow, Cap Shaped, Ex Release, Andrx Logo	Metformin HCl 750 mg	Glucophage XR by Andrx	62037-0577	Antidiabetic
5770 <> BMS	Tab, Coated, Mottled	Diltiazem HCl 90 mg	Cardizem by BMS	00093-5770 Discontinued	Antihypertensive
5771 <> M	Tab, White, Rectangle Shaped, Scored, Box around "M"	Methadone HCl 10 mg	Dolophine by Mallinckrodt	00406-5771	Analgesic; C II
5777 <> DAN50	Tab, White, Round, Scored	Atenolol 50 mg	Tenormin by Schein	00364-2513	Antihypertensive
5777 <> DAN50	Tab, White, Round, Scored	Atenolol 50 mg	Tenormin by Watson	00591-5777	Antihypertensive
5777 <> DAN50	Tab, White, Round, Scored	Atenolol 50 mg	Tenormin by Nat Pharmpak	55154-5211	Antihypertensive
5777 <> DAN50	Tab, White, Round, Scored	Atenolol 50 mg	Tenormin by Danbury	61955-2513	Antihypertensive
5778 <> DAN100	Tab, White, Round	Atenolol 100 mg	Tenormin by Danbury	61955-2514	Antihypertensive
5778 <> DAN100	Tab, White, Round	Atenolol 100 mg	Tenormin by Watson	00591-5778	Antihypertensive
5778 <> DAN100	Tab, White, Round	Atenolol 100 mg	Tenormin by Schein	00364-2514	Antihypertensive
58	Tab, Green, Elongated, Boots Logo 58	Atropine 0.04 mg, Chlorpheniramine 8 mg, Hyoscyamine 0.19 mg, Phenylephrine 25 mg, Phenylpropanolamine 50 mg, Scopolamine 0.01 mg	Ru-Tuss by Eon		Cold Remedy
58 <> 93	Tab, White, Oval	Tramadol HCl 50 mg	Ultram by Teva	00093-0058	Analgesic
58 <> C	Tab, White to Off-White, Barrel-Shaped	Amlodipine Besylate 5 mg	Norvasc by Aurobindo	65862-0102	Antihypertensive
58 <> D	Tab, White to Off White, Cap Shaped, Scored	Perindopril Erbumine 4 mg	Aceon by Aurobindo	65862-0287	Antihypertensive
58 <> G	Tab, White to Off White, Round	Amlodipine Besylate 2.5 mg	Norvasc by Glenmark	68462-0210	Antihypertensive
581 <> WC	Tab, White, Round, Scored, W/C	Ethinyl Estradiol 0.035 mg, Norethindrone 0.4 mg	Ovcon 35 by Warner Chilcott	00430-0582	Oral Contraceptive
5811V	Tab, Film Coated, 5811/V	Salsalate 500 mg	by Vintage	00254-5811	NSAID
5812 <> V	Tab, Turquoise, Coated, Scored, 58 to Left 12 to Right over V	Salsalate 750 mg	Disalcid by Vintage	00254-5812	NSAID
5812 <> V	Tab, Turquoise, Coated, Scored, 58 to Left 12 to Right over V	Salsalate 750 mg	Disalcid by Quality Care	60346-0034	NSAID
5812 <> V	Tab, Turquoise, Coated, Scored, 58 to Left 12 to Right over V	Salsalate 750 mg	Disalcid by Qualitest	00603-5755	NSAID
5812 <> V	Tab, Turquoise, Coated, Scored, 58 to Left 12 to Right over V	Salsalate 750 mg	Disalcid by Vintage	00254-5812	NSAID
5812 <> V	Tab, Turquoise, Coated, Scored, 58 to Left 12 to Right over V	Salsalate 750 mg	Disalcid by Quality Care	60346-0034	NSAID
5814 <> 59911	Tab, White, Oval	Metoclopramide 5 mg	Reglan by ESI Lederle	59911-5814	Gastrointestinal
5814 <> 59911	Tab, White, Oval, Scored	Metoclopramide 5 mg	Reglan by A H Robins	00031-5814	Gastrointestinal
5815 <> 59911	Tab, White, Oblong, Scored	Metoclopramide 10 mg	Reglan by ESI Lederle	59911-5815	Gastrointestinal
5815 <> 59911	Tab, White, Oblong, Scored	Metoclopramide 10 mg	Reglan by A H Robins	00031-5815	Gastrointestinal
5816 <> DAN250	Tab, Green, Round	Naproxen 250 mg	Naprosyn by Watson	00591-5816	NSAID
5816 <> DAN250	Tab, Green, Round	Naproxen 250 mg	Naprosyn by Schein	00364-2562	NSAID
5817 <> DAN375	Tab, Lavender, Cap Shaped	Naproxen 375 mg	Naprosyn by Schein	00364-2563	NSAID
5817 <> DAN375	Tab, Purple, Oblong	Naproxen 375 mg	Naprosyn by Watson	00591-5817	NSAID
5818 <> DAN500	Tab, Light Green, Cap Shaped	Naproxen 500 mg	Naprosyn by Watson	00591-5818	NSAID
5818 <> DAN500	Tab, Light Green, Cap Shaped	Naproxen 500 mg	Naprosyn by Schein	00364-2564	NSAID
581HD	Tab, White, Round	Acetaminophen 500 mg	Tylenol Ex Strength by Halsey	Discontinued	Analgesic
5825	Tab, Light Blue, Round, Film Coated, Hourglass Logo <> 5825	Finasteride 5 mg	Proscar by Teva	00093-5825	Antiandrogen
582HD	Tab, White, Round	Quinidine Gluconate 324 mg	Quinaglute by Halsey	Discontinued	Antiarrhythmic
583 <> MJ	Tab, White, Peach, Round	Ethinyl Estradiol 0.035 mg, Norethindrone 0.4 mg	Ovcon 35 21 by Warner Chilcott	00430-0583	Oral Contraceptive
583 <> MJ	Tab, White, Peach, Round	Ethinyl Estradiol 0.035 mg, Norethindrone 0.4 mg	Ovcon 35 21 by BMS	00087-0583	Oral Contraceptive
583 <> MJ	Tab, White, Peach, Round	Ethinyl Estradiol 0.035 mg, Norethindrone 0.4 mg	Ovcon 35 21 by Physician Total Care	54868-0509	Oral Contraceptive
584 <> MJ	Tab, Yellow, Round	Ethinyl Estradiol 0.05 mg, Norethindrone 1 mg	Ovcon 50 28 by BMS	00087-0579	Oral Contraceptive
584 <> MJ	Tab, Yellow, Round	Ethinyl Estradiol 0.05 mg, Norethindrone 1 mg	Ovcon 50 28 by Physician Total Care	54868-3772	Oral Contraceptive

ID FRONT <> BACK	DESCRIPTION FRONT <> BACK	INGREDIENT & STRENGTH	BRAND (or Generic Equiv.) by FIRM	NDC#	CLASS; SCH.
584 <> MJ	Tab, Yellow, Round	Ethinyl Estradiol 0.05 mg, Norethindrone 1 mg	Ovcon 50 28 by BMS	15548-0579	Oral Contraceptive
584 <> MJ	Tab, Round, Yellow	Ethinyl Estradiol 0.05 mg, Norethindrone 1 mg	Ovcon 50 28 by Warner Chilcott	00430-0585	Oral Contraceptive
5840 <> 59911	Tab, White, Diamond Shaped	Guanfacine HCl 1 mg	Tenex by ESI Lederle	59911-5840	Antihypertensive
5840 <> 59911	Tab, White, Coated	Guanfacine HCl 1.15 mg	Tenex by A H Robins	00031-5840	Antihypertensive
5841 <> 100	Tab, White, Round, Ivax Logo 100 <> 5841	Cilostazol 100 mg	Pletal by Ivax	00172-5841 Discontinued	Antiplatelet
5841 <> 59911	Tab, Yellow, Diamond Shaped	Guanfacine HCl 2 mg	Tenex by ESI Lederle	59911-5841	Antihypertensive
5841 <> 59911	Tab, Light Yellow, Coated	Guanfacine HCl 2.3 mg	Tenex by A H Robins	00031-5841	Antihypertensive
584259911	Cap, Blue & Pink	Acebutolol HCl 200 mg	Sectral by ESI Lederle	59911-5842	Antihypertensive
584BARR	Cap, Clear & Green	Erythromycin 250 mg	by Murfreesboro	51129-1392	Antibiotic
5850 <> BMS	Tab, Coated, Mottled	Diltiazem HCl 120 mg	Cardizem by BMS	00003-5850 Discontinued	Antihypertensive
58552PROTECTPLUSNR	Cap, Purple, Softgel	Coenzyme Q10 30 mg, Alpha-Lipoic Acid 40 mg, Vitamin E 400 IU, Beta Carotene 5,000 IU, Vitamin A 5,000 IU, Vitamin C 500 mg, Vitamin D 400 IU, Grape Seed Extract 500 mcg, Superoxide Dismutase 500 mcg, L-Glutathione 30 mg, Vanadium 50 mcg, Chromium 200 mcg	Protect Plus NR by Gil Pharma	58552-0309	Vitamin
5858 <> DAN50	Tab, White, Round, Scored	Captopril 50 mg	Capoten by Schein	00364-2630	Antihypertensive
5859 <> DAN100	Tab, White, Round, Quadrisected	Captopril 100 mg	Capoten by Schein	00364-2631	Antihypertensive
5871 <> 59911	Tab, White, Scored	Promethazine HCl 12.5 mg	Phenergan by Wyeth	52903-5871	Antiemetic; Antihistamine
5871 <> 59911	Tab, White, Scored	Promethazine HCl 12.5 mg	Phenergan by ESI Lederle	59911-5871	Antiemetic; Antihistamine
5872 <> 59911	Tab, White, Scored	Promethazine HCl 25 mg	Phenergan by Wyeth	52903-5872	Antiemetic; Antihistamine
5872 <> 59911	Tab, White, Scored	Promethazine HCl 25 mg	Phenergan by ESI Lederle	59911-5872	Antiemetic; Antihistamine
5873 <> 59911	Tab, White, Scored	Promethazine HCl 50 mg	Phenergan by Wyeth	52903-5873	Antiemetic; Antihistamine
5873 <> 59911	Tab, White, Scored	Promethazine HCl 50 mg	Phenergan by ESI Lederle	59911-5873	Antiemetic; Antihistamine
5875 <> V	Tab, Light Blue, Oval	Sotalol 80 mg	Betapace by Vintage	00254-5875	Antiarrhythmic
5876 <> V	Tab, Light Blue, Oval	Sotalol 120 mg	Betapace by Vintage	00254-5876	Antiarrhythmic
5876 <> V	Tab, Blue, Oval	Sotalol HCl 120 mg	Betapace by Qualitest	00603-5770	Antiarrhythmic
5877 <> V	Tab, Light Blue, Oval	Sotalol 160 mg	Betapace by Vintage	00254-5877	Antiarrhythmic
5878 <> V	Tab, Light Blue, Oval	Sotalol 240 mg	Betapace by Vintage	00254-5878	Antiarrhythmic
5880 <> V	Tab, White, Round, Film-Coated	Spironolactone 25 mg	Aldactone by Vintage	00254-5880	Diuretic
5881 <> V	Tab, White, Oval, Scored, Film-Coated	Spironolactone 50 mg	Aldactone by Vintage	00254-5881	Diuretic
5882 <> DAN5	Tab, Light Purple, Round	Methylphenidate HCl 5 mg	Ritalin by Watson	00591-5882	Stimulant; C II
5882 <> DAN5	Tab, Light Purple, Round	Methylphenidate HCl 5 mg	Ritalin by Schein	00364-0561	Stimulant; C II
5882 <> V	Tab, White, Round, Scored, Film-Coated	Spironolactone 100 mg	Aldactone by Vintage	00254-5882	Diuretic
5883 <> DAN10	Tab, Light Green, Round, Scored	Methylphenidate HCl 10 mg	Ritalin by Schein	00364-0479	Stimulant; C II
5883 <> DAN10	Tab, Light Green, Round, Scored	Methylphenidate HCl 10 mg	Ritalin by Watson	00591-5883	Stimulant; C II
5884 <> DAN20	Tab, Peach, Round, Scored	Methylphenidate HCl 20 mg	Ritalin by Watson	00591-5884	Stimulant; C II
5884 <> DAN20	Tab, Peach, Round, Scored	Methylphenidate HCl 20 mg	Ritalin by Schein	00364-0562	Stimulant; C II
5895 <> 59911	Tab, White, Ex Release, Scored	Quinidine Sulfate 300 mg	by A H Robins	00031-5895	Antiarrhythmic
5897 <> V	Tab, White to Off-White, Round, Scored	Sulfamethoxazole 400 mg, Trimethoprim 80 mg	Bactrim by Vintage	00254-5897	Antibiotic
5898 <> V	Tab, White to Off-White, Oval, Scored	Sulfamethoxazole 800 mg, Trimethoprim 160 mg	Bactrim DS by Vintage	00254-5898	Antibiotic
589959911	Cap, White, Ex Release	Potassium Chloride 750 mg	by A H Robins	00031-5899	Electrolytes
58P	Cap, Maroon, Soft Gel	Docusate Sodium 100 mg, Casanthranol 30 mg	Peri-colace by Ivax	00182-1418	Laxative
59 <> 59	Tab, Wyeth	Penicillin V Potassium	Pen Vee K by Casa DeAmigos	62138-0059	Antibiotic
59 <> C	Tab, White to Off-White, Round	Amlodipine Besylate 10 mg	Norvasc by Aurobindo	65862-0103	Antihypertensive
59 <> D	Tab, White to Off White, Round, Scored	Perindopril Erbumine 8 mg	Aceon by Aurobindo	65862-0288	Antihypertensive
59 <> R	Tab, White, Round, Scored	Lorazepam 1 mg	Ativan by Nat Pharmpak	55154-1115	Antianxiety; C IV
59 <> R	Tab, White, Round, Scored	Lorazepam 1 mg	Ativan by Actavis	00228-2059	Antianxiety; C IV
59 <> R	Tab, White, Round, Scored	Lorazepam 1 mg	Ativan by Golden State	60429-0512	Antianxiety; C IV
59 <> R	Tab, White, Round, Scored	Lorazepam 1 mg	Ativan by Mylan	55160-0131	Antianxiety; C IV

ID FRONT <> BACK	DESCRIPTION FRONT <> BACK	INGREDIENT & STRENGTH	BRAND (or Generic Equiv.) by FIRM	NDC#	CLASS; SCH.
59 <> WYETH	Tab, White, Round, Scored	Penicillin V Potassium	by Kaiser	00179-0081	Antibiotic
59 <> WYETH	Tab, White, Round, Scored	Penicillin V Potassium	by Wyeth	00008-0059	Antibiotic
59 <> WYETH	Tab, White, Round, Scored	Penicillin V Potassium	by Med Pro	53978-5042	Antibiotic
59010240	Tab, Light Blue, Cap Shaped, Scored	Acetaminophen 650 mg, Butalbital 50 mg	Bupap by ECR	00095-0240	Analgesic
59010240	Tab, Light Blue, Cap Shaped, Scored	Acetaminophen 650 mg, Butalbital 50 mg	Bupap by Mikart	46672-0098	Analgesic
5904V	Tab, Round, Gold, Scored	Sulfasalazine 500 mg	Azulfidine by Vintage	00254-5904	Gastrointestinal
5905 <> V	Tab, Gold, Oval, Enteric Coated	Sulfasalazine EC 500 mg	Sulfazine by Vintage	00254-5905	Gastrointestinal
5905 <> V	Tab, Gold, Oval, Enteric Coated	Sulfasalazine EC 500 mg	Sulfazine by Qualitest	00603-5803	Gastrointestinal
591 <> G	Tab, Blue Round	Pilocarpine HCl 7.5 mg	Salagen by Global	00115-5911	Cholinergic Agonist
5912 <> DAN	Tab, Blue, Oval, Scored	Captopril 50 mg, HCTZ 25 mg	Capozide by Schein	00364-2640	Antihypertensive; Diuretic
591A	Tab, White, Round, Scored, 591-A	Meprobamate 400 mg	Miltown by Schein	00364-0161	Sedative/Hypnotic; C IV
591A	Tab, White, Round, Scored, 591-A	Meprobamate 400 mg	Miltown by Watson	00591-5238	Sedative/Hypnotic; C IV
591B	Tab, White, Round, Scored, 591-B	Meprobamate 200 mg	Miltown by Watson	00591-5239	Sedative/Hypnotic; C IV
591B	Tab, White, Round, Scored, 591-B	Meprobamate 200 mg	Miltown by Schein	00364-0160	Sedative/Hypnotic; C IV
591C	Tab, White, Round, 591 - C	Phenobarbital 15 mg	Phenobarbital by Danbury		Sedative/Hypnotic; C IV
591D	Tab, White, Round, 591 - D	Phenobarbital 30 mg	by Danbury		Sedative/Hypnotic; C IV
591F	Tab, White, Round, 591-F	Acetaminophen 325 mg, Butalbital 50 mg, Caffeine 40 mg	Fioricet by Danbury		Analgesic
591O	Tab, White, Round, 591 - O	Phenobarbital 100 mg	Phenobarbital by Danbury		Sedative/Hypnotic; C IV
591V	Tab, White, Round, 591 - V	Phenobarbital 60 mg	by Danbury		Sedative/Hypnotic; C IV
592 <> G	Tab, White, Round	Pilocarpine HCl 5 mg	Salagen by Global	00115-5922	Cholinergic Agonist
593 <> M	Tab, White, Round, M inside Square, Extended Release	Oxycodone HCl 10 mg	OxyContin by Mallinckrodt	00406-0593	Analgesic; C II
594	Tab, White, Round, Scored, with an A shaped Logo above the 594	Tizanidine HCl 4 mg	Zanaflex by Athena		Muscle Relaxant
594 <> M	Tab, Pink, Round, M inside Square	Oxycodone HCl 20 mg	Oxycodone by Mallinckrodt	00406-0594	Analgesic; C II
595 <> M	Tab, Yellow, Round, M inside square, Ex Release	Oxycodone HCl 40 mg	OxyContin by Mallinckrodt	00406-0595	Analgesic; C II
596 <> M	Tab, Green, Round, M inside Square, Extended Release	Oxycodone HCl 80 mg	OxyContin by Mallinckrodt	00406-0596	Analgesic; C II
597 <> R	Tab, Orange, Round, Film Coated	Indapamide 1.25 mg	Lozol by Caremark	00339-6182	Diuretic
597 <> R	Tab, Orange, Round, Film Coated	Indapamide 1.25 mg	Lozol by Actavis	00228-2597	Diuretic
5971V	Tab, White, Round, Scored, 5971 over V	Trihexyphenidyl 2 mg	Artane by Qualitest	00603-6240	Antiparkinson
5971V	Tab, White, Round, Scored, 5971 over V	Trihexyphenidyl 2 mg	Artane by Vintage	00254-5971	Antiparkinson
5971V	Tab, White, Round, Scored, 5971 over V	Trihexyphenidyl 2 mg	Artane by Richmond	54738-0554	Antiparkinson
5972V	Tab, White, Round, Scored, 5972 over V	Trihexyphenidyl 5 mg	Artane by Vintage	00254-5972	Antiparkinson
59743002	Cap, White & Clear, Black Print, Opaque, Hard Gel	Guaifenesin 250 mg, Pseudoephedrine 120 mg	Sudafed Sinus by Alphagen	59743-0002	Cold Remedy
59743002	Cap, White & Clear, Black Print, Opaque, Hard Gel	Guaifenesin 250 mg, Pseudoephedrine HCl 120 mg	Sudafed Sinus by Pharmafab	62542-0451	Cold Remedy
59743003	Cap, Blue & Clear, Black Print, Hard Gel	Guaifenesin 300 mg, Pseudoephedrine HCl 60 mg	Deconamine SR by Pharmafab	62542-0402	Cold Remedy
59743003	Cap, Blue & Clear, Black Print, Hard Gel	Guaifenesin 300 mg, Pseudoephedrine 60 mg	Sudafed Sinus by Alphagen	59743-0003	Cold Remedy
59743004	Cap, White, Green Print, Hard Gel	Acetaminophen 325 mg, Butalbital 50 mg, Caffeine 40 mg	Fioricet by Alphagen	59743-0004	Analgesic
59743011	Cap, in White Ink	Acetaminophen 500 mg, Hydrocodone Bitartrate 5 mg	Vicodin by Alphagen	59743-0011	Analgesic; C III
59743018	Tab, Green, Cap Shaped	Guaifenesin 600 mg	Robitussin by Alphagen	59743-0018	Expectorant
59743050	Tab, 59743 over 050	Guaifenesin 600 mg, Pseudoephedrine HCl 60 mg	Desal II by Pharmafab	62542-0740	Cold Remedy
59743053	Cap, Blue & Clear, Black Print	Chlorpheniramine Maleate 8 mg, Pseudoephedrine HCl 120 mg	Deconamine SR by Pharmafab	62542-0251	Cold Remedy
59743053	Cap, Blue & Clear, Black Print	Chlorpheniramine Maleate 8 mg, Pseudoephedrine HCl 120 mg	Deconamine SR by Alphagen	59743-0061	Cold Remedy
59743054	Cap, Green, Cap Shaped, Scored	Dextromethorphan 30 mg, Guaifenesin 600 mg	Humibid-DM by Alphagen	59743-0054	Cold Remedy
59743054	Cap, Green, Cap Shaped, Scored	Dextromethorphan 30 mg, Guaifenesin 600 mg	Humibid-DM by Pharmafab	62542-0720	Cold Remedy
59743060	Cap, Light Green & Clear	Brompheniramine Maleate 12 mg, Pseudoephedrine HCl 120 mg	Bromfed by Pharmafab	62542-0153	Cold Remedy
59743060	Cap, Light Green & Clear	Brompheniramine Maleate 12 mg, Pseudoephedrine HCl 120 mg	Bromfed by Alphagen	59743-0060	Cold Remedy
59743060	Cap, Light Green & Clear	Brompheniramine Maleate 6 mg, Pseudoephedrine HCl 60 mg	Bromfed by Qualitest	00603-2505	Cold Remedy
59743060	Cap, Light Green & Clear	Brompheniramine Maleate 6 mg, Pseudoephedrine HCl 60 mg	Bromfed by Ivax	00182-1053	Cold Remedy
59743061	Cap, Dark Green & Clear	Brompheniramine Maleate 6 mg, Pseudoephedrine HCl 60 mg	Bromfed PD by Pharmafab	62542-0103	Cold Remedy

ID FRONT <> BACK	DESCRIPTION FRONT <> BACK	INGREDIENT & STRENGTH	BRAND (or Generic Equiv.) by FIRM	NDC#	CLASS; SCH.
59743061	Cap, Dark Green & Clear	Brompheniramine Maleate 6 mg, Pseudoephedrine HCl 60 mg	Bromfed PD by Ivax	00182-1054	Cold Remedy
59743061	Cap, Dark Green & Clear	Brompheniramine Maleate 6 mg, Pseudoephedrine HCl 60 mg	Bromfed PD by DRX	55045-2297	Cold Remedy
59743061	Cap, Dark Green & Clear	Brompheniramine Maleate 6 mg, Pseudoephedrine HCl 60 mg	Bromfed PD by Alphagen	59743-0061	Cold Remedy
598	Tab, Pink, Round, Schering Logo 598	Perphenazine 2 mg, Amitriptyline HCl 25 mg	Etrafon by Schering		Antipsychotic; Antidepressant
599	Tab, Film Coated, Logo 599	Etodolac 400 mg	Lodine by Caremark	00339-5986	NSAID
59911 <> 3608	Tab, White, Oval	Etodolac 400 mg	Lodine by Hoffmann La Roche	00004-0292	NSAID
59911 <> 3608	Tab, White, Oval	Etodolac 400 mg	Lodine by Wyeth	52903-3608	NSAID
59911 <> 3608	Tab, White, Oval	Etodolac 400 mg	Lodine by ESI Lederle	59911-3608	NSAID
59911 <> 5814	Tab, White, Oval, Scored	Metoclopramide 5 mg	Reglan by A H Robins	00031-5814	Gastrointestinal
59911 <> 5814	Tab, White, Oval, Scored	Metoclopramide 5 mg	Reglan by ESI Lederle	59911-5814	Gastrointestinal
59911 <> 5815	Tab, White, Oblong, Scored	Metoclopramide 10 mg	Reglan by ESI Lederle	59911-5815	Gastrointestinal
59911 <> 5815	Tab, White, Oblong, Scored	Metoclopramide 10 mg	Reglan by A H Robins	00031-5815	Gastrointestinal
59911 <> 5840	Tab, White, Coated	Guanfacine HCl 1.15 mg	Tenex by A H Robins	00031-5840	Antihypertensive
59911 <> 5840	Tab, White, Diamond Shaped	Guanfacine HCl 1 mg	Tenex by ESI Lederle	59911-5840	Antihypertensive
59911 <> 5841	Tab, Light Yellow, Coated	Guanfacine HCl 2 mg	Tenex by A H Robins	00031-5841	Antihypertensive
59911 <> 5841	Tab, Yellow, Diamond Shaped	Guanfacine HCl 2 mg	Tenex by ESI Lederle	59911-5841	Antihypertensive
59911 <> 5871	Tab, White, Scored	Promethazine HCl 12.5 mg	Phenergan by ESI Lederle	59911-5871	Antiemetic; Antihistamine
59911 <> 5871	Tab, White, Scored	Promethazine HCl 12.5 mg	Phenergan by Wyeth	52903-5871	Antiemetic; Antihistamine
59911 <> 5872	Tab, White, Scored	Promethazine HCl 25 mg	Phenergan by Wyeth	52903-5872	Antiemetic; Antihistamine
59911 <> 5872	Tab, White, Scored	Promethazine HCl 25 mg	Phenergan by ESI Lederle	59911-5872	Antiemetic; Antihistamine
59911 <> 5873	Tab, White, Scored	Promethazine HCl 50 mg	Phenergan by ESI Lederle	59911-5873	Antiemetic; Antihistamine
59911 <> 5873	Tab, White, Scored	Promethazine HCl 50 mg	Phenergan by Wyeth	52903-5873	Antiemetic; Antihistamine
59911 <> 5895	Tab, White, Ex Release, Scored	Quinidine Sulfate 300 mg	Quinidex Extentabs by ESI Lederle	59911-5895	Antiarrhythmic
59911 <> 5895	Tab, White, Ex Release, Scored	Quinidine Sulfate 300 mg	Quinidex Extentabs by A H Robins	00031-5895	Antiarrhythmic
59911120MG	Cap, Dark Blue & White, White Print, 59911 over 120 mg	Propranolol HCl 120 mg	Inderal LA by ESI Lederle	59911-5473	Antihypertensive
59911120MG	Cap, Dark Blue & White, White Print, 59911 over 120 mg	Propranolol HCl 120 mg	Inderal LA by Ayerst	00046-5473	Antihypertensive
59911120MG	Cap, Dark Blue & White, White Print, 59911 over 120 mg	Propranolol HCl 120 mg	Inderal LA by Caremark	00339-5756	Antihypertensive
59911160MG	Cap, Dark Blue & White, White Print, 59911 over 160 mg	Propranolol HCl 160 mg	Inderal LA by ESI Lederle	59911-5479	Antihypertensive
59911160MG	Cap, Dark Blue & White, White Print, 59911 over 160 mg	Propranolol HCl 160 mg	Inderal LA by Wyeth	52903-5479	Antihypertensive
59911160MG	Cap, Dark Blue & White, White Print, 59911 over 160 mg	Propranolol HCl 160 mg	Inderal LA by Ayerst	00046-5479	Antihypertensive
59911160MG	Cap, Dark Blue & White, White Print, 59911 over 160 mg	Propranolol HCl 160 mg	Inderal LA by RPR	00801-1101	Antihypertensive
59911160MG	Cap, Dark Blue & White, White Print, 59911 over 160 mg	Propranolol HCl 60 mg	Inderal by Vangard	00615-1331	Antihypertensive
59913606200	Cap, White, Red Print, 59911 over 3606 over 200	Etodolac 200 mg	Lodine by Heartland	61392-0906	NSAID
59913606200	Cap, White, Red Print, 59911 over 3606 over 200	Etodolac 200 mg	Lodine by Ayerst	00046-3606	NSAID
59913606200	Cap, White, Red Print, 59911 over 3606 over 200	Etodolac 200 mg	Lodine by Wyeth	52903-3606	NSAID
59913606200	Cap, White, Red Print, 59911 over 3606 over 200	Etodolac 200 mg	Lodine by Heartland	61392-0862	NSAID
59913606200	Cap, White, Red Print, 59911 over 3606 over 200	Etodolac 200 mg	Lodine by ESI Lederle	59911-3606	NSAID
59913607300	Cap, White, Oblong	Etodolac 300 mg	Lodine by ESI Lederle	59911-3607	NSAID
59913607300	Cap, White, 59911/3607 <> 300	Etodolac 300 mg	Lodine by Heartland	61392-0907	NSAID
59913607300	Cap, White	Etodolac 300 mg	Lodine by Wyeth	52903-3607	NSAID
59913608	Tab, White, Oval	Etodolac 400 mg	Lodine by ESI Lederle		NSAID
59913767	Tab, White, Oval	Etodolac 500 mg	Lodine by ESI Lederle		NSAID
59913787	Tab, White, Black Print, Oval, Film Coated, 59911 over 3787	Etodolac 500 mg	Lodine by Wyeth	52903-3787	NSAID
59913787	Tab, White, Black Print, Oval, Film Coated, 59911 over 3787	Etodolac 500 mg	Lodine by Heartland	61392-0872	NSAID
59915805	Tab, White, Square	Griseofulvin, Ultramicrosize 250 mg	Fulvicin P/G by ESI Lederle		Antifungal
59915806	Tab, White, Oval	Griseofulvin, Ultramicrosize 330 mg	Fulvicin P/G by ESI Lederle		Antifungal
59915807	Cap, Opaque & White	Griseofulvin 250 mg	Fulvicin P/G by ESI Lederle		Antifungal

ID FRONT <> BACK	DESCRIPTION FRONT <> BACK	INGREDIENT & STRENGTH	BRAND (or Generic Equiv.) by FIRM	NDC#	CLASS; SCH.
599115808	Tab, White, Round	Griseofulvin 500 mg	Fulvicin P/G by ESI Lederle		Antifungal
599115814	Tab, White, Elliptical	Metoclopramide 5 mg	Reglan by ESI Lederle		Gastrointestinal
599115815	Tab, White, Oblong	Metoclopramide 10 mg	Reglan by ESI Lederle		Gastrointestinal
599115842	Cap, Blue & Pink	Acebutolol HCl 200 mg	Sectral by ESI Lederle		Antihypertensive
599115842	Cap, Blue & Pink	Acebutolol HCl 200 mg	Sectral by ESI Lederle	52903-5842	Antihypertensive
599115842	Cap, Blue & Pink	Acebutolol HCl 200 mg	Sectral by Wyeth		Antihypertensive
599115844	Cap, Pink & Red	Acebutolol HCl 400 mg	Sectral by ESI Lederle	59911-5844	Antihypertensive
599115844	Cap, Pink & Rose	Acebutolol HCl 400 mg	Sectral by ESI Lederle		Antihypertensive
599115844	Cap, Pink & Red	Acebutolol HCl 400 mg	Sectral by Watson	52903-5844	Antihypertensive
599115869	Cap, Yellow	Minocycline HCl 50 mg	Minocin by ESI Lederle		Antibiotic
599115869	Cap, Yellow	Minocycline HCl 50 mg	Minocin by ESI Lederle	59911-5869	Antibiotic
599115870	Cap, Green & Yellow	Minocycline HCl 100 mg	Minocin by ESI Lederle		Antibiotic
599115870	Cap, Green & Yellow	Minocycline HCl 100 mg	Minocin by ESI Lederle	59911-5870	Antibiotic
599115870	Cap, Green & Yellow	Minocycline HCl 100 mg	Minocin by Murfreesboro	51129-1414	Antibiotic
599115871	Tab, White, Round	Promethazine 12.5 mg	Phenergan by ESI Lederle		Antiemetic; Antihistamine
599115872	Tab, White, Round	Promethazine 25 mg	Phenergan by ESI Lederle		Antiemetic; Antihistamine
599115873	Tab, White, Round	Promethazine 50 mg	Phenergan by ESI Lederle		Antiemetic; Antihistamine
599115876	Cap, Pink & White	Oxazepam 10 mg	Serax by ESI Lederle	59911-5876	Sedative/Hypnotic; C IV
599115876	Cap, Pink & White	Oxazepam 10 mg	Serax by ESI Lederle		Sedative/Hypnotic; C IV
599115876	Cap, Pink & White	Oxazepam 10 mg	Serax by Wyeth	52903-5876	Sedative/Hypnotic; C IV
599115877	Cap, Orange & White	Oxazepam 15 mg	Serax by ESI Lederle	59911-5877	Sedative/Hypnotic; C IV
599115877	Cap, Orange & White	Oxazepam 15 mg	Serax by Murfreesboro	51129-1676	Sedative/Hypnotic; C IV
599115877	Cap, Orange & White	Oxazepam 15 mg	Serax by Wyeth	52903-5877	Sedative/Hypnotic; C IV
599115877	Cap, Orange & White	Oxazepam 15 mg	Serax by ESI Lederle		Sedative/Hypnotic; C IV
599115878	Cap, Blue & White	Oxazepam 30 mg	Serax by Wyeth	52903-5878	Sedative/Hypnotic; C IV
599115878	Cap, Blue & White	Oxazepam 30 mg	Serax by ESI Lederle	59911-5878	Sedative/Hypnotic; C IV
599115878	Cap, Blue & White	Oxazepam 30 mg	Serax by ESI Lederle		Sedative/Hypnotic; C IV
599115887	Cap, Blue & Green & Opaque, Ex Release	Ketoprofen 100 mg	Orudis by Murfreesboro	51129-1601	NSAID
599115887	Cap, Blue & Green	Ketoprofen 100 mg	Orudis by Wyeth	52903-5887	NSAID
599115887	Cap, Blue & Green & Opaque	Ketoprofen 100 mg	Orudis by Murfreesboro	51129-1598	NSAID
599115888	Cap, Blue & Yellow	Ketoprofen 150 mg	Orudis by Wyeth	52903-5888	NSAID
599115888	Cap, Blue & Opaque & Yellow	Ketoprofen 150 mg	Orudis by Murfreesboro	51129-1599	NSAID
599115888	Cap, Blue & Opaque & Yellow, Ex Release	Ketoprofen 150 mg	Orudis by Murfreesboro	51129-1602	NSAID
599115889	Cap, Light Blue & White, Opaque, Ex Release	Ketoprofen 200 mg	Orudis by Murfreesboro	51129-1603	NSAID
599115889	Cap, Light Blue & White, Opaque, Ex Release	Ketoprofen 200 mg	Orudis by Murfreesboro	51129-1600	NSAID
599115889	Cap, Light Blue & White, Opaque, Ex Release	Ketoprofen 200 mg	Orudis by Wyeth	52903-5889	NSAID
599115889	Cap, Blue & White	Ketoprofen 200 mg	Orudis by Wyeth	52903-5889	NSAID
599115889	Cap, Light Blue & White, Opaque, Ex Release	Ketoprofen 200 mg	Orudis by ESI Lederle	59911-5889	NSAID
599115895	Tab, White, Round, Ex Release	Quinidine Sulfate 300 mg	Quinidex by ESI Lederle		Antiarrhythmic
599115899	Cap, White, Ex Release	Potassium Chloride 750 mg	by A H Robins	00031-5899	Electrolytes
599115899	Cap	Potassium Chloride 750 mg	K-Dur by Caremark	00339-6119	Electrolytes
5991160MG	Cap, White, Blue Print, 59911 over 60 mg	Propranolol HCl 60 mg	Inderal by ESI Lederle	59911-5470	Antihypertensive
5991160MG	Cap, White, Blue Print, 59911 over 60	Propranolol HCl 60 mg	Inderal by Caremark	00339-5752	Antihypertensive
5991160MG	Cap, White, Blue Print, 59911 over 60	Propranolol HCl 60 mg	Inderal by Ayerst	00046-5470	Antihypertensive
5991160MG	Cap, Light Blue & White, White Print, 59911 over 60	Propranolol HCl 60 mg	Inderal by Wyeth	52903-5470	Antihypertensive
5991180MG	Cap, Light Blue & White, White Print, 59911 over 80 mg	Propranolol HCl 80 mg	Inderal by Wyeth	52903-5471	Antihypertensive

ID FRONT <> BACK	DESCRIPTION FRONT <> BACK	INGREDIENT & STRENGTH	BRAND (or Generic Equiv.) by FIRM	NDC#	CLASS; SCH.
599118OMG	Cap, Light Blue & White, White Print, 59911 over 80 mg	Propranolol HCl 80 mg	Inderal by ESI Lederle	59911-5471	Antihypertensive
599118OMG	Cap, Light Blue & White, White Print, 59911 over 80 mg	Propranolol HCl 80 mg	Inderal by Ayerst	00046-5471	Antihypertensive
599118OMG	Cap, Light Blue & White, White Print, 59911 over 80 mg	Propranolol HCl 80 mg	Inderal by Caremark	00339-5754	Antihypertensive
599118OMG	Cap, Light Blue & White, White Print, 59911 over 80 mg	Propranolol HCl 80 mg	Inderal by Southwood	58016-0529	Antihypertensive
59911PLUS	Tab, Yellow, Oval, 59911/Plus	Prenatal	by ESI Lederle	Canadian DIN 02221845	Vitamin
5ALTACE	Cap, Red and White, Opaque, Hard Gel	Ramipril 5 mg	Altace by Aventis		Antihypertensive
5AYGESTIN	Tab, White, Oval, Scored, 5 over Aygestin	Norethindrone 5 mg	Aygestin by Wyeth	00046-0894	Hormone
5AYGESTIN	Tab, White, Oval, Scored, 5 over Aygestin	Norethindrone 5 mg	Aygestin by ESI Lederle	59911-5894	Hormone
5AYGESTIN <> B424	Tab, White, Oval, Scored, 5 over Aygestin	Norethindrone 5 mg	Aygestin by Barr	51285-0424	Hormone
5C33	Tab, Yellow, Round	Leucovorin Calcium 5 mg	Wellcovorin by Lederle		Antineoplastic
5CC <> GS	Tab, Red, Cap Shaped, Film Coated	Ropinirole HCl 8 mg	Requip XL by GSK	00007-4888	Antiparkinson
5DAN5606	Tab	Haloperidol 5 mg	Haldol by Allscripts		Antipsychotic
5FE <> PAL	Tab, Red, Round, PAL <> 5Fe	Iron 100 mg, Vitamin C 60 mg, D-biotin 0.3 mg, Pantothenic Acid (B5) 10 mg, Niacinamide (B3) 20 mg, Riboflavin (B2) 1.5 mg, Thiamine HCl (B1) 1.5 mg, Pyridoxine HCl (B6) 50 mg, Cyanocobalamin (B12) 1 mg, Folacin 5 mg	Diatx Fe by Pamlab	00525-0503	Dietary Supplement
5MG	Cap, Blue	Pericyazine 5 mg	by RPR	Canadian	Psychotropic Agent
5MG	Tab, White, Circular, Scored	Bumetanide 5 mg	Burinex by Leo Pharma	Canadian DIN 00728276	Diuretic
5MG <> 4760	Tab, Yellow, Hexagonal, Film-Coated	Prasugrel 5 mg	Effient by Eli Lilly	00002-4760	Antiplatelet
5MG <> APO	Tab, White, Oval, Scored	Cetirizine 5 mg	Zyrtec by Apotex	Canadian DIN 02240910	Antihistamine
5MG <> ETHEX264	Tab, Yellow, Oval, Scored	Buspirone HCl 5 mg	BuSpar by Ethex	58177-0264	Antianxiety
5MG <> RSN	Tab, Yellow, Oval, Film Coated	Risedronate Sodium 5 mg	Actonel by Proc & Gamble	Canadian DIN 02244518	Bisphosphonate
5MG <> RSN	Tab, Yellow, Oval, Film Coated	Risedronate Sodium 5 mg	Actonel by Procter and Gamble	00149-0471	Bisphosphonate
5MG35125MGSB	Cap, Brown & Clear	Dextroamphetamine Sulfate 5 mg	Dexedrine by Int'l Processing	59885-3512	Stimulant; C II
5MGF657	Cap, Red	Anhydrous Tacrolimus 5 mg	Prograf by Astellas	Canadian DIN 02175983	Immunosuppressant
5MGLEDERLEL1	Cap, Green	Loxapine 5 mg	Loxitane by Lederle		Antipsychotic
5MGSB5MG3512	Cap, Brown & Clear	Dextroamphetamine Sulfate 5 mg	Dexedrine by Int'l Processing	59885-3512	Stimulant; C II
5MGSB5MG3512	Cap, Brown & Clear	Dextroamphetamine Sulfate 5 mg	Dexedrine by SKB	00007-3512	Stimulant; C II
5MGSONATA	Cap, Green & Opaque	Zaleplon 5 mg	Sonata by Wyeth	52903-0925	Sedative/Hypnotic; C IV
5MGSONATA	Cap, Green & Opaque	Zaleplon 5 mg	Sonata by URL Mutual	00677-1684	Sedative/Hypnotic; C IV
5MGSONATA	Cap, Green & Opaque	Zaleplon 5 mg	Sonata by Wyeth	00008-0925	Sedative/Hypnotic; C IV
5MGSONATA	Cap, Green & Opaque	Zaleplon 5 mg	Sonata by King	60793-0145	Sedative/Hypnotic; C IV
5MMDC	Tab, White, Square, 5/MMDC	Metoclopramide 5 mg	Reglan by Aventis	Canadian	Gastrointestinal
5R	Cap, Light Pink, Soft Gel	Isotretinoin 10 mg	Sotret by Ranbaxy	63304-0584	Dermatologic
5VALIUM <> ROCHE	Tab, Yellow, Round, Scored	Diazepam 5 mg	Valium by PDRX	55289-0117	Antianxiety; C IV
5VALIUM <> ROCHE	Tab, Yellow, Round, Scored	Diazepam 5 mg	Valium by Caremark	00339-4073	Antianxiety; C IV
5VALIUM <> ROCHE	Tab, Yellow, Round, Scored	Diazepam 5 mg	Valium by Roche	00140-0005	Antianxiety; C IV
5XL	Tab, Yellow, Round	Oxybutynin Chloride 5 mg	Ditropan XL by Janssen-Ortho	Canadian DIN 02243960	Urinary Tract
5XL	Tab, Yellow, Round	Oxybutynin Chloride 5 mg	Ditropan XL by Alza	17314-8500	Urinary Tract
5Z2941	Tab, Light Lavender, Sugar-Coated, 5/Z2941	Trifluoperazine HCl	Stelazine by Physician Total Care	54868-1352	Antipsychotic
6	Tab, Pink, Buccal	Fentanyl 600 mcg	Fentora by Cephalon	63459-0546	Opioid Agonist; C II
6	Tab, White, Round, # and 6	Nitroglycerin 0.6 mg	Nitrostat by Endo	60951-0726	Vasodilator
6	Tab, Green, Oval	Dextrothyroxine Sodium 6 mg	Choloxin by Boots		Thyroid Hormone
6	Tab, Film Coated, Norton	Ibuprofen 600 mg	Motrin by Med Pro	53978-5006	NSAID

ID FRONT <> BACK	DESCRIPTION FRONT <> BACK	INGREDIENT & STRENGTH	BRAND (or Generic Equiv.) by FIRM	NDC#	CLASS; SCH.
6	Tab, White, Oval	Ibuprofen 600 mg	Motrin by Norton	43068-0106	NSAID
6	Tab, White, Round, Vanda Logo <> 6	Iloperidone 6 mg	Fanapt by Vanda	43068-0106	Antipsychotic
6	Tab, White, Round, Sublingual	Nitroglycerin 0.6 mg	Nitrostat by Glenmark	68462-0147	Vasodilator
6	Tab, White, Round, Scored	Medroxyprogesterone Acetate 2.5 mg	by Southwood	58016-0374	Hormone
6 <> B	Tab, White to Off-White, Round	Vitamin B6 25 mg	CitraNatal B-Calm by Mission	50178-0866	Vitamin; Supplement
6 <> CL	Tab, White to Off-White, Rectangle, Sublingual	Nitroglycerin 0.6 mg	Nitrostat by Pliva	50111-0991	Vasodilator
6 <> ETH	Tab, White, Oval	Nitroglycerin 0.6 mg	Nitrostat by PDRX	55289-0302	Vasodilator
6 <> ETH	Tab, White, Oval	Nitroglycerin 0.6 mg	NitroQuick by Ethex	58177-0325	Vasodilator
6 <> N	Tab, White, Round	Nitroglycerin 0.6 mg	Nitrostat by Parke Davis	Canadian DIN 00037621	Vasodilator
6 <> N	Tab, White, Round	Nitroglycerin 0.6 mg	Nitrostat by Parke Davis	00071-0419	Vasodilator
6 <> NOVO	Tab, Green, Round	Bromazepam 6 mg	Lectopam by Novopharm	Canadian DIN 02230585	Sedative; C IV
6 <> SEARLE	Tab, Underlined 6 <> Searle	Ethinyl Estradiol 0.035 mg, Norethindrone 0.5 mg, Norethindrone 1 mg	Tri Noninyl 21 Day by Searle	00025-0272	Oral Contraceptive
6 <> SEARLE	Tab, Underlined 6 <> Searle	Ethinyl Estradiol 0.035 mg, Norethindrone 0.5 mg	Brevicon 21 Day by Searle	00025-0252	Oral Contraceptive
6 <> SP	Tab, Green, Oval	Doxepin 6 mg	Silenor by Somaxon	42847-0106	Sedative/Hypnotic
6 <> WARFARINTARO	Tab, Teal, Cap Shaped	Warfarin Sodium 6 mg	Coumadin by Taro	51672-4033	Anticoagulant
6 <> Z	Tab, Red, Round, Film Coated	Risperidone 0.5 mg	Risperdal by Zydus	68382-0113	Antipsychotic
60	Tab, Light Peach, Andrx Logo 60, Ex Release	Lovastatin 60 mg	Altoprev by Andrx	62202-0630	Antihyperlipidemic
60	Cap, Gray, Oval	Terazosin HCl 1 mg	Hytrin by Teva	00093-0760	Antihypertensive
60	Cap, Gray, Oval	Terazosin HCl 1 mg	Hytrin by RP Scherer	Discontinued 11014-1218	Antihypertensive
60	Tab, Peach, Round	Fexofenadine HCl 60 mg	Allegra by Aventis	Canadian	Antihistamine
60 <> 54933	Tab, White, Round, Sustained Release	Morphine Sulfate 60 mg	Oramorph SR by Xanodyne	66479-0542	Analgesic; C II
60 <> 5660	Tab, Yellow, Round, Scored	Isosorbide Mononitrate 60 mg	Imdur by Ivax	00172-5660	Antianginal
60 <> ABG	Tab, Orange, Round, Film-Coated	Morphine Sulfate 60 mg	MS Contin by Ivax	00172-2164	Analgesic; C II
60 <> ADALATCC	Tab, Reddish Pink, Round, Film Coated, Adalat over CC	Nifedipine 60 mg	Adalat CC by Va Cmop	65243-0054	Antihypertensive
60 <> ADALATCC	Tab, Reddish Pink, Round, Film Coated, Adalat over CC	Nifedipine 60 mg	Adalat CC by Bayer	00026-8851	Antihypertensive
60 <> ADALATCC	Tab, Reddish Pink, Round, Film Coated, Adalat over CC	Nifedipine 60 mg	Adalat CC by Par	49884-0631	Antihypertensive
60 <> ADALATCC	Tab, Reddish Pink, Round, Film Coated, Adalat over CC	Nifedipine 60 mg	Adalat CC by Nat Pharmpak	55154-4809	Antihypertensive
60 <> ADALATCC	Tab, Reddish Pink, Round, Film Coated, Adalat over CC	Nifedipine 60 mg	Adalat CC by Wal Mart	49035-0155	Antihypertensive
60 <> ADALATCC	Tab, Reddish Pink, Round, Film Coated, Adalat over CC	Nifedipine 60 mg	Adalat CC by Med Pro	53978-3034	Antihypertensive
60 <> ADALATCC	Tab, Reddish Pink, Round, Film Coated, Adalat over CC	Nifedipine 60 mg	Adalat CC by Amerisource	62584-0006	Antihypertensive
60 <> ADALATCC	Tab, Reddish Pink, Round, Film Coated, Adalat over CC	Nifedipine 60 mg	Adalat CC by Smiths Food & Drug	58341-0059	Antihypertensive
60 <> ADALATCC	Tab, Reddish Pink, Round, Film Coated, Adalat over CC	Nifedipine 60 mg	Adalat CC by Talbert	44514-0761	Antihypertensive
60 <> AMGEN	Tab, Light Green, Oval, Film Coated	Cinacalcet HCl 60 mg	Sensipar by Amgen	55513-0074	Calcimimetic
60 <> B	Tab, Yellow, Round, Ex Release	Nifedipine 60 mg	Adalat CC by Ivax	00182-8233	Antihypertensive
60 <> B	Tab, Yellow, Round, Ex Release	Nifedipine 60 mg	Adalat CC by Teva	Discontinued 00093-1022	Antihypertensive
60 <> B	Tab, Reddish Brown, Round, Film Coated, Ex Release	Nifedical 60 mg	Procardia XL by Teva	00093-5173	Antihypertensive
60 <> E	Tab, White, Oval, Extended Release	Morphine Sulfate 60 mg	MS Contin by Ethex	58177-0330	Analgesic; C II
60 <> E655	Tab, Orange, Cap Shaped	Morphine Sulfate 60 mg	MS Contin by Endo	60951-0655	Analgesic; C II
60 <> E655	Tab, Orange, Cap Shaped	Morphine Sulfate 60 mg	MS Contin by BMS	00056-0655	Analgesic; C II
60 <> M	Tab, White, Coated, Beveled Edge, 6 on Left, 0 on Right of Score	Maprotiline HCl 25 mg	Ludiomil by Mylan	00378-0060	Antidepressant
60 <> M	Tab, Orange, Round, M inside square <> 60	Morphine Sulfate 60 mg	MS Contin by Mallinckrodt	00406-8380	Analgesic; C II
60 <> MOSSR	Tab, Red, Round, M.O.S.-SR/60	Morphine HCl 60 mg	M.O.S.-S.R. by ICN	Canadian DIN 00776203	Analgesic; C II
60 <> N	Tab, Orange, Round	Morphine Sulfate 60 mg	MS Contin by Novopharm	Canadian DIN 02302780	Analgesic; N

ID FRONT <> BACK	DESCRIPTION FRONT <> BACK	INGREDIENT & STRENGTH	BRAND (or Generic Equiv.) by FIRM	NDC#	CLASS; SCH.
60 <> OC	Tab, Red, Round, CR	Oxycodone HCl 60 mg	OxyContin by Purdue	59011-0860	Analgesic; C II
60 <> STARLIX	Tab, Pink, Round	Nateglinide 60 mg	Starlix by Novartis	Canadian DIN 02245438	Antidiabetic
60 <> STARLIX	Tab, Pink, Round	Nateglinide 60 mg	Starlix by Novartis	00078-0351	Antidiabetic
60 <> WW	Tab, Yellow, Oval	Isosorbide Mononitrate 60 mg	Imdur by West-Ward	00143-2260	Antianginal
600	Cap, Red and White, 600 inside circle	Acetaminophen 500 mg	Tylenol by PDRX		Analgesic
600	Tab, Film Coated, Upjohn Logo and 600	Ibuprofen 600 mg	Motrin by Quality Care	60346-0556	NSAID
600 <> 3RP	Tab, Dark Blue, Cap-Shaped, Film-Coated	Ribavirin 600 mg	Copegus by Three Rivers	66435-0104	Antiviral
600 <> 4348	Tab, White, Oval, Scored, Hourglass Logo / 4348	Oxaprozin 600 mg	Daypro by Ivax	00172-4348 Discontinued	NSAID
600 <> 4443	Tab, White, Oval, Scored, Ivax Logo 4443	Gabapentin 600 mg	Neurontin by Ivax	00093-4443	Anticonvulsant
600 <> A	Tab, Blue & White, Round, Ex Release	Guaifenesin 600 mg	Mucinex by Adams	63824-0008	Expectorant
600 <> ADAMS	Tab, Yellow and White, Oval, Bi-Layer, ER	Guaifenesin 600 mg, Dextromethorphan HBr 30 mg	Mucinex DM by Adams	63824-0056	Cold Remedy
600 <> APO034	Tab, White, Oval, Film Coated	Gemfibrozil 600 mg	Lopid by Apotex	60505-0034	Antihyperlipidemic
600 <> APO034	Tab, White, Oval, Film Coated	Gemfibrozil 600 mg	Lopid by Major	00904-5379	Antihyperlipidemic
600 <> APO034	Tab, White, Oval, Film Coated	Gemfibrozil 600 mg	Lopid by Torpharm	62318-0034	Antihyperlipidemic
600 <> AZL	Tab, White, Oval, Scored, Film Coated, Abbott Logo (a)	Zileuton 600 mg	Zyflo by Abbott	00074-8036	Antiasthmatic
600 <> C102	Tab, White, Oval	Ibuprofen 600 mg	Motrin by Dr. Reddy's	55111-0102	NSAID
600 <> G	Tab, Film Coated	Ibuprofen 600 mg	Motrin by Quality Care	60346-0556	NSAID
600 <> IP132	Tab, White, Oval, Film Coated	Ibuprofen 600 mg	Motrin by Golden State	60429-0093	NSAID
600 <> IP132	Tab, White, Oval, Film Coated	Ibuprofen 600 mg	Motrin by Urgent Care Center	50716-0743	NSAID
600 <> IP132	Tab, White, Oval, Film Coated	Ibuprofen 600 mg	Motrin by Qualitest	00603-4019	NSAID
600 <> IP132	Tab, White, Oval, Film Coated	Ibuprofen 600 mg	Motrin by Major	00904-5186	NSAID
600 <> IP132	Tab, White, Oval, Film Coated	Ibuprofen 600 mg	Motrin by Rx Dispensing	61807-0011	NSAID
600 <> IP132	Tab, White, Oval, Film Coated	Ibuprofen 600 mg	Motrin by Ivax	00182-1810 Discontinued	NSAID
600 <> IP132	Tab, White, Oval, Film Coated	Ibuprofen 600 mg	Motrin by Qualitest	00603-4019	NSAID
600 <> IP132	Tab, White, Oval, Film Coated	Ibuprofen 600 mg	Motrin by Breckenridge	51991-0730	NSAID
600 <> IP132	Tab, White, Oval, Film Coated	Ibuprofen 600 mg	Motrin by Amneal	65162-0569	NSAID
600 <> IP132	Tab, White, Oval, Film Coated	Ibuprofen 600 mg	Motrin by Watson	00591-3465	NSAID
600 <> IP132	Tab, White, Oval, Film Coated	Ibuprofen 600 mg	Motrin by Interpharm	53746-0132	NSAID
600 <> N	Tab, White, Oval, Black Ink	Gabapentin 600 mg	Neurontin by Novopharm	Canadian DIN 02248457	Antiepileptic
600 <> NOVO	Tab, White, Oval	Gemfibrozil 600 mg	Lopid by Novopharm	Canadian DIN 02142074	Antihyperlipidemic
600 <> NOVO	Tab, Green, Oval	Cimetidine 600 mg	Tagamet by Novopharm	Canadian DIN 00603686	Gastrointestinal
600 <> NOVO	Tab, Light Orange, Oval	Ibuprofen 600 mg	Motrin by Novopharm	Canadian DIN 00629359	NSAID
600 <> P	Tab, White, Oblong	Azithromycin 600 mg	by Pharmascience	Canadian DIN 02261642	Antibiotic
600 <> PAL	Tab, Blue, Oval, Coated	L-methylfolate (Metafolin) 5.6 mg, Methylcobalamin 2 mg, N-acetylcysteine 600 mg	Cerefolin NAC by PamLab	00525-0510	Vitamin; Supplement
600 <> PAR163	Tab, Film Coated	Ibuprofen 600 mg	Motrin by Par	49884-0163	NSAID
600 <> PAR163	Tab, Film Coated	Ibuprofen 600 mg	Motrin by Pharmedix	53002-0301	NSAID
600 <> PAR163	Tab, Film Coated	Ibuprofen 600 mg	Motrin by Ivax	00172-3646	NSAID
600 <> TMC	Tab, Orange, Oval, Film Coated	Darunavir 600 mg	Prezista by Tibotec	59676-0562	Antiviral
600 <> WALLACE371601	Tab, Wallace over 37-1601	Meprobamate 600 mg	Miltown by Wallace	00037-1601	Sedative/Hypnotic; C IV
600 <> Z4141	Tab, Orange, Film Coated, 600 and Zenith Logo	Fenoprofen Calcium 600 mg	by Quality Care	60346-0233	NSAID

ID FRONT <> BACK	DESCRIPTION FRONT <> BACK	INGREDIENT & STRENGTH	BRAND (or Generic Equiv.) by FIRM	NDC#	CLASS; SCH.
600 <> Z4141	Tab, Peach, Oblong, Z over 4141	Fenoprofen Calcium 600 mg	Nalfon by Ivax	00172-4141 Discontinued	NSAID
600 <> ZL	Tab, White, Oval, Scored, Film Coated, Abbott Logo ZL	Zileuton 600 mg	by Murfreesboro	51129-1380	Antiasthmatic
60030 <> TRINITY	Tab, Film Coated, Scored	Dextromethorphan HBr 30 mg, Guaifenesin 600 mg	by URL Mutual	00677-1486	Cold Remedy
600MG	Tab, Yellow, Round	Potassium Chloride 600 mg	Klor-Con by Pharmacy Care	65070-0067	Electrolytes
600mg <> TMC	Tab, Orange, Oval, Film Coated	Darunavir 600 mg	Prezista by Janssen-Ortho	Canadian DIN 02324024	Antiviral
600P <> CALTRATE	Tab, Pink, Oblong, Scored	Vitamin D 200 IU, Calcium 600 mg, Magnesium 40 mg, Zinc 7.5 mg, Copper 1 mg, Manganese 1.8 mg, Boron 250 mcg	Caltrate 600 Plus by Wyeth	00005-5556	Vitamin; Supplement
601 <> MYLAN	Tab, Beveled Edge, Coated	Ibuprofen 600 mg	Motrin by Mylan	00378-0601	NSAID
601 <> SINEMETCR	Tab, Pink, Oval, Sustained Release, SINEMET over CR	Carbidopa 25 mg, Levodopa 100 mg	Sinemet CR by BMS	00056-0601	Antiparkinson
601 <> SINEMETCR	Tab, Pink, Oval, Sustained Release, SINEMET over CR	Carbidopa 25 mg, Levodopa 100 mg	Sinemet CR by BMS	Canadian DIN 0208786	Antiparkinson
60274120MG	Cap, Yellow, Black Print, 60274 over 120 mg	Verapamil HCl 120 mg	Verelan SR by Watson	00591-2880	Antihypertensive
60274120MG	Cap, Yellow, Black Print, 60274 over 120 mg	Verapamil HCl 120 mg	Verelan SR by Teva	00480-0948	Antihypertensive
60274120MG	Cap, Yellow, Black Print, 60274 over 120 mg	Verapamil HCl 120 mg	Verelan SR by Schein	00364-2880	Antihypertensive
60274180MG	Cap, Light Gray & Yellow, Opaque, 60274 over 180 mg	Verapamil HCl 180 mg	Verelan SR by Schein	00364-2882	Antihypertensive
60274180MG	Cap, Light Gray & Yellow, Opaque, 60274 over 180 mg	Verapamil HCl 180 mg	Verelan SR by Watson	00591-2882	Antihypertensive
60274240MG	Cap, Dark Blue & Yellow, Black Print, Opaque, 60274 over 240 mg	Verapamil HCl 240 mg	Verelan SR by Watson	00591-2884	Antihypertensive
60274240MG	Cap, Dark Blue & Yellow, Black Print, Opaque, 60274 over 240 mg	Verapamil HCl 240 mg	Verelan SR by Schein	00364-2884	Antihypertensive
60274240MG	Cap, Dark Blue & Yellow, Black Print, Opaque, 60274 over 240 mg	Verapamil HCl 240 mg	Verelan SR by Teva	00480-0958	Antihypertensive
60274360MG	Cap, Purple & Yellow, Black Print, Hard Gel, 60274 over 360 mg	Verapamil HCl 360 mg	Verelan SR by Teva	00480-0960	Antihypertensive
60274360MG	Cap, Purple & Yellow, Black Print, Hard Gel, 60274 over 360 mg	Verapamil HCl 360 mg	Verelan SR by Schein	00364-2886	Antihypertensive
60274360MG	Cap, Purple & Yellow, Black Print, Hard Gel, 60274 over 360 mg	Verapamil HCl 360 mg	Verelan SR by Watson	00591-2886	Antihypertensive
603	Tab, Pink, Cap Shaped	Tetracycline HCl 500 mg	Sumycin by Par	49884-0798	Antibiotic
6036 <> N	Tab, Dark Blue, Oval, Scored	Glyburide 6 mg	Glynase by Teva	00093-3036	Antidiabetic
604 <> SL	Tab, Green, Oblong, Scored, Film Coated	Guaifenesin 600 mg, Pseudoephedrine HCl 120 mg	Entex PSE by Pliva	50111-0604	Cold Remedy
605 <> BP	Tab, White, Round, Scored	Carbinoxamine 4 mg	Palgic by Boca	64376-0605	Cold Remedy
6057	Tab, Pale Yellow, Cap Shaped, Film Coated	Glyburide 1.25 mg, Metformin HCl 250 mg	Glucovance by Par	49884-0967	Antianginal
6057V	Tab, Tan, Round	Thyroid 90 mg	Thyroid by Qualitest	00603-6053	Thyroid Hormone
6058	Tab, Pale Orange, Cap Shaped, Film Coated	Glyburide 2.5 mg, Metformin HCl 500 mg	Glucovance by Par	49884-0968	Antidiabetic
6058V	Tab, Tan, Round	Thyroid 60 mg	Thyroid by Qualitest	00603-6052	Thyroid Hormone
6059	Tab, Yellow, Cap Shaped, Film Coated	Glyburide 5 mg, Metformin HCl 500 mg	Glucovance by Par	49884-0969	Antidiabetic
6059V	Tab, Tan, Round	Thyroid 120 mg	Thyroid by Qualitest	00603-6054	Thyroid Hormone
606 <> R	Tab, White, Round	Acyclovir 400 mg	Zovirax by Actavis	00228-2606	Antiviral
606 <> R	Tab, White, Round	Acyclovir 400 mg	Zovirax by Golden State	60429-0712	Antiviral
6060 <> IMDUR	Tab, Yellow, Oval, Scored	Isosorbide Mononitrate 60 mg	Imdur by Caremark	00339-6003	Antianginal
6060 <> IMDUR	Tab, Yellow, Oval, Scored	Isosorbide Mononitrate 60 mg	Imdur by Nat Pharmpak	55154-3512	Antianginal
6060 <> IMDUR	Tab, Yellow, Oval, Scored	Isosorbide Mononitrate 60 mg	Imdur by Schering	00085-4110	Antianginal
6060 <> IMDUR	Tab, Yellow, Oval, Scored	Isosorbide Mononitrate 60 mg	Imdur by Murfreesboro	51129-1575	Antianginal
6060V	Tab, White, Round	Thyroid 180 mg	Armour Thyroid by Qualitest	00603-6060	Thyroid Hormone
6065 <> 500	Tab, White to Off-White, Cap Shaped, Extended Release	Metformin HCl 500 mg	Glucophage XR by Par	49884-0921	Antidiabetic
606HD	Tab, White, Round	Methyldopa 125 mg	Aldomet by Halsey	Discontinued	Antihypertensive
606PRILOSEC10	Cap, Peach & Purple, Opaque, Hard Gel, Delayed Release	Omeprazole 10 mg	Prilosec by Merck	00006-0606	Gastrointestinal
606PRILOSEC10	Cap, Peach & Purple, Opaque, Hard Gel, Delayed Release	Omeprazole 10 mg	Prilosec by AstraZeneca	00186-0606	Gastrointestinal

ID FRONT <> BACK	DESCRIPTION FRONT <> BACK	INGREDIENT & STRENGTH	BRAND (or Generic Equiv.) by FIRM	NDC#	CLASS; SCH.
606PRILOSEC10	Cap, Peach & Purple, Opaque, Hard Gel, Delayed Release	Omeprazole 10 mg	Prilosec by Kaiser	62224-2226	Gastrointestinal
606PRILOSEC10	Cap, Peach & Purple, Opaque, Hard Gel, Delayed Release	Omeprazole 10 mg	Prilosec by PDRX	55289-0475	Gastrointestinal
6072 <> BMS	Tab, Light Yellow, Cap Shaped, Film Coated	Glyburide 1.25 mg, Metformin 250 mg	Glucovance by BMS	12783-0072	Antidiabetic
6072 <> BMS	Tab, Light Yellow, Cap Shaped, Film Coated	Glyburide 1.25 mg, Metformin 250 mg	Glucovance by BMS	00087-6072	Antidiabetic
6073 <> BMS	Tab, Light Orange, Cap Shaped, Film Coated	Glyburide 2.5 mg, Metformin 500 mg	Glucovance by BMS	00087-6073	Antidiabetic
6073 <> BMS	Tab, Light Orange, Cap Shaped, Film Coated	Glyburide 2.5 mg, Metformin 500 mg	Glucovance by BMS	12783-0073	Antidiabetic
6074 <> BMS	Tab, Yellow, Cap Shaped, Film Coated	Glyburide 5 mg, Metformin 500 mg	Glucovance by BMS	00087-6074	Antidiabetic
6074 <> BMS	Tab, Yellow, Cap Shaped, Film Coated	Glyburide 5 mg, Metformin 500 mg	Glucovance by BMS	12783-0074	Antidiabetic
6077 <> BMS	Tab, White, Oval, Film Coated	Glipizide 2.5 mg, Metformin HCl 500 mg	Metaglip by BMS	00087-6077	Antidiabetic
6078 <> BMS	Tab, Pink, Oval, Film Coated	Glipizide 5 mg, Metformin HCl 500 mg	Metaglip by BMS	00087-6078	Antidiabetic
607HD	Tab, White, Round	Methyldopa 250 mg	Aldomet by Halsey	Discontinued	Antihypertensive
607OR	Tab, Light Pink, Round, OR <> 607	Ranitidine HCl 75 mg	by Schein		Gastrointestinal
608 <> PA	Tab, White, Round, Film Coated	Ketorolac Tromethamine 10 mg	Toradol by Pliva	50111-0608	NSAID
608 <> SL	Tab, White, Round, Film Coated	Ketorolac Tromethamine 10 mg	Toradol by Sidmak		NSAID
6081 <> BMS	Tab, Pink, Oval, Film Coated	Glipizide 2.5 mg, Metformin HCl 250 mg	Metaglip by BMS	00087-6081	Antidiabetic
608HD	Tab, White, Round	Methyldopa 500 mg	Aldomet by Halsey	Discontinued	Antihypertensive
609 <> PLIVA	Tab, Yellow, Black Print, Cap Shaped, Film Coated, Ex Release	Pentoxifylline 400 mg	Trental by Pliva	50111-0609	Anticoagulant
609542	Cap, Green Opaque Body, Blue Opaque Cap	Duloxetine 60 mg	Cymbalta by Eli Lilly	Canadian DIN 02301490	Antidepressant, Anxiolytic, Analgesic
609MJ <> M	Tab, Lower Case M	Fosinopril Sodium 20 mg	Monopril by Quality Care	62682-6026	Antihypertensive
60ADALATCC <> 885MILES60	Tab, Salmon, Film Coated, 885/Miles 60	Nifedipine 60 mg	Adalat CC by Allscripts		Antihypertensive
60MG <> P	Tab, Orange, Round, Sustained Release	Morphine Sulfate 60 mg	MS Contin by Pharmascience	Canadian DIN 02245286	Analgesic
60MG <> PF	Tab, Orange, Round	Morphine Sulfate 60 mg	MS Contin by Purdue	Canadian	Analgesic; C II
60MG1102	Cap, Pink & White	Fexofenadine HCl 60 mg	Allegra by Allscripts	00093-0761	Antihistamine
60P <> DAN	Tab, White, Round, Scored	Phenobarbital 60 mg	by Schein	00364-0697 Discontinued	Sedative/Hypnotic; C IV
61	Cap, Yellow, Oval	Terazosin HCl 2 mg	Hytrin by RP Scherer	11014-1212	Antihypertensive
61	Cap, Yellow, Oval	Terazosin HCl 2 mg	Hytrin by Teva	00093-0761 Discontinued	Antihypertensive
61 <> C	Tab, Light Yellowish-Orange, Elliptical, Film Coated	Cefpodoxime Proxetil 100 mg	Vantin by Aurobindo	65862-0095	Antibiotic
61 <> E	Tab, Blue, Round, Film-Coated	Finasteride 5 mg	Proscar by Aurobindo	65862-0149	Antiandrogen
61 <> OV	Tab, White, Scored	Ethotoin 250 mg	Peganone by Ovation	67386-0601	Anticonvulsant
61 <> SEARLE	Tab, White, Round	Diphenoxylate HCl 2.5 mg	Lomotil by Searle	Canadian DIN 00036323	Antidiarrheal; C V
61 <> SEARLE	Tab, White, Round	Atropine Sulfate 0.025 mg, Diphenoxylate HCl 2.5 mg	Lomotil by St. Mary's Med	60760-0061	Antidiarrheal; C V
61 <> SEARLE	Tab, White, Round	Atropine Sulfate 0.025 mg, Diphenoxylate HCl 2.5 mg	Lomotil by Amerisource	62584-0027	Antidiarrheal; C V
61 <> SEARLE	Tab, White, Round	Atropine Sulfate 0.025 mg, Diphenoxylate HCl 2.5 mg	Lomotil by Med Pro	53978-3088	Antidiarrheal; C V
61 <> SEARLE	Tab, White, Round	Atropine Sulfate 0.025 mg, Diphenoxylate HCl 2.5 mg	Lomotil by Nat Pharmpak	55154-3614	Antidiarrheal; C V
61 <> SEARLE	Tab, White, Round	Atropine Sulfate 0.025 mg, Diphenoxylate HCl 2.5 mg	Lomotil by Searle	00014-0061	Antidiarrheal; C V
61 <> SEARLE	Tab, White, Round	Atropine Sulfate 0.025 mg, Diphenoxylate HCl 2.5 mg	Lomotil by Searle	00025-0061	Antidiarrheal; C V
61 <> SZ	Tab, White, Oval	Carvedilol 3.125 mg	Coreg by Sandoz	00781-5221	Antihypertensive
610HD	Tab, White, Oblong	Acetaminophen 325 mg, Propoxyphene Napsylate 50 mg	Darvocet-N 50 by Halsey	Discontinued	Analgesic; C IV
611 <> MYLAN	Tab, Beige, Round, Film Coated	Methyldopa 250 mg	Aldomet by UDL	51079-0200	Antihypertensive
611 <> MYLAN	Tab, Beige, Round, Film Coated	Methyldopa 250 mg	Aldomet by Murfreesboro	51129-1293	Antihypertensive
611 <> MYLAN	Tab, Beige, Round, Film Coated	Methyldopa 250 mg	Aldomet by Mylan	00378-0611	Antihypertensive
611 <> R	Tab, Yellow, Oblong, Coated, Ex Release	Pentoxifylline 400 mg	Trental by Murfreesboro	51129-1100	Anticoagulant
611 <> R	Tab, Yellow, Oblong, Coated, Ex Release	Pentoxifylline 400 mg	Trental by Caremark	00339-5278	Anticoagulant

For updated data, go to www.IdentADrug.com

ID FRONT <> BACK	DESCRIPTION FRONT <> BACK	INGREDIENT & STRENGTH	BRAND (or Generic Equiv.) by FIRM	NDC#	CLASS; SCH.
611 <> R	Tab, Yellow, Oblong, Coated, Ex Release	Pentoxifylline 400 mg	Trental by Actavis	00228-2611	Anticoagulant
611 <> R	Tab, Yellow, Oblong, Coated, Ex Release	Pentoxifylline 400 mg	Trental by Pharmacy Care	65070-0030	Anticoagulant
611 <> R	Tab, Yellow, Oblong, Coated, Ex Release	Pentoxifylline 400 mg	Trental by Heartland	61392-0833	Anticoagulant
611 <> R	Tab, Yellow, Oblong, Coated, Ex Release	Pentoxifylline 400 mg	Trental by Murfreesboro	51129-1121	Anticoagulant
611 <> R	Tab, Yellow, Oblong, Coated, Ex Release	Pentoxifylline 400 mg	Trental by Pharmafab	62542-0753	Anticoagulant
612 <> UCB	Tab, White, Oval, Scored, Film Coated	Guaifenesin 600 mg, Pseudoephedrine 120 mg	Duratuss by Mikart	46672-0126	Cold Remedy
612 <> UCB	Tab, White, Oval, Scored, Film Coated	Guaifenesin 600 mg, Pseudoephedrine HCl 120 mg	Duratuss by UCB	50474-0612	Cold Remedy
612 <> UCB	Tab, White, Oval, Scored, Film Coated	Guaifenesin 600 mg, Pseudoephedrine HCl 120 mg	Duratuss by Nat Pharmpak	55154-7203	Cold Remedy
612 <> UCB	Tab, White, Oval, Scored, Film Coated	Guaifenesin 600 mg, Pseudoephedrine 120 mg	Duratuss by Physician Total Care	54868-3943	Cold Remedy
612 <> WHITBY	Tab, Film Coated	Guaifenesin 600 mg, Pseudoephedrine 120 mg	Duratuss by UCB	50474-0612	Cold Remedy
612 <> WHITBY	Tab, Film Coated	Guaifenesin 600 mg, Pseudoephedrine 120 mg	Duratuss by CVS	51316-0238	Cold Remedy
6121 <> PAL	Tab, White, Oblong, Scored	Carbinoxamine Maleate 8 mg, Pseudoephedrine HCl 80 mg	Palgic D by Pamlab	005525-6121	Cold Remedy
613	Cap, Dark Green & Light Green, Eon Logo 613	Hydroxyzine Pamoate 25 mg	by Quality Care	60346-0208	Antianxiety; Antihistamine
613 <> R	Tab, White, Oval, Film Coated	Ticlopidine HCl 250 mg	Ticlid by Actavis	00228-2613	Anticoagulant
6131 <> PAL	Tab, White, Cap Shaped, Scored	Carbinoxamine Maleate 8 mg, Pseudoephedrine HCl 80 mg	Palgic D by Pamlab	005525-6131	Cold Remedy
616 <> SL	Tab, White	Tramadol HCl 50 mg	Ultram by Sidmak	Discontinued	Analgesic
617 <> R	Tab, Yellow, Cap Shaped, Enteric Coated, Delayed Release	Naproxen 375 mg	Naprosyn by Actavis	00228-2617	NSAID
618 <> R	Tab, Yellow, Cap Shaped, Enteric Coated, Delayed Release	Naproxen 500 mg	Naprosyn by Actavis	00228-2618	NSAID
618 <> R	Tab, Yellow, Cap Shaped, Enteric Coated, Delayed Release	Naproxen 500 mg	Naprosyn by Orion	52483-0014	NSAID
6180100	Tab, White, Round, 6180/100	Labetalol HCl 100 mg	Trandate by BMS		Antihypertensive
6181200	Tab, White, Round, 6181/200	Labetalol HCl 200 mg	Normodyne by BMS		Antihypertensive
6182300	Tab, White, Round, 6182/300	Labetalol HCl 300 mg	Normodyne by BMS		Antihypertensive
62	Cap, Red, Oval	Terazosin HCl 5 mg	Hytrin by RP Scherer	11014-1213	Antihypertensive
62	Cap, Red, Oval	Terazosin HCl 5 mg	Hytrin by Teva	00093-0762 Discontinued	Antihypertensive
62 <> C	Tab, Coral Red, Elliptical, Film Coated	Cefpodoxime Proxetil 200 mg	Vantin by Aurobindo	65862-0096	Antibiotic
62 <> S	Tab, Pink, Round, Film-Coated	Ethinyl Estradiol 0.03 mg, Levonorgestrel 0.15 mg	Seasonale by Duramed	51285-0058	Oral Contraceptive
62 <> SZ	Tab, White, Oval	Carvedilol 6.25 mg	Coreg by Sandoz	00781-5222	Antihypertensive
62 <> WYETH	Tab, Yellow, Round	Norgestrel 0.075 mg	Ovrette by Wyeth	00008-0062	Oral Contraceptive
620	Tab, Blue, Round, Scored, Logo and 620	Isosorbide Mononitrate 20 mg	Ismo by Murfreesboro	51129-1577	Antianginal
6211 <> V	Tab, Yellow, Oval, Scored, 62 over 11	Guaifenesin 600 mg, Pseudoephedrine HCl 120 mg	by Ivax	00182-1740	Cold Remedy
6211 <> V	Tab, Yellow, Oval, Scored, 62 over 11	Guaifenesin 600 mg, Pseudoephedrine HCl 120 mg	by Quality Care	60346-0933	Cold Remedy
622HD	Tab, White, Oblong	Ibuprofen 800 mg	Motrin by Halsey	Discontinued	NSAID
625	Cap, Yellow	Docusate Potassium 100 mg, Casanthranol 30 mg	Dialose Plus by OHM		Laxative
625	Tab, White & Orange, Round, Film Coated, 62.5	Anhydrous Bosentan 62.5 mg	Tracleer by Actelion	Canadian DIN 02244981	Antihypertensive
625	Tab, White & Orange, Round, Film Coated, 62.5	Anhydrous Bosentan 62.5 mg	Tracleer by Actelion	66215-0101	Antihypertensive
625 <> APO	Tab, White, Oval, Film Coated, APO <> 6.25	Carvedilol 6.25 mg	Apo Carvedilol by Apotex	Canadian DIN 02247934	Antihypertensive
625 <> ETH	Tab, Orange to Rust, Scored	Oxycodone HCl 5 mg	Roxicodone by Ethex	58177-0625	Analgesic; C II
625 <> N	Tab, White, Oval, N <> 6.25	Carvedilol 6.25 mg	Coreg by Novopharm	Canadian DIN 02246530	Antihypertensive
625 <> P	Tab, White, Oval, Film Coated, P <> 6.25	Carvedilol 6.25 mg	Coreg by Pharmascience	Canadian DIN 02245915	Antihypertensive
625 <> V	Tab, White, Oval, Film Coated	Nelfinavir Mesylate 625 mg	Viracept by Agouron	63010-0027	Antiviral
625DPI	Tab, Light Orange, 625/DPI	Estropipate 0.75 mg	by Schein	00364-2600	Hormone
626	Tab, Beige, Oval	Vitamin A 4000 IU, Vitamin C 120 mg, Vitamin D-3 400 IU, Vitamin E 11 IU, Thiamin 1.84 mg, Riboflavin 3 mg, Niacin 20 mg, Vitamin B6 10 mg, Folic Acid 1 mg, Vitamin B12 12 mcg, Calcium 200 mg, Iron 65 mg, Zinc 25 mg, Copper 2 mg	Prenatal 1 Plus 1 by Amneal	65162-0635	Vitamin

ID FRONT <> BACK	DESCRIPTION FRONT <> BACK	INGREDIENT & STRENGTH	BRAND (or Generic Equiv.) by FIRM	NDC#	CLASS; SCH.
63	Cap, Blue, Oval	Terazosin HCl 10 mg	Hytrin by Teva	00093-0763 Discontinued	Antihypertensive
63	Cap, Blue, Oval	Terazosin HCl 10 mg	Hytrin by RP Scherer	11014-1219	Antihypertensive
630HD	Tab, Pink, Oblong	Acetaminophen 650 mg, Propoxyphene Napsylate 100 mg	Darvocet-N 100 by Halsey	Discontinued	Analgesic; C IV
630SJ	Cap, Blue Print, 630 <> S-J	Acetaminophen 500 mg, Hydrocodone Bitartrate 5 mg	Vicodin by Stewart Jackson	45985-0630	Analgesic; C III
631	Tab, Blue, Round, Scored, Logo 631	Isosorbide Mononitrate 10 mg	Ismo by Murfreesboro	51129-1576	Antianginal
631 <> ENDO	Tab, Film Coated	Cimetidine HCl 300 mg	Tagamet by Endo	Discontinued	Gastrointestinal
631PAR	Tab, White, Oval	Penicillin V Potassium 250 mg	by Pharmafab	62542-0710	Antibiotic
632HD	Cap, Flesh & Lavender	Fenoprofen Calcium 200 mg	Nalfon by Halsey	Discontinued	NSAID
632PAR	Tab, White, Oval	Penicillin V Potassium 500 mg	by Pharmafab	62542-0723	Antibiotic
633 <> R	Tab, White, Round	Lovastatin 10 mg	Mevacor by Major	00904-5581	Antihyperlipidemic
633 <> R	Tab, White, Round	Lovastatin 10 mg	Mevacor by Actavis	00228-2633	Antihyperlipidemic
6330 <> VAD	Tab, Blue, Oblong, Scored	Acetaminophen 650 mg, Hydrocodone Bitartrate 10 mg	Lorcet by H J Harkins Co	52959-0403	Analgesic; C III
633HD	Cap, Flesh & Orange	Fenoprofen Calcium 300 mg	Nalfon by Halsey	Discontinued	NSAID
634 <> R	Tab, Pink, Round	Lovastatin 20 mg	Mevacor by Actavis	00228-2634	Antihyperlipidemic
634 <> R	Tab, Pink, Round	Lovastatin 20 mg	Mevacor by Major	00904-5582	Antihyperlipidemic
634HD	Tab, Peach, Oblong	Fenoprofen Calcium 600 mg	Nalfon by Halsey	Discontinued	NSAID
635	Tab, White, Black Print, Round, Sugar Coated	Chlorambucil 2 mg	Leukeran by BW Inc	Canadian	Antineoplastic
635	Tab, White, Black Print, Round, Sugar Coated	Chlorambucil 2 mg	Leukeran by DSM	63552-0635	Antineoplastic
635	Tab, White, Black Print, Round, Sugar Coated	Chlorambucil 2 mg	Leukeran by GSK	00173-0635 Discontinued	Antineoplastic
635 <> PAR	Tab, White, Round	Lisinopril 30 mg	Zestril by Par	49884-0635	Antihypertensive
635 <> R	Tab, Yellow, Round	Lovastatin 40 mg	Mevacor by Major	00904-5583	Antihyperlipidemic
635 <> R	Tab, Yellow, Round	Lovastatin 40 mg	Mevacor by Actavis	00228-2635	Antihyperlipidemic
6350 <> UAD	Tab, Light Blue, Cap Shaped, Scored	Acetaminophen 650 mg, Hydrocodone Bitartrate 10 mg	Lorcet by Nat Pharmpak	55154-7301	Analgesic; C III
6350 <> UAD	Tab, Light Blue, Cap Shaped, Scored	Acetaminophen 650 mg, Hydrocodone Bitartrate 10 mg	Lorcet by Amerisource	62584-0021	Analgesic; C III
6350 <> UAD	Tab, Light Blue, Cap Shaped, Scored	Acetaminophen 650 mg, Hydrocodone Bitartrate 10 mg	Lorcet by Med Pro	53978-2068	Analgesic; C III
6350 <> UAD	Tab, Light Blue, Cap Shaped, Scored	Acetaminophen 650 mg, Hydrocodone Bitartrate 10 mg	Lorcet by DRX	55045-2122	Analgesic; C III
6350 <> UAD	Tab, Light Blue, Cap Shaped, Scored	Acetaminophen 650 mg, Hydrocodone Bitartrate 10 mg	Lorcet by Mikart	46672-0103	Analgesic; C III
6350 <> UAD	Tab, Light Blue, Cap Shaped, Scored	Acetaminophen 650 mg, Hydrocodone Bitartrate 10 mg	Lorcet by Southwood	58016-0232	Analgesic; C III
6350 <> UAD	Tab, Light Blue, Cap Shaped, Scored	Acetaminophen 650 mg, Hydrocodone Bitartrate 10 mg	Lorcet by Forest	00785-6350	Analgesic; C III
639500 <> WATSON	Tab	Chlorzoxazone 500 mg	Parafon Forte by Martec	52555-0263	Muscle Relaxant
640	Cap, Eon Logo 640	Phentermine HCl 30 mg	by Quality Care	62682-7025	Anorexiant; C IV
641 <> R	Tab, Beige, Round, Film Coated	Famotidine 40 mg	by Actavis	00228-2641	Gastrointestinal
643 <> 212	Tab, Pink, Round, 643 <> 2 1/2	Metolazone 2.5 mg	Zaroxolyn by Upstate Pharma	65580-0643	Diuretic
643 <> 54	Tab	Naproxen 250 mg	by Roxane	00054-8641	NSAID
643 <> COPLEY	Tab, Film Coated	Prochlorperazine Maleate 8.26 mg	by H J Harkins Co	52959-0511	Antiemetic
643 <> COPLEY	Tab, Film Coated	Prochlorperazine Maleate 8.26 mg	by Teva	38245-0643	Antiemetic
643 <> COPLEY	Tab, Film Coated, Debossed	Prochlorperazine 5 mg	by Qualitest	00603-5418	Antiemetic
644 <> 5	Tab, Blue, Round	Metolazone 5 mg	Zaroxolyn by Upstate	65580-0644	Diuretic
644DPI	Cap	Acetaminophen 500 mg, Oxycodone HCl 5 mg	Percocet by Schein	00364-2395	Analgesic; C II
647	Cap, Eon Logo 647	Phentermine HCl 30 mg	by Quality Care	62682-7025	Anorexiant; C IV
647 <> SINEMET	Tab, Dark Blue, Oval, Scored	Carbidopa 10 mg, Levodopa 100 mg	Sinemet by BMS	Canadian DIN 00355658	Antiparkinson
647 <> SINEMET	Tab, Dark Blue, Oval, Scored	Carbidopa 10 mg, Levodopa 100 mg	Sinemet by BMS	00056-0647	Antiparkinson
647HD	Cap, Blue & White	Aspirin 325 mg, Butalbital 50 mg, Caffeine 40 mg, Codeine 30 mg	Fiorinal #3 by Halsey	Discontinued	Analgesic; C III
648HD	Cap, Gray & White	Aspirin 325 mg, Butalbital 50 mg, Caffeine 40 mg, Codeine 15 mg	Fiorinal #2 by Halsey	Discontinued	Analgesic; C III
649	Tab, White, Cap Shaped, Scored, 649/649	Guaifenesin 400 mg	Bidex-400 by Stewart Jackson	45985-0654	Cold Remedy
64BI	Cap, Celery	Phendimetrazine Tartrate 105 mg	by Quality Care	60346-0621	Anorexiant; C III

ID FRONT <> BACK	DESCRIPTION FRONT <> BACK	INGREDIENT & STRENGTH	BRAND (or Generic Equiv.) by FIRM	NDC#	CLASS; SCH.
65 <> Z	Tab, White to Off-White, Round	Atenolol 25 mg	Tenormin by Zydus	68382-0022	Antihypertensive
65 <> Z	Tab, White to Off-White, Round	Atenolol 25 mg	Tenormin by Mallinckrodt	00406-2022	Antihypertensive
650 <> OM	Tab, Light Yellow, Capsule-Shaped, Coated, O-M	Tramadol HCl 37.5 mg, Acetaminophen 325 mg	Tramacet by Ivax	00172-6359	Analgesic
650 <> OM	Tab, Yellow, Cap Shaped	Acetaminophen 325 mg, Tramadol HCl 37.5 mg	Ultracet by Ortho-McNeil	00045-0650	Analgesic
650 <> R	Tab, Yellow, Cap Shaped, Film Coated	Bisoprolol 2.5 mg, Hydrochlorothiazide 6.25 mg	Ziac by Actavis	00228-2650	Antihypertensive; Diuretic
650 <> SINEMET	Tab, Yellow, Oval, Scored	Carbidopa 25 mg, Levodopa 100 mg	Sinemet by BMS	00056-0650	Antiparkinson
650 <> SINEMET	Tab, Yellow, Oval, Scored	Carbidopa 25 mg, Levodopa 100 mg	Sinemet by BMS	Canadian DIN 00513997	Antiparkinson
650ICN	Cap, Gelatin Coated	Methoxsalen 10 mg	Oxsoralen Ultra by RP Scherer	11014-1123	Dermatologic
651 <> R	Tab, Pink, Cap Shaped, Film Coated	Bisoprolol 5 mg, Hydrochlorothiazide 6.25 mg	Ziac by Actavis	00228-2651	Antihypertensive; Diuretic
652 <> COPLEY	Tab, Yellow, Round, Film Coated	Prochlorperazine Maleate 10 mg	by Ranbaxy	63304	Antiemetic
652 <> COPLEY	Tab, Yellow, Round, Film Coated	Prochlorperazine Maleate 10 mg	by Teva	00093-9652	Antiemetic
652 <> COPLEY	Tab, Yellow, Round, Film Coated	Prochlorperazine Maleate 16.53 mg	by Physician Total Care	54868-1082	Antiemetic
652 <> COPLEY	Tab, Film Coated	Prochlorperazine Maleate 16.53 mg	by H J Harkins Co	52959-0476	Antiemetic
652 <> COPLEY	Tab, Debossed	Prochlorperazine 10 mg	by Qualitest	00603-5419	Antiemetic
652 <> COPLEY	Tab, Film Coated	Prochlorperazine Maleate 16.53 mg	by Teva	38245-0652	Antiemetic
652 <> R	Tab, White, Cap Shaped, Film Coated	Bisoprolol 10 mg, Hydrochlorothiazide 6.25 mg	Ziac by Actavis	00228-2652	Antihypertensive; Diuretic
654 <> SINEMET	Tab, Light Blue, Oval, Scored	Carbidopa 25 mg, Levodopa 250 mg	Sinemet by BMS	00056-0654	Antiparkinson
654 <> SINEMET	Tab, Light Blue, Oval, Scored	Carbidopa 25 mg, Levodopa 250 mg	Sinemet by BMS	Canadian DIN 00328219	Antiparkinson
655	Cap, Blue and White, Opaque	Mycophenolate Mofetil 250 mg	CellCept by Sandoz	00781-2067	Immunosuppressant
656HD	Cap, Green	Chlordiazepoxide 5 mg, Clidinium Bromide 2.5 mg	Librax by Halsey	Discontinued	Gastrointestinal
657 <> WATSON	Tab, White, Oval, Scored	Buspirone HCl 5 mg	BuSpar by Watson	00591-0657	Antianxiety
658 <> WATSON	Tab, White, Oval, Scored	Buspirone HCl 10 mg	BuSpar by Watson	00591-0658	Antianxiety
659 <> MCNEIL	Tab, White, Cap Shaped, Film Coated	Tramadol HCl 50 mg	Ultram by Teva	00480-0148	Analgesic
659 <> MCNEIL	Tab, White, Cap Shaped, Film Coated	Tramadol HCl 50 mg	Ultram by McNeil	00045-0659	Analgesic
659 <> MCNEIL	Tab, White, Cap Shaped, Film Coated	Tramadol HCl 50 mg	Ultram by Ortho-McNeil	00062-0659	Analgesic
659 <> MCNEIL	Tab, White, Cap Shaped, Film Coated	Tramadol HCl 50 mg	Ultram by Caremark	00339-6099	Analgesic
659 <> MCNEIL	Tab, White, Cap Shaped, Film Coated	Tramadol HCl 50 mg	Ultram by DRX	55045-2219	Analgesic
659 <> MCNEIL	Tab, White, Cap Shaped, Film Coated	Tramadol HCl 50 mg	Ultram by McNeil	52021-0659	Analgesic
659 <> MCNEIL	Tab, White, Cap Shaped, Film Coated	Tramadol HCl 50 mg	Ultram by H J Harkins Co	52959-0414	Analgesic
659 <> MCNEIL	Tab, White, Cap Shaped, Film Coated	Tramadol HCl 50 mg	Ultram by Rx Dispensing	61807-0128	Analgesic
659 <> MCNEIL	Tab, White, Cap Shaped, Film Coated	Tramadol HCl 50 mg	Ultram by Heartland	61392-0625	Analgesic
659 <> MCNEIL	Tab, White, Cap Shaped, Film Coated	Tramadol HCl 50 mg	Ultram by PDRX	55289-0650	Analgesic
659 <> MCNEIL	Tab, White, Cap Shaped, Film Coated	Tramadol HCl 50 mg	Ultram by Northeast	58163-0659	Analgesic
65B	Cap, White, Opaque, Gelatin w/ Dark Blue Print, Organon Logo 65B	Amylase 30,000 USP, Bile Salts 65 mg, Cellulase 2 mg, Lipase 8000 USP, Protease 30,000 USP	Cotazym ECS 65B by Organon	Canadian DIN 00456233	Gastrointestinal
66 <> A	Tab, Pink, Cap Shaped, Film Coated	Amoxicillin 500 mg	Amoxil by Aurobindo	65862-0014	Antibiotic
66 <> MP	Tab, Off-White, ER	Quinidine Gluconate 324 mg	by Quality Care	60346-0555	Antiarrhythmic
66 <> SL	Tab, Pink, Round, Film Coated	Amitriptyline HCl 10 mg	Elavil by Pliva	50111-0366	Antidepressant
66 <> SL	Tab, Pink, Round, Film Coated	Amitriptyline HCl 10 mg	Elavil by Vangard	00615-0828	Antidepressant
66 <> UU	Tab, White, Round, Scored	Pramipexole DiHCl 1 mg	Mirapex by Pharmacia	00009-0006	Antiparkinson
66 <> UU	Tab, White, Round, Scored	Pramipexole DiHCl 1 mg	Mirapex by Boehringer Ingelheim	00597-0090	Antiparkinson
663	Tab, Light Pink, Cap Shaped	Tetracycline HCl 250 mg	Sumycin by Par	49884-0797	Antibiotic
663 <> 93	Tab, White, Oval, Film Coated	Indapamide 1.25 mg	Lozol by Teva	00093-0663	Diuretic
6666 <> 4001	Tab	Medroxyprogesterone Acetate 10 mg	by Apotheca	12634-0108	Hormone
667400 <> WATSON	Tab, 667 over 400 <> Watson	Etodolac 400 mg	by Watson	52544-0667	NSAID
667400 <> WATSON	Tab, 667 over 400 <> Watson	Etodolac 400 mg	by Major	00904-5246	NSAID
667400 <> WATSON	Tab, 667 over 400 <> Watson	Etodolac 400 mg	by Qualitest	00603-3570	NSAID

ID FRONT <> BACK	DESCRIPTION FRONT <> BACK	INGREDIENT & STRENGTH	BRAND (or Generic Equiv.) by FIRM	NDC#	CLASS; SCH.
67 <> A	Tab, Pink, Cap Shaped, Film Coated, Scored, A <> 6/7	Amoxicillin 875 mg	Amoxil by Aurobindo	65862-0015	Antibiotic
67 <> SL	Tab, Green, Black Print, Round, Film Coated	Amitriptyline HCl 25 mg	Elavil by Amerisource	62584-0614	Antidepressant
67 <> SL	Tab, Green, Black Print, Round, Film Coated	Amitriptyline HCl 25 mg	Elavil by St. Mary's Med	60760-0367	Antidepressant
67 <> SL	Tab, Green, Black Print, Round, Film Coated	Amitriptyline HCl 25 mg	Elavil by Rx Dispensing	61807-0129	Antidepressant
67 <> SL	Tab, Green, Black Print, Round, Film Coated	Amitriptyline HCl 25 mg	Elavil by Nat Pharmpak	55154-5814	Antidepressant
67 <> SL	Tab, Green, Black Print, Round, Film Coated	Amitriptyline HCl 25 mg	Elavil by Apothecon	59772-2593	Antidepressant
67 <> SL	Tab, Green, Black Print, Round, Film Coated	Amitriptyline HCl 25 mg	Elavil by Qualitest	00603-2213	Antidepressant
67 <> SL	Tab, Green, Black Print, Round, Film Coated	Amitriptyline HCl 25 mg	Elavil by H J Harkins Co	52959-0348	Antidepressant
67 <> SL	Tab, Green, Black Print, Round, Film Coated	Amitriptyline HCl 25 mg	Elavil by Apotheca	12634-0401	Antidepressant
67 <> SL	Tab, Green, Black Print, Round, Film Coated	Amitriptyline HCl 25 mg	Elavil by Pliva	50111-0367	Antidepressant
67 <> SL	Tab, Green, Black Print, Round, Film Coated	Amitriptyline HCl 25 mg	Elavil by Vangard	00615-0829	Antidepressant
67 <> SL	Tab, Green, Black Print, Round, Film Coated	Amitriptyline HCl 25 mg	Elavil by Ivax	00182-1019	Antidepressant
67 <> SL	Tab, Green, Black Print, Round, Film Coated	Amitriptyline HCl 25 mg	Elavil by Kaiser	00179-1275	Antidepressant
67 <> SL	Tab, Green, Black Print, Round, Film Coated	Amitriptyline HCl 25 mg	Elavil by Baker Cummins	63171-1019	Antidepressant
67 <> SL	Tab, Green, Black Print, Round, Film Coated	Amitriptyline HCl 25 mg	Elavil by Med Pro	53978-0023	Antidepressant
67093	Tab, White, Oval, 670/93	Gemfibrozil 500 mg	by Genpharm	Canadian	Antihyperlipidemic
672 <> PENTOX	Tab, White, Oblong, Film Coated	Pentoxifylline 400 mg	Trental by Blue Ridge	59273-0018	Anticoagulant
672 <> PENTOX	Tab, Film Coated	Pentoxifylline 400 mg	Trental by Merrell	00068-0672	Anticoagulant
672 <> PENTOX	Tab, Film Coated	Pentoxifylline 400 mg	Trental by Teva	38245-0672 Discontinued	Anticoagulant
672COPLEY	Tab, White, Oval, 672/Copley	Pentoxifylline 400 mg	Trental by Copley		Anticoagulant
673 <> PP	Tab, White to Off-White, Oval	Cabergoline 0.5 mg	Dostinex by Par	49884-0673	Antiparkinson
673WC	Tab	Penicillin V Potassium	by Pharmedix	53002-0202	Antibiotic
675 <> PLIVA	Tab, Pale Pink, Round	Fluconazole 50 mg	Diflucan by Par	49884-0935	Antifungal
675 <> POLYVENT	Tab, 6 over 75 <> Poly-vent	Guaifenesin 600 mg, Phenylpropanolamine HCl 75 mg	Entex LA by Pharmafab	62542-0780	Cold Remedy
675 <> POLYVENT	Tab, 6 over 75 <> Poly-Vent	Guaifenesin 600 mg, Phenylpropanolamine HCl 75 mg	Entex LA by Poly	50991-0408	Cold Remedy
678 <> FOREST	Tab	Acetaminophen 500 mg, Butalbital 50 mg, Caffeine 40 mg	by PDRX	55289-0264	Analgesic
678 <> FOREST	Tab, White, Oblong, Scored	Acetaminophen 500 mg, Butalbital 50 mg, Caffeine 40 mg	Esgic Plus by Rx Pak	65084-0195	Analgesic
678 <> FOREST	Tab, White, Oblong, Scored	Acetaminophen 500 mg, Butalbital 50 mg, Caffeine 40 mg	Esgic Plus by Rightpak	65240-0644	Analgesic
678 <> FOREST	Tab	Acetaminophen 500 mg, Butalbital 50 mg, Caffeine 40 mg	by Nat Pharmpak	55154-4602	Analgesic
678 <> FOREST	Tab, White, Cap Shaped, Scored	Acetaminophen 500 mg, Butalbital 50 mg, Caffeine 40 mg	Esgic Plus by Forest	00456-0678	Analgesic
679 <> R	Tab, Yellow, Round, Film Coated	Famotidine 20 mg	by Activis	00228-2679	Gastrointestinal
681	Tab, Yellow, Oval, Film Coated, Ex Release	Bupropion 150 mg	Wellbutrin XL by Global	00115-6811	Antidepressant
682 <> G	Tab, Yellow, Oval, Extended Release	Bupropion HCl 300 mg	Wellbutrin XL by Teva	00093-5351	Antidepressant
682 <> PAR200	Tab, White, Cap Shaped	Ofloxacin 200 mg	Floxin by Par	49884-0682	Antibiotic
682025 <> WATSON	Tab, White, Oval, Scored, 682 0.25 <> Watson	Alprazolam 0.25 mg	Xanax by Allscripts		Antianxiety; C IV
683 <> PAR300	Tab, White, Cap Shaped	Ofloxacin 300 mg	Floxin by Par	49884-0683	Antibiotic
68305 <> WATSON	Tab, Peach, Oval, Scored	Alprazolam 0.5 mg	Xanax by Allscripts		Antianxiety; C IV
6835	Tab, Light Yellow, Oval	Vitamin E 400 IU	Vitamin E by Ivax	00182-8216 Discontinued	Vitamin
684 <> PAR400	Tab, White, Cap Shaped	Ofloxacin 400 mg	Floxin by Par	49884-0684	Antibiotic
6841 <> WATSON	Tab, Blue, Oval, Scored, 684 over 1 <> Watson	Alprazolam 1 mg	Xanax by Apotheca	12634-0523	Antianxiety; C IV
68410 <> WATSON	Tab, Blue, Oval, Scored, 684 1.0 <> Watson	Alprazolam 1 mg	Xanax by Allscripts		Antianxiety; C IV
685550 <> WATSON	Tab, Peach, Round, 685 over 5-50	Amiloride HCl 5 mg, Hydrochlorothiazide 50 mg	Moduretic by Watson	52544-0685	Antihypertensive; Diuretic
685550 <> WATSON	Tab	Amiloride HCl 5 mg, Hydrochlorothiazide 50 mg	Moduretic by Qualitest	00603-2188	Antihypertensive; Diuretic
685550 <> WATSON	Tab	Amiloride HCl 5 mg, Hydrochlorothiazide 50 mg	Moduretic by Major	00904-2114	Antihypertensive; Diuretic
68610 <> WATSON	Tab, 686 over 10	Baclofen 10 mg	Lioresal by Supremus	62114-0120	Muscle Relaxant
68610 <> WATSON	Tab, 686/10 <> Watson	Baclofen 10 mg	Lioresal by Watson	52544-0686	Muscle Relaxant
68610 <> WATSON	Tab, 686/10 <> Watson	Baclofen 10 mg	Lioresal by Major	00904-5216	Muscle Relaxant

ID FRONT <> BACK	DESCRIPTION FRONT <> BACK	INGREDIENT & STRENGTH	BRAND (or Generic Equiv.) by FIRM	NDC#	CLASS; SCH.
68610 <> WATSON	Tab, 686/10 <> Watson	Baclofen 10 mg	Lioresal by Moore	00839-7472	Muscle Relaxant
68610 <> WATSON	Tab, White, Oval, Scored	Baclofen 10 mg	Lioresal by Murfreesboro	51129-1409	Muscle Relaxant
68610 <> WATSON	Tab, White, Oval, Scored	Baclofen 10 mg	Lioresal by DRX	55045-2724	Muscle Relaxant
687	Tab, Blue, Round, Sugar Coated, 68-7	Desipramine HCl 10 mg	Norpramin by Merrell	00068-0007	Antidepressant
687	Tab, Blue, Round, Sugar Coated, 68-7	Desipramine HCl 10 mg	Norpramin by Marion	Canadian	Antidepressant
68720 <> WATSON	Tab, White, Oval, Scored, 687/20 <> Watson	Baclofen 20 mg	Lioresal by Supremus	62114-0122	Muscle Relaxant
68720 <> WATSON	Tab, White, Oval, Scored, 687/20 <> Watson	Baclofen 20 mg	Lioresal by Major		Muscle Relaxant
68720 <> WATSON	Tab, White, Oval, Scored, 687/20 <> Watson	Baclofen 20 mg	Lioresal by Watson	52544-0687	Muscle Relaxant
688 <> 93	Tab, White to Off-White, Round, Chewable	Lamotrigine 5 mg	Lamictal by Teva	00093-0688	Anticonvulsant
688125 <> WATSON	Tab, White, Oblong, Scored, 688 12.5	Captopril 12.5 mg	Capoten by Watson	52544-0688	Antihypertensive
688125 <> WATSON	Tab, White, Oblong, Scored, 688 12.5	Captopril 12.5 mg	Capoten by Qualitest	00603-2555	Antihypertensive
688125 <> WATSON	Tab, White, Oblong, Scored, 688 12.5	Captopril 12.5 mg	Capoten by Major		Antihypertensive
68925 <> WATSON	Tab, White, Round, Scored	Captopril 25 mg	Capoten by Southwood	58016-0166	Antihypertensive
68925 <> WATSON	Tab, White, Round, Scored	Captopril 25 mg	Capoten by Qualitest	00603-2556	Antihypertensive
68925 <> WATSON	Tab, White, Round, Scored	Captopril 25 mg	Capoten by Watson	52544-0689	Antihypertensive
69 <> M	Tab, Dark Pink, Film Coated	Indapamide 1.25 mg	Lozol by Mylan	00378-0069	Diuretic
69 <> Z	Tab, White to Off-White, Oval, Film-Coated	Metformin HCl 850 mg	Glucophage by Mallinckrodt	00406-2029	Antidiabetic
69 <> Z	Tab, White to Off-White, Oval, Film-Coated	Metformin HCl 850 mg	Glucophage by Zydus	68382-0029	Antidiabetic
690	Tab, White, Round	Testolactone 50 mg	Teslac by BMS	00003-0690 Discontinued	Hormone; C III
690	Tab, White, Round	Testolactone 50 mg	Teslac by BMS	64747-0690 Discontinued	Hormone; C III
69050 <> WATSON	Tab	Captopril 50 mg	Capoten by Qualitest	00603-2557	Antihypertensive
69050 <> WATSON	Tab	Captopril 50 mg	Capoten by Major		Antihypertensive
69050 <> WATSON	Tab, Football Shaped	Captopril 50 mg	Capoten by Watson	52544-0690	Antihypertensive
691 <> WATSON	Tab	Captopril 100 mg	Capoten by Major	00904-5048	Antihypertensive
6910AP10MEQ	Tab, Light Orange, Round, Film Coated, 6910 over AP over 10 MEQ	Potassium Chloride 750 mg	K-Dur by Caremark	00339-6120	Electrolytes
6910AP10MEQ	Tab, Light Orange, Round, Film Coated, 6910 over AP over 10 MEQ	Potassium Chloride 750 mg	K-Dur by Apothecon	59772-6910	Electrolytes
691100 <> WATSON	Tab	Captopril 100 mg	Capoten by Watson	52544-0691	Antihypertensive
693500 <> WATSON	Tab, Green, Oblong	Chlorzoxazone 500 mg	by Watson	52544-0693	Muscle Relaxant
693500 <> WATSON	Tab	Chlorzoxazone 500 mg	by Major	00904-0302	Muscle Relaxant
693500 <> WATSON	Tab, Green, Cap Shaped, Scored, "693,500" <> Watson	Chlorzoxazone 500 mg	by Allscripts		Muscle Relaxant
698200 <> WATSON	Tab, White, Oval	Hydroxychloroquine Sulfate 200 mg	Plaquenil by Watson	00591-0698	Antimalarial
698200 <> WATSON	Tab, White, Oval	Hydroxychloroquine Sulfate 200 mg	Plaquenil by Major	00904-5107	Antimalarial
698200 <> WATSON	Tab, White, Oval	Hydroxychloroquine Sulfate 200 mg	Plaquenil by Qualitest	00603-3944	Antimalarial
698200 <> WATSON	Tab, White, Oval	Hydroxychloroquine Sulfate 200 mg	Plaquenil by Moore	00839-7963	Antimalarial
69910 <> WATSON	Tab, Orange, Round, Film Coated	Hydroxyzine HCl 10 mg	by Watson	52544-0699	Antianxiety; Antihistamine
6I	Tab, White, Cap Shaped	Ibuprofen 600 mg	Motrin by Dr. Reddy's	55111-0683	NSAID
6MG	Cap, Light Blue with White Stripe, Opaque	Tizanidine HCl 6 mg	Zanaflex by Acorda	10144-0606	Muscle Relaxant
6R	Cap, Maroon, Soft Gel	Isotretinoin 20 mg	Sotret by Ranbaxy	63304-0585	Dermatologic
6SYCBMZ	Tab, Green, Cylindrical, 6/Syc-BMZ	Bromazepam 6 mg	Lectopam by AltiMed	Canadian DIN 02167824	Sedative; C IV
7 <> A	Tab, Orange, Octagonal, Film Coated	Indapamide 1.25 mg	Lozol by RPR	00801-0777	Diuretic
7 <> A	Tab, Orange, Octagonal, Film Coated	Indapamide 1.25 mg	Lozol by Caremark	00339-6084	Diuretic
7 <> A	Tab, Orange, Octagonal, Film Coated	Indapamide 1.25 mg	Lozol by Arcola	00070-0777 Discontinued	Diuretic
7 <> A	Tab, Orange, Octagonal, Film Coated	Indapamide 1.25 mg	Lozol by Murfreesboro	51129-1536	Diuretic
7 <> CIBA	Tab, Yellow, Round	Methylphenidate HCl 5 mg	by Caremark	00339-4082	Stimulant; C II

ID FRONT <> BACK	DESCRIPTION FRONT <> BACK	INGREDIENT & STRENGTH	BRAND (or Generic Equiv.) by FIRM	NDC#	CLASS; SCH.
7 <> CIBA	Tab, Yellow, Round	Methylphenidate HCl 5 mg	Ritalin by Novartis	00083-0007	Stimulant; C II
7 <> I	Tab, White, Round	Meprobamate 200 mg	Miltown by Dr. Reddy's	55111-0640	Tranquilizer
7 <> R	Tab, Orange, Octagonal, Film Coated	Indapamide 1.25 mg	Lozol by RPR	00075-0700	Diuretic
7 <> R	Tab, Orange, Octagonal, Film Coated	Indapamide 1.25 mg	Lozol by Amerisource	62584-0700	Diuretic
7 <> R	Tab, Orange, Octagonal, Film Coated	Indapamide 1.25 mg	Lozol by Thrift Drug	59198-0263	Diuretic
7 <> R	Tab, Orange, Octagonal, Film Coated	Indapamide 1.25 mg	Lozol by RPR	00801-0700	Diuretic
7 <> SEARLE	Tab, Yellowish Green	Ethinyl Estradiol 0.035 mg, Norethindrone 0.5 mg, Norethindrone 1 mg	Tri Noryl 21 Day by Searle	00025-0272	Oral Contraceptive
7 <> SEARLE	Tab, Yellowish Green	Ethinyl Estradiol 0.035 mg, Norethindrone 1 mg	Noryl 1 35 21 Day by Searle	00025-0257	Oral Contraceptive
7 <> Z	Tab, White to Off-White, Round	Amlodipine Besylate 2.5 mg	Norvasc by Zydus	68382-0121	Antihypertensive
70 <> A	Tab, Green, Cap Shaped, Film Coated	Risperidone 0.5 mg	Risperdal by Aurobindo	65862-0120	Antipsychotic
70 <> N	Tab, White, Oval	Alendronate Sodium 70 mg	Fosamax by Novopharm	Canadian DIN 02261715	Antiosteoporosis
70 <> P	Tab, White, Oval, P logo	Alendronate Sodium 70 mg	Fosamax by Pharmascience	Canadian DIN 02284006	Antiosteoporosis
70 <> Z	Tab, White to Off-White, Round, Film-Coated	Metformin HCl 500 mg	Glucophage by Zydus	68382-0028	Antidiabetic
70 <> Z	Tab, White to Off-White, Round, Film-Coated	Metformin HCl 500 mg	Glucophage by Mallinckrodt	00406-2028	Antidiabetic
700 <> PU	Tab, White, Cap Shaped, Scored	Cabergoline 0.5 mg	Dostinex by Pharmacia	10829-7001	Antiparkinson
700 <> PU	Tab, White, Cap Shaped, Scored	Cabergoline 0.5 mg	Dostinex by Pharmacia	Canadian DIN 02242471	Antiparkinson
700 <> PU	Tab, White, Cap Shaped, Scored	Cabergoline 0.5 mg	Dostinex by Pharmacia	00013-7001	Antiparkinson
70010115	Cap, White	Lipram 4500 Units	by Global	00115-7001	Gastrointestinal
70010115	Cap	Pancrelipase (Amylase, Lipase, Protease) 175.74 mg	Pancreatic Enzyme by Ivax	00182-1968	Gastrointestinal
70010115	Cap	Pancrelipase (Amylase, Lipase, Protease) 175.74 mg	Protilase by Rugby	00536-4509	Gastrointestinal
70025 <> WATSON	Tab, Green, Round, Film Coated	Hydroxyzine HCl 25 mg	by Watson	52544-0700	Antianxiety; Antihistamine
70040115	Cap, White	Lipram 4500 Units	by Global	00115-7004	Gastrointestinal
7005 <> 0115	Tab, White, Round	Mephobarbital 32 mg	by Global	00115-7005	Sedative/Hypnotic; C IV
7006 <> 0115	Tab, White, Round	Mephobarbital 50 mg	by Global	00115-7006	Sedative/Hypnotic; C IV
7007 <> 0115	Tab, White, Round	Mephobarbital 100 mg	by Global	00115-7007	Sedative/Hypnotic; C IV
7008 <> 0115	Tab, Pale Blue-Green, Compressed	Hyoscyamine Sulfate 0.125 mg	Levsin by Global	00115-7008	Gastrointestinal
7009 <> 0115	Tab, White, Compressed	Hyoscyamine Sulfate 0.125 mg	Levsin by Global	00115-7009	Gastrointestinal
701 <> GILEAD	Tab, Blue, Cap Shaped, Film Coated	Emtricitabine 200 mg, Tenofovir Disoproxil Fumarate 300 mg	Truvada by Gilead	61958-0701	Antiviral
701 <> W25	Tab, Peach, Shield Shaped, Scored, W over 25	Venlafaxine 25 mg	Effexor by Wyeth	00008-0701	Antidepressant
7010	Tab, White, Round	Chloroquine Phosphate 500 mg	Aralen Phosphate by Global	00115-7010	Antimalarial
7011 <> 0115	Tab, White, Round	Aminobenzoate Potassium 0.5 mg	Potaba by Global	00115-7011	Antifibrotic
7012015	Cap, Light Gray	Aminobenzoate Potassium 0.5 mg	Potaba by Global	00115-7012	Antifibrotic
7013 <> 0115	Tab, Orange, Oblong	Guaifenesin 600 mg, Pseudoephedrine HCl 120 mg	by Global	00115-7013	Cold Remedy
702 <> MJ	Tab, White, Coated, Speckled	Ascorbic Acid 80 mg, Biotin 0.03 mg, Calcium 200 mg, Copper 3 mg, Cyanocobalamin 2.5 mcg, Folic Acid 1 mg, Iron 54 mg, Magnesium 100 mg, Niacin 17 mg, Pantothenic Acid 7 mg, Pyridoxine HCl 4 mg, Riboflavin 1.6 mg, Thiamine 1.5 mg, Vitamin A 4000 Units, Vitamin D 400 Units, Vitamin E 15 Units, Zinc 25 mg	Natalins Tablets Rx by BMS	00087-0702	Vitamin
7025 <> 0115	Tab, Light Orange, Compressed	Hyoscyamine Sulfate 0.375 mg	Levsin by Global	00115-7025	Gastrointestinal
7026 <> 0115	Tab, White, Tan, Round	Oxycodone HCl 5 mg	by Global	00115-7026	Analgesic; C II
7029	Tab, White, Tan, Round	Pancrelipase 8000 Units	Creon 8 by Major	00904-3472	Gastrointestinal
7029 <> 0115	Tab, White, Round	Pancrelipase 8000 Units	by Global	00115-7029	Gastrointestinal
703 <> W50	Tab, Peach, Shield Shaped, Scored, W over 50	Venlafaxine 50 mg	Effexor by Wyeth	00008-0703	Antidepressant
7033	Tab, White to Off-White, Round, Convex	Fludrocortisone Acetate 0.1 mg	Florinef by Global	00115-7033	Steroid
7037	Tab, White, Round, Scored	Methyltestosterone 10 mg	Methitest by Global	00115-7037	Hormone; C III
7038 <> 0115	Tab, Yellow, Round	Methyltestosterone 25 mg	by Global	00115-7038	Hormone; C III
704 <> R	Tab, Green, Cap Shaped, Film Coated	Fluvoxamine Maleate 25 mg	Luvox by Activis	00228-2704	OCD
704 <> W75	Tab, Peach, Shield Shaped, Scored, W over 75	Venlafaxine 75 mg	Effexor by Wyeth	00008-0704	Antidepressant

ID FRONT <> BACK	DESCRIPTION FRONT <> BACK	INGREDIENT & STRENGTH	BRAND (or Generic Equiv.) by FIRM	NDC#	CLASS; SCH.
704 <> W75	Tab, Peach, Shield Shaped, Scored, W over 75	Venlafaxine 75 mg	Effexor by Caremark	00339-6034	Antidepressant
7045 <> AP	Tab, White, Round, Scored	Captopril 12.5 mg	Capoten by Med Pro	53978-0939	Antihypertensive
7045 <> AP	Tab, White, Round, Scored	Captopril 12.5 mg	Capoten by Nat Pharmpak	55154-7601	Antihypertensive
7045 <> AP	Tab, White, Round, Scored	Captopril 12.5 mg	Capoten by Apothecon	55772-7045	Antihypertensive
7045 <> AP	Tab, White, Round, Scored	Captopril 12.5 mg	Capoten by BMS	15548-0045	Antihypertensive
70450 <> WATSON	Tab, Yellow, Round, Film Coated	Hydroxyzine HCl 50 mg	Atarax by Watson	52544-0704	Antianxiety; Antihistamine
705	Tab, Gray, Round, Schering Logo 705	Perphenazine 2 mg	Trilafon by Schering		Antipsychotic
705 <> MGI	Tab, White, Black Print, Round, Film Coated	Pilocarpine HCl 5 mg	Salagen by MGI	58063-0705	Cholinergic Agonist
705 <> W100	Tab, Peach, Shield Shaped, Scored, W over 100	Venlafaxine 100 mg	Effexor by Wyeth	00008-0705	Antidepressant
706210 <> WATSON	Tab, Blue, Round	Amitriptyline 10 mg, Perphenazine 2 mg	Triavil by Watson	52544-0706	Antidepressant; Antipsychotic
7065 <> 511	Tab, Light Yellow, Round	Bisoprolol 2.5 mg, Hydrochlorothiazide 6.25 mg	Ziac by ESI Lederle	59911-7065	Antihypertensive; Diuretic
7066 <> 511	Tab, Light Pink, Round	Bisoprolol 2.5 mg, Hydrochlorothiazide 6.25 mg	Ziac by ESI Lederle	59911-7066	Antihypertensive; Diuretic
7067 <> 511	Tab, White, Round	Bisoprolol 10 mg, Hydrochlorothiazide 6.25 mg	Ziac by ESI Lederle	59911-7067	Antihypertensive; Diuretic
707 <> SP75	Tab, Pink, Round, Scored, Film Coated, SP 7.5	Moexipril HCl 7.5 mg	Univasc by Schwarz	00091-3707	Antihypertensive
707 <> TONOCARD	Tab, Yellow, Oval, Scored, Film Coated	Tocainide HCl 400 mg	Tonocard by AstraZeneca	00186-0707	Antiarrhythmic
707225 <> WATSON	Tab, Orange, Round	Amitriptyline 25 mg, Perphenazine 2 mg	Triavil by Major	00904-1825	Antidepressant; Antipsychotic
707225 <> WATSON	Tab, Orange, Round	Amitriptyline 25 mg, Perphenazine 2 mg	Triavil by Watson	52544-0707	Antidepressant; Antipsychotic
708410 <> WATSON	Tab, Beige, Round	Amitriptyline 10 mg, Perphenazine 4 mg	Triavil by Watson	52544-0708	Antidepressant; Antipsychotic
709 <> TONOCARD	Tab, Yellow, Oblong, Scored, Film Coated	Tocainide HCl 600 mg	Tonocard by AstraZeneca	00186-0709	Antiarrhythmic
709425 <> WATSON	Tab, Yellow, Round	Amitriptyline 25 mg, Perphenazine 4 mg	Triavil by Watson	52544-0709	Antidepressant; Antipsychotic
71 <> A	Tab, White, Cap Shaped, Film Coated	Risperidone 1 mg	Risperdal by Aurobindo	65862-0121	Antipsychotic
71 <> AN	Tab, White, Round, Film Coated	Hydroxyzine HCl 25 mg	Atarax by Harris	67405-0671	Antianxiety; Antihistamine
71 <> C	Tab, Pink, Oval, Film-Coated	Ondansetron 24 mg	Ondansetron by Aurobindo	65862-0188	Antiemetic
71 <> C	Tab	Atenolol 100 mg, Chlorthalidone 25 mg	Tenoretic by IPR	54921-0117	Antihypertensive; Diuretic
71 <> I	Tab, Yellow, Round	Minocycline 50 mg	Dynacin by Dr. Reddy's	55111-0637	Antibiotic
71 <> SEARLE	Tab, White, Round	Ethinyl Estradiol 50 mcg, Ethynodiol Diacetate 1 mg	Demulen 1/50 by Pharm Util	60491-0183	Oral Contraceptive
71 <> SEARLE	Tab, White, Round	Ethinyl Estradiol 50 mcg, Ethynodiol Diacetate 1 mg	Demulen 1/50 by Searle	00025-0071	Oral Contraceptive
71 <> SEARLE	Tab, White, Round	Ethinyl Estradiol 50 mcg, Ethynodiol Diacetate 1 mg	Demulen 1/50 by Physician Total Care	54868-3790	Oral Contraceptive
710	Tab, White to Off-White, Cap Shaped, 710 <> Bone Image	Alendronate Sodium 70 mg, Cholecalciferol 2800 IU	Fosavance by Merck Frosst	Canadian DIN 02276429	Antiosteoporosis
710	Tab, White to Off-White, Cap Shaped, 710 <> Bone Image	Alendronate Sodium 70 mg, Cholecalciferol 2800 IU	Fosamax Plus D by Merck	00006-0710	Antiosteoporosis
7105 <> WATSON	Tab, 710 over 5	Pindolol 5 mg	by Qualitest	00603-5220	Antihypertensive
7105 <> WATSON	Tab, 710 over 5	Pindolol 5 mg	by Major	00904-7893	Antihypertensive
7105 <> WATSON	Tab, 710 over 5	Pindolol 5 mg	by Moore	00839-7761	Antihypertensive
7105 <> WATSON	Tab, White, Round	Pindolol 5 mg	by Watson	52544-0710	Antihypertensive
711	Tab, Beige, Oval, Scored, Film Coated, Logo and 711	Isosorbide Mononitrate 60 mg	Imdur by Murfreesboro	51129-1572	Antianginal
711	Tab, Beige, Oval, Scored	Isosorbide Mononitrate 60 mg	Imdur by Vangard	00615-4544	Antianginal
711 <> 93	Tab, Coated	Flurbiprofen 100 mg	by Quality Care	60346-0968	NSAID
711 <> AN	Tab, White, Oval	Guanfacine HCl 1 mg	Tenex by Amneal	65162-0711	Antihypertensive
711 <> MYLAN	Tab, Green, Coated, Beveled Edge	Hydrochlorothiazide 25 mg, Methyldopa 250 mg	Aldoril by Mylan	00378-0711	Diuretic; Antihypertensive
711 <> MYLAN	Tab, Coated	Hydrochlorothiazide 25 mg, Methyldopa 250 mg	Aldoril by Allscripts		Diuretic; Antihypertensive
7111 <> Z200	Tab, Coated	Cimetidine HCl 200 mg	Tagamet by Ivax	00172-7111	Gastrointestinal
71110 <> WATSON	Tab, White, Round	Pindolol 10 mg	by Watson	52544-0711	Antihypertensive
7112	Cap, Light Red, Opaque, White Print, Oval, Soft Gel	Docusate Sodium 100 mg	Colace by Rugby	00536-3756	Laxative
7112	Cap, Light Red, Opaque, White Print, Oval, Soft Gel	Docusate Sodium 100 mg	Colace by Cypress	60258-0955	Laxative

ID FRONT <> BACK	DESCRIPTION FRONT <> BACK	INGREDIENT & STRENGTH	BRAND (or Generic Equiv.) by FIRM	NDC#	CLASS; SCH.
7112	Cap, Light Red, Opaque, White Print, Oval, Soft Gel	Docusate Sodium 100 mg	Colace by Ivax	00182-0287 Discontinued	Laxative
7112	Softgel	Docusate Sodium 100 mg	Colace by LNK	50844-0112	Laxative
7113	Cap, Red, White Print, Oblong, Soft Gel	Docusate Sodium 250 mg	Colace by Rugby	00536-3757	Laxative
7113 <> 93	Tab, Mottled Peach, Oblong, Scored, 93 to left of Score <> 7113	Nefazodone HCl 150 mg	Serzone by Teva	00093-7113	Antidepressant
7113 <> M	Tab, White, Round, Scored, M inside square <> 7113 over Score	Meperidine 50 mg	Demerol by Mallinckrodt	00406-7113	Analgesic; C II
7113 <> M	Tab, White, Round, Scored, M inside square <> 7113 over Score	Meperidine 50 mg	Demerol by D M Graham	00756-0286	Analgesic; C II
7114	Cap, Maroon, Oval, Soft Gel	Docusate Sodium 100 mg, Casanthranol 30 mg	Peri-Colace by Rugby	00536-3751	Laxative
7114 <> 93	Tab, Yellow, Round, Film Coated, Scored, 9 / 3	Paroxetine HCl 10 mg	Paxil by Teva	00093-7114 Discontinued	Antidepressant
7115	Cap, Red, Oblong, Soft Gel	Docusate Calcium 240 mg	Surfak by Rugby	00536-3755	Laxative
7115 <> 93	Tab, Pink, Round, Film Coated, Scored, 9 / 3	Paroxetine HCl 20 mg	Paxil by Teva	00093-7115 Discontinued	Antidepressant
7115 <> 93	Tab, Pink, Round, Film Coated, Scored, 9 / 3	Paroxetine HCl 20 mg	Paxil by UDL	51079-0774	Antidepressant
7115 <> M	Tab, White, Round, Scored, M inside square	Meperidine 100 mg	Demerol by Mallinckrodt	00406-7115	Analgesic; C II
7116 <> 93	Tab, Blue, Round, Film Coated	Paroxetine HCl 30 mg	Paxil by Teva	00093-7116 Discontinued	Antidepressant
7117 <> Z300	Tab, White, Round, Z over 300	Cimetidine HCl 300 mg	Tagamet by Ivax	00172-7117	Gastrointestinal
7117 <> Z300	Tab, White, Round, Z over 300	Cimetidine HCl 300 mg	Tagamet by Ivax	00182-1984	Gastrointestinal
7117 <> Z300	Tab, White to Off White, Round	Cimetidine 300 mg	Tagamet by Teva	00172-7117	Gastrointestinal
711ENDO	Tab	Glipizide 5 mg	by BMS	00056-0711	Antidiabetic
712	Tab, Gray, Octagonal, Film-Coated, 7 1/2	Oxymorphone HCl 7.5 mg	Opana ER by Endo	63481-0522	Analgesic; C II
712 <> B775	Tab, Blue, Round, Scored, 7 over 1/2	Mixed Amphetamine Salts 7.5 mg: Dextroamphetamine Saccharate 1.875 mg, Amphetamine Aspartate 1.875 mg, Dextroamphetamine Sulfate 1.875 mg, Amphetamine Sulfate 1.875 mg	Adderall by Barr	00555-0775	Stimulant; C II
712 <> COPLEY	Tab	Atenolol 50 mg	Tenormin by Teva	38245-0712	Antihypertensive
712 <> M	Tab, White, Round	Enalapril Maleate 5 mg, Hydrochlorothiazide 12.5 mg	Vaseretic by Mylan	00378-0712	Antihypertensive; Diuretic
712 <> SP	Tab, Yellow, Oval, Scored, Film Coated	Moexipril HCl 7.5 mg, Hydrochlorothiazide 12.5 mg	Uniretic by Schwarz	00091-3712	Antihypertensive; Diuretic
712 <> WARFARINTARO	Tab, Yellow, Cap Shaped, 7 1/2	Warfarin Sodium 7.5 mg	Coumadin by Taro	51672-4034	Anticoagulant
7121 <> 93	Tab, Green, Round, Film Coated	Paroxetine HCl 40 mg	Paxil by Teva	00093-7121	Antidepressant
7121 <> 93	Tab, Green, Round, Film Coated	Paroxetine HCl 40 mg	Paxil by UDL	51079-0775	Antidepressant
7122212	Tab, Brown, Round, 7122 212	Senna Concentrate 8.6 mg	by RP Scherer	11014-1214	Gastrointestinal
7127 <> 93	Tab, White to Off-White, Oval, Scored	Torsemide 5 mg	Demadex by Teva Pharmaceuticals	00093-7127 Discontinued	Diuretic
7128 <> 93	Tab, White to Off-White, Oval, Scored, 9 over 3 <> 7128	Torsemide 10 mg	Demadex by Teva Pharmaceuticals	00093-7128 Discontinued	Diuretic
7128 <> 93	Tab, White to Off-White, Oval, Scored, 9 over 3 <> 7128	Torsemide 10 mg	Demadex by UDL	51079-0025	Diuretic
7129 <> 93	Tab, White to Off-White, Oval, Scored, 9 over 3 <> 7129	Torsemide 20 mg	Demadex by UDL	51079-0026	Diuretic
7129 <> 93	Tab, White to Off-White, Oval, Scored, 9 over 3 <> 7129	Torsemide 20 mg	Demadex by Teva Pharmaceuticals	00093-7129 Discontinued	Diuretic
713	Tab, White, Oval, Scored, Film Coated, Logo 713	Isosorbide Mononitrate 30 mg	Imdur by Murfreesboro	51129-1571	Antianginal
713 <> AN	Tab, White, Oval	Guanfacine HCl 2 mg	Tenex by Amneal	65162-0713	Antihypertensive
713 <> COPLEY	Tab	Atenolol 100 mg	Tenormin by Teva	38245-0713	Antihypertensive
7130 <> 93	Tab, White to Off-white, Oval, Scored	Torsemide 100 mg	Demadex by Teva Pharmaceuticals	00093-7130 Discontinued	Diuretic
7146 <> 93	Tab, Pink, Mottled, Oval, Film Coated	Azithromycin 250 mg	Zithromax by Teva	00093-7146	Antibiotic

ID FRONT <> BACK	DESCRIPTION FRONT <> BACK	INGREDIENT & STRENGTH	BRAND (or Generic Equiv.) by FIRM	NDC#	CLASS; SCH.
71465650 <> WATSON	Tab, Orange, Cap Shaped, Film Coated, 71465 over 650	Propoxyphene HCl 65 mg, Acetaminophen 650 mg	Wygesic by Watson	00591-0714	Analgesic; C IV
71465650 <> WATSON	Tab, Orange, Cap Shaped, Film Coated, 71465 over 650	Acetaminophen 650 mg, Propoxyphene HCl 65 mg	Wygesic by Qualitest	00603-5463	Analgesic; C IV
7147 <> 93	Tab, White to Off-White, Cap Shaped, Film Coated	Azithromycin 600 mg	Zithromax by Teva	00093-7147	Antibiotic
715 <> 260	Tab, White, Round	Quinine Sulfate 260 mg	Quinamm by Ivax	00182-8615 Discontinued	Antimalarial
715 <> B	Tab, Light Pink, Round	Norethindrone 0.35 mg	Camilla by Barr	00555-0715	Oral Contraceptive
715 <> SP15	Tab, Salmon, Round, Scored, Film Coated	Moexipril HCl 15 mg	Univasc by Schwarz	00091-3715	Antihypertensive
7152 <> 93	Tab, Light Yellow, Round, Film Coated	Simvastatin 5 mg	Zocor by Teva	00093-7152	Antihyperlipidemic
715260 <> WATSON	Tab, White, Round, 715 over 260	Quinine Sulfate 260 mg	Quinamm by RX Pak	65084-0143	Antimalarial
715260 <> WATSON	Tab, White, Round, 715 over 260	Quinine Sulfate 260 mg	Quinamm by Watson	00591-0715	Antimalarial
7153 <> 93	Tab, Light Pink, Round, Film Coated	Simvastatin 10 mg	Zocor by Teva	00093-7153	Antihyperlipidemic
7153 <> 93	Tab, Light Pink, Round, Film Coated	Simvastatin 10 mg	Zocor by UDL	51079-0454	Antihyperlipidemic
7154 <> 93	Tab, Tan, Round, Film Coated	Simvastatin 20 mg	Zocor by UDL	51079-0455	Antihyperlipidemic
7154 <> 93	Tab, Tan, Round, Film Coated	Simvastatin 20 mg	Zocor by Teva	00093-7154	Antihyperlipidemic
7155 <> 93	Tab, Red, Round, Film Coated	Simvastatin 40 mg	Zocor by Teva	00093-7155	Antihyperlipidemic
7155 <> 93	Tab, Red, Round, Film Coated	Simvastatin 40 mg	Zocor by UDL	51079-0456	Antihyperlipidemic
7156 <> 93	Tab, Brick Red, Cap Shaped, Film Coated	Simvastatin 80 mg	Zocor by Teva	00093-7156	Antihyperlipidemic
7157 <> 93	Tab, Yellow, Oval, Film Coated	Clarithromycin 250 mg	Biaxin by Teva	00093-7157	Antibiotic
7157 <> 93	Tab, Yellow, Oval, Film Coated	Clarithromycin 250 mg	Biaxin by UDL	51079-0361 Discontinued	Antibiotic
7158 <> 93	Tab, Light Yellow, Oval, Film Coated	Clarithromycin 500 mg	Biaxin by Teva	00093-7158	Antibiotic
7158 <> 93	Tab, Light Yellow, Oval, Film Coated	Clarithromycin 500 mg	Biaxin by UDL	51079-0362	Antibiotic
7159 <> 93	Tab, Mottled Green, Cap Shaped, Scored, 9 over 3	Pergolide Mesylate 0.25 mg	Permax by UDL	51079-0143 Discontinued	Antiparkinson
7159 <> 93	Tab, Green, Cap Shaped, Scored, 9 over 3	Pergolide Mesylate 0.25 mg	Permax by Teva	00093-7159	Antiparkinson
7160 <> 93	Tab, Ivory, Cap Shaped, Scored, 9 over 3	Pergolide Mesylate 0.05 mg	Permax by Teva	00093-7160 Discontinued	Antiparkinson
7161 <> 93	Tab, Pink, Cap Shaped, Scored, 9 over 3	Pergolide Mesylate 1 mg	Permax by Teva	00093-7161 Discontinued	Antiparkinson
7161 <> 93	Tab, Mottled Pink, Cap Shaped, Scored, 9 over 3	Pergolide Mesylate 1 mg	Permax by UDL	51079-0144 Discontinued	Antiparkinson
7167 <> 93	Tab, White to Off-White, Round	Amlodipine Besylate 5 mg	Norvasc by Teva	00093-7167	Antihypertensive
7168 <> 93	Tab, White to Off-White, Round	Amlodipine Besylate 10 mg	Norvasc by Teva	00093-7168	Antihypertensive
7169 <> 93	Tab, Pink, Mottled, Oval, Film Coated	Azithromycin 500 mg	Zithromax by Teva	00093-7169	Antibiotic
717 <> R	Tab, Yellow, Round, Film Coated, Ex Release	Diclofenac Sodium 100 mg	Voltaren XR by Actavis	00228-2717	NSAID
7171 <> GEIGY	Tab, Grey, Cap Shaped, Scored, Film Coated	Metoprolol Tartrate 100 mg	Lopressor by Novartis	Canadian DIN 00397431	Antihypertensive
7171 <> GEIGY	Tab, Grey, Cap Shaped, Scored, Film Coated	Metoprolol Tartrate 100 mg	Lopressor by Novartis	00078-0459	Antihypertensive
7171 <> M	Tab, White, Cap Shaped	Tramadol HCl 50 mg	Ultram by Mallinckrodt	00406-7171	Analgesic
7171 <> Z400	Tab, White, Oblong, Scored	Cimetidine HCl 400 mg	Tagamet by Ivax	00172-7171	Gastrointestinal
7171 <> Z400	Tab, White, Oblong, Scored	Cimetidine HCl 400 mg	Tagamet by Ivax	00182-1985	Gastrointestinal
7171 <> Z400	Tab, White, Oblong, Scored	Cimetidine HCl 400 mg	Tagamet by Med Pro	53978-2009	Gastrointestinal
7171 <> Z400	Tab, White, Oblong, Scored	Cimetidine HCl 400 mg	Tagamet by Murfreesboro	51129-1336	Gastrointestinal
7171 <> Z400	Tab, White, Oblong, Scored	Cimetidine HCl 400 mg	Tagamet by Golden State	60429-0047	Gastrointestinal
7171 <> Z400	Tab, White to Off-White, Capsule Shaped	Cimetidine 400 mg	Tagamet by Teva	00172-7171	Gastrointestinal
7172 <> 93	Tab, Gray, Oval, Ex Release	Etodolac 500 mg	Lodine XL by Teva	00093-7172	NSAID
7173 <> 93	Tab, White to Off-White, Oval, Film Coated, Scored	Gabapentin 600 mg	Neurontin by Teva	00093-7173 Discontinued	Anticonvulsant

ID FRONT <> BACK	DESCRIPTION FRONT <> BACK	INGREDIENT & STRENGTH	BRAND (or Generic Equiv.) by FIRM	NDC#	CLASS; SCH.
7174 <> 93	Tab, White to Off-White, Oval, Film Coated, Scored	Gabapentin 800 mg	Neurontin by Teva	00093-7174 Discontinued	Anticonvulsant
7175 <> 93	Tab, Light Green, Elliptical, Film-Coated, Scored	Sertraline HCl 25 mg	Zoloft by Teva	00093-7175 Discontinued	Antidepressant
71754 <> WATSON	Tab, 717 over 5.4	Yohimbine HCl 5.4 mg	by Watson	52544-0717	Impotence Agent
71754 <> WATSON	Tab, White, Round, Scored	Yohimbine HCl 5.4 mg	by Southwood	58016-0890	Impotence Agent
7176 <> 93	Tab, Light Blue, Elliptical, Film-Coated, Scored	Sertraline HCl 50 mg	Zoloft by Teva	00093-7176 Discontinued	Antidepressant
7178 <> 93	Tab, Light Pink to Mottled Pink, Oblong	Nefazodone HCl 50 mg	Serzone by Teva	00093-7178	Antidepressant
7180 <> 93	Tab, Light Yellow, Oval, Film Coated	Ofloxacin 200 mg	Floxin by Teva	00093-7180	Antibiotic
7181 <> 93	Tab, White to Off White, Oval, Film Coated	Ofloxacin 300 mg	Floxin by Teva	00093-7181	Antibiotic
7182 <> 93	Tab, Pale Gold, Oval, Film Coated	Ofloxacin 400 mg	Floxin by Teva	00093-7182	Antibiotic
7188 <> 93	Tab, Blue, Oval, Scored, Film Coated	Fluoxetine HCl 10 mg	Prozac by Teva	00093-7188	Antidepressant
72	Tab, Light Blue, Modified Apple Shaped	Finasteride 5 mg	Proscar by Dr. Reddy's	55111-0554	Antiandrogen
72 <> 93	Tab, White, Cap Shaped, Film Coated	Fluvoxamine Maleate 25 mg	Luvox by Teva Pharmaceuticals	00093-0072 Discontinued	OCD
72 <> A	Tab, Light Orange, Cap Shaped, Film Coated	Risperidone 2 mg	Risperdal by Aurobindo	65862-0122	Antipsychotic
72 <> I	Tab, Grey, Round	Minocycline 75 mg	Dynacin by Dr. Reddy's	55111-0638	Antibiotic
720	Tab, Red, Round, Schering Logo 720	Perphenazine 4 mg, Amitriptyline HCl 25 mg	Etrafon-Forte by Schering		Antipsychotic; Antidepressant
720 <> B70	Tab, White, Oval	Alendronate Sodium 70 mg	Fosamax by Barr	00555-0720 Discontinued	Antiosteoporosis
720 <> SP	Tab, White, Oval, Scored, Film Coated	Moexipril HCl 15 mg, Hydrochlorothiazide 12.5 mg	Uniretic by Schwarz	00091-3720	Antihypertensive; Diuretic
7201 <> 93	Tab, Light Yellow, Round	Pravastatin Sodium 20 mg	Pravachol by Teva	00093-7201	Antihyperlipidemic
7201 <> 93	Tab, Light Yellow, Round	Pravastatin Sodium 20 mg	Pravachol by UDL	51079-0458	Antihyperlipidemic
72012 <> WC	Tab, White to Off-White, Round	Estradiol 0.5 mg	Estrace by Warner Chilcott	00430-0720	Hormone
7202 <> 93	Tab, Light Green, Round	Pravastatin Sodium 40 mg	Pravachol by UDL	51079-0782	Antihyperlipidemic
7202 <> 93	Tab, Red, Squared-Oblong, 720/Vaseretic	Pravastatin Sodium 40 mg	Pravachol by Teva Pharmaceuticals	00093-7202 Discontinued	Antihyperlipidemic
7202 <> TEVA	Tab, Light Green, Round	Pravastatin Sodium 40 mg	Pravachol by Teva Pharmaceuticals	00093-7202	Antihyperlipidemic
7206 <> 93	Tab, Round, Yellow, Scored	Mirtazapine 15 mg	Remeron by Teva	00093-7206	Antidepressant
7207 <> 93	Tab, Round, Scored, Red-Brown	Mirtazapine 30 mg	Remeron by Teva	00093-7207	Antidepressant
7208 <> 93	Tab, White to Off-White, Round	Mirtazapine 45 mg	Remeron by Teva	00093-7208	Antidepressant
720VASERETIC	Tab, Red, Squared-Oblong, 720/Vaseretic	Enalapril Maleate 10 mg	Vasotec by Frosst	Canadian	Antihypertensive
721	Tab, White to Off-White, Cap Shaped, Film Coated, Actavis Logo 721	Sertraline HCl 25 mg	Zoloft by Actavis	00228-2721	Antidepressant
721 <> ENDO	Tab, White, Round, Partially Scored	Captopril 12.5 mg	Capoten by Endo	60951-0721	Antihypertensive
721 <> ENDO	Tab, White, Round, Partially Scored	Captopril 12.5 mg	Capoten by BMS	00056-0721	Antihypertensive
7211 <> WC	Tab, Light purple, Oval, Scored	Estradiol 1 mg	Estrace by Warner Chilcott	00430-0721	Hormone
7212 <> 93	Tab, Brick Red, Oval, Mottled, Extended Release	Metformin HCl 750 mg	Glucophage by Teva	00093-7212	Antidiabetic
7214 <> 93	Tab, White to Off-White, Oval, Scored, 9 / 3 <> 72 / 14	Metformin HCl 1000 mg	Glucophage by Teva	00093-7214	Antidiabetic
7215 <> 93	Tab, Pink, Cap Shaped, Mottled	Metolazone 2.5 mg	Zaroxolyn by Teva	00093-7215 Discontinued	Diuretic
7216 <> 93	Tab, Mottled Blue, Cap Shaped	Metolazone 5 mg	Zaroxolyn by Teva	00093-7216 Discontinued	Diuretic
7217 <> 93	Tab, Yellow, Round	Metolazone 10 mg	Zaroxolyn by Teva	00093-7217 Discontinued	Diuretic
7219 <> 93	Tab, Yellow, Cap Shaped	Topiramate 100 mg	Topamax by Teva	00093-7219	Anticonvulsant
722	Tab, Orange, Cap Shaped, Film Coated, Actavis Logo 722	Sertraline HCl 50 mg	Zoloft by Actavis	00228-2722	Antidepressant
7220 <> 93	Tab, Salmon, Cap Shaped	Topiramate 200 mg	Topamax by Teva	00093-7220	Anticonvulsant

ID FRONT <> BACK	DESCRIPTION FRONT <> BACK	INGREDIENT & STRENGTH	BRAND (or Generic Equiv.) by FIRM	NDC#	CLASS; SCH.
7221 <> 93	Tab, White, Oval	Prenatal Optima Advance	Prenate Advance by Optima	00093-7221	Vitamin
7222 <> 93	Tab, White to Off White, Rectangular, Scored, 9 score 3 <> 72 score 22	Fosinopril Sodium 10 mg	Monopril by Teva	00093-7222	Antihypertensive
7222 <> WC	Tab, Green, Oval, Scored	Estradiol 2 mg	Estrace by Warner Chilcott	00430-0722	Hormone
7223 <> 93	Tab, White to Off White, Cap Shaped	Fosinopril Sodium 20 mg	Monopril by Teva	00093-7223	Antihypertensive
7224 <> 93	Tab, White to Off White, Round	Fosinopril Sodium 40 mg	Monopril by Teva	00093-7224	Antihypertensive
723	Tab, Pink, Cap Shaped, Film Coated, Actavis Logo 723	Sertraline HCl 100 mg	Zoloft by Actavis	00228-2723	Antidepressant
723 <> M	Tab, White, Round	Enalapril Maleate 10 mg, Hydrochlorothiazide 25 mg	Vaseretic by Mylan	00378-0723	Antihypertensive; Diuretic
723 <> M	Tab, White, Round	Enalapril Maleate 10 mg, Hydrochlorothiazide 25 mg	Vaseretic by UDL	51079-0977	Antihypertensive; Diuretic
7230 <> 93	Tab, White to Off-White, Pillow Shaped	Cilostazol 50 mg	Pletal by Teva	00093-7230	Antiplatelet
7231 <> 93	Tab, White to Off-White, Round	Cilostazol 100 mg	Pletal by Teva	00093-7231	Antiplatelet
7231 <> 93	Tab, White to Off-White, Round	Cilostazol 100 mg	Pletal by UDL	51079-0424	Antiplatelet
				Discontinued	
7232 <> 93	Tab, Pink, Round, Coated	Ribavirin 200 mg	Copegus by Teva	00093-7232	Antiviral
7234 <> 93	Tab, Cap Shaped, Mottled Yellow	Meloxicam 7.5 mg	Mobic by Teva	00093-7234	NSAID
				Discontinued	
7236 <> 93	Tab, Yellow, Round, Film Coated	Ondansetron HCl 8 mg	Zofran by Teva	00093-7236	Antiemetic
724 <> GG	Tab	Naproxen 250 mg	Naprosyn by Sandoz		NSAID
724 <> W	Tab, White, Oval, Film Coated, Extended Release	Divalproex Sodium 250 mg	Depakote by Wockhardt	64679-0724	Anticonvulsant
7240 <> 93	Tab, White to Off-White, Round, Film Coated	Risperidone 1 mg	Risperdal by Teva	00093-7240	Antipsychotic
7241 <> 93	Tab, Orange, Round, Film Coated	Risperidone 2 mg	Risperdal by Teva	00093-7241	Antipsychotic
7242 <> 93	Tab, Yellow, Round, Film Coated	Risperidone 3 mg	Risperdal by Teva	00093-7242	Antipsychotic
7243 <> 93	Tab, Green, Round, Film Coated	Risperidone 4 mg	Risperdal by Teva	00093-7243	Antipsychotic
7244 <> 93	Tab, Yellow, Oval, Film Coated, Extended Release	Clarithromycin 500 mg	Biaxin XL by Teva	00093-7244	Antibiotic
7247 <> 93	Tab, Cream, Diamond Shaped, Scored, 9 / 3	Lamotrigine 150 mg	Lamictal by Teva	00093-7247	Anticonvulsant
7248 <> 93	Tab, Blue, Diamond Shaped, Scored, 9 / 3	Lamotrigine 200 mg	Lamictal by Teva	00093-7248	Anticonvulsant
724PAR	Cap, Pink & Dark Green	Hydroxyurea 500 mg	Hydrea by Par	49884-0724	Antineoplastic
725 <> SP	Tab, Yellow, Oval, Scored, Film Coated	Moexipril HCl 15 mg, Hydrochlorothiazide 25 mg	Uniretic by Schwarz	00091-3725	Antihypertensive; Diuretic
725 <> SP	Tab, Yellow, Oval, Scored, Film Coated	Moexipril HCl 15 mg, HCTZ 25 mg	Uniretic by Schwarz	51217-3725	Antihypertensive; Diuretic
7251 <> 93	Tab, Peach, Cap Shaped, Film Coated	Fexofenadine HCl 30 mg	Allegra by Teva	00093-7251	Antihistamine
7252 <> 93	Tab, Peach, Round, Film Coated	Fexofenadine HCl 60 mg	Allegra by Teva	00093-7252	Antihistamine
7253 <> 93	Tab, Peach, Round, Film Coated	Fexofenadine HCl 180 mg	Allegra by Teva	00093-7253	Antihistamine
7254 <> 93	Tab, Pink, Mottled, Round, Scored, 9 / 3 <> 72 / 54	Glimepiride 1 mg	Amaryl by Teva	00093-7254	Antidiabetic
7255 <> 93	Tab, Green, Mottled, Round, Scored, 9 / 3 <> 72 / 55	Glimepiride 2 mg	Amaryl by Teva	00093-7255	Antidiabetic
7256 <> 93	Tab, Light Blue, Mottled, Round, Scored, 9 / 3 <> 72 / 56	Glimepiride 4 mg	Amaryl by Teva	00093-7256	Antidiabetic
725725 <> COPLEY	Tab, Pink, Hexagonal	Glyburide 1.5 mg	Micronase by Blue Ridge	59273-0016	Antidiabetic
725725 <> COPLEY	Tab, Pink, Hexagonal	Glyburide 1.5 mg	Micronase by Teva	38245-0725	Antidiabetic
				Discontinued	
725725 <> COPLEY	Tab, Pink, Hexagonal	Glyburide 1.5 mg	Micronase by Merrell	00068-3203	Antidiabetic
7258 <> 93	Tab, Blue, Cap Shaped, Film Coated	Valacyclovir HCl 500 mg	Valtrex by Teva Pharmaceuticals	00093-7258	Antiviral
7259 <> 93	Tab, Blue, Cap Shaped, Film Coated, Scored	Valacyclovir HCl 1000 mg	Valtrex by Teva Pharmaceuticals	00093-7259	Antiviral
725HD	Cap	Doxycycline Hyclate	by Quality Care	60346-0449	Antibiotic
				Discontinued	
7260 <> 93	Tab, Pale Yellow, Oval, Film Coated	Glyburide 1.25 mg, Metformin HCl 250 mg	Glucovance by Teva	00093-7260	Antidiabetic
7261 <> 93	Tab, Pale Orange, Oval, Film Coated	Glyburide 2.5 mg, Metformin HCl 500 mg	Glucovance by Teva	00093-7261	Antidiabetic
7262 <> 93	Tab, Yellow, Film Coated, Yellow	Glyburide 5 mg, Metformin HCl 500 mg	Glucovance by Teva	00093-7262	Antidiabetic
				Discontinued	
72650 <> WATSON	Tab, White, Round, 726 over 50	Meperidine 50 mg	Demerol by Watson	00591-0726	Analgesic; C II
72650 <> WATSON	Tab, White, Round, 726 over 50	Meperidine 50 mg	Demerol by Watson	52544-0726	Analgesic; C II
7267 <> 93	Tab, White, Oval, Extended Release	Metformin HCl 500 mg	Glucophage by UDL	00093-7267	Antidiabetic

ID FRONT <> BACK	DESCRIPTION FRONT <> BACK	INGREDIENT & STRENGTH	BRAND (or Generic Equiv.) by FIRM	NDC#	CLASS; SCH.
726Z	Tab, Buff, Shield, 726/Z	Simvastatin 5 mg	Zocor by Frosst	Canadian	Antihyperlipidemic
727 <> 50N	Tab, Film Coated	Metoprolol Tartrate 50 mg	Lopressor by Ivax	00182-1987	Antihypertensive
727 <> MYLAN	Tab, Blue, Round, Film Coated	Amitriptyline 10 mg, Perphenazine 4 mg	Triavil by Mylan	00378-0042	Antidepressant; Antipsychotic
7270 <> 93	Tab, Off-White to Mottled Grey, Oval	Pravastatin Sodium 80 mg	Pravachol by Teva	00093-7270	Antihyperlipidemic
722100 <> WATSON	Tab, White, Round, 727 over 100	Meperidine 100 mg	Demerol by Watson	52544-0727	Analgesic; C II
722100 <> WATSON	Tab, White, Round, 727 over 100	Meperidine 100 mg	Demerol by Watson	00591-0727	Analgesic; C II
7272 <> LOTENSINHCT	Tab, Light Pink, Oblong, Coated	Benazepril HCl 10 mg, Hydrochlorothiazide 12.5 mg	Lotensin HCT by Novartis	00078-0452	Antihypertensive; Diuretic
7272 <> LOTENSINHCT	Tab, Light Pink, Oblong, Scored	Benazepril HCl 10 mg, Hydrochlorothiazide 12.5 mg	Lotensin HCT by Novartis	00083-0072	Antihypertensive; Diuretic
727N <> 50	Tab, Film Coated, 727/N	Metoprolol Tartrate 50 mg	Lopressor by Schein	00364-2560	Antihypertensive
728 <> B	Tab, Yellow, Round, Film Coated	Doxycycline 50 mg	Adoxa by Doak	10337-0800	Antibiotic
728 <> B	Tab, Yellow, Round, Film Coated	Doxycycline 50 mg	Adoxa by Bradley	62436-0728	Antibiotic
7281 <> 93	Tab, Brown to Dark Brown, Cap Shaped, Film Coated, Scored, 9 / 3 <> 72 / 81	Oxcarbazepine 150 mg	Trileptal by Teva	00093-7281	Anticonvulsant
7282 <> 93	Tab, Brown to Dark Brown, Cap Shaped, Film Coated, Scored, 9 / 3 <> 72 / 82	Oxcarbazepine 300 mg	Trileptal by Teva	00093-7282	Anticonvulsant
7283 <> 93	Tab, Brown to Dark Brown, Cap Shaped, Film Coated, Scored, 9 / 3 <> 72 / 83	Oxcarbazepine 600 mg	Trileptal by Teva	00093-7283	Anticonvulsant
7285 <> 93	Tab, Blue, Oblong, Film Coated, Scored, 9 / 3	Levetiracetam 250 mg	Keppra by Teva	00093-7285	Anticonvulsant
728500 <> WATSON	Tab, Blue, Oblong, Film Coated	Etodolac 500 mg	by Watson	52544-0728	NSAID
7286 <> 93	Tab, Yellow, Oblong, Film Coated, Scored, 9 / 3	Levetiracetam 500 mg	Keppra by Teva	00093-7286	Anticonvulsant
7287 <> 93	Tab, Orange, Oblong, Film Coated, Scored, 9 / 3	Levetiracetam 750 mg	Keppra by Teva	00093-7287	Anticonvulsant
729 <> B	Tab, Yellow, Round, Film Coated	Doxycycline 100 mg	Adoxa by Bradley	62436-0729	Antibiotic
729 <> B	Tab, Yellow, Round, Film Coated	Doxycycline 100 mg	Adoxa by Doak	10337-0802	Antibiotic
7294 <> 93	Tab, White to Off-White, Round	Terbinafine HCl 250 mg	Lamisil by Teva	00093-7294	Antifungal
7295 <> 93	Tab, White, Oval, Film Coated	Carvedilol 12.5 mg	Coreg by Teva	00093-7295	Antihypertensive
7296 <> 93	Tab, White, Oval, Film Coated	Carvedilol 25 mg	Coreg by Teva	00093-7296	Antihypertensive
7299 <> 93	Tab, Pillow Shaped, Mottled Yellow	Meloxicam 15 mg	Mobic by Teva	00093-7299 Discontinued	NSAID
73 <> 93	Tab, Pink, Round, Film Coated	Zolpidem Tartrate 5 mg	Ambien by Teva	00093-0073	Sedative/Hypnotic; C IV
73 <> A	Tab, Yellow, Cap Shaped, Film Coated	Risperidone 3 mg	Risperdal by Aurobindo	65862-0123	Antipsychotic
73 <> I	Tab, Dark Grey, Round	Minocycline 100 mg	Dynacin by Dr. Reddy's	55111-0639	Antibiotic
73 <> MYLAN	Tab, Purple, Round, Coated	Amitriptyline 50 mg, Perphenazine 4 mg	Triavil by Mylan	00378-0073	Antidepressant; Antipsychotic
73 <> RPC	Tab, White, Round	Propantheline Bromide 7.5 mg	by Compumed	00403-5167	Gastrointestinal
730	Tab, White, Round	Tamoxifen Citrate 10 mg	Nolvadex by AstraZeneca	00310-0730 Discontinued	Antiestrogen
730 <> B	Tab, Light Orange, Round, Film Coated	Doxycycline 75 mg	Adoxa by Doak	10337-0801	Antibiotic
730 <> B	Tab, Light Orange, Round, Film Coated	Doxycycline 75 mg	Adoxa by Bradley	62436-0730	Antibiotic
7300	Tab, White, Oblong, Scored, Film Coated, Ex Release, 7300 <> Hourglass Logo	Verapamil HCl 240 mg	Calan SR by Schein	00364-2567	Antihypertensive
7300	Tab, White, Oblong, Scored, Film Coated, Ex Release, 7300 <> Hourglass Logo	Verapamil HCl 240 mg	Calan SR by Ivax	00182-1970	Antihypertensive
7300	Tab, White, Oblong, Scored, Film Coated, Ex Release, 7300 <> Hourglass Logo	Verapamil HCl 240 mg	Calan SR by Kaiser	00179-1161	Antihypertensive
7300	Tab, White, Oblong, Scored, Film Coated, Ex Release, 7300 <> Hourglass Logo	Verapamil HCl 240 mg	Calan SR by Ivax	00172-4280	Antihypertensive
7300	Tab, White, Oblong, Scored, Film Coated, Ex Release, 7300 <> Hourglass Logo	Verapamil HCl 240 mg	Calan SR by Talbert	44514-0905	Antihypertensive
7300	Tab, White, Oblong, Scored, Film Coated, Ex Release, 7300 <> Hourglass Logo	Verapamil HCl 240 mg	Calan SR by Caremark	00339-5808	Antihypertensive

ID FRONT <> BACK	DESCRIPTION FRONT <> BACK	INGREDIENT & STRENGTH	BRAND (or Generic Equiv.) by FIRM	NDC#	CLASS; SCH.
7300	Tab, White, Oblong, Scored, Film Coated, Ex Release, 7300 <> Hourglass Logo	Verapamil HCl 240 mg	Calan SR by Golden State	60429-0198	Antihypertensive
7300	Tab, White, Oblong, Scored, Film Coated, Ex Release, 7300 <> Hourglass Logo	Verapamil HCl 240 mg	Calan SR by Kaiser	62224-8551	Antihypertensive
7301	Tab, Orange, Oblong	Verapamil HCl 180 mg	Calan SR/Isoptin SR by Ivax	00172-7301	Antihypertensive
7301	Tab, Orange, Oblong, Scored, Film Coated, Ex Release	Verapamil HCl 180 mg	Calan SR by Ivax	00172-4286	Antihypertensive
7301	Tab, Orange, Oblong, Scored, Film Coated, Ex Release	Verapamil HCl 180 mg	Calan SR by Schein	00364-2590	Antihypertensive
7301	Tab, Orange, Oblong, Scored, Film Coated, Ex Release	Verapamil HCl 180 mg	Calan SR by Kaiser	00179-1196	Antihypertensive
7301	Tab, Orange, Oblong, Scored, Film Coated, Ex Release	Verapamil HCl 180 mg	Calan SR by Golden State	60429-0237	Antihypertensive
7301	Tab, Orange, Oblong, Scored, Film Coated, Ex Release	Verapamil HCl 180 mg	Calan SR by Heartland	61392-0345	Antihypertensive
7301	Tab, Orange, Oblong, Scored, Film Coated, Ex Release	Verapamil HCl 180 mg	Calan SR by URL Mutual	00677-1518	Antihypertensive
7301	Tab, Orange, Oblong, Scored, Film Coated, Ex Release	Verapamil HCl 180 mg	Calan SR by Caremark	00339-5810	Antihypertensive
7301 <> 93	Tab, White to Off-White, Round, Orally Disintegrating	Ondansetron 4 mg	Zofran ODT by Teva	00093-7301	Antiemetic
7302 <> 93	Tab, White to Off-White, Round, Orally Disintegrating	Ondansetron 8 mg	Zofran ODT by Teva	00093-7302	Antiemetic
7303 <> 93	Tab, White to Off-White, Round	Mirtazapine 15 mg	Remeron SolTab by Teva	00093-7303	Antidepressant
7304 <> 93	Tab, White to Off-White, Round	Mirtazapine 30 mg	Remeron SolTab by Teva	00093-7304	Antidepressant
7305 <> 93	Tab, White to Off-White, Round	Mirtazapine 45 mg	Remeron SolTab by Teva	00093-7305	Antidepressant
731	Tab, White, Round	Tamoxifen Citrate 20 mg	Nolvadex by AstraZeneca	00310-0731 Discontinued	Antiestrogen
7316 <> 93	Tab, White to Off-White, Cap Shaped, Scored, 9/3 <> 7316	Desmopressin Acetate 0.1 mg	DDAVP by Teva	00093-7316	Antidiuretic
7317 <> 93	Tab, White to Off-White, Round, Scored, 9/3 <> 7317	Desmopressin Acetate 0.2 mg	DDAVP by Teva	00093-7317	Antidiuretic
7317 <> 93	Tab, White to Off-White, Round, Scored, 9/3 <> 7317	Desmopressin Acetate 0.2 mg	DDAVP by UDL	51079-0446	Antidiuretic
73173 1MEVACOR	Tab, Light Blue, Octagon, 731/731/Mevacor	Lovastatin 20 mg	Mevacor by MSD	Canadian	Antihyperlipidemic
732 <> M	Tab, White to Off-White, Round, Orally Disintegrating	Ondansetron 4 mg	Zofran ODT by Mylan	00378-7732	Antiemetic
7325 <> 93	Tab, White to Off-White, Mottled Salmon, Cap Shaped, Scored, 9 / 3 <> 7325	Trandolapril 1 mg	Mavik by Teva	00093-7325	Antihypertensive
7326 <> 93	Tab, White to Off-White, Mottled Yellow, Cap Shaped	Trandolapril 2 mg	Mavik by Teva	00093-7326	Antihypertensive
7327 <> 93	Tab, White to Off-White, Mottled Rose, Cap Shaped	Trandolapril 4 mg	Mavik by Teva	00093-7327	Antihypertensive
732MEVACOR	Tab, Green, Octagon, 732/Mevacor	Lovastatin 40 mg	Mevacor by MSD	Canadian	Antihyperlipidemic
733 <> MYLAN	Tab, Light Blue, Film Coated, Beveled Edge	Naproxen 550 mg	by Mylan	00378-0733	NSAID
733 <> MYLAN	Tab, Film Coated	Naproxen 550 mg	by Allscripts		NSAID
7330 <> 93	Tab, Yellow, Round, Film Coated	Fenofibrate 54 mg	Lofibra by Gate	57844-0691	Antihyperlipidemic
7331 <> 93	Tab, White to Off-White, Oval, Film Coated	Fenofibrate 160 mg	Lofibra by Gate	57844-0692	Antihyperlipidemic
734 <> M	Tab, White to Off-White, Round, Orally Disintegrating	Ondansetron 8 mg	Zofran ODT by Mylan	00378-7734	Antiemetic
7340 <> 93	Tab, White, Oval, Ex Release	Divalproex Sodium 500 mg	Depakote ER by Teva	00093-7340	Anticonvulsant
734N <> 100	Tab, Film Coated, 734/N	Metoprolol Tartrate 100 mg	Lopressor by Schein	00364-2561	Antihypertensive
7355 <> 93	Tab, Blue, Cap-Shaped	Finasteride 5 mg	Proscar by Teva	00093-7355	Antiandrogen
735Z	Tab, Peach, Shield, 735/Z	Simvastatin 10 mg	by Frosst	Canadian	Antihyperlipidemic
7364 <> 93	Tab, Light Green, Oval, Film Coated	Losartan Potassium 25 mg	Cozaar by Teva Pharmaceuticals	00093-7364	Antihypertensive
7365 <> 93	Tab, Green, Oval, Film Coated	Losartan Potassium 50 mg	Cozaar by Teva Pharmaceuticals	00093-7365	Antihypertensive
7366 <> 93	Tab, Dark Green, Oval, Film Coated	Losartan Potassium 100 mg	Cozaar by Teva Pharmaceuticals	00093-7366	Antihypertensive
7367 <> 93	Tab, Yellow, Oval, Film Coated	Hydrochlorothiazide 12.5 mg, Losartan Potassium 50 mg	Hyzaar by Teva Pharmaceuticals	00093-7367	Diuretic; Antihypertensive
7368 <> 93	Tab, Light Yellow, Oval, Film Coated	Hydrochlorothiazide 25 mg, Losartan Potassium 100 mg	Hyzaar by Teva Pharmaceuticals	00093-7368	Diuretic; Antihypertensive
7369 <> 93	Tab, White to Off-White, Oval, Film Coated	Hydrochlorothiazide 12.5 mg, Losartan Potassium 100 mg	Hyzaar by Teva Pharmaceuticals	00093-7369	Diuretic; Antihypertensive
737	Cap, Black & Orange	Vitamin A 8000 IU, Vitamin E 50 IU, Ascorbic Acid 150 mg, Zinc Sulfate 80 mg, Magnesium Sulfate 70 mg	Vitacon Forte by Breckenridge	51991-0645	Vitamin
737	Cap	Ascorbic Acid 150 mg, Calcium Pantothenate 10 mg, Cyanocobalamin 10 mcg, Folic Acid 1 mg, Magnesium Sulfate 70 mg, Manganese Chloride 4 mg, Niacinamide 25 mg, Pyridoxine HCl 2 mg, Riboflavin 5 mg, Thiamine Mononitrate 10 mg, Vitamin A 8000 Units, Vitamin E 50 Units, Zinc Sulfate 80 mg	Therapeutic Vit & Min by Contract	10267-0737	Vitamin

ID FRONT <> BACK	DESCRIPTION FRONT <> BACK	INGREDIENT & STRENGTH	BRAND (or Generic Equiv.) by FIRM	NDC#	CLASS; SCH.
7373 <> GEIGY	Tab, White, Mottled Yellow, Cap Shaped, Scored	Hydrochlorothiazide 50 mg, Metoprolol Tartrate 100 mg	Lopressor HCT by Novartis	00078-0462	Diuretic; Antihypertensive
7375BRISTOL250MG	Cap, Printed in White Ink	Cephalexin 250 mg	by Golden State	60429-0036	Antibiotic
7376BRISTOL500MG	Cap, Blue, Blue Body Printed in White Ink <> Blue Cap Written in White Ink	Cephalexin 500 mg	by Golden State	60429-0037	Antibiotic
7380 <> 93	Tab, Peach, Round, Scored, Mottled	Venlafaxine HCl 37.5 mg	Effexor by Teva	00093-7380	Antidepressant
7381 <> 93	Tab, Peach, Round, Scored, Mottled	Venlafaxine HCl 50 mg	Effexor by Teva	00093-7381	Antidepressant
7382 <> 93	Tab, Peach, Round, Scored, Mottled	Venlafaxine HCl 75 mg	Effexor by Teva	00093-7382	Antidepressant
7383 <> 93	Tab, Peach, Round, Scored, Mottled	Venlafaxine HCl 100 mg	Effexor by Teva	00093-7383	Antidepressant
74 <> 93	Tab, White to Off-White, Film Coated, Round	Zolpidem Tartrate 10 mg	Ambien by Teva Pharmaceuticals	00093-0074 Discontinued	Sedative/Hypnotic; C IV
74 <> A	Tab, White, Scored	Difenoxin HCl 1 mg, Atropine Sulfate 0.025 mg	Motofen by West-Ward	00143-9031	Antidiarrheal; C IV
74 <> A	Tab, Green, Cap Shaped, Film Coated	Risperidone 4 mg	Risperdal by Aurobindo	65862-0124	Antipsychotic
74 <> D	Tab, White to Off-White, Round	Terbinafine HCl 250 mg	Lamisil by Aurobindo	65862-0079	Antifungal
74 <> M	Tab, Green, Triangular, Film Coated	Fluphenazine HCl 5 mg	Prolixin by Mylan	00378-6074	Antipsychotic
74 <> M	Tab, Green, Triangular, Film Coated	Fluphenazine HCl 5 mg	Prolixin by UDL	51079-0487	Antipsychotic
74 <> TEVA	Tab, White to Off-White, Film Coated, Round	Zolpidem Tartrate 10 mg	Ambien by Teva Pharmaceuticals	00093-0074	Sedative/Hypnotic; C IV
74 <> ZA	Tab, White	Terazosin 1 mg	by AltiMed	Canadian DIN 02218941	Antihypertensive
74 <> ZB	Tab, Orange	Terazosin 2 mg	by AltiMed	Canadian DIN 02218968	Antihypertensive
74 <> ZC	Tab, Tan	Terazosin 5 mg	by AltiMed	Canadian DIN 02218976	Antihypertensive
74 <> ZD	Tab, Blue	Terazosin 10 mg	by AltiMed	Canadian DIN 02218984	Antihypertensive
74 <> ZE	Tab, Film Coated	Erythromycin 500 mg	by Quality Care	60346-0646	Antibiotic
7401 <> 93	Tab, White, Oval, Scored, 9 / 3 <> 7401	Sotalol HCl 80 mg	Betapace AF by Teva	00093-7401	Antiarrhythmic
7402 <> 93	Tab, White, Oval, Scored, 9 / 3 <> 7402	Sotalol HCl 120 mg	Betapace AF by Teva	00093-7402	Antiarrhythmic
7403 <> 93	Tab, White, Oval, Scored, 9 / 3 <> 7403	Sotalol HCl 160 mg	Betapace AF by Teva	00093-7403	Antiarrhythmic
740EL	Cap, Ex Release	Chlorpheniramine Maleate 8 mg, Pseudoephedrine HCl 120 mg	Colfed A by Pharmafab	62542-0253	Cold Remedy
740EL	Cap	Chlorpheniramine Maleate 8 mg, Pseudoephedrine HCl 120 mg	N D Clear by Seatrace	00551-0147	Cold Remedy
740Z	Tab, Tan, Shield, 740/Z	Simvastatin 20 mg	by Frosst	Canadian	Antihyperlipidemic
741 <> COPLEY	Tab, Light Blue, Film Coated	Naproxen 275 mg	by Teva	38245-0741	NSAID
741 <> S	Tab, White to Off-White, Oval	Gemfibrozil 600 mg	Lopid by Dava	67253-0741	Antihyperlipidemic
741LUCHEM	Tab, Blue & White Specks, Oblong, 7/41 LuChem	Phenylpropanolamine HCl 75 mg, Guaifenesin LA 400 mg	Banex LA by LuChem		Cold Remedy
742 <> HOPE	Tab, White, Round	Atropine Sulfate 0.4 mg	Sal-Tropine by Hope	60267-0742	Gastrointestinal
742 <> HOPE	Tab, White, Round	Atropine Sulfate 0.4 mg	Sal-Tropine by Anabolic	00722-6685	Gastrointestinal
742PRILOSEC20	Cap, Purple, Opaque, Hard Gel, Delayed Release	Omeprazole 20 mg	Prilosec by AstraZeneca	00186-0742	Gastrointestinal
742PRILOSEC20	Cap, Purple, Opaque, Hard Gel, Delayed Release	Omeprazole 20 mg	Prilosec by Amerisource	62584-0451	Gastrointestinal
742PRILOSEC20	Cap, Purple, Opaque, Hard Gel, Delayed Release	Omeprazole 20 mg	Prilosec by Southwood	58016-0327	Gastrointestinal
742PRILOSEC20	Cap, Purple, Opaque, Hard Gel, Delayed Release	Omeprazole 20 mg	Prilosec by PDRX	55289-0477	Gastrointestinal
742PRILOSEC20	Cap, Purple, Opaque, Hard Gel, Delayed Release	Omeprazole 20 mg	Prilosec by Merck	00006-0742	Gastrointestinal
743	Tab, Teal, Round, 743 <> Inverted Triangle	Inert	Ortho-Cyclen by Teva	00093-5316	Oral Contraceptive; Placebo
743	Tab, Teal, Round, 743 <> Inverted Triangle	Inert	Ortho Tri-Cyclen by Teva	00093-5315	Oral Contraceptive; Placebo
743 <> R	Tab, White, Round, Enteric Coated	Diclofenac Sodium 50 mg	Voltaren by Actavis	00228-2743	NSAID
743 <> W	Tab, White, Round	Terbinafine HCl 250 mg	Lamisil by Wockhardt	64679-0743	Antifungal
743PRILOSEC40	Cap, Peach & Purple, Opaque, Hard Gel, Delayed Release	Omeprazole 40 mg	Losec by AstraZeneca	Canadian DIN 02016788	Gastrointestinal
743PRILOSEC40	Cap, Peach & Purple, Opaque, Hard Gel, Delayed Release	Omeprazole 40 mg	Prilosec by Merck	00006-0743	Gastrointestinal

ID FRONT <> BACK	DESCRIPTION FRONT <> BACK	INGREDIENT & STRENGTH	BRAND (or Generic Equiv.) by FIRM	NDC#	CLASS; SCH.
743PRILOSEC40	Cap, Peach & Purple, Opaque, Hard Gel, Delayed Release	Omeprazole 40 mg	Prilosec by AstraZeneca	00186-0743	Gastrointestinal
743PRILOSEC40	Cap, Peach & Purple, Opaque, Hard Gel, Delayed Release	Omeprazole 40 mg	Prilosec by PDRX	55289-0476	Gastrointestinal
744 <> COPLEY	Tab, Film Coated, Debossed	Naproxen 550 mg	Naprosyn by St. Mary's Med	60760-0744	NSAID
744 <> COPLEY	Tab, Film Coated	Naproxen 550 mg	Naprosyn by Teva	38245-0744	NSAID
744 <> R	Tab, White, Round, Enteric Coated	Diclofenac Sodium 75 mg	Voltaren by Actavis	00228-2744	NSAID
7441 <> WATSON	Tab, White, Diamond Shaped, Scored, 744 to left of Score, 1 to right	Estazolam 1 mg	Prosom by Watson	00591-0744	Sedative/Hypnotic; C IV
7447 <> 93	Tab, Purple, Oval, Film Coated	Mycophenolate Mofetil 500 mg	CellCept by Teva	00093-7447	Immunosuppressant
745	Tab, White, Oval	Hydrochlorothiazide 12.5 mg, Losartan Potassium 100 mg	Hyzaar by Merck	00006-0745	Diuretic; Antihypertensive
745 <> R	Tab, Yellow, Cap Shaped, Film Coated, Delayed Release	Naproxen 375 mg	Naprosyn by Actavis	00228-2745	NSAID
7452 <> WATSON	Tab, Pink, Diamond Shaped, Scored, 745 on left of Score, 2 on right	Estazolam 2 mg	Prosom by Watson	00591-0745	Sedative/Hypnotic; C IV
7455 <> 93	Tab, Pink, Cap Shaped, Film Coated	Glipizide 2.5 mg, Metformin HCl 250 mg	Metaglip by Teva	00093-7455	Antidiabetic
7456 <> 93	Tab, White, Cap Shaped, Film Coated	Glipizide 2.5 mg, Metformin HCl 500 mg	Metaglip by Teva	00093-7456	Antidiabetic
7457 <> 93	Tab, Pink, Cap Shaped, Film Coated	Glipizide 5 mg, Metformin HCl 500 mg	Metaglip by Teva	00093-7457	Antidiabetic
746	Tab, White, Round, 746 <> Inverted Triangle	Norgestimate 0.18 mg, Ethinyl Estradiol 0.035 mg	Ortho Tri-Cyclen by Teva	00093-5315	Oral Contraceptive
746 <> R	Tab, Green, Cap Shaped, Film Coated, Delayed Release	Naproxen 500 mg	Naprosyn by Actavis	00228-2746	NSAID
747	Tab, Light Blue, Round, 747 <> Inverted Triangle	Norgestimate 0.215 mg, Ethinyl Estradiol 0.035 mg	Ortho Tri-Cyclen by Teva	00093-5315	Oral Contraceptive
7474 <> LOTENSINHCT	Tab, Grayish Violet, Oblong, Scored	Benazepril HCl 20 mg, Hydrochlorothiazide 12.5 mg	Lotensin HCT by Novartis	00078-0453	Antihypertensive; Diuretic
7474 <> LOTENSINHCT	Tab, Grayish Violet, Oblong, Scored	Benazepril HCl 20 mg, Hydrochlorothiazide 12.5 mg	Lotensin HCT by Novartis	00083-0074	Antihypertensive; Diuretic
748	Tab, Blue, Round, 748 <> Inverted Triangle	Norgestimate 0.25 mg, Ethinyl Estradiol 0.035 mg	Ortho Tri-Cyclen by Teva	00093-5315	Oral Contraceptive
748	Tab, Blue, Round, 748 <> Inverted Triangle	Norgestimate 0.25 mg, Ethinyl Estradiol 0.035 mg	Ortho-Cyclen by Teva	00093-5316	Oral Contraceptive
7485 <> 93	Tab, White to Off-White, Cap-Shaped, Film-Coated	Granisetron HCl 1 mg	Kytril by Teva	00093-7485	Antiemetic
749	Tab, Peach, Shield Shaped	Simvastatin 40 mg	Zocor by Dr. Reddy's	55111-0749	Antihyperlipidemic
7493 <> 93	Tab, White, Oblong, Film Coated, Scored, 9 / 3	Levetiracetam 1000 mg	Keppra by Teva	00093-7493	Anticonvulsant
749Z	Tab, Red, Shield, 749/Z	Simvastatin 40 mg	Zocor by Frosst	Canadian	Antihyperlipidemic
74XX	Tab, Brown, Oblong, Film Coated	Potassium Chloride 750 mg	Slow K by Abbott	60692-7763	Electrolytes
74XX	Tab, Brown, Oblong, Film Coated	Potassium Chloride 750 mg	Slow K by Kaiser	00179-1235	Electrolytes
74XX	Tab, Brown, Oval, Film Coated, Ex Release	Potassium Chloride 750 mg	Slow K by Abbott	00074-7763 Discontinued	Electrolytes
74ZA	Tab, White, Round, 74/ZA	Terazosin HCl 1 mg	Hytrin by AltiMed	Canadian	Antihypertensive
74ZB	Tab, Orange, Round, 74/ZB	Terazosin HCl 2 mg	Hytrin by AltiMed	Canadian	Antihypertensive
74ZC	Tab, Tan, Round, 74/ZC	Terazosin HCl 5 mg	Hytrin by AltiMed	Canadian	Antihypertensive
74ZD	Tab, Blue, Round, 74/ZD	Terazosin HCl 10 mg	Hytrin by AltiMed	Canadian	Antihypertensive
74ZE	Tab, Mottled Pink, Oval	Erythromycin Ethylsuccinate 400 mg	E.E.S. 400 by Abbott	00074-2589	Antibiotic
74ZZ	Tab, Brown, Round, Ex Release	Potassium Chloride 600 mg	Slow K by Abbott	00074-7767 Discontinued	Electrolytes
75	Tab, Pink, Shield-Shaped	Ranitidine HCl 75 mg	Ranitidine by Apotex	Canadian	Gastrointestinal
75	Cap, White, Ex Release, Printed in Red	Theophylline Anhydrous 75 mg	Slo-Bid by RPR	00801-1075	Antiasthmatic
75	Tab, Peach, Round, Hourglass logo <> 75	Ranitidine HCl 75 mg	Zantac by Ivax	00182-2661 Discontinued	Gastrointestinal
75	Tab, Light Yellow, Round, 7.5	Meloxicam 7.5 mg	Mobic by Lupin	68180-0501	NSAID
75	Tab, Pink, Shield-Shaped	Ranitidine HCl 75 mg	Ranitidine by Major	00904-5399	Gastrointestinal
75	Tab, Film Coated	Clopidogrel 75 mg	Plavix by Sanofi Winthrop	53360-1171	Antiplatelet
75	Tab, Orange, Round	Desipramine HCl 75 mg	Apo Desipramine by Apotex	Canadian DIN 02216272	Antidepressant
75	Tab, Salmon, Triangle Shaped, Film Coated, 7.5 <> Servier Logo	Ivabradine 7.5 mg	Procoralan by Servier		Antianginal
75 <> 1171	Tab, Pink, Round, Film Coated	Clopidogrel 75 mg	Plavix by Nat Pharmpak	55154-2016	Antiplatelet
75 <> 1171	Tab, Pink, Round, Film Coated	Clopidogrel 75 mg	Plavix by BMS	63653-1171	Antiplatelet

ID FRONT <> BACK	DESCRIPTION FRONT <> BACK	INGREDIENT & STRENGTH	BRAND (or Generic Equiv.) by FIRM	NDC#	CLASS; SCH.
75 <> 1171	Tab, Pink, Round, Film Coated	Clopidogrel 75 mg	Plavix by Sanofi-Aventis	Canadian DIN 02238682	Antiplatelet
75 <> A	Tab, White, Round, Film Coated	Hydroxyzine HCl 10 mg	Atarax by Harris	67405-0575	Antianxiety; Antihistamine
75 <> AD	Tab, Blue, Round, Scored, 7.5 <> AD	Mixed Amphetamine Salts 7.5 mg: Amphetamine Aspartate 1.875 mg, Amphetamine Sulfate 1.875 mg, Dextroamphetamine Saccharate 1.875 mg, Dextroamphetamine Sulfate 1.875 mg	Adderall by Shire	58521-0075	Stimulant; C II
75 <> APO	Tab, Yellow, Round, Biconvex	Meloxicam 7.5 mg	Mobic by Apotex	Canadian DIN 02248973	NSAID
75 <> CL	Tab, Reddish-Brown, Round, Film Coated	Clopidogrel 75 mg	Plavix by Apotex	60505-0253	Antiplatelet
75 <> DF	Tab, White, Round, Extended Release, DF <> 7.5	Darifenacin 7.5 mg	Enablex by Novartis	Canadian DIN 02273217	Urinary Tract
75 <> DF	Tab, White, Round, Extended Release, DF <> 7.5	Darifenacin 7.5 mg	Enablex by Novartis	00078-0419	Urinary Tract
75 <> DORAL	Tab, Light Orange w/ White Specks, Cap Shaped, 7.5 <> Doral	Quazepam 7.5 mg	Doral by Wallace	00037-9000	Sedative/Hypnotic; C IV
75 <> E	Tab, Blue, Octagonal, 7.5 <> E	Acetaminophen 400 mg, Hydrocodone Bitartrate 7.5 mg	Zydone by West Pharm	52967-0274	Analgesic; C III
75 <> E	Tab, Blue, Octagonal, 7.5 <> E	Acetaminophen 400 mg, Hydrocodone Bitartrate 7.5 mg	Zydone by Endo	63481-0669	Analgesic; C III
75 <> E796	Tab, Peach, Cap Shaped, E796 <> 7.5	Oxycodone HCl 7.5, Acetaminophen 500 mg	Endocet by Endo	60951-0796	Analgesic; C II
75 <> FLINT	Tab, Gray, Round, Scored	Levothyroxine Sodium 75 mcg	Synthroid by Abbott	Canadian DIN 0217209	Thyroid Hormone
75 <> FLINT	Tab, Gray, Round, Scored	Levothyroxine Sodium 75 mcg	Levothroid by Nat Pharmpak	55154-0904	Thyroid Hormone
75 <> FLINT	Tab, Gray, Round, Scored	Levothyroxine Sodium 75 mcg	Synthroid by Rite Aid	11822-5286	Thyroid Hormone
75 <> FLINT	Tab, Gray, Round, Scored	Levothyroxine Sodium 75 mcg	Synthroid by Giant Food	11146-0302	Thyroid Hormone
75 <> FLINT	Tab, Gray, Round, Scored	Levothyroxine Sodium 75 mcg	Synthroid by Abbott	00048-1050	Thyroid Hormone
75 <> FLINT	Tab, Gray, Round, Scored	Levothyroxine Sodium 75 mcg	Synthroid by Forest	00456-0322	Thyroid Hormone
75 <> G	Tab, Peach, Round, G <> 7.5	Meloxicam 7.5 mg	Mobic by Genpharm	15330-0218	NSAID
75 <> G14	Tab, Light Yellow, Round, G14 <> 7.5	Meloxicam 7.5 mg	Mobic by Glenmark	68462-0140	NSAID
75 <> GG333	Tab, Violet, Cap Shaped, Scored, 75 <> GG over 333	Levothyroxine 75 mcg	Levo-T by Alara	64909-0124	Thyroid Hormone
75 <> GG333	Tab, Violet, Cap Shaped, Scored, 75 <> GG over 333	Levothyroxine 75 mcg	Levo-T by Sandoz	00781-5182	Thyroid Hormone
75 <> INV314	Tab, Yellow, Square, Scored, 7.5 <> INV over 314	Warfarin Sodium 7.5 mg	Coumadin by Sandoz	00781-0386	Anticoagulant
75 <> INV314	Tab, Yellow, Square, Scored, 7.5 <> INV over 314	Warfarin Sodium 7.5 mg	Coumadin by Apothecon	59772-0386	Anticoagulant
75 <> L617	Tab, Pink, Round	Ranitidine HCl 75 mg	Zantac by Perrigo	00113-0617	Gastrointestinal
75 <> M	Tab, White to Cream Colored, Pillow-Shaped, M inside square <> 7.5	Mixed Amphetamine Salts 7.5 mg: Amphetamine Aspartate 1.875 mg, Amphetamine Sulfate 1.875 mg, Dextroamphetamine Saccharate 1.875 mg, Dextroamphetamine Sulfate 1.875 mg	Adderall by Mallinckrodt	00406-8884	Stimulant; C II
75 <> N	Tab, Off-White, Round, N <> 7.5	Meloxicam 7.5 mg	Mobicox by Novopharm	Canadian DIN 02258315	NSAID
75 <> N737	Tab, White, Round, N over 737	Diclofenac Sodium 75 mg	Voltaren by Teva	55953-0737 Discontinued	NSAID
75 <> N737	Tab, White, Round, N over 737	Diclofenac Sodium 75 mg	Voltaren by DRX	55045-2247	NSAID
75 <> N737	Tab, White, Round, N over 737	Diclofenac Sodium 75 mg	Voltaren by H J Harkins Co	52959-0423	NSAID
75 <> N737	Tab, White, Round, N over 737	Diclofenac Sodium 75 mg	Voltaren by Allscripts		NSAID
75 <> N737	Tab, White, Round, N over 737	Diclofenac Sodium 75 mg	Voltaren by Warrick	59930-1642	NSAID
75 <> N737	Tab, White, Round, N over 737	Diclofenac Sodium 75 mg	Voltaren by Rx Dispensing	61807-0088	NSAID
75 <> OM	Tab, Yellow-Orange, Round	Tapentadol Hydrochloride 75 mg	Tapentadol Hydrochloride by Janssen-Ortho	50458-0830; C II	Analgesic
75 <> PAL	Tab, Blue, Round, Coated, PAL <> 7.5	L-methylfolate (Metafolin) 7.5 mg	Deplin by PamLab	00525-0410	Supplement
75 <> PAR725	Tab, Off-White, Oval, Scored, 7.5	Buspirone HCl 7.5 mg	Buspar by Par	49884-0725	Antianxiety
75 <> PERCOCET	Tab, Peach, Cap Shaped, 7.5 <> Percocet	Oxycodone HCl 7.5 mg, Acetaminophen 500 mg	Percocet by Endo	63481-0621	Analgesic; C II
75 <> PERCOCET	Tab, Peach, Cap Shaped, 7.5 <> Percocet	Oxycodone HCl 7.5 mg, Acetaminophen 500 mg	Percocet by West Pharm	52967-0279	Analgesic; C II
75 <> SAL	Tab, Blue, Biconvex, Coated, SAL <> 7.5	Pilocarpine HCl 7.5 mg	Salagen by MGI	58063-0775	Cholinergic Agonist
75 <> SYNTHROID	Tab, Violet, Round, Scored	Levothyroxine Sodium 75 mcg	Synthroid by Abbott	00074-5182	Thyroid Hormone
75 <> T4	Tab, Violet, Cap Shaped	Levothyroxine Sodium 75 mcg	Levothroid by Forest	00456-1322	Thyroid Hormone

ID FRONT <> BACK	DESCRIPTION FRONT <> BACK	INGREDIENT & STRENGTH	BRAND (or Generic Equiv.) by FIRM	NDC#	CLASS; SCH.
75 <> TMC	Tab, White, Cap Shaped, Film Coated	Darunavir 75 mg	Prezista by Tibotec	59676-0563	Antiviral
75 <> WATSON364	Tab, Light Beige, Round, Scored, 7.5	Clorazepate Dipotassium 7.5 mg	Tranxene by Major	00904-5160	Antianxiety; C IV
75 <> WATSON364	Tab, Light Beige, Round, Scored, 7.5	Clorazepate Dipotassium 7.5 mg	Tranxene by Ivax	00182-0010	Antianxiety; C IV
75 <> WATSON364	Tab, Light Beige, Round, Scored, 7.5	Clorazepate Dipotassium 7.5 mg	Tranxene by Watson	00591-0364	Antianxiety; C IV
75 <> Z	Tab, Pink, Pentagonal	Ranitidine HCl 75 mg	Zantac by Pfizer		Gastrointestinal
750	Tab, Pink, Cap Shaped, Scored	Polygel Controlled-Release Niacin 750 mg	Slo-Niacin by Upsher Smith	00245-0064	Vitamin
750	Tab, Off White, Capsule Shaped	Nicotinic Acid 750 mg	Niaspan FCT by Sepracor	Canadian DIN 02262355	Antihyperlipidemic
750 <> 4099	Tab, Dark Yellow, Oval, Film Coated, Double-Triangle Logo	Nabumetone 750 mg	Relafen by Par	49884-0650	NSAID
750 <> 5313	Tab, White to Off White, Oval, Ivax Logo 5313 <> 750	Ciprofloxacin 750 mg	Cipro by Ivax	00172-5313	Antibiotic
750 <> 577	Tab, Light Yellow, Cap Shaped, Ex Release, Adrx Logo	Metformin HCl 750 mg	Glucophage XR by Andrx	62037-0577	Antidiabetic
750 <> A	Tab, Coated	Salsalate 750 mg	by Quality Care	60346-0034	NSAID
750 <> B816	Tab, White, Cap Shaped, Film Coated, b816	Ciprofloxacin 750 mg	Cipro by Barr	00555-0816	Antibiotic
750 <> BMS6064	Tab, Pale Red, Cap Shaped, Ex Release	Metformin HCl 750 mg	Glucophage XR by BMS	00087-6064	Antidiabetic
750 <> CIPRO	Tab, White to Light Yellow, Oblong, Film Coated	Ciprofloxacin HCl 750 mg	Cipro by Bayer	00085-1756	Antibiotic
750 <> CIPRO	Tab, White to Light Yellow, Oblong, Film Coated	Ciprofloxacin HCl 750 mg	Cipro by Bayer	Canadian DIN 0215974	Antibiotic
750 <> CIPRO	Tab, White to Light Yellow, Oblong, Film Coated	Ciprofloxacin HCl 750 mg	Cipro by Compumed	00403-4650	Antibiotic
750 <> CIPRO	Tab, White to Light Yellow, Oblong, Film Coated	Ciprofloxacin HCl 750 mg	Cipro by Pharmedix	53002-0268	Antibiotic
750 <> CIPRO	Tab, White to Light Yellow, Oblong, Film Coated	Ciprofloxacin HCl 750 mg	Cipro by H J Harkins Co	52959-0037	Antibiotic
750 <> CIPRO	Tab, White to Light Yellow, Oblong, Film Coated	Ciprofloxacin HCl 750 mg	Cipro by Nat Pharmpak	55154-4807	Antibiotic
750 <> CIPRO	Tab, White to Light Yellow, Oblong, Film Coated	Ciprofloxacin HCl 750 mg	Cipro by Bayer	00026-8514	Antibiotic
750 <> CIPRO	Tab, White to Light Yellow, Oblong, Film Coated	Ciprofloxacin HCl 750 mg	Cipro by Physician Total Care	54868-1184	Antibiotic
750 <> KOS	Tab, White, Cap Shaped, Extended Release	Niacin 750 mg	Niaspan by KOS	60598-0002	Antihyperlipidemic
750 <> KOS	Tab, Orange, Cap Shaped, Film Coated, Extended Release	Niacin 750 mg	Niaspan by KOS	60958-0141	Antihyperlipidemic
750 <> LEVAQUIN	Tab, White, Oblong, Film Coated	Levofloxacin 750 mg	Levaquin by Janssen-Ortho	Canadian DIN 02246804	Antibiotic
750 <> LEVAQUIN	Tab, White, Oblong, Film Coated	Levofloxacin 750 mg	Levaquin by McNeil	00045-1530	Antibiotic
750 <> NOVO	Tab, White, Cap-Shaped, Film Coated	Ciprofloxacin 750 mg	Novo-Ciprofloxacin by Novopharm	Canadian DIN 0216753	Antibiotic
750 <> ODYSSEY	Tab, Off-White, Oval	Nystatin Vaginal 10,000 Units	Mycostatin by Odyssey	65473-0705	Antifungal
750 <> RELAFEN	Tab, Beige, Oblong, Film Coated	Nabumetone 750 mg	Relafen by Rx Dispensing	61807-0059	NSAID
750 <> RELAFEN	Tab, Beige, Oblong, Film Coated	Nabumetone 750 mg	Relafen by SKB	00029-4852	NSAID
750 <> RELAFEN	Tab, Beige, Oblong, Film Coated	Nabumetone 750 mg	Relafen by H J Harkins Co	52959-0373	NSAID
750 <> RELAFEN	Tab, Beige, Oblong, Film Coated	Nabumetone 750 mg	Relafen by SB	59742-4852	NSAID
750 <> RELAFEN	Tab, Beige, Oblong, Film Coated	Nabumetone 750 mg	Relafen by DRX	55045-2440	NSAID
750 <> SP	Tab, Orange, Cap Shaped, Film Coated	Methocarbamol 750 mg	Robaxin by Schwarz		Muscle Relaxant
750 <> UCB	Tab, Orange, Oblong, Scored, Film Coated	Levetiracetam 750 mg	Keppra by UCB	50474-0593	Anticonvulsant
750 <> US	Tab, Blue, Oblong	Salsalate 750 mg	Disalcid by Upsher Smith		NSAID
750A	Tab, Film Coated, 750/A	Salsalate 750 mg	Disalcid by Schein	00364-0833	NSAID
750A	Tab, Orange, Cap Shaped, Film Coated, Extended Release, 750 "Abbott Logo"	Niacin 750 mg	Niaspan by Abbott	00074-3079	Antihyperlipidemic
750MG <> SP2164	Tab, Pink, Oval, Scored, Film Coated	Salsalate 750 mg	Disalcid by Schwarz	00131-2164	NSAID
750MG <> TRYPTAN	Tab, White, Oval, Film Coated	L-Tryptophan 750 mg	Tryptan by Valeant	Canadian DIN 02239327	Supplement
751 <> M	Tab, Brownish Orange, Round	Cyclobenzaprine HCl 10 mg	Flexeril by Mylan	00378-0751	Muscle Relaxant
751 <> M	Tab, Butterscotch Yellow, Round, Film Coated	Cyclobenzaprine HCl 10 mg	Flexeril by Med Pro	53978-1035	Muscle Relaxant
751 <> M	Tab, Butterscotch Yellow, Round, Film Coated	Cyclobenzaprine HCl 10 mg	Flexeril by Pharmedix	53002-0308	Muscle Relaxant
751 <> M	Tab, Butterscotch Yellow, Round, Film Coated	Cyclobenzaprine HCl 10 mg	Flexeril by DJ Pharma	64455-0034	Muscle Relaxant
751 <> M	Tab, Butterscotch Yellow, Round, Film Coated	Cyclobenzaprine HCl 10 mg	Flexeril by Kaiser	62224-7559	Muscle Relaxant

ID FRONT <> BACK	DESCRIPTION FRONT <> BACK	INGREDIENT & STRENGTH	BRAND (or Generic Equiv.) by FIRM	NDC#	CLASS; SCH.
751 <> M	Tab, Butterscotch Yellow, Round, Film Coated	Cyclobenzaprine HCl 10 mg	Flexeril by UDL	51079-0644 Discontinued	Muscle Relaxant
751 <> M	Tab, Butterscotch Yellow, Round, Film Coated	Cyclobenzaprine HCl 10 mg	Flexeril by Physician Total Care	54868-1110	Muscle Relaxant
751 <> M	Tab, Butterscotch Yellow, Round, Film Coated	Cyclobenzaprine HCl 10 mg	Flexeril by Kaiser	00179-1140	Muscle Relaxant
751 <> M	Tab, Butterscotch Yellow, Round, Film Coated	Cyclobenzaprine HCl 10 mg	Flexeril by Mylan	00378-0751	Muscle Relaxant
751 <> M	Tab, Butterscotch Yellow, Round, Film Coated	Cyclobenzaprine HCl 10 mg	Flexeril by PDRX	55289-0567	Muscle Relaxant
751 <> M	Tab, Butterscotch Yellow, Round, Film Coated	Cyclobenzaprine HCl 10 mg	Flexeril by Va Cmop	65243-0022	Muscle Relaxant
752 <> KOS	Tab, Light Orange, Cap Shaped	Lovastatin 20 mg, Niacin 750 mg	Advicor by KOS	60598-0007	Antihyperlipidemic
752 <> M	Tab, Blue, Round, Film Coated	Fexofenadine HCl 30 mg	Allegra by Mylan	00378-0752	Antihistamine
7522	Tab, White, Round	Hydromorphone HCl 2 mg	Dilaudid by BMS	00056-0752	Analgesic; C II
7522	Tab, White, Round	Hydromorphone HCl 2 mg	Dilaudid by Endo	60951-0752	Analgesic; C II
753	Tab, Light Yellow, Round, Scored, Film Coated	Mirtazapine 15 mg	Remeron by Andrx	62037-0753	Antidepressant
753	Cap, Green & Clear, Schering Logo 753	Theophylline Anhydrous LA 250 mg	Theovent by Schering		Antiasthmatic
75325 <> E700	Tab, Peach, Cap Shaped	Oxycodone 7.5 mg, Acetaminophen 325 mg	Endocet by Endo	60951-0700	Analgesic; C II
75325 <> M522	Tab, White to Off-White, Cap Shaped, M522 <> 7.5/325	Oxycodone 7.5 mg, Acetaminophen 325 mg	Percocet by Mallinckrodt	00406-0522	Analgesic; C II
75325 <> PERCOCET	Tab, Peach, Cap Shaped, 7.5 / 325 <> Percocet	Oxycodone HCl 7.5 mg, Acetaminophen 325 mg	Percocet by Endo	63481-0628	Analgesic; C II
754	Tab, Beige, Round, Scored, Film Coated	Mirtazapine 30 mg	Remeron by Andrx	62037-0754	Antidepressant
7540 <> 93	Tab, Light Yellow, Cap Shaped	Topiramate 50 mg	Topamax by Teva	00093-7540	Anticonvulsant
7540 <> WATSON	Tab, White, Round	Ethinyl Estradiol 0.04 mg, Levonorgestrel 0.075 mg	Trivora-28 by Murfreesboro	51129-1633	Oral Contraceptive
7540 <> WATSON	Tab, White, Round	Ethinyl Estradiol 0.04 mg, Levonorgestrel 0.075 mg	Trivora-28 by Watson	52544-0291	Oral Contraceptive
75493	Tab, Blue, Oblong, Film Coated	Diflunisal 250 mg	Dolobid by Teva	00093-0754	NSAID
755	Tab, White, Round, Scored, Film Coated	Mirtazapine 45 mg	Remeron by Andrx	62037-0755	Antidepressant
755 <> R	Tab, Beige, Cap Shaped, Film Coated	Citalopram 10 mg	Celexa by Actavis	00228-2755	Antidepressant
75593	Tab, Blue, Oblong, Film Coated	Diflunisal 500 mg	Dolobid by Duramed	51285-0684	NSAID
75593	Tab, Blue, Oblong, Film Coated	Diflunisal 500 mg	Dolobid by Medirex	57480-0479	NSAID
75593	Tab, Blue, Oblong, Film Coated	Diflunisal 500 mg	Dolobid by PDRX	55289-0460	NSAID
75593	Tab, Blue, Oblong, Film Coated	Diflunisal 500 mg	Dolobid by Murfreesboro	51129-1684	NSAID
75593	Tab, Blue, Oblong, Film Coated	Diflunisal 500 mg	Dolobid by Ivax	00182-1954	NSAID
75593	Tab, Blue, Oblong, Film Coated	Diflunisal 500 mg	Dolobid by Schein	00364-2537	NSAID
75593	Tab, Blue, Oblong, Film Coated	Diflunisal 500 mg	Dolobid by Pharmedix	53002-0303	NSAID
75593	Tab, Blue, Oblong, Film Coated	Diflunisal 500 mg	Dolobid by UDL	51079-0754	NSAID
75593	Tab, Blue, Oblong, Film Coated	Diflunisal 500 mg	Dolobid by Teva	00093-0755	NSAID
755MJ	Tab, Purple, Round, Scored	Estradiol 1 mg	Estrace by Kaiser	62224-0330	Hormone
755MJ	Tab, Purple, Round, Scored	Estradiol 1 mg	Estrace by Rx Pak	65084-0181	Hormone
755MJ	Tab, Purple, Round, Scored	Estradiol 1 mg	Estrace by CVS	51316-0229	Hormone
755MJ	Tab, Purple, Round, Scored	Estradiol 1 mg	Estrace by Amerisource	62584-0755	Hormone
755MJ	Tab, Purple, Round, Scored	Estradiol 1 mg	Estrace by Warner Chilcott	00430-0023	Hormone
756	Tab, White, Cap Shaped, Film Coated, Scored, Andrx Logo 756	Benazepril HCl 5 mg, Hydrochlorothiazide 6.25 mg	Lotensin HCT by Andrx	62037-0756	Antihypertensive; Diuretic
75693	Cap, Olive	Piroxicam 10 mg	Feldene by Quality Care	60346-0737	NSAID
756MJ	Tab, Blue, Round, Scored	Estradiol 2 mg	Estrace by Warner Chilcott	00430-0024	Hormone
756MJ	Tab, Blue, Round, Scored	Estradiol 2 mg	Estrace by Rx Pak	65084-0187	Hormone
756MJ	Tab, Blue, Round, Scored	Estradiol 2 mg	Estrace by Kaiser	62224-0333	Hormone
756MJ	Tab, Blue, Round, Scored	Estradiol 2 mg	Estrace by Physician Total Care	54868-0495	Hormone
756PPP	Cap, White & Orange	Procainamide HCl 375 mg	Pronestyl by BMS	00003-0756	Antiarrhythmic
757	Tab, Purple, Cap Shaped, Film Coated, Scored, Andrx Logo 757	Benazepril HCl 10 mg, Hydrochlorothiazide 12.5 mg	Lotensin HCT by Andrx	62037-0757	Antihypertensive; Diuretic
757 <> M	Tab, White, Round	Atenolol 100 mg	Tenormin by Diversified Healthcare	55887-0998	Antihypertensive
757 <> M	Tab, White, Round	Atenolol 100 mg	Tenormin by UDL	51079-0685	Antihypertensive
757 <> M	Tab, White, Round	Atenolol 100 mg	Tenormin by Mylan	00378-0757	Antihypertensive

ID FRONT <> BACK	DESCRIPTION FRONT <> BACK	INGREDIENT & STRENGTH	BRAND (or Generic Equiv.) by FIRM	NDC#	CLASS; SCH.
7574	Tab, Light Yellow, Round	Hydromorphone HCl 4 mg	Dilaudid by BMS	00056-0757	Analgesic; C II
7574	Tab, Light Yellow, Round	Hydromorphone HCl 4 mg	Dilaudid by Endo	60951-0757	Analgesic; C II
7575 <> DURA	Tab, White, Oblong, Scored, 7.5/7.5 <> Dura	Guaifenesin 600 mg, Phenylpropanolamine HCl 75 mg	Entex LA by CVS	51316-0242	Cold Remedy
7575 <> DURA	Tab, White, Oblong, Scored, 7.5/7.5 <> Dura	Guaifenesin 600 mg, Phenylpropanolamine HCl 75 mg	Entex LA by Med Pro	53978-3337	Cold Remedy
7575 <> DURA	Tab, White, Oblong, Scored, 7.5/7.5 <> Dura	Guaifenesin 600 mg, Phenylpropanolamine HCl 75 mg	Entex LA by DHHS Prog	11819-0049	Cold Remedy
7575 <> DURA	Tab, White, Oblong, Scored, 7.5/7.5 <> Dura	Guaifenesin 600 mg, Phenylpropanolamine HCl 75 mg	Entex LA by Anabolic	00722-6051	Cold Remedy
7575 <> DURA	Tab, White, Oblong, Scored, 7.5/7.5 <> Dura	Guaifenesin 600 mg, Phenylpropanolamine HCl 75 mg	Duravent by Prepackage Specialists	58864-0100	Cold Remedy
7575 <> LOTENSINHCT	Tab, Red, Oblong	Benazepril HCl 20 mg, Hydrochlorothiazide 25 mg	Lotensin HCT by Novartis	00078-0454	Antihypertensive; Diuretic
7575 <> LOTENSINHCT	Tab, Red, Oblong, Scored	Benazepril HCl 20 mg, Hydrochlorothiazide 25 mg	Lotensin HCT by Novartis	00083-0075	Antihypertensive; Diuretic
7575DURA	Tab, White, Oval, 7.5/7.5 Dura	Guaifenesin 600 mg, Phenylpropanolamine HCl 75 mg	Duravent by Dura		Cold Remedy
758	Tab, Pink, Cap Shaped, Film Coated, Scored, Andrx Logo 758	Benazepril HCl 20 mg, Hydrochlorothiazide 12.5 mg	Lotensin HCT by Andrx	62037-0758	Antihypertensive; Diuretic
759	Tab, Red, Cap Shaped, Film Coated, Scored, Andrx Logo 759	Benazepril HCl 20 mg, Hydrochlorothiazide 25 mg	Lotensin HCT by Andrx	62037-0759	Antihypertensive; Diuretic
75FLINT	Tab	Levothyroxine Sodium 0.075 mg	by Med Pro	53978-2034	Thyroid Hormone
75M	Tab	Levothyroxine Sodium 75 mcg	Synthroid by Mova	55370-0127	Thyroid Hormone
75M	Tab	Levothyroxine Sodium 75 mcg	Euthyrox by Em Pharma	63254-0437	Thyroid Hormone
75M <> P	Tab, White, Round, Scored, 7.5 / M	Meloxicam 7.5 mg	Mobicox by Pharmascience	Canadian DIN 02248267	NSAID
75M <> Z	Tab, Purple, Round, Scored	Levothyroxine Sodium 75 mcg	Synthroid by Zoetica	64909-0107	Thyroid Hormone
75MG <> N	Tab, Light Yellow, Triangle Shaped	Azathioprine 75 mg	Azasan by AAI Pharma	66591-0231	Immunosuppressant
75MG <> N	Tab, Triangle-Shaped, Yellow, Scored	Azathioprine 75 mg	Azasan by Salix	65649-0231	Immunosuppressant
75MG <> RSN	Tab, Pink, Oval, Film Coated	Risedronate Sodium 75 mg	Actonel by Procter and Gamble	00149-0477	Bisphosphonate
75N033	Cap, Bright Yellow, 75 <> N over 033	Clomipramine HCl 75 mg	by Teva	55953-0033 Discontinued	OCD
75Z <> P	Tab, Blue, Oval, Scored, Z 7.5	Zopiclone 7.5 mg	Imovane by Pharmascience	Canadian DIN 02240606	Hypnotic
762 <> PAL	Tab, White, Oval, Scored	Pseudoephedrine HCl 45 mg, Guaifenesin 600 mg	Panmist JR by Pamlab	00525-0762 Discontinued	Cold Remedy
762 <> PAL	Tab, White, Oblong	Pseudoephedrine HCl 45 mg, Guaifenesin 600 mg	Panmist Jr by Sovereign	58716-0680	Cold Remedy
7663	Tab, Off-White to Light Grey, Round	Exemestane 25 mg	Aromasin by Pfizer	Canadian DIN 02242705	Aromatase Inhibitor
7663	Tab, Off-White to Light Grey, Round	Exemestane 25 mg	Aromasin by Pfizer	10829-7663	Aromatase Inhibitor
7663	Tab, Off-White to Light Grey, Round	Exemestane 25 mg	Aromasin by Pfizer	00009-7663	Aromatase Inhibitor
769PPP	Tab, Green, Round	Bendroflumethiazide 4 mg, Rauwolfia Serpentina 50 mg	Rauzide by BMS		Antihypertensive; Diuretic
77	Tab, Yellow, Oblong, Coated	Ascorbic Acid 500 mg, Biotin 0.15 mg, Chromic Nitrate 0.1 mg, Cupric Oxide, Cyanocobalamin 50 mcg, Ferrous Fumarate 27 mg, Folic Acid 0.8 mg, Magnesium Oxide 50 mg, Manganese Dioxide 5 mg, Niacin 100 mg, Pantothenic Acid 25 mg, Pyridoxine HCl 25 mg, Riboflavin 20 mg, Thiamine Mononitrate 20 mg, Vitamin A Acetate 5000 Units, Vitamin E Acetate 30 Units	Therobec Plus by Qualitest	00603-5970	Vitamin
77	Tab, White, Oval, 77 <> Bone image	Alendronate Sodium 35 mg	Fosamax by Merck	00006-0077	Antiosteoporosis
77 <> AN	Tab, White, Round, Film Coated	Hydroxyzine HCl 50 mg	Atarax by Harris	67405-0577	Antianxiety; Antihistamine
77 <> E	Tab, White, Round, Film Coated, 77 <> Elan Logo	Frovatriptan 2.5 mg	Frova by Elan	59075-0740	Antimigraine
77 <> E	Tab, White, Round, Film Coated, 77 <> E Logo	Frovatriptan 2.5 mg	Frova by Endo	63481-0025	Antimigraine
770	Cap, White	Acetaminophen 500 mg	Tylenol Ex Strength by ABG	60999-0902	Analgesic
770	Tab, White, Oblong	Acetaminophen 500 mg	Tylenol Ex Strength by JB		Analgesic
770 <> RG	Tab, White to Off-White, Triangular-Shaped, Film-Coated	Finasteride 5 mg	Proscar by Barr	00555-0770 Discontinued	Antiandrogen
770 <> S	Tab, Green, Oval, Scored	Isosorbide Dinitrate 5 mg	Isordil by Zeneca	00310-0770	Antianginal

ID FRONT <> BACK	DESCRIPTION FRONT <> BACK	INGREDIENT & STRENGTH	BRAND (or Generic Equiv.) by FIRM	NDC#	CLASS; SCH.
771	Tab, White	Acetaminophen 325 mg	Tylenol by Paddock	00574-0007	Analgesic
771 <> 93	Tab, Pink, Round	Pravastatin Sodium 10 mg	Pravachol by Teva	00093-0771	Antihyperlipidemic
771 <> M	Tab, Light Blue, Round	Cyclobenzaprine HCl 5 mg	Flexeril by Mylan	00378-0771	Muscle Relaxant
771 <> WW	Tab, White, Round, Scored	Isosorbide Dinitrate 10 mg	Isordil by Heartland	61392-0305	Antianginal
771 <> WW	Tab, White, Round, Scored	Isosorbide Dinitrate 10 mg	Isordil by West-Ward	00143-1771	Antianginal
7711 <> SR180	Tab, Film Coated	Verapamil 180 mg	by Qualitest	00603-6359	Antihypertensive
7711 <> Z800	Tab, White, Oval, Scored, Z over 800	Cimetidine HCl 800 mg	Tagamet by Ivax	00182-1986	Gastrointestinal
7711 <> Z800	Tab, White, Oval, Scored, Z over 800	Cimetidine HCl 800 mg	Tagamet by Ivax	00172-7711	Gastrointestinal
7711 <> Z800	Tab, White, Oval, Scored, Z over 800	Cimetidine HCl 800 mg	Tagamet by Direct Dispensing	57866-6753	Gastrointestinal
7711 <> Z800	Tab, White, Oval, Scored, Z over 800	Cimetidine HCl 800 mg	Tagamet by Golden State	60429-0048	Gastrointestinal
7711 <> Z800	Tab, White to Off White, Oval Shaped, Scored	Cimetidine 800 mg	Tagamet by Teva	00172-7711	Gastrointestinal
711875 <> WATSON	Tab, White, Round, Scored, 771 over 18.75 <> Watson	Pemoline 18.75 mg	by Watson	52544-0771	Stimulant; C IV
772 <> WW	Tab, Green, Round, Scored	Isosorbide Dinitrate 20 mg	Isordil by Heartland	61392-0321	Antianginal
772 <> WW	Tab, Green, Round, Scored	Isosorbide Dinitrate 20 mg	Isordil by West-Ward	00143-1772	Antianginal
7720 <> 250	Tab, Light Orange, Film Coated	Cefprozil 250 mg	Cefzil by BMS	00087-7720	Antibiotic
7720 <> 250	Tab, Light Orange, Film Coated	Cefprozil 250 mg	Cefzil by BMS	Canadian DIN 02163659	Antibiotic
7720BMS250	Cap, Light Orange, 7720/BMS 250	Cefprozil 250 mg	Cefzil by BMS	Canadian	Antibiotic
7721 <> 500	Tab, White, Cap Shaped, Film Coated	Cefprozil 500 mg	Cefzil by BMS	00087-7721	Antibiotic
7721 <> 500	Tab, White, Cap Shaped, Film Coated	Cefprozil 500 mg	Cefzil by BMS	Canadian DIN 02163667	Antibiotic
7721BMS500	Cap, White	Cefprozil 500 mg	Cefzil by BMS	Canadian	Antibiotic
7722 <> SR240	Tab, Off-White, Film Coated	Verapamil HCl 240 mg	Verelan by DRX	55045-2321	Antihypertensive
7722 <> SR240	Tab, Off-White, Film Coated	Verapamil HCl 240 mg	Verelan by Qualitest	00603-6360	Antihypertensive
7722 <> SR240	Tab, Off-White, Film Coated	Verapamil HCl 240 mg	Verelan by URL Mutual	00677-1453	Antihypertensive
772375 <> WATSON	Tab, Peach, Round, Scored, 772 over 37.5 <> Watson	Pemoline 37.5 mg	by Watson	52544-0772	Stimulant; C IV
772WESTWARD	Tab	Isosorbide Dinitrate 20 mg	Isordil by Schein	00364-0509	Antianginal
773	Tab, White, Round	Hyoscyamine Sulfate 0.125 mg	Levsin by Marlop		Gastrointestinal
773 <> S	Tab	Isosorbide Dinitrate 30 mg	Isordil by Zeneca	00310-0773	Antianginal
731875 <> WATSON	Tab, Yellow, Round, Scored, 773 over 18.75 <> Watson	Pemoline 75 mg	by Watson	52544-0773	Stimulant; C IV
774 <> S	Tab, Light Blue, Oval, Scored	Isosorbide Dinitrate 40 mg	Isordil by Zeneca	00310-0774	Antianginal
774 <> WATSON	Tab, White, Round, Scored	Oxycodone HCl 5 mg	Percolone by Watson	52544-0774	Analgesic; C II
747BRL	Tab, Blue, 77/47/BRL	Oxybutynin Chloride 5 mg	by Parke Davis	Canadian DIN 02220067	Urinary Tract
7767100	Cap, White w/ Blue Bands, 7767 over 100	Celecoxib 100 mg	Celebrex by Pfizer	Canadian DIN 02239941	NSAID
7767100	Cap, White w/ Blue Bands, 7767 over 100	Celecoxib 100 mg	Celebrex by Searle	00025-1520	NSAID
7767200	Cap, White w/ Yellow Bands, 7767 over 200	Celecoxib 200 mg	Celebrex by Pfizer	Canadian DIN 02239942	NSAID
7767200	Cap, White w/ Yellow Bands, 7767 over 200	Celecoxib 200 mg	Celebrex by Southwood	58016-0223	NSAID
7767200	Cap, White w/ Yellow Bands, 7767 over 200	Celecoxib 200 mg	Celebrex by Physician Total Care	54868-4101	NSAID
7767200	Cap, White w/ Yellow Bands, 7767 over 200	Celecoxib 200 mg	Celebrex by Searle	00025-1525	NSAID
7767400	Cap, White w/ Green Bands, 7767 over 400	Celecoxib 400 mg	Celebrex by Searle	00025-1530	NSAID
777	Tab, White	Acetaminophen 325 mg	Tylenol by JB		Analgesic
7772 <> 100	Tab, Pale Yellow, Round, Hourglass Logo over 4360	Clozapine 100 mg	Clozaril by Teva Pharmaceuticals	00093-7772	Antipsychotic
778 <> 9393	Tab, Pink w/ Red Specks, Round, Chewable, 93 over 93	Carbamazepine 100 mg	Tegretol by Ivax	00182-1331	Anticonvulsant
778 <> 9393	Tab, Pink w/ Red Specks, Round, Chewable, 93 over 93	Carbamazepine 100 mg	Tegretol by Heartland	61392-0029	Anticonvulsant
778 <> 9393	Tab, Pink w/ Red Specks, Round, Chewable, 93 over 93	Carbamazepine 100 mg	Tegretol by Vangard	00615-4515	Anticonvulsant
778 <> 9393	Tab, Pink w/ Red Specks, Round, Chewable, 93 over 93	Carbamazepine 100 mg	Tegretol by Teva	00093-0778	Anticonvulsant

ID FRONT <> BACK	DESCRIPTION FRONT <> BACK	INGREDIENT & STRENGTH	BRAND (or Generic Equiv.) by FIRM	NDC#	CLASS; SCH.
778 <> 9393	Tab, Pink w/ Red Specks, Round, Chewable, 93 over 93	Carbamazepine 100 mg	Tegretol by UDL	51079-0870 Discontinued	Anticonvulsant
778 <> WATSON	Tab, White, Oblong, Scored	Diltiazem HCl 120 mg	Diltiazem HCl by Watson	52544-0778	Antihypertensive
77C77C	Tab, Yellow, 77C77C <> Boehringer Ingelheim Logo	Meloxicam 15 mg	Mobicox by Boehringer Ingelheim Canada	Canadian DIN 02242786	NSAID
78 <> E	Tab, White to Off-White, Round, Film Coated	Zolpidem Tartrate 5 mg	Ambien by Aurobindo	65862-0159	Sedative/Hypnotic; C IV
78 <> WYETH	Tab, White, Round	Ethinyl Estradiol 0.03 mg, Norgestrel 0.3 mg	Lo Ovral by Dept Health	53808-0028	Oral Contraceptive
78 <> WYETH	Tab, White, Round	Ethinyl Estradiol 0.03 mg, Norgestrel 0.3 mg	Lo Ovral by PDRX	55289-0246	Oral Contraceptive
780 <> GG	Tab, White, Round, Film Coated	Methylphenidate HCl 20 mg	Ritalin by Caremark	00339-4103	Stimulant; C II
780 <> ML	Tab, Round, Peach	Folic Acid 2.5 mg, Vitamin B-12 2 mg, Vitamin B-6 25 mg	Folamin by Midlothian	68308-0780	Vitamin; Supplement
780 <> S	Tab, Yellow, Oval, Scored	Isosorbide Dinitrate 10 mg	Isordil by Zeneca	00310-0780	Antianginal
780 <> SR	Tab, White, Round, Sustained Release	Methylphenidate HCl 20 mg	Ritalin SR by Sandoz	00781-5754	Stimulant; C II
781 <> W375	Tab, Peach, Shield Shaped, Scored, W over 37.5	Venlafaxine 37.5 mg	Effexor by Wyeth	00008-0781	Antidepressant
781 <> W375	Tab, Peach, Shield Shaped, Scored, W over 37.5	Venlafaxine 37.5 mg	Effexor by Caremark	00339-6035	Antidepressant
7815 <> 10	Tab, White, Cap Shaped, Film Coated	Valdecoxib 10 mg	Bextra by Pfizer	Canadian DIN 02246621 Discontinued	COX 2 Inhibitor
7815 <> 20	Tab, White, Cap Shaped, Film Coated	Valdecoxib 20 mg	Bextra by Pfizer	Canadian DIN 02246622 Discontinued	COX 2 Inhibitor
782 <> S	Tab, Light Green, Black Print, Round, Film Coated, 78-2 <> S in Triangle	Thioridazine 10 mg	Mellaril by Novartis	00078-0002	Antipsychotic
78242	Cap, Yellow, Gelatin, 78/242	Cyclosporine 50 mg	Sandimmune by Novartis	00078-0242	Immunosuppressant
7827	Tab, Green, Orange & White, Round, 78-27	Belladonna 0.25 mg, Phenobarbital 50 mg	Belladenal-S by Sandoz	00179-0432	Gastrointestinal; C IV
7828	Tab, White, Round, 78-28	Belladonna 0.25 mg, Phenobarbital 50 mg	Belladenal by Sandoz	55289-0708	Gastrointestinal; C IV
783 <> GG	Tab, Yellow, Round	Methylphenidate HCl 5 mg	by Caremark	00339-4100	Stimulant; C II
783 <> GG	Tab, Yellow, Round	Methylphenidate HCl 5 mg	Ritalin by Sandoz	00781-1748	Stimulant; C II
7831	Tab, Green, Orange & Yellow, Round, Scored, 78-31	Belladonna 0.2 mg, Phenobarbital 40 mg, Ergotamine Tartrate 0.6 mg	by Novartis	00078-0031	Gastrointestinal; C IV
7831	Tab, Green, Orange & Yellow, Round, Scored, 78-31	Belladonna 0.2 mg, Phenobarbital 40 mg, Ergotamine Tartrate 0.6 mg	Bellergal-S by Sandoz	64579-0020	Gastrointestinal; C IV
7840 <> AHR2	Tab, White, Round, Scored	Glycopyrrolate 2 mg	Robinul Forte by ESI Lederle	59911-3787	Gastrointestinal
785	Tab	Ursodiol 250 mg	Urso by Schwarz	00078-0058	Gastrointestinal
785	Tab, Film Coated	Ursodiol 250 mg	Urso by Schering	00982-0785	Gastrointestinal
785 <> WESTWARD	Tab	Aspirin 325 mg, Butalbital 50 mg, Caffeine 40 mg	Fiorinal by Schein	00364-0677	Analgesic; C III
7854 <> SANDOZ	Tab, Orchid, Coated, 78-54 in Black Ink	Methylergonovine Maleate 0.2 mg	by Kaiser	00179-0432	Ergot Alkaloids
7854 <> SANDOZ	Tab, Orchid, Coated, 78-54 in Black Ink	Methylergonovine Maleate 0.2 mg	by PDRX	55289-0708	Ergot Alkaloids
7854 <> SANDOZ	Tab, Orchid, Coated, 78-54 in Black Ink	Methylergonovine Maleate 0.2 mg	Methergine by Neuman	64579-0020	Ergot Alkaloids
7854 <> SANDOZ	Tab, Orchid, Coated, 78-54 in Black Ink	Methylergonovine Maleate 0.2 mg	Methergine by Novartis	00078-0054	Ergot Alkaloids
7858 <> SANDOZ	Tab, Yellow, Black Print, Round, Film Coated	Methysergide Maleate 2 mg	Sansert by Novartis	00078-0058	Antimigraine
7866 <> SANDOZ	Tab, White, Round, Scored	Mazindol 2 mg	by Nat Pharmpak	55154-5545	Anorexiant; C IV
787 <> 93	Tab, White to Off-White, Round, Marbled	Atenolol 25 mg	Tenormin by Teva	00093-0787	Antihypertensive
787 <> PLIVA	Tab, White, Oval, Film Coated	Azithromycin 250 mg	Zithromax by Pliva	50111-0787 Discontinued	Antibiotic
7871 <> SANOREX	Tab, White, Elliptical, 78-71 <> Sanorex	Mazindol 1 mg	by Allscripts		Anorexiant; C IV
788 <> 93	Tab, White to Off-White, Round	Selegiline HCl 5 mg	by Murfreesboro	51129-1111	Antiparkinson
788 <> 93	Tab, White to Off-White, Round	Selegiline HCl 5 mg	by Teva	00093-0788	Antiparkinson
788 <> 93	Tab, White to Off-White, Round	Selegiline HCl 5 mg	by Teva	17372-0788	Antiparkinson
788 <> 93	Tab, White to Off-White, Round	Selegiline HCl 5 mg	by Vangard	00615-4516	Antiparkinson
788 <> PLIVA	Tab, Blue, Cap Shaped, Film Coated	Azithromycin 500 mg	Zithromax by Pliva	50111-0788	Antibiotic

ID FRONT <> BACK	DESCRIPTION FRONT <> BACK	INGREDIENT & STRENGTH	BRAND (or Generic Equiv.) by FIRM	NDC#	CLASS; SCH.
788 <> S	Tab, Pink, Black Print, Round, Film Coated, 78-8 <> S in Triangle	Thioridazine 15 mg	Mellaril by Novartis	00078-0008	Antipsychotic
789 <> GG	Tab, Green, Round, Scored	Methylphenidate HCl 10 mg	Ritalin by Caremark	00339-4101	Stimulant; C II
789 <> PLIVA	Tab, White, Cap Shaped, Film Coated	Azithromycin 600 mg	Zithromax by Pliva	50111-0789	Antibiotic
789RESPA	Cap	Brompheniramine Maleate 6 mg, Pseudoephedrine HCl 60 mg	Respahist by Pharmafab	62542-0102	Cold Remedy
79	Tab, Yellow, Oblong, Coated	Ascorbic Acid 500 mg, Calcium Pantothenate 18 mg, Cyanocobalamin 5 mcg, Folic Acid 0.5 mg, Niacinamide 100 mg, Pyridoxine HCl 4 mg, Riboflavin 15 mg, Thiamine Mononitrate 15 mg	Therobec by Qualitest	00603-5969	Vitamin
79 <> C	Tab, Yellow, Round	Meloxicam 7.5 mg	Mobic by Aurobindo	65862-0097	NSAID
79 <> E	Tab, White to Off-White, Oval, Film Coated	Zolpidem Tartrate 10 mg	Ambien by Aurobindo	65862-0160	Sedative/Hypnotic; C IV
790 <> SZ	Tab, Light Yellow, Round	Methylphenidate HCl 20 mg	Ritalin by Sandoz	00781-5753	Stimulant; C II
791	Tab, White to Off-White, Round, Andrx Logo <> 791	Lovastatin 10 mg	Mevacor by Andrx	62037-0791	Antihyperlipidemic
792	Tab, Peach, Round, Andrx Logo <> 792	Lovastatin 20 mg	Mevacor by Andrx	62037-0792	Antihyperlipidemic
793	Tab, White to Off-White, Round, Andrx Logo over 793	Lovastatin 40 mg	Mevacor by Andrx	62037-0793	Antihyperlipidemic
795	Tab, Pink, Oval, Heart logo <> 795	Vitamin A 4000 IU, Vitamin C 120 mg, Vitamin D 400 IU, Vitamin E 30 IU, Thiamin 1.8 mg, Riboflavin 1.7 mg, Niacin 20 mg, Vitamin B6 2.6 mg, Folic Acid 800 mcg, Vitamin B12 8 mcg, Calcium 200 mg, Iron 28 mg, Zinc 25 mg	Stuart Prenatal by Xanodyne	64731-0795	Vitamin
795 <> SCHERING	Tab, Pink, Oval, Scored	Anisindione 50 mg	Miradon by Schering	00085-0795	Anticoagulant
796	Tab, Pink, Oval, Delayed-Release	Divalproex Sodium 125 mg	Depakote by Caraco	62756-0796	Anticonvulsant
797	Tab, Peach, Oblong, Delayed-Release	Divalproex Sodium 250 mg	Depakote by Caraco	62756-0797	Anticonvulsant
798	Tab, Pink, Oval, Delayed-Release	Divalproex Sodium 500 mg	Depakote by Caraco	62756-0798	Anticonvulsant
798 <> b	Tab, White, Oval, Stylized b, Sublingual	Buprenorphine HCl 2 mg	Subutex by Teva Pharmaceuticals	00093-5378	Detoxification Agent; C III
799 <> b	Tab, White, Oval, Stylized b, Sublingual	Buprenorphine HCl 8 mg	Subutex by Teva Pharmaceuticals	00093-5379	Detoxification Agent; C III
79B <> TEC	Tab, Brown, D-Shaped, Film Coated, Scored	Famotidine 40 mg	Pepcid by AltiMed	Canadian DIN 02242328	Gastrointestinal
79B <> TEC	Tab, Beige, D-Shaped, Film Coated, Scored	Famotidine 20 mg	Pepcid by AltiMed	Canadian DIN 02242327	Gastrointestinal
7R	Cap, Yellow, Soft Gel	Isotretinoin 40 mg	Sotret by Ranbaxy	63304-0586	Dermatologic
8	Tab, Yellow, Buccal	Fentanyl 800 mcg	Fentora by Cephalon	63459-0548	Opioid Agonist; C II
8	Tab, Yellow, Round, Enteric Coated, Raised "8"	Aspirin 81 mg	Aspirin by Perrigo	00113-0535	Analgesic
8	Tab, Yellow, Round, Enteric Coated, Raised "8"	Aspirin 81 mg	Aspirin by Perrigo	00113-0937	Analgesic
8	Tab, White, Oval	Ibuprofen 800 mg	Motrin by Norton		NSAID
8	Tab, Yellow, Round, Enteric Coated, Raised "8"	Aspirin 81 mg	Aspirin by Ivax	00182-1061 Discontinued	Analgesic
8	Tab, White, Round	Perphenazine 8 mg	Apo Perphenazine by Apotex	Canadian DIN 00335118	Antipsychotic
8	Tab, White, Round, Vanda Logo <> 8	Iloperidone 8 mg	Fanapt by Vanda	43068-0108	Antipsychotic
8 <> 3688	Tab, Green, Round, Scored, Hourglass Logo 8	Doxazosin Mesylate 8 mg	Cardura by Ivax	00172-3688	Antihypertensive
8 <> 93	Tab, White, Round, Film Coated	Indapamide 2.5 mg	Lozol by Teva	00093-0008	Diuretic
8 <> AA	Tab, White, Triangular, Scored, double Abbott Logo (aa)	Hydromorphone HCl 8 mg	Dilaudid by Abbott	00074-2426	Analgesic; C II
8 <> COPLEY711	Tab	Guanabenz Acetate 10.28 mg	by Teva	38245-0711 Discontinued	Antihypertensive
8 <> E	Tab, White, Round	Hydromorphone HCl 8 mg	Dilaudid by Ethex	58177-0449	Analgesic; C II
8 <> G	Tab, White, Round	Ondansetron ODT 8 mg	Zofran ODT by Glenmark	68462-0158	Antiemetic
8 <> G1	Tab, Yellow, Oval	Ondansetron HCl 8 mg	Zofran by Glenmark	68462-0106	Antiemetic
8 <> GLAXO	Tab, Yellow, Oval	Ondansetron HCl 8 mg	Zofran by GSK		Antiemetic
8 <> GLAXO	Tab, Dark Yellow, Oval, Film Coated	Ondansetron HCl 8 mg	Zofran by GSK	Canadian DIN 02213575	Antiemetic
8 <> M	Tab, White to Off-White, Arc-Triangle Shaped, Scored	Hydromorphone HCl 8 mg	Dilaudid by Mallinckrodt	00406-3249	Analgesic; C II

ID FRONT <> BACK	DESCRIPTION FRONT <> BACK	INGREDIENT & STRENGTH	BRAND (or Generic Equiv.) by FIRM	NDC#	CLASS; SCH.
8 <> N598	Tab, White to Off-White, Round, Scored, N over 598	Doxazosin Mesylate 8 mg	Cardura by Teva	00093-8123	Antihypertensive
8 <> P	Tab, Yellow, Oval, P logo <> 8	Ondansetron HCl 8 mg	Zofran by Pharmascience	Canadian DIN 02258196	Antiemetic
8 <> PLOND	Tab, White, Oval	Ondansetron 8 mg	Zofran by Sandoz	00781-5258	Antiemetic
8 <> PMS	Tab, White, Round, Scored	Hydromorphone HCl 8 mg	Dilaudid by Pharmascience	Canadian DIN 00885428	Analgesic; C II
8 <> R	Tab, White, Octagonal	Indapamide 2.5 mg	Lozol by Thrift Drug	59198-0174	Diuretic
8 <> R	Tab, White, Octagonal	Indapamide 2.5 mg	Lozol by Pharm Util	60491-0382	Diuretic
8 <> R	Tab, White, Octagonal	Indapamide 2.5 mg	Lozol by Allscripts		Diuretic
8 <> R	Tab, White, Octagonal	Indapamide 2.5 mg	Lozol by RPR	00075-0082	Diuretic
8 <> R	Tab, White, Octagonal	Indapamide 2.5 mg	Lozol by Drug Distr	52985-0062	Diuretic
8 <> R	Tab, White, Octagonal	Indapamide 2.5 mg	Lozol by Nat Pharmpak	55154-4011	Diuretic
8 <> SAMPLE	Tab	Ondansetron HCl 8 mg	Zofran by GSK		Antiemetic
8 <> SB	Tab, Reddish Brown, Pentagonal, Film Coated	Rosiglitazone Maleate 8 mg	Avandia by GSK	Canadian DIN 02241114	Antidiabetic
8 <> SB	Tab, Reddish Brown, Pentagonal	Rosiglitazone Maleate 8 mg	Avandia by SKB	00029-3160	Antidiabetic
8 <> V	Tab, White, Round, Ex Release	Albuterol Sulfate 8 mg	Vospire ER by Odyssey	65473-0758	Antiasthmatic
8 <> V	Tab, White, Round, Ex Release	Albuterol Sulfate 8 mg	Vospire ER by Dava	68774-0601	Antiasthmatic
8 <> VOLMAX	Tab, White, Hexagonal, 8 in Dark Blue	Albuterol Sulfate 8 mg	Volmax by Muro	00451-0399	Antiasthmatic
8 <> VOLMAX	Tab, White, Hexagonal, 8 in Dark Blue	Albuterol Sulfate 8 mg	Volmax by Eckerd	19458-0849	Antiasthmatic
8 <> VOLMAX	Tab, White, Hexagonal, 8 in Dark Blue	Albuterol Sulfate 8 mg	Volmax by Thrift Drug	59198-0355	Antiasthmatic
8 <> ZOFRAN	Tab, Yellow, Oval, Film Coated	Ondansetron HCl 8 mg	Zofran by PDRX	55289-0478	Antiemetic
8 <> ZOFRAN	Tab, Yellow, Oval, Film Coated	Ondansetron HCl 8 mg	Zofran by GSK	00173-0447	Antiemetic
80	Tab, Blue	Acetaminophen 80 mg	Children's Tylenol by Mead Johnson	Canadian DIN 00884561	Analgesic
80 <> 543	Tab, Brick Red, Cap Shaped, Film Coated	Simvastatin 80 mg	Zocor by Merck	00006-0543	Antihyperlipidemic
80 <> 543	Tab, Brick Red, Cap Shaped, Film Coated	Simvastatin 80 mg	Zocor by Merck-Frosst	Canadian DIN 02240332	Antihyperlipidemic
80 <> 59911	Tab, White, Oblong	Propranolol HCl 80 mg	Inderal by Southwood	58016-0526	Antihypertensive
80 <> ABG	Tab, Green, Round, Controlled Release	Oxycodone HCl 80 mg	OxyContin by Ivax	00172-6357	Analgesic; C II
80 <> APO	Tab, Dusty Rose, Oblong	Simvastatin 80 mg	Zocor by Apotex	Canadian DIN 02247015	Antihyperlipidemic
80 <> BMS	Tab, Yellow, Oval	Pravastatin Sodium 80 mg	Pravachol by BMS	00003-5195	Antihyperlipidemic
80 <> BMS	Tab, Yellow, Oval	Pravastatin Sodium 80 mg	Pravigard by BMS	00003-5183 00003-5184	Antihyperlipidemic
80 <> C	Tab, Yellow, Oblong	Meloxicam 15 mg	Mobic by Aurobindo	65862-0098	NSAID
80 <> CALAN	Tab, Light Peach, Oval, Scored	Verapamil HCl 80 mg	Calan by Searle	00025-1851	Antihypertensive
80 <> CALAN	Tab, Light Peach, Oval, Scored	Verapamil HCl 80 mg	Calan by Nat Pharmpak	55154-3603	Antihypertensive
80 <> CALAN	Tab, Light Peach, Oval, Scored	Verapamil HCl 80 mg	Calan by Thrift Drug	59198-0015	Antihypertensive
80 <> CALAN	Tab, Light Peach, Oval, Scored	Verapamil HCl 80 mg	Calan by Amerisource	62584-0852	Antihypertensive
80 <> CALAN	Tab, Light Peach, Oval, Scored	Verapamil HCl 80 mg	Calan by Rightpak	65240-0619	Antihypertensive
80 <> CALAN	Tab, Light Peach, Oval, Scored	Verapamil HCl 80 mg	Calan by Med Pro	53978-3398	Antihypertensive
80 <> DAN5557	Tab, Yellow, Round, Scored, DAN over 5557	Propranolol HCl 80 mg	Inderal by Schein	00364-0760	Antihypertensive
80 <> DAN5557	Tab, Yellow, Round, Scored, DAN over 5557	Propranolol HCl 80 mg	Inderal by Watson	00591-5557	Antihypertensive
80 <> E710	Tab, Green, Round, Coated, Extended Release	Oxycodone HCl 80 mg	OxyContin by Endo	60951-0710	Analgesic; C II
80 <> G	Tab, Yellow, Oval	Pravastatin Sodium 80 mg	Pravachol by Glenmark	68462-0198	Antilipemic Agent
80 <> G5	Tab, Yellow, Oval	Pravastatin Sodium 80 mg	Pravachol by Glenmark	68462-0198	Antihyperlipidemic
80 <> INV238	Tab	Nadolol 80 mg	Nadolol by Sandoz	00781-1183	Antihypertensive
80 <> INV238	Tab	Nadolol 80 mg	Nadolol by Major	00904-5071	Antihypertensive
80 <> INV238	Tab	Nadolol 80 mg	Nadolol by Moore	00839-7871	Antihypertensive

ID FRONT <> BACK	DESCRIPTION FRONT <> BACK	INGREDIENT & STRENGTH	BRAND (or Generic Equiv.) by FIRM	NDC#	CLASS; SCH.
80 <> INV238	Tab	Nadolol 80 mg	Nadolol by Schein	00364-2654	Antihypertensive
80 <> INV238	Tab	Nadolol 80 mg	Nadolol by Ivax	00182-2634	Antihypertensive
80 <> INV238	Tab	Nadolol 80 mg	Nadolol by Invamed	52189-0238	Antihypertensive
80 <> L292	Tab, Pink, Cap-Shaped, Film-Coated	Simvastatin 80 mg	Zocor by Perrigo	45802-0292	Antihyperlipidemic
80 <> LESCOLXL	Tab, Yellow, Round, Film Coated	Fluvastatin Sodium 80 mg	Lescol XL by Novartis	Canadian DIN 02250527	Antihyperlipidemic
80 <> LESCOLXL	Tab, Yellow, Round, Film Coated	Fluvastatin Sodium 80 mg	Lescol XL by Novartis	00078-0354	Antihyperlipidemic
80 <> M	Tab, White, Round, Film Coated	Indapamide 2.5 mg	Lozol by DRX	55045-2385	Diuretic
80 <> M	Tab, White, Round, Film Coated	Indapamide 2.5 mg	Lozol by UDL	51079-0868	Diuretic
80 <> M	Tab, White, Round, Film Coated	Indapamide 2.5 mg	Lozol by Mylan	00378-0080	Diuretic
80 <> MYLAN185	Tab, Yellow, Round, Scored, Mylan over 185	Propranolol HCl 80 mg	Inderal by Mylan	00378-0185	Antihypertensive
80 <> MYLAN185	Tab, Yellow, Round, Scored, Mylan over 185	Propranolol HCl 80 mg	Inderal by UDL	51079-0280	Antihypertensive
80 <> MYLAN232	Tab, White, Round, Scored, Mylan over 232	Furosemide 80 mg	Lasix by Heartland	61392-0254	Diuretic
80 <> MYLAN232	Tab, White, Round, Scored, Mylan over 232	Furosemide 80 mg	Lasix by Mylan	00378-0232	Diuretic
80 <> MYLAN232	Tab, White, Round, Scored, Mylan over 232	Furosemide 80 mg	Lasix by UDL	51079-0527	Diuretic
80 <> N	Tab, Pink, Cap Shaped	Simvastatin 80 mg	Zocor by Novopharm	Canadian DIN 02250187	Antihyperlipidemic
80 <> N	Tab, Light Blue, Cap Shaped, Scored, N <> 8/0	Sotalol HCl 80 mg	Sotacor by Novopharm	Canadian DIN 02231181	Antiarrhythmic
80 <> OC	Tab, Green, Round, Coated	Oxycodone HCl 80 mg	OxyContin by Purdue	59011-0107	Analgesic; C II
80 <> P	Tab, Pink, Cap Shaped	Simvastatin 80 mg	Zocor by Pharmascience	Canadian DIN 02269295	Antihyperlipidemic
80 <> PD158	Tab, White, Oval, Film Coated	Atorvastatin Calcium 80 mg	Lipitor by Parke Davis	Canadian DIN 02243097	Antihyperlipidemic
80 <> PD158	Tab, White, Oval, Film Coated	Atorvastatin Calcium 80 mg	Lipitor by Parke Davis	00071-0158	Antihyperlipidemic
80 <> TAP	Tab, Green, Teardrop Shaped	Febuxostat 80 mg	Uloric by Takeda	64764-0677	Antigout
80 <> TAP	Tab, Green, Teardrop Shaped	Febuxostat 80 mg	Uloric by Takeda	64764-0677	Antigout
80 <> TAP	Tab, Green, Teardrop Shaped	Febuxostat 80 mg	Uloric by Takeda	64764-0677	Antigout
80 <> TAP	Tab, Green, Teardrop Shaped	Febuxostat 80 mg	Uloric by Takeda	64764-0677	Antigout
80 <> TYLENOL	Tab, Pink or Purple, Round, Scored, Chewable	Acetaminophen 80 mg	Children's Tylenol by McNeil	Canadian DIN 02229539	Analgesic
80 <> TYLENOLCOLD	Tab, Pink or Orange, Round, Scored, Chewable	Acetaminophen 80 mg, Chlorpheniramine Maleate 0.5 mg, Pseudoephedrine HCl 7.5 mg	Children's Tylenol Cold by McNeil	Canadian DIN 00743224	Cold Remedy
80 <> TYLENOLCOLDDM	Tab, Pink or Purple, Round, Chewable	Acetaminophen 80 mg, Chlorpheniramine Maleate 0.5 mg, Pseudoephedrine HCl 7.5 mg, Dextromethorphan 3.75 mg	Children's Tylenol Cold Plus Cough by McNeil	Canadian DIN 00870455	Cold Remedy
80 <> US12	Tab, White, Cap Shaped	Sotalol HCl 80 mg	Sorine by Upsher Smith	00245-0012	Antiarrhythmic
80 <> Z4237	Tab, White, Round, Scored, Z over 4237	Nadolol 80 mg	Corgard by Ivax	00093-4237	Antihypertensive
80 <> Z4237	Tab, White, Round, Scored, Z over 4237	Nadolol 80 mg	Corgard by Ivax	00182-2634	Antihypertensive
800	Tab, Film Coated	Ibuprofen 400 mg	Motrin by Quality Care	60346-0030	NSAID
800 <> 4268	Tab, White, Oval, Hourglass Logo 4268	Acyclovir 800 mg	Zovirax by Quality Care	00182-2667 Discontinued	Antiviral
800 <> 4268	Tab, White, Oval, Hourglass Logo 4268	Acyclovir 800 mg	Zovirax by Ivax	00172-4268 Discontinued	Antiviral
800 <> 4444	Tab, White, Oval, Scored, Ivax Logo 4444	Gabapentin 800 mg	Neurontin by Ivax	00093-4444	Anticonvulsant
800 <> A03	Tab, White, Oval	Acyclovir 800 mg	Zovirax by Mova	55370-0556	Antiviral
800 <> C103	Tab, White, Oblong, Film Coated	Ibuprofen 800 mg	Motrin by Dr. Reddy's	55111-0103	NSAID
800 <> G	Tab, Film Coated	Ibuprofen 400 mg	Motrin by Quality Care	60346-0030	NSAID
800 <> IP137	Tab, White, Cap Shaped, Film Coated	Ibuprofen 800 mg	Motrin by Urgent Care Center	50716-0726	NSAID
800 <> IP137	Tab, White, Cap Shaped, Film Coated	Ibuprofen 800 mg	Motrin by Golden State	60429-0094	NSAID
800 <> IP137	Tab, White, Cap Shaped, Film Coated	Ibuprofen 800 mg	Motrin by Rx Dispensing	61807-0012	NSAID
800 <> IP137	Tab, White, Cap Shaped, Film Coated	Ibuprofen 800 mg	Motrin by Major	00904-5187	NSAID

ID FRONT <> BACK	DESCRIPTION FRONT <> BACK	INGREDIENT & STRENGTH	BRAND (or Generic Equiv.) by FIRM	NDC#	CLASS; SCH.
800 <> IP137	Tab, White, Cap Shaped, Film Coated	Ibuprofen 800 mg	Motrin by Interpharm	53746-0137	NSAID
800 <> IP137	Tab, White, Cap Shaped, Film Coated	Ibuprofen 800 mg	Motrin by Ivax	00172-3648 Discontinued	NSAID
800 <> IP137	Tab, White, Cap Shaped, Film Coated	Ibuprofen 800 mg	Motrin by Breckenridge	51991-0740	NSAID
800 <> IP137	Tab, White, Cap Shaped, Film Coated	Ibuprofen 800 mg	Motrin by Qualitest	00603-4020	NSAID
800 <> IP137	Tab, White, Cap Shaped, Film Coated	Ibuprofen 800 mg	Motrin by Ivax	00182-1297 Discontinued	NSAID
800 <> IP137	Tab, White, Cap Shaped, Film Coated	Ibuprofen 800 mg	Motrin by Amneal	65162-0570 Discontinued	NSAID
800 <> IP137	Tab, White, Cap Shaped, Film Coated	Ibuprofen 800 mg	Motrin by Watson	00591-3665	NSAID
800 <> MP99	Tab, Film Coated	Ibuprofen 800 mg	Motrin by URL Mutual	00677-1119	NSAID
800 <> N	Tab, White, Oval, Black Ink	Gabapentin 800 mg	Neurontin by Novopharm	Canadian DIN 02247346	Antiepileptic
800 <> N235	Tab, Coated, N/235	Cimetidine HCl 800 mg	Tagamet by Brightstone	62939-2141	Gastrointestinal
800 <> N235	Tab, Film Coated, Scored	Cimetidine HCl 800 mg	Tagamet by Warrick	59930-1803	Gastrointestinal
800 <> N235	Tab, Coated	Cimetidine HCl 800 mg	Tagamet by URL Mutual	00677-1530	Gastrointestinal
800 <> N305	Tab, White, Oval, Scored, 800 <> N score 305	Cimetidine HCl 800 mg	Tagamet by Teva	00093-8305 Discontinued	Gastrointestinal
800 <> N947	Tab, White, Cap Shaped	Acyclovir 800 mg	Zovirax by Teva	00093-8947	Antiviral
800 <> N947	Tab, White, Cap Shaped	Acyclovir 800 mg	Zovirax by Amerisource	62584-0429	Antiviral
800 <> N947	Tab, White, Cap Shaped	Acyclovir 800 mg	Zovirax by UDL	51079-0878 Discontinued	Antiviral
800 <> N947	Tab, White, Cap Shaped	Acyclovir 800 mg	Zovirax by Teva	55953-0947	Antiviral
800 <> N947	Tab, White, Cap Shaped	Acyclovir 800 mg	Zovirax by Warrick	59930-1584	Antiviral
800 <> NN	Tab, Blue, Elongated, Scored, Compressed tablet	Acyclovir 800 mg	Zovirax by Novopharm	Canadian DIN 02285975	Antiviral
800 <> NOVO	Tab, Green, Oval	Cimetidine 800 mg	Tagamet by Novopharm	Canadian DIN 00663727	Gastrointestinal
800 <> PAR216	Tab, Coated, Par over 216	Ibuprofen 800 mg	Motrin by Nat Pharmpak	55154-5565	NSAID
800 <> PAR216	Tab, White, Cap Shaped, Film-Coated, 800 <> Par over 216	Ibuprofen 800 mg	Motrin by UDL	51079-0596 Discontinued	NSAID
800 <> PAR216	Tab, Coated, Par over 216	Ibuprofen 800 mg	Motrin by Baker Cummins	63171-1297	NSAID
800 <> PAR216	Tab, Film Coated, Par over 216	Ibuprofen 800 mg	Motrin by PDRX	55289-0140	NSAID
800 <> PAR216	Tab, Coated	Ibuprofen 800 mg	Motrin by Par	49884-0216	NSAID
800 <> ZOVIRAX	Tab, Light Blue	Acyclovir 800 mg	Zovirax by Quality Care	60346-0735	Antiviral
800M80	Tab, White, Oblong, Scored	Cimetidine 800 mg	Tagamet by Dava	67253-0342	Gastrointestinal
800M80 <> MOVA	Tab, White, Cap Shaped, Scored	Cimetidine HCl 800 mg	Tagamet by Mova	55370-0137	Gastrointestinal
800M8C <> MOVA	Tab, White, Oblong, Film Coated, 800/M8C <> Mova	Cimetidine HCl 800 mg	Tagamet by Compumed		Gastrointestinal
800MCG <> 286	Tab, Brown	Cerivastatin Sodium 0.8 mg	Baycol by Bayer	00026-2886	Antihyperlipidemic
800MG	Tab	Ibuprofen 800 mg	Motrin by Rite Aid	11822-5213	NSAID
800N <> 235	Tab, Light Green, Coated, 800/N	Cimetidine HCl 800 mg	Tagamet by Schein	00364-2594	Gastrointestinal
801 <> MYLAN	Tab, Coated, Beveled Edge	Ibuprofen 800 mg	Motrin by Mylan	00378-0801	NSAID
803 <> R	Tab, White to Off-White, Round, Film Coated	Spironolactone 25 mg	Aldactone by Purepac	00228-2803	Diuretic
805 <> AP	Tab, Light Green, Cap-Shaped, Film Coated	Esterified Estrogens 0.625 mg, Methyltestosterone 1.25 mg	Estratest by Glenmark	68462-0173	Hormone
805 <> WATSON	Tab, White, Round	Meprobamate 400 mg	by Watson	52544-0805	Sedative/Hypnotic; C IV
8059911	Cap, Blue & White	Propranolol HCl 80 mg	Inderal by ESI Lederle	59911-5471	Antihypertensive
806 <> AP	Tab, Green, Cap Shaped, Film Coated	Esterified Estrogens 1.25 mg, Methyltestosterone 2.5 mg	Estratest by Glenmark	68462-0174	Hormone
80INNOPRANXL	Cap, Gray & White, Ex Release, 80 2 Bands InnoPranXL Reliant Logo	Propranolol HCl 80 mg	InnoPran XL by Reliant	65726-0250	Antihypertensive
80MG <> BERLEX	Tab, White, Cap Shaped, Scored	Sotalol 80 mg	Betapace AF by Berlex	50419-0115	Antiarrhythmic

ID FRONT <> BACK	DESCRIPTION FRONT <> BACK	INGREDIENT & STRENGTH	BRAND (or Generic Equiv.) by FIRM	NDC#	CLASS; SCH.
80MG <> BETAPACE	Tab, Light Blue, Cap Shaped, Scored	Sotalol 80 mg	Betapace by Berlex	50419-0105	Antiarrhythmic
81	Tab, Yellow, Round, Enteric Coated	Aspirin 81 mg	Aspirin by Bayer	00280-2100	Analgesic
81	Tab, Pale Blue, Round, Enteric Coated	Aspirin 81 mg	Aspirin Low Dose by Bayer	Canadian DIN 02237726	Analgesic
810 <> S	Tab, Green, Round, Scored, Chewable	Isosorbide Dinitrate 5 mg	Isordil by Zeneca	00310-0810	Antianginal
8117 <> 93	Tab, White, Round, Film-Coated	Famciclovir 125 mg	Famvir by Teva	00093-8117	Famvir
8118 <> 93	Tab, White, Round, Film-Coated	Famciclovir 250 mg	Famvir by Teva	00093-8118	Antiviral
8119 <> 93	Tab, White, Cap Shaped, Film-Coated	Famciclovir 500 mg	Famvir by Teva	00093-8119	Antiviral
812	Cap, Blue & White	Butalbital 50 mg, Acetaminophen 325 mg, Caffeine 40 mg	Fiogesic by Marlop		Analgesic
814	Tab	Ibuprofen 400 mg	Motrin by Marlop		NSAID
815	Tab, Chewable	Isosorbide Dinitrate 10 mg	Isordil by Pharmedix	53002-1061	Antianginal
815 <> S	Tab, Chewable	Isosorbide Dinitrate 10 mg	Isordil by Zeneca	00310-0815	Antianginal
82	Tab, White, Round	Indapamide 2.5 mg	Lozol by RPR		Diuretic
82 <> W	Tab, White, Round	Primidone 50 mg	Mysoline by West-Ward	00143-1482	Anticonvulsant
82 <> W	Tab, White, Round	Primidone 50 mg	Mysoline by Blu	24658-0150	Anticonvulsant
820	Tab, Red, Oval, 820 <> Schering Logo	Dexchlorpheniramine Maleate 2 mg	Polaramine by Schering	00085-0820	Antihistamine
820 <> S	Tab, Blue, Oval, Scored	Isosorbide Dinitrate 20 mg	Isordil by Zeneca	00310-0820	Antianginal
820 <> S	Tab, Blue, Oval, Scored	Isosorbide Dinitrate 20 mg	Isordil by Nat Pharmpak	55154-4402	Antianginal
828	Tab, Yellow, Oval, Heart logo <> 828	Vitamin A 3000 IU, Calcium 200 mg, Vitamin D 400 IU, Copper 2 mg, Vitamin E 30 mg, Iron 29 mg, Vitamin C 120 mg, Magnesium 25 mg, Folic Acid 1 mg, Zinc 25 mg, Vitamin B1 1.8 mg, Vitamin B2 4 mg, Niacinamide 20 mg, Vitamin B6 25 mg, Vitamin B12 12 mcg	Duet by Xanodyne	64731-0828	Vitamin
83	Tab, Mottled Orange, Heart Shaped, Chewable, Heart logo <> 83	Vitamin A 3000 IU, Calcium 100 mg, Vitamin D 400 IU, Copper 2 mg, Vitamin E 30 mg, Iron 29 mg, Vitamin C 120 mg, Magnesium 25 mg, Folic Acid 1 mg, Zinc 25 mg, Vitamin B1 1.8 mg, Vitamin B2 4 mg, Niacinamide 20 mg, Vitamin B6 25 mg, Vitamin B12 12 mcg	Duet Chewable by Xanodyne	64731-0830	Vitamin
83 <> 93	Tab, White to Off-White, Round	Amlodipine Besylate 2.5 mg	Norvasc by Teva	00093-0083	Antihypertensive
83 <> BI	Tab, White, Round	Pramipexole DiHCl 0.125 mg	Mirapex by Boehringer Ingelheim	00597-0183	Antiparkinson
83 <> R	Tab, White to Off-White, Round, Extended Release	Alprazolam 0.5 mg	Xanax XR by Actavis	00228-3083	Antianxiety; C IV
830	Cap	Hydroxyurea 500 mg	Hydrea by BMS	17101-0830	Antineoplastic
831	Tab, White, Round, Ex Release, Andrx Logo 831	Metoprolol Succinate 50 mg	Toprolol XL by Andrx	62037-0831	Antihypertensive
8311 <> BARR	Tab, Pink, Oval, Scored	Warfarin Sodium 1 mg	Coumadin by Barr	00555-0831	Anticoagulant
8311 <> BARR	Tab, Pink, Oval, Scored	Warfarin Sodium 1 mg	Coumadin by UDL	51079-0908	Anticoagulant
831BM05	Tab	Benztropine Mesylate 0.5 mg	Cogentin by Rosemont	00832-1080	Antiparkinson
832 <> 10	Tab, Butterscotch Yellow, Sugar Coated	Chlorpromazine HCl 10 mg	Thorazine by Qualitest	00603-2808	Antipsychotic
832 <> 10	Tab, Butterscotch Yellow, Sugar Coated	Chlorpromazine HCl 10 mg	Thorazine by Schein	00364-0380	Antipsychotic
832 <> 100	Tab, Butterscotch Yellow, Sugar Coated	Chlorpromazine HCl 100 mg	Thorazine by Schein	00364-0383	Antipsychotic
832 <> 100	Tab, Butterscotch Yellow, Sugar Coated	Chlorpromazine HCl 100 mg	Thorazine by Qualitest	00603-2811	Antipsychotic
832 <> 100	Tab, Sugar Coated	Chlorpromazine HCl 100 mg	Thorazine by URL Mutual	00677-0456	Antipsychotic
832 <> 200	Tab, Coated	Chlorpromazine HCl 200 mg	Thorazine by URL Mutual	00677-0787	Antipsychotic
832 <> 200	Tab, Butterscotch Yellow, Sugar Coated	Chlorpromazine HCl 200 mg	Thorazine by Qualitest	00603-2812	Antipsychotic
832 <> 200	Tab, Butterscotch Yellow, Sugar Coated	Chlorpromazine HCl 200 mg	Thorazine by Schein	00364-0384	Antipsychotic
832 <> 25	Tab, Butterscotch Yellow, Sugar Coated	Chlorpromazine HCl 25 mg	Thorazine by Qualitest	00603-2809	Antipsychotic
832 <> 38	Tab, White, Round, Scored	Oxybutynin Chloride 5 mg	Ditropan by Rosemont	00832-0038	Urinary Tract
832 <> 38	Tab, White, Round, Scored	Oxybutynin Chloride 5 mg	Ditropan by Dixon Shane	17236-0850	Urinary Tract
832 <> 38	Tab, White, Round, Scored	Oxybutynin Chloride 5 mg	Ditropan by UDL	51079-0628	Urinary Tract
832 <> 50	Tab, Sugar Coated	Chlorpromazine HCl 50 mg	by URL Mutual	00677-0455	Antipsychotic
832 <> 50	Tab, Sugar Coated	Chlorpromazine HCl 50 mg	by Schein	00364-0382	Antipsychotic
832 <> 50	Tab, Butterscotch Yellow, Sugar Coated	Chlorpromazine HCl 50 mg	by Qualitest	00603-2810	Antipsychotic
832 <> 86	Tab, Light Green, Round, Scored	Fluoxymesterone 10 mg	Androxy by Upsher-Smith	00832-0086	Steroid; C III

ID FRONT <> BACK	DESCRIPTION FRONT <> BACK	INGREDIENT & STRENGTH	BRAND (or Generic Equiv.) by FIRM	NDC#	CLASS; SCH.
832 <> ALP10	Tab, White, Round	Amlodipine Besylate 10 mg	Norvasc by Upsher-Smith	00832-	Antihypertensive
832 <> ALP212	Tab, White, Round	Amlodipine Besylate 2.5 mg	Norvasc by Upsher-Smith	00832-	Antihypertensive
832 <> ALP5	Tab, White, Round	Amlodipine Besylate 5 mg	Norvasc by Upsher-Smith	00832-	Antihypertensive
832 <> AMT	Tab, Peach, Round	Amantadine HCl 100 mg	Symmetrel by Upsher Smith	00832-0111	Antiviral
832 <> BAC10	Tab, White, Round	Baclofen 10 mg	Lioresal by Qualitest	00603-2408	Muscle Relaxant
832 <> BCL10	Tab, White, Round, Scored, BCL / 10	Bethanechol Chloride 10 mg	Urecholine by Upsher-Smith	00832-0511	Urinary Tract
832 <> BCL25	Tab, Yellow, Round, Scored, BCL / 25	Bethanechol Chloride 25 mg	Urecholine by Upsher-Smith	00832-0512	Urinary Tract
832 <> BCL5	Tab, White, Round, Scored, BCL / 5	Bethanechol Chloride 5 mg	Urecholine by Upsher-Smith	00832-0510	Urinary Tract
832 <> BCL50	Tab, Yellow, Round, Scored, BCL / 50	Bethanechol Chloride 50 mg	Urecholine by Upsher-Smith	00832-0513	Urinary Tract
832 <> G359	Tab	Fluoxymesterone 10 mg	by Qualitest	00603-3645	Steroid; C III
832 <> G463	Tab, White, Round	Medroxyprogesterone Acetate 10 mg	by Qualitest	00603-4368	Hormone
832 <> WRF1	Tab, Pink, Round, Scored	Warfarin Sodium 1 mg	Jantoven by Upsher Smith	00832-1211	Anticoagulant
832 <> WRF10	Tab, White, Round, Scored	Warfarin Sodium 10 mg	Jantoven by Upsher Smith	00832-1219	Anticoagulant
832 <> WRF2	Tab, Lavender, Round, Scored	Warfarin Sodium 2 mg	Jantoven by Upsher Smith	00832-1212	Anticoagulant
832 <> WRF212	Tab, Green, Round, Scored, WRF 2 1/2 <> 832	Warfarin Sodium 2.5 mg	Jantoven by Upsher Smith	00832-1213	Anticoagulant
832 <> WRF3	Tab, Tan, Round, Scored	Warfarin Sodium 3 mg	Jantoven by Upsher Smith	00832-1214	Anticoagulant
832 <> WRF4	Tab, Blue, Round, Scored	Warfarin Sodium 4 mg	Jantoven by Upsher Smith	00832-1215	Anticoagulant
832 <> WRF5	Tab, Peach, Round, Scored	Warfarin Sodium 5 mg	Jantoven by Upsher Smith	00832-1216	Anticoagulant
832 <> WRF6	Tab, Teal, Round, Scored	Warfarin Sodium 6 mg	Jantoven by Upsher Smith	00832-1217	Anticoagulant
832 <> WRF712	Tab, Yellow, Round, Scored, WRF 7 1/2 <> 832	Warfarin Sodium 7.5 mg	Jantoven by Upsher Smith	00832-1218	Anticoagulant
8320420	Tab, Green, Round, 832-0420	Hydroflumethiazide 50 mg, Reserpine 0.125 mg	Salutensin by Rosemont		Diuretic; Antihypertensive
83205	Tab, Pink, Round, 832/05	Oxybutynin Chloride 5 mg	Ditropan by Rosemont		Urinary Tract
83210	Tab, Yellow, Round, Sugar Coated, 832 over 10	Chlorpromazine HCl 10 mg	Thorazine by UDL	51079-0518	Antipsychotic
83210	Tab, Yellow, Round, Sugar Coated, 832 over 10	Chlorpromazine HCl 10 mg	Thorazine by Rosemont	00832-0300	Antipsychotic
832100	Tab, Yellow, Round, Sugar Coated, 832 over 200	Chlorpromazine HCl 100 mg	Thorazine by Ivax	00182-0476	Antipsychotic
832100	Tab, Yellow, Round, Sugar Coated, 832 over 200	Chlorpromazine HCl 100 mg	Thorazine by UDL	51079-0516	Antipsychotic
832100	Tab, Yellow, Round, Sugar Coated, 832 over 200	Chlorpromazine HCl 100 mg	Thorazine by Rosemont	00832-0303	Antipsychotic
83210C	Tab, Blue, Round, 832/10C	Diazepam 10 mg	Valium by Rosemont		Antianxiety; C IV
8322	Tab, Lavender, Round, 832/2	Warfarin Sodium 2 mg	Coumadin by Rosemont		Anticoagulant
832200	Tab, Yellow, Round, Sugar Coated, 832 over 200	Chlorpromazine HCl 200 mg	Thorazine by Rosemont	00832-0304	Antipsychotic
832200	Tab, Yellow, Round, Sugar Coated, 832 over 200	Chlorpromazine HCl 200 mg	Thorazine by UDL	51079-0517	Antipsychotic
832200	Tab, Yellow, Round, Sugar Coated, 832 over 200	Chlorpromazine HCl 200 mg	Thorazine by Ivax	00182-0477	Antipsychotic
832212 <> BARR	Tab, Green, Oval, Scored, 832/2 1/2 <> barr	Warfarin Sodium 2.5 mg	Coumadin by Barr	00555-0832	Anticoagulant
83225	Tab, Orange, Round, 832/2.5	Warfarin Sodium 2.5 mg	Coumadin by Rosemont		Anticoagulant
83225	Tab, Butterscotch, Round, Sugar Coated, 832 over 25	Chlorpromazine HCl 25 mg	Thorazine by Rosemont	00832-0301	Antipsychotic
83225	Tab, Butterscotch, Round, Sugar Coated, 832 over 25	Chlorpromazine HCl 25 mg	Thorazine by UDL	51079-0519	Antipsychotic
83225	Tab, Butterscotch, Round, Sugar Coated, 832 over 25	Chlorpromazine HCl 25 mg	Thorazine by Ivax	00182-0474	Antipsychotic
83225	Cap, 832 over 25	Chlordiazepoxide 25 mg	Librium by Qualitest	00603-2668	Antianxiety; C IV
83225C	Tab, White, Round, 832/2C	Diazepam 2 mg	Valium by Rosemont		Antianxiety; C IV
8322L	Tab, Coated	Cimetidine HCl 200 mg	Tagamet by LEK	48866-0101	Gastrointestinal
8322L	Tab, White, Round, Coated	Cimetidine HCl 200 mg	Tagamet by Rosemont	00832-0101	Gastrointestinal
83238	Tab, Debossed	Oxybutynin Chloride 5 mg	by Major	00904-5223	Urinary Tract
8323L	Tab, Coated	Cimetidine HCl 300 mg	Tagamet by LEK	48866-0102	Gastrointestinal
8323L	Tab, White, Round, Coated	Cimetidine HCl 300 mg	Tagamet by Rosemont	00832-0102	Gastrointestinal
8325	Cap, Green & Yellow, 832/5	Chlordiazepoxide 5 mg	Librium by Rosemont		Antianxiety; C IV
8325	Tab, Pink, Round, 832/5	Warfarin Sodium 5 mg	Coumadin by Rosemont		Anticoagulant
83250	Tab, Butterscotch, Round, Sugar Coated, 832 over 50	Chlorpromazine HCl 50 mg	Thorazine by Ivax	00182-0475	Antipsychotic
83250	Tab, Butterscotch, Round, Sugar Coated, 832 over 50	Chlorpromazine HCl 50 mg	Thorazine by Rosemont	00832-0302	Antipsychotic
83250	Tab, Butterscotch, Round, Sugar Coated, 832 over 50	Chlorpromazine HCl 50 mg	Thorazine by UDL	51079-0130	Antipsychotic

ID FRONT <> BACK	DESCRIPTION FRONT <> BACK	INGREDIENT & STRENGTH	BRAND (or Generic Equiv.) by FIRM	NDC#	CLASS; SCH.
8325C	Tab, Yellow, Round, 832/5C	Diazepam 5 mg	Valium by Rosemont		Antianxiety; C IV
8326113	Tab, White, Round, 832/6113	Carbamazepine 200 mg	Tegretol by Rosemont		Anticonvulsant
8328375C	Tab, Yellow, Round, 832/8375C	Phentermine 37.5 mg	Adipex-P by Rosemont		Anorexiant; C IV
83286	Tab	Fluoxymesterone 10 mg	by URL Mutual	00677-0934	Steroid; C III
8328L	Tab	Cimetidine HCl 800 mg	Tagamet by URL Mutual	00677-1530	Gastrointestinal
8328L	Tab, Coated	Cimetidine HCl 800 mg	Tagamet by LEK	48866-0104	Gastrointestinal
8328L	Tab, Coated, 832 8L	Cimetidine HCl 800 mg	Tagamet by Schein	00364-2594	Gastrointestinal
8328L	Tab, Coated, 832/8L	Cimetidine HCl 800 mg	Tagamet by Rosemont	00832-0104	Gastrointestinal
8328L	Tab, Coated	Cimetidine HCl 800 mg	Tagamet by Apotheca	12634-0497	Gastrointestinal
8328L	Tab	Cimetidine HCl 800 mg	Tagamet by Dixon Shane	17236-0172	Gastrointestinal
832A5	Tab, White, Oval, Scored	Amiloride HCl 5 mg	Midamor by Rosemont		Diuretic
832BAC10	Tab	Baclofen 10 mg	Lioresal by Rosemont	00832-1024	Muscle Relaxant
832BAC10	Tab, 832/BAC10	Baclofen 10 mg	Lioresal by URL Mutual	00677-1259	Muscle Relaxant
832BC20	Tab, White, Round, Scored, 832 BC20	Baclofen 20 mg	Lioresal by Rosemont	00832-1025	Muscle Relaxant
832BC20	Tab, White, Round, Scored, 832 BC20	Baclofen 20 mg	Lioresal by URL Mutual	00677-1260	Muscle Relaxant
832BC20	Tab, White, Round, Scored, 832 BC20	Baclofen 20 mg	Lioresal by Qualitest	00603-2409	Muscle Relaxant
832BC20	Tab, White, Round, Scored, 832 over BM05	Baclofen 20 mg	Lioresal by Boca	64376-0501	Muscle Relaxant
832BM05	Tab, White, Round, Scored, 832 over BM05	Benztropine Mesylate 0.5 mg	Cogentin by UDL	51079-0220	Antiparkinson
832BM1	Tab, White, Oval, Scored	Benztropine Mesylate 1 mg	Cogentin by UDL	51079-0221	Antiparkinson
832BM1	Tab, White, Oval, Scored	Benztropine Mesylate 1 mg	Cogentin by Rosemont	00832-1081	Antiparkinson
832BM1	Tab, White, Oval, Scored	Benztropine Mesylate 1 mg	Cogentin by Dixon Shane	17236-0847	Antiparkinson
832BM2	Tab, White, Round, Scored	Benztropine Mesylate 2 mg	Cogentin by Bryant	63629-0351	Antiparkinson
832BM2	Tab, White, Round, Scored	Benztropine Mesylate 2 mg	Cogentin by UDL	51079-0222	Antiparkinson
832BM2	Tab, White, Round, Scored	Benztropine Mesylate 2 mg	Cogentin by Dixon Shane	17236-0848	Antiparkinson
832BM2	Tab, White, Round, Scored	Benztropine Mesylate 2 mg	Cogentin by Rosemont	00832-1082	Antiparkinson
832C5C	Cap, Blue & Green, 832/C5C	Chlordiazepoxide 5 mg, Clidinium Bromide 2.5 mg	Librax by Rosemont		Gastrointestinal
832D25	Tab, White, Round, 832/D25	Dipyridamole 25 mg	Persantine by Rosemont		Antiplatelet
832D50	Tab, White, Round, 832/D50	Dipyridamole 50 mg	Persantine by Rosemont		Antiplatelet
832D75	Tab, White, Round, 832/D75	Dipyridamole 75 mg	Persantine by Rosemont		Antiplatelet
832FC500	Tab, Peach, Oblong, 832/FC500	Fenoprofen Calcium 600 mg	Nalfon by Rosemont		NSAID
832G133	Tab, White, Round, 832/G133	Carbamazepine 200 mg	Tegretol by Rosemont		Anticonvulsant
832G197	Tab, Blue, Round	Chlorpropamide 250 mg	Diabinese by Rosemont		Antidiabetic
832G198	Tab, Blue, Round, 832/G198	Chlorpropamide 100 mg	Diabinese by Rosemont		Antidiabetic
832G203	Tab, Orange, Round, 832/G203	Chlorthalidone 25 mg	Hygroton by Rosemont		Diuretic
832G204	Tab, Blue, Round, 832/G204	Chlorthalidone 50 mg	Hygroton by Rosemont		Diuretic
832G220C	Cap, White, 832/G220C	Clorazepate Dipotassium 30.75 mg	Tranxene by Rosemont		Antianxiety; C IV
832G221C	Cap, White, 832/G221C	Clorazepate Dipotassium 7.5 mg	Tranxene by Rosemont		Antianxiety; C IV
832G222C	Cap, White, 832/G222C	Clorazepate Dipotassium 15 mg	Tranxene by Rosemont		Antianxiety; C IV
832G254	Tab, Lavender, Round, 832/G254	Desipramine HCl 25 mg	Norpramin by Rosemont		Antidepressant
832G255	Tab, Blue, Round, 832/G255	Desipramine HCl 50 mg	Norpramin by Rosemont		Antidepressant
832G256	Tab, White, Round, 832/G256	Desipramine HCl 75 mg	Norpramin by Rosemont		Antidepressant
832G257	Tab, Butterscotch Yellow, Round, 832/G257	Desipramine HCl 100 mg	Norpramin by Rosemont		Antidepressant
832G31	Tab, White, Oblong, 832/G31	Acetohexamide 250 mg	Dymelor by Rosemont		Antidiabetic
832G32	Tab, White, Oblong, 832/G32	Acetohexamide 500 mg	Dymelor by Rosemont		Antidiabetic

ID FRONT <> BACK	DESCRIPTION FRONT <> BACK	INGREDIENT & STRENGTH	BRAND (or Generic Equiv.) by FIRM	NDC#	CLASS; SCH.
832G359	Tab, 832/G359 Rosemont	Fluoxymesterone 10 mg	by Rugby	00536-3826	Steroid; C III
832G366C	Cap, Blue & White, 832/G366C	Flurazepam HCl 15 mg	Dalmane by Rosemont		Hypnotic; C IV
832G367C	Cap, Blue, 832/G367C	Flurazepam HCl 30 mg	Dalmane by Rosemont		Hypnotic; C IV
832G368	Tab	Folic Acid 1 mg	Folic Acid by Rosemont		Vitamin
832G420	Tab, Green, Round, 832/G420	Hydroflumethiazide 50 mg, Reserpine 0.125 mg	Serpasil by Rosemont		Diuretic; Antihypertensive
832G423	Tab, Purple, Round, 832/G423	Hydroxyzine HCl 10 mg	Atarax by Rosemont		Antianxiety; Antihistamine
832G424	Tab, Purple, Round, 832/G424	Hydroxyzine HCl 25 mg	Atarax by Rosemont		Antianxiety; Antihistamine
832G425	Tab, Lavender, Round, 832/G425	Hydroxyzine HCl 50 mg	Atarax by Rosemont		Antianxiety; Antihistamine
832G463	Tab, 832/G463	Medroxyprogesterone Acetate 10 mg	by URL Mutual	00677-0803	Hormone
832G463	Tab, Coated, 832/G463	Medroxyprogesterone Acetate 10 mg	by Major	00904-2690	Hormone
832G463	Tab, White, Round, 832 over G463	Medroxyprogesterone Acetate 10 mg	Provera by Martec	52555-0463	Hormone
832G506	Tab, Brown, Round, 832/G506	Nystatin 500,000 Units	Mycostatin by Rosemont		Antifungal
832G528C	Tab, Green, Round, 832/G528C	Phendimetrazine HCl 35 mg	Melfiat by Rosemont		Anorexiant; C III
832G528C	Tab, Orange, Round, 832/G528C	Phendimetrazine HCl 35 mg	Melfiat by Rosemont		Anorexiant; C III
832G528C	Tab, Yellow, Round, 832/G528C	Phendimetrazine HCl 35 mg	Melfiat by Rosemont		Anorexiant; C III
832G531C	Tab, White, Round, 832 / G531C	Phenobarbital 15 mg	Phenobarbital by Rosemont		Sedative/Hypnotic; C IV
832G532C	Tab, White, Round, 832 / G532C	Phenobarbital 30 mg	Phenobarbital by Rosemont		Sedative/Hypnotic; C IV
832G533C	Tab, White, Round, 832/G533C	Phenobarbital 60 mg	by Rosemont		Sedative/Hypnotic; C IV
832G536C	Cap, Yellow, 832/G536C	Phentermine 30 mg	Ionamin by Forest		Anorexiant; C IV
832G536C	Cap, Blue & Clear, 832/G536C	Phentermine 30 mg	Fastin by Rosemont		Anorexiant; C IV
832G536C	Cap, Black, 832/G536C	Phentermine 30 mg	Fastin by Forest		Anorexiant; C IV
832G55C	Tab, White, Round, 832/G55C	Amitriptyline 12.5 mg, Chlordiazepoxide 5 mg	Limbitrol by Rosemont		Antianxiety; C IV
832G56C	Tab, Green, Round, 832/G56C	Amitriptyline 25 mg, Chlordiazepoxide 10 mg	Limbitrol by Rosemont		Antianxiety; C IV
832G602	Tab, White, Oblong, 832/G602	Sulfamethoxazole 400 mg, Trimethoprim 80 mg	Bactrim by Rosemont		Antibiotic
832G603	Tab, White, Oblong, 832/G603	Sulfamethoxazole 800 mg, Trimethoprim 160 mg	Bactrim by Rosemont		Antibiotic
832G613	Tab, Tan, Round, 832/G613	Thyroid Hormone 30 mg	Thyroid by Rosemont		Thyroid Hormone
832G614	Tab, Tan, Round, 832/G614	Thyroid 60 mg	Thyroid by Rosemont		Thyroid Hormone
832G615	Tab, Tan, Round, 832/G615	Thyroid 120 mg	Thyroid by Rosemont		Thyroid Hormone
832G616	Tab, Tan, Round, 832/G616	Thyroid 180 mg	Thyroid by Rosemont		Thyroid Hormone
832G618	Tab, White, Round, 832/G618	Tolazamide 100 mg	Tolinase by Rosemont		Antidiabetic
832G621	Tab, White, Round, 832/G621	Tolazamide 500 mg	Tolinase by Rosemont		Antidiabetic
832G622	Tab, White, Round, 832/G622	Tolazamide 250 mg	Tolinase by Rosemont		Antidiabetic
832GC100	Tab, White, Round, 832/GC100	Chlorthalidone 100 mg	Hygroton by Rosemont		Diuretic
832L01	Tab, Yellow, Round	Levothyroxine Sodium 0.1 mg	Synthroid by Rosemont		Thyroid Hormone
832L02	Tab, White, Round	Levothyroxine Sodium 0.2 mg	Synthroid by Rosemont		Thyroid Hormone
832L03	Tab, Green, Round	Levothyroxine Sodium 0.3 mg	Synthroid by Rosemont		Thyroid Hormone
832L15	Tab, Blue, Round	Levothyroxine Sodium 0.15 mg	Synthroid by Rosemont		Thyroid Hormone
832L300	Cap, White, 832/L-300	Lithium Carbonate 300 mg	Eskalith by Rosemont		Antipsychotic
832LR1C	Tab, White, Round, 832/LR1C	Lorazepam 1 mg	Ativan by Rosemont		Antianxiety; C IV
832LR2C	Tab, White, Round, 832/LR2C	Lorazepam 2 mg	Ativan by Rosemont		Antianxiety; C IV
832M400	Tab, Yellow, Round, 832/M400	Tridihexethyl Chloride 25 mg, Meprobamate 400 mg	Pathibamate by Rosemont		Antispasmodic; C IV

ID FRONT <> BACK	DESCRIPTION FRONT <> BACK	INGREDIENT & STRENGTH	BRAND (or Generic Equiv.) by FIRM	NDC#	CLASS; SCH.
832M5	Tab, Orange, Round	Methyclothiazide 5 mg	Enduron by Rosemont		Diuretic; Antihypertensive
832M510	Tab, White, Round, 832/M 510	Metaproterenol Sulfate 10 mg	Alupent by Rosemont		Antiasthmatic
832M520	Tab, White, Round, 832/M 520	Metaproterenol Sulfate 20 mg	Alupent by Rosemont		Antiasthmatic
832MC100	Cap, Maroon & White, 832/MC100	Meclofenamate Sodium 100 mg	Meclomen by Rosemont		NSAID
832MC50	Cap, Maroon & Pink, 832/MC50	Meclofenamate Sodium 50 mg	Meclomen by Rosemont		NSAID
832MS	Tab, Rosemont	Methyclothiazide 5 mg	by Pharmedix	53002-1044	Diuretic; Antihypertensive
832MS10	Tab, White, Round, 832/MS10	Metaproterenol Sulfate 10 mg	Alupent by Rosemont		Antiasthmatic
832MS20	Tab, White, Round, 832/MS20	Metaproterenol Sulfate 20 mg	Alupent by Rosemont		Antiasthmatic
832P10C	Cap, Green & White, 832/P10C	Prazepam 10 mg	Centrax by Rosemont		Sedative/Hypnotic; C IV
832P19C	Tab, White, Oblong, 832/P19C	Acetaminophen 500 mg, Hydrocodone Bitartrate 5 mg	Vicodin by Rosemont		Analgesic; C III
832P375C	Tab, Blue & White, Round, 832/P37.5C	Phentermine 37.5 mg	Adipex-P by Rosemont		Anorexiant; C IV
832P375C	Tab, Yellow, Round, 832/P37.5C	Phentermine HCl 37.5 mg	by Rosemont		Anorexiant; C IV
832P5C	Cap, Green & White, 832/P5C	Prazepam 5 mg	Centrax by Rosemont		Sedative/Hypnotic; C IV
832PPPC	Tab, White, Round, with Red Mottles, 832/PPPC	Phenylpropanolamine HCl 40 mg, Phenylephrine HCl 10 mg, Phentoloxamine 15 mg, Chlorpheniramine 5 mg	Nalspan SR by Rosemont		Cold Remedy
832S500	Tab, Blue, Round	Salsalate 500 mg	Disalcid by Rosemont		NSAID
832S500	Tab, Yellow, Round	Salsalate 500 mg	Disalcid by Rosemont		NSAID
832S750	Tab, Yellow, Oblong	Salsalate 750 mg	Disalcid by Rosemont		NSAID
832S750	Tab, Blue, Oblong	Salsalate 750 mg	Disalcid by Rosemont		NSAID
832T10	Cap, Green & White, 832/T10	Timolol Maleate 10 mg	Blocadren by Rosemont		Antihypertensive
832T20	Cap, Green & White, 832/T20	Timolol Maleate 20 mg	Blocadren by Rosemont		Antihypertensive
832T5	Cap, Green & White, 832/T5	Timolol Maleate 5 mg	Blocadren by Rosemont		Antihypertensive
832TEM15	Cap, Green & White, 832/Tem15	Temazepam 15 mg	Restoril by Rosemont		Sedative/Hypnotic; C IV
832TEM30	Cap, White, 832/Tem30	Temazepam 30 mg	Restoril by Rosemont		Sedative/Hypnotic; C IV
832TM100	Cap, Brown & Green, 832/TM100	Trimipramine Maleate 100 mg	Surmontil by Rosemont		Antidepressant
832TM25	Cap, Orange & Purple, 832/TM25	Trimipramine Maleate 25 mg	Surmontil by Rosemont		Antidepressant
832TM50	Cap, Pink & White, 832/TM50	Trimipramine Maleate 50 mg	Surmontil by Rosemont		Antidepressant
832X25	Tab, White, Round, 832/X25	Minoxidil 2.5 mg	Loniten by Rosemont		Antihypertensive
833	Tab, White, Oblong, Film Coated, Compumed Logo 833	Choline Magnesium Trisalicylate 750 mg	by Compumed	00403-0694	NSAID
8335 <> BARR	Tab, Peach, Oval, Scored	Warfarin Sodium 5 mg	Coumadin by UCB	50474-0935	Anticoagulant
8335 <> BARR	Tab, Peach, Oval, Scored	Warfarin Sodium 5 mg	Coumadin by UDL	51079-0913	Anticoagulant
8335 <> BARR	Tab, Peach, Oval, Scored	Warfarin Sodium 5 mg	Coumadin by Barr	00555-0833	Anticoagulant
834712 <> BARR	Tab, Yellow, Oval, Scored, 834/7 1/2 <> barr	Warfarin Sodium 7.5 mg	Coumadin by Barr	00555-0834	Anticoagulant
834712 <> BARR	Tab, Yellow, Oval, Scored, 834/7 1/2 <> barr	Warfarin Sodium 7.5 mg	Coumadin by UDL	51079-0915	Anticoagulant
83510 <> BARR	Tab, White, Oval, Scored	Warfarin Sodium 10 mg	Coumadin by Barr	00555-0835	Anticoagulant
83510 <> BARR	Tab, White, Oval, Scored	Warfarin Sodium 10 mg	Coumadin by UDL	51079-0916	Anticoagulant
835375 <> WATSON	Tab, Blue, Triangular, Scored	Clorazepate Dipotassium 3.75 mg	by Watson	52544-0835	Antianxiety; C IV
83675 <> WATSON	Tab, Peach, Triangular, Scored, WATSON written down middle <> 836 / 7.5	Clorazepate Dipotassium 7.5 mg	Tranxene by Watson	52544-0836	Antianxiety; C IV
83715 <> WATSON	Tab, Purple, Triangular, Scored	Clorazepate Dipotassium 15 mg	by Watson	52544-0837	Antianxiety; C IV
84 <> R	Tab, Yellow, Round, Extended Release	Alprazolam 1 mg	Xanax XR by Actavis	00228-3084	Antianxiety; C IV
84 <> WW	Tab, White, Round	Primidone 250 mg	Mysoline by Blu	24658-0151	Anticonvulsant
843	Tab, White, Round, Scherring Logo 843	Prednisone 1 mg	Meticorten by Schering		Steroid

ID FRONT <> BACK	DESCRIPTION FRONT <> BACK	INGREDIENT & STRENGTH	BRAND (or Generic Equiv.) by FIRM	NDC#	CLASS; SCH.
847 <> WATSON	Tab, White, Round	Norgestrel 0.3 mg, Ethinyl Estradiol 0.03 mg	Lo-Ogestrel by Watson	52544-0847	Oral Contraceptive
848 <> WATSON	Tab, White, Round	Norgestrel 0.5 mg, Ethinyl Estradiol 0.05 mg	Ogestrel by Watson	52544-0848	Oral Contraceptive
8484 <> BIBI	Tab, White, Oval, Scored	Pramipexole DiHCl 0.25 mg	Mirapex by Boehringer Ingelheim	00597-0184	Antiparkinson
85 <> E	Tab, White to Off-White, Cap Shaped, Film Coated, Scored	Penicillin V Potassium 500 mg	by Aurobindo	65862-0176	Antibiotic
85 <> WYETH	Tab, Coated	Acetaminophen 650 mg, Propoxyphene HCl 65 mg	Wygesic by Wyeth	00008-0085	Analgesic; C IV
850	Tab, White to Off-White, Cap-Shaped, Cobalt Logo <> 850	Metformin HCl 850 mg	Glucophage by Cobalt	Canadian DIN 02257734	Antidiabetic
850 <> 4330	Tab, White, Oval, Hourglass Logo 4330	Metformin HCl 850 mg	Glucophage by Ivax	00172-4330 Discontinued	Antidiabetic
850 <> ANDRX675	Tab, White, Round, Film Coated	Metformin HCl 850 mg	Glucophage by Andrx	62037-0675	Antidiabetic
850 <> APO	Tab, White, Oblong	Metformin HCl 850 mg	Glucophage by Apotex	Canadian DIN 02229785	Antidiabetic
850 <> B386	Tab, White to Off-White, Oval, Film Coated	Metformin HCl 850 mg	Glucophage by Barr	00555-0386	Antidiabetic
850 <> BMS6070	Tab, White to Off-White, Round, Film Coated	Metformin HCl 850 mg	Glucophage by Va Cmop	65243-0047	Antidiabetic
850 <> BMS6070	Tab, White to Off-White, Round, Film Coated	Metformin HCl 850 mg	Glucophage by Nat Pharmpak	55154-5825	Antidiabetic
850 <> BMS6070	Tab, White to Off-White, Round, Film Coated	Metformin HCl 850 mg	Glucophage by BMS	12783-0070	Antidiabetic
850 <> BMS6070	Tab, White to Off-White, Round, Film Coated	Metformin HCl 850 mg	Glucophage by Kaiser	00179-1378	Antidiabetic
850 <> BMS6070	Tab, White to Off-White, Round, Film Coated	Metformin HCl 850 mg	Glucophage by Direct Dispensing	57866-9058	Antidiabetic
850 <> BMS6070	Tab, White to Off-White, Round, Film Coated	Metformin HCl 850 mg	Glucophage by Caremark	00339-6085	Antidiabetic
850 <> BMS6070	Tab, White to Off-White, Round, Film Coated	Metformin HCl 850 mg	Glucophage by BMS	00087-6070	Antidiabetic
850 <> G45	Tab, White, Round	Metformin 850 mg	Glucophage by Glenmark	68462-0160	Antihyperglycemic
850 <> IP176	Tab, White to Off White, Round	Metformin HCl 850 mg	Glucophage by Amneal	65162-0174	Antihyperglycemic
850 <> MJ	Tab, Green, Cap Shaped	Inert	Ovcon 50 28 by Physician Total Care	54868-3772	Oral Contraceptive; Placebo
850 <> MJ	Tab, Green, Cap Shaped	Inert	Ovcon 50 28 by BMS	00087-0579	Oral Contraceptive; Placebo
850 <> MJ	Tab, Green, Cap Shaped	Inert	Ovcon 50 28 by Warner Chilcott	00430-0585	Oral Contraceptive; Placebo
850 <> N	Tab, White, Oval	Metformin HCl 850 mg	Glucophage by Novopharm	Canadian DIN 02230475	Antidiabetic
850 <> NU	Tab, White, Cap Shaped	Metformin HCl 850 mg	by Nu Pharm	Canadian DIN 02229517	Antidiabetic
850 <> P	Tab, White, Cap Shaped, Film Coated	Metformin HCl 850 mg	Glucophage by Pharmascience	Canadian DIN 02242589	Antidiabetic
850 <> PAR	Tab, Off-White to Yellow, Round	Meloxicam 7.5 mg	Mobic by Par	49884-0850	NSAID
8505 <> M	Tab, White, Round, Scored	Flecainide Acetate 50 mg	Tambocor by Mylan	00378-8505	Antiarrhythmic
8505 <> M	Tab, White, Round	Flecainide Acetate 50 mg	Tambocor by UDL	51079-0987 Discontinued	Antiarrhythmic
851 <> 93	Tab, White, Round	Metronidazole 250 mg	Flagyl by Neuman	64579-0181	Antibiotic
851 <> 93	Tab, White, Round	Metronidazole 250 mg	Flagyl by UDL	51079-0122	Antibiotic
851 <> 93	Tab, White, Round	Metronidazole 250 mg	Flagyl by Teva	00093-0851 Discontinued	Antibiotic
851 <> 93	Tab, White, Round	Metronidazole 250 mg	Flagyl by MS State Health	50596-0027	Antibiotic
851 <> 93	Tab, White, Round	Metronidazole 250 mg	Flagyl by Golden State	60429-0128	Antibiotic
851 <> 93	Tab, White, Round	Metronidazole 250 mg	Flagyl by Pharmedix	53002-0221	Antibiotic
851 <> 93	Tab, White, Round	Metronidazole 250 mg	Flagyl by Nat Pharmpak	55154-5509	Antibiotic
851 <> PAR	Tab, Off-White to Yellow, Oval	Meloxicam 15 mg	Mobic by Par	49884-0851	NSAID
8510 <> M	Tab, White, Round, Scored	Flecainide Acetate 100 mg	Tambocor by UDL	51079-0988 Discontinued	Antiarrhythmic
8510 <> M	Tab, White, Round, Scored	Flecainide Acetate 100 mg	Tambocor by Mylan	000378-8510	Antiarrhythmic
8515 <> M	Tab, White, Oval, Scored	Flecainide Acetate 150 mg	Tambocor by Mylan	00378-8515	Antiarrhythmic

ID FRONT <> BACK	DESCRIPTION FRONT <> BACK	INGREDIENT & STRENGTH	BRAND (or Generic Equiv.) by FIRM	NDC#	CLASS; SCH.
852 <> 9393	Tab, White, Oblong, Scored	Metronidazole 500 mg	Flagyl by Pharmedix	53002-0247	Antibiotic
852 <> 9393	Tab, White, Oblong, Scored	Metronidazole 500 mg	Flagyl by Family Health	65149-0126	Antibiotic
852 <> 9393	Tab, White, Oblong, Scored	Metronidazole 500 mg	Flagyl by UDL	51079-0126	Antibiotic
852 <> 9393	Tab, White, Oblong, Scored	Metronidazole 500 mg	Flagyl by Nat Pharmpak	55154-5566	Antibiotic
852 <> 9393	Tab, White, Oblong, Scored	Metronidazole 500 mg	Flagyl by Teva	00093-0852 Discontinued	Antibiotic
852 <> 9393	Tab, White, Oblong, Scored	Metronidazole 500 mg	Flagyl by Prepackage Specialists	58864-0355	Antibiotic
852 <> 9393	Tab, White, Oblong, Scored	Metronidazole 500 mg	Flagyl by Neuman	64579-0107	Antibiotic
852 <> 9393	Tab, White, Oblong, Scored	Metronidazole 500 mg	Flagyl by Golden State	60429-0129	Antibiotic
8522 <> 93	Tab, Light Gray, D Shaped	Naratriptan 1 mg	Amerge by Teva Pharmaceuticals	00093-8522	Antimigraine
8523 <> 93	Tab, Green, D Shaped	Naratriptan 2.5 mg	Amerge by Teva Pharmaceuticals	00093-8523	Antimigraine
853 <> S	Tab	Isosorbide Dinitrate 2.5 mg	Isordil by Zeneca	00310-0853	Antianginal
857 <> DP	Tab, White, Cap Shaped, Scored	Guaifenesin 1200 mg	Robitussin by Duramed	51285-0857	Expectorant
858	Tab, Yellow, Oval, Heart logo <> 858	Vitamin A 3000 IU, Vitamin C 120 mg, Vitamin D 400 IU, Vitamin E 3 mg, Vitamin B1 1.8 mg, Vitamin B2 4 mg, Niacinamide 20 mg, Vitamin B6 25 mg, Folic Acid 1 mg, Vitamin B12 12 mcg, Calcium 200 mg, Iron 29 mg, Magnesium 25 mg, Zinc 25 mg, Copper 2 mg	DuetDHA by Xanodyne	66479-0861	Prenatal Vitamin
8585 <> BIBI	Tab, White, Oval, Scored	Pramipexole DiHCl 0.5 mg	Mirapex by Boehringer Ingelheim	00597-0185	Antiparkinson
859 <> B	Tab, White to Off-White, Round	Flecainide Acetate 50 mg	Tambocor by Barr	00555-0859	Antiarrhythmic
85WMH	Tab, Red, Round, 85-WMH	Dexbrompheniramine Maleate 6 mg, Pseudoephedrine Sulfate 120 mg	Disophrol by Schering		Cold Remedy
86 <> 832	Tab, Light Green, Round, Scored	Fluoxymesterone 10 mg	Androxy by Upsher-Smith	00832-0086	Steroid; C III
86 <> C	Tab, Pink, Round, Film Coated, Scored	Bisoprolol Fumarate 5 mg	Zebeta by Aurobindo	65862-0086	Antihypertensive
86 <> R	Tab, Light Green, Round, Extended Release	Alprazolam 3 mg	Xanax XR by Actavis	00228-3086	Antianxiety; C IV
860100 <> B	Tab, White to Off-White, Oval, Scored, 860 over 100	Flecainide Acetate 100 mg	Tambocor by Barr	00555-0860	Antiarrhythmic
860EL	Cap	Guaifenesin 250 mg, Pseudoephedrine HCl 120 mg	Sudafed Sinus by Econolab	55053-0860	Cold Remedy
860EL	Cap	Guaifenesin 250 mg, Pseudoephedrine HCl 120 mg	Sudafed Sinus by URL Mutual	00677-1503	Cold Remedy
861150 <> B	Tab, White to Off-White, Oval, Scored	Flecainide Acetate 150 mg	Tambocor by Barr	00555-0861	Antiarrhythmic
8632C	Tab, White, Oval	Theophylline Anhydrous 200 mg	Theo-X by Carnrick	00086-0032	Antiasthmatic
8633UNIMED	Tab, White	Oxymetholone 50 mg	Anadrol-50 by Unimed	00051-8633	Steroid; C III
8633UNIMED	Tab	Oxymetholone 50 mg	Anadrol-50 by Oread	63015-0007	Steroid; C III
8648 <> C	Tab, Layered	Phendimetrazine Tartrate 35 mg	Bontril PDM by Carnrick	00086-0048	Anorexiant; C III
8650 <> C	Tab, Purple, Oblong, Scored	Acetaminophen 325 mg, Butalbital 50 mg	by Thrift Drug	59198-0364	Analgesic
8650 <> C	Tab, Purple, Scored	Acetaminophen 325 mg, Butalbital 50 mg	Promacet by Carnrick	00086-0050	Analgesic
8651	Tab, White, Oval	Phenylpropanolamine 25 mg	Propagest by Carnrick		Decongestant; Appetite Suppressant
8656C	Cap	Acetaminophen 650 mg, Acetaminophen 650 mg	Phrenilin Forte by Carnrick	00086-0056	Analgesic
8656C	Cap, Purple	Butalbital 50 mg, Acetaminophen 650 mg	Promacet by Thrift Drug	59198-0365	Analgesic
8657C	Cap	Acetaminophen 500 mg, Hydrocodone Bitartrate 5 mg	Vicodin by Carnrick	00086-0057	Analgesic; C III
866	Tab, White with Blue, Round, Schering Logo 866	Dexbrompheniramine Maleate 2 mg, Pseudoephedrine Sulfate 60 mg	Disophrol by Schering		Cold Remedy
866	Cap, Red	Docusate Calcium 240 mg	Surfak by RP Scherer		Laxative
866	Tab, White, Round	Phenolphthalein 65 mg, Docusate Sodium 100 mg	by Perrigo		Gastrointestinal
8662 <> C	Tab, Lavender, Round, Scored, 86 over 62	Metaxalone 400 mg	Skelaxin by West-Ward	00143-9029	Muscle Relaxant
8662 <> C	Tab, Lavender, Round, Scored, 86 over 62	Metaxalone 400 mg	Skelaxin by King	60793-0135	Muscle Relaxant
8662 <> C	Tab, Lavender, Round, Scored, 86 over 62	Metaxalone 400 mg	Skelaxin by Thrift Drug	59198-0367	Muscle Relaxant
8662 <> C	Tab, Lavender, Round, Scored, 86 over 62	Metaxalone 400 mg	Skelaxin by H J Harkins Co	52959-0410	Muscle Relaxant
8662 <> C	Tab, Lavender, Round, Scored, 86 over 62	Metaxalone 400 mg	Skelaxin by Rx Pak	65084-0167	Muscle Relaxant
8662 <> C	Tab, Lavender, Round, Scored, 86 over 62	Metaxalone 400 mg	Skelaxin by Carnrick	00086-0062	Muscle Relaxant
8662 <> C	Tab, Lavender, Round, Scored, 86 over 62	Metaxalone 400 mg	Skelaxin by Drug Distr	52985-0226	Muscle Relaxant
8662 <> C	Tab, Lavender, Round, Scored, 86 over 62	Metaxalone 400 mg	Skelaxin by CVS	51316-0231	Muscle Relaxant

ID FRONT <> BACK	DESCRIPTION FRONT <> BACK	INGREDIENT & STRENGTH	BRAND (or Generic Equiv.) by FIRM	NDC#	CLASS; SCH.
8662 <> C	Tab, Lavender, Round, Scored, 86 over 62	Metaxalone 400 mg	Skelaxin by Amerisource	62584-0033	Muscle Relaxant
8662 <> C	Tab, Lavender, Round, Scored, 86 over 62	Metaxalone 400 mg	Skelaxin by Direct Dispensing	57866-4637	Muscle Relaxant
8667 <> S	Tab, Pink, Oblong, Scored	Metaxalone 800 mg	Skelaxin by King	60793-0136	Muscle Relaxant
8667 <> S	Tab, Pink, Oblong, Scored	Metaxalone 800 mg	Skelaxin by Elan	59075-0068	Muscle Relaxant
8673 <> C	Tab, White, Oval, Scored	Phenylpropanolamine HCl 75 mg, Guaifenesin 400 mg	by Eckerd	19458-0832	Cold Remedy
8673 <> C	Tab, White with Blue Specks	Guaifenesin 400 mg, Phenylpropanolamine HCl 75 mg	Entex LA by Carnrick	00086-0063	Cold Remedy
8674 <> C	Tab, White, Pentagonal, Scored	Difenoxin HCl 1 mg, Atropine Sulfate 0.025 mg	Motofen by Carnrick	00086-0074	Antidiarrheal; C IV
8674 <> C	Tab, White, Pentagonal, Scored	Difenoxin HCl 1 mg, Atropine Sulfate 0.025 mg	Motofen by DRX	55045-2771	Antidiarrheal; C IV
8674 <> C	Tab, White, Pentagonal, Scored	Atropine Sulfate 0.025 mg, Difenoxin HCl 1 mg	Motofen by Physician Total Care	54868-3510	Antidiarrheal; C IV
8692 <> BARR	Tab, Purple, Oval, Scored	Warfarin Sodium 2 mg	Coumadin by Barr	00555-0869	Anticoagulant
8692 <> BARR	Tab, Purple, Oval, Scored	Warfarin Sodium 2 mg	Coumadin by UCB		Anticoagulant
8692 <> BARR	Tab, Purple, Oval, Scored	Warfarin Sodium 2 mg	Coumadin by UDL	51079-0909	Anticoagulant
87 <> C	Tab, White, Round, Film Coated	Bisoprolol Fumarate 10 mg	Zebeta by Aurobindo	65862-0087	Antihypertensive
87 <> M	Tab, Blue, Round, Scored, Film Coated	Maprotiline HCl 50 mg	Ludiomil by Mylan	00378-0087	Antidepressant
87 <> M	Tab, Blue, Round, Scored, Film Coated	Maprotiline HCl 50 mg	Ludiomil by Murfreesboro	51129-1679	Antidepressant
87 <> R	Tab, Peach, Round, Extended Release	Alprazolam 2 mg	Xanax XR by Actavis	00228-3087	Antianxiety; C IV
870EL	Cap, Ex Release, White Beads	Guaifenesin 300 mg, Pseudoephedrine HCl 60 mg	Sudafed Sinus by Pharmafab	62542-0401	Cold Remedy
871	Tab, Blue, Round, Andrx Logo 871, ER	Glipizide 2.5 mg	Glucotrol XL by Andrx	62037-0871	Antidiabetic
872	Tab, White, Round, Andrx Logo 872, ER	Glipizide 5 mg	Glucotrol XL by Andrx	62037-0872	Antidiabetic
872	Cap	Nifedipine 10 mg	by Sandoz	00781-2504	Antihypertensive
872CARACO	Cap, RP Scherer Logo 872	Nifedipine 10 mg	by Caraco		Antihypertensive
872PAR	Cap, Light Blue Opaque Cap, White Opaque Body	Fluoxetine 40 mg	Prozac by Par	49884-0872	Antidepressant
873	Tab, White, Round, Andrx Logo 873, ER	Glipizide 10 mg	Glucotrol XL by Andrx	62037-0873	Antidiabetic
8733UNIMED	Tab, White, Round, 87 33/Unimed	Oxymetuclor 50 mg	Anadrol by Unimed		Steroid; C III
8744 <> BARR	Tab, Blue, Oval, Scored	Warfarin Sodium 4 mg	Coumadin by UDL	51079-0912	Anticoagulant
8744 <> BARR	Tab, Blue, Oval, Scored	Warfarin Sodium 4 mg	Coumadin by Barr	00555-0874	Anticoagulant
875 <> NN	Tab, White, Oblong, Scored, N / N <> 875	Amoxicillin 875 mg, Clavulanate Potassium 125 mg	Clavulin by Novopharm	Canadian DIN 02248138	Antibiotic
875125 <> AMC	Tab, Off-White, Oblong, Scored, 875/125	Amoxicillin 875 mg, Clavulanate Potassium 125 mg	Augmentin by LEK	66685-1001	Antibiotic
8778	Cap, Light Brown, Oval	Fiber	Metamucil by Watson	00536-1500	Supplement
879	Tab	Acetaminophen 300 mg, Codeine Phosphate 60 mg	Tylenol w/ Codeine by Pharmedix	53002-0103	Analgesic; C III
879	Tab, White, Round	Codeine Sulfate 30 mg	by Halsey		Analgesic; C II
8790155	Cap, Pink	Propoxyphene HCl 65 mg	Prophene-65 by Halsey		Analgesic; C IV
8790158	Cap	Tetracycline HCl 250 mg	by Halsey	00879-0158	Antibiotic
8790158	Cap	Tetracycline HCl 250 mg	by Moore	00839-1656	Antibiotic
879027	Cap, Yellow	Pentobarbital Sodium 100 mg	Nembutal by Halsey		Sedative/Hypnotic; C II
8790364	Cap	Chlordiazepoxide 5 mg	Librium by Ivax	00182-0977	Antianxiety; C IV
8790365	Cap	Chlordiazepoxide 10 mg	Librium by Ivax	00182-0978	Antianxiety; C IV
8790365	Cap	Chlordiazepoxide 10 mg	Librium by Pharmedix	53002-0450	Antianxiety; C IV
87903658790365	Cap, 879/0365 <> 879/0365	Chlordiazepoxide 10 mg	Librium by Kaiser	00179-0134	Antianxiety; C IV
8790366	Cap, Green & White	Chlordiazepoxide 25 mg	Librium by Halsey		Antianxiety; C IV
879129	Tab, White, Round	Prednisone 5 mg	Cortan by Halsey		Steroid
879130	Tab, White, Round	Propylthiouracil 50 mg	by Halsey		Antithyroid
879158	Cap	Tetracycline HCl 250 mg	by Qualitest	00603-5919	Antibiotic
879159	Cap	Tetracycline HCl 500 mg	by Halsey	00879-0159	Antibiotic
879159	Cap	Tetracycline HCl 500 mg	by Moore	00839-5075	Antibiotic
879317	Tab, Yellow, Round	Dextroamphetamine Sulfate 10 mg	Dexedrine by Halsey		Stimulant; C II
879341	Tab	Isoniazid 300 mg	Laniazid by Halsey	00879-0341	Antimycobacterial

ID FRONT <> BACK	DESCRIPTION FRONT <> BACK	INGREDIENT & STRENGTH	BRAND (or Generic Equiv.) by FIRM	NDC#	CLASS; SCH.
879358	Tab, White, Round	Quinidine Sulfate 200 mg	by Halsey		Antiarrhythmic
879360	Tab, White, Round	Triprolidine HCl 2.5 mg, Pseudoephedrine HCl 60 mg	Triposed by Halsey		Cold Remedy
879364	Cap, Green & Yellow	Chlordiazepoxide 5 mg	Librium by Halsey		Antianxiety; C IV
879365	Cap, Black & Green	Chlordiazepoxide 10 mg	Librium by Halsey		Antianxiety; C IV
879366	Cap, Green & White	Chlordiazepoxide 25 mg	Librium by Halsey		Antianxiety; C IV
879452	Cap, Red & White	Acetaminophen 500 mg	Tylenol Ex Strength by Halsey		Analgesic
879453	Tab, White	Acetaminophen 500 mg	Tylenol Ex Strength by Halsey		Analgesic
879501	Cap, White	Chlordiazepoxide 5 mg, Clidinium Bromide 2.5 mg	Librax by Halsey		Gastrointestinal
879525	Cap, Halsey Drug	Doxycycline Hyclate	by URL Mutual	00677-0598	Antibiotic
879525AP0837	Cap	Doxycycline Hyclate 50 mg	by Rachelle	00196-0552	Antibiotic
879526	Tab, Blue, Oblong, 879/526	Doxycycline Hyclate 100 mg	by Urgent Care Center	50716-0522	Antibiotic
879526	Cap, Blue	Doxycycline Hyclate 100 mg	by Dixon Shane	17236-0527	Antibiotic
879526	Tab, Blue, Oblong, 879/526	Doxycycline Hyclate 100 mg	by Prepackage Specialists	58864-0190	Antibiotic
879526	Tab, Blue, Oblong, 879/526	Doxycycline Hyclate 100 mg	by Halsey	00879-0526	Antibiotic
879526	Tab, Blue, Oblong, 879/526	Doxycycline Hyclate 100 mg	by Apotheca	12634-0169	Antibiotic
879526	Tab, Blue, Oblong, 879/526	Doxycycline Hyclate 100 mg	by Southwood	58016-0161	Antibiotic
879G10C2	Tab, White, Round	Acetaminophen 300 mg, Codeine Phosphate 15 mg	Tylenol w/ Codeine by Halsey		Analgesic; C III
879G11C3	Tab, White, Round	Acetaminophen 300 mg, Codeine Phosphate 30 mg	Tylenol w/ Codeine by Halsey		Analgesic; C III
879G122C	Tab, Green, Round	Butabarbital Sodium 30 mg	Sarisol #2 by Halsey		Sedative; C III
879G12C4	Tab, White, Round	Acetaminophen 300 mg, Codeine Phosphate 60 mg	Tylenol w/ Codeine by Halsey		Analgesic; C III
879G180	Tab, Green, Round	Chlorpheniramine Maleate 4 mg	Chlor-Trimeton by Halsey		Antihistamine
879G20C	Tab	Acetaminophen 325 mg, Oxycodone HCl 5 mg	Percocet by Ivax	00182-1465	Analgesic; C II
879G302	Cap, Clear & Pink	Diphenhydramine HCl 25 mg	Benadryl by Halsey		Antihistamine
879G303	Cap, Pink	Diphenhydramine HCl 50 mg	Benadryl by Halsey		Antihistamine
879G368	Tab, Yellow, Round	Folic Acid 1 mg	Folvite by Halsey		Vitamin
879G406	Tab, Peach, Round	Hydrochlorothiazide 25 mg	Hydrodiuril by Halsey		Diuretic; Antihypertensive
879G407	Tab, Peach, Round	Hydrochlorothiazide 50 mg	Hydro-D by Halsey		Diuretic; Antihypertensive
879G41	Tab, White, Round	Aminophylline 100 mg	Aminophylline by Halsey		Antiasthmatic
879G468C	Tab, White, Round	Meperidine HCl 50 mg	Pethadol by Halsey		Analgesic; C II
879G469C	Tab, White, Round	Meperidine HCl 100 mg	Pethadol by Halsey		Analgesic; C II
879G471C	Tab, White, Round, 879 /G471C	Meprobamate 400 mg	Miltown by Halsey		Sedative/Hypnotic; C IV
879G545	Tab, Orange, Round	Prednisolone 5 mg	Cortalone by Halsey		Steroid
879G549	Tab, Peach, Round	Prednisone 20 mg	Cortan by Halsey		Steroid
879G587	Tab, Red, Round	Rauwolfia Serpentina 100 mg	Raudixin by Halsey		Antihypertensive
879G594C	Cap, Reddish-Orange	Secobarbital Sodium 100 mg	Seconal by Halsey		Sedative/Hypnotic; C II
879G650C	Tab, Yellow, Round	Oxycodone HCl 4.5 mg, Oxycodone Terephthalate 0.38 mg, Aspirin 325 mg	Percodan by Halsey		Analgesic; C II
879G85C2	Tab, White, Round	Aspirin 325 mg, Codeine Phosphate 15 mg	Aspirin w/ Codeine by Halsey		Analgesic; C III
879G86C3	Tab, White, Round	Aspirin 325 mg, Codeine Phosphate 30 mg	Aspirin w/ Codeine by Halsey		Analgesic; C III
879G87C4	Tab, White, Round	Aspirin 325 mg, Codeine Phosphate 60 mg	Aspirin w/ Codeine by Halsey		Analgesic; C III
879G88C	Tab, White, Round	Atropine Sulfate 0.025 mg, Diphenoxylate HCl 2.5 mg	Lomotil by Halsey		Antidiarrheal; C V
879G90C	Tab, White, Round	Phenobarbital, Belladonna Alkaloids	Susano by Halsey		Gastrointestinal; C IV

ID FRONT <> BACK	DESCRIPTION FRONT <> BACK	INGREDIENT & STRENGTH	BRAND (or Generic Equiv.) by FIRM	NDC#	CLASS; SCH.
87RH405RELIANT	Cap, Dark Green and Light Green, Segmented Band, Reliant Logo	Fenofibrate 87 mg	Antara by Reliant	65726-0402	Antihyperlipidemic
88 <> FLINT	Tab, Green, Round, Scored	Levothyroxine Sodium 88 mcg	Synthroid by Abbott	Canadian DIN 02172097	Thyroid Hormone
88 <> FLINT	Tab, Green, Round, Scored	Levothyroxine Sodium 88 mcg	Synthroid by Abbott	00048-1060	Thyroid Hormone
88 <> FLINT	Tab, Green, Round, Scored	Levothyroxine Sodium 88 mcg	Synthroid by Forest	00456-0329	Thyroid Hormone
88 <> FLINT	Tab, Olive, Round, Scored	Levothyroxine Sodium 88 mcg	Synthroid by Rightpac	65240-0757	Thyroid Hormone
88 <> FLINT	Tab, Green, Round, Scored	Levothyroxine Sodium 88 mcg	Synthroid by Physician Total Care	54868-2705	Thyroid Hormone
88 <> GG334	Tab, Olive Green, Cap Shaped, Scored, 88 <> GG over 334	Levothyroxine 88 mcg	Levo-T by Alara	64909-0125	Thyroid Hormone
88 <> GG334	Tab, Olive Green, Cap Shaped, Scored, 88 <> GG over 334	Levothyroxine 88 mcg	Levo-T by Sandoz	00781-5183	Thyroid Hormone
88 <> MYLAN	Tab, Purple, Oval, Ex Release	Carbidopa 25 mg, Levodopa 100 mg	Sinemet CR by Mylan	00378-0088	Antiparkinson
88 <> MYLAN	Tab, Purple, Oval, Ex Release	Carbidopa 25 mg, Levodopa 100 mg	Sinemet CR by UDL	51079-0978 Discontinued	Antiparkinson
88 <> PAL	Tab, Light Green, Oblong, Scored	Pseudoephedrine HCl 90 mg, Carbinoxamine Maleate 8 mg, Methscopolamine Nitrate 2.5 mg	Pannaz by PamLab	00525-0880	Cold Remedy
88 <> SYNTHROID	Tab, Green, Round, Scored	Levothyroxine Sodium 88 mcg	Synthroid by Abbott	00074-6594	Thyroid Hormone
88 <> T4	Tab, Mint Green, Cap Shaped	Levothyroxine Sodium 88 mcg	Levothroid by Forest	00456-1329	Thyroid Hormone
88 <> UU	Tab, White, Oval, Scored	Pramipexole DiHCl 0.5 mg	Mirapex by Boehringer Ingelheim	00597-0085	Antiparkinson
88 <> UU	Tab, White, Oval, Scored	Pramipexole DiHCl 0.5 mg	Mirapex by Pharmacia	00009-0008	Antiparkinson
8818 <> AP	Tab	Buspirone HCl 5 mg	Buspar by Apothecon	59772-8818	Antianxiety
8819 <> AP	Tab	Buspirone HCl 10 mg	Buspar by Apothecon	59772-8819	Antianxiety
884 <> MILES30	Tab, Pink	Nifedipine 30 mg	Adalat CC by Direct Dispensing	57866-6719	Antihypertensive
884 <> MILES30	Tab, Film Coated	Nifedipine 30 mg	Adalat CC by Caremark	00339-5976	Antihypertensive
885 <> MILES60	Tab, Film Coated	Nifedipine 60 mg	Adalat CC by Pharm Util	60491-0010	Antihypertensive
885MILES60 <> 60ADALATCC	Tab, Salmon, Film Coated	Nifedipine 60 mg	Adalat CC by Allscripts		Antihypertensive
8861 <> B	Tab, Light Purple, Oval, Scored, 886 over 1	Estradiol 1 mg	Estrace by Barr	00555-0886	Hormone
8861 <> B	Tab, Light Purple, Oval, Scored, 886 over 1	Estradiol 1 mg	Estrace by Halsey	00904-5442	Hormone
8861 <> B	Tab, Light Purple, Oval, Scored, 886 over 1	Estradiol 1 mg	Estrace by DRX	55045-2739	Hormone
8872 <> B	Tab, Green, Oval, Scored, 887 over 2	Estradiol 2 mg	Estrace by Halsey	00904-7738	Hormone
8872 <> B	Tab, Green, Oval, Scored, 887 over 2	Estradiol 2 mg	Estrace by Barr	00555-0887	Hormone
889	Cap, Red & Yellow	Phentermine 30 mg	Fastin by Marlop		Anorexiant; C IV
88M	Tab	Levothyroxine Sodium 88 mcg	Synthroid by Mova	55370-0160	Thyroid Hormone
88M	Tab	Levothyroxine Sodium 88 mcg	Synthroid by Em Pharma	63254-0438	Thyroid Hormone
88M <> Z	Tab, Green, Round, Scored	Levothyroxine Sodium 88 mcg	Synthroid by Zoetica	64909-0115	Thyroid Hormone
88MCG	Tab, Olive, Oval	Levothyroxine Sodium 88 mcg	Synthroid by Physician Total Care	54868-4177	Thyroid Hormone
88MCG	Tab	Levothyroxine Sodium 88 mcg	Synthroid by GSK	53873-0117	Thyroid Hormone
89 <> TARO	Tab, Blue, Oval, Film Coated	Etodolac 500 mg	Lodine by Taro	51672-4036	NSAID
890	Cap, Black	Phendimetrazine Tartrate 105 mg	Prelu-2 by Marlop		Anorexiant; C III
890 <> 93	Tab, Pink, Oblong, Film Coated	Acetaminophen 650 mg, Propoxyphene Napsylate 100 mg	Darvocet-N 100 by Ranbaxy	63304-0714	Analgesic; C IV
890 <> 93	Tab, Pink, Oblong, Film Coated	Acetaminophen 650 mg, Propoxyphene Napsylate 100 mg	Darvocet-N 100 by Heartland	61392-0446	Analgesic; C IV
890 <> 93	Tab, Pink, Oblong, Film Coated	Acetaminophen 650 mg, Propoxyphene Napsylate 100 mg	Darvocet-N 100 by Teva	00093-0890	Analgesic; C IV
890 <> 93	Tab, Pink, Oblong, Film Coated	Acetaminophen 650 mg, Propoxyphene Napsylate 100 mg	Darvocet-N 100 by Ivax	00182-0317	Analgesic; C IV
891 <> AZ10	Tab, Oyster, Round, Film Coated, Ex Release	Nisoldipine 10 mg	Sular by AstraZeneca	00310-0891	Antihypertensive
891 <> G	Tab, Light Blue, Round, Film Coated	Levonorgestrel 0.25 mg, Ethinyl Estradiol 0.05 mg	Preven by Gynetics	63955-0020	Oral Contraceptive
891 <> G	Tab, Light Blue, Round, Film Coated	Levonorgestrel 0.25 mg, Ethinyl Estradiol 0.05 mg	by Barr	00555-0891	Oral Contraceptive
891 <> ZENECA10	Tab, Oyster, Round, Film Coated, Ex Release	Nisoldipine 10 mg	Sular by AstraZeneca	00310-0891	Antihypertensive
891 <> ZENECA10	Tab	Nisoldipine 10 mg	Sular by Bayer	12527-0891	Antihypertensive
892 <> 93	Tab, Pink, Cap Shaped, Film Coated	Etodolac 400 mg	Lodine by Heartland	61392-0911	NSAID
892 <> 93	Tab, Pink, Cap Shaped, Film Coated	Etodolac 400 mg	Lodine by Teva	00093-0892	NSAID

ID FRONT <> BACK	DESCRIPTION FRONT <> BACK	INGREDIENT & STRENGTH	BRAND (or Generic Equiv.) by FIRM	NDC#	CLASS; SCH.
892 <> AZ20	Tab, Yellow Cream, Round, Film Coated, Ex Release	Nisoldipine 20 mg	Sular by AstraZeneca	00310-0892	Antihypertensive
892 <> WATSON	Tab, Lime Green, Round	Norethindrone 0.35 mg	Jolivette by Watson	52544-0892	Oral Contraceptive
892 <> ZENECA20	Tab, Dark Yellow, Round, Film Coated, Ex Release	Nisoldipine 20 mg	Sular by AstraZeneca	00310-0892	Antihypertensive
892 <> ZENECA20	Tab, Dark Yellow, Round	Nisoldipine 20 mg	Sular by Murfreesboro	51129-1278	Antihypertensive
892 <> ZENECA20	Tab, Dark Yellow, Round	Nisoldipine 20 mg	Sular by Bayer	12527-0892	Antihypertensive
893 <> AZ30	Tab, Mustard, Round, Film Coated, Ex Release	Nisoldipine 30 mg	Sular by AstraZeneca	00310-0893	Antihypertensive
893 <> ZENECA30	Tab, Mustard, Round, Film Coated, Ex Release	Nisoldipine 30 mg	Sular by AstraZeneca	00310-0893	Antihypertensive
893 <> ZENECA30	Tab	Nisoldipine 30 mg	Sular by Murfreesboro	51129-1334	Antihypertensive
893 <> ZENECA30	Tab	Nisoldipine 30 mg	Sular by Bayer	12527-0893	Antihypertensive
894 <> AZ40	Tab, Burnt Orange, Round, Film Coated, Ex Release	Nisoldipine 40 mg	Sular by AstraZeneca	00310-0894	Antihypertensive
894 <> ZENECA40	Tab, Burnt Orange, Round, Film Coated, Ex Release	Nisoldipine 40 mg	Sular by AstraZeneca	00310-0894	Antihypertensive
894 <> ZENECA40	Tab, Burnt Orange, Round, Film Coated, Ex Release	Nisoldipine 40 mg	Sular by Bayer	12527-0894	Antihypertensive
896 <> 93	Tab, Beige, Round, Film Coated	Famotidine 20 mg	Pepcid by Teva	00093-0896 Discontinued	Gastrointestinal
896 <> DP	Tab, Blue, Cap Shaped, Scored	Guaifenesin 500 mg, Pseudoephedrine 60 mg	Sudafed Sinus by Duramed	51285-0896	Cold Remedy
8962 <> TISH	Tab, Beige, Oblong	Polycarbophil 500 mg	FiberCon by Rugby	00536-4306	Laxative
897	Cap, Clear Bright Orange, Oval, Soft Gel	Docusate Sodium 100 mg	Colace by Ivax	00182-8363	Laxative
897 <> 93	Tab, Tan, Round, Film Coated	Famotidine 40 mg	Pepcid by Teva	00093-0897 Discontinued	Gastrointestinal
899 <> 54	Tab	Prednisone 10 mg	Deltasone by Med Pro	53978-3037	Steroid
89912 <> B	Tab, White to Off-White, Oval, Scored, 899 over 1/2	Estradiol 0.5 mg	Estrace by Barr	00555-0899	Hormone
8GLAXO	8/Glaxo	Ondansetron HCl 8 mg	Zofran by GSK	Canadian	Antiemetic
8I	Tab, White, Cap Shaped	Ibuprofen 800 mg	Motrin by Dr. Reddy's	55111-0684	NSAID
8MG <> CARDURA	Tab, Green, Oblong, Scored	Doxazosin Mesylate 8 mg	Cardura by Pharm Util	60491-0123	Antihypertensive
8MG <> CARDURA	Tab, Green, Oblong, Scored	Doxazosin Mesylate 8 mg	Cardura by Roerig	00049-2780	Antihypertensive
8MG <> ETH269	Tab, Blue, Oblong	Doxazosin Mesylate 8 mg	Cardura by Ethex	58177-0269	Antihypertensive
8MG <> ETH269	Tab, Blue, Oblong, Scored	Doxazosin Mesylate 8 mg	Cardura by Dava	67253-0387	Antihypertensive
8MG <> MLP19	Tab, Green, Oval	Doxazosin Mesylate 8 mg	Cardura by Dava	67253-0383	Antihypertensive
8MGWATSON152	Cap, White, Opaque, Hard Gelatin	Silodosin 8 mg	Rapaflo by Watson	52544-0152	Alpha Blocker
8MGWATSON152	Cap, White, Opaque, Hard Gelatin	Silodosin 8 mg	Rapaflo by Watson	52544-0152	Alpha Blocker
8R	Cap, Golden Yellow, Soft Gel	Isotretinoin 30 mg	Sotret by Ranbaxy	63304-0447	Dermatologic
8R	Tab, Film Coated, 8 over R	Indapamide 2.5 mg	Lozol by Quality Care	60346-0946	Diuretic
9 <> C	Tab, White, Round	Bromocriptine Mesylate 0.8 mg	Cycloset by Veroscience		Antidiabetic
9 <> M	Tab, Yellow, Triangular, Film Coated	Fluphenazine HCl 2.5 mg	Prolixin by Mylan	00378-6009	Antipsychotic
9 <> M	Tab, Yellow, Triangular, Film Coated	Fluphenazine HCl 2.5 mg	Prolixin by UDL	51079-0486	Antipsychotic
90	Tab, Blue, Elongated, Triangle Logo	Guaifenesin 600 mg, Pseudoephedrine 120 mg	Ru-Tuss DE by Knoll		Cold Remedy
90 <> ADALATCC	Tab, Reddish Brown, Round, Film Coated, Adalat over CC	Nifedipine 90 mg	Adalat CC by Bayer	00026-8861	Antihypertensive
90 <> ADALATCC	Tab, Reddish Brown, Round, Film Coated, Adalat over CC	Nifedipine 90 mg	Adalat CC by Med Pro	53978-3044	Antihypertensive
90 <> AMGEN	Tab, Light Green, Oval, Film Coated	Cinacalcet HCl 90 mg	Sensipar by Amgen	55513-0075	Calcimimetic
90 <> B	Tab, Yellow, Round, Ex Release	Nifedipine 90 mg	Adalat CC by Teva	00093-1023	Antihypertensive
90 <> B	Tab, Yellow, Round, Ex Release	Nifedipine 90 mg	Adalat CC by Ivax	00182-8234 Discontinued	Antihypertensive
901 <> LV	Cap, Yellow, Opaque	Oxycodone 5 mg	by Glenmark	68462-0204	Opiate Agonist
901 <> UCB	Tab, White, Cap Shaped, Scored	Acetaminophen 500 mg, Hydrocodone Bitartrate 2.5 mg	Lortab by UCB	50474-0901	Analgesic; C III
901 <> WHITBY	Tab, White, Oblong, Pink Specks	Acetaminophen 500 mg, Hydrocodone Bitartrate 2.5 mg	Lortab by Alphapharm		Analgesic; C III
901W	Cap, Film Coated	Naproxen 375 mg	Naprelan by Wyeth	00008-0901	NSAID
902 <> UCB	Tab, White, Cap Shaped, Scored	Acetaminophen 500 mg, Hydrocodone Bitartrate 5 mg	Lortab by UCB	50474-0902	Analgesic; C III
902 <> UCB	Tab, White, Cap Shaped, Scored	Acetaminophen 500 mg, Hydrocodone Bitartrate 5 mg	Lortab by Nat Pharmpak	55154-7204	Analgesic; C III
902 <> UCB	Tab, White, Cap Shaped, Scored	Acetaminophen 500 mg, Hydrocodone Bitartrate 5 mg	Lortab by H J Harkins Co	52959-0185	Analgesic; C III

ID FRONT <> BACK	DESCRIPTION FRONT <> BACK	INGREDIENT & STRENGTH	BRAND (or Generic Equiv.) by FIRM	NDC#	CLASS; SCH.
902 <> UCB	Tab, White, Cap Shaped, Scored	Acetaminophen 500 mg, Hydrocodone Bitartrate 5 mg	Lortab by Murfreesboro	51129-1434	Analgesic; C III
902 <> W	Tab, White, Oblong	Naproxen 550 mg	by PDRX	55289-0304	NSAID
902 <> W	Tab, Film Coated	Naproxen 550 mg	by Caremark	00339-6102	NSAID
902 <> W	Tab, Film Coated	Naproxen 550 mg	by Physician Total Care	54868-3973	NSAID
902W	Cap, Film Coated	Naproxen 550 mg	Naprelan by Wyeth	00008-0902	NSAID
903 <> LV	Tab, White, Round, Scored, L/V <> 903	Codeine Sulfate 30 mg	by Glenmark	68462-0193	Analgesic; C II
903 <> UCB	Tab, White, Cap Shaped, Scored	Acetaminophen 500 mg, Hydrocodone Bitartrate 7.5 mg	Lortab by Amerisource	62584-0907	Analgesic; C III
903 <> UCB	Tab, White, Cap Shaped, Scored	Acetaminophen 500 mg, Hydrocodone Bitartrate 7.5 mg	Lortab by Med Pro	53978-2069	Analgesic; C III
903 <> UCB	Tab, White, Cap Shaped, Scored	Acetaminophen 500 mg, Hydrocodone Bitartrate 7.5 mg	Lortab by H J Harkins Co	52959-0186	Analgesic; C III
903 <> UCB	Tab, White, Cap Shaped, Scored	Acetaminophen 500 mg, Hydrocodone Bitartrate 7.5 mg	Lortab by Nat Pharmpak	55154-7201	Analgesic; C III
903 <> UCB	Tab, White, Cap Shaped, Scored	Acetaminophen 500 mg, Hydrocodone Bitartrate 7.5 mg	Lortab by UCB	50474-0907	Analgesic; C III
904 <> BARR	Tab, White, Round	Tamoxifen Citrate 20 mg	Nolvadex by Zeneca	00310-0904	Antiestrogen
904 <> BARR	Tab, White, Round	Tamoxifen Citrate 20 mg	Nolvadex by Barr	00555-0904	Antiestrogen
905 <> CEN	Tab, Yellow, Round, Coated	Folacin 5 mg, Thiamine 1.5 mg, Riboflavin 1.5 mg, Niacinamide 20 mg, Pantothenic Acid 10 mg, Pyridoxine 50 mg, Cyanocobalamin 2 mg, Ascorbic Acid 60 mg, D-biotin 300 mcg, Zinc 25 mg, Copper 1.5 mg	Diatx Zn by Centrix	11528-0905	Vitamin
905 <> SZ	Tab, Off White, Round, Film Coated	Cetirizine HCl 5 mg	Zyrtec by Sandoz	00781-1683	Antihistamine
906 <> LV	Tab, White, Round, Scored, L/V <> 906	Codeine Sulfate 60 mg	by Glenmark	68462-0194	Analgesic; C II
906 <> SZ	Tab, Off White, Round, Film Coated	Cetirizine HCl 10 mg	Zyrtec by Sandoz	00781-1684	Antihistamine
907	Tab, Green, Round, Duramed Logo	Belladonna Alkaloids 0.2 mg, Ergotamine Tartrate 0.6 mg, Phenobarbital 40 mg	Duragal S by Duramed	51285-0907	Gastrointestinal; C IV
9090 <> BIBI	Tab, White, Round, Scored	Pramipexole DiHCl 1 mg	Mirapex by Boehringer Ingelheim	00597-0190	Antiparkinson
91 <> F	Tab, White to Off-White, Oval, Film-Coated	Ondansetron 4 mg	Ondansetron by Aurobindo	65862-0187	Antiemetic
91 <> G	Tab, Purple, Round	Dipyridamole 50 mg	Persantine by Glenmark	68462-0117	Vasodilator
91 <> GG	Tab, White, Round	Lorazepam 0.5 mg	Ativan by Ivax	00182-8237	Antianxiety; C IV
91 <> GG	Tab, White, Round	Lorazepam 0.5 mg	Ativan by Sandoz	00781-1403	Antianxiety; C IV
910 <> STSS	Tab, White, Round, ST/SS	Sulfamethoxazole 400 mg, Trimethoprim 80 mg	by Teva	Discontinued	Antibiotic
910 <> UCB	Tab, Pink, Cap Shaped, Scored	Acetaminophen 500 mg, Hydrocodone Bitartrate 10 mg	Lortab by Nat Pharmpak	55154-7202	Analgesic; C III
910 <> UCB	Tab, Pink, Cap Shaped, Scored	Acetaminophen 500 mg, Hydrocodone Bitartrate 10 mg	Lortab by H J Harkins Co	52959-0453	Analgesic; C III
910 <> UCB	Tab, Pink, Cap Shaped, Scored	Acetaminophen 500 mg, Hydrocodone Bitartrate 10 mg	Lortab by D M Graham	00756-0249	Analgesic; C III
910 <> UCB	Tab, Pink, Cap Shaped, Scored	Acetaminophen 500 mg, Hydrocodone Bitartrate 10 mg	Lortab by Amerisource	62584-0016	Analgesic; C III
910 <> UCB	Tab, Pink, Cap Shaped, Scored	Acetaminophen 500 mg, Hydrocodone Bitartrate 10 mg	Lortab by UCB	50474-0910	Analgesic; C III
9111 <> 93	Tab, Yellowish Tan, Oval, Film Coated	Ascorbic Acid 120 mg, Beta-Carotene 4.2 mg, Calcium Carbonate 490.76 mg, Cholecalciferol 0.49 mg, Cupric Oxide 2.5 mg, Cyanocobalamin 12 mcg, Ferrous Fumarate 197.75 mg, Folic Acid 1 mg, Niacinamide 21 mg, Pyridoxine HCl 10.5 mg, Riboflavin 3.15 mg, Thiamine Mononitrate 1.575 mg, Vitamin A Acetate 8.4 mg, Vitamin E Acetate 44 mg, Zinc Oxide 31.12 mg	Prenatal Plus (Stuartnatal Plus) by Teva	00093-9111 Discontinued	Vitamin
9111 <> VIOKASE	Tab, Tan, Round	Amylase 30,000 Units, Protease 30,000 Units, Lipase 8,000 Units	Viokase by Axcan	58914-0111	Gastrointestinal
9111 <> VIOKASE	Tab, Tan, Round	Amylase 30,000 Units, Protease 30,000 Units, Lipase 8,000 Units	Viokase by Axcan	Canadian DIN 02230019	Gastrointestinal
9111 <> VIOKASEAHR	Tab, Light Brown & White, Round, Viokase over AHR	Amylase 30,000 Units, Lipase 8000 Units, Protease 30,000 Units	Viokase by A H Robins	00031-9111	Gastrointestinal
9111 <> VIOKASEAHR	Tab, Light Brown & White, Round, Viokase over AHR	Amylase 30,000 Units, Lipase 8000 Units, Protease 30,000 Units	Viokase by Eckerd	19458-0871	Gastrointestinal
9111 <> VIOKASEAHR	Tab, Light Brown & White, Round, Viokase over AHR	Amylase 30,000 Units, Lipase 8000 Units, Protease 30,000 Units	Viokase by Paddock	00574-9111	Gastrointestinal
9116 <> V16	Tab, Tan, Oval, '16' in superscript	Amylase 60,000 Units, Protease 60,000 Units, Lipase 16,000 Units	Viokase by Axcan	Canadian DIN 02241933	Gastrointestinal
9116 <> V16	Tab, Tan, Oval, '16' in superscript	Amylase 60,000 Units, Protease 60,000 Units, Lipase 16,000 Units	Viokase by Axcan	58914-0116	Gastrointestinal
912 <> W	Tab, Pink, Round, Scored	Levonorgestrel 0.1 mg, Ethinyl Estradiol 0.02 mg	Alesse 21 by Wyeth	00008-0912	Oral Contraceptive
912 <> W	Tab, Pink, Round, Scored	Levonorgestrel 0.1 mg, Ethinyl Estradiol 0.02 mg	Alesse 28 by Wyeth	00008-2576	Oral Contraceptive
913 <> WATSON	Tab, White w/ Orange Specks, Cap Shaped, Scored	Acetaminophen 325 mg, Hydrocodone Bitartrate 5 mg	Norco by Watson	52544-0913	Analgesic; C III
915 <> LV	Tab, White, Round, Scored	Morphine Sulfate 15 mg	by Glenmark	68462-0202	Analgesic; C II

ID FRONT <> BACK	DESCRIPTION FRONT <> BACK	INGREDIENT & STRENGTH	BRAND (or Generic Equiv.) by FIRM	NDC#	CLASS; SCH.
9152 <> 93	Tab, Yellow, Oval, Film Coated	Ascorbic Acid 200 mg, Biotin 0.15 mg, Calcium Pantothenate 27.17 mg, Chromic Chloride 0.51 mg, Cupric Oxide 3.75 mg, Cyanocobalamin 50 mcg, Ferrous Fumarate 82.2 mg, Folic Acid 0.8 mg, Magnesium Oxide 82.89 mg, Manganese 50 mg, Manganese Sulfate 15.5 mg, Niacinamide Ascorbate 400 mg, Pyridoxine HCl 30.25 mg, Riboflavin 20 mg, Thiamine Mononitrate 20 mg, Vitamin A Acetate 10.75 mg, Vitamin E Acetate 30 mg, Zinc Oxide 27.99 mg	B Complex Vit Plus by Teva	00093-9152	Vitamin
9165 <> 93	Tab, Oval, White	Ascorbic Acid 17.53 mg, Beta-Carotene 0.56 mg, Calcium Carbonate 249.41 mg, Calcium Pantothenate 4.18 mg, Cholecalciferol 0.25 mcg, Cupric Oxide 2.02 mg, Ferrous Fumarate 82.15 mg, Magnesium Oxide 82.93 mg, Niacinamide Ascorbate 8.54 mg, Pyridoxine HCl 2.43 mg, Riboflavin 0.84 mg, Thiamine Mononitrate 1 mg, Vitamin A Acetate 2680 Units, Zinc Oxide 15.56 mg	Enfamil Natalins by Teva	00093-9165 Discontinued	Vitamin
917200 <> B	Tab, White, Round, Scored, 917 over 200 <> b	Amiodarone 200 mg	Cordarone by Barr	00555-0917 Discontinued	Antiarrhythmic
9191 <> BIBI	Tab, White, Round, Scored	Pramipexole DiHCl 1.5 mg	Mirapex by Boehringer Ingelheim	00597-0191	Antiparkinson
92 <> BL	Tab, White, Round	Metoclopramide HCl 5 mg	Reglan by Teva	00093-2204	Gastrointestinal
92 <> BL	Tab, White, Round	Metoclopramide HCl 5 mg	Reglan by UDL	51079-0629	Gastrointestinal
92 <> BL	Tab, White, Round	Metoclopramide HCl 5 mg	Reglan by Murfreesboro	51129-1683	Gastrointestinal
92 <> F	Tab, Yellow, Oval, Film-Coated	Ondansetron 8 mg	Ondansetron by Aurobindo	65862-0188	Antiemetic
92 <> G	Tab, Purple, Round	Dipyridamole 75 mg	Persantine by Glenmark	68462-0118	Antiplatelet
92 <> M	Tab, White, Coated, Beveled Edge	Maprotiline HCl 75 mg	Ludiomil by Mylan	00378-0092	Antidepressant
920	Tab, Pink, Oblong	Estrogen, Methytestosterone	Essian by Prasco		Hormone
9200	Tab, White, Round	Glipizide 10 mg	Glucotrol by Ivax	00172-3650	Antidiabetic
9200	Tab, White, Round	Glipizide 10 mg	Glucotrol by Ivax	00182-1995 Discontinued	Antidiabetic
9200 <> DITROPAN	Tab, Blue, Round, Scored, Ditropan <> 92-00	Oxybutynin Chloride 5 mg	Ditropan by Janssen-Ortho	Canadian DIN 01924761	Urinary Tract
9200 <> DITROPAN	Tab, Blue, Round, Scored, Ditropan <> 92-00	Oxybutynin Chloride 5 mg	Ditropan by Alza	17314-9200	Urinary Tract
9200 <> I	Tab, White, Round, Scored	Glipizide 10 mg	Glucotrol by Teva	00172-3650	Antidiabetic
9201	Tab, White, Round	Glipizide 5 mg	Glucotrol by Ivax	00172-3649 Discontinued	Antidiabetic
9201	Tab, White, Round	Glipizide 5 mg	Glucotrol by Ivax	00182-1994 Discontinued	Antidiabetic
9201 <> I	Tab, White, Round, Scored	Glipizide 5 mg	Glucotrol by Teva	00172-3649	Antidiabetic
923400 <> B	Tab, White, Oval, Scored, Film Coated, 923 over 400	Ethambutol HCl 400 mg	Myambutol by Barr	00555-0923	Antituberculosis
9253 <> BARR	Tab, Tan, Oval, Scored	Warfarin Sodium 3 mg	Coumadin by Truett	11312-0128	Anticoagulant
9253 <> BARR	Tab, Tan, Oval, Scored	Warfarin Sodium 3 mg	Coumadin by UDL	51079-0911	Anticoagulant
9253 <> BARR	Tab, Tan, Oval, Scored	Warfarin Sodium 3 mg	Coumadin by Barr	00555-0925	Anticoagulant
926 <> 93	Tab, Light Peach, Round	Lovastatin 10 mg	Mevacor by Teva	00093-0926	Antihyperlipidemic
9266 <> BARR	Tab, Teal, Oval, Scored	Warfarin Sodium 6 mg	Coumadin by UDL	51079-0898	Anticoagulant
9266 <> BARR	Tab, Teal, Oval, Scored	Warfarin Sodium 6 mg	Coumadin by UCB	50474-0612	Anticoagulant
9266 <> BARR	Tab, Teal, Oval, Scored	Warfarin Sodium 6 mg	Coumadin by Barr	00555-0926	Anticoagulant
92693	Tab, Light Peach, Round	Lovastatin 10 mg	Mevacor by Teva	00093-0926	Antihyperlipidemic
9275 <> B	Tab, Green, Oval, Scored, Film Coated, 927/5 <> b	Methotrexate 5 mg	Trexall by Barr	00555-0927	Antineoplastic
928 <> 93	Tab, Light Green, Round	Lovastatin 40 mg	Mevacor by Teva	00093-0928	Antihyperlipidemic
928712 <> B	Tab, Blue, Oval, Scored, Film Coated, 928/7 1/2 <> b	Methotrexate 7.5 mg	Trexall by Barr	00555-0928	Antineoplastic
92893	Tab, Light Green, Round	Lovastatin 40 mg	Mevacor by Teva	00093-0928	Antihyperlipidemic
929 <> ANDRX	Tab, White, Cap Shaped, Scored, Sustained Release	Phenylephrine HCl 30 mg, Guaifenesin 600 mg	Entex LA by Andrx	62037-0929	Cold Remedy
92910 <> B	Tab, Pink, Oval, Scored, Film Coated, 929/10 <> b	Methotrexate 10 mg	Trexall by Barr	00555-0929	Antineoplastic

ID FRONT <> BACK	DESCRIPTION FRONT <> BACK	INGREDIENT & STRENGTH	BRAND (or Generic Equiv.) by FIRM	NDC#	CLASS; SCH.
93 <> 0863	Tab, White to Off-White, Round, Film Coated	Ciprofloxacin 250 mg	Cipro by Teva	00093-0863 Discontinued	Antibiotic
93 <> 0864	Tab, White to Off-White, Cap Shaped, Film Coated	Ciprofloxacin 500 mg	Cipro by Teva	00093-0864 Discontinued	Antibiotic
93 <> 0865	Tab, White to Off-White, Cap Shaped, Film Coated	Ciprofloxacin 750 mg	Cipro by Teva	00093-0865	Antibiotic
93 <> 0924	Tab, White to Off-White, Cap Shaped, Scored, 9 over 3	Oxaprozin 600 mg	Daypro by Teva	00093-0924	NSAID
93 <> 1024	Tab, White to Off-White, Oblong, Scored, 93 to left of Score <> 1024	Nefazodone HCl 100 mg	Serzone by Teva	00093-1024	Antidepressant
93 <> 1025	Tab, Light Yellow to Yellow, Oblong	Nefazodone HCl 200 mg	Serzone by Teva	00093-1025	Antidepressant
93 <> 1026	Tab, White to Off-White, Oblong	Nefazodone HCl 250 mg	Serzone by Teva	00093-1026	Antidepressant
93 <> 1035	Tab, Peach, Round	Lisinopril 10 mg, HCTZ 12.5 mg	Prinzide by Teva	00093-1035	Antihypertensive; Diuretic
93 <> 1036	Tab, White, Round	Lisinopril 20 mg, HCTZ 12.5 mg	Prinzide by Teva	00093-1036 Discontinued	Antihypertensive; Diuretic
93 <> 1037	Tab, Peach, Round	Lisinopril 20 mg, HCTZ 25 mg	Prinzide by Teva	00093-1037 Discontinued	Antihypertensive; Diuretic
93 <> 1041	Tab, Pink, Round, Film Coated, Ex Release	Diclofenac Sodium 100 mg	Voltaren XR by Biovail	62660-0021	NSAID
93 <> 1041	Tab, Pink, Round, Film Coated, Ex Release	Diclofenac Sodium 100 mg	Voltaren XR by Teva	00093-1041	NSAID
93 <> 1044	Tab, White, Cap Shaped	Enalapril Maleate 5 mg, Hydrochlorothiazide 12.5 mg	Vaseretic by Teva	00093-1044	Antihypertensive; Diuretic
93 <> 1045	Tab, Brown, Cap Shaped, Film Coated	Quinapril 20 mg	Accupril by Teva	00093-1045	Antihypertensive
93 <> 1050	Tab, Brown, Round, Film-Coated, Scored	Quinapril 5 mg	Accupril by Teva	00093-1050	Antihypertensive
93 <> 1051	Tab, Brown, Oval, Film-Coated	Quinapril 10 mg	Accupril by Teva	00093-1051	Antihypertensive
93 <> 1052	Tab, Rust, Cap Shaped	Enalapril Maleate 10 mg, Hydrochlorothiazide 25 mg	Vaseretic by Teva	00093-1052	Antihypertensive; Diuretic
93 <> 1053	Tab, Brown, Oblong, Film-Coated	Quinapril 40 mg	Accupril by Teva	00093-1053	Antihypertensive
93 <> 1073	Tab, White to Off-White, Cap Shaped, Biconvex	Cefuroxime Axetil 250 mg	Ceftin by Teva	00093-1073 Discontinued	Antibiotic
93 <> 1074	Tab, White to Off-White, Cap Shaped, Biconvex	Cefuroxime Axetil 500 mg	Ceftin by Teva	00093-1074	Antibiotic
93 <> 1077	Tab, Round, Light Orange, Film Coated	Cefprozil 250 mg	Cefzil by Teva	00093-1077	Antibiotic
93 <> 1078	Tab, White, Cap Shaped, Film Coated	Cefprozil 500 mg	Cefzil by Teva	00093-1078	Antibiotic
93 <> 1087	Tab, Dark Blue, Oval, Ex Release	Cefaclor 500 mg	Ceclor by Teva	00093-1087	Antibiotic
93 <> 111	Tab, White, Round, Film Coated	Cimetidine HCl 200 mg	Tagamet by Teva	00093-0111	Gastrointestinal
93 <> 1111	Tab, White, Round	Lisinopril 2.5 mg	Prinivil by Teva	00093-1111 Discontinued	Antihypertensive
93 <> 1113	Tab, Red, Round	Lisinopril 10 mg	Prinivil by Teva	00093-1113	Antihypertensive
93 <> 1114	Tab, Red, Cap Shaped	Lisinopril 20 mg	Prinivil by Teva	00093-1114 Discontinued	Antihypertensive
93 <> 1115	Tab, Yellow, Cap Shaped	Lisinopril 40 mg	Prinivil by Teva	00093-1115 Discontinued	Antihypertensive
93 <> 1118	Tab, Light Blue, Oval, Ex Release	Etodolac 600 mg	Lodine XL by Teva	00093-1118	NSAID
93 <> 112	Tab, White, Round, Film Coated	Cimetidine HCl 300 mg	Tagamet by Teva	00093-0012	Gastrointestinal
93 <> 112	Tab, White, Round, Film Coated	Cimetidine HCl 300 mg	Tagamet by PDRX	55289-0799	Gastrointestinal
93 <> 1122	Tab, Orange, Oval, Ex Release	Etodolac 400 mg	Lodine XL by Teva	00093-1122	NSAID
93 <> 1172	Tab, White to Off-White, Oval	Penicillin V Potassium 250 mg	by Teva Pharmaceuticals	00093-1172	Antibiotic
93 <> 1174	Tab, White to Off-White, Oval, Scored	Penicillin V Potassium 500 mg	V-Cillin K by Teva Pharmaceuticals	00093-1174	Antibiotic
93 <> 1177	Tab, Off-White, Round	Neomycin Sulfate 500 mg	Mycifradin by UDL	51079-0015	Antibiotic
93 <> 1177	Tab, Off-White, Round	Neomycin Sulfate 500 mg	Mycifradin by Teva	00093-1177	Antibiotic
93 <> 1215	Tab, Dark Blue, Oval, Ex Release	Cefaclor 375 mg	Ceclor CD by Teva	00093-1215 Discontinued	Antibiotic
93 <> 132	Tab, White to Off-White, Oval, Chewable	Lamotrigine 25 mg	Lamictal by Teva	00093-0132	Anticonvulsant
93 <> 135	Tab, White, Oval, Film Coated	Carvedilol 6.25 mg	Coreg by Teva	00093-0135	Antihypertensive

ID FRONT <> BACK	DESCRIPTION FRONT <> BACK	INGREDIENT & STRENGTH	BRAND (or Generic Equiv.) by FIRM	NDC#	CLASS; SCH.
93 <> 147	Tab, Light Red, Round	Naproxen 250 mg	Naprosyn by Ivax	00182-8240 Discontinued	NSAID
93 <> 147	Tab, Light Red, Round	Naproxen 250 mg	Naprosyn by Teva	00093-0147	NSAID
93 <> 147	Tab, Light Red, Round	Naproxen 250 mg	Naprosyn by Heartland	61392-0289	NSAID
93 <> 147	Tab, Light Red, Round	Naproxen 250 mg	Naprosyn by Brightstone	62939-8311	NSAID
93 <> 148	Tab, Peach, Oval	Naproxen 375 mg	Naprosyn by Otsuka	46602-0004	NSAID
93 <> 148	Tab, Peach, Oval	Naproxen 375 mg	Naprosyn by Teva	00093-0148 Discontinued	NSAID
93 <> 148	Tab, Peach, Oval	Naproxen 375 mg	Naprosyn by Heartland	61392-0292	NSAID
93 <> 148	Tab, Peach, Oval	Naproxen 375 mg	Naprosyn by Brightstone	62939-8321	NSAID
93 <> 149	Tab, Light Red, Oval	Naproxen 500 mg	Naprosyn by Brightstone	62939-8331	NSAID
93 <> 149	Tab, Light Red, Oval	Naproxen 500 mg	Naprosyn by Teva	55953-0399	NSAID
93 <> 149	Tab, Light Red, Oval	Naproxen 500 mg	Naprosyn by Heartland	61392-0295	NSAID
93 <> 149	Tab, Light Red, Oval	Naproxen 500 mg	Naprosyn by Teva	00093-0149	NSAID
93 <> 149	Tab, Light Red, Oval	Naproxen 500 mg	Naprosyn by Vangard	00615-3563	NSAID
93 <> 149	Tab, Light Red, Oval	Naproxen 500 mg	Naprosyn by Ivax	00182-8241 Discontinued	NSAID
93 <> 15	Tab, White, Oval, Film Coated	Nabumetone 500 mg	Relafen by UDL	51079-0989	NSAID
93 <> 15	Tab, White, Oval, Film Coated	Nabumetone 500 mg	Relafen by Teva	00093-1015	NSAID
93 <> 154	Tab, White, Oval, Film Coated	Ticlopidine HCl 250 mg	Ticlid by Pharmascience	Canadian DIN 02243327	Anticoagulant
93 <> 154	Tab, White, Oval, Film Coated	Ticlopidine HCl 250 mg	Ticlid by UDL	51079-0920	Anticoagulant
93 <> 154	Tab, White, Oval, Film Coated	Ticlopidine HCl 250 mg	Ticlid by Teva	00093-0154	Anticoagulant
93 <> 155	Tab, White to Off-White, Cap Shaped	Topiramate 25 mg	Topamax by Teva	00093-0155	Anticonvulsant
93 <> 16	Tab, Beige, Oval, Film Coated	Nabumetone 750 mg	Relafen by Teva	00093-1016	NSAID
93 <> 173	Tab, White, Round, Film Coated	Leflunomide 10 mg	Arava by Teva	00093-0173	Antiarthritic
93 <> 174	Tab, Yellow, Round, Film-Coated	Leflunomide 20 mg	Arava by Teva	00093-0174	Antiarthritic
93 <> 1893	Tab, Blue, Oval, Film Coated	Etodolac 500 mg	Lodine by Teva	00093-1893	NSAID
93 <> 199	Tab, Peach, Round, Scored, Mottled	Venlafaxine HCl 25 mg	Effexor by Teva	00093-0199	Antidepressant
93 <> 2158	Tab, White, Round, Scored, 9 over 3 <> 2158	Trimethoprim 100 mg	Proloprim by Teva	00093-2158	Antibiotic
93 <> 220	Tab, White, Round, Film-Coated	Bicalutamide 50 mg	Casodex by Novopharm	Canadian DIN 02270226	Antiandrogen
93 <> 220	Tab, White to Off White, Round	Bicalutamide 50 mg	Casodex by Teva	00093-0220	Antiandrogen
93 <> 221	Tab, Dark Yellow, Round, Film Coated	Risperidone 0.25 mg	Risperdal by Teva	00093-0221	Antipsychotic
93 <> 222	Tab, White to Off-White, Cap Shaped, Film Coated	Sumatriptan Succinate 25 mg	Imitrex by Teva	00093-0222	Antimigraine
93 <> 223	Tab, White to Off-White, Cap Shaped, Film Coated	Sumatriptan Succinate 50 mg	Imitrex by Teva	00093-0223	Antimigraine
93 <> 2238	Tab, White, Cap Shaped, Scored	Cephalexin 250 mg	Keflex by Teva	00093-2238	Antibiotic
93 <> 224	Tab, Light Pink, Cap Shaped, Film Coated	Sumatriptan Succinate 100 mg	Imitrex by Teva	00093-0224	Antimigraine
93 <> 2240	Tab, White, Cap Shaped, Scored	Cephalexin 500 mg	Keflex by Teva	00093-2240	Antibiotic
93 <> 225	Tab, Reddish Brown, Round, Film Coated	Risperidone 0.5 mg	Risperdal by Teva	00093-0225	Antipsychotic
93 <> 2263	Tab, Off-White, Cap Shaped, Film Coated	Amoxicillin 500 mg	Amoxil by Novopharm	00093-2263	Antibiotic
93 <> 2263	Tab, Off-White, Cap Shaped, Film Coated	Amoxicillin 500 mg	Amoxil by Teva	55953-2263	Antibiotic
93 <> 2267	Tab, White to Off-White, Cap Shaped	Amoxicillin 125 mg	Amoxil by Teva	00093-2267	Antibiotic
93 <> 2268	Tab, White to Off-White, Oblong	Amoxicillin 250 mg	Amoxil by Teva	00093-2268	Antibiotic
93 <> 2270	Tab, Mottled Pink, Oval, Chewable	Amoxicillin 200 mg, Clavulanate Potassium 28.5 mg	Augmentin by Teva	00093-2270	Antibiotic
93 <> 2272	Tab, Mottled Pink, Oval, Chewable	Amoxicillin 400 mg, Clavulanate Potassium 57 mg	Augmentin by Teva	00093-2272	Antibiotic
93 <> 2274	Tab, White, Oblong	Amoxicillin 500 mg, Clavulanate Potassium 125 mg	Augmentin by Teva	00093-2274	Antibiotic
93 <> 2275	Tab, White, Oblong, Scored	Amoxicillin 875 mg, Clavulanate Potassium 125 mg	Augmentin by Teva	00093-2275	Antibiotic
93 <> 233	Tab, White, Round, Film Coated	Ondansetron HCl 4 mg	Zofran by Teva	00093-0233	Antiemetic
93 <> 24	Tab, White, Oval, Film Coated, Extended Release	Oxycodone HCl 10 mg	OxyContin by Teva	00093-0024 Discontinued	Analgesic; C II

ID FRONT <> BACK	DESCRIPTION FRONT <> BACK	INGREDIENT & STRENGTH	BRAND (or Generic Equiv.) by FIRM	NDC#	CLASS; SCH.
93 <> 308	Tab	Clemastine Fumarate 2.5 mg	by H J Harkins Co	52959-0501	Antihistamine
93 <> 31	Tab, Pink, Oval, Film Coated, Extended Release	Oxycodone HCl 20 mg	OxyContin by Teva	00093-0031 Discontinued	Analgesic; C II
93 <> 314	Tab, White, Round, Film Coated	Ketorolac Tromethamine 10 mg	Toradol by Murfreesboro	51129-1604	NSAID
93 <> 314	Tab, White, Round, Film Coated	Ketorolac Tromethamine 10 mg	Toradol by Teva	00093-0314	NSAID
93 <> 314	Tab, White, Round, Film Coated	Ketorolac Tromethamine 10 mg	Toradol by Southwood	58016-0247	NSAID
93 <> 32	Tab, Yellow, Oval, Film Coated, Extended Release	Oxycodone HCl 40 mg	OxyContin by Teva	00093-0032 Discontinued	Analgesic; C II
93 <> 33	Tab, Green, Oval, Film Coated, Extended Release	Oxycodone HCl 80 mg	OxyContin by Teva	00093-0033 Discontinued	Analgesic; C II
93 <> 39	Tab, White to Off-White, Diamond Shaped, Scored, 9 / 3	Lamotrigine 25 mg	Lamictal by Teva	00093-0039	Anticonvulsant
93 <> 4059	Tab, White, Oval, Scored, 9 / 3	Cefadroxil 1000 mg	Duricef by Teva	00093-4059	Antibiotic
93 <> 463	Tab, Peach, Diamond Shaped, Scored, 9 / 3	Lamotrigine 100 mg	Lamictal by Teva	00093-0463	Anticonvulsant
93 <> 4740	Tab, Light Beige, Cap-Shaped	Citalopram HBr 10 mg	Celexa by Teva	00093-4740	Antidepressant
93 <> 4741	Tab, Light Pink, Cap-Shaped, Scored, 9 / 3	Citalopram HBr 20 mg	Celexa by Teva	00093-4741	Antidepressant
93 <> 4742	Tab, White to Off-White, Cap-Shaped, Scored, 9 / 3	Citalopram HBr 40 mg	Celexa by Teva	00093-4742	Antidepressant
93 <> 48	Tab, White to Off-White, Oval	Metformin HCl 500 mg	Glucophage by Teva	00093-1048	Antidiabetic
93 <> 49	Tab, White to Off-White, Oval	Metformin HCl 850 mg	Glucophage by Teva	00093-1049	Antidiabetic
93 <> 51	Tab, White, Oval, Film Coated	Carvedilol 3.125 mg	Coreg by Teva	00093-0051	Antihypertensive
93 <> 5124	Tab, Light Yellow, Triangular, Coated	Benazepril HCl 5 mg	Lotensin by Teva	00093-5124	Antihypertensive
93 <> 5125	Tab, Mustard Yellow, Triangular, Coated	Benazepril HCl 10 mg	Lotensin by Teva	00093-5125	Antihypertensive
93 <> 5126	Tab, Pink, Triangular, Coated	Benazepril HCl 20 mg	Lotensin by Teva	00093-5126	Antihypertensive
93 <> 5127	Tab, Pink to Light Red, Triangular, Coated	Benazepril HCl 40 mg	Lotensin by Teva	00093-5127	Antihypertensive
93 <> 5140	Tab, White to Off-White, Round	Alendronate Sodium 5 mg	Fosamax by Teva	00093-5140	Antiosteoporosis
93 <> 5141	Tab, White to Off-White, Round	Alendronate Sodium 10 mg	Fosamax by Teva	00093-5141	Antiosteoporosis
93 <> 5142	Tab, White to Off-White, Oval	Alendronate Sodium 40 mg	Fosamax by Teva	00093-5142	Antiosteoporosis
93 <> 5150	Tab, Pink, Oval, Scored	Moexipril 15 mg	Univasc by Teva	00093-5150	Antihypertensive
93 <> 5157	Tab, White, Round	Lisinopril 30 mg	Prinivil by Teva	00093-5157 Discontinued	Antihypertensive
93 <> 5171	Tab, White to Off-White, Oval	Alendronate Sodium 70 mg	Fosamax by Teva	00093-5171	Antiosteoporosis
93 <> 5172	Tab, White to Off-White, Pillow-Shaped	Alendronate Sodium 35 mg	Fosamax by Teva	00093-5172	Antiosteoporosis
93 <> 5194	Tab, White, Oval	Penicillin V Potassium 250 mg	V-Cillin K by Teva	00093-5194	Antibiotic
93 <> 5195	Tab, White, Oval	Penicillin V Potassium 500 mg	V-cillin K by Teva	00093-5195 Discontinued	Antibiotic
93 <> 5213	Tab, Yellow, Cap Shaped, Film Coated, Scored, 9 / 3	Moexipril HCl 7.5 mg, Hydrochlorothiazide 12.5 mg	Uniretic by Teva	00093-5213	Antihypertensive; Diuretic
93 <> 5214	Tab, White, Cap Shaped, Film Coated, Scored, 9 / 3	Moexipril HCl 15 mg, Hydrochlorothiazide 12.5 mg	Uniretic by Teva	00093-5214	Antihypertensive; Diuretic
93 <> 5215	Tab, Yellow, Cap Shaped, Film Coated, Scored, 9 / 3	Moexipril HCl 15 mg, Hydrochlorothiazide 25 mg	Uniretic by Teva	00093-5215	Antihypertensive; Diuretic
93 <> 5275	Tab, Blue, Round	Dexmethylphenidate HCl 2.5 mg	Focalin by Teva	00093-5275	Stimulant; C II
93 <> 5276	Tab, Yellow, Round	Dexmethylphenidate HCl 5 mg	Focalin by Teva	00093-5276	Stimulant; C II
93 <> 5277	Tab, White to Off-White, Round	Dexmethylphenidate HCl 10 mg	Focalin by Teva	00093-5277	Stimulant; C II
93 <> 5282	Tab, White, Round, Film Coated	Ropinirole HCl 0.25 mg	Requip by Teva	00093-5282	Antiparkinson
93 <> 5283	Tab, Yellow, Round, Film Coated	Ropinirole HCl 0.5 mg	Requip by Teva	00093-5283	Antiparkinson
93 <> 5284	Tab, Green, Round, Film Coated	Ropinirole HCl 1 mg	Requip by Teva	00093-5284	Antiparkinson
93 <> 5285	Tab, Pink, Round, Film-Coated	Ropinirole HCl 2 mg	Requip by Teva	00093-5285	Antiparkinson
93 <> 5286	Tab, Purple, Round, Film-Coated	Ropinirole HCl 3 mg	Requip by Teva	00093-5286	Antiparkinson
93 <> 5287	Tab, Beige, Round, Film-Coated	Ropinirole HCl 4 mg	Requip by Teva	00093-5287	Antiparkinson
93 <> 5288	Tab, Blue, Round, Film Coated	Ropinirole HCl 5 mg	Requip by Teva	00093-5288	Antiparkinson
93 <> 536	Tab, White, Oval, Film Coated	Naproxen 275 mg	Anaprox by Brightstone	62939-8431	NSAID
93 <> 536	Tab, White, Oval, Film Coated	Naproxen 275 mg	Anaprox by Ivax	00182-1974	NSAID
93 <> 536	Tab, White, Oval, Film Coated	Naproxen 275 mg	Anaprox by Teva	00093-0536	NSAID

ID FRONT <> BACK	DESCRIPTION FRONT <> BACK	INGREDIENT & STRENGTH	BRAND (or Generic Equiv.) by FIRM	NDC#	CLASS; SCH.
93 <> 536	Tab, White, Oval, Film Coated	Naproxen 275 mg	Anaprox by Kaiser	00179-1206	NSAID
93 <> 5360	Tab, White to Off White, Oval, Film Coated	Ursodiol 250 mg	Urso by Teva	00093-5360	Gastrointestinal
93 <> 5361	Tab, White to Off White, Oval, Film Coated, Scored	Ursodiol 500 mg	Urso Forte by Teva	00093-5361	Gastrointestinal
93 <> 537	Tab, White to Off-White, Oval	Naproxen 550 mg	Anaprox DS by Kaiser	00179-1223	NSAID
93 <> 537	Tab, White to Off-White, Oval	Naproxen 550 mg	Anaprox DS by Teva	00093-0537	NSAID
93 <> 537	Tab, White to Off-White, Oval	Naproxen 550 mg	Anaprox DS by Brightstone	62939-8441	NSAID
93 <> 5450	Tab, White, Round, Ex Release	Alprazolam 0.5 mg	Xanax XR by Teva	00093-5450	Antianxiety; C IV
93 <> 5451	Tab, Yellow, Round, Ex Release	Alprazolam 1 mg	Xanax XR by Teva	00093-5451	Antianxiety; C IV
93 <> 5452	Tab, Blue, Oval, Ex Release	Alprazolam 2 mg	Xanax XR by Teva	00093-5452	Antianxiety; C IV
93 <> 5453	Tab, Green, Round, Ex Release	Alprazolam 3 mg	Xanax XR by Teva	00093-5453	Antianxiety; C IV
93 <> 5510	Tab, Round, Pale Yellow to Buff, Scored	Mercaptopurine 50 mg	Purinethol by Teva	00093-5510	Antineoplastic
93 <> 56	Tab, Yellow, Cap Shaped, Film Coated, Scored, 9 / 3	Fluvoxamine Maleate 50 mg	Luvox by Teva	00093-0056	OCD
93 <> 57	Tab, Light Pink to Brick, Cap Shaped, Film Coated, Scored, 9 / 3	Fluvoxamine Maleate 100 mg	Luvox by Teva	00093-0057	OCD
93 <> 576	Tab, Blue, Round	Lovastatin 20 mg	Mevacor by Teva	00093-0576	Antihyperlipidemic
93 <> 58	Tab, White, Oval	Tramadol HCl 50 mg	Ultram by Teva	00093-0058	Analgesic
93 <> 663	Tab, White, Oval, Film Coated	Indapamide 1.25 mg	Lozol by Teva	00093-0663	Diuretic
93 <> 688	Tab, White to Off-White, Round, Chewable	Lamotrigine 5 mg	Lamictal by Teva	00093-0688	Anticonvulsant
93 <> 711	Tab, Coated	Flurbiprofen 100 mg	by Quality Care	60346-0968	NSAID
93 <> 7113	Tab, Mottled Peach, Oblong, Scored, 93 to left of Score <> 7113	Nefazodone HCl 150 mg	Serzone by Teva	00093-7113	Antidepressant
93 <> 7114	Tab, Yellow, Round, Film Coated, Scored, 9 / 3	Paroxetine HCl 10 mg	Paxil by Teva	00093-7114 Discontinued	Antidepressant
93 <> 7115	Tab, Pink, Round, Film Coated, Scored, 9 / 3	Paroxetine HCl 20 mg	Paxil by Teva	00093-7115 Discontinued	Antidepressant
93 <> 7115	Tab, Pink, Round, Film Coated, Scored, 9 / 3	Paroxetine HCl 20 mg	Paxil by UDL	51079-0774	Antidepressant
93 <> 7116	Tab, Blue, Round, Film Coated	Paroxetine HCl 30 mg	Paxil by Teva	00093-7116 Discontinued	Antidepressant
93 <> 7121	Tab, Green, Round, Film Coated	Paroxetine HCl 40 mg	Paxil by Teva	00093-7121	Antidepressant
93 <> 7121	Tab, Green, Round, Film Coated	Paroxetine HCl 40 mg	Paxil by UDL	51079-0775 Discontinued	Antidepressant
93 <> 7127	Tab, White to Off-White, Oval, Scored	Torsemide 5 mg	Demadex by Teva Pharmaceuticals	00093-7127 Discontinued	Diuretic
93 <> 7128	Tab, White to Off-White, Oval, Scored, 9 over 3 <> 7128	Torsemide 10 mg	Demadex by Teva Pharmaceuticals	00093-7128 Discontinued	Diuretic
93 <> 7128	Tab, White to Off-White, Oval, Scored, 9 over 3 <> 7128	Torsemide 10 mg	Demadex by UDL	51079-0025	Diuretic
93 <> 7129	Tab, White to Off-White, Oval, Scored, 9 over 3 <> 7129	Torsemide 20 mg	Demadex by UDL	51079-0026	Diuretic
93 <> 7129	Tab, White to Off-White, Oval, Scored, 9 over 3 <> 7129	Torsemide 20 mg	Demadex by Teva Pharmaceuticals	00093-7129 Discontinued	Diuretic
93 <> 7130	Tab, White to Off-White, Oval, Scored	Torsemide 100 mg	Demadex by Teva Pharmaceuticals	00093-7130 Discontinued	Diuretic
93 <> 7146	Tab, Pink, Mottled, Oval, Film Coated	Azithromycin 250 mg	Zithromax by Teva	00093-7146	Antibiotic
93 <> 7147	Tab, White to Off-White, Cap Shaped, Film Coated	Azithromycin 600 mg	Zithromax by Teva	00093-7147	Antibiotic
93 <> 7152	Tab, Light Yellow, Round, Film Coated	Simvastatin 5 mg	Zocor by Teva	00093-7152	Antihyperlipidemic
93 <> 7153	Tab, Light Pink, Round, Film Coated	Simvastatin 10 mg	Zocor by Teva	00093-7153	Antihyperlipidemic
93 <> 7153	Tab, Light Pink, Round, Film Coated	Simvastatin 10 mg	Zocor by UDL	51079-0454	Antihyperlipidemic
93 <> 7154	Tab, Tan, Round, Film Coated	Simvastatin 20 mg	Zocor by UDL	51079-0455	Antihyperlipidemic
93 <> 7154	Tab, Tan, Round, Film Coated	Simvastatin 20 mg	Zocor by Teva	00093-7154	Antihyperlipidemic
93 <> 7155	Tab, Red, Round, Film Coated	Simvastatin 40 mg	Zocor by Teva	00093-7155	Antihyperlipidemic

ID FRONT <> BACK	DESCRIPTION FRONT <> BACK	INGREDIENT & STRENGTH	BRAND (or Generic Equiv.) by FIRM	NDC#	CLASS; SCH.
93 <> 7155	Tab, Red, Round, Film Coated	Simvastatin 40 mg	Zocor by UDL	51079-0456	Antihyperlipidemic
93 <> 7156	Tab, Brick Red, Cap Shaped, Film Coated	Simvastatin 80 mg	Zocor by Teva	00093-7156	Antihyperlipidemic
93 <> 7157	Tab, Yellow, Oval, Film Coated	Clarithromycin 250 mg	Biaxin by Teva	00093-7157	Antibiotic
93 <> 7157	Tab, Yellow, Oval, Film Coated	Clarithromycin 250 mg	Biaxin by UDL	51079-0361 Discontinued	Antibiotic
93 <> 7158	Tab, Light Yellow, Oval, Film Coated	Clarithromycin 500 mg	Biaxin by Teva	00093-7158	Antibiotic
93 <> 7158	Tab, Light Yellow, Oval, Film Coated	Clarithromycin 500 mg	Biaxin by UDL	51079-0362 Discontinued	Antibiotic
93 <> 7159	Tab, Mottled Green, Cap Shaped, Scored, 9 over 3	Pergolide Mesylate 0.25 mg	Permax by UDL	51079-0143 Discontinued	Antiparkinson
93 <> 7159	Tab, Green, Cap Shaped, Scored, 9 over 3	Pergolide Mesylate 0.25 mg	Permax by Teva	00093-7159	Antiparkinson
93 <> 7160	Tab, Ivory, Cap Shaped, Scored, 9 over 3	Pergolide Mesylate 0.05 mg	Permax by Teva	00093-7160 Discontinued	Antiparkinson
93 <> 7161	Tab, Pink, Cap Shaped, Scored, 9 over 3	Pergolide Mesylate 1 mg	Permax by Teva	00093-7161	Antiparkinson
93 <> 7161	Tab, Mottled Pink, Cap Shaped, Scored, 9 over 3	Pergolide Mesylate 1 mg	Permax by UDL	51079-0144 Discontinued	Antiparkinson
93 <> 7167	Tab, White to Off-White, Round	Amlodipine Besylate 5 mg	Norvasc by Teva	00093-7167	Antihypertensive
93 <> 7168	Tab, White to Off-White, Round	Amlodipine Besylate 10 mg	Norvasc by Teva	00093-7168	Antihypertensive
93 <> 7169	Tab, Pink, Mottled, Oval, Film Coated	Azithromycin 500 mg	Zithromax by Teva	00093-7169	Antibiotic
93 <> 7172	Tab, Gray, Oval, Ex Release	Etodolac 500 mg	Lodine XL by Teva	00093-7172	NSAID
93 <> 7173	Tab, White to Off-White, Oval, Film Coated, Scored	Gabapentin 600 mg	Neurontin by Teva	00093-7173 Discontinued	Anticonvulsant
93 <> 7174	Tab, White to Off-White, Oval, Film Coated, Scored	Gabapentin 800 mg	Neurontin by Teva	00093-7174	Anticonvulsant
93 <> 7175	Tab, Light Green, Elliptical, Film-Coated, Scored	Sertraline HCl 25 mg	Zoloft by Teva	00093-7175	Antidepressant
93 <> 7176	Tab, Light Blue, Elliptical, Film-Coated, Scored	Sertraline HCl 50 mg	Zoloft by Teva	00093-7176 Discontinued	Antidepressant
93 <> 7178	Tab, Light Pink to Mottled Pink, Oblong	Nefazodone HCl 50 mg	Serzone by Teva	00093-7178	Antidepressant
93 <> 7180	Tab, Light Yellow, Oval, Film Coated	Ofloxacin 200 mg	Floxin by Teva	00093-7180	Antibiotic
93 <> 7181	Tab, White to Off White, Oval, Film Coated	Ofloxacin 300 mg	Floxin by Teva	00093-7181	Antibiotic
93 <> 7182	Tab, Pale Gold, Oval, Film Coated	Ofloxacin 400 mg	Floxin by Teva	00093-7182	Antibiotic
93 <> 7188	Tab, Blue, Oval, Scored, Film Coated	Fluoxetine HCl 10 mg	Prozac by Teva	00093-7188	Antidepressant
93 <> 72	Tab, White, Cap Shaped, Film Coated	Fluvoxamine Maleate 25 mg	Luvox by Teva Pharmaceuticals	00093-0072 Discontinued	OCD
93 <> 7201	Tab, Light Yellow, Round	Pravastatin Sodium 20 mg	Pravachol by Teva	00093-7201	Antihyperlipidemic
93 <> 7201	Tab, Light Yellow, Round	Pravastatin Sodium 20 mg	Pravachol by UDL	51079-0458	Antihyperlipidemic
93 <> 7202	Tab, Light Green, Round	Pravastatin Sodium 40 mg	Pravachol by UDL	51079-0782 Discontinued	Antihyperlipidemic
93 <> 7202	Tab, Light Green, Round	Pravastatin Sodium 40 mg	Pravachol by Teva Pharmaceuticals	00093-7202 Discontinued	Antihyperlipidemic
93 <> 7206	Tab, Round, Yellow, Scored	Mirtazapine 15 mg	Remeron by Teva	00093-7206	Antidepressant
93 <> 7207	Tab, Round, Scored, Red-Brown	Mirtazapine 30 mg	Remeron by Teva	00093-7207	Antidepressant
93 <> 7208	Tab, White to Off-White, Round	Mirtazapine 45 mg	Remeron by Teva	00093-7208	Antidepressant
93 <> 7212	Tab, Brick Red, Oval, Mottled, Extended Release	Metformin HCl 750 mg	Glucophage by Teva	00093-7212	Antidiabetic
93 <> 7214	Tab, White to Off-White, Oval, Scored, 9 / 3 <> 72 / 14	Metformin 1000 mg	Glucophage by Teva	00093-7214	Antidiabetic
93 <> 7215	Tab, Pink, Cap Shaped, Mottled	Metolazone 2.5 mg	Zaroxolyn by Teva	00093-7215 Discontinued	Diuretic

ID FRONT <> BACK	DESCRIPTION FRONT <> BACK	INGREDIENT & STRENGTH	BRAND (or Generic Equiv.) by FIRM	NDC#	CLASS; SCH.
93 <> 7216	Tab, Mottled Blue, Cap Shaped	Metolazone 5 mg	Zaroxolyn by Teva	00093-7216 Discontinued	Diuretic
93 <> 7217	Tab, Yellow, Round	Metolazone 10 mg	Zaroxolyn by Teva	00093-7217 Discontinued	Diuretic
93 <> 7219	Tab, Yellow, Cap Shaped	Topiramate 100 mg	Topamax by Teva	00093-7219	Anticonvulsant
93 <> 7220	Tab, Salmon, Cap Shaped	Topiramate 200 mg	Topamax by Teva	00093-7220	Anticonvulsant
93 <> 7221	Tab, White, Oval	Prenatal Optima Advance	Prenate Advance by Teva	00093-7221	Vitamin
93 <> 7222	Tab, White to Off White, Rectangular, Scored, 9 score 3 <> 72 score 22	Fosinopril Sodium 10 mg	Monopril by Teva	00093-7222	Antihypertensive
93 <> 7223	Tab, White to Off White, Cap Shaped	Fosinopril Sodium 20 mg	Monopril by Teva	00093-7223	Antihypertensive
93 <> 7224	Tab, White to Off White, Round	Fosinopril Sodium 40 mg	Monopril by Teva	00093-7224	Antihypertensive
93 <> 7230	Tab, White to Off-White, Pillow Shaped	Cilostazol 50 mg	Pletal by Teva	00093-7230	Antiplatelet
93 <> 7231	Tab, White to Off-White, Round	Cilostazol 100 mg	Pletal by Teva	00093-7231	Antiplatelet
93 <> 7231	Tab, White to Off-White, Round	Cilostazol 100 mg	Pletal by UDL	51079-0424	Antiplatelet
93 <> 7232	Tab, Pink, Round, Coated	Ribavirin 200 mg	Copegus by Teva	00093-7232	Antiviral
93 <> 7234	Tab, Cap Shaped, Mottled Yellow	Meloxicam 7.5 mg	Mobic by Teva	00093-7234 Discontinued	NSAID
93 <> 7236	Tab, Yellow, Round, Film Coated	Ondansetron HCl 8 mg	Zofran by Teva	00093-7236	Antiemetic
93 <> 7240	Tab, White to Off-White, Round, Film Coated	Risperidone 1 mg	Risperdal by Teva	00093-7240	Antipsychotic
93 <> 7241	Tab, Orange, Round, Film Coated	Risperidone 2 mg	Risperdal by Teva	00093-7241	Antipsychotic
93 <> 7242	Tab, Yellow, Round, Film Coated	Risperidone 3 mg	Risperdal by Teva	00093-7242	Antipsychotic
93 <> 7243	Tab, Green, Round, Film Coated	Risperidone 4 mg	Risperdal by Teva	00093-7243	Antipsychotic
93 <> 7244	Tab, Yellow, Oval, Film Coated, Extended Release	Clarithromycin 500 mg	Biaxin XL by Teva	00093-7244	Antibiotic
93 <> 7247	Tab, Cream, Diamond Shaped, Scored, 9 / 3	Lamotrigine 150 mg	Lamictal by Teva	00093-7247	Anticonvulsant
93 <> 7248	Tab, Blue, Diamond Shaped, Scored, 9 / 3	Lamotrigine 200 mg	Lamictal by Teva	00093-7248	Anticonvulsant
93 <> 7251	Tab, Peach, Cap Shaped, Film Coated	Fexofenadine HCl 30 mg	Allegra by Teva	00093-7251	Antihistamine
93 <> 7252	Tab, Peach, Round, Film Coated	Fexofenadine HCl 60 mg	Allegra by Teva	00093-7252	Antihistamine
93 <> 7253	Tab, Peach, Round, Film Coated	Fexofenadine HCl 180 mg	Allegra by Teva	00093-7253	Antihistamine
93 <> 7254	Tab, Pink, Mottled, Round, Scored, 9 / 3 <> 72 / 54	Glimepiride 1 mg	Amaryl by Teva	00093-7254	Antidiabetic
93 <> 7254	Tan, Mottled Pink, Round tablet, Scored, 9 / 3 <> 72 / 54	Glimepiride 1 mg	Novo-Glimepiride by Novopharm	Canadian DIN 02273756	Antidiabetic
93 <> 7255	Tab, Mottled Green, Round, Bisected, 9 / 3 <> 72 / 55	Glimepiride 2 mg	Novo-Glimepiride by Novopharm	Canadian DIN 02273764	Antidiabetic
93 <> 7255	Tab, Green, Mottled, Round, Scored, 9 / 3 <> 72 / 55	Glimepiride 2 mg	Amaryl by Teva	00093-7255	Antidiabetic
93 <> 7256	Tab, Light Blue, Mottled, Round, Scored, 9 / 3 <> 72 / 56	Glimepiride 4 mg	Amaryl by Teva	00093-7256	Antidiabetic
93 <> 7256	Tab, Mottled Blue, Round, Bisected, 9 / 3 <> 72 / 56	Glimepiride 4 mg	Novo-Glimepiride by Novopharm	Canadian DIN 02273772	Antidiabetic
93 <> 7258	Tab, Blue, Cap Shaped, Film Coated	Valacyclovir HCl 500 mg	Valtrex by Teva Pharmaceuticals	00093-7258	Antiviral
93 <> 7259	Tab, Blue, Cap Shaped, Film Coated, Scored	Valacyclovir HCl 1000 mg	Valtrex by Teva Pharmaceuticals	00093-7259	Antiviral
93 <> 7260	Tab, Pale Yellow, Oval, Film Coated	Glyburide 1.25 mg, Metformin HCl 250 mg	Glucovance by Teva	00093-7260	Antidiabetic
93 <> 7261	Tab, Pale Orange, Oval, Film Coated	Glyburide 2.5 mg, Metformin HCl 500 mg	Glucovance by Teva	00093-7261	Antidiabetic
93 <> 7262	Tab, Yellow, Film Coated, Yellow	Glyburide 5 mg, Metformin HCl 500 mg	Glucovance by Teva	00093-7262 Discontinued	Antidiabetic
93 <> 7267	Tab, White, Oval, Extended Release	Metformin HCl 500 mg	Glucophage by Teva	00093-7267	Antidiabetic
93 <> 7270	Tab, Off-White to Mottled Grey, Oval	Pravastatin Sodium 80 mg	Pravachol by Teva	00093-7270	Antihyperlipidemic
93 <> 7281	Tab, Brown to Dark Brown, Cap Shaped, Film Coated, Scored, 9 / 3 <> 72 / 81	Oxcarbazepine 150 mg	Trileptal by Teva	00093-7281	Anticonvulsant
93 <> 7282	Tab, Brown to Dark Brown, Cap Shaped, Film Coated, Scored, 9 / 3 <> 72 / 82	Oxcarbazepine 300 mg	Trileptal by Teva	00093-7282	Anticonvulsant

ID FRONT <> BACK	DESCRIPTION FRONT <> BACK	INGREDIENT & STRENGTH	BRAND (or Generic Equiv.) by FIRM	NDC#	CLASS; SCH.
93 <> 7283	Tab, Brown to Dark Brown, Cap Shaped, Film Coated, Scored, 9 / 3 <> 72 / 83	Oxcarbazepine 600 mg	Trileptal by Teva	00093-7283	Anticonvulsant
93 <> 7285	Tab, Blue, Oblong, Film Coated, Scored, 9 / 3	Levetiracetam 250 mg	Keppra by Teva	00093-7285	Anticonvulsant
93 <> 7286	Tab, Yellow, Oblong, Film Coated, Scored, 9 / 3	Levetiracetam 500 mg	Keppra by Teva	00093-7286	Anticonvulsant
93 <> 7287	Tab, Orange, Oblong, Film Coated, Scored, 9 / 3	Levetiracetam 750 mg	Keppra by Teva	00093-7287	Anticonvulsant
93 <> 7294	Tab, White to Off-White, Round	Terbinafine HCl 250 mg	Lamisil by Teva	00093-7294	Antifungal
93 <> 7295	Tab, White, Oval, Film Coated	Carvedilol 12.5 mg	Coreg by Teva	00093-7295	Antihypertensive
93 <> 7296	Tab, White, Oval, Film Coated	Carvedilol 25 mg	Coreg by Teva	00093-7296	Antihypertensive
93 <> 7299	Tab, Pillow Shaped, Mottled Yellow	Meloxicam 15 mg	Mobic by Teva	00093-7299 Discontinued	NSAID
93 <> 73	Tab, Pink, Round, Film Coated	Zolpidem Tartrate 5 mg	Ambien by Teva	00093-0073	Sedative/Hypnotic; C IV
93 <> 7301	Tab, White to Off-White, Round, Orally Disintegrating	Ondansetron 4 mg	Zofran ODT by Teva	00093-7301	Antiemetic
93 <> 7302	Tab, White to Off-White, Round, Orally Disintegrating	Ondansetron 8 mg	Zofran ODT by Teva	00093-7302	Antiemetic
93 <> 7303	Tab, White to Off-White, Round	Mirtazapine 15 mg	Remeron SolTab by Teva	00093-7303	Antidepressant
93 <> 7304	Tab, White to Off-White, Round	Mirtazapine 30 mg	Remeron SolTab by Teva	00093-7304	Antidepressant
93 <> 7305	Tab, White to Off-White, Round	Mirtazapine 45 mg	Remeron SolTab by Teva	00093-7305	Antidepressant
93 <> 7316	Tab, White to Off-White, Cap Shaped, Scored, 9/3 <> 7316	Desmopressin Acetate 0.1 mg	DDAVP by Teva	00093-7316	Antidiuretic
93 <> 7317	Tab, White to Off-White, Round, Scored, 9/3 <> 7317	Desmopressin Acetate 0.2 mg	DDAVP by Teva	00093-7317	Antidiuretic
93 <> 7317	Tab, White to Off-White, Round, Scored, 9/3 <> 7317	Desmopressin Acetate 0.2 mg	DDAVP by UDL	51079-0446	Antidiuretic
93 <> 7325	Tab, Mottled Salmon, Cap Shaped, Scored, 9 / 3 <> 7325	Trandolapril 1 mg	Mavik by Teva	00093-7325	Antihypertensive
93 <> 7326	Tab, Mottled Yellow, Cap Shaped	Trandolapril 2 mg	Mavik by Teva	00093-7326	Antihypertensive
93 <> 7327	Tab, Mottled Rose, Cap Shaped	Trandolapril 4 mg	Mavik by Teva	00093-7327	Antihypertensive
93 <> 7330	Tab, Yellow, Round, Film Coated	Fenofibrate 54 mg	Lofibra by Gate	57844-0691	Antihyperlipidemic
93 <> 7331	Tab, White to Off-White, Oval, Film Coated	Fenofibrate 160 mg	Lofibra by Gate	57844-0692	Antihyperlipidemic
93 <> 7340	Tab, White, Oval, Ex Release	Divalproex Sodium 500 mg	Depakote ER by Teva	00093-7340	Anticonvulsant
93 <> 7355	Tab, Blue, Cap-Shaped	Finasteride 5 mg	Proscar by Teva	00093-7355	Antiandrogen
93 <> 7364	Tab, Light Green, Oval, Film Coated	Losartan Potassium 25 mg	Cozaar by Teva Pharmaceuticals	00093-7364	Antihypertensive
93 <> 7365	Tab, Green, Oval, Film Coated	Losartan Potassium 50 mg	Cozaar by Teva Pharmaceuticals	00093-7365	Antihypertensive
93 <> 7366	Tab, Dark Green, Oval, Film Coated	Losartan Potassium 100 mg	Cozaar by Teva Pharmaceuticals	00093-7366	Antihypertensive
93 <> 7367	Tab, Yellow, Oval, Film Coated	Hydrochlorothiazide 12.5 mg, Losartan Potassium 50 mg	Hyzaar by Teva Pharmaceuticals	00093-7367	Diuretic; Antihypertensive
93 <> 7368	Tab, Light Yellow, Oval, Film Coated	Hydrochlorothiazide 25 mg, Losartan Potassium 100 mg	Hyzaar by Teva Pharmaceuticals	00093-7368	Diuretic; Antihypertensive
93 <> 7369	Tab, White to Off-White, Oval, Film Coated	Hydrochlorothiazide 12.5 mg, Losartan Potassium 100 mg	Hyzaar by Teva Pharmaceuticals	00093-7369	Diuretic; Antihypertensive
93 <> 7380	Tab, Peach, Round, Scored, Mottled	Venlafaxine HCl 37.5 mg	Effexor by Teva	00093-7380	Antidepressant
93 <> 7381	Tab, Peach, Round, Scored, Mottled	Venlafaxine HCl 50 mg	Effexor by Teva	00093-7381	Antidepressant
93 <> 7382	Tab, Peach, Round, Scored, Mottled	Venlafaxine HCl 75 mg	Effexor by Teva	00093-7382	Antidepressant
93 <> 7383	Tab, Peach, Round, Scored, Mottled	Venlafaxine HCl 100 mg	Effexor by Teva	00093-7383	Antidepressant
93 <> 74	Tab, White to Off-White, Film Coated, Round	Zolpidem Tartrate 10 mg	Ambien by Teva Pharmaceuticals	00093-0074 Discontinued	Sedative/Hypnotic; C IV
93 <> 7401	Tab, White, Oval, Scored, 9 / 3 <> 7401	Sotalol HCl 80 mg	Betapace AF by Teva	00093-7401	Antiarrhythmic
93 <> 7402	Tab, White, Oval, Scored, 9 / 3 <> 7402	Sotalol HCl 120 mg	Betapace AF by Teva	00093-7402	Antiarrhythmic
93 <> 7403	Tab, White, Oval, Scored, 9 / 3 <> 7403	Sotalol HCl 160 mg	Betapace AF by Teva	00093-7403	Antiarrhythmic
93 <> 7447	Tab, Purple, Oval, Film Coated	Mycophenolate Mofetil 500 mg	CellCept by Teva	00093-7447	Immunosuppressant
93 <> 7455	Tab, Pink, Cap Shaped, Film Coated	Glipizide 2.5 mg, Metformin HCl 250 mg	Metaglip by Teva	00093-7455	Antidiabetic
93 <> 7456	Tab, White, Cap Shaped, Film Coated	Glipizide 2.5 mg, Metformin HCl 500 mg	Metaglip by Teva	00093-7456	Antidiabetic
93 <> 7457	Tab, Pink, Cap Shaped, Film Coated	Glipizide 5 mg, Metformin HCl 500 mg	Metaglip by Teva	00093-7457	Antidiabetic
93 <> 7485	Tab, White to Off-White, Cap-Shaped, Film-Coated	Granisetron HCl 1 mg	Kytril by Teva	00093-7485	Antiemetic
93 <> 7493	Tab, White, Oblong, Film Coated, Scored, 9 / 3	Levetiracetam 1000 mg	Keppra by Teva	00093-7493	Anticonvulsant
93 <> 7540	Tab, Light Yellow, Cap Shaped	Topiramate 50 mg	Topamax by Teva	00093-7540	Anticonvulsant
93 <> 771	Tab, Pink, Round	Pravastatin Sodium 10 mg	Pravachol by Teva	00093-0771	Antihyperlipidemic
93 <> 787	Tab, White to Off-White, Round, Marbled	Atenolol 25 mg	Tenormin by Teva	00093-0787	Antihypertensive

ID FRONT <> BACK	DESCRIPTION FRONT <> BACK	INGREDIENT & STRENGTH	BRAND (or Generic Equiv.) by FIRM	NDC#	CLASS; SCH.
93 <> 788	Tab, White to Off-White, Round	Selegiline 5 mg	Eldepryl by Vangard	00615-4516	Antiparkinson
93 <> 788	Tab, White to Off-White, Round	Selegiline 5 mg	Eldepryl by Teva	17372-0788	Antiparkinson
93 <> 788	Tab, White to Off-White, Round	Selegiline 5 mg	Eldepryl by Murfreesboro	51129-1111	Antiparkinson
93 <> 788	Tab, White to Off-White, Round	Selegiline 5 mg	Eldepryl by Teva	00093-0788	Antiparkinson
93 <> 8	Tab, White, Round, Film Coated	Indapamide 2.5 mg	Lozol by Teva	00093-0008	Diuretic
93 <> 8117	Tab, White, Round, Film-Coated	Famciclovir 125 mg	Famvir by Teva	00093-8117	Antiviral
93 <> 8118	Tab, White, Round, Film-Coated	Famciclovir 250 mg	Famvir by Teva	00093-8118	Antiviral
93 <> 8119	Tab, White, Cap Shaped, Film-Coated	Famciclovir 500 mg	Famvir by Teva	00093-8119	Antiviral
93 <> 83	Tab, White to Off-White, Round	Amlodipine Besylate 2.5 mg	Norvasc by Teva	00093-0083	Antihypertensive
93 <> 851	Tab, White, Round	Metronidazole 250 mg	Flagyl by MS State Health	50596-0027	Antibiotic
93 <> 851	Tab, White, Round	Metronidazole 250 mg	Flagyl by Neuman	64579-0181	Antibiotic
93 <> 851	Tab, White, Round	Metronidazole 250 mg	Flagyl by UDL	51079-0122	Antibiotic
93 <> 851	Tab, White, Round	Metronidazole 250 mg	Flagyl by Golden State	60429-0128	Antibiotic
93 <> 851	Tab, White, Round	Metronidazole 250 mg	Flagyl by Nat Pharmpak	55154-5509	Antibiotic
93 <> 851	Tab, White, Round	Metronidazole 250 mg	Flagyl by Pharmedix	53002-0221	Antibiotic
93 <> 851	Tab, White, Round	Metronidazole 250 mg	Flagyl by Teva	00093-0851 Discontinued	Antibiotic
93 <> 8522	Tab, Light Gray, D Shaped	Naratriptan 1 mg	Amerge by Teva Pharmaceuticals	00093-8522	Antimigraine
93 <> 8523	Tab, Green, D Shaped	Naratriptan 2.5 mg	Amerge by Teva Pharmaceuticals	00093-8523	Antimigraine
93 <> 890	Tab, Pink, Oblong, Film Coated	Acetaminophen 650 mg, Propoxyphene Napsylate 100 mg	Darvocet-N 100 by Teva	00093-0890	Analgesic; C IV
93 <> 890	Tab, Pink, Oblong, Film Coated	Acetaminophen 650 mg, Propoxyphene Napsylate 100 mg	Darvocet-N 100 by Ivax	00182-0317	Analgesic; C IV
93 <> 890	Tab, Pink, Oblong, Film Coated	Acetaminophen 650 mg, Propoxyphene Napsylate 100 mg	Darvocet-N 100 by Heartland	61392-0446	Analgesic; C IV
93 <> 890	Tab, Pink, Oblong, Film Coated	Acetaminophen 650 mg, Propoxyphene Napsylate 100 mg	Darvocet-N 100 by Ranbaxy	63304-0714	Analgesic; C IV
93 <> 892	Tab, Pink, Cap Shaped, Film Coated	Etodolac 400 mg	Lodine by Heartland	61392-0911	NSAID
93 <> 892	Tab, Pink, Cap Shaped, Film Coated	Etodolac 400 mg	Lodine by Teva	00093-0892	NSAID
93 <> 896	Tab, Beige, Round	Famotidine 20 mg	Pepcid by Pharmedix	00093-0896 Discontinued	Gastrointestinal
93 <> 897	Tab, Tan, Round	Famotidine 40 mg	Pepcid by Teva	00093-0897 Discontinued	Gastrointestinal
93 <> 9111	Tab, Yellowish Tan, Oval, Film Coated	Ascorbic Acid 120 mg, Beta-Carotene 4.2 mg, Calcium Carbonate 490.76 mg, Cholecalciferol 0.49 mg, Cupric Oxide 2.5 mg, Niacinamide 21 mg, Pyridoxine HCl 10.5 mg, Folic Acid 1 mg, Cyanocobalamin 12 mcg, Ferrous Fumarate 197.75 mg, Riboflavin 3.15 mg, Thiamine Mononitrate 1.575 mg, Vitamin A Acetate 8.4 mg, Vitamin E Acetate 44 mg, Zinc Oxide 31.12 mg	Prenatal Plus (Stuartnatal Plus) by Teva	00093-9111 Discontinued	Vitamin
93 <> 9152	Tab, Yellow, Oval, Film Coated	Ascorbic Acid 200 mg, Biotin 0.15 mg, Calcium Pantothenate 27.17 mg, Chromic Chloride 0.51 mg, Cupric Oxide 3.75 mg, Cyanocobalamin 50 mcg, Ferrous Fumarate 82.2 mg, Folic Acid 0.8 mg, Magnesium Oxide 82.89 mg, Manganese 50 mg, Manganese Sulfate 15.5 mg, Niacinamide Ascorbate 400 mg, Pyridoxine HCl 30.25 mg, Riboflavin 20 mg, Thiamine Mononitrate 20 mg, Vitamin A Acetate 10.75 mg, Vitamin E Acetate 30 mg, Zinc Oxide 27.99 mg	B Complex Vit Plus by Teva	00093-9152	Vitamin
93 <> 9165	Tab, Oval, White	Ascorbic Acid 17.53 mg, Beta-Carotene 0.56 mg, Calcium Carbonate 249.41 mg, Calcium Pantothenate 4.18 mg, Cholecalciferol 0.25 mg, Cupric Oxide 2.02 mg, Ferrous Fumarate 82.15 mg, Magnesium Oxide 82.93 mg, Niacinamide Ascorbate 8.54 mg, Pyridoxine HCl 2.43 mg, Riboflavin 0.84 mg, Thiamine Mononitrate 1 mg, Vitamin A Acetate 2680 Units, Zinc Oxide 15.56 mg	Enfamil Natalins by Teva	00093-9165 Discontinued	Vitamin
93 <> 926	Tab, Light Peach, Round	Lovastatin 10 mg	Mevacor by Teva	00093-0926	Antihyperlipidemic
93 <> 928	Tab, Light Green, Round	Lovastatin 40 mg	Mevacor by Teva	00093-0928	Antihyperlipidemic
93 <> 93778	Tab, Chewable, 93 <> 93/778	Carbamazepine 100 mg	Tegretol by Major	00904-3854	Anticonvulsant

ID FRONT <> BACK	DESCRIPTION FRONT <> BACK	INGREDIENT & STRENGTH	BRAND (or Generic Equiv.) by FIRM	NDC#	CLASS; SCH.
93 <> 9411	Tab, White, Square	Methazolamide 25 mg	Neptazane by Teva	00093-9411	Antiglaucoma Agent
93 <> 9643	Tab, Yellow, Round, Film Coated	Prochlorperazine 5 mg	Compazine by Teva	00093-9643	Antiemetic
93 <> 9652	Tab, Yellow, Round, Film Coated	Prochlorperazine 10 mg	Compazine by Teva	00093-9652	Antiemetic
93 <> 968	Tab, Pink, Round	Famotidine 10 mg	Pepcid by Perrigo	00113-0207	Gastrointestinal
93 <> 968	Tab, Pink, Round	Famotidine 10 mg	Pepcid by Major	00904-4529	Gastrointestinal
93 <> 983	Tab, Brown, Round, Film Coated	Nystatin 500,000 Units	Mycostatin by Schein	00364-2051	Antifungal
93 <> 983	Tab, Brown, Round, Film Coated	Nystatin 500,000 Units	Mycostatin by Teva	00093-0983	Antifungal
93 <> BL	Tab, White, Round, Scored	Metoclopramide HCl 10 mg	Reglan by Vangard	00615-2536	Gastrointestinal
93 <> BL	Tab, White, Round, Scored	Metoclopramide HCl 10 mg	Reglan by Biocraft	00093-2203	Gastrointestinal
93 <> BL	Tab, White, Round, Scored	Metoclopramide HCl 10 mg	Reglan by Neuman	64579-0051	Gastrointestinal
93 <> BL	Tab, White, Round, Scored	Metoclopramide HCl 10 mg	Reglan by Moore	00839-7127	Gastrointestinal
93 <> BL	Tab, White, Round, Scored	Metoclopramide HCl 10 mg	Reglan by Duramed	51285-0805	Gastrointestinal
93 <> BL	Tab, White, Round	Metoclopramide 10 mg	Reglan by UDL	51079-0283	Gastrointestinal
93 <> BL	Tab, White, Round, Scored	Metoclopramide HCl 10 mg	Reglan by Neuman	64579-0049	Gastrointestinal
93 <> BL	Tab, White, Round, Scored	Metoclopramide HCl 10 mg	Reglan by Teva	00093-2203	Gastrointestinal
93 <> C	Tab, White to Off White, Cap Shaped, Film Coated	Ciprofloxacin 750 mg	Cipro by Aurobindo	65862-0078	Antibiotic
930 <> LV	Tab, White, Round, Scored	Morphine Sulfate 30 mg	by Glenmark	68462-0203	Analgesic; C II
930 <> PLIVA	Tab, Light Green, Round, Scored, Film Coated	Sertraline HCl 25 mg	Zoloft by Pliva		Antidepressant
93019	Cap, Blue & White	Phentermine 37.5 mg	Adipex-P by Lemmon	50111-0930	Anorexiant; C IV
		Clemastine Fumarate 1.34 mg	Tavist-1 by Lemmon		Antihistamine
93037	Tab, White, Round, 93/037				
93044	Cap, Dark Blue, 93 over 044	Acyclovir 200 mg	Zovirax by Teva	00093-0044	Antiviral
93064	Cap, Orange & Yellow, 93-064	Tetracycline HCl 250 mg	Achromycin V by Lemmon		Antibiotic
93088	Tab, White, Round, Scored, 93 over 088	Sulfamethoxazole 400 mg, Trimethoprim 80 mg	Septra by Teva	00093-0088 Discontinued	Antibiotic
93088	Tab, White, Round, Scored, 93 over 088	Sulfamethoxazole 400 mg, Trimethoprim 80 mg	Septra by St. Mary's Med	60760-0046	Antibiotic
93088	Tab, White, Round, Scored, 93 over 088	Sulfamethoxazole 400 mg, Trimethoprim 80 mg	Septra by Sovereign	58716-0676	Antibiotic
93089	Tab, White, Oval, Scored, 93 over 089	Sulfamethoxazole 800 mg, Trimethoprim 160 mg	Septra by Teva	00093-0089 Discontinued	Antibiotic
93089	Tab, White, Oval, Scored, 93 over 089	Sulfamethoxazole 800 mg, Trimethoprim 160 mg	Septra by Teva	17372-0089	Antibiotic
93089	Tab, White, Oval, Scored, 93 over 089	Sulfamethoxazole 800 mg, Trimethoprim 160 mg	Septra by St. Mary's Med	60760-0079	Antibiotic
93089	Tab, White, Oval, Scored, 93 over 089	Sulfamethoxazole 800 mg, Trimethoprim 160 mg	Septra by H J Harkins Co	52959-0144	Antibiotic
93089	Tab, White, Oval, Scored, 93 over 089	Sulfamethoxazole 800 mg, Trimethoprim 160 mg	Septra by Heartland	61392-0947	Antibiotic
93089	Tab, White, Oval, Scored, 93 over 089	Sulfamethoxazole 800 mg, Trimethoprim 160 mg	Septra by Golden State	60429-0170	Antibiotic
93089	Tab, White, Oval, Scored, 93 over 089	Sulfamethoxazole 800 mg, Trimethoprim 160 mg	Septra by St. Mary's Med	60760-0135	Antibiotic
93089	Tab, White, Oval, Scored, 93 over 089	Sulfamethoxazole 800 mg, Trimethoprim 160 mg	Septra by Murfreesboro	51129-1335	Antibiotic
93090	Tab, White, Round, 93 over 090	Carbamazepine 200 mg	Tegretol by Lemmon		Anticonvulsant
931	Tab, Yellow, D-Shaped	Cyclobenzaprine HCl 10 mg	Flexeril by Frosst	Canadian	Muscle Relaxant
931 <> PLIVA	Tab, Light Blue, Round, Scored, Film Coated	Sertraline HCl 50 mg	Zoloft by Pliva	50111-0931	Antidepressant
9310	Tab, Blue, Round	Chlorpropamide 100 mg	Diabinese by Lemmon		Antidiabetic
93100	Tab, Light Pink, Round, Film Coated, Scored, 93 over 100	Labetalol HCl 100 mg	Normodyne by Murfreesboro	51129-1612	Antihypertensive
93100	Tab, Light Pink, Round, Film Coated, Scored, 93 over 100	Labetalol HCl 100 mg	Normodyne by Teva	00093-0100 Discontinued	Antihypertensive
931003 <> 555	Tab, White to Off-White, Rectangular, Scored	Buspirone HCl 15 mg	Buspar by Teva Pharmaceuticals	00093-1003	Antianxiety
93102	Tab, Off-White, Round, Film Coated, Scored, 93 over 102	Labetalol HCl 200 mg	Normodyne by Murfreesboro	51129-1613	Antihypertensive
93102	Tab, Off-White, Round, Film Coated, Scored, 93 over 102	Labetalol HCl 200 mg	Normodyne by Teva	00093-0102 Discontinued	Antihypertensive
93106	Tab, Light Purple, Round, Film Coated, 93 over 106	Labetalol HCl 300 mg	Normodyne by Teva	00093-0106 Discontinued	Antihypertensive
931060	Tab, Light Blue, Oval, Scored	Sotalol 120 mg	Betapace by Teva	00093-1060	Antiarrhythmic

ID FRONT <> BACK	DESCRIPTION FRONT <> BACK	INGREDIENT & STRENGTH	BRAND (or Generic Equiv.) by FIRM	NDC#	CLASS; SCH.
93107	Tab, Light Peach, Round	Mebendazole 100 mg	Vermox by Teva	00093-9107	Anthelmintic
93109	Tab	Carbamazepine 200 mg	Tegretol by Teva	17372-0109	Anticonvulsant
9311	Tab, Yellow, Oval, Black Ink	Pantoprazole Sodium 20 mg	Protonix by Teva	00093-0011	Gastrointestinal
931112	Tab, Red, Round, Scored	Lisinopril 5 mg	Prinivil by Teva	00093-1112 Discontinued	Antihypertensive
93113	Tab, White, Oblong, Scored, Film Coated	Cimetidine HCl 400 mg	Tagamet by Teva	00093-0113 Discontinued	Gastrointestinal
93113	Tab, White, Oblong, Scored, Film Coated	Cimetidine HCl 400 mg	Tagamet by Vangard	00615-3566	Gastrointestinal
9312	Tab, Yellow, Oval, Black Ink	Pantoprazole Sodium 40 mg	Protonix by Teva	00093-0012	Gastrointestinal
9312	Tab, Yellow, Oval, Black Ink	Pantoprazole Sodium 40 mg	Protonix by Teva	00093-0012	Gastrointestinal
93122	Tab, White, Oblong, Scored, Film Coated	Cimetidine HCl 800 mg	Tagamet by Teva	00093-0122 Discontinued	Gastrointestinal
93123	Tab, White, Round, 93 12/3	Aspirin 325 mg, Codeine Phosphate 30 mg	Aspirin w/ Codeine by Lemmon		Analgesic; C III
93129	Tab, White, Oval, Scored	Estazolam 1 mg	ProSom by Teva	00093-0129	Sedative/Hypnotic; C IV
93129	Tab, White, Oval	Estazolam 1 mg	by Halsey		Sedative/Hypnotic; C IV
93129	Tab, White, Oval, Double Scored	Estazolam 1 mg	ProSom by Par	49884-0112	Sedative/Hypnotic; C IV
93130	Tab, Coral, Oval, Scored	Estazolam 2 mg	ProSom by Teva	00093-0130	Sedative/Hypnotic; C IV
93130	Tab, Coral, Oval, Single Scored	Estazolam 2 mg	ProSom by Par	49884-0343	Sedative/Hypnotic; C IV
93132	Tab, Caramel & White	Acetaminophen 300 mg, Codeine Phosphate 15 mg	Tylenol w/ Codeine by Lemmon		Analgesic; C III
93134	Tab, White, Round, 93 13/4	Aspirin 325 mg, Codeine Phosphate 60 mg	Aspirin w/ Codeine by Lemmon		Analgesic; C III
93138	Cap, Clear & Pink	Diphenhydramine HCl 25 mg	Benadryl by Lemmon		Antihistamine
93139	Cap, Pink	Diphenhydramine HCl 50 mg	Benadryl by Lemmon		Antihistamine
93143	Tab, Lavender, Round, 93-143	Warfarin Sodium 2 mg	Sofarin by Lemmon		Anticoagulant
93144	Tab, Orange, Round, 93-144	Warfarin Sodium 2.5 mg	Sofarin by Lemmon		Anticoagulant
93145	Tab, Pink, Round, 93-145	Warfarin Sodium 5 mg	Sofarin by Lemmon		Anticoagulant
93147	Tab, Red, Round	Naproxen 250 mg	Naprosyn by Otsuka	46602-0002	NSAID
93147	Tab, Red, Round	Naproxen 250 mg	Naprosyn by Ivax	00182-1971	NSAID
93147	Tab, Red, Round	Naproxen 250 mg	Naprosyn by Novopharm	62528-0734	NSAID
93148	Tab	Naproxen 375 mg	Naprosyn by Ivax	00182-1972	NSAID
93149	Tab, Light Red	Naproxen 500 mg	Naprosyn by St. Mary's Med	60760-0149	NSAID
93149	Tab, Light Red	Naproxen 500 mg	Naprosyn by Ivax	00182-1973	NSAID
93150 <> 3	Tab, White, Round, 93 over 150	Acetaminophen 300 mg, Codeine Phosphate 30 mg	Tylenol w/ Codeine by ABG	60999-0903	Analgesic; C III
93150 <> 3	Tab, White, Round, 93 over 150	Acetaminophen 300 mg, Codeine Phosphate 30 mg	Tylenol w/ Codeine by UDL	51079-0161 Discontinued	Analgesic; C III
93150 <> 3	Tab, White, Round, 93 over 150	Acetaminophen 300 mg, Codeine Phosphate 30 mg	Tylenol w/ Codeine by Teva	00093-0150	Analgesic; C III
93150 <> 3	Tab, White, Round, 93 over 150	Acetaminophen 300 mg, Codeine Phosphate 30 mg	Tylenol w/ Codeine by Nat Pharmpak	55154-5548	Analgesic; C III
93150 <> 3	Tab, White, Round, 93 over 150	Acetaminophen 300 mg, Codeine Phosphate 30 mg	Tylenol w/ Codeine by Major	00904-0175	Analgesic; C III
93150 <> 3	Tab, White, Round, 93 over 150	Acetaminophen 300 mg, Codeine Phosphate 30 mg	Tylenol w/ Codeine by Murfreesboro	51129-0089	Analgesic; C III
93150 <> 3	Tab, White, Round, 93 over 150	Acetaminophen 300 mg, Codeine Phosphate 30 mg	Tylenol w/ Codeine by Urgent Care Center	50716-0465	Analgesic; C III
93150 <> 3	Tab, White, Round, 93 over 150	Acetaminophen 300 mg, Codeine Phosphate 30 mg	Tylenol w/ Codeine by Pharmedix	53002-0101	Analgesic; C III
93152	Cap, Coral & Scarlet	Acetaminophen 300 mg, Codeine Phosphate 30 mg	Tylenol w/ Codeine by Lemmon		Analgesic; C III
93157	Tab, White, Round	Diethylpropion HCl 25 mg	Tenuate by Lemmon		Anorexiant; C IV
93172	Cap, Brown & Gray	Acetaminophen 300 mg, Codeine Phosphate 60 mg	Tylenol w/ Codeine by Lemmon		Analgesic; C III
93175	Tab, White, Round, Film Coated, Ex Release, 93 over 175	Quinidex Sulfate 300 mg	Quinidex Extentabs by Teva	00093-9175	Antiarrhythmic
93176	Tab, White, Round, Scored, 93 over 176	Captopril 25 mg, HCTZ 15 mg	Capozide by Teva	00093-9176	Antihypertensive; Diuretic
93177	Tab, Tan, Round, Scored, 93 over 177	Captopril 25 mg, HCTZ 25 mg	Capozide by Teva	00093-9177	Antihypertensive; Diuretic
93181	Tab, White, Oval, Scored	Captopril 50 mg, HCTZ 15 mg	Capozide by Teva	00093-0181	Antihypertensive; Diuretic

ID FRONT <> BACK	DESCRIPTION FRONT <> BACK	INGREDIENT & STRENGTH	BRAND (or Generic Equiv.) by FIRM	NDC#	CLASS; SCH.
93182	Tab, Tan, Oval, Scored	Captopril 50 mg, HCTZ 25 mg	Capozide by Teva	00093-0182	Antihypertensive; Diuretic
93188	Tab, White, Round	Sulfamethoxazole 400 mg, Trimethoprim 80 mg	Cotrim by Lemmon		Antibiotic
93189	Tab, White, Oval	Sulfamethoxazole 800 mg, Trimethoprim 160 mg	Cotrim DS by Lemmon		Antibiotic
932	Tab	Atenolol 50 mg	Tenormin by Heartland	61392-0543	Antihypertensive
932 <> PLIVA	Tab, Light Yellow, Round, Scored, Film Coated	Sertraline HCl 100 mg	Zoloft by Pliva	50111-0932	Antidepressant
93208	Cap, Orange, Opaque, 93-208	Zinc Acetate 50 mg	Galzin by Teva	00093-0208 Discontinued	Mineral
93208	Cap, Orange, Opaque, 93-208	Zinc Acetate 50 mg	Galzin by Gate	57844-0208	Mineral
93221	Cap, Pink & White, 93 over 21	Diltiazem HCl 60 mg	Cardizem by Teva	00093-0021 Discontinued	Antihypertensive
9321	Cap, Pink & White	Diltiazem HCl 60 mg	Cardizem by Eisai	11071-0812	Antihypertensive
93213	Cap, 93 over 213	Tolmetin Sodium 492 mg	by Teva	00093-0213	NSAID
93213	Cap	Tolmetin Sodium 492 mg	by Quality Care	60346-0615	NSAID
93214	Tab, Coated	Tolmetin Sodium 735 mg	by Teva	00093-0214	NSAID
93214	Tab, Coated	Tolmetin Sodium 735 mg	by Teva	17372-0214	NSAID
93215	Cap, Aqua Blue, Opaque, 93 over 215	Zinc Acetate 25 mg	Galzin by Teva	00093-0215 Discontinued	Mineral
93215	Cap, Aqua Blue, 93-215	Zinc Acetate 25 mg	Galzin by Gate	57844-0215	Mineral
932159	Tab, White, Round, Scored, 93 above Score 2159 below	Trimethoprim 200 mg	Proloprim by Teva	00093-2159	Antibiotic
93218	Tab, White, Round	Phenobarbital 30 mg	by Lemmon		Sedative/Hypnotic; C IV
9322	Cap, Pink & Yellow, 93 over 22	Diltiazem HCl 90 mg	Cardizem by Teva	00093-0022 Discontinued	Antihypertensive
932264	Tab, Off-White, Cap Shaped, Scored	Amoxicillin 875 mg	Amoxil by Teva	00093-2264	Antibiotic
9323	Cap, Orange & Pink, Ex Release	Diltiazem HCl 120 mg	Cardizem by Lemmon		Antihypertensive
9323	Cap, Orange & Pink, 93 over 23	Diltiazem HCl 120 mg	Cardizem by Teva	00093-0023 Discontinued	Antihypertensive
93241	Tab, White, Round	Phenobarbital 15 mg	Phenobarbital by Lemmon		Sedative/Hypnotic; C IV
9326	Tab, Yellow, Oval, Scored	Enalapril Maleate 2.5 mg	Vasotec by Teva	00093-0026	Antihypertensive
9327	Tab, White, Oval, Scored	Enalapril Maleate 5 mg	Vasotec by Teva	00093-0027	Antihypertensive
9328	Tab, Salmon, Oval, 93 over 28	Enalapril Maleate 10 mg	Vasotec by Teva	00093-0028	Antihypertensive
93280	Tab, Yellow, Round, Film Coated, 93 over 280	Bupropion HCl 75 mg	Wellbutrin by Caremark	00339-4056	Antidepressant
93280	Tab, Yellow, Round, Film Coated, 93 over 280	Bupropion HCl 75 mg	Wellbutrin by Teva	00093-0280	Antidepressant
9329	Tab, Peach, Oval, 93 over 29	Enalapril Maleate 20 mg	Vasotec by Teva	00093-0029	Antihypertensive
93290	Tab, Pink, Round, Film Coated, 93 over 290	Bupropion HCl 100 mg	Wellbutrin by Teva	00093-0290	Antidepressant
93290	Tab, Pink, Round, Film Coated, 93 over 290	Bupropion HCl 100 mg	Wellbutrin by Caremark	00339-4104	Antidepressant
93292	Tab, Blue, Round, Scored, 93 over 292	Carbidopa 10 mg, Levodopa 100 mg	Sinemet by Teva	00093-0292	Antiparkinson
93292	Tab, Blue, Round, Scored, 93 over 292	Carbidopa 10 mg, Levodopa 100 mg	Sinemet by Teva	17372-0292	Antiparkinson
93292	Tab, Blue, Round, Scored, 93 over 292	Carbidopa 10 mg, Levodopa 100 mg	Sinemet by Caremark	53978-3059	Antiparkinson
93292	Tab, Blue, Round, Scored, 93 over 292	Carbidopa 10 mg, Levodopa 100 mg	Sinemet by Med Pro	53978-3059	Antiparkinson
93292	Tab, Blue, Round, Scored, 93 over 292	Carbidopa 10 mg, Levodopa 100 mg	Sinemet by Ivax	00182-1948	Antiparkinson
93292	Tab, Blue, Round, Scored, 93 over 292	Carbidopa 10 mg, Levodopa 100 mg	Sinemet by Medirex	57480-0807	Antiparkinson
93292	Tab, Blue, Round, Scored, 93 over 292	Carbidopa 10 mg, Levodopa 100 mg	Sinemet by Amerisource	62584-0641	Antiparkinson
93292	Tab, Blue, Round, Scored, 93 over 292	Carbidopa 10 mg, Levodopa 100 mg	Sinemet by Baker Cummins	63171-1948	Antiparkinson
93292	Tab, Blue, Round, Scored, 93 over 292	Carbidopa 10 mg, Levodopa 100 mg	Sinemet by Major	00904-7718	Antiparkinson
93292	Tab, Blue, Round, Scored, 93 over 292	Carbidopa 10 mg, Levodopa 100 mg	Sinemet by UDL	51079-0755 Discontinued	Antiparkinson
932929	Tab, White, Round, Scored, 93 / 2929	Cyproheptadine HCl 4 mg	Periactin by Teva	00093-2929	Antihistamine
93293	Tab, Yellow, Round, Scored, 93 over 293	Carbidopa 25 mg, Levodopa 100 mg	Sinemet by Nat Pharmpak	55154-5816	Antiparkinson
93293	Tab, Yellow, Round, Scored, 93 over 293	Carbidopa 25 mg, Levodopa 100 mg	Sinemet by Medirex	57480-0808	Antiparkinson

ID FRONT <> BACK	DESCRIPTION FRONT <> BACK	INGREDIENT & STRENGTH	BRAND (or Generic Equiv.) by FIRM	NDC#	CLASS; SCH.
93293	Tab, Yellow, Round, Scored, 93 over 293	Carbidopa 25 mg, Levodopa 100 mg	Sinemet by Amerisource	62584-0642	Antiparkinson
93293	Tab, Yellow, Round, Scored, 93 over 293	Carbidopa 25 mg, Levodopa 100 mg	Sinemet by Caremark	00339-6136	Antiparkinson
93293	Tab, Yellow, Round, Scored, 93 over 293	Carbidopa 25 mg, Levodopa 100 mg	Sinemet by Teva	00093-0293	Antiparkinson
93293	Tab, Yellow, Round, Scored, 93 over 293	Carbidopa 25 mg, Levodopa 100 mg	Sinemet by Vangard	00615-3561	Antiparkinson
93293	Tab, Yellow, Round, Scored, 93 over 293	Carbidopa 25 mg, Levodopa 100 mg	Sinemet by Teva	17372-0293	Antiparkinson
93293	Tab, Yellow, Round, Scored, 93 over 293	Carbidopa 25 mg, Levodopa 100 mg	Sinemet by Ivax	00182-1949	Antiparkinson
93293	Tab, Yellow, Round, Scored, 93 over 293	Carbidopa 25 mg, Levodopa 100 mg	Sinemet by Major	00904-7719	Antiparkinson
93293	Tab, Yellow, Round, Scored, 93 over 293	Carbidopa 25 mg, Levodopa 100 mg	Sinemet by UDL	51079-0756	Antiparkinson
				Discontinued	
93294	Tab, Blue, Round, Scored, 93 over 294	Carbidopa 25 mg, Levodopa 250 mg	Sinemet by Ivax	00182-1950	Antiparkinson
93294	Tab, Blue, Round, Scored, 93 over 294	Carbidopa 25 mg, Levodopa 250 mg	Sinemet by Nat Pharmpak	55154-5536	Antiparkinson
93294	Tab, Blue, Round, Scored, 93 over 294	Carbidopa 25 mg, Levodopa 250 mg	Sinemet by Medirex	57480-0476	Antiparkinson
93294	Tab, Blue, Round, Scored, 93 over 294	Carbidopa 25 mg, Levodopa 250 mg	Sinemet by Amerisource	62584-0643	Antiparkinson
93294	Tab, Blue, Round, Scored, 93 over 294	Carbidopa 25 mg, Levodopa 250 mg	Sinemet by Caremark	00339-6138	Antiparkinson
93294	Tab, Blue, Round, Scored, 93 over 294	Carbidopa 25 mg, Levodopa 250 mg	Sinemet by Teva	17372-0294	Antiparkinson
93294	Tab, Blue, Round, Scored, 93 over 294	Carbidopa 25 mg, Levodopa 250 mg	Sinemet by Teva	00093-0294	Antiparkinson
93294	Tab, Blue, Round, Scored, 93 over 294	Carbidopa 25 mg, Levodopa 250 mg	Sinemet by Vangard	00615-4504	Antiparkinson
93294	Tab, Blue, Round, Scored, 93 over 294	Carbidopa 25 mg, Levodopa 250 mg	Sinemet by UDL	51079-0783	Antiparkinson
93294	Tab, Blue, Round, Scored, 93 over 294	Carbidopa 25 mg, Levodopa 250 mg	Sinemet by Major	00904-7720	Antiparkinson
93307	Tab, 93/307	Clemastine Fumarate 1.34 mg	Tavist-1 by Teva	00093-0307	Antihistamine
93308	Tab, White, Round, Scored, 93 over 308	Clemastine Fumarate 2.68 mg	Tavist-1 by Northeast	58163-0072	Antihistamine
93308	Tab, White, Round, Scored, 93 over 308	Clemastine Fumarate 2.68 mg	Tavist-1 by Teva	00093-0308	Antihistamine
93308	Tab, White, Round, Scored, 93 over 308	Clemastine Fumarate 2.68 mg	Tavist-1 by Ivax	00182-1936	Antihistamine
933107	Cap, Buff & Caramel, 93 over 3107	Amoxicillin 250 mg	Amoxil by Teva	00093-3107	Antibiotic
933107	Cap, Buff & Caramel, 93 over 3107	Amoxicillin 250 mg	Amoxil by Teva	17372-0613	Antibiotic
933109	Cap, Buff, Black Print, 93 over 3109	Amoxicillin 500 mg	Amoxil by Teva	00093-3109	Antibiotic
933109	Cap, Buff, Black Print, 93 over 3109	Amoxicillin 500 mg	Amoxil by UDL	51079-0601	Antibiotic
				Discontinued	
93311	Cap, Dark Brown & Light Brown, White Print, 93 over 311	Loperamide 2 mg	Imodium by Teva	00093-0311	Antidiarrheal
93311	Cap, Dark Brown & Light Brown, White Print, 93 over 311	Loperamide 2 mg	Imodium by Ivax	00182-1505	Antidiarrheal
933111	Cap, Gray & Scarlet, 93 over 3111	Ampicillin 250 mg	Principen by Moore	00839-5087	Antibiotic
933111	Cap, Gray & Scarlet, 93 over 3111	Ampicillin 250 mg	Principen by UDL	51079-0602	Antibiotic
933111	Cap, Gray & Scarlet, 93 over 3111	Ampicillin 250 mg	Principen by Teva	00093-3111	Antibiotic
933113	Cap, Gray & Scarlet, 93 over 3113	Ampicillin 500 mg	Principen by Teva	00093-3113	Antibiotic
				Discontinued	
933115	Cap, Blue, Opaque, 93 over 3115	Oxacillin Sodium Monohydrate 250 mg	by Teva	00093-3115	Antibiotic
933117	Cap, Blue, Opaque, 93 over 3117	Oxacillin Sodium Monohydrate 500 mg	by Teva	00093-3117	Antibiotic
933119	Cap, Dark Green & Scarlet, 93 over 3119	Cloxacillin Sodium 250 mg	by H J Harkins Co	52959-0468	Antibiotic
933119	Cap, Dark Green & Scarlet, 93 over 3119	Cloxacillin Sodium 250 mg	by Teva	00093-3119	Antibiotic
933121	Cap, Dark Green & Scarlet, 93 over 3121	Cloxacillin Sodium 500 mg	by Teva	00093-3121	Antibiotic
				Discontinued	
933123	Cap, Light Green, 93 over 3123	Dicloxacillin Sodium 250 mg	Dynapen by DRX	51079-0610	Antibiotic
933123	Cap, Light Green, 93 over 3123	Dicloxacillin Sodium 250 mg	Dynapen by UDL	51079-0610	Antibiotic
933123	Cap, Light Green, 93 over 3123	Dicloxacillin Sodium 250 mg	Dynapen by Teva	00093-3123	Antibiotic
933125	Cap, Light Green, Black Print, 93 over 3125	Dicloxacillin Sodium 500 mg	Dynapen by Teva	00093-3125	Antibiotic
933125	Cap, Light Green, Black Print, 93 over 3125	Dicloxacillin Sodium 500 mg	Dynapen by UDL	51079-0611	Antibiotic
933127	Cap, Blue & Scarlet, Black Print, Hard Gel, 93 over 3127	Disopyramide Phosphate 100 mg	Norpace by Teva	00093-3127	Antiarrhythmic
933129	Cap, Buff & Scarlet, Black Print, Hard Gel, 93 over 3129	Disopyramide Phosphate 150 mg	Norpace by Teva	00093-3129	Antiarrhythmic

ID FRONT <> BACK	DESCRIPTION FRONT <> BACK	INGREDIENT & STRENGTH	BRAND (or Generic Equiv.) by FIRM	NDC#	CLASS; SCH.
933145	Cap, Gray & Orange, Black Print, 93 over 3145	Cephalexin 250 mg	Keflex by Teva	00093-3145	Antibiotic
933145	Cap, Gray & Orange, Black Print, 93 over 3145	Cephalexin 250 mg	Keflex by Caremark	00339-6166	Antibiotic
933145	Cap, Gray & Orange, Black Print, 93 over 3145	Cephalexin 250 mg	Keflex by UDL	51079-0604 Discontinued	Antibiotic
933147	Cap, Orange, Black Print, 93 over 3147	Cephalexin 500 mg	Keflex by Teva	00093-3147	Antibiotic
933153	Cap, Light Green & Pink, 93 over 3153	Cephradine 250 mg	Velosef by Teva	00093-3153 Discontinued	Antibiotic
933153	Cap, Light Green, 93-3153 <> 93-3153	Cephradine 250 mg	Velosef by UDL	51079-0606	Antibiotic
933155	Cap, Light Green, Opaque, 93 over 3155	Cephradine 500 mg	Velosef by Teva	00093-3155 Discontinued	Antibiotic
933155	Cap, 93-3155	Cephradine 500 mg	Velosef by H J Harkins Co	52959-0032	Antibiotic
933155	Cap, 93-3155	Cephradine 500 mg	Velosef by UDL	51079-0607	Antibiotic
933160	Cap, Lavender and Light Green, Opaque	Cefdinir 300 mg	Omnicef by Teva	00093-3160	Antibiotic
933165	Cap, Pink, Black Print, 93 over 3165	Minocycline HCl 50 mg	Minocin by Teva	00093-3165	Antibiotic
933167	Cap, Maroon & Pink, Black Print, 93 over 3167	Minocycline HCl 100 mg	Minocin by Teva	00093-3167	Antibiotic
933169	Cap, Red, 93-3169	Clindamycin HCl 75 mg	Cleocin HCl by Teva	00093-3169 Discontinued	Antibiotic
933171	Cap, Blue & Red, 93 over 3171	Clindamycin HCl 150 mg	Cleocin HCl by UDL	51079-0598	Antibiotic
933171	Cap, Blue & Red, 93 over 3171	Clindamycin HCl 150 mg	Cleocin HCl by Teva	00093-3171	Antibiotic
93318	Tab, Light Orange, Round, Film Coated, 93 over 318	Diltiazem HCl 30 mg	Cardizem by Lemmon		Antihypertensive
93318	Tab, Light Orange, Round, Film Coated, 93 over 318	Diltiazem HCl 30 mg	Cardizem by Teva	00093-0318	Antihypertensive
93319	Tab, Orange, Round, Scored, Film Coated, 93 over 319	Diltiazem HCl 60 mg	Cardizem by Teva	00093-0319	Antihypertensive
93193	Cap, Blue & Light Blue, Black Print, 93 over 3193	Ketoprofen 50 mg	Orudis by Teva	00093-3193	NSAID
93195	Cap, Blue & White, Black Print, 93 over 3195	Ketoprofen 75 mg	Orudis by Southwood	58016-0380	NSAID
93195	Cap, Blue & White, Black Print, 93 over 3195	Ketoprofen 75 mg	Orudis by Teva	00093-3195	NSAID
93196	Cap, Orange and White, Opaque	Cefadroxil Monohydrate 500 mg	Duricef by Teva	00093-3196	Antibiotic
93320	Tab, Light Orange, Oblong, Scored, Film Coated	Diltiazem HCl 90 mg	Cardizem by Fournier	63924-0002	Antihypertensive
93320	Tab, Light Orange, Oblong, Scored, Film Coated	Diltiazem HCl 90 mg	Cardizem by Teva	00093-0320	Antihypertensive
93320	Tab, Light Orange, Oblong, Scored, Film Coated	Diltiazem HCl 90 mg	Cardizem by Lemmon		Antihypertensive
93321	Tab, Orange, Oblong, Scored, Film Coated	Diltiazem HCl 120 mg	Cardizem by Fournier	63924-0003	Antihypertensive
93321	Tab, Orange, Oblong, Scored, Film Coated	Diltiazem HCl 120 mg	Cardizem by Teva	00093-0321	Antihypertensive
93321	Tab, Orange, Oblong, Scored, Film Coated	Diltiazem HCl 120 mg	Cardizem by Lemmon		Antihypertensive
93325	Tab, Purple, Round	Desipramine HCl 25 mg	Norpramin by Lemmon		Antidepressant
93326	Tab, Blue, Round	Desipramine HCl 50 mg	Norpramin by Lemmon		Antidepressant
93327	Tab, White, Round	Desipramine HCl 75 mg	Norpramin by Lemmon		Antidepressant
93328	Tab, Yellow, Round	Desipramine HCl 100 mg	Norpramin by Lemmon		Antidepressant
93350 <> 4	Tab, White, Round, 93 over 350	Acetaminophen 300 mg, Codeine Phosphate 60 mg	Tylenol w/ Codeine by St. Mary's Med	60760-0350	Analgesic; C III
93350 <> 4	Tab, White, Round, 93 over 350	Acetaminophen 300 mg, Codeine Phosphate 60 mg	Tylenol w/ Codeine by Teva	00093-0350	Analgesic; C III
93350 <> 4	Tab, White, Round, 93 over 350	Acetaminophen 300 mg, Codeine Phosphate 60 mg	Tylenol w/ Codeine by Sandoz	00781-1654	Analgesic; C III
93350 <> 4	Tab, White, Round, 93 over 350	Acetaminophen 300 mg, Codeine Phosphate 60 mg	Tylenol w/ Codeine by UDL	51079-0106 Discontinued	Analgesic; C III
93350 <> 4	Tab, White, Round, 93 over 350	Acetaminophen 300 mg, Codeine Phosphate 60 mg	Tylenol w/ Codeine by Murfreesboro	51129-6662	Analgesic; C III
93350 <> 4	Tab, White, Round, 93 over 350	Acetaminophen 300 mg, Codeine Phosphate 60 mg	Tylenol w/ Codeine by Southwood	58016-0272	Analgesic; C III
9338	Cap, Grey, Hard Gel	Gabapentin 100 mg	Neurontin by UDL	51079-0785	Anticonvulsant
9338	Cap, Grey, Hard Gel	Gabapentin 100 mg	Neurontin by Teva Pharmaceuticals	00093-1038 Discontinued	Anticonvulsant
9339	Cap, Orange, Hard Gel	Gabapentin 300 mg	Neurontin by UDL	51079-0786	Anticonvulsant
9339	Cap, Orange, Hard Gel	Gabapentin 300 mg	Neurontin by Teva Pharmaceuticals	00093-1039	Anticonvulsant
933DP	Tab, White, Oblong, Scored	Hyoscyamine Sulfate 0.375 mg	Levsin by Sovereign	58716-0668	Gastrointestinal

ID FRONT <> BACK	DESCRIPTION FRONT <> BACK	INGREDIENT & STRENGTH	BRAND (or Generic Equiv.) by FIRM	NDC#	CLASS; SCH.
9340	Cap, Caramel, Hard Gel	Gabapentin 400 mg	Neurontin by Teva	00093-1040 Discontinued	Anticonvulsant
934067	Cap, Ivory, Opaque	Prazosin HCl 1 mg	Minipress by Teva	00093-4067	Antihypertensive
934068	Cap, Pink, Opaque	Prazosin HCl 2 mg	Minipress by Teva	00093-4068	Antihypertensive
934069	Cap, Blue	Prazosin HCl 5 mg	Minipress by Teva	00093-4069	Antihypertensive
9341	Tab, White, Round, Scored, 93 over 41	Clomiphene Citrate 50 mg	Clomid by Teva	00093-0041	Infertility
9342	Cap, Powder Blue, Hard Gel, 93 over 42	Fluoxetine HCl 10 mg	Prozac by Teva	00093-1042	Antidepressant
9342	Cap, Powder Blue, Opaque	Fluoxetine 10 mg	Prozac by Teva	00172-1042	Antidepressant
9343	Cap, Powder Blue & White, Hard Gel, 93 over 43	Fluoxetine HCl 20 mg	Prozac by Teva	00093-1043 Discontinued	Antidepressant
93431	Tab, Blue, Round	Chlorthalidone 50 mg	Hygroton by Lemmon		Diuretic
93433	Tab, White, Round	Chlorthalidone 100 mg	Hygroton by Lemmon		Diuretic
93484	Tab, Orange, Round	Doxycycline Hyclate 100 mg	Vibra-Tab by Lemmon		Antibiotic
93486	Tab, White, Round	Ibuprofen 200 mg	Motrin by Lemmon		NSAID
93490	Tab, White, Oblong, Film Coated	Acetaminophen 650 mg, Propoxyphene Napsylate 100 mg	Darvocet-N 100 by Teva	00093-0490	Analgesic; C IV
93490	Tab, White, Oblong, Film Coated	Acetaminophen 650 mg, Propoxyphene Napsylate 100 mg	Darvocet-N 100 by H J Harkins Co	52959-0335	Analgesic; C IV
93490	Tab, White, Oblong, Film Coated	Acetaminophen 650 mg, Propoxyphene Napsylate 100 mg	Darvocet-N 100 by Reese	10956-0745	Analgesic; C IV
93491	Tab, White, Round, 93-491	Ibuprofen 400 mg	Motrin by Lemmon		NSAID
93492	Tab, White, Oval, 93-492	Ibuprofen 600 mg	Motrin by Lemmon		NSAID
93498	Tab, White, Oblong, 93-498	Ibuprofen 800 mg	Motrin by Lemmon		NSAID
935	Tab, White to Off-White, Blue Print, Ex Release, 93-5	Naproxen 375 mg	Naprosyn by Teva	00093-1005	NSAID
9350 <> 2	Tab, White, Round, 93 over 50	Acetaminophen 300 mg, Codeine Phosphate 15 mg	Tylenol w/ Codeine by Teva	00093-0050	Analgesic; C III
935160	Tab, White to Off-White, Round, Scored	Tizanidine HCl 4 mg	Zanaflex by Teva	00093-5160 Discontinued	Muscle Relaxant
935163	Tab, White to Off-White, Round, Scored	Tizanidine HCl 2 mg	Zanaflex by Teva	00093-5163 Discontinued	Muscle Relaxant
935200 <> 101010	Tab, White to Off-White, Rectangular, Trisect Scored	Buspirone HCl 30 mg	BuSpar by Teva	00093-5200	Antianxiety
93525	Tab, Pink, Round	Amitriptyline HCl 10 mg	Elavil by Lemmon		Antidepressant
935256	Cap, Light Blue, Opaque	Clindamycin HCl 300 mg	Cleocin HCl by Teva	00093-5256	Antibiotic
935268	Cap, Blue Green and White, Opaque	Zaleplon 5 mg	Sonata by Teva	00093-5268	Sedative/Hypnotic; C IV
935269	Cap, Blue Green and Aqua Blue, Opaque	Zaleplon 10 mg	Sonata by Teva	00093-5269	Sedative/Hypnotic; C IV
93527	Tab, Green, Round	Amitriptyline HCl 25 mg	Elavil by Lemmon		Antidepressant
93529	Tab, Brown, Round	Amitriptyline HCl 50 mg	Elavil by Lemmon		Antidepressant
9353	Tab, White to Off-White, Round, Scored, 93 over 53	Buspirone HCl 5 mg	Buspar by Teva Pharmaceuticals	00093-0053	Antianxiety
93531	Tab, Purple, Round	Amitriptyline HCl 75 mg	Elavil by Lemmon		Antidepressant
93533	Tab, Orange, Round	Amitriptyline HCl 100 mg	Elavil by Lemmon		Antidepressant
93535	Tab, Peach, Round	Amitriptyline HCl 150 mg	Elavil by Lemmon		Antidepressant
93537	Tab, White, Oval, Scored	Naproxen 550 mg	Naprosyn by Direct Dispensing	57866-6613	NSAID
93537	Tab, Film Coated, 93 537	Naproxen 550 mg	Naprosyn by H J Harkins Co	52959-0271	NSAID
9354	Tab, White to Off-White, Round, Scored, 93 over 54	Buspirone HCl 10 mg	BuSpar by Teva	00093-0054 Discontinued	Antianxiety
93541	Cap, Dark Orange & Gray, 93 over 541	Cephalexin 250 mg	Keflex by Teva	00093-0541 Discontinued	Antibiotic
93542	Tab, White, Oblong, Scored	Chlorzoxazone 500 mg	Parafon Forte by Teva	00093-0542 Discontinued	Muscle Relaxant
93543	Cap, Orange, 93 over 543	Cephalexin 500 mg	Keflex by Teva	00093-0543 Discontinued	Antibiotic

ID FRONT <> BACK	DESCRIPTION FRONT <> BACK	INGREDIENT & STRENGTH	BRAND (or Generic Equiv.) by FIRM	NDC#	CLASS; SCH.
93545	Tab, Green, Round	Chlorzoxazone 250 mg, Acetaminophen 300 mg	Parafon Forte by Lemmon		Muscle Relaxant
93548	Cap, Yellow, 93-548	Amantadine HCl 100 mg	Symmetrel by Lemmon		Antiviral
93585	Cap, Green	Indomethacin 25 mg	Indocin by Lemmon		NSAID
93587	Cap, Green	Indomethacin 50 mg	Indocin by Lemmon		NSAID
93590	Tab, White	Acetaminophen 650 mg, Propoxyphene Napsylate 100 mg	Darvocet-N 100 by Lemmon		Analgesic; C IV
936	Tab, White to Off-White, Blue Print, Ex Release, 93-6	Naproxen 500 mg	Naprosyn by Teva	00093-1006	NSAID
936 <> MRK	Tab, White, Oval	Alendronate Sodium 10 mg	Fosamax by Merck Frosst	Canadian DIN 02201011	Antiosteoporosis
936 <> MRK	Tab, White, Oval	Alendronate Sodium 10 mg	Fosamax by Merck	00006-0936	Antiosteoporosis
9361	Tab, Light Blue, Oval, Scored	Sotalol 80 mg	Betapace by Teva	00480-1061	Antiarrhythmic
9361	Tab, Light Blue, Oval, Scored	Sotalol 80 mg	Betapace by Teva	00093-1061	Antiarrhythmic
93613	Cap, Brown & White, Black Print, 93 over 613	Amoxicillin 250 mg	Amoxil by Teva	00093-0613	Antibiotic
93615	Cap, White, Black Print, 93 over 615	Amoxicillin 500 mg	Amoxil by Teva	00093-0615	Antibiotic
93617	Cap, White	Chlordiazepoxide 5 mg, Clidinium Bromide 2.5 mg	Librax by Lemmon		Gastrointestinal
9362	Tab, Light Blue, Oblong, Scored	Sotalol 160 mg	Betapace by Teva	00480-1062	Antiarrhythmic
9362	Tab, Light Blue, Oblong, Scored	Sotalol 160 mg	Betapace by Teva	00093-1062	Antiarrhythmic
93620	Tab, Blue, Round	Propranolol HCl 20 mg	Inderal by Lemmon		Antihypertensive
93628	Cap, Clear & Lavender, Ex Release, 93-628	Indomethacin 75 mg	Indocin SR by Lemmon		NSAID
9363	Tab, Light Blue, Oblong, Scored	Sotalol 240 mg	Betapace by Teva	00480-1063	Antiarrhythmic
9363	Tab, Light Blue, Oblong, Scored	Sotalol 240 mg	Betapace by Teva	00093-1063	Antiarrhythmic
93637	Tab, White, Round, Scored, Film Coated, 93 over 637	Trazodone HCl 50 mg	Desyrel by Teva	00093-0637	Antidepressant
93638	Tab, White, Round, Scored, Film Coated, 93 over 638	Trazodone HCl 100 mg	Desyrel by Teva	00093-0638	Antidepressant
93640	Tab, Green, Round	Propranolol HCl 40 mg	Inderal by Lemmon		Antihypertensive
93653	Cap, Blue, 93-653	Doxycycline Hyclate 100 mg	Vibramycin by Lemmon		Antibiotic
93657	Cap, Red-Brown & Yellow-Brown, Oval, Opaque, 93 over 657	Calcitriol 0.25 mcg	Rocaltrol by Teva	00093-0657	Vitamin; Mineral
93658	Cap, Brown & Pink, Opaque, 93 over 658	Calcitriol 0.5 mcg	Rocaltrol by Teva	00093-0658	Vitamin; Mineral
93665	Tab, White, Round, Scored, 93 over 665	Albuterol Sulfate 2 mg	Proventil by Teva	00093-0665	Antiasthmatic
93666	Tab, White, Round, Scored, 93 over 666	Albuterol Sulfate 4 mg	Proventil by Teva	00093-0666	Antiasthmatic
93670	Tab, White, Oval, Scored, Film Coated	Gemfibrozil 600 mg	Lopid by Ivax	00182-1956	Antihyperlipidemic
93670	Tab, White, Oval, Scored, Film Coated	Gemfibrozil 600 mg	Lopid by Kaiser	00179-1293	Antihyperlipidemic
93670	Tab, White, Oval, Scored, Film Coated	Gemfibrozil 600 mg	Lopid by Teva	00093-0670	Antihyperlipidemic
93670	Tab, White, Oval, Scored, Film Coated	Gemfibrozil 600 mg	Lopid by Baker Cummins	63171-1956	Antihyperlipidemic
93670	Tab, White, Oval, Scored, Film Coated	Gemfibrozil 600 mg	Lopid by Heartland	61392-0093	Antihyperlipidemic
93670	Tab, White, Oval, Scored, Film Coated	Gemfibrozil 600 mg	Lopid by Medirex	57480-0809	Antihyperlipidemic
93670	Tab, White, Oval, Scored, Film Coated	Gemfibrozil 600 mg	Lopid by Va Cmop	65243-0035	Antihyperlipidemic
93670	Tab, White, Oval, Scored, Film Coated	Gemfibrozil 600 mg	Lopid by Nat Pharmpak by Med Pro	55154-5231	Antihyperlipidemic
93670	Tab, White, Oval, Scored, Film Coated	Gemfibrozil 600 mg	Lopid by UDL	53978-2033	Antihyperlipidemic
93670	Tab, White, Oval, Scored, Film Coated	Gemfibrozil 600 mg	Lopid by Pharmascience	51079-0787 Discontinued	Antihyperlipidemic
93670	Tab, White, Oval, Scored, Film Coated	Gemfibrozil 600 mg	Lopid by Pharmascience	Canadian DIN 02230183	Antihyperlipidemic
93686	Cap, Grey & Red, 93/686	Aspirin 389 mg, Caffeine 32.4 mg, Propoxyphene HCl 65 mg	Propoxyphene Compound 65 by Allscripts		Analgesic; C IV
93686	Cap	Aspirin 389 mg, Caffeine 32.4 mg, Propoxyphene HCl 65 mg	Propoxyphene Compound 65 by Ivax	00182-1673	Analgesic; C IV
93686	Cap, Gray & Red, 93 over 686	Aspirin 389 mg, Caffeine 32.4 mg, Propoxyphene HCl 65 mg	Propoxyphene Compound 65 by Teva	00093-0686 Discontinued	Analgesic; C IV
93686	Cap	Aspirin 389 mg, Caffeine 32.4 mg, Propoxyphene HCl 65 mg	Propoxyphene Compound 65 by Pharmedix	53002-0535	Analgesic; C IV
93691	Cap, Brown & Clear, Ex Release, 93-691	Propranolol HCl 60 mg	Inderal LA by Lemmon		Antihypertensive

ID FRONT <> BACK	DESCRIPTION FRONT <> BACK	INGREDIENT & STRENGTH	BRAND (or Generic Equiv.) by FIRM	NDC#	CLASS; SCH.
93692	Cap, Blue & Clear, Ex Release, 93-692	Propranolol HCl 80 mg	Inderal LA by Lemmon		Antihypertensive
93693	Cap, Blue & Clear, Ex Release, 93-693	Propranolol HCl 120 mg	Inderal LA by Lemmon		Antihypertensive
93694	Cap, Blue & Clear, Ex Release, 93-694	Propranolol HCl 160 mg	Inderal LA by Lemmon		Antihypertensive
93695	Tab, Coated, Debossed, Appears as 93-695	Trazodone HCl 150 mg	Desyrel by Teva	00093-0695	Antidepressant
93695	Cap, Coated, Debossed, Appears as 93-695	Trazodone HCl 150 mg	Desyrel by Teva	17372-0695	Antidepressant
93695	Tab, White, Round	Trazodone HCl 150 mg	Desyrel by Teva	00480-0695	Antidepressant
937	Tab, Blue, Round	Chlorpropamide 250 mg	Diabinese by Lemmon		Antidiabetic
93711	Tab, Blue, Round, Film Coated, 93 over 711	Flurbiprofen 100 mg	Ansaid by Invamed	52189-0394	NSAID
93711	Tab, Blue, Round, Film Coated, 93 over 711	Flurbiprofen 100 mg	Ansaid by Major	00904-5019	NSAID
93711	Tab, Blue, Round, Film Coated, 93 over 711	Flurbiprofen 100 mg	Ansaid by H J Harkins Co	52959-0346	NSAID
93711	Tab, Blue, Round, Film Coated, 93 over 711	Flurbiprofen 100 mg	Ansaid by Teva	00093-0711	NSAID
937120	Cap, Beige, Black Print, Opaque, 93 over 7120	Flutamide 125 mg	Eulexin by Teva	00093-7120 Discontinued	Antiandrogen
937120	Cap, Beige, Opaque	Flutamide 125 mg	Eulexin by Par	49884-0753	Antiandrogen
937162	Cap, Pink and Flesh, Opaque, Hard Gel	Zonisamide 100 mg	Zonegran by Teva	00093-7162 Discontinued	Anticonvulsant
937198	Cap, Blue & Orange, 93 over 7198	Fluoxetine HCl 40 mg	Prozac by Teva	00093-7198	Antidepressant
937225	Cap, Purple, Hard Gel	Fluoxetine 10 mg	Selfemra by Teva	00093-7225	Antidepressant
937226	Cap, Purple and Flesh, Hard Gel	Fluoxetine 20 mg	Selfemra by Teva	00093-7226	Antidepressant
937227	Cap, White, Opaque, Hard Gel	Ribavirin 200 mg	Rebetol by Teva	00093-7227	Antiviral
937227	Cap, Brown & Clear	Papaverine HCl 150 mg	Pavabid by Lemmon		Vasodilator
93728	Tab, Yellow, Round	Sulindac 150 mg	Clinoril by Lemmon		NSAID
93729	Tab, Yellow, Round	Sulindac 200 mg	Clinoril by Lemmon		NSAID
937300	Cap, Light Gray and White	Minocycline HCl 75 mg	Minocin by Teva	00093-7300	Antibiotic
937733	Tab, Pink, Round, Scored, Film Coated, 93 over 733	Metoprolol Tartrate 50 mg	Lopressor by Neuman	64579-0096	Antihypertensive
937733	Tab, Pink, Round, Scored, Film Coated, 93 over 733	Metoprolol Tartrate 50 mg	Lopressor by Teva	00093-0733	Antihypertensive
937334	Cap, Light Blue and Bright Orange, Opaque	Mycophenolate Mofetil 250 mg	CellCept by Teva	00093-7334	Immunosuppressant
937335	Cap, White	Topiramate 15 mg	Topamax Sprinkles by Teva	00093-7335	Anticonvulsant
937336	Cap, White	Topiramate 25 mg	Topamax Sprinkles by Teva	00093-7336	Anticonvulsant
937338	Cap, Light Brown and Buff, Opaque, Hard Gel	Tamsulosin HCl 0.4 mg	Flomax by Teva Pharmaceuticals	00093-7338	Antiadrenergic
937734	Tab, Mottled Blue, Round, Scored, Film Coated, 93 over 734	Metoprolol Tartrate 100 mg	Lopressor by Neuman	64579-0099	Antihypertensive
937734	Tab, Mottled Blue, Round, Scored, Film Coated, 93 over 734	Metoprolol Tartrate 100 mg	Lopressor by Caremark	00339-6191	Antihypertensive
937734	Tab, Mottled Blue, Round, Scored, Film Coated, 93 over 734	Metoprolol Tartrate 100 mg	Lopressor by Teva	00093-0734 Discontinued	Antihypertensive
937350	Cap, Light Blue and Flesh Colored, Opaque, Hard Gel, Delayed Release	Lansoprazole 15 mg	Prevacid by Teva Pharmaceuticals	00093-7350	Gastrointestinal
937351	Cap, Light Gray and Flesh Colored, Opaque, Hard Gel, Delayed Release	Lansoprazole 30 mg	Prevacid by Teva Pharmaceuticals	00093-7351	Gastrointestinal
937370	Cap, White, Opaque	Amlodipine Besylate 2.5 mg, Benazepril HCl 10 mg	Lotrel by Teva	00093-7370	Antihypertensive
937371	Cap, Orange and White, Opaque	Amlodipine Besylate 5 mg, Benazepril HCl 10 mg	Lotrel by Teva	00093-7371	Antihypertensive
937372	Cap, Pink and White, Opaque	Amlodipine Besylate 5 mg, Benazepril HCl 20 mg	Lotrel by Teva	00093-7372	Antihypertensive
937373	Cap, Blue Violet, Opaque	Amlodipine Besylate 10 mg, Benazepril HCl 20 mg	Lotrel by Teva	00093-7373	Antihypertensive
937384	Cap, Light Grey and Buff, Opaque, Ex Release	Venlafaxine HCl 37.5 mg	Effexor XR by Teva Pharmaceuticals	00093-7384	Antidepressant
937385	Cap, Buff, Opaque, Ex Release	Venlafaxine HCl 75 mg	Effexor XR by Teva Pharmaceuticals	00093-7385	Antidepressant
937386	Cap, Light Orange, Opaque, Ex Release	Venlafaxine HCl 150 mg	Effexor XR by Teva Pharmaceuticals	00093-7386	Antidepressant
93741	Cap, Pink, Opaque, 93 over 741	Propoxyphene 65 mg	Darvon by Pharmedix	53002-0574	Analgesic; C IV
93741	Cap, Pink, Opaque, 93 over 741	Propoxyphene 65 mg	Darvon by Med Pro	53978-0531	Analgesic; C IV
93741	Cap, Pink, Opaque, 93 over 741	Propoxyphene 65 mg	Darvon by Kaiser	00179-0679	Analgesic; C IV

ID FRONT <> BACK	DESCRIPTION FRONT <> BACK	INGREDIENT & STRENGTH	BRAND (or Generic Equiv.) by FIRM	NDC#	CLASS; SCH.
93741	Cap, Pink, Opaque, 93 over 741	Propoxyphene 65 mg	Darvon by Teva	00093-0741 Discontinued	Analgesic; C IV
93741	Cap, Pink	Propoxyphene HCl 65 mg	Darvan by Par	49884-0314	Analgesic; C IV
93742	Cap, Blue & White	Doxycycline Hyclate 50 mg	Vibramycin by Lemmon		Antibiotic
93743	Cap, Blue	Doxycycline Hyclate 100 mg	Vibramycin by Lemmon		Antibiotic
937435	Cap, Yellow, Opaque	Ramipril 1.25 mg	Altace by Teva	00093-7435	Antihypertensive
937436	Cap, Light Orange, Opaque	Ramipril 2.5 mg	Altace by Teva	00093-7436	Antihypertensive
937437	Cap, Pink, Opaque	Ramipril 5 mg	Altace by Teva	00093-7437	Antihypertensive
937438	Cap, Blue, Opaque	Ramipril 10 mg	Altace by Teva	00093-7438	Antihypertensive
937439	Tab, Reddish-Brown, Oval, Film Coated	Divalproex Sodium 125 mg	Depakote by Teva	00093-7439	Anticonvulsant
937440	Tab, Beige, Oval, Film Coated	Divalproex Sodium 250 mg	Depakote by Teva	00093-7440	Anticonvulsant
937441	Tab, Dark Pink, Oval, Film Coated	Divalproex Sodium 500 mg	Depakote by Teva	00093-7441	Anticonvulsant
937508	Cap, White, Opaque, Hard Gel	Zonisamide 25 mg	Zonegran by Teva	00093-7508 Discontinued	Anticonvulsant
937509	Cap, Gray, Opaque, Hard Gel	Zonisamide 50 mg	Zonegran by Teva	00093-7509 Discontinued	Anticonvulsant
93752	Tab, White, Round, Scored, 93 over 752	Atenolol 50 mg	Tenormin by Teva	00093-0752	Antihypertensive
93752	Tab, White, Round, Scored, 93 over 752	Atenolol 50 mg	Tenormin by Teva	17372-0752	Antihypertensive
93752	Tab, White, Round, Scored, 93 over 752	Atenolol 50 mg	Tenormin by Med Pro	53978-1199	Antihypertensive
93753	Tab, White, Round, 93 over 753	Atenolol 100 mg	Tenormin by Teva	00093-0753	Antihypertensive
93753	Tab, White, Round, 93 over 753	Atenolol 100 mg	Tenormin by Teva	17372-0753	Antihypertensive
93754	Cap, Blue & Lavender	Diflunisal 250 mg	Dolobid by Lemmon		NSAID
93756	Cap, Dark Green and Olive, 93 over 756	Piroxicam 10 mg	Feldene by Promeco SA	64674-0011	NSAID
93756	Cap, Dark Green and Olive, 93 over 756	Piroxicam 10 mg	Feldene by Teva	00093-0756	NSAID
93756	Cap, Dark Green and Olive, 93 over 756	Piroxicam 10 mg	Feldene by Ivax	00182-1933	NSAID
93757	Cap, Dark Green, 93 over 757	Piroxicam 20 mg	Feldene by Promeco SA	64674-0017	NSAID
93757	Cap, Dark Green, 93 over 757	Piroxicam 20 mg	Feldene by Major	00904-5063	NSAID
93757	Cap, Dark Green, 93 over 757	Piroxicam 20 mg	Feldene by Teva	00093-0757	NSAID
93757	Cap, Dark Green, 93 over 757	Piroxicam 20 mg	Feldene by Ivax	00182-1934	NSAID
93758EPITOL	Tab, Pink, Round, Red Specks, Chewable, 93-758 Epitol	Carbamazepine 100 mg	Tegretol by Lemmon		Anticonvulsant
9376	Tab, Yellow, Round, Scored, Film Coated, 93 over 76	Isosorbide Mononitrate 20 mg	Ismo by Murfreesboro	51129-1578	Antianginal
9376	Tab, Yellow, Round, Scored, Film Coated, 93 over 76	Isosorbide Mononitrate 20 mg	Ismo by Teva	00093-0076 Discontinued	Antianginal
93777	Tab, Peach, Round	Hydrochlorothiazide 25 mg	Hydrodiuril by Lemmon		Diuretic; Antihypertensive
93778 <> 93	Tab, Pink, Round, Scored, Red Specks, Chewable, 93 over 778	Carbamazepine 100 mg	Tegretol by Caremark	00339-6134	Anticonvulsant
93778 <> 93	Tab, Chewable, 93/778 <> 93	Carbamazepine 100 mg	Tegretol by Major	00904-3854	Anticonvulsant
93779	Tab, Peach, Round	Hydrochlorothiazide 50 mg	Hydrodiuril by Lemmon		Diuretic; Antihypertensive
93782	Tab, White to Off-White, Round	Tamoxifen Citrate 20 mg	Nolvadex by Teva	00093-0782	Antiestrogen
93783	Cap, Pink	Propoxyphene 65 mg	Darvon by Lemmon		Analgesic; C IV
93784	Tab, White, Round, 93 over 784	Tamoxifen Citrate 10 mg	Nolvadex by Lemmon	00093-0784	Antiestrogen
93789	Tab, Gray, Round, 93-789	Perphenazine 2 mg	Trilafon by Lemmon		Antipsychotic
93790	Tab, Gray, Round, 93-790	Perphenazine 4 mg	Trilafon by Lemmon		Antipsychotic
93791	Tab, Gray, Round, 93-791	Perphenazine 8 mg	Trilafon by Lemmon		Antipsychotic
93792	Tab, Gray, Round, 93-792	Perphenazine 16 mg	Trilafon by Lemmon		Antipsychotic
93793	Cap, Aqua Blue & White, Gel Coated, Opaque, 93 over 793	Nicardipine HCl 20 mg	Cardene by Teva Pharmaceuticals	00093-0793 Discontinued	Antihypertensive

ID FRONT <> BACK	DESCRIPTION FRONT <> BACK	INGREDIENT & STRENGTH	BRAND (or Generic Equiv.) by FIRM	NDC#	CLASS; SCH.
93794	Cap, Light Blue & White, Gel Coated, Opaque, 93 over 794	Nicardipine HCl 30 mg	Cardene by Teva	00093-0794; Discontinued	Antihypertensive
93798	Cap, Green, 93-798	Indomethacin 25 mg	Indocin by Lemmon		NSAID
93799	Cap, Green, 93-799	Indomethacin 50 mg	Indocin by Lemmon		NSAID
938	Tab, White, Round	Indapamide 2.5 mg	Lozol by Lemmon		Diuretic
93802	Cap, Clear & Green	Atropine Sulfate, Hyoscyamine Sulfate, Phenobarbital, Scopolamine	Donnatal by Lemmon		Gastrointestinal; C IV
93804	Cap, Black & Scarlet	Phentermine HCl 30 mg	by Lemmon		Anorexiant; C IV
93810	Cap, Orange & White, Black Print, 93 over 810	Nortriptyline HCl 10 mg	Pamelor by Teva Pharmaceuticals	00093-0810 Discontinued	Antidepressant
93810	Cap, Orange & White, Black Print, 93 over 810	Nortriptyline HCl 10 mg	Pamelor by Ivax	00182-1190 Discontinued	Antidepressant
93810	Cap, Orange & White, Black Print, 93 over 810	Nortriptyline HCl 10 mg	Pamelor by Major Pharmaceuticals	00904-7939 Discontinued	Antidepressant
93811	Cap, Orange & White, Black Print, 93 over 811	Nortriptyline HCl 25 mg	Pamelor by Teva Pharmaceuticals	00093-0811 Discontinued	Antidepressant
93811	Cap, Orange & White, Black Print, 93 over 811	Nortriptyline HCl 25 mg	Pamelor by Ivax	00182-1191 Discontinued	Antidepressant
93811	Cap, Orange & White, Black Print, 93 over 811	Nortriptyline HCl 25 mg	Pamelor by PDRX	55289-0099 Discontinued	Antidepressant
93811	Cap, Orange & White, Black Print, 93 over 811	Nortriptyline HCl 25 mg	Pamelor by Major Pharmaceuticals	00904-7940 Discontinued	Antidepressant
93812	Cap, White, Black Print, 93 over 812	Nortriptyline HCl 50 mg	Pamelor by H J Harkins Co	52959-0519 Discontinued	Antidepressant
93812	Cap, White, Black Print, 93 over 812	Nortriptyline HCl 50 mg	Pamelor by Teva Pharmaceuticals	00093-0812 Discontinued	Antidepressant
93812	Cap, White, Black Print, 93 over 812	Nortriptyline HCl 50 mg	Pamelor by Ivax	00182-1192 Discontinued	Antidepressant
93812	Cap, White, Black Print, 93 over 812	Nortriptyline HCl 50 mg	Pamelor by Major Pharmaceuticals	00904-7941 Discontinued	Antidepressant
93813	Cap, Orange, Black Print, 93 over 813	Nortriptyline HCl 75 mg	Pamelor by Teva Pharmaceuticals	00093-0813 Discontinued	Antidepressant
93813	Cap, Orange, Black Print, 93 over 813	Nortriptyline HCl 75 mg	Pamelor by Ivax	00182-1193 Discontinued	Antidepressant
93813	Cap, Orange, Black Print, 93 over 813	Nortriptyline HCl 75 mg	Pamelor by Major Pharmaceuticals	00904-7942 Discontinued	Antidepressant
93821	Tab, White, Round	Reserpine 0.25 mg	by Lemmon		Antihypertensive
93824	Tab, White, Round	Pseudoephedrine 60 mg	Sudafed by Lemmon		Decongestant
93827	Tab, White, Round	Reserpine 0.1 mg	by Lemmon		Antihypertensive
93828	Tab, Blue, Round	Urinary Antiseptic Combination	Urinary Antiseptic 3 by Lemmon		Urinary Tract
93832	Tab, Light Yellow, Round, Scored, 93 over 832	Clonazepam 0.5 mg	Klonopin by Teva	00093-0832	Sedative; C IV
93832	Tab, Light Yellow, Round, Scored, 93 over 832	Clonazepam 0.5 mg	Klonopin by Vangard	00615-0456	Sedative; C IV
93832	Tab, Light Yellow, Round, Scored, 93 over 832	Clonazepam 0.5 mg	Klonopin by Caremark	00339-4091	Sedative; C IV
93832	Tab, Light Yellow, Round, Scored, 93 over 832	Clonazepam 0.5 mg	Klonopin by Physician Total Care	54868-3854	Sedative; C IV
93832	Tab, Light Yellow, Round, Scored, 93 over 832	Clonazepam 0.5 mg	Klonopin by Heartland	61392-0825	Sedative; C IV
93832	Tab, Light Yellow, Round, Scored, 93 over 832	Clonazepam 0.5 mg	Klonopin by Ivax	00182-8228 Discontinued	Sedative; C IV
93833	Tab, Green, Round, Scored, 93 over 833	Clonazepam 1 mg	Klonopin by Teva	17372-0833	Sedative; C IV
93833	Tab, Green, Round, Scored, 93 over 833	Clonazepam 1 mg	Klonopin by Physician Total Care	54868-3855	Sedative; C IV
93833	Tab, Green, Round, Scored, 93 over 833	Clonazepam 1 mg	Klonopin by Vangard	00615-0457	Sedative; C IV

ID FRONT <> BACK	DESCRIPTION FRONT <> BACK	INGREDIENT & STRENGTH	BRAND (or Generic Equiv.) by FIRM	NDC#	CLASS; SCH.
93833	Tab, Green, Round, Scored, 93 over 833	Clonazepam 1 mg	Klonopin by Caremark	00339-4000	Sedative; C IV
93833	Tab, Green, Round, Scored, 93 over 833	Clonazepam 1 mg	Klonopin by Apotheca	12634-0677	Sedative; C IV
93833	Tab, Green, Round, Scored, 93 over 833	Clonazepam 1 mg	Klonopin by Teva	00093-0833	Sedative; C IV
93833	Tab, Green, Round, Scored, 93 over 833	Clonazepam 1 mg	Klonopin by Ivax	00182-8229 Discontinued	Sedative; C IV
93834	Tab, White, Round, Scored, 93 over 834	Clonazepam 2 mg	Klonopin by Teva	00093-0834	Sedative; C IV
93834	Tab, White, Round, Scored, 93 over 834	Clonazepam 2 mg	Klonopin by D M Graham	00756-0265	Sedative; C IV
93834	Tab, White, Round, Scored, 93 over 834	Clonazepam 2 mg	Klonopin by Physician Total Care	54868-3861	Sedative; C IV
93834	Tab, White, Round, Scored, 93 over 834	Clonazepam 2 mg	Klonopin by Teva	17372-0834	Sedative; C IV
93834	Tab, White, Round, Scored, 93 over 834	Clonazepam 2 mg	Klonopin by DHHS Prog	11819-0099	Sedative; C IV
93834	Tab, White, Round, Scored, 93 over 834	Clonazepam 2 mg	Klonopin by Ivax	00182-8230 Discontinued	Sedative; C IV
93835	Tab, Purple, Round	Urinary Antiseptic Combination (Veterinary)	Urinary Antiseptic by Lemmon		Veterinary
93841	Cap, Blue	Dicyclomine HCl 10 mg	Bentyl by Lemmon		Gastrointestinal
93845	Tab, Purple, Round	Urinary Antiseptic Combination	Urinary Antiseptic 2 by Lemmon		Urinary Tract
93848	Tab, White, Round	Triprolidine 2.5 mg, Pseudoephedrine 60 mg	Actifed by Lemmon		Cold Remedy
93860	Cap, Yellow	Phentermine HCl 30 mg	by Lemmon		Anorexiant; C IV
93872	Tab, Purple, Round	Butabarbital 15 mg	Butisol Sodium by Lemmon		Sedative/Hypnotic; C III
93873	Tab, Green, Round	Butabarbital 30 mg	Butisol Sodium by Lemmon		Sedative/Hypnotic; C III
93888	Cap, Black	Phentermine HCl 30 mg	by Lemmon		Anorexiant; C IV
93891	Tab, Blue, Round	Dicyclomine HCl 20 mg	Bentyl by Lemmon		Gastrointestinal
9390	Tab	Carbamazepine 200 mg	Tegretol by Teva	17372-0090	Anticonvulsant
93900	Tab, White, Round, Scored, 93 over 900	Ketoconazole 200 mg	Nizoral by Teva	00093-0900	Antifungal
93901	Tab, White, Oval, Scored	Captopril 12.5 mg	Capoten by Teva	00093-0091	Antihypertensive
9391110	Tab, White, Round, 93 911/10	Isoxsuprine HCl 10 mg	Vasodilan by Lemmon		Vasodilator
939131	Tab, Pink, Round, Chewable	Fluoride 1 mg	Luride by Teva	00093-9131	Mineral
9391320	Tab, White, Round, 93 913/20	Isoxsuprine HCl 20 mg	Vasodilan by Lemmon		Vasodilator
939133	Tab, Pink, Round, Scored, 93 over 9133	Amiodarone 200 mg	Cordarone by UDL	51079-0906	Antiarrhythmic
939133	Tab, Pink, Round, Scored, 93 over 9133	Amiodarone 200 mg	Cordarone by Teva	00093-9133	Antiarrhythmic
939158	Tab, Orange, Pink & Purple, Square, Chewable	Ascorbic Acid 34.5 mg, Cyanocobalamin 4.9 mcg, Folic Acid 0.35 mg, Niacinamide 14.16 mg, Pyridoxine HCl 1.1 mg, Riboflavin 1.2 mg, Sodium Ascorbate 32.2 mg, Sodium Fluoride 1.1 mg, Thiamine Mononitrate 1.15 mg, Vitamin A Acetate 5.5 mg, Vitamin D 0.194 mg, Vitamin E Acetate 15.75 mg	Poly-Vi-Flor by Teva	00093-9158	Vitamin
939159	Tab, Purple, Square, Chewable, 93 over 9159	Cholecalciferol 0.194 mg, Cupric Oxide 1.25 mg, Cyanocobalamin 4.9 mcg, Ferrous Fumarate 36.5 mg, Folic Acid 0.35 mg, Niacinamide 14.17 mg, Pyridoxine HCl 1.1 mg, Riboflavin 1.26 mg, Sodium Ascorbate 32.2 mg, Sodium Fluoride 2.21 mg, Thiamine Mononitrate 1.15 mg, Vitamin A Acetate 5.5 mg, Vitamin E 15.75 mg, Zinc Oxide 12.5 mg	Poly-Vi-Flor w/ Iron by Teva	00093-9159	Vitamin
939166	Tab, Orange, Pink & Purple, Square, Chewable	Ascorbic Acid 34.5 mg, Cyanocobalamin 4.9 mcg, Folic Acid 0.35 mg, Niacinamide 14.17 mg, Pyridoxine HCl 1.1 mg, Riboflavin 1.26 mg, Sodium Ascorbate 32.2 mg, Sodium Fluoride 2.21 mg, Thiamine Mononitrate 1.15 mg, Vitamin A Palmitate 5.5 mg, Vitamin D 0.194 mg, Vitamin E Acetate 15.75 mg	Poly-Vi-Flor by Teva	00093-9166	Vitamin

ID FRONT <> BACK	DESCRIPTION FRONT <> BACK	INGREDIENT & STRENGTH	BRAND (or Generic Equiv.) by FIRM	NDC#	CLASS; SCH.
939197	Tab, Pink, Square, Chewable, 93 over 9197	Ascorbic Acid 34.47 mg, Cholecalciferol 0.194 mg, Cupric Oxide 1.25 mg, Cyanocobalamin 4.9 mcg, Ferrous Fumarate 36.48 mg, Folic Acid 0.35 mg, Niacinamide 14.16 mg, Pyridoxine HCl 1.1 mg, Riboflavin 1.258 mg, Sodium Fluoride 1.1 mg, Thiamine Mononitrate 1.15 mg, Vitamin A Acetate 5.5 mg, Vitamin E Acetate 15.75 mg, Zinc Oxide 12.5 mg	Poly-Vi-Flor w/ Iron by Teva	00093-9197	Vitamin
9392	Tab, White, Round, Scored, 93 over 92	Captopril 25 mg	Capoten by Teva	00093-0092	Antihypertensive
9393 <> 778	Tab, Pink w/ Red Specks, Round, Chewable, 93 over 93	Carbamazepine 100 mg	Tegretol by UDL	51079-0870 Discontinued	Anticonvulsant
9393 <> 778	Tab, Pink w/ Red Specks, Round, Chewable, 93 over 93	Carbamazepine 100 mg	Tegretol by Vangard	00615-4515	Anticonvulsant
9393 <> 778	Tab, Pink w/ Red Specks, Round, Chewable, 93 over 93	Carbamazepine 100 mg	Tegretol by Teva	00093-0778	Anticonvulsant
9393 <> 778	Tab, Pink w/ Red Specks, Round, Chewable, 93 over 93	Carbamazepine 100 mg	Tegretol by Heartland	61392-0029	Anticonvulsant
9393 <> 778	Tab, Pink w/ Red Specks, Round, Chewable, 93 over 93	Carbamazepine 100 mg	Tegretol by Ivax	00182-1331	Anticonvulsant
9393 <> 852	Tab, White, Oblong, Scored	Metronidazole 500 mg	Flagyl by Nat Pharmpak	55154-5566	Antibiotic
9393 <> 852	Tab, White, Oblong, Scored	Metronidazole 500 mg	Flagyl by Neuman	64579-0107	Antibiotic
9393 <> 852	Tab, White, Oblong, Scored	Metronidazole 500 mg	Flagyl by Family Health	65149-0126	Antibiotic
9393 <> 852	Tab, White, Oblong, Scored	Metronidazole 500 mg	Flagyl by UDL	51079-0126	Antibiotic
9393 <> 852	Tab, White, Oblong, Scored	Metronidazole 500 mg	Flagyl by Lemmon		Antibiotic
9393 <> 852	Tab, White, Oblong, Scored	Metronidazole 500 mg	Flagyl by Golden State	60429-0129	Antibiotic
9393 <> 852	Tab, White, Oblong, Scored	Metronidazole 500 mg	Flagyl by Prepackage Specialists	58864-0355	Antibiotic
9393 <> 852	Tab, White, Oblong, Scored	Metronidazole 500 mg	Flagyl by Pharmedix	53002-0247	Antibiotic
9393 <> 852	Tab, White, Oblong, Scored	Metronidazole 500 mg	Flagyl by Teva	00093-0852 Discontinued	Antibiotic
9393 <> COTRIM	Tab, White, Round, Scored, 93 over 93 <> Cotrim	Sulfamethoxazole 400 mg, Trimethoprim 80 mg	by Teva	00093-0188	Antibiotic
9393 <> COTRIMDS	Tab, White, Oblong, Scored, 93/93 <> Cotrim DS	Sulfamethoxazole 800 mg, Trimethoprim 160 mg	by Teva	00093-0189	Antibiotic
9393 <> EPITOL	Tab, White, Round, Scored, 93 over 93	Carbamazepine 200 mg	Tegretol by Caremark	00339-6132	Anticonvulsant
9393 <> EPITOL	Tab, White, Round, Scored, 93 over 93	Carbamazepine 200 mg	Tegretol by Teva	00093-0090	Anticonvulsant
939380	Cap, White & Red, Opaque, 93 over 9380	Ursodiol 300 mg	Actigall by Teva	00093-9380	Gastrointestinal
939424	Tab, White, Round, Scored, 93 over 9424	Methazolamide 50 mg	Neptazane by Teva	00093-9424	Antiglaucoma Agent
93943	Tab, Yellow, Diamond, 93-943	Nystatin Vaginal 100,000 Units	Mycostatin by Lemmon		Antifungal
939472	Tab, Peach, Round, Scored, 93 over 9472	Pemoline 75 mg	Cylert by Teva	00093-9472 Discontinued	Stimulant; C IV
93948	Tab, Orange, Round, Film Coated, 93 over 948	Diclofenac Potassium 50 mg	Cataflam by Teva	17372-0948	NSAID
93948	Tab, Orange, Round, Film Coated, 93 over 948	Diclofenac Potassium 50 mg	Cataflam by Teva	00093-0948	NSAID
93948	Tab, Orange, Round, Film Coated, 93 over 948	Diclofenac Potassium 50 mg	Cataflam by DRX	55045-2680	NSAID
939524	Tab, Peach, Round, Scored, 93 over 9524	Pemoline 37.5 mg	Cylert by Teva	00093-9524 Discontinued	Stimulant; C IV
939541	Tab, Peach, Round, Scored, 93 over 9541	Pemoline 18.75 mg	Cylert by Teva	00093-9541 Discontinued	Stimulant; C IV
93956	Cap, Orange & White, 93 over 956	Clomipramine HCl 25 mg	Anafranil by Teva	00093-0956	OCD
93956	Cap, Orange & White, 93 over 956	Clomipramine HCl 25 mg	Anafranil by D M Graham	00756-0215	OCD
93956	Cap, Orange & White, 93 over 956	Clomipramine HCl 25 mg	Anafranil by Teva	17372-0956	OCD
93957	Cap, Green & Yellow	Chlordiazepoxide 5 mg	Librium by Lemmon		Antianxiety; C IV
939577	Tab, Yellow, Square, Scored, Chewable, 93 over 9577	Pemoline 37.5 mg	Cylert by Teva	00093-9577 Discontinued	Stimulant; C IV
93958	Cap, Light Blue & White, 93 over 958	Clomipramine HCl 50 mg	Anafranil by Teva	00093-0958	OCD
93958	Cap, Light Blue & White, 93 over 958	Clomipramine HCl 50 mg	Anafranil by D M Graham	00756-0263	OCD
93958	Cap, Light Blue & White, 93 over 958	Clomipramine HCl 50 mg	Anafranil by Teva	17372-0958	OCD
93959	Cap, Black & Green	Chlordiazepoxide 10 mg	Librium by Lemmon		Antianxiety; C IV
93960	Cap, Brown & White, 93 over 960	Clomipramine HCl 75 mg	Anafranil by Teva	00093-0960	OCD
93960	Cap, Brown & White, 93 over 960	Clomipramine HCl 75 mg	Anafranil by Teva	17372-0960	OCD

ID FRONT <> BACK	DESCRIPTION FRONT <> BACK	INGREDIENT & STRENGTH	BRAND (or Generic Equiv.) by FIRM	NDC#	CLASS; SCH.
93960	Cap, Brown & White, 93 over 960	Clomipramine HCl 75 mg	Anafranil by D M Graham	00756-0264	OCD
93961	Cap, Green & White	Chlordiazepoxide 25 mg	Librium by Lemmon		Antianxiety; C IV
9397	Tab, White, Round, Scored, 93 over 97	Captopril 50 mg	Capoten by Teva	00093-0097	Antihypertensive
939774	Tab, White, Cap Shaped, Film Coated, 93 over 774	Hydroxychloroquine Sulfate 200 mg	Plaquenil by Teva	00093-9774	Antimalarial
9398	Tab, White, Round, Scored, 93 over 98	Captopril 100 mg	Capoten by Teva	00093-0098	Antihypertensive
9398	Tab, White, Round, Scored, 93 over 98	Captopril 100 mg	Capoten by Lemmon		Antihypertensive
93COTRIM	Tab, White, Round	Sulfamethoxazole 400 mg, Trimethoprim 80 mg	Cotrim by Lemmon		Antibiotic
93COTRIMDS	Tab, White, Round	Sulfamethoxazole 800 mg, Trimethoprim 160 mg	Cotrim DS by Lemmon		Antibiotic
93EPITOL	Tab, White, Round	Carbamazepine 200 mg	Tegretol by Lemmon		Anticonvulsant
93T13	Tab, White and Tan, Layered. Film Coated, ER	Fexofenadine HCl 60 mg, Pseudoephedrine HCl 120 mg	Allegra-D by Teva	00093-1130	Cold Remedy
94 <> C	Tab, White to Off White, Cap Shaped, Film Coated	Ciprofloxacin 500 mg	Cipro by Aurobindo	13107-0077	Antibiotic
94 <> C	Tab, White to Off White, Cap Shaped, Film Coated	Ciprofloxacin 500 mg	Cipro by Aurobindo	65862-0077	Antibiotic
94 <> GG	Tab, White, Round, Scored	Albuterol Sulfate 2 mg	Proventil by Sandoz	00781-1671	Antiasthmatic
94 <> MYLAN	Tab, Purple, Oval, Scored, Ex Release, Mylan <> 9/4	Carbidopa 50 mg, Levodopa 200 mg	Sinemet CR by Mylan	00378-0094	Antiparkinson
94 <> MYLAN	Tab, Purple, Oval, Scored, Ex Release, 9/4 <> Mylan	Carbidopa 50 mg, Levodopa 200 mg	Sinemet CR by UDL	51079-0923 Discontinued	Antiparkinson
940	Tab, Gray, Round, Schering Logo over 940	Perphenazine 4 mg	Trilafon by Schering	00085-0940	Antipsychotic
941	Tab, Yellow, Hexagonal	Sulindac 150 mg	by Frosst	Canadian	NSAID
941 <> B	Tab, Light Yellow, Round	Norethindrone 0.5 mg, Ethinyl Estradiol 0.035 mg	Modicon by Barr	00555-9008	Oral Contraceptive
9411 <> 93	Tab, White, Square	Methazolamide 25 mg	Neptazane by Teva	00093-9411	Antiglaucoma Agent
942	Tab, Yellow, Hexagonal	Sulindac 200 mg	by Frosst	Canadian	NSAID
942 <> B	Tab, Blue, Round	Norethindrone 0.75 mg, Ethinyl Estradiol 0.035 mg	Ortho-Novum by Barr	00555-9012	Oral Contraceptive
943 <> B	Tab, Blue, Round	Norethindrone 1 mg, Ethinyl Estradiol 0.035 mg	Ortho-Novum by Barr	00555-9012	Oral Contraceptive
944 <> B	Tab, White, Round	Inert	Ortho-Novum by Barr	00555-9010	Oral Contraceptive; Placebo
944 <> B	Tab, White, Round	Inert	Ortho-Novum by Barr	00555-9012	Oral Contraceptive; Placebo
944 <> B	Tab, White, Round	Inert	Modicon by Barr	00555-9008	Oral Contraceptive; Placebo
944 <> DAN	Tab, White, Round	Colchicine 0.6 mg	by Pharmedix	53002-0444	Antigout
944 <> DAN	Tab, White, Round	Colchicine 0.6 mg	by Heartland	61392-0174	Antigout
944 <> DAN	Tab, White, Round	Colchicine 0.6 mg	by Schein	00364-0074	Antigout
944 <> DAN	Tab, White, Round	Colchicine 0.6 mg	by Watson	00591-0944	Antigout
94515 <> B	Tab, Purple, Oval, Scored, Film Coated, 945/15 <> b	Methotrexate 15 mg	Trexall by Barr	00555-0945	Antineoplastic
948	Tab, White, Mortar and Pestle to Right of Schering Logo 948	Griseofulvin, Microsize 250 mg	Fulvicin P/G by Schering	00085-0948	Antifungal
949 <> B	Tab, Yellow, Round	Norethindrone 1 mg, Ethinyl Estradiol 0.035 mg	Ortho-Novum by Barr	00555-9009	Oral Contraceptive
949 <> B	Tab, Yellow, Round	Norethindrone 1 mg, Ethinyl Estradiol 0.035 mg	Ortho-Novum by Barr	00555-9010	Oral Contraceptive
949 <> WATSON	Tab, White, Round	Levonorgestrel 0.1 mg, Ethinyl Estradiol 0.02 mg	Lutera by Watson	52544-0949	Oral Contraceptive
95 <> B	Tab, Brown, Round, Film Coated	Ethinyl Estradiol 0.03 mg, Levonorgestrel 0.05 mg	Tri-Levlen by Pharm Util	60491-0653	Oral Contraceptive
95 <> B	Tab, Brown, Round, Film Coated	Ethinyl Estradiol 0.03 mg, Levonorgestrel 0.05 mg	Tri-Levlen by Nat Pharmpak	55154-0304	Oral Contraceptive
95 <> B	Tab, Brown, Round, Film Coated	Ethinyl Estradiol 0.03 mg, Levonorgestrel 0.05 mg	Tri-Levlen by Berlex	50419-0195	Oral Contraceptive
95 <> C	Tab, White to Off White, Round, Film Coated	Ciprofloxacin 250 mg	Cipro by Aurobindo	65862-0076	Antibiotic
95 <> C	Tab, White to Off White, Round, Film Coated	Ciprofloxacin 250 mg	Cipro by Aurobindo	13107-0076	Antibiotic
951	Tab, White, Oval, Film Coated	Losartan Potassium 25 mg	Cozaar by Sandoz	00781-5805	Antihypertensive
951	Tab, White, Oval, Film Coated	Losartan Potassium 25 mg	Cozaar by Merck	00006-0951	Antihypertensive
951 <> B	Tab, Light Yellow, Round	Norethindrone 0.5 mg, Ethinyl Estradiol 0.035 mg	Ortho-Novum by Barr	00555-9012	Oral Contraceptive
951 <> MRK	Tab, Light Green, Tear Drop Shaped, Film Coated	Losartan Potassium 25 mg	Cozaar by Nat Pharmpak	55154-5009	Antihypertensive
951 <> MRK	Tab, Light Green, Tear Drop Shaped, Film Coated	Losartan Potassium 25 mg	Cozaar by Merck Frosst	Canadian DIN 02182815	Antihypertensive

ID FRONT <> BACK	DESCRIPTION FRONT <> BACK	INGREDIENT & STRENGTH	BRAND (or Generic Equiv.) by FIRM	NDC#	CLASS; SCH.
952	Tab, White, Oval, Scored, Film Coated	Losartan Potassium 50 mg	Cozaar by Merck	00006-0952	Antihypertensive
952	Tab, White, Oval, Scored, Film Coated	Losartan Potassium 50 mg	Cozaar by Sandoz	00781-5806	Antihypertensive
9525 <> B	Tab, Peach, Round, Scored, 952 over 5	Dextroamphetamine Sulfate 5 mg	Dexedrine by Barr	00555-0952	Stimulant; C II
9531	Tab, White, Round	Methenamine 300 mg, Sodium Biphosphate 500 mg	Uro-Phosphate by Poythress		Antibiotic; Urinary Tract
95310 <> B	Tab, Pink, Round, Scored, 953 over 10	Dextroamphetamine Sulfate 10 mg	Dexedrine by Barr	00555-0953	Stimulant; C II
9532	Tab, White, Round	Aminophylline 130 mg, Potassium Iodide 195 mg,	Mudrane-2 by Poythress		Antiasthmatic
9533	Tab, Green, Round	Aminophylline 130 mg, Guaifenesin 100 mg	Mudrane GG-2 by Poythress		Antiasthmatic
953HOPE	Cap, White	Aminobenzoate Potassium 500 mg	Potaba by Hope	60267-0953	Antifibrotic
954 <> WATSON	Tab, White, Round	Desogestrel 0.15 mg, Ethinyl Estradiol 0.03 mg	Ortho-Cept by Watson	52544-0954	Oral Contraceptive
9540	Tab, Yellow, Round	Atropine Sulfate 0.195 mg, Phenobarbital 16 mg	Anthrocol by Poythress		Gastrointestinal; C IV
955	Tab, White, Round	Famotidine 20 mg	Pepcid by Andrx	62037-0955	Gastrointestinal
9550	Tab, Yellow, Round	Potassium Iodide 195 mg, Aminophylline 130 mg, Phenobarbital 8 mg, Ephedrine 16 mg	Mudrane by Poythress		Antiasthmatic; C IV
9551	Tab, Mottled Yellow, Round	Aminophylline 130 mg, Ephedrine 16 mg, Phenobarbital 8 mg, Guaifenesin 100 mg	Mudrane GG by Poythress		Antiasthmatic
956	Tab, White, Round	Famotidine 40 mg	Pepcid by Andrx	62037-0956	Gastrointestinal
958PAR	Cap, Green and Yellow, Opaque	Chlordiazepoxide 5 mg	Librium by Par	49884-0958	Antianxiety; C IV
959PAR	Cap, Black and Green, Opaque	Chlordiazepoxide 10 mg	Librium by Par	49884-0959	Antianxiety; C IV
96 <> B	Tab, Off-White to White, Round, Film Coated	Ethinyl Estradiol 0.04 mg, Levonorgestrel 0.075 mg	Tri-Levlen by Berlex	50419-0196	Oral Contraceptive
96 <> B	Tab, Off-White to White, Round, Film Coated	Ethinyl Estradiol 0.04 mg, Levonorgestrel 0.075 mg	Tri-Levlen by Pharm Util	60491-0653	Oral Contraceptive
960	Tab, White, Teardrop Shaped, Film Coated	Losartan Potassium 100 mg	Cozaar by Merck	00006-0960	Antihypertensive
960	Tab, White, Tear Drop Shaped, Film Coated	Losartan Potassium 100 mg	Cozaar by Sandoz	00781-5807	Antihypertensive
960 <> MRK	Tab, Dark Green, Teardrop Shaped, Film Coated	Losartan Potassium 100 mg	Cozaar by Merck Frosst	Canadian DIN 02182882	Antihypertensive
960PAR	Cap, Green and White, Opaque	Chlordiazepoxide 25 mg	Librium by Par	49884-0960	Antianxiety; C IV
961 <> PAR	Tab, Blue, Round, Film Coated	Chlordiazepoxide 5 mg, Amitriptyline HCl 12.5 mg	Limbitrol by Par	49884-0961	Antidepressant; Antianxiety
9643 <> 93	Tab, Yellow, Round, Film Coated	Prochlorperazine 5 mg	Compazine by Teva	00093-9643	Antiemetic
965 <> B	Tab, Pink, Round, Film Coated	Ethinyl Estradiol 0.02 mg, Levonorgestrel 0.1 mg	Levlite by Barr	00555-9014	Oral Contraceptive
9652 <> 93	Tab, Yellow, Round, Film Coated	Prochlorperazine 10 mg	Compazine by Teva	00093-9652	Antiemetic
966 <> WATSON	Tab, White, Round	Levonorgestrel 0.15 mg, Ethinyl Estradiol 0.03 mg	Quasense by Watson	52544-0966	Oral Contraceptive
967 <> B	Tab, Off-White, Oval, Film Coated	Fluvoxamine Maleate 25 mg	Luvox by Barr	00555-0967	OCD
968	Tab, Salmon, Round, Schering Logo 968	Acetophenazine Maleate 20 mg	Tindal by Schering		Antipsychotic
968 <> 93	Tab, Pink, Round	Famotidine 10 mg	Pepcid by Major	00904-5529	Gastrointestinal
968 <> 93	Tab, Pink, Round	Famotidine 10 mg	Pepcid by Perrigo	00113-0207	Gastrointestinal
968 <> B3593	Tab, Pink, Round	Famotidine 10 mg	Pepcid by Perrigo	00113-1207	Gastrointestinal
96850 <> B	Tab, Yellow, Oval, Scored, Film Coated	Fluvoxamine Maleate 50 mg	Luvox by Barr	00555-0968	OCD
969100 <> B	Tab, Brown, Oval, Scored, Film Coated	Fluvoxamine Maleate 100 mg	Luvox by Barr	00555-0969	OCD
97 <> B	Tab, Light Yellow, Round, Film Coated	Ethinyl Estradiol 0.03 mg, Levonorgestrel 0.125 mg	Tri-Levlen by Pharm Util	60491-0653	Oral Contraceptive
97 <> B	Tab, Light Yellow, Round, Film Coated	Ethinyl Estradiol 0.03 mg, Levonorgestrel 0.125 mg	Tri-Levlen by Berlex	50419-0197	Oral Contraceptive
97 <> M	Tab, Orange, Triangular, Film Coated	Fluphenazine HCl 10 mg	Prolixin by UDL	51079-0488	Antipsychotic
97 <> M	Tab, Orange, Triangular, Film Coated	Fluphenazine HCl 10 mg	Prolixin by Mylan	00378-6097	Antipsychotic
97 <> M	Tab, Orange, Triangular, Film Coated	Fluphenazine HCl 10 mg	Prolixin by Invamed	52189-0312	Antipsychotic
970	Tab, Lavender, Oval, Sch. Logo 970	Methyltestosterone Buccal 10 mg	Oreton Buccal by Schering		Hormone; C III
970	Tab, Duramed Logo over 970	Digoxin 0.125 mg	Lanoxin by Murfreesboro	51129-1102	Cardiac Agent
970	Tab, Duramed Logo on Top of 970	Digoxin 0.125 mg	Lanoxin by Murfreesboro	51129-1113	Cardiac Agent
970 <> M	Tab, White, Round, M inside square <> 970	Acetaminophen 325 mg, Butalbital 50 mg, Caffeine 40 mg	Fioricet by Mallinckrodt	00406-0970	Analgesic
971	Tab, Logo 971	Digoxin 0.25 mg	Lanoxin by Quality Care	60346-0607	Cardiac Agent
977 <> B	Tab, Light Yellow, Round	Norethindrone Acetate 1 mg, Ethinyl Estradiol 20 mcg	Junel 1/20 Fe by Barr	00555-9026	Oral Contraceptive

ID FRONT <> BACK	DESCRIPTION FRONT <> BACK	INGREDIENT & STRENGTH	BRAND (or Generic Equiv.) by FIRM	NDC#	CLASS; SCH.
977 <> B	Tab, Light Yellow, Round	Norethindrone Acetate 1 mg, Ethinyl Estradiol 20 mcg	Junel 1/20 by Barr	00555-9025	Oral Contraceptive
978 <> B	Tab, Pink, Round	Norethindrone Acetate 1.5 mg, Ethinyl Estradiol 30 mcg	Junel 1.5/30 by Barr	00555-9027	Oral Contraceptive
978 <> B	Tab, Pink, Round	Norethindrone Acetate 1.5 mg, Ethinyl Estradiol 30 mcg	Junel 1.5/30 Fe by Barr	00555-9028	Oral Contraceptive
979 <> BARR	Tab, Beige, Cap Shaped, Scored, Film Coated	Hydroxyurea 1000 mg	Hydrea by Barr	00555-0979	Antineoplastic
983 <> 93	Tab, Brown, Round, Film Coated	Nystatin 500,000 Units	Mycostatin by Schein	00364-2051	Antifungal
983 <> 93	Tab, Brown, Round, Film Coated	Nystatin 500,000 Units	Mycostatin by Teva	00093-0983	Antifungal
985 <> B	Tab, Gray, Round	Norgestimate 0.180 mg, Ethinyl Estradiol 0.035 mg	Tri-Sprintec by Barr	00555-9018	Oral Contraceptive
986 <> B	Tab, Light Blue, Round	Norgestimate 0.215 mg, Ethinyl Estradiol 0.035 mg	Tri-Sprintec by Barr	00555-9018	Oral Contraceptive
987 <> B	Tab, Blue, Round	Norgestimate 0.250 mg, Ethinyl Estradiol 0.035 mg	Tri-Sprintec by Barr	00555-9018	Oral Contraceptive
987 <> B	Tab, Blue, Round	Norgestimate 0.250 mg, Ethinyl Estradiol 0.035 mg	Sprintec by Barr	00555-9016	Oral Contraceptive
99 <> ADIPEX	Tab, White with Blue Specks, Scored, Adipex-P 99	Phentermine 37.5 mg	Adipex-P by Gate	57844-0009	Anorexiant; C IV
99 <> ADIPEX	Tab, White with Blue Specks, Scored, Adipex-P 99	Phentermine HCl 37.5 mg	by Teva	00093-0009 Discontinued	Anorexiant; C IV
99 <> LEMMON	Tab, Mottled Blue & White	Phentermine HCl 37.5 mg	by Allscripts		Anorexiant; C IV
992 <> B	Tab, Pink, Round, Film Coated	Levonorgestrel 0.15 mg, Ethinyl Estradiol 0.03 mg	Nordette by Barr	00555-9020	Oral Contraceptive
992 <> B	Tab, Pink, Round, Film Coated	Levonorgestrel 0.15 mg, Ethinyl Estradiol 0.03 mg	Jolessa by Barr	00555-9123	Oral Contraceptive
992 <> B	Tab, Pink, Round, Film Coated	Levonorgestrel 0.15 mg, Ethinyl Estradiol 0.03 mg	Portia 21 by Apotex	Canadian DIN 02295946	Oral Contraceptive
992 <> B	Tab, Pink, Round, Film Coated	Levonorgestrel 0.15 mg, Ethinyl Estradiol 0.03 mg	Portia 28 by Apotex	Canadian DIN 02295954	Oral Contraceptive
993 <> GG	Tab, White, Round, Film Coated	Leflunomide 10 mg	Arava by Sandoz	00781-5056	Antiarthritic
994 <> GG	Tab, White, Round, Film Coated	Leflunomide 20 mg	Arava by Sandoz	00781-5057	Antiarthritic
996 <> SZ	Tab, Yellow, Round	Simvastatin 5 mg	Zocor by Sandoz	00781-5070	Antihyperlipidemic
997 <> SZ	Tab, Round, Light Pink	Simvastatin 10 mg	Zocor by Sandoz	00781-5071	Antihyperlipidemic
997110 <> B	Tab, Yellow, Oval, Scored, 997 over 1/10	Fludrocortisone 0.1 mg	Florinef by Barr	00555-0997	Steroid
A	Tab, White, Round, Blue Print, Stylized A	Almotriptan Malate 12.5 mg	Axert by Ortho-McNeil	00062-2085	Antimigraine
A	Tab, Yellow, Oval, Film Coated, Abbott logo (a)	Clarithromycin 250 mg	Biaxin BID by Abbott	Canadian DIN 01984853	Antibiotic
A	Tab, Pale Yellow, Oval, Film Coated, Abbott logo (a)	Clarithromycin 500 mg	Biaxin BID by Abbott	Canadian DIN 02126710	Antibiotic
A	Tab, White, Round, Blue Print, Stylized A	Almotriptan Malate 12.5 mg	Axert by Janssen-Ortho	Canadian DIN 02248129	Antimigraine
A	Tab, Pink, Round, Coated, A~, Extended Release	Zolpidem Tartrate 6.25 mg	Ambien CR by Sanofi	00024-5501	Sedative/Hypnotic; C IV
A	Tab, Blue, Round, Coated, A~, Extended Release	Zolpidem Tartrate 12.5 mg	Ambien CR by Sanofi	00024-5521	Sedative/Hypnotic; C IV
A	Tab, Light Red, Round, Speckled, Orally Disintegrating	Desloratadine 5 mg	Clarinex Reditabs by Schering	00085-1384	Antihistamine
A	Tab, Deep Maroon, Round, Film Coated	Phenazopyridine HCl 95 mg	Pyridium by Able	53265-0095 Discontinued	Urinary Analgesic
A	Tab, Orange, Logo/A	Perphenazine 4 mg, Amitriptyline 10 mg	by Schering	Canadian	Antipsychotic; Antidepressant
A	Tab, White, Round	Nylidrin 12 mg	by RPR	Canadian	Vasodilator
A	Tab, White, Round	Nylidrin 6 mg	by RPR	Canadian	Vasodilator
A	Tab, Peach, Round, Uncoated	Phenylpropanolamine HCl 75 mg	by Physician Total Care	54868-4099	Decongestant; Appetite Suppressant
A	Tab, Yellow, Round	Phenylpropanolamine HCl 25 mg, Brompheniramine Sulfate 4 mg	Porcupine by PFI		Cold Remedy
A	Tab, White, Scored	Disulfiram 500 mg	Antabuse by Wyeth	Canadian Discontinued	Antialcoholism
A	Tab, White, Round, Blue Print, Stylized A	Almotriptan Malate 12.5 mg	Axert by Searle	00025-2085	Antimigraine
A	Tab, Orange, Round, Schering Logo/A	Amitriptyline 10 mg, Perphenazine 4 mg	Triavil by Bayer	Canadian	Antidepressant; Antipsychotic

ID FRONT <> BACK	DESCRIPTION FRONT <> BACK	INGREDIENT & STRENGTH	BRAND (or Generic Equiv.) by FIRM	NDC#	CLASS; SCH.
A	Tab, White, Round	Disulfiram 250 mg	Antabuse by Wyeth	Canadian Discontinued	Antialcoholism
A	Tab, Pink, Round	Trimipramine Maleate 12.5 mg	Trimip by Apotex	Canadian DIN 00740799	Antidepressant
A	Cap, Orange, Soft Gel	Valproic Acid 250 mg	Depakene by Abbott	Canadian DIN 00443840	Anticonvulsant
A	Tab, Salmon, Oblong, Enteric Coated	Divalproex Sodium 125 mg	Epival by Abbott	Canadian DIN 00596418	Anticonvulsant
A	Tab, Peach, Oblong, Film Coated	Divalproex Sodium 250 mg	Epival by Abbott	Canadian DIN 00596426	Anticonvulsant
A	Tab, Pink, Oblong, Enteric Coated	Divalproex Sodium 500 mg	Epival by Abbott	Canadian DIN 00596434	Anticonvulsant
A	Tab, White, Round	Captopril 6.25 mg	Capoten by Apotex	Canadian DIN 01999559	Antihypertensive
A <> 002	Tab, Blue, Round, Scored	Dextromethorphan 60 mg, Guaifenesin 1200 mg	Aquatab DM by Adams	63824-0002	Cold Remedy
A <> 003	Tab, Pink, Round	Guaifenesin 1200 mg, Phenylpropanolamine 75 mg	Aquatab D by Prepackage Specialists	58864-0074	Cold Remedy
A <> 004	Tab, Yellow, Round, Scored	Dextromethorphan 60 mg, Guaifenesin 1200 mg, Phenylpropanolamine HCl 75 mg	Aquatab C by Prepackage Specialists	58864-0033	Cold Remedy
A <> 01	Tab, Light Pink, Round, Film Coated	Simvastatin 10 mg	Zocor by Aurobindo	65862-0051	Antihyperlipidemic
A <> 019	Tab, Pink, Round	Guaifenesin 200 mg	Aquabid by Ivax	00182-2614 Discontinued	Expectorant
A <> 02	Tab, Light Pink, Round, Film Coated	Simvastatin 20 mg	Zocor by Aurobindo	65862-0052	Antihyperlipidemic
A <> 03	Tab, Pink, Round, Film Coated	Simvastatin 40 mg	Zocor by Aurobindo	65862-0053	Antihyperlipidemic
A <> 031	Tab, Chewable	Ascorbic Acid 34.5 mg, Cyanocobalamin 4.9 mcg, Folic Acid 0.35 mg, Niacinamide 14.16 mg, Pyridoxine HCl 1.1 mg, Riboflavin 1.2 mg, Sodium Ascorbate 32.2 mg, Sodium Fluoride 1.1 mg, Thiamine Mononitrate 1.15 mg, Vitamin A Acetate 5.5 mg, Vitamin D 0.194 mg, Vitamin E Acetate 15.75 mg	Poly Vitamins by Ivax	00182-1819	Vitamin
A <> 04	Tab, Pink, Cap Shaped, Film Coated	Simvastatin 80 mg	Zocor by Aurobindo	65862-0054	Antihyperlipidemic
A <> 05	Tab, Peach, Round, Film Coated	Citalopram HBr 10 mg	Celexa by Aurobindo	65862-0005	Antidepressant
A <> 05	Tab, Peach, Round, Film Coated	Citalopram HBr 10 mg	Celexa by Aurolife	13107-0005	Antidepressant
A <> 06	Tab, Light Pink, Cap Shaped, Scored, A <> 0 / 6	Citalopram HBr 20 mg	Celexa by Aurolife	13107-0006	Antidepressant
A <> 06	Tab, Light Pink, Cap Shaped, Scored, A <> 0 / 6	Citalopram HBr 20 mg	Celexa by Aurobindo	65862-0006	Antidepressant
A <> 07	Tab, White, Cap Shaped, Film Coated, Scored, A <> 0 / 7	Citalopram HBr 40 mg	Celexa by Aurobindo	65862-0007	Antidepressant
A <> 07	Tab, White, Cap Shaped, Film Coated, Scored, A <> 0 / 7	Citalopram HBr 40 mg	Celexa by Aurolife	13107-0007	Antidepressant
A <> 08	Tab, Yellow, Cap Shaped, Film Coated, Scored, A <> 0 / 8	Mirtazapine 15 mg	Remeron by Aurolife	13107-0031	Antidepressant
A <> 08	Tab, Yellow, Cap Shaped, Film Coated, Scored, A <> 0 / 8	Mirtazapine 15 mg	Remeron by Aurobindo	65862-0031	Antidepressant
A <> 09	Tab, Reddish Brown, Cap Shaped, Film Coated, Scored, A <> 0 / 9	Mirtazapine 30 mg	Remeron by Aurobindo	65862-0003	Antidepressant
A <> 09	Tab, Reddish Brown, Cap Shaped, Film Coated, Scored, A <> 0 / 9	Mirtazapine 30 mg	Remeron by Aurolife	13107-0003	Antidepressant
A <> 1	Tab, Light Yellow	Dextromethorphan HBr 30 mg, Guaifenesin 600 mg, Phenylephrine HCl 15 mg	Albatussin Sr by Anabolic	00722-6211	Cold Remedy
A <> 10	Tab, White, Cap Shaped, Film Coated	Mirtazapine 45 mg	Remeron by Aurobindo	65862-0032	Antidepressant
A <> 10	Tab, White, Cap Shaped, Film Coated	Mirtazapine 45 mg	Remeron by Aurolife	13107-0032	Antidepressant
A <> 107	Tab, Coated	Ascorbic Acid 120 mg, Calcium 200 mg, Copper 2 mg, Cyanocobalamin 12 mcg, Folic Acid 1 mg, Iron 65 mg, Niacinamide 20 mg, Pyridoxine HCl 10 mg, Riboflavin 3 mg, Thiamine Mononitrate 1.84 mg, Vitamin A 4000 Units, Vitamin D 400 Units, Vitamin E 22 mg, Zinc 25 mg	Prenatal Plus by Ivax	00182-4464	Vitamin
A <> 11	Tab, White, Cap Shaped, Film Coated	Mirtazapine 7.5 mg	Remeron by Aurobindo	65862-0001	Antidepressant
A <> 11	Tab, White, Cap Shaped, Film Coated	Mirtazapine 7.5 mg	Remeron by Aurolife	13107-0001	Antidepressant

ID FRONT <> BACK	DESCRIPTION FRONT <> BACK	INGREDIENT & STRENGTH	BRAND (or Generic Equiv.) by FIRM	NDC#	CLASS; SCH.
A <> 111	Tab, Brown, Oval, Film Coated, Scored	Methenamine Mandelate 500 mg	Mandelamine by Murfreesboro	51129-1430	Antibiotic; Urinary Tract
A <> 12	Tab, White, Round, Film Coated	Metformin HCl 500 mg	Glucophage by Aurobindo	65862-0008	Antidiabetic
A <> 13	Tab, White, Round, Film Coated	Metformin HCl 850 mg	Glucophage by Aurobindo	65862-0009	Antidiabetic
A <> 135	Cap, Blue Cap, Yellow Body, Hard Gelatin Cap Contains White Mini Tabs	Choline Fenofibrate 135 mg	Trilipix by Abbott	00074-9189	Treats Cholesterol
A <> 14	Tab, White, Oblong, Film Coated, Scored, A <> 1/4	Metformin HCl 1000 mg	Glucophage by Aurobindo	65862-0010	Antidiabetic
A <> 14	Tab, White, Oblong, Film Coated, Scored, A <> 1/4	Metformin HCl 1000 mg	Glucophage by Eon	00185-0221	Antidiabetic
A <> 15	Tab, Yellow, Round, Film Coated	Simvastatin 5 mg	Zocor by Aurobindo	65862-0050	Antihyperlipidemic
A <> 156	Tab, ER	Hyoscyamine Sulfate 0.375 mg	Levsin by Ivax	00182-2657	Gastrointestinal
A <> 16	Tab, Green, Cap Shaped, Film Coated, A <> 1/6	Sertraline HCl 25 mg	Zoloft by Aurobindo	65862-0011	Antidepressant
A <> 17	Tab, Blue, Cap Shaped, Film Coated, A <> 1/7	Sertraline HCl 50 mg	Zoloft by Aurobindo	65862-0012	Antidepressant
A <> 18	Tab, Yellow, Cap Shaped, Film Coated, A <> 1/8	Sertraline HCl 100 mg	Zoloft by Aurobindo	65862-0013	Antidepressant
A <> 2	Tab, Orange, Round, Abbott Logo (a)	Hydromorphone HCl 2 mg	Dilaudid by Abbott	00074-2415	Analgesic; C II
A <> 20	Tab, White to Off-White, Round	Lisinopril 2.5 mg	Zestril by Aurobindo	65862-0037	Antihypertensive
A <> 21	Tab, Light Red, Round, Scored, A <> 2/1	Lisinopril 5 mg	Zestril by Aurobindo	65862-0038	Antihypertensive
A <> 22	Tab, Light Yellow, Round	Lisinopril 10 mg	Zestril by Aurobindo	65862-0039	Antihypertensive
A <> 23	Tab, Light Yellow, Cap Shaped	Lisinopril 20 mg	Zestril by Aurobindo	65862-0040	Antihypertensive
A <> 237	Tab, White to Off-White, Round	Atropine Sulfate 0.025 mg, Diphenoxylate HCl 2.5 mg	Lomotil by Able	53265-0237 Discontinued	Antidiarrheal; C V
A <> 24	Tab, Light Yellow, Round	Lisinopril 30 mg	Zestril by Aurobindo	65862-0041	Antihypertensive
A <> 25	Tab, Light Yellow, Cap Shaped	Lisinopril 40 mg	Zestril by Aurobindo	65862-0042	Antihypertensive
A <> 253	Tab, Yellow Mottled, Round	Methylphenidate HCl 5 mg	Ritalin by Able	53265-0253 Discontinued	Stimulant; C II
A <> 254	Tab, White to Off-White, Round, Scored	Methylphenidate HCl 10 mg	Ritalin by Able	53265-0254 Discontinued	Stimulant; C II
A <> 255	Tab, Orange Mottled, Round, Scored	Methylphenidate HCl 20 mg	Ritalin by Able	53265-0255 Discontinued	Stimulant; C II
A <> 26	Tab, Light Pink, Round	Lisinopril 10 mg, HCTZ 12.5 mg	Prinzide by Aurobindo	65862-0043	Antihypertensive; Diuretic
A <> 27	Tab, Light Pink, Round	Lisinopril 20 mg, HCTZ 25 mg	Prinzide by Aurobindo	65862-0045	Antihypertensive; Diuretic
A <> 28	Tab, Light Yellow, Round	Lisinopril 20 mg, HCTZ 12.5 mg	Prinzide by Aurobindo	65862-0044	Antihypertensive; Diuretic
A <> 3	Tab, White, Octagonal, Film Coated	Indapamide 2.5 mg	Lozol by Arcola	00070-3000 Discontinued	Diuretic
A <> 3	Tab, Pink, Round, Film Coated, Scored	Guaifenesin 1200 mg, Phenylpropanolamine 75 mg	Aquatab D by Adams	63824-0003	Cold Remedy
A <> 3	Tab, White, Octagonal, Film Coated	Indapamide 2.5 mg	Lozol by Murfreesboro	51129-1537	Diuretic
A <> 3	Tab, White, Octagonal, Film Coated	Indapamide 2.5 mg	Lozol by RPR	00801-3000	Diuretic
A <> 3438	Tab, White, Round, Apotex Logo	Selegiline 5 mg	Eldepryl by Apotex	60505-3438	Antiparkinson
A <> 3438	Tab, White, Round, Apotex Logo	Selegiline 5 mg	Eldepryl by Major	00904-5266	Antiparkinson
A <> 36	Tab, White, Round, Scored, Orally Disintegrating	Mirtazapine 15 mg	Remeron SolTab by Aurobindo	65862-0021	Antidepressant
A <> 37	Tab, White, Round, Scored, Orally Disintegrating	Mirtazapine 30 mg	Remeron SolTab by Aurobindo	65862-0022	Antidepressant
A <> 387	Tab, White to Off White, Round, Film Coated	Hydroxyzine HCl 10 mg	Atarax by Able	53265-0387 Discontinued	Antianxiety; Antihistamine
A <> 388	Tab, White to Off White, Round, Film Coated	Hydroxyzine HCl 25 mg	Atarax by Able	53265-0388 Discontinued	Antianxiety; Antihistamine
A <> 389	Tab, White to Off White, Round, Film Coated	Hydroxyzine HCl 50 mg	Atarax by Able	53265-0389 Discontinued	Antianxiety; Antihistamine
A <> 396	Tab, Light Peach, Mottled, Round,	Methamphetamine HCl 5 mg	Desoxyn by Able	53265-0396 Discontinued	Stimulant; C II
A <> 4	Tab, Yellow, Round, Scored	Guaifenesin 1200 mg, Phenylpropanolamine 75 mg	Aquatab D by Adams	63824-0004	Cold Remedy
A <> 4	Tab, Yellow, Round, Abbott Logo (a)	Hydromorphone HCl 4 mg	Dilaudid by Abbott	00074-2416	Analgesic; C II
A <> 45	Cap, Reddish-Brown Cap, Yellow Body, Hard Gelatin Cap Contains White Mini Tabs	Choline Fenofibrate 45 mg	Trilipix by Abbott	00074-9642	Treats Cholesterol

ID FRONT <> BACK	DESCRIPTION FRONT <> BACK	INGREDIENT & STRENGTH	BRAND (or Generic Equiv.) by FIRM	NDC#	CLASS; SCH.
A <> 46	Tab, Yellow, Cap Shaped, Film Coated	Glyburide 1.25 mg, Metformin 250 mg	Glucovance by Aurobindo	65862-0080	Antidiabetic
A <> 47	Tab, Light Pink, Cap Shaped, Film Coated	Glyburide 2.5 mg, Metformin 500 mg	Glucovance by Aurobindo	65862-0081	Antidiabetic
A <> 48	Tab, Yellow, Cap Shaped, Film Coated	Glyburide 5 mg, Metformin 500 mg	Glucovance by Aurobindo	65862-0082	Antidiabetic
A <> 48	Tab, Green, Yellow, White, Round, Scored	Phendimetrazine Tartrate 35 mg	Bontril PDM by Amarin	65234-0048	Anorexiant; C III
A <> 49	Tab, Yellow, Round, Film Coated	Risperidone 0.25 mg	Risperdal by Aurobindo	65862-0119	Antipsychotic
A <> 5	Tab, White, Round, Flat-Faced, A<>5	Alendronate 5 mg	Fosamax by Apotex	Canadian DIN 0248727	Antiosteoporosis
A <> 50	Tab, Pale Violet, Scored	Acetaminophen 325 mg, Butalbital 50 mg	Phrenilin by Amarin	65234-0050	Analgesic
A <> 50	Tab, Light Pink, Round, Film Coated	Dolasetron 50 mg	Anzemet by Aventis	00088-1202	Antiemetic
A <> 51	Tab, White, Round	Benazepril HCl 5 mg	Lotensin by Amneal	65162-0751	Antihypertensive
A <> 52	Tab, White, Round	Benazepril HCl 10 mg	Lotensin by Amneal	65162-0752	Antihypertensive
A <> 53	Tab, White, Round	Benazepril HCl 20 mg	Lotensin by Amneal	65162-0753	Antihypertensive
A <> 54	Tab, White, Round	Benazepril HCl 40 mg	Lotensin by Amneal	65162-0754	Antihypertensive
A <> 600	Tab, Blue & White, Round, Ex Release	Guaifenesin 600 mg	Mucinex by Adams	63824-0008	Expectorant
A <> 66	Tab, Pink, Cap Shaped, Film Coated	Amoxicillin 500 mg	Amoxil by Aurobindo	65862-0014	Antibiotic
A <> 67	Tab, Pink, Cap Shaped, Film Coated, Scored, A <> 6 / 7	Amoxicillin 875 mg	Amoxil by Aurobindo	65862-0015	Antibiotic
A <> 7	Tab, Orange, Octagonal, Film Coated	Indapamide 1.25 mg	Lozol by RPR	00801-0777	Diuretic
A <> 7	Tab, Orange, Octagonal, Film Coated	Indapamide 1.25 mg	Lozol by Murfreesboro	51129-1536	Diuretic
A <> 7	Tab, Orange, Octagonal, Film Coated	Indapamide 1.25 mg	Lozol by Caremark	00339-6084	Diuretic
A <> 7	Tab, Orange, Octagonal, Film Coated	Indapamide 1.25 mg	Lozol by Arcola	00070-0777 Discontinued	Diuretic
A <> 70	Tab, Green, Cap Shaped, Film Coated	Risperidone 0.5 mg	Risperdal by Aurobindo	65862-0120	Antipsychotic
A <> 71	Tab, White, Cap Shaped, Film Coated	Risperidone 1 mg	Risperdal by Aurobindo	65862-0121	Antipsychotic
A <> 72	Tab, Light Orange, Cap Shaped, Film Coated	Risperidone 2 mg	Risperdal by Aurobindo	65862-0122	Antipsychotic
A <> 73	Tab, Yellow, Cap Shaped, Film Coated	Risperidone 3 mg	Risperdal by Aurobindo	65862-0123	Antipsychotic
A <> 74	Tab, Green, Cap Shaped, Film Coated	Risperidone 4 mg	Risperdal by Aurobindo	65862-0124	Antipsychotic
A <> 74	Tab, White, Scored	Difenoxin HCl 1 mg, Atropine Sulfate 0.025 mg	Motofen by West-Ward	00143-9031	Antidiarrheal; C IV
A <> 75	Tab, White, Round, Film Coated	Hydroxyzine HCl 10 mg	Atarax by Harris	67405-0575	Antianxiety; Antihistamine
A <> 750	Tab, Coated	Salsalate 750 mg	by Quality Care	60346-0034	NSAID
A <> AD	Tab, White, Round, Scored, Abbott Logo (a)	Ethotoin 250 mg	Paganone by Abbott	00074-6902	Anticonvulsant
A <> ADX1	Tab, White, Round, Film Coated, ADX1 <> A with arrowhead attached to right leg of A	Anastrozole 1 mg	Arimidex by AstraZeneca	Canadian DIN 02224135	Antineoplastic
A <> ADX1	Tab, White, Round, Film Coated, ADX1 <> A with arrowhead attached to right leg of A	Anastrozole 1 mg	Arimidex by Murfreesboro	51129-1122	Antineoplastic
A <> ADX1	Tab, White, Round, Film Coated, ADX1 <> A with arrowhead attached to right leg of A	Anastrozole 1 mg	Arimidex by AstraZeneca	00310-0201	Antineoplastic
A <> AF	Tab, Yellow, Round, Abbott Logo (a) <> AF	Colchicine 0.6 mg	by Abbott	00074-3781	Antigout
A <> AMIDE001	Tab, Orange, Pink & Purple, Round, Chewable, AMIDE001 <> A, B, C, or D	Ascorbic Acid 60 mg, Cyanocobalamin 4.5 mcg, Folic Acid 0.3 mg, Niacinamide, Pyridoxine HCl 1.05 mg, Riboflavin 1.2 mg, Sodium Fluoride, Thiamine Mononitrate, Vitamin A Acetate, Vitamin D 400 Units, Vitamin E Acetate	Multi Vita Bets by Amide	52152-0001	Vitamin
A <> AMIDE001	Tab, Orange, Pink & Purple, Round, Chewable, AMIDE001 <> A, B, C, or D	Ascorbic Acid 60 mg, Cyanocobalamin 4.5 mcg, Folic Acid 0.3 mg, Niacinamide, Pyridoxine HCl 1.05 mg, Riboflavin 1.2 mg, Sodium Fluoride, Thiamine Mononitrate, Vitamin A Acetate, Vitamin D 400 Units, Vitamin E Acetate	Multi Vita Bets by Major	00904-5275	Vitamin
A <> AMIDE001	Tab, Orange, Pink & Purple, Round, Chewable, AMIDE001 <> A, B, C, or D	Ascorbic Acid 60 mg, Cyanocobalamin 4.5 mcg, Folic Acid 0.3 mg, Niacinamide, Pyridoxine HCl 1.05 mg, Riboflavin 1.2 mg, Sodium Fluoride, Thiamine Mononitrate, Vitamin A Acetate, Vitamin D 400 Units, Vitamin E Acetate	Multi Vita Bets by Qualitest	00603-4712	Vitamin
A <> AN25	Tab, White, Round, Abbott Logo (a) <> AN over 25	Dicumarol 25 mg	Dicumarol by Abbott	00074-3794 Discontinued	Anticoagulant

ID FRONT <> BACK	DESCRIPTION FRONT <> BACK	INGREDIENT & STRENGTH	BRAND (or Generic Equiv.) by FIRM	NDC#	CLASS; SCH.
A <> ANTABUSE250	Tab, White, Octagonal, Scored	Disulfiram 250 mg	Antabuse by Wyeth	00046-0809	Antialcoholism
A <> AO50	Tab, Pink, Round, Abbott Logo (a) <> AO over 50	Dicumarol 50 mg	by Abbott	00074-3773 Discontinued	Anticoagulant
A <> BPl63	Tab, White, Pentagonal	Lorazepam 0.5 mg	Ativan by DJ Pharma	64455-0063	Antianxiety; C IV
A <> CHEWEZ	Tab, White, Round, Scored, Chewable, Abbott Logo (a)	Erythromycin 200 mg	EryPed Chewable by Abbott	00074-6314 Discontinued	Antibiotic
A <> DF	Tab, White, Round, Abbott Logo (a)	Terazosin HCl 1 mg	Hytrin by Abbott	00074-3322 Discontinued	Antihypertensive
A <> DH	Tab, Orange, Round, Abbott Logo (a)	Terazosin HCl 2 mg	Hytrin by Abbott	00074-3323 Discontinued	Antihypertensive
A <> DI	Tab, Green, Round, Abbott Logo (a)	Terazosin HCl 10 mg	Hytrin by Abbott	00074-3325 Discontinued	Antihypertensive
A <> DJ	Tab, Tan, Round, Abbott Logo (a)	Terazosin HCl 5 mg	Hytrin by Abbott	00074-3324 Discontinued	Antihypertensive
A <> EA	Tab, Pink, Oval, Film Coated, Abbott Logo (a)	Erythromycin 500 mg	Ery-Tab by Abbott	00074-6227	Antibiotic
A <> EA	Tab, Pink, Oval, Film Coated, Abbott Logo (a)	Erythromycin 500 mg	by Allscripts		Antibiotic
A <> EA	Tab, Pink, Oval, Film Coated, Abbott Logo (a)	Erythromycin 500 mg	by Halsey		Antibiotic
A <> EA	Tab, Pink, Oval, Film Coated, Abbott Logo (a)	Erythromycin 500 mg	by Apotheca	12634-0507	Antibiotic
A <> EB	Tab, Pink, Oval, Film Coated, Abbott Logo	Erythromycin 250 mg	Eryc by Abbott	00074-6328	Antibiotic
A <> EC	Tab, White, Oval, Enteric Coated, Delayed Release, Abbott Logo (a)	Erythromycin 250 mg	by Nat Pharmpak	55154-0107	Antibiotic
A <> EC	Tab, White, Oval, Enteric Coated, Delayed Release, Abbott Logo (a)	Erythromycin 250 mg	by Kaiser	00179-1055	Antibiotic
A <> EC	Tab, White, Oval, Enteric Coated, Delayed Release, Abbott Logo (a)	Erythromycin 250 mg	Ery Tab by Pharmedix	53002-0203	Antibiotic
A <> EC	Tab, White, Oval, Enteric Coated, Delayed Release, Abbott Logo (a)	Erythromycin 250 mg	by Amerisource	62584-0372	Antibiotic
A <> EC	Tab, White, Oval, Enteric Coated, Delayed Release, Abbott Logo (a)	Erythromycin 250 mg	Ery-Tab by Abbott	00074-6304	Antibiotic
A <> ED	Tab, White, Oval, Enteric Coated, Delayed Release, Abbott Logo (a <> ED)	Erythromycin 500 mg	Ery Tab by Pharmedix	53002-0205	Antibiotic
A <> ED	Tab, White, Oval, Enteric Coated, Delayed Release, Abbott Logo (a <> ED)	Erythromycin 500 mg	Ery-Tab by Kaiser	00179-1056	Antibiotic
A <> ED	Tab, White, Oval, Enteric Coated, Delayed Release, Abbott Logo (a)	Erythromycin 500 mg	Ery-Tab by Abbott	00074-6321	Antibiotic
A <> EH	Tab, White, Oval, Enteric Coated, Delayed Release, Abbott Logo (a)	Erythromycin 333 mg	Ery Tab by Pharmedix	53002-0204	Antibiotic
A <> EH	Tab, White, Oval, Enteric Coated, Delayed Release, Abbott Logo (a)	Erythromycin 333 mg	Ery-Tab by Abbott	00074-6320	Antibiotic
A <> EH	Tab, White, Oval, Enteric Coated, Delayed Release, Abbott Logo (a)	Erythromycin 333 mg	by Allscripts		Antibiotic
A <> EH	Tab, White, Oval, Enteric Coated, Delayed Release, Abbott Logo (a)	Erythromycin 333 mg	by Med Pro	53978-0089	Antibiotic
A <> ES	Tab, Pink, Round, Film Coated, Abbott Logo (a)	Erythromycin Stearate 250 mg	by Pharmedix	53002-0270	Antibiotic
A <> ES	Tab, Pink, Round, Film Coated, Abbott Logo (a)	Erythromycin Stearate 250 mg	Erythrocin by Abbott	00074-6346	Antibiotic
A <> ET	Tab, Pink, Oval, Film Coated, Abbott Logo (a)	Erythromycin Stearate 500 mg	Erythrocin by Abbott	00074-6316	Antibiotic
A <> ET	Tab, Pink, Oval, Film Coated, Abbott Logo (a)	Erythromycin Stearate 500 mg	by Pharmedix	53002-0269	Antibiotic
A <> ET	Tab, Pink, Oval, Film Coated, Abbott Logo (a)	Erythromycin Stearate 500 mg	by Allscripts		Antibiotic
A <> FI	Tab, Yellow, Abbott Logo <> FI	Fenofibrate 48 mg	TriCor by Abbott	00074-6122	Antihyperlipidemic
A <> FI	Tab, Yellow, Abbott Logo <> FI	Fenofibrate 48 mg	TriCor by Abbott	00074-6122	Antihyperlipidemic

ID FRONT <> BACK	DESCRIPTION FRONT <> BACK	INGREDIENT & STRENGTH	BRAND (or Generic Equiv.) by FIRM	NDC#	CLASS; SCH.
A <> FO	Tab, White, Abbott Logo FO	Fenofibrate 145 mg	TriCor by Abbott	00074-6123	Antihyperlipidemic
A <> FT	Tab, Pink, Round, Scored, Abbott Logo (a)	Trandolapril 1 mg	Mavik by Abbott	00074-2278	Antihypertensive
A <> FX	Tab, Yellow, Round, Abbott Logo (a)	Trandolapril 2 mg	Mavik by Abbott	00074-2279	Antihypertensive
A <> FZ	Tab, Rose, Round, Abbott Logo (a)	Trandolapril 4 mg	Mavik by Abbott	00074-2280	Antihypertensive
A <> GXEH3	Tab, White, Round, Requires refrigeration	Melphalan 2 mg	Alkeran by GSK	Canadian DIN 00004715	Antineoplastic
A <> GXEH3	Tab, White, Round, Requires refrigeration	Melphalan 2 mg	Alkeran by GSK	59572-0302	Antineoplastic
A <> KL	Tab, Yellow, Oval, Film Coated, Abbott Logo (a <> KL), Extended-Release	Clarithromycin 500 mg	Biaxin by Abbott	00074-2586	Antibiotic
A <> KL	Tab, Yellow, Oval, Film Coated, Abbott Logo (a <> KL), Extended-Release	Clarithromycin 500 mg	Biaxin by PDRX	55289-0021	Antibiotic
A <> KL	Tab, Yellow, Oval, Film Coated, Abbott Logo (a <> KL), Extended-Release	Clarithromycin 500 mg	Biaxin by DRX	55045-1865	Antibiotic
A <> KL	Tab, Yellow, Oval, Film Coated, Abbott Logo (a <> KL), Extended-Release	Clarithromycin 500 mg	Biaxin by Amerisource	62584-0317	Antibiotic
A <> KL	Tab, Yellow, Oval, Film Coated, Abbott Logo (a <> KL), Extended-Release	Clarithromycin 500 mg	Biaxin by Nat Pharmpak	55154-0109	Antibiotic
A <> KL	Tab, Yellow, Oval, Film Coated, Abbott Logo (a <> KL), Extended-Release	Clarithromycin 500 mg	Biaxin by Murfreesboro	51129-2586	Antibiotic
A <> KL	Tab, Yellow, Oval, Film Coated, Abbott Logo (a <> KL), Extended-Release	Clarithromycin 500 mg	Biaxin by Promex Med	62301-0001	Antibiotic
A <> KL	Tab, Yellow, Oval, Film Coated, Abbott Logo (a <> KL), Extended-Release	Clarithromycin 500 mg	Biaxin by Med Pro	53978-3038	Antibiotic
A <> KL	Tab, Yellow, Oval, Film Coated, Abbott Logo (a <> KL), Extended-Release	Clarithromycin 500 mg	Biaxin by H J Harkins Co	52959-0230	Antibiotic
A <> KL	Tab, Yellow, Oval, Film Coated, Abbott Logo (a <> KL), Extended-Release	Clarithromycin 500 mg	Prevpac by Tap	00300-3702	Antibiotic
A <> KL	Tab, Yellow, Oval, Film Coated, Abbott Logo (a <> KL), Extended-Release	Clarithromycin 500 mg	Biaxin by Promex Med	62301-0037	Antibiotic
A <> KTAB	Tab, Yellow, Oval, Film Coated, Ex Release, Abbott Logo (a) <> K-TAB	Potassium Chloride 750 mg	K-Tab by Nat Pharmpak	55154-0106	Electrolytes
A <> KTAB	Tab, Yellow, Oval, Film Coated, Ex Release, Abbott Logo (a) <> K-TAB	Potassium Chloride 750 mg	K-Tab by Promex Med	62301-0036	Electrolytes
A <> KTAB	Tab, Yellow, Oval, Film Coated, Ex Release, Abbott Logo (a) <> K-TAB	Potassium Chloride 750 mg	K-Tab by Abbott	00074-7804	Electrolytes
A <> LE	Tab, White, Square, Chewable, Abbott Logo (a)	Trimethadione 150 mg	Tridione Dulcet by Abbott	00074-3753	Anticonvulsant
A <> LS	Tab, Yellow, Square, Scored, Abbott Logo (a)	Methylclothiazide 5 mg, Deserpidine 0.25 mg	Enduronyl by Abbott	00074-6838 Discontinued	Diuretic; Antihypertensive
A <> LT	Tab, Gray, Square, Scored, Abbott Logo (a)	Methylclothiazide 5 mg, Deserpidine 0.5 mg	Enduronyl Forte by Abbott	00074-6854 Discontinued	Diuretic; Antihypertensive
A <> ORETIC	Tab, White, Round, Scored, Abbott Logo (a)	Hydrochlorothiazide 50 mg	Oretic by Kaiser	00179-0352	Diuretic; Antihypertensive
A <> ORETIC	Tab, White, Round, Scored, Abbott Logo (a)	Hydrochlorothiazide 25 mg	Hydrodiuril by Kaiser	00179-0347	Diuretic; Antihypertensive
A <> ORETIC	Tab, White, Round, Scored, Abbott Logo (a)	Hydrochlorothiazide 50 mg	Oretic by Abbott	00074-6985 Discontinued	Diuretic; Antihypertensive
A <> ORETIC	Tab, White, Round, Abbott Logo (a)	Hydrochlorothiazide 25 mg	Hydrodiuril by Abbott	00074-6978 Discontinued	Diuretic; Antihypertensive
A <> SC	Tab, Light Violet, Oval, Film Coated, Abbott Logo (a)	Verapamil HCl 120 mg	Isoptin SR by Abbott	00074-1149	Antihypertensive
A <> SCHERING	Tab, Orange, Round, Film Coated	Amitriptyline HCl 10 mg, Perphenazine 4 mg	Etrafon-A by Pharmascience	Canadian DIN 00176958	Antidepressant; Antipsychotic
A <> TA	Tab, Yellow, Oblong, Abbott Logo (a)	Fenofibrate 54 mg	TriCor by Abbott	00074-4009	Antihyperlipidemic
A <> TC	Tab, White, Oblong, Abbott Logo (a)	Fenofibrate 160 mg	TriCor by Abbott	00074-4013	Antihyperlipidemic

ID FRONT <> BACK	DESCRIPTION FRONT <> BACK	INGREDIENT & STRENGTH	BRAND (or Generic Equiv.) by FIRM	NDC#	CLASS; SCH.
A <> TD	Tab, Tan, Round, A over Mortar and Pestle Logo <> TD	Desiccated Thyroid 30 mg	by DRX	55045-1325	Thyroid Hormone
A <> TD	Tab	Levothyroxine 19 mcg, Liothyronine 4.5 mcg	Armour Thyroid by Amerisource	62584-0457	Thyroid Hormone
A <> TE	Tab, White, Round, Abbott Logo (a)	Methamphetamine HCl 5 mg	Desoxyn by Abbott	00074-3377	Stimulant; C II
A <> TF	Tab, Tan, Round	Levothyroxine 76 mcg, Liothyronine 18 mcg	Armour Thyroid by Amerisource	62584-0461	Thyroid Hormone
A <> TH	Tab, White, Round, Scored, Abbott Logo (a)	Pemoline 18.75 mg	Cylert by Abbott	00074-6025 Discontinued	Stimulant; C IV
A <> TI	Tab, Orange, Round, Scored, Abbott Logo (a)	Pemoline 37.5 mg	Cylert by Abbott	00074-6057 Discontinued	Stimulant; C IV
A <> TJ	Tab, Tan, Round, Scored, Abbott Logo (a)	Pemoline 75 mg	Cylert by Abbott	00074-6073 Discontinued	Stimulant; C IV
A <> TK	Tab, Orange, Square, Scored, Chewable, Abbott Logo (a)	Pemoline 37.5 mg	Cylert Chewable by Abbott	00074-6088 Discontinued	Stimulant; C IV
A <> US200	Tab, White, Round, Scored, U-S over 200	Amiodarone 200 mg	Cordarone by Sandoz	00781-1203	Antiarrhythmic
A <> US200	Tab, White, Round, Scored, U-S over 200	Amiodarone 200 mg	Cordarone by Upsher Smith	00245-1480	Antiarrhythmic
A <> WL02	Tab, White, Cap Shaped	Acetaminophen 500 mg, Pseudoephedrine HCl 60 mg, Triprolidine HCl 2.5 mg	Actifed Plus by Pfizer	Canadian DIN 02239154	Cold Remedy
A <> WL02	Tab, White, Cap Shaped	Acetaminophen 500 mg, Pseudoephedrine HCl 60 mg, Triprolidine HCl 2.5 mg	Actifed Plus by Pfizer	Canadian DIN 02239154	Cold Remedy
A <> WYETH64	Tab, White, Shield Shaped, Scored	Lorazepam 1 mg	Ativan by Med Pro	53978-3086	Antianxiety; C IV
A <> WYETH64	Tab, White, Shield Shaped, Scored	Lorazepam 1 mg	Ativan by Physician Total Care	54868-1339	Antianxiety; C IV
A <> WYETH64	Tab, White, Shield Shaped, Scored	Lorazepam 1 mg	Ativan by Wyeth	00008-0064	Antianxiety; C IV
A <> WYETH64	Tab, White, Shield Shaped, Scored	Lorazepam 1 mg	Ativan by Nat Pharmpak	55154-4204	Antianxiety; C IV
A <> WYETH81	Tab, White, Pentagonal	Lorazepam 0.5 mg	Ativan by Med Pro	53978-3085	Antianxiety; C IV
A <> WYETH81	Tab, White, Pentagonal	Lorazepam 0.5 mg	Ativan by Wyeth	00008-0081	Antianxiety; C IV
A002	Tab, Orange, Pink & Purple, Square, Chewable	Vitamin A 2500 IU, Vitamin D 400 IU, Vitamin C 60 mg, Fluoride 1.0 mg	Tri Vita-Bets by Qualitest	00603-6300	Vitamin
A002	Tab, Orange, Pink & Purple, Square, Chewable	Vitamin A 2500 IU, Vitamin D 400 IU, Vitamin C 60 mg, Fluoride 1.0 mg	Tri Vita-Bets by Amide	52152-0002	Vitamin
A003	Tab, Maroon, Round	Phenazopyridine HCl 100 mg	Pyridium by Major	00904-7922	Urinary Analgesic
A003	Tab, Maroon, Round	Phenazopyridine HCl 100 mg	Pyridium by Murfreesboro	51129-1431	Urinary Analgesic
A003	Tab, Maroon, Round	Phenazopyridine HCl 100 mg	Pyridium by Ivax	00182-0138	Urinary Analgesic
A003	Tab, Maroon, Round	Phenazopyridine HCl 100 mg	Pyridium by Amide	52152-0003	Urinary Analgesic
A003	Tab, Maroon, Round	Phenazopyridine HCl 100 mg	Pyridium by Physician Total Care	54868-0138	Urinary Analgesic
A004	Tab, Maroon, Round	Phenazopyridine HCl 200 mg	Pyridium by Apotheca	12634-0189	Urinary Analgesic
A004	Tab, Maroon, Round	Phenazopyridine HCl 200 mg	Pyridium by Amide	52152-0004	Urinary Analgesic
A004	Tab, Maroon, Round	Phenazopyridine HCl 200 mg	Pyridium by Ivax	00182-0904	Urinary Analgesic
A004	Tab, Maroon, Round	Phenazopyridine HCl 200 mg	Pyridium by Major	00904-7923	Urinary Analgesic
A0062	Tab, Green, Rectangular, Scored, A-006 over 2	Aripiprazole 2 mg	Abilify by BMS	59148-0006	Antipsychotic
A0075	Tab, Blue, Rectangular, Scored, A-007 over 5	Aripiprazole 5 mg	Abilify by BMS	59148-0007	Antipsychotic
A00810	Tab, Pink, Rectangular, A-008 over 10	Aripiprazole 10 mg	Abilify by BMS	59148-0008	Antipsychotic
A00915	Tab, Yellow, Rectangular, A-009 over 15	Aripiprazole 15 mg	Abilify by BMS	59148-0009	Antipsychotic
A01	Tab, Round, Yellow, Scored, Orally Disintegrating	Clozapine 25 mg	Fazaclo by Alamo	68322-0001	Antipsychotic
A01020	Tab, White, Round, A-010 over 20	Aripiprazole 20 mg	Abilify by BMS	59148-0010	Antipsychotic
A01130	Tab, Pink, Round, A-011 over 30	Aripiprazole 30 mg	Abilify by BMS	59148-0011	Antipsychotic
A018	Cap, Green, Opaque	Chlordiazepoxide 5 mg, Clidinium Bromide 2.5 mg	Librax by Watson	00591-4007	Gastrointestinal
A018	Cap, Green	Chlordiazepoxide 5 mg, Clidinium Bromide 2.5 mg	Librax by Ivax	00182-1856	Gastrointestinal
A018	Cap, Green	Chlordiazepoxide 5 mg, Clidinium Bromide 2.5 mg	Librax by Amide	52152-0018	Gastrointestinal
A018	Cap, Green	Chlordiazepoxide 5 mg, Clidinium Bromide 2.5 mg	Librax by URL Mutual	00677-1247	Gastrointestinal
A019	Tab, Pink, Round, Greek A 019	Guaifenesin 200 mg	Aquabid by Lee	23558-5401	Expectorant
A019	Tab, Blue or Yellow, Round	Salsalate 500 mg	Amigesic by Amide	52152-0019	NSAID
A019	Tab, Pink, Round, Greek A 019	Guaifenesin 200 mg	Aquabid by Major	00904-5154	Expectorant
A019	Tab, Pink, Round, Greek A 019	Guaifenesin 200 mg	Aquabid by Alphagen	59743-0019	Expectorant
A02	Tab, Round, Yellow, Scored, Orally Disintegrating	Clozapine 100 mg	Fazaclo by Alamo	68322-0002	Antipsychotic

ID FRONT <> BACK	DESCRIPTION FRONT <> BACK	INGREDIENT & STRENGTH	BRAND (or Generic Equiv.) by FIRM	NDC#	CLASS; SCH.
A02	Tab, White, Cap Shaped	Acyclovir 400 mg	Zovirax by Dava	67253-0101	Antiviral
A02 <> 400	Tab, White, Oval	Acyclovir 400 mg	Zovirax by Mova	55370-0555	Antiviral
A02 <> 400	Tab, White, Oval	Acyclovir 400 mg	Zovirax by Amerisource	62584-0817	Antiviral
A020	Tab, Blue OR Yellow, Cap Shaped	Salsalate 750 mg	Amigesic by Amide	52152-0020	NSAID
A024	Tab, Ivory, Rectangular, Scored	Pergolide Mesylate 0.05 mg	Permax by Amarin	65234-0024 Discontinued	Antiparkinson
A025	Cap, White	Amylase 20,000 Units, Lipase 4500 Units, Protease 25,000 Units	Pancrease by Amide		Gastrointestinal
A025	Tab, Green, Rectangular, Scored	Pergolide Mesylate 0.25 mg	Permax by Amarin	65234-0025 Discontinued	Antiparkinson
A026	Tab, White, Round, Scored, Greek A over 026	Hyoscyamine Sulfate 0.125 mg	Levsin by Alphagen	59743-0026	Gastrointestinal
A026	Tab, White, Round, Scored, Greek A over 026	Hyoscyamine Sulfate 0.125 mg	Levsin by Pharmafab	62542-0350	Gastrointestinal
A026	Tab, Pink, Rectangular, Scored	Pergolide Mesylate 1 mg	Permax by Amarin	65234-0026 Discontinued	Antiparkinson
A027	Tab, White, Round	Calcium Carbonate 420 mg	Os-Cal by Amide	52152-0027	Vitamin, Mineral
A028	Tab, White, Cap Shaped, Scored, Greek A over 028	Guaifenesin 1200 mg	Robitussin by Eli Lilly	00002-3056	Expectorant
A028	Tab, White, Cap Shaped, Scored, Greek A over 028	Guaifenesin 1200 mg	Robitussin by Alphagen	59743-0028	Expectorant
A03	Tab, White, Oval	Acyclovir 800 mg	Zovirax by Dava	67253-0102	Antiviral
A03 <> 800	Tab, White, Oval	Acyclovir 800 mg	Zovirax by Mova	55370-0556	Antiviral
A031	Tab, Orange, Pink & Purple, Square, Chewable	Vitamin A 2500 IU, Vitamin C 60 mg, Vitamin D 400 IU, Vitamin E 15 IU, Thiamin 1.05 mg, Riboflavin 1.2 mg, Niacin 13.5 mg, Vitamin B6 1.05 mg, Folate 0.3 mg, Vitamin B12 4.5 mcg, Fluoride 0.5 mg	Multi-Vit-Fluoride by Qualitest	00603-4711	Vitamin
A031	Tab, Orange, Pink & Purple, Square, Chewable	Vitamin A 2500 IU, Vitamin C 60 mg, Vitamin D 400 IU, Vitamin E 15 IU, Thiamin 1.05 mg, Riboflavin 1.2 mg, Niacin 13.5 mg, Vitamin B6 1.05 mg, Folate 0.3 mg, Vitamin B12 4.5 mcg, Fluoride 0.5 mg	Multivite W Fl by Major	00904-5274	Vitamin
A031	Tab, Orange, Pink & Purple, Square, Chewable	Vitamin A 2500 IU, Vitamin C 60 mg, Vitamin D 400 IU, Vitamin E 15 IU, Thiamin 1.05 mg, Riboflavin 1.2 mg, Niacin 13.5 mg, Vitamin B6 1.05 mg, Folate 0.3 mg, Vitamin B12 4.5 mcg, Fluoride 0.5 mg	Multi Vita-Bets by Amide	52152-0031	Vitamin
A037	Tab, Pink, Rectangular, Chewable	Vitamin A 2500 IU, Vitamin D 400 IU, dl-Alpha Tocopheryl Acetate 15 IU, Ascorbic Acid 60 mg, Folic Acid 0.3 mg, Thiamine 1.05 mg, Riboflavin 1.2 mg, Niacin 13.5 mg, Pyridoxine HCl 1.05 mg, Cyanocobalamin 4.5 mcg, Iron 12 mg, Copper 1 mg, Zinc 10 mg, Fluoride 0.5 mg	Multi Vita-Bets by Amide	52152-0037	Vitamin
A038	Tab, Pink, Square, Chewable	Ascorbic Acid 60 mg, Cupric Oxide 1 mg, Cyanocobalamin 4.5 mcg, Ferrous Fumarate 12 mg, Folic Acid 0.3 mg, Niacin 13.5 mg, Pyridoxine HCl 1.05 mg, Riboflavin 1.2 mg, Sodium Fluoride 1 mg, Thiamine Mononitrate 1.05 mg, Vitamin A Acetate 2500 Units, Vitamin D 400 Units, Vitamin E Acetate 15 Units, Zinc Oxide 10 mg	Multi Vita-Bets by Amide	52152-0038	Vitamin
A039	Cap, White	Acetaminophen 325 mg, Dichloralphenazone 100 mg, Isometheptene Mucate (1:1) 65 mg	Amidrine by Amide	52152-0039	Analgesic; C IV
A04 <> 400	Tab, White, Oblong	Etodolac 400 mg	Lodine by Aventis	55370-0552	NSAID
A04 <> 400	Tab, White, Oblong	Etodolac 400 mg	by Aventis	64734-0003	NSAID
A040	Tab, White, Round	Dimenhydrinate 50 mg	Dramamine by Amide	52152-0040	Antiemetic
A041	Cap, Red & White, Opaque	Oxycodone 5 mg, Acetaminophen 500 mg	Tylox by Amide	52152-0041	Analgesic; C II
A047	Cap, Green & Yellow	Phendimetrazine Tartrate 105 mg	Bontril SR by Amarin	65234-0047	Anorexiant; C III
A048	Tab, Film Coated	Calcium Pantothenate 10 mg, Cyanocobalamin 25 mcg, Ferrous Sulfate 525 mg, Folic Acid 800 mcg, Niacinamide 30 mg, Pyridoxine HCl 5 mg, Riboflavin 6 mg, Sodium Ascorbate 500 mg, Thiamine Mononitrate 6 mg	Multi Ferrous Folic 500 by URL Mutual	00677-0990	Vitamin, Mineral
A05	Tab, Red, Round	Potassium Chloride 300 mg	by Eli Lilly		Electrolytes
A05	Cap, Blue, Black Ink	Acyclovir 200 mg	Zovirax by Dava	67253-0100	Antiviral
A05200	Cap, Blue	Acyclovir 200 mg	Zovirax by Mova	55370-0557	Antiviral
A056	Tab, Yellow, Round	Chlorpheniramine Maleate 4 mg	Chlor-Trimeton by Amide	52152-0056	Antihistamine

ID FRONT <> BACK	DESCRIPTION FRONT <> BACK	INGREDIENT & STRENGTH	BRAND (or Generic Equiv.) by FIRM	NDC#	CLASS; SCH.
A056	Tab, Yellow, Round, Scored, Coated	Chlorpheniramine Maleate 4 mg	Chlor-Trimeton by Sandoz	00781-1148	Antihistamine
A057	Tab, Orange, Cap Shaped	Vitamins & Minerals	Prenatal Care by Amide	52152-0057	Vitamin
A058	Tab, Blue, Cap Shaped	Guaifenesin 400 mg, Phenylpropanolamine HCl 75 mg	Entex LA by Amide	52152-0058	Cold Remedy
A059	Cap, Orange & White, A-059	Guaifenesin 200 mg, Phenylephrine HCl 5 mg, Phenylpropanolamine HCl 45 mg	Entex by Amide	52152-0059	Cold Remedy
A059	Cap, Orange & White, A-059	Guaifenesin 200 mg, Phenylephrine HCl 5 mg, Phenylpropanolamine HCl 45 mg	Entex by Qualitest	00603-5665	Cold Remedy
A059	Cap, Orange & White, A-059	Guaifenesin 200 mg, Phenylephrine HCl 5 mg, Phenylpropanolamine HCl 45 mg	Entex by Physician Total Care	54868-4098	Cold Remedy
A06	Tab, Red, Round	Potassium Iodide 300 mg	by Eli Lilly		Antithyroid
A060	Cap, Pink & White, Opaque, A-060	Ursodiol 300 mg	Actigall by Amide	52152-0060	Gastrointestinal
A060	Cap, Pink & White, Opaque, A-060	Ursodiol 300 mg	Actigall by Qualitest	00603-6320	Gastrointestinal
A060	Cap, Pink & White, Opaque, A-060	Ursodiol 300 mg	Actigall by UDL	51079-0970 Discontinued	Gastrointestinal
A07	Tab, White, Round	Ketoconazole 200 mg	Nizoral by Mova	55370-0558	Antifungal
A07	Tab, White, Round, Scored, A / 07	Ketoconazole 200 mg	Nizoral by Dava	67253-0500	Antifungal
A071	Tab, White, Oblong	Prenatal Vitamin	Zenate by Amide		Vitamin
A07PB	Tab, White, Oblong, A07/pB	Acetaminophen 500 mg, Hydrocodone Bitartrate 5 mg	Vicodin by Martec		Analgesic; C III
A085	Tab, White, Cap Shaped	Choline Magnesium Trisalicylate 750 mg	Trilisate by Amide	52152-0085	NSAID
A089	Cap, Red & Yellow	Docusate Sodium 250 mg	Colace by Amide		Laxative
A1	Tab, White, Round	Guanfacine HCl 1 mg	Tenex by Qualitest	00603-3774	Antihypertensive
A1	Tab, White, Round	Guanfacine HCl 1 mg	Tenex by Amide	52152-0118	Antihypertensive
A1	Tab, White, Round	Guanfacine HCl 1 mg	Tenex by Warner Chilcott	00047-0312	Antihypertensive
A1	Tab, White, Cap Shaped	Iodine 150 mcg, Calcium 250 mg, Elemental Iron 90 mg, Copper 2 mg, Zinc 25 mg, Folic Acid 1 mg, Acetate 4000 IU, Cholecalciferol 400 IU, dl-Alpha Tocopheryl Acetate 30 IU, Ascorbic Acid 120 mg, Thiamine Mononitrate 3 mg, Riboflavin 3.4 mg, Pyridoxine HCl 20 mg, Cyanocobalamin 12 mcg, Niacinamide 20 mg, Docusate Sodium 50 mg	Aminate Fe by Amide	52152-0168	Vitamin
A1	Tab, Coated	Ascorbic Acid 120 mg, Calcium 250 mg, Cholecalciferol 400 Units, Copper 2 mg, Cyanocobalamin 12 mcg, Docusate Sodium 50 mg, Folic Acid 1 mg, Iodine 150 mcg, Iron 90 mg, Niacinamide 20 mg, Pyridoxine HCl 20 mg, Riboflavin 3.4 mg, Thiamine HCl 3 mg, Vitamin A 4000 Units, Vitamin E 30 Units, Zinc 25 mg	Maternity 90 Prenatal Vit & Min by Qualitest	00603-5355	Vitamin
A1	Tab, Coated	Ascorbic Acid 120 mg, Calcium 250 mg, Cholecalciferol 400 Units, Copper 2 mg, Cyanocobalamin 12 mcg, Docusate Sodium 50 mg, Folic Acid 1 mg, Iodine 150 mcg, Iron 90 mg, Niacinamide 20 mg, Pyridoxine HCl 20 mg, Riboflavin 3.4 mg, Thiamine HCl 3 mg, Vitamin A 4000 Units, Vitamin E 30 Units, Zinc 25 mg	Prenatal Fe 90 by Moore	00839-8093	Vitamin
A1	Tab, White, Round	Guanfacine HCl 1 mg	Tenex by Major	00904-5579	Antihypertensive
A1	Tab, White, Oblong, Scored, "TO" logo	Glyburide 2.5 mg	Euglucon by Pharmascience	Canadian DIN 00720933	Antidiabetic
A1	Tab, White to Off White and Blue, Oval, Multilayer, Boehringer Tower Logo <> A1	Telmisartan 40 mg, Amlodipine 5 mg	Twynsta by Boehringer Ingelheim	00597-0124	Antihypertensive
A1	Tab, White, Oblong, Scored, "TO" logo	Tab, White, Oblong, Scored, "TO" logo	Euglucon by Pharmascience	Canadian DIN 02236733	Antidiabetic
A1	Cap, Yellow, Oval	Benzonatate 100 mg	Tessalon Perle by Amneal	65162-0536	Cough Suppressant
A1 <> 06	Tab, Light Green, Oblong, Ex Release	Guaifenesin 600 mg	Robitussin by Ivax	00182-1188	Expectorant
A1 <> ASPIRIN	Tab, White, Round	Aspirin 325 mg	Aspirin by Major	00904-2009	Analgesic
A1 <> CIBA	Tab, White, Round, Film Coated, Scored	Oxprenolol HCl 40 mg	Trasicor by Novartis	Canadian DIN 00402575	Antihypertensive

ID FRONT <> BACK	DESCRIPTION FRONT <> BACK	INGREDIENT & STRENGTH	BRAND (or Generic Equiv.) by FIRM	NDC#	CLASS; SCH.
A1 <> F	Tab	Triamcinolone 1 mg	Aristocort by Astellas	00469-5121	Steroid
A10	Tab, Grayish Pink, Round	Nifedipine 10 mg	Adalat PA by Miles		Antihypertensive
A10	Tab, White to Off-White, Film Coated	Dalfampridine 10 mg	Ampyra by Acorda	10144-0427	Potassium Channel Blocker
A10 <> APO	Tab, White, Round, APO <> A10	Alendronate 10 mg	Fosamax by Apotex	Canadian DIN 02248728	Antiosteoporosis
A10 <> LL	Tab, White, Round, Scored, LL <> A/10	Aminocaproic Acid 500 mg	Amicar by Wyeth	Canadian DIN 02169754 Discontinued	Hemostatic
A10 <> LL	Tab, White, Round, Scored, LL <> A/10	Aminocaproic Acid 500 mg	Amicar by Immunex	58406-0612	Hemostatic
A10 <> M	Tab, Blue, Round	Amlodipine Besylate 10 mg	Norvasc by Mylan	00378-5210	Antihypertensive
A10 <> M	Tab, Blue, Round	Amlodipine Besylate 10 mg	Norvasc by UDL	51079-0452	Antihypertensive
A10 <> TEVA	Tab, White to Off White, Round, Film Coated	Anastrozole 1 mg	Arimidex by Teva Pharmaceuticals	00093-7536	Antineoplastic
A100	Cap, Red	Amantadine HCl 100 mg	Symmetrel by Genpharm	Canadian DIN 02139200	Antiviral
A100 <> G	Tab, White, Round	Atenolol 100 mg	Tenormin by Par	49884-0457	Antihypertensive
A100 <> G	Tab, White, Round, A over 100	Atenolol 100 mg	Tenormin by Amerisource	62584-0621	Antihypertensive
A100 <> G	Tab, White, Round, Flat	Atenolol 100 mg	Tenormin by Genpharm	15330-0029	Antihypertensive
A100020	Tab, Blue, Black Ink, Film Coated, Extended Release, A 1000-20	Simvastatin 20 mg, Niacin 1000 mg	Simcor by Abbott	00074-3455	Antihyperlipidemic
A100040	Tab, Dark Blue, White Ink, Film Coated, Extended Release, A 1000-40	Simvastatin 40 mg, Niacin 1000 mg	Simcor by Abbott	00074-3457	Antihyperlipidemic
A100MGOT	Cap, White, Blue Print and Two Stripes, Oval, Abbott Logo (a)	Cyclosporine 100 mg	Gengraf by Abbott	00074-6479	Immunosuppressant
A100MGPI	Cap, White, Abbott Logo (a)	Ritonavir 100 mg	Norvir by Abbott	00074-9492	Antiviral
A100MGPI	Cap, White, Abbott Logo (a)	Ritonavir 100 mg	Norvir by Physician Total Care	54868-3782	Antiviral
A100MGPI	Cap, White, Abbott Logo (a)	Ritonavir 100 mg	Norvir by DRX	55045-2485	Antiviral
A101	Tab, White to Off-White, Round, Extended Release	Bupropion HCl 150 mg	Wellbutrin XL by Anchen	10370-0101	Antidepressant
A101	Tab, White to Off-White, Round, Extended Release	Bupropion HCl 150 mg	Wellbutrin XL by Teva	00093-5350	Antidepressant
A102	Tab, White to Off-White, Round, Extended Release	Bupropion HCl 300 mg	Wellbutrin XL by Anchen	10370-0102	Antidepressant
A104	Tab, White, Oval	Calcium 200 mg, Vitamin C 100 mg, Iron 29 mg, Docusate Sodium 25 mg, Vitamin E 30 IU, Vitamin B6 20 mg, Zinc 20 mg, Vitamin B3 15 mg, Vitamin B5 7 mg, Vitamin B1 3 mg, Vitamin B2 3 mg, Vitamin B9 1 mg, Vitamin B12 12 mcg, Vitamin A 1000 IU, Vitamin D 400 IU	Prenatal Start by Amide	52152-0104	Vitamin; Mineral
A105	Tab, Pale Yellow, Cap Shaped, Scored, Film Coated, A1 over 05	Naltrexone HCl 50 mg	Revia by Amide	52152-0105	Opioid Antagonist
A106	Tab, Green, Cap Shaped	Guaifenesin 600 mg	Amibid LA by Amide	52152-0106	Expectorant
A11	Tab, Pink, Oval, Scored, Ex Release, A/11	Isosorbide Mononitrate 30 mg	Imdur by Murfreesboro	51129-1579	Antianginal
A11	Tab, Red, Oval, Scored	Isosorbide Mononitrate 30 mg	Imdur by Murfreesboro	51129-1567	Antianginal
A11	Tab, Red, Oval, Scored	Isosorbide Mononitrate 30 mg	Imdur by Warrick	59930-1502	Antianginal
A111	Tab, Brown, Oval	Methenamine Mandelate 500 mg	Mandelamine by Amide	52152-0111	Antibiotic; Urinary Tract
A111	Tab, Brown, Oval	Methenamine Mandelate 500 mg	Mandelamine by Warner Chilcott	00430-0166	Antibiotic; Urinary Tract
A115	Tab, Green, Round, Scored	Belladonna Alkaloids 0.2 mg, Ergotamine Tartrate 0.6 mg, Phenobarbital 40 mg	Bellamine S by Sandoz	00781-1701	Gastrointestinal; C IV
A115	Tab, Green, Round, Scored	Belladonna Alkaloids 0.2 mg, Ergotamine Tartrate 0.6 mg, Phenobarbital 40 mg	Bellamine S by Amide	52152-0115	Gastrointestinal; C IV
A115	Tab, Green, Round, Scored	Belladonna Alkaloids 0.2 mg, Ergotamine Tartrate 0.6 mg, Phenobarbital 40 mg	Bellamine S by DRX	55045-2417	Gastrointestinal; C IV
A115	Tab, Green, Round, Scored	Belladonna Alkaloids 0.2 mg, Ergotamine Tartrate 0.6 mg, Phenobarbital 40 mg	Bellamine S by Major	00904-2548	Gastrointestinal; C IV

ID FRONT <> BACK	DESCRIPTION FRONT <> BACK	INGREDIENT & STRENGTH	BRAND (or Generic Equiv.) by FIRM	NDC#	CLASS; SCH.
A115	Tab, Green, Round, Scored	Belladonna Alkaloids 0.2 mg, Ergotamine Tartrate 0.6 mg, Phenobarbital 40 mg	Bellamine S by Murfreesboro	51129-1374	Gastrointestinal; C IV
A117	Tab, Pink, Round, Chewable	Meclizine 25 mg	Bonine by Ivax	00182-0571 Discontinued	Antiemetic
A117	Tab, Pink, Round, Chewable	Meclizine 25 mg	Bonine by Amide	52152-0117	Antiemetic
A121	Tab, White, Round	Phenylpropanolamine HCl 25 mg	by Amide		Decongestant; Appetite Suppressant
A122	Tab, Yellow, Round	Phenylpropanolamine HCl 50 mg	by Amide		Decongestant; Appetite Suppressant
A124	Tab, Light Peach, Round, Chewable	Fluoride 0.25 mg	Luride by Amide	52152-0124	Mineral
A126	Tab, Blue, Round, Scored, Greek A over 126	Hyoscyamine Sulfate 0.125 mg	Levsin by Alphagen	59743-0126	Gastrointestinal
A126	Tab, Blue, Round, Scored, Greek A over 126	Hyoscyamine Sulfate 0.125 mg	Levsin by Murfreesboro	51129-1506	Gastrointestinal
A127	Tab, Purple, Round	Fluoride 0.5 mg	Luride by Amide	52152-0127	Mineral
A127	Tab, Purple, Round	Fluoride 0.5 mg	Luride by Qualitest	00603-3622	Mineral
A128	Tab, Assorted Colors, Round, Chewable	Fluoride 1 mg	Luride by Amide	52152-0128	Mineral
A128	Tab, Assorted Colors, Round, Chewable	Fluoride 1 mg	Luride by Qualitest	00603-3623	Mineral
A13	Tab, Coated, Abbott Logo	Erythromycin	E-Mycin by Apotheca	12634-0170	Antibiotic
A133	Tab, White, Oval	Glyburide 5 mg	Glynase by Amide	52152-0133	Antidiabetic
A133	Tab, Pale Yellow, Round, Film Coated	Bupropion HCl 150 mg	Wellbutrin SR by Actavis	67767-0133	Antidepressant
A134	Tab, Blue, Oval	Glyburide 3 mg	Glynase by Amide	52152-0134	Antidiabetic
A135	Tab, Yellow, Oval	Glyburide 6 mg	Glynase by Amide	52152-0135	Antidiabetic
A136	Tab, White, Round, A-136	Carisoprodol 350 mg	Soma by Southwood	58016-0261	Muscle Relaxant
A136	Tab, White, Round, A-136	Carisoprodol 350 mg	Soma by Amide	52152-0136	Muscle Relaxant
A137	Tab, Red & White, Round	Carisoprodol 200 mg, Aspirin 325 mg	Soma Compound by Amide	52152-0137	Muscle Relaxant
A137	Tab, White, Lavender	Aspirin 325 mg, Carisoprodol 200 mg	Soma Compound by Qualitest	00603-2583	Analgesic; Muscle Relaxant
A138	Tab, White & Yellow	Aspirin 325 mg, Carisoprodol 200 mg, Codeine 16 mg	Soma Compound/Codeine by Qualitest	00603-2584	Analgesic; C III
A138	Tab, White & Yellow, Round	Carisoprodol 200 mg, Aspirin 325 mg, Codeine Phosphate 16 mg	Soma Compound w/ Codeine by Amide	52152-0138	Analgesic; C III
A139	Tab, Green, Cap Shaped	Dextromethorphan HBr 30 mg, Guaifenesin 600 mg	Amibid DM by Amide	52152-0139	Cold Remedy
A139	Tab, Green, Cap Shaped	Dextromethorphan HBr 30 mg, Guaifenesin 600 mg	Amibid DM by Ivax	00182-1042 Discontinued	Cold Remedy
A139	Tab, Green, Cap Shaped	Dextromethorphan HBr 30 mg, Guaifenesin 600 mg	Amibid DM by Moore	00839-7897	Cold Remedy
A139	Tab, Green, Cap Shaped	Dextromethorphan HBr 30 mg, Guaifenesin 600 mg	Amibid DM by Med Pro	53978-3092	Cold Remedy
A14	Tab, Red, Round	Thyroid 30 mg	by Eli Lilly		Thyroid Hormone
A140	Tab, White, Round	Hydrocodone Bitartrate 5 mg, Homatropine Methylbromide 1.5 mg	Hycodan by Amide	52152-0140	Cold Remedy; C III
A143	Tab, White, Round	Hyoscyamine Sulfate 0.125 mg	Levsin by Major	00904-2496	Gastrointestinal
A143	Tab, White, Round	Hyoscyamine Sulfate 0.125 mg	Levsin by Qualitest	00603-4003	Gastrointestinal
A143	Tab, White, Round	Hyoscyamine Sulfate 0.125 mg	Levsin by Amide	52152-0143	Gastrointestinal
A143	Tab, White, Round	Hyoscyamine Sulfate 0.125 mg	Levsin by Ivax	00182-1607	Gastrointestinal
A145	Tab, Yellow, Round, Scored	Digoxin 0.125 mg	Lanoxin by Compumed	00403-1194	Cardiac Agent
A145	Tab	Digoxin 0.125 mg	Lanoxin by Qualitest	00603-3314	Cardiac Agent
A145	Tab, Yellow, Round	Digoxin 0.125 mg	Lanoxin by Amide	52152-0145	Cardiac Agent
A145	Tab, Yellow, Scored	Digoxin 0.125 mg	Lanoxin by Kaiser	00179-1251	Cardiac Agent
A146	Tab	Digoxin 0.25 mg	Lanoxin by PDRX	55289-0626	Cardiac Agent
A146	Tab, White, Scored	Digoxin 0.25 mg	Lanoxin by Kaiser	00179-1254	Cardiac Agent
A146	Tab	Digoxin 0.25 mg	Lanoxin by Qualitest	00603-3313	Cardiac Agent
A146	Tab, White, Round	Digoxin 0.25 mg	Lanoxin by Amide	52152-0146	Cardiac Agent
A146	Tab, White, Scored	Digoxin 0.25 mg	Lanoxin by Compumed	00403-1196	Cardiac Agent
A147	Tab	Digoxin 0.5 mg	Lanoxin by Amide	52152-0147	Cardiac Agent
A15	Tab, White, Rectangular	Buspirone HCl 15 mg	Buspar by Major	00904-5589	Antianxiety

ID FRONT <> BACK	DESCRIPTION FRONT <> BACK	INGREDIENT & STRENGTH	BRAND (or Generic Equiv.) by FIRM	NDC#	CLASS; SCH.
A15	Tab, White, Rectangular	Buspirone HCl 15 mg	Buspar by Amide	52152-0224	Antianxiety
A15	Tab, Red, Round	Thyroid 60 mg	Westhroid by Eli Lilly		Thyroid Hormone
A15 <> LL50	Tab, Orange, Heptagonal (7 sided), Scored	Amoxapine 50 mg	Asendin by Lederle	00005-5390	Antidepressant
A150	Tab, Orange, Pink & Purple, Round, Chewable	Vitamin A 2500 IU, Ascorbic Acid 60 mg, Vitamin D 400 IU, dl-Alpha Tocopheryl Acetate 15 IU, Pyridoxine HCl 1.05 mg, Cyanocobalamin 4.5 mcg, Thiamine 1.05 mg, Riboflavin 1.2 mg, Niacin 13.5 mg, Fluoride 0.25 mg, Folate 0.3 mg	Multi Vita-Bets by Amide	52152-0150	Vitamin; Supplement
A150	Tab, Orange, Pink & Purple, Round, Chewable	Vitamin A 2500 IU, Ascorbic Acid 60 mg, Vitamin D 400 IU, dl-Alpha Tocopheryl Acetate 15 IU, Pyridoxine HCl 1.05 mg, Cyanocobalamin 4.5 mcg, Thiamine 1.05 mg, Riboflavin 1.2 mg, Niacin 13.5 mg, Fluoride 0.25 mg, Folate 0.3 mg	Polyviflor Chew by Qualitest	00603-4710	Vitamin; Supplement
A150	Tab, Orange, Pink & Purple, Round, Chewable	Vitamin A 2500 IU, Ascorbic Acid 60 mg, Vitamin D 400 IU, dl-Alpha Tocopheryl Acetate 15 IU, Pyridoxine HCl 1.05 mg, Cyanocobalamin 4.5 mcg, Thiamine 1.05 mg, Riboflavin 1.2 mg, Niacin 13.5 mg, Fluoride 0.25 mg, Folate 0.3 mg	Multi Vita-Bets by Major	00904-5340	Vitamin; Supplement
A151	Tab, Yellow, Round, ER	Nifedipine 60 mg	Adalat CC by Actavis	67767-0151	Antihypertensive
A153	Tab, Yellow, Round, ER	Nifedipine 30 mg	Adalat CC by Actavis	67767-0153	Antihypertensive
A155	Tab, Blue, Round, Sublingual	Hyoscyamine Sulfate 0.125 mg	Levsin by Major	00904-5120	Gastrointestinal
A155	Tab, Blue, Round, Sublingual	Hyoscyamine Sulfate 0.125 mg	Levsin by Amide	52152-0155	Gastrointestinal
A155	Tab, Blue, Round, Sublingual	Hyoscyamine Sulfate 0.125 mg	Levsin by Murfreesboro	51129-1495	Gastrointestinal
A155	Tab, Blue, Round, Sublingual	Hyoscyamine Sulfate 0.125 mg	Levsin by URL Mutual	00677-1536	Gastrointestinal
A156	Tab, Orange, Cap Shaped, Extended Release	Hyoscyamine Sulfate 0.375 mg	Levsin by Amide	52152-0156	Gastrointestinal
A156	Tab, Orange, Cap Shaped, Extended Release	Hyoscyamine Sulfate 0.375 mg	Levsin by Qualitest	00603-4005	Gastrointestinal
A156	Tab, Orange, Cap Shaped, Extended Release	Hyoscyamine Sulfate 0.375 mg	Levsin by URL Mutual	00677-1717	Gastrointestinal
A156	Tab, Orange, Cap Shaped, Extended Release	Hyoscyamine Sulfate 0.375 mg	Levsin by Murfreesboro	51129-1496	Gastrointestinal
A157	Tab, White, Round	Meperidine 100 mg	Demerol by Amide	52152-0157	Analgesic; C II
A158	Tab, White, Round	Meperidine 50 mg	Demerol by Amide	52152-0158	Analgesic; C II
A159	Tab, White w/ Blue Specks, Oval, Scored	Phentermine 37.5 mg	Adipex by Amide	52152-0159	Anorexiant; C IV
A159	Tab, White w/ Blue Specks, Oval, Scored	Phentermine 37.5 mg	Adipex by Superior	00144-0740	Anorexiant; C IV
A159	Tab, White w/ Blue Specks, Oval, Scored	Phentermine HCl 37.5 mg	Adipex by Qualitest	00603-5191	Anorexiant; C IV
A159	Tab, White w/ Blue Specks, Oval, Scored	Phentermine 37.5 mg	Adipex by URL Mutual	00677-0829	Anorexiant; C IV
A160	Cap, Yellow, Opaque	Phentermine 30 mg	Fastin by Amide	52152-0160	Anorexiant; C IV
A161	Tab, Peach, Round, Scored	Pemoline 37.5 mg	Cylert by Amide	52152-0161	Stimulant; C IV
A161	Tab, Peach, Round, Scored	Pemoline 37.5 mg	Cylert by Mallinckrodt	00406-1554	Stimulant; C IV
				Discontinued	
A162	Tab, Peach, Round, Scored	Pemoline 75 mg	Cylert by Amide	52152-0162	Stimulant; C IV
				Discontinued	
A162	Tab, Peach, Round, Scored	Pemoline 75 mg	Cylert by Mallinckrodt	00406-1558	Stimulant; C IV
				Discontinued	
A163	Cap, Clear, Ex Release	Hyoscyamine Sulfate 0.375 mg	Levsin by Ivax	00182-1993	Gastrointestinal
A163	Cap, Clear, Ex Release	Hyoscyamine Sulfate 0.375 mg	Levsin by Amide	52152-0163	Gastrointestinal
A163	Cap, Clear, Ex Release	Hyoscyamine Sulfate 0.375 mg	Levsin by URL Mutual	00677-1718	Gastrointestinal
A166	Cap, Aqua & Light Blue	Trimethobenzamide HCl 250 mg	Tigan by Major	00904-3291	Antiemetic
A166	Cap, Aqua & Light Blue	Trimethobenzamide HCl 250 mg	Tigan by H J Harkins Co	52959-0479	Antiemetic
A166	Cap, Aqua & Light Blue	Trimethobenzamide HCl 250 mg	Tigan by Ivax	00182-1396	Antiemetic
A166	Cap, Aqua & Light Blue	Trimethobenzamide HCl 250 mg	Tigan by Amide	52152-0166	Antiemetic
A167	Cap, Blue & White, Opaque	Phentermine 37.5 mg	Adipex-P by Amide	52152-0167	Anorexiant; C IV
A167	Cap, Blue & White, Opaque	Phentermine 37.5 mg	Adipex-P by Physician Total Care	54868-4064	Anorexiant; C IV
A168	Tab, White, Oblong	Prenatal Vitamin, Iron	Prenate 90 by Amide		Vitamin

ID FRONT <> BACK	DESCRIPTION FRONT <> BACK	INGREDIENT & STRENGTH	BRAND (or Generic Equiv.) by FIRM	NDC#	CLASS; SCH.
A16A16 <> ALTIMED	Tab, White, Round, Scored, A16 over A16 <> Altimed	Clobazam 10 mg	by AltiMed	Canadian DIN 02238797	Anticonvulsant
A17 <> LL100	Tab, Greyish Blue, Heptagonal (7 sided), Scored, A over 17 <> LL over 100	Amoxapine 100 mg	Asendin by Lederle	00005-5391	Antidepressant
A17 <> LL100	Tab, Greyish Blue, Heptagonal (7 sided), Scored, A over 17 <> LL over 100	Amoxapine 100 mg	Asendin by Wyeth	Canadian Discontinued	Antidepressant
A171	Tab, White, Oval	Ascorbic Acid 80 mg, Biotin 0.03 mg, Calcium 200 mg, Copper 3 mg, Cyanocobalamin 2.5 mcg, Folic Acid 1 mg, Iron 54 mg, Magnesium 100 mg, Niacin 17 mg, Pantothenic Acid 7 mg, Pyridoxine HCl 4 mg, Riboflavin 1.6 mg, Thiamine 1.5 mg, Vitamin A 4000 Units, Vitamin D 400 Units, Vitamin E 15 Units, Zinc 25 mg	Prenatal Rx by Amide	52152-0171	Vitamin
A172	Tab, Red, Cap Shaped	Codeine Phosphate 10 mg, Guaifenesin 300 mg	Brontex by Amide	52152-0172	Cold Remedy; C III
A173	Cap, Dark Blue and Clear, A-173	Phentermine HCl 30 mg	Phentermine by Amide	52152-0160	Anorexiant; C IV
A177	Tab, White, Cap Shaped	Ascorbic Acid 70 mg, Calcium 200 mg, Cyanocobalamin 2.2 mcg, Folic Acid 1 mg, Iodine 175 mcg, Iron 65 mg, Magnesium 100 mg, Niacin 17 mg, Pyridoxine HCl 2.2 mg, Riboflavin 1.6 mg, Thiamine HCl 1.5 mg, Vitamin A 3000 Units, Vitamin D 400 Units, Vitamin E 10 Units, Zinc 15 mg	New Adv Form Prenatal Z by Amide	52152-0177	Vitamin
A178	Tab, Yellow, Oval	Ascorbic Acid 120 mg, Calcium 200 mg, Copper 2 mg, Cyanocobalamin 12 mcg, Folic Acid 1 mg, Iron 27 mg, Niacinamide 20 mg, Pyridoxine HCl 10 mg, Riboflavin 3 mg, Thiamine HCl 1.84 mg, Vitamin A 4000 Units, Vitamin D 400 Units, Vitamin E 22 mg, Zinc 25 mg	Prenatal Plus by Amide	52152-0178	Vitamin
A178	Tab, Yellow, Oval	Ascorbic Acid 120 mg, Calcium 200 mg, Copper 2 mg, Cyanocobalamin 12 mcg, Folic Acid 1 mg, Iron 27 mg, Niacinamide 20 mg, Pyridoxine HCl 10 mg, Riboflavin 3 mg, Thiamine HCl 1.84 mg, Vitamin A 4000 Units, Vitamin D 400 Units, Vitamin E 22 mg, Zinc 25 mg	Prenatal Plus by Major	00904-5339	Vitamin
A178	Tab, Yellow, Oval	Ascorbic Acid 120 mg, Calcium 200 mg, Copper 2 mg, Cyanocobalamin 12 mcg, Folic Acid 1 mg, Iron 27 mg, Niacinamide 20 mg, Pyridoxine HCl 10 mg, Riboflavin 3 mg, Thiamine HCl 1.84 mg, Vitamin A 4000 Units, Vitamin D 400 Units, Vitamin E 22 mg, Zinc 25 mg	Stuartnatal Plus by Qualitest	00603-5361	Vitamin
A179	Tab, White, Round	Betaxolol HCl 10 mg	Kerlone by Amide	52152-0179	Antihypertensive
A180	Tab, White, Round	Betaxolol HCl 20 mg	Kerlone by Amide	52152-0180	Antihypertensive
A185	Cap, Lavender, Opaque	Trimethobenzamide HCl 300 mg	Tigan by Amide	52152-0185	Antiemetic
A186	Tab, Peach, Square, Scored, Chewable	Pemoline 37.5 mg	Cylert by Amide	52152-0186 Discontinued	Stimulant; C IV
A186	Tab, Peach, Square, Scored, Chewable	Pemoline 37.5 mg	Cylert by Mallinckrodt	00406-8854 Discontinued	Stimulant; C IV
A1861	Tab, White, Oval, Greek Letter A (Alpha)	Pseudoephedrine 48 mg, Guaifenesin 595 mg, Dextromethorphan 32 mg	Panmist DM by Alphagen	59743-	Cold Remedy
A187	Cap, Peach & Brown, Opaque	Oxycodone HCl 5 mg	Roxicodone by Amide	52152-0187	Analgesic; C II
A19	Tab, Red, Round	Diethylstilbestrol Diphosphate 0.1 mg	by Eli Lilly		Hormone
A190	Cap, Red & Clear	Meperidine HCl 50 mg, Promethazine HCl 25 mg	Mepergan Fortis by Amide	52152-0190	Analgesic; C II
A197	Tab, White, Round, Scored	Pemoline 18.75 mg	Cylert by Mallinckrodt	00406-1552 Discontinued	Stimulant; C IV
A197	Tab, Peach, Round, Scored	Pemoline 18.75 mg	Cylert by Amide	52152-0162 Discontinued	Stimulant; C IV
A19LL	Tab, White, Round, A/19-LL	Acetaminophen 500 mg	Tylenol Ex Strength by Lederle		Analgesic
A2	Tab, Off-White, A/2	Chlorpheniramine Maleate 8 mg, Methscopolamine Nitrate 2.5 mg, Phenylephrine HCl 20 mg	Phenacon TR by Anabolic	00722-6227	Cold Remedy
A2	Tab, Yellow, Round	Guanfacine HCl 2 mg	Tenex by Warner Chilcott	00047-0313	Antihypertensive
A2	Tab, Yellow, Round	Guanfacine HCl 2 mg	Tenex by Amide	52152-0119	Antihypertensive
A2	Tab, Yellow, Round	Guanfacine HCl 2 mg	Tenex by Qualitest	00603-3775	Antihypertensive

ID FRONT <> BACK	DESCRIPTION FRONT <> BACK	INGREDIENT & STRENGTH	BRAND (or Generic Equiv.) by FIRM	NDC#	CLASS; SCH.
A2	Tab, White to Off White and Blue, Oval, Multilayer, Boehringer Tower Logo <> A2	Telmisartan 40 mg, Amlodipine 10 mg	Twynsta by Boehringer Ingelheim	00597-0125	Antihypertensive
A2	Cap, Yellow, Oblong, Clear	Benzonatate 200 mg	Tessalon Perle by Amneal	65162-0537	Cough Suppressant
A2 <> ASPIRIN	Tab, White, Round	Aspirin 325 mg	Bayer Aspirin by Qualitest	00603-0031	Analgesic
A2 <> M	Tab, White, Round	Atenolol 25 mg	Tenormin by Mylan	00378-0218	Antihypertensive
A2 <> M	Tab, White, Round	Atenolol 25 mg	Tenormin by UDL	51079-0759	Antihypertensive
A2 <> WYETH65	Tab, White, Pentagonal	Lorazepam 2 mg	Ativan by Wyeth	00008-0065	Antianxiety; C IV
A200	Tab, White, Oblong	Ibuprofen 200 mg	Motrin by Sanofi		NSAID
A200	Cap, White	Ibuprofen 200 mg	Motrin by Bayer	Canadian	NSAID
A206	Tab, Light Blue, a 206	Hyoscyamine Sulfate 0.125 mg SL	Levsin SL by Qualitest	00603-4002	Gastrointestinal
A20A20	Tab, White, Round, A20/A20	Metaproterenol Sulfate 20 mg	Alupent by Boehringer Ingelheim		Antiasthmatic
A21 <> M	Tab, White, Round, Extended-Release	Alprazolam 0.5 mg	Xanax XR by Mylan	00378-5021	Antianxiety; C IV
A211	Tab, Light Yellow, Cap Shaped	Pentazocine HCl 50 mg, Naloxone HCl 0.5 mg	Talwin by Amide	52152-0211	Analgesic; C IV
A213	Tab, Light Blue, Cap Shaped	Pentazocine HCl 25 mg, Acetaminophen 650 mg	Talacen by Amide	52152-0213	Analgesic; C IV
A214	Tab, Green, Round, Scored	Oxycodone HCl 15 mg	Roxicodone by Amide		Analgesic; C II
A215	Tab, Blue, Round, Scored	Oxycodone HCl 30 mg	Roxicodone by Amide	52152-0215	Analgesic; C II
A216	Tab, Dark Purple, Round	Carbetapentane Tannate 60 mg, Chlorpheniramine Tannate 5 mg	Tussi 12 by Amide	52152-0216	Cold Remedy
A219	Cap, Orange	Dantrolene Sodium 25 mg	by Amide	52152-0219	Muscle Relaxant
A21LL	Tab, White, Round, A/21-LL	Acetaminophen 325 mg	Tylenol by Lederle		Analgesic
A22	Tab, Red, Round	Diethylstilbestrol Diphosphate 1 mg	by Eli Lilly		Hormone
A22 <> DAN	Tab, Yellow, Round, Film Coated	Ranitidine HCl 150 mg	by Schein	00364-2633	Gastrointestinal
A22 <> M	Tab, Peach, Round, Extended-Release	Alprazolam 1 mg	Xanax XR by Mylan	00378-5022	Antianxiety; C IV
A225	Cap, White, Opaque, Hard Gel, Abbott Logo 225	Propafenone HCl 225 mg	Rythmol SR by Abbott	00074-6134	Antiarrhythmic
A226	Tab, Yellow, Oval	Mirtazapine 15 mg	Remeron by Amide	52152-0226	Antidepressant
A227	Tab, Tan, Oval, Scored	Mirtazapine 30 mg	Remeron by Amide	52152-0227	Antidepressant
A227	Tab, Tan, Oval, Film Coated, Scored	Mirtazapine 30 mg	Remeron by Cobalt	Canadian DIN 02274361	Antidepressant
A228	Tab, White, Oval	Mirtazapine 45 mg	Remeron by Amide	52152-0228	Antidepressant
A22DAN	Tab, Yellow, Round	Ranitidine 150 mg	by Danbury		Gastrointestinal
A22LL	Tab, White, Oblong, A22-LL	Acetaminophen 500 mg	Tylenol Ex Strength by Lederle		Analgesic
A23 <> DAN	Tab, Yellow, Cap Shaped, Film Coated	Ranitidine HCl 300 mg	by Schein	00364-2634	Gastrointestinal
A23 <> M	Tab, Light Purple, Round, Extended-Release	Alprazolam 2 mg	Xanax XR by Mylan	00378-5023	Antianxiety; C IV
A234	Tab, White, Round	Tizanidine HCl 4 mg	Zanaflex by Amide	52152-0234	Muscle Relaxant
A235	Tab, White to Off-White, Cap Shaped, Scored	Acetaminophen 500 mg, Butalbital 50 mg, Caffeine 40 mg	Esgic Plus by Able	53265-0235 Discontinued	Analgesic
A236	Tab, White to Off-White, Cap Shaped	Acetaminophen 325 mg, Butalbital 50 mg, Caffeine 40 mg	Fioricet by Able	53265-0236 Discontinued	Analgesic
A236	Tab, White, Round	Tizanidine HCl 2 mg	Zanaflex by Amide	52152-0236	Muscle Relaxant
A237	Tab, Yellow, Oval	Vitamin A 3000 IU, Vitamin D 400 IU, Vitamin E 22 mg, Vitamin C 120 mg, Folic Acid 1 mg, Vitamin B1 1.8 mg, Vitamin B2 4 mg, Niacinamide 20 mg, Vitamin B 25 mg, Vitamin B12 12 mcg, Calcium 200 mg, Copper 2 mg, Iron 28 mg, Zinc 25 mg, Magnesium 25 mg	Prenatal Formula 3 by Amide	52152-0248	Vitamin; Mineral
A238	Tab, Peach, Oval	Quinapril HCl 10 mg, Hydrochlorothiazide 12.5 mg	Quinaretic by Amide	52152-0238	Antihypertensive; Diuretic
A239	Tab, Peach, Triangle	Quinapril HCl 20 mg, Hydrochlorothiazide 12.5 mg	Quinaretic by Amide	52152-0239	Antihypertensive; Diuretic
A23DAN	Tab, Yellow, Oblong	Ranitidine 300 mg	by Danbury		Gastrointestinal
A24	Tab, White, Round, A-24	Loratadine 10 mg	Alavert by Wyeth	00573-2620	Antihistamine
A24 <> M	Tab, Pink, Round, Extended-Release	Alprazolam 3 mg	Xanax XR by Mylan	00378-5024	Antianxiety; C IV
A240	Cap, Light Blue, Opaque, Black Print	Acetaminophen 325 mg, Butalbital 50 mg, Caffeine 40 mg, Codeine 30 mg	Fioricet w/ Codeine by Able	53265-0240 Discontinued	Analgesic; C III

ID FRONT <> BACK	DESCRIPTION FRONT <> BACK	INGREDIENT & STRENGTH	BRAND (or Generic Equiv.) by FIRM	NDC#	CLASS; SCH.
A240	Tab, Peach, Round	Quinapril HCl 20 mg, Hydrochlorothiazide 25 mg	Quinaretic by Amide	52152-0240	Antihypertensive; Diuretic
A241	Tab, Brown, Oval, Film Coated, Scored	Quinapril HCl 5 mg	Accupril by Par	49884-0992	Antihypertensive
A242	Tab, Brown, Triangular, Film Coated	Quinapril HCl 10 mg	Accupril by Par	49884-0993	Antihypertensive
A243	Tab, Brown, Round, Film Coated	Quinapril HCl 20 mg	Accupril by Par	49884-0990	Antihypertensive
A244	Tab, Brown, Oval, Film Coated	Quinapril HCl 40 mg	Accupril by Par	49884-0991	Antihypertensive
A245	Tab, White, Cap Shaped, Ex Release	Guaifenesin 1200 mg	Robitussin by Amide	52152-0245	Expectorant
A246	Tab, Blue, Cap Shaped, Ex Release	Guaifenesin 1200 mg, Dextromethorphan HBr 60 mg	Aquatab DM by Amide	52152-0246	Cold Remedy
A247	Tab, White, Cap Shaped, Ex Release	Guaifenesin 1200 mg, Pseudoephedrine HCl 120 mg	Duratus GP by Amide	52152-0247	Cold Remedy
A25 <> P	Tab, White, Round	Atenolol 25 mg	Tenormin by Pharmascience	Canadian DIN 02246581	Antihypertensive
A250	Tab, White, Round	Cilostazol 100 mg	Pletal by Actavis	52152-0250	Antiplatelet
A252	Tab, White, Round, A/252	Dipyridamole 25 mg	Persantine by Schein		Antiplatelet
A253	Tab, White, Cap Shaped	Phenylephrine HCl 30 mg, Guaifenesin 600 mg	Entex LA by Amide	52152-0253	Cold Remedy
A256	Tab, Pink, Cap Shaped, Film Coated	Acetaminophen 650 mg, Propoxyphene Napsylate 100 mg	Darvocet-N 100 by Able	53265-0256 Discontinued	Analgesic; C IV
A257	Tab, Blue & White, Oval, Scored	Phentermine 37.5 mg	Adipex-P by Able	53265-0257 Discontinued	Anorexiant; C IV
A258	Cap, Yellow, Black Print, Opaque	Phentermine 30 mg	Adipex-P by Able	53265-0258 Discontinued	Anorexiant; C IV
A259	Cap, Dark Blue & Clear, Red Print	Phentermine 30 mg	Adipex-P by Able	53265-0259 Discontinued	Anorexiant; C IV
A25MGOR	Cap, White, Blue Print, Oval, Abbott Logo (a)	Cyclosporine 25 mg	Gengraf by Abbott	00074-6463	Immunosuppressant
A261	Tab, White to Off-White, Cap Shaped, Film Coated	Acetaminophen 650 mg, Propoxyphene Napsylate 100 mg	Darvocet-N 100 by Able	53265-0261 Discontinued	Analgesic; C IV
A262	Tab, White, Round, Ex Release	Methylphenidate HCl 20 mg	Ritalin by Able	53265-0262 Discontinued	Stimulant; C II
A263	Cap, White, Opaque	Isradipine 2.5 mg	DynaCirc by Actavis	52152-0263	Antihypertensive
A264	Cap, Flesh, Opaque	Isradipine 5 mg	DynaCirc by Actavis	52152-0264	Antihypertensive
A264	Tab, White to Off-White, Cap Shaped	Methocarbamol 750 mg	Robaxin by Able	53265-0264 Discontinued	Muscle Relaxant
A265	Tab, White to Off-White, Cap Shaped	Methocarbamol 500 mg	Robaxin by Able	53265-0265 Discontinued	Muscle Relaxant
A265	Tab, Yellow, Round, Film-Coated	Dipyridamole 25 mg	Persantine by Actavis	52152-0265	Antiplatelet
A266	Tab, White to Off-White, Round	Carisoprodol 350 mg	Soma by Able	53265-0266 Discontinued	Muscle Relaxant
A266	Tab, Yellow, Round, Film-Coated	Dipyridamole 50 mg	Persantine by Actavis	52152-0266	Antiplatelet
A267	Cap, Light Green, Opaque, Black Ink	Indomethacin 25 mg	Indocin by Able	53265-0267 Discontinued	NSAID
A267	Tab, Yellow, Round, Film-Coated	Dipyridamole 75 mg	Persantine by Actavis	52152-0267	Antiplatelet
A268	Cap, Light Green, Opaque, Black Ink	Indomethacin 50 mg	Indocin by Able	53265-0268 Discontinued	NSAID
A269	Cap, Yellow & Natural, Black Print, Opaque, Ex Release	Indomethacin 75 mg	Indocin SR by Able	53265-0269 Discontinued	NSAID
A270	Cap, Pink, Black Print, Opaque	Lithium Carbonate 300 mg	Eskalith by Able	53265-0270 Discontinued	Antipsychotic
A270	Cap, Pink, Black Print, Opaque	Lithium Carbonate 300 mg	Eskalith by Major	00904-5568 Discontinued	Antipsychotic
A273	Tab, White, Round, A over 273	Tramadol HCl 50 mg	Ultram by Ivax	00172-6515 Discontinued	Analgesic
A273	Tab, White, Round, A over 273	Tramadol HCl 50 mg	Ultram by Able	53265-0273 Discontinued	Analgesic

ID FRONT <> BACK	DESCRIPTION FRONT <> BACK	INGREDIENT & STRENGTH	BRAND (or Generic Equiv.) by FIRM	NDC#	CLASS; SCH.
A283	Tab, White to Off-White, A above 283	Lithium Carbonate 300 mg	Lithobid by Able	53265-0283 Discontinued	Antipsychotic
A283	Tab, White to Off-White, Round, A above 283	Lithium Carbonate 300 mg	Lithobid by UDL	51079-0253 Discontinued	Antipsychotic
A285	Tab, White, Round	Dipyridamole 50 mg	Persantine by Schein		Antiplatelet
A285 <> 3	Tab, White to Off-White, Round	Acetaminophen 300 mg, Codeine Phosphate 30 mg	Tylenol w/ Codeine by Able	53265-0285 Discontinued	Analgesic; C III
A286 <> 4	Tab, White to Off-White, Round	Acetaminophen 300 mg, Codeine Phosphate 60 mg	Tylenol w/ Codeine by Able	53265-0286 Discontinued	Analgesic; C III
A2900	Tab, White, Round, Sustained Release	Glipizide 10 mg	Glucotrol XL by Actavis	00228-2900	Antidiabetic
A2C	Cap	Digoxin 0.05 mg	Lanoxicaps by DSM	63552-0270	Cardiac Agent
A2C	Cap	Digoxin 0.05 mg	Lanoxin by Murfreesboro	51129-1112	Cardiac Agent
A2C	Cap, Red	Digoxin 0.05 mg	Lanoxicaps by GSK	00173-0270	Cardiac Agent
A2C	Cap, Clear & Dark Red	Digoxin 0.05 mg	Lanoxicaps by RP Scherer	11014-0747	Cardiac Agent
A2L	Tab, Pink, A2/L	Triamcinolone 2 mg	Aristocort by Stiefel	Canadian Discontinued	Steroid
A3	Tab, Maroon, Round	Phenazopyridine HCl 100 mg	Pyridium by Sandoz	00781-1510	Urinary Analgesic
A3	Tab, White to Off White and Blue, Oval, Multilayer, Boehringer Tower Logo <> A3	Telmisartan 80 mg, Amlodipine 5 mg	Twynsta by Boehringer Ingelheim	00597-0126	Antihypertensive
A301	Tab, Orange, Round, Film Coated	Cyclobenzaprine HCl 5 mg	Flexeril by Pliva	50111-0820 Discontinued	Muscle Relaxant
A302	Tab, Yellow, Round	Cyclobenzaprine HCl 10 mg	Flexeril by Actavis	52152-0302	Muscle Relaxant
A31	Tab, Red, Round	Potassium Chloride 1000 mg	by Eli Lilly		Electrolytes
A311	Tab, Orange, Round, Film-Coated	Hydroxyzine HCl 10 mg	Atarax by UDL	51079-0530	Antianxiety; Antihistamine
A312	Tab, Green, Round, Film-Coated	Hydroxyzine HCl 25 mg	Atarax by UDL	51079-0531 Discontinued	Antianxiety; Antihistamine
A313	Tab, Yellow, Round, Film Coated	Hydroxyzine HCl 50 mg	Atarax by UDL	51079-0532 Discontinued	Antianxiety; Antihistamine
A32	Tab, White to Off-White, Cap Shaped	Cefuroxime Axetil 125 mg	Ceftin by Aurobindo	65862-0033	Antibiotic
A325	Cap, White, Opaque, Hard Gel, Abbott Logo 325	Propafenone HCl 325 mg	Rythmol SR by Abbott	00074-6135	Antiarrhythmic
A325 <> GPI	Tab, Orange, Round	Diphenhydramine HCl 25 mg	Benadryl by Gemini		Antihistamine
A328	Tab, White to Off-White, Cap Shaped, Scored	Acetaminophen 325 mg, Hydrocodone Bitartrate 10 mg	Norco by Able	53265-0328 Discontinued	Analgesic; C III
A328	Tab, White to Off-White, Cap Shaped, Scored	Acetaminophen 325 mg, Hydrocodone Bitartrate 10 mg	Norco by UDL	51079-0305 Discontinued	Analgesic; C III
A329	Tab, White to Off-White, Cap Shaped, Scored	Acetaminophen 500 mg, Hydrocodone Bitartrate 5 mg	Vicodin by Able	53265-0329 Discontinued	Analgesic; C III
A33	Cap, Light Yellow, Clear, White Ink	Diphenhydramine HCl 25 mg	Benadryl by Rite Aid	11822-0382	Antihistamine
A33	Tab, White to Off-White, Cap Shaped	Cefuroxime Axetil 250 mg	Ceftin by Aurobindo	65862-0034	Antibiotic
A33	Tab, White, Circular, A/33	Metoprolol Tartrate 50 mg	Lopressor by AstraZeneca	Canadian	Antihypertensive
A330	Tab, White, Cap Shaped, Scored	Acetaminophen 500 mg, Hydrocodone Bitartrate 7.5 mg	Lortab by UDL	51079-0867 Discontinued	Analgesic; C III
A330	Tab, Blue and White, Mottled, Cap Shaped	Acetaminophen 500 mg, Hydrocodone Bitartrate 7.5 mg	Lortab by Able	53265-0330 Discontinued	Analgesic; C III
A331	Tab, Blue, Oval, Scored	Acetaminophen 500 mg, Hydrocodone Bitartrate 10 mg	Lortab by Able	53265-0331 Discontinued	Analgesic; C III
A332	Tab, White to Off-White, Cap Shaped, Scored	Acetaminophen 650 mg, Hydrocodone Bitartrate 7.5 mg	Lorcet Plus by Able	53265-0332 Discontinued	Analgesic; C III

ID FRONT <> BACK	DESCRIPTION FRONT <> BACK	INGREDIENT & STRENGTH	BRAND (or Generic Equiv.) by FIRM	NDC#	CLASS; SCH.
A333	Tab, Green, Cap Shaped, Scored	Acetaminophen 650 mg, Hydrocodone Bitartrate 10 mg	Lorcet by Able	53265-0333 Discontinued	Analgesic; C III
A334	Tab, White to Off-White, Cap Shaped, Scored	Acetaminophen 750 mg, Hydrocodone Bitartrate 7.5 mg	Vicodin ES by Able	53265-0334 Discontinued	Analgesic; C III
A334	Tab, White to Off-White, Cap Shaped, Scored	Acetaminophen 750 mg, Hydrocodone Bitartrate 7.5 mg	Vicodin ES by UDL	51079-0748 Discontinued	Analgesic; C III
A335	Tab, Light Yellow, Cap Shaped, Scored	Acetaminophen 325 mg, Hydrocodone Bitartrate 7.5 mg	Anexsia by Able	53265-0335 Discontinued	Analgesic; C III
A335	Tab, Light Yellow, Cap Shaped, Scored	Acetaminophen 325 mg, Hydrocodone Bitartrate 7.5 mg	Anexsia by UDL	51079-0295 Discontinued	Analgesic; C III
A338	Tab, Light Peach, Mottled, Round, Scored, A over 338	Bethanechol Chloride 25 mg	Urecholine by Able	53265-0338 Discontinued	Urinary Tract
A339	Tab, White to Off-White, Round, Scored, A over 339	Bethanechol Chloride 5 mg	Urecholine by Able	53265-0339 Discontinued	Urinary Tract
A34	Tab, White to Off-White, Cap Shaped	Cefuroxime Axetil 500 mg	Ceftin by Aurobindo	65862-0035	Antibiotic
A340	Tab, White to Off-White, Round, Scored, A over 340	Bethanechol Chloride 10 mg	Urecholine by Able	53265-0340 Discontinued	Urinary Tract
A341	Tab, Light Peach, Mottled, Round, Scored, A over 341	Bethanechol Chloride 50 mg	Urecholine by Able	53265-0341 Discontinued	Urinary Tract
A345	Tab, Blue & White, Cap Shaped, Scored	Acetaminophen 325 mg, Hydrocodone Bitartrate 5 mg	Anexsia by UDL	51079-0274 Discontinued	Analgesic; C III
A345	Tab, Blue & White, Cap Shaped, Scored	Acetaminophen 325 mg, Hydrocodone Bitartrate 5 mg	Anexsia by Able	53265-0345 Discontinued	Analgesic; C III
A346	Cap, Gray and Yellow, Opaque	Phentermine 15 mg	Phentermine HCl by Able	53265-0346 Discontinued	Anorexiant; C IV
A352	Tab, Yellow, Oval, Film-Coated	Metronidazole 750 mg ER	Flagyl ER by Able	53265-0352 Discontinued	Antibiotic
A353	Cap, Yellow and Gray, Opaque, Black Ink	Metronidazole 375 mg	Flagyl by Able	53265-0353 Discontinued	Antibiotic
A355	Cap, Buff, Opaque	Lithium Carbonate 150 mg	Eskalith by Able	53265-0355 Discontinued	Antipsychotic
A356	Cap, Buff, Opaque	Lithium Carbonate 600 mg	Eskalith by Able	53265-0356 Discontinued	Antipsychotic
A363	Tab, White to Off-White, Oval, Film Coated	Naproxen 275 mg	Anaprox by Able	53265-0363 Discontinued	NSAID
A364	Tab, White to Off-White, Oval, Film Coated, Scored	Naproxen 550 mg	Anaprox by Able	53265-0364 Discontinued	NSAID
A374	Tab, White to Off-White, Round	Metronidazole 250 mg	Flagyl by Able	53265-0374 Discontinued	Antibiotic
A375	Tab, White to Off-White, Oval	Metronidazole 500 mg	Flagyl by Able	53265-0375 Discontinued	Antibiotic
A379	Tab, White to Off-White, Cap Shaped, Scored, Extended Release	Theophylline Anhydrous 300 mg	Theochron by Able	53265-0379 Discontinued	Antiasthmatic
A380	Tab, White to Off White, Round, Scored, Ex Release	Theophylline Anhydrous 400 mg	Uniphyl by Able	53265-0380 Discontinued	Antiasthmatic
A381	Tab, White to Off-White, Cap Shaped, Scored, Extended Release	Theophylline Anhydrous 450 mg	Theochron by Able	53265-0381 Discontinued	Antiasthmatic
A382	Tab, White to Off White, Oval, Partial Score, Ex Release	Theophylline Anhydrous 600 mg	Uniphyl by Able	53265-0382 Discontinued	Antiasthmatic
A3A <> DARAPRIM	Tab	Pyrimethamine 25 mg	Darapim by DSM	63552-0201	Antiprotozoal
A3A <> DARAPRIM	Tab, White, Scored	Pyrimethamine 25 mg	Darapim by GSK	00173-0201	Antiprotozoal

ID FRONT <> BACK	DESCRIPTION FRONT <> BACK	INGREDIENT & STRENGTH	BRAND (or Generic Equiv.) by FIRM	NDC#	CLASS; SCH.
A4	Tab, Maroon, Round	Phenazopyridine HCl 200 mg	Pyridium by Sandoz	00781-1512	Urinary Analgesic
A4	Tab, White to Off White and Blue, Oval, Multilayer, Boehringer Tower Logo <> A4	Telmisartan 80 mg, Amlodipine 10 mg	Twynsta by Boehringer Ingelheim	00597-0127	Antihypertensive
A4 <> LL	Tab, White, Oblong, Scored	Triamcinolone 4 mg	Aristocort by Astellas	00469-5124	Steroid
A4 <> LL	Tab, White, Oblong, Scored	Triamcinolone 4 mg	Aristocort by Lederle	00005-4406	Steroid
A405	Tab, Light Peach, Round, Scored	Promethazine HCl 12.5 mg	Phenergan by Able	53265-0405 Discontinued	Antiemetic; Antihistamine
A406	Tab, White to Off-White, Round, Scored	Promethazine HCl 25 mg	Phenergan by Able	53265-0406 Discontinued	Antiemetic; Antihistamine
A407	Tab, Light Pink, Round, Scored	Promethazine HCl 50 mg	Phenergan by Able	53265-0407 Discontinued	Antiemetic; Antihistamine
A412	Tab, White to Off-White, Round, A over 412	Atenolol 25 mg	Tenormin by Able	53265-0412 Discontinued	Antihypertensive
A413	Tab, White to Off-White, Round, A over 413, Scored	Atenolol 50 mg	Tenormin by Able	53265-0413 Discontinued	Antihypertensive
A414	Tab, White to Off-White, Round, A over 414	Atenolol 100 mg	Tenormin by Able	53265-0414 Discontinued	Antihypertensive
A415	Tab, White, Oval	Ergoloid Mesylate 1 mg	by B F Ascher		Ergot Alkaloids
A42250MG	Cap, Green, Opaque	Cephalexin 250 mg	Keflex by Aurobindo	65862-0018	Antibiotic
A425	Cap, White, Opaque, Hard Gel, Abbott Logo 425	Propafenone HCl 425 mg	Rythmol SR by Abbott	00074-6136	Antiarrhythmic
A43500MG	Cap, Dark Green and Light Green, Opaque, Black Ink	Cephalexin 500 mg	Keflex by Aurobindo	65862-0019	Antibiotic
A45 <> LL	Tab, White, Round, Scored, A over 45 <> LL	Albuterol Sulfate 2 mg	Proventil by Lederle	00005-3062	Antiasthmatic
A49 <> LL	Tab, White, Round, Scored, A over 49	Atenolol 50 mg	Tenormin by Kaiser	62224-7224	Antihypertensive
A49 <> LL	Tab, White, Round, Scored, A over 49	Atenolol 50 mg	Tenormin by Baker Cummins	63171-1004	Antihypertensive
A49 <> LL	Tab, White, Round, Scored, A over 49	Atenolol 50 mg	Tenormin by Kaiser	00179-1165	Antihypertensive
A49 <> LL	Tab, White, Round, Scored, A over 49	Atenolol 50 mg	Tenormin by Vangard	00615-3532	Antihypertensive
A49 <> LL	Tab, White, Round, Scored, A over 49	Atenolol 50 mg	Tenormin by Lederle	00005-3219	Antihypertensive
A49 <> LL	Tab, White, Round, Scored, A over 49	Atenolol 50 mg	Tenormin by Med Pro	53978-1199	Antihypertensive
A4L	Tab, White, A4/L	Triamcinolone 4 mg	Aristocort by Stiefel	Canadian Discontinued	Steroid
A5	Tab, White, Round, Scored	Oxycodone HCl 5 mg	Roxicodone by Amide	52152-0165	Analgesic; C II
A50 <> G	Tab, White, Round, Flat	Atenolol 50 mg	Tenormin by Genpharm	15330-0028	Antihypertensive
A50 <> G	Tab, White, Round, Scored	Atenolol 50 mg	Tenormin by Par	49884-0456	Antihypertensive
A50 <> G	Tab, White, Round, Scored, A over 50	Atenolol 50 mg	Tenormin by Amerisource	62584-0620	Antihypertensive
A500	Tab, Dark Orange, Oval, Film Coated, A500 <> A500	Propoxyphene Napsylate 100 mg, Acetaminophen 500 mg	Darvocet A500 by Xanodyne	66479-0513	Analgesic; C IV
A500	Tab, Dark Orange, Oval, Film Coated, A500 <> A500	Acetaminophen 500 mg, Propoxyphene Napsylate 100 mg	Darvocet A500 by AAI Pharma	66591-0691	Analgesic; C IV
A500	Tab, Light Turquoise, Round, Film Coated, Scored, A over 500	Salsalate 500 mg	Disalcid by Able	53265-0132 Discontinued	NSAID
A500	Tab, Light Turquoise, Round, Film Coated, Scored, A over 500	Salsalate 500 mg	Disalcid by Superior	00144-1305	NSAID
A50020	Tab, Blue, Black Ink, Film Coated, Extended Release, A 500-20	Simvastatin 20 mg, Niacin 500 mg	Simcor by Abbott	00074-3312	Antihyperlipidemic
A50040	Tab, Dark Blue, White Ink, Film Coated, Extended Release, A 500-40	Simvastatin 40 mg, Niacin 500 mg	Simcor by Abbott	00074-3459	Antihyperlipidemic
A51 <> LL	Tab	Alprazolam 0.25 mg	Xanax by Vangard	00615-0426	Antianxiety; C IV
A51 <> LL	Tab	Alprazolam 0.25 mg	Xanax by Nat Pharmpak	55154-5553	Antianxiety; C IV
A512	Tab, Pink, Round	Phenolphthalein 60 mg	Modane Mild by Adria		Gastrointestinal
A513	Tab, Red, Round	Phenolphthalein 130 mg	Modane by Adria		Gastrointestinal
A515	Tab, Orange, Round	Phenolphthalein 65 mg, Docusate Sodium 100 mg	Modane Plus by Adria		Gastrointestinal
A52 <> LL	Tab	Alprazolam 0.5 mg	Xanax by Vangard	00615-0401	Antianxiety; C IV

ID FRONT <> BACK	DESCRIPTION FRONT <> BACK	INGREDIENT & STRENGTH	BRAND (or Generic Equiv.) by FIRM	NDC#	CLASS; SCH.
A52 <> LL	Tab	Alprazolam 0.5 mg	Xanax by Caremark	00339-4057	Antianxiety; C IV
A53 <> LL	Tab	Alprazolam 1 mg	Xanax by Caremark	00339-4054	Antianxiety; C IV
A4306	Tab, White to Off-White, Oval, Apotex Logo	Acyclovir 400 mg	Zovirax by Apotex	60505-5306	Antiviral
A4307	Tab, White to Off-White, Oval, Apotex Logo	Acyclovir 800 mg	Zovirax by Apotex	60505-5307	Antiviral
A56	Cap, Amethyst, Opaque	Acetaminophen 650 mg, Butalbital 50 mg	Phrenilin Forte by Amarin	65234-0056	Analgesic
A56	Tab, Yellow, Round, Scored	Chlorpheniramine Maleate 4 mg	Chlor-Trimeton by Sandoz	00781-1148	Antihistamine
A585	Tab, Mottled Yellow, Round	Carbidopa 25 mg, Levodopa 100 mg	Sinemet by Lemmon		Antiparkinson
A587	Tab, Mottled Blue, Round	Carbidopa 25 mg, Levodopa 250 mg	Sinemet by Lemmon		Antiparkinson
A59	Tab, Pink, Cap-Shaped, Biconvex, Film-coated	Paroxetine 40 mg	Paroxetine by Aurobindo	65862-0157	Antidepressant
A59025MG	Tab, A590 2.5 mg	Bromocriptine 2.5 mg	Parlodel by Elan	59075-0590	Antiparkinson
A592	Tab, White, Scored	Tizanidine HCl 2 mg	Zanaflex by Elan	59075-0592	Muscle Relaxant
A594	Tab, White, Scored	Tizanidine HCl 4 mg	Zanaflex by Elan	59075-0594	Muscle Relaxant
A594	Tab, White, Round	Tizanidine HCl 4.576 mg	Zanaflex by Shire BioChem	Canadian DIN 02239170	Muscle Relaxant
A60	Cap, White, Opaque	Ursodiol 300 mg	Actigall by Amide	52152-0060	Gastrointestinal
A615	Tab, White, Square, Scored, A over 615	Pergolide Mesylate 0.05 mg	Permax by Eli Lilly	00002-0615 Discontinued	Antiparkinson
A625	Tab, Green, Rectangular	Pergolide Mesylate 0.25 mg	Permax by Eli Lilly	00002-0625 Discontinued	Antiparkinson
A625 <> UC5337	Tab, Green, Round, Scored	Pergolide Mesylate 0.25 mg	Epermax by Pharmacy Care	65070-0513	Antiparkinson
A629	Cap, Red, Soft Gel	Sennosides 8.6 mg, Docusate 50 mg	Senokot-S by Leader	37205-0349	Laxative
A630	Tab, Pink, Round	Pergolide 1 mg	Permax by Eli Lilly	00002-0630 Discontinued	Antiparkinson
A630	Tab	Pergolide Mesylate 1 mg	Permax by Pharm Util	60491-0508 Discontinued	Antiparkinson
A652	Tab, Orange, Round	Sennosides 8.6 mg, Docusate Sodium 50 mg	Senokot-S by Major	00904-5512	Gastrointestinal
A7 <> DAN25	Tab, White, Round, Scored	Captopril 25 mg	Capoten by Schein	00364-2629	Antihypertensive
A7 <> LL	Tab, White, Round	Atenolol 25 mg	Tenormin by Lederle	00005-3218	Antihypertensive
A7 <> LL	Tab, White, Round	Atenolol 25 mg	Tenormin by Med Pro	53978-3055	Antihypertensive
A7 <> LL	Tab, White, Round	Atenolol 25 mg	Tenormin by Ivax	00182-1001	Antihypertensive
A7 <> LL	Tab, White, Round	Atenolol 25 mg	Tenormin by Nat Pharmpak	55154-5511	Antihypertensive
A7 <> M	Tab, White, Round	Alendronate Sodium 10 mg	Fosamax by UDL	51079-0941	Antiosteoporosis
A7 <> M	Tab, White, Round	Alendronate Sodium 10 mg	Fosamax by Mylan	00378-3567	Antiosteoporosis
A71 <> LL	Tab, White, Round, A over 71	Atenolol 100 mg	Tenormin by Kaiser	00179-1166	Antihypertensive
A71 <> LL	Tab, White, Round, A over 71	Atenolol 100 mg	Tenormin by Kaiser	62224-7331	Antihypertensive
A71 <> LL	Tab, White, Round, A over 71	Atenolol 100 mg	Tenormin by Lederle	00005-3220	Antihypertensive
A75	Tab, White, Round	Oxycodone 5 mg, Acetaminophen 325 mg	Percocet by Amide	52152-0075	Analgesic; C II
A75 <> 511	Tab, White, Round	Acyclovir 400 mg	Zovirax by ESI Lederle	59911-3163	Antiviral
A750	Tab, Light Turquoise, Cap Shaped, Film Coated, Scored, A over 750	Salsalate 750 mg	Disalcid by Able	53265-0133 Discontinued	NSAID
A750	Tab, Light Turquoise, Cap Shaped, Film Coated, Scored, A over 750	Salsalate 750 mg	Disalcid by Superior	00144-1307 Discontinued	NSAID
A75020	Tab, Blue, Black Ink, Film Coated, Extended Release, A 750-20	Simvastatin 20 mg, Niacin 750 mg	Simcor by Abbott	00074-3315	Antihyperlipidemic
A77 <> 511	Tab, White, Oval	Acyclovir 800 mg	Zovirax by ESI Lederle	59911-3164	Antiviral
A77 <> W	Tab, Bright Pink, Black Print, Film Coated	Chloroquine Phosphate 500 mg	Aralen Phosphate by Bayer	00280-0084	Antimalarial
A77 <> W	Tab, Bright Pink, Black Print, Film Coated	Chloroquine Phosphate 500 mg	Aralen Phosphate by Allscripts		Antimalarial
A77 <> W	Tab, Bright Pink, Black Print, Film Coated	Chloroquine Phosphate 500 mg	Aralen Phosphate by Sanofi	00024-0084	Antimalarial
A7DAN25	Tab, White, Round, Scored	Captopril 25 mg	Capoten by Caremark	00339-5791	Antihypertensive
A8 <> M	Tab, Blue, Round	Amlodipine Besylate 2.5 mg	Norvasc by Mylan	00378-5208	Antihypertensive

ID FRONT <> BACK	DESCRIPTION FRONT <> BACK	INGREDIENT & STRENGTH	BRAND (or Generic Equiv.) by FIRM	NDC#	CLASS; SCH.
A9 <> M	Tab, Blue, Round	Amlodipine Besylate 5 mg	Norvasc by Mylan	00378-5209	Antihypertensive
A9 <> M	Tab, Blue, Round	Amlodipine Besylate 5 mg	Norvasc by UDL	51079-0451	Antihypertensive
A92	Cap, Red, Soft Gel	Docusate Sodium 100 mg	Colace by Geri-Care	57896-0401	Laxative
A9L	Cap, Blue	Trihexyphenidyl HCl 5 mg	Artane Sequels by Lederle		Antiparkinson
AA	Tab, White, Oval, A/A	Chlorpheniramine 4 mg, Phenylephrine 10 mg, Phenylpropanolamine 50 mg, Pyrilamine 25 mg	Vanex Forte by Abana		Cold Remedy
AA	Tab, White, Oblong	Aspirin SR 800 mg	Aspirin by Able	Discontinued	Analgesic
AA	Tab, Peach, Round, Abbott Logo	Chlorthalidone 25 mg	Hygroton by Abbott		Diuretic
AA <> 150	Tab, Pink, Oblong, A/A <> 150	Choline Magnesium Trisalicylate 500 mg	Trilisate by Schein	00364-3150	NSAID
AA <> 151	Tab, White, Oblong, A/A <> 151	Choline Magnesium Trisalicylate 750 mg	Trilisate by Schein	00364-3151	NSAID
AA <> 152	Tab, Red, Oblong, A/A <> 152	Choline Magnesium Trisalicylate 1000 mg	Trilisate by Schein	00364-3152	NSAID
AA <> 8	Tab, White, Triangular, Scored, double Abbott Logo (aa)	Hydromorphone HCl 8 mg	Dilaudid by Abbott	00074-2426	Analgesic; C II
AA <> 8	Tab, White, Triangular, Scored, double Abbott Logo (aa)	Hydromorphone HCl 8 mg	Dilaudid by Knoll	00044-1028	Analgesic; C II
AA <> PP	Tab, White, Oval, Scored, P logo / P logo <> A / A	Pramipexole DiHCl 0.25 mg	Mirapex by Pharmascience	Canadian DIN 02290111	Antiparkinson
AA <> SK	Tab, Light Pink, Oval, Scored, Film Coated, double Abbott Logo (aa)	Verapamil HCl 180 mg	Isoptin SR by Abbott	00074-1486	Antihypertensive
AA <> ST	Tab, Light Green, Cap Shaped, Scored, Film Coated, double Abbott Logo (aa)	Verapamil HCl 240 mg	Isoptin SR by Abbott	00074-1625	Antihypertensive
AAA	Cap, Dark Red	Vitamin A 18.334 mg	Vitamin A by RP Scherer	11014-1085	Vitamin
AAA50 <> SEARLE1411	Tab, White to Off-White, Round, Film Coated, A's around 50	Diclofenac Sodium 50 mg, Misoprostol 200 mcg	Arthrotec 50 by Pfizer	Canadian DIN 01917056	NSAID
AAA50 <> SEARLE1411	Tab, White to Off-White, Round, Film Coated, A's around 50	Diclofenac Sodium 50 mg, Misoprostol 200 mcg	Arthrotec 50 by Searle	51227-6169	NSAID
AAA50 <> SEARLE1411	Tab, White to Off-White, Round, Film Coated, A's around 50	Diclofenac Sodium 50 mg, Misoprostol 200 mcg	Arthrotec 50 by Searle	00014-1411	NSAID
AAA50 <> SEARLE1411	Tab, White to Off-White, Round, Film Coated, A's around 50	Diclofenac Sodium 50 mg, Misoprostol 200 mcg	Arthrotec 50 by Searle	00025-1411	NSAID
AAA75 <> SEARLE1421	Tab, White to Off-White, Round, A's around 75	Diclofenac Sodium 75 mg, Misoprostol 200 mcg	Arthrotec 75 by Searle	00025-1421	NSAID
AAA75 <> SEARLE1421	Tab, White to Off-White, Round, A's around 75	Diclofenac Sodium 75 mg, Misoprostol 200 mcg	Arthrotec 75 by Searle	00014-1421	NSAID
AAA75 <> SEARLE1421	Tab, White to Off-White, Round, A's around 75	Diclofenac Sodium 75 mg, Misoprostol 200 mcg	Arthrotec 75 by DRX		NSAID
AAA75 <> SEARLE1421	Tab, White to Off-White, Round, A's around 75	Diclofenac Sodium 75 mg, Misoprostol 200 mcg	Arthrotec 75 by Searle	51227-6179	NSAID
AAA75 <> SEARLE1421	Tab, White to Off-White, Round, A's around 75	Diclofenac Sodium 75 mg, Misoprostol 200 mcg	Arthrotec 75 by Searle	Canadian	NSAID
AAA75 <> SEARLE1421	Tab, White to Off-White, Round, A's around 75	Diclofenac Sodium 75 mg, Misoprostol 200 mcg	Arthrotec 75 by Pfizer	Canadian DIN 02229837	NSAID
AAB	Cap, Clear & Dark Red	Vitamin A 36.7 mg	Vitamin A by RP Scherer	11014-1084	Vitamin
AAK	Tab, Red, Oval, Film Coated, Controlled Release, AK over Abbott Logo (a), Abbott Logo (a)	Iron w/ Vitamin C and B-Complex including Folic Acid	Iberet-Folic 500 by Abbott	00074-7125	Mineral
AAR	Cap, White, Abbott Logo	Fenofibrate 134 mg	TriCor by ICN	00187-4052	Antihyperlipidemic
AARP173	Tab, Beige, Round	Ferrous Sulfate 325 mg	Feosol by AARP		Mineral
AARP174	Tab, White, Oblong	Ascorbic Acid 1000 mg	Formula 174 by AARP		Vitamin
AARP201	Tab, White, Round	Aluminum 200 mg, Magnesium Hydroxide 200 mg	by PFI		Gastrointestinal
AARP242	Tab, White, Round	Calcium Carbonate 420 mg	Os-Cal by PFI		Vitamin; Mineral
AARP247	Tab, Off-White, Round	Aluminum 80 mg, Magnesium Hydroxide 80 mg, Sodium Bicarbonate 200 mg	by PFI		Gastrointestinal
AARP263	Tab, White, Round	Magnesium Hydroxide 311 mg	by PFI		Mineral
AARP400	Tab, Beige, Round	Docusate Sodium 100 mg, Phenolphthalein 65 mg	Correctol by PFI		Laxative
AARP428	Tab, White & Yellow, Round	Acetaminophen 325 mg, Phenylephrine HCl 5 mg, Chlorpheniramine Maleate 2 mg	by PFI		Cold Remedy
AARP556	Tab, Green, Oval	Magnesium Salicylate 325 mg	by PFI		Analgesic
AARP562	Tab, White, Round	Ibuprofen 200 mg	Motrin by Danbury		NSAID

ID FRONT <> BACK	DESCRIPTION FRONT <> BACK	INGREDIENT & STRENGTH	BRAND (or Generic Equiv.) by FIRM	NDC#	CLASS; SCH.
AARP5625	Tab, White	Ibuprofen 200 mg	Motrin by Danbury		NSAID
AARP685	Cap, White	Acetaminophen 650 mg	Tylenol by AARP		Analgesic
AB	Tab, Lavender, Round, Abbott Logo	Chlorthalidone 50 mg	Hygroton by Abbott		Diuretic
AB	Tab, White, Oval, Scored, Film Coated, A over B	Metoprolol Succinate 25 mg	Toprol XL by AstraZeneca	00186-1088	Antihypertensive
AB <> CIBA	Tab, Pale Blue, Round, Scored	Methylphenidate HCl 10 mg	Ritalin by Novartis	Canadian DIN 00005606	Stimulant; C II
ABANA217	Cap, White, with Green Beads	Phentermine HCl 37.5 mg	Obenix by Elge	58298-0952	Anorexiant; C IV
ABANA217	Cap, Clear & Green	Phentermine HCl 37.5 mg	Obenix by Abana	12463-0217	Anorexiant; C IV
ABANA250	Cap, Ex Release	Guaifenesin 250 mg, Pseudoephedrine HCl 90 mg	Sudafed Sinus by Sovereign	58716-0005	Cold Remedy
ABANA250	Cap	Guaifenesin 250 mg, Pseudoephedrine HCl 90 mg	Sudafed Sinus by Sovereign	58716-0005	Cold Remedy
ABB	Tab, White, Round, Scored, A over BB	Metoprolol Tartrate 50 mg	Betaloc by AstraZeneca	Canadian DIN 00402605	Antihypertensive
ABB	Tab, White, Round, Scored, A over BB	Metoprolol Tartrate 50 mg	Lopressor by Pharmascience	Canadian DIN 5760654132	Antihypertensive
ABCIBA	Tab, Blue, Round, AB/Ciba	Methylphenidate HCl 10 mg	Ritalin by Ciba	Canadian	Stimulant; C II
ABG <> 10	Tab, White, Round, Controlled Release	Oxycodone HCl 10 mg	OxyContin by Ivax	00172-6354	Analgesic; C II
ABG <> 100	Tab, Green, Capsule-Shaped, Film-Coated, Controlled Release	Morphine Sulfate 100 mg	MS Contin by Ivax	00172-2165	Analgesic; C II
ABG <> 100	Tab, Gray, Round, Convex	Morphine Sulfate 100 mg	MS Contin by Novartis	00043-0143	Analgesic; C II
ABG <> 15	Tab, Blue, Round, Film-Coated, Controlled Release	Morphine Sulfate 15 mg	MS Contin by Neuman	64579-0349	Analgesic; C II
ABG <> 15	Tab, Blue, Round, Film-Coated, Controlled Release	Morphine Sulfate 15 mg	MS Contin by Ivax	00172-2162	Analgesic; C II
ABG <> 20	Tab, Pink, Round, Controlled Release	Oxycodone HCl 20 mg	OxyContin by Ivax	00172-6355	Analgesic; C II
ABG <> 200	Tab, Green, Oblong, Convex, Film Coated	Morphine Sulfate 200 mg	MS Contin by Novartis	00043-0148	Analgesic; C II
ABG <> 30	Tab, Purple, Round, Convex, Film Coated	Morphine Sulfate 30 mg	MS Contin by Neuman	64579-0350	Analgesic; C II
ABG <> 30	Tab, Orange, Round, Film-Coated, Controlled Release	Morphine Sulfate 30 mg	MS Contin by Ivax	00172-2163	Analgesic; C II
ABG <> 40	Tab, Yellow, Round, Controlled Release	Oxycodone HCl 40 mg	OxyContin by Ivax	00172-6356	Analgesic; C II
ABG <> 60	Tab, Orange, Round, Film-Coated	Morphine Sulfate 60 mg	MS Contin by Ivax	00172-2164	Analgesic; C II
ABG <> 60	Tab, Orange, Round, Convex, Film Coated	Morphine Sulfate 60 mg	MS Contin by Neuman	64579-0358	Analgesic; C II
ABG <> 80	Tab, Green, Round, Controlled Release	Oxycodone HCl 80 mg	OxyContin by Ivax	00172-6357	Analgesic; C II
ABN150	Cap, Yellow and Light Yellow, Opaque	Nizatidine 150 mg	Axid by Pharmascience	Canadian DIN 02177714	Gastrointestinal
ABN300	Cap, Orange and Light Yellow, Opaque	Nizatidine 300 mg	Axid by Pharmascience	Canadian DIN 02177722	Gastrointestinal
ABRIKA108	Cap, Brown, Opaque	Isradipine 2.5 mg	DynaCirc by Abrika	67767-0108	Antihypertensive
ABRIKA108	Cap, Brown, Opaque	Isradipine 2.5 mg	DynaCirc by Cobalt	16252-0539	Antihypertensive
ABRIKA109	Cap, Caramel, Opaque	Isradipine 5 mg	DynaCirc by Cobalt	16252-0540	Antihypertensive
ABRIKA109	Cap, Caramel, Opaque	Isradipine 5 mg	DynaCirc by Abrika	67767-0109	Antihypertensive
ABRS123	Tab, White to Off-White, Cap Shaped, Scored, ABRS-123	Potassium Chloride 20 mEq	K-Dur by Andrx	62037-0999	Electrolytes
ABRS123	Tab, White to Off-White, Cap Shaped, Scored, ABRS-123	Potassium Chloride 20 mEq	K-Dur by Par	49884-0392	Electrolytes
AC <> APO	Tab, White, Oblong, Scored, Film Coated	Amoxicillin 875 mg, Clavulanate Potassium 125 mg	Clavulin by Apotex	Canadian DIN 02245623	Antibiotic
AC10	Tab, Film Coated, AC/10	Salicylate 1000 mg	Choline Magnesium Trisalicylate by Rugby	00536-3470	NSAID
AC100 <> G	Tab, White, Round, Film Coated, AC / 100	Acebutolol 100 mg	Monitan by Genpharm	Canadian DIN 02237721	Antihypertensive
AC100 <> G	Tab, White, Shield Shaped, Scored	Acebutolol 100 mg	Sectral by Genpharm	Canadian DIN 02237885	Antihypertensive
AC1000625	Tab, White, Oval, Film Coated, AC 1000 over 62.5	Amoxicillin 1000 mg, Clavulanic Acid 62.5 mg	Augmentin XR by SKB		Antibiotic
AC150GLAXO	Tab, Coated	Ranitidine HCl 150 mg	by Med Pro	53978-0101	Gastrointestinal
AC200 <> G	Tab, White, Oval, Film Coated, AC / 200	Acebutolol 200 mg	Monitan by Genpharm	Canadian DIN 02237722	Antihypertensive

ID FRONT <> BACK	DESCRIPTION FRONT <> BACK	INGREDIENT & STRENGTH	BRAND (or Generic Equiv.) by FIRM	NDC#	CLASS; SCH.
AC200 <> G	Tab, Blue, Shield Shaped, Scored	Acebutolol 200 mg	Sectral by Genpharm	Canadian DIN 02237886	Antihypertensive
AC200G	Cap, Orange & Purple	Acebutolol HCl 200 mg	Sectral by Par	49884-0587	Antihypertensive
AC200G	Cap, Orange & Purple	Acebutolol HCl 200 mg	Sectral by Genpharm	55567-0089	Antihypertensive
AC200G	Cap, Orange & Purple	Acebutolol HCl 200 mg	Sectral by Alphapharm	57315-0025	Antihypertensive
AC400 <> G	Tab, White, Oblong, Film Coated, AC / 400	Acebutolol 400 mg	Monitan by Genpharm	Canadian DIN 02237723	Antihypertensive
AC400 <> G	Tab, White, Shield Shaped, Scored	Acebutolol 400 mg	Sectral by Genpharm	Canadian DIN 02237887	Antihypertensive
AC400G	Cap, Orange & Purple	Acebutolol HCl 400 mg	Sectral by Alphapharm	57315-0026	Antihypertensive
AC400G	Cap, Orange & Purple	Acebutolol HCl 400 mg	Sectral by Genpharm	55567-0090	Antihypertensive
AC400G	Cap, Orange & Purple	Acebutolol HCl 400 mg	Sectral by Par	49884-0588	Antihypertensive
AC50	Tab, White, Oblong	Choline Magnesium Trisalicylate 500 mg	Trilisate by Able	Discontinued	NSAID
AC50	Tab, Yellow, Oblong	Choline Magnesium Trisalicylate 500 mg	Trilisate by Able	Discontinued	NSAID
AC58	Tab	Guaifenesin 400 mg, Phenylpropanolamine HCl 75 mg	Entex LA by Pharmedix	53002-0323	Cold Remedy
AC75	Tab, Blue, Oblong	Choline Magnesium Trisalicylate 750 mg	Trilisate by Able	Discontinued	NSAID
AC75	Tab, White, Oblong	Choline Magnesium Trisalicylate 750 mg	Trilisate by Able	Discontinued	NSAID
ACCOLATE10	Tab, White, Round, Film Coated	Zafirlukast 10 mg	Accolate by AstraZeneca	00310-0401	Antiasthmatic
ACCOLATE20	Tab, White, Round, Film Coated	Zafirlukast 20 mg	Accolate by AstraZeneca	00310-0402	Antiasthmatic
ACCOLATE20	Tab, White, Round, Film Coated	Zafirlukast 20 mg	Accolate by IPR	54921-0402	Antiasthmatic
ACCOLATE20	Tab, White, Round, Film Coated	Zafirlukast 20 mg	Accolate by URL Mutual	00677-1651	Antiasthmatic
ACCOLATE20 <> ZENECA	Tab, White to Off-White, Round, Film-Coated	Zafirlukast 20 mg	Accolate by AstraZeneca	Canadian DIN 02236606	Antiasthmatic
ACCUTANE10ROCHE	Cap, Light Pink, Soft Gel, Accutane over 10 Roche	Isotretinoin 10 mg	Accutane by Hoffmann La Roche	00004-0155	Dermatologic
ACCUTANE20ROCHE	Cap, Maroon, Soft Gel, Accutane over 20 Roche	Isotretinoin 20 mg	Accutane by Hoffmann La Roche	00004-0169	Dermatologic
ACCUTANE40ROCHE	Cap, Yellow, Soft Gel, Accutane over 40 Roche	Isotretinoin 40 mg	Accutane by Hoffmann La Roche	00004-0156	Dermatologic
ACET2	Tab, White, Round, Acet-2	Acetaminophen 300 mg, Codeine Phosphate 15 mg, Caffeine 15 mg	Tylenol w/ Codeine by Pharmascience	Canadian	Analgesic; C III
ACET3	Tab, White, Round, Acet-3	Acetaminophen 300 mg, Codeine Phosphate 30 mg, Caffeine 15 mg	Atasol-30 by Pharmascience	Canadian	Analgesic; C III
ACET30CODEINE	Tab, White, Round, Acet-30-Codeine	Acetaminophen 300 mg, Codeine Phosphate 30 mg	Tylenol w/ Codeine by Pharmascience	Canadian DIN 01999648	Analgesic; C III
ACET60CODEINE	Tab, White, Round, Acet-60 Codeine	Acetaminophen 300 mg, Codeine Phosphate 60 mg	Tylenol w/ Codeine by Pharmascience	Canadian DIN 01999656	Analgesic; C III
ACF <> 004	Tab, White to Off-White, Round, A over CF	Candesartan Cilexetil 4 mg	Atacand by AstraZeneca	00186-0004	Antihypertensive
ACF <> 004	Tab, White to Off-White, Round, A over CF	Candesartan Cilexetil 4 mg	Atacand by AstraZeneca	Canadian DIN 02239090	Antihypertensive
ACF <> 004	Tab, White, Round	Candesartan Cilexetil 4 mg	Atacand by AstraZeneca	17228-0018	Antihypertensive
ACG <> 008	Tab, Light Pink, Round, A over CG	Candesartan Cilexetil 8 mg	Atacand by AstraZeneca	Canadian DIN 02239091	Antihypertensive
ACG <> 008	Tab	Candesartan Cilexetil 8 mg	Atacand by AstraZeneca	17228-0017	Antihypertensive
ACG <> 008	Tab, Light Pink, Round, A over CG	Candesartan Cilexetil 8 mg	Atacand by AstraZeneca	00186-0008	Antihypertensive
ACH <> 016	Tab, Pink, Round, A over CH	Candesartan Cilexetil 16 mg	Atacand by AstraZeneca	00186-0016	Antihypertensive
ACH <> 016	Tab, Pink, Round, A over CH	Candesartan Cilexetil 16 mg	Atacand by AstraZeneca	Canadian DIN 02239092	Antihypertensive
ACH <> 16	Tab	Candesartan Cilexetil 16 mg	by AstraZeneca	17228-0016	Antihypertensive
ACIPHEX20	Tab, Light Yellow, Enteric Coated, Delayed Release	Rabeprazole Sodium 20 mg	Aciphex by Eisai	62856-0243	Gastrointestinal
ACJ <> 322	Tab, Yellow, Oval, A over CJ	Candesartan Cilexetil 32 mg, Hydrochlorothiazide 12.5 mg	Atacand HCT by AstraZeneca	17228-0322	Antihypertensive; Diuretic
ACJ <> 322	Tab, Yellow, Oval, A over CJ	Candesartan Cilexetil 32 mg, Hydrochlorothiazide 12.5 mg	Atacand HCT by AstraZeneca	00186-0322	Antihypertensive; Diuretic
ACKEM	Tab, Scored, ACK/EM	Propesterane 9 mg	Sigh by EST Pharma	99508-7777	Mood Enhancer
ACL <> 032	Tab, Pink, Round, A over CL	Candesartan Cilexetil 32 mg	Atacand by AstraZeneca	00186-0032	Antihypertensive
ACL <> 032	Tab, Pink, Round, A over CL	Candesartan Cilexetil 32 mg	Atacand by AstraZeneca	17228-0032	Antihypertensive

ID FRONT <> BACK	DESCRIPTION FRONT <> BACK	INGREDIENT & STRENGTH	BRAND (or Generic Equiv.) by FIRM	NDC#	CLASS; SCH.
ACN2 <> SLVSLV	Tab, White, Oblong, Scored	Perindopril Erbumine 2 mg	Aceon by Solvay	00032-1101	Antihypertensive
ACN2 <> SLVSLV	Tab, White, Oblong, Scored	Perindopril Erbumine 2 mg	Aceon by Pharmafab	62542-0783	Antihypertensive
ACN2 <> SLVSLV	Tab, White, Oblong, Scored	Perindopril Erbumine 2 mg	Aceon by Pharmafab	62542-0782	Antihypertensive
ACN4 <> SLVSLV	Tab, Pink, Oblong	Perindopril Erbumine 4 mg	Aceon by Solvay	00032-1102	Antihypertensive
ACN4 <> SLVSLV	Tab, Pink, Oblong, Scored	Perindopril Erbumine 4 mg	Aceon by RPR	00801-1102	Antihypertensive
ACN8 <> SLVSLV	Tab, Orange, Oblong, Scored, SLV Score SLV<>ACN 8	Perindopril Erbumine 8 mg	Aceon by RPR	00801-1103	Antihypertensive
ACN8 <> SLVSLV	Tab, Orange, Oblong, Scored, SLV Score SLV<>ACN 8	Perindopril Erbumine 8 mg	Aceon by Solvay	00032-1103	Antihypertensive
ACN8 <> SLVSLV	Tab, Orange, Oblong, Scored, SLV Score SLV<>ACN 8	Perindopril Erbumine 8 mg	Aceon by Pharmafab	62542-0790	Antihypertensive
ACS	Tab, Peach, Oval, Scored, A/CS	Candesartan Cilexetil 16 mg, HCTZ 12.5 mg	Atacand Plus by AstraZeneca	Canadian DIN 02244021	Antihypertensive; Diuretic
ACS <> 162	Tab, Peach, Oval, A over CS	Candesartan Cilexetil 16 mg, Hydrochlorothiazide 12.5 mg	Atacand HCT by AstraZeneca	17228-0162	Antihypertensive; Diuretic
ACS <> 162	Tab, Peach, Oval, A over CS	Candesartan Cilexetil 16 mg, Hydrochlorothiazide 12.5 mg	Atacand HCT by AstraZeneca	00186-0162	Antihypertensive; Diuretic
ACS10	Cap, Pink, Opaque, Hard Gel, Delayed Release	Omeprazole 10 mg	Losec by AstraZeneca	Canadian DIN 02119579	Gastrointestinal
ACTIFEDA2F	Tab, White	Triprolidine HCl 2.5 mg, Pseudoephedrine 60 mg, Dextromethorphan 30 mg	Actifed DM by Warner Wellcome	Canadian	Cold Remedy
ACTIFEDM2A	Tab, White, Round, Scored	Triprolidine 2.5 mg, Pseudoephedrine 60 mg	Actifed by Pfizer	Canadian DIN 02238302	Cold Remedy
ACTIGALL300MG	Cap, White & Pink, Black Print, Opaque	Ursodiol 300 mg	Actigall by Summit	57267-0153	Gastrointestinal
ACTIGALL300MG	Cap, White & Pink, Black Print, Opaque	Ursodiol 300 mg	Actigall by Novartis	00078-0319	Gastrointestinal
ACTIGALL300MG	Cap, White & Pink, Black Print, Opaque	Ursodiol 300 mg	Actigall by Watson	52544-0930	Gastrointestinal
ACTOS <> 15	Tab, White to Off-White, Round	Pioglitazone HCl 15 mg	Actos by Eli Lilly	Canadian DIN 02242572	Antidiabetic
ACTOS <> 15	Tab, White to Off-White, Round	Pioglitazone HCl 15 mg	Actos by Prestige	58056-0337	Antidiabetic
ACTOS <> 15	Tab, White to Off-White, Round	Pioglitazone HCl 15 mg	Actos by Takeda	64764-0151	Antidiabetic
ACTOS <> 30	Tab, White to Off-White, Round	Pioglitazone HCl 30 mg	Actos by Prestige	58056-0338	Antidiabetic
ACTOS <> 30	Tab, White to Off-White, Round	Pioglitazone HCl 30 mg	Actos by Takeda	64764-0301	Antidiabetic
ACTOS <> 30	Tab, White to Off-White, Round	Pioglitazone HCl 30 mg	Actos by Eli Lilly	Canadian DIN 02242573	Antidiabetic
ACTOS <> 45	Tab, White to Off-White, Round	Pioglitazone HCl 45 mg	Actos by Eli Lilly	Canadian DIN 02242574	Antidiabetic
ACTOS <> 45	Tab, White to Off-White, Round	Pioglitazone HCl 45 mg	Actos by Prestige	58056-0339	Antidiabetic
ACTOS <> 45	Tab, White to Off-White, Round	Pioglitazone HCl 45 mg	Actos by Takeda	64764-0451	Antidiabetic
ACV200	Tab, Pink, Round, ACV/200	Acyclovir 200 mg	Zovirax by Ratiopharm	Canadian DIN 02078635	Antiviral
ACV400	Tab, Pink, Round, ACV/400	Acyclovir 400 mg	Zovirax by Ratiopharm	Canadian DIN 02078635	Antiviral
ACV800	Tab, Blue, Oval, ACV/800	Acyclovir 800 mg	Zovirax by Ratiopharm	Canadian DIN 02078651	Antiviral
ACY200	Cap, White	Acyclovir 200 mg	Zovirax by H J Harkins Co	52959-0517	Antiviral
ACY200	Cap	Acyclovir 200 mg	Zovirax by LEK	48866-1220	Antiviral
ACY200	Cap, Opaque & White	Acyclovir 200 mg	Zovirax by Amerisource	62584-0369	Antiviral
ACY200	Cap	Acyclovir 200 mg	Zovirax by Par	49884-0460	Antiviral
ACY200	Cap, White	Acyclovir 200 mg	Zovirax by Compumed	00403-2360	Antiviral
ACY200	Cap	Acyclovir 200 mg	Zovirax by Apotheca	12634-0506	Antiviral
ACY200 <> G	Tab, Blue, Flat, Shield-Shaped	Acyclovir 200 mg	Zovirax by Genpharm	Canadian DIN 02242784	Antiviral
ACY400	Tab	Acyclovir 400 mg	Zovirax by Par	49884-0487	Antiviral
ACY400	Tab	Acyclovir 400 mg	Zovirax by LEK	48866-1140	Antiviral
ACY400	Tab	Acyclovir 400 mg	Zovirax by Schein	00364-2689	Antiviral
ACY400	Tab, White, Oval	Acyclovir 400 mg	Zovirax by Amerisource	62584-0371	Antiviral
ACY400	Tab, White, Oval	Acyclovir 400 mg	Zovirax by Amerisource	62584-0795	Antiviral

ID FRONT <> BACK	DESCRIPTION FRONT <> BACK	INGREDIENT & STRENGTH	BRAND (or Generic Equiv.) by FIRM	NDC#	CLASS; SCH.
ACY400	Tab, White, Oval	Acyclovir 400 mg	Zovirax by Amerisource	62584-0663	Antiviral
ACY400	Tab, Off-White	Acyclovir 400 mg	Zovirax by Quality Care	62682-1020	Antiviral
ACY400 <> G	Tab, Pink, Shield Shaped	Acyclovir 400 mg	Zovirax by Genpharm	Canadian DIN 02242463	Antiviral
ACY800	Tab, White, Rectangle	Acyclovir 800 mg	Zovirax by Amerisource	62584-0674	Antiviral
ACY800	Tab, Bar Shaped	Acyclovir 800 mg	Zovirax by LEK	48866-1180	Antiviral
ACY800	Tab	Acyclovir 800 mg	Zovirax by Mylan	00378-1468	Antiviral
ACY800	Tab	Acyclovir 800 mg	Zovirax by Schein	00364-2690	Antiviral
ACY800	Tab	Acyclovir 800 mg	Zovirax by Par	49884-0474	Antiviral
ACY800 <> G	Tab, Blue, Oval-Shaped, Scored	Acyclovir 800 mg	Zovirax by Genpharm	Canadian DIN 02242464	Antiviral
ACYCLOVIR200STASON	Cap, Opaque & Blue	Acyclovir 200 mg	Zovirax by Amerisource	62584-0784	Antiviral
AD <> 10	Tab, Blue, Round, Scored	Mixed Amphetamine Salts 10 mg: Amphetamine Aspartate 2.5 mg, Amphetamine Sulfate 2.5 mg, Dextroamphetamine Saccharate 2.5 mg, Dextroamphetamine Sulfate 2.5 mg	Adderall by Shire	58521-0032	Stimulant; C II
AD <> 10	Tab, Blue, Round, Scored	Mixed Amphetamine Salts 10 mg: Amphetamine Aspartate 2.5 mg, Amphetamine Sulfate 2.5 mg, Dextroamphetamine Saccharate 2.5 mg, Dextroamphetamine Sulfate 2.5 mg	Adderall by Physician Total Care	54868-3674	Stimulant; C II
AD <> 10	Tab, Blue, Round, Scored	Mixed Amphetamine Salts 10 mg: Amphetamine Aspartate 2.5 mg, Amphetamine Sulfate 2.5 mg, Dextroamphetamine Saccharate 2.5 mg, Dextroamphetamine Sulfate 2.5 mg	Adderall by DRX	55045-2607	Stimulant; C II
AD <> 125	Tab, Orange, Round, Scored, AD <> 12.5	Mixed Amphetamine Salts 12.5 mg: Amphetamine Aspartate 3.125 mg, Amphetamine Sulfate 3.125 mg, Dextroamphetamine Saccharate 3.125 mg, Dextroamphetamine Sulfate 3.125 mg	Adderall by Shire	58521-0125	Stimulant; C II
AD <> 15	Tab, Orange, Oval, Scored	Mixed Amphetamine Salts 15 mg: Amphetamine Aspartate 3.75 mg, Amphetamine Sulfate 3.75 mg, Dextroamphetamine Saccharate 3.75 mg, Dextroamphetamine Sulfate 3.75 mg	Adderall by Shire	58521-0150	Stimulant; C II
AD <> 20	Tab, Orange, Round, Scored	Mixed Amphetamine Salts 20 mg: Amphetamine Aspartate 5 mg, Amphetamine Sulfate 5 mg, Dextroamphetamine Saccharate 5 mg, Dextroamphetamine Sulfate 5 mg	Adderall by DRX	55045-2608	Stimulant; C II
AD <> 20	Tab, Orange, Round, Scored	Mixed Amphetamine Salts 20 mg: Amphetamine Aspartate 5 mg, Amphetamine Sulfate 5 mg, Dextroamphetamine Saccharate 5 mg, Dextroamphetamine Sulfate 5 mg	Adderall by Shire	58521-0033	Stimulant; C II
AD <> 30	Tab, Orange, Round, Scored	Mixed Amphetamine Salts 30 mg: Amphetamine Aspartate 7.5 mg, Amphetamine Sulfate 7.5 mg, Dextroamphetamine Saccharate 7.5 mg, Dextroamphetamine Sulfate 7.5 mg	Adderall by Shire	58521-0034	Stimulant; C II
AD <> 5	Tab, Blue, Round, Scored	Mixed Amphetamine Salts 5 mg: Amphetamine Aspartate 1.25 mg, Amphetamine Sulfate 1.25 mg, Dextroamphetamine Saccharate 1.25 mg, Dextroamphetamine Sulfate 1.25 mg	Adderall by DRX	55045-2606	Stimulant; C II
AD <> 5	Tab, Blue, Round, Scored	Mixed Amphetamine Salts 5 mg: Amphetamine Aspartate 1.25 mg, Amphetamine Sulfate 1.25 mg, Dextroamphetamine Saccharate 1.25 mg, Dextroamphetamine Sulfate 1.25 mg	Adderall by Shire	58521-0031	Stimulant; C II
AD <> 75	Tab, Blue, Round, Scored, AD <> 7.5	Mixed Amphetamine Salts 7.5 mg: Amphetamine Aspartate 1.875 mg, Amphetamine Sulfate 1.875 mg, Dextroamphetamine Saccharate 1.875 mg, Dextroamphetamine Sulfate 1.875 mg	Adderall by Shire	58521-0075	Stimulant; C II
AD <> A	Tab, White, Round, Scored, Abbott Logo (a)	Ethotoin 250 mg	Peganone by Abbott	00074-6902	Anticonvulsant
AD10 <> G	Tab, White, Oval	Alendronate Sodium 10 mg	Fosamax by Genpharm	Canadian DIN 02270129	Antiosteoporosis
AD5 <> G	Tab, White, Round	Alendronate Sodium 5 mg	Fosamax by Genpharm	Canadian DIN 02270110	Antiosteoporosis
AD70 <> G	Tab, White, Oval	Alendronate Sodium 70 mg	Fosamax by Genpharm	Canadian DIN 02286335	Antiosteoporosis

ID FRONT <> BACK	DESCRIPTION FRONT <> BACK	INGREDIENT & STRENGTH	BRAND (or Generic Equiv.) by FIRM	NDC#	CLASS; SCH.
ADALAT	Cap, Brown & Yellow, Adalat/Bayer Cross	Nifedipine 10 mg	Adalat by Bayer	Canadian	Antihypertensive
ADALAT10	Cap, Orange, Black Print, Adalat over 10	Nifedipine 10 mg	Adalat by Bayer	00026-8811	Antihypertensive
ADALAT10	Cap, Orange, Black Print, Adalat over 10	Nifedipine 10 mg	Adalat by Nat Pharmpak	55154-4803	Antihypertensive
ADALAT10	Cap, Orange, Black Print, Adalat over 10	Nifedipine 10 mg	Adalat by RP Scherer	11014-0802	Antihypertensive
ADALAT20	Tab, Dusty Rose, Round	Nifedipine 20 mg	Adalat XL by Bayer	Canadian DIN 02237618	Antihypertensive
ADALAT20	Cap, Pale Orange & Rust Brown, Adalat/20	Nifedipine 20 mg	Adalat by RP Scherer	11014-0894	Antihypertensive
ADALAT30	Tab, Dusty Rose, Round	Nifedipine 30 mg	Adalat XL by Bayer	Canadian DIN 02155907	Antihypertensive
ADALAT5	Cap, Brown & Yellow, Adalat 5/Bayer Cross	Nifedipine 5 mg	Adalat by Bayer	Canadian	Antihypertensive
ADALAT60	Tab, Dusty Rose, Round	Nifedipine 60 mg	Adalat XL by Bayer	Canadian DIN 02155990	Antihypertensive
ADALAT811	Cap	Nifedipine 10 mg	by Med Pro	53978-2048	Antihypertensive
ADALATCC <> 30	Tab, Reddish Pink, Round, Film Coated, Adalat over CC	Nifedipine 30 mg	Adalat CC by Bayer	00026-8841	Antihypertensive
ADALATCC <> 30	Tab, Reddish Pink, Round, Film Coated, Adalat over CC	Nifedipine 30 mg	Adalat CC by Southwood	58016-0120	Antihypertensive
ADALATCC <> 30	Tab, Reddish Pink, Round, Film Coated, Adalat over CC	Nifedipine 30 mg	Adalat CC by Va Cmop	65243-0053	Antihypertensive
ADALATCC <> 30	Tab, Reddish Pink, Round, Film Coated, Adalat over CC	Nifedipine 30 mg	Adalat CC by DRX	55045-2788	Antihypertensive
ADALATCC <> 30	Tab, Reddish Pink, Round, Film Coated, Adalat over CC	Nifedipine 30 mg	Adalat CC by Talbert	44514-0701	Antihypertensive
ADALATCC <> 30	Tab, Reddish Pink, Round, Film Coated, Adalat over CC	Nifedipine 30 mg	Adalat CC by Compumed	00403-4957	Antihypertensive
ADALATCC <> 30	Tab, Reddish Pink, Round, Film Coated, Adalat over CC	Nifedipine 30 mg	Adalat CC by Eckerd	19458-0878	Antihypertensive
ADALATCC <> 30	Tab, Reddish Pink, Round, Film Coated, Adalat over CC	Nifedipine 30 mg	Adalat CC by Amerisource	62584-0841	Antihypertensive
ADALATCC <> 30	Tab, Reddish Pink, Round, Film Coated, Adalat over CC	Nifedipine 30 mg	Adalat CC by Smiths Food & Drug	58341-0058	Antihypertensive
ADALATCC <> 30	Tab, Reddish Pink, Round, Film Coated, Adalat over CC	Nifedipine 30 mg	Adalat CC by Wal Mart	49035-0154	Antihypertensive
ADALATCC <> 30	Tab, Reddish Pink, Round, Film Coated, Adalat over CC	Nifedipine 30 mg	Adalat CC by Med Pro	53978-3033	Antihypertensive
ADALATCC <> 30	Tab, Reddish Pink, Round, Film Coated, Adalat over CC	Nifedipine 30 mg	Adalat CC by Nat Pharmpak	55154-4805	Antihypertensive
ADALATCC <> 30	Tab, Reddish Pink, Round, Film Coated, Adalat over CC	Nifedipine 30 mg	Adalat CC by Allscripts		Antihypertensive
ADALATCC <> 60	Tab, Reddish Pink, Round, Film Coated, Adalat over CC	Nifedipine 60 mg	Adalat CC by Med Pro	53978-3034	Antihypertensive
ADALATCC <> 60	Tab, Reddish Pink, Round, Film Coated, Adalat over CC	Nifedipine 60 mg	Adalat CC by Bayer	00026-8851	Antihypertensive
ADALATCC <> 60	Tab, Reddish Pink, Round, Film Coated, Adalat over CC	Nifedipine 60 mg	Adalat CC by Wal Mart	49035-0155	Antihypertensive
ADALATCC <> 60	Tab, Reddish Pink, Round, Film Coated, Adalat over CC	Nifedipine 60 mg	Adalat CC by Nat Pharmpak	55154-4809	Antihypertensive
ADALATCC <> 60	Tab, Reddish Pink, Round, Film Coated, Adalat over CC	Nifedipine 60 mg	Adalat CC by Va Cmop	65243-0054	Antihypertensive
ADALATCC <> 60	Tab, Reddish Pink, Round, Film Coated, Adalat over CC	Nifedipine 60 mg	Adalat CC by Talbert	44514-0761	Antihypertensive
ADALATCC <> 60	Tab, Reddish Pink, Round, Film Coated, Adalat over CC	Nifedipine 60 mg	Adalat CC by Smiths Food & Drug	58341-0059	Antihypertensive
ADALATCC <> 60	Tab, Reddish Pink, Round, Film Coated, Adalat over CC	Nifedipine 60 mg	Adalat CC by Amerisource	62584-0006	Antihypertensive
ADALATCC <> 60	Tab, Reddish Pink, Round, Film Coated, Adalat over CC	Nifedipine 60 mg	Adalat CC by Par	49884-0631	Antihypertensive
ADALATCC <> 90	Tab, Reddish Brown, Round, Film Coated, Adalat over CC	Nifedipine 90 mg	Adalat CC by Med Pro	53978-3044	Antihypertensive
ADALATCC <> 90	Tab, Reddish Brown, Round, Film Coated, Adalat over CC	Nifedipine 90 mg	Adalat CC by Bayer	00026-8861	Antihypertensive
ADALATMILES821	Cap	Nifedipine 20 mg	Adalat by Med Pro	53978-2050	Antihypertensive
ADAMS <> 006	Tab, Yellow, Oval, Scored	Pseudoephedrine HCl 120 mg, Methscopolamine Nitrate 2.5 mg	Allerx-D by Adams	63824-0006	Cold Remedy
ADAMS <> 007	Tab, Blue, Oval, Scored	Chlorpheniramine Maleate 8 mg, Methscopolamine Nitrate 2.5 mg	Allerx by Adams	63824-0067	Cold Remedy
ADAMS <> 012	Tab	Guaifenesin 600 mg	Robitussin by Nat Pharmpak	55154-5903	Expectorant
ADAMS <> 024	Tab, Yellow	Atropine Sulfate 0.04 mg, Chlorpheniramine Maleate 8 mg, Hyoscyamine Sulfate 0.19 mg, Phenylephrine 25 mg, Phenylpropanolamine 50 mg, Scopolamine 0.01 mg	Atrohist Plus by Medeva	53014-0024	Cold Remedy
ADAMS <> 024	Tab, Adams <> 0/24	Atropine Sulfate 0.04 mg, Chlorpheniramine Maleate 8 mg, Hyoscyamine Sulfate 0.19 mg, Phenylephrine 25 mg, Phenylpropanolamine 50 mg, Scopolamine 0.01 mg	Atrohist Plus by Drug Distr	52985-0227	Cold Remedy
ADAMS <> 063	Tab, Yellow, Oval, Scored	Dextromethorphan 60 mg, Guaifenesin 1200 mg, Pseudoephedrine 60 mg	Aquatab C by Adams	63824-0063	Cold Remedy
ADAMS <> 068	Tab, Green, Oval, Scored	Guaifenesin 1200 mg, Pseudoephedrine 75 mg	Aquatab D by Adams	63824-0068	Cold Remedy
ADAMS <> 077	Tab, Blue, Oblong, Scored	Chlorpheniramine 8 mg, Methscopolamine 2.5 mg	AllerRx PM by Adams	63824-0077	Antihistamine

ID FRONT <> BACK	DESCRIPTION FRONT <> BACK	INGREDIENT & STRENGTH	BRAND (or Generic Equiv.) by FIRM	NDC#	CLASS; SCH.
ADAMS <> 1200	Tab, Green & White, Oval, Ex Release	Guaifenesin 1200 mg	Robitussin by Adams	63824-0052	Expectorant
ADAMS <> 17	Tab	Guaifenesin 600 mg, Pseudoephedrine HCl 60 mg	by Nat Pharmpak	55154-5901	Cold Remedy
ADAMS <> 30	Tab	Dextromethorphan HBr 30 mg, Guaifenesin 600 mg	by Nat Pharmpak	55154-5902	Cold Remedy
ADAMS <> 600	Tab, Yellow and White, Oval, Bi-Layer, ER	Guaifenesin 600 mg, Dextromethorphan HBr 30 mg	Mucinex DM by Adams	63824-0056	Cold Remedy
ADAMS012	Tab, Adams/012	Guaifenesin 600 mg	Robitussin by Amerisource	62584-0012	Expectorant
ADAMS015	Tab, Blue, Oblong	Guaifenesin 400 mg, Pseudoephedrine HCl 120 mg	Sudafed Sinus by Adams		Cold Remedy
ADAMS017	Tab, Dark Blue	Guaifenesin 600 mg, Pseudoephedrine HCl 60 mg	by Adams		Cold Remedy
ADAMS018	Cap, Clear & Green	Guaifenesin 300 mg	Robitussin by Adams		Expectorant
ADAMS019	Cap, Blue & Clear	Phenylephrine 10 mg, Guaifenesin 300 mg	Deconsal Sprinkle by Adams		Cold Remedy
ADAMS022	Cap, Clear & Yellow	Brompheniramine Maleate 2 mg, Phenyltoloxamine 25 mg, Phenylephrine HCl 10 mg	Atrohist Sprinkle by Adams		Cold Remedy
ADAMS024	Tab	Atropine Sulfate 0.04 mg, Chlorpheniramine Maleate 8 mg, Hyoscyamine Sulfate 0.19 mg, Phenylephrine 25 mg, Phenylpropanolamine 50 mg, Scopolamine 0.01 mg	Atrohist Plus by Eckerd	19458-0839	Cold Remedy
ADAMS024	Tab, Adams/024	Atropine Sulfate 0.04 mg, Chlorpheniramine Maleate 8 mg, Hyoscyamine Sulfate 0.19 mg, Phenylephrine 25 mg, Phenylpropanolamine 50 mg, Scopolamine 0.01 mg	Atrohist Plus by Vintage	00254-2162	Cold Remedy
ADAMS030	Tab	Dextromethorphan 30 mg, Guaifenesin 600 mg	Humibid-DM by Drug Distr	52985-0206	Cold Remedy
ADAMS030	Tab, Adams/030	Dextromethorphan HBr 30 mg, Guaifenesin 600 mg	by Amerisource	62584-0030	Cold Remedy
ADAMS034	Cap, Clear & Green	Dextromethorphan 15 mg, Guaifenesin 300 mg	Humibid-DM Sprinkle by Adams		Cold Remedy
ADAMS309	Tab, Oblong	Guaifenesin 600 mg, Pseudoephedrine HCl 30 mg	Syn-RX DM by Adams		Cold Remedy
ADAMS310	Tab, Oblong	Guaifenesin 600 mg, Pseudoephedrine HCl 60 mg	Syn-RX DM by Adams		Cold Remedy
ADDERALLXR10MG	Cap, Blue, Ex Release	Mixed Amphetamine Salts 10 mg: Amphetamine Aspartate 2.5 mg, Amphetamine Sulfate 2.5 mg, Dextroamphetamine Saccharate 2.5 mg, Dextroamphetamine Sulfate 2.5 mg	Adderall XR by Shire	Canadian DIN 02248809	Stimulant; C II
ADDERALLXR10MG	Cap, Blue	Mixed Amphetamine Salts 10 mg: Amphetamine Aspartate 2.5 mg, Amphetamine Sulfate 2.5 mg, Dextroamphetamine Saccharate 2.5 mg, Dextroamphetamine Sulfate 2.5 mg	Adderall XR by Shire	54092-0383	Stimulant; C II
ADDERALLXR15MG	Cap, Blue & White, Ex Release	Mixed Amphetamine Salts 15 mg: Amphetamine Aspartate 3.75 mg, Amphetamine Sulfate 3.75 mg, Dextroamphetamine Saccharate 3.75 mg, Dextroamphetamine Sulfate 3.75 mg	Adderall XR by Shire	54092-0385	Stimulant; C II
ADDERALLXR15MG	Cap, Blue & White, Ex Release	Mixed Amphetamine Salts 15 mg: Amphetamine Aspartate 3.75 mg, Amphetamine Sulfate 3.75 mg, Dextroamphetamine Saccharate 3.75 mg, Dextroamphetamine Sulfate 3.75 mg	Adderall XR by Shire	Canadian DIN 02248810	Stimulant; C II
ADDERALLXR20MG	Cap, Orange, Ex Release	Mixed Amphetamine Salts 20 mg: Amphetamine Aspartate 5 mg, Amphetamine Sulfate 5 mg, Dextroamphetamine Saccharate 5 mg, Dextroamphetamine Sulfate 5 mg	Adderall XR by Shire	Canadian DIN 02248811	Stimulant; C II
ADDERALLXR20MG	Cap, Orange	Mixed Amphetamine Salts 20 mg: Amphetamine Aspartate 5 mg, Amphetamine Sulfate 5 mg, Dextroamphetamine Saccharate 5 mg, Dextroamphetamine Sulfate 5 mg	Adderall XR by Shire	54092-0387	Stimulant; C II
ADDERALLXR25MG	Cap, Orange & White, Ex Release	Mixed Amphetamine Salts 25 mg: Amphetamine Aspartate 6.25 mg, Amphetamine Sulfate 6.25 mg, Dextroamphetamine Saccharate 6.25 mg, Dextroamphetamine Sulfate 6.25 mg	Adderall XR by Shire	54092-0389	Stimulant; C II
ADDERALLXR25MG	Cap, Orange & White, Ex Release	Mixed Amphetamine Salts 25 mg: Amphetamine Aspartate 6.25 mg, Amphetamine Sulfate 6.25 mg, Dextroamphetamine Saccharate 6.25 mg, Dextroamphetamine Sulfate 6.25 mg	Adderall XR by Shire	Canadian DIN 02248812	Stimulant; C II
ADDERALLXR30MG	Cap, Clear & Orange, Ex Release	Mixed Amphetamine Salts 30 mg: Amphetamine Aspartate 7.5 mg, Amphetamine Sulfate 7.5 mg, Dextroamphetamine Saccharate 7.5 mg, Dextroamphetamine Sulfate 7.5 mg	Adderall XR by Shire	Canadian DIN 02248813	Stimulant; C II

ID FRONT <> BACK	DESCRIPTION FRONT <> BACK	INGREDIENT & STRENGTH	BRAND (or Generic Equiv.) by FIRM	NDC#	CLASS; SCH.
ADERALLXR30MG	Cap, Natural and Orange	Mixed Amphetamine Salts 30 mg: Amphetamine Aspartate 7.5 mg, Amphetamine Sulfate 7.5 mg, Dextroamphetamine Saccharate 7.5 mg, Dextroamphetamine Sulfate 7.5 mg	Adderall XR by Shire	54092-0391	Stimulant; C II
ADDERALLXR5MG	Cap, Clear & Blue, Ex Release	Mixed Amphetamine Salts 5 mg: Amphetamine Aspartate 1.25 mg, Amphetamine Sulfate 1.25 mg, Dextroamphetamine Saccharate 1.25 mg, Dextroamphetamine Sulfate 1.25 mg	Adderall XR by Shire	54092-0381	Stimulant; C II
ADDERALLXR5MG	Cap, Clear & Blue, Ex Release	Mixed Amphetamine Salts 5 mg: Amphetamine Aspartate 1.25 mg, Amphetamine Sulfate 1.25 mg, Dextroamphetamine Saccharate 1.25 mg, Dextroamphetamine Sulfate 1.25 mg	Adderall XR by Shire	Canadian DIN 02248808	Stimulant; C II
ADEFLORM <> KENWOOD	Tab	Ascorbic Acid 100 mg, Calcium 250 mg, Calcium Pantothenate 10 mg, Cyanocobalamin 2 mcg, Fluorides 1 mg, Iron 30 mg, Niacinamide 20 mg, Pyridoxine HCl 10 mg, Riboflavin 2.5 mg, Thiamine Mononitrate 1.5 mg, Vitamin A 6000 Units, Vitamin D 400 Units	Adeflor M by Kenwood	00482-0115	Vitamin
ADG <> 10500	Tab, White, Cap Shaped, 10/500	Acetaminophen 500 mg, Oxycodone 10 mg	Percocet by Mikart	46672-0826	Analgesic; C II
ADG <> 25400	Tab, White, Cap Shaped, 2.5/400	Acetaminophen 400 mg, Oxycodone 2.5 mg	Percocet by Mikart	46672-0828	Analgesic; C II
ADH	Tab, Gray, Round, Schering Logo ADH	Perphenazine 2 mg	Trilafon by Schering		Antipsychotic
ADIPEXP <> 99	Tab, White with Blue Specks, Scored, Adipex-P 99	Phentermine 37.5 mg	Adipex-P by Gate	57844-0009	Anorexiant; C IV
ADIPEXP <> 99	Tab, White with Blue Specks, Scored, Adipex-P 99	Phentermine HCl 37.5 mg	by Teva	00093-0009 Discontinued	Anorexiant; C IV
ADIPEXP375	Cap, Bright Blue & White with 2 Dark Blue Stripes, Opaque, Adipex-P over 37.5	Phentermine HCl 37.5 mg	by Teva	00093-0019 Discontinued	Anorexiant; C IV
ADIPEXP375	Cap, Blue & White, Adipex-P 37.5	Phentermine 37.5 mg	Adipex-P by Gate	57844-0019	Anorexiant; C IV
ADJ	Tab, Gray, Round, Schering Logo ADJ	Perphenazine 8 mg	Trilafon by Schering		Antipsychotic
ADK	Tab, Gray, Round, Schering Logo ADK	Perphenazine 4 mg	Trilafon by Schering		Antipsychotic
ADL2698	Cap, Blue, Hard Gel	Alvimopan 12 mg	Entereg by GSK	11227-0010	Gastrointestinal
ADM	Tab, Gray, Round, Schering Logo ADM	Perphenazine 16 mg	Trilafon by Schering		Antipsychotic
ADRIA130	Tab, White, Oblong, Adria/130	Butalbital 50 mg, Aspirin 650 mg	Axotal by Adria		Analgesic
ADRIA200	Tab, Beige, Round, Adria/200	Pancrelipase, Lipase, Protease NLT, Amylase NLT	Ilozyme by Adria		Gastrointestinal
ADRIA217	Tab, Red, Round	Phenolphthalein 130 mg	Evac-Q-Tab by Adria		Gastrointestinal
ADRIA230	Tab, Yellow, Octagonal, Adria/230	Metoclopramide 10 mg	Reglan by Adria		Gastrointestinal
ADRIA231	Tab, White, Round, Adria/231	Choline Bitartrate 25 mg, Dexpanthenol 50 mg	Ilopan-Choline by Adria		Antiflatulent
ADRIA304	Tab, Green, Oblong, Adria/304	Potassium Chloride 10 mEq	Kaon-CL 10 by Adria		Electrolytes
ADRIA307	Tab, Yellow, Round, Adria/307	Potassium Chloride 6.7 mEq	Kaon-CL by Adria		Electrolytes
ADRIA312	Tab, Purple, Round, Adria/312	Potassium Gluconate 5 mEq	Kaon by Adria		Electrolytes
ADRIA412	Tab, Pink, Oblong, Adria/412	Magnesium Salicylate 545 mg	Magan by Adria		Analgesic
ADRIA420	Tab, Yellow, Oblong, Adria/420	Magnesium Lactate 7 mEq	Mag-Tab by Adria		Mineral
ADRIA648	Tab, Peach, Oval	Cyclothiazide 2 mg	Fluidil by Adria		Diuretic; Antihypertensive
ADS100	Cap, White, Black Print, Abbott Logo (a) DS over 100	Ritonavir 100 mg	Norvir by RP Scherer	11014-1233	Antiviral
ADS100	Cap, White, Black Print, Abbott Logo (a) DS over 100	Ritonavir 100 mg	Norvir by Abbott	00074-6633	Antiviral
ADS100	Cap, White, Black Print, Abbott Logo (a) DS over 100	Ritonavir 100 mg	Norvir by Abbott	Canadian DIN 02241480	Antiviral
ADVILAS	Tab, Orange, Cap Shaped, Black Ink, ADVIL A/S	Chlorpheniramine Maleate 2 mg, Ibuprofen 200 mg, Pseudoephedrine HCl 30 mg	Advil Cold and Sinus Plus by Wyeth	Canadian DIN 02248645	Cold Remedy
ADVILCOLDSINUS	Cap, Butterscotch, Oval, Advil Cold & Sinus	Ibuprofen 200 mg, Pseudoephedrine 30 mg	Dristan by Whitehall Robins		Cold Remedy
ADVILFLU	Tab, White, Oval, Enteric Coated, Advil over Flu	Ibuprofen 200 mg, Pseudoephedrine HCl 30 mg	Advil Flu by Whitehall-Robbins		Cold Remedy
ADX1 <> A	Tab, White, Round, Film Coated, ADX1 <> A with arrowhead attached to right leg of A	Anastrozole 1 mg	Arimidex by AstraZeneca	00310-0201	Antineoplastic

ID FRONT <> BACK	DESCRIPTION FRONT <> BACK	INGREDIENT & STRENGTH	BRAND (or Generic Equiv.) by FIRM	NDC#	CLASS; SCH.
ADX1 <> A	Tab, White, Round, Film Coated, ADX1 <> A with arrowhead attached to right leg of A	Anastrozole 1 mg	Arimidex by AstraZeneca	Canadian DIN 02224135	Antineoplastic
ADX1 <> A	Tab, White, Round, Film Coated, ADX1 <> A with arrowhead attached to right leg of A	Anastrozole 1 mg	Arimidex by Murfreesboro	51129-1122	Antineoplastic
AE50	Tab, Yellow, Cap Shaped, Scored	Azathioprine 50 mg	Imuran by Genpharm	Canadian DIN 02231491	Immunosuppressant
AEB	Tab, Pink, Black Print, Oval, Film Coated, Abbott Logo (a)	Erythromycin 250 mg	Ery-Tab by Abbott	00074-6326	Antibiotic
AEB	Tab, Pink, Black Print, Oval, Film Coated, Abbott Logo (aEB)	Erythromycin Stearate	by Apotheca	12634-0163	Antibiotic
AEC	Tab, Pink, Black Print, Oval, Enteric Coated, Abbott Logo (a)	Erythromycin 250 mg	Ery-Tab by Abbott	00074-6304 Discontinued	Antibiotic
AEE	Tab, Pink, Oval, Film Coated, Abbott Logo (a)	Erythromycin Ethylsuccinate 400 mg	E.E.S. 400 by Pharmedix	53002-0295	Antibiotic
AEE	Tab, Pink, Oval, Film Coated, Abbott Logo (a)	Erythromycin Ethylsuccinate 400 mg	E.E.S. 400 by Allscripts		Antibiotic
AEE	Tab, Pink, Oval, Film Coated, Abbott Logo (a)	Erythromycin Ethylsuccinate 400 mg	E.E.S. 400 by Kaiser	00179-1014	Antibiotic
AEE	Tab, Pink, Oval, Film Coated, Abbott Logo (a)	Erythromycin Ethylsuccinate 400 mg	E.E.S. 400 by Murfreesboro	51129-1421	Antibiotic
AEE	Tab, Pink, Oval, Film Coated, Abbott Logo (a)	Erythromycin Ethylsuccinate 400 mg	E.E.S. 400 by Abbott	00074-5729	Antibiotic
AEH	Tab, Abbott Logo	Erythromycin 333 mg	Ery Tab by Apotheca	12634-0407	Antibiotic
AEH <> 20MG	Tab, Light Pink, Oblong, Delayed-Release	Esomeprazole 20 mg	Nexium by AstraZeneca	Canadian DIN 02244521	Proton Pump Inhibitor
AEI <> 40MG	Tab, Pink, Oblong, Delayed-Release	Esomeprazole 40 mg	Nexium by AstraZeneca	Canadian DIN 02244522	Proton Pump Inhibitor
AEK	Tab, White, Oval, Abbott Logo (a) EK	Erythromycin 500 mg	PCE by Abbott	00074-3389	Antibiotic
AER	Cap, Clear & Maroon, White Print, Delayed Release, Abbott Logo (aER)	Erythromycin 250 mg	by Abbott	00074-6301	Antibiotic
AF <> A	Tab, Yellow, Round, AF <> Abbott Logo (a)	Colchicine 0.6 mg	by Abbott	00074-3781	Antigout
AF1	Tab, White & Yellow, Round, AF-1	Phenylephrine 5 mg, Chlorpheniramine 2 mg, Acetaminophen 325 mg	by Perrigo	00113-0414	Cold Remedy
AF120 <> APO	Tab, White to Off-White, Cap Shaped, APO <> AF over 120	Sotalol HCl 120 mg	Betapace AF by Apotex	60505-0223	Antiarrhythmic
AF160 <> APO	Tab, White to Off-White, Cap Shaped, APO <> AF over 160	Sotalol HCl 160 mg	Betapace AF by Apotex	60505-0224	Antiarrhythmic
AF2	Tab, Round	Sodium Fluoride 2.2 mg	Luride by Able	Discontinued	Element
AF80 <> APO	Tab, White to Off-White, Cap Shaped, APO <> AF over 80	Sotalol HCl 80 mg	Betapace AF by Apotex	60505-0222	Antiarrhythmic
AFA	Tab, White	Acetaminophen 325 mg	Tylenol by Whitehall Robins	Canadian	Analgesic
AFA500	Tab, White, AFA/500	Acetaminophen 500 mg	Tylenol Ex Strength by Whitehall Robins	Canadian	Analgesic
AFE	Tab, White, Oblong, Film Coated	Acetaminophen 500 mg, Caffeine 65 mg	Excedrin Extra-Strength by BMS	Canadian DIN 01990675	Analgesic
AFE <> 10	Tab, Reddish Brown, Round, Film Coated, Extended Release	Felodipine 10 mg	Plendil by AstraZeneca	Canadian DIN 00851787	Antihypertensive
AFL <> 25	Tab, Yellow, Round, Film Coated, Extended Release, AFL <> 2.5	Felodipine 2.5 mg	Plendil by AstraZeneca	Canadian DIN 02057778	Antihypertensive
AFM <> 5	Tab, Pink, Round, Film Coated, Extended Release	Felodipine 5 mg	Plendil by AstraZeneca	Canadian DIN 00851779	Antihypertensive
AFR	Cap, Yellow, Black Print, Abbott Logo (a) over FR	Fenofibrate 67 mg	TriCor by Abbott	00074-4342 Discontinued	Antihyperlipidemic
AG <> M	Tab, White, Round	Alendronate Sodium 5 mg	Fosamax by Mylan	00378-3566	Antiosteoporosis
AGA	Tab, Red, Oval, Ex Release, Schering Logo AGA	Dexchlorpheniramine Maleate 4 mg	Polaramine by Schering		Antihistamine
AGB	Tab, Red, Oval, Ex Release, Schering Logo AGB	Dexchlorpheniramine Maleate 6 mg	Polaramine by Schering		Antihistamine
AGT	Tab, Red, Oval, Schering Logo AGT	Dexchlorpheniramine Maleate 2 mg	Polaramine by Schering		Antihistamine
AH	Tab, Rose, Round, Abbott Logo	Hydrochlorothiazide 25 mg, Deserpidine 0.125 mg	Oreticyl Forte by Abbott		Diuretic; Antihypertensive
AH1K	Tab, Pink, Round, AH/1K	Salbutamol Sulfate 2 mg	Ventolin by GSK	Canadian	Antiasthmatic
AH2K	Tab, Pink, Round, AH/2K	Salbutamol Sulfate 4 mg	Ventolin by GSK	Canadian	Antiasthmatic
AHC	Tab, Gray, Blue Print, Oval, Ex Release, Abbott Logo (a)	Divalproex Sodium 500 mg	Depakote by Abbott	00074-7126	Anticonvulsant
AHF	Tab, White, Blue Print, Oval, Ex Release, Abbott Logo (a)	Divalproex Sodium 250 mg	Depakote by Abbott	00074-3826	Anticonvulsant

ID FRONT <> BACK	DESCRIPTION FRONT <> BACK	INGREDIENT & STRENGTH	BRAND (or Generic Equiv.) by FIRM	NDC#	CLASS; SCH.
AHH	Cap, Gray, Black Print, Abbott Logo (a)	Terazosin HCl 1 mg	Hytrin by Allscripts		Antihypertensive
AHH	Cap, Gray, Black Print, Abbott Logo (a)	Terazosin HCl 1 mg	Hytrin by Nat Pharmpak	55154-0115	Antihypertensive
AHH	Cap, Gray, Black Print, Abbott Logo (a)	Terazosin HCl 1 mg	Hytrin by RP Scherer	11014-1031	Antihypertensive
AHH	Cap, Gray, Black Print, Abbott Logo (a)	Terazosin HCl 1 mg	Hytrin by Va Cmop	65243-0088	Antihypertensive
AHH	Cap, Gray, Black Print, Abbott Logo (a)	Terazosin HCl 1 mg	Hytrin by Abbott	00074-3805	Antihypertensive
AHK	Cap, Red, Black Print, Round, Abbott Logo (a)	Terazosin HCl 5 mg	Hytrin by Nat Pharmpak	55154-0116	Antihypertensive
AHK	Cap, Red, Black Print, Round, Abbott Logo (a)	Terazosin HCl 5 mg	Hytrin by Va Cmop	65243-0069	Antihypertensive
AHK	Cap, Red, Black Print, Round, Abbott Logo (a)	Terazosin HCl 5 mg	Hytrin by PDRX	55289-0070	Antihypertensive
AHK	Cap, Red, Black Print, Round, Abbott Logo (a)	Terazosin HCl 5 mg	Hytrin by RP Scherer	11014-1033	Antihypertensive
AHK	Cap, Red, Black Print, Round, Abbott Logo (a)	Terazosin HCl 5 mg	Hytrin by Abbott	00074-3807	Antihypertensive
AHN	Cap, Blue, Black Print, Round, Abbott Logo (a)	Terazosin HCl 10 mg	Hytrin by Abbott	00074-3808	Antihypertensive
AHN	Cap, Blue, Black Print, Round, Abbott Logo (a)	Terazosin HCl 10 mg	Hytrin by RP Scherer	11014-1034	Antihypertensive
AHN	Cap, Blue, Black Print, Round, Abbott Logo (a)	Terazosin HCl 10 mg	Hytrin by Va Cmop	65243-0089	Antihypertensive
AHR	Tab, Blue, Round, Scored	Acetaminophen 325 mg, Phenylephrine 5 mg, Phenylpropanolamine 5 mg	Dimetapp by Whitehall Robins		Cold Remedy
AHR	Tab, White, Round, Bisect	Pseudoephedrine HCl 60 mg	Robidrine by Whitehall Robins		Decongestant
AHR	Tab, White	Pseudoephedrine HCl 60 mg	Robidrine by Whitehall Robins	Canadian	Decongestant
AHR	Tab	Glycopyrrolate 1 mg	Robinul by Pharm Pkg Ctr	54383-0081	Gastrointestinal
AHR	Tab, Pink, Round, Schering Logo AHR	Carisoprodol 350 mg	Rela by Schering		Muscle Relaxant
AHR	Cap, Black & Yellow	Acetaminophen 325 mg, Phenobarbital 16.2 mg, Codeine Phosphate 16.2 mg	Phenaphen by Wyeth	Canadian	Analgesic; C IV
AHR	Cap, Yellow	Attapulgite 300 mg, Pectin 71.4 mg, Opium 12 mg	Donnagel PG by Wyeth	Canadian	Antidiarrheal; C V
AHR	Tab, Green, Round, Scored	Brompheniramine Maleate 4 mg, Phenylpropanolamine HCl 5 mg	Dimetapp by Whitehall Robins		Cold Remedy
AHR	Tab, Peach	Brompheniramine Maleate 4 mg	Dimetane by Whitehall Robins	Canadian Discontinued	Antihistamine
AHR <> DONNATAL	Tab, Film Coated	Atropine Sulfate 0.0582 mg, Hyoscyamine Sulfate 0.3111 mg, Phenobarbital 48.6 mg, Scopolamine 0.0195 mg	Donnatal by Pharmedix	53002-0449	Gastrointestinal; C IV
AHR <> DONNATALEXTENTAB	Tab, Pale Green, Film Coated	Atropine Sulfate 0.0582 mg, Hyoscyamine Sulfate 0.3111 mg, Phenobarbital 48.6 mg, Scopolamine 0.0195 mg	Donnatal by Thrift Drug	59198-0233	Gastrointestinal; C IV
AHR <> ROBAXIN750	Tab, Orange, Film Coated	Methocarbamol 750 mg	Robaxin by Schwarz	00031-7449	Muscle Relaxant
AHR <> ROBAXIN750	Tab, Film Coated, Robaxin-750	Methocarbamol 750 mg	Robaxin by Thrift Drug	59198-0182	Muscle Relaxant
AHR <> ROBAXIN750	Tab, Film Coated, Robaxin over 750	Methocarbamol 750 mg	Robaxin by Amerisource	62584-0450	Muscle Relaxant
AHR <> ROBAXIN750	Tab, Film Coated	Methocarbamol 750 mg	Robaxin by Leiner	59606-0730	Muscle Relaxant
AHR0677	Tab, Orange, Elliptical	B Complex, Ascorbic Acid, Vitamin E	Allbee C-800 by Robins		Vitamin
AHR0678	Tab, Red, Elliptical	B Complex, Ascorbic Acid, Vitamin E, Iron	Allbee C-800 Plus FE by Robins		Vitamin
AHR10 <> REGLAN	Tab, White, Cap Shaped, Scored	Metoclopramide HCl 10 mg	Reglan by Wal Mart	49035-0157	Gastrointestinal
AHR10 <> REGLAN	Tab, White, Cap Shaped, Scored	Metoclopramide HCl 10 mg	Reglan by Thrift Drug	59198-0099	Gastrointestinal
AHR10 <> REGLAN	Tab, White, Cap Shaped, Scored	Metoclopramide HCl 10 mg	Reglan by Nat Pharmpak	55154-3004	Gastrointestinal
AHR1007141	Tab, White, Round, AHR/100 7141	Amoxicillin Veterinary 100 mg	Biomox by Biocraft		Veterinary
AHR1535	Tab, Yellow, Round	Calcium Polycarbophil 500 mg	Mitrolan by A H Robins	00031-1535	Vitamin; Mineral
AHR1843	Tab, Beige to Tan, Black Print, Round, AHR over 1843	Brompheniramine Maleate 12 mg	Dimetane by A H Robins	00031-1843	Cold Remedy
AHR1857	Tab, Round	Brompheniramine Maleate 4 mg	Dimetane by A H Robins		Antihistamine
AHR1868	Tab, Round	Brompheniramine Maleate 8 mg	Dimetane by A H Robins		Antihistamine
AHR2007151	Tab, White, Round, AHR/200 7151	Amoxicillin Veterinary 200 mg	Biomox by Biocraft		Veterinary
AHR2255l	Tab, Purple & Red, Oval	Brompheniramine Maleate 4 mg, Phenylpropanolamine HCl 25 mg	Dimetapp by Whitehall Robins		Cold Remedy
AHR2279	Tab, Orange & Red, Oval	Brompheniramine Maleate 4 mg, Phenylpropanolamine HCl 25 mg, Dextromethorphan HBr 20 mg	Dimetapp by Whitehall Robins		Cold Remedy
AHR2290	Tab, Purple	Brompheniramine Maleate 1 mg, Phenylpropanolamine HCl 6.25 mg	by Whitehall Robins	Canadian Discontinued	Cold Remedy

ID FRONT <> BACK	DESCRIPTION FRONT <> BACK	INGREDIENT & STRENGTH	BRAND (or Generic Equiv.) by FIRM	NDC#	CLASS; SCH.
AHR27840	Tab, Pink, Round, AHR 2/7840	Glycopyrrolate 2 mg	Robinul Forte by A H Robins	00031-7840	Gastrointestinal
AHR4007171	Tab, White, Round, AHR/400 7171	Amoxicillin Veterinary 400 mg	Biomox by Biocraft		Veterinary
AHR4207	Cap, Green & White	Atropine Sulfate, Hyoscyamine Sulfate, Phenobarbital, Scopolamine	Donnatal by A H Robins		Gastrointestinal; C IV
AHR4649	Tab, Green, Round	Combination Enzyme, Antispasmodic	Donnazyme by A H Robins		Digestant
AHR5049	Tab, White, Round	Pancreatin 300 mg, Pepsin 250 mg, Bile Salts 150 mg	Entozyme by A H Robins		Gastrointestinal
AHR507131	Tab, White, Round, AHR/50 7131	Amoxicillin Veterinary 50 mg	Biomox by Biocraft		Veterinary
AHR5449	Tab, Yellow, Round	Benzthiazide 50 mg	Aquatag by A H Robins	Discontinued	Diuretic; Antihypertensive
AHR5720MICROK	Cap, Ex Release	Potassium Chloride 600 mg	Micro K by A H Robins	00031-5720	Electrolytes
AHR5720MICROK	Cap, AHR 5720 <> Micro-K	Potassium Chloride 600 mg	by Med Pro	53978-0155	Electrolytes
AHR5720MICROK	Cap	Potassium Chloride 600 mg	by Thrift Drug	59198-0310	Electrolytes
AHR5720MICROK	Cap	Potassium Chloride 600 mg	Micro K by Leiner	59606-0691	Electrolytes
AHR5720MICROK	Cap, AHR/5720 <> Micro-K	Potassium Chloride 600 mg	by Nat Pharmpak	55154-3010	Electrolytes
AHR5816	Tab, Yellow, Round	Sodium Salicylate 300 mg, Sodium Aminobenzoate 300 mg	Pabalate by A H Robins		Analgesic
AHR5883	Tab, Rose, Round	Potassium Salicylate 300 mg, Potassium Aminobenzoate 300 mg	Pabalate SF by A H Robins		Dermatologic
AHR5MICROK10	Cap	Potassium Chloride 750 mg	by Med Pro	53978-5044	Electrolytes
AHR6242	Cap, Black & Yellow	Acetaminophen 325 mg, Codeine Phosphate 15 mg	Tylenol w/ Codeine by A H Robins		Analgesic; C III
AHR6251	Tab, White, Oblong	Acetaminophen 650 mg, Codeine Phosphate 30 mg	Tylenol w/ Codeine by A H Robins		Analgesic; C III
AHR6257	Cap, Green & Black, White Print	Acetaminophen 325 mg, Codeine Phosphate 30 mg	Tylenol w/ Codeine by A H Robins	00031-6257	Analgesic; C III
AHR6274	Cap, Green & White, White Print	Acetaminophen 325 mg, Codeine Phosphate 60 mg	Tylenol w/ Codeine by A H Robins	00031-6274	Analgesic; C III
AHR6447	Tab, Orange, Round	Fenfluramine HCl 20 mg	Pondimin by A H Robins		Anorexiant; C IV
AHR7824	Tab, White, Round, Scored, AHR over 7824	Glycopyrrolate 1 mg	Robinul by A H Robins		Gastrointestinal
AHR8600	Cap, Red, Oval, AHR-8600	Guaifenesin 200 mg, Dextromethorphan HBr 10 mg, Pseudoephedrine HCl 30 mg	Organidin NR by Whitehall Robins		Cold Remedy
AHR8602	Cap, Amber, Oval, AHR-8602	Guaifenesin 100 mg, Dextromethorphan HBr 10 mg, Pseudoephedrine HCl 30 mg, Acetaminophen 250 mg	Robitussin by Whitehall Robins		Cold Remedy
AHRDONNATAL	Tab, Light Green, Film Coated	Atropine Sulfate 0.0582 mg, Hyoscyamine Sulfate 0.3111 mg, Phenobarbital 48.6 mg, Scopolamine 0.0195 mg	Donnatal by A H Robins	00031-4235	Gastrointestinal; C IV
AHRDONNATAL EXTENTABS	Tab, Pale Green, Film Coated, AHR over Donnatal Extentabs	Atropine Sulfate 0.0582 mg, Hyoscyamine Sulfate 0.3111 mg, Phenobarbital 48.6 mg, Scopolamine 0.0195 mg	Donnatal by Quality Care	60346-0857	Gastrointestinal; C IV
AHRROBICAP8417	Cap	Tetracycline 250 mg	Robitet 250mg by A H Robins		Antibiotic
AHRROBICAP8427	Cap	Tetracycline 500 mg	Robitet 500mg by A H Robins		Antibiotic
AHT	Tab, Peach, Round, Schering Logo AHT	Reserpine 0.1 mg, Trichlormethiazide 4 mg	Naquival by Schering		Antihypertensive; Diuretic
AHY	Cap, Yellow, Round, Black Print, Abbott Symbol and Abbott Code <> HY	Terazosin HCl 2 mg	Hytrin by PDRX	55289-0042	Antihypertensive
AHY	Cap, Yellow, Round, Black Print, Abbott Symbol and Abbott Code <> HY	Terazosin HCl 2 mg	Hytrin by Abbott	00074-3806	Antihypertensive
AHY	Cap, Yellow, Round, Black Print, Abbott Symbol and Abbott Code <> HY	Terazosin HCl 2 mg	Hytrin by RP Scherer	11014-1032	Antihypertensive
AHY	Cap, Yellow, Round, Black Print, Abbott Symbol and Abbott Code <> HY	Terazosin HCl 2 mg	Hytrin by Physician Total Care	54868-3842	Antihypertensive
AHY	Cap, Yellow, Round, Black Print, Abbott Symbol and Abbott Code <> HY	Terazosin HCl 2 mg	Hytrin by Va Cmop	65243-0068	Antihypertensive
AI	Tab, Rose, Round, Abbott Logo	Hydrochlorothiazide 50 mg, Deserpidine 0.125 mg	Oreticyl by Abbott		Diuretic; Antihypertensive
AID	Tab, Yellow, Oval, Scored, A/ID	Isosorbide Mononitrate 60 mg	Imdur by Murfreesboro	51129-1580	Antianginal
AID	Tab, Yellow, Oval, Scored, A/ID	Isosorbide Mononitrate 60 mg	Imdur by AstraZeneca	Canadian DIN 02126559	Antianginal
AID	Tab, Yellow, Oval, Scored, A/ID	Isosorbide Mononitrate 60 mg	Imdur by Warrick	59930-1549	Antianginal

ID FRONT <> BACK	DESCRIPTION FRONT <> BACK	INGREDIENT & STRENGTH	BRAND (or Generic Equiv.) by FIRM	NDC#	CLASS; SCH.
AID	Tab, Yellow, Oval, Scored, A/ID	Isosorbide Mononitrate 60 mg	Imdur by Murfreesboro	51129-1568	Antianginal
AII	Tab, White, Scored, Abbott Logo (a) over II	Phenacemide 500 mg	Phenurone by Abbott	00074-3971	Anticonvulsant
AIRPLANE	Tab, Yellow, Round, Airplane Logo	3,4-Methylenedioxymethamphetamine (MDMA)	Ecstasy by Illegal		Euphoric; Illicit
AJ	Tab, Red, Oval, Film Coated, Abbott Logo (a)	Iron w/ Vitamin C and Folic Acid	Fero-Folic 500 by Abbott	00074-7079	Mineral
AKA	Tab, Yellow, Oval, Film Coated	Lopinavir 200 mg, Ritonavir 50 mg	Kaletra by Abbott	00074-6799	Antiviral
AKA	Tab, Yellow, Oval, Film Coated	Lopinavir 200 mg, Ritonavir 50 mg	Kaletra by Abbott	Canadian DIN 02285533	Antiviral
AKH	Cap, Red, Abbott Logo (a)	Ethchlorvynol 500 mg	Placidyl by Abbott	00074-6685 Discontinued	Hypnotic; C IV
AKJ	Tab, Yellow, Oval, Film Coated, KJ <> Abbott Logo (a)	Clarithromycin 500 mg	Biaxin XL by Abbott	Canadian DIN 02244756	Antibiotic
AKJ	Tab, Yellow, Oval, Film Coated, KJ <> Abbott Logo (a)	Clarithromycin 500 mg	Biaxin XL by Abbott	00074-3165	Antibiotic
AKN	Cap, Green, Abbott Logo (a)	Ethchlorvynol 750 mg	Placidyl by Abbott	00074-6630 Discontinued	Hypnotic; C IV
AKT	Tab, Yellow, Blue Print, Oval, Film Coated, Abbott Logo (a KT)	Clarithromycin 250 mg	by Nat Pharmpak	55154-0122	Antibiotic
AKT	Tab, Yellow, Blue Print, Oval, Film Coated, Abbott Logo (a KT)	Clarithromycin 250 mg	by Physician Total Care	54868-3820	Antibiotic
AKT	Tab, Yellow, Blue Print, Oval, Film Coated, Abbott Logo (a KT)	Clarithromycin 250 mg	by Allscripts		Antibiotic
AKT	Tab, Yellow, Blue Print, Oval, Film Coated, Abbott Logo (a KT)	Clarithromycin 250 mg	Biaxin by H J Harkins Co	52959-0442	Antibiotic
AKT	Tab, Yellow, Blue Print, Oval, Film Coated, Abbott Logo (a KT)	Clarithromycin 250 mg	by DRX	55045-2165	Antibiotic
AKT	Tab, Yellow, Blue Print, Oval, Film Coated, Abbott Logo (a KT)	Clarithromycin 250 mg	Biaxin by Contract	10267-2155	Antibiotic
AKT	Tab, Yellow, Blue Print, Oval, Film Coated, Abbott Logo (a KT)	Clarithromycin 250 mg	by Compumed	00403-4625	Antibiotic
AKT	Tab, Yellow, Blue Print, Oval, Film Coated, Abbott Logo (a KT)	Clarithromycin 250 mg	Biaxin by Abbott	00074-3368	Antibiotic
AL	Tab, Blue, Round, Scored	Clorazepate Dipotassium 3.75 mg	Tranxene by Able	53265-0048 Discontinued	Antianxiety; C IV
AL <> G2	Tab, White, Oblong, /A/L <> /G/2/	Alprazolam 2 mg	Xanax by Par	49884-0400	Antianxiety; C IV
AL <> G2	Tab, White, Oblong, /A/L <> /G/2/	Alprazolam 2 mg	Xanax by Apotheca	12634-0524	Antianxiety; C IV
AL <> G2	Tab, White, Oblong, /A/L <> /G/2/	Alprazolam 2 mg	Xanax by Genpharm	Canadian DIN 02229814	Antianxiety; C IV
AL025 <> G	Tab, White, Oval, Scored, AL 0.25	Alprazolam 0.25 mg	Xanax by Genpharm	Canadian DIN 02137534	Antianxiety; C IV
AL025 <> G	Tab, White, Oval, Scored, AL 0.25	Alprazolam 0.25 mg	Xanax by Par	49884-0448	Antianxiety; C IV
AL025MGG	Tab, AL/0.25MGG	Alprazolam 0.25 mg	Xanax by Qualitest	00603-2346	Antianxiety; C IV
AL025MGG	Tab, Yellow, Oval, AL/0.25 mg G	Alprazolam 0.25 mg	Xanax by Par	49884-0449	Antianxiety; C IV
AL05 <> G	Tab, Pale Orange, Oval, Scored, AL 0.5	Alprazolam 0.5 mg	Xanax by Par	49884-0449	Antianxiety; C IV
AL05 <> G	Tab, Pale Orange, Oval, Scored, AL 0.5	Alprazolam 0.5 mg	Xanax by Genpharm	Canadian DIN 02137542	Antianxiety; C IV
AL05MGG	Tab, AL/0.5MGG	Alprazolam 0.5 mg	Xanax by Qualitest	00603-2347	Antianxiety; C IV
AL05MGG	Tab, Yellow, Oval, AL/0.5 mg G	Alprazolam 0.5 mg	Xanax by Par		Antianxiety; C IV
AL10 <> G	Tab, Mauve, Oval, Scored, AL 1.0	Alprazolam 1 mg	Xanax by Alphapharm	57315-0008	Antianxiety; C IV
AL10 <> G	Tab, Mauve, Oval, Scored, AL 1.0	Alprazolam 1 mg	Xanax by Direct Dispensing	57866-4636	Antianxiety; C IV
AL10 <> G	Tab, Mauve, Oval, Scored, AL 1.0	Alprazolam 1 mg	Xanax by Par	49884-0450	Antianxiety; C IV

ID FRONT <> BACK	DESCRIPTION FRONT <> BACK	INGREDIENT & STRENGTH	BRAND (or Generic Equiv.) by FIRM	NDC#	CLASS; SCH.
AL10 <> G	Tab, Mauve, Oval, Scored, AL 1.0	Alprazolam 1 mg	Xanax by Genpharm	Canadian DIN 02229813	Antianxiety; C IV
AL10MG	Tab, White, Oval, AL/1.0 mg G	Alprazolam 1 mg	Xanax by Par	00603-2348	Antianxiety; C IV
AL10MGG	Tab, White, Oval, AL/1.0MGG	Alprazolam 1 mg	Xanax by Qualitest	68220-0055	Antianxiety; C IV
ALAVEN <> 0055	Tab, White, Round, Scored	Oxymetholone 50 mg	Anadrol-50 by Alaven Pharmaceutical	00573-2660	Steroid; C III
ALAVERTD12	Tab, White, Round, Coated, SR	Loratadine 5 mg, Pseudoephedrine 120 mg	Alavert Allergy Sinus by Wyeth	Canadian DIN 01900927	Cold Remedy
ALBERT <> GLYGLY	Tab, White, Round, Scored, Albert Logo <> Gly over Gly	Glyburide 2.5 mg	by AltiMed	00025-1011	Antidiabetic
ALDACTAZIDE25 <> SEARLE1011	Tab, Tan, Round, Film Coated	Hydrochlorothiazide 25 mg, Spironolactone 25 mg	Aldactazide by Searle	55154-3601	Diuretic; Antihypertensive
ALDACTAZIDE25 <> SEARLE1011	Tab, Tan, Round, Film Coated	Hydrochlorothiazide 25 mg, Spironolactone 25 mg	Aldactazide by Nat Pharmpak	59198-0170	Diuretic; Antihypertensive
ALDACTAZIDE25 <> SEARLE1011	Tab, Tan, Round, Film Coated	Hydrochlorothiazide 25 mg, Spironolactone 25 mg	Aldactazide by Thrift Drug	62584-0011	Diuretic; Antihypertensive
ALDACTAZIDE25 <> SEARLE1011	Tab, Tan, Round, Film Coated	Hydrochlorothiazide 25 mg, Spironolactone 25 mg	Aldactazide by Amerisource	Canadian DIN 00180408	Diuretic; Antihypertensive
ALDACTAZIDE25 <> SEARLE1011	Tab, Tan, Round, Film Coated	Hydrochlorothiazide 25 mg, Spironolactone 25 mg	Aldactazide by Pfizer	51129-1377	Diuretic; Antihypertensive
ALDACTAZIDE25 <> SEARLE1011	Tab, Tan, Round, Film Coated	Hydrochlorothiazide 25 mg, Spironolactone 25 mg	Aldactazide by Murfreesboro	53978-3382	Diuretic; Antihypertensive
ALDACTAZIDE25 <> SEARLE1011	Tab, Tan, Round, Film Coated	Hydrochlorothiazide 25 mg, Spironolactone 25 mg	Aldactazide by Med Pro	65240-0600	Diuretic; Antihypertensive
ALDACTAZIDE25 <> SEARLE1011	Tab, Tan, Round, Film Coated	Hydrochlorothiazide 25 mg, Spironolactone 25 mg	Aldactazide by Rightpak	Canadian DIN 00594377	Diuretic; Antihypertensive
ALDACTAZIDE50 <> SEARLE1021	Tab, Tan, Oblong, Film Coated	Hydrochlorothiazide 50 mg, Spironolactone 50 mg	Aldactazide by Pfizer	00025-1021	Diuretic; Antihypertensive
ALDACTAZIDE50 <> SEARLE1021	Tab, Tan, Oblong, Film Coated	Hydrochlorothiazide 50 mg, Spironolactone 50 mg	Aldactazide by Searle	Canadian DIN 00285455	Diuretic; Antihypertensive
ALDACTONE100 <> SEARLE1031	Tab, Peach, Round, Scored, Film Coated	Spironolactone 100 mg	Aldactone by Pfizer	00025-1031	Diuretic
ALDACTONE100 <> SEARLE1031	Tab, Peach, Round, Scored, Film Coated	Spironolactone 100 mg	Aldactone by Searle	55045-2716	Diuretic
ALDACTONE25 <> SEARLE1001	Tab, Light Yellow, Round, Film Coated	Spironolactone 25 mg	Aldactone by DRX	59198-0001	Diuretic
ALDACTONE25 <> SEARLE1001	Tab, Light Yellow, Round, Film Coated	Spironolactone 25 mg	Aldactone by Thrift Drug	62584-0001	Diuretic
ALDACTONE25 <> SEARLE1001	Tab, Light Yellow, Round, Film Coated	Spironolactone 25 mg	Aldactone by Amerisource	65084-0106	Diuretic
ALDACTONE25 <> SEARLE1001	Tab, Light Yellow, Round, Film Coated	Spironolactone 25 mg	Aldactone by Rx Pak	65240-0601	Diuretic
ALDACTONE25 <> SEARLE1001	Tab, Light Yellow, Round, Film Coated	Spironolactone 25 mg	Aldactone by Rightpak	00025-1001	Diuretic
ALDACTONE25 <> SEARLE1001	Tab, Light Yellow, Round, Film Coated	Spironolactone 25 mg	Aldactone by Searle	55154-3602	Diuretic
ALDACTONE25 <> SEARLE1001	Tab, Light Yellow, Round, Film Coated	Spironolactone 25 mg	Aldactone by Nat Pharmpak	00339-5531	Diuretic
ALDACTONE25 <> SEARLE1001	Tab, Light Yellow, Round, Film Coated	Spironolactone 25 mg	Aldactone by Caremark	Canadian DIN 00028606	Diuretic
ALDACTONE25 <> SEARLE1001	Tab, Light Yellow, Round, Film Coated	Spironolactone 25 mg	Aldactone by Pfizer		Diuretic

ID FRONT <> BACK	DESCRIPTION FRONT <> BACK	INGREDIENT & STRENGTH	BRAND (or Generic Equiv.) by FIRM	NDC#	CLASS; SCH.
ALDACTONE50 <> SEARLE1041	Tab, Light Orange, Oval, Film Coated	Spironolactone 50 mg	Aldactone by Searle	00025-1041	Diuretic
ALDOCLOR <> MSD634	Tab, Green, Oval, Film Coated	Chlorothiazide 250 mg, Methyldopa 250 mg	Aldoclor by Merck	00006-0634	Diuretic; Antihypertensive
ALDOMET <> MSD135	Tab, Yellow, Round	Methyldopa 125 mg	Aldomet by Merck	00006-0135	Antihypertensive
ALDOMET <> MSD401	Tab, Yellow, Round, Film Coated	Methyldopa 250 mg	Aldomet by Merck	00006-0401	Antihypertensive
ALDOMET <> MSD516	Tab, Yellow, Round, Film Coated	Methyldopa 500 mg	Aldomet by Merck	00006-0516	Antihypertensive
ALDOMETMSD135	Tab, Yellow, Biconvex, Aldomet/MSD 135	Methyldopa 125 mg	Aldomet by MSD	Canadian Discontinued	Antihypertensive
ALDORIL <> MSD423	Tab, Salmon, Round, Film Coated	Hydrochlorothiazide 15 mg, Methyldopa 250 mg	Aldoril 15 by Merck	00006-0423	Diuretic; Antihypertensive
ALDORIL <> MSD456	Tab, White, Round, Film Coated	Hydrochlorothiazide 15 mg, Methyldopa 250 mg	Aldoril by Merck	00006-0456	Diuretic; Antihypertensive
ALDORIL <> MSD694	Tab, Salmon, Round	Hydrochlorothiazide 30 mg, Methyldopa 500 mg	Aldoril by Merck	00006-0694	Diuretic; Antihypertensive
ALDORIL <> MSD935	Tab, White, Oval, Film Coated	Hydrochlorothiazide 50 mg, Methyldopa 500 mg	Aldoril by Merck	00006-0935	Diuretic; Antihypertensive
ALE70 <> APO	Tab, White, Oval, Biconvex tablet, APO <> ALE70	Alendronate 70 mg	Fosamax by Apotex	Canadian DIN 02248730	Antiosteoporosis
ALEVECOLD&SINUS	Tab, White, Blue Print, Cap Shaped, Ex Release, ALEVE over COLD & SINUS	Naproxen 220 mg, Pseudoephedrine HCl 120 mg	Aleve by Bayer		NSAID
ALEVESINUS& HEADACHE	Tab, White, Blue Print, Cap Shaped, Ex Release, ALEVE over SINUS & HEADACHE	Naproxen 220 mg, Pseudoephedrine HCl 120 mg	Aleve by Bayer		NSAID
ALKERANA2A	Tab, White, Round, Scored, Alkeran over A2A	Melphalan 2 mg	by GSK	Canadian	Antineoplastic
ALKERANA2A	Tab, White, Round, Scored, Alkeran over A2A	Melphalan 2 mg	Alkeran by DSM	63552-0045	Antineoplastic
ALKERANA2A	Tab, White, Round, Scored, Alkeran over A2A	Melphalan 2 mg	Alkeran by GSK	00173-0045	Antineoplastic
ALL100 <> APO	Tab, White, Round, Biconvex	Allopurinol 100 mg	Zyloprim by Apotex	Canadian DIN 00402818	Antigout
ALL200 <> APO	Tab, Peach, Round, Biconvex	Allopurinol 200 mg	Zyloprim by Apotex	Canadian DIN 00479799	Antigout
ALL300 <> APO	Tab, Orange, Round, APO/300	Allopurinol 300 mg	Zyloprim by Apotex	Canadian DIN 00402796	Antigout
ALLEGRA60MG	Cap, Pink & White, Black Print, allegra over 60 mg	Fexofenadine HCl 60 mg	Allegra by Aventis	00088-1102	Antihistamine
ALLEGRAD	Tab, White and Tan, Layered, Film Coated	Fexofenadine HCl 60 mg, Pseudoephedrine HCl 120 mg	Allegra D by Aventis	Canadian DIN 02239853	Cold Remedy
ALLERGYSINUS-HEADACHE	Cap, Green and Yellow, Gelcap	Diphenhydramine HCl 12.5 mg, Pseudoephedrine HCl 30 mg, Acetaminophen 500 mg	Benadryl Allergy Sinus Headache by Pfizer		Cold Remedy
ALLERGYTOURO	Cap, Ex Release	Brompheniramine Maleate 5.75 mg, Pseudoephedrine HCl 60 mg	Touro Allergy by Pharmafab	62542-0106	Cold Remedy
ALLFEN <> MCR513	Tab, White, Oblong	Guaifenesin 1000 mg	Robitussin by AM Pharms	58605-0513	Expectorant
ALLFEN <> MCR513	Tab, White, Oblong, Scored	Guaifenesin 1000 mg	Robitussin by Pfab	62542-0907	Expectorant
ALLFENDM <> MCR521	Tab, White, Oblong, Scored, MCR over 521 <> Allfen DM	Dextromethorphan HBr 50 mg, Guaifenesin 1000 mg	Allfen DM by AM Pharms	58605-0521	Cold Remedy
ALLFENJR	Tab, White, Scored	Guaifenesin 400 mg	Allfen Jr. by AM Pharms	58605-0530	Cold Remedy
ALLIGATOR	Tab, Green, Mottled, Round, Alligator Logo	3,4-Methylenedioxymethamphetamine (MDMA)	Ecstasy by Illegal		Euphoric; Illicit
ALLIGATOR	Tab, Yellow, Mottled, Round, Alligator Logo	3,4-Methylenedioxymethamphetamine (MDMA)	Ecstasy by Illegal		Euphoric; Illicit
ALOR5 <> AP	Tab, Scored	Aspirin 500 mg, Hydrocodone Bitartrate 5 mg	Alor 5 500 by Atley	59702-0550	Analgesic; C III
ALP10 <> 832	Tab, White, Round	Amlodipine Besylate 10 mg	Norvasc by Upsher-Smith	00832-	Antihypertensive
ALP212 <> 832	Tab, White, Round	Amlodipine Besylate 2.5 mg	Norvasc by Upsher Smith	00832-	Antihypertensive
ALP5 <> 832	Tab, White, Round	Amlodipine Besylate 5 mg	Norvasc by Upsher-Smith	00832-	Antihypertensive
ALPHAMALE	Cap, Black and Green	ALPHA MALE Formula 1500 mg: BIOTEST Nano-Dispersed Gel Extracts (pharmaceutical grade tribulus terrestris, vitex agnus castus, eurycoma longifolia), Lauroyl Macrogol-32 Glycerides	Alpha Male by BioTest Labs		Supplement
ALRA <> K10	Tab, Film Coated, Debossed, Alra <> K+10	Potassium Chloride 750 mg	by PDRX	55289-0359	Electrolytes
ALRA <> K10	Tab, Film Coated, K+10	Potassium Chloride 750 mg	by Golden State	60429-0215	Electrolytes
ALRA <> K8	Tab, Film Coated, K+8	Potassium Chloride 600 mg	by Golden State	60429-0158	Electrolytes
ALRA215	Tab, Orange, Round	Ibuprofen 200 mg	Motrin by Alra	51641-0215	NSAID

ID FRONT <> BACK	DESCRIPTION FRONT <> BACK	INGREDIENT & STRENGTH	BRAND (or Generic Equiv.) by FIRM	NDC#	CLASS; SCH.
ALRAGN	Tab, Green, Round	Clorazepate Dipotassium 15 mg	Tranxene by Alra		Antianxiety; C IV
ALRAGT	Tab, Yellow, Round	Clorazepate Dipotassium 7.5 mg	Tranxene by Alra		Antianxiety; C IV
ALRAGX	Tab, Gray, Round	Clorazepate Dipotassium 30.75 mg	Tranxene by Alra	51641-0242	Antianxiety; C IV
ALRAIF400	Tab, Orange, Round	Ibuprofen 400 mg	Motrin by Alra		NSAID
ALRAIF600	Tab, Orange, Oval	Ibuprofen 600 mg	Motrin by Alra	51641-0213	NSAID
ALRAIF800	Tab, Light Peach, Oval	Ibuprofen 800 mg	Motrin by Alra	51641-0212	NSAID
ALTACE10MGMP	Cap, Blue, Black Print, Altace over 10 mg	Ramipril 10 mg	Altace by King	61570-0120	Antihypertensive
ALTACE10MGMP	Cap, Blue, Black Print, Altace over 10 mg	Ramipril 10 mg	Altace by Aventis	00039-0106	Antihypertensive
ALTACE10MGMP	Cap, Blue, Black Print, Altace over 10 mg	Ramipril 10 mg	Altace by Monarch	00088-0106	Antihypertensive
ALTACE10MGMP	Cap, Blue, Black Print, Altace over 10 mg	Ramipril 10 mg	Altace by Physician Total Care	54868-3846	Antihypertensive
ALTACE125MGMP	Cap, Yellow, Black Print, Altace over 1.25 mg, Hard Gel	Ramipril 1.25 mg	Altace by King	61570-0110	Antihypertensive
ALTACE125MGMP	Cap, Yellow, Black Print, Altace over 1.25 mg, Hard Gel	Ramipril 1.25 mg	Altace by Aventis	00039-0103	Antihypertensive
ALTACE125MGMP	Cap, Yellow, Black Print, Altace over 1.25 mg, Hard Gel	Ramipril 1.25 mg	Altace by Monarch	00088-0103	Antihypertensive
ALTACE25MGMP	Cap, Orange, Black Print, Altace over 2.5 mg	Ramipril 2.5 mg	Altace by Rx Pak	65084-0234	Antihypertensive
ALTACE25MGMP	Cap, Orange, Black Print, Altace over 2.5 mg	Ramipril 2.5 mg	Altace by Aventis	00039-0104	Antihypertensive
ALTACE25MGMP	Cap, Orange, Black Print, Altace over 2.5 mg	Ramipril 2.5 mg	Altace by Monarch	00088-0104	Antihypertensive
ALTACE25MGMP	Cap, Orange, Black Print, Altace over 2.5 mg	Ramipril 2.5 mg	Altace by King	61570-0111	Antihypertensive
ALTACE5MGMP	Cap, Red, Black Print, Altace over 5 mg	Ramipril 5 mg	Altace by Rx Pak	65084-0235	Antihypertensive
ALTACE5MGMP	Cap, Red, Black Print, Altace over 5 mg	Ramipril 5 mg	Altace by Aventis	00039-0105	Antihypertensive
ALTACE5MGMP	Cap, Red, Black Print, Altace over 5 mg	Ramipril 5 mg	Altace by Monarch	00088-0105	Antihypertensive
ALTACE5MGMP	Cap, Red, Black Print, Altace over 5 mg	Ramipril 5 mg	Altace by King	61570-0112	Antihypertensive
ALTI200	Tab, Blue, Round	Acyclovir 200 mg	Zovirax by AltiMed	Canadian DIN 02229707 Discontinued	Antiviral
ALTI200 <> 200	Tab, Pink, Round, Scored	Amiodarone 200 mg	Cordarone by AltiMed	Canadian DIN 0240071	Antiarrhythmic
ALTI400	Tab, Blue, Round	Acyclovir 400 mg	Zovirax by AltiMed	Canadian DIN 02229708 Discontinued	Antiviral
ALTI50	Tab, Off-White & Yellow, Circle	Azathioprine 50 mg	Imuran by AltiMed	Canadian DIN 02236799	Immunosuppressant
ALTI800	Tab, Blue, Oval	Acyclovir 800 mg	Zovirax by AltiMed	Canadian DIN 02229709	Antiviral
ALTIDILT120MG	Cap, Light Turquoise, Alti-Dilt 120 mg	Diltiazem HCl 120 mg	Cardizem by AltiMed	Canadian Discontinued	Antihypertensive
ALTIDILT180MG	Cap, Light Turquoise, Alti-Dilt 180 mg	Diltiazem HCl 180 mg	Cardizem by AltiMed	Canadian Discontinued	Antihypertensive
ALTIDILT240MG	Cap, Light Blue, Alti-Dilt 240 mg	Diltiazem HCl 240 mg	Cardizem by AltiMed	Canadian Discontinued	Antihypertensive
ALTIDILT300MG	Cap, Light Blue & Light Gray, Alti-Dilt 300 mg	Diltiazem HCl 300 mg	Cardizem by AltiMed	Canadian Discontinued	Antihypertensive
ALTIDILTCD120MG	Cap, Light Turquoise, Alti-Dilt CD 120 mg	Diltiazem HCl 120 mg	Cardizem by AltiMed	Canadian DIN 02229781 Discontinued	Antihypertensive
ALTIDILTCD180MG	Cap, Light Blue, Alti-Dilt CD 180 mg	Diltiazem HCl 180 mg	Cardizem by AltiMed	Canadian DIN 02229782 Discontinued	Antihypertensive
ALTIDILTCD240MG	Cap, Light Blue, Alti-Dilt CD 240 mg	Diltiazem HCl 240 mg	Cardizem by AltiMed	Canadian DIN 02229783 Discontinued	Antihypertensive

ID FRONT <> BACK	DESCRIPTION FRONT <> BACK	INGREDIENT & STRENGTH	BRAND (or Generic Equiv.) by FIRM	NDC#	CLASS; SCH.
ALTIDILTCD300MG	Cap, Light Blue & Light Gray, Alti-Dilt CD 300 mg	Diltiazem HCl 300 mg	Cardizem by AltiMed	Canadian DIN 02229784 Discontinued	Antihypertensive
ALTIMED <> A16A16	Tab, White, Round, Scored, A16 over A16 <> Altimed	Clobazam 10 mg	by AltiMed	Canadian DIN 02238797	Anticonvulsant
ALTIMEDM2MIN50MG	Cap, Orange w/ Yellow Powder, AltiMed M2 Min 50 mg	Minocycline HCl 50 mg	Minocin by AltiMed	Canadian DIN 01914138	Antibiotic
ALTIMEDM4MIN100MG	Cap, Orange & Purple, Altimed/M4/Min 100 mg	Minocycline HCl 100 mg	Minocin by AltiMed	Canadian DIN 01914146	Antibiotic
ALTIMEDPC150	Cap, Lavender & Maroon, Gelatin Altimed, PC 150	Clindamycin HCl 150 mg	Cleocin HCl by AltiMed	Canadian DIN 02130033	Antibiotic
ALTIMEDPC300	Cap, Light Blue, Gelatin, Altimed, PC 300	Clindamycin HCl 300 mg	Cleocin HCl by AltiMed	Canadian DIN 02192659	Antibiotic
ALTIPENTOX	Tab, Pink, Oblong, Alti/Pentox	Pentoxifylline 400 mg	Trental by AltiMed	Canadian DIN 01968432	Anticoagulant
ALTITRYP1GM	Tab, White, Oval, Alti-Tryp/1gm	Tryptophan 1 g	by AltiMed	Canadian DIN 02237250	Dietary Supplement
ALTO401	Cap, Blue & Pink	Zinc Sulfate 220 mg	Orazinc by Alto	00731-0401	Mineral
ALUCAP3M	Cap, Green & Red, White Print, Alu-Cap over 3M	Aluminum Hydroxide 400 mg	Amphojel by 3M	00089-0105 Discontinued	Gastrointestinal
ALUCAPRIKER	Cap, Green & Red, Alu-Cap/Riker	Aluminum Hydroxide 400 mg	Amphojel by 3M	00089-0105 Discontinued	Gastrointestinal
ALVA	Tab, Blue, Round, Black Ink, Coated	Caffeine 50 mg, Magnesium Salicylate 162.5 mg	Diurex by Alva		Analgesic; Diuretic
ALVA	Tab, Light Orange, Round, Chewable	Soluable Dietary Fiber 2.1 g	Ultra-Fiber Chewable by Alva		Supplement
ALVA	Tab, Dark Red, Round	Phenazopyridine HCl 95 mg	Uricalm by Alva		Urinary Analgesic
ALVA	Cap, Blue, Translucent, Oval, Soft Gel	Pamabrom 50 mg	Diurex Aquagels by Alva		Diuretic
ALVA	Tab, Light Greenish-Brown, Oval	Proprietary Blend 705 mg: White Bean Extract, Green Tea Leaf Extract, Tumeric Extract	Thinz Carbo Fast by Alva		Supplement
ALVA	Tab, Gold, Cap Shaped	Acetaminophen 500 mg, Pamabrom 25 mg	Backaid by Alva		Analgesic; Diuretic
ALVA	Tab, Pink, Round, Chewable	Dextrose 968 mg, Levulose 175 mg, Sodium Citrate Dihydrate 230 mg	Nauzene by Alva		Gastrointestinal
ALVA	Cap, Clear, White, Blue, Gold Beads, Red ink	Pamabrom 50 mg	Diurex Capsules by Alva		Diuretic
ALVA	Tab, Red, Oval	Acetaminophen 500 mg, Pamabrom 50 mg, Pyrilamine Maleate 15 mg	Diurex PMS by Alva		PMS Relief
ALVA	Tab, Oval, Gray	Buchu 100 mg, Dandelion 300 mg, Guarana 228 mg, Juniper Extract 100 mg	Diurex for Men by Alva		Supplement
ALVA <> 1	Tab, White, Oval	Acetaminophen 250 mg, Caffeine 32.5 mg, Magnesium Salicylate Tetrahydrate 310 mg	Arthiten by Alva		Analgesic
ALVA <> 1	Tab, Light Blue, Oval	Pamabrom 50 mg	Diurex Maximum Relief by Alva		Diuretic
ALVA <> 2	Tab, Dark Red, Round	Magnesium Salicylate 162.5 mg, Pamabrom 25 mg	Diurex Caffeine Free by Alva		Analgesic; Diuretic
ALVA <> 3	Tab, Olive, Cap Shaped	Riboflavin 1 mg, Green Tea Leaf 300 mg	Thinz by Alva		Supplement
ALZA10	Tab, Pink, Oval	Oxybutynin Chloride 10 mg	Ditropan XL by Alza		Urinary Tract
ALZA15	Tab, Gray, Oval	Oxybutynin Chloride 15 mg	Ditropan XL by Alza		Urinary Tract
ALZA18	Tab, Yellow, Barrel Shaped, Ex Release	Methylphenidate HCl 18 mg	Concerta by Janssen-Ortho	Canadian DIN 02247732	Stimulant; C II
ALZA18	Tab, Yellow, Barrel Shaped, Ex Release	Methylphenidate HCl 18 mg	Concerta by Alza	17314-5850	Stimulant; C II
ALZA27	Tab, Gray, Barrel Shaped, Ex Release	Methylphenidate HCl 27 mg	Concerta by Janssen-Ortho	Canadian DIN 02250241	Stimulant; C II
ALZA27	Tab, Gray, Barrel Shaped, Ex Release	Methylphenidate HCl 27 mg	Concerta by Alza	17314-5853	Stimulant; C II
ALZA36	Tab, White, Barrel Shaped, Ex Release	Methylphenidate HCl 36 mg	Concerta by Janssen-Ortho	Canadian DIN 02247733	Stimulant; C II

ID FRONT <> BACK	DESCRIPTION FRONT <> BACK	INGREDIENT & STRENGTH	BRAND (or Generic Equiv.) by FIRM	NDC#	CLASS; SCH.
ALZA36	Tab, White, Barrel Shaped, Ex Release	Methylphenidate HCl 36 mg	Concerta by Alza	17314-5851	Stimulant; C II
ALZA5	Tab, Yellow, Oval	Oxybutynin Chloride 5 mg	Ditropan XL by Alza	Canadian DIN 02247734	Urinary Tract
ALZA54	Tab, Brownish-Red, Barrel Shaped, Ex Release	Methylphenidate HCl 54 mg	Concerta by Janssen-Ortho		Stimulant; C II
ALZA54	Tab, Brownish-Red, Barrel Shaped, Ex Release	Methylphenidate HCl 54 mg	Concerta by Alza	17314-5852	Stimulant; C II
AM	Tab, Peach, Round, Scored	Clorazepate Dipotassium 7.5 mg	Tranxene by Able	53265-0049 Discontinued	Antianxiety; C IV
AM	Cap, White, Abbott Logo	Trimethadione 300 mg	Tridione by Abbott		Anticonvulsant
AM1	Tab, Purple, Oval	Methenamine Mandelate 1000 mg	Mandelamine by Amide	52152-0112	Antibiotic; Urinary Tract
AM1	Tab, Purple, Oval, Film Coated	Methenamine Mandelate 1000 mg	Mandelamine by Nat Pharmpak	55154-9305	Antibiotic; Urinary Tract
AM10	Tab, White, Octagon Shaped, AM10 <> Cobalt Logo	Amlodipine Besylate 10 mg	Norvasc by Cobalt	16252-0546	Antihypertensive
AM102004	Tab, Sugar Coated	Phenazopyridine HCl 200 mg	by Pharmedix	53002-0315	Urinary Analgesic
AM2	Tab, White, Diamond, AM2 <> Cobalt Logo	Amlodipine Besylate 2 mg	Norvasc by Cobalt	16252-0544	Antihypertensive
AM200 <> G	Tab, Pink, Round, Scored, AM / 200	Amiodarone 200 mg	Cordarone by Genpharm	Canadian DIN 02240604	Antiarrhythmic
AM200 <> G	Tab, White, Round, Scored	Amiodarone 200 mg	Cordarone by Alphapharm	57315-0009	Antiarrhythmic
AM200 <> G	Tab, White, Round, Scored	Amiodarone 200 mg	Cordarone by Par	49884-0458	Antiarrhythmic
AM5	Tab, White, Octagon Shaped, AM5 <> Cobalt Logo	Amlodipine Besylate 5 mg	Norvasc by Cobalt	16252-0545	Antihypertensive
AMARYL	Tab, Pink, Oblong, Notched, Scored, AMARYL <> Logo	Glimepiride 1 mg	Amaryl by Aventis	00039-0221	Antidiabetic
AMARYL	Tab, Pink, Oblong, Notched, Scored, AMARYL <> Logo	Glimepiride 1 mg	Amaryl by Murfreesboro	51129-1366	Antidiabetic
AMARYL	Tab, Green, Oblong, Notched, Scored, AMARYL <> Logo	Glimepiride 2 mg	Amaryl by Aventis	00039-0222	Antidiabetic
AMARYL	Tab, Blue, Oblong, Notched, Scored, AMARYL <> Logo	Glimepiride 4 mg	Amaryl by Murfreesboro	51129-1114	Antidiabetic
AMARYL	Tab, Blue, Oblong, Notched, Scored, AMARYL <> Logo	Glimepiride 4 mg	Amaryl by Aventis	00039-0223	Antidiabetic
AMARYL	Tab, Blue, Oblong, Notched, Scored, AMARYL <> Logo	Glimepiride 4 mg	Amaryl by Caremark	00339-6113	Antidiabetic
AMARYL	Tab, Blue, Oblong, Notched, Scored, AMARYL <> Logo	Glimepiride 4 mg	Amaryl by Aventis	Canadian DIN 02245274	Antidiabetic
AMARYL	Tab, Green, Oblong, Notched, Scored, AMARYL <> Logo	Glimepiride 2 mg	Amaryl by Aventis	Canadian DIN 02245273	Antidiabetic
AMARYL	Tab, Pink, Oblong, Notched, Scored, AMARYL <> Logo	Glimepiride 1 mg	Amaryl by Aventis	Canadian DIN 02245272	Antidiabetic
AMB10 <> 5421	Tab, White, Cap Shaped, Film Coated	Zolpidem Tartrate 10 mg	Ambien by Sanofi	00024-5421	Sedative/Hypnotic; C IV
AMB10 <> 5421	Tab, White, Cap Shaped, Film Coated	Zolpidem Tartrate 10 mg	Ambien by Caremark	00339-4065	Sedative/Hypnotic; C IV
AMB10 <> 5421	Tab, White, Cap Shaped, Film Coated	Zolpidem Tartrate 10 mg	Ambien by Searle	00025-5421	Sedative/Hypnotic; C IV
AMB10 <> 5421	Tab, White, Cap Shaped, Film Coated	Zolpidem Tartrate 10 mg	Ambien by PDRX	55289-0792	Sedative/Hypnotic; C IV
AMB10 <> 5421	Tab, White, Cap Shaped, Film Coated	Zolpidem Tartrate 10 mg	Ambien by H J Harkins Co	52959-0363	Sedative/Hypnotic; C IV
AMB115	Tab, White, Cap Shaped, Scored	Pseudoephedrine HCl 45 mg, Guaifenesin 800 mg	AMBI 45/800 by AM Pharms	66870-0115	Cold Remedy
AMB5 <> 5401	Tab, Pink, Cap Shaped, Film Coated	Zolpidem Tartrate 5 mg	Ambien by Sanofi	00024-5401	Sedative/Hypnotic; C IV
AMB5 <> 5401	Tab, Pink, Cap Shaped, Film Coated	Zolpidem Tartrate 5 mg	Ambien by Searle	00025-5401	Sedative/Hypnotic; C IV
AMB5 <> 5401	Tab, Pink, Cap Shaped, Film Coated	Zolpidem Tartrate 5 mg	Ambien by H J Harkins Co	52959-0362	Sedative/Hypnotic; C IV
AMB5 <> 5401	Tab, Pink, Cap Shaped, Film Coated	Zolpidem Tartrate 5 mg	Ambien by Caremark	00339-4064	Sedative/Hypnotic; C IV
AMB5 <> 5401	Tab, Pink, Cap Shaped, Film Coated	Zolpidem Tartrate 5 mg	Ambien by Nat Pharmpak	55154-3617	Sedative/Hypnotic; C IV
AMB118	Tab, White, Cap Shaped	Guaifenesin 800 mg, Pseudoephedrine HCl 80 mg	AMBI 700/80 by AM Pharms	66870-0118	Cold Remedy
AMB119	Tab, White, Cap Shaped	Pseudoephedrine HCl 80 mg, Guaifenesin 700 mg, Dextromethorphan HCl 40 mg	AMBI 80/700/40 by AM Pharms	66870-0119	Cold Remedy
AMB120	Tab, White, Cap Shaped, Scored	Guaifenesin 1000 mg, Dextromethorphan HCl 55 mg	AMBI 1000/55 by AM Pharms	66870-0120	Cold Remedy
AMBIFEDG <> AMBIG	Tab, White, Cap Shaped, Scored, AMBI / G <> AMBIfED G	Pseudoephedrine HCl 60 mg, Guaifenesin 1000 mg	Ambifed-G by AM Pharms	66870-0012	Cold Remedy
AMBIFEDG <> AMBIGDM	Tab, White, Cap Shaped, Scored, AMBI / G DM <> AMBIFED G	Pseudoephedrine HCl 60 mg, Guaifenesin 1000 mg, Dextromethorphan HBr 30 mg	Ambifed-G DM by AM Pharms	66870-0015	Cold Remedy
AMBIG <> AMBIFEDG	Tab, White, Cap Shaped, Scored, AMBI / G <> AMBIfED G	Pseudoephedrine HCl 60 mg, Guaifenesin 1000 mg	Ambifed-G by AM Pharms	66870-0012	Cold Remedy

ID FRONT <> BACK	DESCRIPTION FRONT <> BACK	INGREDIENT & STRENGTH	BRAND (or Generic Equiv.) by FIRM	NDC#	CLASS; SCH.
AMBIGDM <> AMBIFEDG	Tab, White, Cap Shaped, Scored, AMBI / G DM <> AMBIFED G	Pseudoephedrine HCl 60 mg, Guaifenesin 1000 mg, Dextromethorphan HBr 30 mg	Ambifed-G DM by AM Pharms	66870-0015	Cold Remedy
AMC <> 500125	Tab, White, Oblong	Amoxicillin 500 mg, Clavulanate Potassium 125 mg	Augmentin by LEK	66685-1002	Antibiotic
AMC <> 875125	Tab, Off-White, Oblong, Scored, 875/125	Amoxicillin 875 mg, Clavulanate Potassium 125 mg	Augmentin by LEK	66685-1001	Antibiotic
AMD	Tab, White, Oval, A/MD	Metoprolol Tartrate 200 mg	Betaloc by AstraZeneca	Canadian DIN 00497827	Antihypertensive
AME	Tab, White, Round, Scored, A over ME	Metoprolol Tartrate 100 mg	Betaloc by AstraZeneca	Canadian DIN 00402540	Antihypertensive
AME	Tab, Sugar Coated	Hyoscyamine Sulfate 0.12 mg, Methenamine 81.6 mg, Methylene Blue 10.8 mg, Phenyl Salicylate 36.2 mg, Sodium Phosphate, Monobasic 40.8 mg	Disurex DS by Advanced Med	55495-0100	Gastrointestinal
AMEN	Tab, Layered	Medroxyprogesterone Acetate 10 mg	Amen by Carnrick	00086-0049	Hormone
AMEN <> C	Tab	Medroxyprogesterone Acetate 10 mg	by Eckerd	19458-0831	Hormone
AMGEN <> 30	Tab, Light Green, Oval, Film Coated	Cinacalcet HCl 30 mg	Sensipar by Amgen	55513-0073	Calcimimetic
AMGEN <> 30	Tab, Light Green, Oval, Film-Coated	Cinacalcet 30 mg	Sensipar by Amgen	Canadian DIN 02257130	Calcimimetic
AMGEN <> 60	Tab, Light Green, Oval, Film-Coated	Cinacalcet 60 mg	Sensipar by Amgen	Canadian DIN 02257149	Calcimimetic
AMGEN <> 60	Tab, Light Green, Oval, Film Coated	Cinacalcet HCl 60 mg	Sensipar by Amgen	55513-0074	Calcimimetic
AMGEN <> 90	Tab, Light Green, Oval, Film Coated	Cinacalcet HCl 90 mg	Sensipar by Amgen	55513-0075	Calcimimetic
AMGEN <> 90	Tab, Light Green, Oval, Film-Coated	Cinacalcet 90 mg	Sensipar by Amgen	Canadian DIN 02257157	Calcimimetic
AMI200 <> APO	Tab, Pink, Round, Scored, AMI/200	Amiodarone HCl 200 mg	Apo Amiodarone by Apotex	Canadian DIN 02246194	Antiarrhythmic
AMIDE <> 002	Tab, Orange, Pink & Purple, Pillow Shaped, Chewable	Ascorbic Acid 30 mg, Sodium Ascorbate 33 mg, Sodium Fluoride, Vitamin A Acetate, Vitamin D 400 Units	Tri Vitamin Fluoride by Major	00904-7810	Vitamin
AMIDE <> 002	Tab, Orange, Pink & Purple, Pillow Shaped, Chewable	Ascorbic Acid 30 mg, Sodium Ascorbate 33 mg, Sodium Fluoride, Vitamin A Acetate, Vitamin D 400 Units	Tri Vitamin Fluoride by Schein	00364-0846	Vitamin
AMIDE <> 014	Tab, Film Coated	Dexchlorpheniramine Maleate 4 mg	by Schein	00364-0585	Antihistamine
AMIDE <> 084	Tab, Peach, Oblong	Choline Magnesium Trisalicylate 500 mg	Trilisate by Ivax	00182-1899 Discontinued	NSAID
AMIDE <> 085	Tab, White, Oblong	Choline Magnesium Trisalicylate 750 mg	Trilisate by Ivax	00182-1895 Discontinued	NSAID
AMIDE001	Tab, Orange & Pink & Purple, Round	Multivitamin, Fluoride 1 mg	Poly-Vi-Flor by Amide		Vitamin
AMIDE001 <> A	Tab, Orange, Pink & Purple, Round, Chewable, AMIDE001 <> A, B, C, or D	Ascorbic Acid 60 mg, Cyanocobalamin 4.5 mcg, Folic Acid 0.3 mg, Niacinamide, Pyridoxine HCl 1.05 mg, Riboflavin 1.2 mg, Sodium Fluoride, Thiamine Mononitrate, Vitamin A Acetate, Vitamin D 400 Units, Vitamin E Acetate	Multi Vita Bets by Qualitest	00603-4712	Vitamin
AMIDE001 <> A	Tab, Orange, Pink & Purple, Round, Chewable, AMIDE001 <> A, B, C, or D	Ascorbic Acid 60 mg, Cyanocobalamin 4.5 mcg, Folic Acid 0.3 mg, Niacinamide, Pyridoxine HCl 1.05 mg, Riboflavin 1.2 mg, Sodium Fluoride, Thiamine Mononitrate, Vitamin A Acetate, Vitamin D 400 Units, Vitamin E Acetate	Multi Vita Bets by Major	00904-5275	Vitamin
AMIDE001 <> A	Tab, Orange, Pink & Purple, Round, Chewable, AMIDE001 <> A, B, C, or D	Ascorbic Acid 60 mg, Cyanocobalamin 4.5 mcg, Folic Acid 0.3 mg, Niacinamide, Pyridoxine HCl 1.05 mg, Riboflavin 1.2 mg, Sodium Fluoride, Thiamine Mononitrate, Vitamin A Acetate, Vitamin D 400 Units, Vitamin E Acetate	Multi Vita Bets by Amide	52152-0001	Vitamin
AMIDE001 <> B	Tab, Orange, Pink & Purple, Round, Chewable, AMIDE001 <> A, B, C, or D	Ascorbic Acid 60 mg, Cyanocobalamin 4.5 mcg, Folic Acid 0.3 mg, Niacinamide, Pyridoxine HCl 1.05 mg, Riboflavin 1.2 mg, Sodium Fluoride, Thiamine Mononitrate, Vitamin A Acetate, Vitamin D 400 Units, Vitamin E Acetate	Multi Vita Bets by Amide	52152-0001	Vitamin

ID FRONT <> BACK	DESCRIPTION FRONT <> BACK	INGREDIENT & STRENGTH	BRAND (or Generic Equiv.) by FIRM	NDC#	CLASS; SCH.
AMIDE001 <> B	Tab, Orange, Pink & Purple, Round, Chewable, AMIDE001 <> A, B, C, or D	Ascorbic Acid 60 mg, Cyanocobalamin 4.5 mcg, Folic Acid 0.3 mg, Niacinamide, Pyridoxine HCl 1.05 mg, Riboflavin 1.2 mg, Sodium Fluoride, Thiamine Mononitrate, Vitamin A Acetate, Vitamin D 400 Units, Vitamin E Acetate	Multi Vita Bets by Qualitest	00603-4712	Vitamin
AMIDE001 <> B	Tab, Orange, Pink & Purple, Round, Chewable, AMIDE001 <> A, B, C, or D	Ascorbic Acid 60 mg, Cyanocobalamin 4.5 mcg, Folic Acid 0.3 mg, Niacinamide, Pyridoxine HCl 1.05 mg, Riboflavin 1.2 mg, Sodium Fluoride, Thiamine Mononitrate, Vitamin A Acetate, Vitamin D 400 Units, Vitamin E Acetate	Multi Vita Bets by Major	00904-5275	Vitamin
AMIDE001 <> C	Tab, Orange, Pink & Purple, Round, Chewable, AMIDE001 <> A, B, C, or D	Ascorbic Acid 60 mg, Cyanocobalamin 4.5 mcg, Folic Acid 0.3 mg, Niacinamide, Pyridoxine HCl 1.05 mg, Riboflavin 1.2 mg, Sodium Fluoride, Thiamine Mononitrate, Vitamin A Acetate, Vitamin D 400 Units, Vitamin E Acetate	Multi Vita Bets by Amide	52152-0001	Vitamin
AMIDE001 <> C	Tab, Orange, Pink & Purple, Round, Chewable, AMIDE001 <> A, B, C, or D	Ascorbic Acid 60 mg, Cyanocobalamin 4.5 mcg, Folic Acid 0.3 mg, Niacinamide, Pyridoxine HCl 1.05 mg, Riboflavin 1.2 mg, Sodium Fluoride, Thiamine Mononitrate, Vitamin A Acetate, Vitamin D 400 Units, Vitamin E Acetate	Multi Vita Bets by Qualitest	00603-4712	Vitamin
AMIDE001 <> C	Tab, Orange, Pink & Purple, Round, Chewable, AMIDE001 <> A, B, C, or D	Ascorbic Acid 60 mg, Cyanocobalamin 4.5 mcg, Folic Acid 0.3 mg, Niacinamide, Pyridoxine HCl 1.05 mg, Riboflavin 1.2 mg, Sodium Fluoride, Thiamine Mononitrate, Vitamin A Acetate, Vitamin D 400 Units, Vitamin E Acetate	Multi Vita Bets by Major	00904-5275	Vitamin
AMIDE001 <> D	Tab, Orange, Pink & Purple, Round, Chewable, AMIDE001 <> A, B, C, or D	Ascorbic Acid 60 mg, Cyanocobalamin 4.5 mcg, Folic Acid 0.3 mg, Niacinamide, Pyridoxine HCl 1.05 mg, Riboflavin 1.2 mg, Sodium Fluoride, Thiamine Mononitrate, Vitamin A Acetate, Vitamin D 400 Units, Vitamin E Acetate	Multi Vita Bets by Amide	52152-0001	Vitamin
AMIDE001 <> D	Tab, Orange, Pink & Purple, Round, Chewable, AMIDE001 <> A, B, C, or D	Ascorbic Acid 60 mg, Cyanocobalamin 4.5 mcg, Folic Acid 0.3 mg, Niacinamide, Pyridoxine HCl 1.05 mg, Riboflavin 1.2 mg, Sodium Fluoride, Thiamine Mononitrate, Vitamin A Acetate, Vitamin D 400 Units, Vitamin E Acetate	Multi Vita Bets by Qualitest	00603-4712	Vitamin
AMIDE001 <> D	Tab, Orange, Pink & Purple, Round, Chewable, AMIDE001 <> A, B, C, or D	Ascorbic Acid 60 mg, Cyanocobalamin 4.5 mcg, Folic Acid 0.3 mg, Niacinamide, Pyridoxine HCl 1.05 mg, Riboflavin 1.2 mg, Sodium Fluoride, Thiamine Mononitrate, Vitamin A Acetate, Vitamin D 400 Units, Vitamin E Acetate	Multi Vita Bets by Major	00904-5275	Vitamin
AMIDE003	Tab, Sugar Coated	Phenazopyridine HCl 100 mg	Pyridium by URL Mutual	00677-0575	Urinary Analgesic
AMIDE003	Tab, Sugar Coated	Phenazopyridine HCl 100 mg	Pyridium by Pharmedix	53002-0463	Urinary Analgesic
AMIDE004	Tab, Sugar Coated	Phenazopyridine HCl 200 mg	Pyridium by URL Mutual	00677-0804	Urinary Analgesic
AMIDE0046	Tab, Buff	Chlorpheniramine Tannate 8 mg, Phenylephrine Tannate 25 mg, Pyrilamine Tannate 25 mg	Tri Tannate by Amide	52152-0046	Cold Remedy
AMIDE009 <> 10	Tab	Isoxsuprine HCl 10 mg	Vasodilan by Qualitest	00603-4146	Vasodilator
AMIDE009 <> 10	Tab, White, Round	Isoxsuprine HCl 10 mg	Vasodilan by Ivax	00182-1055	Vasodilator
AMIDE009 <> 10	Tab, White, Round	Isoxsuprine HCl 10 mg	Vasodilan by Amide	52152-0009	Vasodilator
AMIDE010 <> 20	Tab, White, Round	Isoxsuprine HCl 20 mg	Vasodilan by Amide	52152-0010	Vasodilator
AMIDE010 <> 20	Tab, White, Round	Isoxsuprine HCl 20 mg	Vasodilan by Ivax	00182-1056	Vasodilator
AMIDE010 <> 20	Tab	Isoxsuprine HCl 20 mg	Vasodilan by Qualitest	00603-4147	Vasodilator
AMIDE013	Tab, White, Round	Ephedrine Sulfate 25 mg, Hydroxyzine HCl 10 mg, Theophylline 130 mg	by Ivax	00182-1344	Antiasthmatic
AMIDE013	Tab, White, Round	Ephedrine Sulfate 25 mg, Hydroxyzine HCl 10 mg, Theophylline 130 mg	Hydroxy Compound by Qualitest	00603-3948	Antiasthmatic
AMIDE013	Tab, White, Round	Ephedrine Sulfate 25 mg, Hydroxyzine HCl 10 mg, Theophylline 130 mg	Ami Rax by Amide	52152-0013	Antianxiety; Antihistamine
AMIDE014	Tab, Yellow, Oval	Dexchlorpheniramine Maleate 4 mg	Polaramine by Qualitest	00603-3198	Antihistamine
AMIDE014	Tab, Yellow, Oval	Dexchlorpheniramine Maleate 4 mg	Polaramine by Amide	52152-0014	Antihistamine
AMIDE014	Tab, Yellow, Oval, Ex Release	Dexchlorpheniramine Maleate 4 mg	Polaramine by Watson	00591-4008	Antihistamine
AMIDE015	Tab, White, Oval	Dexchlorpheniramine Maleate 6 mg	Polaramine by Ivax	00182-1015	Antihistamine
AMIDE015	Tab, White, Oval	Dexchlorpheniramine Maleate 6 mg	Polaramine by Qualitest	00603-3199	Antihistamine
AMIDE015	Tab, White, Oval	Dexchlorpheniramine Maleate 6 mg	Polaramine by Schein	00364-0586	Antihistamine

ID FRONT <> BACK	DESCRIPTION FRONT <> BACK	INGREDIENT & STRENGTH	BRAND (or Generic Equiv.) by FIRM	NDC#	CLASS; SCH.
AMIDE015	Tab, White, Oval	Dexchlorpheniramine Maleate 6 mg	Polaramine by Amide	52152-0015	Antihistamine
AMIDE019	Tab, Yellow, Round, Film Coated	Salsalate 500 mg	Disalcid by Sandoz	00781-1108	NSAID
AMIDE020	Tab, Yellow, Cap Shaped, Scored, Film Coated	Salsalate 750 mg	Disalcid by Sandoz	00781-1109	NSAID
AMIDE022	Tab, Yellow, Oval	Prenatal Vitamins, Beta-Carotene	Stuartnatal by Amide		Vitamin
AMIDE024	Tab, White, Cap Shaped	Guaifenesin 300 mg, Phenylephrine HCl 20 mg	Amidal by Qualitest	00603-5571	Cold Remedy
AMIDE024	Tab, White, Cap Shaped	Guaifenesin 300 mg, Phenylephrine HCl 20 mg	Amidal by Amide	52152-0024	Cold Remedy
AMIDE025	Tab, Green, Cap Shaped, Hexagon marking	Chlorzoxazone 500 mg	Parafon Forte by Amide	52152-0025	Muscle Relaxant
AMIDE026	Tab, Orange & Pink & Purple, Round	Multivitamin, Fluoride DF 1 mg	Poly-Vi-Flor by Amide	52152-0025	Vitamin
AMIDE032	Tab, White, Round, Scored, AMIDE over 032	Yohimbine HCl 5.4 mg	Yocon by Amide	52152-0032	Impotence Agent
AMIDE035	Tab, White, Round	Theophylline Anhydrous 130 mg, Ephedrine HCl 24 mg, Phenobarbital 8 mg	Tedral by Amide		Antiasthmatic; C IV
AMIDE039	Cap, Red & White	Acetaminophen 325 mg, Dichloralantipyrine 100 mg, Isometheptene Mucate (1:1) 65 mg	Migquin by Qualitest	00603-4664	Analgesic; C IV
AMIDE039A039	Cap, Red & White, Amide 039 <> A-039	Sodium Fluoride 2.2 mg	by Allscripts		Element
AMIDE043	Tab, Coated	Ascorbic Acid 120 mg, Calcium 200 mg, Copper 2 mg, Cyanocobalamin 12 mcg, Folic Acid 1 mg, Iron 65 mg, Niacinamide 20 mg, Pyridoxine HCl 10 mg, Riboflavin 3 mg, Thiamine Mononitrate 1.5 mg, Vitamin A Acetate 4000 Units, Vitamin E Acetate 11 Units, Zinc 25 mg	Prenatal 1 Plus 1 by Ivax	00182-4457	Vitamin
AMIDE045	Tab, Coated	Ascorbic Acid 80 mg, Beta-Carotene, Biotin 0.03 mg, Calcium Carbonate, Calcium Pantothenate, Cupric Oxide, Cyanocobalamin 2.5 mcg, Ergocalciferol, Ferrous Fumarate, Folic Acid 1 mg, Magnesium Hydroxide, Niacinamide, Pyridoxine HCl 4 mg, Riboflavin 1.6 mg, Thiamine Mononitrate 1.5 mg, Vitamin A Acetate, Vitamin E Acetate, Zinc Oxide	Prenatal Rx by Ivax	00182-4456	Vitamin
AMIDE046	Tab, Tan, Oblong, Scored	Chlorpheniramine Tannate 8 mg, Phenylephrine Tannate 25 mg, Pyrilamine Tannate 25 mg	Tri Tannate by Compumed		Cold Remedy
AMIDE046	Tab, Buff, Oblong	Chlorpheniramine 8 mg, Phenylephrine 25 mg, Pyrilamine 25 mg	Rynatan by Amide		Cold Remedy
AMIDE053	Tab, Peach, Round	Chlorzoxazone 250 mg	Para-Flex by Ivax	00182-1780	Muscle Relaxant
AMIDE053	Tab, Peach, Round	Chlorzoxazone 250 mg	Para-Flex by Amide	52152-0053	Muscle Relaxant
AMIDE074	Tab, Pink, Round	Phenindamine 24 mg, Chlorpheniramine 4 mg, Phenylpropanolamine 50 mg	Nolamine by Amide		Cold Remedy
AMIDE076	Tab, Green, Oblong	Ascorbic Acid 500 mg, Calcium Pantothenate 18 mg, Cyanocobalamin 5 mcg, Folic Acid 0.5 mg, Niacinamide 100 mg, Pyridoxine HCl 4 mg, Riboflavin 15 mg, Thiamine Mononitrate 15 mg	B Plex by Ivax	00182-4062 Discontinued	Vitamin
AMIDE077	Tab, Mustard, Oval, Film Coated	Ascorbic Acid 500 mg, Biotin 0.15 mg, Chromic Nitrate 0.1 mg, Cupric Oxide, Cyanocobalamin 50 mcg, Ferrous Fumarate 27 mg, Folic Acid 0.8 mg, Magnesium Oxide 50 mg, Manganese Dioxide 5 mg, Niacin 100 mg, Pantothenic Acid 25 mg, Pyridoxine HCl 25 mg, Riboflavin 20 mg, Thiamine Mononitrate 20 mg, Vitamin A Acetate 5000 Units, Vitamin E Acetate 30 Units	B Plex Plus by Ivax	00182-4064	Vitamin
AMIDE077	Tab, Mustard, Oval, Film Coated	Ascorbic Acid 500 mg, Biotin 0.15 mg, Chromic Nitrate 0.1 mg, Cupric Oxide, Cyanocobalamin 50 mcg, Ferrous Fumarate 27 mg, Folic Acid 0.8 mg, Magnesium Oxide 50 mg, Manganese Dioxide 5 mg, Niacin 100 mg, Pantothenic Acid 25 mg, Pyridoxine HCl 25 mg, Riboflavin 20 mg, Thiamine Mononitrate 20 mg, Vitamin A Acetate 5000 Units, Vitamin E Acetate 30 Units	Berroca Plus by Sandoz	00781-1102	Vitamin
AMIDE078	Cap, Black & Orange	Ascorbic Acid 150 mg, Calcium Pantothenate 10 mg, Cyanocobalamin 10 mcg, Folic Acid 1 mg, Magnesium Sulfate 70 mg, Manganese Chloride 4 mg, Niacinamide 25 mg, Pyridoxine HCl 2 mg, Riboflavin 5 mg, Thiamine Mononitrate 10 mg, Vitamin A 8000 Units, Vitamin E 50 Units, Zinc Sulfate 80 mg	Vicon Forte by Amide	52152-0078	Vitamin
AMIDE082	Cap, Blue	Cyclandelate 200 mg	Cyclospasmol by Amide		Vasodilator
AMIDE083	Cap, Blue & Red	Cyclandelate 400 mg	Cyclospasmol by Amide		Vasodilator

ID FRONT <> BACK	DESCRIPTION FRONT <> BACK	INGREDIENT & STRENGTH	BRAND (or Generic Equiv.) by FIRM	NDC#	CLASS; SCH.
AMIDE084	Tab, Peach, Cap Shaped	Choline Magnesium Trisalicylate 500 mg	Trilisate by Amide	52152-0084	NSAID
AML10 <> APO	Tab, White to Off-White, Round	Amlodipine Besylate 10 mg	Norvasc by Vintage	60505-0195	Antihypertensive
AML25 <> APO	Tab, White to Off-White, Round	Amlodipine Besylate 2.5 mg	Norvasc by Vintage	60505-0193	Antihypertensive
AML5 <> APO	Tab, White to Off-White, Round	Amlodipine Besylate 5 mg	Norvasc by Vintage	60505-0194	Antihypertensive
AMNEAL669	Cap, Purple and Orange, Opaque	Acebutolol HCl 200 mg	Sectral by Amneal	65162-0669	Antihypertensive
AMNEAL670	Cap, Purple and Orange, Opaque	Acebutolol HCl 400 mg	Sectral by Amneal	65162-0670	Antihypertensive
AMO	Tab, White, Round, Scored, Film Coated, A over MO	Metoprolol Succinate 50 mg	Toprol XL by Physician Total Care	54868-3587	Antihypertensive
AMO	Tab, White, Round, Scored, Film Coated, A over MO	Metoprolol Succinate 50 mg	Toprol XL by AstraZeneca	17228-0109	Antihypertensive
AMO	Tab, White, Round, Scored, Film Coated, A over MO	Metoprolol Succinate 50 mg	Toprol XL by Neuman	64579-0058	Antihypertensive
AMO	Tab, White, Round, Scored, Film Coated, A over MO	Metoprolol Succinate 50 mg	Toprol XL by AstraZeneca	00186-1090	Antihypertensive
AMOX500	Cap, Yellow	Amoxicillin 500 mg	Amoxil by Mova	55370-0920	Antibiotic
AMOX500BC	Cap	Amoxicillin 500 mg, Amoxicillin Trihydrate 574 mg	by Sandoz	43858-0355	Antibiotic
AMOX500GG849	Cap, Yellow, Hard Shell	Amoxicillin 500 mg	Amoxil by Sandoz	00781-2613	Antibiotic
AMOXIL <> 125	Tab, Chewable	Amoxicillin 125 mg	Amoxil by Quality Care	60346-0100	Antibiotic
AMOXIL <> 250	Tab, Pink, Oval	Amoxicillin 250 mg	Amoxil by Bayer	00280-1060	Antibiotic
AMOXIL <> 250	Tab, Pink, Oval	Amoxicillin 250 mg	Amoxil by SKB	00029-6005	Antibiotic
AMOXIL <> 500	Tab, Pink, Cap Shaped	Amoxicillin 500 mg	Amoxil by SKB	00029-6046	Antibiotic
AMOXIL125	Tab, Rose, Oval, Amoxil/125	Amoxicillin 125 mg	Amoxil by Wyeth	Canadian Discontinued	Antibiotic
AMOXIL125	Tab, Chewable	Amoxicillin 125 mg	Amoxil by Pharmedix	53002-0283	Antibiotic
AMOXIL125	Tab, Pink, Oval	Amoxicillin 125 mg	Amoxil by SKB	00029-6004	Antibiotic
AMOXIL200	Tab, Pale Pink, Round	Amoxicillin 200 mg	Amoxil by SKB	00029-6044	Antibiotic
AMOXIL250	Cap, Pink & Blue, White Print, Amoxil over 250	Amoxicillin 250 mg	Amoxil by SKB	00029-6006	Antibiotic
AMOXIL250	Cap, Pink & Blue, White Print, Amoxil over 250	Amoxicillin 250 mg	Amoxil by Urgent Care Center	50716-0606	Antibiotic
AMOXIL250	Cap, Pink & Blue, White Print, Amoxil over 250	Amoxicillin 250 mg	Amoxil by Wyeth	Canadian Discontinued	Antibiotic
AMOXIL400	Tab, Pale Pink, Round	Amoxicillin 400 mg	Amoxil by SKB	00029-6045	Antibiotic
AMOXIL500	Cap, Pink & Blue, White Print, Amoxil over 500	Amoxicillin 500 mg	Amoxil by SKB	00029-6007	Antibiotic
AMOXIL875	Tab, Pink, Cap Shaped, Amoxil over 875	Amoxicillin 875 mg	Amoxil by SKB	00029-6047	Antibiotic
AMP250	Cap, Light Blue & White, Opaque	Ampicillin 250 mg	Principen by Par	49884-0627	Antibiotic
AMP250	Cap, Light Blue & White, Opaque	Ampicillin 250 mg	Principen by Teva	00093-5145	Antibiotic
AMP500	Cap, Light Blue & White, Opaque	Ampicillin 500 mg	Principen by Par	49884-0628	Antibiotic
AMP500	Cap, Light Blue & White, Opaque	Ampicillin 500 mg	Principen by Teva	00093-5146 Discontinued	Antibiotic
AMPHOJEL	Tab, White, Scored	Aluminum Hydroxide 600 mg	Aurium by Axcan	Canadian DIN 02124971	Gastrointestinal
AMPHOJELPLUS	Tab, White	Aluminum Hydroxide 300 mg, Magnesium Hydroxide 300 mg	Maalox by Axcan	Canadian	Gastrointestinal
AMPI250BC	Cap	Ampicillin 250 mg	Principen by Sandoz	43858-0282	Antibiotic
AMPI500BC	Cap	Ampicillin	Principen by Sandoz	43858-0285	Antibiotic
AMPM	Tab, AM over PM	Guaifenesin 500 mg, Pseudoephedrine HCl 120 mg	Sudafed Sinus by Pharmafab	62542-0901	Cold Remedy
AMPM	Tab, AM over PM	Guaifenesin 500 mg, Pseudoephedrine HCl 120 mg	Sudafed Sinus by Seatrace	00551-0170	Cold Remedy
AMS	Tab, White, Round, Scored, Film Coated, A over MS	Metoprolol Succinate 100 mg	Toprol XL by AstraZeneca	17228-0110	Antihypertensive
AMS	Tab, White, Round, Scored, Film Coated, A over MS	Metoprolol Succinate 100 mg	Toprol XL by AstraZeneca	00186-1092	Antihypertensive
AMT <> 832	Tab, Peach, Round	Amantadine HCl 100 mg	Symmetrel by Upsher Smith	00832-0111	Antiviral
AMX250GG848	Cap, Yellow, Hard Shell	Amoxicillin 250 mg	Amoxil by Sandoz	00781-2020	Antibiotic
AMY	Tab, White, Oval, Scored, Film Coated, A over MY	Metoprolol Succinate 200 mg	Toprol XL by Caremark	00339-5782	Antihypertensive
AMY	Tab, White, Oval, Scored, Film Coated, A over MY	Metoprolol Succinate 200 mg	Toprol XL by AstraZeneca	59252-0111	Antihypertensive
AMY	Tab, White, Oval, Scored, Film Coated, A over MY	Metoprolol Succinate 200 mg	Toprol XL by AstraZeneca	17228-0111	Antihypertensive
AMY	Tab, White, Oval, Scored, Film Coated, A over MY	Metoprolol Succinate 200 mg	Toprol XL by AstraZeneca	00186-1094	Antihypertensive

ID FRONT <> BACK	DESCRIPTION FRONT <> BACK	INGREDIENT & STRENGTH	BRAND (or Generic Equiv.) by FIRM	NDC#	CLASS; SCH.
AN	Tab, White, Round, Scored	Clorazepate Dipotassium 15 mg	Tranxene by Able	53265-0050 Discontinued	Antianxiety; C IV
AN <> 71	Tab, White, Round, Film Coated	Hydroxyzine HCl 25 mg	Atarax by Harris	67405-0671	Antianxiety; Antihistamine
AN <> 711	Tab, White, Oval	Guanfacine HCl 1 mg	Tenex by Amneal	65162-0711	Antihypertensive
AN <> 713	Tab, White, Oval	Guanfacine HCl 2 mg	Tenex by Amneal	65162-0713	Antihypertensive
AN <> 77	Tab, White, Round, Film Coated	Hydroxyzine HCl 50 mg	Atarax by Harris	67405-0577	Antianxiety; Antihistamine
AN1	Tab, Reddish Brown, Round	Phenazopyridine 100 mg	Pyridium by Amneal	65162-0517	Urinary Antiseptic
AN100	Tab, White to Off-White, Round, Scored, Cobalt Logo <> AN / 100	Atenolol 100 mg	Tenormin by Cobalt	Canadian DIN 02255553	Antihypertensive
AN2	Tab, Reddish Brown, Round	Phenazopyridine 200 mg	Pyridium by Amneal	65162-0520	Urinary Antiseptic
AN211	Tab, White, Round, Scored, AN over 211	Acetaminophen 325 mg	Tylenol by UDL	51079-0002 Discontinued	Analgesic
AN24	Tab, Off-White, Round	Colchicine 0.6 mg	Colchicine by Amneal	65162-0227	Antigout
AN25 <> A	Tab, White, Round, AN over 25 <> Abbott Logo (a)	Dicumarol 25 mg	Dicumarol by Abbott	00074-3794 Discontinued	Anticoagulant
AN361	Tab, Light Yellow, Round, Scored	Folic Acid 1 mg	Folvite by Amneal	65162-0361	Vitamin
AN40	Tab, White to Off-White, Arc Triangle Shaped	Alendronate Sodium 40 mg	Fosamax by Cobalt	Canadian DIN 02258102	Antiosteoporosis
AN41	Tab, Round, Light Orange to Deep Yellow , AN / 41	Cyclobenzaprine HCl 10 mg	Flexeril by Amneal		Muscle Relaxant
AN50	Tab, White to Off-White, Round, Scored, Cobalt Logo <> AN / 50	Atenolol 50 mg	Tenormin by Cobalt	Canadian DIN 02255545	Antihypertensive
AN54	Tab, Red, Round	Demeclocycline HCl 150 mg	Declomycin by Amneal	65162-0554	Antibiotic
AN543	Tab, White, Round	Terbinafine HCl 250 mg	Lamisil by Harris	67405-0543	Antifungal
AN543	Tab, White, Round, AN over 543	Terbinafine HCl 250 mg	Lamisil by Amneal	67090-0543	Antifungal
AN55	Tab, Dark Pink, Round	Demeclocycline HCl 300 mg	Declomycin by Amneal	65162-0555	Antibiotic
AN571	Tab, White, Round, Scored	Bethanechol Chloride 5 mg	Urecholine by Amneal	65162-0571	Urinary Tract
AN572	Tab, White, Round, Scored	Bethanechol Chloride 10 mg	Urecholine by Amneal	65162-0572	Urinary Tract
AN573	Tab, Peach, Round, Scored	Bethanechol Chloride 25 mg	Urecholine by Amneal	65162-0573	Urinary Tract
AN574	Tab, Yellow, Round, Scored	Bethanechol Chloride 50 mg	Urecholine by Amneal	65162-0574	Urinary Tract
AN627	Tab, White, Round, AN over 627	Tramadol HCl 50 mg	Ultram by Amneal	65162-0627	Analgesic
AN641	Tab, White, Round	Flecainide Acetate 50 mg	Tambocor by Amneal	65162-0641	Antiarrhythmic
AN642	Tab, White, Round, Scored	Flecainide Acetate 100 mg	Tambocor by Amneal	65162-0642	Antiarrhythmic
AN643	Tab, White, Oval, Scored	Flecainide Acetate 150 mg	Tambocor by Amneal	65162-0643	Antiarrhythmic
AN70	Tab, White to Off-White, Oval, Cobalt Logo <> AN70	Alendronate Sodium 70 mg	Fosamax by Cobalt	Canadian DIN 02258110	Antiosteoporosis
ANA	Tab, Yellow, Round, Schering Logo ANA	Perphenazine 2 mg, Amitriptyline HCl 10 mg	Etrafon by Schering		Antipsychotic; Antidepressant
ANACIN	Tab, White	Aspirin 325 mg, Caffeine 30 mg	by Whitehall Robins	Canadian	Analgesic
ANACIN	Cap, White	Aspirin 325 mg, Caffeine 30 mg	by Whitehall Robins	Canadian	Analgesic
ANACIN500	Tab, White	Aspirin 500 mg, Caffeine 32 mg	Anacin by Whitehall Robins	Canadian	Analgesic
ANACIN500	Cap, White	Aspirin 500 mg, Caffeine 32 mg	Anacin by Whitehall Robins	Canadian	Analgesic
ANAFRANIL25MG	Cap, Ivory & Melon Yellow	Clomipramine HCl 25 mg	Anafranil by Mallinckrodt	00406-9906	OCD
ANAFRANIL50MG	Cap, Ivory & Aqua	Clomipramine HCl 50 mg	Anafranil by Mallinckrodt	00406-9907	OCD
ANAFRANIL50MG	Cap, Ivory & Aqua	Clomipramine HCl 50 mg	Anafranil by Pharm Util	60491-0035	OCD
ANAFRANIL75MG	Cap, Ivory & Yellow	Clomipramine HCl 75 mg	Anafranil by Mallinckrodt	00406-9908	OCD
ANAMINE1234	Cap, Black Print	Chlorpheniramine Maleate 8 mg, Pseudoephedrine HCl 120 mg	Anamine TD by Merz	00259-1234	Cold Remedy
ANANDRON <> 50	Tab, White, Round, Biconvex	Nilutamide 50 mg	Anandron by Aventis	Canadian DIN 02221861	Antiandrogen
ANANDRON100	Tab, White, Biconvex, Anandron/100	Nilutamide 100 mg	Anandron by Aventis	Canadian DIN 02221888	Antiandrogen

ID FRONT <> BACK	DESCRIPTION FRONT <> BACK	INGREDIENT & STRENGTH	BRAND (or Generic Equiv.) by FIRM	NDC#	CLASS; SCH.
ANAPROX <> ROCHE	Tab, Film Coated	Naproxen 275 mg	Anaprox by H J Harkins Co	52959-0015	NSAID
ANAPROXDS	Tab, Film Coated	Naproxen 550 mg	by Amerisource	62584-0276	NSAID
ANAPROXDS <> ROCHE	Tab, Dark Blue, Film Coated, Debossed	Naproxen 550 mg	by Thrift Drug	59198-0244	NSAID
ANAPROXDS <> ROCHE	Tab, Film Coated	Naproxen 550 mg	by Nat Pharmpak	55154-3805	NSAID
ANAPROXDS <> ROCHE	Tab, Blue, Oblong	Naproxen 550 mg	by Med Pro	53978-3369	NSAID
ANAPROXDS <> ROCHE	Tab, Blue, Oblong	Naproxen 550 mg	Anaprox DS by Rightpak	65240-0603	NSAID
ANAPROXDS <> ROCHE	Tab, Dark Blue, Film Coated	Naproxen 550 mg	Anaprox DS by H J Harkins Co	52959-0016	NSAID
ANAPROXDS <> ROCHE	Tab, Dark Blue, Film Coated	Naproxen 550 mg	by Syntex	18393-0276	NSAID
ANAPROXDS	Tab, Film Coated	Naproxen 550 mg	by Allscripts		NSAID
ANAPROXDS <> SYNTEX	Tab, Film Coated	Naproxen 550 mg	by Quality Care	60346-0035 Discontinued	NSAID
ANB	Tab, Orange, Round, Schering Logo ANB	Perphenazine 4 mg, Amitriptyline HCl 10 mg	Etrafon-A by Schering		Antipsychotic; Antidepressant
ANC	Tab, Pink, Round, Schering Logo ANC	Perphenazine 2 mg, Amitriptyline HCl 25 mg	Etrafon by Schering		Antipsychotic; Antidepressant
ANDRX	Cap, Purple and Orange	Phenylephrine HCl 30 mg, Guaifenesin 400 mg	Entex LA by Andrx	62022-0333	Cold Remedy
ANDRX	Cap, White and Blue, Opaque	Pseudoephedrine HCl 120 mg, Guaifenesin 400 mg	Entex PSE by Andrx	62022-0132	Cold Remedy
ANDRX <> 929	Tab, White, Cap Shaped, Scored, Sustained Release	Phenylephrine HCl 30 mg, Guaifenesin 600 mg	Entex LA by Andrx	62037-0929	Cold Remedy
ANDRX132	Cap, White and Blue, Opaque	Pseudoephedrine HCl 120 mg, Guaifenesin 400 mg	Entex PSE by Andrx	62022-0132	Cold Remedy
ANDRX333	Cap, Purple and Orange	Phenylephrine HCl 30 mg, Guaifenesin 400 mg	Entex LA by Andrx	62022-0333	Cold Remedy
ANDRX510100MG	Cap, White, Opaque, Ex Release	Ketoprofen 100 mg	Oruvail by Andrx	62037-0510	NSAID
ANDRX515150MG	Cap, Light Turquoise & White, Opaque, Ex Release	Ketoprofen 150 mg	Oruvail by Andrx	62037-0515	NSAID
ANDRX520200MG	Cap, Light Turquoise, Ex Release	Ketoprofen 200 mg	Oruvail by Andrx	62037-0520	NSAID
ANDRX53810MG	Cap, Blue-Green	Fluoxetine 10 mg	Prozac by Andrx	62037-0538	Antidepressant
ANDRX53920MG	Cap, Ivory & Green	Fluoxetine 20 mg	Prozac by Andrx	62037-0539	Antidepressant
ANDRX548	Cap, White	Diltiazem HCl 120 mg	Diltia XT by Andrx	62037-0548	Antihypertensive
ANDRX548120MG	Cap, White	Diltiazem HCl 120 mg	Diltia XT by F Hoffmann La Roche	12783-0060	Antihypertensive
ANDRX549180MG	Cap, Gray & White	Diltiazem HCl 180 mg	Diltia XT by Kaiser	00179-1375	Antihypertensive
ANDRX549180MG	Cap, Gray & White	Diltiazem HCl 180 mg	Diltia XT by Andrx	62037-0549	Antihypertensive
ANDRX549180MG	Cap, Gray & White	Diltiazem HCl 180 mg	Diltia XT by F Hoffmann La Roche	12806-0800	Antihypertensive
ANDRX550240MG	Cap, Gray	Diltiazem HCl 240 mg	Diltia XT by Andrx	62037-0550	Antihypertensive
ANDRX550240MG	Cap, Gray	Diltiazem HCl 240 mg	Diltia XT by Faulding	50564-0507	Antihypertensive
ANDRX559	Cap, White, Opaque, XR	Potassium Chloride 8 mEq	Micro K by Andrx	62037-0559	Electrolytes
ANDRX560	Cap, Dark Blue, Andrx Logo 560, XR	Potassium Chloride 10 mEq	Micro-K by Andrx	62037-0560	Electrolytes
ANDRX605	Tab, White to Off-White, Oval	Loratadine 10 mg, Pseudoephedrine Sulfate 240 mg	Claritin D 24 Hr. by Perrigo	00113-0165	Cold Remedy
ANDRX674 <> 500	Tab, White, Round, Film Coated	Metformin HCl 500 mg	Glucophage by Andrx	62037-0674	Antidiabetic
ANDRX675 <> 850	Tab, White, Round, Film Coated	Metformin HCl 850 mg	Glucophage by Andrx	62037-0675	Antidiabetic
ANDRX676 <> 1000	Tab, White, Round, Film Coated	Metformin HCl 1000 mg	Glucophage by Andrx	62037-0676	Antidiabetic
ANDRX687120	Cap, White	Diltiazem HCl 120 mg	Cardizem by Heartland	61392-0957	Antihypertensive
ANDRX696120MG	Cap, Pink, Opaque	Diltiazem HCl 120 mg	Taztia XT by Andrx	62037-0696	Antihypertensive
ANDRX697180MG	Cap, Light Blue, Buff Opaque	Diltiazem HCl 180 mg	Taztia XT by Andrx	62037-0697	Antihypertensive
ANDRX698240MG	Cap, Pink and Light Blue, Opaque	Diltiazem HCl 240 mg	Taztia XT by Andrx	62037-0698	Antihypertensive
ANDRX699240MG	Cap, Brown	Diltiazem HCl 240 mg	Cardizem by Heartland	61392-0959	Antihypertensive
ANDRX699300MG	Cap, Pink and Buff, Opaque	Diltiazem HCl 300 mg	Taztia XT by Andrx	62037-0699	Antihypertensive
ANDRX700360MG	Cap, Light Blue, Opaque	Diltiazem HCl 360 mg	Taztia XT by Andrx	62037-0700	Antihypertensive
ANDRX710	Tab, Off-White, Cap Shaped	Potassium Chloride 10 mEq	K-Dur by Andrx	62037-0710	Electrolytes
ANDRX720	Tab, Off-White, Cap Shaped, Scored	Potassium Chloride 20 mEq	K-Dur by Andrx	62037-0720	Electrolytes
ANDRX825	Tab, White, Round	Naproxen Sodium 375 mg	Naprelan by Andrx	62037-0825	NSAID
ANDRX826	Tab, White, Cap Shaped	Naproxen Sodium 500 mg	Naprelan by Andrx	62037-0826	NSAID
ANDRX827	Cap, Orange, Opaque	Phenylephrine 30 mg, Guaifenesin 400 mg	Entex LA by Andrx	62037-0827	Cold Remedy

ID FRONT <> BACK	DESCRIPTION FRONT <> BACK	INGREDIENT & STRENGTH	BRAND (or Generic Equiv.) by FIRM	NDC#	CLASS; SCH.
ANE	Tab, Red, Round, Schering Logo ANE	Perphenazine 4 mg, Amitriptyline HCl 25 mg	Etrafon-Forte by Schering		Antipsychotic; Antidepressant
ANE	Tab, Yellow, Oblong	Niacin 500 mg	Nicolar by RPR		Vitamin
ANEXSIA <> 5361	Tab, White, Cap Shaped, Scored	Acetaminophen 500 mg, Hydrocodone Bitartrate 5 mg	Anexsia by Mallinckrodt	00406-5361	Analgesic; C III
ANEXSIA <> 5362	Tab, White, Cap Shaped, Scored	Acetaminophen 650 mg, Hydrocodone Bitartrate 7.5 mg	Anexsia by Mallinckrodt	00406-5362	Analgesic; C III
ANEXSIA <> 5363	Tab	Acetaminophen 660 mg, Hydrocodone Bitartrate 10 mg	Vicodin HP by Mallinckrodt	00406-5363	Analgesic; C III
ANEXSIA <> MPC188	Tab, White, Cap Shaped, Scored	Acetaminophen 650 mg, Hydrocodone Bitartrate 7.5 mg	Lorcet Plus by Nat Pharmpak	55154-7101	Analgesic; C III
ANEXSIA <> MPC188	Tab, White, Cap Shaped, Scored	Acetaminophen 650 mg, Hydrocodone Bitartrate 7.5 mg	Lorcet Plus by King	60793-0843	Analgesic; C III
ANEXSIA <> MPC188	Tab, White, Cap Shaped, Scored	Acetaminophen 650 mg, Hydrocodone Bitartrate 7.5 mg	Lorcet Plus by Med Pro	53978-3309	Analgesic; C III
ANEXSIA <> MPC207	Tab, White, Round, Scored	Acetaminophen 500 mg, Hydrocodone Bitartrate 5 mg	Vicodin by King	60793-0842	Analgesic; C III
ANJ	Tab, Green, Oval, Film Coated, Abbott Logo (a)	B-Complex, Folic Acid, Vitamin E w/ 750 mg Vitamin C	Cefol by Abbott	00074-6089	Vitamin
ANK	Tab, Pink, Round, Schering Logo ANK	Anisindione 50 mg	Miradon by Schering		Anticoagulant
ANR	Tab, Peach, Oval, Abbott Logo (a)	Divalproex Sodium 250 mg	Depakote by Amerisource	62584-0356	Anticonvulsant
ANR	Tab, Peach, Oval, Abbott Logo (a)	Divalproex Sodium 250 mg	Depakote by Abbott	00074-6214	Anticonvulsant
ANS	Tab, Lavender (Appears Pink), Oval, Abbott Logo (a)	Divalproex Sodium 500 mg	Depakote by Abbott	00074-6215	Anticonvulsant
ANSAID	Tab, White, Oval, Film Coated	Flurbiprofen 50 mg	Ansaid by Pfizer	Canadian DIN 00647942	NSAID
ANSAID	Tab, Blue, Oval, Film Coated	Flurbiprofen 100 mg	Ansaid by Pfizer	Canadian DIN 00600792	NSAID
ANSAID100MG	Tab, Blue, Black Print, Oval, Film Coated, Ansaid over 100 mg	Flurbiprofen 100 mg	Ansaid by Med Pro	53978-3379	NSAID
ANSAID100MG	Tab, Blue, Black Print, Oval, Film Coated, Ansaid over 100 mg	Flurbiprofen 100 mg	Ansaid by Leiner	59606-0604	NSAID
ANSAID100MG	Tab, Blue, Black Print, Oval, Film Coated, Ansaid over 100 mg	Flurbiprofen 100 mg	Ansaid by Amerisource	62584-0305	NSAID
ANSAID100MG	Tab, Blue, Black Print, Oval, Film Coated, Ansaid over 100 mg	Flurbiprofen 100 mg	Ansaid by Pharmacia	Canadian DIN 00600792	NSAID
ANSAID100MG	Tab, Blue, Black Print, Oval, Film Coated, Ansaid over 100 mg	Flurbiprofen 100 mg	Ansaid by Thrift Drug	59198-0125	NSAID
ANSAID100MG	Tab, Blue, Black Print, Oval, Film Coated, Ansaid over 100 mg	Flurbiprofen 100 mg	Ansaid by Invamed	52189-0393	NSAID
ANSAID100MG	Tab, Blue, Black Print, Oval, Film Coated, Ansaid over 100 mg	Flurbiprofen 100 mg	Ansaid by Allscripts		NSAID
ANSAID100MG	Tab, Blue, Black Print, Oval, Film Coated, Ansaid over 100 mg	Flurbiprofen 100 mg	Ansaid by Pharmacia	00009-0305	NSAID
ANSAID50	Tab, White, Oval, Film Coated	Flurbiprofen 50 mg	Ansaid by Pharmacia	Canadian DIN 00647942	NSAID
ANSAID50	Tab, White, Oval, Film Coated	Flurbiprofen 50 mg	Ansaid by Pharmacia	00009-0170	NSAID
ANT	Tab, Pink, Blue Print, Oval, Abbott Logo (a)	Divalproex Sodium 125 mg	Depakote by Abbott	00074-6212	Anticonvulsant
ANTABUSE250 <> A	Tab, White, Octagonal, Scored	Disulfiram 250 mg	Antabuse by Wyeth	00046-0809	Antialcoholism
ANTIVERT <> 210	Tab, Blue & White, Oblong	Meclizine HCl 12.5 mg	Antivert by Roerig	00662-2100	Antiemetic
ANTIVERT <> 210	Tab, Blue & White, Oblong	Meclizine HCl 12.5 mg	Antivert by Roerig	00049-2100	Antiemetic
ANTIVERT <> 211	Tab, White & Yellow, Oblong	Meclizine HCl 25 mg	Antivert by Roerig	00662-2110	Antiemetic
ANTIVERT <> 211	Tab, White & Yellow, Oblong	Meclizine HCl 25 mg	Antivert by Rightpak	65240-0605	Antiemetic
ANTIVERT <> 211	Tab, White & Yellow, Oblong	Meclizine HCl 25 mg	Antivert by Roerig	00049-2110	Antiemetic
ANTIVERT <> 214	Tab, Blue & Yellow, Oblong	Meclizine HCl 50 mg	Antivert by Roerig	00049-2140	Antiemetic
ANTIVERT210	Tab, Blue, Oval	Meclizine HCl 12.5 mg	Antivert by Rightpak	65240-0659	Antiemetic
ANZEMET <> 100	Tab, Pink, Oval, Film Coated	Dolasetron 100 mg	Anzemet by Aventis	Canadian DIN 02231379	Antiemetic
ANZEMET <> 100	Tab, Pink, Oval, Film Coated	Dolasetron 100 mg	Anzemet by Aventis	00088-1203	Antiemetic

ID FRONT <> BACK	DESCRIPTION FRONT <> BACK	INGREDIENT & STRENGTH	BRAND (or Generic Equiv.) by FIRM	NDC#	CLASS; SCH.
ANZEMET <> 100	Tab, Pink, Oval, Film Coated	Dolasetron 100 mg	Anzemet by Merrell	00068-1203	Antiemetic
ANZEMET <> 50	Tab, Light Pink, Round, Film Coated	Dolasetron 50 mg	Anzemet by Merrell	00068-1202	Antiemetic
ANZEMET50	Tab, Light Pink, Round, Film Coated	Dolasetron 50 mg	Anzemet by Aventis	Canadian DIN 02231378	Antiemetic
AO <> 20	Tab, Coated	Salsalate 750 mg	Disalcid by Quality Care	60346-0034	NSAID
AO50 <> A	Tab, Pink, Round, AO over 50 <> Abbott Logo (a)	Dicumarol 50 mg	by Abbott	00074-3773 Discontinued	Anticoagulant
AO58	Tab, Ex Release, AO over 58	Guaifenesin 400 mg, Phenylpropanolamine HCl 75 mg	Entex LA by Quality Care	60346-0339	Cold Remedy
AOM20	Cap, Pink and Reddish-Brown, Opaque, Hard Gel, Delayed Release	Omeprazole 20 mg	Losec by AstraZeneca	Canadian DIN 00846503	Gastrointestinal
AP <> 009	Tab, Orange, Round, Chewable	Aspirin 81 mg	Bayer Aspirin-Children by Qualitest	00603-0024	Analgesic
AP <> 009	Tab, Orange, Round, Scored, p inside A	Aspirin 81 mg	Aspirin by Rugby	00536-3297	Analgesic
AP <> 110	Tab, Light Blue, Cap Shaped, Scored	Acetaminophen 650 mg, Butalbital 50 mg	Promacet by Atley	59702-0650	Analgesic
AP <> 112	Tab, Blue, Round	Hyoscyamine Sulfate 0.125 mg	Levsin by Alaven Pharmaceutical	68220-0112	Gastrointestinal
AP <> 113	Tab, Blue, Round, Sublingual	Hyoscyamine Sulfate 0.125 mg	Levsin by Alaven Pharmaceutical	68220-0113	Gastrointestinal
AP <> 115	Tab, White, Cap Shaped, Extended Release	Hyoscyamine Sulfate 0.375 mg	Levbid by Alaven Pharmaceutical	68220-0115	Gastrointestinal
AP <> 133	Tab, Blue, Oblong, AP logo (Upside down V over p) <> 133	Acetaminophen 500 mg, Diphenhydramine HCl 25 mg	Tylenol PM by Advance		Cold Remedy
AP <> 152	Tab, Purple, Cap Shaped, Scored, Chewable	Pseudoephedrine HCl 15 mg, Chlorpheniramine Maleate 2 mg	Pediox by Atley	59702-0152	Cold Remedy
AP <> 304	Tab, Purple, Chewable, A/P <> 30/4	Pseudoephedrine HCl 30 mg, Chlorpheniramine Maleate 4 mg	Sudal 12 by Atley	59702-0809	Cold Remedy
AP <> 5162	Tab, White, Oval, Scored	Captopril 50 mg, HCTZ 15 mg	Capozide by Apothecon	59772-5162	Antihypertensive; Diuretic
AP <> 5163	Tab, Peach, Oval, Scored	Captopril 50 mg, HCTZ 25 mg	Capozide by Apothecon	59772-5163	Antihypertensive; Diuretic
AP <> 7045	Tab, White, Round, Scored	Captopril 12.5 mg	Capoten by Nat Pharmpak	55154-7601	Antihypertensive
AP <> 7045	Tab, White, Round, Scored	Captopril 12.5 mg	Capoten by Apothecon	59772-7045	Antihypertensive
AP <> 7045	Tab, White, Round, Scored	Captopril 12.5 mg	Capoten by BMS	15548-0045	Antihypertensive
AP <> 7045	Tab, White, Round, Scored	Captopril 12.5 mg	Capoten by Med Pro	53978-0939	Antihypertensive
AP <> 805	Tab, Light Green, Cap-Shaped, Film Coated	Esterified Estrogens 0.625 mg, Methyltestosterone 1.25 mg	Estratest by Interpharm	68462-0173	Hormone
AP <> 805	Cap, Light Green	Esterified Estrogens 0.625mg, Methyltestosterone 1.25mg	Estratest HS by Glenmark	68462-0173	Hormones
AP <> 806	Capsule, Dark Green	Esterified Estrogens 1.25 mg, Methyltestosterone 2.5 mg	Estratest HS by Glenmark	68462-0174	Hormones
AP <> 806	Tab, Green, Cap Shaped, Film Coated	Esterified Estrogens 1.25 mg, Methyltestosterone 2.5 mg	Estratest by Interpharm	68462-0174	Hormone
AP <> 8818	Tab	Buspirone HCl 5 mg	Buspar by Apothecon	59772-8818	Antianxiety
AP <> 8819	Tab	Buspirone HCl 10 mg	Buspar by Apothecon	59772-8819	Antianxiety
AP <> ALOR5	Tab, A Bisect P	Aspirin 500 mg, Hydrocodone Bitartrate 5 mg	Alor 5 500 by Atley	59702-0550	Analgesic; C III
AP <> NU	Tab, Round, White, AP <> nu, Chewable	Hyoscyamine Sulfate 0.125 mg	NuLev Chewable Melt by Alaven Pharmaceutical	68220-0118	Gastrointestinal
AP <> REGLAN5	Tab, Green, Elliptical-Shaped	Metoclopramide 5 mg	Reglan by Alaven Pharmaceutical	68220-0150	Gastrointestinal
AP <> SUDAL60	Tab, White, Cap Shaped, Scored	Guaifenesin 500 mg, Pseudoephedrine HCl 60 mg	Sudafed Sinus by Martec		Cold Remedy
AP <> SUDAL60	Tab, White, Cap Shaped, Scored	Guaifenesin 500 mg, Pseudoephedrine HCl 60 mg	Sudafed Sinus by Atley	59702-0060	Cold Remedy
AP <> SUDAL60	Tab, White, Cap Shaped, Scored	Guaifenesin 500 mg, Pseudoephedrine HCl 60 mg	Sudafed Sinus by Anabolic	00722-6395	Cold Remedy
AP <> SUDALDM	Tab, White, Cap Shaped, Scored	Guaifenesin 500 mg, Dextromethorphan HBr 30 mg	GFN 500 DTMH 30 by Martec		Cold Remedy
AP <> SUDALDM	Tab, White, Cap Shaped, Scored	Guaifenesin 500 mg, Dextromethorphan HBr 30 mg	Sudal DM by Atley	59702-0305	Cold Remedy
AP <> SUDALSR	Tab, White, Cap Shaped, Scored	Pseudoephedrine HCl 50 mg, Guaifenesin 1200 mg	Cephadyn by Atley	59702-0050	Cold Remedy
AP011	Tab, Orange, Round	Aspirin 325 mg	Aspirin by Rugby	00536-3313	Analgesic
AP016	Tab, Light Yellow, Round, Scored, p inside A over 016	Chlorpheniramine Maleate 4 mg	Chlor-Trimeton by Rugby	00536-3467	Antihistamine
AP016	Tab, Light Yellow, Round, Scored, p inside A over 016	Chlorpheniramine Maleate 4 mg	Chlor-Trimeton by Amneal	65162-0116	Antihistamine
AP019	Tab, White, Round	Simethicone 80 mg	Mylanta Gas by Qualitest	00603-0210	Antiflatulent
AP019	Tab, White, Round	Simethicone 80 mg	Mylanta by Rugby	00536-4533	Antiflatulent
AP025	Tab, White, Round, Scored, AP over 025	Estradiol 0.5 mg	Estrace by BMS	59772-0025	Hormone
AP025	Tab, White, Round	Calcium Carbonate 648 mg	Os-Cal by Rugby		Vitamin; Mineral
AP025	Tab, White, Round, Scored, AP over 025	Estradiol 0.5 mg	Estrace by Apothecon	59772-0025	Hormone

ID FRONT <> BACK	DESCRIPTION FRONT <> BACK	INGREDIENT & STRENGTH	BRAND (or Generic Equiv.) by FIRM	NDC#	CLASS; SCH.
AP026	Tab, Lavender, Round, Scored, AP over 026	Estradiol 1 mg	Estrace by Apothecon	59772-0026	Hormone
AP026	Tab, Lavender, Round, Scored, AP over 026	Estradiol 1 mg	Estrace by BMS		Hormone
AP027	Tab, Turquoise, Round, Scored, AP over 027	Estradiol 2 mg	Estrace by Apothecon	59772-0027	Hormone
AP027	Tab, Turquoise, Round, Scored, AP over 027	Estradiol 2 mg	Estrace by BMS		Hormone
AP027	Tab, Off-White, Round	Aluminum Hydroxide 200 mg, Magnesium Hydroxide 200 mg	Maalox by Rugby	00536-4496	Antacid
AP040	Tab, White, Round	Simethicone 125 mg	Mylanta Gas by Qualitest	00603-0211	Antiflatulent
AP040	Tab, White, Round	Simethicone 125 mg	Mylanta Gas Ex Strength by Rugby	00536-4534	Antiflatulent
AP042	Tab, Pink, Oblong	Diphenhydramine 25 mg	Benadryl by Qualitest	00603-0239	Antihistamine
AP043	Tab, Multi Colored, Round	Calcium Carbonate 500 mg	Tums by Rugby	00536-4742	Antacid
AP044	Tab, Light Purple, Round, Scored	Acetaminophen 80 mg	Children's Tylenol by Rugby	00536-3234	Analgesic
AP045	Tab, Light Pink, Round	Bismuth Subsalicylate 262.5 mg	Pepto Bismol by Rugby	00536-4301	Gastrointestinal
AP045	Tab, Pink, Round	Bismuth 262 mg	Pepto Bismol by Qualitest	00603-0235	Gastrointestinal
AP051	Tab, Pink, Round, Scored	Acetaminophen 80 mg	Children's Tylenol by Rugby	00536-3233	Analgesic
AP0812	Tab, Light Orange, Round, Film Coated	Doxycycline Hyclate 100 mg	Vibramycin Hyclate by Mutual	53489-0120	Antibiotic
AP0812	Tab, Light Orange, Round, Film Coated	Doxycycline Hyclate 100 mg	Vibramycin Hyclate by BMS	00003-0812 Discontinued	Antibiotic
AP0812	Tab, Light Orange, Round, Film Coated	Doxycycline Hyclate 100 mg	Vibramycin Hyclate by Apothecon	59772-0803	Antibiotic
AP0814	Cap, Light Blue, Opaque	Doxycycline Hyclate 100 mg	Vibramycin Hyclate by Apothecon	59772-0940	Antibiotic
AP0814	Cap, Light Blue, Opaque	Doxycycline Hyclate 100 mg	Vibramycin Hyclate by BMS	00003-0814 Discontinued	Antibiotic
AP0814	Cap, Light Blue, Opaque	Doxycycline Hyclate 100 mg	Vibramycin Hyclate by Mutual	53489-0119	Antibiotic
AP0837	Cap, Light Blue & White, Opaque	Doxycycline Hyclate 50 mg	Vibramycin Hyclate by BMS	00003-8708	Antibiotic
AP0837	Cap, Light Blue & White, Opaque	Doxycycline Hyclate 50 mg	Vibramycin Hyclate by Mutual	53489-0118	Antibiotic
AP0837	Cap, Light Blue & White, Opaque	Doxycycline Hyclate 50 mg	Vibramycin Hyclate by Rachelle	00196-0552	Antibiotic
AP0837	Cap, Light Blue & White, Opaque	Doxycycline Hyclate 50 mg	Vibramycin Hyclate by Apothecon	59772-0808	Antibiotic
AP1	Tab, Maroon, White Print, Round, Sugar Coated	Phenazopyridine HCl 100 mg	Pyridium by Able	53265-0196	Urinary Analgesic
AP1	Tab, Maroon, White Print, Round, Sugar Coated	Phenazopyridine HCl 100 mg	Pyridium by Schein	00364-0286 Discontinued	Urinary Analgesic
AP10 <> REGLAN	Tab, White, Cap Shaped, Scored	Metoclopramide 10 mg	Reglan by Alaven Pharmaceutical	68220-0151	Gastrointestinal
AP121	Tab, Yellow, Round, A (upside down V) over P	Aspirin 81 mg	Ecotrin Adult Low-Dose by Qualitest	00603-0025	Analgesic
AP18	Tab, White, Coated, Scored	Folacin (Folic Acid) 2.05 mg, Hydroxocobalamin (B12a) 425 mcg, Pyridoxine (B6) 25 mg, D-alpha Tocopheryl Succinate (Vitamin E) 100 IU, Magnesium Oxide 100 mg	Folpace RX by Alaven Pharmaceutical	68220-0018	Supplement
AP2	Tab, Maroon, White Print, Round, Sugar Coated	Phenazopyridine HCl 200 mg	Pyridium by Schein	00364-0321 Discontinued	Urinary Analgesic
AP2	Tab, Maroon, White Print, Round, Sugar Coated	Phenazopyridine HCl 200 mg	Pyridium by Able	53265-0197 Discontinued	Urinary Analgesic
AP20	Cap, Pink & White	Diphenhydramine 25 mg	Benadryl by Qualitest	00603-0240	Antihistamine
AP20	Cap, Pink & Clear	Diphenhydramine 25 mg	Benadryl Cap by Qualitest	00603-3337	Antihistamine
AP20	Cap, Pink & White	Diphenhydramine 25 mg	Benadryl by Amneal	65162-0156	Antihistamine
AP21	Cap, Pink	Diphenhydramine 50 mg	Benadryl Cap by Qualitest	00603-3338	Antihistamine
AP21	Cap, Pink, Black Print	Diphenhydramine 50 mg	Benadryl by Amneal	65162-0518	Antihistamine
AP2461	Tab, White, Round, Scored, AP over 2461	Nadolol 20 mg	Nadolol by Apothecon	59772-2461	Antihypertensive
AP2462	Tab, White, Round, Scored, AP over 2462	Nadolol 40 mg	Nadolol by Qualitest	59772-2462	Antihypertensive
AP2462	Tab, White, Round, Scored, AP over 2462	Nadolol 40 mg	Nadolol by Mead Johnson	00015-2462	Antihypertensive
AP2463	Tab, White, Round, Scored, AP over 2463	Nadolol 80 mg	Nadolol by Apothecon	59772-2463	Antihypertensive
AP2464	Tab, White, Round, Scored, AP over 2464	Nadolol 120 mg	Nadolol by Apothecon	59772-2464	Antihypertensive
AP2465	Tab, White, Round, Scored, AP over 2465	Nadolol 160 mg	Nadolol by Apothecon	59772-2465	Antihypertensive
AP2472	Tab, White, Round	Nadolol 40 mg, Bendroflumethiazide 5 mg	by Apothecon	59772-2472	Antihypertensive; Diuretic

ID FRONT <> BACK	DESCRIPTION FRONT <> BACK	INGREDIENT & STRENGTH	BRAND (or Generic Equiv.) by FIRM	NDC#	CLASS; SCH.
AP2472	Tab, White, Round	Bendroflumethiazide 5 mg, Nadolol 40 mg	Corzide by Apothecon		Diuretic; Antihypertensive
AP2473	Tab, White, Round	Nadolol 80 mg, Bendroflumethiazide 5 mg	by Apothecon	59772-2473	Antihypertensive; Diuretic
AP2473	Tab, White, Round	Bendroflumethiazide 5 mg, Nadolol 80 mg	Corzide by Apothecon		Diuretic; Antihypertensive
AP3171 <> 505050	Tab, Off-White, Rectangular, Scored	Trazodone HCl 150 mg	Desyrel by Apothecon	59772-3171	Antidepressant
AP35	Cap, Red & Yellow	Docusate Sodium 240 mg	Colace by Advance		Laxative
AP4165	Tab, White, Round	Acyclovir 400 mg	Zovirax by BMS		Antiviral
AP4166	Tab, White, Oblong	Acyclovir 800 mg	Zovirax by BMS		Antiviral
AP4168	Cap, Blue & White	Acyclovir 200 mg	Zovirax by BMS		Antiviral
AP5160	Tab, White, Square, Scored, AP over 5160	Captopril 25 mg, HCTZ 15 mg	Capozide by Apothecon	59772-5160	Antihypertensive; Diuretic
AP5161	Tab, Peach, Square, Scored, AP over 5161	Captopril 25 mg, HCTZ 25 mg	Capozide by Apothecon	59772-5161	Antihypertensive; Diuretic
AP6910	Tab, Orange, Round	Potassium Chloride 10 mEq	K-Tab by BMS		Electrolytes
AP7046	Tab, White, Round, Scored, AP over 7046	Captopril 25 mg	Capoten by Sandoz	00781-7046	Antihypertensive
AP7046	Tab, White, Round, Scored, AP over 7046	Captopril 25 mg	Capoten by Ivax	00182-2623	Antihypertensive
AP7046	Tab, White, Round, Scored, AP over 7046	Captopril 25 mg	Capoten by Caremark	00339-5877	Antihypertensive
AP7046	Tab, White, Round, Scored, AP over 7046	Captopril 25 mg	Capoten by Nat Pharmpak	55154-7602	Antihypertensive
AP7046	Tab, White, Round, Scored, AP over 7046	Captopril 25 mg	Capoten by Apothecon	59772-7046	Antihypertensive
AP7046	Tab, White, Round, Scored, AP over 7046	Captopril 25 mg	Capoten by Southwood	58016-0166	Antihypertensive
AP7046	Tab, White, Round, Scored, AP over 7046	Captopril 25 mg	Capoten by Med Pro	53978-0236	Antihypertensive
AP7046	Tab, White, Round, Scored, AP over 7046	Captopril 25 mg	Capoten by BMS	15548-0046	Antihypertensive
AP7047	Tab, White, Round, Scored, AP over 7047	Captopril 50 mg	Capoten by Southwood	58016-0165	Antihypertensive
AP7047	Tab, White, Round, Scored, AP over 7047	Captopril 50 mg	Capoten by Apothecon	59772-7047	Antihypertensive
AP7047	Tab, White, Round, Scored, AP over 7047	Captopril 50 mg	Capoten by BMS	15548-0047	Antihypertensive
AP7047	Tab, White, Round, Scored, AP over 7047	Captopril 50 mg	Capoten by Murfreesboro	51129-1309	Antihypertensive
AP7047	Tab, White, Round, Scored, AP over 7047	Captopril 50 mg	Capoten by Sandoz	00781-7047	Antihypertensive
AP7048	Tab, White, Round, Scored, AP over 7048	Captopril 100 mg	Capoten by Sandoz	00781-7048	Antihypertensive
AP7048	Tab, White, Round, Scored, AP over 7047	Captopril 100 mg	Capoten by BMS	15548-0048	Antihypertensive
AP7048	Tab, White, Round, Scored, AP over 7048	Captopril 100 mg	Capoten by Apothecon	59772-7048	Antihypertensive
AP7491250MG	Cap, Blue & White, AP 7491/250 mg	Cefaclor 250 mg	Ceclor by Apothecon		Antibiotic
AP7491250MG	Cap, Blue & White, AP 7491/250 mg	Cefaclor 250 mg	Ceclor by Golden State	60429-0701	Antibiotic
AP7491250MG	Cap, Blue & White, AP 7491/250 mg	Cefaclor 250 mg	Ceclor by Apothecon	59772-7491	Antibiotic
AP7494500MG	Cap, Blue & Gray, AP 7494/500 mg	Cefaclor 500 mg	Ceclor CD by Golden State	60429-0702	Antibiotic
AP7494500MG	Cap, Blue & Gray, AP 7494/500 mg	Cefaclor 500 mg	by Apothecon	59772-7494	Antibiotic
AP7494500MG	Cap, Blue & Gray, AP 7494/500 mg	Cefaclor 500 mg	Ceclor CD by Apothecon		Antibiotic
AP812	Tab, Beige, Round	Doxycycline Hyclate 100 mg	Vibramycin by BMS		Antibiotic
AP88	Tab, Purple, Oval, Scored, Film Coated	Vitamin D3 400 IU, Vitamin E 10 IU, Vitamin B1 1.5 mg, Vitamin B2 1.6 mg, Vitamin B3 17 mg, Vitamin B6 50 mg, Folic Acid 1 mg, Vitamin B12 12 mg, Biotin 30 mcg, Vitamin B5 10 mg, Iron (Polysaccharide Iron Complex 22 mg, Heme Iron Polypeptide 6 mg), Iodine 175 mcg, Zinc 15 mg, Selenium 65 mcg, Copper 0.8 mg	PreferaOB by Alaven Pharmaceutical	68220-0088	Prenatal Vitamin
AP8819	Tab, White, Round	Buspirone HCl 10 mg	Buspar by BMS		Antianxiety
AP908	Tab, White, Round	Selegiline 5 mg	Eldepryl by BMS		Antiparkinson
AP99	Tab, White, Oval, Coated	Folic Acid 1.6 mg, Hydroxocobalamin (B12a) 425 mcg, Pyridoxine (B6) 25 mg, Calcium Carbonate 600 mg, Cholecalciferol (D3) 400 IU, Policosanol 5 mg	Calafol Rx by Alaven Pharmaceutical	68220-0099	Supplement
APCE	Tab, Pink Speckled, Abbott Logo	Erythromycin 333 mg	by Abbott		Antibiotic
APCE	Tab, Pink w/ White Specks, Oval, Abbott Logo (a)	Erythromycin 333 mg	PCE by Abbott	00074-6290	Antibiotic
APCE	Tab, Pink w/ White Specks, Oval, Abbott Logo (a)	Erythromycin 333 mg	PCE by Pharmedix	53002-0253	Antibiotic
APCE	Tab, Pink w/ White Specks, Oval, Abbott Logo (a)	Erythromycin 333 mg	PCE by Allscripts		Antibiotic

ID FRONT <> BACK	DESCRIPTION FRONT <> BACK	INGREDIENT & STRENGTH	BRAND (or Generic Equiv.) by FIRM	NDC#	CLASS; SCH.
APHRODYNE	Tab, Aqua, Cap Shaped, Scored	Yohimbine HCl 5.4 mg	Aphrodyne by Star	00076-0401	Impotence Agent
APIS <> NOVO291	Tab, White, Round, Film Coated	Estradiol 0.5 mg, Norethindrone Acetate 0.1 mg	Activelle LD by Novo Nordisk	Canadian DIN 02309009	Estrogenic and Progestin Hormones
APK	Cap, Orange, Black Print, Soft Gel, Abbott Logo (a)	Lopinavir 133.3 mg, Ritonavir 33.3 mg	Kaletra by Abbott	00074-3959	Antiviral
APK	Cap, Orange, Black Print, Soft Gel, Abbott Logo (a)	Lopinavir 133.3 mg, Ritonavir 33.3 mg	Kaletra by Abbott	Canadian DIN 02243643	Antiviral
APO	Tab, White, Round, Cross-Scored, "A", "P", and "O" in different segments	Mefloquine HCl 250 mg	Lariam by Apotex	Canadian DIN 02244366	Antiprotozoal
APO <> 025	Tab, Blue, Round	Clonidine 0.025 mg	Dixarit by Apotex	Canadian DIN 02248732	Antihypertensive
APO <> 05	Tab, White, Round, APO/0.5	Lorazepam 0.5 mg	Ativan by Apotex	Canadian DIN 00655740	Antianxiety; C IV
APO <> 083	Tab, White to Off-White, Oval, Film Coated	Paroxetine HCl 20 mg	Paxil by Apotex	60505-0083	Antidepressant
APO <> 084	Tab, White to Off-White, Oval, Film Coated	Paroxetine HCl 30 mg	Paxil by Apotex	60505-0084	Antidepressant
APO <> 093	Tab, White, Round	Doxazosin Mesylate 1 mg	Cardura by Major	00904-5522	Antihypertensive
APO <> 093	Tab, White, Round	Doxazosin Mesylate 1 mg	Cardura by Apotex	60505-0093	Antihypertensive
APO <> 094	Tab, White, Cap Shaped	Doxazosin Mesylate 2 mg	Cardura by Major	60505-0094	Antihypertensive
APO <> 094	Tab, White, Cap Shaped	Doxazosin Mesylate 2 mg	Cardura by Major	00904-5523	Antihypertensive
APO <> 095	Tab, White, Cap Shaped	Doxazosin Mesylate 4 mg	Cardura by Apotex	60505-0095	Antihypertensive
APO <> 095	Tab, White, Cap Shaped	Doxazosin Mesylate 4 mg	Cardura by Apotex	00904-5524	Antihypertensive
APO <> 096	Tab, White, Cap Shaped	Doxazosin Mesylate 8 mg	Cardura by Apotex	60505-0096	Antihypertensive
APO <> 096	Tab, White, Cap Shaped	Doxazosin Mesylate 8 mg	Cardura by Major	00904-5525	Antihypertensive
APO <> 097	Tab, White to Off-White, Oval, Film Coated	Paroxetine HCl 10 mg	Paxil by Apotex	60505-0097	Antidepressant
APO <> 10	Tab, White, Round, Biconvex	Domperidone 10 mg	Apo Domperidone by Apotex	Canadian DIN 02103613	Gastrointestinal
APO <> 10	Tab, White, Cap Shaped, Film Coated	Zolpidem Tartrate 10 mg	Ambien by Apotex	60505-2605	Sedative/Hypnotic; C IV
APO <> 10	Tab, Yellow, Round, APO/10	Oxazepam 10 mg	Apo Oxazepam by Apotex	Canadian DIN 00402680	Sedative/Hypnotic; C IV
APO <> 10	Tab, Grayish Pink, Round	Nifedipine 10 mg	Nifed PA by Apotex	Canadian DIN 02197448	Antihypertensive
APO <> 10	Tab, Yellow, Oblong	Paroxetine HCl 10 mg	Paxil by Apotex	Canadian DIN 02240907	Antidepressant
APO <> 10	Tab, Pink, Shield-Shaped	Simvastatin 10 mg	Zocor by Apotex	Canadian DIN 02247012	Antihyperlipidemic
APO <> 10025	Tab, White, Round, Scored, Film Coated	Atenolol 100 mg, Chlorthalidone 25 mg	Tenoretic by Apotex	Canadian DIN 02248764	Antihypertensive; Diuretic
APO <> 101	Tab, White to Off-White, Oval, Film Coated	Paroxetine HCl 40 mg	Paxil by Apotex	60505-0101	Antidepressant
APO <> 10125	Tab, Pink, Oval, APO <> 10 over 12.5	Lisinopril 10 mg, HCTZ 12.5 mg	Prinzide by Apotex	60505-0205	Antihypertensive; Diuretic
APO <> 10125	Tab, Pink, Round	Hydrochlorothiazide 12.5 mg, Lisinopril 10 mg	Zestoretic by Apotex	Canadian DIN 02261979	Diuretic; Antihypertensive
APO <> 10MG	Tab, White, Ovoid, Scored	Cetirizine HCl 10 mg	Reactine by Apotex	Canadian DIN 02231603	Antihistamine
APO <> 125	Tab, Orange, Round, APO <> 1.25	Indapamide 1.25 mg	Lozol by Apotex	Canadian DIN 02245246	Diuretic
APO <> 125	Tab, White, Oblong, APO <> 12.5	Captopril 12.5 mg	Capoten by Apotex	Canadian DIN 00083595	Antihypertensive
APO <> 125	Tab, Red, Oval, Biconvex	Divalproex Sodium 125 mg	Depakote by Apotex	Canadian DIN 02239698	Anticonvulsant
APO <> 125	Tab, White, Oval, Film Coated, APO <> 12.5	Carvedilol 12.5 mg	Apo Carvedilol by Apotex	Canadian DIN 02247935	Antihypertensive

ID FRONT <> BACK	DESCRIPTION FRONT <> BACK	INGREDIENT & STRENGTH	BRAND (or Generic Equiv.) by FIRM	NDC#	CLASS; SCH.
APO <> 20	Tab, White, Oval, Film Coated	Citalopram 20 mg	Celexa by Apotex	Canadian DIN 02246056	Antidepressant
APO <> 20	Tab, Grayish Pink, Round	Nifedipine 20 mg	Nifed PA by Apotex	Canadian DIN 02181525	Antihypertensive
APO <> 20	Tab, Pink, Oblong, Scored	Paroxetine HCl 20 mg	Paxil by Apotex	Canadian DIN 02240908	Antidepressant
APO <> 20	Tab, Peach, Shield-Shaped	Simvastatin 20 mg	Zocor by Apotex	Canadian DIN 02247013	Antihyperlipidemic
APO <> 20	Tab, Yellow, Oval, Film Coated	Tenoxicam 20 mg	Mobiflex by Apotex	Canadian DIN 02230661	NSAID
APO <> 200	Tab, Pink, Round	Amiodarone HCl 200 mg	Pacerone by Apotex	Canadian	Antiarrhythmic
APO <> 200	Tab, White, Round, Biconvex, SR	Ketoprofen 200 mg	Orudis by Apotex	Canadian DIN 02172577	NSAID
APO <> 200	Tab, Light Yellow, Oval	Ofloxacin 200 mg	Apo Ofloxacin by Apotex	Canadian DIN 02231529	Antibiotic
APO <> 20050	Tab, Peach, Oval, Scored	Carbidopa 50 mg Levodopa 200 mg	Sinemet by Apotex	Canadian DIN 02245211	Antiparkinson
APO <> 20125	Tab, White, Round	Lisinopril 20 mg, HCTZ 12.5 mg	Zestoretic by Apotex	Canadian DIN 02261987	Antihypertensive; Diuretic
APO <> 20125	Tab, White to Off-White, Oval, APO <> 20 over 12.5	Lisinopril 20 mg, HCTZ 12.5 mg	Prinzide by Apotex	60505-0206	Antihypertensive; Diuretic
APO <> 2025	Tab, Pink, Oval, APO <> 20 over 25	Lisinopril 20 mg, HCTZ 25 mg	Prinzide by Apotex	60505-0207	Antihypertensive; Diuretic
APO <> 2025	Tab, Pink, Round, APO <> 20 over 25	Lisinopril 20 mg, HCTZ 25 mg	Zestoretic by Apotex	Canadian DIN 02261995	Antihypertensive; Diuretic
APO <> 25	Tab, White, Shield Shaped	Lamotrigine 25 mg	Lamictal by Apotex	Canadian DIN 02245208	Anticonvulsant
APO <> 25	Tab, White to Off-White, Round, APO <> 2.5	Lisinopril 2.5 mg	Zestril by Apotex	60505-0184	Antihypertensive
APO <> 250	Tab, Peach, Oval, Biconvex	Divalproex Sodium 250 mg	Depakote by Apotex	Canadian DIN 02239699	Anticonvulsant
APO <> 250	Tab, White, Round, Biconvex, Enteric Coated	Naproxen 250 mg	Naprosyn by Apotex	Canadian DIN 02246699	NSAID
APO <> 250	Tab, White, Oval	Ticlopidine HCl 250 mg	Ticlopidine by Apotex	Canadian DIN 02237701	Anticoagulant
APO <> 250125	Tab, White, Oval, Film Coated	Amoxicillin 250 mg, Clavulanate Potassium 125 mg	Clavulin by Apotex	Canadian DIN 02243350	Antibiotic
APO <> 30	Tab, Blue, Oblong	Paroxetine HCl 30 mg	Paxil by Apotex	Canadian DIN 02240909	Antidepressant
APO <> 300	Tab, White, Oval	Ofloxacin 300 mg	Oflox by Apotex	Canadian DIN 02231531	Antibiotic
APO <> 325	Tab, White, Cap Shaped	Acetaminophen 325 mg	Tylenol by Apotex	Canadian DIN 02229873	Analgesic
APO <> 375	Tab, White, Cap Shaped, Biconvex, Enteric Coated	Naproxen 375 mg	Naprosyn by Apotex	Canadian DIN 02246700	NSAID
APO <> 40	Tab, White, Oval, Film Coated	Citalopram 40 mg	Celexa by Apotex	Canadian DIN 02246057	Antidepressant
APO <> 40	Tab, Dusty Rose, Shield-Shaped	Simvastatin 40 mg	Zocor by Apotex	Canadian DIN 02247014	Antihyperlipidemic
APO <> 400	Tab, Pink, Oblong	Pentoxifylline 400 mg	Trental by Apotex	Canadian DIN 02230090	Anticoagulant
APO <> 400	Tab, Yellow, Oval	Ofloxacin 400 mg	Oflox by Apotex	Canadian DIN 02231532	Antibiotic
APO <> 5	Tab, Yellow, Shield-Shaped	Simvastatin 5 mg	Zocor by Apotex	Canadian DIN 02247011	Antihyperlipidemic

ID FRONT <> BACK	DESCRIPTION FRONT <> BACK	INGREDIENT & STRENGTH	BRAND (or Generic Equiv.) by FIRM	NDC#	CLASS; SCH.
APO <> 50	Tab, White, Round	Fluvoxamine Maleate 50 mg	Luvox by Apotex	Canadian DIN 02231329	OCD
APO <> 500	Tab, White, Cap Shaped, Biconvex, Enteric Coated	Naproxen 500 mg	Naprosyn by Apotex	Canadian DIN 02246701	NSAID
APO <> 500	Tab, Pink, Oval, Biconvex	Divalproex Sodium 500 mg	Depakote by Apotex	Canadian DIN 02239700	Anticonvulsant
APO <> 500	Tab, White, Cap Shaped	Acetaminophen 500 mg	Tylenol by Apotex	Canadian DIN 02229977	Analgesic
APO <> 500	Tab, White, Oval	Nabumetone 500 mg	Nabumetone by Apotex	Canadian DIN 02238639	NSAID
APO <> 500125	Tab, White, Oval, Film Coated, 500-125	Amoxicillin 500 mg, Clavulanate Potassium 125 mg	Clavulin by Apotex	Canadian DIN 02243351	Antibiotic
APO <> 5025	Tab, White, Round, Scored, Film Coated	Atenolol 50 mg, Chlorthalidone 25 mg	Tenoretic by Apotex	Canadian DIN 02248763	Antihypertensive; Diuretic
APO <> 5125	Tab, Pink, Oval, Scored, 5 / 12.5	Cilazapril 5 mg, Hydrochlorothiazide 12.5 mg	Inhibace Plus by Apotex	Canadian DIN 02284987	Antihypertensive
APO <> 5MG	Tab, White, Oval, Scored	Cetirizine 5 mg	Zyrtec by Apotex	Canadian DIN 02240910	Antihistamine
APO <> 625	Tab, White, Oval, Film Coated, APO <> 6.25	Carvedilol 6.25 mg	Apo Carvedilol by Apotex	Canadian DIN 02247934	Antihypertensive
APO <> 75	Tab, Yellow, Round, Biconvex	Meloxicam 7.5 mg	Mobic by Apotex	Canadian DIN 02248973	NSAID
APO <> 80	Tab, Dusty Rose, Oblong	Simvastatin 80 mg	Zocor by Apotex	Canadian DIN 02247015	Antihyperlipidemic
APO <> 850	Tab, White, Oblong	Metformin HCl 850 mg	Glucophage by Apotex	Canadian DIN 02229785	Antidiabetic
APO <> A10	Tab, White, Round, APO <> A10	Alendronate 10 mg	Fosamax by Apotex	Canadian DIN 02248728	Antiosteoporosis
APO <> AC	Tab, White, Oblong, Scored, Film Coated	Amoxicillin 875 mg, Clavulanate Potassium 125 mg	Clavulin by Apotex	Canadian DIN 02245623	Antibiotic
APO <> AF120	Tab, White to Off-White, Cap Shaped, APO <> AF over 120	Sotalol HCl 120 mg	Betapace AF by Apotex	60505-0223	Antiarrhythmic
APO <> AF160	Tab, White to Off-White, Cap Shaped, APO <> AF over 160	Sotalol HCl 160 mg	Betapace AF by Apotex	60505-0224	Antiarrhythmic
APO <> AF80	Tab, White to Off-White, Cap Shaped, APO <> AF over 80	Sotalol HCl 80 mg	Betapace AF by Apotex	60505-0222	Antiarrhythmic
APO <> ALE70	Tab, White, Oval, Biconvex tablet, APO <> ALE70	Alendronate 70 mg	Fosamax by Apotex	Canadian DIN 02248730	Antiosteoporosis
APO <> ALL100	Tab, White, Round, Biconvex	Allopurinol 100 mg	Zyloprim by Apotex	Canadian DIN 00402818	Antigout
APO <> ALL200	Tab, Peach, Round, Biconvex	Allopurinol 200 mg	Zyloprim by Apotex	Canadian DIN 00479799	Antigout
APO <> ALL300	Tab, Orange, Round, APO/300	Allopurinol 300 mg	Zyloprim by Apotex	Canadian DIN 00402796	Antigout
APO <> AMI200	Tab, Pink, Round, Scored, AMI/200	Amiodarone HCl 200 mg	Apo Amiodarone by Apotex	Canadian DIN 02246194	Antiarrhythmic
APO <> AML10	Tab, White to Off-White, Round	Amlodipine Besylate 10 mg	Norvasc by Vintage	60505-0195	Antihypertensive
APO <> AML25	Tab, White to Off-White, Round	Amlodipine Besylate 2.5 mg	Norvasc by Vintage	60505-0193	Antihypertensive
APO <> AML5	Tab, White to Off-White, Round	Amlodipine Besylate 5 mg	Norvasc by Vintage	60505-0194	Antihypertensive
APO <> ATE100	Tab, White, Round, ATE/100	Atenolol 100 mg	Tenormin by Apotex	Canadian DIN 00773697	Antihypertensive
APO <> ATE50	Tab, White, Round, ATE/50	Atenolol 50 mg	Tenormin by Apotex	Canadian DIN 00773689	Antihypertensive

ID FRONT <> BACK	DESCRIPTION FRONT <> BACK	INGREDIENT & STRENGTH	BRAND (or Generic Equiv.) by FIRM	NDC#	CLASS; SCH.
APO <> AZ250	Tab, Dark Pink, Oval, Film Coated	Azithromycin 250 mg	Zithromax by Apotex	Canadian DIN 02247423	Antibiotic
APO <> AZ250	Tab, Pale Yellow, Peanut Shaped, Scored	Azathioprine 50 mg	Imuran by Apotex	Canadian DIN 02242907	Immunosuppressant
APO <> BE10	Tab, Yellow, Round, Film Coated	Benazepril HCl 10 mg	Lotensin by Apotex	Canadian DIN 02290340	Antihypertensive
APO <> BE10	Tab, Yellow, Round, Film Coated	Benazepril HCl 10 mg	Lotensin by Apotex	60505-0266	Antihypertensive
APO <> BE20	Tab, Light Pink, Round, Film Coated	Benazepril HCl 20 mg	Lotensin by Apotex	60505-0267	Antihypertensive
APO <> BE20	Tab, Light Pink, Round, Film Coated	Benazepril HCl 20 mg	Lotensin by Apotex	Canadian DIN 02273918	Antihypertensive
APO <> BE40	Tab, Pink, Round, Film Coated	Benazepril HCl 40 mg	Lotensin by Apotex	60505-0268	Antihypertensive
APO <> BE5	Tab, Light Yellow, Round, Film Coated	Benazepril HCl 5 mg	Lotensin by Apotex	60505-0265	Antihypertensive
APO <> BE5	Tab, Light Yellow, Round, Film Coated	Benazepril HCl 5 mg	Lotensin by Apotex	Canadian DIN 02290332	Antihypertensive
APO <> BI10	Tab, White, Round, Film-Coated	Bisoprolol Fumarate 10 mg	Apo-Bisoprolol by Apotex	Canadian DIN 02256177	Antihypertensive
APO <> BI5	Tab, Salmon Pink, Round, Film-Coated, Scored	Bisoprolol Fumarate 5 mg	Apo-Bisoprolol by Apotex	Canadian DIN 02256134	Antihypertensive
APO <> BIC50	Tab, White, Round, Film Coated	Bicalutamide 50 mg	Casodex by Apotex	Canadian DIN 02296063	Antineoplastic
APO <> BU10	Tab, White, Pillow Shaped, Scored	Buspirone HCl 10 mg	Buspar by Apotex	Canadian DIN 02211076	Antianxiety
APO <> C25	Tab, White, Oval, Film Coated	Carvedilol 25 mg	Apo Carvedilol by Apotex	Canadian DIN 02247936	Antihypertensive
APO <> C250	Tab, White to Off-White, Oblong	Cefuroxime Axetil 250 mg	Ceftin by Apotex	Canadian DIN 02244393	Antibiotic
APO <> C250	Tab, White to Off-White, Oblong	Cefuroxime Axetil 250 mg	Ceftin by Apotex	60505-1202	Antibiotic
APO <> C3	Tab, White, Oval, Film Coated	Carvedilol 3.125 mg	Apo Carvedilol by Apotex	Canadian DIN 02247933	Antihypertensive
APO <> C500	Tab, White to Off-White, Oblong	Cefuroxime Axetil 500 mg	Ceftin by Apotex	Canadian DIN 02244394	Antibiotic
APO <> C500	Tab, White to Off-White, Oblong	Cefuroxime Axetil 500 mg	Ceftin by Apotex	60505-1201	Antibiotic
APO <> CI10	Tab, Beige-Pink, Oval	Citalopram HBr 10 mg	Celexa by Apotex	60505-2518	Antidepressant
APO <> CI20	Tab, Pink, Oval	Citalopram HBr 20 mg	Celexa by Apotex	60505-2519	Antidepressant
APO <> CI40	Tab, White, Oval	Citalopram HBr 40 mg	Celexa by Apotex	60505-2520	Antidepressant
APO <> CIL100	Tab, White, Round, CIL/100 <> APO	Cilostazol 100 mg	Pletal by Apotex	60505-2522	Antiplatelet
APO <> CIL50	Tab, White, Round, CIL/50 <> APO	Cilostazol 50 mg	Pletal by Apotex	60505-2521	Antiplatelet
APO <> CIP250	Tab, White to Off-White, Round, CIP over 250	Ciprofloxacin 250 mg	Cipro by Apotex	60505-1308	Antibiotic
APO <> CIP500	Tab, White to Off-White, Cap Shaped	Ciprofloxacin 500 mg	Cipro by Apotex	60505-1309	Antibiotic
APO <> CIP750	Tab, White to Off-White, Cap Shaped	Ciprofloxacin 750 mg	Cipro by Apotex	60505-1310	Antibiotic
APO <> CL75	Tab, Pink, Round	Clopidogrel 75 mg	Plavix by Apotex	Canadian DIN 02274744	Antiplatelet
APO <> CLA250	Tab, Pale Yellow, Oval	Clarithromycin 250 mg	Biaxin by Apotex	Canadian DIN 02274744	Antibiotic
APO <> CLA250	Tab, Pale Yellow, Cap Shaped	Clarithromycin 250 mg	Biaxin by Apotex	60505-2616	Antibiotic
APO <> CLA500	Tab, Pale Yellow, Cap Shaped	Clarithromycin 500 mg	Biaxin by Apotex	60505-2615	Antibiotic
APO <> CLA500	Tab, Pale Yellow, Cap Shaped	Clarithromycin 500 mg	Biaxin by Apotex	Canadian DIN 02274752	Antibiotic
APO <> CLO10	Tab, White, Round, Scored, CLO / 10	Clobazam 10 mg	Frisium by Apotex	Canadian DIN 02244638	Anticonvulsant
APO <> CP250	Tab, Light Orange, Cap Shaped	Cefprozil 250 mg	Cefzil by Apotex	Canadian DIN 02292998	Antibiotic

ID FRONT <> BACK	DESCRIPTION FRONT <> BACK	INGREDIENT & STRENGTH	BRAND (or Generic Equiv.) by FIRM	NDC#	CLASS; SCH.
APO <> CPZ500	Tab, White, Cap Shaped	Cefprozil 500 mg	Cefzil by Apotex	Canadian DIN 02293005	Antibiotic
APO <> CYP50	Tab, White, Round, Scored	Cyproterone Acetate 50 mg	Androcur by Apotex	Canadian DIN 02245898	Antiandrogen
APO <> CZ1	Tab, Yellow, Oval, Scored, CZ / 1	Cilazapril 1 mg	Inhibace by Apotex	Canadian DIN 02291134	Antihypertensive
APO <> CZ2.5	Tab, Rose, Oval, Scored, CZ / 2.5	Cilazapril 2.5 mg	Inhibace by Apotex	Canadian DIN 02291142	Antihypertensive
APO <> CZ5	Tab, Reddish-Brown, Oval, Scored, CZ / 5	Cilazapril 5 mg	Inhibace by Apotex	Canadian DIN 02291150	Antihypertensive
APO <> D1	Tab, White, Round, Biconvex	Doxazosin Mesylate 1 mg	Cardura by Apotex	Canadian DIN 02240588	Antihypertensive
APO <> D2	Tab, White, Cap Shaped, Biconvex, Scored	Doxazosin Mesylate 2 mg	Cardura by Apotex	Canadian DIN 02240589	Antihypertensive
APO <> D250	Tab, Light Orange, Cap Shaped	Diflunisal 250 mg	Apo Diflunisal by Apotex	Canadian DIN 02039486	NSAID
APO <> D4	Tab, White, Diamond Shaped, Biconvex, Scored	Doxazosin Mesylate 4 mg	Cardura by Apotex	Canadian DIN 02240590	Antihypertensive
APO <> D500	Tab, Orange, Cap Shaped	Diflunisal 500 mg	Apo Diflunisal by Apotex	Canadian DIN 02039494	NSAID
APO <> DES01	Tab, White to Off-White, Round, Scored, DES / 0.1	Desmopressin Acetate 0.1 mg	DDAVP by Apotex	Canadian DIN 02284030	Antidiuretic
APO <> DES01	Tab, White to Off-White, Round, Scored, DES / 0.1	Desmopressin Acetate 0.1 mg	DDAVP by Apotex	60505-0257	Antidiuretic
APO <> DES02	Tab, White to Off-White, Round, Scored, DES / 0.2	Desmopressin Acetate 0.2 mg	DDAVP by Apotex	60505-0258	Antidiuretic
APO <> DIG	Tab, Pink, Round	Digoxin 62.5 mcg	Lanoxin by Apotex	Canadian DIN 02281236	Cardiac Agent
APO <> DIG125	Tab, Yellow, Round, Scored, APO <> DIG .125	Digoxin 125 mcg	Lanoxin by Apotex	Canadian DIN 02281228	Cardiac Agent
APO <> DIG25	Tab, White, Round, Scored, APO <> DIG .25	Digoxin 250 mcg	Lanoxin by Apotex	Canadian DIN 02281201	Cardiac Agent
APO <> EN25	Tab, White, Oval, Scored, EN / 2.5	Enalapril Maleate 2.5 mg	Vasotec by Apotex	Canadian DIN 02020025	Antihypertensive
APO <> F25	Tab, White to Off-White, Round	Fluvoxamine Maleate 25 mg	Luvox by Apotex	60505-0164	OCD
APO <> F50	Tab, Gold, Round	Fluvoxamine Maleate 50 mg	Luvox by Apotex	60505-0165	OCD
APO <> FAM125	Tab, White, Round	Famciclovir 125 mg	Famvir by Apotex	Canadian DIN 02292025	Antiviral
APO <> FAM250	Tab, White, Round	Famciclovir 250 mg	Famvir by Apotex	Canadian DIN 02292041	Antiviral
APO <> FAM500	Tab, White, Oval	Famciclovir 500 mg	Famvir by Apotex	Canadian DIN 02292068	Antiviral
APO <> FCN100	Tab, Pink, Round	Fluconazole 100 mg	Diflucan by Apotex	60505-0120	Antifungal
APO <> FCN150	Tab, Pink, Round	Fluconazole 150 mg	Diflucan by Apotex	60505-0121	Antifungal
APO <> FCN200	Tab, Pink, Round	Fluconazole 200 mg	Diflucan by Apotex	60505-0122	Antifungal
APO <> FCN50	Tab, Pink, Round	Fluconazole 50 mg	Diflucan by Apotex	60505-0119	Antifungal
APO <> FEN160	Tab, White, Oval, Film Coated	Fenofibrate 160 mg	Apo-Feno Super by Apotex	Canadian DIN 02246860	Antihyperlipidemic
APO <> FLA200	Tab, White, Round, Coated	Flavoxate HCl 200 mg	Apo Flavoxate by Apotex	Canadian DIN 02244842	Antispasmodic
APO <> FLE100	Tab, White, Round, Scored	Flecainide Acetate 100 mg	Tambocor by Apotex	Canadian 02275546	Antiarrhythmic
APO <> FLE50	Tab, White, Round	Flecainide Acetate 50 mg	Tambocor by Apotex	Canadian DIN 02275538	Antiarrhythmic

ID FRONT <> BACK	DESCRIPTION FRONT <> BACK	INGREDIENT & STRENGTH	BRAND (or Generic Equiv.) by FIRM	NDC#	CLASS; SCH.
APO <> FLO200	Tab, White, Round, Biconvex	Floctafenine 200 mg	Idarac by Apotex	Canadian DIN 02244680	Anti-Inflammatory
APO <> FLO400	Tab, White, Round, Biconvex	Floctafenine 400 mg	Idarac by Apotex	Canadian DIN 02244681	Anti-Inflammatory
APO <> FLU100	Tab, Reddish Brown, Pillow Shaped	Fluvoxamine Maleate 100 mg	Luvox by Apotex	60505-0166	OCD
APO <> FLUT250	Tab, Pale Yellow, Round, Scored	Flutamide 250 mg	Apo Flutamide by Apotex	Canadian DIN 02238560	Antiandrogen
APO <> FOS10	Tab, White, Cap Shaped, Notched, APO <> FOS-10	Fosinopril Sodium 10 mg	Monopril by Apotex	Canadian DIN 02266008	Antihypertensive
APO <> FOS20	Tab, White, Oval, APO <> FOS-20	Fosinopril Sodium 20 mg	Monopril by Apotex	Canadian DIN 02266016	Antihypertensive
APO <> FSO10	Tab, White, Cap Shaped, Notched on Top and Bottom, APO <> FSO - 10	Fosinopril 10 mg	Monopril by Apotex	60505-2510	Antihypertensive
APO <> FSO20	Tab, White, Oval, APO <> FSO - 20	Fosinopril 20 mg	Monopril by Apotex	60505-2511	Antihypertensive
APO <> FSO40	Tab, White, Round, APO <> FSO - 40	Fosinopril 40 mg	Monopril by Apotex	60505-2512	Antihypertensive
APO <> GAB600	Tab, White, Oval, Scored, "GAB" and "600" curved around edges	Gabapentin 600 mg	Neurontin by Apotex	60505-2551	Anticonvulsants
APO <> GLP10	Tab, White to Off-White	Glipizide 10 mg	Glucotrol by Apotex	60505-0142	Antidiabetic
APO <> GLP10	Tab, White, Round, Scored	Glipizide 10 mg	Glucotrol by Major	00904-7925	Antidiabetic
APO <> GLP5	Tab, White, Round, Scored	Glipizide 5 mg	Glucotrol by Major	00904-7924	Antidiabetic
APO <> GLP5	Tab, White to Off-White	Glipizide 5 mg	Glucotrol by Apotex	60505-0141	Antidiabetic
APO <> GR1	Tab, White to Off White, Triangular, Film Coated	Granisetron 1 mg	Apo-Granisetron by Apotex	Canadian DIN 02308894	Antiemetic
APO <> HCQ200	Tab, White, Cap Shaped, Film Coated	Hydroxychloroquine Sulfate 200 mg	Apo Hydroxyquine by Apotex	Canadian DIN 02246691	Antimalarial
APO <> ISO60	Tab, Yellow, Oval	Isosorbide Mononitrate 60 mg	Apo-ISMN by Apotex	Canadian DIN 02272830	Antianginal
APO <> KE10	Tab, White, Round, Biconvex	Ketorolac Tromethamine 10 mg	Toradol by Apotex	Canadian DIN 02229080	NSAID
APO <> KET200	Tab, White to Off-White, KET over 200	Ketoconazole 200 mg	Nizoral by Apotex	60505-0092	Antifungal
APO <> L10	Tab, Reddish Brown, Oval	Lisinopril 10 mg	Zestril by Apotex	60505-0186	Antihypertensive
APO <> L20	Tab, Reddish Brown, Oval	Lisinopril 20 mg	Zestril by Apotex	60505-0187	Antihypertensive
APO <> L30	Tab, Reddish Brown, Oval	Lisinopril 30 mg	Zestril by Apotex	60505-0188	Antihypertensive
APO <> L40	Tab, Yellow, Oval	Lisinopril 40 mg	Zestril by Apotex	60505-0189	Antihypertensive
APO <> L5	Tab, Reddish Brown, Oval, Scored	Lisinopril 5 mg	Zestril by Apotex	60505-0185	Antihypertensive
APO <> LAB100	Tab, Orange, Cap Shaped, Film Coated, Scored	Labetalol HCl 100 mg	Trandate by Apotex	Canadian DIN 02243538	Antihypertensive
APO <> LAB200	Tab, White, Cap Shaped, Film Coated, Scored	Labetalol HCl 200 mg	Trandate by Apotex	Canadian DIN 02243539	Antihypertensive
APO <> LAM100	Tab, Peach, Shield Shaped, Scored, LAM / 100	Lamotrigine 100 mg	Apo Lamotrigine by Apotex	Canadian DIN 02245209	Anticonvulsant
APO <> LAM150	Tab, Cream, Shield Shaped, Scored, LAM / 150	Lamotrigine 150 mg	Apo Lamotrigine by Apotex	Canadian DIN 02245210	Anticonvulsant
APO <> LE10	Tab, White, Round, APO <> LE over 10	Leflunomide 10 mg	Arava by Apotex	Canadian DIN 02256495	Antiarthritic
APO <> LE10	Tab, White, Round, APO <> LE over 10	Leflunomide 10 mg	Arava by Apotex	60505-2502	Antiarthritic
APO <> LE20	Tab, White, Triangular, APO <> LE over 20	Leflunomide 20 mg	Arava by Apotex	Canadian DIN 02256509	Antiarthritic
APO <> LEV250	Tab, Blue, Oval, Film Coated	Levetiracetam 250 mg	Keppra by Apotex	Canadian DIN 02285924	Anticonvulsant

ID FRONT <> BACK	DESCRIPTION FRONT <> BACK	INGREDIENT & STRENGTH	BRAND (or Generic Equiv.) by FIRM	NDC#	CLASS; SCH.
APO <> LEV500	Tab, Tan, Oval, Film Coated	Levetiracetam 500 mg	Keppra by Apotex	Canadian DIN 02285932	Anticonvulsant
APO <> LEV750	Tab, Pink, Oval, Film Coated	Levetiracetam 750 mg	Keppra by Apotex	Canadian DIN 02285940	Anticonvulsant
APO <> LIT300	Tab, White, Round, Scored	Lithium Carbonate 300 mg	Duralith by Apotex	Canadian DIN 02266695	Antipsychotic
APO <> LO10	Tab, White, Oval, Scored, LO / 10	Loratadine 10 mg	Claritin by Apotex	Canadian DIN 02243880	Antihistamine
APO <> LOVA20	Tab, Light Blue, Octagonal, APO/Lova 20	Lovastatin 20 mg	Lovastatin by Apotex	Canadian DIN 02220172	Antihyperlipidemic
APO <> LOVA40	Tab, Light Green, Octagonal, APO/Lova 40	Lovastatin 40 mg	Lovastatin by Apotex	Canadian DIN 02220180	Antihyperlipidemic
APO <> LOX10	Tab, Green, Round	Loxapine 10 mg	Loxitane by Apotex	Canadian DIN 02237652	Antipsychotic
APO <> LOX25	Tab, Pink, Round	Loxapine 25 mg	Loxitane by Apotex	Canadian DIN 02237653	Antipsychotic
APO <> LOX5	Tab, Yellow, Round	Loxapine 5 mg	Loxitane by Apotex	Canadian DIN 02237651	Antipsychotic
APO <> LOX50	Tab, White, Round	Loxapine 50 mg	Loxitane by Apotex	Canadian DIN 02237654	Antipsychotic
APO <> LTR1000	Tab, White, Oval	Tryptophan 1000 mg	Tryptan by Apotex	Canadian DIN 02248539	Antidepressant
APO <> LTR500	Tab, White, Oval	Tryptophan 500 mg	Tryptan by Apotex	Canadian DIN 02248538	Antidepressant
APO <> M500	Tab, White, Round, APO/M500	Metformin 500 mg	Metformin by Apotex	Canadian DIN 02167786	Antidiabetic
APO <> ME25	Tab, White, Oval	Metoprolol Tartrate 25 mg	Lopressor by Apotex	Canadian DIN 02246010	Antihypertensive
APO <> MED10	Tab, White, Round, Scored, MED / 10	Medroxyprogesterone Acetate 10 mg	Provera by Apotex	Canadian DIN 02277298	Hormone
APO <> MED100	Tab, White, Round, Scored, MED / 100	Medroxyprogesterone Acetate 100 mg	Provera by Apotex	Canadian DIN 02267640	Hormone
APO <> MED25	Tab, Orange, Round, APO <> MED 2.5	Medroxyprogesterone Acetate 2.5 mg	Provera by Apotex	Canadian DIN 02244726	Hormone
APO <> MED5	Tab, Blue, Round	Medroxyprogesterone Acetate 5 mg	Provera by Apotex	Canadian DIN 02244727	Hormone
APO <> MEL15	Tab, Yellow, Round	Meloxicam 15 mg	Mobic by Apotex	Canadian DIN 02248974	NSAID
APO <> MEL15	Tab, Light Yellow, Round	Meloxicam 15 mg	Mobic by Apotex	60505-2554	NSAID
APO <> MEL75	Tab, Light Yellow, Round, APO <> MEL 7.5	Meloxicam 7.5 mg	Mobic by Apotex	60505-2553	NSAID
APO <> MI15	Tab, Light Yellow, Oval, Film Coated, Scored	Mirtazapine 15 mg	Remeron by Apotex	Canadian DIN 02286610	Antidepressant
APO <> MI30	Tab, Pink, Oval, Film Coated, Scored	Mirtazapine 30 mg	Remeron by Apotex	Canadian DIN 02286629	Antidepressant
APO <> MI45	Tab, White, Oval, Film Coated, Scored	Mirtazapine 45 mg	Remeron by Apotex	Canadian DIN 02286637	Antidepressant
APO <> MID10	Tab, Light Blue, Round, Scored	Midodrine HCl 10 mg	Proamatine by Apotex	60505-1325	Antihypotensive
APO <> MID25	Tab, White, Round, Scored	Midodrine HCl 2.5 mg	Amatine by Apotex	Canadian DIN 02278677	Antihypotensive
APO <> MID5	Tab, Orange, Round, Scored	Midodrine HCl 5 mg	Amatine by Apotex	Canadian DIN 02278685	Antihypotensive

ID FRONT <> BACK	DESCRIPTION FRONT <> BACK	INGREDIENT & STRENGTH	BRAND (or Generic Equiv.) by FIRM	NDC#	CLASS; SCH.
APO <> MISO100	Tab, White, Round	Misoprostol 100 mcg	Cytotec by Apotex	Canadian DIN 02244022	Gastrointestinal
APO <> MISO200	Tab, White, Hexagonal	Misoprostol 200 mcg	Cytotec by Apotex	Canadian DIN 02244023	Gastrointestinal
APO <> MOD100	Tab, White, Round	Modafinil 100 mg	Alertec by Apotex	Canadian DIN 02285398	Stimulant; C IV
APO <> MTP10	Tab, Pale Green, Round, Scored	Methylphenidate HCl 10 mg	Ritalin by Apotex	Canadian DIN 02249324	Stimulant; C II
APO <> MTP20	Tab, Yellow, Round, Scored	Methylphenidate HCl 20 mg	Ritalin by Apotex	Canadian DIN 02249332	Stimulant; C II
APO <> MTP5	Tab, Peach, Round	Methylphenidate HCl 5 mg	Ritalin by Apotex	Canadian DIN 02273950	Stimulant; C II
APO <> MZ50	Tab, White, Round, Biconvex	Methazolamide 50 mg	Neptazane by Apotex	Canadian DIN 02245882	Antiglaucoma Agent
APO <> NIT10	Tab, Round, White	Nitrazepam 10 mg	Apo Nitrazepam by Apotex	Canadian DIN 02245231	Sedative; Hypnotic; C IV
APO <> NIT5	Tab, Round, White	Nitrazepam 5 mg	Apo Nitrazepam by Apotex	Canadian DIN 02245230	Sedative; Hypnotic; C IV
APO <> OND4	Tab, Yellow, Oval, Film Coated	Ondansetron HCl 4 mg	Zofran by Apotex	Canadian DIN 02288184	Antiemetic
APO <> OND8	Tab, Yellow, Oval, Film Coated	Ondansetron HCl 8 mg	Zofran by Apotex	Canadian DIN 02288192	Antiemetic
APO <> OX15	Tab, Yellow, Round, Scored	Oxazepam 15 mg	Serax by Apotex	Canadian DIN 00402745	Sedative/Hypnotic; C IV
APO <> OXA600	Tab, White to Off-White, Cap Shaped, Scored, Film Coated	Oxaprozin 600 mg	Daypro by Apotex	Canadian DIN 02243661	NSAID
APO <> OXA600	Tab, White to Off-White, Cap Shaped, Scored, Film Coated	Oxaprozin 600 mg	Daypro by Apotex	60505-0176	NSAID
APO <> OXC150	Tab, Yellow, Oval, Film Coated, Scored	Oxcarbazepine 150 mg	Trileptal by Apotex	Canadian DIN 02284294	Anticonvulsant
APO <> OXC300	Tab, Yellow, Oval, Film Coated, Scored	Oxcarbazepine 300 mg	Trileptal by Apotex	Canadian DIN 02284308	Anticonvulsant
APO <> OXC600	Tab, Yellow, Oval, Film Coated, Scored	Oxcarbazepine 600 mg	Trileptal by Apotex	Canadian DIN 02284316	Anticonvulsant
APO <> P1015	Tab, White, Round	Pioglitazone 15 mg	Actos by Apotex	Canadian DIN 02302942	Antidiabetic
APO <> P1030	Tab, White, Round	Pioglitazone 30 mg	Actos by Apotex	Canadian DIN 02302950	Antidiabetic
APO <> P1045	Tab, White, Round	Pioglitazone 45 mg	Actos by Apotex	Canadian DIN 02302977	Antidiabetic
APO <> P20	Tab, Yellow, Oval, Coated	Pantoprazole Sodium 20 mg	Pantoloc by Apotex	Canadian DIN 02292912	Gastrointestinal
APO <> P40	Tab, Yellow, Oval, Coated	Pantoprazole Sodium 40 mg	Pantoloc by Apotex	Canadian DIN 02292920	Gastrointestinal
APO <> PE8	Tab, Green, Round	Perindopril Erbumine 8 mg	Coversyl by Apotex	Canadian DIN 02289296	Antihypertensive
APO <> PIM2	Tab, White, Round, Scored	Pimozide 2 mg	ORAP by Apotex	Canadian DIN 02245432	Antipsychotic
APO <> PIM4	Tab, Green, Round, Scored	Pimozide 4 mg	Apo Pimozide by Apotex	Canadian DIN 02245433	Antipsychotic
APO <> PR1	Tab, White, Round, Scored	Pramipexole DiHCl 1 mg	Mirapex by Apotex	Canadian DIN 02292394	Antiparkinson

ID FRONT <> BACK	DESCRIPTION FRONT <> BACK	INGREDIENT & STRENGTH	BRAND (or Generic Equiv.) by FIRM	NDC#	CLASS; SCH.
APO <> PR15	Tab, White, Round, Scored, APO <> PR / 1.5	Pramipexole DiHCl 1.5 mg	Mirapex by Apotex	Canadian DIN 02292408	Antiparkinson
APO <> PR25	Tab, White, Oval, Scored, APO <> PR / .25	Pramipexole DiHCl 0.25 mg	Mirapex by Apotex	Canadian DIN 02292378	Antiparkinson
APO <> PR5	Tab, White, Oval, Scored, APO <> PR / .5	Pramipexole DiHCl 0.50 mg	Mirapex by Apotex	Canadian DIN 02292386	Antiparkinson
APO <> PRA10	Tab, Pink to Peach, Rounded Square	Pravastatin Sodium 10 mg	Apo Pravastatin by Apotex	Canadian DIN 02243506	Antihyperlipidemic
APO <> PRA10	Tab, Light Pink, Round	Pravastatin Sodium 10 mg	Pravachol by Apotex	60505-0168	Antihyperlipidemic
APO <> PRA20	Tab, Off-White to Yellow, Round	Pravastatin Sodium 20 mg	Pravachol by Apotex	60505-0169	Antihyperlipidemic
APO <> PRA20	Tab, Yellow, Rounded Square	Pravastatin Sodium 20 mg	Apo Pravastatin by Apotex	Canadian DIN 02243507	Antihyperlipidemic
APO <> PRA40	Tab, Green, Rounded Square	Pravastatin Sodium 40 mg	Apo Pravastatin by Apotex	Canadian DIN 02243508	Antihyperlipidemic
APO <> PRA40	Tab, Light Green, Round	Pravastatin Sodium 40 mg	Pravachol by Apotex	60505-0170	Antihyperlipidemic
APO <> Q5	Tab, Reddish-Brown, Cap Shaped, Scored, Film Coated, Q / 5	Quinapril 5 mg	Accupril by Apotex	60505-0172	Antihypertensive
APO <> QU10	Tab, Reddish-Brown, Cap Shaped, Film Coated	Quinapril 10 mg	Accupril by Apotex	60505-0173	Antihypertensive
APO <> QU20	Tab, Reddish-Brown, Cap Shaped, Film Coated	Quinapril 20 mg	Accupril by Apotex	60505-0174	Antihypertensive
APO <> QU40	Tab, Reddish-Brown, Cap Shaped, Film Coated	Quinapril 40 mg	Accupril by Apotex	60505-0175	Antihypertensive
APO <> RAN150	Tab, White to Off-White, Round, Film Coated	Ranitidine HCl 150 mg	Zantac by Apotex	60505-0025	Gastrointestinal
APO <> RAN300	Tab, White to Off-White, Cap Shaped, Film Coated	Ranitidine HCl 300 mg	Zantac by Apotex	60505-0026	Gastrointestinal
APO <> RI1	Tab, White, Cap Shaped, Scored	Risperidone 1 mg	Risperdal by Apotex	Canadian DIN 02282135	Antipsychotic
APO <> RI2	Tab, Peach, Cap Shaped, Scored	Risperidone 2 mg	Risperdal by Apotex	Canadian DIN 02282143	Antipsychotic
APO <> RI25	Tab, Yellowish-Orange, Cap Shaped, APO <> RI .25	Risperidone 0.25 mg	Risperdal by Apotex	Canadian DIN 02282119	Antipsychotic
APO <> RI3	Tab, Yellow, Cap Shaped, Scored	Risperidone 3 mg	Risperdal by Apotex	Canadian DIN 02282151	Antipsychotic
APO <> RI4	Tab, Green, Cap Shaped, Scored	Risperidone 4 mg	Risperdal by Apotex	Canadian DIN 02282178	Antipsychotic
APO <> RI5	Tab, Reddish-Brown, Cap Shaped, Scored, APO <> RI .5	Risperidone 0.50 mg	Risperdal by Apotex	Canadian DIN 02282127	Antipsychotic
APO <> SE25	Tab, Light Green, Oval, Scored, Film Coated, SE / 25	Sertraline HCl 25 mg	Zoloft by Apotex	60505-0180	Antidepressant
APO <> SE50	Tab, Bluish Purple, Oval, Scored, Film Coated, SE / 50	Sertraline HCl 50 mg	Zoloft by Apotex	60505-0181	Antidepressant
APO <> SER100	Tab, Yellow, Oval, Scored, Film Coated, SER / 100	Sertraline HCl 100 mg	Zoloft by Apotex	60505-0182	Antidepressant
APO <> SOT120	Tab, White to Off-White, Cap Shaped, APO <> SOT over 120	Sotalol HCl 120 mg	Betapace by Apotex	60505-0159	Antiarrhythmic
APO <> SOT160	Tab, White to Off-White, Cap Shaped, APO <> SOT over 160	Sotalol HCl 160 mg	Betapace by Apotex	60505-0081	Antiarrhythmic
APO <> SOT240	Tab, White to Off-White, Cap Shaped, APO <> SOT over 240	Sotalol HCl 240 mg	Betapace by Apotex	60505-0082	Antiarrhythmic
APO <> SOT80	Tab, White to Off-White, Cap Shaped, APO <> SOT over 80	Sotalol HCl 80 mg	Betapace by Apotex	60505-0080	Antiarrhythmic
APO <> SR20	Tab, White, Round, SR	Methylphenidate HCl 20 mg	Ritalin SR by Apotex	Canadian DIN 02266687	Stimulant; C II
APO <> SRM100	Tab, Orange, Round, SR	Metoprolol Tartrate 100 mg	Lopresor SR by Apotex	Canadian DIN 02285169	Antihypertensive
APO <> SRM200	Tab, Light Yellow, Round, SR	Metoprolol Tartrate 200 mg	Lopresor SR by Apotex	Canadian DIN 02285177	Antihypertensive
APO <> SUM100	Tab, Pink, Triangle Shaped	Sumatriptan Succinate 100 mg	Imitrex DF by Apotex	Canadian DIN 02268396	Antimigraine
APO <> SUM50	Tab, White, Triangle Shaped	Sumatriptan Succinate 50 mg	Imitrex DF by Apotex	Canadian DIN 02268388	Antimigraine

ID FRONT <> BACK	DESCRIPTION FRONT <> BACK	INGREDIENT & STRENGTH	BRAND (or Generic Equiv.) by FIRM	NDC#	CLASS; SCH.
APO <> T1	Tab, White, Round	Terazosin HCl 1 mg	Terazosin by Apotex	Canadian DIN 02234502	Antihypertensive
APO <> T10	Tab, Blue, Round	Terazosin HCl 10 mg	Hytrin by Apotex	Canadian DIN 02234505	Antihypertensive
APO <> T2	Tab, Orange, Round	Terazosin HCl 2 mg	Hytrin by Apotex	Canadian DIN 02234503	Antihypertensive
APO <> T5	Tab, Tan, Round	Terazosin HCl 5 mg	Hytrin by Apotex	Canadian DIN 02234504	Antihypertensive
APO <> T5	Tab, White to Off-White, Cap Shaped, Scored, APO <> T / 5	Torsemide 5 mg	Demadex by Apotex	60505-0232	Diuretic
APO <> TAM10	Tab, White, Round	Tamoxifen Citrate 10 mg	Nolvadex by Apotex	Canadian DIN 00812404	Antiestrogen
APO <> TAM20	Tab, White, Hexagonal, Scored	Tamoxifen Citrate 20 mg	Nolvadex by Apotex	Canadian DIN 00812390	Antiestrogen
APO <> TER250	Tab, White, Round, Scored	Terbinafine HCl 250 mg	Lamisil by Apotex	Canadian DIN 02239893	Antifungal
APO <> THE100	Tab, White, Round, The/100	Theophylline Anhydrous 100 mg	Theo LA by Apotex	Canadian DIN 00692689	Antiasthmatic
APO <> THE200	Tab, White, Oval	Theophylline Anhydrous 200 mg	Theo LA by Apotex	Canadian DIN 00692697	Antiasthmatic
APO <> THE300	Tab, White, Cap Shaped, Scored	Theophylline 300 mg	Theo-DUR by Apotex	Canadian DIN 00692700	Muscle Relaxant
APO <> TMB100	Tab, White, Round, Scored	Trimebutine Maleate 100 mg	Modulon by Apotex	Canadian DIN 02245663	Motility Regulator
APO <> TMB200	Tab, White, Round, Scored	Trimebutine Maleate 100 mg	Modulon by Apotex	Canadian DIN 02245664	Motility Regulator
APO <> TO10	Tab, White to Off-White, Cap Shaped, Scored, APO <> TO / 10	Torsemide 10 mg	Demadex by Apotex	60505-0233	Diuretic
APO <> TO20	Tab, White to Off-White, Cap Shaped, Scored, APO <> TO / 20	Torsemide 20 mg	Demadex by Apotex	60505-0234	Diuretic
APO <> TOR100	Tab, White to Off-White, Cap Shaped, Scored, APO <> TOR / 100	Torsemide 100 mg	Demadex by Apotex	60505-0235	Diuretic
APO <> TP100	Tab, Mustard, Round	Topiramate 100 mg	Topamax by Apotex	Canadian DIN 02279630	Anticonvulsant
APO <> TP200	Tab, Pink, Round	Topiramate 200 mg	Topamax by Apotex	Canadian DIN 02279649	Anticonvulsant
APO <> TP25	Tab, White, Round	Topiramate 25 mg	Topamax by Apotex	Canadian DIN 02279614	Anticonvulsant
APO <> TR50	Tab, White to Off-White, Oblong	Tramadol HCl 50 mg	Ultram by Apotex	60505-0171	Analgesic
APO <> TR50	Tab, White to Off-White, Oblong	Tramadol HCl 50 mg	Ultram by Major	00904-5556	Analgesic
APO <> TRI100	Tab, White, Round, Scored, TRI / 100	Trimethoprim 100 mg	Apo Trimethoprim by Apotex	Canadian DIN 02243116	Antibiotic
APO <> TRI200	Tab, Yellow, Round, Scored, TRI / 200	Trimethoprim 200 mg	Apo Trimethoprim by Apotex	Canadian DIN 02243117	Antibiotic
APO <> VAL500	Tab, Blue, Cap Shaped, Film Coated	Valacyclovir 500 mg	Valtrex by Apotex	Canadian DIN 02295822	Antiviral
APO <> VSR120	Tab, White, Round, Film Coated	Verapamil HCl 120 mg	Apo Verapamil by Apotex	Canadian DIN 02246893	Antihypertensive
APO <> VSR180	Tab, Pink, Oval, Scored	Verapamil HCl 180	Apo Verapamil by Apotex	Canadian DIN 02246894	Antihypertensive
APO <> VSR240	Tab, Off-White, Cap Shaped, Scored, Film Coated	Verapamil HCl 240 mg	Apo Verapamil by Apotex	Canadian DIN 02246895	Antihypertensive

ID FRONT <> BACK	DESCRIPTION FRONT <> BACK	INGREDIENT & STRENGTH	BRAND (or Generic Equiv.) by FIRM	NDC#	CLASS; SCH.
APO <> WAR1	Tab, Pink, Round, Scored, WAR / 1	Warfarin Sodium 1 mg	Apo Warfarin by Apotex	Canadian DIN 02242924	Anticoagulant
APO <> WAR10	Tab, White, Round, Scored, WAR / 10	Warfarin Sodium 10 mg	Apo Warfarin by Apotex	Canadian DIN 02242929	Anticoagulant
APO <> WAR2	Tab, Lavender, Round, Scored, WAR / 2	Warfarin Sodium 2 mg	Apo Warfarin by Apotex	Canadian DIN 02242925	Anticoagulant
APO <> WAR25	Tab, Green, Round, Scored, WAR / 2.5	Warfarin Sodium 2.5 mg	Apo Warfarin by Apotex	Canadian DIN 02242926	Anticoagulant
APO <> WAR3	Tab, Tan, Round, Scored, WAR / 3	Warfarin Sodium 3 mg	Apo Warfarin by Apotex	Canadian DIN 02245618	Anticoagulant
APO <> WAR4	Tab, Blue, Round, Scored, WAR / 4	Warfarin Sodium 4 mg	Apo Warfarin by Apotex	Canadian DIN 02242927	Anticoagulant
APO <> WAR5	Tab, Round, Peach, Scored, WAR / 5	Warfarin Sodium 5 mg	Apo Warfarin by Apotex	Canadian DIN 02242928	Anticoagulant
APO <> XR500	Tab, White, Cap Shaped, Extended Release	Metformin HCl 500 mg	Glucophage XR by Apotex	60505-0260	Antidiabetic
APO <> ZOL5	Tab, Pink, Cap Shaped, Film Coated	Zolpidem Tartrate 5 mg	Ambien by Apotex	60505-2604	Sedative/Hypnotic; C IV
APO <> ZOP5	Tab, White, Round	Zopiclone 5 mg	Imovane by Apotex	Canadian DIN 02245077	Sedative; Hypnotic
APO007	Cap, White, Extended Release	Diltiazem HCl 120 mg	Cardizem CD by Apotex	60505-0007	Antihypertensive
APO008	Cap, Blue and White, Extended Release	Diltiazem HCl 180 mg	Cardizem CD by Apotex	60505-0008	Antihypertensive
APO009	Cap, Light Blue and White, Extended Release	Diltiazem HCl 240 mg	Cardizem CD by Apotex	60505-0009	Antihypertensive
APO01	Tab, White, Round, APO/0.1	Clonidine HCl 0.1 mg	Apo Clonidine by Apotex	Canadian DIN 00868949	Antihypertensive
APO0010	Cap, Pink and Reddish Brown, Opaque, Black Ink, Delayed Release	Omeprazole 10 mg	Prilosec by Apotex	60505-0145	Gastrointestinal
APO0010	Cap, Light Gray and White, Extended Release	Diltiazem HCl 300 mg	Cardizem CD by Apotex	60505-0010	Antihypertensive
APO0014	Cap, Orange & White, Opaque, Ex Release	Diltiazem HCl 120 mg	Dilacor XR by Apotex	60505-0014	Antihypertensive
APO0015	Cap, Bright Orange & White, Ex Release	Diltiazem HCl 180 mg	Dilacor XR by Apotex	60505-0015	Antihypertensive
APO0016	Cap, Brown & White, Ex Release	Diltiazem HCl 240 mg	Dilacor XR by Apotex	60505-0016	Antihypertensive
APO0016	Cap, Brown & White, Ex Release	Diltiazem HCl 240 mg	Dilacor XR by Major	00904-5382	Antihypertensive
APO0018	Tab, Green, Round, Film Coated, APO over 018	Cimetidine HCl 200 mg	Tagamet by Major	00904-5445	Gastrointestinal
APO0018	Tab, Green, Round, Film Coated, APO over 018	Cimetidine HCl 200 mg	Tagamet by Compumed	00403-1209	Gastrointestinal
APO0018	Tab, Green, Round, Film Coated, APO over 018	Cimetidine HCl 200 mg	Tagamet by Apotex	60505-0018	Gastrointestinal
APO0019	Tab, Green, Round, Film Coated, APO over 019	Cimetidine HCl 300 mg	Tagamet by Apotex	60505-0019	Gastrointestinal
APO0019	Tab, Green, Round, Film Coated, APO over 019	Cimetidine HCl 300 mg	Tagamet by Compumed	00403-1312	Gastrointestinal
APO02	Tab, Orange, Round, APO/0.2	Clonidine HCl 0.2 mg	Apo Clonidine by Apotex	Canadian DIN 00868957	Antihypertensive
APO0020	Tab, Green, Oval, Scored	Cimetidine HCl 400 mg	Tagamet by Apotex	60505-0020	Gastrointestinal
APO0020	Tab, Green, Oval, Scored	Cimetidine HCl 400 mg	Tagamet by Compumed	00403-1334	Gastrointestinal
APO0020	Cap, Pink and Reddish Brown, Opaque, Black Ink, Delayed Release	Omeprazole 20 mg	Prilosec by Apotex	60505-0065	Gastrointestinal
APO0021	Tab, Green, Oval, Scored	Cimetidine HCl 800 mg	Tagamet by Apotex	60505-0021	Gastrointestinal
APO0021	Tab, Green, Oval, Scored	Cimetidine HCl 800 mg	Tagamet by Compumed	00403-1335	Gastrointestinal
APO0025	Tab, White to Off-White, Round, Film Coated	Ranitidine HCl 150 mg	Zantac by Major	00904-5261	Gastrointestinal
APO0025	Tab, White to Off-White, Round, Film Coated	Ranitidine HCl 150 mg	Zantac by Golden State	60429-0704	Gastrointestinal
APO0025	Tab, Powder Blue, Oval, APO/0.25	Triazolam 0.25 mg	Apo Triazo by Apotex	Canadian DIN 00808571	Sedative/Hypnotic; C IV
APO027	Tab, White, Cap Shaped	Ticlopidine HCl 250 mg	Ticlid by Apotex	60505-0027	Anticoagulant
APO027	Tab, White, Cap Shaped	Ticlopidine HCl 250 mg	Ticlid by Major	00904-5378	Anticoagulant
APO033	Tab, White, Oval, Extended Release	Pentoxifylline 400 mg	Trental by Major	00904-5448	Anticoagulant
APO033	Tab, White, Oval, Extended Release	Pentoxifylline 400 mg	Trental by Pharmafab	62542-0744	Anticoagulant

ID FRONT <> BACK	DESCRIPTION FRONT <> BACK	INGREDIENT & STRENGTH	BRAND (or Generic Equiv.) by FIRM	NDC#	CLASS; SCH.
APO033	Tab, White, Oval, Extended Release	Pentoxifylline 400 mg	Trental by Apotex	60505-0033	Anticoagulant
APO034 <> 600	Tab, White, Oval, Film Coated	Gemfibrozil 600 mg	Lopid by Major	00904-5379	Antihyperlipidemic
APO034 <> 600	Tab, White, Oval, Film Coated	Gemfibrozil 600 mg	Lopid by Apotex	60505-0034	Antihyperlipidemic
APO034 <> 600	Tab, White, Oval, Film Coated	Gemfibrozil 600 mg	Lopid by Torpharm	62318-0034	Antihyperlipidemic
APO039	Cap, White, Light Grey	Etodolac 200 mg	Lodine by Apotex	60505-0039	NSAID
APO040	Cap, White, Light Grey	Etodolac 300 mg	Lodine by Apotex	60505-0040	NSAID
APO041 <> 400	Tab, White to Off-White, Oblong	Etodolac 400 mg	Lodine by Apotex	60505-0041	NSAID
APO042	Cap, Aqua Blue and White, Opaque	Acyclovir 200 mg	Zovirax by Apotex	60505-0042	Antiviral
APO046 <> 125	Tab, White to Off-White, Oval	Divalproex Sodium 125 mg	Depakote by Apotex	60505-3065	Anticonvulsant
APO047 <> 250	Tab, White to Off-White, Oval	Divalproex Sodium 250 mg	Depakote by Apotex	60505-3066	Anticonvulsant
APO048 <> 500	Tab, White to Off-White, Oval	Divalproex Sodium 500 mg	Depakote by Apotex	60505-3067	Anticonvulsant
APO05	Tab, Peach, Oval, APO/0.5	Alprazolam 0.5 mg	Xanax by Apotex	Canadian DIN 00865400	Antianxiety; C IV
APO05	Tab, White, Round, APO/0.5	Haloperidol 0.5 mg	Haldol by Apotex	Canadian DIN 00396796	Antipsychotic
APO055	Cap, Aqua Blue & White	Selegiline 5 mg	Eldepryl by Apotex	60505-0055	Antiparkinson
APO083	Tab, White, Round, Scored	Paroxetine HCl 20 mg	Paxil by Major	00904-5677	Antidepressant
APO084	Tab, White, Round	Paroxetine HCl 30 mg	Paxil by Major	00904-5678	Antidepressant
APO097	Tab, White, Round, Scored	Paroxetine HCl 10 mg	Paxil by Major	00904-5676	Antidepressant
APO1	Tab, Lavender, Oval, Scored, APO/1	Alprazolam 1 mg	Xanax by Apotex	Canadian DIN 02243611	Antianxiety; C IV
APO1	Tab, White, Round, APO/1	Prednisone 1 mg	by AltiMed	Canadian	Steroid
APO1	Tab, White, Round, APO/1	Prednisone 1 mg	Apo Prednisone by Apotex	Canadian DIN 00598194	Steroid
APO1	Tab, Yellow, Round, APO/1	Haloperidol 1 mg	Haldol by Apotex	Canadian DIN 00396818	Antipsychotic
APO1	Cap, White, Oval	Lorazepam 1 mg	Ativan by Apotex	Canadian DIN 00655759	Antianxiety; C IV
APO10	Tab, White, Round	Ketorolac Tromethamine 10 mg	Toradol by Apotex	Canadian	NSAID
APO10	Tab, Pale Yellow, Round, APO/10	Guanethidine Monosulfate 10 mg	Apo Guanethidine by Apotex	Canadian	Antihypertensive
APO10	Tab, White, Round	Domperidone 10 mg	Motilium by Apotex	Canadian	Gastrointestinal
APO10	Cap, Black & Green	Chlordiazepoxide 10 mg	Librium by Apotex	Canadian DIN 00522988	Antianxiety; C IV
APO10	Tab, Blue, Round, APO/10	Diazepam 10 mg	Apo Diazepam by Apotex	Canadian	Antianxiety; C IV
APO10	Cap, Mustard	Nifedipine 10 mg	Apo Nifed by Apotex	Canadian DIN 00755907	Antihypertensive
APO10	Cap, White & Yellow	Nortriptyline HCl 10 mg	Nortriptyline by Apotex	Canadian DIN 02223511	Antidepressant
APO10	Tab, Orange, Round, APO/10	Propranolol HCl 10 mg	Inderal by Apotex	Canadian DIN 00402788	Antihypertensive
APO10	Cap, Blue & Maroon	Piroxicam 10 mg	Feldene by Apotex	Canadian DIN 00642886	NSAID
APO10	Tab, Blue, Round	Diazepam 10 mg	Valium by Apotex	Canadian DIN 00405337	Antianxiety; C IV
APO10	Tab, Yellow, D-Shaped, APO/10	Cyclobenzaprine HCl 10 mg	Apo Cyclobenzaprine by Apotex	Canadian DIN 02177145	Muscle Relaxant
APO10	Cap, Pink & Scarlet	Doxepin HCl 10 mg	Apo Doxepin by Apotex	Canadian DIN 02049996 Discontinued	Antidepressant
APO10	Cap, Gray & Green	Fluoxetine HCl 10 mg	Prozac by Apotex	Canadian DIN 02216353	Antidepressant

ID FRONT <> BACK	DESCRIPTION FRONT <> BACK	INGREDIENT & STRENGTH	BRAND (or Generic Equiv.) by FIRM	NDC#	CLASS; SCH.
APO10	Tab, Light Green, Round, APO/10	Haloperidol 10 mg	Haldol by Apotex	Canadian DIN 00463698	Antipsychotic
APO10	Cap, Blue and White, Opaque	Ramipril 10 mg	Altace by Apotex	Canadian DIN 02251582	Antihypertensive
APO10	Tab, Orange, Round	Prochlorperazine Maleate 10 mg	Stemetil by Apotex	Canadian DIN 00886432	Antiemetic
APO100	Tab, White, Round, APO/100	Chlorthalidone 100 mg	Apo Chlorthalidone by Apotex	Canadian DIN 00360287	Diuretic
APO100	Tab, White, Round, APO/100	Chlorpropamide 100 mg	Apo Chlorpropam by Apotex	Canadian DIN 00399302	Antidiabetic
APO100	Tab, White, Round, APO/100	Theophylline Anhydrous 100 mg	Apo Theo LA by Apotex	Canadian	Antiasthmatic
APO100	Tab, Pink, Round, APO/100	Oxtriphylline 100 mg	Apo Oxtriphylline by Apotex	Canadian DIN 00441724	Antiasthmatic
APO100	Tab, White, Round, APO/100	Sulfinpyrazone 100 mg	Apo Sulfinpyrazone by Apotex	Canadian	Uricosuric
APO100	Cap, Opaque & White	Zidovudine 100 mg	Retrovir by Apotex	Canadian Discontinued	Antiviral
APO100	Cap, Red and White, Opaque	Zonisamide 100 mg	Zonegran by Apotex	60505-2547	Anticonvulsant
APO100	Cap, White, Blue Print	Gabapentin 100 mg	Neurontin by Apotex	Canadian DIN 02244304	Anticonvulsant
APO100	Tab, White, Round, Biconvex, Film-Coated, Scored	Acebutolol 100 mg	Apo-Acebutolol by Apotex	Canadian DIN 02147602	Antihypertensive
APO100	Cap, Orange, Oval, Soft Gel	Docusate Sodium 100 mg	Colace by Apotex	Canadian DIN 02245079	Laxative
APO100	Tab, Pink, Round, APO/100	Trimipramine 100 mg	Trimip by Apotex	Canadian DIN 00740829	Antidepressant
APO100	Tab, White, Oval, APO-100	Captopril 100 mg	Capoten by Apotex	Canadian DIN 00893625	Antihypertensive
APO100	Tab, Pink, Round, APO/100	Diclofenac Sodium 100 mg	Apo Diclo SR by Apotex	Canadian DIN 02091194	NSAID
APO100	Tab, White, Round, APO/100	Acebutolol HCl 100 mg	Sectral by Apotex	Canadian DIN 02147602	Antihypertensive
APO100	Tab, Pink, Round, APO/100	Hydrochlorothiazide 100 mg	Apo Hydro by Apotex	Canadian DIN 00644552	Diuretic; Antihypertensive
APO100	Tab, White, Oval	Fluvoxamine Maleate 100 mg	Luvox by Apotex	Canadian DIN 02231330	OCD
APO100	Tab, Pink, Trapezoid	Fluconazole 100 mg	Fluconazole by Apotex	Canadian DIN 02237371	Antifungal
APO100	Cap, Blue & Flesh	Doxepin HCl 100 mg	Apo Doxepin by Apotex	Canadian DIN 02050048	Antidepressant
APO100	Cap, Pale Blue	Doxycycline Hyclate 100 mg	Apo Doxy by Apotex	Canadian DIN 00740713	Antibiotic
APO100	Cap, White	Fenofibrate 100 mg	Fenofibrate by Apotex	Canadian DIN 02225980	Antihyperlipidemic
APO100	Tab, Blue, Oval, APO-100	Flurbiprofen 100 mg	Apo Flurbiprofen by Apotex	Canadian DIN 01912038	NSAID
APO100	Tab, Yellow, Round, APO/100	Ketoprofen 100 mg	Orudis by Apotex	Canadian DIN 00842664	NSAID
APO100	Cap, Orange & Purple	Minocycline HCl 100 mg	Minocin by Apotex	Canadian DIN 02084104	Antibiotic
APO100	Tab, Orange, Oval	Moclobemide 100 mg	Moclobemide by Apotex	Canadian DIN 02232148	Antidepressant

ID FRONT <> BACK	DESCRIPTION FRONT <> BACK	INGREDIENT & STRENGTH	BRAND (or Generic Equiv.) by FIRM	NDC#	CLASS; SCH.
APO100	Cap, Orange, Opaque	Sertraline HCl 100 mg	Zoloft by Apotex	Canadian DIN 02238282	Antidepressant
APO1000	Tab, White to Off-White, Oblong, Scored	Metformin HCl 1000 mg	Glucophage by Apotex	60505-0192	Antidiabetic
APO10010	Tab, Blue, Oval, Biconvex, APO Score 100 over 10	Levodopa 100 mg, Carbidopa 10 mg	Sinemet by Apotex	Canadian DIN 02195933	Antiparkinson
APO10025	Tab, Yellow, Oval, APO Score 100 over 25	Levodopa 100 mg, Carbidopa 25 mg	Sinemet by Apotex	Canadian DIN 02195941	Antiparkinson
APO101	Tab, White, Round, Scored	Paroxetine HCl 40 mg	Paxil by Major	00904-5679	Antidepressant
APO102 <> 500	Tab, White to Off-White, Oblong	Etodolac 500 mg	Lodine by Apotex	60505-0102	NSAID
APO112	Cap, White, Opaque	Gabapentin 100 mg	Neurontin by Apotex	60505-0112	Anticonvulsant
APO113	Cap, White and Yellow, Opaque	Gabapentin 300 mg	Neurontin by Apotex	60505-0113	Anticonvulsant
APO114	Cap, White and Orange, Opaque	Gabapentin 400 mg	Neurontin by Apotex	60505-0114	Anticonvulsant
APO115	Cap, Beige, Opaque	Terazosin HCl 1 mg	Hytrin by Apotex	60505-0115	Antihypertensive
APO115	Cap, Beige, Opaque	Terazosin HCl 1 mg	Hytrin by Major	00904-5650	Antihypertensive
APO116	Cap, Yellow, Opaque	Terazosin HCl 2 mg	Hytrin by Major	00904-5651	Antihypertensive
APO116	Cap, Yellow, Opaque	Terazosin HCl 2 mg	Hytrin by Apotex	60505-0116	Antihypertensive
APO117	Cap, Red, Opaque	Terazosin HCl 5 mg	Hytrin by Apotex	60505-0117	Antihypertensive
APO117	Cap, Red, Opaque	Terazosin HCl 5 mg	Hytrin by Major	00904-5652	Antihypertensive
APO118	Cap, Blue, Opaque	Terazosin HCl 10 mg	Hytrin by Major	00904-5653	Antihypertensive
APO118	Cap, Blue, Opaque	Terazosin HCl 10 mg	Hytrin by Apotex	60505-0118	Antihypertensive
APO120	Tab, White, Oblong, APO/120	Terfenadine 120 mg	Apo Terfenadine by Apotex	Canadian Discontinued	Antihistamine
APO120	Tab, Rose, Round, APO/120	Propranolol HCl 120 mg	Inderal LA by Apotex	Canadian DIN 00504335	Antihypertensive
APO120	Cap, Light Turquoise	Diltiazem HCl 120 mg	Diltiaz CD by Apotex	Canadian DIN 02230997	Antihypertensive
APO120	Cap, Caramel & Chocolate Brown	Diltiazem HCl 120 mg	Diltiaz SR by Apotex	Canadian DIN 02222973	Antihypertensive
APO125	Tab, White, Oblong, APO/12.5	Captopril 12.5 mg	Capoten by Apotex	Canadian	Antihypertensive
APO125	Tab, Light Green, Oval	Naproxen 125 mg	Apo Naproxen by Apotex	Canadian DIN 00522678	NSAID
APO125	Tab, Yellow, Round, APO/125	Methyldopa 125 mg	Apo Methyldopa by Apotex	Canadian DIN 00360252	Antihypertensive
APO125	Tab, White, Round, APO/125	Primidone 125 mg	Apo Primidone by Apotex	Canadian DIN 00399310	Anticonvulsant
APO125	Tab, Violet, Oval, APO/.125	Triazolam 0.125 mg	Apo Triazo by Apotex	Canadian DIN 00808563	Sedative/Hypnotic; C IV
APO125	Cap, Yellow and White, Opaque, APO 1.25	Ramipril 1.25 mg	Altace by Apotex	Canadian DIN 02251515	Antihypertensive
APO131	Tab, Reddish Brown, Round, Sustained Release	Carbidopa 25 mg, Levodopa 100 mg	Sinemet by Apotex	60505-0131	Antiparkinson
APO132	Tab, Buff to Light Brown, Round, Scored, Sustained Release	Carbidopa 50 mg, Levodopa 200 mg	Sinemet by Apotex	60505-0132	Antiparkinson
APO13325	Cap, Reddish Brown, Opaque	Cyclosporine 25 mg	Sandimmune by Apotex	60505-0133	Immunosuppressant
APO134100	Cap, Reddish Brown, Opaque	Cyclosporine 100 mg	Sandimmune by Apotex	60505-0134	Immunosuppressant
APO15	Tab, Orange & Yellow, Round, APO/15	Oxazepam 15 mg	Apo Oxazepam by Apotex	Canadian	Sedative/Hypnotic; C IV
APO15	Tab, Pink, Round, APO/15	Methyldopa, Hydrochlorothiazide 15 mg	Apo Methazide by Apotex	Canadian DIN 00441708	Antihypertensive; Diuretic
APO15	Cap, Ivory & Orange	Flurazepam HCl 15 mg	Apo Flurazepam by Apotex	Canadian DIN 00521698	Hypnotic; C IV
APO15	Cap, Gray	Clorazepate Dipotassium 15 mg	Apo Clorazepate by Apotex	Canadian DIN 00860697	Antianxiety; C IV

ID FRONT <> BACK	DESCRIPTION FRONT <> BACK	INGREDIENT & STRENGTH	BRAND (or Generic Equiv.) by FIRM	NDC#	CLASS; SCH.
APO15	Cap, Flesh & Maroon	Temazepam 15 mg	Restoril by Apotex	Canadian DIN 02225964	Sedative/Hypnotic; C IV
APO150	Cap, Dark Yellow & Pale Yellow	Nizatidine 150 mg	Axid by Apotex	60505-0230	Gastrointestinal
APO150	Cap, Pale Yellow and Dark Yellow	Nizatidine 150 mg	Apo Nizatidine by Apotex	Canadian DIN 02220156	Gastrointestinal
APO150	Cap, Pink	Doxepin HCl 150 mg	Apo Doxepin by Apotex	Canadian DIN 02050056	Antidepressant
APO150	Tab, Pale Yellow, Oval	Moclobemide 150 mg	Moclobemide by Apotex	Canadian DIN 02232150	Antidepressant
APO150	Cap, Orange and White	Lithium Carbonate 150 mg	Eskalith by Apotex	Canadian DIN 02242837	Antipsychotic
APO150	Cap, Maroon and Lavender, Hard Gel	Clindamycin HCl 150 mg	Cleocin HCl by Apotex	Canadian DIN 02245232	Antibiotic
APO150	Tab, White, Round, APO/150	Ranitidine HCl 150 mg	Apo Ranitidine by Apotex	Canadian DIN 00733059	Gastrointestinal
APO150	Tab, Yellow, Hexagonal, APO/150	Sulindac 150 mg	Apo Sulin by Apotex	Canadian DIN 00778354	NSAID
APO150 <> 50252550	Tab, Pale Orange, Rectangular, Scored, APO-150 <> 50/25/25/50	Trazodone HCl 150 mg	Apo Trazodone by Apotex	Canadian DIN 02147653	Antidepressant
APO15050252550	Tab, Pale Orange, Rectangular, APO-150 50 25 25 50	Trazodone HCl 150 mg	Desyrel by Apotex	Canadian	Antidepressant
APO160	Tab, Blue, Oblong, APO-160	Sotalol HCl 160 mg	Sotalol by Apotex	Canadian DIN 02167794	Antiarrhythmic
APO160	Tab, Blue, Cap Shaped, Scored	Nadolol 160 mg	Apo Nadol by Apotex	Canadian DIN 00782475	Antihypertensive
APO160	Tab, White, Oval	Megestrol Acetate 160 mg	Megestrol by Apotex	Canadian DIN 02195925	Hormone
APO180	Cap, Light Blue & Light Turquoise	Diltiazem HCl 180 mg	Diltiaz CD by Apotex	Canadian DIN 02230998	Antihypertensive
APO1G	Tab, White, Oblong, APO-1 g	Sucralfate 1 g	Apo Sucralfate by Apotex	Canadian DIN 02125250	Gastrointestinal
APO2	Tab, White, Rectangular, Scored, A over P over O over 2	Alprazolam 2 mg	Xanax by Apotex	Canadian DIN 02243612	Antianxiety; C IV
APO2	Tab, White, Round, APO/2	Benztropine Mesylate 2 mg	Cogentin by Apotex	Canadian DIN 00426857	Antiparkinson
APO2	Tab, White, Round, APO/2	Diazepam 2 mg	Apo Diazepam by Apotex	Canadian DIN 00405329	Antianxiety; C IV
APO2	Cap, Light Green	Loperamide HCl 2 mg	Loperamide by Apotex	Canadian DIN 02212005	Antidiarrheal
APO2	Tab, White, Oval	Lorazepam 2 mg	Ativan by Apotex	Canadian DIN 00655767	Antianxiety; C IV
APO2	Tab, Pink, Round, APO/2	Haloperidol 2 mg	Haldol by Apotex	Canadian DIN 00396826	Antipsychotic
APO2	Tab, Light Purple, Round, APO/2	Salbutamol Sulfate 2 mg	Salvent by Apotex	Canadian DIN 02146843	Antiasthmatic
APO20	Tab, Yellow, Oval, APO/20	Tenoxicam 20 mg	Tenoxicam by Apotex	Canadian	NSAID
APO20	Tab, Blue, Round, APO/20	Trifluoperazine HCl 20 mg	Apo Trifluoperaz by Apotex	Canadian DIN 00595942	Antipsychotic
APO20	Tab, Blue, Hexagonal, APO/20	Propranolol HCl 20 mg	Inderal by Apotex	Canadian DIN 00663719	Antihypertensive
APO20	Cap, Maroon	Piroxicam 20 mg	Feldene by Apotex	Canadian DIN 00642894	NSAID

ID FRONT <> BACK	DESCRIPTION FRONT <> BACK	INGREDIENT & STRENGTH	BRAND (or Generic Equiv.) by FIRM	NDC#	CLASS; SCH.
APO20	Cap, Green & Ivory	Fluoxetine HCl 20 mg	Prozac by Apotex	Canadian DIN 02216361	Antidepressant
APO20	Tab, White, Round, APO/20	Furosemide 20 mg	Apo Furosemide by Apotex	Canadian DIN 00396788	Diuretic
APO20	Tab, Beige, D-Shaped, APO/20	Famotidine 20 mg	Apo Famotidine by Apotex	Canadian DIN 01953842	Gastrointestinal
APO200	Tab, White to Off-White, Round	Carbamazepine 200 mg	Tegretol by Apotex	60505-0183	Anticonvulsant
APO200	Tab, White to Off-White, Round, APO over 200	Carbamazepine 200 mg	Tegretol by Major	00904-3855	Anticonvulsant
APO200	Tab, Yellow, Round, Biconvex	Oxtriphylline 200 mg	Apo Oxtruphylline by Apotex	Canadian DIN 00441732	Antiasthmatic
APO200	Tab, White to Grey, Round, Scored	Ketoconazole 200 mg	Nizoral by Apotex	Canadian DIN 02237235	Antifungal
APO200	Cap, Light Grey and Dark Grey	Etodolac 200 mg	Lodine by Apotex	Canadian DIN 02232317	NSAID
APO200	Cap, Orange, Black Print	Fenofibrate 200 mg	TriCor by Apotex	Canadian DIN 02239864	Antihyperlipidemic
APO200	Tab, Yellow, Hexagonal, Scored, APO/200	Sulindac 200 mg	Apo Sulin by Apotex	Canadian DIN 00778362	NSAID
APO200	Tab, White, Round, Scored, APO/200	Tiaprofenic Acid 200 mg	Apo Tiaprofenic by Apotex	Canadian DIN 02136112	NSAID
APO200	Tab, Blue, Round, APO over 200	Acyclovir 200 mg	Zovirax by Apotex	Canadian DIN 02207621	Antiviral
APO200	Tab, White, Oval, Scored, APO over 200	Acebutolol 200 mg	Sectral by Apotex	Canadian DIN 02147610	Antihypertensive
APO200	Tab, Pale Green, Round	Cimetidine HCl 200 mg	Tagamet by Apotex	Canadian DIN 00584215	Gastrointestinal
APO200	Tab, White to Off-White, Round, APO over 200	Carbamazepine 200 mg	Tegretol by Apotex	Canadian DIN 00402699	Anticonvulsant
APO200	Tab, White, Oval, Biconvex, Film-Coated, Scored	Acebutolol 200 mg	Apo-Acebutolol by Apotex	Canadian DIN 02147610	Antihypertensive
APO200	Cap, White, Opaque	Quinine Sulfate 200 mg	by Apotex	Canadian DIN 02254514	Antimalarial
APO200	Tab, White, Round	Sulfinpyrazone 200 mg	Anturan by Apotex	Canadian DIN 00441767	Uricosuric
APO200	Tab, White, Round	Sulfinpyrazone 200 mg	Anturan by Apotex	Canadian DIN 00441767	Uricosuric
APO240	Cap, Red, Oblong, Soft Gel	Docusate Calcium 240 mg	Surfak by Apotex	Canadian DIN 02245080	Laxative
APO240	Cap, Light Blue	Diltiazem HCl 240 mg	Diltiaz CD by Apotex	Canadian DIN 02230999	Antihypertensive
APO25	Cap, Green & White	Chlordiazepoxide 25 mg	Librium by Apotex	Canadian DIN 00522996	Antianxiety; C IV
APO25	Tab, White, Oval, APO/.25	Alprazolam 0.25 mg	Xanax by Apotex	Canadian DIN 00865397	Antianxiety; C IV
APO25	Tab, Yellow, Round, APO/2.5	Enalapril Maleate 2.5 mg	Vasotec by Apotex	Canadian	Antihypertensive
APO25	Tab, White, Round, APO/25	Methyldopa, Hydrochlorothiazide 25 mg	Apo Methazide by Apotex	Canadian DIN 00441716	Antihypertensive, Diuretic
APO25	Cap, White, Opaque	Zonisamide 25 mg	Zonegran by Apotex	60505-2545	Anticonvulsant
APO25	Cap, Yellow & White	Nortriptyline HCl 25 mg	Nortriptyline by Apotex	Canadian DIN 02223538	Antidepressant

ID FRONT <> BACK	DESCRIPTION FRONT <> BACK	INGREDIENT & STRENGTH	BRAND (or Generic Equiv.) by FIRM	NDC#	CLASS; SCH.
APO25	Tab, Pink, Round, Scored	Hydrochlorothiazide 25 mg	Apo Hydro by Apotex	Canadian DIN 00326844	Diuretic; Antihypertensive
APO25	Cap, Blue and White	Indomethacin 25 mg	Indocin by Apotex	Canadian DIN 00611158	NSAID
APO25	Tab, Yellow, Round	Methotrimeprazine Maleate 25 mg	Methoprazine by Apotex	Canadian DIN 02238405	Antipsychotic
APO25	Tab, White, Round, APO/2.5	Glyburide 2.5 mg	Apo Glyburide by Apotex	Canadian DIN 01913654	Antidiabetic
APO25	Tab, Pale Pink, Round, APO/25	Hydrochlorothiazide 25 mg	Hydrodiuril by Apotex	Canadian DIN 00326844	Diuretic; Antihypertensive
APO25	Tab, White, Square, APO/25	Captopril 25 mg	Capoten by Apotex	Canadian DIN 00893609	Antihypertensive
APO25	Tab, White, Oval, APO/2.5	Bromocriptine 2.5 mg	Parlodel by Apotex	Canadian DIN 02087324	Antiparkinson
APO25	Cap, Blue & Pink	Doxepin HCl 25 mg	Apo Doxepin by Apotex	Canadian DIN 02050005 Discontinued	Antidepressant
APO25	Cap, Yellow, Opaque	Sertraline HCl 25 mg	Zoloft by Apotex	Canadian DIN 02238280	Antidepressant
APO25	Cap, Orange and White, APO 2.5	Ramipril 2.5 mg	Altace by Apotex	Canadian DIN 02251531	Antihypertensive
APO250	Tab, Orange, Oblong, APO-250	Cephalexin 250 mg	Apo Cephalex by Apotex	Canadian DIN 00768723	Antibiotic
APO250	Tab, White, Oval	Chlorpropamide 250 mg	Apo Chlorpropam by Apotex	Canadian DIN 00312711	Antidiabetic
APO250	Cap, Black & Red	Ampicillin 250 mg	Principen by Apotex	Canadian DIN 00603279	Antibiotic
APO250	Tab, Pink, Round, APO/250	Erythromycin Stearate 250 mg	Apo Erythro-S by Apotex	Canadian DIN 02238048	Antibiotic
APO250	Cap, Yellow	Procainamide HCl 250 mg	Apo Procainamide by Apotex	Canadian	Antiarrhythmic
APO250	Tab, White, Round, APO/250	Primidone 250 mg	Apo Primidone by Apotex	Canadian DIN 00396761	Anticonvulsant
APO250	Cap, Orange, Gel, Colorless Liquid-Filled	Valproic Acid 250 mg	Depakene by Apotex	Canadian DIN 02238048	Anticonvulsant
APO250	Cap, Orange & Yellow	Tetracycline HCl 250 mg	Tetracyn by Apotex	Canadian DIN 00580929	Antibiotic
APO250	Tab, Bright Pink, Round	Erythromycin Stearate 250 mg	Erythrocin by Apotex	Canadian DIN 00545678	Antibiotic
APO250	Tab, White, Round, Film Coated	Ciprofloxacin HCl 250 mg	Cipro by Apotex	Canadian DIN 02229521	Antibiotic
APO250	Cap, Clear & Orange	Erythromycin 250 mg	Apo Erythro E-C by Apotex	Canadian DIN 00726672	Antibiotic
APO250	Tab, Pink, Oval, APO-250	Erythromycin 250 mg	Apo Erythro Base by Apotex	Canadian DIN 00682020	Antibiotic
APO250	Cap, Blue & Yellow	Mefenamic Acid 250 mg	Pnostel by Apotex	Canadian DIN 02229452	NSAID
APO250	Tab, Yellow, Round, APO/250	Methyldopa 250 mg	Apo Methyldopa by Apotex	Canadian DIN 00360260	Antihypertensive
APO250	Tab, Yellow, Oval, APO-250	Naproxen 250 mg	Apo Naproxen by Apotex	Canadian DIN 00522651	NSAID
APO250	Tab, White, Round, APO/250	Metronidazole 250 mg	Apo Metronidazole by Apotex	Canadian DIN 00545066	Antibiotic

ID FRONT <> BACK	DESCRIPTION FRONT <> BACK	INGREDIENT & STRENGTH	BRAND (or Generic Equiv.) by FIRM	NDC#	CLASS; SCH.
APO250	Cap, Gold & Scarlet, APO/250	Amoxicillin 250 mg	Amoxil by Apotex	Canadian DIN 00628115	Antibiotic
APO250	Tab, White, Round, APO over 250	Acetazolamide 250 mg	Diamox by Apotex	Canadian DIN 00545015	Antiglaucoma Agent
APO250	Cap, Purple & White	Cefaclor 250 mg	Ceclor by Apotex	Canadian DIN 02230263	Antibiotic
APO250	Cap, Black & Orange	Cloxacillin Sodium 250 mg	Apo Cloxi by Apotex	Canadian DIN 00618292	Antibiotic
APO25025	Tab, Blue, Oval, APO Score 250 over 25	Levodopa 250 mg, Carbidopa 25 mg	Sinemet by Apotex	Canadian DIN 02195968	Antiparkinson
APO26	Tab, White to Off-White, Cap Shaped, Film Coated	Ranitidine HCl 300 mg	Zantac by Major	00904-5262	Gastrointestinal
APO275	Tab, Blue, Oval, APO-275	Naproxen 275 mg	Apo Napro-Na by Apotex	Canadian DIN 00784354	NSAID
APO30	Cap, Ivory & Red	Flurazepam HCl 30 mg	Apo Flurazepam by Apotex	Canadian DIN 00521701	Hypnotic; C IV
APO30	Tab, White, Round, APO/30	Oxazepam 30 mg	Serax by Apotex	Canadian DIN 00402737	Sedative/Hypnotic; C IV
APO30	Cap, Blue & Maroon	Temazepam 30 mg	Restoril by Apotex	Canadian DIN 02225972	Sedative/Hypnotic; C IV
APO300	Tab, White, Oblong	Theophylline Anhydrous 300 mg	Apo Theo LA by Apotex	Canadian	Antiasthmatic
APO300	Cap, White and Light Brown	Nizatidine 300 mg	Axid by Apotex	60505-0231	Gastrointestinal
APO300	Tab, White, Round, APO/300	Oxtriphylline 300 mg	Apo Oxtriphylline by Apotex	Canadian DIN 00511692	Antiasthmatic
APO300	Cap, Pale Yellow and Reddish Brown	Nizatidine 300 mg	Apo Nizatidine by Apotex	Canadian DIN 02220164	Gastrointestinal
APO300	Cap, Flesh	Lithium Carbonate 300 mg	Eskalith by Apotex	60505-2504	Antipsychotic
APO300	Cap, Light Gray	Etodolac 300 mg	Etodolac by Apotex	Canadian	NSAID
APO300	Cap, Maroon & White	Gemfibrozil 300 mg	Apo Gemfibrozil by Apotex	Canadian DIN 01979574	Antihyperlipidemic
APO300	Tab, Pale Green, Round, APO/300	Ferrous Gluconate 300 mg	Apo Ferrous Gluco by Apotex	Canadian DIN 00545031	Mineral
APO300	Tab, White, Round, APO/300	Ibuprofen 300 mg	Motrin by Apotex	Canadian DIN 00441651	NSAID
APO300	Cap, Light Blue & Light Gray	Diltiazem HCl 300 mg	Diltiaz CD by Apotex	Canadian DIN 02229526	Antihypertensive
APO300	Tab, Pale Green, Round, APO/300	Cimetidine HCl 300 mg	Tagamet by Apotex	Canadian DIN 00487872	Gastrointestinal
APO300	Tab, White, Oval, Scored	Moclobemide 300 mg	Apo Moclobemide by Apotex	Canadian DIN 02240456	Antidepressant
APO300	Cap, Flesh	Lithium Carbonate 300 mg	Eskalith by Apotex	Canadian DIN 02242838	Antipsychotic
APO300	Cap, Light Grey	Etodolac 300 mg	Lodine by Apotex	Canadian DIN 02232318	NSAID
APO300	Cap, Light Blue, Hard Gel	Clindamycin HCl 300 mg	Cleocin HCl by Apotex	Canadian DIN 02245233	Antibiotic
APO300	Cap, Yellow	Gabapentin 300 mg	Neurontin by Apotex	Canadian DIN 02244305	Anticonvulsant
APO300	Tab, Orange, Round, APO/300	Penicillin V Potassium 300 mg	Apo Pen VK by Apotex	Canadian DIN 00642215	Antibiotic
APO300	Tab, White, Oblong, APO-300	Ranitidine HCl 300 mg	Apo Ranitidine by Apotex	Canadian DIN 00733067	Gastrointestinal

ID FRONT <> BACK	DESCRIPTION FRONT <> BACK	INGREDIENT & STRENGTH	BRAND (or Generic Equiv.) by FIRM	NDC#	CLASS; SCH.
APO300	Tab, White, Round, APO/300	Tiaprofenic Acid 300 mg	Apo Tiaprofenic by Apotex	Canadian DIN 02136120	NSAID
APO300	Cap, White, Opaque	Quinine Sulfate 300 mg	by Apotex	Canadian DIN 02254522	Antimalarial
APO325	Tab, White, Round, APO/325	Acetaminophen 325 mg	Tylenol by Apotex	Canadian DIN 00544981	Analgesic
APO325	Cap, White, Cap-Shaped, Biconvex, Film-Coated	Acetaminophen 325 mg	Apo-Acetaminophen by Apotex	Canadian DIN 02229873	Analgesic
APO333	Cap, Clear & Yellow	Erythromycin 333 mg	by Parke Davis	Canadian	Antibiotic
APO333	Cap, Clear & Yellow	Erythromycin 333 mg	Erythro E-C by Apotex	Canadian DIN 01925938	Antibiotic
APO375	Cap, Orange & White	Procainamide HCl 375 mg	Apo Procainamide by Apotex	Canadian	Antiarrhythmic
APO375	Tab, Peach, Oblong	Naproxen 375 mg	Apo Naproxen by Apotex	Canadian DIN 00600806	NSAID
APO375	Cap, Gray & White, APO/3.75	Clorazepate Dipotassium 3.75 mg	Apo Clorazepate by Apotex	Canadian DIN 00860689	Antianxiety; C IV
APO4	Tab, Light Purple, Round, APO/4	Salbutamol Sulfate 4 mg	Salvent by Apotex	Canadian DIN 02146851	Antiasthmatic
APO4	Tab, White, Pentagon-Shaped, Scored	Dexamethasone 4 mg	Decadron by Apotex	Canadian DIN 02250055	Steroid
APO40	Tab, Green, Round, APO/40	Propranolol HCl 40 mg	Inderal by Apotex	Canadian DIN 00402753	Antihypertensive
APO40	Tab, Light Blue, Round, APO/40	Megestrol Acetate 40 mg	Megestrol by Apotex	Canadian DIN 02195917	Hormone
APO40	Tab, Light Brown, D-Shaped	Famotidine 40 mg	Famotidine by Apotex	Canadian DIN 01953834	Gastrointestinal
APO40	Tab, Yellow, Round, APO/40	Furosemide 40 mg	Apo Furosemide by Apotex	Canadian DIN 00362166	Diuretic
APO400	Tab, White, Oval	Norfloxacin 400 mg	Norflox by Apotex	Canadian DIN 02229524	Antibiotic
APO400	Tab, Pink, Oblong, APO/400	Pentoxifylline 400 mg	Trental by Apotex	Canadian	Anticoagulant
APO400	Cap, Orange	Gabapentin 400 mg	Neurontin by Apotex	Canadian DIN 02244306	Anticonvulsant
APO400	Tab, Orange, Round, APO/400	Ibuprofen 400 mg	Motrin by Apotex	Canadian DIN 00506052	NSAID
APO400	Tab, Pale Green, Oblong, APO-400	Cimetidine HCl 400 mg	Tagamet by Apotex	Canadian DIN 00600059	Gastrointestinal
APO400	Tab, White, Oblong, APO/400	Acebutolol HCl 400 mg	Sectral by Apotex	Canadian DIN 02147629	Antihypertensive
APO400	Tab, Pink, Round, APO over 400	Acyclovir 400 mg	Zovirax by Apotex	Canadian DIN 02207648	Antiviral
APO40080	Tab, White, Round, APO/400-80	Sulfamethoxazole 400 mg, Trimethoprim 80 mg	Apo Sulfatrim by Apotex	Canadian DIN 00445274	Antibiotic
APO5	Cap, Green & Yellow	Chlordiazepoxide 5 mg	Librium by Apotex	Canadian DIN 00522724	Antianxiety; C IV
APO5	Tab, Yellow, Round, APO/5	Diazepam 5 mg	Apo Diazepam by Apotex	Canadian DIN 00362158	Antianxiety; C IV
APO5	Cap, Caramel & White	Bromocriptine 5 mg	Parlodel by Apotex	Canadian DIN 02230454	Antiparkinson
APO5	Tab, Green, Round, APO/5	Haloperidol 5 mg	Haldol by Apotex	Canadian DIN 00396834	Antipsychotic

ID FRONT <> BACK	DESCRIPTION FRONT <> BACK	INGREDIENT & STRENGTH	BRAND (or Generic Equiv.) by FIRM	NDC#	CLASS; SCH.
APO5	Cap, White	Glyburide 5 mg	Apo Glyburide by Apotex	Canadian DIN 01913662	Antidiabetic
APO5	Tab, Yellow, Round, APO/5	Folic Acid 5 mg	Apo Folic by Apotex	Canadian DIN 00426849	Vitamin
APO5	Tab, White, Round, APO/5	Trihexyphenidyl HCl 5 mg	Apo Trihex by Apotex	Canadian DIN 00545074	Antiparkinson
APO5	Tab, Blue, Round	Oxybutynin Chloride 5 mg	Ditropan by Apotex	Canadian DIN 02163543	Urinary Tract
APO5	Tab, White, Round, APO/5	Prednisone 5 mg	Apo Prednisone by Apotex	Canadian DIN 00312770	Steroid
APO5	Tab, Light Yellow, Pentagon-Shaped, Scored, APO .5	Dexamethasone 0.5 mg	Decadron by Apotex	Canadian DIN 02261081	Steroid
APO5	Tab, Yellow, Diamond-Shaped, Biconvex	Amiloride 5 mg	Apo-Amiloride by Apotex	Canadian DIN 02249510	Diuretic
APO5	Cap, Red and Grey	Flunarizine HCl 5 mg	Apo Flunarizine by Apotex	Canadian DIN 02246082	Entry Blocker
APO5	Cap, Red, Opaque	Ramipril 5 mg	Altace by Apotex	Canadian DIN 02251574	Antihypertensive
APO5	Tab, Orange, Round	Prochlorperazine Maleate 5 mg	Stemetil by Apotex	Canadian DIN 00886440	Antiemetic
APO50	Cap, Grey and White, Opaque	Zonisamide 50 mg	Zonegran by Apotex	60505-2546	Anticonvulsant
APO50	Tab, White, Round	Fluvoxamine Maleate 50 mg	Luvox by Apotex	Canadian	OCD
APO50	Tab, Yellow, Round, APO/50	Chlorthalidone 50 mg	Apo Chlorthalidone by Apotex	Canadian DIN 00360279	Diuretic
APO50	Tab, White, Round, APO/50	Clomipramine HCl 50 mg	Apo Clomipramine by Apotex	Canadian DIN 02040751	OCD
APO50	Tab, White, Oval, APO-50	Captopril 50 mg	Capoten by Apotex	Canadian DIN 00893617	Antihypertensive
APO50	Cap, Flesh & Pink	Doxepin HCl 50 mg	Apo Doxepin by Apotex	Canadian DIN 02050013	Antidepressant
APO50	Tab, Orange, Round, APO/50	Dimenhydrinate 50 mg	Apo Dimenhydrin by Apotex	Canadian DIN 00363766	Antiemetic
APO50	Tab, Pink, Trapezoid	Fluconazole 50 mg	Fluconazole by Apotex	Canadian DIN 02237370	Antifungal
APO50	Tab, White, Oval, APO-50	Flurbiprofen 50 mg	Apo Flurbiprofen by Apotex	Canadian DIN 01912046	NSAID
APO50	Tab, Pink, Round, APO/50	Hydrochlorothiazide 50 mg	Apo Hydro by Apotex	Canadian DIN 00312800	Diuretic; Antihypertensive
APO50	Tab, Yellow, Round	Methotrimeprazine Maleate 50 mg	Methoprazine by Apotex	Canadian DIN 02238406	Antipsychotic
APO50	Cap, Orange, APO/50	Minocycline HCl 50 mg	Minocin by Apotex	Canadian DIN 02084090	Antibiotic
APO50	Cap, Green & Ivory	Ketoprofen 50 mg	Orudis by Apotex	Canadian DIN 00790427	NSAID
APO50	Cap, Blue & White	Indomethacin 50 mg	Indocin by Apotex	Canadian DIN 00611166	NSAID
APO50	Tab, White, Round, APO/50	Prednisone 50 mg	Apo Prednisone by Apotex	Canadian DIN 00550957	Steroid
APO50	Tab, Rose, Round	Trimipramine Maleate 50 mg	Apo Trimipramine by Apotex	Canadian DIN 00740810	Antidepressant
APO50	Cap, Yellow and White, Opaque	Sertraline HCl 50 mg	Zoloft by Apotex	Canadian DIN 02238281	Antidepressant

ID FRONT <> BACK	DESCRIPTION FRONT <> BACK	INGREDIENT & STRENGTH	BRAND (or Generic Equiv.) by FIRM	NDC#	CLASS; SCH.
APO500	Cap, Orange & Yellow	Procainamide HCl 500 mg	Apo Procainamide by Apotex	Canadian	Antiarrhythmic
APO500	Tab, White, Round, Scored, APO/500	Acetaminophen 500 mg	Tylenol by Apotex	Canadian DIN 00545007	Analgesic
APO500	Cap, Gold & Scarlet, APO/500	Amoxicillin 500 mg	Apo Amoxil by Apotex	Canadian DIN 00628123	Antibiotic
APO500	Cap, Black & Red	Ampicillin 500 mg	Principen by Apotex	Canadian DIN 00603295	Antibiotic
APO500	Cap, Black & Orange	Cloxacillin Sodium 500 mg	Apo Cloxi by Apotex	Canadian DIN 00618284	Antibiotic
APO500	Tab, Orange, Cap Shaped, Scored	Cephalexin 500 mg	Cephalex by Apotex	Canadian DIN 00768715	Antibiotic
APO500	Cap, Gray & Purple	Cefaclor 500 mg	Ceclor CD by Apotex	Canadian DIN 02230264	Antibiotic
APO500	Tab, Yellow, Oblong	Naproxen 500 mg	Apo Naproxen by Apotex	Canadian DIN 00592277	NSAID
APO500	Tab, Yellow, Round, APO/500	Methyldopa 500 mg	Apo Methyldopa by Apotex	Canadian DIN 00426830	Antihypertensive
APO500	Tab, White, Oval, APO-500	Erythromycin 500 mg	Erythro S by Apotex	Canadian DIN 00688568	Antibiotic
APO500	Tab, White, Cap Shaped, Film Coated	Ciprofloxacin HCl 500 mg	Cipro by Apotex	Canadian DIN 02229522	Antibiotic
APO500	Cap, Red and White	Cefadroxil 500 mg	Duricef by Apotex	Canadian DIN 02240774	Antibiotic
APO500	Cap, Pink and Turquoise	Hydroxyurea 500 mg	Apo Hydroxyurea by Apotex	Canadian DIN 02247937	Antineoplastic
APO500	Cap, Pale Green and Light Grey	Metronidazole 500 mg	Flagyl by Apotex	Canadian DIN 02248562	Antibiotic
APO500	Cap, White, Cap-shaped, Biconvex, Film-Coated	Acetaminophen 500 mg	Apo-Acetaminophen by Apotex	Canadian DIN 02229977	Analgesic
APO500	Cap, White, Opaque	Tryptophan 500 mg	Tryptan by Apotex	Canadian DIN 02248540	Antidepressant
APO500 <> MET	Tab, White to Off-White, Oblong	Metformin HCl 500 mg	Glucophage by Apotex	60505-0190	Antidiabetic
APO5025	Tab, Yellow, Round, APO/50-25	Triamterene 50 mg, Hydrochlorothiazide 25 mg	Apo Triazide by Apotex	Canadian DIN 00441775	Antihypertensive; Diuretic
APO550	Tab, Peach, Diamond, APO/5/50	Hydrochlorothiazide 50 mg, Amiloride 5 mg	Apo Amilzide by Apotex	Canadian DIN 00784400	Diuretic; Antihypertensive
APO550	Tab, Blue, Oval, APO-550	Naproxen 550 mg	Apo Napro-Na by Apotex	Canadian DIN 01940309	NSAID
APO60	Tab, White, Round, APO/60	Terfenadine 60 mg	Apo Terfenadine by Apotex	Canadian Discontinued	Antihistamine
APO60	Cap, Chocolate Brown & Ivory	Diltiazem HCl 60 mg	Dilitiaz SR by Apotex	Canadian DIN 02222957	Antihypertensive
APO600	Tab, Pale Green, Oblong, APO-600	Cimetidine HCl 600 mg	Tagamet by Apotex	Canadian DIN 00600067	Gastrointestinal
APO600	Tab, Light Orange, Oval, APO-600	Ibuprofen 600 mg	Motrin by Apotex	Canadian DIN 00585114	NSAID
APO600	Tab, Yellow, Oval, APO-600	Erythromycin 600 mg	Apo Erythro-ES by Apotex	Canadian DIN 00637416	Antibiotic
APO600	Tab, White, Oval, APO-600	Gemfibrozil 600 mg	Apo Gemfibrozil by Apotex	Canadian DIN 01979582	Antihyperlipidemic
APO67	Cap, Yellow, Black Print	Fenofibrate 67 mg	TriCor by Apotex	Canadian DIN 02243180	Antihyperlipidemic

ID FRONT <> BACK	DESCRIPTION FRONT <> BACK	INGREDIENT & STRENGTH	BRAND (or Generic Equiv.) by FIRM	NDC#	CLASS; SCH.
APO75	Tab, Blue, Oval, APO 7.5	Zopiclone 7.5 mg	Rhovane by Apotex	Canadian DIN 02218313	Hypnotic
APO75	Cap, Dark Pink and Light Pink	Trimipramine Maleate 75 mg	Apo Trimipramine by Apotex	Canadian DIN 02070987	Antidepressant
APO75	Tab, Light Brown, Round, APO/75	Imipramine HCl 75 mg	Tofranil by Apotex	Canadian DIN 00644579	Antidepressant
APO75	Cap, Gray & Maroon, APO 7.5	Clorazepate Dipotassium 7.5 mg	Apo Clorazepate by Apotex	Canadian DIN 00860700	Antianxiety; C IV
APO75	Cap, Flesh & Flesh	Doxepin HCl 75 mg	Apo Doxepin by Apotex	Canadian DIN 02050021	Antidepressant
APO75	Tab, Pink, Triangular	Diclofenac Sodium 75 mg	Diclo SR by Apotex	Canadian DIN 02162814	NSAID
APO75	Tab, Orange, Round	Amitriptyline HCl 75 mg	Elavil by Apotex	Canadian DIN 00754129	Antidepressant
APO750	Tab, Peach, Cap Shaped	Naproxen 750 mg	Naproxen SR by Apotex	Canadian DIN 02177072	NSAID
APO750	Tab, White, Cap Shaped, Film Coated	Ciprofloxacin HCl 750 mg	Cipro by Apotex	Canadian DIN 02229523	Antibiotic
APO80	Tab, White, Round	Gliclazide 80 mg	Apo Gliclazide by Apotex	Canadian DIN 02245247	Antidiabetic
APO80	Tab, Yellow, Round, APO/80	Propranolol HCl 80 mg	Inderal by Apotex	Canadian DIN 00402761	Antihypertensive
APO80	Tab, Blue, Oblong, APO-80	Sotalol HCl 80 mg	Satalol by Apotex	Canadian DIN 02210428	Antiarrhythmic
APO80	Tab, Yellow, Cap Shaped, APO/80	Furosemide 80 mg	Apo Furosemide by Apotex	Canadian DIN 00707570	Diuretic
APO800	Tab, Blue, Oval, APO over 800	Acyclovir 800 mg	Zovirax by Apotex	Canadian DIN 02207656	Antiviral
APO800	Tab, Pale Green, Oblong, APO-800	Cimetidine HCl 800 mg	Tagamet by Apotex	Canadian DIN 00749494	Gastrointestinal
APO850	Tab, White, Oblong	Metformin HCl 850 mg	Glucophage by Apotex	60505-0191	Antidiabetic
APO90	Cap, Chocolate Brown & Gold	Diltiazem HCl 90 mg	Diltiaz SR by Apotex	Canadian DIN 02222965	Antihypertensive
APOAPO <> GLM1	Tab, Pink, Cap Shaped, Notched, Scored	Glimepiride 1 mg	Amaryl by Apotex	Canadian DIN 02295377	Antidiabetic
APOAPO <> GLM2	Tab, Green, Cap Shaped, Notched, Scored	Glimepiride 2 mg	Amaryl by Apotex	Canadian DIN 02295385	Antidiabetic
APOAPO <> GLM4	Tab, Blue, Cap Shaped, Notched, Scored	Glimepiride 4 mg	Amaryl by Apotex	Canadian DIN 02295393	Antidiabetic
APOB10	Tab, White, Oval, APO/B10	Baclofen 10 mg	Lioresal by Apotex	Canadian DIN 02139332	Muscle Relaxant
APOB15	Tab, White, Round, APO/B-1.5	Bromazepam 1.5 mg	Lectopam by Apotex	Canadian DIN 02177153	Sedative; C IV
APOB20	Tab, White, Oblong, APO/B20	Baclofen 20 mg	Lioresal by Apotex	Canadian DIN 02139391	Muscle Relaxant
APOB3	Tab, Pink, Round, APO/B-3	Bromazepam 3 mg	Lectopam by Apotex	Canadian DIN 02177161	Sedative; C IV
APOB6	Tab, Green, Round, APO/B-6	Bromazepam 6 mg	Lectopam by Apotex	Canadian DIN 02177188	Sedative; C IV
APOC05	Tab, Orange, Round, APO/C-0.5	Clonazepam 0.5 mg	Klonopin by Apotex	60505-0066	Sedative; C IV
APOC05	Tab, Orange, Round, APO/C-0.5	Clonazepam 0.5 mg	Klonopin by Major	00904-5342	Sedative; C IV

ID FRONT <> BACK	DESCRIPTION FRONT <> BACK	INGREDIENT & STRENGTH	BRAND (or Generic Equiv.) by FIRM	NDC#	CLASS; SCH.
APOC05	Tab, Orange, Round, APO/C-0.5	Clonazepam 0.5 mg	Klonopin by Apotex	Canadian DIN 02177889	Sedative; C IV
APOC1	Tab, Blue, Round, APO/C-1	Clonazepam 1 mg	Klonopin by Major	60505-0067	Sedative; C IV
APOC1	Tab, Blue, Round, APO/C-1	Clonazepam 1 mg	Klonopin by Major	00904-5343	Sedative; C IV
APOC2	Tab, White to Off-White, Round, APO/C-2	Clonazepam 2 mg	Klonopin by Major	00904-5344	Sedative; C IV
APOC2	Tab, White to Off-White, Round, APO/C-2	Clonazepam 2 mg	Klonopin by Apotex	60505-0068	Sedative; C IV
APOC2	Tab, White to Off-White, Round, APO/C-2	Clonazepam 2 mg	Klonopin by Apotex	Canadian DIN 02177897	Sedative; C IV
APOCAL	Tab, Light Green, Oblong, APO-CAL	Calcium 500 mg	Apo Cal by Apotex	Canadian DIN 00682039	Vitamin; Mineral
APOCAL	Tab, Light Green, Biconvex, APO over CAL	Calcium 250 mg	Apo Cal by Apotex	Canadian DIN 00682047	Vitamin; Mineral
APOD30	Tab, Light Green, Round, APO/D30	Diltiazem HCl 30 mg	Apo Diltiaz by Apotex	Canadian DIN 00771376	Antihypertensive
APOD60	Tab, Yellow, Round, APO/D60	Diltiazem HCl 60 mg	Apo Diltiaz by Apotex	Canadian DIN 00771384	Antihypertensive
APODOXY100	Tab, Orange, Round, APO-Doxy 100	Doxycycline Hyclate 100 mg	Apo Doxy Tabs by Apotex	Canadian DIN 00874256	Antibiotic
APODS	Tab, White, Oblong	Sulfamethoxazole 800 mg, Trimethoprim 160 mg	Sulfatrim by Apotex	Canadian DIN 00445282	Antibiotic
APOE10	Tab, Pink & Red, Barrel, APO/E10	Enalapril Maleate 10 mg	Vasotec by Apotex	Canadian	Antihypertensive
APOE20	Tab, Peach, Barrel, APO/E20	Enalapril Maleate 20 mg	Vasotec by Apotex	Canadian	Antihypertensive
APOE5	Tab, White, Barrel, APO/E5	Enalapril Maleate 5 mg	Vasotec by Apotex	Canadian	Antihypertensive
APOEN10	Tab, Red, Triangular, Scored	Enalapril Maleate 10 mg	Vasotec by Apotex	Canadian DIN 02019892	Antihypertensive
APOEN20	Tab, Peach, Triangular, Scored	Enalapril Maleate 20 mg	Vasotec by Apotex	Canadian DIN 02019906	Antihypertensive
APOEN5	Tab, White, Triangular, Scored	Enalapril Maleate 5 mg	Vasotec by Apotex	Canadian DIN 02019884	Antihypertensive
APOF150	Cap, White, Opaque	Fluconazole 150 mg	Apo Fluconazole by Apotex	Canadian DIN 02241895	Antifungal
APOH10	Tab, Yellow, Round, APO/H10	Hydralazine HCl 10 mg	Apo Hydralazine by Apotex	Canadian DIN 00441619	Antihypertensive
APOI30	Tab, White, Round, APO/I30	Isosorbide Dinitrate 30 mg	Isordil by Apotex	Canadian DIN 00441694	Antianginal
APOI30	Tab, White, Round, APO/I30	Isosorbide Dinitrate 10 mg	Isordil by Apotex	Canadian DIN 00441686	Antianginal
APOK600	Tab, Orange, Round, APO/K600	Potassium Chloride 600 mg	Apo K by Apotex	Canadian DIN 00602884	Electrolytes
APOL10	Tab, Pink, Oval, Biconvex	Lisinopril 10 mg	Zestril by Major	00904-5639	Antihypertensive
APOL10	Tab, Pink, Oval, Biconvex	Lisinopril 10 mg	Zestril by Apotex	Canadian DIN 02217503	Antihypertensive
APOL20	Tab, Deep Pink, Oval, Biconvex	Lisinopril 20 mg	Zestril by Major	00904-5640	Antihypertensive
APOL20	Tab, Deep Pink, Oval, Biconvex	Lisinopril 20 mg	Zestril by Apotex	Canadian DIN 02217511	Antihypertensive
APOL40	Tab, Yellow, Oval	Lisinopril 40 mg	Zestril by Major	00904-5642	Antihypertensive
APOL5	Tab, Pink, Oval, APO/L5	Lisinopril 5 mg	Prinivil by Major	00904-5638	Antihypertensive
APOL5	Tab, Pink, Oval, APO/L5	Lisinopril 5 mg	Prinivil by Apotex	Canadian DIN 02217481	Antihypertensive
APOM10	Tab, White, Round, APO/M10	Metoclopramide HCl 10 mg	Reglan by Apotex	Canadian DIN 00842834	Gastrointestinal

ID FRONT <> BACK	DESCRIPTION FRONT <> BACK	INGREDIENT & STRENGTH	BRAND (or Generic Equiv.) by FIRM	NDC#	CLASS; SCH.
APOM100	Tab, White, Round, APO/M100	Metoprolol Tartrate 100 mg	Lopressor by Apotex	Canadian DIN 00618640	Antihypertensive
APOM5	Tab, White, Square, APO/M5	Metoclopramide HCl 5 mg	Emex by Apotex	Canadian DIN 00842826	Gastrointestinal
APOM50	Tab, White, Round, APO/M50	Metoprolol Tartrate 50 mg	Lopressor by Apotex	Canadian DIN 00618632	Antihypertensive
APON40	Tab, White, Round, APO/N40	Nadolol 40 mg	Apo Nadol by Apotex	Canadian DIN 00782505	Antihypertensive
APON80	Tab, White, Round, APO/N80	Nadolol 80 mg	Apo Nadol by Apotex	Canadian DIN 00782467	Antihypertensive
APOO20	Cap, Pink and Reddish Brown, Opaque	Omeprazole 20 mg	Apo Omeprazole by Apotex	Canadian DIN 02245058	Gastrointestinal
APOP1	Tab, Peach, Oblong	Prazosin HCl 1 mg	Apo Prazo by Apotex	Canadian DIN 00882801	Antihypertensive
APOP10	Tab, White, Round, APO/P10	Pindolol 10 mg	Apo Pindol by Apotex	Canadian DIN 00755885	Antihypertensive
APOP15	Tab, White, Round, APO/P15	Pindolol 15 mg	Apo Pindol by Apotex	Canadian DIN 00755893	Antihypertensive
APOP150	Tab, White, Round	Propafenone HCl 150 mg	Rythmol by Apotex	Canadian DIN 02243324	Antiarrhythmic
APOP2	Tab, White, Round, APO/P2	Prazosin HCl 2 mg	Apo Prazo by Apotex	Canadian DIN 00882828	Antihypertensive
APOP300	Tab, White, Round, Scored	Propafenone HCl 300 mg	Rythmol by Apotex	Canadian DIN 02243325	Antiarrhythmic
APOP5	Tab, White, Round, Scored	Pindolol 5 mg	Visken by Apotex	Canadian DIN 00755877	Antihypertensive
APOP5	Tab, White, Diamond, APO/P5	Prazosin HCl 5 mg	Apo Prazo by Apotex	Canadian DIN 00882836	Antihypertensive
APOP500	Cap, Yellow and Orange	Procainamide 500 mg	Procan by Apotex	Canadian DIN 00713341	Antiarrhythmic
APOPED	Tab, White, Round, APO/PED	Sulfamethoxazole 100 mg, Trimethoprim 20 mg	Sulfatrim by Apotex	Canadian DIN 00445266	Antibiotic
APOT10	Tab, White, Round	Tamoxifen Citrate 10 mg	Nolvadex by Apotex	Canadian	Antiestrogen
APOT10	Tab, Blue, Round	Timolol Maleate 10 mg	Apo Timol by Apotex	Canadian DIN 00755850	Antihypertensive
APOT100	Tab, White, APO/T100	Trazodone HCl 100 mg	Desyrel by Apotex	Canadian DIN 02147645	Antidepressant
APOT150 <> 505050	Tab, White, Oval, Scored	Trazodone HCl 150 mg	Desyrel by Apotex	60505-2655	Antidepressant
APOT20	Tab, White, Octagonal, APO/T20	Tamoxifen Citrate 20 mg	Nolvadex by Apotex	Canadian	Antiestrogen
APOT20	Tab, Light Blue, Oblong, APO/T20	Timolol Maleate 20 mg	Apo Timol by Apotex	Canadian DIN 00755869	Antihypertensive
APOT5	Tab, White, Round, APO/T5	Timolol Maleate 5 mg	Apo Timol by Apotex	Canadian DIN 00755842	Antihypertensive
APOT50	Tab, Round, APO/T50	Trazodone HCl 50 mg	Desyrel by Apotex	Canadian DIN 02147637	Antidepressant
APOTI2	Tab, White, Round, Scored, APO over TI-2	Tizanidine HCl 2 mg	Zanaflex by Apotex	60505-0251	Muscle Relaxant
APOTI4	Tab, White, Round, Scored, APO over TI-4	Tizanidine HCl 4 mg	Zanaflex by Apotex	60505-0252	Muscle Relaxant
APOTI4	Tab, White, Round, Scored, APO over TI-4	Tizanidine HCl 4 mg	Zanaflex by Apotex	Canadian DIN 02259893	Muscle Relaxant
APOTOL	Tab, White, Round, APO/TOL	Tolbutamide 500 mg	Apo Tolbutamide by Apotex	Canadian DIN 00312762	Antidiabetic

ID FRONT <> BACK	DESCRIPTION FRONT <> BACK	INGREDIENT & STRENGTH	BRAND (or Generic Equiv.) by FIRM	NDC#	CLASS; SCH.
APOTRM	Tab, White, Round, APO/TRM	Trihexyphenidyl HCl 2 mg	Apo Trihex by Apotex	Canadian DIN 00545058	Antiparkinson
APOV120	Tab, White, Round, APO/V120	Verapamil HCl 120 mg	Apo Verap by Apotex	Canadian DIN 00782491	Antihypertensive
APOV80	Tab, Yellow, Round, APO/V80	Verapamil HCl 80 mg	Apo Verap by Apotex	Canadian DIN 00782483	Antihypertensive
APOZ100	Cap, White, Opaque	Zidovudine 100 mg	Retrovir by Apotex	Canadian DIN 01946323	Antiviral
APP784DURICEF500	Cap	Cefadroxil Monohydrate 500 mg	Duricef by Pharmedix	53002-0284	Antibiotic
APSE	Tab, Yellow, Cap Shaped	Pseudoephedrine HCl 120 mg, Guaifenesin 600 mg	Ami-tex PSE by Amide	52152-0130	Cold Remedy
APSE	Tab, Yellow, Cap Shaped	Pseudoephedrine HCl 120 mg, Guaifenesin 600 mg	Ami-tex PSE by H J Harkins Co	52959-0397	Cold Remedy
APT <> JMI	Tab, Sugar Coated	Thyroid 3 g	Westhroid Apt 2 by JMI Canton	00252-7505	Thyroid Hormone
APT <> JMI	Tab, Sugar Coated	Thyroid 3 g	Westhroid Apt 2 by Jones	52604-7505	Thyroid Hormone
AQUAPURE028	Cap, Red	Lipase 16,000 Units, Amylase 48,000 Units, Protease 48,000 Units	Pangestyme MT 16 by Ethex	58177-0028	Gastrointestinal
AQUAPURE029	Cap, Pink & Natural	Lipase 10,000 Units, Amylase 33,200 Units, Protease 37,500 Units	Pangestyme CN 10 by Ethex	58177-0029	Gastrointestinal
AQUAPURE050	Cap, Clear & Green	Lipase 20,000 Units, Amylase 65,000 Units, Protease 65,000 Units	Pangestyme UL 20 by Ethex	58177-0050	Gastrointestinal
AR102	Cap, Clear, Black Ink	Quinine Sulfate 324 mg	Qualaquin by AR Scientific	13310-0153	Antimalarial
AR374	Tab, Purple, Cap Shaped, Film Coated, Scored	Colchicine 0.6 mg	Colcrys by AR Scientific	13310-0119	Antigout
ARA	Cap, White, Abbott Logo (a) over AR	Fenofibrate 134 mg	TriCor by Abbott	00074-6447 Discontinued	Antihyperlipidemic
ARACEPT10	Tab, Yellow, Aracept/10	Donepezil HCl 10 mg	Aricept by Pfizer	Canadian	Antialzheimers
ARACEPT5	Tab, White, Aracept/5	Donepezil HCl 5 mg	Aricept by Pfizer	Canadian	Antialzheimers
ARICEPT <> 10	Tab, Yellow, Round, Film Coated	Donepezil HCl 10 mg	Aricept by Eisai	62856-0246	Antialzheimers
ARICEPT <> 10	Tab, Yellow, Round, Film Coated	Donepezil HCl 10 mg	Aricept by Pfizer	Canadian DIN 02232044	Antialzheimers
ARICEPT <> 10	Tab, Yellow, Round, Orally Disintegrating	Donepezil HCl 10 mg	Aricept RDT by Pfizer	Canadian DIN 02269465	Antialzheimers
ARICEPT <> 5	Tab, White, Round, Orally Disintegrating	Donepezil HCl 5 mg	Aricept ODT by Eisai	62856-0832	Antialzheimers
ARICEPT <> 5	Tab, White, Round, Orally Disintegrating	Donepezil HCl 5 mg	Aricept ODT by Eisai	62856-0831	Antialzheimers
ARICEPT <> 5	Tab, White, Round, Orally Disintegrating	Donepezil HCl 5 mg	Aricept RDT by Pfizer	Canadian DIN 02269457	Antialzheimers
ARICEPT <> 5	Tab, White, Round, Film Coated	Donepezil HCl 5 mg	Aricept by Pfizer	Canadian DIN 02232043	Antialzheimers
ARM	Tab, Yellow, Cap Shaped	Pseudoephedrine HCl 60 mg, Chlorpheniramine Maleate 4 mg	A.R.M. by B F Ascher	62856-0245	Antialzheimers
ARMOURATO	Tab, Tan, Round, Armour A/ TO	Thyroid 30 mg	Thyrar by RPR	00225-0575	Cold Remedy
ARMOURATP	Tab, Tan, Round, Armour A/ TP	Thyroid 60 mg	Thyrar by RPR		Thyroid Hormone
ARROW	Tab, White, Round, Arrow Logo	3,4-Methylenedioxymethamphetamine (MDMA)	Ecstasy by Illegal		Euphoric; Illicit
ARTANE2 <> LLA11	Tab, White, Round, Scored, Artane over 2 <> LL over A11	Trihexyphenidyl HCl 2 mg	Artane by Amerisource	62584-0434	Antiparkinson
ARTANE2 <> LLA11	Tab, White, Round, Scored, Artane over 2 <> LL over A11	Trihexyphenidyl HCl 2 mg	Artane by Thrift Drug	59198-0006	Antiparkinson
ARTANE2 <> LLA11	Tab, White, Round, Scored, Artane over 2 <> LL over A11	Trihexyphenidyl HCl 2 mg	Artane by UDL	51079-0115	Antiparkinson
ARTANE2 <> LLA11	Tab, White, Round, Scored, Artane over 2 <> LL over A11	Trihexyphenidyl HCl 2 mg	Artane by Lederle	00005-4434	Antiparkinson
ARTANE2 <> LLA11	Tab, White, Round, Scored, Artane over 2 <> LL over A11	Trihexyphenidyl HCl 2 mg	Artane by Wyeth	Canadian	Antiparkinson
ARTANE5 <> LLA12	Tab, White, Round, Scored, Artane over 5 <> LL over A12	Trihexyphenidyl HCl 5 mg	Artane by Wyeth	Canadian	Antiparkinson
ARTANE5 <> LLA12	Tab, White, Round, Scored, Artane over 5 <> LL over A12	Trihexyphenidyl HCl 5 mg	Artane by UDL	51079-0124	Antiparkinson
ARTANE5 <> LLA12	Tab, White, Round, Scored, Artane over 5 <> LL over A12	Trihexyphenidyl HCl 5 mg	Artane by Lederle	00005-4436	Antiparkinson
AS200	Tab, Yellow, Round, Scored	Amiodarone HCl 200 mg	Pacerone by Aurobindo	13107-0056 Discontinued	Antiarrhythmic
AS400	Tab, Yellow, Oval, Scored	Amiodarone HCl 400 mg	Pacerone by Aurobindo	13107-0088	Antiarrhythmic

ID FRONT <> BACK	DESCRIPTION FRONT <> BACK	INGREDIENT & STRENGTH	BRAND (or Generic Equiv.) by FIRM	NDC#	CLASS; SCH.
ASACOL800	Tab, Reddish Brown, Cap-Shaped, Enteric Coated	Mesalazine 800 mg	Asacol 800 by Proc & Gamble	Canadian DIN 02267217	Gastrointestinal
ASACOLNE	Tab, Reddish Brown, Cap Shaped, Delayed Release	Mesalamine 400 mg	Asacol by Caremark	00339-6026	Gastrointestinal
ASACOLNE	Tab, Reddish Brown, Cap Shaped, Delayed Release	Mesalamine 400 mg	Asacol by Procter and Gamble	00149-0752	Gastrointestinal
ASACOLNE	Tab, Reddish Brown, Cap Shaped, Enteric-Coated	Mesalamine 400 mg	Asacol by Proc & Gamble	Canadian DIN 01997580	Gastrointestinal
ASAPHEN80	Tab, Orange, Round, Scored, Chewable	Aspirin 80 mg	Asaphen by Pharmascience	Canadian DIN 02009013	Analgesic
ASAPHEN81	Tab, Orange, Round, Scored, Chewable	Aspirin 81 mg	Asaphen by Pharmascience	Canadian DIN 02243974	Analgesic
ASCOLD	Tab, Blue, Oblong, AS + Cold	Acetaminophen 325 mg, Chlorpheniramine Maleate 2 mg, Pseudoephedrine HCl 30 mg	Alka Seltzer Plus Liquid Gels by Medeva	53014-0004	Cold Remedy
ASF2	Tab, White, A/SF/2	Nitroglycerin 2 mg	Nitrogard SR by AstraZeneca	Canadian	Vasodilator
ASI1	Tab, White, A/SI/1	Nitroglycerin 1 mg	Nitrogard SR by AstraZeneca	Canadian	Vasodilator
ASN3	Tab, White, A/SN/3	Nitroglycerin 3 mg	Nitrogard SR by AstraZeneca	Canadian	Vasodilator
ASPIRIN <> 44157	Tab, White, Round, Film Coated, Aspirin <> 44 over 157	Aspirin 325 mg	Aspirin by UDL	51079-0005	Analgesic
ASPIRIN <> 500	Tab, White, Round	Aspirin 500 mg	Aspirin by Perrigo	00113-0448	Analgesic
ASPIRIN <> A1	Tab, White, Round	Aspirin 325 mg	Aspirin by Major	00904-2009	Analgesic
ASPIRIN <> A2	Tab, White, Round	Aspirin 325 mg	Bayer Aspirin by Qualitest	00603-0031	Analgesic
ASPIRIN <> BAYER	Tab, Peach, Round	Aspirin 80 mg	Aspirin Children's Size by Bayer	Canadian DIN 02150352	Analgesic
ASPIRIN <> K48	Tab, White Round	Aspirin 325 mg	Aspirin by McKesson	63739-0024	Analgesic
ASPIRIN44157	Tab, White, Round, Aspirin/44/157	Aspirin 325 mg	Aspirin by LNK		Analgesic
ASPIRIN44157	Tab, White, Round, Aspirin 44-157	Aspirin 325 mg	Aspirin by Ivax	00182-0444 Discontinued	Analgesic
ASPIRINL	Tab, White, Round, Aspirin -L	Aspirin 325 mg	Aspirin by Perrigo	00113-0416	Analgesic
ASPIRINL	Tab, White, Round, Aspirin -L	Aspirin 325 mg	Aspirin by Perrigo	00113-0411	Analgesic
ASPIRINL	Tab, White, Round, Aspirin -L	Aspirin 325 mg	Aspirin by Perrigo	00113-2416	Analgesic
ASR	Cap, Orange, Abbott Logo (a) over SR	Fenofibrate 200 mg	TriCor by Abbott	00074-6415 Discontinued	Antihyperlipidemic
AST10 <> JANSSEN	Tab, White, Round, AST over 10 <> Janssen	Astemizole 10 mg	Hismanal by Kaiser	00179-1234 Discontinued	Antihistamine
AST10 <> JANSSEN	Tab, White, Round, AST over 10 <> Janssen	Astemizole 10 mg	Hismanal by Pharmedix	53002-0642 Discontinued	Antihistamine
AST10 <> JANSSEN	Tab, White, Round, AST over 10 <> Janssen	Astemizole 10 mg	Hismanal by Janssen	50458-0510 Discontinued	Antihistamine
AST10 <> JANSSEN	Tab, White, Round, AST over 10 <> Janssen	Astemizole 10 mg	Hismanal by Johnson & Johnson	59604-0510 Discontinued	Antihistamine
AST10 <> JANSSEN	Tab, White, Round, AST over 10 <> Janssen	Astemizole 10 mg	Hismanal by PDRX	55289-0527	Antihistamine
AST10 <> JANSSEN	Tab, White, Round, AST over 10 <> Janssen	Astemizole 10 mg	Hismanal by Direct Dispensing	57866-6480	Antihistamine
AST10 <> JANSSEN	Tab, White, Round, AST over 10 <> Janssen	Astemizole 10 mg	Hismanal by Ortho-McNeil	00062-0510 Discontinued	Antihistamine
AST10 <> JANSSEN	Tab, White, Round, AST over 10 <> Janssen	Astemizole 10 mg	Hismanal by St. Mary's Med	60760-0510 Discontinued	Antihistamine
AST10 <> JANSSEN	Tab, White, Round, AST over 10 <> Janssen	Astemizole 10 mg	Hismanal by Janssen	Discontinued	Antihistamine
AST10 <> JANSSEN	Tab, White, Round, AST over 10 <> Janssen	Astemizole 10 mg	Hismanal by Amerisource	62584-0510 Discontinued	Antihistamine
AST5	Tab, White, A/ST/5	Nitroglycerin 5 mg	Nitrogard SR by AstraZeneca	Canadian	Vasodilator

ID FRONT <> BACK	DESCRIPTION FRONT <> BACK	INGREDIENT & STRENGTH	BRAND (or Generic Equiv.) by FIRM	NDC#	CLASS; SCH.
ASTRA <> CARDURA1	Tab, White, Round, Cardura 1/Astra	Doxazosin Mesylate 1 mg	Cardura by AstraZeneca	Canadian DIN 01958100	Antihypertensive
ASTRA <> CARDURA2	Tab, White, Oval, Cardura 2/Astra	Doxazosin Mesylate 2 mg	Cardura by AstraZeneca	Canadian DIN 01958097	Antihypertensive
ASTRA <> CARDURA4	Tab, White	Doxazosin Mesylate 4 mg	Cardura by AstraZeneca	Canadian DIN 01958119	Antihypertensive
ASTRA <> CARDURA4	Tab, White, Diamond, Cardura 4/Astra	Doxazosin Mesylate 4 mg	Cardura by AstraZeneca	Canadian DIN 01958100	Antihypertensive
AT	Tab, Round, Abbott Logo	Pipobroman 25 mg	Vercyte by Abbott		Antineoplastic
AT05056	Tab, White, Round, AT 0.5/056	Lorazepam 0.5 mg	Ativan by ATI		Antianxiety; C IV
AT053	Cap, White	Clorazepate Dipotassium 30.75 mg	Tranxene by ATI		Antianxiety; C IV
AT054	Cap, Orange	Clorazepate Dipotassium 7.5 mg	Tranxene by ATI		Antianxiety; C IV
AT055	Cap, Red	Clorazepate Dipotassium 15 mg	Tranxene by ATI		Antianxiety; C IV
AT083	Cap, Orange	Danazol 200 mg	Danocrine by ATI		Steroid
AT096	Tab, Green, Hexagonal	Chlorzoxazone 250 mg, Acetaminophen 300 mg	Parafon Forte by ATI		Muscle Relaxant
AT098	Tab, Yellow, Oblong	Theranatal Plus One	by ATI		Vitamin
AT100	Tab, Golden Yellow, Oblong	Therapeutic Vitamin Plus	Berocca Plus by ATI		Vitamin
AT100 <> G	Tab, White, Round, Scored	Atenolol 100 mg	Tenormin by Genpharm	Canadian DIN 02147432	Antihypertensive
AT10058	Tab, White, Round, AT 1.0/058	Lorazepam 1 mg	Ativan by ATI		Antianxiety; C IV
AT101	Cap, Orange	Meclofenamate Sodium 50 mg	Meclomen by ATI		NSAID
AT102	Cap, Orange	Meclofenamate Sodium 100 mg	Meclomen by ATI		NSAID
AT109	Cap, Clear & Pink, AT-109	Oxazepam 10 mg	Serax by ATI		Sedative/Hypnotic; C IV
AT110	Cap, Clear & Orange, AT-110	Oxazepam 15 mg	Serax by ATI		Sedative/Hypnotic; C IV
AT113	Cap, Clear & White, AT-113	Oxazepam 30 mg	Serax by ATI		Sedative/Hypnotic; C IV
AT121	Tab, White, Round	Trazodone HCl 50 mg	Desyrel by ATI		Antidepressant
AT125	Tab, White, Round	Trazodone HCl 100 mg	Desyrel by ATI		Antidepressant
AT133	Tab, Yellow, Oblong	Therapeutic Vitamin	Berocca by ATI		Vitamin
AT135	Tab, White, Round	Methocarbamol 500 mg	Robaxin by ATI		Muscle Relaxant
AT137	Tab, White, Oblong	Methocarbamol 750 mg	Robaxin by ATI		Muscle Relaxant
AT141	Tab, White, Round	Prednisone 5 mg	Deltasone by ATI		Steroid
AT142	Tab, White, Round	Prednisone 10 mg	Deltasone by ATI		Steroid
AT143	Tab, White, Round	Prednisone 20 mg	Deltasone by ATI		Steroid
AT145	Tab, White, Round	Quinine Sulfate 260 mg	Quinamm by ATI		Antimalarial
AT146	Tab, White, Round	Quinine Sulfate 325 mg	by ATI		Antimalarial
AT147	Tab, Peach, Oblong	Fenoprofen Calcium 600 mg	Nalfon by ATI		NSAID
AT148	Tab, Orange, Round	Clonidine HCl 0.1 mg	Catapres by ATI		Antihypertensive
AT149	Tab, White, Round	Clonidine HCl 0.2 mg	Catapres by ATI		Antihypertensive
AT150	Tab, White, Round	Clonidine HCl 0.3 mg	Catapres by ATI		Antihypertensive
AT151	Cap, Orange & Yellow	Thiothixene 1 mg	Navane by ATI		Antipsychotic
AT152	Cap, Green & Yellow	Thiothixene 2 mg	Navane by ATI		Antipsychotic
AT153	Cap, Orange & White	Thiothixene 5 mg	Navane by ATI		Antipsychotic

ID FRONT <> BACK	DESCRIPTION FRONT <> BACK	INGREDIENT & STRENGTH	BRAND (or Generic Equiv.) by FIRM	NDC#	CLASS; SCH.
AT154	Cap, Green & White	Thiothixene 10 mg	Navane by ATI		Antipsychotic
AT155	Cap, Blue & White	Thiothixene 20 mg	Navane by ATI		Antipsychotic
AT156	Tab, Blue, Round	Clorazepate Dipotassium 3.75 mg	Tranxene by ATI		Antianxiety; C IV
AT157	Tab, Peach, Round	Clorazepate Dipotassium 7.5 mg	Tranxene by ATI		Antianxiety; C IV
AT158	Tab, Pink, Round	Clorazepate Dipotassium 15 mg	Tranxene by ATI		Antianxiety; C IV
AT164	Tab, Yellow, Round, AT-164	Hydrochlorothiazide 50 mg, Triamterene 75 mg	Maxzide by ATI		Diuretic; Antihypertensive
AT165	Tab, White, Round	Metaproterenol Sulfate 10 mg	Alupent by ATI		Antiasthmatic
AT166	Tab, White, Round	Metaproterenol Sulfate 20 mg	Alupent by ATI		Antiasthmatic
AT167	Tab, Orange, Round	Maprotiline 25 mg	Ludiomil by ATI		Antidepressant
AT168	Tab, Orange, Round	Maprotiline 50 mg	Ludiomil by ATI		Antidepressant
AT169	Tab, White, Round	Maprotiline 75 mg	Ludiomil by ATI		Antidepressant
AT172	Tab, White, Round	Albuterol Sulfate 2 mg	Proventil by ATI		Antiasthmatic
AT174	Tab, Green, Oblong	Chlorzoxazone 500 mg	Parafon by ATI		Muscle Relaxant
AT177	Tab, White, Round	Albuterol Sulfate 4 mg	Proventil by ATI		Antiasthmatic
AT178	Cap, Light Brown	Fenoprofen Calcium 200 mg	Nalfon by ATI		NSAID
AT182	Cap, White	Prazosin HCl 1 mg	Minipress by ATI		Antihypertensive
AT184	Cap, Pink	Prazosin HCl 2 mg	Minipress by ATI		Antihypertensive
AT187	Cap, Blue	Prazosin HCl 5 mg	Minipress by ATI		Antihypertensive
AT190	Cap, Yellow	Fenoprofen Calcium 300 mg	Nalfon by ATI		NSAID
AT20060	Tab, White, Round, AT 2.0/060	Lorazepam 2 mg	Ativan by ATI		Antianxiety; C IV
AT2012	Tab, White, Round, AT 201/2	Acetaminophen 300 mg, Codeine Phosphate 15 mg	Tylenol w/ Codeine by ATI		Analgesic; C III
AT2023	Tab, White, Round, AT 202/3	Acetaminophen 300 mg, Codeine Phosphate 30 mg	Tylenol w/ Codeine by ATI		Analgesic; C III
AT2034	Tab, White, Round, AT 203/4	Acetaminophen 300 mg, Codeine Phosphate 60 mg	Tylenol w/ Codeine by ATI		Analgesic; C III
AT211	Tab, White, Oval	Theralins RX	Natalin RX by ATI		Vitamin
AT25 <> G	Tab, White, Round	Atenolol 25 mg	Tenormin by Genpharm	Canadian DIN 02303647	Antihypertensive
AT250	Tab, Pink, Cap-Shaped, Film-Coated, Cobalt Logo <> AT250	Azithromycin 250 mg	Zithromax by Cobalt	Canadian DIN 02255340	Antibiotic
AT4312	Tab, Orange & Pink & Purple, Round, AT-4312	Poly Vitamins, Fluoride 0.5 mg	Poly-Vi-Flor by ATI		Vitamin
AT50 <> G	Tab, White, Round, Scored	Atenolol 50 mg	Tenormin by Genpharm	Canadian DIN 02146894	Antihypertensive
AT600	Tab, White to Off-White, Oval, Film-Coated, Scored, Cobalt Logo <> AT / 600	Azithromycin 600 mg	Zithromax by Cobalt	Canadian DIN 02256088	Antibiotic
ATA <> GEIGY	Tab, Brownish-Red, Round, Sugar Coated	Imipramine HCl 75 mg	Tofranil by Novartis	Canadian DIN 00306487	Antidepressant
ATARAX10	Tab, Orange, Triangular	Hydroxyzine HCl 10 mg	Atarax by Roerig	00049-5600	Antianxiety; Antihistamine
ATARAX100	Tab, Red, Triangular	Hydroxyzine HCl 100 mg	Atarax by Roerig	00049-5630	Antianxiety; Antihistamine
ATARAX25	Tab, Green, Triangular	Hydroxyzine HCl 25 mg	Atarax by Urgent Care Center	50716-0516	Antianxiety; Antihistamine
ATARAX25	Tab, Green, Triangular	Hydroxyzine HCl 25 mg	Atarax by Roerig	00049-5610	Antianxiety; Antihistamine
ATARAX50	Tab, Yellow, Triangular	Hydroxyzine HCl 50 mg	Atarax by Roerig	00049-5620	Antianxiety; Antihistamine
ATASOL	Tab, White, Round, Scored	Acetaminophen 325 mg	Atasol by Church and Dwight	Canadian DIN 00293482	Analgesic
ATASOL <> FORTE	Tab, White, Shield-Shaped, Scored	Acetaminophen 500 mg	Atasol by Church and Dwight	Canadian DIN 00013668	Analgesic

ID FRONT <> BACK	DESCRIPTION FRONT <> BACK	INGREDIENT & STRENGTH	BRAND (or Generic Equiv.) by FIRM	NDC#	CLASS; SCH.
ATASOL15	Tab, Light Yellow, Round, Atasol/15	Acetaminophen 325 mg, Codeine Phosphate 15 mg, Caffeine Citrate 30 mg	Atasol-15 by Church and Dwight	Canadian DIN 00293504	Analgesic; C III
ATASOL30	Tab, Green, Round, Atasol/30	Acetaminophen 325 mg, Codeine Phosphate 30 mg, Caffeine Citrate 30 mg	Atasol by Church and Dwight	Canadian DIN 00293512	Analgesic; C III
ATASOL8	Tab, Light Peach, Round, Atasol/8	Acetaminophen 325 mg, Codeine Phosphate 8 mg, Caffeine Citrate 30 mg	Atasol-8 by Church and Dwight	Canadian DIN 00293490	Analgesic; C III
ATC	Tab, Light Tan, Round, Scored, A over TC	Levothyroxine 9.5 mcg, Liothyronine 2.25 mcg	Armour Thyroid by Forest	00456-0457	Thyroid Hormone
ATC	Tab, Light Tan, Round, Scored, A over TC	Levothyroxine 9.5 mcg, Liothyronine 2.25 mcg	Armour Thyroid by Allscripts		Thyroid Hormone
ATD	Tab, Light Tan, Round, Scored, A/TD	Levothyroxine 19 mcg, Liothyronine 4.5 mcg	Armour Thyroid by Forest	00456-0458	Thyroid Hormone
ATD	Tab, Light Tan, Round, Scored, A/TD	Levothyroxine 19 mcg, Liothyronine 4.5 mcg	Armour Thyroid by Wal Mart	49035-0180	Thyroid Hormone
ATE	Tab, Light Tan, Round, A/TE	Levothyroxine 38 mcg, Liothyronine 9 mcg	Armour Thyroid by Murfreesboro	51129-1635	Thyroid Hormone
ATE	Tab, Light Tan, Round, Scored, A over TE	Levothyroxine 38 mcg, Liothyronine 9 mcg	Armour Thyroid by Amerisource	62584-0459	Thyroid Hormone
ATE	Tab, Light Tan, Round, A/TE	Levothyroxine 38 mcg, Liothyronine 9 mcg	Armour Thyroid by Forest	00456-0459	Thyroid Hormone
ATE	Tab, Light Tan, Round, A/TE	Levothyroxine 38 mcg, Liothyronine 9 mcg	Armour Thyroid by Wal Mart	49035-0181	Thyroid Hormone
ATE100 <> APO	Tab, White, Round, ATE/100	Atenolol 100 mg	Tenormin by Apotex	Canadian DIN 00773697	Antihypertensive
ATE50 <> APO	Tab, White, Round, ATE/50	Atenolol 50 mg	Tenormin by Apotex	Canadian DIN 00773689	Antihypertensive
ATENOLOL <> P100	Tab, White, Round, Scored	Atenolol 100 mg	Tenormin by Pharmascience	Canadian DIN 02237601	Antihypertensive
ATENOLOL <> P50	Tab, White, Round, Scored	Atenolol 50 mg	Tenormin by Pharmascience	Canadian DIN 02237600	Antihypertensive
ATF	Tab, Light Tan, Round, Scored, A over TF	Levothyroxine 76 mcg, Liothyronine 18 mcg	Armour Thyroid by Wal Mart	49035-0182	Thyroid Hormone
ATF	Tab, Light Tan, Round, Scored, A over TF	Levothyroxine 76 mcg, Liothyronine 18 mcg	Armour Thyroid by Forest	00456-0461	Thyroid Hormone
ATG	Tab, Light Tan, Round, Scored, A over TG	Levothyroxine 114 mcg, Liothyronine 27 mcg	Armour Thyroid by Wal Mart	49035-0183	Thyroid Hormone
ATG	Tab, Light Tan, Round, Scored, A over TG	Levothyroxine 114 mcg, Liothyronine 27 mcg	Armour Thyroid by Forest	00456-0462	Thyroid Hormone
ATH	Tab, Light Tan, Round, Scored, A over TH	Levothyroxine 152 mcg, Liothyronine 36 mcg	Armour Thyroid by Forest	00456-0463	Thyroid Hormone
ATI	Tab, Light Tan, Round, Scored, A over TI	Levothyroxine 190 mcg, Liothyronine 45 mcg	Armour Thyroid by Forest	00456-0464	Thyroid Hormone
ATI076	Cap, White	Chlordiazepoxide 5 mg, Clidinium Bromide 2.5 mg	Librax by ATI		Gastrointestinal
ATIVAN <> 1	Tab, White, Oblong, I/Ativan	Lorazepam 1 mg	Ativan by Wyeth	Canadian DIN 02041421	Antianxiety; C IV
ATIVAN <> 2	Tab, White, Oval	Lorazepam 2 mg	Ativan by Wyeth	Canadian DIN 02041448	Antianxiety; C IV
ATJ	Tab, Light Tan, Round, Scored, A over TJ	Levothyroxine 57 mcg, Liothyronine 13.5 mcg	Armour Thyroid by Forest	00456-0460	Thyroid Hormone
ATL <> T	Tab, Blue, _/ Shaped, Scored, Abbott Logo (aTL <> T)	Clorazepate Dipotassium 3.75 mg	Tranxene T-Tab by Ovation		Antianxiety; C IV
ATM <> T	Tab, Peach, _/ Shaped, Scored, Abbott Logo (aTM <> T)	Clorazepate Dipotassium 7.5 mg	Tranxene T-Tab by Med Pro	53978-3079	Antianxiety; C IV
ATN <> T	Tab, Lavender, _/ Shaped, Scored, Abbott Logo (aTN <> T)	Clorazepate Dipotassium 15 mg	Tranxene T-Tab by Ovation		Antianxiety; C IV
ATRAL250MG	Cap	Tetracycline HCl 250 mg	by Quality Care	60346-0609	Antibiotic
ATRAL250MG	Cap, Warner Chilcott	Tetracycline HCl 250 mg	by Pharmedix	53002-0225	Antibiotic
ATRAL250MG	Cap, Light Green	Cephalexin 250 mg	Keflex by Lab A		Antibiotic
ATRAL250MG	Cap, Pink	Amoxicillin 250 mg	Amoxil by Lab A		Antibiotic
ATRAL500MG	Cap, Pink	Amoxicillin 500 mg	Amoxil by Lab A		Antibiotic
ATRAL500MG	Cap, Gray & Orange	Cephalexin 500 mg	Keflex by Lab A		Antibiotic
ATRIANGLE <> ZOVIRAX	Tab, Shield Shaped	Acyclovir 400 mg	Zovirax by DRX	55045-2293	Antiviral
ATROMIDS500	Cap, Dark Orange, White Print	Clofibrate 500 mg	Atromid-S by Ayerst	00046-0243	Antihyperlipidemic
ATT	Tab, Yellow, Round	Tocainide HCl 400 mg	Tonocard by AstraZeneca	Canadian	Antiarrhythmic
AUC	Tab, White, Rectangular, Scored, Abbott Logo (a) over UC	Estazolam 1 mg	ProSom by Abbott	00074-3735	Sedative/Hypnotic; C IV
AUD	Tab, Pink, Rectangular, Scored, Abbott Logo (a) over UD	Estazolam 2 mg	Prosom by Abbott	00074-3736	Sedative/Hypnotic; C IV
AUF	Tab, White, Round, Schering Logo AUF	Griseofulvin 250 mg	Fulvicin P/G by Schering	00085-0948	Antifungal

ID FRONT <> BACK	DESCRIPTION FRONT <> BACK	INGREDIENT & STRENGTH	BRAND (or Generic Equiv.) by FIRM	NDC#	CLASS; SCH.
AUG	Tab, White, Round, Schering Logo	Griseofulvin 500 mg	Fulvicin P/G by Schering	00085-0496	Antifungal
AUGMENTIN <> 250125	Tab, White, Oblong, Film Coated, 250/125	Amoxicillin 250 mg, Clavulanate Potassium 125 mg	Augmentin by Southwood	58016-0107	Antibiotic
AUGMENTIN <> 250125	Tab, White, Oblong, Film Coated, 250/125	Amoxicillin 250 mg, Clavulanate Potassium 125 mg	Augmentin by Casa DeAmigos	62138-6075	Antibiotic
AUGMENTIN <> 250125	Tab, White, Oblong, Film Coated, 250/125	Amoxicillin 250 mg, Clavulanate Potassium 125 mg	Augmentin by Pharmedix	53002-0250	Antibiotic
AUGMENTIN <> 250125	Tab, White, Oblong, Film Coated, 250/125	Amoxicillin 250 mg, Clavulanate Potassium 125 mg	Augmentin by Bayer	00280-1001	Antibiotic
AUGMENTIN <> 250125	Tab, White, Oblong, Film Coated, 250/125	Amoxicillin 250 mg, Clavulanate Potassium 125 mg	Augmentin by SKB	00029-6075	Antibiotic
AUGMENTIN <> 500125	Tab, White, Oblong, Film Coated, 500/125	Amoxicillin 500 mg, Clavulanate Potassium 125 mg	Augmentin by Pharmedix	53002-0239	Antibiotic
AUGMENTIN <> 500125	Tab, White, Oblong, Film Coated, 500/125	Amoxicillin 500 mg, Clavulanate Potassium 125 mg	Augmentin by SKB	00029-6080	Antibiotic
AUGMENTIN <> 500125	Tab, White, Oblong, Film Coated, 500/125	Amoxicillin 500 mg, Clavulanate Potassium 125 mg	Augmentin by H J Harkins Co	52959-0021	Antibiotic
AUGMENTIN <> 500125	Tab, White, Oblong, Film Coated, 500/125	Amoxicillin 500 mg, Clavulanate Potassium 125 mg	Augmentin by Amerisource	62584-0312	Antibiotic
AUGMENTIN <> 500125	Tab, White, Oblong, Film Coated, 500/125	Amoxicillin 500 mg, Clavulanate Potassium 125 mg	Augmentin by Casa DeAmigos	62138-6080	Antibiotic
AUGMENTIN <> 500125	Tab, White, Oblong, Film Coated, 500/125	Amoxicillin 500 mg, Clavulanate Potassium 125 mg	Augmentin by PDRX	55289-0296	Antibiotic
AUGMENTIN <> 500125	Tab, White, Oblong, Film Coated, 500/125	Amoxicillin 500 mg, Clavulanate Potassium 125 mg	Augmentin by Bayer	00280-1011	Antibiotic
AUGMENTIN200	Tab, Pink, Round	Amoxicillin 200 mg, Clavulanate Potassium 28.5	Augmentin by SKB	00029-6071	Antibiotic
AUGMENTIN400	Tab, Pink, Round	Amoxicillin 400 mg, Clavulanate Potassium 57 mg	Augmentin by SKB	00029-6072	Antibiotic
AUGMENTIN875	Tab, White, Oblong, Scored, Film Coated, Augmentin over 875	Amoxicillin 875 mg, Clavulanate Potassium 125 mg	Augmentin by H J Harkins Co	52959-0478	Antibiotic
AUGMENTIN875	Tab, White, Oblong, Scored, Film Coated, Augmentin over 875	Amoxicillin 875 mg, Clavulanate Potassium 125 mg	Augmentin by Bayer	00280-1091	Antibiotic
AUGMENTIN875	Tab, White, Oblong, Scored, Film Coated, Augmentin over 875	Amoxicillin 875 mg, Clavulanate Potassium 125 mg	Augmentin by SKB	00029-6086	Antibiotic
AUGMENTINXR	Tab, White, Oval, Film Coated, AC 1000 over 62.5	Amoxicillin 1000 mg, Clavulanic Acid 62.5 mg	Augmentin XR by GSK	00029-6096	Antibiotic
AVENTYLH17	Cap, White and Yellow, Opaque	Nortriptyline 10 mg	Aventyl by Pharmascience	Canadian DIN 00015229	Antidepressant
AVENTYLH19	Cap, White and Yellow, Opaque	Nortriptyline 25 mg	Aventyl by Pharmascience	Canadian DIN 00015237	Antidepressant
AVINZA120MG508	Cap, Blue-Violet & White, AVINZA on cap, 120MG508 on body, Extended Release	Morphine Sulfate 120 mg	Avinza by King	60793-0608	Analgesic; C II
AVINZA30MG505	Cap, Yellow & White, AVINZA imprinted on cap and 30MG505 on body, Extended Release	Morphine Sulfate 30 mg	Avinza by King	60793-0605	Analgesic; C II
AVINZA60MG506	Cap, Blue & White, AVINZA on cap, 60MG506 on body, Extended Release	Morphine Sulfate 60 mg	Avinza by King	60793-0606	Analgesic; C II
AVINZA90MG507	Cap, Red & White, AVINZA on cap, 90MG507 on body, Extended Release	Morphine Sulfate 90 mg	Avinza by King	60793-0607	Analgesic; C II
AX <> 3438	Tab, White, Round, Mottled, Apotex Logo	Selegiline HCl 5 mg	Selegiline HCl by SB	59742-3160	Antiparkinson
AX3438	Tab, White, Round	Selegiline 5 mg	Eldepryl by Caraco		Antiparkinson
AXID300MGLILLY3145	Cap, Brown & Pale Yellow, Black Print, Opaque	Nizatidine 300 mg	Axid by Eli Lilly	00002-3145	Gastrointestinal
AXID3144AXID150MG	Cap, Yellow and Light Yellow, Opaque	Nizatidine 150 mg	Axid by Pharmascience	Canadian DIN 00778338	Gastrointestinal
AXID3145AXID300MG	Cap, Orange and Light Yellow, Opaque	Nizatidine 300 mg	Axid by Pharmascience	Canadian DIN 00778346	Gastrointestinal
AYC	Tab, Violet & White, Round	Levothyroxine 12.5 mcg, Liothyronine 3.1 mcg	Thyrolar by Forest	00456-0040	Thyroid Hormone
AYD	Tab, Peach & White, Round	Levothyroxine 25 mcg, Liothyronine 6.25 mcg	Thyrolar by Forest	00456-0045	Thyroid Hormone
AYE	Tab, Pink & White, Round	Levothyroxine 50 mcg, Liothyronine 12.5 mcg	Thyrolar by Forest	00456-0050	Thyroid Hormone
AYERST	Tab, White, Round	Magaldrate 480 mg	Riopan by Whitehall Robins		Gastrointestinal
AYERST	Tab, Blue	Metoclopramide 10 mg	Reglan by Wyeth	Canadian	Gastrointestinal
AYERST	Tab, Orange	Fenfluramine HCl 20 mg	Pondimin by Wyeth	Canadian	Anorexiant; C IV
AYERST	Tab, Pink	Glycopyrrolate 2 mg	Robinul Forte by Wyeth	Canadian	Gastrointestinal
AYERST	Tab, Pink	Glycopyrrolate 1 mg	Robinul by Wyeth	Canadian	Gastrointestinal
AYERST	Cap, Green & White	Aspirin 325 mg, Phenobarbital 16.2 mg, Codeine Phosphate 64.8 mg	Phenaphen by Wyeth	Canadian	Analgesic; C III

ID FRONT <> BACK	DESCRIPTION FRONT <> BACK	INGREDIENT & STRENGTH	BRAND (or Generic Equiv.) by FIRM	NDC#	CLASS; SCH.
AYERST	Cap, Black & Green	Aspirin 325 mg, Phenobarbital 16.2 mg, Codeine Phosphate 32.4 mg	Phenaphen by Wyeth	Canadian	Analgesic; C III
AYERST	Tab, Orange, Oblong	B Complex Vitamin	Beminal by Whitehall Robins		Vitamin
AYERST	Cap, Red	Clofibrate 1 g	Atromid-S by Wyeth	Canadian Discontinued	Antihyperlipidemic
AYERST	Cap, Orange	Clofibrate 500 mg	Atromid-S by Wyeth	Canadian Discontinued	Antihyperlipidemic
AYERST	Tab, White, Round, Scored	Dapsone 100 mg	Avlosulfon by Wyeth	Canadian Discontinued	Antimycobacterial
AYERST	Tab, White, Round	Primidone 250 mg	by Wyeth	Canadian	Anticonvulsant
AYERST250	Tab, Caramel & Red	Amoxicillin 250 mg	Amoxil by Ayerst		Antibiotic
AYERST252	Cap, Black	Vitamin Combination	Mediatric by Ayerst		Vitamin; C III
AYERST500	Cap, Caramel & Red	Amoxicillin 500 mg	Amoxil by Ayerst		Antibiotic
AYERST5REGLAN	Tab, Blue, Oblong, Ayerst 5/Reglan	Metoclopramide 5 mg	Reglan by Wyeth	Canadian	Gastrointestinal
AYERST752	Tab, Orange, Oblong	Vitamin Combination	Mediatric by Ayerst		Vitamin; C III
AYERST783	Tab, Yellow, Round	Sulfamethizole 500 mg, Phenazopyridine 50 mg	Thiosulfil-A Forte by Ayerst		Antibiotic; Urinary Analgesic
AYERST784	Tab, Red, Round	Sulfamethizole 250 mg, Phenazopyridine 50 mg	Thiosulfil-A by Ayerst		Antibiotic; Urinary Analgesic
AYERST786	Tab, White, Oval	Sulfamethizole 500 mg	Thiosulfil Forte by Ayerst		Antibiotic
AYERST878	Tab, Maroon, Round	Conjugated Estrogens 0.625 mg, Methyltestosterone 5 mg	Premarin w Methyltes by Ayerst		Hormone
AYERST879	Tab, Yellow, Round	Conjugated Estrogens 1.25 mg, Methyltestosterone 10 mg	Premarin w Methyltes by Ayerst		Hormone
AYERST880	Tab, Green, Oblong	Conjugated Estrogens 0.45 mg, Meprobamate 200 mg	PMB 200 by Ayerst		Hormone
AYERST881	Tab, Pink, Oblong	Conjugated Estrogens 0.45 mg, Meprobamate 400 mg	PMB 400 by Ayerst		Hormone
AYERSTMICROK	Cap, Orange, Ayerst/Micro-K	Potassium Chloride 600 mg	by Key	Canadian	Electrolytes
AYERSTMICROK10	Cap, Orange & White, Ayerst/Micro-K-10	Potassium Chloride 750 mg	by Key	Canadian	Electrolytes
AYF	Tab, Green & White, Round	Levothyroxine 100 mcg, Liothyronine 25 mcg	Thyrolar by Forest	00456-0055	Thyroid Hormone
AYGESTIN	Tab, White, Oval	Norethindrone Acetate 5 mg	by ESI Lederle		Hormone
AYH	Tab, White & Yellow, Round	Levothyroxine 150 mcg, Liothyronine 37.5 mcg	Thyrolar by Forest	00456-0060	Thyroid Hormone
AZ	Tab, Yellow, Round, Scored	Azathioprine 50 mg	Imuran by Genpharm	55567-0084	Immunosuppressant
AZ	Tab, Yellow, Round, Scored	Azathioprine 50 mg	Imuran by Mylan	00378-1005	Immunosuppressant
AZ	Tab, Yellow, Round, Scored	Azathioprine 50 mg	Imuran by Sandoz	00781-5075	Immunosuppressant
AZ	Tab, Yellow, Round, Scored	Azathioprine 50 mg	Imuran by UDL	51079-0620	Immunosuppressant
AZ010	Tab, White, Round	Acetaminophen 325 mg	Tylenol by URL	00677-1974	Analgesic
AZ012	Tab, White, Oblong	Acetaminophen 500 mg	Tylenol by A & Z Pharma		Analgesic
AZ036	Tab, White, Round	Calcium Carbonate 420 mg	Tums by Edwards Medical Supply		Antacid
AZ10 <> 891	Tab, Oyster, Round, Film Coated, Ex Release	Nisoldipine 10 mg	Sular by AstraZeneca	00310-0891	Antihypertensive
AZ20 <> 892	Tab, Yellow Cream, Round, Film Coated, Ex Release	Nisoldipine 20 mg	Sular by AstraZeneca	00310-0892	Antihypertensive
AZ234	Tab, White, Round, AZ over 234	Acetaminophen 325 mg	Tylenol by A & Z Pharma		Analgesic
AZ250 <> APO	Tab, Dark Pink, Oval, Film Coated	Azithromycin 250 mg	Zithromax by Apotex	Canadian DIN 02247423	Antibiotic
AZ261	Tab, White, Round	Acetaminophen 500 mg, Phenylephrine 5 mg	by A & Z Pharma		Cold Remedy
AZ30 <> 893	Tab, Mustard, Round, Film Coated, Ex Release	Nisoldipine 30 mg	Sular by AstraZeneca	00310-0893	Antihypertensive
AZ40 <> 894	Tab, Burnt Orange, Round, Film Coated, Ex Release	Nisoldipine 40 mg	Sular by AstraZeneca	00310-0894	Antihypertensive
AZ50 <> APO	Tab, Pale Yellow, Peanut Shaped, Scored	Azathioprine 50 mg	Imuran by Apotex	Canadian DIN 02242907	Immunosuppressant
AZA	Cap, Gray, Oval, Soft Gel	Paricalcitol 1 mcg	Zemplar by Abbott	00074-4317	Thyroid
AZF	Cap, Orange-Brown, Oval, Soft Gel	Paricalcitol 2 mcg	Zemplar by Abbott	00074-4314	Thyroid

ID FRONT <> BACK	DESCRIPTION FRONT <> BACK	INGREDIENT & STRENGTH	BRAND (or Generic Equiv.) by FIRM	NDC#	CLASS; SCH.
AZK	Cap, Gold, Oval, Soft Gel	Paricalcitol 4 mcg	Zemplar by Abbott	00074-4315	Thyroid
AZL <> 600	Tab, White, Oval, Scored, Film Coated, Abbott Logo (a)	Zileuton 600 mg	Zyflo by Abbott	00074-8036	Antiasthmatic
B	Tab, Orange, Round	Ascorbic Acid 200 mg, Natural Citrus Bioflavonoid Complex Hesperidin Complex 150 mg, Hesperidin Methyl Chalcone 50 mg	Peridin-C by Beutlich	00283-0597	Dietary Supplement
B	Tab, Orange, Cap Shaped, Enteric Coated	Aspirin 650 mg	Aspirin Arthritis by Bayer	Canadian DIN 02237900	Analgesic
B	Tab, White, Cap-Shaped, Bi-Layer	Aspirin 325 mg	Bufferin by BMS	Canadian DIN 01990667	Analgesic
B	Tab, White, Oval, Lower Case "b"	Aspirin 81 mg	Pravigard PAC by BMS		Analgesic
B	Tab, White, Round	Aspirin 325 mg	Pravigard PAC by BMS		Analgesic
B	Tab, Beveled Edge, Debossed	Isosorbide Dinitrate 2.5 mg	Isordil by Barr	00555-0172	Antianginal
B	Cap, Light Yellow, Round, Soft Gel	Benzonatate 200 mg	Tessalon by Zydus	68382-0248	Antitussive
B	Cap, Light Yellow, Soft Gelatin	Benzonatate 200 mg	Tessalon by Blu	00406-2248	Antitussive
B <> 066100	Tab, White to Off-White, Round, Scored, 066 over 100	Isoniazid 100 mg	Laniazid by UDL	51079-0082 Discontinued	Antimycobacterial
B <> 066100	Tab, White to Off-White, Round, Scored, 066 over 100	Isoniazid 100 mg	Laniazid by Barr	00555-0066	Antimycobacterial
B <> 071300	Tab, White to Off-White, Oval, Scored, 071 over 300	Isoniazid 300 mg	Laniazid by Barr	00555-0071	Antimycobacterial
B <> 071300	Tab, White to Off-White, Oval, Scored, 071 over 300	Isoniazid 300 mg	Laniazid by UDL	51079-0083	Antimycobacterial
B <> 107	Tab, White, Oblong, b <> 107, Extended Release	Metformin HCl 750 mg	Glucophage XR by Barr	00555-0107 Discontinued	Antidiabetic
B <> 11	Tab, Light Green, Round, Film Coated	Inert	Tri-Levlen 28 by Berlex	50419-0111	Oral Contraceptive; Placebo
B <> 120	Tab, White, Cap Shaped, Ex Release	Diltiazem HCl 120 mg	Cardizem LA by Biovail	64455-0100	Antihypertensive
B <> 120	Tab, White, Cap Shaped, Ex Release	Diltiazem HCl 120 mg	Tiazac XC by Biovail	Canadian DIN 02256738	Antihypertensive
B <> 14	Tab, Light Yellow, Round, b <> 14	Ethinyl Estradiol 35 mcg, Ethynodiol Diacetate 1 mg	Demulen by Barr	00555-9064	Oral Contraceptive
B <> 143	Tab, White, Round	Inert	Demulen by Barr	00555-9064	Oral Contraceptive; Placebo
B <> 143	Tab, White, Round	Inert	Tri-Sprintec by Barr	00555-9018	Oral Contraceptive; Placebo
B <> 143	Tab, White, Round	Inert	Sprintec by Barr	00555-9016	Oral Contraceptive; Placebo
B <> 180	Tab, White, Cap Shaped, Ex Release	Diltiazem HCl 180 mg	Cardizem LA by Biovail	64455-0101	Antihypertensive
B <> 180	Tab, White, Cap Shaped, Ex Release	Diltiazem HCl 180 mg	Tiazac XC by Biovail	Canadian DIN 02256746	Antihypertensive
B <> 20110	Tab, Beige, Oval, Scored, Film Coated	Fluoxetine HCl 10 mg	Prozac by Barr	00555-0201	Antidepressant
B <> 208	Tab, White, Round	Inert	Levlite by Barr	00555-9014	Oral Contraceptive; Placebo
B <> 208	Tab, White, Round	Inert	Portia by Barr	00555-9020	Oral Contraceptive; Placebo
B <> 208	Tab, White, Round	Inert	Jolessa by Barr	00555-9123	Oral Contraceptive; Placebo
B <> 208	Tab, White, Round	Inert	Tri-Lo-Sprintec by Barr	00555-9065	Oral Contraceptive; Placebo
B <> 208	Tab, White, Round, Stylized b	Inert	Gianvi by Teva Pharmaceuticals	00093-5661	Oral Contraceptive; Placebo
B <> 21	Tab, Light Orange, Round	Ethinyl Estradiol 0.03 mg, Levonorgestrel 0.15 mg	Levlen 28 by Berlex	50419-0411	Oral Contraceptive
B <> 21	Tab, Light Orange, Round	Ethinyl Estradiol 0.03 mg, Levonorgestrel 0.15 mg	Levlen 21 by Berlex	50419-0410	Oral Contraceptive
B <> 2115	Tab, White, Oval, Scored	Norethindrone Acetate 5 mg	Aygestin by Barr	00555-0211	Hormone
B <> 22	Tab, Pink, Round	Ethinyl Estradiol 0.02 mg, Levonorgestrel 0.1 mg	Levlite by Schering	64259-1165	Oral Contraceptive
B <> 22	Tab, Pink, Round, Coated	Ethinyl Estradiol 0.02 mg, Levonorgestrel 0.1 mg	Levlite 28 by Berlex	50419-0022	Oral Contraceptive

ID FRONT <> BACK	DESCRIPTION FRONT <> BACK	INGREDIENT & STRENGTH	BRAND (or Generic Equiv.) by FIRM	NDC#	CLASS; SCH.
B <> 22	Tab, Sugar Coated	Ethinyl Estradiol 0.02 mg, Levonorgestrel 0.1 mg	Levlite by Schering	12866-1163	Oral Contraceptive
B <> 240	Tab, White, Cap Shaped, Ex Release	Diltiazem HCl 240 mg	Cardizem LA by Biovail	64455-0102	Antihypertensive
B <> 240	Tab, White, Cap Shaped, Ex Release	Diltiazem HCl 240 mg	Tiazac XC by Biovail	Canadian DIN 02256754	Antihypertensive
B <> 247	Tab, Brown, Round	Ferrous Fumarate	Junel 1/20 Fe by Barr	00555-9026	Oral Contraceptive; Placebo
B <> 247	Tab, Brown, Round	Ferrous Fumarate	Junel 1.5/30 Fe by Barr	00555-9028	Oral Contraceptive; Placebo
B <> 25	Tab, Bright Pink, Cap Shaped	Diphenhydramine HCl 25 mg	Benadryl by Warner Lambert	00501-2002	Antihistamine
B <> 252	Tab, White, Round	Dipyridamole 25 mg	Persantine by Major	00904-1086	Antiplatelet
B <> 252	Tab, White, Round, Film Coated	Dipyridamole 25 mg	Persantine by Kaiser	00179-1153	Antiplatelet
B <> 252	Tab, White, Round, Film Coated	Dipyridamole 25 mg	Persantine by Qualitest	00603-3383	Antiplatelet
B <> 252	Tab, White, Round, Film Coated	Dipyridamole 25 mg	Persantine by Genpharm	55567-0088	Antiplatelet
B <> 252	Tab, White, Round, Film Coated	Dipyridamole 25 mg	Persantine by Schein	00364-2491	Antiplatelet
B <> 252	Tab, White, Round, Film Coated	Dipyridamole 25 mg	Persantine by Barr	00555-0252	Antiplatelet
B <> 252	Tab, White, Round, Film Coated	Dipyridamole 25 mg	Persantine by Ivax	00182-1568	Antiplatelet
B <> 252	Tab, White, Round, Film Coated	Dipyridamole 25 mg	Persantine by UDL	51079-0068	Antiplatelet
B <> 252	Tab, White, Round, Film Coated	Dipyridamole 25 mg	Persantine by Sandoz	00781-1890	Antiplatelet
B <> 252	Tab, White, Round, Film Coated	Dipyridamole 25 mg	Persantine by Heartland	61392-0549	Antiplatelet
B <> 257	Tab, Pink, Round, Film Coated, Stylized b	Drospirenone 3 mg, Ethinyl Estradiol 0.02 mg	Gianvi by Teva Pharmaceuticals	00093-5661	Oral Contraceptive
B <> 28	Tab, Orange, Round	Levonorgestrel 0.10 mg, Ethinyl Estradiol 0.02 mg	Lo Seasonique by Duramed	51285-0092	Oral Contraceptive
B <> 28	Tab, Pink, Round	Inert	Levlen 28 by Berlex	50419-0028	Oral Contraceptive; Placebo
B <> 28	Tab, Light Pink, Round	Inert	Levlen 28 by Berlex	50419-0411	Oral Contraceptive; Placebo
B <> 285	Tab, White, Round	Dipyridamole 50 mg	Persantine by Major	00904-1087	Antiplatelet
B <> 285	Tab, White, Round, Film Coated	Dipyridamole 50 mg	Persantine by Barr	00555-0285	Antiplatelet
B <> 285	Tab, White, Round, Film Coated	Dipyridamole 50 mg	Persantine by Ivax	00182-1569	Antiplatelet
B <> 285	Tab, White, Round, Film Coated	Dipyridamole 50 mg	Persantine by UDL	51079-0069 Discontinued	Antiplatelet
B <> 29	Tab, White, Round, Coated	Inert	Levlite 28 by Berlex	50419-0029	Oral Contraceptive; Placebo
B <> 30	Tab, Yellow, Round, Extended Release	Nifedipine 30 mg	Adalat CC by Teva	00093-5272	Antihypertensive
B <> 30	Tab, Yellow, Round, Extended Release	Nifedipine 30 mg	Adalat CC by Ivax	00182-8232 Discontinued	Antihypertensive
B <> 30	Tab, Reddish Brown, Round, Film Coated, Ex Release	Nifedical 30 mg	Procardia XL by Teva	00093-0819	Antihypertensive
B <> 300	Tab, White, Cap Shaped, Ex Release	Diltiazem HCl 300 mg	Tiazac XC by Biovail	Canadian DIN 02256762	Antihypertensive
B <> 300	Tab, White, Cap Shaped, Ex Release	Diltiazem HCl 300 mg	Cardizem LA by Biovail	64455-0103	Antihypertensive
B <> 332	Tab, Round, Orange, Coated	Desogestrel 0.125 mg, Ethinyl Estradiol 0.025 mg	Velivet by Barr	00555-9051	Oral Contraceptive
B <> 333	Tab, Round, Beige, Coated	Desogestrel 0.1 mg, Ethinyl Estradiol 0.025 mg	Velivet by Barr	00555-9051	Oral Contraceptive
B <> 334	Tab, Round, White	Inert	Velivet by Barr	00555-9051	Oral Contraceptive; Placebo
B <> 335	Tab, Round, Pink, Coated	Desogestrel 0.15 mg, Ethinyl Estradiol 0.025 mg	Velivet by Barr	00555-9051	Oral Contraceptive
B <> 34	Tab, White, Round, Film Coated, Stylized b	Estradiol 1 mg, Norethindrone Acetate 0.5 mg	Mimvey by Teva Pharmaceuticals	00093-5455	Hormone
B <> 341	Tab, Light Yellow, Round	Norethindrone 0.5 mg, Ethinyl Estradiol 0.035 mg	Aranelle by Barr	00555-9066	Oral Contraceptive
B <> 342	Tab, White, Round	Norethindrone 1 mg, Ethinyl Estradiol 0.035 mg	Aranelle by Barr	00555-9066	Oral Contraceptive
B <> 343	Tab, Peach, Round	Inert	Aranelle by Barr	00555-9066	Oral Contraceptive; Placebo
B <> 344	Tab, Yellow, Round	Norethindrone 0.35 mg	Errin by Barr	00555-0344	Oral Contraceptive
B <> 345	Tab, Off White, Round, Film Coated, Biconvex	Lithium Carbonate 300 mg	Lithobid by Barr	00555-0345	Antipsychotic

ID FRONT <> BACK	DESCRIPTION FRONT <> BACK	INGREDIENT & STRENGTH	BRAND (or Generic Equiv.) by FIRM	NDC#	CLASS; SCH.
B <> 360	Tab, White, Cap Shaped, Ex Release	Diltiazem HCl 360 mg	Cardizem LA by Biovail	64455-0104	Antihypertensive
B <> 360	Tab, White, Cap Shaped, Ex Release	Diltiazem HCl 360 mg	Tiazac XC by Biovail	Canadian DIN 02256770	Antihypertensive
B <> 40	Tab, White, Round, Film Coated, Heart Outline around B	Bisoprolol 10 mg, Hydrochlorothiazide 6.25 mg	Ziac by Duramed	51285-0040	Antihypertensive; Diuretic
B <> 420	Tab, White, Cap Shaped, Ex Release	Diltiazem HCl 420 mg	Cardizem LA by Biovail	64455-0105	Antihypertensive
B <> 451	Tab, Gray, Round, Film Coated	Norgestimate 0.18 mg, Ethinyl Estradiol 0.025 mg	Tri-Lo-Sprintec by Barr	00555-9065	Oral Contraceptive
B <> 452	Tab, Light Blue, Round, Film Coated	Norgestimate 0.215 mg, Ethinyl Estradiol 0.025 mg	Tri-Lo-Sprintec by Barr	00555-9065	Oral Contraceptive
B <> 453	Tab, Blue, Round, Film Coated	Norgestimate 0.25 mg, Ethinyl Estradiol 0.025 mg	Tri-Lo-Sprintec by Barr	00555-9065	Oral Contraceptive
B <> 484	Tab, White, Round	Leucovorin Calcium 5 mg	Wellcovorin by Major	00904-2315	Antineoplastic
B <> 484	Tab, White, Round	Leucovorin Calcium 5 mg	Wellcovorin by Qualitest	00603-4183	Antineoplastic
B <> 484	Tab, White, Round	Leucovorin Calcium 5 mg	Wellcovorin by Supergen	62701-0900	Antineoplastic
B <> 484	Tab, White, Round	Leucovorin Calcium 5 mg	Wellcovorin by Barr	00555-0484	Antineoplastic
B <> 484	Tab, White, Round	Leucovorin Calcium 5 mg	Wellcovorin by UDL	51079-0581	Antineoplastic
B <> 485	Tab, Pale Green, Round	Leucovorin Calcium 25 mg	Wellcovorin by Supergen	62701-0901	Antineoplastic
B <> 485	Tab, Pale Green, Round	Leucovorin Calcium 25 mg	Wellcovorin by Qualitest	00603-4184	Antineoplastic
B <> 485	Tab, Pale Green, Round	Leucovorin Calcium 25 mg	Wellcovorin by UDL	51079-0582	Antineoplastic
B <> 485	Tab, Pale Green, Round	Leucovorin Calcium 25 mg	Wellcovorin by Barr	00555-0485	Antineoplastic
B <> 50	Tab, Pink, Round, Film Coated, Heart Outline around B	Bisoprolol 5 mg, Hydrochlorothiazide 6.25 mg	Ziac by Duramed	51285-0050	Antihypertensive; Diuretic
B <> 50	Tab, White, Cap Shaped, Film Coated	Diphenhydramine HCl 50 mg	Benadryl by Pfizer	Canadian DIN 02239138	Antihistamine
B <> 50902	Tab, Beige, Round, Scored, Film Coated, 50 over 902	Naltrexone HCl 50 mg	ReVia by Barr	00555-0902	Opioid Antagonist
B <> 555	Tab, Light Blue-Green, Round, Film Coated	Levonorgestrel 0.15 mg, Ethinyl Estradiol 0.03 mg	Seasonique by Duramed	51285-0087	Oral Contraceptive
B <> 555606	Tab, White, Round, Scored, 555 over 606	Megestrol Acetate 20 mg	Megace by Major	00904-3570	Hormone
B <> 555606	Tab, White, Round, Scored, 555 over 606	Megestrol Acetate 20 mg	Megace by UDL	51079-0434	Hormone
B <> 555606	Tab, White, Round, Scored, 555 over 606	Megestrol Acetate 20 mg	Megace by Barr	00555-0606	Hormone
B <> 555779	Tab, White, Round, Scored, 555 over 779	Medroxyprogesterone Acetate 10 mg	Provera by Major	00904-2690	Hormone
B <> 555779	Tab, White, Round, Scored, 555 over 779	Medroxyprogesterone Acetate 10 mg	Provera by Qualitest	00603-4367	Hormone
B <> 555779	Tab, White, Round, Scored, 555 over 779	Medroxyprogesterone Acetate 10 mg	Provera by URL Mutual	00677-1619	Hormone
B <> 555779	Tab, White, Round, Scored, 555 over 779	Medroxyprogesterone Acetate 10 mg	Provera by Barr	00555-0779	Hormone
B <> 555779	Tab, White, Round, Scored, 555 over 779	Medroxyprogesterone Acetate 10 mg	Provera by Nat Pharmpak	55154-5575	Hormone
B <> 555872	Tab, White, Round, Scored, 555 over 872	Medroxyprogesterone Acetate 2.5 mg	Provera by Nat Pharmpak	55154-5569	Hormone
B <> 555872	Tab, White, Round, Scored, 555 over 872	Medroxyprogesterone Acetate 2.5 mg	Provera by Southwood	58016-0374	Hormone
B <> 555872	Tab, White, Round, Scored, 555 over 872	Medroxyprogesterone Acetate 2.5 mg	Provera by Major	00904-5227	Hormone
B <> 555872	Tab, White, Round, Scored, 555 over 872	Medroxyprogesterone Acetate 2.5 mg	Provera by Barr	00555-0872	Hormone
B <> 555872	Tab, White, Round, Scored, 555 over 872	Medroxyprogesterone Acetate 2.5 mg	Provera by Murfreesboro	51129-1373	Hormone
B <> 555872	Tab, White, Round, Scored, 555 over 872	Medroxyprogesterone Acetate 2.5 mg	Provera by Qualitest	00603-4365	Hormone
B <> 555873	Tab, White, Round, Scored, 555 over 873	Medroxyprogesterone Acetate 5 mg	Provera by URL Mutual	00677-1617	Hormone
B <> 555873	Tab, White, Round, Scored, 555 over 873	Medroxyprogesterone Acetate 5 mg	Provera by URL Mutual	00677-1618	Hormone
B <> 555873	Tab, White, Round, Scored, 555 over 873	Medroxyprogesterone Acetate 5 mg	Provera by Qualitest	00603-4366	Hormone
B <> 555873	Tab, White, Round, Scored, 555 over 873	Medroxyprogesterone Acetate 5 mg	Provera by Barr	00555-0873	Hormone
B <> 555873	Tab, White, Round, Scored, 555 over 873	Medroxyprogesterone Acetate 5 mg	Provera by Major	00904-5228	Hormone
B <> 555873	Tab, White, Round, Scored, 555 over 873	Medroxyprogesterone Acetate 5 mg	Provera by Nat Pharmpak	55154-5571	Hormone
B <> 556	Tab, Yellow, Round, Film Coated	Ethinyl Estradiol 0.01 mg	Seasonique by Duramed	51285-0087	Oral Contraceptive
B <> 556	Tab, Yellow, Round	Ethinyl Estradiol 0.01 mg	Lo Seasonique by Duramed	51285-0092	Oral Contraceptive
B <> 572	Tab, Coated	Methotrexate 2.5 mg	Rheumatrex by Qualitest	00603-4499	Antineoplastic
B <> 6	Tab, White to Off-White, Round	Vitamin B6 25 mg	CitraNatal B-Calm by Mission	00178-0866	Vitamin; Supplement
B <> 60	Tab, Yellow, Round, Ex Release	Nifedipine 60 mg	Adalat CC by Ivax	00182-8233 Discontinued	Antihypertensive
B <> 60	Tab, Yellow, Round, Ex Release	Nifedipine 60 mg	Adalat CC by Teva	00093-1022	Antihypertensive
B <> 60	Tab, Reddish Brown, Round, Film Coated, Ex Release	Nifedical 60 mg	Procardia XL by Teva	00093-5173	Antihypertensive

ID FRONT <> BACK	DESCRIPTION FRONT <> BACK	INGREDIENT & STRENGTH	BRAND (or Generic Equiv.) by FIRM	NDC#	CLASS; SCH.
B <> 715	Tab, Light Pink, Round	Norethindrone 0.35 mg	Camilla by Barr	00555-0715	Oral Contraceptive
B <> 728	Tab, Yellow, Round, Film Coated	Doxycycline 50 mg	Adoxa by Bradley	62436-0728	Antibiotic
B <> 728	Tab, Yellow, Round, Film Coated	Doxycycline 50 mg	Adoxa by Doak	10337-0800	Antibiotic
B <> 729	Tab, Yellow, Round, Film Coated	Doxycycline 100 mg	Adoxa by Doak	10337-0802	Antibiotic
B <> 729	Tab, Yellow, Round, Film Coated	Doxycycline 100 mg	Adoxa by Bradley	62436-0729	Antibiotic
B <> 730	Tab, Light Orange, Round, Film Coated	Doxycycline 75 mg	Adoxa by Doak	10337-0801	Antibiotic
B <> 730	Tab, Light Orange, Round, Film Coated	Doxycycline 75 mg	Adoxa by Bradley	62436-0730	Antibiotic
b <> 798	Tab, White, Oval, Stylized b, Sublingual	Buprenorphine HCl 2 mg	Subutex by Teva Pharmaceuticals	00093-5378	Detoxification Agent; C III
b <> 799	Tab, White, Oval, Stylized b, Sublingual	Buprenorphine HCl 8 mg	Subutex by Teva Pharmaceuticals	00093-5379	Detoxification Agent; C III
B <> 859	Tab, White to Off-White, Round	Flecainide Acetate 50 mg	Tambocor by Barr	00555-0859	Antiarrhythmic
B <> 860100	Tab, White to Off-White, Oval, Scored, 860 over 100	Flecainide Acetate 100 mg	Tambocor by Barr	00555-0860	Antiarrhythmic
B <> 861150	Tab, White to Off-White, Oval, Scored	Flecainide Acetate 150 mg	Tambocor by Barr	00555-0861	Antiarrhythmic
B <> 8861	Tab, Light Purple, Oval, Scored, 886 over 1	Estradiol 1 mg	Estrace by Halsey	00904-5442	Hormone
B <> 8861	Tab, Light Purple, Oval, Scored, 886 over 1	Estradiol 1 mg	Estrace by Barr	00555-0886	Hormone
B <> 8861	Tab, Light Purple, Oval, Scored, 886 over 1	Estradiol 1 mg	Estrace by DRX	55045-2739	Hormone
B <> 8872	Tab, Green, Oval, Scored, 887 over 2	Estradiol 2 mg	Estrace by Barr	00555-0887	Hormone
B <> 8872	Tab, Green, Oval, Scored, 887 over 2	Estradiol 2 mg	Estrace by Halsey	00904-7738	Hormone
B <> 89912	Tab, White to Off-White, Oval, Scored, 899 over 1/2	Estradiol 0.5 mg	Estrace by Barr	00555-0899	Hormone
B <> 90	Tab, Yellow, Round, Ex Release	Nifedipine 90 mg	Adalat CC by Teva	00093-1023	Antihypertensive
B <> 90	Tab, Yellow, Round, Ex Release	Nifedipine 90 mg	Adalat CC by Ivax	00182-8234 Discontinued	Antihypertensive
B <> 917200	Tab, White, Round, Scored, b <> 917 over 200	Amiodarone 200 mg	Cordarone by Barr	00555-0917 Discontinued	Antiarrhythmic
B <> 923400	Tab, White, Oval, Scored, Film Coated, 923 over 400	Ethambutol HCl 400 mg	Myambutol by Barr	00555-0923	Antituberculosis
B <> 9275	Tab, Green, Oval, Scored, Film Coated, b <> 927/5	Methotrexate 5 mg	Trexall by Barr	00555-0927	Antineoplastic
B <> 928712	Tab, Blue, Oval, Scored, Film Coated, b <> 928/7 1/2	Methotrexate 7.5 mg	Trexall by Barr	00555-0928	Antineoplastic
B <> 92910	Tab, Pink, Oval, Scored, Film Coated, b <> 929/10	Methotrexate 10 mg	Trexall by Barr	00555-0929	Antineoplastic
B <> 941	Tab, Light Yellow, Round	Norethindrone 0.5 mg, Ethinyl Estradiol 0.035 mg	Modicon by Barr	00555-9008	Oral Contraceptive
B <> 942	Tab, Blue, Round	Norethindrone 0.75 mg, Ethinyl Estradiol 0.035 mg	Ortho-Novum by Barr	00555-9012	Oral Contraceptive
B <> 943	Tab, Blue, Round	Norethindrone 1 mg, Ethinyl Estradiol 0.035 mg	Ortho-Novum by Barr	00555-9012	Oral Contraceptive
B <> 944	Tab, White, Round	Inert	Ortho-Novum by Barr	00555-9012	Oral Contraceptive; Placebo
B <> 944	Tab, White, Round	Inert	Ortho-Novum by Barr	00555-9010	Oral Contraceptive; Placebo
B <> 944	Tab, White, Round	Inert	Modicon by Barr	00555-9008	Oral Contraceptive; Placebo
B <> 94515	Tab, Purple, Oval, Scored, Film Coated, b <> 945/15	Methotrexate 15 mg	Trexall by Barr	00555-0945	Antineoplastic
B <> 949	Tab, Yellow, Round	Norethindrone 1 mg, Ethinyl Estradiol 0.035 mg	Ortho-Novum by Barr	00555-9009	Oral Contraceptive
B <> 949	Tab, Yellow, Round	Norethindrone 1 mg, Ethinyl Estradiol 0.035 mg	Ortho-Novum by Barr	00555-9010	Oral Contraceptive
B <> 95	Tab, Brown, Round, Film Coated	Ethinyl Estradiol 0.03 mg, Levonorgestrel 0.05 mg	Tri-Levlen by Nat Pharmpak	55154-0304	Oral Contraceptive
B <> 95	Tab, Brown, Round, Film Coated	Ethinyl Estradiol 0.03 mg, Levonorgestrel 0.05 mg	Tri-Levlen by Pharm Util	60491-0653	Oral Contraceptive
B <> 95	Tab, Brown, Round, Film Coated	Ethinyl Estradiol 0.03 mg, Levonorgestrel 0.05 mg	Tri-Levlen by Berlex	50419-0195	Oral Contraceptive
B <> 951	Tab, Light Yellow, Round	Norethindrone 0.5 mg, Ethinyl Estradiol 0.035 mg	Ortho-Novum by Barr	00555-9012	Oral Contraceptive
B <> 9525	Tab, Peach, Round, Scored, 952 over 5	Dextroamphetamine Sulfate 5 mg	Dexedrine by Barr	00555-0952	Stimulant; C II
B <> 95310	Tab, Pink, Round, Scored, 953 over 10	Dextroamphetamine Sulfate 10 mg	Dexedrine by Barr	00555-0953	Stimulant; C II
B <> 96	Tab, Off-White to White, Round, Film Coated	Ethinyl Estradiol 0.04 mg, Levonorgestrel 0.075 mg	Tri-Levlen by Pharm Util	60491-0653	Oral Contraceptive
B <> 96	Tab, Off-White to White, Round, Film Coated	Ethinyl Estradiol 0.04 mg, Levonorgestrel 0.075 mg	Tri-Levlen by Berlex	50419-0196	Oral Contraceptive
B <> 965	Tab, Pink, Round, Film Coated	Ethinyl Estradiol 0.02 mg, Levonorgestrel 0.1 mg	Levlite by Barr	00555-9014	Oral Contraceptive
B <> 967	Tab, Off-White, Oval, Film Coated	Fluvoxamine Maleate 25 mg	Luvox by Barr	00555-0967	OCD
B <> 96850	Tab, Yellow, Oval, Scored, Film Coated	Fluvoxamine Maleate 50 mg	Luvox by Barr	00555-0968	OCD

ID FRONT <> BACK	DESCRIPTION FRONT <> BACK	INGREDIENT & STRENGTH	BRAND (or Generic Equiv.) by FIRM	NDC#	CLASS; SCH.
B <> 969100	Tab, Brown, Oval, Scored, Film Coated	Fluvoxamine Maleate 100 mg	Luvox by Barr	00555-0969	OCD
B <> 97	Tab, Light Yellow, Round, Film Coated	Ethinyl Estradiol 0.03 mg, Levonorgestrel 0.125 mg	Tri-Levlen by Berlex	50419-0197	Oral Contraceptive
B <> 97	Tab, Light Yellow, Round, Film Coated	Ethinyl Estradiol 0.03 mg, Levonorgestrel 0.125 mg	Tri-Levlen by Pharm Util	60491-0653	Oral Contraceptive
B <> 977	Tab, Light Yellow, Round	Norethindrone Acetate 1 mg, Ethinyl Estradiol 20 mcg	Junel 1/20 Fe by Barr	00555-9026	Oral Contraceptive
B <> 977	Tab, Light Yellow, Round	Norethindrone Acetate 1 mg, Ethinyl Estradiol 20 mcg	Junel 1/20 by Barr	00555-9025	Oral Contraceptive
B <> 978	Tab, Pink, Round	Norethindrone Acetate 1.5 mg, Ethinyl Estradiol 30 mcg	Junel 1.5/30 by Barr	00555-9027	Oral Contraceptive
B <> 978	Tab, Pink, Round	Norethindrone Acetate 1.5 mg, Ethinyl Estradiol 30 mcg	Junel 1.5/30 Fe by Barr	00555-9028	Oral Contraceptive
B <> 985	Tab, Gray, Round	Norgestimate 0.180 mg, Ethinyl Estradiol 0.035 mg	Tri-Sprintec by Barr	00555-9018	Oral Contraceptive
B <> 986	Tab, Light Blue, Round	Norgestimate 0.215 mg, Ethinyl Estradiol 0.035 mg	Tri-Sprintec by Barr	00555-9018	Oral Contraceptive
B <> 987	Tab, Blue, Round	Norgestimate 0.250 mg, Ethinyl Estradiol 0.035 mg	Tri-Sprintec by Barr	00555-9018	Oral Contraceptive
B <> 987	Tab, Blue, Round	Norgestimate 0.250 mg, Ethinyl Estradiol 0.035 mg	Sprintec by Barr	00555-9016	Oral Contraceptive
B <> 992	Tab, Pink, Round, Film Coated	Levonorgestrel 0.15 mg, Ethinyl Estradiol 0.03 mg	Nordette by Barr	00555-9020	Oral Contraceptive
B <> 992	Tab, Pink, Round, Film Coated	Levonorgestrel 0.15 mg, Ethinyl Estradiol 0.03 mg	Jolessa by Barr	00555-9123	Oral Contraceptive
B <> 992	Tab, Pink, Round, Film Coated	Levonorgestrel 0.15 mg, Ethinyl Estradiol 0.03 mg	Portia 28 by Apotex	Canadian DIN 02295954	Oral Contraceptive
B <> 992	Tab, Pink, Round, Film Coated	Levonorgestrel 0.15 mg, Ethinyl Estradiol 0.03 mg	Portia 21 by Apotex	Canadian DIN 02295946	Oral Contraceptive
B <> 997110	Tab, Yellow, Oval, Scored, 997 over 1/10	Fludrocortisone 0.1 mg	Florinef by Barr	00555-0997	Steroid
B <> AMIDE001	Tab, Orange, Pink & Purple, Round, Chewable, AMIDE001 <> A, B, C, or D	Ascorbic Acid 60 mg, Cyanocobalamin 4.5 mcg, Folic Acid 0.3 mg, Niacinamide, Pyridoxine HCl 1.05 mg, Riboflavin 1.2 mg, Sodium Fluoride, Thiamine Mononitrate, Vitamin A Acetate, Vitamin D 400 Units, Vitamin E Acetate	Multi Vita Bets by Amide	52152-0001	Vitamin
B <> AMIDE001	Tab, Orange, Pink & Purple, Round, Chewable, AMIDE001 <> A, B, C, or D	Ascorbic Acid 60 mg, Cyanocobalamin 4.5 mcg, Folic Acid 0.3 mg, Niacinamide, Pyridoxine HCl 1.05 mg, Riboflavin 1.2 mg, Sodium Fluoride, Thiamine Mononitrate, Vitamin A Acetate, Vitamin D 400 Units, Vitamin E Acetate	Multi Vita Bets by Qualitest	00603-4712	Vitamin
B <> AMIDE001	Tab, Orange, Pink & Purple, Round, Chewable, AMIDE001 <> A, B, C, or D	Ascorbic Acid 60 mg, Cyanocobalamin 4.5 mcg, Folic Acid 0.3 mg, Niacinamide, Pyridoxine HCl 1.05 mg, Riboflavin 1.2 mg, Sodium Fluoride, Thiamine Mononitrate, Vitamin A Acetate, Vitamin D 400 Units, Vitamin E Acetate	Multi Vita Bets by Major	00904-5275	Vitamin
B <> C2	Tab, White, Round, Stylized "b" <> C2	Pramipexole DiHCl 0.125 mg	Mirapex by Barr	00555-0617	Antiparkinson
B <> C3	Tab, White, Oval, Scored, Stylized "b" <> C/3	Pramipexole DiHCl 0.25 mg	Mirapex by Barr	00555-0612	Antiparkinson
B <> C4	Tab, White, Oval, Scored, Stylized "b" <> C/4	Pramipexole DiHCl 0.5 mg	Mirapex by Barr	00555-0613	Antiparkinson
B <> C5	Tab, White, Round, Scored, Stylized "b" <> C/5	Pramipexole DiHCl 1 mg	Mirapex by Barr	00555-0614	Antiparkinson
B <> C6	Tab, White, Round, Scored, Stylized "b" <> C/6	Pramipexole DiHCl 1.5 mg	Mirapex by Barr	00555-0615	Antiparkinson
B <> KERLONE20	Tab, White, Round, Film Coated, Kerlone over 20 <> Greek Letter Beta	Betaxolol HCl 20 mg	Kerlone by Sanofi	00024-2300	Antihypertensive
B <> KERLONE20	Tab, White, Round, Film Coated, Kerlone over 20 <> Greek Letter Beta	Betaxolol HCl 20 mg	Kerlone by Searle	00025-5201	Antihypertensive
B <> WL25	Tab, Bright Pink	Diphenhydramine HCl 25 mg	Benadryl by Pfizer	00501-2009	Antihistamine
B <> WL26	Tab, White	Diphenhydramine HCl 12.5 mg, Pseudoephedrine HCl 30 mg, Acetaminophen 500 mg	Benadryl Allergy-Cold by Pfizer	00501-2006	Cold Remedy
B <> WL26	Tab, Green, Cap Shaped	Diphenhydramine HCl 12.5 mg, Pseudoephedrine HCl 30 mg, Acetaminophen 500 mg	Benadryl Allergy Sinus Headache by Pfizer	00501-2005	Cold Remedy
B <> WL26	Tab, Green, Cap Shaped	Diphenhydramine HCl 12.5 mg, Pseudoephedrine HCl 30 mg, Acetaminophen 500 mg	Benadryl Total Allergy by Pfizer	Canadian DIN 02255472	Cold Remedy
B <> WL28	Tab, Blue, Cap Shaoed	Diphenhydramine HCl 25 mg, Pseudoephedrine HCl 30 mg, Acetaminophen 500 mg	Benadryl Total Allergy Ex Strength by Pfizer	Canadian DIN 02250993	Cold Remedy
B <> WL28	Tab, Blue, Cap Shaped	Diphenhydramine HCl 25 mg, Pseudoephedrine HCl 30 mg, Acetaminophen 500 mg	Benadryl Severe Allergy Sinus Headache by Pfizer	00501-2030	Cold Remedy
B003	Tab, Pink w/ white specks, Round, Chewable	Acetaminophen 80 mg	Children's Tylenol by Breckenridge		Analgesic

ID FRONT <> BACK	DESCRIPTION FRONT <> BACK	INGREDIENT & STRENGTH	BRAND (or Generic Equiv.) by FIRM	NDC#	CLASS; SCH.
B01	Tab, Yellow, Round	Bisacodyl 5 mg	Dulcolax by Upsher Smith		Gastrointestinal
B01	Tab, Yellow, Round	Bisacodyl 5 mg	Dulcolax by Boehringer Ingelheim		Gastrointestinal
B01 <> LL	Tab, Blue, Hexagonal	Lisinopril 10 mg, HCTZ 12.5 mg	Prinzide by Lupin	68180-0518	Antihypertensive; Diuretic
B02 <> LL	Tab, Yellow, Round	Lisinopril 20 mg, HCTZ 12.5 mg	Prinzide by Lupin	68180-0519	Antihypertensive; Diuretic
B027	Tab, Blue, Round, B-027	Methenamine 40.8 mg, Phenyl Salicylate 18.1 mg, Methylene Blue 5.4 mg, Benzoic Acid 4.5 mg	Urised by Breckenridge	51991-0027	Urinary Tract
B03 <> LL	Tab, Pink, Round	Lisinopril 20 mg, HCTZ 25 mg	Prinzide by Lupin	68180-0520	Antihypertensive; Diuretic
B035	Tab, Light Green, Oblong, B-035	Chlorpheniramine Maleate 8 mg, Phenylephrine 25 mg, Phenylpropanolamine HCl 50 mg	Ru-tuss by Breckenridge	51991-0250	Cold Remedy
B042	Cap, White, B-042	Phenylpropanolamine HCl 25 mg	Polyhistine D pediatric by Breckenridge	51991-0042	Decongestant; Appetite Suppressant
B042	Cap, Opaque White, B-042	Phenylpropanolamine HCl 25 mg, Phenyltoloxamine Citrate 8 mg, Pheniramine Maleate 8 mg, Pyrilamine Maleate 8 mg	PPAH PTC PNM PRM PD by Prepackage Specialists	58864-0029	Cold Remedy
B058	Tab, White, Oblong, B-058	Pseudoephedrine HCl 120 mg, Guaifenesin 1200 mg	by Pharmafab	62542-0764	Cold Remedy
B060	Tab, Violet, Oval, B-060	Carbinoxamine Maleate 8 mg, Pseudoephedrine HCl 120 mg	Coldec TR by Breckenridge	51991-0060 Discontinued	Cold Remedy
B074	Cap, Blue and Yellow	Aspirin 325 mg, Butalbital 50 mg, Caffeine 40 mg, Codeine 30 mg	Ascomp w/ Codeine by Breckenridge	51991-0074	Analgesic; C III
B080	Cap, Reddish Brown, Oval, Gelatin, B-080	Chloral Hydrate 500 mg	Somnote by Breckenridge	51991-0080	Sedative/Hypnotic; C IV
B082	Tab, Yellow, Cap Shaped, Film Coated	Folic Acid 5 mg, Cyanocobalamin (B12) 1 mg, Thiamine HCl 1.5 mg, Riboflavin (B2) 1.5 mg, Pyridoxine HCl (B6) 50 mg, Niacinamide (Niacin) 20 mg, Ascorbic Acid (Vitamin C) 60 mg, Calcium Pantothenate (Pantothenic Acid) 10 mg, Biotin 300 mcg	Folbee Plus by Breckenridge	51991-0082	Vitamin; Supplement
B084	Tab, Peach, Oval	Folic Acid 2.5 mg, Pyridoxine HCl (B6) 25 mg, Cyanocobalamin (B12) 1 mg	Folbee by Breckenridge	51991-0084	Vitamin; Supplement
B1 <> 15	Tab, White, Round, B1 <> 1 over 5	Penicillin V Potassium 250 mg	V-Cillin K by Teva	00093-1171	Antibiotic
B1 <> 17	Tab, White, Round, B1 <> 1 over 7	Penicillin V Potassium 500 mg	V-Cillin K by Teva	00093-1173	Antibiotic
B1 <> LL	Tab, Pink, Heart Shaped, Film Coated, Scored	Bisoprolol Fumarate 5 mg	Zebeta by Duramed	51285-0060	Antihypertensive
B1 <> LL	Tab, Pink, Heart Shaped, Scored, Film Coated	Bisoprolol Fumarate 5 mg	Zebeta by Lederle	00005-3816	Antihypertensive
B1 <> LL	Tab, Pink, Heart Shaped, Scored, Film Coated	Bisoprolol Fumarate 5 mg	Zebeta by Ayerst	00046-3816	Antihypertensive
B10 <> G	Tab, White, Barrel Shaped, Scored	Buspirone HCl 10 mg	Buspar by Genpharm	Canadian DIN 02230874	Antianxiety
B11	Tab, White, Black Print, Round, Film Coated	Sparfloxacin 200 mg	Zagam by Bertek	62794-0011	Antibiotic
B1114	Tab, White, Round, Scored	Benztropine Mesylate 0.5 mg	Cogentin by Pliva	50111-0393	Antiparkinson
B1115	Tab, White, Oval, Scored	Benztropine Mesylate 1 mg	Cogentin by Pliva	50111-0394	Antiparkinson
B12 <> LL	Tab, Yellow, Round	Bisoprolol 2.5 mg, Hydrochlorothiazide 6.25 mg	Ziac by Lederle	00005-3238	Antihypertensive; Diuretic
B12 <> LL	Tab, Yellow, Round, Film Coated, Script LL inside heart	Bisoprolol 2.5 mg, Hydrochlorothiazide 6.25 mg	Ziac by Duramed	51285-0047	Antihypertensive; Diuretic
B13 <> LL	Tab, Pink, Round, Film Coated, Script LL inside heart	Bisoprolol 5 mg, Hydrochlorothiazide 6.25 mg	Ziac by Duramed	51285-0048	Antihypertensive; Diuretic
B13 <> LL	Tab, Pink, Round	Bisoprolol 5 mg, Hydrochlorothiazide 6.25 mg	Ziac by Lederle	00005-3234	Antihypertensive; Diuretic
B131	Tab, White to Off-White, Round, Scored	Tizanidine HCl 2 mg	Zanaflex by Barr	00555-0131	Muscle Relaxant
B132	Tab, White to Off-White, Round, Scored	Tizanidine HCl 4 mg	Zanaflex by Barr	00555-0132	Muscle Relaxant
B133	Tab, White, Round, Scored	Pyridostigmine Bromide 60 mg	Mestinon by Barr	00555-0133	Muscle Stimulant
B14 <> LL	Tab, White, Round, Film Coated, Script LL inside heart	Bisoprolol 10 mg, Hydrochlorothiazide 6.25 mg	Ziac by Duramed	51285-0049	Antihypertensive; Diuretic
B14 <> LL	Tab, White, Round	Bisoprolol 10 mg, Hydrochlorothiazide 6.25 mg	Ziac by Lederle	00005-3235	Antihypertensive; Diuretic
B145	Tab, Yellow, Round, Scored, B over 145	Digoxin 0.125 mg	Digitek by Bertek	62794-0145 Discontinued	Cardiac Agent
B145	Tab, Yellow, Round, Scored, B over 145	Digoxin 0.125 mg	Digitek by UDL	51079-0945 Discontinued	Cardiac Agent
B146	Tab, Sugar Coated, B-146	Phenazopyridine HCl 100 mg	by Lini	58215-0313 Discontinued	Urinary Analgesic
B146	Tab, White, Round, Scored, B over 146	Digoxin 0.25 mg	Digitek by Bertek	62794-0146 Discontinued	Cardiac Agent

ID FRONT <> BACK	DESCRIPTION FRONT <> BACK	INGREDIENT & STRENGTH	BRAND (or Generic Equiv.) by FIRM	NDC#	CLASS; SCH.
B146	Tab, White, Round, Scored, B over 146	Digoxin 0.25 mg	Digitek by UDL	51079-0946 Discontinued	Cardiac Agent
B147	Tab, Sugar Coated	Phenazopyridine HCl 200 mg	by Lini	58215-0314 Discontinued	Urinary Analgesic
B147	Tab, Sugar Coated	Phenazopyridine HCl 200 mg	by Breckenridge	51991-0525	Urinary Analgesic
B147	Tab, Sugar Coated	Phenazopyridine HCl 200 mg	by Apotheca	12634-0189	Urinary Analgesic
B15 <> G	Tab, White, Round, Scored, B / 1.5	Bromazepam 1.5 mg	Lectopam by Genpharm	Canadian DIN 0192705	Sedative; C IV
B154	Tab, White, Oval, B-154	Elemental Iron 90 mg, Calcium 200 mg, Zinc 25 mg, Vitamin A 2700 IU, Vitamin D3 400 IU, Vitamin E 30 IU, Vitamin C 120 mg, Vitamin B6 20 mg, Docusate Sodium 50 mg	Prenate Ultra by Breckenridge	51991-0154	Vitamin; Mineral
B156	Tab, Sugar Coated	Dexchlorpheniramine Maleate 4 mg	by Lini	58215-0311 Discontinued	Antihistamine
B156	Tab, Sugar Coated	Dexchlorpheniramine Maleate 4 mg	by Breckenridge	51991-0470	Antihistamine
B157	Tab, Sugar Coated	Dexchlorpheniramine Maleate 6 mg	by Lini	58215-0312 Discontinued	Antihistamine
B157	Tab, Sugar Coated	Dexchlorpheniramine Maleate 6 mg	by URL Mutual	00677-0669	Antihistamine
B158	Tab, White, Oval, B-158	Vitamin A 4000 IU, Vitamin C 80 mg, Vitamin D 400 IU, Vitamin E 15 IU, Niacin 17 mg, Calcium 200 mg, Iron 54 mg, Magnesium 100 mg, Zinc 25 mg, Copper 3 mg	Natalins Rx by Breckenridge	51991-0158	Vitamin
B15G	Tab, White, Round, B/1.5/G	Bromazepam 1.5 mg	Lectopam by Genpharm	Canadian	Sedative; C IV
B167	Tab, Ex Release, B on One Side of Bisect and 167 on Other Side	Chlorpheniramine Maleate 8 mg, Methscopolamine Nitrate 2.5 mg, Phenylephrine HCl 20 mg	Guaivent DA by Lini	58215-0327 Discontinued	Cold Remedy
B168	Tab, Delayed Release, B-168	Atropine Sulfate 0.04 mg, Chlorpheniramine Maleate 8 mg, Hyoscyamine Sulfate 0.19 mg, Phenylephrine 25 mg, Phenylpropanolamine 50 mg, Scopolamine 0.01 mg	Atrohist Plus by Lini	58215-0326 Discontinued	Cold Remedy
B17	Tab, Orange, Oval, Scored	Clonidine HCl 0.2 mg	by Physician Total Care	54868-0931	Antihypertensive
B170	Cap, Red, White Ink	Chlorpheniramine Maleate 12 mg, Pseudoephedrine HCl 120 mg	Histade by Breckenridge	51991-0170	Cold Remedy
B171	Tab, White, Oval, Scored	Mefloquine HCl 250 mg	Lariam by Barr	00555-0171	Antimalarial
B172	Tab, Yellow, Round	Isosorbide Dinitrate Sublingual 2.5 mg	Isordil by Barr		Antianginal
B173	Tab, Pink, Round	Isosorbide Dinitrate Sublingual 5.0 mg	Isordil by Barr		Antianginal
B198	Cap, Maroon, Opaque, B-198	Polysaccharide Iron Complex 150 mg, Folic Acid 1 mg, Vitamine B12 25 mcg	Niferex 150 Forte by Breckenridge	51991-0198	Vitamin
B2	Tab, White, Oval, B2 <> Sword Logo	Buprenorphine 2 mg	Subutex by Reckitt Benckiser	12496-1278	Detoxification Agent; C III
B2	Tab, B2	Ergotamine Tartrate 2 mg	Ergomar Sublingual by New River	59417-0120	Analgesic
B200	Tab, White, Round	Ibuprofen 200 mg	Motrin by Barr		NSAID
B200	Tab, Blue, Oval, Film Coated	Polysaccharide Iron Complex 60 mg, Folic Acid 1 mg, Ascorbic Acid 1 mg, Vitamin B12 3mcg, Vitamin A 4000 IU, Vitamin D 400 IU, Thiamine 3 mg, Riboflavin 3 mg, Vitamin B6 2 mg, Niacinamide 10 mg, Calcium 125 mg, Zinc 18 mg	Niferex PC by Breckenridge	51991-0200	Vitamin
B202	Tab, White, Oval, B-202	Polysaccharide Iron Complex 60 mg, Folic Acid 1 mg, Vitamin B12 12 mcg, Vitamin A 5000 IU, Vitamin D 400 IU, Thiamine 3 mg, Riboflavin 3.4 mg, Vitamin B6 4 mg, Niacinamide 20 mg, Calcium 250 mg, Zinc 25 mg, Vitamin E 30 IU, Iodine 0.2 mg, Magnesium 10 mg, Copper 2 mg	Niferex PC Forte by Breckenridge	51991-0202	Vitamin
B203	Cap, Brown & Red, B-203	Polysaccharide Iron Complex 150 mg	Niferex 150 by Breckenridge	51991-0203	Vitamin
B203	Cap, Brown & Red, B-203	Polysaccharide Iron Complex 150 mg	Niferex 150 by Major	00904-5395	Vitamin
B236	Tab, White, Oblong	Phenylephrine 30 mg, Guaifenesin 600 mg	Crantex LA by Breckenridge	51991-0236	Cold Remedy
B237	Tab, Pink, Triangle	Amitriptyline 25 mg, Perphenazine 2 mg	Triavil by Barr		Antidepressant; Antipsychotic
B238	Tab, Light Green, Round	Amitriptyline 25 mg, Perphenazine 4 mg	Triavil by Barr		Antidepressant; Antipsychotic

ID FRONT <> BACK	DESCRIPTION FRONT <> BACK	INGREDIENT & STRENGTH	BRAND (or Generic Equiv.) by FIRM	NDC#	CLASS; SCH.
B241	Tab, White to Off-White, Round, Orally Disintegrating	Mirtazapine 15 mg	RemeronSolTab by Barr	00555-0241	Antidepressant
B242	Tab, White to Off-White, Round, Orally Disintegrating	Mirtazapine 30 mg	RemeronSolTab by Barr	00555-0242	Antidepressant
B245	Tab, White, Triangle	Amitriptyline 10 mg, Perphenazine 2 mg	Triavil by Barr		Antidepressant; Antipsychotic
B246	Tab, Salmon, Triangle	Amitriptyline 10 mg, Perphenazine 4 mg	Triavil by Barr		Antidepressant; Antipsychotic
B260	Tab, Beige, Round	Thioridazine 10 mg	Mellaril by Barr		Antipsychotic
B261	Tab, Yellow, Round	Thioridazine 25 mg	Mellaril by Barr		Antipsychotic
B277	Tab, White, Round	Isosorbide Dinitrate Sublingual 10 mg	Isordil by Barr		Antianginal
B292	Tab, Brown, Oval, Scored	Oxcarbazepine 150 mg	Trileptal by Breckenridge	51991-0292	Anticonvulsant
B293	Tab, Brown, Oval, Scored	Oxcarbazepine 300 mg	Trileptal by Breckenridge	51991-0293	Anticonvulsant
B294	Tab, Brown, Oval, Scored	Oxcarbazepine 600 mg	Trileptal by Breckenridge	51991-0294	Anticonvulsant
B2C	Cap, Yellow, Clear	Digoxin 0.1 mg	Lanoxicaps by DSM	63552-0272	Cardiac Agent
B2C	Cap, Yellow, Clear	Digoxin 0.1 mg	Lanoxicaps by GSK	53873-0272	Cardiac Agent
B2C	Cap, Yellow, Clear	Digoxin 0.1 mg	Lanoxicaps by GSK	00173-0272	Cardiac Agent
B2C	Cap, Yellow, Clear	Digoxin 0.1 mg	Lanoxicaps by Murfreesboro	51129-1246	Cardiac Agent
B2C	Cap, Yellow, Clear	Digoxin 0.1 mg	Lanoxicaps by RP Scherer	11014-0748	Cardiac Agent
B3	Tab, Red, Round, B over 3	Ferrous Sulfate 324 mg	Feosol by Paddock	00574-0608	Mineral
B3 <> G	Tab, Pink, Round, Scored, B / 3	Bromazepam 3 mg	Lectopam by Genpharm	Canadian DIN 0219 2713	Sedative; C IV
B3 <> LL	Tab, White, Heart Shaped, Scored	Bisoprolol Fumarate 10 mg	Zebeta by Lederle	00005-3817	Antihypertensive
B3 <> LL	Tab, White, Heart Shaped, Film Coated, Scored	Bisoprolol Fumarate 10 mg	Zebeta by Duramed	51285-0061	Antihypertensive
B303 <> 3	Tab, White, Round, B/303 <> 3	Acetaminophen 300 mg, Codeine Phosphate 30 mg	Tylenol w/ Codeine by Barr	00555-0303 Discontinued	Analgesic; C III
B303 <> 3	Tab, White, Round, B/303 <> 3	Acetaminophen 300 mg, Codeine Phosphate 30 mg	Tylenol w/ Codeine by Duramed	51285-0303	Analgesic; C III
B304 <> 4	Tab, White, Round, Scored	Acetaminophen 300 mg, Codeine Phosphate 60 mg	Tylenol w/ Codeine by Barr	00555-0304	Analgesic; C III
B305 <> 2	Tab, White, Round, Scored	Acetaminophen 300 mg, Codeine Phosphate 15 mg	Tylenol w/ Codeine by Barr	00555-0305	Analgesic; C III
B329	Tab, Blue, Round	Thioridazine 15 mg	Mellaril by Barr		Antipsychotic
B336	Cap, White, Black Ink	Phenylephrine 30 mg, Guaifenesin 400 mg	Crantex LA by Breckenridge	51991-0336	Cold Remedy
B351 <> 10	Tab, White, Round, Film Coated, b over 351	Leflunomide 10 mg	Arava by Barr	00555-0351	Antiarthritic
B352 <> 20	Tab, Yellow, Round, Film Coated	Leflunomide 20 mg	Arava by Barr	00555-0352	Antiarthritic
B3593 <> 968	Tab, Pink, Round	Famotidine 10 mg	Pepcid by Perrigo	00113-1207	Gastrointestinal
B384	Tab, Rose, Oval	Folic Acid 2.5 mg, Vitamin B6 25 mg, Vitamin B12 2 mg	Folbic by Breckenridge	51991-0384	Vitamin
B385 <> 500	Tab, White to Off-White, Oval, Film Coated	Metformin HCl 500 mg	Glucophage by Barr	00555-0385	Antidiabetic
B386 <> 850	Tab, White to Off-White, Oval, Film Coated	Metformin HCl 850 mg	Glucophage by Barr	00555-0386	Antidiabetic
B387 <> 1000	Tab, White to Off-White, Oval, Scored, Film Coated	Metformin HCl 1000 mg	Glucophage by Barr	00555-0387	Antidiabetic
B396	Cap, Blue	Phenylbutazone 100 mg	Butazolidin by Barr		Anti-Inflammatory
B397	Tab, Yellow, Round	Clonidine HCl 0.1 mg	Catapres by Barr		Antihypertensive
B398	Tab, White, Round	Clonidine HCl 0.2 mg	Catapres by Barr		Antihypertensive
B399	Tab, Green, Round	Clonidine HCl 0.3 mg	Catapres by Barr		Antihypertensive
B3G	Tab, Pink, Round, B/3/G	Bromazepam 3 mg	Lectopam by Genpharm	Canadian	Sedative; C IV
B404	Tab, Yellow, Round	Meloxicam 7.5 mg	Mobic by Breckenridge	51991-0404	NSAID
B419	Tab, Yellow, Cap Shaped	Meloxicam 15 mg	Mobic by Breckenridge	51991-0419	NSAID
B424 <> 5AYGESTIN	Tab, White, Oval, Scored, 5 over Aygestin	Norethindrone 5 mg	Aygestin by Barr	51285-0424	Hormone
B477	Tab, White, Round	Haloperidol 0.5 mg	Haldol by Barr		Antipsychotic
B478	Tab, Yellow, Round	Haloperidol 1 mg	Haldol by Barr		Antipsychotic
B479	Tab, White, Round	Haloperidol 2 mg	Haldol by Barr		Antipsychotic

ID FRONT <> BACK	DESCRIPTION FRONT <> BACK	INGREDIENT & STRENGTH	BRAND (or Generic Equiv.) by FIRM	NDC#	CLASS; SCH.
B480	Tab, Green, Round	Haloperidol 5 mg	Haldol by Barr	00182-1869	Antipsychotic
B484	Tab	Leucovorin Calcium	Wellcovorin by Ivax	00182-1870	Antineoplastic
B485	Tab	Leucovorin Calcium	Wellcovorin by Ivax		Antineoplastic
B491 <> 05	Tab, White, Round, b over 491 <> 0.5, Ex Release	Alprazolam 0.5 mg	Xanax XR by Barr	00555-0491	Antianxiety; C IV
B492 <> 1	Tab, Yellow, Round, b over 492, Ex Release	Alprazolam 1 mg	Xanax XR by Barr	00555-0492	Antianxiety; C IV
B493 <> 2	Tab, Blue, Round, b over 493, Ex Release	Alprazolam 2 mg	Xanax XR by Barr	00555-0493	Antianxiety; C IV
B494 <> 3	Tab, Green, Round, b over 494, Ex Release	Alprazolam 3 mg	Xanax XR by Barr	00555-0494	Antianxiety; C IV
B5 <> PMS	Tab, White, Round, Scored	Buspirone HCl 5 mg	Buspar by Pharmascience	Canadian DIN 5760609410	Antianxiety
B52	Cap, Red	Vitamin A 50,000 Units	Alphalin by Eli Lilly		Vitamin
B527	Tab, Off-White, Round	Doxycycline Hyclate 100 mg	Vibra-Tab by Martec	00781-1076	Antibiotic
B572	Tab, Yellow, Oval, Scored, Film Coated, b over 572	Methotrexate 2.5 mg	Rheumatrex by Sandoz	00839-7905	Antineoplastic
B572	Tab, Yellow, Oval, Scored, Film Coated, b over 572	Methotrexate 2.5 mg	Rheumatrex by Moore	00904-1749	Antineoplastic
B572	Tab, Yellow, Oval, Scored, Film Coated, b over 572	Methotrexate 2.5 mg	Rheumatrex by Major	00182-1539	Antineoplastic
B572	Tab, Yellow, Oval, Scored, Film Coated, b over 572	Methotrexate 2.5 mg	Rheumatrex by Ivax	00555-0572	Antineoplastic
B572	Tab, Yellow, Oval, Scored, Film Coated, b over 572	Methotrexate 2.5 mg	Rheumatrex by Supergen	62701-0940	Antineoplastic
B6 <> G	Tab, Pale Green, Round, Scored, B / 6	Bromazepam 6 mg	Lectopam by Genpharm	Canadian DIN 02192721	Sedative; C IV
B60	Cap, Brown	Ergocalciferol 50,000 Units	Deltalin by Eli Lilly		Vitamin
B6G	Tab, Green, Round, B/6/G	Bromazepam 6 mg	Lectopam by Genpharm	Canadian	Sedative; C IV
B70 <> 720	Tab, White, Oval	Alendronate Sodium 70 mg	Fosamax by Barr	00555-0720 Discontinued	Antiosteoporosis
B700	Cap, Ex Release	Chlorpheniramine Maleate 4 mg, Methscopolamine Nitrate 1.25 mg, Phenylephrine HCl 10 mg	Extendryl Jr by Lini	58215-0325 Discontinued	Cold Remedy
B701	Tab	Dextrompheniramine Maleate 6 mg, Pseudoephedrine Sulfate 120 mg	Pharmadrine by Breckenridge	51991-0175	Cold Remedy
B701	Tab	Dextrompheniramine Maleate 6 mg, Pseudoephedrine Sulfate 120 mg	Drixoral Type by Lini	58215-0111 Discontinued	Cold Remedy
B701 <> 150	Tab, Pink, Round, Film Coated, b over 701	Demeclocycline HCl 150 mg	Declomycin by Barr	00555-0701	Antibiotic
B702 <> 300	Tab, Pink, Round, Film Coated, b over 702	Demeclocycline HCl 300 mg	Declomycin by Barr	00555-0702	Antibiotic
B71 <> 511	Tab, Orange, Round	Bupropion HCl 75 mg	Wellbutrin by ESI Lederle	59911-5861	Antidepressant
B736	Tab, Light Yellow, Cap Shaped, Scored, B/736	Acetaminophen 750 mg, Hydrocodone Bitartrate 7.5 mg	Vicodin ES by Barr	00555-0736	Analgesic; C III
B77 <> 511	Tab, Orange, Oval	Bupropion HCl 100 mg	Wellbutrin by ESI Lederle	59911-5862	Antidepressant
B775 <> 712	Tab, Blue, Round, Scored, 7 over 1/2	Mixed Amphetamine Salts 7.5 mg: Dextroamphetamine Saccharate 1.875 mg, Amphetamine Aspartate 1.875 mg, Dextroamphetamine Sulfate 1.875 mg, Amphetamine Sulfate 1.875 mg	Adderall by Barr	00555-0775	Stimulant; C II
B776 <> 1212	Tab, Peach, Oval, Scored, 12 over 1/2	Mixed Amphetamine Salts 12.5 mg: Dextroamphetamine Saccharate 3.125 mg, Amphetamine Aspartate 3.125 mg, Dextroamphetamine Sulfate 3.125 mg, Amphetamine Sulfate 3.125 mg	Adderall by Barr	00555-0776	Stimulant; C II
B777 <> 15	Tab, Peach, Round, Scored, 1 over 5	Mixed Amphetamine Salts 15 mg: Dextroamphetamine Saccharate 3.75 mg, Amphetamine Aspartate 3.75 mg, Dextroamphetamine Sulfate 3.75 mg, Amphetamine Sulfate 3.75 mg	Adderall by Barr	00555-0777	Stimulant; C II
B8	Tab, White, Oval, B8 <> Sword Logo	Buprenorphine 8 mg	Subutex by Reckitt Benckiser	12496-1310	Detoxification Agent; C III
B814 <> 250	Tab, Round, Film Coated, Biconvex	Ciprofloxacin HCl 250 mg	Cipro by Barr	00555-0814	Antibiotic
B815 <> 500	Tab, White, Cap Shaped, Film Coated, b815	Ciprofloxacin 500 mg	Cipro by Barr	00555-0815	Antibiotic
B816 <> 750	Tab, White, Cap Shaped, Film Coated, b816	Ciprofloxacin 750 mg	Cipro by Barr	00555-0816	Antibiotic
B8861	Tab, Light Purple, Oval, B 886/1	Estradiol 1 mg	Estrace by Barr		Hormone
B8872	Tab, Green, Oval, B 887/2	Estradiol 2 mg	Estrace by Barr		Hormone
B895	Tab, Peach, Cap Shaped, Scored, B/895	Acetaminophen 650 mg, Hydrocodone Bitartrate 7.5 mg	Lorcet Plus by Barr	00555-0895	Analgesic; C III

ID FRONT <> BACK	DESCRIPTION FRONT <> BACK	INGREDIENT & STRENGTH	BRAND (or Generic Equiv.) by FIRM	NDC#	CLASS; SCH.
B896	Tab, Light Pink, Cap Shaped, Scored, B/896	Acetaminophen 500 mg, Hydrocodone Bitartrate 2.5 mg	by Barr	00555-0896	Analgesic; C III
B897	Tab, Light Green, Cap Shaped, Scored, B/897	Acetaminophen 500 mg, Hydrocodone Bitartrate 7.5 mg	Lortab by Barr	00555-0897	Analgesic; C III
B898	Tab, Blue, Cap Shaped, Scored, B/898	Acetaminophen 650 mg, Hydrocodone Bitartrate 10 mg	by Barr	00555-0898	Analgesic; C III
B89912	Tab, White, Oval, B 899 1/2	Estradiol 0.5 mg	Estrace by Barr		Hormone
B915	Tab, White, Cap Shaped, Scored, B/915	Acetaminophen 500 mg, Hydrocodone Bitartrate 5 mg	by Barr	00555-0915	Analgesic; C III
B919	Tab, Light Beige, Cap Shaped, Scored, b/919	Acetaminophen 500 mg, Hydrocodone Bitartrate 10 mg	by Barr	00555-0919 Discontinued	Analgesic; C III
B94 <> 18	Tab, White to Off-White, Round, 1/8, b over 94, Orally Disintegrating	Clonazepam 0.125 mg	Klonopin Wafers by Barr	00555-0094	Sedative; C IV
B95 <> 14	Tab, White, Round, Orally Disintegrating, 1/4	Clonazepam 0.25 mg	Klonopin Wafers by Barr	00555-0095	Sedative; C IV
B96 <> 12	Tab, White, Round, Orally Disintegrating, 1/2	Clonazepam 0.5 mg	Klonopin Wafers by Barr	00555-0096	Sedative; C IV
B97 <> 1	Tab, White, Round, Orally Disintegrating	Clonazepam 1 mg	Klonopin Wafers by Barr	00555-0097	Sedative; C IV
B971 <> 5	Tab, Blue, Oval, Scored, b over 971	Mixed Amphetamine Salts 5 mg: Amphetamine Aspartene 1.25 mg, Amphetamine Sulfate 1.25 mg, Dextroamphetamine Saccharate 1.25 mg, Dextroamphetamine Sulfate 1.25 mg	Adderall by Barr	00555-0971	Stimulant; C II
B972 <> 10	Tab, Blue, Oval, Scored, b over 972	Mixed Amphetamine Salts 10 mg: Amphetamine Aspartene 2.5 mg, Amphetamine Sulfate 2.5 mg, Dextroamphetamine Saccharate 2.5 mg, Dextroamphetamine Sulfate 2.5 mg	Adderall by Barr	00555-0972	Stimulant; C II
B973 <> 20	Tab, Peach, Oval, Scored, b over 973, 2 over 0	Mixed Amphetamine Salts 20 mg: Amphetamine Aspartene 5 mg, Amphetamine Sulfate 5 mg, Dextroamphetamine Saccharate 5 mg, Dextroamphetamine Sulfate 5 mg	Adderall by Barr	00555-0973	Stimulant; C II
B974 <> 30	Tab, Peach, Oval, Scored, b over 974, 3 over 0	Mixed Amphetamine Salts 30 mg: Amphetamine Aspartene 7.5 mg, Amphetamine Sulfate 7.5 mg, Dextroamphetamine Saccharate 7.5 mg, Dextroamphetamine Sulfate 7.5 mg	Adderall by Barr	00555-0974	Stimulant; C II
BAC10	Tab, BAC over 10	Baclofen 10 mg	Lioresal by Rosemont	00832-1024	Muscle Relaxant
BAC10 <> 832	Tab, White, Round	Baclofen 10 mg	Lioresal by Qualitest	00603-2408	Muscle Relaxant
BAC10832	Tab, White, Round, Scored, BAC over 10/832	Baclofen 10 mg	Lioresal by Martec	52555-0695	Muscle Relaxant
BACLOFEN <> PMS10	Tab, White, Oval, Scored	Baclofen 10 mg	Lioresal by Pharmascience	Canadian DIN 02063735	Muscle Relaxant
BACLOFEN <> PMS20	Tab, White, Cap Shaped, Scored	Baclofen 20 mg	Lioresal by Pharmascience	Canadian DIN 02063743	Muscle Relaxant
BACLOFENPMS10	Cap, White, Oval, Scored	Baclofen 10 mg	Lioresal by Pharmascience	Canadian DIN 5760637352	Muscle Relaxant
BACLOFENPMS20	Cap, White, Oblong, Scored	Baclofen 20 mg	Lioresal by Pharmascience	Canadian DIN 5760637432	Muscle Relaxant
BACTRIM	Tab, White, Round, Scored	Sulfamethoxazole 400 mg, Trimethoprim 80 mg	Bactrim by AR Scientific	13310-0145	Antibiotic
BACTRIM <> WFHC	Tab, White, Round, Scored	Sulfamethoxazole 400 mg, Trimethoprim 80 mg	Bactrim by Women First HealthCare	64248-0004	Antibiotic
BACTRIMDS	Tab, White, Oval, Scored	Sulfamethoxazole 800 mg, Trimethoprim 160 mg	Bactrim DS by AR Scientific	13310-0146	Antibiotic
BACTRIMDS <> ROCHE	Tab, White, Oblong, Bactrim-DS	Sulfamethoxazole 800 mg, Trimethoprim 160 mg	Bactrim DS by Med Pro	53978-3380	Antibiotic
BACTRIMDS <> ROCHE	Tab, White, Oblong, Bactrim-DS	Sulfamethoxazole 800 mg, Trimethoprim 160 mg	Bactrim DS by Rightpak	65240-0612	Antibiotic
BACTRIMDS <> ROCHE	Tab, White, Oblong, Bactrim-DS	Sulfamethoxazole 800 mg, Trimethoprim 160 mg	Bactrim DS by Thrift Drug	59198-0258	Antibiotic
BACTRIMDS <> ROCHE	Tab, White, Oblong, Bactrim-DS	Sulfamethoxazole 800 mg, Trimethoprim 160 mg	Bactrim DS by St. Mary's Med	60760-0102	Antibiotic
BACTRIMDS <> ROCHE	Tab, White, Oblong, Bactrim-DS	Sulfamethoxazole 800 mg, Trimethoprim 160 mg	Bactrim DS by DRX	55045-2291	Antibiotic
BACTRIMDS <> ROCHE	Tab, White, Oblong, Bactrim-DS	Sulfamethoxazole 800 mg, Trimethoprim 160 mg	Bactrim DS by Amerisource	62584-0117	Antibiotic
BACTRIMDS <> ROCHE	Tab, White, Oblong, Bactrim-DS	Sulfamethoxazole 800 mg, Trimethoprim 160 mg	Bactrim DS by Nat Pharmpak	55154-3101	Antibiotic
BACTRIMDS <> ROCHE	Tab, White, Oblong, Bactrim-DS	Sulfamethoxazole 800 mg, Trimethoprim 160 mg	Bactrim DS by Hoffmann La Roche	00004-0117	Antibiotic
BACTRIMDS <> WFHC	Tab, White, Oval, Scored	Sulfamethoxazole 800 mg, Trimethoprim 160 mg	Bactrim DS by Women First Healthcare	64248-0117	Antibiotic
BAR159	Cap, Black Print, White Powder	Chlordiazepoxide 25 mg	Librium by Major	00904-0092	Antianxiety; C IV
BARR <> 0546	Tab, Dark Orange, Cap Shaped, Film Coated	Cephalexin 500 mg	by Barr	00555-0546 Discontinued	Antibiotic

ID FRONT <> BACK	DESCRIPTION FRONT <> BACK	INGREDIENT & STRENGTH	BRAND (or Generic Equiv.) by FIRM	NDC#	CLASS; SCH.
BARR <> 219	Tab, Pink, Cap Shaped, Film Coated	Erythromycin Stearate 500 mg	by Barr	00555-0219 Discontinued	Antibiotic
BARR <> 23201	Tab, White, Oval, Scored, barr <> 232/0.1	Desmopressin Acetate 0.1 mg	DDAVP by Barr	00555-0232	Antidiuretic
BARR <> 23302	Tab, White, Oval, Scored, barr <> 233/0.2	Desmopressin Acetate 0.2 mg	DDAVP by Barr	00555-0233	Antidiuretic
BARR <> 259	Tab, Beige, Oval, Film Coated	Erythromycin Ethylsuccinate 400 mg	by Barr	00555-0259 Discontinued	Antibiotic
BARR <> 262	Tab, Coated	Thioridazine HCl 50 mg	by Barr	00555-0262	Antipsychotic
BARR <> 263	Tab, Coated	Thioridazine HCl 100 mg	by Barr	00555-0263	Antipsychotic
BARR <> 286	Tab, White, Round	Dipyridamole 75 mg	Persantine by Major	00904-1088	Antiplatelet
BARR <> 286	Tab, White, Round, Film Coated	Dipyridamole 75 mg	Persantine by Barr	00555-0286	Antiplatelet
BARR <> 286	Tab, White, Round, Film Coated	Dipyridamole 75 mg	Persantine by UDL	51079-0070	Antiplatelet
BARR <> 286	Tab, White, Round, Film Coated	Dipyridamole 75 mg	Persantine by Ivax	00182-1570 Discontinued	Antiplatelet
BARR <> 382	Tab, White, Round	Meperidine 100 mg	Demerol by Barr	00555-0382	Analgesic; C II
BARR <> 419	Tab, White, Round, Film Coated	Ibuprofen 400 mg	Motrin by Barr	00555-0419 Discontinued	NSAID
BARR <> 420	Tab, White, Oval, Film Coated	Ibuprofen 600 mg	Motrin by Barr	00555-0420 Discontinued	NSAID
BARR <> 446	Tab, White, Round	Tamoxifen Citrate 10 mg	Nolvadex by Barr	00555-0446	Antiestrogen
BARR <> 446	Tab, White, Round	Tamoxifen Citrate 10 mg	Nolvadex by Zeneca	00310-0446	Antiestrogen
BARR <> 446	Tab, White, Round	Tamoxifen Citrate 10 mg	Nolvadex by Haines	59564-0144	Antiestrogen
BARR <> 499	Tab, White, Oval, Film Coated	Ibuprofen 800 mg	Motrin by Barr	00555-0499 Discontinued	NSAID
BARR <> 545	Tab, Light Orange, Cap Shaped, Film Coated	Cephalexin 250 mg	Keflex by Barr	00555-0545	Antibiotic
BARR <> 555013	Tab, Pink, Round, Film Coated	Erythromycin Stearate 250 mg	Erythrocin by Barr	00555-0013 Discontinued	Antibiotic
BARR <> 555163	Tab, White, Round, Scored, 555 over 163	Diazepam 2 mg	Valium by Southwood	58016-0274	Antianxiety; C IV
BARR <> 555163	Tab, White, Round, Scored, 555 over 163	Diazepam 2 mg	Valium by Barr	00555-0163 Discontinued	Antianxiety; C IV
BARR <> 555164	Tab, Blue, Round, Scored, 555 over 164	Diazepam 10 mg	Valium by Barr	00555-0164	Antianxiety; C IV
BARR <> 555164	Tab, Blue, Round, Scored, 555 over 164	Diazepam 10 mg	Valium by Southwood	58016-0273	Antianxiety; C IV
BARR <> 555271	Tab, White, Round, Scored, 555 over 271	Sulfinpyrazone 100 mg	Anturane by Barr	00555-0271	Uricosuric
BARR <> 555363	Tab, Yellow, Round, Scored, Barr <> 555/363	Diazepam 5 mg	Valium by Barr	00555-0363 Discontinued	Antianxiety; C IV
BARR <> 555363	Tab, Yellow, Round, Scored	Diazepam 5 mg	Valium by Southwood	58016-0275	Antianxiety; C IV
BARR <> 555427	Tab, White, Round, Scored, Barr <> 555/427	Hydrochlorothiazide 25 mg, Propranolol HCl 40 mg	by Barr	00555-0427	Diuretic; Antihypertensive
BARR <> 555428	Tab, White, Round, Scored, Barr <> 555/428	Hydrochlorothiazide 25 mg, Propranolol HCl 80 mg	by Barr	00555-0428	Diuretic; Antihypertensive
BARR <> 555444	Tab, Yellow, Oval, Scored, barr <> 555/444	Hydrochlorothiazide 50 mg, Triamterene 75 mg	Maxzide by Barr	00555-0444	Diuretic; Antihypertensive
BARR <> 555444	Tab, Yellow, Oval, Scored, barr <> 555/444	Hydrochlorothiazide 50 mg, Triamterene 75 mg	Maxzide by Major	00904-1965	Diuretic; Antihypertensive
BARR <> 555444	Tab, Yellow, Oval, Scored, barr <> 555/444	Hydrochlorothiazide 50 mg, Triamterene 75 mg	Maxzide by PDRX	55289-0488	Diuretic; Antihypertensive
BARR <> 555483	Tab, Light Yellow, Round, Scored, barr <> 555 over 483	Amiloride HCl 5 mg, Hydrochlorothiazide 50 mg	Moduretic by Barr	00555-0483 Discontinued	Antihypertensive; Diuretic
BARR <> 555489	Tab, White, Round, Scored, barr <> 555 over 489	Trazodone HCl 50 mg	Desyrel by Nat Pharmpak	55154-1406	Antidepressant
BARR <> 555489	Tab, White, Round, Scored, barr <> 555 over 489	Trazodone HCl 50 mg	Desyrel by UDL	51079-0427 Discontinued	Antidepressant
BARR <> 555489	Tab, White, Round, Scored, barr <> 555 over 489	Trazodone HCl 50 mg	Desyrel by Barr	00555-0489	Antidepressant
BARR <> 555490	Tab, White, Round, Scored, barr <> 555 over 490	Trazodone HCl 100 mg	Desyrel by UDL	51079-0428 Discontinued	Antidepressant
BARR <> 555490	Tab, White, Round, Scored, barr <> 555 over 490	Trazodone HCl 100 mg	Desyrel by Murfreesboro	511291-1131	Antidepressant
BARR <> 555490	Tab, White, Round, Scored, barr <> 555 over 490	Trazodone HCl 100 mg	Desyrel by Barr	00555-0490	Antidepressant
BARR <> 555585	Tab, Light Green, Round, Scored, barr <> 555 over 585	Chlorzoxazone 500 mg	Parafon Forte by Barr	00555-0585	Muscle Relaxant

ID FRONT <> BACK	DESCRIPTION FRONT <> BACK	INGREDIENT & STRENGTH	BRAND (or Generic Equiv.) by FIRM	NDC#	CLASS; SCH.
BARR <> 555585	Tab, Light Green, Round, Scored, barr <> 555 over 585	Chlorzoxazone 500 mg	Parafon Forte by UDL	51079-0476	Muscle Relaxant
BARR <> 555585	Tab, Light Green, Round, Scored, barr <> 555 over 585	Chlorzoxazone 500 mg	Parafon Forte by Direct Dispensing	57866-3444	Muscle Relaxant
BARR <> 555585	Tab, Light Green, Round, Scored, barr <> 555 over 585	Chlorzoxazone 500 mg	Parafon Forte by PDRX	55289-0633	Muscle Relaxant
BARR <> 555607	Tab, White, Round, Scored, 555 over 607	Megestrol Acetate 40 mg	Megace by Qualitest	00603-4392	Hormone
BARR <> 555607	Tab, White, Round, Scored, 555 over 607	Megestrol Acetate 40 mg	Megace by CVS	00894-6651	Hormone
BARR <> 555607	Tab, White, Round, Scored, 555 over 607	Megestrol Acetate 40 mg	Megace by Supergen	62701-0920	Hormone
BARR <> 555607	Tab, White, Round, Scored, 555 over 607	Megestrol Acetate 40 mg	Megace by UDL	51079-0435	Hormone
BARR <> 555607				Discontinued	
BARR <> 555607	Tab, White, Round, Scored, 555 over 607	Megestrol Acetate 40 mg	Megace by Major		Hormone
BARR <> 555607	Tab, White, Round, Scored, 555 over 607	Megestrol Acetate 40 mg	Megace by CVS	51316-0239	Hormone
BARR <> 555607	Tab, White, Round, Scored, 555 over 607	Megestrol Acetate 40 mg	Megace by Barr	00555-0607	Hormone
BARR <> 555607	Tab, White, Round, Scored, 555 over 607	Megestrol Acetate 40 mg	Megace by Warner Chilcott	00047-0108	Hormone
BARR <> 555607	Tab, White, Round, Scored, 555 over 607	Megestrol Acetate 40 mg	Megace by URL Mutual	00677-1206	Hormone
BARR <> 555643	Tab, Green, Oval, Scored, barr <> 555/643	Hydrochlorothiazide 25 mg, Triamterene 37.5 mg	Maxzide by Barr	00555-0643	Diuretic; Antihypertensive
BARR <> 555727	Tab, Yellow, Round, Scored, 555 over 727	Estropipate 0.75 mg	Ogen by Heartland	61392-0617	Hormone
BARR <> 555727	Tab, Yellow, Round, Scored, 555 over 727	Estropipate 0.75 mg	Ogen by Barr	00555-0727	Hormone
BARR <> 555728	Tab, Peach, Round, Scored, 555 over 728	Estropipate 1.5 mg	Ogen by Barr	00555-0728	Hormone
BARR <> 555728				Discontinued	
BARR <> 555728	Tab, Peach, Round, Scored, 555 over 728	Estropipate 1.5 mg	Ogen by Heartland	61392-0707	Hormone
BARR <> 555729	Tab, Blue, Round, Scored, 555 over 729	Estropipate 3 mg	Ogen by Heartland	61392-0715	Hormone
BARR <> 555729	Tab, Blue, Round, Scored, 555 over 729	Estropipate 3 mg	Ogen by Barr	00555-0729	Hormone
BARR <> 555831	Tab, Pink, Oval, Scored	Warfarin Sodium 1 mg	Coumadin by Barr	00555-0831	Anticoagulant
BARR <> 555832	Tab, Green, Oval, Scored, Barr <> 555/832	Warfarin Sodium 2.5 mg	Coumadin by Barr	00555-0832	Anticoagulant
BARR <> 555832				Discontinued	
BARR <> 555833	Tab, Peach, Oval, Scored, Barr <> 555/833	Warfarin Sodium 5 mg	Coumadin by Barr	Discontinued	Anticoagulant
BARR <> 555834	Tab, Yellow, Oval, Scored, Barr <> 555/834	Warfarin Sodium 7.5 mg	Coumadin by Barr	Discontinued	Anticoagulant
BARR <> 555835	Tab, White, Oval, Scored, Barr <> 555/835	Warfarin Sodium 10 mg	Coumadin by Barr	Discontinued	Anticoagulant
BARR <> 555869	Tab, Lavender, Oval, Scored, Barr <> 555/869	Warfarin Sodium 2 mg	Coumadin by Barr	00555-0869	Anticoagulant
BARR <> 555874	Tab, Blue, Oval, Scored, Barr <> 555/874	Warfarin Sodium 4 mg	Coumadin by Barr	Discontinued	Anticoagulant
BARR <> 8311	Tab, Pink, Oval, Scored	Warfarin Sodium 1 mg	Coumadin by UDL	51079-0908	Anticoagulant
BARR <> 8311	Tab, Pink, Oval, Scored	Warfarin Sodium 1 mg	Coumadin by Barr	00555-0831	Anticoagulant
BARR <> 832212	Tab, Green, Oval, Scored, barr <> 832/2 1/2	Warfarin Sodium 2.5 mg	Coumadin by Barr	00555-0832	Anticoagulant
BARR <> 8335	Tab, Peach, Oval, Scored	Warfarin Sodium 5 mg	Coumadin by Barr	00555-0833	Anticoagulant
BARR <> 8335	Tab, Peach, Oval, Scored	Warfarin Sodium 5 mg	Coumadin by UDL	51079-0913	Anticoagulant
BARR <> 8335	Tab, Peach, Oval, Scored	Warfarin Sodium 5 mg	Coumadin by UCB	50474-0935	Anticoagulant
BARR <> 834712	Tab, Yellow, Oval, Scored, barr <> 834/7 1/2	Warfarin Sodium 7.5 mg	Coumadin by Barr	00555-0834	Anticoagulant
BARR <> 834712	Tab, Yellow, Oval, Scored, barr <> 834/7 1/2	Warfarin Sodium 7.5 mg	Coumadin by UDL	51079-0915	Anticoagulant
BARR <> 83510	Tab, White, Oval, Scored	Warfarin Sodium 10 mg	Coumadin by Barr	00555-0835	Anticoagulant
BARR <> 83510	Tab, White, Oval, Scored	Warfarin Sodium 10 mg	Coumadin by UDL	51079-0916	Anticoagulant
BARR <> 8692	Tab, Purple, Oval, Scored	Warfarin Sodium 2 mg	Coumadin by UDL	51079-0909	Anticoagulant
BARR <> 8692	Tab, Purple, Oval, Scored	Warfarin Sodium 2 mg	Coumadin by Barr	00555-0869	Anticoagulant
BARR <> 8744	Tab, Blue, Oval, Scored	Warfarin Sodium 4 mg	Coumadin by Barr	00555-0874	Anticoagulant
BARR <> 8744	Tab, Blue, Oval, Scored	Warfarin Sodium 4 mg	Coumadin by UDL	51079-0912	Anticoagulant
BARR <> 904	Tab, White, Round	Tamoxifen Citrate 20 mg	Nolvadex by Zeneca	00310-0904	Antiestrogen
BARR <> 904	Tab, White, Round	Tamoxifen Citrate 20 mg	Nolvadex by Barr	00555-0904	Antiestrogen
BARR <> 9253	Tab, Tan, Oval, Scored	Warfarin Sodium 3 mg	Coumadin by UDL	51079-0911	Anticoagulant
BARR <> 9253	Tab, Tan, Oval, Scored	Warfarin Sodium 3 mg	Coumadin by Barr	00555-0925	Anticoagulant
BARR <> 9253	Tab, Tan, Oval, Scored	Warfarin Sodium 3 mg	Coumadin by Truett	11312-0128	Anticoagulant

ID FRONT <> BACK	DESCRIPTION FRONT <> BACK	INGREDIENT & STRENGTH	BRAND (or Generic Equiv.) by FIRM	NDC#	CLASS; SCH.
BARR <> 9266	Tab, Teal, Oval, Scored	Warfarin Sodium 6 mg	Coumadin by UCB	50474-0612	Anticoagulant
BARR <> 9266	Tab, Teal, Oval, Scored	Warfarin Sodium 6 mg	Coumadin by UDL	51079-0898	Anticoagulant
BARR <> 9266	Tab, Teal, Oval, Scored	Warfarin Sodium 6 mg	Coumadin by Barr	00555-0926	Anticoagulant
BARR <> 979	Tab, Beige, Cap Shaped, Scored, Film Coated	Hydroxyurea 1000 mg	Hydrea by Barr	00555-0979	Antineoplastic
BARR <> EBASE333MG	Tab, White, Green Print, Cap Shaped, Enteric Coated, Barr <> E-Base over 333 mg	Erythromycin 333 mg	E-Mycin by Barr	00555-0495 Discontinued	Antibiotic
BARR <> EBASE333MG	Tab, White, Blue Print, Cap Shape, Enteric Coated, Barr <> E-Base 333 mg	Erythromycin 333 mg	E-Mycin by Barr	00555-0532 Discontinued	Antibiotic
BARR <> EBASE500MG	Tab, White, Red Print, Cap Shaped, Enteric Coated, Barr <> E-Base 500 mg	Erythromycin 500 mg	E-Mycin by Barr	00555-0533 Discontinued	Antibiotic
BARR010	Cap, Black & Yellow, White Print, Opaque, Hard Gel	Tetracycline HCl 500 mg	Sumycin by Pharmedix	53002-0217	Antibiotic
BARR010	Cap, Black & Yellow, White Print, Opaque, Hard Gel	Tetracycline HCl 500 mg	Sumycin by Barr	00555-0010	Antibiotic
BARR010	Cap, Black & Yellow, White Print, Opaque, Hard Gel	Tetracycline HCl 500 mg	Sumycin by H J Harkins Co	52959-0336	Antibiotic
BARR011	Cap, Orange & Yellow, Black Print, Opaque, Hard Gel	Tetracycline HCl 250 mg	Sumycin by Southwood	58016-0102	Antibiotic
BARR011	Cap, Orange & Yellow, Black Print, Opaque, Hard Gel	Tetracycline HCl 250 mg	Sumycin by Major	00904-2416	Antibiotic
BARR011	Cap, Orange & Yellow, Black Print, Opaque, Hard Gel	Tetracycline HCl 250 mg	Sumycin by Barr	00555-0011	Antibiotic
BARR011	Cap, Orange & Yellow, Black Print, Opaque, Hard Gel	Tetracycline HCl 250 mg	Sumycin by Pharmedix	53002-0225	Antibiotic
BARR011	Cap, Orange & Yellow, Black Print, Opaque, Hard Gel	Tetracycline HCl 250 mg	Sumycin by Southwood	58016-0101	Antibiotic
BARR011	Cap, Orange & Yellow, Black Print, Opaque, Hard Gel	Tetracycline HCl 250 mg	Sumycin by Med Pro	53978-5048	Antibiotic
BARR033	Cap, Black & Green	Chlordiazepoxide 10 mg	Librium by UDL	51079-0375	Antianxiety; C IV
BARR033	Cap, Black & Green, White Print, Opaque, Hard Gel, barr033	Chlordiazepoxide 10 mg	Librium by Ivax	00182-0978	Antianxiety; C IV
BARR033	Cap, Black & Green	Chlordiazepoxide 10 mg	Librium by Sandoz	00781-2082	Antianxiety; C IV
BARR033	Cap, Black & Green, White Print, Opaque, Hard Gel, barr033	Chlordiazepoxide 10 mg	Librium by Barr	00555-0033	Antianxiety; C IV
BARR033	Cap, Black & Green	Chlordiazepoxide 10 mg	Librium by Med Pro	53978-3175	Antianxiety; C IV
BARR058	Cap, Clear & Pink	Diphenhydramine HCl 25 mg	Benadryl by Barr	00555-0058	Antihistamine
BARR059	Cap, Pink, Black Print, Hard Gel	Diphenhydramine HCl 50 mg	Benadryl by Barr	00555-0059	Antihistamine
BARR059	Cap, Pink	Diphenhydramine HCl 50 mg	Benadryl by UDL	51079-0066 Discontinued	Antihistamine
BARR05MG101	Cap, Ivory, Opaque	Anagrelide HCl 0.5 mg	Agrylin by Barr	00555-0101 Discontinued	Antiplatelet
BARR071 <> 300	Tab, White, Round, Scored, Barr over 071	Isoniazid 300 mg	Laniazid by Schein	00364-0151	Antimycobacterial
BARR071 <> 300	Tab, White, Round, Scored, Barr over 071	Isoniazid 300 mg	Laniazid by Barr	Discontinued	Antimycobacterial
BARR100MG829	Cap, Orange, Opaque, Black Ink	Zonisamide 100 mg	Zonegran by Barr	00555-0829	Anticonvulsant
BARR10MG876	Cap, Blue & Yellow, Black Print, Opaque, barr over 10 mg	Fluoxetine HCl 10 mg	Prozac by Barr	00603-2666	Antidepressant
BARR10MG876	Cap, Blue Opaque Cap, Yellow Opaque Body	Fluoxetine 10 mg	Prozac by Teva	00555-0876	Antidepressant
BARR115	Tab, Salmon, Round	Hydralazine 25 mg, Hydrochlorothiazide 15 mg, Reserpine 0.1 mg	Serapes by Barr	00555-0876	Antihypertensive; Diuretic
BARR128	Cap, White Print	Dicyclomine HCl 10 mg	by Barr	00555-0128	Gastrointestinal
BARR158	Cap, Green & Yellow	Chlordiazepoxide 5 mg	Librium by UDL	51079-0374	Antianxiety; C IV
BARR158	Cap, Aqua Green & Yellow, Black Print, Opaque, Hard Gel, barr158	Chlordiazepoxide 5 mg	Librium by Ivax	00182-0977	Antianxiety; C IV
BARR158	Cap, Aqua Green & Yellow, Black Print, Opaque, Hard Gel, barr158	Chlordiazepoxide 5 mg	Librium by Sandoz	00555-0158	Antianxiety; C IV
BARR158	Cap, Green & Yellow	Chlordiazepoxide 5 mg	Librium by Sandoz	00781-2080	Antianxiety; C IV
BARR158	Cap, Green & Yellow	Chlordiazepoxide 5 mg	Librium by Qualitest	00603-2666	Antianxiety; C IV
BARR158	Cap, Green & Yellow	Chlordiazepoxide 5 mg	Librium by Physician Total Care	54868-2463	Antianxiety; C IV
BARR159	Cap, Aqua Green & White, Black Print, Opaque, Hard Gel, barr159	Chlordiazepoxide 25 mg	Librium by Sandoz	00781-2084	Antianxiety; C IV
BARR159	Cap, Aqua Green & White, Black Print, Opaque, Hard Gel, barr159	Chlordiazepoxide 25 mg	Librium by Barr	00555-0159	Antianxiety; C IV
BARR159	Cap, Green & White	Chlordiazepoxide 25 mg	Librium by PDRX	55289-0126	Antianxiety; C IV

ID FRONT <> BACK	DESCRIPTION FRONT <> BACK	INGREDIENT & STRENGTH	BRAND (or Generic Equiv.) by FIRM	NDC#	CLASS; SCH.
BARR159	Cap, Green & White	Chlordiazepoxide 25 mg	Librium by UDL	51079-0141	Antianxiety; C IV
BARR159	Cap, Aqua Green & White, Black Print, Opaque, Hard Gel, barr159	Chlordiazepoxide 25 mg	Librium by Ivax	00182-0979	Antianxiety; C IV
BARR170	Tab, White, Oval	Furosemide 20 mg	Lasix by Barr		Diuretic
BARR198 <> 3	Tab	Acetaminophen 300 mg, Codeine Phosphate 30 mg	Tylenol w/ Codeine by Pharmedix	53002-0101	Analgesic; C III
BARR198 <> 3	Tab, Barr/198 <> 3	Acetaminophen 300 mg, Codeine Phosphate 30 mg	Tylenol w/ Codeine by Barr	00555-0198	Analgesic; C III
BARR1MG102	Cap, Light Gray, Opaque, Black Ink	Anagrelide HCl 1.0 mg	Agrylin by Barr	00555-0102 Discontinued	Antiplatelet
BARR200MG588	Cap, Green and White, Opaque, Delayed-Release	Didanosine 200 mg	Videx by Barr	00555-0588	Antiviral
BARR20MG	Cap, Blue and Gray, Opaque	Fluoxetine 20 mg	Prozac by Teva	00555-0877	Antidepressant
BARR20MG877	Cap, Blue & Gray, Black Print, Opaque, barr over 20 mg	Fluoxetine HCl 20 mg	Prozac by Barr	00555-0877 Discontinued	Antidepressant
BARR214	Cap, Green & White	Chlordiazepoxide 5 mg, Clidinium Bromide 2.5 mg	Librax by Barr		Gastrointestinal
BARR2172	Tab, White, Round, Barr 217/2	Acetaminophen 300 mg, Codeine Phosphate 15 mg	Tylenol w/ Codeine by Barr		Analgesic; C III
BARR219	Tab, Pink, Oblong	Erythromycin Stearate 500 mg	Erythrocin by Barr		Antibiotic
BARR229 <> 4	Tab	Acetaminophen 300 mg, Codeine Phosphate 60 mg	Tylenol w/ Codeine by Pharmedix	53002-0103	Analgesic; C III
BARR230	Cap, Reddish Orange, Opaque, Barr over 230	Erythromycin Estolate 250 mg	by Barr	00555-0230	Antibiotic
BARR234	Cap, Red & Ivory, Black Print, Opaque	Erythromycin Estolate 125 mg	by Barr	00555-0234	Antibiotic
BARR243	Tab, White, Round	Amitriptyline 25 mg, Chlordiazepoxide 10 mg	Limbitrol by Barr		Antianxiety; C IV
BARR244	Tab, Peach, Round	Amitriptyline 12.5 mg, Chlordiazepoxide 5 mg	Limbitrol by Barr		Antianxiety; C IV
BARR248	Tab, White, Round, Barr/248	Methyldopa 500 mg	Aldomet by Barr		Antihypertensive
BARR250MG589	Cap, Blue and White, Opaque, Delayed-Release	Didanosine 250 mg	Videx by Barr	00555-0589	Antiviral
BARR259	Tab, Coated	Erythromycin Ethylsuccinate 400 mg	by Pharmedix	53002-0206	Antibiotic
BARR25MG827	Cap, White, Opaque, Black Ink	Zonisamide 25 mg	Zonegran by Barr	00555-0827	Anticonvulsant
BARR260	Tab, Coated	Thioridazine HCl 10 mg	by Pharmedix	53002-1065	Antipsychotic
BARR2643	Tab, White, Round, Barr 264/3	Aspirin 325 mg, Codeine Phosphate 30 mg	Aspirin w/ Codeine by Barr		Analgesic; C III
BARR267	Tab, Yellow, Round	Chlorthalidone 25 mg	Hygroton by Barr		Diuretic
BARR268	Tab, Green, Round	Chlorthalidone 50 mg	Hygroton by Barr		Diuretic
BARR272	Cap, Orange, Black Print, Opaque, Hard Gel	Sulfinpyrazone 200 mg	by Barr	00555-0272	Uricosuric
BARR276	Tab, White, Round, Barr/276	Chlorpropamide 250 mg	Diabinese by Barr		Antidiabetic
BARR2804	Tab, White, Round	Aspirin 325 mg, Codeine Phosphate 60 mg	Aspirin w/ Codeine by Barr		Analgesic; C III
BARR288	Tab, Yellow, Round	Isosorbide Dinitrate 40 mg	Isordil by Barr		Antianginal
BARR2942	Tab, White, Round, Barr 294/2	Aspirin 325 mg, Codeine Phosphate 15 mg	Aspirin w/ Codeine by Barr		Analgesic; C III
BARR30250	Cap, Light Yellow & Maroon, Black Print, Opaque, Hard Gel, barr over 302	Hydroxyzine Pamoate 50 mg	Vistaril by Barr	00555-0302	Antianxiety; Antihistamine
BARR30250	Cap, Light Yellow & Maroon, Black Print, Opaque, Hard Gel, barr over 302	Hydroxyzine Pamoate 50 mg	Vistaril by Murfreesboro	51129-1483	Antianxiety; Antihistamine
BARR30250	Cap, Light Yellow & Maroon, Black Print, Opaque, Hard Gel, barr over 302	Hydroxyzine Pamoate 50 mg	Vistaril by UDL	51079-0078	Antianxiety; Antihistamine
BARR321	Tab, White, Oblong, Barr/321	Sulfamethoxazole 400 mg, Trimethoprim 80 mg	Septra by Barr		Antibiotic
BARR322	Tab, White, Oval, Barr/322	Sulfamethoxazole 800 mg, Trimethoprim 160 mg	Septra by Barr		Antibiotic
BARR32325	Cap, Light Yellow & Pink, Black Print, Opaque, Hard Gel, barr over 323	Hydroxyzine Pamoate 25 mg	Vistaril by Barr	00555-0323	Antianxiety; Antihistamine
BARR32325	Cap, Light Yellow & Pink, Black Print, Opaque, Hard Gel, barr over 323	Hydroxyzine Pamoate 25 mg	Vistaril by Qualitest	00603-3994	Antianxiety; Antihistamine
BARR32325	Cap, Light Yellow & Pink, Black Print, Opaque, Hard Gel, barr over 323	Hydroxyzine Pamoate 25 mg	Vistaril by UDL	51079-0077	Antianxiety; Antihistamine

ID FRONT <> BACK	DESCRIPTION FRONT <> BACK	INGREDIENT & STRENGTH	BRAND (or Generic Equiv.) by FIRM	NDC#	CLASS; SCH.
BARR324100	Cap, Light Yellow & Pink, Black Print, Opaque, Hard Gel, barr over 324	Hydroxyzine Pamoate 100 mg	Vistaril by Barr	00555-0324	Antianxiety; Antihistamine
BARR325	Tab	Acetaminophen 500 mg, Hydrocodone Bitartrate 5 mg	Vicodin by Pharmedix	53002-0119	Analgesic; C III
BARR327	Tab, Green, Round	Thioridazine 150 mg	Mellaril by Barr	00555-0327	Antipsychotic
BARR328	Tab, Orange, Round	Thioridazine 200 mg	Mellaril by Barr	00555-0328	Antipsychotic
BARR331	Cap, Blue & Red	Disopyramide Phosphate 100 mg	Norpace by Barr	00555-0331	Antiarrhythmic
BARR332	Cap, Ivory & Red	Disopyramide Phosphate 150 mg	Norpace by Barr	00555-0332	Antiarrhythmic
BARR336	Cap, Green & Green, Barr/336	Indomethacin 25 mg	Indocin by Barr	00555-0326	NSAID
BARR337	Cap, Green & Green, Barr/337	Indomethacin 50 mg	Indocin by Barr	00555-0327	NSAID
BARR349	Tab, Blue, Round	Chlorpropamide 100 mg	Diabinese by Barr	00555-0349	Antidiabetic
BARR350	Tab, Blue, Round	Chlorpropamide 250 mg	Diabinese by Barr	00555-0350	Antidiabetic
BARR357	Tab, White, Round	Methyldopa 125 mg	Aldomet by Barr	00555-0357	Antihypertensive
BARR358	Tab, White, Round	Methyldopa 250 mg	Aldomet by Barr	00555-0358	Antihypertensive
BARR374	Cap, White	Oxazepam 10 mg	Serax by Barr	00555-0374	Sedative/Hypnotic; C IV
BARR375	Cap, Red	Oxazepam 15 mg	Serax by Barr	00555-0375	Sedative/Hypnotic; C IV
BARR376	Cap, Maroon	Oxazepam 30 mg	Serax by Barr	00555-0376	Sedative/Hypnotic; C IV
BARR377	Cap, Blue & White, Barr/377	Flurazepam HCl 15 mg	Dalmane by Barr	00555-0377	Hypnotic; C IV
BARR378	Cap, Blue, Barr/378	Flurazepam HCl 30 mg	Dalmane by Barr	00555-0378	Hypnotic; C IV
BARR383	Tab, White, Round	Ergoloid Mesylate 1 mg	Hydergine by Barr	00555-0383	Ergot Alkaloids
BARR388	Tab, Orange, Round	Hydralazine HCl 10 mg	Apresoline by Barr	00555-0388	Antihypertensive
BARR389	Tab, Orange, Round, Barr/389	Hydralazine HCl 100 mg	Apresoline by Barr	00555-0389	Antihypertensive
BARR395	Tab, Orange & Red, Round	Phenylbutazone 100 mg	Butazolidin by Barr	00555-0395	Anti-Inflammatory
BARR396	Cap, Green & White	Phenylbutazone 100 mg	Butazolidin by Barr	00555-0396	Anti-Inflammatory
BARR400MG590	Cap, Red and White, Opaque, Delayed-Release	Didanosine 400 mg	Videx by Barr	00555-0590	Antiviral
BARR404	Cap, Ivory	Doxepin HCl 25 mg	Sinequan by Barr	00555-0404	Antidepressant
BARR405	Cap, Ivory	Doxepin HCl 50 mg	Sinequan by Barr	00555-0405	Antidepressant
BARR406	Cap, Green	Doxepin HCl 75 mg	Sinequan by Barr	00555-0406	Antidepressant
BARR407	Cap, Green & White	Doxepin HCl 100 mg	Sinequan by Barr	00555-0407	Antidepressant
BARR415	Tab, White, Round	Tolazamide 100 mg	Tolinase by Barr	00555-0415	Antidiabetic
BARR416	Tab, White, Round	Tolazamide 250 mg	Tolinase by Barr	00555-0416	Antidiabetic
BARR417	Tab, White, Oval	Tolazamide 500 mg	Tolinase by Barr	00555-0417	Antidiabetic
BARR419	Tab, Coated	Ibuprofen 400 mg	Motrin by Pharmedix	53002-0337	NSAID
BARR420	Tab, Film Coated	Ibuprofen 600 mg	Motrin by Pharmedix	53002-0301	NSAID
BARR425	Tab, Beige, Round, Barr/425	Verapamil HCl 80 mg	Isoptin, Calan by Barr	00555-0425	Antihypertensive
BARR442	Tab, White, Oval, Scored	Acetohexamide 250 mg	Dymelor by Barr	00555-0442	Antidiabetic
BARR443	Tab, White, Cap Shaped, Scored	Acetohexamide 500 mg	Dymelor by Barr	00555-0443	Antidiabetic
BARR443	Tab, White, Cap Shaped, Scored	Acetohexamide 500 mg	Dymelor by Amerisource	62584-0049	Antidiabetic
BARR454	Cap, Orange, Opaque	Isotretinoin 30 mg	Claravis by Barr	00555-1056	Dermatologic
BARR486	Tab, Blue, Round	Chlorthalidone 50 mg	Hygroton by Barr	00555-0486	Diuretic
BARR487	Cap, Green & White, Barr/487	Temazepam 15 mg	Restoril by Barr	00555-0487	Sedative/Hypnotic; C IV
BARR488	Cap, White, Barr/488	Temazepam 30 mg	Restoril by Barr	00555-0487	Sedative/Hypnotic; C IV
BARR499	Tab, Coated	Ibuprofen 800 mg	Motrin by Pharmedix	53002-0398	NSAID
BARR50302	Cap, in Black Ink	Hydroxyzine Pamoate 85.22 mg	Vistaril by Qualitest	00603-3995	Antianxiety; Antihistamine
BARR513	Cap, Orange, Opaque, Black Ink, Extended Release	Acetazolamide 500 mg	Diamox Sequels by Barr	00555-0513	Antiglaucoma Agent
BARR514	Cap, Red & Tan w/ Black Print	Cephalexin 250 mg	by Warner Chilcott	00047-0938	Antibiotic
BARR514	Cap, Red & Tan w/ Black Print	Cephalexin 250 mg	by ESI Lederle	59911-5933	Antibiotic
BARR514	Cap, Grey & Red, Black Print, Opaque, Hard Gel	Cephalexin 250 mg	by Barr	00555-0514	Antibiotic
BARR515	Cap, Red, Opaque, Hard Gel	Cephalexin 500 mg	by Barr	00555-0515	Antibiotic
BARR515	Cap, Red	Cephalexin 500 mg	by ESI Lederle	59911-5934	Antibiotic
BARR515	Cap, Red	Cephalexin 500 mg	by Warner Chilcott	00047-0939	Antibiotic

ID FRONT <> BACK	DESCRIPTION FRONT <> BACK	INGREDIENT & STRENGTH	BRAND (or Generic Equiv.) by FIRM	NDC#	CLASS; SCH.
BARR546	Tab, Orange, Oblong	Cephalexin 500 mg	Keflex by Barr	00555-0546	Antibiotic
BARR550	Cap, Green & Pink	Cephradine 250 mg	Velosef by Barr	00555-0550	Antibiotic
BARR550	Cap, Light Green & Pink, Black Print, Opaque, Hard Gel	Cephradine 250 mg	by Barr	00555-0550 Discontinued	Antibiotic
BARR551	Cap, Light Green, Opaque, Hard Gel	Cephradine 500 mg	by Barr	00555-0551 Discontinued	Antibiotic
BARR551	Cap, Green & Green	Cephradine 500 mg	Velosef by Barr	00555-0551	Antibiotic
BARR554	Cap, Maroon & Pink	Meclofenamate Sodium 50 mg	Meclomen by Barr	00555-0554	NSAID
BARR555	Cap, Maroon & White	Meclofenamate Sodium 100 mg	Meclomen by Barr	00555-0555	NSAID
BARR555196	Tab, White, Round, Barr 555/196	Furosemide 80 mg	Lasix by Barr	00555-0196	Diuretic
BARR555363	Tab	Diazepam 5 mg	by Pharmedix	53002-0334	Antianxiety; C IV
BARR555483	Tab, Barr/455/483	Amiloride HCl 5 mg, Hydrochlorothiazide 50 mg	Moduretic by Qualitest	00603-2188	Antihypertensive; Diuretic
BARR555483	Tab	Amiloride HCl 5 mg, Hydrochlorothiazide 50 mg	Moduretic by Ivax	00182-1877	Antihypertensive; Diuretic
BARR582	Cap, Brown & White, Black Print, Opaque, Hard Gel	Cefadroxil Monohydrate 500 mg	Duricef by Barr	00555-0582 Discontinued	Antibiotic
BARR582	Cap, Brown & White, Black Print, Opaque, Hard Gel	Cefadroxil Monohydrate 500 mg	Duricef by Caremark	00339-6154	Antibiotic
BARR584	Cap, Clear & Dark Green, Black Print	Erythromycin 250 mg	E-Mycin by PDRX	55289-0645	Antibiotic
BARR584	Cap, Clear & Dark Green, Black Print	Erythromycin 250 mg	E-Mycin by Barr	00555-0584	Antibiotic
BARR584	Cap, Clear & Dark Green, Black Print	Erythromycin 250 mg	E-Mycin by UDL	51079-0671	Antibiotic
BARR584	Cap, Clear & Dark Green, Black Print	Erythromycin 250 mg	E-Mycin by DRX	55045-2076	Antibiotic
BARR584	Cap, Clear & Dark Green, Black Print	Erythromycin 250 mg	E-Mycin by Major	00904-2465	Antibiotic
BARR584	Cap, Clear & Dark Green, Black Print	Erythromycin 250 mg	E-Mycin by Pharmedix	53002-0252	Antibiotic
BARR584	Cap, Clear & Dark Green, Black Print	Erythromycin 250 mg	E-Mycin by Murfreesboro	51129-1392	Antibiotic
BARR633	Cap, Yellow & White, Black Print, Opaque, Hard Gel	Danazol 50 mg	Danocrine by Barr	00555-0633	Steroid
BARR634	Cap, Yellow & Clear, Black Print, Opaque, Hard Gel	Danazol 100 mg	Danocrine by Barr	00555-0634	Steroid
BARR635	Cap, Orange & Clear, Black Print, Opaque	Danazol 200 mg	Danocrine by Ivax	00182-1880	Steroid
BARR635	Cap, Orange & Clear, Black Print, Opaque	Danazol 200 mg	Danocrine by Barr	00555-0635	Steroid
BARR651	Cap, Light Yellow & Red, Black Print, Opaque	Oxycodone 5 mg, Acetaminophen 500 mg	Percocet by Barr	00555-0651	Analgesic; C II
BARR658	Cap, Red and White, Opaque	Acetaminophen 500 mg, Oxycodone 5 mg	Tylox by Barr	00555-0658	Analgesic; C II
BARR732 <> 505050	Tab, White, Oval, Scored	Trazodone HCl 150 mg	Desyrel by Teva	00480-0290	Antidepressant
BARR732 <> 505050	Tab, White, Oval, Scored	Trazodone HCl 150 mg	Desyrel by Barr	00555-0732	Antidepressant
BARR733 <> 100100100	Tab, White, Oval, Scored	Trazodone HCl 300 mg	Desyrel by Barr	00555-0733	Antidepressant
BARR733 <> 100100100	Tab, White, Oval, Scored	Trazodone HCl 300 mg	Desyrel by Teva	00480-0292	Antidepressant
BARR808	Cap, Brown and Dark Yellow, Opaque	Tretinoin 10 mg	Vesanoid by Barr	00555-0808	Retinoid
BARR870	Cap, Brown & White, Black Print, Opaque	Flutamide 125 mg	Eulexin by Barr	00555-0870	Antiandrogen
BARR875	Cap, Peach & White, Black Print, Opaque, Hard Gel	Hydrochlorothiazide 25 mg, Triamterene 37.5 mg	by Barr	00555-0875	Diuretic; Antihypertensive
BARR882	Cap, Pink & Purple, Black Print, Opaque, Hard Gel	Hydroxyurea 500 mg	Hydrea by Barr	00555-0882	Antineoplastic
BARR932	Cap, Brown & Olive, Black Print, Hard Gel	Minocycline HCl 50 mg	Minocin by Barr	00555-0932	Antibiotic
BARR933	Cap, Olive & White, Black Print, Hard Gel	Minocycline HCl 100 mg	Minocin by Barr	00555-0933	Antibiotic
BARR934	Cap, Light Gray, Opaque, Red Print	Isotretinoin 10 mg	Claravis by Barr	00555-1054	Dermatologic
BARR935	Cap, Brown, Opaque, White Print	Isotretinoin 20 mg	Claravis by Barr	00555-1055	Dermatologic
BARR936	Cap, Light Orange, Opaque, Black Print	Isotretinoin 40 mg	Claravis by Barr	00555-1057	Dermatologic
BARR947	Cap, Green & Pink, Black Print, Opaque, Hard Gel	Hydroxyurea 250 mg	Hydrea by Barr	00555-0947	Antineoplastic
BARR954	Cap, Beige, Black Print, Opaque, Hard Gel, Extended Release	Dextroamphetamine Sulfate 5 mg	Dexedrine by Barr	00555-0954	Stimulant; C II
BARR955	Cap, Brown & Clear, Black Print, Opaque, Hard Gel, Extended Release	Dextroamphetamine Sulfate 10 mg	Dexedrine by Barr	00555-0955	Stimulant; C II
BARR956	Cap, Dark Brown & Clear, Black Print, Opaque, Hard Gel, Extended Release	Dextroamphetamine Sulfate 15 mg	Dexedrine by Barr	00555-0956	Stimulant; C II

ID FRONT <> BACK	DESCRIPTION FRONT <> BACK	INGREDIENT & STRENGTH	BRAND (or Generic Equiv.) by FIRM	NDC#	CLASS; SCH.
BAYER	Tab, White, Cap Shaped, Scored	Aspirin 325 mg	Aspirin by Bayer	Canadian DIN 02150328	Analgesic
BAYER	Cap, White, Oblong, Scored	Acetaminophen 325 mg	Tylenol by Bayer	Canadian	Analgesic
BAYER <> 10	Tab, Orange, Round, Film-Coated, BAYER BAYER in cross	Vardenafil HCl 10 mg	Levitra by Bayer	Canadian DIN 02250470	Impotence Agent
BAYER <> 10	Tab, Orange, Round, Film-Coated, BAYER BAYER in cross	Vardenafil HCl 10 mg	Levitra by Bayer	00026-8730	Impotence Agent
BAYER <> 20	Tab, Orange, Round, Film-Coated, BAYER BAYER in cross	Vardenafil HCl 20 mg	Levitra by Bayer	00026-8740	Impotence Agent
BAYER <> 20	Tab, Orange, Round, Film-Coated, BAYER BAYER in cross	Vardenafil HCl 20 mg	Levitra by Bayer	Canadian DIN 02250489	Impotence Agent
BAYER <> 200	Tab, Red, Round, Film Coated, Bayer Cross <> 200	Sorafenib 200 mg	Nexavar by Bayer	Canadian DIN 02284227	Cancer Treatment
BAYER <> 200	Tab, Red, Round, Film Coated, Bayer Cross <> 200	Sorafenib 200 mg	Nexavar by Bayer	00026-8488	Cancer Treatment
BAYER <> 25	Tab, Orange, Round, Film-Coated, 2.5	Vardenafil HCl 2.5 mg	Levitra by Bayer	00026-8710	Impotence Agent
BAYER <> 5	Tab, Orange, Round, Film-Coated	Vardenafil HCl 5 mg	Levitra by Bayer	00026-8720	Impotence Agent
BAYER <> 5	Tab, Orange, Round, Film-Coated	Vardenafil HCl 5 mg	Levitra by Bayer	Canadian DIN 02250462	Impotence Agent
BAYER <> ASPIRIN	Tab, Peach, Round	Aspirin 80 mg	Aspirin Children's Size by Bayer	Canadian DIN 02150352	Analgesic
BAYER <> C1000QD	Tab, White to Yellow, Oblong, Film Coated	Ciprofloxacin HCl 1000 mg	Cipro XL by Bayer	Canadian DIN 02251787	Antibiotic
BAYER <> C1000QD	Tab, White to Yellow, Oblong, Film Coated, Ex Release	Ciprofloxacin HCl 1000 mg	Cipro XR by Bayer	00026-8897	Antibiotic
BAYER <> C500QD	Tab, White to Yellow, Oblong, Film Coated, Ex Release	Ciprofloxacin HCl 500 mg	Cipro XR by Bayer	00026-8889	Antibiotic
BAYER <> C500QD	Tab, White to Yellow, Oblong, Film Coated, Ex Release	Ciprofloxacin HCl 500 mg	Cipro XL by Bayer	Canadian DIN 02247916	Antibiotic
BAYER <> LG	Tab, White, Oblong, Film Coated, Triple Score	Praziquantel 600 mg	Biltricide by Bayer	Canadian DIN 02230897	Antihelmintic
BAYER <> LG	Tab, White, Coated, with Orange Tint <> Triple Score on Side 1	Praziquantel 600 mg	Biltricide by Bayer	00085-1747	Antihelmintic
BAYER <> M400	Tab, Red, Oblong, Film Coated	Moxifloxacin HCl 400 mg	Avelox by Bayer	Canadian DIN 02242965	Antibiotic
BAYER <> M400	Tab, Red, Oblong, Film Coated	Moxifloxacin HCl 400 mg	Avelox by Bayer	00026-8581	Antibiotic
BAYER <> M400	Tab, Red, Oblong, Film Coated	Moxifloxacin HCl 400 mg	Avelox by Bayer	12527-8581	Antibiotic
BAYER10	Tab, Dusty Rose, Round, Bayer/10	Nifedipine 10 mg	Adalat PA 10 by Bayer	Canadian Discontinued	Antihypertensive
BAYER20	Tab, Dusty Rose, Round, Bayer/20	Nifedipine 20 mg	Adalat PA by Bayer	Canadian Discontinued	Antihypertensive
BAYER325	Tab, Pale Yellow, Cap Shaped, Enteric Coated, Brown Ink	Aspirin 325 mg	Aspirin (Coated) by Bayer	Canadian DIN 02150417	Analgesic
BAYER325	Cap, Yellow	Acetaminophen 325 mg	Tylenol by Bayer	Canadian	Analgesic
BAYER500	Cap, Yellow	Acetaminophen 500 mg	Tylenol Ex Strength by Bayer	Canadian	Analgesic
BAYER500	Tab, Pale Yellow, Cap Shaped, Enteric Coated, Brown Ink	Aspirin 500 mg	Aspirin Ex Strength (Coated) by Bayer	Canadian DIN 02150425	Analgesic
BAYER855	Cap, Ivory, Soft Gel	Nimodipine 30 mg	Nimotop by Bayer	Canadian 55154-4804	Antihypertensive
BAYER855	Cap, Ivory, Soft Gel	Nimodipine 30 mg	by Nat Pharmpak	Canadian 55154-4804	Antihypertensive
BAYERBAYER	Tab, White, Round, Red Ink	Aspirin 500 mg	Aspirin Ex Strength by Bayer	Canadian DIN 02150336	Analgesic
BAYERBAYER	Tab, White, Round, Bayer Cross on both sides	Aspirin 325 mg	Aspirin by Bayer	Canadian DIN 02150328	Analgesic
BAYERBAYER <> G100	Tab, Off-White, Round, Scored, G100 <> Bayer Cross	Acarbose 100 mg	Glucobay by Bayer	Canadian DIN 02190893	Antidiabetic

ID FRONT <> BACK	DESCRIPTION FRONT <> BACK	INGREDIENT & STRENGTH	BRAND (or Generic Equiv.) by FIRM	NDC#	CLASS; SCH.
BAYERBAYER <> G50	Tab, Off-White, Round, G50 over Bayer Cross	Acarbose 50 mg	Glucobay by Bayer	Canadian DIN 02190885	Antidiabetic
BAYERCROSS	Tab, White, Bayer Logo	Acetaminophen 325 mg	Tylenol by Bayer	Canadian	Analgesic
BAYERCROSS	Tab, Peach, Scored	Acetaminophen 325 mg	Tylenol by Bayer	Canadian	Analgesic
BAYERCROSS <> 10TRIANGLE	Tab, Light Red, Round, Film Coated	Rivaroxaban 10 mg	Xarelto by Bayer	Canadian DIN 02316986	Anticoagulant
BAYERLG	Tab, White, Oblong, Bayer/LG	Praziquantel 600 mg	Biltricide by Bayer	Canadian	Antihelmintic
BAYERPLUS	Tab, White, Round, Film Coated, Blue Ink	Aspirin 325 mg, Calcium Carbonate 160 mg, Magnesium Carbonate 34 mg, Magnesium Oxide 63 mg	Aspirin with Stomach Guard by Bayer	Canadian DIN 02229980	Analgesic
BAYERPLUS500	Tab, White, Cap Shaped, Film Coated, Blue Ink, BAYERPLUS <> 500	Aspirin 500 mg, Calcium Carbonate 246.2 mg, Magnesium Carbonate 52.3 mg, Magnesium Oxide 96.9 mg	Aspirin with Stomach Guard Ex Strength by Bayer	Canadian DIN 02229967	Analgesic
BB <> PP	Tab, White, Oval, Scored, P logo / P logo <> B / B	Pramipexole DiHCl 0.5 mg	Mirapex by Pharmascience	Canadian DIN 02290138	Antiparkinson
BB455	Tab, Orange, Oval, B/B 455	Verapamil HCl 120 mg	Isoptin, Calan by Barr		Antihypertensive
BBA	Tab, Salmon, Round, Schering Logo BBA	Acetophenazine Maleate 20 mg	Tindal by Schering		Antipsychotic
BC <> SANDOZ	Tab, Ivory, Round, Sugar Coated	Pizotifen 0.5 mg	Sandomigran by Novartis	Canadian DIN 00329320	Antimigraine
BC20832	Tab, White, Round, Scored, BC over 20/832	Baclofen 20 mg	Lioresal by Martec	52555-0696	Muscle Relaxant
BC50 <> G	Tab, White, Round, Film Coated	Bicalutamide 50 mg	Casodex by Genpharm	Canadian DIN 02302403	Antineoplastic
BCAMPI250	Cap	Ampicillin 250 mg	Principen by Sandoz	43858-0282	Antibiotic
BCAMPI500	Cap	Ampicillin	Principen by Sandoz	43858-0285	Antibiotic
BCI	Cap, Yellow, Oval, Soft Gel	Doxercalciferol 2.5 mcg	Hectorol by Genzyme	58468-0121	Calcium Metabolism
BCI	Cap, Yellow, Oval, Soft Gel	Doxercalciferol 2.5 mcg	Hectorol by RP Scherer	11014-1235	Calcium Metabolism
BCI	Cap, Citrus Orange, Oval, Soft Gel	Doxercalciferol 0.5 mcg	Hectorol by Genzyme	58468-0120	Calcium Metabolism
BCI	Cap, Yellow, Oval, Soft Gelatin	Doxercalciferol 2.5 mcg	Hectorol by Shire BioChem	Canadian DIN 02243790	Calcium Metabolism
BCL10 <> 832	Tab, White, Round, Scored, BCL / 10	Bethanechol Chloride 10 mg	Urecholine by Upsher-Smith	00832-0511	Urinary Tract
BCL25 <> 832	Tab, Yellow, Round, Scored, BCL / 25	Bethanechol Chloride 25 mg	Urecholine by Upsher-Smith	00832-0512	Urinary Tract
BCL5 <> 832	Tab, White, Round, Scored, BCL / 5	Bethanechol Chloride 5 mg	Urecholine by Upsher-Smith	00832-0510	Urinary Tract
BCL50 <> 832	Tab, Yellow, Round, Scored, BCL / 50	Bethanechol Chloride 50 mg	Urecholine by Upsher-Smith	00832-0513	Urinary Tract
BCT212	Tab, White, Round, Scored, BCT 2 1/2	Bromocriptine 2.5 mg	Parlodel by LEK	66685-5905	Antiparkinson
BCT212	Tab, White, Round, Scored, BCT 2 1/2	Bromocriptine 2.5 mg	Parlodel by Rosemont	00832-0105	Antiparkinson
BCT25	Tab, White, Oblong, Scored, BCT 2.5	Bromocriptine 2.5 mg	Parlodel by Pharmascience	Canadian DIN 02231702	Antiparkinson
BCT5MGP	Cap, Beige and Brown	Bromocriptine 5 mg	Parlodel by Pharmascience	Canadian DIN 02236949	Antiparkinson
BDA	Tab, Pink, Round, Schering Logo BDA	Betamethasone 0.6 mg	Celestone by Schering	00085-0011	Steroid
BE	Tab, Lavender, Oval, Schering Logo BE	Methyltestosterone Buccal 10 mg	Oreton Buccal by Schering		Hormone; C III
BE10 <> APO	Tab, Yellow, Round, Film Coated	Benazepril HCl 10 mg	Lotensin by Apotex	Canadian DIN 02290340	Antihypertensive
BE10 <> APO	Tab, Yellow, Round, Film Coated	Benazepril HCl 10 mg	Lotensin by Apotex	60505-0266	Antihypertensive
BE20 <> APO	Tab, Light Pink, Round, Film Coated	Benazepril HCl 20 mg	Lotensin by Apotex	60505-0267	Antihypertensive
BE20 <> APO	Tab, Light Pink, Round, Film Coated	Benazepril HCl 20 mg	Lotensin by Apotex	Canadian DIN 02273918	Antihypertensive
BE40 <> APO	Tab, Pink, Round, Film Coated	Benazepril HCl 40 mg	Lotensin by Apotex	60505-0268	Antihypertensive
BE5 <> APO	Tab, Light Yellow, Round, Film Coated	Benazepril HCl 5 mg	Lotensin by Apotex	60505-0265	Antihypertensive
BE5 <> APO	Tab, Light Yellow, Round, Film Coated	Benazepril HCl 5 mg	Lotensin by Apotex	Canadian DIN 02290332	Antihypertensive
BEACH <> 1114	Tab, Yellow, Oblong, Film Coated	Methenamine Mandelate 500 mg, Sodium Phosphate, Monobasic 500 mg	Uroqid Acid No. 2 by Neogen	59051-0090	Antibiotic; Urinary Tract

ID FRONT <> BACK	DESCRIPTION FRONT <> BACK	INGREDIENT & STRENGTH	BRAND (or Generic Equiv.) by FIRM	NDC#	CLASS; SCH.
BEACH <> 1114	Tab, Yellow, Oblong, Film Coated	Methenamine Mandelate 500 mg, Sodium Phosphate, Monobasic 500 mg	Uroqid Acid No. 2 by West-Ward	00143-9023	Antibiotic; Urinary Tract
BEACH <> 1114	Tab, Yellow, Oblong, Film Coated	Methenamine Mandelate 500 mg, Sodium Phosphate, Monobasic, Monohydrate 500 mg	Uroqid Acid No. 2 by Pharmaceutical Assoc	00121-0352	Antibiotic; Urinary Tract
BEACH <> 1114	Tab, Yellow, Oblong, Film Coated	Methenamine Mandelate 500 mg, Sodium Phosphate, Monobasic, Monohydrate 500 mg	Uroqid Acid No. 2 by Beach	00486-1114	Antibiotic; Urinary Tract
BEACH <> 1134	Tab, White, Oblong, Scored, Film Coated	Sodium Phosphate, Dibasic, Anhydrous 852 mg, Potassium Phosphate, Tribasic 155 mg, Sodium Phosphate, Monobasic, Monohydrate 130 mg	K-Phos No 2 by West-Ward	00143-9024	Electrolytes
BEACH <> 1134	Tab, White, Oblong, Scored, Film Coated	Sodium Phosphate, Dibasic, Anhydrous 852 mg, Potassium Phosphate, Tribasic 155 mg, Sodium Phosphate, Monobasic, Monohydrate 130 mg	K-Phos No 2 by Beach	00486-1134	Electrolytes
BEACH <> 1134	Tab, White, Oblong, Scored, Film Coated	Sodium Phosphate, Dibasic, Anhydrous 852 mg, Potassium Phosphate, Tribasic 155 mg, Sodium Phosphate, Monobasic, Monohydrate 130 mg	K-Phos No 2 by Pharm Assoc	00121-0386	Electrolytes
BEACH <> 1136	Tab, White, Cap Shaped	Potassium Citrate Anhydrous 50 mg, Sodium Citrate, Anhydrous 950 mg	Citrolith by Beach	00486-1136	Electrolytes
BEACH <> 1136	Tab, White, Cap Shaped	Potassium Citrate Anhydrous 50 mg, Sodium Citrate, Anhydrous 950 mg	Citrolith by Pharmaceutical Assoc	00121-0374	Electrolytes
BEACH1111	Tab, White, Scored	Potassium Phosphate, Monobasic 500 mg	K Phos Original by West-Ward	00143-9001	Electrolytes
BEACH1111	Tab, White	Potassium Phosphate, Monobasic 500 mg	K Phos Original by Beach	00486-1111	Electrolytes
BEACH1112	Tab, Yellow, Round	Methenamine Mandelate 350 mg, Sodium Acid Phosphate 200 mg	Uroquid-Acid by Beach	00486-1112	Antibiotic; Urinary Tract
BEACH1115	Tab, Green, Oblong	Methenamine Mandelate 500 mg, Potassium Acid Phosphate 250 mg	Thiacide by Beach	00486-1115	Antibiotic; Urinary Tract
BEACH1135	Tab, White, Round	Potassium Phosphate, Monobasic 155 mg, Sodium Phosphate, Monobasic 350 mg	K Phos MF by West-Ward	00143-9002	Electrolytes
BEACH1135	Tab, White, Round	Potassium Phosphate, Monobasic 155 mg, Sodium Phosphate, Monobasic 350 mg	K-Phos MF by Beach	00486-1135	Electrolytes
BEB <> CG	Tab, Light Red, Round, Film Coated	Oxprenolol HCl 80 mg	Slow Trasicor by Novartis	Canadian DIN 00534579	Antihypertensive
BEECHAM <> 185	Tab	Penicillin V Potassium	by SKB		Antibiotic
BEECHAM186	Tab, White, Oval	Penicillin V Potassium 500 mg	Beepen-VK by SKB		Antibiotic
BEECHAMFASTIN	Cap, Blue & White Beads	Phentermine 30 mg	Fastin by H J Harkins Co	52959-0430	Anorexiant; C IV
BEECHAMFASTIN	Cap, Blue & Clear, Blue & White Beads	Phentermine HCl 30 mg	by PDRX	55289-0180	Anorexiant; C IV
BEECHAMFASTIN	Cap, Blue & White Beads	Phentermine 30 mg	Fastin by King	60793-0836	Anorexiant; C IV
BEECHAMFASTIN	Cap, Beecham in White Ink <> R Inside Circle to Right of Fastin in Red Ink	Phentermine 30 mg	Fastin by SKB	00029-2205	Anorexiant; C IV
BEMINAL	Tab, Brown, Oval	B Complex Vitamin	Beminal by Whitehall Robins		Vitamin
BEMINALC	Cap, Brown & Yellow	B Complex Vitamin	Beminal by Whitehall Robins		Vitamin
BENADRYL	Tab, Light Green, Cap Shaped	Diphenhydramine HCl 12.5 mg, Pseudoephedrine HCl 30 mg, Acetaminophen 500 mg	Benadryl Allergy/Sinus Headache by Pfizer	Canadian DIN 02229367	Cold Remedy
BENADRYL	Tab, Pink, Cap Shaped, Film Coated	Diphenhydramine HCl 25 mg	Benadryl by Pfizer	Canadian DIN 02017849	Antihistamine
BENADRYL	Tab, Blue	Diphenhydramine 25 mg, Pseudoephedrine HCl 60 mg	Benadryl Allergy and Sinus by Pfizer	00501-2062	Cold Remedy
BENADRYL	Cap, Pink and White	Diphenhydramine HCl 25 mg	Benadryl by Pfizer	00501-2000	Antihistamine
BENADRYL125	Tab, Light Purple, Mottled, Round, Scored, Chewable, BENADRYL / 12.5	Diphenhydramine HCl 12.5 mg	Benadryl by Pfizer	Canadian DIN 02061287	Antihistamine
BENADRYL50MG	Cap, Pink and White	Diphenhydramine HCl 50 mg	Benadryl by Pfizer	Canadian DIN 02019671	Antihistamine
BENTYL10	Cap, Blue, Bentyl over 10	Dicyclomine HCl 10 mg	Bentyl by Merrell	00068-0120	Gastrointestinal
BENTYL20	Tab, Blue, Round, Bentyl over 20	Dicyclomine HCl 20 mg	Bentyl by H J Harkins Co	52959-0390	Gastrointestinal
BENTYL20	Tab, Blue, Round, Bentyl over 20	Dicyclomine HCl 20 mg	Bentyl by Aventis	00068-0123	Gastrointestinal
BENYLIN	Tab, Green, Cap Shaped	Dextromethorphan HBr 15 mg, Pseudoephedrine HCl 30 mg, Guaifenesin 100 mg, Acetaminophen 500 mg	Benylin by Pfizer	Canadian DIN 02218186	Cold Remedy
BERLEX <> 120MG	Tab, White, Cap Shaped, Scored	Sotalol 120 mg	Betapace AF by Berlex	50419-0119	Antiarrhythmic
BERLEX <> 160MG	Tab, White, Cap Shaped, Scored	Sotalol 160 mg	Betapace AF by Berlex	50419-0116	Antiarrhythmic
BERLEX <> 80MG	Tab, White, Cap Shaped, Scored	Sotalol 80 mg	Betapace by Promex Med	62301-0051	Antiarrhythmic

ID FRONT <> BACK	DESCRIPTION FRONT <> BACK	INGREDIENT & STRENGTH	BRAND (or Generic Equiv.) by FIRM	NDC#	CLASS; SCH.
BERLEX <> 80MG	Tab, White, Cap Shaped, Scored	Sotalol 80 mg	Betapace AF by Berlex	50419-0115	Antiarrhythmic
BERLEX181	Cap, Blue & Yellow	Chlorpheniramine Maleate 8 mg, Pseudoephedrine HCl 120 mg	Deconamine SR by Berlex		Cold Remedy
BERLEX184	Tab, White, Round	Chlorpheniramine Maleate 4 mg, Pseudoephedrine HCl 60 mg	Deconamine by Berlex		Cold Remedy
BERTEK560BERTEK560	Cap, Light Lavender & White	Phenytoin Sodium 100 mg	Dilantin Kapseals by Mylan	Discontinued	Anticonvulsant
BERTEK560BERTEK560	Cap, Purple & White	Phenytoin Sodium 100 mg	by Physician Total Care	54868-0040	Anticonvulsant
BERTEK670BERTEK670	Cap, Blue, Black Print, Opaque, Hard Gel, BERTEK over 670	Extended Phenytoin Sodium 200 mg	Phenytek by Bertek	62794-0670	Anticonvulsant
BERTEK750BERTEK750	Cap, Blue, Black Print, Opaque, Hard Gel, BERTEK over 750	Extended Phenytoin Sodium 300 mg	Phenytek by Bertek	62794-0750	Anticonvulsant
BERTEX560	Cap, Opaque & Purple, Bertex over 560	Phenytoin Sodium 100 mg	by Prepackage Specialists	58864-0397	Anticonvulsant
BETAPACE <> 120MG	Tab, Light Blue, Cap Shaped, Scored	Sotalol 120 mg	Betapace by Berlex	50419-0109	Antiarrhythmic
BETAPACE <> 160MG	Tab, Light Blue, Cap Shaped, Scored	Sotalol 160 mg	Betapace by Berlex	50419-0106	Antiarrhythmic
BETAPACE <> 240MG	Tab, Light Blue, Cap Shaped, Scored	Sotalol 240 mg	Betapace by Berlex	50419-0107	Antiarrhythmic
BETAPACE <> 80MG	Tab, Light Blue, Cap Shaped, Scored	Sotalol 80 mg	Betapace by Berlex	50419-0105	Antiarrhythmic
BGL	Tab, White, Round, BGL/Logo	Clobazam 10 mg	Frisium by Aventis	Canadian	Anticonvulsant
BHIOM	Tab	Aconite 5 X, Calcium Sulfide 10 X, Capsicum 6 X, Chamomile 4 X, Ferric Phosphate 10 X, Plantain 4 X, Potassium Chlorate 6 X, Pulsatilla 4 X	by Heel	50114-2279	Homeopathic
BHIOM	Tab	Acetic Acid 6 X, Aranea Diadema 8 X, Arsenic Trioxide 6 X, Asafoetida 6 X, Bryonia 30 X, Calcium Phosphate 10 X, Carbo Vegetabilis 10 X, Cinchona Officinalis 4 X, Condurango 4 X, Curare 10 X, Ergot 6 X, Kalmia Latifolia 8 X, Lycopodium 6 X, Mercuric Oxide Red 10 X, Phosphoric Acid 6 X, Pulsatilla 4 X, Silicea 10 X, Sodium Sulfate 6 X, Strychnine Nitrate 8 X, Uranyl Nitrate 12 X	Migrane by Heel	50114-2236	Homeopathic
BI	Tab, White and Red, Oblong, Two Layered, Boehringer Logo	Telmisartan 80 mg, Hydrochlorothiazide 12.5 mg	Micardis Plus by Boehringer Ingelheim	Canadian DIN 02244344	Antihypertensive; Diuretic
BI <> 18	Tab, Sugar Coated	Dipyridamole 50 mg	by Nat Pharmpak	55154-0402	Antiplatelet
BI <> 18	Tab, Reddish Orange, Sugar Coated	Dipyridamole 50 mg	Persantine-50 by Boehringer Ingelheim	00597-0018	Antiplatelet
BI <> 19	Tab, Sugar Coated	Dipyridamole 75 mg	Persantine-75 by Boehringer Ingelheim	00597-0019	Antiplatelet
BI <> 83	Tab, White, Round	Pramipexole DiHCl 0.125 mg	Mirapex by Boehringer Ingelheim	00597-0183	Antiparkinson
BI10	Tab	Chlorthalidone 15 mg, Clonidine HCl 0.3 mg	Combipres by Boehringer Ingelheim	00597-0010	Antihypertensive; Diuretic
BI10	Tab, Coated	Mesoridazine Besylate 10 mg	Serentil by Boehringer Ingelheim	00597-0020	Antipsychotic
BI10 <> APO	Tab, White, Round, Film-Coated	Bisoprolol Fumarate 10 mg	Apo-Bisoprolol by Apotex	Canadian DIN 02256177	Antihypertensive
BI100	Tab, Red, Round	Mesoridazine Besylate 100 mg	Serentil by Boehringer Ingelheim	00597-0023	Antipsychotic
BI11	Tab, Peach, Oval, Scored	Clonidine HCl 0.3 mg	Catapres by Boehringer Ingelheim	00597-0011	Antihypertensive
BI11	Tab, Peach, Oval, Scored	Clonidine HCl 0.3 mg	Catapres by DHHS Prog	11819-0111	Antihypertensive
BI12	Tab, Yellow, Round, BI/12	Bisacodyl 5 mg	Dulcolax by Boehringer Ingelheim		Gastrointestinal
BI17	Tab, Orange, Round, Sugar Coated, BI/17	Dipyridamole 25 mg	Persantine by Boehringer Ingelheim	00597-0017	Antiplatelet
BI17	Tab, Orange, Round, Sugar Coated, BI/17	Dipyridamole 25 mg	Persantine by GSK		Antiplatelet
BI17	Tab, Orange, Round, Sugar Coated, BI/17	Dipyridamole 25 mg	Persantine by Genpharm	55667-0092	Antiplatelet
BI18	Tab, Orange, Round, Sugar Coated, BI/18	Dipyridamole 50 mg	Persantine by Amerisource	62584-0018	Antiplatelet
BI18	Tab, Orange, Round, Sugar Coated, BI/18	Dipyridamole 50 mg	Persantine by GSK		Antiplatelet
BI18	Tab, Orange, Round, Sugar Coated, BI/18	Dipyridamole 50 mg	Persantine by Boehringer Ingelheim	00597-0018	Antiplatelet
BI19	Tab, Orange, Round, Sugar Coated, BI/19	Dipyridamole 75 mg	Persantine by Boehringer Ingelheim	00597-0019	Antiplatelet
BI19	Tab, Orange, Round, Sugar Coated, BI/19	Dipyridamole 75 mg	Persantine by Leiner	59606-0718	Antiplatelet
BI19	Tab, Orange, Round, Sugar Coated, BI/19	Dipyridamole 75 mg	Persantine by Pharm Util	60491-0507	Antiplatelet
BI25	Tab, Magenta, Round, Coated	Mesoridazine Besylate 25 mg	Serentil by Boehringer Ingelheim	00597-0021	Antipsychotic
BI28	Tab, Yellow, Round, BI/28	Thiethylperazine Maleate 10 mg	Torecan by Boehringer Ingelheim		Antiemetic
BI48	Tab, White, Round, BI/48	Theophylline Anhydrous 250 mg	Respbid by Boehringer Ingelheim		Antiasthmatic
BI49	Tab, White, Oblong, BI/49	Theophylline Anhydrous 500 mg	Respbid by Boehringer Ingelheim		Antiasthmatic

ID FRONT <> BACK	DESCRIPTION FRONT <> BACK	INGREDIENT & STRENGTH	BRAND (or Generic Equiv.) by FIRM	NDC#	CLASS; SCH.
BI5 <> APO	Tab, Salmon Pink, Round, Film-Coated, Scored	Bisoprolol Fumarate 5 mg	Apo-Bisoprolol by Apotex	Canadian DIN 02256134	Antihypertensive
BI50	Tab, Coated	Mesoridazine Besylate 50 mg	Serentil by Boehringer Ingelheim	00597-0022	Antipsychotic
BI58FLOMAX04MG	Cap, Olive Green, Gelatin Coated, Flomax over 0.4 mg <> BI 58	Tamsulosin HCl 0.4 mg	Flomax by Astellas	12838-0058	Antiadrenergic
BI58FLOMAX04MG	Cap, Olive Green, Gelatin Coated, Flomax over 0.4 mg <> BI 58	Tamsulosin HCl 0.4 mg	Flomax by Boehringer Ingelheim	00597-0058	Antiadrenergic
BI58FLOMAX04MG	Cap, Olive Green, Gelatin Coated, Flomax over 0.4 mg <> BI 58	Tamsulosin HCl 0.4 mg	Flomax by Astellas	51248-0058	Antiadrenergic
BI6	Tab, Tan, Oval, Scored	Clonidine HCl 0.1 mg	Catapres by Boehringer Ingelheim	00597-0006	Antihypertensive
BI6	Tab, Tan, Oval, Scored	Clonidine HCl 0.1 mg	Catapres by DHHS Prog	11819-0101	Antihypertensive
BI62	Tab, Pink, Round, BI/62	Phendimetrazine HCl 75 mg	Preludin Endurets by Boehringer Ingelheim		Appetite Suppressant; C II
BI64	Cap, Celery	Phendimetrazine Tartrate 105 mg	by Quality Care	60346-0621	Anorexiant; C III
BI64	Cap, Green	Phendimetrazine Tartrate 105 mg	by Allscripts		Anorexiant; C III
BI66	Cap, Brown & Red	Mexiletine 150 mg	Mexitil by Boehringer Ingelheim	00597-0066	Antiarrhythmic
BI66	Cap, Brown & Red	Mexiletine HCl 150 mg	Mexitil by Roxane	00054-0066	Antiarrhythmic
BI67	Cap, Red, BI/67	Mexiletine 200 mg	Mexitil by Boehringer Ingelheim	00597-0067	Antiarrhythmic
BI67	Cap, Red, BI/67	Mexiletine HCl 200 mg	Mexitil by Roxane	00054-0067	Antiarrhythmic
BI68	Cap, Aqua Green & Red, BI/68	Mexiletine HCl 250 mg	Mexitil by Roxane	00054-0068	Antiarrhythmic
BI68	Cap, Aqua Green & Red, BI/68	Mexiletine 250 mg	Mexitil by Boehringer Ingelheim	00597-0068	Antiarrhythmic
BI7	Tab, Orange, Oval, Scored	Clonidine HCl 0.2 mg	Catapres by Boehringer Ingelheim	00597-0007	Antihypertensive
BI7	Tab, Orange, Oval, Scored	Clonidine HCl 0.2 mg	Catapres by DHHS Prog	11819-0102	Antihypertensive
BI72	Tab	Metaproterenol Sulfate 20 mg	Alupent by Boehringer Ingelheim	00597-0072	Antiasthmatic
BI74	Tab	Metaproterenol Sulfate 10 mg	Alupent by Boehringer Ingelheim	00597-0074	Antiasthmatic
BI76	Tab, White, Kidney Shaped, BI/76	Chlorthalidone 25 mg	Thalitone by Boehringer Ingelheim		Diuretic
BI77	Tab, White, Kidney Shaped, BI/77	Chlorthalidone 15 mg	Thalitone by Boehringer Ingelheim		Diuretic
BI8	Tab, Pink, Oval	Chlorthalidone 15 mg, Clonidine HCl 0.1 mg	Combipres by Boehringer Ingelheim	00597-0008	Antihypertensive; Diuretic
BI9	Tab, Blue, Oval	Chlorthalidone 15 mg, Clonidine HCl 0.2 mg	Combipres by Boehringer Ingelheim	00597-0009	Antihypertensive; Diuretic
BIBI <> 8484	Tab, White, Oval, Scored	Pramipexole DiHCl 0.25 mg	Mirapex by Boehringer Ingelheim	00597-0184	Antiparkinson
BIBI <> 8585	Tab, White, Oval, Scored	Pramipexole DiHCl 0.5 mg	Mirapex by Boehringer Ingelheim	00597-0185	Antiparkinson
BIBI <> 9090	Tab, White, Round, Scored	Pramipexole DiHCl 1 mg	Mirapex by Boehringer Ingelheim	00597-0190	Antiparkinson
BIBI <> 9191	Tab, White, Round, Scored	Pramipexole DiHCl 1.5 mg	Mirapex by Boehringer Ingelheim	00597-0191	Antiparkinson
BIBI <> P11P11	Tab, White, Round, Scored	Pramipexole DiHCl 1.5 mg	Mirapex by Boehringer Ingelheim Canada	Canadian DIN 02237147	Antiparkinson
BIBI <> P7P7	Tab, White, Oval, Scored	Pramipexole DiHCl 0.25 mg	Mirapex by Boehringer Ingelheim Canada	Canadian DIN 02237145	Antiparkinson
BIBI <> P8P8	Tab, White, Oval, Scored	Pramipexole DiHCl 0.5 mg	Mirapex by Boehringer Ingelheim Canada	Canadian DIN 02241594	Antiparkinson
BIBI <> P9P9	Tab, White, Round, Scored	Pramipexole DiHCl 1 mg	Mirapex by Boehringer Ingelheim Canada	Canadian DIN 02237146	Antiparkinson
BIC50 <> APO	Tab, White, Round, Film Coated	Bicalutamide 50 mg	Casodex by Apotex	Canadian DIN 02296063	Antineoplastic
BIC50 <> P	Tab, White, Round	Bicalutamide 50 mg	Casodex by Pharmascience	Canadian DIN 02275589	Antineoplastic
BIOCRAFT <> 105105	Tab, White, Oblong, Scored	Sucralfate 1 g	Carafate by Golden State	60429-0706	Gastrointestinal
BIOCRAFT <> 105105	Tab, White, Oblong, Scored	Sucralfate 1 g	Carafate by UDL	51079-0871	Gastrointestinal
BIOCRAFT <> 105105	Tab, White, Oblong, Scored	Sucralfate 1 g	Carafate by Teva	00093-2210	Gastrointestinal
BIOCRAFT <> 105105	Tab, White, Oblong, Scored	Sucralfate 1 g	Carafate by Murfreesboro	51129-1266	Gastrointestinal
BIOCRAFT <> 105105	Tab, White, Oblong, Scored	Sucralfate 1 g	Carafate by Vangard	00615-4517	Gastrointestinal
BIOCRAFT <> 16	Tab, White, Oval	Penicillin V Potassium 250 mg	V-Cillin K by Teva	Discontinued	Antibiotic

ID FRONT <> BACK	DESCRIPTION FRONT <> BACK	INGREDIENT & STRENGTH	BRAND (or Generic Equiv.) by FIRM	NDC#	CLASS; SCH.
BIOCRAFT <> 16	Tab, White, Oval	Penicillin V Potassium 250 mg	by Major	00904-2450	Antibiotic
BIOCRAFT <> 16	Tab, White, Oval	Penicillin V Potassium 250 mg	by Qualitest	00603-5067	Antibiotic
BIOCRAFT <> 16	Tab, White, Oval	Penicillin V Potassium 250 mg	by Apotheca	12634-0468	Antibiotic
BIOCRAFT <> 16	Tab, White, Oval	Penicillin V Potassium 250 mg	by Moore	00839-5188	Antibiotic
BIOCRAFT <> 16	Tab, White, Oval	Penicillin V Potassium 250 mg	by Southwood	58016-0146	Antibiotic
BIOCRAFT <> 16	Tab, White, Oval	Penicillin V Potassium 250 mg	by Vangard	00615-0170	Antibiotic
BIOCRAFT <> 33	Tab	Sulfamethoxazole 800 mg, Trimethoprim 160 mg	by Ivax	00182-8844	Antibiotic
BIOCRAFT <> 33	Tab	Sulfamethoxazole 800 mg, Trimethoprim 160 mg	by Nat Pharmpak	55154-5805	Antibiotic
BIOCRAFT <> 33	Tab	Sulfamethoxazole 800 mg, Trimethoprim 160 mg	by Teva	Discontinued	Antibiotic
BIOCRAFT <> 34	Tab, White, Round, Scored, Biocraft <> 3 over 4	Trimethoprim 100 mg	by Moore	00839-7284	Antibiotic
BIOCRAFT <> 34	Tab, White, Round, Scored, Biocraft <> 3 over 4	Trimethoprim 100 mg	by Major	00904-1646	Antibiotic
BIOCRAFT <> 34	Tab, White, Round, Scored, Biocraft <> 3 over 4	Trimethoprim 100 mg	by Ivax	00182-1536	Antibiotic
BIOCRAFT <> 34	Tab, White, Round, Scored, Biocraft <> 3 over 4	Trimethoprim 100 mg	by DRX	55045-2302	Antibiotic
BIOCRAFT <> 34	Tab, White, Round, Scored, Biocraft <> 3 over 4	Trimethoprim 100 mg	by Murfreesboro	51129-1204	Antibiotic
BIOCRAFT <> 49	Tab, White, Oval, Scored	Penicillin V Potassium 500 mg	by Apotheca	12634-0422	Antibiotic
BIOCRAFT <> 49	Tab, White, Oval, Scored	Penicillin V Potassium 500 mg	by Rx Dispensing	61807-0004	Antibiotic
BIOCRAFT <> 49	Tab, White, Oval, Scored	Penicillin V Potassium 500 mg	by Ivax	00182-1537	Antibiotic
BIOCRAFT <> 49	Tab, White, Oval, Scored	Penicillin V Potassium 500 mg	by Teva	Discontinued	Antibiotic
BIOCRAFT01	Cap, Buff & Caramel, Black Print, Biocraft over 01	Amoxicillin 250 mg	Amoxil by Teva	00093-3107	Antibiotic
BIOCRAFT01	Cap, Buff & Caramel, Black Print, Biocraft over 01	Amoxicillin 250 mg	Amoxil by Pharmedix	53002-0208	Antibiotic
BIOCRAFT01	Cap, Buff & Caramel, Black Print, Biocraft over 01	Amoxicillin 250 mg	Amoxil by Med Pro	53978-5002	Antibiotic
BIOCRAFT01	Cap, Buff & Caramel, Black Print, Biocraft over 01	Amoxicillin 250 mg	Amoxil by Qualitest	00603-2266	Antibiotic
BIOCRAFT01	Cap, Buff & Caramel, Black Print, Biocraft over 01	Amoxicillin 250 mg	Amoxil by Biocraft	00332-3107	Antibiotic
BIOCRAFT01	Cap, Buff & Caramel, Black Print, Biocraft over 01	Amoxicillin 250 mg	Amoxil by Teva	17372-0613	Antibiotic
BIOCRAFT02	Cap, Light Green & Medium Green, Black Print, biocraft over 02	Dicloxacillin Sodium 250 mg	Dynapen by Qualitest	00603-2267	Antibiotic
BIOCRAFT02	Cap, Light Green & Medium Green, Black Print, biocraft over 02	Dicloxacillin Sodium 250 mg	Dynapen by Teva	00093-0123 Discontinued	Antibiotic
BIOCRAFT02	Cap, Light Green & Medium Green, Black Print, biocraft over 02	Dicloxacillin Sodium 250 mg	Dynapen by Ivax	00182-1506	Antibiotic
BIOCRAFT02	Cap, Light Green & Medium Green, Black Print, biocraft over 02	Dicloxacillin Sodium 250 mg	Dynapen by H J Harkins Co	52959-0048	Antibiotic
BIOCRAFT02	Cap, Light Green & Medium Green, Black Print, biocraft over 02	Dicloxacillin Sodium 250 mg	Dynapen by Kaiser	00179-1048	Antibiotic
BIOCRAFT02	Cap, Light Green & Medium Green, Black Print, biocraft over 02	Dicloxacillin Sodium 250 mg	Dynapen by Warner Chilcott	00047-0945	Antibiotic
BIOCRAFT02	Cap, Light Green & Medium Green, Black Print, biocraft over 02	Dicloxacillin Sodium 250 mg	Dynapen by Urgent Care Center	50716-0222	Antibiotic
BIOCRAFT02	Cap, Light Green & Medium Green, Black Print, biocraft over 02	Dicloxacillin Sodium 250 mg	Dynapen by Pharmedix	53002-0220	Antibiotic
BIOCRAFT02	Cap, Light Green & Medium Green, Black Print, biocraft over 02	Dicloxacillin Sodium 250 mg	Dynapen by Apotheca	12634-0439	Antibiotic
BIOCRAFT02	Cap, Light Green & Medium Green, Black Print, biocraft over 02	Dicloxacillin Sodium 250 mg	Dynapen by UDL	51079-0610	Antibiotic
BIOCRAFT02	Cap, Green & Light Green	Dicloxacillin Sodium 250 mg	Dynapen by Biocraft	00332-3123	Antibiotic
BIOCRAFT02	Cap, Light Green & Medium Green, Black Print, biocraft over 02	Dicloxacillin Sodium 250 mg	Dynapen by Rx Dispensing	61807-0038	Antibiotic
BIOCRAFT02	Cap, Light Green & Medium Green, Black Print, biocraft over 02	Dicloxacillin Sodium 250 mg	Dynapen by Southwood	58016-0121	Antibiotic
BIOCRAFT03	Cap, Buff, Black Print, Biocraft over 03	Amoxicillin 500 mg	Amoxil by Ivax	00182-1071	Antibiotic
BIOCRAFT03	Cap, Buff, Black Print, Biocraft over 03	Amoxicillin 500 mg	Amoxil by Pharmedix	53002-0216	Antibiotic

ID FRONT <> BACK	DESCRIPTION FRONT <> BACK	INGREDIENT & STRENGTH	BRAND (or Generic Equiv.) by FIRM	NDC#	CLASS; SCH.
BIOCRAFT03	Cap, Buff, Black Print, Biocraft over 03	Amoxicillin 500 mg	Amoxil by Med Pro	53978-5003	Antibiotic
BIOCRAFT03	Cap, Buff, Black Print, Biocraft over 03	Amoxicillin 500 mg	Amoxil by Teva	00093-3109	Antibiotic
BIOCRAFT03	Cap, Buff, Black Print, Biocraft over 03	Amoxicillin 500 mg	Amoxil by Biocraft	00093-3109	Antibiotic
BIOCRAFT03	Cap, Buff, Black Print, Biocraft over 03	Amoxicillin 500 mg	Amoxil by Diversified Healthcare	55887-0982	Antibiotic
BIOCRAFT04	Cap, Light Green, Biocraft over 04	Dicloxacillin Sodium 500 mg	by Warner Chilcott	00047-0946	Antibiotic
BIOCRAFT04	Cap, Light Green, Biocraft over 04	Dicloxacillin Sodium 500 mg	by Ivax	00182-1507	Antibiotic
BIOCRAFT04	Cap, Light Green, Biocraft over 04	Dicloxacillin Sodium 500 mg	by UDL	51079-0611	Antibiotic
BIOCRAFT04	Cap, Light Green, Biocraft over 04	Dicloxacillin Sodium 500 mg	by Teva		Antibiotic
BIOCRAFT04	Cap, Light Green, Biocraft over 04	Dicloxacillin Sodium 500 mg	by Allscripts		Antibiotic
BIOCRAFT04	Cap, Light Green, Biocraft over 04	Dicloxacillin Sodium 500 mg	by H J Harkins Co	52959-0049	Antibiotic
BIOCRAFT04	Cap, Light Green, Biocraft over 04	Dicloxacillin Sodium 500 mg	by Moore	00839-6614	Antibiotic
BIOCRAFT05	Cap, Gray & Scarlet, Biocraft over 05	Ampicillin 250 mg	Principen by UDL	51079-0602	Antibiotic
BIOCRAFT05	Cap, Gray & Scarlet, Biocraft over 05	Ampicillin 250 mg	Principen by Moore	00839-5087	Antibiotic
BIOCRAFT05	Cap, Gray & Scarlet, Biocraft over 05	Ampicillin 250 mg	Principen by Pharmedix	53002-0230	Antibiotic
BIOCRAFT05	Cap, Gray & Scarlet, Biocraft over 05	Ampicillin 250 mg	Principen by Apotheca	12634-0417	Antibiotic
BIOCRAFT05	Cap, Gray & Scarlet, Biocraft over 05	Ampicillin 250 mg	Principen by Sandoz	00781-2555	Antibiotic
BIOCRAFT05	Cap, Gray & Scarlet, Biocraft over 05	Ampicillin 250 mg	Principen by Teva	00093-3111 Discontinued	Antibiotic
BIOCRAFT05	Cap, Gray & Scarlet, Biocraft over 05	Ampicillin 250 mg	Principen by Southwood	58016-0148	Antibiotic
BIOCRAFT05	Cap, Gray & Scarlet, Biocraft over 05	Ampicillin 250 mg	Principen by Ivax	00182-0163	Antibiotic
BIOCRAFT05	Cap, Gray & Scarlet, Biocraft over 05	Ampicillin 250 mg	Principen by Qualitest	00603-2290	Antibiotic
BIOCRAFT05	Cap, Gray & Scarlet, Biocraft over 05	Ampicillin 250 mg	Principen by Signal Health	62125-0415	Antibiotic
BIOCRAFT05	Cap, Gray & Scarlet, Biocraft over 05	Ampicillin 250 mg	Principen by Kaiser	00179-0085	Antibiotic
BIOCRAFT06	Cap, Gray & Scarlet, Biocraft over 06	Ampicillin 500 mg	Principen by Qualitest	00603-2291	Antibiotic
BIOCRAFT06	Cap, Gray & Scarlet, Biocraft over 06	Ampicillin 500 mg	Principen by Ivax	00182-0641	Antibiotic
BIOCRAFT06	Cap, Gray & Scarlet, Biocraft over 06	Ampicillin 500 mg	Principen by Teva	00093-3113 Discontinued	Antibiotic
BIOCRAFT06	Cap, Gray & Scarlet, Biocraft over 06	Ampicillin 500 mg	Principen by PDRX	55289-0024	Antibiotic
BIOCRAFT06	Cap, Gray & Scarlet, Biocraft over 06	Ampicillin 500 mg	Principen by Major	00904-2073	Antibiotic
BIOCRAFT06	Cap, Gray & Scarlet, Biocraft over 06	Ampicillin 500 mg	Principen by Sandoz	00781-2999	Antibiotic
BIOCRAFT06	Cap, Gray & Scarlet, Biocraft over 06	Ampicillin 500 mg	Principen by Med Pro	53978-5019	Antibiotic
BIOCRAFT06	Cap, Gray & Scarlet, Biocraft over 06	Ampicillin 500 mg	Principen by H J Harkins Co	52959-0389	Antibiotic
BIOCRAFT06	Cap, Gray & Scarlet, Biocraft over 06	Ampicillin 500 mg	Principen by Apotheca	12634-0168	Antibiotic
BIOCRAFT112	Cap, Light Green & Pink, Opaque, Biocraft over 112	Cephradine 250 mg	by UDL	51079-0606	Antibiotic
BIOCRAFT112	Cap, Light Green & Pink, Opaque, Biocraft over 112	Cephradine 250 mg	by Schein	00364-2141	Antibiotic
BIOCRAFT112	Cap, Light Green & Pink, Opaque, Biocraft over 112	Cephradine 250 mg	by Teva	00093-3153 Discontinued	Antibiotic
BIOCRAFT112	Cap, Light Green & Pink, Opaque, Biocraft over 112	Cephradine 250 mg	by Carlsbad	61442-0103	Antibiotic
BIOCRAFT112	Cap, Light Green & Pink, Opaque, Biocraft over 112	Cephradine 250 mg	by Rx Dispensing	61807-0048	Antibiotic
BIOCRAFT112	Cap, Light Green & Pink, Opaque, Biocraft over 112	Cephradine 250 mg	by Ivax	00182-1253	Antibiotic
BIOCRAFT112	Cap, Light Green & Pink, Opaque, Biocraft over 112	Cephradine 250 mg	by Pharmedix	53002-0248	Antibiotic
BIOCRAFT113	Cap, Light Green, Opaque, Biocraft over 113	Cephradine 500 mg	by PDRX	55289-0597	Antibiotic
BIOCRAFT113	Cap, Light Green, Opaque, Biocraft over 113	Cephradine 500 mg	by H J Harkins Co	52959-0032	Antibiotic
BIOCRAFT113	Cap, Light Green, Opaque, Biocraft over 113	Cephradine 500 mg	by UDL	51079-0607	Antibiotic
BIOCRAFT113	Cap, Light Green, Opaque, Biocraft over 113	Cephradine 500 mg	by Ivax	00182-1254	Antibiotic
BIOCRAFT113	Cap, Light Green, Opaque, Biocraft over 113	Cephradine 500 mg	by Pharmedix	53002-0249	Antibiotic
BIOCRAFT113	Cap, Light Green, Opaque, Biocraft over 113	Cephradine 500 mg	by Teva	00093-3155 Discontinued	Antibiotic
BIOCRAFT113	Cap, Light Green, Opaque, Biocraft over 113	Cephradine 500 mg	by Schein	00364-2142	Antibiotic
BIOCRAFT114	Cap, Yellow	Cefadroxil Monohydrate 500 mg	Duricef by Biocraft		Antibiotic

ID FRONT <> BACK	DESCRIPTION FRONT <> BACK	INGREDIENT & STRENGTH	BRAND (or Generic Equiv.) by FIRM	NDC#	CLASS; SCH.
BIOCRAFT115	Cap, Gray & Orange, Biocraft over 115	Cephalexin 250 mg	Keflex by Qualitest	00603-2595	Antibiotic
BIOCRAFT115	Cap, Gray & Orange, Biocraft over 115	Cephalexin 250 mg	Keflex by Pharmedix	53002-0226	Antibiotic
BIOCRAFT115	Cap, Gray & Orange, Biocraft over 115	Cephalexin 250 mg	Keflex by Ivax	00182-1278	Antibiotic
BIOCRAFT115	Cap, Gray & Orange, Biocraft over 115	Cephalexin 250 mg	Keflex by Apotheca	12634-0433	Antibiotic
BIOCRAFT115	Cap, Gray & Orange, Biocraft over 115	Cephalexin 250 mg	Keflex by Moore	00839-7311	Antibiotic
BIOCRAFT115	Cap, Gray & Orange, Biocraft over 115	Cephalexin 250 mg	Keflex by Talbert	44514-0490	Antibiotic
BIOCRAFT115	Cap, Gray & Orange, Biocraft over 115	Cephalexin 250 mg	Keflex by Med Pro	53978-5020	Antibiotic
BIOCRAFT115	Cap, Gray & Orange, Biocraft over 115	Cephalexin 250 mg	Keflex by Signal Health	62125-0317	Antibiotic
BIOCRAFT115	Cap, Gray & Orange, Biocraft over 115	Cephalexin 250 mg	Keflex by PDRX	55289-0057	Antibiotic
BIOCRAFT115	Cap, Gray & Orange, Biocraft over 115	Cephalexin 250 mg	Keflex by Signal Health	62125-0318	Antibiotic
BIOCRAFT115	Cap, Gray & Orange, Biocraft over 115	Cephalexin 250 mg	Keflex by Teva	00093-3145 Discontinued	Antibiotic
BIOCRAFT115	Cap, Gray & Orange, Biocraft over 115	Cephalexin 250 mg	Keflex by Caremark	00339-6167	Antibiotic
BIOCRAFT115	Cap, Gray & Orange, Biocraft over 115	Cephalexin 250 mg	Keflex by Darby Group	66467-0120	Antibiotic
BIOCRAFT117	Cap, Orange, Biocraft over 117	Cephalexin 500 mg	Keflex by Darby Group	66467-0130	Antibiotic
BIOCRAFT117	Cap, Orange, Biocraft over 117	Cephalexin 500 mg	Keflex by Nat Pharmpak	55154-5522	Antibiotic
BIOCRAFT117	Cap, Orange, Biocraft over 117	Cephalexin 500 mg	Keflex by Signal Health	62125-0320	Antibiotic
BIOCRAFT117	Cap, Orange, Biocraft over 117	Cephalexin 500 mg	Keflex by Signal Health	62125-0319	Antibiotic
BIOCRAFT117	Cap, Orange, Biocraft over 117	Cephalexin 500 mg	Keflex by Biocraft	00332-3147	Antibiotic
BIOCRAFT117	Cap, Orange, Biocraft over 117	Cephalexin 500 mg	Keflex by PDRX	55289-0057	Antibiotic
BIOCRAFT117	Cap, Orange, Biocraft over 117	Cephalexin 500 mg	Keflex by Urgent Care Center	50716-0144	Antibiotic
BIOCRAFT117	Cap, Orange, Biocraft over 117	Cephalexin 500 mg	Keflex by Med Pro	53978-5021	Antibiotic
BIOCRAFT117	Cap, Orange, Biocraft over 117	Cephalexin 500 mg	Keflex by Apotheca	12634-0434	Antibiotic
BIOCRAFT117	Cap, Orange, Biocraft over 117	Cephalexin 500 mg	Keflex by Talbert	44514-0491	Antibiotic
BIOCRAFT117	Cap, Orange, Biocraft over 117	Cephalexin 500 mg	Keflex by Amerisource	62584-0328	Antibiotic
BIOCRAFT117	Cap, Orange, Biocraft over 117	Cephalexin 500 mg	Keflex by Qualitest	00603-2596	Antibiotic
BIOCRAFT117	Cap, Orange, Biocraft over 117	Cephalexin 500 mg	Keflex by Ivax	00182-1279	Antibiotic
BIOCRAFT117	Cap, Orange, Biocraft over 117	Cephalexin 500 mg	Keflex by Pharmedix	53002-0218	Antibiotic
BIOCRAFT117	Cap, Orange, Biocraft over 117	Cephalexin 500 mg	Keflex by Teva	00093-3147 Discontinued	Antibiotic
BIOCRAFT117	Cap, Orange, Biocraft over 117	Cephalexin 500 mg	Keflex by Moore	00839-7312	Antibiotic
BIOCRAFT12	Cap, Blue, Opaque, Biocraft over 12	Oxacillin 250 mg	Prostaphlin by Teva	00093-3115	Antibiotic
BIOCRAFT12	Cap, Blue, Opaque, Biocraft over 12	Oxacillin 250 mg	Prostaphlin by Biocraft		Antibiotic
BIOCRAFT134	Cap, Pink, Biocraft over 134	Minocycline HCl 50 mg	Minocin by Teva	00093-3165 Discontinued	Antibiotic
BIOCRAFT134	Cap, Pink, Biocraft over 134	Minocycline HCl 50 mg	Minocin by Ivax	00182-1102	Antibiotic
BIOCRAFT134	Cap, Pink, Biocraft over 134	Minocycline HCl 50 mg	Minocin by URL Mutual	00677-1435	Antibiotic
BIOCRAFT134	Cap, Pink, Biocraft over 134	Minocycline HCl 50 mg	Minocin by Qualitest	00603-4678	Antibiotic
BIOCRAFT135	Cap, Maroon & Pink, Biocraft over 135	Minocycline HCl 100 mg	Minocin by Qualitest	00603-4679	Antibiotic
BIOCRAFT135	Cap, Maroon & Pink, Biocraft over 135	Minocycline HCl 100 mg	Minocin by Major	00904-7683	Antibiotic
BIOCRAFT135	Cap, Maroon & Pink, Biocraft over 135	Minocycline HCl 100 mg	Minocin by Ivax	00182-1103	Antibiotic
BIOCRAFT135	Cap, Maroon & Pink, Biocraft over 135	Minocycline HCl 100 mg	Minocin by Teva	00093-3167 Discontinued	Antibiotic
BIOCRAFT14	Cap, Blue, Opaque, Biocraft over 14	Oxacillin Sodium 500 mg	by Ivax	00182-1341	Antibiotic
BIOCRAFT14	Cap, Blue, Opaque, Biocraft over 14	Oxacillin Sodium 500 mg	by Qualitest	00603-4928	Antibiotic
BIOCRAFT14	Cap, Blue, Opaque, Biocraft over 14	Oxacillin Sodium 500 mg	by Teva	00093-3117	Antibiotic
BIOCRAFT148	Cap, Red, Biocraft over 148	Clindamycin HCl 75 mg	Cleocin HCl by Biocraft		Antibiotic
BIOCRAFT148	Cap, Red, Biocraft over 148	Clindamycin HCl 75 mg	Cleocin HCl by Teva	00093-3169 Discontinued	Antibiotic
BIOCRAFT149	Cap	Clindamycin HCl 150 mg	Cleocin HCl by Nat Pharmpak	55154-5546	Antibiotic

ID FRONT <> BACK	DESCRIPTION FRONT <> BACK	INGREDIENT & STRENGTH	BRAND (or Generic Equiv.) by FIRM	NDC#	CLASS; SCH.
BIOCRAFT149	Cap	Clindamycin HCl 150 mg	Cleocin HCl by Biocraft		Antibiotic
BIOCRAFT149	Cap	Clindamycin HCl 150 mg	Cleocin HCl by Ivax	00182-1202	Antibiotic
BIOCRAFT149	Cap	Clindamycin HCl 150 mg	Cleocin HCl by Pharmedix	53002-0232	Antibiotic
BIOCRAFT149	Cap	Clindamycin HCl 150 mg	Cleocin HCl by Major	00904-3838	Antibiotic
BIOCRAFT149	Cap	Clindamycin HCl 150 mg	Cleocin HCl by Apotheca	12634-0092	Antibiotic
BIOCRAFT149	Cap, Blue & Red, Biocraft over 149	Clindamycin HCl 150 mg	Cleocin HCl by Teva	00093-3171 Discontinued	Antibiotic
BIOCRAFT163	Cap, Blue & Yellow	Cinoxacin 250 mg	Cinobac by Biocraft		Antibiotic
BIOCRAFT164	Cap, Blue & Yellow	Cinoxacin 500 mg	Cinobac by Biocraft		Antibiotic
BIOCRAFT177	Cap	Potassium Chloride 600 mg	by Teva	00093-3189	Electrolytes
BIOCRAFT178	Cap	Potassium Chloride 750 mg	by Teva	00093-3190	Electrolytes
BIOCRAFT185	Cap, White	Ketoprofen 25 mg	Orudis by Biocraft		NSAID
BIOCRAFT187	Cap	Ketoprofen 50 mg	Orudis by Ivax	00182-1959	NSAID
BIOCRAFT187	Cap, Blue & Light Blue, Biocraft over 187	Ketoprofen 50 mg	Orudis by Teva	00093-3193 Discontinued	NSAID
BIOCRAFT187	Cap	Ketoprofen 50 mg	Orudis by Pharmedix	53002-0588	NSAID
BIOCRAFT187	Cap, Light Blue	Ketoprofen 50 mg	Orudis by Qualitest	00603-4177	NSAID
BIOCRAFT192	Cap, Blue & White, Biocraft over 192	Ketoprofen 75 mg	Orudis by Ivax	00182-1960	NSAID
BIOCRAFT192	Cap, Blue & White, Biocraft over 192	Ketoprofen 75 mg	Orudis by Teva	00093-3195 Discontinued	NSAID
BIOCRAFT192	Cap, Blue & White, Biocraft over 192	Ketoprofen 75 mg	Orudis by Pharmedix	53002-0531	NSAID
BIOCRAFT192	Cap, Blue & White, Biocraft over 192	Ketoprofen 75 mg	Orudis by Med Pro	53978-2082	NSAID
BIOCRAFT192	Cap, Blue & White, Biocraft over 192	Ketoprofen 75 mg	Orudis by Murfreesboro	51129-1103	NSAID
BIOCRAFT192	Cap, Blue & White, Biocraft over 192	Ketoprofen 75 mg	Orudis by Qualitest	00603-4178	NSAID
BIOCRAFT223	Cap, Gray & White	Cefaclor 250 mg	Ceclor by Biocraft	00332-3206	Antibiotic
BIOCRAFT224	Cap, Red & White	Cefaclor 500 mg	Ceclor CD by Biocraft		Antibiotic
BIOCRAFT28	Cap, Dark Green & Scarlet, Biocraft over 28	Cloxacillin Sodium 250 mg	by Ivax	00182-1358	Antibiotic
BIOCRAFT28	Cap, Dark Green & Scarlet, Biocraft over 28	Cloxacillin Sodium 250 mg	by Qualitest	00603-3029	Antibiotic
BIOCRAFT28	Cap, Dark Green & Scarlet, Biocraft over 28	Cloxacillin Sodium 250 mg	by H J Harkins Co	52959-0468	Antibiotic
BIOCRAFT28	Cap, Dark Green & Scarlet, Biocraft over 28	Cloxacillin Sodium 250 mg	by Teva	00093-3119 Discontinued	Antibiotic
BIOCRAFT30	Cap, Dark Green & Scarlet, Biocraft over 30	Cloxacillin Sodium 500 mg	by Teva	00093-3121 Discontinued	Antibiotic
BIOCRAFT30	Cap	Cloxacillin Sodium 500 mg	by Ivax	00182-1359	Antibiotic
BIOCRAFT33	Tab	Sulfamethoxazole 800 mg, Trimethoprim 160 mg	by Ivax	00182-1408	Antibiotic
BIOCRAFT33	Tab, White, Oval, Scored	Sulfamethoxazole 800 mg, Trimethoprim 160 mg	by Allscripts		Antibiotic
BIOCRAFT33	Tab	Sulfamethoxazole 800 mg, Trimethoprim 160 mg	by URL Mutual	00677-0784	Antibiotic
BIOCRAFT33	Tab	Sulfamethoxazole 800 mg, Trimethoprim 160 mg	by Apotheca	12634-0177	Antibiotic
BIOCRAFT40	Cap, Blue & Scarlet, Black Print, Hard Gel, Biocraft over 40	Disopyramide Phosphate 100 mg	Norpace by Teva	00093-3127	Antiarrhythmic
BIOCRAFT40	Cap, Blue & Scarlet, Black Print, Hard Gel, Biocraft over 40	Disopyramide Phosphate 100 mg	Norpace by Ivax	00182-1743	Antiarrhythmic
BIOCRAFT41	Cap, Scarlet & Buff, Black Print, Hard Gel, Biocraft over 41	Disopyramide Phosphate 150 mg	Norpace by Teva	00093-3129	Antiarrhythmic
BIOCRAFT41	Cap, Scarlet & Buff, Black Print, Hard Gel, Biocraft over 41	Disopyramide Phosphate 150 mg	Norpace by Ivax	00182-1744	Antiarrhythmic
BIOCRAFT94	Tab, White, Oblong, Biocraft/94	Cyclacillin 250 mg	Cylcapen by Biocraft		Antibiotic
BIOCRAFT95	Tab, White, Oblong, Biocraft/95	Cyclacillin 500 mg	Cylcapen by Biocraft		Antibiotic
BIOHIST	Tab, White, Oval, Scored, Ex Release	Chlorpheniramine Maleate 12 mg, Pseudoephedrine HCl 120 mg	Deconamine SR by Ivax Labs	59310-0112	Cold Remedy
BIOHIST	Tab, White, Oval, Scored, Ex Release	Chlorpheniramine Maleate 12 mg, Pseudoephedrine HCl 120 mg	Deconamine SR by Sovereign	58716-0662	Cold Remedy
BIPHENTIN10MG	Cap, White and Turquoise Blue, Controlled Release	Methylphenidate HCl 10 mg.	Biphentin by Purdue Pharma	Canadian DIN 02277166	Stimulant

ID FRONT <> BACK	DESCRIPTION FRONT <> BACK	INGREDIENT & STRENGTH	BRAND (or Generic Equiv.) by FIRM	NDC#	CLASS; SCH.
BIPHENTIN15MG	Cap, White and Orange, Controlled Release	Methylphenidate HCl 15 mg	Biphentin by Purdue Pharma	Canadian DIN 02277131	Stimulant
BIPHENTIN20MG	Cap, White and Yellow, Controlled Release	Methylphenidate HCl 20 mg.	Biphentin by Purdue Pharma	Canadian DIN 02277158	Stimulant
BIPHENTIN30MG	Cap, White and Blue Violet, Controlled Release	Methylphenidate HCl 30 mg	Biphentin by Purdue Pharma	Canadian DIN 02277174	Stimulant
BIPHENTIN40MG	Cap, White and Pink, Controlled Release	Methylphenidate HCl 40 mg	Biphentin by Purdue Pharma	Canadian DIN 02277182	Stimulant
BIPHENTIN50MG	Cap, White and Light Green, Controlled Release	Methylphenidate HCl 50 mg	Biphentin by Purdue Pharma	Canadian DIN 02277190	Stimulant
BIPHENTIN60MG	Cap, White and Iron Grey, Controlled Release	Methylphenidate HCl 60 mg	Biphentin by Purdue Pharma	Canadian DIN 02277204	Stimulant
BIPHENTIN80MG	Cap, White and Reddish Orange, Controlled Release	Methylphenidate HCl 80 mg	Biphentin by Purdue Pharma	Canadian DIN 02277212	Stimulant
BL <> 130	Tab, White, Round, Scored	Albuterol Sulfate 2 mg	Proventil by Teva	00093-2226	Antiasthmatic
BL <> 131	Tab, White, Round, Scored	Albuterol Sulfate 4 mg	Proventil by Teva	00093-2228	Antiasthmatic
BL <> 132	Tab, White, Round, Scored	Metaproterenol Sulfate 10 mg	by Nat Pharmpak	55154-5586	Antiasthmatic
BL <> 133	Tab, Buff, Round, Scored	Metaproterenol Sulfate 20 mg	by Teva	00093-2232 Discontinued	Antiasthmatic
BL <> 136	Tab, White, Cap Shaped, Scored	Cephalexin 250 mg	Keflex by Teva	00093-2238	Antibiotic
BL <> 137	Tab, White, Cap Shaped, Scored	Cephalexin 500 mg	Keflex by Teva	00093-2240	Antibiotic
BL <> 15	Tab, White, Round, Scored	Penicillin V Potassium 250 mg	by PDRX	55289-0206	Antibiotic
BL <> 15	Tab, White, Round, Scored	Penicillin V Potassium 250 mg	by Diversified Healthcare	55887-0980	Antibiotic
BL <> 15	Tab, White, Round, Scored	Penicillin V Potassium 250 mg	by Pharmedix	53002-0201	Antibiotic
BL <> 15	Tab, White, Round, Scored	Penicillin V Potassium 250 mg	V-Cillin K by Biocraft	58016-0146	Antibiotic
BL <> 15	Tab, White, Round, Scored	Penicillin V Potassium 250 mg	by Teva	00093-1171 Discontinued	Antibiotic
BL <> 15	Tab, White, Round, Scored	Penicillin V Potassium 250 mg	Pen*Vee K by UDL	51079-0615	Antibiotic
BL <> 17	Tab, White, Round, Scored	Penicillin V Potassium 500 mg	V-Cillin K by Biocraft		Antibiotic
BL <> 17	Tab, White, Round, Scored	Penicillin V Potassium 500 mg	by Pharmafab	62542-0724	Antibiotic
BL <> 17	Tab, White, Round, Scored	Penicillin V Potassium 500 mg	by Teva	00093-1173 Discontinued	Antibiotic
BL <> 17	Tab, White, Round, Scored	Penicillin V Potassium 500 mg	Pen*Vee K by UDL	51079-0616	Antibiotic
BL <> 17	Tab, White, Round, Scored	Penicillin V Potassium 500 mg	by Talbert	44514-0645	Antibiotic
BL <> 17	Tab, White, Round, Scored	Penicillin V Potassium 500 mg	by Moore	00839-1766	Antibiotic
BL <> 17	Tab, White, Round, Scored	Penicillin V Potassium 500 mg	by Qualitest	00603-5068	Antibiotic
BL <> 17	Tab, White, Round, Scored	Penicillin V Potassium 500 mg	by St. Mary's Med	60760-0174	Antibiotic
BL <> 17	Tab, White, Round, Scored	Penicillin V Potassium 500 mg	by Pharmedix	53002-0202	Antibiotic
BL <> 18	Tab, Off-White, Round	Neomycin Sulfate 500 mg	by Teva	00093-1177 Discontinued	Antibiotic
BL <> 19	Tab, Yellow, Round	Imipramine HCl 10 mg	Tofranil by Teva	00093-2111	Antidepressant
BL <> 20	Tab, Salmon, Round	Imipramine HCl 25 mg	Tofranil by Schein	00364-0406	Antidepressant
BL <> 20	Tab, Salmon, Round	Imipramine HCl 25 mg	Tofranil by Teva	00093-2113	Antidepressant
BL <> 20	Tab, Salmon, Round	Imipramine HCl 25 mg	Tofranil by UDL	51079-0080	Antidepressant
BL <> 21	Tab, Green, Round	Imipramine HCl 50 mg	Tofranil by Teva	00093-2117	Antidepressant
BL <> 21	Tab, Green, Round	Imipramine HCl 50 mg	Tofranil by UDL	51079-0081	Antidepressant
BL <> 22	Tab, Pink, Round, Coated	Amitriptyline HCl 10 mg	Elavil by Teva	00093-2120	Antidepressant
BL <> 221	Tab, White to Off-White, Oblong, Chewable	Amoxicillin 125 mg	Amoxil by Teva	00093-2267	Antibiotic
BL <> 222	Tab, White to Off-White, Oblong, Scored, Chewable	Amoxicillin 250 mg	Amoxil by St. Mary's Med	60760-0268	Antibiotic

ID FRONT <> BACK	DESCRIPTION FRONT <> BACK	INGREDIENT & STRENGTH	BRAND (or Generic Equiv.) by FIRM	NDC#	CLASS; SCH.
BL <> 222	Tab, White to Off-White, Oblong, Scored, Chewable	Amoxicillin 250 mg	Amoxil by Teva	00093-2268	Antibiotic
BL <> 222	Tab, White to Off-White, Oblong, Scored, Chewable	Amoxicillin 250 mg	Amoxil by DRX	55045-2004	Antibiotic
BL <> 222	Tab, White to Off-White, Oblong, Scored, Chewable	Amoxicillin 250 mg	Amoxil by Casa DeAmigos	62138-6005	Antibiotic
BL <> 23	Tab, Light Green, Round, Coated	Amitriptyline HCl 25 mg	Elavil by Teva	00093-2122	Antidepressant
BL <> 24	Tab, Brown, Round, Coated	Amitriptyline HCl 50 mg	Elavil by Teva	00093-2124	Antidepressant
BL <> 25	Tab, Lavender, Round, Coated	Amitriptyline HCl 75 mg	Elavil by Teva	00093-2126	Antidepressant
BL <> 26	Tab, Orange, Round, Coated, Scored	Amitriptyline HCl 100 mg	Elavil by Teva	00093-2128	Antidepressant
BL <> 32	Tab	Sulfamethoxazole 400 mg, Trimethoprim 80 mg	by PDRX	55289-0457	Antibiotic
BL <> 35	Tab, White, Round, Scored	Trimethoprim 200 mg	by Teva	Discontinued	Antibiotic
BL <> 92	Tab, White, Round	Metoclopramide HCl 5 mg	Reglan by UDL	51079-0629	Gastrointestinal
BL <> 92	Tab, White, Round	Metoclopramide HCl 5 mg	Reglan by Murfreesboro	51129-1683	Gastrointestinal
BL <> 92	Tab, White, Round	Metoclopramide HCl 5 mg	Reglan by Teva	00093-2204	Gastrointestinal
BL <> 93	Tab, White, Round, Scored	Metoclopramide HCl 10 mg	Reglan by Vangard	00615-2536	Gastrointestinal
BL <> 93	Tab, White, Round, Scored	Metoclopramide HCl 10 mg	Reglan by Teva	00093-2203	Gastrointestinal
BL <> 93	Tab, White, Round, Scored	Metoclopramide HCl 10 mg	Reglan by Biocraft	00093-2203	Gastrointestinal
BL <> 93	Tab, White, Round, Scored	Metoclopramide HCl 10 mg	Reglan by Neuman	64579-0051	Gastrointestinal
BL <> 93	Tab, White, Round, Scored	Metoclopramide HCl 10 mg	Reglan by Moore	00839-7127	Gastrointestinal
BL <> 93	Tab, White, Round, Scored	Metoclopramide HCl 10 mg	Reglan by Duramed	51285-0805	Gastrointestinal
BL <> 93	Tab, White, Round, Scored	Metoclopramide HCl 10 mg	Reglan by Neuman	64579-0049	Gastrointestinal
BL <> 93	Tab, White, Round	Metoclopramide 10 mg	Reglan by UDL	51079-0283	Gastrointestinal
BL <> L1	Tab	Mitotane 500 mg	Lysodren by Anabolic	00722-5240	Antineoplastic
BL01	Tab, Orange, Oblong, Scored	Vitamin A 28,640 IU, Vitamin C 452 mg, Vitamin E 400 IU, Zinc 69.6 mg, Copper 1.6 mg	Ocuvite PreserVision by Bausch & Lomb	24208-4326 24208-4327	Vitamin; Mineral
BL07	Tab, White, Round	Penicillin G Potassium 200,000 Units	Pentids by Biocraft	00839-7485	Antibiotic
BL09	Tab, White, Round	Penicillin G Potassium 250,000 Units	Pentids by Biocraft		Antibiotic
BL10	Tab, White, Round	Penicillin G Potassium 400,000 Units	Pentids by Biocraft		Antibiotic
BL10 <> BUSPAR	Tab, White, Rectangular	Buspirone HCl 10 mg	Buspar by BMS	Canadian DIN 00603821	Antianxiety
BL131	Tab	Albuterol Sulfate 4 mg	Proventil by Ivax	00182-1012	Antiasthmatic
BL132	Tab, White, Round	Metaproterenol 10 mg	Metaprel by Teva	00093-2230	Antiasthmatic
BL132	Tab, White, Round	Metaproterenol 10 mg	Metaprel by Moore	Discontinued	Antiasthmatic
BL132	Tab, White, Round	Metaproterenol 10 mg	Metaprel by Major	00904-2878	Antiasthmatic
BL132	Tab, White, Round	Metaproterenol 10 mg	Metaprel by Qualitest	00603-4464	Antiasthmatic
BL133	Tab, BL/133	Metaproterenol 20 mg	Metaprel by Qualitest	00603-4465	Antiasthmatic
BL133	Tab, BL/133	Metaproterenol 20 mg	Metaprel by Moore	00839-7486	Antiasthmatic
BL136	Tab, White, Cap Shaped, Coated, BL/136	Cephalexin 250 mg	Keflex by Diversified Healthcare	55887-0991	Antibiotic
BL136	Cap	Cephalexin 250 mg	Keflex by IDE Inter	00814-1605	Antibiotic
BL136	Cap	Cephalexin 250 mg	Keflex by Darby Group	66467-0120	Antibiotic
BL137	Tab, Coated	Cephalexin 500 mg	Keflex by Ivax	00182-1887	Antibiotic
BL137	Tab, Coated	Cephalexin 500 mg	Keflex by Pharmedix	53002-0298	Antibiotic
BL14	Cap	Oxacillin Sodium	Prostaphlin by URL Mutual	00677-0933	Antibiotic
BL141	Tab, White, Round, Scored, BL over 141	Baclofen 10 mg	Lioresal by Teva	00093-2234	Muscle Relaxant
BL141	Tab, White, Round, Scored, BL over 141	Baclofen 10 mg	Lioresal by Vangard	00615-3541	Muscle Relaxant
BL142	Tab, White, Round, Scored, BL over 142	Baclofen 20 mg	Lioresal by Vangard	00615-3542	Muscle Relaxant
BL142	Tab, White, Round, Scored, BL over 142	Baclofen 20 mg	Lioresal by Teva	00093-2236	Muscle Relaxant
BL170	Tab, White, Round	Amoxicillin Veterinary 50 mg	Biomox by Biocraft		Veterinary
BL171	Tab, White, Round	Amoxicillin Veterinary 100 mg	Biomox by Biocraft		Veterinary
BL172	Tab, White, Round	Amoxicillin Veterinary 200 mg	Biomox by Biocraft		Veterinary

ID FRONT <> BACK	DESCRIPTION FRONT <> BACK	INGREDIENT & STRENGTH	BRAND (or Generic Equiv.) by FIRM	NDC#	CLASS; SCH.
BL173	Tab, White, Round	Amoxicillin Veterinary 400 mg	Biomox by Biocraft		Veterinary
BL18	Tab, White, Round	Neomycin Sulfate 500 mg	Neomycin Sulfate by Ivax	00182-0673	Antibiotic
BL18	Tab, White, Round	Neomycin Sulfate 500 mg	Neomycin Sulfate by Biocraft		Antibiotic
BL19	Tab, Yellow, Round, Film Coated	Imipramine HCl 10 mg	Tofranil by Moore	00839-1370	Antidepressant
BL19	Tab, Yellow, Round, Film Coated	Imipramine HCl 10 mg	Tofranil by PDRX	55289-0149	Antidepressant
BL19	Tab, Yellow, Round, Film Coated	Imipramine HCl 10 mg	Tofranil by Allscripts		Antidepressant
BL19	Tab, Yellow, Round, Film Coated	Imipramine HCl 10 mg	Tofranil by Heartland	61392-0025	Antidepressant
BL19	Tab, Yellow, Round, Film Coated	Imipramine HCl 10 mg	Tofranil by Qualitest	00603-4043	Antidepressant
BL19	Tab, Yellow, Round, Film Coated	Imipramine HCl 10 mg	Tofranil by Biocraft		Antidepressant
BL19	Tab, Yellow, Round, Film Coated	Imipramine HCl 10 mg	Tofranil by Schein	00364-0443	Antidepressant
BL20	Tab, Salmon, Round, Film Coated	Imipramine HCl 25 mg	Tofranil by Biocraft		Antidepressant
BL20	Tab, Salmon, Round, Film Coated	Imipramine HCl 25 mg	Tofranil by Qualitest	00603-4044	Antidepressant
BL20	Tab, Salmon, Round, Film Coated	Imipramine HCl 25 mg	Tofranil by Heartland	61392-0026	Antidepressant
BL20	Tab, Salmon, Round, Film Coated	Imipramine HCl 25 mg	Tofranil by Kaiser	62224-3440	Antidepressant
BL207 <> CORGARD40	Tab, Grey, Round, Scored, BL over 207	Nadolol 40 mg	Corgard by Nat Pharmpak	55154-0605	Antihypertensive
BL207 <> CORGARD40	Tab, Grey, Round, Scored, BL over 207	Nadolol 40 mg	Corgard by Repack Co of America	55306-0207	Antihypertensive
BL207 <> CORGARD40	Tab, Grey, Round, Scored, BL over 207	Nadolol 40 mg	Corgard by Thrift Drug	59198-0375	Antihypertensive
BL207 <> CORGARD40	Tab, Grey, Round, Scored, BL over 207	Nadolol 40 mg	Corgard by King	00003-0207	Antihypertensive
BL207 <> CORGARD40	Tab, Grey, Round, Scored, BL over 207	Nadolol 40 mg	Corgard by BMS	Canadian DIN	Antihypertensive
BL207 <> CORGARD40	Tab, Grey, Round, Scored, BL over 207	Nadolol 40 mg	Corgard by Pharmedix	53002-1018	Antihypertensive
BL208 <>	Tab, Light Blue	Nadolol 120 mg	Corgard by King	00003-0208	Antihypertensive
CORGARD120MG					
BL21	Tab, Green, Round, BL/21	Imipramine HCl 50 mg	Tofranil by Biocraft		Antidepressant
BL21	Tab, Coated	Imipramine HCl 50 mg	Tofranil by Med Pro	53978-0073	Antidepressant
BL21	Tab, BL/21	Imipramine HCl 50 mg	Tofranil by Schein	00364-0435	Antidepressant
BL21	Tab, Coated, BL/21	Imipramine HCl 50 mg	Tofranil by Kaiser	62224-3444	Antidepressant
BL21	Tab	Imipramine HCl 50 mg	Tofranil by Heartland	61392-0027	Antidepressant
BL21	Tab, Film Coated	Imipramine HCl 50 mg	Tofranil by Qualitest	00603-4045	Antidepressant
BL21	Tab, Coated	Imipramine HCl 50 mg	Tofranil by Pharmedix	53002-1066	Antidepressant
BL21	Tab, Coated, BL/21	Imipramine HCl 50 mg	Tofranil by Moore	00839-1372	Antidepressant
BL22	Tab, Pink, Round, BL/22	Amitriptyline HCl 10 mg	Elavil by Biocraft		Antidepressant
BL22	Tab, Coated	Amitriptyline HCl 10 mg	Elavil by Pharmedix	53002-0491	Antidepressant
BL222	Tab, Chewable	Amoxicillin 250 mg	Amoxil by Ivax	00182-1962	Antibiotic
BL222	Tab, Chewable	Amoxicillin 250 mg	Amoxil by Med Pro	53978-1257	Antibiotic
BL23	Tab, Green, Round, BL/23	Amitriptyline HCl 25 mg	Elavil by Biocraft		Antidepressant
BL232 <> CORGARD20	Tab, BL over 232	Nadolol 20 mg	Corgard by King	00003-0232	Antihypertensive
BL24	Tab, Brown, Round, BL/24	Amitriptyline HCl 50 mg	Elavil by Biocraft		Antidepressant
BL241 <> CORGARD80	Tab, Grey, Round, Scored, BL over 241	Nadolol 80 mg	Corgard by Nat Pharmpak	55154-0604	Antihypertensive
BL241 <> CORGARD80	Tab, Grey, Round, Scored, BL over 241	Nadolol 80 mg	Corgard by King	00003-0241	Antihypertensive
BL241 <> CORGARD80	Tab, Grey, Round, Scored, BL over 241	Nadolol 80 mg	Corgard by BMS	Canadian	Antihypertensive
BL246 <>	Tab, Dark Blue	Nadolol 160 mg	Corgard by King	00003-0246	Antihypertensive
CORGARD160MG					
BL25	Tab, Lavender, Round, BL/25	Amitriptyline HCl 75 mg	Elavil by Biocraft		Antidepressant
BL26	Tab, Orange, Round	Amitriptyline HCl 100 mg	Elavil by Biocraft		Antidepressant
BL283 <> CORZIDE405	Tab, Bluish White to White, Dark Blue Specks, BL over 283	Bendroflumethiazide 5 mg, Nadolol 40 mg	Corzide by BMS	00003-0283	Diuretic; Antihypertensive
BL284 <> CORZIDE805	Tab, Bluish White to White, Dark Blue Specks, BL over 284 <> Corzide 80/5	Bendroflumethiazide 5 mg, Nadolol 80 mg	Corzide by BMS	00003-0284	Diuretic; Antihypertensive

ID FRONT <> BACK	DESCRIPTION FRONT <> BACK	INGREDIENT & STRENGTH	BRAND (or Generic Equiv.) by FIRM	NDC#	CLASS; SCH.
BL32	Tab	Sulfamethoxazole 400 mg, Trimethoprim 80 mg	by Ivax	00182-1478	Antibiotic
BL32	Tab	Sulfamethoxazole 400 mg, Trimethoprim 80 mg	by URL Mutual	00677-0783	Antibiotic
BL35	Tab, BL/35	Trimethoprim 200 mg	by Pharmedix	53002-0291	Antibiotic
BL35	Tab, BL/35	Trimethoprim 200 mg	by Qualitest	00603-6265	Antibiotic
BL35	Tab, BL/35	Trimethoprim 200 mg	by Moore	00839-7433	Antibiotic
BL38	Tab, White, Round	Chloroquine Phosphate 250 mg	Aralen Phosphate by Biocraft		Antimalarial
BL42	Tab, Green, Oval, BL/42	Thioridazine 10 mg	Mellaril by Biocraft		Antipsychotic
BL46	Tab, Light Green, Oval, BL/46	Thioridazine 100 mg	Mellaril by Biocraft		Antipsychotic
BL512	Tab, Yellow, Rectangular	Theophylline Anhydrous 300 mg	Quibron T by BMS		Antiasthmatic
BL519	Tab, White, Rectangular	Theophylline Anhydrous SR 300 mg	Quibron T SR by BMS		Antiasthmatic
BL52	Tab, Yellow, Round, BL/52	Amiloride HCl 5 mg, Hydrochlorothiazide 50 mg	Moduretic by Biocraft		Antihypertensive; Diuretic
BL53	Tab, White, Oblong, BL/53	Furosemide (Veterinary) 12.5 mg	by Biocraft		Veterinary
BL54	Tab, White, Oblong, BL/54	Furosemide (Veterinary) 50 mg	by Biocraft		Veterinary; Diuretic
BL71	Tab, Brown, Round, BL/71	Clonidine HCl 0.1 mg	Catapres by Biocraft		Antihypertensive
BL72	Tab, Purple, Round, BL/72	Clonidine HCl 0.2 mg	Catapres by Biocraft		Antihypertensive
BL73	Tab, Pink, Round, BL/73	Clonidine HCl 0.3 mg	Catapres by Biocraft		Antihypertensive
BL92	Tab, White, Round	Metoclopramide HCl 5 mg	Reglan by Neuman	64579-0047	Gastrointestinal
BL92	Tab, White, Round	Metoclopramide HCl 5 mg	Reglan by Nat Pharmpak	55154-5226	Gastrointestinal
BL92	Tab, White, Round	Metoclopramide HCl 5 mg	Reglan by Duramed	51285-0834	Gastrointestinal
BL92	Tab, White, Round	Metoclopramide HCl 5 mg	Reglan by Nat Pharmpak	55154-5526	Gastrointestinal
BL92	Tab, White, Round	Metoclopramide HCl 5 mg	Reglan by Major	00904-1069	Gastrointestinal
BLAINE	Tab, White	Magnesium Oxide 400 mg	Mag-Ox 400 by Blaine	00165-0022	Mineral
BLAINE0054	Cap, White	Magnesium Oxide 140 mg	Uro-Mag by Central		Mineral
BLAINE0054	Cap, White	Magnesium Oxide 140 mg	Uro-Mag by Blaine		Mineral
BLANSETT30	Cap, Ex Release, Printed in Red Ink	Guaifenesin 250 mg, Pseudoephedrine HCl 120 mg	Sudafed Sinus by Sovereign	58716-0010	Cold Remedy
BLANSETT33NALEXJR	Cap, Ex Release, BLANSETT 33 Green Ink <> NALEX JR White Ink	Guaifenesin 300 mg, Pseudoephedrine HCl 60 mg	Sudafed Sinus by Sovereign	58716-0006	Cold Remedy
BLBL <> 505050	Tab, Orange, Rectangular, Scored, Trisected	Trazodone HCl 150 mg	Desyrel by BMS	Canadian DIN 00702277	Antidepressant
BLC1	Tab, Yellow, Oblong	Cefadroxil 1 g	Ultracef by BMS		Antibiotic
BLKLOTRIX10MEQ770	Tab, Orange, Round, BL Klotrix 10mEq 770	Potassium Chloride ER 10 mEq	Klotrix by Apothecon		Electrolytes
BLL1	Tab, Engraved, BL over L1	Mitotane 500 mg	Lysodren by Mead Johnson	00015-3080	Antineoplastic
BLL1	Tab, White, Round, Scored	Mitotane 500 mg	Lysodren by BMS	Canadian DIN 0463221	Antineoplastic
BLLLD9	Cap, Coral, BL-LL-D9	Demeclocycline HCl 150 mg	Declomycin by Lederle		Antibiotic
BLN1 <> NALDECON	Tab, White, Red Specks, BL over N1	Chlorpheniramine Maleate 5 mg, Phenylephrine HCl 10 mg, Phenylpropanolamine HCl 40 mg, Phenyltoloxamine Citrate 15 mg	Naldecon by Mead Johnson	00015-5600 Discontinued	Cold Remedy
BLNI	Tab, Pink, Round	Phenylpropanolamine HCl 40 mg, Phenylephrine HCl 10 mg, Phentoloxamine 15 mg, Chlorpheniramine 5 mg	Naldecon by BMS		Cold Remedy
BLOCADREN <> MSD136	Tab, White, Round, Scored, MSD over 136	Timolol Maleate 10 mg	Blocadren by Merck	00006-0136	Antihypertensive
BLOCADREN <> MSD437	Tab, Light Blue, Cap Shaped	Timolol Maleate 20 mg	Blocadren by Merck	00006-0437	Antihypertensive
BLOCADREN <> MSD59	Tab, Light Blue, Round	Timolol Maleate 5 mg	Blocadren by Merck	00006-0059	Antihypertensive
BLPV	Cap, Rust, Soft Gel	Vitamin A 14,320 IU, Vitamin C 226 mg, Vitamin E 200 IU, Zinc 34.8 mg, Copper 0.8 mg	PreserVision by Bausch & Lomb		Supplement
BLS1	Tab, Green, Round	Hydroflumethiazide 50 mg, Reserpine 0.125 mg	Salutensin by BMS		Diuretic; Antihypertensive
BLS2	Tab, White, Round	Hydroflumethiazide 50 mg	Diucardin by BMS		Diuretic; Antihypertensive

ID FRONT <> BACK	DESCRIPTION FRONT <> BACK	INGREDIENT & STRENGTH	BRAND (or Generic Equiv.) by FIRM	NDC#	CLASS; SCH.
BLS3	Tab, Yellow, Round	Hydroflumethiazide 25 mg, Reserpine 0.125 mg	Salutensin-Demi by BMS		Antihypertensive; Diuretic
BLV1	Tab, White, Round, Film Coated, BL over V1	Penicillin V Potassium 250 mg	Veetids by Sandoz	00003-0115	Antibiotic
BLV2	Tab, White, Round, Film Coated, BL over V2	Penicillin V Potassium 500 mg	Veetids by Sandoz	00003-0116	Antibiotic
BM <> D9	Tab, White, Round, Sustained Release	Bezafibrate 400 mg	Bezalip by Roche	Canadian DIN 02083523	Antihyperlipidemic
BM102	Tab, Off-White to White, BM Logo/102	Torsemide 5 mg	Demadex by Boehringer Mannheim	53169-0102	Diuretic
BM103	Tab, Off-White to White, BM Logo/103	Torsemide 10 mg	Demadex by Boehringer Mannheim	53169-0103	Diuretic
BM103	Tab, BM Logo	Torsemide 10 mg	Demadex by Boehringer Mannheim	12871-3775	Diuretic
BM104	Tab, Off-White to White, BM Logo/104	Torsemide 20 mg	Demadex by Boehringer Mannheim	53169-0104	Diuretic
BM104	Tab, BM Logo	Torsemide 20 mg	Demadex by Boehringer Mannheim	12871-6507	Diuretic
BM105	Tab, Off-White to White, Beveled Edge, BM Logo/105	Torsemide 100 mg	Demadex by Boehringer Mannheim	53169-0105	Diuretic
BM105	Tab, BM Logo	Torsemide 100 mg	Demadex by Boehringer Mannheim	12871-6531	Diuretic
BM8 <> MAXZIDE	Tab, Light Yellow, Bowtie Shaped, Scored	Hydrochlorothiazide 50 mg, Triamterene 75 mg	Maxzide by Mylan	00378-7550	Diuretic; Antihypertensive
BM8 <> MAXZIDE	Tab, Light Yellow, Bowtie Shaped, Scored	Hydrochlorothiazide 50 mg, Triamterene 75 mg	Maxzide by Bertek	62794-0460	Diuretic; Antihypertensive
BM9 <> MAXZIDE	Tab, Light Green, Bowtie Shaped, Scored	Hydrochlorothiazide 25 mg, Triamterene 37.5 mg	Maxzide 25 by Caremark	00339-6094	Diuretic; Antihypertensive
BM9 <> MAXZIDE	Tab, Light Green, Bowtie Shaped, Scored	Hydrochlorothiazide 25 mg, Triamterene 37.5 mg	Maxzide 25 by Direct Dispensing	57866-6801	Diuretic; Antihypertensive
BM9 <> MAXZIDE	Tab, Light Green, Bowtie Shaped, Scored	Hydrochlorothiazide 25 mg, Triamterene 37.5 mg	Maxzide 25 by Bertek	62794-0464	Diuretic; Antihypertensive
BM9 <> MAXZIDE	Tab, Teal, Bow Tie Shaped	Triamterene 37.5 mg, HCl 25 mg	Maxzide by Mylan	00378-3725	Diuretic; Antihypertensive
BMB7	Cap, White, Opaque, Black Ink	Clodronate Disodium 400 mg	Ostac by Roche	Canadian DIN 01927078	Bisphosphonate
BMBU <> BMBU	Tab, White, Oblong, Scored	Glyburide 5 mg	Pro-Glyburide by Pro Doc Limitee	Canadian DIN 02316544	Oral Hypoglycemic Agent
BMEU	Tab, White, Oblong, BMEU	Glyburide 5 mg	by Boehringer Mannheim	Canadian	Antidiabetic
BMEU <> BMEU	Tab, White, Oblong, Scored	Glyburide 5 mg	Euglucon by Pharmascience	Canadian DIN 00720941	Antidiabetic
BMEU <> BMEU	Tab, White, Oblong, Scored	Glyburide 5 mg	Euglucon by Pharmascience	Canadian DIN 02236734	Antidiabetic
BMG6	Tab, White, Round, BM/G6	Bezafibrate 200 mg	Bezalip by Roche	Canadian	Antihyperlipidemic
BMP <> 202	Tab, Blue, Round	Amoxicillin 100 mg	Amoxil by Pfizer		Antibiotic
BMP <> 203	Tab, Pink, Round	Amoxicillin 200 mg	Amoxil by Pfizer		Antibiotic
BMP112	Cap, Yellow	Atropine Sulfate 0.13, Aspirin 130, Caffeine 8, Ipecac 3, Camphor 15	Dasin by SKB		Gastrointestinal
BMP121	Cap, Pink	Multivitamin Combination	Livitamin by SKB		Vitamin
BMP122	Cap, Green	Multivitamin Combination	Livitamin with IF by SKB		Vitamin
BMP123	Tab, Orange	Multivitamin	Livitamin Chewable by SKB		Vitamin
BMP125	Tab, Yellow, Oblong	Esterified Estrogens 0.3 mg	Menest by SKB		Hormone
BMP125	Tab, Yellow, Oblong	Esterified Estrogens 0.3 mg	Menest by Monarch	61570-0072	Hormone
BMP126	Tab, Orange, Oblong	Esterified Estrogens 0.625 mg	Menest by Monarch	61570-0073	Hormone
BMP126	Tab, Orange, Oblong	Esterified Estrogens 0.625 mg	Menest by SKB	00029-2810	Hormone
BMP127	Tab, Coated	Esterified Estrogens 1.25 mg	Menest by SKB	00029-2820	Hormone
BMP127	Tab, Green, Oblong	Esterified Estrogens 1.25 mg	Menest by Monarch	61570-0074	Hormone
BMP128	Tab, Coated	Esterified Estrogens 2.5 mg	Menest by King	60793-0840	Hormone
BMP128	Tab, Coated	Esterified Estrogens 2.5 mg	Menest by SKB	00029-2830	Hormone
BMP141	Cap, Brown & Orange	Ampicillin 500 mg	Principen by SKB		Antibiotic
BMP143	Cap, Brown & Yellow	Oxacillin Sodium 250 mg	Bactocill by SKB		Antibiotic
BMP144	Cap, Brown & Yellow	Oxacillin Sodium 500 mg	Bactocill by SKB		Antibiotic
BMP145	Tab, White, Round	Oxyphencyclimine HCl 10 mg	Daricon by SKB		Antispasmodic
BMP165	Cap, Blue & Cream, Black Print, Bmp over 165	Dicloxacillin Sodium 250 mg	Dycill by SKB		Antibiotic

ID FRONT <> BACK	DESCRIPTION FRONT <> BACK	INGREDIENT & STRENGTH	BRAND (or Generic Equiv.) by FIRM	NDC#	CLASS; SCH.
BMP166	Cap, Blue & Cream	Dicloxacillin Sodium 500 mg	Dycill by SKB		Antibiotic
BMP169	Cap, Beige & Lime	Cloxacillin Sodium 250 mg	Cloxapen by SKB		Antibiotic
BMP170	Cap, Beige & Lime	Cloxacillin Sodium 500 mg	Cloxapen by SKB		Antibiotic
BMP182	Cap, Clear & Green	Codeine Phosphate 20 mg, Pseudoephedrine HCl 60 mg	Nucofed by Monarch	61570-0018	Cold Remedy; C III
BMP182	Cap	Codeine Phosphate 20 mg, Pseudoephedrine HCl 60 mg	Nucofed by King	60793-0852	Cold Remedy; C III
BMP188	Tab, BMP/188	Acetaminophen 650 mg, Hydrocodone Bitartrate 7.5 mg	Lorcet Plus by Nat Pharmpak	55154-7101	Analgesic; C III
BMP189	Tab, Chewable	Amoxicillin 125 mg, Clavulanate Potassium 31.25 mg	Augmentin by H J Harkins Co	52959-0470	Antibiotic
BMP190	Tab, Mottled Yellow, Round, Chewable	Amoxicillin 250 mg, Clavulanate Potassium 125 mg	Augmentin by Bayer		Antibiotic
BMP192	Tab, Blue, Round	Metoclopramide 10 mg	Reglan by SKB	00280-1070	Gastrointestinal
BMP207	Tab, White, Round	Acetaminophen 500 mg, Hydrocodone Bitartrate 5 mg	Anexsia by SKB		Analgesic; C III
BMP210	Tab, White, Oblong	Phenylephrine 10 mg, Guaifenesin 100 mg, DM 15 mg, Acetaminophen 300 mg	Conar-A by SKB		Cold Remedy
BMRGP	Cap	Acetaminophen 300 mg, Phenyltoloxamine Citrate 20 mg, Salicylamide 200 mg	by Pharmakon	55422-0411	Analgesic
BMRGP	Cap	Acetaminophen 300 mg, Phenyltoloxamine Citrate 20 mg, Salicylamide 200 mg	by Seatrace	00551-0411	Analgesic
BMS	Tab, White, Hexagonal	Nefazodone HCl 100 mg	Serzone by Va Cmop	65243-0102	Antidepressant
BMS <> 1611	Tab, White to Off-White, Triangular	Entecavir 0.5 mg	Baraclude by BMS	Canadian DIN 02282224	Antiviral
BMS <> 1611	Tab, White to Off-White, Triangular	Entecavir 0.5 mg	Baraclude by BMS	00003-1611	Antiviral
BMS <> 1612	Tab, Pink, Triangular	Entecavir 1 mg	Baraclude by BMS	00003-1612	Antiviral
BMS <> 524	Tab, White to Off-White, Round, Film Coated	Dasatinib 70 mg	Sprycel by BMS	Canadian DIN 02293145	Cancer Treatment
BMS <> 524	Tab, Coated, Mottled	Dasatinib 70 mg	Sprycel by BMS	00003-0524	Cancer Treatment
BMS <> 5250		Diltiazem HCl 30 mg	Cardizem by BMS	00003-5250 Discontinued	Antihypertensive
BMS <> 527	Tab, White to Off-White, Round, Film Coated	Dasatinib 20 mg	Sprycel by BMS	00003-0527	Cancer Treatment
BMS <> 527	Tab, White to Off-White, Round, Film Coated	Dasatinib 20 mg	Sprycel by BMS	Canadian DIN 02293129	Cancer Treatment
BMS <> 528	Tab, White to Off-White, Oval, Film Coated	Dasatinib 50 mg	Sprycel by BMS	Canadian DIN 02293137	Cancer Treatment
BMS <> 528	Tab, White to Off-White, Oval, Film Coated	Dasatinib 50 mg	Sprycel by BMS	00003-0528	Cancer Treatment
BMS <> 5550	Tab, Mottled Clear, Film Coated, Scored	Diltiazem HCl 60 mg	Cardizem by BMS	00003-5550 Discontinued	Antihypertensive
BMS <> 5550	Tab, Mottled Clear, Film Coated, Scored	Diltiazem HCl 60 mg	Cardizem by Med Pro	53978-1235 Discontinued	Antihypertensive
BMS <> 5770	Tab, Coated, Mottled	Diltiazem HCl 90 mg	Cardizem by BMS	00003-5770 Discontinued	Antihypertensive
BMS <> 5850	Tab, Coated, Mottled	Diltiazem HCl 120 mg	Cardizem by BMS	00003-5850 Discontinued	Antihypertensive
BMS <> 6072	Tab, Light Yellow, Cap Shaped, Film Coated	Glyburide 1.25 mg, Metformin 250 mg	Glucovance by BMS	00087-6072	Antidiabetic
BMS <> 6072	Tab, Light Yellow, Cap Shaped, Film Coated	Glyburide 1.25 mg, Metformin 250 mg	Glucovance by BMS	12783-0072	Antidiabetic
BMS <> 6073	Tab, Light Orange, Cap Shaped, Film Coated	Glyburide 2.5 mg, Metformin 500 mg	Glucovance by BMS	12783-0073	Antidiabetic
BMS <> 6073	Tab, Light Orange, Cap Shaped, Film Coated	Glyburide 2.50 mg, Metformin 500 mg	Glucovance by BMS	00087-6073	Antidiabetic
BMS <> 6074	Tab, Yellow, Cap Shaped, Film Coated	Glyburide 5 mg, Metformin 500 mg	Glucovance by BMS	00087-6074	Antidiabetic
BMS <> 6074	Tab, Yellow, Cap Shaped, Film Coated	Glyburide 5 mg, Metformin 500 mg	Glucovance by BMS	12783-0074	Antidiabetic
BMS <> 6077	Tab, White, Oval, Film Coated	Glipizide 2.5 mg, Metformin HCl 500 mg	Metaglip by BMS	00087-6077	Antidiabetic
BMS <> 6078	Tab, Pink, Oval, Film Coated	Glipizide 5 mg, Metformin HCl 500 mg	Metaglip by BMS	00087-6078	Antidiabetic
BMS <> 6081	Tab, Pink, Oval, Film Coated	Glipizide 2.5 mg, Metformin HCl 250 mg	Metaglip by BMS	00087-6081	Antidiabetic

ID FRONT <> BACK	DESCRIPTION FRONT <> BACK	INGREDIENT & STRENGTH	BRAND (or Generic Equiv.) by FIRM	NDC#	CLASS; SCH.
BMS <> 80	Tab, Yellow, Oval	Pravastatin Sodium 80 mg	Pravigard by BMS	00003-5183 00003-5184	Antihyperlipidemic
BMS <> 80	Tab, Yellow, Oval	Pravastatin Sodium 80 mg	Pravachol by BMS	00003-5195	Antihyperlipidemic
BMS <> MONOPRIL10	Tab, White, Diamond Shaped, Monopril over 10	Fosinopril Sodium 10 mg	Monopril by BMS	Canadian DIN 01907107	Antihypertensive
BMS <> MONOPRIL10	Tab, White, Diamond Shaped, Monopril over 10	Fosinopril Sodium 10 mg	Monopril by Caremark	00339-5745	Antihypertensive
BMS <> MONOPRIL10	Tab, White, Diamond Shaped, Monopril over 10	Fosinopril Sodium 10 mg	Monopril by Direct Dispensing	57866-3800	Antihypertensive
BMS <> MONOPRIL10	Tab, White, Diamond Shaped, Monopril over 10	Fosinopril Sodium 10 mg	Monopril by Allscripts		Antihypertensive
BMS <> MONOPRIL10	Tab, White, Diamond Shaped, Monopril over 10	Fosinopril Sodium 10 mg	Monopril by Va Cmop	65243-0092	Antihypertensive
BMS <> MONOPRIL10	Tab, White, Diamond Shaped, Monopril over 10	Fosinopril Sodium 10 mg	Monopril by BMS	00087-0158	Antihypertensive
BMS <> MONOPRIL20	Tab, White, Oblong, Monopril over 20	Fosinopril Sodium 20 mg	Monopril by Direct Dispensing	57866-3803	Antihypertensive
BMS <> MONOPRIL20	Tab, White, Oblong, Monopril over 20	Fosinopril Sodium 20 mg	Monopril by BMS	Canadian DIN 01907115	Antihypertensive
BMS <> MONOPRIL20	Tab, White, Oblong, Monopril over 20	Fosinopril Sodium 20 mg	Monopril by Va Cmop	65243-0093	Antihypertensive
BMS <> MONOPRIL20	Tab, White, Oblong, Monopril over 20	Fosinopril Sodium 20 mg	Monopril by Allscripts		Antihypertensive
BMS <> MONOPRIL20	Tab, White, Oblong, Monopril over 20	Fosinopril Sodium 20 mg	Monopril by BMS	00087-0609	Antihypertensive
BMS <> MONOPRIL20	Tab, White, Oblong, Monopril over 20	Fosinopril Sodium 20 mg	Monopril by BMS	15548-0609	Antihypertensive
BMS <> MONOPRIL20	Tab, White, Oblong, Monopril over 20	Fosinopril Sodium 20 mg	Monopril by JB	51111-0471	Antihypertensive
BMS <> MONOPRIL40	Tab, White, Hexagonal, Monopril over 40	Fosinopril Sodium 40 mg	Monopril by Va Cmop	65243-0094	Antihypertensive
BMS <> MONOPRIL40	Tab, White, Hexagonal, Monopril over 40	Fosinopril Sodium 40 mg	Monopril by BMS	00087-1202	Antihypertensive
BMS <> MONOPRIL40	Tab, White, Hexagonal, Monopril over 40	Fosinopril Sodium 40 mg	Monopril by BMS	15548-0202	Antihypertensive
BMS <> TEQUIN200	Tab, White, Almond Shaped, Film Coated	Gatifloxacin 200 mg	Tequin by Mead Johnson	00015-1117 Discontinued	Antibiotic
BMS <> TEQUIN200	Tab, White, Almond Shaped, Film Coated	Gatifloxacin 200 mg	Tequin by BMS	12783-0117 Discontinued	Antibiotic
BMS <> TEQUIN400	Tab, White, Biconvex, Film Coated	Gatifloxacin 400 mg	Tequin by BMS	12783-0177 Discontinued	Antibiotic
BMS <> TEQUIN400	Tab, White, Biconvex, Film Coated	Gatifloxacin 400 mg	Tequin by Mead Johnson	00015-1177 Discontinued	Antibiotic
BMS <> W921	Tab	Metoprolol Tartrate 50 mg	Lopressor by Apothecon	59772-3692	Antihypertensive
BMS <> W933	Tab	Metoprolol Tartrate 100 mg	Lopressor by Apothecon	59772-3693	Antihypertensive
BMS100 <> 32	Tab, White, Hexagonal, Scored	Nefazodone HCl 100 mg	Serzone by BMS	15548-0032	Antidepressant
BMS100 <> 32	Tab, White, Hexagonal, Scored	Nefazodone HCl 100 mg	Serzone by Kaiser	00179-1241	Antidepressant
BMS100 <> 32	Tab, White, Hexagonal, Scored	Nefazodone HCl 100 mg	Serzone by BMS	00087-0032	Antidepressant
BMS100 <> 32	Tab, White, Hexagonal, Scored	Nefazodone HCl 100 mg	Serzone by BMS	Canadian	Antidepressant
BMS100 <> 32	Tab, White, Hexagonal, Scored	Nefazodone HCl 100 mg	Serzone by Direct Dispensing	57866-0912	Antidepressant
BMS100MG1558	Cap, Yellow, BMS 100 mg, Extended Release	Stavudine 100 mg	Zerit XR by BMS	00003-1558	Antiviral
BMS100MG3623	Cap, Blue and White, White and Blue print	Atazanavir 100 mg	Reyataz by BMS	00003-3623	Antiviral
BMS125MG6671	Cap, White, Tan Print, Delayed Release, Opaque	Didanosine 125 mg	Videx EC by BMS	00087-6671	Antiviral
BMS125MG6671	Cap, White, Tan Print, Delayed Release, Opaque	Didanosine 125 mg	Videx EC by BMS	Canadian DIN 02244596	Antiviral
BMS150 <> 39	Tab, Peach, Hexagonal, Scored	Nefazodone HCl 150 mg	Serzone by BMS	Canadian	Antidepressant
BMS150 <> 39	Tab, Peach, Hexagonal, Scored	Nefazodone HCl 150 mg	Serzone by BMS	00087-0039	Antidepressant
BMS150 <> 39	Tab, Peach, Hexagonal, Scored	Nefazodone HCl 150 mg	Serzone by Kaiser	00179-1242	Antidepressant
BMS150 <> 39	Tab, Peach, Hexagonal, Scored	Nefazodone HCl 150 mg	Serzone by Par	49884-0569	Antidepressant
BMS150 <> 39	Tab, Peach, Hexagonal, Scored	Nefazodone HCl 150 mg	Serzone by Allscripts		Antidepressant
BMS150 <> 39	Tab, Peach, Hexagonal, Scored	Nefazodone HCl 150 mg	Serzone by BMS	15548-0039	Antidepressant
BMS150MG3624	Cap, Blue and Powder Blue, White and Blue print	Atazanavir 150 mg	Reyataz by BMS	00003-3624	Antiviral
BMS150MG3624	Cap, Blue and Powder Blue, White and Blue print	Atazanavir 150 mg	Reyataz by BMS	Canadian DIN 02248610	Antiviral

ID FRONT <> BACK	DESCRIPTION FRONT <> BACK	INGREDIENT & STRENGTH	BRAND (or Generic Equiv.) by FIRM	NDC#	CLASS; SCH.
BMS196415	Cap, Dark Red & Light Yellow, Black Print, BMS over 1964	Stavudine 15 mg	Zerit by BMS	Canadian DIN 02216086	Antiviral
BMS196415	Cap, Dark Red & Light Yellow, Black Print, BMS over 1964	Stavudine 15 mg	Zerit by BMS	00003-1964	Antiviral
BMS196520	Cap, Light Brown, Black Print, BMS over 1965	Stavudine 20 mg	Zerit by Murfreesboro	51129-1396	Antiviral
BMS196520	Cap, Light Brown, Black Print, BMS over 1965	Stavudine 20 mg	Zerit by BMS	Canadian DIN 02216094	Antiviral
BMS196520	Cap, Light Brown, Black Print, BMS over 1965	Stavudine 20 mg	Zerit by BMS	00003-1965	Antiviral
BMS196630	Cap, Dark Orange & Light Orange, Black Print, BMS over 1966	Stavudine 30 mg	Zerit by BMS	Canadian DIN 02216108	Antiviral
BMS196630	Cap, Dark Orange & Light Orange, Black Print, BMS over 1966	Stavudine 30 mg	Zerit by BMS	00003-1966	Antiviral
BMS196740	Cap, Dark Orange, Black Print, BMS over 1967	Stavudine 40 mg	Zerit by BMS	Canadian DIN 02216116	Antiviral
BMS196740	Cap, Dark Orange, Black Print, BMS over 1967	Stavudine 40 mg	Zerit by BMS	00003-1967	Antiviral
BMS200 <> 33	Tab, Light Yellow, Hexagonal	Nefazodone HCl 200 mg	Serzone by BMS	Canadian	Antidepressant
BMS200 <> 33	Tab, Light Yellow, Hexagonal	Nefazodone HCl 200 mg	Serzone by BMS	00087-0033	Antidepressant
BMS200 <> 33	Tab, Light Yellow, Hexagonal	Nefazodone HCl 200 mg	by Kaiser	00179-1243	Antidepressant
BMS200 <> 33	Tab, Light Yellow, Hexagonal	Nefazodone HCl 200 mg	Serzone by BMS	15548-0033	Antidepressant
BMS200MG3631	Cap, Blue, White print	Atazanavir 200 mg	Reyataz by BMS	Canadian DIN 02248611	Antiviral
BMS200MG3631	Cap, Blue, White print	Atazanavir 200 mg	Reyataz by BMS	00003-3631	Antiviral
BMS200MG6672	Cap, White, Green Print, Delayed Release, Opaque	Didanosine 200 mg	Videx EC by BMS	00087-6672	Antiviral
BMS200MG6672	Cap, White, Green Print, Delayed Release, Opaque	Didanosine 200 mg	Videx EC by BMS	Canadian DIN 02244597	Antiviral
BMS250 <> 41	Tab, White, Hexagonal	Nefazodone HCl 250 mg	Serzone by BMS	00087-0041	Antidepressant
BMS250 <> 41	Tab, White, Hexagonal	Nefazodone HCl 250 mg	by Kaiser	00179-1244	Antidepressant
BMS250 <> 41	Tab, White, Hexagonal	Nefazodone HCl 250 mg	Serzone by Par	49884-0574	Antidepressant
BMS250 <> 41	Tab, White, Hexagonal	Nefazodone HCl 250 mg	Serzone by BMS	15548-0041	Antidepressant
BMS250MG6673	Cap, White, Blue Print, Delayed Release, Opaque	Didanosine 250 mg	Videx EC by BMS	Canadian DIN 02244598	Antiviral
BMS250MG6673	Cap, White, Blue Print, Delayed Release, Opaque	Didanosine 250 mg	Videx EC by BMS	00087-6673	Antiviral
BMS30034	Tab, Peach, Hexagonal, BMS 300/34	Nefazodone HCl 300 mg	Serzone by BMS	Canadian	Antidepressant
BMS300MG3622	Cap, Red and Blue, White Print	Atazanavir Sulfate 300 mg	Reyataz by BMS	00003-3622	Antiviral
BMS303	Cap, Green and Pink, Opaque	Hydroxyurea 500 mg	Hydrea by BMS	Canadian DIN 00465283	Antineoplastic
BMS37	Tab, Pink, Round	Amoxicillin 125 mg	Amoxil by Apothecon	59772-0037	Antibiotic
BMS375MG1555	Cap, Red and Yellow, BMS 37.5 mg, Extended Release	Stavudine 37.5 mg	Zerit XR by BMS	00003-1555	Antiviral
BMS38	Tab, Pink, Round	Amoxicillin 250 mg	Amoxil by Apothecon	59772-0038	Antibiotic
BMS400MG6674	Cap, White, Red Print, Delayed Release, Opaque	Didanosine 400 mg	Videx EC by BMS	00087-6674	Antiviral
BMS400MG6674	Cap, White, Red Print, Delayed Release, Opaque	Didanosine 400 mg	Videx EC by BMS	Canadian DIN 02244599	Antiviral
BMS50 <> 31	Tab, Light Pink, Hexagonal	Nefazodone HCl 50 mg	Serzone by BMS	Canadian	Antidepressant
BMS50 <> 31	Tab, Light Pink, Hexagonal	Nefazodone HCl 50 mg	Serzone by Direct Dispensing by Murfreesboro	57866-0911	Antidepressant
BMS50 <> 31	Tab, Light Pink, Hexagonal	Nefazodone HCl 50 mg	Serzone by BMS	51129-1106	Antidepressant
BMS50 <> 31	Tab, Light Pink, Hexagonal	Nefazodone HCl 50 mg	Serzone by BMS	00087-0031	Antidepressant
BMS50 <> 31	Tab, Light Pink, Hexagonal	Nefazodone HCl 50 mg	Serzone by BMS	15548-0031	Antidepressant
BMS5040	Tab, Off-White, Round	Atenolol 50 mg	Tenormin by BMS	Discontinued	Antihypertensive
BMS50MG1556	Cap, Orange, BMS 50 mg, Extended Release	Stavudine 50 mg	Zerit XR by BMS	00003-1556	Antiviral
BMS5240	Tab, Off-White, Round	Atenolol 100 mg	Tenormin by BMS	00003-5240	Antihypertensive
				Discontinued	

ID FRONT <> BACK	DESCRIPTION FRONT <> BACK	INGREDIENT & STRENGTH	BRAND (or Generic Equiv.) by FIRM	NDC#	CLASS; SCH.
BMS5250	Tab, Coated	Diltiazem HCl 30 mg	Cardizem by Med Pro	53978-2064	Antihypertensive
BMS5550	Tab, Film Coated	Diltiazem HCl 60 mg	Cardizem by Med Pro	53978-1235	Antihypertensive
BMS6060 <> 500	Tab, White to Off-White, Round, Film Coated	Metformin HCl 500 mg	Glucophage by BMS	00087-6060	Antidiabetic
BMS6060 <> 500	Tab, White to Off-White, Round, Film Coated	Metformin HCl 500 mg	Glucophage by PDRX	55289-0211	Antidiabetic
BMS6060 <> 500	Tab, White to Off-White, Round, Film Coated	Metformin HCl 500 mg	Glucophage by Heartland	61392-0717	Antidiabetic
BMS6063 <> 500	Tab, White to Off-White, Cap Shaped, Film Coated, Ex Release	Metformin HCl 500 mg	Glucophage XR by BMS	00087-6063	Antidiabetic
BMS6064 <> 750	Tab, Pale Red, Cap Shaped, Ex Release	Metformin HCl 750 mg	Glucophage XR by BMS	00087-6064	Antidiabetic
BMS6070 <> 850	Tab, White to Off-White, Round, Film Coated	Metformin HCl 850 mg	Glucophage by Va Cmop	65243-0047	Antidiabetic
BMS6070 <> 850	Tab, White to Off-White, Round, Film Coated	Metformin HCl 850 mg	Glucophage by Direct Dispensing	57866-9058	Antidiabetic
BMS6070 <> 850	Tab, White to Off-White, Round, Film Coated	Metformin HCl 850 mg	Glucophage by BMS	00087-6070	Antidiabetic
BMS6070 <> 850	Tab, White to Off-White, Round, Film Coated	Metformin HCl 850 mg	Glucophage by Kaiser	00179-1378	Antidiabetic
BMS6070 <> 850	Tab, White to Off-White, Round, Film Coated	Metformin HCl 850 mg	Glucophage by Caremark	00339-6085	Antidiabetic
BMS6070 <> 850	Tab, White to Off-White, Round, Film Coated	Metformin HCl 850 mg	Glucophage by Nat Pharmpak	55154-5825	Antidiabetic
BMS6070 <> 850	Tab, White to Off-White, Round, Film Coated	Metformin HCl 850 mg	Glucophage by Nat Pharmpak	55154-5824	Antidiabetic
BMS6070 <> 850	Tab, White to Off-White, Round, Film Coated	Metformin HCl 850 mg	Glucophage by BMS	12783-0070	Antidiabetic
BMS6071 <> 1000	Tab, White, Cap Shaped, Scored, Film Coated	Metformin HCl 1000 mg	Glucophage by Caremark	00339-6173	Antidiabetic
BMS6071 <> 1000	Tab, White, Cap Shaped, Scored, Film Coated	Metformin HCl 1000 mg	Glucophage by BMS	00087-6071	Antidiabetic
BMS6071 <> 1000	Tab, White, Cap Shaped, Scored, Film Coated	Metformin HCl 1000 mg	Glucophage by Direct Dispensing	57866-9057	Antidiabetic
BMS7491250	Cap, Blue & White, BMS 7491/250	Cefaclor 250 mg	Ceclor by BMS		Antibiotic
BMS7494500	Cap, Blue & Gray, BMS 7494/500	Cefaclor 500 mg	Ceclor CD by BMS		Antibiotic
BMS75MG1557	Cap, Red, BMS 75 mg, Extended Release	Stavudine 75 mg	Zerit XR by BMS	00003-1557	Antiviral
BMS7720250	Tab, Film Coated	Cefprozil 250 mg	Cefzil by BMS	55961-0720	Antibiotic
BMS7721500	Tab, Film Coated	Cefprozil 500 mg	Cefzil by BMS	55961-0721	Antibiotic
BMS97	Tab, Pink, Round	Amoxicillin 125 mg	Amoxil by Apothecon		Antibiotic
BN <> 51	Tab, White, Round	Ephedrine HCl 25 mg, Guaifenesin 200 mg	Ephedrine Plus Tabs by Neil Labs	60242-0225	Cold Remedy
BN10 <> G	Tab, White, Round, BN / 10	Baclofen 10 mg	Lioresal by UDL	51079-0668 Discontinued	Muscle Relaxant
BN10 <> G	Tab, White, Round, BN / 10	Baclofen 10 mg	Lioresal by Genpharm	15330-0245	Muscle Relaxant
BN10 <> G	Tab, White, Round, BN / 10	Baclofen 10 mg	Lioresal by Mylan	00378-6010	Muscle Relaxant
BN10 <> G	Tab, White, Round, BN / 10	Baclofen 10 mg	Lioresal by Genpharm	Canadian DIN 02088398	Muscle Relaxant
BN10G	Tab, White, BN/10/G	Baclofen 10 mg	Lioresal by BDH	Canadian	Muscle Relaxant
BN20 <> G	Tab, White, Round, BN / 20	Baclofen 20 mg	Lioresal by Genpharm	15330-0246	Muscle Relaxant
BN20 <> G	Tab, White, Round, BN / 20	Baclofen 20 mg	Lioresal by Genpharm	Canadian DIN 02088401	Muscle Relaxant
BN20 <> G	Tab, White, Round, BN / 20	Baclofen 20 mg	Lioresal by UDL	51079-0669 Discontinued	Muscle Relaxant
BN20 <> G	Tab, White, Round	Baclofen 20 mg	Lioresal by Mylan	00378-6020	Muscle Relaxant
BN20G	Tab, White, BN/20/G	Baclofen 20 mg	Lioresal by BDH	Canadian	Muscle Relaxant
BNB <> CG	Tab, White, Round, Film Coated	Oxprenolol HCl 160 mg	Slow Trasicor by Novartis	Canadian DIN 00534587	Antihypertensive
BNP6000	Cap, Clear & Orange	Diazoxide 50 mg	Proglycem by Baker		Antihypoglycemic
BNP7400	Cap, Orange	Tolmetin Sodium 400 mg	Tolectin DS by Baker		NSAID
BNP7600	Cap, White, Gelatin Coated	Pentosan Polysulfate Sodium 100 mg	Elmiron by Baker Cummins	Canadian	Analgesic
BNP7600	Cap, White, Gelatin Coated	Pentosan Polysulfate Sodium 100 mg	Elmiron by Ivax	00575-7600	Analgesic
BNP7600	Cap, White, Gelatin Coated	Pentosan Polysulfate Sodium 100 mg	Elmiron by Alza	17314-9300	Analgesic
BNP7600	Cap, White, Gelatin Coated	Pentosan Polysulfate Sodium 100 mg	Elmiron by Janssen-Ortho	Canadian DIN 02029448	Analgesic

ID FRONT <> BACK	DESCRIPTION FRONT <> BACK	INGREDIENT & STRENGTH	BRAND (or Generic Equiv.) by FIRM	NDC#	CLASS; SCH.
BNVA <> 150	Tab, White, Oblong, Film-Coated	Ibandronate Sodium 150 mg	Boniva by Hoffmann La Roche	00004-0186	Bisphosphonate
BOCA <> 121	Tab, White, Ex Release	Guaifenesin 600 mg, Pseudoephedrine HCl 45 mg	by Boca	64376-0030	Cold Remedy
BOCA <> 122	Tab, White, Oblong, Scored	Dextromethorphan HBr 60 mg, Guaifenesin 1000 mg	Dex GG by Boca	64376-0031	Cold Remedy
BOCA <> 123	Tab, White, Ex Release	Pseudoephedrine HCl 120 mg, Chlorpheniramine Maleate 8 mg, Methscopolamine Nitrate 2.5 mg	by Boca	64376-0032	Cold Remedy
BOCA <> 124	Tab, White, Cap Shaped, Extended Release	Guaifenesin 595 mg, Pseudoephedrine HCl 48 mg	Pseudo GG TR by Boca	64376-0033	Cold Remedy
BOCA <> 125	Tab, White, Round, SR	Chlorpheniramine Maleate 12 mg, Pseudoephedrine HCl 20 mg, Methscopolamine Nitrate 2.5 mg	PCM Allergy by Boca	64376-0036	Cold Remedy
BOCA <> 131	Tab, Purple, Oval, Chewable	Phenylephrine HCl 10 mg, Methscopolamine Nitrate 1.25 mg, Chlorpheniramine Maleate 2 mg	PCM Chewable by Boca	64376-0530	Cold Remedy
BOCA <> 132	Tab, White, Cap Shaped	Pseudoephedrine HCl 50 mg, Guaifenesin 1200 mg	Sudal SR by Boca	64376-0531	Cold Remedy
BOCA <> 133	Tab, Purple, Oval	Chlorpheniramine Maleate 2 mg, Pseudoephedrine HCl 15 mg	Pediox by Boca	64376-0532	Cold Remedy
BOCA <> 134	Tab, White, Cap Shaped	Pseudoephedrine HCl 80 mg, Dextromethorphan HBr 40 mg, Guaifenesin 700 mg	Maxifed DMX by Boca	64376-0533	Cold Remedy
BOCA <> 135	Tab, Green, Cap Shaped	Pseudoephedrine HCl 80 mg, Guaifenesin 700 mg	Maxifed by Boca	64376-0538	Cold Remedy
BOCK	Cap, ER, in Black Ink with White Beads	Pheniramine Maleate 16 mg, Phenylpropanolamine HCl 50 mg, Phenyltoloxamine Citrate 16 mg, Pyrilamine Maleate 16 mg	Poly Histine D by Sanofi	00024-1656	Cold Remedy
BOCK	Cap, Black Ink with White Beads	Pheniramine Maleate 8 mg, Phenylpropanolamine HCl 25 mg, Phenyltoloxamine Citrate 8 mg, Pyrilamine Maleate 8 mg	Poly Histine D by Sanofi	00024-1658	Cold Remedy
BOCK <> PN90	Tab, PN/90	Ascorbic Acid 120 mg, Calcium 250 mg, Cholecalciferol 10 mcg, Copper 2 mg, Cyanocobalamin 12 mcg, Docusate Sodium 50 mg, Folic Acid 1 mg, Iodine 150 mcg, Iron 90 mg, Niacinamide 20 mg, Pyridoxine HCl 20 mg, Riboflavin 3.4 mg, Thiamine Mononitrate 3 mg, Vitamin A Acetate 1.2 mg, Vitamin E Acetate 30 mg, Zinc 25 mg	by Physician Total Care	54868-2703	Vitamin
BOCK330	Tab, Beige, Round	Ferrous Fumarate 110 mg, Docusate Na 20 mg, Vitamin C 200 mg	Hemaspan by Sanofi		Mineral
BOCK460	Tab, Blue, Oval, Scored	Guaifenesin 400 mg, Pseudoephedrine HCl 60 mg	Zephrex by Midland Pharms	45255-2070	Cold Remedy
BOCK460	Tab, Bock over 460	Guaifenesin 400 mg, Pseudoephedrine HCl 60 mg	Zephrex by Sanofi	00024-2624	Cold Remedy
BOCKHS33	Tab, Tan, Oblong	Ferrous Fumarate 335 mg, Vitamin C 200 mg, Docusate Na 20 mg	Hemaspan by KV Pharma		Mineral
BOCKPN	Tab, White, Oval	Prenatal Vitamin	Prenate Ultra by Sanofi		Vitamin
BOCKZLA	Tab, Orange, Oval, Bock Z/LA	Guaifenesin 600 mg, Pseudoephedrine HCl 120 mg	Zephrex LA by Sanofi		Cold Remedy
BOLAR227	Cap, Red	Hydrochlorothiazide 25 mg, Triamterene 50 mg	Dyazide by Circa		Diuretic; Antihypertensive
BOLAR277	Cap, Red	Hydrochlorothiazide 25 mg, Triamterene 50 mg	Dyazide by Circa		Diuretic; Antihypertensive
BONEFOS	Cap, Yellow, Hard Gel	Clodronate Disodium 400 mg	Bonefos by Berlex	Canadian DIN 01984845	Bisphosphonate
BOOTS0051	Tab, White, Round	Allopurinol 100 mg	Zyloprim by Boots		Antigout
BOOTS0052	Tab, Orange, Round	Allopurinol 300 mg	Zyloprim by Boots		Antigout
BP <> 132	Tab, Yellow, Round	Magnesium 600 mg, Vitamin B-6 25 mg	Beelith by Beach	00486-1132	Mineral; Vitamin
BP <> 539	Tab, Layered, Round	Guaifenesin 275 mg, Phenylephrine HCl 25 mg	Guaiphen-PD by Boca	64376-0539	Cold Remedy
BP <> 540	Tab, White, Oval	Guaifenesin 600 mg, Phenylephrine HCl 40 mg	Liquibid-D by Boca	64376-0540	Cold Remedy
BP <> 541	Tab, Cap Shaped, Coated, Scored	Guaifenesin 1200 mg, Phenylephrine HCl 40 mg	Guaiphen-PD by Boca	64376-0541	Cold Remedy
BP <> 542	Tab, Red Speckled, Cap Shaped	Guaifenesin 1200 mg, Dextromethorphan HBr 60 mg	Tussi-Bid by Boca	64376-0542	Cold Remedy
BP <> 605	Tab, White, Round, Scored	Carbinoxamine 4 mg	Palgic by Boca	64376-0605	Cold Remedy
BP0004	Tab, White, Round	Primidone 250 mg	Mysoline by Circa		Anticonvulsant
BP0005	Tab, White, Round	Methocarbamol 500 mg	Robaxin by Circa		Muscle Relaxant
BP0007	Tab, White, Round	Trihexyphenidyl HCl 2 mg	Artane by Circa		Antiparkinson
BP0011	Tab, Yellow, Round	Furosemide 12.5 mg	Lasix by Circa		Veterinary; Diuretic
BP0012	Tab, Yellow, Oblong	Furosemide 50 mg	Lasix by Circa		Veterinary; Diuretic

ID FRONT <> BACK	DESCRIPTION FRONT <> BACK	INGREDIENT & STRENGTH	BRAND (or Generic Equiv.) by FIRM	NDC#	CLASS; SCH.
BP0017	Tab, Green, Round	Pentaerythritol Tetranitrate SR 80 mg	Peritrate SA by Circa		Antianginal
BP0024	Tab, White, Round	Trihexyphenidyl HCl 5 mg	Artane by Circa		Antiparkinson
BP0026	Tab, Green, Round	Isosorbide Dinitrate SA 40 mg	Isordil by Circa		Antianginal
BP0036	Tab, White, Round	Chlorothiazide 250 mg	Diuril by Circa		Diuretic; Antihypertensive
BP0037	Tab, White, Round	Orphenadrine Citrate SR 100 mg	Norflex by Circa		Muscle Relaxant
BP0045	Tab, Pink, Round	Warfarin Sodium 5 mg	Coumadin by Circa		Anticoagulant
BP0049	Tab, Green, Round	Isosorbide Dinitrate Oral 20 mg	Isordil by Circa		Antianginal
BP0052	Tab, White, Round	Ergoloid Mesylate 0.5 mg	Hydergine by Circa		Ergot Alkaloids
BP0058	Tab, Orange, Round	Hydrochlorothiazide 100 mg	Hydrodiuril by Circa		Diuretic; Antihypertensive
BP0059	Tab, Brownish Yellow, Round	Sulfasalazine 500 mg	Azulfidine by Major	00904-1152	Gastrointestinal
BP0065	Cap, White	Hydralazine 25 mg, Hydrochlorothiazide 25 mg	Apresazide by Circa		Antihypertensive; Diuretic
BP0066	Cap, Black & White	Hydralazine 50 mg, Hydrochlorothiazide 50 mg	Apresazide by Circa		Antihypertensive; Diuretic
BP0069	Tab, White, Oval	Ergoloid Mesylate 1 mg	Hydergine by Circa		Ergot Alkaloids
BP0073	Tab, White, Round	Bethanechol Chloride 5 mg	Urecholine by Circa		Urinary Tract
BP0074	Tab, Pink, Round	Bethanechol Chloride 10 mg	Urecholine by Circa		Urinary Tract
BP0075	Tab, Yellow, Round	Bethanechol Chloride 25 mg	Urecholine by Circa		Urinary Tract
BP0083	Tab, Orange, Round	Hydralazine 25 mg, Hydrochlorothiazide 15 mg	Apresoline-Esidrix by Circa		Antihypertensive; Diuretic
BP0084	Cap, White, Ex Release	Phenytoin Sodium 100 mg	Dilantin by Circa		Anticonvulsant
BP0093	Tab, Chartreuse, Round	Prochlorperazine 10 mg	Compazine by Circa		Antiemetic
BP0094	Tab, White, Round	Carisoprodol 350 mg	Soma by Circa		Muscle Relaxant
BP0111	Tab, Chartreuse, Round	Prochlorperazine 5 mg	Compazine by Circa		Antiemetic
BP0129	Tab, White, Round	Hydrochlorothiazide 25 mg, Spironolactone 25 mg	Aldactazide by Circa		Diuretic; Antihypertensive
BP0139	Tab, Green, Round	Fluoxymesterone 10 mg	Halotestin by Circa		Steroid; C III
BP0149	Tab, White, Round	Acepromazine Maleate (Veterinary) 10 mg	by Circa		Veterinary
BP0150	Tab, Yellow, Round	Acepromazine Maleate (Veterinary) 25 mg	by Circa		Veterinary
BP0187	Tab, Pink, Oblong	Procainamide HCl SR 1000 mg	Procan SR by Circa		Antiarrhythmic
BP0211	Tab, Blue, Round	Maprotiline 25 mg	Ludiomil by Circa		Antidepressant
BP0212	Tab, Yellow, Round	Maprotiline 50 mg	Ludiomil by Circa		Antidepressant
BP0213	Tab, White, Round	Maprotiline 75 mg	Ludiomil by Circa		Antidepressant
BP095	Tab, Lavender & White, Round	Carisoprodol 200 mg, Aspirin 325 mg	Soma Compound by Circa		Muscle Relaxant
BP1	Tab, Green, Oblong	Thioridazine 10 mg	Mellaril by Circa		Antipsychotic
BP100	Cap, Green	Hydroxyzine Pamoate 25 mg	Vistaril by Circa		Antianxiety; Antihistamine
BP1007	Tab, White, Round	Trazodone HCl 50 mg	Desyrel by Circa		Antidepressant
BP1008	Tab, White, Round	Trazodone HCl 100 mg	Desyrel by Circa		Antidepressant
BP101	Cap, Green & White	Hydroxyzine Pamoate 50 mg	Vistaril by Circa		Antianxiety; Antihistamine
BP1015	Cap, Yellow	Nitrofurantoin 100 mg	Macrodantin by Circa		Antibiotic
BP1016	Cap, White & Yellow	Nitrofurantoin 50 mg	Macrodantin by Circa		Antibiotic
BP102	Cap, Gray & Green	Hydroxyzine Pamoate 100 mg	Vistaril by Circa		Antianxiety; Antihistamine
BP1027	Cap, Pink	Amantadine HCl 100 mg	Symmetrel by Circa		Antiviral
BP111	Tab, Chartreuse, Round	Prochlorperazine 5 mg	Compazine by Circa		Antiemetic

ID FRONT <> BACK	DESCRIPTION FRONT <> BACK	INGREDIENT & STRENGTH	BRAND (or Generic Equiv.) by FIRM	NDC#	CLASS; SCH.
BP112	Tab, Chartreuse, Round	Prochlorperazine 25 mg	Compazine by Circa		Antiemetic
BP117	Tab, Red, Round	Trifluoperazine HCl 5 mg	Stelazine by Circa		Antipsychotic
BP118	Tab, Buff, Oblong	Thioridazine 25 mg	Mellaril by Circa		Antipsychotic
BP119	Tab, White, Oblong	Thioridazine 50 mg	Mellaril by Circa		Antipsychotic
BP120	Tab, Yellow, Oblong	Thioridazine 100 mg	Mellaril by Circa		Antipsychotic
BP121	Tab, Yellow, Oblong	Thioridazine 150 mg	Mellaril by Circa		Antipsychotic
BP122	Tab, Pink, Oblong	Thioridazine 200 mg	Mellaril by Circa		Antipsychotic
BP123	Tab, Peach, Round	Propranolol HCl 10 mg	Inderal by Circa		Antihypertensive
BP124	Tab, Blue, Round	Propranolol HCl 20 mg	Inderal by Circa		Antihypertensive
BP125	Tab, Green, Round	Propranolol HCl 40 mg	Inderal by Circa		Antihypertensive
BP126	Tab, Yellow, Round	Propranolol HCl 80 mg	Inderal by Circa		Antihypertensive
BP127	Tab, Yellow, Round	Hydroflumethiazide 25 mg, Reserpine 0.125 mg	Salutensin-Demi by Circa		Antihypertensive; Diuretic
BP128	Tab, Green, Round	Hydroflumethiazide 50 mg, Reserpine 0.125 mg	Salutensin by Circa		Diuretic; Antihypertensive
BP13	Tab, White, Round	Chlorothiazide 500 mg	Diuril by Circa		Diuretic; Antihypertensive
BP131	Tab, Brownish Orange, Round	Sulfasalazine 500 mg	Azulfidine EN-tabs by Circa		Gastrointestinal
BP132	Tab, Pink, Round	Chlorothiazide 500 mg, Reserpine 0.125 mg	Diupres by Circa		Diuretic; Antihypertensive
BP133	Tab, White, Round	Allopurinol 100 mg	Zyloprim by Circa		Antigout
BP134	Tab, Peach, Round	Allopurinol 300 mg	Zyloprim by Circa		Antigout
BP135	Tab, Orange, Round	Guanethidine Monosulfate 10 mg	Ismelin by Circa		Antihypertensive
BP136	Tab, White, Round	Guanethidine Monosulfate 25 mg	Ismelin by Circa		Antihypertensive
BP137	Tab, Peach, Round	Fluoxymesterone 2 mg	Halotestin by Circa		Steroid; C III
BP138	Tab, Green, Round	Fluoxymesterone 5 mg	Halotestin by Circa		Steroid; C III
BP144	Tab, Lavender & White, Round	Carisoprodol 200 mg, Aspirin 325 mg	Soma Compound by Circa		Muscle Relaxant
BP145	Cap, Green	Indomethacin 25 mg	Indocin by Circa		NSAID
BP146	Cap, Green	Indomethacin 50 mg	Indocin by Circa		NSAID
BP151	Tab, Red, Round	Trifluoperazine HCl 10 mg	Stelazine by Circa		Antipsychotic
BP152	Tab, Blue, Oval	Procainamide HCl SR 250 mg	Procan SR by Circa		Antiarrhythmic
BP153	Tab, Pink, Oval	Procainamide HCl SR 500 mg	Procan SR by Circa		Antiarrhythmic
BP154	Tab, Buff, Oval	Procainamide HCl SR 750 mg	Procan SR by Circa		Antiarrhythmic
BP157	Tab, Gray, Round	Methylclothiazide 5 mg, Deserpidine 0.5 mg	Enduronyl Forte by Circa		Diuretic; Antihypertensive
BP158	Tab, Yellow, Round	Methylclothiazide 5 mg, Deserpidine 0.25 mg	Enduronyl by Circa		Diuretic; Antihypertensive
BP163	Tab, White, Round	Fluphenazine HCl 1 mg	Prolixin by Circa		Antipsychotic
BP164	Tab, Beige, Round	Fluphenazine HCl 2.5 mg	Prolixin by Circa		Antipsychotic
BP165	Tab, Blue, Round	Fluphenazine HCl 5 mg	Prolixin by Circa		Antipsychotic
BP166	Tab, Red, Round	Fluphenazine HCl 10 mg	Prolixin by Circa		Antipsychotic
BP167	Tab, Blue, Round	Chlorpropamide 100 mg	Diabinese by Circa		Antidiabetic
BP168	Tab, Blue, Round	Chlorpropamide 250 mg	Diabinese by Circa		Antidiabetic
BP171	Tab, Red, Round	Trifluoperazine HCl 1 mg	Stelazine by Circa		Antipsychotic
BP172	Tab, Red, Round	Trifluoperazine HCl 2 mg	Stelazine by Circa		Antipsychotic
BP181	Tab, White, Round	Lorazepam 1 mg	Ativan by Circa		Antianxiety; C IV

ID FRONT <> BACK	DESCRIPTION FRONT <> BACK	INGREDIENT & STRENGTH	BRAND (or Generic Equiv.) by FIRM	NDC#	CLASS; SCH.
BP182	Tab, White, Round	Lorazepam 2 mg	Ativan by Circa		Antianxiety; C IV
BP187	Tab, Pink, Oblong	Procainamide HCl SR 1000 mg	Procan SR by Circa		Antiarrhythmic
BP2	Tab, White, Round	Lorazepam 0.5 mg	Ativan by Circa		Antianxiety; C IV
BP2005	Cap, Orange & White	Disopyramide Phosphate 100 mg	Norpace by Circa		Antiarrhythmic
BP2006	Cap, Brown & Orange	Disopyramide Phosphate 150 mg	Norpace by Circa		Antiarrhythmic
BP2014	Tab, White, Round	Methyldopa 125 mg	Aldomet by Circa		Antihypertensive
BP2015	Tab, White, Round	Methyldopa 250 mg	Aldomet by Circa		Antihypertensive
BP2016	Tab, White, Round	Methyldopa 500 mg	Aldomet by Circa		Antihypertensive
BP2023	Cap, Blue	Dicyclomine HCl 10 mg	Bentyl by Circa		Gastrointestinal
BP2024	Cap, Maroon & Pink	Meclofenamate Sodium 50 mg	Meclomen by Circa		NSAID
BP2025	Cap, Maroon & White	Meclofenamate Sodium 100 mg	Meclomen by Circa		NSAID
BP2026	Tab, Blue, Round	Dicyclomine HCl 20 mg	Bentyl by Circa		Gastrointestinal
BP2027	Tab, White, Round	Metoclopramide HCl 10 mg	Reglan by Circa		Gastrointestinal
BP2036	Tab, Chartreuse, Round	Hydrochlorothiazide 15 mg, Methyldopa 250 mg	Aldoril by Circa		Diuretic; Antihypertensive
BP2037	Tab, Pink, Round	Hydrochlorothiazide 25 mg, Methyldopa 250 mg	Aldoril by Circa		Diuretic; Antihypertensive
BP2038	Tab, Chartreuse, Oval	Hydrochlorothiazide 30 mg, Methyldopa 500 mg	Aldoril by Circa		Diuretic; Antihypertensive
BP2039	Tab, Pink, Oval	Hydrochlorothiazide 50 mg, Methyldopa 500 mg	Aldoril by Circa		Diuretic; Antihypertensive
BP2042	Tab, White, Round	Verapamil HCl 80 mg	Isoptin by Circa		Antihypertensive
BP2043	Tab, White, Round	Verapamil HCl 120 mg	Isoptin by Circa		Antihypertensive
BP2047	Tab, Green, Round	Hydrochlorothiazide 25 mg, Reserpine 0.125 mg	Hydropres by Circa		Diuretic; Antihypertensive
BP2048	Tab, Green, Round	Hydrochlorothiazide 50 mg, Reserpine 0.125 mg	Hydropres by Circa		Diuretic; Antihypertensive
BP2049	Tab, White, Round	Hydralazine 25 mg, Hydrochlorothiazide 15 mg, Reserpine 0.1 mg	Ser-Ap-Es by Circa		Antihypertensive; Diuretic
BP2053	Tab, Orange, Round	Amitriptyline 25 mg, Perphenazine 2 mg	Triavil by Circa		Antidepressant; Antipsychotic
BP2054	Tab, Yellow, Round	Amitriptyline 25 mg, Perphenazine 4 mg	Triavil by Circa		Antidepressant; Antipsychotic
BP2055	Tab, Orange, Round	Amitriptyline 50 mg, Perphenazine 4 mg	Triavil by Circa		Antidepressant; Antipsychotic
BP2056	Tab, Blue, Round	Amitriptyline 10 mg, Perphenazine 2 mg	Triavil by Circa		Antidepressant; Antipsychotic
BP2057	Tab, Salmon, Round	Amitriptyline 10 mg, Perphenazine 4 mg	Triavil by Circa		Antidepressant; Antipsychotic
BP2060	Tab, Pink, Round	Propranolol HCl 60 mg	Inderal by Circa		Antihypertensive
BP2062	Tab, White, Round	Tolbutamide 250 mg	Orinase by Circa		Antidiabetic
BP2063	Tab, White, Round	Tolbutamide 500 mg	Orinase by Circa		Antidiabetic
BP2064	Tab, Green, Round	Pentaerythritol Tetranitrate 10 mg	Peritrate by Circa		Antianginal
BP2066	Cap, Pink & White	Lithium Carbonate 300 mg	Eskalith by Circa		Antipsychotic
BP2067	Tab, Green, Round	Pentaerythritol Tetranitrate 20 mg	Peritrate by Circa		Antianginal
BP2068	Tab, White, Round	Tolazamide 100 mg	Tolinase by Circa		Antidiabetic
BP2069	Tab, White, Round	Tolazamide 250 mg	Tolinase by Circa		Antidiabetic
BP2070	Tab, White, Round	Tolazamide 500 mg	Tolinase by Circa		Antidiabetic
BP2074	Tab, White, Oblong	Colchicine 0.5 mg, Probenecid 500 mg	ColBenemid by Circa		Antigout

ID FRONT <> BACK	DESCRIPTION FRONT <> BACK	INGREDIENT & STRENGTH	BRAND (or Generic Equiv.) by FIRM	NDC#	CLASS; SCH.
BP2075	Tab, Yellow, Round	Nitrofurantoin 50 mg	Furadantin by Circa		Antibiotic
BP2076	Cap, Yellow	Procainamide HCl 250 mg	Pronestyl by Circa		Antiarrhythmic
BP2078	Cap, Orange & Yellow	Procainamide HCl 500 mg	Pronestyl by Circa		Antiarrhythmic
BP2080	Tab, Yellow, Round	Nitrofurantoin 100 mg	Furadantin by Circa		Antibiotic
BP2081	Cap, Green & White	Flurazepam HCl 15 mg	Dalmane by Circa		Hypnotic; C IV
BP2082	Cap, Green & White	Flurazepam HCl 30 mg	Dalmane by Circa		Hypnotic; C IV
BP2085	Tab, Pink, Oblong	Acetaminophen 325 mg, Propoxyphene Napsylate 50 mg	Darvocet-N 50 by Circa		Analgesic; C IV
BP2086	Tab, Pink, Oblong	Acetaminophen 650 mg, Propoxyphene Napsylate 100 mg	Darvocet-N 100 by Circa		Analgesic; C IV
BP2087	Cap, Pink	Temazepam 15 mg	Restoril by Circa		Sedative/Hypnotic; C IV
BP2088	Cap, Pink & Yellow	Temazepam 30 mg	Restoril by Circa		Sedative/Hypnotic; C IV
BP2092	Tab, Lavender, Round	Trichlormethiazide 4 mg, Reserpine 0.1 mg	Naquival by Circa		Diuretic; Antihypertensive
BP2093	Tab, Orange, Round	Hydrochlorothiazide 25 mg	Hydrodiuril by Circa		Diuretic; Antihypertensive
BP2094	Tab, Orange, Round	Hydrochlorothiazide 50 mg	Hydrodiuril by Circa		Diuretic; Antihypertensive
BP211	Tab, Blue, Round	Maprotiline 25 mg	Ludiomil by Circa		Antidepressant
BP2118	Cap, Purple & Yellow, Ex Release	Disopyramide Phosphate 100 mg	Norpace CR by Circa		Antiarrhythmic
BP2119	Cap, Orange & Purple, Controlled Release	Disopyramide Phosphate 150 mg	Norpace CR by Circa		Antiarrhythmic
BP212	Tab, Yellow, Round	Maprotiline 50 mg	Ludiomil by Circa		Antidepressant
BP2126	Cap, White	Potassium Chloride 750 mg	Micro K 10 by Circa		Electrolytes
BP213	Tab, White, Round	Maprotiline 75 mg	Ludiomil by Circa		Antidepressant
BP2150	Tab, White, Round	Isoniazid 100 mg	Laniazid by Circa		Antimycobacterial
BP2155	Tab, White, Round	Isoniazid 300 mg	Laniazid by Circa		Antimycobacterial
BP28	Tab, Brown, Round	Imipramine HCl 25 mg	Tofranil by Circa		Antidepressant
BP3000	Tab, White, Round	Quinaglute Gluconate SR 324 mg	Quinaglute Duratabs by Circa		Antiarrhythmic
BP3020	Tab, Blue, Round	Trichlormethiazide 4 mg	Naqua by Circa		Diuretic; Antihypertensive
BP31	Tab, Pink, Oblong	Thioridazine 15 mg	Mellaril by Circa		Antipsychotic
BP32	Tab, Blue, Pentagon	Dexamethasone 0.75 mg	Decadron by Circa		Steroid
BP33	Tab, Peach, Round	Chlorthalidone 25 mg	Hygroton by Circa		Diuretic
BP34	Tab, Blue, Round	Chlorthalidone 50 mg	Hygroton by Circa		Diuretic
BP35	Tab, White, Round	Chlorthalidone 100 mg	Hygroton by Circa		Diuretic
BP39	Tab, Yellow, Triangular	Imipramine HCl 10 mg	Tofranil by Circa		Antidepressant
BP40	Tab, Green, Round	Imipramine HCl 50 mg	Tofranil by Circa		Antidepressant
BP41	Tab, White, Round	Ergoloid Mesylate 1 mg	Hydergine by Circa		Ergot Alkaloids
BP42	Tab, White, Round	Acetazolamide 250 mg	Diamox by Circa		Antiglaucoma Agent
BP44	Tab, Orange, Round	Warfarin Sodium 2.5 mg	Coumadin by Circa		Anticoagulant
BP46	Tab, Yellow, Round	Warfarin Sodium 7.5 mg	Coumadin by Circa		Anticoagulant
BP47	Tab, White, Round	Warfarin Sodium 10 mg	Coumadin by Circa		Anticoagulant
BP50	Tab, Lavender, Round	Warfarin Sodium 2 mg	Coumadin by Circa		Anticoagulant
BP500	Tab, Yellow and Red, Gelcap	Acetaminophen 500 mg	Tylenol by Leiner	49035-0027	Analgesic
BP500	Cap, Dark Purple Opaque and Purple	Phenylephrine 7.5 mg, Brompheniramine 6 mg	Bromfenex by Brighton	10914-0500	Cold Remedy
BP5000	Tab, White, Round	Spironolactone 25 mg	Aldactone by Circa		Diuretic

ID FRONT <> BACK	DESCRIPTION FRONT <> BACK	INGREDIENT & STRENGTH	BRAND (or Generic Equiv.) by FIRM	NDC#	CLASS; SCH.
BP5010	Tab, Yellow, Round	Bethanechol Chloride 50 mg	Urecholine by Circa		Urinary Tract
BP543	Tab, White, Cap Shaped	Brompheniramine 6 mg	Lodrane 12HR by Boca	64376-0543	Cold Remedy
BP544	Tab, White, Cap Shaped	Brompheniramine 6 mg, Pseudoephedrine 45 mg	Lodrane 12D by Boca	64376-0544	Cold Remedy
BP56	Tab, Pink, Round	Chlorothiazide 250 mg, Reserpine 0.125 mg	Diupres by Circa		Diuretic; Antihypertensive
BP6	Tab, White, Oblong	Methocarbamol 750 mg	Robaxin by Circa		Muscle Relaxant
BP60	Tab, White, Round	Liothyronine Sodium 25 mcg	Cytomel by Circa		Thyroid Hormone
BP62	Tab, Orange, Round	Methyclothiazide 2.5 mg	Enduron by Circa		Diuretic; Antihypertensive
BP63	Tab, Reddish Orange, Round	Methyclothiazide 5 mg	Enduron by Circa		Diuretic; Antihypertensive
BP64	Cap, Blue	Hydralazine 100 mg, Hydrochlorothiazide 50 mg	Apresazide by Circa		Antihypertensive; Diuretic
BP72	Tab, White, Round	Hydroflumethiazide 50 mg	Diucardin by Circa		Diuretic; Antihypertensive
BP76	Tab, Red, Round	Oxtriphylline 100 mg	Choledyl by Circa		Antiasthmatic
BP77	Tab, Yellow, Round	Oxtriphylline 200 mg	Choledyl by Circa		Antiasthmatic
BP78	Tab, White, Round	Cyproheptadine HCl 4 mg	Periactin by Circa		Antihistamine
BP79	Tab, White, Round	Clonidine HCl 0.1 mg	Catapres by Circa		Antihypertensive
BP80	Tab, Orange, Round	Clonidine HCl 0.2 mg	Catapres by Circa		Antihypertensive
BP81	Tab, Peach, Round	Clonidine HCl 0.3 mg	Catapres by Circa		Antihypertensive
BR87	Tab, Green, Round	Sulfamethoxazole 500 mg	Gantanol by Circa		Antibiotic
BP88	Tab, White, Round	Primidone (Veterinary) 250 mg	by Circa		Veterinary
BP9000	Tab, White, Round	Quinine Sulfate 260 mg	Quinamm by Circa		Antimalarial
BP93	Tab, Chartreuse, Round	Prochlorperazine 10 mg	Compazine by Circa		Antiemetic
BP955	Cap	Chlorpheniramine Maleate 12 mg	Chlor-Trimeton by Brighton	10914-0955	Antihistamine
BR956	Tab, White, Oblong	Methyltestosterone Buccal 5 mg	Android 5 by Heather		Hormone; C III
BR958	Tab, Green, Square	Methyltestosterone 10 mg	Android 10 by Heather		Hormone; C III
BR996	Tab, Orange, Square	Methyltestosterone 25 mg	Android 25 by Heather		Hormone; C III
BR998	Tab, White, Round	Fluoxymesterone 10 mg	Android F by Heather		Steroid; C III
BRI63 <> A	Tab, White, Pentagonal	Lorazepam 0.5 mg	Ativan by DJ Pharma	64455-0063	Antianxiety; C IV
BPl2	Tab, White, Round	Acetaminophen 300 mg, Codeine Phosphate 15 mg	Tylenol w/ Codeine by Noramco		Analgesic; C III
BPM189	Tab, Yellow, Round, Chewable	Amoxicillin 125 mg, Clavulanate Potassium 31.25 mg	Augmentin by SKB	00029-6073	Antibiotic
BPM190	Tab, Yellow, Round, Chewable	Amoxicillin 250 mg, Clavulanate Potassium 62.5 mg	Augmentin by SKB	00029-6074	Antibiotic
BPMPSE	Cap, Clear & Green, in Black	Brompheniramine Maleate 12 mg, Pseudoephedrine HCl 120 mg	BPM PSEH 08 by Bryant	63629-4488	Cold Remedy
BR174	Tab, White to Off-White, Round, Extended Release	Bupropion HBr 174 mg	Aplenzin by Biovail		Antidepressant
BR2 <> GG	Tab, Brownish Orange, Oblong, Scored, CR	Carbamazepine 200 mg	Tegretol CR by Genpharm	Canadian DIN 02241882	Anticonvulsant
BR348	Tab, White to Off-White, Round, Extended Release	Bupropion HBr 348 mg	Aplenzin by Biovail		Antidepressant
BR4 <> GG	Tab, Brownish Orange, Oblong, Scored, CR	Carbamazepine 400 mg	Tegretol CR by Genpharm	Canadian DIN 02241883	Anticonvulsant
BR522	Tab, White to Off-White, Round, Extended Release	Bupropion HBr 522 mg	Aplenzin by Biovail		Antidepressant
BRA200	Tab, White, Round	Calcium Acetate 667 mg	PhosLo by Braintree	52268-0200	Vitamin; Mineral
BREON100	Cap, Brown & White	Theophylline Anhydrous 100 mg	Bronkodyl by Sanofi		Antiasthmatic
BREON200	Cap, Green & White	Theophylline Anhydrous 200 mg	Bronkodyl by Sanofi		Antiasthmatic
BREON200	Cap, Red	Guaifenesin 200 mg	Aquabid by Sanofi		Expectorant
BREONT100	Tab, Peach, Oblong	Chlormezanone 100 mg	Trancopal by Sanofi		Antihistamine

ID FRONT <> BACK	DESCRIPTION FRONT <> BACK	INGREDIENT & STRENGTH	BRAND (or Generic Equiv.) by FIRM	NDC#	CLASS; SCH.
BREONT200	Tab, Green, Oblong	Chlormezanone 200 mg	Trancopal by Sanofi		Antihistamine
BRISTOL	Cap	Amoxicillin 500 mg	Amoxil by Talbert	44514-0077	Antibiotic
BRISTOL1257892	Cap, Light Blue & White	Dicloxacillin Sodium 125 mg	by Apothecon		Antibiotic
BRISTOL278	Cap, Burgundy & Salmon	Amoxicillin 250 mg	Amoxil by BMS		Antibiotic
BRISTOL303010MG	Cap, White, Bristol over 3030	Lomustine 10 mg	Ceenu by BMS	Canadian DIN 00360430	Antineoplastic
BRISTOL303010MG	Cap, White, Bristol over 3030	Lomustine 10 mg	Ceenu by Mead Johnson	00015-3030	Antineoplastic
BRISTOL303010MG	Cap, White & Green, Bristol over 3031	Lomustine 40 mg	Ceenu Dose Pack by Mead Johnson	00015-3034	Antineoplastic
BRISTOL303140MG	Cap, White & Green, Bristol over 3031	Lomustine 40 mg	Ceenu Dose Pack by Mead Johnson	00015-3034	Antineoplastic
BRISTOL303140MG	Cap, White & Green, Bristol over 3031	Lomustine 40 mg	Ceenu by BMS	Canadian DIN 00360422	Antineoplastic
BRISTOL303140MG	Cap, White & Green, Bristol over 3031	Lomustine 40 mg	Ceenu by Mead Johnson	00015-3031	Antineoplastic
BRISTOL303100MG	Cap, Green, Bristol over 3032	Lomustine 100 mg	Ceenu by BMS	Canadian DIN 00360414	Antineoplastic
BRISTOL303100MG	Cap, Green, Bristol over 3032	Lomustine 100 mg	Ceenu by Mead Johnson	00015-3032	Antineoplastic
BRISTOL303100MG	Cap, Green, Bristol over 3032	Lomustine 100 mg	Ceenu Dose Pack by Mead Johnson	00015-3034	Antineoplastic
BRISTOL3091	Cap, Pink, Black Print, Bristol over 3091	Etoposide 50 mg	Vepesid by Mead Johnson	00015-3091	Antineoplastic
BRISTOL3506	Cap, White	Kanamycin Sulfate 500 mg	Kantrex by Mead Johnson	00015-3506	Antibiotic
BRISTOL515	Cap, White & Yellow	Theophylline Anhydrous 300 mg, Guaifenesin 180 mg	Quibron 300 by BMS		Antiasthmatic
BRISTOL516	Cap, Yellow, Black Print, Bristol over 516	Theophylline Anhydrous 130 mg, Ephedrine HCl 24 mg, Phenobarbital 8 mg	Quibron by King	00087-0516	Antiasthmatic; C IV
BRISTOL7271	Cap, Black & Blue	Cefadroxil Monohydrate 500 mg	Duricef by Sandoz	00781-7271	Antibiotic
BRISTOL7271	Cap, Black & Blue	Cefadroxil Monohydrate 500 mg	by Rx Dispensing	61807-0123	Antibiotic
BRISTOL7271	Cap, Black & Blue	Cefadroxil Monohydrate 500 mg	by DRX	55045-2426	Antibiotic
BRISTOL7271	Cap, Black & Blue	Cefadroxil Monohydrate 500 mg	by Nat Pharmpak	55154-7604	Antibiotic
BRISTOL7271	Cap, Black & Blue	Cefadroxil Monohydrate 500 mg	by Apothecon	59772-7271	Antibiotic
BRISTOL7271	Cap, Black & Blue	Cefadroxil Monohydrate 500 mg	Ultracef by BMS		Antibiotic
BRISTOL7278	Cap, Maroon & Flesh, Black Print, Bristol over 7278	Amoxicillin 250 mg	Trimox by Sandoz	00003-0101	Antibiotic
BRISTOL7279	Cap, Flesh & Red, Black Print, Bristol over 7279	Amoxicillin 500 mg	Trimox by Sandoz	00003-0109	Antibiotic
BRISTOL7279	Cap, Flesh & Red, Black Print, Bristol over 7279	Amoxicillin 500 mg	Prevpac by Tap	00300-3702	Antibiotic
BRISTOL732ENKAID-25MG	Cap	Encainide HCl 25 mg	Enkaid by BMS	00087-0732 Discontinued	Antiarrhythmic
BRISTOL734ENKAID-35MG	Cap	Encainide HCl 35 mg	Enkaid by BMS	00087-0734 Discontinued	Antiarrhythmic
BRISTOL7375	Cap, Blue & Purple, Bristol over 7375	Cephalexin 250 mg	Keflex by BMS	00087-7375 Discontinued	Antibiotic
BRISTOL7376	Cap, Blue, Bristol over 7376	Cephalexin 500 mg	Keflex by BMS	00087-7376 Discontinued	Antibiotic
BRISTOL7496	Cap, Black & Orange	Cloxacillin Sodium 500 mg	Tegopen by BMS		Antibiotic
BRISTOL7578	Cap	Amoxicillin 250 mg	Amoxil by Med Pro	53978-5002	Antibiotic
BRISTOL7658500	Cap, Blue & White, Bristol 7658/500	Dicloxacillin Sodium 500 mg	Dynapen by BMS		Antibiotic
BRISTOL7892125	Cap, Blue & White, Bristol 7892/125	Dicloxacillin Sodium 125 mg	Dynapen by BMS		Antibiotic
BRISTOL7893250	Cap, Blue & White, Bristol 7893/250	Dicloxacillin Sodium 250 mg	Dynapen by BMS		Antibiotic
BRISTOL7922	Cap, Gray & Scarlet	Ampicillin 250 mg	Principen by BMS		Antibiotic
BRISTOL7923	Cap, Gray & Scarlet	Ampicillin 500 mg	Principen by BMS		Antibiotic
BRISTOL7935	Cap, Black & Orange	Cloxacillin Sodium 250 mg	Tegopen by BMS		Antibiotic
BRISTOL7936	Cap, Black & Orange	Cloxacillin Sodium 250 mg	Tegopen by BMS		Antibiotic
BRISTOL7977	Cap, Pink	Oxacillin Sodium 250 mg	Prostaphlin by BMS		Antibiotic

ID FRONT <> BACK	DESCRIPTION FRONT <> BACK	INGREDIENT & STRENGTH	BRAND (or Generic Equiv.) by FIRM	NDC#	CLASS; SCH.
BRISTOL7982	Cap, Pink	Oxacillin Sodium 500 mg	Prostaphlin by BMS	00015-7992 Discontinued	Antibiotic
BRISTOL7992	Cap, Gray & Red, Black Print, Bristol over 7992	Ampicillin 250 mg	Principen by Mead Johnson		Antibiotic
BRISTOL7992	Cap, Gray & Red, Black Print, Bristol over 7992	Ampicillin 250 mg	Principen by Apotheca	12634-0417	Antibiotic
BRISTOL7992	Cap, Gray & Red, Black Print, Bristol over 7992	Ampicillin 250 mg	Principen by Med Pro	53978-5018	Antibiotic
BRISTOL7992	Cap, Gray & Red, Black Print, Bristol over 7992	Ampicillin 250 mg	Principen by Sandoz	00003-0122	Antibiotic
BRISTOL7993	Cap, Gray & Red, Black Print, Bristol over 7993	Ampicillin 500 mg	Principen by Sandoz	00781-0134	Antibiotic
BRISTOLBRISTOL	Cap, Maroon and White, Hard Gel	Cefadroxil 500 mg	Duricef by BMS	Canadian DIN 00507245	Antibiotic
BRL <> 1127	Tab, White, Oblong, Scored	Sucralfate 1 g	Carafate by Blue Ridge	59273-0001	Gastrointestinal
BRL <> 1127	Tab, White, Oblong, Scored	Sucralfate 1 g	Carafate by SKB	00135-0176	Gastrointestinal
BRL120 <> 3104	Tab, White, Oblong	Diltiazem HCl 120 mg	Cardizem by Endo		Antihypertensive
BRL120 <> 3104	Tab, White, Oblong, Scored	Diltiazem HCl 120 mg	Cardizem by Blue Ridge	59273-0005	Antihypertensive
BRL120 <> 3104	Tab, White, Oblong, Scored	Diltiazem HCl 120 mg	Cardizem by Rugby	52544-0778	Antihypertensive
BRL30 <> 3101	Tab, Light Blue, Round, BRL over 30	Diltiazem HCl 30 mg	Cardizem by Blue Ridge	59273-0002	Antihypertensive
BRL30 <> 3101	Tab, Light Blue, Round, BRL over 30	Diltiazem HCl 30 mg	Cardizem by Elan Hold	60274-0884	Antihypertensive
BRL4777	Tab, Blue, Round	Oxybutynin Chloride 5 mg	Ditropan by Rugby		Urinary Tract
BRL60 <> 3102	Tab, White, Round, Scored, BRL over 60	Diltiazem HCl 60 mg	Cardizem by Blue Ridge	59273-0003	Antihypertensive
BRL90 <> 3103	Tab, Light Blue, Oblong, Scored	Diltiazem HCl 90 mg	Cardizem by Blue Ridge	59273-0004	Antihypertensive
BROMFEDMURO12120	Cap, Clear & Green, Bromfed Muro 12-120	Brompheniramine Maleate 12 mg, Pseudoephedrine HCl 120 mg	Bromfed by Bryant	63629-2200	Cold Remedy
BROMFEDMURO12120	Cap, Light Green, Ex Release, <> Muro 12-120	Brompheniramine Maleate 12 mg, Pseudoephedrine HCl 120 mg	Bromfed by Thrift Drug	59198-0190	Cold Remedy
BROMFEDMURO12120	Cap, Bromfed <> Muro 12-120	Brompheniramine Maleate 12 mg, Pseudoephedrine HCl 120 mg	Bromfed by Muro	00451-4000	Cold Remedy
BROMFEDPDMURO660	Cap, Dark Green, Ex Release, Bromfed-PD <> Muro 6-60	Brompheniramine Maleate 6 mg, Pseudoephedrine HCl 60 mg	Bromfed PD by Thrift Drug	59198-0189	Cold Remedy
BROMFEDPDMURO660	Cap, Clear & Green, Bromfed-PD <> Muro 6 60, Contains White Beads	Brompheniramine Maleate 6 mg, Pseudoephedrine HCl 60 mg	Bromfed PD by Capellon		Cold Remedy
BROMFEDPDMURO660	Cap, Clear & Green, Bromfed-PD <> Muro 6 60, Contains White Beads	Brompheniramine Maleate 6 mg, Pseudoephedrine HCl 60 mg	Bromfed PD by Capellon	64543-	Cold Remedy
BROMFEDPDMURO660	Cap, Clear & Green, Bromfed-PD <> Muro 6 60, Contains White Beads	Brompheniramine Maleate 6 mg, Pseudoephedrine HCl 60 mg	Bromfed by Nat Pharmpak	55154-4301	Cold Remedy
BROMFEDPDMURO660	Cap, Clear & Green, Bromfed-PD <> Muro 6 60, Contains White Beads	Brompheniramine Maleate 6 mg, Pseudoephedrine HCl 60 mg	Bromfed PD by Muro	00451-4001	Cold Remedy
BRONTEX	Tab, Red, Oblong	Codeine Phosphate 10 mg, Guaifenesin 300 mg	Brontex by Dixon Shane	17236-0375	Cold Remedy; C III
BRONTEX	Tab, Red, Cap Shaped	Codeine Phosphate 10 mg, Guaifenesin 300 mg	Brontex by Kenwood	00482-0440	Cold Remedy; C III
BTG <> 10	Tab, White, Cap Shaped	Oxandrolone 10 mg	Oxandrin by BTG	54396-0110	Steroid; C III
BTG <> 1111	Tab, White, Oval	Oxandrolone 2.5 mg	Oxandrin by BTG	54396-0111	Steroid; C III
BU10	Tab, White to Off-White, Rectangular, Scored, Cobalt Logo <> BU / 10	Buspirone 10 mg	BuSpar by Cobalt	Canadian DIN 02262916	Antianxiety
BU10 <> APO	Tab, White, Pillow Shaped, Scored	Buspirone HCl 10 mg	Buspar by Apotex	Canadian DIN 02211076	Antianxiety
BU10 <> NU	Tab, White, Rectangular, Scored	Buspirone HCl 10 mg	Buspar by Nu Pharm	Canadian DIN 02207672	Antianxiety
BU10APO	Tab, White, Pillow, BU 10/APO	Buspirone HCl 10 mg	Buspar by Apotex	Canadian	Antianxiety
BU5APO	Tab, White, Pillow, BU 5/APO	Buspirone HCl 5 mg	Buspar by Apotex	Canadian	Antianxiety
BUCETUAD307	Cap, White, Opaque, UAD in circle over 307	Acetaminophen 650 mg, Butalbital 50 mg	Bucet by Forest	00785-2307	Analgesic
BULL	Tab, White, Novo Nordisk Bull Logo	Repaglinide 0.5 mg	Prandin by Novo Nordisk	00169-0081	Antidiabetic
BULL	Tab, Yellow, Novo Nordisk Bull Logo	Repaglinide 1 mg	Prandin by Novo Nordisk	00169-0082	Antidiabetic
BULL	Tab, Peach, Novo Nordisk Bull Logo	Repaglinide 2 mg	Prandin by Novo Nordisk	00169-0084	Antidiabetic
BULLSYMBOL <> 1MG500MG	Tab, Yellow	Repaglinide 1 mg, Metformin 500 mg	PrandiMet by Novo Nordisk	00169-0093	Diabetic Glycemic Control

ID FRONT <> BACK	DESCRIPTION FRONT <> BACK	INGREDIENT & STRENGTH	BRAND (or Generic Equiv.) by FIRM	NDC#	CLASS; SCH.
BULLSYMBOL <> 2MG500MG	Tab, Pink	Repaglinide 2 mg, Metformin 500 mg	PrandiMet by Novo Nordisk	00169-0092	Diabetic Glycemic Control
BUMEX05 <> ROCHE	Tab, Green, Oval, Bumex over 0.5 <> Roche	Bumetanide 0.5 mg	Bumex by Med Pro	53978-3386	Diuretic
BUMEX05 <> ROCHE	Tab, Green, Oval, Bumex over 0.5 <> Roche	Bumetanide 0.5 mg	Bumex by Rightpak	65240-0698	Diuretic
BUMEX05 <> ROCHE	Tab, Green, Oval, Bumex over 0.5 <> Roche	Bumetanide 0.5 mg	Bumex by Amerisource	62584-0125	Diuretic
BUMEX05 <> ROCHE	Tab, Green, Oval, Bumex over 0.5 <> Roche	Bumetanide 0.5 mg	Bumex by Hoffmann La Roche	00004-0125	Diuretic
BUMEX05 <> ROCHE	Tab, Green, Oval, Bumex over 0.5 <> Roche	Bumetanide 0.5 mg	Bumex by Nat Pharmpak	55154-3103	Diuretic
BUMEX05 <> ROCHE	Tab, Green, Oval, Bumex over 0.5 <> Roche	Bumetanide 0.5 mg	Bumex by Thrift Drug	59198-0257	Diuretic
BUMEX1 <> ROCHE	Tab, Yellow, Oval, Bumex over 1 <> Roche	Bumetanide 1 mg	Bumex by Thrift Drug	59198-0256	Diuretic
BUMEX1 <> ROCHE	Tab, Yellow, Oval, Bumex over 1 <> Roche	Bumetanide 1 mg	Bumex by Capellon	64543-0131	Diuretic
BUMEX1 <> ROCHE	Tab, Yellow, Oval, Bumex over 1 <> Roche	Bumetanide 1 mg	Bumex by Nat Pharmpak	55154-3104	Diuretic
BUMEX1 <> ROCHE	Tab, Yellow, Oval, Bumex over 1 <> Roche	Bumetanide 1 mg	Bumex by Hoffmann La Roche	00004-0121	Diuretic
BUMEX1 <> ROCHE	Tab, Yellow, Oval, Bumex over 1 <> Roche	Bumetanide 1 mg	Bumex by Med Pro	53978-0241	Diuretic
BUMEX1 <> ROCHE	Tab, Yellow, Oval, Bumex over 1 <> Roche	Bumetanide 1 mg	Bumex by Amerisource	62584-0121	Diuretic
BUMEX1 <> ROCHE	Tab, Yellow, Oval, Bumex over 1 <> Roche	Bumetanide 1 mg	Bumex by Physician Total Care	54868-1293	Diuretic
BUMEX1 <> ROCHE	Tab, Yellow, Oval, Bumex over 1 <> Roche	Bumetanide 1 mg	Bumex by Rightpak	65240-0610	Diuretic
BUMEX1 <> ROCHE	Tab, Yellow, Oval, Bumex over 1 <> Roche	Bumetanide 1 mg	Bumex by Capellon	64543-0131	Diuretic
BUMEX2 <> ROCHE	Tab, Peach, Oval, Bumex over 2 <> Roche	Bumetanide 2 mg	Bumex by Drug Distr	52985-0222	Diuretic
BUMEX2 <> ROCHE	Tab, Peach, Oval, Bumex over 2 <> Roche	Bumetanide 2 mg	Bumex by Leiner	59606-0716	Diuretic
BUMEX2 <> ROCHE	Tab, Peach, Oval, Bumex over 2 <> Roche	Bumetanide 2 mg	Bumex by Caraco	57664-0219	Diuretic
BUMEX2 <> ROCHE	Tab, Peach, Oval, Bumex over 2 <> Roche	Bumetanide 2 mg	Bumex by Thrift Drug	59198-0101	Diuretic
BUMEX2 <> ROCHE	Tab, Peach, Oval, Bumex over 2 <> Roche	Bumetanide 2 mg	Bumex by Nat Pharmpak	55154-3105	Diuretic
BUMEX2 <> ROCHE	Tab, Peach, Oval, Bumex over 2 <> Roche	Bumetanide 2 mg	Bumex by Med Pro	53978-2035	Diuretic
BUMEX2 <> ROCHE	Tab, Peach, Oval, Bumex over 2 <> Roche	Bumetanide 2 mg	Bumex by Hoffmann La Roche	00004-0162	Diuretic
BUMEX2 <> ROCHE	Tab, Peach, Oval, Bumex over 2 <> Roche	Bumetanide 2 mg	Bumex by Amerisource	62584-0162	Diuretic
BUSPAR <> BL10	Tab, White, Rectangular	Buspirone HCl 10 mg	Buspar by BMS	Canadian DIN 0060382	Antianxiety
BUSPAR <> MJ10	Tab, White, Barrel Shaped, Scored	Buspirone HCl 10 mg	Buspar by Caremark	00339-4109	Antianxiety
BUSPAR <> MJ10	Tab, White, Barrel Shaped, Scored	Buspirone HCl 15 mg	Buspar by PDRX	55289-0556	Antianxiety
BUSPAR <> MJ10	Tab, White, Barrel Shaped, Scored	Buspirone HCl 10 mg	Buspar by Heartland	61392-0602	Antianxiety
BUSPAR <> MJ10	Tab, White, Barrel Shaped, Scored	Buspirone HCl 10 mg	Buspar by Amerisource	62584-0819	Antianxiety
BUSPAR <> MJ10	Tab, White, Barrel Shaped, Scored	Buspirone HCl 10 mg	Buspar by Rightpak	65240-0618	Antianxiety
BUSPAR <> MJ10	Tab, White, Barrel Shaped, Scored	Buspirone HCl 10 mg	Buspar by BMS	00087-0819	Antianxiety
BUSPAR <> MJ10	Tab, White, Barrel Shaped, Scored	Buspirone HCl 10 mg	Buspar by Nat Pharmpak	55154-2010	Antianxiety
BUSPAR <> MJ10	Tab, White, Barrel Shaped, Scored	Buspirone HCl 10 mg	Buspar by Allscripts		Antianxiety
BUSPAR <> MJ10	Tab, White, Barrel Shaped, Scored	Buspirone HCl 10 mg	Buspar by Med Pro	53978-3024	Antianxiety
BUSPAR <> MJ10	Tab, White, Barrel Shaped, Scored	Buspirone HCl 10 mg	Buspar by BMS	15548-0819	Antianxiety
BUSPAR <> MJ10	Tab, White, Barrel Shaped, Scored	Buspirone HCl 10 mg	Buspar by CVS	00894-5215	Antianxiety
BUSPAR <> MJ10	Tab, White, Barrel Shaped, Scored	Buspirone HCl 10 mg	Buspar by Pharmedix	53002-1017	Antianxiety
BUSPAR <> MJ10	Tab, White, Barrel Shaped, Scored	Buspirone HCl 10 mg	Buspar by Drug Distr	52985-0156	Antianxiety
BUSPAR <> MJ10	Tab, White, Barrel Shaped, Scored	Buspirone HCl 5 mg	Buspar by Heartland	61392-0601	Antianxiety
BUSPAR <> MJ5	Tab, White, Barrel Shaped, Scored	Buspirone HCl 5 mg	Buspar by Amerisource	62584-0818	Antianxiety
BUSPAR <> MJ5	Tab, White, Barrel Shaped, Scored	Buspirone HCl 5 mg	Buspar by Rightpak	65240-0617	Antianxiety
BUSPAR <> MJ5	Tab, White, Barrel Shaped, Scored	Buspirone HCl 5 mg	Buspar by Direct Dispensing	57866-0902	Antianxiety
BUSPAR <> MJ5	Tab, White, Barrel Shaped, Scored	Buspirone HCl 5 mg	Buspar by Med Pro	53978-2044	Antianxiety
BUSPAR <> MJ5	Tab, White, Barrel Shaped, Scored	Buspirone HCl 5 mg	Buspar by Nat Pharmpak	55154-2008	Antianxiety
BUSPAR <> MJ5	Tab, White, Barrel Shaped, Scored	Buspirone HCl 5 mg	Buspar by Drug Distr	52985-0155	Antianxiety
BUSPAR <> MJ5	Tab, White, Barrel Shaped, Scored	Buspirone HCl 5 mg	Buspar by BMS	15548-0818	Antianxiety
BUSPAR <> MJ5	Tab, White, Barrel Shaped, Scored	Buspirone HCl 5 mg	Buspar by BMS	00087-0818	Antianxiety
BUSPARBL	Tab, White, Pillow, Buspar/BL Bristol Logo	Buspirone HCl 10 mg	Buspar by BMS	Canadian	Antianxiety

ID FRONT <> BACK	DESCRIPTION FRONT <> BACK	INGREDIENT & STRENGTH	BRAND (or Generic Equiv.) by FIRM	NDC#	CLASS; SCH.
BUSPIRONE <> PMS10MG	Tab, White, Cap Shaped, Scored	Buspirone HCl 10 mg	Buspar by Pharmascience	Canadian DIN 02230942	Antianxiety
BUSPIRONEPMS10MG	Tab, White, Cap Shaped, Buspirone/pms/10 mg	Buspirone HCl 10 mg	Buspar by Pharmascience	Canadian	Antianxiety
BUTEXFORTE070	Cap, White, Opaque	Acetaminophen 650 mg, Butalbital 50 mg	Butex Forte by Alphapharm	57315-0013	Analgesic
BUTIBEL <> 37046	Tab, Red, Round, Butibel <> 37 over 046	Belladonna Extract 15 mg, Butabarbital Sodium 15 mg	Butibel by Wallace	00037-0046	Gastrointestinal; C IV
BUTISOLSODIUM <> 37112	Tab, Lavender, Scored, Butisol Sodium <> 37 over 112	Butabarbital 15 mg	Butisol Sodium by Wallace	00037-0112	Sedative/Hypnotic; C III
BUTISOLSODIUM <> 37113	Tab, Blue-Green, Round, Scored, Butisol over Sodium <> 37 over 113	Butabarbital 30 mg	Butisol Sodium by Wallace	00037-0113	Sedative/Hypnotic; C III
BUTISOLSODIUM <> 37114	Tab, Orange, Scored, Butisol Sodium <> 37 over 114	Butabarbital 50 mg	Butisol Sodium by Wallace	00037-0114	Sedative/Hypnotic; C III
BUTTERFLY	Tab, White, Blue Specks, Butterfly Logo Imprint	3,4-Methylenedioxymethamphetamine (MDMA) 88.8 mg	Ecstasy by Illegal		Euphoric; Illicit
BV	Tab, White, Round, BV in Hexagon, Scored	Cyproterone Acetate 50 mg	Androcur by Pharmascience	Canadian DIN 00704431	Antiandrogen
BVF <> 0117	Tab, White, Oblong, Ex Release	Pentoxifylline 400 mg	Trental by Teva	00093-5116	Anticoagulant
BVF <> 0117	Tab, White, Oblong, Ex Release	Pentoxifylline 400 mg	Trental by Pharmafab	62542-0725	Anticoagulant
BVF <> 0117	Tab, White, Oblong, Ex Release	Pentoxifylline 400 mg	Trental by Vangard	00615-4523	Anticoagulant
BVF120	Cap, Light Green, Opaque, Ex Release, BVF over 120	Diltiazem HCl 120 mg	Cardizem CD by Teva	00093-5112	Antihypertensive
BVF120	Cap, Light Green, Opaque, Ex Release, BVF over 120	Diltiazem HCl 120 mg	Tiazac by Biovail Corp.	Canadian DIN 02231150	Antihypertensive
BVF120	Cap, Light Green, Opaque, Ex Release, BVF over 120	Diltiazem HCl 120 mg	Cardizem CD by Ivax	00182-8225	Antihypertensive
BVF120	Cap, Light Green, Opaque, Ex Release, BVF over 120	Diltiazem HCl 120 mg	Cardizem CD by Biovail	62660-0007	Antihypertensive
BVF120	Cap, Light Green, Opaque, Ex Release, BVF over 120	Diltiazem HCl 120 mg	Cardizem CD by Crystaal	Canadian	Antihypertensive
BVF180	Cap, Light Green & Dark Green, Opaque, Ex Release, BVF over 180	Diltiazem HCl 180 mg	Cardizem CD by Crystaal	Canadian	Antihypertensive
BVF180	Cap, Light Green & Dark Green, Opaque, Ex Release, BVF over 180	Diltiazem HCl 180 mg	Cardizem CD by Biovail	62660-0008	Antihypertensive
BVF180	Cap, Light Green & Dark Green, Opaque, Ex Release, BVF over 180	Diltiazem HCl 180 mg	Cardizem CD by Ivax	00182-8226	Antihypertensive
BVF180	Cap, Light Green & Dark Green, Opaque, Ex Release, BVF over 180	Diltiazem HCl 180 mg	Tiazac by Biovail Corp.	Canadian DIN 02231151	Antihypertensive
BVF180	Cap, Light Green & Dark Green, Opaque, Ex Release, BVF over 180	Diltiazem HCl 180 mg	Cardizem CD by Teva	00093-5117	Antihypertensive
BVF240	Cap, Dark Green, Opaque, Ex Release, BVF over 240	Diltiazem HCl 240 mg	Cardizem CD by Teva	00093-5118	Antihypertensive
BVF240	Cap, Dark Green, Opaque, Ex Release, BVF over 240	Diltiazem HCl 240 mg	Tiazac by Biovail Corp.	Canadian DIN 02231152	Antihypertensive
BVF240	Cap, Dark Green, Opaque, Ex Release, BVF over 240	Diltiazem HCl 240 mg	Cardizem CD by Ivax	00182-8227	Antihypertensive
BVF240	Cap, Dark Green, Opaque, Ex Release, BVF over 240	Diltiazem HCl 240 mg	Cardizem CD by Biovail	62660-0009	Antihypertensive
BVF240	Cap, Dark Green, Opaque, Ex Release, BVF over 240	Diltiazem HCl 240 mg	Cardizem CD by Crystaal	Canadian	Antihypertensive
BVF300	Cap, Ivory & Dark Green, Opaque, Ex Release, BVF over 300	Diltiazem HCl 300 mg	Cardizem CD by Biovail	62660-0010	Antihypertensive
BVF300	Cap, Ivory & Dark Green, Opaque, Ex Release, BVF over 300	Diltiazem HCl 300 mg	Tiazac by Biovail Corp.	Canadian DIN 02231154	Antihypertensive
BVF300	Cap, Ivory & Dark Green, Opaque, Ex Release, BVF over 300	Diltiazem HCl 300 mg	Cardizem CD by Teva	00093-5119	Antihypertensive
BVF360	Cap, Blue & Green, Opaque, Ex Release, BVF over 360	Diltiazem HCl 360 mg	Tiazac by Biovail Corp.	Canadian DIN 02231155	Antihypertensive
BVF360	Cap, Blue & Green	Diltiazem HCl 300 mg	Cardizem CD by Crystaal	Canadian	Antihypertensive
BX <> SEARLE	Tab, Blue, Round	Norethindrone 0.5 mg, Ethinyl Estradiol 0.035 mg	Synphasic 28 day by Pfizer	Canadian DIN 02187116	Oral Contraceptive

ID FRONT <> BACK	DESCRIPTION FRONT <> BACK	INGREDIENT & STRENGTH	BRAND (or Generic Equiv.) by FIRM	NDC#	CLASS; SCH.
BX <> SEARLE	Tab, Blue, Round	Norethindrone 0.5 mg, Ethinyl Estradiol 0.035 mg	Synphasic 21 day by Pfizer	Canadian DIN 02187108	Oral Contraceptive
BX <> SEARLE	Tab, White, Round	Norethindrone 1 mg, Ethinyl Estradiol 0.035 mg	Synphasic 28 day by Pfizer	Canadian DIN 0218716	Oral Contraceptive
BX <> SEARLE	Tab, White, Round	Norethindrone 1 mg, Ethinyl Estradiol 0.035 mg	Synphasic 21 day by Pfizer	Canadian DIN 0218708	Oral Contraceptive
BX <> SEARLE	Tab, Blue, Round	Norethindrone 0.5 mg, Ethinyl Estradiol 0.035 mg	Brevicon 5/35 21 day by Pfizer	Canadian DIN 02187086	Oral Contraceptive
BX <> SEARLE	Tab, Blue, Round	Norethindrone 0.5 mg, Ethinyl Estradiol 0.035 mg	Brevicon 5/35 28 day by Pfizer	Canadian DIN 02187094	Oral Contraceptive
BX <> SEARLE	Tab, White, Round	Norethindrone 1 mg, Ethinyl Estradiol 0.035 mg	Select 1/35 21 day by Pfizer	Canadian DIN 02197502	Oral Contraceptive
BX <> SEARLE	Tab, White, Round	Norethindrone 1 mg, Ethinyl Estradiol 0.035 mg	Brevicon 1/35 28 day by Pfizer	Canadian DIN 02189062	Oral Contraceptive
BX <> SEARLE	Tab, White, Round	Norethindrone 1 mg, Ethinyl Estradiol 0.035 mg	Select 1/35 28 day by Pfizer	Canadian DIN 02199297	Oral Contraceptive
BX <> SEARLE	Tab, White, Round	Norethindrone 1 mg, Ethinyl Estradiol 0.035 mg	Brevicon 1/35 21 day by Pfizer	Canadian DIN 02189054	Oral Contraceptive
C	Tab, White, ER, C in Flask <> Clock Design, Imprint 4 Triangles in Square Around Clock	Quinidine Gluconate 324 mg	Quinaglute Duratabs by RX Pak	65084-0127	Antiarrhythmic
C	Tab, White, ER, C in Flask <> Clock Design, Imprint 4 Triangles in Square Around Clock	Quinidine Gluconate 324 mg	Quinaglute Duratabs by Amerisource	62584-0101	Antiarrhythmic
C	Tab, White, ER, C in Flask <> Clock Design, Imprint 4 Triangles in Square Around Clock	Quinidine Gluconate 324 mg	Quinaglute Duratabs by Caremark	00339-5327	Antiarrhythmic
C	Tab, White, ER, C in Flask <> Clock Design, Imprint 4 Triangles in Square Around Clock	Quinidine Gluconate 324 mg	Quinaglute Duratabs by Med Pro	53978-0739	Antiarrhythmic
C	Tab, White, ER, C in Flask <> Clock Design, Imprint 4 Triangles in Square Around Clock	Quinidine Gluconate 324 mg	Quinaglute Duratabs by CVS	51316-0024	Antiarrhythmic
C	Tab, White, ER, C in Flask <> Clock Design, Imprint 4 Triangles in Square Around Clock	Quinidine Gluconate 324 mg	Quinaglute Duratabs by Rightpac	65240-0727	Antiarrhythmic
C	Tab, White, Cap Shaped	Pseudoephedrine HCl 60 mg, Guaifenesin 400 mg	Congestac by B F Ascher	00225-0580	Cold Remedy
C	Tab, White, ER, C in Flask <> Clock Design, Imprint 4 Triangles in Square Around Clock	Quinidine Gluconate 324 mg	Quinaglute Duratabs by Berlex	50419-0101	Antiarrhythmic
C	Tab, White, ER, C in Flask <> Clock Design, Imprint 4 Triangles in Square Around Clock	Quinidine Gluconate 324 mg	Quinaglute Duratabs by Nat Pharmpak	55154-0303	Antiarrhythmic
C	Tab, White, Black Print, Oval, Film Coated	Phenylpropanolamine HCl 75 mg	by Physician Total Care	54868-4107	Decongestant; Appetite Suppressant
C	Tab, Lime Green, Round, Film Coated, Delayed Release	Mycophenolic Acid 180 mg	Myfortic by Novartis	Canadian DIN 02264560	Immunosuppressant
C	Tab, Pink, Round, Orally Disintegrating	Desloratadine 5 mg	Clarinex RediTabs by Schering-Plough	00085-1280	Antihistamine
C	Tab, Lime Green, Round, Film Coated, Delayed Release	Mycophenolic Acid 180 mg	Myfortic by Novartis	00078-0385	Immunosuppressant
C	Tab, Peach, Round, Film Coated	Citalopram HBr 10 mg	Celexa by Caraco	57664-0507	Antidepressant
C	Tab, Yellow, Round, Film Coated	Mirtazapine 7.5 mg	Remeron by Caraco	57664-0510	Antidepressant
C	Tab, White, Round, Orally Disintegrating	Loratadine 10 mg	Claritin Redi-Tab by Schering	11523-7157	Cold Remedy
C	Tab, White, Round	Atenolol 25 mg	Tenormin by IPR		Antihypertensive
C	Tab, White, Elongated, Scored	Carglumic Acid 200 mg	Carbaglu by Orphan Europe		Antihyperammonemia
C <> 0170	Cap, Yellow, Oval, Scored, C <> 01 70	Oxaprozin 600 mg	Daypro by Dr. Reddy's	55111-0170	NSAID
C <> 103103	Tab, Blue, Round, 103 over 103 <> Caraco Logo	Salsalate 500 mg	Disalcid by Caraco	57664-0103	NSAID
C <> 200	Tab, Pink, Round	Amiodarone 200 mg	Cordarone by Wyeth	52903-4188	Antiarrhythmic
C <> 205	Tab, White, Round	Armodafinil 50 mg	Nuvigil by Cephalon	63459-0205	Stimulant; C IV
C <> 215	Tab, White, Oval	Armodafinil 150 mg	Nuvigil by Cephalon	63459-0215	Stimulant; C IV

ID FRONT <> BACK	DESCRIPTION FRONT <> BACK	INGREDIENT & STRENGTH	BRAND (or Generic Equiv.) by FIRM	NDC#	CLASS: SCH.
C <> 225	Tab, White, Oval	Armodafinil 250 mg	Nuvigil by Cephalon	63459-0225	Stimulant; C IV
C <> 317	Tab, Mottled White, Oblong	Guaifenesin 300 mg, Phenylpropanolamine HCl 20 mg	Miraphen PE by Martec		Cold Remedy
C <> 32	Tab, White to Off White, Round	Sumatriptan Succinate 25 mg	Imitrex by Aurobindo	65862-0146	Antimigraine
C <> 33	Tab, White to Off White, Cap Shaped	Sumatriptan Succinate 50 mg	Imitrex by Aurobindo	65862-0147	Antimigraine
C <> 34	Tab, White to Off White, Cap Shaped	Sumatriptan Succinate 100 mg	Imitrex by Aurobindo	65862-0148	Antimigraine
C <> 355	Tab, Mottled Green, Cap Shaped	Guaifenesin 600 mg, Dextromethorphan HBr 30 mg	Humibid DM by Caraco	57664-0355	Cold Remedy
C <> 402	Tab, Peach, Round, Film Coated	Tiagabine 2 mg	Gabitril by Cephalon	63459-0402	Anticonvulsant
C <> 404	Tab, Yellow, Round, Film Coated	Tiagabine 4 mg	Gabitril by Cephalon	63459-0404	Anticonvulsant
C <> 41	Tab, White to Off White, Oval, Scored	Torsemide 5 mg	Demadex by Aurobindo	65862-0125	Diuretic
C <> 412	Tab, Green, Oval, Film Coated	Tiagabine 12 mg	Gabitril by Cephalon	63459-0412	Anticonvulsant
C <> 416	Tab, Blue, Oval, Film Coated	Tiagabine 16 mg	Gabitril by Cephalon	63459-0416	Anticonvulsant
C <> 42	Tab, White to Off White, Oval, Scored	Torsemide 10 mg	Demadex by Aurobindo	65862-0126	Diuretic
C <> 420	Tab, Pink, Oval, Film Coated	Tiagabine 20 mg	Gabitril by Cephalon	63459-0420	Anticonvulsant
C <> 424	Tab, Blue, Film Coated, Cap Shaped	Paroxetine 30 mg	Paxil by Caraco	57664-0424	Antidepressant
C <> 425	Tab, Green, Film Coated, Cap Shaped	Paroxetine 40 mg	Paxil by Caraco	57664-0425	Antidepressant
C <> 43	Tab, White to Off White, Oval, Scored	Torsemide 20 mg	Demadex by Aurobindo	65862-0127	Diuretic
C <> 44	Tab, White to Off White, Cap Shaped, Scored	Torsemide 100 mg	Demadex by Aurobindo	65862-0128	Diuretic
C <> 51	Tab	Atenolol 50 mg, Chlorthalidone 25 mg	Tenoretic by IPR	54921-0115	Antihypertensive; Diuretic
C <> 540	Tab, White, Barrel Shaped	Cetirizine HCl 5 mg	Zyrtec by Caraco	57664-0540	Antihistamine
C <> 541	Tab, White, Barrel Shaped	Cetirizine HCl 10 mg	Zyrtec by Caraco	57664-0541	Antihistamine
C <> 56	Tab, Pink, Cap-Shaped, Film-Coated, Biconvex	Paroxetine 20 mg	Paroxetine by Aurobindo	65862-0155	Antidepressant
C <> 57	Tab, White to Off-White, Round	Amlodipine Besylate 2.5 mg	Norvasc by Aurobindo	65862-0101	Antihypertensive
C <> 58	Tab, White to Off-White, Barrel-Shaped	Amlodipine Besylate 5 mg	Norvasc by Aurobindo	65862-0102	Antihypertensive
C <> 59	Tab, White to Off-White, Round	Amlodipine Besylate 10 mg	Norvasc by Aurobindo	65862-0103	Antihypertensive
C <> 61	Tab, Light Yellowish-Orange, Elliptical, Film Coated	Cefpodoxime Proxetil 100 mg	Vantin by Aurobindo	65862-0095	Antibiotic
C <> 62	Tab, Coral Red, Elliptical, Film Coated	Cefpodoxime Proxetil 200 mg	Vantin by Aurobindo	65862-0096	Antibiotic
C <> 71	Tab, Pink, Oval, Film-Coated	Ondansetron 24 mg	Ondansetron by Aurobindo	65862-0188	Antiemetic
C <> 71	Tab	Atenolol 100 mg, Chlorthalidone 25 mg	Tenoretic by IPR	54921-0117	Antihypertensive; Diuretic
C <> 79	Tab, Yellow, Round	Meloxicam 7.5 mg	Mobic by Aurobindo	65862-0097	NSAID
C <> 80	Tab, Yellow, Oblong	Meloxicam 15 mg	Mobic by Aurobindo	65862-0098	NSAID
C <> 86	Tab, Pink, Round, Film Coated, Scored	Bisoprolol Fumarate 5 mg	Zebeta by Aurobindo	65862-0086	Antihypertensive
C <> 8648	Tab, Layered	Phendimetrazine Tartrate 35 mg	Bontril PDM by Carnrick	00086-0048	Anorexiant; C III
C <> 8650	Tab, Purple, Oblong, Scored	Acetaminophen 325 mg, Butalbital 50 mg	by Thrift Drug	59198-0364	Analgesic
C <> 8650	Tab, Purple, Scored	Acetaminophen 325 mg, Butalbital 50 mg	Promacet by Carnrick	00086-0050	Analgesic
C <> 8656	Tab, Purple, Round, Scored	Acetaminophen 325 mg, Butalbital 50 mg	Promacet by Able	Discontinued	Analgesic
C <> 8662	Tab, Lavender, Round, Scored, 86 over 62	Metaxalone 400 mg	Skelaxin by CVS	51316-0231	Muscle Relaxant
C <> 8662	Tab, Lavender, Round, Scored, 86 over 62	Metaxalone 400 mg	Skelaxin by Amerisource	62584-0033	Muscle Relaxant
C <> 8662	Tab, Lavender, Round, Scored, 86 over 62	Metaxalone 400 mg	Skelaxin by Direct Dispensing	57866-4637	Muscle Relaxant
C <> 8662	Tab, Lavender, Round, Scored, 86 over 62	Metaxalone 400 mg	Skelaxin by Drug Distr	52985-0226	Muscle Relaxant
C <> 8662	Tab, Lavender, Round, Scored, 86 over 62	Metaxalone 400 mg	Skelaxin by Carnrick	00086-0062	Muscle Relaxant
C <> 8662	Tab, Lavender, Round, Scored, 86 over 62	Metaxalone 400 mg	Skelaxin by Thrift Drug	59198-0367	Muscle Relaxant
C <> 8662	Tab, Lavender, Round, Scored, 86 over 62	Metaxalone 400 mg	Skelaxin by Rx Pak	65084-0167	Muscle Relaxant
C <> 8662	Tab, Lavender, Round, Scored, 86 over 62	Metaxalone 400 mg	Skelaxin by H J Harkins Co	52959-0410	Muscle Relaxant
C <> 8662	Tab, Lavender, Round, Scored, 86 over 62	Metaxalone 400 mg	Skelaxin by West-Ward	00143-9029	Muscle Relaxant
C <> 8662	Tab, Lavender, Round, Scored, 86 over 62	Metaxalone 400 mg	Skelaxin by King	60793-0135	Muscle Relaxant
C <> 8673	Tab, White, Oval, Scored	Phenylpropanolamine HCl 75 mg, Guaifenesin 400 mg	by Eckerd	19458-0832	Cold Remedy
C <> 8673	Tab, White with Blue Specks	Guaifenesin 400 mg, Phenylpropanolamine HCl 75 mg	Entex LA by Carnrick	00086-0063	Cold Remedy
C <> 8674	Tab, White, Pentagonal, Scored	Atropine Sulfate 0.025 mg, Difenoxin HCl 1 mg	Motofen by Physician Total Care	54868-3510	Antidiarrheal; C IV
C <> 8674	Tab, White, Pentagonal, Scored	Difenoxin HCl 1 mg, Atropine Sulfate 0.025 mg	Motofen by Carnrick	00086-0074	Antidiarrheal; C IV
C <> 87	Tab, White, Round, Film Coated	Bisoprolol Fumarate 10 mg	Zebeta by Aurobindo	65862-0087	Antihypertensive

ID FRONT <> BACK	DESCRIPTION FRONT <> BACK	INGREDIENT & STRENGTH	BRAND (or Generic Equiv.) by FIRM	NDC#	CLASS; SCH.
C <> 9	Tab, White, Round	Bromocriptine Mesylate 0.8 mg	Cycloset by Veroscience	65862-0078	Antidiabetic
C <> 93	Tab, White to Off White, Cap Shaped, Film Coated	Ciprofloxacin 750 mg	Cipro by Aurobindo	65862-0078	Antibiotic
C <> 94	Tab, White to Off White, Cap Shaped, Film Coated	Ciprofloxacin 500 mg	Cipro by Aurobindo	13107-0077	Antibiotic
C <> 94	Tab, White to Off White, Cap Shaped, Film Coated	Ciprofloxacin 500 mg	Cipro by Aurobindo	65862-0077	Antibiotic
C <> 95	Tab, White to Off White, Round, Film Coated	Ciprofloxacin 250 mg	Cipro by Aurobindo	65862-0076	Antibiotic
C <> 95	Tab, White to Off White, Round, Film Coated	Ciprofloxacin 250 mg	Cipro by Aurobindo	13107-0076	Antibiotic
C <> AMEN	Tab	Medroxyprogesterone Acetate 10 mg	by Eckerd	19458-0831	Hormone
C <> AMIDE001	Tab, Orange, Pink & Purple, Round, Chewable, AMIDE001 <> A, B, C, or D	Ascorbic Acid 60 mg, Cyanocobalamin 4.5 mcg, Folic Acid 0.3 mg, Niacinamide, Pyridoxine HCl 1.05 mg, Riboflavin 1.2 mg, Sodium Fluoride, Thiamine Mononitrate, Vitamin A Acetate, Vitamin D 400 Units, Vitamin E Acetate	Multi Vita Bets by Amide	52152-0001	Vitamin
C <> AMIDE001	Tab, Orange, Pink & Purple, Round, Chewable, AMIDE001 <> A, B, C, or D	Ascorbic Acid 60 mg, Cyanocobalamin 4.5 mcg, Folic Acid 0.3 mg, Niacinamide, Pyridoxine HCl 1.05 mg, Riboflavin 1.2 mg, Sodium Fluoride, Thiamine Mononitrate, Vitamin A Acetate, Vitamin D 400 Units, Vitamin E Acetate	Multi Vita Bets by Qualitest	00603-4712	Vitamin
C <> AMIDE001	Tab, Orange, Pink & Purple, Round, Chewable, AMIDE001 <> A, B, C, or D	Ascorbic Acid 60 mg, Cyanocobalamin 4.5 mcg, Folic Acid 0.3 mg, Niacinamide, Pyridoxine HCl 1.05 mg, Riboflavin 1.2 mg, Sodium Fluoride, Thiamine Mononitrate, Vitamin A Acetate, Vitamin D 400 Units, Vitamin E Acetate	Multi Vita Bets by Major	00904-5275	Vitamin
C <> CLOCK	Tab, White, Round	Quinidine Gluconate SR 324 mg	Quinaglute Duratabs by RX Pak	65084-0132	Antiarrhythmic
C <> CYCRIN	Tab, Peach, Oval, Scored	Medroxyprogesterone Acetate 10 mg	by Southwood	58016-0926	Hormone
C <> CYCRIN	Tab, Purple, Oval, Scored	Medroxyprogesterone Acetate 5 mg	by Kaiser	62224-4334	Hormone
C <> NVR	Tab, White to Yellowish, Round, Marbled	Everolimus 0.25 mg	Zortress by Novartis Consumer Health, Inc.	00078-0417	Immunosuppressant
C <> SCORED	Tab	Conjugated Estrogens 0.625 mg, Medroxyprogesterone Acetate 2.5 mg	Prempro by Pharm Util	60491-0904	Hormone
C01 <> LL	Tab, Tan, Round, Film Coated	Simvastatin 5 mg	Zocor by Lupin	68180-0482	Antihyperlipidemic
C02 <> LL	Tab, Peach, Oval, Film Coated	Simvastatin 10 mg	Zocor by Lupin	68180-0478	Antihyperlipidemic
C03 <> LL	Tab, Tan, Oval, Film Coated	Simvastatin 20 mg	Zocor by Lupin	68180-0479	Antihyperlipidemic
C04 <> LL	Tab, Brick Red, Oval, Film-Coated	Simvastatin 40 mg	Zocor by Lupin	68180-0480	Antihyperlipidemic
C05 <> LL	Tab, Brick Red, Cap Shaped, Film-Coated	Simvastatin 80 mg	Zocor by Lupin	68180-0481	Antihyperlipidemic
C1	Tab, Blue, Round	Bendroflumethiazide 100 mg, Rauwolfia Serpentina 50 mg	Rauzide by Econlab		Diuretic; Antihypertensive
C1	Tab, Pink, Cap Shaped	Choline Magnesium Trisalicylate 1000 mg	Trilisate by Amide	52152-0086	NSAID
C1	Tab, Film Coated	Salicylate 1000 mg	Choline Magnesium Trisalicylate by Rugby	00536-3470	NSAID
C1	Tab, Coated	Bendroflumethiazide 4 mg, Rauwolfia Serpentina 50 mg	Rauzide by Rugby	00536-4502	Antihypertensive; Diuretic
C10	Cap, Black & Green	Chlordiazepoxide 10 mg	Librium by Sandoz		Antianxiety; C IV
C10	Tab, Yellow, Almond Shaped	Tadalafil 10 mg	Cialis by Eli Lilly	Canadian DIN 02248088	Impotence Agent
C10	Tab, Yellow, Almond Shaped	Tadalafil 10 mg	Cialis by Eli Lilly	00002-4463	Impotence Agent
C10 <> NN	Tab, White, Round, Scored, N / N <> C10	Clobazam 10 mg	Frisium by Novopharm	Canadian DIN 02238334	Anticonvulsant
C100	Tab, White, Round, C > 100	Ciprofloxacin HCl 100 mg	Cipro by Abrika		Antibiotic
C100	Tab, White, Round, Scored	Clozapine 100 mg	Clozaril by Apotex	Canadian DIN 02248035	Antipsychotic
C100 <> G	Tab, White, Oval, Scored	Captopril 100 mg	Capoten by Genpharm	Canadian DIN 02163594	Antihypertensive
C1000J	Tab, White, C 1000/J	Sulfadiazine 820 mg, Trimethoprim 180 mg	Coptin by Jouveinal	Canadian	Antibiotic
C1000QD <> BAYER	Tab, White to Yellow, Oblong, Film Coated	Ciprofloxacin HCl 1000 mg	Cipro XL by Bayer	Canadian DIN 02251787	Antibiotic
C1000QD <> BAYER	Tab, White to Yellow, Oblong, Film Coated	Ciprofloxacin HCl 1000 mg	Cipro XR by Bayer	00026-8897	Antibiotic
C100G	Tab, White, Oval, C 100/G	Captopril 100 mg	Capoten by Genpharm	Canadian	Antihypertensive
C101 <> 400	Tab, White, Round, Film Coated	Ibuprofen 400 mg	Motrin by Dr. Reddy's	55111-0101	NSAID

ID FRONT <> BACK	DESCRIPTION FRONT <> BACK	INGREDIENT & STRENGTH	BRAND (or Generic Equiv.) by FIRM	NDC#	CLASS; SCH.
C102 <> 600	Tab, White, Oval	Ibuprofen 600 mg	Motrin by Dr. Reddy's	55111-0102	NSAID
C103	Tab, Blue, Round, Coated, C/103	Salsalate 500 mg	by Duramed	51285-0296	NSAID
C103 <> 800	Tab, White, Oblong, Film Coated	Ibuprofen 800 mg	Motrin by Dr. Reddy's	55111-0103	NSAID
C105	Tab, Blue, Cap Shaped, Coated, C/105	Salsalate 750 mg	by Duramed	51285-0297	NSAID
C108	Tab, Yellow, Round, Film Coated	Ranitidine 150 mg	Zantac by Dr. Reddy's	55111-0420	Gastrointestinal
C11 <> LU	Tab, White, Round, Scored	Perindopril 2 mg	Aceon by Lupin	68180-0235	Antihypertensive
C11 <> M	Tab, Green, Round, Scored	Clozapine 100 mg	Clozaril by Mylan	00378-0860	Antipsychotic
C11 <> M	Tab, Green, Round, Scored	Clozapine 100 mg	Clozaril by UDL	51079-0922	Antipsychotic
C110	Tab, Blue, Round, Scored	Clonazepam 1 mg	Ceberclon by Cebert	64019-0110	Sedative; C IV
C111	Cap, Yellow		Atromid-S by Rosemont		Antihyperlipidemic
C118	Tab, Pink, Round	Famotidine 10 mg	Pepcid by Dr. Reddy's	55111-0118	Gastrointestinal
C119	Tab, Yellow, Round, Film Coated	Famotidine 20 mg	Pepcid by Major	00904-5551	Gastrointestinal
C119	Tab, Yellow, Round, Film Coated	Famotidine 20 mg	Pepcid by Dr. Reddy's	55111-0119	Gastrointestinal
C119	Tab, Yellow, Round, Film Coated	Famotidine 20 mg	Pepcid by Par	49884-0608	Gastrointestinal
C12	Tab, White, Oval, Scored	Citalopram 20 mg	Celexa by Novopharm	Canadian DIN 02293218	Antidepressant
C12 <> LU	Tab, White, Cap Shaped, Scored	Perindopril 4 mg	Aceon by Lupin	68180-0236	Antihypertensive
C12 <> SANKYO	Tab, Yellow, Round, Film Coated	Olmesartan Medoxomil 5 mg	Benicar by Sankyo	65597-0101	Antihypertensive
C120	Tab, Yellow, Round, Film Coated	Famotidine 40 mg	Pepcid by Par	49884-0609	Gastrointestinal
C120	Tab, Yellow, Round, Film Coated	Famotidine 40 mg	Pepcid by Dr. Reddy's	55111-0120	Gastrointestinal
C120	Tab, Yellow, Round, Film Coated	Famotidine 40 mg	Pepcid by Major	00904-5554	Gastrointestinal
C122	Cap, Yellow, C-122	Amantadine HCl 100 mg	Symmetrel by Upsher Smith	00832-1015	Antiviral
C122	Cap, Yellow, Black Print, Soft Gel, C-122	Amantadine HCl 100 mg	Symmetrel by Warner Chilcott	00047-0853	Antiviral
C122	Cap, Yellow, Black Print, Soft Gel, C-122	Amantadine HCl 100 mg	Symmetrel by Rosemont	00832-1015	Antiviral
C122	Cap, Yellow, Black Print, Soft Gel, C-122	Amantadine HCl 100 mg	Symmetrel by URL Mutual	00677-1128	Antiviral
C122	Cap, Yellow, Black Print, Soft Gel, C-122	Amantadine HCl 100 mg	Symmetrel by Duramed	51285-0839	Antiviral
C122	Cap, Yellow, Black Print, Soft Gel, C-122	Amantadine HCl 100 mg	Symmetrel by UDL	51079-0481	Antiviral
C122	Cap, Yellow, Black Print, Soft Gel, C-122	Amantadine HCl 100 mg	Symmetrel by Allscripts	54569-0084	Antiviral
C122	Cap, Yellow, Black Print, Soft Gel, C-122	Amantadine HCl 100 mg	Symmetrel by HJ Harkins Co	52959-0007	Antiviral
C122	Cap, Yellow, Black Print, Soft Gel, C-122	Amantadine HCl 100 mg	Symmetrel by Banner Pharma	10888-3185	Antiviral
C122	Cap, Yellow, Black Print, Soft Gel, C-122	Amantadine HCl 100 mg	Symmetrel by Dixon Shane	17236-0849	Antiviral
C122	Cap, Yellow, Black Print, Soft Gel, C-122	Amantadine HCl 100 mg	Symmetrel by Apotheca	12634-0536	Antiviral
C122	Cap, Yellow, Black Print, Soft Gel, C-122	Amantadine HCl 100 mg	Symmetrel by Direct Dispensing	57866-3090	Antiviral
C125 <> G	Tab, White, Oblong, Scored, G <> C 12.5	Captopril 12.5 mg	Capoten by Genpharm	Canadian DIN 02163551	Antihypertensive
C125SYC	Tab, White, Oblong, C 12.5/Syc	Captopril 12.5 mg	Capoten by AltiMed	Canadian DIN 00851639	Antihypertensive
C13 <> LU	Tab, White, Round, Scored	Perindopril 8 mg	Aceon by Lupin	68180-0237	Antihypertensive
C13 <> M	Tab, Yellow, Round, Scored, C over 13	Clonazepam 0.5 mg	Klonopin by UDL	51079-0881	Sedative; C IV
C13 <> M	Tab, Yellow, Round, Scored, C over 13	Clonazepam 0.5 mg	Klonopin by Mylan	00378-1910	Sedative; C IV
C13 <> M	Tab, Yellow, Round, Scored, C over 13	Clonazepam 0.5 mg	Klonopin by D M Graham	00756-0266	Sedative; C IV
C133	Cap, Yellow, Soft Gel, C-133	Valproic Acid 250 mg	Depakene by Banner Pharma	00832-1007	Anticonvulsant
C133	Cap, Yellow, Soft Gel, C-133	Valproic Acid 250 mg	Depakene by Rosemont		Anticonvulsant
C133	Tab, White, Round	Enalapril Maleate 5 mg, Hydrochlorothiazide 12.5 mg	Vaseretic by Par	49884-0686	Antihypertensive; Diuretic
C133	Tab, White, Round	Enalapril Maleate 5 mg, Hydrochlorothiazide 12.5 mg	Vaseretic by Dr. Reddy's	55111-0133	Antihypertensive; Diuretic
C134	Tab, White, Round	Enalapril Maleate 10 mg, Hydrochlorothiazide 25 mg	Vaseretic by Par	49884-0687	Antihypertensive; Diuretic
C134	Tab, White, Round	Enalapril Maleate 10 mg, Hydrochlorothiazide 25 mg	Vaseretic by Dr. Reddy's	55111-0134	Antihypertensive; Diuretic
C135	Tab, Peach, Round	Norethindrone 1 mg, Ethinyl Estradiol 0.035 mg	Ortho 7/7/7 21 by Janssen-Ortho	Canadian DIN 00602957	Oral Contraceptive

ID FRONT <> BACK	DESCRIPTION FRONT <> BACK	INGREDIENT & STRENGTH	BRAND (or Generic Equiv.) by FIRM	NDC#	CLASS; SCH.
C135	Tab, Peach, Round	Norethindrone 1 mg, Ethinyl Estradiol 0.035 mg	Ortho 7/7/7 28 by Janssen-Ortho	Canadian DIN 00602965	Oral Contraceptive
C135	Tab, Peach, Round	Norethindrone 1 mg, Ethinyl Estradiol 0.035 mg	Ortho 1/35 21 by Janssen-Ortho	Canadian DIN 00372846	Oral Contraceptive
C135	Tab, Peach, Round	Norethindrone 1 mg, Ethinyl Estradiol 0.035 mg	Ortho 1/35 28 by Janssen-Ortho	Canadian DIN 00372838	Oral Contraceptive
C135	Tab, White, Oval	Doxylamine Succinate 25 mg	Unisom by Ivax	00182-1178	Sleep Aid
C135	Tab, White, Oval	Doxylamine Succinate 25 mg	Unisom by Perrigo		Sleep Aid
C14	Tab, Grey, Oval, Scored	Citalopram 40 mg	Celexa by Novopharm	Canadian DIN 02293226	Antidepressant
C14	Tab, White, Round	Olmesartan Medoxomil 20 mg	Olmetec by Schering-Plough	Canadian DIN 02318660	Antihypertensive
C14 <> M	Tab, Light Green, Round, Scored, C over 14	Clonazepam 1 mg	Klonopin by Mylan	00378-1912	Sedative; C IV
C14 <> M	Tab, Light Green, Round, Scored, C over 14	Clonazepam 1 mg	Klonopin by D M Graham	00756-0267	Sedative; C IV
C14 <> M	Tab, Light Green, Round, Scored, C over 14	Clonazepam 1 mg	Klonopin by UDL	51079-0882	Sedative; C IV
C14 <> SANKYO	Tab, White, Round, Film Coated	Olmesartan Medoxomil 20 mg	Benicar by Sankyo	65597-0103	Antihypertensive
C15	Tab, White, Oval	Olmesartan Medoxomil 40 mg	Olmetec by Schering-Plough	Canadian DIN 02318679	Antihypertensive
C15 <> M	Tab, White, Round, Scored, C over 15	Clonazepam 2 mg	Klonopin by Mylan	00378-1914	Sedative; C IV
C15 <> M	Tab, White, Round, Scored, C over 15	Clonazepam 2 mg	Klonopin by D M Graham	00756-0268	Sedative; C IV
C15 <> M	Tab, White, Round, Scored, C over 15	Clonazepam 2 mg	Klonopin by UDL	51079-0883 Discontinued	Sedative; C IV
C15 <> SANKYO	Tab, White, Oval, Film Coated	Olmesartan Medoxomil 40 mg	Benicar by Sankyo	65597-0104	Antihypertensive
C150	Tab, Pink, Round	Ranitidine 150 mg	Zantac by Dr. Reddy's	55111-0404	Gastrointestinal
C151	Tab, White, Round, Scored	Buspirone HCl 5 mg	BuSpar by Ranbaxy	63304-0500	Antianxiety
C152	Tab, White, Round, Scored	Buspirone HCl 10 mg	BuSpar by Ranbaxy	63304-0501	Antianxiety
C16	Tab, Orange, Cap-Shaped, Biconvex, Film-Coated	Cefprozil 250 mg	Cefprozil by Aurobindo	65862-0068	Antibiotic
C162	Cap, Black, Oval, Soft Gel	Vitamin C 100 mg, Folic Acid 1 mg, Niacin 20 mg, Thiamin 1.5 mg, Riboflavin 1.7 mg, Vitamin B6 10 mg, Vitamin B12 6 mg, Pantothenic Acid 5 mg, Biotin 150 mg	Renal Caps by Cypress	60258-0162	Vitamin; Supplement
C17	Tab, White, Cap Shaped, Film Coated	Cefprozil 500 mg	Cefprozil by Aurobindo	65862-0069	Antibiotic
C17 <> M	Tab, White, Round	Bicalutamide 50 mg	Casodex by UDL	51079-0692	Antiandrogen
C177	Tab, Light Blue, Round	Brompheniramine Maleate 12 mg, Phenylpropanolamine HCl 75 mg	Dimetapp by Teva	00093-9177	Cold Remedy
C177	Tab, Light Blue, Round	Brompheniramine Maleate 12 mg, Phenylpropanolamine HCl 75 mg	Dimetapp by Perrigo	00113-0451	Cold Remedy
C180	Tab, White, Round	Norgestimate 0.18 mg, Ethinyl Estradiol 0.035 mg	Tri-Cyclen 21 by Janssen-Ortho	Canadian DIN 02028700	Oral Contraceptive
C180	Tab, White, Round	Norgestimate 0.18 mg, Ethinyl Estradiol 0.035 mg	Tri-Cyclen 28 by Janssen-Ortho	Canadian DIN 02029421	Oral Contraceptive
C19 <> RBX	Tab, White, Oblong	Ciprofloxacin 750 mg	Cipro by Ranbaxy	Canadian DIN 02267950	Antibiotic
C1M	Tab, M to the Right of the Score and C1 to the Left of the Score	Captopril 12.5 mg	Capoten by Heartland	61392-0604	Antihypertensive
C2 <> B	Tab, White, Round, Stylized "b" <> C2	Pramipexole DiHCl 0.125 mg	Mirapex by Barr	00555-0617	Antiparkinson
C20	Tab, Yellow, Almond Shaped	Tadalafil 20 mg	Cialis by Eli Lilly	Canadian DIN 02248089	Impotence Agent
C20	Tab, Yellow, Almond Shaped	Tadalafil 20 mg	Cialis by Eli Lilly	00002-4464	Impotence Agent
C20	Tab, White, Round, Scored	Carbamazepine 200 mg	Tegretol by Novopharm	Canadian DIN 00782718	Anticonvulsant
C20 <> PL	Tab, Mottled Pink, Round	Amoxicillin 200 mg, Clavulanate Potassium 20 mg	Augmentin by Ivax	00172-7401	Antibiotic
C200	Tab, Pink, Round, Scored, 200 inside C	Amiodarone HCl 200 mg	Cordarone by Wyeth Canada	Canadian DIN 02036282	Antiarrhythmic

ID FRONT <> BACK	DESCRIPTION FRONT <> BACK	INGREDIENT & STRENGTH	BRAND (or Generic Equiv.) by FIRM	NDC#	CLASS; SCH.
C200 <> WYETH4188	Tab, Pink, Round, Scored, 200 inside C <> Wyeth over 4188	Amiodarone 200 mg	Cordarone by Wyeth	Canadian	Antiarrhythmic
C200 <> WYETH4188	Tab, Pink, Round, Scored, 200 inside C <> Wyeth over 4188	Amiodarone 200 mg	Cordarone by Wyeth	00008-4188	Antiarrhythmic
C200 <> WYETH4188	Tab, Pink, Round, Scored, 200 inside C <> Wyeth over 4188	Amiodarone 200 mg	Cordarone by Nat Pharmpak	55154-4202	Antiarrhythmic
C200 <> WYETH4188	Tab, Pink, Round, Scored, 200 inside C <> Wyeth over 4188	Amiodarone 200 mg	Cordarone by Med Pro	53978-2092	Antiarrhythmic
C200 <> WYETH4188	Tab, Pink, Round, Scored, 200 inside C <> Wyeth over 4188	Amiodarone 200 mg	Cordarone by Caremark	00339-6082	Antiarrhythmic
C200 <> WYETH4188	Tab, Pink, Round, Scored, 200 inside C <> Wyeth over 4188	Amiodarone 200 mg	Cordarone by Amerisource	62584-0345	Antiarrhythmic
C21	Tab, White, Oval, with Pink Specks	Acetaminophen 500 mg, Hydrocodone Bitartrate 5 mg	Azdone by Schwarz		Analgesic; C III
C21 <> M	Tab, Yellow, Round, C over 21	Citalopram HBr 10 mg	Celexa by Mylan	00378-1921	Antidepressant
C215	Tab, Light Blue, Round	Norgestimate 0.215 mg, Ethinyl Estradiol 0.035 mg	Tri-Cyclen 28 by Janssen-Ortho	Canadian DIN 02029421	Oral Contraceptive
C215	Tab, Light Blue, Round	Norgestimate 0.215 mg, Ethinyl Estradiol 0.035 mg	Tri-Cyclen 21 by Janssen-Ortho	Canadian DIN 02028700	Oral Contraceptive
C22	Tab, Reddish Yellow, Round, Film Coated	Hydrochlorothiazide 12.5 mg, Olmesartan Medoxomil 20 mg	Olmetec Plus by Schering-Plough	Canadian DIN 02319616	Diuretic
C22 <> M	Tab, Yellow, Round, Scored, C over 22	Citalopram HBr 20 mg	Celexa by Mylan	00378-1922	Antidepressant
C22 <> SANKYO	Tab, Reddish-Yellow, Round, Film Coated	Hydrochlorothiazide 12.5 mg, Olmesartan Medoxomil 20 mg	Benicar HCT by Sankyo	65597-0105	Antihypertensive; Diuretic
C229	Tab, Blue, Round	Dexbrompheniramine Maleate 6 mg, Pseudoephedrine Sulfate 120 mg	Drixoral by Granutec		Cold Remedy
C23	Tab, Reddish Yellow, Oval, Film Coated	Hydrochlorothiazide 12.5 mg, Olmesartan Medoxomil 40 mg	Olmetec Plus by Schering-Plough	Canadian DIN 02319624	Diuretic
C23 <> SANKYO	Tab, Reddish-Yellow, Oval, Film Coated	Hydrochlorothiazide 12.5 mg, Olmesartan Medoxomil 40 mg	Benicar HCT by Sankyo	65597-0106	Antihypertensive; Diuretic
C24 <> M	Tab, Yellow, Round, Scored, C over 24	Citalopram HBr 40 mg	Celexa by Mylan	00378-1924	Antidepressant
C25	Cap, Green & White	Chlordiazepoxide 25 mg	Librium by Sandoz		Antianxiety; C IV
C25	Tab, White, Square	Captopril 25 mg	Capoten by Genpharm	Canadian DIN 02163578	Antihypertensive
C25	Tab, Light Yellow, Round, Scored	Clozapine 25 mg	Clozaril by Apotex	Canadian DIN 02248034	Antipsychotic
C25	Tab, Pink, Oval, Film Coated	Hydrochlorothiazide 25 mg, Olmesartan Medoxomil 40 mg	Olmetec Plus by Schering-Plough	Canadian DIN 02319632	Diuretic
C25 <> APO	Tab, White, Oval, Film Coated	Carvedilol 25 mg	Apo Carvedilol by Apotex	Canadian DIN 02247936	Antihypertensive
C25 <> SANKYO	Tab, Pink, Oval, Film Coated	Hydrochlorothiazide 25 mg, Olmesartan Medoxomil 40 mg	Benicar HCT by Sankyo	65597-0107	Antihypertensive; Diuretic
C250	Tab, White, Round, C > 250	Ciprofloxacin HCl 250 mg	Cipro by Abrika		Antibiotic
C250	Tab, Blue, Round	Norgestimate 0.25 mg, Ethinyl Estradiol 0.035 mg	Tri-Cyclen 28 by Janssen-Ortho	Canadian DIN 02029421	Oral Contraceptive
C250	Tab, Blue, Round	Norgestimate 0.25 mg, Ethinyl Estradiol 0.035 mg	Tri-Cyclen 21 by Janssen-Ortho	Canadian DIN 02028700	Oral Contraceptive
C250	Tab, Blue, Round	Norgestimate 0.25 mg, Ethinyl Estradiol 0.035 mg	Cyclen by Janssen-Ortho	Canadian DIN 01968440	Oral Contraceptive
C250 <> APO	Tab, White to Off-White, Oblong	Cefuroxime Axetil 250 mg	Ceftin by Apotex	Canadian DIN 02244393	Antibiotic
C250 <> APO	Tab, White to Off-White, Oblong	Cefuroxime Axetil 250 mg	Ceftin by Apotex	60505-1202	Antibiotic
C250 <> G	Tab, White, Capsule Shaped	Clarithromycin 250 mg	Biaxin by Mylan	00378-8250	Antibiotic
C250 <> G	Tab, White, Capsule Shaped	Clarithromycin 250 mg	Biaxin by UDL	51079-0672	Antibiotic
C250 <> G	Tab, Yellow, Oval, Film Coated	Clarithromycin 250 mg	Biaxin by Genpharm	Canadian DIN 02248856	Antibiotic
C25SYC	Tab, White, Square, C 25/Syc	Captopril 25 mg	Capoten by AltiMed	Canadian DIN 00851833	Antihypertensive
C27	Cap, Clear & Red, C-27	Docusate Sodium 100 mg	Colace by Chase		Laxative
C27	Cap, Orange & Red	Docusate Sodium 100 mg	Colace by Chase		Laxative

ID FRONT <> BACK	DESCRIPTION FRONT <> BACK	INGREDIENT & STRENGTH	BRAND (or Generic Equiv.) by FIRM	NDC#	CLASS; SCH.
C275 <> PF	Tab, Round, White, Scored	Quinidine Polygalacturonate 275 mg	Cardioquin by Purdue	00034-5470 Discontinued	Antiarrhythmic
C29	Cap, Red	Docusate Sodium 250 mg	Colace by Chase		Laxative
C29	Cap, Orange & Red	Docusate Sodium 250 mg	Colace by Chase		Laxative
C29	Cap, Clear & Orange, C-29	Docusate Sodium 250 mg	Colace by Chase		Laxative
C29 <> RBX	Tab, White, Oblong	Ciprofloxacin 500 mg	Cipro by Ranbaxy	Canadian DIN 02267942	Antibiotic
C2C	Cap, Green, Clear, Softgel	Digoxin 0.2 mg	Lanoxicaps by DSM	63552-0274	Cardiac Agent
C2C	Cap, Green, Clear, Softgel	Digoxin 0.2 mg	Lanoxicaps by GSK	53873-0274	Cardiac Agent
C2C	Cap, Green, Clear, Softgel	Digoxin 0.2 mg	Lanoxicaps by GSK	00173-0274	Cardiac Agent
C2C	Cap, Green, Clear, Softgel	Digoxin 0.2 mg	Lanoxicaps by RP Scherer	11014-0749	Cardiac Agent
C3 <> APO	Tab, White, Oval, Film Coated	Carvedilol 3.125 mg	Apo Carvedilol by Apotex	Canadian DIN 02247933	Antihypertensive
C3 <> B	Tab, White, Oval, Scored, Stylized "b" <> C/3	Pramipexole DiHCl 0.25 mg	Mirapex by Barr	00555-0612	Antiparkinson
C31	Tab, Orange, Round	Clonazepam 0.5 mg	Rivotril by Cobalt	Canadian DIN 02270641	Sedative; C IV
C31	Tab, Orange, Round	Clonazepam 0.5 mg	by ICN	Canadian	Sedative; C IV
C31 <> LU	Tab, White, Round	Myambutol 100 mg	Myambutol by Lupin	68180-0280	Antimycobacterial
C31 <> M	Tab, Blue, Round, Film Coated	Carvedilol 3.125 mg	Coreg by UDL	51079-0771	Antihypertensive
C3148	Cap, Yellow	Clofibrate 500 mg	Atromid-S by Chase		Antihyperlipidemic
C32	Tab, Green, Round	Clonazepam 1 mg	by ICN	Canadian	Sedative; C IV
C32	Tab, Green, Round	Clonazepam 1 mg	Rivotril by Cobalt	Canadian DIN 02270668	Sedative; C IV
C32 <> LU	Tab, White, Round	Myambutol 400 mg	Myambutol by Lupin	68180-0281	Antimycobacterial
C32 <> M	Tab, White to Off-White, Round, Film Coated	Carvedilol 6.25 mg	Coreg by UDL	51079-0930	Antihypertensive
C3227	Cap, White, C-3227	Nifedipine 10 mg	Procardia by Chase		Antihypertensive
C33	Tab, White, Round	Clonazepam 2 mg	Rivotril by Cobalt	Canadian DIN 02270676	Sedative; C IV
C33	Tab, White, Round	Clonazepam 2 mg	by ICN	Canadian	Sedative; C IV
C33 <> LL	Tab	Leucovorin Calcium 5 mg	Wellcovorin by Immunex	58406-0624	Antineoplastic
C33 <> M	Tab, White, Round, Film Coated	Carvedilol 12.5 mg	Coreg by UDL	51079-0931	Antihypertensive
C34 <> LL	Tab	Leucovorin Calcium 16.2 mg	Wellcovorin by Immunex	58406-0626	Antineoplastic
C34 <> M	Tab, White, Round, Film Coated	Carvedilol 25 mg	Coreg by UDL	51079-0932	Antihypertensive
C3453	Cap, White, C-3453	Nifedipine 20 mg	Procardia by Chase		Antihypertensive
C350	Tab, White, Round, C-350	Cestemenol-350 (Passiflora incarnate, Abies balsamea L. extracts) 150 mg	Resolve by The Winning Combination		Supplement
C3543	Cap, White, C-3543	Nifedipine 20 mg	Procardia by Chase		Antihypertensive
C36	Cap, Dark Orange and Light Orange, Opaque	Stavudine 30 mg	Zerit by Aurobindo	65862-0046	Antiviral
C360LL	Tab, Orange, Oblong, C/360-LL	Calcium, Vitamin D	Caltrate Jr w/D by Lederle		Vitamin; Mineral
C37	Cap, Dark Orange, Opaque	Stavudine 40 mg	Zerit by Aurobindo	65862-0047	Antiviral
C39	Cap, Red	Docusate Sodium 100 mg, Casanthranol 30 mg	Peri-Colace by Chase		Laxative
C39	Cap, Light Blue Opaque Cap and Light Green Transparent Body	Clindamycin HCl 150 mg	Cleocin by Aurobindo	65862-0185	Antibiotic
C39 <> RBX	Tab, White, Round, Film Coated	Ciprofloxacin 250 mg	Cipro by Ranbaxy	Canadian DIN 02267934	Antibiotic
C4 <> B	Tab, White, Oval, Scored, Stylized "b" <> C/4	Pramipexole DiHCl 0.5 mg	Mirapex by Barr	00555-0613	Antiparkinson
C40	Cap, Light Blue, Opaque	Clindamycin HCl 300 mg	Cleocin by Aurobindo	65862-0186	Antibiotic
C40	Tab, Oval, White, Scored, Film-Coated, Cobalt Logo <> C / 40	Citalopram 40 mg	Celexa by Cobalt	Canadian DIN 02248051	Antidepressant

ID FRONT <> BACK	DESCRIPTION FRONT <> BACK	INGREDIENT & STRENGTH	BRAND (or Generic Equiv.) by FIRM	NDC#	CLASS; SCH.
C40LL	Tab, Brown, Oblong, C/40 LL	Calcium 600 mg, Vitamin D	Caltrate 600 w/D by Lederle	00339-6148	Vitamin; Mineral
C42 <> LL	Tab, Blue, Round, Scored, C over 42	Clonidine HCl 0.1 mg	Catapres by Caremark	00005-3180	Antihypertensive
C42 <> LL	Tab, Blue, Round, Scored, C over 42	Clonidine HCl 0.1 mg	Catapres by Lederle	00005-3180	Antihypertensive
C428	Tab, White	Isosorbide Dinitrate 20 mg	Isordil by GSK	Canadian	Antianginal
C43 <> LL	Tab, Yellow, Round, Scored, C over 43	Clonidine HCl 0.2 mg	Catapres by Lederle	00005-3181	Antihypertensive
C45	Tab, White, Round	Atenolol 50 mg	Tenormin by IPR	Canadian	Antihypertensive
C45LL	Tab, Red, Oblong, C/45 LL	Calcium 600 mg, Iron	Caltrate 600 w/Fe by Lederle		Vitamin; Mineral
C474	Tab, White, Oval, Film-Coated, Scored	Metformin HCl 1000 mg	Glucophage by Caraco	57664-0474	Antidiabetic
C5	Tab, Yellow, Almond Shaped	Tadalafil 5 mg	Cialis by Eli Lilly	00002-4462	Impotence Agent
C5	Tab, Light Blue, Round, Film Coated	Desloratadine 5 mg	Clarinex by Schering	00085-1264	Antihistamine
C5	Tab, White, Cap, Shaped, Scored, C / 5 <> two Cobalt Logos	Cabergoline 0.5 mg	Dostinex by Cobalt	Canadian DIN 02301407	Antiparkinson
C5 <> B	Tab, White, Round, Scored, Stylized "b" <> C/5	Pramipexole DiHCl 1 mg	Mirapex by Barr	00555-0614	Antiparkinson
C50 <> G	Tab, White, Oval, Scored	Captopril 50 mg	Capoten by Genpharm	Canadian DIN 02163586	Antihypertensive
C50 <> NN	Tab, White, Round, Biconvex, Film-Coated	Chlorpromazine 50 mg	Largactil by Novopharm	Canadian DIN 00232807	Antipsychotic; Antiemetic
C500	Cap, Maroon and White, Opaque	Cefadroxil Monohydrate 500 mg	Duricef by Northstar RX	68820-0043	Antibiotic
C500 <> APO	Tab, White to Off-White, Oblong	Cefuroxime Axetil 500 mg	Ceftin by Apotex	Canadian DIN 02244394	Antibiotic
C500 <> APO	Tab, White to Off-White, Oblong	Cefuroxime Axetil 500 mg	Ceftin by Apotex	60505-1201	Antibiotic
C500 <> G	Tab, Pale Yellow, Oval, Film Coated	Clarithromycin 500 mg	Biaxin by Genpharm	Canadian DIN 02248857	Antibiotic
C500 <> G	Tab, White-White, Capsule Shaped	Clarithromycin 500 mg	Biaxin by UDL	51079-0673	Antibiotic
C500 <> G	Tab, White, Capsule Shaped	Clarithromycin 500 mg	Biaxin by Mylan	00378-8500	Antibiotic
C500 <> NOVO	Tab, White, Oblong	Acetaminophen 500 mg	Tylenol by Novopharm	Canadian DIN 00482323	Analgesic
C500J	Tab, White, C 500/J	Sulfadiazine 410 mg, Trimethoprim 90 mg	Coptin by Jouveinal	Canadian	Antibiotic
C500QD <> BAYER	Tab, White to Yellow, Oblong, Film Coated, Ex Release	Ciprofloxacin HCl 500 mg	Cipro XL by Bayer	Canadian DIN 02247916	Antibiotic
C500QD <> BAYER	Tab, White to Yellow, Oblong, Film Coated, Ex Release	Ciprofloxacin HCl 500 mg	Cipro XR by Bayer	00026-8889	Antibiotic
C50G	Tab, White, Oval, C 50/G	Captopril 50 mg	Capoten by Genpharm	Canadian	Antihypertensive
C51	Tab, Orange and White	Olmesartan Medoxomil 20 mg, Amlodipine 5 mg, Hydrochlorothiazide 12.5 mg	Tribenzor by Daiichi Sankyo	65597-0114	Antihypertensive
C52	Tab, White, Round, Scored	Promethazine HCl 25 mg	Phenergan by Global	00115-1041	Antiemetic; Antihistamine
C53	Tab, Light Yellow	Olmesartan Medoxomil 40 mg, Amlodipine 5 mg, Hydrochlorothiazide 12.5 mg	Tribenzor by Daiichi Sankyo	65597-0115	Antihypertensive
C535	Tab, White, Round	Norethindrone 0.5 mg, Ethinyl Estradiol 0.035 mg	Ortho 0.5/35 21 by Janssen-Ortho	Canadian DIN 00317047	Oral Contraceptive
C535	Tab, White, Round	Norethindrone 0.5 mg, Ethinyl Estradiol 0.035 mg	Ortho 0.5/35 28 by Janssen-Ortho	Canadian DIN 00340731	Oral Contraceptive
C535	Tab, White, Round	Norethindrone 0.5 mg, Ethinyl Estradiol 0.035 mg	Ortho 7/7/7 21 by Janssen-Ortho	Canadian DIN 00602957	Oral Contraceptive
C535	Tab, White, Round	Norethindrone 0.5 mg, Ethinyl Estradiol 0.035 mg	Ortho 7/7/7 28 by Janssen-Ortho	Canadian DIN 00602965	Oral Contraceptive
C54	Cap, Blue & Pink	Cefaclor 250 mg	Ceclor by Lederle		Antibiotic.
C54	Tab, Light Yellow	Olmesartan Medoxomil 40 mg, Amlodipine 5 mg, Hydrochlorothiazide 25 mg	Tribenzor by Daiichi Sankyo	65597-0116	Antihypertensive
C55	Tab, Grayish Red	Olmesartan Medoxomil 40 mg, Amlodipine 10 mg, Hydrochlorothiazide 12.5 mg	Tribenzor by Daiichi Sankyo	65597-0117	Antihypertensive
C55	Tab, Yellow, Cap-Shaped, Film-Coated	Paroxetine 10 mg	Paroxetine by Aurobindo	65862-0154	Antidepressant
C57	Tab, Grayish Red	Olmesartan Medoxomil 40 mg, Amlodipine 10 mg, Hydrochlorothiazide 25 mg	Tribenzor by Daiichi Sankyo	65597-0118	Antihypertensive
C58	Cap, Blue & Lavender	Cefaclor 500 mg	Ceclor CD by Lederle		Antibiotic

ID FRONT <> BACK	DESCRIPTION FRONT <> BACK	INGREDIENT & STRENGTH	BRAND (or Generic Equiv.) by FIRM	NDC#	CLASS; SCH.
C582	Cap, Red & White, Black Print, Opaque, Hard Gel	Cefadroxil Monohydrate 500 mg	Duricef by Ranbaxy	63304-0582	Antibiotic
C582	Cap, Red & White, Black Print, Opaque, Hard Gel	Cefadroxil Monohydrate 500 mg	Duricef by Barr	00555-0582	Antibiotic
C6 <> B	Tab, White, Round, Scored, Stylized "b" <> C/6	Pramipexole DiHCl 1.5 mg	Mirapex by Barr	00555-0615	Antiparkinson
C600LL	Tab, White, Oblong, C/600-LL	Calcium 600 mg	Caltrate 600 by Lederle		Vitamin; Mineral
C66 <> SKF	Tab, Yellow-Green, Coated	Prochlorperazine Maleate 8.1 mg	by Allscripts	60346-0860	Antiemetic
C67 <> SKF	Tab, Yellow-Green, Coated	Prochlorperazine Maleate 16.2 mg	by Quality Care		Antiemetic
C6BVP	Tab, Off-White, Round, C6 B/VP	Cefadroxil 100 mg	Cef-Tab by BMS		Antibiotic
C7 <> M	Tab, Peach, Round, Scored	Clozapine 25 mg	Clozaril by UDL	51079-0921	Antipsychotic
C7 <> M	Tab, Peach, Round, Scored	Clozapine 25 mg	Clozaril by Mylan	00378-0825	Antipsychotic
C73	Tab, White	Amlodipine 5 mg, Olmesartan Medoxomil 20 mg	Azor by Daiichi Sankyo	65597-0110	Antihypertensive
C73	Tab, White, Round, Scored, Film Coated	Metoprolol Tartrate 25 mg	Lopressor by Aurobindo	65862-0062	Antihypertensive
C73 <> M	Tab, Green, Round, Scored	Clozapine 200 mg	Clozaril by UDL	51079-0749	Antipsychotic
C735	Tab, Light Peach, Round	Norethindrone 0.75 mg, Ethinyl Estradiol 0.035 mg	Ortho 7/7/7 21 by Janssen-Ortho	Canadian DIN 00602957	Oral Contraceptive
C735	Tab, Light Peach, Round	Norethindrone 0.75 mg, Ethinyl Estradiol 0.035 mg	Ortho 7/7/7 28 by Janssen-Ortho	Canadian DIN 00602965	Oral Contraceptive
C74	Tab, Pink, Round, Scored, Film Coated	Metoprolol Tartrate 50 mg	Lopressor by Aurobindo	65862-0063	Antihypertensive
C74	Tab, Grayish Orange	Amlodipine 10 mg, Olmesartan Medoxomil 20 mg	Azor by Daiichi Sankyo	65597-0111	Antihypertensive
C75	Tab, Cream	Amlodipine 5 mg, Olmesartan Medoxomil 40 mg	Azor by Daiichi Sankyo	65597-0112	Antihypertensive
C75	Tab, Light Blue, Round, Scored, Film Coated	Metoprolol Tartrate 100 mg	Lopressor by Aurobindo	65862-0064	Antihypertensive
C76	Cap, Pink, Hard Gel, Black Ink	Minocycline HCl 50 mg	Minocin by Aurobindo	65862-0209	Antibiotic
C77	Cap, White and Grey, Hard Gel, Black Ink	Minocycline HCl 75 mg	Minocin by Aurobindo	65862-0210	Antibiotic
C77	Tab, Brownish Red	Amlodipine 10 mg, Olmesartan Medoxomil 40 mg	Azor by Daiichi Sankyo	65597-0113	Antihypertensive
C78	Cap, Maroon and Pink, Hard Gel, Black Ink	Minocycline HCl 100 mg	Minocin by Aurobindo	65862-0211	Antibiotic
C84	Tab, Peach, Round	Fosinopril Sodium 10 mg, Hydrochlorothiazide 12.5 mg	Monopril HCT by Aurobindo	65862-0308	Antihypertensive; Diuretic
C85	Tab, Peach, Round	Fosinopril Sodium 20 mg, Hydrochlorothiazide 12.5 mg	Monopril HCT by Aurobindo	65862-0309	Antihypertensive; Diuretic
C86120	Cap, Pink Band	Acetaminophen 325 mg, Dichloralantipyrine 100 mg, Isometheptene Mucate (2:1) 65 mg	Midrin by Carnrick	00086-0120	Analgesic; C IV
C86120	Cap, Purple Band	Acetaminophen 325 mg, Dichloralantipyrine 100 mg, Isometheptene Mucate (2:1) 65 mg	Midrin by Pharmedix	53002-0545	Analgesic; C IV
C86120	Cap, Red, with Pink Band, C/86120	Acetaminophen 325 mg, Chloralantipyrine 100 mg, Isometheptene Mucate (1:1) 65 mg	by Allscripts		Analgesic; C IV
C86204	Tab, Pink, Round	Phenindamine 24 mg, Chlorpheniramine 4 mg, Phenylpropanolamine 50 mg	Nolamine by Carnrick		Cold Remedy
C8631	Tab, White, Round	Theophylline Anhydrous 100 mg	Theo-X by Carnrick	00086-0031	Antiasthmatic
C8633	Tab, White, Oblong	Theophylline Anhydrous 300 mg	Theo-X by Carnrick	00086-0033	Antiasthmatic
C8647	Cap, Clear Yellow	Phendimetrazine Tartrate 105 mg	Bontril by Carnrick	00086-0047	Anorexiant; C III
C8647	Cap	Phendimetrazine Tartrate 105 mg	Bontril by Quality Care	62682-1034	Anorexiant; C III
C8647	Cap	Phendimetrazine Tartrate 105 mg	Bontril Sr by D M Graham	00756-0250	Anorexiant; C III
C8650	Cap, Opaque & Purple	Acetaminophen 650 mg, Butalbital 50 mg	Phrenilin Forte by American Pharm		Analgesic
C8652	Tab, White, Oblong	Phenindamine Tartrate 25 mg	Nolahist by Carnrick		Antihistamine
C8655	Cap, Amethyst & White	Butalbital 50 mg, Acetaminophen 650 mg, Codeine Phosphate 30 mg	Phrenlin #3 by Carnrick		Analgesic; C III
C8656	Cap, Purple	Butalbital 50 mg, Acetaminophen 650 mg	Promacet by Thrift Drug	59198-0365	Analgesic
C8656	Cap	Acetaminophen 650 mg, Butalbital 50 mg	Phrenilin Forte by Carnrick	00086-0056	Analgesic
C8657	Cap	Acetaminophen 500 mg, Hydrocodone Bitartrate 5 mg	Vicodin by Carnrick	00086-0057	Analgesic
C8662	Tab	Metaxalone 400 mg	Skelaxin by Pharmedix	53002-0459	Muscle Relaxant
C8666	Tab, Peach, Round	Acetaminophen 650 mg, Chlorpheniramine 4 mg, Phenylpropanolamine HCl 25 mg	Sinulin by Carnrick		Cold Remedy
C8671	Tab, White, Round	Salsalate 500 mg	Salflex by Carnrick	00086-0071	NSAID
C8672	Tab, White, Oval	Salsalate 750 mg	Salflex by Carnrick	00086-0072	NSAID

ID FRONT <> BACK	DESCRIPTION FRONT <> BACK	INGREDIENT & STRENGTH	BRAND (or Generic Equiv.) by FIRM	NDC#	CLASS; SCH.
C90	Tab, White, Round	Atenolol 100 mg	Tenormin by IPR	Canadian	Antihypertensive
C9BZYLOPRIM	Tab, Peach, Round, C9B/Zyloprim	Allopurinol 300 mg	Zyloprim by GSK	Canadian DIN 02248050	Antigout
CA	Tab, Oval, White, Scored, Film-Coated, Cobalt Logo <> C / A	Citalopram 20 mg	Celexa by Cobalt	Canadian DIN 00176095	Antidepressant
CAFERGOT	Tab, White, Black Print, Round, Film Coated	Caffeine 100 mg, Ergotamine Tartrate 1 mg	by Novartis	00078-0349	Antimigraine
CAFERGOT	Tab, White, Black Print, Round, Film Coated	Caffeine 100 mg, Ergotamine Tartrate 1 mg	Cafergot by Novartis	00339-5410	Antimigraine
CAFFEINEGPI30	Cap, Pink & White	Caffeine 200 mg	by Caremark	10956-0661	Stimulant
CAFFEINEGPI30	Cap, Pink & White, Bullet Shaped, Caffeine/GPI 30	Caffeine 200 mg	Keep Alert by Reese	00025-1771	Stimulant
CALAN <> 40	Tab, Pink, Round, Coated	Verapamil HCl 40 mg	Calan by Searle	62584-0852	Antihypertensive
CALAN <> 80	Tab, Light Peach, Oval, Scored	Verapamil HCl 80 mg	Calan by Amerisource	59198-0015	Antihypertensive
CALAN <> 80	Tab, Light Peach, Oval, Scored	Verapamil HCl 80 mg	Calan by Thrift Drug	55154-3603	Antihypertensive
CALAN <> 80	Tab, Light Peach, Oval, Scored	Verapamil HCl 80 mg	Calan by Nat Pharmpak	00025-1851	Antihypertensive
CALAN <> 80	Tab, Light Peach, Oval, Scored	Verapamil HCl 80 mg	Calan by Searle	65240-0619	Antihypertensive
CALAN <> 80	Tab, Light Peach, Oval, Scored	Verapamil HCl 80 mg	Calan by Rightpak	53978-3398	Antihypertensive
CALAN <> 80	Tab, Light Peach, Oval, Scored	Verapamil HCl 80 mg	Calan by Med Pro	00025-1901	Antihypertensive
CALAN <> SR120	Tab, Light Violet, Oval, Film Coated	Verapamil HCl 120 mg	Calan SR by Searle	55154-3616	Antihypertensive
CALAN <> SR180	Tab, Light Pink, Oval, Scored, Film Coated	Verapamil HCl 180 mg	Calan SR by Nat Pharmpak	00025-1911	Antihypertensive
CALAN <> SR180	Tab, Light Pink, Oval, Scored, Film Coated	Verapamil HCl 180 mg	Calan SR by Searle	65084-0141	Antihypertensive
CALAN <> SR240	Tab, Light Green, Oblong, Scored, Film Coated	Verapamil HCl 240 mg	Calan SR by Rx Pak	00014-1891	Antihypertensive
CALAN <> SR240	Tab, Light Green, Oblong, Scored, Film Coated	Verapamil HCl 240 mg	Calan SR by Searle	55154-3615	Antihypertensive
CALAN <> SR240	Tab, Light Green, Oblong, Scored, Film Coated	Verapamil HCl 240 mg	Calan SR by Nat Pharmpak	00480-0788	Antihypertensive
CALAN <> SR240	Tab, Light Green, Oblong, Scored, Film Coated	Verapamil HCl 240 mg	Calan SR by Teva	00025-1891	Antihypertensive
CALAN <> SR240	Tab, Light Green, Oblong, Scored, Film Coated	Verapamil HCl 240 mg	Calan SR by Searle	53978-0588	Antihypertensive
CALAN <> SR240	Tab, Light Green, Oblong, Scored, Film Coated	Verapamil HCl 240 mg	Calan SR by Med Pro	00025-1861	Antihypertensive
CALAN120	Tab, Reddish Brown, Oval, Scored, Film Coated, Calan over 120	Verapamil HCl 120 mg	Calan by Searle		Antihypertensive
CALAN120	Tab, Reddish Brown, Oval, Scored, Film Coated, Calan over 120	Verapamil HCl 120 mg	Calan by Amerisource	62584-0861	Antihypertensive
CALCET <> MPC	Tab, Yellow, Rectangular, Film Coated	Vitamin D 200 IU, Calcium 300 mg	Calcet by Mission	00178-0251	Vitamin; Supplement
CALCICHEW <> RD05	Tab, White, Round, Scored, CALCI-CHEW, Chewable	Calcium Carbonate 1250 mg	Calci-Chew Cherry by Watson	54391-0025	Vitamin; Mineral
CALCICHEW <> RD35	Tab, White, Round, CALCI-CHEW, Chewable	Calcium Carbonate 1250 mg	Calci-Chew Orange by Watson	54391-0325	Vitamin; Mineral
CALTRATE <> 600P	Tab, Pink, Oblong, Scored	Vitamin D 200 IU, Calcium 600 mg, Magnesium 40 mg, Zinc 7.5 mg, Copper 1 mg, Manganese 1.8 mg, Boron 250 mcg	Caltrate 600 Plus by Wyeth	00005-5556	Vitamin; Supplement
CANESORAL	Cap, White, Hard Gel, Pink Ink	Fluconazole 150 mg	CanesOral by Bayer	Canadian DIN 02311690	Antifungal
CAP	Tab, Red, Octagonal, Film Coated, CAP and Star Logo	Guaifenesin 600 mg, Phenylephrine HCl 40 mg, Dextromethorphan HBr 60 mg	Certuss-D by Capellon	64543-0175	Cold Remedy
CAPOTEN <> 125	Tab, White, Cap Shaped, Capoten <> 12.5	Captopril 12.5 mg	Capoten by BMS	Canadian DIN 00695661	Antihypertensive
CAPOTEN <> 125	Tab, White, Cap Shaped, Capoten <> 12.5	Captopril 12.5 mg	Capoten by Par	49884-0793	Antihypertensive
CAPOTEN <> 125	Tab, White, Cap Shaped, Capoten <> 12.5	Captopril 12.5 mg	Capoten by Med Pro	53978-0939	Antihypertensive
CAPOTEN <> 125	Tab, White, Cap Shaped, Capoten <> 12.5	Captopril 12.5 mg	Capoten by Par	00003-0450	Antihypertensive
CAPOTEN <> 125	Tab, White, Cap Shaped, Capoten <> 12.5	Captopril 12.5 mg	Capoten by Nat Pharmpak	55154-3706	Antihypertensive
CAPOTEN100	Tab, White, Oval, Scored, Capoten over 100	Captopril 100 mg	Capoten by BMS	Canadian DIN 00546305	Antihypertensive
CAPOTEN100	Tab, White, Oval, Scored, Capoten over 100	Captopril 100 mg	Capoten by Par	00003-0485	Antihypertensive
CAPOTEN100	Tab, White, Oval, Scored, Capoten over 100	Captopril 100 mg	Capoten by Par	49884-0796	Antihypertensive
CAPOTEN25	Tab, White, Square, Scored, Capoten over 25	Captopril 25 mg	Capoten by Par	49884-0794	Antihypertensive
CAPOTEN25	Tab, White, Square, Scored, Capoten over 25	Captopril 25 mg	Capoten by Med Pro	53978-0236	Antihypertensive

ID FRONT <> BACK	DESCRIPTION FRONT <> BACK	INGREDIENT & STRENGTH	BRAND (or Generic Equiv.) by FIRM	NDC#	CLASS; SCH.
CAPOTEN25	Tab, White, Square, Scored, Capoten over 25	Captopril 25 mg	Capoten by Nat Pharmpak	55154-3707	Antihypertensive
CAPOTEN25	Tab, White, Square, Scored, Capoten over 25	Captopril 25 mg	Capoten by BMS	Canadian DIN 00546283	Antihypertensive
CAPOTEN25	Tab, White, Square, Scored, Capoten over 25	Captopril 25 mg	Capoten by Par	00003-0452	Antihypertensive
CAPOTEN50	Tab, White, Oval, Scored, Capoten over 50	Captopril 50 mg	Capoten by Nat Pharmpak	55154-3708	Antihypertensive
CAPOTEN50	Tab, White, Oval, Scored, Capoten over 50	Captopril 50 mg	Capoten by BMS	Canadian DIN 00546291	Antihypertensive
CAPOTEN50	Tab, White, Oval, Scored, Capoten over 50	Captopril 50 mg	Capoten by Par	00003-0482	Antihypertensive
CAPOTEN50	Tab, White, Oval, Scored, Capoten over 50	Captopril 50 mg	Capoten by Par	49884-0795	Antihypertensive
CAPOZIDE2515	Tab, White to Off-White w/ Orange Specks, Capozide over 25/15	Captopril 25 mg, HCTZ 15 mg	Capozide by Par	49884-0815	Antihypertensive; Diuretic
CAPOZIDE2515	Tab, White to Off-White w/ Orange Specks, Capozide over 25/15	Captopril 25 mg, HCTZ 15 mg	Capozide by BMS	00003-0338	Antihypertensive; Diuretic
CAPOZIDE2525	Tab, Mottled, Capozide over 25/25	Captopril 25 mg, HCTZ 25 mg	Capozide by BMS	00003-0349	Antihypertensive; Diuretic
CAPOZIDE2525	Tab, Peach, Capozide over 25/25	Captopril 25 mg, HCTZ 25 mg	Capozide by Par	49884-0816	Antihypertensive; Diuretic
CAPOZIDE5015	Tab, White, Orange Mottling, Capozide over 50/15	Captopril 50 mg, HCTZ 15 mg	Capozide by Par	49884-0817	Antihypertensive; Diuretic
CAPOZIDE5015	Tab, White to Off-White, Capozide over 50/15	Captopril 50 mg, HCTZ 15 mg	Capozide by BMS	00003-0384	Antihypertensive; Diuretic
CAPOZIDE5025	Tab, Mottled White, Capozide over 50/25	Captopril 50 mg, HCTZ 25 mg	Capozide by BMS	00003-0390	Antihypertensive; Diuretic
CAPOZIDE5025	Tab, Peach, Capozide over 25/25	Captopril 50 mg, HCTZ 25 mg	Capozide by Par	49884-0818	Antihypertensive; Diuretic
CAPTOPRIL100 <> PP	Tab, White, Oval	Captopril 100 mg	Capoten by Pharmascience	Canadian DIN 02230206	Antihypertensive
CAPTOPRIL25	Tab, White, Square, Scored	Captopril 25 mg	Capoten by Pharmascience	Canadian DIN 02230204	Antihypertensive
CAPTOPRIL50 <> PP	Tab, White, Oval, Scored	Captopril 50 mg	Capoten by Pharmascience	Canadian DIN 02230205	Antihypertensive
CARACO <> 105105	Tab, Film Coated, Caraco <> 105/105	Salsalate 750 mg	by Allscripts		NSAID
CARACO <> 152	Tab	Guaifenesin 600 mg	Robitussin by Caraco	57664-0152	Expectorant
CARACO <> 152	Tab, Green, Oblong, Scored	Guaifenesin LA 600 mg	by Med Pro	53978-3361	Expectorant
CARACO <> 157	Tab	Guaifenesin 400 mg, Phenylpropanolamine HCl 75 mg	Entex LA by Caraco	57664-0157	Cold Remedy
CARACO <> 222	Tab, Mottled Yellow, Cap Shaped, Scored	Guaifenesin 600 mg, Pseudoephedrine HCl 120 mg	Miraphen by Caraco	57664-0222	Cold Remedy
CARACO166	Tab, White, Oblong	Metoprolol Tartrate 50 mg	Lopressor by Major	00904-7946	Antihypertensive
CARACO166	Tab, White, Oblong	Metoprolol Tartrate 50 mg	Lopressor by Caraco		Antihypertensive
CARACO167	Tab, White, Oblong	Metoprolol Tartrate 100 mg	Lopressor by Caraco		Antihypertensive
CARACO167	Tab, White, Oblong	Metoprolol Tartrate 100 mg	Lopressor by Major	00904-7947	Antihypertensive
CARACO199	Tab, White, Round	Yohimbine HCl 5.4 mg	Yocon by Caraco		Impotence Agent
CARACO872	Cap	Nifedipine 10 mg	by Qualitest	00603-4759	Antihypertensive
CARACO872	Cap, RP Scherer Logo 872	Nifedipine 10 mg	by Caraco		Antihypertensive
CARACO872	Cap, Caraco/872	Nifedipine 10 mg	by RP Scherer	11014-0956	Antihypertensive
CARACO873	Cap	Nifedipine 20 mg	by Qualitest	00603-4760	Antihypertensive
CARACO873	Cap, Reddish Brown	Nifedipine 20 mg	by RP Scherer	11014-0966	Antihypertensive
CARAFATE <> 1712	Tab, Light Pink, Oblong, Scored	Sucralfate 1 g	Carafate by Murfreesboro	51129-1166	Gastrointestinal
CARAFATE <> 1712	Tab, Light Pink, Oblong, Scored	Sucralfate 1 g	Carafate by Aventis	00088-1712	Gastrointestinal
CARAFATE <> 1712	Tab, Light Pink, Oblong, Scored	Sucralfate 1 g	Carafate by Med Pro	53978-0305	Gastrointestinal
CARAFATE <> 1712	Tab, Light Pink, Oblong, Scored	Sucralfate 1 g	Carafate by H J Harkins Co	52959-0052	Gastrointestinal
CARAFATE <> 1712	Tab, Light Pink, Oblong, Scored	Sucralfate 1 g	Carafate by Heartland	61392-0606	Gastrointestinal
CARAFATE <> 1712	Tab, Light Pink, Oblong, Scored	Sucralfate 1 g	Carafate by Nat Pharmpak	55154-2207	Gastrointestinal
CARAFATE <> 1712	Tab, Light Pink, Oblong, Scored	Sucralfate 1 g	Carafate by Amerisource	62584-0712	Gastrointestinal
CARAFATE <> 1712	Tab, Light Pink, Oblong, Scored	Sucralfate 1 g	Carafate by Giant Food	11146-0041	Gastrointestinal
CARBEX	Tab, Coated	Selegiline 5 mg	Carbex by BMS	00056-0408	Antiparkinson

ID FRONT <> BACK	DESCRIPTION FRONT <> BACK	INGREDIENT & STRENGTH	BRAND (or Generic Equiv.) by FIRM	NDC#	CLASS; SCH.
CARBEX	Tab, White, Oval	Selegiline 5 mg	Carbex by Endo	63481-0408	Antiparkinson
CARDENE20MGROCHE	Cap, White w/ Blue Band, Opaque, Hard Gel	Nicardipine HCl 20 mg	Cardene by Repack Co of America	55306-2437	Antihypertensive
CARDENE20MGROCHE	Cap, White w/ Blue Band, Opaque, Hard Gel	Nicardipine HCl 20 mg	Cardene by Murfreesboro	51129-1125	Antihypertensive
CARDENE20MGROCHE	Cap, White w/ Blue Band, Opaque, Hard Gel	Nicardipine HCl 20 mg	Cardene by Hoffmann La Roche	00004-0183	Antihypertensive
CARDENE20MGROCHE	Cap, White w/ Blue Band, Opaque, Hard Gel	Nicardipine HCl 20 mg	Cardene by Syntex	18393-0437	Antihypertensive
CARDENE20MG-SYNTEX2437	Cap, White, Pink Print, Blue Band, Cardene 20 mg over Syntex 2437	Nicardipine HCl 20 mg	Cardene by Roche	Canadian Discontinued	Antihypertensive
CARDENE30MGROCHE	Cap, Blue, Opaque, Hard Gel	Nicardipine HCl 30 mg	Cardene by Syntex	18393-0438	Antihypertensive
CARDENE30MGROCHE	Cap, Blue, Opaque, Hard Gel	Nicardipine HCl 30 mg	Cardene by Repack Co of America	55306-2438	Antihypertensive
CARDENE30MGROCHE	Cap, Blue, Opaque, Hard Gel	Nicardipine HCl 30 mg	Cardene by Valeant Puerto Rico	64158-0437	Antihypertensive
CARDENE30MGROCHE	Cap, Blue, Opaque, Hard Gel	Nicardipine HCl 30 mg	Cardene by Hoffmann La Roche	00004-0184	Antihypertensive
CARDENE30MGROCHE	Cap, Blue, Opaque, Hard Gel	Nicardipine HCl 30 mg	Cardene by Murfreesboro	51129-1206	Antihypertensive
CARDENE30MG-SYNTEX2438	Cap, Light Blue & Dark Blue, Cardene 30 mg over Sytnex 2438	Nicardipine HCl 30 mg	Cardene by Roche	Canadian Discontinued	Antihypertensive
CARDENE30MG-SYNTEX2438	Cap, Blue & Opaque	Nicardipine HCl 30 mg	Cardene by Par	49884-0579	Antihypertensive
CARDENESR30M-GROCHE	Cap, Pink, Opaque, Hard Gel	Nicardipine HCl 30 mg	Cardene SR by Physician Total Care	54868-3817	Antihypertensive
CARDENESR30M-GROCHE	Cap, Pink, Opaque, Hard Gel	Nicardipine HCl 30 mg	Cardene SR by Hoffmann La Roche	00004-0180	Antihypertensive
CARDENESR45M-GROCHE	Cap, Blue, Opaque, Hard Gel	Nicardipine HCl 45 mg	Cardene SR by Hoffmann La Roche	00004-0181	Antihypertensive
CARDENESR60M-GROCHE	Cap, Light Blue & White, Opaque, Hard Gel	Nicardipine HCl 60 mg	Cardene SR by Hoffmann La Roche	00004-0182	Antihypertensive
CARDIZEMCD120MG	Cap, Light Blue, Blue Print, cardizem CD over 120 mg	Diltiazem HCl 120 mg	Cardizem CD by Wyeth	00008-1795	Antihypertensive
CARDIZEMCD120MG	Cap, Light Blue, SR	Diltiazem HCl 120 mg	Cardizem CD by Biovail Corp.	64455-0795	Antihypertensive
CARDIZEMCD120MG	Cap, Light Blue, SR	Diltiazem HCl 120 mg	Cardizem CD by Biovail Corp.	Canadian DIN 02271605	Antihypertensive
CARDIZEMCD120MG	Cap, Light Blue, Blue Print, cardizem CD over 120 mg	Diltiazem HCl 120 mg	Cardizem CD by Nat Pharmpak	55154-2212	Antihypertensive
CARDIZEMCD120MG	Cap, Light Blue, Blue Print, cardizem CD over 120 mg	Diltiazem HCl 120 mg	Cardizem CD by Elan Hold	60274-0100	Antihypertensive
CARDIZEMCD120MG	Cap, Light Blue, Blue Print, cardizem CD over 120 mg	Diltiazem HCl 120 mg	Cardizem CD by Elan	56125-0065	Antihypertensive
CARDIZEMCD120MG	Cap, Light Blue, Blue Print, cardizem CD over 120 mg	Diltiazem HCl 120 mg	Cardizem CD by Aventis	Canadian	Antihypertensive
CARDIZEMCD180MG	Cap, Dark Blue & Light Blue, Blue Print, cardizem CD over 180 mg	Diltiazem HCl 180 mg	Cardizem CD by Allscripts		Antihypertensive
CARDIZEMCD180MG	Cap, Dark Blue & Light Blue, Blue Print, cardizem CD over 180 mg	Diltiazem HCl 180 mg	Cardizem CD by Nat Pharmpak	55154-2208	Antihypertensive
CARDIZEMCD180MG	Cap, Dark Blue & Light Blue, Blue Print, cardizem CD over 180 mg	Diltiazem HCl 180 mg	Cardizem CD by Egis	48581-5112	Antihypertensive
CARDIZEMCD180MG	Cap, Dark Blue & Light Blue, Blue Print, cardizem CD over 180 mg	Diltiazem HCl 180 mg	Cardizem CD by Rightpak	65240-0607	Antihypertensive
CARDIZEMCD180MG	Cap, Dark Blue & Light Blue, Blue Print, cardizem CD over 180 mg	Diltiazem HCl 180 mg	Cardizem CD by Rx Pak	65084-0114	Antihypertensive
CARDIZEMCD180MG	Cap, Dark Blue & Light Blue, Blue Print, cardizem CD over 180 mg	Diltiazem HCl 180 mg	Cardizem CD by Wal Mart	49035-0187	Antihypertensive
CARDIZEMCD180MG	Cap, Dark Blue & Light Blue, Blue Print, cardizem CD over 180 mg	Diltiazem HCl 180 mg	Cardizem CD by Elan Hold	60274-0200	Antihypertensive
CARDIZEMCD180MG	Cap, Dark Blue & Light Blue, Blue Print, cardizem CD over 180 mg	Diltiazem HCl 180 mg	Cardizem CD by Pharm Util	60491-0120	Antihypertensive
CARDIZEMCD180MG	Cap, Dark Blue & Light Blue, Blue Print, cardizem CD over 180 mg	Diltiazem HCl 180 mg	Cardizem CD by Amerisource	62584-0796	Antihypertensive

ID FRONT <> BACK	DESCRIPTION FRONT <> BACK	INGREDIENT & STRENGTH	BRAND (or Generic Equiv.) by FIRM	NDC#	CLASS; SCH.
CARDIZEMCD180MG	Cap, Dark Blue & Light Blue, Blue Print, cardizem CD over 180 mg	Diltiazem HCl 180 mg	Cardizem CD by Eckerd	19458-0899	Antihypertensive
CARDIZEMCD180MG	Cap, Blue, Light Blue, SR	Diltiazem HCl 180 mg	Cardizem CD by Biovail Corp.	Canadian DIN 02271613	Antihypertensive
CARDIZEMCD180MG	Cap, Blue, Light Blue, SR	Diltiazem HCl 180 mg	Cardizem CD by Biovail Corp.	64455-0796	Antihypertensive
CARDIZEMCD240MG	Cap, Blue, White Print, cardizem CD over 240 mg	Diltiazem HCl 240 mg	Cardizem CD by Biovail Corp.	64455-0797	Antihypertensive
CARDIZEMCD240MG	Cap, Blue, White Print, cardizem CD over 240 mg	Diltiazem HCl 240 mg	Cardizem CD by Biovail Corp.	Canadian DIN 02271621	Antihypertensive
CARDIZEMCD240MG	Cap, Blue, White Print, cardizem CD over 240 mg	Diltiazem HCl 240 mg	Cardizem CD by Elan Hold	60274-0300	Antihypertensive
CARDIZEMCD240MG	Cap, Blue, White Print, cardizem CD over 240 mg	Diltiazem HCl 240 mg	Cardizem CD by Nat Pharmpak	55154-2210	Antihypertensive
CARDIZEMCD240MG	Cap, Blue, White Print, cardizem CD over 240 mg	Diltiazem HCl 240 mg	Cardizem CD by Allscripts		Antihypertensive
CARDIZEMCD240MG	Cap, Blue, White Print, cardizem CD over 240 mg	Diltiazem HCl 240 mg	Cardizem CD by Med Pro	53978-3062	Antihypertensive
CARDIZEMCD300MG	Cap, Blue & Gray, White Print, cardizem CD over 300 mg	Diltiazem HCl 300 mg	Cardizem CD by Nat Pharmpak	55154-2211	Antihypertensive
CARDIZEMCD300MG	Cap, Blue & Gray, White Print, cardizem CD over 300 mg	Diltiazem HCl 300 mg	Cardizem CD by Murfreesboro	51129-9732	Antihypertensive
CARDIZEMCD300MG	Cap, Blue & Gray, White Print, cardizem CD over 300 mg	Diltiazem HCl 300 mg	Cardizem CD by Eckerd	19458-0895	Antihypertensive
CARDIZEMCD300MG	Cap, Blue, Light Gray, SR	Diltiazem HCl 300 mg	Cardizem CD by Biovail Corp.	Canadian DIN 02271648	Antihypertensive
CARDIZEMCD300MG	Cap, Blue, Light Gray, SR	Diltiazem HCl 300 mg	Cardizem CD by Biovail Corp.	64455-0798	Antihypertensive
CARDIZEMCD360MG	Cap, Light Blue, White, SR	Diltiazem HCl 360 mg	Cardizem CD by Biovail Corp.	64455-0799	Antihypertensive
CARDIZEMSR120MG	Cap, Brown, cardizem SR over 120 mg	Diltiazem HCl 120 mg	Cardizem SR by Egis	48581-5111	Antihypertensive
CARDIZEMSR180MG	Cap, Blue & Turquoise	Diltiazem HCl 180 mg	Cardizem SR by Aventis	Canadian	Antihypertensive
CARDIZEMSR240MG	Cap, Light Blue	Diltiazem HCl 240 mg	Cardizem SR by Aventis	Canadian	Antihypertensive
CARDIZEMSR300MG	Cap, Light Blue & Light Gray	Diltiazem HCl 300 mg	Cardizem SR by Aventis	Canadian	Antihypertensive
CARDIZEMSR60MG	Cap, Brown & Ivory, cardizem SR over 60 mg	Diltiazem HCl 60 mg	Cardizem SR by Eckerd	19458-0905	Antihypertensive
CARDIZEMSR60MG	Cap, Brown & Ivory, cardizem SR over 60 mg	Diltiazem HCl 60 mg	Cardizem SR by Elan	56125-0006	Antihypertensive
CARDIZEMSR90MG	Cap, Brown & Gold, cardizem SR over 90 mg	Diltiazem HCl 90 mg	Cardizem SR by Elan	56125-0006	Antihypertensive
CARDIZEMSR90MG	Cap, Brown & Gold, cardizem SR over 90 mg	Diltiazem HCl 90 mg	Cardizem SR by Allscripts		Antihypertensive
CARDIZEMSR90MG	Cap, Brown & Gold, cardizem SR over 90 mg	Diltiazem HCl 90 mg	Cardizem SR by Eckerd	19458-0906	Antihypertensive
CARDIZEMSR90MG	Cap, Brown & Gold, cardizem SR over 90 mg	Diltiazem HCl 90 mg	Cardizem SR by Aventis	Canadian	Antihypertensive
CARDURA <> 1MG	Tab, White, Oblong, Scored	Doxazosin Mesylate 1 mg	Cardura by Roerig	00049-2750	Antihypertensive
CARDURA <> 2MG	Tab, Yellow, Oblong, Scored	Doxazosin Mesylate 2 mg	Cardura by H J Harkins Co	52959-0003	Antihypertensive
CARDURA <> 2MG	Tab, Yellow, Oblong, Scored	Doxazosin Mesylate 2 mg	Cardura by Roerig	00049-2760	Antihypertensive
CARDURA <> 4MG	Tab, Orange, Oblong, Scored	Doxazosin Mesylate 4 mg	Cardura by Nat Pharmpak	55154-3216	Antihypertensive
CARDURA <> 4MG	Tab, Orange, Oblong, Scored	Doxazosin Mesylate 4 mg	Cardura by Roerig	00049-2770	Antihypertensive
CARDURA <> 8MG	Tab, Green, Oblong, Scored	Doxazosin Mesylate 8 mg	Cardura by Pharm Util	60491-0123	Antihypertensive
CARDURA <> 8MG	Tab, Green, Oblong, Scored	Doxazosin Mesylate 8 mg	Cardura by Roerig	00049-2780	Antihypertensive
CARDURA1 <> ASTRA	Tab, White, Round, Cardura 1/Astra	Doxazosin Mesylate 1 mg	Cardura by AstraZeneca	Canadian DIN 01958100	Antihypertensive
CARDURA2 <> ASTRA	Tab, White, Oval, Cardura 2/Astra	Doxazosin Mesylate 2 mg	Cardura by AstraZeneca	Canadian DIN 01958097	Antihypertensive
CARDURA2MG	Tab	Doxazosin Mesylate 2 mg	Cardura by Med Pro	53978-3071	Antihypertensive
CARDURA4 <> ASTRA	Tab, White, Diamond, Cardura 4/Astra	Doxazosin Mesylate 4 mg	Cardura by AstraZeneca	Canadian DIN 01958100	Antihypertensive
CARDURA4 <> ASTRA	Tab, White	Doxazosin Mesylate 4 mg	Cardura by AstraZeneca	Canadian DIN 01958119	Antihypertensive
CARNITORST	Tab, White	Levocarnitine 330 mg	Carnitor by Sigma Tau	54482-0144	Supplement
CARRX	Tab, Orange, Oval, Coated, CAR / RX	Folic Acid 2 mg, Vitamin B-12 500 mcg, Vitamin B-6 50 mg, L-Arginine HCl 500 mg	Cardiotek-RX by Stewart Jackson	45985-0651	Vitamin
CATAFLAM <> 50	Tab, Light Brown, Round, Sugar Coated	Diclofenac Potassium 50 mg	Cataflam by Novartis	00078-0436	NSAID

ID FRONT <> BACK	DESCRIPTION FRONT <> BACK	INGREDIENT & STRENGTH	BRAND (or Generic Equiv.) by FIRM	NDC#	CLASS; SCH.
CATAFLAM <> 50	Tab, Light Brown, Round, Sugar Coated	Diclofenac Potassium 50 mg	Cataflam by Direct Dispensing	57866-1182	NSAID
CATAFLAM <> 50	Tab, Light Brown, Round, Sugar Coated	Diclofenac Potassium 50 mg	Cataflam by H J Harkins Co	52959-0344	NSAID
CATAFLAM <> 50	Tab, Light Brown, Round, Sugar Coated	Diclofenac Potassium 50 mg	Cataflam by PDRX	55289-0818	NSAID
CATAFLAM <> 50	Tab, Light Brown, Round, Sugar Coated	Diclofenac Potassium 50 mg	Cataflam by Novartis	00028-0151	NSAID
CATAFLAM <> 50	Tab, Light Brown, Round, Sugar Coated	Diclofenac Potassium 50 mg	Cataflam by Novartis	17088-0151	NSAID
CATAFLAM <> 50	Tab, Light Brown, Round, Sugar Coated	Diclofenac Potassium 50 mg	Cataflam by DRX	55045-2225	NSAID
CATAFLAM <> 50	Tab, Light Brown, Round, Sugar Coated	Diclofenac Potassium 50 mg	Cataflam by Allscripts		NSAID
CB300	Tab, Pale, Film Coated	Cimetidine HCl 300 mg	Tagamet by Penn	58437-0001	Gastrointestinal
CB400	Tab, Film Coated	Cimetidine HCl 400 mg	Tagamet by Allscripts		Gastrointestinal
CB400	Tab, Pale, Film Coated	Cimetidine HCl 400 mg	Tagamet by Penn	58437-0002	Gastrointestinal
CB800	Tab, Pale, Film Coated	Cimetidine HCl 800 mg	Tagamet by Penn	58437-0003	Gastrointestinal
CBF	Tab, White, Film Coated	Ascorbic Acid 120 mg, Beta-Carotene 4000 Units, Calcium 200 mg, Cyanocobalamin 8 mcg, Folic Acid 1 mg, Iodine 150 mcg, Iron 50 mg, Niacin 20 mg, Pyridoxine HCl 3 mg, Riboflavin 3 mg, Thiamine HCl 3 mg, Vitamin D 400 Units, Vitamin E 30 Units, Zinc 15 mg	Nestabs CBF by Fielding	00421-1997	Vitamin
CBF	Tab, White, Film Coated	Ascorbic Acid 120 mg, Beta-Carotene 4000 Units, Calcium 200 mg, Cyanocobalamin 8 mcg, Folic Acid 1 mg, Iodine 150 mcg, Iron 50 mg, Niacin 20 mg, Pyridoxine HCl 3 mg, Riboflavin 3 mg, Thiamine HCl 3 mg, Vitamin D 400 Units, Vitamin E 30 Units, Zinc 15 mg	Nestabs CBF by JB	51111-0004	Vitamin
CBP <> 01	Tab, Yellow, Oblong, Scored, CBP <> / 01	Pseudoephedrine HCl 120 mg, Methscopolamine 2.5 mg	RhinaClear by Amneal	65162-0550	Cold Remedy
CBP <> 02	Tab, Blue, Oblong, Scored, CBP <> / 02	Chlorpheniramine Maleate 8 mg, Methscopolamine 2.5 mg	RhinaClear by Amneal	65162-0550	Cold Remedy
CC	Tab, Green, Round	Inert	Ortho 7/7/7 28 by Janssen-Ortho	Canadian DIN 00602965	Oral Contraceptive; Placebo
CC	Tab, Green, Round	Inert	Tri-Cyclen 28 by Janssen-Ortho	Canadian DIN 02029421	Oral Contraceptive; Placebo
CC	Tab, Green, Round	Inert	Ortho 0.5/35 28 by Janssen-Ortho	Canadian DIN 00340731	Oral Contraceptive; Placebo
CC	Tab, Green, Round	Inert	Ortho 1/35 28 by Janssen-Ortho	Canadian DIN 00372838	Oral Contraceptive; Placebo
CC	Tab, Green, Round	Inert	Cyclen by Janssen-Ortho	Canadian DIN 01992872	Oral Contraceptive; Placebo
CC	Tab, Gray & Green, Round, C/C	Chlorophyllin Copper Complex Sodium 14 mg	Chloresium by Rystan		Gastrointestinal
CC <> 105	Tab, Blue, Cap Shaped, Scored, C C on opposite sides of Score	Salsalate 750 mg	Disalcid by Caraco	57664-0105	NSAID
CC <> PP	Tab, White, Round, Scored, P logo / P logo <> C / C	Pramipexole DiHCl 1 mg	Mirapex by Pharmascience	Canadian DIN 02290146	Antiparkinson
CC0147	Cap, Black	Phentermine 30 mg	Fastin by Qualitest	00603-5190	Anorexiant; C IV
CC0147	Cap, Black	Phentermine 30 mg	Fastin by DRX	55045-1264	Anorexiant; C IV
CC0147	Cap, C-C in a Box	Phentermine HCl 30 mg	Phentride by Jones	52604-0010	Anorexiant; C IV
CC0147	Cap, Black	Phentermine 30 mg	Fastin by DRX	55045-2231	Anorexiant; C IV
CC0147	Cap, Black	Phentermine 30 mg	Fastin by Jones	52604-9151	Anorexiant; C IV
CC0147	Cap, Black	Phentermine 30 mg	Fastin by Jones	52604-9152	Anorexiant; C IV
CC0147	Cap, Black	Phentermine 30 mg	Fastin by Jones	52604-9153	Anorexiant; C IV
CC0147	Cap, Black	Phentermine 30 mg	Fastin by JMI Canton	00252-9151	Anorexiant; C IV
CC0147	Cap, Black	Phentermine 30 mg	Fastin by JMI Canton	00252-9152	Anorexiant; C IV
CC101	Tab, Yellow, Oval	Meclizine HCl 25 mg	Antivert by Camall		Antiemetic
CC102	Tab	Phentermine 8 mg	Fastin by Allscripts		Anorexiant; C IV
CC102	Tab	Phentermine 8 mg	Fastin by DRX	55045-1688	Anorexiant; C IV
CC102	Tab, C-C/102, C-C is in a Box	Phentermine 8 mg	Fastin by Jones	52604-9161	Anorexiant; C IV
CC102	Tab, Green, Round, Flat, Scored	Phentermine 8 mg	Fastin by Physician Total Care	54868-4067	Anorexiant; C IV

ID FRONT <> BACK	DESCRIPTION FRONT <> BACK	INGREDIENT & STRENGTH	BRAND (or Generic Equiv.) by FIRM	NDC#	CLASS; SCH.
CC102	Tab, Green, Round, Flat, Scored	Phentermine 8 mg	Fastin by Physician Total Care	54868-4076	Anorexiant; C IV
CC102	Tab, Green, Round, Flat, Scored	Phentermine 8 mg	Fastin by Ivax	00182-0204	Anorexiant; C IV
CC102	Tab, Green, Round, Flat, Scored	Phentermine 8 mg	Fastin by PDRX	55289-0803	Anorexiant; C IV
CC102	Tab, Green, Round, Flat, Scored	Phentermine 8 mg	Fastin by Macnary	55982-0003	Anorexiant; C IV
CC102	Tab, Green, Round, Flat, Scored	Phentermine 8 mg	Fastin by Ems Disp	62792-0102	Anorexiant; C IV
CC105	Tab, Pink, Round, Scored	Phendimetrazine Tartrate 35 mg	Plegine by Physician Total Care	54868-1341	Anorexiant; C III
CC105	Tab, C-C in a Box 105	Phendimetrazine Tartrate 35 mg	Plegine by Jones	52604-9143	Anorexiant; C III
CC105	Tab, Gray, Round	Phendimetrazine Tartrate 35 mg	Plegine by Camall		Anorexiant; C III
CC105	Tab, White, Round	Phendimetrazine Tartrate 35 mg	Plegine by Camall		Anorexiant; C III
CC105	Tab, Yellow, Round	Phendimetrazine Tartrate 35 mg	Plegine by Camall		Anorexiant; C III
CC105	Tab, Pink, Round	Phendimetrazine Tartrate 35 mg	Plegine by Camall		Anorexiant; C III
CC105	Tab, White, Round, Double Scored	Phendimetrazine Tartrate 35 mg	Plegine by PDRX	55289-0300	Anorexiant; C III
CC105	Tab, Gray, Round, Double Scored	Phendimetrazine Tartrate 35 mg	Plegine by PDRX	55289-0285	Anorexiant; C III
CC107	Tab, C-C in a Box/107	Phendimetrazine Tartrate 35 mg	Plegine by JMI Canton	00252-9145	Anorexiant; C III
CC107	Tab	Phendimetrazine Tartrate 35 mg	Plegine by Allscripts		Anorexiant; C III
CC107	Tab, Yellow, Round, Scored	Phendimetrazine Tartrate 35 mg	Plegine by Physician Total Care	54868-1288	Anorexiant; C III
CC107	Tab, C-C/107, C-C is in a Box	Phendimetrazine Tartrate 35 mg	Plegine by Jones	52604-9145	Anorexiant; C III
CC107	Tab, Yellow, Round, Scored	Phendimetrazine Tartrate 35 mg	Plegine by Physician Total Care	54868-1502	Anorexiant; C III
CC107	Tab	Phendimetrazine Tartrate 35 mg	Plegine by DRX	55045-2010	Anorexiant; C III
CC107	Tab, Compressed, CC 107	Phendimetrazine Tartrate 35 mg	Plegine by Macnary	55982-0001	Anorexiant; C III
CC107	Tab	Phendimetrazine Tartrate 35 mg	Plegine by URL Mutual	00677-1499	Anorexiant; C III
CC108	Tab	Hydrochlorothiazide 50 mg	Hydrodiuril by Sandoz	00781-1481	Diuretic; Antihypertensive
CC108	Tab	Hydrochlorothiazide 50 mg	Hydrodiuril by Qualitest	00603-3859	Diuretic; Antihypertensive
CC109	Tab, White, Round	Diethylpropion HCl 25 mg	by BMS	00056-0623	Anorexiant; C IV
CC109	Tab, Blue, Round	Diethylpropion HCl 25 mg	by BMS	00056-0627	Anorexiant; C IV
CC109	Tab, C-C/109	Diethylpropion HCl 25 mg	by Jones	52604-9159	Anorexiant; C IV
CC109	Tab, C-C/109, C-C is in a Box	Diethylpropion HCl 25 mg	by JMI Canton	00252-9159	Anorexiant; C IV
CC109	Tab	Diethylpropion HCl 25 mg	by Ivax	00182-1436	Anorexiant; C IV
CC109	Tab	Diethylpropion HCl 25 mg	Radtue by Macnary	55982-0002	Anorexiant; C IV
CC109	Tab	Diethylpropion HCl 25 mg	by PDRX	55289-0794	Anorexiant; C IV
CC109 <> CC109	Tab, Blue, Round	Diethylpropion HCl 25 mg	by Southwood	58016-0835	Anorexiant; C IV
CC116	Tab, Pink, Round, C-C over 116	Hydrochlorothiazide 25 mg	Hydrodiuril by Qualitest	00603-3858	Diuretic; Antihypertensive
CC116	Tab, Pink, Round, C-C over 116	Hydrochlorothiazide 25 mg	Hydrodiuril by URL Mutual	00677-0346	Diuretic; Antihypertensive
CC116	Tab, Pink, Round, C-C over 116	Hydrochlorothiazide 25 mg	Hydrodiuril by Sandoz	00781-1480	Diuretic; Antihypertensive
CC116	Tab, Pink, Round, C-C over 116	Hydrochlorothiazide 25 mg	Hydrodiuril by Talbert	44514-0410	Diuretic; Antihypertensive
CC116	Tab, Pink, Round, C-C over 116	Hydrochlorothiazide 25 mg	Hydrodiuril by Apotheca	12634-0445	Diuretic; Antihypertensive
CC116	Tab, Pink, Round, C-C over 116	Hydrochlorothiazide 25 mg	Hydrodiuril by Heartland	61392-0011	Diuretic; Antihypertensive
CC116	Tab, Pink, Round, C-C over 116	Hydrochlorothiazide 25 mg	Hydrodiuril by Camall	00147-0116	Diuretic; Antihypertensive
CC123	Tab	Hydrochlorothiazide 25 mg	Hydrodiuril by URL Mutual	00677-0346	Diuretic; Antihypertensive
CC124	Tab, Pink, Round, CC Inside Rectangle and 124	Hydralazine HCl 25 mg, Hydrochlorothiazide 15 mg, Reserpine 0.1 mg	Uni Serp by RX Pak	65084-0184	Antihypertensive; Diuretic
CC124	Tab, Salmon	Hydralazine HCl 25 mg, Hydrochlorothiazide 15 mg, Reserpine 0.1 mg	by Ivax	00182-1820	Antihypertensive; Diuretic
CC124	Tab	Hydralazine HCl 25 mg, Hydrochlorothiazide 15 mg, Reserpine 0.1 mg	Uni Serp by URL Mutual	00677-0415	Antihypertensive; Diuretic
CC124	Tab, CC-124	Hydralazine HCl 25 mg, Hydrochlorothiazide 15 mg, Reserpine 0.1 mg	by Qualitest		Antihypertensive; Diuretic
CC125	Tab, Green, Round	Hydrochlorothiazide 50 mg, Hydrochlorothiazide 0.125 mg	Hydropres-50 by Camall	00603-3807	Diuretic; Antihypertensive
CC135	Tab, White, with Green Specks	Phendimetrazine Tartrate 35 mg	Obezine by Jones	52604-9142	Anorexiant; C III
CC135	Tab, Green & White, Oblong, Double Scored	Phendimetrazine Tartrate 35 mg	by PDRX	55289-0294	Anorexiant; C III
CC136	Tab	Phentermine HCl 8 mg	by DRX	55045-2274	Anorexiant; C IV
CC136	Tab	Phentermine HCl 8 mg	by PDRX	55289-0801	Anorexiant; C IV

ID FRONT <> BACK	DESCRIPTION FRONT <> BACK	INGREDIENT & STRENGTH	BRAND (or Generic Equiv.) by FIRM	NDC#	CLASS; SCH.
CC137	Tab, Blue, Oval	Meclizine HCl 12.5 mg	Antivert by Camall		Antiemetic
CC143	Tab, Aqua, Round	Trichlormethiazide 4 mg	Naquival by PDRX	55289-0795	Diuretic; Antihypertensive
CC143	Tab, Aqua, Round	Trichlormethiazide 4 mg	Naquival by Ivax	00182-0517	Diuretic; Antihypertensive
CC166	Tab, Green, Round	Phendimetrazine Tartrate 35 mg	Plegine by Camall		Anorexiant; C III
CC1875	Cap, CC 18.75	Phentermine HCl 18.75 mg	by Camall	00147-0249	Anorexiant; C IV
CC1875	Cap, CC 18.75	Phentermine HCl 18.75 mg	by Ems Disp	62792-0249	Anorexiant; C IV
CC1875	Cap, Logo CC 18.75	Phentermine HCl 18.75 mg	by Apotheca	12634-0517	Anorexiant; C IV
CC227	Tab, Tan, Round	Thyroid 3 g	by Camall		Thyroid Hormone
CC232	Tab, White, with Blue Specks	Phentermine HCl 37.5 mg	Pbw Phentride by JMI Canton	00252-9156	Anorexiant; C IV
CC232	Tab	Phentermine HCl 37.5 mg	by Ivax	00182-0205	Anorexiant; C IV
CC232	Tab, Blue Specks	Phentermine HCl 37.5 mg	by Camall	00147-0248	Anorexiant; C IV
CC232	Tab, White, with Blue Specks	Phentermine HCl 37.5 mg	Phentride by Jones	52604-9156	Anorexiant; C IV
CC232	Tab	Phentermine HCl 37.5 mg	by Allscripts		Anorexiant; C IV
CC232	Tab	Phentermine HCl 37.5 mg	by PDRX	55289-0865	Anorexiant; C IV
CC232	Tab, White, with Blue Specks	Phentermine HCl 37.5 mg	by Physician Total Care	54868-4091	Anorexiant; C IV
CC232	Tab, Yellow, Oblong, Scored	Phentermine HCl 37.5 mg	by Compumed	00403-5312	Anorexiant; C IV
CC232	Tab, Blue Specks	Phentermine HCl 37.5 mg	by PDRX	55289-0701	Anorexiant; C IV
CC232	Tab, White w/ Blue Specks, Oval, Scored	Phentermine HCl 37.5 mg	Adipex by Qualitest	00603-5191	Anorexiant; C IV
CC232 <> CC232	Tab, White, w/ Blue Specks	Phentermine HCl 37.5 mg	by Allscripts		Anorexiant; C IV
CC236	Tab, White, Round	Cyproheptadine HCl 4 mg	Periactin by Camall		Antihistamine
CC238	Tab, White, Round	Potassium Gluconate 500 mg	Potassium Gluconate by Camall	00147-0238	Electrolytes
CC242	Tab, Tan, Round	Thyroid 0.5 g	by Camall		Thyroid Hormone
CC243	Tab, Tan, Round	Thyroid 1 g	by Camall		Thyroid Hormone
CC244	Tab, Tan, Round	Thyroid 2 g	by Camall		Thyroid Hormone
CC245	Tab, Pink, Oval	Chromium Picolinate 200 mcg	Pichrome by Camall		Supplement
CC250	Tab, White, Oblong	Vitamin Combination	by Camall		Vitamin
CC255	Tab, Orange, Round	Hydralazine HCl 10 mg	by Camall	00147-0255	Antihypertensive
CC255	Tab, Orange, Round	Hydralazine HCl 10 mg	Apresoline by Camall		Antihypertensive
CC256	Tab, Orange, Round	Hydralazine HCl 25 mg	by Camall	00147-0256	Antihypertensive
CC256	Tab, Orange, Round	Hydralazine HCl 25 mg	Apresoline by Camall		Antihypertensive
CC257	Tab, Orange, Round	Hydralazine HCl 50 mg	Apresoline by Camall		Antihypertensive
CC257	Tab, Orange, Round	Hydralazine HCl 50 mg	by Camall	00147-0257	Antihypertensive
CC258	Tab, Orange, Round	Hydralazine HCl 100 mg	by Camall	00147-0258	Antihypertensive
CC258	Tab, Orange, Round	Hydralazine HCl 100 mg	Apresoline by Camall		Antihypertensive
CC270	Tab, Yellow, Oval	Phenylpropanolamine HCl 37.5 mg	by Camall		Decongestant; Appetite Suppressant
CC270	Tab, Gray, Oval	Phenylpropanolamine HCl 37.5 mg	by Camall		Decongestant; Appetite Suppressant
CC270	Tab, Pink, Oval	Phenylpropanolamine HCl 37.5 mg	by Camall		Decongestant; Appetite Suppressant
CC270	Tab, Blue, Oval	Phenylpropanolamine HCl 37.5 mg	by Camall		Decongestant; Appetite Suppressant
CC270	Tab, Green, Oval	Phenylpropanolamine HCl 37.5 mg	by Camall		Decongestant; Appetite Suppressant
CC270	Tab, Peach, Oval	Phenylpropanolamine HCl 37.5 mg	by Camall		Decongestant; Appetite Suppressant

ID FRONT <> BACK	DESCRIPTION FRONT <> BACK	INGREDIENT & STRENGTH	BRAND (or Generic Equiv.) by FIRM	NDC#	CLASS; SCH.
CC270	Tab, White, Oval	Phenylpropanolamine HCl 37.5 mg	by Camall		Decongestant; Appetite Suppressant
CC375	Cap, Clear, with Orange & White Beads, CC 37.5	Phentermine HCl 37.5 mg	Phentride by Jones	52604-9155	Anorexiant; C IV
CC375	Cap, Logo CC 37.5	Phentermine HCl 37.5 mg	by DRX	55045-2294	Anorexiant; C IV
CC375	Cap, Orange & White Beads, CC 37.5	Phentermine HCl 37.5 mg	by DRX	55045-2289	Anorexiant; C IV
CC375	Cap, Clear, with Orange & White Beads, CC 37.5	Phentermine HCl 37.5 mg	Pbc Phentride by JMI Canton	00252-9155	Anorexiant; C IV
CC375	Cap, Black & Red, CC 37.5	Phentermine HCl 37.5 mg	by Camall		Anorexiant; C IV
CC375	Cap, Brown & Clear, CC 37.5	Phentermine HCl 37.5 mg	by Camall		Anorexiant; C IV
CC375	Cap, Black, CC 37.5	Phentermine HCl 37.5 mg	by Camall	00147-0253	Anorexiant; C IV
CC375	Cap, Black & Yellow, CC 37.5	Phentermine HCl 37.5 mg	by Camall		Anorexiant; C IV
CC375	Cap, Yellow, CC 37.5	Phentermine HCl 37.5 mg	by Camall		Anorexiant; C IV
CC375	Cap, CC 37.5	Phentermine HCl 37.5 mg	by Apotheca	12634-0515	Anorexiant; C IV
CC375	Tab, CC 37.5	Phentermine HCl 37.5 mg	by Ems Disp	62792-0231	Anorexiant; C IV
CC375	Cap, Clear & Green, CC 37.5	Phentermine 37.5 mg	by Physician Total Care	54868-4059	Anorexiant; C IV
CC375P	Tab, Pink, Round, CC 37.5P	Phenylpropanolamine 37.5 mg	by Camall		Decongestant; Appetite Suppressant
CC375P	Tab, Peach, Round, CC 37.5P	Phenylpropanolamine 37.5 mg	by Camall		Decongestant; Appetite Suppressant
CC375P	Tab, Gray, Round, CC 37.5P	Phenylpropanolamine 37.5 mg	by Camall		Decongestant; Appetite Suppressant
CC375P	Tab, White, Round, CC 37.5P	Phenylpropanolamine 37.5 mg	by Camall		Decongestant; Appetite Suppressant
CC375P	Tab, White, Round, Green Specks, CC 37.5P	Phenylpropanolamine 37.5 mg	by Camall		Decongestant; Appetite Suppressant
CC375P	Tab, Yellow, Round, CC 37.5P	Phenylpropanolamine 37.5 mg	by Camall		Decongestant; Appetite Suppressant
CC375P	Tab, Green, Round, CC 37.5P	Phenylpropanolamine 37.5 mg	by Camall		Decongestant; Appetite Suppressant
CC525	Tab, Purple, Oval	Zinc 15 mg, Chromium 200 mcg	by Camall		Mineral; Supplement
CC75P	Cap, Blue & Clear	Phenylpropanolamine 75 mg	by Camall		Decongestant; Appetite Suppressant
CC75P	Cap, Black	Phenylpropanolamine 75 mg	by Camall		Decongestant; Appetite Suppressant
CC75P	Cap, Black & Yellow	Phenylpropanolamine 75 mg	by Camall		Decongestant; Appetite Suppressant
CC75P	Cap, Yellow	Phenylpropanolamine 75 mg	by Camall		Decongestant; Appetite Suppressant
CCAD	Cap, Green	Activated Charcoal 260 mg	CharcoCaps by Requa	10961-0302	Gastrointestinal
CCC	Tab, Red, Round, C over C + C	Chlorpheniramine Maleate 4 mg, Dextromethorphan Hydrobromide 30 mg	Coricidin HBP Cough and Cold by Schering-Plough		Cold Remedy
CCHF	Tab, Pink, Cap Shaped	Activated Charcoal 260 mg	CharcoCaps by Requa	10961-0200	Gastrointestinal
CD129	Cap, Light Brown, Black Print, Opaque, Hard Gel	Ranitidine HCl 150 mg	Zantac by Par	49884-0647	Gastrointestinal
CD129	Cap, Light Brown, Black Print, Opaque, Hard Gel	Ranitidine HCl 150 mg	Zantac by Dr. Reddy's	55111-0129	Gastrointestinal
CD130	Cap, Light Brown, Black Print, Opaque, Hard Gel	Ranitidine HCl 300 mg	Zantac by Par	49884-0648	Gastrointestinal
CD130	Cap, Light Brown, Black Print, Opaque, Hard Gel	Ranitidine HCl 300 mg	Zantac by Dr. Reddy's	55111-0130	Gastrointestinal
CDAY	Cap, Yellow, C-Day	Acetaminophen 650 mg, Pseudoephedrine HCl 60 mg, Dextromethorphan HBr 30 mg	Tylenol Cold Ex Strength by SKB	Canadian	Cold Remedy
CDAY	Tab, Yellow, Oblong, C-Day	Acetaminophen 650 mg, Pseudoephedrine HCl 60 mg, Dextromethorphan HBr 30 mg	Tylenol Cold Ex Strength by SKB	Canadian	Cold Remedy

ID FRONT <> BACK	DESCRIPTION FRONT <> BACK	INGREDIENT & STRENGTH	BRAND (or Generic Equiv.) by FIRM	NDC#	CLASS; SCH.
CDC <> GEIGY	Tab, Light Yellow, Round, Film Coated	Metoprolol Tartrate 200 mg	Lopressor by Novartis	Canadian DIN 00534560	Antihypertensive
CDC322	Tab, CDC/322	Yohimbine HCl 5.4 mg	Thybine Blue by JMI Canton	00252-3223	Impotence Agent
CDN <> 10	Tab, White, Round, Unscored, Biconvex	Oxycodone HCl 10 mg	OxyContin by Purdue Pharma	Canadian DIN 02202441	Analgesic
CDN <> 20	Tab, Pink, Round, Unscored, Biconvex	Oxycodone HCl 20 mg	OxyContin by Purdue Pharma	Canadian DIN 02202468	Analgesic
CDN <> 40	Tab, Yellow, Round, Unscored, Biconvex	Oxycodone HCl 40 mg	OxyContin by Purdue Pharma	Canadian DIN 02202476	Analgesic
CDN <> 5	Tab, Pale Blue, Round, Unscored, Biconvex tablet	Oxycodone HCl 5 mg	OxyContin by Purdue Pharma	Canadian DIN 02258129	Analgesic
CDN <> 80	Tab, Green, Round, Unscored, Biconvex	Oxycodone HCl 80 mg	OxyContin by Purdue Pharma	Canadian DIN 02202484	Analgesic
CDT051 <> PFIZER	Tab, White, Oval	Amlodipine Besylate 5 mg, Atorvastatin Calcium 10 mg	Caduet by Pfizer	Canadian DIN 02273233	Antihypertensive; Antihyperlipidemic
CDT051 <> PFIZER	Tab, White, Oval	Amlodipine Besylate 5 mg, Atorvastatin Calcium 10 mg	Caduet by Pfizer	00069-2150	Antihypertensive; Antihyperlipidemic
CDT052 <> PFIZER	Tab, White, Oval	Amlodipine Besylate 5 mg, Atorvastatin Calcium 20 mg	Caduet by Pfizer	00069-2170	Antihypertensive; Antihyperlipidemic
CDT052 <> PFIZER	Tab, White, Oval	Amlodipine Besylate 5 mg, Atorvastatin Calcium 20 mg	Caduet by Pfizer	Canadian DIN 02273241	Antihypertensive; Antihyperlipidemic
CDT054 <> PFIZER	Tab, White, Oval	Amlodipine Besylate 5 mg, Atorvastatin Calcium 40 mg	Caduet by Pfizer	00069-2190	Antihypertensive; Antihyperlipidemic
CDT058 <> PFIZER	Tab, White, Oval	Amlodipine Besylate 5 mg, Atorvastatin Calcium 80 mg	Caduet by Pfizer	00069-2260	Antihypertensive; Antihyperlipidemic
CDT058 <> PFIZER	Tab, White, Oval	Amlodipine Besylate 5 mg, Atorvastatin Calcium 80 mg	Caduet by Pfizer	Canadian DIN 02273276	Antihypertensive; Antihyperlipidemic
CDT101 <> PFIZER	Tab, Blue, Oval	Amlodipine Besylate 10 mg, Atorvastatin Calcium 10 mg	Caduet by Pfizer	Canadian DIN 02273284	Antihypertensive; Antihyperlipidemic
CDT101 <> PFIZER	Tab, Blue, Oval	Amlodipine Besylate 10 mg, Atorvastatin Calcium 10 mg	Caduet by Pfizer	00069-2160	Antihypertensive; Antihyperlipidemic
CDT102 <> PFIZER	Tab, Blue, Oval	Amlodipine Besylate 10 mg, Atorvastatin Calcium 20 mg	Caduet by Pfizer	00069-2180	Antihypertensive; Antihyperlipidemic
CDT102 <> PFIZER	Tab, Blue, Oval	Amlodipine Besylate 10 mg, Atorvastatin Calcium 20 mg	Caduet by Pfizer	Canadian DIN 02273292	Antihypertensive; Antihyperlipidemic
CDT104 <> PFIZER	Tab, Blue, Oval	Amlodipine Besylate 10 mg, Atorvastatin Calcium 40 mg	Caduet by Pfizer	Canadian DIN 02273306	Antihypertensive; Antihyperlipidemic
CDT104 <> PFIZER	Tab, Blue, Oval	Amlodipine Besylate 10 mg, Atorvastatin Calcium 40 mg	Caduet by Pfizer	00069-2250	Antihypertensive; Antihyperlipidemic
CDT108 <> PFIZER	Tab, Blue, Oval	Amlodipine Besylate 10 mg, Atorvastatin Calcium 80 mg	Caduet by Pfizer	00069-2270	Antihypertensive; Antihyperlipidemic
CDT108 <> PFIZER	Tab, Blue, Oval	Amlodipine Besylate 10 mg, Atorvastatin Calcium 80 mg	Caduet by Pfizer	Canadian DIN 02273314	Antihypertensive; Antihyperlipidemic
CDT251 <> PFIZER	Tab, White, Oval	Amlodipine Besylate 2.5 mg, Atorvastatin Calcium 10 mg	Caduet by Pfizer	00069-2960	Antihypertensive; Antihyperlipidemic
CDT252 <> PFIZER	Tab, White, Oval	Amlodipine Besylate 2.5 mg, Atorvastatin Calcium 20 mg	Caduet by Pfizer	00069-2970	Antihypertensive; Antihyperlipidemic
CDT254 <> PFIZER	Tab, White, Oval	Amlodipine Besylate 2.5 mg, Atorvastatin Calcium 40 mg	Caduet by Pfizer	00069-2980	Antihypertensive; Antihyperlipidemic
CDX50	Tab, White, Film Coated, CDX50 <> Casodex Logo	Bicalutamide 50 mg	Casodex by AstraZeneca	Canadian DIN 02184478	Antiandrogen
CDX50	Tab, White, Film Coated, CDX50 <> Casodex Logo	Bicalutamide 50 mg	Casodex by Zeneca	62311-0705	Antiandrogen

ID FRONT <> BACK	DESCRIPTION FRONT <> BACK	INGREDIENT & STRENGTH	BRAND (or Generic Equiv.) by FIRM	NDC#	CLASS; SCH.
CDX50	Tab, White, Film Coated, CDX50 <> Casodex Logo	Bicalutamide 50 mg	Casodex by Zeneca	Canadian	Antiandrogen
CDX50	Tab, White, Film Coated, CDX50 <> Casodex Logo	Bicalutamide 50 mg	Casodex by AstraZeneca	00310-0705	Antiandrogen
CECLOR250LILLY3061	Cap, Purple and White	Cefaclor 250 mg	Ceclor by Pharmedix	53002-0211	Antibiotic
CECLOR250MGLILLY-3061	Cap, Purple and White	Cefaclor 250 mg	Ceclor by Eli Lilly	00002-3061	Antibiotic
CECLOR250MGLILLY-3061	Cap, Purple and White	Cefaclor 250 mg	Ceclor by H J Harkins Co	52959-0027	Antibiotic
CECLOR500MGLILLY-3062	Cap, Purple and Gray	Cefaclor 500 mg	Ceclor CD by Pharmedix	53002-0244	Antibiotic
CECLOR500MGLILLY-3062	Cap, Purple and Gray	Cefaclor 500 mg	Ceclor by Eli Lilly	00002-3062	Antibiotic
CECLORCD375MG	Tab	Cefaclor 375 mg	Ceclor CD by Dura	51479-0036	Antibiotic
CECLORCD500LILL	Tab	Cefaclor 500 mg	by Allscripts		Antibiotic
CECLORCD500MG	Tab	Cefaclor 500 mg	Ceclor CD by Dura	51479-0035	Antibiotic
CEDAX400	Cap, White	Ceftibuten Dihydrate 400 mg	Cedax by Schering	00085-0691	Antibiotic
CEDAX400	Cap, White, Opaque	Ceftibuten Dihydrate 400 mg	Cedax by Biovail	64455-0691	Antibiotic
CEFACLOR250MG-2614SCHEIN	Cap, Purple	Cefaclor 250 mg	Ceclor by Schein	00364-2614	Antibiotic
CEFACLOR250MG-LEDERLEC54	Cap	Cefaclor 250 mg	Ceclor by UDL	51079-0617	Antibiotic
CEFACLOR250-ZENITH4760	Cap	Cefaclor 250 mg	Ceclor by PDRX	55289-0749	Antibiotic
CEFACLOR500MG-2615SCHEIN	Cap, Purple & Yellow	Cefaclor 500 mg	by Schein	00364-2615	Antibiotic
CEFACLOR500MG-LEDERLEC58	Cap, Lavender	Cefaclor 500 mg	Ceclor CD by UDL	51079-0618	Antibiotic
CELGENE	Cap, White, Hard Gel	Thalidomide 50 mg	Thalomid by Celgene	59572-0105	Immunomodulator
CELGENE	Cap, White	Thalidomide 50 mg	Thalomid by Penn	63069-0630	Immunomodulator
CELGENE100MG	Cap, Tan, CELGENE/100MG and "Do Not Get Pregnant" Logo	Thalidomide 100 mg	Thalomid by Celgene	59572-0210	Immunomodulator
CELGENE200MG	Cap, Blue, CELGENE/200MG and "Do Not Get Pregnant" Logo	Thalidomide 200 mg	Thalomid by Celgene	59572-0220	Immunomodulator
CELGENE50MG	Cap, White, Opaque, CELGENE/50MG and "Do Not Get Pregnant" Logo	Thalidomide 50 mg	Thalomid by Celgene	59572-0205	Immunomodulator
CELLCEPT250ROCHE	Cap, Blue & Brown, Hard Gel, Cellcept over 250 over Roche	Mycophenolate Mofetil 250 mg	CellCept by Valeant Puerto Rico	64158-0920	Immunosuppressant
CELLCEPT250ROCHE	Cap, Blue & Brown, Hard Gel, Cellcept over 250 over Roche	Mycophenolate Mofetil 250 mg	CellCept by Syntex	18393-0259	Immunosuppressant
CELLCEPT250ROCHE	Cap, Blue & Brown, Hard Gel, Cellcept over 250 over Roche	Mycophenolate Mofetil 250 mg	CellCept by Murfreesboro	51129-1358	Immunosuppressant
CELLCEPT250ROCHE	Cap, Blue & Brown, Hard Gel, Cellcept over 250 over Roche	Mycophenolate Mofetil 250 mg	CellCept by Roche	Canadian DIN 02192748	Immunosuppressant
CELLCEPT250ROCHE	Tab, Lavender, Black Print, Cap Shaped, Film Coated, Cellcept over 500	Mycophenolate Mofetil 250 mg	CellCept by Hoffmann La Roche	00004-0259	Immunosuppressant
CELLCEPT500 <> ROCHE	Tab, Lavender, Black Print, Cap Shaped, Film Coated, Cellcept over 500	Mycophenolate Mofetil 500 mg	CellCept by Syntex	18393-0923	Immunosuppressant
CELLCEPT500 <> ROCHE	Tab, Lavender, Black Print, Cap Shaped, Film Coated, Cellcept over 500	Mycophenolate Mofetil 500 mg	CellCept by Roche	Canadian DIN 02237484	Immunosuppressant
CELLCEPT500 <> ROCHE	Tab, Lavender, Black Print, Cap Shaped, Film Coated, Cellcept over 500	Mycophenolate Mofetil 500 mg	CellCept by Hoffmann La Roche	00004-0260	Immunosuppressant
CELLCEPT500 <> ROCHE	Tab, Lavender, Black Print, Cap Shaped, Film Coated, Cellcept over 500	Mycophenolate Mofetil 500 mg	CellCept by Novartis		Immunosuppressant
CELLTECH57410MG	Cap, Green and White	Methylphenidate HCl 10 mg	Metadate CD by Celltech	53014-0574	Stimulant; C II
CELLTECH57520MG	Cap, Blue & White, Black & White Print, Ex Release	Methylphenidate HCl 20 mg	Metadate CD by Celltech	53014-0575	Stimulant; C II
CELLTECH57630MG	Cap, Reddish Brown and White	Methylphenidate HCl 30 mg	Metadate CD by Celltech	53014-0576	Stimulant; C II

ID FRONT <> BACK	DESCRIPTION FRONT <> BACK	INGREDIENT & STRENGTH	BRAND (or Generic Equiv.) by FIRM	NDC#	CLASS; SCH.
CEN <> 905	Tab, Yellow, Round, Coated	Folacin 5 mg, Thiamine 1.5 mg, Riboflavin 1.5 mg, Niacinamide 20 mg, Pantothenic Acid 10 mg, Pyridoxine 50 mg, Cyanocobalamin 2 mg, Ascorbic Acid 60 mg, D-biotin 300 mcg, Zinc 25 mg, Copper 1.5 mg	Diatx Zn by Centrix	11528-0905	Vitamin
CENTRAL130MG	Cap, Clear	Theophylline Anhydrous 130 mg	Theoclear LA-130 by Schwarz		Antiasthmatic
CENTRAL13105	Tab, Blue, Oval, Central 131/05	Vitamin Combination	Niferex-PN by Schwarz		Vitamin
CENTRAL13107	Tab, Red, Round, Central 131/07	Prednisone 5 mg	Prednicen-M by Schwarz		Steroid
CENTRAL260MG	Cap, Clear	Theophylline Anhydrous 260 mg	Theoclear LA-260 by Schwarz		Antiasthmatic
CENTRAL40	Cap, Clear & Red	Chlorpheniramine Maleate 8 mg, Pseudoephedrine HCl 120 mg	Codimal LA by Schwarz		Cold Remedy
CENTRAL4220	Cap, Clear & Orange	Vitamin Combination	Niferex-150 by Schwarz		Vitamin
CENTRAL4330	Cap, Clear & Red	Vitamin Combination	Niferex-150 Forte by Schwarz		Vitamin
CENTRAL44	Cap, Brown & Red	Vitamin Combination	Niferex-150 Forte by Schwarz		Vitamin
CENTRAL5005	Tab, White, Oval, Central 500/5	Acetaminophen 500 mg, Hydrocodone Bitartrate 5 mg	Co-Gesic by Schwarz		Analgesic; C III
CENTRAL500MG	Tab, Pink, Round	Salsalate 500 mg	Mono-Gesic by Schwarz		NSAID
CENTRAL604	Cap, Clear, Central 60/4	Chlorpheniramine Maleate 4 mg, Pseudoephedrine HCl 60 mg	Codimal LA Half by Schwarz		Cold Remedy
CENTRAL750MG	Tab, Pink, Oval	Salsalate 750 mg	Mono-Gesic by Schwarz		NSAID
CENTRALC	Cap, Red & White	Chlorpheniramine Maleate 2 mg, Pseudoephedrine HCl 30 mg, Acetaminophen 325 mg	Codimal by Schwarz		Cold Remedy
CENTRUM <> CHEW	Tab, Orange, Oval, Chewable	Vitamin A 3500 IU, Vitamin C 60 mg, Vitamin D 400 IU, Vitamin E 30 IU, Vitamin K 10 mg, Thiamin 1.5 mg, Riboflavin 1.7 mg, Niacin 20 mg, Vitamin B6 2 mg, Folic Acid 400 mcg, Vitamin B12 6 mcg, Biotin 45 mcg, Pantothenic Acid 10 mg, Calcium 108 mg, Iron 18 mg, Phosphorus 50 mg, Iodine 150 mcg, Magnesium 40 mg, Zinc 15 mg, Copper 2 mg, Manganese 1 mg, Chromium 20 mcg, Molybdenum 20 mcg	Centrum Advanced Formula by Wyeth		Vitamin
CEPHALON15MG	Cap, Orange, Blue Ink, Dashed Band on Cap, Extended Release	Cyclobenzaprine HCl 15 mg	Amrix by Cephalon	63459-0700	Muscle Relaxant
CEPHALON30MG	Cap, Orange and Blue, White Ink, Dashed Band on Cap, Extended Release	Cyclobenzaprine HCl 30 mg	Amrix by Cephalon	63459-0701	Muscle Relaxant
CERTUSS	Tab, Red and White, Cap Shaped, Scored	Guaifenesin 1200 mg, Carbetapentane Citrate 60 mg	Certuss by Capellon	64543-0180	Cold Remedy
CF	Cap, Transparent & Orange, CF over Abbott Logo (a)	Pentobarbital Sodium 50 mg	Nembutal by Abbott	00074-3150 Discontinued	Sedative/Hypnotic; C II
CF <> HYL	Tab, White, Cap Shaped	Passiflora 1X, Avena Sativa 1X, Humulus lupulus 1X, Chamomilla 2X, Calcarea Phosphorica 3X, Ferrum Phosphorica 3X, Kali Phosphorica 3X, Natrum Phosphoricum 3X, Magnesia Phosphoricum 3X	Calm's Forte by Hyland's		Homeopathic
CF250 <> G	Tab, White to Off-White, Round, Coated	Ciprofloxacin 250 mg	Cipro by Par	49884-0637	Antibiotic
CF250 <> G	Tab, White, Round, Film Coated	Ciprofloxacin 250 mg	Cipro by Genpharm	Canadian DIN 02245647	Antibiotic
CF500 <> G	Tab, White to Off-White, Cap Shaped, Coated	Ciprofloxacin 500 mg	Cipro by Genpharm	Canadian DIN 02245648	Antibiotic
CF500 <> G	Tab, White to Off-White, Cap Shaped, Coated	Ciprofloxacin 500 mg	Cipro by Par	49884-0638	Antibiotic
CF750 <> G	Tab, White to Off-White, Cap Shaped, Coated	Ciprofloxacin 750 mg	Cipro by Par	49884-0639	Antibiotic
CF750 <> G	Tab, White to Off-White, Cap Shaped, Coated	Ciprofloxacin 750 mg	Cipro by Genpharm	Canadian DIN 02245649	Antibiotic
CG <> BEB	Tab, Light Red, Round, Film Coated	Oxprenolol HCl 80 mg	Slow Trasicor by Novartis	Canadian DIN 00534579	Antihypertensive
CG <> BNB	Tab, White, Round, Film Coated	Oxprenolol HCl 160 mg	Slow Trasicor by Novartis	Canadian DIN 00534587	Antihypertensive
CG <> CG	Tab, Light Yellow, Round, Film Coated, Scored	Oxprenolol HCl 80 mg	Trasicor by Novartis	Canadian DIN 00402583	Antihypertensive

ID FRONT <> BACK	DESCRIPTION FRONT <> BACK	INGREDIENT & STRENGTH	BRAND (or Generic Equiv.) by FIRM	NDC#	CLASS; SCH.
CG <> FV	Tab, Dark Yellow, Round, Film Coated	Letrozole 2.5 mg	Femara by Novartis	Canadian DIN 02231384	Antineoplastic
CG <> FV	Tab, Dark Yellow, Round, Film Coated	Letrozole 2.5 mg	Femara by Novartis	00078-0249	Antineoplastic
CG <> HC	Tab, Beige & Orange, Oval, Scored	Carbamazepine 200 mg	Tegretol by Novartis	Canadian DIN 00773611	Anticonvulsant
CG <> HGH	Tab, Light Orange, Oval, Film Coated	Hydrochlorothiazide 12.5 mg, Valsartan 80 mg	Diovan HCT by Novartis	00078-0314	Diuretic; Antihypertensive
CG <> HGH	Tab, Light Orange, Oval, Film Coated	Hydrochlorothiazide 12.5 mg, Valsartan 80 mg	Diovan HCT by Novartis	Canadian DIN 02241900	Diuretic; Antihypertensive
CG <> HGH	Tab, Light Orange, Oval, Film Coated	Valsartan 80 mg, Hydrochlorothiazide 12.5 mg	Diovan HCT by Allscripts		Antihypertensive; Diuretic
CG <> HGH	Tab, Light Orange, Oval, Film Coated	Hydrochlorothiazide 12.5 mg, Valsartan 80 mg	Diovan HCT by Novartis	17088-3932	Diuretic; Antihypertensive
CG <> HHH	Tab, Dark Red, Oval, Film Coated	Hydrochlorothiazide 12.5 mg, Valsartan 160 mg	Diovan HCT by Novartis	17088-3933	Diuretic; Antihypertensive
CG <> HHH	Tab, Dark Red, Oval, Film Coated	Hydrochlorothiazide 12.5 mg, Valsartan 160 mg	Diovan HCT by Novartis	00078-0315	Diuretic; Antihypertensive
CG <> HHH	Tab, Dark Red, Oval, Film Coated	Hydrochlorothiazide 12.5 mg, Valsartan 160 mg	Diovan HCT by Novartis	Canadian DIN 02241901	Diuretic; Antihypertensive
CG <> HO	Tab, Dark Yellow, Cap Shaped, Film Coated	Benazepril HCl 10 mg	Lotensin by Novartis	Canadian DIN 00885843	Antihypertensive
CG <> HP	Tab, Reddish-Orange, Cap Shaped, Film Coated	Benazepril HCl 20 mg	Lotensin by Novartis	Canadian DIN 00885851	Antihypertensive
CG <> HP	Tab, Light Orange, Round, Film-Coated	Benazepril HCl 20 mg	Lotensin by Novartis	Canadian DIN 00885851	Antihypertensive
CG <> LV	Tab, Light Yellow, Cap Shaped, Film Coated	Benazepril HCl 5 mg	Lotensin by Geigy	Canadian DIN 00885835	Antihypertensive
CG <> NC	Tab, Yellow, Round, Scored	Artemether 20 mg, Lumefantrine 120 mg	Coartem by Novartis International AG	00078-0568	Antimalarial
CG <> TD	Tab, Pale Grey-Green, Oval, Scored, Film Coated	Oxcarbazepine 150 mg	Trileptal by Novartis	Canadian DIN 02242067	Anticonvulsant
CG <> TD	Tab, Pale Grey-Green, Oval, Scored, Film Coated	Oxcarbazepine 150 mg	Trileptal by Novartis	00078-0456	Anticonvulsant
CG503	Tab, White	Ferrous Sulfate 160 mg	by Kaiser	Canadian	Mineral
CG622	White, Oblong	Terazosin HCl 1 mg	by Geigy	00179-1359	Antihypertensive
CGCG <> ENEENE	Tab, Brownish-Orange, Oval, Scored	Carbamazepine 400 mg	Tegretol by Geigy	Canadian DIN 00755583	Anticonvulsant
CGCG <> TETE	Tab, Yellow, Oval, Scored, Film Coated	Oxcarbazepine 300 mg	Trileptal by Novartis	17088-0011	Anticonvulsant
CGCG <> TETE	Tab, Yellow, Oval, Scored, Film Coated	Oxcarbazepine 300 mg	Trileptal by Novartis	00078-0337	Anticonvulsant
CGCG <> TETE	Tab, Yellow, Oval, Scored, Film Coated	Oxcarbazepine 300 mg	Trileptal by Novartis	Canadian DIN 02244068	Anticonvulsant
CGCG <> TFTF	Tab, Light Pink, Oval, Scored, Film Coated	Oxcarbazepine 600 mg	Trileptal by Novartis	Canadian DIN 02242069	Anticonvulsant
CGCG <> TFTF	Tab, Light Pink, Oval, Scored, Film Coated	Oxcarbazepine 600 mg	Trileptal by Novartis	00078-0457	Anticonvulsant
CGCS	Cap, Brown & Red, CG/CS	Rifampin 300 mg	Rifadin by Novartis	Canadian	Antibiotic
CGFXF	Cap, Clear, Gelatin w/ White Powder	Formoterol Fumarate 12 mg	Foradil by Novartis	Canadian DIN 02230898	Antiasthmatic
CGFZF	Cap, Pink & Gray, Black Print, Opaque, CG over FZF	Valsartan 80 mg	Diovan by Novartis	Canadian DIN 02236808	Antihypertensive
CGFZF	Cap, Pink & Gray, Black Print, Opaque, CG over FZF	Valsartan 80 mg	Diovan by Novartis	00083-4000	Antihypertensive
CGGOG	Cap, Gray & Pink, White Print, Opaque, CG over GOG	Valsartan 160 mg	Diovan by Novartis	Canadian DIN 02236809	Antihypertensive
CGGOG	Cap, Gray & Pink, White Print, Opaque, CG over GOG	Valsartan 160 mg	Diovan by Novartis	00083-4001	Antihypertensive
CGGOG	Cap	Valsartan 160 mg	Diovan by Novartis	17088-4001	Antihypertensive
CGJZ	Cap, Brown & Red, CG/JZ	Rifampin 150 mg	Rifadin by Novartis	Canadian	Antibiotic
CGLV	Tab, Light Yellow, Oblong, CG/LV	Benazepril HCl 5 mg	Lotensin by Novartis	Canadian	Antihypertensive
CGPI40	Cap, Beige, Opaque	Doxycycline 40 mg	Oracea by Collagenex	64682-0009	Antibiotic

ID FRONT <> BACK	DESCRIPTION FRONT <> BACK	INGREDIENT & STRENGTH	BRAND (or Generic Equiv.) by FIRM	NDC#	CLASS; SCH.
CH	Cap, Yellow, CH over Abbott Logo (a)	Pentobarbital Sodium 100 mg	Nembutal by Abbott	00074-3114 Discontinued	Sedative/Hypnotic; C II
CH <> NVR	Tab, White to Yellowish, Round, Marbled	Everolimus 0.5 mg	Zortress by Novartis Consumer Health, Inc.	00078-0414	Immunosuppressant
CHEMET100	Cap, Filled with White Beads	Succimer 100 mg	Chemet by Sanofi	00024-0333	Chelating Agent
CHEMET100	Cap, Filled with White Beads	Succimer 100 mg	Chemet by Ovation	67386-0201	Chelating Agent
CHEW <> CENTRUM	Tab, Orange, Oval, Chewable	Vitamin A 3500 IU, Vitamin C 60 mg, Vitamin D 400 IU, Vitamin E 30 IU, Vitamin K 10 mcg, Thiamin 1.5 mg, Riboflavin 1.7 mg, Niacin 20 mg, Vitamin B6 2 mg, Folic Acid 400 mcg, Vitamin B12 6 mcg, Biotin 45 mcg, Pantothenic Acid 10 mg, Calcium 108 mg, Iron 18 mg, Phosphorus 50 mg, Iodine 150 mcg, Magnesium 40 mg, Zinc 15 mg, Copper 2 mg, Manganese 1 mg, Chromium 20 mcg, Molybdenum 20 mcg	Centrum Advanced Formula by Wyeth		Vitamin
CHEW <> DURA	Tab, Chewable	Chlorpheniramine Maleate 2 mg, Methscopolamine Nitrate 1.25 mg, Phenylephrine HCl 10 mg	D A Chewable by Anabolic	00722-6219	Cold Remedy
CHEWEZ	Tab, Chewable, Chew over EZ <> Abbott Logo	Erythromycin Ethylsuccinate	by Quality Care	60346-0032	Antibiotic
CHEWEZ <> A	Tab, White, Round, Scored, Chewable, Abbott Logo (a)	Erythromycin 200 mg	EryPed Chewable by Abbott	00074-6314 Discontinued	Antibiotic
CHICKENFOOTPRINT	Tab, White, Round, W/ logo	3,4-Methylenedioxymethamphetamine (MDMA)	Ecstasy by Illegal		Euphoric; Illicit
CHLORAFEDHS-ROBERTS135	Cap, White Beads, Black Print	Chlorpheniramine Maleate 4 mg, Pseudoephedrine HCl 60 mg	Chlorafed by Roberts		Cold Remedy
CHLORAFED-ROBERTS136	Cap, Black Print, White Beads	Chlorpheniramine Maleate 8 mg, Pseudoephedrine HCl 120 mg	Chlorafed by Roberts		Cold Remedy
CHX05 <> PFIZER	Tab, White to Off-White, Film Coated, CHX 0.5	Varenicline 0.5 mg	Chantix by Pfizer	00069-0471; 00069-0469	Smoking Cessation
CHX05 <> PFIZER	Tab, White to Off-White, Film Coated, CHX 0.5	Varenicline 0.5 mg	Champix by Pfizer	Canadian DIN 02291177	Smoking Cessation
CHX05 <> PFIZER	Tab, White to Off-White, Film Coated, CHX 0.5	Varenicline 0.5 mg	Chantix by Pfizer	00069-0468	Smoking Cessation
CHX10 <> PFIZER	Tab, Light Blue, Cap Shaped, Film Coated, CHX 1.0	Varenicline 1 mg	Champix by Pfizer	Canadian DIN 02291185	Smoking Cessation
CHX10 <> PFIZER	Tab, Light Blue, Cap Shaped, Film Coated, CHX 1.0	Varenicline 1 mg	Chantix by Pfizer	00069-0469; 00069-0471	Smoking Cessation
CI1 <> G	Tab, Yellow, Oval, Scored	Cilazapril 1 mg	Inhibace by Genpharm	Canadian DIN 02283778	Antihypertensive
CI10 <> APO	Tab, Beige-Pink, Oval	Citalopram HBr 10 mg	Celexa by Apotex	60505-2518	Antidepressant
CI10G	Tab, Yellow, Triangular, CI/10/G	Clomipramine HCl 10 mg	Gen Clomipramine by Genpharm	Canadian	OCD
CI20 <> APO	Tab, Pink, Oval	Citalopram HBr 20 mg	Celexa by Apotex	60505-2519	Antidepressant
CI25 <> G	Tab, Pinkish Brown, Oval, Scored, CI / 2.5	Cilazapril 2.5 mg	Inhibace by Genpharm	Canadian DIN 02283786	Antihypertensive
CI25G	Tab, Yellow, Biconvex, CI/25/G	Clomipramine HCl 25 mg	Gen Clomipramine by Genpharm	Canadian	OCD
CI40 <> APO	Tab, White, Oval	Citalopram HBr 40 mg	Celexa by Apotex	60505-2520	Antidepressant
CI5 <> G	Tab, Reddish Brown, Oval, Scored, CI / 5	Cilazapril 5 mg	Inhibace by Genpharm	Canadian DIN 02283794	Antihypertensive
CI50G	Tab, White, Biconvex, CI/50/G	Clomipramine HCl 50 mg	Gen Clomipramine by Genpharm	Canadian	OCD
CIBA <> 110	Tab, Orange, Oval, Scored	Maprotiline 25 mg	Ludiomil by Ciba	00083-0110	Antidepressant
CI10G	Tab, Orange, Oval, Scored	Maprotiline HCl 25 mg	by Novartis		Antidepressant
CIBA <> 16	Tab, White, Round, Film Coated	Methylphenidate HCl 20 mg	Ritalin by Novartis	Canadian DIN 00632775	Stimulant; C II
CIBA <> 16	Tab, White, Round, Coated	Methylphenidate HCl 20 mg	Ritalin by Caremark	00339-4084	Stimulant; C II
CIBA <> 16	Tab, White, Round, Coated	Methylphenidate HCl 20 mg	Ritalin SR by Novartis	00083-0016	Stimulant; C II
CIBA <> 26	Tab, Orange, Round, Scored	Maprotiline 50 mg	Ludiomil by Ciba		Antidepressant
CIBA <> 26	Tab, Orange, Round, Scored	Maprotiline HCl 50 mg	by Novartis	00083-0026	Antidepressant

ID FRONT <> BACK	DESCRIPTION FRONT <> BACK	INGREDIENT & STRENGTH	BRAND (or Generic Equiv.) by FIRM	NDC#	CLASS; SCH.
CIBA <> 3	Tab, Pale Green, Round, Scored	Methylphenidate HCl 10 mg	Ritalin by Caremark	00339-4083	Stimulant; C II
CIBA <> 3	Tab, Pale Green, Round, Scored	Methylphenidate HCl 10 mg	Ritalin by Novartis	00083-0003	Stimulant; C II
CIBA <> 34	Tab, Pale Yellow, Round, Scored	Methylphenidate HCl 20 mg	Ritalin by Novartis	00083-0034	Stimulant; C II
CIBA <> 34	Tab, Pale Yellow, Round, Scored	Methylphenidate HCl 20 mg	Ritalin by Physician Total Care	54868-2762	Stimulant; C II
CIBA <> 34	Tab, Pale Yellow, Round, Scored	Methylphenidate HCl 20 mg	Ritalin by Caremark	00339-4085	Stimulant; C II
CIBA <> 46	Tab, Tan, Round, Scored	Hydrochlorothiazide 50 mg	Esidrix by Ciba	14656-0046	Diuretic; Antihypertensive
CIBA <> 7	Tab, Yellow, Round	Methylphenidate HCl 5 mg	by Caremark	00339-4082	Stimulant; C II
CIBA <> 7	Tab, Yellow, Round	Methylphenidate HCl 5 mg	Ritalin by Novartis	00083-0007	Stimulant; C II
CIBA <> A1	Tab, White, Round, Film Coated, Scored	Oxprenolol HCl 40 mg	Trasicor by Novartis	Canadian DIN 00402575	Antihypertensive
CIBA <> AB	Tab, Pale Blue, Round, Scored	Methylphenidate HCl 10 mg	Ritalin by Novartis	Canadian DIN 00005606	Stimulant; C II
CIBA <> CO	Tab, Cream, Round, Film Coated	Maprotiline 10 mg	Ludiomil by Ciba	Canadian DIN 00641855	Antidepressant
CIBA <> DP	Tab, Brownish-Orange, Round, Film Coated	Maprotiline 25 mg	Ludiomil by Ciba	Canadian DIN 00360481	Antidepressant
CIBA <> ER	Tab, Brownish-Yellow, Round, Film Coated	Maprotiline 50 mg	Ludiomil by Ciba	Canadian DIN 00360503	Antidepressant
CIBA <> FA	Tab, White, Scored	Hydralazine HCl 10 mg	Apresoline by Novartis	Canadian DIN 00005525	Antihypertensive
CIBA <> GF	Tab, Blue, Round, Coated	Hydralazine HCl 25 mg	Apresoline by Novartis	Canadian DIN 00005533	Antihypertensive
CIBA <> HG	Tab, Pink, Round, Coated	Hydralazine HCl 50 mg	Apresoline by Novartis	Canadian DIN 00005541	Antihypertensive
CIBA <> NR	Tab, Tan, Round	Ferrous Sulfate (Dried) 160 mg	Slow FE by Novartis	00067-0125	Supplement
CIBA <> PN	Tab, Pale Yellow, Round, Scored	Methylphenidate HCl 20 mg	Ritalin by Novartis	Canadian DIN 00005614	Stimulant; C II
CIBA101	Tab, Peach, Round	Hydralazine HCl 100 mg	Apresoline by Ciba		Antihypertensive
CIBA103	Tab, White, Round	Guanethidine Monosulfate 25 mg	Ismil by Ciba		Antihypertensive
CIBA104	Tab, Yellow, Round	Reserpine 0.2 mg, Hydralazine HCl 50 mg	Serpasil-Apresoline2 by Ciba		Antihypertensive
CIBA129	Tab, Orange, Round	Hydralazine 25 mg, Hydrochlorothiazide 15 mg	Apresoline-Esidrix by Ciba		Antihypertensive; Diuretic
CIBA13	Tab, Orange, Round	Reserpine 0.1 mg, Hydrochlorothiazide 25 mg	Hydropres-25 by Ciba		Antihypertensive; Diuretic
CIBA130	Tab, White, Round, Ciba/130	Metyrapone 250 mg	Metopirone by Ciba	Canadian	Diagnostic
CIBA130	Tab, White, Round	Metyrapone 250 mg	Metopirone by Ciba		Diagnostic
CIBA135	Tab, White, Oval	Maprotiline 75 mg	Ludiomil by Ciba	00083-0135	Antidepressant
CIBA154	Cap, Caramel & Red, White Print, Ciba over 154	Rifampin 300 mg	by Sandoz	00781-2018	Antibiotic
CIBA154	Cap, Caramel & Red, White Print, Ciba over 154	Rifampin 300 mg	Rimactane by Ciba	14656-0154	Antibiotic
CIBA154	Cap, Caramel & Red, White Print, Ciba over 154	Rifampin 300 mg	Rimactane by Novartis	17088-7189	Antibiotic
CIBA154	Cap, Caramel & Red, White Print, Ciba over 154	Rifampin 300 mg	by Novartis	00083-0154	Antibiotic
CIBA16	Tab, White, Round	Methylphenidate HCl 20 mg	Ritalin SR by Novartis	00083-0016	Stimulant; C II
CIBA16	Tab, White, Round	Methylphenidate HCl 20 mg	Ritalin SR by Caremark	00339-4084	Stimulant; C II
CIBA165	Tab, Orange, Round	Potassium Chloride 600 mg (8 mEq)	Slow K by Ciba		Electrolytes
CIBA192	Tab, Blue, Round	Hydrochlorothiazide 100 mg	Esidrix by Ciba		Diuretic; Antihypertensive
CIBA22	Tab	Hydrochlorothiazide 25 mg	Hydrodiuril by Ciba	14656-0022	Diuretic; Antihypertensive
CIBA24	Tab, White, Round, Scored	Aminoglutethimide 250 mg	Cytadren by Novartis	61615-0103	Sedative; C II
CIBA24	Tab, White, Round, Scored	Aminoglutethimide 250 mg	Cytadren by Ciba	00083-0024	Sedative; C II
CIBA30	Tab, White, Round	Methyltestosterone 10 mg	Metandren by Ciba		Hormone; C III
CIBA32	Tab, Yellow, Round	Methyltestosterone 25 mg	Metandren by Ciba		Hormone; C III

ID FRONT <> BACK	DESCRIPTION FRONT <> BACK	INGREDIENT & STRENGTH	BRAND (or Generic Equiv.) by FIRM	NDC#	CLASS; SCH.
CIBA34 <> CIBA34	Tab, Pale Yellow, Round, Scored	Methylphenidate HCl 20 mg	Ritalin SR by Physician Total Care	54868-2418	Stimulant; C II
CIBA35	Tab, White, Round	Reserpine 0.1 mg	Serpasil by Ciba		Antihypertensive
CIBA36	Tab, White, Round	Reserpine 0.25 mg	Serpasil by Ciba		Antihypertensive
CIBA37	Tab, Yellow, Round	Hydralazine HCl 10 mg	Apresoline by Ciba		Antihypertensive
CIBA39	Tab, Blue, Round	Hydralazine HCl 25 mg	Apresoline by Ciba		Antihypertensive
CIBA40	Tab, Yellow, Round	Reserpine 0.1 mg, Hydralazine HCl 25 mg	Serpasil-Apresoline1 by Ciba		Antihypertensive
CIBA47	Tab, White, Round	Guanethidine Monosulfate 10 mg, Hydrochlorothiazide 25 mg	Esimil by Ciba		Antihypertensive; Diuretic
CIBA49	Tab, Yellow, Round	Guanethidine Monosulfate 10 mg	Esimil by Ciba		Antihypertensive
CIBA51	Tab, White, Oval	Methyltestosterone Sublingual 5 mg	Metandren Linguets by Ciba		Hormone; C III
CIBA64	Tab, Yellow, Oval	Methyltestosterone Sublingual 10 mg	Metandren Linguets by Ciba		Hormone; C III
CIBA65	Tab, Peach, Round	Lithium Carbonate 300 mg	Eskalith by Ciba		Antipsychotic
CIBA71	Tab, Pink, Round	Hydralazine 25 mg, Hydrochlorothiazide 15 mg, Reserpine 0.1 mg	Ser-Ap-Es by Ciba		Antihypertensive; Diuretic
CIBA73	Tab, Blue, Round	Hydralazine HCl 50 mg	Apresoline by Physician Total Care	54868-3369	Antihypertensive
CIBA97	Tab, Orange, Round	Reserpine 0.1 mg, Hydrochlorothiazide 50 mg	Hydropres-50 by Ciba		Antihypertensive; Diuretic
CIBAAC	Tab, Pink, Round, Ciba/AC	Reserpine 0.1 mg, Hydralazine 25 mg, Hydrochlorothiazide 15 mg	by Novartis	Canadian	Antihypertensive
CIBAAAC	Tab, Pink, Round, Ciba/AC	Reserpine Hydralazine HCl 15 mg	Ser-Ap-Es by Novartis	Canadian	Antihypertensive
CIBAAI	Tab, White, Round, Ciba/AI	Oxprenolol HCl 40 mg	Trasicor by Ciba	Canadian	Antihypertensive
CIBABNB	Tab, White, Round, Ciba/BNB	Oxprenolol HCl 160 mg	Slow-Trasicor by Ciba	Canadian	Antihypertensive
CIBACG	Tab, Light Yellow, Round, Ciba/CG	Oxprenolol HCl 80 mg	Trasicor by Ciba	Canadian	Antihypertensive
CIBACO	Tab, Cream, Round, Ciba/CO	Maprotiline 10 mg	Ludiomil by Novartis	Canadian	Antidepressant
CIBADP	Tab, Brown & Yellow, Round, Ciba/DP	Maprotiline 25 mg	Ludiomil by Novartis	Canadian	Antidepressant
CIBAFS	Tab, Brown & Red, Round, Ciba/FS	Maprotiline 75 mg	Ludiomil by Novartis	Canadian	Antidepressant
CIBAGG	Tab, White, Round, Ciba/GG	Aminoglutethimide 250 mg	Cytadren by Ciba	Canadian	Sedative; C II
CIBAJL	Tab, White, Round, Ciba/JL	Methyltestosterone 10 mg	Metandren by Novartis	Canadian	Hormone; C III
CIBAKM	Tab, White, Round, Ciba/KM	Methyltestosterone 25 mg	Metandren by Novartis	Canadian	Hormone; C III
CIBALJ	Tab, Blue, Round, Ciba/LJ	Tripelennamine HCl 50 mg	PBZ by Novartis	Canadian	Antihistamine
CIBASP	Tab, White, Round, Ciba/SP	Reserpine 0.25 mg	Serpasil by Ciba	Canadian	Antihypertensive
CIBATP	Tab, Yellow, Ciba/TP	Ferrous Sulfate 160 mg, Folic Acid 400 mcg	Slow-Fe Folic by Ciba	Canadian	Mineral
CIBATRASICOR20	Tab, White, Round, Ciba/Trasicor/20	Oxprenolol HCl 20 mg	Trasicor by Novartis	Canadian	Antihypertensive
CIBATRASICOR20	Tab, White, Round, Ciba/Trasicor 20	Oxprenolol HCl 20 mg	Trasicor by Ciba	Canadian	Antihypertensive
CIL1	Tab, Yellow, Oval, Scored	Cilazapril 1 mg	Inhibace by Roche	Canadian DIN 01911465	Antihypertensive
CIL100 <> APO	Tab, White, Round, CIL/100 <> APO	Cilostazol 100 mg	Pletal by Apotex	60505-2522	Antiplatelet
CIL25	Tab, Reddish Brown & Pink, Oval, Cil 2.5	Cilazapril 2.5 mg	Inhibace by Roche	Canadian DIN 01911473	Antihypertensive
CIL5	Tab, Reddish Brown, Oval	Cilazapril 5 mg	Inhibace by Roche	Canadian DIN 01911481	Antihypertensive
CIL50 <> APO	Tab, White, Round, CIL/50 <> APO	Cilostazol 50 mg	Pletal by Apotex	60505-2521	Antiplatelet
CIL5125	Tab, Pink, Oval, Scored	Cilazapril 5 mg, Hydrochlorothiazide 12.5 mg	Inhibace Plus by Roche	Canadian DIN 02181479	Antihypertensive
CIP250 <> APO	Tab, White to Off-White, Round, CIP over 250	Ciprofloxacin 250 mg	Cipro by Apotex	60505-1308	Antibiotic
CIP500 <> APO	Tab, White to Off-White, Cap Shaped	Ciprofloxacin 500 mg	Cipro by Apotex	60505-1309	Antibiotic
CIP750 <> APO	Tab, White to Off-White, Cap Shaped	Ciprofloxacin 750 mg	Cipro by Apotex	60505-1310	Antibiotic
CIPRO <> 100	Tab, Yellow, Round, Film Coated	Ciprofloxacin HCl 100 mg	by Compumed	00403-2558	Antibiotic
CIPRO <> 100	Tab, Yellow, Round, Film Coated	Ciprofloxacin HCl 100 mg	Ciprobay by Bayer	00026-8511	Antibiotic
CIPRO <> 250	Tab, White to Light Yellow, Round, Film Coated	Ciprofloxacin HCl 250 mg	Cipro by H J Harkins Co	52959-0171	Antibiotic
CIPRO <> 250	Tab, White to Light Yellow, Round, Film Coated	Ciprofloxacin HCl 250 mg	by Compumed	00403-4258	Antibiotic

ID FRONT <> BACK	DESCRIPTION FRONT <> BACK	INGREDIENT & STRENGTH	BRAND (or Generic Equiv.) by FIRM	NDC#	CLASS; SCH.
CIPRO <> 250	Tab, White to Light Yellow, Round, Film Coated	Ciprofloxacin HCl 250 mg	Cipro by Bayer	Canadian DIN 02155958	Antibiotic
CIPRO <> 250	Tab, White to Light Yellow, Round, Film Coated	Ciprofloxacin HCl 250 mg	Cipro by Direct Dispensing	57866-6250	Antibiotic
CIPRO <> 250	Tab, White to Light Yellow, Round, Film Coated	Ciprofloxacin HCl 250 mg	by Allscripts		Antibiotic
CIPRO <> 250	Tab, White to Light Yellow, Round, Film Coated	Ciprofloxacin HCl 250 mg	Cipro by Apotheca	12634-0423	Antibiotic
CIPRO <> 250	Tab, White to Light Yellow, Round, Film Coated	Ciprofloxacin HCl 250 mg	Ciprobay by Bayer	00026-8512	Antibiotic
CIPRO <> 250	Tab, White to Light Yellow, Round, Film Coated	Ciprofloxacin HCl 250 mg	Cipro by Pharmedix	53002-0279	Antibiotic
CIPRO <> 250	Tab, White to Light Yellow, Round, Film Coated	Ciprofloxacin HCl 250 mg	by Nat Pharmpak	55154-4806	Antibiotic
CIPRO <> 250	Tab, White to Light Yellow, Round, Film Coated	Ciprofloxacin HCl 250 mg	by Amerisource	62584-0335	Antibiotic
CIPRO <> 250	Tab, White to Light Yellow, Round, Film Coated	Ciprofloxacin HCl 250 mg	Cipro by Bayer	00085-1758	Antibiotic
CIPRO <> 500	Tab, White to Light Yellow, Oblong, Film Coated	Ciprofloxacin HCl 500 mg	Cipro by Bayer	00085-1754	Antibiotic
CIPRO <> 500	Tab, White to Light Yellow, Oblong, Film Coated	Ciprofloxacin HCl 500 mg	by St. Mary's Med	60760-0513	Antibiotic
CIPRO <> 500	Tab, White to Light Yellow, Oblong, Film Coated	Ciprofloxacin HCl 500 mg	Cipro by H J Harkins Co	52959-0036	Antibiotic
CIPRO <> 500	Tab, White to Light Yellow, Oblong, Film Coated	Ciprofloxacin HCl 500 mg	Ciprobay by Bayer	00026-8513	Antibiotic
CIPRO <> 500	Tab, White to Light Yellow, Oblong, Film Coated	Ciprofloxacin HCl 500 mg	by Amerisource	62584-0336	Antibiotic
CIPRO <> 500	Tab, White to Light Yellow, Oblong, Film Coated	Ciprofloxacin HCl 500 mg	Cipro by Rx Dispensing	61807-0035	Antibiotic
CIPRO <> 500	Tab, White to Light Yellow, Oblong, Film Coated	Ciprofloxacin HCl 500 mg	by Compumed	00403-4522	Antibiotic
CIPRO <> 500	Tab, White to Light Yellow, Oblong, Film Coated	Ciprofloxacin HCl 500 mg	by Med Pro	53978-3075	Antibiotic
CIPRO <> 500	Tab, White to Light Yellow, Oblong, Film Coated	Ciprofloxacin HCl 500 mg	by Nat Pharmpak	55154-4801	Antibiotic
CIPRO <> 500	Tab, White to Light Yellow, Oblong, Film Coated	Ciprofloxacin HCl 500 mg	by Physician Total Care	54868-0939	Antibiotic
CIPRO <> 500	Tab, White to Light Yellow, Oblong, Film Coated	Ciprofloxacin HCl 500 mg	by PDRX	55289-0371	Antibiotic
CIPRO <> 500	Tab, White to Light Yellow, Oblong, Film Coated	Ciprofloxacin HCl 500 mg	Cipro by Bayer	Canadian DIN 02155966	Antibiotic
CIPRO <> 500	Tab, White to Light Yellow, Oblong, Film Coated	Ciprofloxacin HCl 500 mg	by Allscripts		Antibiotic
CIPRO <> 750	Tab, White to Light Yellow, Oblong, Film Coated	Ciprofloxacin HCl 750 mg	Cipro by H J Harkins Co	52959-0037	Antibiotic
CIPRO <> 750	Tab, White to Light Yellow, Oblong, Film Coated	Ciprofloxacin HCl 750 mg	by Nat Pharmpak	55154-4807	Antibiotic
CIPRO <> 750	Tab, White to Light Yellow, Oblong, Film Coated	Ciprofloxacin HCl 750 mg	by Physician Total Care	54868-1184	Antibiotic
CIPRO <> 750	Tab, White to Light Yellow, Oblong, Film Coated	Ciprofloxacin HCl 750 mg	Cipro by Pharmedix	53002-0268	Antibiotic
CIPRO <> 750	Tab, White to Light Yellow, Oblong, Film Coated	Ciprofloxacin HCl 750 mg	Cipro by Bayer	Canadian DIN 02155974	Antibiotic
CIPRO <> 750	Tab, White to Light Yellow, Oblong, Film Coated	Ciprofloxacin HCl 750 mg	by Compumed	00403-4650	Antibiotic
CIPRO <> 750	Tab, White to Light Yellow, Oblong, Film Coated	Ciprofloxacin HCl 750 mg	Ciprobay by Bayer	00026-8514	Antibiotic
CIPRO <> 750	Tab, White to Light Yellow, Oblong, Film Coated	Ciprofloxacin HCl 750 mg	Cipro by Bayer	00085-1756	Antibiotic
CIPRO100	Tab, Yellow, Round, Film Coated	Ciprofloxacin HCl 100 mg	Cipro by Bayer	Canadian	Antibiotic
CIR3MG	Cap, Light Gray & Pink, Opaque	Budesonide 3 mg	Entocort by AstraZeneca	Canadian DIN 02229293	Steroid
CIS20JANSSEN	Tab, Beige & White, Circular, CIS/20/Janssen	Cisapride 20 mg	Propulsid by Janssen	Canadian	Gastrointestinal
CIS5JANSSEN	Tab, Beige & White, Circular, CIS/5/Janssen	Cisapride 5 mg	Propulsid by Janssen	Canadian	Gastrointestinal
CITRACAL <> 250	Tab, White, Modified Rectangle, Film Coated	Calcium Citrate 250 mg, Vitamin D 62.5 IU	Citracal 250 mg + D by Mission	00178-0837	Vitamin; Supplement
CITRACAL <> MPC	Tab, White, Barrel Shaped, Film Coated	Calcium Citrate 200 mg	Citracal by Mission	Canadian DIN 02150220	Vitamin; Supplement
CITRACAL <> MPC	Tab, White, Barrel Shaped, Film Coated	Calcium Citrate 200 mg	Citracal by Mission	00178-0800	Vitamin; Supplement
CITRACAL <> PLUS	Tab, White, Modified Rectangle, Film Coated	Calcium Citrate, Vitamin D, Magnesium	Citracal Plus by Mission	00178-0825	Vitamin; Supplement
CITRACALD	Tab, White, Cap Shaped, CITRACAL +D <> Score, Film Coated	Calcium Citrate 315 mg, Vitamin D 200 IU	Citracal +D by Mission	00178-0815	Vitamin; Supplement
CITRACALD	Tab, White, Cap Shaped, CITRACAL +D <> Score, Film Coated	Calcium Citrate 315 mg, Vitamin D 200 IU	Citracal +D by Mission	Canadian DIN 02150158	Vitamin; Supplement
CK	Tab, Pink, Round, Film Coated, CK inside a Hexagon	Drospirenone 0.5 mg, Estradiol 1 mg	Angeliq by Berlex	50419-0483	Hormone
CK	Tab, Pink, Round, Ck Logo	3,4-Methylenedioxymethamphetamine (MDMA)	Ecstasy by Illegal		Euphoric; Illicit
CL	Tab, Green & Light Green	Pentaerythritol Tetranitrate 80 mg	Peritrate by Parke Davis	Canadian	Antianginal

ID FRONT <> BACK	DESCRIPTION FRONT <> BACK	INGREDIENT & STRENGTH	BRAND (or Generic Equiv.) by FIRM	NDC#	CLASS; SCH.
CL	Tab, Green	Pentaerythritol Tetranitrate 80 mg	Peritrate by Parke Davis	Canadian	Antianginal
CL <> 020	Tab, White, Round	Colchicine 0.6 mg	Colchicine by Concord	20254-0020	Antigout
CL <> 3	Tab, White to Off-White, Rectangle, Sublingual	Nitroglycerin 0.3 mg	Nitrostat by Pliva	50111-0992	Vasodilator
CL <> 4	Tab, White to Off-White, Rectangle, Sublingual	Nitroglycerin 0.4 mg	Nitrostat by Pliva	50111-0989	Vasodilator
CL <> 6	Tab, White to Off-White, Rectangle, Sublingual	Nitroglycerin 0.6 mg	Nitrostat by Pliva	50111-0991	Vasodilator
CL <> 75	Tab, Reddish-Brown, Round, Film Coated	Clopidogrel 75 mg	Plavix by Apotex	60505-0253	Antiplatelet
CL <> NVR	Tab, White to Yellowish, Round, Marbled	Everolimus 0.75 mg	Zortress by Novartis Consumer Health, Inc.	00078-0415	Immunosuppressant
CL1	Tab, Yellow, Round, CL/1	Isosorbide Dinitrate SL 2.5 mg	Isordil by Sandoz		Antianginal
CL100 <> G	Tab, White, Round	Cilostazol 100 mg	Pletal by Andrx	62037-0541	Antiplatelet
CL125	Tab, White, Cylindrical, CL 12.5	Tetrabenazine 12.5 mg	Xenazine by Prestwick	18722-0001	Anti-Chorea Agent
CL15	Tab, White, Round	Nylidrin 12 mg	Arlidin by Sandoz		Vasodilator
CL2	Tab, Pinkish-Brown, Oval, Film-Coated, Scored	Cilazapril 2.5 mg	Inhibace by Cobalt	Canadian DIN 02285215	Antihypertensive
CL205	Tab, White, Round	Sodium Bicarbonate 5 g	by Rugby	00536-4540	Antacid
CL205	Tab, White, Round	Sodium Bicarbonate 5 g	by Concord	20254-0205	Antacid
CL206	Tab, White, Round, Scored	Sodium Bicarbonate 650 mg	Sodium Bicarbonate by URL	00677-0131	Antacid
CL209	Tab, Brown, Round	Senna Concentrate 187 mg	Senna-Gen by Concord		Gastrointestinal
CL215	Tab, Brown, Round	Sennosides 8.6 mg	Senokot by Rugby	00536-5904	Gastrointestinal
CL219	Tab, White, Round, CL 219 <> +	Guaifenesin 200 mg, Ephedrine 25 mg	by Concord		Cold Remedy
CL220 <> TCL081	Tab, Orange, Round	Sennosides 8.6 mg, Docusate Sodium 50 mg	Senokot-S by Ivax	00182-1113	Gastrointestinal
CL228	Tab, Orange, Round	Acetaminophen 325 mg, Phenyltoloxamine Citrate 30 mg	Percogesic by Rugby	00536-3014	Analgesic
CL25	Tab, Yellowish, Cylindrical	Tetrabenazine 25 mg	Xenazine by Prestwick	18722-0002	Anti-Chorea Agent
CL284	Tab, White, Round	Isoxsuprine HCl 20 mg	Vasodilan by Sandoz		Vasodilator
CL3	Tab, Reddish-Brown, Oval, Film-Coated, Scored	Cilazapril 5 mg	Inhibace by Cobalt	Canadian DIN 02285223	Antihypertensive
CL300	Cap, Maroon & White	Gemfibrozil 300 mg	by AltiMed	Canadian	Antihyperlipidemic
CL400	Tab, Beige, Black Print, Round, CL over 400	Ergotamine Tartrate 1 mg, Caffeine 100 mg	by Allscripts		Antimigraine
CL400	Tab, Beige, Black Print, Round, CL over 400	Caffeine 100 mg, Ergotamine Tartrate 1 mg	Cafergot by Sandoz	00781-1995	Antimigraine
CL50 <> G	Tab, White, Round	Cilostazol 50 mg	Pletal by Andrx	62037-0540	Antiplatelet
CL512	Cap, Green & Yellow	Nitroglycerin SR 9 mg	Nitrobid by Sandoz		Vasodilator
CL555	Tab, Lavender, Round, CL55/5	Trifluoperazine HCl 5 mg	Stelazine by Cord		Antipsychotic
CL564	Cap, Green, Clear	Niacin 250 mg	Niacin by Major	00904-0629	Vitamin
CL600	Tab, White	Gemfibrozil 600 mg	by AltiMed	Canadian	Antihyperlipidemic
CL75 <> APO	Tab, Pink, Round	Clopidogrel 75 mg	Plavix by Apotex		Antiplatelet
CLA250 <> APO	Tab, Pale Yellow, Oval	Clarithromycin 250 mg	Biaxin by Apotex	Canadian DIN 02274744	Antibiotic
CLA250 <> APO	Tab, Pale Yellow, Oval	Clarithromycin 250 mg	Biaxin by Apotex	60505-2616	Antibiotic
CLA500 <> APO	Tab, Pale Yellow, Cap Shaped	Clarithromycin 500 mg	Biaxin by Apotex	60505-2615	Antibiotic
CLA500 <> APO	Tab, Pale Yellow, Cap Shaped	Clarithromycin 500 mg	Biaxin by Apotex	Canadian DIN 02274752	Antibiotic
CLARITIN10 <> 458	Tab, White, Round, Claritin over 10	Loratadine 10 mg	Claritin by Nat Pharmpak	55154-3513	Antihistamine
CLARITIN10 <> 458	Tab, White, Round, Claritin over 10	Loratadine 10 mg	Claritin by Compumed	00403-4369	Antihistamine
CLARITIN10 <> 458	Tab, White, Round, Claritin over 10	Loratadine 10 mg	Claritin by Schering	00085-0458	Antihistamine
CLARITIN10 <> 458	Tab, White, Round, Claritin over 10	Loratadine 10 mg	Claritin by Amerisource	62584-0458	Antihistamine
CLARITIN10 <> 458	Tab, White, Round, Claritin over 10	Loratadine 10 mg	Claritin by Allscripts		Antihistamine
CLARITIN10 <> 458	Tab, White, Round, Claritin over 10	Loratadine 10 mg	Claritin by Direct Dispensing	57866-3500	Antihistamine
CLARITIN10 <> 458	Tab, White, Round, Claritin over 10	Loratadine 10 mg	Claritin by Urgent Care Center	50716-0267	Antihistamine
CLARITIN10 <> 458	Tab, White, Round, Claritin over 10	Loratadine 10 mg	Claritin by H J Harkins Co	52959-0452	Antihistamine

ID FRONT <> BACK	DESCRIPTION FRONT <> BACK	INGREDIENT & STRENGTH	BRAND (or Generic Equiv.) by FIRM	NDC#	CLASS; SCH.
CLARITIN10 <> 458	Tab, White, Round, Claritin over 10	Loratadine 10 mg	Claritin by Mylan	00378-3358	Antihistamine
CLARITIN10 <> 458	Tab, White, Round, Claritin over 10	Loratadine 10 mg	Claritin by Southwood	58016-0560	Antihistamine
CLARITIN10 <> 458	Tab, White, Round, Claritin over 10	Loratadine 10 mg	Claritin by Patient First	57575-0100	Antihistamine
CLARITIN10 <> 458	Tab, White, Round, Claritin over 10	Loratadine 10 mg	Claritin by Neuman	64579-0251	Antihistamine
CLARITIND	Tab, White, Green Print, Round, Film Coated, Ex Release	Loratadine 5 mg, Pseudoephedrine Sulfate 120 mg	Claritin D by Schering	00085-0635	Cold Remedy
CLARITIND	Tab, White, Green Print, Round, Film Coated, Ex Release	Loratadine 5 mg, Pseudoephedrine Sulfate 120 mg	Claritin D by Caremark	00339-6021	Cold Remedy
CLARITIND	Tab, White, Green Print, Round, Film Coated, Ex Release	Loratadine 5 mg, Pseudoephedrine Sulfate 120 mg	Claritin D by Allscripts		Cold Remedy
CLARITIND	Tab, White, Green Print, Round, Film Coated, Ex Release	Loratadine 5 mg, Pseudoephedrine Sulfate 120 mg	Claritin D by DRX	55045-2263	Cold Remedy
CLARITIND	Tab, White, Green Print, Round, Film Coated, Ex Release	Loratadine 5 mg, Pseudoephedrine Sulfate 120 mg	Claritin D by H J Harkins Co	52959-0443	Cold Remedy
CLARITIND	Tab, White, Green Print, Round, Film Coated, Ex Release	Loratadine 5 mg, Pseudoephedrine Sulfate 120 mg	Claritin D by Direct Dispensing	57866-3401	Cold Remedy
CLARITIND	Tab, White, Green Print, Round, Film Coated, Ex Release	Loratadine 5 mg, Pseudoephedrine Sulfate 120 mg	Claritin D by Compumed	00403-5323	Cold Remedy
CLARITIND12	Tab, White, Round, Film Coated, Ex Release	Loratadine 5 mg, Pseudoephedrine Sulfate 120 mg	Claritin D by Schering	11523-7162	Cold Remedy
CLARITIND24HOUR	Tab, White, Black Print, Oval, Film Coated, Claritin D over 24 HOUR	Loratadine 10 mg, Pseudoephedrine 240 mg	Claritin D 24 Hr by Murfreesboro	51129-1555	Cold Remedy
CLARITIND24HOUR	Tab, White, Black Print, Oval, Film Coated, Claritin D over 24 HOUR	Loratadine 10 mg, Pseudoephedrine Sulfate 240 mg	Claritin D 24 Hr by Schering	00085-1233	Cold Remedy
CLARITIND24HOUR	Tab, White, Black Print, Oval, Film Coated, Claritin D over 24 HOUR	Loratadine 10 mg, Pseudoephedrine Sulfate 240 mg	Claritin D 24 Hr by Caremark	00339-6110	Cold Remedy
CLARITIND24HOUR	Tab, White, Black Print, Oval, Film Coated, Claritin D over 24 HOUR	Loratadine 10 mg, Pseudoephedrine Sulfate 240 mg	Claritin D 24 Hr by Allscripts		Cold Remedy
CLARITIND24HOUR	Tab, White, Black Print, Oval, Film Coated, Claritin D over 24 HOUR	Loratadine 10 mg, Pseudoephedrine Sulfate 240 mg	Claritin D 24 Hr by Compumed	00403-0915	Cold Remedy
CLEOCIN150MG	Cap, Light Blue & Green	Clindamycin HCl 150 mg	Cleocin HCl by Pharmacia	00009-0225	Antibiotic
CLEOCIN300MG	Cap, Light Blue	Clindamycin HCl 300 mg	Cleocin HCl by Nat Pharmpak	55154-3923	Antibiotic
CLEOCIN300MG	Cap, Light Blue	Clindamycin HCl 300 mg	Cleocin HCl by Pharmacia	00009-0395	Antibiotic
CLEOCIN75MG	Cap, Green	Clindamycin HCl 75 mg	Cleocin HCl by Pharmacia	00009-0331	Antibiotic
CLIN150	Cap, Scarlet and Purple	Clindamycin HCl 150 mg	Dalacin C by Genpharm	Canadian DIN 02258331	Antibiotic
CLIN300	Cap, Light Blue	Clindamycin HCl 300 mg	Dalacin C by Genpharm	Canadian DIN 02258358	Antibiotic
CLINORIL <> MSD941	Tab, Bright Yellow, Hexagonal	Sulindac 200 mg	Clinoril by Merck	00006-0941	NSAID
CLINORIL <> MSD942	Tab, Bright Yellow, Hexagonal	Sulindac 200 mg	Clinoril by Merck	00006-0942	NSAID
CLINORIL <> MSD942	Tab, Bright Yellow, Hexagonal	Sulindac 150 mg	Clinoril by Merck	62904-0941	NSAID
CLINORIL <> MSD942	Tab, Bright Yellow, Hexagonal	Sulindac 200 mg	Clinoril by Merck	62904-0942	NSAID
CLL <> NVR	Tab, Pale Yellow, Oval, Film Coated	Aliskiren 150 mg, HCTZ 25 mg	Tekturna HCT by Novartis	00078-0522	Antihypertensive; Diuretic
CLO10 <> APO	Tab, White, Round, Scored, CLO / 10	Clobazam 10 mg	Frisium by Apotex	Canadian DIN 02244638	Anticonvulsant
CLOM25	Cap, Light Blue & Dark Blue, Black Print	Clomipramine HCl 25 mg	Anafranil by Taro	51672-4011	OCD
CLOM50	Cap, Yellow, Black Print	Clomipramine HCl 50 mg	Anafranil by Taro	51672-4012	OCD
CLOM75	Cap, White, Black Print	Clomipramine HCl 75 mg	Anafranil by Taro	51672-4013	OCD
CLOMID50	Tab, White, Round	Clomiphene Citrate 50 mg	Clomid by Merrell	00068-0226	Infertility
CLONAZEPAM	Tab, Blue, Round	Clonazepam 0.25 mg	Rivotril by Pharmascience	Canadian DIN 02179660	Sedative; C IV
CLONAZEPAM <> PMS05	Tab, Orange, Round, Scored, pms over 0.5	Clonazepam 0.5 mg	Rivotril by Pharmascience	Canadian DIN 02048701	Sedative; C IV
CLONAZEPAM <> PMS05	Tab, Orange, Round, Scored, pms over 0.5	Clonazepam 0.5 mg	Rivotril by Pharmascience	Canadian DIN 02207818	Sedative; C IV
CLONAZEPAM <> PMS10	Tab, Pink, Round, pms 1.0	Clonazepam 1 mg	Rivotril by Pharmascience	Canadian DIN 02048728	Sedative; C IV
CLONAZEPAM <> PMS20	Tab, White, Round, Scored, pms over 2.0	Clonazepam 2 mg	Rivotril by Pharmascience	Canadian DIN 02048736	Sedative; C IV

ID FRONT <> BACK	DESCRIPTION FRONT <> BACK	INGREDIENT & STRENGTH	BRAND (or Generic Equiv.) by FIRM	NDC#	CLASS; SCH.
CLOZARIL <> 100	Tab, Yellow, Round, Scored	Clozapine 100 mg	Clozaril by Dixon Shane	17236-0303	Antipsychotic
CLOZARIL <> 100	Tab, Yellow, Round, Scored	Clozapine 100 mg	Clozaril by Novartis	00078-0127	Antipsychotic
CLOZARIL <> 100	Tab, Yellow, Round, Scored	Clozapine 100 mg	Clozaril by Physician Total Care	54868-3576	Antipsychotic
CLOZARIL <> 100	Tab, Pale Yellow, Round, Scored	Clozapine 100 mg	Clozaril by Novartis	Canadian DIN 00894745	Antipsychotic
CLOZARIL <> 25	Tab, Yellow, Round, Scored	Clozapine 25 mg	Clozaril by Direct Dispensing	57866-4421	Antipsychotic
CLOZARIL <> 25	Tab, Yellow, Round, Scored	Clozapine 25 mg	by Nat Pharmpak	55154-3412	Antipsychotic
CLOZARIL <> 25	Tab, Yellow, Round, Scored	Clozapine 25 mg	Clozaril by Novartis	Canadian DIN 00894737	Antipsychotic
CLOZARIL <> 25	Tab, Yellow, Round, Scored	Clozapine 25 mg	Clozaril by Novartis	00078-0126	Antipsychotic
CLOZARIL <> 25	Tab, Yellow, Round, Scored	Clozapine 25 mg	Clozaril by Dista Prod		Antipsychotic
CM20 <> G	Tab, White, Oval, Scored, Film Coated	Citalopram 20 mg	Celexa by Genpharm	Canadian DIN 02246594	Antidepressant
CM300 <> G	Tab, Light Green, Round, Film Coated	Cimetidine 300 mg	Tagamet by Genpharm	Canadian DIN 02227444	Gastrointestinal
CM40 <> G	Tab, White, Oval, Scored, Film Coated	Citalopram 40 mg	Celexa by Genpharm	Canadian DIN 02246595	Antidepressant
CM400 <> G	Tab, Light Green, Elliptical, Film Coated	Cimetidine 400 mg	Tagamet by Genpharm	Canadian DIN 02227452	Gastrointestinal
CM600 <> G	Tab, Light Green, Elliptical, Film Coated	Cimetidine 600 mg	Tagamet by Genpharm	Canadian DIN 02227460	Gastrointestinal
CM800 <> G	Tab, Light Green, Elliptical, Film Coated	Cimetidine 800 mg	Tagamet by Genpharm	Canadian DIN 02227479	Gastrointestinal
CN	Tab, White, Oval, Film-Coated, Scored	Citalopram 20 mg	Celexa by Lundbeck	Canadian DIN 02239607	Antidepressant
CN	Tab, White, Oval, Film-Coated Scored	Citalopram 40 mg	Celexa by Lundbeck	Canadian DIN 02239608	Antidepressant
CN05 <> G	Tab, Light Yellow, Round, Scored, CN/0.5	Clonazepam 0.5 mg	Klonopin by Alphapharm	57315-0017	Sedative; C IV
CN05 <> G	Tab, Light Yellow, Round, Scored, CN/0.5	Clonazepam 0.5 mg	Klonopin by Par	49884-0495	Sedative; C IV
CN1 <> G	Tab, Yellow, Round, Scored	Clonazepam 1 mg	Klonopin by Par	49884-0496	Sedative; C IV
CN1 <> G	Tab, Yellow, Round, Scored	Clonazepam 1 mg	Klonopin by Alphapharm	57315-0018	Sedative; C IV
CN2 <> G	Tab, White, Round, Scored	Clonazepam 2 mg	Klonopin by Alphapharm	57315-0019	Sedative; C IV
CN2 <> G	Tab, White, Round, Scored	Clonazepam 2 mg	Klonopin by Par	49884-0497	Sedative; C IV
CN90	Tab, White, Oval, Scored	Vitamin C 120 mg, Calcium 200 mg, Iron 90 mg, Vitamin D3 400 IU, Vitamin E 30 IU, Thiamin 3 mg, Riboflavin 3.4 mg, Niacinamide 20 mg, Vitamin B6 20 mg, Folic Acid 1 mg, Iodine 150 mcg, Zinc 25 mg, Copper 2 mg, Docusate Sodium 50 mg, Docosahexaenoic acid (DHA) 250 mg, Eicosapentaenoic Acid (EPA) not more than 0.625 mg	CitraNatal 90 DHA by Mission	00178-0885 Discontinued	Vitamin
CN90 <> 0829	Tab, White, Oval, Scored, 08 / 29	Vitamin C 120 mg, Calcium 160 mg, Iron 90 mg, Vitamin D3 400 IU, Vitamin E 30 IU, Thiamin 3 mg, Riboflavin 3.4 mg, Niacinamide 20 mg, Vitamin B6 20 mg, Folic Acid 1 mg, Iodine 150 mcg, Zinc 25 mg, Copper 2 mg, Docusate Sodium 50 mg	CitraNatal 90 DHA by Mission	00178-0829	Vitamin
CNIGHT	Tab, Blue, C-Night	Acetaminophen 650 mg, Pseudoephedrine HCl 60 mg, Diphenhydramine HCl 50 mg	Contac Night Allergy Relief by SKB	Canadian	Cold Remedy
CNRX	Tab, White, Oval, Scored	Vitamin C 120 mg, Calcium 125 mg, Iron 27 mg, Vitamin D3 400 IU, Vitamin E 30 IU, Thiamin 3 mg, Riboflavin 3.4 mg, Niacinamide 20 mg, Vitamin B6 20 mg, Folic Acid 1 mg, Iodine 150 mcg, Zinc 25 mg, Copper 2 mg, Docusate Sodium 50 mg	CitraNatal DHA by Mission	00178-0898	Vitamin; Supplement

ID FRONT <> BACK	DESCRIPTION FRONT <> BACK	INGREDIENT & STRENGTH	BRAND (or Generic Equiv.) by FIRM	NDC#	CLASS; SCH.
CNRX	Tab, White, Oval, Scored	Vitamin C 120 mg, Calcium 125 mg, Iron 27 mg, Vitamin D3 400 IU, Vitamin E 30 IU, Thiamin 3 mg, Riboflavin 3.4 mg, Niacinamide 20 mg, Vitamin B6 20 mg, Folic Acid 1 mg, Iodine 150 mg, Zinc 25 mg, Copper 2 mg, Docusate Sodium 50 mg	CitraNatal Rx by Mission	00178-0859	Vitamin; Supplement
CO <> CIBA	Tab, Cream, Round, Film Coated	Maprotiline 10 mg	Ludiomil by Ciba	Canadian DIN 00641855	Antidepressant
COBALT LOGO <> 100	Tab, Pink, Trapezoidal, Cobalt Logo	Fluconazole 100 mg	Co Fluconazole by Cobalt	Canadian DIN 02281279	Antifungal
COBALTLOGO <> 50	Tab, Pink, Trapezoidal	Fluconazole 50 mg	Co Fluconazole by Cobalt	Canadian DIN 02281260	Antifungal
COGENTIN <> MSD60	Tab, White, Round	Benztropine Mesylate 2 mg	Cogentin by Merck	00006-0060	Antiparkinson
COGENTIN <> MSD635	Tab, White, Oval	Benztropine Mesylate 1 mg	Cogentin by Merck	00006-0635	Antiparkinson
COGNEX10	Cap, Bluish Green & Yellow, Black Print, Cognex over 10	Tacrine HCl 10 mg	Cognex by Horizon	59630-0190	Antialzheimers
COGNEX10	Cap, Bluish Green & Yellow, Black Print, Cognex over 10	Tacrine HCl 10 mg	Cognex by Parke Davis	00071-0096	Antialzheimers
COGNEX20	Cap, Bluish Green & Yellow, Black Print, Cognex over 20	Tacrine HCl 20 mg	Cognex by Parke Davis	00071-0097	Antialzheimers
COGNEX20	Cap, Bluish Green & Yellow, Black Print, Cognex over 20	Tacrine HCl 20 mg	Cognex by Horizon	59630-0191	Antialzheimers
COGNEX30	Cap, Orange & Yellow, Black Print, Cognex over 30	Tacrine HCl 30 mg	Cognex by Horizon	59630-0192	Antialzheimers
COGNEX30	Cap, Orange & Yellow, Black Print, Cognex over 30	Tacrine HCl 30 mg	Cognex by Parke Davis	00071-0095	Antialzheimers
COGNEX40	Cap, Lavender & Yellow, Black Print, Cognex over 40	Tacrine HCl 40 mg	Cognex by Parke Davis	00071-0098	Antialzheimers
COGNEX40	Cap, Lavender & Yellow, Black Print, Cognex over 40	Tacrine HCl 40 mg	Cognex by Horizon	59630-0193	Antialzheimers
COMHIST <> RPC066	Tab	Chlorpheniramine Maleate 2 mg, Phenylephrine HCl 10 mg, Phenyltoloxamine Citrate 25 mg	Comhist by Roberts	54092-0066	Cold Remedy
COMHISTLAROBERTS	Cap	Chlorpheniramine Maleate 4 mg, Phenylephrine HCl 20 mg, Phenyltoloxamine Citrate 50 mg	Comhist LA by Roberts	54092-0065	Cold Remedy
COMPOZ	Tab, White, Oblong	Diphenhydramine HCl 50 mg	Compoz by Medtech		Antihistamine
COMTAN	Tab, Brownish-Orange, Oval, Film Coated	Entacapone 200 mg	Comtan by Haines	59564-0197	Antiparkinson
COMTAN	Tab, Brownish-Orange, Oval, Film Coated	Entacapone 200 mg	Comtan by Novartis	00078-0327	Antiparkinson
COMTAN	Tab, Brownish-Orange, Oval, Film Coated	Entacapone 200 mg	Comtan by Halsey	00904-5171	Antiparkinson
COMTAN	Tab, Brownish-Orange, Oval, Film Coated	Entacapone 200 mg	Comtan by Novartis	Canadian DIN 02243763	Antiparkinson
CONTACT	Cap, Gray & Red	Chlorpheniramine Maleate 12 mg, Phenylpropanolamine 75 mg	Ornade by SKB	Canadian Discontinued	Cold Remedy
CONTACTC	Cap, Gray & White, Contact-C	Pseudoephedrine HCl 120 mg	by SKB	Canadian	Decongestant
COP <> 006	Tab, Pink, Round	Sodium Fluoride 1 mg	Luride by Colgate	00126-0006	Element
COP <> 014	Tab, Chewable	Sodium Fluoride 1.1 mg	Luride Half Strength by Colgate	00126-0014	Element
COP <> 186	Tab, Chewable	Fluoride Ion .25 mg	Luride by Colgate	00126-0186	Mineral
COPEY <> 150	Tab	Naproxen 500 mg	by Qualitest	00603-4732	NSAID
COPEY <> 443	Tab	Naproxen 375 mg	by Qualitest	00603-4731	NSAID
COPLEY <> 111	Tab, Yellowish Tan, Coated	Ascorbic Acid 120 mg, Beta-Carotene 4.2 mg, Calcium Carbonate 490.76 mg, Cholecalciferol 0.49 mg, Cupric Oxide 2.5 mg, Cyanocobalamin 12 mcg, Ferrous Fumarate 197.75 mg, Folic Acid 1 mg, Niacinamide 21 mg, Pyridoxine HCl 10.5 mg, Riboflavin 3.15 mg, Thiamine Mononitrate 1.575 mg, Vitamin A Acetate 8.4 mg, Vitamin E Acetate 44 mg, Zinc Oxide 31.12 mg	by Teva	38245-0111 Discontinued	Vitamin
COPLEY <> 113	Tab, Buff	Chlorpheniramine Tannate 8 mg, Phenylephrine Tannate 25 mg, Pyrilamine Tannate 25 mg	R-Tannate by Schein	00364-2196	Cold Remedy
COPLEY <> 114	Tab, Light Orange, Cap Shaped, Scored, Film Coated, Ex Release	Procainamide HCl 750 mg	Procan SR by Teva	00093-9114 Discontinued	Antiarrhythmic
COPLEY <> 114	Tab, Light Orange, Cap Shaped, Scored, Film Coated, Ex Release	Procainamide HCl 750 mg	Procan SR by Ivax	00182-1709	Antiarrhythmic

ID FRONT <> BACK	DESCRIPTION FRONT <> BACK	INGREDIENT & STRENGTH	BRAND (or Generic Equiv.) by FIRM	NDC#	CLASS: SCH.
COPLEY <> 114	Tab, Light Orange, Cap Shaped, Scored, Film Coated, Ex Release	Procainamide HCl 750 mg	Procan SR by Moore	00839-7029	Antiarrhythmic
COPLEY <> 114	Tab, Light Orange, Cap Shaped, Scored, Film Coated, Ex Release	Procainamide HCl 750 mg	Procan SR by Murfreesboro	51129-1174	Antiarrhythmic
COPLEY <> 1166	Tab, Orange, Pink & Purple, Chewable	Ascorbic Acid 34.5 mg, Cyanocobalamin 4.9 mcg, Folic Acid 0.35 mg, Niacinamide 14.17 mg, Pyridoxine HCl 1.1 mg, Riboflavin 1.26 mg, Sodium Ascorbate 32.2 mg, Sodium Fluoride 2.21 mg, Thiamine Mononitrate 1.15 mg, Vitamin A Palmitate 5.5 mg, Vitamin D 0.194 mg, Vitamin E Acetate 15.75 mg	Polyvitamin by Schein	00364-1075	Vitamin
COPLEY <> 136	Tab	Metoprolol Tartrate 50 mg	Lopressor by Teva	38245-0136	Antihypertensive
COPLEY <> 150	Tab, White, Oblong	Naproxen 500 mg	by Southwood	58016-0289	NSAID
COPLEY <> 150	Tab, Film Coated	Naproxen 550 mg	by Rx Dispensing	61807-0021	NSAID
COPLEY <> 150	Tab, Off-White, Cap Shaped	Naproxen 500 mg	by Teva	38245-0150	NSAID
COPLEY <> 150	Tab, White, Oblong	Naproxen 500 mg	by Nutramax	38206-0400	NSAID
COPLEY <> 152	Tab, Film Coated	Ascorbic Acid 200 mg, Biotin 0.15 mg, Calcium Pantothenate 27.17 mg, Chromic Chloride 0.51 mg, Cupric Oxide 3.75 mg, Cyanocobalamin 50 mcg, Ferrous Fumarate 82.2 mg, Folic Acid 0.8 mg, Magnesium Oxide 82.89 mg, Manganese 50 mg, Manganese Sulfate 15.5 mg, Niacinamide Ascorbate 400 mg, Pyridoxine HCl 30.25 mg, Riboflavin 20 mg, Thiamine Mononitrate 20 mg, Vitamin A Acetate 10.75 mg, Vitamin E Acetate 30 mg, Zinc Oxide 27.99 mg	Berplex Plus by Schein	00364-0814	Vitamin
COPLEY <> 152	Tab, Golden Yellow, Film Coated	Ascorbic Acid 200 mg, Biotin 0.15 mg, Calcium Pantothenate 27.17 mg, Chromic Chloride 0.51 mg, Cupric Oxide 3.75 mg, Cyanocobalamin 50 mcg, Ferrous Fumarate 82.2 mg, Folic Acid 0.8 mg, Magnesium Oxide 82.89 mg, Manganese 50 mg, Manganese Sulfate 15.5 mg, Niacinamide Ascorbate 400 mg, Pyridoxine HCl 30.25 mg, Riboflavin 20 mg, Thiamine Mononitrate 20 mg, Vitamin A Acetate 10.75 mg, Vitamin E Acetate 30 mg, Zinc Oxide 27.99 mg	by Teva	38245-0152 Discontinued	Vitamin
COPLEY <> 152	Tab, Yellow, Oval, Film Coated	Ascorbic Acid 200 mg, Biotin 0.15 mg, Calcium Pantothenate 27.17 mg, Chromic Chloride 0.51 mg, Cupric Oxide 3.75 mg, Cyanocobalamin 50 mcg, Ferrous Fumarate 82.2 mg, Folic Acid 0.8 mg, Magnesium Oxide 82.89 mg, Manganese 50 mg, Manganese Sulfate 15.5 mg, Niacinamide Ascorbate 400 mg, Pyridoxine HCl 30.25 mg, Riboflavin 20 mg, Thiamine Mononitrate 20 mg, Vitamin A Acetate 10.75 mg, Vitamin E Acetate 30 mg, Zinc Oxide 27.99 mg	B Complex Vit Plus by Teva	00093-9152	Vitamin
COPLEY <> 158	Tab, Chewable	Ascorbic Acid 34.5 mg, Cyanocobalamin 4.9 mcg, Folic Acid 0.35 mg, Niacinamide 14.16 mg, Pyridoxine HCl 1.1 mg, Riboflavin 1.2 mg, Sodium Ascorbate 32.2 mg, Sodium Fluoride 1.1 mg, Thiamine Mononitrate 1.15 mg, Vitamin A Acetate 5.5 mg, Vitamin D 0.194 mg, Vitamin E Acetate 15.75 mg	Polyvitamin by Schein	00364-1157	Vitamin
COPLEY <> 159	Tab, Chewable	Cholecalciferol 0.194 mg, Cupric Oxide 1.25 mg, Cyanocobalamin 4.9 mcg, Ferrous Fumarate 36.5 mg, Folic Acid 0.35 mg, Niacinamide 14.17 mg, Pyridoxine HCl 1.1 mg, Riboflavin 1.26 mg, Sodium Ascorbate 32.2 mg, Sodium Fluoride 2.21 mg, Thiamine Mononitrate 1.15 mg, Vitamin A Acetate 5.5 mg, Vitamin E 15.75 mg, Zinc Oxide 12.5 mg	Polyvitamin by Schein	00364-0770	Vitamin
COPLEY <> 165	Tab, Oval, White	Ascorbic Acid 17.53 mg, Beta-Carotene 0.56 mg, Calcium Carbonate 249.41 mg, Calcium Pantothenate 4.18 mg, Cholecalciferol 0.25 mg, Cupric Oxide 2.02 mg, Ferrous Fumarate 82.15 mg, Magnesium Oxide 82.93 mg, Niacinamide Ascorbate 8.54 mg, Pyridoxine HCl 2.43 mg, Riboflavin 0.84 mg, Thiamine Mononitrate 1 mg, Vitamin A Acetate 2680 Units, Zinc Oxide 15.56 mg	Enfamil Natalins by Teva	38245-0165 Discontinued	Vitamin

ID FRONT <> BACK	DESCRIPTION FRONT <> BACK	INGREDIENT & STRENGTH	BRAND (or Generic Equiv.) by FIRM	NDC#	CLASS; SCH.
COPLEY <> 165	Tab, Oval, White	Ascorbic Acid 17.53 mg, Beta-Carotene 0.56 mg, Calcium Carbonate 249.41 mg, Calcium Pantothenate 4.18 mg, Cholecalciferol 0.25 mg, Cupric Oxide 2.02 mg, Ferrous Fumarate 82.15 mg, Magnesium Oxide 82.93 mg, Niacinamide Ascorbate 8.54 mg, Pyridoxine HCl 2. 43 mg, Riboflavin 0.84 mg, Thiamine Mononitrate 1 mg, Vitamin A Acetate 2680 Units, Zinc Oxide 15.56 mg	Enfamil Natalins by Teva	00093-9165 Discontinued	Vitamin
COPLEY <> 188	Tab, Pink, Cap Shaped, Scored, Film Coated, Ex Release	Procainamide HCl 500 mg	Procan SR by Teva	00093-9188 Discontinued	Antiarrhythmic
COPLEY <> 188	Tab, Pink, Cap Shaped, Scored, Film Coated, Ex Release	Procainamide HCl 500 mg	Procan SR by URL Mutual	00677-0987	Antiarrhythmic
COPLEY <> 188	Tab, Pink, Cap Shaped, Scored, Film Coated, Ex Release	Procainamide HCl 500 mg	Procan SR by Moore	00839-7028	Antiarrhythmic
COPLEY <> 188	Tab, Pink, Cap Shaped, Scored, Film Coated, Ex Release	Procainamide HCl 500 mg	Procan SR by Qualitest	00603-5411	Antiarrhythmic
COPLEY <> 188	Tab, Pink, Cap Shaped, Scored, Film Coated, Ex Release	Procainamide HCl 500 mg	Procan SR by Ivax	00182-1708	Antiarrhythmic
COPLEY <> 197	Tab, Dark Red, Chewable	Ascorbic Acid 34.47 mg, Cholecalciferol 0.194 mg, Cupric Oxide 1.25 mg, Cyanocobalamin 4.9 mcg, Ferrous Fumarate 36.48 mg, Folic Acid 0.35 mg, Niacinamide 14.16 mg, Pyridoxine HCl 1.1 mg, Riboflavin 1.258 mg, Sodium Fluoride 1.1 mg, Thiamine Mononitrate 1.15 mg, Vitamin A Acetate 5.5 mg, Vitamin E Acetate 15.75 mg, Zinc Oxide 12.5 mg	Polyvitamin by Schein	00364-2506	Vitamin
COPLEY <> 217	Tab, White, Oval	Prenatal Vitamins	Prenatal Optima Tablet by Teva	00093-9217	Vitamin; Mineral
COPLEY <> 225	Tab, Film Coated	Potassium Chloride 600 mg	by Schein	00364-0861	Electrolytes
COPLEY <> 381381	Tab, Green, Hexagonal, Scored	Micronized Glyburide 3 mg	by Neuman	64579-0222	Antidiabetic
COPLEY <> 381381	Tab, Green, Hexagonal, Scored	Micronized Glyburide 3 mg	by Neuman	64579-0223	Antidiabetic
COPLEY <> 381381	Tab, Green, Hexagonal, Scored	Micronized Glyburide 3 mg	by Neuman	64579-0187	Antidiabetic
COPLEY <> 381381	Tab, Green, Hexagonal, Scored	Micronized Glyburide 3 mg	by Blue Ridge	59273-0017	Antidiabetic
COPLEY <> 381381	Tab, Green, Hexagonal, Scored	Micronized Glyburide 3 mg	by Kaiser	00179-1336	Antidiabetic
COPLEY <> 381381	Tab, Green, Hexagonal, Scored	Micronized Glyburide 3 mg	by Blue Ridge	59273-0016	Antidiabetic
COPLEY <> 381381	Tab, Green, Hexagonal, Scored	Micronized Glyburide 3 mg	by Teva	38245-0381	Antidiabetic
COPLEY <> 411	Tab, White, Square	Methazolamide 25 mg	Neptazane by Teva	38245-0411 Discontinued	Antiglaucoma Agent
COPLEY <> 417	Tab, Light Blue	Metoprolol Tartrate 100 mg	Lopressor by Teva	38245-0417	Antihypertensive
COPLEY <> 443	Tab, Off-White, Cap Shaped	Naproxen 375 mg	by Teva	38245-0443	NSAID
COPLEY <> 443	Tab, White, Oblong	Naproxen 375 mg	by Nutramax	38206-0201	NSAID
COPLEY <> 443	Tab, White, Oblong	Naproxen 375 mg	by Southwood	58016-0267	NSAID
COPLEY <> 643	Tab, Debossed	Prochlorperazine 5 mg	by Qualitest	00603-5418	Antiemetic
COPLEY <> 643	Tab, Film Coated	Prochlorperazine Maleate 8.26 mg	by H J Harkins Co	52959-0511	Antiemetic
COPLEY <> 643	Tab, Film Coated	Prochlorperazine Maleate 8.26 mg	by Teva	38245-0643	Antiemetic
COPLEY <> 652	Tab, Yellow, Round, Film Coated	Prochlorperazine Maleate 10 mg	by Kaiser	63304	Antiemetic
COPLEY <> 652	Tab, Yellow, Round, Film Coated	Prochlorperazine Maleate 10 mg	by Ranbaxy	54868-1082	Antiemetic
COPLEY <> 652	Tab, Yellow, Round, Film Coated	Prochlorperazine Maleate 16.53 mg	by Physician Total Care	38245-0652	Antiemetic
COPLEY <> 652	Tab, Yellow, Round, Film Coated	Prochlorperazine Maleate 16.53 mg	by Teva	38245-0652 Discontinued	Antiemetic
COPLEY <> 652	Tab, Yellow, Round, Film Coated	Prochlorperazine Maleate 16.53 mg	by H J Harkins Co	52959-0476	Antiemetic
COPLEY <> 652	Tab, Yellow, Round, Film Coated	Prochlorperazine 10 mg	by Qualitest	00603-5419	Antiemetic
COPLEY <> 652	Tab, Yellow, Round, Film Coated	Prochlorperazine Maleate 10 mg	by Teva	00093-9652	Antiemetic
COPLEY <> 712	Tab	Atenolol 50 mg	Tenormin by Teva	38245-0712	Antihypertensive
COPLEY <> 713	Tab	Atenolol 100 mg	Tenormin by Teva	38245-0713	Antihypertensive
COPLEY <> 725725	Tab, Pink, Hexagonal	Micronized Glyburide	by Neuman	64579-0206	Antidiabetic
COPLEY <> 725725	Tab, Pink, Hexagonal	Glyburide 1.5 mg	by Teva	38245-0725 Discontinued	Antidiabetic
COPLEY <> 725725	Tab, Pink, Hexagonal	Glyburide 1.5 mg	Micronized by Merrell	00068-3203	Antidiabetic
COPLEY <> 725725	Tab, Pink, Hexagonal	Glyburide 1.5 mg	by Blue Ridge	59273-0016	Antidiabetic
COPLEY <> 741	Tab, Light Blue, Film Coated	Naproxen 275 mg	by Teva	38245-0741	NSAID
COPLEY <> 744	Tab, Film Coated, Debossed	Naproxen 550 mg	by St. Mary's Med	60760-0744	NSAID

ID FRONT <> BACK	DESCRIPTION FRONT <> BACK	INGREDIENT & STRENGTH	BRAND (or Generic Equiv.) by FIRM	NDC#	CLASS; SCH.
COPLEY <> 744	Tab, Film Coated	Naproxen 550 mg	by Teva	38245-0744	NSAID
COPLEY0159	Tab, Square, Purple, Chewable	Cholecalciferol 0.194 mg, Cupric Oxide 1.25 mg, Cyanocobalamin 4.9 mcg, Ferrous Fumarate 36.5 mg, Folic Acid 0.35 mg, Niacinamide 14.17 mg, Pyridoxine HCl 1.1 mg, Riboflavin 1.26 mg, Sodium Ascorbate 32.2 mg, Sodium Fluoride 2.21 mg, Thiamine Mononitrate 1.15 mg, Vitamin A Acetate 5.5 mg, Vitamin E 15.75 mg, Zinc Oxide 12.5 mg	by Teva	00093-9159 Discontinued	Vitamin
COPLEY0519	Tab, Square	Vitamin and Fluoride Combination (Chewable) 1 mg	Poly-Vi-Flor by Copley		Vitamin
COPLEY107	Tab, Light Peach, Round, Chewable, Copley over 107	Mebendazole 100 mg	Vermox by Teva	00093-9107	Antihelmintic
COPLEY107	Tab, Light Peach, Round, Chewable, Copley over 107	Mebendazole 100 mg	Vermox by Teva	38245-0107	Antihelmintic
COPLEY107	Tab, Light Peach, Round, Chewable, Copley over 107	Mebendazole 100 mg	Vermox by DRX	55045-2742	Antihelmintic
COPLEY107	Tab, Light Peach, Round, Chewable, Copley over 107	Mebendazole 100 mg	Vermox by Physician Total Care	54868-3732	Antihelmintic
COPLEY111	Tab, Coated	Ascorbic Acid 120 mg, Beta-Carotene 4.2 mg, Calcium Carbonate 490.76 mg, Cholecalciferol 0.49 mg, Cupric Oxide 2.5 mg, Cyanocobalamin 12 mcg, Ferrous Fumarate 197.75 mg, Folic Acid 1 mg, Niacinamide 21 mg, Pyridoxine HCl 10.5 mg, Riboflavin 3.15 mg, Thiamine Mononitrate 1.575 mg, Vitamin A Acetate 8.4 mg, Vitamin E Acetate 44 mg, Zinc Oxide 31.12 mg	Prenatal 1 Mg Plus Iron by Ivax	00182-4463	Vitamin
COPLEY113	Tab, Buff	Chlorpheniramine Tannate 8 mg, Phenylephrine Tannate 25 mg, Pyrilamine Tannate 25 mg	R Tannate by Pharmedix	53002-0480	Cold Remedy
COPLEY113	Tab, Buff	Chlorpheniramine Tannate 8 mg, Phenylephrine Tannate 25 mg, Pyrilamine Tannate 25 mg	by Teva	38245-0113 Discontinued	Cold Remedy
COPLEY114	Tab, Buff, Film Coated	Procainamide HCl 750 mg	by Qualitest	00603-5412	Antiarrhythmic
COPLEY114	Tab, Buff, Film Coated	Procainamide HCl 750 mg	by URL Mutual	00677-0988	Antiarrhythmic
COPLEY117	Tab, Red, Cap Shaped, Scored, Film Coated, Ex Release	Procainamide HCl 1000 mg	Procan SR by Teva	00093-9117 Discontinued	Antiarrhythmic
COPLEY123	Tab, Purple, Round	Sodium Fluoride 0.5 mg	Luride by Copley		Element
COPLEY126	Tab, Pink, Oblong	Multivitamin, Folic Acid 500	Iberet Folic 500 by Copley		Vitamin
COPLEY131	Tab, Pink, Round, Chewable	Sodium Fluoride 2.2 mg	by Teva	00093-0131	Element
COPLEY131	Tab, Pink, Round, Chewable	Fluoride 1 mg	Luride by Teva	00093-9131	Mineral
COPLEY133	Tab, Pink, Round, Copley over 133	Amiodarone 200 mg	Cordarone by Teva	38245-0133 Discontinued	Antiarrhythmic
COPLEY133	Tab, Pink, Round, Scored	Amiodarone 200 mg	Cordarone by Apotheca	12634-0552	Antiarrhythmic
COPLEY133	Tab, Pink, Round, Scored, Copley over 133	Amiodarone 200 mg	Cordarone by Teva	38245-9133	Antiarrhythmic
COPLEY143	Tab, Aqua, Oblong	Salsalate 500 mg	Disalcid by Copley		NSAID
COPLEY144	Tab, Aqua, Oblong	Salsalate 750 mg	Disalcid by Copley		NSAID
COPLEY146	Tab, Off-White	Naproxen 250 mg	by Copley	38245-0146	NSAID
COPLEY146	Tab, Off-White, Round, Copley over 146	Naproxen 250 mg	by Teva	38245-0146	NSAID
COPLEY146	Tab	Naproxen 250 mg	by Qualitest	00603-4730	NSAID
COPLEY146	Tab, White, Round	Naproxen 250 mg	by Southwood	58016-0314	NSAID
COPLEY151	Tab, Green	B Complex Vitamins	Berocca by Copley		Vitamin
COPLEY158	Tab, Orange, Pink & Purple, Chewable	Ascorbic Acid 34.5 mg, Cyanocobalamin 4.9 mcg, Folic Acid 0.35 mg, Niacinamide 14.16 mg, Pyridoxine HCl 1.1 mg, Riboflavin 1.2 mg, Sodium Ascorbate 32.2 mg, Sodium Fluoride 1.1 mg, Thiamine Mononitrate 1.15 mg, Vitamin A Acetate 5.5 mg, Vitamin D 0.194 mg, Vitamin E Acetate 15.75 mg	Polyvitamin by Teva	00093-9158 Discontinued	Vitamin
COPLEY166	Tab, Orange, Pink & Purple, Square, Chewable	Ascorbic Acid 34.5 mg, Cyanocobalamin 4.9 mcg, Folic Acid 0.35 mg, Niacinamide 14.17 mg, Pyridoxine HCl 1.1 mg, Riboflavin 1.26 mg, Sodium Ascorbate 32.2 mg, Sodium Fluoride 2.21 mg, Thiamine Mononitrate 1.15 mg, Vitamin A Palmitate 5.5 mg, Vitamin D 0.194 mg, Vitamin E Acetate 15.75 mg	Polyvitamin by Teva	00093-9166 Discontinued	Vitamin

ID FRONT <> BACK	DESCRIPTION FRONT <> BACK	INGREDIENT & STRENGTH	BRAND (or Generic Equiv.) by FIRM	NDC#	CLASS; SCH.
COPLEY169	Tab, White, Oval	Prenatal Vitamin RX	Natalins RX by Copley	38245-0169	Vitamin
COPLEY170	Tab, Blue, Oblong	Prenatal Vitamin, Folic Acid	Pramet FA by Copley		Vitamin
COPLEY175	Tab, White Round, Film Coated, Ex Release, Copley over 175	Quinidine Sulfate 300 mg	Quinidex Extentabs by Teva	00093-9175	Antiarrhythmic
COPLEY176	Tab, Orange & Pink & Purple, Pillow	Triple Vitamins 1 mg, Fluoride 1 mg	Tri-Vi-Flor by Copley		Vitamin
COPLEY177	Tab, Blue, Round	Brompheniramine, Phenylephrine, Phenylpropanolamine	Dimetapp by Copley		Cold Remedy
COPLEY192	Tab, Blue, Oblong	Prenatal Vitamins, Zinc	Zenate by Copley		Vitamin
COPLEY197	Tab, Chewable	Ascorbic Acid 34.47 mg, Cholecalciferol 0.194 mg, Cupric Oxide 1.25 mg, Cyanocobalamin 4.9 mcg, Ferrous Fumarate 36.48 mg, Folic Acid 0.35 mg, Niacinamide 14.16 mg, Pyridoxine HCl 1.1 mg, Riboflavin 1.258 mg, Sodium Fluoride 1.1 mg, Thiamine Mononitrate 1.15 mg, Vitamin A Acetate 5.5 mg, Vitamin E Acetate 15.75 mg, Zinc Oxide 12.5 mg	by DRX	55045-1949	Vitamin
COPLEY197	Tab, Chewable	Ascorbic Acid 34.47 mg, Cholecalciferol 0.194 mg, Cupric Oxide 1.25 mg, Cyanocobalamin 4.9 mcg, Ferrous Fumarate 36.48 mg, Folic Acid 0.35 mg, Niacinamide 14.16 mg, Pyridoxine HCl 1.1 mg, Riboflavin 1.258 mg, Sodium Fluoride 1.1 mg, Thiamine Mononitrate 1.15 mg, Vitamin A Acetate 5.5 mg, Vitamin E Acetate 15.75 mg, Zinc Oxide 12.5 mg	by Teva	00093-0197 Discontinued	Vitamin
COPLEY206	Tab, Blue, Round	Amitriptyline HCl 10 mg	Elavil by Copley		Antidepressant
COPLEY207	Tab, Yellow, Round	Amitriptyline HCl 25 mg	Elavil by Copley		Antidepressant
COPLEY208	Tab, Beige, Round	Amitriptyline HCl 50 mg	Elavil by Copley		Antidepressant
COPLEY209	Tab, Orange, Round	Amitriptyline HCl 75 mg	Elavil by Copley		Antidepressant
COPLEY210	Tab, Pink, Round	Amitriptyline HCl 100 mg	Elavil by Copley		Antidepressant
COPLEY211	Tab, Blue, Oblong	Amitriptyline HCl 150 mg	Elavil by Copley		Antidepressant
COPLEY225	Tab, Orange, Round, Film Coated, Copley over 225	Potassium Chloride 600 mg	Slow-K by Murfreesboro	51129-8245	Electrolytes
COPLEY225	Tab, Orange, Round, Film Coated, Copley over 225	Potassium Chloride 600 mg	Slow-K by UDL	51079-0744	Electrolytes
COPLEY225	Tab, Orange, Round, Film Coated, Copley over 225	Potassium Chloride 600 mg	Slow-K by Pharmedix	53002-1039	Electrolytes
COPLEY225	Tab, Orange, Round, Film Coated, Copley over 225	Potassium Chloride 600 mg	Slow-K by Teva	00093-9225 Discontinued	Electrolytes
COPLEY225	Tab, Orange, Round, Film Coated, Copley over 225	Potassium Chloride 600 mg	Slow-K by URL Mutual	00677-1096	Electrolytes
COPLEY231	Tab, Peach, Oblong	Choline Magnesium Trisalicylate 500 mg	Trilisate by Copley		NSAID
COPLEY233	Tab, White, Oblong	Choline Magnesium Trisalicylate 750 mg	Trilisate by Copley		NSAID
COPLEY299-ACYCLOVIR200	Cap, Blue, Opaque	Acyclovir 200 mg	Zovirax by Teva	38245-0299	Antiviral
COPLEY301	Tab, Blue, Cap Shaped	Acyclovir 800 mg	Zovirax by Copley	38245-0310	Antiviral
COPLEY312	Tab	Captopril 50 mg	Capoten by Teva	38245-0312	Antihypertensive
COPLEY327	Tab, Blue, Round	Acyclovir 400 mg	Zovirax by Copley	38245-0327	Antiviral
COPLEY380-URSODIOL300MG	Cap, Red & White	Ursodiol 300 mg	by Teva	38245-0380	Gastrointestinal
COPLEY381	Tab, Green, Hexagonal	Glyburide 3 mg	Glynase by Copley	38245-0381	Antidiabetic
COPLEY381381	Tab	Glyburide 3 mg	by DRX	55045-2267	Antidiabetic
COPLEY411	Tab, White, Round	Methazolamide 25 mg	Neptazane by Qualitest	00603-4470	Antiglaucoma Agent
COPLEY424	Tab, White, Round	Methazolamide 50 mg	Neptazane by Qualitest	00603-4471	Antiglaucoma Agent
COPLEY424	Tab, White, Round	Methazolamide 50 mg	Neptazane by Teva	38245-0424	Antiglaucoma Agent
COPLEY427	Tab	Diclofenac Sodium 75 mg	by Teva	38245-0427	NSAID
COPLEY431	Tab	Diclofenac Sodium 25 mg	by Teva	38245-0431	NSAID
COPLEY447	Tab, Orange, Round	Iodinated Glycerol 30 mg	Organidin by Copley		Expectorant
COPLEY457	Tab, Orange, Oblong	Magnesium Gluconate	by Copley		Mineral

ID FRONT <> BACK	DESCRIPTION FRONT <> BACK	INGREDIENT & STRENGTH	BRAND (or Generic Equiv.) by FIRM	NDC#	CLASS; SCH.
COPLEY471	Tab	Captopril 25 mg	Capoten by Teva	38245-0471	Antihypertensive
COPLEY472	Tab, Peach, Round, Scored	Pemoline 75 mg	Pemoline by Pharmafab	62542-0410	Stimulant; C IV
COPLEY474	Tab	Diclofenac Sodium 50 mg	by Teva	38245-0474	NSAID
COPLEY474	Tab, Pink, Round	Diclofenac Sodium 50 mg	Diclofenac Sodium by H J Harkins Co	52959-0436	NSAID
COPLEY524	Tab, White, Round	Pemoline 37.5 mg	by Teva	38245-0577	Stimulant; C IV
COPLEY524	Tab, White, Round, Scored	Pemoline 37.5 mg	Pemoline by Pharmafab	62542-0453	Stimulant; C IV
COPLEY541	Tab, Peach, Round, Scored	Pemoline 18.75 mg	by Teva	38245-0541	Stimulant; C IV
COPLEY577	Tab, Yellow, Square, Scored, Chewable, 93 over 9577	Pemoline 37.5 mg	Cylert by Teva	00093-9577 Discontinued	Stimulant; C IV
COPLEY631	Tab	Diltiazem HCl 30 mg	Cardizem by Medirex	57480-0489	Antihypertensive
COPLEY631	Tab	Diltiazem HCl 30 mg	Cardizem by Sandoz	00781-1158	Antihypertensive
COPLEY631	Tab, Film Coated	Diltiazem HCl 30 mg	Cardizem by Qualitest	00603-3319	Antihypertensive
COPLEY631	Tab	Diltiazem HCl 30 mg	Cardizem by Teva	38245-0631	Antihypertensive
COPLEY653	Tab	Captopril 100 mg	Capoten by Teva	38245-0653 Discontinued	Antihypertensive
COPLEY662	Tab, White, Round Scored	Diltiazem HCl 60 mg	Cardizem by Medirex	57480-0490	Antihypertensive
COPLEY662	Tab, Film Coated, Copley 662	Diltiazem HCl 60 mg	Cardizem by Qualitest	00603-3320	Antihypertensive
COPLEY662	Tab	Diltiazem HCl 60 mg	Cardizem by Teva	38245-0662 Discontinued	Antihypertensive
COPLEY662	Tab, Film Coated	Diltiazem HCl 60 mg	Cardizem by Med Pro	53978-1235	Antihypertensive
COPLEY662	Tab	Diltiazem HCl 60 mg	Cardizem by Sandoz	00781-1159	Antihypertensive
COPLEY691	Tab, Film Coated, Copley 720	Diltiazem HCl 90 mg	Cardizem by Medirex	57480-0491	Antihypertensive
COPLEY691	Tab, Pale Blue	Diltiazem HCl 90 mg	Cardizem by Teva	38245-0691 Discontinued	Antihypertensive
COPLEY691	Tab	Diltiazem HCl 90 mg	Cardizem by Sandoz	00781-1174	Antihypertensive
COPLEY711 <> 8	Tab	Guanabenz Acetate 10.28 mg	by Teva	38245-0711 Discontinued	Antihypertensive
COPLEY717 <> 4	Tab	Guanabenz Acetate 5.14 mg	by Teva	38245-0717 Discontinued	Antihypertensive
COPLEY720	Tab, White, Cap Shaped, Film Coated, Scored	Diltiazem HCl 120 mg	Cardizem by Medirex	57480-0492	Antihypertensive
COPLEY720	Tab	Diltiazem HCl 120 mg	Cardizem by Teva	38245-0720	Antihypertensive
COPLEY720	Tab, Film Coated, Copley 720	Diltiazem HCl 120 mg	Cardizem by Qualitest	00603-3322	Antihypertensive
COPLEY720	Tab	Diltiazem HCl 120 mg	Cardizem by Sandoz	00781-1175	Antihypertensive
COPLEY724	Tab	Nadolol 80 mg	by Teva	38245-0724 Discontinued	Antihypertensive
COPLEY725	Tab, Pink, Hexagonal	Glyburide 1.5 mg	Glynase by Copley	38245-0725	Antidiabetic
COPLEY727	Tab	Nadolol 120 mg	by Teva	38245-0727 Discontinued	Antihypertensive
COPLEY731	Tab	Nadolol 160 mg	by Teva	38245-0731 Discontinued	Antihypertensive
COPLEY743	Tab	Captopril 12.5 mg	Capoten by Teva	38245-0743	Antihypertensive
COPLEY774	Tab, White, Cap Shaped, Film Coated, Copley over 774	Hydroxychloroquine Sulfate 201 mg	by Moore	00839-7963	Antimalarial
COPLEY774	Tab, White, Cap Shaped, Film Coated, Copley over 774	Hydroxychloroquine Sulfate 200 mg	by Physician Total Care	54868-3821	Antimalarial
COPLEY774	Tab, White, Cap Shaped, Film Coated, Copley over 774	Hydroxychloroquine Sulfate 200 mg	by Teva	38245-0774	Antimalarial
COPLEY774	Tab, White, Cap Shaped, Film Coated, Copley over 774	Hydroxychloroquine Sulfate 200 mg	by Murfreesboro	51129-1468	Antimalarial
COPLEY774	Tab, White, Cap Shaped, Film Coated, Copley over 774	Hydroxychloroquine Sulfate 200 mg	Plaquenil by Teva	00093-9774	Antimalarial
COR <> 111	Tab, Orange, Round, Film Coated	Rimantadine HCl 100 mg	Flumadine by Sandoz	00781-5029	Antiviral
COR <> 124	Tab, Light Yellow, Round, Scored	Glyburide 2.5 mg	Micronase by Ivax	00182-2646	Antidiabetic
COR <> 125	Tab, Light Green, Round, Scored	Glyburide 5 mg	Micronase by Ivax	00182-2647 Discontinued	Antidiabetic
COR <> 160	Tab, White, Round	Levocarnitine 330 mg	Carnitor by Rising	64980-0130	Supplement

ID FRONT <> BACK	DESCRIPTION FRONT <> BACK	INGREDIENT & STRENGTH	BRAND (or Generic Equiv.) by FIRM	NDC#	CLASS; SCH.
COR <> 201	Tab, White, Round, Coated	Ropinirole HCl 0.25 mg	Requip by CorePharma	64720-0201	Antiparkinson
COR <> 202	Tab, Yellow, Round	Ropinirole HCl 0.5 mg	Requip by CorePharma	64720-0202	Antiparkinson
COR <> 203	Tab, Green, Round, Coated	Ropinirole HCl 1 mg	Requip by CorePharma	64720-0203	Antiparkinson
COR103	Tab, White, Round	Carisoprodol 350 mg	Soma by Sandoz	00781-5005	Muscle Relaxant
COR106	Tab, White, Round, Scored	Tizanidine HCl 2 mg	Zanaflex by Deca	68552-0740	Muscle Relaxant
COR106	Tab, White, Round, Scored	Tizanidine HCl 2 mg	Zanaflex by Amneal	65162-0106	Muscle Relaxant
				Discontinued	
COR108	Tab, Yellow, Round, COR over 108	Salsalate 500 mg	by OHM		NSAID
COR116	Tab, White, Oval	Acetaminophen 650 mg	Tylenol Ex Strength by CorePharma		Analgesic
COR119	Tab, White, Round	Phenobarbital 30 mg	by OHM		Sedative/Hypnotic; C IV
COR123	Tab, White, Round, Scored	Glyburide 1.25 mg	Micronase by Sandoz	00781-1138	Antidiabetic
COR124	Tab, Yellow, Round, Scored	Glyburide 2.5 mg	Micronase by Sandoz	00781-1146	Antidiabetic
COR125	Tab, Light Green, Round, Scored	Glyburide 5 mg	Micronase by Sandoz	00781-1191	Antidiabetic
COR127	Tab, White, Round	Tramadol HCl 50 mg	Ultram by Deca	68552-0701	Analgesic
COR127	Tab, White, Round	Tramadol HCl 50 mg	Ultram by Amneal	65162-0127	Analgesic
COR128	Tab, White, Round, Scored	Pyridostigmine Bromide 60 mg	Mestinon by Sandoz	00781-5015	Muscle Stimulant
COR130	Tab, Blue, Round, Scored	Mixed Amphetamine Salts 5 mg; Amphetamine Aspartate 1.25 mg, Amphetamine Sulfate 1.25 mg, Dextroamphetamine Saccharate 1.25 mg, Dextroamphetamine Sulfate 1.25 mg	Adderall by Ranbaxy	63304-0908	Stimulant; C II
COR132	Tab, Blue, Round, Scored	Mixed Amphetamine Salts 10 mg; Amphetamine Aspartate 2.5 mg, Amphetamine Sulfate 2.5 mg, Dextroamphetamine Saccharate 2.5 mg, Dextroamphetamine Sulfate 2.5 mg	Adderall by Ranbaxy	63304-0909	Stimulant; C II
COR135	Tab, Pink, Round, Scored	Mixed Amphetamine Salts 20 mg; Amphetamine Aspartate 5 mg, Amphetamine Sulfate 5 mg, Dextroamphetamine Saccharate 5 mg, Dextroamphetamine Sulfate 5 mg	Adderall by Ranbaxy	63304-0910	Stimulant; C II
COR135	Tab, Pink, Round, Scored	Mixed Amphetamine Salts 20 mg; Amphetamine Aspartate 5 mg, Amphetamine Sulfate 5 mg, Dextroamphetamine Saccharate 5 mg, Dextroamphetamine Sulfate 5 mg	Adderall by CorePharma	64720-0135	Stimulant; C II
COR136	Tab, Pink, Round, Scored	Mixed Amphetamine Salts 30 mg; Amphetamine Aspartate 7.5 mg, Amphetamine Sulfate 7.5 mg, Dextroamphetamine Saccharate 7.5 mg, Dextroamphetamine Sulfate 7.5 mg	Adderall by Ranbaxy	63304-0911	Stimulant; C II
COR137	Tab, White, Round, Film Coated	Pilocarpine HCl 5 mg	Salagen by Sandoz	00781-5100	Cholinergic Agonist
COR138	Tab, White, Round, Scored	Tizanidine HCl 4 mg	Zanaflex by Deca	68552-0750	Muscle Relaxant
COR138	Tab, White, Round, Scored	Tizanidine HCl 4 mg	Zanaflex by Amneal	65162-0138	Muscle Relaxant
				Discontinued	
COR139	Tab, Peach, Oval, Scored, COR / 139	Methenamine Hippurate 1 g	Hiprex by Rising	64980-0119	Antibiotic; Urinary Tract
COR140	Tab, Light Yellow, Round	Glyburide 1.25 mg, Metformin 250 mg	Glucovance by Sandoz	00781-5170	Antidiabetic
COR141	Tab, Orange, Round	Glyburide 2.5 mg, Metformin 500 mg	Glucovance by Sandoz	00781-5171	Antidiabetic
COR142	Tab, Yellow, Round	Glyburide 5 mg, Metformin HCl 500 mg	Glucovance by Sandoz	00781-5172	Antidiabetic
COR143	Tab, White, Round	Benztropine Mesylate 0.5 mg	Congentin by Rising	64980-0111	Antiparkinson
COR144	Tab, White, Oval	Benztropine Mesylate 1 mg	Congentin by Rising	64980-0112	Antiparkinson
COR144	Tab, White, Oval	Benztropine Mesylate 1 mg	Congentin by Amneal	65162-0012	Antiparkinson
COR145	Tab, White, Round	Benztropine Mesylate 2 mg	Congentin by Rising	64980-0113	Antiparkinson
COR145	Tab, White, Round	Benztropine Mesylate 2 mg	Congentin by Amneal	65162-0016	Antiparkinson
COR150	Tab, White, Round	Cyproheptadine HCl 4 mg	Periactin by Rising	64980-0123	Antihistamine
COR152	Tab, White, Round, Film Coated	Doxycycline Hyclate 20 mg	Periostat by Sandoz	00781-5115	Antibiotic
COR153	Cap, Light Blue, Black Ink, COR / 153	Clindamycin HCl 150 mg	Cleocin HCl by Sandoz	00781-2112	Antibiotic
COR154	Cap, Light Blue, Black Ink, COR / 154	Clindamycin HCl 300 mg	Cleocin HCl by Sandoz	00781-2113	Antibiotic
COR155	Tab, White, Round	Glycopyrrolate 1 mg	Robinul by Rising	64980-0131	Gastrointestinal
COR156	Tab, White, Round	Glycopyrrolate 2 mg	Robinul by Rising	64980-0132	Gastrointestinal

ID FRONT <> BACK	DESCRIPTION FRONT <> BACK	INGREDIENT & STRENGTH	BRAND (or Generic Equiv.) by FIRM	NDC#	CLASS; SCH.
COR158	Tab, White, Round	Cilostazol 50 mg	Pletal by Sandoz	00781-5095	Antiplatelet
COR159	Tab, White, Round	Cilostazol 100 mg	Pletal by Sandoz	00781-5096	Antiplatelet
COR164	Tab, Pink, Round, Scored	Glimepiride 1 mg	Amaryl by Sandoz	00781-5045	Antidiabetic
COR164	Tab, White, Round, Scored	Benztropine Mesylate 0.5 mg	Cogentin by Major	00904-1055	Antiparkinson
COR165	Tab, Light Green, Round, Scored	Glimepiride 2 mg	Amaryl by Sandoz	00781-5046	Antidiabetic
COR166	Tab, Blue, Round, Scored	Glimepiride 4 mg	Amaryl by Sandoz	00781-5047	Antidiabetic
COR167	Tab, Pink, Round, Film Coated	Glipizide 2.5 mg, Metformin HCl 250 mg	Metaglip by Sandoz	00781-5304	Antidiabetic
COR168	Tab, Pink, Round, Film Coated	Glipizide 2.5 mg, Metformin HCl 500 mg	Metaglip by Sandoz	00781-5305	Antidiabetic
COR169	Tab, Pink, Round, Film Coated	Glipizide 5 mg, Metformin HCl 500 mg	Metaglip by Sandoz	00781-5306	Antidiabetic
COR170	Tab, Pink, Round, Film Coated, COR / 170	Citalopram HBr 10 mg	Celexa by Sandoz	00781-5157	Antidepressant
COR171	Tab, Pink, Round, Film Coated, Scored, COR / 171	Citalopram HBr 20 mg	Celexa by Sandoz	00781-5158	Antidepressant
COR172	Tab, White, Round, Film Coated, Scored, COR / 172	Citalopram HBr 40 mg	Celexa by Sandoz	00781-5159	Antidepressant
COR175	Tab, Yellow, Round	Meloxicam 7.5 mg	Mobic by Corepharma	00781-5195	NSAID
COR176	Tab, Pastel Yellow, Round	Meloxicam 15 mg	Mobic by Corepharma	00781-5196	NSAID
COR177	Cap, Dark Green, Opaque	Zonisamide 25 mg	Zonegran by Corepharma	64720-0177	Anticonvulsant
COR178	Cap, Dark Green and White, Opaque	Zonisamide 50 mg	Zonegran by Corepharma	64720-0178	Anticonvulsant
COR179	Cap, Orange and White, Opaque	Zonisamide 100 mg	Zonegran by Corepharma	64720-0179	Anticonvulsant
COR187	Tab, White, Round, COR / 187, Extended Release	Alprazolam 0.5 mg	Xanax XR by CorePharma	64980-0140	Antianxiety; C IV
COR188	Tab, Yellow, Round, COR / 188, Extended Release	Alprazolam 1 mg	Xanax XR by CorePharma	64980-0141	Antianxiety; C IV
COR189	Tab, Light Blue, Round, COR / 189, Ex Release	Alprazolam 2 mg	Xanax XR by CorePharma	64720-0189	Antianxiety; C IV
COR189	Tab, Light Blue, Round, COR / 189, Ex Release	Alprazolam 2 mg	Xanax XR by CorePharma	64980-0142	Antianxiety; C IV
COR190	Tab, Green, Round, COR / 190, Extended Release	Alprazolam 3 mg	Xanax XR by CorePharma	64980-0143	Antianxiety; C IV
COR204	Tab, Light Peach, Round	Ropinirole HCl 2 mg	Requip by CorePharma	64720-0204	Antiparkinson
COR205	Tab, Purple, Round	Ropinirole HCl 3 mg	Requip by CorePharma	64720-0205	Antiparkinson
COR206	Tab, Brown, Round, Coated	Ropinirole HCl 4 mg	Requip by CorePharma	64720-0206	Antiparkinson
COR207	Tab, Blue, Round, Coated	Ropinirole HCl 5 mg	Requip by CorePharma	64720-0207	Antiparkinson
CORGARD120MG <> BL208	Tab, Light Blue	Nadolol 120 mg	Corgard by King	00003-0208	Antihypertensive
CORGARD160MG <> BL246	Tab, Dark Blue	Nadolol 160 mg	Corgard by King	00003-0246	Antihypertensive
CORGARD160SQUIBB	Tab, Blue, Oblong, Corgard 160/Squibb	Nadolol 160 mg	Corgard by BMS	Canadian	Antihypertensive
CORGARD20 <> BL232	Tab, BL over 232	Nadolol 20 mg	Corgard by King	00003-0232	Antihypertensive
CORGARD40 <> BL207	Tab, Grey, Round, Scored, BL over 207	Nadolol 40 mg	Corgard by Repack Co of America	55306-0207	Antihypertensive
CORGARD40 <> BL207	Tab, Grey, Round, Scored, BL over 207	Nadolol 40 mg	Corgard by Nat Pharmpak	55154-0605	Antihypertensive
CORGARD40 <> BL207	Tab, Grey, Round, Scored, BL over 207	Nadolol 40 mg	Corgard by Pharmedix	53002-1018	Antihypertensive
CORGARD40 <> BL207	Tab, Grey, Round, Scored, BL over 207	Nadolol 40 mg	Corgard by King	00003-0207	Antihypertensive
CORGARD40 <> BL207	Tab, Grey, Round, Scored, BL over 207	Nadolol 40 mg	Corgard by BMS	Canadian	Antihypertensive
CORGARD40 <> BL207	Tab, Grey, Round, Scored, BL over 207	Nadolol 40 mg	Corgard by Thrift Drug	59198-0375	Antihypertensive
CORGARD80 <> BL241	Tab, Grey, Round, Scored, BL over 241	Nadolol 80 mg	Corgard by BMS	Canadian	Antihypertensive
CORGARD80 <> BL241	Tab, Grey, Round, Scored, BL over 241	Nadolol 80 mg	Corgard by Nat Pharmpak	55154-0604	Antihypertensive
CORGARD80 <> BL241	Tab, Grey, Round, Scored, BL over 241	Nadolol 80 mg	Corgard by King	00003-0241	Antihypertensive
CORRECTOL	Tab, Pink, Round, Enteric Coated	Bisacodyl 5 mg	Correctol by Schering-Plough Health Care		Laxative
CORTEF10	Tab, White, Round, Scored, Cortef over 10	Hydrocortisone 10 mg	Cortef by Pfizer	Canadian DIN 00030910	Steroid
CORTEF10	Tab, White, Round, Scored, Cortef over 10	Hydrocortisone 10 mg	Cortef by Pharmacia	00009-0031	Steroid
CORTEF20	Tab, White, Round, Scored, Cortef over 20	Hydrocortisone 20 mg	Cortef by Pharmacia	00009-0044	Steroid
CORTEF20	Tab, White, Round, Scored, Cortef over 20	Hydrocortisone 20 mg	Cortef by Pfizer	Canadian DIN 00030929	Steroid
CORTEF20	Tab, White, Round, Scored, Cortef over 20	Hydrocortisone 20 mg	Cortef by Murfreesboro	51129-9004	Steroid
CORTEF5	Tab, White, Round, Scored, Cortef over 5	Hydrocortisone 5 mg	Cortef by Physician Total Care	54868-3924	Steroid

ID FRONT <> BACK	DESCRIPTION FRONT <> BACK	INGREDIENT & STRENGTH	BRAND (or Generic Equiv.) by FIRM	NDC#	CLASS; SCH.
CORTEF5	Tab, White, Round, Scored, Cortef over 5	Hydrocortisone 5 mg	Cortef by Pharmacia	00009-0012	Steroid
CORTONE <> MSD219	Tab	Cortisone Acetate 25 mg	by Merck	00006-0219	Steroid
CORZIDE405 <> BL283	Tab, Bluish White to White w/ Dark Blue Specks, BL over 283	Bendroflumethiazide 5 mg, Nadolol 40 mg	Corzide by King		Diuretic; Antihypertensive
CORZIDE805 <> BL284	Tab, Bluish White to White w/ Dark Blue Specks, BL over 284	Bendroflumethiazide 5 mg, Nadolol 80 mg	Corzide by King		Diuretic; Antihypertensive
COTAZYM65B	Cap, White, Blue Ink	Lipase 8000 Units, Amylase 30,000 Units, Protease 30,000 Units	Cotazym by Organon	Canadian DIN 00456233	Gastrointestinal
COTAZYMECS20	Cap, Orange, Gelatin w/ Dark Blue Print, Organon Logo Cotazym ECS 20	Amylase 55000 USP, Lipase 20,000 USP, Protease 55000 USP	Cotazym ECS 20 by Organon	Canadian DIN 00821373	Gastrointestinal
COTAZYMECS4	Cap, Clear & Pink, Gelatin w/ Dark Blue Print, Organon Logo Cotazym ECS 4	Amylase 11000 USP, Lipase 4000 USP, Protease 11000 USP	Cotazym ECS 4 by Organon	Canadian DIN 02181215	Gastrointestinal
COTAZYMECS8	Cap, Clear, Gelatin w/ Dark Blue Print, Organon Logo Cotazym ECS 8	Amylase 30,000 USP, Lipase 8000 USP, Protease 30,000 USP	Cotazym ECS 8 by Organon	Canadian DIN 00502790	Gastrointestinal
COTRIM <> 9393	Tab, White, Round, Scored, Cotrim <> 93 over 93	Sulfamethoxazole 400 mg, Trimethoprim 80 mg	by Teva	00093-0188	Antibiotic
COTRIMDS <> 9393	Tab, White, Oblong, Scored, Cotrim DS <> 93/93	Sulfamethoxazole 800 mg, Trimethoprim 160 mg	by Teva	00093-0189	Antibiotic
COUMADIN1	Tab, Pink, Round, Scored, Coumadin over 1	Warfarin Sodium 1 mg	Coumadin by BMS	00056-0169	Anticoagulant
COUMADIN1	Tab, Pink, Round, Scored, Coumadin over 1	Warfarin Sodium 1 mg	Coumadin by BMS	Canadian DIN 01918311	Anticoagulant
COUMADIN10	Tab, White, Round, Scored, Coumadin over 10	Warfarin Sodium 10 mg	Coumadin by BMS	00056-0174	Anticoagulant
COUMADIN10	Tab, White, Round, Scored, Coumadin over 10	Warfarin Sodium 10 mg	Coumadin by BMS	Canadian DIN 01918362	Anticoagulant
COUMADIN2	Tab, Lavender, Round, Scored, Coumadin over 2	Warfarin Sodium 2 mg	Coumadin by BMS	00056-0170	Anticoagulant
COUMADIN2	Tab, Lavender, Round, Scored, Coumadin over 2	Warfarin Sodium 2 mg	Coumadin by BMS	Canadian DIN 01918338	Anticoagulant
COUMADIN212	Tab, Green, Round, Scored, Coumadin over 2 1/2	Warfarin Sodium 2.5 mg	Coumadin by BMS	00056-0176	Anticoagulant
COUMADIN212	Tab, Green, Round, Scored, Coumadin over 2 1/2	Warfarin Sodium 2.5 mg	Coumadin by BMS	Canadian DIN 01918346	Anticoagulant
COUMADIN3	Tab, Tan, Round, Scored, Coumadin over 3	Warfarin Sodium 3 mg	Coumadin by BMS	00056-0188	Anticoagulant
COUMADIN3	Tab, Tan, Round, Scored, Coumadin over 3	Warfarin Sodium 3 mg	Coumadin by BMS	Canadian DIN 02240205	Anticoagulant
COUMADIN4	Tab, Blue, Round, Scored, Coumadin over 4	Warfarin Sodium 4 mg	Coumadin by BMS	00056-0168	Anticoagulant
COUMADIN4	Tab, Blue, Round, Scored, Coumadin over 4	Warfarin Sodium 4 mg	Coumadin by BMS	Canadian DIN 02007959	Anticoagulant
COUMADIN5	Tab, Peach, Round, Scored, Coumadin over 5	Warfarin Sodium 5 mg	Coumadin by BMS	00056-0172	Anticoagulant
COUMADIN5	Tab, Peach, Round, Scored, Coumadin over 5	Warfarin Sodium 5 mg	Coumadin by BMS	Canadian DIN 01918354	Anticoagulant
COUMADIN6	Tab, Teal, Round, Scored, Coumadin over 6	Warfarin Sodium 6 mg	Coumadin by BMS	00056-0189	Anticoagulant
COUMADIN6	Tab, Teal, Round, Scored, Coumadin over 6	Warfarin Sodium 6 mg	Coumadin by BMS	Canadian DIN 02240206	Anticoagulant
COUMADIN712	Tab, Yellow, Round, Scored, Coumadin over 7 1/2	Warfarin Sodium 7.5 mg	Coumadin by BMS	00056-0173	Anticoagulant
COVERAHS2011	Tab, Lavender, Round, Film Coated, Covera-HS 2011	Verapamil HCl 180 mg	Covera HS by Searle	00025-2011	Antihypertensive
COVERAHS2011	Tab, Lavender, Round, Film Coated, Covera-HS 2011	Verapamil HCl 180 mg	Covera HS by Pfizer	Canadian DIN 02231676	Antihypertensive
COVERAHS2021	Tab, Pale Yellow, Black Print, Round, Film Coated, Covera-HS 2021	Verapamil HCl 240 mg	Covera HS by Pfizer	Canadian DIN 02231677	Antihypertensive
COVERAHS2021	Tab, Pale Yellow, Black Print, Round, Film Coated, Covera-HS 2021	Verapamil HCl 240 mg	Covera HS by Searle	00025-2021	Antihypertensive
COVERAHS2021	Tab, Pale Yellow, Black Print, Round, Film Coated, Covera-HS 2021	Verapamil HCl 240 mg	Covera HS by Caremark	00339-5884	Antihypertensive
COZAAR <> MRK952	Tab, Green, Tear Drop Shaped, Film Coated	Losartan Potassium 50 mg	Cozaar by Merck Frosst	Canadian DIN 02182874	Antihypertensive
COZAAR <> MRK952	Tab, Green, Tear Drop Shaped, Film Coated	Losartan Potassium 50 mg	Cozaar by Nat Pharmpak	55154-5016	Antihypertensive

ID FRONT <> BACK	DESCRIPTION FRONT <> BACK	INGREDIENT & STRENGTH	BRAND (or Generic Equiv.) by FIRM	NDC#	CLASS; SCH.
COZAAR <> MRK952	Tab, Green, Tear Drop Shaped, Film Coated	Losartan Potassium 50 mg	Cozaar by Physician Total Care	54868-3726	Antihypertensive
CP <> 200	Tab, Light Green, Oblong, Scored	Guaifenesin 600 mg, Potassium Guaiacolsulfonate 300 mg	Humibid LA by Carolina	68249-0200	Cold Remedy
CP <> 266	Tab, Coated, Imprinted in Black Ink	Thioridazine HCl 25 mg	by Heartland	61392-0463	Antipsychotic
CP <> 270	Tab, Coated	Thioridazine HCl 200 mg	by Creighton	50752-0270	Antipsychotic
CP <> 275	Tab	Acetaminophen 325 mg, Butalbital 50 mg, Caffeine 40 mg	Fioricet by Creighton	50752-0275	Analgesic
CP252	Cap, Green & Yellow	Nortriptyline HCl 50 mg	Pamelor by Creighton		Antidepressant
CP253	Cap, Green	Nortriptyline HCl 75 mg	Aventyl HCl by Novartis		Antidepressant
CP253	Cap, Green	Nortriptyline HCl 75 mg	Pamelor by Sandoz	00781-2633	Antidepressant
CP262	Tab, White, Round	Bromocriptine 2.5 mg	Parlodel by Novartis		Antiparkinson
CP264	Tab, Yellow Green, Round	Thioridazine 10 mg	Mellaril by Creighton		Antipsychotic
CP265	Tab, White, Round	Thioridazine 15 mg	Mellaril by Creighton		Antipsychotic
CP267	Tab, White, Round	Thioridazine 50 mg	Mellaril by Creighton		Antipsychotic
CP268	Tab, Coated	Thioridazine HCl 100 mg	by Creighton	50752-0268	Antipsychotic
CP269	Tab, Yellow, Round	Thioridazine 150 mg	Mellaril by Creighton		Antipsychotic
CP271	Cap, Pink & White	Temazepam 7.5 mg	Restoril by Creighton		Sedative/Hypnotic; C IV
CP272	Cap, Aqua & White	Temazepam 15 mg	Restoril by Creighton		Sedative/Hypnotic; C IV
CP273	Cap, Aqua	Temazepam 30 mg	Restoril by Creighton		Sedative/Hypnotic; C IV
CP277	Tab, White, Round	Butalbital 50 mg, Aspirin 325 mg, Caffeine 40 mg	Fiorinal by Creighton	00781-2120	Analgesic; C III
CP278	Cap, Green	Butalbital 50 mg, Aspirin 325 mg, Caffeine 40 mg	Fiorinal by Novartis	00781-2221	Analgesic; C III
CP278	Cap, Green & Lime Green	Butalbital 50 mg, Aspirin 325 mg, Caffeine 40 mg	Fiorinal by Sandoz		Analgesic; C III
CP279	Cap, Blue & Yellow	Aspirin 325 mg, Butalbital 50 mg, Caffeine 40 mg, Codeine Phosphate 30 mg	Fiorinal w/ Codeine by Sandoz		Analgesic; C III
CP279	Cap, Blue & Yellow	Aspirin 325 mg, Butalbital 50 mg, Caffeine 40 mg, Codeine Phosphate 30 mg	Fiorinal w/ Codeine by Novartis		Analgesic; C III
CP800	Cap, Gray & Red, Opaque	Ampicillin 250 mg	Principen by Bayer	12527-2885	Antibiotic
CP800	Cap	Ampicillin 250 mg	Principen by Medpharm	62780-0657	Antibiotic
CP800	Cap, Scarlet	Ampicillin 250 mg	Principen by Consolidated Pharma	61423-0800	Antibiotic
CP805	Cap, Scarlet	Ampicillin 500 mg	Principen by Consolidated Pharma	61423-0805	Antibiotic
CP820	Cap, Buff and Caramel	Amoxicillin 250 mg	Amoxil by Consolidated Pharma	61423-0820	Antibiotic
CP820	Cap	Amoxicillin 250 mg	Amoxil by Richmond	54738-0108	Antibiotic
CP820	Cap, Beige & Caramel	Amoxicillin 250 mg	Amoxil by Medpharm	62780-0658	Antibiotic
CP820	Cap	Amoxicillin 250 mg	Amoxil by Qualitest	00603-2266	Antibiotic
CP825	Cap, Buff	Amoxicillin 500 mg	Amoxil by Qualitest	00603-2267	Antibiotic
CP825	Cap, Buff	Amoxicillin 500 mg	Amoxil by Richmond	54738-0110	Antibiotic
CP825	Cap, Buff	Amoxicillin 500 mg	Amoxil by Consolidated Pharma	61423-0825	Antibiotic
CP840	Tab, White, Oval	Penicillin V Potassium 250 mg	by Pharmafab	62542-0691	Antibiotic
CP840	Tab	Penicillin V Potassium	by Richmond	54738-0122	Antibiotic
CP840	Tab	Penicillin V Potassium	by Medpharm	62780-0659	Antibiotic
CP840	Tab	Penicillin V Potassium	by Consolidated Pharma	61423-0840	Antibiotic
CP845	Tab	Penicillin V Potassium	by Consolidated Pharma	61423-0845	Antibiotic
CP845	Tab	Penicillin V Potassium	by Richmond	54738-0123	Antibiotic
CP845	Tab	Penicillin V Potassium 500 mg	by Pharmafab	62542-0704	Antibiotic
CPC1027	Tab, Yellow, Oblong	Multi-Vitamins	Berocca Plus by Major	00904-7929	Vitamin
CPC1027	Tab, Yellow, Oblong	Multi-Vitamins	Berocca Plus by Qualitest	00603-5970	Vitamin
CPC1121	Tab, White, Oval, CPC 11/21	Elemental Iron 90 mg, Calcium 200 mg, Zinc 25 mg, Vitamin A 4000 IU, Vitamin D3 400 IU, Vitamin E 30 IU, Vitamin C 120 mg, Docusate Sodium 50 mg	Prenate 90 by Breckenridge	51991-0152	Vitamin; Mineral
CPC1125	Tab, White	Prenatal Vitamins	Vernate Advanced by Rugby		Vitamin
CPC1167	Tab, Brown, Round	Phenazopyridine HCl 95 mg	UTI Relief by Consumers Choice Systems	61814-9505	Urinary Analgesic

ID FRONT <> BACK	DESCRIPTION FRONT <> BACK	INGREDIENT & STRENGTH	BRAND (or Generic Equiv.) by FIRM	NDC#	CLASS; SCH.
CPC1190	Tab, White, Oval	Acetaminophen 500 mg	Tylenol Ex Strength by Contract	10267-1190	Analgesic
CPC120	Tab, Yellow, Round	Folic Acid 1 mg	by Contract	10267-0120	Vitamin
CPC1277	Tab, Brown, Round	Cascara Sagrada 325 mg	Cascara Sagrada by Rugby	00536-3440	Laxative
CPC1325	Tab, Blue, Cap Shaped	Vitamin C 200 mg, Iron 106 mg, Thiamine 10 mg, Riboflavin 6 mg, Niacin 30 mg, Vitamin B6 5 mg, Folic Acid 1 mg, Vitamin B12 15 mcg, Pantothenic Acid 10 mg, Magnesium 6.9 mg, Zinc 18.2 mg, Copper 0.8 mg, Manganese 1.3 mg	Hematinic Plus by Cypress	60258-0180	Vitamin; Supplement
CPC1327	Tab, Blue, Round	Iron 106 mg, Folic Acid 1 mg	Hematinic with Folic Acid by Cypress	60258-0181	Vitamin; Supplement
CPC1620	Cap, Brown & White Beads	Hyoscyamine Sulfate 0.375 mg	Levsin by URL Mutual	00677-1507	Gastrointestinal
CPC1620	Cap, Clear & Coral	Hyoscyamine Sulfate 0.375 mg	Levsin by Lini	58215-0305 Discontinued	Gastrointestinal
CPC1620	Cap, Clear & Coral	Hyoscyamine Sulfate 0.375 mg	Levsin by Pecos		Gastrointestinal
CPC1620	Cap, Clear & Coral	Hyoscyamine Sulfate 0.375 mg	Levsin by Mutual	53489-0240	Gastrointestinal
CPC1620	Cap, Clear & Coral	Hyoscyamine Sulfate 0.375 mg	Levsin by Pecos	59879-0109	Gastrointestinal
CPC1620	Cap, Brown & White Beads	Hyoscyamine Sulfate 0.375 mg	Levsin by Major	00904-7833	Gastrointestinal
CPC1667	Tab, Maroon, Round	Phenazopyridine HCl 95 mg	Azo-Standard by Alphagen	59743-0115	Urinary Analgesic
CPC1667	Tab, Maroon, Round	Phenazopyridine HCl 95 mg	Azo-Standard by Reese	10956-0551	Urinary Analgesic
CPC1724	Tab, Blue, Round, Film Coated	Methenamine 40.8 mg, Benzoic Acid 4.5 mg, Phenyl Salicylate 18.1 mg, Methylene Blue 5.4 mg, Hyoscyamine Sulfate 0.03 mg, Atropine Sulfate 0.03 mg	by Contract	10267-1724	Antibiotic; Urinary Tract
CPC1991	Tab, Beige, Oval	Vitamin A 5000 IU, Vitamin D3 400 IU, Vitamin E 30 IU, Vitamin C 120 mg, Calcium 200 mg	Materna by Breckenridge	51991-0155	Vitamin
CPC2069	Tab, Beige, Oval, Film Coated	Vitamin Combination	Prenatal Plus by Contract Pharmacal	10267-2069	Vitamin
CPC231	Cap, White	Quinine Sulfate 325 mg	Quinamm by Contract Pharmacal	10267-0231	Antimalarial
CPC2365	Tab, White, Round	Magnesium 64 mg, Calcium 106 mg	Mag-SR by Cypress	60258-0174	Vitamin; Supplement
CPC2369	Tab, White, Oval	Dibasic Sodium Phosphate 852 mg, Monobasic Potassium Phosphate 155 mg, Monobasic Sodium Phosphate 130 mg	Phospha 250 Neutral by Rising	64980-0104	Urinary Tract
CPC2465	Tab, Maroon, Cap Shaped	Ferrous Sulfate 105 mg, Vitamin C 500 mg, Folic Acid 0.8 mg	Folitab by Rising	64980-0105	Vitamin
CPC2826	Tab, White, Oblong, Film Coated	Acetaminophen 500 mg, Pamabrom 25 mg, Pyrilamine 15 mg	Midol by Contract	10267-2826	PMS Relief
CPC365	Cap, Orange & Yellow	Acetaminophen 325 mg, Phenylpropanolamine HCl 12.5 mg, Chlorpheniramine 2 mg, Dextromethorphan HBr 10 mg	Multi Symptom Cold Relief by Contract		Cold Remedy
CPC3712	Cap, White, CPC 37 1/2	Phenylpropanolamine HCl 37.5 mg	Phenylpropanolamine by Quality Care		Decongestant; Appetite Suppressant
CPC464	Cap, Brown & Red	Multivitamin, Mineral	Trinsicon by Moore		Vitamin
CPC464	Cap, Brown & Red	Liver Stomach Concentrate 240 mg, Cyanocobalamin 15 mcg, Iron 110 mg, Ascorbic Acid 75 mg, Folic Acid 0.5 mg	Ferocon by Breckenridge	51991-0635	Vitamin
CPC465	Cap, Orange	Phenylpropanolamine HCl (Timed Release) 75 mg	Just-One-Per-Day by Reese	10956-0603	Decongestant; Appetite Suppressant
CPC490	Tab, Orange, Round	Sennosides 8.6 mg, Docusate Sodium 50 mg	Senokot-S by Cypress	60258-0951	Laxative
CPC490	Tab, Orange, Round	Sennosides 8.6 mg, Docusate Sodium 50 mg	Senokot-S by Major	00904-5512	Gastrointestinal
CPC737	Cap, Black & Orange	Ascorbic Acid 150 mg, Calcium Pantothenate 10 mg, Cyanocobalamin 10 mcg, Folic Acid 1 mg, Magnesium Sulfate 70 mg, Manganese Chloride 4 mg, Niacinamide 25 mg, Pyridoxine HCl 2 mg, Riboflavin 5 mg, Thiamine Mononitrate 10 mg, Vitamin A 8000 Units, Vitamin E 50 Units, Zinc Sulfate 80 mg	Vica-Forte by Qualitest	00603-6381	Vitamin
CPC752	Tab, Aqua, Oblong	Acetaminophen 500 mg, Diphenhydramine 25 mg	Tylenol PM by Contract		Cold Remedy
CPC835	Cap, White and Pink, Red Band	Diphenhydramine 25 mg	Benadryl by Contract	10267-0835	Antihistamine
CPC836	Cap, Pink	Diphenhydramine HCl 50 mg	Benadryl by Contract		Antihistamine
CPC860	Cap, Red	Phenazopyridine HCl 200 mg	by Breckenridge	51991-0525	Urinary Analgesic
CPC860	Tab, Red, Cap Shaped	Phenazopyridine HCl 200 mg	Pyridium by Breckenridge	51991-0525	Urinary Analgesic

ID FRONT <> BACK	DESCRIPTION FRONT <> BACK	INGREDIENT & STRENGTH	BRAND (or Generic Equiv.) by FIRM	NDC#	CLASS; SCH.
CPC997	Tab, Round, Yellow	Chlorpheniramine Maleate 4 mg	Chlor-Trimeton by Contract	10267-0997	Antihistamine
CPI	Tab, CPI Logo	Phenobarbital 7.5 mg	by Century	00436-0864	Sedative/Hypnotic; C IV
CPI	Tab, CPI Logo	Aprobarbital 25 mg, Butabarbital Sodium 50 mg, Phenobarbital 25 mg	Triple Barbital by Century	00436-0198	Sedative; C IV
CPI <> 2	Tab, CPI Logo	Phenobarbital 30 mg	by Century	00436-0869	Sedative/Hypnotic; C IV
CPI <> 2	Tab, CPI Logo	Phenobarbital 30 mg	by Century	00436-0870	Sedative/Hypnotic; C IV
CPI <> 2	Tab, CPI Logo	Phenobarbital 30 mg	by Century	00436-0129	Sedative/Hypnotic; C IV
CPI <> 4	Tab, CPI Logo	Phenobarbital 16.2 mg	by Century	00436-0867	Sedative/Hypnotic; C IV
CPI <> 4	Tab, CPI Logo	Phenobarbital 16.2 mg	by Century	00436-0866	Sedative/Hypnotic; C IV
CPI107	Tab, Peach, Round	Mebendazole 100 mg	Vermox by Copley		Antihelmintic
CPI111	Tab, Yellow, Oval	Prenatal Vitamin + Iron 1 mg	Stuartnatal Plus by Copley		Vitamin
CPI113	Tab, Off-White, Oblong	Chlorpheniramine 8 mg, Phenylephrine 25 mg, Pyrilamine 25 mg	Rynatan by Copley		Cold Remedy
CPI114	Tab, Orange, Oblong	Procainamide HCl ER 750 mg	Procan SR by Copley		Antiarrhythmic
CPI117	Tab, Red, Oblong	Procainamide HCl ER 1000 mg	Procan SR by Copley		Antiarrhythmic
CPI131	Tab, Pink, Round	Sodium Fluoride 2.2 mg	Luride by Copley		Element
CPI135	Tab, White, Oval	Doxylamine Succinate 25 mg	Unisom by Copley		Sleep Aid
CPI146	Tab, Off-White, Round	Naproxen 250 mg	Naprosyn by Copley		NSAID
CPI150	Tab, Off-White, Oblong	Naproxen 500 mg	Naprosyn by Copley		NSAID
CPI152	Tab, Yellow, Oval	B Complex Vitamin Plus	Berocca Plus by Copley		Vitamin
CPI158	Tab, Orange or Pink or Purple, Square	Multivitamins, Fluoride 0.5 mg	Poly-Vi-Flor 0.5mg by Copley		Vitamin
CPI159	Tab, Purple, Square	Multivitamins 1 mg, Fluoride + Iron 1 mg	Poly-Vi-Flor w Iron by Copley		Vitamin
CPI166	Tab, Orange or Pink or Purple, Square	Multivitamins 1 mg, Fluoride 1 mg	Poly-Vi-Flor 1mg by Copley		Vitamin
CPI169	Tab, White, Oval	Prenatal Vitamin RX	Natalins RX by Copley		Vitamin
CPI175	Tab, White, Round, Ex Release	Quinidine Sulfate 300 mg	Quinidex by Copley		Antiarrhythmic
CPI188	Tab, Orange, Oblong	Procainamide HCl ER 500 mg	Procan SR by Copley		Antiarrhythmic
CPI197	Tab, Pink, Square	Multivitamin, Fluoride + Iron 0.5 mg	Poly-Vi-Flor w Iron by Copley		Vitamin
CPI225	Tab, Orange, Round	Potassium Chloride ER 600 mg (8 mEq)	Slow K by Copley		Electrolytes
CPI312	White	Captopril 50 mg	Capoten by Copley		Antihypertensive
CPI381	Tab, Green, Hexagonal	Glyburide 3 mg	Glynase by Copley		Antidiabetic
CPI411	Tab, White, Square	Methazolamide 25 mg	Neptazane by Copley		Antiglaucoma Agent
CPI424	Tab, White, Round	Methazolamide 50 mg	Neptazane by Copley		Antiglaucoma Agent
CPI443	Tab, Off-White, Oblong	Naproxen 375 mg	Naprosyn by Copley		NSAID
CPI471	Tab, White, Round	Captopril 25 mg	Capoten by Copley		Antihypertensive
CPI514	Tab, White, Oval	Prenatal Vitamin, Zinc	Zenate by Copley		Vitamin
CPI631	Tab, Blue, Round	Diltiazem HCl 30 mg	Cardizem by Copley		Antihypertensive
CPI643	Tab, Yellow, Round	Prochlorperazine 5 mg	Compazine by Copley		Antiemetic
CPI652	Tab, Yellow, Round	Prochlorperazine 10 mg	Compazine by Copley		Antiemetic
CPI653	White	Captopril 100 mg	Capoten by Copley		Antihypertensive
CPI662	Tab, White, Round	Diltiazem HCl 60 mg	Cardizem by Copley		Antihypertensive
CPI691	Tab, Blue, Oblong	Diltiazem HCl 90 mg	Cardizem by Copley		Antihypertensive
CPI711	Tab, Peach, Square	Guanabenz Acetate 8 mg	Wytensin by Copley		Antihypertensive
CPI717	Tab, Peach, Square	Guanabenz Acetate 4 mg	Wytensin by Copley		Antihypertensive
CPI720	Tab, White, Oblong	Diltiazem HCl 120 mg	Cardizem by Copley		Antihypertensive

ID FRONT <> BACK	DESCRIPTION FRONT <> BACK	INGREDIENT & STRENGTH	BRAND (or Generic Equiv.) by FIRM	NDC#	CLASS; SCH.
CPI724	Tab, Blue, Round	Nadolol 80 mg	Corgard by Copley		Antihypertensive
CPI725	Tab, Pink, Hexagonal	Glyburide 1.5 mg	Glynase by Copley		Antidiabetic
CPI727	Tab, Blue, Oblong	Nadolol 120 mg	Corgard by Copley		Antihypertensive
CPI731	Tab, Blue, Oblong	Nadolol 160 mg	Corgard by Copley		Antihypertensive
CPI743	Tab, White, Round	Captopril 12.5 mg	Capoten by Copley		Antihypertensive
CPI774	Tab, White, Oblong	Hydroxychloroquine Sulfate 200 mg	Plaquenil by Copley		Antimalarial
CPL	Tab, Blue & Green, Round, CPL Logo	Chlorpheniramine Maleate 2 mg, Phenylephrine HCl 5 mg	Hista Tab Plus by Century	00436-0633	Cold Remedy
CPM12CPM12	Cap, Green & Clear	Chlorpheniramine 12 mg	Teldrin by Qualitest	00603-2785	Antihistamine
CPMPSE	Cap, Blue & Clear, CPM over PSE	Chlorpheniramine Maleate 8 mg, Pseudoephedrine HCl 120 mg	by Pfab	62542-0260	Cold Remedy
CPMPSE	Cap, Blue & Clear	Chlorpheniramine Maleate 8 mg, Pseudoephedrine HCl 120 mg	by Compumed	00403-0010	Cold Remedy
CPMPSE	Cap, Blue & Clear, CPM over PSE	Chlorpheniramine Maleate 8 mg, Pseudoephedrine HCl 120 mg	by Allscripts		Cold Remedy
CPW5088	Cap, Blue & Clear, Blue & White Beads, CPW 50-88	Caffeine 200 mg	Fastlene by BDI		Stimulant
CPW50888	Cap, Black, CPW 50-888	Caffeine 200 mg	Dextrophin by Clifton		Stimulant
CPW50888	Cap, Black, CPW 50-888	Caffeine 250 mg	Dextrophin by Clifton		Stimulant
CPW50888	Cap, Black, CPW 50-888	Caffeine 350 mg	Dextrophin by Clifton		Stimulant
CPZ250 <> APO	Tab, Light Orange, Cap Shaped	Cefprozil 250 mg	Cefzil by Apotex	Canadian DIN 02292998	Antibiotic
CPZ500 <> APO	Tab, White, Cap Shaped	Cefprozil 500 mg	Cefzil by Apotex	Canadian DIN 02293005	Antibiotic
CR250	Tab, White, Round, CR 250 over Cobalt Logo	Ciprofloxacin HCl 250 mg	Cipro by Cobalt	Canadian DIN 02247339	Antibiotic
CR250	Tab, White, Round, CR 250 over >	Ciprofloxacin HCl 250 mg	Cipro by Cobalt	16252-0514	Antibiotic
CR250	Tab, White, Round, CR 250 over >	Ciprofloxacin HCl 250 mg	Cipro by Abrika	67767-0137	Antibiotic
CR500	Tab, White, Cap Shaped, CR 500 over >	Ciprofloxacin HCl 500 mg	Cipro by Cobalt	16252-0515	Antibiotic
CR500	Tab, White, Cap Shaped, CR 500 over Cobalt Logo	Ciprofloxacin HCl 500 mg	Cipro by Cobalt	Canadian DIN 02247340	Antibiotic
CR500	Tab, White, Cap Shaped, CR 500 over >	Ciprofloxacin HCl 500 mg	Cipro by Abrika	67767-0138	Antibiotic
CR750	Tab, White, Cap Shaped, CR 750 over >	Ciprofloxacin HCl 750 mg	Cipro by Abrika	67767-0139	Antibiotic
CR750	Tab, White, Cap Shaped, CR 750 over Cobalt Logo	Ciprofloxacin HCl 750 mg	Cipro by Cobalt	Canadian DIN 02247341	Antibiotic
CR750	Tab, White, Cap Shaped, CR 750 over >	Ciprofloxacin HCl 750 mg	Cipro by Cobalt	16252-0516	Antibiotic
CR750	Tab, White, Cap Shaped, CR 750 over >	Ciprofloxacin HCl 750 mg	Cipro by Ivax	00182-2722 Discontinued	Antibiotic
CRD400	Tab, Blue, Cap Shaped	Calcium 500 mg, Vitamin D3 400 IU	Carbocal D by Euro-Pharm	Canadian DIN 02245511	Supplement
CRESTOR <> 40	Tab, Pink, Oval, Coated	Rosuvastatin 40 mg	Crestor by AstraZeneca	00310-0754	Antihyperlipidemic
CRESTOR10	Tab, Pink, Round, Coated	Rosuvastatin 10 mg	Crestor by AstraZeneca	00310-0751	Antihyperlipidemic
CRESTOR20	Tab, Pink, Round, Coated	Rosuvastatin 20 mg	Crestor by AstraZeneca	00310-0752	Antihyperlipidemic
CRESTOR5	Tab, Yellow, Round, Coated	Rosuvastatin 5 mg	Crestor by AstraZeneca	00310-0755	Antihyperlipidemic
CRIXIVAN100MG	Cap, White, Green Print, Opaque	Indinavir Sulfate 100 mg	Crixivan by Merck	00006-0570	Antiviral
CRIXIVAN200MG	Cap, White, Blue Print, Opaque	Indinavir Sulfate 200 mg	Crixivan by Merck	00006-0571	Antiviral
CRIXIVAN200MG	Cap, White, Blue Print, Opaque	Indinavir Sulfate 200 mg	Crixivan by Merck Frosst	Canadian DIN 02229161	Antiviral
CRIXIVAN333MG	Cap, White, Red Print, Opaque	Indinavir Sulfate 333 mg	Crixivan by Merck	00006-0574	Antiviral
CRIXIVAN400MG	Cap, White, Green Print, Opaque	Indinavir Sulfate 400 mg	Crixivan by Merck Frosst	Canadian DIN 02229196	Antiviral
CRIXIVAN400MG	Cap, White, Green Print, Opaque	Indinavir Sulfate 400 mg	Crixivan by Merck	00006-0573	Antiviral
CS11SILVER	Tab, Gray, Oblong, CS 11-Silver	Multivitamin, Minerals	Centrum Silver by Lederle		Vitamin

ID FRONT <> BACK	DESCRIPTION FRONT <> BACK	INGREDIENT & STRENGTH	BRAND (or Generic Equiv.) by FIRM	NDC#	CLASS; SCH.
CSCOTT <> 110	Tab, Sugar Coated, C Scott	Thyroid 1 g	by JMI Canton	00252-7007	Thyroid Hormone
CSF <> NVR	Tab, Dark Yellow, Oval, Film Coated	Amlodipine 5 mg, Valsartan 320 mg	Exforge by Novartis	00078-0490	Antihypertensive
CT	Tab, Orange-Red, Oval, Film Coated, Delayed Release	Mycophenolic Acid 360 mg	Myfortic by Novartis	Canadian DIN 02264579	Immunosuppressant
CT	Tab, Orange-Red, Oval, Film Coated, Delayed Release	Mycophenolic Acid 360 mg	Myfortic by Novartis	00078-0386	Immunosuppressant
CT15	Tab, White, Scored	Codeine Phosphate 15 mg	by Pharmascience	Canadian DIN 5760601231	Analgesic; C II
CT2	Tab, Red and White, Oblong, Film-Coated, Tri-Layered, Extended Release	Zileuton 600 mg	Zyflo CR by Clinical Therapeutics	68734-0710	Antiasthmatic
CT30	Tab, White, Scored	Codeine Phosphate 30 mg	by Pharmascience	Canadian DIN 5760601233	Analgesic; C II
CT937	Tab, White, Round	Calcium Lactate 10 g	by Fresh		Vitamin; Mineral
CTD <> 200	Tab, White, Oblong	Cimetidine HCl 200 mg	QC Heartburn by Chain Drug	63868-0519	Gastrointestinal
CTI <> NVR	Tab, Yellow, Oval	Hydrochlorothiazide 25 mg, Valsartan 320 mg	Diovan HCT by Novartis	00078-0472	Antihypertensive; Diuretic
CTI101	Tab, White, Round	Diclofenac Sodium 25 mg	by DRX	55045-2681	NSAID
CTI102	Tab, White, Round	Diclofenac Sodium 50 mg	by DRX	55045-2682	NSAID
CTI103	Tab, White, Round	Diclofenac Sodium 75 mg	by DRX	55045-2685	NSAID
CTI112	Tab, White, Oval	Acyclovir 400 mg	Zovirax by Amerisource	62584-0798	Antiviral
CTI113	Tab, White, Oval	Acyclovir 800 mg	Zovirax by Amerisource	62584-0816	Antiviral
CTX088	Tab, Peach & White, Oblong, Scored, Film Coated	Acetaminophen 500 mg, Phenylephrine HCl 40 mg, Chlorpheniramine Maleate 8 mg	Histex SR by Alphapharm	57315-0012	Cold Remedy
CVI <> NVR	Tab, Violet and White, Oval, Film Coated	Aliskiren 300 mg, HCTZ 12.5 mg	Tekturna HCT by Novartis	00078-0523	Antihypertensive; Diuretic
CVT500	Tab, Light Orange, Oblong, Film Coated, Extended Release	Ranolazine 500 mg	Ranexa by CVT	67159-0112	Antianginal
CVV <> NVR	Tab, Light Yellow, Oval, Film Coated	Aliskiren 300 mg, HCTZ 25 mg	Tekturna HCT by Novartis	00078-0524	Antihypertensive; Diuretic
CY	Tab, White, Cap Shaped, Film Coated, CY engraved in arcs	Tranexamic Acid 500 mg	by Pharmacia	Canadian DIN 02064405	Hemostatic
CY	Tab, White, Round	Tranexamic Acid 500 mg	Cyklokapron by Pharmacia		Hemostatic
CY250	Cap, Green, Opaque, CY250, Two Blue Partial Lines	Ganciclovir Sodium 250 mg	Cytovene by Roche	Canadian DIN 02186802	Antiviral
CY4	Tab, White, Round, Scored	Cyproheptadine HCl 4 mg	by Pharmascience	Canadian DIN 5760677132	Antihistamine
CY500	Cap, Yellow and Green, Opaque, CY500, Two Blue Partial Lines	Ganciclovir Sodium 500 mg	Cytovene by Roche	Canadian DIN 02240362	Antiviral
CYCRIN	Tab, Peach, Oval	Medroxyprogesterone Acetate 10 mg	Cycrin by ESI Lederle		Hormone
CYCRIN <> C	Tab, Peach, Oval, Scored	Medroxyprogesterone Acetate 10 mg	by Southwood	58016-0926	Hormone
CYCRIN <> C	Tab, Light Purple, Oval	Medroxyprogesterone Acetate 5 mg	Cycrin by ESI Lederle	59911-5897	Hormone
CYCRIN <> C	Tab, Purple, Oval, Opposing C	Medroxyprogesterone Acetate 5 mg	by Nat Pharmpak	55154-5577	Hormone
CYCRIN <> C	Tab, Purple, Oval, Scored	Medroxyprogesterone Acetate 5 mg	by Kaiser	62224-4334	Hormone
CYCRIN <> OPPOSINGCS	Tab, Debossed, Cycrin <> Opposing C's	Medroxyprogesterone Acetate 10 mg	by Kaiser	62224-4331	Hormone
CYP	Tab, Round, Scored	Cyproheptadine HCl 4 mg	Periactin by Cypress	60258-0850	Antihistamine
CYP105	Tab, Purple, Oval	Magnesium Salicylate 600 mg, Phenyltoloxamine Citrate 25 mg	Tetra-Mag by Cypress	60258-0105	Analgesic
CYP106	Tab, Yellow, Round	Magnesium Salicylate 600 mg	MST 600 by Cypress	60258-0106	Analgesic
CYP160	Tab, Yellow, Round	Vitamin C 60 mg, Thiamin 1.5 mg, Riboflavin 1.7 mg, Niacin 20 mg, Vitamin B6 10 mg, Folic Acid 800 mcg, Vitamin B12 6 mcg, d-Biotin 300 mcg, Pantothenic Acid 10 mg	Rena-Vite by Cypress	60258-0160	Vitamin; Supplement
CYP161	Tab, Yellow, Round	Vitamin C 60 mg, Thiamin 1.5 mg, Riboflavin 1.7 mg, Niacin 20 mg, Vitamin B6 10 mg, Folic Acid 1 mg, Vitamin B12 6 mcg, d-Biotin 300 mcg, Pantothenic Acid 10 mg	Rena-Vite Rx by Cypress	60258-0161	Vitamin; Supplement

ID FRONT <> BACK	DESCRIPTION FRONT <> BACK	INGREDIENT & STRENGTH	BRAND (or Generic Equiv.) by FIRM	NDC#	CLASS; SCH.
CYP176	Tab, White, Oval	Calcium 200 mg, Folic Acid 1 mg, Iodine 150 mcg, Iron 29 mg, Niacin 20 mg, Vitamin B1 3 mg, Vitamin B12 8 mcg, Vitamin B2 3 mg, Vitamin B6 3 mg, Vitamin D 400 IU, Vitamin E 30 IU, Zinc 15 mg	Prenatabs OBN by Cypress	60258-0176	Vitamin; Supplement
CYP177	Tab, Speckled White, Round	Biotin 50 mcg, Folic Acid 0.2 mg, Niacin 10 mg, Pantothenic Acid 10 mg, Riboflavin 1.2 mg, Vitamin A 9,000 IU, Vitamin B12 12 mcg, Vitamin B6 1.5 mg, Vitamin C 60 mg, Vitamin D 400 IU, Vitamin E 150 IU, Zinc 7.5 mg, Vitamin B1 1.3 mg, Vitamin K 150 mcg	CF Vite by Cypress	60258-0177	Vitamin; Supplement
CYP178	Tab, Pink, Oval	Calcium 200 mg, Folic Acid 1 mg, Iodine 150 mcg, Iron 17 mg, Niacin 20 mg, Vitamin A 4,000 IU, Vitamin B1 3 mg, Vitamin B12 8 mcg, Vitamin B2 3 mg, Vitamin B6 3 mg, Vitamin C 120 mg, Vitamin D 400 IU, Vitamin E 30 IU, Zinc 15 mg	Prenafirst by Cypress	60258-0178	Vitamin; Supplement
CYP179	Tab, Blue-Violet, Cap Shaped	Iron 106.5 mg, Vitamin C 200 mg, Vitamin B1 10 mg, Riboflavin 6 mg, Vitamin B6 5 mg, Vitamin B12 15 mcg, Folic Acid 1 mg, Niacinamide 30 mg, Pantothenic Acid 10 mg, Manganese 1.3 mg, Copper 0.8 mg	Prenatal U by Cypress	60258-0179	Vitamin; Supplement
CYP187	Tab, White, Cap Shaped	Iron 106.5 mg, Vitamin C 200 mg, Vitamin B1 10 mg, Vitamin B2 6 mg, Vitamin B6 5 mg, Vitamin B12 15 mcg, Folic Acid 1 mg, Niacinamide 30 mg, Pantothenic Acid 10 mg, Zinc 18.2 mg, Magnesium 6.9 mg, Manganese 1.3 mg, Copper 0.8 mg	Prenatal H by Cypress	60258-0187	Vitamin; Supplement
CYP190	Tab, Pink, Oval	Vitamin A 4000 IU, Vitamin C 120 mg, Calcium 200 mg, Iron 29 mg, Vitamin D 400 IU, Vitamin E 30 IU, Thiamin 3 mg, Riboflavin 3 mg, Niacin 20 mg, Vitamin B6 3 mg, Folic Acid 1 mg, Vitamin B12 8 mcg, Iodine 150 mcg, Zinc 15 mg	Prenatabs FA by Cypress	60258-0190	Vitamin; Supplement
CYP191	Tab, White, Oval	Vitamin A 4000 IU, Vitamin C 120 mg, Calcium 200 mg, Iron 50 mg, Vitamin D 400 IU, Vitamin E 30 IU, Thiamin 3 mg, Riboflavin 3 mg, Niacin 20 mg, Vitamin B6 3 mg, Folate 1 mg, Vitamin B12 8 mcg, Iodine 150 mcg, Zinc 15 mg	Prenatabs CBF by Cypress	60258-0191	Vitamin; Supplement
CYP192	Tab, White, Cap Shaped	Vitamin A 3000 IU, Vitamin C 120 mg, Calcium 200 mg, Iron 28 mg, Vitamin D 400 IU, Vitamin E 22 IU, Thiamin 1.8 mg, Riboflavin 4 mg, Niacin 20 mg, Vitamin B6 25 mg, Folic Acid 1 mg, Vitamin B12 12 mcg, Zinc 25 mg, Copper 2 mg, Magnesium 25 mg	Trinate by Cypress	60258-0192	Vitamin; Supplement
CYP193	Tab, White, Cap Shaped	Vitamin A 4000 IU, Vitamin C 120 mg, Calcium 200 mg, Iron 29 mg, Vitamin D 400 IU, Vitamin E 30 IU, Thiamin 3 mg, Riboflavin 3 mg, Niacin 20 mg, Vitamin B6 3 mg, Folic Acid 1 mg, Vitamin B12 8 mcg, Biotin 30 mcg, Pantothenic Acid 7 mg, Iodine 150 mcg, Magnesium 100 mg, Zinc 15 mg, Copper 3 mg	Prenatabs Rx by Cypress	60258-0193	Vitamin; Supplement
CYP194	Tab, White, Cap Shaped	Vitamin A 2700 IU, Vitamin C 120 mg, Calcium 200 mg, Iron 90 mg, Vitamin D3 400 IU, Vitamin E 30 IU, Thiamin 3 mg, Riboflavin 3.4 mg, Niacin 20 mg, Vitamin B6 20 mg, Folic Acid 1 mg, Vitamin B12 12 mcg, Magnesium 30 mg, Zinc 25 mg, Copper 2 mg, Docusate Sodium 50 mg	Prenatal AD by Cypress	60258-0194	Vitamin; Supplement
CYP232	Tab, White, Cap Shaped	Chlorpheniramine Maleate 8 mg, Methscopolamine Nitrate 2.5 mg, Phenylephrine HCl 40 mg	Ralix by Cypress	60258-0232	Cold Remedy
CYP241	Tab, White, Cap Shaped, Sustained Release	Dextromethorphan HBr 60 mg, Guaifenesin 600 mg, Phenylephrine HCl 40 mg	Anextuss by Cypress	60258-0241	Cold Remedy
CYP242	Tab, White, Cap Shaped	Guaifenesin 600 mg, Phenylephrine HCl 10 mg	Pendex by Cypress	60258-0242	Cold Remedy
CYP248	Tab, White, Caplet, Extended Release	Dextromethorphan HBr 30 mg, Guaifenesin 600 mg, Phenylephrine HCl 10 mg	Dacex-PE by Cypress	60258-0248	Cold Remedy
CYP250	Tab, White, Cap Shaped, Extended Release	Chlorpheniramine Maleate 8 mg, Methscopolamine Nitrate 1.25 mg, Phenylephrine HCl 20 mg	CPM 8/PE 20/MSC 1.25 by Cypress	60258-0250	Cold Remedy
CYP252	Tab, White, Cap Shaped	Guaifenesin 1200 mg, Phenylephrine HCl 40 mg, Dextromethorphan HBr 20 mg	GFN 1200/DM 20/PE 40 by Cypress	60258-0252	Cold Remedy
CYP253	Tab, White, Cap Shaped	Guaifenesin 795 mg, Pseudoephedrine HCl 85 mg	GFN 795/PSE 85 by Cypress	60258-0253	Cold Remedy
CYP254	Tab, White, Cap Shaped	Guaifenesin 800 mg, Pseudoephedrine HCl 60 mg	GFN 800/PSE 60 by Cypress	60258-0254	Cold Remedy

ID FRONT <> BACK	DESCRIPTION FRONT <> BACK	INGREDIENT & STRENGTH	BRAND (or Generic Equiv.) by FIRM	NDC#	CLASS; SCH.
CYP255	Tab, White, Cap Shaped	Guaifenesin 1200 mg, Pseudoephedrine HCl 50 mg	GFN 1200/PSE 50 by Cypress	60258-0255	Cold Remedy
CYP263	Tab, White, Caplet	Guaifenesin 1200 mg, Dextromethorphan HBr 60 mg	GFN 1200/DM 60 by Cypress	60258-0263	Cold Remedy
CYP264	Tab, White, Cap Shaped	Guaifenesin 600 mg, Pseudoephedrine HCl 60 mg, Dextromethorphan HBr 30 mg	GFN 600/PSE 60/DM 30 by Cypress	60258-0264	Cold Remedy
CYP266	Tab, White, Cap Shaped, Scored	Guaifenesin 1200 mg, Pseudoephedrine HCl 120 mg	Duratuss by Cypress	60258-0266	Cold Remedy
CYP267	Tab, White, Cap Shaped	Guaifenesin 1000 mg, Dextromethorphan HBr 60 mg	GFN 1000/DM 60 by Cypress	60258-0267	Cold Remedy
CYP268	Tab, White, Caplet	Guaifenesin 1200 mg, Pseudoephedrine HCl 60 mg, Dextromethorphan HBr 60 mg	GFN 1200/DM 60/PSE 60 by Cypress	60258-0268	Cold Remedy
CYP269	Tab, White, Cap Shaped	Guaifenesin 600 mg, Phenylephrine HCl 20 mg	GFN 600/Phenylephrine 20 by Cypress	60258-0269	Cold Remedy
CYP274	Tab, White, Cap Shaped	Guaifenesin 600 mg, Phenylephrine HCl 40 mg	GFN 600/Phenylephrine 40 by Cypress	60258-0274	Cold Remedy
CYP276	Tab, White, Cap Shaped	Guaifenesin 595 mg, Pseudoephedrine HCl 48 mg, Dextromethorphan 32 mg	GFN 595/PSE 48/DM 32 by Cypress	60258-0276	Cold Remedy
CYP277	Tab, White, Caplet	Guaifenesin 1200 mg, Pseudoephedrine HCl 75 mg	G/P 1200/75 by Cypress	60258-0277	Cold Remedy
CYP279	Tab, White, Cap Shaped	Guaifenesin 550 mg, Pseudoephedrine HCl 60 mg	GFN 550/PSE 60 by Cypress	60258-0279	Cold Remedy
CYP280	Tab, White, Cap Shaped	Chlorpheniramine Maleate 8 mg, Methscopolamine Nitrate 1.25 mg, Pseudoephedrine HCl 60 mg	PCM LA by Cypress	60258-0280	Cold Remedy
CYP281	Tab, White, Cap Shaped	Methscopolamine Nitrate 2.5 mg, Pseudoephedrine HCl 120 mg	PSE 120/MSC 2.5 by Cypress	60258-0281	Cold Remedy
CYP282	Tab, White, Caplet	Chlorpheniramine Maleate 8 mg, Pseudoephedrine 90 mg, Methscopolamine Nitrate 2.5 mg	CPM 8/PSE 90/MSC 2.5 by Cypress	60258-0282	Cold Remedy
CYP283	Tab, White, Cap Shaped, Sustained-Release	Phenylephrine HCl 20 mg, Chlorpheniramine Maleate 4 mg, Phenyltoloxamine Citrate 40 mg	Chlorex-A by Cypress	60258-0283	Cold Remedy
CYP284	Tab, White, Caplet	Guaifenesin 1200 mg, Phenylephrine HCl 40 mg	GFN 1200/Phenylephrine 40 by Cypress	60258-0284	Cold Remedy
CYP285	Tab, White, Cap Shaped	Guaifenesin 595 mg, Pseudoephedrine HCl 48 mg	GFN 595/PSE 48 by Cypress	60258-0285	Cold Remedy
CYP286	Tab, White, Cap Shaped	Dextromethorphan HBr 30 mg, Guaifenesin 500 mg	GFN 500/DM 30 by Cypress	60258-0286	Cold Remedy
CYP287	Tab, White, Cap Shaped	Guaifenesin 550 mg, Pseudoephedrine HCl 60 mg, Dextromethorphan HBr 30 mg	GFN 550/PSE 60/DM 30 by Cypress	60258-0287	Cold Remedy
CYP288	Tab, White, Cap Shaped	Guaifenesin 1000 mg, Dextromethorphan HBr 50 mg	GFN 1000/DM 50 by Cypress	60258-0288	Cold Remedy
CYP291	Tab, White, Cap Shaped	Guaifenesin 800 mg, Pseudoephedrine HCl 60 mg, Dextromethorphan HBr 30 mg	GFN 800/PSE 60/DM 30 by Cypress	60258-0291	Cold Remedy
CYP292	Tab, White, Cap Shaped	Guaifenesin 800 mg, Dextromethorphan HBr 30 mg	GFN 800/DM 30 by Cypress	60258-0292	Cold Remedy
CYP293	Tab, Tan, Speckled, Cap Shaped	Dextromethorphan HBr 30 mg, Guaifenesin 650 mg	Extuss LA by Cypress	60258-0293	Cold Remedy
CYP294	Tab, White, Cap Shaped, Sustained Release	Guaifenesin 800 mg, Phenylephrine HCl 25 mg	GFN 800/Phenylephrine 25 by Cypress	60258-0294	Cold Remedy
CYP295	Tab, Red, Round, Chewable	Chlorpheniramine Maleate 2 mg, Pseudoephedrine HCl 15 mg	PSE 15/CPM 2 by Cypress	60258-0295	Cold Remedy
CYP297	Tab, White, Cap Shaped	Guaifenesin 650 mg, Phenylephrine HCl 25 mg	Nasex by Cypress	60258-0297	Cold Remedy
CYP298	Tab, White, Caplet	Dextromethorphan HBr 25 mg, Guaifenesin 550 mg, Phenylephrine HCl 20 mg	Dexcon-PE by Cypress	60258-0298	Cold Remedy
CYP299	Tab, White, Cap Shaped	Guaifenesin 275 mg, Phenylephrine HCl 25 mg	Nescon PD by Cypress	60258-0299	Cold Remedy
CYP303	Tab, Tan, Speckled, Cap Shaped	Carbetapentane Tannate 60 mg, Chlorpheniramine Tannate 5 mg	Tannic-12 by Cypress	60258-0303	Cold Remedy
CYP329	Tab, White, Cap Shaped, Sustained Release	Chlorpheniramine Maleate 8 mg, Phenylephrine HCl 20 mg	Relera by Cypress	60258-0329	Cold Remedy
CYP351	Tab, White, Cap Shaped, Sustained-Release	Carbinoxamine Maleate 8 mg, Methscopolamine Nitrate 2.5 mg, Pseudoephedrine HCl 90 mg	Nacon by Cypress	60258-0351 Discontinued	Cold Remedy
CYP362	Tab, White	Chlorpheniramine 12 mg, Methscopolamine 2.5 mg, Phenylephrine 20 mg	Chlor-mes by Cypress	60258-0362	Cold Remedy
CYP449	Tab, White, Cap Shaped, Sustained Release	Phenylephrine HCl 20 mg, Chlorpheniramine Maleate 8 mg, Hyoscyamine Sulfate 0.19 mg, Atropine Sulfate 0.04 mg, Scopolamine HBr 0.01 mg	Bellahist-D LA by Cypress	60258-0449	Cold Remedy
CYP470	Tab, White, Modified Oval	Brompheniramine Maleate 6 mg, Pseudoephedrine HCl 45 mg	Bidhist-D by Cypress	60258-0470	Cold Remedy
CYP471	Tab, White, Modified Oval	Brompheniramine Maleate 6 mg	Bidhist by Cypress	60258-0471	Cold Remedy
CYP50 <> APO	Tab, White, Round, Scored	Cyproterone Acetate 50 mg	Androcur by Apotex	Canadian DIN 02245898	Antiandrogen
CYP512	Tab, Round, Blue	Hyoscyamine Sulfate 0.12 mg, Methenamine 81.6 mg, Phenyl Salicylate 36.2 mg, Sodium Bisphosphonate 40.8 mg, Methylene Blue 10.8 mg	Utira by Hawthorn	63717-0512	Urinary

ID FRONT <> BACK	DESCRIPTION FRONT <> BACK	INGREDIENT & STRENGTH	BRAND (or Generic Equiv.) by FIRM	NDC#	CLASS; SCH.
CYP513	Tab, Maroon, Round	Hyoscyamine HBr 0.3 mg, Phenazopyridine HCl 150 mg, Butabarbital 15 mg	Urelief Plus by Cypress	60258-0513	Urinary Tract
CYP514	Tab, Blue, Round, Sugar Coated	Hyoscyamine Sulfate 0.12 mg, Methenamine 81 mg, Methylene Blue 10 mg, Phenyl Salicylate 36 mg, Sodium Biphosphate 40 mg	Uro Blue by Cypress	60258-0514	Gastrointestinal
CYP515	Tab, Green, Round	Hyoscyamine Sulfate 0.03 mg, Atropine Sulfate 0.03 mg, Methenamine 40.8 mg, Methylene Blue 5.4 mg, Phenyl Salicylate 18.1 mg, Benzoic Acid 4.5 mg	Urised by Cypress	60258-0515	Urinary Tract
CYP516	Tab, Light Blue, Cap Shaped	Hyoscyamine Sulfate 0.06 mg, Atropine Sulfate 0.06 mg, Methenamine 81.6 mg, Methylene Blue 10.8 mg, Phenyl Salicylate 36.2 mg, Benzoic Acid 9 mg	Uritact DS by Cypress	60258-0516	Urinary Tract
CYP804	Tab, Green, Round	Atropine Sulfate 0.0582 mg, Hyoscyamine Sulfate 0.3111 mg, Scoplamine HBr 0.0195 mg, Phenobarbital 48.6 mg	Donnatal Extentabs by Cypress	60258-0804	Gastrointestinal; C IV
CYP810	Cap, Green and Yellow	Lipase 1200 Units, Amylase 15,000 Units, Protease 15,000 Units	Lapase by Cypress	60258-0810	Gastrointestinal
CYP811	Cap, Green and White, Opaque	Lipase 2400 Units, Amylase 30,000 Units, Protease 30,000 Units	Dygase by Cypress	60258-0811	Gastrointestinal
CYP840	Cap, White, Opaque	Aminobenzoate Potassium 0.5 gm	Potaba by Cypress	60258-0840	Antifibrotic
CYSTA50MYLAN	Cap, Cysta over 50	Cysteamine Bitartrate 50 mg	Cystagon by Mylan	00378-9040	Nephropathic Cystimosis
CYSTAGON150MYLAN	Cap, Cystagon over 150	Cysteamine Bitartrate 150 mg	Cystagon by Mylan	00378-9045	Nephropathic Cystimosis
CYTOVENE250MG ROCHE	Cap, Green w/ 2 Blue Lines, Blue Print, Cytovene over 250 mg over Roche	Ganciclovir Sodium 250 mg	Cytovene by Hoffmann La Roche	00004-0269	Antiviral
CYTOVENE250MG ROCHE	Cap, Green w/ 2 Blue Lines, Blue Print, Cytovene over 250 mg over Roche	Ganciclovir Sodium 250 mg	Cytovene by Syntex	18393-0269	Antiviral
CYTOVENE500ROCHE	Cap, Yellow & Green w/ 2 Blue Lines, Opaque, Hard Gel	Ganciclovir Sodium 500 mg	Cytovene by Hoffmann La Roche	00004-0278	Antiviral
CYTOVENE500ROCHE	Cap, Yellow & Green w/ 2 Blue Lines, Opaque, Hard Gel	Ganciclovir Sodium 500 mg	Cytovene by Syntex	18393-0914	Antiviral
CZ	Cap, Beige, Black Print	Balsalazide Disodium 750 mg	Colazal by Salix	65649-0101	Gastrointestinal
CZ1 <> APO	Tab, Yellow, Oval, Scored, CZ / 1	Cilazapril 1 mg	Inhibace by Apotex	Canadian DIN 02291134	Antihypertensive
CZ25 <> APO	Tab, Rose, Oval, Scored, CZ / 2.5	Cilazapril 2.5 mg	Inhibace by Apotex	Canadian DIN 02291142	Antihypertensive
CZ5 <> APO	Tab, Reddish-Brown, Oval, Scored, CZ / 5	Cilazapril 5 mg	Inhibace by Apotex	Canadian DIN 02291150	Antihypertensive
D	Tab, Yellow, Round, Chewable	Bismuth Subgallate 200 mg	Devrom by Parthenon		Gastrointestinal
D	Tab, Dark Green, Round, Scored	Chlorophyllin Copper Complex Sodium 100 mg	Derfil by West-Ward	00143-9045	Gastrointestinal
D	Tab, Yellow, Chewable	Bismuth Subgallate 200 mg	Devrom by Parthenon	Canadian DIN 00452696	Gastrointestinal
D	Tab, Pink, Logo/D	Perphenazine 2 mg, Amitriptyline 25 mg	by Schering	Canadian	Antipsychotic; Antidepressant
D	Tab, White, Round	Lactose Enzyme 3000 FCC	by Blistex		Gastrointestinal
D	Tab, Green, Round	Chlorophyllin Copper Complex Sodium 100 mg	Derfil by Rystan		Gastrointestinal
D	Tab, Pink, Round, Schering Logo/D	Amitriptyline 25 mg, Perphenazine 2 mg	Triavil by Bayer	Canadian	Antidepressant; Antipsychotic
D <> 10	Tab, White, D-Shaped	Dexmethylphenidate HCl 10 mg	Focalin by Novartis	00078-0382	Stimulant; C II
D <> 11	Tab, White, Round, Film Coated	Zidovudine 300 mg	Retrovir by Aurobindo	65862-0024	Antiviral
D <> 18	Tab, Pink, Oval, Scored	Hydrochlorothiazide 12.5 mg, Quinapril 10 mg	Accuretic by Aurobindo	65862-0161	Diuretic; Antihypertensive
D <> 19	Tab, Pink, Round, Film Coated	Hydrochlorothiazide 12.5 mg, Quinapril 20 mg	Accuretic by Aurobindo	65862-0162	Diuretic; Antihypertensive
D <> 20	Tab, Pink, Round, Film Coated	Hydrochlorothiazide 25 mg, Quinapril 20 mg	Accuretic by Aurobindo	65862-01623	Diuretic; Antihypertensive
D <> 21	Tab, White to Off White, Round	Atenolol 25 mg	Tenormin by Aurobindo	65862-0168	Antihypertensive
D <> 22	Tab, White to Off White, Round, Scored	Atenolol 50 mg	Tenormin by Aurobindo	65862-0169	Antihypertensive
D <> 23	Tab, White to Off White, Round, Scored	Atenolol 100 mg	Tenormin by Aurobindo	65862-0170	Antihypertensive
D <> 25	Tab, Blue, D-Shaped, D <> 2.5	Dexmethylphenidate HCl 2.5 mg	Focalin by Novartis	00078-0380	Stimulant; C II
D <> 31	Tab, White, Round	Carisoprodol 350 mg	Soma by Aurobindo	65862-0158	Muscle Relaxant
D <> 5	Tab, Yellow, D-Shaped	Dexmethylphenidate HCl 5 mg	Focalin by Novartis	00078-0381	Stimulant; C II

ID FRONT <> BACK	DESCRIPTION FRONT <> BACK	INGREDIENT & STRENGTH	BRAND (or Generic Equiv.) by FIRM	NDC#	CLASS; SCH.
D <> 57	Tab, White to Off White, Round, Scored	Perindopril Erbumine 2 mg	Aceon by Aurobindo	65862-0286	Antihypertensive
D <> 58	Tab, White to Off White, Cap Shaped, Scored	Perindopril Erbumine 4 mg	Aceon by Aurobindo	65862-0287	Antihypertensive
D <> 59	Tab, White to Off White, Round, Scored	Perindopril Erbumine 8 mg	Aceon by Aurobindo	65862-0288	Antihypertensive
D <> 74	Tab, White to Off-White, Round	Terbinafine HCl 250 mg	Lamisil by Aurobindo	65862-0079	Antifungal
D <> AMIDE001	Tab, Orange, Pink & Purple, Round, Chewable, AMIDE001 <> A, B, C, or D	Ascorbic Acid 60 mg, Cyanocobalamin 4.5 mcg, Folic Acid 0.3 mg, Niacinamide, Pyridoxine HCl 1.05 mg, Riboflavin 1.2 mg, Sodium Fluoride, Thiamine Mononitrate, Vitamin A Acetate, Vitamin D 400 Units, Vitamin E Acetate	Multi Vita Bets by Amide	52152-0001	Vitamin
D <> AMIDE001	Tab, Orange, Pink & Purple, Round, Chewable, AMIDE001 <> A, B, C, or D	Ascorbic Acid 60 mg, Cyanocobalamin 4.5 mcg, Folic Acid 0.3 mg, Niacinamide, Pyridoxine HCl 1.05 mg, Riboflavin 1.2 mg, Sodium Fluoride, Thiamine Mononitrate, Vitamin A Acetate, Vitamin D 400 Units, Vitamin E Acetate	Multi Vita Bets by Qualitest	00603-4712	Vitamin
D <> AMIDE001	Tab, Orange, Pink & Purple, Round, Chewable, AMIDE001 <> A, B, C, or D	Ascorbic Acid 60 mg, Cyanocobalamin 4.5 mcg, Folic Acid 0.3 mg, Niacinamide, Pyridoxine HCl 1.05 mg, Riboflavin 1.2 mg, Sodium Fluoride, Thiamine Mononitrate, Vitamin A Acetate, Vitamin D 400 Units, Vitamin E Acetate	Multi Vita Bets by Major	00904-5275	Vitamin
D <> DV	Tab, Yellow, Oval, Film-Coated	Clarithromycin 500 mg	Biaxin by Dava	68774-0122	Antibiotic
D01	Tab, White, Oval, Scored	Desmopressin Acetate 0.1 mg	DDAVP by Novopharm	Canadian DIN 02287730	Antidiuretic
D01 <> LU	Tab, Green, Cap Shaped, Film Coated, Scored, L/U	Sertraline HCl 25 mg	Zoloft by Lupin	68180-0351	Antidepressant
D02	Tab, White, Round, Scored	Desmopressin Acetate 0.2 mg	DDAVP by Novopharm	Canadian DIN 02287749	Antidiuretic
D02	Cap, White, Hard Gel, Black Ink	Gabapentin 100 mg	Neurontin by Aurobindo	65862-0198	Anticonvulsant
D02 <> LU	Tab, Blue, Cap Shaped, Film Coated, Scored, L/U	Sertraline HCl 50 mg	Zoloft by Lupin	68180-0352	Antidepressant
D03	Cap, Yellow, Hard Gel, Black Ink	Gabapentin 300 mg	Neurontin by Aurobindo	65862-0199	Anticonvulsant
D03 <> LU	Tab, Yellow, Cap Shaped, Film Coated, Scored, L/U	Sertraline HCl 100 mg	Zoloft by Lupin	68180-0353	Antidepressant
D04	Cap, Orange, Hard Gel, Black Ink	Gabapentin 400 mg	Neurontin by Aurobindo	65862-0200	Anticonvulsant
D09	Cap, White, Delayed Release	Didanosine 400 mg	Videx by Aurobindo	65862-0313	Antiviral
D1 <> APO	Tab, White, Round, Biconvex	Doxazosin Mesylate 1 mg	Cardura by Apotex	Canadian DIN 02240588	Antihypertensive
D10	Cap, White, Delayed Release	Didanosine 250 mg	Videx by Aurobindo	65862-0312	Antiviral
D100	Tab, White, Oval, Yellow Pellets, Delayed Release	Doxycycline 100 mg	Doryx by Warner Chilcott	00430-0112	Antibiotic
D11 <> LL	Tab, Dark Pink, Round	Demeclocycline HCl 150 mg	Declomycin by Wyeth	Canadian	Antibiotic
D11 <> LL	Tab, Dark Pink, Round	Demeclocycline HCl 150 mg	Declomycin by Lederle	00005-9218	Antibiotic
D12	Tab, Blue and White, Oval, Bi-Layer, Extended Release	Desloratadine 2.5 mg, Pseudoephedrine Sulfate 120 mg	Clarinex-D by Schering	00085-1322	Cold Remedy
D12 <> LL	Tab, Dark Pink, Round	Demeclocycline HCl 300 mg	Declomycin by Wyeth	Canadian	Antibiotic
D12 <> LL	Tab, Dark Pink, Round	Demeclocycline HCl 300 mg	Declomycin by Lederle	00005-9270	Antibiotic
D1200	Tab, White, Oblong, D-1200	Guaifenesin SR 1200 mg	Duratuss by SDA Labs	66424-0600	Expectorant
D14 <> JMI	Tab, White, Round	Liothyronine Sodium 5 mcg	Cytomel by Jones	52604-3414	Thyroid Hormone
D147	Cap	Phentermine HCl 30 mg	by URL Mutual	00677-0460	Anorexiant; C IV
D150	Tab, Orange, Round	Desogestrel 0.15 mg, Ethinyl Estradiol 0.03 mg	Ortho-Cept 21 by Janssen-Ortho	Canadian DIN 02042541	Oral Contraceptive
D150	Tab, Orange, Round	Desogestrel 0.15 mg, Ethinyl Estradiol 0.03 mg	Ortho-Cept 28 by Janssen-Ortho	Canadian DIN 02042533	Oral Contraceptive
D150	Tab	Desogestrel 0.15 mg, Ethinyl Estradiol 0.03 mg	Ortho-Cept 28 by Dept Health	53808-0042	Oral Contraceptive
D150 <> ORTHO	Tab, Orange	Desogestrel 0.15 mg, Ethinyl Estradiol 0.03 mg	Ortho-Cept 28 by Ortho-McNeil	00062-1796	Oral Contraceptive
D150 <> ORTHO	Tab, Peach, Round	Desogestrel 0.15 mg, Ethinyl Estradiol 0.03 mg	Ortho-Cept 21 by Ortho-McNeil	00062-1795	Oral Contraceptive
D2 <> APO	Tab, White, Cap Shaped, Biconvex, Scored	Doxazosin Mesylate 2 mg	Cardura by Apotex	Canadian DIN 02240589	Antihypertensive
D24	Tab, Light Blue, Oval, Coated, Black Ink, Extended Release	Desloratadine 5 mg, Pseudoephedrine 240 mg	Clarinex-D by Schering	00085-1317	Cold Remedy

ID FRONT <> BACK	DESCRIPTION FRONT <> BACK	INGREDIENT & STRENGTH	BRAND (or Generic Equiv.) by FIRM	NDC#	CLASS; SCH.
D250 <> APO	Tab, Light Orange, Cap Shaped	Diflunisal 250 mg	Apo Diflunisal by Apotex	Canadian DIN 02039486	NSAID
D27	Tab, Light Pink, Round, Scored, D / 27	Hydrochlorothiazide 25 mg	Hydrodiuril by Aurobindo	65862-0133	Diuretic; Antihypertensive
D28	Tab, Light Pink, Round, Scored, D / 28	Hydrochlorothiazide 50 mg	Hydrodiuril by Aurobindo	65862-0134	Diuretic; Antihypertensive
D31	Tab, Pink, Round	Meperidine 50 mg, Acetaminophen 300 mg	Demerol APAP by Sanofi		Analgesic; C II
D32	Tab, Yellow, 5-Sided, D-Shaped, Film Coated	Cyclobenzaprine HCl 10 mg	Flexeril by Aurobindo	65862-0191	Muscle Relaxant
D35 <> W	Tab, Coated, D/35	Meperidine 50 mg	Demerol by Bayer	00280-0335	Analgesic; C II
D35 <> W	Tab, D/35	Meperidine 50 mg	Demerol by Sanofi	00024-0335	Analgesic; C II
D37 <> W	Tab, D/37	Meperidine 100 mg	Demerol by Sanofi	00024-0337	Analgesic; C II
D37 <> W	Tab, Coated, D/37	Meperidine 100 mg	Demerol by Bayer	00280-0337	Analgesic; C II
D4 <> APO	Tab, White, Diamond Shaped, Biconvex, Scored	Doxazosin Mesylate 4 mg	Cardura by Apotex	Canadian DIN 02240590	Antihypertensive
D44 <> LL	Tab, Purple, Round, D over 44	Dipyridamole 25 mg	Persantine by Lederle	00005-3743	Antiplatelet
D44 <> LL	Tab, Purple, Round, D over 44	Dipyridamole 25 mg	Persantine by PDRX	55289-0748	Antiplatelet
D45 <> LL	Tab, Purple, Round, D over 45	Dipyridamole 50 mg	Persantine by Caremark	00339-5107	Antiplatelet
D45 <> LL	Tab, Purple, Round, D over 45	Dipyridamole 50 mg	Persantine by Nat Pharmpak	55154-5506	Antiplatelet
D45 <> LL	Tab, Purple, Round, D over 45	Dipyridamole 50 mg	Persantine by Lederle	00005-3790	Antiplatelet
D46 <> LL	Tab, Purple, Round, D over 46	Dipyridamole 75 mg	Persantine by Nat Pharmpak	55154-5507	Antiplatelet
D46 <> LL	Tab, Purple, Round, D over 46	Dipyridamole 75 mg	Persantine by Caremark	00339-5109	Antiplatelet
D46 <> LL	Tab, Purple, Round, D over 46	Dipyridamole 75 mg	Persantine by Lederle	00005-3791	Antiplatelet
D50	Tab, Brown, Round	Dipyridamole 50 mg	Dipyridamone by Apotex	Canadian DIN 00895652	Antiplatelet
D500 <> APO	Tab, Orange, Cap Shaped	Diflunisal 500 mg	Apo Diflunisal by Apotex	Canadian DIN 02039494	NSAID
D500 <> NU	Tab, Orange, Cap Shaped, Film Coated	Diflunisal 500 mg	by Nu Pharm	Canadian DIN 02058413	NSAID
D51 <> LL	Tab, White, Round, Scored, D over 51	Diazepam 2 mg	Valium by Lederle	00005-3128	Antianxiety; C IV
D52 <> LL	Tab, Tan, Round, Scored, D over 52	Diazepam 5 mg	Valium by Nat Pharmpak	55154-5554	Antianxiety; C IV
D52 <> LL	Tab, Tan, Round, Scored, D over 52	Diazepam 5 mg	Valium by Lederle	50053-3129	Antianxiety; C IV
D52 <> LL	Tab, Tan, Round, Scored, D over 52	Diazepam 5 mg	Valium by Southwood	58016-0275	Antianxiety; C IV
D53 <> LL	Tab, Green, Round, Scored, D over 53	Diazepam 10 mg	Valium by Lederle	00005-3130	Antianxiety; C IV
D53 <> LL	Tab, Green, Round, Scored, D over 53	Diazepam 10 mg	Valium by Southwood	58016-0273	Antianxiety; C IV
D600	Tab, White, Oval	Carbinoxamine 4 mg, Pseudoephedrine 60 mg	Rondamine by Major	00904-3248 Discontinued	Cold Remedy
D69	Cap, White, Delayed Release	Didanosine 200 mg	Videx EC by Aurobindo	65862-0311	Antiviral
D70	Tab, Pink, Black Print, Round, Schering Logo over D70	Ethinyl Estradiol 0.05 mg	by Amerisource	62584-0299	Oral Contraceptive
D70	Tab, Pink, Black Print, Round, Schering Logo over D70	Ethinyl Estradiol 0.05 mg	Estinyl by Schering	00085-0070	Hormone
D70	Cap, White, Delayed Release	Didanosine 125 mg	Videx EC by Aurobindo	65862-0310	Antiviral
D71 <> LL	Tab, Light Blue, Round, Scored	Diltiazem HCl 30 mg	Cardizem by Amerisource	62584-0366	Antihypertensive
D71 <> LL	Tab, Light Blue, Round, Scored	Diltiazem HCl 30 mg	Cardizem by Nat Pharmpak	55154-5504	Antihypertensive
D72 <> LL	Tab, Light Blue, Round, Scored	Diltiazem HCl 60 mg	Cardizem by Lederle	00005-3334	Antihypertensive
D75	Tab, White, Oval, Yellow Pellets, Delayed Release	Doxycycline 75 mg	Doryx by Warner Chilcott	00430-0111	Antibiotic
D75	Tab, Red, Round	Dipyridamole 75 mg	Dipyridamone by Apotex	Canadian DIN 00895660	Antiplatelet
D75 <> LL	Tab, Light Blue, Cap Shaped, Scored	Diltiazem HCl 90 mg	Cardizem by Lederle	00005-3335	Antihypertensive
D75 <> LL	Tab, Light Blue, Cap Shaped, Scored	Diltiazem HCl 90 mg	Cardizem by Eckerd	19458-0896	Antihypertensive
D75 <> LL	Tab, Light Blue, Cap Shaped, Scored	Diltiazem HCl 90 mg	Cardizem by PDRX	55289-0893	Antihypertensive
D75 <> LL	Tab, Light Blue, Cap Shaped, Scored	Diltiazem HCl 90 mg	Cardizem by Ivax	00182-1939	Antihypertensive
D77 <> LL	Tab, Light Blue, Cap Shaped	Diltiazem HCl 120 mg	Cardizem by Ivax	00182-1940	Antihypertensive
D77 <> LL	Tab, Light Blue, Cap Shaped	Diltiazem HCl 120 mg	Cardizem by Lederle	00005-3336	Antihypertensive

ID FRONT <> BACK	DESCRIPTION FRONT <> BACK	INGREDIENT & STRENGTH	BRAND (or Generic Equiv.) by FIRM	NDC#	CLASS; SCH.
D87	Tab, Yellowish Orange, 5-Sided, D-Shaped, Film Coated	Cyclobenzaprine HCl 5 mg	Flexeril by Aurobindo	65862-0190	Muscle Relaxant
D9 <> BM	Tab, White, Round, Sustained Release	Bezafibrate 400 mg	Bezalip by Roche	Canadian DIN 02083523	Antihyperlipidemic
D92W	Cap, Green, White Print, Soft Gel, W in circle	Ergocalciferol 1.25 mg	Drisdol by RP Scherer	11014-0890	Vitamin
D92W	Cap, Green, White Print, Soft Gel, W in circle	Ergocalciferol 1.25 mg	Drisdol by Sanofi	00024-0392	Vitamin
D92W	Cap, Green, White Print, Soft Gel, W in circle	Ergocalciferol 1.25 mg	Drisdol by Bayer	00280-0392	Vitamin
D93	Tab, White to Off-White, Shield Shaped, Scored	Lamotrigine 25 mg	Lamictal by Aurobindo	65862-0227	Anticonvulsant
D94	Tab, Peach, Shield Shaped, Scored	Lamotrigine 100 mg	Lamictal by Aurobindo	65862-0228	Anticonvulsant
D95	Tab, Cream Colored, Shield Shaped, Scored	Lamotrigine 150 mg	Lamictal by Aurobindo	65862-0229	Anticonvulsant
D96	Tab, Blue, Shield Shaped, Scored	Lamotrigine 150 mg	Lamictal by Aurobindo	65862-0230	Anticonvulsant
DA <> DURA	Tab, D/A <> DU/RA	Chlorpheniramine Maleate 8 mg, Methscopolamine Nitrate 2.5 mg, Phenylephrine HCl 20 mg	Dura Vent by Anabolic	00722-6072	Cold Remedy
DAII <> DURA	Tab	Chlorpheniramine Maleate 4 mg, Methscopolamine Nitrate 1.25 mg, Phenylephrine HCl 10 mg	DA II by Anabolic	00722-6354	Cold Remedy
DALLERGY	Tab, Off-White	Chlorpheniramine Maleate 8 mg, Methscopolamine Nitrate 2.5 mg, Phenylephrine HCl 20 mg	Dallergy by Anabolic	00722-6273	Cold Remedy
DALLERGY	Tab	Mivacurium Chloride 8 mg, Methscopolamine Nitrate 2.5 mg, Phenylephrine HCl 20 mg	Dallergy IR by Anabolic	00722-6457	Antihistamine
DALLERGY <> 12H	Tab, White, Cap Shaped, Scored	Chlorpheniramine Maleate 8 mg, Methscopolamine Nitrate 2.5 mg, Phenylephrine HCl 20 mg	Dallergy ER by Laser	00277-0180 Discontinued	Cold Remedy
DALLERGY <> 12H	Tab, White, Cap Shaped, Scored, Ex Release	Chlorpheniramine Maleate 12 mg, Methscopolamine Nitrate 2.5 mg, Phenylephrine HCl 20 mg	Dallergy by Laser	00277-0182	Cold Remedy
DALLERGY <> LASER	Tab, White, Round, Scored	Chlorpheniramine Maleate 4 mg, Methscopolamine Nitrate 1.25 mg, Phenylephrine HCl 10 mg	Dallergy by Laser	00277-0160	Cold Remedy
DALLERGYJRLASER176	Cap, Maize, Opaque, Ex Release, Dallergy JR <> Laser over 176	Brompheniramine Maleate 6 mg, Pseudoephedrine HCl 60 mg	Dallergy Jr by Sovereign	58716-0028	Cold Remedy
DALLERGYJRLASER176	Cap, Maize, Opaque	Brompheniramine Maleate 6 mg, Pseudoephedrine HCl 60 mg	Dallergy Jr by Laser	00277-0176 Discontinued	Cold Remedy
DALLERGYJRLASER176	Cap, Maize, Opaque, Ex Release, Dallergy JR <> Laser over 176	Chlorpheniramine Maleate 4 mg, Phenylephrine HCl 20 mg	Dallergy Jr by Laser	00277-0183	Cold Remedy
DALMANE15ROCHE	Cap, Orange, Dalmane/15 Roche	Flurazepam HCl 15 mg	Dalmane by Roche	Canadian	Hypnotic; C IV
DALMANE30ROCHE	Cap, Ivory & Red, Dalmane/30 Roche	Flurazepam HCl 30 mg	Dalmane by Roche	Canadian	Hypnotic; C IV
DAN <> 100P	Tab, White, Round, Scored	Phenobarbital 100 mg	Phenobarbital by Schein	00364-0206	Sedative/Hypnotic; C IV
DAN <> 15P	Tab, White, Round, Scored	Phenobarbital 15 mg	Phenobarbital by Schein	00364-2444	Sedative/Hypnotic; C IV
DAN <> 30P	Tab, White, Round, Scored	Phenobarbital 30 mg	Phenobarbital by Schein	00364-0203	Sedative/Hypnotic; C IV
DAN <> 5050	Tab, Orange, Round, Film Coated	Hydralazine HCl 25 mg	by Schein	00364-0144	Antihypertensive
DAN <> 5319	Tab, White, Round	Promethazine HCl 50 mg	Phenergan by Schein	00364-0345	Antiemetic; Antihistamine
DAN <> 5319	Tab, White, Round	Promethazine HCl 50 mg	Phenergan by Watson	00591-5319	Antiemetic; Antihistamine
DAN <> 5373	Tab	Isosorbide Dinitrate 10 mg	Isordil by Watson	00591-5373	Antianginal
DAN <> 5385	Tab	Isosorbide Dinitrate 5 mg	Isordil by Watson	00591-5385	Antianginal
DAN <> 5385	Tab, White, Round	Isosorbide Dinitrate 5 mg	Isordil by Schein	00364-0368	Antianginal
DAN <> 5387	Tab, Yellow, Round	Isosorbide Dinitrate 2.5 mg	Isordil by Watson	00591-5387	Antianginal
DAN <> 5387	Tab, Yellow, Round	Isosorbide Dinitrate 2.5 mg	Isordil by Schein	00364-0367	Antianginal
DAN <> 5428	Tab, Light Yellow, Round	Reserpine 0.1 mg, Hydralazine HCl 25 mg, Hydrochlorothiazide 15 mg	by Schein	00364-0361	Antihypertensive; Diuretic
DAN <> 5444	Tab, White, Round, Scored	Chlorthiazide 250 mg	Diuril by Schein	00364-0389	Diuretic; Antihypertensive
DAN <> 5501	Tab, White, Oval, Sublingual	Ergoloid Mesylate 1 mg	by Schein	00364-0446	Ergot Alkaloids
DAN <> 5502	Tab, White, Round, Sublingual	Ergoloid Mesylate 0.5 mg	by Schein	00364-0415	Ergot Alkaloids
DAN <> 5503	Tab, Amber-Yellow, Round	Sulfasalazine 500 mg	by Schein	00364-0444	Gastrointestinal
DAN <> 5504	Tab, White, Round	Ergoloid Mesylate 1 mg	by Schein	00364-0622	Ergot Alkaloids
DAN <> 5507	Tab, Yellow, Round	Chlorthalidone 25 mg	by Schein	00364-0564	Diuretic
DAN <> 5507	Tab, Yellow, Round	Chlorthalidone 25 mg	by Schein	00364-0592	Diuretic

ID FRONT <> BACK	DESCRIPTION FRONT <> BACK	INGREDIENT & STRENGTH	BRAND (or Generic Equiv.) by FIRM	NDC#	CLASS; SCH.
DAN <> 5513	Tab, White, Round	Carisoprodol 350 mg	Soma by Schein	00364-0475	Muscle Relaxant
DAN <> 5513	Tab, White, Round	Carisoprodol 350 mg	Soma by Watson	00591-5513	Muscle Relaxant
DAN <> 5513	Tab, White, Round	Carisoprodol 350 mg	Soma by Pharmedix	53002-0356	Muscle Relaxant
DAN <> 5513	Tab, White, Round	Carisoprodol 350 mg	Soma by Urgent Care Center	50716-0202	Muscle Relaxant
DAN <> 5513	Tab, White, Round	Carisoprodol 350 mg	Soma by Kaiser	00179-1349	Muscle Relaxant
DAN <> 5513	Tab, White, Round	Carisoprodol 350 mg	Soma by Heartland	61392-0949	Muscle Relaxant
DAN <> 5516	Tab, White, Round	Quinine Sulfate 260 mg	Quinamm by Schein	00364-0560	Antimalarial
DAN <> 5518	Tab, Light Green, Round	Chlorthalidone 50 mg	Hygroton by Schein	00364-0593	Diuretic
DAN <> 5518	Tab, Light Green, Round	Chlorthalidone 50 mg	Hygroton by Schein	00364-0528	Diuretic
DAN <> 5522	Tab, Orange, Round, Film Coated	Hydroxyzine HCl 10 mg	Atarax by Heartland	61392-0012	Antianxiety; Antihistamine
DAN <> 5522	Tab, Orange, Round, Film Coated	Hydroxyzine HCl 10 mg	Atarax by Schein	00364-0494	Antianxiety; Antihistamine
DAN <> 5522	Tab, Orange, Round, Film Coated	Hydroxyzine HCl 10 mg	Atarax by Watson	00591-5522	Antianxiety; Antihistamine
DAN <> 5523	Tab, Green, Round, Film Coated	Hydroxyzine HCl 25 mg	Atarax by Nat Pharmpak	55154-5203	Antianxiety; Antihistamine
DAN <> 5523	Tab, Green, Round, Film Coated	Hydroxyzine HCl 25 mg	Atarax by Vangard	00615-1526	Antianxiety; Antihistamine
DAN <> 5523	Tab, Green, Round, Film Coated	Hydroxyzine HCl 25 mg	Atarax by Watson	00591-5523	Antianxiety; Antihistamine
DAN <> 5523	Tab, Green, Round, Film Coated	Hydroxyzine HCl 25 mg	Atarax by Heartland	61392-0013	Antianxiety; Antihistamine
DAN <> 5523	Tab, Green, Round, Film Coated	Hydroxyzine HCl 25 mg	Atarax by Med Pro	53978-3066	Antianxiety; Antihistamine
DAN <> 5523	Tab, Green, Round, Film Coated	Hydroxyzine HCl 25 mg	Atarax by Schein	00364-0495	Antianxiety; Antihistamine
DAN <> 5538	Tab, Off-White, Round, Ex Release	Quinidine Gluconate 324 mg	Quinaglute by Watson	00591-5538	Antiarrhythmic
DAN <> 5538	Tab, Off-White, Round, Ex Release	Quinidine Gluconate 324 mg	Quinaglute by Schein	00364-0604	Antiarrhythmic
DAN <> 5540	Tab, Off-White to White, Round	Metronidazole 250 mg	Flagyl by Schein	00591-5595	Antibiotic
DAN <> 5540	Tab, Off-White to White, Round	Metronidazole 250 mg	Flagyl by Watson	00591-5540	Antibiotic
DAN <> 5540	Tab, Off-White to White, Round	Metronidazole 250 mg	Flagyl by Med Pro	53978-0215	Antibiotic
DAN <> 5540	Tab, Off-White to White, Round	Metronidazole 250 mg	Flagyl by Nat Pharmpak	55154-5212	Antibiotic
DAN <> 5549	Tab, White, Round, Film Coated	Chloroquine Phosphate 500 mg	Aralen Phosphate by Schein	00364-2431	Antimalarial
DAN <> 5552	Tab	Metronidazole 500 mg	by Nat Pharmpak	55154-5234	Antibiotic
DAN <> 5553	Tab, Light Orange, Round, Film Coated	Doxycycline Hyclate 100 mg	Vibramycin by Schein	00591-2063	Antibiotic
DAN <> 5553	Tab, Light Orange, Round, Film Coated	Doxycycline Hyclate 100 mg	Vibramycin by Med Pro	53978-3028	Antibiotic
DAN <> 5553	Tab, Light Orange, Round, Film Coated	Doxycycline Hyclate 100 mg	Vibramycin by Watson	00591-5553	Antibiotic
DAN <> 5553	Tab, Light Orange, Round, Film Coated	Doxycycline Hyclate 100 mg	Vibramycin by Pharmedix	53002-0271	Antibiotic
DAN <> 5553	Tab, Light Orange, Round, Film Coated	Doxycycline Hyclate 100 mg	Vibramycin by Murfreesboro	51129-1357	Antibiotic
DAN <> 5562	Tab, White, Oval, Film Coated, Ex Release	Procainamide HCl 250 mg	by Watson	00591-5562	Antiarrhythmic
DAN <> 5562	Tab, White, Oval, Film Coated, Ex Release	Procainamide HCl 250 mg	by Schein	00364-0715	Antiarrhythmic
DAN <> 5565	Tab, Yellow, Round, Film Coated	Hydroxyzine HCl 50 mg	Atarax by Watson	00591-5565	Antianxiety; Antihistamine
DAN <> 5565	Tab, Coated	Hydroxyzine HCl 50 mg	Atarax by Med Pro	53978-3186	Antianxiety; Antihistamine
DAN <> 5565	Tab, Sugar Coated	Hydroxyzine HCl 50 mg	by Allscripts		Antianxiety; Antihistamine
DAN <> 5565	Tab, Yellow, Round, Film Coated	Hydroxyzine HCl 50 mg	Atarax by Schein	00364-0496	Antianxiety; Antihistamine
DAN <> 5569	Tab, Orange, Round, Film Coated	Thioridazine HCl 100 mg	by Schein	00364-0670	Antipsychotic
DAN <> 5572	Tab, White, Round, Film Coated	Thioridazine HCl 15 mg	by Schein	00364-0669	Antipsychotic
DAN <> 5580	Tab, Orange, Round, Film Coated	Thioridazine HCl 150 mg	by Schein	00364-0723	Antipsychotic
DAN <> 5581	Tab, Reddish Pink, Round, Film Coated	Thioridazine HCl 200 mg	by Schein	00364-0724	Antipsychotic
DAN <> 5584	Tab, White, Round, Film Coated	Ibuprofen 400 mg	Motrin by Schein	00364-0765	NSAID
DAN <> 5585	Tab, White, Round, Film Coated	Ibuprofen 200 mg	Motrin by Schein	00364-2145	NSAID
DAN <> 5587	Tab, White, Round, Film Coated	Methyldopa 500 mg	by Schein	00364-0708	Antihypertensive
DAN <> 5588	Tab, White, Round, Film Coated	Methyldopa 250 mg	by Schein	00364-0707	Antihypertensive
DAN <> 5589	Tab, White, Round, Scored	Metoclopramide HCl 10 mg	Reglan by Danbury		Gastrointestinal
DAN <> 5601	Tab, Film Coated	Verapamil HCl 80 mg	Verelan by Nat Pharmpak	55154-5227	Antihypertensive
DAN <> 5644	Tab, White, Oval, Film Coated	Ibuprofen 800 mg	Motrin by Schein	00364-2137	NSAID
DAN <> 5658	Tab, White, Round, Film Coated	Cyclobenzaprine HCl 10 mg	Flexeril by Danbury	61955-2348	Muscle Relaxant
DAN <> 5658	Tab, White, Round, Film Coated	Cyclobenzaprine HCl 10 mg	Flexeril by DJ Pharma	64455-0013	Muscle Relaxant

ID FRONT <> BACK	DESCRIPTION FRONT <> BACK	INGREDIENT & STRENGTH	BRAND (or Generic Equiv.) by FIRM	NDC#	CLASS; SCH.
DAN <> 5658	Tab, White, Round, Film Coated	Cyclobenzaprine HCl 10 mg	Flexeril by Southwood	58016-0234	Muscle Relaxant
DAN <> 5658	Tab, White, Round, Film Coated	Cyclobenzaprine HCl 10 mg	Flexeril by PDRX	55289-0567	Muscle Relaxant
DAN <> 5658	Tab, White, Round, Film Coated	Cyclobenzaprine HCl 10 mg	Flexeril by Watson	00591-5658	Muscle Relaxant
DAN <> 5658	Tab, White, Round, Film Coated	Cyclobenzaprine HCl 10 mg	Flexeril by Schein	00364-2348	Muscle Relaxant
DAN <> 5658	Tab, White, Round, Film Coated	Cyclobenzaprine HCl 10 mg	Flexeril by Pharmedix	53002-0308	Muscle Relaxant
DAN <> 5658	Tab, White, Round, Film Coated	Cyclobenzaprine HCl 10 mg	Flexeril by Vangard	00615-3520	Muscle Relaxant
DAN <> 5658	Tab, White, Round, Film Coated	Cyclobenzaprine HCl 10 mg	Flexeril by Nat Pharmpak	55154-5217	Muscle Relaxant
DAN <> 5658	Tab, White, Round, Film Coated	Cyclobenzaprine HCl 10 mg	Flexeril by Heartland	61392-0830	Muscle Relaxant
DAN <> 5658	Tab, White, Round, Film Coated	Cyclobenzaprine HCl 10 mg	Flexeril by Heartland	61392-0098	Muscle Relaxant
DAN <> 5658	Tab, White, Round, Film Coated	Cyclobenzaprine HCl 10 mg	Flexeril by Amerisource	62584-0354	Muscle Relaxant
DAN <> 5661	Tab, Yellow, Round	Sulindac 150 mg		61392-0954	NSAID
DAN <> 5661	Tab, Yellow, Round	Sulindac 150 mg	Clinoril by Heartland	57866-4621	NSAID
DAN <> 5661	Tab, Yellow, Round	Sulindac 150 mg	Clinoril by Direct Dispensing	60760-0290	NSAID
DAN <> 5661	Tab, Yellow, Round	Sulindac 150 mg	Clinoril by St. Mary's Med	00591-5661	NSAID
DAN <> 5661	Tab, Yellow, Round	Sulindac 150 mg	Clinoril by Watson	00364-2441	NSAID
DAN <> 5662	Tab, Off-White, Oval, Scored	Nalidixic Acid 1 g	Clinoril by Schein	00364-2325	Antibiotic
DAN <> 5678	Tab, White, Round, Film Coated	Amitriptyline 25 mg, Chlordiazepoxide 10 mg	by Schein	00364-2158	Antianxiety; C IV
DAN <> 5679	Tab, Light Green, Round, Film Coated	Amitriptyline 12.5 mg, Chlordiazepoxide 5 mg	Limbitrol by Schein	00364-2157	Antianxiety; C IV
DAN <> 5912	Tab, Blue, Oval, Scored	Captopril 50 mg, HCTZ 25 mg	Limbitrol by Schein	00364-2640	Antihypertensive; Diuretic
DAN <> 60P	Tab, White, Round, Scored	Phenobarbital 60 mg	Capozide by Schein	00364-0697	Sedative/Hypnotic; C IV
DAN <> 944	Tab, White, Round	Colchicine 0.6 mg	by Schein	53002-0444	Antigout
DAN <> 944	Tab, White, Round	Colchicine 0.6 mg	by Pharmedix	00364-0074	Antigout
DAN <> 944	Tab, White, Round	Colchicine 0.6 mg	by Schein	00591-0944	Antigout
DAN <> 944	Tab, White, Round	Colchicine 0.6 mg	by Watson	61392-0174	Antigout
DAN <> A22	Tab, Yellow, Round, Film Coated	Ranitidine HCl 150 mg	by Heartland	00364-2633	Gastrointestinal
DAN <> A23	Tab, Yellow, Cap Shaped, Film Coated	Ranitidine HCl 300 mg	by Schein	00364-2634	Gastrointestinal
DAN025 <> 5449	Tab, Orange, Pentagonal, Scored, Dan 0.25 <> 5449	Dexamethasone 0.25 mg	by Schein	00364-0397	Steroid
DAN03 <> 5613	Tab, Light Blue, Pentagonal, Scored, Dan 0.3 <> 5613	Clonidine HCl 0.3 mg	by Schein	00364-0824	Antihypertensive
DAN05 <> 5605	Tab, White, Round, Scored, Dan 0.5 <> 5605	Haloperidol 0.5 mg	Haldol by Schein	00364-2204	Antipsychotic
DAN05 <> 5625	Tab, White, Round, Scored, Dan 0.5 <> 5625	Lorazepam 0.5 mg	Ativan by Schein	00364-0793	Antianxiety; C IV
DAN050 <> 5450	Tab, Yellow, Pentagonal, Scored, Dan over 0.50	Dexamethasone 0.5 mg	by Schein	00364-0398	Steroid
DAN075 <> 5361	Tab, Light Blue, Round, Scored, Dan 0.75 <> 5361	Dexamethasone 0.75 mg	by Schein	00364-0098	Steroid
DAN1 <> 5624	Tab, White, Round, Scored	Lorazepam 1 mg	Ativan by Schein	00364-0794	Antianxiety; C IV
DAN10 <> 5566	Tab, Yellow-Green, Triangular	Thioridazine HCl 10 mg	by Schein	00364-2317	Antipsychotic
DAN10 <> 5620	Tab, Light Blue, Round, Scored	Diazepam 10 mg	by Schein	00364-0776	Antianxiety; C IV
DAN10 <> 5724	Tab, White, Round, Scored	Metaproterenol Sulfate 10 mg	by Schein	00364-2283	Antiasthmatic
DAN10 <> 5737	Tab, White, Round, Scored	Timolol Maleate 10 mg	Blocadren by Schein	00364-2358	Antihypertensive
DAN10 <> 5883	Tab, Light Green, Round, Scored	Methylphenidate HCl 10 mg	Ritalin by Watson	00591-5883	Stimulant; C II
DAN10 <> 5883	Tab, Light Green, Round, Scored	Methylphenidate HCl 10 mg	Ritalin by Schein	00364-0479	Stimulant; C II
DAN100 <> 5715	Tab, Blue, Round, Scored, DAN over 100	Amoxapine 100 mg	Asendin by Watson	00591-5715	Antidepressant
DAN100 <> 5715	Tab, Blue, Round, Scored, DAN over 100	Amoxapine 100 mg	Asendin by Schein	00364-2434	Antidepressant
DAN100 <> 5778	Tab, White, Round	Atenolol 100 mg	Tenormin by Schein	00364-2514	Antihypertensive
DAN100 <> 5778	Tab, White, Round	Atenolol 100 mg	Tenormin by Watson	00591-5778	Antihypertensive
DAN100 <> 5778	Tab, White, Round	Atenolol 100 mg	Tenormin by Danbury	61955-2514	Antihypertensive
DAN100 <> 5859	Tab, White, Round, Quadrisected	Captopril 100 mg	Capoten by Schein	00364-2631	Antihypertensive
DAN1005778	Tab, Coated, Dan/100/5778	Atenolol 100 mg	Tenormin by Duramed	51285-0838	Antihypertensive
DAN1005859	Tab, White, Round, Scored	Captopril 100 mg	Capoten by Caremark		Antihypertensive
DAN105724	Tab, White, Round	Metaproterenol Sulfate 10 mg	Alupent by Danbury	00339-5851	Antiasthmatic
DAN105730	Tab, White, Round, Dan-10, 5730	Baclofen 10 mg	Lioresal by Danbury		Muscle Relaxant

436

For updated data, go to www.IdentADrug.com

ID FRONT <> BACK	DESCRIPTION FRONT <> BACK	INGREDIENT & STRENGTH	BRAND (or Generic Equiv.) by FIRM	NDC#	CLASS; SCH.
DAN1153	Tab, White, Round	Carisoprodol 350 mg	Soma by Danbury		Muscle Relaxant
DAN1255856	Tab, White, Round, Scored, Dan 12.5 5856	Captopril 12.5 mg	Capoten by Caremark	00339-5781	Antihypertensive
DAN15 <> 5451	Tab, White, Pentagonal, Scored, Dan 1.5 <> 5451	Dexamethasone 1.5 mg	by Schein	00364-0399	Steroid
DAN15 <> 5607	Tab, White, Round, Film Coated	Methyldopa 250 mg, Hydrochlorothiazide 15 mg	by Schein	00364-0827	Antihypertensive; Diuretic
DAN150 <> 5716	Tab, Orange, Round, Scored	Amoxapine 150 mg	Asendin by Schein	00364-2435	Antidepressant
DAN150 <> 5716	Tab, Orange, Round, Scored	Amoxapine 150 mg	Asendin by Watson	00591-5716	Antidepressant
DAN2 <> 5603	Tab, Yellow, Round, Scored	Haloperidol 2 mg	Haldol by Schein	00364-2206	Antipsychotic
DAN2 <> 5621	Tab, White, Round, Scored	Diazepam 2 mg	by Schein	00364-0774	Antianxiety; C IV
DAN2 <> 5622	Tab, White, Round, Scored	Lorazepam 2 mg	Ativan by Schein	00364-0795	Antianxiety; C IV
DAN2 <> 5710	Tab, White, Round, Scored	Albuterol Sulfate 2 mg	Proventil by Schein	00364-2438	Antiasthmatic
DAN20 <> 5725	Tab, White, Round, Scored	Metaproterenol Sulfate 20 mg	by Schein	00364-2284	Antiasthmatic
DAN20 <> 5738	Tab, White, Cap Shaped, Scored	Timolol Maleate 20 mg	Blocadren by Schein	00364-2359	Antihypertensive
DAN20 <> 5884	Tab, Peach, Round, Scored	Methylphenidate HCl 20 mg	Ritalin by Schein	00364-0562	Stimulant; C II
DAN20 <> 5884	Tab, Peach, Round, Scored	Methylphenidate HCl 20 mg	Ritalin by Watson	00591-5884	Stimulant; C II
DAN205725	Tab, White, Round	Metaproterenol Sulfate 20 mg	Alupent by Danbury		Antiasthmatic
DAN205731	Tab, White, Round, Dan-20, 5731	Baclofen 20 mg	Lioresal by Danbury		Muscle Relaxant
DAN205738	Tab, White, Oblong, Dan/20 5738	Timolol Maleate 20 mg	Blocadren by Danbury		Antihypertensive
DAN25 <> 5542	Tab, Beige, Triangular, Film Coated	Thioridazine HCl 25 mg	by Schein	00364-0662	Antipsychotic
DAN25 <> 5608	Tab, White, Round, Film Coated	Methyldopa 250 mg, Hydrochlorothiazide 25 mg	by Schein	00364-0828	Antihypertensive; Diuretic
DAN25 <> 5713	Tab, White, Round, Scored	Amoxapine 25 mg	Asendin by Schein	00591-5713	Antidepressant
DAN25 <> 5713	Tab, White, Round, Scored	Amoxapine 25 mg	Asendin by Schein	00364-2432	Antidepressant
DAN25 <> A7	Tab, White, Round, Scored	Captopril 25 mg	Capoten by Schein	00364-2629	Antihypertensive
DAN2505816	Cap, Light Green, Round	Naproxen 250 mg	Naprosyn by Schein	00364-2562	NSAID
DAN2505816	Cap, Light Green, Round	Naproxen 250 mg	Naprosyn by Watson	00591-5816	NSAID
DAN30 <> 5611	Tab, White, Round, Film Coated	Methyldopa 500 mg, Hydrochlorothiazide 30 mg	by Schein	00364-2400	Antihypertensive; Diuretic
DAN3120	Cap, Pink, Opaque	Clindamycin 300 mg	Cleocin HCl by Watson	00591-3120	Antibiotic
DAN375 <> 5817	Tab, Purple, Oblong	Naproxen 375 mg	Naprosyn by Watson	00591-5817	NSAID
DAN375 <> 5817	Tab, Lavender, Cap Shaped	Naproxen 375 mg	Naprosyn by Schein	00364-2563	NSAID
DAN4 <> 5711	Tab, White, Round, Scored	Albuterol Sulfate 4 mg	Proventil by Schein	00364-2439	Antiasthmatic
DAN5 <> 5606	Tab, Blue, Round, Scored	Haloperidol 5 mg	Haldol by Schein	00364-2357	Antipsychotic
DAN5 <> 5736	Tab, White, Round	Timolol Maleate 5 mg	by Schein	00364-0561	Antihypertensive
DAN5 <> 5882	Tab, Purple, Round	Methylphenidate HCl 5 mg	Ritalin by Schein	00591-5882	Stimulant; C II
DAN5 <> 5882	Tab, Light Purple, Round	Methylphenidate HCl 5 mg	Ritalin by Watson	00364-2318	Stimulant; C II
DAN50 <> 5568	Tab, White, Triangular, Film Coated	Thioridazine HCl 50 mg	by Schein	00364-2401	Antipsychotic
DAN50 <> 5610	Tab, White, Round, Film Coated, Scored	Methyldopa 500 mg, Hydrochlorothiazide 50 mg	by Schein	00364-2433	Antihypertensive; Diuretic
DAN50 <> 5714	Tab, Red, Round, Scored, DAN over 50	Amoxapine 50 mg	Asendin by Schein	00591-5714	Antidepressant
DAN50 <> 5714	Tab, Red, Round, Scored, DAN over 50	Amoxapine 50 mg	Asendin by Watson	00364-2513	Antidepressant
DAN50 <> 5777	Tab, White, Round, Scored	Atenolol 50 mg	Tenormin by Schein	00591-5777	Antihypertensive
DAN50 <> 5777	Tab, White, Round, Scored	Atenolol 50 mg	Tenormin by Watson	61955-2513	Antihypertensive
DAN50 <> 5777	Tab, White, Round, Scored	Atenolol 50 mg	Tenormin by Danbury	55154-5211	Antihypertensive
DAN50 <> 5777	Tab, White, Round, Scored	Atenolol 50 mg	Tenormin by Nat Pharmpak	00364-2630	Antihypertensive
DAN50 <> 5858	Tab, White, Round, Scored	Captopril 50 mg	Capoten by Schein	00364-2255	Antihypertensive
DAN500 <> 5706	Tab, Light Green, Round, Scored	Chlorzoxazone 500 mg	by Schein	00364-2564	Muscle Relaxant
DAN500 <> 5818	Tab, Light Green, Cap Shaped	Naproxen 500 mg	Naprosyn by Schein	00591-5818	NSAID
DAN500 <> 5818	Tab, Light Green, Cap Shaped	Naproxen 500 mg	Naprosyn by Watson		NSAID
DAN5002	Cap, Clear & Pink	Diphenhydramine HCl 25 mg	Benadryl by Danbury		Antihistamine
DAN5003	Cap, Pink	Diphenhydramine HCl 50 mg	Benadryl by Danbury		Antihistamine
DAN5005706	Tab, Green, Round, Dan-500, 5706	Chlorzoxazone 500 mg	Parafon Forte DSC by Danbury		Muscle Relaxant

ID FRONT <> BACK	DESCRIPTION FRONT <> BACK	INGREDIENT & STRENGTH	BRAND (or Generic Equiv.) by FIRM	NDC#	CLASS; SCH.
DAN5026	Cap, Yellow, Black Print, DAN over 5026	Procainamide HCl 250 mg	by Schein	00364-0219	Antiarrhythmic
DAN5026	Cap, Yellow, Black Print, DAN over 5026	Procainamide HCl 250 mg	by Watson	00591-5026	Antiarrhythmic
DAN5028	Cap, Clear, Black Print, DAN over 5028	Quinine Sulfate 5 g	by Schein	00364-0230	Antimalarial
DAN5050	Tab, Orange, Round	Hydralazine HCl 25 mg	Apresoline by Danbury		Antihypertensive
DAN5055	Tab, Orange, Round	Hydralazine HCl 50 mg	Apresoline by Danbury		Antihypertensive
DAN505777	Tab, White, Round, Dan/50/5777	Atenolol 50 mg	Tenormin by Duramed	51285-0837	Antihypertensive
DAN5058	Tab, Bluish Green, Round, Dan/5058	Tripelennamine HCl 50 mg	PBZ by Danbury		Antihistamine
DAN505858	Tab, White, Round, Scored	Captopril 50 mg	Capoten by Caremark	00339-5840	Antihypertensive
DAN5162	Cap	Tetracycline HCl 500 mg	by Med Pro	53978-5048	Antibiotic
DAN5162	Cap	Tetracycline HCl 250 mg	by Talbert	44514-0884	Antibiotic
DAN5183	Tab, White, Round	Hydrocortisone 20 mg	Cortone by Danbury		Steroid
DAN5196	Cap, Brown & Clear	Papaverine HCl 150 mg	Pavabid by Danbury		Vasodilator
DAN5204	Tab, White, Round	Pseudoephedrine 60 mg	Sudafed by Danbury		Decongestant
DAN526	Tab, White, Round	Isoniazid 300 mg	Laniazid by Danbury		Antimycobacterial
DAN5304	Tab, Gray, Round	Promethazine HCl 12.5 mg	Phenergan by Danbury		Antiemetic; Antihistamine
DAN5316	Tab, White, Round, (Veterinary)	Phenylbutazone 100 mg	Butazolidin by Danbury		Veterinary; Anti-Inflammatory
DAN5326	Tab, White, Oblong	Colchicine 0.5 mg, Probenecid 500 mg	ColBenemid by Danbury		Antigout
DAN5333	Cap	Procainamide HCl 500 mg	by Watson	00591-5333	Antiarrhythmic
DAN5342	Tab, White, Round	Nylidrin 6 mg	Arlidin by Danbury		Vasodilator
DAN5345	Tab, Peach, Round	Hydrochlorothiazide 50 mg	Esidrix by Danbury		Diuretic; Antihypertensive
DAN5350	Cap, Orange & White, Black Print, DAN over 5350	Procainamide HCl 375 mg	by Watson	00591-5350	Antiarrhythmic
DAN5350	Cap, Orange & White, Black Print, DAN over 5350	Procainamide HCl 375 mg	by Schein	00364-0343	Antiarrhythmic
DAN5361075	Tab, Blue, Round, Dan 5361 0.75	Dexamethasone 0.75 mg	Decadron by Danbury		Steroid
DAN5368	Tab, White, Round, Dan/5368	Disulfiram 500 mg	Antabuse by Danbury		Antialcoholism
DAN5376	Tab, White, Round, Dan/5376	Disulfiram 250 mg	Antabuse by Danbury		Antialcoholism
DAN5388	Tab, White, Oblong, Dan/5388	Triamcinolone 4 mg	Aristocort by Danbury		Steroid
DAN5390	Tab, White, Round	Nylidrin 12 mg	Arlidin by Danbury		Vasodilator
DAN5406	Tab, Green, Round, Dan/5406	Hydrochlorothiazide 25 mg, Reserpine 0.125 mg	Hydropres by Danbury		Diuretic; Antihypertensive
DAN5407	Tab, Green, Round, Dan/5407	Hydrochlorothiazide 50 mg, Reserpine 0.125 mg	Hydropres by Danbury		Diuretic; Antihypertensive
DAN5428	Tab, Yellow, Round	Hydralazine 25 mg, Hydrochlorothiazide 15 mg, Reserpine 0.1 mg	Ser-Ap-Es by Danbury		Antihypertensive; Diuretic
DAN5434	Tab, White, Round	Triprolidine 2.5 mg, Pseudoephedrine 60 mg	Actifed by Danbury		Cold Remedy
DAN5440	Cap, Blue, Black Print, DAN over 5440	Doxycycline Hyclate 100 mg	Vibramycin by Schein	00364-2033	Antibiotic
DAN5440	Cap, Blue, Black Print, DAN over 5440	Doxycycline Hyclate 100 mg	Vibramycin by Pharmedix	53002-0212	Antibiotic
DAN5440	Cap, Blue, Black Print, DAN over 5440	Doxycycline Hyclate 100 mg	Vibramycin by Danbury	61955-2033	Antibiotic
DAN5440	Cap, Blue, Black Print, DAN over 5440	Doxycycline Hyclate 100 mg	Vibramycin by H J Harkins Co	52959-0467	Antibiotic
DAN5440	Cap, Blue, Black Print, DAN over 5440	Doxycycline Hyclate 100 mg	Vibramycin by Watson	00591-5440	Antibiotic
DAN5444	Tab, White, Round	Chlorothiazide 250 mg	Diuril by Danbury		Diuretic; Antihypertensive
DAN5449025	Tab, Orange, Pentagonal, Dan 5449 0.25	Dexamethasone 0.25 mg	Decadron by Danbury		Steroid
DAN545115	Tab, White, Pentagonal, Dan 5451 1.5	Dexamethasone 1.5 mg	Decadron by Danbury		Steroid
DAN5453	Tab, White, Round	Quinidine Sulfate 100 mg	Quinidine Sulfate by Danbury		Antiarrhythmic
DAN5455	Tab, Blue, Round	Chlorpropamide 250 mg	Diabinese by Danbury		Antidiabetic
DAN5479	Cap, Ivory & Orange, Dan/5479	Erythromycin Estolate 250 mg	Ilosone by Danbury		Antibiotic
DAN5484	Tab, White, Round	Cyproheptadine HCl 4 mg	Periactin by Danbury		Antihistamine

ID FRONT <> BACK	DESCRIPTION FRONT <> BACK	INGREDIENT & STRENGTH	BRAND (or Generic Equiv.) by FIRM	NDC#	CLASS; SCH.
DAN5490	Tab, White, Round	Prednisone 50 mg	Deltasone by Danbury		Steroid
DAN5495	Tab, Peach, Round	Chlorzoxazone 250 mg	Parafon by Danbury		Muscle Relaxant
DAN5501	Tab, White, Round	Ergoloid Mesylate 1 mg	Hydergine by Danbury		Ergot Alkaloids
DAN5502	Tab, White, Round	Ergoloid Mesylate 0.5 mg	Hydergine by Danbury		Ergot Alkaloids
DAN5503	Tab, Butterscotch, Round, Dan/5503	Sulfasalazine 500 mg	Azulfidine by Danbury		Gastrointestinal
DAN5504	Tab, White, Round	Ergoloid Mesylate 1 mg	Hydergine by Danbury		Ergot Alkaloids
DAN5506	Tab, Red, Round	Pseudoephedrine 30 mg	Sudafed by Danbury		Decongestant
DAN5510	Tab, White, Round	Dipyridamole 25 mg	Persantine by Danbury		Antiplatelet
DAN5511	Tab, White, Round	Dipyridamole 50 mg	Persantine by Danbury		Antiplatelet
DAN5512	Tab, White, Round	Dipyridamole 75 mg	Persantine by Danbury		Antiplatelet
DAN5514	Tab, White, Round	Sulfinpyrazone 100 mg	Anturane by Danbury		Uricosuric
DAN5515	Tab, Yellow, Round	Bethanechol Chloride 50 mg	Urecholine by Danbury		Urinary Tract
DAN5516	Tab, Red, Round	Quinine Sulfate 260 mg	Quinamm by Danbury		Antimalarial
DAN5520	Cap, Black & Yellow	Tetracycline HCl 500 mg	Achromycin V by Danbury		Antibiotic
DAN5532	Tab, Film Coated	Hydroxyzine HCl 25 mg	Vistaril by Direct Dispensing	57866-3874	Antianxiety; Antihistamine
DAN5535	Cap, Blue & White, Black Print, DAN over 5535	Doxycycline Hyclate 50 mg	Vibramycin by Danbury	61955-2032	Antibiotic
DAN5535	Cap, Blue & White, Black Print, DAN over 5535	Doxycycline Hyclate 50 mg	Vibramycin by Schein	00364-2032	Antibiotic
DAN5535	Cap, Light Blue & White	Doxycycline Hyclate 50 mg	Vibramycin by Watson	00591-5535	Antibiotic
DAN5548	Tab, White, Round, Dan/5548	Chloroquine Phosphate 250 mg	Aralen Phosphate by Danbury		Antimalarial
DAN5549	Tab, White, Round	Chloroquine Phosphate 500 mg	Aralen Phosphate by Danbury		Antimalarial
DAN5554 <> 10	Tab, Orange, Round, Scored, DAN over 5554	Propranolol HCl 10 mg	Inderal by Schein	00364-0756	Antihypertensive
DAN5554 <> 10	Tab, Orange, Round, Scored, DAN over 5554	Propranolol HCl 10 mg	Inderal by Med Pro	53978-0034	Antihypertensive
DAN5554 <> 10	Tab, Orange, Round, Scored, DAN over 5554	Propranolol HCl 10 mg	Inderal by Watson	00591-5554	Antihypertensive
DAN5555 <> 20	Tab, Blue, Round, Scored, DAN over 5555	Propranolol HCl 20 mg	Inderal by Rx Pak	65084-0101	Antihypertensive
DAN5555 <> 20	Tab, Blue, Round, Scored, DAN over 5555	Propranolol HCl 20 mg	Inderal by Vangard	00615-2562	Antihypertensive
DAN5555 <> 20	Tab, Blue, Round, Scored, DAN over 5555	Propranolol HCl 20 mg	Inderal by Watson	00591-5555	Antihypertensive
DAN5555 <> 20	Tab, Blue, Round, Scored, DAN over 5555	Propranolol HCl 20 mg	Inderal by Schein	00364-0757	Antihypertensive
DAN5556 <> 40	Tab, Green, Round, Scored, DAN over 5556	Propranolol HCl 40 mg	Inderal by Schein	00364-0758	Antihypertensive
DAN5556 <> 40	Tab, Green, Round, Scored, DAN over 5556	Propranolol HCl 40 mg	Inderal by Vangard	00615-2563	Antihypertensive
DAN5556 <> 40	Tab, Green, Round, Scored, DAN over 5556	Propranolol HCl 40 mg	Inderal by Rx Pak	65084-0102	Antihypertensive
DAN5556 <> 40	Tab, Green, Round, Scored, DAN over 5556	Propranolol HCl 40 mg	Inderal by Watson	00591-5556	Antihypertensive
DAN5557 <> 80	Tab, Yellow, Round, Scored, DAN over 80	Propranolol HCl 80 mg	Inderal by Watson	00591-5557	Antihypertensive
DAN5557 <> 80	Tab, Yellow, Round, Scored, DAN over 80	Propranolol HCl 80 mg	Inderal by Schein	00364-0760	Antihypertensive
DAN5560	Cap, Orange, Opaque	Disopyramide Phosphate 100 mg	Norpace by Schein	00364-0739	Antiarrhythmic
DAN5560	Cap, Orange, Opaque	Disopyramide Phosphate 100 mg	Norpace by Watson	00591-5560	Antiarrhythmic
DAN5561	Cap, Brown, Opaque	Disopyramide Phosphate 150 mg	Norpace by Watson	00591-5561	Antiarrhythmic
DAN5569	Tab, Orange, Round	Thioridazine 100 mg	Mellaril by Danbury		Antipsychotic
DAN5572	Tab, White, Round	Thioridazine 15 mg	Mellaril by Danbury		Antipsychotic
DAN5576	Tab, White, Round	Furosemide 20 mg	Lasix by Danbury		Diuretic
DAN5582	Tab, White, Round	Tolazamide 250 mg	Tolinase by Danbury		Antidiabetic
DAN5584	Tab, White, Round	Ibuprofen 400 mg	Motrin by Danbury		NSAID
DAN5586	Tab, White, Oval	Ibuprofen 600 mg	Motrin by Danbury		NSAID
DAN5592	Cap, Light Green, Black Print, DAN over 5592	Thiothixene 2 mg	by Watson	00591-5592	Antipsychotic
DAN5592	Cap, Light Green, Black Print, DAN over 5592	Thiothixene 2 mg	by Schein	00364-2167	Antipsychotic
DAN5593	Cap, Yellow, Black Print, DAN over 5593	Thiothixene 1 mg	by Schein	00364-2166	Antipsychotic

ID FRONT <> BACK	DESCRIPTION FRONT <> BACK	INGREDIENT & STRENGTH	BRAND (or Generic Equiv.) by FIRM	NDC#	CLASS; SCH.
DAN5593	Cap, Yellow, Black Print, DAN over 5593	Thiothixene 1 mg	by Watson	00591-5593	Antipsychotic
DAN5594	Cap, White, Black Print, DAN over 5594	Thiothixene 10 mg	by Schein	00364-2169	Antipsychotic
DAN5594	Cap, White, Black Print, DAN over 5594	Thiothixene 10 mg	by Watson	00591-5594	Antipsychotic
DAN5595	Cap, Orange, Black Print, DAN over 5595	Thiothixene 5 mg	by Watson	00591-5595	Antipsychotic
DAN5595	Cap, Orange, Black Print, DAN over 5595	Thiothixene 5 mg	by Schein	00364-2168	Antipsychotic
DAN5595	Cap, Orange, Black Print, DAN over 5595	Thiothixene 5 mg	by Taro	52549-4032	Antipsychotic
DAN5601	Tab, Film Coated	Verapamil HCl 80 mg	Verelan by Pharmedix	53002-1027	Antihypertensive
DAN5602	Tab, Coated	Verapamil HCl 120 mg	by Pharmedix	53002-1074	Antihypertensive
DAN56032	Tab, Yellow, Round, Dan 5603/2	Haloperidol 2 mg	Haldol by Danbury		Antipsychotic
DAN5604 <> 1	Tab, Peach, Round, Scored, DAN over 5604	Haloperidol 1 mg	Haldol by Danbury		Antipsychotic
DAN5604 <> 1	Tab, Peach, Round, Scored, DAN over 5604	Haloperidol 1 mg	Haldol by Schein	00364-2205	Antipsychotic
DAN560505	Tab, White, Round, Dan 5605 0.5	Haloperidol 0.5 mg	Haldol by Danbury		Antipsychotic
DAN56065	Tab, Blue, Round, Dan 5606/5	Haloperidol 5 mg	Haldol by Danbury		Antipsychotic
DAN560715	Tab, White, Round	Hydrochlorothiazide 15 mg, Methyldopa 250 mg	Aldoril 15 by Danbury		Diuretic; Antihypertensive
DAN560825	Tab, White, Round	Hydrochlorothiazide 25 mg, Methyldopa 250 mg	Aldoril 25 by Danbury		Diuretic; Antihypertensive
DAN5609 <> 01	Tab, White, Pentagonal, Scored, Dan over 5609 <> 0.1	Clonidine HCl 0.1 mg	by Watson	00591-5609	Antihypertensive
DAN561050	Tab, White, Round	Hydrochlorothiazide 50 mg, Methyldopa 500 mg	Aldoril D50 by Danbury		Diuretic; Antihypertensive
DAN561130	Tab, White, Round	Hydrochlorothiazide 30 mg, Methyldopa 500 mg	Aldoril D30 by Danbury		Diuretic; Antihypertensive
DAN5612 <> 02	Tab, Yellow, Pentagonal, Scored, Dan over 5612 <> 0.2	Clonidine HCl 0.2 mg	by Schein	00364-0821	Antihypertensive
DAN5612 <> 02	Tab, Yellow, Pentagonal, Scored, Dan over 5612 <> 0.2	Clonidine HCl 0.2 mg	by Watson	00591-5612	Antihypertensive
DAN5613 <> 03	Tab, Dan 5613 <> 0.3	Clonidine HCl 0.3 mg	by Watson	00591-5613	Antihypertensive
DAN561303	Tab, Blue, Pentagonal, Dan 5613/0.3	Clonidine HCl 0.3 mg	Catapres by Danbury		Antihypertensive
DAN5614	Cap, Blue & White	Flurazepam HCl 15 mg	Dalmane by Danbury		Hypnotic; C IV
DAN5615	Cap	Flurazepam HCl 30 mg	by Quality Care	60346-0762	Hypnotic; C IV
DAN5616	Cap, Red	Oxazepam 15 mg	Serax by Danbury		Sedative/Hypnotic; C IV
DAN5617	Cap, White	Oxazepam 10 mg	Serax by Danbury		Sedative/Hypnotic; C IV
DAN5618	Cap, Maroon	Oxazepam 30 mg	Serax by Danbury		Sedative/Hypnotic; C IV
DAN5619 <> 5	Tab, Yellow, Round, Scored, Dan over 5619	Diazepam 5 mg	Valium by Schein	00364-0775	Antianxiety; C IV
DAN5619 <> 5	Tab, Yellow, Round, Scored, Dan over 5619	Diazepam 5 mg	Valium by Vangard	00615-1533	Antianxiety; C IV
DAN5619 <> 5	Tab, Yellow, Round, Scored, Dan over 5619	Diazepam 5 mg	Valium by Watson	00591-5619	Antianxiety; C IV
DAN5619 <> 5	Tab, Yellow, Round, Scored, Dan over 5619	Diazepam 5 mg	Valium by St. Mary's Med	60760-0775	Antianxiety; C IV
DAN5619 <> 5	Tab, Yellow, Round, Scored, Dan over 5619	Diazepam 5 mg	Valium by DRX	55045-2656	Antianxiety; C IV
DAN5620 <> 10	Tab, Light Blue, Round, Scored	Diazepam 10 mg	Valium by Watson	00591-5620	Antianxiety; C IV
DAN5620 <> 10	Tab, Light Blue, Round, Scored	Diazepam 10 mg	Valium by St. Mary's Med	60760-0776	Antianxiety; C IV
DAN5621 <> 2	Tab, White, Round, Scored	Diazepam 2 mg	Valium by DRX	55045-2652	Antianxiety; C IV
DAN5621 <> 2	Tab, White, Round, Scored	Diazepam 2 mg	Valium by Murfreesboro	51129-1302	Antianxiety; C IV
DAN5621 <> 2	Tab, White, Round, Scored	Diazepam 2 mg	Valium by Vangard	00615-1532	Antianxiety; C IV
DAN5621 <> 2	Tab, White, Round, Scored	Diazepam 2 mg	Valium by Watson	00591-5621	Antianxiety; C IV
DAN56222	Tab, White, Round, Dan 5622/2	Lorazepam 2 mg	Ativan by Danbury		Antianxiety; C IV
DAN562360	Tab, Red, Round, Dan 5623/60	Propranolol HCl 60 mg	Inderal by Danbury		Antihypertensive
DAN56241	Tab, White, Round, Dan 5624/1	Lorazepam 1 mg	Ativan by Danbury		Antianxiety; C IV
DAN562505	Tab, White, Round, Dan 5625/0.5	Lorazepam 0.5 mg	Ativan by Danbury		Antianxiety; C IV
DAN5629	Cap, Beige, Black Print, DAN over 5629	Doxepin HCl 10 mg	Sinequan by H J Harkins Co	52959-0369	Antidepressant
DAN5629	Cap, Beige, Black Print, DAN over 5629	Doxepin HCl 10 mg	Sinequan by Heartland	61392-0120	Antidepressant
DAN5629	Cap, Beige, Black Print, DAN over 5629	Doxepin HCl 10 mg	Sinequan by H J Harkins Co	52959-0246	Antidepressant
DAN5629	Cap, Beige, Black Print, DAN over 5629	Doxepin HCl 10 mg	Sinequan by H J Harkins Co	52959-0366	Antidepressant

ID FRONT <> BACK	DESCRIPTION FRONT <> BACK	INGREDIENT & STRENGTH	BRAND (or Generic Equiv.) by FIRM	NDC#	CLASS; SCH.
DAN5629	Cap, Beige, Black Print, DAN over 5629	Doxepin HCl 10 mg	Sinequan by Schein	00364-2113	Antidepressant
DAN5629	Cap, Beige, Black Print, DAN over 5629	Doxepin HCl 10 mg	Sinequan by Watson	00591-5629	Antidepressant
DAN5630	Cap, White & Yellow, Black Print, DAN over 5630	Doxepin HCl 25 mg	Sinequan by Schein	00364-2114	Antidepressant
DAN5630	Cap, White & Yellow, Black Print, DAN over 5630	Doxepin HCl 25 mg	Sinequan by Watson	00591-5630	Antidepressant
DAN5630	Cap, White & Yellow, Black Print, DAN over 5630	Doxepin HCl 25 mg	Sinequan by Schein	00364-2114	Antidepressant
DAN5630	Cap, White & Yellow, Black Print, DAN over 5630	Doxepin HCl 25 mg	Sinequan by H J Harkins Co	52959-0377	Antidepressant
DAN5631	Cap, Yellow, Black Print, DAN over 5631	Doxepin HCl 50 mg	Sinequan by H J Harkins Co	52959-0012	Antidepressant
DAN5631	Cap, Yellow, Black Print, DAN over 5631	Doxepin HCl 50 mg	Sinequan by H J Harkins Co	52959-0391	Antidepressant
DAN5631	Cap, Yellow, Black Print, DAN over 5631	Doxepin HCl 50 mg	Sinequan by Schein	00364-2115	Antidepressant
DAN5631	Cap, Yellow, Black Print, DAN over 5631	Doxepin HCl 50 mg	Sinequan by Watson	00591-5631	Antidepressant
DAN5632	Cap, Green, Black Print, DAN over 5632	Doxepin HCl 75 mg	Sinequan by Watson	00591-5632	Antidepressant
DAN5632	Cap, Green, Black Print, DAN over 5632	Doxepin HCl 75 mg	Sinequan by Schein	00364-2116	Antidepressant
DAN5632	Cap, Green, Black Print, DAN over 5632	Doxepin HCl 75 mg	Sinequan by Heartland	61392-0933	Antidepressant
DAN5632	Cap, Green, Black Print, DAN over 5632	Doxepin HCl 75 mg	Sinequan by Schein	00364-2116	Antidepressant
DAN5633	Cap, Light Green & White, Opaque	Doxepin HCl 100 mg	Sinequan by Schein	00364-2117	Antidepressant
DAN5633	Cap, Light Green & White, Opaque	Doxepin HCl 100 mg	Sinequan by Watson	00591-5633	Antidepressant
DAN563590	Tab, Lavender, Round, Dan 5635/90	Propranolol HCl 90 mg	Inderal by Danbury		Antihypertensive
DAN5636	Cap, Coral	Meclofenamate Sodium 50 mg	Meclomen by Watson	00591-5636	NSAID
DAN5636	Cap, Coral	Meclofenamate Sodium 50 mg	Meclomen by Schein	00364-2155	NSAID
DAN5637	Cap, Red & White, Black Print	Meclofenamate Sodium 100 mg	Meclomen by Schein	00364-2156	NSAID
DAN5637	Cap, Red & White, Black Print	Meclofenamate Sodium 100 mg	Meclomen by Pharmedix	53002-0400	NSAID
DAN5637	Cap, Red & White, Black Print	Meclofenamate Sodium 100 mg	Meclomen by Watson	00591-5637	NSAID
DAN5642 <> 25	Tab, White, Round, Scored, Dan over 5642 <> 2.5	Minoxidil 2.5 mg	Rogaine by Schein	00364-2172	Antihypertensive
DAN5642 <> 25	Tab, White, Round, Scored, Dan over 5642 <> 2.5	Minoxidil 2.5 mg	Rogaine by Watson	00591-5642	Antihypertensive
DAN5643 <> 10	Tab, White, Round, Scored, Dan over 5643	Minoxidil 10 mg	Rogaine by Watson	00591-5643	Antihypertensive
DAN5643 <> 10	Tab, White, Round, Scored, Dan over 5643	Minoxidil 10 mg	Rogaine by Schein	00364-2173	Antihypertensive
DAN5644	Tab, White, Oval	Ibuprofen 800 mg	Motrin by Danbury		NSAID
DAN5658	Tab, White, Round, Film Coated	Cyclobenzaprine HCl 10 mg	Flexeril by Ivax	00182-1919 Discontinued	Muscle Relaxant
DAN5658	Tab, White, Round, Film Coated	Cyclobenzaprine HCl 10 mg	Flexeril by Major	00904-7809 Discontinued	Muscle Relaxant
DAN5662	Tab, Off-White, Oval, Dan/5662	Nalidixic Acid 1 g	NegGram by Danbury		Antibiotic
DAN5677	Tab, Off-White, Round, Dan/5677	Nalidixic Acid 500 mg	NegGram by Danbury		Antibiotic
DAN5678	Tab, White, Round	Amitriptyline 25 mg, Chlordiazepoxide 10 mg	Limbitrol by Danbury		Antianxiety; C IV
DAN5679	Tab, Green, Round	Amitriptyline 12.5 mg, Chlordiazepoxide 5 mg	Limbitrol by Danbury		Antianxiety; C IV
DAN5682	Tab, Light Yellow, Round, Scored, DAN over 5682	Hydrochlorothiazide 25 mg, Triamterene 50 mg	by Med Pro	53978-5009	Diuretic; Antihypertensive
DAN5682	Tab, Light Yellow, Round, Scored, DAN over 5682	Hydrochlorothiazide 50 mg, Triamterene 75 mg	by Kaiser	00179-1132	Diuretic; Antihypertensive
DAN5682	Tab, Light Yellow, Round, Scored, DAN over 5682	Hydrochlorothiazide 50 mg, Triamterene 75 mg	by Watson	00591-5682	Diuretic; Antihypertensive
DAN5682	Tab, Light Yellow, Round, Scored, DAN over 5682	Hydrochlorothiazide 50 mg, Triamterene 75 mg	by Heartland	61392-0965	Diuretic; Antihypertensive
DAN5682	Tab, Light Yellow, Round, Scored, DAN over 5682	Triamterene 75 mg, Hydrochlorothiazide 50 mg	by Schein	00364-2242	Diuretic; Antihypertensive
DAN5693	Cap, Orange	Prazosin HCl 5 mg	Minipress by Danbury		Antihypertensive
DAN5696	Cap, Gray	Prazosin HCl 2 mg	Minipress by Danbury		Antihypertensive
DAN5697	Cap,	Prazosin HCl	by Pharmedix	53002-0499	Antihypertensive
DAN5708	Cap, Gray & Pink, Black Print, DAN over 5708	Clindamycin HCl 150 mg	Cleocin HCl by St. Mary's Med	60760-0337	Antibiotic
DAN5708	Cap, Gray & Pink, Black Print, DAN over 5708	Clindamycin HCl 150 mg	Cleocin HCl by Schein	00364-2337	Antibiotic
DAN5708	Cap, Gray & Pink, Black Print, DAN over 5708	Clindamycin HCl 150 mg	Cleocin HCl by Watson	00591-5708	Antibiotic
DAN57102	Tab, White, Round, Dan-5710, 2	Albuterol Sulfate 2 mg	Ventolin by Danbury		Antiasthmatic
DAN57114	Tab, White, Round, Dan-5711, 4	Albuterol Sulfate 4 mg	Proventil by Danbury		Antiasthmatic

ID FRONT <> BACK	DESCRIPTION FRONT <> BACK	INGREDIENT & STRENGTH	BRAND (or Generic Equiv.) by FIRM	NDC#	CLASS; SCH.
DAN571325	Tab, White, Round	Amoxapine 25 mg	Asendin by Danbury		Antidepressant
DAN571450	Tab, Orange, Round	Amoxapine 50 mg	Asendin by Danbury		Antidepressant
DAN571510	Tab, Blue, Round	Amoxapine 100 mg	Asendin by Danbury		Antidepressant
DAN5716150	Tab, Orange, Round	Amoxapine 150 mg	Asendin by Danbury		Antidepressant
DAN5726	Cap, Dark Green & Light Green, Black Print, DAN over 5726	Hydroxyzine Pamoate 25 mg	Vistaril by Watson	00591-5726	Antianxiety; Antihistamine
DAN5726	Cap, Dark Green & Light Green, Black Print, DAN over 5726	Hydroxyzine Pamoate 25 mg	Vistaril by Heartland	61392-0801	Antianxiety; Antihistamine
DAN5726	Cap, Dark Green & Light Green, Black Print, DAN over 5726	Hydroxyzine Pamoate 25 mg	Vistaril by Schein	00364-0483	Antianxiety; Antihistamine
DAN5730 <> 10	Tab, White, Round, Scored	Baclofen 10 mg	Lioresal by Watson	00591-5730	Muscle Relaxant
DAN5730 <> 10	Tab, White, Round, Scored	Baclofen 10 mg	Lioresal by Schein	00364-2312	Muscle Relaxant
DAN5730 <> 10	Tab, White, Round, Scored	Baclofen 10 mg	Lioresal by Heartland	61392-0090	Muscle Relaxant
DAN5730 <> 10	Tab, White, Round, Scored	Baclofen 10 mg	Lioresal by Amerisource	62584-0623	Muscle Relaxant
DAN5730 <> 10	Tab, White, Round, Scored	Baclofen 10 mg	Lioresal by Amerisource	61392-0706	Muscle Relaxant
DAN5731 <> 20	Tab, White, Round, Scored	Baclofen 20 mg	Lioresal by Amerisource	62584-0624	Muscle Relaxant
DAN5731 <> 20	Tab, White, Round, Scored	Baclofen 20 mg	Lioresal by Watson	00591-5731	Muscle Relaxant
DAN5731 <> 20	Tab, White, Round, Scored	Baclofen 20 mg	Lioresal by Schein	00364-2313	Muscle Relaxant
DAN57365	Tab, White, Round	Timolol Maleate 5 mg	Blocadren by Danbury		Antihypertensive
DAN573710	Tab, White, Round	Timolol Maleate 10 mg	Blocadren by Danbury		Antihypertensive
DAN577750	Tab, White, Round, Dan-5777, 50	Atenolol 50 mg	Tenormin by Danbury		Antihypertensive
DAN5778100	Tab, White, Round, Dan-5778, 100	Atenolol 100 mg	Tenormin by Danbury		Antihypertensive
DAN5782	Tab, White, Round, Scored	Atenolol 50 mg, Chlorthalidone 25 mg	Tenoretic by Schein	00364-2527	Antihypertensive; Diuretic
DAN5782	Tab, White, Round, Scored	Atenolol 50 mg, Chlorthalidone 25 mg	Tenoretic by Watson	00591-5782	Antihypertensive; Diuretic
DAN5783	Tab, White, Round, Scored	Atenolol 100 mg, Chlorthalidone 25 mg	Tenoretic by Schein	00364-2528	Antihypertensive; Diuretic
DAN5783	Tab, White, Round, Scored	Atenolol 100 mg, Chlorthalidone 25 mg	Tenoretic by Watson	00591-5783	Antihypertensive; Diuretic
DAN5912	Tab	Captopril 50 mg, HCTZ 25 mg	Capozide by Watson	00591-5912	Antihypertensive; Diuretic
DAN937	Tab, White, Round	Papaverine HCl 60 mg	by Danbury		Vasodilator
DAN938	Tab, White, Round	Papaverine HCl 100 mg	by Danbury		Vasodilator
DANA15	Tab, Light Orange, Round, Film Coated	Famotidine 20 mg	by Watson	00591-3123	Gastrointestinal
DANA17	Tab, Beige, Round, Film Coated	Famotidine 40 mg	by Watson	00591-3124	Gastrointestinal
DANA22	Tab, Film Coated	Ranitidine HCl 167.5 mg	by Ranbaxy	63304-0745	Gastrointestinal
DANA22	Tab, Film Coated	Ranitidine HCl 167.5 mg	by Watson	00591-8013	Gastrointestinal
DANA22	Tab, Yellow, Round, Film Coated	Ranitidine HCl 150 mg	by Dixon Shane	17236-0741	Gastrointestinal
DANA23	Tab, Coated	Ranitidine HCl 336 mg	by Ranbaxy	63304-0746	Gastrointestinal
DANA23	Tab, Yellow	Ranitidine HCl 336 mg	by Apotheca	12634-0560	Gastrointestinal
DANA23	Tab, Coated	Ranitidine HCl 336 mg	by Watson	00591-8014	Gastrointestinal
DANAND5538	Tab, White, Round	Quinidine Gluconate 324 mg	by Heartland	61392-0952	Antiarrhythmic
DANBURY5373	Tab	Isosorbide Dinitrate 10 mg	Isordil by Pharmedix	53002-0451	Antianginal
DANDAN <> 5052	Tab, White, Round, Scored	Prednisone 5 mg	Deltasone by Merz	00259-0390	Steroid
DANDAN <> 5052	Tab, White, Round, Scored	Prednisone 5 mg	Deltasone by Danbury	61955-0218	Steroid
DANDAN <> 5052	Tab, White, Round, Scored	Prednisone 5 mg	Deltasone by WA Butler	11695-1801	Steroid
DANDAN <> 5052	Tab, White, Round, Scored	Prednisone 5 mg	Deltasone by Vedco	50989-0601	Steroid
DANDAN <> 5052	Tab, White, Round, Scored	Prednisone 5 mg	Deltasone by Nat Pharmpak	55154-5208	Steroid
DANDAN <> 5052	Tab, White, Round, Scored	Prednisone 5 mg	Deltasone by Southwood	58016-0216	Steroid
DANDAN <> 5052	Tab, White, Round, Scored	Prednisone 5 mg	Deltasone by Schein	00364-0218	Steroid
DANDAN <> 5052	Tab, White, Round, Scored	Prednisone 5 mg	Deltasone by Watson	00591-5052	Steroid
DANDAN <> 5058	Tab, Blue-Green, Round, Scored	Tripelennamine HCl 50 mg	by Schein	00364-0281	Antihistamine
DANDAN <> 5059	Tab, Peach, Round, Scored	Prednisolone 5 mg	Prednisolone by Watson	00591-5059	Steroid
DANDAN <> 5059	Tab, Peach, Round, Scored	Prednisolone 5 mg	Prednisolone by Schein	00364-0217	Steroid
DANDAN <> 5059	Tab, Peach, Round, Scored	Prednisolone 5 mg	Prednisolone by Vedco	50989-0600	Steroid

ID FRONT <> BACK	DESCRIPTION FRONT <> BACK	INGREDIENT & STRENGTH	BRAND (or Generic Equiv.) by FIRM	NDC#	CLASS; SCH.
DANDAN <> 5059	Tab, Peach, Round, Scored	Prednisolone 5 mg	Prednisolone by WA Butler	11695-1800	Steroid
DANDAN <> 5059	Tab, Peach, Round, Scored	Prednisolone 5 mg	Prednisolone by Darby Group	66467-4346	Steroid
DANDAN <> 5059	Tab, Peach, Round, Scored	Prednisolone 5 mg	Prednisolone by Danbury		Steroid
DANDAN <> 5216	Tab, Tan, Round, Scored	Folic Acid 1 mg	Folvite by Amerisource	62584-0708	Vitamin
DANDAN <> 5216	Tab, Tan, Round, Scored	Folic Acid 1 mg	Folvite by JB	51111-0087	Vitamin
DANDAN <> 5216	Tab, Tan, Round, Scored	Folic Acid 1 mg	Folvite by Vangard	00615-0664	Vitamin
DANDAN <> 5216	Tab, Tan, Round, Scored	Folic Acid 1 mg	Folvite by Schein	00364-0137	Vitamin
DANDAN <> 5216	Tab, Tan, Round, Scored	Folic Acid 1 mg	Folvite by Watson	00591-5216	Vitamin
DANDAN <> 526	Tab, White, Round, Scored	Isoniazid 300 mg	Laniazid by Schein	00364-0151	Antimycobacterial
DANDAN <> 5307	Tab, White, Round, Scored	Promethazine HCl 25 mg	Miltown by Watson	00591-5307	Antiemetic; Antihistamine
DANDAN <> 5307	Tab, White, Round, Scored	Promethazine HCl 25 mg	Miltown by Schein	00364-0222	Antiemetic; Antihistamine
DANDAN <> 5307	Tab, White, Round, Scored	Promethazine HCl 25 mg	Phenergan by Pharmedix	53002-0402	Antiemetic; Antihistamine
DANDAN <> 5321	Tab, White, Round, Scored	Primidone 250 mg	Mysoline by Vangard	00615-2521	Anticonvulsant
DANDAN <> 5321	Tab, White, Round, Scored	Primidone 250 mg	Mysoline by Watson	00591-5321	Anticonvulsant
DANDAN <> 5321	Tab, White, Round, Scored	Primidone 250 mg	Mysoline by Schein	00364-0366	Anticonvulsant
DANDAN <> 5325	Tab, White, Cap Shaped, Scored	Colchicine 0.5 mg, Probenecid 500 mg	ColBenemid by Watson	00591-5325	Antigout
DANDAN <> 5325	Tab, White, Cap Shaped, Scored	Colchicine 0.5 mg, Probenecid 500 mg	ColBenemid by Schein	00364-0315	Antigout
DANDAN <> 5335	Tab, White, Round, Scored	Trihexyphenidyl HCl 2 mg	Artane by Heartland	61392-0634	Antiparkinson
DANDAN <> 5335	Tab, White, Round, Scored	Trihexyphenidyl HCl 2 mg	Artane by Schein	00364-0408	Antiparkinson
DANDAN <> 5335	Tab, White, Round, Scored	Trihexyphenidyl HCl 2 mg	Artane by Vangard	00615-0675	Antiparkinson
DANDAN <> 5335	Tab, White, Round, Scored	Trihexyphenidyl HCl 2 mg	Artane by Watson	00591-5335	Antiparkinson
DANDAN <> 5335	Tab, White, Round, Scored	Trihexyphenidyl HCl 2 mg	Artane by Octofoil	63467-0301	Antiparkinson
DANDAN <> 5335	Tab, White, Round, Scored	Trihexyphenidyl HCl 2 mg	Artane by Amerisource	62584-0886	Antiparkinson
DANDAN <> 5335	Tab, White, Round, Scored	Trihexyphenidyl HCl 2 mg	Artane by Danbury	61955-0408	Antiparkinson
DANDAN <> 5337	Tab, White, Round, Scored	Trihexyphenidyl HCl 5 mg	Artane by Schein	00364-0409	Antiparkinson
DANDAN <> 5337	Tab, White, Round, Scored	Trihexyphenidyl HCl 5 mg	Artane by Danbury	61955-0409	Antiparkinson
DANDAN <> 5337	Tab, White, Round, Scored	Trihexyphenidyl HCl 5 mg	Artane by Amerisource	62584-0887	Antiparkinson
DANDAN <> 5337	Tab, White, Round, Scored	Trihexyphenidyl HCl 5 mg	Artane by Watson	00591-5337	Antiparkinson
DANDAN <> 5337	Tab, White, Round, Scored	Trihexyphenidyl HCl 5 mg	Artane by Heartland	61392-0956	Antiparkinson
DANDAN <> 5342	Tab, White, Round, Scored	Nylidrin 6 mg	by Schein	00364-0391	Vasodilator
DANDAN <> 5345	Tab, Peach, Round, Scored	Hydrochlorothiazide 50 mg	Hydrodiuril by Talbert	44514-0411	Diuretic; Antihypertensive
DANDAN <> 5345	Tab, Peach, Round, Scored	Hydrochlorothiazide 50 mg	Hydrodiuril by Schein	00364-0328	Diuretic; Antihypertensive
DANDAN <> 5347	Tab, Yellow, Cap Shaped, Scored, Film Coated	Probenecid 500 mg	Benemid by Watson	00591-5347	Antigout
DANDAN <> 5347	Tab, Yellow, Cap Shaped, Scored, Film Coated	Probenecid 500 mg	Benemid by Pharmedix	53002-0397	Antigout
DANDAN <> 5347	Tab, Yellow, Cap Shaped, Scored, Film Coated	Probenecid 500 mg	Benemid by Schein	00364-0314	Antigout
DANDAN <> 5368	Tab, Off-White, Round, Scored	Disulfiram 500 mg	Antabuse by Schein	00364-0337	Antialcoholism
DANDAN <> 5369	Tab, White, Round, Scored	Bethanechol Chloride 10 mg	Urecholine by Bryant	63629-1164	Urinary Tract
DANDAN <> 5369	Tab, White, Round, Scored	Bethanechol Chloride 10 mg	Urecholine by Watson	00591-5369	Urinary Tract
DANDAN <> 5369	Tab, White, Round, Scored	Bethanechol Chloride 10 mg	Urecholine by Schein	00364-0349	Urinary Tract
DANDAN <> 5373	Tab, White, Round, Scored	Isosorbide Dinitrate 10 mg	Isordil by Schein	00364-0341	Antianginal
DANDAN <> 5374	Tab, White, Round, Scored	Isosorbide Dinitrate 5 mg	Isordil by Schein	00364-0340	Antianginal
DANDAN <> 5374	Tab, White, Round, Scored	Isosorbide Dinitrate 5 mg	Isordil by Watson	00591-5374	Antianginal
DANDAN <> 5381	Tab, White, Round, Scored	Methocarbamol 500 mg	Robaxin by Kaiser	00179-0446	Muscle Relaxant
DANDAN <> 5381	Tab, White, Round, Scored	Methocarbamol 500 mg	Robaxin by Schein	00364-0346	Muscle Relaxant
DANDAN <> 5381	Tab, White, Round, Scored	Methocarbamol 500 mg	Robaxin by Pharmedix	53002-0304	Muscle Relaxant
DANDAN <> 5381	Tab, White, Round, Scored	Methocarbamol 500 mg	Robaxin by Watson	00591-5381	Muscle Relaxant
DANDAN <> 5381	Tab, White, Round, Scored	Methocarbamol 500 mg	Robaxin by Talbert	44514-0557	Muscle Relaxant
DANDAN <> 5382	Tab, White, Cap Shaped, Scored	Methocarbamol 750 mg	Robaxin by Schein	00364-0347	Muscle Relaxant
DANDAN <> 5382	Tab, White, Cap Shaped, Scored	Methocarbamol 750 mg	Robaxin by Kaiser	00179-0447	Muscle Relaxant
DANDAN <> 5382	Tab, White, Cap Shaped, Scored	Methocarbamol 750 mg	Robaxin by Watson	00591-5382	Muscle Relaxant

ID FRONT <> BACK	DESCRIPTION FRONT <> BACK	INGREDIENT & STRENGTH	BRAND (or Generic Equiv.) by FIRM	NDC#	CLASS; SCH.
DANDAN <> 5382	Tab, White, Cap Shaped, Scored	Methocarbamol 750 mg	Robaxin by Talbert	44514-0558	Muscle Relaxant
DANDAN <> 5388	Tab, White, Cap Shaped, Scored	Triamcinolone 4 mg	by Schein	00364-0352	Steroid
DANDAN <> 5390	Tab, White, Round, Scored	Nylidrin 12 mg	by Schein	00364-0392	Vasodilator
DANDAN <> 5402	Tab, Tan, Round, Scored	Bethanechol Chloride 25 mg	Urecholine by Watson	00591-5402	Urinary Tract
DANDAN <> 5402	Tab, Tan, Round, Scored	Bethanechol Chloride 25 mg	Urecholine by Schein	00364-0410	Urinary Tract
DANDAN <> 5406	Tab, Green, Round, Scored	Reserpine 0.125 mg, Hydrochlorothiazide 25 mg	by Schein	00364-0354	Antihypertensive; Diuretic
DANDAN <> 5407	Tab, Green, Round, Scored	Reserpine 0.125 mg, Hydrochlorothiazide 50 mg	by Schein	00364-0355	Antihypertensive; Diuretic
DANDAN <> 5430	Tab, White, Round, Scored	Acetazolamide 250 mg	Diamox by Amerisource	62584-0043	Antiglaucoma Agent
DANDAN <> 5430	Tab, White, Round, Scored	Acetazolamide 250 mg	Diamox by Schein	00364-0400	Antiglaucoma Agent
DANDAN <> 5430	Tab, White, Round, Scored	Acetazolamide 250 mg	Diamox by Watson	00591-5430	Antiglaucoma Agent
DANDAN <> 5430	Tab, White, Round, Scored	Acetazolamide 250 mg	Diamox by Compumed	00403-0058	Antiglaucoma Agent
DANDAN <> 5438	Tab, White, Round, Scored	Quinidine Sulfate 200 mg	by Heartland	61392-0953	Antiarrhythmic
DANDAN <> 5438	Tab, White, Round, Scored	Quinidine Sulfate 200 mg	Quinidine Sulfate by Watson	00591-5438	Antiarrhythmic
DANDAN <> 5438	Tab, White, Round, Scored	Quinidine Sulfate 200 mg	Quinidine Sulfate by Schein	00364-0229	Antiarrhythmic
DANDAN <> 5442	Tab, White, Round, Scored	Prednisone 10 mg	Deltasone by Heartland	61392-0417	Steroid
DANDAN <> 5442	Tab, White, Round, Scored	Prednisone 10 mg	Deltasone by Merz	00259-0364	Steroid
DANDAN <> 5442	Tab, White, Round, Scored	Prednisone 10 mg	Deltasone by Danbury	61955-0461	Steroid
DANDAN <> 5442	Tab, White, Round, Scored	Prednisone 10 mg	Deltasone by Schein	00364-0461	Steroid
DANDAN <> 5442	Tab, White, Round, Scored	Prednisone 10 mg	Deltasone by Watson	00591-5442	Steroid
DANDAN <> 5442	Tab, White, Round, Scored	Prednisone 10 mg	Deltasone by Med Pro	53978-3037	Steroid
DANDAN <> 5442	Tab, White, Round, Scored	Prednisone 10 mg	Deltasone by Nat Pharmpak	55154-5215	Steroid
DANDAN <> 5442	Tab, White, Round, Scored	Prednisone 10 mg	Deltasone by Amerisource	62584-0833	Steroid
DANDAN <> 5443	Tab, Peach, Round, Scored	Prednisone 20 mg	Deltasone by Vangard	00615-1542	Steroid
DANDAN <> 5443	Tab, Peach, Round, Scored	Prednisone 20 mg	Deltasone by Watson	00591-5443	Steroid
DANDAN <> 5443	Tab, Peach, Round, Scored	Prednisone 20 mg	Deltasone by H J Harkins Co	52959-0127	Steroid
DANDAN <> 5443	Tab, Peach, Round, Scored	Prednisone 20 mg	Deltasone by Schein	00364-0442	Steroid
DANDAN <> 5443	Tab, Peach, Round, Scored	Prednisone 20 mg	Deltasone by WA Butler	11695-1802	Steroid
DANDAN <> 5443	Tab, Peach, Round, Scored	Prednisone 20 mg	Deltasone by Vedco	50989-0602	Steroid
DANDAN <> 5443	Tab, Peach, Round, Scored	Prednisone 20 mg	Deltasone by Qualitest	00603-2551	Steroid
DANDAN <> 5443	Tab, Peach, Round, Scored	Prednisone 20 mg	Deltasone by Danbury	61955-0442	Steroid
DANDAN <> 5454	Tab, White, Round, Scored	Quinidine Sulfate 300 mg	Quinidine Sulfate by Schein	00364-0582	Antiarrhythmic
DANDAN <> 5454	Tab, White, Round, Scored	Quinidine Sulfate 300 mg	Quinidine Sulfate by Watson	00591-5454	Antiarrhythmic
DANDAN <> 5455	Tab, Blue, Tab, Blue, Round, Scored	Chlorpropamide 250 mg	by Schein	00364-0510	Antidiabetic
DANDAN <> 5496	Tab, Buff, Round, Scored	Hydrochlorothiazide 25 mg, Spironolactone 25 mg	Aldactazide by Schein	00364-0513	Diuretic; Antihypertensive
DANDAN <> 5508	Tab, White, Round, Scored	Tolbutamide 500 mg	by Schein	00364-0477	Antidiabetic
DANDAN <> 5515	Tab, Yellow, Round, Scored	Bethanechol Chloride 50 mg	Urecholine by Schein	00364-0590	Urinary Tract
DANDAN <> 5515	Tab, Yellow, Round, Scored	Bethanechol Chloride 50 mg	Urecholine by Watson	00591-5515	Urinary Tract
DANDAN <> 5543	Tab, White, Round, Scored	Allopurinol 100 mg	Zyloprim by Nat Pharmpak	55154-5239	Antigout
DANDAN <> 5543	Tab, White, Round, Scored	Allopurinol 100 mg	Zyloprim by Danbury	61955-0632	Antigout
DANDAN <> 5543	Tab, White, Round, Scored	Allopurinol 100 mg	Zyloprim by Schein	00364-0632	Antigout
DANDAN <> 5543	Tab, White, Round, Scored	Allopurinol 100 mg	Zyloprim by Watson	00591-5543	Antigout
DANDAN <> 5544	Tab, Orange, Round, Scored	Allopurinol 300 mg	Zyloprim by Danbury	61955-0633	Antigout
DANDAN <> 5544	Tab, Orange, Round, Scored	Allopurinol 300 mg	Zyloprim by Apotheca	12634-0498	Antigout
DANDAN <> 5544	Tab, Orange, Round, Scored	Allopurinol 300 mg	Zyloprim by Schein	00364-0633	Antigout
DANDAN <> 5544	Tab, Orange, Round, Scored	Allopurinol 300 mg	Zyloprim by Watson	00591-5544	Antigout
DANDAN <> 5544	Tab, Orange, Round, Scored	Allopurinol 300 mg	Zyloprim by Nat Pharmpak	55154-5216	Antigout
DANDAN <> 5544	Tab, Orange, Round, Scored	Allopurinol 300 mg	Zyloprim by Med Pro	53978-5001	Antigout
DANDAN <> 5546	Tab, White, Round, Scored	Sulfamethoxazole 400 mg, Trimethoprim 80 mg	Septra by St. Mary's Med	60760-0004	Antibiotic
DANDAN <> 5546	Tab, White, Round, Scored	Sulfamethoxazole 400 mg, Trimethoprim 80 mg	Septra by Schein	00364-2068	Antibiotic
DANDAN <> 5546	Tab, White, Round, Scored	Sulfamethoxazole 400 mg, Trimethoprim 80 mg	Septra by Watson	00591-5546	Antibiotic

ID FRONT <> BACK	DESCRIPTION FRONT <> BACK	INGREDIENT & STRENGTH	BRAND (or Generic Equiv.) by FIRM	NDC#	CLASS; SCH.
DAN DAN <> 5547	Tab, White, Oval, Scored	Sulfamethoxazole 800 mg, Trimethoprim 160 mg	Septra by Amerisource	62584-0399	Antibiotic
DAN DAN <> 5547	Tab, White, Oval, Scored	Sulfamethoxazole 800 mg, Trimethoprim 160 mg	Septra by Va Cmop	65243-0067	Antibiotic
DAN DAN <> 5547	Tab, White, Oval, Scored	Sulfamethoxazole 800 mg, Trimethoprim 160 mg	Septra by Southwood	58016-0109	Antibiotic
DAN DAN <> 5547	Tab, White, Oval, Scored	Sulfamethoxazole 800 mg, Trimethoprim 160 mg	Septra by Pharmedix	53002-0210	Antibiotic
DAN DAN <> 5547	Tab, White, Oval, Scored	Sulfamethoxazole 800 mg, Trimethoprim 160 mg	Septra by Nat Pharmpak	55154-5205	Antibiotic
DAN DAN <> 5547	Tab, White, Oval, Scored	Sulfamethoxazole 800 mg, Trimethoprim 160 mg	Septra by Schein	00364-2069	Antibiotic
DAN DAN <> 5547	Tab, White, Oval, Scored	Sulfamethoxazole 800 mg, Trimethoprim 160 mg	Septra by Watson	00591-5547	Antibiotic
DAN DAN <> 5548	Tab, White to Off-White, Round, Scored	Chloroquine Phosphate 250 mg	Aralen Phosphate by Schein	00364-0470	Antimalarial
DAN DAN <> 5552	Tab, White to Off-White, Round, Scored	Metronidazole 500 mg	Flagyl by Watson	00591-5552	Antibiotic
DAN DAN <> 5552	Tab, White to Off-White, Round, Scored	Metronidazole 500 mg	Flagyl by Schein	00364-0687	Antibiotic
DAN DAN <> 5563	Tab, White, Oval, Scored, Film Coated, Ex Release	Procainamide HCl 500 mg	Procanbid by Schein	00364-0716	Antiarrhymic
DAN DAN <> 5564	Tab, White, Oval, Film Coated, Scored, Ex Release	Procainamide HCl 750 mg	Procanbid by Schein	00364-0717	Antiarrhymic
DAN DAN <> 5571	Tab, White, Oval, Scored	Trimethoprim 100 mg	Trimpex by Schein	00364-0649	Antibiotic
DAN DAN <> 5571	Tab, White, Oval, Scored	Trimethoprim 100 mg	Trimpex by Watson	00591-5571	Antibiotic
DAN DAN <> 5575	Tab, White, Round, Scored	Furosemide 40 mg	by Schein	00364-0514	Diuretic
DAN DAN <> 5579	Tab, Blue, Round, Scored	Chlorpropamide 100 mg	by Schein	00364-0699	Antidiabetic
DAN DAN <> 5582	Tab, White, Round, Scored	Tolazamide 250 mg	by Schein	00364-0720	Antidiabetic
DAN DAN <> 5589	Tab, White, Round, Scored	Metoclopramide HCl 10 mg	Reglan by Schein	00364-0769	Gastrointestinal
DAN DAN <> 5589	Tab, White, Round, Scored	Metoclopramide HCl 10 mg	Reglan by Med Pro	53978-5011	Gastrointestinal
DAN DAN <> 5589	Tab, White, Round, Scored	Metoclopramide HCl 10 mg	Reglan by Watson	00591-5589	Gastrointestinal
DAN DAN <> 5589	Tab, White, Round, Scored	Metoclopramide HCl 10 mg	Reglan by Nat Pharmpak	55154-5202	Gastrointestinal
DAN DAN <> 5590	Tab, White, Round, Scored	Tolazamide 500 mg	by Schein	00364-0722	Antidiabetic
DAN DAN <> 5591	Tab, White, Round, Scored	Tolazamide 100 mg	by Schein	00364-0721	Antidiabetic
DAN DAN <> 5597	Tab, White, Cap Shaped, Scored	Acetohexamide 500 mg	Dymelor by Watson	00591-5597	Antidiabetic
DAN DAN <> 5597	Tab, White, Cap Shaped, Scored	Acetohexamide 500 mg	Dymelor by Schein	00364-2233	Antidiabetic
DAN DAN <> 5598	Tab, White, Cap Shaped, Scored	Acetohexamide 250 mg	Dymelor by Schein	00364-2232	Antidiabetic
DAN DAN <> 5598	Tab	Acetohexamide 250 mg	Dymelor by Watson	00591-5598	Antidiabetic
DAN DAN <> 5599	Tab, White, Round, Scored, Film Coated	Trazodone HCl 100 mg	Desyrel by Schein	00364-2110	Antidepressant
DAN DAN <> 5599	Tab, White, Round, Scored, Film Coated	Trazodone HCl 100 mg	Desyrel by Watson	00591-5599	Antidepressant
DAN DAN <> 5600	Tab, White, Round, Scored, Film Coated	Trazodone HCl 50 mg	Desyrel by Schein	00364-2109	Antidepressant
DAN DAN <> 5600	Tab, White, Round, Scored, Film Coated	Trazodone HCl 50 mg	Desyrel by Watson	00591-5600	Antidepressant
DAN DAN <> 5601	Tab, Film Coated	Verapamil HCl 80 mg	Verelan by Amerisource	62584-0888	Antihypertensive
DAN DAN <> 5601	Tab, White, Round, Film Coated, Scored	Verapamil HCl 80 mg	by Schein	00364-2111	Antihypertensive
DAN DAN <> 5601	Tab, Film Coated	Verapamil HCl 80 mg	by Watson	00591-5601	Antihypertensive
DAN DAN <> 5602	Tab, Coated	Verapamil HCl 120 mg	Verelan by Amerisource	62584-0889	Antihypertensive
DAN DAN <> 5602	Tab, Coated	Verapamil HCl 120 mg	by Watson	00591-5602	Antihypertensive
DAN DAN <> 5602	Tab, White, Round, Coated, Scored	Verapamil HCl 120 mg	by Schein	00364-2112	Antihypertensive
DAN DAN <> 5602	Tab, Dan/Dan <> 5602	Clonidine HCl 0.2 mg	by Nat Pharmpak	55154-5229	Antihypertensive
DAN DAN <> 5659	Tab, White, Round, Scored	Furosemide 80 mg	by Schein	00364-0700	Diuretic
DAN DAN <> 5660	Tab, Yellow, Round, Scored	Sulindac 200 mg	Clinoril by Heartland	61392-0955	NSAID
DAN DAN <> 5660	Tab, Yellow, Round, Scored	Sulindac 200 mg	Clinoril by H J Harkins Co	52959-0195	NSAID
DAN DAN <> 5660	Tab, Yellow, Round, Scored	Sulindac 200 mg	Clinoril by Pharmedix	53002-0388	NSAID
DAN DAN <> 5660	Tab, Yellow, Round, Scored	Sulindac 200 mg	Clinoril by Schein	00364-2442	NSAID
DAN DAN <> 5660	Tab, Yellow, Round, Scored	Sulindac 200 mg	Clinoril by Watson	00591-5660	NSAID
DAN DAN <> 5660	Tab, Yellow, Round, Scored	Sulindac 200 mg	Clinoril by St. Mary's Med	60760-0424	NSAID
DAN DAN <> 5660	Tab, Yellow, Round, Scored	Sulindac 200 mg	Clinoril by PDRX	55289-0930	NSAID
DAN DAN <> 5677	Tab, Off-White, Round, Scored	Nalidixic Acid 500 mg	by Schein	00364-2324	Antibiotic
DAN DAN <> 5704	Tab, White, Cap Shaped, Film Coated, Scored	Fenoprofen Calcium 600 mg	by Schein	00364-2316	NSAID
DANDAN5443	Tab	Prednisone 20 mg	by Amerisource	62584-0834	Steroid
DANDAN5564	Tab, White, Oval, Dan/Dan 5564	Procainamide HCl SR 750 mg	Procan SR by Danbury		Antiarrhymic

ID FRONT <> BACK	DESCRIPTION FRONT <> BACK	INGREDIENT & STRENGTH	BRAND (or Generic Equiv.) by FIRM	NDC#	CLASS; SCH.
DANDAN5704	Tab, White, Dan/Dan 5704	Fenoprofen Calcium 600 mg	Nalfon by Danbury		NSAID
DANP100	Tab, White, Round, Dan-P 100	Phenobarbital 100 mg	Phenobarbital by Danbury		Sedative/Hypnotic; C IV
DANP15	Tab, White, Round, Dan-P 15	Phenobarbital 15 mg	Phenobarbital by Danbury		Sedative/Hypnotic; C IV
DANP30	Tab, White, Round, Dan-P 30	Phenobarbital 30 mg	by Danbury		Sedative/Hypnotic; C IV
DANP60	Tab, White, Round, Dan-P 60	Phenobarbital 60 mg	by Danbury		Sedative/Hypnotic; C IV
DANTRIUM100MG-01490033	Cap, Orange & Tan, Opaque	Dantrolene Sodium 100 mg	Dantrium by Proc & Gamble	Canadian DIN 0197602	Muscle Relaxant
DANTRIUM100MG-01490033	Cap, Orange & Tan, Opaque	Dantrolene Sodium 100 mg	Dantrium by Procter and Gamble	00149-0033	Muscle Relaxant
DANTRIUM25MG-01490030	Cap, Orange & Tan, Opaque	Dantrolene Sodium 25 mg	Dantrium by Proctor and Gamble	Canadian DIN 0197602	Muscle Relaxant
DANTRIUM25MG-01490030	Cap, Orange & Tan, Opaque	Dantrolene Sodium 25 mg	Dantrium by Drug Distr	52985-0231	Muscle Relaxant
DANTRIUM25MG-01490030	Cap, Orange & Tan, Opaque	Dantrolene Sodium 25 mg	Dantrium by Procter and Gamble	00149-0030	Muscle Relaxant
DANTRIUM50MG-01490031	Cap, Orange & Tan, Opaque	Dantrolene Sodium 50 mg	Dantrium by Procter and Gamble	00149-0031	Muscle Relaxant
DARANIDE <> MSD49	Tab, Yellow, Round	Dichlorphenamide 50 mg	Daranide by Merck	Discontinued	Carbonic Anhydrase Inhibitor
DARAPRIM <> A3A	Tab, White, Scored	Pyrimethamine 25 mg	Daraprim by GSK	00173-0201	Antiprotozoal
DARAPRIM <> A3A	Tab	Pyrimethamine 25 mg	Daraprim by DSM	63552-0201	Antiprotozoal
DARAPRIMA3A	Tab, White, Round, Scored, Biconvex	Pyrimethamine 25 mg	Daraprim by GSK	Canadian DIN 00004774	Antiprotozoal
DARVOCETN100	Tab, Film Coated, Darvocet-N 100	Acetaminophen 650 mg, Propoxyphene Napsylate 100 mg	Darvocet-N 100 by Caremark	00339-4045	Analgesic; C IV
DARVOCETN100	Tab, Dark Orange, Cap Shaped, Film Coated	Propoxyphene Napsylate 100 mg, Acetaminophen 650 mg	Darvocet N by AAI Pharma	66591-0641	Analgesic; C IV
DARVOCETN100	Tab, Dark Orange, Cap Shaped, Film-Coated	Propoxyphene Napsylate 100 mg, Acetaminophen 650 mg	Darvocet-N 100 by Xanodyne	66479-0515	Analgesic; C IV
DARVOCETN100 <> LILLY	Tab, Film Coated, Darvocet-N 100	Acetaminophen 650 mg, Propoxyphene Napsylate 100 mg	Darvocet-N 100 by Eli Lilly	00002-0363	Analgesic; C IV
DARVOCETN100 <> LILLY	Tab, Film Coated	Acetaminophen 650 mg, Propoxyphene Napsylate 100 mg	Darvocet-N 100 by Nat Pharmpak	55154-1807	Analgesic; C IV
DARVOCETN50	Tab, Dark Orange, Cap Shaped, Film Coated	Propoxyphene Napsylate 50 mg, Acetaminophen 325 mg	Darvocet N by AAI Pharma	66591-0651	Analgesic; C IV
DARVOCETN50	Tab, Dark Orange, Cap Shaped, Film-Coated	Propoxyphene Napsylate 50 mg, Acetaminophen 325 mg	Darvocet-N 50 by Xanodyne	66479-0514	Analgesic; C IV
DARVONCOMP65	Cap, Red, Opaque, Darvon Comp-65	Propoxyphene HCl 65 mg, Aspirin 389 mg, Caffeine 32.4 mg	Darvon Compound 65 by AAI Pharma	66591-0612	Analgesic; C IV
DARVONCOMP65-LILLY3111	Cap, Darvon Comp 65 <> Lilly 3111	Aspirin 389 mg, Caffeine 32.4 mg, Propoxyphene HCl 65 mg	Propoxyphene Compound 65 by Med Pro	53978-3083	Analgesic; C IV
DARVONCOMP65-LILLY3111	Cap, Darvon Comp 65 <> Lilly 3111	Aspirin 389 mg, Caffeine 32.4 mg, Propoxyphene 65 mg	Darvon Compound 65 by Eli Lilly	00002-3111	Analgesic; C IV
DARVONN100	Tab, Buff, Elliptical, Film Coated, Darvon-N 100	Propoxyphene Napsylate 100 mg	Darvon-N by AAI Pharma	66591-0631	Analgesic; C IV
DAVA	Tab, Yellow, Oval, Film-Coated, Blue Imprint	Clarithromycin 250 mg	Biaxin by Dava	68774-0120	Antibiotic
DAYPRO <> 1381	Tab, White, Cap Shaped, Scored, Film Coated	Oxaprozin 600 mg	Daypro by PF	48692-0013	NSAID
DAYPRO <> 1381	Tab, White, Cap Shaped, Scored, Film Coated	Oxaprozin 600 mg	Daypro by Amerisource	62584-0381	NSAID
DAYPRO <> 1381	Tab, White, Cap Shaped, Scored, Film Coated	Oxaprozin 600 mg	Daypro by Rx Dispensing	61807-0079	NSAID
DAYPRO <> 1381	Tab, White, Cap Shaped, Scored, Film Coated	Oxaprozin 600 mg	Daypro by St. Mary's Med	6076-0381	NSAID
DAYPRO <> 1381	Tab, White, Cap Shaped, Scored, Film Coated	Oxaprozin 600 mg	Daypro by Pharmacia	Canadian DIN 02027860	NSAID
DAYPRO <> 1381	Tab, White, Cap Shaped, Scored, Film Coated	Oxaprozin 600 mg	Daypro by Searle	00025-1381	NSAID
DAYPRO <> 1381	Tab, White, Cap Shaped, Scored, Film Coated	Oxaprozin 600 mg	Daypro by Searle	00014-1381	NSAID
DAYPRO <> 1381	Tab, White, Cap Shaped, Scored, Film Coated	Oxaprozin 600 mg	Daypro by H J Harkins Co	52959-0252	NSAID
DAYPRO <> 1381	Tab, White, Cap Shaped, Scored, Film Coated	Oxaprozin 600 mg	Daypro by Allscripts		NSAID
DAYPRO <> 1381	Tab, White, Cap Shaped, Scored, Film Coated	Oxaprozin 600 mg	Daypro by DRX	55045-2120	NSAID
DAYPRO <> 1381	Tab, White, Cap Shaped, Scored, Film Coated	Oxaprozin 600 mg	Daypro by Perrigo		NSAID

ID FRONT <> BACK	DESCRIPTION FRONT <> BACK	INGREDIENT & STRENGTH	BRAND (or Generic Equiv.) by FIRM	NDC#	CLASS; SCH.
DAYPRO <> 1381	Tab, White, Cap Shaped, Scored, Film Coated	Oxaprozin 600 mg	Daypro by Caremark	00339-5881	NSAID
DAYQ	Cap, Orange, Oval, Liquid Filled, DayQ	Acetaminophen 325 mg, Dextromethorphan HBr 15 mg, Pseudoephedrine HCl 30 mg	DayQuil by P & G Health	37000-0537	Cold Remedy
DBETHEX <> 260	Tab, Coated, Scored	Ascorbic Acid 100 mg, Biotin 30 mcg, Calcium Carbonate, Precipitated 250 mg, Chromic Chloride 25 mcg, Cupric Oxide 2 mg, Cyanocobalamin 12 mcg, Ferrous Fumarate 60 mg, Folic Acid 1 mg, Magnesium Oxide 25 mg, Manganese Sulfate 5 mg, Niacinamide 20 mg, Pantothenic Acid 10 mg, Potassium Iodide 150 mcg, Pyridoxine HCl 10 mg, Riboflavin 3.4 mg, Sodium Molybdate 25 mcg, Thiamine HCl 3 mg, Vitamin A 5000 Units, Vitamin D 400 Units, Vitamin E 30 Units, Zinc Oxide 25 mg	Prenatal MTR by Ethex	58177-0260 Discontinued	Vitamin
DCIPANCRECARBMS16	Cap, Clear, Hard Gel, Blue Ink	Lipase 16,000 Units, Amylase 52,000 Units, Protease 52,000 Units	Pancrecarb MS-16 by Digestive Care	59767-0003	Gastrointestinal
DCIPANCRECARBMS4	Cap, Delayed Release, Blue Ink	Amylase 25,000 Units, Lipase 4000 Units, Protease 25,000 Units	Pancrecarb Ms-4 by Digestive Care	59767-0002	Gastrointestinal
DCIPANCRECARBMS8	Cap, Delayed Release	Amylase 40,000 Units, Lipase 8000 Units, Protease 45,000 Units	Pancrecarb Ms-8 by Digestive Care	59767-0001	Gastrointestinal
DD	Tab, Dark Yellow, Round, Film-Coated, "DD" inside a hexagon	Estradiol Valerate 3 mg	Natazia by Berlex	50419-0409	Oral Contraceptive
DD <> PP	Tab, White, Round, Scored, P logo / P logo <> D / D	Pramipexole DiHCl 1.5 mg	Mirapex by Pharmascience	Canadian DIN 02290154	Antiparkinson
DDAVP01 <> RPR	Tab, White, Oblong, Scored, DDAVP0.1 <> RPR Logo	Desmopressin Acetate 0.1 mg	DDAVP by Aventis	00075-0016	Antidiuretic
DDAVP02 <> RPR	Tab, White, Round, Scored, DDAVP over 0.2 <> RPR Logo	Desmopressin Acetate 0.2 mg	DDAVP by Promex Med	62301-0030	Antidiuretic
DDAVP02 <> RPR	Tab, White, Round, Scored, DDAVP over 0.2 <> RPR Logo	Desmopressin Acetate 0.2 mg	DDAVP by Aventis	00075-0026	Antidiuretic
DDS080	Tab, Yellowish-Beige, Cap-Shaped, Ex-Release, Coated, Scored	Trazodone HCl 150 mg	Oleptro by Labopharm	43595-0080	Antidepressant
DDS081	Tab, Beige-Orange, Cap-Shaped, Ex-Release, Coated, Scored	Trazodone HCl 300 mg	Oleptro by Labopharm	43595-0081	Antidepressant
DE	Cap, Black, D & E	Caffeine 325 mg	by D & E Pharma		Stimulant
DE	Tab, White, Oblong	Lactose Enzyme 3000 FCC	by Blistex		Gastrointestinal
DE160	Cap, Blue, White Print	Caffeine 175 mg	Small Blues by D&E Pharma		Stimulant
DE200	Tab, Pink, Heart Shaped	Caffeine 200 mg	by D & E Pharma		Stimulant
DE225	Tab, Pink, Oval	Caffeine 200 mg	Pink Footballs by D&E Pharma		Stimulant
DE260	Cap, Red and Black, White Print	Caffeine 200 mg	Red and Blacks by D&E Pharma		Stimulant
DECADRON <> MSD41	Tab, Yellow, Pentagonal	Dexamethasone 0.5 mg	Decadron by Merck	00006-0041	Steroid
DECADRON <> MSD63	Tab, Bluish-Green, Pentagon Shaped	Dexamethasone 0.75 mg	Decadron by Merck	00006-0063	Steroid
DECII <> 017	Tab, Dark Blue, Scored	Guaifenesin 600 mg, Pseudoephedrine HCl 60 mg	Deconsal II by Celltech	53014-0017	Cold Remedy
DEES25	Cap, Yellow, Gray Print, D & E ES25	Ephedrine Sulfate 25 mg	Diet and Energy Herbal Caps by D & E Pharma		Supplement
DEFEN	Tab	Guaifenesin 600 mg, Pseudoephedrine HCl 60 mg	Defen LA by Anabolic	00722-6298	Cold Remedy
DELTASONE10	Tab, White, Round, Scored	Prednisone 10 mg	Deltasone by Pharmacia	00009-0193	Steroid
DELTASONE20	Tab, Peach, Round, Scored	Prednisone 20 mg	Deltasone by Pharmacia	00009-0165	Steroid
DELTASONE25	Tab, Pink, Round, Scored, DELTASONE 2.5	Prednisone 2.5 mg	Deltasone by Pharmacia	00009-0032	Steroid
DELTASONE5	Tab, White, Round, Scored	Prednisone 5 mg	Deltasone by Pharmacia	00009-0045	Steroid
DELTASONE5	Tab, White, Round, Scored	Prednisone 5 mg	Deltasone by Urgent Care Center	50716-0305	Steroid
DELTASONE5	Tab, White, Round, Scored	Prednisone 5 mg	Deltasone by Qualitest	00603-2542	Steroid
DELTASONE50	Tab, White, Round, Scored	Prednisone 50 mg	Deltasone by Pharmacia	00009-0388	Steroid
DEMOLE	Cap, White, Black Print, D&E M o l E	Caffeine 165 mg	Mole by D&E Pharma		Stimulant
DEPADE <> 100	Tab, Beige, Cap Shaped, Film Coated	Naltrexone HCl 100 mg	Depade by Mallinckrodt	00406-0119	Opioid Antagonist
DEPADE <> 25	Tab, Pink, Cap Shaped, Film Coated	Naltrexone HCl 25 mg	Depade by Mallinckrodt	00406-0089	Opioid Antagonist
DEPADE <> 50	Tab, Pale Yellow, Cap Shaped, Scored, Film Coated	Naltrexone HCl 50 mg	Depade by Mallinckrodt	00406-0092	Opioid Antagonist; Antialcoholism

ID FRONT <> BACK	DESCRIPTION FRONT <> BACK	INGREDIENT & STRENGTH	BRAND (or Generic Equiv.) by FIRM	NDC#	CLASS; SCH.
DEPAKENE	Cap, Orange, Soft Gelatin	Valproic Acid 250 mg	Depakene by Abbott	00074-5681	Anticonvulsant
DEPAKENE	Cap, Orange, Soft Gelatin, Abbott (a)	Valproic Acid 250 mg	Depakene by Abbott	00074-5681	Anticonvulsant
DEPLIN <> 15MG	Tab, Orange, Oval, Coated	L-methylfolate (Metafolin) 15 mg	Deplin by PAMLAB, LLC.	00525-0450	Supplement
DES01 <> APO	Tab, White to Off-White, Round, Scored, DES / 0.1	Desmopressin Acetate 0.1 mg	DDAVP by Apotex	Canadian DIN 02284030	Antidiuretic
DES01 <> APO	Tab, White to Off-White, Round, Scored, DES / 0.1	Desmopressin Acetate 0.1 mg	DDAVP by Apotex	60505-0257	Antidiuretic
DES02 <> APO	Tab, White to Off-White, Round, Scored, DES / 0.2	Desmopressin Acetate 0.2 mg	DDAVP by Apotex	60505-0258	Antidiuretic
DESPECSR <> 44	Tab, Green, Oblong, Scored	Guaifenesin 600 mg, Phenylpropanolamine HCl 75 mg	Entex LA by Med Pro	53978-3315	Cold Remedy
DESPECSR <> SR80	Tab, White, Scored	Pseudoephedrine HCl 800 mg, Guaifenesin 120 mg	Despec SR by Int'l Ethical Labs	11584-0442	Cold Remedy
DESPEDDM <> DMI81	Tab, White, Oval, Scored, Extended Release	Guaifenesin 800 mg, Pseudoephedrine HCl 120 mg, Dextromethorphan HBr 60 mg	Despec DM by Int'l Ethical Labs	11584-0105	Cold Remedy
DESYRELBL	Tab, Orange, Round, Scored	Trazodone HCl 50 mg	Desyrel by BMS	Canadian DIN 00579351	Antidepressant
DESYRELBL	Tab, White to Off-White, Round, Scored	Trazodone HCl 100 mg	Desyrel by BMS	Canadian DIN 00579378	Antidepressant
DESYRELMJ775	Tab, Orange, Round, Scored	Trazodone HCl 50 mg	Desyrel by BMS	00087-0775	Antidepressant
DESYRELMJ775	Tab, Orange, Round, Scored	Trazodone HCl 50 mg	Desyrel by Amerisource	62584-0775	Antidepressant
DESYRELMJ775	Tab, Orange, Round, Scored	Trazodone HCl 50 mg	Desyrel by Nat Pharmpak	55154-2001	Antidepressant
DESYRELMJ775	Tab, Orange, Round, Scored	Trazodone HCl 50 mg	Desyrel by Leiner	59606-0629	Antidepressant
DESYRELMJ775	Tab, Orange, Round, Scored	Trazodone HCl 50 mg	Desyrel by Rightpak	65240-0629	Antidepressant
DESYRELMJ775	Tab, Orange, Round, Scored	Trazodone HCl 50 mg	Desyrel by Rx Pak	65084-0233	Antidepressant
DESYRELMJ776	Tab, White, Round, Scored, Film Coated	Trazodone HCl 100 mg	Desyrel by Teva	00480-0536	Antidepressant
DESYRELMJ776	Tab, White, Round, Scored, Film Coated	Trazodone HCl 100 mg	Desyrel by Amerisource	62584-0776	Antidepressant
DESYRELMJ776	Tab, White, Round, Scored, Film Coated	Trazodone HCl 100 mg	Desyrel by Rightpak	65240-0630	Antidepressant
DESYRELMJ776	Tab, White, Round, Scored, Film Coated	Trazodone HCl 100 mg	Desyrel by BMS	00087-0776	Antidepressant
DEVROM	Cap, Yellow	Bismuth Subgallate 200 mg	Devrom by Parthenon		Gastrointestinal
DEWNM2	Cap, Yellow, Black Print	Caffeine 200 mg	Wait No More by D&E Pharma		Stimulant
DF <> 15	Tab, Light Peach, Round, Extended Release	Darifenacin 15 mg	Enablex by Novartis	Canadian DIN 02273225	Urinary Tract
DF <> 15	Tab, Light Peach, Round, Extended Release	Darifenacin 15 mg	Enablex by Novartis	00078-0420	Urinary Tract
DF <> 75	Tab, White, Round, Extended Release, DF <> 7.5	Darifenacin 7.5 mg	Enablex by Novartis	00078-0419	Urinary Tract
DF <> 75	Tab, White, Round, Extended Release, DF <> 7.5	Darifenacin 7.5 mg	Enablex by Novartis	Canadian DIN 02273217	Urinary Tract
DF <> A	Tab, White, Round, Abbott Logo (a)	Terazosin HCl 1 mg	Hytrin by Abbott	00074-3322 Discontinued	Antihypertensive
DG033	Tab, White, Oblong, Scored	Pseudoephedrine 90 mg, Guaifenesin 1200 mg	Dynex by Athlon	66813-0033	Cold Remedy
DH	Tab, Light Yellow, Round, Film-Coated, "DH" inside a hexagon	Estradiol Valerate 2 mg, Estradiol Dienogest 3 mg	Natazia by Berlex	50419-0409	Oral Contraceptive
DH <> A	Tab, Orange, Round, Abbott Logo (a)	Terazosin HCl 2 mg	Hytrin by Abbott	00074-3323 Discontinued	Antihypertensive
DHA250	Cap, Light Yellow to Dark Orange, Clear, Oval, Leaf encircles DHA-250	Docosahexaenoic Acid (DHA) 250 mg	OptiNate by Horizon	59630-0412	Prenatal Vitamin
DI <> A	Tab, Green, Round, Abbott Logo (a)	Terazosin HCl 10 mg	Hytrin by Abbott	00074-3325 Discontinued	Antihypertensive
DIA30	Tab, White, Oblong	Gliclazide 30 mg	Diamicron MR by Servier	Canadian DIN 02242987	Antidiabetic
DIAB <> HOECHST	Tab, Light Pink, Oblong, Scored	Glyburide 2.5 mg	Diabeta by Drug Distr	52985-0221	Antidiabetic
DIAB <> HOECHST	Tab, Light Green, Oblong, Scored	Glyburide 5 mg	Diabeta by Nat Pharmpak	55154-1201	Antidiabetic
DIAB <> HOECHST	Tab, Light Green, Oblong, Scored	Glyburide 5 mg	Diabeta by Coventry	61372-0578	Antidiabetic
DIAB <> HOECHST	Tab, Light Green, Oblong, Scored	Glyburide 5 mg	Diabeta by Merrell	00068-1212	Antidiabetic

ID FRONT <> BACK	DESCRIPTION FRONT <> BACK	INGREDIENT & STRENGTH	BRAND (or Generic Equiv.) by FIRM	NDC#	CLASS; SCH.
DIAB <> HOECHST	Tab, Light Green, Oblong, Scored	Glyburide 5 mg	Diabeta by Aventis	00039-0052	Antidiabetic
DIAB <> HOECHST	Tab, Light Green, Oblong, Scored	Glyburide 5 mg	Diabeta by Thrift Drug	59198-0023	Antidiabetic
DIAB <> HOECHST	Tab, Light Green, Oblong, Scored	Glyburide 5 mg	Diabeta by Rite Aid	11822-5186	Antidiabetic
DIAB <> HOECHST	Tab, Peach, Oblong, Scored	Glyburide 1.25 mg	Diabeta by Aventis	00039-0053	Antidiabetic
DIAB <> HOECHST	Tab, Peach, Oblong, Scored	Glyburide 1.25 mg	Diabeta by Merrell	00068-1210	Antidiabetic
DIAB <> HOECHST	Tab, Light Pink, Oblong, Scored	Glyburide 2.5 mg	Diabeta by Merrell	00068-1211	Antidiabetic
DIAB <> HOECHST	Tab, Light Pink, Oblong, Scored	Glyburide 2.5 mg	Diabeta by Nat Pharmpak	55154-1206	Antidiabetic
DIAB <> HOECHST	Tab, Light Pink, Oblong, Scored	Glyburide 2.5 mg	Diabeta by Amerisource	62584-0361	Antidiabetic
DIAB <> HOECHST	Tab, Light Pink, Oblong, Scored	Glyburide 2.5 mg	Diabeta by Thrift Drug	59198-0022	Antidiabetic
DIAB <> HOECHST	Tab, Light Pink, Oblong, Scored	Glyburide 2.5 mg	Diabeta by Aventis	00039-0051	Antidiabetic
DIAMOX125 <> LLD1	Tab, White, Round, Scored	Acetazolamide 125 mg	Diamox by Lederle	00005-4398	Antiglaucoma Agent
DIAMOX250 <> LLD2	Tab, White, Round, Scored	Acetazolamide 250 mg	Diamox by Lederle	00005-4469	Antiglaucoma Agent
DIAMOX250 <> LLD2	Tab, Diamox 250 <> LL in Upper Right Quad, D2 in Lower Left Quadrant	Acetazolamide 250 mg	Diamox by Thrift Drug	59198-0186	Antiglaucoma Agent
DIAMOX250 <> LLD2	Tab	Acetazolamide 250 mg	Diamox by Storz	57706-0755	Antiglaucoma Agent
DIAMOXD3	Cap, Orange, Black Print, Diamox over D3	Acetazolamide 500 mg	Diamox by Haines	59564-0142	Antiglaucoma Agent
DIAMOXD3	Cap, Orange, Black Print, Diamox over D3	Acetazolamide 500 mg	Diamox by Storz	Canadian	Antiglaucoma Agent
DIAMOXD3	Cap, Orange, Black Print, Diamox over D3	Acetazolamide 500 mg	Diamox by Lederle	00005-0753	Antiglaucoma Agent
DIAZEPAM10 <> PAR192	Tab	Diazepam 10 mg	Valium by Par	49884-0192	Antianxiety; C IV
DIAZEPAM2 <> PAR190	Tab	Diazepam 2 mg	Valium by Par	49884-0190	Antianxiety; C IV
DIAZEPAM5 <> PAR191	Tab	Diazepam 5 mg	Valium by Par	49884-0191	Antianxiety; C IV
DIDREX50	Tab, Light Pink, Round, Scored	Benzphetamine HCl 50 mg	Didrex by Pharmacia	00009-0024	Sympathomimetic; C III
DIDREX50	Tab, Light Pink, Round, Scored	Benzphetamine HCl 50 mg	Didrex by Compumed	00403-0059	Sympathomimetic; C III
DIFILG <> MD305	Tab, White, Round, Scored	Guaifenesin 200 mg, Dyphylline 200 mg	Difil G by Stewart-Jackson	45985-0644	Antiasthmatic; Expectorant
DIFILG <> MD305	Tab, White, Round, Scored	Guaifenesin 200 mg, Dyphylline 200 mg	Difil G by Co Med Pharma	45565-0305	Antiasthmatic; Expectorant
DIFLUCAN100 <> PFIZER	Tab, Pink, Trapezoidal	Fluconazole 100 mg	Diflucan by Pfizer	Canadian DIN 00891819	Antifungal
DIFLUCAN100 <> ROERIG	Tab, Pink, Trapezoidal, Diflucan over 100	Fluconazole 100 mg	Diflucan by Roerig	00049-3420	Antifungal
DIFLUCAN100 <> ROERIG	Tab, Pink, Trapezoidal, Diflucan over 100	Fluconazole 100 mg	Diflucan by Med Pro	53978-3012	Antifungal
DIFLUCAN100 <> ROERIG	Tab, Pink, Trapezoidal, Diflucan over 100	Fluconazole 100 mg	Diflucan by Nat Pharmpak	55154-3214	Antifungal
DIFLUCAN100 <> ROERIG	Tab, Pink, Trapezoidal, Diflucan over 100	Fluconazole 100 mg	Diflucan by Amerisource	62584-0362	Antifungal
DIFLUCAN150 <> ROERIG	Tab, Pink, Oval, Diflucan over 150	Fluconazole 150 mg	Diflucan by Roerig	00049-3500	Antifungal
DIFLUCAN200 <> ROERIG	Tab, Pink, Trapezoidal, Diflucan over 200	Fluconazole 200 mg	Diflucan by Nat Pharmpak	55154-3215	Antifungal
DIFLUCAN200 <> ROERIG	Tab, Pink, Trapezoidal, Diflucan over 200	Fluconazole 200 mg	Diflucan by Amerisource	62584-0363	Antifungal
DIFLUCAN200 <> ROERIG	Tab, Pink, Trapezoidal, Diflucan over 200	Fluconazole 200 mg	Diflucan by Roerig	00049-3430	Antifungal
DIFLUCAN200 <> ROERIG	Tab, Pink, Trapezoidal, Diflucan over 200	Fluconazole 200 mg	Diflucan by Med Pro	53978-3105	Antifungal
DIFLUCAN50 <> PFIZER	Tab, Pink, Trapezoid	Fluconazole 50 mg	Diflucan by Pfizer	Canadian DIN 00891800	Antifungal
DIFLUCAN50 <> ROERIG	Tab, Pink, Trapezoidal, Diflucan over 50	Fluconazole 50 mg	Diflucan by Pharm Util	60491-0194	Antifungal
DIFLUCAN50 <> ROERIG	Tab, Pink, Trapezoidal, Diflucan over 50	Fluconazole 50 mg	Diflucan by Roerig	00049-3410	Antifungal
DIG <> APO	Tab, Pink, Round	Digoxin 62.5 mcg	Lanoxin by Apotex	Canadian DIN 02281236	Cardiac Agent

ID FRONT <> BACK	DESCRIPTION FRONT <> BACK	INGREDIENT & STRENGTH	BRAND (or Generic Equiv.) by FIRM	NDC#	CLASS; SCH.
DIG125 <> APO	Tab, Yellow, Round, Scored, APO <> DIG .125	Digoxin 125 mcg	Lanoxin by Apotex	Canadian DIN 02281228	Cardiac Agent
DIG25 <> APO	Tab, White, Round, Scorec, APO <> DIG .25	Digoxin 250 mcg	Lanoxin by Apotex	Canadian DIN 02281201	Cardiac Agent
DILACORXR120MG	Cap, Pink & Flesh, Black Print, Opaque, Watson logo DILACOR XR over 120 mg	Diltiazem HCl 120 mg	Dilacor XR by Watson	52544-0482	Antihypertensive
DILACORXR180MG	Cap, Lavender & Flesh, Black Print, Opaque, Watson logo DILACOR XR over 180 mg	Diltiazem HCl 180 mg	Dilacor XR by Rx Pak	65084-0240	Antihypertensive
DILACORXR180MG	Cap, Lavender & Flesh, Black Print, Opaque, Watson logo DILACOR XR over 180 mg	Diltiazem HCl 180 mg	Dilacor XR by Kaiser	62224-9339	Antihypertensive
DILACORXR180MG	Cap, Lavender & Flesh, Black Print, Opaque, Watson logo DILACOR XR over 180 mg	Diltiazem HCl 180 mg	Dilacor XR by Watson	52544-0483	Antihypertensive
DILACORXR240MG	Cap, Blue & Flesh, Black Print, Opaque, Watson logo DILACOR XR over 240 mg	Diltiazem HCl 240 mg	Dilacor XR by Watson	52544-0484	Antihypertensive
DILACORXR240MG	Cap, Blue & Flesh, Black Print, Opaque, Watson logo DILACOR XR over 240 mg	Diltiazem HCl 240 mg	Dilacor XR by Rx Pak	65084-0242	Antihypertensive
DILANTIN100MG	Cap, Clear w/ Orange Band, Black Print, Ex Release, Dilantin over 100 mg	Phenytoin Sodium 100 mg	Dilantin by Parke Davis	00071-0369	Anticonvulsant
DILEXG	Tab, White, Round	Dyphylline 200 mg, Guaifenesin 200 mg	Dilex-G by Poly Pharms	50991-0400	Antiasthmatic; Expectorant
DiltHClER120	Cap, Purple, White Ink, Extended-Release	Diltiazem 120 mg	Novo-Diltiazem HCl ER by Novopharm	Canadian DIN 02271605	Antihypertensive
DiltHClER180	Cap, Blue-Green and White, Black Ink	Diltiazem 180 mg	Novo-Diltiazem HCl ER by Novopharm	Canadian DIN 02271613	Antihypertensive
DiltHClER240	Cap, Purple and Blue-Green, White Ink	Diltiazem 240 mg	Novo-Diltiazem HCl ER by Novopharm	Canadian DIN 02271621	Antihypertensive
DiltHClER300	Cap, Purple and White, Black Ink	Diltiazem 300 mg	Novo-Diltiazem HCl ER by Novopharm	Canadian DIN 02271648	Antihypertensive
DiltHClER360	Cap, Blue-Green, White Ink	Diltiazem 360 mg	Novo-Diltiazem HCl ER by Novopharm	Canadian DIN 02271656	Antihypertensive
DIOVOL	Cap, Blue	Aluminum Hydroxide 200 mg	by Homer	Canadian	Gastrointestinal
DIOVOL	Cap, Blue, Oval, Convex, Beveled Edged, Opaque, Film-Coated, Mint-Flavored	Aluminum Hydroxide 200 mg, Magnesium Hydroxide 200 mg	Diovol by Church and Dwight	Canadian DIN 01910620	Gastrointestinal
DIOVOLEX	Tab, White, Round	Aluminum Hydroxide 600 mg	Amphojel by Homer	Canadian	Gastrointestinal
DIPENTUM250MG	Cap, Beige	Olsalazine Sodium 250 mg	Dipentum by Celltech	53014-0726	Gastrointestinal
DIPENTUM250MG	Cap, Beige, Black Print, Dipentum over 250 mg	Olsalazine Sodium 250 mg	Dipentum by Pharmacia	00013-0105	Gastrointestinal
DIPENTUM250MG	Cap, Beige, Black Print, Dipentum over 250 mg	Olsalazine Sodium 250 mg	Dipentum by Pharmacia	59632-0105	Gastrointestinal
DIPENTUM250MG	Cap, Beige, Black Print, Dipentum over 250 mg	Olsalazine Sodium 250 mg	Dipentum by Pharmacia	Canadian DIN 02063808	Gastrointestinal
DIPENTUM250MG	Cap, Beige, Hard Gelatin, Black Print, Dipentum over 250 mg	Olsalazine Sodium 250 mg	Dipentum by Lundbeck	Canadian DIN 02063808	Gastrointestinal
DIPENTUM250MG	Cap, Beige, Black Print, Dipentum over 250 mg	Olsalazine Sodium 250 mg	Dipentum by Alaven Pharmaceutical	68220-0160	Gastrointestinal
DISALCID750 <> 3M	Tab, Film Coated	Salsalate 750 mg	Disalcid by Leiner	59606-0635	NSAID
DISALCID750 <> 3M	Tab, Film Coated, Embossed	Salsalate 750 mg	by Amerisource	62584-0151	NSAID
DISALCID750 <> 3M	Tab, Film Coated	Salsalate 750 mg	Disalcid by Thrift Drug	59198-0121	NSAID
DISALCID750 <> 3M	Tab, Aqua, Cap Shaped, Bisected, Film Coated	Salsalate 750 mg	Disalcid by 3M	00089-0151	NSAID
DISALCID750 <> 3M	Tab, Film Coated	Salsalate 750 mg	by Nat Pharmpak	55154-2902	NSAID
DISALCID750 <> 3M	Tab, Aqua, Oblong, Scored, Film Coated	Salsalate 750 mg	Disalcid by RX Pak	65084-0216	NSAID
DISALCID750 <> 3M	Tab, Blue, Oblong, Film Coated, Bisected	Salsalate 750 mg	Disalcid by Rx Pak	65084-0212	NSAID
DISTA3104PROZAC10	Cap, Green, Opaque	Fluoxetine HCl 10 mg	Prozac Pulvule by Heartland	61392-0234	Antidepressant
DISTA3104PROZAC10	Cap, Green, Opaque	Fluoxetine HCl 10 mg	Prozac Pulvule by Kaiser	62224-1115	Antidepressant
DISTA3104PROZAC10	Cap, Green, Opaque	Fluoxetine HCl 10 mg	Prozac Pulvule by Kaiser	00179-1252	Antidepressant

ID FRONT <> BACK	DESCRIPTION FRONT <> BACK	INGREDIENT & STRENGTH	BRAND (or Generic Equiv.) by FIRM	NDC#	CLASS; SCH.
DISTA3104PROZAC10	Cap, Green, Opaque	Fluoxetine HCl 10 mg	Prozac Pulvule by Eli Lilly	00002-3104	Antidepressant
DISTA3104PROZAC10	Cap, Green, Opaque	Fluoxetine HCl 10 mg	Prozac Pulvule by Dista Prod	00777-3104	Antidepressant
DISTA3104PROZAC10	Cap, Green, Opaque	Fluoxetine HCl 10 mg	Prozac Pulvule by Invamed	52189-0310	Antidepressant
DISTA3104PROZAC10MG	Cap, Gray & Green, Dista 3104/Prozac 10 mg	Fluoxetine HCl 10 mg	Prozac by Eli Lilly	Canadian DIN 02018985	Antidepressant
DISTA3105PROZAC20MG	Cap, Green & White, Dista 3105/Prozac 20 mg	Fluoxetine HCl 20 mg	Prozac by Eli Lilly	Canadian DIN 00636622	Antidepressant
DISTA3105PROZAC20MG	Cap, Green & White, Black Print, Opaque, Dista over 3105 & Prozac over 20 mg	Fluoxetine HCl 20 mg	Prozac Pulvule by Invamed	52189-0262	Antidepressant
DISTA3105PROZAC20MG	Cap, Green & White, Black Print, Opaque, Dista over 3105 & Prozac over 20 mg	Fluoxetine HCl 20 mg	Prozac Pulvule by Southwood	58016-0828	Antidepressant
DISTA3105PROZAC20MG	Cap, Green & White, Black Print, Opaque, Dista over 3105 & Prozac over 20 mg	Fluoxetine HCl 20 mg	Prozac Pulvule by Va Cmop	65243-0031	Antidepressant
DISTA3105PROZAC20MG	Cap, Green & White, Black Print, Opaque, Dista over 3105 & Prozac over 20 mg	Fluoxetine HCl 20 mg	Prozac Pulvule by Heartland	61392-0235	Antidepressant
DISTA3105PROZAC20MG	Cap, Green & White, Black Print, Opaque, Dista over 3105 & Prozac over 20 mg	Fluoxetine HCl 20 mg	Prozac Pulvule by Promex Med	62301-0008	Antidepressant
DISTA3105PROZAC20MG	Cap, Green & White, Black Print, Opaque, Dista over 3105 & Prozac over 20 mg	Fluoxetine HCl 20 mg	Prozac Pulvule by Eli Lilly	00002-3105	Antidepressant
DISTA3105PROZAC20MG	Cap, Green & White, Black Print, Opaque, Dista over 3105 & Prozac over 20 mg	Fluoxetine HCl 20 mg	Prozac Pulvule by Kaiser	00179-1159	Antidepressant
DISTA3105PROZAC20MG	Cap, Green & White, Black Print, Opaque, Dista over 3105 & Prozac over 20 mg	Fluoxetine HCl 20 mg	Prozac Pulvule by Dista Prod	00777-3105	Antidepressant
DISTA3105PROZAC20MG	Cap, Green & White, Black Print, Opaque, Dista over 3105 & Prozac over 20 mg	Fluoxetine HCl 20 mg	Prozac Pulvule by Pharmedix	53002-1016	Antidepressant
DISTA3105PROZAC20MG	Cap, Green & White, Black Print, Opaque, Dista over 3105 & Prozac over 20 mg	Fluoxetine HCl 20 mg	Prozac Pulvule by Med Pro	53978-1033	Antidepressant
DISTA3107PROZAC40MG	Cap, Green & Orange, Opaque	Fluoxetine HCl 40 mg	Prozac Pulvule by Dista Prod	00777-3107	Antidepressant
DISTA3107PROZAC40MG	Cap, Green & Orange, Opaque	Fluoxetine HCl 40 mg	Prozac Pulvule by Invamed	52189-0309	Antidepressant
DISTA3123	Cap, Green & Yellow, Oval	Chlorpheniramine Maleate 4 mg, Pseudoephedrine HCl 60 mg	Co-Pyronil 2 by Eli Lilly		Cold Remedy
DISTAH71KEFLEX500MG	Cap, Dark Green & Light Green	Cephalexin 500 mg	Keflex by Carlsbad	61442-0102	Antibiotic
DISTAH71KEFLEX500MG	Cap, Dark Green & Light Green	Cephalexin 500 mg	Keflex by Dista	00777-0871	Antibiotic
DISTAH74	Cap, Blue	Ethinamate 500 mg	Valmid by Dista		Hypnotic; C IV
DISTAH77NALFON	Cap	Fenoprofen Calcium 300 mg	by Physician Total Care	54868-0856	NSAID
DISTAH77NALFON	Cap	Fenoprofen Calcium 300 mg	Nalfon by Dista Prod	00777-0877	NSAID
DISTANALFON	Yellow, Oblong, Dista/Nalfon	Fenoprofen Calcium 600 mg	Nalfon by Eli Lilly		NSAID
DISTAU26	Tab, Coated	Erythromycin Estolate 500 mg	Ilosone by Dista Prod	00777-2126	Antibiotic
DITROPAN <> 1375	Tab, 13/75	Oxybutynin Chloride 5 mg	Ditropan by Ortho-McNeil	00088-1375	Urinary Tract
DITROPAN <> 1375	Tab, 13/75	Oxybutynin Chloride 5 mg	Ditropan by Nat Pharmpak	55154-2209	Urinary Tract
DITROPAN <> 9200	Tab, Blue, Round, Scored, Ditropan <> 92-00	Oxybutynin Chloride 5 mg	Ditropan by Alza	17314-9200	Urinary Tract
DITROPAN <> 9200	Tab, Blue, Round, Scored, Ditropan <> 92-00	Oxybutynin Chloride 5 mg	Ditropan by Janssen-Ortho	Canadian DIN 01924761	Urinary Tract
DIUCARDIN50	Tab, White, Oval	Hydroflumethiazide 50 mg	Diucardin by Ayerst	00046-0702	Diuretic; Antihypertensive
DIUPRES <> MSD405	Tab	Chlorothiazide 500 mg, Reserpine 0.125 mg	Diupres by Merck	00006-0405	Diuretic; Antihypertensive
DIURIL <> MSD214	Tab, White, Round, Scored, MSD over 214	Chlorothiazide 250 mg	Diuril by Merck	00006-0214	Diuretic; Antihypertensive
DJ	Tab, Red, Round, Film-Coated, "DJ" inside a hexagon	Estradiol Valerate 2 mg, Estradiol Dienogest 2 mg	Natazia by Berlex	50419-0409	Oral Contraceptive
DJ <> A	Tab, Tan, Round, Abbott Logo (a)	Terazosin HCl 5 mg	Hytrin by Abbott	00074-3324 Discontinued	Antihypertensive
DL <> NVR	Tab, White, Round	Tegaserod Maleate 2 mg	Zelnorm by Novartis	00078-0355	Gastrointestinal
DLANOXINX3A	Tab	Digoxin 0.25 mg	Lanoxin by Med Pro	53978-0177	Cardiac Agent

ID FRONT <> BACK	DESCRIPTION FRONT <> BACK	INGREDIENT & STRENGTH	BRAND (or Generic Equiv.) by FIRM	NDC#	CLASS; SCH.
DMI <> 500	Tab, Blue, Oval, Film Coated, Extended Release	Ciprofloxacin 500 mg	Proquin XR by Depomed	13913-0001	Antibiotic
DMI81 <> DESPEDDM	Tab, White, Oval, Scored, Extended Release	Guaifenesin 800 mg, Pseudoephedrine HCl 120 mg, Dextromethorphan HBr 60 mg	Despec DM by Int'l Ethical Labs	11584-0105	Cold Remedy
DMSP <> 272	Tab	Carbidopa 25 mg, Levodopa 100 mg	by Murfreesboro	51129-1127	Antiparkinson
DMSP019	Tab, White, Oval	Cimetidine HCl 200 mg	Tagamet by BMS		Gastrointestinal
DMSP050	Tab, White, Oval	Cimetidine HCl 300 mg	Tagamet by BMS		Gastrointestinal
DMSP087	Tab, White, Oval	Cimetidine HCl 400 mg	Tagamet by BMS		Gastrointestinal
DMSP088	Tab, White, Oval	Cimetidine HCl 800 mg	Tagamet by BMS		Gastrointestinal
DMSP251	Tab, Dapple Blue, Oval	Carbidopa 25 mg, Levodopa 250 mg	Sinemet by BMS		Antiparkinson
DMSP271	Tab, Dapple Blue, Oval	Carbidopa 10 mg, Levodopa 100 mg	Sinemet by BMS		Antiparkinson
DMSP272	Tab, Yellow, Oval	Carbidopa 25 mg, Levodopa 100 mg	Sinemet by BMS		Antiparkinson
DN	Tab, White, Oblong	Inosine Pranobex 500 mg	Imunovir by Rivex Pharma	Canadian DIN 02240713	Antiviral
DN	Tab, Dark Red, Round, Film-Coated, "DN" inside a hexagon	Estradiol Valerate 1 mg	Natazia by Berlex	50419-0409	Oral Contraceptive
DO	Tab, Yellow, Round, Film Coated, DO inside hexagon	Drospirenone 3 mg, Ethinyl Estradiol 0.03 mg	Yasmin by Berlex	50419-0402	Oral Contraceptive
DO	Tab, Yellow, Round, Film Coated, DO inside hexagon	Drospirenone 3 mg, Ethinyl Estradiol 0.03 mg	Yasmin 21 by Bayer	Canadian DIN 02261723	Oral Contraceptive
DO	Tab, Yellow, Round, Film Coated, DO inside hexagon	Drospirenone 3 mg, Ethinyl Estradiol 0.03 mg	Yasmin 28 by Bayer	Canadian DIN 02261731	Oral Contraceptive
DO <> NVR	Tab, Yellow, Oval	Valsartan 40 mg	Diovan by Novartis	Canadian DIN 02270528	Antihypertensive
DO <> NVR	Tab, Yellow, Oval	Valsartan 40 mg	Diovan by Novartis	00078-0423	Antihypertensive
DOH	Cap, Yellow, Medium Gel	Hydroacytonin 0.3 mg	Acytox by Feeder Labs	99569-0000	Relaxant
DOLACETROBERTS138	Cap	Acetaminophen 500 mg, Hydrocodone Bitartrate 5 mg	Vicodin by Mikart	46672-0247	Analgesic; C III
DOLACETROBERTS138	Cap	Acetaminophen 500 mg, Hydrocodone Bitartrate 5 mg	Vicodin by Roberts	54092-0138	Analgesic; C III
DOLOBID	Tab, Orange, Oblong	Diflunisal 500 mg	by Frosst	Canadian	NSAID
DOLOBID <> MSD675	Tab, Peach, Cap Shaped, Film Coated	Diflunisal 250 mg	by Frosst	Canadian	NSAID
DOLOBID <> MSD675	Tab, Peach, Cap Shaped, Film Coated	Diflunisal 250 mg	Dolobid by Merck	00006-0675	NSAID
DOLOBID <> MSD697	Tab, Orange, Cap Shaped	Diflunisal 500 mg	Dolobid by Merck	00006-0697	NSAID
DOLOBID <> MSD697	Tab, Orange, Cap Shaped	Diflunisal 500 mg	Dolobid by Allscripts		NSAID
DONNATAL <> AHR	Tab, Film Coated	Atropine Sulfate 0.0582 mg, Hyoscyamine Sulfate 0.0195 mg, Phenobarbital 48.6 mg, Scopolamine 0.3111 mg	Donnatal by Pharmedix	53002-0449	Gastrointestinal; C IV
DONNATALEXTENTA <> AHR	Tab, Pale Green, Film Coated	Atropine Sulfate 0.0582 mg, Hyoscyamine Sulfate 0.0195 mg, Phenobarbital 48.6 mg, Scopolamine 0.3111 mg	Donnatal by Thrift Drug	59198-0233	Gastrointestinal; C IV
DORAL <> 15	Tab, Light Orange w/ White Speckles, Capsule-shaped, Doral <> 15	Quazepam 15 mg	Doral by Wallace	00037-9002	Sedative/Hypnotic; C IV
DORAL <> 75	Tab, Light Orange w/ White Specks, Cap Shaped, Doral <> 7.5	Quazepam 7.5 mg	Doral by Wallace	00037-9000	Sedative/Hypnotic; C IV
DORMIN25MG	Cap, Pink	Diphenhydramine HCl 25 mg	Dormin by Randob		Antihistamine
DORYX	Cap, White Print	Doxycycline Hyclate 100 mg	Doryx by Pharm Util	60491-0215	Antibiotic
DORYX	Cap, Clear	Doxycycline Hyclate 100 mg	by Physician Total Care	54868-1491	Antibiotic
DORYX75MG	Cap, Green and Orange	Doxycycline 75 mg	Doryx by Warner	00430-0836	Antibiotic
DORYXDORYX	Cap, White Print	Doxycycline Hyclate 100 mg	Doryx by Faulding	50546-0400	Antibiotic
DORYXPD	Cap, Yellow & Blue	Doxycycline Hyclate 100 mg	by Parke Davis	Canadian	Antibiotic
DORYXPD	Cap, Yellow & Blue	Doxycycline Hyclate 100 mg	Doryx by Parke Davis	00071-0838	Antibiotic
DORYXWC	Cap, Blue and Yellow, White Print	Doxycycline Hyclate 100 mg	Doryx by Warner Chilcott	00430-0838	Antibiotic
DOXA <> P	Tab, White, Lozenge-Shaped	Doxazosin Mesylate 4 mg	Cardura by Pharmascience	Canadian DIN 02244529	Antihypertensive

ID FRONT <> BACK	DESCRIPTION FRONT <> BACK	INGREDIENT & STRENGTH	BRAND (or Generic Equiv.) by FIRM	NDC#	CLASS; SCH.
DOXA <> P2	Tab, White, Oblong, Scored	Doxazosin Mesylate 2 mg	Cardura by Pharmascience	Canadian DIN 02244528	Antihypertensive
DOXA1 <> P	Tab, White, Round	Doxazosin Mesylate 1 mg	Cardura by Pharmascience	Canadian DIN 02244527	Antihypertensive
DOXY100	Tab, Orange, Round, Scored	Doxycycline Hyclate 100 mg	Vibra-Tabs by Pharmascience	Canadian DIN 02289466	Antibiotic
DOXYCAPBARR296	Cap, Doxy-Cap <> Barr over 296	Doxycycline Hyclate	by Barr	00555-0296	Antibiotic
DOXYCAPBARR297	Cap, Doxy-Cap <> Barr over 297	Doxycycline Hyclate	by Barr	00555-0297	Antibiotic
DOXYCIN100	Tab, Orange	Doxycycline Hyclate 100 mg	Doxycin by Genpharm	Canadian 00860751	Antibiotic
DOXYTAB <> BARR295	Tab, Coated, Doxy-Tab <> Barr 295	Doxycycline Hyclate	by Barr	00555-0295	Antibiotic
DOXYTEC100	Tab, Light Orange, Round, Film Coated, Scored, Doxytec over 100	Doxycycline Hyclate 100 mg	by AltiMed	Canadian DIN 02091232 Discontinued	Antibiotic
DOZZY	Tab, Yellow, Oblong	Acetaminophen 100 mg	Tylenol by EST		Pain Reliever
DP	Tab, White, Round, Film Coated, DP inside hexagon	Inert	Yaz by Berlex	50419-0405	Oral Contraceptive; Placebo
DP	Tab, White, Round, Film Coated, DP inside hexagon	Inert	Yasmin by Berlex	50419-0402	Oral Contraceptive; Placebo
DP	Tab, White, Round, Film Coated, DP inside hexagon	Inert	Yasmin 28 by Bayer	Canadian DIN 02261731	Oral Contraceptive; Placebo
DP <> 016	Tab, Orange, Round	Levonorgestrel 0.10 mg, Ethinyl Estradiol 0.02 mg	Aviane by Duramed	51285-0017	Oral Contraceptive
DP <> 016	Tab, Orange, Round	Levonorgestrel 0.10 mg, Ethinyl Estradiol 0.02 mg	Aviane by Barr	00555-9045	Oral Contraceptive
DP <> 016	Tab, Orange, Round	Levonorgestrel 0.10 mg, Ethinyl Estradiol 0.02 mg	Aviane by Apotex	Canadian DIN 02298538	Oral Contraceptive
DP <> 016	Tab, Orange, Round	Levonorgestrel 0.10 mg, Ethinyl Estradiol 0.02 mg	Aviane by Apotex	Canadian DIN 02298546	Oral Contraceptive
DP <> 021	Tab, White, Round	Desogestrel 0.15 mg, Ethinyl Estradiol 0.02 mg	Kariva by Barr	00555-9050	Oral Contraceptive
DP <> 022	Tab, Light Blue, Round	Ethinyl Estradiol 0.01 mg	Kariva by Barr	00555-9050	Oral Contraceptive
DP <> 200	Tab	Levothyroxine Sodium 200 mcg	Levoxyl by Jones	52604-1112	Thyroid Hormone
DP <> 331	Tab, Light Green, Round	Inert	Kariva by Barr	00555-9050	Oral Contraceptive; Placebo
DP <> 331	Tab, Light Green, Round	Inert	Lo Ovral by Barr	00555-9049	Oral Contraceptive; Placebo
DP <> 402	Tab, Yellow, Cap Shaped, Scored	Pseudoephedrine HCl 120 mg, Guaifenesin 600 mg	by Duramed	51285-0402	Cold Remedy
DP <> 41	Tab, Green, Round, Film Coated, dp <> 41	Conjugated Estrogens 0.3 mg	Cenestin by Barr	51285-0441	Hormone
DP <> 417	Tab, Green, Oblong, Scored, Film Coated, Duramed Logo	Guaifenesin 600 mg	Robitussin by Eli Lilly	00110-4117	Expectorant
DP <> 42	Tab, Red, Round, Film Coated, dp <> 42	Conjugated Estrogens 0.625 mg	Cenestin by Barr	51285-0442	Hormone
DP <> 43	Tab, White, Round, Film Coated, dp <> 43	Conjugated Estrogens 0.9 mg	Cenestin by Barr	51285-0443	Hormone
DP <> 44	Tab, Blue, Round, Film Coated	Conjugated Estrogens 1.25 mg	Cenestin by Duramed	51285-0444	Hormone
DP <> 46	Tab, Orange, Round, Film Coated, 46 <> dp	Conjugated Estrogens 0.45 mg	Cenestin by Barr	51285-0446	Hormone
DP <> 501	Tab, Lavender, Round, Duramed Logo	Estradiol 0.5 mg	by Duramed	51285-0501	Hormone
DP <> 502	Tab, Rose, Round, Duramed Logo	Estradiol 1 mg	by Duramed	51285-0502	Hormone
DP <> 504	Tab, Duramed Logo	Estradiol 2 mg	by Duramed	51285-0504	Hormone
DP <> 510	Tab, Pink, Round, Film Coated	Levonorgestrel 0.050 mg, Ethinyl Estradiol 0.03 mg	Triphasil by Barr	51285-0514	Oral Contraceptive
DP <> 510	Tab, Pink, Round, Film Coated	Levonorgestrel 0.050 mg, Ethinyl Estradiol 0.03 mg	Triphasil by Barr	00555-9047	Oral Contraceptive
DP <> 511	Tab, White, Round, Film Coated	Levonorgestrel 0.075 mg, Ethinyl Estradiol 0.04 mg	Triphasil by Barr	00555-9047	Oral Contraceptive
DP <> 511	Tab, White, Round, Film Coated	Levonorgestrel 0.075 mg, Ethinyl Estradiol 0.04 mg	Triphasil by Barr	51285-0514	Oral Contraceptive
DP <> 512	Tab, Orange, Round, Film Coated	Levonorgestrel 0.125 mg, Ethinyl Estradiol 0.03 mg	Triphasil by Barr	51285-0514	Oral Contraceptive
DP <> 512	Tab, Orange, Round, Film Coated	Levonorgestrel 0.125 mg, Ethinyl Estradiol 0.03 mg	Triphasil by Barr	00555-9047	Oral Contraceptive

ID FRONT <> BACK	DESCRIPTION FRONT <> BACK	INGREDIENT & STRENGTH	BRAND (or Generic Equiv.) by FIRM	NDC#	CLASS; SCH.
DP <> 519	Tab, Light Green, Round, Film Coated	Inert	Triphasil by Barr	00555-9047	Oral Contraceptive; Placebo
DP <> 519	Tab, Light Green, Round, Film Coated	Inert	Triphasil by Barr	51285-0514	Oral Contraceptive; Placebo
DP <> 519	Tab, Light Green, Round, Film Coated	Inert	Aviane by Barr	00555-9045	Oral Contraceptive; Placebo
DP <> 521	Tab, Orange, Round	Prochlorperazine 5 mg	Compazine by Barr	00555-0521 Discontinued	Antiemetic
DP <> 522	Tab, Yellow, Round	Prochlorperazine 10 mg	Compazine by Barr	00555-0522 Discontinued	Antiemetic
DP <> 543	Tab, White, Round, Film Coated	Ethinyl Estradiol 0.03 mg, Norgestrel 0.3 mg	Lo Ovral by Barr	51285-0546	Oral Contraceptive
DP <> 543	Tab, White, Round, Film Coated	Ethinyl Estradiol 0.03 mg, Norgestrel 0.3 mg	Lo Ovral by Barr	00555-9049	Oral Contraceptive
DP <> 570	Tab, White, Round	Inert	Apri 28 Day by Duramed	51285-0576	Oral Contraceptive; Placebo
DP <> 570	Tab, White, Round	Inert	Ortho-Cept by Barr	00555-9043	Oral Contraceptive; Placebo
DP <> 570	Tab, White, Round	Inert	Ortho-Cept by Allscripts		Oral Contraceptive; Placebo
DP <> 575	Tab, Rose, Round	Desogestrel 0.15 mg, Ethinyl Estradiol 0.03 mg	Ortho-Cept by Allscripts		Oral Contraceptive
DP <> 575	Tab, Rose, Round	Desogestrel 0.15 mg, Ethinyl Estradiol 0.03 mg	Ortho-Cept by Barr	00555-9043	Oral Contraceptive
DP <> 857	Tab, White, Cap Shaped, Scored	Guaifenesin 1200 mg	Robitussin by Duramed	51285-0857	Expectorant
DP <> 896	Tab, Blue, Cap Shaped, Scored	Guaifenesin 500 mg, Pseudoephedrine 60 mg	Sudafed Sinus by Duramed	51285-0896	Cold Remedy
DP <> CIBA	Tab, Brownish-Orange, Round, Film Coated	Maprotiline 25 mg	Ludiomil by Ciba	Canadian DIN 00360481	Antidepressant
DP <> M	Tab	Aspirin 500 mg, Hydrocodone Bitartrate 5 mg	Lortab ASA by Mason	12758-0057	Analgesic; C III
DP <> TOUROCC	Tab, White, Cap Shaped, Scored	Guaifenesin 575 mg, Pseudoephedrine HCl 60 mg, Dextromethorphan HBr 30 mg	Touro CC by Pfab	62542-0770	Cold Remedy
DP <> TOUROCC	Tab, White, Cap Shaped, Scored	Guaifenesin 575 mg, Pseudoephedrine HCl 60 mg, Dextromethorphan HBr 30 mg	Touro CC by Dartmouth	58869-0441	Cold Remedy
DP01	Tab, Tan, Round	Clonidine HCl 0.1 mg	Catapres by Duramed		Antihypertensive
DP02	Tab, Orange, Round	Clonidine HCl 0.2 mg	Catapres by Duramed		Antihypertensive
DP03	Tab, Peach, Round	Clonidine HCl 0.3 mg	Catapres by Duramed		Antihypertensive
DP082 <> TUSSIGON	Tab, Blue, Round, Scored, dp/082	Homatropine Methylbromide 1.5 mg, Hydrocodone Bitartrate 5 mg	Tussigon by JMI Daniels	00689-0082	Cold Remedy; C III
DP10	Tab, Peach, Round	Propranolol HCl 10 mg	Inderal by Duramed		Antihypertensive
DP100 <> LEVOXYL	Tab, Yellow, Oval	Levothyroxine Sodium 100 mcg	Levoxyl by Jones	52604-5100	Thyroid Hormone
DP11	Tab, Lavender, Round	Trifluoperazine HCl 1 mg	Stelazine by Duramed		Antipsychotic
DP112 <> LEVOXYL	Tab, Pink, Oval	Levothyroxine Sodium 112 mcg	Levoxyl by Jones	52604-5112	Thyroid Hormone
DP12	Tab, Lavender, Round	Trifluoperazine HCl 2 mg	Stelazine by Duramed		Antipsychotic
DP125 <> LEVOXYL	Tab, Brown, Oval	Levothyroxine Sodium 125 mcg	Levoxyl by Jones	52604-5125	Thyroid Hormone
DP13	Tab, Lavender, Round	Trifluoperazine HCl 5 mg	Stelazine by Duramed		Antipsychotic
DP137 <> LEVOXYL	Tab, Dark Blue, Oval	Levothyroxine Sodium 137 mcg	Levoxyl by Jones	52604-5137	Thyroid Hormone
DP14	Tab, Lavender, Round	Trifluoperazine HCl 10 mg	Stelazine by Duramed		Antipsychotic
DP150 <> LEVOXYL	Tab, Blue, Oval	Levothyroxine Sodium 150 mcg	Levoxyl by Jones	52604-5150	Thyroid Hormone
DP1625	Tab	Estropipate 0.75 mg	by URL Mutual	00677-1508	Hormone
DP175 <> LEVOXYL	Tab, Turquoise	Levothyroxine Sodium 175 mcg	Levoxyl by Jones	52604-5175	Thyroid Hormone
DP20	Tab, Blue, Round	Propranolol HCl 20 mg	Inderal by Duramed		Antihypertensive
DP200 <> LEVOXYL	Tab, Pink, Oval	Levothyroxine Sodium 200 mcg	Levoxyl by Jones	52604-5200	Thyroid Hormone
DP223	Tab, White, Round	Aminophylline 100 mg	Aminophylline by Duramed		Antiasthmatic

ID FRONT <> BACK	DESCRIPTION FRONT <> BACK	INGREDIENT & STRENGTH	BRAND (or Generic Equiv.) by FIRM	NDC#	CLASS; SCH.
DP224	Tab, White, Round	Aminophylline 200 mg	Aminophylline by Duramed		Antiasthmatic
DP225	Tab, White, Round	Haloperidol 0.5 mg	Haldol by Duramed		Antipsychotic
DP226	Tab, Yellow, Round	Haloperidol 1 mg	Haldol by Duramed		Antipsychotic
DP227	Tab, Lavender, Round	Haloperidol 2 mg	Haldol by Duramed		Antipsychotic
DP228	Tab, Green, Round	Haloperidol 5 mg	Haldol by Duramed		Antipsychotic
DP229	Tab, Aqua, Round	Haloperidol 10 mg	Haldol by Duramed		Antipsychotic
DP230	Tab, Salmon, Round	Haloperidol 20 mg	Haldol by Duramed		Antipsychotic
DP241	Tab, Yellow, Oval	Choline Magnesium Trisalicylate 500 mg	Trilisate by Duramed		NSAID
DP242	Tab, Blue, Oval	Choline Magnesium Trisalicylate 750 mg	Trilisate by Duramed		NSAID
DP246	Tab, White, Round	Cyproheptadine HCl 4 mg	Periactin by Duramed		Antihistamine
DP25 <> LEVOXYL	Tab, dp/25	Levothyroxine Sodium 25 mcg	Levoxyl by Jones	52604-1117	Thyroid Hormone
DP25 <> LEVOXYL	Tab, Orange, Oval, Scored, dp/25 <> Levoxyl	Levothyroxine Sodium 25 mcg	Levoxyl by JMI Daniels	00689-1117	Thyroid Hormone
DP25 <> LEVOXYL	Tab, Orange, Oval	Levothyroxine Sodium 25 mcg	Levoxyl by Jones	52604-5025	Thyroid Hormone
DP251	Tab, Blue, Round	Chlorpropamide 250 mg	Diabinese by Duramed		Antidiabetic
DP252	Tab, Blue, Round, dp-252	Chlorpropamide 100 mg	Diabinese by Duramed		Antidiabetic
DP265	Cap, Green, Oblong	Hydroxyzine Pamoate 25 mg	Vistaril by Duramed		Antianxiety; Antihistamine
DP266	Cap, Green & White, Oblong	Hydroxyzine Pamoate 50 mg	Vistaril by Duramed		Antianxiety; Antihistamine
DP267	Cap, Gray & Green, Oblong	Hydroxyzine Pamoate 100 mg	Vistaril by Duramed		Antianxiety; Antihistamine
DP274	Tab, White, Round	Isoniazid 100 mg	Laniazid by Duramed		Antimycobacterial
DP275	Cap, Green, Oblong	Indomethacin 25 mg	Indocin by Duramed		NSAID
DP276	Cap, Green	Indomethacin 50 mg	Indocin by Duramed		NSAID
DP277	Tab	Isoniazid 300 mg	Laniazid by Ivax	00182-1356	Antimycobacterial
DP277	Tab, White, Round	Isoniazid 300 mg	Laniazid by Duramed	51285-0277	Antimycobacterial
DP293	Cap, Beige & Orange	Guaifenesin 200 mg, Phenylephrine HCl 5 mg, Phenylpropanolamine HCl 45 mg	Entex by Qualitest	00603-5665	Cold Remedy
DP293	Cap, Beige & Orange	Guaifenesin 200 mg, Phenylephrine HCl 5 mg, Phenylpropanolamine HCl 45 mg	Entex by Duramed	51285-0293	Cold Remedy
DP294	Tab, Ex Release, Duramed Logo 294	Guaifenesin 400 mg, Phenylpropanolamine HCl 75 mg	Entex LA by Duramed	53002-0323	Cold Remedy
DP295	Tab	Guaifenesin 400 mg, Phenylpropanolamine HCl 75 mg	Entex LA by Pharmedix	51285-0295	Cold Remedy
DP295	Tab, Blue, Oval	Guaifenesin 400 mg, Phenylpropanolamine HCl 75 mg	Entex LA by Duramed		Cold Remedy
DP296	Tab, Yellow, Cap Shaped, Coated	Salsalate 500 mg	by Duramed	51285-0858	NSAID
DP297	Tab, Yellow, Oblong	Salsalate 750 mg	Disalcid by Amide		NSAID
DP297	Tab, Yellow, Cap Shaped	Salsalate 750 mg	by Duramed	51285-0859	NSAID
DP298	Tab, Yellow, Round	Salsalate 500 mg	Disalcid by Duramed		NSAID
DP299	Tab, Yellow, Oblong	Salsalate 750 mg	Disalcid by Duramed		NSAID
DP3	Tab	Acetaminophen 300 mg, Codeine Phosphate 30 mg	Tylenol w/ Codeine by Major	00904-0175	Analgesic; C III
DP30	Tab, White, Round	Conjugated Estrogens 0.3 mg	Premarin by Duramed		Hormone
DP300 <> LEVOXYL	Tab, Green, Oval	Levothyroxine Sodium 300 mcg	Levoxyl by Jones	52604-5300	Thyroid Hormone
DP301	Tab, White, Oval, Scored, Film Coated	Methylprednisolone 4 mg	Medrol by Duramed	00555-0301	Steroid
DP301	Tab, White, Oval, Scored, Film Coated	Methylprednisolone 4 mg	Medrol by Qualitest	00603-4593	Steroid
DP301	Tab, White, Oval, Scored, Film Coated	Methylprednisolone 4 mg	Medrol by Neuman	64579-0039	Steroid
DP301	Tab, White, Oval, Scored, Film Coated	Methylprednisolone 4 mg	Medrol by Schein	00364-0467	Steroid
DP301	Tab, White, Oval, Scored, Film Coated	Methylprednisolone 4 mg	Medrol by Duramed	51285-0301	Steroid
DP301	Tab, White, Oval, Scored, Film Coated	Methylprednisolone 4 mg	Medrol by Pharmedix	53002-0312	Steroid
DP301	Tab, White, Oval, Scored, Film Coated	Methylprednisolone 4 mg	Medrol by URL Mutual	00677-0565	Steroid

ID FRONT <> BACK	DESCRIPTION FRONT <> BACK	INGREDIENT & STRENGTH	BRAND (or Generic Equiv.) by FIRM	NDC#	CLASS; SCH.
DP301	Tab, White, Oval, Scored, Film Coated	Methylprednisolone 4 mg	Medrol by Moore	00839-6224	Steroid
DP31	Tab, White, Round	Conjugated Estrogens 0.625 mg	Premarin by Duramed		Hormone
DP311 <> TOURODM	Tab, Light Blue, Cap Shaped, Scored	Dextromethorphan HBr 30 mg, Guaifenesin 575 mg	Touro DM by Dartmouth	58869-0411	Cold Remedy
DP311 <> TOURODM	Tab, Light Blue, Scored	Dextromethorphan HBr 30 mg, Guaifenesin 575 mg	Touro DM by Anabolic	00722-6297	Cold Remedy
DP312	Tab, White, Round	Prednisone 10 mg	Deltasone by Duramed		Steroid
DP313	Tab, Orange, Round	Prednisone 20 mg	Deltasone by Duramed		Steroid
DP314	Tab, Yellow, Round	Prochlorperazine 5 mg	Compazine by Duramed		Antiemetic
DP315	Tab, Yellow, Round	Prochlorperazine 10 mg	Compazine by Duramed		Antiemetic
DP316	Tab, Yellow, Round	Prochlorperazine 25 mg	Compazine by Duramed		Antiemetic
DP32	Tab, White, Round	Conjugated Estrogens 1.25 mg	Premarin by Duramed		Hormone
DP321 <> TOUROEX	Tab, DP/321 <> Touro EX	Guaifenesin 575 mg	Robitussin by Anabolic	00722-6394 Discontinued	Expectorant
DP321 <> TOUROEX	Tab, DP/321 <> Touro EX	Guaifenesin 600 mg	Robitussin by Anabolic	00722-6282 Discontinued	Expectorant
DP321 <> TOUROEX	Tab, White, Ex Release	Guaifenesin 575 mg	Robitussin by Dartmouth	58869-0421 Discontinued	Expectorant
DP325	Tab, White, Round	Tolazamide 100 mg	Tolinase by Duramed		Antidiabetic
DP327	Tab, White, Round	Tolazamide 500 mg	Tolinase by Duramed		Antidiabetic
DP332	Tab, Yellow, Round	Hydrochlorothiazide 25 mg, Propranolol HCl 40 mg	Inderide by Duramed		Diuretic; Antihypertensive
DP333	Tab, Yellow, Round	Hydrochlorothiazide 25 mg, Propranolol HCl 80 mg	Inderide by Duramed		Diuretic; Antihypertensive
DP34	Tab, White, Round	Conjugated Estrogens 2.5 mg	Premarin by Duramed		Hormone
DP364	Cap, Scarlet & White	Acetaminophen 325 mg, Dichloralphenazone 100 mg, Isometheptene Mucate 65 mg	Midrin by Amide		Analgesic; C IV
DP371	Tab, White, Round	Methyldopa 250 mg	Aldomet by Duramed		Antihypertensive
DP372	Tab, White, Round	Methyldopa 500 mg	Aldomet by Duramed		Antihypertensive
DP40	Tab	Propranolol HCl 40 mg	Inderal by Pharmedix	53002-0495	Antihypertensive
DP401	Tab, Yellow, Cap Shaped, Film Coated	Guaifenesin 600 mg, Pseudoephedrine HCl 120 mg	by Duramed	51285-0401	Cold Remedy
DP406 <> TA	Tab, White, Sustained-Release	Pseudoephedrine HCl 45 mg, Brompheniramine Maleate 6 mg	Touro Allergy by Dartmouth	58869-0406	Cold Remedy
DP417	Tab, Green, Cap Shaped, Film Coated	Guaifenesin 600 mg	Robitussin by Duramed	51285-0417	Expectorant
DP42	Tab, Red, Round, Duramed Logo and 42	Synthetic Conjugated Estrogens 0.625 mg	by Duramed	51285-0442	Hormone
DP420	Tab, White, Cap Shaped	Dextromethorphan HBr 30 mg, Guaifenesin 600 mg	by Duramed	51285-0420	Cold Remedy
DP421 <> TOUROEX	Tab, White, Oblong, Scored	Guaifenesin 575 mg	Robitussin by Pfab	62542-0705	Expectorant
DP436 <> TOUROLA	Tab, White, Cap Shaped	Pseudoephedrine HCl 120 mg, Guaifenesin 500 mg	Touro LA by Dartmouth	58869-0536 Discontinued	Cold Remedy
DP445 <> TOUROCCLD	Tab, Scored	Dextromethorphan 30 mg, Pseudoephedrine 25 mg, Guaifenesin 575 mg	Touro CC-LD by Dartmouth	58869-0445	Cold Remedy
DP480	Tab, Light Pink, Cap Shaped	Verapamil HCl SR 120 mg	Isoptin SR by Duramed	51285-0480	Antihypertensive
DP482	Tab, Light Pink, Cap Shaped	Verapamil HCl SR 240 mg	Isoptin SR by Duramed	51285-0482	Antihypertensive
DP50 <> LEVOXYL	Tab, White, Oval	Levothyroxine Sodium 50 mcg	Levoxyl by Jones	52604-5050	Thyroid Hormone
DP50 <> LEVOXYL	Tab, White, Oval, Scored, dp/50 <> Levoxyl	Levothyroxine Sodium 50 mcg	Levoxyl by JMI Daniels	00689-1118	Thyroid Hormone
DP50 <> LEVOXYL	Tab, dp/50 <> Levoxyl	Levothyroxine Sodium 50 mcg	Levoxyl by Jones	52604-1118	Thyroid Hormone
DP501	Tab, Purple, Round, Scored, D over P 501	Estradiol 0.5 mg	by Heartland	61392-0176	Hormone
DP504	Tab, Blue, Round, Scored, D over P 504	Estradiol 2 mg	by Heartland	61392-0121	Hormone
DP504	Tab, Blue, Round, Scored, D over P 504	Estradiol 2 mg	Estrace by Martec	52555-0718	Hormone
DP509	Tab, Yellow, Oval, Scored	Methotrexate 2.5 mg	Rheumatrex by Kiel	59063-0114	Antineoplastic
DP509	Tab, Yellow, Round	Methotrexate Sodium 2.5 mg	Rheumatrex by Kiel	51285-0509	Antineoplastic
DP548	Cap, Buff & Dark Green	Hydroxyurea 500 mg	Hydrea by Duramed	51285-0548	Antineoplastic
DP575	Tab, Medium Rose, Round	Desogestrel 0.15 mg, Ethinyl Estradiol 0.03 mg	Apri 28 Day by Duramed	51285-0576	Oral Contraceptive

ID FRONT <> BACK	DESCRIPTION FRONT <> BACK	INGREDIENT & STRENGTH	BRAND (or Generic Equiv.) by FIRM	NDC#	CLASS; SCH.
DP575	Tab, Medium Rose, Round	Desogestrel 0.15 mg, Ethinyl Estradiol 0.03 mg	Apri 21 Day by Duramed	51285-0575	Oral Contraceptive
DP581 <> TOUROHC	Tab, White, Cap Shaped, Scored	Hydrocodone Bitartrate 5 mg, Guaifenesin 575 mg	Touro HC by Dartmouth	58869-0581	Cold Remedy; C III
DP60	Tab, Pink, Round	Propranolol HCl 60 mg	Inderal by Duramed		Antihypertensive
DP610	Tab, Off-White, Round	Oxycodone 5 mg, Acetaminophen 325 mg	Percocet by Duramed	51285-0610	Analgesic; C II
DP622	Tab, Yellow, Round	Diazepam 5 mg	Valium by Duramed		Antianxiety; C IV
DP623	Tab, Blue, Round	Diazepam 10 mg	Valium by Duramed		Antianxiety; C IV
DP635 <> TOUROLALD	Tab, Scored	Pseudoephedrine 50 mg, Guaifenesin 525 mg	Touro LA-LD by Dartmouth	58869-0635	Cold Remedy
DP636 <> TOUROLA	Tab, White, Oblong, Scored	Guaifenesin 525 mg, Pseudoephedrine HCl 120 mg	Sudafed Sinus by Pfab	62542-0755	Cold Remedy
DP636 <> TOUROLA	Tab, White, Oblong	Guaifenesin 525 mg, Pseudoephedrine HCl 120 mg	Sudafed Sinus by Dartmouth Pharms	58869-0636	Cold Remedy
DP651	Cap, Blue & Clear	Phentermine 30 mg	Fastin by Duramed		Anorexiant; C IV
DP660	Cap, Green & White	Temazepam 15 mg	Restoril by Duramed		Sedative/Hypnotic; C IV
DP661	Cap, White	Temazepam 30 mg	Restoril by Duramed		Sedative/Hypnotic; C IV
DP70	Yellow, Scored	Digoxin 0.125 mg	Lanoxin by Eckerd	19458-0892	Cardiac Agent
DP75 <> LEVOXYL	Tab	Levothyroxine Sodium 75 mcg	Synthroid by Jones	52604-1119	Thyroid Hormone
DP75 <> LEVOXYL	Tab, Purple, Oval, Scored, dp/75 <> Levoxyl	Levothyroxine Sodium 75 mcg	Synthroid by JMI Daniels	00689-1119	Thyroid Hormone
DP75 <> LEVOXYL	Tab, Purple, Oval	Levothyroxine Sodium 75 mcg	Synthroid by Jones	52604-5075	Thyroid Hormone
DP80	Tab, Yellow, Round, dp/80	Propranolol HCl 80 mg	Inderal by Duramed		Antihypertensive
DP825	Tab, Beige, Cap Shaped	Chlorpheniramine Tannate 8 mg, Phenylephrine Tannate 25 mg, Pyrilamine Tannate 25 mg	Triotann by Duramed	51285-0825	Cold Remedy
DP832	Tab, Pale Pink, Cap Shaped	Choline Magnesium Trisalicylate 500 mg	Trilisate by Amide	51285-0902	NSAID
DP833	Tab, White, Cap Shaped, Film Coated	Salicylate 750 mg	Choline Magnesium Trisalicylate by Duramed	51285-0903	NSAID
DP849	Tab, White, Cap Shaped	Acetaminophen 325 mg, Butalbital 50 mg, Caffeine 40 mg	Fioricet by Mikart		Analgesic
DP877	Tab, White, Round	Yohimbine HCl 5.4 mg	by Duramed	51285-0877	Impotence Agent
DP88 <> LEVOXYL	Tab, Green, Oval	Levothyroxine Sodium 88 mcg	Synthroid by Jones	52604-5088	Thyroid Hormone
DP88 <> LEVOXYL	Tab, Olive, Oval, Scored, dp/88 <> Levoxyl	Levothyroxine Sodium 88 mcg	Synthroid by JMI Daniels	00689-1132	Thyroid Hormone
DP88 <> LEVOXYL	Tab	Levothyroxine Sodium 88 mcg	Synthroid by Jones	52604-1132	Thyroid Hormone
DP896	Tab, Blue, Cap Shaped	Guaifenesin 600 mg, Pseudoephedrine HCl 60 mg	Deconsal II by Sovereign	51285-0293	Cold Remedy
DP90	Tab, Lavender, Round	Propranolol HCl 90 mg	Inderal by Duramed		Antihypertensive
DP914	Tab, White, Round	Digoxin 0.125 mg	Lanoxin by Jerome Stevens	51285-0914	Cardiac Agent
DP915	Tab, White, Round	Digoxin 0.25 mg	Lanoxin by Jerome Stevens	51285-0915	Cardiac Agent
DP915	Tab, White, Round	Digoxin 0.25 mg	Lanoxin by Duramed	51285-0915	Cardiac Agent
DP932	Tab, White, Round	Hyoscyamine Sulfate 0.125 mg	Levsin by Rugby		Gastrointestinal
DP932	Tab, White, Round	Hyoscyamine Sulfate 0.125 mg	Levsin by Amide	51285-0932	Gastrointestinal
DP933	Tab, White, Oblong, Scored	Hyoscyamine Sulfate 0.375 mg	Levsin by Duramed	51285-0937	Gastrointestinal
DP933	Tab, Orange, Cap Shaped, Ex Release	Hyoscyamine Sulfate 0.375 mg	Levsin by Duramed	51285-0933	Gastrointestinal
DP935	Tab, Blue, Round	Hyoscyamine Sulfate 0.125 mg	Levsin SL by Amide	51285-0935	Gastrointestinal
DP935	Tab, White, Round	Hyoscyamine Sulfate 0.125 mg	Levsin by Rugby		Gastrointestinal
DP970	Tab, Yellow, Round	Digoxin 0.125 mg	Lanoxin by Duramed	51285-0970	Cardiac Agent
DP971	Tab, White, Round	Digoxin 0.25 mg	Lanoxin by Duramed	51285-0971	Cardiac Agent
DP972	Tab, Green, Round	Digoxin 0.5 mg	Lanoxin by Amide	51285-0972	Cardiac Agent
DPi <> 4	Tab	Acetaminophen 300 mg, Codeine Phosphate 60 mg	Tylenol w/ Codeine by Quality Care	60346-0632 Discontinued	Analgesic; C III
DP1125	Tab, White, Diamond Shaped	Estropipate 1.5 mg	by Duramed	51285-0876	Hormone
DPi2	Tab, White, Round	Acetaminophen 300 mg, Codeine Phosphate 15 mg	Tylenol w/ Codeine by Duramed	51285-0600	Analgesic; C III
DPi2	Tab, White, Round	Acetaminophen 300 mg, Codeine Phosphate 15 mg	Tylenol w/ Codeine by URL Mutual	00677-0611	Analgesic; C III
DPi2	Tab, White, Round	Acetaminophen 300 mg, Codeine Phosphate 15 mg	Tylenol w/ Codeine by Ivax	00182-1268	Analgesic; C III
DPi2	Tab, White, Round	Acetaminophen 300 mg, Codeine Phosphate 15 mg	Tylenol w/ Codeine by McNeil	52021-0600	Analgesic; C III

ID FRONT <> BACK	DESCRIPTION FRONT <> BACK	INGREDIENT & STRENGTH	BRAND (or Generic Equiv.) by FIRM	NDC#	CLASS; SCH.
DPI2	Tab, White, Round	Acetaminophen 300 mg, Codeine Phosphate 15 mg	Tylenol w/ Codeine by Major	00904-0571	Analgesic; C III
DPI2	Tab, White, Round	Acetaminophen 300 mg, Codeine Phosphate 15 mg	Tylenol w/ Codeine by Elge	58298-0954	Analgesic; C III
DPI3	Tab, White, Round	Acetaminophen 300 mg, Codeine Phosphate 30 mg	Tylenol w/ Codeine by Elge	58298-0953	Analgesic; C III
DPI3	Tab, White, Round	Acetaminophen 300 mg, Codeine Phosphate 30 mg	Tylenol w/ Codeine by URL Mutual	00677-0612	Analgesic; C III
DPI3	Tab, White, Round	Acetaminophen 300 mg, Codeine Phosphate 30 mg	Tylenol w/ Codeine by McNeil	52021-0601	Analgesic; C III
DPI3	Tab, White, Round	Acetaminophen 300 mg, Codeine Phosphate 30 mg	Tylenol w/ Codeine by Noramco		Analgesic; C III
DPI3	Tab, White, Round	Acetaminophen 300 mg, Codeine Phosphate 30 mg	Tylenol w/ Codeine by Duramed	51285-0601	Analgesic; C III
DPI364	Cap, Scarlet & White, Black Print, Hard Gel	Acetaminophen 325 mg, Dichloralphenazone 100 mg, Isometheptene mucate 65 mg	Duradrin by Duramed	51285-0364	Analgesic; C IV
DPI364	Cap, Scarlet, Black Print	Acetaminophen 325 mg, Dichloralantipyrine 100 mg, Isometheptene Mucate (1:1) 65 mg	by Kaiser	00179-1222	Analgesic; C IV
DPI364	Cap, Scarlet, DPI or DP	Acetaminophen 325 mg, Dichloralantipyrine 100 mg, Isometheptene Mucate (1:1) 65 mg	Midchlor by Schein	00364-2342	Analgesic; C IV
DPI364	Cap, Scarlet & White, Black Print, Hard Gel	Acetaminophen 325 mg, Dichloralphenazone 100 mg, Isometheptene mucate 65 mg	Duradrin by Barr	00555-0364	Analgesic; C IV
DPI4	Tab, White, Round	Acetaminophen 300 mg, Codeine Phosphate 60 mg	Tylenol w/ Codeine by Prepackage Specialists	58864-0005	Analgesic; C III
DPI4	Tab, White, Round	Acetaminophen 300 mg, Codeine Phosphate 60 mg	Tylenol w/ Codeine by Noramco		Analgesic; C III
DPI4	Tab, White, Round	Acetaminophen 300 mg, Codeine Phosphate 60 mg	Tylenol w/ Codeine by Duramed	51285-0602	Analgesic; C III
DPI4	Tab, White, Round	Acetaminophen 300 mg, Codeine Phosphate 60 mg	Tylenol w/ Codeine by Elge	58298-0951	Analgesic; C III
DPI4	Tab, White, Round	Acetaminophen 300 mg, Codeine Phosphate 60 mg	Tylenol w/ Codeine by McNeil	52021-0602	Analgesic; C III
DPI4	Tab, White, Round	Acetaminophen 300 mg, Codeine Phosphate 60 mg	Tylenol w/ Codeine by Major	00904-3916	Analgesic; C III
DPI4	Tab, White, Round	Acetaminophen 300 mg, Codeine Phosphate 60 mg	Tylenol w/ Codeine by Ivax	00182-1338	Analgesic; C III
DPI4	Tab, White, Round	Acetaminophen 300 mg, Codeine Phosphate 60 mg	Tylenol w/ Codeine by URL Mutual	00677-0632	Analgesic; C III
DPI488	Cap, Opaque & White	Hydrochlorothiazide 25 mg, Triamterene 37.5 mg	Dyazide by Duramed	51285-0488	Diuretic; Antihypertensive
DPI625	Tab, Light Orange, Diamond Shaped	Estropipate 0.75 mg	by Duramed	51285-0875	Hormone
DPI644	Cap, Red & White	Acetaminophen 500 mg, Oxycodone HCl 5 mg	Percocet by Duramed	51285-0644	Analgesic; C II
DPI644	Cap, Red & White	Acetaminophen 500 mg, Oxycodone HCl 5 mg	Percocet by McNeil	52021-0644	Analgesic; C II
DPI644	Cap	Acetaminophen 500 mg, Oxycodone HCl 5 mg	Percocet by Schein	00364-2395	Analgesic; C II
DPI644	Cap, Red & White	Acetaminophen 500 mg, Oxycodone HCl 5 mg	Percocet by Ivax	00182-9175	Analgesic; C II
DPI658	Cap, Red & White	Acetaminophen 500 mg, Oxycodone HCl 5 mg	Percocet by Duramed	51285-0658	Analgesic; C II
DPI855	Cap, Clear & White	Guaifenesin 250 mg, Pseudoephedrine HCl 120 mg	Sudafed Sinus by Duramed	51285-0855	Cold Remedy
DPI856	Cap, Blue & Clear	Guaifenesin 300 mg, Pseudoephedrine HCl 60 mg	Sudafed Sinus by Duramed	51285-0856	Cold Remedy
DPI894	Cap, White	Guaifenesin 250 mg, Pseudoephedrine HCl 120 mg	Sudafed Sinus by Pfab	62542-0454	Cold Remedy
DPI895	Cap, Blue	Guaifenesin 300 mg, Pseudoephedrine HCl 60 mg	Sudafed Sinus by Pfab	62542-0406	Cold Remedy
DQ <> X732	Tab, Green, Scored	Pseudoacline 10 mg	Sudaamox by TRC Chem	99598-9999	Anti-Congestion
DRISTANNDESEF	Cap, Yellow	Acetaminophen 500 mg, Pseudoephedrine 30 mg	Sudafed Sinus by Whitehall Robins		Cold Remedy
DRISTANSINUS1	Cap, White, Oval	Ibuprofen 200 mg, Pseudoephedrine 30 mg	Dristan by Whitehall Robins		Cold Remedy
DRIXORAL	Tab, Green, Black Print, Round	Dexbrompheniramine Maleate 6 mg, Pseudoephedrine Sulfate 120 mg	Drixoral by Schering	Canadian	Cold Remedy
DRIXORAL	Tab, Green, Black Print, Round	Dexbrompheniramine Maleate 6 mg, Pseudoephedrine Sulfate 120 mg	Drixoral by Schering	00085-0147	Cold Remedy
DRIXORALND	Tab, Yellow, Round, Drixoral N. D.	Pseudoephedrine Sulfate 120 mg	Drixoral N.D. by Schering	Canadian	Decongestant
DRL100 <> 2	Tab, White, Oval	Nefazodone HCl 100 mg	Serzone by Dr. Reddy's	55111-0139	Antidepressant
DRL100 <> 2	Tab, White, Oval	Nefazodone HCl 100 mg	Serzone by Par	49884-0917	Antidepressant
DRL150 <> 3	Tab, White, Oval	Nefazodone HCl 150 mg	Serzone by Par	49884-0918	Antidepressant
DRL150 <> 3	Tab, White, Oval	Nefazodone HCl 150 mg	Serzone by Dr. Reddy's	55111-0140	Antidepressant
DRL200 <> 4	Tab, White, Oval	Nefazodone HCl 200 mg	Serzone by Dr. Reddy's	55111-0141	Antidepressant
DRL200 <> 4	Tab, White, Oval	Nefazodone HCl 200 mg	Serzone by Par	49884-0919	Antidepressant
DRL250 <> 5	Tab, White, Oval	Nefazodone HCl 250 mg	Serzone by Par	49884-0920	Antidepressant
DRL250 <> 5	Tab, White, Oval	Nefazodone HCl 250 mg	Serzone by Dr. Reddy's	55111-0142	Antidepressant

ID FRONT <> BACK	DESCRIPTION FRONT <> BACK	INGREDIENT & STRENGTH	BRAND (or Generic Equiv.) by FIRM	NDC#	CLASS; SCH.
DRL50 <> 1	Tab, White, Oval	Nefazodone HCl 50 mg	Serzone by Dr. Reddy's	55111-0138	Antidepressant
DRL50 <> 1	Tab, White, Oval	Nefazodone HCl 50 mg	Serzone by Par	49884-0916	Antidepressant
DROXIA6335	Cap, Blue-Green, Black Print, Opaque, Hard Gel, Droxia over 6335	Hydroxyurea 200 mg	Droxia by BMS	00003-6335	Antineoplastic
DROXIA6336	Cap, Purple, Black Print, Opaque, Hard Gel, Droxia over 6336	Hydroxyurea 300 mg	Droxia by BMS	00003-6336	Antineoplastic
DROXIA6337	Cap, Reddish-Orange, Black Print, Opaque, Hard Gel, Droxia over 6337	Hydroxyurea 400 mg	Droxia by BMS	00003-6337	Antineoplastic
DS	Tab, Light Pink, Round, Film Coated, DS inside hexagon	Drospirenone 3.0 mg, Ethinyl Estradiol 0.02 mg	Yaz by Berlex	50419-0405	Oral Contraceptive
DT	Tab, White, Round	Tolterodine 2 mg	Detrol by Physician Total Care	54868-2824	Urinary Tract
DT	Tab, White, Round	Tolterodine 2 mg	Detrol by Pharmacia	10829-4544	Urinary Tract
DT	Tab, White, Round	Tolterodine 2 mg	Detrol by Pharmacia	00009-4544	Urinary Tract
DT	Tab, White, Round	Tolterodine 2 mg	Detrol by Pharmacia	Canadian DIN 02239065	Urinary Tract
DT	Tab, White, Round, Film-Coated, "DT" inside a hexagon	Inert	Natazia by Berlex	50419-0409	Oral Contraceptive; Placebo
DT30G	Tab, Green, Round, DT 30/G	Diltiazem HCl 30 mg	Cardizem by Genpharm	Canadian	Antihypertensive
DT60	Tab, Yellow, Round	Diltiazem HCl 60 mg	Cardizem by Genpharm	Canadian	Antihypertensive
DUNHALL0805	Cap, Red	Doxycycline Hyclate 100 mg	Doxy-D by Dunhall		Antibiotic
DUNHALL2811	Cap, Orange & White	Acetaminophen 325 mg, Butalbital 50 mg	Promacet by Dunhall		Analgesic
DUNHALL2829	Cap, Red & Yellow	Carbetapentane Tannate 20 mg, Phenylephrine Tannate 10 mg, Phenylpropanolamine HCl 10 mg, Potassium Guaiacolsulfonate 45 mg	Cophene-X by Dunhall		Cold Remedy
DUOTAB <> SYMAX	Tab, Purple and White, Cap-Shaped, Bilayered	Hyoscyamine Sulfate 0.125 mg IR, Hyoscyamine Sulfate 0.250 mg ER	Symax DuoTab by Capellon	64543-0118	Gastrointestinal
DUPHAR313	Tab, White, Oval	Fluvoxamine Maleate 100 mg	Luvox by Solvay	Canadian	OCD
DUPONT <> 11	Tab, Pale Yellow, Cap Shaped, Scored, Film Coated	Naltrexone HCl 50 mg	Revia by Dupont	Canadian	Opioid Antagonist
DUPONT <> HYCODAN	Tab, White, Round, Scored	Hydrocodone Bitartrate 5 mg, Homatropine Methylbromide 1.5 mg	by DRX	55045-2728	Cold Remedy; C III
DUPONT <> MOBAN10	Tab, Lavender, Round, Moban over 10	Molindone HCl 10 mg	Moban by BMS	00056-0073	Antipsychotic
DUPONT <> NTR	Tab, White w/ Orange Specks, Round, Scored	Naltrexone HCl 50 mg	Revia by Dupont	Canadian	Opioid Antagonist
DUPONT <> NTR	Tab, White w/ Orange Specks, Round, Scored	Naltrexone HCl 50 mg	by BMS	00056-0079	Opioid Antagonist
DUPONT <> PERCOCET	Tab	Acetaminophen 325 mg, Oxycodone HCl 5 mg	Percocet by BMS	00590-0127	Analgesic; C II
DUPONT <> PERCODANDEMI	Tab, Dupont <> Percodan-Demi	Aspirin 325 mg, Oxycodone HCl 2.25 mg	Percodan by BMS	00590-0166	Analgesic; C II
DUPONT <> TREXAN	Tab, White w/ Brown Specks, Round, Scored	Naltrexone HCl 50 mg	Trexan by BMS	00056-0080	Opioid Antagonist
DUPONTHYCODAN	Tab	Homatropine Methylbromide 1.5 mg, Hydrocodone Bitartrate 5 mg	Hycodan by BMS	00056-0042	Cold Remedy; C III
DUPONTHYCOMINE	Tab, Coral, Dupont/Hycomine	Acetaminophen 250 mg, Caffeine 30 mg, Chlorpheniramine Maleate 2 mg, Hydrocodone Bitartrate 5 mg, Phenylephrine HCl 10 mg	Hycomine Compound by BMS	00056-0048	Cold Remedy; C III
DUPONTZYDONE	Cap, White, Red Band, Red Print	Acetaminophen 500 mg, Hydrocodone Bitartrate 5 mg	Vicodin by BMS	00056-0091	Analgesic; C III
DURA <> 009	Tab, Blue, Oblong, Scored	Guaifenesin 600 mg	Robitussin by Med Pro	53978-3363	Expectorant
DURA <> 009	Tab, Light Blue, DU-RA	Guaifenesin 600 mg	Robitussin by Anabolic	00722-6139	Expectorant
DURA <> 15	Tab, White, Oblong, Scored	Guaifenesin 600 mg, Pseudoephedrine 120 mg	Guai Vent PSE by Anabolic	00722-6310	Cold Remedy
DURA <> 15	Tab, White, Scored	Guaifenesin 600 mg, Pseudoephedrine HCl 120 mg	by DJ Pharma	64455-0015	Cold Remedy
DURA <> 7575	Tab, Dura <> 7.5/7.5	Guaifenesin 600 mg, Phenylpropanolamine HCl 75 mg	Entex LA by CVS	51316-0242	Cold Remedy
DURA <> 7575	Tab, White, Oblong, Scored, Dura <> 7.5/7.5	Guaifenesin 600 mg, Phenylpropanolamine HCl 75 mg	Entex LA by Med Pro	53978-3334	Cold Remedy
DURA <> 7575	Tab, Dura <> 7.5/7.5	Guaifenesin 600 mg, Phenylpropanolamine HCl 75 mg	Entex LA by Anabolic	00722-6051	Cold Remedy
DURA <> 7575	Tab, Dura <> 7.5/7.5	Guaifenesin 600 mg, Phenylpropanolamine HCl 75 mg	Entex LA by DHHS Prog	11819-0049	Cold Remedy
DURA <> CHEW	Tab, Orange, Scored	Methscopolamine Nitrate 1.25 mg, Phenylephrine HCl 10 mg, Dextromethorphan Hydrobromide 25 mg	DA Chewable by Neuman	64579-0015	Cold Remedy
DURA <> CHEW	Tab, Chewable	Chlorpheniramine Maleate 2 mg, Methscopolamine Nitrate 1.25 mg, Phenylephrine HCl 10 mg	D A Chewable by Anabolic	00722-6219	Cold Remedy

ID FRONT <> BACK	DESCRIPTION FRONT <> BACK	INGREDIENT & STRENGTH	BRAND (or Generic Equiv.) by FIRM	NDC#	CLASS; SCH.
DURA <> DA	Tab, DU/RA <> D/A	Chlorpheniramine Maleate 8 mg, Methscopolamine Nitrate 2.5 mg, Phenylephrine HCl 20 mg	Dura Vent by Anabolic	00722-6072	Cold Remedy
DURA <> DA	Tab, Brown, Oblong, Scored	Methscopolamine Nitrate 2.5 mg, Phenylephrine HCl 20 mg, Chlorpheniramine Maleate 8 mg	Dura Vent DA by Neuman	64579-0016	Cold Remedy
DURA <> DAII	Tab, White, Oblong	Chlorpheniramine Maleate 4 mg, Methscopolamine Nitrate 1.25 mg, Phenylephrine HCl 10 mg	DA II by Neuman	64579-0014	Cold Remedy
DURA <> DAII	Tab	Chlorpheniramine Maleate 4 mg, Methscopolamine Nitrate 1.25 mg, Phenylephrine HCl 10 mg	DA II by Anabolic	00722-6354	Cold Remedy
DURA <> FDM014	Tab, DU/RA <> FDM 014	Dextromethorphan HBr 30 mg, Guaifenesin 600 mg	Fenesin DM by Anabolic	00722-6275	Cold Remedy
DURA <> FDM014	Tab, Film Coated	Dextromethorphan HBr 30 mg, Guaifenesin 600 mg	by PDRX	55289-0625	Cold Remedy
DURA015	Tab, White, Oblong	Guaifenesin 600 mg, Pseudoephedrine HCl 120 mg	Guai-Vent/PSE by Dura		Cold Remedy
DURA017	Tab, Pink, Oval	Brompheniramine Maleate 4 mg, Pseudoephedrine HCl 60 mg	Rondec Chewable by Dura		Cold Remedy
DURADAJR	Tab, Orange	Chlorpheniramine Maleate 2 mg, Methscopolamine 1.25 mg, Phenylephrine 10 mg	Duravent by Dura		Cold Remedy
DURADAJR	Tab, Orange	Chlorpheniramine Maleate 2 mg, Methscopolamine 1.25 mg, Phenylephrine 10 mg	Duravent DA Chew by Dura		Cold Remedy
DUVOID10 <> WPC004	Tab, White, Round	Bethanechol Chloride 10 mg	Urecholine by Abrika	67767-0144	Urinary Tract
DUVOID25 <> WPC005	Tab, White, Round	Bethanechol Chloride 25 mg	Urecholine by Abrika	67767-0145	Urinary Tract
DUVOID50 <> WPC006	Tab, Tan, Round	Bethanechol Chloride 50 mg	Urecholine by Abrika	67767-0146	Urinary Tract
DV <> D	Tab, Yellow, Oval, Film-Coated	Clarithromycin 500 mg	Biaxin by Dava	68774-0122	Antibiotic
DV <> NVR	Tab, Pale Red, Round	Valsartan 80 mg	Diovan by Novartis	Canadian DIN 02244781	Antihypertensive
DV <> NVR	Tab, Pale Red, Almond Shaped	Valsartan 80 mg	Diovan by Novartis	00078-0358	Antihypertensive
DV350	Tab, White, Round, Scored	Codeine Sulfate 30 mg	Codeine Sulfate by Dava	67253-0350	Analgesic
DV351	Tab, White, Round, Scored	Codeine Sulfate 60 mg	Codeine Sulfate by Dava	67253-0351	Analgesic
DX <> 31	Tab, Yellow, Oblong	Isosorbide Mononitrate 60 mg	Imdur by Ivax	00182-2687	Antianginal
DX <> NVR	Tab, Greyish Orange, Oblong	Valsartan 160 mg	Diovan by Novartis	Canadian DIN 02244782	Antihypertensive
DX <> NVR	Tab, Greyish Orange, Almond Shaped	Valsartan 160 mg	Diovan by Novartis	00078-0359	Antihypertensive
DX1 <> G	Tab, White, Round	Doxazosin Mesylate 1 mg	Cardura by Par	49884-0552	Antihypertensive
DX2 <> G	Tab, White, Cap Shaped Scored, DX over 2	Doxazosin Mesylate 2 mg	Cardura by Par	49884-0553	Antihypertensive
DX4 <> G	Tab, White, Cap Shaped Scored, DX over 4	Doxazosin Mesylate 4 mg	Cardura by Par	49884-0554	Antihypertensive
DX41	Tab, Pink, Round, Extended Release	Diclofenac Sodium 100 mg	Voltaren XR by Watson	00591-0676	NSAID
DX8 <> G	Tab, White, Cap Shaped Scored, DX over 8	Doxazosin Mesylate 8 mg	Cardura by Par	49884-0555	Antihypertensive
DXL <> NVR	Tab, Dark Greyish Violet, Almond Shaped	Valsartan 320 mg	Diovan by Novartis	00078-0360	Antihypertensive
DYAZIDESB	Cap, Red & White, Black Print, Opaque, Dyazide over SB	Hydrochlorothiazide 25 mg, Triamterene 37.5 mg	Dyazide by Teva	00480-0733	Diuretic; Antihypertensive
DYAZIDESB	Cap, Red & White, Black Print, Opaque, Dyazide over SB	Hydrochlorothiazide 25 mg, Triamterene 37.5 mg	by Amerisource	62584-0365	Diuretic; Antihypertensive
DYAZIDESB	Cap, Red & White, Black Print, Opaque, Dyazide over SB	Hydrochlorothiazide 25 mg, Triamterene 37.5 mg	Dyazide by Wal Mart	49035-0170	Diuretic; Antihypertensive
DYAZIDESB	Cap, Red & White, Black Print, Opaque, Dyazide over SB	Hydrochlorothiazide 25 mg, Triamterene 37.5 mg	by Physician Total Care	54868-3366	Diuretic; Antihypertensive
DYAZIDESB	Cap, Red & White, Black Print, Opaque, Dyazide over SB	Hydrochlorothiazide 25 mg, Triamterene 37.5 mg	by Allscripts		Diuretic; Antihypertensive
DYAZIDESB	Cap, Red & White, Black Print, Opaque, Dyazide over SB	Hydrochlorothiazide 25 mg, Triamterene 37.5 mg	by Murfreesboro	51129-1385	Diuretic; Antihypertensive
DYAZIDESB	Cap, Red & White, Black Print, Opaque, Dyazide over SB	Hydrochlorothiazide 25 mg, Triamterene 37.5 mg	by Repack Co of America	55306-3650	Diuretic; Antihypertensive
DYAZIDESB	Cap, Red & White, Black Print, Opaque, Dyazide over SB	Hydrochlorothiazide 25 mg, Triamterene 37.5 mg	Dyazide by Wal Mart	49035-0170	Diuretic; Antihypertensive
DYAZIDESB	Cap, Red & White, Black Print, Opaque, Dyazide over SB	Hydrochlorothiazide 25 mg, Triamterene 37.5 mg	Dyazide by SKB	00007-3650	Diuretic; Antihypertensive
DYFLEXG	Tab, White, Round, Scored, Dyflex/G	Dyphylline 200 mg, Guaifenesin 200 mg	Dyflex G by Emrex Econo	38130-0012	Antiasthmatic; Expectorant
DYN045	Tab, Gray, Coated, DYN-045, Extended Release	Minocycline HCl 45 mg	Solodyn by Medicis	99207-0460	Antibiotic
DYN090	Tab, Yellow, Coated, DYN-090, Extended Release	Minocycline HCl 90 mg	Solodyn by Medicis	99207-0461	Antibiotic
DYN135	Tab, Brownish Orange, Coated, DYN-135, Extended Release	Minocycline HCl 135 mg	Solodyn by Medicis	99207-0462	Antibiotic
DYNABACUC5364	Tab, White, Oval, Enteric Coated	Dirithromycin 250 mg	Dynabac by Eli Lilly	00002-0490	Antibiotic
DYNABACUC5364	Tab, White, Oval, Enteric Coated	Dirithromycin 250 mg	Dynabac by Sanofi	00024-0490	Antibiotic
DYNABACUC5364	Tab, White, Oval, Enteric Coated	Dirithromycin 250 mg	Dynabac by Muro	00451-0490	Antibiotic

ID FRONT <> BACK	DESCRIPTION FRONT <> BACK	INGREDIENT & STRENGTH	BRAND (or Generic Equiv.) by FIRM	NDC#	CLASS; SCH.
DYNACIN100MG498	Cap, Gray & White	Minocycline HCl 100 mg	Minocin by Nat Pharmpak	55154-9101	Antibiotic
DYNACIN100MG498	Cap, Gray & White	Minocycline HCl 100 mg	Dynacin by Wal Mart	49035-0186	Antibiotic
DYNACIN50MG497	Cap, White	Minocycline HCl 50 mg	Dynacin by Nat Pharmpak	55154-9102	Antibiotic
DYNACIN75MG499	Cap, Gray	Minocycline HCl 75 mg	Dynacin by Neuman	64579-0307	Antibiotic
DYNACIN75MG499	Cap, Gray	Minocycline HCl 75 mg	Dynacin by Eckerd	19458-0914	Antibiotic
DYNACIN75MG499	Cap, Gray	Minocycline HCl 75 mg	Dynacin by Rx Pak	65084-0236	Antibiotic
DYNACIRCCR10	Tab, DR, in Red Ink	Isradipine 10 mg	Dynacirc CR by Novartis	00078-0236	Antihypertensive
DYNACIRCCR10	Tab, Beige, Round, Film Coated, "DynaCircCR" in semi-circle with "10" inside circle	Isradipine 10 mg	DynaCirc CR by Reliant	65726-0236	Antihypertensive
DYNACIRCCR5	Tab, Light Pink, Round, Film Coated, "DynaCircCR" in semi-circle with "5" inside circle	Isradipine 5 mg	DynaCirc CR by Reliant	65726-0235	Antihypertensive
DYNACIRCCR5	Tab, DR, in Red Ink	Isradipine 5 mg	Dynacirc CR by Novartis	00078-0235	Antihypertensive
DYNACN0499	Cap, Gray	Minocycline HCl 75 mg	Dynacin by Wal Mart	49035-0195	Antibiotic
DYRENIUM100MGDYRENIUMWPC003	Cap, Red, Opaque	Triamterene 100 mg	Dyrenium by Wellspring	65197-0003	Diuretic
DYRENIUM100SKF	Cap, Red, White Print, Dyrenium over 100 SKF	Triamterene 100 mg	Dyrenium by SKB	00108-3807	Diuretic
DYRENIUM50MGDYRENIUMWPC002	Cap, Red, Opaque	Triamterene 50 mg	Dyrenium by Wellspring	65197-0002	Diuretic
DYRENIUM50SKF	Cap, Red, White Print, Dyrenium over 50 SKF	Triamterene 50 mg	Dyrenium by SKB	00108-3806	Diuretic
E	Tab, White, Round	Selegilline 5 mg	Eldepryl by Draxis	Canadian DIN 02123312 Discontinued	Antiparkinson
E	Tab, Light Yellow, Rounded E logo	3,4-Methylenedioxymethamphetamine (MDMA)	Ecstasy by Illegal		Euphoric; Illicit
E	Cap, White, Round, Opaque, Soft Gel	Benzonatate 100 mg	Tessalon Pearles by Ethex	58177-0091	Antitussive
E <> 01	Tab, White to Off-White, Oval, Film Coated	Carvedilol 3.125 mg	Coreg by Aurobindo	65862-0142	Antihypertensive
E <> 018	Tab, Peach, Oblong, Film Coated, Scripted E	Fexofenadine HCl 180 mg	Allegra by Aventis	00088-1109	Antihistamine
E <> 02	Tab, White to Off-White, Oval, Film Coated	Carvedilol 6.25 mg	Coreg by Aurobindo	65862-0143	Antihypertensive
E <> 03	Tab, White to Off-White, Oval, Film Coated	Carvedilol 12.5 mg	Coreg by Aurobindo	65862-0144	Antihypertensive
E <> 03	Tab, Peach, Round, Film Coated, Scripted E	Fexofenadine HCl 30 mg	Allegra by Aventis	00088-1106	Antihistamine
E <> 04	Tab, White to Off-White, Oval, Film Coated	Carvedilol 25 mg	Coreg by Aurobindo	65862-0145	Antihypertensive
E <> 06	Tab, Peach, Oblong, Film Coated, Scripted E, 06 is underlined	Fexofenadine HCl 60 mg	Allegra 12 hr by Aventis	Canadian DIN 02231462	Antihistamine
E <> 06	Tab, Peach, Oblong, Film Coated, Scripted E	Fexofenadine HCl 60 mg	Allegra by Aventis	00088-1107	Antihistamine
E <> 10	Tab, Red, Octagonal	Acetaminophen 400 mg, Hydrocodone Bitartrate 10 mg	Zydone by Endo	63481-0698	Analgesic; C III
E <> 10	Tab, Red, Octagonal	Acetaminophen 400 mg, Hydrocodone Bitartrate 10 mg	Zydone by West Pharm	52967-0275	Analgesic; C III
E <> 100	Tab, Grey, Oval, Extended Release	Morphine Sulfate 200 mg	MS Contin by Ethex	58177-0340	Analgesic; C II
E <> 1111	Tab, Light Pink, Round, Sustained Release	Bupropion HCl 200 mg	Wellbutrin SR by Eon	00185-1111	Antidepressant
E <> 15	Tab, Green, Oval, Extended Release	Morphine Sulfate 15 mg	MS Contin by Ethex	58177-0310	Analgesic; C II
E <> 15	Tab, Dark Yellow, Round	Benazepril HCl 10 mg	Lotensin by Aurobindo	65862-0116	Antihypertensive
E <> 16	Tab, Pink, Round	Benazepril HCl 20 mg	Lotensin by Aurobindo	65862-0117	Antihypertensive
E <> 17	Tab, Dark Pink, Round	Benazepril HCl 40 mg	Lotensin by Aurobindo	65862-0118	Antihypertensive
E <> 2	Tab, Blue, Round, Film Coated	Hydromorphone HCl 2 mg	Dilaudid by Ethex	58177-0298	Analgesic; C II
E <> 200	Tab, Brown, Oval, Extended Release	Morphine Sulfate 200 mg	MS Contin by Ethex	58177-0380	Analgesic; C II
E <> 22	Tab, White, Round, Film Coated	Topiramate 25 mg	Topiramate by Aurobindo	65862-0171	Anticonvulsant
E <> 23	Tab, Dark Yellow, Round, Film Coated	Topiramate 100 mg	Topiramate by Aurobindo	65862-0173	Anticonvulsant
E <> 24	Tab, Pink, Round, Film Coated	Topiramate 200 mg	Topiramate by Aurobindo	65862-0174	Anticonvulsant
E <> 25	Tab, White, Round, Film Coated, 2.5 <> Elan Logo	Frovatriptan 2.5 mg	Frova by Endo	63481-0025	Antimigraine
E <> 3	Tab, Oval, Pink, Film Coated	Conjugated Estrogens 0.625 mg	Enjuvia by Barr	51285-0408	Hormone
E <> 30	Tab, Pink, Oval, Extended Release	Morphine Sulfate 30 mg	MS Contin by Ethex	58177-0320	Analgesic; C II
E <> 33	Tab, Light Yellow, Round, Film Coated	Topiramate 50 mg	Topiramate by Aurobindo	65862-0172	Anticonvulsant

ID FRONT <> BACK	DESCRIPTION FRONT <> BACK	INGREDIENT & STRENGTH	BRAND (or Generic Equiv.) by FIRM	NDC#	CLASS; SCH.
E <> 35	Tab, Salmon, Round, Scored, E above score <> 35	Trandolapril 1 mg	Mavik by Aurobindo	65862-0164	Antihypertensive
E <> 36	Tab, Yellow, Round	Trandolapril 2 mg	Mavik by Aurobindo	65862-0165	Antihypertensive
E <> 37	Tab, Rose, Round	Trandolapril 4 mg	Mavik by Aurobindo	65862-0166	Antihypertensive
E <> 4	Tab, Yellow, Oval, Film Coated	Conjugated Estrogens 1.25 mg	Enjuvia by Barr	51285-0410	Hormone
E <> 4	Tab, Tan, Film Coated	Hydromorphone HCl 4 mg	Dilaudid by Ethex	58177-0299	Analgesic; C II
E <> 423	Tab, White, Round	Hyoscyamine Sulfate 0.125 mg	NuLev by Ethex	58177-0423	Gastrointestinal
E <> 5	Tab, Yellow, Octagonal	Acetaminophen 400 mg, Hydrocodone Bitartrate 5 mg	Zydone by West Pharm	52967-0273	Analgesic; C III
E <> 5	Tab, Yellow, Octagonal	Acetaminophen 400 mg, Hydrocodone Bitartrate 5 mg	Zydone by Endo	63481-0668	Analgesic; C III
E <> 536	Tab, White, Oval	Amlodipine Besylate 2.5 mg	Norvasc by Ethex	58177-0536	Antihypertensive
E <> 537	Tab, White, Oval	Amlodipine Besylate 5mg	Norvasc by Ethex	58177-0537	Antihypertensive
E <> 538	Tab, White, Oval	Amlodipine Besylate 10 mg	Norvasc by Pfizer	58177-0538	Antihypertensive
E <> 60	Tab, White, Oval, Extended Release	Morphine Sulfate 60 mg	MS Contin by Ethex	58177-0330	Analgesic; C II
E <> 61	Tab, Blue, Round, Film-Coated	Finasteride 5 mg	Proscar by Aurobindo	65862-0149	Antiandrogen
E <> 75	Tab, Blue, Octagonal, E <> 7.5	Acetaminophen 400 mg, Hydrocodone Bitartrate 7.5 mg	Zydone by West Pharm	52967-0274	Analgesic; C III
E <> 75	Tab, Blue, Octagonal, E <> 7.5	Acetaminophen 400 mg, Hydrocodone Bitartrate 7.5 mg	Zydone by Endo	63481-0669	Analgesic; C III
E <> 77	Tab, White, Round, Film Coated, 77 <> Elan Logo	Frovatriptan 2.5 mg	Frova by Endo	63481-0025	Antimigraine
E <> 77	Tab, White, Round, Film Coated, 77 <> Elan Logo	Frovatriptan 2.5 mg	Frova by Elan	59075-0740	Antimigraine
E <> 78	Tab, White to Off-White, Round, Film Coated	Zolpidem Tartrate 5 mg	Ambien by Aurobindo	65862-0159	Sedative/Hypnotic; C IV
E <> 79	Tab, White to Off-White, Oval, Film Coated	Zolpidem Tartrate 10 mg	Ambien by Aurobindo	65862-0160	Sedative/Hypnotic; C IV
E <> 8	Tab, White, Round	Hydromorphone HCl 8 mg	Dilaudid by Ethex	58177-0449	Analgesic; C II
E <> 85	Tab, White to Off White, Cap Shaped, Film Coated, Scored	Penicillin V Potassium 500 mg	by Aurobindo	65862-0176	Antibiotic
E0019	Tab, Blue, Round	Desipramine HCl 25 mg	Norpramin by Eon		Antidepressant
E1 <> 511	Tab, Off-White, Round, Scored	Estradiol 0.5 mg	Estrace by Ayerst	00046-5879	Hormone
E1 <> 511	Tab, Off-White, Round, Scored	Estradiol 0.5 mg	Estrace by ESI Lederle	59911-5879	Hormone
E10	Tab, White, Round, Scored, Film Coated, E over 10	Labetalol HCl 100 mg	Normodyne by Eon	00185-0010	Antihypertensive
E10	Tab, White, Round, Scored, Film Coated, E over 10	Labetalol HCl 100 mg	Trandate by UDL	51079-0928	Antihypertensive
E10	Tab, Blue, Oval, Film Coated	Levetiracetam 250 mg	Keppra by Aurobindo	65862-0245	Anticonvulsant
E101	Tab, Pink, Oval	Lisinopril 10 mg	Zestril by Eon	00185-0101	Antihypertensive
E102	Tab, Peach, Oval	Lisinopril 20 mg	Zestril by Eon	00185-0102	Antihypertensive
E103	Tab, Red, Oval	Lisinopril 30 mg	Zestril by Eon	00185-0103	Antihypertensive
E104	Tab, Yellow, Oval	Lisinopril 40 mg	Zestril by Eon	00185-0104	Antihypertensive
E11	Tab, Yellow, Oval, Film Coated	Levetiracetam 500 mg	Keppra by Aurobindo	65862-0246	Anticonvulsant
E111	Tab, Dark Blue, Round, E over 111	Mixed Amphetamine Salts 10 mg; Amphetamine Aspartate 2.5 mg, Amphetamine Sulfate 2.5 mg, Dextroamphetamine Saccharate 2.5 mg, Dextroamphetamine Sulfate 2.5 mg	Adderall by Eon	00185-0111	Stimulant; C II
E112	Tab, White, Oval, Scored	Sulfamethoxazole 800 mg, Trimethoprim 160 mg	Bactrim DS by Eon	00185-0112	Antibiotic
E1125	Cap, Brown & White, Black Print, Opaque	Flutamide 125 mg	Eulexin by Eon	00185-1125	Antiandrogen
E114	Tab, Yellow, Round, E over 114	Enalapril Maleate 2.5 mg	Vasotec by Eon	00185-0114	Antihypertensive
E115	Tab, White, Oval	Ticlopidine HCl 250 mg	Ticlid by Eon	00185-0115	Anticoagulant
E117	Tab, White, Round, Scored, Film Coated	Labetalol HCl 200 mg	Trandate by UDL	51079-0929	Antihypertensive
E117	Tab, White, Round, E over 117	Labetalol HCl 200 mg	Normodyne by Eon	00185-0117	Antihypertensive
E118	Tab, White, Round, E over 118	Labetalol HCl 300 mg	Normodyne by Eon	00185-0118	Antihypertensive
E12	Tab, Orange, Oval, Film Coated	Levetiracetam 750 mg	Keppra by Aurobindo	65862-0247	Anticonvulsant
E120	Tab, White, Oval, Film Coated, Ex Release	Isosorbide Mononitrate 120 mg	Imdur by Ethex	58177-0201	Antianginal
E120MG508	Cap, Blue-Violet & White, Ligand Logo on cap, 120MG508 on body, Extended Release	Morphine Sulfate 120 mg	Avinza by Ligand	64365-0508	Analgesic; C II
E121	Tab, White, Round, Scored	Captopril 12.5 mg	Capoten by Par	49884-0619	Antihypertensive
E121	Tab, White, Round, Scored, E over 121	Captopril 12.5 mg	Capoten by Caremark	00339-5948	Antihypertensive
E121	Tab, White, Round, Scored, E over 121	Captopril 12.5 mg	Capoten by Caremark	00339-5918	Antihypertensive
E1217	Cap, Green & Yellow, White Print, Ex Release	Nitroglycerin 9 mg	Nitrobid by Eon	00185-1217	Vasodilator

ID FRONT <> BACK	DESCRIPTION FRONT <> BACK	INGREDIENT & STRENGTH	BRAND (or Generic Equiv.) by FIRM	NDC#	CLASS; SCH.
E122	Tab, White, Round, Scored	Captopril 25 mg	Capoten by Par	49884-0620	Antihypertensive
E122	Cap, Black and Ivory, Opaque	Nitrofurantoin 100 mg	Macrobid by Eon	00185-0122	Antibiotic
E122	Tab, White, Round, Scored	Captopril 25 mg	Capoten by Caremark	00339-6112	Antihypertensive
E122	Tab, White, Round, Scored, E over 123	Captopril 25 mg	Capoten by Caremark	00339-5920	Antihypertensive
E123	Tab, White, Round, Scored	Captopril 50 mg	Capoten by Caremark	00339-5944	Antihypertensive
E123	Tab, White, Round, Scored	Captopril 50 mg	Capoten by Par	49884-0621	Antihypertensive
E1235	Cap, Blue & Yellow, Red Print, Ex Release	Nitroglycerin 6.5 mg	Nitrobid by Eon	00185-1235	Vasodilator
E124	Tab, White, Round, Scored	Captopril 100 mg	Capoten by Par	49884-0622	Antihypertensive
E124	Tab, Off-White, Oblong, Eon Logo	Benazepril HCl 5 mg, HCTZ 6.25 mg	Lotensin HCT by Eon	00185-0124	Antihypertensive; Diuretic
E124	Tab, White, Round, Scored	Captopril 100 mg	Capoten by Caremark	00339-5946	Antihypertensive
E124	Tab, White, Round, Scored	Captopril 100 mg	Capoten by Caremark	00339-6127	Antihypertensive
E126	Tab, Light Yellow, Cap Shaped, Eon Logo	Nefazodone HCl 200 mg	Serzone by Eon	00185-0126	Antidepressant
E127	Tab, White, Round, E over 127	Enalapril Maleate 5 mg	Vasotec by Eon	00185-0127	Antihypertensive
E128	Tab, Green, Round, Scored, E over 128	Bumetanide 0.5 mg	Bumex by UDL	51079-0891	Diuretic
E128	Tab, Green, Round, Scored, E over 128	Bumetanide 0.5 mg	Bumex by Eon	00185-0128	Diuretic
E128	Tab, Green, Round, Scored, E over 128	Bumetanide 0.5 mg	Bumex by Mylan	00378-0245	Diuretic
E129	Tab, Yellow, Round, Scored, E over 129	Bumetanide 1 mg	Bumex by Mylan	00378-0370	Diuretic
E129	Tab, Yellow, Round, Scored, E over 129	Bumetanide 1 mg	Bumex by UDL	51079-0892	Diuretic
E129	Tab, Yellow, Round, Scored, E over 129	Bumetanide 1 mg	Bumex by Eon	00185-0129	Diuretic
E12SKF	Cap	Dextroamphetamine Sulfate 5 mg	Dexedrine by Physician Total Care	54868-3402	Stimulant; C II
E13	Tab, Green	Ferrous Sulfate 325 mg	by Eon	00185-0013	Mineral
E13	Tab, White to Off White, Oval, Film Coated	Levetiracetam 1000 mg	Keppra by Aurobindo	65662-0315	Anticonvulsant
E130	Tab, Beige to Light Brown, Round, Scored, E over 130	Bumetanide 2 mg	Bumex by UDL	51079-0893	Diuretic
E130	Tab, Beige to Light Brown, Round, Scored, E over 130	Bumetanide 2 mg	Bumex by Eon	00185-0130	Diuretic
E130	Tab, Beige to Light Brown, Round, Scored, E over 130	Bumetanide 2 mg	Bumex by Mylan	00378-0417	Diuretic
E1303	Cap, Clear	Quinine Sulfate 325 mg	by Eon		Antimalarial
E1303	Cap, Clear	Quinine Sulfate 325 mg	by Eon		Antimalarial
E1304	Cap, Dark Blue & Clear, Black Print, Ex Release	Chlorpheniramine Maleate 8 mg, Pseudoephedrine HCl 120 mg	Novafed by Eon	00185-1304	Cold Remedy
E131	Tab, White, Round	Methadone HCl 10 mg	Dolophine by Eon	00185-0131	Analgesic; C II
E131	Tab, White, Round, Eon Logo over 131	Methadone HCl 10 mg	Dolophine by Nat Pharmpak	55154-6905	Analgesic; C II
E132	Tab, White, Quadrisected	Methadone HCl 40 mg	Dolophine by Eon	00185-0132	Analgesic; C II
E132	Tab, White, Scored, E over 132	Methadone HCl 40 mg	Dolophine by Nat Pharmpak	55154-5826	Analgesic; C II
E134	Tab, White, Round, Scored, E over 134	Reserpine 0.25 mg	Serpasil by Eon	00185-0134	Antihypertensive
E139	Tab, White, Oval	Etodolac 500 mg	Lodine by Eon	00185-0139	NSAID
E14	Tab, Yellow	Chlorpheniramine Maleate 4 mg	by Eon	00185-1064	Antihistamine
E140	Tab, White, Oval, Film Coated	Etodolac 400 mg	Lodine by Eon	00185-0140	NSAID
E141	Tab, White, Cap Shaped	Oxaprozin 600 mg	Daypro by Eon	00185-0141	NSAID
E144	Tab, Yellow, Round, Scored, E over 144	Amiodarone 200 mg	Cordarone by Eon	00185-0144	Antiarrhythmic
E145	Tab, White, Oval	Nabumetone 500 mg	Relafen by Eon	00185-0145	NSAID
E146	Tab, White, Oval, Slanted E 146	Nabumetone 750 mg	Relafen by Eon	00185-0146	NSAID
E147	Tab, Salmon, Round, E over 147	Enalapril Maleate 10 mg	Vasotec by Eon	00185-0147	Antihypertensive
E149	Tab, Blue-Gray, Round, Eon Logo	Midodrine HCl 10 mg	ProAmatine by Eon	00185-0149	Antihypotensive
E150	Cap, White & Yellow, Black Print	Nizatidine 150 mg	Axid by Eon	00185-0150	Gastrointestinal
E151	Tab, Green, Round	Enalapril Maleate 5 mg, Hydrochlorothiazide 12.5 mg	Vaseretic by Eon	00185-0151	Antihypertensive; Diuretic
E152	Tab, White, Round, E over 152	Lisinopril 20 mg, HCTZ 12.5 mg	Prinzide by Eon	00185-0152	Antihypertensive; Diuretic
E153	Tab, Light Blue, Oval, Film Coated	Sertraline HCl 50 mg	Zoloft by Sandoz	00185-0153	Antidepressant
E155	Cap, White, Opaque	Anagrelide HCl 0.5 mg	Agrylin by Eon	00185-0155	Antiplatelet
E156	Cap, Gray, Opaque	Anagrelide HCl 1.0 mg	Agrylin by Eon	00185-0156	Antiplatelet
E157	Tab, Beige, Round, E over 157	Fluvoxamine Maleate 100 mg	Luvox by Eon	00185-0157	OCD
E16	Tab, White, Cap Shaped, Scored, Eon Logo	Nefazodone HCl 100 mg	Serzone by Eon	00185-0016	Antidepressant

ID FRONT <> BACK	DESCRIPTION FRONT <> BACK	INGREDIENT & STRENGTH	BRAND (or Generic Equiv.) by FIRM	NDC#	CLASS; SCH.
E17	Tab, White, Round, E over 17	Fluvoxamine Maleate 25 mg	Luvox by Eon	00185-0017	OCD
E170	Tab, Blue, Cap Shaped	Sotalol 120 mg	Betapace by Eon	00185-0170	Antiarrhythmic
E171	Tab, Blue, Cap Shaped	Sotalol 80 mg	Betapace by Eon	00185-0171	Antiarrhythmic
E172	Tab, Salmon, Round	Enalapril Maleate 10 mg, Hydrochlorothiazide 25 mg	Vaseretic by Eon	00185-0172	Antihypertensive; Diuretic
E173	Tab, Light Pink, Round, E over 173	Lisinopril 20 mg, HCTZ 25 mg	Prinzide by Eon	00185-0173	Antihypertensive; Diuretic
E174	Tab, Blue, Cap Shaped	Sotalol 240 mg	Betapace by Eon	00185-0174	Antiarrhythmic
E175	Tab, Orange, Round	Bupropion HCl 75 mg	Wellbutrin by Eon	00185-0175	Antidepressant
E176	Tab, Red, Round	Bupropion HCl 100 mg	Wellbutrin by Eon	00185-0176	Antidepressant
E177	Tab, Blue, Cap Shaped	Sotalol 160 mg	Betapace by Eon	00185-0177	Antiarrhythmic
E19	Tab, Light Blue, Round, E over 19	Desipramine HCl 25 mg	Norpramin by Eon	00185-0019	Antidepressant
E19	Cap, Green and Pale Green, Opaque	Zaleplon 5 mg	Sonata by Aurobindo	65862-0214	Sedative/Hypnotic; C IV
E19 <> SKF	Tab, Orange, Triangular	Dextroamphetamine Sulfate 5 mg	Dexedrine by Abbott	00074-3241	Stimulant; C II
E193	Cap, Reddish Orange and Light Grey, Opaque	Zonisamide 25 mg	Zonegran by Sandoz	00185-0193	Anticonvulsant
E195	Tab, White, Round, E over 195, Ex Release	Alprazolam 0.5 mg	Xanax XR by Sandoz	00185-0195	Antianxiety; C IV
E196	Tab, Yellow, Oblong, Ex Release	Alprazolam 1 mg	Xanax XR by Sandoz	00185-0196	Antianxiety; C IV
E197	Tab, Blue, Oblong, Ex Release	Alprazolam 2 mg	Xanax XR by Sandoz	00185-0197	Antianxiety; C IV
E198	Tab, Green, Round, E over 198, Ex Release	Alprazolam 3 mg	Xanax XR by Sandoz	00185-0198	Antianxiety; C IV
E199	Cap, Light Grey	Zonisamide 50 mg	Zonegran by Sandoz	00185-0199	Anticonvulsant
E2	Cap, White, Oval, Opaque, Soft Gel	Benzonatate 200 mg	Tessalon Pearles by Ethex	58177-0092	Antitussive
E20	Tab, Yellow, Round, E over 20	Mirtazapine 15 mg	Remeron by Eon	00185-0020	Antidepressant
E20	Cap, Green and Light Green, Opaque	Zaleplon 10 mg	Sonata by Aurobindo	65862-0215	Sedative/Hypnotic; C IV
E200	Cap, Reddish Orange, Opaque	Zonisamide 100 mg	Zonegran by Sandoz	00185-0200	Anticonvulsant
E204	Tab, Pink, Oblong, Eon Logo	Benazepril HCl 10 mg, HCTZ 12.5 mg	Lotensin HCT by Eon	00185-0204	Antihypertensive; Diuretic
E205	Tab, White, Round, E over 205	Methimazole 5 mg	Tapazole by Eon	00185-0205	Antithyroid
E21	Tab, White, Round, Eon Logo over 21	Methadone HCl 5 mg	Dolophine by Nat Pharmpak	55154-6904	Analgesic; C II
E21	Tab, White, Round	Methadone HCl 5 mg	Dolophine by Eon	00185-0021	Analgesic; C II
E210	Tab, White, Round, E over 210	Methimazole 10 mg	Tapazole by Eon	00185-0210	Antithyroid
E211	Tab, Lavender, Oblong, Eon Logo	Benazepril HCl 20 mg, HCTZ 12.5 mg	Lotensin HCT by Eon	00185-0211	Antihypertensive; Diuretic
E212	Tab, Reddish Brown, Round	Mirtazapine 30 mg	Remeron by Eon	00185-0212	Antidepressant
E213	Tab, White to Off-White, Round, E over 213	Metformin HCl 500 mg	Glucophage by Eon	00185-0213	Antidiabetic
E214	Tab, Peach, Round, E over 214	Enalapril Maleate 20 mg	Vasotec by Eon	00185-0214	Antihypertensive
E215	Tab, White to Off-White, Round, E over 215	Metformin HCl 850 mg	Glucophage by Eon	00185-0215	Antidiabetic
E216	Tab, Yellow, Oblong	Doxycycline Monohydrate 100 mg	Adoxa by Sandoz	00185-0216	Antibiotic
E217	Tab, Light Yellow, Oval	Amiodarone 400 mg	Cordarone by Eon	00185-0217	Antiarrhythmic
E22	Tab, White, Round, Ex Release, E over 22	Orphenadrine Citrate 100 mg	Norflex by Eon	00185-0022	Muscle Relaxant
E220	Tab, Sugar Coated, Stylized E	Atropine Sulfate 0.03 mg, Benzoic Acid 4.5 mg, Hyoscyamine 0.03 mg, Methenamine 40.8 mg, Methylene Blue 5.4 mg, Phenyl Salicylate 18.1 mg	by PDRX	55289-0518	Antiseptic
E221	Tab, White to Off-White, Oval, Scored	Metformin HCl 1000 mg	Glucophage by Eon	00185-0221	Antidiabetic
E222	Tab, White, Round, Eon Logo over 222	Mirtazapine 45 mg	Remeron by Eon	00185-0222	Antidepressant
E223	Tab, White, Round, Eon Logo over 223	Cilostazol 100 mg	Pletal by Eon	00185-0223	Antiplatelet
E230	Tab, Blue, Round	Urinary Antiseptic #2	Hexalol by Eon	00185-0230	Urinary Tract
E24	Tab, White, Round, E over 24	Atropine Sulfate 0.025 mg, Diphenoxylate HCl 2.5 mg	Lomotil by Eon	00185-0024	Antidiarrheal; C V
E241	Tab, Pink, Round, Enteric Coated	Rabeprazole Sodium 10 mg	Pariet by Janssen-Ortho	Canadian DIN 02243796	Gastrointestinal
E243	Tab, Light Yellow, Round, Enteric Coated	Rabeprazole Sodium 20 mg	Pariet by Janssen-Ortho	Canadian DIN 02243797	Gastrointestinal
E243	Tab, Yellow, Round	Rabeprazole Sodium 20 mg	Aciphex by RX Pak	65084-0145	Gastrointestinal
E243	Tab, Yellow, Round	Rabeprazole Sodium 20 mg	Aciphex by RX Pak	65084-0147	Gastrointestinal
E25	Tab, White, Oval	Lisinopril 2.5 mg	Zestril by Eon	00185-0025	Antihypertensive
E26	Cap, Red, E-26	Docusate Calcium 240 mg	Surfak by Chase		Laxative

ID FRONT <> BACK	DESCRIPTION FRONT <> BACK	INGREDIENT & STRENGTH	BRAND (or Generic Equiv.) by FIRM	NDC#	CLASS; SCH.
E262	Tab, Pink, Oblong, Film Coated, Eisai Logo 262	Rufinamide 200 mg	Banzel by Eisai	62856-0582	Antiepileptic
E263	Tab, Pink, Oblong, Film Coated	Rufinamide 400 mg	Banzel by Eisai	62856-0583	Antiepileptic
E265	Tab, Light Yellow, Oval, Film Coated	Sertraline HCl 100 mg	Zoloft by Sandoz	00185-0265	Antidepressant
E27	Tab, Yellow, Round, E over 27	Fluvoxamine Maleate 50 mg	Luvox by Eon	00185-0027	OCD
E271	Tab, White, Oval	Oxandrolone 2.5 mg	Oxandrin by Sandoz	00185-0271	Steroid; C III
E272	Tab, White, Oblong	Oxandrolone 10 mg	Oxandrin by Sandoz	00185-0272	Steroid; C III
E277	Tab, Maroon, Oblong, Eon Logo	Benazepril HCl 20 mg, HCTZ 25 mg	Lotensin HCT by Eon	00185-0277	Antihypertensive; Diuretic
E281	Tab, White, Oval, Scored, E over 281, Ex Release	Metoprolol 25 mg	Toprol XL by Sandoz	00185-0281	Antihypertensive
E282	Tab, White, Football-Shaped, Scored, Extended Release	Metoprolol Succinate 50 mg	Toprol XL by Eon	00185-0282	Antihypertensive
E29	Cap, Orange & Red, E-29	Docusate Sodium 250 mg	Colace by Chase		Laxative
E29	Tab, White, Round, E over 29	Desipramine HCl 10 mg	Norpramin by Eon	00185-0029	Antidepressant
E2NOM <> 190JC	Tab, White, Round, E2/N O-M <> 1/90 J-C	Estradiol 1 mg, Norgestimate 0.09 mg	Ortho-Prefest by Ortho-McNeil	00062-1840	Hormone
E2OM <> 1JC	Tab, Pink, Round, E2 O-M <> 1 J-C	Estradiol 1 mg	Ortho-Prefest by Ortho-McNeil	00062-1840	Hormone
E3 <> M	Tab, White, Round, Flat, Scored, Uncoated	Estradiol 0.5 mg	Estrace by Mylan	00378-1452	Hormone
E3 <> M	Tab, White, Round, Flat, Scored, Uncoated	Estradiol 0.5 mg	Estrace by Heartland	61392-0122	Hormone
E30	Tab, Reddish Pink, Oval, Film Coated, Ex Release	Isosorbide Mononitrate 30 mg	Imdur by Ethex	58177-0222	Antianginal
E300	Cap, White & Peach, Black Print	Nizatidine 300 mg	Axid by Eon	00185-0300	Gastrointestinal
E30MG505	Cap, Yellow & White, Ligand Logo on cap, 30MG505 on body, Extended Release	Morphine Sulfate 30 mg	Avinza by Ligand	64365-0505	Analgesic; C II
E31	Tab, White, Round	Captopril 12.5 mg	Capoten by Eon	00185-0031	Antihypertensive
E311	Tab, White, Round, E over 311	Tramadol HCl 50 mg	Ultram by Eon	00185-0311	Analgesic
E32	Tab, White, Round, Scored, E over 32	Reserpine 0.1 mg	Serpasil by Eon	00185-0032	Antihypertensive
E34	Tab, White, Round, E over 34	Tizanidine HCl 2 mg	Zanaflex by Eon	00185-0034	Muscle Relaxant
E341	Tab, Light Pink, Round	Fosinopril Sodium 10 mg, HCTZ 12.5 mg	Monopril HCT by Sandoz	00185-0341	Antihypertensive; Diuretic
E342	Tab, Dark Pink, Round	Fosinopril Sodium 20 mg, HCTZ 12.5 mg	Monopril HCT by Sandoz	00185-0342	Antihypertensive; Diuretic
E345	Cap, Clear & White	Caramiphen Edisylate 40 mg, Phenylpropanolamine HCl 75 mg	Ordrine AT by Eon	00185-0345	Cold Remedy
E36	Tab, Yellow, Oblong	Doxycycline Monohydrate 50 mg	Adoxa by Sandoz	00185-0036	Antibiotic
E371	Tab, Orange, Cap Shaped, Eon Logo	Citalopram HBr 10 mg	Celexa by Eon	00185-0371	Antidepressant
E372	Tab, Dark Pink, Cap Shaped, Eon Logo	Citalopram HBr 20 mg	Celexa by Eon	00185-0372	Antidepressant
E373	Tab, White, Cap Shaped, Eon Logo	Citalopram HBr 40 mg	Celexa by Eon	00185-0373	Antidepressant
E38	Tab, Light Pink, Cap Shaped, Eon Logo	Nefazodone HCl 50 mg	Serzone by Eon	00185-0038	Antidepressant
E39	Tab, White, Cap Shaped, E over 39	Naltrexone HCl 50 mg	Revia by Eon	00185-0039	Opioid Antagonist
E4	Tab, Blue, Round	Hydromorphone HCl 4 mg	Dilaudid by KV Pharma		Analgesic; C II
E4 <> M	Tab, Pink, Round, Flat, Scored, Uncoated	Estradiol 1 mg	Estrace by Heartland	61392-0149	Hormone
E4 <> M	Tab, Pink, Round, Scored, E over 4	Estradiol 1 mg	Estrace by Mylan	00378-1454	Hormone
E40	Tab, White, Round, Eon Logo	Midodrine HCl 2.5 mg	ProAmatine by Eon	00185-0040	Antihypotensive
E401	Tab, Dark Orange, Round, E over 401	Mixed Amphetamine Salts 20 mg: Amphetamine Aspartate 5 mg, Amphetamine Sulfate 5 mg, Dextroamphetamine Saccharate 5 mg, Dextroamphetamine Sulfate 5 mg	Adderall by Eon	00185-0401	Stimulant; C II
E404	Tab, Dark Orange, Round, E over 404	Mixed Amphetamine Salts 30 mg: Amphetamine Aspartate 7.5 mg, Amphetamine Sulfate 7.5 mg, Dextroamphetamine Saccharate 7.5 mg, Dextroamphetamine Sulfate 7.5 mg	Adderall by Eon	00185-0404	Stimulant; C II
E41	Tab, White, Oval	Fosinopril Sodium 10 mg	Monopril by Eon	00185-0041	Antihypertensive
E410	Tab, Blue, Round, ER	Bupropion HCl 100 mg	Wellbutrin SR by Eon	00185-0410	Antidepressant
E415	Tab, Plum, Round, ER	Bupropion HCl 150 mg	Wellbutrin SR by Eon	00185-0415	Antidepressant
E42	Tab, White, Cap Shaped	Fosinopril Sodium 20 mg	Monopril by Eon	00185-0042	Antihypertensive
E421	Tab, Orange-Red, Oval, Ex Release	Etodolac 400 mg	Lodine XL by Eon	00185-0421	NSAID
E422	Tab, Gray-Green, Oval, Ex Release	Etodolac 500 mg	Lodine XL by Eon	00185-0422	NSAID
E423	Tab, Light Green Oval, Ex Release	Etodolac 600 mg	Lodine XL by Eon	00185-0423	NSAID
E43	Tab, Orange, Round	Midodrine HCl 5 mg	ProAmatine by Eon	00185-0043	Antihypotensive

ID FRONT <> BACK	DESCRIPTION FRONT <> BACK	INGREDIENT & STRENGTH	BRAND (or Generic Equiv.) by FIRM	NDC#	CLASS; SCH.
E435	Tab	Isoniazid 100 mg	Laniazid by Med Pro	53978-3065	Antimycobacterial
E4350	Tab, White, Round, Scored, E over 4350	Isoniazid 300 mg	Laniazid by Eon	00185-4350	Antimycobacterial
E4354	Tab, White, Round, Scored, E over 4354	Isoniazid 100 mg	Laniazid by Eon	00185-4351	Antimycobacterial
E44	Tab, White, Round, E over 44	Tizanidine HCl 4 mg	Zanaflex by Eon	00185-4400	Muscle Relaxant
E4416	Tab, White, Oblong, Extended Release	Metformin HCl 500 mg	Glucophage XR by Eon	00185-4416	Antidiabetic
E442	Tab, White, Round, Eon Logo	Ciprofloxacin HCl 250 mg	Cipro by Eon	00185-0442	Antibiotic
E451	Tab, White, Cap Shaped, Eon Logo	Ciprofloxacin HCl 500 mg	Cipro by Eon	00185-0451	Antibiotic
E47	Tab, White, Round	Fosinopril Sodium 40 mg	Monopril by Eon	00185-0047	Antihypertensive
E470	Tab, White, Cap Shaped, Eon Logo	Ciprofloxacin HCl 750 mg	Cipro by Eon	00185-0470	Antibiotic
E471	Tab, Round, Eon Logo	Captopril 50 mg	Capoten by Eon	00185-0471	Antihypertensive
E474	Tab	Acetaminophen 500 mg, Hydrocodone Bitartrate 5 mg	Vicodin by Eon	00185-0474	Analgesic; C III
E475	Tab	Acetaminophen 750 mg, Hydrocodone Bitartrate 7.5 mg	Vicodin ES by Eon	00185-0475	Analgesic; C III
E48	Tab, Red, Round, E over 48	Benazepril HCl 40 mg	Lotensin by Eon	00185-0048	Antihypertensive
E491	Tab, White, Round	Captopril 100 mg	Capoten by Eon	00185-0491	Antihypertensive
E5	Tab, Yellow-Orange, Round, E over 5	Benazepril HCl 5 mg	Lotensin by Eon	00185-0505	Antihypertensive
E5 <> M	Tab, Pale Blue, Round, Scored, E over 5	Estradiol 2 mg	Estrace by Mylan	00378-1458	Hormone
E50	Cap, Dark Pink, Opaque, Soft Gel	Etoposide 50 mg	VePesid by UDL	51079-0965	Antineoplastic
E50	Tab, Pink, Oval	Metolazone 2.5 mg	Zaroxolyn by Eon	00185-5050	Diuretic
E50	Cap, Dark Pink, Opaque, Soft Gel	Etoposide 50 mg	VePesid by Genpharm	55567-0050	Antineoplastic
E5000	Cap, Blue & Clear	Phentermine 30 mg	Fastin by Eon	00185-5000	Anorexiant; C IV
E51	Tab, White, Round	Doxazosin Mesylate 1 mg	Cardura by Eon	00185-0051	Antihypertensive
E511	Tab, White, Round, Scored, E over 511	Quinidine Sulfate 200 mg	Quinora by Eon	00185-4346	Antiarrhythmic
E512	Tab, White, Round, Scored, E over 512	Quinidine Sulfate 300 mg	Quinora by Eon	00185-1047	Antiarrhythmic
E5156	Cap, Brown & Clear, Black Print, Slow Release	Papaverine HCl 150 mg	Pavabid by Eon	00185-5156	Vasodilator
E5174	Cap, Amethyst & Clear, Black Print, Oval, Ex Release	Nitroglycerin 2.5 mg	Nitrobid by Eon	00185-5174	Vasodilator
E52	Tab, Yellow, Round	Doxazosin Mesylate 2 mg	Cardura by Eon	00185-0052	Antihypertensive
E5254E5254	Cap, Brown & Clear	Phendimetrazine Tartrate 105 mg	Plegine by Eon	00185-5254	Anorexiant; C III
E53	Tab, Orange, Round, E over 53	Benazepril HCl 10 mg	Lotensin by Eon	00185-0053	Antihypertensive
E530 <> 10	Tab, White, Round	Isoxsuprine HCl 10 mg	Vasodilan by Eon	00185-0530	Vasodilator
E531 <> 20	Tab, White, Round	Isoxsuprine HCl 20 mg	Vasodilan by Eon	00185-0531	Vasodilator
E535	Tab, White, Round	Tolbutamide 500 mg	Orinase by Eon		Antidiabetic
E5380	Cap, Red & Scarlet, White Print, Opaque	Ascorbic Acid 75 mg, Cyanocobalamin 15 mcg, Ferrous Fumarate 110 mg, Folic Acid 0.5 mg, Liver-Stomach 240 mg	Trinsicon by Eon	00185-5380	Vitamin
E5385	Cap, Clear & Red	Ferrous Sulfate SR 250 mg	by Eon		Mineral
E54	Tab, Pink, Oval	Lisinopril 5 mg	Zestril by Eon	00185-5400	Antihypertensive
E55	Tab, Blue, Oval	Metolazone 5 mg	Zaroxolyn by Eon	00185-0055	Diuretic
E550	Cap, Light Blue and Clear	Itraconazole 100 mg	Sporanox by Eon	00185-0550	Antifungal
E555	Tab, Compressed, Eon Logo	Metronidazole 500 mg	by Quality Care	60346-0507 Discontinued	Antibiotic
E56	Tab, Yellow, Oval	Metolazone 10 mg	Zaroxolyn by Eon	00185-5600	Diuretic
E57	Tab, Light Green, Oval, Film Coated	Sertraline HCl 25 mg	Zoloft by Sandoz	00185-0057	Antidepressant
E58	Tab, Orange, Round	Doxazosin Mesylate 4 mg	Cardura by Eon	00185-0058	Antihypertensive
E59	Tab, Green, Round	Doxazosin Mesylate 8 mg	Cardura by Eon	00185-0059	Antihypertensive
E591	Tab, Round, Eon Logo	Captopril 100 mg	Capoten by Eon	00185-0591	Antihypertensive
E6	Tab, White, Round, Film Coated	Ethambutol HCl 100 mg	Myambutol by Heritage	23155-0100	Antituberculosis
E60	Tab, Yellow, Oval, Scored, Film Coated, Ex Release	Isosorbide Mononitrate 60 mg	Imdur by Ethex	58177-0238	Antianginal
E60MG506	Cap, Blue & White, Ligand Logo on cap, 60MG506 on body, Extended Release	Morphine Sulfate 60 mg	Avinza by Ligand	64365-0506	Analgesic; C II
E61	Tab, White, Round	Captopril 25 mg	Capoten by Eon	00185-0061	Antihypertensive
E6125	Tab, Blue, Round, E612 over 5	Oxymorphone HCl 5 mg	Opana by Endo	63481-0612	Analgesic; C II

ID FRONT <> BACK	DESCRIPTION FRONT <> BACK	INGREDIENT & STRENGTH	BRAND (or Generic Equiv.) by FIRM	NDC#	CLASS; SCH.
E613	Cap, Dark Green & Light Green, Black Print	Hydroxyzine Pamoate 25 mg	Vistaril by Eon	00185-0613	Antianxiety; Antihistamine
E61310	Tab, Red, round, E613 over 10	Oxymorphone HCl 10 mg	Opana by Endo	63481-0613	Analgesic; C II
E615	Cap, Dark Green & White, Black Print	Hydroxyzine Pamoate 50 mg	Vistaril by Eon	00185-0615	Antianxiety; Antihistamine
E616	Tab	Dicyclomine HCl 20 mg	by Chelsea	46193-0115	Gastrointestinal
E616	Tab, Blue, Round	Dicyclomine HCl 20 mg	by Endo	60951-0616	Gastrointestinal
E617	Cap, White	Chlordiazepoxide 5 mg, Clidinium Bromide 2.5 mg	Librax by Eon	00185-0617	Gastrointestinal
E61720	Tab, Light Green, Octagonal, Film Coated, E617 over 20, Extended Release	Oxymorphone HCl 20 mg	Opana ER by Endo	63481-0617 Discontinued	Analgesic; C II
E620	Tab, Coated	Selegiline 5 mg	Carbex by Endo	63481-0408	Antiparkinson
E63	Tab, Light Yellow, Round, E over 63	Clonazepam 0.5 mg	Klonopin by Eon	00185-0063	Sedative; C IV
E64	Tab, Light Blue, Round, E over 64	Clonazepam 1 mg	Klonopin by Eon	00185-0064	Sedative; C IV
E644	Cap, Gray & Yellow	Phentermine 15 mg	Ionamin by Eon		Anorexiant; C IV
E647	Cap, Yellow, Black Print	Phentermine 30 mg	Fastin by Eon	00185-0647	Anorexiant; C IV
E648	Cap, Clear & Pink, Black Print	Diphenhydramine HCl 25 mg	Benadryl by Eon	00185-0648	Antihistamine
E649	Cap, Pink, Black Print	Diphenhydramine HCl 50 mg	Benadryl by Eon	00185-0649	Antihistamine
E649	Cap, Pink, Black Print	Diphenhydramine HCl 50 mg	Benadryl by Major	00904-2056	Antihistamine
E65	Tab, White, Round, E over 65	Clonazepam 2 mg	Klonopin by Eon	00185-0065	Sedative; C IV
E652 <> 15	Tab, Blue, Round	Morphine Sulfate 15 mg	MS Contin by Endo	60951-0652	Analgesic; C II
E653 <> 30	Tab, Green, Round	Morphine Sulfate 30 mg	MS Contin by Endo	60951-0653	Analgesic; C II
E655 <> 60	Tab, Orange, Cap Shaped	Morphine Sulfate 60 mg	MS Contin by Endo	60951-0655	Analgesic; C II
E655 <> 60	Tab, Orange, Cap Shaped	Morphine Sulfate 60 mg	MS Contin by BMS	00056-0655	Analgesic; C II
E658 <> 100	Tab, Blue, Cap Shaped, Ex Release	Morphine Sulfate 100 mg	MS Contin by Endo	60951-0658	Analgesic; C II
E659 <> 200	Tab, Green, Oval, Ex Release	Morphine Sulfate 200 mg	MS Contin by Endo	60951-0659	Analgesic; C II
E660	Cap, Orange	Acetaminophen 500 mg, Oxycodone HCl 5 mg	Percocet by BMS	00056-0660	Analgesic; C II
E660	Cap, Orangish Red	Acetaminophen 500 mg, Oxycodone HCl 5 mg	Percocet by Endo	60951-0660	Analgesic; C II
E670	Cap, Orange & Yellow	Tetracycline HCl 250 mg	Sumycin by Eon		Antibiotic
E67410	Tab, Light Orange, Octagonal, Film Coated, E674 over 10, Extended Release	Oxymorphone HCl 10 mg	Opana ER by Endo	63481-0674 Discontinued	Analgesic; C II
E675	Cap, Blue & Yellow, Red Print, Cap Shaped	Aspirin 325 mg, Butalbital 50 mg, Caffeine 40 mg, Codeine Phosphate 30 mg	Fiorinal w/ Codeine by Endo	60951-0675	Analgesic; C III
E675	Cap, Blue & Yellow, Red Print, Cap Shaped	Aspirin 325 mg, Butalbital 50 mg, Caffeine 40 mg, Codeine Phosphate 30 mg	Fiorinal w/ Codeine by Caremark	00339-5299	Analgesic; C III
E693	Tab, Coated	Salsalate 500 mg	by Major	00904-5072	NSAID
E69340	Tab, Yellow, Octagonal, Film Coated, E693 over 40, Extended Release	Oxymorphone HCl 40 mg	Opana ER by Endo	63481-0693 Discontinued	Analgesic; C II
E694	Tab, Coated	Salsalate 750 mg	by Major	00904-5073	NSAID
E7	Tab, White, Round, Film Coated, Scored, E / 7	Ethambutol HCl 400 mg	Myambutol by Heritage	23155-0101	Antituberculosis
E7	Tab, Tan, Oblong	Chlorpheniramine 8 mg, Phenylephrine 20 mg, Methscopolamine 2.5 mg	Rynatan by Eon		Cold Remedy
E7 <> 511	Tab, Off-White, Round, Scored	Estradiol 1 mg	Estrace by ESI Lederle	59911-5880	Hormone
E7 <> 511	Tab, Off-White, Round, Scored	Estradiol 1 mg	Estrace by Ayerst	00046-5880	Hormone
E70	Tab, Peach, Round, E over 70	Lovastatin 10 mg	Mevacor by Eon	00185-0070	Antihyperlipidemic
E700 <> 75325	Tab, Peach, Cap Shaped	Oxycodone 7.5 mg, Acetaminophen 325 mg	Endocet by Eon	60951-0700	Analgesic; C II
E701	Tab, Orange, Round, E over 701	Bisoprolol 2.5 mg, Hydrochlorothiazide 6.25 mg	Ziac by Eon	00185-0701	Antihypertensive; Diuretic
E702 <> 10	Tab, White, Round, Coated, Extended Release	Oxycodone HCl 10 mg	OxyContin by Endo	60951-0702	Analgesic; C II
E703 <> 20	Tab, Pink, Round, Coated, Extended Release	Oxycodone HCl 20 mg	OxyContin by Endo	60951-0703	Analgesic; C II
E704	Tab, Red, Round, E over 704	Bisoprolol 5 mg, Hydrochlorothiazide 6.25 mg	Ziac by Eon	00185-0704	Antihypertensive; Diuretic
E705 <> 40	Tab, Yellow, Round, Coated, Extended Release	Oxycodone HCl 40 mg	OxyContin by Endo	60951-0705	Analgesic; C II
E707	Tab, White, Round, E over 707	Bisoprolol 10 mg, Hydrochlorothiazide 6.25 mg	Ziac by Eon	00185-0707	Antihypertensive; Diuretic
E71	Tab, Light Pink, Round, E over 71	Lisinopril 10 mg, HCTZ 12.5 mg	Prinzide by Eon	00185-7100	Antihypertensive; Diuretic
E710 <> 80	Tab, Green, Round, Coated, Extended Release	Oxycodone HCl 80 mg	OxyContin by Endo	60951-0710	Analgesic; C II
E712 <> 10325	Tab, Yellow, Oval	Oxycodone 10 mg, Acetaminophen 325 mg	Endocet by Endo	60951-0712	Analgesic; C II

ID FRONT <> BACK	DESCRIPTION FRONT <> BACK	INGREDIENT & STRENGTH	BRAND (or Generic Equiv.) by FIRM	NDC#	CLASS; SCH.
E713	Tab, Green & White, Round, E over 713	Aspirin 385 mg, Caffeine 30 mg, Orphenadrine Citrate 25 mg	Norgesic by Eon	00185-0713	Analgesic; Muscle Relaxant
E714	Tab, Green & White, Cap Shaped, Scored	Aspirin 770 mg, Caffeine 60 mg, Orphenadrine Citrate 50 mg	Norgesic Forte by Eon	00185-0714	Analgesic
E716	Tab, White, Round, E over 716	Meprobamate 200 mg	Miltown by Eon	00185-0716	Sedative/Hypnotic; C IV
E717	Tab, White, Round, E over 717	Meprobamate 400 mg	Miltown by Eon	00185-0717	Sedative/Hypnotic; C IV
E72	Tab, Light Blue, Round, E over 72	Lovastatin 20 mg	Mevacor by Eon	00185-0072	Antihyperlipidemic
E720	Cap, Clear & Green, Black Print, Ex Release	Indomethacin 75 mg	Indocin SR by Eon	00185-0720	NSAID
E721	Tab, Blue, Round, E over 721	Desipramine HCl 50 mg	Norpramin by Eon	00185-0721	Antidepressant
E722	Tab, Light Blue, Round, E over 722	Desipramine HCl 75 mg	Norpramin by Eon	00185-0722	Antidepressant
E724	Tab, Lavender & White, Round, E over 724	Aspirin 325 mg, Carisoprodol 200 mg	Soma Compound by Eon	00185-0724	Analgesic; Muscle Relaxant
E736	Tab, Blue, Round, E over 736	Desipramine HCl 100 mg	Norpramin by Eon	00185-0736	Antidepressant
E74	Tab, Green, Round, E over 74	Lovastatin 40 mg	Mevacor by Eon	00185-0074	Antihyperlipidemic
E745	Tab, Light Blue, Oval	Phenylpropanolamine HCl 75 mg, Guaifenesin 400 mg	Guaipax SR by Eon	00185-0745	Cold Remedy
E749	Tab, White & Yellow, Round, E over 749	Carisoprodol 200 mg, Aspirin 325 mg, Codeine Phosphate 16 mg	Soma Compound w/ Codeine by Eon	00185-0749	Analgesic; C III
E750	Tab, Brown, Round	Nystatin 500,000 Units	Mycostatin by Eon	00185-0750	Antifungal
E757	Tab, White, Cap Shaped	Sulfadiazine 500 mg	by Eon	00185-0757	Antibiotic
E76	Tab, Light Yellow, Round, Scored, E over 76	Phendimetrazine Tartrate 35 mg	Plegine by Eon	00185-4057	Anorexiant; C III
E76	Cap, Dark Red and Light Yellow, Opaque	Stavudine 15 mg	Zerit by Aurobindo	65862-0111	Antiviral
E760	Tab, White, Round, E over 760	Desipramine HCl 150 mg	Norpramin by Eon	00185-0760	Antidepressant
E761	Tab, Yellow, Oblong	Salsalate 500 mg	Disalcid by Eon	00185-0761	NSAID
E762	Tab, Yellow, Oblong	Salsalate 750 mg	Disalcid by Eon	00185-0762	NSAID
E77	Cap, Light Brown, Opaque	Stavudine 20 mg	Zerit by Aurobindo	65862-0112	Antiviral
E77 <> 511	Tab, Off-White, Round, Scored	Estradiol 2 mg	Estrace by ESI Lederle	59911-5882	Hormone
E77 <> 511	Tab, Off-White, Round, Scored	Estradiol 2 mg	Estrace by Ayerst	00046-5882	Hormone
E771	Tab, Pink, Round, E over 771	Bisoprolol Fumarate 5 mg	Zebeta by Eon	00185-0771	Antihypertensive
E771	Tab, Pink, Round, E over 771	Bisoprolol Fumarate 5 mg	Sandoz Bisoprolol by Sandoz	Canadian DIN 02247439	Antihypertensive
E774	Tab, White, Round, E over 774	Bisoprolol Fumarate 10 mg	Zebeta by Eon	00185-0774	Antihypertensive
E774	Tab, White, Round, E over 774	Bisoprolol Fumarate 10 mg	Sandoz Bisoprolol by Sandoz	Canadian DIN 02247440	Antihypertensive
E784	Tab, White, Oval, Scored	Guaifenesin 600 mg, Pseudoephedrine HCl 120 mg	Entex PSE by Eon	00185-0784	Cold Remedy
E796 <> 75	Tab, Peach, Cap Shaped, E796 <> 7.5	Oxycodone HCl 7.5, Acetaminophen 500 mg	Endocet by Endo	60951-0796	Analgesic; C II
E797 <> 10	Tab, Yellow, Oval	Oxycodone HCl 10 mg, Acetaminophen 650 mg	Endocet by Endo	60951-0797	Analgesic; C II
E799	Cap, Red	Rifampin 300 mg	Rifadin by UDL	51079-0890	Antibiotic
E799	Cap, Red, Black Print	Rifampin 300 mg	Rifadin by Eon	00185-0799	Antibiotic
E80	Cap, Light Green, Black Print, Opaque	Fluoxetine HCl 10 mg	Prozac by Eon	00185-0080	Antidepressant
E801	Cap, Orange, Black Print	Rifampin 150 mg	Rifadin by Eon	00185-0801	Antibiotic
E805	Cap, Yellow, Black Print	Doxycycline Monohydrate 50 mg	Monodox by Eon	00185-0805	Antibiotic
E81	Tab, Peach, Cap Shaped, Scored, Eon Logo	Nefazodone HCl 150 mg	Serzone by Eon	00185-0081	Antidepressant
E81	Cap, White, Black Ink	Ribavirin 200 mg	Rebetol by Aurobindo	65862-0290	Antiviral
E810	Cap, Brown, White Print	Doxycycline Monohydrate 100 mg	Monodox by Eon	00185-0810	Antibiotic
E814	Cap, Dark Green and Green	Doxycycline Hyclate 75 mg	Doryx by Sandoz	00781-2268	Antibiotic
E815	Cap, Light Green and Green	Doxycycline Hyclate 100 mg	Doryx by Sandoz	00781-2269	Antibiotic
E82	Tab, Pink, Round	Benazepril HCl 20 mg	Lotensin by Eon	00185-0820	Antihypertensive
E839	Cap, Red, E-839	Docusate Sodium 100 mg, Casanthranol 30 mg	Peri-Colace by Chase		Laxative
E84	Tab, Dark Blue, Round, E over 84	Mixed Amphetamine Salts 5 mg: Amphetamine Aspartate 1.25 mg, Amphetamine Sulfate 1.25 mg, Dextroamphetamine Saccharate 1.25 mg, Dextroamphetamine Sulfate 1.25 mg	Adderall by Eon	00185-0084	Stimulant; C II
E84	Tab, White to Off White, Round, Film Coated, Scored	Penicillin V Potassium 250 mg	by Aurobindo	65862-0175	Antibiotic

ID FRONT <> BACK	DESCRIPTION FRONT <> BACK	INGREDIENT & STRENGTH	BRAND (or Generic Equiv.) by FIRM	NDC#	CLASS; SCH.
E85	Cap, Light Green & White, Black Print, Opaque	Fluoxetine HCl 20 mg	Prozac by Eon	0185-0085	Antidepressant
E856	Tab, Blue, Oblong	Salsalate 500 mg	Disalcid by Eon		NSAID
E857	Tab, Blue, Oblong	Salsalate 750 mg	Disalcid by Eon		NSAID
E88	Cap, Green, Opaque	Fluoxetine 10 mg	Prozac by Aurobindo	65862-0192	Antidepressant
E882E882	Cap, Gray & Yellow, Black Print	Phentermine 15 mg	Fastin by Eon	00185-0644	Anorexiant; C IV
E9075	Tab, Pink, Octagonal, Film Coated, E907 over 5, Extended Release	Oxymorphone HCl 5 mg	Opana ER by Endo	63481-0907 Discontinued	Analgesic; C II
E90MG507	Cap, Red & White, Ligand Logo on cap, 90MG507 on body, Extended Release	Morphine Sulfate 90 mg	Avinza by Ligand	64365-0507	Analgesic; C II
E91	Cap, White Opaque and Clear	Gabapentin 100 mg	Neurontin by Eon	00185-0091	Anticonvulsant
E91	Cap, Green and White, Opaque	Fluoxetine 20 mg	Prozac by Aurobindo	65862-0193	Antidepressant
E92	Cap, Green and Orange, Opaque	Fluoxetine 40 mg	Prozac by Aurobindo	65862-0194	Antidepressant
E93	Cap, Yellow Opaque and Yellow Clear	Gabapentin 300 mg	Neurontin by Eon	00185-0093	Anticonvulsant
E932	Cap, Clear, Soft Gel	Cyclosporine 25 mg	Neoral by Eon	00185-0932	Immunosuppressant
E933	Cap, Clear, Soft Gel	Cyclosporine 100 mg	Neoral by Eon	00185-0933	Immunosuppressant
E94	Cap, Orange, Opaque and Clear, Black Ink	Gabapentin 400 mg	Neurontin by Eon	00185-0094	Anticonvulsant
E968	Cap, Light Green	Chlordiazepoxide 5 mg, Clidinium Bromide 2.5 mg	Librax by Eon	00185-0968	Gastrointestinal
E988	Tab, White, Round	Quinine Sulfate 260 mg	Quinamm by Eon		Antimalarial
E99	Cap, Lavender and Turquoise, Opaque	Cefdinir 300 mg	Omnicef by Aurobindo	65862-0177	Antibiotic
E998	Tab, White, Round, Scored, E over 998	Yohimbine HCl 5.4 mg	Yocon by Eon	00185-0998	Impotence Agent
EA <> A	Tab, Pink, Oval, Film Coated, Abbott Logo (a)	Erythromycin 500 mg	Erythromycin by Abbott	00074-6227	Antibiotic
EA <> A	Tab, Pink, Oval, Film Coated, Abbott Logo (a)	Erythromycin 500 mg	by Apotheca	12634-0507	Antibiotic
EATON036	Tab, Yellow, Round	Nitrofurantoin 50 mg	Furadantin by Norwich		Antibiotic
EATON037	Tab, Yellow, Round	Nitrofurantoin 100 mg	Furadantin by Norwich		Antibiotic
EATON072	Tab, Brown, Round	Furazolidone 100 mg	Furoxone by Norwich		Antibiotic
EB <> A	Tab, Pink, Oval, Film Coated, Abbott Logo	Erythromycin 250 mg	Eryc by Abbott	00074-6328	Antibiotic
EBASE333MG <> BARR	Tab, White, Blue Print, Cap Shape, Enteric Coated, E-Base 333 mg <> Barr	Erythromycin 333 mg	by Barr	00555-0532 Discontinued	Antibiotic
EBASE333MG <> BARR	Tab, White, Green Print, Cap Shaped, Enteric Coated, E-Base over 333 mg <> barr	Erythromycin 333 mg	by Barr	00555-0495 Discontinued	Antibiotic
EBASE500MG <> BARR	Tab, White, Red Print, Cap Shaped, Enteric Coated, E-Base 500 mg <> Barr	Erythromycin 500 mg	by Barr	00555-0533 Discontinued	Antibiotic
EC <> A	Tab, White, Oval, Enteric Coated, Delayed Release, Abbott Logo (a)	Erythromycin 250 mg	Ery Tab by Pharmedix	53002-0203	Antibiotic
EC <> A	Tab, White, Oval, Enteric Coated, Delayed Release, Abbott Logo (a)	Erythromycin 250 mg	by Allscripts		Antibiotic
EC <> A	Tab, White, Oval, Enteric Coated, Delayed Release, Abbott Logo (a)	Erythromycin 250 mg	by Nat Pharmpak	55154-0107	Antibiotic
EC <> A	Tab, White, Oval, Enteric Coated, Delayed Release, Abbott Logo (a)	Erythromycin 250 mg	by Amerisource	62584-0372	Antibiotic
EC <> A	Tab, White, Oval, Enteric Coated, Delayed Release, Abbott Logo (a)	Erythromycin 250 mg	by Kaiser	00179-1055	Antibiotic
EC <> A	Tab, White, Oval, Enteric Coated, Delayed Release, Abbott Logo (a)	Erythromycin 250 mg	Ery-Tab by Abbott	00074-6304	Antibiotic
ECE <> NVR	Tab, Light Yellow, Oval, Film Coated	Amlodipine 5 mg, Valsartan 160 mg	Exforge by Novartis	00078-0488	Antihypertensive
ECNAPROSYN <> 375	Tab, White, Cap Shaped, Enteric Coated	Naproxen 375 mg	EC-Naprosyn by Hoffmann La Roche	00004-6415	NSAID
ECNAPROSYN <> 375	Tab, White, Cap Shaped	Naproxen 375 mg	Naprosyn by Syntex	18393-0255	NSAID
ECNAPROSYN <> 375	Tab, White, Cap Shaped	Naproxen 375 mg	Naprosyn by DRX	55045-2425	NSAID
ECNAPROSYN <> 375	Tab, White, Cap Shaped	Naproxen 375 mg	Naprosyn by PDRX	55289-0267	NSAID

ID FRONT <> BACK	DESCRIPTION FRONT <> BACK	INGREDIENT & STRENGTH	BRAND (or Generic Equiv.) by FIRM	NDC#	CLASS; SCH.
ECNAPROSYN <> 500	Tab, White, Cap Shaped	Naproxen 500 mg	Naprosyn by DRX	55045-2441	NSAID
ECNAPROSYN <> 500	Tab, White, Cap Shaped	Naproxen 500 mg	Naprosyn by PDRX	55289-0693	NSAID
ECNAPROSYN <> 500	Tab, White, Cap Shaped	Naproxen 500 mg	Naprosyn by Par	49884-0568	NSAID
ECNAPROSYN <> 500	Tab, White, Cap Shaped	Naproxen 500 mg	Naprosyn by H J Harkins Co	52959-0456	NSAID
ECNAPROSYN <> 500	Tab, White, Cap Shaped	Naproxen 500 mg	Naprosyn by Compumed	00403-0717	NSAID
ECNAPROSYN <> 500	Tab, White, Cap Shaped	Naproxen 500 mg	Naprosyn by Syntex	18393-0256	NSAID
ECNAPROSYN <> 500	Tab, White, Cap Shaped, Enteric Coated	Naproxen 500 mg	EC-Naprosyn by Hoffmann La Roche	00004-6416	NSAID
ECR0141	Tab, White, Oval, Scored, ECR/0141	Acetaminophen 500 mg, Hydrocodone Bitartrate 5 mg	Vicodin by Schwarz	00131-2057	Analgesic; C III
ECR15	Cap, Orange, White Band, Extended Release	Cyclobenzaprine HCl 15 mg	Amrix by ECR	00095-0150	Muscle Relaxant
ECR25	Tab, White, Cap Shaped, Scored, ECR 2.5	Guaifenesin 300 mg, Hydrocodone Bitartrate 2.5 mg	Pneumotussin by ECR	00095-0066 Discontinued	Analgesic; Expectorant; C III
ECR30	Cap, Blue and Orange, Two White Bands	Cyclobenzaprine HCl 30 mg	Amrix by ECR	00095-0300	Muscle Relaxant
ECR6	Tab, White, Cap Shaped, Scored	Brompheniramine Maleate 6 mg	Lodrane by ECR	00095-0006	Cold Remedy
ECR600	Tab, Ex Release, ECR/600	Guaifenesin 600 mg	Robitussin by Sovereign	58716-0603	Expectorant
ECR6006	Cap, Clear, Ex Release, ECR over 6006	Brompheniramine Maleate 6 mg, Pseudoephedrine HCl 60 mg	Lodrane LD by Sovereign	58716-0027	Cold Remedy
ECR6006	Cap, Clear, Ex Release, ECR over 6006	Brompheniramine Maleate 6 mg, Pseudoephedrine HCl 60 mg	Lodrane LD by ECR	00095-6006	Cold Remedy
ECR645	Tab, White, Scored, Ex Release	Brompheniramine Maleate 6 mg, Pseudoephedrine HCl 45 mg	Lodrane 12 D by ECR	00095-0645	Cold Remedy
ECR86	Tab, Pink, Pentagonal, Scored	Dexamethasone 1.5 mg	DexPak by ECR	00095-0088	Steroid
ECR86	Tab, Pink, Round, Scored, 54 over 943	Dexamethasone 1.5 mg	DexPak by ECR	00095-0087	Steroid
ECR89	Tab, Pink, Pentagonal, Scored	Dexamethasone 1.5 mg	DexPak TaperPak by ECR	00095-0089	Steroid
ED	Tab	Chlorpheniramine Maleate 8 mg, Phenylephrine HCl 20 mg	Ed A Hist by Anabolic	00722-6287	Cold Remedy
ED <> A	Tab, White, Oval, Enteric Coated, Delayed Release, Abbott Logo (a <> ED)	Erythromycin 500 mg	Ery Tab by Pharmedix	53002-0205	Antibiotic
ED <> A	Tab, White, Oval, Enteric Coated, Delayed Release, Abbott Logo (a <> ED)	Erythromycin 500 mg	Ery Tab by Kaiser	00179-1056	Antibiotic
ED <> A	Tab, White, Oval, Enteric Coated, Delayed Release, Abbott Logo (a)	Erythromycin 500 mg	Ery-Tab by Abbott	00074-6321	Antibiotic
ED2	Tab, Off-White, Rectangular-Shaped, Cobalt Logo <> ED2	Etidronate Disodium 200 mg	Didronel by Cobalt	Canadian DIN 02248686	Calcium Metabolism
ED200 <> G	Tab, White, Rectangular	Etidronate Disodium 200 mg	Didronel by Genpharm	15330-0094	Calcium Metabolism
ED200 <> G	Tab, White, Rectangular Shaped	Etidronate 200 mg	Didronel by Mylan	00378-3286	Calcium Metabolism
ED4	Tab, Off White, Cap Shaped, Scored, ED / 4 <> Cobalt Cobalt Logo	Etidronate Disodium 400 mg	Didrocal by Cobalt	Canadian DIN 02263866	Antiosteporosis
ED400 <> G	Tab, White, Capsule Shaped	Etidronate 400 mg	Didronel by Mylan	00378-3288	Calcium Metabolism
ED400 <> G	Tab, White, Cap Shaped	Etidronate Disodium 400 mg	Didronel by Genpharm	15330-0095	Calcium Metabolism
EDAHIST	Tab, Peach, Oblong, Controlled Release	Chlorpheniramine 8 mg, Phenylephrine 20 mg	Ed A-Hist by Edwards	00485-0054	Cold Remedy
EDECRIN <> MSD65	Tab, White, Cap Shaped, Scored	Ethacrynic Acid 25 mg	Edecrin by Merck	00006-0065	Diuretic
EDECRIN <> MSD90	Tab, Green, Cap Shaped, Scored	Ethacrynic Acid 50 mg	Edecrin by Merck	00006-0090	Diuretic
EDEPRYL5MG	Cap, Blue, Somer Logo/ Edepryl 5 mg	Selegiline HCl 5 mg	by Somerset		Antiparkinson
EDFLEX	Cap, ED-Flex	Acetaminophen 300 mg, Phenyltoloxamine Citrate 20 mg, Salicylamide 200 mg	Durabac by Seatrace	00551-0066	Analgesic
EDFLEX	Cap, ED-Flex	Acetaminophen 300 mg, Phenyltoloxamine Citrate 20 mg, Salicylamide 200 mg	Durabac by Edwards	00485-0066	Analgesic
EF	Tab, White, Round, Abbott Logo	Erythromycin Ethylsuccinate 200 mg	EES Chewable by Abbott		Antibiotic
EFF <> 20	Tab, White, Round, Debossed	Methazolamide 50 mg	Neptazane by Duramed	51285-0969	Antiglaucoma Agent
EFF <> 20	Tab, White, Round, Scored	Methazolamide 50 mg	Neptazane by Lederle	55806-0020	Antiglaucoma Agent
EFF <> 20	Tab	Methazolamide 50 mg	Neptazane by Mikart	46672-0109	Antiglaucoma Agent
EFF <> 21	Tab, White, Round, Debossed	Methazolamide 25 mg	Neptazane by Duramed	51285-0988	Antiglaucoma Agent
EFF <> 21	Tab, White, Round, Debossed	Methazolamide 25 mg	Neptazane by Lederle	55806-0021	Antiglaucoma Agent
EFF <> 26	Tab, White, Round	Isoniazid 100 mg	Laniazid by Mikart	46672-0158	Antimycobacterial

ID FRONT <> BACK	DESCRIPTION FRONT <> BACK	INGREDIENT & STRENGTH	BRAND (or Generic Equiv.) by FIRM	NDC#	CLASS; SCH.
EFF <> 27	Tab, White, Round	Isoniazid 300 mg	Laniazid by Mikart	46672-0159	Antimycobacterial
EFF12	Tab, White, Round, Scored, EFF / 12	Pyrazinamide 500 mg	by Mikart	55806-0012	Antibiotic
EFF20	Tab	Methazolamide 50 mg	Neptazane by Ivax	00182-1076	Antiglaucoma Agent
EFF21	Tab	Methazolamide 25 mg	Neptazane by Ivax	00182-1075	Antiglaucoma Agent
EGIS111	Cap, Light Blue & Red	Piroxicam 10 mg	Feldene by Ranbaxy	63304-0690	NSAID
EGIS111PIROXICAM	Cap, Blue & Red	Piroxicam 10 mg	Feldene by Prestige	58056-0344	NSAID
EGIS111-PIROXICAM10MG	Cap, Blue & Red	Piroxicam 10 mg	Feldene by Prestige	58056-0347	NSAID
EGIS112	Cap, Red	Piroxicam 20 mg	Feldene by Ranbaxy	63304-0691	NSAID
EGIS112-PIROXICAM20MG	Cap, Red	Piroxicam 20 mg	Feldene by Prestige	58056-0345	NSAID
EGIS112-PIROXICAM20MG	Cap, Red	Piroxicam 20 mg	Feldene by Promeco SA	64674-0006	NSAID
EH <> A	Tab, White, Oval, Enteric Coated, Delayed Release, Abbott Logo (a)	Erythromycin 333 mg	Ery Tab by Pharmedix	53002-0204	Antibiotic
EH <> A	Tab, White, Oval, Enteric Coated, Delayed Release, Abbott Logo (a)	Erythromycin 333 mg	by Allscripts		Antibiotic
EH <> A	Tab, White, Oval, Enteric Coated, Delayed Release, Abbott Logo (a)	Erythromycin 333 mg	by Med Pro	53978-0089	Antibiotic
EH <> A	Tab, White, Oval, Enteric Coated, Delayed Release, Abbott Logo (a)	Erythromycin 333 mg	Ery-Tab by Abbott	00074-6320	Antibiotic
EH <> NVR	Tab, White, Round	Tegaserod Maleate 6 mg	Zelnorm by Novartis	00078-0356	Gastrointestinal
EH <> NVR	Tab, White, Round	Tegaserod Maleate 6 mg	Zelnorm by Novartis	Canadian DIN 02245566	Gastrointestinal
EH <> NVR	Tab, White, Round	Tegaserod Maleate 6 mg	Zelnorm by Novartis	00078-0426	Gastrointestinal
EHYDROGESIC	Cap, Edwards Logo <> Hydrogesic	Acetaminophen 500 mg, Hydrocodone Bitartrate 5 mg	Vicodin by Edwards	00485-0050	Analgesic; C III
EI <> KTAB	Tab, K-Tab, Film Coated	Potassium Chloride 750 mg	by Heartland	61392-0900	Electrolytes
EK25	Tab, Lime	Potassium 977.5 mg (25 mEq)	Effer-K by Nomax	51801-0002	Electrolytes
EK25	Tab, Orange	Potassium 977.5 mg (25 mEq)	Effer-K by Nomax	51801-0001	Electrolytes
EL	Tab, White, Oval, Film-Coated, Scored	Escitalopram 10 mg	Cipralex by Lundbeck	Canadian DIN 02263238	Antidepressant
EL	Tab, White, Oval, Scored, Film-Coated	Escitalopram 20 mg	Cipralex by Lundbeck	Canadian DIN 02263254	Antidepressant
EL <> 130	Tab	Hyoscyamine Sulfate 0.125 mg	Levsin by Anabolic	00722-6294	Gastrointestinal
EL040	Tab, Light Green, Ex Release, EL/040	Guaifenesin 600 mg	Robitussin by Theraids	59037-6159	Expectorant
EL069	Tab, Blue, Round	Bendroflumethiazide 4 mg, Rauwolfia Serpentina 50 mg	Rauzide by Econolab		Diuretic; Antihypertensive
EL073	Tab, Green, Oval	Atropine 0.04 mg, Chlorpheniramine 8 mg, Hyoscyamine 0.19 mg, Phenylephrine 25 mg, Phenylpropanolamine 50 mg, Scopolamine 0.01 mg	Ru-tuss by Econolab		Cold Remedy
EL077	Tab, Violet, Oval	Carbinoxamine Maleate 8 mg, Pseudoephedrine HCl 120 mg	Rondec TR by Economed	Discontinued	Cold Remedy
EL082	Tab, White, Oval	Carbinoxamine Maleate 4 mg, Pseudoephedrine HCl 60 mg	Rondec by Economed	Discontinued	Cold Remedy
EL090	Tab, Green	Guaifenesin 600 mg, Dextromethorphan HBr 60 mg	by Econolab		Cold Remedy
EL10	Tab, Salmon, Barrel Shaped, Scored, EL / 10 <> Cobalt Logo	Enalapril Maleate 10 mg	Vasotec by Cobalt	Canadian DIN 02291894	Antihypertensive
EL111	Tab, Blue, Round	Hyoscyamine Sulfate 0.15 mg	Levsin by Econolab		Gastrointestinal
EL122	Tab, Pink, Oval	Carbetapentane Tannate 60 mg, Chlorpheniramine Tannate 5 mg, Ephedrine Tannate 10 mg, Phenylephrine Tannate 10 mg	Rynatuss by Econolab		Cold Remedy
EL124	Tab, Blue, Round, Scored	Belladonna Alkaloids 0.2 mg, Ergotamine Tartrate 0.6 mg, Phenobarbital 40 mg	Spastrin by Anabolic	00722-6307	Gastrointestinal; C IV
EL124	Tab, Blue, Round, Cross Scored	Phenobarbital 40 mg, Ergotamine Tartrate 0.6 mg, Belladonna Alkaloids 0.2 mg	Bel Tabs by URL Mutual	00677-1660	Antimigraine; C IV

ID FRONT <> BACK	DESCRIPTION FRONT <> BACK	INGREDIENT & STRENGTH	BRAND (or Generic Equiv.) by FIRM	NDC#	CLASS; SCH.
EL125	Cap, Blue & Clear	Brompheniramine Maleate 6 mg, Pseudoephedrine HCl 60 mg	Bromfed PD by Econolab		Cold Remedy
EL140	Tab, Blue	Guaifenesin 600 mg, Pseudoephedrine HCl 60 mg	Deconsal II by Econolab		Cold Remedy
EL158	Tab, Beige, OTC, EL 158	Polycarbophil 625 mg	Fibercon by Breckenridge		Laxative
EL175	Tab, Pink, Round	Meprobamate 400 mg, Benactyzine HCl 1 mg	Deprol by Econolab	51991-0007	Sedative/Hypnotic; C IV
EL191	Tab, Beige, Oval	Chlorpheniramine 8 mg, Phenylephrine 25 mg, Pyrilamine 25 mg	Rynatan by Econolab		Cold Remedy
EL20	Tab, Peach, Barrel Shaped, Scored, EL / 20 <> Cobalt Logo	Enalapril Maleate 20 mg	Vasotec by Cobalt	Canadian DIN 02291908	Antihypertensive
EL222	Cap, Ex Release, EL-222	Brompheniramine Maleate 6 mg, Pseudoephedrine HCl 60 mg	Nalfed PD by Sovereign	58716-0031	Cold Remedy
EL25	Tab, Yellow, Barrel Shaped, Scored, EL / 25 <> Cobalt Logo	Enalapril Maleate 2.5 mg	Vasotec by Cobalt	Canadian DIN 02291878	Antihypertensive
EL270	Tab, Pink, Round	Guaifenesin 200 mg	Aquabid by Econolab		Expectorant
EL310	Cap, ER, EL-310	Hyoscyamine Sulfate 0.375 mg	Levsin by Major	00904-7833	Gastrointestinal
EL310	Cap, ER, EL-310	Hyoscyamine Sulfate 0.375 mg	Levsin by Pharmafab	62542-0310	Gastrointestinal
EL320	Tab, Cream, Round, Scored	Lipase 8000 Units, Protease 30,000 Units, Amylase 30,000 Units	by Murfreesboro	51129-1428	Gastrointestinal
EL320	Tab, Off-White, Round, EL 320	Amylase 30,000 Units, Lipase 8000 Units, Protease 30,000 Units	Viokase by Breckenridge	51991-0520	Gastrointestinal
EL320	Tab, EL/320	Amylase 30,000 Units, Lipase 8000 Units, Protease 30,000 Units	Pancrelipase by Anabolic	00722-6089	Gastrointestinal
EL323	Cap, Clear & White	Amylase 20,000 Units, Lipase 4500 Units, Protease 25,000 Units	Pancrease by Econolab		Gastrointestinal
EL323	Cap	Amylase 20,000 Units, Lipase 4500 Units, Protease 25,000 Units	Pancrease by Anabolic		Gastrointestinal
EL410	Tab, ER	Hyoscyamine Sulfate 0.375 mg	Levsin by Pegasus	55246-0970	Gastrointestinal
EL410	Tab, ER	Hyoscyamine Sulfate 0.375 mg	Levsin by Econolab	55053-0410	Gastrointestinal
EL410	Tab, Orange, Oblong, Scored	Hyoscyamine Sulfate 0.375 mg	Levsin by Murfreesboro	51129-1488	Gastrointestinal
EL444	Cap, Light Blue	Trimethobenzamide HCl 250 mg	Tigan by Breckenridge	51991-0625	Antiemetic
EL444	Cap, Dark Blue & Light Blue	Trimethobenzamide HCl 250 mg	by Anabolic	00722-6149	Antiemetic
EL444	Cap	Trimethobenzamide HCl 250 mg	by URL Mutual	00677-1383	Antiemetic
EL5	Tab, White to Off-White, Barrel Shaped, Scored, EL / 5 <> Cobalt Logo	Enalapril Maleate 5 mg	Vasotec by Cobalt	Canadian DIN 02291886	Antihypertensive
EL518	Tab, Pink, Oval	Pseudoephedrine 60 mg, Chlorpheniramine 4 mg, Acetaminophen 650 mg	by Econolab		Cold Remedy
EL522	Tab, White, Round, Scored	Dyphylline 200 mg, Guaifenesin 200 mg	Dyphylline GG by H J Harkins Co	52959-0482	Antiasthmatic; Expectorant
EL522	Tab	Dyphylline 200 mg, Guaifenesin 200 mg	by Econolab	55053-0522	Antiasthmatic; Expectorant
EL522	Tab	Dyphylline 200 mg, Guaifenesin 200 mg	by Pegasus	55246-0953	Antiasthmatic; Expectorant
EL524	Cap, Clear & Yellow	Chlorpheniramine Maleate 4 mg, Phenylephrine HCl 50 mg, Phenyltoloxamine Citrate 20 mg	Comhist LA by Econolab		Cold Remedy
EL525	Tab, Coated, EL/525	Belladonna Alkaloid Malate 125 mcg, Caffeine 100 mg, Ergotamine Tartrate 1 mg, Pentobarbital Sodium 30 mg	Micomp PB by Anabolic	00722-6090	Gastrointestinal; C III
EL717	Tab	Hyoscyamine Sulfate 0.125 mg	Levsin by Pegasus	55246-0949	Gastrointestinal
EL717	Tab, Light Blue Green	Hyoscyamine Sulfate 0.125 mg	Levsin by Econolab	55053-0717	Gastrointestinal
EL717	Tab	Hyoscyamine Sulfate 0.125 mg	Levsin by URL Mutual	00677-1536	Gastrointestinal
EL730	Tab, EL-730	Yohimbine HCl 5.4 mg	by Major	00904-3255	Impotence Agent
EL730	Tab	Yohimbine HCl 5.4 mg	by Pegasus	55246-0947	Impotence Agent
EL740	Cap, Ex Release	Chlorpheniramine Maleate 8 mg, Pseudoephedrine HCl 120 mg	Colfed A by Pharmafab	62542-0253	Cold Remedy
EL740	Cap, Black Print, White Beads	Chlorpheniramine Maleate 8 mg, Pseudoephedrine HCl 120 mg	Colfed A by Econolab	55053-0740	Cold Remedy
EL740	Cap	Chlorpheniramine Maleate 8 mg, Pseudoephedrine HCl 120 mg	N D Clear by Seatrace	00551-0147	Cold Remedy
EL740	Cap, Black Print, White Beads	Chlorpheniramine Maleate 8 mg, Pseudoephedrine HCl 120 mg	by Moore	00839-7178	Cold Remedy
EL740	Cap	Chlorpheniramine Maleate 8 mg, Pseudoephedrine HCl 120 mg	by Ivax	00182-1151	Cold Remedy
EL800	Cap, Clear, Red Beads, EL-800	Chlorpheniramine Maleate 4 mg, Pseudoephedrine HCl 60 mg	Dynahist ER by Breckenridge	51991-0217	Cold Remedy
EL800	Cap, Ex Release	Chlorpheniramine Maleate 4 mg, Pseudoephedrine HCl 60 mg	Dynafed by Pharmafab	62542-0201	Cold Remedy

ID FRONT <> BACK	DESCRIPTION FRONT <> BACK	INGREDIENT & STRENGTH	BRAND (or Generic Equiv.) by FIRM	NDC#	CLASS; SCH.
EL840	Tab, Coated	Ascorbic Acid 120 mg, Calcium 250 mg, Copper 2 mg, Cyanocobalamin 12 mcg, Docusate Sodium 50 mg, Folic Acid 1 mg, Iodine 0.15 mg, Iron 90 mg, Niacinamide 20 mg, Pyridoxine HCl 20 mg, Riboflavin 3.4 mg, Thiamine Mononitrate 3 mg, Vitamin A Acetate 4000 Units, Vitamin D 400 Units, Vitamin E 30 Units, Zinc 25 mg	Obnate 90 by Intertech	60917-0001	Vitamin
EL860	Cap	Guaifenesin 250 mg, Pseudoephedrine HCl 120 mg	Sudafed Sinus by URL Mutual	00677-1503	Cold Remedy
EL860	Cap	Guaifenesin 250 mg, Pseudoephedrine HCl 120 mg	Sudafed Sinus by Econolab	55053-0860	Cold Remedy
EL860	Cap, Ex Release	Guaifenesin 250 mg, Pseudoephedrine HCl 120 mg	Sudafed Sinus by Pharmafab	62542-0452	Cold Remedy
EL870	Cap, Ex Release	Guaifenesin 300 mg, Pseudoephedrine HCl 60 mg	Sudafed Sinus by Pharmafab	62542-0401	Cold Remedy
EL870	Cap, Black Print, White Beads	Guaifenesin 300 mg, Pseudoephedrine HCl 60 mg	Sudafed Sinus by Econolab	55053-0870	Cold Remedy
EL880	Cap, Clear & White	Lipase, Protease, Amylase	Creon-10 by Econolab		Gastrointestinal
EL890	Tab, Coated	Ascorbic Acid 100 mg, Biotin 30 mcg, Calcium 250 mg, Chromium 25 mcg, Copper 2 mg, Cyanocobalamin 12 mcg, Folic Acid 1 mg, Iodine 150 mcg, Iron 60 mg, Magnesium 25 mg, Manganese 5 mg, Molybdenum 25 mcg, Niacinamide 20 mg, Pantothenic Acid 10 mg, Pyridoxine HCl 10 mg, Riboflavin 3.4 mg, Thiamine Mononitrate 3 mg, Vitamin A Acetate 5000 Units, Vitamin D 400 Units, Vitamin E Acetate 30 Units, Zinc 25 mg	Preterna by Intertech	60917-0002	Vitamin
EL950	Tab, Film Coated	Ascorbic Acid 70 mg, Calcium 200 mg, Cyanocobalamin 2.2 mcg, Folic Acid 1 mg, Iodine 175 mcg, Iron 65 mg, Magnesium 100 mg, Niacin 17 mg, Pyridoxine HCl 2.2 mg, Riboflavin 1.6 mg, Selenium 65 mcg, Thiamine Mononitrate 1.5 mg, Vitamin A 4000 Units, Vitamin D 400 Units, Vitamin E 10 Units, Zinc 15 mg	Zitamin by Intertech	60917-0003	Vitamin
ELAVIL <> 40	Tab, Blue, Round, Film Coated	Amitriptyline HCl 10 mg	Elavil by Zeneca	00310-0040	Antidepressant
ELAVIL <> 40	Tab, Blue, Round, Film Coated	Amitriptyline HCl 10 mg	Elavil by H J Harkins Co	52959-0396	Antidepressant
ELAVIL <> 41	Tab, Beige, Round, Film Coated	Amitriptyline HCl 50 mg	Elavil by Zeneca	00310-0041	Antidepressant
ELAVIL <> 42	Tab, Orange, Round, Film Coated	Amitriptyline HCl 75 mg	Elavil by Zeneca	00310-0042	Antidepressant
ELAVIL <> 43	Tab, Mauve, Round, Film Coated	Amitriptyline HCl 100 mg	Elavil by Zeneca	00310-0043	Antidepressant
ELAVIL <> 43	Tab, Film Coated	Amitriptyline HCl 100 mg	Elavil by Merck	00006-0435	Antidepressant
ELAVIL <> 45	Tab, Yellow, Round	Amitriptyline HCl 25 mg	Elavil by Rightpak	65240-0637	Antidepressant
ELAVIL <> 45	Tab, Yellow, Round, Film Coated	Amitriptyline HCl 25 mg	Elavil by Zeneca	00310-0045	Antidepressant
ELAVIL <> 45	Tab, Film Coated	Amitriptyline HCl 25 mg	Elavil by Physician Total Care	54868-0409	Antidepressant
ELAVIL <> 47	Tab, Blue, Cap Shaped, Film Coated	Amitriptyline HCl 150 mg	Elavil by Zeneca	00310-0047	Antidepressant
ELAVILSTUART45	Tab, Film Coated	Amitriptyline HCl 25 mg	Elavil by Allscripts		Antidepressant
ELDEPRYL5MG	Cap, Aqua Blue, Opaque, Eldepryl/5 mg <> Somerset Logo	Selegiline 5 mg	Eldepryl by UDL	51079-0887	Antiparkinson
ELDEPRYL5MG	Cap, Aqua Blue, Opaque, Eldepryl/5 mg <> Somerset Logo	Selegiline 5 mg	Eldepryl by Somerset	39506-0022	Antiparkinson
ELDER600	Cap, Salmon	Methoxsalen 10 mg	Oxsoralen by ICN		Dermatologic
ELN30	Tab, Brownish-Red, Round, Ex Release, ELN over 30	Nifedipine 30 mg	Procardia XL by Teva	00093-1021	Antihypertensive
ELN30	Tab, Brownish-Red, Round, Ex Release, ELN over 30	Nifedipine 30 mg	Adalat CC by Watson	00591-3193	Antihypertensive
ELN60	Tab, Brownish-Red, Round, Ex Release, ELN over 60	Nifedipine 60 mg	Adalat CC by Watson	00591-3194	Antihypertensive
ELP10	Tab, Pink, Round	Enalapril Maleate 10 mg	Vasotec by Mova	55370-0924	Antihypertensive
ELP10	Tab, Pink, Round	Enalapril Maleate 10 mg	Vasotec by LEK	66685-0303	Antihypertensive
ELP20	Tab, Gray, Round	Enalapril Maleate 20 mg	Vasotec by Mova	55370-0925	Antihypertensive
ELP20	Tab, Gray, Round	Enalapril Maleate 20 mg	Vasotec by LEK	66685-0304	Antihypertensive
ELP212	Tab, Light Yellow, Round, Scored	Enalapril Maleate 2.5 mg	Vasotec by Mova	55370-0922	Antihypertensive
ELP212	Tab, Light Yellow, Round, Scored	Enalapril Maleate 2.5 mg	Vasotec by LEK	66685-0301	Antihypertensive
ELP5	Tab, Pink, Round, Scored	Enalapril Maleate 5 mg	Vasotec by LEK	66685-0302	Antihypertensive
ELP5	Tab, Pink, Round, Scored	Enalapril Maleate 5 mg	Vasotec by Mova	55370-0923	Antihypertensive
EM	Tab, White, Round	Dyphylline 200 mg	Dyflex by Lemmon		Antiasthmatic
EM	Tab, Pink, Round, Schering Logo EM	Ethinyl Estradiol 0.05 mg	Estinyl by Schering		Hormone
EM10	Tab, White to Off-White, Round, Scored, EM over 10	Methimazole 10 mg	Tapazole by Par	49884-0641	Antithyroid

ID FRONT <> BACK	DESCRIPTION FRONT <> BACK	INGREDIENT & STRENGTH	BRAND (or Generic Equiv.) by FIRM	NDC#	CLASS; SCH.
EM100	Tab, Off-White, Round, Scored	Levothyroxine Sodium 100 mcg	Novothyrox by Genpharm	55567-0134	Thyroid Hormone
EM100	Tab, Yellow, Round, Scored	Levothyroxine Sodium 100 mcg	Novothyrox by Ivax	00182-2711 Discontinued	Thyroid Hormone
EM100	Tab, Yellow, Round, Scored	Levothyroxine Sodium 100 mcg	Levoxyl by Genpharm	15330-0191	Thyroid Hormone
EM100	Tab, Yellow, Round, Scored	Levothyroxine Sodium 100 mcg	Euthyrox by Genpharm	Canadian DIN 02264374	Thyroid Hormone
EM112	Tab, Rose, Round, Scored	Levothyroxine Sodium 112 mcg	Euthyrox by Genpharm	Canadian DIN 02264390	Thyroid Hormone
EM112	Tab, Rose, Round, Scored	Levothyroxine Sodium 112 mcg	Levoxyl by Genpharm	15330-0192	Thyroid Hormone
EM112	Tab, Rose, Round, Scored	Levothyroxine Sodium 112 mcg	Novothyrox by Ivax	00182-2712 Discontinued	Thyroid Hormone
EM112	Tab, Off-White, Round, Scored	Levothyroxine Sodium 112 mcg	Novothyrox by Genpharm	55567-0135	Thyroid Hormone
EM125	Tab, Off-White, Round, Scored	Levothyroxine Sodium 125 mcg	Novothyrox by Genpharm	55567-0136	Thyroid Hormone
EM125	Tab, Brown, Round, Scored	Levothyroxine Sodium 125 mcg	Novothyrox by Ivax	00182-2713 Discontinued	Thyroid Hormone
EM125	Tab, Brown, Round, Scored	Levothyroxine Sodium 125 mcg	Levoxyl by Genpharm	15330-0193	Thyroid Hormone
EM125	Tab, Brown, Round, Scored	Levothyroxine Sodium 125 mcg	Euthyrox by Genpharm	Canadian DIN 02264404	Thyroid Hormone
EM137	Tab, Blue, Round, Scored	Levothyroxine Sodium 137 mcg	Euthyrox by Genpharm	Canadian DIN 02264412	Thyroid Hormone
EM137	Tab, Off-White, Round, Scored	Levothyroxine Sodium 137 mcg	Novothyrox by Genpharm	55567-0137	Thyroid Hormone
EM150	Tab, Off-White, Round, Scored	Levothyroxine Sodium 150 mcg	Novothyrox by Genpharm	55567-0138	Thyroid Hormone
EM150	Tab, Blue, Round, Scored	Levothyroxine Sodium 150 mcg	Euthyrox by Genpharm	Canadian DIN 02264420	Thyroid Hormone
EM150	Tab, Blue, Round, Scored	Levothyroxine Sodium 150 mcg	Levoxyl by Genpharm	15330-0195	Thyroid Hormone
EM150	Tab, Blue, Round, Scored	Levothyroxine Sodium 150 mcg	Novothyrox by Ivax	00182-2714 Discontinued	Thyroid Hormone
EM175	Tab, Lilac, Round, Scored	Levothyroxine Sodium 175 mcg	Novothyrox by Ivax	00182-2715 Discontinued	Thyroid Hormone
EM175	Tab, Lilac, Round, Scored	Levothyroxine Sodium 175 mcg	Levoxyl by Genpharm	15330-0196	Thyroid Hormone
EM175	Tab, Lilac, Round, Scored	Levothyroxine Sodium 175 mcg	Euthyrox by Genpharm	Canadian DIN 02264439	Thyroid Hormone
EM175	Tab, Off-White, Round, Scored	Levothyroxine Sodium 175 mcg	Novothyrox by Genpharm	55567-0139	Thyroid Hormone
EM20	Tab, White to Off-White, Round, EM over 20	Methimazole 20 mg	Tapazole by Par	49884-0689	Antithyroid
EM200	Tab, Off-White, Round, Scored	Levothyroxine Sodium 200 mcg	Novothyrox by Genpharm	55567-0140	Thyroid Hormone
EM200	Tab, Pink, Round, Scored	Levothyroxine Sodium 200 mcg	Euthyrox by Genpharm	Canadian DIN 02264447	Thyroid Hormone
EM200	Tab, Pink, Round, Scored	Levothyroxine Sodium 200 mcg	Levoxyl by Genpharm	15330-0197	Thyroid Hormone
EM200	Tab, Pink, Round, Scored	Levothyroxine Sodium 200 mcg	Novothyrox by Ivax	00182-2716 Discontinued	Thyroid Hormone
EM25	Tab, Orange, Round, Scored	Levothyroxine Sodium 25 mcg	Novothyrox by Ivax	00182-2707 Discontinued	Thyroid Hormone
EM25	Tab, Orange, Round, Scored	Levothyroxine Sodium 25 mcg	Levoxyl by Genpharm	15330-0187	Thyroid Hormone
EM25	Tab, Orange, Round, Scored	Levothyroxine Sodium 25 mcg	Euthyrox by Genpharm	Canadian DIN 02264323	Thyroid Hormone
EM25	Tab, Off-White, Round, Scored	Levothyroxine Sodium 25 mcg	Novothyrox by Genpharm	55567-0130	Thyroid Hormone
EM300	Tab, Off-White, Round, Scored	Levothyroxine Sodium 300 mcg	Novothyrox by Genpharm	55567-0141	Thyroid Hormone
EM300	Tab, Green, Round, Scored	Levothyroxine Sodium 300 mcg	Euthyrox by Genpharm	Canadian DIN 02264455	Thyroid Hormone
EM300	Tab, Green, Round, Scored	Levothyroxine Sodium 300 mcg	Levoxyl by Genpharm	15330-0198	Thyroid Hormone

ID FRONT <> BACK	DESCRIPTION FRONT <> BACK	INGREDIENT & STRENGTH	BRAND (or Generic Equiv.) by FIRM	NDC#	CLASS; SCH.
EM300	Tab, Green, Round, Scored	Levothyroxine Sodium 300 mcg	Novothyrox by Ivax	00182-2717 Discontinued	Thyroid Hormone
EM5	Tab, White to Off-White, Round, Scored, EM over 5	Methimazole 5 mg	Tapazole by Par	49884-0640	Antithyroid
EM50	Tab, White, Round, Scored	Levothyroxine Sodium 50 mcg	Novothyrox by Ivax	00182-2708 Discontinued	Thyroid Hormone
EM50	Tab, White, Round, Scored	Levothyroxine Sodium 50 mcg	Levoxyl by Genpharm	15330-0188	Thyroid Hormone
EM50	Tab, White, Round, Scored	Levothyroxine Sodium 50 mcg	Euthyrox by Genpharm	Canadian DIN 02264331	Thyroid Hormone
EM50	Tab, Off-White, Round, Scored	Levothyroxine Sodium 50 mcg	Novothyrox by Genpharm	55567-0131	Thyroid Hormone
EM75	Tab, Off-White, Round, Scored	Levothyroxine Sodium 75 mcg	Novothyrox by Genpharm	55567-0132	Thyroid Hormone
EM75	Tab, Violet, Round, Scored	Levothyroxine Sodium 75 mcg	Euthyrox by Genpharm	Canadian DIN 02264358	Thyroid Hormone
EM75	Tab, Violet, Round, Scored	Levothyroxine Sodium 75 mcg	Levoxyl by Genpharm	15330-0189	Thyroid Hormone
EM75	Tab, Violet, Round, Scored	Levothyroxine Sodium 75 mcg	Novothyrox by Ivax	00182-2709 Discontinued	Thyroid Hormone
EM88	Tab, Olive, Round, Scored	Levothyroxine Sodium 88 mcg	Levoxyl by Genpharm	15330-0190	Thyroid Hormone
EM88	Tab, Olive, Round, Scored	Levothyroxine Sodium 88 mcg	Euthyrox by Genpharm	Canadian DIN 02264366	Thyroid Hormone
EM88	Tab, Olive, Round, Scored	Levothyroxine Sodium 88 mcg	Novothyrox by Ivax	00182-2710 Discontinued	Thyroid Hormone
EM88	Tab, Off-White, Round, Scored	Levothyroxine Sodium 88 mcg	Novothyrox by Genpharm	55567-0133	Thyroid Hormone
EMBEDA100	Cap, Dark Green Cap and Light Green Body, Opaque, Grey Band and Circle	Morphine 100 mg, Naltrexone HCl 4 mg	Embeda by King	60793-0437	Opioid Analgesic; C II
EMBEDA20	Cap, Dark Yellow Cap and Light Yellow Body, Opaque, Grey Band and Circle	Morphine 20 mg, Naltrexone HCl 0.8 mg	Embeda by King	60793-0430	Opioid Analgesic; C II
EMBEDA30	Cap, Dark Blue Violate Cap and Light Blue Violet Body, Opaque, Grey Band and Circle	Morphine 30 mg, Naltrexone HCl 1.2 mg	Embeda by King	60793-0431	Opioid Analgesic; C II
EMBEDA50	Cap, Dark Blue Cap and Light Blue Body, Opaque, Grey Band and Circle	Morphine 50 mg, Naltrexone HCl 2 mg	Embeda by King	60793-0433	Opioid Analgesic; C II
EMBEDA60	Cap, Dark Pink Cap and Light Pink Body, Opaque, Grey Band and Circle	Morphine 60 mg, Naltrexone HCl 2.4 mg	Embeda by King	60793-0434	Opioid Analgesic; C II
EMBEDA80	Cap, Dark Peach Cap and Light Peach Body, Opaque, Grey Band and Circle	Morphine 80 mg, Naltrexone HCl 3.2 mg	Embeda by King	60793-0435	Opioid Analgesic; C II
EMBEL320	Tab	Amylase 30,000 Units, Lipase 8000 Units, Protease 30,000 Units	Pancrelipase by Ivax	00182-1741	Gastrointestinal
EMPRACET30K9B	Tab, Peach, Round	Acetaminophen 300 mg, Codeine Phosphate 30 mg	Tylenol w/ Codeine by GSK	Canadian	Analgesic; C III
EMPRACET60L9B	Tab, Peach, Round	Acetaminophen 300 mg, Codeine Phosphate 60 mg	Tylenol w/ Codeine by GSK	Canadian	Analgesic; C III
EMTEC30	Tab, Peach, Round, Scored, Emtec-30	Acetaminophen 300 mg, Codeine Phosphate 30 mg	Tylenol w/ Codeine by AltiMed	Canadian DIN 00608882	Analgesic; C III
EMYCIN250MG	Tab, Black Print	Erythromycin 250 mg	E Mycin by PDRX	52289-0120	Antibiotic
EMYCIN250MG	Tab, Black Print	Erythromycin 250 mg	E Mycin by Casa DeAmigos	62138-6304	Antibiotic
EMYCIN333MG	Tab, White, Orange Print, Round	Erythromycin 333 mg	E Mycin by Rx Pak	65084-0223	Antibiotic
EMYCIN333MG	Tab, White, Orange Print, Round	Erythromycin 333 mg	E Mycin by Amerisource	62584-0208	Antibiotic
EMYCIN333MG	Tab, White, Orange Print, Round	Erythromycin 333 mg	E Mycin by Drug Distr	52985-0180	Antibiotic
EMYCIN333MG	Tab, White, Orange Print, Round	Erythromycin 333 mg	E Mycin by Urgent Care Center	50716-0376	Antibiotic
EMYCIN333MG	Tab, White, Orange Print, Round	Erythromycin 333 mg	E Mycin by Prestige	58056-0194	Antibiotic
EMYCIN333MG	Tab, White, Orange Print, Round	Erythromycin 333 mg	E Mycin by Nat Pharmpak	55154-0504	Antibiotic
EMYCIN333MG	Tab, White, Orange Print, Round	Erythromycin 333 mg	E Mycin by Rightpak	65240-0645	Antibiotic
EN10 <> G	Tab, Orangish-Red, Oval	Enalapril Maleate 10 mg	Vasotec by Par	49884-0593	Antihypertensive
EN20 <> G	Tab, Peach, Oval, Scored	Enalapril Maleate 20 mg	Vasotec by Par	49884-0594	Antihypertensive
EN25 <> APO	Tab, White, Oval, Scored, EN / 2.5	Enalapril Maleate 2.5 mg	Vasotec by Apotex	Canadian DIN 02020025	Antihypertensive

ID FRONT <> BACK	DESCRIPTION FRONT <> BACK	INGREDIENT & STRENGTH	BRAND (or Generic Equiv.) by FIRM	NDC#	CLASS; SCH.
EN25 <> G	Tab, White, Round, Scored, EN/2.5	Enalapril Maleate 2.5 mg	Vasotec by Par	49884-0591	Antihypertensive
EN5 <> GG	Tab, White, Oval, Scored, G / G <> EN5	Enalapril Maleate 5 mg	Vasotec by Par	49884-0592	Antihypertensive
ENDO	Tab, Yellow	Oxycodone 5 mg, Aspirin 325 mg	Percodan by Dupont	Canadian	Analgesic; C II
ENDO	Tab, White	Oxycodone 5 mg, Acetaminophen 325 mg	Percocet by Dupont	Canadian	Analgesic; C II
ENDO	Tab, White, Oval	Selegiline 5 mg	Eldepryl by BMS	00056-0620	Antiparkinson
ENDO	Tab, White, Oval	Selegiline 5 mg	Eldepryl by Endo	60951-0620	Antiparkinson
ENDO <> 631	Tab, Film Coated	Cimetidine HCl 300 mg	Tagamet by Endo		Gastrointestinal
ENDO <> 721	Tab, Coated	Captopril 12.5 mg	Capoten by BMS	00056-0721	Antihypertensive
ENDO <> 721	Tab, White, Round, Partially Scored	Captopril 12.5 mg	Capoten by Endo	60951-0721	Antihypertensive
ENDO10010	Tab, Blue, Oval, Endo/100/10	Levodopa 100 mg, Carbidopa 10 mg	Sinemet by Endo	Canadian	Antiparkinson
ENDO10025	Tab, Yellow, Oval, Endo/100/25	Levodopa 100 mg, Carbidopa 25 mg	Sinemet by Endo	Canadian	Antiparkinson
ENDO25025	Tab, Light Blue, Oval, Endo/250/25	Levodopa 250 mg, Carbidopa 25 mg	Sinemet by Endo	Canadian	Antiparkinson
ENDO602	Tab, White, Round, Scored	Acetaminophen 325 mg, Oxycodone HCl 5 mg	Endocet by BMS	00590-0602	Analgesic; C II
ENDO602	Tab, White, Round, Scored	Acetaminophen 325 mg, Oxycodone HCl 5 mg	Endocet by Endo	60951-0602	Analgesic; C II
ENDO603	Tab, Dark Blue, Oval, Scored	Carbidopa 10 mg, Levodopa 100 mg	Sinemet by Endo	60951-0603	Antiparkinson
ENDO605	Tab, Yellow, Oval, Scored	Carbidopa 25 mg, Levodopa 100 mg	Sinemet by Endo	60951-0605	Antiparkinson
ENDO607	Tab, Light Blue, Oval, Scored	Carbidopa 25 mg, Levodopa 250 mg	Sinemet by Endo	60951-0607	Antiparkinson
ENDO610	Tab, Yellow, Round, Scored	Aspirin 325 mg, Oxycodone HCl 4.5 mg	Percodan by BMS	00590-0610	Analgesic; C II
ENDO610	Tab, Yellow, Round, Scored	Aspirin 325 mg, Oxycodone HCl 4.5 mg	Percodan by Endo	60951-0610	Analgesic; C II
ENDO630	Tab, White, Oval	Cimetidine HCl 200 mg	Tagamet by Endo	60951-0630	Gastrointestinal
ENDO631	Tab, White, Oval	Cimetidine HCl 300 mg	Tagamet by Endo	60951-0631	Gastrointestinal
ENDO631	Tab, White, Oval	Cimetidine HCl 300 mg	Tagamet by Amerisource	62584-0631	Gastrointestinal
ENDO631	Tab, White, Oval	Cimetidine HCl 300 mg	Tagamet by BMS	00056-0631	Gastrointestinal
ENDO632	Tab, White, Oval, Scored, Film Coated	Cimetidine HCl 400 mg	Tagamet by BMS	00056-0632	Gastrointestinal
ENDO632	Tab, White, Oval, Scored, Film Coated	Cimetidine HCl 400 mg	Tagamet by Amerisource	62584-0632	Gastrointestinal
ENDO632	Tab, White, Oval, Scored, Film Coated	Cimetidine HCl 400 mg	Tagamet by Endo	60951-0632	Gastrointestinal
ENDO632	Tab, White, Oval, Scored, Film Coated	Cimetidine HCl 400 mg	Tagamet by Med Pro	53978-2009	Gastrointestinal
ENDO633	Tab, White, Oval, Scored, Film Coated	Cimetidine HCl 800 mg	Tagamet by Endo	60951-0633	Gastrointestinal
ENDO688	Cap, Gelatin Coated	Etodolac 200 mg	by Endo	60951-0688	NSAID
ENDO688	Cap, Gelatin	Etodolac 200 mg	by BMS	00056-0688	NSAID
ENDO689	Cap, Gelatin Coated, Imprinted in Red	Etodolac 300 mg	by Endo	60951-0689	NSAID
ENDO689	Cap, Gelatin	Etodolac 300 mg	by BMS	00056-0689	NSAID
ENDO711	Tab, White, Round	Glipizide 5 mg	by Endo	60951-0711	Antidiabetic
ENDO714	Tab	Glipizide 10 mg	by BMS	00056-0714	Antidiabetic
ENDO714	Tab, White, Round	Glipizide 10 mg	by Endo	60951-0714	Antidiabetic
ENDO722	Tab, White, Round, Scored	Captopril 25 mg	Capoten by Direct Dispensing	57866-6106	Antihypertensive
ENDO722	Tab, White, Round, Scored	Captopril 25 mg	Capoten by Endo	60951-0722	Antihypertensive
ENDO722	Tab, White, Round, Scored	Captopril 25 mg	Capoten by BMS	00056-0722	Antihypertensive
ENDO724	Tab, White, Round, Scored	Captopril 50 mg	Capoten by BMS	00056-0724	Antihypertensive
ENDO724	Tab, White, Round, Scored	Captopril 50 mg	Capoten by Endo	60951-0724	Antihypertensive
ENDO727	Tab, White, Round, Scored	Captopril 100 mg	Capoten by BMS	00056-0727	Antihypertensive
ENDO727	Tab, White, Round, Scored	Captopril 100 mg	Capoten by Endo	60951-0727	Antihypertensive
ENDO731	Tab, Peach, Round, Scored	Captopril 50 mg, HCTZ 25 mg	Capozide by BMS	00056-0731	Antihypertensive; Diuretic
ENDO731	Tab, Peach, Round, Scored	Captopril 50 mg, HCTZ 25 mg	Capozide by Endo	60951-0731	Antihypertensive; Diuretic
ENDO733	Tab, White, Round, Scored	Captopril 25 mg, HCTZ 15 mg	Capozide by Endo	60951-0733	Antihypertensive; Diuretic
ENDO733	Tab, White, Round, Scored	Captopril 25 mg, HCTZ 15 mg	Capozide by BMS	00056-0733	Antihypertensive; Diuretic
ENDO739	Tab, White, Round, Scored	Captopril 50 mg, HCTZ 15 mg	Capozide by BMS	00056-0739	Antihypertensive; Diuretic
ENDO739	Tab, White, Round, Scored	Captopril 50 mg, HCTZ 15 mg	Capozide by Endo	60951-0739	Antihypertensive; Diuretic
ENDO741	Tab, Peach, Round, Scored	Captopril 25 mg, HCTZ 25 mg	Capozide by Endo	60951-0741	Antihypertensive; Diuretic
ENDO741	Tab, Peach, Round, Scored	Captopril 25 mg, HCTZ 25 mg	Capozide by BMS	00056-0741	Antihypertensive; Diuretic

ID FRONT <> BACK	DESCRIPTION FRONT <> BACK	INGREDIENT & STRENGTH	BRAND (or Generic Equiv.) by FIRM	NDC#	CLASS; SCH.
ENDO744	Tab, Pale Yellow, Oval	Etodolac 400 mg	Lodine by Endo	60951-0744	NSAID
ENDO744	Tab, Pale Yellow, Oval	Etodolac 400 mg	Lodine by BMS	00056-0744	NSAID
ENDURONA	Tab, Orange, Square, Scored, Enduron over Abbott Logo (a)	Methyclothiazide 2.5 mg	Enduron by Abbott	00074-6827 Discontinued	Diuretic; Antihypertensive
ENDURONA	Tab, Salmon, Square, Scored, Enduron over Abbott Logo (a)	Methyclothiazide 5 mg	Enduron by Abbott	00074-6812 Discontinued	Diuretic; Antihypertensive
ENE <> PP	Tab, Brown-Orange, Scored	Carbamazepine 400 mg	Tegretol by Pharmascience	Canadian DIN 02231544	Anticonvulsant
ENEENE <> CGCG	Tab, Brownish-Orange, Oval, Scored	Carbamazepine 400 mg	Tegretol by Geigy	Canadian DIN 00755583	Anticonvulsant
ENT	Tab, Ex Release	Brompheniramine Maleate 12 mg, Phenylpropanolamine HCl 75 mg	E N T by Sovereign	58716-0641	Cold Remedy
ENTEX01490412	Cap	Guaifenesin 200 mg, Phenylephrine HCl 5 mg, Phenylpropanolamine HCl 45 mg	Entex by Amerisource	62584-0412	Cold Remedy
ENTEX51479030	Tab	Guaifenesin 200 mg, Phenylephrine HCl 5 mg, Phenylpropanolamine HCl 45 mg	Entex by Welpharm	63375-6378	Cold Remedy
ENTEX51479030	Cap, Orange & White	Guaifenesin 200 mg, Phenylephrine HCl 5 mg, Phenylpropanolamine HCl 45 mg	Entex by Dura	51479-0030	Cold Remedy
ENTEXLA	Tab, Yellow, Cap-Shaped, Scored	Pseudoephedrine HCl 120 mg, Guaifenesin 600 mg	Entex LA by Purdue Pharma	Canadian DIN 02246971	Decongestant; Expectorant
ENTEXLA <> 01490436	Tab, Ex Release	Guaifenesin 400 mg, Phenylpropanolamine HCl 75 mg	Entex LA by Leiner	59606-0641	Cold Remedy
ENTEXLA <> 01490436	Tab	Guaifenesin 400 mg, Phenylpropanolamine HCl 75 mg	Entex LA by Nat Pharmpak	55154-2303	Cold Remedy
ENTEXLA <> 01490436	Tab	Guaifenesin 400 mg, Phenylpropanolamine HCl 75 mg	Entex LA by Urgent Care Center	50716-0436	Cold Remedy
ENTEXLA <> 01490436	Tab	Guaifenesin 400 mg, Phenylpropanolamine HCl 75 mg	Entex LA by Amerisource	62584-0436	Cold Remedy
ENTEXLA <> 01490436	Tab	Guaifenesin 400 mg, Phenylpropanolamine HCl 75 mg	Entex LA by Caremark	00339-5128	Cold Remedy
ENTEXLA <> 033033	Tab, Film Coated	Guaifenesin 400 mg, Phenylpropanolamine HCl 75 mg	Entex LA by Welpharm	63375-6377	Cold Remedy
ENTEXLA <> 033033	Tab, Orange, Scored	Guaifenesin 400 mg, Phenylpropanolamine HCl 75 mg	Entex LA by Dura	51479-0033	Cold Remedy
ENTEXLA <> 033033	Tab, Orange, Oblong, Scored	Guaifenesin 400 mg, Phenylpropanolamine HCl 75 mg	Entex LA by Martec		Cold Remedy
ENTEXPSE <> 032032	Tab, Film Coated, Entex PSE <> 032 over 032	Guaifenesin 600 mg, Pseudoephedrine HCl 120 mg	Entex PSE by Welpharm	63375-6376	Cold Remedy
ENTEXPSE <> 032032	Tab, Yellow, Scored, Film Coated	Guaifenesin 600 mg, Pseudoephedrine HCl 120 mg	Entex PSE by Dura	51479-0032	Cold Remedy
ENTOCORTEC3MG	Cap, Light Grey & Pink, Opaque, Hard Gel	Budesonide 3 mg	Entocort EC by AstraZeneca	00186-0702	Steroid
ENTROPHEN325MG	Tab, Brown, Round, Film Coated	Acetaminophen 325 mg	Entrophen by Johnson & Johnson	Canadian DIN 0010332	Analgesic
ENTROPHEN325MG	Cap, Yellow, Film Coated	Acetaminophen 325 mg	Entrophen by Johnson & Johnson	Canadian DIN 02050161	Analgesic
ENTROPHEN500MG	Tab, Pink, Oval, Film Coated	Acetaminophen 500 mg	Tylenol Ex Strength by Johnson & Johnson	Canadian DIN 00852015	Analgesic
ENTROPHEN650MG	Cap, Orange, Film Coated	Acetaminophen 650 mg	Tylenol by Johnson & Johnson	Canadian DIN 01905392	Analgesic
ENTROPHEN650MG	Tab, Orange, Oval, Film Coated	Acetaminophen 650 mg	Tylenol by Johnson & Johnson	Canadian DIN 00010340	Analgesic
ENTROPHEN975MG	Tab, Yellow, Oval	Acetaminophen 975 mg	Tylenol by Johnson & Johnson	Canadian	Analgesic
EON720	Cap, Green & Clear, Eon Logo 720	Indomethacin 75 mg	Indocin SR by Allscripts		NSAID
EP	Tab, Peach, Round, Schering Logo EP	Ethinyl Estradiol 0.5 mg	Estinyl by Schering		Hormone
EP102	Tab, Green, Round, Scored	Belladonna Alkaloids 0.2 mg, Ergotamine Tartrate 0.6 mg, Phenobarbital 40 mg	Bellamine S by Qualitest	00603-2424	Gastrointestinal; C IV
EP102	Tab, Green, Round, Scored	Belladonna Alkaloids 0.2 mg, Ergotamine Tartrate 0.6 mg, Phenobarbital 40 mg	Bellamine S by Excellium	64125-0102	Gastrointestinal; C IV
EP103	Tab, White, Round, Scored	Pseudoephedrine HCl 60 mg	by RX Pak	65084-0107	Decongestant
EP103	Tab, White, Round, Scored	Pseudoephedrine HCl 60 mg	by RX Pak	65084-0108	Decongestant
EP104	Tab, White, Round	Colchicine 0.6 mg	Colchicine by Excellium	64125-0104	Antigout

ID FRONT <> BACK	DESCRIPTION FRONT <> BACK	INGREDIENT & STRENGTH	BRAND (or Generic Equiv.) by FIRM	NDC#	CLASS; SCH.
EP104	Tab, White, Round	Colchicine 0.6 mg	Colchicine by URL	00677-1683	Antigout
EP104	Tab, White, Round, EP 104	Colchicine 0.6 mg	by DJ Pharma	64455-0005	Antigout
EP104	Tab, White, Round	Colchicine 0.6 mg	by Dixon Shane	17236-0655	Antigout
EP105	Tab, Green, Oval	Magnesium Salicylate 600 mg, Phenyltoloxamine 25 mg	by Nat Pharmpak	55154-5237	Analgesic
EP105	Tab, Green, Oblong, Bisected	Magnesium Salicylate 600 mg, Phenyltoloxamine 25 mg	by Nat Pharmpak	55154-5241	Analgesic
EP105	Tablet, White, Oblong, Scored	Phenyltoloxamine 25 mg, Magnesium Salicylate 600 mg	Mag-Phen by Rising	64980-0101	Analgesic
EP105	Tab, Green, Oblong, Bisected	Phenyltoloxamine Citrate 25 mg, Magnesium Salicylate Tetrahydrate Citrate 600 mg	by Physician Total Care	54868-2469	Cold Remedy
EP106	Tab, White, Oval, EP-106	Aspirin 800 mg	ZORprin Tablets by Excellium	64125-0106	Analgesic
EP106	Tab, White, Oval, EP-106	Aspirin 800 mg	Zero-Order by Cypress	60258-0052	Analgesic
EP107	Tab, White, Round, Scored	Acetaminophen 500 mg	Tylenol by Excellium	64125-0107	Analgesic
EP107	Cap, Orange Opaque Body, Hard Gelatin, Filled with White to Off White Pellets, Extended Release	Acetazolamide 500 mg	Diamox by Zydus	68382-0261	Antiglaucoma Agent
EP110	Tab, Orange, Cap Shaped, ER	Hyoscyamine Sulfate 0.375 mg	Levbid by Excellium	64125-0110	Gastrointestinal
EP112	Tab, White, Oval	Magnesium Salicylate Tetrahydrate 600 mg, Phenyltoloxamine 25 mg	Mag-Sal by Excellium	64125-0112	Supplement
EP112	Tab, White, Oval	Magnesium Salicylate Tetrahydrate 600 mg, Phenyltoloxamine 25 mg	MagPhen by Rising	64980-0101	Supplement
EP116	Tab, White, Round	Furosemide 20 mg	Lasix by Excellium	64125-0116	Diuretic
EP120	Cap, White	Quinine Sulfate 325 mg	Quinine SO4 by Excellium	64125-0120	Antimalarial
EP121	Tab, White, Round	Quinine Sulfate 260 mg	Quinine SO4 by Excellium	64125-0121	Antimalarial
EP125	Tab, White, Round, Scored, EP 12.5	Ephedrine 12.5 mg, Guaifenesin 200 mg	by Ultratab		Cold Remedy
EP126	Tab, Off White, Cap Shaped	Guaifenesin 1200, Dextromethorphan HBr 60 mg	Aquatab DM by Excellium	64125-0126	Cold Remedy
EP128	Tab, White, Round	Belladonna, Phenobarbital 16.2 mg	Donnatal by Excellium	64125-0128	Gastrointestinal; C IV
EP128	Tab, White, Round	Belladonna, Phenobarbital 16.2 mg	Haponal by URL	00677-1685	Gastrointestinal; C IV
EP225	Tab, White, Round	Ephedrine HCl 25 mg, Guaifenesin 200 mg	Ephedrine Plus Tabs by Ultratab	62959-0320	Cold Remedy
EP901	Tab, White, Round, Scored	Phenobarbital 30 mg	Phenobarb by Excellium	64125-0901	Sedative/Hypnotic; C IV
EP902	Tab, White, Round, Scored	Phenobarbital 60 mg	Phenobarb by Excellium	64125-0902	Sedative/Hypnotic; C IV
EP903	Tab, White, Round, Scored	Phenobarbital 100 mg	Phenobarb Tabs by Excellium	64125-0903	Sedative/Hypnotic; C IV
EP905 <> 1	Tab, White, Round	Lorazepam 1 mg	Ativan by Excellium	64125-0905	Antianxiety; C IV
EP915	Tab, White, Round	Phenobarbital 15 mg	Phenobarbital by Excellium	64125-0915	Sedative/Hypnotic; C IV
EP915	Tab, White, Round	Phenobarbital 15 mg	Phenobarbital by URL Mutual	00677-1731	Sedative/Hypnotic; C IV
EPH325224/3850	Cap, Crimson, EPH 325 224/3850	Ephedra 325 mg	Ephedra 325 by NVE		Supplement
EPI101	Cap, Red & White	Dichloralphenazone 100 mg, Acetaminophen 325 mg, Isometheptene Mucate 65 mg	Migratine by Excellium	64125-0101	Antimigraine; C IV
EPI132 <> 5	Tab, White, Round, Scored, EPI over 132 <> 5	Oxycodone HCl 5 mg	Percolone by Endo	63481-0132	Analgesic; C II
EPI132 <> 5	Tab, White, Round, Scored, EPI over 132 <> 5	Oxycodone HCl 5 mg	Percolone by BMS	00056-0132	Analgesic; C II
EPITOL <> 9393	Tab, White, Round, Scored, 93 over 93	Carbamazepine 200 mg	Tegretol by Teva	00093-0090	Anticonvulsant
EPITOL <> 9393	Tab, White, Round, Scored, 93 over 93	Carbamazepine 200 mg	Tegretol by Caremark	00339-6132	Anticonvulsant
EQUAGESIC	Tab, White & Yellow, Equa-Gesic	Aspirin 75 mg, Ethoheptazine 250 mg, Meprobamate 200 mg	Equagesic by Wyeth	Canadian	Sedative/Hypnotic; C IV
EQUANIL400	Tab, White	Meprobamate 400 mg	Equanil by Wyeth	Canadian	Sedative/Hypnotic; C IV
ER	Tab, Beige, Round, Schering Logo ER	Ethinyl Estradiol 0.02 mg	Estinyl by Schering		Hormone
ER <> 0375	Tab, White to Off White, Round, Ex Release, "0.375" <> ER	Pramipexole DiHCl 0.375 mg	Mirapex ER by Boehringer Ingelheim	00597-0109	Antiparkinson
ER <> 075	Tab, White to Off White, Round, Ex Release, "0.75" <> ER	Pramipexole DiHCl 0.75 mg	Mirapex ER by Boehringer Ingelheim	00597-0285	Antiparkinson
ER <> 15	Tab, White to Off-White, Oval, Ex Release, "1.5" <> ER	Pramipexole DiHCl 1.5 mg	Mirapex ER by Boehringer Ingelheim	00597-0113	Antiparkinson
ER <> 30	Tab, White to Off-White, Oval, Ex Release, "3.0" <> ER	Pramipexole DiHCl 3.0 mg	Mirapex ER by Boehringer Ingelheim	00597-0115	Antiparkinson
ER <> 45	Tab, White to Off-White, Oval, Ex Release, "4.5" <> ER	Pramipexole DiHCl 4.5 mg	Mirapex ER by Boehringer Ingelheim	00597-0116	Antiparkinson
ER <> CIBA	Tab, Brownish-Yellow, Round, Film Coated	Maprotiline 50 mg	Ludiomil by Novartis	Canadian DIN 00360503	Antidepressant
ERCIBA	Tab, Brown & Yellow, Round, ER/Ciba	Maprotiline 50 mg	Ludiomil by Ciba	Canadian	Antidepressant
EREX	Tab	Yohimbine HCl 5.4 mg	Erex by Sovereign	58716-0613	Impotence Agent
ERVA54	Tab, White, Round, Erva 5.4	Yohimbine HCl 5.4 mg	by Royce	51875-0361	Impotence Agent

ID FRONT <> BACK	DESCRIPTION FRONT <> BACK	INGREDIENT & STRENGTH	BRAND (or Generic Equiv.) by FIRM	NDC#	CLASS; SCH.
ERYC250MG	Cap, Orange and Clear, Orange and White Beads	Erythromycin 250 mg	Eryc by Warner Chilcott	00430-0696	Antibiotic
ERYC333MG-PARKEDAVIS	Cap, Clear & Yellow, Eryc/333 mg	Erythromycin 333 mg	Eryc by Pfizer	Canadian DIN 00873454	Antibiotic
ERYCPD696	Cap, P-D 696	Erythromycin 250 mg	by Allscripts		Antibiotic
ERYCPD696	Cap, P-D 696	Erythromycin 250 mg	Eryc by Parke Davis	00071-0696	Antibiotic
ERYCPD696	Cap, Clear & Orange	Erythromycin 250 mg	by Murfreesboro	51129-1422	Antibiotic
ERYCPD696	Cap, Clear & Orange, Opaque	Erythromycin 250 mg	Eryc by Parke Davis	Canadian DIN 00607142	Antibiotic
ES <> A	Tab, Pink, Round, Film Coated, Abbott Logo (a)	Erythromycin Stearate 250 mg	by Pharmedix	53002-0270	Antibiotic
ES <> A	Tab, Pink, Round, Film Coated, Abbott Logo (a)	Erythromycin Stearate 250 mg	by Allscripts		Antibiotic
ES <> A	Tab, Pink, Round, Film Coated, Abbott Logo (a)	Erythromycin Stearate 250 mg	Erythrocin by Abbott	00074-6346	Antibiotic
ESB	Tab, White, Oval	Aspirin 500 mg	Bufferin by BMS	19810-0717	Analgesic
ESB	Tab, White, Oval	Aspirin 500 mg	Bufferin Extra Strength by BMS	Canadian DIN 01990691	Analgesic
ESH	Tab, White, Oblong	Acetaminophen 325 mg, Phenylephrine HCl 5 mg	Excedrin Sinus Headache by Novartis		Cold Remedy
ESKALITHSB	Cap, Gray & Yellow	Lithium Carbonate 300 mg	Eskalith by Mylan	00378-0423	Antipsychotic
ESKALITHSB	Cap, Gray & Yellow, Eskalith/SB	Lithium Carbonate 300 mg	Eskalith by SKB	00007-4007	Antipsychotic
ESMAALOXPLUS	Tab, Pink, Round	Magnesium Hydroxide 350 mg	by Novartis	Canadian	Mineral
ESTAC500	Cap, Blue, Film Coated	Acetaminophen 500 mg, Chlorzoxazone 250 mg	Extra Strength Tylenol Aches & Strains by McNeil	Canadian DIN 02155214	Analgesic; Muscle Relaxant
ET <> A	Tab, Pink, Oval, Film Coated, Abbott Logo (a)	Erythromycin Stearate 500 mg	by Pharmedix	53002-0269	Antibiotic
ET <> A	Tab, Pink, Oval, Film Coated, Abbott Logo (a)	Erythromycin Stearate 500 mg	Erythrocin by Abbott	00074-6316	Antibiotic
ET500 <> G	Tab, Blue, Oval, Film Coated	Etodolac 500 mg	by Genpharm	55567-0032	NSAID
ET500 <> G	Tab, Light Blue, Oval, Film Coated	Etodolac 500 mg	Lodine by Par	49884-0596	NSAID
ET7	Tab	Chlorpheniramine Tannate 8 mg, Phenylephrine Tannate 25 mg, Pyrilamine Tannate 25 mg	Tritan by Eon	00185-0700	Cold Remedy
ETH	Tab, Red, Cap Shaped	Acetaminophen 500 mg, Caffeine 65 mg	Excedrin Tension Headache by BMS		Analgesic
ETH <> 15	Tab, Brown, Round, Scored, Immediate Release	Morphine Sulfate 15 mg	MSIR by Ethex	58177-0313	Analgesic; C II
ETH <> 20	Tab, White, Cap Shaped, Scored, Ex Release	Potassium Chloride 20 mEq	by Ethex	58177-0202	Electrolytes
ETH <> 274	Tab, White, Oval, Partially Scored, Film Coated	Hyoscyamine Sulfate 0.125 mg	Levsin by Ethex	58177-0274	Gastrointestinal
ETH <> 3	Tab, White, Oval	Nitroglycerin 0.3 mg	NitroQuick by Ethex	58177-0323	Vasodilator
ETH <> 3	Tab, White, Oval	Nitroglycerin 0.3 mg	Nitrostat by PDRX	55289-0308	Vasodilator
ETH <> 315	Tab, Orange, Scored	Oxycodone HCl 5 mg	Roxicodone by Ethex	58177-0315	Analgesic; C II
ETH <> 331	Tab, White, Round, Scored, Film Coated	Propafenone HCl 150 mg	Rythmol by Ethex	58177-0331	Antiarrhythmic
ETH <> 332	Tab, White, Round, Scored, Film Coated	Propafenone HCl 225 mg	Rythmol by Ethex	58177-0332	Antiarrhythmic
ETH <> 333	Tab, White, Round, Scored, Film Coated	Propafenone HCl 300 mg	Rythmol by Ethex	58177-0333	Antiarrhythmic
ETH <> 341	Tab, White, Round	Benazepril HCl 5 mg	Lotensin by Ethex	58177-0341	Antihypertensive
ETH <> 342	Tab, Red, Round	Benazepril HCl 10 mg	Lotensin by Ethex	58177-0342	Antihypertensive
ETH <> 343	Tab, Grey, Round	Benazepril HCl 20 mg	Lotensin by Ethex	58177-0343	Antihypertensive
ETH <> 344	Tab, Blue, Round	Benazepril HCl 40 mg	Lotensin by Ethex	58177-0344	Antihypertensive
ETH <> 383	Tab, Light Orange, Oval, Scored, ETH to left of Score <> 383	Carbidopa 50 mg, Levodopa 200 mg	Sinemet CR by Ethex	58177-0383	Antiparkinson
ETH <> 4	Tab, White, Oval	Nitroglycerin 0.4 mg	Nitrostat by PDRX	55289-0309	Vasodilator
ETH <> 4	Tab, White, Oval	Nitroglycerin 0.4 mg	NitroQuick by Ethex	58177-0324	Vasodilator
ETH <> 416	Tab, Tan, Round	Lipase 8000 Units, Amylase 30,000 Units, Protease 30,000 Units	Plaretase by Ethex	58177-0416	Gastrointestinal
ETH <> 432	Tab, Yellow, Round, Chewable, Vanilla Flavor	Fluoride Ion 0.25 mg	Luride by Ethex	58177-0432	Mineral
ETH <> 433	Tab, White, Round, Chewable, Grape Flavor	Fluoride Ion 0.50 mg	EtheDent by Ethex	58177-0433	Mineral
ETH <> 434	Tab, Red, Round, Chewable, Cherry Flavor	Fluoride Ion 1.0 mg	Luride by Ethex	58177-0434	Mineral
ETH <> 440	Tab, Tan, Oval, Film Coated, Scored	Folic Acid 2.2 mg, Vitamin B6 25 mg, Vitamin B12 500 mcg	ComBgen by Ethex	58177-0440	Vitamin
ETH <> 445	Tab, Yellow, Round, Scored	Oxycodone HCl 15 mg	Roxicodone by Ethex	58177-0445	Analgesic; C II

ID FRONT <> BACK	DESCRIPTION FRONT <> BACK	INGREDIENT & STRENGTH	BRAND (or Generic Equiv.) by FIRM	NDC#	CLASS; SCH.
ETH <> 446	Tab, White, Round, Scored	Oxycodone HCl 30 mg	Roxicodone by Ethex	58177-0446	Analgesic; C II
ETH <> 461	Tab, Pink, Round, Scored	Oxycodone HCl 10 mg	OxyContin by Ethex	58177-0461	Analgesic; C II
ETH <> 462	Tab, Grey, Round, Scored	Oxycodone HCl 20 mg	Oxycodone by Ethex	58177-0462	Analgesic; C II
ETH <> 6	Tab, White, Oval	Nitroglycerin 0.6 mg	Nitrostat by PDRX	55289-0302	Vasodilator
ETH <> 6	Tab, White, Oval	Nitroglycerin 0.6 mg	NitroQuick by Ethex	58177-0325	Vasodilator
ETH <> 625	Tab, Orange, Round, Scored	Oxycodone HCl 5 mg	Roxicodone by Ethex	58177-0625	Analgesic; C II
ETH042	Cap, Maroon, Soft Gel	Ferrous Fumarate 200 mg, Ascorbic Acid 250 mg, Cyanocobalamin 10 mcg, Desiccated Stomach Substance 100 mg	Anemagen by Ethex	58177-0042 Discontinued	Mineral
ETH042	Cap, Maroon, Soft Gel	Ferrous Fumarate 200 mg, Ascorbic Acid 250 mg, Cyanocobalamin 10 mcg, Desiccated Stomach Substance 100 mg	Anemagen by Accucaps	61474-4070	Vitamin
ETH043	Cap, Brown & Green, Soft Gel	Ferrous Fumarate 200 mg, Ascorbic Acid 250 mg, Cyanocobalamin 10 mcg, Folic Acid 1 mg	Anemagen FA by Ethex	58177-0043 Discontinued	Mineral
ETH052	Cap, Green, Soft Gel	Vitamin C 60 mg, Calcium 200 mg, Iron 28 mg, Vitamin D3 400 IU, Vitamin E 30 IU, Vitamin B1 1.6 mg, Vitamin B2 1.8 mg, Vitamin B6 20 mg, Vitamin B12 12 mcg, Docusate Calcium 25 mg, Folic Acid 1 mg	Anemagen OB by Ethex	58177-0052	Vitamin
ETH227	Tab, Brown, Cap Shaped, Scored, Ex Release	Chlorpheniramine Maleate 8 mg, Methscopolamine 2.5 mg, Phenylephrine 20 mg	Hista-Vent DA by Ethex	58177-0227	Cold Remedy
ETH255	Tab, White, Peppermint Flavor	Hyoscyamine Sulfate 0.125 mg	Levsin by Ethex	58177-0255	Gastrointestinal
ETH266 <> 1MG	Tab, Gray, Oblong	Doxazosin Mesylate 1 mg	Cardura by Ethex	58177-0266	Antihypertensive
ETH267 <> 2MG	Tab, Yellow, Oblong	Doxazosin Mesylate 2 mg	Cardura by Ethex	58177-0267	Antihypertensive
ETH268 <> 4MG	Tab, Pink, Oblong	Doxazosin Mesylate 4 mg	Cardura by Ethex	58177-0268	Antihypertensive
ETH269 <> 8MG	Tab, Blue, Oblong	Doxazosin Mesylate 8 mg	Cardura by Ethex	58177-0269	Antihypertensive
ETH269 <> 8MG	Tab, Blue, Oblong, Scored	Doxazosin Mesylate 8 mg	Cardura by Dava	67253-0387	Antihypertensive
ETH30	Cap, Brown, ETH/30	Morphine Sulfate IR 30 mg	MS Contin by KV Pharma		Analgesic; C II
ETH301	Tab, White, Round	Ketorolac Tromethamine 10 mg	Toradol by Syntex		NSAID
ETH309 <> 555	Tab, Yellow, Cap Shaped, Scored	Buspirone HCl 15 mg	BuSpar by Ethex	58177-0309	Antianxiety
ETHEX <> 205	Tab, White, Oblong, Ex Release	Guaifenesin 600 mg	Guaifenex LA by Ethex	58177-0205 Discontinued	Expectorant
ETHEX <> 208	Tab, White, Cap Shaped, Ex Release	Guaifenesin 600 mg, Pseudoephedrine 120 mg	Duratuss by Ethex	58177-0208	Cold Remedy
ETHEX <> 208	Tab, White, Cap Shaped, Ex Release	Guaifenesin 600 mg, Pseudoephedrine 120 mg	Duratuss by Murfreesboro	51129-1390	Cold Remedy
ETHEX <> 212	Tab, Pink, Oval, Film Coated	Ascorbic Acid 120 mg, Calcium 250 mg, Copper 2 mg, Cyanocobalamin 12 mcg, Docusate Sodium 50 mg, Folic Acid 1 mg, Iodine 0.15 mg, Iron 90 mg, Niacinamide 20 mg, Pyridoxine HCl 20 mg, Riboflavin 3.4 mg, Thiamine Mononitrate 3 mg, Vitamin A 4000 Units, Vitamin D 400 Units, Vitamin E 30 Units, Zinc 25 mg	Prenatal MR 90 by Ethex	58177-0212	Vitamin
ETHEX <> 213	Tab, Green, Cap Shaped, Ex Release	Dextromethorphan 30 mg, Guaifenesin 600 mg	Guaifenex PM by Ethex	58177-0213 Discontinued	Cold Remedy
ETHEX <> 213	Tab, Green, Cap Shaped, Ex Release	Dextromethorphan 30 mg, Guaifenesin 600 mg	Humibid-DM by DRX	55045-2623	Cold Remedy
ETHEX <> 214	Tab, Blue, Cap Shaped, Scored	Guaifenesin 600 mg, Pseudoephedrine HCl 60 mg	Guaifenex AM by Ethex	58177-0214 Discontinued	Cold Remedy
ETHEX <> 216	Tab, White, Oval	Ascorbic Acid 80 mg, Beta-Carotene 0.4 mg, Biotin 30 mcg, Calcium 200 mg, Copper 3 mg, Cyanocobalamin 2.5 mg, Folic Acid 1 mg, Iron 60 mg, Magnesium 100 mg, Niacinamide 17 mg, Pantothenic Acid 7 mg, Pyridoxine HCl 4.86 mg, Riboflavin 1.6 mg, Thiamine 1.5 mg, Vitamin A 0.8 mg, Vitamin D 10 mcg, Vitamin E 10 mg, Zinc 25 mg	Natalins Rx by Ethex	58177-0216	Vitamin
ETHEX <> 223	Tab, Red, Oval	Codeine Phosphate 10 mg, Guaifenesin 300 mg	Brontex by Ethex	58177-0223	Cold Remedy; C III
ETHEX <> 225	Tab, Pink, Oval, Scored	Ascorbic Acid 120 mg, Calcium 200 mg, Copper 2 mg, Cyanocobalamin 12 mcg, Folic Acid 1 mg, Iron 27 mg, Niacinamide 20 mg, Pyridoxine HCl 10 mg, Riboflavin 3 mg, Thiamine HCl 1.84 mg, Vitamin A 4000 Units, Vitamin D 400 Units, Vitamin E 22 mg, Zinc 25 mg	NatalCare Plus by Ethex	58177-0225	Vitamin

ID FRONT <> BACK	DESCRIPTION FRONT <> BACK	INGREDIENT & STRENGTH	BRAND (or Generic Equiv.) by FIRM	NDC#	CLASS; SCH.
ETHEX <> 232	Tab, Peach, Film Coated	Ascorbic Acid 50 mg, Calcium 250 mg, Copper 2 mg, Folic Acid 1 mg, Iron 40 mg, Magnesium 50 mg, Pyridoxine HCl 2 mg, Vitamin D 6 mcg, Vitamin E 3.5 mg, Zinc 15 mg	Natalcare by Ethex	58177-0232 Discontinued	Vitamin
ETHEX <> 234	Tab, Buff, Cap Shaped	Phenylephrine HCl 25 mg	Sudafed PE by Ethex	58177-0234 Discontinued	Decongestant
ETHEX <> 237	Tab, White, Ex Release	Hyoscyamine Sulfate 0.375 mg	Levbid by Ethex	58177-0237	Gastrointestinal
ETHEX <> 257	Tab, Blue, Oval, Film Coated	Ascorbic Acid 50 mg, Calcium 125 mg, Cyanocobalamin 3 mcg, Folic Acid 1 mg, Iron 60 mg, Niacinamide 10 mg, Pyridoxine HCl 2 mg, Riboflavin 3 mg, Thiamine Mononitrate 3 mg, Vitamin A 4000 Units, Vitamin D 400 Units, Zinc 18 mg	Niferex PN by Ethex	58177-0257	Vitamin
ETHEX <> 258	Tab, White, Oval, Film Coated	Ascorbic Acid 80 mg, Calcium 250 mg, Copper 2 mg, Cyanocobalamin 12 mcg, Folic Acid 1 mg, Iodine 0.2 mg, Iron 60 mg, Magnesium 10 mg, Niacinamide 20 mg, Pyridoxine HCl 4 mg, Riboflavin 3.4 mg, Thiamine 3 mg, Vitamin A Acetate 5000 Units, Vitamin D 400 Units, Vitamin E 30 Units, Zinc 25 mg	Niferex PN Forte by Ethex	58177-0258	Vitamin
ETHEX <> 275	Tab, White, Film Coated	Ascorbic Acid 70 mg, Calcium 200 mg, Cyanocobalamin 2.2 mcg, Folic Acid 1 mg, Iodine 175 mcg, Iron 65 mg, Magnesium 100 mg, Niacin 17 mg, Pyridoxine HCl 2.2 mg, Riboflavin 1.6 mg, Thiamine HCl 1.5 mg, Vitamin A 3000 Units, Vitamin D 400 Units, Vitamin E 10 Units, Zinc 15 mg	Prenatal Z by Ethex	58177-0275	Vitamin
ETHEX <> 292	Tab, Beige, Oval, Scored, Film Coated	Ascorbic Acid 120 mg, Calcium 200 mg, Cholecalciferol 400 Units, Copper 2 mg, Cyanocobalamin 12 mcg, Docusate Sodium 50 mg, Folic Acid 1 mg, Iodine 150 mcg, Iron 90 mg, Niacinamide 20 mg, Pyridoxine HCl 20 mg, Riboflavin 3.4 mg, Thiamine HCl 3 mg, Vitamin A 2700 Units, Vitamin E 30 Units, Zinc 25 mg	Ultra Natalcare by Ethex	58177-0292	Vitamin
ETHEX <> 30	Tab, Brown, Cap Shaped, Scored, Immediate Release	Morphine Sulfate 30 mg	MSIR by Ethex	58177-0314	Analgesic; C II
ETHEX <> 301	Tab, White, Red Print, Round, Film Coated	Ketorolac Tromethamine 10 mg	Toradol by Ethex	58177-0301	NSAID
ETHEX <> 301	Tab, White, Red Print, Round, Film Coated	Ketorolac Tromethamine 10 mg	Toradol by Murfreesboro	51129-1437	NSAID
ETHEX <> 301	Tab, White, Red Print, Round, Film Coated	Ketorolac Tromethamine 10 mg	Toradol by Compumed	00403-4136	NSAID
ETHEX <> 301	Tab, White, Red Print, Round, Film Coated	Ketorolac Tromethamine 10 mg	Toradol by Syntex	18393-0301	NSAID
ETHEX <> 308	Tab, White, Cap Shaped, Scored, Ex Release	Guaifenesin 1200 mg	Guaifenex G by Ethex	58177-0308 Discontinued	Expectorant
ETHEX <> 312	Tab, Orange, Round, Scored	Dextroamphetamine Sulfate 10 mg	Dexedrine by Ethex	58177-0312	Stimulant; C II
ETHEX <> 316	Tab, Tan, Scored, Film Coated	Ascorbic Acid 120 mg, Biotin 30 mcg, Calcium 200 mg, Chromium 25 mcg, Copper 2 mg, Cyanocobalamin 12 mcg, Folic Acid 1 mg, Iodine 150 mcg, Iron 27 mg, Magnesium 25 mg, Manganese 5 mg, Molybdenum 25 mcg, Niacinamide 20 mg, Pantothenic Acid 10 mg, Pyridoxine HCl 10 mg, Riboflavin 3.4 mg, Selenium 20 mcg, Thiamine HCl 3 mg, Retinol 5000 Units, Vitamin D 400 Units, Alpha-tocopherol 30 mg, Zinc 25 mg	Prenatal MTR by Ethex	58177-0316	Vitamin
ETHEX <> 317	Tab, White, Oval	Vitamin A 4000 IU, Vitamin C 80 mg, Calcium 200 mg, Iron 54 mg, Vitamin D 400 IU, Vitamin E 15 IU, Thiamine 1.5 mg, Riboflavin 1.6 mg, Niacin 17 mg, Vitamin B6 4 mg, Folate 1 mg, Vitamin B12 2.5 mcg, Biotin 30 mcg, Pantothenic Acid 7 mg, Magnesium 100 mg, Zinc 25 mg, Copper 3 mg	Enfamil Natalins by Ethex	58177-0317	Vitamin
ETHEX <> 322	Tab, Orange, Oval, Film Coated	Vitamin A 1000 Units, Ascorbic Acid 120 mg, Iron 60 mg, Cholecalciferol, Vitamin E, Thiamine 2 mg, Riboflavin 3 mg, Niacinamide 20 mg, Pyridoxine HCl 10 mg, Folic Acid 1 mg, Cyanocobalamin 12 mcg	NatalCare by Ethex	58177-0322 Discontinued	Vitamin
ETHEX <> 322	Tab, Orange, Oval, Film Coated	Vitamin A 1000 Units, Ascorbic Acid 120 mg, Iron 60 mg, Cholecalciferol, Vitamin E, Thiamine 2 mg, Riboflavin 3 mg, Niacinamide 20 mg, Pyridoxine HCl 10 mg, Folic Acid 1 mg, Cyanocobalamin 12 mcg	NatalCare by Thrift Drug	59198-0320	Vitamin

ID FRONT <> BACK	DESCRIPTION FRONT <> BACK	INGREDIENT & STRENGTH	BRAND (or Generic Equiv.) by FIRM	NDC#	CLASS; SCH.
ETHEX <> 328	Tab, White, Oval	Vitamin A 4,000 IU, Vitamin C 120 mg, Calcium 200 mg, Iron 50 mg, Vitamin D 400 IU, Vitamin E 30 IU, Vitamin B1 3 mg, Vitamin B2 3 mg, Niacin 20 mg, Vitamin B6 3 mg, Folic Acid 1 mg, Vitamin B12 8 mcg, Iodine 150 mcg, Zinc 15 mg	Nata Tab CFe by Ethex	58177-0328	Vitamin
ETHEX <> 329	Tab, Purple, Oval	Vitamin A 4,000 IU, Vitamin C 120 mg, Calcium 200 mg, Iron 29 mg, Vitamin D3 400 IU, Vitamin E 30 IU, Vitamin B1 3 mg, Vitamin B2 3 mg, Niacin 20 mg, Vitamin B6 3 mg, Folic Acid 1 mg, Vitamin B12 8 mcg, Iodine 150 mcg, Zinc 15 mg	Nata Tab FA by Ethex	58177-0329	Vitamin
ETHEX <> 350	Tab, White, Oval	Vitamin A 2700 Units, Ascorbic Acid 120 mg, Calcium 200 mg, Iron 90 mg, Vitamin D 400 Units, Thiamine HCl 3 mg, Riboflavin 3.4 mg, Niacinamide 20 mg, Pyridoxine HCl 20 mg, Folic Acid 1 mg, Cyanocobalamin 12 mcg, Zinc 25 mg, Copper 2 mg, Magnesium 30 mg, Docusate Sodium	Prenate Advance by Ethex	58177-0350	Vitamin
ETHEX <> 351	Tab, Mottled White, Round	Vitamin A 1000 Units, Cholecalciferol 400 Units, Vitamin E 11 Units, Ascorbic Acid 120 mg, Folic Acid 1 mg, Thiamine Mononitrate 2 mg, Riboflavin 3 mg, Niacinamide 20 mg, Pyridoxine HCl 10 mg, Cyanocobalamin 12 mcg, Iron 29 mg	Nutrinate Chewable by Ethex	58177-0351	Vitamin
ETHEX <> 373	Tab, White, Oval, Film Coated, Ex Release	Guaifenesin 1200 mg, Pseudoephedrine HCl 120 mg	Aquabid D by Ethex	58177-0373	Cold Remedy
ETHEX <> 375	Tab, Pink & Beige, Oval	Prenatal Multivitamin	Stuartnatal Plus 3 by Ethex	58177-0375	Vitamin
ETHEX <> 376	Tab, Yellow, Oval	Vitamin A 4,000 IU, Vitamin D 400 IU, Vitamin E 30 IU, Vitamin C 120 mg, Folic Acid 1 mg, Vitamin B1 3 mg, Vitamin B2 3 mg, Niacin 20 mg, Vitamin B6 3 mg, Vitamin B12 8 mcg, Biotin 30 mcg, Pantothenic Acid 7 mg, Calcium 200 mg, Iodine 150 mcg, Zinc 15 mg, Magnesium 100 mg, Iron 29 mg, Copper 3 mg	NataTab by Ethex	58177-0376	Vitamin
ETHEX <> 413	Tab, White, Cap Shaped, Scored	Guaifenesin 800 mg, Pseudoephedrine HCl 80 mg	Panmist LA by Ethex	58177-0413	Cold Remedy
ETHEX <> 414	Tab, White, Cap Shaped	Guaifenesin 600 mg, Pseudoephedrine HCl 45 mg, Dextromethorphan HBr 30 mg	Pseudovent DM by Ethex	58177-0414	Cold Remedy
ETHEX <> 415	Tab, Pink & Beige, Oval	Vitamin A 3,000 IU, Vitamin D 400 IU, Vitamin E 22 mg, Vitamin C 120 mg, Folic Acid 1 mg, Vitamin B1 1.8 mg, Vitamin B2 4 mg, Niacinamide 20 mg, Vitamin B6 25 mg, B12 12 mcg, Calcium 200 mg, Copper 2 mg, Iron 28 mg, Zinc 25 mg, Magnesium 25 mg	NatalCare 3 by Ethex	58177-0415	Vitamin
ETHEX <> 418	Tab, Pink, Oval, Gloss Coated	Prenatal Multivitamin	Natalcare GlossTabs by Ethex	58177-0418	Vitamin
ETHEX <> 426	Tab, White, Oblong, Scored	Chlorpheniramine Maleate 8 mg, Pseudoephedrine HCl 120 mg, Methscopolamine Nitrate 2.5 mg	Hista-Vent PSE by Ethex	58177-0426	Cold Remedy
ETHEX <> 427	Tab, Yellow, Cap Shaped, Scored	Pseudoephedrine HCl 120 mg, Methscopolamine Nitrate 2.5 mg	HistaClear by Ethex	58177-0427 Discontinued	Cold Remedy
ETHEX <> 435	Tab, Yellow, Oval	Vitamin C 60 mg, Iron 90 mg, Vitamin D3 400 IU, Vitamin E 30 IU, Vitamin B1 2 mg, Vitamin B2 3 mg, Vitamin B6 3 mg, Folic Acid 1 mg, Magnesium 25 mg, Zinc 20 mg, Copper 2 mg, Vitamin A 3500 IU, Vitamin B12 12 mcg, Dioctylsulfosuccinate Sodium 50 mg	Care Nate 600 by Ethex	58177-0437	Vitamin; Supplement
ETHEX <> 436	Tab, Yellow, Round, Chewable	Calcium Carbonate 600 mg	Care Nate 600 by Ethex	58177-0437	Vitamin; Supplement
ETHEX <> 438	Tab, White Cap Shaped	Guaifenesin 595 mg, Pseudoephedrine HCl 48 mg, Dextromethorphan HBr 32 mg	Pseudovent DM by Ethex	58177-0438	Cold Remedy
ETHEX <> 439	Tab, White, Oval, Scored	Vitamin A 2700 IU, Vitamin C 120 mg, Calcium Citrate 125 mg, Iron 27 mg, Vitamin D3 400 IU, Vitamin E 30 IU, Thiamine 3 mg, Riboflavin 3.4 mg, Niacinamide 20 mg, Vitamin B6 20 mg, Folic Acid 1 mg, Iodine 150 mcg, Zinc 25 mg, Copper 2 mg, Docusate Sodium 50 mg	Cal-Nate by Ethex	58177-0439	Vitamin
ETHEX <> 444	Tab, White, Cap Shaped, Film Coated, Scored	Guaifenesin 1200 mg, Phenylephrine HCl 40 mg	PhenaVent D by Ethex	58177-0444	Cold Remedy
ETHEX <> 458	Tab, White, Oval	Vitamin C 120 mg, Calcium Carbonate 200 mg, Elemental Iron 90 mg, Vitamin D3 400 IU, Vitamin E 30 IU, Vitamin B1 3 mg, Vitamin B2 3.4 mg, Niacinamide 20 mg, Vitamin B6 20 mg, Folic Acid 1 mg, Vitamin B12 12 mcg, Zinc 25 mg, Copper 2 mg, Magnesium 30 mg, Docusate Sodium 50 mg	Advanced-RF NatalCare by Ethex	58177-0458	Vitamin

ID FRONT <> BACK	DESCRIPTION FRONT <> BACK	INGREDIENT & STRENGTH	BRAND (or Generic Equiv.) by FIRM	NDC#	CLASS; SCH.
ETHEX <> 463	Tab, Blue, Cap Shaped	Vitamin D3 400 IU, Vitamin E 30 IU, Vitamin C 120 mg, Folic Acid 1 mg, Vitamin B1 3 mg, Vitamin B2 3 mg, Niacin 20 mg, Vitamin B6 3 mg, Vitamin B12 8 mcg, Calcium 200 mg, Iodine 150 mcg, Zinc 15 mg, Iron 29 mg	NutriSpire by Ethex	58177-0463	Vitamin
ETHEX001	Cap, Clear, Pink Print, Hard Gel, Ex Release, Ethex over 001	Potassium Chloride 10mEq (750 mg)	Micro-K 10 by Vangard	00615-1318	Electrolytes
ETHEX001	Cap, Clear, Pink Print, Hard Gel, Ex Release, Ethex over 001	Potassium Chloride 10mEq (750 mg)	Micro-K 10 by Heartland	61392-0402	Electrolytes
ETHEX001	Cap, Clear, Pink Print, Hard Gel, Ex Release, Ethex over 001	Potassium Chloride 10mEq (750 mg)	Micro-K 10 by Promeco SA	64674-0018	Electrolytes
ETHEX001	Cap, Clear, Pink Print, Hard Gel, Ex Release, Ethex over 001	Potassium Chloride 10mEq (750 mg)	Micro-K 10 by Med Pro	53978-5044	Electrolytes
ETHEX001	Cap, Clear, Pink Print, Hard Gel, Ex Release, Ethex over 001	Potassium Chloride 10mEq (750 mg)	Micro-K 10 by Ethex	58177-0001	Electrolytes
ETHEX001	Cap, Clear, Pink Print, Hard Gel, Ex Release, Ethex over 001	Potassium Chloride 10mEq (750 mg)	Micro-K 10 by Major Pharmaceuticals	00904-2295	Electrolytes
ETHEX002	Cap, Orange & Purple, Ex Release	Disopyramide Phosphate 150 mg	Norpace CR by Ethex	58177-0002	Antiarrhythmic
ETHEX003	Cap, Purple & Yellow, Ex Release	Disopyramide Phosphate 100 mg	Norpace CR by Ethex	58177-0003	Antiarrhythmic
ETHEX004	Cap, Clear & Lavender w/ White Beads, Ex Release	Nitroglycerin 2.5 mg	Nitrobid by Ethex	58177-0004 Discontinued	Vasodilator
ETHEX005	Cap, Blue & Orange, Ex Release	Nitroglycerin 6.5 mg	Nitrobid by Ethex	58177-0005 Discontinued	Vasodilator
ETHEX005	Cap, Blue & Orange, Ex Release	Nitroglycerin 6.5 mg	Nitrobid by Physician Total Care	54868-0689 Discontinued	Vasodilator
ETHEX006	Cap, Clear w/ White Beads, Ex Release	Nitroglycerin 9 mg	Nitrobid by Ethex	58177-0006 Discontinued	Vasodilator
ETHEX015	Cap, Blue & Clear with White Beads	Guaifenesin 300 mg, Pseudoephedrine HCl 60 mg	Nalex JR by Ethex	58177-0046	Cold Remedy
ETHEX015	Cap, Blue & Clear	Phenylpropanolamine HCl 60 mg, Guaifenesin 300 mg	Guaifed-PD by Ethex	58177-0015 Discontinued	Cold Remedy
ETHEX016	Cap, Clear & White w/ White Beads, Ex Release	Guaifenesin 250 mg, Pseudoephedrine HCl 120 mg	Guaifed by Ethex	58177-0045	Cold Remedy
ETHEX017	Cap, Clear, Ex Release	Hyoscyamine Sulfate 0.375 mg	Levsinex by Ethex	58177-0017	Gastrointestinal
ETHEX019	Cap, Clear & Green w/ White Beads, Ex Release	Pseudoephedrine HCl 120 mg, Brompheniramine Maleate 12 mg	Bromfenex by Ethex	58177-0019	Decongestant
ETHEX020	Cap, Clear & Green w/ White Beads, Ex Release	Pseudoephedrine HCl 60 mg, Brompheniramine Maleate 6 mg	Bromfenex PD by Ethex	58177-0020	Decongestant
ETHEX022	Cap, Clear & Pink	Phenylpropanolamine HCl 50 mg, Phenyltoloxamine Citrate 16 mg, Pyrilamine Maleate 16 mg, Pheniramine Maleate 16 mg	Quadra-Hist D by Ethex	58177-0022	Cold Remedy
ETHEX023	Cap, Clear, Ethex/023	Phenylpropanolamine HCl 25 mg, Phenyltoloxamine Citrate 8 mg, Pyrilamine Maleate 8 mg, Pheniramine Maleate 8 mg	Quadra-Hist D PED by Ethex	58177-0023	Cold Remedy
ETHEX024	Cap, Orange, Opaque	Iron 150 mg	FE-Tinic 150 by Ethex	58177-0024 Discontinued	Mineral
ETHEX024	Cap, Orange, Opaque	Iron 150 mg	FE-Tinic 150 by DJ Pharma	64455-0009	Mineral
ETHEX025	Cap, Maroon, Opaque	Cyanocobalamin 25 mcg, Folic Acid 1 mg, Iron 150 mg	Fe-Tinic 150 Forte by Ethex	58177-0025	Vitamin
ETHEX027	Cap, Maroon, Opaque	Meperidine HCl 50 mg, Promethazine HCl 25 mg	Meprozine by Ethex	58177-0027	Analgesic; C II
ETHEX028	Cap, Red	Lipase 16,000 Units, Amylase 48,000 Units, Protease 48,000 Units	Pangestyme MT 16 by Ethex	58177-0028	Gastrointestinal
ETHEX029	Cap, Pink & Natural	Lipase 10,000 Units, Amylase 33,200 Units, Protease 37,500 Units	Pangestyme CN 10 by Ethex	58177-0029	Gastrointestinal
ETHEX037	Cap, Green, Opaque	Trimethobenzamide HCl 250 mg	Tigan by Ethex	58177-0037 Discontinued	Antiemetic
ETHEX041	Cap, Beige & Opaque & White, in Black Ink	Oxycodone HCl 5 mg	OxyIR by Ethex	58177-0041	Analgesic; C II
ETHEX041	Cap, Beige & Opaque & White, in Black Ink	Oxycodone HCl 5 mg	OxyIR by Pharmafab	62542-0257	Analgesic; C II
ETHEX044	Cap, Brown, White Print	Liver Concentrate 240 mg, Ascorbic Acid 75 mg, Cyanocobalamin 15 mcg, Iron 110 mg, Folic Acid 0.5 mg	Conison by Ethex	58177-0044	Deficiency Anemias
ETHEX048	Cap, Blue & Clear	Lipase 12,000 Units, Amylase 39,000 Units, Protease 39,000 Units	Pangestyme UL 12 by Ethex	58177-0048	Gastrointestinal
ETHEX049	Cap, Blue	Lipase 18,000 Units, Amylase 58,500 Units, Protease 58,500 Units	Pangestyme UL 18 by Ethex	58177-0049	Gastrointestinal

ID FRONT <> BACK	DESCRIPTION FRONT <> BACK	INGREDIENT & STRENGTH	BRAND (or Generic Equiv.) by FIRM	NDC#	CLASS: SCH.
ETHEX050	Cap, Clear & Green	Lipase 20,000 Units, Amylase 65,000 Units, Protease 65,000 Units	Pangestyme UL 20 by Ethex	58177-0050	Gastrointestinal
ETHEX056	Cap, Pink & White	Pseudoephedrine HCl 80 mg, Phenyltoloxamine Citrate 16 mg, Pyrilamine Maleate 16 mg, Pheniramine Maleate 16 mg	Quadra-Hist D by Ethex	58177-0056 Discontinued	Cold Remedy
ETHEX057	Cap, White	Pseudoephedrine HCl 40 mg, Phenyltoloxamine Citrate 8 mg, Pyrilamine Maleate 8 mg, Pheniramine Maleate 8 mg	Quadra-Hist D by Ethex	58177-0057 Discontinued	Cold Remedy
ETHEX061	Cap, Maroon, Opaque, Black Ink, Extended Release	Diltiazem HCl 120 mg	Tiazac by Ethex	58177-0061	Antihypertensive
ETHEX062	Cap, Maroon and Ivory, Opaque, Black Ink, Extended Release	Diltiazem HCl 180 mg	Tiazac by Ethex	58177-0062	Antihypertensive
ETHEX063	Cap, Ivory and Caramel, Opaque, Black Ink, Extended Release	Diltiazem HCl 240 mg	Tiazac by Ethex	58177-0063	Antihypertensive
ETHEX064	Cap, Caramel and Maroon, Opaque, Black Ink, Extended Release	Diltiazem HCl 300 mg	Tiazac by Ethex	58177-0064	Antihypertensive
ETHEX065	Cap, Caramel, Opaque, Black Ink	Diltiazem HCl 360 mg	Tiazac by Ethex	58177-0065	Antihypertensive
ETHEX066	Cap, Ivory, Opaque, Black Ink, Extended Release	Diltiazem HCl 420 mg	Tiazac by Ethex	58177-0066	Antihypertensive
ETHEX073	Cap, Yellow and White, Black Ink	Ferrous Fumarate 324 mg, Vitamin C 200 mg, Vitamin B1 10 mg, Vitamin B2 6 mg, Vitamin B6 5 mg, Vitamin B12 15 mcg, Folic Acid 1 mg, Niacinamide 30 mg, Pantothenic Acid 10 mg, Manganese 1.3 mg, Copper 0.8 mg	NataCaps by Ethex	58177-0073	Vitamin; Supplement
ETHEX076	Cap, Green and Clear, Black Ink	Phenylephrine HCl 7.5 mg, Brompheniramine Maleate 6 mg	Bromfenex by Ethex	58177-0076	Cold Remedy
ETHEX077	Cap, Light Green and Clear	Phenylephrine HCl 15 mg, Brompheniramine Maleate 12 mg	Bromfenex PE by Ethex	58177-0077	Cold Remedy
ETHEX078	Cap, White Opaque, Clear, Black Ink	Phenylephrine HCl 15 mg, Guaifenesin 400 mg	PhenaVent by Ethex	58177-0078	Cold Remedy
ETHEX079	Cap, Blue and White	Phenylephrine HCl 7.5 mg, Guaifenesin 200 mg	PhenaVent PED by Ethex	58177-0079	Cold Remedy
ETHEX095	Cap, Blue and Light Blue, Opaque, Black Ink	Guaifenesin 400 mg, Phenylephrine HCl 30 mg	PhenaVent LA by Ethex	58177-0095	Cold Remedy
ETHEX096	Cap, Maroon and Light Blue, Opaque, Black Ink	Pseudoephedrine HCl 120 mg, Guaifenesin 400 mg	Pseudovent by Ethex	58177-0096	Cold Remedy
ETHEX1	Cap, Clear, Hard Gel	Potassium Chloride 750 mg	by Eckerd	19458-0877	Electrolytes
ETHEX204	Tab, White, Oval	Guaifenesin 600 mg, Phenylpropanolamine 75 mg	Duravent by Ethex	58177-0204	Cold Remedy
ETHEX264 <> 5MG	Tab, Yellow, Oval, Scored	Buspirone HCl 5 mg	BuSpar by Ethex	58177-0264	Antianxiety
ETHEX265 <> 10MG	Tab, Yellow, Oval, Scored	Buspirone HCl 10 mg	BuSpar by Ethex	58177-0265	Antianxiety
ETHEX302	Tab, White, Enteric Coated	Naproxen 375 mg	Naprosyn by Ethex	58177-0302	NSAID
ETHEX302	Tab, White, Enteric Coated	Naproxen 375 mg	Naprosyn by Syntex	18393-0257	NSAID
ETHEX303	Tab, White, Enteric Coated	Naproxen 500 mg	Naprosyn by Syntex	18393-0258	NSAID
ETHEX303	Tab, White, Enteric Coated	Naproxen 500 mg	Naprosyn by PDRX	55289-0307	NSAID
ETHEX303	Tab, White, Enteric Coated	Naproxen 500 mg	Naprosyn by Ethex	58177-0303	NSAID
ETHEX311	Tab, Orange, Round, Scored	Dextroamphetamine Sulfate 5 mg	Dexedrine by Ethex	58177-0311	Stimulant; C II
ETHEX312	Tab, Orange, Round, Scored	Dextroamphetamine Sulfate 10 mg	Dextrostat by Ethex	58177-0312	Stimulant; C II
ETHEX667	Cap, Pale Orange, Extended Release	Potassium Chloride 8 mEq	Micro-K by Ethex	58177-0667	Electrolytes
ETHEXAQUAPURE030	Cap, Red & Clear	Lipase 20,000 Units, Amylase 66,400 Units, Protease 75,000 Units	Pangestyme CN 20 by Ethex	58177-0030	Gastrointestinal
ETHEXAQUAPURE031	Cap, White	Lipase 4500 Units, Amylase 20,000 Units, Protease 25,000 Units	Pangestyme EC by Ethex	58177-0031	Gastrointestinal
ETHMOZINE200 <> ROBERTS	Tab, Light Green, Oval, Film Coated	Moricizine HCl 200 mg	Ethmozine by Roberts	54092-0046	Antiarrhythmic
ETHMOZINE250 <> ROBERTS	Tab, Light Orange, Oval, Film Coated	Moricizine HCl 250 mg	Ethmozine by Roberts	54092-0047	Antiarrhythmic
ETHMOZINE300 <> ROBERTS	Tab, Light Blue, Oval, Film Coated	Moricizine HCl 300 mg	Ethmozine by Roberts	54092-0048	Antiarrhythmic
ETO200MG	Cap, Dark Pink, Black Writing	Etodolac 200 mg	Lodine by Taro	51672-4016	NSAID
ETO300MG	Cap, Light Pink, Black Writing	Etodolac 300 mg	Lodine by Taro	51672-4017	NSAID
EUBM <> BMEU	Tab, White, Oblong, Scored	Glyburide 5 mg	by Pharmascience	Canadian DIN 5760667341	Antidiabetic
EUFLEX <> SPSP	Tab, Yellow, Round, Scored, SP logo	Flutamide 250 mg	Euflex by Schering	Canadian DIN 00637726	Antiandrogen
EURAND10	Cap, Yellow and White, Opaque, Blue print	Lipase 10,000 Units, Protease 34,000 Units, Amylase 55,000 Units	Zenpep by Eurand	42865-0101	Gastrointestinal

ID FRONT <> BACK	DESCRIPTION FRONT <> BACK	INGREDIENT & STRENGTH	BRAND (or Generic Equiv.) by FIRM	NDC#	CLASS; SCH.
EURAND15	Cap, Red and White, Opaque, Blue print	Lipase 15,000 Units, Protease 51,000 Units, Amylase 82,000 Units	Zenpep by Eurand	42865-0102	Gastrointestinal
EURAND20	Cap, Green and White, Opaque, Blue print	Lipase 20,000 Units, Protease 68,000 Units, Amylase 109,000 Units	Zenpep by Eurand	42865-0103	Gastrointestinal
EURAND5	Cap, White, Opaque, Blue print	Lipase 5000 Units, Protease 17,000 Units, Amylase 27,000 Units	Zenpep by Eurand	42865-0100	Gastrointestinal
EV0066	Tab, Light Brown, Chewable	Calcium (elemental) 500 mg, Vitamin D3 200 IU, Magnesium 50 mg, Boron 1 mg, Folic Acid 1.6 mg, Vitamin B6 10 mg, Vitamin B12 25 mcg	Calcifol by Everett	00642-0066	Supplement
EV0072	Tab, Film Coated	Ascorbic Acid 60 mg, Calcium 125 mg, Cyanocobalamin 5 mcg, Folic Acid 1 mg, Iron 65 mg, Niacin 15 mg, Pyridoxine HCl 2.5 mg, Riboflavin 1.8 mg, Thiamine Mononitrate 1.1 mg, Vitamin A 6000 Units, Vitamin D 400 Units, Vitamin E 30 Units	Vitafol by Lini	58215-0301 Discontinued	Vitamin
EV0078	Tab, Film Coated	Ascorbic Acid 60 mg, Calcium 125 mg, Cyanocobalamin 5 mcg, Folic Acid 1 mg, Iron 65 mg, Magnesium 25 mg, Niacin 15 mg, Pyridoxine HCl 2.5 mg, Riboflavin 1.8 mg, Selenium 65 mcg, Thiamine HCl 1.6 mg, Vitamin A 4000 Units, Vitamin D 400 Units, Vitamin E 30 Units, Zinc 15 mg	Vitafol PN by Lini	58215-0121 Discontinued	Vitamin
EV0078	Tab, Film Coated	Ascorbic Acid 60 mg, Calcium 125 mg, Cyanocobalamin 5 mcg, Folic Acid 1 mg, Iron 65 mg, Magnesium 25 mg, Niacin 15 mg, Pyridoxine HCl 2.5 mg, Riboflavin 1.8 mg, Thiamine HCl 1.6 mg, Vitamin A 4000 Units, Vitamin D 400 Units, Vitamin E 30 Units, Zinc 15 mg	Vitafol PN by Lini	58215-0134 Discontinued	Vitamin
EV0078	Tab, Blue, Film Coated	Ascorbic Acid 60 mg, Calcium 125 mg, Cyanocobalamin 5 mcg, Folic Acid 1 mg, Iron 65 mg, Magnesium 25 mg, Niacin 15 mg, Pyridoxine HCl 2.5 mg, Riboflavin 1.8 mg, Thiamine HCl 1.6 mg, Vitamin A 4000 Units, Vitamin D 400 Units, Vitamin E 30 Units, Zinc 15 mg	Vitafol PN by Everett	00642-0078	Vitamin
EV0204	Tab, Film Coated	Ascorbic Acid 500 mg, Biotin 0.15 mg, Chromium 0.1 mg, Copper 3 mg, Cyanocobalamin 50 mcg, Folic Acid 0.8 mg, Iron 10 mg, Magnesium 50 mg, Molybdenum 25 mcg, Niacin 100 mg, Pantothenic Acid 25 mg, Pyridoxine HCl 25 mg, Riboflavin 20 mg, Selenium 50 mcg, Thiamine HCl 20 mg, Vitamin A 4000 Units, Vitamin E 60 Units, Zinc 15 mg	Strovite Forte by Lini	58215-0328 Discontinued	Vitamin
EV0204	Tab, Green, Film Coated	Ascorbic Acid 500 mg, Biotin 0.15 mg, Chromium 0.1 mg, Copper 3 mg, Cyanocobalamin 50 mcg, Folic Acid 0.8 mg, Iron 10 mg, Magnesium 50 mg, Molybdenum 25 mcg, Niacin 100 mg, Pantothenic Acid 25 mg, Pyridoxine HCl 25 mg, Riboflavin 20 mg, Selenium 50 mcg, Thiamine HCl 20 mg, Vitamin A 4000 Units, Vitamin E 60 Units, Zinc 15 mg	Strovite Forte by Everett	00642-0204	Vitamin
EV0204	Tab, Dark Green, Oblong, Scored	Vitamin A Acetate, Beta Carotene, Vitamin E Acetate, Ergocalciferol, Folic Acid 1.0 mg, Ascorbic Acid 500 mg, Thiamine Mononitrate 20 mg, Riboflavin 20 mg, Pyridoxine HCl 25 mg, Cyanocobalamin 50 mcg, Niacinamide 100 mg, Biotin 0.15 mg, Calcium Pantothenate 25 mg, Ferrous Fumarate 10 mg, Sodium Selenate 50 mcg, Magnesium Oxide 50 mg, Zinc Oxide 15 mg, Sodium Molybdate 20 mcg, Cupric Oxide 3 mg, Chromium Nitrate 0.05 mg	Strovite Forte by West-Ward	00143-9038	Vitamin
EV0208	Tab, White, Cap Shaped	Carotenoids (Alpha-Carotene, Beta-Carotene, Cryptoxanthin, Lutein, Zeaxanthin) 3000 IU, Vitamin E (Succinate) 100 IU, Vitamin D3 400 IU, Vitamin C (Ascorbic Acid) 300 mg, Vitamin B1 20 mg, Vitamin B2 (Riboflavin) 5 mg, Vitamin B12 50 mcg, Vitamin B6 25 mg, Folic Acid 1 mg, Biotin 100 mcg, Pantothenic Acid 15 mg, Niacin (Niacinamide) 25 mg, Minerals, Magnesium (Magnesium Oxide) 50 mg, Manganese (Manganese Sulfate) 1.5 mg, Zinc (Zinc Oxide) 25 mg, Selenium (Sodium Selenate) 100 mcg, Chromium (Chromic Chloride) 50 mcg, Copper (Cupric Sulfate) 1.5 mg, Other Nutrients, Alpha Lipoic Acid 15 mg, Lutein 5 mg	Strovite Advance by Everett	00642-0208	Vitamin; Mineral

ID FRONT <> BACK	DESCRIPTION FRONT <> BACK	INGREDIENT & STRENGTH	BRAND (or Generic Equiv.) by FIRM	NDC#	CLASS; SCH.
EV0300	Cap, White, Film Coated	Biotin 300 mcg, Chromium 200 mcg, Folic Acid 2.5 mg, Niacin 20 mg, Pantothenic Acid 10 mg, Selenium 70 mcg, Vitamin B1 3 mg, Vitamin B2 2 mg, Vitamin B6 15 mg, Vitamin B12 12 mcg, Vitamin C 50 mg, Vitamin E 35 IU, Zinc 20 mg	Renax by Everett	00642-0300	Vitamin
EV0650	Tab, White, Oblong, Scored	Guaifenesin 600 mg, Pseudoephedrine HCl 60 mg, Dextromethorphan Hydrobromide 30 mg	by Pfab	62542-0771	Cold Remedy
EV201	Tab, Film Coated	Ascorbic Acid 500 mg, Biotin 0.15 mg, Chromium 0.1 mg, Copper 3 mg, Cyanocobalamin 50 mcg, Folic Acid 0.8 mg, Iron 27 mg, Magnesium 50 mg, Manganese 5 mg, Niacin 100 mg, Pantothenic Acid 25 mg, Pyridoxine HCl 25 mg, Riboflavin 20 mg, Thiamine Mononitrate 20 mg, Vitamin A 5000 Units, Vitamin E 30 Units, Zinc 22.5 mg	Bacmin by Marnel	00682-3000	Vitamin
EV201	Tab, Dark Red, Film Coated	Ascorbic Acid 500 mg, Biotin 0.15 mg, Chromium 0.1 mg, Copper 3 mg, Cyanocobalamin 50 mcg, Folic Acid 0.8 mg, Iron 27 mg, Magnesium 50 mg, Manganese 5 mg, Niacin 100 mg, Pantothenic Acid 25 mg, Pyridoxine HCl 25 mg, Riboflavin 20 mg, Thiamine HCl 20 mg, Vitamin A 5000 Units, Vitamin E 30 Units, Zinc 22.5 mg	Strovite Plus by Everett	00642-0201	Vitamin
EV201	Tab, Dark Red, Film Coated	Ascorbic Acid 500 mg, Biotin 0.15 mg, Chromium 0.1 mg, Copper 3 mg, Cyanocobalamin 50 mcg, Folic Acid 0.8 mg, Iron 27 mg, Magnesium 50 mg, Manganese 5 mg, Niacin 100 mg, Pantothenic Acid 25 mg, Pyridoxine HCl 25 mg, Riboflavin 20 mg, Thiamine Mononitrate 20 mg, Vitamin A 5000 Units, Vitamin E 30 Units, Zinc 22.5 mg	Bacmin by Lini	58215-0316 Discontinued	Vitamin
EV201	Tab, Film Coated	Ascorbic Acid 500 mg, Biotin 0.15 mg, Chromium 0.1 mg, Copper 3 mg, Cyanocobalamin 50 mcg, Folic Acid 0.8 mg, Iron 27 mg, Magnesium 50 mg, Manganese 5 mg, Niacin 100 mg, Pantothenic Acid 25 mg, Pyridoxine HCl 25 mg, Riboflavin 20 mg, Thiamine HCl 20 mg, Vitamin A 5000 Units, Vitamin E 30 Units, Zinc 22.5 mg	Strovite Plus by Lini	58215-0330 Discontinued	Vitamin
EVERETT0072	Tab, Maroon, Oblong	Multivitamin, Iron, Folic Acid	Vitafol by Everett		Vitamin
EVERETT0078	Tab, Blue, Oblong	Prenatal Vitamin	by Everett		Vitamin
EVERETT0201	Tab, Pink, Oblong	Multivitamin, Minerals	Strovite Plus by Everett		Vitamin
EVERETT0204	Tab, Green, Oblong	Multivitamin, Minerals	Strovite Forte by Everett		Vitamin
EVERETT162	Tab, White, Round	Butalbital 50 mg, Caffeine 40 mg, Acetaminophen 325 mg	Repan by Everett		Analgesic
EVERETT164	Cap, White	Butalbital 50 mg, Caffeine 40 mg, Acetaminophen 325 mg	Repan by Everett		Analgesic
EVERETT166	Tab, Blue	Butalbital 50 mg, Acetaminophen 650 mg	Repan CF by Everett	00642-0166	Analgesic
EVO078	Cap, Blue, Scored	Magnesium Oxide, Zinc Gluconate, Cyanocobalamin, Folic Acid, Thiamine Mononitrate, Pyridoxine HCl, Riboflavin, Calcium Carbonate, Tocopheryl Acetate, Beta-Carotene, Niacinamide, Ascorbic Acid, Ferrous Fumarate	by Nat Pharmpak	55154-4921	Mineral
EVOXAC30MG	Cap, White, Hard Gel	Cevimeline HCl 30 mg	Evoxac by Daiichi	63395-0201	Cholinergic Agonist
EWGEIGY	Tab, Peach, Round, EW/Geigy	Desipramine HCl 25 mg	Pertofrane by Geigy	Canadian	Antidepressant
EXELON15MG	Cap, Yellow, Red Print, Exelon over 1.5 mg	Rivastigmine 1.5 mg	Exelon by Novartis	00078-0323	Antialzheimers
EXELON15MG	Cap, Yellow, Red Print, Exelon over 1.5 mg	Rivastigmine 1.5 mg	Exelon by Novartis	17088-0018	Antialzheimers
EXELON15MG	Cap, Yellow, Red Print, Exelon over 1.5 mg	Rivastigmine 1.5 mg	Exelon by Novartis	Canadian DIN 02242115	Antialzheimers
EXELON3MG	Cap, Orange, Red Print, Exelon over 3 mg	Rivastigmine 3 mg	Exelon by Novartis	Canadian DIN 02242116	Antialzheimers
EXELON3MG	Cap, Orange, Red Print, Exelon over 3 mg	Rivastigmine 3 mg	Exelon by Novartis	17088-0019	Antialzheimers
EXELON3MG	Cap, Orange, Red Print, Exelon over 3 mg	Rivastigmine 3 mg	Exelon by Novartis	00078-0324	Antialzheimers
EXELON45MG	Cap, Red, White Print, Exelon over 4.5 mg	Rivastigmine 4.5 mg	Exelon by Novartis	17088-0020	Antialzheimers
EXELON45MG	Cap, Red, White Print, Exelon over 4.5 mg	Rivastigmine 4.5 mg	Exelon by Novartis	00078-0325	Antialzheimers

ID FRONT <> BACK	DESCRIPTION FRONT <> BACK	INGREDIENT & STRENGTH	BRAND (or Generic Equiv.) by FIRM	NDC#	CLASS; SCH.
EXELON45MG	Cap, Red, White Print, Exelon over 4.5 mg	Rivastigmine 4.5 mg	Exelon by Novartis	Canadian DIN 02242117	Antialzheimers
EXELON6MG	Cap, Orange & Red, Red Print, Exelon over 6 mg	Rivastigmine 6 mg	Exelon by Novartis	Canadian DIN 02242118	Antialzheimers
EXELON6MG	Cap, Orange & Red, Red Print, Exelon over 6 mg	Rivastigmine 6 mg	Exelon by Novartis	00078-0326	Antialzheimers
EXELON6MG	Cap, Orange & Red, Red Print, Exelon over 6 mg	Rivastigmine 6 mg	Exelon by Novartis	17088-0021	Antialzheimers
EXH12	Tab, Dark Yellow, Round, Ex Release	Hydromorphone HCl 12 mg	Exalgo by Mallinckrodt	23635-0412	Analgesic; C II
EXH16	Tab, Yellow, Round, Ex Release	Hydromorphone HCl 16 mg	Exalgo by Mallinckrodt	23635-0416	Analgesic; C II
EXH8	Tab, Red, Round, Ex Release	Hydromorphone HCl 8 mg	Exalgo by Mallinckrodt	23635-0408	Analgesic; C II
EXTRA	Tab, Orange, Film Coated, Scored	Vitamin A 1000 IU, Vitamin C 300 mg, Vitamin E 100 IU, Lutein 2 mg, Zinc 40 mg, Copper 2 mg, Riboflavin 3 mg, Manganese 5 mg, Selenium 55 mcg, Niacinamide 40 mg, L-glutathione 5 mg	Ocuvite Extra by Bausch and Lomb	24208-3881	Vitamin; Supplement
EZOL	Cap, Green Print	Acetaminophen 325 mg, Butalbital 50 mg, Caffeine 40 mg	Fioricet by Stewart Jackson	45985-0578	Analgesic
F	Cap, Black	Ascorbic Acid 100 mg, Biotin 150 mcg, Cyanocobalamin 6 mcg, Folic Acid 1 mg, Niacin 20 mg, Pantothenic Acid 5 mg, Pyridoxine HCl 10 mg, Riboflavin 1.7 mg, Thiamine Mononitrate 1.5 mg	Nephrocaps Vit by Fleming	00256-0185	Vitamin
F	Tab, Pink, Round, Schering Logo/F	Amitriptyline 4 mg, Perphenazine 25 mg	Triavil by Bayer	Canadian	Antidepressant; Antipsychotic
F	Tab, Salmon, Oval, Scored	Propoxyphene HCl 65 mg, Aspirin 375 mg, Caffeine 30 mg	by Frosst	Canadian	Analgesic; C IV
F	Tab, Scored	Propoxyphene HCl 65 mg	by Frosst	Canadian	Analgesic; C IV
F	Tab, Red, Logo/F	Perphenazine 4 mg, Amitriptyline 25 mg	by Schering	Canadian	Antipsychotic; Antidepressant
F <> 12	Tab, Blue, Cap Shaped, Film Coated	Paroxetine HCl 30 mg	Paxil by Aurobindo	65862-0156	Antidepressant
F <> 18	Tab, White to Off-White, Round	Alendronate Sodium 10 mg	Fosamax by Aurobindo	65862-0327	Antiosteoporosis
F <> 19	Tab, White to Off-White, Oval	Alendronate Sodium 35 mg	Fosamax by Aurobindo	65862-0328	Antiosteoporosis
F <> 21	Tab, White to Off-White, Oval	Alendronate Sodium 70 mg	Fosamax by Aurobindo	65862-0329	Antiosteoporosis
F <> 91	Tab, White to Off-White, Oval, Film-Coated	Ondansetron 4 mg	Ondansetron by Aurobindo	65862-0187	Antiemetic
F <> 92	Tab, Yellow, Oval, Film-Coated	Ondansetron 8 mg	Ondansetron by Aurobindo	65862-0188	Antiemetic
F <> A1	Tab, Yellow, Oblong	Triamcinolone 1 mg	Aristocort by Astellas	00469-5121	Steroid
F <> L	Tab, Pink, Round, Film Coated	Milnacipran HCl 12.5 mg	Savella by Forest	00456-1512	Antidepressant; Antifibromyalgia
F01 <> LU	Tab, Yellow, Oval, Film Coated, Scored, L / U	Quinapril 5 mg	Accupril by Lupin	68180-0556	Antihypertensive
F01CPI	Tab, Yellow, Round, F01/CPI	Folic Acid 1 mg	Folvite by Charlotte		Vitamin
F02 <> LU	Tab, Yellow, Round, Film Coated	Quinapril 10 mg	Accupril by Lupin	68180-0557	Antihypertensive
F03 <> LU	Tab, Yellow, Round, Film Coated	Quinapril 20 mg	Accupril by Lupin	68180-0558	Antihypertensive
F04	Cap, Gray & Red	Cycloserine 250 mg	Seromycin by Eli Lilly		Antibiotic
F04 <> LU	Tab, Yellow, Oblong, Film Coated	Quinapril 40 mg	Accupril by Lupin	68180-0559	Antihypertensive
F05	Tab, Chewable, F over 0.5	Fluoride Ion	Fluoritab by Century	00436-0776	Mineral
F05	Tab, Chewable, F over 0.5	Fluoride Ion	Fluoritab by Century	00436-0778	Mineral
F05	Tab, Chewable, F over 0.5	Fluoride Ion	Fluoritab by Century	00436-0777	Mineral
F1	Tab, Chewable, F/1	Fluoride Ion	Fluoritab by Century	00436-0774	Mineral
F1	Tab, Mottled Pink, Round, Quick Dissolve, Fruit Flavor	Acetaminophen 80 mg	Children's Tylenol by Perrigo	00113-0115	Analgesic
F1	Tab, Mottled Purple, Round, Quick Dissolve, Fruit Flavor	Acetaminophen 80 mg	Children's Tylenol by Perrigo	00113-0122	Analgesic
F1	Tab, Chewable, F/1	Sodium Fluoride 1.1 mg	Fluoritab by Century	00436-0772	Element
F1	Tab, Chewable, F over 1	Sodium Fluoride 1.1 mg	Fluoritab by Century	00436-0770	Element
F10	Tab, Blue, Round, Scored	Mixed Amphetamine Salts 10 mg: Dextroamphetamine Saccharate 2.5 mg, Amphetamine Aspartate 2.5 mg, Dextroamphetamine Sulfate 2.5 mg, Amphetamine Sulfate 2.5 mg	Adderall by Abrika	67767-0103	Stimulant; C II
F10	Tab, White, Diamond Shaped, Notched	Fosinopril Sodium 10 mg	Monopril by Pharmascience	Canadian DIN 02255944	Antihypertensive

ID FRONT <> BACK	DESCRIPTION FRONT <> BACK	INGREDIENT & STRENGTH	BRAND (or Generic Equiv.) by FIRM	NDC#	CLASS; SCH.
F100	Tab, White, Black Print	Flurbiprofen 100 mg	Froben by Abbott	Canadian	NSAID
F100 <> RG	Tab, White to Off-White, Rectangular, Rounded	Fluconazole 100 mg	Diflucan by Barr	00555-0772	Antifungal
F11 <> LL	Tab	Furosemide 20 mg	by Lederle		Diuretic
F12 <> M	Tab, Yellow, Round, Film Coated, Extended Release	Felodipine 5 mg	Plendil by UDL	51079-0467	Antihypertensive
F13 <> M	Tab, Blue, Round, Film Coated, Extended Release	Felodipine 10 mg	Plendil by UDL	51079-0468	Antihypertensive
F14	Cap, Yellow	Ephedrine Sulfate 25 mg, Amobarbital 50 mg	Ephedrine & Amytal by Eli Lilly		Antiasthmatic; C II
F15	Cap, Red	Combination Liver Stomach Concentrate, Iron, B Vitamins	Lextron by Eli Lilly		Digestant
F150 <> RG	Tab, White to Off-White, Rectangular, Rounded	Fluconazole 150 mg	Diflucan by Barr	00555-0773	Antifungal
F15500	Cap, Red, Black Ink, F and Degree Symbol, 15/500	Fahrenheit Formula 750 mg: A7-E Liquid Thermogenic Complex 15/500 (3;17-dihydroxy-delta-5-etiocholane-7-one diethylcarbonate, Sclaremax Proprietary Liquid [sclareolide], Proprietary Guggulsterone), Caffeine	Fahrenheit by BioTest Labs		Supplement
F16	Cap, Red	Combination Liver Stomach Concentrate, Iron, B Vitamins	Lextron Ferrous by Eli Lilly		Digestant
F19	Cap, Brown	Liver Stomach Concentrate	Extralin by Eli Lilly		Hematinic
F2	Tab, Pink, Round	Acetaminophen 160 mg	Children's Tylenol by Perrigo	00113-0222	Analgesic
F2	Tab, Purple, Round	Acetaminophen 160 mg	Children's Tylenol by Perrigo	00113-0271	Analgesic
F2	Tab, Chewable, F/2	Sodium Fluoride 2.2 mg	Fluoritab by Century	00436-0771	Element
F20	Tab, Blue, Round, Scored	Mixed Amphetamine Salts 20 mg: Dextroamphetamine Saccharate 5 mg, Amphetamine Aspartate 5 mg, Dextroamphetamine Sulfate 5 mg, Amphetamine Sulfate 5 mg	Adderall by Abrika	67767-0106	Stimulant; C II
F20	Tab, White to Off-White, Oval	Fosinopril 20 mg	Monopril by Pharmascience	Canadian DIN 02255952	Antihypertensive
F200 <> RG	Tab, White to Off-White, Rectangular, Rounded	Fluconazole 200 mg	Diflucan by Barr	00555-0774	Antifungal
F22 <> LL	Tab, White, Oblong, Scored	Fenoprofen Calcium 600 mg	Nalfon by Lederle	00005-3559	NSAID
F22 <> LL	Tab, White, Oblong, Scored	Fenoprofen Calcium 600 mg	by UDL	51079-0477	NSAID
F23	Cap, Blue	Amobarbital Sodium 60 mg	Amytal by Eli Lilly		Sedative/Hypnotic; C II
F25	Cap, Pink	Ephedrine Sulfate 50 mg	by Eli Lilly		Antiasthmatic
F25 <> APO	Tab, White to Off-White, Round	Fluvoxamine Maleate 25 mg	Luvox by Apotex	60505-0164	OCD
F2F	Cap, White	Triprolidine HCl 2.5 mg, Pseudoephedrene 60 mg, Acetaminophen 500 mg	Actifed Plus ES by Warner Wellcome	Canadian	Cold Remedy
F3 <> M	Tab, Yellow, Round	Fluconazole 50 mg	Diflucan by Mylan	00378-2514	Antifungal
F30	Tab, Blue, Round, Scored	Mixed Amphetamine Salts 30 mg: Dextroamphetamine Saccharate 7.5 mg, Amphetamine Aspartate 7.5 mg, Dextroamphetamine Sulfate 7.5 mg, Amphetamine Sulfate 7.5 mg	Adderall by Abrika	67767-0107	Stimulant; C II
F33	Cap, Blue	Amobarbital Sodium 200 mg	Amytal by Eli Lilly		Sedative/Hypnotic; C II
F34	Cap, Pink	Arsenic Extract 250 mg	Carbarsone by Eli Lilly		Veterinary
F36	Cap, Clear	Papaverine 15 mg, Codeine 15 mg	Copavin by Eli Lilly		Analgesic; C III
F39	Cap, Pink	Quinidine Sulfate 200 mg	Quinidine Sulfate by Eli Lilly		Antiarrhythmic
F40	Cap, Orange	Secobarbital Sodium 100 mg	Seconal by Eli Lilly		Sedative/Hypnotic; C II
F42	Cap, Orange	Secobarbital Sodium 50 mg	Seconal by Eli Lilly		Sedative/Hypnotic; C II
F5	Tab, White, Round, F/5	Warfarin Sodium 5 mg	by Frosst	Canadian	Anticoagulant
F5	Tab, Blue, Round, Scored	Mixed Amphetamine Salts 5 mg: Dextroamphetamine Saccharate 1.25 mg, Amphetamine Aspartate 1.25 mg, Dextroamphetamine Sulfate 1.25 mg, Amphetamine Sulfate 1.25 mg	Adderall by Abrika	67767-0101	Stimulant; C II
F5	Tab, Green, Modified Rectangle-Shaped, Film-Coated	Iron 90 mg, Folic Acid 1 mg, Vitamin B12 12 mcg, Vitamin C 120 mg, Docusate Sodium 50 mg	Ferralet 90 by Mission	00178-0083 Discontinued	Supplement
F5	Tab, Blue, Round, Film Coated, F5 <> Crescent Moon Logo	Finasteride 5 mg	Proscar by Actavis	52152-0500	Antiandrogen
F50	Tab, White, Black Print	Flurbiprofen 50 mg	Froben by Abbott	Canadian DIN 02223066	NSAID
F50 <> APO	Tab, Gold, Round	Fluvoxamine Maleate 50 mg	Luvox by Apotex	60505-0165	OCD

ID FRONT <> BACK	DESCRIPTION FRONT <> BACK	INGREDIENT & STRENGTH	BRAND (or Generic Equiv.) by FIRM	NDC#	CLASS; SCH.
F50 <> RG	Tab, White to Off-White, Rectangular, Rounded	Fluconazole 50 mg	Diflucan by Barr	00555-0771	Antifungal
F6	Tab, Green, Modified Rectangle-Shaped, Film-Coated	Iron 90 mg, Folic Acid 1 mg, Vitamin B12 12 mcg, Vitamin C 120 mg, Docusate Sodium 50 mg	Ferralet 90 by Mission	00178-0089	Supplement
F617IMG	Cap, White	Tacrolimus 1 mg	Prograf by Astellas	00469-0617	Immunosuppressant
F64	Cap, Blue & Orange	Amobarbital Sodium 25 mg, Secobarbital Sodium 25 mg	Tuinal by Eli Lilly		Sedative/Hypnotic; C II
F65	Cap, Blue & Orange	Amobarbital Sodium 50 mg, Secobarbital Sodium 50 mg	Tuinal by Eli Lilly		Sedative/Hypnotic; C II
F6575MG	Cap, Pink	Tacrolimus 5 mg	Prograf by Astellas	00469-0657	Immunosuppressant
F66	Cap, Blue & Orange	Amobarbital Sodium 100 mg, Secobarbital Sodium 100 mg	Tuinal by Eli Lilly		Sedative/Hypnotic; C II
F66LL	Tab, Beige, Oblong, F/66-LL	Polycarbophil 500 mg	Fibercon by Lederle		Laxative
F74	Cap, Red	Vitamin Combination	Tycopan by Eli Lilly		Vitamin
F82	Tab, Blue, Cap Shaped, Film Coated	Valacyclovir HCl 500 mg	Valtrex by Aurobindo	65862-0448	Antiviral
F83	Tab, Blue, Cap Shaped, Film Coated, Scored	Valacyclovir HCl 1000 mg	Valtrex by Aurobindo	65862-0449	Antiviral
F96	Cap, Brown	Liver Stomach Concentrate, Vitamin Combination	Reticulex by Eli Lilly		Hematinic
F9BZYLOPRIM	Tab, White, Round, F9B/Zyloprim	Allopurinol 200 mg	Zyloprim by GSK	Canadian	Antigout
FA	Tab, Yellow, Oval	Beta-Carotene 4000 Units, Ascorbic Acid 120 mg, Thiamine HCl 3 mg, Riboflavin 3 mg, Pyridoxine HCl 3 mg, Cyanocobalamin 8 mcg, Niacin 20 mg, Vitamin D 400 Units, Vitamin E 30 Units, Folic Acid 1 mg, Calcium 200 mg, Iodine 150 mcg, Iron 29 mg, Zinc 15 mg	Nestabs FA by JB	51111-0008	Vitamin
FA	Tab, Yellow, Oval	Beta-Carotene 4000 Units, Ascorbic Acid 120 mg, Thiamine HCl 3 mg, Riboflavin 3 mg, Pyridoxine HCl 3 mg, Cyanocobalamin 8 mcg, Niacin 20 mg, Vitamin D 400 Units, Vitamin E 30 Units, Folic Acid 1 mg, Calcium 200 mg, Iodine 150 mcg, Iron 29 mg, Zinc 15 mg	Nestabs FA by Fielding	00421-1594	Vitamin
FA <> CIBA	Tab, White, Scored	Hydralazine HCl 10 mg	Apresoline by Novartis	Canadian DIN 00005525	Antihypertensive
FA2	Tab, Pink, Oblong	Triamcinolone 2 mg	Aristocort by Astellas		Steroid
FA8	Tab, Yellow, Oblong	Triamcinolone 8 mg	Aristocort by Astellas		Steroid
FACE	Tab, White, Round, Rastafarian Face Logo	3,4-Methylenedioxymethamphetamine (MDMA)	Ecstasy by Illegal		Euphoric; Illicit
FAM125 <> APO	Tab, White, Round	Famciclovir 125 mg	Famvir by Apotex	Canadian DIN 02292025	Antiviral
FAM250 <> APO	Tab, White, Round	Famciclovir 250 mg	Famvir by Apotex	Canadian DIN 02292041	Antiviral
FAM500 <> APO	Tab, White, Oval	Famciclovir 500 mg	Famvir by Apotex	Canadian DIN 02292068	Antiviral
FAMVIR <> 125	Tab, White, Round, Film Coated	Famciclovir 125 mg	Famvir by Apotheca	12634-0508	Antiviral
FAMVIR <> 125	Tab, White, Round, Film Coated	Famciclovir 125 mg	Famvir by Allscripts		Antiviral
FAMVIR <> 125	Tab, White, Round, Film Coated	Famciclovir 125 mg	Famvir by SKB	00007-4115	Antiviral
FAMVIR <> 125	Tab, White, Round, Film Coated	Famciclovir 125 mg	Famvir by Novartis	00078-0366	Antiviral
FAMVIR <> 125	Tab, White, Round, Film Coated	Famciclovir 125 mg	Famvir by SKB	60351-4115	Antiviral
FAMVIR <> 125	Tab, White, Round, Film Coated	Famciclovir 125 mg	Famvir by Physician Total Care	54868-3882	Antiviral
FAMVIR <> 125	Tab, White, Round, Film Coated	Famciclovir 125 mg	Famvir by Novartis	Canadian DIN 02229110	Antiviral
FAMVIR <> 250	Tab, White, Round, Film Coated	Famciclovir 250 mg	Famvir by Physician Total Care	54868-3969	Antiviral
FAMVIR <> 250	Tab, White, Round, Film Coated	Famciclovir 250 mg	Famvir by SKB	00007-4116	Antiviral
FAMVIR <> 250	Tab, White, Round, Film Coated	Famciclovir 250 mg	Famvir by Novartis	00078-0367	Antiviral
FAMVIR <> 250	Tab, White, Round, Film Coated	Famciclovir 250 mg	Famvir by Novartis	Canadian DIN 02229129	Antiviral
FAMVIR <> 250	Tab, White, Round, Film Coated	Famciclovir 250 mg	Famvir by SKB	60351-4116	Antiviral

ID FRONT <> BACK	DESCRIPTION FRONT <> BACK	INGREDIENT & STRENGTH	BRAND (or Generic Equiv.) by FIRM	NDC#	CLASS; SCH.
FAMVIR <> 500	Tab, White, Oblong, Film Coated	Famciclovir 500 mg	Famvir by Novartis	Canadian DIN 02177102	Antiviral
FAMVIR <> 500	Tab, White, Oblong, Film Coated	Famciclovir 500 mg	Famvir by SKB	00007-4117	Antiviral
FAMVIR <> 500	Tab, White, Oblong, Film Coated	Famciclovir 500 mg	Famvir by SKB	60351-4117	Antiviral
FAMVIR <> 500	Tab, White, Oblong, Film Coated	Famciclovir 500 mg	Famvir by Novartis	00078-0368	Antiviral
FANSIDARROCHE	Tab, White, Round, Scored, FANSIDAR and Roche Logo over ROCHE	Pyrimethamine 25 mg, Sulfadoxine 500 mg	Fansidar by Hoffmann La Roche	00004-0161	Antimalarial
FANSIDARROCHE	Tab, Scored	Pyrimethamine 25 mg, Sulfadoxine 500 mg	Fansidar by F Hoffmann La Roche	12806-0161	Antimalarial
FASTAB <> SYMAX	Tab, Light Blue, Round	Hyoscyamine Sulfate 0.125 mg	Symax FasTab by Capellon by PDRX	64543-0114	Gastrointestinal
FASTINBEECHAM	Cap, Blue & Clear	Phentermine HCl 30 mg		55289-0180	Anorexiant; C IV
FASTINBEECHAM	Cap, Blue & White Beads	Phentermine 30 mg	Fastin by H J Harkins Co	52959-0430	Anorexiant; C IV
FASTINBEECHAM	Cap, Blue & White Beads	Phentermine 30 mg	Fastin by King	60793-0836	Anorexiant; C IV
FASTINBEECHAM	Cap, R inside Circle to Right of Fastin in Red Ink <> Beecham in White Ink	Phentermine 30 mg	Fastin by SKB	00029-2205	Anorexiant; C IV
FC	Tab, White, Oval, Abbott Logo	Temafloxacin HCl 400 mg	Omniflox by Abbott		Antibiotic
FC100 <> G	Tab, White, Round, Scored, FC_100	Flecainide Acetate 100 mg	Tambocor by Par	49884-0695	Antiarrhythmic
FC119	Cap, Tan	Psyllium 0.52 g	Metamucil by Equate	68163-0119	Supplement
FC150 <> G	Tab, White, Oval, Scored	Flecainide Acetate 150 mg	Tambocor by Par	49884-0696	Antiarrhythmic
FC1SANDOZ78105	Cap, Red & Yellow, F-C #1 Sandoz 78-105	Aspirin 325 mg, Butalbital 50 mg, Caffeine 40 mg, Codeine 7.5 mg	Fiorinal #1 by Sandoz		Analgesic; C III
FC2SANDOZ78106	Cap, Gray & Yellow, F-C #2 Sandoz 78-106	Aspirin 325 mg, Butalbital 50 mg, Caffeine 40 mg, Codeine 15 mg	Fiorinal #2 by Sandoz		Analgesic; C III
FC50 <> G	Tab, White, Round	Flecainide Acetate 50 mg	Tambocor by Par	49884-0694	Antiarrhythmic
FCN100 <> APO	Tab, Pink, Round	Fluconazole 100 mg	Diflucan by Apotex	60505-0120	Antifungal
FCN150 <> APO	Tab, Pink, Round	Fluconazole 150 mg	Diflucan by Apotex	60505-0121	Antifungal
FCN200 <> APO	Tab, Pink, Round	Fluconazole 200 mg	Diflucan by Apotex	60505-0122	Antifungal
FCN50 <> APO	Tab, Pink, Round	Fluconazole 50 mg	Diflucan by Apotex	60505-0119	Antifungal
FCSANDOZ78107	Cap, Sandoz Logo F-C <> Sandoz 78-107	Aspirin 325 mg, Butalbital 50 mg, Caffeine 40 mg, Codeine Phosphate 30 mg	Fiorinal w/ Codeine by Allscripts		Analgesic; C III
FDM014 <> DURA	Tab, Blue, Oblong, Scored	Dextromethorphan HBr 30 mg, Guaifenesin 600 mg	Fenesin DM by DRX	55045-2621	Cold Remedy
FDM014 <> DURA	Tab, Blue, Oblong, Scored	Dextromethorphan HBr 30 mg, Guaifenesin 600 mg	Fenesin DM by Anabolic	00722-6275	Cold Remedy
FDM014 <> DURA	Tab, Blue, Oblong, Scored	Dextromethorphan HBr 30 mg, Guaifenesin 600 mg	Fenesin DM by PDRX	55289-0625	Cold Remedy
FE	Tab, Red, Round, Film Coated	Ferrous Sulfate 300 mg	Feratab by Upsher Smith	00245-0053	Mineral
FE	Tab, Green, Round, Sugar Coated	Ferrous Gluconate 300 mg	Fergon by Upsher Smith	00245-0061	Mineral
FELDENEPFIZER322	Cap, Maroon & Blue	Piroxicam 10 mg	Feldene by Pfizer	Canadian DIN 00525596	NSAID
FELDENEPFIZER322	Cap, Maroon & Blue	Piroxicam 10 mg	Feldene by Pfizer	00069-3220	NSAID
FELDENEPFIZER323	Cap, Maroon	Piroxicam 20 mg	Feldene by Pfizer	Canadian DIN 00525618	NSAID
FELDENEPFIZER323	Cap, Maroon	Piroxicam 20 mg	Feldene by Prestige	58056-0340	NSAID
FELDENEPFIZER323	Cap, Maroon	Piroxicam 20 mg	Feldene by Amerisource	62584-0230	NSAID
FELDENEPFIZER323	Cap, Maroon	Piroxicam 20 mg	Feldene by Nat Pharmpak	55154-2702	NSAID
FELDENEPFIZER323	Cap, Maroon	Piroxicam 20 mg	Feldene by Pharmedix	53002-0389	NSAID
FELDENEPFIZER323	Cap, Maroon	Piroxicam 20 mg	Feldene by Pfizer	00069-3230	NSAID
FEN160 <> APO	Tab, White, Oval, Film Coated	Fenofibrate 160 mg	Apo-Feno Super by Apotex	Canadian DIN 02246860	Antihyperlipidemic
FH <> GEIGY	Tab, Cream, Round, Sugar Coated	Clomipramine HCl 25 mg	Anafranil by Cobalt	Canadian DIN 02244817	OCD
FH <> GEIGY	Tab, Cream, Round, Sugar Coated	Clomipramine HCl 25 mg	Anafranil by Novartis	Canadian DIN 00324019	OCD
FH10 <> 440	Tab, Oyster, Round, Film Coated, Extended Release	Nisoldipine 10 mg	Sular by Horizon	59630-0440	Antihypertensive
FH20 <> 441	Tab, Yellow, Round, Film Coated, Extended Release	Nisoldipine 20 mg	Sular by Horizon	59630-0441	Antihypertensive
FH30 <> 442	Tab, Mustard, Round, Film Coated, Extended Release	Nisoldipine 30 mg	Sular by Horizon	59630-0442	Antihypertensive

For updated data, go to www.IdentADrug.com

ID FRONT <> BACK	DESCRIPTION FRONT <> BACK	INGREDIENT & STRENGTH	BRAND (or Generic Equiv.) by FIRM	NDC#	CLASS; SCH.
FH40 <> 443	Tab, Burnt Orange, Round, Film Coated, Extended Release	Nisoldipine 40 mg	Sular by Horizon	59630-0443	Antihypertensive
FHPC400PONSTEL	Cap, Ivory w/ Blue Bands, a Logo	Mefenamic Acid 250 mg	Ponstel by Horizon	59630-0400	NSAID
FI <> A	Tab, Yellow, Abbott Logo <> FI	Fenofibrate 48 mg	TriCor by Abbott	00074-6122	Antihyperlipidemic
FIII	Cap, ER, White Beads in Capsule	Theophylline Anhydrous 65 mg	Aerolate III by Fleming	00256-0150	Antiasthmatic
FIORICET	Tab, Light Blue, Round, Three Head Profile	Acetaminophen 325 mg, Butalbital 50 mg, Caffeine 40 mg	FIORICET by Watson	52544-0957	Analgesic
FIORICETCODEINE	Tab, Dark Blue & Gray, Opaque, Red Print, Four-Head Profile	Acetaminophen 325 mg, Butalbital 50 mg, Caffeine 40 mg, Codeine Phosphate 30 mg	Fioricet w/ Codeine by Novartis	00078-0243	Analgesic; C III
FIORICETCODEINE	Cap, Dark Blue & Gray, Opaque, Red Print, Four-Head Profile	Acetaminophen 325 mg, Butalbital 50 mg, Caffeine 40 mg, Codeine Phosphate 30 mg	Fioricet w/ Codeine by Watson	52544-0958	Analgesic; C III
FIORICETS	Tab, Blue, Round, Fioricet over S in Triangle <> 3 Headed Profile	Acetaminophen 325 mg, Butalbital 50 mg, Caffeine 40 mg	Fioricet by Prestige	58056-0349	Analgesic
FIORICETS	Tab, Blue, Round, Fioricet over S in Triangle <> 3 Headed Profile	Acetaminophen 325 mg, Butalbital 50 mg, Caffeine 40 mg	Fioricet by Amerisource	62584-0084	Analgesic
FIORICETS	Tab, Blue, Round, Fioricet over S in Triangle <> 3 Headed Profile	Acetaminophen 325 mg, Butalbital 50 mg, Caffeine 40 mg	Fioricet by Novartis	00078-0084	Analgesic
FIORICETS	Tab, Blue, Round, Fioricet over S in Triangle <> 3 Headed Profile	Acetaminophen 325 mg, Butalbital 50 mg, Caffeine 40 mg	Fioricet by Repack Co of America	55306-0084	Analgesic
FIORICETS	Tab, Blue, Round, Fioricet over S in Triangle <> 3 Headed Profile	Acetaminophen 325 mg, Butalbital 50 mg, Caffeine 40 mg	Fioricet by Leiner	59606-0649	Analgesic
FIORICETS	Tab, Blue, Round, Fioricet over S in Triangle <> 3 Headed Profile	Acetaminophen 325 mg, Butalbital 50 mg, Caffeine 40 mg	Fioricet by Able	Discontinued	Analgesic
FIORICETS	Tab, Blue, Round, Fioricet over S in Triangle <> 3 Headed Profile	Acetaminophen 325 mg, Butalbital 50 mg, Caffeine 40 mg	Fioricet by Allscripts		Analgesic
FIORICETS	Tab, Blue, Round, Fioricet over S in Triangle <> 3 Headed Profile	Acetaminophen 325 mg, Butalbital 50 mg, Caffeine 40 mg	Fioricet by CVS	00894-6131	Analgesic
FIORICETS	Tab, Blue, Round, Fioricet over S in Triangle <> 3 Headed Profile	Acetaminophen 325 mg, Butalbital 50 mg, Caffeine 40 mg	Fioricet by Rightpak	65240-0649	Analgesic
FIORINAL <> S	Tab, White, Round, Fiorinal <> S in a Triangle	Butalbital 50 mg, Caffeine 40 mg, Aspirin 330 mg	Fiorinal by Novartis	Canadian DIN 00275328	Analgesic; C III
FIORINAL78103	Cap, Green	Butalbital 50 mg, Caffeine 40 mg, Aspirin 325 mg	Fiorinal by Med Pro	53978-3395	Analgesic; C III
FIORINAL78103	Cap, Dark Green & Light Green, Fiorinal 78-103 <> Fiorinal 78-103	Aspirin 325 mg, Butalbital 50 mg, Caffeine 40 mg	Fiorinal by Novartis	00078-0103	Analgesic; C III
FIORINAL955	Cap, Kelly Green and Lime Green	Butalbital 50 mg, Aspirin 325 mg, Caffeine 40 mg	Fiorinal by Watson	52544-0955	Analgesic; C III
FIORINALC12S	Cap, Blue & Light Blue, Gelatin, Fiorinal C 1/2 S in a Triangle	Butalbital 50 mg, Caffeine 40 mg, Aspirin 330 mg	Fiorinal by Novartis	Canadian DIN 00176206	Analgesic; C III
FIORINALC14S	Cap, Blue & White, Gelatin, Fiorinal C 1/4 S in a Triangle	Butalbital 50 mg, Caffeine 40 mg, Aspirin 330 mg	Fiorinal by Novartis	Canadian DIN 00176192	Analgesic; C III
FIORINALCODEINE-WATSON956	Cap, Blue Cap, Yellow Body	Butalbital 50 mg, Aspirin 325 mg, Caffeine 40 mg, Codeine 30 mg	Fiorinal w/ Codeine by Watson	52544-0956	Analgesic
FIORINALS	Cap, Blue & Purple, Gelatin, Fiorinal w/ S inside a Triangle	Butalbital 50 mg, Caffeine 40 mg, Aspirin 330 mg	Fiorinal by Novartis	Canadian DIN 00226327	Analgesic; C III
FISH	Tab, White, Mottled Red, ><> Fish Logo	3,4-Methylenedioxymethamphetamine (MDMA)	Ecstasy by Illegal		Euphoric; Illicit
FISONS101	Cap, Clear	Sodium Cromoglycate 100 mg	by RPR	Canadian	Antiasthmatic
FISONSINTALP	Cap, Clear & Yellow, Fisons/Intal-p	Sodium Cromoglycate 20 mg	by RPR	Canadian	Antiasthmatic
FJR	Cap, Clear & Red, Ex Release, with White Beads, F in Triangle Symbol	Theophylline Anhydrous 130 mg	Aerolate Jr by Fleming	00256-0114	Antiasthmatic
FJR	Cap, White Beads	Chlorpheniramine Maleate 4 mg, Methscopolamine Nitrate 1.25 mg, Phenylephrine HCl 10 mg	Extendryl Jr by Fleming	00256-0177	Cold Remedy
FJR	Cap, Green & Red, F in Triangle Logo JR	Chlorpheniramine Maleate 4 mg, Phenylephrine HCl 10 mg, Methscopolamine 1.25 mg	Extendryl Jr by Fleming		Cold Remedy
FJR	Cap, Clear & Red, F in Triangle Logo JR	Theophylline Anhydrous 130 mg	Aerolate JR by Fleming		Antiasthmatic

For updated data, go to www.IdentADrug.com

ID FRONT <> BACK	DESCRIPTION FRONT <> BACK	INGREDIENT & STRENGTH	BRAND (or Generic Equiv.) by FIRM	NDC#	CLASS; SCH.
FJR	Cap, Blue & Clear, F in Triangle JR	Guaifenesin 125 mg, Pseudoephedrine 60 mg	Aquabid D by Fleming	62542-0420	Cold Remedy
FJR	Cap, Ex Release, Logo F and JR	Guaifenesin 125 mg, Pseudoephedrine HCl 60 mg	Aquabid D by Pharmatab	00256-0174	Cold Remedy
FJR	Cap, White Beads	Guaifenesin 125 mg, Pseudoephedrine HCl 60 mg	Aquabid D by Fleming		Cold Remedy
FL	Cap, Clear & White, Black Print, Two Black Hearts	Chlorpheniramine Maleate 8 mg, Pseudoephedrine HCl 120 mg	Kronofed A by Ferndale	00496-0382	Cold Remedy
FL	Cap, Clear & White, Red Print, Two Red Hearts	Chlorpheniramine Maleate 4 mg, Pseudoephedrine HCl 60 mg	Kronofed A Jr by Ferndale	00496-0434	Cold Remedy
FL <> 10	Tab, Pinkish-Purple, Triangular	Nebivolol HCl 10 mg	Bystolic by Forest	00456-1410	Antihypertensive
FL <> 10	Tab, White to Off-White, Round, Scored, Film Coated, F over L <> 10	Escitalopram Oxalate 10 mg	Lexapro by Forest	00456-2010	Antidepressant
FL <> 10	Tab, Gray, Cap Shaped, Film Coated	Memantine HCl 10 mg	Namenda Titration Pak by Forest	00456-3200	Antialzheimers
FL <> 10	Tab, Gray, Cap Shaped, Film Coated	Memantine HCl 10 mg	Namenda by Forest	00456-3210	Antialzheimers
FL <> 100	Tab, Blue, Oval, Film Coated	Milnacipran HCl 100 mg	Savella by Forest	00456-1510	Antidepressant; Antifibromyalgia
FL <> 15	Tab, Purple, Cap Shaped, Film Coated	Memantine 15 mg	Namenda by Forest	00456-3215	Antialzheimers
FL <> 20	Tab, White to Off-White, Round, Scored, Film Coated	Escitalopram Oxalate 20 mg	Lexapro by Forest	00456-2020	Antidepressant
FL <> 212	Tab, Light Blue, Triangular, FL <> 2 1/2	Nebivolol HCl 2.5 mg	Bystolic by Forest	00456-1402	Antihypertensive
FL <> 25	Tab, White, Round, Film Coated	Milnacipran HCl 25 mg	Savella by Forest	00456-1525	Antidepressant; Antifibromyalgia
FL <> 5	Tab, Beige, Triangular	Nebivolol HCl 5 mg	Bystolic by Forest	00456-1405	Antihypertensive
FL <> 5	Tab, White to Off-White, Round, Film Coated	Escitalopram Oxalate 5 mg	Lexapro by Forest	00456-2005	Antidepressant
FL <> 5	Tab, Tan, Cap Shaped, Film Coated	Memantine HCl 5 mg	Namenda by Forest	00456-3205	Antialzheimers
FL <> 5	Tab, Tan, Cap Shaped, Film Coated	Memantine HCl 5 mg	Namenda Titration Pak by Forest	00456-3200	Antialzheimers
FL <> 50	Tab, Green, Oval, Film-Coated	Milnacipran HCl 50 mg	Savella by Forest	00456-1550	Antidepressant; Antifibromyalgia
FI <> A	Tab, Yellow, Abbott Logo <> Fl	Fenofibrate 48 mg	TriCor by Abbott	00074-6122	Antihyperlipidemic
FL10 <> G	Tab, White, Oval, Scored, Film Coated, G <> FL over 10	Fluoxetine HCl 10 mg	Prozac by Alphapharm	57315-0051	Antidepressant
FL10 <> TARO	Tab, White, Oval, Scored, Film Coated, G <> FL over 10	Fluoxetine HCl 10 mg	Prozac by Par	49884-0734	Antidepressant
FL100 <> G	Tab, Pink, Rectangular	Fluconazole 100 mg	Diflucan by Par	49884-0939	Antifungal
FL100 <> TARO	Tab, Pink, Rectangular	Fluconazole 100 mg	Diflucan by Taro	51672-4065	Antifungal
FL100 <> TARO	Tab, Pink, Rectangular	Fluconazole 100 mg	Diflucan by Taro	Canadian DIN 02249308	Antifungal
FL1033	Tab, Aqua, Round	Belladonna Alkaloids 0.2 mg, Ergotamine Tartrate 0.6 mg, Phenobarbital 40 mg	Bellamine S by Ivax	00182-1990	Gastrointestinal; C IV
FL150 <> G	Tab, Pink, Oval	Fluconazole 150 mg	Diflucan by Par	49884-0940	Antifungal
FL150 <> TARO	Tab, Pink, Rectangular	Fluconazole 150 mg	Diflucan by Taro	51672-4066	Antifungal
FL20 <> G	Tab, White, Oval, Scored, Film Coated, G <> FL over 20	Fluoxetine HCl 20 mg	Prozac by Alphapharm	57315-0052	Antidepressant
FL20 <> G	Tab, White, Oval, Scored, Film Coated, G <> FL over 20	Fluoxetine HCl 20 mg	Prozac by Par	49884-0735	Antidepressant
FL200 <> G	Tab, Pink, Rectangular	Fluconazole 200 mg	Diflucan by Par	49884-0941	Antifungal
FL200 <> TARO	Tab, Pink, Rectangular	Fluconazole 200 mg	Diflucan by Taro	51672-4067	Antifungal
FL50 <> TARO	Tab, Pink, Rectangular	Fluconazole 50 mg	Diflucan by Taro	51672-4064	Antifungal
FL50 <> TARO	Tab, Pink, Rectangular	Fluconazole 50 mg	Diflucan by Taro	Canadian DIN 02249294	Antifungal
FL88	Tab, Blue, Round	Levothyroxine Sodium 88 mcg	Synthroid by Forest		Thyroid Hormone
FL99	Cap, White	Chlorpheniramine Maleate 4 mg, Pseudoephedrine HCl 60 mg	Kronofed A JR by Collagenex	64682-0007	Cold Remedy
FLA200 <> APO	Tab, White, Round, Coated	Flavoxate HCl 200 mg	Apo Flavoxate by Apotex	Canadian DIN 02244842	Antispasmodic
FLAGYL <> 500	Tab, Blue, Oblong, Film Coated	Metronidazole 500 mg	Flagyl by Thrift Drug	59198-0030	Antibiotic
FLAGYL <> 500	Tab, Blue, Oblong, Film Coated	Metronidazole 500 mg	Flagyl by Neuman	64579-0118	Antibiotic
FLAGYL <> 500	Tab, Blue, Oblong, Film Coated	Metronidazole 500 mg	Flagyl by Searle	00025-1821	Antibiotic
FLAGYL250 <> SEARLE1831	Tab, Blue, Round, Film Coated	Metronidazole 250 mg	Flagyl by Thrift Drug	59198-0311	Antibiotic

ID FRONT <> BACK	DESCRIPTION FRONT <> BACK	INGREDIENT & STRENGTH	BRAND (or Generic Equiv.) by FIRM	NDC#	CLASS; SCH.
FLAGYL250 <> SEARLE1831	Tab, Blue, Round, Film Coated	Metronidazole 250 mg	Flagyl by Amerisource	62584-0831	Antibiotic
FLAGYL250 <> SEARLE1831	Tab, Blue, Round, Film Coated	Metronidazole 250 mg	Flagyl by Searle	00025-1831	Antibiotic
FLAGYL375	Cap, Green & Gray	Metronidazole 375 mg	Flagyl by Physician Total Care	54868-3786	Antibiotic
FLAGYL375	Cap, Green & Gray	Metronidazole 375 mg	Flagyl by Searle	00025-1942	Antibiotic
FLAGYLER <> SEARLE1961	Tab, Blue, Oval, Film Coated, Ex Release	Metronidazole 750 mg	Flagyl by Mova	55370-0562	Antibiotic
FLAGYLER <> SEARLE1961	Tab, Blue, Oval, Film Coated, Ex Release	Metronidazole 750 mg	Flagyl by Searle	00025-1961	Antibiotic
FLE100 <> APO	Tab, White, Round, Scored	Flecainide Acetate 100 mg	Tambocor by Apotex	Canadian 02275546	Antiarrhythmic
FLE50 <> APO	Tab, White, Round	Flecainide Acetate 50 mg	Tambocor by Apotex	Canadian DIN 02275538	Antiarrhythmic
FLEX5 <> FLEXERIL	Tab, Yellow-Orange, D-Shaped, Film Coated, FLEX over 5	Cyclobenzaprine HCl 5 mg	Flexeril by McNeil	50580-0280	Muscle Relaxant
FLEXERIL	Tab, Butterscotch Yellow, D-Shaped, Film Coated	Cyclobenzaprine HCl 10 mg	Flexeril by McNeil	50580-0874	Muscle Relaxant
FLEXERIL <> FLEX5	Tab, Yellow-Orange, D-Shaped, Film Coated, FLEX over 5	Cyclobenzaprine HCl 5 mg	Flexeril by McNeil	50580-0280	Muscle Relaxant
FLEXERIL <> MSD931	Tab, Butterscotch Yellow, D-Shaped, Film Coated	Cyclobenzaprine HCl 10 mg	by Allscripts		Muscle Relaxant
FLEXERIL <> MSD931	Tab, Butterscotch Yellow, D-Shaped, Film Coated	Cyclobenzaprine HCl 10 mg	Flexeril by Merck	00006-0931	Muscle Relaxant
FLEXERIL <> MSD931	Tab, Butterscotch Yellow, D-Shaped, Film Coated	Cyclobenzaprine HCl 10 mg	by Nat Pharmpak	55154-5007	Muscle Relaxant
FLI14MG	Cap, Yellow and Dark Green, Opaque	Memantine HCl 14 mg	Namenda XR by Forest	00456-3414	Antialzheimers
FLI21MG	Cap, White to Off White and Green, Opaque	Memantine HCl 21 mg	Namenda XR by Forest	00456-3421	Antialzheimers
FLI28MG	Cap, Dark Green, Opaque	Memantine HCl 28 mg	Namenda XR by Forest	00456-3428	Antialzheimers
FLI7MG	Cap, Yellow, Opaque, Black Ink, Extended Release	Memantine HCl 7 mg	Namenda XR by Forest	00456-3407	Antialzheimers
FLINT <> 100	Tab, Yellow, Round, Scored	Levothyroxine Sodium 100 mcg	Synthroid by Abbott	00048-1070	Thyroid Hormone
FLINT <> 100	Tab, Yellow, Round, Scored	Levothyroxine Sodium 100 mcg	Synthroid by Pharmedix	53002-1056	Thyroid Hormone
FLINT <> 100	Tab, Yellow, Round, Scored	Levothyroxine Sodium 100 mcg	Synthroid by Med Pro	53978-1038	Thyroid Hormone
FLINT <> 100	Tab, Yellow, Round, Scored	Levothyroxine Sodium 100 mcg	Synthroid by Giant Food	11146-0305	Thyroid Hormone
FLINT <> 100	Tab, Yellow, Round, Scored	Levothyroxine Sodium 100 mcg	Synthroid by Rite Aid	11822-5193	Thyroid Hormone
FLINT <> 100	Tab, Yellow, Round, Scored	Levothyroxine Sodium 100 mcg	Synthroid by Nat Pharmpak	55154-0906	Thyroid Hormone
FLINT <> 100	Tab, Yellow, Round, Scored	Levothyroxine Sodium 100 mcg	Synthroid by Abbott	Canadian DIN 02172100	Thyroid Hormone
FLINT <> 100	Tab, Yellow, Round, Scored	Levothyroxine Sodium 100 mcg	Synthroid by Amerisource	62584-0014	Thyroid Hormone
FLINT <> 100	Tab, Yellow, Round, Scored	Levothyroxine Sodium 100 mcg	Synthroid by Forest	00456-0323	Thyroid Hormone
FLINT <> 100	Tab, Yellow, Round, Scored	Levothyroxine Sodium 100 mcg	Synthroid by Murfreesboro	51129-1665	Thyroid Hormone
FLINT <> 100	Tab, Yellow, Round, Scored	Levothyroxine Sodium 100 mcg	Synthroid by Kaiser	00179-0458	Thyroid Hormone
FLINT <> 100MCG	Tab, Debossed	Levothyroxine Sodium 100 mcg	Synthroid by Amerisource	62584-0070	Thyroid Hormone
FLINT <> 100MCG	Tab, Yellow, Round, Scored	Levothyroxine Sodium 100 mcg	Synthroid by Rightpac	65240-0742	Thyroid Hormone
FLINT <> 100MCG	Tab, Yellow, Round, Scored	Levothyroxine Sodium 100 mcg	Synthroid by Wal Mart	49035-0194	Thyroid Hormone
FLINT <> 112	Tab, Rose, Round, Scored	Levothyroxine Sodium 112 mcg	Synthroid by CVS	51316-0201	Thyroid Hormone
FLINT <> 112	Tab, Rose, Round, Scored	Levothyroxine Sodium 112 mcg	Synthroid by Repack Co Of America	55306-1080	Thyroid Hormone
FLINT <> 112	Tab, Rose, Round, Scored	Levothyroxine Sodium 112 mcg	Synthroid by Nat Pharmpak	55154-0911	Thyroid Hormone
FLINT <> 112	Tab, Rose, Round, Scored	Levothyroxine Sodium 112 mcg	Synthroid by Abbott	00048-1080	Thyroid Hormone
FLINT <> 112	Tab, Rose, Round, Scored	Levothyroxine Sodium 112 mcg	Synthroid by Forest	00456-0330	Thyroid Hormone
FLINT <> 112	Tab, Rose, Round, Scored	Levothyroxine Sodium 112 mcg	Synthroid by Abbott	Canadian DIN 02171228	Thyroid Hormone
FLINT <> 112MCG	Tab, Debossed	Levothyroxine Sodium 112 mcg	Synthroid by Amerisource	62584-0080	Thyroid Hormone
FLINT <> 112MCG	Tab, Round, Scored	Levothyroxine Sodium 112 mcg	Synthroid by Rightpac	65240-0743	Thyroid Hormone
FLINT <> 125	Tab, Light Brown, Round, Scored	Levothyroxine Sodium 125 mcg	Synthroid by Nat Pharmpak	55154-0909	Thyroid Hormone
FLINT <> 125	Tab, Light Brown, Round, Scored	Levothyroxine Sodium 125 mcg	Synthroid by Giant Food	11146-0303	Thyroid Hormone

ID FRONT <> BACK	DESCRIPTION FRONT <> BACK	INGREDIENT & STRENGTH	BRAND (or Generic Equiv.) by FIRM	NDC#	CLASS; SCH.
FLINT <> 125	Tab, Light Brown, Round, Scored	Levothyroxine Sodium 125 mcg	Synthroid by Rite Aid	11822-5285	Thyroid Hormone
FLINT <> 125	Tab, Light Brown, Round, Scored	Levothyroxine Sodium 125 mcg	Synthroid by Kaiser	00179-1210	Thyroid Hormone
FLINT <> 125	Tab, Light Brown, Round, Scored	Levothyroxine Sodium 125 mcg	Synthroid by Abbott	00048-1130	Thyroid Hormone
FLINT <> 125	Tab, Light Brown, Round, Scored	Levothyroxine Sodium 125 mcg	Synthroid by Abbott	Canadian DIN 02172119	Thyroid Hormone
FLINT <> 125	Tab, Light Brown, Round, Scored	Levothyroxine Sodium 125 mcg	Synthroid by Forest	00456-0324	Thyroid Hormone
FLINT <> 125	Tab, Light Brown, Round, Scored	Levothyroxine Sodium 125 mcg	Synthroid by Murfreesboro	51129-1653	Thyroid Hormone
FLINT <> 125MCG	Tab, Debossed	Levothyroxine Sodium 125 mcg	Synthroid by Amerisource	62584-0130	Thyroid Hormone
FLINT <> 125MCG	Tab, Brown, Round, Scored	Levothyroxine Sodium 125 mcg	Synthroid by Rightpac	65240-0744	Thyroid Hormone
FLINT <> 137	Tab, Blue, Round, Scored	Levothyroxine Sodium 137 mcg	Synthroid by Forest	00456-0331	Thyroid Hormone
FLINT <> 137	Tab, Blue, Round, Scored	Levothyroxine Sodium 137 mcg	Synthroid by Abbott	Canadian DIN 02233852	Thyroid Hormone
FLINT <> 150	Tab, Light Blue, Round, Scored	Levothyroxine Sodium 150 mcg	Synthroid by Abbott	Canadian DIN 02172127	Thyroid Hormone
FLINT <> 150	Tab, Light Blue, Round, Scored	Levothyroxine Sodium 150 mcg	Synthroid by Forest	00456-0325	Thyroid Hormone
FLINT <> 150	Tab, Light Blue, Round, Scored	Levothyroxine Sodium 150 mcg	Synthroid by Amerisource	62584-0015	Thyroid Hormone
FLINT <> 150	Tab, Light Blue, Round, Scored	Levothyroxine Sodium 150 mcg	Synthroid by Rx Pak	65084-0182	Thyroid Hormone
FLINT <> 150	Tab, Light Blue, Round, Scored	Levothyroxine Sodium 150 mcg	Synthroid by Med Pro	53978-0999	Thyroid Hormone
FLINT <> 150	Tab, Light Blue, Round, Scored	Levothyroxine Sodium 150 mcg	Synthroid by Nat Pharmpak	55154-0905	Thyroid Hormone
FLINT <> 150	Tab, Light Blue, Round, Scored	Levothyroxine Sodium 150 mcg	Synthroid by Giant Food	11146-0304	Thyroid Hormone
FLINT <> 150	Tab, Light Blue, Round, Scored	Levothyroxine Sodium 150 mcg	Synthroid by Rite Aid	11822-5210	Thyroid Hormone
FLINT <> 150	Tab, Light Blue, Round, Scored	Levothyroxine Sodium 150 mcg	Synthroid by Kaiser	00179-0459	Thyroid Hormone
FLINT <> 150	Tab, Light Blue, Round, Scored	Levothyroxine Sodium 150 mcg	Synthroid by Abbott	00048-1090	Thyroid Hormone
FLINT <> 150MCG	Tab, Blue, Round, Scored	Levothyroxine Sodium 150 mcg	Synthroid by Wal Mart	49035-0193	Thyroid Hormone
FLINT <> 150MCG	Tab, Debossed	Levothyroxine Sodium 150 mcg	Synthroid by Amerisource	62584-0090	Thyroid Hormone
FLINT <> 175	Tab, Lilac, Round, Scored	Levothyroxine Sodium 175 mcg	Synthroid by Abbott	00048-1100	Thyroid Hormone
FLINT <> 175	Tab, Lilac, Round, Scored	Levothyroxine Sodium 175 mcg	Synthroid by Murfreesboro	51129-1643	Thyroid Hormone
FLINT <> 175	Tab, Lilac, Round, Scored	Levothyroxine Sodium 175 mcg	Synthroid by Forest	00456-0326	Thyroid Hormone
FLINT <> 175	Tab, Lilac, Round, Scored	Levothyroxine Sodium 175 mcg	Synthroid by Abbott	Canadian DIN 02172135	Thyroid Hormone
FLINT <> 175MCG	Tab, Purple, Round, Scored	Levothyroxine Sodium 175 mcg	Synthroid by Rightpac	65240-0758	Thyroid Hormone
FLINT <> 200	Tab, Pink, Round, Scored	Levothyroxine Sodium 200 mcg	Synthroid by Rx Pak	65084-0160	Thyroid Hormone
FLINT <> 200	Tab, Pink, Round, Scored	Levothyroxine Sodium 200 mcg	Synthroid by Wal Mart	49035-0172	Thyroid Hormone
FLINT <> 200	Tab, Pink, Round, Scored	Levothyroxine Sodium 200 mcg	Synthroid by Med Pro	53978-0856	Thyroid Hormone
FLINT <> 200	Tab, Pink, Round, Scored	Levothyroxine Sodium 200 mcg	Synthroid by Abbott	00048-1140	Thyroid Hormone
FLINT <> 200	Tab, Pink, Round, Scored	Levothyroxine Sodium 200 mcg	Synthroid by Kaiser	00179-0460	Thyroid Hormone
FLINT <> 200	Tab, Pink, Round, Scored	Levothyroxine Sodium 200 mcg	Synthroid by Rite Aid	11822-5194	Thyroid Hormone
FLINT <> 200	Tab, Pink, Round, Scored	Levothyroxine Sodium 200 mcg	Synthroid by Giant Food	11146-0306	Thyroid Hormone
FLINT <> 200	Tab, Pink, Round, Scored	Levothyroxine Sodium 200 mcg	Synthroid by Nat Pharmpak	55154-0907	Thyroid Hormone
FLINT <> 200	Tab, Pink, Round, Scored	Levothyroxine Sodium 200 mcg	Synthroid by Abbott	Canadian DIN 02172143	Thyroid Hormone
FLINT <> 200	Tab, Pink, Round, Scored	Levothyroxine Sodium 200 mcg	Synthroid by Murfreesboro	51129-1654	Thyroid Hormone
FLINT <> 200	Tab, Pink, Round, Scored	Levothyroxine Sodium 200 mcg	Synthroid by Forest	00456-0327	Thyroid Hormone
FLINT <> 200MCG	Tab, Debossed	Levothyroxine Sodium 200 mcg	Synthroid by Amerisource	62584-0140	Thyroid Hormone
FLINT <> 25	Tab, Orange, Round, Scored	Levothyroxine Sodium 25 mcg	Synthroid by Abbott	00048-1020	Thyroid Hormone
FLINT <> 25	Tab, Orange, Round, Scored	Levothyroxine Sodium 25 mcg	Synthroid by Rx Pak	65084-0174	Thyroid Hormone
FLINT <> 25	Tab, Orange, Round, Scored	Levothyroxine Sodium 25 mcg	Synthroid by Haines	59564-0115	Thyroid Hormone
FLINT <> 25	Tab, Orange, Round, Scored	Levothyroxine Sodium 25 mcg	Synthroid by Rite Aid	11822-5287	Thyroid Hormone
FLINT <> 25	Tab, Orange, Round, Scored	Levothyroxine Sodium 25 mcg	Synthroid by Forest	00456-0320	Thyroid Hormone
FLINT <> 25	Tab, Orange, Round, Scored	Levothyroxine Sodium 25 mcg	Synthroid by Nat Pharmpak	55154-0910	Thyroid Hormone

ID FRONT <> BACK	DESCRIPTION FRONT <> BACK	INGREDIENT & STRENGTH	BRAND (or Generic Equiv.) by FIRM	NDC#	CLASS; SCH.
FLINT <> 25	Tab, Orange, Round, Scored	Levothyroxine Sodium 25 mcg	Synthroid by Abbott	Canadian DIN 02172062	Thyroid Hormone
FLINT <> 25MCG	Tab, Debossed	Levothyroxine Sodium 25 mcg	Synthroid by Amerisource	62584-0020	Thyroid Hormone
FLINT <> 25MCG	Tab, Orange, Round, Scored	Levothyroxine Sodium 25 mcg	Synthroid by Rightpac	65240-0739	Thyroid Hormone
FLINT <> 300	Tab, Green, Round, Scored	Levothyroxine Sodium 300 mcg	Synthroid by Abbott	00048-1170	Thyroid Hormone
FLINT <> 300	Tab, Green, Round, Scored	Levothyroxine Sodium 300 mcg	Synthroid by Thrift Drug	59198-0298	Thyroid Hormone
FLINT <> 300	Tab, Green, Round, Scored	Levothyroxine Sodium 300 mcg	Synthroid by CVS	51316-0246	Thyroid Hormone
FLINT <> 300	Tab, Green, Round, Scored	Levothyroxine Sodium 300 mcg	Synthroid by Amerisource	62584-0170	Thyroid Hormone
FLINT <> 300	Tab, Green, Round, Scored	Levothyroxine Sodium 300 mcg	Synthroid by Abbott	Canadian DIN 02172151	Thyroid Hormone
FLINT <> 50	Tab, White, Round, Scored	Levothyroxine Sodium 50 mcg	Synthroid by Abbott	Canadian DIN 02172070	Thyroid Hormone
FLINT <> 50	Tab, White, Round, Scored	Levothyroxine Sodium 0.05 mg	Synthroid by Murfreesboro	51129-1657	Thyroid Hormone
FLINT <> 50	Tab, White, Round, Scored	Levothyroxine Sodium 50 mcg	Synthroid by Amerisource	62584-0013	Thyroid Hormone
FLINT <> 50	Tab, White, Round, Scored	Levothyroxine Sodium 50 mcg	Synthroid by Forest	00456-0321	Thyroid Hormone
FLINT <> 50	Tab, White, Round, Scored	Levothyroxine Sodium 50 mcg	Synthroid by Kaiser	00179-0457	Thyroid Hormone
FLINT <> 50	Tab, White, Round, Scored	Levothyroxine Sodium 50 mcg	Synthroid by Abbott	00048-1040	Thyroid Hormone
FLINT <> 50	Tab, White, Round, Scored	Levothyroxine Sodium 50 mcg	Synthroid by Med Pro	53978-0589	Thyroid Hormone
FLINT <> 50	Tab, White, Round, Scored	Levothyroxine Sodium 50 mcg	Synthroid by Knoll	55445-0104	Thyroid Hormone
FLINT <> 50	Tab, White, Round, Scored	Levothyroxine Sodium 50 mcg	Synthroid by Physician Total Care	54868-1011	Thyroid Hormone
FLINT <> 50	Tab, White, Round, Scored	Levothyroxine Sodium 50 mcg	Synthroid by Giant Food	11146-0301	Thyroid Hormone
FLINT <> 50MCG	Tab, Debossed	Levothyroxine Sodium 50 mcg	Synthroid by Amerisource	62584-0040	Thyroid Hormone
FLINT <> 50MCG	Tab, White, Round, Scored	Levothyroxine Sodium 50 mcg	Synthroid by Rightpac	65240-0740	Thyroid Hormone
FLINT <> 50MCG	Tab, White, Round, Scored	Levothyroxine Sodium 50 mcg	Synthroid by Murfreesboro	51129-1659	Thyroid Hormone
FLINT <> 75	Tab, Gray, Round, Scored	Levothyroxine Sodium 75 mcg	Synthroid by Rite Aid	11822-5286	Thyroid Hormone
FLINT <> 75	Tab, Gray, Round, Scored	Levothyroxine Sodium 75 mcg	Synthroid by Giant Food	11146-0302	Thyroid Hormone
FLINT <> 75	Tab, Gray, Round, Scored	Levothyroxine Sodium 75 mcg	Synthroid by Abbott	00048-1050	Thyroid Hormone
FLINT <> 75	Tab, Gray, Round, Scored	Levothyroxine Sodium 75 mcg	Synthroid by Nat Pharmpak	55154-0904	Thyroid Hormone
FLINT <> 75	Tab, Gray, Round, Scored	Levothyroxine Sodium 75 mcg	Synthroid by Forest	00456-0322	Thyroid Hormone
FLINT <> 75	Tab, Gray, Round, Scored	Levothyroxine Sodium 75 mcg	Synthroid by Abbott	Canadian DIN 02172089	Thyroid Hormone
FLINT <> 88	Tab, Green, Round, Scored	Levothyroxine Sodium 88 mcg	Synthroid by Abbott	Canadian DIN 02172097	Thyroid Hormone
FLINT <> 88	Tab, Green, Round, Scored	Levothyroxine Sodium 88 mcg	Synthroid by Forest	00456-0329	Thyroid Hormone
FLINT <> 88	Tab, Green, Round, Scored	Levothyroxine Sodium 88 mcg	Synthroid by Abbott	00048-1060	Thyroid Hormone
FLINT <> 88	Tab, Green, Round, Scored	Levothyroxine Sodium 88 mcg	Synthroid by Rightpac	65240-0757	Thyroid Hormone
FLINT <> 88	Tab, Green, Round, Scored	Levothyroxine Sodium 88 mcg	Synthroid by Physician Total Care	54868-2705	Thyroid Hormone
FLINT100MCG	Tab, Yellow, Round, Scored	Levothyroxine Sodium 100 mcg	Synthroid by Murfreesboro	51129-1660	Thyroid Hormone
FLINT112MCG	Tab, Rose	Levothyroxine Sodium 112 mcg	Synthroid by Thrift Drug	59198-0303	Thyroid Hormone
FLINT125MCG	Tab, Brown, Round, Scored	Levothyroxine Sodium 125 mcg	Synthroid by Murfreesboro	51129-1662	Thyroid Hormone
FLINT175MCG	Tab, Purple, Round, Scored	Levothyroxine Sodium 175 mcg	Synthroid by Murfreesboro	51129-1639	Thyroid Hormone
FLINT175MCG	Tab, Blue, Round, Scored	Levothyroxine Sodium 175 mcg	Synthroid by Rx Pak	65084-0196	Thyroid Hormone
FLINT25MCG	Tab, Orange, Round, Scored	Levothyroxine Sodium 25 mcg	Synthroid by Thrift Drug	59198-0337	Thyroid Hormone
FLINT300MCG	Tab, Green, Round, Scored	Levothyroxine Sodium 300 mcg	Synthroid by Murfreesboro	51129-1663	Thyroid Hormone
FLINT3P1093	Tab, Blue, Round, Scored	Levothyroxine Sodium 150 mcg	Synthroid by Rightpac	65240-0745	Thyroid Hormone
FLINT3P1143	Tab, Pink, Round, Scored	Levothyroxine Sodium 0.2 mg	Synthroid by Rightpac	65240-0746	Thyroid Hormone
FLINT3P1173	Tab, Green, Round, Scored	Levothyroxine Sodium 0.3 mg	Synthroid by Rightpac	65240-0747	Thyroid Hormone
FLINT75MCG	Tab, Purple, Round	Levothyroxine Sodium 0.075 mg	Synthroid by Physician Total Care	54868-2005	Thyroid Hormone
FLINT75MCG	Tab, Purple, Round, Scored	Levothyroxine Sodium 75 mcg	Synthroid by Murfreesboro	51129-1661	Thyroid Hormone
FLINT88MCG	Tab, Green, Round, Scored	Levothyroxine Sodium 88 mcg	Synthroid by Murfreesboro	51129-1641	Thyroid Hormone

ID FRONT <> BACK	DESCRIPTION FRONT <> BACK	INGREDIENT & STRENGTH	BRAND (or Generic Equiv.) by FIRM	NDC#	CLASS; SCH.
FLINT88MCG	Tab, Green, Round, Scored	Levothyroxine Sodium 88 mcg	Synthroid by Murfreesboro	51129-1667	Thyroid Hormone
FLINT88MCG	Tab, Green, Round, Scored	Levothyroxine Sodium 0.088 mg	Synthroid by Rx Pak	65084-0222	Thyroid Hormone
FLM50	Tab, White, Round, Scored	Fluvoxamine Maleate 50 mg	Luvox by Pharmascience	Canadian DIN 02240682	OCD
FLO200 <> APO	Tab, White, Round, Biconvex	Floctafenine 200 mg	Idarac by Apotex	Canadian DIN 02244680	Anti-Inflammatory
FLO400 <> APO	Tab, White, Round, Biconvex	Floctafenine 400 mg	Idarac by Apotex	Canadian DIN 02244681	Anti-Inflammatory
FLOMAX04MGBI58	Cap, Olive Green, Gelatin Coated, Flomax over 0.4 mg <> BI 58	Tamsulosin HCl 0.4 mg	Flomax by Boehringer Ingelheim	00597-0058	Antiadrenergic
FLOMAX04MGBI58	Cap, Olive Green, Gelatin Coated, Flomax over 0.4 mg <> BI 58	Tamsulosin HCl 0.4 mg	Flomax by Astellas	51248-0058	Antiadrenergic
FLOMAX04MGBI58	Cap, Olive Green, Gelatin Coated, Flomax over 0.4 mg <> BI 58	Tamsulosin HCl 0.4 mg	Flomax by Caremark	00339-5560	Antiadrenergic
FLOMAX04MGBI58	Cap, Olive Green, Gelatin Coated, Flomax over 0.4 mg <> BI 58	Tamsulosin HCl 0.4 mg	Flomax by Astellas	12838-0058	Antiadrenergic
FLORAZOLEER <> 750MG	Tab, Blue, Oval, Film-Coated, Extended-Release	Metronidazole 750 mg	Florazole ER by Ferring	Canadian DIN 02244405	Antiprotozoal
FLOXIN200	Tab, Light Yellow, Oval, Film Coated, Floxin over 200	Ofloxacin 200 mg	Floxin by Ortho-McNeil	00062-1540	Antibiotic
FLOXIN200	Tab, Light Yellow, Oval, Film Coated, Floxin over 200	Ofloxacin 200 mg	by Med Pro	53978-3014	Antibiotic
FLOXIN300	Tab, White, Oval, Film Coated, Floxin over 300	Ofloxacin 300 mg	Floxin by Ortho-McNeil	00062-1541	Antibiotic
FLOXIN300	Tab, White, Oval, Film Coated, Floxin over 300	Ofloxacin 300 mg	by Med Pro	53978-3018	Antibiotic
FLOXIN300	Tab, White, Oval, Film Coated, Floxin over 300	Ofloxacin 300 mg	Floxin by Janssen-Ortho	Canadian DIN 01968416	Antibiotic
FLOXIN400	Tab, Pale Gold, Oval, Film Coated, Floxin over 400	Ofloxacin 400 mg	Floxin by Janssen-Ortho	Canadian DIN 01968408	Antibiotic
FLOXIN400	Tab, Pale Gold, Oval, Film Coated, Floxin over 400	Ofloxacin 400 mg	Floxin by Ortho-McNeil	00062-1542	Antibiotic
FLU100 <> APO	Tab, Reddish Brown, Pillow Shaped	Fluvoxamine Maleate 100 mg	Luvox by Apotex	60505-0166	OCD
FLUMADINE100 <> FOREST	Tab, Orange, Oval, Film Coated	Rimantadine HCl 100 mg	Flumadine by H J Harkins Co	52959-0490	Antiviral
FLUMADINE100 <> FOREST	Tab, Orange, Oval, Film Coated	Rimantadine HCl 100 mg	Flumadine by Forest	00456-0521	Antiviral
FLUMADINE100 <> FOREST	Tab, Orange, Oval, Film Coated	Rimantadine HCl 100 mg	Flumadine by DRX	55045-2085	Antiviral
FLUORIDE1MG	Tab, Chewable	Sodium Fluoride 2.21 mg	Fluorabon by IVC Ind	00417-0672	Element
FLUORIDE1MG	Tab, Chewable	Sodium Fluoride 2.21 mg	Fluorabon by IVC Ind	00417-0318	Element
FLUORIDE1MG	Tab, Chewable	Sodium Fluoride 2.21 mg	Fluorabon by IVC Ind	00417-0317	Element
FLUORIDE1MG	Tab, Chewable	Sodium Fluoride 2.21 mg	Fluorabon by IVC Ind	00417-0229	Element
FLUORIDE1MG	Tab	Sodium Fluoride 2.2 mg	Fluorabon by IVC Ind	00417-1699	Element
FLUORIDE1MG	Tab	Sodium Fluoride 2.2 mg	Fluorabon by IVC Ind	00417-1599	Element
FLUORIDE1MG	Tab, Off-White	Ascorbic Acid 60 mg, Sodium Fluoride 2.2 mg, Vitamin A 3000 Units, Vitamin D 400 Units	Flor-Dac by IVC Ind	00417-1899	Vitamin
FLUOXETINE40MGR149	Cap, White & Blue, Black Print, Fluoxetine 40 mg on cap, R149 on body	Fluoxetine HCl 40 mg	Prozac by Par	49884-0743	Antidepressant
FLUOXETINER147	Cap, Light Blue, Opaque	Fluoxetine 10 mg	Prozac by Dr. Reddy's	55111-0147	Antidepressant
FLUOXETINER148	Cap, Light Blue and Light Turquoise, Opaque	Fluoxetine 20 mg	Prozac by Dr. Reddy's	55111-0148	Antidepressant
FLUOXETINER149	Cap, Light Blue and White, Opaque	Fluoxetine 40 mg	Prozac by Dr. Reddy's	55111-0149	Antidepressant
FLURAZEPAM15 <> WESTWARD	Tab, Blue & White, Oblong	Flurazepam HCl 15 mg	by Southwood	58016-0811	Hypnotic; C IV
FLURAZEPAM15-WESTWARD	Cap Black Print	Flurazepam HCl 15 mg	by Kaiser	00179-1098	Hypnotic; C IV

ID FRONT <> BACK	DESCRIPTION FRONT <> BACK	INGREDIENT & STRENGTH	BRAND (or Generic Equiv.) by FIRM	NDC#	CLASS; SCH.
FLURAZEPAM30 <> WESTWARD	Tab, Blue, Oblong	Flurazepam HCl 30 mg	by Southwood	58016-0812	Hypnotic; C IV
FLURAZEPAM30-WESTWARD	Cap, Black Print	Flurazepam HCl 30 mg	by Kaiser	00179-1099	Hypnotic; C IV
FLUT250 <> APO	Tab, Pale Yellow, Round, Scored	Flutamide 250 mg	Apo Flutamide by Apotex	Canadian DIN 02238560	Antiandrogen
FLUTAMIDE <> P250	Tab, Pale Yellow, Round, Scored	Flutamide 250 mg	by Pharmascience	Canadian DIN 02230104	Antiandrogen
FLZ100	Tab, Pink, Trapezoidal	Fluconazole 100 mg	Diflucan by Greenstone	59762-5016	Antifungal
FLZ150	Tab, Pink, Oval	Fluconazole 150 mg	Diflucan by Greenstone	59762-5017	Antifungal
FLZ200	Tab, Pink, Trapezoidal	Fluconazole 200 mg	Diflucan by Greenstone	59762-5018	Antifungal
FLZ50	Tab, Pink, Trapezoidal	Fluconazole 50 mg	Diflucan by Greenstone	59762-5015	Antifungal
FM	Tab, Blue, Oval, Film Coated	Tiagabine 16 mg	Gabitril by Abbott	60692-3960	Anticonvulsant
FM20G	Tab, Beige, D-Shaped, FM 20/G	Famotidine 20 mg	by Genpharm	Canadian	Gastrointestinal
FM40G	Tab, Light Brown, D-Shaped, FM 40/G	Famotidine 40 mg	by Genpharm	Canadian	Gastrointestinal
FN	Tab, Pink, Oval, Film Coated	Tiagabine 20 mg	Gabitril by Abbott	60692-3982	Anticonvulsant
FO <> A	Tab, White, Abbott Logo FO	Fenofibrate 145 mg	TriCor by Abbott	00074-6123	Antihyperlipidemic
FO1CPI	Tab, Yellow, Round, FO1/CPI	Folic Acid 1 mg	Folvite by Charlotte		Vitamin
FOREST <> 678	Cap	Acetaminophen 500 mg, Hydrocodone Bitartrate 5 mg	Vicodin by Pharmedix	53002-0120	Analgesic; C III
FOREST <> 678	Tab, White, Cap Shaped, Scored	Acetaminophen 500 mg, Butalbital 50 mg, Caffeine 40 mg	by Nat Pharmpak	55154-4602	Analgesic
FOREST <> 678	Tab, White, Cap Shaped, Scored	Acetaminophen 500 mg, Butalbital 50 mg, Caffeine 40 mg	Esgic Plus by Rightpak	65240-0644	Analgesic
FOREST <> 678	Tab, White, Cap Shaped, Scored	Acetaminophen 500 mg, Butalbital 50 mg, Caffeine 40 mg	Esgic Plus by Rx Pak	65084-0195	Analgesic
FOREST <> 678	Tab, White, Cap Shaped, Scored	Acetaminophen 500 mg, Butalbital 50 mg, Caffeine 40 mg	by PDRX	55289-0264	Analgesic
FOREST <> 678	Tab, White, Cap Shaped, Scored	Acetaminophen 500 mg, Butalbital 50 mg, Caffeine 40 mg	Esgic Plus by Forest	00456-0678	Analgesic
FOREST <> FLUMADINE100	Tab, Orange, Oval, Film Coated	Rimantadine HCl 100 mg	Flumadine by DRX	55045-2085	Antiviral
FOREST <> FLUMADINE100	Tab, Orange, Oval, Film Coated	Rimantadine HCl 100 mg	Flumadine by Forest	00456-0521	Antiviral
FOREST <> FLUMADINE100	Tab, Orange, Oval, Film Coated	Rimantadine HCl 100 mg	Flumadine by H J Harkins Co	52959-0490	Antiviral
FOREST0372-ESGICPLUS	Cap, Red, White Print	Acetaminophen 500 mg, Butalbital 50 mg, Caffeine 40 mg	Esgic Plus by Forest	00456-0679	Analgesic
FOREST0372-ESGICPLUS	Cap, Red, White Print	Acetaminophen 500 mg, Butalbital 50 mg, Caffeine 40 mg	Esgic Plus by Med Pro	53978-3396	Analgesic
FOREST0372-ESGICPLUS	Cap, Red, White Print	Acetaminophen 500 mg, Butalbital 50 mg, Caffeine 40 mg	Esgic Plus by Eckerd	19458-0844	Analgesic
FOREST0372-ESGICPLUS	Cap, Red, White Print	Acetaminophen 500 mg, Butalbital 50 mg, Caffeine 40 mg	Esgic Plus by Mikart	46672-0273	Analgesic
FOREST0372-ESGICPLUS	Cap, Red, White Print	Acetaminophen 500 mg, Butalbital 50 mg, Caffeine 40 mg	Esgic Plus by Thrift Drug	59198-0332	Analgesic
FOREST100	Tab, White, Round	Theophylline Anhydrous 100 mg	Duraphyl by Forest		Antiasthmatic
FOREST1054	Cap, Blue & Pink	Racemethionine 200 mg	Pedameth by Forest		Urinary Tract
FOREST150	Tab, Burgundy, Round	Guaifenesin 200 mg	Aquabid by Forest		Expectorant
FOREST161	Tab, White, Round	Powdered Opium 1.23 mg, Bismuth Subcarbonate 125 mg, Calcium Carb. 125 mg	Diabismul by Forest		Gastrointestinal; C V
FOREST200	Tab, White, Oblong	Theophylline Anhydrous 200 mg	Duraphyl by Forest		Antiasthmatic
FOREST251	Tab, Blue, Oblong	Sulfamethazole 500 mg	Proklar by Forest		Antibiotic
FOREST281	Tab, Green, Round	Dehydrocholic Acid 125 mg, Phenobarbital 8 mg, Homatropine Methylbromide 2.5 mg	G.B.S. by Forest		Gastrointestinal; C IV

ID FRONT <> BACK	DESCRIPTION FRONT <> BACK	INGREDIENT & STRENGTH	BRAND (or Generic Equiv.) by FIRM	NDC#	CLASS; SCH.
FOREST295	Tab, Pink, Sugar Coated	Potassium Iodide 135 mg, Niacinamide Hydroiodide 25 mg	Iodo-Niacin by Forest	00456-0295	Expectorant
FOREST300	Tab, White, Oblong	Theophylline Anhydrous 300 mg	Duraphyl by Forest		Antiasthmatic
FOREST346	Tab, Blue, Round	Rauwolfia Serpentina 50 mg	Rauverid by Forest		Antihypertensive
FOREST355	Cap, Blue & Pink	Racemethionine 200 mg	Pedameth by Forest	00456-0355	Urinary Tract
FOREST372	Tab, Brown, Round	Ferrous Fumarate 100 mg (33 mg elemental iron)	Feostat by Forest	00456-0372	Mineral
FOREST416	Tab, Green, Round	Acetaminophen 500 mg, Hydrocodone Bitartrate 5 mg	Vicodin by Forest	00456-0416	Analgesic; C III
FOREST429	Tab, White, Round	Phenobarbital 16 mg, Sodium Nitrate 65 mg	Soniphen by Forest		Sedative/Hypnotic; C IV
FOREST452	Cap, Orange & Yellow	Tetracycline HCl 250 mg	by Forest		Antibiotic
FOREST4910	Cap, Black & Blue, Forest/4910	Butalbital 50 mg, Caffeine 40 mg, Acetaminophen 500 mg, Codeine 30 mg	by Forest		Analgesic; C III
FOREST4922	Cap, Blue & White, Forest/4922	Butalbital 50 mg, Caffeine 40 mg, Acetaminophen 500 mg, Codeine 7.5 mg	by Forest		Analgesic; C III
FOREST4924	Cap, Blue & White, Forest/4924	Butalbital 50 mg, Caffeine 40 mg, Acetaminophen 500 mg, Codeine 10 mg	by Forest		Analgesic; C III
FOREST4930	Cap, Red & White, Forest/4930	Caffeine 30 mg, Acetaminophen 356.4 mg, Hydrocodone 5 mg	by Forest		Analgesic; C III
FOREST516	Tab, Green, Round	Phendimetrazine 35 mg	by Forest		Anorexiant; C III
FOREST536	Tab, Orange, Round	Rauwolfia Serpentina 100 mg	Wolfina 100 by Forest		Antihypertensive
FOREST546	Cap, Red & White	Butalbital 50 mg, Acetaminophen 325 mg	Bancap by Forest	00456-0546	Analgesic
FOREST573	Cap, Brown & Red	Opium 3 mg, Bismuth Subcarbonate 60 mg, Kaolin 350 mg	KBP/O by Forest		Gastrointestinal; C V
FOREST591	Tab, Orange, Round	Dextromethorphan HBr 15 mg, Guaifenesin 100 mg	Queltuss by Forest		Cold Remedy
FOREST606	Cap, Black	Phentermine HCl 30 mg	Obermine by Forest		Anorexiant; C IV
FOREST610A	Cap, Orange & Yellow, Opaque	Acetaminophen 500 mg, Hydrocodone Bitartrate 5 mg	Vicodin by Forest	00456-0601	Analgesic; C III
FOREST617	Cap, Clearish Red	Chlorpheniramine Maleate 4 mg, Acetaminophen 325 mg, Phenylpropanolamine HCl 25 mg, Powdered Opium 2 mg	Hista-Derfule by Forest	00456-0617	Analgesic
FOREST621	Tab, White, Oblong	Hyoscyamine Sulfate 0.125 mg	Levsin by Forest		Gastrointestinal
FOREST624	Tab, Green, Oblong	Phenylpropanolamine 25 mg, Chlorpheniramine 4 mg, Acetaminophen 325 mg	Conex by Forest		Cold Remedy
FOREST627	Tab, Chartreuse, Round	Phenylpropanolamine 37.5 mg, Chlorpheniramine 4 mg	Conex DA by Forest		Cold Remedy
FOREST628	Cap, Clear & Orange	Chlorpheniramine Maleate 8 mg, Phenylpropanolamine HCl 75 mg	Dehist by Forest	00456-0628	Cold Remedy
FOREST630	Tab, White, Round	Acetaminophen 325 mg, Butalbital 50 mg, Caffeine 40 mg	Fioricet by Forest	00456-0629	Analgesic
FOREST641	Tab, Green, Round	Acetaminophen 500 mg, Hydrocodone Bitartrate 5 mg	Anodynos DHC by Forest		Analgesic; C III
FOREST642	Cap, White, Soft-Gel	Theophylline Anhydrous 100 mg	Elixophyllin DF by Forest	00456-0642	Antiasthmatic
FOREST643	Cap, White, Soft-Gel	Theophylline Anhydrous 200 mg	Elixophyllin DF by Forest	00456-0643	Antiasthmatic
FOREST646	Cap, Clear, with White Nonpareils	Theophylline Anhydrous 125 mg	Elixophyllin SR by Forest	00456-0646	Antiasthmatic
FOREST647	Cap, Clear, with White Nonpareils	Theophylline Anhydrous 250 mg	Elixophyllin SR by Forest	00456-0647	Antiasthmatic
FOREST674	Tab, White, Round	Butalbital 50 mg, Acetaminophen 325 mg	Esgic CF by Forest	00456-0674	Analgesic
FOREST677	Cap, Black & Blue	Acetaminophen 325 mg, Butalbital 50 mg, Caffeine 40 mg, Codeine Phosphate 30 mg	Esgic with Codeine by Forest	00456-0677	Analgesic
FOREST707	Cap, Blue & Clear	Sucrose 75%, Starch 25%	Cebocap 1 by Forest	00456-0707	Placebo
FOREST708	Cap, Clear & Green	Sucrose 75%, Starch 25%	Cebocap 2 by Forest	00456-0708	Placebo
FOREST709	Cap, Clear & Orange	Sucrose 75%, Starch 25%	Cebocap 3 by Forest	00456-0709	Placebo
FOREST766	Cap, Yellow	Phentermine HCl 30 mg	Obermine by Forest		Anorexiant; C IV
FORTE <> ATASOL	Tab, White, Shield-Shaped, Scored	Acetaminophen 500 mg	Atasol by Church and Dwight	Canadian DIN 00013668	Analgesic
FOS10 <> APO	Tab, White, Cap Shaped, Notched, APO <> FOS-10	Fosinopril Sodium 10 mg	Monopril by Apotex	Canadian DIN 02266008	Antihypertensive
FOS20 <> APO	Tab, White, Oval, APO <> FOS-20	Fosinopril Sodium 20 mg	Monopril by Apotex	Canadian DIN 02266016	Antihypertensive
FOSAMAX <> MRK212	Tab, White, Triangular	Alendronate Sodium 40 mg	Fosamax by Merck Frosst	Canadian DIN 02201038	Antiosteoporosis

ID FRONT <> BACK	DESCRIPTION FRONT <> BACK	INGREDIENT & STRENGTH	BRAND (or Generic Equiv.) by FIRM	NDC#	CLASS; SCH.
FOSAMAX <> MRK212	Tab, White, Triangular	Alendronate Sodium 40 mg	Fosamax by Merck	00006-0212	Antiosteoporosis
FOSAMAX <> MRK936	Tab, White, Round, Bone Logo on both sides	Alendronate Sodium 10 mg	Fosamax by Physician Total Care	54868-3857	Antiosteoporosis
FOSAMAX <> MRK936	Tab, White, Round, Bone Logo on both sides	Alendronate Sodium 10 mg	Fosamax by Heartland	61392-0854	Antiosteoporosis
FOSAMAX <> MRK936	Tab, White, Round, Bone Logo on both sides	Alendronate Sodium 10 mg	Fosamax by MSD	Canadian	Antiosteoporosis
FOSTEUM52003	Cap, Off-White, Blue Imprint	Genistein (isolated and purified from soy) 27 mg, Zinc Chelazome 20 mg, Cholecalciferol (Vitamin D3) 200 IU	Fosteum by Primus	68040-0603	Supplement
FP <> 10MG	Tab, Beige, Oval, Scored, Film Coated	Citalopram 10 mg	Celexa by Forest	00456-4010	Antidepressant
FP <> 20MG	Tab, Pink, Oval, Scored, Film Coated	Citalopram 20 mg	Celexa by Compumed	00403-4894	Antidepressant
FP <> 20MG	Tab, Pink, Oval, Scored, Film Coated	Citalopram 20 mg	Celexa by Forest	00456-4020	Antidepressant
FP <> 20MG	Tab, Pink, Oval, Scored, Film Coated	Citalopram 20 mg	Celexa by Forest	63711-0120	Antidepressant
FP <> 40MG	Tab, White, Oval, Scored, Film Coated	Citalopram 40 mg	Celexa by Forest	00456-4040	Antidepressant
FP <> 5400	Tab, White to Off-White, Cap Shaped, Scored, F / P <> 5400	Oxycodone HCl 5 mg, Ibuprofen 400 mg	Combunox by Forest	00456-5200	Analgesic; NSAID; C II
FR	Cap, Yellow, Black Print, Abbott Logo (a over FR)	Fenofibrate 67 mg	TriCor by Fournier	63924-0001	Antihyperlipidemic
FR1	Tab, White, Round	Acetaminophen 500 mg	Tylenol Ex Strength by Ultratab		Analgesic
FR14	Tab, White, Round	Acetaminophen 500 mg, Pseudoephedrine 30 mg	Tylenol Sinus by Ultratab	62959-	Cold Remedy
FR2	Tab, Light Blue, Round	Acetaminophen 325 mg, Phenylephrine HCl 5 mg	Dilotab II by Zee		Cold Remedy
FR4	Tab, Red, Round	Pseudoephedrine HCl 30 mg	Sudafed by Medique	47682-	Decongestant
FROSST	Tab, White	Timolol Maleate 5 mg	Blocadren by Frosst	Canadian Discontinued	Antihypertensive
FROSST	Tab, Light Blue, Oblong	Timolol Maleate 20 mg	Blocarden by Frosst	Canadian Discontinued	Antihypertensive
FROSST222AFR	Tab, White, Round, Frosst/222AF-R	Acetaminophen 325 mg	Tylenol by Frosst	Canadian	Analgesic
FROSST222AFX	Tab, White, Round, Frosst/222AF-X	Acetaminophen 500 mg	Tylenol Ex Strength by Frosst	Canadian	Analgesic
FROSST412	Tab, White, Discoid	Bethanechol Chloride 10 mg	Urecholine by Frosst	Canadian	Urinary Tract
FROSST67	Tab, Light Blue, Hexagonal	Timolol Maleate 10 mg	Blocarden by Frosst	Canadian Discontinued	Antihypertensive
FROSST893	Tab, White, Round, Frosst/893	Acetaminophen 300 mg, Codeine Phosphate 30 mg, Caffeine Citrate 8 mg	Atasol-30 by Frosst	Canadian	Analgesic; C III
FROSST894	Tab, White, Round, Frosst/894	Acetaminophen 300 mg, Codeine Phosphate 30 mg, Caffeine Citrate 15 mg	Atasol-30 by Frosst	Canadian	Analgesic; C III
FROSST895	Tab, White, Round, Frosst/895	Acetaminophen 300 mg, Codeine Phosphate 30 mg, Caffeine Citrate 30 mg	Atasol-30 by Frosst	Canadian	Analgesic; C III
FS	Tab, White, Oval, Abb. Logo	Temafloxacin HCl 600 mg	Omniflox by Abbott	Discontinued	Antibiotic
FS	Tab, Light Blue, Oval, Film Coated	Fesoterodine Fumarate 4 mg	Toviaz by Pfizer	00069-0242	Urinary Tract
FSCIBA	Tab, Reddish Brown, Round, FS/Ciba	Maprotiline 75 mg	Ludiomil by Ciba	Canadian	Antidepressant
FSO10 <> APO	Tab, White, Cap Shaped, Notched on Top and Bottom, APO <> FSO - 10	Fosinopril 10 mg	Monopril by Apotex	60505-2510	Antihypertensive
FSO20 <> APO	Tab, White, Oval, APO <> FSO - 20	Fosinopril 20 mg	Monopril by Apotex	60505-2511	Antihypertensive
FSO40 <> APO	Tab, White, Round, APO <> FSO - 40	Fosinopril 40 mg	Monopril by Apotex	60505-2512	Antihypertensive
FSR	Cap, Clear & Red, Ex Release, with White Beads, F in Triangle	Theophylline Anhydrous 260 mg	Aerolate Sr by Fleming	00256-0115	Antiasthmatic
FSR	Cap, Green & Red	Phenylephrine HCl 20 mg, Methscopolamine Nitrate 2.5 mg, Chlorpheniramine Maleate 8 mg	by DRX	55045-2601	Cold Remedy
FSR	Cap, Blue & Clear, F in Triangle SR	Guaifenesin 250 mg, Pseudoephedrine HCl 120 mg	Sudafed Sinus by Fleming		Cold Remedy
FSR	Cap,	Guaifenesin 250 mg, Pseudoephedrine HCl 120 mg	Sudafed Sinus by Fleming	00256-0173	Cold Remedy
FSR	Cap, Clear & Red, F in Triangle Logo SR	Theophylline Anhydrous 260 mg	Aerolate SR by Fleming	00256-0115	Antiasthmatic
FSR	Cap, F in Triangle	Chlorpheniramine Maleate 8 mg, Methscopolamine Nitrate 2.5 mg, Phenylephrine HCl 20 mg	Extendryl SR by Fleming	00256-0111	Cold Remedy
FSR	Cap, Green & Red, F in Triangle Logo SR	Chlorpheniramine Maleate 8 mg, Phenylephrine HCl 20 mg, Methscopolamine 2.5 mg	Extendryl SR by Fleming		Cold Remedy
FSR	Cap, Yellow, Black Print, Opaque	Flurbiprofen 200 mg	Froben SR by Abbott	Canadian DIN 02223082	NSAID
FT	Tab, Blue, Oval, Film Coated	Fesoterodine Fumarate 8 mg	Toviaz by Pfizer	00069-0242	Urinary Tract

ID FRONT <> BACK	DESCRIPTION FRONT <> BACK	INGREDIENT & STRENGTH	BRAND (or Generic Equiv.) by FIRM	NDC#	CLASS; SCH.
FT <> A	Tab, Salmon, Round, Scored, Abbott Logo (a)	Trandolapril 1 mg	Mavik by Abbott	00074-2278	Antihypertensive
FULVICINPG	Tab, White, Oval, Fulvicin P/G	Griseofulvin, Ultramicrosize 165 mg	Fulvicin P/G by Schering	60491-0275	Antifungal
FULVICINPG <> 352	Tab, Off White, Fulvicin P/G	Griseofulvin, Ultramicrocrystalline 330 mg	Fulvicin P/G by Pharm Util	Canadian DIN 02231384	Antifungal
FV <> CG	Tab, Dark Yellow, Round, Film Coated	Letrozole 2.5 mg	Femara by Novartis	Canadian	Antineoplastic
FV <> CG	Tab, Dark Yellow, Round, Film Coated	Letrozole 2.5 mg	Femara by Novartis	00078-0249	Antineoplastic
FV100	Tab, White, Oval, Scored, Film-Coated, Cobalt Logo <> FV / 100	Fluvoxamine Maleate 100 mg	Luvox by Cobalt	Canadian DIN 02255537	OCD
FV50	Tab, White, Round, Scored, Film-Coated, Cobalt Logo <> FV / 50	Fluvoxamine Maleate 50 mg	Luvox by Cobalt	Canadian DIN 02255529	OCD
FVCG	Tab, Yellow, Round, FV/CG	Letrozole 2.5 mg	Femara by Novartis	Canadian	Antineoplastic
FWH200	Tab, Light Yellow, Round, FWH/200	Cimetidine HCl 200 mg	Tagamet by Horner	Canadian	Gastrointestinal
FWH300	Tab, Blue, Round, FWH/300	Cimetidine HCl 300 mg	Tagamet by Horner	Canadian	Gastrointestinal
FWH400	Tab, Peach, Round, FWH/400	Cimetidine HCl 400 mg	Tagamet by Horner	Canadian	Gastrointestinal
FWH600	Tab, Blue, Ellipsoid	Cimetidine HCl 600 mg	Tagamet by Horner	Canadian	Gastrointestinal
FWH800	Tab, Peach, Ellipsoid	Cimetidine HCl 800 mg	Tagamet by Horner	Canadian	Gastrointestinal
FX <> A	Tab, Yellow, Round, Abbott Logo (a)	Trandolapril 2 mg	Mavik by Abbott	00074-2279	Antihypertensive
FZ <> A	Tab, Rose, Round, Abbott Logo (a)	Trandolapril 4 mg	Mavik by Abbott	00074-2280	Antihypertensive
G	Tab, Light Yellow, Rectangular, Scored	Pergolide Mesylate 0.05 mg	Permax by Ivax	00172-4520	Antiparkinson
G	Tab, Light Green, Rectangular, Scored	Pergolide Mesylate 0.25 mg	Permax by Ivax	00172-4521	Antiparkinson
G	Tab, Pink, Rectangular, Scored	Pergolide Mesylate 1 mg	Permax by Ivax	00172-4522	Antiparkinson
G	Tab, White, Round	Carvedilol 3.125 mg	Coreg by Glenmark	68462-0162	Antihypertensive
G <> 0030	Tab, White to Off-White, Round, Film Coated, G <> 00 / 30	Ranitidine HCl 150 mg	Zantac by Genpharm	15330-0030	Gastrointestinal
G <> 0030	Tab, Off-White, Film Coated, G <> 00 over 30	Ranitidine HCl 150 mg	by Genpharm	55567-0030	Gastrointestinal
G <> 0031	Tab, Film Coated	Ranitidine HCl 300 mg	by Genpharm	55567-0031	Gastrointestinal
G <> 0031	Tab, White to Off-White, Cap Shaped, Film Coated	Ranitidine HCl 300 mg	Zantac by Genpharm	15330-0031	Gastrointestinal
G <> 0037	Tab, Blue, Oval	Acyclovir 800 mg	Zovirax by Genpharm	55567-0037	Antiviral
G <> 0037	Tab, Blue, Oval	Acyclovir 800 mg	Zovirax by Par	49884-0567	Antiviral
G <> 0053	Tab, White, Oval, Scored, Film Coated	Oxaprozin 600 mg	Daypro by Par	49884-0723	NSAID
G <> 05	Tab, White, Pentagonal, G <> 0.5, Ex Release	Alprazolam 0.5 mg	Xanax XR by Greenstone	59762-0057	Antianxiety; C IV
G <> 05	Tab, G <> 0.5	Estradiol 0.5 mg	by AAI Pharma	27280-0004	Hormone
G <> 05	Tab, White, Oval, Scored, G <> 0.5	Estradiol 0.5 mg	by Teva	00093-1057	Hormone
G <> 1	Tab, White, Hexagonal, Scored	Estradiol 1 mg	by AAI Pharma	27280-0005	Hormone
G <> 1	Tab, White, Hexagonal, Scored	Estradiol 1 mg	by Teva	00093-1058	Hormone
G <> 1	Tab, Yellow, Square, Ex Release	Alprazolam 1 mg	Xanax XR by Greenstone	59762-0059	Antianxiety; C IV
G <> 1189500	Tab	Chlorzoxazone 500 mg	by Royce	51875-0239	Muscle Relaxant
G <> 12	Tab, Purple, Round	Dipyridamole 25 mg	Persantine by Glenmark	68462-0116	Antiplatelet
G <> 13	Tab, White, Oval	Gabapentin 800 mg	Neurontin by Glenmark	68462-0127	Anticonvulsant
G <> 137	Tab, Yellow, Oval, Scored	Oxcarbazepine 150 mg	Trileptal by Glenmark	68462-0137	Anticonvulsant
G <> 139	Tab, Yellow, Oval, Scored	Oxcarbazepine 600 mg	Trileptal by Glenmark	68462-0139	Anticonvulsant
G <> 15	Tab, Peach, Round	Meloxicam 15 mg	Mobic by Genpharm	15330-0219	NSAID
G <> 164	Tab, White, Oblong	Carvedilol 12.5 mg	Coreg by Glenmark	68462-0164	Antihypertensive
G <> 180605	Tab, G <> 1806 0.5	Lorazepam 0.51 mg	Ativan by Royce	51875-0240	Antianxiety; C IV
G <> 18071	Tab, G <> 1807 1	Lorazepam 1 mg	Ativan by Royce	51875-0241	Antianxiety; C IV
G <> 18082	Tab, G <> 1808 2	Lorazepam 2 mg	Ativan by Royce	51875-0242	Antianxiety; C IV

ID FRONT <> BACK	DESCRIPTION FRONT <> BACK	INGREDIENT & STRENGTH	BRAND (or Generic Equiv.) by FIRM	NDC#	CLASS; SCH.
G <> 181	Tab, White, Round	Flavoxate HCl 100 mg	Urispas by Global	00115-1811	Antispasmodic
G <> 1911	Tab, Orange, Oval, Film Coated	Rimantadine HCl 10 mg	Flumadine by Global	00115-1911	Antiviral
G <> 2	Tab, Blue, Round, Ex Release	Alprazolam 2 mg	Xanax XR by Greenstone	59762-0066	Antianxiety; C IV
G <> 2	Tab, White, Round, Scored	Estradiol 2 mg	by Teva	00093-1059 Discontinued	Hormone
G <> 2	Tab	Estradiol 2 mg	by AAI Pharma	27280-0006	Hormone
G <> 2011	Tab, White, Round, Extended Release	Orphenadrine Citrate 100 mg	Norflex by Global	00115-2011	Muscle Relaxant
G <> 2111	Tab, Red, Round, Film Coated	Demeclocycline HCl 150 mg	Declomycin by Global	00115-2111	Antibiotic
G <> 2122	Tab, Red, Round, Film Coated	Demeclocycline HCl 300 mg	Declomycin by Global	00115-2122	Antibiotic
G <> 2442	Tab, Yellow, Round, Film Coated	Bupropion HCl 100 mg	Wellbutrin SR by Teva	00093-5501	Antidepressant
G <> 2444	Tab, Light Yellow, Round, Film Coated, Sustained Release	Bupropion HCl 150 mg	Wellbutrin SR by Teva	00093-5502	Antidepressant
G <> 2444	Tab, Light Yellow, Round, Film Coated, Sustained Release	Bupropion HCl 150 mg	Zyban by Teva	00093-5703	Antidepressant
G <> 250	Tab, Dark Pink, Cap Shaped, Film Coated	Azithromycin 250 mg	Zithromax by Genpharm	Canadian DIN 02278359	Antibiotic
G <> 2611	Tab, White, Football Shaped	Terbutaline Sulfate 2.5 mg	Brethine by Global	00115-2611	Antiasthmatic
G <> 2622	Tab, White, Round	Terbutaline Sulfate 5.0 mg	Brethine by Global	00115-2622	Antiasthmatic
G <> 2711	Tab, Light Blue, Cap Shaped	Sotalol 80 mg	Betapace by Global	00115-2711	Antiarrhythmic
G <> 2722	Tab, Light Blue, Cap Shaped	Sotalol 120 mg	Betapace by Global	00115-2722	Antiarrhythmic
G <> 2733	Tab, Light Blue, Cap Shaped	Sotalol 160 mg	Betapace by Global	00115-2733	Antiarrhythmic
G <> 2744	Tab, Light Blue, Cap Shaped	Sotalol 240 mg	Betapace by Global	00115-2744	Antiarrhythmic
G <> 3	Tab, Green, Triangular, Ex Release	Alprazolam 3 mg	Xanax XR by Greenstone	59762-0068	Antianxiety; C IV
G <> 30	Tab, White, Round, Film Coated	Ranitidine HCl 150 mg	by Mylan	00378-3252	Gastrointestinal
G <> 3060	Tab, Pink, Cap Shaped, Film Coated	Azithromycin 250 mg	Zithromax by Greenstone	59762-3060	Antibiotic
G <> 3070	Tab, Pink, Cap Shaped, Film Coated	Azithromycin 500 mg	Zithromax by Greenstone	59762-3070	Antibiotic
G <> 3080	Tab, White, Oval, Film Coated	Azithromycin 600 mg	Zithromax by Greenstone	59762-3080	Antibiotic
G <> 31	Tab, White, Oblong, Film Coated	Ranitidine HCl 300 mg	by Mylan	00378-3254	Gastrointestinal
G <> 31	Tab, White, Oval	Gabapentin 600 mg	Neurontin by Glenmark	68462-0126	Anticonvulsant
G <> 351	Tab, Yellow, Oval, Film Coated	Fenofibrate 54 mg	Lofibra by Global	00115-5511	Antihyperlipidemic
G <> 391	Tab, Purple, Oval, Convex	Carbidopa 50 mg, Levodopa 200 mg	Sinemet CR by Global	00115-3911	Antiparkinson
G <> 392	Tab, Purple, Oval, Convex	Carbidopa 25 mg, Levodopa 100 mg	Sinemet CR by Global	00115-3922	Antiparkinson
G <> 4	Tab, White, Round	Ondansetron ODT 4 mg	Zofran ODT by Glenmark	68462-0157	Antiemetic
G <> 40	Tab, Orange, Oval, Film Coated	Etodolac 400 mg	Lodine by Genpharm	55567-0040	NSAID
G <> 41	Tab, White, Round	Carvedilol 6.25 mg	Coreg by Glenmark	68462-0163	Antihypertensive
G <> 5011	Tab, Light Yellow, Round	Spironolactone 25 mg	Aldactone by Greenstone	59762-5011	Diuretic
G <> 5012	Tab, Orange, Oval, Scored	Spironolactone 50 mg	Aldactone by Greenstone	59762-5012	Diuretic
G <> 5013	Tab, Peach, Round, Scored	Spironolactone 100 mg	Aldactone by Greenstone	59762-5013	Diuretic
G <> 5014	Tab, Tan, Round	Hydrochlorothiazide 25 mg, Spironolactone 25 mg	Aldactazide by Greenstone	59762-5014	Diuretic; Antihypertensive
G <> 53511	Tab, Gilbert Logo	Acetaminophen 325 mg, Butalbital 50 mg, Caffeine 40 mg	Fioricet by Nat Pharmpak	55154-4601	Analgesic
G <> 58	Tab, White to Off White, Round	Amlodipine Besylate 2.5 mg	Norvasc by Glenmark	68462-0210	Antihypertensive
G <> 591	Tab, Blue Round	Pilocarpine HCl 7.5 mg	Salagen by Global	00115-5911	Cholinergic Agonist
G <> 592	Tab, White, Round	Pilocarpine HCl 5 mg	Salagen by Global	00115-5922	Cholinergic Agonist
G <> 600	Tab, Film Coated	Ibuprofen 600 mg	Motrin by Quality Care	60346-0556	NSAID
G <> 682	Tab, Yellow, Oval, Extended Release	Bupropion HCl 300 mg	Wellbutrin XL by Teva	00093-5351	Antidepressant
G <> 75	Tab, Peach, Round, G <> 7.5	Meloxicam 7.5 mg	Mobic by Genpharm	15330-0218	NSAID
G <> 8	Tab, White, Round	Ondansetron ODT 8 mg	Zofran ODT by Glenmark	68462-0158	Antiemetic
G <> 80	Tab, Yellow, Oval	Pravastatin Sodium 80 mg	Pravachol by Glenmark	68462-0198	Antilipemic Agent
G <> 800	Tab, Film Coated	Ibuprofen 400 mg	Motrin by Quality Care	60346-0030	NSAID
G <> 891	Tab, Light Blue, Round, Film Coated	Levonorgestrel 0.25 mg, Ethinyl Estradiol 0.05 mg	by Barr	00555-0891	Oral Contraceptive
G <> 891	Tab, Light Blue, Round, Film Coated	Levonorgestrel 0.25 mg, Ethinyl Estradiol 0.05 mg	Preven by Gynetics	63955-0020	Oral Contraceptive
G <> 91	Tab, Purple, Round	Dipyridamole 50 mg	Persantine by Glenmark	68462-0117	Vasodilator

ID FRONT <> BACK	DESCRIPTION FRONT <> BACK	INGREDIENT & STRENGTH	BRAND (or Generic Equiv.) by FIRM	NDC#	CLASS; SCH.
G <> 92	Tab, Purple, Round	Dipyridamole 75 mg	Persantine by Glenmark	68462-0118	Antiplatelet
G <> A100	Tab, White, Round, Flat	Atenolol 100 mg	Tenormin by Genpharm	15330-0029	Antihypertensive
G <> A100	Tab, White, Round, A over 100	Atenolol 100 mg	Tenormin by Amerisource	62584-0621	Antihypertensive
G <> A100	Tab, White, Round	Atenolol 100 mg	Tenormin by Par	49884-0457	Antihypertensive
G <> A50	Tab, White, Round, Scored	Atenolol 50 mg	Tenormin by Par	49884-0456	Antihypertensive
G <> A50	Tab, White, Round, Scored, A over 50	Atenolol 50 mg	Tenormin by Amerisource	62584-0620	Antihypertensive
G <> A50	Tab, White, Round, Flat	Atenolol 50 mg	Tenormin by Genpharm	15330-0028	Antihypertensive
G <> AC100	Tab, White, Round, Film Coated, AC / 100	Acebutolol 100 mg	Monitan by Genpharm	Canadian DIN 02237721	Antihypertensive
G <> AC100	Tab, White, Shield Shaped, Scored	Acebutolol 100 mg	Sectral by Genpharm	Canadian DIN 02237885	Antihypertensive
G <> AC200	Tab, Blue, Shield Shaped, Scored	Acebutolol 200 mg	Sectral by Genpharm	Canadian DIN 02237886	Antihypertensive
G <> AC200	Tab, White, Oval, Film Coated, AC / 200	Acebutolol 200 mg	Monitan by Genpharm	Canadian DIN 02237722	Antihypertensive
G <> AC400	Tab, White, Oblong, Film Coated, AC / 400	Acebutolol 400 mg	Monitan by Genpharm	Canadian DIN 02237723	Antihypertensive
G <> AC400	Tab, White, Shield Shaped, Scored	Acebutolol 400 mg	Sectral by Genpharm	Canadian DIN 02237887	Antihypertensive
G <> ACY200	Tab, Blue, Flat, Shield-Shaped	Acyclovir 200 mg	Zovirax by Genpharm	Canadian DIN 02242784	Antiviral
G <> ACY400	Tab, Pink, Shield Shaped	Acyclovir 400 mg	Zovirax by Genpharm	Canadian DIN 02242463	Antiviral
G <> ACY800	Tab, Blue, Oval-Shaped, Scored	Acyclovir 800 mg	Zovirax by Genpharm	Canadian DIN 02242464	Antiviral
G <> AD10	Tab, White, Oval	Alendronate Sodium 10 mg	Fosamax by Genpharm	Canadian DIN 02270129	Antiosteoporosis
G <> AD5	Tab, White, Round	Alendronate Sodium 5 mg	Fosamax by Genpharm	Canadian DIN 02270110	Antiosteoporosis
G <> AD70	Tab, White, Oval	Alendronate Sodium 70 mg	Fosamax by Genpharm	Canadian DIN 02286335	Antiosteoporosis
G <> AL025	Tab, White, Oval, Scored, AL 0.25	Alprazolam 0.25 mg	Xanax by Genpharm	Canadian DIN 02137534	Antianxiety; C IV
G <> AL25	Tab, White, Oval, Scored, AL 0.25	Alprazolam 0.25 mg	Xanax by Par	49884-0448	Antianxiety; C IV
G <> AL05	Tab, Pale Orange, Oval, Scored, AL 0.5	Alprazolam 0.5 mg	Xanax by Par	49884-0449	Antianxiety; C IV
G <> AL05	Tab, Pale Orange, Oval, Scored, AL 0.5	Alprazolam 0.5 mg	Xanax by Genpharm	Canadian DIN 02137542	Antianxiety; C IV
G <> AL10	Tab, Mauve, Oval, Scored, AL 1.0	Alprazolam 1 mg	Xanax by Genpharm	Canadian DIN 02229813	Antianxiety; C IV
G <> AL10	Tab, Mauve, Oval, Scored, AL 1.0	Alprazolam 1 mg	Xanax by Alphapharm	57315-0008	Antianxiety; C IV
G <> AL10	Tab, Mauve, Oval, Scored, AL 1.0	Alprazolam 1 mg	Xanax by Direct Dispensing	57866-4636	Antianxiety; C IV
G <> AL10	Tab, Mauve, Oval, Scored, AL 1.0	Alprazolam 1 mg	Xanax by Par	49884-0450	Antianxiety; C IV
G <> AM200	Tab, White, Round, Scored	Amiodarone 200 mg	Cordarone by Alphapharm	57315-0009	Antiarrhythmic
G <> AM200	Tab, White, Round, Scored	Amiodarone 200 mg	Cordarone by Par	49884-0458	Antiarrhythmic
G <> AM200	Tab, Pink, Round, Scored, AM / 200	Amiodarone 200 mg	Cordarone by Genpharm	Canadian DIN 02240604	Antiarrhythmic
G <> AT100	Tab, White, Round, Scored	Atenolol 100 mg	Tenormin by Genpharm	Canadian DIN 02147432	Antihypertensive
G <> AT25	Tab, White, Round	Atenolol 25 mg	Tenormin by Genpharm	Canadian DIN 02303647	Antihypertensive

ID FRONT <> BACK	DESCRIPTION FRONT <> BACK	INGREDIENT & STRENGTH	BRAND (or Generic Equiv.) by FIRM	NDC#	CLASS; SCH.
G <> AT50	Tab, White, Round, Scored	Atenolol 50 mg	Tenormin by Genpharm	Canadian DIN 02146894	Antihypertensive
G <> B10	Tab, White, Barrel Shaped, Scored	Buspirone HCl 10 mg	Buspar by Genpharm	Canadian DIN 02230874	Antianxiety
G <> B15	Tab, White, Round, Scored, B / 1.5	Bromazepam 1.5 mg	Lectopam by Genpharm	Canadian DIN 02192705	Sedative; C IV
G <> B3	Tab, Pink, Round, Scored, B / 3	Bromazepam 3 mg	Lectopam by Genpharm	Canadian DIN 02192713	Sedative; C IV
G <> B6	Tab, Pale Green, Round, Scored, B / 6	Bromazepam 6 mg	Lectopam by Genpharm	Canadian DIN 02192721	Sedative; C IV
G <> BC50	Tab, White, Round, Film Coated	Bicalutamide 50 mg	Casodex by Genpharm	Canadian DIN 02302403	Antineoplastic
G <> BN10	Tab, White, Round, BN / 10	Baclofen 10 mg	Lioresal by Genpharm	Canadian DIN 02088398	Muscle Relaxant
G <> BN10	Tab, White, Round	Baclofen 10 mg	Lioresal by Mylan	00378-6010	Muscle Relaxant
G <> BN10	Tab, White, Round, BN / 10	Baclofen 10 mg	Lioresal by UDL	51079-0668 Discontinued	Muscle Relaxant
G <> BN10	Tab, White, Round, BN / 10	Baclofen 10 mg	Lioresal by Genpharm	15330-0245	Muscle Relaxant
G <> BN20	Tab, White, Round, BN / 20	Baclofen 20 mg	Lioresal by Genpharm	15330-0246	Muscle Relaxant
G <> BN20	Tab, White, Round, BN / 20	Baclofen 20 mg	Lioresal by UDL	51079-0669 Discontinued	Muscle Relaxant
G <> BN20	Tab, White, Round	Baclofen 20 mg	Lioresal by Mylan	00378-6020	Muscle Relaxant
G <> BN20	Tab, White, Round, BN / 20	Baclofen 20 mg	Lioresal by Genpharm	Canadian DIN 02088401	Muscle Relaxant
G <> C100	Tab, White, Oval, Scored	Captopril 100 mg	Capoten by Genpharm	Canadian DIN 02163594	Antihypertensive
G <> C125	Tab, White, Oblong, Scored, G <> C 12.5	Captopril 12.5 mg	Capoten by Genpharm	Canadian DIN 02163551	Antihypertensive
G <> C250	Tab, Yellow, Oval, Film Coated	Clarithromycin 250 mg	Biaxin by Genpharm	Canadian DIN 02248856	Antibiotic
G <> C250	Tab, White, Capsule Shaped	Clarithromycin 250 mg	Biaxin by Mylan	00378-8250	Antibiotic
G <> C250	Tab, White, Capsule Shaped	Clarithromycin 250 mg	Biaxin by UDL	51079-0672	Antibiotic
G <> C50	Tab, White, Oval, Scored	Captopril 50 mg	Capoten by Genpharm	Canadian DIN 02163586	Antihypertensive
G <> C500	Tab, Pale Yellow, Oval, Film Coated	Clarithromycin 500 mg	Biaxin by Genpharm	Canadian DIN 02248857	Antibiotic
G <> C500	Tab, White-White, Capsule Shaped	Clarithromycin 500 mg	Biaxin by UDL	51079-0673	Antibiotic
G <> C500	Tab, White, Capsule Shaped	Clarithromycin 500 mg	Biaxin by Mylan	00378-8500	Antibiotic
G <> CF250	Tab, White, Round, Film Coated	Ciprofloxacin 250 mg	Cipro by Genpharm	Canadian DIN 02245647	Antibiotic
G <> CF250	Tab, White to Off-White, Round, Coated	Ciprofloxacin 250 mg	Cipro by Par	49884-0637	Antibiotic
G <> CF500	Tab, White to Off-White, Cap Shaped, Coated	Ciprofloxacin 500 mg	Cipro by Par	49884-0638	Antibiotic
G <> CF500	Tab, White to Off-White, Cap Shaped, Coated	Ciprofloxacin 500 mg	Cipro by Genpharm	Canadian DIN 02245648	Antibiotic
G <> CF750	Tab, White to Off-White, Cap Shaped, Coated	Ciprofloxacin 750 mg	Cipro by Genpharm	Canadian DIN 02245649	Antibiotic
G <> CF750	Tab, White to Off-White, Cap Shaped, Coated	Ciprofloxacin 750 mg	Cipro by Par	49884-0639	Antibiotic
G <> Cl1	Tab, Yellow, Oval, Scored	Cilazapril 1 mg	Inhibace by Genpharm	Canadian DIN 02283778	Antihypertensive
G <> Cl25	Tab, Pinkish Brown, Oval, Scored, Cl / 2.5	Cilazapril 2.5 mg	Inhibace by Genpharm	Canadian DIN 02283786	Antihypertensive

ID FRONT <> BACK	DESCRIPTION FRONT <> BACK	INGREDIENT & STRENGTH	BRAND (or Generic Equiv.) by FIRM	NDC#	CLASS; SCH.
G <> CI5	Tab, Reddish Brown, Oval, Scored, CI / 5	Cilazzapril 5 mg	Inhibace by Genpharm	Canadian DIN 02283794	Antihypertensive
G <> CL100	Tab, White, Round	Cilostazol 100 mg	Pletal by Andrx	62037-0541	Antiplatelet
G <> CL50	Tab, White, Round	Cilostazol 50 mg	Pletal by Andrx	62037-0540	Antiplatelet
G <> CM20	Tab, White, Oval, Scored, Film Coated	Citalopram 20 mg	Celexa by Genpharm	Canadian DIN 02246594	Antidepressant
G <> CM300	Tab, Light Green, Round, Film Coated	Cimetidine 300 mg	Tagamet by Genpharm	Canadian DIN 02227444	Gastrointestinal
G <> CM40	Tab, White, Oval, Scored, Film Coated	Citalopram 40 mg	Celexa by Genpharm	Canadian DIN 02246595	Antidepressant
G <> CM400	Tab, Light Green, Elliptical, Film Coated	Cimetidine 400 mg	Tagamet by Genpharm	Canadian DIN 02227452	Gastrointestinal
G <> CM600	Tab, Light Green, Elliptical, Film Coated	Cimetidine 600 mg	Tagamet by Genpharm	Canadian DIN 02227460	Gastrointestinal
G <> CM800	Tab, Light Green, Elliptical, Film Coated	Cimetidine 800 mg	Tagamet by Genpharm	Canadian DIN 02227479	Gastrointestinal
G <> CN05	Tab, Light Yellow, Round, Scored, CN/0.5	Clonazepam 0.5 mg	Klonopin by Par	49884-0495	Sedative; C IV
G <> CN05	Tab, Light Yellow, Round, Scored, CN/0.5	Clonazepam 0.5 mg	Klonopin by Alphapharm	57315-0017	Sedative; C IV
G <> CN1	Tab, Yellow, Round, Scored	Clonazepam 1 mg	Klonopin by Alphapharm	57315-0018	Sedative; C IV
G <> CN1	Tab, Yellow, Round, Scored	Clonazepam 1 mg	Klonopin by Par	49884-0496	Sedative; C IV
G <> CN2	Tab, White, Round, Scored	Clonazepam 2 mg	Klonopin by Par	49884-0497	Sedative; C IV
G <> CN2	Tab, White, Round, Scored	Clonazepam 2 mg	Klonopin by Alphapharm	57315-0019	Sedative; C IV
G <> DX1	Tab, White, Round	Doxazosin Mesylate 1 mg	Cardura by Par	49884-0552	Antihypertensive
G <> DX2	Tab, White, Cap Shaped, Scored, DX over 2	Doxazosin Mesylate 2 mg	Cardura by Par	49884-0553	Antihypertensive
G <> DX4	Tab, White, Cap Shaped, Scored, DX over 4	Doxazosin Mesylate 4 mg	Cardura by Par	49884-0554	Antihypertensive
G <> DX8	Tab, White, Cap Shaped, Scored, DX over 8	Doxazosin Mesylate 8 mg	Cardura by Par	49884-0555	Antihypertensive
G <> ED200	Tab, White, Rectangular	Etidronate Disodium 200 mg	Didronel by Genpharm	15330-0094	Calcium Metabolism
G <> ED400	Tab, White, Cap Shaped	Etidronate Disodium 400 mg	Didronel by Genpharm	15330-0095	Calcium Metabolism
G <> EN10	Tab, Orangish-Red, Oval	Enalapril Maleate 10 mg	Vasotec by Par	49884-0593	Antihypertensive
G <> EN20	Tab, Peach, Oval, Scored	Enalapril Maleate 20 mg	Vasotec by Par	49884-0594	Antihypertensive
G <> EN25	Tab, White, Round, Scored, EN/2.5	Enalapril Maleate 2.5 mg	Vasotec by Par	49884-0591	Antihypertensive
G <> ET500	Tab, Light Blue, Oval	Etodolac 500 mg	Lodine by Par	49884-0596	NSAID
G <> ET500	Tab, Light Blue, Oval	Etodolac 500 mg	Lodine by Genpharm	55567-0032	NSAID
G <> ET500	Tab, Light Blue, Oval	Etodolac 500 mg	Lodine by Heartland	61392-0916	NSAID
G <> FC100	Tab, White, Round, Scored, FC_100	Flecainide Acetate 100 mg	Tambocor by Par	49884-0695	Antiarrhythmic
G <> FC150	Tab, White, Oval, Scored	Flecainide Acetate 150 mg	Tambocor by Par	49884-0696	Antiarrhythmic
G <> FC50	Tab, White, Round	Flecainide Acetate 50 mg	Tambocor by Par	49884-0694	Antiarrhythmic
G <> FL10	Tab, White, Oval, Scored, Film Coated, G <> FL over 10	Fluoxetine HCl 10 mg	Prozac by Par	49884-0734	Antidepressant
G <> FL10	Tab, White, Oval, Scored, Film Coated, G <> FL over 10	Fluoxetine HCl 10 mg	Prozac by Alphapharm	57315-0051	Antidepressant
G <> FL100	Tab, Pink, Rectangular	Fluconazole 100 mg	Diflucan by Par	49884-0939	Antifungal
G <> FL150	Tab, Pink, Oval	Fluconazole 150 mg	Diflucan by Par	49884-0940	Antifungal
G <> FL20	Tab, White, Oval, Scored, Film Coated, G <> FL over 20	Fluoxetine HCl 20 mg	Prozac by Alphapharm	57315-0052	Antidepressant
G <> FL20	Tab, White, Oval, Scored, Film Coated, G <> FL over 20	Fluoxetine HCl 20 mg	Prozac by Par	49884-0735	Antidepressant
G <> FL200	Tab, Pink, Rectangular	Fluconazole 200 mg	Diflucan by Par	49884-0941	Antifungal
G <> GP10	Tab	Glipizide 10 mg	by Par	49884-0452	Antidiabetic
G <> GP5	Tab	Glipizide 5 mg	by Par	49884-0451	Antidiabetic
G <> GT12	Tab, White, Round, Film Coated	Galantamine 12 mg	Razadyne by UDL	51079-0471	Antialzheimers
G <> GT4	Tab, White, Round, Film Coated	Galantamine 4 mg	Razadyne by UDL	51079-0469 Discontinued	Antialzheimers
G <> GT4	Tab, White, Round	Galantamine 4 mg	Razadyne by Mylan	00378-8104	Antialzheimers
G <> GT8	Tab, White, Round, Film Coated	Galantamine 8 mg	Razadyne by UDL	51079-0470	Antialzheimers

ID FRONT <> BACK	DESCRIPTION FRONT <> BACK	INGREDIENT & STRENGTH	BRAND (or Generic Equiv.) by FIRM	NDC#	CLASS; SCH.
G <> GU1	Tab, White, Oval	Guanfacine HCl 1 mg	Tenex by Genpharm	55567-0051	Antihypertensive
G <> GU1	Tab, White, Oval	Guanfacine HCl 1 mg	Tenex by Par	49884-0572	Antihypertensive
G <> GU2	Tab, White, Oval	Guanfacine HCl 2 mg	Tenex by Par	49884-0573	Antihypertensive
G <> GU2	Tab, White, Oval	Guanfacine HCl 2 mg	Tenex by Genpharm	55567-0052	Antihypertensive
G <> IE125	Tab, Orange, Round, Film Coated, IE over 1.25	Indapamide 1.25 mg	Lozol by Par	49884-0589	Diuretic
G <> IE25	Tab, White, Round, Film Coated, IE over 2.5	Indapamide 2.5 mg	Lozol by Par	49884-0590	Diuretic
G <> L10	Tab, White, Round, G <> L over 10	Loratadine 10 mg	Claritin by Leiner	12333-0911	Antihistamine
G <> LV10	Tab, Peach, Round, LV over 10	Lovastatin 10 mg	Mevacor by Par	49884-0754	Antihyperlipidemic
G <> LV20	Tab, Light Blue, Round, LV over 20	Lovastatin 20 mg	Mevacor by Par	49884-0755	Antihyperlipidemic
G <> LV40	Tab, Green, Round, LV over 40	Lovastatin 40 mg	Mevacor by Par	49884-0756	Antihyperlipidemic
G <> LY25	Tab, White, Round, Chewable, Dispersible	Lamotrigine 25 mg	Lamictal by Mylan	00378-6925	Anticonvulsant
G <> LY5	Tab, White, Round, Chewable, Dispersible	Lamotrigine 5 mg	Lamictal by Mylan	00378-6905	Anticonvulsant
G <> MF1	Tab, White to Off-White, Round, Film Coated	Metformin HCl 500 mg	Glucophage by Par	49884-0739	Antidiabetic
G <> MF1	Tab, White to Off-White, Round, Film Coated	Metformin HCl 500 mg	Gen-Metformin by Genpharm	Canadian DIN 02148765	Antidiabetic
G <> MF2	Tab, White, Round, Film Coated, MF over 2	Metformin HCl 850 mg	Gen-Metformin by Genpharm	Canadian DIN 02229656	Antidiabetic
G <> MF2	Tab, White, Round, Film Coated, MF over 2	Metformin HCl 850 mg	Glucophage by Par	49884-0740	Antidiabetic
G <> MF3	Tab, White, Oblong, Scored, Film Coated, MF, Score, 3	Metformin HCl 1000 mg	Glucophage by Par	49884-0741	Antidiabetic
G <> MR15	Tab, Round, Yellow, Scored, Film Coated	Mirtazapine 15 mg	Remeron by Par	49884-0655	Antidepressant
G <> MR30	Tab, Round, Buff, Scored, Film Coated	Mirtazapine 30 mg	Remeron by Par	49884-0656	Antidepressant
G <> MR45	Tab, White, Round, Film Coated	Mirtazapine 45 mg	Remeron by Par	49884-0873	Antidepressant
G <> P1	Tab, White, Round, Film Coated	Paroxetine HCl 10 mg	Paxil by Watson	62037-0845	Antidepressant
G <> P10	Tab, White, Round	Pindolol 10 mg	by Genpharm	55567-0016	Antihypertensive
G <> P10	Tab, White, Round	Pindolol 10 mg	by URL Mutual	00677-1458	Antihypertensive
G <> P10	Tab, White, Round	Pindolol 10 mg	by Par	49884-0443	Antihypertensive
G <> P2	Tab, White, Round, Film Coated	Paroxetine HCl 20 mg	Paxil by Watson	62037-0846	Antidepressant
G <> P3	Tab, White, Round, Film Coated	Paroxetine HCl 30 mg	Paxil by Andrx	62037-0847	Antidepressant
G <> P4	Tab, White, Round, Film Coated	Paroxetine HCl 40 mg	Paxil by Andrx	62037-0848	Antidepressant
G <> P5	Tab	Pindolol 5 mg	by Genpharm	55567-0015	Antihypertensive
G <> P5	Tab	Pindolol 5 mg	by URL Mutual	00677-1457	Antihypertensive
G <> P5	Tab	Pindolol 5 mg	by Par	49884-0442	Antihypertensive
G <> PR10	Tab, Pink, Rounded Rectangular, PR over 10	Pravastatin Sodium 10 mg	Pravachol by Par	49884-0176	Antihyperlipidemic
G <> PR10	Tab, White, Square	Pravastatin Sodium 10 mg	Pravachol by Mylan	00378-8210	Antihyperlipidemic
G <> PR20	Tab, White, Square	Pravastatin Sodium 20 mg	Pravachol by Mylan	00378-8220	Antihyperlipidemic
G <> PR20	Tab, Yellow, Rounded Rectangular, PR over 20	Pravastatin Sodium 20 mg	Pravachol by Par	49884-0179	Antihyperlipidemic
G <> PR40	Tab, Green, Rounded Rectangular, PR over 40	Pravastatin Sodium 40 mg	Pravachol by Par	49884-0180	Antihyperlipidemic
G <> PR40	Tab, White, Square	Pravastatin Sodium 40 mg	Pravachol by Mylan	00378-8240	Antihyperlipidemic
G <> S120	Tab, White, Cap Shaped, Scored, S/120	Sotalol HCl 120 mg	Betapace by Genpharm	15330-0209	Antiarrhythmic
G <> S120	Tab, White, Cap Shaped, Scored	Sotalol HCl 120 mg	Betapace by Genpharm	55567-0076	Antiarrhythmic
G <> S120	Tab, White, Cap Shaped, Scored	Sotalol HCl 120 mg	Betapace by Par	49884-0583	Antiarrhythmic
G <> S160	Tab, White, Cap Shaped, Scored	Sotalol HCl 160 mg	Betapace by Par	49884-0584	Antiarrhythmic
G <> S160	Tab, White, Cap Shaped, Scored, S/160	Sotalol HCl 160 mg	Betapace by Genpharm	15330-0210	Antiarrhythmic
G <> S240	Tab, White, Cap Shaped, Scored	Sotalol HCl 240 mg	Betapace by Par	49884-0585	Antiarrhythmic
G <> S240	Tab, White, Cap Shaped, Scored	Sotalol HCl 240 mg	Betapace by Genpharm	55567-0059	Antiarrhythmic
G <> S5E	Tab, White, Round	Selegiline 5 mg	Eldepryl by Par	49884-0610	Antiparkinson
G <> S80	Tab, White, Cap Shaped, Scored	Sotalol HCl 80 mg	Betapace by Par	49884-0582	Antiarrhythmic
G <> S80	Tab, White, Cap Shaped, Scored, S/80	Sotalol HCl 80 mg	Betapace by Genpharm	15330-0208	Antiarrhythmic
G <> SE5	Tab, White, Round, SE over 5	Selegiline HCl 5 mg	by Draxis	Canadian	Antiparkinson
G <> SE5	Tab, White, Round, SE over 5	Selegiline HCl 5 mg	Selegiline HCl by Schein		Antiparkinson

ID FRONT <> BACK	DESCRIPTION FRONT <> BACK	INGREDIENT & STRENGTH	BRAND (or Generic Equiv.) by FIRM	NDC#	CLASS; SCH.
G <> T250	Tab, White to Off-White, Oval, Film Coated	Ticlopidine 250 mg	Ticlid by Par	49884-0599	Anticoagulant
G <> TI	Tab, White, Scored	Tizanidine HCl 2 mg	Zanaflex by Genpharm	15330-0247	Muscle Relaxant
G <> TL50	Tab, White, Film Coated	Tramadol HCl 50 mg	Ultram by Par	49884-0742	Analgesic
G <> TR125	Tab, White, Oval	Triazolam 0.125 mg	Halcion by Genpharm	15330-0249	Sedative/Hypnotic; C IV
G <> TR125	Tab, White, Oval	Triazolam 0.125 mg	Halcion by Par	49884-0453	Sedative/Hypnotic; C IV
G <> TR125	Tab, White, Oval	Triazolam 0.125 mg	Halcion by Qualitest	00603-6186	Sedative/Hypnotic; C IV
G <> TR250	Tab, Pale Yellow, Oval	Triazolam 0.25 mg	Halcion by Par	49884-0454	Sedative/Hypnotic; C IV
G <> TR250	Tab, Pale Yellow, Oval	Triazolam 0.25 mg	Halcion by Qualitest	00603-6187	Sedative/Hypnotic; C IV
G <> TR250	Tab, Pale Yellow, Oval	Triazolam 0.25 mg	Halcion by Genpharm	15330-0250	Sedative/Hypnotic; C IV
G <> WF1	Tab, Dark Pink, Round, Scored	Warfarin Sodium 1 mg	Coumadin by Genpharm	15330-0100	Anticoagulant
G <> WF10	Tab, White, Round, Scored	Warfarin Sodium 10 mg	Coumadin by Genpharm	15330-0108	Anticoagulant
G <> WF2	Tab, Lavender, Round, Scored	Warfarin Sodium 2 mg	Coumadin by Genpharm	15330-0101	Anticoagulant
G <> WF25	Tab, Green, Round, Scored, WF / 2.5	Warfarin Sodium 2.5 mg	Coumadin by Genpharm	15330-0102	Anticoagulant
G <> WF3	Tab, Brown, Round, Scored	Warfarin Sodium 3 mg	Coumadin by Genpharm	15330-0266	Anticoagulant
G <> WF4	Tab, Blue, Round, Scored	Warfarin Sodium 4 mg	Coumadin by Genpharm	15330-0267	Anticoagulant
G <> WF5	Tab, Peach, Round, Scored	Warfarin Sodium 5 mg	Coumadin by Genpharm	15330-0268	Anticoagulant
G <> WF6	Tab, Dark Green, Round, Scored	Warfarin Sodium 6 mg	Coumadin by Genpharm	15330-0106	Anticoagulant
G <> WF75	Tab, Yellow, Round, Scored, WF / 7.5	Warfarin Sodium 7.5 mg	Coumadin by Genpharm	15330-0107	Anticoagulant
G0	Tab, Blue, Oblong, Scored	Naproxen 550 mg	Anaprox by Glenmark	68462-0179	NSAID
G0 <> 275	Tab, Blue, Oval	Naproxen 275 mg	Anaprox by Glenmark	68462-0178	NSAID
G00	Tab, White, Round	Levonorgestrel 1.5 mg	Plan B One-Step by Duramed	51285-0942	Oral Contraceptive
G0034	Cap, Aqua Blue, Black Print, Opaque	Acyclovir 200 mg	Zovirax by Par	49884-0565	Antiviral
G0034	Cap, Aqua Blue, Black Print, Opaque	Acyclovir 200 mg	Zovirax by Amerisource	62584-0736	Antiviral
G0034	Cap, Aqua Blue, Black Print, Opaque	Acyclovir 200 mg	Zovirax by Genpharm	55567-0034	Antiviral
G0036	Tab, White, Pentagonal, G over 0036	Acyclovir 400 mg	Zovirax by Genpharm	55567-0036	Antiviral
G0036	Tab, White, Pentagonal, G over 0036	Acyclovir 400 mg	Zovirax by Amerisource	62584-0749	Antiviral
G0036	Tab, White, Pentagonal, G over 0036	Acyclovir 400 mg	Zovirax by Par	49884-0566	Antiviral
G004	Tab, Red, Oval	Docusate Sodium 100 mg	by Group Health	58087-0110	Laxative
G0041	Cap, White & Light Blue	Nicardipine HCl 20 mg	Cardene by Par	49884-0498	Antihypertensive
G0041	Cap, White & Light Blue	Nicardipine HCl 20 mg	Cardene by Genpharm	55567-0041	Antihypertensive
G0041	Cap, White and Light Blue, Opaque, Hard Gel	Nicardipine HCl 20 mg	Cardene by Genpharm	15330-0041	Antihypertensive
G0042	Cap, Light Blue, Opaque, Hard Gel	Nicardipine HCl 30 mg	Cardene by Genpharm	15330-0042	Antihypertensive
G0042	Cap, Light Blue	Nicardipine HCl 30 mg	Cardene by Genpharm	55567-0042	Antihypertensive
G0042	Cap, Light Blue	Nicardipine HCl 30 mg	Cardene by Par	49884-0499	Antihypertensive
G01 <> LU	Tab, Light Green, Oval	Lovastatin 10 mg	Mevacor by Lupin	68180-0467	Antihyperlipidemic
G0104	Cap, Black & Purple, G-0104	Phenylpropanolamine HCl 75 mg, Caramiphen Edisylate 40 mg	Tuss Ornade by Pioneer	Canadian	Cold Remedy
G0131	Cap, Clear	Quinine Sulfate 325 mg	by Nutro Laboratories		Antimalarial
G019 <> 10	Tab, Brown, Triangular, Film Coated	Quinapril HCl 10 mg	Accupril by Greenstone	59762-5020	Antihypertensive
G02 <> LU	Tab, Light Green, Round	Lovastatin 20 mg	Mevacor by Lupin	68180-0468	Antihyperlipidemic
G020 <> 20	Tab, Brown, Round, Film Coated	Quinapril HCl 20 mg	Accupril by Greenstone	59762-5021	Antihypertensive
G021 <> 40	Tab, Brown, Elliptical, Film Coated	Quinapril HCl 40 mg	Accupril by Greenstone	59762-5022	Antihypertensive
G022 <> 5	Tab, Brown, Elliptical, Scored, Film Coated	Quinapril HCl 5 mg	Accupril by Greenstone	59762-5019	Antihypertensive
G026	Cap, Dark Green & Olive	Piroxicam 10 mg	Feldene by Genpharm	55567-0026	NSAID
G026	Cap	Piroxicam 10 mg	Feldene by Par	49884-0440	NSAID
G026	Cap	Piroxicam 10 mg	Feldene by Par	49884-0440	NSAID
G027	Cap	Piroxicam 20 mg	Feldene by Par	49884-0441	NSAID
G027	Cap, 027	Piroxicam 20 mg	Feldene by Genpharm	55567-0027	NSAID
G027	Cap, Maroon	Piroxicam 20 mg	Feldene by Genpharm	Canadian	NSAID
G03 <> LU	Tab, Light Green, Round	Lovastatin 40 mg	Mevacor by Lupin	68180-0469	Antihyperlipidemic
G0506	Tab, White, Round, G-0506	Reserpine 0.1 mg, Hydralazine HCl 25 mg, Hydrochlorothiazide 15 mg	Ser-Ap-Es by Ivax		Antihypertensive; Diuretic

ID FRONT <> BACK	DESCRIPTION FRONT <> BACK	INGREDIENT & STRENGTH	BRAND (or Generic Equiv.) by FIRM	NDC#	CLASS; SCH.
G0507	Tab, Yellow, Round	Folic Acid 1 mg	Folvite by West-Ward		Vitamin
G0511	Cap, Light Yellow, Opaque, Black Ink	Fenofibrate 67 mg	Lofibra by Global	00115-0511	Antihyperlipidemic
G0522	Cap, White, Opaque, Black Ink	Fenofibrate 134 mg	Lofibra by Global	00115-0522	Antihyperlipidemic
G0533	Cap, Orange, Opaque, Black Ink	Fenofibrate 200 mg	Lofibra by Global	00115-0533	Antihyperlipidemic
G06	Tab	Hydralazine HCl 100 mg	by Ivax	00182-1553	Antihypertensive
G063	Cap, White, Opaque	Anagrelide HCl 0.5 mg	Agrylin by Genpharm	Canadian DIN 02253054	Antiplatelet
G07	Tab, Sugar Coated	Hydroxyzine HCl 10 mg	by Ivax	00182-1492	Antianxiety; Antihistamine
G08	Tab, Sugar Coated	Hydroxyzine HCl 25 mg	by Ivax	00182-1493	Antianxiety; Antihistamine
G09	Tab, Sugar Coated	Hydroxyzine HCl 50 mg	Atarax by Ivax	00182-1494	Antianxiety; Antihistamine
G1	Tab, White, Round	Glycopyrrolate 1 mg	Robinul by URL	00677-1931	Gastrointestinal
G1	Tab, White, Cap Shaped, Scored	Glyburide 1.5 mg	Glynase by West-Ward	00143-9918	Antidiabetic
G1	Tab, White, Round	Glycopyrrolate 1 mg	Robinul by URL Mutual	00677-1931	Gastrointestinal
G1 <> 4	Tab, White, Oval	Ondansetron HCl 4 mg	Zofran by Glenmark	68462-0105	Antiemetic
G1 <> 8	Tab, Yellow, Oval	Ondansetron HCl 8 mg	Zofran by Glenmark	68462-0106	Antiemetic
G10	Tab, White, Oval	Medroxyprogesterone Acetate 10 mg	by Genpharm	Canadian	Hormone
G100 <> BAYERBAYER	Tab, Off-White, Round, Scored, G100 <> Bayer Cross	Acarbose 100 mg	Glucobay by Bayer	Canadian DIN 02190893	Antidiabetic
G1043	Tab	Amoxapine 25 mg	Asendin by Ivax	00182-1043	Antidepressant
G1044	Tab, Salmon, Round	Amoxapine 50 mg	Asendin by Watson		Antidepressant
G1094	Tab, Red, Round	Phenylpropanolamine HCl 40 mg, Phenylephrine HCl 10 mg, Phentoloxamine 15 mg, Chlorpheniramine 5 mg	Naldecon by Rosemont		Cold Remedy
G1098Z2911	Cap, Green & White	Hydroxyzine Pamoate 50 mg	Vistaril by Ivax		Antianxiety; Antihistamine
G1099Z2909	Cap, Green & White	Hydroxyzine Pamoate 25 mg	Vistaril by Ivax		Antianxiety; Antihistamine
G11 <> MYLAN	Tab, White, Oval	Glimepiride 1 mg	Amaryl by Mylan	00378-4011	Antidiabetic
G1140	Tab, Flesh, Oblong	Amitriptyline HCl 150 mg	Elavil by MD		Antidepressant
G1161	Tab, White, Round	Furosemide 40 mg	Lasix by Watson		Diuretic
G1170	Tab	Furosemide 20 mg	by Med Pro	53978-5031	Diuretic
G1189	Tab	Chlorzoxazone 500 mg	by Ivax	00182-1189	Muscle Relaxant
G12	Tab, Tan, Oblong	Prenatal Plus	Stuart by Amneal	65162-0668	Vitamin
G12 <> JANSSEN	Tab, Orange-Brown, Round, Film Coated	Galantamine 12 mg	Reminyl by Janssen-Ortho	Canadian DIN 02244300	Antialzheimers
G12 <> JANSSEN	Tab, Orange-Brown, Round, Film Coated	Galantamine 12 mg	Razadyne by Janssen	50458-0392	Antialzheimers
G12 <> MYLAN	Tab, Light Yellow, Oval, Scored, G/12	Glimepiride 2 mg	Amaryl by UDL	51079-0425	Antidiabetic
G12 <> MYLAN	Tab, Light Green, Oval	Glimepiride 2 mg	Amaryl by Mylan	00378-4012	Antidiabetic
G13	Tab, White, Oval, Scored	Gabapentin 800 mg	Neurontin by Blu	24658-0121	Anticonvulsant
G13	Tab, White, Oval, Scored	Gabapentin 800 mg	Neurontin by Glenmark	68462-0127	Anticonvulsant
G13 <> MYLAN	Tab, Peach, Oval, Scored, G/13	Glimepiride 4 mg	Amaryl by UDL	51079-0426	Antidiabetic
G13 <> MYLAN	Tab, Light Pink, Oval	Glimepiride 4 mg	Amaryl by Mylan	00378-4013	Antidiabetic
G1300	Tab, White, Round	Verapamil HCl 80 mg	Isoptin by Watson		Antihypertensive
G1301	Tab, White, Round	Verapamil HCl 120 mg	Isoptin by Watson		Antihypertensive
G1330 <> Z2971	Tab, White, Round, Z over 2791	Metronidazole 250 mg	Flagyl by Ivax	00172-4291	Antibiotic
G135	Tab, White, Round	Doxylamine Succinate 25 mg	Unisom by Granutec		Sleep Aid
G14	Tab, Light Blue, Round	Naproxen 220 mg	Aleve by Safeway		NSAID
G14	Tab, White, Oval	Ondansetron HCl 4 mg	Zofran by Glenmark	68462-0105	Antiemetic
G14 <> 15	Tab, Light Yellow, Oval	Meloxicam 15 mg	Mobic by Glenmark	68462-0141	NSAID
G14 <> 75	Tab, Light Yellow, Round, G14 <> 7.5	Meloxicam 7.5 mg	Mobic by Glenmark	68462-0140	NSAID
G1410	Tab, White, Round	Acetaminophen 325 mg	Tylenol by Granutec		Analgesic

ID FRONT <> BACK	DESCRIPTION FRONT <> BACK	INGREDIENT & STRENGTH	BRAND (or Generic Equiv.) by FIRM	NDC#	CLASS; SCH.
G1457	Tab, White, Round	Acetaminophen 500 mg	Tylenol Ex Strength by Ivax		Analgesic
G150	Tab, White, Round, G/150	Ranitidine 150 mg	by Genpharm	Canadian	Gastrointestinal
G150MG3328	Cap, Light Blue & Green, G 150 mg on blue half, 3328 on green half	Clindamycin HCl 150 mg	Cleocin HCl by Greenstone	59762-3328	Antibiotic
G150MG3328	Cap, G 150 MG	Clindamycin HCl 150 mg	Cleocin HCl by Quality Care	60346-0018	Antibiotic
G150MG3328	Cap, Light Blue & Green, G 150 mg on blue half, 3328 on green half	Clindamycin HCl 150 mg	Cleocin HCl by Allscripts		Antibiotic
G1520 <> 25	Tab, White, Diamond-Shaped	Amlodipine Besylate 2.5 mg	Norvasc by Greenstone	59762-1520	Antihypertensive
G1530 <> 5	Tab, White, Elongated Octagon-Shaped	Amlodipine Besylate 5 mg	Norvasc by Greenstone	59762-1530	Antihypertensive
G1540 <> 10	Tab, White, Round	Amlodipine Besylate 10 mg	Norvasc by Greenstone	59762-1540	Antihypertensive
G16	Cap, Pink, Opaque, Extended Release	Galantamine 16 mg	Reminyl ER by Janssen-Ortho	Canadian DIN 02266725	Antialzheimers
G161	Tab, White, Round, Film Coated,	Oxycodone HCl 10 mg	Oxycontin by Dava	68774-0161	Analgesic; C II
G162	Tab, Orange, Round, Film Coated, Ex Release	Oxycodone HCl 20 mg	Oxycontin by Dava	68774-0162	Analgesic; C II
G163	Tab, Purple, Round, Film-Coated	Oxycodone HCl 40 mg	Oxycontin by Dava	68774-0163	Analgesic; C II
G164	Tab, Beige, Round, Film-Coated, Ex Release	Oxycodone HCl 80 mg	Oxycontin by Dava	68774-0164	Analgesic; C II
G164	Tab, Beige, Round, Film-Coated	Oxycodone HCl 80 mg	Oxycontin by Global	00115-1644	Analgesic; C II
G17	Tab, Light Blue, Oval	Naproxen 220 mg	by Novopharm		NSAID
G17 <> LL	Tab, Film Coated	Gemfibrozil 600 mg	by Vangard	00615-3559	Antihyperlipidemic
G1724	Tab, White, Round	Quinidine Sulfate 300 mg	Quinidine Sulfate by Eon		Antiarrhythmic
G1736	Tab	Furosemide 80 mg	by Ivax	00182-1736	Diuretic
G1789	Tab	Metoclopramide HCl 10 mg	Reglan by Med Pro	53978-5011	Gastrointestinal
G18	Tab, White, Oval	Ondansetron HCl 4 mg	Zofran by Glenmark	68462-0106	Antiemetic
G1802	Tab, Yellow, Round	Salsalate 500 mg	Disalcid by Rosemont		NSAID
G1803	Tab, Yellow, Oblong	Salsalate 750 mg	Disalcid by Rosemont		NSAID
G180605	Tab, White, Round, G 1806/0.5	Lorazepam 0.5 mg	Ativan by Royce		Antianxiety; C IV
G1808	Tab	Lorazepam 2 mg	Ativan by Ivax	00182-1808	Antianxiety; C IV
G1839	Tab, Film Coated	Potassium Chloride 600 mg	by Ivax	00182-1839	Electrolytes
G1872	Tab, Yellow, Round	Hydrochlorothiazide 50 mg, Triamterene 75 mg	Maxzide by Watson		Diuretic; Antihypertensive
G1919	Tab, Film Coated	Cyclobenzaprine HCl 10 mg	by Invamed	52189-0252	Muscle Relaxant
G1G1	Tab, Pink Cap-Shaped, Scored, Cobalt Logo <> G1 / G1	Glimepiride 1 mg	Amaryl by Cobalt	Canadian DIN 02274248	Antidiabetic
G1LL	Tab, Brown, Oblong, G1-LL	Vitamin, Mineral	Gevral by Lederle		Vitamin
G2	Tab, White, Round, G-2	Triprolidine 2.5 mg, Pseudoephedrine 60 mg	Actifed by K.C.		Cold Remedy
G2	Tab, Blue, Oblong, Scored	Glyburide 3 mg	Glynase by West-Ward	00143-9919	Antidiabetic
G2	Tab, White, Round	Glycopyrrolate 2 mg	Robinul Forte by URL Mutual	00677-1932	Gastrointestinal
G2 <> 250	Tab, White, Round	Terbinafine HCl 250 mg	Lamisil by Glenmark	68462-0136	Antifungal
G2 <> AL	Tab, White, Oblong, /A/L <> /G/2/	Alprazolam 2 mg	Xanax by Genpharm	Canadian DIN 02229814	Antianxiety; C IV
G2 <> AL	Tab, White, Oblong, /A/L <> /G/2/	Alprazolam 2 mg	Xanax by Par	49884-0400	Antianxiety; C IV
G21	Tab, Pink, Round, Film Coated	Amitriptyline HCl 10 mg	Elavil by Ivax	00182-1018	Antidepressant
G21	Tab, White, Elliptical Shaped, Scored, Film Coated	Gabapentin 600 mg	Neurontin by Greenstone	59762-5023	Anticonvulsant
G21 <> M	Tab, Blue	Galantamine 4 mg	Razadyne by UDL	51079-0852	Antialzheimers
G2152	Tab, White, Oblong	Acetaminophen 500 mg	Tylenol Ex Strength by Ivax		Analgesic
G22	Tab, Green, Round	Amitriptyline HCl 25 mg	Elavil by Ivax	00182-1019	Antidepressant
G22	Tab, White, Elliptical Shaped, Scored, Film Coated	Gabapentin 800 mg	Neurontin by Greenstone	59762-5024	Anticonvulsant
G22 <> M	Tab, Blue	Galantamine 8 mg	Razadyne by UDL	51079-0853	Antialzheimers
G23	Tab, Brown, Round	Amitriptyline HCl 50 mg	Elavil by Ivax	00182-1020	Antidepressant

ID FRONT <> BACK	DESCRIPTION FRONT <> BACK	INGREDIENT & STRENGTH	BRAND (or Generic Equiv.) by FIRM	NDC#	CLASS; SCH.
G23 <> M	Tab, Blue	Galantamine 12 mg	Razadyne by UDL	51079-0854	Antialzheimers
G237	Cap, Green	Chloral Hydrate 500 mg	Chloral Hydrate by R. P. Scherer		Sedative/Hypnotic; C IV
G24	Tab, Purple, Round	Amitriptyline HCl 75 mg	Elavil by Ivax	00182-1021	Antidepressant
G24	Tab, Turquoise, Cap Shaped	Diphenhydramine HCl 25 mg, Pseudoephedrine HCl 60 mg	Benadryl-D by Leiner	49035-0289	Cold Remedy
G24	Cap, Caramel Opaque, Extended Release	Galantamine 24 mg	Reminyl ER by Janssen-Ortho	Canadian DIN 02266733	Antialzheimers
G24100	Cap, Light Green and White, Opaque, Scripted G	Zonisamide 100 mg	Zonegran by Glenmark	68462-0130	Anticonvulsant
G2425	Cap, White and Light Blue	Zonisamide 25 mg	Zonegran by Glenmark	68462-0128	Anticonvulsant
G2450	Cap, Yellow and White, Opaque, Scripted G	Zonisamide 50 mg	Zonegran by Glenmark	68462-0129	Anticonvulsant
G246	Cap, White, Opaque, Black Ink	Fenofibrate 50 mg	Lipofen by Kowa Pharmaceuticals	66869-0137	Antihyperlipidemic
G248150	Cap, White, Opaque, Green Ink	Fenofibrate 150 mg	Lipofen by Kowa Pharmaceuticals	66869-0147	Antihyperlipidemic
G25	Tab, White, Round, Flat	Atenolol 25 mg	Tenormin by Genpharm	15330-0025	Antihypertensive
G25	Tab, White, Round, Flat	Atenolol 25 mg	Tenormin by Par	49884-0944	Antihypertensive
G25	Tab, Orange, Round	Amitriptyline HCl 100 mg	Elavil by Ivax	00182-1063	Antidepressant
G25	Tab, Peach, Oval, G 2.5	Medroxyprogesterone Acetate 2.5 mg	by Genpharm	Canadian	Hormone
G252100	Tab, White, Blue Ink, Extended-Release	Tramadol HCl 100 mg	Ultram ER by Galephar	66277-0252	Analgesic
G253200	Tab, White, Violet Ink, Extended-Release	Tramadol HCl 200 mg	Ultram ER by Galephar	66277-0253	Analgesic
G254300	Tab, White, Red Ink, Extended-Release	Tramadol HCl 300 mg	Ultram ER by Galephar	66277-0254	Analgesic
G283	Cap, Natural & Pink	Diphenhydramine HCl 25 mg	by PFI		Antihistamine
G284	Cap, Blue	Pseudoephedrine 60 mg, Diphenhydramine 25 mg	by PFI		Cold Remedy
G29	Tab	Chlorpropamide 250 mg	by Ivax	00182-1852	Antidiabetic
G297	Cap	Chloral Hydrate 500 mg	Chloral Hydrate by URL Mutual	00677-0225	Sedative/Hypnotic; C IV
G297	Cap, Clear & Light Green	Chloral Hydrate 500 mg	Chloral Hydrate by RP Scherer	11014-0918	Sedative/Hypnotic; C IV
G2G2	Tab, Green, Cap-Shaped, Scored, Cobalt Logo <> G2 / G2	Glimepiride 2 mg	Amaryl by Cobalt	Canadian DIN 02274256	Antidiabetic
G2LL	Tab, Maroon, Oblong, G2-LL	Vitamin, Mineral	Gevral T by Lederle	64376-0802	Vitamin
G3	Tab, Red, Oval	Iron 100 mg, Vitamin C 250 mg, Vitamin B-12 0.025 mg, Folic Acid 1 mg	FE C Tab Plus by UDL	51079-0472	Vitamin
G3 <> M	Tab, White, Round	Granisetron HCl 1 mg	Kytril by UDL	00378-	Antiemetic
G3 <> M	Tab, White, Round	Granisetron HCl 1 mg	Kytril by Mylan		Antiemetic
G30	Tab	Chlorthalidone 25 mg	by Ivax	00182-1434	Diuretic
G300	Tab, White, Oblong, G/300	Ranitidine 300 mg	by Genpharm	Canadian	Gastrointestinal
G300MG5010	Cap, Blue, White Print, G300 mg on Cap, 5010 on Body	Clindamycin HCl 300 mg	Cleocin HCl by Greenstone	59762-5010	Antibiotic
G31	Tab, White, Oval	Gabapentin 600 mg	Neurontin by Glenmark	68462-0126	Anticonvulsant
G31	Tab, White, Oval	Gabapentin 600 mg	Neurontin by Blu	24658-0120	Anticonvulsant
G31 <> M	Tab, White, Round	Glipizide 2.5 mg, Metformin HCl 250 mg	MetaGlip by Mylan	00378-3131	Antidiabetic
G32 <> 250	Tab, Pink, Round, G-32 <> 250	Naproxen 250 mg	Naprosyn by Glenmark	68462-0188	NSAID
G32 <> 375	Tab, Pink, Cap Shaped	Naproxen 375 mg	Naprosyn by Glenmark	68462-0189	NSAID
G32 <> 500	Tab, Off White to Light Pink, Cap Shaped	Naproxen 500 mg	Naprosyn by Glenmark	68462-0190	NSAID
G32 <> M	Tab, White, Oval	Glipizide 2.5 mg, Metformin HCl 500 mg	MetaGlip by Mylan	00378-3132	Antidiabetic
G324	Cap, Red	Chloral Hydrate 500 mg	Chloral Hydrate by R. P. Scherer		Sedative/Hypnotic; C IV
G33 <> M	Tab, Peach, Cap Shaped	Glipizide 5 mg, Metformin HCl 500 mg	MetaGlip by Mylan	00378-3133	Antidiabetic
G341	Tab, Purple, Round, Film Coated, Extended Release	Oxybutynin Chloride 5 mg	Ditropan XL by Teva	00093-5206	Urinary Tract
G342	Tab, Pink, Round, Film Coated, Extended Release	Oxybutynin Chloride 10 mg	Ditropan XL by Mylan	00093-5207	Urinary Tract
G343	Tab, Off-White, Round, Film Coated, Extended Release	Oxybutynin Chloride 15 mg	Ditropan XL by Teva	00093-5208	Urinary Tract
G3511	Tab, Off-White, Round	Pyridostigmine Bromide 60 mg	Mestinon by Global	00115-3511	Muscle Stimulant
G352	Tab, White to Off White, Caps Shaped, Film Coated	Fenofibrate 160 mg	Lofibra by Global	00115-5522	Antihyperlipidemic
G359 <> 832	Tab	Fluoxymesterone 10 mg	by Qualitest	00603-3645	Steroid; C III
G3717	Tab, White, Oval, Scored	Triazolam 0.125 mg	Halcion by Greenstone	59762-3717	Sedative/Hypnotic; C IV
G3717	Tab, White, Oval, Scored	Triazolam 0.125 mg	Halcion by DRX	55045-2550	Sedative/Hypnotic; C IV

ID FRONT <> BACK	DESCRIPTION FRONT <> BACK	INGREDIENT & STRENGTH	BRAND (or Generic Equiv.) by FIRM	NDC#	CLASS; SCH.
G3717	Tab, White, Oval, Scored	Triazolam 0.125 mg	Halcion by St. Mary's Med	60760-0717	Sedative/Hypnotic; C IV
G3717	Tab, White, Oval, Scored	Triazolam 0.125 mg	Halcion by Pharmacia	00009-3717	Sedative/Hypnotic; C IV
G3717	Tab, White, Oval, Scored	Triazolam 0.125 mg	Halcion by H J Harkins Co	52959-0401	Sedative/Hypnotic; C IV
G3718	Tab, Blue, Oval, Scored	Triazolam 0.25 mg	Halcion by H J Harkins Co	52959-0402	Sedative/Hypnotic; C IV
G3718	Tab, Blue, Oval, Scored	Triazolam 0.25 mg	Halcion by Pharmacia	00009-3718	Sedative/Hypnotic; C IV
G3718	Tab, Blue, Oval, Scored	Triazolam 0.25 mg	Halcion by Greenstone	59762-3718	Sedative/Hypnotic; C IV
G3719	Tab, White, Oval, Scored	Alprazolam 0.25 mg	Xanax by Greenstone	59762-3719	Antianxiety; C IV
G3720	Tab, Peach, Oval, Scored	Alprazolam 0.5 mg	Xanax by H J Harkins Co	52959-0457	Antianxiety; C IV
G3720	Tab, Peach, Oval, Scored	Alprazolam 0.5 mg	Xanax by Greenstone	59762-3720	Antianxiety; C IV
G3721	Tab, Blue, Oval, Scored	Alprazolam 1 mg	Xanax by Golden State	60429-0504	Antianxiety; C IV
G3721	Tab, Blue, Oval, Scored	Alprazolam 1 mg	Xanax by Greenstone	59762-3721	Antianxiety; C IV
G3721	Tab, Blue, Oval, Scored	Alprazolam 1 mg	Xanax by Physician Total Care	54868-3005	Antianxiety; C IV
G3722	Tab, White, Rectangular, Scored	Alprazolam 2 mg	Xanax by Golden State	60429-0505	Antianxiety; C IV
G3722	Tab, White, Rectangular, Scored	Alprazolam 2 mg	Xanax by Greenstone	59762-3722	Antianxiety; C IV
G3723	Tab, White, Oval	Flurbiprofen 50 mg	Ansaid by Greenstone	59762-3723	NSAID
G3724	Tab, Blue, Oval	Flurbiprofen 100 mg	Ansaid by Greenstone	59762-3724	NSAID
G3724	Tab, Blue, Oval	Flurbiprofen 100 mg	Ansaid by Repack Co of America	55306-3724	NSAID
G3725	Tab, White, Round, Scored	Glyburide 1.25 mg	Micronase by Greenstone	59762-3725	Antidiabetic
G3726	Tab, Pink, Round, Scored	Glyburide 2.5 mg	Diabeta by DRX	55045-2322	Antidiabetic
G3726	Tab, Pink, Round, Scored	Glyburide 2.5 mg	Micronase by Greenstone	59762-3726	Antidiabetic
G3726	Tab, Pink, Round, Scored	Glyburide 2.5 mg	Diabeta by Direct Dispensing	57866-6408	Antidiabetic
G3726	Tab, Pink, Round, Scored	Glyburide 2.5 mg	Diabeta by Caremark	00339-5912	Antidiabetic
G3727	Tab, Blue, Round, Scored	Glyburide 5 mg	Micronase by Greenstone	59762-3727	Antidiabetic
G3727	Tab, Blue, Round, Scored	Glyburide 5 mg	Diabeta by Caremark	00339-5914	Antidiabetic
G3727	Tab, Blue, Round, Scored	Glyburide 5 mg	Diabeta by DRX	55045-2138	Antidiabetic
G3727	Tab, Blue, Round, Scored	Glyburide 5 mg	Diabeta by H J Harkins Co	52959-0449	Antidiabetic
G3727	Tab, Blue, Round, Scored	Glyburide 5 mg	Diabeta by Direct Dispensing	57866-6409	Antidiabetic
G3740	Tab, Orange, Round, Scored	Medroxyprogesterone Acetate 2.5 mg	Provera by Pharmacia	00009-3740	Hormone
G3740	Tab, Orange, Round, Scored	Medroxyprogesterone Acetate 2.5 mg	Provera by Kaiser	00179-1201	Hormone
G3740	Tab, Orange, Round, Scored	Medroxyprogesterone Acetate 2.5 mg	Provera by Apotheca	12634-0432	Hormone
G3740	Tab, Orange, Round, Scored	Medroxyprogesterone Acetate 2.5 mg	Provera by Greenstone	59762-3740	Hormone
G3741	Tab, White, Hexagonal, Scored	Medroxyprogesterone Acetate 5 mg	Provera by Greenstone	59762-3741	Hormone
G3741	Tab, White, Hexagonal, Scored	Medroxyprogesterone Acetate 5 mg	Provera by PDRX	55289-0908	Hormone
G3741	Tab, White, Hexagonal, Scored	Medroxyprogesterone Acetate 5 mg	Provera by Kaiser	00179-1202	Hormone
G3741	Tab, White, Hexagonal, Scored	Medroxyprogesterone Acetate 5 mg	Provera by Pharmacia	00009-3741	Hormone
G3742	Tab, White, Round, Scored	Medroxyprogesterone Acetate 10 mg	Provera by Pharmacia	00009-3742	Hormone
G3742	Tab, White, Round, Scored	Medroxyprogesterone Acetate 10 mg	Provera by Kaiser	00179-1117	Hormone
G3742	Tab, White, Round, Scored	Medroxyprogesterone Acetate 10 mg	Provera by Nat Pharmpak	55154-5568	Hormone
G3742	Tab, White, Round, Scored	Medroxyprogesterone Acetate 10 mg	Provera by Greenstone	59762-3742	Hormone
G3781	Tab, White, Oval, Scored	Glyburide 1.5 mg	Micronase by Greenstone	59762-3781	Antidiabetic
G3782	Tab, Blue, Oval, Scored	Glyburide 3 mg	Micronase by Greenstone	59762-3782	Antidiabetic
G3783	Tab, Yellow, Oval, Scored	Glyburide 6 mg	Micronase by Greenstone	59762-3783	Antidiabetic
G3783	Tab, Yellow, Oval, Scored	Glyburide 6 mg	Micronase by Kaiser	00179-1325	Antidiabetic
G38	Cap, Gray	Etodolac 200 mg	Lodine by Genpharm	55567-0038	NSAID
G383	Cap, Red	Guaifenesin	Robitussin by Granutec		Expectorant
G39	Cap, Gray	Etodolac 300 mg	Lodine by Genpharm	55567-0039	NSAID
G4	Tab, Yellow, Oblong, Scored	Oxcarbazepine 300 mg	Trileptal by Glenmark	68462-0138	Anticonvulsant
G4	Tab, White, Round, Orally Disintegrating	Ondansetron 4 mg	Zofran ODT by Glenmark	68462-0157	Antiemetic
G4 <> JANSSEN	Tab, Off-White, Round, Film Coated	Galantamine 4 mg	Reminyl by Janssen-Ortho	Canadian DIN 02244298	Antialzheimers

ID FRONT <> BACK	DESCRIPTION FRONT <> BACK	INGREDIENT & STRENGTH	BRAND (or Generic Equiv.) by FIRM	NDC#	CLASS; SCH.
G4 <> JANSSEN	Tab, Off-White, Round, Film Coated	Galantamine 4 mg	Razadyne by Janssen	50458-0390	Antialzheimers
G4 <> M	Tab, White, Round	Guanfacine HCl 1 mg	Tenex by Mylan	00378-1160	Antihypertensive
G400	Tab, White, Round, Film Coated	Ibuprofen 400 mg	Motrin by Rx Dispensing	61807-0027	NSAID
G400	Tab, White, Round, Film Coated	Ibuprofen 400 mg	Motrin by Pharmacia	00009-7378	NSAID
G400	Tab, White, Round, Film Coated	Ibuprofen 400 mg	Motrin by Caremark	00339-6076	NSAID
G400	Tab, White, Round, Film Coated	Ibuprofen 400 mg	Motrin by Apotheca	12634-0171	NSAID
G400	Tab, White, Round, Film Coated	Ibuprofen 400 mg	Motrin by Greenstone	59762-7378	NSAID
G403	Cap, White with Blue Print, Gelatin	Sevelamer HCl 403 mg	Renagel by Genzyme	58468-4709	Phosphate Binder
G41 <> 25	Tab, White, Round	Carvedilol 25 mg	Coreg by Glenmark	68462-0165	Antihypertensive
G42	Cap, Clear & Red	Docusate Sodium 100 mg	Colace by Goldcaps		Laxative
G421	Tab, White, Round, Scored	Midodrine HCl 2.5 mg	ProAmatine by Global	00115-4211	Antihypotensive
G422	Tab, Light Orange, Round, Scored	Midodrine HCl 5 mg	ProAmatine by Global	00115-4222	Antihypotensive
G423	Tab, Light Green, Round, Scored	Midodrine HCl 10 mg	ProAmatine by Global	00115-4233	Antihypotensive
G43	Cap, Maroon, Soft Gel, G-43	Docusate Sodium 100 mg, Casanthranol 30 mg	Peri-Colace by Ivax	00182-8616	Laxative
G441	Cap, Yellow and Green, Opaque	Dantrolene Sodium 25 mg	Dantrium by Global	00115-4411	Muscle Relaxant
G442	Cap, Yellow and Light Blue, Opaque	Dantrolene Sodium 50 mg	Dantrium by Global	00115-4422	Muscle Relaxant
G443	Cap, Yellow and Reddish Orange, Opaque	Dantrolene Sodium 100 mg	Dantrium by Global	00115-4433	Muscle Relaxant
G45 <> 1000	Tab, White, Round	Metformin 1000 mg	Glucophage by Glenmark	68462-0161	Antihyperglycemic
G45 <> 500	Tab, White, Round	Metformin 500 mg	Glucophage by Glenmark	68462-0159	Antihyperglycemic
G45 <> 850	Tab, White, Round	Metformin 850 mg	Glucophage by Glenmark	68462-0160	Antihyperglycemic
G461	Cap, White and Gray, Opaque	Anagrelide HCl 0.5 mg	Agrylin by Global	00115-4611	Antiplatelet
G462	Cap, White and Gray, Opaque	Anagrelide HCl 1 mg	Agrylin by Global	00115-4622	Antiplatelet
G463 <> 832	Tab, White, Round	Medroxyprogesterone Acetate 10 mg	Provera by Qualitest	00603-4368	Hormone
G465832	Tab, White, Round, G 465/832	Megestrol Acetate 20 mg	Megace by Rosemont		Hormone
G466832	Tab, White, Round, G 466/832	Megestrol Acetate 40 mg	Megace by Rosemont		Hormone
G4900 <> 50MG	Tab, Light Blue, Cap Shaped, Scored	Sertraline HCl 50 mg	Zoloft by Greenstone	59762-4900	Antidepressant
G4910 <> 100MG	Tab, Light Yellow, Cap Shaped, Scored	Sertraline HCl 100 mg	Zoloft by Greenstone	59762-4910	Antidepressant
G4960 <> 25MG	Tab, Light Green, Cap Shaped, Scored	Sertraline HCl 25 mg	Zoloft by Greenstone	59762-4960	Antidepressant
G4G4	Tab, Blue, Cap-Shaped, Scored, Cobalt Logo <> G2 / G2	Glimepiride 4 mg	Amaryl by Cobalt	Canadian DIN 02274272	Antidiabetic
G5	Tab, Blue, Oval	Medroxyprogesterone Acetate 5 mg	Provera by Genpharm	Canadian	Hormone
G5	Tab, Red & Yellow, Oblong, Scored	Acetaminophen 500 mg	Tylenol Ex Strength by Goldline		Analgesic
G5 <> 10	Tab, Yellow, Circular	Pravastatin Sodium 10 mg	Pravachol by Glenmark	68462-0195	Antihyperlipidemic
G5 <> 20	Tab, Yellow, Rounded Rectangular	Pravastatin Sodium 20 mg	Pravachol by Glenmark	68462-0196	Antihyperlipidemic
G5 <> 40	Tab, Green, Rounded Rectangular	Pravastatin Sodium 40 mg	Pravachol by Glenmark	68462-0197	Antihyperlipidemic
G5 <> 80	Tab, Yellow, Oval	Pravastatin Sodium 80 mg	Pravachol by Glenmark	68462-0198	Antihyperlipidemic
G5 <> M	Tab	Guanfacine HCl 2 mg	Tenex by Mylan	00378-1190	Antihypertensive
G50 <> BAYERBAYER	Tab, Off-White, Round, G50 over Bayer Cross	Acarbose 50 mg	Glucobay by Bayer	Canadian DIN 02190885	Antidiabetic
G500	Tab, Orange, Round, Scored	Sulfasalazine 500 mg	Azulfidine by Greenstone	59762-5000	Gastrointestinal
G5002	Tab, White, Cap Shaped, Scored	Oxaprozin 600 mg	Daypro by Greenstone	59762-5002 Discontinued	NSAID
G5007	Tab, White, Round	Misoprostol 100 mg	Cytotec by Greenstone	59762-5007	Gastrointestinal
G5008	Tab, White, Hexagonal, Scored	Misoprostol 200 mg	Cytotec by Greenstone	59762-5008	Gastrointestinal
G5026	Cap, White, Hard Gel, G <> 5026	Gabapentin 100 mg	Neurontin by Greenstone	59762-5026	Anticonvulsant
G5027	Cap, Yellow, Hard Gel, G <> 5027	Gabapentin 300 mg	Neurontin by Greenstone	59762-5027	Anticonvulsant
G5028	Cap, Orange, Hard Gel, G <> 5028	Gabapentin 400 mg	Neurontin by Greenstone	59762-5028	Anticonvulsant
G52	Tab, Pink, Round	Ranitidine HCl 75 mg	Zantac by RX Pak	65084-0173	Gastrointestinal
G56	Tab, Orange & Red, Round	Acetaminophen 500 mg	Tylenol Ex Strength by Banner Pharma		Analgesic

ID FRONT <> BACK	DESCRIPTION FRONT <> BACK	INGREDIENT & STRENGTH	BRAND (or Generic Equiv.) by FIRM	NDC#	CLASS; SCH.
G58 <> 10	Tab, White to Off White, Round	Amlodipine Besylate 10 mg	Norvasc by Glenmark	68462-0212	Antihypertensive
G58 <> 5	Tab, White to Off White, Round	Amlodipine Besylate 5 mg	Norvasc by Glenmark	68462-0211	Antihypertensive
G600	Tab, White, Cap Shaped	Ibuprofen 600 mg	Motrin by Greenstone	59762-7379	NSAID
G600	Tab, White, Cap Shaped	Ibuprofen 600 mg	Motrin by Med Pro	53978-5006	NSAID
G600	Tab, White, Cap Shaped	Ibuprofen 600 mg	Motrin by Apotheca	12634-0191	NSAID
G600	Tab, White, Cap Shaped	Ibuprofen 600 mg	Motrin by Pharmacia	00009-7379	NSAID
G600	Tab, White, Cap Shaped	Ibuprofen 600 mg	Motrin by Caremark	00339-6077	NSAID
G600 <> P	Tab, White, Elliptical	Gabapentin 600 mg	Neurontin by Pharmascience	Canadian DIN 02255898	Anticonvulsant
G600 <> TTC	Tab	Guaifenesin 600 mg	Robitussin by URL Mutual	00677-1475	Expectorant
G8	Cap, White, Opaque, Extended Release	Galantamine 8 mg	Reminyl ER by Janssen-Ortho	Canadian DIN 02266717	Antialzheimers
G8	Tab, White, Round, Orally Disintegrating	Ondansetron 8 mg	Zofran ODT by Glenmark	68462-0158	Antiemetic
G8 <> JANSSEN	Tab, Pink, Round, Film Coated	Galantamine 8 mg	Reminyl by Janssen-Ortho	Canadian DIN 02244299	Antialzheimers
G8 <> JANSSEN	Tab, Pink, Round, Film Coated	Galantamine 8 mg	Razadyne by Janssen	50458-0391	Antialzheimers
G800	Tab, White, Cap Shaped	Ibuprofen 800 mg	Motrin by Greenstone	59762-7380	NSAID
G800	Tab, White, Cap Shaped	Ibuprofen 800 mg	Motrin by Pharmacia	00009-7380	NSAID
G800	Tab, White, Cap Shaped	Ibuprofen 800 mg	Motrin by Caremark	00339-6078	NSAID
G800	Tab, White, Cap Shaped	Ibuprofen 800 mg	Motrin by Med Pro	53978-5007	NSAID
G800 <> P	Tab, White, Elliptical	Gabapentin 800 mg	Neurontin by Pharmascience	Canadian DIN 02255901	Anticonvulsant
G91	Tab, Purple, Round	Dipyridamole 50 mg	Persantine by Glenmark	68462-0117	Antiplatelet
GA100	Tab, Coated	Atenolol 100 mg	Tenormin by Ivax	00182-1005	Antihypertensive
GA100	Cap, White, Opaque, Blue Ink, Cobalt Logo	Gabapentin 100 mg	Neurontin by Cobalt	Canadian DIN 02256142	Anticonvulsant
GA300	Cap, Yellow, Opaque, Blue Ink, Cobalt Logo	Gabapentin 300 mg	Neurontin by Cobalt	Canadian DIN 02256150	Anticonvulsant
GA400	Cap, Orange, Opaque, Blue Ink, Cobalt Logo	Gabapentin 400 mg	Neurontin by Cobalt	Canadian DIN 02256169	Anticonvulsant
GA50	Tab	Atenolol 50 mg	Tenormin by Ivax	00182-1004	Antihypertensive
GA50	Tab	Atenolol 50 mg	Tenormin by Med Pro	53978-1199	Antihypertensive
GAB600 <> APO	Tab, White, Oval, Scored, "GAB" and "600" curved around edges	Gabapentin 600 mg	Neurontin by Apotex	60505-2551	Anticonvulsants
GABAPENTIN100MGP	Cap, White, Opaque, Hard Gel	Gabapentin 100 mg	Neurontin by Pharmascience	Canadian DIN 02243446	Anticonvulsant
GABAPENTIN300MGP	Cap, Yellow, Opaque, Hard Gel	Gabapentin 300 mg	Neurontin by Pharmascience	Canadian DIN 02243447	Anticonvulsant
GABAPENTIN400MGP	Cap, Orange, Opaque, Hard Gel	Gabapentin 400 mg	Neurontin by Pharmascience	Canadian DIN 02243448	Anticonvulsant
GAC200	Cap, Orange & Purple	Acebutolol HCl 200 mg	Sectral by Par	49884-0587	Antihypertensive
GAC200	Cap, Orange & Purple	Acebutolol HCl 200 mg	Sectral by Genpharm	55567-0089	Antihypertensive
GAC200	Cap, Orange & Purple	Acebutolol HCl 200 mg	Sectral by Alphapharm	57315-0025	Antihypertensive
GAC400	Cap, Orange & Purple	Acebutolol HCl 400 mg	Sectral by Alphapharm	57315-0026	Antihypertensive
GAC400	Cap, Orange & Purple	Acebutolol HCl 400 mg	Sectral by Genpharm	55567-0090	Antihypertensive
GAC400	Cap, Orange & Purple	Acebutolol HCl 400 mg	Sectral by Par	49884-0588	Antihypertensive
GAL16	Cap, Pink, Opaque, Extended Release	Galantamine HBr 16 mg	Razadyne by Ortho-McNeil	50458-0388	Antialzheimers
GAL24	Cap, Caramel, Opaque, Extended Release	Galantamine HBr 24 mg	Razadyne by Ortho-McNeil	50458-0389	Antialzheimers
GAL8	Cap, White, Opaque, Extended Release	Galantamine HBr 8 mg	Razadyne by Ortho-McNeil	50458-0387	Antialzheimers
GANTACID	Tab, White, Round, G/Antacid	Calcium Carbonate 585 mg, Magnesium Hydroxide 120 mg, Simethicone 30 mg	Gastrozepin by Boehringer Ingelheim	Canadian	Vitamin; Mineral

ID FRONT <> BACK	DESCRIPTION FRONT <> BACK	INGREDIENT & STRENGTH	BRAND (or Generic Equiv.) by FIRM	NDC#	CLASS; SCH.
GAT100	Tab, White, Round, G/AT/100	Atenolol 100 mg	Tenormin by Genpharm	Canadian	Antihypertensive
GAT100	Tab, White, Round, G/AT/100	Atenolol 100 mg	Tenormin by Genpharm	Canadian	Antihypertensive
GAT50	Tab, White, Round, G/AT/50	Atenolol 50 mg	Tenormin by Genpharm	Canadian	Antihypertensive
GAT60	Tab, White, Round, G/AT/60	Atenolol 60 mg	Tenormin by Genpharm	Canadian	Antihypertensive
GATE <> MOBAN10	Tab, Purple, Round, Scored	Molindone HCl 10 mg	Moban by Gate	57844-0915	Antipsychotic
GATE <> MOBAN100	Tab, Tan, Round, Scored	Molindone HCl 100 mg	Moban by Gate	57844-0918	Antipsychotic
GATE <> MOBAN25	Tab, Green, Round, Scored	Molindone HCl 25 mg	Moban by Gate	57844-0916	Antipsychotic
GATE <> MOBAN5	Tab, Orange, Round, Scored	Molindone HCl 5 mg	Moban by Gate	57844-0914	Antipsychotic
GATE <> MOBAN50	Tab, Blue, Round, Scored	Molindone HCl 50 mg	Moban by Gate	57844-0917	Antipsychotic
GAVISCONEXTRA	Tab, White, Round, Gaviscon/Extra	Alginic Acid 400 mg	Gaviscon by SKB	Canadian	Gastrointestinal
GAX250	Cap, Red and Gold, Opaque	Amoxicillin 250 mg	Amoxil by Genpharm	Canadian DIN 02238171	Antibiotic
GAX500	Cap, Red and Gold, Opaque	Amoxicillin 500 mg	Amoxil by Genpharm	Canadian DIN 02238172	Antibiotic
GBN10	Tab, White, Round, G BN/10	Baclofen 10 mg	Lioresal by Genpharm		Muscle Relaxant
GBN20	Tab, White, Round, G BN/20	Baclofen 20 mg	Lioresal by Genpharm		Muscle Relaxant
GC125	Tab, White, Oblong, G/C 12.5	Captopril 12.5 mg	Capoten by Genpharm	Canadian	Antihypertensive
GDC <> 111	Tab, White, Round	Calcium Carbonate, Magnesium Hydroxide	MI-Acid by Major	00904-5115	Gastrointestinal
GDC <> 122	Tab, Pink, Round	Bismuth 262 mg	Pepto-Bismol by Ivax	00182-1091	Gastrointestinal
GDC103	Tab, White, Round	Simethicone 80 mg	Mylicon by Walsh Dist.	Discontinued 64899-0003	Antiflatulent
GDC113	Tab, White, Round	Calcium Carbonate 500 mg	Tums by Qualitest	00603-0095	Gastrointestinal
GDC119	Tab, White, Round	Aluminum 80 mg, Magnesium 20 mg	Gaviscon by Qualitest	00603-0186	Gastrointestinal
GDC119	Tab, White, Round, Chewable	Aluminum Hydroxide 80 mg, Magnesium Trisilicate 20 mg	Gaviscon by Rugby	00536-3013	Gastrointestinal
GDC119	Tab, White, Round, Chewable	Aluminum Hydroxide 80 mg, Magnesium Trisilicate 20 mg	Gaviscon by Ivax	00182-2220	Antacid
GDC122	Tab, Multi-Colored, Round, GDC/122	Bismuth 262 mg	Pepto-Bismol by Major	Discontinued 00904-1315	Gastrointestinal
GDC122	Tab, Multi-Colored, Round, GDC/122	Bismuth 262 mg	Pepto-Bismol by Ivax	00182-1091	Gastrointestinal
GDC126	Tab, Multi Colored, Round	Calcium Carbonate 500 mg	Tums by Ivax	Discontinued 00182-1139	Vitamin; Mineral
GDC127	Tab, Assorted Colors, Round	Calcium Carbonate 750 mg	Tums EX by Qualitest	00603-0096	Gastrointestinal
GDC127	Tab, Multi-Colored, Round	Calcium Carbonate 750 mg	Tums E-X by Guardian		Vitamin; Mineral
GDC127	Tab, Multi Colored, Round, Chewable	Calcium Carbonate 750 mg	Tums Ex Strength by Ivax	00182-1136 Discontinued	Vitamin; Mineral
GDC128	Tab, White, Round	Aluminum, Magnesium, Alginic Acid, Sodium Bicarbonate	Gaviscon EX Strength by Qualitest	00603-0187	Gastrointestinal
GDC128	Tab, White, Round	Aluminum, Magnesium, Alginic Acid, Sodium Bicarbonate	Gaviscon EX Strength by Major	00904-5365	Gastrointestinal
GDC143	Tab, Pink, Round	Bisacodyl 5 mg	Correctol by Major	00904-5312	Gastrointestinal
GDC143	Tab, Pink, Round	Bisacodyl 5 mg	Correctol by Qualitest	00603-0129	Gastrointestinal
GDC144	Tab, White, Round	Calcium Carbonate 750 mg	Tums EX by Qualitest	00603-0097	Gastrointestinal
GDC152	Tab, White & Yellow	Aluminum 200 mg, Magnesium 200 mg, Simethicone 25 mg	Maalox Plus by Qualitest	00603-0011	Gastrointestinal
GDC172	Tab, Pink, Cap Shaped	Bismuth Subsalicylate 262 mg	Pepto-Bismol Caps by Guardian		Gastrointestinal
GDC183	Tab, Yellow, Round, Chewable	Calcium Carbonate 600 mg	Tums by Major	00904-5411	Gastrointestinal
GDS50	Tab, Light Brown, Delayed Release	Diclofenac Sodium 50 mg	Voltaren XR by UDL	51079-0466	NSAID
GDS75	Tab, Pale Pink, Delayed Release	Diclofenac Sodium 75 mg	Voltaren XR by UDL	51079-0224	NSAID
GE320	Tab, White to Off-White, Oval, Film Coated, Scored, imprint on both sides	Gemifloxacin 320 mg	Factive by Oscient	67707-0320	Antibiotic
GE320	Tab, White to Off-White, Oval, Film Coated, Scored, imprint on both sides	Gemifloxacin 320 mg	Factive by Abbott	Canadian DIN 02248968	Antibiotic
GE5GG	Tab, White, Oblong, GE/5/G/G	Glyburide 5 mg	Gen Glybe by Genpharm	Canadian	Antidiabetic
GEIGEY136	Tab, Orange, Round	Imipramine HCl 50 mg	Tofranil by Novartis	61615-0106	Antidepressant

ID FRONT <> BACK	DESCRIPTION FRONT <> BACK	INGREDIENT & STRENGTH	BRAND (or Generic Equiv.) by FIRM	NDC#	CLASS; SCH.
GEIGEY32	Tab, Orange, Triangle	Imipramine HCl 10 mg	Tofranil by Novartis	61615-0104	Antidepressant
GEIGY	Tab, White, Round, Scored	Carbamazepine 200 mg	Tegretol by Novartis	Canadian DIN 00010405	Anticonvulsant
GEIGY	Cap	Clofazimine 50 mg	Lamprene by Novartis	17088-0108	Antileprosy
GEIGY	Tab, White, Round, Scored	Acenocoumarol 4 mg	Sintrom by Geigy	Canadian DIN 00010391	Anticoagulant
GEIGY <> 3535	Tab, White, Mottled Blue, Cap Shaped, Scored	Hydrochlorothiazide 25 mg, Metoprolol Tartrate 50 mg	Lopressor HCT by Novartis	00078-0460	Diuretic; Antihypertensive
GEIGY <> 5151	Tab, Reddish Pink, Cap Shaped, Scored, Film Coated	Metoprolol Tartrate 50 mg	Lopressor by Novartis	Canadian DIN 00397423	Antihypertensive
GEIGY <> 5151	Tab, Reddish Pink, Cap Shaped, Scored, Film Coated	Metoprolol Tartrate 50 mg	Lopressor by Nat Pharmpak	55154-1009	Antihypertensive
GEIGY <> 5151	Tab, Reddish Pink, Cap Shaped, Scored, Film Coated	Metoprolol Tartrate 50 mg	Lopressor by Novartis	00078-0458	Antihypertensive
GEIGY <> 5151	Tab, Reddish Pink, Cap Shaped, Scored, Film Coated	Metoprolol Tartrate 50 mg	Lopressor by Caremark	00339-5213	Antihypertensive
GEIGY <> 5151	Tab, Reddish Pink, Cap Shaped, Scored, Film Coated	Metoprolol Tartrate 50 mg	Lopressor by Wal Mart	49035-0179	Antihypertensive
GEIGY <> 5353	Tab, White, Mottled Pink, Cap Shaped, Scored	Hydrochlorothiazide 25 mg, Metoprolol Tartrate 100 mg	Lopressor HCT by Pharm Util	60491-0371	Diuretic; Antihypertensive
GEIGY <> 5353	Tab, White, Mottled Pink, Cap Shaped, Scored	Hydrochlorothiazide 25 mg, Metoprolol Tartrate 100 mg	Lopressor HCT by Novartis	00078-0461	Diuretic; Antihypertensive
GEIGY <> 7171	Tab, Grey, Cap Shaped, Scored, Film Coated	Metoprolol Tartrate 100 mg	Lopressor by Novartis	Canadian DIN 0037431	Antihypertensive
GEIGY <> 7171	Tab, Grey, Cap Shaped, Scored, Film Coated	Metoprolol Tartrate 100 mg	Lopressor by Novartis	00078-0459	Antihypertensive
GEIGY <> 7373	Tab, White, Mottled Yellow, Cap Shaped, Scored	Hydrochlorothiazide 50 mg, Metoprolol Tartrate 100 mg	Lopressor HCT by Novartis	00078-0462	Diuretic; Antihypertensive
GEIGY <> ATA	Tab, Brownish-Red, Round, Sugar Coated	Imipramine HCl 75 mg	Tofranil by Novartis	Canadian DIN 00306487	Antidepressant
GEIGY <> CDC	Tab, Light Yellow, Round, Film Coated	Metoprolol Tartrate 200 mg	Lopressor by Novartis	Canadian DIN 00534560	Antihypertensive
GEIGY <> FH	Tab, Cream, Round, Sugar Coated	Clomipramine HCl 25 mg	Anafranil by Novartis	Canadian DIN 00324019	OCD
GEIGY <> FH	Tab, Cream, Round, Sugar Coated	Clomipramine HCl 25 mg	Anafranil by Cobalt	Canadian DIN 02244817	OCD
GEIGY <> GW	Tab, White to Off-White, Cap Shaped, Scored	Baclofen 20 mg	Lioresal by Geigy	Canadian DIN 00636576	Muscle Relaxant
GEIGY <> KJ	Tab, White to Off-White, Oval, Scored	Baclofen 10 mg	Lioresal by Geigy	Canadian DIN 00455881	Muscle Relaxant
GEIGY <> KR100	Tab, Brownish-Orange, Round, Film Coated	Metoprolol Tartrate 100 mg	Lopressor by Novartis	Canadian DIN 00665855	Antihypertensive
GEIGY <> LB	Tab, Brownish-Red, Round, Sugar Coated	Imipramine HCl 50 mg	Tofranil by Novartis	Canadian DIN 00010480	Antidepressant
GEIGY <> LP	Tab, White, Round, Film Coated	Clomipramine HCl 50 mg	Anafranil by Novartis	Canadian DIN 00402591	OCD
GEIGY <> LP	Tab, White, Round, Film Coated	Clomipramine HCl 50 mg	Anafranil by Cobalt	Canadian DIN 02244818	OCD
GEIGY <> MR	Tab, White w/ Red Specks, Round, Scored	Carbamazepine 100 mg	Tegretol by Novartis	Canadian DIN 00369810	Anticonvulsant
GEIGY <> PU	Tab, White w/ Red Specks, Oval, Scored	Carbamazepine 200 mg	Tegretol by Novartis	Canadian DIN 00665088	Anticonvulsant
GEIGY <> SJ	Tab, Peach, Round	Desipramine HCl 50 mg	Norpramin by Geigy		Antidepressant
GEIGY105	Tab, White, Round, Scored, Geigy over 105	Terbutaline Sulfate 5 mg	Brethine by Rightpak	65240-0614	Antiasthmatic
GEIGY105	Tab, White, Round, Scored, Geigy over 105	Terbutaline Sulfate 5.0 mg	Brethine by Rightpak	00028-0105	Antiasthmatic
GEIGY105	Tab, White, Round, Scored, Geigy over 105	Terbutaline Sulfate 5 mg	by Physician Total Care	54868-1240	Antiasthmatic
GEIGY105	Tab, White, Round, Scored, Geigy over 105	Terbutaline Sulfate 5 mg	Brethine by Drug Distr	52985-0114	Antiasthmatic
GEIGY105	Tab, White, Round, Scored, Geigy over 105	Terbutaline Sulfate 5 mg	by Amerisource	62584-0105	Antiasthmatic
GEIGY105	Tab, White, Round, Scored, Geigy over 105	Terbutaline Sulfate 5 mg	by Thrift Drug	59198-0012	Antiasthmatic
GEIGY105	Tab, White, Round, Scored, Geigy over 105	Terbutaline Sulfate 5 mg	by Nat Pharmpak	55154-1002	Antiasthmatic

ID FRONT <> BACK	DESCRIPTION FRONT <> BACK	INGREDIENT & STRENGTH	BRAND (or Generic Equiv.) by FIRM	NDC#	CLASS; SCH.
GEIGY105	Tab, White, Round, Scored, Geigy over 105	Terbutaline Sulfate 5 mg	by Syntex	18393-0150	Antiasthmatic
GEIGY108	Cap, Brown	Clofazimine 50 mg	Lamprene by Geigy		Antileprosy
GEIGY109	Cap, Brown	Clofazimine 100 mg	Lamprene by Geigy		Antileprosy
GEIGY111	Tab, White, Round	Tripelennamine HCl 25 mg	PBZ by Geigy		Antihistamine
GEIGY117	Tab	Tripelennamine HCl 50 mg	PBZ by Novartis	00028-0117	Antihistamine
GEIGY136	Tab, Coral, Black Print, Round, Sugar Coated	Imipramine HCl 50 mg	Tofranil by Novartis	00028-0136	Antidepressant
-GEIGY14	Tab, Red, Round	Phenylbutazone 100 mg	Butazolidin by Geigy		Anti-Inflammatory
GEIGY140	Tab, Coral, Black Print, Round, Sugar Coated	Imipramine HCl 25 mg	Tofranil by Novartis	00028-0140	Antidepressant
GEIGY23	Tab, White, Oval	Baclofen 10 mg	Lioresal by Geigy		Muscle Relaxant
GEIGY32	Tab, Coral, Black Print, Triangular, Sugar Coated	Imipramine HCl 10 mg	Tofranil by Novartis	00028-0032	Antidepressant
GEIGY33	Tab, White, Oblong	Baclofen 20 mg	Lioresal by Geigy		Muscle Relaxant
GEIGY42	Tab, Pink, Oval	Theophylline Anhydrous 200 mg	Constant-T by Geigy		Antiasthmatic
GEIGY47	Tab, White, Round, Red Specks, Chewable	Carbamazepine 100 mg	Tegretol by Geigy		Anticonvulsant
GEIGY48	Tab, Lavender, Round	Tripelennamine HCl SR 100 mg	PBZ-SR by Geigy		Antihistamine
GEIGY51	Tab, Film Coated	Metoprolol Tartrate 50 mg	Lopressor by Med Pro	53978-2058	Antihypertensive
GEIGY52	Tab, White, Round, Red Specks, Chewable	Carbamazepine 100 mg	Tegretol by Geigy		Anticonvulsant
GEIGY57	Tab, Blue, Oval	Theophylline Anhydrous 300 mg	Constant-T by Geigy		Antiasthmatic
GEIGY72	Tab, White, Oval, Scored, Geigy over 72	Terbutaline Sulfate 2.5 mg	Brethine by Rightpak	65240-0613	Antiasthmatic
GEIGY72	Tab, White, Oval, Scored, Geigy over 72	Terbutaline Sulfate 2.5 mg	Brethine by Novartis	00028-0072	Antiasthmatic
GEIGY72	Tab, White, Oval, Scored, Geigy over 72	Terbutaline Sulfate 2.5 mg	Brethine by Drug Distr	52985-0113	Antiasthmatic
GEIGY72	Tab, White, Oval, Scored, Geigy over 72	Terbutaline Sulfate 2.5 mg	by Thrift Drug	59198-0134	Antiasthmatic
GEIGY72	Tab, White, Oval, Scored, Geigy over 72	Terbutaline Sulfate 2.5 mg	by Nat Pharmpak	55154-1001	Antiasthmatic
GEIGY72	Tab, White, Oval, Scored, Geigy over 72	Terbutaline Sulfate 2.5 mg	by Rite Aid	11822-5296	Antiasthmatic
GEIGY72	Tab, White, Oval, Scored, Geigy over 72	Terbutaline Sulfate 2.5 mg	by Syntex	18393-0149	Antiasthmatic
GEIGYANTURAN	Tab, White, Round, Geigy/Anturan	Sulfinpyrazone 200 mg	Anturan by Novartis	Canadian Discontinued	Uricosuric
GEIGYDK	Tab, Cream, Triangular, Geigy/DK	Clomipramine HCl 10 mg	Anafranil by Novartis	Canadian	OCD
GEIGYDK	Tab, Cream, Triangular	Clomipramine HCl 10 mg	Anafranil by Geigy		OCD
GEIGYFH	Tab, Cream, Round	Clomipramine HCl 25 mg	Anafranil by Geigy		OCD
GEIGYFK	Tab, White, Round, Geigy/FK	Sulfinpyrazone 100 mg	Anturan by Novartis	Canadian Discontinued	Uricosuric
GEIGYFP	Tab, White, Round	Phenylbutazone 100 mg	Alka Butazolidin by Geigy		Anti-Inflammatory
GEIGYFT	Tab, Brown & Red, Triangle, Geigy/FT	Imipramine HCl 10 mg	Tofranil by Geigy		Antidepressant
GEIGYFT	Tab, Brown & Red, Triangular, Geigy/FT	Imipramine HCl 10 mg	Tofranil by Novartis	Canadian	Antidepressant
GEIGYKJ	Tab, White, Oval, Geigy/KJ	Baclofen 10 mg	Lioresal by Novartis	Canadian	Muscle Relaxant
GEIGYLP	Tab, Cream, Round	Clomipramine HCl 50 mg	Anafranil by Geigy	Canadian	OCD
GEIGYPU	Tab, White, Oval, Geigy/PJU	Carbamazepine 200 mg	Tegretol by Geigy	Canadian	Anticonvulsant
GEIGYZA	Tab, Beige & Yellow, Round, Geigy/ZA	Chlorthalidone 50 mg	Hygroton by Novartis	Canadian	Diuretic
GF <> CIBA	Tab, Blue, Round, Coated	Hydralazine HCl 25 mg	Apresoline by Novartis	Canadian DIN 00005533	Antihypertensive
GF1200	Tab, White, Oblong, Scored	Guaifenesin 1200 mg	Robitussin by Eli Lilly	00002-1095	Expectorant
GF1200	Tab, White, Oblong, Scored	Guaifenesin 1200 mg	Robitussin by Pfab	62542-0711	Expectorant
GF1200	Tab, White, Oblong, Scored	Guaifenesin 1200 mg	Robitussin by Eli Lilly	00110-4116	Expectorant
GF200	Tab, Pink, Oblong, Scored	Guaifenesin 200 mg	Aquabid by Eli Lilly	00110-3105	Expectorant
GF200	Tab, Pink, Oblong, Scored	Guaifenesin 200 mg	Aquabid by Lex	49523-0124	Expectorant
GF600	Tab, Green, Oblong, Scored	Guaifenesin 600 mg	Robitussin by Eli Lilly	00002-1094	Expectorant
GF600	Tab, Green, Oblong, Scored	Guaifenesin 600 mg	Robitussin by Eli Lilly	00110-3107	Expectorant

ID FRONT <> BACK	DESCRIPTION FRONT <> BACK	INGREDIENT & STRENGTH	BRAND (or Generic Equiv.) by FIRM	NDC#	CLASS; SCH.
GFDM	Tab, Green, Oblong, Scored, GF over DM	Guaifenesin 600 mg, Dextromethorphan Hydriodide 30 mg	GFN DTMH 03 by McNeil	52021-0645	Cold Remedy
GFDM	Tab, Green, Oblong, Scored	Guaifenesin 600 mg, Pseudoephedrine HCl 30 mg	by Med Pro	53978-3341	Cold Remedy
GFL10	Cap, Light Violet & Light Green	Fluoxetine HCl 10 mg	Prozac by Par	49884-0732	Antidepressant
GFL20	Cap, Light Violet & Light Green	Fluoxetine HCl 20 mg	Prozac by Par	49884-0733	Antidepressant
GFNPSE	Cap, Blue & Clear, Black Print	Guaifenesin 300 mg, Pseudoephedrine HCl 60 mg	Sudafed Sinus by Martec		Cold Remedy
GFNPSE	Cap, Blue & Clear, Opaque	Guaifenesin 300 mg, Pseudoephedrine HCl 60 mg	Sudafed Sinus by Martec		Cold Remedy
GFP120	Tab, Yellow, Oblong, Scored	Guaifenesin 600 mg, Pseudoephedrine HCl 120 mg	by Med Pro	53978-3350	Cold Remedy
GFP120	Cap, Yellow, Scored	Guaifenesin 600 mg, Pseudoephedrine HCl 120 mg	by Med Pro	53978-3344	Cold Remedy
GFP120	Tab, White, Caplet	Guaifenesin 600 mg, Pseudoephedrine HCl 120 mg	GFN 600/PSE 120 by Cypress	60258-0275	Cold Remedy
GFP60	Tab, Blue, Oblong, Scored	Guaifenesin 600 mg, Pseudoephedrine HCl 60 mg	by Med Pro	53978-3342	Cold Remedy
GFP60	Tab, Blue, Oblong, Scored	Guaifenesin 600 mg, Pseudoephedrine HCl 60 mg	by Med Pro	53978-3345	Cold Remedy
GFP60	Tab, Blue, Oblong, Scored	Guaifenesin 600 mg, Pseudoephedrine HCl 60 mg	by Pfab	62542-0745	Cold Remedy
GFPP	Tab, White, Oblong, Scored	Guaifenesin 600 mg, Phenylpropanolamine HCl 75 mg	Entex LA by Med Pro	53978-3319	Cold Remedy
GFPP	Tab, White, Oblong, Scored	Guaifenesin 600 mg, Phenylpropanolamine HCl 75 mg	Entex LA by Med Pro	53978-3317	Cold Remedy
GG	Tab	Meclizine HCl 25 mg	by Patient First	57575-0065	Antiemetic
GG	Tab	Acetaminophen 300 mg, Codeine Phosphate 30 mg	Tylenol w/ Codeine by Patient First	57575-0026	Analgesic; C III
GG	Cap	Cephalexin 500 mg	by Patient First	57575-0082	Antibiotic
GG <> 100	Tab, White, Cap Shaped, Scored	Cabergoline 0.5 mg	Dostinex by Greenstone	59762-0100	Antiparkinson
GG <> 101	Tab, White, Scored	Methocarbamol 750 mg	Robaxin by Sandoz	00781-1750	Muscle Relaxant
GG <> 123	Tab, Yellow, Round, Scored	Haloperidol 1 mg	Haldol by Sandoz	00781-1392	Antipsychotic
GG <> 190	Tab, White, Round, Scored	Methocarbamol 500 mg	Robaxin by Sandoz	00781-1760	Muscle Relaxant
GG <> 191	Tab, Blue, Round	Amoxapine 100 mg	Asendin by Sandoz	00781-1846	Antidepressant
GG <> 30	Tab, Reddish-Orange, Round, Film Coated	Thioridazine 10 mg	Mellaril by Sandoz	00781-1319	Antipsychotic
GG <> 38	Tab, Lavender, Film Coated	Hydroxyzine HCl 25 mg	by Sandoz	00781-1604	Antianxiety; Antihistamine
GG <> 4	Tab	Atropine Sulfate 0.025 mg, Diphenoxylate HCl 2.5 mg	Lomotil by Sandoz		Antidiarrheal; C V
GG <> 41	Tab, Yellow, Round, Film Coated	Imipramine HCl 10 mg	Tofranil by Sandoz	00781-1762	Antidepressant
GG <> 42	Tab, Green, Round, Film Coated	Imipramine HCl 50 mg	Tofranil by Sandoz	00781-1766	Antidepressant
GG <> 429	Tab, Green, Cap Shaped, Film Coated	Cimetidine HCl 400 mg	Tagamet by Sandoz	00781-1449	Gastrointestinal
GG <> 430	Tab, Green, Cap Shaped	Cimetidine HCl 800 mg	Tagamet by Sandoz	00781-1444	Gastrointestinal
GG <> 438	Tab, White, Round, Scored, Compressed	Pindolol 5 mg	Visken by Sandoz	00781-1168	Antihypertensive
GG <> 439	Tab, White, Round, Scored, Compressed	Pindolol 10 mg	Visken by Sandoz	00781-1169	Antihypertensive
GG <> 47	Tab, Beige, Round, Film Coated	Imipramine HCl 25 mg	Tofranil by Sandoz	00781-1764	Antidepressant
GG <> 724	Tab	Naproxen 250 mg	by Sandoz		NSAID
GG <> 76	Tab, Coated	Flurbiprofen 100 mg	by Sandoz		NSAID
GG <> 780	Tab, White, Round, Film Coated	Methylphenidate HCl 20 mg	Ritalin by Caremark	00339-4103	Stimulant; C II
GG <> 783	Tab, Yellow, Round	Methylphenidate HCl 5 mg	by Caremark	00339-4100	Stimulant; C II
GG <> 783	Tab, Yellow, Round	Methylphenidate HCl 5 mg	Ritalin by Sandoz	00781-1748	Stimulant; C II
GG <> 789	Tab, Green, Round, Scored	Methylphenidate HCl 10 mg	Ritalin by Caremark	00339-4101	Stimulant; C II
GG <> 91	Tab, White, Round	Lorazepam 0.5 mg	Ativan by Sandoz	00781-1403	Antianxiety; C IV
GG <> 91	Tab, White, Round	Lorazepam 0.5 mg	Ativan by Ivax	00182-8237	Antianxiety; C IV
GG <> 94	Tab, White, Round, Scored	Albuterol Sulfate 2 mg	Proventil by Sandoz	00781-1671	Antiasthmatic
GG <> 993	Tab, White, Round, Film Coated	Leflunomide 10 mg	Arava by Sandoz	00781-5056	Antiarthritic
GG <> 994	Tab, White, Round, Film Coated	Leflunomide 20 mg	Arava by Sandoz	00781-5057	Antiarthritic
GG <> BR2	Tab, Brownish Orange, Oblong, Scored, CR	Carbamazepine 200 mg	Tegretol CR by Genpharm	Canadian DIN 02241882	Anticonvulsant
GG <> BR4	Tab, Brownish Orange, Oblong, Scored, CR	Carbamazepine 400 mg	Tegretol CR by Genpharm	Canadian DIN 02241883	Anticonvulsant
GG <> EN5	Tab, White, Oval, Scored, G / G <> EN5	Enalapril Maleate 5 mg	Vasotec by Par	49884-0592	Antihypertensive
GG <> MF3	Tab, White, Oblong, Scored, Film Coated	Metformin HCl 1000 mg	Glucophage by BMS		Antidiabetic

ID FRONT <> BACK	DESCRIPTION FRONT <> BACK	INGREDIENT & STRENGTH	BRAND (or Generic Equiv.), by FIRM	NDC#	CLASS; SCH.
GG <> MF3	Tab, White, Oblong, Scored, Film Coated	Metformin HCl 1000 mg	Glucophage by Par	49884-0738	Antidiabetic
GG03	Tab	Captopril 12.5 mg	Capoten by Med Pro	53978-0939	Antihypertensive
GG1	Tab, Yellow, Round	Isosorbide Dinitrate SL 2.5 mg	Isordil by Sandoz		Antianginal
GG100	Tab, Coated	Acetaminophen 650 mg, Propoxyphene Napsylate 100 mg	Darvocet-N 100 by Sandoz	00781-1720	Analgesic; C IV
GG101	Tab, White, Cap Shaped, Scored	Methocarbamol 750 mg	Robaxin by Sandoz	00781-1750	Muscle Relaxant
GG103	Tab, Film Coated	Metronidazole 250 mg	by Sandoz	00781-1742	Antibiotic
GG104	Tab, White, Round	Methyldopa 125 mg	Aldomet by Sandoz		Antihypertensive
GG105	Tab, White, Round, Scored	Haloperidol 0.5 mg	Haldol by Sandoz	00781-1391	Antipsychotic
GG106	Tab	Amiloride HCl 5 mg, Hydrochlorothiazide 50 mg	Moduretic by Sandoz	00781-1119	Antihypertensive; Diuretic
GG107	Tab, White, Round, Film Coated, GG over 107	Perphenazine 4 mg	Trilafon by Sandoz	00781-1047	Antipsychotic
GG108	Tab, White, Round, Film Coated, GG over 108	Perphenazine 8 mg	Trilafon by Sandoz	00781-1048	Antipsychotic
GG109	Tab, White, Round, Film Coated, GG over 109	Perphenazine 16 mg	Trilafon by Sandoz	00781-1049	Antipsychotic
GG11	Tab, Coated	Chlorthalidone 25 mg	by Sandoz	00781-1726	Diuretic
GG110	Tab, Green, Round	Chlorzoxazone 250 mg, Acetaminophen 300 mg	Parafon Forte by Sandoz		Muscle Relaxant
GG111	Tab, White, Round, GG over 111	Methyldopa 250 mg	by Sandoz	00781-1320	Antihypertensive
GG112	Tab, Coated	Acetaminophen 650 mg, Propoxyphene HCl 65 mg	Wygesic by Sandoz	00781-1378	Analgesic; C IV
GG114	Tab, White, Round	Ergoloid Mesylate 1 mg	Hydergine by Danbury		Ergot Alkaloids
GG115	Tab, White, Oval	Ergoloid Mesylate 1 mg	Hydergine by Danbury		Ergot Alkaloids
GG116	Tab, White, Round	Ergoloid Mesylate 0.5 mg	Hydergine by Danbury		Ergot Alkaloids
GG118	Tab, White w/ Blue Specks, Round	Chlorpheniramine Maleate 5 mg, Phenylephrine HCl 10 mg, Phenylpropanolamine HCl 40 mg, Phenyltoloxamine Citrate 15 mg	by Sandoz	00781-1576	Cold Remedy
GG119	Tab, White, Round	Butalbital 50 mg, Aspirin 325 mg, Caffeine 40 mg	Fiorinal by Sandoz		Analgesic; C III
GG12	Tab, White, Round	Medroxyprogesterone Acetate 10 mg	Provera by Solvay		Hormone
GG1214	Tab, White, Round, GG 121/4	Acetaminophen 300 mg, Codeine Phosphate 60 mg	Tylenol w/ Codeine by Sandoz		Analgesic; C III
GG122	Tab, Brownish Yellow	Sulfasalazine 500 mg	Azulfidine by Circa		Gastrointestinal
GG124	Tab, Pink, Round, Scored, GG over 124	Haloperidol 2 mg	Haldol by Sandoz	00781-1393	Antipsychotic
GG125	Tab, Green, Round, Scored, GG over 125	Haloperidol 5 mg	Haldol by Sandoz	00781-1396	Antipsychotic
GG126	Tab, Light Green, Round, Scored, GG over 126	Haloperidol 10 mg	Haldol by Sandoz	00781-1397	Antipsychotic
GG127	Tab, White, Round	Quinine Sulfate 260 mg	by Sandoz		Antimalarial
GG130	Tab, White, Round, Scored, GG over 130	Aminophylline 100 mg	Aminophylline by Sandoz	00781-1214	Antiasthmatic
GG132	Tab, White, Round, Scored, Film Coated, GG over 132	Verapamil HCl 80 mg	Isoptin by Sandoz	00781-1016	Antihypertensive
GG133	Tab, White, Round, Scored, Film Coated, GG over 133	Verapamil HCl 120 mg	Isoptin by Sandoz	00781-1017	Antihypertensive
GG134	Tab, Coral, Round, Scored, GG over 134	Haloperidol 20 mg	Haldol by Sandoz	00781-1398	Antipsychotic
GG1343	Tab, White, Round	Hydralazine 25 mg, Hydrochlorothiazide 15 mg, Reserpine 0.1 mg	Ser-Ap-Es by Danbury		Antihypertensive; Diuretic
GG14	Tab, Peach, Round	Prednisolone 5 mg	Delta Cortef by Sandoz		Steroid
GG141	Tab, Blue, Oval, Scored	Meclizine HCl 12.5 mg	Antivert by Sandoz	00781-1345	Antiemetic
GG142	Tab, White, Round	Tolbutamide 500 mg	Orinase by Sandoz		Antidiabetic
GG144	Tab, White, Round, Scored, GG over 144	Chlorpropamide 250 mg	by Pharmedix	53002-0347	Antidiabetic
GG145	Tab, Yellow, Round	Dimenhydrinate 50 mg	Dramamine by Sandoz		Antiemetic
GG15	Tab, White, Round	Nylidrin 12 mg	Arlidin by Sandoz		Vasodilator
GG150	Tab	Meprobamate 400 mg	by DRX	55045-1753	Sedative/Hypnotic; C IV
GG1513	Tab	Aspirin 325 mg, Codeine Phosphate 30 mg	Aspirin w/ Codeine by Sandoz	00781-1660	Analgesic; C III
GG153	Tab	Hydrochlorothiazide 25 mg, Propranolol HCl 40 mg	by Sandoz	00781-1431	Diuretic; Antihypertensive
GG154	Tab	Hydrochlorothiazide 25 mg, Propranolol HCl 80 mg	by Sandoz	00781-1432	Diuretic; Antihypertensive
GG155	Tab, Peach, Round	Prednisone 20 mg	Deltasone by Sandoz		Steroid
GG156	Tab, White, Round	Prednisone 10 mg	Deltasone by Sandoz		Steroid

ID FRONT <> BACK	DESCRIPTION FRONT <> BACK	INGREDIENT & STRENGTH	BRAND (or Generic Equiv.) by FIRM	NDC#	CLASS; SCH.
GG157	Tab, White, Round	Prednisone 50 mg	Deltasone by Sandoz		Steroid
GG158	Tab, White, Round	Sulfisoxazole 500 mg	Gantrisin by Sandoz		Antibiotic
GG159	Tab, White, Cap Shaped, Scored	Clemastine Fumarate 1.34 mg	Tavist by Sandoz	00781-1358	Antihistamine
GG160	Tab, White, Round, Scored, GG over 160	Clemastine Fumarate 2.68 mg	Tavist by Sandoz	00781-1359	Antihistamine
GG1614	Tab	Aspirin 325 mg, Codeine Phosphate 60 mg	Aspirin w/ Codeine by Sandoz	00781-1875	Analgesic; C III
GG162	Tab, White, Scored	Triazolam 0.125 mg	Halcion by Sandoz	00781-1441	Sedative/Hypnotic; C IV
GG163	Tab, Blue, Scored	Triazolam 0.25 mg	Halcion by Sandoz	00781-1442	Sedative/Hypnotic; C IV
GG165	Tab, Green, Round, Scored, GG over 165	Hydrochlorothiazide 25 mg, Triamterene 37.5 mg	Maxzide 25 by Sandoz	00781-1123	Diuretic; Antihypertensive
GG166	Tab, White, Round, Film Coated, GG over 166	Desipramine HCl 75 mg	Norpramin by Sandoz	00781-1974	Antidepressant
GG167	Tab, White, Round, Film Coated, GG over 167	Desipramine HCl 100 mg	Norpramin by Sandoz	00781-1975	Antidepressant
GG168	Tab, White, Round, Film Coated, GG over 168	Desipramine HCl 150 mg	Norpramin by Sandoz	00781-1976	Antidepressant
GG169	Tab, White, Round, Film Coated, GG over 169	Verapamil HCl 40 mg	Isoptin by Sandoz	00781-1014	Antihypertensive
GG172	Tab, Yellow, Round, Scored, GG over 172	Hydrochlorothiazide 50 mg, Triamterene 75 mg	Maxzide by Sandoz	00781-1008	Diuretic; Antihypertensive
GG174	Tab, White, Round	Sulfamethoxazole 400 mg, Trimethoprim 80 mg	Bactrim by Sandoz		Antibiotic
GG175	Tab, White, Oval	Sulfamethoxazole 800 mg, Trimethoprim 160 mg	Bactrim DS by Sandoz		Antibiotic
GG177	Tab, White, Round, Scored, GG over 177	Captopril 25 mg	Capoten by Sandoz	00781-1829	Antihypertensive
GG178	Tab, White, Round, Scored, GG over 178	Captopril 50 mg	Capoten by Sandoz	00781-1838	Antihypertensive
GG179	Tab, White, Round, Scored, GG over 179	Captopril 100 mg	Capoten by Sandoz	00781-1839	Antihypertensive
GG18	Tab, White, Round, Film Coated, GG over 18	Perphenazine 2 mg	Trilafon by Sandoz	00781-1046	Antipsychotic
GG180	Tab, White, Round	Aminophylline 200 mg	Aminophylline by Sandoz	00781-1318	Antiasthmatic
GG181	Tab, White, Round, Scored, GG over 181	Methazolamide 50 mg	Neptazane by Sandoz	00781-1071	Antiglaucoma Agent
GG182	Tab	Timolol Maleate 10 mg	Blocadren by Sandoz	00781-1127	Antihypertensive
GG183	Tab	Timolol Maleate 20 mg	Blocadren by Sandoz	00781-1128	Antihypertensive
GG185	Tab, White, Round	Glutethimide 500 mg	Doriden by Sandoz		Hypnotic; C II
GG190	Tab, White, Round, Scored, GG over 190	Methocarbamol 500 mg	Robaxin by Sandoz	00781-1760	Muscle Relaxant
GG191	Tab, Blue, Round	Amoxapine 100 mg	Asendin by Sandoz		Antidepressant
GG192	Tab, Light Orange, Round, Scored	Amoxapine 150 mg	Asendin by Sandoz	00781-1847	Antidepressant
GG195	Tab, Film Coated	Metronidazole 500 mg	by Sandoz	00781-1747	Antibiotic
GG196	Tab, Light Yellow, Round, Scored, GG over 196	Chlorpheniramine Maleate 4 mg	Chlor-Trimeton by Sandoz	00781-1140	Antihistamine
GG197	Tab, White, Oval	Acetohexamide 250 mg	Dymelor by Rosemont		Antidiabetic
GG198	Tab, White, Oblong	Acetohexamide 500 mg	Dymelor by Rosemont		Antidiabetic
GG199	Tab, White, Round	Acetaminophen 325 mg	Tylenol by Sandoz		Analgesic
GG2	Tab	Isosorbide Dinitrate 5 mg	Isordil by Sandoz	00781-1565	Antianginal
GG200	Tab, Pink, Oblong	Acetaminophen 650 mg, Propoxyphene Napsylate 100 mg	Darvocet-N 100 by Circa		Analgesic; C IV
GG201	Tab, White, Round, Scored, GG over 201	Furosemide 40 mg	Lasix by Sandoz	00781-1966	Diuretic
GG202	Tab, White, Round, Scored	Paroxetine HCl 20 mg	Paxil by Sandoz	00781-1991	Antidepressant
GG203	Tab, White, Round	Paroxetine HCl 30 mg	Paxil by Sandoz	00781-1992	Antidepressant
GG21	Tab, White, Round, Scored, GG over 21	Furosemide 20 mg	Lasix by Sandoz	00781-1818	Diuretic
GG210	Tab, Yellow, Cap Shaped	Azathioprine 50 mg	Imuran by Sandoz	00781-1059	Immunosuppressant
GG211	Tab, White, Round, Scored, GG over 211	Bromocriptine 2.5 mg	Parlodel by Sandoz	00781-1817	Antiparkinson
GG213	Tab, Blue, Round, Film Coated, GG over 213	Amitriptyline 10 mg, Perphenazine 2 mg	Triavil by Sandoz	00781-1265	Antidepressant; Antipsychotic
GG214	Tab, Orange, Round, Film Coated	Amitriptyline 25 mg, Perphenazine 2 mg	Triavil by Sandoz	00781-1273	Antidepressant; Antipsychotic
GG215	Tab, Coated	Amitriptyline 10 mg, Perphenazine 4 mg	Triavil by Sandoz	00781-1266	Antidepressant; Antipsychotic
GG216	Tab, Yellow, Round	Amitriptyline 25 mg, Perphenazine 4 mg	Triavil by Sandoz	00781-1267	Antidepressant; Antipsychotic

ID FRONT <> BACK	DESCRIPTION FRONT <> BACK	INGREDIENT & STRENGTH	BRAND (or Generic Equiv.) by FIRM	NDC#	CLASS; SCH.
GG217	Tab, Orange, Round, Film Coated	Amitriptyline 50 mg, Perphenazine 4 mg	Triavil by Sandoz	00781-1268	Antidepressant; Antipsychotic
GG2182	Tab, White, Round, GG 218/2	Acetaminophen 300 mg, Codeine Phosphate 15 mg, Methyldopa 250 mg	Tylenol w/ Codeine by KV Pharma		Analgesic; C III
GG219	Tab, Film Coated	Hydrochlorothiazide 15 mg, Pseudoephedrine 60 mg	by Sandoz	00781-1809	Diuretic; Antihypertensive
GG22	Tab, White, Round, Scored, GG over 22	Pseudoephedrine 60 mg	Sudafed by Sandoz	00781-1535	Decongestant
GG220	Tab	Acetaminophen 300 mg, Codeine Phosphate 30 mg	Tylenol w/ Codeine by Sandoz	00781-1752	Analgesic; C III
GG224	Tab, White, Oblong	Guaifenesin 400 mg, Phenylpropanolamine HCl 75 mg	Entex LA by Amide		Cold Remedy
GG225	Tab, White, Round, Scored, GG over 225	Promethazine HCl 25 mg	Phenergan by Sandoz	00781-1830	Antiemetic; Antihistamine
GG225	Tab, White, Round, Scored, GG over 225	Promethazine HCl 25 mg	Phenergan by Ivax	00182-8222 Discontinued	Antiemetic; Antihistamine
GG226	Tab, Blue, Oval	Lovastatin 20 mg	Mevacor by Sandoz	00781-1210	Antihyperlipidemic
GG227	Tab, Green, Round, Scored, GG over 227	Isosorbide Dinitrate 20 mg	Isordil by Sandoz		Antianginal
GG229	Tab, Yellow, Round	Isosorbide Dinitrate 40 mg	Isordil by Sandoz	00781-1695	Antianginal
GG232	Tab, White, Oblong	Acetaminophen 500 mg, Hydrocodone Bitartrate 5 mg	Vicodin by Rosemont		Analgesic; C III
GG234	Tab, White, Oval	Methylprednisolone 4 mg	Medrol by Duramed		Steroid
GG235	Tab, Pink, Round, GG over 235	Promethazine HCl 50 mg	Phenergan by Sandoz	00781-1832	Antiemetic; Antihistamine
GG236	Tab, Yellow, Round, Scored, GG over 236	Sulindac 150 mg	Clinoril by Sandoz	00781-1811	NSAID
GG237	Tab, Yellow, Round, Scored, GG over 237	Sulindac 200 mg	Clinoril by Sandoz	00781-1812	NSAID
GG238	Tab, White, Round	Glyburide 1.25 mg	Diabeta by Greenstone		Antidiabetic
GG239	Tab, Dark Pink, Round, Scored	Glyburide 2.5 mg	Micronase R.N. by Sandoz	00781-1456	Antidiabetic
GG24	Tab, White, Round	Ephedrine 24 mg, Phenobarbital 8 mg, Theophylline 130 mg	Marax by Sandoz		Antiasthmatic; C IV
GG240	Tab	Glyburide 5 mg	by Golden State	60429-0085	Antidiabetic
GG240	Tab	Glyburide 5 mg	by Med Pro	53978-0694	Antidiabetic
GG242	Tab	Methylclothiazide 5 mg	by Sandoz	00781-1810	Diuretic; Antihypertensive
GG243	Tab, Film Coated	Hydrochlorothiazide 30 mg, Methyldopa 500 mg	by Sandoz	00781-1843	Diuretic; Antihypertensive
GG244	Tab	Methylclothiazide 2.5 mg	by Sandoz	00781-1803	Diuretic; Antihypertensive
GG245	Tab, White, Round	Minoxidil 10 mg	Loniten by Quantum		Antihypertensive
GG249	Tab, White, Rectangular, Scored	Alprazolam 2 mg	Xanax by Sandoz	00781-1089	Antianxiety; C IV
GG25	Tab, White, Round	Triprolidine 2.5 mg, Pseudoephedrine 60 mg	Actifed by Sandoz		Cold Remedy
GG250	Tab, Ex Release	Quinidine Gluconate 324 mg	by Sandoz	00781-1804	Antiarrhythmic
GG251	Tab	Carbidopa 10 mg, Levodopa 100 mg	by Sandoz	00781-1626	Antiparkinson
GG252	Tab	Carbidopa 25 mg, Levodopa 100 mg	by Sandoz	00781-1627	Antiparkinson
GG254	Tab	Fenoprofen Calcium 600 mg	by Sandoz	00781-1863	NSAID
GG255	Tab, White, Black Print, Round, Film Coated, GG over 255	Dexbrompheniramine Maleate 6 mg, Pseudoephedrine Sulfate 120 mg	Drixoral by Sandoz	00781-1600	Cold Remedy
GG256	Tab, White, Oval, Scored, GG over 256	Alprazolam 0.25 mg	Xanax by Sandoz	00781-1061	Antianxiety; C IV
GG257	Tab, Peach, Oval, Scored	Alprazolam 0.5 mg	Xanax by Sandoz	00781-1077	Antianxiety; C IV
GG258	Tab, Light Blue, Oval, Scored	Alprazolam 1 mg	Xanax by Sandoz	00781-1079	Antianxiety; C IV
GG259	Tab, Pink, Round, Scored, GG over 259	Isosorbide Dinitrate 5 mg	Isordil by Sandoz	00781-1635	Antianginal
GG26	Tab, White, Round, Scored, GG over 26	Isosorbide Dinitrate 10 mg	Isordil by Sandoz	00781-1556	Antianginal
GG260	Tab, White, Round, Scored, Film Coated, GG over 260	Hydroxychloroquine Sulfate 200 mg	Plaquenil by Sandoz	00781-1407	Antimalarial
GG261	Tab, Yellow, Oval, Scored, GG over 261	Meclizine HCl 25 mg	Antivert by Sandoz	00781-1375	Antiemetic
GG263	Tab, White, Round, Scored, GG over 263	Atenolol 50 mg	Tenormin by Sandoz	00781-1506	Antihypertensive
GG263	Tab, White, Round, Scored, GG over 263	Atenolol 50 mg	Tenormin by Ivax	00182-8236	Antihypertensive
GG264	Tab, White, Round, GG over 264	Atenolol 100 mg	Tenormin by Sandoz	00781-1507	Antihypertensive
GG265	Tab, Film Coated	Hydrochlorothiazide 25 mg, Methyldopa 250 mg	by Sandoz	00781-1819	Diuretic; Antihypertensive
GG27	Tab, Peach, Round	Hydrochlorothiazide 50 mg	Hydrodiuril by Sandoz		Diuretic; Antihypertensive
GG270	Tab	Tolazamide 100 mg	by Sandoz	00781-1922	Antidiabetic
GG271	Tab	Tolazamide 250 mg	by Sandoz	00781-1932	Antidiabetic

ID FRONT <> BACK	DESCRIPTION FRONT <> BACK	INGREDIENT & STRENGTH	BRAND (or Generic Equiv.) by FIRM	NDC#	CLASS; SCH.
GG272	Tab	Tolazamide 500 mg	by Sandoz	00781-1942	Antidiabetic
GG274	Tab, White, Round, Scored, GG over 274	Isoxsuprine HCl 10 mg	Vasodilan by Sandoz	00781-1840	Vasodilator
GG28	Tab, Peach, Round	Hydrochlorothiazide 25 mg	Hydrodiuril by Sandoz		Diuretic; Antihypertensive
GG284	Tab, White, Round, Scored, GG over 284	Isoxsuprine HCl 20 mg	Vasodilan by Sandoz	00781-1842	Vasodilator
GG285	Tab	Quinidine Sulfate 200 mg	Quinidine Sulfate by Sandoz	00781-1900	Antiarrhythmic
GG286	Tab	Quinidine Sulfate 300 mg	Quinidine Sulfate by Sandoz	00781-1902	Antiarrhythmic
GG288	Tab, Butterscotch Yellow, Round, Film Coated, GG over 288	Cyclobenzaprine HCl 10 mg	Flexeril by Sandoz	00781-1324	Muscle Relaxant
GG289	Tab, Film Coated	Hydrochlorothiazide 50 mg, Methyldopa 500 mg	by Sandoz	00781-1853	Diuretic; Antihypertensive
GG291	Tab, White, Round	Ibuprofen 400 mg	Motrin by Ciba		NSAID
GG293	Tab, White, Round	Ibuprofen 200 mg	Motrin by Sandoz		NSAID
GG294	Tab, White, Oblong	Ibuprofen 800 mg	Motrin by Sandoz		NSAID
GG295	Tab, White, Round, Scored	Albuterol Sulfate 4 mg	Proventil by Sandoz	00781-1672	Antiasthmatic
GG296	Tab, White, Round	Loratadine 10 mg	Claritin by Sandoz	00067-6069	Antihistamine
GG296	Tab, White, Round	Loratadine 10 mg	Claritin by Sandoz	00781-5077	Antihistamine
GG298	Tab, Beige, Round, Film Coated, GG over 298	Famotidine 20 mg	Pepcid by Sandoz	00781-1736	Gastrointestinal
GG299	Tab, Tan, Round, Film Coated, GG over 299	Famotidine 40 mg	Pepcid by Sandoz	00781-1746	Gastrointestinal
GG300	Cap, Maroon & White, G/G 300	Gemfibrozil 300 mg	by Genpharm	Canadian	Antihyperlipidemic
GG31 <> 15	Tab, Orange, Round, Film Coated, GG over 31	Thioridazine 15 mg	Mellaril by Sandoz	00781-1614	Antipsychotic
GG32 <> 25	Tab, Orange, Round, Film Coated, GG over 32	Thioridazine 25 mg	Mellaril by Sandoz	00781-1624	Antipsychotic
GG33 <> 50	Tab, Orange, Round, Film Coated, GG over 33	Thioridazine 50 mg	Mellaril by Sandoz	00781-1634	Antipsychotic
GG330 <> 125	Tab, Turquoise, Cap Shaped, Scored, 125 <> GG over 330	Levothyroxine 137 mcg	Levo-T by Alara	64909-0140	Thyroid Hormone
GG330 <> 137	Tab, Turquoise, Cap Shaped, Scored, 137 <> GG over 330	Levothyroxine 137 mcg	Levo-T by Sandoz	00781-5191	Thyroid Hormone
GG331 <> 25	Tab, Orange, Cap Shaped, Scored, 25 <> GG over 331	Levothyroxine 25 mcg	Levo-T by Sandoz	00781-5180	Thyroid Hormone
GG331 <> 25	Tab, Orange, Cap Shaped, Scored, 25 <> GG over 331	Levothyroxine 25 mcg	Levo-T by Alara	64909-0121	Thyroid Hormone
GG332 <> 50	Tab, White, Cap Shaped, Scored, 50 <> GG over 332	Levothyroxine 50 mcg	Levo-T by Alara	64909-0122	Thyroid Hormone
GG332 <> 50	Tab, White, Cap Shaped, Scored, 50 <> GG over 332	Levothyroxine 50 mcg	Levo-T by Sandoz	00781-5181	Thyroid Hormone
GG333 <> 75	Tab, Violet, Cap Shaped, Scored, 75 <> GG over 333	Levothyroxine 75 mcg	Levo-T by Sandoz	00781-5182	Thyroid Hormone
GG333 <> 75	Tab, Violet, Cap Shaped, Scored, 75 <> GG over 333	Levothyroxine 75 mcg	Levo-T by Alara	64909-0124	Thyroid Hormone
GG334 <> 88	Tab, Olive Green, Cap Shaped, Scored, 88 <> GG over 334	Levothyroxine 88 mcg	Levo-T by Alara	64909-0125	Thyroid Hormone
GG334 <> 88	Tab, Olive Green, Cap Shaped, Scored, 88 <> GG over 334	Levothyroxine 88 mcg	Levo-T by Sandoz	00781-5183	Thyroid Hormone
GG335 <> 100	Tab, Yellow, Cap Shaped, Scored, 100 <> GG over 335	Levothyroxine 100 mcg	Levo-T by Sandoz	00781-5184	Thyroid Hormone
GG335 <> 100	Tab, Yellow, Cap Shaped, Scored, 100 <> GG over 335	Levothyroxine 100 mcg	Levo-T by Alara	64909-0126	Thyroid Hormone
GG336 <> 112	Tab, Rose, Cap Shaped, Scored, 112 <> GG over 336	Levothyroxine 112 mcg	Levo-T by Alara	64909-0127	Thyroid Hormone
GG336 <> 112	Tab, Rose, Cap Shaped, Scored, 112 <> GG over 336	Levothyroxine 112 mcg	Levo-T by Sandoz	00781-5185	Thyroid Hormone
GG337 <> 125	Tab, Brown, Cap Shaped, Scored, 125 <> GG over 337	Levothyroxine 125 mcg	Levo-T by Sandoz	00781-5186	Thyroid Hormone
GG337 <> 125	Tab, Brown, Cap Shaped, Scored, 125 <> GG over 337	Levothyroxine 125 mcg	Levo-T by Alara	64909-0129	Thyroid Hormone
GG338 <> 150	Tab, Blue, Cap Shaped, Scored, 150 <> GG over 338	Levothyroxine 150 mcg	Levo-T by Alara	64909-0141	Thyroid Hormone
GG338 <> 150	Tab, Blue, Cap Shaped, Scored, 150 <> GG over 338	Levothyroxine 150 mcg	Levo-T by Sandoz	00781-5187	Thyroid Hormone
GG339 <> 175	Tab, Lilac, Cap Shaped, Scored, 175 <> GG over 339	Levothyroxine 175 mcg	Levo-T by Sandoz	00781-5188	Thyroid Hormone
GG339 <> 175	Tab, Lilac, Cap Shaped, Scored, 175 <> GG over 339	Levothyroxine 175 mcg	Levo-T by Alara	64909-0142	Thyroid Hormone
GG34 <> 100	Tab, Orange, Round, Film Coated, GG over 34	Thioridazine 100 mg	Mellaril by Sandoz	00781-1644	Antipsychotic
GG340 <> 200	Tab, Pink, Cap Shaped, Scored, 200 <> GG over 340	Levothyroxine 200 mcg	Levo-T by Alara	64909-0144	Thyroid Hormone
GG340 <> 200	Tab, Pink, Cap Shaped, Scored, 200 <> GG over 340	Levothyroxine 200 mcg	Levo-T by Sandoz	00781-5189	Thyroid Hormone
GG341 <> 300	Tab, Green, Cap Shaped, Scored, 300 <> GG over 341	Levothyroxine 300 mcg	Levo-T by Sandoz	00781-5190	Thyroid Hormone
GG341 <> 300	Tab, Green, Cap Shaped, Scored, 300 <> GG over 341	Levothyroxine 300 mcg	Levo-T by Alara	64909-0145	Thyroid Hormone
GG35	Tab, Orange, Cap Shaped, Film Coated, GG over 35	Thioridazine 150 mg	Mellaril by Sandoz	00781-1664	Antipsychotic
GG36	Tab, Orange, Round, Film Coated, GG over 36	Thioridazine 200 mg	Mellaril by Sandoz	00781-1674	Antipsychotic
GG364	Tab, White, Oval	Benazepril 5 mg, HCTZ 6.25 mg	Lotensin HCT by Sandoz	00781-5131	Antihypertensive; Diuretic
GG365	Tab, Light Pink, Oval	Benazepril 10 mg, HCTZ 12.5 mg	Lotensin HCT by Sandoz	00781-5132	Antihypertensive; Diuretic

ID FRONT <> BACK	DESCRIPTION FRONT <> BACK	INGREDIENT & STRENGTH	BRAND (or Generic Equiv.) by FIRM	NDC#	CLASS; SCH.
GG366	Tab, Grayish Violet, Oval	Benazepril 20 mg, HCTZ 12.5 mg	Lotensin HCT by Sandoz	00781-5133	Antihypertensive; Diuretic
GG367	Tab, Red, Oval	Benazepril 20 mg, HCTZ 25 mg	Lotensin HCT by Sandoz	00781-5134	Antihypertensive; Diuretic
GG37	Tab, Lavender, Round	Hydroxyzine HCl 10 mg	Atarax by Sandoz		Antianxiety; Antihistamine
GG39	Tab, Purple, Round	Hydroxyzine HCl 50 mg	Atarax by Sandoz		Antianxiety; Antihistamine
GG4	Tab, White, Round, GG over 4	Atropine Sulfate 0.025 mg, Diphenoxylate HCl 2.5 mg	Lonox by Sandoz	00781-1262	Antidiarrheal; C V
GG40	Tab, Pink, Round, Film Coated, GG over 40	Amitriptyline HCl 10 mg	Elavil by Sandoz	00781-1486	Antidepressant
GG405	Tab, White, Round	Acetaminophen 500 mg	Tylenol Ex Strength by Sandoz		Analgesic
GG407 <> 50	Tab, Yellow, Round, GG over 407	Chlorpromazine HCl 50 mg	Thorazine by Sandoz	00781-1717	Antipsychotic
GG411	Tab, White, Round, GG over 411	Carisoprodol 350 mg	Soma by Sandoz	00781-1050	Muscle Relaxant
GG414	Tab, White, Round, Scored, Film Coated	Metoprolol Tartrate 50 mg	Lopressor by Sandoz	00781-1223	Antihypertensive
GG415	Tab, White, Round, Scored, Film Coated	Metoprolol Tartrate 100 mg	Lopressor by Sandoz	00781-1228	Antihypertensive
GG416	Tab, Green, Round	Hydralazine HCl 50 mg	Apresoline by Sandoz		Antihypertensive
GG417	Tab, Yellow, Oval	Naproxen 275 mg	Anaprox by Sandoz	00781-1187	NSAID
GG418	Tab, White, Oval	Naproxen 550 mg	Anaprox by Sandoz	00781-1188	NSAID
GG419	Tab, White, Round, Scored, Film Coated	Trazodone HCl 50 mg	Desyrel by Sandoz	00781-1807	Antidepressant
GG420	Tab, White, Round, Scored, Film Coated	Trazodone HCl 100 mg	Desyrel by Sandoz	00781-1808	Antidepressant
GG421	Tab, Peach, Round, Scored, GG over 421	Chlorzoxazone 250 mg	by Sandoz	00781-1303	Muscle Relaxant
GG422	Tab	Chlorzoxazone 500 mg	by Sandoz	00781-1304	Muscle Relaxant
GG427	Tab, Green, Round, Film Coated	Cimetidine HCl 200 mg	Tagamet by Sandoz	00781-1447	Gastrointestinal
GG428	Tab, Green, Round, Film Coated, GG over 428	Cimetidine HCl 300 mg	Tagamet by Sandoz	00781-1448	Gastrointestinal
GG429	Tab, Green, Oblong, Film Coated, Scored	Cimetidine HCl 400 mg	Tagamet by Murfreesboro	51129-1347	Gastrointestinal
GG429	Tab, Green, Oblong, Scored, Film Coated	Cimetidine HCl 400 mg	Tagamet by Compumed	00403-2021	Gastrointestinal
GG430	Tab, Film Coated	Cimetidine HCl 800 mg	Tagamet by H J Harkins Co	52959-0376	Gastrointestinal
GG431	Tab, Brown, Round, Film Coated, GG over 431	Amitriptyline HCl 50 mg	Elavil by Sandoz	00781-1488	Antidepressant
GG431	Tab, Brown, Round, Film Coated, GG over 431	Amitriptyline HCl 50 mg	Elavil by Golden State	60429-0017	Antidepressant
GG432	Tab, White, Round	Conjugated Estrogens 0.3 mg	Premarin by Duramed		Hormone
GG433	Tab, White, Round	Conjugated Estrogens 0.625 mg	Premarin by Duramed		Hormone
GG434	Tab, White, Round	Conjugated Estrogens 1.25 mg	Premarin by Duramed		Hormone
GG435	Tab, White, Round	Conjugated Estrogens 2.5 mg	Premarin by Duramed		Hormone
GG436	Tab, Brown, Round	Nystatin Oral 500,000 Units	Mycostatin Oral by Eon		Antifungal
GG437 <> 100	Tab, Yellow, Round, GG over 437	Chlorpromazine HCl 100 mg	Thorazine by Sandoz	00781-1718	Antipsychotic
GG44	Tab, Lt. Green, Round, Film Coated, GG over 44	Amitriptyline HCl 25 mg	Elavil by Sandoz	00781-1487	Antidepressant
GG441	Tab, Cream & Orange Specks, Round, Chewable	Vitamin, Fluoride 0.5 mg	Poly-Vi-Flor by Amide		Vitamin
GG441	Tab, Debossed	Carisoprodol 350 mg	by Golden State	60429-0035	Muscle Relaxant
GG444	Tab, White, Round	Dexbrompheniramine Maleate 6 mg, Pseudoephedrine Sulfate 120 mg	Drixoral by Sandoz		Cold Remedy
GG445	Tab, Yellow, Round, Scored, GG over 445	Enalapril Maleate 2.5 mg	Vasotec by Sandoz	00781-1229	Antihypertensive
GG447	Tab, Blue, Round	Brompheniramine Sulfate 12 mg, Phenylpropanolamine HCl 75 mg	Dimetapp Ext. by Sandoz		Cold Remedy
GG45	Tab, White, Black Print, Round, GG over 45	Dipyridamole 50 mg	Persantine by Sandoz	00781-1678	Antiplatelet
GG450	Tab, Lt. Green, Cap Shaped, Film Coated, GG over 450	Amitriptyline HCl 150 mg	Elavil by Sandoz	00781-1491	Antidepressant
GG451	Tab, Purple, Round, Film Coated, GG over 451	Amitriptyline HCl 75 mg	Elavil by Sandoz	00781-1489	Antidepressant
GG455 <> 10	Tab, Yellow, Round, Film Coated, GG over 455	Chlorpromazine HCl 10 mg	Thorazine by Sandoz	00781-1715	Antipsychotic
GG457 <> 200	Tab, Yellow, Round, Film Coated, GG over 457	Chlorpromazine HCl 200 mg	Thorazine by Sandoz	00781-1719	Antipsychotic
GG458	Tab, White, Oblong	Acetaminophen 500 mg	Tylenol Ex Strength by Sandoz		Analgesic
GG459	Tab, White, Oblong	Acetaminophen 325 mg	Tylenol by Sandoz		Analgesic
GG461	Tab, Orange, Round, Film Coated, GG over 461	Amitriptyline HCl 100 mg	Elavil by Sandoz	00781-1490	Antidepressant
GG464	Tab, White, Black Print, Round, GG over 464	Dipyridamole 75 mg	by Sandoz	00781-1478	Antiplatelet
GG471	Tab, Film Coated	Methyldopa 500 mg	Methyldopa by Sandoz	00781-1322	Antihypertensive

ID FRONT <> BACK	DESCRIPTION FRONT <> BACK	INGREDIENT & STRENGTH	BRAND (or Generic Equiv.) by FIRM	NDC#	CLASS; SCH.
GG472	Tab, White, Oblong	Procainamide HCl SR 250 mg	Procan SR by Sandoz		Antiarrhythmic
GG473	Tab, White, Oblong	Procainamide HCl SR 500 mg	Procan SR by Sandoz		Antiarrhythmic
GG474	Tab, White, Oblong	Procainamide HCl SR 750 mg	Procan SR by Danbury		Antiarrhythmic
GG475	Tab, White, Round	Hydralazine HCl 10 mg	Apresoline by Sandoz		Antihypertensive
GG476 <> 25	Tab, Yellow, Round, GG over 476	Chlorpromazine HCl 25 mg	Thorazine by Heartland	61392-0040	Antipsychotic
GG476 <> 25	Tab, Yellow, Round, GG over 476	Chlorpromazine HCl 25 mg	Thorazine by Sandoz	00781-1716	Antipsychotic
GG477	Tab, Blue, Round	Brompheniramine Maleate 12 mg, Phenylephrine HCl 15 mg, Phenylpropanolamine HCl 15 mg	Dimetapp by Sandoz		Cold Remedy
GG48	Tab, Red, Round, GG over 48	Pseudoephedrine 30 mg	Sudafed by Sandoz		Decongestant
GG480	Tab, White, Oblong	Prenatal Vitamins, Zinc	Stuart 1+1 Zinc by Amide		Vitamin
GG481	Tab, Tan, Oblong	Prenatal Vitamin, Zinc Improved	Stuart 1+1 by Amide		Vitamin
GG482	Tab, White, Round, Scored, GG over 482	Enalapril Maleate 5 mg	Vasotec by Sandoz	00781-1231	Antihypertensive
GG483	Tab, Salmon, Round, GG over 483	Enalapril Maleate 10 mg	Vasotec by Sandoz	00781-1232	Antihypertensive
GG484	Tab, Peach, Round, GG over 484	Enalapril Maleate 20 mg	Vasotec by Sandoz	00781-1233	Antihypertensive
GG485	Tab, Green, Round	Hydralazine HCl 25 mg	Apresoline by Sandoz		Antihypertensive
GG487	Tab, White, Oblong	Colchicine 0.5 mg, Probenecid 500 mg	ColBenemid by Danbury		Antigout
GG488	Tab, Orange, Round, Film Coated, GG over 488	Fluphenazine HCl 2.5 mg	Prolixin by Sandoz	00781-1437	Antipsychotic
GG489	Tab, Orange, Round, Film Coated, GG over 489	Fluphenazine HCl 5 mg	Prolixin by Sandoz	00781-1438	Antipsychotic
GG49	Tab, Film Coated	Dipyridamole 25 mg	by Sandoz	00781-1890	Antiplatelet
GG490	Tab, Orange, Round, Film Coated, GG over 490	Fluphenazine HCl 10 mg	Prolixin by Sandoz	00781-1439	Antipsychotic
GG501	Cap, Blue & Yellow	Nitroglycerin SR 6.5 mg	Nitrobid by Sandoz		Vasodilator
GG503	Cap, Brown & Clear	Papaverine HCl TD 150 mg	Pavabid by Sandoz		Vasodilator
GG505	Cap, White, Black & Pink Bands, Opaque	Oxazepam 10 mg	Serax by Sandoz	00781-2809	Sedative/Hypnotic; C IV
GG506	Cap, White, Black & Red Bands, Opaque	Oxazepam 15 mg	Serax by Sandoz	00781-2810	Sedative/Hypnotic; C IV
GG507	Cap, White, Black & Maroon Bands, Opaque	Oxazepam 30 mg	Serax by Sandoz	00781-2811	Sedative/Hypnotic; C IV
GG51 <> 1	Tab, Lavender, Round, GG over 51	Trifluoperazine HCl 1 mg	Stelazine by Sandoz	00781-1030	Antipsychotic
GG51 <> 1	Tab, Lavender, Round, GG over 51	Trifluoperazine HCl 1 mg	by Apotheca	12634-0678	Antipsychotic
GG512	Cap, Green & Yellow, Black Print, GG over 512	Nitroglycerin SR 9 mg	Nitrobid by Sandoz	00781-2798	Vasodilator
GG515	Cap, Clear	Quinine Sulfate 5 gr	by Sandoz		Antimalarial
GG517	Cap, Light Green	Indomethacin 25 mg	Indocin by Quality Care	60346-0684 Discontinued	NSAID
GG517	Cap, Teal Green, Black Print, GG over 517	Indomethacin 25 mg	Indocin by Sandoz	00781-2325	NSAID
GG518	Cap, Teal Green, Black Print, GG over 518	Indomethacin 50 mg	Indocin by Sandoz	00781-2350	NSAID
GG52	Tab, Yellow, Round	Levothyroxine Sodium 0.1 mg	Synthroid by Rosemont		Thyroid Hormone
GG522	Cap, Blue & White	Flurazepam HCl 15 mg	Dalmane by Par		Hypnotic; C IV
GG523	Cap, Blue	Flurazepam HCl 30 mg	Dalmane by Par		Hypnotic; C IV
GG524	Cap	Meclofenamate Sodium	by Sandoz	00781-2702	NSAID
GG525	Cap	Meclofenamate Sodium	by Sandoz	00781-2703	NSAID
GG526	Cap, White Bands	Clorazepate Dipotassium 30.75 mg	Tranxene by Sandoz		Antianxiety; C IV
GG527	Cap, White Bands	Clorazepate Dipotassium 7.5 mg	Tranxene by Sandoz		Antianxiety; C IV
GG527	Tab, White, Round	Prednisone 50 mg	Deltasone by Sandoz		Steroid
GG528	Cap, White Bands	Clorazepate Dipotassium 15 mg	Tranxene by Sandoz		Antianxiety; C IV
GG53 <> 2	Tab, Lavender, Round, Film Coated, GG over 53	Trifluoperazine HCl 2 mg	Stelazine by Sandoz	00781-1032	Antipsychotic
GG530	Cap, White, with Green Bands	Loperamide 2 mg	Imodium by Sandoz	00781-2761	Antidiarrheal
GG531	Cap, Green & White, Black Print, GG over 531	Temazepam 15 mg	Restoril by Sandoz	00781-2201	Sedative/Hypnotic; C IV
GG531	Cap, Green & White	Temazepam 15 mg	Restoril by St. Mary's Med	60760-0552	Sedative/Hypnotic; C IV

ID FRONT <> BACK	DESCRIPTION FRONT <> BACK	INGREDIENT & STRENGTH	BRAND (or Generic Equiv.) by FIRM	NDC#	CLASS; SCH.
GG532	Cap, White, Black Print, GG over 532	Temazepam 30 mg	Restoril by Sandoz	00781-2202	Sedative/Hypnotic; C IV
GG533	Cap, Pink & White, Black Print, GG over 533	Diphenhydramine HCl 25 mg	by Sandoz	00781-2458	Antihistamine
GG535	Cap, White & Yellow, Black Print, GG over 535	Nitrofurantoin 50 mg	by Sandoz		Antibiotic
GG535	Cap, White & Yellow, Black Print, GG over 535	Nitrofurantoin 50 mg	Macrodantin by Sandoz	00781-2502	Antibiotic
GG536	Cap, Yellow, Black Print, GG over 536	Nitrofurantoin 100 mg	Macrodantin by Sandoz	00781-2503	Antibiotic
GG537	Cap, Yellow & White, Black Print, GG over 537	Bromocriptine 5 mg	Parlodel by Sandoz	00781-2819	Antiparkinson
GG538	Cap	Nitrofurantoin 25 mg	by Sandoz	00781-2501	Antibiotic
GG54	Tab, White, Round	Levothyroxine Sodium 0.2 mg	Synthroid by Rosemont		Thyroid Hormone
GG540	Cap, White, Opaque, Single Orange Band	Fluoxetine HCl 40 mg	Prozac by Sandoz	00781-2824	Antidepressant
GG541	Cap, GG over 541	Diphenhydramine HCl 50 mg	by Sandoz		Antihistamine
GG541	Cap	Diphenhydramine HCl 50 mg	by Sandoz	00781-2498	Antihistamine
GG549	Cap, Pink & White, GG over 549	Ursodiol 300 mg	Actigall by Sandoz	00781-2848	Gastrointestinal
GG55 <> 5	Tab, Lavender, Round, Film Coated, GG over 55	Trifluoperazine HCl 5 mg	Stelazine by Sandoz	00781-1034	Antipsychotic
GG550	Cap, White, Opaque, Single Black Band	Fluoxetine HCl 20 mg	Prozac by Sandoz	00781-2822	Antidepressant
GG551	Cap, Yellow	Procainamide HCl 250 mg	Pronestyl by Sandoz		Antiarrhythmic
GG552	Cap, Orange & White	Procainamide HCl 375 mg	Pronestyl by Sandoz		Antiarrhythmic
GG553	Cap, Orange & Yellow	Procainamide HCl 500 mg	Pronestyl by Sandoz		Antiarrhythmic
GG553	Cap	Diphenhydramine HCl 25 mg	by PDRX	55289-0479	Antihistamine
GG554	Cap, Black & Clear	Niacin SR 125 mg	Nicobid by Eon		Vitamin
GG556	Cap, Gray & Orange	Cephalexin 250 mg	Keflex by Novopharm		Antibiotic
GG558	Cap, Black, Gold & White	Fenoprofen Calcium 200 mg	Nalfon by Sandoz		NSAID
GG559	Cap, Gold Bands	Fenoprofen Calcium 300 mg	by DRX	55045-2450	NSAID
GG559	Cap, Gold Bands	Fenoprofen Calcium 300 mg	by Sandoz	00781-2862	NSAID
GG56	Cap	Disopyramide Phosphate	by Sandoz	00781-2110	Antiarrhythmic
GG564	Cap, Clear & Green	Niacin SR 250 mg	Nicobid by Eon		Vitamin
GG565	Cap, White, Black and Orange Bands	Nortriptyline HCl 10 mg	Pamelor by Sandoz	00781-2630	Antidepressant
GG566	Cap, White, Black & Orange Bands	Nortriptyline HCl 25 mg	Pamelor by Sandoz	00781-2631	Antidepressant
GG567	Cap, White, Black Bands	Nortriptyline HCl 50 mg	Pamelor by Sandoz	00781-2632	Antidepressant
GG568	Cap, Orange Ink Bands	Nortriptyline HCl 75 mg	by Sandoz	00781-2633	Antidepressant
GG57	Cap	Disopyramide Phosphate	by Sandoz	00781-2115	Antiarrhythmic
GG570	Cap, Clear & Green	Chlorpheniramine Maleate TD 8 mg	Teldrin by Sandoz		Antihistamine
GG571	Cap, White, Blue & Green Band	Chlordiazepoxide 5 mg, Clidinium Bromide 2.5 mg	Librax by Sandoz		Gastrointestinal
GG572	Cap	Doxepin HCl	Sinequan by Sandoz	00781-2801	Antidepressant
GG573	Cap	Doxepin HCl	Sinequan by Sandoz	00781-2802	Antidepressant
GG574	Cap	Doxepin HCl	Sinequan by Sandoz	00781-2803	Antidepressant
GG575	Cap, White, Green Print, GG over 575	Fluoxetine HCl 10 mg	Prozac by Sandoz	00781-2823	Antidepressant
GG576	Cap	Doxepin HCl	Sinequan by Sandoz		Antidepressant
GG577	Cap	Doxepin HCl 100 mg	Sinequan by Sandoz	00781-2800	Antidepressant
GG58 <> 10	Tab, Lavender, Round, Film Coated, GG over 58	Trifluoperazine HCl 10 mg	Stelazine by Sandoz	00781-1036	Antipsychotic
GG580	Cap, Red, White Print, GG over 580	Hydrochlorothiazide 25 mg, Triamterene 50 mg	Dyazide by Sandoz	00781-2715	Diuretic; Antihypertensive
GG589	Cap, White, Orange & Yellow Print, GG over 589	Thiothixene 1 mg	Navane by Sandoz	00781-2226	Antipsychotic
GG59	Tab, White, Round, Scored, GG over 59	Allopurinol 100 mg	Zyloprim by Sandoz	00781-1080	Antigout
GG590	Cap, Clear & Green	Chlorpheniramine Maleate 12 mg	Chlor-Trimeton by Sandoz		Antihistamine
GG591	Cap	Propoxyphene HCl 65 mg	by Sandoz	00781-2140	Analgesic; C IV
GG592	Cap, Black & White bands	Prazosin HCl 1 mg	Minipress by Sandoz		Antihypertensive
GG593	Cap, Black & Pink & White Bd	Prazosin HCl 2 mg	Minipress by Sandoz		Antihypertensive

ID FRONT <> BACK	DESCRIPTION FRONT <> BACK	INGREDIENT & STRENGTH	BRAND (or Generic Equiv.) by FIRM	NDC#	CLASS; SCH.
GG594	Cap, Black & Pink & White Bd	Prazosin HCl 5 mg	Minipress by Sandoz		Antihypertensive
GG596	Cap, White, Blue & Yellow Print, GG over 596	Thiothixene 2 mg	Navane by Sandoz	00781-2227	Antipsychotic
GG597	Cap, White, Black & Orange Print, GG over 597	Thiothixene 5 mg	Navane by Sandoz	00781-2228	Antipsychotic
GG598	Cap, White, Black & Blue Print, GG over 598	Thiothixene 10 mg	Navane by Sandoz	00781-2229	Antipsychotic
GG60	Tab, Peach, Round, Scored, GG over 60	Allopurinol 300 mg	Zyloprim by Sandoz	00781-1082	Antigout
GG606	Cap, White, Black Print, Black Bands, GG over 606	Hydrochlorothiazide 25 mg, Triamterene 37.5 mg	Dyazide by Sandoz	00781-2074	Diuretic; Antihypertensive
GG608	Cap, White, Opaque, Blue Print	Ribavirin 200 mg	Rebetol by Sandoz	00781-2043	Antiviral
GG61	Tab, White, Round	Chlorpropamide 100 mg	Diabinese by Sandoz		Antidiabetic
GG614	Cap, Caramel, White Print, GG over 614	Ranitidine HCl 150 mg	Zantac by Sandoz	00781-2855	Gastrointestinal
GG615	Cap, Caramel, White Print, GG over 615	Ranitidine HCl 300 mg	Zantac by Sandoz	00781-2865	Gastrointestinal
GG62	Tab, Pink, Round	Sodium Fluoride 2.2 mg	Luride by Trinity		Element
GG621	Cap, White, Black Print, GG over 621	Terazosin HCl 1 mg	Hytrin by Sandoz	00781-2051	Antihypertensive
GG622	Cap, Yellow, Black Print, GG over 622	Terazosin HCl 2 mg	Hytrin by Sandoz	00781-2052	Antihypertensive
GG623	Cap, Pink, Black Print, GG over 623	Terazosin HCl 5 mg	Hytrin by Sandoz	00781-2053	Antihypertensive
GG624	Cap, Auqa, Black Print, GG over 624	Terazosin HCl 10 mg	Hytrin by Sandoz	00781-2054	Antihypertensive
GG63	Tab, White, Round, Film Coated, GG over 63	Desipramine HCl 10 mg	Norpramin by Sandoz	00781-1971	Antidepressant
GG633	Cap, Red & Caramel	Rifampin 300 mg	Rimactane by Sandoz	00781-2077	Antibiotic
GG634	Cap, Red, White Print	Amantadine HCl 100 mg	Symmetrel by Sandoz	00781-2048	Antiviral
GG64	Tab, White, Round, Film Coated, GG over 64	Desipramine HCl 25 mg	Norpramin by Sandoz	00781-1972	Antidepressant
GG65	Tab, White, Round, Film Coated, GG over 65	Desipramine HCl 50 mg	Norpramin by Sandoz	00781-1973	Antidepressant
GG66	Tab	Diazepam 2 mg	by Sandoz	00781-1482	Antianxiety; C IV
GG67	Tab	Diazepam 5 mg	by Sandoz	00781-1483	Antianxiety; C IV
GG68	Tab	Diazepam 10 mg	by Sandoz	00781-1484	Antianxiety; C IV
GG705	Tab, Pink, Round, Film Coated, GG over 705	Ranitidine 150 mg	Zantac by Sandoz	00781-1883	Gastrointestinal
GG705	Tab, Pink, Round, Film Coated, GG over 705	Ranitidine HCl 150 mg	Zantac by UDL	51079-0879	Gastrointestinal
GG706	Tab, Orange, Round, GG over 706	Ranitidine 300 mg	Zantac by Sandoz	00781-1884	Gastrointestinal
GG71	Tab, Peach, Round	Propranolol HCl 10 mg	Inderal by Sandoz		Antihypertensive
GG72	Tab, Blue, Round	Propranolol HCl 20 mg	Inderal by Sandoz		Antihypertensive
GG721	Tab, White, Round, GG over 721	Terazosin HCl 1 mg	Hytrin by Sandoz	00781-1551	Antihypertensive
GG722	Tab, Orange, Round, GG over 722	Terazosin HCl 2 mg	Hytrin by Sandoz	00781-1561	Antihypertensive
GG723	Tab, Tan, Round, GG over 723	Terazosin HCl 5 mg	Hytrin by Sandoz	00781-1571	Antihypertensive
GG724	Tab, Yellow, Round, GG over 724	Naproxen 250 mg	Naprosyn by Sandoz	00781-1163	NSAID
GG725	Tab, Orange, Cap Shaped	Naproxen 375 mg	Naprosyn by Sandoz	00781-1164	NSAID
GG726	Tab, Yellow, Cap Shaped	Naproxen 500 mg	Naprosyn by Sandoz	00781-1165	NSAID
GG73	Tab, Green, Round	Propranolol HCl 40 mg	Inderal by Sandoz		Antihypertensive
GG733	Tab, Green, Round	Salsalate 500 mg	Disalcid by Sandoz		NSAID
GG734	Tab, Green, Oblong	Salsalate 750 mg	Disalcid by Sandoz		NSAID
GG735	Tab, White, Oval	Flurbiprofen 50 mg	Ansaid by Greenstone		NSAID
GG736	Tab, Blue, Round, Film Coated	Flurbiprofen 100 mg	Ansaid by Sandoz	00781-1129	NSAID
GG737	Tab, Yellow, Black Print, Round, Film Coated, GG over 737	Diclofenac Sodium 25 mg	Voltaren by Sandoz	00781-1785	NSAID
GG738	Tab, Brown, Black Print, Round, Film Coated, GG over 738	Diclofenac Sodium 50 mg	Voltaren by Sandoz	00781-1787	NSAID
GG739	Tab, Yellow, Black Print, Round, Film Coated, GG over 739	Diclofenac Sodium 75 mg	Voltaren by Sandoz	00781-1789	NSAID
GG74	Tab, Salmon, Round	Propranolol HCl 60 mg	Inderal by Sandoz		Antihypertensive
GG741	Tab, White, Round	Ciprofloxacin 250 mg	Cipro by Sandoz	00781-1763	Antibiotic
GG742	Cap, White	Ciprofloxacin 500 mg	Cipro by Sandoz	00781-1765	Antibiotic
GG743	Tab, White, Cap Shaped	Ciprofloxacin 750 mg	Cipro by Sandoz	00781-1767	Antibiotic
GG746	Tab, Light Yellow, Round	Benazepril HCl 5 mg	Lotensin by Sandoz	00781-1891	Antihypertensive
GG747	Tab, Dark Yellow, Round	Benazepril HCl 10 mg	Lotensin by Sandoz	00781-1892	Antihypertensive

ID FRONT <> BACK	DESCRIPTION FRONT <> BACK	INGREDIENT & STRENGTH	BRAND (or Generic Equiv.) by FIRM	NDC#	CLASS; SCH.
GG748	Tab, Pink, Round	Benazepril HCl 20 mg	Lotensin by Sandoz	00781-1893	Antihypertensive
GG749	Tab, Dark Rose, Round	Benazepril HCl 40 mg	Lotensin by Sandoz	00781-1894	Antihypertensive
GG75	Tab, Yellow, Round	Propranolol HCl 80 mg	Inderal by Sandoz		Antihypertensive
GG759	Tab, Light Brown, Black Print, Round, GG over 759	Diclofenac Potassium 50 mg	by DRX	55045-2675	NSAID
GG759	Tab, Light Brown, Black Print, Round, GG over 759	Diclofenac Potassium 50 mg	Cataflam IR by Sandoz	00781-1297 Discontinued	NSAID
GG76	Tab, Green, Round	Levothyroxine Sodium 0.3 mg	Synthroid by Rosemont		Thyroid Hormone
GG77	Tab, Blue, Round	Levothyroxine Sodium 0.15 mg	Synthroid by Rosemont		Thyroid Hormone
GG770	Tab, White, Round	Lovastatin 10 mg	Mevacor by Sandoz	00781-1323	Antihyperlipidemic
GG771	Tab, White, Round, Scored, GG over 771	Glipizide 5 mg	Glucotrol by Sandoz	00781-1452	Antidiabetic
GG772	Tab, White, Round, Scored, GG over 772	Glipizide 10 mg	Glucotrol by Sandoz	00781-1453	Antidiabetic
GG773	Tab, Green, Oval	Lovastatin 40 mg	Mevacor by Sandoz	00781-1213	Antihyperlipidemic
GG774	Tab, Film Coated	Etodolac 400 mg	by Sandoz	00781-1234	NSAID
GG78	Tab, White, Round, GG over 78	Methazolamide 25 mg	Neptazane by Sandoz	00781-1072	Antiglaucoma Agent
GG780	Tab, White, Round, SR	Methylphenidate HCl 20 mg SR	Ritalin SR by Sandoz	00781-1754	Stimulant; C II
GG781	Tab, White, Round	Paroxetine HCl 10 mg	Paxil by Sandoz	00781-1967	Antidepressant
GG789	Tab, Pale Green, Round, Scored	Methylphenidate HCl 10 mg	Ritalin by Sandoz	00781-1749	Stimulant; C II
GG79	Tab, White, Round	Prednisone 5 mg	Meticorten by Sandoz		Steroid
GG790	Tab, Light Yellow, Round, Scored	Methylphenidate HCl 20 mg	Ritalin by Sandoz	00781-1753	Stimulant; C II
GG793	Tab, White, Oval	Paroxetine HCl 40 mg	Paxil by Sandoz	00781-1969	Antidepressant
GG795	Tab, Off-White, Round	Fluconazole 50 mg	Diflucan by Sandoz	00781-1927	Antifungal
GG796	Tab, Off-White, Round	Fluconazole 100 mg	Diflucan by Sandoz	00781-1929	Antifungal
GG797	Tab, Off-White, Round	Fluconazole 150 mg	Diflucan by Sandoz	00781-1921	Antifungal
GG798	Tab, Off-White, Round	Fluconazole 200 mg	Diflucan by Sandoz	00781-1931	Antifungal
GG8	Tab, White, Round	Nylidrin 6 mg	Arlidin by Sandoz		Vasodilator
GG80	Tab, White, Round, Scored	Furosemide 80 mg	Lasix by Sandoz	00781-1446	Diuretic
GG801	Cap	Ketoprofen 75 mg	Orudis by Sandoz	00781-2411	NSAID
GG802	Cap, White	Ketoprofen 50 mg	Orudis by Sandoz		NSAID
GG807	Cap, Orange, Oblong	Guaifenesin 200 mg, Phenylephrine HCl 5 mg, Phenylpropanolamine HCl 45 mg	Entex by Amide		Cold Remedy
GG81	Tab	Clonidine HCl 0.1 mg	by Sandoz	00781-1471	Antihypertensive
GG82	Tab	Clonidine HCl 0.2 mg	by Sandoz	00781-1472	Antihypertensive
GG822	Cap, White, Orange & Yellow Print, GG over 822	Clomipramine HCl 25 mg	Anafranil by Sandoz	00781-2027	OCD
GG823	Cap, White, Blue & Yellow Print, GG over 823	Clomipramine HCl 50 mg	Anafranil by Sandoz	00781-2037	OCD
GG824	Cap, White, Yellow Print, GG over 824	Clomipramine HCl 75 mg	Anafranil by Sandoz	00781-2047	OCD
GG825	Cap, White, Caramel & Red Bands	Mexiletine 150 mg	Mexitil by Sandoz	00781-2130	Antiarrhythmic
GG826	Cap, White, Red Print, GG over 826	Mexiletine 200 mg	Mexitil by Sandoz	00781-2131	Antiarrhythmic
GG827	Cap, White, Aqua and Red Bands	Mexiletine 250 mg	Mexitil by Sandoz	00781-2132	Antiarrhythmic
GG83	Tab	Clonidine HCl 0.3 mg	by Sandoz	00781-1473	Antihypertensive
GG832	Cap, Gray & Black Bands, White Powder	Etodolac 200 mg	by Sandoz	00781-2012	NSAID
GG84	Tab	Timolol Maleate 5 mg	by Sandoz	00781-1126	Antihypertensive
GG85	Tab, White, Round, Scored, GG over 85	Spironolactone 25 mg	Aldactone by Sandoz	00781-1599	Diuretic
GG850	Cap, White	Ampicillin 250 mg	Principen by Sandoz	00781-2144	Antibiotic
GG851	Cap, White	Ampicillin 500 mg	Principen by Sandoz	00781-2145	Antibiotic
GG854	Cap, Light Blue	Dicloxacillin Sodium 250 mg	Dynapen by Sandoz	00781-2248	Antibiotic
GG855	Cap, Blue	Dicloxacillin Sodium 500 mg	Dynapen by Sandoz	00781-2258	Antibiotic
GG89	Tab, White, Round, Scored	Amoxapine 25 mg	Asendin by Sandoz	00781-1844	Antidepressant
GG90	Tab, Orange, Round, Scored	Amoxapine 50 mg	Asendin by Sandoz	00781-1845	Antidepressant

ID FRONT <> BACK	DESCRIPTION FRONT <> BACK	INGREDIENT & STRENGTH	BRAND (or Generic Equiv.) by FIRM	NDC#	CLASS; SCH.
GG904	Tab, Light Pink, Round, Film Coated, Ex Release, GG over 904	Diclofenac Sodium 100 mg	Voltaren SR by DRX	55045-2698	NSAID
GG904	Tab, Light Pink, Round, Film Coated, Ex Release, GG over 904	Diclofenac Sodium 100 mg	Voltaren SR by Sandoz	00781-1381	NSAID
GG92	Tab, White, Round, Scored, GG over 92	Lorazepam 1 mg	Ativan by Sandoz	00781-1404	Antianxiety; C IV
GG92	Tab, White, Round, Scored, GG over 92	Lorazepam 1 mg	Ativan by Ivax	00182-8238 Discontinued	Antianxiety; C IV
GG929	Tab, Lavender, Round, Film Coated, GG over 929	Bupropion HCl 75 mg	Wellbutrin by Sandoz	00781-1053	Antidepressant
GG93	Tab, White, Round, Scored, GG over 93	Lorazepam 2 mg	Ativan by Sandoz	00781-1405	Antianxiety; C IV
GG93	Tab, White, Round, Scored, GG over 93	Lorazepam 2 mg	Ativan by Ivax	00182-8239 Discontinued	Antianxiety; C IV
GG930	Tab, Lavender, Round, Film Coated, GG over 930	Bupropion HCl 100 mg	Wellbutrin by Sandoz	00781-1064	Antidepressant
GG931	Tab, White, Round, Ex Release, GG over 931	Orphenadrine Citrate 100 mg	Norflex by Sandoz	00781-1649	Muscle Relaxant
GG932	Tab, White, Round, Scored, GG over 932	Pemoline 18.75 mg	Cylert by Sandoz	00781-1731 Discontinued	Stimulant; C IV
GG933	Tab, White, Round, Scored, GG over 933	Pemoline 37.5 mg	Cylert by Sandoz	00781-1741 Discontinued	Stimulant; C IV
GG934	Tab, White, Round, Scored, GG over 934	Pemoline 75 mg	Cylert by Sandoz	00781-1751 Discontinued	Stimulant; C IV
GG935	Tab, White, Cap Shaped, Film Coated, Ex Release	Naproxen 375 mg	Naprosyn EC by Sandoz	00781-1646	NSAID
GG936	Tab, White, Cap Shaped, Film Coated, Ex Release	Naproxen 500 mg	Naprosyn EC by Sandoz	00781-1653	NSAID
GG949 <> PVK250	Tab, Off-White, Round, Scored, Film Coated	Penicillin 250 mg	Pen Vee K by Sandoz	00781-1205	Antibiotic
GG95	Tab, White, Round	Hydrochlorothiazide 25 mg, Spironolactone 25 mg	Aldactazide by Sandoz		Diuretic; Antihypertensive
GG950 <> PVK500	Tab, Off-White, Oblong	Penicillin V Potassium 500 mg	Pen Vee K by Sandoz	00781-1655	Antibiotic
GG952 <> 5	Tab, Pale Yellow, Round	Prochlorperazine 5 mg	Compazine by Sandoz	00781-5020	Antiemetic
GG953 <> 10	Tab, Pale Yellow, Round	Prochlorperazine 10 mg	Compazine by Sandoz	00781-5021	Antiemetic
GG957	Tab, White	Methylprednisolone 4 mg	Medrol by Sandoz	00781-5022	Steroid
GG958	Tab, White, Round	Metoclopramide 5 mg	Reglan by Sandoz	00781-5030	Gastrointestinal
GG961	Tab, White, Oblong, Film Coated	Amoxicillin 500 mg	Amoxil by Sandoz	00781-5060	Antibiotic
GG962	Tab, White, Oblong, Film Coated	Amoxicillin 875 mg	Amoxil by Sandoz	00781-5061	Antibiotic
GG963250	Tab, Off White, Oval	Cefuroxime Axetil 250 mg	Ceftin by Sandoz	00781-5065	Antibiotic
GG964500	Tab, Off White, Oval	Cefuroxime Axetil 500 mg	Ceftin by Sandoz	00781-5066	Antibiotic
GG97	Tab, Orange, Round, Film Coated, GG over 97	Fluphenazine HCl 1 mg	Prolixin by Invamed	52189-0313	Antipsychotic
GG97	Tab, Orange, Round, Film Coated, GG over 97	Fluphenazine HCl 1 mg	Prolixin by Sandoz	00781-1436	Antipsychotic
GG977	Tab, White, Round, Film Coated	Diclofenac Potassium 50 mg	Cataflam by Sandoz	00781-5017	NSAID
GGAVISCON	Tab, White, Round, G/Gaviscon	Alginic Acid 200 mg	Gaviscon by SKB	Canadian	Gastrointestinal
GGC1	Tab, Light Green, Round, GG over C1	Terazosin HCl 10 mg	Hytrin by Sandoz	00781-1541	Antihypertensive
GGC3	Tab, White, Round, Scored, GG over C3	Captopril 12.5 mg	Capoten by Golden State	60429-0029	Antihypertensive
GGC3	Tab, White, Round, Scored, GG over C3	Captopril 12.5 mg	Capoten by Sandoz	00781-1828	Antihypertensive
GGC6	Tab, White, Oval, Film Coated, Immediate Release	Clarithromycin 250 mg	Biaxin by Sandoz	00781-1961	Antibiotic
GGC9	Tab, White, Oval, Film Coated, Immediate Release	Clarithromycin 500 mg	Biaxin by Sandoz	00781-1962	Antibiotic
GGD6	Tab, White, Oval	Azithromycin 250 mg	Zithromax by Sandoz	00781-1496	Antibiotic
GGD7	Tab, White, Oval	Azithromycin 600 mg	Zithromax by Sandoz	00781-1497	Antibiotic
GGD8	Tab, White, Oval	Azithromycin 500MG	Zithromax by Sandoz	00781-1941	Antibiotic
GGG5	Cap, Orange, Red & Yellow	Acetaminophen 500 mg	Tylenol Ex Strength by Granutec		Analgesic
GGL7	Tab, White, Round, GG over L7	Atenolol 25 mg	Tenormin by Golden State	60429-0211	Antihypertensive
GGL7	Tab, White, Round, GG over L7	Atenolol 25 mg	Tenormin by Sandoz	00781-1078	Antihypertensive
GGL7	Tab, White, Round, GG over L7	Atenolol 25 mg	Tenormin by Ivax	00182-8235	Antihypertensive
GGM	Cap, Brown	Clofazimine 100 mg	Lamprene by Geigy		Antileprosy
GGN2	Tab, Pink, Round, Chewable	Amoxicillin 200 mg, Clavulanate Potassium 28.5 mg	Augmentin by Sandoz	00781-1619	Antibiotic

ID FRONT <> BACK	DESCRIPTION FRONT <> BACK	INGREDIENT & STRENGTH	BRAND (or Generic Equiv.) by FIRM	NDC#	CLASS; SCH.
GGN4	Tab, Pink, Round, Chewable	Amoxicillin 400 mg, Clavulanate Potassium 57 mg	Augmentin by Sandoz	00781-1643	Antibiotic
GGN5	Tab, White, Oblong, Film Coated	Amoxicillin 250 mg, Clavulanate Potassium 125 mg	Augmentin by Sandoz	00781-1874	Antibiotic
GGN6	Tab, White to Light Yellow, Oblong	Amoxicillin 500 mg, Clavulanate Potassium 125 mg	Augmentin by Sandoz	00781-1831	Antibiotic
GGN7	Tab, White to Yellow, Oblong, Scored	Amoxicillin 875 mg, Clavulanate Potassium 125 mg	Augmentin by Sandoz	00781-1852	Antibiotic
GIL05	Tab, White to Off-White, Round, GIL 0.5	Rasagiline 0.5 mg	Azilect by Teva	68546-0142	Antiparkinson
GIL1	Tab, White to Off-White, Round	Rasagiline 1 mg	Azilect by Teva	68546-0229	Antiparkinson
GIL307	Tab, Scored	Phenylephrine HCl 10 mg	Gilchew by Gil Pharm	58552-0307	Decongestant
GIL307	Tab, Scored	Phenylephrine HCl 10 mg	Gilchew IR by Nadin	14836-0307	Decongestant
GILEAD <> 701	Tab, Blue, Cap Shaped, Film Coated	Emtricitabine 200 mg, Tenofovir Disoproxil Fumarate 300 mg	Truvada by Gilead	61958-0701	Antiviral
GILEAD4331 <> 300	Tab, Light Blue, Almond Shaped, Film Coated	Tenofovir Disoproxil Fumarate 300 mg	Viread by Gilead	Canadian DIN 02247128	Antiretroviral Agent
GILGIL <> 303303	Tab, White, Oval, Scored	Guaifenesin 600 mg, Dextromethorphan HBr 30 mg, Phenylephrine HCl 20 mg	Giltuss TR by Gil Pharma	58552-0303	Cold Remedy
GILGIL <> 303303	Tab, White, Oval	Guaifenesin 600 mg, Dextromethorphan HBr 30 mg, Phenylephrine HCl 20 mg	Giltuss by Gil Pharm	58552-0303	Cold Remedy
GILGIL <> 303303	Tab, White, Oval, Scored	Guaifenesin 600 mg, Dextromethorphan HBr 30 mg, Phenylephrine HCl 20 mg	Giltuss by Sovereign	58716-0646	Cold Remedy
GILGIL <> 304304	Tab, White, Oblong, Scored	Guaifenesin 600 mg, Phenylephrine HCl 25 mg	Gilphex TR by Gil Pharma	58552-0304	Cold Remedy
GILGIL <> 305305	Tab, White, Cap Shaped, Scored	Chlorpheniramine 8 mg, Phenylephrine HCl 20 mg	Phenabid by Gil Pharma	58552-0305	Cold Remedy
GILGIL <> 306306	Tab, White, Cap Shaped, Scored	Chlorpheniramine 8 mg, Dextromethorphan HBr 30 mg, Phenylephrine HCl 20 mg	Phenabid DM by Gil Pharma	58552-0306	Cold Remedy
GILLEAD4331 <> 300	Tab, Light Blue, Almond Shaped, Film Coated	Tenofovir Disoproxil Fumarate 300 mg	Viread by Gilead	61958-0401	Antiviral
GL <> 53511	Tab, White, Oblong, Scored	Butalbital 50 mg, Acetaminophen 325 mg, Caffeine 40 mg	Esgic by Rx Pak	65084-0126	Analgesic
GL <> 53511	Tab, Gilbert Logo G with overlaid L <> 535-11	Acetaminophen 325 mg, Butalbital 50 mg, Caffeine 40 mg	Fioricet by Prestige	58056-0354	Analgesic
GL500	Tab, White, Round, GL over 500	Metformin HCl 500 mg	Glucophage by Caremark	00339-6022	Antidiabetic
GL53511	Tab, White, Cap Shaped, Scored, GL 535-11	Acetaminophen 325 mg, Butalbital 50 mg, Caffeine 40 mg	Fioricet by Forest	51947-8121	Analgesic
GL53512	Cap, White, Opaque, GL 535-12	Acetaminophen 325 mg, Butalbital 50 mg, Caffeine 40 mg	Esgic by Forest	62584-0325	Analgesic
GL850	Tab, White, Oblong	Metformin HCl 850 mg	Glucophage by BMS	55154-1109	Antidiabetic
GLAXO <> 250	Tab, White, Oblong	Cefuroxime Axetil 250 mg	Ceftin by GSK	00173-7004	Antibiotic
GLAXO <> 387	Tab, Light Blue, Cap Shaped, Film Coated	Cefuroxime Axetil 250 mg	Ceftin by Med Pro	53978-2088	Antibiotic
GLAXO <> 387	Tab, Light Blue, Cap Shaped, Film Coated	Cefuroxime Axetil 250 mg	Ceftin by Allscripts		Antibiotic
GLAXO <> 387	Tab, Light Blue, Cap Shaped, Film Coated	Cefuroxime Axetil 250 mg	Ceftin by GSK	51947-8121	Antibiotic
GLAXO <> 387	Tab, Light Blue, Cap Shaped, Film Coated	Cefuroxime Axetil 250 mg	Ceftin by Amerisource	62584-0325	Antibiotic
GLAXO <> 387	Tab, Light Blue, Cap Shaped, Film Coated	Cefuroxime Axetil 250 mg	Ceftin by Nat Pharmpak	55154-1109	Antibiotic
GLAXO <> 387	Tab, Light Blue, Cap Shaped, Film Coated	Cefuroxime Axetil 250 mg	Ceftin by GSK	Discontinued	Antibiotic
GLAXO <> 394	Tab, Dark Blue, Cap Shaped, Film Coated	Cefuroxime Axetil 500 mg	Ceftin by Nat Pharmpak	55154-1111	Antibiotic
GLAXO <> 394	Tab, Dark Blue, Cap Shaped, Film Coated	Cefuroxime Axetil 500 mg	Ceftin by GSK	Discontinued	Antibiotic
GLAXO <> 395	Tab, White, Cap Shaped, Film Coated	Cefuroxime Axetil 125 mg	Ceftin by GSK	00173-0395	Antibiotic
GLAXO <> 4	Tab, Yellow, Oval, Film Coated	Ondansetron HCl 4 mg	Zofran by GSK	Canadian DIN 02213567	Antiemetic
GLAXO <> 4	Tab, White, Oval, Film Coated	Ondansetron HCl 4 mg	Zofran by GSK	00173-7005	Antiemetic
GLAXO <> 500	Tab, White, Oblong	Cefuroxime Axetil 500 mg	Ceftin by GSK		Antibiotic
GLAXO <> 8	Tab, Yellow, Oval	Ondansetron HCl 8 mg	Zofran by GSK		Antiemetic
GLAXO <> 8	Tab, Dark Yellow, Oval, Film Coated	Ondansetron HCl 8 mg	Zofran by GSK	Canadian DIN 02213575	Antiemetic
GLAXO <> ZANTAC150	Tab, Peach, Pentagon, Film Coated	Ranitidine HCl 150 mg	Zantac by Pharmedix	53002-0552	Gastrointestinal
GLAXO <> ZANTAC150	Tab, Peach, Pentagon, Film Coated	Ranitidine HCl 150 mg	Zantac by GSK	00173-0344	Gastrointestinal
GLAXO <> ZANTAC150	Tab, Peach, Pentagon, Film Coated	Ranitidine HCl 150 mg	by Nat Pharmpak	55154-1110	Gastrointestinal
GLAXO <> ZANTAC150	Tab, Peach, Pentagon, Film Coated	Ranitidine HCl 150 mg	by Kaiser	00179-1079	Gastrointestinal
GLAXO <> ZANTAC150	Tab, Film Coated	Ranitidine HCl	by Med Pro	53978-2075	Gastrointestinal

ID FRONT <> BACK	DESCRIPTION FRONT <> BACK	INGREDIENT & STRENGTH	BRAND (or Generic Equiv.) by FIRM	NDC#	CLASS; SCH.
GLAXO <> ZANTAC150	Tab, White, Round, Glaxo <> Zantac/150	Ranitidine HCl 150 mg	Zantac by GSK	Canadian DIN 02212331	Gastrointestinal
GLAXO <> ZANTAC150	Tab, Peach, Pentagon, Film Coated	Ranitidine HCl 150 mg	by Amerisource	62584-0488	Gastrointestinal
GLAXO <> ZANTAC150	Tab, Peach, Pentagon, Film Coated	Ranitidine HCl 150 mg	Zantac by Rx Dispensing	61807-0054	Gastrointestinal
GLAXO <> ZANTAC150	Tab, Peach, Pentagon, Film Coated	Ranitidine HCl 150 mg	by Nat Pharmpak	55154-1107	Gastrointestinal
GLAXO <> ZANTAC300	Tab, White, Oblong, Glaxo <> Zantac 300	Ranitidine HCl 300 mg	Zantac by GSK	Canadian DIN 02212358	Gastrointestinal
GLAXO <> ZANTAC300	Tab, Film Coated	Ranitidine HCl 300 mg	by Kaiser	00179-1211	Gastrointestinal
GLAXO <> ZANTAC300	Tab	Ranitidine HCl 336 mg	Zantac by Pharmedix	53002-1028	Gastrointestinal
GLAXO <> ZANTAC300	Tab, Yellow, Cap Shaped, Film Coated	Ranitidine HCl 300 mg	Zantac by GSK	00173-0393	Gastrointestinal
GLAXO <> ZANTAC300	Tab	Ranitidine HCl 336 mg	by Allscripts		Gastrointestinal
GLAXO <> ZANTAC300	Tab, Embossed	Ranitidine HCl 336 mg	by Amerisource	62584-0393	Gastrointestinal
GLAXO268	Tab, Blue & Clear	Theophylline Anhydrous 260 mg	Theobid Duracap by GSK		Antiasthmatic
GLAXO281	Tab, Yellow, Oval	Ethaverine HCl 100 mg	Ethatab by GSK		Vasodilator
GLAXO295	Cap, Blue & Clear	Theophylline Anhydrous 130 mg	Theobid Jr Duracap by GSK		Antiasthmatic
GLAXO309	Cap, Clear & Pink	Phenylpropanolamine 75 mg, Chlorpheniramine 8 mg	Histabid Duracaps by GSK		Cold Remedy
GLAXO316	Cap, Black & Orange	Vitamin Combination	Vicon Forte by GSK		Vitamin
GLAXO371	Tab, Peach, Oval	Labetalol HCl 100 mg, Hydrochlorothiazide 25 mg	Trandate HCT by GSK		Antihypertensive; Diuretic
GLAXO372	Tab, White, Oval	Labetalol HCl 200 mg, Hydrochlorothiazide 25 mg	Trandate HCT by GSK		Antihypertensive; Diuretic
GLAXO373	Tab, Peach, Oval	Labetalol HCl 300 mg, Hydrochlorothiazide 25 mg	Trandate HCT by GSK		Antihypertensive; Diuretic
GLAXO387	Tab, Coated	Cefuroxime Axetil 250 mg	Ceftin by Pharmedix	53002-0275	Antibiotic
GLAXO394	Tab, Coated	Cefuroxime Axetil 500 mg	Ceftin by Pharmedix	53002-0267	Antibiotic
GLAXO4	Tab, Yellow, Oval, Glaxo/4	Ondansetron HCl 4 mg	Zofran by GSK	Canadian	Antiemetic
GLAXO4	Tab, White, Oval, Glaxo/4	Ondansetron HCl 4 mg	Zofran by GSK	00173-0341	Antiemetic
GLAXOGLAXO <> VENTOLIN2	Tab, Glaxo over Glaxo <> Ventolin over 2	Albuterol Sulfate 2 mg	Ventolin by GSK	00173-0342	Antiasthmatic
GLAXOGLAXO <> VENTOLIN4	Tab, Glaxo over Glaxo <> Ventolin over 4	Albuterol Sulfate 4 mg	Ventolin by GSK	00173-0428	Antiasthmatic
GLAXOWELLCOME-ZANTAC150	Cap, Blue Ink	Ranitidine HCl 150 mg	Zantac Geldose by GSK	00173-0481	Gastrointestinal
GLAXOWELLCOME-ZANTAC150	Cap, Blue Ink	Ranitidine HCl 150 mg	Zantac Geldose by GSK	00173-0429	Gastrointestinal
GLAXOWELLCOME-ZANTAC300	Cap, Blue Ink	Ranitidine HCl 300 mg	Zantac Geldose by GSK	59762-5033	Gastrointestinal
GLIPIZIDEXL10	Tab, White, Round, Extended Release	Glipizide 10 mg	Glucotrol XL by Greenstone	59762-5031	Antidiabetic
GLIPIZIDEXL25	Tab, Blue, Round, Extended Release	Glipizide 2.5 mg	Glucotrol XL by Greenstone	59762-5032	Antidiabetic
GLIPIZIDEXL5	Tab, White, Round, Extended Release	Glipizide 5 mg	Glucotrol XL by Greenstone	Canadian DIN 02295377	Antidiabetic
GLM1 <> APOAPO	Tab, Pink, Cap Shaped, Notched, Scored	Glimepiride 1 mg	Amaryl by Apotex	Canadian DIN 02295385	Antidiabetic
GLM2 <> APOAPO	Tab, Green, Cap Shaped, Notched, Scored	Glimepiride 2 mg	Amaryl by Apotex	Canadian DIN 02295393	Antidiabetic
GLM4 <> APOAPO	Tab, Blue, Cap Shaped, Notched, Scored	Glimepiride 4 mg	Amaryl by Apotex	00904-7925	Antidiabetic
GLP10 <> APO	Tab, White, Round, Scored	Glipizide 10 mg	Glucotrol by Major	60505-0142	Antidiabetic
GLP10 <> APO	Tab, White to Off-White	Glipizide 10 mg	Glucotrol by Apotex	60505-0141	Antidiabetic
GLP5 <> APO	Tab, White to Off-White	Glipizide 5 mg	Glucotrol by Apotex	00904-7924	Antidiabetic
GLP5 <> APO	Tab, White, Round, Scored	Glipizide 5 mg	Glucotrol by Major		Antidiabetic

ID FRONT <> BACK	DESCRIPTION FRONT <> BACK	INGREDIENT & STRENGTH	BRAND (or Generic Equiv.) by FIRM	NDC#	CLASS; SCH.
GLUCOTROLXL10	Tab, White, Black Print, Round, Ex Release, Glucotrol XL over 10	Glipizide 10 mg	Glucotrol XL by Allscripts		Antidiabetic
GLUCOTROLXL10	Tab, White, Black Print, Round, Ex Release, Glucotrol XL over 10	Glipizide 10 mg	Glucotrol XL by Roerig	00049-1560	Antidiabetic
GLUCOTROLXL25	Tab, Blue, Black Print, Round, Ex Release, Glucotrol XL over 2.5	Glipizide 2.5 mg	Glucotrol XL by Roerig	00049-1620	Antidiabetic
GLUCOTROLXL5	Tab, White, Black Print, Round, Ex Release, Glucotrol XL over 5	Glipizide 5 mg	Glucotrol XL by Roerig	00049-1550	Antidiabetic
GLUTOFAC	Tab, Green, Caplet	Vitamin-B Complex	Glutofac by Kenwood	00482-0154	Vitamin; Mineral
GLUTOFACMX1	Tab, Light Purple, Cap Shaped, Film Coated	Folic Acid 800 mcg, Magnesium 205 mg, Pantothenic Acid 25 mg, Biotin 300 mcg, Calcium Carbonate 200 mg, Calcium Phosphate 110 mg, Cyanocobalamin 10 mcg, Potassium Chloride 40 mg	Glutofac-MX 1 by Kenwood	00482-0157	Vitamin; Mineral
GLUTOFACMX2	Tab, Dark Purple, Cap Shaped, Film Coated	Iron 15 mg, Zinc 35 mg, Selenium 100 mg, Chromium 200 mcg, Copper 5 mg, Manganese 5 mg, Magnesium 210 mg, Calcium Carbonate 225 mg, Iodine 150 mcg, Molybdenum 75 mcg, Calcium Phosphate 20 mg, Diostyl Sodium Sulfosuccinate 10 mg, Nickel 5 mcg, Tin 10 mcg, Vanadium 10 mcg, Boron Aspartate 150 mcg, Ascorbic Acid 100 mg, Potassium Chloride 40 mg	Glutofac-MX 2 by Kenwood	00482-0157	Vitamin; Mineral
GLUTOFACZX	Tab, Light Green, Cap Shaped	Vitamin A 5000 Units, Vitamin D 400 Units, Vitamin E 50 Units, Vitamin C 500 mg, Vitamin B1 20 mg, Vitamin B2 20 mg, Niacin 100 mg, Vitamin B6 25 mg, Vitamin B12 50 mcg, Folic Acid 1000 mcg, Pantothenic Acid 25 mg, Biotin 200 mg, Zinc 20 mg, Copper 2.5 mg, Magnesium 50 mg, Manganese 5 mg, Selenium 50 mcg, Chromium 200 mcg, Calcium 66 mg	Glutofac-ZX by Kenwood	00482-0158	Vitamin; Mineral
GLY	Tab, White, Round, Gly/Logo	Glyburide 2.5 mg	Glynase by Aventis	Canadian	Antidiabetic
GLYBUR	Tab, White, Oblong, Scored	Glyburide 1.25 mg	DiaBeta by Teva Pharmaceuticals	00093-9477	Antidiabetic
GLYBUR	Tab, Pink, Oblong, Scored	Glyburide 2.5 mg	DiaBeta by Teva Pharmaceuticals	00093-9433	Antidiabetic
GLYBUR	Tab, Light Blue, Oblong, Scored	Glyburide 5 mg	DiaBeta by Teva Pharmaceuticals	00093-9364	Antidiabetic
GLYBUR <> 364364	Tab, Light Blue, Oblong, Scored	Glyburide 5 mg	DiaBeta by Teva	38245-0364 Discontinued	Antidiabetic
GLYBUR <> 364364	Tab, Light Blue, Oblong, Scored	Glyburide 5 mg	DiaBeta by Blue Ridge	59273-0015	Antidiabetic
GLYBUR <> 364364	Tab, Light Blue, Oblong, Scored	Glyburide 5 mg	DiaBeta by Merrell	00068-3202	Antidiabetic
GLYBUR <> 364364	Tab, Light Blue, Oblong, Scored	Glyburide 5 mg	DiaBeta by PDRX	55289-0892	Antidiabetic
GLYBUR <> 364364	Tab, Light Blue, Oblong, Scored	Glyburide 5 mg	DiaBeta by Copley	38245-0364	Antidiabetic
GLYBUR <> 433433	Tab, Pink, Oblong, Scored	Glyburide 2.5 mg	DiaBeta by Blue Ridge	59273-0015	Antidiabetic
GLYBUR <> 433433	Tab, Pink, Oblong, Scored	Glyburide 2.5 mg	DiaBeta by Merrell	00068-3201	Antidiabetic
GLYBUR <> 433433	Tab, Pink, Oblong, Scored	Glyburide 2.5 mg	DiaBeta by Blue Ridge	59273-0014	Antidiabetic
GLYBUR <> 433433	Tab, Pink, Oblong, Scored	Glyburide 2.5 mg	DiaBeta by Teva	38245-0433	Antidiabetic
GLYBUR <> 433433	Tab, Pink, Oblong, Scored	Glyburide 2.5 mg	DiaBeta by Coventry	61372-0577	Antidiabetic
GLYBUR <> 477477	Tab, White, Oblong, Scored	Glyburide 1.25 mg	DiaBeta by Merrell	00068-3200	Antidiabetic
GLYBUR <> 477477	Tab, White, Oblong, Scored	Glyburide 1.25 mg	DiaBeta by Blue Ridge	59273-0013	Antidiabetic
GLYBUR <> 477477	Tab, White, Oblong, Scored	Glyburide 1.25 mg	DiaBeta by Coventry	61372-0576	Antidiabetic
GLYBUR <> 477477	Tab, White, Oblong, Scored	Glyburide 1.25 mg	DiaBeta by Teva	38245-0477	Antidiabetic
GLYBUR <> 477477	Tab, White, Oblong, Scored	Glyburide 1.25 mg	DiaBeta by Blue Ridge	59273-0015	Antidiabetic
GLYGLY <> ALBERT	Tab, White, Round, Scored, Gly over Gly <> Albert Logo	Glyburide 2.5 mg	Glynase by AltiMed	Canadian DIN 01900927	Antidiabetic
GLYNASE15 <> PT	Tab, White, Oval, Scored, Glynase over 1.5	Glyburide 1.5 mg	Glynase by Pharmacia	00009-0341	Antidiabetic
GLYNASE3 <> PTPT	Tab, Blue, Oblong, Scored, Film Coated, Glynase over 3	Glyburide 3 mg	Glynase by Kiel	59063-0111	Antidiabetic
GLYNASE3 <> PTPT	Tab, Blue, Oblong, Scored, Film Coated, Glynase over 3	Glyburide 3 mg	Glynase by Amerisource	62584-0352	Antidiabetic
GLYNASE3 <> PTPT	Tab, Blue, Oblong, Scored, Film Coated, Glynase over 3	Glyburide 3 mg	Glynase by Nat Pharmpak	55154-3909	Antidiabetic
GLYNASE3 <> PTPT	Tab, Blue, Oblong, Scored, Film Coated, Glynase over 3	Glyburide 3 mg	Glynase by Pharmacia	00009-0352	Antidiabetic

ID FRONT <> BACK	DESCRIPTION FRONT <> BACK	INGREDIENT & STRENGTH	BRAND (or Generic Equiv.) by FIRM	NDC#	CLASS; SCH.
GLYNASE3 <> PTPT	Tab, Blue, Oblong, Scored, Film Coated, Glynase over 3	Glyburide 3 mg	Glynase by Thrift Drug	59198-0171	Antidiabetic
GLYNASE3 <> PTPT	Tab, Blue, Oblong, Scored, Film Coated, Glynase over 3	Glyburide 3 mg	Glynase by Allscripts		Antidiabetic
GLYNASE3 <> PTPT	Tab, Blue, Oblong, Scored, Film Coated, Glynase over 3	Glyburide 3 mg	Glynase by Drug Distr	52985-0224	Antidiabetic
GLYNASE3 <> PTPT	Tab, Blue, Oblong, Scored, Film Coated, Glynase over 3	Glyburide 3 mg	Glynase by Physician Total Care	54868-3017	Antidiabetic
GLYNASE3 <> PTPT	Tab, Blue, Oblong, Scored, Film Coated, Glynase over 3	Glyburide 3 mg	Glynase by Pharmacia	00009-3449	Antidiabetic
GLYNASE6 <> PTPT	Tab, Yellow to Light Green, Oblong, Scored, Glynase over 6	Glyburide 6 mg	Glynase by Kaiser	00179-1332	Antidiabetic
GLYNASE6 <> PTPT	Tab, Yellow to Light Green, Oblong, Scored, Glynase over 6	Glyburide 6 mg	Glynase by Nat Pharmpak	55154-3917	Antidiabetic
GLYNASE6 <> PTPT	Tab, Yellow to Light Green, Oblong, Scored, Glynase over 6	Glyburide 6 mg	Glynase by Drug Distr	52985-0225	Antidiabetic
GLYNASE6 <> PTPT	Tab, Yellow to Light Green, Oblong, Scored, Glynase over 6	Glyburide 6 mg	Glynase by DRX	55045-2338	Antidiabetic
GLYNASE6 <> PTPT	Tab, Yellow to Light Green, Oblong, Scored, Glynase over 6	Glyburide 6 mg	Glynase by Repack Co of America	55306-3449	Antidiabetic
GLYNASE6 <> PTPT	Tab, Yellow to Light Green, Oblong, Scored, Glynase over 6	Glyburide 6 mg	Glynase by Physician Total Care	54868-3711	Antidiabetic
GLYNASE6 <> PTPT	Tab, Yellow to Light Green, Oblong, Scored, Glynase over 6	Glyburide 6 mg	Glynase by Compumed	00403-4629	Antidiabetic
GLYNASE6 <> PTPT	Tab, Yellow to Light Green, Oblong, Scored, Glynase over 6	Glyburide 6 mg	Glynase by Thrift Drug	59198-0003	Antidiabetic
GLYNASE6 <> PTPT	Tab, Yellow to Light Green, Oblong, Scored, Glynase over 6	Glyburide 6 mg	Glynase by Allscripts		Antidiabetic
GLYNASE6 <> PTPT	Tab, Yellow to Light Green, Oblong, Scored, Glynase over 6	Glyburide 6 mg	Glynase by Rightpac	65240-0723	Antidiabetic
GLYNASE6 <> PTPT	Tab, Yellow to Light Green, Oblong, Scored, Glynase over 6	Glyburide 6 mg	Glynase by Leiner	59606-0723	Antidiabetic
GLYNASE6 <> PTPT	Tab, Yellow to Light Green, Oblong, Scored, Glynase over 6	Glyburide 6 mg	Glynase by Amerisource	62584-0449	Antidiabetic
GLYNASE6 <> PTPT	Tab, Yellow to Light Green, Oblong, Scored, Glynase over 6	Glyburide 6 mg	Glynase by Kaiser	62224-7447	Antidiabetic
GLYSET <> 100	Tab, White, Round	Miglitol 100 mg	Glyset by Pharmacia	00009-5014	Antidiabetic
GLYSET <> 25	Tab, White, Round	Miglitol 25 mg	Glyset by Pharmacia	00009-5012	Antidiabetic
GLYSET <> 50	Tab, White, Round	Miglitol 50 mg	Glyset by Pharmacia	00009-5013	Antidiabetic
GM1	Tab, White, Cap Shaped	Chlorpheniramine Maleate 2 mg, Phenylephrine HCl 10 mg, Pyrilamine Maleate 10 mg	Phena-Plus by GM Pharma	58809-0281	Cold Remedy
GMZ <> 500	Tab, Blue, Oval, Film Coated	Metformin HCl 500 mg	Glumetza by Depomed	13913-0002	Antidiabetic
GP0026	Cap, Blue and White, Black Print	Cefaclor 250 mg	Ceclor by Ivax	00172-4770	Antibiotic
GP0027	Cap, Blue and Gray, Black Print	Cefaclor 500 mg	Ceclor by Ivax	00172-4771	Antibiotic
GP10	Tab, White, Round, G/P 10	Pindolol 10 mg	Visken by Par		Antihypertensive
GP10 <> G	Tab	Glipizide 10 mg	by Par	49884-0452	Antidiabetic
GP10G	Tab, White, Oval	Glipizide 10 mg	Glucotrol by Par		Antidiabetic
GP111	Tab, White, Round	Lisinopril 2.5 mg	Prinivil by Sandoz	00781-1669	Antihypertensive
GP112	Tab, Pink, Round	Lisinopril 5 mg	Prinivil by Sandoz	00781-1665	Antihypertensive
GP113	Tab, White, Round	Lisinopril 10 mg	Prinivil by Sandoz	00781-1666	Antihypertensive
GP114	Tab, Peach, Round	Lisinopril 20 mg	Prinivil by Sandoz	00781-1667	Antihypertensive
GP115	Tab, Rose, Round	Lisinopril 40 mg	Prinivil by Sandoz	00781-1668	Antihypertensive
GP118	Tab, White, Round, Scored, GP over 118	Mefloquine HCl 250 mg	Lariam by Sandoz	00781-5076	Antiprotozoal
GP121	Tab, Blue, Round	Lisinopril 10 mg, HCTZ 12.5 mg	Prinzide by Sandoz	00781-1848	Antihypertensive; Diuretic
GP122	Tab, Yellow, Round	Lisinopril 20 mg, HCTZ 12.5 mg	Prinzide by Sandoz	00781-1176	Antihypertensive; Diuretic
GP123	Tab, Peach, Round	Lisinopril 20 mg, HCTZ 25 mg	Prinzide by Sandoz	00781-1178	Antihypertensive; Diuretic
GP124	Tab, White, Round, Film Coated, GP over 124	Metformin HCl 500 mg	Glucophage by Sandoz	00781-5050	Antidiabetic
GP127	Tab, White, Round, Film Coated, GP over 127	Metformin HCl 850 mg	Glucophage by Sandoz	00781-5051	Antidiabetic
GP128	Tab, White, Oval, Scored, Film Coated, GP / 128	Metformin HCl 1000 mg	Glucophage by Sandoz	00781-5052	Antidiabetic
GP141	Tab, White, Round, Film Coated, GP over 141	Fluvoxamine Maleate 25 mg	Luvox by Sandoz	00781-5040	OCD
GP142	Tab, White, Round, Film Coated, GP over 142	Fluvoxamine Maleate 50 mg	Luvox by Sandoz	00781-5041	OCD
GP143	Tab, White, Round, Film Coated, GP over 142	Fluvoxamine Maleate 100 mg	Luvox by Sandoz	00781-5042	OCD
GP147	Tab, Yellow, Oval	Bisoprolol 2.5 mg, Hydrochlorothiazide 6.25 mg	Ziac by Sandoz	00781-1841	Antihypertensive; Diuretic
GP148	Tab, Tan, Oval	Bisoprolol 5 mg, Hydrochlorothiazide 6.25 mg	Ziac by Sandoz	00781-1824	Antihypertensive; Diuretic
GP149	Tab, White, Oval	Bisoprolol 10 mg, Hydrochlorothiazide 6.25 mg	Ziac by Sandoz	00781-1833	Antihypertensive; Diuretic
GP150	Tab, Peach, Round	Lisinopril 30 mg	Prinivil by Sandoz	00781-1673	Antihypertensive
GP151	Tab, White, Round, Scored,	Doxazosin Mesylate 1 mg	Cardura by Sandoz	00781-5001	Antihypertensive

ID FRONT <> BACK	DESCRIPTION FRONT <> BACK	INGREDIENT & STRENGTH	BRAND (or Generic Equiv.) by FIRM	NDC#	CLASS; SCH.
GP152	Tab, Yellow, Round, Scored	Doxazosin Mesylate 2 mg	Cardura by Sandoz	00781-5002	Antihypertensive
GP153	Tab, Beige, Round, Scored	Doxazosin Mesylate 4 mg	Cardura by Sandoz	00781-5003	Antihypertensive
GP154	Tab, Light Green, Round, Scored	Doxazosin Mesylate 8 mg	Cardura by Sandoz	00781-5004	Antihypertensive
GP158	Tab, White, Oval, Film Coated	Nabumetone 500 mg	Relafen by Sandoz	00781-1306	NSAID
GP159	Tab, White, Oval, Film Coated	Nabumetone 750 mg	Relafen by Sandoz	00781-1308	NSAID
GP160	Tab, White, Round	Flecainide Acetate 50 mg	Tambocor by Sandoz	00781-5062	Antiarrhythmic
GP161	Tab, White, Round, Scored	Flecainide Acetate 100 mg	Tambocor by Sandoz	00781-5063	Antiarrhythmic
GP162	Tab, White, Oval, Scored	Flecainide Acetate 150 mg	Tambocor by Sandoz	00781-5064	Antiarrhythmic
GP3	Tab, Peach, Round, Film Coated	Cephalexin 250 mg	by Pharmascience	Canadian DIN 5760677812	Antibiotic
GP300	Cap, Maroon	Vitamin, Iron	Ferrogen by Tishcon		Vitamin
GP4	Tab, Peach, Oval, Scored, Film Coated	Cephalexin 500 mg	by Pharmascience	Canadian	Antibiotic
GP400	Tab, White, Round	Magnesium Oxide 400 mg	Magnesium Oxide by Rising	68585-0006	Supplement
GP5	Tab, White, Round, G/P 5	Pindolol 5 mg	Gen Pindolol by Genpharm	Canadian	Antihypertensive
GP5	Tab, White, Round, G/P 5	Pindolol 5 mg	Visken by Par		Antihypertensive
GP5 <> G	Tab,	Glipizide 5 mg	by Par	49884-0451	Antidiabetic
GP5G	Tab, White, Oval	Glipizide 5 mg	Glucotrol by Par		Antidiabetic
GPCM200	Tab, Green, Round, G/p CM 200	Cimetidine HCl 200 mg	Tagamet by Genpharm	Canadian	Gastrointestinal
GPCM300	Tab, Green, Round, G/p CM 300	Cimetidine HCl 300 mg	Tagamet by Genpharm	Canadian	Gastrointestinal
GPCM400	Tab, Green, Ellipsoid, G/p CM 400	Cimetidine HCl 400 mg	Tagamet by Genpharm	Canadian	Gastrointestinal
GPCM600	Tab, Green, Ellipsoid, G/p CM 600	Cimetidine HCl 600 mg	Tagamet by Genpharm	Canadian	Gastrointestinal
GPCM800	Tab, Green, Ellipsoid, G/p CM 800	Cimetidine HCl 800 mg	Tagamet by Genpharm	Canadian	Gastrointestinal
GPI <> A325	Tab, Orange, Round	Diphenhydramine HCl 25 mg	Benadryl by Gemini		Antihistamine
GPI <> S1	Tab, White with Green Specks	Acetaminophen 325 mg, Phenylephrine HCl 5 mg, Chlorpheniramine Maleate 2 mg	Super Cold Tabs by Reese	10956-0771	Cold Remedy
GPI <> W2	Tab, Light Brown, Round	Sennosides 8.6 mg	Senokot by Amneal	65162-0440	Gastrointestinal
GPIA325	Tab, White, Round	Acetaminophen 325 mg	Tylenol by Amneal	65162-0350	Analgesic
GPIA5	Tab, White, Round, Scored, GPI / A5	Acetaminophen 500 mg	Tylenol ES by Amneal	65162-0602 Discontinued	Analgesic
GPIA5	Tab, White, Oblong	Acetaminophen 500 mg	Tylenol ES by Amneal		Analgesic
GPILB	Tab, White, Round, Chewable	Simethicone 80 mg	Mylicon-80 by Amneal	65162-0443	Antiflatulent
GR1 <> APO	Tab, White to Off White, Triangular, Film Coated	Granisetron 1 mg	Apo-Granisetron by Apotex	Canadian DIN 02308894	Antiemetic
GRISACTIN <> 330	Tab	Griseofulvin 330 mg	Grisactin Ultra by Pharm Util	60491-0290	Antifungal
GRISACTIN250	Cap	Griseofulvin 250 mg	Fulvicin P/G by Pharmedix	53002-0277	Antifungal
GRISACTIN500	Tab, Pink, Round	Griseofulvin 500 mg	Grisactin by Ayerst	00046-0444	Antifungal
GRISACTINULTRA250	Tab, White, Rounded Square, Grisactin over Ultra over 250	Griseofulvin, Ultramicrosize 250 mg	Fulvicin P/G by Ayerst	00046-0435	Antifungal
GRISPEG <> 125	Tab, White, Elliptical, Film Coated, Scored	Griseofulvin 125 mg	Gris-PEG by Allergan	00023-0763	Antifungal
GRISPEG <> 125	Tab, White, Elliptical, Film Coated, Scored	Griseofulvin 125 mg	Fulvicin P/G by Novartis	00043-0800	Antifungal
GRISPEG <> 250	Tab, White, Cap Shaped, Film Coated, Gris-Peg <> 250, Scored	Griseofulvin 250 mg	Fulvicin P/G by Novartis	00043-0801	Antifungal
GRISPEG <> 250	Tab, White, Cap Shaped, Film Coated, Gris-Peg <> 250, Scored	Griseofulvin 250 mg	Fulvicin P/G by Allergan	00023-0773	Antifungal
GRISPEG <> 250	Tab, White, Cap Shaped, Film Coated, Gris-Peg <> 250, Scored	Griseofulvin 250 mg	Fulvicin P/G by Amerisource	62584-0773	Antifungal
GRISPEG <> 250	Tab, White, Cap Shaped, Film Coated, Gris-Peg <> 250, Scored	Griseofulvin 250 mg	Fulvicin P/G by Leiner	59606-0654	Antifungal
GS	Tab	Metronidazole 500 mg	by Patient First	57575-0089	Antibiotic

ID FRONT <> BACK	DESCRIPTION FRONT <> BACK	INGREDIENT & STRENGTH	BRAND (or Generic Equiv.) by FIRM	NDC#	CLASS; SCH.
G/S	Tab, Blue, Round, Scored	Bisacodyl 5 mg, Docusate Sodium 50 mg	Gentlax S by Purdue Pharma	Canadian DIN 02252872	Laxative
GS <> 25C	Tab, White to Pale Yellow, Round, Effervescent	Ranitidine HCl 25 mg	Zantac Efferdose by GSK	00173-0734	Gastrointestinal
GS <> 3V2	Tab, Pink, Cap Shaped, Film Coated	Ropinirole HCl 2 mg	Requip XL by GSK	00007-4885	Antiparkinson
GS <> 5CC	Tab, Red, Cap Shaped, Film Coated	Ropinirole HCl 8 mg	Requip XL by GSK	00007-4888	Antiparkinson
GS <> K2C	Tab, Pale Pink, Square, Film Coated	Ambrisentan 5 mg	Volibris by GSK	Canadian DIN 02307065	Antihypertensive
GS <> KE3	Tab, Deep Pink, Oval, Film Coated	Ambrisentan 10 mg	Volibris by GSK	Canadian DIN 02307073	Antihypertensive
GS <> S160	Tab, White, Oblong	Sotalol HCl 160 mg	by Genpharm	55567-0058	Antiarrhythmic
GS <> WXG	Tab, Light Brown, Cap Shaped, Film Coated	Ropinirole HCl 4 mg	Requip XL by GSK	00007-4887	Antiparkinson
GS160	Tab, Blue, Oblong, G/S/160	Sotalol HCl 160 mg	by Genpharm	Canadian	Antiarrhythmic
GS240	Tab, Blue, Oblong, G/S/240	Sotalol HCl 240 mg	by Genpharm	Canadian	Antiarrhythmic
GS7CZ	Cap, Brown and Orange, Oblong	Dutasteride 0.5 mg, Tamsulosin HCl 0.4 mg	Jalyn by GlaxoSmithKline (GSK)	00173-0809	Androgen Hormone Inhibitor; Antiadrenergic
GS80	Tab, Blue, Oblong, G/S/80	Sotalol HCl 80 mg	by Genpharm	Canadian	Antiarrhythmic
GSCL2 <> 5	Tab, White to Off-White, Oblong	Lamotrigine 5 mg	Lamictal by GSK	Canadian DIN 02240115	Anticonvulsant
GSFC2	Tab, Orange, Cap Shaped, Film Coated	Abacavir Sulfate 600 mg, Lamivudine 300 mg	Kivexa by GSK	Canadian DIN 02269341	Antiviral
GSFC2	Tab, Orange, Cap Shaped, Film Coated	Abacavir Sulfate 600 mg, Lamivudine 300 mg	Epzicom by GSK	00173-0742	Antiviral
GSI <> 5	Tab, Pale Pink, Square	Ambrisentan 5 mg	Letairis by Gilead	61958-0801	Antihypertensive
GSJT	Tab, Gray, Cap Shaped, Film Coated	Pazopanib 200 mg	Votrient by GSK	Canadian	Cancer Treatment
GSJT	Tab, Gray, Cap Shaped, Film Coated	Pazopanib 200 mg	Votrient by GSK	00173-0804	Cancer Treatment
GSK <> 1500	Tab, Yellow, Oval, Film Coated, 1/500	Metformin HCl 500 mg, Rosiglitazone 1 mg	Avandamet by GSK	Canadian DIN 02247085	Antidiabetic
GSK <> 1500	Tab, Yellow, Oval, Film Coated, 1/500	Metformin HCl 500 mg, Rosiglitazone 1 mg	Avandamet by SKB	00007-3166	Antidiabetic
GSK <> 21000	Tab, Yellow, Oval, Film Coated, 2/1000	Metformin HCl 1000 mg, Rosiglitazone 2 mg	Avandamet by SKB	00007-3163	Antidiabetic
GSK <> 21000	Tab, Yellow, Oval, Film Coated, 2/1000	Metformin HCl 1000 mg, Rosiglitazone 2 mg	Avandamet by GSK	Canadian DIN 02248440	Antidiabetic
GSK <> 2500	Tab, Pink, Oval, Film Coated, 2/500	Metformin HCl 500 mg, Rosiglitazone 2 mg	Avandamet by GSK	Canadian DIN 02247086	Antidiabetic
GSK <> 2500	Tab, Pink, Oval, Film Coated, 2/500	Metformin HCl 500 mg, Rosiglitazone 2 mg	Avandamet by SKB	00007-3167	Antidiabetic
GSK <> 41	Tab, Yellow, Triangular (Rounded), GSK <> 4/1	Rosiglitazone Maleate 4 mg, Glimepiride 1 mg	Avandaryl by GSK	00007-3151	Antidiabetic
GSK <> 41	Tab, Yellow, Triangular (Rounded), GSK <> 4/1	Rosiglitazone Maleate 4 mg, Glimepiride 1 mg	Avandaryl by GSK	Canadian DIN 02258781	Antidiabetic
GSK <> 41000	Tab, Pink, Oval, Film Coated, 4/1000	Metformin HCl 1000 mg, Rosiglitazone 4 mg	Avandamet by GSK	Canadian DIN 02248441	Antidiabetic
GSK <> 41000	Tab, Pink, Oval, Film Coated, 4/1000	Metformin HCl 1000 mg, Rosiglitazone 4 mg	Avandamet by SKB	00007-3164	Antidiabetic
GSK <> 42	Tab, Orange, Triangular (Rounded), GSK <> 4/2	Rosiglitazone Maleate 4 mg, Glimepiride 2 mg	Avandaryl by GSK	00007-3152	Antidiabetic
GSK <> 42	Tab, Orange, Triangular (Rounded), GSK <> 4/2	Rosiglitazone Maleate 4 mg, Glimepiride 2 mg	Avandaryl by GSK	Canadian DIN 02258803	Antidiabetic
GSK <> 44	Tab, Pink, Triangular (Rounded), GSK <> 4/4	Rosiglitazone Maleate 4 mg, Glimepiride 4 mg	Avandaryl by GSK	Canadian DIN 02258811	Antidiabetic
GSK <> 44	Tab, Pink, Triangular (Rounded), GSK <> 4/4	Rosiglitazone Maleate 4 mg, Glimepiride 4 mg	Avandaryl by GSK	00007-3153	Antidiabetic
GSK <> 4500	Tab, Orange, Oval, Film Coated, 4/500	Metformin HCl 500 mg, Rosiglitazone 4 mg	Avandamet by GSK	Canadian DIN 02247087	Antidiabetic
GSK <> 4500	Tab, Orange, Oval, Film Coated, 4/500	Metformin HCl 500 mg, Rosiglitazone 4 mg	Avandamet by SKB	00007-3168	Antidiabetic
GSKCOREGCR10MG	Cap, White and Green	Carvedilol 10 mg	Coreg CR by GSK	00007-3370	Antihypertensive
GSKCOREGCR20MG	Cap, White and Yellow	Carvedilol 20 mg	Coreg CR by GSK	00007-3371	Antihypertensive
GSKCOREGCR40MG	Cap, Yellow and Green	Carvedilol 40 mg	Coreg CR by GSK	00007-3372	Antihypertensive

ID FRONT <> BACK	DESCRIPTION FRONT <> BACK	INGREDIENT & STRENGTH	BRAND (or Generic Equiv.) by FIRM	NDC#	CLASS; SCH.
GSKCOREGCR80MG	Cap, White	Carvedilol 80 mg	Coreg CR by GSK	00007-3373	Antihypertensive
GSNX325	Tab, Orange, Round, Film Coated	Eltrombopag 25 mg	Promacta by GSK	00007-4640	Clotting Agent
GSR	Cap, Orange, Abbott Logo	Fenofibrate 200 mg	Tricor Micronized by Integrity	64731-0187	Antihyperlipidemic
GSUFU50	Tab, Blue, Round, Film Coated	Eltrombopag 50 mg	Promacta by GSK	00007-4641	Clotting Agent
GSUHL	Tab, Yellow, Cap Shaped, Film Coated	Pazopanib 400 mg	Votrient by GSK	00173-0805	Cancer Treatment
GSXJG	Tab, Orange, Oval, Film Coated	Lapatinib 250 mg	Tykerb by GSK	00173-0752	Cancer Treatment
GSYYG	Tab, Blue, Film Coated	Sumatriptan Succinate 119 mg, Naproxen Sodium 500 mg	Treximet by GSK	00173-0750	Anti-inflammatory
GT12 <> G	Tab, White, Round, Film Coated	Galantamine 12 mg	Razadyne by UDL	51079-0471	Antialzheimers
GT4 <> G	Tab, White, Round, Film Coated	Galantamine 4 mg	Razadyne by UDL	51079-0469 Discontinued	Antialzheimers
GT4 <> G	Tab, White, Round	Galantamine 4 mg	Razadyne by Mylan	00378-8104	Antialzheimers
GT8 <> G	Tab, White, Round, Film Coated	Galantamine 8 mg	Razadyne by UDL	51079-0470	Antialzheimers
GTN10	Tab, White, Round, G TN/10	Tamoxifen Citrate 10 mg	Nolvadex by Genpharm		Antiestrogen
GTN20	Tab, White, Octagonal, G TN/20	Tamoxifen Citrate 20 mg	Nolvadex by Genpharm		Antiestrogen
GU1 <> G	Tab, White, Oval	Guanfacine HCl 1 mg	Tenex by Par	49884-0572	Antihypertensive
GU1 <> G	Tab, White, Oval	Guanfacine HCl 1 mg	Tenex by Genpharm	55567-0051	Antihypertensive
GU2 <> G	Tab, White, Oval	Guanfacine HCl 2 mg	Tenex by Par	49884-0573	Antihypertensive
GU2 <> G	Tab, White, Oval	Guanfacine HCl 2 mg	Tenex by Genpharm	55567-0052	Antihypertensive
GUAIFEDMURO120250	Cap, Clear & White, Ex Release	Guaifenesin 250 mg, Pseudoephedrine HCl 120 mg	Sudafed Sinus by Thrift Drug	59198-0192	Cold Remedy
GUAIFEDMURO120250	Cap, Clear & White, Ex Release	Guaifenesin 250 mg, Pseudoephedrine HCl 120 mg	Sudafed Sinus by Muro	00451-4002	Cold Remedy
GUAIFEDMURO120250	Cap, Clear & White, Ex Release	Guaifenesin 250 mg, Pseudoephedrine HCl 120 mg	Sudafed Sinus by Nat Pharmpak	55154-4302	Cold Remedy
GUAIFEDMURO120250	Cap, Clear & White, Ex Release	Guaifenesin 250 mg, Pseudoephedrine HCl 120 mg	Sudafed Sinus by Rx Pak	65084-0213	Cold Remedy
GUAIFEDPDMURO60300	Cap, Blue & Clear	Guaifenesin 300 mg, Pseudoephedrine HCl 60 mg	Sudafed Sinus by Thrift Drug	59198-0191	Cold Remedy
GUAIFEDPDMURO60300	Cap, Blue & Clear	Guaifenesin 300 mg, Pseudoephedrine HCl 60 mg	Sudafed Sinus by Muro	00451-4003	Cold Remedy
GUAIFEDPDMURO60300	Cap, Blue & Clear	Guaifenesin 300 mg, Pseudoephedrine HCl 60 mg	Sudafed Sinus by Martec		Cold Remedy
GUAIFEDPDMURO60300	Cap, Blue & Clear	Guaifenesin 300 mg, Pseudoephedrine HCl 60 mg	Sudafed Sinus by Pharmedix	53002-0623	Cold Remedy
GUAIFEDPDMURO60300	Cap, Blue & Clear	Guaifenesin 300 mg, Pseudoephedrine HCl 60 mg	Sudafed Sinus by Martec		Cold Remedy
GUAIFEDPDMURO60300	Cap, Blue & Clear	Guaifenesin 300 mg, Pseudoephedrine HCl 120 mg	Sudafed Sinus by Nat Pharmpak	55154-4303	Cold Remedy
GUAIMAXD <> SP2055	Tab, White to Off-White, Cap Shaped, Scored	Guaifenesin 600 mg, Pseudoephedrine HCl 120 mg	Guaimax-D by Schwarz	00131-2055	Cold Remedy
GW <> GEIGY	Tab, White to Off-White, Cap Shaped, Scored	Baclofen 20 mg	Lioresal by Geigy	Canadian DIN 00636576	Muscle Relaxant
GX623	Tab, Yellow, Oblong, Convex, Film Coated	Abacavir Sulfate 300 mg	Ziagen by Abbott	60692-3870	Antiviral
GX623	Tab, Yellow, Oblong, Convex, Film Coated	Abacavir Sulfate 300 mg	Ziagen by Abbott	60692-3869	Antiviral
GX623	Tab, Yellow, Cap Shaped, Film Coated	Abacavir 300 mg	Ziagen by GSK	Canadian DIN 02240357	Antiviral
GX623	Tab, Yellow, Cap Shaped, Film Coated	Abacavir 300 mg	Ziagen by GSK	00173-0661	Antiviral
GXCC1	Cap, White to Off-White, Opaque	Amprenavir 50 mg	Agenerase by GSK	00173-0679	Antiviral
GXCC1	Cap, White to Off-White, Opaque	Amprenavir 50 mg	Agenerase by GSK	Canadian DIN 02243541	Antiviral
GXCC1	Cap, White to Off-White, Opaque	Amprenavir 50 mg	Agenerase by Block Drug	10158-0428	Antiviral
GXCC2	Cap, White to Off-White, Opaque	Amprenavir 150 mg	Agenerase by Biovail	62660-0025	Antiviral
GXCC2	Cap, White to Off-White, Opaque	Amprenavir 150 mg	Agenerase by GSK	Canadian DIN 02243542	Antiviral
GXCC2	Cap, White to Off-White, Opaque	Amprenavir 150 mg	Agenerase by GSK	00173-0672	Antiviral
GXCE2	Cap, Oblong, Opaque, Yellow, Gelatin	Dutasteride 0.5 mg	Avodart by GSK	00173-0712	Androgen Hormone Inhibitor
GXCE2	Cap, Oblong, Opaque, Yellow, Gelatin	Dutasteride 0.5 mg	Avodart by GSK	Canadian DIN 02247813	Androgen Hormone Inhibitor
GXCE3	Tab, D Shaped, White, Film Coated	Naratriptan HCl 1 mg	Amerge by GSK	Canadian DIN 02237820	Antimigraine

ID FRONT <> BACK	DESCRIPTION FRONT <> BACK	INGREDIENT & STRENGTH	BRAND (or Generic Equiv.) by FIRM	NDC#	CLASS; SCH.
GXCE3	Tab, D Shaped, White, Film Coated	Naratriptan HCl 1 mg	Amerge by GSK	00173-0561	Antimigraine
GXCE3	Tab, D Shaped, White, Film Coated	Naratriptan HCl 1 mg	Amerge by GSK	51947-8291	Antimigraine
GXCE5	Tab, D-Shaped, Green, Film Coated	Naratriptan HCl 2.5 mg	Amerge by GSK	00173-0562	Antimigraine
GXCE5	Tab, D-Shaped, Green, Film Coated	Naratriptan HCl 2.5 mg	Amerge by GSK	51947-8290	Antimigraine
GXCE5	Tab, D-Shaped, Green, Film Coated	Naratriptan HCl 2.5 mg	Amerge by GSK	Canadian DIN 02237821	Antimigraine
GXCF2	Tab, White, Cap Shaped, Film Coated	Valacyclovir HCl 1000 mg	Valtrex by GSK	Canadian DIN 02246559	Antiviral
GXCF7 <> 24	Tab, Pink, Oval	Ondansetron HCl 24 mg	Zofran by GSK	00173-0680	Antiemetic
GXCG5	Tab, Butterscotch, Film Coated, Cap Shaped	Lamivudine 100 mg	Heptovir by GSK	Canadian DIN 02239193	Antiviral
GXCG5	Tab, Butterscotch, Film Coated, Cap Shaped	Lamivudine 100 mg	Epivir by GSK	00173-0662	Antiviral
GXCG5	Tab, Butterscotch, Film Coated, Cap Shaped	Lamivudine 100 mg	Epivir by GSK	53873-0662	Antiviral
GXCG5	Tab, Butterscotch, Film Coated, Cap Shaped	Lamivudine 100 mg	Epivir by Murfreesboro	51129-1623	Antiviral
GXCG5	Tab, Butterscotch, Film Coated, Cap Shaped	Lamivudine 100 mg	Epivir by Murfreesboro	51129-1621	Antiviral
GXCG7	Tab, Pink, Round	Atovaquone 62.5 mg, Proguanil HCl 25 mg	Malarone by GSK	00173-0676	Antiprotozoal
GXCG7	Tab, Pink, Round	Atovaquone 62.5 mg, Proguanil HCl 25 mg	Malarone by GSK	53873-0676	Antiprotozoal
GXCG7	Tab, Pink, Round	Atovaquone 62.5 mg, Proguanil HCl 25 mg	Malarone by GSK	Canadian DIN 02264935	Antiprotozoal
GXCJ7	Tab, White, Diamond Shaped, Film Coated	Lamivudine 150 mg	Epivir by Murfreesboro	51129-1619	Antiviral
GXCJ7	Tab, White, Diamond Shaped, Film Coated	Lamivudine 150 mg	Epivir by GSK	00173-0470	Antiviral
GXCJ7	Tab, White, Diamond Shaped, Film Coated	Lamivudine 150 mg	Epivir by Physician Total Care	54868-3693	Antiviral
GXCJ7	Tab, White, Diamond Shaped, Film Coated	Lamivudine 150 mg	Epivir by St. Mary's Med	60760-0470	Antiviral
GXCJ7	Tab, White, Diamond Shaped, Film Coated	Lamivudine 150 mg	Epivir by Compumed	00403-4977	Antiviral
GXCJ7	Tab, White, Diamond Shaped, Film Coated	Lamivudine 150 mg	Epivir by Murfreesboro	51129-1624	Antiviral
GXCJ7	Tab, White, Diamond Shaped, Scored, Film Coated	Lamivudine 150 mg	3TC by GSK	Canadian DIN 02192683	Antiviral
GXCK3	Tab, White & Yellow, Round	Grepafloxacin HCl 200 mg	Raxar by GSK	Canadian	Antibiotic
GXCK3	Tab, Film Coated	Grepafloxacin HCl 200 mg	Raxar by GSK	00173-0566	Antibiotic
GXCK3	Tab, Film Coated	Grepafloxacin HCl 200 mg	Raxar by Otsuka	46602-0003	Antibiotic
GXCK5	Tab, Pale Yellow to White, Film Coated	Grepafloxacin HCl 400 mg	Raxar by GSK	00173-0657	Antibiotic
GXCK5	Tab, Pale Yellow to White, Film Coated	Grepafloxacin HCl 400 mg	Itmd Raxar Aqfc by GSK	51947-8295	Antibiotic
GXCK7	Tab, Film Coated	Grepafloxacin HCl 600 mg	Itmd Raxar Aqfc by GSK	51947-8296	Antibiotic
GXCK7	Tab, Pale Yellow to White, Film Coated	Grepafloxacin HCl 600 mg	Raxar by GSK	00173-0658	Antibiotic
GXCL2	Tab, White, Cap Shaped, Chewable	Lamotrigine 5 mg	Lamictal by GSK	00173-0526	Anticonvulsant
GXCL5	Tab, White, Oval, Chewable	Lamotrigine 25 mg	Lamictal by GSK	00173-0527	Anticonvulsant
GXCL7	Tab, White, Oval, Chewable	Lamotrigine 100 mg	Lamictal by GSK	00173-0539	Anticonvulsant
GXCM3	Tab, Pink, Round, Film Coated	Atovaquone 250 mg, Proguanil HCl 100 mg	Malarone by GSK	Canadian DIN 02238151	Antiprotozoal
GXCM3	Tab, Pink, Round, Film Coated	Atovaquone 250 mg, Proguanil HCl 100 mg	Malarone by GSK	00173-0675	Antiprotozoal
GXCM3	Tab, Pink, Round, Film Coated	Atovaquone 250 mg, Proguanil HCl 100 mg	Malarone by GSK	53873-0675	Antiprotozoal
GXCT1	Tab, Blue, Oval, Film Coated	Alosetron 1 mg	Lotronex by GSK	00173-0690	Gastrointestinal
GXCW3 <> 300	Tab, White, Round, Film Coated	Zidovudine 300 mg	Retrovir by DSM	63552-0501	Antiviral
GXCW3 <> 300	Tab, White, Round, Film Coated	Zidovudine 300 mg	Retrovir by GSK	00173-0501	Antiviral
GXCW3 <> 300	Tab, White, Round, Film Coated	Zidovudine 300 mg	Retrovir by DRX	55045-2488	Antiviral
GXCW3 <> 300	Tab, White, Round, Film Coated	Zidovudine 300 mg	Retrovir by Allscripts		Antiviral
GXEF3 <> M	Tab, White, Film-Coated, Round	Busulfan 2 mg	Myleran by GSK	Canadian DIN 00004618	Antineoplastic
GXEG2	Tab, White, Cap Shaped	Cefuroxime Axetil 500 mg	Ceftin by GSK	Canadian DIN 02212285	Antibiotic

ID FRONT <> BACK	DESCRIPTION FRONT <> BACK	INGREDIENT & STRENGTH	BRAND (or Generic Equiv.) by FIRM	NDC#	CLASS; SCH.
GXEG2	Tab, White, Cap Shaped	Cefuroxime Axetil 500 mg	Ceftin by GSK	00173-0394	Antibiotic
GXEG2	Tab, White, Cap Shaped	Cefuroxime Axetil 500 mg	Ceftin by Dava	67253-0781	Antibiotic
GXEG2	Tab, White, Cap Shaped	Cefuroxime Axetil 500 mg	Ceftin by Ivax	00182-2690 Discontinued	Antibiotic
GXEG3 <> L	Tab, Brown, Round, Film Coated, Needs to be Refrigerated	Chlorambucil 2 mg	Leukeran by GSK	Canadian DIN 00004626	Antineoplastic
GXEG3 <> L	Tab, Brown, Round, Film Coated, Needs to be Refrigerated	Chlorambucil 2 mg	Leukeran by GSK	00173-0635	Antineoplastic
GXEH3 <> A	Tab, White, Round, Requires refrigeration	Melphalan 2 mg	Alkeran by GSK	Canadian DIN 00004715	Antineoplastic
GXEH3 <> A	Tab, White, Round, Requires refrigeration	Melphalan 2 mg	Alkeran by GSK	59572-0302	Antineoplastic
GXEJ7	Tab, Gray, Diamond Shaped, Film Coated	Lamivudine 300 mg	Epivir by GSK	00173-0714	Antiviral
GXEJ7	Tab, Gray, Diamond Shaped, Film Coated	Lamivudine 300 mg	3TC by GSK	Canadian DIN 02247825	Antiviral
GXES7	Tab, White, Cap Shaped	Cefuroxime Axetil 250 mg	Ceftin by GSK	Canadian DIN 02212277	Antibiotic
GXES7	Tab, White, Cap Shaped	Cefuroxime Axetil 250 mg	Ceftin by Ivax	00182-2689 Discontinued	Antibiotic
GXES7	Tab, White, Cap Shaped	Cefuroxime Axetil 250 mg	Ceftin by Dava	67253-0780	Antibiotic
GXES7	Tab, White, Cap Shaped	Cefuroxime Axetil 250 mg	Ceftin by GSK	00173-0387	Antibiotic
GXEX1	Tab, White, Oval, Film Coated	Alosetron 0.5 mg	Lotronex by GSK	00173-0738	Gastrointestinal
GXFC3	Tab, White, Cap Shaped, Film Coated	Lamivudine 150 mg, Zidovudine 300 mg	Combivir by GSK	Canadian DIN 02239213	Antiviral
GXFC3	Tab, White, Cap Shaped, Film Coated	Lamivudine 150 mg, Zidovudine 300 mg	Combivir by GSK	00173-0595	Antiviral
GXLL1	Tab, Blue-Green, Cap Shaped, Film Coated	Abacavir Sulfate 300 mg, Lamivudine 150 mg, Zidovudine 300 mg	Trizivir by GSK	Canadian DIN 02244757	Antiviral
GXLL1	Tab, Blue-Green, Cap Shaped, Film Coated	Abacavir Sulfate 300 mg, Lamivudine 150 mg, Zidovudine 300 mg	Trizivir by GSK	00173-0691	Antiviral
GXLL7	Tab, Pink, Cap Shaped, Film Coated	Fosamprenavir 700 mg	Lexiva by GSK	00173-0721	Antiviral
GXLL7	Tab, Pink, Cap Shaped, Film Coated	Fosamprenavir 700 mg	Telzir by GSK	Canadian DIN 02261545	Antiviral
GZA10	Cap, White, Opaque	Zaleplon 10 mg	Sonata by Mylan	00378-6810	Sedative/Hypnotic
GZA5	Cap, Pink, Opaque	Zaleplon 5 mg	Sonata by Mylan	00378-6805	Sedative/Hypnotic
GZN100	Cap, Light Blue and Powder Blue	Zonisamide 100 mg	Zonegran by Genpharm	15330-0105	Anticonvulsant
GZN25	Cap, Light Blue and Powder Blue	Zonisamide 25 mg	Zonegran by Genpharm	15330-0103	Anticonvulsant
GZN50	Cap, Light Blue and Powder Blue	Zonisamide 50 mg	Zonegran by Genpharm	15330-0104	Anticonvulsant
H	Tab, White, Round	Black Cohosh (Cimicifuga Racemosa), Wild Yam (Dioscorea Villosa), Cuttlefish (Sepia), Adrenalin (Adrenalinum), Ovary (Oophorinum), Testis (Orchitinum), Bushmaster (Lachesis Mutis)	Estrex by Lake Consumer Products		Homeopathic
H	Tab, Coated	Ascorbic Acid 100 mg, Biotin, D- 300 mcg, Cyanocobalamin 6 mcg, Folic Acid 1000 mcg, Niacinamide 20 mg, Pantothenic Acid 10 mg, Pyridoxine HCl 10 mg, Riboflavin 1.7 mg, Thiamine Mononitrate 1.5 mg	Dailyvite Multi Vit by Hillestad	10542-0010	Vitamin
H <> 121	Tab, White, Round, Film Coated	Ropinirole HCl 0.25 mg	Requip by Heritage	23155-0121	Antiparkinson
H <> 122	Tab, Yellow, Round, Film Coated	Ropinirole HCl 0.5 mg	Requip by Heritage	23155-0122	Antiparkinson
H <> 123	Tab, Green, Round, Film Coated	Ropinirole HCl 1 mg	Requip by Heritage	23155-0123	Antiparkinson
H <> 124	Tab, Peach, Round, Film Coated	Ropinirole HCl 2 mg	Requip by Heritage	23155-0124	Antiparkinson
H <> 125	Tab, Purple, Round, Film Coated	Ropinirole HCl 3 mg	Requip by Heritage	23155-0125	Antiparkinson
H <> 126	Tab, Pale Brown, Round, Film Coated	Ropinirole HCl 4 mg	Requip by Heritage	23155-0126	Antiparkinson
H <> 127	Tab, Blue, Round, Film Coated	Ropinirole HCl 5 mg	Requip by Heritage	23155-0127	Antiparkinson
H <> HALDOL10MCNEIL	Tab, Aqua, H <> Haldol 10 McNeil	Haloperidol 10 mg	Haldol by McNeil	00045-0246	Antipsychotic
H <> HALDOL12MCNEIL	Tab, White, H <> Haldol 1/2 McNeil	Haloperidol 0.5 mg	Haldol by McNeil	00045-0240	Antipsychotic
H <> HALDOL1MCNEIL	Tab, Yellow, H <> Haldol 1 McNeil	Haloperidol 1 mg	Haldol by McNeil	00045-0241	Antipsychotic
H <> HALDOL20MCNEIL	Tab, Salmon, H <> Haldol 20 McNeil	Haloperidol 20 mg	Haldol by McNeil	00045-0248	Antipsychotic

ID FRONT <> BACK	DESCRIPTION FRONT <> BACK	INGREDIENT & STRENGTH	BRAND (or Generic Equiv.) by FIRM	NDC#	CLASS; SCH.
H <> HALDOL2MCNEIL	Tab, Pink, H <> Haldol 2 McNeil	Haloperidol 2 mg	Haldol by McNeil	00045-0242	Antipsychotic
H <> HALDOL5MCNEIL	Tab, Green, H <> Haldol 5 McNeil	Haloperidol 5 mg	Haldol by McNeil	00045-0245	Antipsychotic
H01 <> LU	Tab, Pink, Round, Scored	Trandolapril 1 mg	Mavik by Lupin	68180-0566	Antihypertensive
H02 <> LU	Tan, Yellow, Round	Trandolapril 2 mg	Mavik by Lupin	68180-0567	Antihypertensive
H03 <> LU	Tab, Brick Red, Round	Trandolapril 4 mg	Mavik by Lupin	68180-0568	Antihypertensive
H04	Tab, White, Round	Meperidine HCl 50 mg	Pethadol by Halsey		Analgesic; C II
H05	Tab, White, Round	Meperidine HCl 100 mg	Pethadol by Halsey		Analgesic; C II
H09	Cap, Brown & Orange	Erythromycin Estolate 250 mg	Ilosone by Eli Lilly		Antibiotic
H1	Tab, White, Cap Shaped	Naproxen 275 mg	Anaprox by Mova	55370-0918	NSAID
H1	Tab, White, Oblong, Film Coated	Naproxen 275 mg	Anaprox by West-Ward	00143-9916	NSAID
H1	Tab, Film Coated	Naproxen 275 mg	by AL Hikma	59115-0002	NSAID
H1	Tab, White, Round	Captopril 12.5 mg	Capoten by Hallmark		Antihypertensive
H1	Tab, White, Round	Captopril 12.5 mg	Capoten by Duramed	51285-0950	Antihypertensive
H10	Cap, Blue & Pink	Vitamin Combination	En-cebrin F by Eli Lilly		Vitamin
H105	Tab, White, Round, Film Coated	Hydroxyzine HCl 10 mg	Atarax by Heritage	23155-0105	Antianxiety; Antihistamine
H106	Tab, White, Round, Film Coated	Hydroxyzine HCl 25 mg	Atarax by Heritage	23155-0106	Antianxiety; Antihistamine
H107	Tab, White, Round, Film Coated	Hydroxyzine HCl 50 mg	Atarax by Heritage	23155-0107	Antianxiety; Antihistamine
H108	Cap, White, Soft Gel	Nimodipine 30 mg	Nimotop by Heritage	23155-0108	Antihypertensive
H11	Tab, White, Round	Captopril 25 mg	Capoten by Hallmark		Antihypertensive
H11	Tab, White, Round	Captopril 25 mg	Capoten by Duramed	51285-0951	Antihypertensive
H11 <> LL	Tab, Film Coated	Hydralazine HCl 25 mg	by Amerisource	62584-0733	Antihypertensive
H11 <> LL	Tab, Film Coated	Hydralazine HCl 25 mg	by Caremark	00339-5145	Antihypertensive
H11 <> LL	Tab, Film Coated	Hydralazine HCl 25 mg	by PDRX	55289-0133	Antihypertensive
H11 <> LL	Tab, Film Coated	Hydralazine HCl 25 mg	by Med Pro	53978-3051	Antihypertensive
H11 <> LU	Tab, White, Diamond-Shaped	Amlodipine Besylate 2.5 mg	Norvasc by Lupin	68180-0750	Antihypertensive
H111	Tab, Light Blue, H over 111	Hyoscyamine Sulfate 0.15 mg	Levsin by Econolab	55053-0111	Gastrointestinal
H111	Tab, White, Round	Captopril 50 mg	Capoten by Duramed	51285-0952	Antihypertensive
H112	Tab, White, Round	Captopril 100 mg	Capoten by Hallmark		Antihypertensive
H114	Tab, White, Round	Glipizide 5 mg	by Duramed	51285-0598	Antidiabetic
H115	Tab, White, Round	Glipizide 10 mg	by Duramed	51285-0599	Antidiabetic
H12	Tab, White, Round	Captopril 100 mg	Capoten by Duramed	51285-0953	Antihypertensive
H12 <> LL	Tab, Coated	Hydralazine HCl 50 mg	by UDL		Antihypertensive
H12 <> LU	Tab, White, Octagonal	Amlodipine Besylate 5 mg	Norvasc by Lupin	68180-0751	Antihypertensive
H124	Tab, Peach, Round	Hydrochlorothiazide 50 mg	Hydrodiuril by Heather		Diuretic; Antihypertensive
H12PF	Cap, Orange, H12/PF	Hydromorphone HCl 12 mg	by Purdue	Canadian	Analgesic; C II
H13 <> LU	Tab, White, Round	Amlodipine Besylate 10 mg	Norvasc by Lupin	68180-0752	Antihypertensive
H14 <> LL	Tab, Peach, Round, Scored, H over 14	Hydrochlorothiazide 25 mg	Hydrodiuril by Nat Pharmpak	55154-5574	Diuretic; Antihypertensive
H14 <> LL	Tab, Peach, Round, Scored, H over 14	Hydrochlorothiazide 25 mg	Hydrodiuril by Lederle	00005-3752	Diuretic; Antihypertensive
H14 <> LL	Tab, Peach, Round, Scored, H over 14	Hydrochlorothiazide 25 mg	Hydrodiuril by Murfreesboro	51129-1201	Diuretic; Antihypertensive
H14 <> LL	Tab, Peach, Round, Scored, H over 14	Hydrochlorothiazide 25 mg	Hydrodiuril by UDL	51079-0049	Diuretic; Antihypertensive
H15	Loz, Orange	Benzocaine 15 mg	Bi-Zets by Reese	10956-0713	Topical Anesthetic
H15	Loz, Cherry	Benzocaine 15 mg, Dextromethorphan HBr 10 mg	Tetra-Formula by Reese	10956-0749	Topical Anesthetic
H15 <> LL	Tab, Peach, Round, Scored, H over 15	Hydrochlorothiazide 50 mg	Hydrodiuril by Lederle	00005-3753	Diuretic; Antihypertensive
H15 <> LL	Tab, Peach, Round, Scored, H over 15	Hydrochlorothiazide 50 mg	Hydrodiuril by UDL	51079-0111	Diuretic; Antihypertensive
H15 <> LL	Tab, Peach, Round, Scored, H over 15	Hydrochlorothiazide 50 mg	Hydrodiuril by Amerisource	62584-0737	Diuretic; Antihypertensive
H17	Cap, White & Yellow	Nortriptyline HCl 10 mg	Aventyl HCl by Eli Lilly		Antidepressant
H17	Cap, White & Yellow	Nortriptyline HCl 10 mg	by Eli Lilly	Canadian	Antidepressant

ID FRONT <> BACK	DESCRIPTION FRONT <> BACK	INGREDIENT & STRENGTH	BRAND (or Generic Equiv.) by FIRM	NDC#	CLASS; SCH.
H187	Tab, Salmon, Round	Prednisolone 5 mg	Sterane by Heather		Steroid
H193	Tab, White, Round	Methocarbamol 500 mg	Robaxin by Heather		Muscle Relaxant
H196	Tab, Brown, Oblong	Methenamine Mandelate 500 mg	Mandelamine by Heather		Antibiotic; Urinary Tract
H2	Tab, White, Cap Shaped, Film Coated	Naproxen 550 mg	Anaprox by West-Ward	00143-9908	NSAID
H2	Tab, White, Cap Shaped, Film Coated	Naproxen 550 mg	Anaprox by AL Hikma	59115-0001	NSAID
H2	Tab, Peach, Round, Scored	Hydrochlorothiazide 25 mg	Hydrodiuril by Heritage	23155-0008	Diuretic; Antihypertensive
H202	Tab, White, Round	Sulfisoxazole 500 mg	Gantrisin by Heather		Antibiotic
H203	Cap, Black & Yellow	Tetracycline HCl 500 mg	Achromycin V by Heather		Antibiotic
H214	Cap, Orange & Yellow	Tetracycline HCl 250 mg	Achromycin V by Heather		Antibiotic
H214	Cap, Blue & Yellow	Tetracycline HCl 250 mg	Achromycin V by Heather		Antibiotic
H22	Tab, White, Round, Film Coated	Ciprofloxacin 250 mg	Cipro by West-Ward	00143-9927	Antibiotic
H23	Tab, White, Oblong	Ciprofloxacin 500 mg	Cipro by West-Ward	00143-9928	Antibiotic
H24	Tab, White, Cap Shaped, Film Coated	Ciprofloxacin 750 mg	Cipro by West-Ward	00143-9929	Antibiotic
H24PF	Cap, Gray, H24/PF	Hydromorphone HCl 24 mg	by Purdue	Canadian	Analgesic; C II
H25 <> M	Tab, Blue	Hydroxyzine HCl 25 mg	Atarax by UDL	51079-0806	Antianxiety; Antihistamine
H3	Tab, Peach, Round, Scored	Hydrochlorothiazide 50 mg	Hydrodiuril by Heritage	23155-0009	Diuretic; Antihypertensive
H303	Tab, White, Round	Acetaminophen 300 mg, Codeine 30 mg	Tylenol w/ Codeine by Ivax	00182-0948	Analgesic; C III
H304 <> 4	Tab, White, Round, Scored	Acetaminophen 300 mg, Codeine Phosphate 60 mg	Tylenol w/ Codeine by Barr	51285-0304	Analgesic; C III
H30PF	Cap, Red, H30/PF	Hydromorphone HCl 30 mg	by Purdue	Canadian	Analgesic; C II
H33	Tab, Chewable	Nickel Sulfate 1 X, Potassium Bromate 1 X, Zinc Bromide 4 X	Psorizide Ultra by Loma Lux	61480-0124	Supplement
H3647 <> 400	Tab, Light Orange, Oval, Film Coated	Telithromycin 400 mg	Ketek by Aventis	00088-2225	Antibiotic
H373	Tab, Film Coated, H 373	Guaifenesin 400 mg, Phenylpropanolamine HCl 75 mg	Entex LA by Huckaby	58407-0374	Cold Remedy
H3PF	Cap, Green, H3/PF	Hydromorphone HCl 3 mg	Hydromor Contin by Purdue	Canadian	Analgesic; C II
H4	Tab, White and Red, Oblong, Two Layered, Boehringer Logo H4	Telmisartan 40 mg, Hydrochlorothiazide 12.5 mg	Micardis HCT by Boehringer Ingelheim	00597-0043	Antihypertensive; Diuretic
H403	Tab, Green, Round	Sulfamethoxazole 500 mg	Gantanol by Heather		Antibiotic
H5	Tab, Yellow, Cap Shaped, Scored	Glyburide 6 mg	Glynase by West-Ward	00143-9920	Antidiabetic
H50 <> M	Tab, Blue	Hydroxyzine HCl 50 mg	Atarax by UDL	51079-0816	Antianxiety; Antihistamine
H501	Tab, White, Oblong	Methocarbamol 750 mg	Robaxin by Heather		Muscle Relaxant
H503	Tab, Purple, Oval	Methenamine Mandelate 1 g	Mandelamine by Heather		Antibiotic; Urinary Tract
H510	Tab, White, Oval	Methylprednisolone 4 mg	Medrol by Heather		Steroid
H513	Tab, White, Round	Cortisone Acetate 25 mg	Cortone Acetate by Heather		Steroid
H527	Tab, White, Round	Prednisone 50 mg	Deltasone by Heather		Steroid
H539	Cap, Aqua	Doxycycline Hyclate 100 mg	Doxycin by Genpharm	Canadian DIN 00817120	Antibiotic
H64	Cap, Pink	Propoxyphene Napsylate 100 mg	by Eli Lilly	Canadian	Analgesic; C IV
H69	Cap, Green & White	Cephalexin 250 mg	Keflex by Eli Lilly		Antibiotic
H6PF	Cap, Pink, H6/PF	Hydromorphone HCl 6 mg	by Purdue	Canadian	Analgesic; C II
H71	Cap, Green	Cephalexin 500 mg	Keflex by Eli Lilly		Antibiotic
H72	Cap, Black	Vitamin Combination	Theracebrin by Eli Lilly		Vitamin
H74	Cap, Blue	Ethinamate 500 mg	Valmid by Eli Lilly		Hypnotic; C IV
H76	Cap, White & Yellow	Fenoprofen Calcium 200 mg	Nalfon by Eli Lilly		NSAID
H77	Cap, Yellow	Fenoprofen Calcium 300 mg	Nalfon by Eli Lilly		NSAID
H8	Tab, White and Red, Oblong, Two Layered, Boehringer Logo H8	Telmisartan 80 mg, Hydrochlorothiazide 12.5 mg	Micardis HCT by Boehringer Ingelheim	00597-0044	Antihypertensive; Diuretic

ID FRONT <> BACK	DESCRIPTION FRONT <> BACK	INGREDIENT & STRENGTH	BRAND (or Generic Equiv.) by FIRM	NDC#	CLASS; SCH.
H9	Tab, White and Yellow, Oblong, Two Layered, Boehringer Logo H9	Telmisartan 80 mg, Hydrochlorothiazide 25 mg	Micardis HCT by Boehringer Ingelheim	00597-0042	Antihypertensive; Diuretic
HALCION0125	Tab, White, Oval, HALCION 0.125	Triazolam 0.125 mg	Halcion by Pharmedix	53002-0634	Sedative/Hypnotic; C IV
HALCION0125	Tab, White, Oval, HALCION 0.125	Triazolam 0.125 mg	Halcion by Pharmacia	00009-0010	Sedative/Hypnotic; C IV
HALCION025	Tab, Blue, Oval, Scored, HALCION 0.25	Triazolam 0.25 mg	Halcion by Pharmacia	00009-0017	Sedative/Hypnotic; C IV
HALCION025	Tab, Blue, Oval, Scored, HALCION 0.25	Triazolam 0.25 mg	Halcion by PDRX	55289-0128	Sedative/Hypnotic; C IV
HALCION025	Tab, Blue, Oval, Scored, HALCION 0.25	Triazolam 0.25 mg	Halcion by Pharmedix	53002-0380	Sedative/Hypnotic; C IV
HALDOL10MCNEIL <> H	Tab, Haldol 10 McNeil <> H	Haloperidol 10 mg	Haldol by McNeil	00045-0246	Antipsychotic
HALDOL12MCNEIL <> H	Tab, Haldol 1/2 McNeil <> H	Haloperidol 0.5 mg	Haldol by McNeil	00045-0240	Antipsychotic
HALDOL1MCNEIL <> H	Tab, Haldol 1 McNeil <> H	Haloperidol 1 mg	Haldol by McNeil	00045-0241	Antipsychotic
HALDOL20MCNEIL <> H	Tab, Salmon, Haldol 20 McNeil <> H	Haloperidol 20 mg	Haldol by McNeil	00045-0248	Antipsychotic
HALDOL2MCNEIL <> H	Tab, Haldol 2 McNeil <> H	Haloperidol 2 mg	Haldol by McNeil	00045-0242	Antipsychotic
HALDOL5MCNEIL <> H	Tab, Haldol 5 McNeil <> H	Haloperidol 5 mg	Haldol by McNeil	00045-0245	Antipsychotic
HALFAN	Tab, White to Off-White, Cap Shaped	Halofantrine HCl 250 mg	Halfan by SKB	Canadian	Antimalarial
HALFAN	Tab, White to Off-White, Cap Shaped	Halofantrine HCl 250 mg	Halfan by King	60793-0880	Antimalarial
HALFAN	Tab, White to Off-White, Cap Shaped	Halofantrine HCl 250 mg	Halfan by SKB	00007-4195	Antimalarial
HALOTESTIN10	Tab, Green, Round, Scored, Halotestin over 10	Fluoxymesterone 10 mg	Halotestin by Pharmacia	00009-0036 Discontinued	Steroid; C III
HALOTESTIN2	Tab, Peach, Round, Halotestin over 2	Fluoxymesterone 2 mg	Halotestin by Pharmacia	00009-0014	Steroid; C III
HALOTESTIN5	Tab, Light Green, Round, Scored, Halotestin over 5	Fluoxymesterone 5 mg	Halotestin by Pharmacia	00009-0019	Steroid; C III
HAUCK053	Cap, Maroon & Pink, Hauck Logo 053	Phendimetrazine Tartrate 35 mg	Wehless by W.E.Hauck		Anorexiant; C III
HAUCK087	Tab, Orange	Hydrocodone Bitartrate 5 mg, Guaifenesin 300 mg	Entuss by W.E.Hauck		Analgesic; C III
HAUCK202BESTA	Cap, Orange	Vitamin Combination	Besta by W.E.Hauck		Vitamin
HAUCK258	Tab, White	Hydrocodone Bitartrate 5 mg, Guaifenesin 300 mg, Pseudoephedrine HCl 30 mg	Entuss-D by W.E.Hauck		Analgesic; C III
HAW <> 500	Tab, White, Oval, Scored	Methscopolamine Nitrate 2.5 mg, Chlorpheniramine Maleate 8 mg, Pseudoephedrine HCl 120 mg	Xiral by Hawthorn	63717-0500	Cold Remedy
HAW112	Cap, Red	Vitamin C 320 mg, Folic Acid 1 mg, Vitamin B12 25 mcg, Iron 100 mg	Icar-C Plus by Hawthorn	63717-0112	Vitamin
HAW125	Tab, Peach, Oval, Scored	Vitamin A 4000 IU, Vitamin C 120 mg, Vitamin D3 200 IU, Vitamin E 30 IU, Thiamin 3 mg, Riboflavin 3.4 mg, Niacin 20 mg, Vitamin B6 10 mg, Folate 1 mg, Vitamin B12 12 mcg, Biotin 30 mcg, Pantothenic Acid 5 mg, Iodine 150 mcg, Iron 29 mg, Magnesium 225 mg, Zinc 15 mg, Copper 2 mg, Vitamin K 65 mcg, Selenium 75 mcg, Manganese 2 mg, Chromium 100 mcg, Molybdenum 75 mcg, Boron 1 mg	Icar Prenatal by Hawthorn	63717-0150	Vitamin
HAW240	Tab, White, Cap Shaped, Scored	Guaifenesin 600 mg, Carbetapentane Citrate 60 mg	Xpect-AT by Hawthorn	63717-0240	Cold Remedy
HAW251	Tab, White, Oblong	Guaifenesin 400 mg	Xpect by Hawthorn	63717-0251	Cold Remedy
HAW260	Tab, Pink, Orally Disintegrating	Phenylephrine HCl 10 mg	Nasop by Hawthorn	63717-0260	Cold Remedy
HAW301	Tab, Oblong, Scored	Pseudoephedrine HCl 90 mg, Guaifenesin 600 mg	H 9600 SR by RX Pak by Med Pro	65084-0111	Cold Remedy
HAW301	Tab, White, Oblong, Scored	Guaifenesin 600 mg, Pseudoephedrine HCl 90 mg		53978-3354	Cold Remedy
HAW571	Tab, Oval, Scored, Chewable	Diphenhydramine 25 mg	Dytan by Hawthorn	63717-0571	Cold Remedy
HAW577	Tab, Blue, Triangular, Scored, Chewable	Diphenhydramine Tannate 25 mg, Phenylephrine Tannate 10 mg	Dytan-D by Hawthorn	63717-0577	Cold Remedy
HAW581	Tab, White to Tan, Oval, Scored	Diphenhydramine Tannate 25 mg, Phenylephrine Tannate 10 mg, Carbetapentane Tannate 30 mg	Dytan-CS by Hawthorn	63717-0581	Cold Remedy
HAW705	Tab, White	Hydrocodone Bitartrate 5 mg, Guaifenesin 600 mg	Xpect-HC by Hawthorn	63717-0705	Cold Remedy; C III
HAW810	Tab, Purple, Round, Scored	Atropine Sulfate 0.4 mg	Atreza by Hawthorn	63717-0810	Gastrointestinal
HAW840	Tab, Yellow, Scored	Scopolamine HBr 0.4 mg	Maldemar by Hawthorn	63717-840	Antiemetic
HB93614	Tab, Green, Round	Phenobarbital 16.2 mg, Belladonna Extract 10.8 mg	Belap by Lemmon		Gastrointestinal; C IV
HC <> CG	Tab, Beige & Orange, Oval, Scored	Carbamazepine 200 mg	Tegretol by Novartis	Canadian DIN 00773611	Anticonvulsant
HCQ	Tab, White to Off-White, Film Coated, Black Ink	Hydroxychloroquine Sulfate 200 mg	Hydroxychloroquine by Sanofi	00955-0790	Antimalarial

ID FRONT <> BACK	DESCRIPTION FRONT <> BACK	INGREDIENT & STRENGTH	BRAND (or Generic Equiv.) by FIRM	NDC# Canadian DIN	CLASS; SCH.
HCQ200 <> APO	Tab, White, Cap Shaped, Film Coated	Hydroxychloroquine Sulfate 200 mg	Apo Hydroxyquine by Apotex	02246691	Antimalarial
HD <> 512	Tab	Acetaminophen 325 mg, Oxycodone HCl 5 mg	Percocet by Schein	00364-0605 Discontinued	Analgesic; C II
HD <> 567	Tab	Acetaminophen 325 mg, Butalbital 50 mg, Caffeine 40 mg	Fioricet by Schein	00364-2297	Analgesic;
HD004	Tab, White, Round	Meperidine 50 mg	Demerol by Halsey	Discontinued	Analgesic; C II
HD005	Tab, White, Round	Meperidine 100 mg	Demerol by Halsey	Discontinued	Analgesic; C II
HD0656	Cap, Green	Chlordiazepoxide 5 mg, Clidinium Bromide 2.5 mg	Librax by Halsey	Discontinued	Gastrointestinal
HD157	Cap, Clear	Quinine Sulfate 325 mg	by Halsey	Discontinued	Antimalarial
HD4	Tab, White, Round	Meperidine HCl 50 mg	Pethadol by Halsey	Discontinued	Analgesic; C II
HD5	Tab, White, Round	Meperidine HCl 100 mg	Pethadol by Halsey	Discontinued	Analgesic; C II
HD512	Tab	Acetaminophen 325 mg, Oxycodone HCl 5 mg	Percocet by Qualitest	00603-4998 Discontinued	Analgesic; C II
HD532	Cap, Buff & Scarlet, HD532 <> HD532	Acetaminophen 500 mg, Oxycodone HCl 5 mg	Percocet by Ivax	00182-9175 Discontinued	Analgesic; C II
HD532	Cap, Buff & Scarlet, HD532 <> HD532	Acetaminophen 500 mg, Oxycodone HCl 5 mg	Percocet by Qualitest	00603-4997 Discontinued	Analgesic; C II
HD532	Cap, Buff & Scarlet, HD532 <> HD532	Acetaminophen 500 mg, Oxycodone HCl 5 mg	Percocet by Parmed	00349-8659 Discontinued	Analgesic; C II
HD532	Cap, Buff & Scarlet, HD532 <> HD532	Acetaminophen 500 mg, Oxycodone HCl 5 mg	Percocet by Superior	00144-0630 Discontinued	Analgesic; C II
HD532	Cap, Buff & Scarlet, HD532 <> HD532	Acetaminophen 500 mg, Oxycodone HCl 5 mg	Percocet by Rugby	00536-3219 Discontinued	Analgesic; C II
HD532	Cap, Buff & Scarlet, HD532 <> HD532	Acetaminophen 500 mg, Oxycodone HCl 5 mg	Percocet by Halsey	00879-0532 Discontinued	Analgesic; C II
HD532	Cap, Buff & Scarlet, HD532 <> HD532	Acetaminophen 500 mg, Oxycodone HCl 5 mg	Percocet by Mallinckrodt	00406-0532 Discontinued	Analgesic; C II
HD567	Tab, White, Round	Acetaminophen 325 mg, Butalbital 50 mg, Caffeine 40 mg	Fioricet by Murfreesboro	51129-7401	Analgesic
HD567	Tab, White, Round	Acetaminophen 325 mg, Butalbital 50 mg, Caffeine 40 mg	Fioricet by DRX	55045-1582	Analgesic
HD567	Tab, White, Round	Acetaminophen 325 mg, Butalbital 50 mg, Caffeine 40 mg	Fioricet by Kaiser	00179-1278	Analgesic
HD567	Tab, White, Round	Acetaminophen 325 mg, Butalbital 50 mg, Caffeine 40 mg	Fioricet by Warner Chilcott	00047-0106	Analgesic
HD567	Tab, White, Round	Acetaminophen 325 mg, Butalbital 50 mg, Caffeine 40 mg	Fioricet by URL Mutual	00677-1242	Analgesic
HD567	Tab, White, Round	Acetaminophen 325 mg, Butalbital 50 mg, Caffeine 40 mg	Fioricet by Medeva	53014-0003	Analgesic
HD567	Tab, White, Round	Acetaminophen 325 mg, Butalbital 50 mg, Caffeine 40 mg	Fioricet by Watson	52544-0485	Analgesic
HD567	Tab, White, Round	Acetaminophen 325 mg, Butalbital 50 mg, Caffeine 40 mg	Fioricet by Danbury	00591-0485	Analgesic
HD711	Tab, White	Acetaminophen 650 mg, Propoxyphene Napsylate 100 mg	Darvocet-N 100 by Halsey	Discontinued	Analgesic; C IV
HD7152	Tab, White, Round, HD 715/#2	Hydromorphone HCl 2 mg	Dilaudid by Halsey	Discontinued	Analgesic; C II
HD7174	Tab, White, Round, HD 717/#4	Hydromorphone HCl 4 mg	Dilaudid by Halsey	Discontinued	Analgesic; C II
HD724	Tab, Beige, Round	Doxycycline Hyclate 50 mg	Vibra-Tab by Halsey	Discontinued	Antibiotic
HD725	Tab, Yellow Interior, Film Coated	Doxycycline Hyclate	by Kaiser	00179-1170 Discontinued	Antibiotic
HD725	Cap	Doxycycline Hyclate	by Quality Care	60346-0449 Discontinued	Antibiotic
HD765	Tab	Acetaminophen 500 mg, Hydrocodone Bitartrate 5 mg	Vicodin by Halsey	00879-0765 Discontinued	Analgesic; C III
HD765	Tab, White, Oval, Scored	Acetaminophen 500 mg, Hydrocodone Bitartrate 5 mg	Vicodin by UDL	51079-0933 Discontinued	Analgesic; C III
HD778	Tab	Acetaminophen 650 mg, Hydrocodone Bitartrate 10 mg	Lorcet by Halsey	00879-0778 Discontinued	Analgesic; C III
HD779	Tab	Acetaminophen 750 mg, Hydrocodone Bitartrate 7.5 mg	Vicodin ES by Halsey	00879-0779 Discontinued	Analgesic; C III

ID FRONT <> BACK	DESCRIPTION FRONT <> BACK	INGREDIENT & STRENGTH	BRAND (or Generic Equiv.) by FIRM	NDC#	CLASS; SCH.
HD780	Tab	Acetaminophen 650 mg, Hydrocodone Bitartrate 7.5 mg	Lorcet Plus by Halsey	00879-0780 Discontinued	Analgesic; C III
HD813	Cap, Maroon, HD over 813	Hydrocodone Bitartrate 5 mg, Pseudoephedrine HCl 30 mg, Chlorpheniramine Maleate 2 mg	Atuss HD by Atley	59702-0813	Cold Remedy; C III
HDU <> NVR	Tab, Light Red, Oval, Film-Coated	Aliskiren 150 mg, Valsartan 160 mg	Valturna by Novartis Consumer Health, Inc.	00078-0572	Antihypertensive
HEAD	Tab, White, Round, Rastafarian Head Logo	3,4-Methylenedioxymethamphetamine (MDMA)	Ecstasy by Illegal		Euphoric; Illicit
HEART	Tab, Yellow, Round, Enteric Coated, Raised Heart Logo	Aspirin 81 mg	Bayer Low Dose by Time Caps	49483-0070	Analgesic
HEART	Tab, Peach, Round, Enteric Coated, Raised Heart Logo	Aspirin 81 mg	St. Joseph's Aspirin by Time Caps	49483-0107	Analgesic
HEART	Tab, Round, Peach, Coated, Heart Logo	Folacin (Folic Acid) 2.5 mg, Pyridoxine (B6) 25 mg, Cyanocobalamin (B12) 2 mg	Folbalin Plus by Red River Pharma	12593-0047	Vitamin; Supplement
HEXALEN50MGUSB001	Cap, Clear	Altretamine 50 mg	Hexalen by US Bioscience	58178-0001	Antineoplastic
HEXALEN50MGUSB001	Cap	Altretamine 50 mg	Hexalen by AAI Pharma	27280-0001	Antineoplastic
HF <> ZEE	Tab, Bright Orange, Round, ZEE <> H/F	Acetaminophen 325 mg, Dextromethorphan 10 mg, Pseudoephedrine 30 mg	Histenol Forte by Zee		Cold Remedy
HFC	Tab, Pink, Circular, H/FC	Felodipine 5 mg	Renedil by Aventis	Canadian	Antihypertensive
HFC	Tab, Brown & Red, Circular, H/FC	Felodipine 10 mg	Renedil by Aventis	Canadian	Antihypertensive
HFF	Tab, Yellow, Circular, H/FF	Felodipine 2.5 mg	Renedil by Aventis	Canadian	Antihypertensive
HG <> CIBA	Tab, Pink, Round, Coated	Hydralazine HCl 50 mg	Apresoline by Novartis	Canadian DIN 00005541	Antihypertensive
HGH <> CG	Tab, Light Orange, Oval, Film Coated	Hydrochlorothiazide 12.5 mg, Valsartan 80 mg	Diovan HCT by Novartis	Canadian DIN 02241900	Diuretic; Antihypertensive
HGH <> CG	Tab, Light Orange, Oval, Film Coated	Hydrochlorothiazide 12.5 mg, Valsartan 80 mg	Diovan HCT by Novartis	00078-0314	Diuretic; Antihypertensive
HGH <> CG	Tab, Light Orange, Oval, Film Coated	Hydrochlorothiazide 12.5 mg, Valsartan 80 mg	Diovan HCT by Novartis	17088-3932	Diuretic; Antihypertensive
HGH <> CG	Tab, Light Orange, Oval, Film Coated	Valsartan 80 mg, Hydrochlorothiazide 12.5 mg	by Allscripts		Antihypertensive; Diuretic
HHA	Cap, Gray, Black Print, Abbott Logo (a)	Terazosin HCl 1 mg	Hytrin by Nat Pharmpak	55154-0115	Antihypertensive
HHA	Cap, Gray, Black Print, Abbott Logo (a)	Terazosin HCl 1 mg	Hytrin by Va Cmop	65243-0088	Antihypertensive
HHA	Cap, Gray, Black Print, Abbott Logo (a)	Terazosin HCl 1 mg	Hytrin by RP Scherer	11014-1031	Antihypertensive
HHA	Cap, Gray, Black Print, Abbott Logo (a)	Terazosin HCl 1 mg	Hytrin by Abbott	00074-3805	Antihypertensive
HHDP	Cap, Clear, Imprinted in Black	Phenyltoloxamine Citrate 8 mg, Pheniramine Maleate 8 mg, Pyrilamine Maleate 8 mg, Phenylpropanolamine HCl 25 mg	Highland Histine D PED by Prepackage Specialists	58864-0359	Cold Remedy
HHH <> CG	Tab, Dark Red, Oval, Film Coated	Hydrochlorothiazide 12.5 mg, Valsartan 160 mg	Diovan HCT by Novartis	17088-3933	Diuretic; Antihypertensive
HHH <> CG	Tab, Dark Red, Oval, Film Coated	Hydrochlorothiazide 12.5 mg, Valsartan 160 mg	Diovan HCT by Novartis	Canadian DIN 02241901	Diuretic; Antihypertensive
HHH <> CG	Tab, Dark Red, Oval, Film Coated	Hydrochlorothiazide 12.5 mg, Valsartan 160 mg	Diovan HCT by Novartis	00078-0315	Diuretic; Antihypertensive
HIGHLAND	Cap, Clear & Red, in Black	Phenyltoloxamine Citrate 16 mg, Pheniramine Maleate 16 mg, Pyrilamine Maleate 16 mg, Phenylpropanolamine HCl 50 mg	Highland Histine D by Prepackage Specialists	58864-0149	Cold Remedy
HIL <> NVR	Tab, Pink, Oval	Hydrochlorothiazide 12.5 mg, Valsartan 320 mg	Diovan HCT by Novartis	00078-0471	Antihypertensive; Diuretic
HIVID0375 <> ROCHE	Tab, Beige, Black Print, Oval, Film Coated, Hivid over 0.375	Zalcitabine 0.375 mg	Hivid by Roche	Canadian	Antiviral
HIVID0375 <> ROCHE	Tab, Beige, Black Print, Oval, Film Coated, Hivid over 0.375	Zalcitabine 0.375 mg	Hivid by Hoffmann La Roche	00004-0220	Antiviral
HIVID0375 <> ROCHE	Tab, Beige, Black Print, Oval, Film Coated, Hivid over 0.375	Zalcitabine 0.375 mg	Hivid by Pharm Util	60491-0296	Antiviral
HIVID0750 <> ROCHE	Tab, Beige, Black Print, Oval, Film Coated, Hivid over 0.750	Zalcitabine 0.75 mg	Hivid by Pharm Util	60491-0297	Antiviral
HIVID0750 <> ROCHE	Tab, Beige, Black Print, Oval, Film Coated, Hivid over 0.750	Zalcitabine 0.750 mg	Hivid by Hoffmann La Roche	00004-0221	Antiviral
HKA	Cap, Red, Black Print, Round, Abbott Logo (a)	Terazosin HCl 5 mg	Hytrin by Nat Pharmpak	55154-0116	Antihypertensive
HKA	Cap, Red, Black Print, Round, Abbott Logo (a)	Terazosin HCl 5 mg	Hytrin by PDRX	55289-0070	Antihypertensive
HKA	Cap, Red, Black Print, Round, Abbott Logo (a)	Terazosin HCl 5 mg	Hytrin by Va Cmop	65243-0069	Antihypertensive
HKA	Cap, Red, Black Print, Round, Abbott Logo (a)	Terazosin HCl 5 mg	Hytrin by RP Scherer	11014-1033	Antihypertensive
HKA	Cap, Red, Black Print, Round, Abbott Logo (a)	Terazosin HCl 5 mg	Hytrin by Abbott	00074-3807	Antihypertensive
HL	Tab, Green, Round	Herbal Laxative 486 mg	by PFI		Laxative
HLP10	Tab, Light Brown, Round	Pravastatin Sodium 10 mg	Pravachol by Sandoz	00781-5231	Antihyperlipidemic
HLP20	Tab, Light Brown, Round	Pravastatin Sodium 20 mg	Pravachol by Sandoz	00781-5232	Antihyperlipidemic
HLP40	Tab, Light Brown, Round	Pravastatin Sodium 40 mg	Pravachol by Sandoz	00781-5234	Antihyperlipidemic

ID FRONT <> BACK	DESCRIPTION FRONT <> BACK	INGREDIENT & STRENGTH	BRAND (or Generic Equiv.) by FIRM	NDC#	CLASS; SCH.
HLT41	Tab, Grayish Brown, Round, HL over T41	Trimeprazine Tartrate 2.5 mg	Temaril by Forest		Antipruritic
HLT50	Cap, Gray & Natural	Trimeprazine Tartrate 5 mg	Temaril Spansule by Forest		Antipruritic
HMR <> 60	Tab, Light Yellow, Scored	Diltiazem 60 mg	Cardizem by Biovail Corp.	Canadian DIN 02097389	Antihypertensive
HMR <> SULCRATE	Tab, White, Cap Shape	Sucralfate 1 g	Sulcrate by Axcan	Canadian DIN 02100622	Gastrointestinal
HNA	Cap, Blue, Black Print, Round, Abbott Logo (a)	Terazosin HCl 10 mg	Hytrin by RP Scherer	11014-1034	Antihypertensive
HNA	Cap, Blue, Black Print, Round, Abbott Logo (a)	Terazosin HCl 10 mg	Hytrin by Va Cmop	65243-0089	Antihypertensive
HNA	Cap, Blue, Black Print, Round, Abbott Logo (a)	Terazosin HCl 10 mg	Hytrin by Abbott	00074-3808	Antihypertensive
HO <> CG	Tab, Dark Yellow, Cap Shaped, Film Coated	Benazepril HCl 10 mg	Lotensin by Novartis	Canadian DIN 00885843	Antihypertensive
HOECHST <> DIAB	Tab, Light Green, Oblong, Scored	Glyburide 5 mg	Diabeta by Rite Aid	11822-5186	Antidiabetic
HOECHST <> DIAB	Tab, Light Green, Oblong, Scored	Glyburide 5 mg	Diabeta by Thrift Drug	59198-0023	Antidiabetic
HOECHST <> DIAB	Tab, Light Green, Oblong, Scored	Glyburide 5 mg	Diabeta by Merrell	00068-1212	Antidiabetic
HOECHST <> DIAB	Tab, Light Green, Oblong, Scored	Glyburide 5 mg	Diabeta by Nat Pharmpak	55154-1201	Antidiabetic
HOECHST <> DIAB	Tab, Peach, Oblong, Scored, DIA and Beta character	Glyburide 1.25 mg	Diabeta by Aventis	00039-0053	Antidiabetic
HOECHST <> DIAB	Tab, Light Green, Oblong, Scored, DIA and Beta character	Glyburide 5 mg	Diabeta by Aventis	00039-0052	Antidiabetic
HOECHST <> DIAB	Tab, Light Pink, Oblong, Scored, DIA and Beta character	Glyburide 2.5 mg	Diabeta by Aventis	00039-0051	Antidiabetic
HOECHST <> DIAB	Tab, Peach, Oblong, Scored	Glyburide 1.25 mg	Diabeta by Merrell	00068-1210	Antidiabetic
HOECHST <> DIAB	Tab, Light Green, Oblong, Scored	Glyburide 5 mg	Diabeta by Allscripts		Antidiabetic
HOECHST <> DIAB	Tab, Light Pink, Oblong, Scored	Glyburide 2.5 mg	Diabeta by Nat Pharmpak	55154-1206	Antidiabetic
HOECHST <> DIAB	Tab, Light Green, Oblong, Scored	Glyburide 5 mg	Diabeta by Coventry	61372-0578	Antidiabetic
HOECHST <> DIAB	Tab, Light Pink, Oblong, Scored	Glyburide 2.5 mg	Diabeta by Drug Distr	52985-0221	Antidiabetic
HOECHST <> DIAB	Tab, Light Pink, Oblong, Scored	Glyburide 2.5 mg	Diabeta by Amerisource	62584-0361	Antidiabetic
HOECHST <> DIAB	Tab, Light Pink, Oblong, Scored	Glyburide 2.5 mg	Diabeta by Merrell	00068-1211	Antidiabetic
HOECHST <> DIAB	Tab, Light Pink, Oblong, Scored	Glyburide 2.5 mg	Diabeta by Thrift Drug	59198-0022	Antidiabetic
HOECHST <> LASIX	Tab, White, Oval	Furosemide 20 mg	Lasix by Caremark	00339-5203	Diuretic
HOECHST <> LASIX	Tab, White, Oval	Furosemide 20 mg	Lasix by Aventis	00039-0067	Diuretic
HOECHST <> LASIX	Tab, White, Oval	Furosemide 20 mg	Lasix by Merrell	00068-1215	Diuretic
HOECHST <> LASIX	Tab, White, Oval	Furosemide 20 mg	Lasix by Drug Distr	52985-0072	Diuretic
HOECHST <> LASIX	Tab, White, Oval	Furosemide 20 mg	Lasix by Thrift Drug	59198-0224	Diuretic
HOECHST <> LASIX	Tab, White, Oval	Furosemide 20 mg	Lasix by Leiner	59606-0679	Diuretic
HOECHST <> LASIX	Tab, White, Oval	Furosemide 20 mg	Lasix by Amerisource	62584-0067	Diuretic
HOECHST <> LASIX	Tab, White, Oval	Furosemide 20 mg	Lasix by Pharm Util	60491-0359	Diuretic
HOECHST <> TRENTAL	Tab, Pink, Oblong, Film Coated	Pentoxifylline 400 mg	Trental by DRX	55045-2327	Anticoagulant
HOECHST <> TRENTAL	Tab, Pink, Oblong, Film Coated	Pentoxifylline 400 mg	Trental by Nat Pharmpak	55154-1205	Anticoagulant
HOECHST <> TRENTAL	Tab, Pink, Oblong, Film Coated	Pentoxifylline 400 mg	Trental by Amerisource	62584-0078	Anticoagulant
HOECHST <> TRENTAL	Tab, Pink, Oblong, Film Coated	Pentoxifylline 400 mg	Trental by Med Pro	53978-0374	Anticoagulant
HOECHST <> TRENTAL	Tab, Pink, Oblong, Film Coated	Pentoxifylline 400 mg	Trental by Aventis	00039-0078	Anticoagulant
HOECHST <> TRENTAL	Tab, Pink, Oblong, Film Coated	Pentoxifylline 400 mg	Trental by Merrell	00068-0780	Anticoagulant
HOECHST <> TRENTAL	Tab, Pink, Oblong, Film Coated	Pentoxifylline 400 mg	Trental by Pharmedix	53002-1040	Anticoagulant
HOESCHT72	Tab, White, Round	Digestive Enzymes	Festal II by Aventis		Digestant
HOESCHT73	Tab, Orange, Round	Digestive Enzymes, Atropine Methyl Nitrate	Festalan by Aventis		Digestant
HOLD	Tab, Red, Round, Lozenge	Dextromethorphan HBr 5 mg	Hold by B F Ascher	00225-0630	Antitussive
HOLD	Tab, Amber, Round	Dextromethorphan HBr 5 mg	Hold by B F Ascher	00225-0640	Antitussive
HOLD	Tab, Yellow, Round	Dextromethorphan HBr 5 mg	Hold by B F Ascher	00225-0620	Antitussive
HOPE <> 301	Tab, White, Round	Scopolamine Hydrobromide 0.4 mg	Scopace by Anabolic	00722-6383	Antiemetic
HOPE <> 301	Tab, White, Round	Scopolamine Hydrobromide 0.4 mg	Scopace by Hope	60267-0301	Antiemetic
HOPE <> 742	Tab, White, Round	Atropine Sulfate 0.4 mg	Sal-Tropine by Hope	60267-0742	Gastrointestinal

ID FRONT <> BACK	DESCRIPTION FRONT <> BACK	INGREDIENT & STRENGTH	BRAND (or Generic Equiv.) by FIRM	NDC#	CLASS; SCH.
HOPE <> 742	Tab, White, Round	Atropine Sulfate 0.4 mg	Sal-Tropine by Anabolic	00722-6685	Gastrointestinal
HOPE953	Cap, White, Round	Aminobenzoate Potassium 500 mg	Potaba by Hope	60267-0953	Antifibrotic
HORIZON205	Tab, White, Scored	Glycopyrrolate 2 mg	Robinul Forte by Horizon	59630-0250	Gastrointestinal
HORIZON205	Tab, White, Round, Scored	Glycopyrrolate 2 mg	Robinul Forte by Horizon	59630-0205	Gastrointestinal
HORNER	Tab, Salmon, Shield	Tolbutamide 500 mg	Mobenol by Horner	Canadian	Antidiabetic
HORNER15MG	Tab, White, Oval, Horner/15/mg	Flurazepam HCl 15 mg	Somnol by Horner	Canadian	Hypnotic; C IV
HORNER200MG	Cap, White	Ibuprofen 200 mg	Motrin by Horner		NSAID
HORNER300MG	Cap, Yellow	Ibuprofen 300 mg	Motrin by Horner		NSAID
HORNER30MG	Tab, Light Blue, Oval, Horner/30/mg	Flurazepam HCl 30 mg	Somnol by Horner	Canadian	Hypnotic; C IV
HORNER400MG	Cap, Scarlet	Ibuprofen 400 mg	Motrin by Horner		NSAID
HOTROX50700	Cap, Black and Red with a White Band, HOT-ROX, 50/700	Thiamin (vitamin B1) 20 mg, Niacin (vitamin B3) 20 mg, Pantothenic Acid 20 mg, Pyridoxal-5-Phosphate 50 mg, Vitamin B12 (methylcobalamin) 995 mcg, HOT-ROX Thermogenic Formula 950 mg: N-Acetyl-L-Tyrosine, MDX complex: Androst-5-ene-7-one-317-diethl-carbonate, Sclaremax proprietary Salvia Sclarea extract, Guggulsterone Z, Guggulsterone E; Caffeine, 5-Hydroxy - L-Tryptophan	Hot-Rox by BioTest Labs		Supplement
HOYT <> 006	Tab, Pink, Round, Chewable	Sodium Fluoride 2.2 mg	Luride Cherry by Colgate	00126-0006	Element
HOYT007	Tab, White, Round	Sodium Fluoride 1 mg	Luride SF by Colgate	00126-0007	Element
HOYT013	Tab, Blue, Round	Sodium Fluoride 0.5 mg	Luride by Colgate	00126-0013	Element
HOYT014	Tab, Purple, Round	Sodium Fluoride 0.5 mg	Luride by Colgate	00126-0014	Element
HOYT140	Tab, Green, Round	Sodium Fluoride 1 mg	Luride by Colgate	00126-0140	Element
HOYT141	Tab, Yellow, Round	Sodium Fluoride 1 mg	Luride by Colgate	00126-0141	Element
HOYT142	Tab, Orange, Round	Sodium Fluoride 1 mg	Luride by Colgate	00126-0142	Element
HOYT186	Tab, Beige, Round	Sodium Fluoride 0.25 mg	Luride by Colgate	00126-0186	Element
HP <> CG	Tab, Light Orange, Round, Film-Coated	Benazepril HCl 20 mg	Lotensin by Novartis	Canadian DIN 00885851	Antihypertensive
HP <> CG	Tab, Reddish-Orange, Cap Shaped, Film Coated	Benazepril HCl 20 mg	Lotensin by Novartis	Canadian DIN 00885851	Antihypertensive
HP1	Tab, Pink, Round, Film Coated	Hydralazine HCl 10 mg	Apresoline by Heritage	23155-0001	Antihypertensive
HP12	Cap, Bright Pink, Opaque	Propoxyphene HCl 65 mg	Darvon by Heritage	23155-0012	Analgesic; C IV
HP146	Cap, Light Blue and Aqua Blue, Oval, Opaque	Acyclovir 200 mg	Zovirax by Heritage	23155-0146	Antiviral
HP15	Tab, White, Round, Scored, Film Coated	Chlorpheniramine Maleate 8 mg, Methscopolamine Nitrate 2.5 mg, Pseudoephedrine HCl 120 mg	Mescolor by Horner	59630-0150	Cold Remedy
HP15	Tab, White, Round, Scored, Film Coated	Chlorpheniramine Maleate 8 mg, Methscopolamine Nitrate 2.5 mg, Pseudoephedrine HCl 120 mg	Mescolor by Anabolic	00722-6293	Cold Remedy
HP2	Tab, Pink, Round	Hydralazine HCl 25 mg	Apresoline by Heritage	23155-0002	Antihypertensive
HP3	Tab, Pink, Round	Hydralazine HCl 50 mg	Apresoline by Heritage	23155-0003	Antihypertensive
HP38	Cap, Dark Blue and White, Opaque, Black Ink	Paromomycin Sulfate 250 mg	Humatin by Heritage	23155-0038	Antibiotic
HP4	Tab, Pink, Round, Film Coated	Hydralazine HCl 100 mg	Apresoline by Heritage	23155-0004	Antihypertensive
HP5	Tab, Bright Yellow, Round, Scored, HP / 5	Sulindac 150 mg	Clinoril by Heritage	23155-0005	NSAID
HP6	Tab, Bright Yellow, Round, Scored, HP / 6	Sulindac 200 mg	Clinoril by Heritage	23155-0006	NSAID
HPC170	Cap, Red, White Print, A logo	Acetaminophen 500 mg, Butalbital 50 mg, Caffeine 40 mg	Zebutal by Horizon	59630-0170	Analgesic
HPC200	Tab, White, Round, Scored	Glycopyrrolate 1 mg	Robinul by Horizon	59630-0200	Gastrointestinal
HPS	Tab, White, Round	Ergonovine Maleate 0.2 mg	by Pharmafab	62542-0902	Ergot Alkaloids
HPS	Tab, White, Round	Ergonovine Maleate 0.2 mg	by Home Prescription	63704-0001	Ergot Alkaloids
HPS	Tab, White, Round	Ergonovine Maleate 0.2 mg	by Halsey	00904-5387	Ergot Alkaloids
HPS	Tab, White, Round	Ergonovine Maleate 0.2 mg	Ergonovine by Halsey	00904-5386	Ergot Alkaloids
HR	Tab, Brown, Round, Scored	Ginkgo Biloba Extract	Ginkgo Biloba by BDI		Supplement
HR	Tab, Yellow, Round, Scored	Melatonin 3 mg	Melatonin by BDI		Supplement

ID FRONT <> BACK	DESCRIPTION FRONT <> BACK	INGREDIENT & STRENGTH	BRAND (or Generic Equiv.) by FIRM	NDC#	CLASS; SCH.
HR	Tab, White, Round, Scored	Caffeine 200 mg	Overtime by BDI		Stimulant
HR	Tab, Pink, Heart Shaped	Caffeine 200 mg	Valentine by BDI		Stimulant
HR2020	Tab, White, Cap Shaped, Blue, Pink & Yellow Specks, HR/20/20	Caffeine 200 mg	Caffeine by BDI		Stimulant
HR225 <> MINI	Tab, White, Round, HR 225/Mini	Ephedrine HCl 25 mg, Guaifenesin 200 mg	Mini Two-Way Action by BDI		Cold Remedy
HS33	Tab, Beige, Round	Ferrous Fumarate 110 mg, Docusate Na 20 mg, Vitamin C 200 mg	Hemaspan by Sanofi		Mineral
HT15	Loz, Cherry	Benzocaine 15 mg, Dextromethorphan HBr 7.5 mg	Tetra-Formula by Reese	10956-0714	Topical Anesthetic
HT250	Cap, Light Blue and Green, Opaque	Amoxicillin 250 mg	Amoxicillin by Holt Labs	12307-0341	Antibiotic
HT500	Cap, Purple, Opaque	Amoxicillin 500 mg	Amoxicillin by Holt Labs	12307-0342	Antibiotic
HTI76	Tab, White, Kidney Shape, <> HTI over 76	Chlorthalidone 25 mg	Thalitone by Monarch	61570-0023	Diuretic
HTI77	Tab, White, Kidney, HTI/77	Chlorthalidone 15 mg	Thalitone by Monarch	61570-0024	Diuretic
HUMDM <> 030	Tab, Dark Green, Cap Shaped, Scored	Dextromethorphan 30 mg, Guaifenesin 600 mg	Humibid-DM by Celltech	53014-0030	Cold Remedy
HUMLA <> 012	Tab, Light Green, Scored	Guaifenesin 600 mg	Robitussin by Celltech	53014-0012	Expectorant
HUMLA <> 012	Tab, Light Green, Scored	Guaifenesin 600 mg	Robitussin by Celltech	53014-0012	Expectorant
HX814	Cap, Maroon and White, HX over 814	Hydrocodone Bitartrate 5 mg, Guaifenesin (sustained release) 100 mg, Guaifenesin (immediate-release) 200 mg	Atuss HX by Atley	59702-0814	Cold Remedy; C III
HXH <> NVR	Tab, Brownish Orange, Oval	Hydrochlorothiazide 25 mg, Valsartan 160 mg	Diovan HCT by Novartis	Canadian DIN 02246955	Diuretic; Antihypertensive
HXH <> NVR	Tab, Brownish Orange, Oval	Hydrochlorothiazide 25 mg, Valsartan 160 mg	Diovan HCT by Novartis	00078-0383	Diuretic; Antihypertensive
HYA	Cap, Yellow, Round, Black Print, Round, Abbott Logo <> HY	Terazosin HCl 2 mg	Hytrin by Physician Total Care	54868-3842	Antihypertensive
HYA	Cap, Yellow, Round, Black Print, Round, Abbott Logo <> HY	Terazosin HCl 2 mg	Hytrin by Va Cmop	65243-0068	Antihypertensive
HYA	Cap, Yellow, Round, Black Print, Round, Abbott Logo <> HY	Terazosin HCl 2 mg	Hytrin by RP Scherer	11014-1032	Antihypertensive
HYA	Cap, Yellow, Round, Black Print, Round, Abbott Logo <> HY	Terazosin HCl 2 mg	Hytrin by Abbott	00074-3806	Antihypertensive
HYCAMTIN025MG	Cap, White to Yellowish-White, Opaque	Topotecan HCl 0.25 mg	Hycamtin by SmithKline Beecham	00007-4205	Cancer Treatment
HYCAMTIN1MG	Cap, Pink, Opaque	Topotecan HCl 1 mg	Hycamtin by SmithKline Beecham	00007-4207	Cancer Treatment
HYCODAN	Tab, White, Round, Scored	Homatropine Methylbromide 1.5 mg, Hydrocodone Bitartrate 5 mg	Hycodan by DRX	55045-2728	Cold Remedy; C III
HYCODAN	Tab, White, Round, Scored	Homatropine Methylbromide 1.5 mg, Hydrocodone Bitartrate 5 mg	Hycodan by Endo	63481-0042	Cold Remedy; C III
HYCODAN	Tab, White, Round, Scored	Hydrocodone Bitartrate 5 mg	Hycodan by BMS	Canadian DIN 01916599	Cold Remedy; C III
HYCOMINE	Tab, Coral Pink, Round, Scored	Acetaminophen 250 mg, Caffeine 30 mg, Chlorpheniramine Maleate 2 mg, Hydrocodone Bitartrate 5 mg, Phenylephrine HCl 10 mg	Hycomine Compound by Endo	63481-0048	Cold Remedy; C III
HYDERGINE <> S	Tab, White, Round	Ergoloid Mesylate 1 mg	Hydergine by Novartis	61615-0102	Ergot Alkaloids
HYDREA830	Cap, Pink & Green, Black Print, Opaque, Hydrea over 830	Hydroxyurea 500 mg	Hydrea by BMS	00003-0830	Antineoplastic
HYDROCORTONE <> MSD619	Tab, White, Oval, Scored	Hydrocortisone 10 mg	Hydrocortone by Merck	00006-0619	Steroid
HYDRODIURIL <> MSD105	Tab, Peach, Round, Scored, MSD on Left, 105 on Right	Hydrochlorothiazide 50 mg	Hydrodiuril by Merck	00006-0105	Diuretic; Antihypertensive
HYDRODIURIL <> MSD42	Tab, Peach, Round, Scored	Hydrochlorothiazide 25 mg	Hydrodiuril by Merck	00006-0042	Diuretic; Antihypertensive
HYDROXYCUT	Cap, White, Red Print	Hydroxagen 2000 mg, Ma Huang extract 334 mg, Guarana extract 910 mg, Willow Bark extract 100 mg, L-Carnitine 100 mg, Chromium Picolinate 300 mcg	Hydroxy-Cut by Muscletech		Supplement
HYL <> CF	Tab, White, Cap Shaped	Passiflora 1X, Avena Sativa 1X, Humulus lupulus 1X, Chamomilla 2X, Calcarea Phosphorica 3X, Ferrum Phosphorica 3X, Kali Phosphorica 3X, Natrum Phosphoricum 3X, Magnesia Phosphoricum 3X	Calm's Forte by Hyland's		Homeopathic
HYL <> LC	Tab, White, Oblong, Red Specks	Viscum Album 3X, Gnaphalium 3X, Rhus Tox. 6X, Aconitum Nap. 6X, Ledum Pal. 6X, Magnesium Phosphate 6X, Cinchona Off. 3X	Hyland's Leg Cramps by Hyland's		Homeopathic
HYL <> NT	Tab, White, Oblong	Calcarea Phosphorica 3X, Ferrum Phosphorica 3X, Kali Phosphoricum 3X, Natrum Phosphoricum 3X, Magnesia Phosphoricum 3X	Hyland's Nerve Tonic by Hyland's	54973-1129	Homeopathic
HYLOREL10	Tab	Guanadrel Sulfate 10 mg	Hylorel by Medeva	53014-0787	Antihypertensive
HYLOREL25	Tab, White, Oval	Guanadrel Sulfate 25 mg	Hylorel by Medeva	53014-0788	Antihypertensive

ID FRONT <> BACK	DESCRIPTION FRONT <> BACK	INGREDIENT & STRENGTH	BRAND (or Generic Equiv.) by FIRM	NDC#	CLASS; SCH.
HYZAAR <> MRK717	Tab, Yellow, Teardrop Shaped, Film Coated	Hydrochlorothiazide 12.5 mg, Losartan Potassium 50 mg	Hyzaar by Merck	00006-0717	Diuretic; Antihypertensive
HYZAAR <> MRK717	Tab, Yellow, Teardrop Shaped, Film Coated	Hydrochlorothiazide 12.5 mg, Losartan Potassium 50 mg	Hyzaar by Nat Pharmpak	55154-3011	Diuretic; Antihypertensive
HYZAAR <> MRK717	Tab, Yellow, Teardrop Shaped, Film Coated	Hydrochlorothiazide 12.5 mg, Losartan Potassium 50 mg	Hyzaar by Merck Frosst	Canadian DIN 02230047	Diuretic; Antihypertensive
HYZAAR <> MRK747	Tab, Light Yellow, Teardrop Shaped	Hydrochlorothiazide 25 mg, Losartan Potassium 100 mg	Hyzaar by Merck	00006-0747	Diuretic; Antihypertensive
HYZAAR <> MRK747	Tab, Light Yellow, Teardrop Shaped	Hydrochlorothiazide 25 mg, Losartan Potassium 100 mg	Hyzaar by Merck Frosst	Canadian DIN 02241007	Diuretic; Antihypertensive
I	Tab, White to Off-White, Oval, Scored	Sodium Phosphate Monobasic Monohydrate 1.102 g, Sodium Phosphate Dibasic Anhydrous 0.398 g	Visicol by Salix	65649-0601	Gastrointestinal
I	Cap, Yellow	Benzonatate 100 mg	Tessalon by Inwood		Antitussive
I <> 21	Tab, White, Round, Scored	Glycopyrrolate 1 mg	Robinul by Dr. Reddy's	55111-0648	Anticholinergic Agent
I <> 22	Tab, White, Round, Scored	Glycopyrrolate 2 mg	Robinul by Dr. Reddy's	55111-0649	Anticholinergic Agent
I <> 25	Tab, White, Triangular, Film Coated	Sumatriptan Succinate 25 mg	Imitrex by GSK	Canadian DIN 02239738	Antimigraine
I <> 25	Tab, White, Triangular, Film Coated	Sumatriptan Succinate 25 mg	Imitrex by GSK	00173-0735	Antimigraine
I <> 25	Tab, White, Triangular, Film Coated	Sumatriptan Succinate 25 mg	Imitrex by GSK	00173-0460	Antimigraine
I <> 25	Tab, White, Triangular, Film Coated	Sumatriptan Succinate 25 mg	Imitrex by Physician Total Care	54868-3777	Antimigraine
I <> 3759	Tab, White, Oval, Scored	Lisinopril 10 mg	Prinivil by Ivax	00172-3759	Antihypertensive
I <> 4	Tab, White, Round	Meprobamate 400 mg	Miltown by Dr. Reddy's	55111-0641	Tranquilizer
I <> 7	Tab, White, Round	Meprobamate 200 mg	Miltown by Dr. Reddy's	55111-0640	Tranquilizer
I <> 71	Tab, Yellow, Round	Minocycline 50 mg	Dynacin by Dr. Reddy's	55111-0637	Antibiotic
I <> 72	Tab, Grey, Round	Minocycline 75 mg	Dynacin by Dr. Reddy's	55111-0638	Antibiotic
I <> 73	Tab, Dark Grey, Round	Minocycline 100 mg	Dynacin by Dr. Reddy's	55111-0639	Antibiotic
I <> 9200	Tab, White, Round, Scored	Glipizide 10 mg	Glucotrol by Teva	00172-3650	Antidiabetic
I <> 9201	Tab, White, Round, Scored	Glipizide 5 mg	Glucotrol by Teva	00172-3649	Antidiabetic
I <> INDERAL10	Tab, Peach, Hexagonal, Scored, Inderal over 10	Propranolol HCl 10 mg	Inderal by RP Scherer SA	64566-0001	Antihypertensive
I <> INDERAL10	Tab, Peach, Hexagonal, Scored, Inderal over 10	Propranolol HCl 10 mg	Inderal by Med Pro	53978-0034	Antihypertensive
I <> INDERAL10	Tab, Peach, Hexagonal, Scored, Inderal over 10	Propranolol HCl 10 mg	Inderal by Drug Distr	52985-0036	Antihypertensive
I <> INDERAL10	Tab, Peach, Hexagonal, Scored, Inderal over 10	Propranolol HCl 10 mg	Inderal by Leiner	59606-0660	Antihypertensive
I <> INDERAL10	Tab, Peach, Hexagonal, Scored, Inderal over 10	Propranolol HCl 10 mg	Inderal by Nat Pharmpak	55154-0204	Antihypertensive
I <> INDERAL10	Tab, Peach, Hexagonal, Scored, Inderal over 10	Propranolol HCl 10 mg	Inderal by Thrift Drug	59198-0038	Antihypertensive
I <> INDERAL10	Tab, Peach, Hexagonal, Scored, Inderal over 10	Propranolol HCl 10 mg	Inderal by Ayerst	00046-0421	Antihypertensive
I <> INDERAL10	Tab, Peach, Hexagonal, Scored, Inderal over 10	Propranolol HCl 10 mg	Inderal by Amerisource	62584-0421	Antihypertensive
I <> INDERAL20	Tab, Blue, Hexagonal, Scored, Inderal over 20	Propranolol HCl 20 mg	Inderal by Thrift Drug	59198-0039	Antihypertensive
I <> INDERAL20	Tab, Blue, Hexagonal, Scored, Inderal over 20	Propranolol HCl 20 mg	Inderal by PDRX	55289-0131	Antihypertensive
I <> INDERAL20	Tab, Blue, Hexagonal, Scored, Inderal over 20	Propranolol HCl 20 mg	Inderal by Amerisource	62584-0422	Antihypertensive
I <> INDERAL20	Tab, Blue, Hexagonal, Scored, Inderal over 20	Propranolol HCl 20 mg	Inderal by Nat Pharmpak	55154-0205	Antihypertensive
I <> INDERAL20	Tab, Blue, Hexagonal, Scored, Inderal over 20	Propranolol HCl 20 mg	Inderal by Ayerst	00046-0422	Antihypertensive
I <> INDERAL20	Tab, Blue, Hexagonal, Scored, Inderal over 20	Propranolol HCl 20 mg	Inderal by Caremark	00339-5167	Antihypertensive
I <> INDERAL20	Tab, Blue, Hexagonal, Scored, Inderal over 20	Propranolol HCl 20 mg	Inderal by Leiner	59606-0661	Antihypertensive
I <> INDERAL20	Tab, Blue, Hexagonal, Scored, Inderal over 20	Propranolol HCl 20 mg	Inderal by Drug Distr	52985-0037	Antihypertensive
I <> INDERAL20	Tab, Blue, Hexagonal, Scored, Inderal over 20	Propranolol HCl 20 mg	Inderal by Right Pak	65240-0668	Antihypertensive
I <> INDERAL20	Tab, Blue, Hexagonal, Scored, Inderal over 20	Propranolol HCl 20 mg	Inderal by RP Scherer SA	64566-0002	Antihypertensive
I <> INDERAL40	Tab, Green, Hexagonal, Scored, Inderal over 40	Propranolol HCl 40 mg	Inderal by Rightpak	65240-0662	Antihypertensive
I <> INDERAL40	Tab, Green, Hexagonal, Scored, Inderal over 40	Propranolol HCl 40 mg	Inderal by Drug Distr	52985-0019	Antihypertensive
I <> INDERAL40	Tab, Green, Hexagonal, Scored, Inderal over 40	Propranolol HCl 40 mg	Inderal by Nat Pharmpak	55154-0206	Antihypertensive
I <> INDERAL40	Tab, Green, Hexagonal, Scored, Inderal over 40	Propranolol HCl 40 mg	Inderal by Leiner	59606-0662	Antihypertensive
I <> INDERAL40	Tab, Green, Hexagonal, Scored, Inderal over 40	Propranolol HCl 40 mg	Inderal by Thrift Drug	59198-0040	Antihypertensive
I <> INDERAL40	Tab, Green, Hexagonal, Scored, Inderal over 40	Propranolol HCl 40 mg	Inderal by Ayerst	00046-0424	Antihypertensive
I <> INDERAL40	Tab, Green, Hexagonal, Scored, Inderal over 40	Propranolol HCl 40 mg	Inderal by Amerisource	62584-0424	Antihypertensive

ID FRONT <> BACK	DESCRIPTION FRONT <> BACK	INGREDIENT & STRENGTH	BRAND (or Generic Equiv.) by FIRM	NDC#	CLASS; SCH.
I <> INDERAL40	Tab, Green, Hexagonal, Scored, Inderal over 40	Propranolol HCl 40 mg	Inderal by Respa	60575-0087	Antihypertensive
I <> INDERAL60	Tab, Pink, Hexagonal, Scored, Inderal over 60	Propranolol HCl 60 mg	Inderal by Ayerst	00046-0426	Antihypertensive
I <> INDERAL80	Tab, Light Yellow, Hexagonal, Scored, Inderal over 80	Propranolol HCl 80 mg	Inderal by Ayerst	00046-0428	Antihypertensive
I <> INDERAL80	Tab, Light Yellow, Hexagonal, Scored, Inderal over 80	Propranolol HCl 80 mg	Inderal by Nat Pharmpak	55154-0208	Antihypertensive
I <> INDERAL80	Tab, Light Yellow, Hexagonal, Scored, Inderal over 80	Propranolol HCl 80 mg	Inderal by Pharm Util	60491-0319	Antihypertensive
I <> INDERAL80	Tab, Light Yellow, Hexagonal, Scored, Inderal over 80	Propranolol HCl 80 mg	Inderal by Amerisource	62584-0428	Antihypertensive
I <> INDERAL80	Tab, Light Yellow, Hexagonal, Scored, Inderal over 80	Propranolol HCl 80 mg	Inderal by Thrift Drug	59198-0041	Antihypertensive
I <> INDERAL80	Tab, Light Yellow, Hexagonal, Scored, Inderal over 80	Propranolol HCl 80 mg	Inderal by Murfreesboro	51129-1304	Antihypertensive
I <> INDERAL80	Tab, Light Yellow, Hexagonal, Scored, Inderal over 80	Propranolol HCl 80 mg	Inderal by Caremark	00339-5171	Antihypertensive
I <> INDERAL80	Tab, Light Yellow, Hexagonal, Scored, Inderal over 80	Propranolol HCl 80 mg	Inderal by Leiner	59606-0663	Antihypertensive
I <> INDERIDE4025	Tab, Off-White, Round	Hydrochlorothiazide 25 mg, Propranolol HCl 40 mg	Inderide by Ayerst	00046-0484	Diuretic; Antihypertensive
I <> INDERIDE8025	Tab, Off-White, Hexagonal, Scored	Hydrochlorothiazide 25 mg, Propranolol HCl 80 mg	Inderide by Ayerst	00046-0488	Diuretic; Antihypertensive
I <> L	Tab, White, Round	Lorazepam 0.5 mg	Ativan by Teva	00093-4820	Antianxiety; C IV
I <> SMP	Tab, Coated	Sumatriptan Succinate 25 mg	Imitrex by GSK	00173-0460	Antimigraine
1 <> 4821	Tab, White, Round, Scored	Lorazepam 1 mg	Ativan by Teva	00093-4821	Antianxiety; C IV
I10	Tab, Red, Oval	Amnesteem (Isotretinoin) 10 mg	Accutane by Mylan	00378-6611	Dermatologic
I2	Tab, Reddish Brown, Round, Film Coated, I-2	Ibuprofen 200 mg	Motrin by Perrigo	00113-0604	Analgesic
I2	Tab, Reddish Brown, Round, Film Coated, I-2	Ibuprofen 200 mg	Motrin by Perrigo	00113-2604	Analgesic
I2	Tab, Reddish Brown, Round, Film Coated, I-2	Ibuprofen 200 mg	Motrin by Perrigo	00113-0647	Analgesic
I2	Tab, White, Cap Shaped, I-2	Ibuprofen 200 mg	Motrin by Perrigo	00113-0669	Analgesic
I2	Tab, Reddish Brown, Round, Film Coated, I-2	Ibuprofen 200 mg	Motrin by Interpharm	53746-0143	NSAID
I2	Tab, Reddish Brown, Round, Film Coated, I-2	Ibuprofen 200 mg	Motrin by Perrigo	00113-0995	NSAID
I2	Tab, Reddish Brown, Round, Film Coated, I-2	Ibuprofen 200 mg	Motrin by Perrigo	00113-0488	NSAID
I2	Tab, Brown, Cap Shaped, Film Coated, I-2	Ibuprofen 200 mg	Motrin by Major	00904-5323	Analgesic
I2	Tab, White, Cap Shaped, I-2	Ibuprofen 200 mg	Motrin by Major	00904-7914	NSAID
I2	Tab, Brown, Cap Shaped, Film Coated, I-2	Ibuprofen 200 mg	Motrin by Major	00904-7912	Analgesic
I2	Tab, Reddish Brown, Round, Film Coated, I-2	Ibuprofen 200 mg	Motrin by Major	00904-7915	NSAID
I2	Tab, White, Cap Shaped, I-2	Ibuprofen 200 mg	Motrin by Major	00904-1747	Analgesic
I2	Tab, White, Cap Shaped, I-2	Ibuprofen 200 mg	Motrin by Perrigo	00113-0628	NSAID
I2	Tab, Reddish Brown, Round, Film Coated, I-2	Ibuprofen 200 mg	Motrin by Murfreesboro	51129-1508	NSAID
I2 <> 4822	Tab, White, Round, Scored	Lorazepam 2 mg	Ativan by Teva	00093-4822	Antianxiety; C IV
I20	Tab, White to Off White, Oval	Amnesteem (Isotretinoin) 20 mg	Accutane by Mylan	00378-6612	Dermatologic
I25	Tab, Peach, Round, Scored	Hydrochlorothiazide 50 mg	Hydrodiuril by Heritage	23155-0139	Antihypertensive; Diuretic
I26	Tab, Peach, Round, Scored	Hydrochlorothiazide 25 mg	Hydrodiuril by Heritage	23155-0138	Antihypertensive; Diuretic
I40	Tab, Pink, Oval	Amnesteem (Isotretinoin) 40 mg	Accutane by Mylan	00378-6614	Dermatologic
I43361MG	Cap, White, Opaque, Black Print	Terazosin HCl 1 mg	Hytrin by Teva	00093-4336	Antihypertensive
I4372MG	Cap, Yellow and White, Opaque, Black Print	Terazosin HCl 2 mg	Hytrin by Teva	00093-4337	Antihypertensive
I43385MG	Cap, Orange and White, Opaque, Black Print	Terazosin HCl 5 mg	Hytrin by Teva	00093-4338	Antihypertensive
I43910MG	Cap, Blue and White, Opaque, Black Print	Terazosin HCl 10 mg	Hytrin by Teva	00093-4339	Antihypertensive
I67	Tab, Purple, Oval, Film Coated	Carbinoxamine Maleate 8 mg, Pseudoephedrine HCl 120 mg	Cardec by Ivax	00182-1130 Discontinued	Cold Remedy
I8	Tab, White, Cap Shaped	Ibuprofen 800 mg	Motrin by Dr. Reddy's	55111-0684	NSAID
IAA	Tab, Gray, Oval, Film Coated, IA over Abbott Logo (a)	Carteolol HCl 2.5 mg	Cartrol by Abbott	00074-1664	Antihypertensive
IB	Tab, Brown, Round, Film Coated	Ibuprofen 200 mg	Motrin by Barr	00555-0809 Discontinued	NSAID
IB	Tab, White, Cap Shaped, Film Coated	Ibuprofen 200 mg	Motrin by Barr	00555-0810 Discontinued	NSAID
IB	Tab, White, Round, Film Coated	Ibuprofen 200 mg	Motrin by Barr	00555-0811 Discontinued	NSAID
IB	Tab, Brown, Cap Shaped, Film Coated	Ibuprofen 200 mg	Motrin by Barr	00555-0812 Discontinued	NSAID

ID FRONT <> BACK	DESCRIPTION FRONT <> BACK	INGREDIENT & STRENGTH	BRAND (or Generic Equiv.) by FIRM	NDC#	CLASS; SCH.
IB2	Tab, Brown, Round	Ibuprofen 200 mg	Motrin by Perrigo	00113-0488	NSAID
IB2	Tab, White, Oblong	Ibuprofen 200 mg	Motrin by Par		NSAID
IB2	Tab, White, Round	Ibuprofen 200 mg	Motrin by Par		NSAID
IBU <> 200	Tab, Yellow, Cap Shaped, Biconvex	Ibuprofen 200 mg	Motrin by Apotex	Canadian DIN 00441643	NSAID
IBU200	Tab, Yellow, Round, Biconvex	Ibuprofen 200 mg	Motrin by Apotex	Canadian DIN 00441643	NSAID
IBU400	Tab, White, Oval, Black Print, Film Coated	Ibuprofen 400 mg	Motrin by Par	49884-0777	NSAID
IBU400	Tab, White, Oval, Black Print, Film Coated	Ibuprofen 400 mg	Motrin by UDL	51079-0281 Discontinued	NSAID
IBU400	Tab, White, Oval, Black Print, Film Coated	Ibuprofen 400 mg	Motrin by Sandoz	00781-1352	NSAID
IBU400	Tab, White, Oval, Black Print, Film Coated	Ibuprofen 400 mg	Motrin by BASF	10117-0467	NSAID
IBU400	Tab, White, Oval, Black Print, Film Coated	Ibuprofen 400 mg	Motrin by Talbert	44514-0574	NSAID
IBU400	Tab, White, Oval, Black Print, Film Coated	Ibuprofen 400 mg	Motrin by Baker Cummins	63171-1809	NSAID
IBU400	Tab, White, Oval, Black Print, Film Coated	Ibuprofen 400 mg	Motrin by Vangard	00615-2525	NSAID
IBU400	Tab, White, Oval, Black Print, Film Coated	Ibuprofen 400 mg	Motrin by Par	49884-0467	NSAID
IBU400	Tab, White, Oval, Black Print, Film Coated	Ibuprofen 400 mg	Motrin by Golden State	60429-0092	NSAID
IBU400	Tab, White, Oval, Black Print, Film Coated	Ibuprofen 400 mg	Motrin by Murfreesboro	51129-1519	NSAID
IBU600	Tab, White, Black Print, Cap Shaped, Film Coated	Ibuprofen 600 mg	Motrin by Baker Cummins	63171-1810	NSAID
IBU600	Tab, White, Black Print, Cap Shaped, Film Coated	Ibuprofen 600 mg	Motrin by Sandoz	00781-1362	NSAID
IBU600	Tab, White, Black Print, Cap Shaped, Film Coated	Ibuprofen 600 mg	Motrin by BASF	10117-0468	NSAID
IBU600	Tab, White, Black Print, Cap Shaped, Film Coated	Ibuprofen 600 mg	Motrin by Amerisource	62584-0747	NSAID
IBU600	Tab, White, Black Print, Cap Shaped, Film Coated	Ibuprofen 600 mg	Motrin by Murfreesboro	51129-1518	NSAID
IBU600	Tab, White, Black Print, Cap Shaped, Film Coated	Ibuprofen 600 mg	Motrin by Golden State	60429-0093	NSAID
IBU600	Tab, White, Black Print, Cap Shaped, Film Coated	Ibuprofen 600 mg	Motrin by Par	49884-0468	NSAID
IBU600	Tab, White, Black Print, Cap Shaped, Film Coated	Ibuprofen 600 mg	Motrin by Vangard	00615-2526	NSAID
IBU600	Tab, White, Black Print, Cap Shaped, Film Coated	Ibuprofen 600 mg	Motrin by Par	49884-0778	NSAID
IBU600	Tab, White, Black Print, Cap Shaped, Film Coated	Ibuprofen 600 mg	Motrin by UDL	51079-0282 Discontinued	NSAID
IBU800	Tab, White, Cap Shaped, Black Print, Film Coated	Ibuprofen 800 mg	Motrin by UDL	51079-0596 Discontinued	NSAID
IBU800	Tab, White, Cap Shaped, Black Print, Film Coated	Ibuprofen 800 mg	Motrin by Par	49884-0779	NSAID
IBU800	Tab, White, Cap Shaped, Black Print, Film Coated	Ibuprofen 800 mg	Motrin by Moore	00839-7239	NSAID
IBU800	Tab, White, Cap Shaped, Black Print, Film Coated	Ibuprofen 800 mg	Motrin by BASF	10117-0173	NSAID
IBU800	Tab, White, Cap Shaped, Black Print, Film Coated	Ibuprofen 800 mg	Motrin by Major	00904-1760	NSAID
IBU800	Tab, White, Cap Shaped, Black Print, Film Coated	Ibuprofen 800 mg	Motrin by Sandoz	00781-1363	NSAID
IBU800	Tab, White, Cap Shaped, Black Print, Film Coated	Ibuprofen 800 mg	Motrin by Moore	00839-7236	NSAID
IBU800	Tab, White, Cap Shaped, Black Print, Film Coated	Ibuprofen 800 mg	Motrin by IDE Inter	00814-3816	NSAID
IBU800	Tab, White, Cap Shaped, Black Print, Film Coated	Ibuprofen 800 mg	Motrin by Golden State	60429-0094	NSAID
IBU800	Tab, White, Cap Shaped, Black Print, Film Coated	Ibuprofen 800 mg	Motrin by Vangard	00615-2528	NSAID
IBU800	Tab, White, Cap Shaped, Black Print, Film Coated	Ibuprofen 800 mg	Motrin by Warner Chilcott	00047-0914	NSAID
IBU800	Tab, White, Cap Shaped, Black Print, Film Coated	Ibuprofen 800 mg	Motrin by Schein	00364-2137	NSAID
IBU800	Tab, White, Cap Shaped, Black Print, Film Coated	Ibuprofen 800 mg	Motrin by Par	49884-0469	NSAID
IBU800	Tab, White, Cap Shaped, Black Print, Film Coated	Ibuprofen 800 mg	Motrin by Murfreesboro	51129-1520	NSAID
IBU800	Tab, White, Cap Shaped, Black Print, Film Coated	Ibuprofen 800 mg	Motrin by Med Pro	53978-5007	NSAID
ICA	Tab, White, Oval, Film Coated, IC over Abbott Logo (a)	Carteolol HCl 5 mg	Cartrol by Abbott	00074-1665	Antihypertensive
ICAPS	Tab, Off-White, Cap Shaped	Ascorbic Acid, Zinc Acetate, Vitamin E Acetate, Manganese Hydrolyzed vegetable Protein Chelate, Copper Hydrolyzed Vegetable Protein Chelate, Riboflavin, Beta Carotene, Selenium Hydrolyzed Vegetable Protein Chelate	ICAPS by Alcon	Canadian	Vitamin

ID FRONT <> BACK	DESCRIPTION FRONT <> BACK	INGREDIENT & STRENGTH	BRAND (or Generic Equiv.) by FIRM	NDC#	CLASS; SCH.
ICAPS	Tab, Yellow, Cap Shaped	Ascorbic Acid, Zinc Acetate, Vitamin E Acetate, Manganese Hydrolyzed vegetable Protein Chelate, Copper Hydrolyzed Vegetable Protein Chelate, Riboflavin, Beta Carotene, Selenium Hydrolyzed Vegetable Protein Chelate	ICAPS by Alcon	Canadian	Vitamin
ICN	Cap	Methoxsalen 10 mg	Oxsoralen by Pharm Util	60491-0826	Dermatologic
ICN <> 303	Tab, White, Round, ICN/303	Trioxsalen 5 mg	Trisoralen by ICN	Canadian DIN 01966383	Psoralen
ICN <> 303	Tab, White, Round	Trioxsalen 5 mg	Trisoralen by ICN	00187-0303	Psoralen
ICN <> M21	Tab, White, Round, Film Coated	Metformin HCl 500 mg	Glycon by Valeant	Canadian DIN 02229516	Antidiabetic
ICN <> PROSTIGMIN15	Tab, White, Round, Scored	Neostigmine Bromide 15 mg	Prostigmin by ICN	Canadian DIN 00869945	Muscle Stimulant
ICN <> W1	Tab, White, Round	Prednisone 1 mg	Winpred by ICN	Canadian DIN 00271373	Steroid
ICN021	Tab, Blue, Round	Oxybutynin Chloride 5 mg	Oxybutyn by ICN	Canadian DIN 02220059	Urinary Tract
ICN0901	Cap, Red	Methyltestosterone 10 mg	Android by Valeant	00187-0902	Hormone; C III
ICN122	Tab, White, Round, Scored	Isoniazid 300 mg	Laniazid by ICN	Canadian DIN 00272655	Antimycobacterial
ICN3100	Tab, White, Round	Neostigmine Bromide 15 mg	Prostigmin by Roche	Canadian DIN 00548375	Muscle Stimulant
ICN3101	Cap, Blue and White, Opaque	Nabilone 1 mg	Cesamet by Valeant	Canadian DIN 00548375	Antiemetic; C II
ICN3102	Cap, Red and White, Opaque	Nabilone 0.5 mg	Cesamet by Valeant	Canadian DIN 02256193	Antiemetic; C II
ICN311	Tab, White, Round	Methyltestosterone 10 mg	Android 10 by Schering		Hormone; C III
ICN499	Tab, Peach, Round	Methyltestosterone 25 mg	Android 25 by Schering		Hormone; C III
ICN60	Tab, White, Round	Pyridostigmine Bromide 60 mg	Mestinon by Roche		Muscle Stimulant
ICN600	Cap, Pink	Methoxsalen 10 mg	8-MOP by ICN	00187-0651	Dermatologic
ICN600	Cap, Light Pink	Methoxsalen 10 mg	Oxsoralen by ICN	Canadian DIN 01946374	Dermatologic
ICN650	Cap, Green, ICN/650	Methoxsalen 10 mg	Oxsoralen Ultra by RP Scherer	11014-1123	Dermatologic
ICN650	Cap, Green, ICN/650	Methoxsalen 10 mg	Oxsoralen Ultra by Banner Pharma	10888-4554	Dermatologic
ICN650	Cap, Green, ICN/650	Methoxsalen 10 mg	Oxsoralen Ultra by ICN	Canadian DIN 00252654	Dermatologic
ICN650	Cap, Green, ICN/650	Methoxsalen 10 mg	Oxsoralen Ultra by ICN	00187-0650	Dermatologic
ICNA17	Cap, Light Blue & Pink	Diphenhydramine HCl 25 mg	Allerdryl by ICN		Antihistamine
ICNA17	Cap, Light Blue & Pink	Diphenhydramine HCl 25 mg	Allerdryl by Valeant	Canadian DIN 00370517	Antihistamine
ICNA18	Cap, Pink & White	Diphenhydramine HCl 50 mg	Allerdryl by Valeant	Canadian DIN 00271411	Antihistamine
ICNA18	Cap, Pink & White	Diphenhydramine HCl 50 mg	Allerdryl by ICN		Antihistamine
ICNA21	Tab, White, Round	Allopurinol 100 mg	Zyloprim by ICN		Antigout
ICNA22	Tab, Orange, Rectangular	Allopurinol 200 mg	Zyloprim by ICN		Antigout
ICNA23	Tab, Orange, Round	Allopurinol 300 mg	Zyloprim by ICN		Antigout
ICNB11	Tab, White, Round	Probenecid 500 mg	Benuryl by ICN	Canadian DIN 00294926	Antigout
ICNB4	Tab, Yellow, Round, Enteric Coated	Bisacodyl 5 mg	Bisacolax by ICN	Canadian DIN 00714488	Laxative

ID FRONT <> BACK	DESCRIPTION FRONT <> BACK	INGREDIENT & STRENGTH	BRAND (or Generic Equiv.) by FIRM	NDC#	CLASS; SCH.
ICNC11	Cap, Orange & White	Lithium Carbonate 150 mg	Carbolith by ICN	Canadian DIN 00461733	Antipsychotic
ICNC12	Cap, Flesh	Lithium Carbonate 300 mg	Carbolith by ICN	Canadian DIN 00236683	Antipsychotic
ICNC13	Cap, Blue & Opaque	Lithium Carbonate 600 mg	Carbolith by ICN	Canadian DIN 02011239	Antipsychotic
ICNC21	Cap, Green	Chlordiazepoxide 5 mg, Clidinium Bromide 2.5 mg	Corium by ICN	Canadian DIN 00391077	Gastrointestinal; C IV
ICNC23	Tab, White, Round, Scored	Cortisone Acetate 25 mg	Cortisone Acetate by ICN	Canadian DIN 00280437	Steroid
ICND11	Tab, Yellow, Oval, Scored	Dexamethasone 0.5 mg	Dexasone by ICN	Canadian DIN 00295094	Steroid
ICND12	Tab, Blue, Oval, Scored	Dexamethasone 0.75 mg	Dexasone by ICN	Canadian DIN 00285471	Steroid
ICND13	Tab, Green, Oval, Scored	Dexamethasone 4 mg	Dexasone by ICN	Canadian DIN 00489158	Steroid
ICNE12	Tab, Blue, Round, Scored	Ethambutol HCl 400 mg	Etibi by ICN	Canadian DIN 00247979	Antituberculosis
ICNF11	Cap, Blue, Clear	Dicyclomine HCl 10 mg	Formulex by ICN	Canadian DIN 00361933	Gastrointestinal
ICNI22	Tab, White, Scored, Compressed	Isoniazid 300 mg	Isotamine by Valeant	Canadian DIN 00272655	Antimycobacterial
ICNL4	Tab, Orange, Round, Film Coated	Amitriptyline HCl 75 mg	Levate by ICN	Canadian DIN 00405612	Antidepressant
ICNM180	Tab, Straw, Cap Shaped	Pyridostigmine Bromide 180 mg	Mestinon by ICN	Canadian DIN 00869953	Muscle Stimulant
ICNM180	Tab, Straw, Cap Shaped	Pyridostigmine Bromide 180 mg	Mestinon by Roche		Muscle Stimulant
ICNN11	Tab, White, Round	Aminosalicylate 500 mg	Nemasol Sodium by ICN	Canadian DIN 00236691	Antimycobacterial
ICNN14	Tab, White, Round, Scored	Niacin 50 mg	Niacin by ICN	Canadian DIN 00268593	Vitamin
ICNN15	Tab, White, Round, Scored	Niacin 100 mg	Niacin by ICN	Canadian DIN 00268585	Vitamin
ICNN16	Tab, White, Round, Scored	Niacin 500 mg	Niacin by ICN	Canadian DIN 00294950	Vitamin
ICNN21	Tab, White, Round, Scored	Nitrazepam 5 mg	Nitrazadon by Valeant	Canadian DIN 02229654	Sedative; Hypnotic; C IV
ICNN22	Tab, White, Round, Scored	Nitrazepam 10 mg	Nitrazadon by Valeant	Canadian DIN 02229655	Sedative; Hypnotic; C IV
ICNN31	Cap, White & Yellow	Nortriptyline HCl 10 mg	by ICN	Canadian	Antidepressant
ICNN32	Cap, White & Yellow	Nortriptyline HCl 25 mg	by ICN	Canadian	Antidepressant
ICNP17	Tab, Maroon, Round	Phenazopyridine HCl 100 mg	Phenazo by ICN	Canadian DIN 00271489	Urinary Analgesic
ICNP18	Tab, Maroon, Round	Phenazopyridine HCl 200 mg	Phenazo by ICN	Canadian DIN 00454583	Urinary Analgesic
ICNP6	Tab, White	Procyclidine HCl 5 mg	Procyclid by ICN	Canadian DIN 00306290	Antiparkinson
ICNP8	Tab, Peach, Round	Propantheline Bromide 15 mg	Propanthel by ICN	Canadian DIN 00294837	Gastrointestinal
ICNR11	Cap, Opaque & Scarlet	Rifampin 150 mg	Rofact by ICN	Canadian DIN 00393444	Antibiotic

ID FRONT <> BACK	DESCRIPTION FRONT <> BACK	INGREDIENT & STRENGTH	BRAND (or Generic Equiv.) by FIRM	NDC#	CLASS; SCH.
ICNR12	Cap, Brown & Scarlet	Rifampin 300 mg	Rofact by ICN	Canadian DIN 00343617	Antibiotic
ICNS11	Tab, Brown & Yellow, Round	Sulfasalazine 500 mg	SAS by ICN	Canadian DIN	Gastrointestinal
ICNS14	Tab, Brown & Yellow, Oval	Sulfasalazine 500 mg	SAS by ICN	Canadian DIN 00445126	Gastrointestinal
ICNS31	Tab, Light Blue, Oblong	Sotalol HCl 80 mg	Sotacor by ICN	Canadian DIN	Antiarrhythmic
ICNS31	Tab, Light Blue, Oblong, Scored	Sotalol HCl 80 mg	Sotacor by Cobalt	Canadian DIN 02270625	Antiarrhythmic
ICNS32	Tab, Light Blue, Oblong, Scored	Sotalol HCl 160 mg	Sotacor by Cobalt	Canadian DIN 02270633	Antiarrhythmic
ICNS32	Tab, Light Blue, Oblong	Sotalol HCl 160 mg	Sotacor by ICN	Canadian DIN	Antiarrhythmic
ICNS33	Tab, Light Blue, Oblong	Sotalol HCl 240 mg	by ICN	Canadian DIN	Antiarrhythmic
ICNT11	Tab, White, Round, Scored	Pyrazinamide 500 mg	Tebrazid by ICN	Canadian DIN 00283991	Antibiotic
ICNT17	Cap, White, Opaque	L-Tryptophan 500 mg	Tryptan by ICN	Canadian DIN 00718149	Supplement
ICNT21	Tab, Orange	Trazodone HCl 50 mg	Desyrel by ICN	Canadian DIN	Antidepressant
ICNT22	Tab, White	Trazodone HCl 100 mg	Desyrel by ICN	Canadian DIN	Antidepressant
ICNT23	Tab, Orange	Trazodone HCl 150 mg	Desyrel by ICN	Canadian DIN	Antidepressant
ICNV1	Tab, White, Round, Scored	Pyridoxine HCl 25 mg	Vitamin B6 by ICN	Canadian DIN 00268607	Vitamin
ICNV2	Tab, White, Round, Scored	Pyridoxine HCl 50 mg	Vitamin B6 by ICN	Canadian DIN 00252689	Vitamin
ICNV21	Tab, White, Round, Scored	Thiamine HCl 50 mg	Vitamin B1 by ICN	Canadian DIN 00268631	Vitamin
ICNV22	Tab, White, Round, Scored	Thiamine HCl 100 mg	Vitamin B1 by ICN	Canadian DIN 00294853	Vitamin
ICNV3	Tab, White, Round, Scored	Pyridoxine HCl 100 mg	Vitamin B6 by ICN	Canadian DIN 00263958	Vitamin
ID <> 175	Tab, White, Cap Shaped, Scored	Guaifenesin 600 mg	Robitussin by Iopharm	61646-0125	Expectorant
ID111	Tab, Coated, ID/111	Yohimbine HCl 5.4 mg	by Sovereign	58716-0653	Impotence Agent
ID112	Tab, Ex Release	Dextromethorphan HBr 30 mg, Guaifenesin 600 mg, Pseudoephedrine HCl 60 mg	Med Rx DM by Iopharm	61646-0701	Cold Remedy
ID112	Tab, Ex Release	Dextromethorphan HBr 30 mg, Guaifenesin 600 mg	Iobid DM by Sovereign	58716-0654	Cold Remedy
ID121	Tab, Ex Release	Guaifenesin 600 mg, Pseudoephedrine HCl 120 mg	Iotex PSE by Sovereign	58716-0657	Cold Remedy
ID122	Tab, Ex Release	Guaifenesin 600 mg, Pseudoephedrine HCl 60 mg	Decongest II by Qualitest	00603-3116	Cold Remedy
ID122	Tab, Ex Release	Guaifenesin 600 mg, Pseudoephedrine HCl 60 mg	Med Rx by Iopharm	61646-0700	Cold Remedy
ID122	Tab, Ex Release	Guaifenesin 600 mg, Pseudoephedrine HCl 60 mg	Iosal II by Sovereign	58716-0655	Cold Remedy
ID122	Tab, Ex Release	Dextromethorphan HBr 30 mg, Guaifenesin 600 mg, Pseudoephedrine HCl 60 mg	Med Rx DM by Iopharm	61646-0701	Cold Remedy
ID125	Tab, Ex Release	Guaifenesin 600 mg, Pseudoephedrine HCl 60 mg	Med Rx by Iopharm	61646-0700	Cold Remedy
ID125	Tab, White, Oblong, Scored	Guaifenesin 600 mg	Robitussin by Martec	52555-0628	Expectorant
ID125	Tab, Ex Release	Guaifenesin 600 mg	Robitussin by Sovereign	58716-0656	Expectorant
ID152	Tab, Green, Film Coated	Dexbrompheniramine Maleate 6 mg, Pseudoephedrine Sulfate 120 mg	Drexophed Sr by Qualitest	00603-3505	Cold Remedy
ID152	Tab, Green, Round, Film Coated	Dexbrompheniramine Maleate 6 mg, Pseudoephedrine Sulfate 120 mg	Dexaphen SA by Major	00904-0667	Cold Remedy
ID155	Tab, Ex Release	Hyoscyamine Sulfate 0.375 mg	Levsin by Sovereign	58716-0673	Gastrointestinal
ID155	Tab, Ex Release	Hyoscyamine Sulfate 0.375 mg	Levsin by Iopharm	61646-0155	Gastrointestinal
ID155	Tab, Ex Release	Hyoscyamine Sulfate 0.375 mg	Levsin by URL Mutual	00677-1611	Gastrointestinal
ID156	Tab	Hyoscyamine Sulfate 0.125 mg	Levsin by Iopharm	61646-0156	Gastrointestinal
ID156	Tab	Hyoscyamine Sulfate 0.125 mg	Levsin by Sovereign	58716-0675	Gastrointestinal
ID156	Tab	Hyoscyamine Sulfate 0.125 mg	Levsin by Sovereign	58716-0651	Gastrointestinal

ID FRONT <> BACK	DESCRIPTION FRONT <> BACK	INGREDIENT & STRENGTH	BRAND (or Generic Equiv.) by FIRM	NDC#	CLASS; SCH.
ID172	Tab, White, Oblong, Scored	Guaifenesin 1200 mg	Robitussin by Iopharm Labs	61646-0172	Expectorant
ID172	Tab, White, Oblong, Scored	Guaifenesin 1200 mg	Robitussin by New River	59417-0403	Expectorant
ID300	Cap, Ex Release	Chlorpheniramine Maleate 8 mg, Pseudoephedrine HCl 120 mg	Deconomed Sr by Sovereign	58716-0044	Cold Remedy
ID301	Cap, Ex Release	Brompheniramine Maleate 12 mg, Pseudoephedrine HCl 120 mg	by Physician Total Care	54868-3989	Cold Remedy
ID301	Cap, Green and Clear	Brompheniramine Maleate 12 mg, Pseudoephedrine HCl 120 mg	by Qualitest	00603-2505	Cold Remedy
ID301	Cap	Brompheniramine Maleate 12 mg, Pseudoephedrine HCl 120 mg	Iofed by Sovereign	58716-0045	Cold Remedy
ID301	Cap, Ex Release	Brompheniramine Maleate 12 mg, Pseudoephedrine HCl 120 mg	Iofed by Sovereign	58716-0045	Cold Remedy
ID302	Cap, Ex Release	Brompheniramine Maleate 6 mg, Pseudoephedrine HCl 60 mg	Iofed PD by Sovereign	58716-0046	Cold Remedy
ID302	Cap, Dark Green	Brompheniramine Maleate 6 mg, Pseudoephedrine HCl 60 mg	Bromfed PD by Qualitest	00603-2506	Cold Remedy
ID308	Cap	Trimethobenzamide HCl 250 mg	by Sovereign	58716-0055	Antiemetic
ID311	Cap, Ex Release	Chlorpheniramine Maleate 8 mg	by Sovereign	58716-0051	Antihistamine
ID312	Cap, Ex Release	Chlorpheniramine Maleate 12 mg	Chlor-Trimeton by Sovereign	58716-0049	Antihistamine
IE125 <> G	Tab, Orange, Round, Film Coated, IE over 1.25	Indapamide 1.25 mg	Lozol by Par	49884-0589	Diuretic
IE25 <> G	Tab, White, Round, Film Coated, IE over 2.5	Indapamide 2.5 mg	Lozol by Par	49884-0590	Diuretic
IEL650 <> RELAGESIC	Tab, White, Oblong, Scored	Phenyltoloxamine Citrate 50 mg, Acetaminophen 650 mg	Relagesic by Int'l Ethical Labs	11584-0476	Cold Remedy
IG <> 200	Tab, White, Round, Scored	Fosinopril Sodium 10 mg	Monopril by Deca	68552-0221	Antihypertensive
IG <> 200	Tab, White, Round, Scored	Fosinopril Sodium 10 mg	Monopril by Zydus	24658-0100	Antihypertensive
IG <> 201	Tab, White, Round	Fosinopril Sodium 20 mg	Monopril by Zydus	24658-0101	Antihypertensive
IG <> 201	Tab, White, Round	Fosinopril Sodium 20 mg	Monopril by Deca	68552-0222	Antihypertensive
IG <> 202	Tab, White, Round	Fosinopril Sodium 40 mg	Monopril by Deca	68552-0223	Antihypertensive
IG <> 202	Tab, White, Round	Fosinopril Sodium 40 mg	Monopril by Blu	24658-0102	Antihypertensive
IG <> 203	Tab, Pink, Round, I / G	Glimepiride 1 mg	Amaryl by Perrigo	10768-7150	Antidiabetic
IG <> 204	Tab, Green, Round, I / G	Glimepiride 2 mg	Amaryl by Perrigo	10768-7475	Antidiabetic
IG <> 205	Tab, Blue, Round, I / G	Glimepiride 4 mg	Amaryl by Perrigo	10768-7700	Antidiabetic
IG <> 206	Tab, Beige, Round, Coated	Citalopram HBr 10 mg	Celexa by Blu	24658-0140	Antidepressant
IG <> 207	Tab, Pink, Round, Scored, Coated	Citalopram HBr 20 mg	Celexa by Blu	24658-0141	Antidepressant
IG <> 208	Tab, White, Round, Scored, Coated	Citalopram HBr 40 mg	Celexa by Blu	24658-0142	Antidepressant
IG <> 209	Tab, White, Round	Terbinafine 250 mg	Lamisil by Interpharm	68462-0136	Antifungal
IG <> 209	Tab, White, Round	Terbinafine HCl 250 mg	Lamisil by Glenmark	68462-0136	Antifungal
IG <> 209	Tab, White, Round	Terbinafine HCl 250 mg	Lamisil by Blu	24658-0180	Antifungal
IG <> 225	Tab, White, Capsule Shaped	Gemfibrozil 600 mg	Lopid by Blu	24658-130	Antihyperlipidemic
IG <> 225	Tab, White, Cap Shaped, Film Coated, Scored	Gemfibrozil 600 mg	Lopid by Zydus	68382-0100	Antihyperlipidemic
IG <> 237	Tab, White, Round	Amlodipine Besylate 2.5 mg	Norvasc by Blu	24658-0190	Antihypertensive
IG <> 238	Tab, White, Round	Amlodipine Besylate 5 mg	Norvasc by Blu	24658-0191	Antihypertensive
IG <> 239	Tab, White, Round	Amlodipine Besylate 10 mg	Norvasc by Blu	24658-0192	Antihypertensive
IG <> 246	Tab, Blue, Cap Shaped, Scored, I / G <> 246	Levetiracetam 250 mg	Keppra by Glenmark	68462-0545	Antiepileptic
IG <> 247	Tab, Yellow, Cap Shaped, Scored, I / G	Levetiracetam 500 mg	Keppra by Glenmark	68462-0546	Antiepileptic
IG <> 248	Tab, Pink, Cap Shaped, Scored	Levetiracetam 750 mg	Keppra by Glenmark	68462-0547	Antiepileptic
IG <> 257	Tab, White, Oval	Nabumetone 500 mg	Relafen by Glenmark	68462-0358	NSAID
IG <> 258	Tab, White to Light Pink, Oval	Nabumetone 750 mg	Relafen by Glenmark	68462-0359	NSAID
IG <> 259	Tab, Pink, Oval	Zolpidem Tartrate 5 mg	Ambien by Glenmark	68462-0279	Sedative/Hypnotic; C IV
IG <> 260	Tab, White, Oval	Zolpidem Tartrate 10 mg	Ambien by Glenmark	68462-0280	Sedative/Hypnotic; C IV
IG <> 267	Tab, Brown, Round	Quinapril 5 mg	Accupril by Dr. Reddy's	55111-0621	Antihypertensive
IG <> 268	Tab, Brown, Round	Quinapril 10 mg	Accupril by Dr. Reddy's	55111-0622	Antihypertensive
IG <> 269	Tab, Brown, Round	Quinapril 20 mg	Accupril by Dr. Reddy's	55111-0623	Antihypertensive
IG <> 270	Tab, Brown, Oval	Quinapril 40 mg	Accupril by Dr. Reddy's	55111-0624	Antihypertensive
IG <> 275	Tab, White, Round	Hydroxyzine 10 mg	Atarax by Glenmark	68462-0360	Antianxiety; Antihistamine
IG <> 276	Tab, White, Round	Hydroxyzine 25 mg	Atarax by Glenmark	68462-0361	Antianxiety; Antihistamine
IG <> 277	Tab, White, Round	Hydroxyzine 50 mg	Atarax by Glenmark	68462-0362	Antianxiety; Antihistamine
IG <> 278	Tab, White, Round	Topiramate 25 mg	Topamax by Invagen	31722-0278	Anticonvulsant

ID FRONT <> BACK	DESCRIPTION FRONT <> BACK	INGREDIENT & STRENGTH	BRAND (or Generic Equiv.) by FIRM	NDC#	CLASS; SCH.
IG <> 279	Tab, Yellow, Round	Topiramate 50 mg	Topamax by Invagen	31722-0279	Anticonvulsant
IG <> 280	Tab, Light Yellow, Round	Topiramate 100 mg	Topamax by Invagen	31722-0280	Anticonvulsant
IG <> 281	Tab, Pink, Round	Topiramate 200 mg	Topamax by Invagen	31722-0281	Anticonvulsant
IG207	Tab, Pink, Round	Citalopram 20 mg	Celexa by Perrigo		Antidepressant
IG271125MG	Cap, Yellow	Ramipril 1.25 mg	Altace by Blu	24658-0200	Antihypertensive
IG27225MG	Cap, Orange	Ramipril 2.5 mg	Altace by Blu	24658-0201	Antihypertensive
IG2735MG	Cap, Red	Ramipril 5 mg	Altace by Blu	24658-0202	Antihypertensive
IG27410MG	Cap, Blue	Ramipril 10 mg	Altace by Blu	24658-0203	Antihypertensive
IKA11	Tab, White, Round	Clomiphene Citrate 50 mg	Serophene by Serono	44087-8090	Infertility
IL	Cap, Clear, Round, Soft Gel	Benzonatate 100 mg	Tessalon by H J Harkins Co	52959-0411	Antitussive
IL	Cap, Clear, Round, Soft Gel	Benzonatate 100 mg	Tessalon by Inwood	00258-3654	Antitussive
IL	Cap, Clear, Round, Soft Gel	Benzonatate 100 mg	Tessalon by Teva	00093-0060	Antitussive
IL	Cap, Clear, Round, Soft Gel	Benzonatate 100 mg	Tessalon by RP Scherer	11014-1200	Antitussive
IL	Cap, Clear, Round, Soft Gel	Benzonatate 100 mg	Tessalon by RP Scherer	11014-0732	Antitussive
IL	Cap, Clear, Round, Soft Gel	Benzonatate 100 mg	Tessalon by Boca	64376-0502	Antitussive
IL <> 10MG	Tab, Beige, Oval, Film Coated	Citalopram HBr 10 mg	Celexa by Inwood	00258-3695	Antidepressant
IL <> 20MG	Tab, Pink, Oval, Scored, Film Coated, I / L	Citalopram HBr 20 mg	Celexa by Inwood	00258-3696	Antidepressant
IL <> 3613	Tab, Peach, Round, Scored, Ex Release	Isosorbide Dinitrate 40 mg	Isochron by Forest	00456-0637	Antianginal
IL <> 40MG	Tab, White, Oval, Scored, Film Coated, I / L	Citalopram HBr 40 mg	Celexa by Inwood	00258-3697	Antidepressant
IL <> NVR	Tab, Light Pink, Round	Aliskiren 150 mg	Rasilez by Novartis	Canadian DIN 02302063	Antihypertensive
IL <> NVR	Tab, Light Pink, Round	Aliskiren 150 mg	Tekturna by Novartis	00078-0485	Antihypertensive
IL3531	Tab	Theophylline Anhydrous 300 mg	by Med Pro	53978-0320	Antiasthmatic
IL3575	Cap, Clear & White, IL3575	Isosorbide Dinitrate 40 mg	Isordil by Inwood	00258-3575	Antianginal
IL3577	Cap, Clear & White, IL3577	Pentaerythritol Tetranitrate CR 80 mg	Peritrate by Inwood		Antianginal
IL3581	Tab, White, Cap Shaped, Scored, Ex Release, IL Inside Triangle	Theophylline Anhydrous 300 mg	Theo-Dur by Ivax	00182-1400	Antiasthmatic
IL3581	Tab, White, Cap Shaped, Scored, Ex Release, IL Inside Triangle	Theophylline Anhydrous 300 mg	Theo-Dur by Schein	00364-0660	Antiasthmatic
IL3581	Tab, White, Cap Shaped, Scored, Ex Release, IL Inside Triangle	Theophylline Anhydrous 300 mg	Theo-Dur by Inwood	00258-3581	Antiasthmatic
IL3581	Tab, White, Cap Shaped, Scored, Ex Release, IL Inside Triangle	Theophylline Anhydrous 300 mg	Theo-Dur by Teva	00093-0589	Antiasthmatic
IL3581	Tab, White, Cap Shaped, Scored, Ex Release, IL Inside Triangle	Theophylline Anhydrous 300 mg	Theo-Dur by Major	00904-1612	Antiasthmatic
IL3581	Tab, White, Cap Shaped, Scored, Ex Release, IL Inside Triangle	Theophylline Anhydrous 300 mg	Theochron by Forest	00456-4330	Antiasthmatic
IL3581	Tab, White, Capsule Shaped	Theophylline 300 mg	Theodur by URL Mutual	00677-0817	Antiasthmatic
IL3583	Tab, White, Oval, Scored, Ex Release, IL inside Diamond	Theophylline Anhydrous 200 mg	Theo-Dur by Major	00904-1611	Antiasthmatic
IL3583	Tab, White, Oval, Scored, Ex Release, IL inside Diamond	Theophylline Anhydrous 200 mg	Theo-Dur by Schein	00364-0681	Antiasthmatic
IL3583	Tab, White, Oval, Scored, Ex Release, IL inside Diamond	Theophylline Anhydrous 200 mg	Theo-Dur by Qualitest	00603-5945	Antiasthmatic
IL3583	Tab, White, Oval, Scored, Ex Release, IL inside Diamond	Theophylline Anhydrous 200 mg	Theo-Dur by Forest	00456-4320	Antiasthmatic
IL3583	Tab, White, Oval, Scored, Ex Release, IL inside Diamond	Theophylline Anhydrous 200 mg	Theo-Dur by Teva	00093-0588	Antiasthmatic
IL3583	Tab, White, Oval, Scored, Ex Release, IL inside Diamond	Theophylline Anhydrous 200 mg	Theo-Dur by Inwood	00258-3583	Antiasthmatic
IL3583	Tab, White, Oval, Scored, Ex Release, IL inside Diamond	Theophylline Anhydrous 200 mg	Theo-Dur by Ivax	00182-1590	Antiasthmatic
IL3583	Tab, White, Oval, Scored, Ex Release, IL inside Diamond	Theophylline Anhydrous 200 mg	Theo-Dur by URL Mutual	00677-0846	Antiasthmatic
IL3584	Tab, White, Round, Scored, Ex Release, IL Inside Triangle	Theophylline Anhydrous 100 mg	Theo-Dur by Ivax	00182-1589	Antiasthmatic
IL3584	Tab, White, Round, Scored, Ex Release, IL Inside Triangle	Theophylline Anhydrous 100 mg	Theo-Dur by Inwood	00258-3584	Antiasthmatic
IL3584	Tab, White, Round, Scored, Ex Release, IL Inside Triangle	Theophylline Anhydrous 100 mg	Theo-Dur by Schein	00364-0680	Antiasthmatic
IL3584	Tab, White, Round, Scored, Ex Release, IL Inside Triangle	Theophylline Anhydrous 100 mg	Theo-Dur by Forest	00456-4310	Antiasthmatic

ID FRONT <> BACK	DESCRIPTION FRONT <> BACK	INGREDIENT & STRENGTH	BRAND (or Generic Equiv.) by FIRM	NDC#	CLASS; SCH.
IL3584	Tab, White, Round, Scored, Ex Release, IL Inside Triangle	Theophylline Anhydrous 100 mg	Theo-Dur by Teva	00093-0599	Antiasthmatic
IL3584	Tab, White, Round, Scored, Ex Release, IL Inside Triangle	Theophylline Anhydrous 100 mg	Theo-Dur by Major	00904-1610	Antiasthmatic
IL3587	Tab, White, Round	Carbamazepine 200 mg	Tegretol by Inwood	00258-3587	Anticonvulsant
IL3587	Tab, White, Round	Carbamazepine 200 mg	Tegretol by Qualitest	00603-2563	Anticonvulsant
IL3607	Cap, Lavender, Ex Release	Indomethacin 75 mg	Indocin SR by Qualitest	00603-4070	NSAID
IL3607	Cap, Lavender, Ex Release	Indomethacin 75 mg	Indocin SR by Ivax	00182-1469	NSAID
IL3607	Cap, Lavender, Ex Release	Indomethacin 75 mg	Indocin SR by Inwood	00258-3607	NSAID
IL3607	Cap, Lavender, Ex Release	Indomethacin 75 mg	Indocin SR by Schein	00364-2211	NSAID
IL3609	Cap, Brown & Clear, Opaque, Ex Release, IL over 3609	Propranolol HCl 60 mg	Inderal by Ivax	00182-1926	Antihypertensive
IL3609	Cap, Brown & Clear, Opaque, Ex Release, IL over 3609	Propranolol HCl 60 mg	Inderal by Teva	00093-0691	Antihypertensive
IL3609	Cap, Brown & Clear, Opaque, Ex Release, IL over 3609	Propranolol HCl 60 mg	Inderal by Inwood	00258-3609	Antihypertensive
IL3609	Cap, Ex Release	Propranolol HCl 60 mg	Inderal by Qualitest	00603-5497	Antihypertensive
IL3610	Cap, Blue & Clear, Opaque, Ex Release, IL over 3610	Propranolol HCl 80 mg	Inderal by Teva	00093-0692	Antihypertensive
IL3610	Cap, Blue & Clear, Opaque, Ex Release, IL over 3610	Propranolol HCl 80 mg	Inderal by Ivax	00182-1927	Antihypertensive
IL3610	Cap, Blue & Clear, Opaque, Ex Release, IL over 3610	Propranolol HCl 80 mg	Inderal by Qualitest	00603-5498	Antihypertensive
IL3611	Cap, Ex Release	Propranolol HCl 120 mg	Inderal LA by Qualitest	00603-5499	Antihypertensive
IL3611	Cap, Ex Release	Propranolol HCl 120 mg	Inderal LA by URL Mutual	00677-1365	Antihypertensive
IL3611	Cap, Ex Release	Propranolol HCl 120 mg	Inderal LA by Ivax	00182-1928	Antihypertensive
IL3611	Cap, Ex Release	Hydromorphone HCl 2 mg	by Vintage	00254-3611	Analgesic; C II
IL3612	Cap, Blue & Clear, Opaque, Ex Release, IL over 3612	Propranolol HCl 160 mg	Inderal LA by Inwood	00258-3612	Antihypertensive
IL3612	Cap, Blue & Clear, Opaque, Ex Release, IL over 3612	Propranolol HCl 160 mg	Inderal LA by Teva	00093-0694	Antihypertensive
IL3612	Cap, Blue & Clear, Opaque, Ex Release, IL over 3612	Propranolol HCl 160 mg	Inderal LA by Ivax	00182-1929	Antihypertensive
IL3612	Cap, Blue & Clear, Opaque, Ex Release, IL over 3612	Propranolol HCl 160 mg	Inderal LA by Qualitest	00603-5500	Antihypertensive
IL3614	Cap, Off-White, Cap Shaped, Scored, Ex Release	Theophylline Anhydrous 450 mg	by Inwood	00258-3614	Antiasthmatic
IL3614450	Tab, Off-White, Ex Release	Theophylline Anhydrous 450 mg	by Major	00904-1613	Antiasthmatic
IL3622	Tab, White, Cap Shaped	Acetaminophen 650 mg, Hydrocodone Bitartrate 7.5 mg	Lorcet Plus by Inwood	00258-3622	Analgesic; C III
IL3622	Tab, White, Cap Shaped	Acetaminophen 650 mg, Hydrocodone Bitartrate 7.5 mg	Lorcet Plus by Moore	00839-8061	Analgesic; C III
IL3625	Cap, Clear & White, Opaque, Ex Release	Theophylline Anhydrous 300 mg	Theo-Dur by Major	00904-7849	Antiasthmatic
IL3625	Cap, Clear & White, Opaque, Ex Release	Theophylline Anhydrous 300 mg	Theo-Dur by Qualitest	00603-5952	Antiasthmatic
IL3625	Cap, Clear & White, Opaque, Ex Release	Theophylline Anhydrous 300 mg	Theo-Dur by Inwood	00258-3625	Antiasthmatic
IL3625	Cap, Clear & White, Opaque, Ex Release	Theophylline Anhydrous 300 mg	Theo-Dur by Teva	00093-0940	Antiasthmatic
IL3625	Cap, Clear & White, Opaque, Ex Release	Theophylline Anhydrous 300 mg		Discontinued	
IL3634	Cap, Clear & White, Ex Release	Theophylline Anhydrous 200 mg	Theocap by Forest	00456-4303	Antiasthmatic
IL3634	Cap, Clear & White, Ex Release	Theophylline Anhydrous 200 mg	Theocap by Forest	00456-4302	Antiasthmatic
IL3634	Cap, Clear & White, Ex Release	Theophylline Anhydrous 200 mg	Theo-Dur by Qualitest	00603-5951	Antiasthmatic
IL3634	Cap, Clear & White, Ex Release	Theophylline Anhydrous 200 mg	Theo-Dur by Teva	00093-0938	Antiasthmatic
IL3634	Cap, Clear & White, Ex Release	Theophylline Anhydrous 200 mg		Discontinued	
IL3625	Cap, Clear & White, Ex Release	Theophylline Anhydrous 200 mg	Theo-Dur by Inwood	00258-3634	Antiasthmatic
IL3637	Cap, Clear & White, Ex Release	Theophylline Anhydrous 100 mg	Theo-Dur by Inwood	00258-3637	Antiasthmatic
IL3638	Cap, Clear, Ex Release	Theophylline Anhydrous 125 mg	Theo-Dur by Teva	00093-0936	Antiasthmatic
IL3638	Cap, Clear, Ex Release	Theophylline Anhydrous 125 mg		Discontinued	
IL3638	Cap, Clear, Ex Release	Theophylline Anhydrous 125 mg	Theo-Dur by Inwood	00258-3638	Antiasthmatic
IL3638	Cap, Clear, Ex Release	Theophylline Anhydrous 125 mg	Theo-Dur by Qualitest	00603-5950	Antiasthmatic
IL3638	Cap, Clear, Ex Release	Theophylline Anhydrous 125 mg	Theocap by Forest	00456-4301	Antiasthmatic
IL3657	Tab, White, Oblong, Scored	Acetaminophen 500 mg, Butalbital 50 mg, Caffeine 40 mg	Esgic Plus by Mikart	46672-0059	Analgesic
IL3657	Tab, White, Oblong, Scored	Acetaminophen 500 mg, Butalbital 50 mg, Caffeine 40 mg	Esgic Plus by Inwood	00258-3657	Analgesic
IL3657	Tab, White, Oblong, Scored	Acetaminophen 500 mg, Butalbital 50 mg, Caffeine 40 mg	Esgic Plus by Caremark	00339-5021	Analgesic
IL3658	Tab, Blue, Cap Shaped	Acetaminophen 650 mg, Hydrocodone Bitartrate 10 mg	Lorcet by Inwood	00258-3658	Analgesic; C III
IL3660	Tab, White	Acetaminophen 750 mg, Hydrocodone Bitartrate 7.5 mg	Vicodin ES by Inwood	00258-3660	Analgesic; C III
IL3660	Tab, White	Acetaminophen 750 mg, Hydrocodone Bitartrate 7.5 mg	Vicodin ES by Forest		Analgesic; C III

ID FRONT <> BACK	DESCRIPTION FRONT <> BACK	INGREDIENT & STRENGTH	BRAND (or Generic Equiv.) by FIRM	NDC#	CLASS; SCH.
IL3661	Tab, White	Acetaminophen 660 mg, Hydrocodone Bitartrate 10 mg	Vicodin HP by Forest		Analgesic; C III
IL3661	Tab, White	Acetaminophen 660 mg, Hydrocodone Bitartrate 10 mg	Vicodin HP by Inwood	00258-3661	Analgesic; C III
IL3662	Tab, White	Acetaminophen 650 mg, Hydrocodone Bitartrate 7.5 mg	Lorcet Plus by Inwood	00258-3662	Analgesic; C III
IL3662	Tab, White	Acetaminophen 650 mg, Hydrocodone Bitartrate 7.5 mg	Lorcet Plus by Forest		Analgesic; C III
IL3665	Tab, White, Cap Shaped	Acetaminophen 325 mg, Butalbital 50 mg, Caffeine 40 mg	Fioricet by Inwood	00258-3665	Analgesic
IL3711	Tab, Orange, Oval, Film Coated	Rimantadine HCl 100 mg	Flumadine by RX Pak	65084-0189	Antiviral
IL3853	Tab, Ex Release, Inwood	Theophylline Anhydrous 200 mg	by Moore	00839-6729	Antiasthmatic
ILOSONE250MGH09	Cap, Red and Ivory, Opaque, Ilosone 250 mg/H09	Erythromycin Estolate 250 mg	Ilosone by Eli Lilly	Canadian	Antibiotic
ILOSONE250MGH09	Cap, Red and Ivory, Opaque, Ilosone 250 mg/H09	Erythromycin Estolate 250 mg	Ilosone by Dista Prod	00777-0809	Antibiotic
ILXB12	Tab, Red, Caplet, I.L.X B12	Iron 37.5 mg	ILXB12 Caplet by Kenwood	00482-0110	Vitamin; Mineral
IMAX100	Cap, Red	Acetaminophen 325 mg, Dichloralphenazone 100 mg, Isometheptene Mucate 65 mg	Migraine by Major	00904-7622	Analgesic; C IV
IMAX100	Cap, Red	Acetaminophen 325 mg, Dichloralphenazone 100 mg, Isometheptene Mucate 65 mg	Midrin by Breckenridge	51991-0395	Analgesic; C IV
IMDUR <> 120	Tab, White, Oval	Isosorbide Mononitrate 120 mg	Imdur by Schering	00085-1153	Antianginal
IMDUR <> 120	Tab, White, Oval	Isosorbide Mononitrate 120 mg	Imdur by Murfreesboro	51129-1574	Antianginal
IMDUR <> 120	Tab, White, Oval	Isosorbide Mononitrate 120 mg	Imdur by Pharm Util	60491-0314	Antianginal
IMDUR <> 3030	Tab, Light Red, Oval, Scored	Isosorbide Mononitrate 30 mg	Imdur by AstraZeneca	17228-3306	Antianginal
IMDUR <> 3030	Tab, Light Red, Oval, Scored	Isosorbide Mononitrate 30 mg	Imdur by Murfreesboro	51129-1573	Antianginal
IMDUR <> 3030	Tab, Light Red, Oval, Scored	Isosorbide Mononitrate 30 mg	Imdur by Schering	00085-3306	Antianginal
IMDUR <> 3030	Tab, Light Red, Oval, Scored	Isosorbide Mononitrate 30 mg	Imdur by Caremark	00339-6002	Antianginal
IMDUR <> 6060	Tab, Yellow, Oval, Scored	Isosorbide Mononitrate 60 mg	Imdur by Schering	00085-4110	Antianginal
IMDUR <> 6060	Tab, Yellow, Oval, Scored	Isosorbide Mononitrate 60 mg	Imdur by Caremark	00339-6003	Antianginal
IMDUR <> 6060	Tab, Yellow, Oval, Scored	Isosorbide Mononitrate 60 mg	Imdur by Murfreesboro	51129-1575	Antianginal
IMDUR <> 6060	Tab, Yellow, Oval, Scored	Isosorbide Mononitrate 60 mg	Imdur by Nat Pharmpak	55154-3512	Antianginal
IMITREX <> 100	Tab, Pink, Triangular Shaped, Film Coated	Sumatriptan Succinate 100 mg	Imitrex by GSK	00173-0450	Antimigraine
IMITREX <> 50	Tab, White, Triangular, Coated	Sumatriptan Succinate 50 mg	Imitrex by GSK	00173-0459	Antimigraine
IMITREX <> 50	Tab, White, Triangular, Coated	Sumatriptan Succinate 50 mg	Imitrex by Physician Total Care	54868-3852	Antimigraine
IMITREX <> 50	Tab, White, Triangular, Coated	Sumatriptan Succinate 50 mg	Imitrex by Pharm Util	60491-0318	Antimigraine
IMITREX100	Tab, Pink, Triangular, Film Coated, IMITREX100 <> ^	Sumatriptan Succinate 100 mg	Imitrex by GSK	00173-0737	Antimigraine
IMITREX100	Tab, Pink, Triangular, Film Coated, IMITREX100 <> ^	Sumatriptan Succinate 100 mg	Imitrex by GSK	Canadian DIN 02212161	Antimigraine
IMITREX50	Tab, White, Triangular, Film Coated, IMITREX50 <> ^	Sumatriptan Succinate 50 mg	Imitrex by GSK	Canadian DIN 02212153	Antimigraine
IMITREX50	Tab, White, Triangular, Film Coated, IMITREX50 <> ^	Sumatriptan Succinate 50 mg	Imitrex by GSK	00173-0736	Antimigraine
IMO <> 2125	Tab, White, Cap Shaped, 2 over 125	Loperamide HCl 2 mg, Simethicone 125 mg	Imodium by McNeil Consumer		Antidiarrheal; Antiflatulent
IMODIUM2125	Tab, Green, Round, Scored, Chewable, Imodium 2/125	Loperamide 2 mg, Simethicone 125 mg	Imodium by McNeil	Canadian DIN 02237297	Antidiarrheal
IMODIUMAD <> 2MG	Tab, Light Green, Cap Shaped, Scored, Imodium A-D 2 mg	Loperamide 2 mg	Imodium by McNeil	Canadian DIN 02183862	Antidiarrheal
IMOVANE	Tab, Blue, Oval, Logo	Zopiclone 7.5 mg	Rhovane by Rhodiapharm	Canadian	Hypnotic
IMOVANE5 <> RPR	Tab, White, Round	Zopiclone 5 mg	Imovane 5 by ICN	Canadian DIN 02216167	Hypnotic
IMURAN50	Tab, Off-White, Peanut Shaped, Scored, Imuran over 50	Azathioprine 50 mg	Imuran by Pharmedix	53002-0486	Immunosuppressant
IMURAN50	Tab, Off-White, Peanut Shaped, Scored, Imuran over 50	Azathioprine 50 mg	Imuran by GSK	00173-0597	Immunosuppressant
IMURAN50	Tab, Off-White, Peanut Shaped, Scored, Imuran over 50	Azathioprine 50 mg	Imuran by DSM	63552-0597	Immunosuppressant
IMURAN50	Tab, Off-White, Peanut Shaped, Scored, Imuran over 50	Azathioprine 50 mg	Imuran by GSK	Canadian DIN 00004596	Immunosuppressant
IN125 <> PMS	Tab, Orange, Round, Coated, IN 12.5	Indapamide 1.25 mg	Lozide by Pharmascience	Canadian DIN 02239619	Diuretic

ID FRONT <> BACK	DESCRIPTION FRONT <> BACK	INGREDIENT & STRENGTH	BRAND (or Generic Equiv.) by FIRM	NDC#	CLASS; SCH.
IN25 <> P	Tab, Pink, Round	Indapamide 2.5 mg	Lozide by Pharmascience	Canadian DIN 02239620	Antihypertensive; Diuretic
IND25	Cap, Cream	Indomethacin 25 mg	Indocin by Rhodiapharm	Canadian	NSAID
IND50	Cap, Light Brown	Indomethacin 50 mg	Indocin by Rhodiapharm	Canadian	NSAID
INDERAL10 <> I	Tab, Peach, Hexagonal, Scored, Inderal over 10	Propranolol HCl 10 mg	Inderal by Amerisource	62584-0421	Antihypertensive
INDERAL10 <> I	Tab, Peach, Hexagonal, Scored, Inderal over 10	Propranolol HCl 10 mg	Inderal by Nat Pharmpak	55154-0204	Antihypertensive
INDERAL10 <> I	Tab, Peach, Hexagonal, Scored, Inderal over 10	Propranolol HCl 10 mg	Inderal by Drug Distr	52985-0036	Antihypertensive
INDERAL10 <> I	Tab, Peach, Hexagonal, Scored, Inderal over 10	Propranolol HCl 10 mg	Inderal by Thrift Drug	59198-0038	Antihypertensive
INDERAL10 <> I	Tab, Peach, Hexagonal, Scored, Inderal over 10	Propranolol HCl 10 mg	Inderal by Leiner	59606-0660	Antihypertensive
INDERAL10 <> I	Tab, Peach, Hexagonal, Scored, Inderal over 10	Propranolol HCl 10 mg	Inderal by Ayerst	00046-0421	Antihypertensive
INDERAL10 <> I	Tab, Peach, Hexagonal, Scored, Inderal over 10	Propranolol HCl 10 mg	Inderal by Med Pro	53978-0034	Antihypertensive
INDERAL10 <> I	Tab, Peach, Hexagonal, Scored, Inderal over 10	Propranolol HCl 10 mg	Inderal by RP Scherer SA	64566-0001	Antihypertensive
INDERAL20 <> I	Tab, Blue, Hexagonal, Scored, Inderal over 20	Propranolol HCl 20 mg	Inderal by Right Pak	65240-0668	Antihypertensive
INDERAL20 <> I	Tab, Blue, Hexagonal, Scored, Inderal over 20	Propranolol HCl 20 mg	Inderal by Nat Pharmpak	55154-0205	Antihypertensive
INDERAL20 <> I	Tab, Blue, Hexagonal, Scored, Inderal over 20	Propranolol HCl 20 mg	Inderal by PDRX	55289-0131	Antihypertensive
INDERAL20 <> I	Tab, Blue, Hexagonal, Scored, Inderal over 20	Propranolol HCl 20 mg	Inderal by Leiner	59606-0661	Antihypertensive
INDERAL20 <> I	Tab, Blue, Hexagonal, Scored, Inderal over 20	Propranolol HCl 20 mg	Inderal by Amerisource	62584-0422	Antihypertensive
INDERAL20 <> I	Tab, Blue, Hexagonal, Scored, Inderal over 20	Propranolol HCl 20 mg	Inderal by Drug Distr	52985-0037	Antihypertensive
INDERAL20 <> I	Tab, Blue, Hexagonal, Scored, Inderal over 20	Propranolol HCl 20 mg	Inderal by Thrift Drug	59198-0039	Antihypertensive
INDERAL20 <> I	Tab, Blue, Hexagonal, Scored, Inderal over 20	Propranolol HCl 20 mg	Inderal by Ayerst	00046-0422	Antihypertensive
INDERAL20 <> I	Tab, Blue, Hexagonal, Scored, Inderal over 20	Propranolol HCl 20 mg	Inderal by Caremark	00339-5167	Antihypertensive
INDERAL20 <> I	Tab, Blue, Hexagonal, Scored, Inderal over 20	Propranolol HCl 20 mg	Inderal by RP Scherer SA	64566-0002	Antihypertensive
INDERAL40 <> I	Tab, Green, Hexagonal, Scored, Inderal over 40	Propranolol HCl 40 mg	Inderal by Ayerst	00046-0424	Antihypertensive
INDERAL40 <> I	Tab, Green, Hexagonal, Scored, Inderal over 40	Propranolol HCl 40 mg	Inderal by Rightpak	65240-0662	Antihypertensive
INDERAL40 <> I	Tab, Green, Hexagonal, Scored, Inderal over 40	Propranolol HCl 40 mg	Inderal by Drug Distr	52985-0019	Antihypertensive
INDERAL40 <> I	Tab, Green, Hexagonal, Scored, Inderal over 40	Propranolol HCl 40 mg	Inderal by Amerisource	62584-0424	Antihypertensive
INDERAL40 <> I	Tab, Green, Hexagonal, Scored, Inderal over 40	Propranolol HCl 40 mg	Inderal by Nat Pharmpak	55154-0206	Antihypertensive
INDERAL40 <> I	Tab, Green, Hexagonal, Scored, Inderal over 40	Propranolol HCl 40 mg	Inderal by Thrift Drug	59198-0040	Antihypertensive
INDERAL40 <> I	Tab, Green, Hexagonal, Scored, Inderal over 40	Propranolol HCl 40 mg	Inderal by Leiner	59606-0662	Antihypertensive
INDERAL40 <> I	Tab, Green, Hexagonal, Scored, Inderal over 40	Propranolol HCl 40 mg	Inderal by Respa	60575-0087	Antihypertensive
INDERAL60 <> I	Tab, Pink, Hexagonal, Scored, Inderal over 60	Propranolol HCl 60 mg	Inderal by Ayerst	00046-0426	Antihypertensive
INDERAL80 <> I	Tab, Light Yellow, Hexagonal, Scored, Inderal over 80	Propranolol HCl 80 mg	Inderal by Ayerst	00046-0428	Antihypertensive
INDERAL80 <> I	Tab, Light Yellow, Hexagonal, Scored, Inderal over 80	Propranolol HCl 80 mg	Inderal by Murfreesboro	51129-1304	Antihypertensive
INDERAL80 <> I	Tab, Light Yellow, Hexagonal, Scored, Inderal over 80	Propranolol HCl 80 mg	Inderal by Nat Pharmpak	55154-0208	Antihypertensive
INDERAL80 <> I	Tab, Light Yellow, Hexagonal, Scored, Inderal over 80	Propranolol HCl 80 mg	Inderal by Leiner	59606-0663	Antihypertensive
INDERAL80 <> I	Tab, Light Yellow, Hexagonal, Scored, Inderal over 80	Propranolol HCl 80 mg	Inderal by Amerisource	62584-0428	Antihypertensive
INDERAL80 <> I	Tab, Light Yellow, Hexagonal, Scored, Inderal over 80	Propranolol HCl 80 mg	Inderal by Thrift Drug	59198-0041	Antihypertensive
INDERAL80 <> I	Tab, Light Yellow, Hexagonal, Scored, Inderal over 80	Propranolol HCl 80 mg	Inderal by Pharm Util	60491-0319	Antihypertensive
INDERAL80 <> I	Tab, Light Yellow, Hexagonal, Scored, Inderal over 80	Propranolol HCl 80 mg	Inderal by Caremark	00339-5171	Antihypertensive
INDERALLA120	Cap, Dark Blue & Light Blue, White Print, Ex Release	Propranolol HCl 120 mg	Inderal LA by RX Pak	65084-0104	Antihypertensive
INDERALLA120	Cap, Dark Blue & Light Blue, White Print, Ex Release	Propranolol HCl 120 mg	Inderal LA by Rightpak	65240-0666	Antihypertensive
INDERALLA120	Cap, Dark Blue & Light Blue, White Print, Ex Release	Propranolol HCl 120 mg	Inderal LA by Ayerst	00046-0473	Antihypertensive
INDERALLA120	Cap, Dark Blue & Light Blue, White Print, Ex Release	Propranolol HCl 120 mg	Inderal LA by Physician Total Care	54868-1442	Antihypertensive
INDERALLA120	Cap, Dark Blue & Light Blue, White Print, Ex Release	Propranolol HCl 120 mg	Inderal LA by Thrift Drug	59198-0043	Antihypertensive
INDERALLA120	Cap, Dark Blue & Light Blue, White Print, Ex Release	Propranolol HCl 120 mg	Inderal LA by Nat Pharmpak	55154-0202	Antihypertensive
INDERALLA120	Cap, Dark Blue & Light Blue, White Print, Ex Release	Propranolol HCl 120 mg	Inderal LA by Amerisource	62584-0473	Antihypertensive
INDERALLA120	Cap, Dark Blue & Light Blue, White Print, Ex Release	Propranolol HCl 120 mg	Inderal LA by Wyeth	Canadian DIN 02042266	Antihypertensive
INDERALLA160	Cap, Blue, White Print, Ex Release	Propranolol HCl 160 mg	Inderal LA by Ayerst	00046-0479	Antihypertensive
INDERALLA160	Cap, Blue, White Print, Ex Release	Propranolol HCl 160 mg	Inderal LA by Thrift Drug	59198-0044	Antihypertensive

ID FRONT <> BACK	DESCRIPTION FRONT <> BACK	INGREDIENT & STRENGTH	BRAND (or Generic Equiv.) by FIRM	NDC#	CLASS; SCH.
INDERALLA160	Cap, Blue, White Print, Ex Release	Propranolol HCl 160 mg	Inderal LA by Amerisource	62584-0479	Antihypertensive
INDERALLA160	Cap, Blue, White Print, Ex Release	Propranolol HCl 160 mg	Inderal LA by Pharm Util	60491-0323	Antihypertensive
INDERALLA160	Cap, Blue, White Print, Ex Release	Propranolol HCl 160 mg	Inderal LA by Nat Pharmpak	55154-0203	Antihypertensive
INDERALLA160	Cap, Blue, White Print, Ex Release	Propranolol HCl 160 mg	Inderal LA by Wyeth	Canadian DIN 02042274	Antihypertensive
INDERALLA60	Cap, White & Light Blue, White Print, Ex Release	Propranolol HCl 60 mg	Inderal LA by Ayerst	00046-0470	Antihypertensive
INDERALLA60	Cap, White & Light Blue, White Print, Ex Release	Propranolol HCl 60 mg	Inderal LA by RX Pak	65084-0105	Antihypertensive
INDERALLA60	Cap, White & Light Blue, White Print, Ex Release	Propranolol HCl 60 mg	Inderal LA by Respa	60575-0733	Antihypertensive
INDERALLA60	Cap, White & Light Blue, White Print, Ex Release	Propranolol HCl 60 mg	Inderal LA by Thrift Drug	59198-0226	Antihypertensive
INDERALLA60	Cap, White & Light Blue, White Print, Ex Release	Propranolol HCl 60 mg	Inderal LA by Leiner	59606-0664	Antihypertensive
INDERALLA60	Cap, White & Light Blue, White Print, Ex Release	Propranolol HCl 60 mg	Inderal LA by Rightpak	65240-0664	Antihypertensive
INDERALLA60	Cap, White & Light Blue, White Print, Ex Release	Propranolol HCl 60 mg	Inderal LA by Wyeth	Canadian DIN 02042231	Antihypertensive
INDERALLA80	Cap, Blue, White Print, Ex Release	Propranolol HCl 80 mg	Inderal LA by Rightpak	65240-0665	Antihypertensive
INDERALLA80	Cap, Blue, White Print, Ex Release	Propranolol HCl 80 mg	Inderal LA by Ayerst	00046-0471	Antihypertensive
INDERALLA80	Cap, Blue, White Print, Ex Release	Propranolol HCl 80 mg	Inderal LA by RX Pak	65084-0103	Antihypertensive
INDERALLA80	Cap, Blue, White Print, Ex Release	Propranolol HCl 80 mg	Inderal LA by Amerisource	62584-0471	Antihypertensive
INDERALLA80	Cap, Blue, White Print, Ex Release	Propranolol HCl 80 mg	Inderal LA by Nat Pharmpak	55154-0201	Antihypertensive
INDERALLA80	Cap, Blue, White Print, Ex Release	Propranolol HCl 80 mg	Inderal LA by Repack Co of America	55306-0080	Antihypertensive
INDERALLA80	Cap, Blue, White Print, Ex Release	Propranolol HCl 80 mg	Inderal LA by Physician Total Care	54868-0680	Antihypertensive
INDERALLA80	Cap, Blue, White Print, Ex Release	Propranolol HCl 80 mg	Inderal LA by Thrift Drug	59198-0042	Antihypertensive
INDERALLA80	Cap, Blue, White Print, Ex Release	Propranolol HCl 80 mg	Inderal LA by Wyeth	Canadian DIN 02042258	Antihypertensive
INDERIDE4025 <> I	Tab, Off-White, Hexagonal	Hydrochlorothiazide 25 mg, Propranolol HCl 40 mg	Inderide by Ayerst	00046-0484	Diuretic; Antihypertensive
INDERIDE8025 <> I	Tab, Off-White, Hexagonal, Scored	Hydrochlorothiazide 25 mg, Propranolol HCl 80 mg	Inderide by Ayerst	00046-0488	Diuretic; Antihypertensive
INDERIDELA12050	Cap, Ex Release, Inderide LA 120/50	Hydrochlorothiazide 50 mg, Propranolol HCl 120 mg	Inderide LA by Pharm Util	60491-0328	Diuretic; Antihypertensive
INDERIDELA16050	Cap, Ex Release, Inderide LA 160/50	Hydrochlorothiazide 50 mg, Propranolol HCl 160 mg	Inderide LA by Pharm Util	60491-0329	Diuretic; Antihypertensive
INDOCINSR695	Cap, Clear, Indocin SR over 695, Black Ink	Indomethacin 75 mg	Indocin SR by Murfreesboro	51129-1550	NSAID
INDOCINSR695	Cap, Clear, Indocin SR over 695, Black Ink	Indomethacin 75 mg	Indocin SR by Murfreesboro	51129-1551	NSAID
INDOCINSRMSD693	Cap, Blue & Clear & Opaque, Indocin SR Containing Blue & White Pellets	Indomethacin 75 mg	Indocin SR by Murfreesboro	51129-1548	NSAID
INDOTEC25TEC	Cap, Blue & White, Indotec 25/TEC	Indomethacin 25 mg	Indocin by Technilab	Canadian DIN 02143364	NSAID
INDOTEC50TEC	Cap, Blue & White, Indotec 50/TEC	Indomethacin 50 mg	Indocin by Technilab	Canadian DIN 02143372	NSAID
INGELHEIMTOWER-LOGO	Tab, Orange & Red, Round	Dipyridamole 75 mg	by Boehringer Ingelheim	Canadian Discontinued	Antiplatelet
INGELHEIMTOWER-LOGO	Tab, Red, Round	Dipyridamole 50 mg	Persantine by Boehringer Ingelheim	Canadian Discontinued	Antiplatelet
INGELHEIMTOWER-LOGO	Tab, White, Round	Dipyridamole 100 mg	by Boehringer Ingelheim	Canadian Discontinued	Antiplatelet
INGELHEIMTOWER-LOGO	Tab, Orange, Round	Dipyridamole 25 mg	by Boehringer Ingelheim	Canadian Discontinued	Antiplatelet
INOR	Tab, White, Round	Levonorgestrel 0.75 mg	Plan B by Womens Capital	64836-0000	Oral Contraceptive
INOR	Tab, White, Round	Levonorgestrel 0.75 mg	Plan B by Barr	51285-0038	Oral Contraceptive
INV <> 205	Tab, Film Coated	Hydrochlorothiazide 15 mg, Methyldopa 250 mg	by Qualitest	00603-4543	Diuretic; Antihypertensive
INV <> 206	Tab, Film Coated	Hydrochlorothiazide 25 mg, Methyldopa 250 mg	by Qualitest	00603-4544	Diuretic; Antihypertensive
INV <> 250	Tab, Film Coated	Hydroxychloroquine Sulfate 200 mg	by Invamed	52189-0250	Antimalarial
INV <> 250	Tab, White, Oblong, Film Coated	Hydroxychloroquine Sulfate 200 mg	by Murfreesboro	51129-1426	Antimalarial
INV <> 250	Tab, White, Oblong, Film Coated	Hydroxychloroquine Sulfate 200 mg	by DRX	55045-2766	Antimalarial
INV <> 252	Tab, Film Coated	Cyclobenzaprine HCl 10 mg	by Physician Total Care	54868-1110	Muscle Relaxant

ID FRONT <> BACK	DESCRIPTION FRONT <> BACK	INGREDIENT & STRENGTH	BRAND (or Generic Equiv.) by FIRM	NDC#	CLASS; SCH.
INV <> 259	Tab	Atenolol 25 mg	Tenormin by Invamed	52189-0259	Antihypertensive
INV <> 259	Tab	Atenolol 25 mg	Tenormin by Apothecon	62269-0259	Antihypertensive
INV <> 261	Tab, White, Round	Methazolamide 25 mg	Neptazane by Apothecon	62269-0261	Antiglaucoma Agent
INV <> 261	Tab, White, Round	Methazolamide 25 mg	Neptazane by Invamed	52189-0261	Antiglaucoma Agent
INV <> 271	Tab, Scored	Captopril 12.5 mg	Capoten by Invamed	52189-0271	Antihypertensive
INV <> 271	Tab, Scored	Captopril 12.5 mg	Capoten by Schein	00364-2628	Antihypertensive
INV <> 278	Tab, Purple, Round, Film Coated	Trifluoperazine HCl 1 mg	Stelazine by Invamed	52189-0278	Antipsychotic
INV <> 278	Tab, Purple, Round, Film Coated	Trifluoperazine HCl 1 mg	by Apothecon	62269-0278	Antipsychotic
INV100274	Tab, White, Oval	Captopril 100 mg	Capoten by Invamed		Antihypertensive
INV101	Tab, White, Round	Aluminum Hydroxide 80 mg, Magnesium Trilisate 20 mg	Gaviscon by Invamed	Discontinued	Gastrointestinal
INV208	Tab, White, Round, Scored, INV over 208	Benztropine Mesylate 0.5 mg	Cogentin by Apothecon	62269-0208	Antiparkinson
INV208	Tab, White, Round, Scored, INV over 208	Benztropine Mesylate 0.5 mg	Cogentin by Heartland	61392-0167	Antiparkinson
INV208	Tab, White, Round, Scored, INV over 208	Benztropine Mesylate 0.5 mg	Cogentin by Invamed	52189-0208	Antiparkinson
INV209	Tab, White, Oval	Benztropine Mesylate 1 mg	Cogentin by Heartland	61392-0170	Antiparkinson
INV209	Tab, White, Oval	Benztropine Mesylate 1 mg	Cogentin by Golden State	60429-0027	Antiparkinson
INV209	Tab, White, Oval	Benztropine Mesylate 1 mg	Cogentin by Apothecon	62269-0209	Antiparkinson
INV209	Tab, Scored, INV over 209	Benztropine Mesylate 1 mg	Cogentin by Invamed	52189-0209	Antiparkinson
INV210	Tab, White, Round, Scored, INV over 210	Benztropine Mesylate 2 mg	Cogentin by Apothecon	62269-0210	Antiparkinson
INV210	Tab, White, Round, Scored, INV over 210	Benztropine Mesylate 2 mg	Cogentin by Golden State	60429-0028	Antiparkinson
INV210	Tab, White, Round, Scored, INV over 210	Benztropine Mesylate 2 mg	Cogentin by Invamed	52189-0210	Antiparkinson
INV210	Tab, White, Round, Scored, INV over 210	Benztropine Mesylate 2 mg	Cogentin by Med Pro	53978-2093	Antiparkinson
INV210	Tab, White, Round, Scored, INV over 210	Benztropine Mesylate 2 mg	Cogentin by Sandoz	00781-1367	Antiparkinson
INV211	Cap, Red, White Print, INV over 211	Amantadine HCl 100 mg	Symmetrel by Apotheca	12634-0538	Antiviral
INV211	Cap, Red, White Print, INV over 211	Amantadine HCl 100 mg	Symmetrel by Apotheca	12634-0539	Antiviral
INV211	Cap, Red, White Print, INV over 211	Amantadine HCl 100 mg	Symmetrel by Invamed	52189-0211	Antiviral
INV211	Cap, Red, White Print, INV over 211	Amantadine HCl 100 mg	Symmetrel by Qualitest	00603-2164	Antiviral
INV211	Cap, Red, White Print, INV over 211	Amantadine HCl 100 mg	Symmetrel by Caremark	00339-5780	Antiviral
INV211	Cap, Red, White Print, INV over 211	Amantadine HCl 100 mg	Symmetrel by Apothecon	62269-0211	Antiviral
INV220	Tab, Yellow, Round, Enteric Coated, Delayed Release	Aspirin 15 g	Easprin by Duramed	00781-1367	Analgesic
INV221	Tab, White, Round	Ibuprofen 200 mg	Motrin by Sandoz	00781-1349	NSAID
INV221	Tab, White, Round	Ibuprofen 200 mg	Motrin by Invamed		NSAID
INV221	Tab, White, Round	Ibuprofen 200 mg	Motrin by Schein	00364-2145	NSAID
INV228	Tab, Film Coated, INV over 228	Cimetidine HCl 200 mg	Tagamet by Invamed	52189-0228	Gastrointestinal
INV228	Tab, Film Coated, INV over 228	Cimetidine HCl 200 mg	Tagamet by Apothecon	62269-0228	Gastrointestinal
INV229	Tab, Film Coated, INV over 229	Cimetidine HCl 300 mg	Tagamet by Apothecon	62269-0229	Gastrointestinal
INV229	Tab, Film Coated, INV over 229	Cimetidine HCl 300 mg	Tagamet by Invamed	52189-0229	Gastrointestinal
INV230	Tab, Film Coated, Scored	Cimetidine HCl 400 mg	Tagamet by Invamed	52189-0230	Gastrointestinal
INV230	Tab, Film Coated, INV/230	Cimetidine HCl 400 mg	Tagamet by Apothecon	62269-0230	Gastrointestinal
INV231	Tab, Film Coated, INV/231	Cimetidine HCl 800 mg	Tagamet by Apothecon	62269-0231	Gastrointestinal
INV231	Tab, Film Coated, Scored	Cimetidine HCl 800 mg	Tagamet by Invamed	52189-0231	Gastrointestinal
INV232	Tab, White, Oblong	Aspirin SR 800 mg	Aspirin by Duramed		Analgesic
INV234	Tab	Chlorpheniramine Tannate 8 mg, Phenylephrine Tannate 25 mg, Pyrilamine Tannate 25 mg	R Tannamine by Qualitest	00603-5687	Cold Remedy
INV234	Tab	Chlorpheniramine Tannate 8 mg, Phenylephrine Tannate 25 mg, Pyrilamine Tannate 25 mg	by Physician Total Care	54868-2189	Cold Remedy
INV236 <> 20	Tab	Nadolol 20 mg	Nadolol by Major	00904-5069	Antihypertensive
INV236 <> 20	Tab, Engraved INV Above and 236 Below the Bisect	Nadolol 20 mg	Nadolol by Invamed	52189-0236	Antihypertensive
INV236 <> 20	Tab	Nadolol 20 mg	Nadolol by Schein	00364-2652	Antihypertensive
INV236 <> 20	Tab, INV/236 <> 20	Nadolol 20 mg	Nadolol by Sandoz	00781-1181	Antihypertensive

ID FRONT <> BACK	DESCRIPTION FRONT <> BACK	INGREDIENT & STRENGTH	BRAND (or Generic Equiv.) by FIRM	NDC#	CLASS; SCH.
INV236 <> 20	Tab	Nadolol 20 mg	Nadolol by Moore	00839-7869	Antihypertensive
INV237 <> 40	Tab	Nadolol 40 mg	Nadolol by Moore	00839-7870	Antihypertensive
INV237 <> 40	Tab	Nadolol 40 mg	Nadolol by Sandoz	00781-1182	Antihypertensive
INV237 <> 40	Tab	Nadolol 40 mg	Nadolol by Major	00904-5070	Antihypertensive
INV237 <> 40	Tab, Engraved INV Above and 237 Below the Bisect	Nadolol 40 mg	Nadolol by Invamed	52189-0237	Antihypertensive
INV237 <> 40	Tab	Nadolol 40 mg	Nadolol by Schein	00364-2653	Antihypertensive
INV238 <> 80	Tab, Engraved INV Above and 238 Below the Bisect	Nadolol 80 mg	Nadolol by Invamed	52189-0238	Antihypertensive
INV238 <> 80	Tab	Nadolol 80 mg	Nadolol by Major	00904-5071	Antihypertensive
INV238 <> 80	Tab	Nadolol 80 mg	Nadolol by Moore	00839-7871	Antihypertensive
INV238 <> 80	Tab	Nadolol 80 mg	Nadolol by Schein	00364-2654	Antihypertensive
INV238 <> 80	Tab	Nadolol 80 mg	Nadolol by Sandoz	00781-1183	Antihypertensive
INV241	Tab, Yellow, Oblong	Choline Magnesium Trisalicylate 500 mg	Trilisate by Invamed		NSAID
INV241	Tab, White, Oval	Choline Magnesium Trisalicylate 500 mg	Trilisate by Duramed		NSAID
INV242	Tab, White, Oval	Choline Magnesium Trisalicylate 750 mg	Trilisate by Duramed		NSAID
INV242	Cap, Blue, INV/242	Choline Magnesium Trisalicylate 750 mg	Trilisate by Invamed		NSAID
INV244	Tab, Coated, INV and 244	Salsalate 750 mg	by Quality Care	60346-0034	NSAID
INV246	Tab, Film Coated, Engraved INV Above 246	Indapamide 1.25 mg	Lozol by Invamed	52189-0246	Diuretic
INV246	Tab, Film Coated, Engraved INV Above 246	Indapamide 1.25 mg	Lozol by Apothecon	62269-0246	Diuretic
INV247	Tab, Film Coated, INV Above 247	Indapamide 2.5 mg	Lozol by Apothecon	62269-0247	Diuretic
INV247	Tab, Film Coated, INV Above 247	Indapamide 2.5 mg	Lozol by Invamed	52189-0247	Diuretic
INV250	Tab, Film Coated	Hydroxychloroquine Sulfate 200 mg	by Apothecon	62269-0250	Antimalarial
INV252	Tab, Film Coated	Cyclobenzaprine HCl 10 mg	by Urgent Care Center	50716-0932	Muscle Relaxant
INV252	Tab, Film Coated, INV over 252	Cyclobenzaprine HCl 10 mg	by Invamed	52189-0252	Muscle Relaxant
INV252	Tab, Film Coated, INV over 252	Cyclobenzaprine HCl 10 mg	by Apothecon	62269-0252	Muscle Relaxant
INV25272	Tab, White, Round	Captopril 25 mg	Capoten by Invamed		Antihypertensive
INV256	Tab, INV over 256	Atenolol 50 mg	Tenormin by Apothecon	62269-0256	Antihypertensive
INV256	Tab, Scored, INV over 256	Atenolol 50 mg	Tenormin by Invamed	52189-0256	Antihypertensive
INV256	Tab	Atenolol 50 mg	Tenormin by Med Pro	53978-1199	Antihypertensive
INV257	Tab, INV over 257	Atenolol 100 mg	Tenormin by Apothecon	62269-0257	Antihypertensive
INV257	Tab, INV over 257	Atenolol 100 mg	Tenormin by Invamed	52189-0257	Antihypertensive
INV260	Tab, White, Round, Scored	Methazolamide 50 mg	Neptazane by Invamed	52189-0260	Antiglaucoma Agent
INV260	Tab, White, Round, Scored	Methazolamide 50 mg	Neptazane by Apothecon	62269-0260	Antiglaucoma Agent
INV260	Tab, White, Round	Methazolamide 50 mg	Neptazane by Invamed		Antiglaucoma Agent
INV261	Tab, White, Round	Methazolamide 25 mg	Neptazane by Invamed		Antiglaucoma Agent
INV262	Tab, Brown, Oblong, Film	Ibuprofen 200 mg	Motrin by Murfreesboro	51129-1517	NSAID
INV263	Tab, INV over 263	Metoclopramide 5 mg	Reglan by URL Mutual	00677-1323	Gastrointestinal
INV263	Tab, INV over 263	Metoclopramide 5 mg	Reglan by Ivax	00182-1898	Gastrointestinal
INV263	Tab, INV over 263	Metoclopramide 5 mg	Reglan by Invamed	52189-0263	Gastrointestinal
INV263	Tab, White, Round, INV over 263	Metoclopramide 5 mg	Reglan by Apothecon	62269-0263	Gastrointestinal
INV264	Tab, INV Above and 264 Below Bisect	Metoclopramide 10 mg	Reglan by Invamed	52189-0264	Gastrointestinal
INV264	Tab, INV Above and 264 Below Bisect	Metoclopramide 10 mg	Reglan by Apothecon	62269-0264	Gastrointestinal
INV265	Tab, Green & White, Round	Orphenadrine Citrate 25 mg, Aspirin 385 mg, Caffeine 30 mg	by Apothecon	62269-0265	Muscle Relaxant
INV265	Tab, Green & White, Round	Orphenadrine Citrate 25 mg, Aspirin 325 mg, Caffeine 30 mg	Norgesic by Invamed		Muscle Relaxant
INV265	Tab, Green & White, Round	Orphenadrine Citrate 25 mg, Aspirin 428 mg, Caffeine 30 mg	Invagesic by Invamed	52189-0265	Muscle Relaxant
INV266	Tab, Green & White, Cap Shaped	Orphenadrine Citrate 50 mg, Aspirin 750 mg, Caffeine 60 mg	by Apothecon	62269-0266	Muscle Relaxant
INV266	Tab, Green & White, Oblong, Scored	Orphenadrine Citrate 50 mg, Aspirin 856 mg, Caffeine 60 mg	Invagesic Forte by Invamed	52189-0266	Muscle Relaxant
INV266	Tab, Green & White, Oblong, Scored	Orphenadrine Citrate 50 mg, Caffeine 60 mg, Aspirin 856 mg	by DRX	55045-2777	Muscle Relaxant
INV266	Tab, Green & White, Oblong	Orphenadrine 50 mg, Aspirin 770 mg, Caffeine 60 mg	Norgesic Forte by Invamed		Muscle Relaxant

ID FRONT <> BACK	DESCRIPTION FRONT <> BACK	INGREDIENT & STRENGTH	BRAND (or Generic Equiv.) by FIRM	NDC#	CLASS; SCH.
INV272 <> 25	Tab, INV over 272	Captopril 25 mg	Capoten by Schein	00364-2629	Antihypertensive
INV272 <> 25	Tab, Quadrisected, INV over 272 <> 25	Captopril 25 mg	Capoten by Invamed	52189-0272	Antihypertensive
INV273 <> 50	Tab, Scored	Captopril 50 mg	Capoten by Invamed	52189-0273	Antihypertensive
INV274 <> 100	Tab, Scored	Captopril 100 mg	Capoten by Invamed	52189-0274	Antihypertensive
INV275 <> 5	Tab, Pale Yellow, Round, Film Coated, INV over 275 <> 5	Prochlorperazine 5 mg	by Apothecon	62269-0275	Antiemetic
INV275 <> 5	Tab, Yellow, Round, Film Coated	Prochlorperazine Maleate 5 mg	by Murfreesboro	51129-1427	Antiemetic
INV275 <> 5	Tab, Yellow, Round, Film Coated	Prochlorperazine Maleate 5 mg	by Invamed	52189-0275	Antiemetic
INV2755	Tab, Pale Yellow, Round	Prochlorperazine 5 mg	Compazine by Invamed		Antiemetic
INV276 <> 10	Tab, Yellow, Round, Film Coated	Prochlorperazine Maleate 10 mg	by Invamed	52189-0276	Antiemetic
INV276 <> 10	Tab, Yellow, Round, Film Coated	Prochlorperazine Maleate 10 mg	by Apotheca	12634-0676	Antiemetic
INV276 <> 10	Tab, Pale Yellow, Round, Film Coated, INV over 276 <> 10	Prochlorperazine 10 mg	by Apothecon	62269-0276	Antiemetic
INV27610	Tab, Yellow, Round	Prochlorperazine 10 mg	Compazine by Invamed		Antiemetic
INV277 <> 25	Tab, Yellow, Round, Film Coated	Prochlorperazine Maleate 25 mg	by Invamed	52189-0277	Antiemetic
INV27725	Tab, Yellow, Round	Prochlorperazine 25 mg	Compazine by Invamed	52152-0188	Antiemetic
INV278	Tab, Lavender, Round, Film Coated	Trifluoperazine HCl 1 mg	Stelazine by Apothecon	62269-0278	Antipsychotic
INV278	Tab, Lavender, Round, Film Coated	Trifluoperazine HCl 1 mg	Stelazine by Sandoz	00781-0278	Antipsychotic
INV278	Tab, Purple, Round, Film Coated	Trifluoperazine HCl 2 mg	Stelazine by Apothecon	62269-0279	Antipsychotic
INV279 <> 2	Tab, Purple, Round, Film Coated	Trifluoperazine HCl 2 mg	Stelazine by Invamed	52189-0279	Antipsychotic
INV280	Tab, Purple, Round, Film Coated	Trifluoperazine HCl 10 mg	by Apothecon	62269-0281	Antipsychotic
INV280	Tab, Lavender, Round	Trifluoperazine HCl 5 mg	Stelazine by Invamed		Antipsychotic
INV280 <> 5	Tab, Purple, Round, Film Coated	Trifluoperazine HCl 5 mg	Stelazine by Apothecon	62269-0280	Antipsychotic
INV280 <> 5	Tab, Purple, Round, Film Coated	Trifluoperazine HCl 5 mg	Stelazine by Invamed	52189-0280	Antipsychotic
INV281 <> 10	Tab, Purple, Round, Film Coated	Trifluoperazine HCl 10 mg	by Invamed	52189-0281	Antipsychotic
INV286	Tab, Light Blue, Coated	Naproxen 275 mg	Naprosyn by Qualitest	00603-4733	NSAID
INV286	Tab, Coated	Naproxen 275 mg	Naprosyn by Apothecon	62269-0286	NSAID
INV286	Tab, Coated	Naproxen 275 mg	Naprosyn by Invamed	52189-0286	NSAID
INV286	Tab, Coated	Naproxen 275 mg	Naprosyn by Ivax	00182-1974	NSAID
INV287	Tab, Light Blue, Film Coated	Naproxen 550 mg	Naprosyn by Qualitest	00603-4734	NSAID
INV287	Tab, Coated	Naproxen 550 mg	Naprosyn by Invamed	52189-0287	NSAID
INV287	Tab, White, Oval	Naproxen 550 mg	Naprosyn by Apothecon	62269-0287	NSAID
INV289	Tab, White, Oblong, Film Coated	Naproxen 375 mg	Naprosyn by Invamed	52189-0289	NSAID
INV289	Tab, White, Oblong, Film Coated	Naproxen 375 mg	Naprosyn by Apothecon	62269-0289	NSAID
INV290	Cap, White	Naproxen 500 mg	Naprosyn by Invamed	52189-0290	NSAID
INV290	Cap, White	Naproxen 500 mg	Naprosyn by Apothecon	62269-0290	NSAID
INV291	Tab, Scored	Glipizide 5 mg	by Invamed	52189-0291	Antidiabetic
INV291	Tab	Glipizide 5 mg	by Apothecon	62269-0291	Antidiabetic
INV292	Tab, Scored	Glipizide 10 mg	by Invamed	52189-0292	Antidiabetic
INV292	Tab, INV/292	Glipizide 10 mg	by Apothecon	62269-0292	Antidiabetic
INV293	Tab, White, Round, Scored	Glyburide 1.5 mg	by Invamed	52189-0293	Antidiabetic
INV293	Tab, White, Round	Glyburide 1.5 mg	by BMS		Antidiabetic
INV293	Tab, White, Round	Glyburide 1.5 mg	Glynase by Invamed		Antidiabetic
INV293	Tab, White, Round, Scored	Glyburide 1.5 mg	by Apothecon	62269-0293	Antidiabetic
INV294	Tab, Blue, Round	Glyburide 3 mg	by BMS		Antidiabetic
INV294	Tab, Blue, Round, Scored	Glyburide 3 mg	by Invamed	52189-0294	Antidiabetic
INV294	Tab, Blue, Round, Scored	Glyburide 3 mg	by Apothecon	62269-0294	Antidiabetic
INV294	Tab, Blue, Round	Glyburide 3 mg	Glynase by Invamed		Antidiabetic
INV296	Tab, Blue, Round	Salsalate 500 mg	Disalcid by Duramed		NSAID
INV297	Tab, Blue, Oblong	Salsalate 750 mg	Disalcid by Duramed		NSAID

ID FRONT <> BACK	DESCRIPTION FRONT <> BACK	INGREDIENT & STRENGTH	BRAND (or Generic Equiv.) by FIRM	NDC#	CLASS; SCH.
INV309	Tab, Pink, Square, Scored, INV over 309	Warfarin Sodium 1 mg	Coumadin by Sandoz	00781-0352	Anticoagulant
INV309	Tab, Pink, Square, Scored, INV over 309	Warfarin Sodium 1 mg	Coumadin by Apothecon	59772-0352	Anticoagulant
INV310 <> 2	Tab, Lavender, Square, Scored, INV over 310	Warfarin Sodium 2 mg	Coumadin by Apothecon	59772-0363	Anticoagulant
INV310 <> 2	Tab, Lavender, Square, Scored, INV over 310	Warfarin Sodium 2 mg	Coumadin by Sandoz	00781-0363	Anticoagulant
INV311 <> 25	Tab, Green, Square, Scored, INV over 311 <> 2.5	Warfarin Sodium 2.5 mg	Coumadin by Sandoz	00781-0364	Anticoagulant
INV311 <> 25	Tab, Green, Square, Scored, INV over 311 <> 2.5	Warfarin Sodium 2.5 mg	Coumadin by Apothecon	59772-0364	Anticoagulant
INV312 <> 4	Tab, Blue, Square, Scored, INV over 312	Warfarin Sodium 4 mg	Coumadin by Apothecon	59772-0369	Anticoagulant
INV312 <> 4	Tab, Blue, Square, Scored, INV over 312	Warfarin Sodium 4 mg	Coumadin by Sandoz	00781-0369	Anticoagulant
INV313 <> 5	Tab, Peach, Square, Scored, INV over 313	Warfarin Sodium 5 mg	Coumadin by Sandoz	00781-0377	Anticoagulant
INV313 <> 5	Tab, Peach, Square, Scored, INV over 313	Warfarin Sodium 5 mg	Coumadin by Apothecon	59772-0377	Anticoagulant
INV314 <> 75	Tab, Yellow, Square, Scored, INV over 314 <> 7.5	Warfarin Sodium 7.5 mg	Coumadin by Apothecon	59772-0386	Anticoagulant
INV314 <> 75	Tab, Yellow, Square, Scored, INV over 314 <> 7.5	Warfarin Sodium 7.5 mg	Coumadin by Sandoz	00781-0386	Anticoagulant
INV315 <> 10	Tab, White, Square, Scored, INV over 315	Warfarin Sodium 10 mg	Coumadin by Sandoz	00781-0387	Anticoagulant
INV315 <> 10	Tab, White, Square, Scored, INV over 315	Warfarin Sodium 10 mg	Coumadin by Apothecon	59772-0387	Anticoagulant
INV320	Tab, White, Oval, Scored, Film Coated	Gemfibrozil 600 mg	by Kaiser	00179-1292	Antihyperlipidemic
INV320	Tab, Film Coated, INV to Left, 320 to Right of Score	Gemfibrozil 600 mg	by Golden State	60429-0081	Antihyperlipidemic
INV320	Tab, Film Coated, Scored	Gemfibrozil 600 mg	by Invamed	52189-0320	Antihyperlipidemic
INV320	Tab, Film Coated, Scored	Gemfibrozil 600 mg	by Apothecon	62269-0320	Antihyperlipidemic
INV321	Cap, Orange & White	Clomipramine HCl 25 mg	Anafranil by Invamed		OCD
INV321	Cap, White & Yellow, Gelatin	Clomipramine HCl 25 mg	by Invamed	52189-0321	OCD
INV321	Cap, White & Yellow, Hard Gel	Clomipramine HCl 25 mg	by Apothecon	62269-0321	OCD
INV322	Cap, Blue	Clomipramine HCl 50 mg	Anafranil by Invamed		OCD
INV322	Cap, Blue & White, Gelatin	Clomipramine HCl 50 mg	by Invamed	52189-0322	OCD
INV322	Cap, Blue & White	Clomipramine HCl 50 mg	by Apothecon	62269-0322	OCD
INV323	Cap, White & Yellow	Clomipramine HCl 75 mg	by Invamed	52189-0323	OCD
INV323	Cap, White & Yellow	Clomipramine HCl 75 mg	by Apothecon	62269-0323	OCD
INV323	Cap, Yellow	Clomipramine HCl 75 mg	Anafranil by Invamed		OCD
INV328	Cap, Green & White	Nortriptyline 10 mg	Pamelor by Invamed		Antidepressant
INV329	Cap, Green & White	Nortriptyline 25 mg	Pamelor by Invamed		Antidepressant
INV330	Cap, White	Nortriptyline 50 mg	Pamelor by Invamed		Antidepressant
INV331	Cap, Green	Nortriptyline 75 mg	Pamelor by Invamed		Antidepressant
INV336	Tab, White, Round	Orphenadrine Citrate 100 mg	by Apothecon	62269-0336	Muscle Relaxant
INV336	Tab, White, Round	Orphenadrine Citrate 100 mg	Norflex by Invamed		Muscle Relaxant
INV336	Tab, White, Round	Orphenadrine Citrate 100 mg	by Invamed	52189-0336	Muscle Relaxant
INV350	Tab, Yellow, Oval, Film Coated	Etodolac 400 mg	by Apothecon	62269-0350	NSAID
INV350	Tab, Yellow, Oval, Film Coated	Etodolac 400 mg	by Physician Total Care	54868-3955	NSAID
INV350	Tab, Yellow, Oval, Film Coated	Etodolac 400 mg	by Invamed	52189-0350	NSAID
INV351	Tab, White, Oval, Scored	Methylprednisolone 4 mg	Medrol by Invamed	52189-0351	Steroid
INV351	Tab, White, Oval, Scored	Methylprednisolone 4 mg	Medrol by Apothecon	62269-0351	Steroid
INV353	Tab, Yellow, Round, Scored	Clonazepam 0.5 mg	by Invamed	52189-0353	Sedative; C IV
INV353	Tab, Yellow, Round, Scored	Clonazepam 0.5 mg	by Apothecon	62269-0353	Sedative; C IV
INV354	Tab, Green, Round, Scored	Clonazepam 1 mg	by Invamed	52189-0354	Sedative; C IV
INV354	Tab, Green, Round, Scored	Clonazepam 1 mg	by Apothecon	62269-0354	Sedative; C IV
INV354	Tab, Green, Round	Clonazepam 1 mg	by BMS		Sedative; C IV
INV354	Tab, Green, Round	Clonazepam 1 mg	Klonopin by Invamed		Sedative; C IV
INV355	Tab, White, Round, Scored	Clonazepam 2 mg	by Apothecon	62269-0355	Sedative; C IV
INV355	Tab, White, Round, Scored	Clonazepam 2 mg	by Invamed	52189-0355	Sedative; C IV
INV359	Cap, Gray & White	Etodolac 200 mg	by Invamed	52189-0359	NSAID

ID FRONT <> BACK	DESCRIPTION FRONT <> BACK	INGREDIENT & STRENGTH	BRAND (or Generic Equiv.) by FIRM	NDC#	CLASS; SCH.
INV359	Cap, Gray & White	Etodolac 200 mg	Lodine by Invamed		NSAID
INV359	Cap, Gray & White	Etodolac 200 mg	by Apothecon	62269-0359	NSAID
INV360	Cap, Gray	Etodolac 300 mg	by Apothecon	62269-0360	NSAID
INV360	Cap, Gray	Etodolac 300 mg	by Invamed	52189-0360	NSAID
INV360	Cap, Gray	Etodolac 300 mg	by BMS		NSAID
INV360	Cap, Gray	Etodolac 300 mg	Lodine by Invamed	55045-2592	NSAID
INV360	Cap, Gray	Etodolac 300 mg	by DRX		NSAID
INV361	Tab, Lavender, Round, Film Coated	Bupropion HCl 75 mg	Wellbutrin by Invamed	52189-0361	Antidepressant
INV362	Tab, Lavender, Round, Film Coated	Bupropion HCl 100 mg	Wellbutrin by Invamed	52189-0362	Antidepressant
INV375	Tab, Orange, Round, Film, INV over 375	Ticlopidine HCl 250 mg	by Taro	52549-4035	Anticoagulant
INV375	Tab, Light Orange, Round	Ticlopidine HCl 250 mg	Ticlid by Sandoz	00781-1514	Anticoagulant
INV383	Tab, White, Round, Film, INV over 383	Diclofenac Potassium 50 mg	by DRX	55045-2672	NSAID
INV391	Tab, White, Round, Scored	Pemoline 18.75 mg	by Apothecon	62269-0391	Stimulant; C IV
INV391	Tab, White, Round, Scored	Pemoline 18.75 mg	by Invamed	52189-0391	Stimulant; C IV
INV392	Tab, White, Round	Pemoline 37.5 mg	Pemoline by Pharmafab	62542-0460	Stimulant; C IV
INV393	Tab, White, Round, INV Above 393	Pemoline 75 mg	Pemoline by Pharmafab	62542-0690	Stimulant; C IV
INV394	Tab, Peach, Round, Scored, INV 394	Leucovorin Calcium 15 mg	Wellcovorin by Murfreesboro	51129-1627	Antineoplastic
INV423 <> 3	Tab, Tan, Square, Scored, INV over 423	Warfarin Sodium 3 mg	Coumadin by Sandoz	00781-0366	Anticoagulant
INV424 <> 6	Tab, Teal, Square, Scored, INV over 424	Warfarin Sodium 6 mg	Coumadin by Sandoz	00781-0381	Anticoagulant
INV50273	Tab, White, Oval	Captopril 50 mg	Capoten by Invamed		Antihypertensive
INV535	Tab, Yellow, Round, INV/535	Clonazepam 0.5 mg		52189-0535	Sedative; C IV
INV75NORTRIPTYLINE	Cap, Green	Nortriptyline HCl 75 mg	by Apothecon	62269-0331	Antidepressant
INV75NORTRIPTYLINE	Cap, Green	Nortriptyline HCl 75 mg	by Invamed	52189-0331	Antidepressant
IONAMIN15	Cap, Gray & Yellow, Ex Release	Phentermine Resin 15 mg	by PDRX	55289-0987	Anorexiant; C IV
IONAMIN15	Cap, Gray & Yellow, Ex Release	Phentermine 15 mg	Ionamin by H J Harkins Co	52959-0418	Anorexiant; C IV
IONAMIN15	Cap, Gray & Yellow, Ex Release	Phentermine 15 mg	Ionamin by Physician Total Care		Anorexiant; C IV
IONAMIN15	Cap, Gray & Yellow, Ex Release	Phentermine 15 mg	Ionamin by Medeva	53014-0903	Anorexiant; C IV
IONAMIN15	Cap, Gray & Yellow, Ex Release	Phentermine Resin 15 mg	by Allscripts		Anorexiant; C IV
IONAMIN30	Cap, Yellow, Ex Release	Phentermine Resin 30 mg	by DRX	55045-2295	Anorexiant; C IV
IONAMIN30	Cap, Yellow, Ex Release	Phentermine Resin 30 mg	by PDRX	55289-0731	Anorexiant; C IV
IONAMIN30	Cap, Yellow, Ex Release	Phentermine Resin 30 mg	by DRX	55045-2443	Anorexiant; C IV
IONAMIN30	Cap, Yellow, Ex Release	Phentermine 30 mg	Ionamin by Medeva	53014-0904	Anorexiant; C IV
IONAMIN30	Cap, Yellow, Ex Release	Phentermine Resin 30 mg	by Compumed	00403-1069	Anorexiant; C IV
IONAMIN30	Cap, Yellow, Ex Release	Phentermine Resin 30 mg	by Nat Pharmpak	55154-6302	Anorexiant; C IV
IP001	Tab, White, Round	Acetaminophen 500 mg	Tylenol Ex Strength by Interpharm	53746-0001	Analgesic
IP011	Tab, White, Round	Acetaminophen 325 mg	Tylenol by Interpharm	53746-0011	Analgesic
IP018	Tab, White, Oblong	Acetaminophen 500 mg	Tylenol Ex Strength by Interpharm	53746-0018	Analgesic
IP029	Tab	Aspirin 800 mg	Aspirin by URL Mutual	00677-1172	Analgesic
IP037	Tab, Yellow, Round	Chlorpheniramine Maleate 4 mg	Chlor-Trimeton by Interpharm	53746-0037	Antihistamine
IP050	Tab, Pink, Round	Acetaminophen 325 mg, Pseudoephedrine HCl 30 mg	Sinutab by Interpharm	53746-0050	Cold Remedy
IP064	Cap, Pink & White	Diphenhydramine HCl 25 mg	Benadryl by Interpharm		Antihistamine
IP10	Tab, Green, Round, ER	Alprazolam 1 mg	Xanax XR by Amneal	65162-0810	Antianxiety; C IV
IP101	Cap, White, Opaque, Hard Gel	Gabapentin 100 mg	Neurontin by Amneal	53746-0101	Anticonvulsant
IP102	Cap, Buff, Opaque, Hard Gel	Gabapentin 300 mg	Neurontin by Amneal	53746-0102	Anticonvulsant
IP103	Cap, Light Caramel, Opaque, Hard Gel	Gabapentin 400 mg	Neurontin by Amneal	53746-0103	Anticonvulsant
IP109	Tab, White to Off-White, Oblong, Scored	Acetaminophen 325 mg, Hydrocodone Bitartrate 5 mg	Norco by Interpharm	53746-0109	Analgesic; C III
IP110	Tab, White to Off-White, Oblong, Scored	Acetaminophen 325 mg, Hydrocodone Bitartrate 10 mg	Norco by Interpharm	53746-0110	Analgesic; C III
IP111	Tab, White to Off-White, Oblong, Scored, IP / 111	Acetaminophen 500 mg, Hydrocodone Bitartrate 5 mg	Vicodin by Interpharm	53746-0111	Analgesic; C III

ID FRONT <> BACK	DESCRIPTION FRONT <> BACK	INGREDIENT & STRENGTH	BRAND (or Generic Equiv.) by FIRM	NDC#	CLASS; SCH.
IP112	Tab, White to Off-White, Oblong, Scored	Acetaminophen 500 mg, Hydrocodone Bitartrate 7.5 mg	Lortab by Interpharm	53746-0112	Analgesic; C III
IP113	Tab, White to Off-White, Oblong, Scored	Acetaminophen 650 mg, Hydrocodone Bitartrate 7.5 mg	Lorcet Plus by Interpharm	53746-0113	Analgesic; C III
IP114	Tab, White to Off-White, Oblong, Scored	Hydrocodone Bitartrate 10 mg, Acetaminophen 650 mg	Lorcet by Interpharm	53746-0114	Analgesic; C III
IP118	Tab, White to Off-White, Oblong, Scored	Acetaminophen 750 mg, Hydrocodone Bitartrate 7.5 mg	Vicodin ES by Interpharm	53746-0118	Analgesic; C III
IP119	Tab, White, Oval, Scored	Acetaminophen 500 mg, Hydrocodone Bitartrate 10 mg	Vicodin by Interpharm	53746-0118	Analgesic; C III
IP12	Tab, Blue, Round, ER	Alprazolam 2 mg	Xanax XR by Amneal	65162-0812	Antianxiety; C IV
IP13	Tab, White, Round, ER	Alprazolam 3 mg	Xanax XR by Amneal	65162-0813	Antianxiety; C IV
IP131 <> 400	Tab, White, Round, Film Coated	Ibuprofen 400 mg	Motrin by Watson	00591-3464	NSAID
IP131 <> 400	Tab, White, Round, Film Coated	Ibuprofen 400 mg	Motrin by Amneal	65162-0568	NSAID
IP131 <> 400	Tab, White, Round, Film Coated	Ibuprofen 400 mg	Motrin by Interpharm	53746-0131	NSAID
IP131 <> 400	Tab, White, Round, Film Coated	Ibuprofen 400 mg	Motrin by Ivax	00182-1809 Discontinued	NSAID
IP131 <> 400	Tab, White, Round, Film Coated	Ibuprofen 400 mg	Motrin by Major	00904-1748	NSAID
IP131 <> 400	Tab, White, Round, Film Coated	Ibuprofen 400 mg	Motrin by Golden State	60429-0092	NSAID
IP131 <> 400	Tab, White, Round, Film Coated	Ibuprofen 400 mg	Motrin by Rx Dispensing	61807-0027	NSAID
IP131 <> 400	Tab, White, Round, Film Coated	Ibuprofen 400 mg	Motrin by Qualitest	00603-4018	NSAID
IP132 <> 600	Tab, White, Oval, Film Coated	Ibuprofen 600 mg	Motrin by Interpharm	53746-0132	NSAID
IP132 <> 600	Tab, White, Oval, Film Coated	Ibuprofen 600 mg	Motrin by Breckenridge	51991-0730	NSAID
IP132 <> 600	Tab, White, Oval, Film Coated	Ibuprofen 600 mg	Motrin by Urgent Care Center	50716-0743	NSAID
IP132 <> 600	Tab, White, Oval, Film Coated	Ibuprofen 600 mg	Motrin by Golden State	60429-0093	NSAID
IP132 <> 600	Tab, White, Oval, Film Coated	Ibuprofen 600 mg	Motrin by Rx Dispensing	61807-0011	NSAID
IP132 <> 600	Tab, White, Oval, Film Coated	Ibuprofen 600 mg	Motrin by Major	00904-5186	NSAID
IP132 <> 600	Tab, White, Oval, Film Coated	Ibuprofen 600 mg	Motrin by Qualitest	00603-4019	NSAID
IP132 <> 600	Tab, White, Oval, Film Coated	Ibuprofen 600 mg	Motrin by Amneal	65162-0569	NSAID
IP132 <> 600	Tab, White, Oval, Film Coated	Ibuprofen 600 mg	Motrin by Watson	00591-3465	NSAID
IP132 <> 600	Tab, White, Oval, Film Coated	Ibuprofen 600 mg	Motrin by Ivax	00182-1810 Discontinued	NSAID
IP135	Tab, White, Round	Ibuprofen 200 mg	Advil by Ivax	00182-2401	Analgesic
IP135	Tab, White, Round	Ibuprofen 200 mg	Advil by Rugby	00536-3939	NSAID
IP135	Tab, White, Round	Ibuprofen 200 mg	Advil by Major	00904-7914	NSAID
IP135	Tab, White, Round	Ibuprofen 200 mg	Advil by Interpharm	53746-0135	NSAID
IP135	Tab, White, Round	Ibuprofen 200 mg	Advil by Amneal	65162-0565	NSAID
IP136	Cap, Red	Acetaminophen 325 mg, Dichloralphenazone 100 mg, Isometheptene Mucate 65 mg	Midrin by Interpharm		Analgesic; C IV
IP137 <> 800	Tab, White, Cap Shaped, Film Coated	Ibuprofen 800 mg	Motrin by Urgent Care Center	50716-0726	NSAID
IP137 <> 800	Tab, White, Cap Shaped, Film Coated	Ibuprofen 800 mg	Motrin by Ivax	00182-1297 Discontinued	NSAID
IP137 <> 800	Tab, White, Cap Shaped, Film Coated	Ibuprofen 800 mg	Motrin by Ivax	00172-3648 Discontinued	NSAID
IP137 <> 800	Tab, White, Cap Shaped, Film Coated	Ibuprofen 800 mg	Motrin by Rx Dispensing	61807-0012	NSAID
IP137 <> 800	Tab, White, Cap Shaped, Film Coated	Ibuprofen 800 mg	Motrin by Qualitest	00603-4020	NSAID
IP137 <> 800	Tab, White, Cap Shaped, Film Coated	Ibuprofen 800 mg	Motrin by Murfreesboro	51129-1528	NSAID
IP137 <> 800	Tab, White, Cap Shaped, Film Coated	Ibuprofen 800 mg	Motrin by Breckenridge	51991-0740	NSAID
IP137 <> 800	Tab, White, Cap Shaped, Film Coated	Ibuprofen 800 mg	Motrin by Golden State	60429-0094	NSAID
IP137 <> 800	Tab, White, Cap Shaped, Film Coated	Ibuprofen 800 mg	Motrin by Major	00904-5187	NSAID
IP137 <> 800	Tab, White, Cap Shaped, Film Coated	Ibuprofen 800 mg	Motrin by Watson	00591-3665	NSAID
IP137 <> 800	Tab, White, Cap Shaped, Film Coated	Ibuprofen 800 mg	Motrin by Amneal	65162-0570 Discontinued	NSAID
IP137 <> 800	Tab, White, Cap Shaped, Film Coated	Ibuprofen 800 mg	Motrin by Interpharm	53746-0137	NSAID
IP138 <> 200	Tab, White, Oblong, Film Coated	Ibuprofen 200 mg	Advil by Interpharm	53746-0138	NSAID

ID FRONT <> BACK	DESCRIPTION FRONT <> BACK	INGREDIENT & STRENGTH	BRAND (or Generic Equiv.) by FIRM	NDC#	CLASS; SCH.
IP138 <> 400	Tab, White, Round, Film Coated	Ibuprofen 400 mg	Motrin by Breckenridge	51991-0720	NSAID
IP140	Tab, Brown, Round, Coated	Ibuprofen 200 mg	Advil by Interpharm	53746-0140	NSAID
IP141	Cap, Red, Opaque	Isometheptene Mucate 65 mg, Dichloralphenazone 100 mg, Acetaminophen 325 mg	Migrin-A by Prasco	66993-0601	Analgesic; C IV
IP141	Cap, Red	Acetaminophen 325 mg, Dichloralphenazone 100 mg, Isometheptene Mucate 65 mg	Midrin by Interpharm	53746-0141	Analgesic; C IV
IP141	Cap, Red	Acetaminophen 325 mg, Dichloralantipyrine 100 mg, Isometheptene Mucate (1:1) 65 mg	Midrin by Ivax	00182-1234	Analgesic; C IV
IP142	Tab, Brown	Ibuprofen 200 mg	Advil by Interpharm	53746-0142	NSAID
IP144	Tab, Reddish Brown, Cap Shaped, Film Coated	Ibuprofen 200 mg	Motrin by Interpharm	53746-0144	NSAID
IP145	Tab, White, Round, IP over 145	Hydrocodone 7.5 mg, Ibuprofen 200 mg	Vicoprofen by Watson	00591-3168	Analgesic; C III
IP145	Tab, White, Round, IP over 145	Hydrocodone 7.5 mg, Ibuprofen 200 mg	Vicoprofen by Interpharm	53746-0145	Analgesic; C III
IP146	Tab, White, Oval, Scored, Film Coated, IP / 146	Hydrocodone Bitartrate 5 mg, Ibuprofen 200 mg	Reprexain by Watson	52544-0969	Analgesic; C III
IP175 <> 500	Tab, White to Off White, Round	Metformin HCl 500 mg	Glucophage by Amneal	65162-0175	Antihyperglycemic
IP176 <> 850	Tab, White to Off White, Round	Metformin HCl 850 mg	Glucophage by Amneal	65162-0174	Antihyperglycemic
IP177 <> 1000	Tab, White to Off White, Oval, Scored	Metformin HCl 1000 mg	Glucophage by Amneal	65162-0177	Antihyperglycemic
IP178	Tab, White, Oblong, ER	Metformin HCl 500 mg	Glucophage XR by Amneal	53746-0178	Antihyperglycemic
IP179	Tab, White, Oblong, ER	Metformin HCl 750 mg	Glucophage XR by Amneal	53746-0179	Antihyperglycemic
IP188 <> 250	Tab, White, Round	Naproxen 250 mg	Naprosyn by Interpharm	53746-0188	NSAID
IP188 <> 250	Tab, White, Round	Naproxen 250 mg	Naprosyn by Dr. Reddy's	55111-0366	NSAID
IP188 <> 250	Tab, White, Round	Naproxen 250 mg	Naprosyn by Amneal	65162-0076	NSAID
				Discontinued	
IP189 <> 375	Tab, White, Oblong	Naproxen 375 mg	Naprosyn by Amneal	65162-0077	NSAID
				Discontinued	
IP189 <> 375	Tab, White, Oblong	Naproxen 375 mg	Naprosyn by Dr. Reddy's	55111-0367	NSAID
IP189 <> 375	Tab, White, Oblong	Naproxen 375 mg	Naprosyn by Interpharm	53746-0189	NSAID
IP190 <> 500	Tab, White, Oblong	Naproxen 500 mg	Naprosyn by Interpharm	53746-0190	NSAID
IP190 <> 500	Tab, White, Oblong	Naproxen 500 mg	Naprosyn by Dr. Reddy's	55111-0368	NSAID
IP190 <> 500	Tab, White, Oblong	Naproxen 500 mg	Naprosyn by Amneal	65162-0078	NSAID
				Discontinued	
IP191	Tab, Film Coated	Ascorbic Acid 60 mg, Biotin 300 mcg, Cyanocobalamin 6 mcg, Folic Acid 1 mg, Niacinamide 20 mg, Pantothenic Acid 10 mg, Pyridoxine HCl 10 mg, Riboflavin 1.7 mg, Thiamine Mononitrate 1.5 mg	Nephro Vite Rx by Interpharm	53746-0191	Vitamin
IP193	Tab, Blue, Oval	Naproxen Sodium 275 mg	Anaprox by Amneal	53746-0193	NSAID
IP194	Tab, Blue, Oval, Partially Scored	Naproxen Sodium 550 mg	Anaprox DS by Amneal	53746-0194	NSAID
IP203	Tab, White to Off-White, Round, Scored	Oxycodone 5 mg, Acetaminophen 325 mg	Percocet by Interpharm	53746-0203	Analgesic; C II
IP204	Tab, White to Off-White, Cap Shaped	Oxycodone 10 mg, Acetaminophen 325 mg	Percocet by Interpharm	53746-0204	Analgesic; C II
IP205	Tab, White to Off-White, Cap-Shaped	Oxycodone 7.5 mg, Acetaminophen 500 mg	Percocet by Interpharm	53746-0205	Analgesic; C II
IP206	Tab, White to Off-White, Cap-Shaped	Oxycodone 10 mg, Acetaminophen 650 mg	Percocet by Interpharm	53746-0206	Analgesic; C II
IP211	Tab, Pink, Oblong	Acetaminophen 650 mg, Chlorpheniramine 4 mg, Pseudoephedrine HCl 60 mg	Singlet by Interpharm	53746-0211	Cold Remedy
IP221	Tab, Compressed, IP/221	Pseudoephedrine 60 mg	Sudafed by Kaiser	00179-0659	Decongestant
IP221	Tab, White	Pseudoephedrine 60 mg	Sudafed by Interpharm	53746-0221	Cold Remedy
IP251	Tab, White, Round	Quinine Sulfate 260 mg	Quinamm by Interpharm		Antimalarial
IP253	Tab, Orange, Round, Film Coated	Ranitidine HCl 150 mg	Zantac by Interpharm	53746-0253	Gastrointestinal
IP254	Tab, Yellow, Cap Shaped, Film Coated	Ranitidine HCl 300 mg	Zantac by Interpharm	53746-0254	Gastrointestinal
IP271	Tab, White, Round, Scored	Sulfamethoxazole 400 mg, Trimethoprim 80 mg	Bactrim by Interpharm	53746-0271	Antibiotic
IP271	Tab, White, Round, Scored	Sulfamethoxazole 400 mg, Trimethoprim 80 mg	Bactrim by Lannett	00527-1442	Antibiotic
IP272	Tab, White, Oval, Scored	Sulfamethoxazole 800 mg, Trimethoprim 160 mg	Bactrim by Lannett	00527-1443	Antibiotic
IP272	Tab, White, Oval, Scored	Sulfamethoxazole 800 mg, Trimethoprim 160 mg	Bactrim by Interpharm	53746-0272	Antibiotic

ID FRONT <> BACK	DESCRIPTION FRONT <> BACK	INGREDIENT & STRENGTH	BRAND (or Generic Equiv.) by FIRM	NDC#	CLASS; SCH.
IP274	Tab, Pink, Round	Simethicone 80 mg	Mylicon by Interpharm		Antiflatulent
IP276	Tab, Blue, Round	Salsalate 500 mg	Disalcid by Interpharm		NSAID
IP277	Tab, Film Coated, Debossed	Salsalate 750 mg	by Golden State	60429-0207	NSAID
IP288	Tab, White, Scored, IP/288	Triprolidine 2.5 mg, Pseudoephedrine 60 mg	Actifed by Kaiser	00179-0820	Cold Remedy
IP288	Tab, White	Triprolidine 2.5 mg, Pseudoephedrine 60 mg	Actifed by Interpharm	53746-0288	Cold Remedy
IP464	Tab, White, Round	Ibuprofen 400 mg	Motrin by Amneal	53746-0464	NSAID
IP465	Tab, White, Oblong	Ibuprofen 600 mg	Motrin by Amneal	53746-0465	NSAID
IP466	Tab, White, Oblong	Ibuprofen 800 mg	Motrin by Amneal	53746-0466	NSAID
IP52	Tab, Light Orange, Oval	Citalopram HBr 10 mg	Celexa by Amneal	65162-0052	Antidepressant
IP53	Tab, Pink, Oval, Scored	Citalopram HBr 20 mg	Celexa by Amneal	65162-0053	Antidepressant
IP54	Tab, White, Oval, Scored	Citalopram HBr 40 mg	Celexa by Amneal	65162-0054	Antidepressant
IP6	Tab, White, Round	Amlodipine Besylate 2.5 mg	Norvasc by Amneal	65162-0006	Antihypertensive
IP7	Tab, White, Round	Amlodipine Besylate 5 mg	Norvasc by Amneal	65162-0007	Antihypertensive
IP77	Tab, Blue, Oblong	Esterified Estrogens 0.625 mg, Methyltestosterone 1.25 mg	Estratest by Amneal	53746-0077	Hormone Replacement
IP78	Tab, Green, Oblong	Esterified Estrogens 1.25 mg, Methyltestosterone 2.5 mg	Estratest by Amneal	53746-0078	Hormone Replacement
IP8	Tab, White, Round	Amlodipine Besylate 10 mg	Norvasc by Amneal	65162-0008	Antihypertensive
IP9	Tab, Green, Round, ER	Alprazolam 0.5 mg	Xanax XR by Amneal	65162-0809	Antianxiety; C IV
IP94	Tab, White, Oval	Guaifenesin 600 mg, Phenylpropanolamine 75 mg	Duravent by Interpharm		Cold Remedy
IP94	Tab, White, Oval	Guaifenesin 600 mg, Phenylpropanolamine 75 mg	Duravent by Breckenridge	51991-0049	Expectorant
IP95	Tab, White, Oblong	Guaifenesin 600 mg, Pseudoephedrine 120 mg	Duratuss by Interpharm		Cold Remedy
IP96	Tab, Blue, Oval, IP/96	Guaifenesin 400 mg, Phenylpropanolamine HCl 75 mg	Entex LA by Martec		Cold Remedy
IP96	Tab, Blue, Oval, IP/96	Guaifenesin 400 mg, Phenylpropanolamine HCl 75 mg	Entex LA by Interpharm	53746-0096	Cold Remedy
IP97	Tab, Yellow, Oval	Guaifenesin 600 mg, Pseudoephedrine HCl 120 mg	Entex PSE by Breckenridge	51991-0245	Cold Remedy
IP98	Tab	Guaifenesin 600 mg, Pseudoephedrine HCl 60 mg	by Ivax	00182-1037	Cold Remedy
IP99	Tab, Green, Oblong	Guaifenesin 600 mg, Dextromethorphan HBr 30 mg	by Med Pro	53978-3183	Cold Remedy
IP99	Tab, Green, Cap Shaped	Dextromethorphan 30 mg, Guaifenesin 600 mg	Guiadrine DM by Breckenridge	51991-0285	Expectorant
IRCON	Tab, Orange, Round	Ferrous Fumarate 200 mg	Ircon Tablets by Kenwood	00482-0628	Vitamin; Mineral
IRCONFA	Tab, Red, Round	Ferrous Fumarate 250 mg, Folic Acid 0.8 mg	Ircon-FA Tablet by Kenwood	00482-0932	Vitamin; Mineral
IRESSA250	Tab, Brown, Round, Film Coated	Gefitinib 250 mg	Iressa by AstraZeneca	00310-0482	Cancer Treatment
IRESSA250	Tab, Brown, Round, Film Coated	Gefitinib 250 mg	Iressa by AstraZeneca	Canadian DIN 02248676	Cancer Treatment
ISMO20	Tab, Yellowish Orange, Round, Scored, ISMO over 20	Isosorbide Mononitrate 20 mg	Ismo by Reddy Pharma	67857-0702	Antianginal
ISMO20	Tab, Yellowish Orange, Round, Scored, ISMO over 20	Isosorbide Mononitrate 20 mg	Ismo by Wyeth	Canadian	Antianginal
ISMO20	Tab, Yellowish Orange, Round, Scored, ISMO over 20	Isosorbide Mononitrate 20 mg	Ismo by Physician Total Care	54868-3001	Antianginal
ISMO20	Tab, Yellowish Orange, Round, Scored, ISMO over 20	Isosorbide Mononitrate 20 mg	Ismo by Nat Pharmpak	55154-4206	Antianginal
ISMO20	Tab, Yellowish Orange, Round, Scored, ISMO over 20	Isosorbide Mononitrate 20 mg	Ismo by Wyeth	00008-0771	Antianginal
ISMO20	Tab, Yellowish Orange, Round, Scored, ISMO over 20	Isosorbide Mononitrate 20 mg	Ismo by A H Robins	00031-0771	Antianginal
ISO60 <> APO	Tab, Yellow, Oval	Isosorbide Mononitrate 60 mg	Apo-ISMN by Apotex	Canadian DIN 02272830	Antianginal
ISODRIL10	Tab, White	Isosorbide Dinitrate 10 mg	Isordil by Wyeth	Canadian	Antianginal
ISODRIL30	Tab, White	Isosorbide Dinitrate 30 mg	Isordil by Wyeth	Canadian	Antianginal
ISONIAZID300	Tab, White, Round, Scored	Isoniazid 300 mg	Laniazid by Pharmascience	Canadian DIN 00577804	Antimycobacterial
ISOPTIN120 <> KNOLL	Tab, Film Coated	Verapamil HCl 120 mg	Isoptin by Knoll	00044-1823 Discontinued	Antihypertensive
ISOPTIN80 <> KNOLL	Tab, Film Coated	Verapamil HCl 80 mg	Isoptin by Knoll	00044-1822 Discontinued	Antihypertensive
ISOPTIN80 <> KNOLL	Tab, Film Coated	Verapamil HCl 80 mg	Verelan by Amerisource	62584-0822 Discontinued	Antihypertensive

ID FRONT <> BACK	DESCRIPTION FRONT <> BACK	INGREDIENT & STRENGTH	BRAND (or Generic Equiv.) by FIRM	NDC#	CLASS; SCH.
ISOPTIN80 <> KNOLL	Tab, Film Coated	Verapamil HCl 80 mg	by Med Pro	53978-7001 Discontinued	Antihypertensive
ISOPTINSR	Tab, Light Green, Cap Shaped, Scored, Film Coated,	Verapamil HCl 240 mg	Isoptin SR by Abbott	00044-1826	Antihypertensive
ISOPTINSR <> 180MG	Tab, Light Pink, Oval, Scored, Film Coated	Verapamil HCl 180 mg	Isoptin SR by Abbott	00044-1825	Antihypertensive
ISORDIL10	Tab, White	Isosorbide Dinitrate 10 mg	Isordil by Wyeth	Canadian	Antianginal
IT <> L3	Tab, White, Oblong, Film-Coated	Ibandronate Sodium 2.5 mg	Boniva by Hoffmann La Roche	00004-0185	Bisphosphonate
IU <> NVR	Tab, Light Red, Oval	Aliskiren 300 mg	Rasilez by Novartis	Canadian DIN 02302071	Antihypertensive
IU <> NVR	Tab, Light Red, Oval	Aliskiren 300 mg	Tekturna by Novartis	00078-0486	Antihypertensive
IVAX101	Cap, Orange, Black Ink	Polypodium Leucotomos Extract 240 mg	Heliocare by Ivax	13613-0101	Supplement
J	Tab, White	Trimebutine Maleate 100 mg	Modulon by Jouveinal	Canadian	Motility Regulator
J	Tab, White	Trimebutine Maleate 200 mg	Modulon by Jouveinal	Canadian	Motility Regulator
J02	Tab, White, Round	Atropine Sulfate 0.4 mg	Sal-Tropine by Eli Lilly		Gastrointestinal
J09	Tab, White, Round	Codeine Sulfate 15 mg	by Eli Lilly		Analgesic; C II
J1	Cap, Dark Green and White, Opaque	Cephalexin 250 mg	Keflex by West-Ward	00143-9898	Antibiotic
J1 <> LL	Tab, White, Square	Methazolamide 25 mg	Neptazane by Lederle	00005-3519	Antiglaucoma Agent
J10	Tab, White, Round	Codeine Sulfate 30 mg	by Eli Lilly		Analgesic; C II
J11	Tab, White, Round	Codeine Sulfate 60 mg	by Eli Lilly		Analgesic; C II
J125 <> NVR	Tab, Off-White, Round, Tablet for Oral Suspension	Deferasirox 125 mg	Exjade by Novartis	00078-0468	Chelating Agent
J125 <> NVR	Tab, Off-White, Round, Tablet for Oral Suspension	Deferasirox 125 mg	Exjade by Novartis	Canadian DIN 02287420	Chelating Agent
J13	Tab, White, Round	Colchicine 0.6 mg	by Eli Lilly		Antigout
J2	Cap, Dark Green and Light Green, Opaque	Cephalexin 500 mg	Keflex by West-Ward	00143-9897	Antibiotic
J2 <> LL	Tab, White, Round, Scored	Methazolamide 50 mg	Neptazane by Lederle	00005-3520	Antiglaucoma Agent
J2 <> LL	Tab, J Above & 2 Below Score <> LL --Lederle	Methazolamide 50 mg	Neptazane by Allscripts		Antiglaucoma Agent
J20	Tab, White, Round	Quinidine Sulfate 200 mg	Quinidine Sulfate by Eli Lilly		Antiarrhythmic
J25	Tab, Brown, Round	Thyroid 60 mg	by Eli Lilly		Thyroid Hormone
J250 <> NVR	Tab, Off-White, Round, Tablet for Oral Suspension	Deferasirox 250 mg	Exjade by Novartis	00078-0469	Chelating Agent
J250 <> NVR	Tab, Off-White, Round, Tablet for Oral Suspension	Deferasirox 250 mg	Exjade by Novartis	Canadian DIN 02287439	Chelating Agent
J26	Tab, Brown, Round	Thyroid 120 mg	by Eli Lilly		Thyroid Hormone
J29	Tab, Brown, Round	Thyroid 30 mg	by Eli Lilly		Thyroid Hormone
J31	Tab, White, Round	Phenobarbital 15 mg	Phenobarbital by Eli Lilly		Sedative/Hypnotic; C IV
J32	Tab, White, Round	Phenobarbital 30 mg	Phenobarbital by Eli Lilly		Sedative/Hypnotic; C IV
J33	Tab, White, Round	Phenobarbital 100 mg	Phenobarbital by Eli Lilly		Sedative/Hypnotic; C IV
J36	Tab, White, Round	Ergonovine Maleate 0.2 mg	Ergotrate Maleate by Eli Lilly		Ergot Alkaloids
J37	Tab, White, Round	Phenobarbital 60 mg	by Eli Lilly		Sedative/Hypnotic; C IV
J500 <> NVR	Tab, Off-White, Round, Tablet for Oral Suspension	Deferasirox 500 mg	Exjade by Novartis	Canadian DIN 02287447	Chelating Agent
J500 <> NVR	Tab, Off-White, Round, Tablet for Oral Suspension	Deferasirox 500 mg	Exjade by Novartis	00078-0470	Chelating Agent
J52	Tab, White, Round	Diethylstilbestrol Diphosphate 1 mg	by Eli Lilly		Hormone
J54	Tab, White, Round	Diethylstilbestrol Diphosphate 5 mg	by Eli Lilly		Hormone
J60	Tab, Pink, Round	Digitoxin 0.1 mg	Crystodigin by Eli Lilly		Cardiac Agent
J61	Tab, White, Round	Papaverine HCl 30 mg	by Eli Lilly		Vasodilator
J62	Tab, White, Round	Papaverine HCl 60 mg	by Eli Lilly		Vasodilator

ID FRONT <> BACK	DESCRIPTION FRONT <> BACK	INGREDIENT & STRENGTH	BRAND (or Generic Equiv.) by FIRM	NDC#	CLASS; SCH.
J64	Tab, White, Round	Methadone HCl 5 mg	Dolophine by Eli Lilly		Analgesic; C II
J69	Tab, White, Round	Propylthiouracil 50 mg	by Eli Lilly		Antithyroid
J72	Tab, White, Round	Methadone HCl 10 mg	Dolophine by Eli Lilly		Analgesic; C II
J73	Tab, White, Oblong	Methyltestosterone 10 mg	by Eli Lilly		Hormone; C III
J74	Tab, White, Round	Methyltestosterone 25 mg	by Eli Lilly		Hormone; C III
J75	Tab, White, Round	Isoproterenol HCl 10 mg	Isuprel by Sanofi		Antiasthmatic
J75	Tab, Orange, Round	Digitoxin 0.05 mg	Crystodigin by Eli Lilly		Cardiac Agent
J76	Tab, Yellow, Round	Digitoxin 0.15 mg	Crystodigin by Eli Lilly		Cardiac Agent
J77	Tab, White, Round	Isoproterenol HCl 15 mg	Isuprel by Sanofi		Antiasthmatic
J94	Tab, White, Round, Scored	Methimazole 5 mg	Tapazole by Neuman	64579-0001	Antithyroid
J94	Tab, White, Round, Scored	Methimazole 5 mg	Tapazole by Jones	52604-1094	Antithyroid
J94	Tab, White, Round, Scored	Methimazole 5 mg	Tapazole by King	60793-0104	Antithyroid
J95	Tab, White, Round, Scored	Methimazole 10 mg	Tapazole by King	60793-0105	Antithyroid
J95	Tab, White, Round, Scored	Methimazole 10 mg	Tapazole by Jones	52604-1095	Antithyroid
J96	Tab, White, Round	Methyltestosterone 5 mg, Diethylstilbestrol 0.25 mg	Tylosterone by Eli Lilly		Hormone; C III
JACOBUS <> 100101	Tab, Scored, Jacobus <> 100/101	Dapsone 100 mg	Dapsone by Jacobus	49938-0101	Antimycobacterial
JACOBUS <> 100101	Tab, Scored, Jacobus <> 100/101	Dapsone 100 mg	Dapsone by Physician Total Care	54868-3801	Antimycobacterial
JACOBUS <> 25102	Tab, White, Round, 25 over 102	Dapsone 25 mg	Dapsone by Jacobus	49938-0102	Antimycobacterial
JACOBUS <> 25102	Tab, White, Round, 25 over 102	Dapsone 25 mg	Dapsone by PDRX	55289-0188	Antimycobacterial
JACOBUS0704	Tab, Tan, Jacobus 107-04	Aminosalicylic Acid Granules DR 4 g	Paser(R) by Jacobus		Antimycobacterial
JANSSEN	Tab, Chewable	Mebendazole 100 mg	by Dept Health	53808-0003	Anthelmintic
JANSSEN <> AST10	Tab, White, Round, AST over 10 <> Janssen	Astemizole 10 mg	Hismanal by Pharmedix	53002-0642 Discontinued	Antihistamine
JANSSEN <> AST10	Tab, White, Round, AST over 10 <> Janssen	Astemizole 10 mg	Hismanal by Janssen	50458-0510 Discontinued	Antihistamine
JANSSEN <> AST10	Tab, White, Round, AST over 10 <> Janssen	Astemizole 10 mg	Hismanal by Amerisource	62584-0510 Discontinued	Antihistamine
JANSSEN <> AST10	Tab, White, Round, AST over 10 <> Janssen	Astemizole 10 mg	Hismanal by Ortho-McNeil	00062-0510 Discontinued	Antihistamine
JANSSEN <> AST10	Tab, White, Round, AST over 10 <> Janssen	Astemizole 10 mg	Hismanal by Kaiser	00179-1234 Discontinued	Antihistamine
JANSSEN <> AST10	Tab, White, Round, AST over 10 <> Janssen	Astemizole 10 mg	Hismanal by Janssen	Discontinued	Antihistamine
JANSSEN <> AST10	Tab, White, Round, AST over 10 <> Janssen	Astemizole 10 mg	Hismanal by Direct Dispensing	57866-6480 Discontinued	Antihistamine
JANSSEN <> AST10	Tab, White, Round, AST over 10 <> Janssen	Astemizole 10 mg	Hismanal by St. Mary's Med	60760-0510 Discontinued	Antihistamine
JANSSEN <> AST10	Tab, White, Round, AST over 10 <> Janssen	Astemizole 10 mg	Hismanal by Johnson & Johnson	59604-0510 Discontinued	Antihistamine
JANSSEN <> AST10	Tab, White, Round, AST over 10 <> Janssen	Astemizole 10 mg	Hismanal by PDRX	55289-0527 Discontinued	Antihistamine
JANSSEN <> G12	Tab, Orange-Brown, Round, Film Coated	Galantamine 12 mg	Razadyne by Janssen	50458-0392	Antialzheimers
JANSSEN <> G12	Tab, Orange-Brown, Round, Film Coated	Galantamine 12 mg	Reminyl by Janssen-Ortho	Canadian DIN 02244300	Antialzheimers
JANSSEN <> G4	Tab, Off-White, Round, Film Coated	Galantamine 4 mg	Reminyl by Janssen-Ortho	Canadian DIN 02244298	Antialzheimers
JANSSEN <> G4	Tab, Off-White, Round, Film Coated	Galantamine 4 mg	Razadyne by Janssen	50458-0390	Antialzheimers
JANSSEN <> G8	Tab, Pink, Round, Film Coated	Galantamine 8 mg	Reminyl by Janssen-Ortho	Canadian DIN 02244299	Antialzheimers

ID FRONT <> BACK	DESCRIPTION FRONT <> BACK	INGREDIENT & STRENGTH	BRAND (or Generic Equiv.) by FIRM	NDC#	CLASS; SCH.
JANSSEN <> G8	Tab, Pink, Round, Film Coated	Galantamine 8 mg	Razadyne by Janssen	50458-0391	Antialzheimers
JANSSEN <> L50	Tab, Coated, L over 50	Levamisole 50 mg	Ergamisol by Janssen	50458-0270	Immunomodulator
JANSSEN <> ME100	Tab, Orange, Round, Scored, Me/100	Mebendazole 100 mg	Vermox by Janssen-Ortho	Canadian DIN 00556734	Anthelmintic
JANSSEN <> NIZORAL	Tab, White, Scored	Ketoconazole 200 mg	Nizoral by Direct Dispensing	57866-6570	Antifungal
JANSSEN <> NIZORAL	Tab, White, Scored	Ketoconazole 200 mg	Nizoral by Pharm Util	60491-0454	Antifungal
JANSSEN <> NIZORAL	Tab, White, Scored	Ketoconazole 200 mg	Nizoral by Johnson & Johnson	59604-0220	Antifungal
JANSSEN <> NIZORAL	Tab, White, Scored	Ketoconazole 200 mg	Nizoral by H J Harkins Co	52959-0197	Antifungal
JANSSEN <> NIZORAL	Tab, White, Scored	Ketoconazole 200 mg	Nizoral by Janssen	50458-0220	Antifungal
JANSSEN <> P10	Tab, White, Round, Scored, Janssen <> P/10	Cisapride 10 mg	Propulsid by Johnson & Johnson	59604-0430	Gastrointestinal
JANSSEN <> P10	Tab, White, Round, Scored, Janssen <> P/10	Cisapride 10 mg	by PDRX	55289-0105	Gastrointestinal
JANSSEN <> P10	Tab, White, Round, Scored, Janssen <> P/10	Cisapride 10 mg	by Pharm Pkg Ctr	54383-0077	Gastrointestinal
JANSSEN <> P10	Tab, White, Round, Scored, Janssen <> P/10	Cisapride 10 mg	by Nat Pharmpak	55154-1402	Gastrointestinal
JANSSEN <> P10	Tab, White, Round, Scored, Janssen <> P/10	Cisapride 10 mg	by Allscripts	50458-0220	Gastrointestinal
JANSSEN <> P20	Tab, Blue, Oval, P/20 <> Janssen	Cisapride 20 mg	Propulsid by Caremark	00339-6024	Gastrointestinal
JANSSEN <> P20	Tab, Blue, Oval, P/20 <> Janssen	Cisapride 20 mg	Propulsid by Janssen	50458-0440	Gastrointestinal
JANSSEN <> P20	Tab, Blue, Oval, P/20 <> Janssen	Cisapride 20 mg	Propulsid by Johnson & Johnson	59604-0440	Gastrointestinal
JANSSEN <> R1	Tab, White, Cap Shaped, Scored	Risperidone 1 mg	Risperdal by Janssen	50458-0300	Antipsychotic
JANSSEN <> R2	Tab, Orange, Cap Shaped	Risperidone 2 mg	Risperdal by Janssen	50458-0320	Antipsychotic
JANSSEN <> R3	Tab, Yellow, Cap Shaped	Risperidone 3 mg	Risperdal by Janssen	50458-0330	Antipsychotic
JANSSEN <> R4	Tab, Green, Cap Shaped	Risperidone 4 mg	Risperdal by Janssen	50458-0350	Antipsychotic
JANSSEN <> RIS025	Tab, Dark Yellow, Cap Shaped, Ris 0.25	Risperidone 0.25 mg	Risperdal by Janssen	50458-0301	Antipsychotic
JANSSEN <> RIS025	Tab, Dark Yellow, Cap Shaped, Ris 0.25	Risperidone 0.25 mg	Risperdal by Janssen-Ortho	Canadian DIN 02240551	Antipsychotic
JANSSEN <> RIS05	Tab, Red-Brown, Cap Shaped, Ris 0.5	Risperidone 0.5 mg	Risperdal by Janssen-Ortho	Canadian DIN 02240552	Antipsychotic
JANSSEN <> RIS05	Tab, Red-Brown, Cap Shaped, Ris 0.5	Risperidone 0.5 mg	Risperdal by Janssen	50458-0302	Antipsychotic
JANSSEN <> RIS05	Tab, Red-Brown, Ris 0.5	Risperidone 0.5 mg	Risperdal by Janssen	65084-0191	Antipsychotic
JANSSEN <> VERMOX	Tab, Chewable	Mebendazole 100 mg	Vermox by Janssen	50458-0110	Anthelmintic
JANSSEN1	Tab, White, Round	Risperidone 1 mg	by Apotheca	12634-0679	Antipsychotic
JANSSENAST10	Tab, White, Round	Astemizole 10 mg	Hismanal by Johnson & Johnson	Canadian	Antihistamine
JANSSENIMODIUM	Cap	Loperamide 2 mg	Imodium by Nat Pharmpak	55154-1401	Antidiarrheal
JANSSENIMODIUM	Cap, Dark Green & Light Green	Loperamide 2 mg	Imodium by Janssen	50458-0400	Antidiarrheal
JANSSENIMODIUM	Cap, Dark Green & Light Green	Loperamide 2 mg	Imodium by Johnson & Johnson	59604-0400	Antidiarrheal
JANSSENP <> 10	Tab, Janssen/P <> 10	Cisapride 10 mg	Propulsid by Janssen	50458-0430	Gastrointestinal
JANSSENP10	Tab	Cisapride 10 mg	by Med Pro	53978-2062	Gastrointestinal
JANSSENP10	Tab, Janssen P/10	Cisapride 10 mg	by Caremark	00339-5887	Gastrointestinal
JANSSENP10	Tab, White, Scored	Cisapride 10 mg	by Compumed	00403-4662	Gastrointestinal
JANSSENR1	Tab, Coated	Risperidone 1 mg	by Nat Pharmpak	55154-1405	Antipsychotic
JANSSENR1	Tab, White, Scored	Risperidone 1 mg	Risperdal by RX Pak	65084-0198	Antipsychotic
JANSSENR4	Tab, Green, Oblong, Coated	Risperidone 4 mg	by Physician Total Care	54868-3515	Antipsychotic
JANSSENSPORANOX100	Cap, Blue & Pink, White Print, Janssen over Sporanox over 100	Itraconazole 100 mg	Sporanox by Janssen	50458-0290	Antifungal
JANSSENSPORANOX100	Cap, Blue & Pink, White Print, Janssen over Sporanox over 100	Itraconazole 100 mg	Sporanox by Janssen-Ortho	Canadian DIN 02047454	Antifungal
JANSSENSPORANOX100	Cap, Blue & Pink, White Print, Janssen over Sporanox over 100	Itraconazole 100 mg	Sporanox by Janssen	12578-0290	Antifungal
JC <> SANOREX	Tab, Peach, Round, Scored	Mazindol 2 mg	Sanorex by Novartis	Canadian DIN 00285544	Anorexiant; C IV

ID FRONT <> BACK	DESCRIPTION FRONT <> BACK	INGREDIENT & STRENGTH	BRAND (or Generic Equiv.) by FIRM	NDC#	CLASS; SCH.
JC <> TP	Tab, Light Yellow, Cap Shaped, Film Coated, J-C <> T/P	Tramadol HCl 37.5 mg, Acetaminophen 325 mg	Tramacet by Janssen-Ortho	Canadian DIN 02264846	Analgesic
JCA	Tab, White, Round, Scored, Film Coated, JC over Abbott Logo (a)	Propafenone HCl 150 mg	Rythmol by Abbott	00074-1628	Antiarrhythmic
JD	Tab, White, Round, Schering Logo JD	Methyltestosterone 10 mg	Oreton by Schering		Hormone; C III
JE	Tab, Peach, Round, Schering Logo JE	Methyltestosterone 25 mg	Oreton by Schering		Hormone; C III
JIA	Tab, White, Round, Scored, Film Coated, JI over Abbott Logo (a)	Propafenone HCl 225 mg	Rythmol by Abbott	00074-1732	Antiarrhythmic
JIMINT1	Tab, Tan, Round, Jimi/NT 1	Thyroid 64.8 mg	Westhroid by Jones		Thyroid Hormone
JIMITH1	Tab, Red, Round, Jimi TH-1	Thyroid 64.8 mg	Westhroid by Jones		Thyroid Hormone
JIMITH1	Tab, Yellow, Round, Jimi TH-1	Thyroid 64.8 mg	Westhroid by Jones		Thyroid Hormone
JIMITH1	Tab, Blue, Round, Jimi TH-1	Thyroid 64.8 mg	Westhroid by Jones		Thyroid Hormone
JIMITH1	Tab, Pink, Round, Jimi TH-1	Thyroid 64.8 mg	Westhroid by Jones		Thyroid Hormone
JMI <> APT	Tab, Sugar Coated	Thyroid 3 g	Westhroid Apt 2 by Jones	52604-7505	Thyroid Hormone
JMI <> APT	Tab, Sugar Coated	Thyroid 3 g	Westhroid Apt 2 by JMI Canton	00252-7505	Thyroid Hormone
JMI <> D14	Tab, White, Round	Liothyronine Sodium 5 mcg	Cytomel by Jones	52604-3414	Thyroid Hormone
JMI <> NT112	Tab, NT over 1 1/2	Thyroid 97.2 mg	Nature Thyroid by JMI Canton	00252-3304	Thyroid Hormone
JMI <> NT112	Tab, NT over 1 1/2	Thyroid 97.2 mg	Nature Thyroid by Jones	52604-3304	Thyroid Hormone
JMI <> NT12	Tab, NT over 1 1/2	Thyroid 32.4 mg	Nature Thyroid by JMI Canton	00252-3299	Thyroid Hormone
JMI <> NT12	Tab, NT over 1 1/2	Thyroid 32.4 mg	Nature Thyroid by Jones	52604-3299	Thyroid Hormone
JMI <> NT3	Tab	Thyroid 3 g	Nature Thyroid by Jones	52604-3312	Thyroid Hormone
JMI3166	Tab, Green & Pink & Yellow, JMI/3166	Phenobarbital 30 mg	by JMI Canton	00252-3166	Sedative/Hypnotic; C IV
JMI4450	Tab, Salmon, Round	Guaifenesin 200 mg	Aquabid by Jones		Expectorant
JMI627	Tab, Sugar Coated, JMI/627	Thyroid 64.8 mg	by JMI Canton	00252-0627	Thyroid Hormone
JMI627	Tab, JMI/3166	Thyroid 64.8 mg	by Jones	52604-0627	Thyroid Hormone
JMI628	Tab, Sugar Coated, JMI/627	Thyroid 129.6 mg	by JMI Canton	00252-0628	Thyroid Hormone
JMI628	Tab, JMI/628	Thyroid 129.6 mg	by Jones	52604-0628	Thyroid Hormone
JMI629	Tab, Sugar Coated, JMI/627	Thyroid 194.4 mg	by JMI Canton	00252-0629	Thyroid Hormone
JMI629	Tab, Sugar Coated, JMI/629	Thyroid 194.4 mg	by Jones	52604-0629	Thyroid Hormone
JMI674	Tab, JMI/674	Thyroid 64.8 mg	by Jones	52604-0674	Thyroid Hormone
JMI674	Tab, JMI/674	Thyroid 64.8 mg	by JMI Canton	00252-0674	Thyroid Hormone
JMI675	Tab, JMI/675	Thyroid 129.6 mg	by Jones	52604-0675	Thyroid Hormone
JMI675	Tab, JMI/675	Thyroid 129.6 mg	by JMI Canton	00252-0675	Thyroid Hormone
JMI6792	Tab, Embossed, JMI/6792	Atropine Sulfate 0.0194 mg, Hyoscyamine Sulfate 0.1037 mg, Phenobarbital 16.2 mg, Scopolamine 0.0065 mg	Donnatal by Alphagen	59743-0027	Gastrointestinal; C IV
JMI6792	Tab, JMI/6792	Atropine Sulfate 0.0194 mg, Hyoscyamine Sulfate 0.1037 mg, Phenobarbital 16.2 mg, Scopolamine 0.0065 mg	Donnatal by JMI Canton	00252-6792	Gastrointestinal; C IV
JMI6792	Tab, JMI/6792	Atropine Sulfate 0.0194 mg, Hyoscyamine Sulfate 0.1037 mg, Phenobarbital 16.2 mg, Scopolamine 0.0065 mg	Donnatal by Jones	52604-6792	Gastrointestinal; C IV
JMI686	Tab, JMI/686	Thyroid 32.4 mg	by Jones	52604-0626	Thyroid Hormone
JMI686	Tab, JMI/686	Thyroid 32.4 mg	by Jones	52604-0686	Thyroid Hormone
JMI686	Tab, JMI/686	Thyroid 32.4 mg	by JMI Canton	00252-0686	Thyroid Hormone
JMI686	Tab, Sugar Coated, JMI/686	Thyroid 32.4 mg	by JMI Canton	00252-0626	Thyroid Hormone
JMI7070	Tab, JMI/7070	Thyroid 0.5 g	Westhroid Th 1/2 by JMI Canton	00252-7070	Thyroid Hormone
JMI7070	Tab, JMI/7070	Thyroid 0.5 g	Westhroid Th 1/2 by Jones	52604-7070	Thyroid Hormone
JMI7073	Tab, JMI/7073	Thyroid 1 g	Westhroid Th 1 by JMI Canton	00252-7073	Thyroid Hormone
JMI7073	Tab, JMI/7073	Thyroid 1 g	Westhroid Th 1 by Jones	52604-7073	Thyroid Hormone
JMI7080	Tab, JMI/7080	Thyroid 2 g	Westhroid Th 2 by JMI Canton	00252-7080	Thyroid Hormone
JMI7080	Tab, JMI/7080	Thyroid 2 g	Westhroid Th 2 by Jones	52604-7080	Thyroid Hormone

ID FRONT <> BACK	DESCRIPTION FRONT <> BACK	INGREDIENT & STRENGTH	BRAND (or Generic Equiv.) by FIRM	NDC#	CLASS; SCH.
JMI7087	Tab, JMI7087	Thyroid 3 g	Westhroid Th 3 by JMI Canton	00252-7087	Thyroid Hormone
JMI7087	Tab, JMI7087	Thyroid 3 g	Westhroid Th 3 by JMI Canton	52604-7087	Thyroid Hormone
JMI7090	Tab, Tan, with Green, Red, Yellow Specks, JMI7090	Thyroid 3 g	Westhroid Thv 3 by JMI Canton	00252-7090	Thyroid Hormone
JMI7092	Tab, JMI7092	Thyroid 4 g	Westhroid Th 4 by JMI Canton	00252-7092	Thyroid Hormone
JMI7092	Tab, JMI7092	Thyroid 4 g	Westhroid Th 4 by Jones	52604-7092	Thyroid Hormone
JMI7095	Tab, JMI7095	Thyroid 5 g	Westhroid Th 5 by JMI Canton	00252-7095	Thyroid Hormone
JMI7095	Tab, JMI7095	Thyroid 5 g	Westhroid Th 5 by Jones	52604-7095	Thyroid Hormone
JMI776	Tab	Thyroid 32.4 mg	by Jones	52604-7004	Thyroid Hormone
JMI776	Tab	Thyroid 32.4 mg	by URL Mutual	00677-0150	Thyroid Hormone
JMI776	Tab, JMI776	Thyroid 32.4 mg	by Jones	52604-0776	Thyroid Hormone
JMI776	Tab, JMI776	Thyroid 32.4 mg	by JMI Canton	00252-7004	Thyroid Hormone
JMI777	Tab, JMI 777	Thyroid 64.8 mg	by Jones	52604-0777	Thyroid Hormone
JMI777	Tab	Thyroid 64.8 mg	by URL Mutual	00677-0151	Thyroid Hormone
JMI777	Tab, JMI 777	Thyroid 64.8 mg	by JMI Canton	00252-0777	Thyroid Hormone
JMI777	Tab, JMI 777	Thyroid 64.8 mg	by JMI Canton	00252-7006	Thyroid Hormone
JMI777	Tab, JMI 777	Thyroid 65 mg	Etwon by Macnary	55982-0013	Thyroid Hormone
JMI777	Tab, JMI 777	Levothyroxine 38 mcg, Liothyronine 9 mcg	Armour Thyroid by Qualitest	00603-6046	Thyroid Hormone
JMI778	Tab, JMI 778	Levothyroxine Sodium 76 mcg, Liothyronine 18 mcg	Armour Thyroid by Qualitest	00603-6047	Thyroid Hormone
JMI778	Tab, JMI 778	Thyroid 129.6 mg	by JMI Canton	00252-0778	Thyroid Hormone
JMI778	Tab	Thyroid 129.6 mg	by URL Mutual	00677-0153	Thyroid Hormone
JMI778	Tab, JMI 778	Thyroid 194.4 mg	by Jones	52604-0778	Thyroid Hormone
JMI779	Tab, JMI 779	Thyroid 194.4 mg	by JMI Canton	00252-7023	Thyroid Hormone
JMI779	Tab, JMI 779	Levothyroxine 114 mcg, Liothyronine 27 mcg	Armour Thyroid by Qualitest	00603-6048	Thyroid Hormone
JMID16	Tab, White, Round, Scored, JMI over D16	Liothyronine Sodium 25 mcg	Cytomel by Jones	52604-3416	Thyroid Hormone
JMID17	Tab, White, Round	Liothyronine Sodium 50 mcg	Cytomel by Jones	52604-3417	Thyroid Hormone
JMIK	Tab, Off-White, JMI/K	Potassium Bicarbonate 648 mg	Quic K by JMI Canton	00252-5745	Electrolytes
JMIK	Tab, Off-White, JMI/K	Potassium Bicarbonate 648 mg	Quic K by Jones	52604-5745	Electrolytes
JMINT1	Tab, JMI over NT1	Thyroid 1 g	Nature Thyroid by Jones	52604-3300	Thyroid Hormone
JMINT1	Tab, JMI/NT1	Thyroid 1 g	Nature Thyroid by JMI Canton	00252-3300	Thyroid Hormone
JMINT2	Tab, JMI/NT2	Thyroid 2 g	Parloid Thyroid Rn2 by JMI Canton	00252-3308	Thyroid Hormone
JMINT2	Tab, Tan, Round, JMI over NT2	Thyroid 2 g	Nature Thyroid by Jones	52604-3308	Thyroid Hormone
JMITH1	Tab, Sugar Coated, JMI/TH-1	Thyroid 1 g	Westhroid Thb 1 by Jones	52604-7074	Thyroid Hormone
JMITH1	Tab, Sugar Coated, JMI/TH-1	Thyroid 1 g	Westhroid Thr 1 by Jones	52604-7075	Thyroid Hormone
JMITH1	Tab, Sugar Coated, JMI/TH-1	Thyroid 1 g	Westhroid Thb 1 by JMI Canton	00252-7075	Thyroid Hormone
JMITH1	Tab, Sugar Coated, JMI/TH-1	Thyroid 1 g	Westhroid Thy 1 by JMI Canton	00252-7076	Thyroid Hormone
JMITH1	Tab, Sugar Coated, JMI/TH-1	Thyroid 1 g	Westhroid Thp 11 by JMI Canton	00252-7077	Thyroid Hormone
JMITH1	Tab, Sugar Coated, JMI/TH-1	Thyroid 1 g	Westhroid Thp 11 by Jones	52604-7077	Thyroid Hormone
JMITH1	Tab, Sugar Coated, JMI/TH-1	Thyroid 1 g	Westhroid Thy 1 by Jones	52604-7076	Thyroid Hormone
JMITH1	Tab, Sugar Coated, JMI/TH-1	Thyroid 1 g	Westhroid Thb 1 by JMI Canton	00252-7074	Thyroid Hormone
JMITH2	Tab, Sugar Coated, JMI/TH-2	Thyroid 2 g	Westhroid Thp 21 by JMI Canton	00252-7084	Thyroid Hormone
JMITH2	Tab, Sugar Coated, JMI/TH-2	Thyroid 2 g	Westhroid Thp 21 by Jones	52604-7084	Thyroid Hormone
JMITH2	Tab, Sugar Coated, JMI/TH-2	Thyroid 2 g	Westhroid Thy 2 by Jones	52604-7083	Thyroid Hormone
JMITH2	Tab, Red, Round, Sugar Coated, JMI/TH-2	Thyroid 2 g	Westhroid Thr 2 by Jones	52604-7082	Thyroid Hormone
JMITH2	Tab, Blue, Round, Sugar Coated, JMI/TH-2	Thyroid 2 g	Westhroid Thb 2 by Jones	52604-7081	Thyroid Hormone
JMITH2	Tab, Yellow, Round, Sugar Coated, JMI/TH-2	Thyroid 2 g	Westhroid Thb 2 by JMI Canton	00252-7081	Thyroid Hormone
JMITH2	Tab, Pink, Round, Sugar Coated, JMI/TH-2	Thyroid 2 g	Westhroid Thy 2 by JMI Canton	00252-7083	Thyroid Hormone
JMITH2	Tab, Sugar Coated, JMI/TH-2	Thyroid 2 g	Westhroid Thr 2 by JMI Canton	00252-7082	Thyroid Hormone
JMITH3	Tab, Sugar Coated, JMI/TH-3	Thyroid 3 g	Westhroid Thg 32 by JMI Canton	00252-7088	Thyroid Hormone
JMITH3	Tab, Sugar Coated, JMI/TH-3	Thyroid 3 g	Westhroid Thb 33 by JMI Canton	00252-7089	Thyroid Hormone
JMITH3	Tab, Green, Round, Sugar Coated, JMI/TH-3	Thyroid 3 g	Westhroid Thg 32 by Jones	52604-7088	Thyroid Hormone

ID FRONT <> BACK	DESCRIPTION FRONT <> BACK	INGREDIENT & STRENGTH	BRAND (or Generic Equiv.) by FIRM	NDC#	CLASS; SCH.
JMITH3	Tab, Blue, Round, Sugar Coated, JMI/TH-3	Thyroid 3 g	Westhroid Thb 3 by Jones	52604-7089	Thyroid Hormone
JMITH4	Tab, Fuchsia, Round, Sugar Coated, JMI/TH-4	Thyroid 4 g	Westhroid Thf 4 by Jones	52604-7093	Thyroid Hormone
JMITH4	Tab, Fuchsia, Sugar Coated, JMI/TH-4	Thyroid 4 g	Westhroid Thf 4 by JMI Canton	00252-7093	Thyroid Hormone
JMITH5	Tab, Blue, Round, Sugar Coated, JMI/TH-5	Thyroid 5 g	Westhroid Thb 5 by Jones	52604-7097	Thyroid Hormone
JMITH5	Tab, Sugar Coated, JMI/TH-5	Thyroid 5 g	Westhroid Thb 5 by JMI Canton	00252-7097	Thyroid Hormone
JMIY	Tab, White, JMI/Y	Yohimbine HCl 5.4 mg	Yocon by JMI Canton	00252-3245	Impotence Agent
JNA	Tab, White, Round, Scored, Film Coated, JN over Abbott Logo (a)	Propafenone HCl 300 mg	Rythmol by Abbott	00074-1831	Antiarrhythmic
JPI406	Tab, White, Oval, Scored	Chlorpheniramine Maleate 8 mg, Phenylephrine HCl 20 mg, Methscopolamine Nitrate 2.5 mg	Drize-R by Jones	52604-0406	Cold Remedy
JPI406	Tab, White, Oval, Scored	Chlorpheniramine Maleate 8 mg, Methscopolamine Nitrate 2.5 mg, Phenylephrine HCl 20 mg	Vanex Forte-D by Anabolic	00722-6447	Cold Remedy
JPI406	Tab, White, Oval, Scored	Chlorpheniramine Maleate 8 mg, Methscopolamine Nitrate 2.5 mg, Phenylephrine HCl 20 mg	Vanex Forte-D by Jones	52604-0127	Cold Remedy
JSP <> 513	Tab, Peach, Round, Scored	Levothyroxine Sodium 0.025 mg	Unithroid by Watson	52544-0902	Thyroid Hormone
JSP <> 513	Tab, Peach, Round, Scored	Levothyroxine Sodium 0.025 mg	Synthroid by Ivax	00182-1529	Thyroid Hormone
JSP <> 513	Tab, Peach, Round, Scored	Levothyroxine Sodium 0.025 mg	Synthroid by Jerome Stevens	50564-0513	Thyroid Hormone
JSP <> 513	Tab, Peach, Round	Levothyroxine Sodium 25 mcg	Synthroid by Lannett	00527-1341	Thyroid Hormone
JSP <> 514	Tab, White, Round	Levothyroxine Sodium 50 mcg	Synthroid by Lannett	00527-1342	Thyroid Hormone
JSP <> 514	Tab, White, Round, Scored	Levothyroxine Sodium 0.05 mg	Synthroid by Jerome Stevens	50564-0514	Thyroid Hormone
JSP <> 514	Tab, White, Round, Scored	Levothyroxine Sodium 0.05 mg	Unithroid by Watson	52544-0903	Thyroid Hormone
JSP <> 515	Tab, Purple, Round, Scored	Levothyroxine Sodium 75 mcg	Synthroid by Watson	52544-0904	Thyroid Hormone
JSP <> 515	Tab, Purple, Round, Scored	Levothyroxine Sodium 75 mcg	Unithroid by Pharm Pkg Ctr	54383-0086	Thyroid Hormone
JSP <> 515	Tab, Purple, Round, Scored	Levothyroxine Sodium 75 mcg	Unithroid by Jerome Stevens	50564-0515	Thyroid Hormone
JSP <> 515	Tab, Purple, Round	Levothyroxine Sodium 75 mcg	Synthroid by Lannett	00527-1343	Thyroid Hormone
JSP <> 516	Tab, Yellow, Round, Scored	Levothyroxine Sodium 100 mcg	Unithroid by Lannett	00527-1345	Thyroid Hormone
JSP <> 516	Tab, Yellow, Round, Scored	Levothyroxine Sodium 100 mcg	Unithroid by Jerome Stevens	50564-0516	Thyroid Hormone
JSP <> 516	Tab, Yellow, Round, Scored	Levothyroxine Sodium 0.1 mg	by Jones	52604-7701	Thyroid Hormone
JSP <> 516	Tab, Yellow, Round, Scored	Levothyroxine Sodium 100 mcg	Unithroid by Watson	52544-0906	Thyroid Hormone
JSP <> 516	Tab, Yellow, Round, Scored	Levothyroxine Sodium 100 mcg	Unithroid by URL Mutual	00677-0078	Thyroid Hormone
JSP <> 519	Tab, Tan, Round, Scored	Levothyroxine Sodium 0.125 mg	Unithroid by Ivax	00182-1516	Thyroid Hormone
JSP <> 519	Tab, Tan, Round, Scored	Levothyroxine Sodium 0.125 mg	Unithroid by Jerome Stevens	50564-0519	Thyroid Hormone
JSP <> 519	Tab, Tan, Round, Scored	Levothyroxine Sodium 0.125 mg	Unithroid by Watson	52544-0908	Thyroid Hormone
JSP <> 519	Tab, Tan, Round	Levothyroxine Sodium 125 mcg	Unithroid by Lannett	00527-1347	Thyroid Hormone
JSP <> 520	Tab, Blue, Round, Scored	Levothyroxine Sodium 150 mcg	Unithroid by Lannett	00527-1349	Thyroid Hormone
JSP <> 520	Tab, Blue, Round, Scored	Levothyroxine Sodium 150 mcg	Unithroid by Watson	52544-0909	Thyroid Hormone
JSP <> 520	Tab, Blue, Round, Scored	Levothyroxine Sodium 150 mcg	Unithroid by URL Mutual	00677-0992	Thyroid Hormone
JSP <> 520	Tab, Blue, Round, Scored	Levothyroxine Sodium 0.15 mg	by JMI Canton	00252-7700	Thyroid Hormone
JSP <> 520	Tab, Blue, Round, Scored	Levothyroxine Sodium 150 mcg	Unithroid by Ivax	00182-1117	Thyroid Hormone
JSP <> 520	Tab, Debossed	Levothyroxine Sodium 0.15 mg	Estre by Macnary	55982-0015	Thyroid Hormone
JSP <> 520	Tab, Blue, Round, Scored	Levothyroxine Sodium 150 mcg	Unithroid by Jerome Stevens	50564-0520	Thyroid Hormone
JSP <> 522	Tab, Pink, Round, Scored	Levothyroxine Sodium 200 mcg	Unithroid by URL Mutual	00677-0079	Thyroid Hormone
JSP <> 522	Tab, Pink, Round, Scored	Levothyroxine Sodium 200 mcg	Unithroid by Watson	52544-0911	Thyroid Hormone
JSP <> 522	Tab, Pink, Round, Scored	Levothyroxine Sodium 200 mcg	Unithroid by Jerome Stevens	50564-0522	Thyroid Hormone
JSP <> 522	Tab, Pink, Round, Scored	Levothyroxine Sodium 200 mcg	Unithroid by Lannett	00527-1351	Thyroid Hormone
JSP <> 523	Tab, Green, Round, Scored	Levothyroxine Sodium 300 mcg	Unithroid by Lannett	00527-1352	Thyroid Hormone
JSP <> 523	Tab, Green, Round, Scored	Levothyroxine Sodium 300 mcg	Unithroid by Ivax	00182-1119	Thyroid Hormone
JSP <> 523	Tab, Green, Round, Scored	Levothyroxine Sodium 300 mcg	Unithroid by Jerome Stevens	50564-0523	Thyroid Hormone
JSP <> 523	Tab, Green, Round, Scored	Levothyroxine Sodium 300 mcg	Unithroid by Watson	52544-0912	Thyroid Hormone
JSP <> 561	Tab, Green, Round, Scored	Levothyroxine Sodium 88 mcg	Synthroid by Watson	52544-0905	Thyroid Hormone

ID FRONT <> BACK	DESCRIPTION FRONT <> BACK	INGREDIENT & STRENGTH	BRAND (or Generic Equiv.) by FIRM	NDC#	CLASS; SCH.
JSP <> 561	Tab, Green, Round, Scored	Levothyroxine Sodium 88 mcg	Synthroid by Lannett	00527-1344	Thyroid Hormone
JSP <> 562	Tab, Pink, Round, Scored	Levothyroxine Sodium 112 mcg	Unithroid by Lannett	00527-1346	Thyroid Hormone
JSP <> 562	Tab, Pink, Round, Scored	Levothyroxine Sodium 112 mcg	Unithroid by Watson	52544-0907	Thyroid Hormone
JSP <> 563	Tab, Purple, Round, Scored	Levothyroxine Sodium 175 mcg	Unithroid by Watson	52544-0910	Thyroid Hormone
JSP <> 563	Tab, Purple, Round, Scored	Levothyroxine Sodium 175 mcg	Unithroid by Lannett	00527-1350	Thyroid Hormone
JSP125	Tab, Debossed, Color Coded	Levothyroxine Sodium 0.125 mg	by PDRX	55289-0858	Thyroid Hormone
JSP485	Tab, Mustard Yellow, Coated, JSP-485	Ascorbic Acid 120 mg, Calcium Phosphate 64.4 mg, Calcium Sulfate 215 mg, Copper, Cyanocobalamin 12 mcg, Ergocalciferol, Folic Acid 1.21 mg, Iron 199 mg, Niacinamide 20 mg, Pyridoxine HCl 10 mg, Riboflavin 9 mg, Thiamine Mononitrate 4.5 mg, Vitamin A Acetate 8 mg, Vitamin E 22 mg, Zinc Oxide 31 mg	Prenatal 1+ Improved by Jerome Stevens	50564-0485	Vitamin
JSP490	Tab, Pink & White, Round	Aspirin 325 mg, Methocarbamol 400 mg	Robaxisal by Jerome Stevens		Analgesic; Muscle Relaxant
JSP507	Cap, Blue & Yellow	Aspirin 325 mg, Butalbital 50 mg, Caffeine 40 mg, Codeine Phosphate 30 mg	Fiorinal #3 by Jerome Stevens		Analgesic; C III
JSP507	Tab, Blue & Yellow, Oblong	Codeine 30 mg, Butalbital 50 mg, Caffeine 40 mg, Aspirin 325 mg	by Dixon Shane	17236-0358	Analgesic; C III
JSP507	Tab, Blue & Yellow, Oblong	Codeine 30 mg, Butalbital 50 mg, Caffeine 40 mg, Aspirin 325 mg	by Dixon Shane	17236-0359	Analgesic; C III
JSP507	Cap, Yellow & Blue	Aspirin 325 mg, Butalbital 50 mg, Caffeine 40 mg, Codeine Phosphate 30 mg	Fiorinal w/ Codeine by Lannett	00527-1312	Analgesic; C III
JSP508	Cap	Acetaminophen 325 mg, Dichloralantipyrine 100 mg, Isometheptene Mucate (1:1) 65 mg	by Jerome Stevens	50564-0508	Analgesic; C IV
JSP508	Cap	Acetaminophen 325 mg, Dichloralantipyrine 100 mg, Isometheptene Mucate (1:1) 65 mg	by Physician Total Care	54868-1514	Analgesic; C IV
JSP510	Cap	Chlorpheniramine Maleate 8 mg, Pseudoephedrine HCl 120 mg	by Ivax	00182-1151	Cold Remedy
JSP510	Cap, JSP-510	Chlorpheniramine Maleate 8 mg, Pseudoephedrine HCl 120 mg	Decongestant Sr by Jerome Stevens	50564-0510	Cold Remedy
JSP526	Cap, Dark Green, JSP-526	Brompheniramine Maleate 6 mg, Pseudoephedrine HCl 60 mg	Nasal Decongestant by Jerome Stevens	50564-0526	Cold Remedy
JSP527	Cap, Light Green, JSP-527	Brompheniramine Maleate 12 mg, Pseudoephedrine HCl 120 mg	Nasal Decongestant by Jerome Stevens	50564-0527	Cold Remedy
JSP533	Tab, Ex Release	Isosorbide Dinitrate 40 mg	Isordil by Qualitest	00603-4120	Antianginal
JSP533	Tab, Ex Release	Isosorbide Dinitrate 40 mg	Isordil by Jerome Stevens	50564-0533	Antianginal
JSP539	Tab	Hyoscyamine Sulfate 0.125 mg	Levsin by Jerome Stevens	50564-0539	Gastrointestinal
JSP540	Tab, Film Coated	Methenamine Mandelate 500 mg	Mandelamine by Jerome Stevens	50564-0540	Antibiotic; Urinary Tract
JSP541	Tab, Film Coated	Methenamine Mandelate 1000 mg	Mandelamine by Jerome Stevens	50564-0541	Antibiotic; Urinary Tract
JSP544	Tab, Yellow, Round, Scored, JSP over 544	Digoxin 0.125 mg	Lanoxin by Jerome Stevens	50564-0544	Cardiac Agent
JSP544	Tab, Yellow, Round, Scored, JSP over 544	Digoxin 0.125 mg	Lanoxin by Lannett	00527-1324	Cardiac Agent
JSP545	Tab, White, Round, Scored, JSP over 545	Digoxin 0.25 mg	Lanoxin by Lannett	00527-1325	Cardiac Agent
JSP545	Tab, White, Round, Scored, JSP over 545	Digoxin 0.25 mg	Lanoxin by Jerome Stevens	50564-0545	Cardiac Agent
JSP547	Tab, White, Round	Yohimbine HCl 5.4 mg	Yocon by Jerome Stevens		Impotence Agent
JSP548	Tab, JSP-548	Guaifenesin 600 mg	Robitussin by Jerome Stevens	50564-0548	Expectorant
JSP551	Tab, Yellow, Oval	Prenatal Vitamin Plus	Stuartnatal Plus by Jerome Stevens		Vitamin
JSP552	Tab, Green, Round	Hyoscyamine Sulfate 0.125 mg	Levsin SL by Jerome Stevens		Gastrointestinal
JSP553	Tab	Codeine Phosphate 10 mg, Guaifenesin 300 mg	by Pecos	59879-0512	Cold Remedy; C III
JSP553	Tab	Codeine Phosphate 10 mg, Guaifenesin 300 mg	by Ivax	00182-0151	Cold Remedy; C III
JSP553	Tab, JSP-553	Codeine Phosphate 10 mg, Guaifenesin 300 mg	by Jerome Stevens	50564-0553	Cold Remedy; C III
JU <> VISKEN15	Tab, White, Round, Scored	Pindolol 15 mg	Visken by Novartis	Canadian DIN 00417289	Antihypertensive
JUL42 <> PAL	Tab, White, Scored	Pseudoephedrine HCl 85 mg, Guaifenesin 795 mg	Panmist LA by Sovereign	58716-0692	Cold Remedy
JUVISKEN15	Tab, White, JU/Visken 15	Pindolol 15 mg	Visken by Sandoz	Canadian	Antihypertensive
K	Tab, Effervescent	Potassium Bicarbonate 0.5 g, Potassium Chloride 1.5 g	Efferv Potassium Chloride by Qualitest	00603-3508	Electrolytes
K	Tab, Orange, Round	Potassium Bicarbonate 0.5 g, Potassium Chloride 1.5 g	Efferv Potassium Chloride by Tower	50201-1300	Electrolytes
K	Tab, Red, Round, Effervescent	Potassium Bicarbonate 0.5 g, Potassium Chloride 1.5 g	Efferv Potassium Chloride by Bajamar	44184-0025	Electrolytes
K	Tab, Pink, Round	Vitamin B Complex	Apatate by Kenwood		Vitamin

ID FRONT <> BACK	DESCRIPTION FRONT <> BACK	INGREDIENT & STRENGTH	BRAND (or Generic Equiv.) by FIRM	NDC#	CLASS; SCH.
K	Cap, Orange	Valproic Acid 250 mg	Depakene by AltiMed	Canadian DIN 02140047	Anticonvulsant
K	Cap, Orange	Valproic Acid 250 mg	Depakene by Kenral	Canadian	Anticonvulsant
K	Tab, Orange, Round	Aspirin 325 mg	Ecotrin by Rugby	00536-3313	Analgesic
K	Tab, Yellow, Round	Aspirin 81 mg	Aspirin by Rugby	00536-3086	Analgesic
K	Tab, Maroon, Round	Phenazopyridine 95 mg	Azo-Gesic by Major	00904-5025	Urinary Analgesic
K	Tab, Orange, Round Enteric Coated, arrow on end of K upper leg	Aspirin 325 mg	Ecotrin by Major	00904-2013	Analgesic
K	Tab, Orange, Round Enteric Coated, arrow on end of K upper leg	Aspirin 325 mg	Ecotrin by Qualitest	00603-0166	Analgesic
K	Tab, Light Red, Round, Speckled, Orally Disintegrating	Desloratadine 2.5 mg	Clarinex Reditabs by Schering	00085-1408	Antihistamine
K	Tab, Pink w/ White Specks, Round, Chewable	Attapulgite 300 mg	Kaopectate by Johnson & Johnson	Canadian DIN 02229948	Antidiarrheal
K	Tab, Light Pink, Round, Chewable	Kaopectate 300 mg	Kaopectate by Upjohn		Antidiarrheal
K	Tab, Yellow, Enteric Coated	Aspirin 81 mg	Bayer by URL Mutual	00677-1972	Analgesic
K <> 102	Tab, Orange, Round, K with Arrow Logo	Bisacodyl 5 mg	Dulcolax Laxative by Qualitest	00603-0054	Gastrointestinal
K <> 102	Tab, Orange, Round, K with Arrow Logo	Bisacodyl 5 mg	Dulcolax by Watson	00536-3381	Gastrointestinal
K <> 200	Tab, White, Round	Oxandrolone 2.5 mg	Oxandrin by Par	49884-0301	Steroid; CIII
K <> 201	Tab, White, Round	Oxandrolone 10 mg	Oxandrin by Par	49884-0301	Steroid; CIII
K <> 250	Tab, Dark Pink, Round, Film Coated	Tranylcypromine Sulfate 10 mg	Parnate by Par	49884-0032	Antidepressant
K0	Tab, White, Round, Scored	Acetaminophen 325 mg	Tylenol by Rugby	00536-3222	Analgesic
K0	Tab, White, Round, Scored	Acetaminophen 325 mg	Tylenol by Major	00904-1982	Analgesic
K0183	Tab, Chewable	Chlorpheniramine Maleate 1 mg, Pseudoephedrine HCl 15 mg	Children's Deconamine by Kenwood	00482-0183	Cold Remedy
K0183	Tab, Chewable	Chlorpheniramine Maleate 1 mg, Pseudoephedrine HCl 15 mg	Children's Deconamine by Lini	58215-0324	Cold Remedy
K0659	Tab, White, Oval	Ergoloid Mesylate 1 mg	Hydergine by KV Pharma	Discontinued	Ergot Alkaloids
K0849	Cap, Brown & Clear	Papaverine HCl SR 150 mg	Pavabid by KV Pharma		Vasodilator
K1	Tab, White, Triangular, Film Coated	Granisetron HCl 1.12 mg	Kytril by Roche	00004-0241	Antiemetic
K1	Tab, White, Triangular, Film Coated	Granisetron HCl 1 mg	Kytril by Roche	Canadian DIN 02185881	Antiemetic
K1	Tab, White, Round, Orally Disintegrating	Ondansetron 4 mg	Zofran by Barr	50111-0945	Antiemetic
K1	Tab, White, Triangular, Film Coated	Granisetron HCl 1.12 mg	Kytril by SKB	60351-4151	Antiemetic
K1	Tab, White, Triangular, Film Coated	Granisetron HCl 1.12 mg	Kytril by SKB	00029-4151	Antiemetic
K1	Tab, Green, Round	Hydromorphone HCl 1 mg	Dilaudid by Knoll		Analgesic; C II
K1	Tab, Blue, Round	Medroxyprogesterone Acetate 5 mg	by AltiMed	Canadian DIN 02148560	Hormone
K10	Tab, White, Oblong	Acetaminophen 500 mg	Tylenol Ex Strength by Major	00904-1983	Analgesic
K10	Tab, White, Round	Acetaminophen 500 mg	Tylenol Ex Strength by Major	00904-1988	Analgesic
K10	Tab, White, Oblong	Acetaminophen 500 mg	Tylenol Ex Strength by Rugby	00536-3218	Analgesic
K10	Tab, White, Round	Acetaminophen 500 mg	Tylenol Ex Strength by Rugby	00536-3231	Analgesic
K10	Tab, White, Oblong	Acetaminophen 500 mg	Tylenol Ex Strength by Ivax		Analgesic
K10	Cap, Clear w/ One Black Band	Morphine Sulfate 50 mg	Kadian by Abbott	Canadian DIN 02242163	Analgesic; C II
K10 <> ALRA	Tab, Film Coated, Debossed, K+10 <> Alra	Potassium Chloride 750 mg	by PDRX	55289-0359	Electrolytes
K10 <> ALRA	Tab, Film Coated, K+19	Potassium Chloride 750 mg	by Golden State	60429-0215	Electrolytes
K100	Tab, White, Oblong	Ranitidine HCl 336 mg	Ranitidine by Kenral	Canadian DIN 00828688	Gastrointestinal
K100	Tab, White, Oblong	Ranitidine 300 mg	by AltiMed	Canadian	Gastrointestinal
K100	Cap, Clear w/ Four Black Bands	Morphine Sulfate 100 mg	Kadian by Abbott	Canadian DIN 02184451	Analgesic; C II

ID FRONT <> BACK	DESCRIPTION FRONT <> BACK	INGREDIENT & STRENGTH	BRAND (or Generic Equiv.) by FIRM	NDC#	CLASS; SCH.
K101	Tab, White, Round	Ranitidine HCl 168 mg	Ranitidine by Kenral	Canadian DIN 00828823	Gastrointestinal
K101	Tab, White, Round	Ranitidine 150 mg	by AltiMed	Canadian	Gastrointestinal
K104	Tab, White, Elliptical	Flurbiprofen 50 mg	by AltiMed	Canadian DIN 00675202	NSAID
K104	Tab, White, Elliptical	Flurbiprofen 50 mg	Flurbiprofen by Kenral	Canadian	NSAID
K105	Tab, Blue, Elliptical	Flurbiprofen 100 mg	Flurbiprofen by Kenral	Canadian	NSAID
K105	Tab, Blue, Elliptical	Flurbiprofen 100 mg	by AltiMed	Canadian DIN 00675199	NSAID
K105	Tab, Greenish Brown, Round	Sennosides 8.6 mg	Senna by Major	00904-5165	Gastrointestinal
K105	Tab, Brown, Round	Sennosides 8.6 mg	Senokot by Qualitest	00603-0280	Gastrointestinal
K105	Tab, Brown, Round	Sennosides 8.6 mg	Senokot by Rugby	00536-5904	Gastrointestinal
K106	Tab, Red, Round	Docusate Sodium 50 mg, Sennosides 8.6 mg	Senokot-S by Rugby	00536-0355	Gastrointestinal
K106	Tab, Red, Round	Docusate Sodium 50 mg, Sennosides 8.6 mg	Senokot-S by Major	00904-5643	Gastrointestinal
K107	Tab, Orange, Round	Aspirin 500 mg	Aspirin by Major	00904-2014	Analgesic
K108	Tab, Yellow, Round	Desipramine HCl 25 mg	by AltiMed	Canadian DIN 01948784	Antidepressant
K108	Tab, Yellow, Round	Desipramine HCl 25 mg	Desipramine by Kenral	Canadian	Antidepressant
K109	Tab, Green, Round	Desipramine HCl 50 mg	Desipramine by Kenral	Canadian	Antidepressant
K109	Tab, Green, Round	Desipramine HCl 50 mg	by AltiMed	Canadian DIN 01948792	Antidepressant
K110	Tab, Orange, Round	Desipramine HCl 75 mg	by AltiMed	Canadian DIN 01948806	Antidepressant
K110	Tab, Orange, Round	Desipramine HCl 75 mg	Desipramine by Kenral	Canadian	Antidepressant
K111	Tab, White, Round, K-111, Ex Release	Orphenadrine Citrate 100 mg	Norflex by Alphagen	59743-0201	Muscle Relaxant
K113	Tab, White	Domperidone 10 mg	by Kenral	Canadian	Gastrointestinal
K113	Tab, White	Domperidone 10 mg	by AltiMed	Canadian DIN 01912070	Gastrointestinal
K115	Cap, Pink & Clear	Diphenhydramine HCl 25 mg	Benadryl by Rugby	00536-3594	Antihistamine
K124	Tab, Orange	Doxycycline Hyclate 100 mg	by AltiMed	Canadian Discontinued	Antibiotic
K140	Tab, Light Yellow, Round, Scored	Chlorpheniramine Maleate 4 mg	Chlor-Trimeton by Rugby	00536-3467	Antihistamine
K17	Tab, Orange	Prazosin HCl 1 mg	by AltiMed	Canadian DIN 02139979 Discontinued	Antihypertensive
K18	Tab, White, Round	Prazosin HCl 2 mg	by AltiMed	Canadian Discontinued	Antihypertensive
K18	Tab, White, Round	Prazosin HCl 2 mg	by AltiMed	Canadian DIN 02139987 Discontinued	Antihypertensive
K182	Tab, Coated, K Underlined	Guaifenesin 300 mg, Hydrocodone Bitartrate 5 mg, Pseudoephedrine HCl 30 mg	Tussi-Organidin DM NR by Kenwood	00482-0182	Cold Remedy; C III
K19	Tab, White, Diamond	Prazosin HCl 5 mg	by AltiMed	Canadian DIN 02139995 Discontinued	Antihypertensive
K19	Tab, Blue, Oblong	Acetaminophen 500 mg, Diphenhydramine 25 mg	Tylenol PM by PDK		Cold Remedy
K2	Tab, White, Round, Orally Disintegrating	Ondansetron 8 mg	Zofran by Barr	50111-0946	Antiemetic
K2	Tab, Orange, Round	Hydromorphone HCl 2 mg	Dilaudid by Knoll		Analgesic; C II
K20	Tab, Blue, Round	Desipramine HCl 10 mg	Desipramine by Kenral	Canadian	Antidepressant
K20	Tab, Blue, Round	Desipramine HCl 10 mg	by AltiMed	Canadian DIN 01948776	Antidepressant

ID FRONT <> BACK	DESCRIPTION FRONT <> BACK	INGREDIENT & STRENGTH	BRAND (or Generic Equiv.) by FIRM	NDC#	CLASS; SCH.
K20	Cap, Clear w/ Two Black Bands	Morphine Sulfate 20 mg	Kadian by Abbott	Canadian DIN 02184435	Analgesic; C II
K200	Tab, White, Round	Dimenhydrinate 50 mg	Dramamine by Rugby	00536-3745	Antiemetic
K200	Tab, White, Round	Oxandrolone 2.5 mg	Oxandrin by Par	49884-0301	Steroid; CIII
K21	Tab, Light Green, Oblong	Loperamide 2 mg	Imodium by Kenral	Canadian	Antidiarrheal
K211	Tab	Morphine Sulfate 30 mg	MS Contin by King	60793-0211	Analgesic; C II
K212	Tab	Morphine Sulfate 15 mg	MS Contin by King	60793-0212	Analgesic; C II
K25	Tab, White, Blue Specks, Oval, Scored	Phentermine HCl 37.5 mg	Adipex by KVK-Tech	10702-0025	Anorexiant; C IV
K250	Tab, White, Circular	Erythromycin 250 mg	by AltiMed	Canadian	Antibiotic
K250	Tab, White	Erythromycin 250 mg	Erythromycin by Kenral	Canadian	Antibiotic
K27	Tab, White, Round	Pseudoephedrine HCl 60 mg	by PDK		Decongestant
K27	Cap, Yellow	Phentermine 30 mg	Adipex by KVK-Tech	10702-0027	Anorexiant; C IV
K28	Tab, Orange, Round	Aspirin 81 mg	Children's Bayer by Rugby	00536-3297	Analgesic
K29	Tab, White, Oval, Scored	Alprazolam 0.25 mg	Xanax by AltiMed	Canadian DIN 00677485	Antianxiety; C IV
K2A <> MYLERAN	Tab, White, Film Coated	Busulfan 2 mg	Myleran by GSK	00173-0713	Antineoplastic
K2A <> MYLERAN	Tab, White, Film Coated	Busulfan 2 mg	Myleran by DSM	63552-0713	Antineoplastic
K2C <> GS	Tab, Pale Pink, Square, Film Coated	Ambrisentan 5 mg	Volibris by GSK	Canadian DIN 02307065	Antihypertensive
K2H <> ORGANON	Tab, Green, Round, "2" set below K & H	Inert	Linessa 28 by Organon	Canadian DIN 02257238	Oral Contraceptive
K3	Tab, Pink, Round	Hydromorphone HCl 3 mg	Dilaudid by Knoll		Analgesic; C II
K3	Tab, White, Round	Medroxyprogesterone Acetate 10 mg	by AltiMed	Canadian DIN 02148579	Hormone
K3	Tab, White, Round, Cross-Scored	Promethazine HCl 25 mg	Phenergan by KVK-Tech	10702-0003	Antiemetic; Antihistamine
K30	Tab, White, Round	Codeine Sulfate 30 mg	by Knoll	00044-0623 Discontinued	Analgesic; C II
K30	Tab, White, Cap Shaped	Acetaminophen 500 mg	Tylenol Ex Strength by Ivax	00182-1832 Discontinued	Analgesic
K300	Tab, White	Ibuprofen 300 mg	Motrin by Kenral	Canadian	NSAID
K300	Tab, White, Circular	Ibuprofen 300 mg	Motrin by AltiMed	Canadian	NSAID
K38	Tab, White, K with Arrow on End	Acetaminophen	Tylenol by PDK		Analgesic
K39	Tab, White, Round, 44-104	Acetaminophen 325 mg	Tylenol by Ivax	00182-1000 Discontinued	Analgesic
K398	Tab, White, Oblong, Scored	Meclizine HCl 12.5 mg	Antivert by Rugby	00536-3985	Antiemetic
K399	Tab, Pink, Round, Scored	Meclizine HCl 25 mg	Antivert by Rugby	00536-3990	Antiemetic
K4	Tab, Blue, K/4	Triazolam 0.25 mg	Halcion by Kenral	Canadian	Sedative/Hypnotic; C IV
K4	Tab, Powder Blue, Elliptical, K/4	Triazolam 0.25 mg	Halcion by AltiMed	Canadian Discontinued	Sedative/Hypnotic; C IV
K4	Tab, Yellow, Round	Hydromorphone HCl 4 mg	Dilaudid by Knoll		Analgesic; C II
K4	Tab, Pink, Round	Promethazine 50 mg	Phenergan by KVK-Tech	10702-0004	Antiemetic; Antihistamine
K40	Tab, Pink, Oblong	Diphenhydramine 25 mg	Benadryl by Amneal	65162-0156	Antihistamine
K400	Tab, Orange	Ibuprofen 400 mg	Motrin by Kenral	Canadian	NSAID
K400	Tab, Orange, Circular	Ibuprofen 400 mg	Motrin by AltiMed	Canadian	NSAID
K400	Tab, White, Round	Glycopyrrolate 1 mg	Robinul by Par	49884-0065	Gastrointestinal
K401	Tab, White, Round	Glycopyrrolate Forte 2 mg	Robinul Forte by Par	49884-0066	Gastrointestinal
K48 <> ASPIRIN	Tab, White Round	Aspirin 325 mg	Aspirin by McKesson	63739-0024	Analgesic
K5	Tab, White, Circular, Scored	Prednisone 5 mg	Prednisone by Kenral	Canadian	Steroid
K5	Tab, White, Circular	Prednisone 5 mg	by AltiMed	Canadian	Steroid
K5	Tab, White, Round, Rapidly Disintegrating	Clonazepam ODT .125 mg	Klonopin by Par	49884-0306	Sedative

ID FRONT <> BACK	DESCRIPTION FRONT <> BACK	INGREDIENT & STRENGTH	BRAND (or Generic Equiv.) by FIRM	NDC#	CLASS; SCH.
K50	Cap, Clear w/ Three Black Bands	Morphine Sulfate 50 mg	Kadian by Abbott	Canadian DIN 02184443	Analgesic; C II
K55	Tab, Peach, Oval, Scored	Alprazolam 0.5 mg	Xanax by AltiMed	Canadian DIN 00677477	Antianxiety; C IV
K56	Tab, White, Round	Acetaminophen 250 mg, Aspirin 250 mg, Caffeine 64 mg	Excedrin Migraine by PHK Labs		Analgesic
K56	Tab, Pink, Round	Oxycodone 10 mg	OxyContin by KVK-Tech	10702-0056	Analgesic; C II
K6	Tab, Orange, Round	Medroxyprogesterone Acetate 2.5 mg	by AltiMed	Canadian DIN 02148552	Hormone
K6	Tab, Blue, Round, Scored	Diphenhydramine HCl 50 mg	Compoz by Rugby	00536-3772	Antihistamine
K6	Cap, Pink	Diphenhydramine HCl 50 mg	Benadryl by URL	00677-1857	Antihistamine
K6	Tab, White, Round, Rapidly Disintegrating	Clonazepam ODT .25 mg	Klonopin by Par	49884-0306	Sedative
K60	Tab, White, Round	Codeine Sulfate 60 mg	by Knoll	00044-0626 Discontinued	Analgesic; C II
K600	Cap, Peach	Ibuprofen 600 mg	Motrin by AltiMed	Canadian	NSAID
K600	Tab, Peach	Ibuprofen 600 mg	Motrin by Kenral	Canadian	NSAID
K634	Cap, Clear & Lavender, K-634	Nitroglycerin TD 2.5 mg	Nitrobid by KV Pharma		Vasodilator
K635	Cap, Blue & Yellow, K-635	Nitroglycerin TD 6.5 mg	Nitrobid by KV Pharma		Vasodilator
K698	Cap, Clear	Nitroglycerin TD 9 mg	Nitrobid by KV Pharma		Vasodilator
K7	Tab, White, Round	Clonazepam ODT .5 mg	Klonopin by Par	49884-0308	Sedative
K713	Cap, Blue & Maroon	Piroxicam 10 mg	Feldene by Kenral	Canadian	NSAID
K713	Cap, Blue & Maroon	Piroxicam 10 mg	Feldene by AltiMed	Canadian DIN 02139952 Discontinued	NSAID
K714	Cap, Maroon & Opaque	Piroxicam 20 mg	Feldene by AltiMed	Canadian DIN 02139960 Discontinued	NSAID
K714	Cap, Maroon & Opaque	Piroxicam 20 mg	Feldene by Kenral	Canadian	NSAID
K715	Cap, Pink & Scarlet	Doxepin HCl 10 mg	by AltiMed	Canadian DIN 02140071 Discontinued	Antidepressant
K716	Cap, Blue & Pink	Doxepin HCl 25 mg	by AltiMed	Canadian DIN 02140098 Discontinued	Antidepressant
K717	Cap, Flesh & Pink	Doxepin HCl 50 mg	by AltiMed	Canadian DIN 02140101 Discontinued	Antidepressant
K718	Cap, Flesh	Doxepin HCl 75 mg	by AltiMed	Canadian DIN 02140128 Discontinued	Antidepressant
K718	Cap, Flesh	Domperidone 75 mg	by AltiMed	Canadian	Gastrointestinal
K750	Cap, Blue	Doxycycline Hyclate 100 mg	by AltiMed	Canadian Discontinued	Antibiotic
K8	Tab, Orange, Round	Potassium Chloride SA 600 mg	Slow K by Alra	51641-0175	Electrolytes
K8	Tab, Light Violet, Elliptical, K/8	Triazolam 0.125 mg	by AltiMed	Canadian Discontinued	Sedative/Hypnotic; C IV
K8	Tab, Violet, K/8	Triazolam 0.125 mg	Triazolam by Kenral	Canadian	Sedative/Hypnotic; C IV
K8	Tab, White, Round	Clonazepam ODT 1 mg	Klonopin by Par	49884-0309	Sedative
K8 <> ALRA	Tab, Film Coated, K+8	Potassium Chloride 600 mg	by Golden State	60429-0158	Electrolytes
K9	Tab, White, Round	Clonazepam ODT 2 mg	Klonopin by Par	49884-0310	Sedative
KADIAN100MG	Cap, Green, Opaque, Ex Release	Morphine Sulfate 100 mg	Kadian by Actavis	00228-2055	Analgesic; C II

ID FRONT <> BACK	DESCRIPTION FRONT <> BACK	INGREDIENT & STRENGTH	BRAND (or Generic Equiv.) by FIRM	NDC#	CLASS; SCH.
KADIAN100MG	Cap, Green, Opaque, Ex Release	Morphine Sulfate 100 mg	Kadian by Actavis	63857-0324	Analgesic; C II
KADIAN20MG	Cap, Yellow, Opaque, Ex Release	Morphine Sulfate 20 mg	Kadian by Actavis	00228-2043	Analgesic; C II
KADIAN20MG	Cap, Yellow, Opaque, Ex Release	Morphine Sulfate 20 mg	Kadian by Faulding	63857-0322	Analgesic; C II
KADIAN30MG	Cap, Blue Violet, Opaque, Ex Release	Morphine Sulfate 30 mg	Kadian by Actavis	63857-0325	Analgesic; C II
KADIAN50MG	Cap, Blue, Opaque, Ex Release	Morphine Sulfate 50 mg	Kadian by Actavis	00228-2045	Analgesic; C II
KADIAN50MG	Cap, Blue, Opaque, Ex Release	Morphine Sulfate 50 mg	Kadian by Actavis	63857-0323	Analgesic; C II
KADIAN60MG	Cap, Pink, Opaque, Ex Release	Morphine Sulfate 60 mg	Kadian by Actavis	63857-0326	Analgesic; C II
KALI <> 083	Tab, Reddish Orange, Round	Acetaminophen 325 mg, Tramadol 37.5 mg	Ultracet by Kali	66893-	Analgesic
KALI <> 083	Tab, Orange, Capsule Shaped, Film Coated	Tramadol HCl 37.5 mg, Acetaminophen 325 mg	Ultracet by Par	49884-0946	Analgesic
KALI <> 280	Tab, Beige, Round	Citalopram HBr 10 mg	Celexa by Perrigo	10768-7060	Antidepressant
KALI <> 281	Tab, Pink, Round	Citalopram HBr 20 mg	Celexa by Perrigo	10768-7191	Antidepressant
KALI <> 282	Tab, White, Round	Citalopram HBr 40 mg	Celexa by Perrigo	10768-7616	Antidepressant
KAO600	Tab, White, Elliptical	Attapulgite 600 mg	Kaopectate by Johnson & Johnson	Canadian DIN 02229953	Antidiarrheal
KAO750	Tab, White, Cap Shaped	Attapulgite 750 mg	Kaopectate by Johnson & Johnson	Canadian DIN 02229949	Antidiarrheal
KBI2	Tab, White, Round	Acetaminophen 750 mg, Hydrocodone Bitartrate 7.5 mg	Vicodin ES by Heartland	61392-0921	Analgesic; C III
KC <> 1	Tab, White, Round, Film Coated	Pitavastatin 1 mg	Livalo by Kowa Pharmaceuticals	00002-4770	Antihyperlipidemic
KC <> 2	Tab, White, Round, Film Coated	Pitavastatin 2 mg	Livalo by Kowa Pharmaceuticals	00002-4771	Antihyperlipidemic
KC <> 4	Tab, White, Round, Film Coated	Pitavastatin 4 mg	Livalo by Kowa Pharmaceuticals	00002-4772	Antihyperlipidemic
KC10	Tab, Yellow, Round, Film Coated	Potassium Chloride 10 mEq	Klor-Con by Upsher Smith	00245-0041	Electrolytes
KC8	Tab, Light Blue, Round, Film Coated	Potassium Chloride 8 mEq	Klor-Con by Upsher Smith	00245-0040	Electrolytes
KCl10BOLARKV	Cap, Clear, KCl 10/Bolar/KV	Potassium Chloride 10 mEq	Micro K 10 by Circa		Electrolytes
KCM10	Tab, White, Oblong, Ex Release	Potassium Chloride 10 mEq	Klor-Con M10 by Upsher Smith	00245-0057	Electrolytes
KCM20	Tab, White, Oblong, Scored, Ex Release	Potassium Chloride 20 mEq	Klor-Con M20 by Upsher Smith	00245-0058	Electrolytes
KDUR10	Tab, Ex Release, K-DUR 10	Potassium Chloride 750 mg	by Amerisource	62584-0404	Electrolytes
KDUR10	Tab, Ex Release, K-DUR 10	Potassium Chloride 750 mg	by Nat Pharmpak	55154-1505	Electrolytes
KDUR10	Tab, ER	Potassium Chloride 750 mg	by Med Pro	53978-2060	Electrolytes
KDUR10	Tab, White, Oblong, K-DUR 10	Potassium Chloride 750 mg	K-Dur 10 ER by Schering	00085-0263	Electrolytes
KDUR20	Tab, White, Cap Shaped, Scored, K-DUR 20	Potassium Chloride 20 mEq	K Dur 20 by Rightpak	65240-0675	Electrolytes
KDUR20	Tab, White, Cap Shaped, Scored, K-DUR 20	Potassium Chloride 20 mEq	by Schering	00085-0787	Electrolytes
KDUR20	Tab, White, Cap Shaped, Scored, K-DUR 20	Potassium Chloride 20 mEq	by Nat Pharmpak	55154-1504	Electrolytes
KDUR20	Tab, White, Cap Shaped, Scored, K-DUR 20	Potassium Chloride 20 mEq	by PDRX	55289-0079	Electrolytes
KDUR20	Tab, White, Cap Shaped, Scored, K-DUR 20	Potassium Chloride 20 mEq	by Amerisource	62584-0787	Electrolytes
KDUR20	Tab, White, Cap Shaped, Scored, K-DUR 20	Potassium Chloride 20 mEq	by Pharmascience	Canadian DIN 56219211100	Electrolytes
KDUR20	Tab, White, Cap Shaped, Scored, K-DUR 20	Potassium Chloride 20 mEq	K-Dur by Schering	Canadian DIN 00713376	Electrolytes
KE10 <> APO	Tab, White, Round, Biconvex	Ketorolac Tromethamine 10 mg	Toradol by Apotex	Canadian DIN 02229080	NSAID
KE3 <> GS	Tab, Deep Pink, Oval, Film Coated	Ambrisentan 10 mg	Volibris by GSK	Canadian DIN 02307073	Antihypertensive
KEENE7788	Cap, Green Print, Keene/7788	Acetaminophen 325 mg, Butalbital 50 mg, Caffeine 40 mg	Fioricet by Keene	00588-7788	Analgesic
KEFLEX250DISTAH69	Cap	Cephalexin 250 mg	Keflex by Eli Lilly	00110-0869	Antibiotic
KEFLEX250DISTAH69	Cap	Cephalexin 250 mg	Keflex by Dista Prod	00777-0869	Antibiotic
KEFLEX250MG	Cap, White and Dark Green, Opaque, Black Ink	Cephalexin 250 mg	Keflex by MiddleBrook	11042-0112	Antibiotic
KEFLEX333MG	Cap, Light Green, Opaque, Black Ink	Cephalexin 333 mg	Keflex by MiddleBrook	11042-0114	Antibiotic
KEFLEX500MG	Cap, Light Green and Dark Green, Opaque, Black Ink	Cephalexin 500 mg	Keflex by MiddleBrook	11042-0113	Antibiotic
KEFLEX750MG	Cap, Dark Green, Opaque, White Ink	Cephalexin 750 mg	Keflex by MiddleBrook	11042-0115	Antibiotic
KEFTAB500	Tab	Cephalexin 500 mg	Keftab by Dista Prod	00777-4143	Antibiotic

ID FRONT <> BACK	DESCRIPTION FRONT <> BACK	INGREDIENT & STRENGTH	BRAND (or Generic Equiv.) by FIRM	NDC#	CLASS; SCH.
KEFTAB500	Tab, Green, Oval	Cephalexin 500 mg	Keftab by Carlsbad	61442-0101	Antibiotic
KEM	Tab, White, Round, Schering Logo KEM	Prednisone 1 mg	Meticorten by Schering		Steroid
KEMADRINS3A	Tab, White, Round, Scored, Kemadrin over S3A	Procyclidine HCl 5 mg	by GSK	Canadian	Antiparkinson
KEMADRINS3A	Tab, White, Round, Scored, Kemadrin over S3A	Procyclidine HCl 5 mg	Kemadrin by DSM	63552-0604	Antiparkinson
KEMADRINS3A	Tab, White, Round, Scored, Kemadrin over S3A	Procyclidine HCl 5 mg	Kemadrin by Monarch	61570-0059	Antiparkinson
KENWOOD <> ADEFLORM	Tab	Ascorbic Acid 100 mg, Calcium 250 mg, Calcium Pantothenate 10 mg, Cyanocobalamin 2 mcg, Fluorides 1 mg, Iron 30 mg, Niacinamide 20 mg, Pyridoxine HCl 10 mg, Riboflavin 2.5 mg, Thiamine Mononitrate 1.5 mg, Vitamin A 6000 Units, Vitamin D 400 Units	Adeflor M by Kenwood	00482-0115	Vitamin
KENWOOD181	Cap, Blue & Yellow	Chlorpheniramine Maleate 8 mg, Pseudoephedrine HCl 120 mg	Deconamine SR by Thrift Drug	59198-0183	Cold Remedy
KENWOOD181	Cap, Blue & Yellow	Chlorpheniramine Maleate 8 mg, Pseudoephedrine HCl 120 mg	Deconamine SR by Nat Pharmpak	55154-6401	Cold Remedy
KENWOOD181	Cap, Blue & Yellow	Chlorpheniramine Maleate 8 mg, Pseudoephedrine HCl 120 mg	Deconamine SR by Kenwood	00482-0181	Cold Remedy
KENWOOD184	Tab, White, Scored	Chlorpheniramine Maleate 4 mg, Pseudoephedrine HCl 60 mg	Deconamine by Kenwood	00482-0184	Cold Remedy
KERLONE10	Tab, White, Round, Scored, Film Coated, Kerlone over 10	Betaxolol HCl 10 mg	Kerlone by Searle	00025-5101	Antihypertensive
KERLONE20 <> B	Tab, White, Round, Film Coated, Kerlone over 20 <> Greek Letter Beta	Betaxolol HCl 20 mg	Kerlone by Searle	00025-5201	Antihypertensive
KERLONE20 <> B	Tab, White, Round, Film Coated, Kerlone over 20 <> Greek Letter Beta	Betaxolol HCl 20 mg	Kerlone by Sanofi	00024-2300	Antihypertensive
KET10	Tab, White, Round	Ketorolac Tromethamine 10 mg	Toradol by Roche	Canadian	NSAID
KET200 <> APO	Tab, White to Off-White, KET over 200	Ketoconazole 200 mg	Nizoral by Apotex	60505-0092	Antifungal
KETOPROFENER-200MGSHN	Cap, ER, KETOPROFEN ER 200 MG	Ketoprofen 200 mg	Orudis by Schein	00364-2667	NSAID
KETOPROFENER-200MGSHN	Cap, ER, KETOPROFEN ER 200 MG	Ketoprofen 200 mg	Orudis by Watson	00591-8847	NSAID
KETOPROFENER-200MGSHN	Cap, Blue & Opaque & White, KETOPROFEN ER 200 MG	Ketoprofen 200 mg	Orudis by Murfreesboro	51129-1596	NSAID
KETOPROFENER-200MGSHN	Cap, ER, KETOPROFEN ER 200 MG	Ketoprofen 200 mg	Orudis by Elan	56125-0102	NSAID
KETOTIFEN <> P	Tab, White, Round, Scored	Ketotifen Fumarate 1 mg	by Pharmascience	Canadian DIN 5760616809	Antiasthmatic
KH2 <> ORGANON	Tab, Green, Film Coated, KH over 2 <> Organon	Inert	Cesia by Prasco	66993-0615	Oral Contraceptive; Placebo
KH2 <> ORGANON	Tab, Green, Round	Inert	Cyclessa by Organon	00052-0283	Oral Contraceptive; Placebo
KH2 <> ORGANON	Tab, Green, Round	Inert	Marvelon 28 by Organon	Canadian DIN 02042479	Oral Contraceptive; Placebo
KH2 <> ORGANON	Tab, KH over 2	Desogestrel 0.15 mg, Ethinyl Estradiol 0.03 mg	Desogen by Organon	60889-0261	Oral Contraceptive
KH2 <> ORGANON	Tab, Green, Film Coated, K H over 2 <> Organon	Inert	Desogen by Organon	00052-0261	Oral Contraceptive; Placebo
KH2 <> ORGANON	Tab, Green, Film Coated, KH over 2 <> Organon	Inert	Mircette by Organon	00052-0281	Oral Contraceptive; Placebo
KH2 <> ORGANON	Tab, Film Coated, K H over 2 <> Organon	Inert	Mircette by NV Organon	12860-0281	Oral Contraceptive; Placebo
KH2 <> PRASCO	Tab, Green, Round, PRASCO <> KH / 2	Inert	Solia by Prasco	66993-0611	Oral Contraceptive; Placebo
KJ <> GEIGY	Tab, White to Off-White, Oval, Scored	Baclofen 10 mg	Lioresal by Geigy	Canadian DIN 00455881	Muscle Relaxant
KL	Tab, K/L	Yohimbine HCl 5.4 mg	Yohimex by JMI Canton	00252-3230	Impotence Agent
KL <> A	Tab, Yellow, Oval, Film Coated, Abbott Logo (a <> KL), Extended-Release	Clarithromycin 500 mg	Biaxin by Promex Med	62301-0037	Antibiotic

ID FRONT <> BACK	DESCRIPTION FRONT <> BACK	INGREDIENT & STRENGTH	BRAND (or Generic Equiv.) by FIRM	NDC#	CLASS; SCH.
KL <> A	Tab, Yellow, Oval, Film Coated, Abbott Logo (a <> KL), Extended-Release	Clarithromycin 500 mg	Prevpac by Tap	00300-3702	Antibiotic
KL <> A	Tab, Yellow, Oval, Film Coated, Abbott Logo (a <> KL), Extended-Release	Clarithromycin 500 mg	Biaxin by Abbott	00074-2586	Antibiotic
KL <> A	Tab, Yellow, Oval, Film Coated, Abbott Logo (a <> KL), Extended-Release	Clarithromycin 500 mg	Biaxin by PDRX	55289-0021	Antibiotic
KL <> A	Tab, Yellow, Oval, Film Coated, Abbott Logo (a <> KL), Extended-Release	Clarithromycin 500 mg	Biaxin by Amerisource	62584-0317	Antibiotic
KL <> A	Tab, Yellow, Oval, Film Coated, Abbott Logo (a <> KL), Extended-Release	Clarithromycin 500 mg	Biaxin by Promex Med	62301-0001	Antibiotic
KL <> A	Tab, Yellow, Oval, Film Coated, Abbott Logo (a <> KL), Extended-Release	Clarithromycin 500 mg	Biaxin by Nat Pharmpak	55154-0109	Antibiotic
KL <> A	Tab, Yellow, Oval, Film Coated, Abbott Logo (a <> KL), Extended-Release	Clarithromycin 500 mg	Biaxin by Med Pro	53978-3038	Antibiotic
KL <> A	Tab, Yellow, Oval, Film Coated, Abbott Logo (a <> KL), Extended-Release	Clarithromycin 500 mg	Biaxin by H J Harkins Co	52959-0230	Antibiotic
KL <> A	Tab, Yellow, Oval, Film Coated, Abbott Logo (a <> KL), Extended-Release	Clarithromycin 500 mg	Biaxin by DRX	55045-1865	Antibiotic
KL <> A	Tab, Yellow, Oval, Film Coated, Abbott Logo (a <> KL), Extended-Release	Clarithromycin 500 mg	Biaxin by Murfreesboro	51129-2586	Antibiotic
KL107	Tab, Ex Release, KL-107	Guaifenesin 600 mg	Robitussin by Kiel	59063-0107	Expectorant
KL107	Tab, Ex Release, KL-107	Guaifenesin 600 mg	Robitussin by WE	59196-0008	Expectorant
KL107	Tab, Ex Release	Guaifenesin 600 mg	Robitussin by Warner Kiel	62291-0102	Expectorant
KL109	Tab, Ex Release, KL-109	Guaifenesin 600 mg, Phenylpropanolamine HCl 75 mg	Entex LA by WE	59196-0001	Cold Remedy
KL109	Tab, Ex Release, KL-109	Guaifenesin 600 mg, Phenylpropanolamine HCl 75 mg	Entex LA by Alphagen	59743-0049	Cold Remedy
KL109	Tab, Ex Release, KL-109	Guaifenesin 600 mg, Phenylpropanolamine HCl 75 mg	Entex LA by Kiel	59063-0109	Cold Remedy
KL110	Tab, Blue & Green, Cap Shaped, Film Coated	Guaifenesin 600 mg	Robitussin by Duramed	51285-0588	Expectorant
KL110	Tab, Light Blue, Cap Shaped	Dextromethorphan HBr 30 mg, Guaifenesin 600 mg	S Pack DM by Duramed	51285-0589	Cold Remedy
KL110	Tab, Light Blue, Cap Shaped, KL-110	Dextromethorphan HBr 30 mg, Guaifenesin 600 mg	Deconsal II by Kiel	51285-0565	Cold Remedy
KL111	Tab, White, Round, Ex Release	Orphenadrine Citrate 100 mg	Norgesic by Schein	00364-2830	Muscle Relaxant
KL111	Tab, White, Round, Ex Release	Orphenadrine Citrate 100 mg	Norgesic by Watson	00591-2830	Muscle Relaxant
KL111	Tab, White, Round, Ex Release	Orphenadrine Citrate 100 mg	Norgesic by Perrigo	00113-	Muscle Relaxant
KL112	Tab, KL-112	Carbinoxamine Maleate 8 mg, Pseudoephedrine HCl 120 mg	Carbodec by Rugby	00536-4453 Discontinued	Cold Remedy
KL119	Tab, Tan to Brown, Cap Shaped, Scored	Carbetapentane Tannate 60 mg, Chlorpheniramine Tannate 5 mg, Phenylephrine Tannate 10 mg	Xiratuss by Hawthorn	63717-0551	Cold Remedy
KL142	Tab, Tan to Brown	Phenylephrine Tannate 25 mg, Chlorpheniramine Tannate 9 mg	R-Tanna by Prasco	66993-0532	Cold Remedy
KLORCON10	Tab, Yellow, Round, Ex Release, KLOR-CON over 10	Potassium Chloride 10 mEq	Klor-Con 10 by Caremark	00339-6011	Electrolytes
KLORCON10	Tab, Yellow, Round, KLOR-CON 10, Ex Release	Potassium Chloride 10 mEq	Klor-Con 10 by Upsher Smith	00245-0041	Electrolytes
KLORCON8	Tab, Blue, Round, Ex Release, KLOR-CON over 8	Potassium Chloride 8 mEq	Klor-Con 8 by Kaiser	00179-1164	Electrolytes
KLORCON8	Tab, Blue, Round, Ex Release, KLOR-CON over 8	Potassium Chloride 8 mEq	Klor-Con 8 by Upsher Smith	00245-0040	Electrolytes
KLOTRIX10MEQ770BL	Tab, Black Print, Ex Release, KLOTRIX 10 MEQ 770 over BL	Potassium Chloride 750 mg	Klotrix by BMS	00087-0770	Electrolytes
KLX140	Cap, Green and White, Opaque	Cephalexin 250 mg	Keflex by Karalex	42043-0140	Antibiotic
KLX141	Cap, Light Green and Dark Green, Opaque	Cephalexin 500 mg	Keflex by Karalex	42043-0141	Antibiotic
KNOLL <> 120SR	Tab, Light Violet, Oval, Film Coated	Verapamil HCl 120 mg	Isoptin SR by Abbott	00044-1827	Antihypertensive
KNOLL <> 120SR	Tab, Light Violet, Oval, Film Coated	Verapamil HCl 120 mg	Isoptin SR by Abbott	Canadian DIN 01907123	Antihypertensive
KNOLL <> ISOPTIN120	Tab, Film Coated	Verapamil HCl 120 mg	Isoptin by Knoll	00044-1823 Discontinued	Antihypertensive

ID FRONT <> BACK	DESCRIPTION FRONT <> BACK	INGREDIENT & STRENGTH	BRAND (or Generic Equiv.) by FIRM	NDC#	CLASS; SCH.
KNOLL <> ISOPTIN80	Tab, Film Coated	Verapamil HCl 80 mg	Isoptin by Knoll	00044-1822 Discontinued	Antihypertensive
KNOLL <> ISOPTIN80	Tab, Film Coated	Verapamil HCl 80 mg	Isoptin by Med Pro	53978-7001 Discontinued	Antihypertensive
KNOLL <> ISOPTIN80	Tab, Film Coated	Verapamil 80 mg	Isoptin by Amerisource	62584-0822 Discontinued	Antihypertensive
KNOLL <> SR180	Tab, Pink, Oval, Scored	Verapamil HCl 180 mg	Isoptin SR by Abbott	Canadian DIN 01934317	Antihypertensive
KNOLL1	Tab, Salmon, Round, Scored	Trandolapril 1 mg	Mavik by Abbott	00048-5805	Antihypertensive
KNOLL2	Tab, Yellow, Round	Trandolapril 2 mg	Mavik by Abbott	00048-5806	Antihypertensive
KNOLL4	Tab, Rose, Round	Trandolapril 4 mg	Mavik by Abbott	00048-5807	Antihypertensive
KOK	Tab, White, Round, KO/K with Arrow	Acetaminophen 325 mg	Tylenol by PDK		Analgesic
KOS <> 021	Tab, Blue, Extended Release	Niacin 500 mg, Simvastatin 20mg	Simcor by Abbott	00074-3312	Antihyperlipidemic
KOS <> 022	Tab, Blue, Extended Release	Niacin 750 mg, Simvastatin 20mg	Simcor by Abbott	00074-3315	Antihyperlipidemic
KOS <> 023	Tab, Blue, Extended Release	Niacin 1000 mg, Simvastatin 20mg	Simcor by Abbott	00074-3316	Antihyperlipidemic
KOS <> 1000	Tab, Orange, Cap Shaped, Film Coated, Extended Release	Niacin 1000 mg	Niaspan by KOS	60958-0142	Antihyperlipidemic
KOS <> 1000	Tab, White, Cap Shaped	Niacin 1000 mg	Niaspan by KOS	60598-0003	Antihyperlipidemic
KOS <> 1002	Tab, Dark Pink and Light Purple, Cap Shaped	Lovastatin 20 mg, Niacin 1000 mg	Advicor by KOS	60598-0008	Antihyperlipidemic
KOS <> 1002	Tab, White, Cap Shaped, Extended Release	Niacin 500 mg	Niaspan by Allscripts	54569-5267	Antihyperlipidemic
KOS <> 500	Tab, White, Cap Shaped, Extended Release	Niacin 500 mg	Niaspan by KOS	60598-0001	Antihyperlipidemic
KOS <> 500	Tab, Orange, Cap Shaped, Film Coated, Extended Release	Niacin 500 mg	Niaspan by KOS	60958-0140	Antihyperlipidemic
KOS <> 502	Tab, Light Yellow, Cap Shaped	Lovastatin 20 mg, Niacin 500 mg	Advicor by KOS	60598-0006	Antihyperlipidemic
KOS <> 750	Tab, White, Cap Shaped, Extended Release	Niacin 750 mg	Niaspan by KOS	60598-0002	Antihyperlipidemic
KOS <> 750	Tab, Orange, Cap Shaped, Film Coated, Extended Release	Niacin 750 mg	Niaspan by KOS	60958-0141	Antihyperlipidemic
KOS <> 752	Tab, Light Orange, Cap Shaped	Lovastatin 20 mg, Niacin 750 mg	Advicor by KOS	60598-0007	Antihyperlipidemic
KP <> 101	Tab, Yellowish Orange, Round, Scored	Sulfasalazine 500 mg	Azulfidine by Pharmacia		Gastrointestinal
KP1026	Cap	Codeine Phosphate 20 mg, Pseudoephedrine HCl 60 mg	Kg Fed by King	60793-0026	Cold Remedy; C III
KP112	Tab	Acetaminophen 750 mg, Hydrocodone Bitartrate 7.5 mg	Vicodin ES by Mallinckrodt	00406-0360 Discontinued	Analgesic; C III
KPH <> 101	Tab, Gold, Round, Scored	Sulfasalazine 500 mg	Azulfidine by Amerisource	62584-0005	Gastrointestinal
KPH <> 101	Tab, Gold, Round, Scored	Sulfasalazine 500 mg	Azulfidine by Pharmacia	00013-0101	Gastrointestinal
KPH <> 101	Tab, Gold, Round, Scored	Sulfasalazine 500 mg	Azulfidine by Pharmacia	Canadian DIN 02064480	Gastrointestinal
KPH <> 101	Tab, Gold, Round, Scored	Sulfasalazine 500 mg	Azulfidine by Pharmacia	59632-0101	Gastrointestinal
KPH <> 101	Tab, Gold, Round, Scored	Sulfasalazine 500 mg	Azulfidine by Thrift Drug	59198-0010	Gastrointestinal
KPH <> 102	Tab, Gold, Oval, Film Coated	Sulfasalazine 500 mg	Azulfidine EN Tabs by Pharmacia	Canadian DIN 02064472	Gastrointestinal
KPH <> 102	Tab, Gold, Oval, Film Coated	Sulfasalazine 500 mg	Azulfidine EN Tabs by Pharmacia	00013-0102	Gastrointestinal
KPH <> 102	Tab, Gold, Oval, Film Coated	Sulfasalazine 500 mg	Azulfidine EN Tabs by Pharmacia	59632-0102	Gastrointestinal
KPH <> 102	Tab, Gold, Oval, Film Coated	Sulfasalazine 500 mg	Azulfidine EN Tabs by Thrift Drug	59198-0230	Gastrointestinal
KPH <> 102	Tab, Gold, Oval, Film Coated	Sulfasalazine 500 mg	Azulfidine EN Tabs by Nat Pharmpak	55154-2801	Gastrointestinal
KPH <> 102	Tab, Gold, Oval, Film Coated	Sulfasalazine 500 mg	Azulfidine EN Tabs by Wal Mart	49035-0167	Gastrointestinal
KPH <> 102	Tab, Gold, Oval, Film Coated	Sulfasalazine 500 mg	Azulfidine EN Tabs by Rx Pak	65084-0171	Gastrointestinal
KPI <> 115	Tab, Round, Light Gray	Liothyronine Sodium 5 mcg	Cytomel by King	52604-3414	Thyroid Hormone
KPI <> 13	Tab, Light Green, Oval, Ex Release	Guaifenesin 600 mg	Robitussin by Monarch	61570-0026	Expectorant
KPI1	Tab, White, Round, KPI 1	Acetaminophen 500 mg, Hydrocodone Bitartrate 5 mg	Vicodin by King	60793-0844	Analgesic; C III
KPI1	Tab, White, Round, KPI 1	Acetaminophen 500 mg, Hydrocodone Bitartrate 5 mg	Vicodin by Endo	60951-0639	Analgesic; C III
KPI115	Tab, White to Off-White, Round	Liothyronine Sodium 5 mcg	Cytomel by King	60793-0115	Thyroid Hormone
KPI116	Tab, White to Off-White, Round, Scored	Liothyronine Sodium 25 mcg	Cytomel by King	60793-0116	Thyroid Hormone
KPI117	Tab, White to Off-White, Round, Scored	Liothyronine Sodium 50 mcg	Cytomel by King	60793-0117	Thyroid Hormone

ID FRONT <> BACK	DESCRIPTION FRONT <> BACK	INGREDIENT & STRENGTH	BRAND (or Generic Equiv.) by FIRM	NDC#	CLASS; SCH.
KPI13	Tab, Light Green	Guaifenesin 600 mg	Robitussin by King	60793-0850	Expectorant
KPI13	Tab, Ex Release	Guaifenesin 600 mg	Robitussin by King	60793-0049	Expectorant
KPI14	Tab, Ex Release, Embossed	Dextromethorphan HBr 30 mg, Guaifenesin 600 mg	Monafed DM by King	60793-0851	Cold Remedy
KPI14	Tab, Ex Release, Embossed	Dextromethorphan HBr 30 mg, Guaifenesin 600 mg	by King	60793-0050	Cold Remedy
KPI14	Tab, Green, Oval, Ex Release	Dextromethorphan HBr 30 mg, Guaifenesin 600 mg	Monafed DM by Monarch	61570-0027	Cold Remedy
KPI2	Tab, White, Round, Scored	Acetaminophen 750 mg, Hydrocodone Bitartrate 7.5 mg	Vicodin ES by Sandoz	00781-1532	Analgesic; C III
KPI2	Tab, White, Round	Acetaminophen 750 mg, Hydrocodone Bitartrate 7.5 mg	Vicodin ES by Endo	60951-0641	Analgesic; C III
KPI2	Tab	Acetaminophen 750 mg, Hydrocodone Bitartrate 7.5 mg	Vicodin ES by King	60793-0846	Analgesic; C III
KPI2	Tab, Light Blue, Round	Acetaminophen 750 mg, Hydrocodone Bitartrate 7.5 mg	Vicodin ES by King		Analgesic; C III
KPI33	Cap	Phentermine HCl 30 mg		60793-0009	Anorexiant; C IV
KPI4	Tab, White, Oblong	Acetaminophen 650 mg, Hydrocodone Bitartrate 7.5 mg	Lorcet Plus by Mallinckrodt	00406-0359 Discontinued	Analgesic; C III
KPI4	Tab, White, Oblong	Acetaminophen 650 mg, Hydrocodone Bitartrate 7.5 mg	Lorcet Plus by Heartland	61392-0922	Analgesic; C III
KPI4	Tab, White, Oblong	Acetaminophen 650 mg, Hydrocodone Bitartrate 7.5 mg	Lorcet Plus by Sandoz	00781-1523	Analgesic; C III
KPI4	Tab, White, Oblong	Acetaminophen 650 mg, Hydrocodone Bitartrate 7.5 mg	Lorcet Plus by King	60793-0845	Analgesic; C III
KPI4	Tab, White, Oblong	Acetaminophen 650 mg, Hydrocodone Bitartrate 7.5 mg	Lorcet Plus by Endo	60951-0640	Analgesic; C III
KR100 <> GEIGY	Tab, Brownish-Orange, Round, Film Coated	Metoprolol Tartrate 100 mg	Lopressor by Novartis	Canadian DIN 00658855	Antihypertensive
KREMERSURBAN055	Cap, Clear	Pseudoephedrine HCl 120 mg, Chlorpheniramine 8 mg	Fedahist Timecaps by Schwarz		Cold Remedy
KREMERSURBAN320	Cap, Clear & Violet, Kremers-Urban 320	Nitroglycerin SR 2.5 mg	Nitrocine Timecaps by Schwarz		Vasodilator
KREMERSURBAN330	Cap, Blue & Orange, Kremers-Urban 330	Nitroglycerin SR 6.5 mg	Nitrocine Timecaps by Schwarz		Vasodilator
KREMERSURBAN340	Cap, Clear, Kremers-Urban 340	Nitroglycerin SR 9 mg	Nitrocine Timecaps by Schwarz		Vasodilator
KREMERSURBAN475	Cap, Green & White	Enzyme Combination	Kutrase by Schwarz		Gastrointestinal
KREMERSURBAN505	Cap, Orange & White, Red Print, Kremers over Urban	Lactase 250 mg	Lactaid by Rivex Pharma	Canadian	Gastrointestinal
KREMERSURBAN505	Cap, Orange & White, Red Print, Kremers over Urban	Lactase Enzyme 250 mg	Lactrase by Schwarz	00091-3505	Gastrointestinal
KREMERSURBAN522	Cap, White & Yellow	Amylase 30 mg, Cellulase 2 mg, Protease 6 mg, Lipase 75 mg	Ku-Zyme by Schwarz		Gastrointestinal
KREMERSURBAN525	Cap, White	Amylase 30,000 Units, Lipase 8000 Units, Protease 30,000 Units	Ku-Zyme HP by Schwarz		Gastrointestinal
KREMERSURBAN537	Cap, Brown & Clear	Hyoscyamine Sulfate 0.375 mg	Levsin by Schwarz		Gastrointestinal
KREMERSURBAN539	Cap, Clear & Pink, Kremers-Urban 539	Hyoscyamine Sulfate 0.375 mg, Phenobarbital 45 mg	Levsinex Pb Timecaps by Schwarz		Gastrointestinal; C IV
KREMERSURBANE537	Cap, ER	Hyoscyamine Sulfate 0.375 mg	Levsin by Drug Distr	52985-0228	Gastrointestinal
KS2 <> ORGANON	Tab, Yellow, Film Coated, Organon <> K S over 2	Ethinyl Estradiol 0.01 mg	Mircette by Organon	00052-0281	Oral Contraceptive
KS2 <> ORGANON	Tab, Film Coated, K S over 2 <> Organon	Ethinyl Estradiol 0.01 mg	Mircette by NV Organon	12860-0281	Oral Contraceptive
KTAB <> A	Tab, Yellow, Oval, Film Coated, Ex Release, K-TAB <> Abbott Logo (a)	Potassium Chloride 750 mg	K-Tab by Nat Pharmpak	55154-0106	Electrolytes
KTAB <> A	Tab, Yellow, Oval, Film Coated, Ex Release, K-TAB <> Abbott Logo (a)	Potassium Chloride 750 mg	K-Tab by Promex Med	62301-0036	Electrolytes
KTAB <> A	Tab, Yellow, Oval, Film Coated, Ex Release, K-TAB <> Abbott Logo (a)	Potassium Chloride 750 mg	K-Tab by Abbott	00074-7804	Electrolytes
KTAB <> EI	Tab, Film Coated, K-Tab	Potassium Chloride 750 mg	by Heartland	61392-0900	Electrolytes
KU <> 101	Tab, White, Round, Scored	Hyoscyamine Sulfate 0.125 mg	Levsin by Murfreesboro	51129-1501	Gastrointestinal
KU <> 101	Tab, White, Round, Scored	Hyoscyamine Sulfate 0.125 mg	Levsin by Kremers Urban	62175-0101	Gastrointestinal
KU <> 102	Tab, White, Round, Scored, Sublingual	Hyoscyamine Sulfate 0.125 mg	Levsin by Kremers Urban	62175-0102	Gastrointestinal
KU <> 102	Tab, White, Round, Scored, Sublingual	Hyoscyamine Sulfate 0.125 mg	Levsin by Murfreesboro	51129-1503	Gastrointestinal
KU050	Tab, White, Oval	Pseudoephedrine HCl 60 mg, Chlorpheniramine Maleate 4 mg	Fedahist by Schwarz		Cold Remedy
KU1	Tab, Yellow, Oval	Ergocalciferol 1.25 mg	Calciferol by Schwarz		Vitamin
KU103	Cap, Brown & Clear	Hyoscyamine Sulfate 0.375 mg	Levsin by Murfreesboro	51129-1505	Gastrointestinal
KU103	Cap, Brown & White, Ex Release	Hyoscyamine Sulfate 0.375 mg	Levsin by Kremers Urban	62175-0103	Gastrointestinal
KU106 <> 10	Tab, White, Round, Scored	Isosorbide Mononitrate 10 mg	Ismo by Kremers Urban	62175-0106	Antianginal

ID FRONT <> BACK	DESCRIPTION FRONT <> BACK	INGREDIENT & STRENGTH	BRAND (or Generic Equiv.) by FIRM	NDC#	CLASS; SCH.
KU107 <> 20	Tab, White, Round, Scored	Isosorbide Mononitrate 20 mg	Ismo by Physician Total Care	54868-3822	Antianginal
KU107 <> 20	Tab, White, Round, Scored	Isosorbide Mononitrate 20 mg	Ismo by Kremers Urban	62175-0107	Antianginal
KU108	Tab, Light Orange, Cap Shaped, Scored, Ex Release	Hyoscyamine Sulfate 0.375 mg	Levsin by Kremers Urban	62175-0108	Gastrointestinal
KU108	Tab, Light Orange, Cap Shaped, Scored, Ex Release	Hyoscyamine Sulfate 0.375 mg	Levsin by Murfreesboro	51129-1502	Gastrointestinal
KU114	Cap, White, Opaque, Black Ink, Delayed Release	Omeprazole 10 mg	Prilosec by Kremers Urban	62175-0114	Gastrointestinal
KU118	Cap, White & Gold, Opaque, Delayed Release	Omeprazole 20 mg	Prilosec by Kremers Urban	62175-0118	Gastrointestinal
KU119	Tab, White, Cap Shaped, Scored, Ex Release	Isosorbide Mononitrate 60 mg	Imdur by Kremers Urban	62175-0119	Antianginal
KU120	Cap	Pseudoephedrine 120 mg, Chlorpheniramine 8 mg	GG-Cen by Kremers Urban		Cold Remedy
KU128	Tab, White, Cap Shaped, Scored, Ex Release	Isosorbide Mononitrate 30 mg	Imdur by Kremers Urban	62175-0128	Antianginal
KU129	Tab, White, Cap Shaped, Scored, Ex Release	Isosorbide Mononitrate 120 mg	Imdur by Kremers Urban	62175-0129	Antianginal
KU171	Tab, White, Oval	Aspirin 325 mg, Acetaminophen 325 mg	Gemnisyn by Schwarz		Analgesic
KU202	Tab, Gray, Round	Belladona Extract 15 mg, Phenobarbital 15 mg	Chardonna-2 by Schwarz		Gastrointestinal; C IV
KU261	Tab, Pink, Round	Nifedipine 60 mg	Gen-Nifedipine Extended Release by Genpharm	Canadian DIN 02321149	Antihypertensive, Antianginal
KU531	Tab, White, Round, K-U 531	Hyoscyamine Sulfate 0.125 mg	Levsin by Schwarz		Gastrointestinal
KU531	Tab, White, K-U/531	Hyoscyamine Sulfate 0.125 mg	Levsin by Rivex Pharma	Canadian	Gastrointestinal
KU534	Tab, Pink, Round, K-U 534	Hyoscyamine Sulfate 0.125 mg, Phenobarbital 15 mg	Levsin Pb by Schwarz		Gastrointestinal; C IV
L	Tab, Orange, Round	Iodinated Glycerol 30 mg	Organidin by LuChem		Expectorant
L	Tab, Off-White, Hexagonal	Hydrochlorothiazide 25 mg, Propranolol HCl 40 mg	Inderide by Wyeth	Canadian	Diuretic; Antihypertensive
L	Tab, Off-White, Hexagonal	Hydrochlorothiazide 25 mg, Propranolol HCl 80 mg	Inderide by Wyeth	Canadian	Diuretic; Antihypertensive
L	Tab, Yellow, Round, Scored, Enteric Coated	Aspirin 81 mg	Aspirin by Major	00904-7704	Analgesic
L	Tab, White, Round, Flat on one side, Convex on the other, Buccal	Miconazole 50 mg	Oravig by Strativa	49884-0082	Antifungal
L <> 5	Tab, White, Oval, Film-Coated	Simvastatin 5 mg	Zocor by Perrigo	45802-0924	Antihyperlipidemic
L <> F	Tab, Pink, Round, Film Coated	Milnacipran HCl 12.5 mg	Savella by Forest	00456-1512	Antidepressant; Antifibromyalgia
L <> GXEG3	Tab, Brown, Round, Film Coated, Needs to be Refrigerated	Chlorambucil 2 mg	Leukeran by GSK	Canadian DIN 00004626	Antineoplastic
L <> GXEG3	Tab, Brown, Round, Film Coated, Needs to be Refrigerated	Chlorambucil 2 mg	Leukeran by GSK	00173-0635	Antineoplastic
L <> l	Tab, White, Round	Lorazepam 0.5 mg	Ativan by Teva	00093-4820	Antianxiety; C IV
L <> RG	Tab, White to Off-White, Round, Film-Coated	Bicalutamide 50 mg	Casodex by Cobalt	Canadian DIN 02274337	Antiandrogen
L005	Tab, Pink, Oval, Coated, Delayed Release	Divalproex Sodium 125 mg	Depakote by Lupin	68180-0265	Anticonvulsant
L006	Tab, Pink, Oval, Coated, Delayed Release	Divalproex Sodium 250 mg	Depakote by Lupin	68180-0266	Anticonvulsant
L007	Tab, Lavender, Oval, Enteric Coated, Delayed Release	Divalproex Sodium 500 mg	Depakote ER by Lupin	68180-0267	Anticonvulsant
L010	Tab, White, Cap Shaped	Acetaminophen 500 mg	Tylenol by Perrigo	00113-0010	Analgesic
L010	Tab, White, Round, Scored	Acetaminophen 325 mg	Tylenol by Leiner		Analgesic
L011	Tab, White, Cap Shaped, Scored	Ibuprofen 100 mg	Motrin by Perrigo	00113-0011	NSAID
L012	Tab, White, Round	Aspirin 325 mg	Aspirin by Leiner		Analgesic
L014	Tab, White, Oblong	Acetaminophen 500 mg	Tylenol Ex Strength by Leiner		Analgesic
L015	Tab, Yellow, Cap Shaped	Pseudoephedrine HCl 30 mg, Guaifenesin 200 mg, Dextromethorphan HBr 15 mg, Acetaminophen 325 mg	Severe Cold by Perrigo	00113-0015	Cold Remedy
L016	Tab, White, Round	Acetaminophen 500 mg	Tylenol Ex Strength by Leiner		Analgesic
L017	Tab, White & Green, Gel Tab, L017 inside Perrigo Symbol	Acetaminophen 500 mg, Pseudoephedrine 30 mg	Sudafed Sinus by Perrigo	00113-0017	Cold Remedy
L021	Tab, Brown, Round	Sennosides 8.6 mg	Senna Laxative by Time Caps	00113-0021	Gastrointestinal
L021	Tab, Brown, Round	Sennosides 8.6 mg	Senna Laxative by Perrigo	51660-0021	Gastrointestinal
L021	Tab, Yellow, Round	Chlorpheniramine Maleate 4 mg	by Leiner		Antihistamine
L022	Tab, White, Oval	Cimetidine HCl 200 mg	Tagamet by Perrigo	00113-0022	Gastrointestinal

ID FRONT <> BACK	DESCRIPTION FRONT <> BACK	INGREDIENT & STRENGTH	BRAND (or Generic Equiv.) by FIRM	NDC#	CLASS; SCH.
L022	Tab, White, Round	Cimetidine HCl 200 mg	Tagamet by Major	00904-5336	Gastrointestinal
L024	Cap, Aqua, Soft Gel	Diphenhydramine HCl 50 mg	Sleep Aid by RP Scherer	00113-0024	Antihistamine
L030	Tab, Light Green, Cap Shaped	Acetaminophen 500 mg, Diphenhydramine HCl 12.5 mg, Pseudoephedrine HCl 30 mg	Allergy, Sinus, Headache by Perrigo	00113-0030	Cold Remedy
L030	Tab, Yellow, Oblong	Phenylpropanolamine 75 mg	by Leiner		Decongestant; Appetite Suppressant
L036	Cap, Light Blue	Diphenhydramine HCl 25 mg	Ex Stre Non A PM by Leiner		Antihistamine
L039	Tab, Yellow, Round	Meclizine HCl 25 mg	Antivert by Perrigo		Antiemetic
L040	Tab, Blue, Round	Diphenhydramine HCl 25 mg	Diphenhydramine by Leiner		Antihistamine
L052	Tab, White, Football Shaped, Black Specks	Calcium Polycarbophil 625 mg	by Leiner		Vitamin; Mineral
L054	Tab, White, Cap Shaped	Pseudoephedrine HCl 120 mg	Sudafed 12 Hr by Perrigo	00113-0054	Cold Remedy
L054	Cap, White	Pseudoephedrine HCl 120 mg	Sudafed 12 Hr by Perrigo	00113-0286	Cold Remedy
L077	Tab, Orange, Cap Shaped	Acetaminophen 500 mg, Pseudoephedrine 30 mg	Sudafed Sinus by Perrigo	00113-0077	Cold Remedy
L079	Cap, Orange & Beige, Gel Caps	Acetaminophen 325 mg, Dextromethorphan HBr 15 mg, Pseudoephedrine HCl 30 mg	Tylenol Cold by Perrigo	00113-0079	Cold Remedy
L091	Tab, Mottled Pink, Round, Chewable, Bubblegum Flavor	Acetaminophen 80 mg	Children's Tylenol by Perrigo	00113-0091	Analgesic
L093 <> 10	Tab, Peach, Oval, Film-Coated	Simvastatin 10 mg	Zocor by Perrigo	45802-0093	Antihyperlipidemic
L094	Tab, Yellow & Red, Round	Acetaminophen 500 mg	Tylenol Ex Strength by Leiner		Analgesic
L1	Tab, Green, Round	Ferrous Sulfate 65 mg	by Perrigo		Mineral
L1	Tab, White, Round	Famotidine 20 mg	Pepcid by Dr. Reddy's	55111-0396	Gastrointestinal
L1 <> BL	Tab	Mitotane 500 mg	Lysodren by Anabolic	00722-5240	Antineoplastic
L10	Tab, Pink, Round, Scored, L/10 <> Cobalt logo	Lisinopril 10 mg	Zestril by Cobalt	Canadian DIN 02271451	Antihypertensive
L10 <> APO	Tab, Reddish Brown, Oval	Lisinopril 10 mg	Zestril by Apotex	60505-0186	Antihypertensive
L10 <> G	Tab, White, Round, G <> L over 10	Loratadine 10 mg	Claritin by Leiner	12333-0911	Antihistamine
L10 <> M	Tab, Gray, Oblong, Scored, M <> L over 10	Levothyroxine Sodium 125 mcg	Unithroid by Mylan	00378-1813	Thyroid Hormone
L10 <> M	Tab, Gray, Oblong, Scored, M <> L over 10	Levothyroxine Sodium 125 mcg	Unithroid by UDL	51079-0443	Thyroid Hormone
L10 <> P	Tab, Green, Round, Scored	Loxapine Succinate 10 mg	Loxapac by Pharmascience	Canadian DIN 02230838	Antipsychotic
L101	Cap, Green & White	Pseudoephedrine 30 mg, Acetaminophen 500 mg	Non-Aspirin Sinus by Perrigo		Cold Remedy
L105	Tab, White to Off White, Round, Scored	Meprobamate 400 mg	Equanil by Heritage	23155-0129	Sedative/Hypnotic; C IV
L11 <> M	Tab, Blue, Oblong, Scored, M <> L over 11	Levothyroxine Sodium 150 mcg	Unithroid by UDL	51079-0445	Thyroid Hormone
L11 <> M	Tab, Blue, Oblong, Scored, M <> L over 11	Levothyroxine Sodium 150 mcg	Unithroid by Mylan	00378-1815	Thyroid Hormone
L110	Tab, Red	Yohimbine HCl 5.4 mg	by Ivax	00182-1625	Impotence Agent
L113	Tab, White, Oblong	Lactase Enzyme 60 mg	Lactrase by Major	00904-5224	Gastrointestinal
L113	Tab, White, Oblong	Lactase Enzyme 60 mg	by Perrigo	00113-0113	Gastrointestinal
L114	Tab, Bright Yellow, Round	Caffeine 200 mg	Stay Awake by Leiner	Discontinued	Stimulant
L12	Tab, White, Oblong, Scored	Guaifenesin 1200 mg	Robitussin by Capellon	64543-0121	Expectorant
L12	Tab, White, Oblong, Scored	Guaifenesin 1200 mg	Robitussin by Sovereign	58716-0683	Expectorant
L12	Tab, White, Oblong, Scored	Guaifenesin 1200 mg	Robitussin by Eckerd	19458-0913	Expectorant
L12 <> LL	Tab, Pink	Levothyroxine Sodium 0.2 mg	by ESI Lederle	59911-3451	Thyroid Hormone
L12 <> M	Tab, Purple, Oblong, Scored, M <> L over 12	Levothyroxine Sodium 175 mcg	Unithroid by Mylan	00378-1817	Thyroid Hormone
L121	Tab, White to Off-White, Round	Naproxen 250 mg	Naprosyn by Perrigo	10768-7121	NSAID
L124 <> 200	Tab, White, Oval	Cimetidine HCl 200 mg	Tagamet by Perrigo	00113-0124	Gastrointestinal
L125	Tab, White to Off White, Round, Scored	Meprobamate 200 mg	Equanil by Heritage	23155-0128	Sedative/Hypnotic; C IV
L126	Tab, White, Cap Shaped	Pseudoephedrine HCl 30 mg, Dextromethorphan HBr 15 mg, Acetaminophen 325 mg	Non Aspirin Cold Caps by Perrigo	00113-0126	Cold Remedy
L128	Cap, Blue & White	Calcium Carbonate 311 mg, Magnesium Carbonate 232 mg	by Perrigo	00113-0128	Vitamin; Mineral
L13 <> M	Tab, Pink, Oblong, Scored, M <> L over 13	Levothyroxine Sodium 200 mcg	Unithroid by Mylan	00378-1819	Thyroid Hormone

For updated data, go to www.IdentADrug.com

ID FRONT <> BACK	DESCRIPTION FRONT <> BACK	INGREDIENT & STRENGTH	BRAND (or Generic Equiv.) by FIRM	NDC#	CLASS; SCH.
L137	Tab, Pink, Round, Chewable	Acetaminophen 160 mg	Children's Tylenol by Perrigo	00113-0137	Analgesic
L14 <> M	Tab, Green, Oblong, Scored, M <> L over 14	Levothyroxine Sodium 300 mcg	Unithroid by Mylan	00378-1821	Thyroid Hormone
L143	Tab, Pink, Round, Chewable, Fruit Splash Flavor	Acetaminophen 80 mg	Children's Tylenol by Perrigo	00113-0143	Analgesic
L148	Tab, Pink, Round, Chewable, Cherry Flavor	Acetaminophen 80 mg, Chlorpheniramine Maleate 0.5 mg, Dextromethorphan HBr 2.5 mg, Pseudoephedrine HCl 7.5 mg	Children's Tylenol Cold Plus Cough by Perrigo	00113-0148	Cold Remedy
L15 <> M	Tab, Blue, Capsule Shaped	Levothyroxine Sodium 137 mcg	Synthroid by Mylan	00378-1823	Thyroid Hormone
L156	Tab, Pink, Hexagonal	Ranitidine 75 mg	Zantac by Perrigo	00113-2156	Gastrointestinal
L156	Tab, Pink, Hexagonal	Ranitidine 75 mg	Zantac by Perrigo	00113-0156	Gastrointestinal
L159	Tab, White & Aqua, Cap Shaped, Gel Cap	Calcium Carbonate 311 mg, Magnesium Carbonate 232 mg	by Perrigo	00113-0159	Vitamin; Mineral
L164	Tab, Brown, Cap Shaped	Ibuprofen 200 mg	Advil by Perrigo	00113-0164	NSAID
L167	Tab, White, Oval	Ibuprofen 600 mg	Motrin by Perrigo	10768-7167	NSAID
L17 <> M	Tab, White to Off-White, Round	Loratadine 10 mg	Claritin by UDL	51079-0538	Antihistamine
L171	Cap, White, Blue Band	Acetaminophen 500 mg, Diphenhydramine HCl 25 mg	Tylenol PM by Perrigo	00113-0171	Cold Remedy
L172	Tab, Pink, Round	Acetaminophen 160 mg	Children's Tylenol by Perrigo	00113-0172	Analgesic
L173	Cap, Green & Yellow	Chlorpheniramine Maleate 2 mg, Pseudoephedrine HCl 30 mg, Acetaminophen 500 mg	by Perrigo	00113-0173	Cold Remedy
L179	Tab, Yellow, Red, Orange or Green, Round	Calcium Carbonate 750 mg	Tums Ex Strength by Perrigo	00113-0179	Vitamin; Mineral
L179	Tab, Yellow, Red, Orange or Green, Round	Calcium Carbonate 750 mg	Tums Ex Strength by Major	00904-7695	Vitamin; Mineral
L185	Tab, Blue & White, Cap Shaped, Gel Cap	Acetaminophen 500 mg, Diphenhydramine HCl 25 mg	Tylenol PM by Perrigo	00113-0185	Cold Remedy
L187	Tab, Red & Yellow, Round, Gel Cap, L sometimes in Perrigo symbol	Acetaminophen 500 mg	Tylenol Ex Strength by Perrigo	00113-0187	Analgesic
L193	Cap, Green, Soft Gel	Pseudoephedrine HCl 30 mg, Doxylamine Succinate 6.25 mg, Acetaminophen 250 mg, Dextromethorphan HBr 10 mg	Nite Time Liquid Capsules by Perrigo	00113-0193	Cold Remedy
L194	Tab, White, Round	Famotidine 20 mg	Pepcid by Major Pharmaceuticals	00904-5553	Gastrointestinal
L198	Tab, Green & Yellow, Cap Shaped, Gel Cap	Acetaminophen 500 mg, Chlorpheniramine Maleate 2 mg, Pseudoephedrine HCl 30 mg	Tylenol Allergy/Sinus Ex Strength by Perrigo	00113-0198	Cold Remedy
L2	Tab, Green, Cap Shaped, Easy Open	Loperamide 2 mg	Imodium by Perrigo	00113-0960	Antidiarrheal
L2	Tab, Green, Cap Shaped	Loperamide 2 mg	Imodium by Perrigo	00113-1554	Antidiarrheal
L2	Tab, Green, Oblong, L-2	Loperamide 2 mg	Imodium by Major	00904-7725	Antidiarrheal
L2	Tab, Green, Cap Shaped	Loperamide 2 mg	Imodium by Perrigo	00113-0224	Antidiarrheal
L2	Tab, Green, Oblong, L-2	Loperamide 2 mg	Imodium by Novopharm		Antidiarrheal
L20	Tab, Pink, Round, Scored, L / 20 <> Cobalt logo	Lisinopril 20 mg	Zestril by Cobalt	Canadian DIN 02271478	Antihypertensive
L20 <> APO	Tab, Reddish Brown, Oval	Lisinopril 20 mg	Zestril by Apotex	60505-0187	Antihypertensive
L203	Tab, Red, Cap Shaped	Phenylpropanolamine HCl 75 mg	by Perrigo	00113-0203	Decongestant
L211	Tab, Green, Cap Shaped	Acetaminophen 325 mg, Guaifenesin 200 mg, Pseudoephedrine HCl 30 mg	Tylenol Sinus by Perrigo	00113-0211	Cold Remedy
L216	Tab, Purple, Round	Acetaminophen 80 mg, Chlorpheniramine Maleate 0.5 mg, Pseudoephedrine HCl 7.5 mg	Children's Tylenol Cold by Perrigo	00113-0216	Cold Remedy
L22 <> M	Tab, Light Blue, Round, L over 22	Lisinopril 2.5 mg	Prinivil by Mylan	00378-2072	Antihypertensive
L223	Tab, Dark Yellow, Oval	Acetaminophen 500 mg, Chlorpheniramine Maleate 2 mg, Phenylephrine 5 mg	Maximum Pain Relief Allergy Sinus by Perrigo	00113-0223	Cold Remedy
L226	Cap, Red, Soft Gel	Pseudoephedrine 30 mg, Dextromethorphan 10 mg, Guaifenesin 200 mg	by Perrigo	00113-0226	Cold Remedy
L227	Tab, Red, Round	Acetaminophen 500 mg	Tylenol by Perrigo		Analgesic
L228	Cap, Green & White	Acetaminophen 500 mg, Pseudoephedrine 30 mg	Sudafed Sinus by Perrigo	00113-0228	Cold Remedy
L23 <> M	Tab, Peach, Round	Lisinopril 5 mg	Prinivil by Mylan	00378-2073	Antihypertensive
L235	Tab, White, Round	Dihydroxyaluminum Sodium Carbonate 300 mg	Rolaids by Perrigo	00113-0235	Gastrointestinal
L24 <> M	Tab, White, Round, L over 24	Lisinopril 10 mg	Zestril by UDL	51079-0982 Discontinued	Antihypertensive
L24 <> M	Tab, White, Round, L over 24	Lisinopril 10 mg	Zestril by Mylan	00378-2074 Discontinued	Antihypertensive

ID FRONT <> BACK	DESCRIPTION FRONT <> BACK	INGREDIENT & STRENGTH	BRAND (or Generic Equiv.) by FIRM	NDC#	CLASS; SCH.
L240	Tab, Beige, Round	Phenolphthalein 90 mg	by Perrigo	00113-0240	Gastrointestinal
L25 <> M	Tab, Yellow, Round, L over 25	Lisinopril 20 mg	Zestril by Mylan	00378-2075	Antihypertensive
L25 <> M	Tab, Yellow, Round, L over 25	Lisinopril 20 mg	Zestril by UDL	51079-0983	Antihypertensive
L25 <> P	Tab, White, Oblong, Scored	Metoprolol Tartrate 25 mg	Lopressor by Pharmascience	Canadian DIN 02248855	Antihypertensive
L25 <> P	Tab, Blue, Round, Scored, L / 2.5	Loxapine Succinate 2.5 mg	Loxapac by Pharmascience	Canadian DIN 02242868	Antipsychotic
L253	Tab, White, Caplet	Naproxen Sodium 220 mg, Pseudoephedrine HCl 120 mg	Naproxen Cold Caplet by Perrigo	00113-0253	Cold Remedy
L254	Cap, Orange	Methylcellulose 500 mg	Methylcellulose by Perrigo	00113-0254	Gastrointestinal
L259	Tab, Round	Aspirin 81 mg	Aspirin by Perrigo	00113-0259	Analgesic
L26 <> M	Tab, Green, Round	Lisinopril 40 mg	Zestril by UDL	51079-0984	Antihypertensive
L26 <> M	Tab, Green, Round, L over 26	Lisinopril 40 mg	Prinivil by Mylan	00378-2076	Antihypertensive
L267	Cap, Red & White	Acetaminophen 500 mg, Dextromethorphan HBr 15 mg, Pseudoephedrine HCl 30 mg	Tylenol Flu Ex Strength by Perrigo	00113-0267	Cold Remedy
L27 <> M	Tab, Light Blue, Round, L over 27	Lisinopril 30 mg	Prinivil by Mylan	00378-2077	Antihypertensive
L274	Tab, Pink, Round, Chewable	Aspirin 81 mg	Children's Aspirin by Perrigo	00113-0274	Analgesic
L277	Tab, Peach, Round, Enteric Coated	Aspirin 81 mg	Aspirin by Time Caps	49483-0102	Analgesic
L277	Tab, Peach, Round, Enteric Coated	Aspirin 81 mg	Aspirin by Perrigo	00113-0102	Analgesic
L282	Tab, Off-White, Oblong	Clemastine Fumarate 1.34 mg	Tavist-1 by Major	00904-7729	Antihistamine
L282	Tab, Off-White, Oblong	Clemastine Fumarate 1.34 mg	Tavist-1 by Perrigo	00113-0282	Antihistamine
L292 <> 80	Tab, Pink, Cap-Shaped, Film-Coated	Simvastatin 80 mg	Zocor by Perrigo	45802-0292	Antihyperlipidemic
L299	Tab, White, Oblong	Acetaminophen 500 mg, Calcium Carbonate 250 mg	by Perrigo	00112-0299	Analgesic
L3 <> IT	Tab, White, Oblong, Film-Coated	Ibandronate Sodium 2.5 mg	Boniva by Hoffmann La Roche	00004-0185	Bisphosphonate
L30 <> APO	Tab, Reddish Brown, Oval	Lisinopril 30 mg	Zestril by Apotex	60505-0188	Antihypertensive
L314	Tab, Yellow, Cap Shaped	Acetaminophen 500 mg, Diphenhydramine HCl 12.5 mg	Tylenol Sinus Ex Strength by Perrigo	00113-0314	Cold Remedy
L326	Tab, Green & Yellow, Round	Acetaminophen 500 mg, Chlorpheniramine Maleate 2 mg, Pseudoephedrine HCl 30 mg	Tylenol Allergy/Sinus Ex Strength by Perrigo	00113-0326	Cold Remedy
L326	Tab, Green & Yellow, Round	Acetaminophen 500 mg, Chlorpheniramine Maleate 2 mg, Pseudoephedrine HCl 30 mg	Tylenol Allergy Sinus by Perrigo	00113-1326	Cold Remedy
L326P	Tab, Green & Yellow, Round, L326 inside Perrigo Logo	Acetaminophen 500 mg, Chlorpheniramine Maleate 2 mg, Pseudoephedrine HCl 30 mg	Tylenol Allergy Sinus by Perrigo	00113-1326	Cold Remedy
L326P	Tab, Green & Yellow, Round, L326 inside Perrigo Logo	Acetaminophen 500 mg, Chlorpheniramine Maleate 2 mg, Pseudoephedrine HCl 30 mg	Tylenol Allergy/Sinus Ex Strength by Perrigo	00113-0326	Cold Remedy
L33	Tab, White, Round	Aspirin 325 mg, Codeine Phosphate 60 mg	Aspirin w/ Codeine by Lee		Analgesic; C III
L33	Tab, White, Round	Aspirin 325 mg, Codeine Phosphate 30 mg	Aspirin w/ Codeine by Lee		Analgesic; C III
L348	Cap, Green, Oblong, Soft Gel	Acetaminophen 325 mg, Pseudoephedrine HCl 30 mg, Dextromethorphan HBr 15 mg, Doxylamine Succinate 6.25 mg	Nitetime 6 hr Softgel by Accucaps	00113-0348	Cold Remedy
L355PM	Tab, Light Blue, Round	Acetaminophen 500 mg, Diphenhydramine HCl 25 mg	Tylenol PM Ex Strength by Perrigo	00113-0355	Cold Remedy
L368	Tab, Light Blue, Oval	Naproxen Sodium 220 mg	Naprosyn by Perrigo	00113-0368	NSAID
L368	Tab, Light Blue, Oval	Naproxen Sodium 220 mg	Naprosyn by Perrigo	00113-0140	NSAID
L368	Tab, Light Blue, Oval	Naproxen Sodium 220 mg	Naprosyn by Major	00904-5230	NSAID
L368	Tab, Light Blue, Oval	Naproxen 220 mg	Aleve by Ivax	00182-1106 Discontinued	NSAID
L373	Tab, White, Round	Ibuprofen 400 mg	Motrin by Perrigo	45802-0184	NSAID
L374	Tab, White, Cap Shaped	Acetaminophen 250 mg, Aspirin 250 mg, Caffeine 65 mg	Excedrin Migraine by Perrigo	00113-0374	Analgesic
L378	Tab, White, Round	Aspirin 325 mg, Chlorpheniramine Maleate 2 mg, Phenylpropanolamine 24.08 mg	Excedrin Migraine by Perrigo	00113-0378	Analgesic
L381	Tab, White, Cap Shaped	Acetaminophen 250 mg, Aspirin 250 mg, Caffeine 65 mg	Excedrin Migraine by Perrigo	00113-0381	Analgesic
L389	Cap, Orange, Soft Gel	Dextromethorphan 10 mg, Pseudoephedrine 30 mg	Sudafed Cold/Flu by Perrigo	00113-0389	Cold Remedy
L4	Tab, Green, Oblong	Prenatal Vitamin	by Perrigo		Vitamin

ID FRONT <> BACK	DESCRIPTION FRONT <> BACK	INGREDIENT & STRENGTH	BRAND (or Generic Equiv.) by FIRM	NDC#	CLASS; SCH.
L4 <> M	Tab, Peach, Oblong, Scored, M <> L over 4	Levothyroxine Sodium 25 mcg	Unithroid by Mylan	00378-1800	Thyroid Hormone
L4 <> M	Tab, Peach, Oblong, Scored, M <> L over 4	Levothyroxine Sodium 25 mcg	Unithroid by UDL	51079-0444	Thyroid Hormone
L40 <> APO	Tab, Yellow, Oval	Lisinopril 40 mg	Zestril by Apotex	60505-0189	Antihypertensive
L403 <> 325MG	Tab, White, Round	Acetaminophen 325 mg	Tylenol by Perrigo	00113-0403	Analgesic
L405 <> 500MG	Tab, White, Round	Acetaminophen 500 mg	Tylenol Ex Strength by Perrigo	00113-0405	Analgesic
L406 <> 325MG	Tab, Light Blue, Round	Diphenhydramine HCl 25 mg	Benadryl by Perrigo	00113-0406	Antihistamine
L407 <> 500MG	Tab, Pink, Cap Shaped	Pseudoephedrine 120 mg	Sudafed 12 Hr by Perrigo	00113-0407	Decongestant
L409	Tab, Yellow, Round	Caffeine 200 mg	by Perrigo	00113-0409	Stimulant
L410	Tab, Orange, Cap Shaped	Acetaminophen 500 mg, Pseudoephedrine 30 mg	Sudafed Sinus by Perrigo	00113-0410	Cold Remedy
L415	Tab, White, Round	Aspirin 400 mg, Caffeine 32 mg	Anacin by Perrigo	00113-0415	Analgesic
L416	Tab, White, Round	Aspirin 325 mg	Aspirin by Perrigo	00113-2416	Analgesic
L418	Cap, Blue, Soft Gel	Guaifenesin 200 mg, Pseudoephedrine 30 mg	Sudafed Sinus by Perrigo	00113-0418	Cold Remedy
L419	Tab, White, Round	Phenylpropanolamine HCl 15 mg, Diphenhydramine HCl 38.33 mg, Aspirin 325 mg	by Perrigo	00113-0419	Cold Remedy
L420	Tab, Yellow, Round	Pseudoephedrine HCl 30 mg, Dextromethorphan HBr 10 mg, Acetaminophen HCl 325 mg, Chlorpheniramine 2 mg	by Perrigo	00113-0420	Cold Remedy
L421	Tab, White, Round	Aspirin 325 mg, Sodium Bicarbonate 1916 mg, Citric Acid 1000 mg	Pain Relief Effervescent by Perrigo	00113-0421	Analgesic
L421	Tab, White, Round	Aspirin 325 mg, Sodium Bicarbonate 1916 mg, Citric Acid 1000 mg	Pain Relief Effervescent by Major	00904-7948	Analgesic
L421	Tab, White, Round	Aspirin 325 mg, Sodium Bicarbonate 1916 mg, Citric Acid 1000 mg	Pain Relief Effervescent by Perrigo	00113-2421	Analgesic
L427	Tab, White & Yellow, Round	Acetaminophen 500 mg, Chlorpheniramine Maleate 2 mg, Pseudoephedrine HCl 30 mg	Tylenol Allergy/Sinus Ex Strength by Perrigo	00113-0427	Cold Remedy
L427	Tab, Yellow, Caplet	Acetaminophen 500 mg, Chlorpheniramine Maleate 2 mg, Pseudoephedrine HCl 30 mg	Tylenol Allergy/Sinus Ex Strength by Perrigo	00113-2427	Cold Remedy
L428	Cap, Green, Soft Gel	Simethicone 125 mg	Mylicon by Perrigo	00113-0428	Antiflatulent
L429	Tab, Orange, Round	Aspirin 325 mg	Aspirin by Perrigo	00113-0429	Analgesic
L430	Tab, White, Round	Acetaminophen 250 mg, Aspirin 250 mg, Caffeine 65 mg	Excedrin Migraine by Perrigo	00113-0430	Analgesic
L431	Tab, Blue, Cap Shaped	Diphenhydramine HCl 25 mg	Benadryl by Perrigo	00113-0431	Antihistamine
L431	Tab, Blue, Cap Shaped	Diphenhydramine HCl 25 mg	Benadryl by Perrigo	00113-1431	Antihistamine
L432	Tab, Red, Round	Pseudoephedrine 30 mg	Sudafed by Perrigo	00113-0432	Decongestant
L432	Tab, Red, Round	Pseudoephedrine 30 mg	Sudafed by Today's Health	38309-0432	Decongestant
L432	Tab, Red, Round	Pseudoephedrine 30 mg	Sudafed by Perrigo	00113-2432	Decongestant
L434	Tab, White, Round	Triprolidine 2.5 mg, Pseudoephedrine 60 mg	Actifed by Perrigo	00113-0434	Cold Remedy
L435	Tab, Yellow, Cap Shaped	Acetaminophen 325 mg, Chlorpheniramine Maleate 2 mg, Pseudoephedrine HCl 30 mg, Dextromethorphan HBr 15 mg	Alka Seltzer Plus Liquid Gels by Perrigo	00113-0435	Cold Remedy
L437 <> PM	Tab, Light Blue, Cap Shaped	Acetaminophen 500 mg, Diphenhydramine HCl 25 mg	Tylenol PM by Major Pharmaceuticals	00904-7651	Analgesic; Sleep Aid
L437 <> PM	Tab, Light Blue, Cap Shaped	Acetaminophen 500 mg, Diphenhydramine HCl 25 mg	Tylenol PM by Perrigo	00113-0437	Analgesic; Sleep Aid
L438	Tab, Light Green, Cap Shaped	Acetaminophen 500 mg, Pseudoephedrine HCl 30 mg	Tylenol Sinus by Major	00904-7954	Cold Remedy
L438	Tab, Light Green, Cap Shaped	Acetaminophen 500 mg, Pseudoephedrine HCl 30 mg	Tylenol Sinus by Perrigo	00113-0438	Cold Remedy
L438	Tab, Light Green, Cap Shaped	Acetaminophen 500 mg, Pseudoephedrine HCl 30 mg	Tylenol Sinus by Perrigo	00113-2438	Cold Remedy
L441	Tab, Blue, Cap Shaped	Doxylamine Succinate 25 mg	Unisom by Perrigo	00113-0441	Sleep Aid
L447	Tab, Orange, Cap Shaped	Acetaminophen 500 mg, Pseudoephedrine HCl 30 mg	Tylenol Sinus by Perrigo	00113-0447	Cold Remedy
L449	Tab, Purple, Round, Scored, Chewable	Acetaminophen 160 mg	Tylenol Ex Strength by Perrigo	00113-0449	Analgesic
L450	Tab, White, Round	Chlorpheniramine 4 mg, Pseudoephedrine 60 mg	Sudafed Cold/Allergy by Perrigo	00113-0450	Cold Remedy
L452	Tab, White, Round	Aspirin 325 mg, Aluminum Hydroxide 50 mg, Magnesium Hydroxide 50 mg	Ascriptin by Perrigo	00113-0452	Analgesic
L453	Tab, White, Cap Shaped	Acetaminophen 325 mg	Tylenol by Perrigo	00113-0453	Analgesic
L458	Tab, Light Yellow, Cap Shaped	Phenylpropanolamine HCl 75 mg	by Perrigo	00113-0458	Decongestant; Appetite Suppressant
L459	Tab, Yellow, Oblong	Phenylpropanolamine HCl 25 mg, Chlorpheniramine 4 mg	by Perrigo	00113-0459	Cold Remedy
L461	Tab, Light Orange, Chewable	Ibuprofen 100 mg	Advil by Today's Health	00113-0461	Analgesic
L462	Cap, Pink, Red Band	Diphenhydramine HCl 25 mg	Benadryl by Today's Health	38309-0462	Antihistamine
L462	Cap, Pink, Red Band	Diphenhydramine HCl 25 mg	Benadryl by Perrigo	00113-0462	Antihistamine

ID FRONT <> BACK	DESCRIPTION FRONT <> BACK	INGREDIENT & STRENGTH	BRAND (or Generic Equiv.) by FIRM	NDC#	CLASS; SCH.
L463	Tab, Yellow, Round	Chlorpheniramine Maleate 4 mg	Chlor-Trimeton by Perrigo	00113-0463	Antihistamine
L465 <> PM	Tab, Blue, Round	Acetaminophen 500 mg, Diphenhydramine HCl 25 mg	Tylenol PM by Perrigo	00113-0465	Analgesic; Sleep Aid
L467	Tab, Light Orange, Round, Chewable	Aspirin 81 mg	Children's Aspirin by Perrigo	00113-0259	Analgesic
L467	Tab, Orange, Round, Chewable	Aspirin 81 mg	Aspirin by Perrigo	00113-0467	Analgesic
L468	Tab, Red, Yellow, White OR Orange, Round	Calcium Carbonate 750 mg	Tums by Perrigo	00113-0468	Gastrointestinal
L469	Tab, Pink, Round	Bismuth Subsalicylate 262 mg	Pepto Bismol by Perrigo	00113-0469	Gastrointestinal
L470	Cap, Yellow, with 1 Red Band	Acetaminophen 500 mg	Tylenol Ex Strength by Perrigo	00113-0470	Analgesic
L477	Tab, Light Brown, Cap Shaped	Polycarbophil Calcium 625 mg, Polycarbophil 500 mg	by Perrigo	00113-0477	Gastrointestinal
L478	Tab, Red, Green, Yellow OR Orange, Round	Calcium Carbonate 500 mg	Tums by Major	00904-1258	Vitamin; Mineral
L478	Tab, Red, Green, Yellow OR Orange, Round	Calcium Carbonate 500 mg	Tums by Perrigo	00113-0478	Vitamin; Mineral
L479 <> 25	Tab, Pink, Cap Shaped	Diphenhydramine HCl 25 mg	Benadryl by Perrigo	00113-0479	Antihistamine
L480	Tab, Yellow, Oval	Pseudoephedrine 30 mg, Chlorpheniramine 2 mg, Acetaminophen 500 mg	by Perrigo	00113-0480	Cold Remedy
L481	Tab, Purple, Round, Grape Flavor	Acetaminophen 80 mg	Children's Tylenol by Perrigo	00113-0481	Analgesic
L482	Cap, Clear	Phenylpropanolamine 75 mg, Chlorpheniramine 8 mg	Contac by Perrigo	00113-0482	Cold Remedy
L484	Tab, White, Caplet	Acetaminophen 500 mg	Tylenol Ex Strength by Perrigo	00113-0484	Analgesic
L484	Tab, White, Caplet	Acetaminophen 500 mg	Tylenol Ex Strength by Perrigo	00113-2484	Analgesic
L485	Tab, White, Round	Calcium Carbonate 500 mg	Tums by Perrigo	00113-0485	Vitamin; Mineral
L485	Tab, White, Round	Calcium Carbonate 500 mg	Tums by Major	00904-1257	Vitamin; Mineral
L486	Cap, Red & Beige, Oval, Soft Gel	Docusate Sodium 100 mg	Colace by Perrigo	00113-0486	Laxative
L489	Tab, Pink, Purple, OR Dark Pink, Round, Chewable, Fruit Flavor	Calcium Carbonate 750 mg	Tums by Perrigo	00113-0489	Analgesic
L490	Tab, Light Blue, Round	Naproxen 220 mg	Naprosyn by Major	00904-5229	NSAID
L490	Tab, Light Blue, Round	Naproxen 220 mg	Naprosyn by Perrigo	00113-9490	NSAID
L492	Tab, Pink, Round	Acetaminophen 80 mg	Children's Tylenol by Perrigo	00113-0492	Analgesic
L494	Tab, White, Round	Phenylpropanolamine HCl 15 mg, Chlorpheniramine Maleate 2 mg, Aspirin 325 mg	by Perrigo	00113-0494	Cold Remedy
L495	Cap, Dark Red, Oval, Soft Gel	Docusate Sodium 100 mg, Casanthranol 31.5 mg	Peri-Colace by Perrigo	00113-0495	Laxative
L496	Tab, Blue, Round	Phenylpropanolamine 25 mg, Brompheniramine 4 mg	by Perrigo	00113-0496	Cold Remedy
L5	Cap, Red and Blue, Grey Band	Acetaminophen 500 mg	Tylenol Extra Strength Rapid Release Gel by Leiner		Analgesic
L5	Tab, Pink, Round, Scored, L / 5 <> Cobalt Logo	Lisinopril 5 mg	Zestril by Cobalt	Canadian DIN 02271443	Antihypertensive
L5 <> APO	Tab, Reddish Brown, Oval, Scored	Lisinopril 5 mg	Zestril by Apotex	60505-0185	Antihypertensive
L5 <> M	Tab, White, Oblong, Scored, M <> L over 5	Levothyroxine Sodium 50 mcg	Unithroid by Mylan	00378-1803	Thyroid Hormone
L5 <> M	Tab, White, Oblong, Scored, M <> L over 5	Levothyroxine Sodium 50 mcg	Unithroid by UDL	51079-0440	Thyroid Hormone
L5 <> P	Tab, Yellow, Round, Scored	Loxapine Succinate 5 mg	Loxapac by Pharmascience	Canadian DIN 02230837	Antipsychotic
L50 <> JANSSEN	Tab, Coated, L over 50	Levamisole 50 mg	Ergamisol by Janssen	50458-0270	Immunomodulator
L50 <> P	Tab, White, Round, Scored	Loxapine Succinate 50 mg	Loxapac by Pharmascience	Canadian DIN 02230840	Antipsychotic
L501	Tab, Blue, Cap Shaped	Phenylpropanolamine HCl 12.5 mg, Dextromethorphan HBr 15 mg, Acetaminophen 500 mg, Chlorpheniramine 2 mg	Tylenol Cold Ex Strength by Perrigo	00113-0501	Cold Remedy
L507	Tab, Purple, Round	Phenylpropanolamine 6.25 mg, Brompheniramine 1 mg	by Perrigo	00113-0507	Cold Remedy
L50JANSSEN	Tab, White, L50/Janssen	Levamisole 50 mg	Ergamisol by Janssen	Canadian	Immunomodulator
L51 <> M	Tab, White to Off-White, Round, Scored	Lamotrigine 25 mg	Lamictal by UDL	51079-0598	Anticonvulsant
L511	Tab, Orange, Round, Enteric Coated	Aspirin 500 mg	Aspirin by Perrigo	00113-0511	Analgesic
L512	Cap, Clear with Brownish Powder	Psyllium Husk 520 mg	NVP Cap by Perrigo	00113-0512	Gastrointestinal
L522	Tab, White, Oblong	Ibuprofen 800 mg	Motrin by Perrigo	10768-	NSAID
L524	Tab, White, Round	Acetaminophen 325 mg, Pseudoephedrine HCl 30 mg	Tylenol Sinus Non-Drowsy by Perrigo	Discontinued	Cold Remedy
L525	Tab, Yellow, Round	Acetaminophen 500 mg, Chlorpheniramine Maleate 2 mg, Dextromethorphan HBr 15 mg, Pseudoephedrine HCl 30 mg	Tylenol Cold by Major	00904-3650	Cold Remedy

ID FRONT <> BACK	DESCRIPTION FRONT <> BACK	INGREDIENT & STRENGTH	BRAND (or Generic Equiv.) by FIRM	NDC#	CLASS; SCH.
L525	Tab, Yellow, Round	Acetaminophen 500 mg, Chlorpheniramine Maleate 2 mg, Dextromethorphan HBr 15 mg, Pseudoephedrine HCl 30 mg	by Perrigo	00113-0525	Cold Remedy
L527	Tab, White, Round	Calcium Carbonate 550 mg, Magnesium Hydroxide 110 mg	by Perrigo	00113-0527	Vitamin; Mineral
L528	Tab, Green, Round	Calcium Carbonate 750 mg	Os-Cal by Perrigo	00113-0528	Gastrointestinal
L530	Tab, Light Blue, Cap Shaped	Acetaminophen 500 mg, Chlorpheniramine Maleate 2 mg, Dextromethorphan HBr 15 mg, Pseudoephedrine HCl 30 mg	by Perrigo	00113-0530	Cold Remedy
L534	Tab, White to Off-White, Cap Shaped	Naproxen 375 mg	Naprosyn by Perrigo	10768-7534	NSAID
L535	Tab, Yellow, Round	Aspirin 81 mg	Aspirin by Time Caps	00113-0937	Analgesic
L535	Tab, Yellow, Round	Aspirin 81 mg	Aspirin by Perrigo	00113-0535	Analgesic
L537	Cap, Green, Soft Gel	Pseudoephedrine HCl 30 mg, Guaifenesin 200 mg	by Perrigo	00113-0537	Cold Remedy
L540 <> 20	Tab, Orange, Oval, Film-Coated	Simvastatin 20 mg	Zocor by Perrigo	45802-0384	Antihyperlipidemic
L544	Tab, White, Cap Shaped	Acetaminophen 650 mg	Tylenol by Perrigo	00113-0544	Analgesic
L544	Tab, White, Cap Shaped	Acetaminophen 650 mg	Tylenol by Perrigo	00113-1544	Analgesic
L556	Tab, White, Round	Brompheniramine Maleate 2 mg, Aspirin 500 mg, Dextromethorphan HBr 10 mg, Phenylpropanolamine HCl 12.5 mg	by Perrigo	00113-0556	Cold Remedy
L562	Cap, Orange, Softgel	Acetaminophen 250 mg, Guaifenesin 100 mg, Dextromethorphan HBr 10 mg, Pseudoephedrine HCl 30 mg	Tylenol Cold by Perrigo	00113-0562	Cold Remedy
L562	Cap, Orange, Soft Gel, White Ink	Pseudoephedrine HCl 30 mg, Guaifenesin 100 mg, Dextromethorphan HBr 10 mg, Acetaminophen 250 mg	Suphedrine Cold/Cough by Perrigo	00113-0080	Cold Remedy
L576	Cap, Orange & Yellow	Pseudoephedrine HCl 30 mg, Dextromethorphan HBr 15 mg, Acetaminophen 325 mg	Non Aspirin Cold Caps by Perrigo	00113-0576	Cold Remedy
L582	Tab, White, Cap Shaped	Aspirin 325 mg	Aspirin by Perrigo	00113-0582	Analgesic
L595	Tab, Green, Yellow, Red OR Orange, Round	Calcium Carbonate 1000 mg	Os-Cal by Perrigo	00113-0595	Vitamin; Mineral
L596	Tab, White, Cap Shaped	Pseudoephedrine HCl 30 mg, Dextromethorphan HBr 15 mg, Acetaminophen 500 mg	by Perrigo	00113-0596	Cold Remedy
L6 <> M	Tab, Violet, Oblong, Scored, M <> L over 6	Levothyroxine Sodium 75 mcg	Unithroid by Mylan	00378-1805	Thyroid Hormone
L6 <> M	Tab, Violet, Oblong, Scored, M <> L over 6	Levothyroxine Sodium 75 mcg	Unithroid by UDL	51079-0441	Thyroid Hormone
L609	Tab, Green, Oblong	Atropine 0.04 mg, Chlorpheniramine 8 mg, Hyoscyamine 0.19 mg, Phenylephrine 25 mg, Phenylpropanolamine 50 mg, Scopolamine 0.01 mg	Ru-tuss by Norton		Cold Remedy
L612	Tab, White, Oval	Loratadine 10 mg	Claritin by Perrigo	00113-0612	Antihistamine
L615	Cap, Red, Soft Gel	Docusate Sodium 100 mg	Colace by Perrigo	00113-0615	Laxative
L617 <> 75	Tab, Pink, Round	Ranitidine HCl 75 mg	Zantac by Perrigo	00113-0617	Gastrointestinal
L631	Tab, White, Oval	Naproxen 500 mg	Aleve by Perrigo		NSAID
L642	Tab, White, Round	Aspirin 325 mg	Aspirin by Perrigo	00113-0642	Analgesic
L643	Tab, White, Round	Pseudoephedrine HCl 30 mg, Acetaminophen 500 mg	Suphedrine Ex Strength by Perrigo	00113-0643	Cold Remedy
L657	Cap, Orange, Oval, Soft Gel	Simethicone 180 mg	Mylanta Gas by Perrigo	00113-0657	Antiflatulent
L670	Tab, White, Round	Quinine Sulfate 260 mg	Quinamm by LuChem		Antimalarial
L685	Tab, Beige	Thyroid 32.5 mg	by Taro	52549-4034	Thyroid Hormone
L686	Tab	Thyroid 1 g	by Pharmedix	53002-1029	Thyroid Hormone
L687	Tab, Tan, Round	Thyroid 120 mg	Synthroid by LuChem		Thyroid Hormone
L7 <> M	Tab, Light Green, Oblong, Scored, M <> L over 7	Levothyroxine Sodium 88 mcg	Unithroid by Mylan	00378-1807	Thyroid Hormone
L754	Tab, Green, Oblong	Guaifenesin 300 mg, Phenylephrine HCl 20 mg	Endal by Norton		Cold Remedy
L8 <> M	Tab, Yellow, Oblong, Scored, M <> L over 8	Levothyroxine Sodium 100 mcg	Unithroid by Mylan	00378-1809	Thyroid Hormone
L8 <> M	Tab, Yellow, Oblong, Scored, M <> L over 8	Levothyroxine Sodium 100 mcg	Unithroid by UDL	51079-0442	Thyroid Hormone
L814	Cap, Clear, Soft Gel	Diphenhydramine HCl 25 mg	Benadryl by Perrigo	00113-0814	Antihistamine
L821	Tab, White, Cap Shaped	Acetaminophen 500 mg, Pamabrom Maleate 25 mg	by Perrigo	00113-0821	PMS Relief
L835	Tab, White, Cap Shaped	Acetaminophen 325 mg, Dextromethorphan HBr 15 mg, Pseudoephedrine HCl 30 mg	Tylenol Cold by Perrigo	00113-0835	Cold Remedy
L837P	Tab, Blue & White, Round, L837 inside Perrigo symbol	Acetaminophen 500 mg, Diphenhydramine HCl 25 mg	Tylenol PM by Perrigo	00113-0837	Cold Remedy
L855	Cap, Red, Soft Gel	Simethicone 131.5 mg	Mylanta Gas by Perrigo	00113-0855	Antiflatulent

ID FRONT <> BACK	DESCRIPTION FRONT <> BACK	INGREDIENT & STRENGTH	BRAND (or Generic Equiv.) by FIRM	NDC#	CLASS; SCH.
L860	Tab, White, Round	Phenylpropanolamine HCl 75 mg, Clemastine Fumarate 1.34 mg	Tavist-D by Perrigo	00113-0860	Cold Remedy
L867	Cap, Orange, Oblong	Pseudoephedrine HCl 30 mg, Dextromethorphan HBr 15 mg	Daytime 6 hr Softgel by Accucaps	00113-0867	Cold Remedy
L870	Tab, White, Round	Acetaminophen 250 mg, Chlorpheniramine Maleate 2 mg, Phenylephrine HCl 5 mg	Alka-Seltzer PLUS by Perrigo	00113-0870	Cold Remedy
L870	Tab, White, Round	Acetaminophen 250 mg, Chlorpheniramine Maleate 2 mg, Phenylephrine HCl 5 mg	Alka-Seltzer PLUS by Perrigo	00113-1870	Cold Remedy
L877	Tab, Reddish-Orange, Cap Shaped	Acetaminophen 500 mg	Tylenol Ex Strength by Perrigo	00113-0877	Analgesic
L879 <> 40	Tab, Light Pink, Oval, Film-Coated	Simvastatin 40 mg	Zocor by Perrigo	45802-0879	Antihyperlipidemic
L880	Tab, White, Round	Aluminum Hydroxide 160 mg, Magnesium Carbonate 105 mg	Maalox by Perrigo	00113-0880	Gastrointestinal
L890	Tab, White, Round	Dimenhydrinate 50 mg	Dramamine by Perrigo	00113-0890	Antiemetic
L9 <> M	Tab, Dark Pink, Oblong, Scored, M <> L over 9	Levothyroxine Sodium 112 mcg	Unithroid by Mylan	00378-1811	Thyroid Hormone
L965	Tab, Green, Round	Dexbrompheniramine Maleate 6 mg, Pseudoephedrine Sulfate 120 mg	Drixoral by Perrigo	00113-0965	Cold Remedy
L976	Tab, White and Red, Caplet, L976 <> L976	Acetaminophen 500 mg	Tylenol Ex Strength by Perrigo	00113-0976	Analgesic
L995	Tab, White, Round	Ibuprofen 200 mg	Motrin by Murfreesboro	51129-1521	NSAID
LAB100 <> APO	Tab, Orange, Cap Shaped, Film Coated, Scored	Labetalol HCl 100 mg	Trandate by Apotex	Canadian DIN 02243538	Antihypertensive
LAB200 <> APO	Tab, White, Cap Shaped, Film Coated, Scored	Labetalol HCl 200 mg	Trandate by Apotex	Canadian DIN 02243539	Antihypertensive
LACTAID	Tab, White, Cap Shaped, Chewable	Lactase 3000 Units	Regular Strength Lactaid Tables by McNeil	Canadian DIN 02230653	Gastrointestinal
LACTAID	Tab, White, Cap Shaped	Lactase 5000 Units	Lactaid Ultra by McNeil	Canadian DIN 02231507	Gastrointestinal
LACTAID	Tab, White, Round, Chewable	Lactase 9,000 Units	by McNeil	Canadian DIN 02239664	Gastrointestinal
LACTAID	Tab, White, Round, Chewable	Lactase 9000 Units	Lactaid Ultra Chewable Tablets by McNeil	Canadian DIN 02231507	Gastrointestinal
LACTAIDES	Tab, White, Cap Shaped, Chewable	Lactase 4500 Units	Lactaid by McNeil	Canadian DIN 02230654	Gastrointestinal
LAM150 <> APO	Tab, Cream, Shield Shaped, Scored, LAM / 150	Lamotrigine 150 mg	Apo Lamotirgine by Apotex	Canadian DIN 02245210	Anticonvulsant
LAMICTAL <> 100	Tab, White, Round, Orally Disintegrating	Lamotrigine 100 mg	Lamictal ODT by GSK	00173-0776	Anticonvulsant
LAMICTAL <> 200	Tab, White, Round, Orally Disintegrating	Lamotrigine 200 mg	Lamictal ODT by GSK	00173-0777	Anticonvulsant
LAMICTAL100	Tab, Peach, Shield Shaped, Scored	Lamotrigine 100 mg	Lamictal by GSK	Canadian DIN 02142104	Anticonvulsant
LAMICTAL100	Tab, Peach, Shield Shaped, Scored	Lamotrigine 100 mg	Lamictal Starter Kit by GSK	00173-0594	Anticonvulsant
LAMICTAL100	Tab, Peach, Shield Shaped, Scored	Lamotrigine 100 mg	Lamictal by BW Inc	Canadian	Anticonvulsant
LAMICTAL100	Tab, Peach, Shield Shaped, Scored	Lamotrigine 100 mg	Lamictal by DSM	63552-0642	Anticonvulsant
LAMICTAL100	Tab, Peach, Shield Shaped, Scored	Lamotrigine 100 mg	Lamictal by GSK	00173-0642	Anticonvulsant
LAMICTAL150	Tab, Cream, Shield Shaped, Scored	Lamotrigine 150 mg	Lamictal by DSM	63552-0643	Anticonvulsant
LAMICTAL150	Tab, Cream, Shield Shaped, Scored	Lamotrigine 150 mg	Lamictal by BW Inc	Canadian	Anticonvulsant
LAMICTAL150	Tab, Cream, Shield Shaped, Scored	Lamotrigine 150 mg	Lamictal by GSK	00173-0643	Anticonvulsant
LAMICTAL150	Tab, Cream, Shield Shaped, Scored	Lamotrigine 150 mg	Lamictal by GSK	Canadian DIN 02142112	Anticonvulsant
LAMICTAL200	Tab, Blue, Shield Shaped, Scored	Lamotrigine 200 mg	Lamictal by DSM	63552-0644	Anticonvulsant
LAMICTAL200	Tab, Blue, Shield Shaped, Scored	Lamotrigine 200 mg	Lamictal by GSK	00173-0644	Anticonvulsant
LAMICTAL25	Tab, White, Shield Shaped, Scored	Lamotrigine 25 mg	Lamictal by BW Inc	Canadian	Anticonvulsant
LAMICTAL25	Tab, White, Shield Shaped, Scored	Lamotrigine 25 mg	Lamictal by DSM	63552-0633	Anticonvulsant
LAMICTAL25	Tab, White, Shield Shaped, Scored	Lamotrigine 25 mg	Lamictal by GSK	00173-0633	Anticonvulsant
LAMICTAL25	Tab, White, Shield Shaped, Scored	Lamotrigine 25 mg	Lamictal by GSK	Canadian DIN 02142082	Anticonvulsant

ID FRONT <> BACK	DESCRIPTION FRONT <> BACK	INGREDIENT & STRENGTH	BRAND (or Generic Equiv.) by FIRM	NDC#	CLASS; SCH.
LAMICTAL25	Tab, White, Shield Shaped, Scored	Lamotrigine 25 mg	Lamictal Starter Kit by GSK	00173-0594	Anticonvulsant
LAMICTALXR100	Tab, Orange and White, Round	Lamotrigine 100 mg	Lamictal XR by GSK	00173-0760	Anticonvulsant
LAMICTALXR200	Tab, Blue and White, Round	Lamotrigine 200 mg	Lamictal XR by GSK	00173-0759	Anticonvulsant
LAMICTALXR25	Tab, White and Yellow, Round	Lamotrigine 25 mg	Lamictal XR by GSK	00173-0760	Anticonvulsant
LAMICTALXR50	Tab, Green and White, Round	Lamotrigine 50 mg	Lamictal XR by GSK	00173-0760	Anticonvulsant
LAMISIL <> 250	Tab, White, Round	Terbinafine HCl 250 mg	by Allscripts		Antifungal
LAMISIL <> 250	Tab, White, Round	Terbinafine HCl 250 mg	Lamisil by Novartis	00078-0179	Antifungal
LAMISIL125	Tab, White & Yellow, Round	Terbinafine HCl 125 mg	Lamisil by Sandoz	Canadian	Antifungal
LAMISIL250	Tab, White, Round	Terbinafine HCl 250 mg	Lamisil by Novartis	Canadian DIN 02031116	Antifungal
LAMP	Tab, White, Round, Genie Lamp Logo	3,4-Methylenedioxymethamphetamine (MDMA)	Ecstasy by Illegal		Euphoric; Illicit
LAN	Cap, Blue	Dicyclomine HCl 10 mg	Bentyl by Mova	55370-0854	Gastrointestinal
LAN <> 1313	Tab, White, Round	Pilocarpine HCl 5 mg	Salagen by Lannett	00527-1313	Cholinergic Agonist
LAN0586	Cap, Blue	Dicyclomine HCl 10 mg	Bentyl by Mova	55370-0854	Gastrointestinal
LAN0586	Cap, Blue	Dicyclomine HCl 10 mg	Bentyl by DRX	55045-2729	Gastrointestinal
LAN0586	Cap, Blue	Dicyclomine HCl 10 mg	Bentyl by Teva	55953-0555	Gastrointestinal
LAN0586	Cap, Blue	Dicyclomine HCl 10 mg	Bentyl by Kaiser	62224-9119	Gastrointestinal
LAN0586	Cap, Blue	Dicyclomine HCl 10 mg	Bentyl by Ivax	00182-0519	Gastrointestinal
LAN0586	Cap, Blue	Dicyclomine HCl 10 mg	Bentyl by Qualitest	00603-3265	Gastrointestinal
LAN0586	Cap, Blue	Dicyclomine HCl 10 mg	Bentyl by Lannett	00527-0586	Gastrointestinal
LAN0586	Cap, Blue	Dicyclomine HCl 10 mg	Bentyl by URL Mutual	00677-0341	Gastrointestinal
LAN0586	Cap, Blue	Dicyclomine HCl 10 mg	Bentyl by Duramed	51285-0929	Gastrointestinal
LAN1050	Tab, White, Round, Scored	Acetazolamide 250 mg	Diamox by Lannett	00527-1050	Antiglaucoma Agent
LAN1109	Tab, White, Round	Isoniazide 300 mg	INH by Lannett	Discontinued	Antimycobacterial
LAN1152	Tab, White, Cap Shaped	Methocarbamol 750 mg	Robaxin by Lannett	00527-1152	Muscle Relaxant
LAN1170	Tab, White, Round, LAN over 1170	Atropine Sulfate 0.025 mg, Diphenoxylate HCl 2.5 mg	Lomotil by Lannett	00527-1170	Antidiarrheal; C V
LAN1201	Tab, Light Orange, Round, Scored, LAN over 1201	Prednisolone 5 mg	by Lannett	00527-1201	Steroid
LAN1231	Tab, White, Round, Scored, LAN over 1231	Primidone 250 mg	Mysoline by Lannett	00527-1231	Anticonvulsant
LAN1231	Tab, White, Round, Scored, Lan over 1231	Primidone 250 mg	by Duramed	51285-0939	Anticonvulsant
LAN1231	Tab, White, Round, Scored, Lan over 1231	Primidone 250 mg	by URL Mutual	00677-0354	Anticonvulsant
LAN1231	Tab, White, Round, Scored, Lan over 1231	Primidone 250 mg	Mysoline by Qualitest	00603-5370	Anticonvulsant
LAN1231	Tab, White, Round, Scored, Lan over 1231	Primidone 250 mg	by Dixon Shane	17236-0547	Anticonvulsant
LAN1231	Tab, White, Round, Scored, Lan over 1231	Primidone 250 mg	by Teva	55953-0527	Anticonvulsant
LAN1231	Tab, White, Round, Scored, Lan over 1231	Primidone 250 mg	Mysoline by Mova	55370-0888	Anticonvulsant
LAN1231	Tab, White, Round, Scored, Lan over 1231	Primidone 250 mg	Mysoline by Major	00904-0560	Anticonvulsant
LAN1231	Tab, White, Round, Scored, LAN over 1231	Primidone 250 mg	Mysoline by Amneal	65162-0547	Anticonvulsant
LAN1282	Tab, White, Round, Scored	Dicyclomine HCl 20 mg	Bentyl by Lannett	00527-1282	Gastrointestinal
LAN1290	Tab, Light Blue, Round	Pseudoephedrine HCl 60 mg	by Lannett	00527-1290	Decongestant
LAN1301	Tab, White, Round, Scored, LAN over 1290	Primidone 50 mg	Mysoline by Lannett	00527-1301	Anticonvulsant
LAN1301	Tab, White, Round, Scored, LAN over 1301	Primidone 50 mg	Mysoline by Major	00904-5559	Anticonvulsant
LAN1301	Tab, White, Round, Scored, LAN over 1301	Primidone 50 mg	Mysoline by Qualitest	00603-5369	Anticonvulsant
LAN1301	Tab, White, Round, Scored, LAN over 1301	Primidone 50 mg	Mysoline by Amneal	65162-0545	Anticonvulsant
LAN1302	Tab, White, Round, Scored	Methocarbamol 500 mg	Robaxin by Lannett	00527-1302	Muscle Relaxant
LAN1305	Tab, White, Round, LAN over 1305	Pseudoephedrine 30 mg	Sudafed by Lannett	00527-1305	Decongestant
LAN1317	Tab, Blue, Speckled, Cap Shaped	Phentermine HCl 37.5 mg	Adipex-P By Lannett	00527-1317	Anorexiant; C IV
LANNET05271552	Cap, Dark Green & Light Green, 0527 over 1552	Aspirin 325 mg, Butalbital 50 mg, Caffeine 40 mg	Fiorinal by Lannett	00527-1552	Analgesic; C III
LANNETT05271552	Cap, Green & Clear	Aspirin 325 mg, Butalbital 50 mg, Caffeine 40 mg	Fiorinal Cap by Qualitest	00603-2550	Analgesic; C III
LANNETT0597	Cap, Black	Phentermine HCl 30 mg	by Lannett	00527-0597	Anorexiant; C IV
LANNETT1308	Cap, Natural and Blue	Phentermine HCl 30 mg	by Lannett	00527-1308	Anorexiant; C IV

ID FRONT <> BACK	DESCRIPTION FRONT <> BACK	INGREDIENT & STRENGTH	BRAND (or Generic Equiv.) by FIRM	NDC#	CLASS; SCH.
LANNETT1310	Cap, Yellow	Phentermine HCl 30 mg	by Lannett	00527-1310	Anorexiant; C IV
LANOXINU3A	Tab, Peach, Round	Digoxin 0.0625 mg	Lanoxin by GSK	Canadian	Cardiac Agent
LANOXINX3A	Tab, White, Round, Scored, Lanoxin over X3A	Digoxin 0.25 mg	Lanoxin by GSK	00179-0404	Cardiac Agent
LANOXINX3A	Tab, White, Round, Scored, Lanoxin over X3A	Digoxin 0.25 mg	Lanoxin by Kaiser	55154-0702	Cardiac Agent
LANOXINX3A	Tab, White, Round, Scored, Lanoxin over X3A	Digoxin 0.25 mg	Lanoxin by Nat Pharmpak	65243-0024	Cardiac Agent
LANOXINX3A	Tab, White, Round, Scored, Lanoxin over X3A	Digoxin 0.25 mg	Lanoxin by Va Cmop	Canadian	Cardiac Agent
LANOXINX3A	Tab, White, Round, Scored, Lanoxin over X3A	Digoxin 0.25 mg	Lanoxin by GSK	62584-0249	Cardiac Agent
LANOXINX3A	Tab, White, Round, Scored, Lanoxin over X3A	Digoxin 0.25 mg	Lanoxin by Amerisource	63552-0249	Cardiac Agent
LANOXINX3A	Tab, White, Round, Scored, Lanoxin over X3A	Digoxin 0.25 mg	Lanoxin by DSM	59198-0373	Cardiac Agent
LANOXINX3A	Tab, White, Round, Scored, Lanoxin over X3A	Digoxin 0.25 mg	Lanoxin by Thrift Drug	51316-0245	Cardiac Agent
LANOXINX3A	Tab, White, Round, Scored, Lanoxin over X3A	Digoxin 0.25 mg	Lanoxin by CVS	00173-0249	Cardiac Agent
LANOXINX3A	Tab, White, Round, Scored, Lanoxin over X3A	Digoxin 0.25 mg	Lanoxin by GSK	00339-5202	Cardiac Agent
LANOXINX3A	Tab, White, Round, Scored, Lanoxin over X3A	Digoxin 0.25 mg	Lanoxin by Caremark	00615-0518	Cardiac Agent
LANOXINX3A	Tab, White, Round, Scored, Lanoxin over X3A	Digoxin 0.25 mg	Lanoxin by Vangard	53978-3060	Cardiac Agent
LANOXINX3A	Tab, White, Round, Scored, Lanoxin over X3A	Digoxin 0.25 mg	Lanoxin by Med Pro	44514-0499	Cardiac Agent
LANOXINX3A	Tab, White, Round, Scored, Lanoxin over X3A	Digoxin 0.25 mg	Lanoxin by Talbert	51129-1311	Cardiac Agent
LANOXINX3A	Tab, White, Round, Scored, Lanoxin over X3A	Digoxin 0.25 mg	Lanoxin by Allscripts	53002-0366	Cardiac Agent
LANOXINX3A	Tab, White, Round, Scored, Lanoxin over X3A	Digoxin 0.25 mg	Lanoxin by Murfreesboro	59606-0678	Cardiac Agent
LANOXINX3A	Tab, White, Round, Scored, Lanoxin over X3A	Digoxin 0.25 mg	Lanoxin by Pharmedix	44514-0498	Cardiac Agent
LANOXINX3A	Tab, White, Round, Scored, Lanoxin over X3A	Digoxin 0.25 mg	Lanoxin by Leiner	19458-0885	Cardiac Agent
LANOXINY3B	Tab, Light Yellow, Round, Scored, Lanoxin over Y3B	Digoxin 0.125 mg	Lanoxin by Talbert	55045-2130	Cardiac Agent
LANOXINY3B	Tab, Light Yellow, Round, Scored, Lanoxin over Y3B	Digoxin 0.125 mg	Lanoxin by Eckerd	00339-5198	Cardiac Agent
LANOXINY3B	Tab, Light Yellow, Round, Scored, Lanoxin over Y3B	Digoxin 0.125 mg	Lanoxin by Allscripts	00615-0547	Cardiac Agent
LANOXINY3B	Tab, Light Yellow, Round, Scored, Lanoxin over Y3B	Digoxin 0.125 mg	Lanoxin by DRX	63552-0242	Cardiac Agent
LANOXINY3B	Tab, Light Yellow, Round, Scored, Lanoxin over Y3B	Digoxin 0.125 mg	Lanoxin by Caremark	65243-0023	Cardiac Agent
LANOXINY3B	Tab, Light Yellow, Round, Scored, Lanoxin over Y3B	Digoxin 0.125 mg	Lanoxin by Vangard	62584-0242	Cardiac Agent
LANOXINY3B	Tab, Light Yellow, Round, Scored, Lanoxin over Y3B	Digoxin 0.125 mg	Lanoxin by DSM	00173-0242	Cardiac Agent
LANOXINY3B	Tab, Light Yellow, Round, Scored, Lanoxin over Y3B	Digoxin 0.125 mg	Lanoxin by Va Cmop	59198-0232	Cardiac Agent
LANOXINY3B	Tab, Light Yellow, Round, Scored, Lanoxin over Y3B	Digoxin 0.125 mg	Lanoxin by Amerisource	59606-0677	Cardiac Agent
LANOXINY3B	Tab, Light Yellow, Round, Scored, Lanoxin over Y3B	Digoxin 0.125 mg	Lanoxin by GSK	00179-0377	Cardiac Agent
LANOXINY3B	Tab, Light Yellow, Round, Scored, Lanoxin over Y3B	Digoxin 0.125 mg	Lanoxin by Thrift Drug	53978-0202	Cardiac Agent
LANOXINY3B	Tab, Light Yellow, Round, Scored, Lanoxin over Y3B	Digoxin 0.125 mg	Lanoxin by Leiner	55154-0701	Cardiac Agent
LANOXINY3B	Tab, Light Yellow, Round, Scored, Lanoxin over Y3B	Digoxin 0.125 mg	Lanoxin by Kaiser	Canadian DIN 02242322	Cardiac Agent
LANOXINY3B	Tab, Light Yellow, Round, Scored, Lanoxin over Y3B	Digoxin 0.125 mg	Lanoxin by Med Pro		
LANOXINY3B	Tab, Light Yellow, Round, Scored, Lanoxin over Y3B	Digoxin 0.125 mg	Lanoxin by Nat Pharmpak		
LANOXINY3B	Tab, Light Yellow, Round, Scored, Lanoxin over Y3B	Digoxin 0.125 mg	Lanoxin by GSK		
LARIAM250 <> ROCHE	Tab, White, Round, Scored	Mefloquine HCl 250 mg	Lariam by PDRX	55289-0780	Antiprotozoal
LARIAM250 <> ROCHE	Tab, White, Round, Scored	Mefloquine HCl 250 mg	Lariam by DRX	55045-2459	Antiprotozoal
LARIAM250 <> ROCHE	Tab, White, Round, Scored	Mefloquine HCl 250 mg	Lariam by Hoffmann La Roche	00004-0172	Antiprotozoal
LARODOPA100 <> ROCHE	Tab, Pink, Oval, Scored	Levodopa 100 mg	Larodopa by Hoffmann La Roche	00004-0072	Antiparkinson
LARODOPA250 <> ROCHE	Tab, Pink, Round, Scored	Levodopa 250 mg	Larodopa by Hoffmann La Roche	00004-0057	Antiparkinson
LARODOPA500	Tab, Pink, Oblong, Scored	Levodopa 500 mg	Larodopa by Hoffmann La Roche	00004-0056	Antiparkinson
LASER <> DALLERGY	Tab, White, Round, Scored	Chlorpheniramine Maleate 4 mg, Methscopolamine Nitrate 1.25 mg, Phenylephrine HCl 10 mg	Dallergy by Laser	00277-0160	Cold Remedy
LASER0169	Cap, Clear & Orange	Guaifenesin 250 mg, Pseudoephedrine HCl 120 mg	Sudafed Sinus by Laser	00277-0169	Cold Remedy
LASER0172	Cap, Orange & Red	Multihematinic	Fumatinic by Laser		Vitamin
LASER0174	Cap, Clear & Green, Opaque	Guaifenesin 200 mg, Pseudoephedrine HCl 60 mg	Sudafed Sinus by Marnel	00682-1445	Cold Remedy
LASER0174	Cap, Clear & Green	Guaifenesin 200 mg, Pseudoephedrine HCl 60 mg	Sudafed Sinus by Laser	00277-0174	Cold Remedy

ID FRONT <> BACK	DESCRIPTION FRONT <> BACK	INGREDIENT & STRENGTH	BRAND (or Generic Equiv.) by FIRM	NDC#	CLASS; SCH.
LASER0181	Cap, Clear & Maroon	Multihematinic, Vitamin B 12, Vitamin C	Fumatinic by Allscripts	54569-4858	Vitamin
LASER0181	Cap	Ascorbic Acid 60 mg, Cyanocobalamin 5 mcg, Ferrous Fumarate 200 mg	Fumatinic by JLM	63369-0181	Vitamin
LASER0181	Cap, Clear & Maroon	Ascorbic Acid 60 mg, Cyanocobalamin 5 mcg, Ferrous Fumarate 200 mg	Fumatinic by Laser	00277-0181	Vitamin
LASER173	Tab, Film Coated	Ascorbic Acid 100 mg, Calcium Carbonate 200 mg, Cupric Sulfate, Anhydrous 2 mg, Cyanocobalamin 12 mcg, Ferrous Fumarate 65 mg, Folic Acid 1 mg, Magnesium Oxide 10 mg, Niacinamide 20 mg, Potassium Iodide 0.15 mg, Pyridoxine HCl 5 mg, Riboflavin 3.4 mg, Thiamine Mononitrate 3 mg, Vitamin A Acetate 4000 Units, Vitamin D 400 Units, Vitamin E 30 Units, Zinc Sulfate 15 mg	Lactocal F by JLM	63369-0179	Vitamin
LASER173	Tab, White, Oval, Film Coated	Ascorbic Acid 100 mg, Calcium Carbonate 200 mg, Cupric Sulfate, Anhydrous 2 mg, Cyanocobalamin 12 mcg, Ferrous Fumarate 65 mg, Folic Acid 1 mg, Magnesium Oxide 10 mg, Niacinamide 20 mg, Potassium Iodide 0.15 mg, Pyridoxine HCl 5 mg, Riboflavin 3.4 mg, Thiamine Mononitrate 3 mg, Vitamin A Acetate 4000 Units, Vitamin D 400 Units, Vitamin E 30 Units, Zinc Sulfate 15 mg	Lactocal F by Laser	00277-0179	Vitamin
LASER35	Tab, Orange, Round	Phendimetrazine Tartrate 35 mg	Trimstat by Laser		Anorexiant; C III
LASIX	Tab, White, Oval	Furosemide 20 mg	Lasix by Aventis	00039-0067	Diuretic
LASIX <> HOECHST	Tab, White, Oval	Furosemide 20 mg	Lasix by Drug Distr	52985-0072	Diuretic
LASIX <> HOECHST	Tab, White, Oval	Furosemide 20 mg	Lasix by Aventis	00039-0067	Diuretic
LASIX <> HOECHST	Tab, White, Oval	Furosemide 20 mg	Lasix by Merrell	00068-1215	Diuretic
LASIX <> HOECHST	Tab, White, Oval	Furosemide 20 mg	Lasix by Caremark	00339-5203	Diuretic
LASIX <> HOECHST	Tab, White, Oval	Furosemide 20 mg	Lasix by Leiner	59606-0679	Diuretic
LASIX <> HOECHST	Tab, White, Oval	Furosemide 20 mg	Lasix by Thrift Drug	59198-0224	Diuretic
LASIX <> HOECHST	Tab, White, Oval	Furosemide 20 mg	Lasix by Amerisource	62584-0067	Diuretic
LASIX <> HOECHST	Tab, White, Oval	Furosemide 20 mg	Lasix by Pharm Util	60491-0359	Diuretic
LASIX40	Tab, White, Round, Scored, Lasix40 <> Hoechst Logo or just Lasix40	Furosemide 40 mg	Lasix by Amerisource	62584-0060	Diuretic
LASIX40	Tab, White, Round, Scored, Lasix40 <> Hoechst Logo or just Lasix40	Furosemide 40 mg	Lasix by Aventis	00039-0060	Diuretic
LASIX40	Tab, White, Round, Scored, Lasix40 <> Hoechst Logo or just Lasix40	Furosemide 40 mg	Lasix by Merrell	00068-1216	Diuretic
LASIX40	Tab, White, Round, Scored, Lasix40 <> Hoechst Logo or just Lasix40	Furosemide 40 mg	Lasix by Allscripts		Diuretic
LASIX40	Tab, White, Round, Scored, Lasix40 <> Hoechst Logo or just Lasix40	Furosemide 40 mg	Lasix by Drug Distr	52985-0220	Diuretic
LASIX40	Tab, White, Round, Scored, Lasix40 <> Hoechst Logo or just Lasix40	Furosemide 40 mg	Lasix by Wal Mart	49035-0156	Diuretic
LASIX40	Tab, White, Round, Scored, Lasix40 <> Hoechst Logo or just Lasix40	Furosemide 40 mg	Lasix by Thrift Drug	59198-0068	Diuretic
LASIX40	Tab, White, Round, Scored, Lasix40 <> Hoechst Logo or just Lasix40	Furosemide 40 mg	Lasix by Nat Pharmpak	55154-1203	Diuretic
LASIX80	Tab, White, Round, Lasix80 <> Hoechst Logo or just Lasix80	Furosemide 80 mg	Lasix by Wal Mart	49035-0171	Diuretic
LASIX80	Tab, White, Round, Lasix80 <> Hoechst Logo or just Lasix80	Furosemide 80 mg	Lasix by Merrell	00068-1217	Diuretic
LASIX80	Tab, White, Round, Lasix80 <> Hoechst Logo or just Lasix80	Furosemide 80 mg	Lasix by Aventis	00039-0066	Diuretic
LASIX80	Tab, White, Round, Lasix80 <> Hoechst Logo or just Lasix80	Furosemide 80 mg	Lasix by Thrift Drug	59198-0024	Diuretic
LASIX80	Tab, White, Round, Lasix80 <> Hoechst Logo or just Lasix80	Furosemide 80 mg	Lasix by Pharm Util	60491-0361	Diuretic
LB <> GEIGY	Tab, Brownish-Red, Round, Sugar Coated	Imipramine HCl 50 mg	Tofranil by Novartis	Canadian DIN 00010480	Antidepressant
LB <> VISKEN	Tab, White, Round, Scored	Pindolol 5 mg	Visken by Novartis	Canadian DIN 00417270	Antihypertensive
LB2	Tab, Green, Round	Ergotamine Tartrate 2 mg	Ergomar Sublingual by New River	59417-0120	Analgesic

ID FRONT <> BACK	DESCRIPTION FRONT <> BACK	INGREDIENT & STRENGTH	BRAND (or Generic Equiv.) by FIRM	NDC#	CLASS; SCH.
LB210	Tab, Blue, Triangular, LB 2-10	Amitriptyline 10 mg, Perphenazine 2 mg	Triavil by New River	59417-0401	Antidepressant; Antipsychotic
LB225	Tab, Light Orange, Triangular, LB/2-25	Amitriptyline 25 mg, Perphenazine 2 mg	Triavil by Watson		Antidepressant; Antipsychotic
LB225	Tab, Orange, Triangular, LB 2-25	Amitriptyline 25 mg, Perphenazine 2 mg	Triavil by New River	59417-0402	Antidepressant; Antipsychotic
LB410	Tab, Beige, Triangle, Convex	Amitriptyline 10 mg, Perphenazine 4 mg	Triavil by Pharmafab	62542-0915	Antidepressant; Antipsychotic
LB425	Tab, Yellow, Triangular, LB 4-25	Amitriptyline 25 mg, Perphenazine 4 mg	Triavil by New River	59417-0404	Antidepressant; Antipsychotic
LB975	Tab, White, Oval, Green Ink, LB-975	Aspirin 975 mg	Aspirin by New River	59417-0975	Analgesic
LBSO1	Tab, Yellow, Round	Mecamylamine HCl 2.5 mg	Inversine by Layton	65525-0626	Antihypertensive
LBSO1	Tab, Yellow, Round	Mecamylamine HCl 2.5 mg	Inversine by Oread	63015-0626	Antihypertensive
LBSO1 <> LBSO1	Tab, Yellow, Round	Mecamylamine HCl 2.5 mg	Inversine by Siegfried CMS	17205-0626	Antihypertensive
LBVISKEN5	Tab, White, Round, LB/Visken 5	Pindolol 5 mg	Visken by Novartis		Antihypertensive
LC <> HYL	Tab, White, Oblong, Red Specks	Viscum Album 3X, Gnaphalium 3X, Rhus Tox. 6X, Aconitum Nap. 6X, Ledum Pal. 6X, Magnesium Phosphate 6X, Cinchona Off. 3X	Hyland's Leg Cramps by Hyland's	Canadian	Homeopathic
LC738	Tab, LC/738	Propranolol HCl 10 mg	Inderal by LC		Antihypertensive
LC739	Tab, LC/739	Propranolol HCl 20 mg	Inderal by LC		Antihypertensive
LC740	Tab, LC/740	Propranolol HCl 40 mg	Inderal by LC		Antihypertensive
LC741	Tab, LC/741	Propranolol HCl 80 mg	Inderal by LC		Antihypertensive
LC770	Cap, LC/770	Phenytoin Sodium 100 mg	by LC		Anticonvulsant
LCE100	Tab, Brownish or Greyish Red, Oval, Film Coated	Carbidopa 25 mg, Entacapone 200 mg, Levodopa 100 mg	Stalevo by Novartis	00078-0408	Antiparkinson
LCE150	Tab, Brownish or Greyish Red, Oval, Film Coated	Carbidopa 37.5 mg, Entacapone 200 mg, Levodopa 150 mg	Stalevo by Novartis	00078-0409	Antiparkinson
LCE50	Tab, Brownish or Greyish Red, Round, Film Coated	Carbidopa 12.5 mg, Entacapone 200 mg, Levodopa 50 mg	Stalevo by Novartis	00078-0407	Antiparkinson
LCI <> 1335	Tab, Yellow, Round	Doxycycline 50 mg	Adoxa by Lannett	00527-1335	Antibiotic
LCI <> 1367	Tab, Yellow, Cap Shaped	Probenecid 500 mg	Benemid by Lannett	00527-1367	Antigout
LCI <> 1445	Tab, Blue, Speckled, Cap Shaped, Scored	Phentermine HCl 37.5 mg	Adipex-P by Lannett	00527-1445	Anorexiant; C IV
LCI <> NVR	Tab, White, Oval, Film Coated	Aliskiren 150 mg, HCTZ 12.5 mg	Tekturna HCT by Novartis	00078-0521	Antihypertensive; Diuretic
LCI1311	Tab, White, Round, Scored	Terbutaline Sulfate 5 mg	Brethine by Lannett	00527-1311	Antiasthmatic
LCI1318	Tab, White, Oval, Scored	Terbutaline Sulfate 2.5 mg	Brethine by Lannett	00527-1318	Antiasthmatic
LCI1336	Tab, White, Round	Doxycycline Hyclate 20 mg	Periostat by Lannett	00527-1336	Antibiotic
LCI1337	Tab, White, Round, Scored, LCI over 1337	Baclofen 20 mg	Lioresal by Lannett	00527-1337	Muscle Relaxant
LCI1338	Tab, Yellow, Cap Shaped	Doxycycline 100 mg	Adoxa by Lannett	00527-1338	Antibiotic
LCI1353	Tab, White, Round	Hydromorphone HCl 2 mg	Dilaudid by Lannett	00527-1353	Analgesic; C II
LCI1354	Tab, White, Round	Hydromorphone HCl 4 mg	Dilaudid by Lannett	00527-1354	Analgesic; C II
LCI1369	Cap, Orange	Danazol 200 mg	Danocrine by Lannett	00527-1369	Steroid
LCI1382	Cap, Light Green and Light Blue	Clindamycin HCl 150 mg	Cleocin HCl by Lannett	00527-1382	Antibiotic
LCI1383	Cap, Light Blue, Opaque	Clindamycin HCl 300 mg	Cleocin HCl by Lannett	00527-1383	Antibiotic
LCI1409	Tab, Dark Green, Cap Shaped	Methyltestosterone 2.5 mg, Esterified Estrogens 1.25m	Estratest by Lannett	00527-1409	Hormone
LCI1410	Tab, Light Green, Oval	Methyltestosterone 1.25 mg, Esterified Estrogens 0.625 mg	Estratest by Lannett	00527-1410	Hormone
LCI1417	Tab, White, Round	Chloride 287 mg, Sodium 180 mg, Potassium 15 mg	Thermotabs by Lannett	00527-1417	Supplement
LDBT	Tab, Green and White, Cap-Shaped, Bilayered, Scored	Guaifenesin 1200 mg, Phenylephrine HCl 40 mg	Duomax by Capellon	64543-0142	Cold Remedy
LDM	Tab, Mottled Pink, Cap Shaped, Scored	Dextromethorphan HBr 60 mg, Guaifenesin 1200 mg	Tussibid by Capellon	64543-0171	Cold Remedy
LDM	Tab, Mottled Pink, Cap Shaped, Scored	Dextromethorphan HBr 60 mg, Guaifenesin 1200 mg	Tussibid by Sovereign	58716-0694	Cold Remedy
LDT	Tab, White to Yellowish, Oval, Film Coated	Telbivudine 600 mg	Tyzeka by Novartis	24108-0101	Antiviral
LDT	Tab, White Yellowish, Ovaloid Shaped, Film Coated	Telbivudine 600 mg	Sebivo by Novartis	Canadian DIN 02288389	Antiviral
LDY	Tab, White, Round	Glyburide 2.5 mg	Diabeta by Aventis	Canadian	Antidiabetic

ID FRONT <> BACK	DESCRIPTION FRONT <> BACK	INGREDIENT & STRENGTH	BRAND (or Generic Equiv.) by FIRM	NDC#	CLASS; SCH.
LE <> A	Tab, White, Square, Chewable, Abbott Logo (a)	Trimethadione 150 mg	Tridione Dulcet by Abbott	00074-3753	Anticonvulsant
LE10 <> APO	Tab, White, Round, APO <> LE over 10	Leflunomide 10 mg	Arava by Apotex	Canadian DIN 02256495	Antiarthritic
LE20 <> APO	Tab, White, Triangular, APO <> LE over 20	Leflunomide 20 mg	Arava by Apotex	Canadian DIN 02256509	Antiarthritic
LE250	Tab, Blue, Oval, Scored, Cobalt Logo <> LE / 250	Levetiracetam 250 mg	Keppra by Cobalt	Canadian DIN 02274183	Antiepileptic
LE500	Tab, Yellow, Oval, Scored, Cobalt Logo <> LE / 500	Levetiracetam 500 mg	Keppra by Cobalt	Canadian DIN 02274191	Antiepileptic
LE750	Tab, Orange, Oval, Scored, Cobalt Logo <> LE / 750	Levetiracetam 750 mg	Keppra by Cobalt	Canadian DIN 02274205	Antiepileptic
LEDERLE100MG-LEDERLEM46	Cap, Green, LEDERLE over 100 mg over LEDERLE over M46	Minocycline HCl 100 mg	Minocin by Lederle	00005-5344	Antibiotic
LEDERLE100MG-LEDERLEM46	Cap, Green, LEDERLE over 100 mg over LEDERLE over M46	Minocycline HCl 100 mg	Minocin by Neuman	64579-0304	Antibiotic
LEDERLE119	Cap, Pink	Indomethacin 25 mg	Indocin by Southwood	58016-0235	NSAID
LEDERLE250A31	Cap, Green & White	Ampicillin 250 mg	Principen by Lederle		Antibiotic
LEDERLE250MG-LEDERLEA3	Cap, Yellow & Dark Blue, Lederle over 250 mg on yellow half, Lederle over A3 on blue half	Tetracycline HCl 250 mg	Achromycin V by Lederle	00005-4880	Antibiotic
LEDERLE4516	Tab, White, Round	Diethylcarbamazine Citrate 50 mg	Hetrazan by Wyeth	Canadian	Antiparasitic
LEDERLE500A32	Cap, Green & White	Ampicillin 500 mg	Principen by Lederle		Antibiotic
LEDERLE500MG-LEDERLEA5	Cap, Yellow & Blue, Lederle over 500 mg on yellow half, Lederle over A5 on blue half	Tetracycline HCl 500 mg	by Lederle	00005-4875	Antibiotic
LEDERLE50MG-LEDERLEM45	Cap, Yellow & Green, LEDERLE over 50 mg over LEDERLE over M45	Minocycline HCl 50 mg	Minocin by Lederle	00005-5343	Antibiotic
LEDERLEA20	Cap, Blue, Lederle/A20	Acetaminophen 500 mg	Tylenol Ex Strength by Lederle		Analgesic
LEDERLEA33	Cap, Gray & White	Amoxicillin 250 mg	Amoxil by Lederle		Antibiotic
LEDERLEA34	Cap	Amoxicillin 500 mg	Amoxil by Lederle		Antibiotic
LEDERLEC10	Cap, Black & Green	Chlordiazepoxide 10 mg	Librium by Lederle		Antianxiety; C IV
LEDERLEC11	Cap, Green & White	Chlordiazepoxide 25 mg	Librium by Lederle		Antianxiety; C IV
LEDERLEC17	Cap, Green & Natural	Chlorpheniramine Maleate TD 8 mg	Teldrin by Lederle		Antihistamine
LEDERLEC18	Cap, Green & Natural	Chlorpheniramine Maleate TD 12 mg	Teldrin by Lederle		Antihistamine
LEDERLEC54-CEFACLOR250MG	Cap	Cefaclor 250 mg	Ceclor by UDL	51079-0617	Antibiotic
LEDERLEC55	Cap, Lavender & White	Clorazepate Dipotassium 30.75 mg	Tranxene by Lederle		Antianxiety; C IV
LEDERLEC56	Cap, Lavender & Maroon	Clorazepate Dipotassium 7.5 mg	Tranxene by Lederle		Antianxiety; C IV
LEDERLEC57	Cap, Lavender	Clorazepate Dipotassium 15 mg	Tranxene by Lederle		Antianxiety; C IV
LEDERLEC58-CEFACLOR500MG	Cap, Lavender	Cefaclor 500 mg	Ceclor CD by UDL	51079-0618	Antibiotic
LEDERLEC61	Cap, Green & Pink	Cephradine 250 mg	Velosef by Lederle		Antibiotic
LEDERLEC62	Cap, Green	Cephradine 500 mg	Velosef by Lederle		Antibiotic
LEDERLEC62	Cap, Light Green	Cephradine 500 mg	by Lederle		Antibiotic
LEDERLEC64	Cap, Gray & Red	Cephalexin 250 mg	Keflex by Lederle		Antibiotic
LEDERLEC65	Cap, Red	Cephalexin 500 mg	Keflex by Lederle		Antibiotic
LEDERLEC9	Cap, Green & Yellow	Chlordiazepoxide 5 mg	Librium by Lederle		Antianxiety; C IV
LEDERLED16	Cap, Green	Dicloxacillin Sodium 250 mg	Dynapen by Lederle		Antibiotic

ID FRONT <> BACK	DESCRIPTION FRONT <> BACK	INGREDIENT & STRENGTH	BRAND (or Generic Equiv.) by FIRM	NDC#	CLASS; SCH.
LEDERLED17	Cap, Green	Dicloxacillin Sodium 500 mg	Dynapen by Lederle		Antibiotic
LEDERLED22	Cap, Brown & Green	Doxycycline Hyclate 50 mg	Vibramycin by Lederle		Antibiotic
LEDERLED23	Cap, Blue	Dicyclomine HCl 10 mg	Bentyl by Lederle		Gastrointestinal
LEDERLED25	Cap, Brown	Doxycycline Hyclate 100 mg	Vibramycin by Lederle		Antibiotic
LEDERLED3	Cap, Orange	Acetazolamide 500 mg	Diamox by Lederle		Antiglaucoma Agent
LEDERLED35	Tab, Pink, Oval	Acetaminophen 650 mg, Propoxyphene HCl 65 mg	Wygesic by Lederle		Analgesic; C IV
LEDERLED36	Cap, Pink	Propoxyphene 65 mg	Darvon by Lederle		Analgesic; C IV
LEDERLED43	Cap, Buff & Red	Disopyramide Phosphate 150 mg	Norpace by Lederle		Antiarrhythmic
LEDERLED47	Cap, Ivory & White	Doxepin HCl 25 mg	Sinequan by Lederle		Antidepressant
LEDERLED48	Cap, Ivory	Doxepin HCl 50 mg	Sinequan by Lederle		Antidepressant
LEDERLED49	Cap, Green	Doxepin HCl 75 mg	Sinequan by Lederle		Antidepressant
LEDERLED50	Cap, Buff	Doxepin HCl 10 mg	Sinequan by Lederle		Antidepressant
LEDERLED54	Cap, Green & White	Doxepin HCl 100 mg	Sinequan by Lederle		Antidepressant
LEDERLED55	Cap, Gray & Orange	Doxepin HCl 150 mg	Sinequan by Lederle		Antidepressant
LEDERLED62	Cap, Blue & Red	Disopyramide Phosphate 100 mg	Norpace by Lederle		Antiarrhythmic
LEDERLEF15	Cap, Blue & White	Flurazepam HCl 15 mg	Dalmane by Lederle		Hypnotic; C IV
LEDERLEF30	Cap, Blue	Flurazepam HCl 30 mg	Dalmane by Lederle		Hypnotic; C IV
LEDERLEI19	Cap, Pink & White	Indomethacin 25 mg	Indocin by Caremark	00339-5471	NSAID
LEDERLEI20	Cap, Pink & White	Indomethacin 50 mg	Indocin by Caremark	00339-5473	NSAID
LEDERLEK1	Cap, Green	Ketoprofen 25 mg	Orudis by Lederle	00005-3284	NSAID
LEDERLEK2	Cap, Light Green, Blue Print, Lederle over K2	Ketoprofen 50 mg	Orudis by Lederle	00005-3285	NSAID
LEDERLEK2	Cap, Light Green, Blue Print, Lederle over K2	Ketoprofen 50 mg	Orudis by Physician Total Care	54868-2414	NSAID
LEDERLEK2	Cap, Light Green, Blue Print, Lederle over K2	Ketoprofen 50 mg	Orudis by PDRX	55289-0287	NSAID
LEDERLEK2	Cap, Light Green, Blue Print, Lederle over K2	Ketoprofen 50 mg	Orudis by Direct Dispensing	57866-4638	NSAID
LEDERLEK3	Cap, White, Blue Print, Lederle over K3	Ketoprofen 75 mg	Orudis by Physician Total Care	54868-2415	NSAID
LEDERLEK3	Cap, White, Blue Print, Lederle over K3	Ketoprofen 75 mg	Orudis by Lederle	00005-3286	NSAID
LEDERLEL15MG	Cap, Green, Lederle over L1 on one end, 5 mg on the other	Loxapine 5 mg	Loxitane by Watson		Antipsychotic
LEDERLEL15MG	Cap, Green, Lederle over L1 on one end, 5 mg on the other	Loxapine 5 mg	Loxitane by Lederle	00005-5359	Antipsychotic
LEDERLEL210MG	Cap, Green & Yellow, Lederle over L2 on one end, 10 mg on the other	Loxapine 10 mg	Loxitane by Lederle	00005-5360	Antipsychotic
LEDERLEL210MG	Cap, Green & Yellow, Lederle over L2 on one end, 10 mg on the other	Loxapine 10 mg	Loxitane by Watson		Antipsychotic
LEDERLEL325MG	Cap, Light Green & Dark Green, Lederle over L3 on one end, 25 mg on the other	Loxapine 25 mg	Loxitane by Watson		Antipsychotic
LEDERLEL325MG	Cap, Light Green & Dark Green, Lederle over L3 on one end, 25 mg on the other	Loxapine 25 mg	Loxitane by Lederle	00005-5361	Antipsychotic
LEDERLEL450MG	Cap, Blue & Dark Green, Lederle over L4 on one end, 50 mg on the other	Loxapine 50 mg	Loxitane by Watson		Antipsychotic
LEDERLEL450MG	Cap, Blue & Dark Green, Lederle over L4 on one end, 50 mg on the other	Loxapine 50 mg	Loxitane by Lederle	00005-5362	Antipsychotic
LEDERLELLC81	Tab, White, Oval	Cephalexin 250 mg	Keflex by Lederle		Antibiotic
LEDERLELLC82	Tab, White, Oval	Cephalexin 500 mg	Keflex by Lederle		Antibiotic
LEDERLEM2MINOCIN	Cap, Orange & Purple, Lederle M2/Minocin	Minocycline HCl 100 mg	Minocin by Wyeth	Canadian	Antibiotic
LEDERLEM2MINOCIN	Cap, Orange, Lederle M2/Minocin	Minocycline HCl 50 mg	Minocin by Wyeth	Canadian	Antibiotic
LEDERLEM41	Cap, Coral	Meclofenamate Sodium 50 mg	Meclomen by Lederle		NSAID

ID FRONT <> BACK	DESCRIPTION FRONT <> BACK	INGREDIENT & STRENGTH	BRAND (or Generic Equiv.) by FIRM	NDC#	CLASS; SCH.
LEDERLEM42	Cap, Coral & White	Meclofenamate Sodium 100 mg	Meclomen by Lederle		NSAID
LEDERLEN20	Cap, Natural & Purple	Nitroglycerin SR 2.5 mg	Nitrobid by Lederle		Vasodilator
LEDERLEN21	Cap, Blue & Yellow	Nitroglycerin SR 6.5 mg	Nitrobid by Lederle		Vasodilator
LEDERLEN22	Cap, Amber & Green	Nitroglycerin SR 9 mg	Nitrobid by Lederle		Vasodilator
LEDERLEP11	Cap, Brown & Natural	Papaverine HCl TD 150 mg	Pavabid by Lederle		Vasodilator
LEDERLEP29	Cap, Yellow	Procainamide HCl 250 mg	Pronestyl by Lederle		Antiarrhythmic
LEDERLEP30	Cap, Orange & White	Procainamide HCl 375 mg	Pronestyl by Lederle		Antiarrhythmic
LEDERLEP31	Cap, Orange & Yellow	Procainamide HCl 500 mg	Pronestyl by Lederle		Antiarrhythmic
LEDERLEP53	Cap, Transparent, Ex Release	Phenytoin Sodium 100 mg	Dilantin by Lederle		Anticonvulsant
LEDERLEP69	Cap, Light Pink, Black Print, Opaque	Prazosin HCl 1 mg	Minipress by Lederle	00005-3473	Antihypertensive
LEDERLEP70	Cap, Pink, Black Print, Opaque	Prazosin HCl 2 mg	Minipress by Lederle	00005-3474	Antihypertensive
LEDERLEP71	Cap, Light Blue, Black Print, Opaque	Prazosin HCl 5 mg	Minipress by Lederle	00005-3475	Antihypertensive
LEDERLEQ15	Cap, Transparent	Quinine Sulfate 325 mg	by Lederle		Antimalarial
LEDERLES5	Cap, Brown	Vitamin, Mineral	Stresscaps by Lederle		Vitamin
LEDERLET32	Cap, Peach	Temazepam 15 mg	Restoril by Lederle		Sedative/Hypnotic; C IV
LEDERLET33	Cap, Yellow	Temazepam 30 mg	Restoril by Lederle		Sedative/Hypnotic; C IV
LEDERLEU21-CENTRUMJR	Cap, Orange, Pink & Purple, Oval, Lederle U21/Centrum Jr	12 Vitamins & Minerals	Centrum by Whitehall Robins		Vitamin
LEDERLEU22-CENTRUMJR	Cap, Orange & Pink, Oval, Lederle U22/Centrum Jr	17 Vitamins & Minerals	Centrum by Whitehall Robins		Vitamin
LEDERLEV6-VERELAN360	Cap, ER, Lederle over V6 on Left <> Verelan over 360 on Right	Verapamil HCl 360 mg	Verelan by Elan Hold	60274-0360	Antihypertensive
LEDERLEV7-VERELAN180	Cap, ER, Lederle over V7 on Left <> Verelan over 180 on Right	Verapamil HCl 180 mg	Verelan by Elan Hold	60274-0180	Antihypertensive
LEDERLEV8-VERELAN120MG	Cap, Yellow, Black Print, Ex Release, Lederle over V8, Verelan over 120	Verapamil HCl 120 mg	Verelan by Elan Hold	60274-0120	Antihypertensive
LEDERLEV8-VERELAN120MG	Cap, Yellow, Black Print, Ex Release, Lederle over V8, Verelan over 120	Verapamil HCl 120 mg	Verelan by Lederle	00005-2490	Antihypertensive
LEDERLEV9-VERELAN240	Cap, ER, Lederle over V9 on Left <> Verelan over 240 on Right	Verapamil HCl 240 mg	Verelan by Elan Hold	60274-0240	Antihypertensive
LEKCT3	Tab, White, Round	Cimetidine HCl 300 mg	Tagamet by Ivax		Gastrointestinal
LEKCT3	Tab, Off-White, Round, Scored	Cimetidine HCl 300 mg	Tagamet by LEK	66685-1702	Gastrointestinal
LEKCT4	Tab, Off-White, Cap Shaped, Scored	Cimetidine HCl 400 mg	Tagamet by Schein	00364-2593	Gastrointestinal
LEKCT4	Tab, Off-White, Cap Shaped, Scored	Cimetidine HCl 400 mg	Tagamet by URL Mutual	00677-1529	Gastrointestinal
LEKCT4	Tab, White, Oblong	Cimetidine HCl 400 mg	Tagamet by Ivax		Gastrointestinal
LEKCT4	Tab, Off-White, Cap Shaped, Scored	Cimetidine HCl 400 mg	Tagamet by Rosemont	00832-0103	Gastrointestinal
LEKCT4	Tab, Off-White, Cap Shaped, Scored	Cimetidine HCl 400 mg	Tagamet by LEK	66685-1703	Gastrointestinal
LEKCT8	Tab, White, Oval, Scored	Cimetidine HCl 800 mg	Tagamet by Ivax		Gastrointestinal
LEKCT8	Tab, Off-White, Oval, Scored	Cimetidine HCl 800 mg	Tagamet by LEK	66685-1704	Gastrointestinal
LEMMON	Tab, Blue, Round	Promethazine HCl 25 mg	Phenergan by Lemmon		Antiemetic; Antihistamine
LEMMON	Tab, Yellow, Oblong	Hydralazine HCl 25 mg	Dralzine by Lemmon		Antihypertensive
LEMMON <> 99	Tab, Mottled Blue & White	Phentermine HCl 37.5 mg	Adipex-P by Allscripts		Anorexiant; C IV
LEMMON <> LEMMON	Tab	Acetaminophen 300 mg, Codeine Phosphate 30 mg	Tylenol w/ Codeine by Kaiser	00179-0038	Analgesic; C III
LEMMON <> ORAP2	Tab, White, Oval, Scored, Lemmon <> Orap/2	Pimozide 2 mg	Orap by Gate	57844-0187	Antipsychotic
LEMMON <> ORAP2	Tab, White, Oval, Scored, Lemmon <> Orap/2	Pimozide 2 mg	Orap by Teva	00093-0187 Discontinued	Antipsychotic

ID FRONT <> BACK	DESCRIPTION FRONT <> BACK	INGREDIENT & STRENGTH	BRAND (or Generic Equiv.) by FIRM	NDC#	CLASS; SCH.
LEMMON110	Tab, White, Round	Acetaminophen 300 mg, Salicylamide 300 mg, Phenylpropanol 60 mg, Chlorpheniramine 4 mg	Rhinex D-Lay by Lemmon		Analgesic
LEMMON128	Tab, White, Round	Dyphylline 200 mg, Guaifenesin 200 mg	Neothylline-GG by Lemmon		Antiasthmatic; Expectorant
LEMMON133	Cap, Clear & Green	Dextroamphetamine Sulfate 15 mg	Dexedrine by Lemmon		Stimulant; C II
LEMMON169	Tab, Yellow, Round	Opium, Bismuth Sulgal, Pectin, Kaolin, Zinc Phenolsulf	B.P.P. by Lemmon		Gastrointestinal; C V
LEMMON178	Tab, Pink, Oblong	Methamphetamine HCl 10 mg	Desoxyn by Lemmon		Stimulant; C II
LEMMON179	Tab, Blue, Oblong	Dextroamphetamine Sulfate 5 mg	Dexedrine by Lemmon		Stimulant; C II
LEMMON180	Tab, Pink, Oblong	Dextroamphetamine Sulfate 10 mg	Dexedrine by Lemmon		Stimulant; C II
LEMMON277	Cap, Green & White	Phendimetrazine Tartrate 35 mg	Statobex by Lemmon		Anorexiant; C III
LEMMON30	Tab, White, Round	Dyphylline 200 mg	Neothylline by Lemmon		Antiasthmatic
LEMMON368	Cap, Blue	Pheniramine, Pyrilamine, Phenpropanol, Phenylephrine	Allerstat by Lemmon		Cold Remedy
LEMMON37	Tab, White, Oblong	Dyphylline 400 mg	Neothylline by Lemmon		Antiasthmatic
LEMMON71	Tab, Oblong, Green & White Specks	Phendimetrazine tartrate 35 mg	Statobex by Lemmon		Anorexiant; C III
LEMMON714	Tab, White, Round	Methaqualone HCl 300 mg	Quaalude by Lemmon	Discontinued	Hypnotic; C I
LEMMON77	Tab, Green, Oblong	Phendimetrazine Tartrate 35 mg	Statobex-G by Lemmon		Anorexiant; C III
LEMMON86	Tab, White, Round	Secobarbital 50 mg, Butabarbital 30 mg, Phenobarbital 15 mg	S.B.P. by Lemmon		Sedative/Hypnotic; C III
LEMMON9	Tab, Blue & White, Oblong	Phentermine 37.5 mg	Adipex-P by Lemmon		Anorexiant; C IV
LEMMON93205	Tab, Pink, Round	Phenobarbital, Hyoscyamine, Atropine, Scopolamine	Donphen by Lemmon		Gastrointestinal; C IV
LEMMON9393	Tab, Blue & White	Phentermine HCl 37.5 mg	by Lemmon		Anorexiant; C IV
LEMMON99	Tab, Blue & White, Oblong, Scored	Phentermine 37.5 mg	Adipex-P By Physician Total Care		Anorexiant; C IV
LEOPHARMALOGO	Tab, White, Oval, Film Coated, Leo Pharma Logo=Assyrian Lion	Pivampicillin 500 mg	Pondocillin by Leo Pharma	Canadian DIN 00582247	Antibiotic
LEOPHARMALOGO	Tab, White, Film Coated, Leo Pharma Logo=Assyrian Lion	Pivmecillinam HCl 200 mg	Selexid by Leo Pharma	Canadian DIN 00657212	Antibiotic
LEOPHARMALOGO	Tab, White, Round, Scored, Leo Pharma Logo=Assyrian Lion	Bumetanide 2 mg	Burinex by Novartis	Canadian DIN 02176076	Diuretic
LEOPHARMALOGO	Tab, White, Round, Scored, Leo Pharma Logo=Assyrian Lion	Bumetanide 1 mg	Burinex by Novartis	Canadian DIN 00728284	Diuretic
LESCOLXL <> 80	Tab, Yellow, Round, Film Coated	Fluvastatin Sodium 80 mg	Lescol XL by Novartis	00078-0354	Antihyperlipidemic
LESCOLXL <> 80	Tab, Yellow, Round, Film Coated	Fluvastatin Sodium 80 mg	Lescol XL by Novartis	Canadian DIN 02250527	Antihyperlipidemic
LEV250 <> APO	Tab, Blue, Oval, Film Coated	Levetiracetam 250 mg	Keppra by Apotex	Canadian DIN 02285924	Anticonvulsant
LEV500 <> APO	Tab, Tan, Oval, Film Coated	Levetiracetam 500 mg	Keppra by Apotex	Canadian DIN 02285932	Anticonvulsant
LEV750 <> APO	Tab, Pink, Oval, Film Coated	Levetiracetam 750 mg	Keppra by Apotex	Canadian DIN 02285940	Anticonvulsant
LEVAQUIN <> 250	Tab, Pink, Rectangular, Film Coated	Levofloxacin 250 mg	Levaquin by Janssen-Ortho	Canadian DIN 02236841	Antibiotic
LEVAQUIN <> 250	Tab, Pink, Rectangular, Film Coated	Levofloxacin 250 mg	Levaquin by McNeil	00045-1520	Antibiotic
LEVAQUIN <> 250	Tab, Pink, Rectangular, Film Coated	Levofloxacin 250 mg	Levaquin by Physician Total Care	54868-4175	Antibiotic
LEVAQUIN <> 500	Tab, Peach, Rectangular, Film Coated	Levofloxacin 500 mg	Levaquin by Physician Total Care	54868-3923	Antibiotic
LEVAQUIN <> 500	Tab, Peach, Rectangular, Film Coated	Levofloxacin 500 mg	Levaquin by Janssen-Ortho	Canadian DIN 02236842	Antibiotic
LEVAQUIN <> 500	Tab, Peach, Rectangular, Film Coated	Levofloxacin 500 mg	Levaquin by McNeil	00045-1525	Antibiotic
LEVAQUIN <> 750	Tab, White, Oblong, Film Coated	Levofloxacin 750 mg	Levaquin by McNeil	00045-1530	Antibiotic

ID FRONT <> BACK	DESCRIPTION FRONT <> BACK	INGREDIENT & STRENGTH	BRAND (or Generic Equiv.) by FIRM	NDC#	CLASS; SCH.
LEVAQUIN <> 750	Tab, White, Oblong, Film Coated	Levofloxacin 750 mg	Levaquin by Janssen-Ortho	Canadian DIN 02246804	Antibiotic
LEVOT100M	Tab, Yellow, Round, Levo-T/100/M	Levothyroxine Sodium 100 mcg	by Pharmascience	Canadian	Thyroid Hormone
LEVOT125M	Tab, Brown, Round, Levo-T/125/M	Levothyroxine Sodium 0.125 mg	by Pharmascience	Canadian	Thyroid Hormone
LEVOT150M	Tab, Blue, Round, Levo-T/150/M	Levothyroxine Sodium 0.15 mg	by Pharmascience	Canadian	Thyroid Hormone
LEVOT200M	Tab, Pink, Round, Levo-T/200/M	Levothyroxine Sodium 0.2 mg	by Pharmascience	Canadian	Thyroid Hormone
LEVOT25M	Tab, Orange, Round, Levo-T/25/M	Levothyroxine Sodium 0.025 mg	Synthroid by Pharmascience	Canadian	Thyroid Hormone
LEVOT300M	Tab, Green, Round, Levo-T/300/M	Levothyroxine Sodium 0.3 mg	by Pharmascience	Canadian	Thyroid Hormone
LEVOT50M	Tab, White, Round, Levo-T/50/M	Levothyroxine Sodium 0.05 mg	Synthroid by Pharmascience	Canadian	Thyroid Hormone
LEVOT75M	Tab, Violet, Round, Levo-T/75/M	Levothyroxine Sodium 0.075 mg	by Pharmascience	Canadian	Thyroid Hormone
LEVOXYL <> DP100	Tab, Yellow, Oval	Levothyroxine Sodium 100 mcg	Levoxyl by Jones	52604-5100	Thyroid Hormone
LEVOXYL <> DP112	Tab, Pink, Oval	Levothyroxine Sodium 112 mcg	Levoxyl by Jones	52604-5112	Thyroid Hormone
LEVOXYL <> DP125	Tab, Brown, Oval	Levothyroxine Sodium 125 mcg	Levoxyl by Jones	52604-5125	Thyroid Hormone
LEVOXYL <> DP137	Tab, Dark Blue, Oval	Levothyroxine Sodium 137 mcg	Levoxyl by Jones	52604-5137	Thyroid Hormone
LEVOXYL <> DP150	Tab, Blue, Oval	Levothyroxine Sodium 150 mcg	Levoxyl by Jones	52604-5150	Thyroid Hormone
LEVOXYL <> DP175	Tab, Turquoise	Levothyroxine Sodium 175 mcg	Levoxyl by Jones	52604-5175	Thyroid Hormone
LEVOXYL <> DP200	Tab, Pink, Oval	Levothyroxine Sodium 200 mcg	Levoxyl by Jones	52604-5200	Thyroid Hormone
LEVOXYL <> DP25	Tab, Orange, Oval	Levothyroxine Sodium 25 mcg	Levoxyl by Jones	52604-5025	Thyroid Hormone
LEVOXYL <> DP300	Tab, Green, Oval	Levothyroxine Sodium 300 mcg	Levoxyl by Jones	52604-5300	Thyroid Hormone
LEVOXYL <> DP50	Tab, White, Oval	Levothyroxine Sodium 50 mcg	Levoxyl by Jones	52604-5050	Thyroid Hormone
LEVOXYL <> DP75	Tab, Purple, Oval	Levothyroxine Sodium 75 mcg	Synthroid by Jones	52604-5075	Thyroid Hormone
LEVOXYL <> DP88	Tab, Green, Oval	Levothyroxine Sodium 88 mcg	Synthroid by Jones	52604-5088	Thyroid Hormone
LEXXEL155	Tab, Film Coated, MERCK	Enalapril Maleate 5 mg, Felodipine 5 mg	Lexxel by Promex Med	62301-0027	Antihypertensive
LEXXEL155	Tab, White, Round, Film Coated, Ex Release, Lexxel 1, 5-5	Enalapril Maleate 5 mg, Felodipine 5 mg	Lexxel by AstraZeneca	00186-0001	Antihypertensive
LEXXEL2525	Tab, White, Round, Film Coated, Ex Release, Lexxel 2, 5-2.5	Enalapril Maleate 5 mg, Felodipine 2.5 mg	Lexxel by AstraZeneca	00186-0002	Antihypertensive
LF	Tab, White, Round, Abb. Logo	Warfarin Sodium 10 mg	Panwarfin by Abbott		Anticoagulant
LG <> BAYER	Tab, White, Coated, with Orange Tinge <> Triple Score on Side 1	Praziquantel 600 mg	Biltricide by Bayer	00085-1747	Antihelmintic
LG <> BAYER	Tab, White, Oblong, Film Coated, Triple Score	Praziquantel 600 mg	Biltricide by Bayer	Canadian DIN 02230897	Antihelmintic
LH	Cap	Chlorpheniramine Maleate 4 mg, Phenylephrine HCl 20 mg, Phenyltoloxamine Citrate 50 mg	Linhist LA by Pharmedix	53002-0355	Cold Remedy
LH1 <> M	Tab, White, Round	Lisinopril 10 mg, HCTZ 12.5 mg	Prinzide by Mylan	00378-1012	Antihypertensive; Diuretic
LH12	Tab, White, Oblong	Brompheniramine 6 mg	Lohist 12 by Larken	68047-0121	Cold Remedy
LH12D	Tab, White, Oblong	Brompheniramine 6 mg, Pseudoephedrine 45 mg	Lohist 12D by Larken	68047-0122	Cold Remedy
LH2 <> M	Tab, Light Yellow, Round	Lisinopril 20 mg, HCTZ 12.5 mg	Prinzide by Mylan	00378-2012	Antihypertensive; Diuretic
LH3 <> M	Tab, Light Green, Round	Lisinopril 20 mg, HCTZ 25 mg	Prinzide by Mylan	00378-2025	Antihypertensive; Diuretic
LH524	Cap	Chlorpheniramine Maleate 4 mg, Phenylephrine HCl 20 mg, Phenyltoloxamine Citrate 50 mg	by Ivax	00182-1574	Cold Remedy
LIBRAX	Cap, Light Green, Opaque, Black Ink	Chlordiazepoxide 5 mg, Clidinium Bromide 2.5 mg	Librax by Valeant	Canadian DIN 00115630	Gastrointestinal
LIBRAXROCHE	Cap, Librax over Roche <> Librax over Roche	Chlordiazepoxide 5 mg, Clidinium Bromide 2.5 mg	Librax by Roche	00140-0007	Gastrointestinal
LILLY <> 4116	Tab, White, Round, Film Coated, Imprint in Blue Ink	Olanzapine 7.5 mg	Zyprexa by PDRX		Antipsychotic
LILLY <> 4117	Tab, White, Round, Film Coated, Imprint in Blue Ink	Olanzapine 10 mg	Zyprexa by PDRX		Antipsychotic
LILLY <> DARVOCETN100	Tab, Dark Orange, Film Coated, Lilly <> Darvocet-N 100	Acetaminophen 650 mg, Propoxyphene Napsylate 100 mg	Darvocet-N 100 by Eli Lilly	00002-0363	Analgesic; C IV
LILLY <> DARVOCETN100	Tab, Film Coated	Acetaminophen 650 mg, Propoxyphene Napsylate 100 mg	Darvocet-N 100 by Nat Pharmpak	55154-1807	Analgesic; C IV
LILLY300490MG	Cap, Clear & Green, Opaque	Fluoxetine HCl 90 mg	Prozac Weekly by Eli Lilly	00002-3004	Antidepressant

ID FRONT <> BACK	DESCRIPTION FRONT <> BACK	INGREDIENT & STRENGTH	BRAND (or Generic Equiv.) by FIRM	NDC#	CLASS; SCH.
LILLY3061CECLOR250	Cap, Purple & White	Cefaclor 250 mg	Ceclor by Pharmedix	53002-0211	Antibiotic
LILLY3061CECLOR-250MG	Cap, Purple & White	Cefaclor 250 mg	Ceclor by Eli Lilly	00002-3061	Antibiotic
LILLY3061CECLOR-250MG	Cap, Purple & White	Cefaclor 250 mg	Ceclor by H J Harkins Co	52959-0027	Antibiotic
LILLY3062CECLOR-250MG	Cap	Cefaclor 500 mg	by Pharmedix	53002-0244	Antibiotic
LILLY3062CECLOR-500MG	Cap	Cefaclor 500 mg	Ceclor CD by Eli Lilly	00002-3062	Antibiotic
LILLY3111-DARVONCOMP65	Cap, Lilly 3111 <> Darvon Comp 65	Aspirin 389 mg, Caffeine 32.4 mg, Propoxyphene 65 mg	Darvon Compound 65 by Eli Lilly	00002-3111	Analgesic; C IV
LILLY3111-DARVONCOMP65	Cap, Lilly 3111 <> Darvon Comp 65	Aspirin 389 mg, Caffeine 32.4 mg, Propoxyphene HCl 65 mg	Propoxyphene Compound 65 by Med Pro	53978-3083	Analgesic; C IV
LILLY3125-VANCOCINHCL125	Cap, Also Imprinted "3125MG"	Vancomycin HCl	by Nat Pharmpak	55154-1805	Antibiotic
LILLY3144AXID150MG	Cap, Dark Yellow & Pale Yellow, Opaque, Black Ink, Lilly over 3144 on dark yellow half, Axid over 150 mg on pale yellow half	Nizatidine 150 mg	Axid by Promex Med	62301-0047	Gastrointestinal
LILLY3144AXID150MG	Cap, Dark Yellow & Pale Yellow, Opaque, Black Ink, Lilly over 3144 on dark yellow half, Axid over 150 mg on pale yellow half	Nizatidine 150 mg	Axid by Eli Lilly	00002-3144	Gastrointestinal
LILLY3144AXID150MG	Cap, Dark Yellow & Pale Yellow, Opaque, Black Ink, Lilly over 3144 on dark yellow half, Axid over 150 mg on pale yellow half	Nizatidine 150 mg	Axid by Nat Pharmpak	55154-1803	Gastrointestinal
LILLY3144AXID150MG	Cap, Dark Yellow & Pale Yellow, Opaque, Black Ink, Lilly over 3144 on dark yellow half, Axid over 150 mg on pale yellow half	Nizatidine 150 mg	Axid by Murfreesboro	51129-3144	Gastrointestinal
LILLY3144AXID150MG	Cap, Dark Yellow & Pale Yellow, Opaque, Black Ink, Lilly over 3144 on dark yellow half, Axid over 150 mg on pale yellow half	Nizatidine 150 mg	Axid by Med Pro	53978-2079	Gastrointestinal
LILLY3144AXID150MG	Cap, Dark Yellow & Pale Yellow, Opaque, Black Ink, Lilly over 3144 on dark yellow half, Axid over 150 mg on pale yellow half	Nizatidine 150 mg	Axid by PDRX	55289-0348	Gastrointestinal
LILLY3144AXID150MG	Cap, Dark Yellow & Pale Yellow, Opaque, Black Ink, Lilly over 3144 on dark yellow half, Axid over 150 mg on pale yellow half	Nizatidine 150 mg	Axid by Pharmedix	53002-1041	Gastrointestinal
LILLY3145AXID300MG	Cap, Brown & Pale Yellow, Opaque, Black Ink	Nizatidine 300 mg	Axid by Eli Lilly	00002-3145	Gastrointestinal
LILLY3170LORABID-200MG	Cap, Blue & Gray, Lilly 3170 <> Lorabid 200 mg	Loracarbef 200 mg	Lorabid by Eli Lilly	00002-3170	Antibiotic
LILLY3170LORABID-200MG	Cap, Blue-Gray, Bullet Shaped	Loracarbef 200 mg	Lorabid by Allscripts		Antibiotic
LILLY3171LORABID-400MG	Cap, Blue & Pink, Lilly 3171 <> Lorabid 400 mg	Loracarbef 400 mg	Lorabid by Eli Lilly	00002-3171	Antibiotic
LILLY3171LORABID-400MG	Cap, Coated, Lilly 3171 <> Lorabid 400 mg	Loracarbef 400 mg	by Allscripts		Antibiotic
LILLY3210	Cap, Pink & Purple	Fluoxetine HCl 10 mg	Prozac by Eli Lilly	00002-3210	Antidepressant
LILLY322020MG	Cap, Pink & Purple	Fluoxetine HCl 20 mg	by Eli Lilly	00002-3220	Antidepressant
LILLY322710MG	Cap, White, Opaque	Atomoxetine 10 mg	Strattera by Eli Lilly	00002-3227	Non-Stimulant Anti-ADHD
LILLY322710MG	Cap, White, Opaque	Atomoxetine 10 mg	Strattera by Eli Lilly	Canadian DIN 02262800	Non-Stimulant Anti-ADHD
LILLY322825MG	Cap, Blue & White, Opaque	Atomoxetine 25 mg	Strattera by Eli Lilly	00002-3228	Non-Stimulant Anti-ADHD

ID FRONT <> BACK	DESCRIPTION FRONT <> BACK	INGREDIENT & STRENGTH	BRAND (or Generic Equiv.) by FIRM	NDC#	CLASS; SCH.
LILLY322825MG	Cap, Blue & White, Opaque	Atomoxetine 25 mg	Strattera by Eli Lilly	Canadian DIN 02262827	Non-Stimulant Anti-ADHD
LILLY322940MG	Cap, Blue, Opaque	Atomoxetine 40 mg	Strattera by Eli Lilly	00002-3229	Non-Stimulant Anti-ADHD
LILLY322940MG	Cap, Blue, Opaque	Atomoxetine 40 mg	Strattera by Eli Lilly	Canadian DIN 02262835	Non-Stimulant Anti-ADHD
LILLY3231625	Cap, Mustard Yellow and Light Yellow, 6/25	Olanzapine 6 mg, Fluoxetine 25 mg	Symbyax by Eli Lilly	00002-3231	Antidepressant
LILLY32321225	Cap, Red and Light Yellow, 12/25	Olanzapine 12 mg, Fluoxetine 25 mg	Symbyax by Eli Lilly	00002-3232	Antidepressant
LILLY3233650	Cap, Mustard Yellow and Light Grey, 6/50	Olanzapine 6 mg, Fluoxetine 50 mg	Symbyax by Eli Lilly	00002-3233	Antidepressant
LILLY32341250	Cap, Red and Light Grey	Olanzapine 12 mg, Fluoxetine 50 mg	Symbyax by Eli Lilly	00002-3234	Antidepressant
LILLY323520MG	Cap, Green, Opaque	Duloxetine HCl 20 mg	Cymbalta by Eli Lilly	00002-3235	Antidepressant
LILLY323760MG	Cap, Green and Blue, Opaque	Duloxetine HCl 60 mg	Cymbalta by Eli Lilly	00002-3237	Antidepressant
LILLY323818MG	Cap, White & Gold, Opaque	Atomoxetine 18 mg	Strattera by Eli Lilly	00002-3238	Non-Stimulant Anti-ADHD
LILLY323818MG	Cap, White & Gold, Opaque	Atomoxetine 18 mg	Strattera by Eli Lilly	Canadian DIN 02262819	Non-Stimulant Anti-ADHD
LILLY323960MG	Cap, Blue & Gold, Opaque	Atomoxetine 60 mg	Strattera by Eli Lilly	00002-3239	Non-Stimulant Anti-ADHD
LILLY323960MG	Cap, Blue & Gold, Opaque	Atomoxetine 60 mg	Strattera by Eli Lilly	Canadian DIN 02262843	Non-Stimulant Anti-ADHD
LILLY324030MG	Cap, White and Blue, Opaque	Duloxetine HCl 30 mg	Cymbalta by Eli Lilly	00002-3240	Antidepressant
LILLY325080MG	Cap, Brown and White, Opaque	Atomoxetine 80 mg	Strattera by Eli Lilly	00002-3250	Non-Stimulant Anti-ADHD
LILLY325100MG	Cap, Brown, Opaque	Atomoxetine 100 mg	Strattera by Eli Lilly	00002-3251	Non-Stimulant Anti-ADHD
LILLY4112	Tab, White, Blue Print, Round, Film Coated, Lilly over 4112	Olanzapine 2.5 mg	Zyprexa by Eli Lilly	Canadian DIN 02229250	Antipsychotic
LILLY4112	Tab, White, Blue Print, Round, Film Coated, Lilly over 4112	Olanzapine 2.5 mg	Zyprexa by Pharmacy Care	65070-0192	Antipsychotic
LILLY4112	Tab, White, Blue Print, Round, Film Coated, Lilly over 4112	Olanzapine 2.5 mg	Zyprexa by Eli Lilly	00110-4112	Antipsychotic
LILLY4112	Tab, White, Blue Print, Round, Film Coated, Lilly over 4112	Olanzapine 2.5 mg	Zyprexa by Eli Lilly	00002-4112	Antipsychotic
LILLY4115	Tab, White, Blue Print, Round, Lilly over 4115	Olanzapine 5 mg	Zyprexa by Eli Lilly	Canadian DIN 02229269	Antipsychotic
LILLY4115	Tab, White, Blue Print, Round, Lilly over 4115	Olanzapine 5 mg	Zyprexa by Heartland	61392-0858	Antipsychotic
LILLY4115	Tab, White, Blue Print, Round, Lilly over 4115	Olanzapine 5 mg	Zyprexa by Med Pro	53978-3371	Antipsychotic
LILLY4115	Tab, White, Blue Print, Round, Lilly over 4115	Olanzapine 5 mg	Zyprexa by Eli Lilly	00110-4115	Antipsychotic
LILLY4115	Tab, White, Blue Print, Round, Lilly over 4115	Olanzapine 5 mg	Zyprexa by PDRX	55289-0462	Antipsychotic
LILLY4116	Tab, White, Blue Print, Round, Lilly over 4116	Olanzapine 7.5 mg	Zyprexa by Eli Lilly	Canadian DIN 02229277	Antipsychotic
LILLY4116	Tab, White, Blue Print, Round, Lilly over 4116	Olanzapine 7.5 mg	Zyprexa by Eli Lilly	00002-4116	Antipsychotic
LILLY4117	Tab, White, Blue Print, Round, Lilly over 4117	Olanzapine 10 mg	Zyprexa by Eli Lilly	00002-4117	Antipsychotic
LILLY4117	Tab, White, Blue Print, Round, Lilly over 4117	Olanzapine 10 mg	Zyprexa by Eli Lilly	Canadian DIN 02229285	Antipsychotic
LILLY4131	Tab, Ivory, Rectangular	Pergolide Mesylate 0.05 mg	Permax by Eli Lilly	Discontinued	Antiparkinson
LILLY4133	Tab, Pink, Rectangular	Pergolide Mesylate 0.25 mg	Permax by Eli Lilly	Discontinued	Antiparkinson
LILLY4135	Tab, Pink, Rectangular	Pergolide Mesylate 1 mg	Permax by Eli Lilly	Discontinued	Antiparkinson
LILLY4165	Tab, White, Blue Print, Oval, Lilly over 4165	Raloxifene HCl 60 mg	Evista by Eli Lilly	00002-4165	Antiosteoporosis
LILLY4165	Tab, White, Blue Print, Oval, Lilly over 4165	Raloxifene HCl 60 mg	Evista by Eli Lilly	00110-4165	Antiosteoporosis
LILLY4415	Tab, Blue, Oval, Lilly over 4415	Olanzapine 15 mg	Zyprexa by Eli Lilly	00002-4415	Antipsychotic
LILLY4415	Tab, Blue, Oval, Lilly over 4415	Olanzapine 15 mg	Zyprexa by PDRX	55289-0458	Antipsychotic
LILLY4415	Tab, Blue, Oval, Lilly over 4415	Olanzapine 15 mg	Zyprexa by Eli Lilly	Canadian DIN 02238850	Antipsychotic
LILLY4420	Tab, Pink, Elliptical	Olanzapine 20 mg	Zyprexa by Eli Lilly	00002-4420	Antipsychotic
LILLYDARVOCETN100	Tab, Orange, Oblong, Lilly/Darvocet-N 100	Acetaminophen 650 mg, Propoxyphene Napsylate 100 mg	Darvocet-N 100 by Eli Lilly		Analgesic; C IV
LILLYDARVOCETN50	Tab, Orange, Oblong, Coated, Lilly Darvocet N50	Acetaminophen 325 mg, Propoxyphene Napsylate 50 mg	Darvocet-N 50 by Eli Lilly	00002-0351	Analgesic; C IV

ID FRONT <> BACK	DESCRIPTION FRONT <> BACK	INGREDIENT & STRENGTH	BRAND (or Generic Equiv.) by FIRM	NDC#	CLASS; SCH.
LILLYDARVONN100	Tab, Buff, Black Print, Oval, Lilly over Darvon-N 100	Propoxyphene Napsylate 100 mg	Darvon N by Eli Lilly	00002-0353	Analgesic; C IV
LILLYDARVONN100	Tab, Buff, Black Print, Oval, Lilly over Darvon-N 100	Propoxyphene Napsylate 100 mg	by Med Pro	53978-3082	Analgesic; C IV
LILLYDYNABAC4215	Tab	Dirithromycin 250 mg	Dynabac by Eli Lilly	00002-4215	Antibiotic
LILLYF40	Cap	Secobarbital Sodium 100 mg	by Eli Lilly	00002-0640	Sedative/Hypnotic; C II
LILLYF47	Cap, Blue & Orange	Aminophylline 130 mg, Ephedrine 25 mg, Amobarbital 25 mg	Amesec by Eli Lilly		Antiasthmatic; C III
LILLYF65	Cap, Lilly F65	Amobarbital Sodium 50 mg, Secobarbital Sodium 50 mg	Tuinal by Eli Lilly	00002-0665	Sedative/Hypnotic; C II
LILLYH02	Cap, Pink	Propoxyphene 32 mg	Darvon by Eli Lilly		Analgesic; C IV
LILLYH03DARVON	Cap, Pink, with Dark Pink Band <> in Edible Black Ink	Propoxyphene 65 mg	Darvon by Eli Lilly	00002-0803	Analgesic; C IV
LILLYH17	Cap, White & Yellow	Nortriptyline HCl 10 mg	Aventyl HCl by Eli Lilly	00002-0817	Antidepressant
LILLYH19	Cap, White & Yellow, Black Print, Lilly over H19	Nortriptyline HCl 25 mg	Aventyl HCl by Eli Lilly	Canadian	Antidepressant
LILLYH19	Cap, White & Yellow, Black Print, Lilly over H19	Nortriptyline HCl 25 mg	Aventyl HCl by Eli Lilly	00002-0819	Antidepressant
LILLYJ31	Tab	Phenobarbital 15 mg	Phenobarbital by Eli Lilly	00002-1031	Sedative/Hypnotic; C IV
LILLYJ32	Tab	Phenobarbital 30 mg	by Eli Lilly	00002-1032	Sedative/Hypnotic; C IV
LILLYJ33	Tab	Phenobarbital 100 mg	Phenobarbital by Eli Lilly	00002-1033	Sedative/Hypnotic; C IV
LILLYJ37	Tab	Phenobarbital 60 mg	by Eli Lilly	00002-1037	Sedative/Hypnotic; C IV
LILLYJ64	Tab	Methadone HCl 5 mg	Dolophine by Eli Lilly	00002-1064	Analgesic; C II
LILLYJ72	Tab	Methadone HCl 10 mg	Dolophine by Eli Lilly	00002-1072	Analgesic; C II
LILLYJ94	Tab, White, Round, Scored	Methimazole 5 mg	Tapazole by Neuman	64579-0002	Antithyroid
LILLYJ95	Tab, White, Round, Scored, Lilly over J95	Methimazole 10 mg	Tapazole by Jones	52604-1095	Antithyroid
LILLYJ95	Tab, White, Round, Scored, Lilly over J95	Methimazole 10 mg	Tapazole by DRX	55045-2749	Antithyroid
LILLYJ95	Tab, White, Round, Scored, Lilly over J95	Methimazole 10 mg	Tapazole by Neuman	64579-0003	Antithyroid
LILLYNALFON	Tab, Yellow, Oblong, Lilly/Nalfon	Fenoprofen Calcium 600 mg	Nalfon by Eli Lilly		NSAID
LILLYT24	Tab, White, Round	Sodium Chloride 1 g	by Eli Lilly	Canadian	Electrolytes
LILLYT29	Tab, White, Round	Sodium Bicarbonate 10 g	by Eli Lilly		Antacid
LILLYU03	Tab, Lilly U03	Acetohexamide 250 mg	Dymelor by Eli Lilly	00002-2103	Antidiabetic
LILLYU53	Tab	Methadone HCl 40 mg	Dolophine by Eli Lilly	00002-2153	Analgesic; C II
LIMBREL52001	Cap, Teal	Flavocoxid 250 mg	Limbrel by Primus	68040-0601	Antiosteoporosis
LINK6094	Cap, Yellow & Blue	Aspirin 325 mg, Butalbital 50 mg, Caffeine 40 mg, Codeine Phosphate 30 mg	Fiorinal w/ Codeine by Major	00904-5140	Analgesic; C III
LIPIDIL100MG	Cap, Orange	Fenofibrate 100 mg	by Fournier	Canadian	Antihyperlipidemic
LIPIDILMICRO	Cap, Orange, Hard Gel	Fenofibrate 200 mg	Lipidil Micro by Fournier	Canadian DIN 02146959	Antihyperlipidemic
LIPIDILMICRO	Cap, Yellow, Hard Gel	Fenofibrate 67 mg	Lipidil Micro by Fournier	Canadian DIN 02230283	Antihyperlipidemic
LIQUIBID	Tab, White, Oblong, Scored	Guaifenesin 600 mg	Robitussin by Sovereign	58716-0604	Expectorant
LIQUIBID	Tab, White, Oblong, Scored	Guaifenesin 600 mg	Robitussin by ION	11808-0300 Discontinued	Expectorant
LIQUIBID	Tab, White, Oblong, Scored	Guaifenesin 600 mg	Robitussin by Eckerd	19458-0834	Expectorant
LIQUIBID	Tab, White, Oblong, Scored	Guaifenesin 600 mg	Robitussin by Capellon	64543-0131	Expectorant
LIQUIBIDD	Tab, Blue and White, Cap Shaped, Bilayered, Scored	Guaifenesin 250 mg IR, Guaifenesin 400 mg SR, Phenylephrine 40 mg SR	Liquibid-D by Capellon	64543-0150	Cold Remedy
LIQUIBIDD	Tab, White, Oval, Scored	Guaifenesin 600 mg, Phenylephrine 40 mg	Liquibid-D by Sovereign	58716-0648	Cold Remedy
LIQUIBIDD	Tab, White, Oval, Scored	Guaifenesin 600 mg, Phenylephrine 40 mg	Liquibid-D by Med Pro	53978-3313	Cold Remedy
LIT300 <> APO	Tab, White, Round, Scored	Lithium Carbonate 300 mg	Duralith by Apotex	Canadian DIN 02266695	Antipsychotic
LITHIZINE150	Cap, Aqua & Green	Lithium Carbonate 150 mg	Eskalith by Technilab	Canadian	Antipsychotic
LITHIZINE300	Cap, Aqua & Green	Lithium Carbonate 300 mg	Eskalith by Technilab	Canadian	Antipsychotic
LITHOBID300	Tab, Peach, Round, Slow-Release	Lithium Carbonate 300 mg	Lithobid by Solvay	68968-4492	Antipsychotic
LK	Tab, Salmon, Round, Abbott Logo	Deserpidine 0.25 mg	Harmonyl by Abbott		Antihypertensive
LL	Tab, Gray, Round, Abb. Logo	Hydrochlorothiazide 25 mg, Deserpidine 0.25 mg	Oreticyl Forte by Abbott		Diuretic; Antihypertensive
LL <> A10	Tab, White, Round, Scored, LL <> A10	Aminocaproic Acid 500 mg	Amicar by Immunex	58406-0612	Hemostatic

ID FRONT <> BACK	DESCRIPTION FRONT <> BACK	INGREDIENT & STRENGTH	BRAND (or Generic Equiv.) by FIRM	NDC#	CLASS; SCH.
LL <> A10	Tab, White, Round, Scored, LL <> A10	Aminocaproic Acid 500 mg	Amicar by Wyeth	Canadian DIN 02169754 Discontinued	Hemostatic
LL <> A4	Tab, White, Oblong, Scored	Triamcinolone 4 mg	Aristocort by Astellas	00469-5124	Steroid
LL <> A4	Tab, White, Oblong, Scored	Triamcinolone 4 mg	Aristocort by Lederle	00005-4406	Steroid
LL <> A45	Tab, White, Round, Scored, A over 45	Albuterol Sulfate 2 mg	Proventil by Lederle	00005-3062	Antiasthmatic
LL <> A49	Tab, White, Round, Scored, A over 49	Atenolol 50 mg	Tenormin by Lederle	53978-1199	Antihypertensive
LL <> A49	Tab, White, Round, Scored, A over 49	Atenolol 50 mg	Tenormin by Med Pro	00615-3532	Antihypertensive
LL <> A49	Tab, White, Round, Scored, A over 49	Atenolol 50 mg	Tenormin by Vangard	00179-1165	Antihypertensive
LL <> A49	Tab, White, Round, Scored, A over 49	Atenolol 50 mg	Tenormin by Baker Cummins	63171-1004	Antihypertensive
LL <> A49	Tab, White, Round, Scored, A over 49	Atenolol 50 mg	Tenormin by Kaiser	62224-7224	Antihypertensive
LL <> A51	Tab	Alprazolam 0.25 mg	Xanax by Vangard	00615-0426	Antianxiety; C IV
LL <> A51	Tab	Alprazolam 0.25 mg	Xanax by Nat Pharmpak	55154-5553	Antianxiety; C IV
LL <> A52	Tab	Alprazolam 0.5 mg	Xanax by Vangard	00615-0401	Antianxiety; C IV
LL <> A52	Tab	Alprazolam 0.5 mg	Xanax by Caremark	00339-4057	Antianxiety; C IV
LL <> A53	Tab	Alprazolam 1 mg	Xanax by Caremark	00339-4054	Antianxiety; C IV
LL <> A7	Tab, White, Round	Atenolol 25 mg	Tenormin by Ivax	00182-1001	Antihypertensive
LL <> A7	Tab, White, Round	Atenolol 25 mg	Tenormin by Lederle	00005-3218	Antihypertensive
LL <> A7	Tab, White, Round	Atenolol 25 mg	Tenormin by Med Pro	53978-3055	Antihypertensive
LL <> A7	Tab, White, Round	Atenolol 25 mg	Tenormin by Nat Pharmpak	55154-5511	Antihypertensive
LL <> A71	Tab, White, Round, A over 71	Atenolol 100 mg	Tenormin by Kaiser	62224-7331	Antihypertensive
LL <> A71	Tab, White, Round, A over 71	Atenolol 100 mg	Tenormin by Kaiser	00179-1166	Antihypertensive
LL <> A71	Tab, White, Round, A over 71	Atenolol 100 mg	Tenormin by Lederle	00005-3220	Antihypertensive
LL <> B01	Tab, Blue, Hexagonal	Lisinopril 10 mg, HCTZ 12.5 mg	Prinzide by Lupin	68180-0518	Antihypertensive; Diuretic
LL <> B02	Tab, Yellow, Round	Lisinopril 20 mg, HCTZ 12.5 mg	Prinzide by Lupin	68180-0519	Antihypertensive; Diuretic
LL <> B03	Tab, Pink, Round	Lisinopril 20 mg, HCTZ 25 mg	Prinzide by Lupin	68180-0520	Antihypertensive; Diuretic
LL <> B1	Tab, Pink, Heart Shaped, Film Coated, Scored	Bisoprolol Fumarate 5 mg	Zebeta by Duramed	51285-0060	Antihypertensive
LL <> B1	Tab, Pink, Heart Shaped, Scored, Film Coated	Bisoprolol Fumarate 5 mg	Zebeta by Lederle	00005-3816	Antihypertensive
LL <> B1	Tab, Pink, Heart Shaped, Scored, Film Coated	Bisoprolol Fumarate 5 mg	Zebeta by Ayerst	00046-3816	Antihypertensive
LL <> B12	Tab, Yellow, Round	Bisoprolol 2.5 mg, Hydrochlorothiazide 6.25 mg	Ziac by Lederle	00005-3238	Antihypertensive; Diuretic
LL <> B12	Tab, Yellow, Round, Film Coated, Script LL inside heart	Bisoprolol 2.5 mg, Hydrochlorothiazide 6.25 mg	Ziac by Duramed	51285-0047	Antihypertensive; Diuretic
LL <> B13	Tab, Pink, Round, Film Coated, Script LL inside heart	Bisoprolol 5 mg, Hydrochlorothiazide 6.25 mg	Ziac by Duramed	51285-0048	Antihypertensive; Diuretic
LL <> B13	Tab, Pink, Round	Bisoprolol 5 mg, Hydrochlorothiazide 6.25 mg	Ziac by Lederle	00005-3234	Antihypertensive; Diuretic
LL <> B14	Tab, White, Round	Bisoprolol 10 mg, Hydrochlorothiazide 6.25 mg	Ziac by Lederle	00005-3235	Antihypertensive; Diuretic
LL <> B14	Tab, White, Round, Film Coated, Script LL inside heart	Bisoprolol 10 mg, Hydrochlorothiazide 6.25 mg	Ziac by Duramed	51285-0049	Antihypertensive; Diuretic
LL <> B3	Tab, White, Heart Shaped, Film Coated, Scored	Bisoprolol Fumarate 10 mg	Zebeta by Duramed	51285-0061	Antihypertensive
LL <> B3	Tab, White, Heart Shaped, Scored	Bisoprolol Fumarate 10 mg	Zebeta by Lederle	00005-3817	Antihypertensive
LL <> C01	Tab, Tan, Round, Film Coated	Simvastatin 5 mg	Zocor by Lupin	68180-0482	Antihyperlipidemic
LL <> C02	Tab, Peach, Oval, Film Coated	Simvastatin 10 mg	Zocor by Lupin	68180-0478	Antihyperlipidemic
LL <> C03	Tab, Tan, Oval, Film Coated	Simvastatin 20 mg	Zocor by Lupin	68180-0479	Antihyperlipidemic
LL <> C04	Tab, Brick Red, Oval, Film-Coated	Simvastatin 40 mg	Zocor by Lupin	68180-0480	Antihyperlipidemic
LL <> C05	Tab, Brick Red, Cap Shaped, Film-Coated	Simvastatin 80 mg	Zocor by Lupin	68180-0481	Antihyperlipidemic
LL <> C33	Tab	Leucovorin Calcium 5 mg	Wellcovorin by Immunex	58406-0624	Antineoplastic
LL <> C34	Tab	Leucovorin Calcium 16.2 mg	Wellcovorin by Immunex	58406-0626	Antineoplastic
LL <> C42	Tab, Blue, Round, Scored, C over 42	Clonidine HCl 0.1 mg	Catapres by Lederle	00005-3180	Antihypertensive
LL <> C42	Tab, Blue, Round, Scored, C over 42	Clonidine HCl 0.1 mg	Catapres by Caremark	00339-6148	Antihypertensive
LL <> C43	Tab, Yellow, Round, Scored, C over 43	Clonidine HCl 0.2 mg	Catapres by Lederle	00005-3181	Antihypertensive
LL <> D11	Tab, Dark Pink, Round	Demeclocycline HCl 150 mg	Declomycin by Wyeth	Canadian	Antibiotic
LL <> D11	Tab, Dark Pink, Round	Demeclocycline HCl 150 mg	Declomycin by Lederle	00005-9218	Antibiotic

ID FRONT <> BACK	DESCRIPTION FRONT <> BACK	INGREDIENT & STRENGTH	BRAND (or Generic Equiv.) by FIRM	NDC#	CLASS; SCH.
LL <> D12	Tab, Dark Pink, Round	Demeclocycline HCl 300 mg	Declomycin by Wyeth	Canadian	Antibiotic
LL <> D12	Tab, Dark Pink, Round	Demeclocycline HCl 300 mg	Declomycin by Lederle	00005-9270	Antibiotic
LL <> D44	Tab, Purple, Round, D over 44	Dipyridamole 25 mg	Persantine by PDRX	55289-0748	Antiplatelet
LL <> D44	Tab, Purple, Round, D over 44	Dipyridamole 25 mg	Persantine by Lederle	00005-3743	Antiplatelet
LL <> D45	Tab, Purple, Round, D over 45	Dipyridamole 50 mg	Persantine by Nat Pharmpak	55154-5506	Antiplatelet
LL <> D45	Tab, Purple, Round, D over 45	Dipyridamole 50 mg	Persantine by Caremark	00339-5107	Antiplatelet
LL <> D45	Tab, Purple, Round, D over 45	Dipyridamole 50 mg	Persantine by Lederle	00005-3790	Antiplatelet
LL <> D46	Tab, Purple, Round, D over 46	Dipyridamole 75 mg	Persantine by Nat Pharmpak	55154-5507	Antiplatelet
LL <> D46	Tab, Purple, Round, D over 46	Dipyridamole 75 mg	Persantine by Lederle	00005-3791	Antiplatelet
LL <> D46	Tab, Purple, Round, D over 46	Dipyridamole 75 mg	Persantine by Caremark	00339-5109	Antiplatelet
LL <> D51	Tab, White, Round, Scored, D over 51	Diazepam 2 mg	Valium by Lederle	00005-3128	Antianxiety; C IV
LL <> D52	Tab, Tan, Round, Scored, D over 52	Diazepam 5 mg	Valium by Lederle	50053-3129	Antianxiety; C IV
LL <> D52	Tab, Tan, Round, Scored, D over 52	Diazepam 5 mg	Valium by Nat Pharmpak	55154-5554	Antianxiety; C IV
LL <> D52	Tab, Tan, Round, Scored, D over 52	Diazepam 5 mg	Valium by Southwood	58016-0275	Antianxiety; C IV
LL <> D53	Tab, Green, Round, Scored, D over 53	Diazepam 10 mg	Valium by Lederle	00005-5130	Antianxiety; C IV
LL <> D53	Tab, Green, Round, Scored, D over 53	Diazepam 10 mg	Valium by Southwood	58016-0273	Antianxiety; C IV
LL <> D71	Tab, Light Blue, Round, Scored	Diltiazem HCl 30 mg	Cardizem by Amerisource	62584-0366	Antihypertensive
LL <> D71	Tab, Light Blue, Round, Scored	Diltiazem HCl 30 mg	Cardizem by Nat Pharmpak	55154-5504	Antihypertensive
LL <> D72	Tab, Light Blue, Round, Scored	Diltiazem HCl 60 mg	Cardizem by Excellium	64125-0105	Antihypertensive
LL <> D72	Tab, Light Blue, Round, Scored	Diltiazem HCl 60 mg	Cardizem by Lederle	00005-3334	Antihypertensive
LL <> D75	Tab, Light Blue, Cap Shaped, Scored	Diltiazem HCl 90 mg	Cardizem by Eckerd	19458-0896	Antihypertensive
LL <> D75	Tab, Light Blue, Cap Shaped, Scored	Diltiazem HCl 90 mg	Cardizem by Ivax	00182-1939	Antihypertensive
LL <> D75	Tab, Light Blue, Cap Shaped, Scored	Diltiazem HCl 90 mg	Cardizem by PDRX	55289-0893	Antihypertensive
LL <> D75	Tab, Light Blue, Cap Shaped, Scored	Diltiazem HCl 90 mg	Cardizem by Lederle	00005-3335	Antihypertensive
LL <> D77	Tab, Light Blue, Cap Shaped	Diltiazem HCl 120 mg	Cardizem by Lederle	00005-3336	Antihypertensive
LL <> D77	Tab, Light Blue, Cap Shaped	Diltiazem HCl 120 mg	Cardizem by Ivax	00182-1940	Antihypertensive
LL <> F11	Tab, Lederle	Furosemide 20 mg	by Lederle		Diuretic
LL <> F22	Tab, White, Oblong, Scored	Fenoprofen Calcium 600 mg	by UDL	51079-0477	NSAID
LL <> F22	Tab, White, Oblong, Scored	Fenoprofen Calcium 600 mg	Nalfon by Lederle	00005-3559	NSAID
LL <> G17	Tab, Film Coated	Gemfibrozil 600 mg	by Vangard	00615-3559	Antihyperlipidemic
LL <> H11	Tab, Film Coated	Hydralazine HCl 25 mg	Apresoline by Caremark	00339-5145	Antihypertensive
LL <> H11	Tab, Film Coated	Hydralazine HCl 25 mg	Apresoline by Med Pro	53978-3051	Antihypertensive
LL <> H11	Tab, Film Coated	Hydralazine HCl 25 mg	Apresoline by PDRX	55289-0133	Antihypertensive
LL <> H11	Tab, Film Coated	Hydralazine HCl 25 mg	Apresoline by Amerisource	62584-0733	Antihypertensive
LL <> H12	Tab, Coated	Hydralazine HCl 50 mg	Apresoline by UDL		Antihypertensive
LL <> H14	Tab, Peach, Round, Scored, H over 14	Hydrochlorothiazide 25 mg	Hydrodiuril by UDL	51079-0049	Diuretic; Antihypertensive
LL <> H14	Tab, Peach, Round, Scored, H over 14	Hydrochlorothiazide 25 mg	Hydrodiuril by Lederle	00005-3752	Diuretic; Antihypertensive
LL <> H14	Tab, Peach, Round, Scored, H over 14	Hydrochlorothiazide 25 mg	Hydrodiuril by Nat Pharmpak	55154-5574	Diuretic; Antihypertensive
LL <> H14	Tab, Peach, Round, Scored, H over 14	Hydrochlorothiazide 25 mg	Hydrodiuril by Murfreesboro	51129-1201	Diuretic; Antihypertensive
LL <> H15	Tab, Peach, Round, Scored, H over 15	Hydrochlorothiazide 50 mg	Hydrodiuril by Amerisource	62584-0737	Diuretic; Antihypertensive
LL <> H15	Tab, Peach, Round, Scored, H over 15	Hydrochlorothiazide 50 mg	Hydrodiuril by UDL	51079-0111	Diuretic; Antihypertensive
LL <> H15	Tab, Peach, Round, Scored, H over 15	Hydrochlorothiazide 50 mg	Hydrodiuril by Lederle	00005-3753	Diuretic; Antihypertensive
LL <> J1	Tab, White, Square	Methazolamide 25 mg	Neptazane by Lederle	00005-3519	Antiglaucoma Agent
LL <> J2	Tab, White, Round, Scored	Methazolamide 50 mg	Neptazane by Lederle	00005-3520	Antiglaucoma Agent
LL <> M1	Tab, White to Off-White, Round, Scored, M over 1	Methotrexate 2.5 mg	Rheumatrex by Lederle	00005-4507	Antineoplastic
LL <> M19	Tab, White, Round, Scored, M over 19	Methocarbamol 500 mg	Robaxin by UDL	51079-0091	Muscle Relaxant
LL <> M19	Tab, White, Round, Scored, M over 19	Methocarbamol 500 mg	Robaxin by Nat Pharmpak	55154-5541	Muscle Relaxant
LL <> M19	Tab, White, Round, Scored, M over 19	Methocarbamol 500 mg	Robaxin by Lederle	00005-3562	Muscle Relaxant
LL <> M19	Tab, White, Round, Scored, M over 19	Methocarbamol 500 mg	Robaxin by Neuman	64579-0010	Muscle Relaxant
LL <> M20	Tab, White, Cap Shaped, Scored	Methocarbamol 750 mg	Robaxin by Neuman	64579-0008	Muscle Relaxant

ID FRONT <> BACK	DESCRIPTION FRONT <> BACK	INGREDIENT & STRENGTH	BRAND (or Generic Equiv.) by FIRM	NDC#	CLASS; SCH.
LL <> M20	Tab, White, Cap Shaped, Scored	Methocarbamol 750 mg	Robaxin by UDL	51079-0092	Muscle Relaxant
LL <> M20	Tab, White, Cap Shaped, Scored	Methocarbamol 750 mg	Robaxin by Physician Total Care	54868-1103	Muscle Relaxant
LL <> M20	Tab, White, Cap Shaped, Scored	Methocarbamol 750 mg	Robaxin by Lederle	00005-3563	Muscle Relaxant
LL <> M22	Tab, Peach, Round	Methyldopa 250 mg	Aldomet by Lederle	00005-3850	Antihypertensive
LL <> M22	Tab, Peach, Round	Methyldopa 250 mg	Aldomet by Neuman	64579-0018	Antihypertensive
LL <> M23	Tab, Peach, Round	Methyldopa 500 mg	Aldomet by Neuman	64579-0019	Antihypertensive
LL <> M23	Tab, Peach, Round	Methyldopa 500 mg	Aldomet by Lederle	00005-3851	Antihypertensive
LL <> M23	Tab, Peach, Round	Methyldopa 500 mg	Aldomet by Caremark	00339-5231	Antihypertensive
LL <> M6	Tab, White, Round	Ethambutol HCl 100 mg	Myambutol by Lederle	00005-5015	Antituberculosis
LL <> M6	Tab, White, Round	Ethambutol HCl 100 mg	Myambutol by Dura	51479-0046	Antituberculosis
LL <> M6	Tab, White, Round	Ethambutol HCl 100 mg	by Heartland	61392-0718	Antituberculosis
LL <> M7	Tab, White, Round, Scored, Film Coated	Ethambutol HCl 400 mg	Myambutol by Nat Pharmpak	55154-1709	Antituberculosis
LL <> M7	Tab, White, Round, Scored, Film Coated, M to left of Score, 7 to right	Ethambutol HCl 400 mg	Myambutol by Dura	51479-0047	Antituberculosis
LL <> M7	Tab, White, Round, Scored, Film Coated	Ethambutol HCl 400 mg	Myambutol by Wyeth	Canadian	Antituberculosis
LL <> M7	Tab, White, Round, Scored, Film Coated	Ethambutol HCl 400 mg	Myambutol by Lederle	00005-5084	Antituberculosis
LL <> M7	Tab, White, Round, Scored, Film Coated	Ethambutol HCl 400 mg	Myambutol by Dept Health	53808-0006	Antituberculosis
LL <> M7	Tab, White, Round, Scored, Film Coated	Ethambutol HCl 400 mg	Myambutol by DRX	55045-2763	Antituberculosis
LL <> N1	Tab, White, Round, Scored	Methazolamide 50 mg	Neptazane by Lederle	00005-4570	Antiglaucoma Agent
LL <> N11	Tab, White, Round	Naproxen 250 mg	Naprosyn by Lederle	00005-3300	NSAID
LL <> N11	Tab, White, Oblong	Naproxen 375 mg	Naprosyn by Lederle	00005-3301	NSAID
LL <> N17	Tab, White, Oblong	Naproxen 375 mg	Naprosyn by Physician Total Care	54868-2965	NSAID
LL <> N77	Tab, White, Oblong	Naproxen 500 mg	Naprosyn by St. Mary's Med	60760-0452	NSAID
LL <> N77	Tab, White, Oblong	Naproxen 500 mg	Naprosyn by Lederle	00005-3302	NSAID
LL <> P33	Tab, White, Round, Scored, P over 33	Propylthiouracil 50 mg	Propylthiouracil by Lederle	00005-4609	Antithyroid
LL <> P33	Tab, White, Round, Scored, P over 33	Propylthiouracil 50 mg	Propylthiouracil by Physician Total Care	54868-1752	Antithyroid
LL <> P36	Tab, White, Round, Scored, P over 36	Pyrazinamide 500 mg	by Lederle	00005-5093	Antibiotic
LL <> P36	Tab, White, Round, Scored, P over 36	Pyrazinamide 500 mg	by PDRX	55289-0283	Antibiotic
LL <> P36	Tab, White, Round, Scored, P over 36	Pyrazinamide 500 mg	by UDL	51079-0691	Antibiotic
LL <> P36	Tab, White, Round, Scored, P over 36	Pyrazinamide 500 mg	by Amerisource	62584-0848	Antibiotic
LL <> P44	Tab, Gray, Round, Scored	Propranolol HCl 10 mg	Inderal by Lederle	00005-3109	Antihypertensive
LL <> Q11	Tab, White, Round, Scored, Q over 11	Quinidine Sulfate 200 mg	by UDL	51079-0031	Antiarrhythmic
LL <> Q11	Tab, White, Round, Scored, Q over 11	Quinidine Sulfate 200 mg	Quinidine Sulfate by Lederle	00005-3558	Antiarrhythmic
LL <> S11	Tab, White, Round, Scored	Selegiline 5 mg	Eldepryl by ESI Lederle	59911-3254	Antiparkinson
LL <> S16	Tab	Sulindac 150 mg	by Caremark	00339-5696	NSAID
LL <> S16	Tab	Sulindac 150 mg	by Lederle	00005-3550	NSAID
LL <> S17	Tab	Sulindac 200 mg	by Lederle		NSAID
LL <> T1	Tab, Dark Red, Coated	Ascorbic Acid 600 mg, Cobalamin Concentrate 25 mcg, Docusate Sodium 50 mg, Ferrous Fumarate 350 mg, Folic Acid 1 mg, Intrinsic Factor 75 mg, Tocopheryl Succinate 30 Units	Trihemic 600 by Lederle	00005-4590	Vitamin
LL077		Diltiazem HCl 120 mg	Cardizem by Lederle		Antihypertensive
LL100	Tab, Blue, Round	Levothyroxine Sodium 100 mcg	Levo-T by Lederle		Thyroid Hormone
LL100 <> A17	Tab, Yellow, Round	Amoxapine 100 mg	Asendin by Wyeth	Canadian Discontinued	Antidepressant
LL100 <> A17	Tab, Greyish Blue, Heptagonal (7 sided), Scored, LL over 100 <> A over 17	Amoxapine 100 mg	Asendin by Lederle	00005-5391	Antidepressant
LL10X2	Tab, Greyish Blue, Heptagonal (7sided), Scored, LL over 100 <> A over 17	Loxapine 10 mg	by Wyeth	Canadian	Antipsychotic
LL112	Tab, Light Green, Round, LL/10/x/2	Furosemide 40 mg	by Med Pro	53978-5032	Diuretic
LL125	Tab, LL 1/12	Levothyroxine Sodium 125 mcg	Levo-T by Lederle		Thyroid Hormone
	Tab, Beige, Round				

ID FRONT <> BACK	DESCRIPTION FRONT <> BACK	INGREDIENT & STRENGTH	BRAND (or Generic Equiv.) by FIRM	NDC#	CLASS; SCH.
LL150	Tab, Blue, Round	Levothyroxine Sodium 150 mcg	Levo-T by Lederle		Thyroid Hormone
LL15C35	Tab, Yellow, Oval	Leucovorin Calcium 15 mg	Wellcovorin by Lederle		Antineoplastic
LL15C35	Tab, Yellow, Oval, LL15/C35	Leucovorin 15 mg	Wellcovorin by Immunex	58406-0626	Antineoplastic
LL200	Tab, Pink, Round	Levothyroxine Sodium 200 mcg	Levo-T by Lederle		Thyroid Hormone
LL200 <> SUPRAX	Tab, White, Rectangular, Scored	Cefixime 200 mg	Suprax by Lederle	00005-3899	Antibiotic
LL25	Tab, Peach, Round	Levothyroxine Sodium 25 mcg	Levo-T by Lederle		Thyroid Hormone
LL25A13	Tab, White, Heptagonal, LL25/A13	Amoxapine 25 mg	Asendin by Wyeth	Canadian Discontinued	Antidepressant
LL25X3	Tab, Pink, Round, LL/25/x/3	Loxapine 25 mg	by Wyeth	Canadian	Antipsychotic
LL300	Tab, Green, Round	Levothyroxine Sodium 300 mcg	Levo-T by Lederle		Thyroid Hormone
LL400 <> SUPRAX	Tab, White, Rectangular, Scored	Cefixime 400 mg	Suprax by PDRX	55289-0954	Antibiotic
LL400 <> SUPRAX	Tab, White, Rectangular, Scored	Cefixime 400 mg	Suprax by Lederle	00005-3897	Antibiotic
LL400 <> SUPRAX	Tab, White, Rectangular, Scored	Cefixime 400 mg	Suprax by Physician Total Care	54868-1383	Antibiotic
LL400 <> SUPRAX	Tab, White, Rectangular, Scored	Cefixime 400 mg	Suprax by Dept Health	53808-0062	Antibiotic
LL50	Tab, White, Round	Levothyroxine Sodium 50 mcg	Levo-T by Lederle		Thyroid Hormone
LL50	Tab, Light Blue, Oblong	Phenylephrine 10 mg, Guaifenesin 600 mg	Exefen PD by Larken	68047-0150	Cold Remedy
LL50 <> A15	Tab, Orange, Heptagonal (7 sided), Scored	Amoxapine 50 mg	Asendin by Lederle	00005-5390	Antidepressant
LL50 <> A15	Tab	Amoxapine 50 mg	Asendin by Lederle	00005-5390	Antidepressant
LL50A15	Tab, Orange, Heptagonal, LL50/A15	Amoxapine 50 mg	Asendin by Wyeth	Canadian Discontinued	Antidepressant
LL50X4	Tab, White, Round, LL/50/x/4	Loxapine 50 mg	by Wyeth	Canadian	Antipsychotic
LL51	Tab, White, Oblong	Dextromethorphan 55 mg, Guaifenesin 1000 mg	Exefen DM by Larken	68047-0151	Cold Remedy
LL5C33	Tab, Yellow, Round, LL5/C33	Leucovorin 5 mg	Wellcovorin by Immunex		Antineoplastic
LL5U2	Tab, Round, Light Yellow, Scored tablet	Leucovorin 5 mg	Lederle Leucovorin Calcium by Wyeth Canada	Canadian DIN 02170493	Vitamin
LL5X1	Tab, Yellow, Round, LL/5/x/1	Loxapine 5 mg	by Wyeth	Canadian	Antipsychotic
LL60	Tab, White, Oblong, Scored	Chlorpheniramine Maleate 8 mg, Phenylephrine Hydrochloride 20 mg	NoHist by Larken	68047-0160	Cold Remedy
LL61	Tab, Blue, Oblong, Scored	Chlorpheniramine Maleate 8 mg, Methscopolamine Nitrate 2.5 mg	NoHist EXT by Larken	68047-0161	Cold Remedy
LL75	Tab, Lavender, Round	Levothyroxine Sodium 75 mcg	Synthroid by Lederle		Thyroid Hormone
LLA1	Tab, Yellow, Oblong	Triamcinolone 1 mg	Aristocort by Lederle		Steroid
LLA10	Tab, White, Round	Aminocaproic Acid 500 mg	Amicar by Lederle		Hemostatic
LLA11 <> ARTANE2	Tab, White, Round, Scored, LL over A11 <> Artane over 2	Trihexyphenidyl HCl 2 mg	Artane by UDL	51079-0115	Antiparkinson
LLA11 <> ARTANE2	Tab, White, Round, Scored, LL over A11 <> Artane over 2	Trihexyphenidyl HCl 2 mg	Artane by Amerisource	62584-0434	Antiparkinson
LLA11 <> ARTANE2	Tab, White, Round, Scored, LL over A11 <> Artane over 2	Trihexyphenidyl HCl 2 mg	Artane by Thrift Drug	59198-0006	Antiparkinson
LLA11 <> ARTANE2	Tab, White, Round, Scored, LL over A11 <> Artane over 2	Trihexyphenidyl HCl 2 mg	Artane by Lederle	00005-4434	Antiparkinson
LLA11 <> ARTANE2	Tab, White, Round, Scored, LL over A11 <> Artane over 2	Trihexyphenidyl HCl 2 mg	Artane by Wyeth	Canadian	Antiparkinson
LLA12 <> ARTANE5	Tab, White, Round, Scored, LL over A12 <> Artane over 5	Trihexyphenidyl HCl 5 mg	Artane by Lederle	Canadian	Antiparkinson
LLA12 <> ARTANE5	Tab, White, Round, Scored, LL over A12 <> Artane over 5	Trihexyphenidyl HCl 5 mg	Artane by Lederle	00005-4436	Antiparkinson
LLA12 <> ARTANE5	Tab, White, Round, Scored, LL over A12 <> Artane over 5	Trihexyphenidyl HCl 5 mg	by UDL	51079-0124	Antiparkinson
LLA14	Tab, Yellow, Round, LL-A14	Amiloride HCl 5 mg, Hydrochlorothiazide 50 mg	Moduretic by Lederle		Antihypertensive; Diuretic
LLA16	Tab, White, Oblong	Triamcinolone 16 mg	Aristocort by Lederle		Steroid
LLA2	Tab, White, Oblong, LL/A2	Triamcinolone 2 mg	Aristocort by Glades	Canadian Discontinued	Steroid
LLA2	Tab, Pink, Oblong	Triamcinolone 2 mg	Aristocort by Lederle		Steroid
LLA23	Tab, White, Round	Acetaminophen 300 mg, Codeine Phosphate 30 mg	Tylenol w/ Codeine by Lederle		Analgesic; C III
LLA24	Tab, Pink, Round	Amitriptyline HCl 10 mg	Elavil by Lederle		Antidepressant

ID FRONT <> BACK	DESCRIPTION FRONT <> BACK	INGREDIENT & STRENGTH	BRAND (or Generic Equiv.) by FIRM	NDC#	CLASS; SCH.
LLA25	Tab, Green, Round	Amitriptyline HCl 25 mg	Elavil by Lederle		Antidepressant
LLA26	Tab, Brown, Round	Amitriptyline HCl 50 mg	Elavil by Lederle		Antidepressant
LLA27	Tab, Purple, Round	Amitriptyline HCl 75 mg	Elavil by Lederle		Antidepressant
LLA28	Tab, Orange, Round	Amitriptyline HCl 100 mg	Elavil by Lederle		Antidepressant
LLA353	Tab, White, Round, LLA 35-3	Aspirin 325 mg, Codeine Phosphate 30 mg	Aspirin w/ Codeine by Lederle		Analgesic; C III
LLA36	Tab, White, Round, LL-A36	Ascorbic Acid 250 mg	Vitamin C by Lederle		Vitamin
LLA37	Tab, White, Round, LL-A37	Ascorbic Acid 500 mg	Vitamin C by Lederle		Vitamin
LLA38	Tab, White, Round, LL-A38	Ascorbic Acid 1000 mg	Vitamin C by Lederle		Vitamin
LLA4	Tab, Red, Oblong, LL/A4	Triamcinolone 4 mg	Aristocort by Glades	Canadian Discontinued	Steroid
LLA4	Tab, White, Oblong	Triamcinolone 4 mg	Aristocort by Lederle		Steroid
LLA43	Tab, White, Round	Allopurinol 100 mg	Zyloprim by Lederle		Antigout
LLA44	Tab, White, Round	Allopurinol 300 mg	Zyloprim by Lederle		Antigout
LLA46	Tab, White, Round, LL-A46	Albuterol Sulfate 4 mg	Proventil by Lederle		Antiasthmatic
LLA52	Tab	Alprazolam 0.5 mg	Xanax by Ivax	00182-0028	Antianxiety; C IV
LLA53	Tab	Alprazolam 1 mg	Xanax by Ivax	00182-0029	Antianxiety; C IV
LLA54	Tab, Green, Rectangular	Alprazolam 2 mg	Xanax by Lederle		Antianxiety; C IV
LLA7	Tab	Atenolol 25 mg	Tenormin by PDRX	55289-0227	Antihypertensive
LLA7	Tab, White, Round	Atenolol 50 mg	Tenormin by Southwood	58016-0333	Antihypertensive
LLA8	Tab, Yellow, Oblong	Triamcinolone 8 mg	Aristocort by Lederle		Steroid
LLB10	Tab, White, Oval	Benztropine Mesylate 1 mg	Cogentin by Lederle		Antiparkinson
LLB11	Tab, White, Round	Benztropine Mesylate 2 mg	Cogentin by Lederle		Antiparkinson
LLB14	Tab, White, Round	Bisoprolol 10 mg, Hydrochlorothiazide 6.25 mg	Ziac by Lederle		Antihypertensive; Diuretic
LLC13	Tab, White, Round	Chlorothiazide 250 mg	Diuril by Lederle		Diuretic; Antihypertensive
LLC14	Tab, White, Round	Chlorothiazide 500 mg	Diuril by Lederle		Diuretic; Antihypertensive
LLC15	Tab, Blue, Round	Chlorthalidone 50 mg	Hygroton by Lederle		Diuretic
LLC16	Tab, Yellow, Round	Chlorpheniramine Maleate 4 mg	Chlor-Trimeton by Lederle		Antihistamine
LLC19	Tab, Yellow, Round	Chlorzoxazone 250 mg, Acetaminophen 300 mg	Parafon Forte by Lederle		Muscle Relaxant
LLC22	Tab, Tan, Round	Chlorpromazine HCl 25 mg	Thorazine by Lederle		Antipsychotic
LLC23	Tab, Tan, Round	Chlorpromazine HCl 50 mg	Thorazine by Lederle		Antipsychotic
LLC24	Tab, Tan, Round	Chlorpromazine HCl 100 mg	Thorazine by Lederle		Antipsychotic
LLC25	Tab, Tan, Round	Chlorpromazine HCl 200 mg	Thorazine by Lederle		Antipsychotic
LLC37	Tab, Green, Round	Chlorpropamide 100 mg	Diabinese by Lederle		Antidiabetic
LLC38	Tab, Green, Round	Chlorpropamide 250 mg	Diabinese by Lederle		Antidiabetic
LLC44	Tab, Green, Round	Clonidine HCl 0.3 mg	Catapres by Lederle		Antihypertensive
LLC66	Tab, White, Round	Carbamazepine 200 mg	Tegretol by Lederle		Anticonvulsant
LLC67	Tab, Green, Round	Amitriptyline 12.5 mg, Chlordiazepoxide 5 mg	Limbitrol by Lederle		Antianxiety; C IV
LLC68	Tab, White, Round	Amitriptyline 25 mg, Chlordiazepoxide 10 mg	Limbitrol by Lederle		Antianxiety; C IV
LLC69	Tab, Blue, Round	Clorazepate Dipotassium 30.75 mg	Tranxene by Lederle		Antianxiety; C IV
LLC7	Tab, Orange, Round	Chlorthalidone 25 mg	Hygroton by Lederle		Diuretic
LLC70	Tab, Peach, Round	Clorazepate Dipotassium 7.5 mg	Tranxene by Lederle		Antianxiety; C IV

ID FRONT <> BACK	DESCRIPTION FRONT <> BACK	INGREDIENT & STRENGTH	BRAND (or Generic Equiv.) by FIRM	NDC#	CLASS; SCH.
LLC71	Tab, Lavender, Round	Clorazepate Dipotassium 15 mg	Tranxene by Lederle		Antianxiety; C IV
LLD1 <> DIAMOX125	Tab, White, Round, Scored	Acetazolamide 125 mg	Diamox by Lederle	00005-4398	Antiglaucoma Agent
LLD2 <> DIAMOX250	Tab, White, Round, Scored	Acetazolamide 250 mg	Diamox by Lederle	00005-4469	Antiglaucoma Agent
LLD2 <> DIAMOX250	Tab, LL in Upper Right Quadrant, D2 in Lower Left Quadrant <> Diamox 250	Acetazolamide 250 mg	Diamox by Thrift Drug	59198-0186	Antiglaucoma Agent
LLD2 <> DIAMOX250	Tab	Acetazolamide 250 mg	Diamox by Storz	57706-0755	Antiglaucoma Agent
LLD24	Tab, Blue, Round	Dicyclomine HCl 20 mg	Bentyl by Lederle		Gastrointestinal
LLD27	Tab, White, Round	Ergoloid Mesylate 0.5 mg	Hydergine by Lederle		Ergot Alkaloids
LLD2DIAMOX250	Tab, White, Round, LLD2/Diamox 250	Acetazolamide 250 mg	Diamox by Storz	Canadian	Antiglaucoma Agent
LLD31	Tab, White, Round	Atropine Sulfate 0.025 mg, Diphenoxylate HCl 2.5 mg	Lomotil by Lederle		Antidiarrheal; C V
LLD32	Cap, Red	Docusate Sodium 100 mg	Colace by Lederle		Laxative
LLD34	Cap, Maroon	DSS 100 mg, Casanthranol 30 mg	Peri-Colace by Lederle		Laxative
LLD41	Tab, Green, Round	Doxycycline Hyclate 100 mg	Vibra-Tab by Lederle		Antibiotic
LLD71	Tab, Coated	Diltiazem HCl 30 mg	Cardizem by Med Pro	53978-2064	Antihypertensive
LLD71	Tab, Film Coated	Diltiazem HCl 30 mg	Cardizem by Ivax	00182-1937	Antihypertensive
LLD71	Tab, Light Blue, Film Coated	Diltiazem HCl 30 mg	Cardizem by PDRX	55289-0335	Antihypertensive
LLD72	Tab, Film Coated	Diltiazem HCl 60 mg	Cardizem by Ivax	00182-1938	Antihypertensive
LLD72	Tab, Film Coated	Diltiazem HCl 60 mg	Cardizem by Nat Pharmpak	55154-5523	Antihypertensive
LLD72	Tab, Film Coated	Diltiazem HCl 60 mg	Cardizem by Med Pro	53978-1235	Antihypertensive
LLE10	Tab, Beige, Oblong	Erythromycin Ethylsuccinate 400 mg	EES 400 by Lederle		Antibiotic
LLE2	Tab, Pink, Round	Erythromycin Stearate 250 mg	Erythrocin by Lederle		Antibiotic
LLE27	Tab, White, Round	Ergoloid Mesylate 0.5 mg	Hydergine by Lederle		Ergot Alkaloids
LLE28	Tab, White, Oval	Ergoloid Mesylate 1 mg	Hydergine by Lederle		Ergot Alkaloids
LLE3	Tab, White, Round	Ergoloid Mesylate 1 mg	Hydergine by Lederle		Ergot Alkaloids
LLE5	Tab, Yellow, Oval	Erythromycin Stearate 500 mg	Erythrocin by Lederle		Antibiotic
LLF1	Tab, Orange, Round	Folic Acid 1 mg	Folvite by Lederle		Vitamin
LLF13	Tab	Furosemide 80 mg	by Med Pro	53978-0927	Diuretic
LLF2	Tab, Green, Oblong, LL-F2	Vitamin, Mineral	Ferro-Sequels by Lederle		Vitamin
LLF20	Tab, Green, Round, LL/F20	Ferrous Sulfate 300 mg	Feosol by Lederle		Mineral
LLF21	Tab, White, Round, LL/F21	Ferrous Gluconate 300 mg	Fergon by Lederle		Mineral
LLF4	Tab, Pink, Oblong, LL-F4	Prenatal Vitamin, Mineral	Filibon by Lederle		Vitamin
LLF5	Tab, Pink, Oblong	Prenatal Vitamin Combination	Filibon FA by Lederle		Vitamin
LLF6	Tab, Pink, Oblong	Prenatal Vitamin Combination	Filibon Forte by Lederle		Vitamin
LLF7	Tab, Pink, Oblong, LL-F7	Prenatal Vitamin, Mineral	Filibon OT by Lederle		Vitamin
LLH1	Tab, White, Round	Quinethazone 50 mg	Hydromox by Lederle		Diuretic
LLH17	Tab, Lavender, Round	Hydroxyzine HCl 10 mg	Atarax by Lederle		Antianxiety; Antihistamine
LLH18	Tab, Fuchsia, Round	Hydroxyzine HCl 25 mg	Atarax by Lederle		Antianxiety; Antihistamine
LLH2	Tab, Yellow, Round	Quinethazone 50 mg, Reserpine 0.125 mg	Hydromox R by Lederle		Diuretic; Antihypertensive
LLH21	Tab, Purple, Round	Hydroxyzine HCl 50 mg	Atarax by Lederle		Antianxiety; Antihistamine
LLH22	Tab, Brown, Round	Hydralazine 25 mg, Hydrochlorothiazide 15 mg, Reserpine 0.1 mg	Ser-Ap-Es by Lederle		Antihypertensive; Diuretic
LLH25	Tab, Orange, Round	Haloperidol 0.5 mg	Haldol by Lederle		Antipsychotic
LLH26	Tab, Orange, Round	Haloperidol 1 mg	Haldol by Lederle		Antipsychotic
LLH27	Tab, Orange, Round	Haloperidol 2 mg	Haldol by Lederle		Antipsychotic

ID FRONT <> BACK	DESCRIPTION FRONT <> BACK	INGREDIENT & STRENGTH	BRAND (or Generic Equiv.) by FIRM	NDC#	CLASS; SCH.
LLH28	Tab, Orange, Round	Haloperidol 5 mg	Haldol by Lederle		Antipsychotic
LLH29	Tab, Green, Round	Haloperidol 10 mg	Haldol by Lederle		Antipsychotic
LLH5	Tab, White, Round	Diethylcarbamazine Citrate 50 mg	Hetrazan by Lederle		Antiparasitic
LLI11	Tab, Yellow, Round	Imipramine HCl 10 mg	Tofranil by Lederle		Antidepressant
LLI12	Tab, Salmon, Round	Imipramine HCl 25 mg	Tofranil by Lederle		Antidepressant
LLI13	Tab, Green, Round	Imipramine HCl 50 mg	Tofranil by Lederle		Antidepressant
LLI15	Tab, Pink, Round	Isosorbide Dinitrate 5 mg	Isordil by Lederle		Antianginal
LLI16	Tab, White, Round	Isosorbide Dinitrate 10 mg	Isordil by Lederle		Antianginal
LLI21	Tab, White, Round	Isoxsuprine HCl 10 mg	Vasodilan by Lederle		Vasodilator
LLI22	Tab, White, Round	Isoxsuprine HCl 20 mg	Vasodilan by Lederle		Vasodilator
LLI23	Tab, Green, Round	Isosorbide Dinitrate SA 40 mg	Isordil by Lederle		Antianginal
LLI24	Tab, Green, Round	Isosorbide Dinitrate 20 mg	Isordil by Lederle		Antianginal
LLI27	Tab, Orange, Round	Ibuprofen 200 mg	Motrin by Lederle		NSAID
LLI28	Tab, White, Round	Ibuprofen 400 mg	Motrin by Lederle		NSAID
LLI29	Tab, White, Oval	Ibuprofen 600 mg	Motrin by Lederle		NSAID
LLI30	Tab, White, Oblong	Ibuprofen 800 mg	Motrin by Lederle		NSAID
LLL10	Tab, Brown, Round, LL/L10	Potassium Phenoxymethyl Penicillin 400,000 Units	Ledercillin VK by Wyeth	Canadian	Antibiotic
LLL10	Tab, White, Round	Penicillin V Potassium 250 mg	Ledercillin by Lederle		Antibiotic
LLL17	Tab, Blue, Round	Levothyroxine Sodium 0.15 mg	Synthroid by Lederle		Thyroid Hormone
LLL30	Tab, White, Round	Lorazepam 0.5 mg	Ativan by Lederle		Antianxiety; C IV
LLL31	Tab, White, Round	Lorazepam 1 mg	Ativan by Lederle		Antianxiety; C IV
LLL32	Tab, White, Round	Lorazepam 2 mg	Ativan by Lederle		Antianxiety; C IV
LLL6	Cap, White, LL/L6	Vitamin	Lederplex by Lederle		Vitamin
LLL9	Tab, White, Round	Penicillin V Potassium 500 mg	Ledercillin by Lederle		Antibiotic
LLM	Tab	Ethambutol HCl 400 mg	Myambutol by Leiner	59606-0737	Antituberculosis
LLM12	Tab, Yellow, Oval	Meclizine HCl 12.5 mg	Antivert by Lederle		Antiemetic
LLM13	Tab, White & Yellow, Oval	Meclizine HCl 25 mg	Antivert by Lederle		Antiemetic
LLM21	Tab, Peach, Round	Methyldopa 125 mg	Aldomet by Lederle		Antihypertensive
LLM25	Tab, Blue, Round	Methylclothiazide 5 mg	Enduron by Lederle		Diuretic; Antihypertensive
LLM26	Tab, White, Round	Metronidazole 250 mg	Flagyl by Lederle		Antibiotic
LLM27	Tab, White, Oval	Metronidazole 500 mg	Flagyl by Lederle		Antibiotic
LLM28	Tab, White, Round	Metoclopramide 10 mg	Reglan by Lederle		Gastrointestinal
LLM3	Tab, Orange, Round	Minocycline HCl 50 mg	Minocin by Lederle		Antibiotic
LLM35	Tab, White, Round	Medroxyprogesterone Acetate 10 mg	Provera by Lederle		Hormone
LLM36	Tab, Chartreuse, Round	Hydrochlorothiazide 15 mg, Methyldopa 250 mg	Aldoril by Lederle		Diuretic; Antihypertensive
LLM37	Tab, Pink, Round	Hydrochlorothiazide 25 mg, Methyldopa 250 mg	Aldoril by Lederle		Diuretic; Antihypertensive
LLM5	Tab, Orange, Round	Minocycline HCl 100 mg	Minocin by Lederle		Antibiotic
LLM8 <> MAXZIDE	Tab, Off-White, Bone Shaped, Scored	Hydrochlorothiazide 50 mg, Triamterene 75 mg	by Nat Pharmpak	55154-1705	Diuretic; Antihypertensive
LLM8 <> MAXZIDE	Tab, Off-White, Bone Shaped, Scored	Hydrochlorothiazide 50 mg, Triamterene 75 mg	by Lederle	00005-4460	Diuretic; Antihypertensive
LLM9 <> MAXZIDE	Tab, Bowtie Shaped	Hydrochlorothiazide 25 mg, Triamterene 37.5 mg	by Lederle		Diuretic; Antihypertensive
LLN23	Tab, White, Round	Nylidrin 6 mg	Arlidin by Lederle		Vasodilator

ID FRONT <> BACK	DESCRIPTION FRONT <> BACK	INGREDIENT & STRENGTH	BRAND (or Generic Equiv.) by FIRM	NDC#	CLASS; SCH.
LLN24	Tab, White, Round	Nylidrin 12 mg	Arlidin by Lederle		Vasodilator
LLN5	Tab, Pink, Round	Nystatin Oral 500,000 Units	Nilstat by Lederle		Antifungal
LLN6	Tab, Yellow, Oval	Nystatin Vaginal 100,000 Units	Nilstat by Lederle		Antifungal
LLO4LEDERLE	Tab, Red & White, Oval	Vitamin, Mineral	Ocuvite by Lederle		Vitamin
LLP	Tab, White, Round	Scopolamine Hydrobromide 0.0065 mg, Hyoscyamine Sulfate 0.1037 mg, Atropine Sulfate 0.0194 mg	Colytrol by Llorens Pharm	54859-0704	Gastrointestinal
LLP	Tab, White, Round	Scopolamine Hydrobromide 0.0065 mg, Hyoscyamine Sulfate 0.1037 mg, Atropine Sulfate 0.0194 mg	Colytrol by Lex	49523-0169	Gastrointestinal
LLP13	Tab, White, Round	Papaverine HCl 100 mg	by Lederle		Vasodilator
LLP24	Tab, White, Round	Prednisone 5 mg	Deltasone by Lederle		Steroid
LLP25	Tab, Orange, Oblong	Probenecid 500 mg	Benemid by Lederle		Antigout
LLP26	Tab, White, Oblong	Colchicine 0.5 mg, Probenecid 500 mg	ColBenemid by Lederle		Antigout
LLP34	Tab, White, Round	Pseudoephedrine 60 mg	Sudafed by Lederle		Decongestant
LLP35	Tab, Red, Round	Pseudoephedrine 30 mg	Sudafed by Lederle		Decongestant
LLP37	Tab, White, Round, LL-P37	Pyridoxine HCl 25 mg	Betalin by Lederle		Vitamin
LLP38	Tab, White, Round, LL-P38	Pyridoxine HCl 50 mg	Hexa Betalin by Lederle		Vitamin
LLP39	Tab, White, Oblong	Acetaminophen 650 mg, Propoxyphene Napsylate 100 mg	Darvocet-N 100 by Lederle		Analgesic; C IV
LLP4	Tab, Pink, Round	Tridihexethyl Chloride 25 mg	Pathilon by Lederle		Antispasmodic
LLP45	Tab, Lavender, Round	Propranolol HCl 20 mg	Inderal by Lederle		Antihypertensive
LLP46	Tab, Brown, Round	Propranolol HCl 40 mg	Inderal by Lederle		Antihypertensive
LLP47	Tab, Blue, Round	Propranolol HCl 80 mg	Inderal by Lederle		Antihypertensive
LLP48	Tab, Blue, Oval	Procainamide HCl SR 250 mg	Procan SR by Lederle		Antiarrhythmic
LLP49	Tab, Pink, Oval	Procainamide HCl SR 500 mg	Procan SR by Lederle		Antiarrhythmic
LLP50	Tab, Tan, Oval	Procainamide HCl SR 750 mg	Procan SR by Lederle		Antiarrhythmic
LLP65	Tab, White, Round	Propranolol HCl 60 mg	Inderal by Lederle		Antihypertensive
LLP67	Tab, White, Round	Hydrochlorothiazide 25 mg, Propranolol HCl 40 mg	Inderide by Lederle		Diuretic; Antihypertensive
LLP68	Tab, White, Round	Hydrochlorothiazide 25 mg, Propranolol HCl 80 mg	Inderide by Lederle		Diuretic; Antihypertensive
LLP7	Cap, Red	Vitamin Combination, Stool Softener	Perihemin by Lederle		Vitamin
LLP72	Tab, Blue, Round	Amitriptyline 10 mg, Perphenazine 2 mg	Triavil by Lederle		Antidepressant; Antipsychotic
LLP73	Tab, Orange, Round	Amitriptyline 25 mg, Perphenazine 2 mg	Triavil by Lederle		Antidepressant; Antipsychotic
LLP74	Tab, Salmon, Round	Amitriptyline 10 mg, Perphenazine 4 mg	Triavil by Lederle		Antidepressant; Antipsychotic
LLP75	Tab, Yellow, Round	Amitriptyline 25 mg, Perphenazine 4 mg	Triavil by Lederle		Antidepressant; Antipsychotic
LLP76	Tab, Orange, Round	Amitriptyline 50 mg, Perphenazine 4 mg	Triavil by Lederle		Antidepressant; Antipsychotic
LLP8	Tab, Maroon, Oblong	Vitamin, Mineral	Peritinic by Lederle		Vitamin
LLP9	Cap, White	Vitamin Combination	Pronemia by Lederle		Vitamin
LLQ13	Tab, White, Round	Quinidine Gluconate SR 324 mg	Quinaglute by Lederle		Antiarrhythmic
LLS1	Tab, Orange, Oblong	Vitamin	Stresstab 600 by Lederle		Vitamin
LLS12	Tab, White, Round	Hydrochlorothiazide 25 mg, Spironolactone 25 mg	Aldactazide by Lederle		Diuretic; Antihypertensive

ID FRONT <> BACK	DESCRIPTION FRONT <> BACK	INGREDIENT & STRENGTH	BRAND (or Generic Equiv.) by FIRM	NDC#	CLASS; SCH.
LLS13	Tab, White, Round	Spironolactone 25 mg	Aldactone by Lederle		Diuretic
LLS14	Tab, Brown, Round	Sulfasalazine 500 mg	Azulfidine by Lederle		Gastrointestinal
LLS2	Tab, Red, Oblong	Vitamin, Mineral	Stresstab 600 FE by Lederle		Vitamin
LLS3	Tab, Peach, Oblong	Vitamin, Mineral	Stresstab 600 Zn by Lederle		Vitamin
LLT1	Tab, Red, Oblong	Vitamin Combination	Trihemic 600 by Lederle		Vitamin
LLT10	Tab, Orange, Round	Thioridazine 10 mg	Mellaril by Lederle		Antipsychotic
LLT11	Tab, White, Round	Thiamine HCl 50 mg	Betalin by Lederle		Vitamin
LLT12	Tab, White, Round	Thiamine HCl 100 mg	Betalin by Lederle		Vitamin
LLT13	Tab, White, Round	Sulfamethoxazole 400 mg, Trimethoprim 80 mg	Bactrim by Lederle		Antibiotic
LLT14	Tab, Tan, Round	Thyroid 65 mg	by Lederle		Thyroid Hormone
LLT16	Tab, White, Oval	Sulfamethoxazole 800 mg, Trimethoprim 160 mg	Bactrim DS by Lederle		Antibiotic
LLT17	Tab, White, Round	Tolbutamide 500 mg	Orinase by Lederle		Antidiabetic
LLT19	Tab, White, Round	Tolazamide 100 mg	Tolinase by Lederle		Antidiabetic
LLT20	Tab, White, Round	Tolazamide 250 mg	Tolinase by Lederle		Antidiabetic
LLT22	Tab, White, Round	Tolazamide 500 mg	Tolinase by Lederle		Antidiabetic
LLT23	Tab, White, Round	Triprolidine 2.5 mg, Pseudoephedrine 60 mg	Actifed by Lederle		Cold Remedy
LLT25	Tab, Orange, Round	Thioridazine 25 mg	Mellaril by Lederle		Antipsychotic
LLT29	Tab, White, Round	Trazodone HCl 50 mg	Desyrel by Lederle		Antidepressant
LLT30	Tab, White, Round	Trazodone HCl 100 mg	Desyrel by Lederle		Antidepressant
LLT3150100	Tab, White, Rectangular, LL T31-50/100	Trazodone HCl 150 mg	Desyrel by Lederle		Antidepressant
LLT34	Tab, White, Round	Theophylline Anhydrous CR 100 mg	Theo-Dur by Lederle		Antiasthmatic
LLT35	Tab, White, Oval	Theophylline Anhydrous CR 200 mg	Theo-Dur by Lederle		Antiasthmatic
LLT36	Tab, White, Oblong	Theophylline Anhydrous CR 300 mg	Theo-Dur by Lederle		Antiasthmatic
LLU1	Tab, Yellow, Round	Folic Acid 5 mg	Folvite by Wyeth	Canadian	Vitamin
LLU13	Tab, White, Round, LL/U13	Calcium Carbimide 50 mg	Temposil by Wyeth	Canadian	Vitamin; Mineral
LLU4	Tab, White, Round	Aminophylline 100 mg	Aminophylline by Lederle		Antiasthmatic
LLU5	Tab, White, Round	Aminophylline 200 mg	Aminophylline by Lederle		Antiasthmatic
LLV4	Tab, White, Round	Verapamil HCl 80 mg	Isoptin by Lederle		Antihypertensive
LLV5	Tab, White, Round	Verapamil HCl 120 mg	Isoptin by Lederle		Antihypertensive
LM	Tab, Lavender, Round, Abbott Logo	Warfarin Sodium 2 mg	Panwarfin by Abbott		Anticoagulant
LMT <> 25	Tab, White, Round, Orally Disintegrating	Lamotrigine 25 mg	Lamictal ODT by GSK	00173-0772	Anticonvulsant
LMT <> 50	Tab, White, Round, Orally Disintegrating	Lamotrigine 50 mg	Lamictal ODT by GSK	00173-0774	Anticonvulsant
LMT100 <> TARO	Tab, Peach, Round	Lamotrigine 100 mg	Lamictal by Taro	51672-4131	Anticonvulsant
LMT150 <> TARO	Tab, Off White, Round	Lamotrigine 150 mg	Lamictal by Taro	51672-4132	Anticonvulsant
LMT200 <> TARO	Tab, Light Blue, Round	Lamotrigine 200 mg	Lamictal by Taro	51672-4133	Anticonvulsant
LMT25 <> TARO	Tab, White, Round	Lamotrigine 25 mg	Lamictal by Taro	51672-4130	Anticonvulsant
LN	Tab, Orange, Round, Abb. Logo	Warfarin Sodium 2.5 mg	Panwarfin by Abbott		Anticoagulant
LN	Tab, Salmon Pink, Film Coated	Fludarabine Phosphate 10 mg	Fludarabine Phosphate by Bayer by URL Mutual	45414-1311	Cancer Treatment
LN144500	Cap	Cephalexin 500 mg	Amoxil by URL Mutual	00677-1159	Antibiotic
LN259724	Cap	Amoxicillin 250 mg	Amoxil by URL Mutual	00677-0660	Antibiotic
LN382	Cap, Yellow	Clofibrate 500 mg	Atromid-S by Novopharm	43806-0382	Antihyperlipidemic
LN716500	Cap	Amoxicillin 500 mg	Amoxil by URL Mutual	00677-0661	Antibiotic
LN72Y250	Cap	Amoxicillin 250 mg	Amoxil by Sandoz	Discontinued	Antibiotic

ID FRONT <> BACK	DESCRIPTION FRONT <> BACK	INGREDIENT & STRENGTH	BRAND (or Generic Equiv.) by FIRM	NDC#	CLASS; SCH.
LNK25	Cap, Pink & Natural	Diphenhydramine HCl 25 mg	Benadryl by Ivax	00182-0492 Discontinued	Antihistamine
LNK50	Cap	Diphenhydramine HCl 50 mg	Benadryl by Ivax	00182-0135	Antihistamine
LNK50	Cap	Diphenhydramine HCl 50 mg	Benadryl by LNK	50844-0108	Antihistamine
LO	Tab, Peach, Round, Abbott Logo	Warfarin Sodium 5 mg	Panwarfin by Abbott		Anticoagulant
LO10 <> APO	Tab, White, Oval, Scored, LO / 10	Loratadine 10 mg	Claritin by Apotex	Canadian DIN 02243880	Antihistamine
LOBAC0176SEATRACE	Cap, Egg Shell, Lobac-0176 <> Seatrace	Acetaminophen 300 mg, Phenyltoloxamine Citrate 20 mg, Salicylamide 200 mg	Durabac by Seatrace	00551-0176	Analgesic
LODINE200	Cap, Gray w/ Red Bands	Etodolac 200 mg	Lodine by Wyeth	52903-0738	NSAID
LODINE200	Cap, Gray w/ Red Bands	Etodolac 200 mg	Lodine by Ayerst	00046-0738	NSAID
LODINE300	Cap, Gray w/ Red Bands	Etodolac 200 mg	Lodine by Ayerst	00046-0739	NSAID
LODINE300	Cap, Gray w/ Red Bands	Etodolac 300 mg	Lodine by Wyeth	52903-0739	NSAID
LODINE300	Cap, Gray w/ Red Bands	Etodolac 300 mg	Lodine by Heartland	61392-0909	NSAID
LODINE400	Tab, Yellowish Orange, Oval	Etodolac 400 mg	Lodine by Wyeth	52903-0761	NSAID
LODINE400	Tab, Yellowish Orange, Oval	Etodolac 400 mg	Lodine by PDRX	55289-0644	NSAID
LODINE400	Tab, Yellowish Orange, Oval	Etodolac 400 mg	Lodine by Wyeth	00046-0761	NSAID
LODINE500	Tab, Blue, Black Print, Oval	Etodolac 500 mg	Lodine by H J Harkins Co	52959-0445	NSAID
LODINE500	Tab, Blue, Black Print, Oval	Etodolac 500 mg	Lodine by Ayerst	00046-0787	NSAID
LODINE500	Tab, Blue, Black Print, Oval	Etodolac 500 mg	Lodine by PDRX	55289-0197	NSAID
LODINE500	Tab, Blue, Black Print, Oval	Etodolac 500 mg	Lodine by Wyeth	52903-0787	NSAID
LODINE500	Tab, Blue, Black Print, Oval	Etodolac 500 mg	Lodine by Physician Total Care	54868-3856	NSAID
LODINEXL400	Tab, Red, Black Print, Oval, Film Coated, Lodine XL over 400	Etodolac 400 mg	Lodine XL by Murfreesboro	51129-1145	NSAID
LODINEXL400	Tab, Red, Black Print, Oval, Film Coated, Lodine XL over 400	Etodolac 400 mg	Lodine XL by Ayerst	00046-0829	NSAID
LODINEXL400	Tab, Red, Black Print, Oval, Film Coated, Lodine XL over 400	Etodolac 400 mg	Lodine XL by Physician Total Care	54868-3901	NSAID
LODINEXL400	Tab, Red, Black Print, Oval, Film Coated, Lodine XL over 400	Etodolac 400 mg	Lodine XL by PDRX	55289-0237	NSAID
LODINEXL400	Tab, Red, Black Print, Oval, Film Coated, Lodine XL over 400	Etodolac 400 mg	Lodine XL by Caremark	00339-5710	NSAID
LODINEXL400	Tab, Red, Black Print, Oval, Film Coated, Lodine XL over 400	Etodolac 400 mg	Lodine XL by Compumed	00403-0561	NSAID
LODINEXL500	Tab, Grayish Green, Black Print, Oval, Film Coated, Lodine XL over 500	Etodolac 500 mg	Lodine XL by Wyeth	52903-0839	NSAID
LODINEXL500	Tab, Grayish Green, Black Print, Oval, Film Coated, Lodine XL over 500	Etodolac 500 mg	Lodine XL by Ayerst	00046-0839	NSAID
LODINEXL600	Tab, Light Gray, Oval, Film Coated, Lodine XL over 600	Etodolac 600 mg	Lodine XL by Wyeth	52903-0831	NSAID
LODINEXL600	Tab, Light Gray, Oval, Film Coated, Lodine XL over 600	Etodolac 600 mg	Lodine XL by Ayerst	00046-0831	NSAID
LODOSYN <> 511	Tab, Orange, Round, Scored	Carbidopa 25 mg	Lodosyn by BMS	00056-0511	Antiparkinson
LODRANE24	Cap, White, Extended Release, "Lodrane 24" on both cap and body	Brompheniramine Maleate 12 mg	Lodrane 24 by ECR	00095-1200	Cold Remedy
LODRANE24D	Cap, Extended Release	Brompheniramine Maleate 12 mg, Pseudoephedrine HCl 90 mg	Lodrane 24D by ECR	00095-1290	Cold Remedy
LOFIBRA134MGGATE323	Cap, Light Blue, Lofibra <> 134 mg on cap, Gate 323 on body	Fenofibrate 134 mg	Lofibra by Gate	57844-0323	Antihyperlipidemic
LOFIBRA200MGGATE324	Cap, Orange, N <> 412 on cap, 200 on body	Fenofibrate 200 mg	Lofibra by Gate	57844-0324	Antihyperlipidemic
LOFIBRA67MGGATE322	Cap, Pink, Lofibra <> 67 mg on cap, Gate 322 on body	Fenofibrate 67 mg	Lofibra by Gate	57844-0322	Antihyperlipidemic
LOGO <> 3875500	Tab, 387 5 over 500	Acetaminophen 500 mg, Hydrocodone Bitartrate 5 mg	Vicodin by Quality Care	60346-0442	Analgesic; C III
LOGO063	Tab, White, Round, Scored, Logo 063	Lorazepam 2 mg	Ativan by Nat Pharmpak	55154-1350	Antianxiety; C IV
LONITEN10	Tab, White, Round, Scored, Loniten over 10	Minoxidil 10 mg	Loniten by Pharmacia	00009-0137	Antihypertensive

ID FRONT <> BACK	DESCRIPTION FRONT <> BACK	INGREDIENT & STRENGTH	BRAND (or Generic Equiv.) by FIRM	NDC#	CLASS: SCH.
LOP <> 2MG	Tab, Light Green, Cap Shaped	Loperamide 2 mg	Imodium by Novopharm	Canadian DIN 02213591	Antidiarrheal
LOPERAMIDE <> P2MG	Tab, Green, Cap Shaped, Scored, P/2 mg	Loperamide 2 mg	Imodium by Pharmascience	Canadian DIN 02228351	Antidiarrheal
LOPID <> PD737	Tab, White, Blue Print, Oval, Scored, Film Coated	Gemfibrozil 600 mg	Lopid by Parke Davis	00071-0737	Antihyperlipidemic
LOPID600MG <> PARKEDAVIS	Tab, White, Ellipsoid, Film Coated	Gemfibrozil 600 mg	by Parke Davis	Canadian DIN 00659606	Antihyperlipidemic
LORABID200MG-LILLY3170	Cap, Blue & Gray, Lorabid 200 mg <> Lilly 3170	Loracarbef 200 mg	Lorabid by Eli Lilly	00002-3170	Antibiotic
LORABID400MG-LILLY3171	Cap, Lorabid 400 mg <> Lilly 3171	Loracarbef 400 mg	Lorabid by Eli Lilly	00002-3171	Antibiotic
LORABID400MG-LILLY3171	Cap, Coated, Lorabid 400 mg <> Lilly 3171	Loracarbef 400 mg	by Allscripts		Antibiotic
LORELCO250	Tab, White, Black Print, Round, Lorelco over 250	Probucol 250 mg	by Merrell	00068-0051	Antihyperlipidemic
LORELCO250	Tab, White, Black Print, Round, Lorelco over 250	Probucol 250 mg	Lorelco by Marion	Canadian	Antihyperlipidemic
LOSEC10	Tab, Pink, Round, Delayed Release	Omeprazole 10 mg	Losec by AstraZeneca	Canadian DIN 02230737	Gastrointestinal
LOSEC20	Tab, Brown & Red, Round, Delayed Release	Omeprazole 20 mg	Losec by AstraZeneca	Canadian DIN 02190915	Gastrointestinal
LOTENSIN <> 10	Tab, Dark Yellow, Round, Film Coated	Benazepril HCl 10 mg	Lotensin by Southwood	58016-0420	Antihypertensive
LOTENSIN <> 10	Tab, Dark Yellow, Round, Film Coated	Benazepril HCl 10 mg	Lotensin by DRX	55045-2374	Antihypertensive
LOTENSIN <> 10	Tab, Dark Yellow, Round, Film Coated	Benazepril HCl 10 mg	Lotensin by Amerisource	62584-0063	Antihypertensive
LOTENSIN <> 10	Tab, Dark Yellow, Round, Film Coated	Benazepril HCl 10 mg	Lotensin by PDRX	55289-0109	Antihypertensive
LOTENSIN <> 10	Tab, Dark Yellow, Round, Film Coated	Benazepril HCl 10 mg	Lotensin by Pharm Util	60491-0383	Antihypertensive
LOTENSIN <> 10	Tab, Dark Yellow, Round, Film Coated	Benazepril HCl 10 mg	Lotensin by Novartis	00078-0448	Antihypertensive
LOTENSIN <> 20	Tab, Beige, Round, Film Coated	Benazepril HCl 20 mg	Lotensin by Amerisource	62584-0079	Antihypertensive
LOTENSIN <> 20	Tab, Beige, Round, Film Coated	Benazepril HCl 20 mg	Lotensin by PDRX	55289-0086	Antihypertensive
LOTENSIN <> 20	Tab, Beige, Round, Film Coated	Benazepril HCl 20 mg	Lotensin by Novartis	00078-0449	Antihypertensive
LOTENSIN <> 40	Tab, Rose, Round, Film Coated	Benazepril HCl 40 mg	Lotensin by Physician Total Care	54868-2352	Antihypertensive
LOTENSIN <> 40	Tab, Rose, Round, Film Coated	Benazepril HCl 40 mg	Lotensin by Novartis	00078-0450	Antihypertensive
LOTENSIN <> 5	Tab, Light Yellow, Round	Benazepril HCl 5 mg	Lotensin by Southwood	58016-0264	Antihypertensive
LOTENSIN <> 5	Tab, Light Yellow, Round	Benazepril HCl 5 mg	Lotensin by Novartis	00078-0447	Antihypertensive
LOTENSINHCT <> 57	Tab, White, Oblong, Scored	Benazepril HCl 5 mg, Hydrochlorothiazide 6.25 mg	Lotensin HCT by Novartis	00083-0057	Antihypertensive; Diuretic
LOTENSINHCT <> 57	Tab, White, Oblong, Coated	Benazepril HCl 5 mg, Hydrochlorothiazide 6.25 mg	Lotensin HCT by Novartis	00083-0451	Antihypertensive; Diuretic
LOTENSINHCT <> 7272	Tab, Light Pink, Oblong, Scored	Benazepril HCl 10 mg, Hydrochlorothiazide 12.5 mg	Lotensin HCT by Novartis	00083-0072	Antihypertensive; Diuretic
LOTENSINHCT <> 7272	Tab, Light Pink, Oblong, Coated	Benazepril HCl 10 mg, Hydrochlorothiazide 12.5 mg	Lotensin HCT by Novartis	00083-0452	Antihypertensive; Diuretic
LOTENSINHCT <> 7474	Tab, Greyish Violet, Oblong, Scored	Benazepril HCl 20 mg, Hydrochlorothiazide 12.5 mg	Lotensin HCT by Novartis	00083-0074	Antihypertensive; Diuretic
LOTENSINHCT <> 7474	Tab, Greyish Violet, Oblong, Scored	Benazepril HCl 20 mg, Hydrochlorothiazide 12.5 mg	Lotensin HCT by Novartis	00078-0453	Antihypertensive; Diuretic
LOTENSINHCT <> 7575	Tab, Red, Oblong, Scored	Benazepril HCl 20 mg, Hydrochlorothiazide 25 mg	Lotensin HCT by Novartis	00083-0075	Antihypertensive; Diuretic
LOTENSINHCT <> 7575	Tab, Red, Oblong, Scored	Benazepril HCl 20 mg, Hydrochlorothiazide 25 mg	Lotensin HCT by Novartis	00078-0454	Antihypertensive; Diuretic
LOTREL0364	Cap, Purple, Black Print, 2 White Bands, LOTREL over 0364	Amlodipine Besylate 10 mg, Benazepril HCl 20 mg	Lotrel by Novartis	00078-0364	Antihypertensive
LOTREL0379	Cap, Dark Blue, Two White Bands	Amlodipine Besylate 10 mg, Benazepril HCl 20 mg	Lotrel by Novartis	00078-0379	Antihypertensive
LOTREL0384	Cap, Light Blue, Two White Bands	Amlodipine Besylate 5 mg, Benazepril HCl 40 mg	Lotrel by Novartis	00078-0384	Antihypertensive
LOTREL2255	Cap, White, Black Print, 2 Yellow Bands, Lotrel over 2255	Amlodipine Besylate 2.5 mg, Benazepril HCl 10 mg	Lotrel by Sandoz	00781-2271	Antihypertensive
LOTREL2255	Cap, White, Black Print, 2 Yellow Bands, Lotrel over 2255	Amlodipine Besylate 2.5 mg, Benazepril HCl 10 mg	Lotrel by Pharm Util	60491-0807	Antihypertensive
LOTREL2255	Cap, White, Black Print, 2 Yellow Bands, Lotrel over 2255	Amlodipine Besylate 2.5 mg, Benazepril HCl 10 mg	Lotrel by Novartis	00078-0404	Antihypertensive
LOTREL2260	Cap, Light Brown, Black Print, 2 White Bands, Lotrel over 2260	Amlodipine Besylate 5 mg, Benazepril HCl 10 mg	Lotrel by Novartis	00078-0405	Antihypertensive
LOTREL2260	Cap, Light Brown, Black Print, 2 White Bands, Lotrel over 2260	Amlodipine Besylate 5 mg, Benazepril HCl 10 mg	Lotrel by Caremark	00339-6100	Antihypertensive
LOTREL2265	Cap, Pink, Black Print, Lotrel over 2265	Amlodipine Besylate 5 mg, Benazepril HCl 20 mg	Lotrel by Novartis	00078-0406	Antihypertensive

ID FRONT <> BACK	DESCRIPTION FRONT <> BACK	INGREDIENT & STRENGTH	BRAND (or Generic Equiv.) by FIRM	NDC#	CLASS; SCH.
LOVA20 <> APO	Tab, Light Blue, Octagonal, APO/Lova 20	Lovastatin 20 mg	Lovastatin by Apotex	Canadian DIN 02220172	Antihyperlipidemic
LOVA20 <> P	Tab, Blue, Octagonal, Scored	Lovastatin 20 mg	Mevacor by Pharmascience	Canadian DIN 02246013	Antihyperlipidemic
LOVA40 <> APO	Tab, Light Green, Octagonal, APO/Lova 40	Lovastatin 40 mg	Lovastatin by Apotex	Canadian DIN 02220180	Antihyperlipidemic
LOVA40 <> P	Tab, Green, Octagonal	Lovastatin 40 mg	Mevacor by Pharmascience	Canadian DIN 02246014	Antihyperlipidemic
LOX10 <> APO	Tab, Green, Round	Loxapine 10 mg	Loxitane by Apotex	Canadian DIN 02237652	Antipsychotic
LOX10 <> NU	Tab, Green, Round, Film Coated, Scored, Lox over 10 <> NU	Loxapine Succinate 10 mg	by Nu Pharm	Canadian DIN 02237535	Antipsychotic
LOX25 <> APO	Tab, Pink, Round	Loxapine 25 mg	Loxitane by Apotex	Canadian DIN 02237653	Antipsychotic
LOX25 <> NU	Tab, Pink, Round, Film Coated, Scored, Lox over 25 <> NU	Loxapine Succinate 25 mg	by Nu Pharm	Canadian DIN 02237535	Antipsychotic
LOX5 <> APO	Tab, Yellow, Round	Loxapine 5 mg	Loxitane by Apotex	Canadian DIN 02237651	Antipsychotic
LOX5 <> NU	Tab, Yellow, Round, Film Coated, Scored, Lox over 5 <> NU	Loxapine Succinate 5 mg	by Nu Pharm	Canadian DIN 02237534	Antipsychotic
LOX50 <> APO	Tab, White, Round	Loxapine 50 mg	Loxitane by Apotex	Canadian DIN 02237654	Antipsychotic
LOX50 <> NU	Tab, White, Round, Film Coated, Scored, Lox over 50 <> NU	Loxapine Succinate 50 mg	by Nu Pharm	Canadian DIN 02237536	Antipsychotic
LP <> GEIGY	Tab, White, Round, Film Coated	Clomipramine HCl 50 mg	Anafranil by Novartis	Canadian DIN 00402591	OCD
LP <> GEIGY	Tab, White, Round, Film Coated	Clomipramine HCl 50 mg	Anafranil by Cobalt	Canadian DIN 02244818	OCD
LR	Tab, Yellow, Round, Abbott Logo	Warfarin Sodium 7.5 mg	Panwarfin by Abbott		Anticoagulant
LS <> A	Tab, Yellow, Square, Scored, Abbott Logo (a)	Methylclothiazide 5 mg, Deserpidine 0.25 mg	Enduronyl by Abbott	00074-6838 Discontinued	Diuretic; Antihypertensive
LS10	Tab, Pink, Round	Lisinopril 10 mg	Zestril by Pharmascience	Canadian DIN 02292211	Antihypertensive
LS20	Tab, Pink, Round	Lisinopril 20 mg	Zestril by Pharmascience	Canadian DIN 02292238	Antihypertensive
LS20	Tab, Blue, Octagonal, Scored, Cobalt Logo <> LS / 20	Lovastatin 20 mg	Mevacor by Cobalt	Canadian DIN 02248572	Antihyperlipidemic
LS40	Tab, Green, Octagonal, Scored, Cobalt Logo <> LS / 40	Lovastatin 40 mg	Mevacor by Cobalt	Canadian DIN 02248573	Antihyperlipidemic
LS5	Tab, Pink, Round, Scored	Lisinopril 5 mg	Zestril by Pharmascience	Canadian DIN 02292203	Antihypertensive
LSP10	Tab, Yellow, Round	Lisinopril 10 mg	Zestril by LEK	66685-0703	Antihypertensive
LSP20	Tab, Light Grey, Round	Lisinopril 20 mg	Zestril by LEK	66685-0704	Antihypertensive
LSP212	Tab, Light Yellow, Round, LSP 2 1/2	Lisinopril 2.5 mg	Zestril by LEK	66685-0701	Antihypertensive
LSP30	Tab, Light Grey, Round	Lisinopril 30 mg	Zestril by LEK	66685-0705	Antihypertensive
LSP40	Tab, Light Grey, Round	Lisinopril 40 mg	Zestril by LEK	66685-0706	Antihypertensive
LSP5	Tab, Green, Round, Scored	Lisinopril 5 mg	Zestril by LEK	66685-0702	Antihypertensive
LT <> A	Tab, Gray, Square, Scored, Abbott Logo (a)	Methylclothiazide 5 mg, Deserpidine 0.5 mg	Enduronyl Forte by Abbott	00074-6854 Discontinued	Diuretic; Antihypertensive
LTG2	Tab, White to Off-White, Round, Chewable, LTG over 2	Lamotrigine 2 mg	Lamictal by GSK	00173-0699	Anticonvulsant

ID FRONT <> BACK	DESCRIPTION FRONT <> BACK	INGREDIENT & STRENGTH	BRAND (or Generic Equiv.) by FIRM	NDC#	CLASS; SCH.
LTG2	Tab, White to Off-White, Round, Chewable, LTG over 2	Lamotrigine 2 mg	Lamictal by GSK	Canadian DIN 02243803	Anticonvulsant
LTR1000 <> APO	Tab, White, Oval	Tryptophan 1000 mg	Tryptan by Apotex	Canadian DIN 02248539	Antidepressant
LTR500 <> APO	Tab, White, Oval	Tryptophan 500 mg	Tryptan by Apotex	Canadian DIN 02248538	Antidepressant
LU	Tab, Yellow, Oblong, Abbott Logo	Estropipate 0.625 mg	Ogen by Abbott		Hormone
LU <> C11	Tab, White, Round, Scored	Perindopril 2 mg	Aceon by Lupin	68180-0235	Antihypertensive
LU <> C12	Tab, White, Cap Shaped, Scored	Perindopril 4 mg	Aceon by Lupin	68180-0236	Antihypertensive
LU <> C13	Tab, White, Round, Scored	Perindopril 8 mg	Aceon by Lupin	68180-0237	Antihypertensive
LU <> C31	Tab, White, Round	Myambutol 100 mg	Myambutol by Lupin	68180-0280	Antimycobacterial
LU <> C32	Tab, White, Round	Myambutol 400 mg	Myambutol by Lupin	68180-0281	Antimycobacterial
LU <> D01	Tab, Green, Cap Shaped, Film Coated, Scored, L / U	Sertraline HCl 25 mg	Zoloft by Lupin	68180-0351	Antidepressant
LU <> D02	Tab, Blue, Cap Shaped, Film Coated, Scored, L / U	Sertraline HCl 50 mg	Zoloft by Lupin	68180-0352	Antidepressant
LU <> D03	Tab, Yellow, Cap Shaped, Film Coated, Scored, L / U	Sertraline HCl 100 mg	Zoloft by Lupin	68180-0353	Antidepressant
LU <> F01	Tab, Yellow, Oval, Film Coated, Scored, L / U	Quinapril 5 mg	Accupril by Lupin	68180-0556	Antihypertensive
LU <> F02	Tab, Yellow, Round, Film Coated	Quinapril 10 mg	Accupril by Lupin	68180-0557	Antihypertensive
LU <> F03	Tab, Yellow, Round, Film Coated	Quinapril 20 mg	Accupril by Lupin	68180-0558	Antihypertensive
LU <> F04	Tab, Yellow, Oblong, Film Coated	Quinapril 40 mg	Accupril by Lupin	68180-0559	Antihypertensive
LU <> G01	Tab, Light Green, Oval	Lovastatin 10 mg	Mevacor by Lupin	68180-0467	Antihyperlipidemic
LU <> G02	Tab, Light Green, Round	Lovastatin 20 mg	Mevacor by Lupin	68180-0468	Antihyperlipidemic
LU <> G03	Tab, Light Green, Round	Lovastatin 40 mg	Mevacor by Lupin	68180-0469	Antihyperlipidemic
LU <> H01	Tab, Pink, Round, Scored	Trandolapril 1 mg	Mavik by Lupin	68180-0566	Antihypertensive
LU <> H02	Tan, Yellow, Round	Trandolapril 2 mg	Mavik by Lupin	68180-0567	Antihypertensive
LU <> H03	Tab, Brick Red, Round	Trandolapril 4 mg	Mavik by Lupin	68180-0568	Antihypertensive
LU <> H11	Tab, White, Diamond-Shaped	Amlodipine Besylate 2.5 mg	Norvasc by Lupin	68180-0750	Antihypertensive
LU <> H12	Tab, White, Octagonal	Amlodipine Besylate 5 mg	Norvasc by Lupin	68180-0751	Antihypertensive
LU <> H13	Tab, White, Round	Amlodipine Besylate 10 mg	Norvasc by Lupin	68180-0752	Antihypertensive
LU <> M42	Tab, White, Oval, Film Coated	Losartan 100 mg, Hydrochlorothiazide 12.5 mg	Hyzaar by Lupin	68180-0216	Antihypertensive; Diuretic
LU <> N01	Tab, Yellow, Cap Shaped, Film Coated	Pravastatin Sodium 10 mg	Pravachol by Lupin	68180-0485	Antihyperlipidemic
LU <> N02	Tab, Yellow, Cap Shaped, Film Coated	Pravastatin Sodium 20 mg	Pravachol by Lupin	68180-0486	Antihyperlipidemic
LU <> N03	Tab, Yellow, Cap Shaped, Film Coated	Pravastatin Sodium 40 mg	Pravachol by Lupin	68180-0487	Antihyperlipidemic
LU <> N04	Tab, Yellow, Oval, Film Coated	Pravastatin Sodium 80 mg	Pravachol by Lupin	68180-0488	Antihyperlipidemic
LU <> X01	Tab, Blue, Oblong, Film Coated, Scored	Levetiracetam 250 mg	Keppra by Lupin	68180-0112	Anticonvulsant
LU <> X02	Tab, Yellow, Oblong, Scored, Film Coated	Levetiracetam 500 mg	Keppra by Lupin	68180-0113	Anticonvulsant
LU <> X03	Tab, Orange, Oblong, Scored, Film Coated	Levetiracetam 750 mg	Keppra by Lupin	68180-0114	Anticonvulsant
LU <> X04	Tab, White, Oblong, Scored, Film Coated	Levetiracetam 1 g	Keppra by Lupin	68180-0115	Anticonvulsant
LUCHEM110	Tab, White, Oblong, with Pink Specks, Luchem Logo 110	Yohimbine HCl 5.4 mg	Yocon by LuChem		Impotence Agent
LUCHEM5	Tab, White, Oblong	Acetaminophen 500 mg, Hydrocodone Bitartrate 5 mg	Vicodin by LuChem		Analgesic; C III
LUCHEM5	Tab	Acetaminophen 500 mg, Hydrocodone Bitartrate 5 mg	Vicodin by Pharmedix	53002-0119	Analgesic; C III
LUCHEM649	Tab, Green, Round	Dexbrompheniramine Maleate 6 mg, Pseudoephedrine Sulfate 120 mg	Drixoral by Norton		Cold Remedy
LUCHEM663	Cap	Acetaminophen 500 mg, Hydrocodone Bitartrate 5 mg	Vicodin by Ivax	00182-0156	Analgesic; C III
LUCHEM663	Cap, Black & Red	Acetaminophen 500 mg, Hydrocodone Bitartrate 5 mg	Zydone by LuChem		Analgesic; C III
LUCHEM741	Tab, Blue, Oval	Guaifenesin 400 mg, Phenylpropanolamine HCl 75 mg	Entex LA by LuChem		Cold Remedy
LUCHEM743	Tab	Chlorpheniramine Tannate 8 mg, Phenylephrine Tannate 25 mg, Pyrilamine Tannate 25 mg	by Ivax	00182-1912	Cold Remedy
LUCHEM746	Cap	Guaifenesin 200 mg, Phenylephrine HCl 5 mg, Phenylpropanolamine HCl 45 mg	Entex by Pharmedix	53002-0518	Cold Remedy
LUCHEM992	Cap, Clear & Green	Chlorpheniramine Maleate 12 mg	Chlor-Trimeton by LuChem		Antihistamine

ID FRONT <> BACK	DESCRIPTION FRONT <> BACK	INGREDIENT & STRENGTH	BRAND (or Generic Equiv.) by FIRM	NDC#	CLASS; SCH.
LUE11	Cap, White, Opaque	Amlodipine Besylate 2.5 mg, Benazepril HCl 10 mg	Lotrel by Lupin	68180-0755	Antihypertensive
LUE12	Cap, Light Brown to Yellow, Opaque	Amlodipine Besylate 5 mg, Benazepril HCl 10 mg	Lotrel by Lupin	68180-0756	Antihypertensive
LUE13	Cap, Flesh, Opaque	Amlodipine Besylate 5 mg, Benazepril HCl 20 mg	Lotrel by Lupin	68180-0757	Antihypertensive
LUE14	Cap, Purple	Amlodipine Besylate 10 mg, Benazepril HCl 20 mg	Lotrel by Lupin	68180-0758	Antihypertensive
LUF <> NVR	Tab, Dark Yellow, Oval, Film Coated	Amlodipine 10 mg, Valsartan 320 mg	Exforge by Novartis	00078-0491	Antihypertensive
LUF11	Cap, Maroon and White	Cefadroxil 500 mg	Duricef by Lupin	68180-0180	Antibiotic
LUNSCO	Cap, Green Print	Acetaminophen 325 mg, Butalbital 50 mg, Caffeine 40 mg	Fioricet by Lunsco	10892-0116	Analgesic
LUNSCO <> 0127	Tab, Film Coated	Acetaminophen 500 mg, Chlorpheniramine Maleate 8 mg, Phenylephrine HCl 40 mg	by Mikart	46672-0161	Cold Remedy
LUNSCO <> 0127	Tab, Film Coated	Acetaminophen 500 mg, Chlorpheniramine Maleate 8 mg, Phenylephrine HCl 40 mg	Protid by Lunsco	10892-0127	Cold Remedy
LUNSCO151	Cap	Acetaminophen 300 mg, Phenyltoloxamine Citrate 20 mg, Salicylamide 200 mg	Durabac by Seatrace	00551-0151	Analgesic
LUNSCO151	Cap	Acetaminophen 300 mg, Phenyltoloxamine Citrate 20 mg, Salicylamide 200 mg	Durabac by Lunsco	10892-0151	Analgesic
LUNSCO151	Cap	Acetaminophen 300 mg, Phenyltoloxamine Citrate 20 mg, Salicylamide 200 mg	Durabac by Lunsco	10892-0151	Analgesic
LUPIN <> 10	Tab, Pink, Round	Lisinopril 10 mg	Zestril by Lupin	68180-0514	Antihypertensive
LUPIN <> 20	Tab, Dark Pink, Round	Lisinopril 20 mg	Zestril by Lupin	68180-0515	Antihypertensive
LUPIN <> 25	Tab, White to Off-White, Round, LUPIN <> 2.5	Lisinopril 2.5 mg	Zestril by Lupin	68180-0512	Antihypertensive
LUPIN <> 250	Tab, Light Orange, Oval, Film Coated	Cefprozil 250 mg	Cefzil by Lupin	68180-0403	Antibiotic
LUPIN <> 30	Tab, Red, Round	Lisinopril 30 mg	Zestril by Lupin	68180-0516	Antihypertensive
LUPIN <> 302	Tab, White, Oblong	Cefuroxime Axetil 250 mg	Ceftin by Watson	00591-3224	Antibiotic
LUPIN <> 302	Tab, White, Oblong	Cefuroxime Axetil 250 mg	Ceftin by Lupin	68180-0302	Antibiotic
LUPIN <> 303	Tab, White, Oblong	Cefuroxime Axetil 500 mg	Ceftin by Lupin	68180-0303	Antibiotic
LUPIN <> 303	Tab, White, Oblong	Cefuroxime Axetil 500 mg	Ceftin by Watson	00591-3225	Antibiotic
LUPIN <> 40	Tab, Yellow, Round	Lisinopril 40 mg	Zestril by Lupin	68180-0517	Antihypertensive
LUPIN <> 500	Tab, White, Oval, Film Coated	Cefprozil 500 mg	Cefzil by Lupin	68180-0404	Antibiotic
LUPIN500	Cap, Dark Green and Light Green	Cephalexin 500 mg	Keflex by Lupin	68180-0122	Antibiotic
LUPINLUPINCEFDINIR	Cap, Blue and Purple	Cefdinir 300 mg	Omnicef by Lupin	68180-0711	Antibiotic
LUPINRAMIPRIL10MG	Cap, Light Blue	Ramipril 10 mg	Altace by Lupin	68180-0591	Antihypertensive
LUPINRAMIPRIL125MG	Cap, Yellow	Ramipril 1.25 mg	Altace by Lupin	68180-0588	Antihypertensive
LUPINRAMIPRIL25MG	Cap, Orange	Ramipril 2.5 mg	Altace by Lupin	68180-0589	Antihypertensive
LUPINRAMIPRIL5MG	Cap, Red	Ramipril 5 mg	Altace by Lupin	68180-0590	Antihypertensive
LUU01	Cap, Brownish Orange	Imipramine Pamoate 75 mg	Tofranil-PM by Lupin	68180-0314	Antidepressant
LUU02	Cap, Brownish Orange and Yellow	Imipramine Pamoate 100 mg	Tofranil-PM by Lupin	68180-0315	Antidepressant
LUU03	Cap, Brownish Orange and Light Yellow	Imipramine Pamoate 125 mg	Tofranil-PM by Lupin	68180-0316	Antidepressant
LUU04	Cap, Brownish Orange	Imipramine Pamoate 150 mg	Tofranil-PM by Lupin	68180-0317	Antidepressant
LV	Tab, Peach, Oblong, Abbott Logo	Estropipate 1.25 mg	Ogen by Abbott		Hormone
LV <> 901	Cap, Yellow, Opaque	Oxycodone 5 mg	by Glenmark	68462-0204	Opiate Agonist
LV <> 903	Tab, White, Round, Scored, L/V <> 903	Codeine Sulfate 30 mg	by Glenmark	68462-0193	Analgesic; C II
LV <> 906	Tab, White, Round, Scored, L/V <> 906	Codeine Sulfate 60 mg	by Glenmark	68462-0194	Analgesic; C II
LV <> 915	Tab, White, Round, Scored	Morphine Sulfate 15 mg	by Glenmark	68462-0202	Analgesic; C II
LV <> 930	Tab, White, Round, Scored	Morphine Sulfate 30 mg	by Glenmark	68462-0203	Analgesic; C II
LV <> CG	Tab, Light Yellow, Cap Shaped, Film Coated	Benazepril HCl 5 mg	Lotensin by Geigy	Canadian DIN 00885835	Antihypertensive
LV10 <> G	Tab, Peach, Round, LV over 10	Lovastatin 10 mg	Mevacor by Par	49884-0754	Antihyperlipidemic
LV20 <> G	Tab, Light Blue, Round, LV over 20	Lovastatin 20 mg	Mevacor by Par	49884-0755	Antihyperlipidemic
LV250	Tab, Blue, Oblong	Levetiracetam 250 mg	Keppra by Pharmascience	Canadian DIN 02296101	Anticonvulsant

ID FRONT <> BACK	DESCRIPTION FRONT <> BACK	INGREDIENT & STRENGTH	BRAND (or Generic Equiv.) by FIRM	NDC#	CLASS; SCH.
LV40 <> G	Tab, Green, Round, LV over 40	Lovastatin 40 mg	Mevacor by Par	49884-0756	Antihyperlipidemic
LV500	Tab, Yellow, Oblong	Levetiracetam 500 mg	Keppra by Pharmascience	Canadian DIN 02296128	Anticonvulsant
LV750	Tab, Peach, Oblong	Levetiracetam 750 mg	Keppra by Pharmascience	Canadian DIN 02296136	Anticonvulsant
LV901	Cap, Yellow and White, Opaque	Oxycodone 5 mg	Oxycodone by Glenmark	68462-0204	Analgesic; C II
LX	Tab, Blue, Oblong, Abbott Logo	Estropipate 2.5 mg	Ogen by Abbott		Hormone
LY	Tab, Green, Oblong, Abbott Logo	Estropipate 5 mg	Ogen by Abbott		Hormone
LY25 <> G	Tab, White, Round, Chewable, Dispersible	Lamotrigine 25 mg	Lamictal by Mylan	00378-6925	Anticonvulsant
LY5 <> G	Tab, White, Round, Chewable, Dispersible	Lamotrigine 5 mg	Lamictal by Mylan	00378-6905	Anticonvulsant
M	Tab, Yellow, Round, M <> Boehringer Ingelheim Logo	Meloxicam 7.5 mg	Mobic by Boehringer Ingelheim	00597-0029	NSAID
M	Tab, Yellow, Round, M <> Boehringer Ingelheim Logo	Meloxicam 7.5 mg	Mobic by Boehringer Ingelheim	12714-0126	NSAID
M	Tab, Pink, Round, M underlined Logo	Benzocaine 10 mg, Cetylpyridinium Chloride 0.4 mg	Max Lozenger by Century	00436-0663	Anesthetic; Antiseptic
M	Tab, White	Theophylline Anhydrous 118 mg, Ephedrine 24 mg, Phenobarbital 8 mg	Tedral by Parke Davis	Canadian	Antiasthmatic; C IV
M	Tab, Yellow, Round	Vitamin Combination with Iron	Daily-Vite by Watson	00536-3546	Vitamin; Mineral
M	Tab, Yellow, Round, M <> Boehringer Ingelheim Logo	Meloxicam 7.5 mg	Mobicox by Boehringer Ingelheim Canada	Canadian DIN 02247785	NSAID
M	Tab, White, Oblong, Scored, Ex Release, Andrx Logo / M	Metoprolol Succinate 25 mg	Toprolol XL by Andrx	62037-0830	Antihypertensive
M <> 0552	Tab, White, Round, Scored, M in square	Oxycodone HCl 5 mg	Roxicodone by Mallinckrodt	00406-0552	Analgesic; C II
M <> 057	Tab, White, Oblong, Scored	Sucralfate 1 g	by SKB	00029-4153	Gastrointestinal
M <> 10	Tab, White, Diamond Shaped, Scored, M inside square <> 10	Dextroamphetamine Sulfate 10 mg	Dexedrine by Mallinckrodt	00406-8959	Stimulant; C II
M <> 10	Tab, Coral, Triangular, Film Coated, M inside a Box	Imipramine HCl 10 mg	Tofranil by Mallinckrodt	00406-9920	Antidepressant
M <> 10	Tab, White to Cream Colored, Pillow-Shaped, M inside square	Mixed Amphetamine Salts 10 mg: Dextroamphetamine Saccharate 2.5 mg, Amphetamine Aspartate 2.5 mg, Dextroamphetamine Sulfate 2.5 mg, Amphetamine Sulfate 2.5 mg	Adderall by Mallinckrodt	00406-8892	Stimulant; C II
M <> 10	Tab, White, Round, M in a double circle <> 10	Dicyclomine HCl 10 mg	Bentylol by Axcan	Canadian DIN 02103087	Gastrointestinal
M <> 10	Tab, White, Round, Scored	Methylphenidate HCl 10 mg	Ritalin by D M Graham	00756-0284	Stimulant; C II
M <> 10	Tab, White, Round, Scored	Methylphenidate HCl 10 mg	Ritalin by Mallinckrodt	00406-1122	Stimulant; C II
M <> 100	Tab, Gray, Round, M inside square <> 100	Morphine Sulfate 100 mg	MS Contin by Mallinckrodt	00406-8390	Analgesic; C II
M <> 1202MJ	Tab	Fosinopril Sodium 40 mg	Monopril by BMS	15548-0202	Antihypertensive
M <> 125	Tab, White to Cream Colored, Octagon, M inside square <> 12.5	Mixed Amphetamine Salts 12.5 mg: Dextroamphetamine Saccharate 3.125 mg, Amphetamine Aspartate 3.125 mg, Dextroamphetamine Sulfate 3.125 mg, Amphetamine Sulfate 3.125 mg	Adderall by Mallinckrodt	00406-8886	Stimulant; C II
M <> 1423	Tab, White, Round, Ex Release, M inside square, Extended Release	Methylphenidate HCl 10 mg	Ritalin by Mallinckrodt	00406-1423	Stimulant; C II
M <> 1423	Tab, White, Round, Ex Release, M inside square, Extended Release	Methylphenidate HCl 10 mg	Ritalin by D M Graham	00756-0285	Stimulant; C II
M <> 144	Tab, White, Round	Tamoxifen Citrate 10 mg	Nolvadex by Mylan	00378-0144	Antiestrogen
M <> 1451	Tab, White, Round, M inside Box, Ex Release	Methylphenidate HCl 20 mg	Ritalin by Mallinckrodt	00406-1451	Stimulant; C II
M <> 15	Tab, Blue, Round, M inside square <> 15	Morphine Sulfate 15 mg	MS Contin by Mallinckrodt	00406-8315	Analgesic; C II
M <> 15	Tab, Yellow, Oblong	Meloxicam 15 mg	Mobic by Boehringer Ingelheim	00597-0030	NSAID
M <> 15	Tab, White to Cream Colored, Octagon, M inside square	Mixed Amphetamine Salts 15 mg: Dextroamphetamine Saccharate 3.75 mg, Amphetamine Aspartate 3.75 mg, Dextroamphetamine Sulfate 3.75 mg, Amphetamine Sulfate 3.75 mg	Adderall by Mallinckrodt	00406-8885	Stimulant; C II
M <> 15	Tab, Light Green, Round, Convex, Scored, M inside square	Oxycodone HCl 15 mg	Roxicodone by Mallinckrodt	00406-8515	Analgesic; C II
M <> 151	Tab, White, Round	Finasteride 5 mg	Proscar by Mylan	00378-3151	Antiandrogen
M <> 151	Tab, White, Round	Finasteride 5 mg	Proscar by UDL	51079-0520	Antiandrogen
M <> 17	Tab, Orange, Round, Scored, M <> 1 / 7	Quinapril HCl 5 mg	Accupril by Mylan	00378-1117	Antihypertensive
M <> 172	Tab, White, Round	Metolazone 2.5 mg	Zaroxolyn by Mylan	00378-6172	Diuretic

ID FRONT <> BACK	DESCRIPTION FRONT <> BACK	INGREDIENT & STRENGTH	BRAND (or Generic Equiv.) by FIRM	NDC#	CLASS; SCH.
M <> 172	Tab, White, Round	Metolazone 2.5 mg	Zaroxolyn by UDL	51079-0023	Diuretic
M <> 1721	Tab, White, Oval, M inside square <> 1721	Acetaminophen 650 mg, Propoxyphene Napsylate 100 mg	Darvocet-N 100 by Mallinckrodt	00406-1721	Analgesic; C IV
M <> 173	Tab, Orange, Round	Metolazone 5 mg	Zaroxolyn by UDL	51079-0024	Diuretic
M <> 173	Tab, Orange, Round	Metolazone 5 mg	Zaroxolyn by Mylan	00378-6173	Diuretic
M <> 174	Tab, Light Green, Round	Metolazone 10 mg	Zaroxolyn by Mylan	00378-6174	Diuretic
M <> 1772	Tab, Pink, Oval, M inside square	Acetaminophen 650 mg, Propoxyphene Napsylate 100 mg	Darvocet-N 100 by Mallinckrodt	00406-1772	Analgesic; C IV
M <> 2	Tab, White, Round, M inside a square <> 2	Acetaminophen 300 mg, Codeine Phosphate 15 mg	Tylenol w/ Codeine by Mallinckrodt	00406-0483	Analgesic; C III
M <> 2	Tab, White, Round	Hydromorphone HCl 2 mg	Dilaudid by Mallinckrodt	00406-3243	Analgesic; C II
M <> 2	Tab, White, Round	Hydromorphone HCl 2 mg	Dilaudid by Murfreesboro	51129-1465	Analgesic; C II
M <> 20	Tab, White, Round, Scored, M inside square <> 20 above Score	Methylphenidate HCl 20 mg	Ritalin by Mallinckrodt	00406-1124	Stimulant; C II
M <> 20	Tab, White, Round, Scored, M in a double circle <> 20	Dicyclomine HCl 20 mg	Bentylol by Axcan	Canadian DIN 02103095	Gastrointestinal
M <> 20	Tab, White to Cream Colored, Octagon, M inside square	Mixed Amphetamine Salts 20 mg: Dextroamphetamine Saccharate 5 mg, Amphetamine Aspartate 5 mg, Dextroamphetamine Sulfate 5 mg, Amphetamine Sulfate 5 mg	Adderall by Mallinckrodt	00406-8893	Stimulant; C II
M <> 20	Tab, White, Round, Scored, M inside square <> 20 above Score	Methylphenidate HCl 20 mg	Ritalin by Neuman		Stimulant; C II
M <> 200	Tab, Green, Oblong, M inside square <> 200	Morphine Sulfate 200 mg	MS Contin by Mallinckrodt	00406-8320	Analgesic; C II
M <> 204	Tab, White, Round	Diclofenac Sodium 50 mg	by Martec	65413-0001	NSAID
M <> 205	Tab, White, Round	Diclofenac Sodium 75 mg	by Martec	65413-0002	NSAID
M <> 21	Tab, White, Round, Scored, M inside square	Methylphenidate HCl 20 mg	Methylin by Neuman	64579-0034	Stimulant; C II
M <> 22	Tab, White, Round	Albuterol Sulfate 4 mg	VoSpire ER by Mylan	00378-4122	Antiasthmatic
M <> 226	Tab, Orange, Round, Scored	Quinapril HCl 10 mg	Accupril by Mylan	00378-0226	Antihypertensive
M <> 231	Tab, White, Round, Scored	Atenolol 50 mg	Tenormin by Heartland	61392-0543	Antihypertensive
M <> 231	Tab, White, Round, Scored	Atenolol 50 mg	Tenormin by Mylan	00378-0231	Antihypertensive
M <> 231	Tab, White, Round, Scored	Atenolol 50 mg	Tenormin by UDL	51079-0684	Antihypertensive
M <> 234	Tab, White, Round, Film Coated	Metformin HCl 500 mg	Glucophage by UDL	51079-0972	Antidiabetic
				Discontinued	
M <> 234	Tab, White, Round, Film Coated	Metformin HCl 500 mg	Glucophage by Mylan	00378-0234	Antidiabetic
M <> 24	Tab, Blue, Round	Albuterol Sulfate 8 mg	VoSpire ER by Mylan	00378-4124	Antiasthmatic
M <> 240	Tab, White, Round, Film Coated	Metformin HCl 850 mg	Glucophage by Mylan	00378-0240	Antidiabetic
M <> 240	Tab, White, Round, Film Coated	Metformin HCl 850 mg	Glucophage by UDL	51079-0973	Antidiabetic
M <> 25	Tab, Coral, Round, Biconvex, Film Coated, M inside Box	Imipramine HCl 25 mg	Tofranil by Mallinckrodt	00406-9921	Antidepressant
M <> 254	Tab, Orange, Round, Scored	Quinapril HCl 20 mg	Accupril by Mylan	00378-0254	Antihypertensive
M <> 272	Tab, Orange, Round, Scored	Quinapril HCl 40 mg	Accupril by Mylan	00378-0272	Antihypertensive
M <> 274	Tab, White to Off-White, Round	Tamoxifen Citrate 20 mg	Nolvadex by Mylan	00378-0274	Antiestrogen
M <> 28	Tab	Nadolol 20 mg	Nadolol by Qualitest	00603-4740	Antihypertensive
M <> 3	Tab, White, Round, M inside square <> 3	Acetaminophen 300 mg, Codeine Phosphate 30 mg	Tylenol w/ Codeine by Mallinckrodt	00406-0484	Analgesic; C III
M <> 30	Tab, Purple, Round, M inside square <> 30	Morphine Sulfate 30 mg	MS Contin by Mallinckrodt	00406-8330	Analgesic; C II
M <> 30	Tab, White to Cream Colored, Octagon, M inside square	Mixed Amphetamine Salts 30 mg: Dextroamphetamine Saccharate 7.5 mg, Amphetamine Aspartate 7.5 mg, Dextroamphetamine Sulfate 7.5 mg, Amphetamine Sulfate 7.5 mg	Adderall by Mallinckrodt	00406-8894	Stimulant; C II
M <> 30	Tab, Light Blue, Round, Convex, Scored, M inside square	Oxycodone HCl 30 mg	Roxicodone by Mallinckrodt	00406-8530	Analgesic; C II
M <> 315	Tab, White	Ondansetron HCl 4 mg	Zofran by UDL	51079-0524	Antiemetic
M <> 315	Tab, White, Round	Ondansetron HCl 4 mg	Zofran by Mylan	00378-7732	Antiemetic
M <> 317	Tab, Green, Shield Shaped, Film Coated	Cimetidine HCl 300 mg	Tagamet by Murfreesboro	51129-1181	Gastrointestinal
M <> 317	Tab, Green, Shield Shaped, Film Coated	Cimetidine HCl 300 mg	Tagamet by UDL	51079-0807 Discontinued	Gastrointestinal
M <> 317	Tab, Green, Shield Shaped, Film Coated	Cimetidine HCl 300 mg	Tagamet by H J Harkins Co	52959-0345	Gastrointestinal

ID FRONT <> BACK	DESCRIPTION FRONT <> BACK	INGREDIENT & STRENGTH	BRAND (or Generic Equiv.) by FIRM	NDC#	CLASS; SCH.
M <> 317	Tab, Green, Shield Shaped, Film Coated	Cimetidine HCl 300 mg	Tagamet by Nat Pharmpak	55154-5560	Gastrointestinal
M <> 317	Tab, Green, Shield Shaped, Film Coated	Cimetidine HCl 300 mg	Tagamet by Heartland	61392-0197	Gastrointestinal
M <> 317	Tab, Green, Shield Shaped, Film Coated	Cimetidine HCl 300 mg	Tagamet by Mylan	00378-0317	Gastrointestinal
M <> 317	Tab, Green, Shield Shaped, Film Coated	Cimetidine HCl 300 mg	Tagamet by Qualitest	00603-2891	Gastrointestinal
M <> 321	Tab, White, Round	Lorazepam 0.5 mg	Ativan by Vangard	00615-0450	Antianxiety; C IV
M <> 321	Tab, White, Round	Lorazepam 0.5 mg	Ativan by UDL	51079-0417 Discontinued	Antianxiety; C IV
M <> 321	Tab, White, Round	Lorazepam 0.5 mg	Ativan by Murfreesboro	51129-1344	Antianxiety; C IV
M <> 321	Tab, White, Round	Lorazepam 0.5 mg	Ativan by Nat Pharmpak	55154-5550	Antianxiety; C IV
M <> 321	Tab, White, Round	Lorazepam 0.5 mg	Ativan by Caremark	00339-4018	Antianxiety; C IV
M <> 321	Tab, White, Round	Lorazepam 0.5 mg	Ativan by Mylan	00378-0321	Antianxiety; C IV
M <> 322	Tab, Orange, Round	Ciprofloxacin 250 mg	Cipro by Mylan	00378-1322	Antibiotic
M <> 322	Tab, Orange, Round, Film Coated	Ciprofloxacin 250 mg	Cipro by UDL	51079-0402	Antibiotic
M <> 3354	Tab, White & Yellow, Round	Orphenadrine Citrate 25 mg, Aspirin 385 mg, Caffeine 30 mg	Norgesic by Mylan	00378-3354	Muscle Relaxant
M <> 3356	Tab, White & Yellow	Orphenadrine Citrate 25 mg, Aspirin 770 mg, Caffeine 60 mg	Norgesic Forte by Mylan	00378-3356	Muscle Relaxant
M <> 3356	Tab, White & Yellow, Oblong, Scored	Orphenadrine Citrate 50 mg, Aspirin 770 mg, Caffeine 60 mg	Norgesic Forte by Perrigo	00113-0454	Muscle Relaxant
M <> 3358	Tab, White, Round	Orphenadrine Citrate ER 100 mg	Norflex by 3M	00089-1221	Muscle Relaxant
M <> 3358	Tab, White, Round	Orphenadrine Citrate 100 mg	Norflex by Mylan	00378-3358	Muscle Relaxant
M <> 3358	Tab, White, Round	Orphenadrine Citrate 100 mg	Norflex by Physician Total Care	54868-4102	Muscle Relaxant
M <> 34	Tab, White	Anastrozole 1 mg	Arimidex by UDL	51079-0323	Antineoplastic
M <> 341	Tab, Orange & Red, Round, Film	Ranitidine HCl 150 mg	Ranitidine by RX Pak	65084-0170	Gastrointestinal
M <> 344	Tab, Orange	Ondansetron HCl 8 mg	Zofran by UDL	51079-0525	Antiemetic
M <> 361	Tab, Blue, Oblong, Scored	Acetaminophen 650 mg, Hydrocodone Bitartrate 10 mg	by Southwood	58016-0232	Analgesic; C III
M <> 372	Tab, Green, Pentagonal, Scored, Film Coated	Cimetidine HCl 400 mg	Tagamet by Nat Pharmpak	55154-5555	Gastrointestinal
M <> 372	Tab, Green, Pentagonal, Scored, Film Coated	Cimetidine HCl 400 mg	Tagamet by H J Harkins Co	52959-0375	Gastrointestinal
M <> 372	Tab, Green, Pentagonal, Scored, Film Coated	Cimetidine HCl 400 mg	Tagamet by UDL	51079-0808 Discontinued	Gastrointestinal
M <> 372	Tab, Green, Pentagonal, Scored, Film Coated	Cimetidine HCl 400 mg	Tagamet by Mylan	00378-0372	Gastrointestinal
M <> 372	Tab, Green, Pentagonal, Scored, Film Coated	Cimetidine HCl 400 mg	Tagamet by Murfreesboro	51129-1179	Gastrointestinal
M <> 373	Tab, White, Round, Film Coated	Hydroxychloroquine Sulfate 200 mg	Plaquenil by Mylan	00378-0373	Antimalarial
M <> 4	Tab, White, Round	Hydromorphone HCl 4 mg	Dilaudid by Mallinckrodt	00406-3244	Analgesic; C II
M <> 4	Tab, White, Round	Hydromorphone HCl 4 mg	Dilaudid by Murfreesboro	51129-1466	Analgesic; C II
M <> 4	Tab, White, Triangular, Film Coated	Fluphenazine HCl 1 mg	Prolixin by UDL	51079-0485	Antipsychotic
M <> 4	Tab, White, Triangular, Film Coated	Fluphenazine HCl 1 mg	Prolixin by Mylan	00378-6004	Antipsychotic
M <> 4	Tab, White, Round, M inside square <> 4	Acetaminophen 300 mg, Codeine Phosphate 60 mg	Tylenol w/ Codeine by Mallinckrodt	00406-0485	Analgesic; C III
M <> 423	Tab, Orange & Red, Round, Film	Ranitidine HCl 300 mg	Ranitidine by RX Pak	65084-0172	Gastrointestinal
M <> 433	Tab, Peach, Round, Film Coated	Bupropion HCl 75 mg	Wellbutrin by Mylan	00378-0433	Antidepressant
M <> 433	Tab, Peach, Round, Film Coated	Bupropion HCl 75 mg	Wellbutrin by UDL	51079-0943	Antidepressant
M <> 435	Tab, Light Blue, Round, Film Coated	Bupropion HCl 100 mg	Wellbutrin by UDL	51079-0944	Antidepressant
M <> 435	Tab, Light Blue, Round, Film Coated	Bupropion HCl 100 mg	Wellbutrin by Mylan	00378-0435	Antidepressant
M <> 441	Tab, White, Round, Film Coated	Benazepril HCl 5 mg	Lotensin by Mylan	00378-0441	Antihypertensive
M <> 443	Tab, White, Round, Film Coated	Benazepril HCl 10 mg	Lotensin by Mylan	00378-0443	Antihypertensive
M <> 443	Tab, White, Round, Film Coated	Benazepril HCl 10 mg	Lotensin by UDL	51079-0145	Antihypertensive
M <> 454	Tab, Round	Pindolol 5 mg	by Merckle	58107-0004	Antihypertensive
M <> 455	Tab, Round	Pindolol 10 mg	by Merckle	58107-0005	Antihypertensive
M <> 5	Tab, White to Cream Colored, Pillow-Shaped, M inside square	Mixed Amphetamine Salts 5 mg: Dextroamphetamine Saccharate 1.25 mg, Amphetamine Aspartate 1.25 mg, Dextroamphetamine Sulfate 1.25 mg, Amphetamine Sulfate 1.25 mg	Adderall by Mallinckrodt	00406-8891	Stimulant; C II
M <> 5	Tab, White, Triangular, Scored, M inside square <> over 5	Dextroamphetamine Sulfate 5 mg	Dexedrine by Mallinckrodt	00406-8958	Stimulant; C II
M <> 5	Tab, White, Round, M inside square	Methylphenidate HCl 5 mg	Methylin by Mallinckrodt	00406-1121	Stimulant; C II

ID FRONT <> BACK	DESCRIPTION FRONT <> BACK	INGREDIENT & STRENGTH	BRAND (or Generic Equiv.) by FIRM	NDC#	CLASS; SCH.
M <> 5	Tab, White, Round	Methylin Methylphenidate HCl 5 mg	Ritalin by Mallinckrodt	00406-1121	Stimulant; CII
M <> 50	Tab, Coral, Round, Biconvex, Film Coated, M inside Box	Imipramine HCl 50 mg	Tofranil by Mallinckrodt	00406-9922	Antidepressant
M <> 501	Tab, Orange, Round, Film Coated	Bisoprolol 2.5 mg, Hydrochlorothiazide 6.25 mg	Ziac by Mylan	00378-0501	Antihypertensive; Diuretic
M <> 501	Tab, Orange, Round, Film Coated	Bisoprolol 2.5 mg, Hydrochlorothiazide 6.25 mg	Ziac by UDL	51079-0954 Discontinued	Antihypertensive; Diuretic
M <> 503	Tab, Blue, Round, Film Coated	Bisoprolol 5 mg, Hydrochlorothiazide 6.25 mg	Ziac by UDL	51079-0955 Discontinued	Antihypertensive; Diuretic
M <> 503	Tab, Blue, Round, Film Coated	Bisoprolol 5 mg, Hydrochlorothiazide 6.25 mg	Ziac by Mylan	00378-0503	Antihypertensive; Diuretic
M <> 505	Tab, White, Round, Film Coated	Bisoprolol 10 mg, Hydrochlorothiazide 6.25 mg	Ziac by Mylan	00378-0505	Antihypertensive; Diuretic
M <> 505	Tab, White, Round, Film Coated	Bisoprolol 10 mg, Hydrochlorothiazide 6.25 mg	Ziac by UDL	51079-0956 Discontinued	Antihypertensive; Diuretic
M <> 523	Tab, Pink, Round Scored, M <> 523 to side of score	Bisoprolol Fumarate 5 mg	Zebeta by Mylan	00378-0523	Antihypertensive
M <> 524	Tab, White, Round	Bisoprolol Fumarate 10 mg	Zebeta by Mylan	00378-0524	Antihypertensive
M <> 53	Tab, Green, Pentagonal, Film Coated	Cimetidine HCl 200 mg	Tagamet by H J Harkins Co	52959-0374	Gastrointestinal
M <> 53	Tab, Green, Pentagonal, Film Coated	Cimetidine HCl 200 mg	Tagamet by Heartland	61392-0194	Gastrointestinal
M <> 53	Tab, Green, Pentagonal, Film Coated	Cimetidine HCl 200 mg	Tagamet by Murfreesboro	51129-1177	Gastrointestinal
M <> 53	Tab, Green, Pentagonal, Film Coated	Cimetidine HCl 200 mg	Tagamet by Mylan	00378-0053	Gastrointestinal
M <> 53	Tab, Green, Pentagonal, Film Coated	Cimetidine HCl 200 mg	Tagamet by Qualitest	00603-2890	Gastrointestinal
M <> 537	Tab, Light Blue, Film Coated	Naprosyn 275 mg	Naprosyn by Mylan	00378-0537	NSAID
M <> 537	Tab, Light Blue, Film Coated	Naprosyn 275 mg	Naprosyn by H J Harkins Co	52959-0357	NSAID
M <> 57	Tab, White, Oblong, Scored	Sucralfate 1000 mg	by Merckle	58107-0001	Gastrointestinal
M <> 57	Tab, White, Oblong, Scored	Sucralfate 1000 mg	by Warrick	59930-1532	Gastrointestinal
M <> 5755	Tab, White, Rectangle Shaped, Scored, M inside of Box	Methadone HCl 5 mg	Dolophine by Mallinckrodt	00406-5755	Analgesic; C II
M <> 5771	Tab, White, Rectangle Shaped, Scored, Box around "M"	Methadone HCl 10 mg	Dolophine by Mallinckrodt	00406-5771	Analgesic; C II
M <> 593	Tab, White, Round, M inside Square, Extended Release	Oxycodone HCl 10 mg	OxyContin by Mallinckrodt	00406-0593	Analgesic; C II
M <> 594	Tab, Pink, Round, M inside Square	Oxycodone HCl 20 mg	OxyContin by Mallinckrodt	00406-0594	Analgesic; C II
M <> 595	Tab, Yellow, Round, M inside square, Ex Release	Oxycodone HCl 40 mg	OxyContin by Mallinckrodt	00406-0595	Analgesic; C II
M <> 596	Tab, Green, Round, M inside Square, Extended Release	Oxycodone HCl 80 mg	OxyContin by Mallinckrodt	00406-0596	Analgesic; C II
M <> 60	Tab, Orange, Round, M inside square <> 60	Morphine Sulfate 60 mg	MS Contin by Mallinckrodt	00406-8380	Analgesic; C II
M <> 60	Tab, White, Beveled Edge, Coated, 6 on Left, 0 on Right of Score	Maprotiline HCl 25 mg	Ludiomil by Mylan	00378-0060	Antidepressant
M <> 609MJ	Tab, Lower Case M	Fosinopril Sodium 20 mg	Monopril by Quality Care	62682-6026	Antihypertensive
M <> 69	Tab, Dark Pink, Film Coated	Indapamide 1.25 mg	Lozol by Mylan	00378-0069	Diuretic
M <> 7113	Tab, White, Round, Scored	Meperidine 50 mg	Demerol by D M Graham	00756-0286	Analgesic; C II
M <> 7113	Tab, White, Round, Scored, M inside square <> 7113 over Score	Meperidine 50 mg	Demerol by Mallinckrodt	00406-7113	Analgesic; C II
M <> 7115	Tab, White, Round, Scored, M inside square	Meperidine 100 mg	Demerol by Mallinckrodt	00406-7115	Analgesic; C II
M <> 712	Tab, White, Round	Enalapril Maleate 5 mg, Hydrochlorothiazide 12.5 mg	Vaseretic by Mylan	00378-0712	Antihypertensive; Diuretic
M <> 7171	Tab, White, Cap Shaped	Tramadol HCl 50 mg	Ultram by Mallinckrodt	00406-7171	Analgesic
M <> 723	Tab, White, Round	Enalapril Maleate 10 mg, Hydrochlorothiazide 25 mg	Vaseretic by Mylan	00378-0723	Antihypertensive; Diuretic
M <> 723	Tab, White, Round	Enalapril Maleate 10 mg, Hydrochlorothiazide 25 mg	Vaseretic by Mylan	51079-0977 Discontinued	Antihypertensive; Diuretic
M <> 732	Tab, White to Off-White, Round, Orally Disintegrating	Ondansetron 4 mg	Zofran ODT by Mylan	00378-7732	Antiemetic
M <> 733	Tab, Light Blue, Beveled Edge, Film Coated	Naproxen 550 mg	Naprosyn by Mylan	00378-0733	NSAID
M <> 734	Tab, White, Round, Orally Disintegrating	Ondansetron 8 mg	Zofran ODT by Mylan	00378-7734	Antiemetic
M <> 74	Tab, Green, Triangular, Film Coated	Fluphenazine HCl 5 mg	Prolixin by Mylan	00378-6074	Antipsychotic
M <> 74	Tab, Green, Triangular, Film Coated	Fluphenazine HCl 5 mg	Prolixin by UDL	51079-0487	Antipsychotic
M <> 75	Tab, White to Cream Colored, Pillow-Shaped, M inside square <> 7.5	Mixed Amphetamine Salts 7.5 mg: Amphetamine Aspartate 1.875 mg, Amphetamine Sulfate 1.875 mg, Dextroamphetamine Saccharate 1.875 mg, Dextroamphetamine Sulfate 1.875 mg	Adderall by Mallinckrodt	00406-8884	Stimulant; C II

ID FRONT <> BACK	DESCRIPTION FRONT <> BACK	INGREDIENT & STRENGTH	BRAND (or Generic Equiv.) by FIRM	NDC#	CLASS; SCH.
M <> 751	Tab, Brownish Orange, Round	Cyclobenzaprine HCl 10 mg	Flexeril by Mylan	00378-0751	Muscle Relaxant
M <> 751	Tab, Butterscotch Yellow, Round, Film Coated	Cyclobenzaprine HCl 10 mg	Flexeril by Kaiser	62224-7559	Muscle Relaxant
M <> 751	Tab, Butterscotch Yellow, Round, Film Coated	Cyclobenzaprine HCl 10 mg	Flexeril by UDL	51079-0644 Discontinued	Muscle Relaxant
M <> 751	Tab, Butterscotch Yellow, Round, Film Coated	Cyclobenzaprine HCl 10 mg	Flexeril by PDRX	55289-0567	Muscle Relaxant
M <> 751	Tab, Butterscotch Yellow, Round, Film Coated	Cyclobenzaprine HCl 10 mg	Flexeril by DJ Pharma	64455-0034	Muscle Relaxant
M <> 751	Tab, Butterscotch Yellow, Round, Film Coated	Cyclobenzaprine HCl 10 mg	Flexeril by Va Cmop	65243-0022	Muscle Relaxant
M <> 751	Tab, Butterscotch Yellow, Round, Film Coated	Cyclobenzaprine HCl 10 mg	Flexeril by Kaiser	00179-1140	Muscle Relaxant
M <> 751	Tab, Butterscotch Yellow, Round, Film Coated	Cyclobenzaprine HCl 10 mg	Flexeril by Mylan	00378-0751	Muscle Relaxant
M <> 751	Tab, Butterscotch Yellow, Round, Film Coated	Cyclobenzaprine HCl 10 mg	Flexeril by Physician Total Care	54868-1110	Muscle Relaxant
M <> 751	Tab, Butterscotch Yellow, Round, Film Coated	Cyclobenzaprine HCl 10 mg	Flexeril by Med Pro	53978-1035	Muscle Relaxant
M <> 751	Tab, Butterscotch Yellow, Round, Film Coated	Cyclobenzaprine HCl 10 mg	Flexeril by Pharmedix	53002-0308	Muscle Relaxant
M <> 752	Tab, Blue, Round, Film Coated	Fexofenadine HCl 30 mg	Allegra by Mylan	00378-0752	Antihistamine
M <> 757	Tab, White, Round	Atenolol 100 mg	Tenormin by Mylan	00378-0757	Antihypertensive
M <> 757	Tab, White, Round	Atenolol 100 mg	Tenormin by Diversified Healthcare	55887-0998	Antihypertensive
M <> 757	Tab, White, Round	Atenolol 100 mg	Tenormin by UDL	51079-0685	Antihypertensive
M <> 771	Tab, Light Blue, Round	Cyclobenzaprine HCl 5 mg	Flexeril by Mylan	00378-0771	Muscle Relaxant
M <> 8	Tab, White to Off-White, Arc-Triangle Shaped, Scored	Hydromorphone HCl 8 mg	Dilaudid by Mallinckrodt	00406-3249	Analgesic; C II
M <> 80	Tab, White, Round, Film Coated	Indapamide 2.5 mg	Lozol by DRX	55045-2385	Diuretic
M <> 80	Tab, White, Round, Film Coated	Indapamide 2.5 mg	Lozol by Mylan	00378-0080	Diuretic
M <> 80	Tab, White, Round, Film Coated	Indapamide 2.5 mg	Lozol by UDL	51079-0868	Diuretic
M <> 8505	Tab, White, Round, Scored	Flecainide Acetate 50 mg	Tambocor by Mylan	000378-8505	Antiarrhythmic
M <> 8505	Tab, White, Round	Flecainide Acetate 50 mg	Tambocor by UDL	51079-0987	Antiarrhythmic
M <> 8510	Tab, White, Round, Scored	Flecainide Acetate 100 mg	Tambocor by Mylan	51079-0988 Discontinued	Antiarrhythmic
M <> 8510	Tab, White, Round, Scored	Flecainide Acetate 100 mg	Tambocor by Mylan	00378-8510	Antiarrhythmic
M <> 8515	Tab, White, Oval, Scored	Flecainide Acetate 150 mg	Tambocor by Mylan	000378-8515	Antiarrhythmic
M <> 87	Tab, Blue, Round, Scored, Film Coated	Maprotiline HCl 50 mg	Ludiomil by Mylan	00378-0087	Antidepressant
M <> 87	Tab, Blue, Round, Scored, Film Coated	Maprotiline HCl 50 mg	Ludiomil by Murfreesboro	51129-1679	Antidepressant
M <> 9	Tab, Yellow, Triangular, Film Coated	Fluphenazine HCl 2.5 mg	Prolixin by UDL	51079-0486	Antipsychotic
M <> 9	Tab, Yellow, Triangular, Film Coated	Fluphenazine HCl 2.5 mg	Prolixin by Mylan	00378-6009	Antipsychotic
M <> 92	Tab, White, Beveled Edge, Coated, 9 to Left, 2 to Right of Score	Maprotiline HCl 75 mg	Ludiomil by Mylan	00378-0092	Antidepressant
M <> 97	Tab, Orange, Triangular, Film Coated	Fluphenazine HCl 10 mg	Prolixin by Invamed	52189-0312	Antipsychotic
M <> 97	Tab, Orange, Triangular, Film Coated	Fluphenazine HCl 10 mg	Prolixin by Mylan	00378-6097	Antipsychotic
M <> 97	Tab, Orange, Triangular, Film Coated	Fluphenazine HCl 10 mg	Prolixin by UDL	51079-0488	Antipsychotic
M <> 970	Tab, White, Round, M inside square <> 970	Acetaminophen 325 mg, Butalbital 50 mg, Caffeine 40 mg	Fioricet by Mallinckrodt	00406-0970	Analgesic
M <> A10	Tab, Blue, Round	Amlodipine Besylate 10 mg	Norvasc by UDL	51079-0452	Antihypertensive
M <> A10	Tab, Blue, Round	Amlodipine Besylate 10 mg	Norvasc by Mylan	00378-5210	Antihypertensive
M <> A2	Tab, White, Round	Atenolol 25 mg	Tenormin by Mylan	00378-0218	Antihypertensive
M <> A2	Tab, White, Round	Atenolol 25 mg	Tenormin by UDL	51079-0759	Antihypertensive
M <> A21	Tab, White, Round, Extended-Release	Alprazolam 0.5 mg	Xanax XR by Mylan	00378-5021	Antianxiety; C IV
M <> A22	Tab, Peach, Round, Extended-Release	Alprazolam 1 mg	Xanax XR by Mylan	00378-5022	Antianxiety; C IV
M <> A23	Tab, Light Purple, Round, Extended-Release	Alprazolam 2 mg	Xanax XR by Mylan	00378-5023	Antianxiety; C IV
M <> A24	Tab, Pink, Round, Extended-Release	Alprazolam 3 mg	Xanax XR by Mylan	00378-5024	Antianxiety; C IV
M <> A7	Tab, White, Round	Alendronate Sodium 10 mg	Fosamax by Mylan	00378-3567	Antiosteoporosis
M <> A7	Tab, White, Round	Alendronate Sodium 10 mg	Fosamax by UDL	51079-0941	Antiosteoporosis
M <> A8	Tab, Blue, Round	Amlodipine Besylate 2.5 mg	Norvasc by Mylan	00378-5208	Antihypertensive
M <> A9	Tab, Blue, Round	Amlodipine Besylate 5 mg	Norvasc by Mylan	00378-5209	Antihypertensive

ID FRONT <> BACK	DESCRIPTION FRONT <> BACK	INGREDIENT & STRENGTH	BRAND (or Generic Equiv.) by FIRM	NDC#	CLASS; SCH.
M <> A9	Tab, Blue, Round	Amlodipine Besylate 5 mg	Novasc by UDL	51079-0451	Antihypertensive
M <> AG	Tab, White, Round	Alendronate Sodium 5 mg	Fosamax by Mylan	00378-3566	Antiosteoporosis
M <> C11	Tab, Green, Round, Scored	Clozapine 100 mg	Clozaril by Mylan	00378-0860	Antipsychotic
M <> C11	Tab, Green, Round, Scored	Clozapine 100 mg	Clozaril by UDL	51079-0922	Antipsychotic
M <> C13	Tab, Yellow, Round, Scored, C over 13	Clonazepam 0.5 mg	Klonopin by D M Graham	00756-0266	Sedative; C IV
M <> C13	Tab, Yellow, Round, Scored, C over 13	Clonazepam 0.5 mg	Klonopin by Mylan	00378-1910	Sedative; C IV
M <> C13	Tab, Yellow, Round, Scored, C over 13	Clonazepam 0.5 mg	Klonopin by UDL	51079-0881	Sedative; C IV
M <> C14	Tab, Light Green, Round, Scored, C over 14	Clonazepam 1 mg	Klonopin by Mylan	00378-1912	Sedative; C IV
M <> C14	Tab, Light Green, Round, Scored, C over 14	Clonazepam 1 mg	Klonopin by UDL	51079-0882	Sedative; C IV
M <> C14	Tab, Light Green, Round, Scored, C over 14	Clonazepam 1 mg	Klonopin by D M Graham	00756-0267	Sedative; C IV
M <> C15	Tab, White, Round, Scored, C over 15	Clonazepam 2 mg	Klonopin by Mylan	00378-1914	Sedative; C IV
M <> C15	Tab, White, Round, Scored, C over 15	Clonazepam 2 mg	Klonopin by UDL	51079-0883 Discontinued	Sedative; C IV
M <> C15	Tab, White, Round, Scored, C over 15	Clonazepam 2 mg	Klonopin by D M Graham	00756-0268	Sedative; C IV
M <> C17	Tab, White, Round	Bicalutamide 50 mg	Casodex by UDL	51079-0692	Antiandrogen
M <> C21	Tab, Yellow, Round, C over 21	Citalopram HBr 10 mg	Celexa by Mylan	00378-1921	Antidepressant
M <> C22	Tab, Yellow, Round, Scored, C over 22	Citalopram HBr 20 mg	Celexa by Mylan	00378-1922	Antidepressant
M <> C24	Tab, Yellow, Round, Scored, C over 24	Citalopram HBr 40 mg	Celexa by Mylan	00378-1924	Antidepressant
M <> C31	Tab, Blue, Round, Film Coated	Carvedilol 3.125 mg	Coreg by UDL	51079-0771	Antihypertensive
M <> C32	Tab, White to Off-White, Round, Film Coated	Carvedilol 6.25 mg	Coreg by UDL	51079-0930	Antihypertensive
M <> C33	Tab, White, Round, Film Coated	Carvedilol 12.5 mg	Coreg by UDL	51079-0931	Antihypertensive
M <> C34	Tab, White, Round, Film Coated	Carvedilol 25 mg	Coreg by UDL	51079-0932	Antihypertensive
M <> C7	Tab, Peach, Round, Scored	Clozapine 25 mg	Clozaril by Mylan	00378-0825	Antipsychotic
M <> C7	Tab, Peach, Round, Scored	Clozapine 25 mg	Clozaril by UDL	51079-0921	Antipsychotic
M <> C73	Tab, Green, Round, Scored	Clozapine 200 mg	Clozaril by UDL	51079-0749	Antipsychotic
M <> D5	Tab, White	Diclofenac Potassium 50 mg	by Mylan		NSAID
M <> DP	Tab	Aspirin 500 mg, Hydrocodone Bitartrate 5 mg	Lortab ASA by Mason	12758-0057	Analgesic; C III
M <> E3	Tab, White to Off-White, Round, Scored, M <> E over 3	Estradiol 0.5 mg	Estrace by Mylan	00378-1452	Hormone
M <> E4	Tab, Pink, Round, Scored, E over 4	Estradiol 1 mg	Estrace by Heartland	61392-0149	Hormone
M <> E4	Tab, Pink, Round, Scored, E over 4	Estradiol 1 mg	Estrace by Mylan	00378-1454	Hormone
M <> E5	Tab, Pale Blue, Round, Scored, E over 5	Estradiol 2 mg	Estrace by Mylan	00378-1458	Hormone
M <> F12	Tab, Yellow, Round, Film Coated, Extended Release	Felodipine 5 mg	Plendil by UDL	51079-0467	Antihypertensive
M <> F13	Tab, Blue, Round, Film Coated, Extended Release	Felodipine 10 mg	Plendil by UDL	51079-0468	Antihypertensive
M <> F3	Tab, Yellow, Round	Fluconazole 50 mg	Diflucan by Mylan	00378-2514	Antifungal
M <> G21	Tab, Blue	Galantamine 4 mg	Razadyne by UDL	51079-0852	Antialzheimers
M <> G22	Tab, Blue	Galantamine 8 mg	Razadyne by UDL	51079-0853	Antialzheimers
M <> G23	Tab, Blue	Galantamine 12 mg	Razadyne by UDL	51079-0854	Antialzheimers
M <> G3	Tab, White, Round	Granisetron HCl 1 mg	Kytril by UDL	51079-0472	Antiemetic
M <> G3	Tab, White, Round	Granisetron HCl 1 mg	Kytril by Mylan	00378-	Antiemetic
M <> G31	Tab, White, Oval	Glipizide 2.5 mg, Metformin HCl 250 mg	MetaGlip by Mylan	00378-3131	Antidiabetic
M <> G32	Tab, White, Oval	Glipizide 2.5 mg, Metformin HCl 500 mg	MetaGlip by Mylan	00378-3132	Antidiabetic
M <> G33	Tab, Peach, Cap Shaped	Glipizide 5 mg, Metformin HCl 500 mg	MetaGlip by Mylan	00378-3133	Antidiabetic
M <> G4	Tab, White, Round	Guanfacine HCl 1 mg	Tenex by Mylan	00378-1160	Antihypertensive
M <> G5	Tab, Blue	Guanfacine HCl 2 mg	Tenex by Mylan	00378-1190	Antihypertensive
M <> GXEF3	Tab, White, Film-Coated, Round	Busulfan 2 mg	Myleran by GSK	Canadian DIN 00004618	Antineoplastic
M <> H25	Tab, Blue	Hydroxyzine HCl 25 mg	Atarax by UDL	51079-0806	Antianxiety; Antihistamine
M <> H50	Tab, Blue	Hydroxyzine HCl 50 mg	Atarax by UDL	51079-0816	Antianxiety; Antihistamine
M <> L10	Tab, Gray, Oblong, Scored, M <> L over 10	Levothyroxine Sodium 125 mcg	Unithroid by UDL	51079-0443	Thyroid Hormone
M <> L10	Tab, Gray, Oblong, Scored, M <> L over 10	Levothyroxine Sodium 125 mcg	Unithroid by Mylan	00378-1813	Thyroid Hormone

ID FRONT <> BACK	DESCRIPTION FRONT <> BACK	INGREDIENT & STRENGTH	BRAND (or Generic Equiv.) by FIRM	NDC#	CLASS; SCH.
M <> L11	Tab, Blue, Oblong, Scored, M <> L over 11	Levothyroxine Sodium 150 mcg	Unithroid by Mylan	00378-1815	Thyroid Hormone
M <> L11	Tab, Blue, Oblong, Scored, M <> L over 11	Levothyroxine Sodium 150 mcg	Unithroid by UDL	51079-0445	Thyroid Hormone
M <> L12	Tab, Purple, Oblong, Scored, M <> L over 12	Levothyroxine Sodium 175 mcg	Unithroid by Mylan	00378-1817	Thyroid Hormone
M <> L13	Tab, Pink, Oblong, Scored, M <> L over 13	Levothyroxine Sodium 200 mcg	Unithroid by Mylan	00378-1819	Thyroid Hormone
M <> L14	Tab, Green, Oblong, Scored, M <> L over 14	Levothyroxine Sodium 300 mcg	Unithroid by Mylan	00378-1821	Thyroid Hormone
M <> L15	Tab, Blue, Capsule Shaped	Levothyroxine Sodium 137 mcg	Synthroid by Mylan	00378-1823	Thyroid Hormone
M <> L17	Tab, White to Off-White, Round	Loratadine 10 mg	Claritin by UDL	51079-0538	Antihistamine
M <> L22	Tab, Light Blue, Round, L over 22	Lisinopril 2.5 mg	Prinivil by Mylan	00378-2072	Antihypertensive
M <> L23	Tab, Peach, Round	Lisinopril 5 mg	Prinivil by Mylan	00378-2073	Antihypertensive
M <> L24	Tab, White, Round, L over 24	Lisinopril 10 mg	Zestril by Mylan	00378-2074	Antihypertensive
M <> L24	Tab, White, Round, L over 24	Lisinopril 10 mg	Zestril by UDL	51079-0982 Discontinued	Antihypertensive
M <> L25	Tab, Light Yellow, Round, L over 25	Lisinopril 20 mg	Zestril by UDL	51079-0983 Discontinued	Antihypertensive
M <> L25	Tab, Light Yellow, Round, L over 25	Lisinopril 20 mg	Zestril by Mylan	00378-2075	Antihypertensive
M <> L26	Tab, Green, Round, L over 26	Lisinopril 40 mg	Prinivil by Mylan	00378-2076	Antihypertensive
M <> L26	Tab, Green, Round	Lisinopril 40 mg	Zestril by UDL	51079-0984	Antihypertensive
M <> L27	Tab, Light Blue, Round, L over 27	Lisinopril 30 mg	Prinivil by Mylan	00378-2077	Antihypertensive
M <> L4	Tab, Peach, Oblong, Scored, M <> L over 4	Levothyroxine Sodium 25 mcg	Unithroid by Mylan	00378-1800	Thyroid Hormone
M <> L4	Tab, Peach, Oblong, Scored, M <> L over 4	Levothyroxine Sodium 25 mcg	Unithroid by UDL	51079-0444	Thyroid Hormone
M <> L5	Tab, White, Oblong, Scored, M <> L over 5	Levothyroxine Sodium 50 mcg	Unithroid by UDL	51079-0440	Thyroid Hormone
M <> L5	Tab, White, Oblong, Scored, M <> L over 5	Levothyroxine Sodium 50 mcg	Unithroid by Mylan	00378-1803	Thyroid Hormone
M <> L51	Tab, White to Off-White, Round, Scored	Lamotrigine 25 mg	Lamictal by UDL	51079-0598	Anticonvulsant
M <> L6	Tab, Violet, Oblong, Scored, M <> L over 6	Levothyroxine Sodium 75 mcg	Unithroid by Mylan	00378-1805	Thyroid Hormone
M <> L6	Tab, Violet, Oblong, Scored, M <> L over 6	Levothyroxine Sodium 75 mcg	Unithroid by UDL	51079-0441	Thyroid Hormone
M <> L7	Tab, Light Green, Oblong, Scored, M <> L over 7	Levothyroxine Sodium 88 mcg	Unithroid by Mylan	00378-1807	Thyroid Hormone
M <> L8	Tab, Yellow, Oblong, Scored, M <> L over 8	Levothyroxine Sodium 100 mcg	Unithroid by Mylan	00378-1809	Thyroid Hormone
M <> L8	Tab, Yellow, Oblong, Scored, M <> L over 8	Levothyroxine Sodium 100 mcg	Unithroid by UDL	51079-0442	Thyroid Hormone
M <> L9	Tab, Dark Pink, Oblong, Scored, M <> L over 9	Levothyroxine Sodium 112 mcg	Unithroid by Mylan	00378-1811	Thyroid Hormone
M <> LH1	Tab, White, Round	Lisinopril 10 mg, HCTZ 12.5 mg	Prinzide by Mylan	00378-1012	Antihypertensive; Diuretic
M <> LH2	Tab, Light Yellow, Round	Lisinopril 20 mg, HCTZ 12.5 mg	Prinzide by Mylan	00378-2012	Antihypertensive; Diuretic
M <> LH3	Tab, Light Green, Round	Lisinopril 20 mg, HCTZ 25 mg	Prinzide by Mylan	00378-2025	Antihypertensive; Diuretic
M <> MH1	Tab, White, Round, Scored, MH over 1	Midodrine HCl 2.5 mg	ProAmatine by Mylan	00378-1901	Antihypotensive
M <> MH2	Tab, White, Round, Scored, MH over 2	Midodrine HCl 5 mg	ProAmatine by Mylan	00378-1902	Antihypotensive
M <> MH2	Tab, White, Round, Scored, MH over 2	Midodrine HCl 5 mg	ProAmatine by UDL	51079-0453	Antihypotensive
M <> MH3	Tab, White, Round, Scored, MH over 3	Midodrine HCl 10 mg	ProAmatine by Mylan	00378-1903	Antihypotensive
M <> MJ158	Tab, White, Diamond Shaped, MJ over 158	Fosinopril Sodium 10 mg	Monopril by Mead Johnson		Antihypertensive
M <> MJ158	Tab, White, Diamond Shaped, MJ over 158	Fosinopril Sodium 10 mg	Monopril by Allscripts		Antihypertensive
M <> MJ609	Tab, White, Cap Shaped, MJ over 609	Fosinopril Sodium 20 mg	Monopril by Allscripts		Antihypertensive
M <> MSD917	Tab, Peach, Diamond Shaped, Scored	Amiloride HCl 5 mg, Hydrochlorothiazide 50 mg	Moduretic by Merck	00006-0917	Antihypertensive; Diuretic
M <> MYSOLINE250	Tab	Primidone 250 mg	Mysoline by Wal Mart	49035-0169	Anticonvulsant
M <> MYSOLINE250	Tab	Primidone 250 mg	Mysoline by Thrift Drug	59198-0181	Anticonvulsant
M <> MYSOLINE250	Tab	Primidone 250 mg	Mysoline by Murfreesboro	51129-1168	Anticonvulsant
M <> N1	Tab, Blue, Capsule Shaped	Paroxetine 10 mg	Paxil by Mylan	00378-7001	Antidepressant
M <> N10	Tab, Green, Round	Ropinirole HCl 1 mg	Requip by Mylan	00378-5501	Antiparkinson
M <> N2	Tab, Blue, Capsule Shaped	Paroxetine 20 mg	Paxil by Mylan	00378-7002	Antidepressant
M <> N20	Tab, Peach, Round	Ropinirole HCl 2 mg	Requip by Mylan	00378-5502	Antiparkinson
M <> N22	Tab, Pink, Round	Nisoldipine ER 20 mg	Sular by Mylan	00378-2222	Antihypertensive
M <> N23	Tab, Pink, Round	Nisoldipine ER 30 mg	Sular by Mylan	00378-2223-	Antihypertensive
M <> N24	Tab, Orange, Round	Nisoldipine ER 40 mg	Sular by Mylan	00378-2224	Antihypertensive

ID FRONT <> BACK	DESCRIPTION FRONT <> BACK	INGREDIENT & STRENGTH	BRAND (or Generic Equiv.), by FIRM	NDC#	CLASS; SCH.
M <> N25	Tab, White, Round	Ropinirole HCl 0.25 mg	Requip by Mylan	00378-5525	Antiparkinson
M <> N30	Tab, Purple, Round	Ropinirole HCl 3 mg	Requip by Mylan	00378-5503	Antiparkinson
M <> N40	Tab, Grey, Round	Ropinirole HCl 4 mg	Requip by Mylan	00378-5504	Antiparkinson
M <> N5	Tab, Yellow, Round	Ropinirole HCl 0.5 mg	Requip by Mylan	00378-5550	Antiparkinson
M <> N50	Tab, Blue, Round	Ropinirole HCl 5 mg	Requip by Mylan	00378-5505	Antiparkinson
M <> N52	Tab, White, Round, Scored, M <> N / 52	Nefazodone HCl 100 mg	Serzone by Mylan	00378-2052	Antidepressant
M <> N53	Tab, White, Round, Scored, M <> N / 53	Nefazodone HCl 150 mg	Serzone by Mylan	00378-2053	Antidepressant
M <> N54	Tab, White, Round, M <> N / 54	Nefazodone HCl 200 mg	Serzone by Mylan	00378-2054	Antidepressant
M <> N55	Tab, White, Round, M <> N / 55	Nefazodone HCl 250 mg	Serzone by Mylan	00378-2055	Antidepressant
M <> P1	Tab, Maroon, Round, Film Coated	Prochlorperazine 5 mg	Compazine by UDL	51079-0541 Discontinued	Antiemetic
M <> P1	Tab, Maroon, Round, Film Coated	Prochlorperazine 5 mg	Compazine by Mylan	00378-5105	Antiemetic
M <> P2	Tab, Maroon, Round, Film Coated	Prochlorperazine 10 mg	Compazine by Mylan	00378-5110	Antiemetic
M <> P2	Tab, Maroon, Round, Film Coated	Prochlorperazine 10 mg	Compazine by UDL	51079-0542 Discontinued	Antiemetic
M <> PAL	Tab, Purple, Round, Coated	L-methylfolate Calcium (Metafolin) 3 mg, Pyridoxal-5'-Phosphate 35 mg, Methylcobalamin 2 mg	Metanx by PAMLAB, LLC.	00525-8019	Supplement
M <> PT	Tab, Peach, Round	Tramadol HCl 37.5 mg, Acetaminophen 325 mg	Ultracet by Mylan	00378-8088	Analgesic
M <> R	Tab, White, Round	Risperidone .25 mg	Risperdal by Mylan	00378-3502	Antipsychotic
M <> R	Tab, White, Round, Film Coated	Risperidone 0.25 mg	Risperdal by UDL	51079-0460	Antipsychotic
M <> R11	Tab, White, Round, Film-Coated	Risperidone 1 mg	Risperdal by UDL	51079-0462	Antipsychotic
M <> R11	Tab, White, Round	Risperidone 1 mg	Risperdal by Mylan	00378-3511	Antipsychotic
M <> R12	Tab, Pink, Round	Risperidone 2 mg	Risperdal by Mylan	00378-3512	Antipsychotic
M <> R12	Tab, Beige, Round, Film-Coated	Risperidone 2 mg	Risperdal by UDL	51079-0463	Antipsychotic
M <> R13	Tab, White, Round, Film-Coated	Risperidone 3 mg	Risperdal by UDL	51079-0464	Antipsychotic
M <> R13	Tab, White, Round	Risperidone 3 mg	Risperdal by Mylan	00378-3513	Antipsychotic
M <> R14	Tab, Pink, Round	Risperidone 4 mg	Risperdal by Mylan	00378-3514	Antipsychotic
M <> R14	Tab, Beige, Round, Film-Coated	Risperidone 4 mg	Risperdal by UDL	51079-0465	Antipsychotic
M <> R5	Tab, Beige, Round, Film-Coated	Risperidone 0.5 mg	Risperdal by UDL	51079-0461	Antipsychotic
M <> R5	Tab, Pink, Round	Risperidone .5 mg	Risperdal by Mylan	00378-3505	Antipsychotic
M <> T3	Tab, Purple, Round, Film Coated	Trifluoperazine HCl 1 mg	Stelazine by UDL	51079-0572	Antipsychotic
M <> T3	Tab, Purple, Round, Film Coated	Trifluoperazine HCl 1 mg	Stelazine by Dixon Shane	17236-0296	Antipsychotic
M <> T4	Tab, Purple, Round, Film Coated	Trifluoperazine HCl 2 mg	Stelazine by Mylan	00378-2402	Antipsychotic
M <> T4	Tab, Purple, Round, Film Coated	Trifluoperazine HCl 2 mg	Stelazine by UDL	51079-0573	Antipsychotic
M <> T4	Tab, White, Round, Film Coated	Trifluoperazine HCl 2 mg	Stelazine by Dixon Shane	17236-0293	Antipsychotic
M <> T41	Tab, White, Oblong, Scored, M <> T / 41	Trandolapril 1 mg	Mavik by Mylan	00378-3241	Antihypertensive
M <> T42	Tab, White, Round	Trandolapril 2 mg	Mavik by Mylan	00378-3242	Antihypertensive
M <> T43	Tab, Peach, Round	Trandolapril 4 mg	Mavik by Mylan	00378-3243	Antihypertensive
M <> T5	Tab, Purple, Round, Film Coated	Trifluoperazine HCl 5 mg	Stelazine by UDL	51079-0574	Antipsychotic
M <> T5	Tab, Purple, Round, Film Coated	Trifluoperazine HCl 5 mg	Stelazine by Dixon Shane	17236-0296	Antipsychotic
M <> T5	Tab, Purple, Round, Film Coated	Trifluoperazine HCl 5 mg	Stelazine by Mylan	00378-2405	Antipsychotic
M <> T6	Tab, Purple, Round, Film Coated	Trifluoperazine HCl 10 mg	Stelazine by Mylan	00378-2410	Antipsychotic
M <> T6	Tab, Purple, Round, Film Coated	Trifluoperazine HCl 10 mg	Stelazine by Dixon Shane	17236-0334	Antipsychotic
M <> T6	Tab, Purple, Round, Film Coated	Trifluoperazine HCl 10 mg	Stelazine by UDL	51079-0575	Antipsychotic
M <> T7	Tab, White, Round, Film Coated	Tramadol HCl 50 mg	Ultram by UDL	51079-0991 Discontinued	Analgesic
M <> T7	Tab, White, Round, Film Coated	Tramadol HCl 50 mg	Ultram by Mylan	00378-4151	Analgesic
M <> V1	Tab, Yellow, Round, Scored	Venlafaxine 25 mg	Effexor by Mylan	00378-4881	Antidepressant
M <> V2	Tab, Yellow, Round, Scored	Venlafaxine 37.5 mg	Effexor by Mylan	00378-4882	Antidepressant
M <> V2	Tab, Yellow, Round, Scored	Venlafaxine 37.5 mg	Effexor by UDL	51079-0480	Antidepressant

ID FRONT <> BACK	DESCRIPTION FRONT <> BACK	INGREDIENT & STRENGTH	BRAND (or Generic Equiv.) by FIRM	NDC#	CLASS; SCH.
M <> V3	Tab, Yellow, Round, Scored	Venlafaxine 50 mg	Effexor by Mylan	00378-4883	Antidepressant
M006	Tab, White, Round	Atenolol 50 mg	Tenormin by Mylan		Antihypertensive
M007	Tab, White, Round	Atenolol 100 mg	Tenormin by Mylan		Antihypertensive
M01 <> MOVA	Tab, White, Oval, Scored	Captopril 12.5 mg	Capoten by Mova	55370-0164	Antihypertensive
M010	Tab, Peach, Round, Film Coated, Extended Release	Oxybutynin Chloride 10 mg	Ditropan XL by Mylan	00378-6610	Urinary Tract
M017	Tab, Grey, Round, Extended Release	Oxybutynin Chloride 15 mg	Ditropan XL by Mylan	00378-6015	Urinary Tract
M018	Cap, Clear & Green	Codeine Phosphate 20 mg, Pseudoephedrine HCl 60 mg	Nucofed by King	61570-0018	Cold Remedy; C III
M019	Tab, White	Theophylline Anhydrous 300 mg	Quibron-T/SR by King	61570-0019	Antiasthmatic
M020	Tab, Ivory	Theophylline Anhydrous 300 mg	Quibron-T by King	61570-0020	Antiasthmatic
M022	Cap, Opaque & Yellow	Theophylline Anhydrous 150 mg, Guaifenesin 90 mg	Quibron by Roberts	54092-0067	Antiasthmatic
M022	Cap, Yellow	Theophylline Anhydrous 150 mg, Guaifenesin 90 mg	Quibron by Talbert	44514-0469	Antiasthmatic
M024	Tab, White, Oval, M over 024	Chlorthalidone 15 mg	Thaliton by Monarch	61570-0024	Diuretic
M024	Tab, White, Oval, M over 024	Chlorthalidone 15 mg	Hygroton by Compumed	00403-0044	Diuretic
M0315	Tab, White, Oval, Scored, M03 / 1.5	Glyburide 1.5 mg	Glynase by Dava	67253-0460	Antidiabetic
M0315 <> Z	Tab, White, Oval, Scored	Glyburide 1.5 mg	Glycron by Mova	55370-0592	Antidiabetic
M0361	Tab, Blue, Cap Shaped, Scored	Acetaminophen 650 mg, Hydrocodone Bitartrate 10 mg	Lorcet by Sandoz	00781-1524	Analgesic; C III
M0361	Tab, M on One Side of the Score and 0361 on the Opposite Side	Acetaminophen 650 mg, Hydrocodone Bitartrate 10 mg	Lorcet by King	60793-0849	Analgesic; C III
M0362	Tab, White, Oblong, M/0362	Acetaminophen 660 mg, Hydrocodone Bitartrate 10 mg	Vicodin HP by Mallinckrodt	00406-0421	Analgesic; C III
M0421	Cap, Blue & Clear	Chlorpheniramine Maleate 12 mg, Phenylpropanolamine 75 mg	Ornade by Mallinckrodt	Discontinued	Cold Remedy
M0421	Tab, Blue & Clear, M/0421	Chlorpheniramine Maleate 12 mg, Phenylpropanolamine 75 mg	Ornade by Mallinckrodt		Cold Remedy
M0430	Tab, Light Blue, Oval, Scored, MOVA <> M04 / 3.0	Glyburide 3 mg	Glynase by Dava	67253-0461	Antidiabetic
M0430 <> Z	Tab, Blue, Oval, Scored	Glyburide 3 mg	Glycron by Mova	55370-0594	Antidiabetic
M05	Tab, Grey, Round, Extended Release	Oxybutynin Chloride 5 mg	Ditropan XL by Mylan	00378-6605	Urinary Tract
M05	Tab, Light Green, Round, Film Coated, Extended Release	Oxybutynin Chloride 5 mg	Ditropan XL by UDL	51079-0722	Urinary Tract
M052	Tab, Pink, Round, Scored	Sulfamethoxazole 400 mg, Trimethoprim 80 mg	Septra by King	61570-0052	Antibiotic
M053	Tab, Pink, Oval, Scored	Sulfamethoxazole 800 mg, Trimethoprim 160 mg	Septra DS by King	61570-0053	Antibiotic
M057	Tab, White, Oblong, Scored	Sucralfate 1 g	Carafate by Martec	52555-0057	Gastrointestinal
M057	Tab, White, Oblong, Scored	Sucralfate 1 g	Carafate by Prasco	66993-0830	Gastrointestinal
M057	Tab, White, Oblong, Scored	Sucralfate 1 g	Carafate by Major	00904-5438	Gastrointestinal
M057	Tab, White, Oblong, Scored	Sucralfate 1 g	Carafate by Eon	00185-2100	Gastrointestinal
M057	Tab, White, Oblong, Scored	Sucralfate 1 g	Carafate by Amneal	65162-0546	Gastrointestinal
M0645 <> Z	Tab, Green, Oval, Scored	Glyburide 4.5 mg	Glycron by Mova	55370-0595	Antidiabetic
M0661	Cap, Light Green, Opaque, Hard Gel, M inside Square	Fluoxetine HCl 10 mg	Prozac by Mallinckrodt	00406-0661	Antidepressant
M0663	Cap, Green & White, Opaque, Hard Gel	Fluoxetine HCl 20 mg	Prozac by Mallinckrodt	00406-0663	Antidepressant
M0760 <> Z	Tab, Yellow, Oval, Scored	Glyburide 6 mg	Glycron by Mova	55370-0596	Antidiabetic
M0765	Tab, Yellow, Oval, Scored, M07 / 6.5	Glyburide 6 mg	Glynase by Dava	67253-0462	Antidiabetic
M1	Tab, Yellow, Round, Scored, M over Score, 1 below	Methotrexate 2.5 mg	Rheumatrex by Dava	67253-0580	Antineoplastic
M1	Tab, Purple, Oval, Film Coated	Methenamine Mandelate 1 mg	Mandelamine by Nat Pharmpak	55154-9002	Antibiotic; Urinary Tract
M1	Tab, Yellow, Round, Scored, M over 1	Chlorthalidone 15 mg, Clonidine HCl 0.1 mg	Clorpres by Bertek	62794-0001	Diuretic; Antihypertensive
M1	Tab, Yellow, Round, Scored	Chlorthalidone 15 mg, Clonidine HCl 0.1 mg	Clorpres by Mylan	00378-0001	Diuretic; Antihypertensive
M1	Tab, Yellow, Round, Scored	Chlorthalidone 15 mg, Clonidine HCl 0.1 mg	Clorpres by Med Pro	53978-0851	Diuretic; Antihypertensive
M1 <> LL	Tab, White to Off-White, Round, Scored, M over 1	Methotrexate 2.5 mg	Rheumatrex by Lederle	00005-4507	Antineoplastic
M10	Tab, Orange, Round	Propranolol HCl 10 mg	Inderal by Martec		Antihypertensive
M10	Tab	Buspirone HCl 10 mg	Buspar by Med Pro	53978-2036	Antianxiety
M10	Tab, White, Round, Scored	Methimazole 10 mg	Tapazole by Jones	00689-1085	Antithyroid

ID FRONT <> BACK	DESCRIPTION FRONT <> BACK	INGREDIENT & STRENGTH	BRAND (or Generic Equiv.) by FIRM	NDC#	CLASS; SCH.
M10 <> P	Tab, White, Round, Scored	Metoclopramide HCl 10 mg	Maxeran by Pharmascience	Canadian DIN 02230432	Gastrointestinal
M100	Tab	Levothyroxine Sodium 100 mcg	Euthyrox by Em Pharma	63254-0439	Thyroid Hormone
M100	Tab, Yellow, Scored	Levothyroxine Sodium 100 mcg	by AltiMed	Canadian DIN 02237216	Thyroid Hormone
M100	Cap, White, Film Coated, Scored	Ibuprofen 100 mg	Children's Motrin by McNeil	Canadian DIN 02240527	NSAID
M100	Tab, Film Coated	Ibuprofen 100 mg	Motrin by McNeil	50580-0445	NSAID
M100	Tab, White, Round, Film Coated, Extended Release, Scripted M	Metoprolol Succinate 100 mg	Toprol XL by Par	49884-0406	Antihypertensive
M1000	Tab, White, Oval, Film Coated, Extended Release	Metformin HCl 1000 mg	Glumetza by Depomed	13913-0003	Antidiabetic
M10061	Tab, Film Coated, M 100 61	Thioridazine HCl 100 mg	by Med Pro	53978-2007	Antipsychotic
M100G	Cap, Orange, M 100/G	Minocycline HCl 100 mg	Minocin by Genpharm	Canadian	Antibiotic
M100LEVOT	Tab, Yellow, Round	Levothyroxine Sodium 0.1 mg	Synthroid by Mova		Thyroid Hormone
M101	Tab, Oval, Reddish Brown, Scored	Mirtazapine 30 mg	Remeron by Sandoz	00185-5999	Antidepressant
M11	Tab	Penicillin V Potassium 250 mg	by Rx Dispensing	61807-0003	Antibiotic
M11	Tab	Penicillin V Potassium 250 mg	by Mylan	00378-0111	Antibiotic
M112	Tab, Rose, Scored	Levothyroxine Sodium 112 mcg	by AltiMed	Canadian DIN 02237217	Thyroid Hormone
M113	Tab, White, Oblong, Scored	Glyburide 1.5 mg	Glynase Press-Tabs by Mylan	00378-1113	Antidiabetic
M118	Tab, Light Yellow, Cap Shaped, Scored	Pentazocine HCl 50 mg, Naloxone HCl 0.5 mg	Talwin by OHM	51660-0506	Analgesic; C IV
M118	Tab, Light Yellow, Cap Shaped, Scored	Pentazocine HCl 50 mg, Naloxone HCl 0.5 mg	Talwin by Mallinckrodt	00406-3118	Analgesic; C IV
M118	Tab, Light Yellow, Cap Shaped, Scored	Pentazocine HCl 50 mg, Naloxone HCl 0.5 mg	Talwin by Ranbaxy	63304-0506	Analgesic; C IV
M12	Tab, Film Coated, M 12	Verapamil HCl 80 mg	by Med Pro	53978-7001	Antihypertensive
M12	Tab, M to Left, 12 to Right of Score	Penicillin V Potassium 500 mg	by Mylan	00378-0112	Antibiotic
M12	Tab, Film Coated	Penicillin V Potassium	by Med Pro	53978-5055	Antibiotic
M125	Tab, Light Yellow, Oblong, Scored	Glyburide 3 mg	Glynase Press-Tabs by Mylan	00378-1125	Antidiabetic
M125	Tab, Brown, Scored	Levothyroxine Sodium 125 mcg	by AltiMed	Canadian DIN 02237218	Thyroid Hormone
M125	Tab, Tan, Round	Levothyroxine Sodium 0.125 mg	Synthroid by Duramed		Thyroid Hormone
M125LEVOT	Tab, Brown, Round	Levothyroxine Sodium 0.125 mg	Synthroid by Mova		Thyroid Hormone
M127	Tab, White, Round, M Above Score, 127 Below	Pindolol 10 mg	Visken by Mylan	55160-0133	Antihypertensive
M127	Tab, White, Round, M Above Score, 127 Below	Pindolol 10 mg	Visken by Mylan	00378-0127	Antihypertensive
M13	Tab, White, Round, Scored	Tolbutamide 500 mg	Orinase by UDL	51079-0560	Antidiabetic
M13	Tab, White, Round	Tolbutamide 500 mg	Orinase by Mylan		Antidiabetic
M13	Tab, White, Round, Scored	Tolbutamide 500 mg	Orinase by Kaiser	00179-0198	Antidiabetic
M13	Tab, White, Round, Scored	Tolbutamide 500 mg	Orinase by Mylan	00378-0215	Antidiabetic
M13	Tab, White, Round, Scored	Tolbutamide 500 mg	Orinase by Pharmedix	53002-0519	Antidiabetic
M132	Tab, Yellow, Round, Scored, M over 132	Nadolol 80 mg	Corgard by Med Pro	53978-2019	Antihypertensive
M132	Tab, Yellow, Round, Scored, M over 132	Nadolol 80 mg	Corgard by Physician Total Care	54868-3721	Antihypertensive
M132	Tab, Yellow, Round, Scored, M over 132	Nadolol 80 mg	Corgard by Mylan	00378-1132	Antihypertensive
M132	Tab, Yellow, Round, Scored, M over 132	Nadolol 80 mg	Corgard by Qualitest	00603-4742	Antihypertensive
M132	Tab, Yellow, Round, Scored, M over 132	Nadolol 80 mg	Corgard by UDL	51079-0814 Discontinued	Antihypertensive
M134	Tab, White, Beveled Edge, Film Coated, M over 134	Ketorolac Tromethamine 10 mg	Toradol by Mylan	00378-1134	NSAID
M135	Tab, White, Cap Shaped, Scored, Film Coated	Diltiazem HCl 90 mg	Cardizem by Heartland	61392-0146	Antihypertensive
M135	Tab, White, Cap Shaped, Scored, Film Coated	Diltiazem HCl 90 mg	Cardizem by Heartland	61392-0055	Antihypertensive
M135	Tab, White, Cap Shaped, Scored, Film Coated	Diltiazem HCl 90 mg	Cardizem by Mylan	00378-0135	Antihypertensive
M135	Tab, White, Cap Shaped, Scored, Film Coated	Diltiazem HCl 90 mg	Cardizem by UDL	51079-0747	Antihypertensive
M135	Tab, White, Cap Shaped, Scored, Film Coated	Diltiazem HCl 90 mg	Cardizem by Egis	48581-6123	Antihypertensive

ID FRONT <> BACK	DESCRIPTION FRONT <> BACK	INGREDIENT & STRENGTH	BRAND (or Generic Equiv.) by FIRM	NDC#	CLASS; SCH.
M139	Tab, White, Round, M-139	Sulfamethoxazole 400 mg, Trimethoprim 80 mg	Bactrim by Mylan		Antibiotic
M14	Tab, Orange, Round, Scored, M over 14	Methotrexate Sodium 2.5 mg	Rheumatrex by Mylan	00378-0014	Antineoplastic
M14	Tab, Orange, Round, Scored, M over 14	Methotrexate Sodium 2.5 mg	Rheumatrex by UDL	51079-0670	Antineoplastic
M140	Tab, White, Round, M-140	Sulfamethoxazole 800 mg, Trimethoprim 160 mg	Bactrim DS by Mylan		Antibiotic
M142	Tab, Teal, Oval, Scored	Glyburide 6 mg	Glynase by Mylan	00378-1142	Antidiabetic
M146	Tab, White, Round	Spironolactone 25 mg	Aldactone by Mylan	00378-2146	Diuretic
M15	Tab, White, Oblong, Scored, Extended Release	Potassium Chloride 15 mEq	Klor-Con M15 by Upsher Smith	00245-0150	Electrolytes
M15	Tab, White, Round, M over 15	Atropine Sulfate 0.025 mg, Diphenoxylate HCl 2.5 mg	Lomotil by Nat Pharmpak	55154-5563	Antidiarrheal; C V
M15	Tab, White, Round, M over 15	Atropine Sulfate 0.025 mg, Diphenoxylate HCl 2.5 mg	Lomotil by Kaiser	00179-0276	Antidiarrheal; C V
M15	Tab, White, Round, M over 15	Atropine Sulfate 0.025 mg, Diphenoxylate HCl 2.5 mg	Lomotil by Mylan	00378-0415	Antidiarrheal; C V
M15	Tab, White, Round, M over 15	Atropine Sulfate 0.025 mg, Diphenoxylate HCl 2.5 mg	Lomotil by Vangard	00615-0429	Antidiarrheal; C V
M15	Tab, White, Round, M over 15	Atropine Sulfate 0.025 mg, Diphenoxylate HCl 2.5 mg	Lomotil by Murfreesboro	51129-1343	Antidiarrheal; C V
M15	Tab, White, Round, M over 15	Atropine Sulfate 0.025 mg, Diphenoxylate HCl 2.5 mg	Lomotil by Urgent Care Center	50716-0477	Antidiarrheal; C V
M15	Tab, White, Round, M over 15	Atropine Sulfate 0.025 mg, Diphenoxylate HCl 2.5 mg	Lomotil by Patient First	57575-0074	Antidiarrheal; C V
M15	Tab, White, Round, M over 15	Atropine Sulfate 0.025 mg, Diphenoxylate HCl 2.5 mg	Lomotil by Physician Total Care	54868-0032	Antidiarrheal; C V
M15	Tab, White, Round, M over 15	Atropine Sulfate 0.025 mg, Diphenoxylate HCl 2.5 mg	Lomotil by UDL	51079-0067 Discontinued	Antidiarrheal; C V
M15	Tab, Tan to Yellow, Modified Rectangle Shaped	Potassium Citrate 15 mEq	Urocit K by Mission	00178-0615	Electrolytes
M15 <> PF	Tab, Blue, Round	Morphine Sulfate 15 mg	MS Contin by Purdue	59011-0260	Analgesic; C II
M150	Tab, Blue, Scored	Levothyroxine Sodium 150 mcg	by AltiMed	Canadian DIN 02237219	Thyroid Hormone
M150	Tab, Blue, Round	Levothyroxine Sodium 0.15 mg	Synthroid by Duramed		Thyroid Hormone
M150LEVOT	Tab, Blue, Round	Levothyroxine Sodium 0.15 mg	Synthroid by Mova		Thyroid Hormone
M158	Tab, White, Diamond	Fosinopril Sodium 10 mg	Monopril by Mead Johnson		Antihypertensive
M170LORABID200MG	Cap, Blue and Gray	Loracarbef 200 mg	Lorabid by Monarch	61570-0170	Antibiotic
M171	Tab, Yellow, Round, Scored, M over 171	Nadolol 40 mg	Corgard by Med Pro	53978-2018	Antihypertensive
M171	Tab, Yellow, Round, Scored, M over 171	Nadolol 40 mg	Corgard by UDL	51079-0813	Antihypertensive
M171	Tab, Yellow, Round, Scored, M over 171	Nadolol 40 mg	Corgard by Mylan	00378-1171	Antihypertensive
M171	Tab, Yellow, Round, Scored, M over 171	Nadolol 40 mg	Corgard by Qualitest	00603-4741	Antihypertensive
M171LORABID400MG	Cap, Blue and Pink	Loracarbef 400 mg	Lorabid by Monarch	61570-0171	Antibiotic
M1743	Tab, Orange, Cap Shaped, Ex Release	Ciprofloxacin 500 mg	Cipro XR by Mylan	00378-1743	Antibiotic
M1745	Tab, Orange, Cap Shaped, Ex Release	Ciprofloxacin 1000 mg	Cipro XR by Mylan	00378-1745	Antibiotic
M175	Tab, Lilac, Scored	Levothyroxine Sodium 175 mcg	Synthroid by AltiMed	Canadian DIN 02237220	Thyroid Hormone
M177	Tab, White, Round, Film Coated, Extended Release	Divalproex Sodium 250 mg	Depakote E.R. by UDL	51079-0766	Anticonvulsant
M177	Tab, White, Round, Film Coated, Extended Release	Divalproex Sodium 250 mg	Depakote E.R. by Mylan	00378-0472	Anticonvulsant
M18	Tab, White, Round, M18/+	Guaifenesin 200 mg, Ephedrine 25 mg	by PDK		Cold Remedy
M18	Tab, White, Round, Scored	Metoprolol Tartrate 25 mg	Lopressor by UDL	51079-0255	Antihypertensive
M18	Tab, White, Round, Scored	Metoprolol Tartrate 25 mg	Lopressor by Mylan	00378-0018	Antihypertensive
M18TIGAN	Cap, Blue, Opaque	Trimethobenzamide HCl 250 mg	Tigan by Roberts	54092-0186	Antiemetic
M18TIGAN	Cap, Blue, Opaque	Trimethobenzamide HCl 250 mg	Tigan by Monarch	61570-0187	Antiemetic
M19 <> LL	Tab, White, Round, Scored, M over 19	Methocarbamol 500 mg	Robaxin by Lederle	00005-3562	Muscle Relaxant
M19 <> LL	Tab, White, Round, Scored, M over 19	Methocarbamol 500 mg	Robaxin by Nat Pharmpak	55154-5541	Muscle Relaxant
M19 <> LL	Tab, White, Round, Scored, M over 19	Methocarbamol 500 mg	Robaxin by Neuman	64579-0010	Muscle Relaxant
M19 <> LL	Tab, White, Round, Scored, M over 19	Methocarbamol 500 mg	Robaxin by UDL	51079-0091	Muscle Relaxant
M1LL	Tab, Yellow, Round, M1/LL	Methotrexate 2.5 mg	Rheumatrex by Wyeth	Canadian	Antineoplastic
M2	Tab, White, Round	Furosemide 20 mg	Lasix by PDRX	55289-0593	Diuretic
M2	Tab, White, Round	Furosemide 20 mg	Lasix by Martec		Diuretic
M2	Tab, White, Round	Furosemide 20 mg	Lasix by Kaiser	62224-1220	Diuretic

ID FRONT <> BACK	DESCRIPTION FRONT <> BACK	INGREDIENT & STRENGTH	BRAND (or Generic Equiv.) by FIRM	NDC#	CLASS; SCH.
M2	Tab, White, Round	Furosemide 20 mg	Lasix by Heartland	61392-0256	Diuretic
M2	Tab, White, Round	Furosemide 20 mg	Lasix by Diversified Healthcare	55887-0997	Diuretic
M2	Tab, White, Round	Furosemide 20 mg	Lasix by Mylan	00378-0208	Diuretic
M2	Tab, White, Round	Furosemide 20 mg	Lasix by JB	51111-0480	Diuretic
M2	Tab, White, Round	Furosemide 20 mg	Lasix by UDL	51079-0072 Discontinued	Diuretic
M20	Tab, Blue, Round	Propranolol HCl 20 mg	Inderal by Martec		Antihypertensive
M20 <> LL	Tab, White, Cap Shaped, Scored	Methocarbamol 750 mg	Robaxin by Physician Total Care	54868-1103	Muscle Relaxant
M20 <> LL	Tab, White, Cap Shaped, Scored	Methocarbamol 750 mg	Robaxin by Neuman	64579-0008	Muscle Relaxant
M20 <> LL	Tab, White, Cap Shaped, Scored	Methocarbamol 750 mg	Robaxin by UDL	51079-0092	Muscle Relaxant
M20 <> LL	Tab, White, Cap Shaped, Scored	Methocarbamol 750 mg	Robaxin by Lederle	00005-3563	Muscle Relaxant
M200	Tab, Pink, Scored	Levothyroxine Sodium 200 mcg	by AltiMed	Canadian DIN 02237221	Thyroid Hormone
M200	Tab	Levothyroxine Sodium 200 mcg	Euthyrox by Em Pharma	63254-0444	Thyroid Hormone
M200	Tab, White, Oval, Film Coated, Extended Release, Scripted M	Metoprolol Succinate 200 mg	Toprol XL by Par	49884-0407	Antihypertensive
M200 <> PF	Tab, Green, Cap Shaped, Ex Release	Morphine Sulfate 200 mg	Ms Contin by Purdue	59011-0264	Analgesic; C II
M200LEVOT	Tab, Pink, Round	Levothyroxine Sodium 0.2 mg	Synthroid by Mova		Thyroid Hormone
M204	Tab, White, Round, M/204	Diclofenac Sodium 50 mg	Voltaren by Martec	52555-0204	NSAID
M205	Tab, White, Round, Delayed Release, M/205	Diclofenac Sodium 75 mg	Voltaren by Martec	52555-0205	NSAID
M21	Tab, White, Round	Penicillin G Potassium 250,000 Units	Pentids by Mylan		Antibiotic
M21 <> ICN	Tab, White, Round, Film Coated	Metformin HCl 500 mg	Glycon by Valeant	Canadian DIN 02229516	Antidiabetic
M21ICN	Tab, White, Round, M21/ICN	Metformin HCl 500 mg	Glucophage by ICN	Canadian	Antidiabetic
M22 <> LL	Tab, Peach, Round	Methyldopa 250 mg	Aldomet by Lederle	00005-3850	Antihypertensive
M22 <> LL	Tab, Peach, Round	Methyldopa 250 mg	Aldomet by Neuman	64579-0018	Antihypertensive
M221	Tab, Green, Round, Scored, M over 221	Timolol Maleate 10 mg	Blocarden by Teva	00480-0088	Antihypertensive
M221	Tab, Green, Round, Scored, M over 221	Timolol Maleate 10 mg	Blocarden by Mylan	00378-0221	Antihypertensive
M221	Tab, Green, Round, Scored, M over 221	Timolol Maleate 10 mg	Blocarden by Med Pro	53978-2021	Antihypertensive
M23	Tab, White, Round, Film Coated, M over 23	Diltiazem HCl 30 mg	Cardizem by Heartland	61392-0053	Antihypertensive
M23	Tab, White, Round, Film Coated, M over 23	Diltiazem HCl 30 mg	Cardizem by Elan Hold	60274-0880	Antihypertensive
M23	Tab, White, Round, Film Coated, M over 23	Diltiazem HCl 30 mg	Cardizem by Mylan	00378-0023	Antihypertensive
M23	Tab, White, Round, Film Coated, M over 23	Diltiazem HCl 30 mg	Cardizem by Vangard	00615-3548	Antihypertensive
M23	Tab, White, Round, Film Coated, M over 23	Diltiazem HCl 30 mg	Cardizem by PDRX	55289-0335	Antihypertensive
M23	Tab, White, Round, Film Coated, M over 23	Diltiazem HCl 30 mg	Cardizem by UDL	51079-0745	Antihypertensive
M23 <> LL	Tab, Peach, Round	Methyldopa 500 mg	Aldomet by Caremark	00339-5231	Antihypertensive
M23 <> LL	Tab, Peach, Round	Methyldopa 500 mg	Aldomet by Lederle	00005-3851	Antihypertensive
M23 <> LL	Tab, Peach, Round	Methyldopa 500 mg	Aldomet by Neuman	64579-0019	Antihypertensive
M243	Tab, White, Round, Scored, Film Coated, M over 243	Spironolactone 50 mg	Aldactone by Mylan	00378-0243	Diuretic
M243	Tab, White, Round, Scored, Film Coated, M over 243	Spironolactone 50 mg	Aldactone by UDL	51079-0979	Diuretic
M244	Tab, White, Oval, Scored, Film Coated	Metformin HCl 1000 mg	Glucophage by Mylan	00378-0244	Antidiabetic
M244	Tab, White, Oval, Scored, Film Coated	Metformin HCl 1000 mg	Glucophage by UDL	51079-0995	Antidiabetic
M25	Tab	Methyclothiazide 5 mg	by Med Pro	53978-2016	Diuretic; Antihypertensive
M25	Tab, Yellow, Round, M 2.5	Methotrexate 2.5 mg	Rheumatrex by Faulding	Canadian	Antineoplastic
M25	Tab, Peach, Round	Levothyroxine Sodium 25 mcg	Synthroid by AltiMed	Canadian DIN 02237213	Thyroid Hormone
M25	Tab, Peach, Round	Levothyroxine Sodium 25 mcg	Synthroid by Duramed		Thyroid Hormone
M25	Tab, Yellow, Round, M 2.5	Methotrexate 2.5 mg	Rheumatrex by Apotex	Canadian DIN 02182963	Antineoplastic
M253	Tab, White, Round	Acyclovir 400 mg	Zovirax by Mylan	00378-0253	Antiviral

ID FRONT <> BACK	DESCRIPTION FRONT <> BACK	INGREDIENT & STRENGTH	BRAND (or Generic Equiv.) by FIRM	NDC#	CLASS; SCH.
M2540	Tab, Orange, Speckled, Rounded Rectangular, Scored, For Suspension	Methadone HCl 40 mg	Diskets by Mallinckrodt	00406-2540	Analgesic; C II
M255	Tab, White, Round, Scored, M over 255	Albuterol Sulfate 2 mg	Proventil by Mylan	00378-0255	Antiasthmatic
M255	Tab, White, Round, Scored, M over 255	Albuterol Sulfate 2 mg	Proventil by UDL	51079-0657	Antiasthmatic
M2558	Tab, Film Coated	Thioridazine HCl 25 mg	by Med Pro	53978-2005	Antipsychotic
M259MONODOX100	Cap, Brown & Yellow	Doxycycline Monohydrate 100 mg	Monodox by Oclassen	55515-0259	Antibiotic
M259MONODOX100MG	Cap, Brown & Yellow	Doxycycline Monohydrate 100 mg	Monodox by Vintage	00254-4316	Antibiotic
M259MONODOX100MG	Cap, Brown & Yellow	Doxycycline Monohydrate 100 mg	Monodox by Eckerd	19458-0838	Antibiotic
M259MONODOX100MG	Cap, Brown & Yellow	Doxycycline Monohydrate 100 mg	Monodox by Thrift Drug	59198-0363	Antibiotic
M259MONODOX100MG	Cap, Brown & Yellow	Doxycycline Monohydrate 100 mg	Monodox by West Pharm	52967-0302	Antibiotic
M260MONODOX50	Cap, White & Yellow	Doxycycline Monohydrate 50 mg	Monodox by West Pharm	52967-0301	Antibiotic
M260MONODOX50	Cap, White & Yellow	Doxycycline Monohydrate 50 mg	Monodox by Vintage	00254-4315	Antibiotic
M260MONODOX50	Cap, White & Yellow	Doxycycline Monohydrate 50 mg	Monodox by Oclassen	55515-0260	Antibiotic
M261	Tab, White, Round, Scored, M over 261	Ketoconazole 200 mg	Nizoral by Mylan	00378-0026	Antibiotic
M27	Tab, Yellow, Round, Scored, M over 27	Chlorthalidone 15 mg, Clonidine HCl 0.2 mg	Clopres by Bertek	62794-0027	Diuretic; Antihypertensive
M27	Tab, Yellow, Round, Scored, M over 27	Chlorthalidone 15 mg, Clonidine HCl 0.2 mg	Clopres by Mylan	00378-0027	Diuretic; Antihypertensive
M27	Tab, Yellow, Round, Scored, M over 27	Chlorthalidone 15 mg, Clonidine HCl 0.2 mg	Clopres by Med Pro	53978-2030	Diuretic; Antihypertensive
M28	Tab, Yellow, Round, Scored, M over 28	Nadolol 20 mg	Corgard by Mylan	00378-0028	Antihypertensive
M28	Tab, Yellow, Round, Scored, M over 28	Nadolol 20 mg	Corgard by Med Pro	53978-2017	Antihypertensive
M28	Tab, Yellow, Round, Scored, M over 28	Nadolol 20 mg	Corgard by UDL	51079-0812	Antihypertensive
M29	Tab, Blue, Beveled Edge, M Above Score, 29 Below	Methyclothiazide 5 mg	Enduron by Mylan	00378-0160	Diuretic; Antihypertensive
M29	Tab	Methyclothiazide 5 mg	by Pharmedix	53002-1044	Diuretic; Antihypertensive
M2A357344	Tab, White, Round, M2A3 over 57344	Acetaminophen 325 mg	Tylenol by Marlex	10135-0123	Analgesic
M2A457344	Tab, White, Cap Shaped	Acetaminophen 500 mg	Tylenol by AAA		Analgesic
M2MIN50MG	Cap, Orange, M2/MIN 50 mg	Minocycline 50 mg	Minocin by AltiMed	Canadian	Antibiotic
M3	Tab, Orange, Round, Enteric Coated	Aspirin 325 mg	Aspirin by Amneal	65162-0382	Analgesic
M30	Tab, Blue, Round, Scored, M over 30	Clorazepate Dipotassium 3.75 mg	Tranxene by Allscripts		Antianxiety; C IV
M30	Tab, Blue, Round, Scored, M over 30	Clorazepate Dipotassium 3.75 mg	Tranxene by Mylan	00378-0030	Antianxiety; C IV
M30	Tab, Blue, Round, Scored, M over 30	Clorazepate Dipotassium 3.75 mg	Tranxene by UDL	51079-0633 Discontinued	Antianxiety; C IV
M30 <> PF	Tab, Lavender, Round	Morphine Sulfate 30 mg	MS Contin by Purdue	59011-0261	Analgesic; C II
M300	Tab, Green, Scored	Levothyroxine Sodium 0.3 mg	Synthroid by AltiMed	Canadian DIN 02237222	Thyroid Hormone
M300	Tab, Green, Round	Levothyroxine Sodium 0.3 mg	Synthroid by Duramed		Thyroid Hormone
M300LEVOT	Tab, Green, Round	Levothyroxine Sodium 0.3 mg	Synthroid by Mova		Thyroid Hormone
m305	Tab, Peach, Round	Sotalol HCl	Betaspace by Mylan	00378-0305	Antiarrhythmic
M31	Tab, White, Round, Scored	Allopurinol 100 mg	Zyloprim by UDL	51079-0205	Antigout
M31	Tab, White, Round, Scored	Allopurinol 100 mg	Zyloprim by Kaiser	62224-7111	Antigout
M31	Tab, White, Round, Scored	Allopurinol 100 mg	Zyloprim by Heartland	61392-0103	Antigout
M31	Tab, White, Round, Scored	Allopurinol 100 mg	Zyloprim by Nat Pharmpak	55154-5534	Antigout
M31	Tab, White, Round, Scored	Allopurinol 100 mg	Zyloprim by Mylan	00378-0137	Antigout
M31	Tab, White, Round, Scored	Mephobarbital 32 mg	Mebaral by Ovation	67386-0801	Sedative/Hypnotic; C IV
M310	Tab, Peach, Round	Sotalol HCl 120 mg	Betaspace by Mylan	00378-0310	Antiarrhythmic
M312	Tab, Blue, Oval, Scored, Film Coated, Ex Release	Verapamil HCl 180 mg	Isoptin SR by Thrift Drug	59198-0319	Antihypertensive
M312	Tab, Blue, Oval, Scored, Film Coated, Ex Release	Verapamil HCl 180 mg	Isoptin SR by Mylan	00378-1180	Antihypertensive
M312	Tab, Blue, Oval, Scored, Film Coated, Ex Release	Verapamil HCl 180 mg	Isoptin SR by UDL	51079-0899	Antihypertensive
M313	Tab, Beige, Oval, Film Coated	Tolmetin Sodium 600 mg	Tolectin by Teva	00480-0102	NSAID
M313	Tab, Beige, Oval, Film Coated	Tolmetin Sodium 600 mg	Tolectin by Teva	00480-0106	NSAID
M313	Tab, Beige, Oval, Film Coated	Tolmetin Sodium 600 mg	Tolectin by Mylan	00378-0313	NSAID

ID FRONT <> BACK	DESCRIPTION FRONT <> BACK	INGREDIENT & STRENGTH	BRAND (or Generic Equiv.) by FIRM	NDC#	CLASS; SCH.
M314	Tab, Peach, Round	Sotalol HCl 160 mg	Betaspace by Mylan	00378-0314	Antiarrhythmic
M32	Tab, White, Round	Mephobarbital 50 mg	Mebaral by Ovation	67386-0802	Sedative/Hypnotic; C IV
M32	Tab, Pink, Round, Scored, Film Coated, M over 32	Metoprolol Tartrate 50 mg	Lopressor by Caremark	00339-5861	Antihypertensive
M32	Tab, Pink, Round, Scored, Film Coated, M over 32	Metoprolol Tartrate 50 mg	Lopressor by Mylan	00378-0032	Antihypertensive
M32	Tab, Pink, Round, Scored, Film Coated, M over 32	Metoprolol Tartrate 50 mg	Lopressor by Kaiser	62224-4446	Antihypertensive
M32	Tab, Pink, Round, Scored, Film Coated, M over 32	Metoprolol Tartrate 50 mg	Lopressor by Med Pro	53978-2058	Antihypertensive
M32	Tab, Pink, Round, Scored, Film Coated, M over 32	Metoprolol Tartrate 50 mg	Lopressor by Nat Pharmpak	55154-5512	Antihypertensive
M32	Tab, Pink, Round, Scored, Film Coated, M over 32	Metoprolol Tartrate 50 mg	Lopressor by Heartland	61392-0286	Antihypertensive
M32	Tab, Pink, Round, Scored, Film Coated, M over 32	Metoprolol Tartrate 50 mg	Lopressor by Bayer	00280-1232	Antihypertensive
M32	Tab, Pink, Round, Scored, Film Coated, M over 32	Metoprolol Tartrate 50 mg	Lopressor by UDL	51079-0801	Antihypertensive
				Discontinued	
M33	Tab, Coated, M 33	Mephobarbital 100 mg	Mebaral by Bayer	00280-1233	Sedative/Hypnotic; C IV
M33	Tab, Scored	Chlorothiazide 250 mg, Reserpine 0.125 mg	Diupres by Mylan	00378-0175	Diuretic; Antihypertensive
M33	Tab, White, Round	Mephobarbital 100 mg	Mebaral by Ovation	67386-0803	Sedative/Hypnotic; C IV
M35	Tab, Yellow, Round	Chlorthalidone 25 mg	Hygroton by UDL	51079-0058	Diuretic
M35	Tab, Yellow, Round	Chlorthalidone 25 mg	Hygroton by Med Pro	53978-0032	Diuretic
M35	Tab, Yellow, Round	Chlorthalidone 25 mg	Hygroton by Mylan	00378-0222	Diuretic
M350	Tab, Tan, Oval, Extended-Release	Metformin HCl 750 mg	Glucophage XR by UDL	51079-0627	Antidiabetic
				Discontinued	
M350	Tab, Yellow Orange Speckled, Capsule Shaped	Metformin HCl 750 mg	Glucophage XR by Mylan	00378-0350	Antidiabetic
M352	Tab, Tan, Oval, Extended-Release	Metformin HCl 500 mg	Glucophage XR by UDL	51079-0626	Antidiabetic
M352	Tab, Yellow Orange Speckled, Capsule Shaped	Metformin HCl Extended Release 500 mg	Glucophage XR by Mylan	00378-0352	Antidiabetic
M355	Tab, Yellow, Round, M over 355, Extended Release	Diclofenac Sodium 100 mg	Voltaren XR by Mylan	00378-0355	NSAID
M357	Tab, White, Cap Shaped, Scored	Acetaminophen 500 mg, Hydrocodone Bitartrate 5 mg	Vicodin by Sandoz	00781-1606	Analgesic; C III
M357	Tab, White, Cap Shaped, Scored	Acetaminophen 500 mg, Hydrocodone Bitartrate 5 mg	Vicodin by Mallinckrodt	00406-0357	Analgesic; C III
M357	Tab, White, Cap Shaped, Scored	Acetaminophen 500 mg, Hydrocodone Bitartrate 5 mg	Vicodin by Murfreesboro	51129-1445	Analgesic; C III
M357	Tab, White, Cap Shaped, Scored	Acetaminophen 500 mg, Hydrocodone Bitartrate 5 mg	Vicodin by D M Graham	00756-0276	Analgesic; C III
M358	Tab, White, Cap Shaped, Scored	Acetaminophen 500 mg, Hydrocodone Bitartrate 7.5 mg	Lortab by Murfreesboro	51129-1455	Analgesic; C III
M358	Tab, White, Cap Shaped, Scored	Acetaminophen 500 mg, Hydrocodone Bitartrate 7.5 mg	Lortab by D M Graham	00756-0282	Analgesic; C III
M358	Tab, White, Cap Shaped, Scored	Acetaminophen 500 mg, Hydrocodone Bitartrate 7.5 mg	Lortab by Sandoz	00781-1513	Analgesic; C III
M358	Tab, White, Cap Shaped, Scored	Acetaminophen 500 mg, Hydrocodone Bitartrate 7.5 mg	Lortab by King	60793-0889	Analgesic; C III
M358	Tab, White, Cap Shaped, Scored	Acetaminophen 500 mg, Hydrocodone Bitartrate 7.5 mg	Lortab by Mallinckrodt	00406-0358	Analgesic; C III
M359	Tab, White, Cap Shaped, Scored	Acetaminophen 650 mg, Hydrocodone Bitartrate 7.5 mg	Lortab by Mallinckrodt	00406-0359	Analgesic; C III
M359	Tab, White, Cap Shaped, Scored	Acetaminophen 650 mg, Hydrocodone Bitartrate 7.5 mg	Lorcet Plus by Mallinckrodt	00756-0281	Analgesic; C III
M359	Tab, White, Cap Shaped, Scored	Acetaminophen 650 mg, Hydrocodone Bitartrate 7.5 mg	Lorcet Plus by D M Graham		Analgesic; C III
M36	Tab, Brown, Round, Film Coated, M over 36	Amitriptyline HCl 50 mg	Elavil by Mylan	00378-2650	Antidepressant
M36	Tab, Brown, Round, Film Coated, M over 36	Amitriptyline HCl 50 mg	Elavil by UDL	51079-0133	Antidepressant
M360	Tab, White, Cap Shaped, Scored	Acetaminophen 750 mg, Hydrocodone Bitartrate 7.5 mg	Vicodin ES by Mallinckrodt	00406-0360	Analgesic; C III
M360	Tab, White, Cap Shaped, Scored	Acetaminophen 750 mg, Hydrocodone Bitartrate 7.5 mg	Vicodin ES by D M Graham	00756-0280	Analgesic; C III
M361	Tab, Blue, Cap Shaped, Scored	Acetaminophen 650 mg, Hydrocodone Bitartrate 10 mg	Lorcet by D M Graham	00756-0279	Analgesic; C III
M361	Tab, Blue, Cap Shaped, Scored	Acetaminophen 650 mg, Hydrocodone Bitartrate 10 mg	Lorcet by Mallinckrodt	00406-0361	Analgesic; C III
M362	Tab, White, Cap Shaped, Scored	Acetaminophen 660 mg, Hydrocodone Bitartrate 10 mg	Vicodin HP by Mallinckrodt	00406-0362	Analgesic; C III
M362	Tab, White, Cap Shaped, Scored	Acetaminophen 660 mg, Hydrocodone Bitartrate 10 mg	Vicodin HP by D M Graham	00756-0278	Analgesic; C III
M363	Tab, White, Cap Shaped, Scored	Acetaminophen 500 mg, Hydrocodone Bitartrate 10 mg	Lortab by King	60793-0890	Analgesic; C III
M363	Tab, White, Cap Shaped, Scored	Acetaminophen 500 mg, Hydrocodone Bitartrate 10 mg	Lortab by D M Graham	00756-0277	Analgesic; C III
M363	Tab, White, Cap Shaped, Scored	Acetaminophen 500 mg, Hydrocodone Bitartrate 10 mg	Lortab by Mallinckrodt	00406-0363	Analgesic; C III
M364	Tab, White, Oval, Scored	Hydrocodone Bitartrate 10 mg, Acetaminophen 750 mg	Maxidone by Mallinckrodt	00406-0364	Analgesic; C III
M365	Tab, White, Cap Shaped, Scored	Acetaminophen 325 mg, Hydrocodone Bitartrate 5 mg	Norco by Mallinckrodt	00406-0365	Analgesic; C III
M366	Tab, White, Cap Shaped	Acetaminophen 325 mg, Hydrocodone Bitartrate 7.5 mg	Norco by Mallinckrodt	00406-0366	Analgesic; C III
M367	Tab, White, Cap Shaped, Scored	Acetaminophen 325 mg, Hydrocodone Bitartrate 10 mg	Norco by Mallinckrodt	00406-0367	Analgesic; C III
M37	Tab, Blue, Round, Film Coated, M over 37	Amitriptyline HCl 75 mg	Elavil by Mylan	00378-2675	Antidepressant

ID FRONT <> BACK	DESCRIPTION FRONT <> BACK	INGREDIENT & STRENGTH	BRAND (or Generic Equiv.) by FIRM	NDC#	CLASS; SCH.
M37	Tab, Blue, Round, Film Coated, M over 37	Amitriptyline HCl 75 mg	Elavil by Caremark	00339-5016	Antidepressant
M37	Tab, Blue, Round, Film Coated, M over 37	Amitriptyline HCl 75 mg	Elavil by UDL	51079-0147	Antidepressant
M372	Tab, Film Coated, M/372	Cimetidine HCl 400 mg	Tagamet by Heartland	61392-0200	Gastrointestinal
M372	Tab, Coated, M/372	Cimetidine HCl 400 mg	Tagamet by Qualitest	00603-2892	Gastrointestinal
M38	Tab, Orange, Round, Film Coated, M over 38	Amitriptyline HCl 100 mg	Elavil by UDL	51079-0563	Antidepressant
M38	Tab, Orange, Round, Film Coated, M over 38	Amitriptyline HCl 100 mg	Elavil by Mylan	00378-2685	Antidepressant
M38	Tab, Orange, Round, Film Coated, M over 38	Amitriptyline HCl 100 mg	Elavil by Caremark	00339-5018	Antidepressant
M39	Tab, Flesh, Cap Shaped, Film Coated	Amitriptyline HCl 150 mg	Elavil by Mylan	00378-2695	Antidepressant
M39	Tab, Flesh, Cap Shaped, Film Coated	Amitriptyline HCl 150 mg	Elavil by UDL	51079-0564 Discontinued	Antidepressant
M4	Tab, White, Round, M/4	Hydromorphone HCl 4 mg	Dilaudid by Mallinckrodt		Analgesic; C II
M4	Tab, Coated	Fluphenazine HCl 1 mg	by Heartland	61392-0057	Antipsychotic
M4	Tab, White, Oblong, Scored	Mesna 400 mg	Mesnex by BMS	00015-3565	Detoxification Agent
M4	Tab, Pink, Cap Shaped, Film Coated	Magnesium Carbonate 400 mg, Calcium Carbonate 200 mg, Folic Acid 1 mg	MagneBind by Nephro-Tech	59528-0416	Vitamin; Supplement
M40	Tab, Peach, Round, Scored, M over 40	Clorazepate Dipotassium 7.5 mg	Tranxene by UDL	51079-0634 Discontinued	Antianxiety; C IV
M40	Tab, Peach, Round, Scored, M over 40	Clorazepate Dipotassium 7.5 mg	Tranxene by Murfreesboro	51129-1355	Antianxiety; C IV
M40	Tab, Peach, Round, Scored, M over 40	Clorazepate Dipotassium 7.5 mg	Tranxene by Mylan	00378-0040	Antianxiety; C IV
M40	Tab, Beige, Oblong, Film Coated	Erythromycin Ethylsuccinate 400 mg	by Direct Dispensing	57866-0351	Antibiotic
M400	Tab, Film Coated	Erythromycin Ethylsuccinate 400 mg	by Allscripts		Antibiotic
M400	Tab, Film Coated	Erythromycin Ethylsuccinate 400 mg	by Med Pro	53978-0022	Antibiotic
M400	Tab, Film Coated	Erythromycin Ethylsuccinate 400 mg	by Physician Total Care	54868-0018	Antibiotic
M400	Tab, Peach, Film Coated	Erythromycin Ethylsuccinate 400 mg	by Mylan	00378-6400	Antibiotic
M400 <> BAYER	Tab, Red, Oblong, Film Coated	Moxifloxacin HCl 400 mg	Avelox by Bayer	12527-8581	Antibiotic
M400 <> BAYER	Tab, Red, Oblong, Film Coated	Moxifloxacin HCl 400 mg	Avelox by Bayer	00026-8581	Antibiotic
M400 <> BAYER	Tab, Red, Oblong, Film Coated	Moxifloxacin HCl 400 mg	Avelox by Bayer	Canadian DIN 02242965	Antibiotic
M407	Tab, Orange, Oval, Film Coated	Fluvoxamine Maleate 25 mg	Luvox by Mylan	00378-0407	OCD
M41	Tab, Ivory, Round, Scored, M over 41	Hydrochlorothiazide 25 mg, Spironolactone 25 mg	Aldactazide by Mylan	00378-0141	Diuretic; Antihypertensive
M41	Tab, Ivory, Round, Scored, M over 41	Hydrochlorothiazide 25 mg, Spironolactone 25 mg	Aldactazide by UDL	51079-0104	Diuretic; Antihypertensive
M411	Tab, Blue, Cap Shaped, Film Coated, Ex Release	Verapamil HCl 240 mg	Isoptin SR by Teva	00480-1005	Antihypertensive
M411	Tab, Blue, Cap Shaped, Film Coated, Ex Release	Verapamil HCl 240 mg	Isoptin SR by Direct Dispensing	57866-6914	Antihypertensive
M411	Tab, Blue, Cap Shaped, Film Coated, Ex Release	Verapamil HCl 240 mg	Isoptin SR by Compumed	00403-5198	Antihypertensive
M411	Tab, Blue, Cap Shaped, Film Coated, Ex Release	Verapamil HCl 240 mg	Isoptin SR by Mylan	00378-0411	Antihypertensive
M411	Tab, Blue, Cap Shaped, Film Coated, Ex Release	Verapamil HCl 240 mg	Isoptin SR by UDL	51079-0869 Discontinued	Antihypertensive
M412	Tab, Orange, Oval, Scored, Film Coated	Fluvoxamine Maleate 50 mg	Luvox by Mylan	00378-0412	OCD
M412	Tab, Orange, Oval, Scored, Film Coated	Fluvoxamine Maleate 50 mg	Luvox by UDL	51079-0992	OCD
M414	Tab, Orange, Oval, Scored, Film Coated	Fluvoxamine Maleate 100 mg	Luvox by UDL	51079-0993	OCD
M414	Tab, Orange, Oval, Scored, Film Coated	Fluvoxamine Maleate 100 mg	Luvox by Mylan	00378-0414	OCD
M42	Tab, White, Round, Scored	Bromocriptine 2.5 mg	Parlodel by Mylan	00378-2042	Antiparkinson
M42 <> LU	Tab, White, Oval, Film Coated	Losartan 100 mg, Hydrochlorothiazide 12.5 mg	Hyzaar by Lupin	68180-0216	Antihypertensive; Diuretic
M424	Tab, Peach, Round, Scored, M over 424	Metoprolol Tartrate 50 mg, HCTZ 25 mg	Lopressor HCT by Mylan	00378-0424	Antihypertensive; Diuretic
M43	Tab, Scored	Chlorothiazide 500 mg, Reserpine 0.125 mg	Diupres by Mylan	00378-0176	Diuretic; Antihypertensive
M434	Tab, Peach, Oval, Scored, M over 434	Metoprolol Tartrate 100 mg, HCTZ 25 mg	Lopressor HCT by Mylan	00378-0434	Antihypertensive; Diuretic
M4357	Cap, Maroon, Hard Gel, M inside square	Acetaminophen 500 mg, Hydrocodone Bitartrate 5 mg	Lorcet by Mallinckrodt	00406-4357	Analgesic; C III
M4357	Cap, Maroon, Hard Gel	Acetaminophen 500 mg, Hydrocodone Bitartrate 5 mg	Lorcet by D M Graham	00756-0253	Analgesic; C III
M4358	Cap, White, Hard Gel, M Inside a Square and 4358 Imprinted in Red	Acetaminophen 500 mg, Hydrocodone Bitartrate 5 mg	Vicodin by Murfreesboro	51129-1444	Analgesic; C III
M437	Tab, White, Round, Scored, Film Coated, M over 437	Spironolactone 100 mg	Aldactone by UDL	51079-0980	Diuretic

ID FRONT <> BACK	DESCRIPTION FRONT <> BACK	INGREDIENT & STRENGTH	BRAND (or Generic Equiv.) by FIRM	NDC#	CLASS; SCH.
M437	Tab, White, Round, Scored, Film Coated, M over 437	Spironolactone 100 mg	Aldactone by Mylan	00378-0437	Diuretic
M44	Tab, White, Round	Cyproheptadine HCl 4 mg	Periactin by Mylan		Antihistamine
M444	Tab, White, Round, Film Coated, M over 444	Benazepril HCl 20 mg	Lotensin by UDL	51079-0146	Antihypertensive
M444	Tab, White, Round	Benazepril HCl 20 mg	Lotensin by Mylan	00378-0444	Antihypertensive
M445	Tab, Peach, Cap Shaped, Scored, M over 445	Metoprolol Tartrate 100 mg, HCTZ 50 mg	Lopressor HCT by Mylan	00378-0445	Antihypertensive; Diuretic
M447	Tab, White, Oval	Benazepril HCl 40 mg	Lotensin by Mylan	00378-0447	Antihypertensive
M45	Tab, White, Round, Scored, Film Coated, M over 45	Diltiazem HCl 60 mg	Cardizem by Vangard	00615-3549	Antihypertensive
M45	Tab, White, Round, Scored, Film Coated, M over 45	Diltiazem HCl 60 mg	Cardizem by UDL	51079-0746	Antihypertensive
M45	Tab, White, Round, Scored, Film Coated, M over 45	Diltiazem HCl 60 mg	Cardizem by Med Pro	53978-1235	Antihypertensive
M45	Tab, White, Round, Scored, Film Coated, M over 45	Diltiazem HCl 60 mg	Cardizem by Nat Pharmpak	55154-5523	Antihypertensive
M45	Tab, White, Round, Scored, Film Coated, M over 45	Diltiazem HCl 60 mg	Cardizem by Kaiser	62224-9337	Antihypertensive
M45	Tab, White, Round, Scored, Film Coated, M over 45	Diltiazem HCl 60 mg	Cardizem by Amerisource	62584-0367	Antihypertensive
M45	Tab, White, Round, Scored, Film Coated, M over 45	Diltiazem HCl 60 mg	Cardizem by Elan Hold	60274-0882	Antihypertensive
M45	Tab, White, Round, Scored, Film Coated, M over 45	Diltiazem HCl 60 mg	Cardizem by Heartland	61392-0054	Antihypertensive
M45	Tab, White, Round, Scored, Film Coated, M over 45	Diltiazem HCl 60 mg	Cardizem by Mylan	00378-0045	Antihypertensive
M450	Tab, White, Round, Film Coated	Atenolol 50 mg, Chlorthalidone 25 mg	Tenoretic by Merckle	58107-0002	Antihypertensive; Diuretic
M450	Tab, White, Round, Scored	Atenolol 50 mg, Chlorthalidone 25 mg	Tenoretic by Martec	52555-0450	Antihypertensive; Diuretic
M451	Tab, White, Round, Film Coated	Atenolol 100 mg, Chlorthalidone 25 mg	Tenoretic by Merckle	58107-0003	Antihypertensive; Diuretic
M451	Tab, White, Round	Atenolol 100 mg, Chlorthalidone 25 mg	Tenoretic by Martec	52555-0451	Antihypertensive; Diuretic
M454	Tab, White, Round, Scored	Pindolol 5 mg	Visken by Martec	52555-0454	Antihypertensive
M455	Tab, White, Round, Scored	Pindolol 10 mg	Visken by Martec	52555-0455	Antihypertensive
M47	Tab, Light Blue, Round, Scored, Film Coated, M over 47	Metoprolol Tartrate 100 mg	Lopressor by Kaiser	62224-4442	Antihypertensive
M47	Tab, Light Blue, Round, Scored, Film Coated, M over 47	Metoprolol Tartrate 100 mg	Lopressor by Mylan	00378-0047	Antihypertensive
M47	Tab, Light Blue, Round, Scored, Film Coated, M over 47	Metoprolol Tartrate 100 mg	Lopressor by Heartland	61392-0280	Antihypertensive
M47	Tab, Light Blue, Round, Scored, Film Coated, M over 47	Metoprolol Tartrate 100 mg	Lopressor by UDL	51079-0802	Antihypertensive
M471	Tab, Light Orange, Oblong, Scored, Film Coated	Fenoprofen Calcium 600 mg	Nalfon by Mylan	00378-0471	NSAID
M471	Tab, Light Orange, Oblong, Scored, Film Coated	Fenoprofen Calcium 600 mg	Nalfon by St. Mary's Med	60760-0471	NSAID
M471	Tab, Light Orange, Oblong, Scored, Film Coated	Fenoprofen Calcium 600 mg	Nalfon by H J Harkins Co	52959-0067	NSAID
M471	Tab, Light Orange, Oblong, Scored, Film Coated	Fenoprofen Calcium 600 mg	Nalfon by UDL	51079-0477	NSAID
M473	Tab, White, Oval, Film-Coated	Divalproex Sodium 500 mg	Depakote E.R. by Mylan	00378-0473	Anticonvulsant
M473	Tab, White, Oval, Film-Coated	Divalproex Sodium 500 mg	Depakote E.R. by UDL	51079-0767	Anticonvulsant
M475	Tab, Pink, Round, Film Coated, Ex Release, M over 475	Nifedipine 30 mg	Procardia XL by Mylan	00378-3475	Antihypertensive
M475	Tab, Pink, Round, Film Coated, Ex Release, M over 475	Nifedipine 30 mg	Procardia XL by UDL	51079-0940	Antihypertensive
M482	Tab, Pink, Round, Film Coated, Ex Release, M over 482	Nifedipine 60 mg	Procardia XL by Mylan	51079-0968	Antihypertensive
M482	Tab, Pink, Round, Film Coated, Ex Release, M over 482	Nifedipine 60 mg	Procardia XL by UDL	00378-3482	Antihypertensive
M495	Tab, Pink, Round, Film Coated, Ex Release, M over 495	Nifedipine 90 mg	Procardia XL by Mylan	00378-3495	Antihypertensive
M495	Tab, Pink, Round, Film Coated, Ex Release, M over 495	Nifedipine 90 mg	Procardia XL by UDL	51079-0969	Antihypertensive
M5	Tab, White, Round, Scored	Methenamine Mandelate 0.5 g	Mandelamine by Able	53265-0159 Discontinued	Antithyroid
M5	Tab, White, Round, Scored	Methenamine Mandelate 0.5 g	Mandelamine by Jones	00689-1084	Antithyroid
M5 <> P	Tab, White, Square	Metoclopramide HCl 5 mg	Maxeran by Pharmascience	Canadian DIN 02230431	Gastrointestinal
M5 <> PAL	Tab, Blue, Round, Coated	L-methylfolate 5.635 mg, Riboflavin 5 mg, Pyridoxine 50 mg, Cyanocobalamin 1 mg	Cerefolin by PamLab	00525-0503	Vitamin; Supplement
M50	Tab, White, Scored	Levothyroxine Sodium 50 mcg	by AltiMed	Canadian DIN 02237214	Thyroid Hormone
M50	Tab, White, Round, Scored	Chlorothiazide 250 mg	Diuril by Mylan	00378-0150	Diuretic; Antihypertensive
M50	Tab, White, Round, Scored	Chlorothiazide 250 mg	Diuril by UDL	51079-0060 Discontinued	Diuretic; Antihypertensive

ID FRONT <> BACK	DESCRIPTION FRONT <> BACK	INGREDIENT & STRENGTH	BRAND (or Generic Equiv.) by FIRM	NDC#	CLASS; SCH.
M50	Tab, White, Round, Film Coated, Extended Release, Scripted M	Metoprolol Succinate 50 mg	Toprol XL by Par	49884-0405	Antihypertensive
M500	Tab, White, Oval, Film-Coated	Metformin 500 mg	Glumetza by Biovail Corp.	Canadian DIN 02268493	Antidiabetic
M500 <> APO	Tab, White, Round, APO/M500	Metformin 500 mg	Metformin by Apotex	Canadian DIN 02167786	Antidiabetic
M5059	Tab, Film Coated	Thioridazine HCl 50 mg	by Med Pro	53978-2006	Antipsychotic
M50G	Cap, Orange, M/50/G	Minocycline HCl 50 mg	Minocin by Genpharm	Canadian	Antibiotic
M50LEVOT	Tab, White, Round	Levothyroxine Sodium 0.05 mg	Synthroid by Mova		Thyroid Hormone
M51	Tab, Green, Round, Film Coated, M over 51	Amitriptyline HCl 25 mg	Elavil by Rx Dispensing	61807-0129	Antidepressant
M51	Tab, Green, Round, Film Coated, M over 51	Amitriptyline HCl 25 mg	Elavil by Diversified Healthcare	55887-0986	Antidepressant
M51	Tab, Green, Round, Film Coated, M over 51	Amitriptyline HCl 25 mg	Elavil by Mylan	00378-2625	Antidepressant
M51	Tab, Green, Round, Film Coated, M over 51	Amitriptyline HCl 25 mg	Elavil by Caremark	00339-5015	Antidepressant
M51	Tab, Green, Round, Film Coated, M over 51	Amitriptyline HCl 25 mg	Elavil by UDL	51079-0107	Antidepressant
M515	Tab, Beige, Round	Mirtazapine 15 mg	Remeron by UDL	51079-0086	Antidepressant
M515	Tab, Pink, Round	Mirtazapine 15 mg	Remeron by Mylan	00378-3515	Antidepressant
M52	Tab, White, Round, Scored, Film Coated, M over 52	Pindolol 5 mg	Visken by Mylan	55160-0132	Antihypertensive
M52	Tab, White, Round, Scored, Film Coated, M over 52	Pindolol 5 mg	Visken by Mylan	00378-0052	Antihypertensive
M522 <> 75325	Tab, White to Off-White, Cap Shaped, M522 <> 7.5/325	Oxycodone 7.5 mg, Acetaminophen 325 mg	Percocet by Mallinckrodt	00406-0522	Analgesic; C II
M523 <> 10325	Tab, White to Off-White, Cap Shaped, M523 <> 10/325	Oxycodone 10 mg, Acetaminophen 325 mg	Percocet by Mallinckrodt	00406-0523	Analgesic; C II
M525	Tab, White, Oblong, Scored, Film Coated	Diltiazem HCl 120 mg	Cardizem by Heartland	61392-0056	Antihypertensive
M525	Tab, White, Oblong, Scored, Film Coated	Diltiazem HCl 120 mg	Cardizem by Mylan	00378-0525	Antihypertensive
M525	Tab, White, Oblong, Scored, Film Coated	Diltiazem HCl 120 mg	Cardizem by Heartland	61392-0145	Antihypertensive
M530	Tab, Beige, Round	Mirtazapine 30 mg	Remeron by UDL	51079-0087	Antidepressant
M530	Tab, Pink, Round	Mirtazapine 30 mg	Remeron by Mylan	00378-3530	Antidepressant
M532	Tab, Beige & Red, Hard Gel, M Inside a Square and 532	Acetaminophen 500 mg, Oxycodone HCl 5 mg	Tylox by Pharmafab	62542-0255	Analgesic; C II
M532	Tab, Beige & Red, Hard Gel, M Inside a Square and 532	Acetaminophen 500 mg, Oxycodone HCl 5 mg	Tylox by Mallinckrodt	00406-0532	Analgesic; C II
M533	Tab, Blue, Round	Azithromycin 250 mg	Zithromax by UDL	51079-0591	Antibiotic
M533	Tab, Blue, Round	Azithromycin 250 mg	Zithromax by Mylan	00378-1533	Antibiotic
M534	Tab, Blue, Oblong	Azithromycin 500 mg	Zithromax by Mylan	00378-1534	Antibiotic
M535	Tab, Blue, Oval	Azithromycin 600 mg	Zithromax by Mylan	00378-1535	Antibiotic
M536	Tab, White, Round	Atenolol 25 mg	Tenormin by Major	00904-5392	Antihypertensive
M54 <> 10	Tab, Orange, Round, Film Coated, M/541	Thioridazine 10 mg	Mellaril by Vangard	00615-2504	Antipsychotic
M54 <> 10	Tab, Orange, Round, Film Coated, M/54	Thioridazine 10 mg	Mellaril by UDL	51079-0565	Antipsychotic
M54 <> 10	Tab, Orange, Round, Film Coated, M/54	Thioridazine 10 mg	Mellaril by Dixon Shane	17236-0318	Antipsychotic
M54 <> 10	Tab, Orange, Round, Film Coated, M/54	Thioridazine 10 mg	Mellaril by Mylan	00378-0612	Antipsychotic
M54 <> 10	Tab, Orange, Round, Film Coated, M/54	Thioridazine 10 mg	Mellaril by Qualitest	00603-5992	Antipsychotic
M541	Tab, Green, Oval, Scored, Film Coated, M/541	Cimetidine HCl 800 mg	Tagamet by Mylan	00378-0541	Gastrointestinal
M541	Tab, Green, Oval, Scored, Film Coated, M/541	Cimetidine HCl 800 mg	Tagamet by Qualitest	00603-2893	Gastrointestinal
M541	Tab, Green, Oval, Scored, Film Coated, M/541	Cimetidine HCl 800 mg	Tagamet by Murfreesboro	51129-1178	Gastrointestinal
M541	Tab, Green, Oval, Scored, Film Coated, M/541	Cimetidine HCl 800 mg	Tagamet by UDL	51079-0809 Discontinued	Gastrointestinal
M541	Tab, Green, Oval, Scored, Film Coated, M/541	Cimetidine HCl 800 mg	Tagamet by Heartland	61392-0203	Gastrointestinal
M5410	Tab, Film Coated	Thioridazine 10 mg	Mellaril by Med Pro	53978-2004	Antipsychotic
M542	Tab, Pink, Round, Scored, M over 542	HCTZ 12.5 mg, Quinapril HCl 10 mg	Accuretic by Mylan	00378-0542	Diuretic; Antihypertensive
M543	Tab, Yellow, Round, Scored, M over 543	HCTZ 12.5 mg, Quinapril HCl 20 mg	Accuretic by Mylan	00378-0543	Diuretic; Antihypertensive
M544	Tab, Pink, Round, M over 544	HCTZ 25 mg, Quinapril HCl 25 mg	Accuretic by Mylan	00378-0544	Diuretic; Antihypertensive
M545	Tab, Beige, Round	Mirtazapine 45 mg	Remeron by Mylan	51079-0088	Antidepressant
M547	Tab, White, Round, Scored	Mercaptopurine 50 mg	Purinethol by Mylan	00378-3547	Antineoplastic
M55	Tab, Green, Beveled Edge, M over 55	Timolol Maleate 5 mg	Blocarden by Mylan	00378-0055	Antihypertensive

ID FRONT <> BACK	DESCRIPTION FRONT <> BACK	INGREDIENT & STRENGTH	BRAND (or Generic Equiv.) by FIRM	NDC#	CLASS; SCH.
M55	Tab, Green, Round, M 55	Timolol Maleate 5 mg	Blocarden by Teva	00480-0076	Antihypertensive
M55 <> MATERNA	Tab, Beige, Oblong	Vitamin Combination	Materna by Wyeth	00005-5586	Vitamin
M562	Tab, White to Off-White, Cap Shaped	Acetaminophen 650 mg, Oxycodone HCl 10 mg	Percocet by Mallinckrodt	00406-0562	Analgesic; C II
M571	Tab, White, Capsule Shaped	Terbinafine HCl 250 mg	Lamisil by Mylan	00378-5710	Antifungal
M572	Tab, White, Round, Scored, M over 572	Albuterol Sulfate 4 mg	Proventil by Mylan	00378-0572	Antiasthmatic
M572	Tab, White, Round, Scored, M over 572	Albuterol Sulfate 4 mg	Proventil by UDL	51079-0658	Antiasthmatic
M577	Tab, Light Orange, Round, Scored, M over 577	Amiloride HCl 5 mg, HCTZ 50 mg	Moduretic by Mylan	00378-0577	Antihypertensive; Diuretic
M577	Tab, Light Orange, Round, Scored, M over 577	Amiloride HCl 5 mg, HCTZ 50 mg	Moduretic by UDL	51079-0421 Discontinued	Antihypertensive; Diuretic
M577	Tab, Light Orange, Round, Scored, M over 577	Amiloride HCl 5 mg, HCTZ 50 mg	Moduretic by Kaiser	62224-7115	Antihypertensive; Diuretic
M58 <> 25	Tab, Orange, Round, Film Coated, M over 58	Thioridazine 25 mg	Mellaril by Mylan	00378-0614	Antipsychotic
M58 <> 25	Tab, Orange, Round, Film Coated, M over 58	Thioridazine 25 mg	Mellaril by Dixon Shane	17236-0301	Antipsychotic
M58 <> 25	Tab, Orange, Round, Film Coated, M over 58	Thioridazine 25 mg	Mellaril by Vangard	00615-2506	Antipsychotic
M58 <> 25	Tab, Orange, Round, Film Coated, M over 58	Thioridazine 25 mg	Mellaril by UDL	51079-0566	Antipsychotic
M582	Tab, White to Off-White, Oval	Acetaminophen 500 mg, Oxycodone HCl 7.5 mg	Percocet by Mallinckrodt	00406-0582	Analgesic; C II
M59 <> 50	Tab, Orange, Round, Film Coated, M over 59	Thioridazine 50 mg	Mellaril by Mylan	00378-0616	Antipsychotic
M59 <> 50	Tab, Orange, Round, Film Coated, M over 59	Thioridazine 50 mg	Mellaril by UDL	51079-0567	Antipsychotic
M59 <> 50	Tab, Orange, Round, Film Coated, M over 59	Thioridazine 50 mg	Mellaril by Qualitest	00603-5994	Antipsychotic
M59 <> 50	Tab, Orange, Round, Film Coated, M over 59	Thioridazine 50 mg	Mellaril by Vangard	00615-2507	Antipsychotic
M59 <> 50	Tab, Orange, Round, Film Coated, M over 59	Thioridazine 50 mg	Mellaril by Dixon Shane	17236-0302	Antipsychotic
M5MG0554	Cap, Brown & Light Brown, Black Print, Opaque, 0554/M over 5 mg	Oxycodone HCl 5 mg	Roxicodone by Mallinckrodt	00406-0554	Analgesic; C II
M6	Tab, Pink, Round	Erythromycin Stearate 250 mg	Erythrocin by Mylan		Antibiotic
M6	Tab, Yellow, Round	Erythromycin Stearate 250 mg	Erythrocin by Mylan		Antibiotic
M6 <> LL	Tab, White, Round	Ethambutol HCl 100 mg	Myambutol by Dura	51479-0046	Antituberculosis
M6 <> LL	Tab, White, Round	Ethambutol HCl 100 mg	Myambutol by Heartland	61392-0718	Antituberculosis
M6 <> LL	Tab, White, Round	Ethambutol HCl 100 mg	Myambutol by Lederle	00005-5015	Antituberculosis
M60 <> PF	Tab, Orange, Round	Morphine Sulfate 60 mg	MS Contin by Purdue	59011-0262	Analgesic; C II
M61 <> 100	Tab, Orange, Round, Film Coated, M over 61	Thioridazine 100 mg	Mellaril by UDL	51079-0580	Antipsychotic
M61 <> 100	Tab, Orange, Round, Film Coated, M over 61	Thioridazine 100 mg	Mellaril by Mylan	00378-0618	Antipsychotic
M61 <> 100	Tab, Orange, Round, Film Coated, M over 61	Thioridazine 100 mg	Mellaril by Dixon Shane	17236-0305	Antipsychotic
M61 <> 100	Tab, Orange, Round, Film Coated, M over 61	Thioridazine 100 mg	Mellaril by Vangard	00615-2508	Antipsychotic
M61 <> 100	Tab, Orange, Round, Film Coated, M over 61	Thioridazine 100 mg	Mellaril by Qualitest	00603-5995	Antipsychotic
M613	Tab, White to Off-White, Scored, Film Coated	Levetiracetam 250 mg	Keppra by UDL	51079-0820	Anticonvulsant
M615	Tab, White to Off White, Cap Shaped, Scored, M / 615	Levetiracetam 500 mg	Keppra by UDL	51079-0821	Anticonvulsant
M615	Tab, White to Off White, Cap Shaped, Scored, M / 615	Levetiracetam 500 mg	Keppra by Mylan	00378-0615	Anticonvulsant
M617	Tab, White, Cap Shaped, Scored, M / 617	Levetiracetam 750 mg	Keppra by UDL	51079-0822	Anticonvulsant
M619	Tab, White	Levetiracetam 1000 mg	Keppra by UDL	51079-0860	Anticonvulsant
M62	Tab, White, Round	Chlorothiazide 500 mg	Diuril by Mylan		Diuretic; Antihypertensive
M63	Tab, White, Scored, M over 63	Atenolol 50 mg, Chlorthalidone 25 mg	Tenoretic by Caremark	00339-5839	Antihypertensive; Diuretic
M63	Tab, White, Scored, M over 63	Atenolol 50 mg, Chlorthalidone 25 mg	Tenoretic by Mylan	00378-2063	Antihypertensive; Diuretic
M64	Tab, White, M over 64	Atenolol 100 mg, Chlorthalidone 25 mg	Tenoretic by Mylan	00378-2064	Antihypertensive; Diuretic
M65	Tab, Orange, Oblong	Acetaminophen 650 mg, Propoxyphene HCl 65 mg	Wygesic by Mylan		Analgesic; C IV
M66	Tab, Yellow, Round	Meloxicam 7.5 mg	Mobic by UDL	51079-0457	NSAID
M66	Tab, White, Round	Meloxicam 7.5 mg	Mobic by Mylan	00378-1066	Anti-inflammatory
M663	Tab, White, Round	Ciprofloxacin 250 mg	Cipro by Martec	52555-0769	Antibiotic
M664	Tab, White, Oblong	Ciprofloxacin 500 mg	Cipro by Martec	52555-0770	Antibiotic
M665	Tab, White, Oblong	Ciprofloxacin 750 mg	Cipro by Martec	52555-0771	Antibiotic
M7	Tab, Pink, Oval	Erythromycin Stearate 500 mg	Erythrocin by Mylan		Antibiotic

ID FRONT <> BACK	DESCRIPTION FRONT <> BACK	INGREDIENT & STRENGTH	BRAND (or Generic Equiv.) by FIRM	NDC#	CLASS; SCH.
M7	Tab, Yellow, Oval	Erythromycin Stearate 500 mg	Erythrocin by Mylan		Antibiotic
M7 <> LL	Tab, White, Round, Scored, Film Coated	Ethambutol HCl 400 mg	Myambutol by DRX	55045-2763	Antituberculosis
M7 <> LL	Tab, White, Round, Scored, Film Coated	Ethambutol HCl 400 mg	Myambutol by Lederle	00005-5084	Antituberculosis
M7 <> LL	Tab, White, Round, Scored, Film Coated	Ethambutol HCl 400 mg	Myambutol by Nat Pharmpak	55154-1709	Antituberculosis
M7 <> LL	Tab, White, Round, Scored, Film Coated, M to left of Score, 7 to right	Ethambutol HCl 400 mg	Myambutol by Dura	51479-0047	Antituberculosis
M7 <> LL	Tab, White, Round, Scored, Film Coated	Ethambutol HCl 400 mg	Myambutol by Dept Health	53808-0006	Antituberculosis
M7 <> LL	Tab, White, Round, Scored, Film Coated	Ethambutol HCl 400 mg	Myambutol by Wyeth	Canadian	Antituberculosis
M70	Tab, White, Round, Scored, M over 70	Clorazepate Dipotassium 15 mg	Tranxene by Compumed	00403-3466	Antianxiety; C IV
M70	Tab, White, Round, Scored, M over 70	Clorazepate Dipotassium 15 mg	Tranxene by Murfreesboro	51129-1354	Antianxiety; C IV
M70	Tab, White, Round, Scored, M over 70	Clorazepate Dipotassium 15 mg	Tranxene by Mylan	00378-0070	Antianxiety; C IV
M70	Tab, White, Round, Scored, M over 70	Clorazepate Dipotassium 15 mg	Tranxene by UDL	51079-0635 Discontinued	Antianxiety; C IV
M71	Tab, White, Round, Scored	Allopurinol 300 mg	Zyloprim by Kaiser	62224-7113	Antigout
M71	Tab, White, Round, Scored	Allopurinol 300 mg	Zyloprim by Heartland	61392-0104	Antigout
M71	Tab, White, Round, Scored	Allopurinol 300 mg	Zyloprim by UDL	51079-0206	Antigout
M71	Tab, White, Round, Scored	Allopurinol 300 mg	Zyloprim by Mylan	00378-0181	Antigout
M715	Tab, Green, Beveled Edge, M to Left, 715 to Right of Score	Timolol Maleate 20 mg	Blocadren by Mylan	00378-0715	Antihypertensive
M715	Tab, Green, Beveled Edge, M to Left, 715 to Right of Score	Timolol Maleate 20 mg	Blocadren by Med Pro	53978-2022	Antihypertensive
M72	Tab, Yellow, Oblong, Film Coated	Esterified Estrogens 0.3 mg	Menest by King	61570-0072	Hormone
M72	Tab, Yellow, Round, Scored, M over 72	Chlorthalidone 15 mg, Clonidine HCl 0.3 mg	Clorpres by Bertek	62794-0072	Diuretic; Antihypertensive
M72	Tab, Yellow, Round, Scored, M over 72	Chlorthalidone 15 mg, Clonidine HCl 0.3 mg	Clorpres by Mylan	00378-0072	Diuretic; Antihypertensive
M722	Tab, White to Off-White, Round, Scored, M over 722	Tizanidine HCl 2 mg	Zanaflex by Mylan	00378-0722	Muscle Relaxant
M724	Tab, White to Off-White, Round, Scored, M over 724	Tizanidine HCl 4 mg	Zanaflex by Mylan	00378-0724	Muscle Relaxant
M724	Tab, White to Off-White, Round, Scored, M over 724	Tizanidine HCl 4 mg	Zanaflex by UDL	51079-0998	Muscle Relaxant
M725	Tab, Beige, Oval, Scored	Benazepril HCl 5 mg, Hydrochlorothiazide 6.25 mg	Lotensin HCT by Mylan	00378-4725	Antihypertensive; Diuretic
M73	Tab, Orange, Oblong, Film Coated	Esterified Estrogens 0.625 mg	Menest by King	61570-0073	Hormone
M735	Tab, Beige, Round, Scored, M over 735	Benazepril HCl 10 mg, Hydrochlorothiazide 12.5 mg	Lotensin HCT by Mylan	00378-4735	Antihypertensive; Diuretic
M74	Tab, Green, Oblong, Film Coated	Esterified Estrogens 1.25 mg	Menest by King	61570-0074	Hormone
M745	Tab, Beige, Oval, Scored	Benazepril HCl 20 mg, Hydrochlorothiazide 12.5 mg	Lotensin HCT by Mylan	00378-4745	Antihypertensive; Diuretic
M75	Tab, Green, Round, Scored	Chlorthalidone 50 mg	Hygroton by Mylan	00378-0213	Diuretic
M75	Tab, Pink, Oblong, Film Coated	Esterified Estrogens 2.5 mg	Menest by King	61570-0075	Hormone
M75	Tab, Violet, Scored	Levothyroxine Sodium 75 mcg	Synthroid by AltiMed	Canadian DIN 0223721S	Thyroid Hormone
M75	Tab, Green, Round, Scored	Chlorthalidone 50 mg	Hygroton by UDL	51079-0059 Discontinued	Diuretic
M753	Tab, Blue, Round, Film Coated	Fexofenadine HCl 60 mg	Allegra by UDL	51079-0529	Antihistamine
M753	Tab, Blue, Round, Film Coated	Fexofenadine HCl 60 mg	Allegra by Mylan	51079-0753	Antihistamine
M755	Tab, Blue, Cap Shaped	Fexofenadine HCl 180 mg	Allegra by UDL	51079-0526	Antihistamine
M755	Tab, Blue, Cap Shaped	Fexofenadine HCl 180 mg	Allegra by Mylan	51079-0755	Antihistamine
M76	Tab, Beige, Round, Film Coated, M over 76	Flurbiprofen 50 mg	Ansaid by Mylan	00378-0076	NSAID
M76	Tab, Beige, Round, Film Coated, M over 76	Flurbiprofen 50 mg	Ansaid by Allscripts		NSAID
M76	Tab, Beige, Round, Film Coated, M over 76	Flurbiprofen 100 mg	Ansaid by PDRX	55289-0561	NSAID
M77	Tab, White, Round, Film Coated	Amitriptyline HCl 10 mg	Elavil by Mylan	00378-2610	Antidepressant
M77	Tab, White, Round, Film Coated	Amitriptyline HCl 10 mg	Elavil by UDL	51079-0131	Antidepressant
M775	Tab, Beige, Oval, Scored	Benazepril HCl 20 mg, Hydrochlorothiazide 25 mg	Lotensin HCT by Mylan	00378-4775	Antihypertensive; Diuretic
M81	Tab, White, Oval, Scored	Buspirone HCl 5 mg	BuSpar by Mylan	00378-0140	Antianxiety
M81	Tab, White, Round, Scored	Captopril 25 mg, HCTZ 15 mg	Capozide by Mylan	00378-0081	Antihypertensive; Diuretic
M82	Tab, White, Oval, Scored	Buspirone HCl 10 mg	BuSpar by Mylan	00378-1150	Antianxiety
M83	Tab, Peach, Round, Scored	Captopril 25 mg, HCTZ 25 mg	Capozide by Mylan	00378-0083	Antihypertensive; Diuretic

ID FRONT <> BACK	DESCRIPTION FRONT <> BACK	INGREDIENT & STRENGTH	BRAND (or Generic Equiv.) by FIRM	NDC#	CLASS; SCH.
M84	Tab, White, Oblong, Scored	Captopril 50 mg, HCTZ 15 mg	Capozide by Mylan	00378-0084	Antihypertensive; Diuretic
M86	Tab, Peach, Oblong, Scored	Captopril 50 mg, HCTZ 25 mg	Capozide by Mylan	00378-0086	Antihypertensive; Diuretic
M87 <> W	Tab, M/87 <>	Ambenonium Chloride 10 mg	Mytelase by Sanofi	00024-1287	Myasthenia Gravis
M87 <> W	Tab, Coated, M/87 <> W	Ambenonium Chloride 10 mg	Mytelase by Bayer	00280-1287	Myasthenia Gravis
M89	Tab, Yellow, Round	Meloxicam 15 mg	Mobic by UDL	51079-0459	NSAID
M89	Tab, White, Round	Meloxicam 15 mg	Mobic by Mylan	00378-1089	Anti-inflammatory
M89605MG	Cap, White, Opaque, M inside square on cap, 8960 5mg on body, Blue Ink	Dextroamphetamine Sulfate 5 mg	Dexedrine by Mallinckrodt	00406-8960	Stimulant; C II
M896110MG	Cap, White, Opaque, M inside square on cap, 8961 10 mg on body, Blue ink	Dextroamphetamine Sulfate 10 mg	Dexedrine by Mallinckrodt	00406-8961	Stimulant; C II
M896215MG	Cap, White, Opaque, M inside square on cap, 8962 15mg on body, Pink Ink	Dextroamphetamine Sulfate 15 mg	Dexedrine by Mallinckrodt	00406-8962	Stimulant; C II
M93	Tab, Beige, Round, Film Coated, M over 93	Flurbiprofen 100 mg	Ansaid by Physician Total Care	54868-3362	NSAID
M93	Tab, Beige, Round, Film Coated, M over 93	Flurbiprofen 100 mg	Ansaid by Allscripts		NSAID
M93	Tab, Beige, Round, Film Coated, M over 93	Flurbiprofen 100 mg	Ansaid by Mylan	00378-0093	NSAID
M93	Tab, Beige, Round, Film Coated, M over 93	Flurbiprofen 100 mg	Ansaid by UDL	51079-0815 Discontinued	NSAID
M944	Tab, Blue, Round, Delayed Release	Divalproex Sodium 250 mg	Depakote by Mylan	00378-0472	Anticonvulsant
M944	Tab, Blue, Round, Delayed Release	Divalproex Sodium 250 mg	Depakote by Mylan	51079-0474	Anticonvulsant
M945	Tab, Blue, Round, Delayed Release	Divalproex Sodium 500 mg	Depakote by UDL	51079-0475	Anticonvulsant
M945	Tab, Blue, Round, Delayed Release	Divalproex Sodium 500 mg	Depakote by Mylan	00378-0473	Anticonvulsant
M95	Tab, M to Left, 95 to Right of Score	Penicillin V Potassium	by Mylan	00378-0195	Antibiotic
M96	Tab, Light Yellow, Round	Nadolol 40 mg, Bendroflumethiazide 5 mg	Corzide by Mylan	00378-0096	Antihypertensive
M970	Tab, White, Round, M/970	Acetaminophen 325 mg, Butalbital 50 mg, Caffeine 40 mg	Fioricet by Mallinckrodt		Analgesic
M98	Tab	Penicillin V Potassium	by Mylan	00378-0198	Antibiotic
M98	Tab	Penicillin V Potassium	by Rx Dispensing	61807-0004	Antibiotic
M99	Tab, Light Yellow, Round	Nadolol 80 mg, Bendroflumethiazide 5 mg	Corzide by Mylan	00378-0099	Antihypertensive
M9B <> MAXZIDE	Tab, Bowtie Shaped, B on the Left and M9 on the Right of the Score	Hydrochlorothiazide 25 mg, Triamterene 37.5 mg	by Eckerd	19458-0845	Diuretic; Antihypertensive
MA11	Tab, White, Capsule Shaped	Alendronate Sodium 35 mg	Fosamax by Mylan	00378-3568	Antiosteoporosis
MA12	Tab, White, Capsule Shaped	Alendronate Sodium 70 mg	Fosamax by Mylan	00378-3569	Antiosteoporosis
MA12	Tab, White, Cap Shaped	Alendronate Sodium 70 mg	Fosamax by UDL	51079-0942	Antiosteoporosis
MAALOXAG150	Tab, Pink, Round	Simethicone 150 mg	Maalox by Ciba	Canadian	Antiflatulent
MAALOXAG80	Tab, Pink, Round	Simethicone 80 mg	Maalox by Ciba	Canadian	Antiflatulent
MAALOXHRF	Tab, Green, Round	Alginate Compound 250 mg	Maalox by Ciba	Canadian	Gastrointestinal
MAALOXTC	Tab, White, Round, Mallox TC/Novartis Logo	Aluminum Hydroxide 300 mg	Amphojel by Novartis	Canadian	Gastrointestinal
MACROBID-NORWICHEATON	Cap, Black & Yellow, Opaque	Nitrofurantoin 100 mg	Macrobid by DRX	55045-2341	Antibiotic
MACROBID-NORWICHEATON	Cap, Black & Yellow, Opaque	Nitrofurantoin 100 mg	Macrobid by Promex Med	62301-0039	Antibiotic
MACROBID-NORWICHEATON	Cap, Black & Yellow, Opaque	Nitrofurantoin 100 mg	Macrobid by Southwood	58016-0260	Antibiotic
MACROBID-NORWICHEATON	Cap, Black & Yellow, Opaque	Nitrofurantoin 100 mg	Macrobid by Procter and Gamble	00149-0710	Antibiotic
MACROBID-NORWICHEATON	Cap, Black and Yellow, Opaque, Hard Shell Gelatin	Nitrofurantoin 100 mg	MacroBID by Proc & Gamble	Canadian DIN 02063662	Antibiotic
MACRODANTIN-100MG01149009	Cap, Yellow, Opaque, Three Black Lines encircling the cap	Nitrofurantoin 100 mg	Macrodantin by Rightpak	65240-0688	Antibiotic
MACRODANTIN-100MG01149009	Cap, Yellow, Opaque, Three Black Lines encircling the cap	Nitrofurantoin 100 mg	Macrodantin by Amerisource	62584-0009	Antibiotic

ID FRONT <> BACK	DESCRIPTION FRONT <> BACK	INGREDIENT & STRENGTH	BRAND (or Generic Equiv.) by FIRM	NDC#	CLASS; SCH.
MACRODANTIN-100MG01490009	Cap, Yellow, Opaque, Three Black Lines encircling the cap	Nitrofurantoin 100 mg	Macrodantin by Pharmedix	53002-0273	Antibiotic
MACRODANTIN-100MG01490009	Cap, Yellow, Opaque, Three Black Lines encircling the cap	Nitrofurantoin 100 mg	Macrodantin by Pharm Util	60491-0389	Antibiotic
MACRODANTIN-100MG01490009	Cap, Yellow, Opaque, Three Black Lines encircling the cap	Nitrofurantoin 100 mg	Macrodantin by Thrift Drug	59198-0057	Antibiotic
MACRODANTIN-100MG01490009	Cap, Yellow, Opaque, Three Black Lines encircling the cap	Nitrofurantoin 100 mg	Macrodantin by Procter and Gamble	00149-0009	Antibiotic
MACRODANTIN-25MG01490007	Cap, White, Opaque, One Black Line encircling the cap	Nitrofurantoin 25 mg	Macrodantin by Procter and Gamble	00149-0007	Antibiotic
MACRODANTIN-50MG01490008	Cap, White & Yellow, Opaque, Two Black Lines encircling the cap	Nitrofurantoin 50 mg	Macrodantin by PDRX	55289-0239	Antibiotic
MACRODANTIN-50MG01490008	Cap, White & Yellow, Opaque, Two Black Lines encircling the cap	Nitrofurantoin 50 mg	Macrodantin by Nat Pharmpak	55154-2301	Antibiotic
MACRODANTIN-50MG01490008	Cap, White & Yellow, Opaque, Two Black Lines encircling the cap	Nitrofurantoin 50 mg	Macrodantin by Thrift Drug	59198-0056	Antibiotic
MACRODANTIN-50MG01490008	Cap, White & Yellow, Opaque, Two Black Lines encircling the cap	Nitrofurantoin 50 mg	Macrodantin by Amerisource	62584-0008	Antibiotic
MACRODANTIN-50MG01490008	Cap, White & Yellow, Opaque, Two Black Lines encircling the cap	Nitrofurantoin 50 mg	Macrodantin by Med Pro	53978-3397	Antibiotic
MACRODANTIN-50MG01490008	Cap, White & Yellow, Opaque, Two Black Lines encircling the cap	Nitrofurantoin 50 mg	Macrodantin by Rightpak	65240-0687	Antibiotic
MACRODANTIN-50MG01490008	Cap, White & Yellow, Opaque, Two Black Lines encircling the cap	Nitrofurantoin 50 mg	Macrodantin by Procter and Gamble	00149-0008	Antibiotic
MAG64	Tab, White, Round	Calcium 220 mg, Magnesium 64 mg	Mag 64 by Rising	68585-0005	Supplement
MAG64	Tab, White, Round	Calcium 220 mg, Magnesium 64 mg	Mag 64 by Major	00904-7911	Supplement
MAGNUM	Tab, Pink, Bullet Shaped	Caffeine 200 mg	Magnum 357 by D&E Pharma		Stimulant
MAJOR0058	Cap, Ex Release	Chlorpheniramine Maleate 8 mg, Pseudoephedrine HCl 120 mg	Pseudo Chlor by Sovereign	58716-0014	Cold Remedy
MAMPHETSALTS10MG	Cap, Blue, Extended Release	Mixed Amphetamine Salts 10 mg: Amphetamine Aspartate 2.5 mg, Amphetamine Sulfate 2.5 mg, Dextroamphetamine Saccharate 2.5 mg, Dextroamphetamine Sulfate 2.5 mg	Adderall XR by Teva	00555-0787	Stimulant; C II
MAMPHETSALTS15MG	Cap, Blue and White	Mixed Amphetamine Salts 15 mg: Amphetamine Aspartate 3.75 mg, Amphetamine Sulfate 3.75 mg, Dextroamphetamine Saccharate 3.75 mg, Dextroamphetamine Sulfate 3.75 mg	Adderall XR by Teva	00555-0791	Stimulant; C II
MAMPHETSALTS20MG	Cap, Orange	Mixed Amphetamine Salts 20 mg: Amphetamine Aspartate 5 mg, Amphetamine Sulfate 5 mg, Dextroamphetamine Saccharate 5 mg, Dextroamphetamine Sulfate 5 mg	Adderall XR by Teva	00555-0788	Stimulant; C II
MAMPHETSALTS25MG	Cap, Orange and White	Mixed Amphetamine Salts 25 mg: Amphetamine Aspartate 6.25 mg, Amphetamine Sulfate 6.25 mg, Dextroamphetamine Saccharate 6.25 mg, Dextroamphetamine Sulfate 6.25 mg	Adderall XR by Teva	00555-0792	Stimulant; C II
MAMPHETSALTS30MG	Cap, Natural and Orange	Mixed Amphetamine Salts 30 mg: Amphetamine Aspartate 7.5 mg, Amphetamine Sulfate 7.5 mg, Dextroamphetamine Saccharate 7.5 mg, Dextroamphetamine Sulfate 7.5 mg	Adderall XR by Teva	00555-0789	Stimulant; C II
MAMPHETSALTS5MG	Cap, Clear and Blue	Mixed Amphetamine Salts 5 mg: Amphetamine Aspartate 1.25 mg, Amphetamine Sulfate 1.25 mg, Dextroamphetamine Saccharate 1.25 mg, Dextroamphetamine Sulfate 1.25 mg	Adderall XR by Teva	00555-0790	Stimulant; C II
MANPLAYINGFLUTE	Tab, Peach, Round, Greek-god like figure playing horn	3,4-Methylenedioxymethamphetamine (MDMA)	Ecstasy by Illegal		Euphoric; Illicit
MANPLAYINGTRUMPET	Tab, Peach, Round, Greek-god like figure playing horn	3,4-Methylenedioxymethamphetamine (MDMA)	Ecstasy by Illegal		Euphoric; Illicit
MARAX <> ROERIG254	Tab	Ephedrine 25 mg, Hydroxyzine 10 mg, Theophylline 130 mg	Marax by Roerig	00049-2540	Antiasthmatic
MARCPM	Tab, Off-White, MAR-CPM	Chlorpheniramine Maleate 8 mg, Methscopolamine Nitrate 2.5 mg, Phenylephrine HCl 20 mg	Prehist by Anabolic	00722-6280	Cold Remedy

ID FRONT <> BACK	DESCRIPTION FRONT <> BACK	INGREDIENT & STRENGTH	BRAND (or Generic Equiv.) by FIRM	NDC#	CLASS; SCH.
MAREZINE	Tab, Round	Cyclizine HCl 50 mg	Marezine by Himmel		Antiemetic
MARGESICH	Cap, White Print	Acetaminophen 500 mg, Hydrocodone Bitartrate 5 mg	Vicodin by Marnel	00682-0808	Analgesic; C III
MARGESICMARNEL	Cap, Green Print	Acetaminophen 325 mg, Butalbital 50 mg, Caffeine 40 mg	Fioricet by Marnel	00682-0804	Analgesic
MARION <> 1772	Tab, Coated	Diltiazem HCl 60 mg	Cardizem by Drug Distr	52985-0191	Antihypertensive
MARION1375	Tab, Blue, Round	Oxybutynin Chloride 5 mg	Ditropan by Marion		Urinary Tract
MARION1555	Cap, Brown & Clear	Papaverine HCl 150 mg	Pavabid by Aventis		Vasodilator
MARION1712	Tab, Pink, Oblong, Marion/1712	Sucralfate 1 g	Carafate by Marion		Gastrointestinal
MARNATALF	Tab, Film Coated, Marnatal-F	Ascorbic Acid 100 mg, Calcium 250 mg, Copper 2 mg, Cyanocobalamin 12 mcg, Folic Acid 1 mg, Iodine 0.2 mg, Iron 60 mg, Magnesium 25 mg, Niacinamide 20 mg, Pyridoxine HCl 5 mg, Riboflavin 3.4 mg, Thiamine HCl 3 mg, Vitamin A 4000 Units, Vitamin D 400 Units, Vitamin E 30 Units, Zinc 25 mg	Marnatal F by Lini	58215-0309 Discontinued	Vitamin
MARSAM0530	Cap, Purple	Cefaclor 250 mg	Ceclor by Marsam		Antibiotic
MARSAM0531	Cap, Purple & Yellow	Cefaclor 500 mg	Ceclor CD by Marsam		Antibiotic
MARSAM530	Cap, Purple	Cefaclor 250 mg	Ceclor by Schein		Antibiotic
MARTEC972	Cap, Ivory & Red, Martec/972	Piroxicam 10 mg	Feldene by Martec	52555-0972	NSAID
MARTEC973	Cap	Piroxicam 20 mg	Feldene by Med Pro	53978-1255	NSAID
MARTEC973	Cap, Red, Martec/973	Piroxicam 20 mg	Feldene by Martec	52555-0973	NSAID
MATERNA <> M55	Tab, Beige, Oblong	Vitamin Combination	Materna by Wyeth	00005-5586	Vitamin
MATERNAU24	Tab, Pink, Oval	Multi Vitamin	Materna by Wyeth	Canadian	Vitamin
MATULANEROCHEMAT-ULANEROCHE	Cap, Matulane/Roche	Procarbazine HCl 50 mg	Matulane by Hoffmann La Roche	00004-0053	Antineoplastic
MATULANESIGMATAU	Cap, Ivory	Procarbazine HCl 50 mg	Matulane by Ranbaxy	54907-0608	Antineoplastic
MATULANESIGMATAU	Cap, Ivory	Procarbazine HCl 50 mg	Matulane by Sigma-Tau	54482-0053	Antineoplastic
MAXALT <> MRK267	Tab, Light Pink, Cap Shaped	Rizatriptan Benzoate 10 mg	Maxalt by Merck	00006-0267	Antimigraine
MAXALT <> MSD267	Tab, Pale Pink, Cap-Shaped	Rizatriptan 10 mg	Maxalt by Merck Frosst	Canadian DIN 02240521	Antimigraine
MAXAQUIN400	Tab, White, Oval, Film Coated	Lomefloxacin 400 mg	Maxaquin by Searle	00025-5501	Antibiotic
MAXAQUIN400	Tab, White, Oval, Scored	Lomefloxacin 400 mg	Maxaquin by West Pharm	52967-0283	Antibiotic
MAXAQUIN400	Tab, White, Oval, Film Coated	Lomefloxacin 400 mg	Maxaquin by Unimed	00051-1651	Antibiotic
MAXIDONE634	Tab, Yellow, Cap Shaped, Scored	Acetaminophen 750 mg, Hydrocodone Bitartrate 10 mg	Maxidone by Watson	52544-0634	Analgesic; C III
MAXIFED <> MCR520	Tab, Green, Oblong, Scored	Pseudoephedrine HCl 80 mg, Guaifenesin 700 mg	Maxifed by AM Pharms	58605-0520	Cold Remedy
MAXIFEDDM	Tab, White, Cap Shaped, Scored	Pseudoephedrine HCl 60 mg, Guaifenesin 580 mg, Dextromethorphan HBr 30 mg	Maxifed DM by AM Pharms	58605-0626	Cold Remedy
MAXIFEDDM <> MCR526	Tab, Scored	Guaifenesin 500 mg, Pseudoephedrine HCl 60 mg, Dextromethorphan HBr 30 mg	Maxifed DM by AM Pharms	58605-0526	Cold Remedy
MAXIFEDDM <> MCR526	Tab, Scored	Guaifenesin 500 mg, Pseudoephedrine HCl 60 mg, Dextromethorphan HBr 30 mg	by Pfab	62542-0772	Cold Remedy
MAXIFEDG <> MCR514	Tab, White, Cap Shaped	Pseudoephedrine HCl 60 mg, Guaifenesin 550 mg	Maxifed-G by AM Pharms	58605-0514	Cold Remedy
MAXZIDE <> BM8	Tab, Light Yellow, Bowtie Shaped, Scored	Hydrochlorothiazide 50 mg, Triamterene 75 mg	Maxzide by Bertek	62794-0460	Diuretic; Antihypertensive
MAXZIDE <> BM8	Tab, Light Yellow, Bowtie Shaped, Scored	Hydrochlorothiazide 50 mg, Triamterene 75 mg	Maxzide by Mylan	00378-7550	Diuretic; Antihypertensive
MAXZIDE <> BM9	Tab, Light Green, Bowtie Shaped, Scored	Hydrochlorothiazide 25 mg, Triamterene 37.5 mg	Maxzide 25 by Eckerd	19458-0845	Diuretic; Antihypertensive
MAXZIDE <> BM9	Tab, Light Green, Bowtie Shaped, Scored	Hydrochlorothiazide 25 mg, Triamterene 37.5 mg	Maxzide 25 by Bertek	62794-0464	Diuretic; Antihypertensive
MAXZIDE <> BM9	Tab, Light Green, Bowtie Shaped, Scored	Hydrochlorothiazide 25 mg, Triamterene 37.5 mg	Maxzide 25 by Direct Dispensing	57866-6801	Diuretic; Antihypertensive
MAXZIDE <> BM9	Tab, Light Green, Bowtie Shaped, Scored	Hydrochlorothiazide 25 mg, Triamterene 37.5 mg	Maxzide 25 by Caremark	00339-6094	Diuretic; Antihypertensive
MAXZIDE <> BM9	Tab, Teal, Bow Tie Shaped	Triamterene 37.5 mg, HCl 25 mg	Maxzide by Mylan	00378-3725	Diuretic; Antihypertensive
MAXZIDE <> LLM8	Tab, Off-White, Bone Shaped, Scored	Triamterene 75 mg, HCTZ 50 mg	by Lederle	00005-4460	Antihypertensive; Diuretic
MAXZIDE <> LLM8	Tab, Off-White, Bone Shaped, Scored	Triamterene 75 mg, HCTZ 50 mg	by Nat Pharmpak	55154-1705	Antihypertensive; Diuretic

ID FRONT <> BACK	DESCRIPTION FRONT <> BACK	INGREDIENT & STRENGTH	BRAND (or Generic Equiv.) by FIRM	NDC#	CLASS; SCH.
MB	Tab, White, Oval, Scored, Film Coated, Extended Release, Scripted M over Greek Letter Beta	Metoprolol Succinate 25 mg	Toprol XL by Par	49884-0404	Antihypertensive
MB1	Tab, White, Oval, Scored	Buspirone HCl 5 mg	BuSpar by UDL	51079-0985	Antianxiety
MB-111	Tab, Blue, Oval, Film-Coated	Amoxicillin 775 mg	Moxatag by MiddleBrook	11042-0142	Antibacterial
MB2	Tab, White, Oval, Scored	Buspirone HCl 10 mg	BuSpar by UDL	51079-0986	Antianxiety
MB3 <> 555	Tab, White, Cap Shaped, Scored	Buspirone HCl 15 mg	BuSpar by Mylan	00378-1165	Antianxiety
MB3 <> 555	Tab, White, Cap Shaped, Scored	Buspirone HCl 15 mg	BuSpar by UDL	51079-0960	Antianxiety
MB4 <> 101010	Tab, White, Cap Shaped, Scored	Buspirone HCl 30 mg	BuSpar by Mylan	00378-1175	Antianxiety
MB4 <> 101010	Tab, White, Cap Shaped, Scored	Buspirone HCl 30 mg	BuSpar by UDL	51079-0994	Antianxiety
MC <> 10	Tab, White, Round, Scored	Isoxsuprine HCl 10 mg	Vasodilan by Murfreesboro	51129-1584	Vasodilator
MC <> 20	Tab, White, Round, Scored	Isoxsuprine HCl 20 mg	Vasodilan by Shire	58521-0576	Vasodilator
MC <> 20	Tab, White, Round, Scored	Isoxsuprine HCl 20 mg	Vasodilan by Murfreesboro	51129-1585	Vasodilator
MC1	Tab, White, Oval, Scored	Captopril 12.5 mg	Capoten by Mylan	00378-3007	Antihypertensive
MC1	Tab, White, Oval, Scored	Captopril 12.5 mg	Capoten by UDL	51079-0863	Antihypertensive
MC2	Tab, White, Round, Scored, M over C2	Captopril 25 mg	Capoten by Direct Dispensing	57866-6106	Antihypertensive
MC2	Tab, White, Round, Scored, M over C2	Captopril 25 mg	Capoten by Mylan	00378-3012	Antihypertensive
MC2	Tab, White, Round, Scored, M over C2	Captopril 25 mg	Capoten by UDL	51079-0864	Antihypertensive
MC3	Tab, White, Round, Scored	Captopril 50 mg	Capoten by Southwood	58016-0165	Antihypertensive
MC3	Tab, White, Round, Scored	Captopril 50 mg	Capoten by Heartland	61392-0147	Antihypertensive
MC3	Tab, White, Round, Scored, M over C3	Captopril 50 mg	Capoten by Mylan	00378-3017	Antihypertensive
MC4	Tab, White, Round, Scored, M over C4	Captopril 100 mg	Capoten by Mylan	00378-3022	Antihypertensive
MC41	Tab, White, Round	Cilostazol 50 mg	Pletal by Mylan	00378-2979	Antiplatelet
MC42	Tab, White, Round	Cilostazol 100 mg	Pletal by Mylan	00378-2980	Antiplatelet
MC42	Tab, White, Round	Cilostazol 100 mg	Pletal by UDL	51079-0213	Antiplatelet
MC51	Tab, Blue, Round	Carbidopa 10 mg, Levodopa 100 mg	Parcopa by Mylan	00378-5051	Antiparkinson
MC52	Tab, Blue, Round	Carbidopa 25 mg, Levodopa 100 mg	Parcopa by Mylan	00378-5052	Antiparkinson
MC53	Tab, Blue, Round	Carbidopa 25 mg, Levodopa 250 mg	Parcopa by Mylan	00378-5053	Antiparkinson
MCG219	Cap	Phenylpropanolamine 75 mg, Chlorpheniramine 8 mg, Methscop. 2.5 mg	Rhinolar by McGregor		Cold Remedy
MCL1	Tab, Blue	Carbidopa 10 mg, Levodopa 100 mg	Sinemet by UDL	51079-0861	Antiparkinson
MCL2	Tab, Yellow	Carbidopa 25 mg, Levodopa 100 mg	Sinemet by UDL	51079-0884	Antiparkinson
MCNEIL	Tab, Peach, Round	Pimozide 10 mg	Orap by McNeil	Canadian	Antipsychotic
MCNEIL	Tab, White, Round	Pimozide 2 mg	Orap by McNeil	Canadian	Antipsychotic
MCNEIL	Tab, Green, Round	Pimozide 4 mg	Orap by McNeil	Canadian	Antipsychotic
MCNEIL	Tab, Green, Round	Chlorzoxazone 250 mg	Parafon Forte by McNeil	Canadian	Muscle Relaxant
MCNEIL	Tab, Light Green, Round, Scored	Acetaminophen 300 mg, Chlorzoxazone 250 mg	Parafon Forte by Johnson & Johnson	Canadian DIN 02229946	Analgesic
MCNEIL	Tab	Acetaminophen 300 mg, Codeine Phosphate 30 mg	Tylenol w/ Codeine by Nat Pharmpak	55154-1908	Analgesic; C III
MCNEIL <> 2	Tab, White, Round, McNeil	Acetaminophen 300 mg, Caffeine 15 mg, Codeine Phosphate 15 mg	Tylenol w/ Codeine by Janssen-Ortho	Canadian DIN 02163934	Analgesic; C III
MCNEIL <> 2	Tab, White, Flat-Faced, Beveled	Acetaminophen 300 mg, Caffeine 15 mg, Codeine Phosphate 15 mg	Tylenol with Codeine No. 2 by McNeil Consumer Heal	Canadian DIN 02163934	Analgesic
MCNEIL <> 3	Tab, White, Round, Flat-Faced, Beveled	Acetaminophen 300 mg, Caffeine 15 mg, Codeine Phosphate 30 mg	Tylenol with Codeine No. 3 by McNeil Consumer Heal	Canadian DIN 02163926	Analgesic
MCNEIL <> 3	Tab, White, Round, McNeil	Acetaminophen 300 mg, Caffeine 15 mg, Codeine Phosphate 30 mg	Tylenol w/ Codeine by Janssen-Ortho	Canadian DIN 02163926	Analgesic; C III
MCNEIL <> 4	Tab, White, Round, McNeil	Acetaminophen 300 mg, Codeine Phosphate 60 mg	Tylenol w/ Codeine by Janssen-Ortho	Canadian DIN 02163918	Analgesic; C III
MCNEIL <> 4	Tab, Round, White, Flat-Faced, Beveled	Acetaminophen 300 mg, Codeine Phosphate 60 mg	Tylenol with Codeine No. 4 by McNeil Consumer Heal	Canadian DIN 02163918	Analgesic
MCNEIL <> 659	Tab, White, Cap Shaped, Film Coated	Tramadol HCl 50 mg	Ultram by McNeil	00045-0659	Analgesic

ID FRONT <> BACK	DESCRIPTION FRONT <> BACK	INGREDIENT & STRENGTH	BRAND (or Generic Equiv.) by FIRM	NDC#	CLASS; SCH.
MCNEIL <> 659	Tab, White, Cap Shaped, Film Coated	Tramadol HCl 50 mg	Ultram by Ortho-McNeil	00062-0659	Analgesic
MCNEIL <> 659	Tab, White, Cap Shaped, Film Coated	Tramadol HCl 50 mg	Ultram by Teva	00480-0148	Analgesic
MCNEIL <> 659	Tab, White, Cap Shaped, Film Coated	Tramadol HCl 50 mg	Ultram by Caremark	00339-6099	Analgesic
MCNEIL <> 659	Tab, White, Cap Shaped, Film Coated	Tramadol HCl 50 mg	Ultram by Northeast	58163-0659	Analgesic
MCNEIL <> 659	Tab, White, Cap Shaped, Film Coated	Tramadol HCl 50 mg	Ultram by DRX	55045-2219	Analgesic
MCNEIL <> 659	Tab, White, Cap Shaped, Film Coated	Tramadol HCl 50 mg	Ultram by PDRX	55289-0650	Analgesic
MCNEIL <> 659	Tab, White, Cap Shaped, Film Coated	Tramadol HCl 50 mg	Ultram by Rx Dispensing	61807-0128	Analgesic
MCNEIL <> 659	Tab, White, Cap Shaped, Film Coated	Tramadol HCl 50 mg	Ultram by Heartland	61392-0625	Analgesic
MCNEIL <> 659	Tab, White, Cap Shaped, Film Coated	Tramadol HCl 50 mg	Ultram by H J Harkins Co	52959-0414	Analgesic
MCNEIL <> 659	Tab, White, Cap Shaped, Film Coated	Tramadol HCl 50 mg	Ultram by McNeil	52021-0659	Analgesic
MCNEIL <> PARAFONFORTEDSC	Tab, Light Green, Cap Shaped, Scored	Chlorzoxazone 500 mg	Parafon Forte DSC by Rightpac	65240-0715	Muscle Relaxant
MCNEIL <> PARAFONFORTEDSC	Tab, Light Green, Cap Shaped, Scored	Chlorzoxazone 500 mg	Parafon Forte DSC by McNeil	00045-0325	Muscle Relaxant
MCNEIL <> PARAFONFORTEDSC	Tab, Light Green, Cap Shaped, Scored	Chlorzoxazone 500 mg	Parafon Forte DSC by Compumed	00403-0261	Muscle Relaxant
MCNEIL <> PARAFONFORTEDSC	Tab, Light Green, Cap Shaped, Scored	Chlorzoxazone 500 mg	Parafon Forte DSC by Nat Pharmpak	55154-1907	Muscle Relaxant
MCNEIL <> PARAFONFORTEDSC	Tab, Light Green, Cap Shaped, Scored	Chlorzoxazone 500 mg	Parafon Forte DSC by Thrift Drug	59198-0089	Muscle Relaxant
MCNEIL <> TOLECTIN200	Tab, White, Round, Scored, Tolectin over 200	Tolmetin Sodium 246 mg	Tolectin 200 by McNeil	00045-0412	NSAID
MCNEIL <> TOLECTIN200	Tab, White, Round, Scored, Tolectin over 200	Tolmetin Sodium 200 mg		Canadian	NSAID
MCNEIL <> TYLCODEINE3	Tab, White, Tyl over Codeine 3	Acetaminophen 300 mg, Codeine Phosphate 30 mg	Tylenol w/ Codeine by McNeil		Analgesic; C III
MCNEIL <> TYLENOL3CODEINE	Tab, White, Round	Acetaminophen 300 mg, Codeine Phosphate 30 mg	Tylenol w/ Codeine by McNeil	00045-0513	Analgesic; C III
MCNEIL <> TYLENOL4CODEINE	Tab, White, Round	Acetaminophen 300 mg, Codeine Phosphate 60 mg	Tylenol w/ Codeine by McNeil	00045-0515	Analgesic; C III
MCNEIL <> TYLENOLCODEINE2	Tab	Acetaminophen 300 mg, Codeine Phosphate 15 mg	Tylenol w/ Codeine by Murfreesboro	51129-1393	Analgesic; C III
MCNEIL <> TYLENOLCODEINE2	Tab, White	Acetaminophen 300 mg, Codeine Phosphate 15 mg	Tylenol w/ Codeine by McNeil	00045-0511	Analgesic; C III
MCNEIL <> TYLENOLCODEINE3	Tab	Acetaminophen 300 mg, Codeine Phosphate 30 mg	Tylenol w/ Codeine by Med Pro	53978-3087	Analgesic; C III
MCNEIL <> TYLENOLCODEINE3	Tab	Acetaminophen 300 mg, Codeine Phosphate 30 mg	Tylenol w/ Codeine by Allscripts		Analgesic; C III
MCNEIL <> TYLENOLCODEINE4	Tab	Acetaminophen 300 mg, Codeine Phosphate 60 mg	Tylenol w/ Codeine by Med Pro	53978-3094	Analgesic; C III
MCNEIL <> TYLENOLCODEINE4	Tab, White, Round	Acetaminophen 300 mg, Codeine Phosphate 60 mg	Tylenol w/ Codeine by Nat Pharmpak	55154-1916	Analgesic; C III
MCNEIL1520 <> 250	Tab, Coated	Levofloxacin 250 mg	Levaquin by McNeil	00045-1520	Antibiotic
MCNEIL1520 <> 250	Tab, Pink, Modified Rectangular, Film Coated	Levofloxacin 250 mg	Levaquin by Ortho-McNeil	00062-1520	Antibiotic
MCNEIL1520 <> 250	Tab, Film Coated	Levofloxacin 250 mg	Levaquin by Johnson & Johnson	59604-0520	Antibiotic
MCNEIL1525 <> 500	Tab, Peach, Oblong, Film Coated	Levofloxacin 500 mg	Levaquin by McNeil	00045-1525	Antibiotic
MCNEIL1525 <> 500	Tab, Peach, Oblong, Film Coated	Levofloxacin 500 mg	Levaquin by Johnson & Johnson	59604-0525	Antibiotic
MCNEIL1525 <> 500	Tab, Peach, Oblong, Film Coated	Levofloxacin 500 mg	Levaquin by Ortho-McNeil	00062-1525	Antibiotic
MCNEIL1525 <> 500	Tab, Peach, Oblong, Film Coated	Levofloxacin 500 mg	Levaquin by Murfreesboro	51129-1629	Antibiotic
MCNEIL425200	Tab, White, Round, McNeil 425/200	Theophylline Anhydrous 100 mg	Duraphyl by Forest	00456-0632	Antiasthmatic
MCNEIL426200	Tab, White, Cap Shaped, McNeil 426/200	Theophylline Anhydrous 200 mg	Duraphyl by Forest	00456-0633	Antiasthmatic

ID FRONT <> BACK	DESCRIPTION FRONT <> BACK	INGREDIENT & STRENGTH	BRAND (or Generic Equiv.) by FIRM	NDC#	CLASS; SCH.
MCNEIL427200	Tab, White, Cap Shaped, McNeil 427/200	Theophylline Anhydrous 300 mg	Duraphyl by Forest	00456-0634	Antiasthmatic
MCNEILHALDOL05MG	Tab, H Symbol, McNeil Haldol 0.5 mg	Haloperidol 0.5 mg	Haldol by McNeil	52021-0240	Antipsychotic
MCNEILHALDOL1	Tab, H Symbol	Haloperidol 1 mg	Haldol by H J Harkins Co	52959-0356	Antipsychotic
MCNEILHALDOL10	Tab, H Symbol	Haloperidol 10 mg	Haldol by McNeil	52021-0246	Antipsychotic
MCNEILHALDOL1MG	Tab, H Symbol	Haloperidol 1 mg	Haldol by McNeil	52021-0241	Antipsychotic
MCNEILHALDOL20	Tab, H Symbol	Haloperidol 20 mg	Haldol by McNeil	52021-0248	Antipsychotic
MCNEILHALDOL2MG	Tab, H Symbol	Haloperidol 2 mg	Haldol by McNeil	52021-0242	Antipsychotic
MCNEILHALDOL5MG	Tab, H Symbol	Haloperidol 5 mg	Haldol by McNeil	52021-0245	Antipsychotic
MCNEILNO1	Cap, White, Film Coated, McNeil <> No. 1	Acetaminophen 300 mg, Caffeine 15 mg, Codeine Phosphate 8 mg	Tylenol w/ Codeine by McNeil	Canadian DIN 02181061	Analgesic; C III
MCNEILNO1FORTE	Cap, White, Film Coated, McNeil <> No. 1 Forte	Acetaminophen 500 mg, Caffeine 15 mg, Codeine Phosphate 8 mg	Tylenol No. 1 Forte by McNeil	Canadian DIN 02181088	Analgesic; C III
MCNEILPANCREASE	Cap, Clear & Natural, McNeil-Pancrease	Lipase 4500 Units, Amylase 20,000 Units, Protease 25,000 Units	Pancrease by McNeil	Canadian	Gastrointestinal
MCNEIL-PANCREASEMT20	Cap, White, Yellow Band, Yellow Beads	Amylase 56,000 Units, Lipase 20,000 Units, Protease 44,000 Units	Pancrease Mt 20 by McNeil	00045-0346	Gastrointestinal
MCNEIL-PANCREASEMT20	Cap, Yellow Band	Amylase 56,000 Units, Lipase 20,000 Units, Protease 44,000 Units	Pancrease Mt 20 by McNeil	52021-0346	Gastrointestinal
MCNEILPANCREASEMT4	Cap, Clear & Yellow	Amylase 12,000 Units, Lipase 4000 Units, Protease 12,000 Units	Pancrease Mt 4 by McNeil	00045-0341	Gastrointestinal
MCNEILPANCREASEMT4	Cap	Amylase 12,000 Units, Lipase 4000 Units, Protease 12,000 Units	Pancrease Mt 4 by McNeil	52021-0341	Gastrointestinal
MCR513 <> ALLFEN	Tab, White, Oblong	Guaifenesin 1000 mg	Robitussin by AM Pharms	58605-0513	Expectorant
MCR513 <> ALLFEN	Tab, White, Oblong, Scored	Guaifenesin 1000 mg	Robitussin by Pfab	62542-0907	Expectorant
MCR514 <> MAXIFEDG	Tab, White, Oblong, Scored	Guaifenesin 550 mg, Pseudoephedrine HCl 60 mg	Sudafed Sinus by Pfab	62542-0750	Cold Remedy
MCR514 <> MAXIFEDG	Tab, White, Oblong	Pseudoephedrine HCl 60 mg, Guaifenesin 550 mg	Maxifed G by RX Pak	65084-0109	Cold Remedy
MCR514 <> MAXIFEDG	Tab, White, Cap Shaped	Pseudoephedrine HCl 60 mg, Guaifenesin 550 mg	Maxifed-G by AM Pharms	58605-0514	Cold Remedy
MCR520 <> MAXIFED	Tab, Green, Oblong, Scored	Pseudoephedrine HCl 80 mg, Guaifenesin 700 mg	Maxifed by AM Pharms	58605-0520	Cold Remedy
MCR520 <> MAXIFED	Tab, Green, Oblong, Scored	Pseudoephedrine HCl 80 mg, Guaifenesin 700 mg	Maxifed by RX Pak	65084-0110	Cold Remedy
MCR520 <> MAXIFED	Tab, Green, Oblong, Scored	Guaifenesin 700 mg, Pseudoephedrine HCl 80 mg	by Med Pro	53978-3359	Cold Remedy
MCR521 <> ALLFENDM	Tab, White, Oblong, Scored, MCR over 521<> Alfen DM	Dextromethorphan HBr 50 mg, Guaifenesin 1000 mg	by DRX	55045-2650	Cold Remedy
MCR521 <> ALLFENDM	Tab, White, Oblong, Scored, MCR over 521<> Alfen DM	Dextromethorphan HBr 50 mg, Guaifenesin 1000 mg	Alfen DM by AM Pharms	58605-0521	Cold Remedy
MCR524 <> PROMACET	Tab, Blue, Oblong, Scored	Butalbital 50 mg, Acetaminophen 650 mg	Promacet by AM Pharms	58605-0524	Analgesic
MCR526 <> MAXIFEDDM	Tab, Scored	Guaifenesin 500 mg, Pseudoephedrine HCl 60 mg, Dextromethorphan HBr 30 mg	by Pfab	62542-0772	Cold Remedy
MCR526 <> MAXIFEDDM	Tab, Scored	Guaifenesin 500 mg, Pseudoephedrine HCl 60 mg, Dextromethorphan HBr 30 mg	Maxifed DM by AM Pharms	58605-0526	Cold Remedy
MCRTIMEHIST	Cap, Time Hist Printed in Red, Ex Release	Chlorpheniramine Maleate 8 mg, Pseudoephedrine HCl 120 mg	Time Hist by Sovereign	58716-0016	Cold Remedy
MD <> 450	Tab	Diethylpropion HCl 75 mg	by Jones	52604-9160	Anorexiant; C IV
MD <> 502	Tab, Dark Green	Dextromethorphan HBr 30 mg, Guaifenesin 600 mg	Humigen DM by MD	43567-0502	Cold Remedy
MD <> 530	Tab, Light Blue, Round, Scored	Methylphenidate HCl 10 mg	by AltiMed	Canadian DIN 02230321	Stimulant; C II
MD <> 530	Tab, Light Blue, Round, Scored	Methylphenidate HCl 10 mg	Ritalin by Qualitest	00603-4570	Stimulant; C II
MD <> 530	Tab, Light Blue, Round, Scored	Methylphenidate HCl 10 mg	Ritalin by Apothecon	59772-8841	Stimulant; C II
MD <> 530	Tab, Blue & Green, Round, Scored	Methylphenidate HCl 10 mg	Ritalin by Sandoz	00781-8841	Stimulant; C II
MD <> 531	Tab	Methylphenidate HCl 5 mg	by Qualitest	00603-4569	Stimulant; C II
MD <> 532	Tab, Orange, Round, Scored	Methylphenidate HCl 20 mg	Ritalin by Apothecon	59772-8842	Stimulant; C II
MD <> 532	Tab, Orange, Round, Scored	Methylphenidate HCl 20 mg	Ritalin by AltiMed	Canadian DIN 02230322	Stimulant; C II
MD <> 562	Tab, White, Extended Release	Methylphenidate HCl 20 mg	Ritalin by Medeva	53014-0562	Stimulant; C II
MD10	Tab, Pink, Round, Scored, M over D10	Doxazosin Mesylate 2 mg	Cardura by UDL	51079-0958	Antihypertensive
MD10	Tab, Pink, Round, Scored, M over D10	Doxazosin Mesylate 2 mg	Cardura by Mylan	00378-4022	Antihypertensive
MD11	Tab, Blue, Round, Scored, M over D11	Doxazosin Mesylate 4 mg	Cardura by Mylan	00378-4024	Antihypertensive
MD11	Tab, Blue, Round, Scored, M over D11	Doxazosin Mesylate 4 mg	Cardura by UDL	51079-0959	Antihypertensive

ID FRONT <> BACK	DESCRIPTION FRONT <> BACK	INGREDIENT & STRENGTH	BRAND (or Generic Equiv.) by FIRM	NDC#	CLASS; SCH.
MD12	Tab, Lavender, Round, Scored	Doxazosin Mesylate 8 mg	Cardura by Mylan	00378-4028	Antihypertensive
MD20	Tab, Purple, Coated, Imprinted MD-20	Hyoscyamine Sulfate 0.12 mg, Methenamine 81.6 mg, Methylene Blue 10.8 mg, Phenyl Salicylate 36.2 mg, Sodium Phosphate, Monobasic 40.8 mg	Urimar T by Shire	58521-0945	Gastrointestinal
MD20	Tab, Purple, Coated, Imprinted MD-20	Hyoscyamine Sulfate 0.12 mg, Methenamine 81.6 mg, Methylene Blue 10.8 mg, Phenyl Salicylate 36.2 mg, Sodium Phosphate, Monobasic 40.8 mg	Urimar T by Marnel	00682-0333	Gastrointestinal
MD20	Tab, Purple, Coated, Imprinted MD-20	Hyoscyamine Sulfate 0.12 mg, Methenamine 81.6 mg, Methylene Blue 10.8 mg, Phenyl Salicylate 36.2 mg, Sodium Phosphate, Monobasic 40.8 mg	Uro Blue by RA McNeil	12830-0301	Gastrointestinal
MD20	Tab, Purple, Coated, Imprinted MD-20	Hyoscyamine Sulfate 0.12 mg, Methenamine 81.6 mg, Methylene Blue 10.8 mg, Phenyl Salicylate 36.2 mg, Sodium Phosphate, Monobasic 40.8 mg	Urogesic Blue by Edwards	00485-0051	Gastrointestinal
MD20	Tab, Purple, Coated, Imprinted MD-20	Hyoscyamine Sulfate 0.12 mg, Methenamine 81.6 mg, Methylene Blue 10.8 mg, Phenyl Salicylate 36.2 mg, Sodium Phosphate, Monobasic 40.8 mg	Urogesic Blue by Murfreesboro	51129-1504	Gastrointestinal
MD305 <> DIFILG	Tab, White, Round, Scored	Guaifenesin 200 mg, Dyphylline 200 mg	Difil G by Co Med Pharma	45565-0305	Antiasthmatic; Expectorant
MD305 <> DIFILG	Tab, White, Round, Scored	Guaifenesin 200 mg, Dyphylline 200 mg	Difil G by Stewart-Jackson	45985-0644	Antiasthmatic; Expectorant
MD451	Tab, Blue, Oblong, MD/451	Guaifenesin 600 mg, Pseudoephedrine HCl 120 mg	Entex PSE by MD		Cold Remedy
MD5	Tab, White, Round, M over D5	Diclofenac Potassium 50 mg	Cataflam by Quality Care	00378-2474	NSAID
MD518	Tab, MD over 518	Diethylpropion HCl 25 mg	by Quality Care	60346-0060	Anorexiant; C IV
MD531	Tab, Yellow, Round, Scored	Methylphenidate HCl 5 mg	Ritalin by Sandoz	00781-8840	Stimulant; C II
MD532	Tab, Orange, Round, Scored	Methylphenidate HCl 20 mg	Ritalin by Sandoz	00781-8842	Stimulant; C II
MD535	Tab, White	Diphenoxylate HCl 2.5 mg, Atropine Sulfate 0.025 mg	by Qualitest	00603-3360	Antidiarrheal; C V
MD538	Tab, Pink, Round	Amitriptyline HCl 10 mg	Elavil by MD		Antidepressant
MD539	Tab, Green, Round	Amitriptyline HCl 25 mg	Elavil by MD		Antidepressant
MD540	Tab, Brown, Round	Amitriptyline HCl 50 mg	Elavil by MD		Antidepressant
MD541	Tab, Purple, Round	Amitriptyline HCl 75 mg	Elavil by MD		Antidepressant
MD542	Tab, Orange, Round	Amitriptyline HCl 100 mg	Elavil by MD		Antidepressant
MD543	Tab, Flesh, Round	Amitriptyline HCl 150 mg	Elavil by MD		Antidepressant
MD561	Tab, White, Oval, Ex Release	Methylphenidate HCl 10 mg	Metadate ER by Celltech	53014-0593	Stimulant; C II
MD561	Tab, White, Oval, Ex Release	Methylphenidate HCl 10 mg	Ritalin by Medeva	43567-0561	Stimulant; C II
MD562	Tab, White, Round, Scored, Ex Release	Methylphenidate HCl 20 mg	Ritalin by Sandoz	00781-8843	Stimulant; C II
MD6	Tab, Blue, Round, M over D6	Dicyclomine HCl 20 mg	Bentyl by UDL	51079-0119	Gastrointestinal
MD6	Tab, Blue, Round, M over D6	Dicyclomine HCl 20 mg	Bentyl by Mylan	00378-1620	Gastrointestinal
MD711	Tab, White, Round	Triprolidine 2.5 mg, Pseudoephedrine 60 mg	Actifed by MD		Cold Remedy
MD9	Tab, White to Off-White, Round, Scored, M over D9	Doxazosin Mesylate 1 mg	Cardura by Mylan	00378-4021	Antihypertensive
MD9	Tab, White to Off-White, Round, Scored, M over D9	Doxazosin Mesylate 1 mg	Cardura by UDL	51079-0957	Antihypertensive
MDC	Tab, Blue, Round, M D-C	Acetaminophen 500 mg, Hydrocodone Bitartrate 5 mg	Doucet by Mason		Analgesic; C III
MDP	Tab, Pink, Round, M D-P	Hydrocodone Bitartrate 5 mg, Aspirin 224 mg, Caffeine 32 mg	Damason-P by Mason		Analgesic; C III
ME100 <> JANSSEN	Tab, Orange, Round, Scored, Me/100	Mebendazole 100 mg	Vermox by Janssen-Ortho	Canadian DIN 00556734	Anthelmintic
ME15	Tab, White, Round, Scored, M over E15	Enalapril Maleate 2.5 mg	Vasotec by Mylan	00378-1051	Antihypertensive
ME15	Tab, White, Round, Scored, M over E15	Enalapril Maleate 2.5 mg	Vasotec by UDL	51079-0950	Antihypertensive
ME16	Tab, White, Round, Scored, M over E16	Enalapril Maleate 5 mg	Vasotec by UDL	51079-0951	Antihypertensive
ME16	Tab, White, Round, Scored, M over E16	Enalapril Maleate 5 mg	Vasotec by Mylan	00378-1052	Antihypertensive

ID FRONT <> BACK	DESCRIPTION FRONT <> BACK	INGREDIENT & STRENGTH	BRAND (or Generic Equiv.) by FIRM	NDC#	CLASS; SCH.
ME17	Tab, Light Blue, Round, M over E17	Enalapril Maleate 10 mg	Vasotec by Mylan	00378-1053	Antihypertensive
ME17	Tab, Light Blue, Round, M over E17	Enalapril Maleate 10 mg	Vasotec by UDL	51079-0952	Antihypertensive
ME18	Tab, Medium Blue, Round, M over E18	Enalapril Maleate 20 mg	Vasotec by UDL	51079-0953	Antihypertensive
ME18	Tab, Medium Blue, Round, M over E18	Enalapril Maleate 20 mg	Vasotec by Mylan	00378-1054	Antihypertensive
ME25 <> APO	Tab, White, Oval	Metoprolol Tartrate 25 mg	Lopressor by Apotex	Canadian DIN 02246010	Antihypertensive
ME7	Tab, Yellow, Round, Scored	Estropipate 0.75 mg	Ogen by Mylan	00378-4551	Hormone
ME7	Tab, Yellow, Round, Scored	Estropipate 0.75 mg	Ogen by Mylan	55160-0134	Hormone
ME8	Tab, Peach, Round, Scored	Estropipate 1.5 mg	Ogen by Mylan	00378-4553	Hormone
ME8	Tab, Peach, Round, Scored	Estropipate 1.5 mg	Ogen by Mylan	55160-0135	Hormone
ME9	Tab, Blue, Round, Scored	Estropipate 3 mg	Ogen by Mylan	00378-4555	Hormone
ME9	Tab, Blue, Round, Scored	Estropipate 3 mg	Ogen by Mylan	55160-0136	Hormone
MED10 <> APO	Tab, White, Round, Scored, MED / 10	Medroxyprogesterone Acetate 10 mg	Provera by Apotex	Canadian DIN 02277298	Hormone
MED100 <> APO	Tab, White, Round, Scored, MED / 100	Medroxyprogesterone Acetate 100 mg	Provera by Apotex	Canadian DIN 02267640	Hormone
MED25 <> APO	Tab, Orange, Round, APO <> MED 2.5	Medroxyprogesterone Acetate 2.5 mg	Provera by Apotex	Canadian DIN 02244726	Hormone
MED5 <> APO	Tab, Blue, Round	Medroxyprogesterone Acetate 5 mg	Provera by Apotex	Canadian DIN 02244727	Hormone
MEDEVA <> 012	Tab, Green, Oblong, Scored,	Guaifenesin 600 mg	Robitussin by Eli Lilly	00110-0894	Expectorant
MEDEVA <> 012	Tab, Light Green, Scored	Guaifenesin 600 mg	Robitussin by Medeva	53014-0012	Expectorant
MEDEVA <> 015	Tab, Light Blue, Scored	Guaifenesin 400 mg, Pseudoephedrine HCl 120 mg	Sudafed Sinus by Medeva	53014-0015	Cold Remedy
MEDEVA <> 017	Tab, Dark Blue, Scored	Guaifenesin 600 mg, Pseudoephedrine HCl 60 mg	Deconsal II by Medeva	53014-0017	Cold Remedy
MEDEVA <> 030	Tab, Green, Oblong, Scored	Dextromethorphan HBr 30 mg, Guaifenesin 600 mg	by DRX	55045-2634	Cold Remedy
MEDEVA <> 030	Tab, Dark Green, Scored	Dextromethorphan 30 mg, Guaifenesin 600 mg	Humibid-DM by Medeva	53014-0030	Cold Remedy
MEDEVA <> 12	Tab, Green, Oblong, Scored	Guaifenesin 600 mg	Syn Rx by Adams	63824-0308	Cold Remedy
MEDEVA <> 12	Tab, Green, Oblong, Scored	Guaifenesin 600 mg	Robitussin by Compumed	00403-1009	Expectorant
MEDEVA <> 12	Tab, Green, Oblong, Scored	Guaifenesin 600 mg	Robitussin by Physician Total Care	54868-1777	Expectorant
MEDEVA <> 12	Tab, Green, Oblong, Scored	Guaifenesin 600 mg	Robitussin by Adams	63824-0012	Expectorant
MEDEVA <> 15	Tab, Blue, Scored	Guaifenesin 400 mg, Pseudoephedrine HCl 120 mg	Sudafed Sinus by Adams	63824-0015	Cold Remedy
MEDEVA <> 17	Tab, Blue, Scored	Guaifenesin 600 mg, Pseudoephedrine HCl 60 mg	Deconsal LA by Adams	63824-0017	Cold Remedy
MEDEVA <> 17	Tab, Blue, Oblong, Scored	Guaifenesin 600 mg, Pseudoephedrine 60 mg	Syn Rx by Adams	63824-0308	Cold Remedy
MEDEVA <> 30	Tab, Green, Oblong, Scored	Dextromethorphan 30 mg, Guaifenesin 600 mg	Humibid-DM by Adams	63824-0030	Cold Remedy
MEDEVA <> 309	Tab, Yellow, Oblong, Scored	Guaifenesin 600 mg, Pseudoephedrine 60 mg	Syn Rx by Adams	63824-0311	Cold Remedy
MEDEVA <> 309	Tab, Yellow, Scored, p.m. tab	Dextromethorphan 30 mg, Guaifenesin 600 mg, Pseudoephedrine 60 mg	Syn Rx DM by Medeva	53014-0311	Cold Remedy
				Discontinued	
MEDEVA <> 310	Tab, Light Blue, Scored, a.m. tab	Dextromethorphan 30 mg, Guaifenesin 600 mg, Pseudoephedrine 60 mg	Syn Rx DM by Medeva	53014-0311	Cold Remedy
MEDEVA <> 310	Tab, Blue, Oblong, Scored	Guaifenesin 600 mg, Pseudoephedrine 60 mg	Syn Rx by Adams	63824-0311	Cold Remedy
MEDEVA017	Tab, Blue, Medeva/017	Guaifenesin 600 mg, Pseudoephedrine HCl 60 mg	Deconsal II by Medeva	Discontinued	Cold Remedy
MEDEVA024	Tab, Yellow, Medeva/0 24	Atropine Sulfate 0.04 mg, Chlorpheniramine Maleate 8 mg, Hyoscyamine Sulfate 0.19 mg, Phenylephrine 25 mg, Phenylpropanolamine 50 mg, Scopolamine 0.01 mg	Atrohist Plus by Medeva	53014-0024	Cold Remedy
MEDEVA400	Cap, White & Yellow	Chlorpheniramine Maleate 4 mg, Pseudoephedrine HCl 60 mg	Atrohist by Adams	63824-0400	Cold Remedy
MEDEVA400	Cap, White & Yellow	Chlorpheniramine Maleate 4 mg, Pseudoephedrine HCl 60 mg	Atrohist Ped by Medeva	53014-0400	Cold Remedy
MEDEVA401	Cap, Blue & Clear, with White Beads	Phenylephrine HCl 10 mg, Guaifenesin 300 mg	Deconsal Ped by Medeva	53014-0401	Cold Remedy
MEDEVA402	Cap, Clear & Green, White Beads	Guaifenesin 300 mg	Robitussin by Medeva	53014-0402	Expectorant
MEDEVA402	Cap, Clear & Green	Guaifenesin 300 mg	Robitussin by Adams	63824-0402	Expectorant
MEDEVA575	Cap, Blue & White, Black & White Print, Ex Release	Methylphenidate HCl 20 mg	Metadate by Medeva	53014-0575	Stimulant; C II

ID FRONT <> BACK	DESCRIPTION FRONT <> BACK	INGREDIENT & STRENGTH	BRAND (or Generic Equiv.) by FIRM	NDC#	CLASS; SCH.
MEDEVASEMPREXD	Cap, Printed in White Ink <> Semprex-D	Acrivastine 8 mg, Pseudoephedrine HCl 60 mg	Semprex D by DSM	63552-0404	Cold Remedy
MEDEVASEMPREXD	Cap, Dark Green & White, Yellow Band	Acrivastine 8 mg, Pseudoephedrine HCl 60 mg	Semprex D by Medeva	53014-0404	Cold Remedy
MEDICIS049750MG	Cap, 0497 50MG	Minocycline 50 mg	Minocin by Thrift Drug	59198-0276	Antibiotic
MEDICIS049750MG	Cap	Minocycline HCl 50 mg	Minocin by Thrift Drug	59198-0276	Antibiotic
MEDICIS0498100MG	Cap	Minocycline HCl 100 mg	Minocin by Thrift Drug	59198-0277	Antibiotic
MEDICIS0498100MG	Cap, 0498 100MG	Minocycline HCl 100 mg	Minocin by Thrift Drug	59198-0277	Antibiotic
MEDICIS0498100MG	Cap, 0498 100 MG	Minocycline HCl 50 mg	Minocin by Medicis	99207-0498	Antibiotic
MEDICIS0498100MG	Cap	Minocycline HCl 50 mg	Minocin by Medicis	99207-0498	Antibiotic
MEDROL16	Tab, White, Half Oval, Scored, Medrol over 16	Methylprednisolone 16 mg	Medrol by Pfizer	Canadian DIN 00036129	Steroid
MEDROL16	Tab, White, Half Oval, Scored, Medrol over 16	Methylprednisolone 16 mg	Medrol by Pharmacia	00009-0073	Steroid
MEDROL2	Tab, Pink, Oval, Scored	Methylprednisolone 2 mg	Medrol by Pharmacia	00009-0049	Steroid
MEDROL24	Tab, Yellow, Half Oval, Scored	Methylprednisolone 24 mg	Medrol by Pharmacia	00009-0155 Discontinued	Steroid
MEDROL32	Tab, Peach, Half Oval, Scored	Methylprednisolone 32 mg	Medrol by Pharmacia	00009-0176	Steroid
MEDROL4	Tab, White, Oval, Scored, Medrol over 4	Methylprednisolone 4 mg	Medrol by Pharmacia	00009-0056	Steroid
MEDROL8	Tab, Peach, Half Oval, Scored	Methylprednisolone 8 mg	Medrol by Pharmacia	00009-0022	Steroid
MEDROL8	Tab, Peach, Half Oval, Scored	Methylprednisolone 8 mg	Medrol by Allscripts		Steroid
MEDTEK	Tab, MED/TEK	Meclizine HCl 30 mg	Medivert by Anabolic	00722-6312	Antiemetic
MEDTEK	Tab, MED/TEK	Hyoscyamine Sulfate 0.125 mg	Levsin by Anabolic	00722-6352	Gastrointestinal
MEDTEK	Tab, Med/Tek	Acetaminophen 500 mg, Chlorpheniramine Maleate 2 mg, Pseudoephedrine HCl 30 mg	Lorsin by Pharmafab	62542-0800	Cold Remedy
MEDTEK	Tab, Med/Tek	Acetaminophen 500 mg, Chlorpheniramine Maleate 2 mg, Pseudoephedrine HCl 30 mg	Sinumed by Anabolic	00722-6315	Cold Remedy
MEGACE <> 40	Tab, Light Blue, Round, Scored	Megestrol Acetate 40 mg	Megace by Mead Johnson	00015-0596	Hormone
MEGESTROL40 <> PCH	Tab, White, Scored, Megestrol over 40 <> PCH	Megestrol Acetate 40 mg	by Teva	00093-5138 Discontinued	Hormone
MEGESTROL40 <> PCH	Tab, White, Scored	Megestrol Acetate 40 mg	by Pharmachemie	57527-0513	Hormone
MEL15 <> APO	Tab, Yellow, Round	Meloxicam 15 mg	Mobic by Apotex	Canadian DIN 02248974	NSAID
MEL15 <> APO	Tab, Light Yellow, Round	Meloxicam 15 mg	Mobic by Apotex	60505-2554	NSAID
MEL75 <> APO	Tab, Light Yellow, Round, APO <> MEL 7.5	Meloxicam 7.5 mg	Mobic by Apotex	60505-2553	NSAID
MELLARIL100 <> S	Tab, Light Yellow, Black Print, Round, Film Coated, Mellaril over 100 <> S in Triangle	Thioridazine 100 mg	Mellaril by Novartis	00078-0005	Antipsychotic
MELLARIL150 <> S	Tab, Yellow, Black Print, Round, Film Coated, Mellaril over 150 <> S in Triangle	Thioridazine 150 mg	Mellaril by Novartis	00078-0006	Antipsychotic
MELLARIL200 <> S	Tab, Purple, Black Print, Round, Film Coated, Mellaril over 200 <> S in Triangle	Thioridazine 200 mg	Mellaril by Novartis	00078-0007	Antipsychotic
MELLARIL25 <> S	Tab, Brown, Black Print, Round, Film Coated, Mellaril over 25 <> S in Triangle	Thioridazine 25 mg	Mellaril by Novartis	00078-0003	Antipsychotic
MELLARIL50 <> S	Tab, White, Black Print, Round, Film Coated, Mellaril over 50 <> S in Triangle	Thioridazine 50 mg	Mellaril by Novartis	00078-0004	Antipsychotic
MEPHYTON <> MSD43	Tab, Yellow, Round, Scored	Vitamin K 5 mg	Mephyton by Merck	00006-0043	Vitamin
MEPHYTON <> MSD43	Tab, Yellow, Round, Scored	Vitamin K 5 mg	Mephyton by PDRX	55289-0793	Vitamin
MEPROSPAN200	Cap, Yellow	Meprobamate 200 mg	Meprospan by Wallace	00037-1401	Sedative/Hypnotic; C IV
MEPROSPAN400	Cap, Blue	Meprobamate 400 mg	Meprospan by Wallace	00037-1301	Sedative/Hypnotic; C IV
MERICON	Tab, Tan, Mericon Logo	Ginkgo Biloba 60 mg	Ginkgo by Mericon		Supplement
MERICON220	Cap, Pink	Zinc Sulfate 220 mg	Orazinc by Mericon		Mineral
MERICONLOGO	Tab, Brown	Zinc 10 mg	Orazinc by Mericon		Mineral
MERIDIA10	Cap, Blue & White, White Print, MERIDIA over 10	Sibutramine HCl 10 mg	by PDRX	55289-0375	Anorexiant; C IV

ID FRONT <> BACK	DESCRIPTION FRONT <> BACK	INGREDIENT & STRENGTH	BRAND (or Generic Equiv.) by FIRM	NDC#	CLASS; SCH.
MERIDIA10	Cap, Blue & White, White Print, MERIDIA over 10	Sibutramine HCl 10 mg	by DRX	55045-2555	Anorexiant; C IV
MERIDIA10	Cap, Blue & White, White Print, MERIDIA over 10	Sibutramine HCl 10 mg	by BASF	10117-0610	Anorexiant; C IV
MERIDIA10	Cap, Blue & White, White Print, MERIDIA over 10	Sibutramine HCl 10 mg	by Compumed	00403-5373	Anorexiant; C IV
MERIDIA10	Cap, Blue & White, White Print, MERIDIA over 10	Sibutramine 10 mg	Meridia by Abbott	00048-0610	Anorexiant; C IV
MERIDIA10	Cap, Blue & White, White Print, MERIDIA over 10	Sibutramine 10 mg	Meridia by Abbott	00074-2457	Anorexiant; C IV
MERIDIA10	Cap, Blue & White, White Print, MERIDIA over 10	Sibutramine HCl 10 mg	Meridia by Abbott	Canadian DIN 02243163	Anorexiant; C IV
MERIDIA15	Cap, Yellow & White, Gray Print, MERIDIA over 15	Sibutramine HCl 15 mg	by PDRX	55289-0380	Anorexiant; C IV
MERIDIA15	Cap, Yellow & White, Gray Print, MERIDIA over 15	Sibutramine 15 mg	Meridia by BASF	10117-0615	Anorexiant; C IV
MERIDIA15	Cap, Yellow & White, Gray Print, MERIDIA over 15	Sibutramine HCl 15 mg	by Compumed	00403-5375	Anorexiant; C IV
MERIDIA15	Cap, Yellow & White, Gray Print, MERIDIA over 15	Sibutramine 15 mg	Meridia by Abbott	00074-2458	Anorexiant; C IV
MERIDIA15	Cap, Yellow & White, Gray Print, MERIDIA over 15	Sibutramine 15 mg	Meridia by Abbott	00048-0615	Anorexiant; C IV
MERIDIA15	Cap, Yellow & White, Gray Print, MERIDIA over 15	Sibutramine HCl 15 mg	Meridia by Abbott	Canadian DIN 02243164	Anorexiant; C IV
MERIDIA5	Cap, Blue & Yellow, Red Print, MERIDIA over 5	Sibutramine HCl 5 mg	by PDRX	55289-0377	Anorexiant; C IV
MERIDIA5	Cap, Blue & Yellow, Red Print, MERIDIA over 5	Sibutramine HCl 5 mg	by Compumed	00403-5371	Anorexiant; C IV
MERIDIA5	Cap, Blue & Yellow, Red Print, MERIDIA over 5	Sibutramine HCl 5 mg	by BASF	10117-0605	Anorexiant; C IV
MERIDIA5	Cap, Blue & Yellow, Red Print, MERIDIA over 5	Sibutramine 5 mg	Meridia by Abbott	00048-0605	Anorexiant; C IV
MERIDIA5	Cap, Blue & Yellow, Red Print, MERIDIA over 5	Sibutramine 5 mg	Meridia by Abbott	00074-2456	Anorexiant; C IV
MERRELL277	Tab, Light Yellow, Oblong, Scored, Merrell over 277	Methenamine Hippurate 1 g	Hiprex by Merrell	00068-0277	Antibiotic; Urinary Tract
MERRELL37	Tab, Yellow, Round	Metenzolate Bromide 25 mg	Cantil by Merrell	00068-0037	Antispasmodic
MERRELL547 <> W	Tab, White, Round, Merrell over 547	Quinine Sulfate 260 mg	Quinamm by Merrell	00068-0547	Antimalarial
MERRELL62	Tab, Pink, Round	Trichlormethiazide 2 mg	Metahydrin by Aventis		Diuretic; Antihypertensive
MERRELL63	Tab, Blue, Round	Trichlormethiazide 4 mg	Metahydrin by Aventis		Diuretic; Antihypertensive
MERRELL64	Tab, Yellow, Round	Trichlormethiazide 2 mg, Reserpine 0.1 mg	Metatensin #2 by Aventis		Diuretic; Antihypertensive
MERRELL65	Tab, Blue & Yellow, Red Print, MERIDIA over 5	Trichlormethiazide 4 mg, Reserpine 0.1 mg	Metatensin #4 by Aventis		Diuretic; Antihypertensive
MERRELL69	Cap, Clear & Green	Chlorotrianisene 12 mg	TACE by RP Scherer	11014-0152	Hormone
MERRELL690	Cap, Clear & Forest Green, Gelatin	Chlorotrianisene 12 mg	TACE by RP Scherer	11014-1224	Hormone
MERRELL691	Cap, Green	Chlorotrianisene 25 mg	TACE by Merrell		Hormone
MERRELL692	Cap, Green & Yellow	Chlorotrianisene 72 mg	TACE by Merrell		Hormone
MERRELL697	Tab, White, Round	Diethylpropion HCl 25 mg	Tenuate by Merrell	00068-0697	Anorexiant; C IV
MERRELL698	Tab, White, Cap Shaped	Diethylpropion HCl 75 mg	Tenuate by Merrell	00068-0698	Anorexiant; C IV
MERRELL725	Tab, White, Round	Terbutaline Sulfate 2.5 mg	Bricanyl by Merrell		Antiasthmatic
MESLON10	Cap, White, M-Eslon 10	Morphine Sulfate 10 mg	MS Contin by RPR	Canadian	Analgesic; C II
MESLON100	Cap, White, M-Eslon 100	Morphine Sulfate 100 mg	MS Contin by RPR	Canadian	Analgesic; C II
MESLON30	Cap, White, M-Eslon 30	Morphine Sulfate 30 mg	MS Contin by RPR	Canadian	Analgesic; C II
MESLON60	Cap, White, M-Eslon 60	Morphine Sulfate 60 mg	MS Contin by RPR	Canadian	Analgesic; C II
MESTINON60ICN	Tab, White, Mestinon 60-ICN	Pyridostigmine Bromide 60 mg	Mestinon by ICN	Canadian DIN 00869961	Muscle Stimulant
MET <> APO500	Tab, White to Off-White, Oblong	Metformin HCl 500 mg	Glucophage by Apotex	60505-0190	Antidiabetic
MET10832	Tab, White, Round, MET-10/832	Metoclopramide HCl 10 mg	Reglan by Rosemont		Gastrointestinal
MET500 <> P	Tab, White, Round, Scored, Film Coated	Metformin HCl 500 mg	Glucophage by Pharmascience	Canadian DIN 02223562	Antidiabetic
METAC	Cap, Brown Stripe	Psyllium 2.1 g, Calcium Carbonate 300 mg	Metamucil Plus Calcium by P & G Health	37000-4650	Supplement
METHADOSE10	Tab, White, Round, Scored	Methadone HCl 10 mg	Methadose by Mallinckrodt	00406-3454	Analgesic; C II
METHADOSE40	Tab, White, Round, Scored	Methadone HCl 40 mg	Methadose by Mallinckrodt	00406-0540	Analgesic; C II
METHADOSE5	Tab, White, Round, Scored	Methadone HCl 5 mg	Methadose by Mallinckrodt	00406-6974	Analgesic; C II

ID FRONT <> BACK	DESCRIPTION FRONT <> BACK	INGREDIENT & STRENGTH	BRAND (or Generic Equiv.) by FIRM	NDC#	CLASS; SCH.
METOPL <> PMS100	Tab, Pale Blue, Cap Shaped, Scored, Film Coated	Metoprolol Succinate 100 mg	Toprol XL by Pharmascience	Canadian DIN 02230804	Antihypertensive
METOPL <> PMS50	Tab, Pink, Oblong, Scored	Metoprolol Tartrate 50 mg	Lopressor by Pharmascience	Canadian DIN 02230803	Antihypertensive
MEVACOR <> MSD730	Tab, Peach, Octagonal, MSD over 730	Lovastatin 10 mg	Mevacor by Nat Pharmpak	55154-3618	Antihyperlipidemic
MEVACOR <> MSD730	Tab, Peach, Octagonal, MSD over 730	Lovastatin 10 mg	Mevacor by Kaiser	00179-1209	Antihyperlipidemic
MEVACOR <> MSD730	Tab, Peach, Octagonal, MSD over 730	Lovastatin 10 mg	Mevacor by Merck	00006-0730	Antihyperlipidemic
MEVACOR <> MSD731	Tab, Blue, Octagonal, MSD over 731	Lovastatin 20 mg	Mevacor by Allscripts		Antihyperlipidemic
MEVACOR <> MSD731	Tab, Blue, Octagonal, MSD over 731	Lovastatin 20 mg	Mevacor by Pharmedix	53002-0570	Antihyperlipidemic
MEVACOR <> MSD731	Tab, Blue, Octagonal, MSD over 731	Lovastatin 20 mg	Mevacor by Nat Pharmpak	55154-5004	Antihyperlipidemic
MEVACOR <> MSD731	Tab, Blue, Octagonal, MSD over 731	Lovastatin 20 mg	Mevacor by Va Cmop	65243-0045	Antihyperlipidemic
MEVACOR <> MSD731	Tab, Blue, Octagonal, MSD over 731	Lovastatin 20 mg	Mevacor by Amerisource	62584-0426	Antihyperlipidemic
MEVACOR <> MSD731	Tab, Blue, Octagonal, MSD over 731	Lovastatin 20 mg	Mevacor by Merck	00006-0731	Antihyperlipidemic
MEVACOR <> MSD731	Tab, Blue, Octagonal, MSD over 731	Lovastatin 20 mg	Mevacor by Merck Frosst	Canadian DIN 00795860	Antihyperlipidemic
MEVACOR <> MSD732	Tab, Light Green, Octagonal, MSD over 732	Lovastatin 40 mg	Mevacor by Merck Frosst	Canadian DIN 00795852	Antihyperlipidemic
MEVACOR <> MSD732	Tab, Light Green, Octagonal, MSD over 732	Lovastatin 40 mg	Mevacor by PDRX	55289-0548	Antihyperlipidemic
MEVACOR <> MSD732	Tab, Light Green, Octagonal, MSD over 732	Lovastatin 40 mg	Mevacor by Merck	00006-0732	Antihyperlipidemic
MEVACOR <> MSD732	Tab, Light Green, Octagonal, MSD over 732	Lovastatin 40 mg	Mevacor by Allscripts		Antihyperlipidemic
MF	Tab, Light Yellow, Round	Mifepristone 200 mg	Mifeprex by Danco	64875-0001	Antiprogestational
MF1	Tab, Yellow, Round, Film Coated, M over F1	Famotidine 20 mg	Pepcid by UDL	51079-0966	Gastrointestinal
MF1	Tab, Yellow, Round, Film Coated, M over F1	Famotidine 20 mg	Pepcid by Mylan	00378-3020	Gastrointestinal
MF1 <> G	Tab, White to Off-White, Round, Film Coated	Metformin HCl 500 mg	Gen-Metformin by Genpharm	Canadian DIN 0214876	Antidiabetic
MF1 <> G	Tab, White to Off-White, Round, Film Coated	Metformin HCl 500 mg	Glucophage by Par	49884-0739	Antidiabetic
MF2	Tab, Green, Round, Film Coated, M over F2	Famotidine 40 mg	Pepcid by Mylan	00378-3040	Gastrointestinal
MF2 <> G	Tab, White, Round, Film Coated, MF over 2	Metformin HCl 850 mg	Glucophage by Par	49884-0740	Antidiabetic
MF2 <> G	Tab, White, Round, Film Coated, MF over 2	Metformin HCl 850 mg	Gen-Metformin by Genpharm	Canadian DIN 02229656	Antidiabetic
MF3 <> G	Tab, White, Oblong, Scored, Film Coated, MF, Score, 3	Metformin HCl 1000 mg	Glucophage by Par	49884-0738	Antidiabetic
MF3 <> G	Tab, White, Oblong, Scored, Film Coated, MF, Score, 3	Metformin HCl 1000 mg	Glucophage by Par	49884-0741	Antidiabetic
MF3 <> GG	Tab, White, Oblong	Metformin HCl 1000 mg	Glucophage by BMS		Antidiabetic
MF4	Tab, Yellow, Round, M over F4	Fluconazole 100 mg	Diflucan by Mylan	00378-2516	Antifungal
MF5	Tab, Yellow, Round, M over F5	Fluconazole 150 mg	Diflucan by Mylan	00378-2518	Antifungal
MF6	Tab, Yellow, Round, M over F6	Fluconazole 200 mg	Diflucan by Mylan	00378-2520	Antifungal
MF6	Tab, Yellow, Round, M over F6	Fluconazole 200 mg	Diflucan by UDL	51079-0773	Antifungal
MFG	Tab, White, MF/G	Metformin HCl 500 mg	Glucophage by BDH	Canadian	Antidiabetic
MG	Cap, Light Blue Opaque with Black Band, Hard Gelatin	Mesalamine .375 mg	Apriso by Salix	65649-0103	Locally-Acting Aminosalicylate
MG	Cap, Light Blue Opaque with Black Band, Hard Gelatin	Mesalamine .375	Apriso by Salix	65649-0103	Locally-Acting Aminosalicylate
MGH	Cap, Lavender, White Print	Acetaminophen 500 mg, Hydrocodone Bitartrate 5 mg	Vicodin by A G Marin	12539-0984	Analgesic; C III
MGI <> 705	Tab, White, Black Print, Round, Film Coated	Pilocarpine HCl 5 mg	Salagen by MGI	58063-0705	Cholinergic Agonist
MGI532	Cap, Red and Beige, Hard Gel	Acetaminophen 500 mg, Oxycodone HCl 5 mg	Percocet by Mallinckrodt	00406-2535	Analgesic; C II
MH <> 123	Tab, Beige, Round, Film Coated	Ergotamine Tartrate 1 mg, Caffeine 100 mg	Cafergot by Mikart	46672-0198	Antimigraine
MH1 <> M	Tab, White, Round, Scored, MH over 1	Midodrine HCl 2.5 mg	ProAmatine by Mylan	00378-1901	Antihypotensive
MH2 <> M	Tab, White, Round, Scored, MH over 2	Midodrine HCl 5 mg	ProAmatine by Mylan	00378-1902	Antihypotensive
MH2 <> M	Tab, White, Round, Scored, MH over 2	Midodrine HCl 5 mg	ProAmatine by UDL	51079-0453	Antihypotensive
MH3 <> M	Tab, White, Round, Scored, MH over 3	Midodrine HCl 10 mg	ProAmatine by Mylan	00378-1903	Antihypotensive

For updated data, go to www.IdentADrug.com

ID FRONT <> BACK	DESCRIPTION FRONT <> BACK	INGREDIENT & STRENGTH	BRAND (or Generic Equiv.) by FIRM	NDC#	CLASS; SCH.
MI15 <> APO	Tab, Light Yellow, Oval, Film Coated, Scored	Mirtazapine 15 mg	Remeron by Apotex	Canadian DIN 02286610	Antidepressant
MI15 <> PF	Tab, White, Round, Scored	Morphine Sulfate 15 mg	MSIR by Purdue	00034-0518	Analgesic; C II
MI30 <> APO	Tab, Pink, Oval, Film Coated, Scored	Mirtazapine 30 mg	Remeron by Apotex	Canadian DIN 02286629	Antidepressant
MI30 <> PF	Tab, White, Cap Shaped, Scored	Morphine Sulfate 30 mg	MSIR by Purdue	00034-0519	Analgesic; C II
MI45 <> APO	Tab, White, Oval, Film Coated, Scored	Mirtazapine 45 mg	Remeron by Apotex	Canadian DIN 02286637	Antidepressant
MIA <> 093	Tab	Chlorpheniramine Tannate 8 mg, Phenylephrine Tannate 25 mg, Pyrilamine Tannate 25 mg	Histatan by Ivax	00172-4376	Cold Remedy
MIA <> 093	Tab	Chlorpheniramine Tannate 8 mg, Phenylephrine Tannate 25 mg, Pyrilamine Tannate 25 mg	by Ivax	00182-1912	Cold Remedy
MIA <> 093	Tab	Chlorpheniramine 8 mg, Phenylephrine 25 mg, Pyrilamine 25 mg	Rhinatate by Major	00904-1669	Cold Remedy
MIA <> 116	Tab, Orange, Cap Shaped, Scored	Acetaminophen 325 mg, Hydrocodone 7.5 mg	Vicodin by Mikart	46672-0147	Analgesic; C III
MIA093	Tab, Beige, Cap Shaped, MIA/093	Phenylephrine HCl 25 mg, Chlorpheniramine Tannate 8 mg, Pyrilamine Tannate 25 mg	Tanamine by Mikart	46672-0093	Cold Remedy
MIA102	Tab, White, Cap Shaped, Scored	Acetaminophen 650 mg, Codeine Phosphate 30 mg	Tylenol w/ Codeine by Mikart	46672-0054	Analgesic; C III
MIA106	Tab, White, Cap Shaped, Scored	Acetaminophen 325 mg, Butalbital 50 mg	Phrenilin by Qualitest	00603-2540	Analgesic
MIA106	Tab, White, Cap Shaped, Scored	Acetaminophen 325 mg, Butalbital 50 mg	Promacet by Marnel	00682-1400	Analgesic
MIA106	Tab, White, Cap Shaped, Scored	Acetaminophen 325 mg, Butalbital 50 mg	Butapap by Mikart	46672-0099	Analgesic
MIA108	Tab, White, Cap Shaped, Scored	Acetaminophen 500 mg, Hydrocodone Bitartrate 5 mg	Vicodin by Mikart	46672-0052	Analgesic; C III
MIA108	Tab, White, Cap Shaped, Scored	Acetaminophen 500 mg, Hydrocodone Bitartrate 5 mg	Vicodin by Inwood	00258-3666	Analgesic; C III
MIA110	Tab, White, Cap Shaped, Scored	Acetaminophen 325 mg, Butalbital 50 mg, Caffeine 40 mg	Fioricet by Qualitest	00603-2547	Analgesic
MIA110	Tab, White, Cap Shaped, Scored	Acetaminophen 325 mg, Butalbital 50 mg, Caffeine 40 mg	Fioricet by Sandoz	00781-1901	Analgesic
MIA110	Tab, White, Cap Shaped, Scored	Acetaminophen 325 mg, Butalbital 50 mg, Caffeine 40 mg	Fioricet by Ivax	00182-1274	Analgesic
MIA110	Tab, White, Cap Shaped, Scored	Acetaminophen 325 mg, Butalbital 50 mg, Caffeine 40 mg	Fioricet by Diversified Healthcare	55887-0988	Analgesic
MIA110	Tab, White, Cap Shaped, Scored	Acetaminophen 325 mg, Butalbital 50 mg, Caffeine 40 mg	Fioricet by Mikart	46672-0053	Analgesic
MIA110	Tab, White, Cap Shaped, Scored	Acetaminophen 325 mg, Butalbital 50 mg, Caffeine 40 mg	Fioricet by Physician Total Care	54868-1075	Analgesic
MIA111	Tab, White, Round	Yohimbine HCl 5.4 mg	Yocon by Mikart		Impotence Agent
MIA112	Tab, Blue, Cap Shaped, MIA/112	Acetaminophen 650 mg, Butalbital 50 mg	Promacet by Mikart	46672-0098	Analgesic
MIA112	Tab, Blue, Cap Shaped, MIA/112	Acetaminophen 650 mg, Butalbital 50 mg	Promacet by Andrx	62022-0073	Analgesic
MIA113	Tab, Blue, Cap Shaped, Scored	Hydrocodone Bitartrate 5 mg, Acetaminophen 500 mg	Vicodin by Mikart	46672-0070	Analgesic; C III
MIA253	Cap, White Print	Acetaminophen 325 mg, Dichloralantipyrine 100 mg, Isometheptene Mucate (1:1) 65 mg	Migratine by Major		Analgesic; C IV
MIA253	Cap, Red & White	Acetaminophen 325 mg, Dichloralantipyrine 100 mg, Isometheptene Mucate (1:1) 65 mg	Migquin by Qualitest	00603-4664	Analgesic; C IV
MIA253	Cap, White Print	Acetaminophen 325 mg, Dichloralantipyrine 100 mg, Isometheptene Mucate (2:1) 65 mg	Midrin by Carnrick	00086-0120	Analgesic; C IV
MICROK10AHR5730	Cap, Orange & White, Black Print, Ex Release, Micro-K over 10 on orange half, AHR over 5730 on white half	Potassium Chloride 750 mg	Micro K 10 by Amerisource	62584-0730	Electrolytes
MICROK10AHR5730	Cap, Orange & White, Black Print, Ex Release, Micro-K over 10 on orange half, AHR over 5730 on white half	Potassium Chloride 750 mg	Micro K 10 by Leiner	59606-0772	Electrolytes
MICROK10AHR5730	Cap, Orange & White, Black Print, Ex Release, Micro-K over 10 on orange half, AHR over 5730 on white half	Potassium Chloride 750 mg	Micro K 10 by Thrift Drug	59198-0229	Electrolytes
MICROK10AHR5730	Cap, Orange & White, Black Print, Ex Release, Micro-K over 10 on orange half, AHR over 5730 on white half	Potassium Chloride 750 mg	Micro K 10 by PDRX	55289-0899	Electrolytes
MICROK10AHR5730	Cap, Orange & White, Black Print, Ex Release, Micro-K over 10 on orange half, AHR over 5730 on white half	Potassium Chloride 750 mg	Micro K 10 by Nat Pharmpak	55154-3009	Electrolytes
MICROK10AHR5730	Cap, Orange & White, Black Print, Ex Release, Micro-K over 10 on orange half, AHR over 5730 on white half	Potassium Chloride 750 mg	Micro K 10 by Nat Pharmpak	55154-3012	Electrolytes

ID FRONT <> BACK	DESCRIPTION FRONT <> BACK	INGREDIENT & STRENGTH	BRAND (or Generic Equiv.) by FIRM	NDC#	CLASS; SCH.
MICROK10AHR5730	Cap, Orange & White, Black Print, Ex Release, Micro-K over 10 on orange half, AHR over 5730 on white half	Potassium Chloride 750 mg	Micro K 10 by Rx Pak	65084-0193	Electrolytes
MICROK10AHR5730	Cap, Orange & White, Black Print, Ex Release, Micro-K over 10 on orange half, AHR over 5730 on white half	Potassium Chloride 750 mg	Micro K 10 by A H Robins	00031-5730	Electrolytes
MICROK10AHR5730	Cap, Orange & White, Black Print, Ex Release, Micro-K over 10 on orange half, AHR over 5730 on white half	Potassium Chloride 750 mg	Micro K 10 by Med Pro	53978-5044	Electrolytes
MICROK10AHR5730	Cap, Orange & White, Black Print, Ex Release, Micro-K over 10 on orange half, AHR over 5730 on white half	Potassium Chloride 750 mg	Micro K 10 by Wal Mart	49035-0153	Electrolytes
MICROK10THERRX009	Cap, Orange & White, Black Print, Opaque, Gelatin, Micro-K 10 Ther-Rx 009	Potassium Chloride 750 mg	Micro K 10 by Ther Rx	64011-0009	Electrolytes
MICROKAHR5720	Cap, Pale Orange, Ex Release	Potassium Chloride 600 mg	Micro K by Caremark	00339-5239	Electrolytes
MICROKAHR5720	Cap, Pale Orange, Ex Release	Potassium Chloride 600 mg	Micro K by Nat Pharmpak	55154-3010	Electrolytes
MICROKAHR5720	Cap, Pale Orange, Ex Release	Potassium Chloride 600 mg	Micro K by Amerisource	62584-0720	Electrolytes
MICROKAHR5720	Cap, Pale Orange, Ex Release	Potassium Chloride 600 mg	Micro K by Promeco SA	64674-0019	Electrolytes
MICROKAHR5720	Cap, Pale Orange, Ex Release	Potassium Chloride 600 mg	Micro K by Leiner	59606-0691	Electrolytes
MICROKAHR5720	Cap, Pale Orange, Ex Release	Potassium Chloride 600 mg	Micro K by Med Pro	53978-0155	Electrolytes
MICROKAHR5720	Cap, Pale Orange, Ex Release	Potassium Chloride 600 mg	Micro K by Thrift Drug	59198-0310	Electrolytes
MICROKAYERST	Cap, Orange, Hard Gelatin	Potassium Chloride 600 mg	Micro-K Extencaps by Wyeth Canada	Canadian DIN 02042304	Electrolytes
MICROKTHERRX010	Cap, Orange, Black Print, Micro-K Ther-Rx 010	Potassium Chloride 600 mg	Micro K by KV Pharma	64011-0010	Electrolytes
MICRONASE125	Tab, White, Oval, Scored, 1.25	Glyburide 1.25 mg	Micronase by Pharmacia	00009-0131	Antidiabetic
MICRONASE25	Tab, Peach, Round, Scored, Micronase over 2.5	Glyburide 2.5 mg	Micronase by Nat Pharmpak	55154-3916	Antidiabetic
MICRONASE25	Tab, Peach, Round, Scored, Micronase over 2.5	Glyburide 2.5 mg	Micronase by Med Pro	53978-0693	Antidiabetic
MICRONASE25	Tab, Peach, Round, Scored, Micronase over 2.5	Glyburide 2.5 mg	Micronase by Pharmacia	00009-0141	Antidiabetic
MICRONASE5	Tab, Light Blue, Round, Scored	Glyburide 5 mg	Micronase by Kiel	59063-0113	Antidiabetic
MICRONASE5	Tab, Light Blue, Round, Scored	Glyburide 5 mg	Micronase by Rightpak	65240-0690	Antidiabetic
MICRONASE5	Tab, Light Blue, Round, Scored	Glyburide 5 mg	Micronase by Nat Pharmpak	55154-3905	Antidiabetic
MICRONASE5	Tab, Light Blue, Round, Scored	Glyburide 5 mg	Micronase by Med Pro	53978-3000	Antidiabetic
MICRONASE5	Tab, Light Blue, Round, Scored	Glyburide 5 mg	Micronase by H J Harkins Co	52959-0177	Antidiabetic
MICRONASE5	Tab, Light Blue, Round, Scored	Glyburide 5 mg	Micronase by Pharmacia	00009-0171	Antidiabetic
MICRONASE5	Tab, Light Blue, Round, Scored	Glyburide 5 mg	Micronase by Amerisource	62584-0171	Antidiabetic
MICRONASE5	Tab, Light Blue, Round, Scored	Glyburide 5 mg	Micronase by Thrift Drug	59198-0335	Antidiabetic
MICRONASE5	Tab, Light Blue, Round, Scored	Glyburide 5 mg	Micronase by Pharmedix	53002-0417	Antidiabetic
MICROZIDE125	Cap, Teal w/ Black Print	Hydrochlorothiazide 12.5 mg	by Caremark	00339-6188	Diuretic; Antihypertensive
MICROZIDE125MG	Cap, Teal, Opaque, Microzide 12.5 mg	Microzide 12.5 mg	Microzide by Watson	52544-0622	Diuretic
MID10 <> APO	Tab, Light Blue, Round, Scored	Midodrine HCl 10 mg	Proamatine by Apotex	60505-1325	Antihypotensive
MID25 <> APO	Tab, White, Round, Scored	Midodrine HCl 2.5 mg	Amatine by Apotex	Canadian DIN 02278677	Antihypotensive
MID5 <> APO	Tab, Orange, Round, Scored	Midodrine HCl 5 mg	Amatine by Apotex	Canadian DIN 02278685	Antihypotensive
MIDAMOR <> MSD92	Tab, Yellow, Diamond Shaped	Amiloride HCl 5 mg	Midamor by Merck	00006-0092	Diuretic
MIDOL	Tab, White, Cap Shaped, Orange Ink	Acetaminophen 500 mg, Pamabrom 25 mg, Pyrilamine 15 mg	Midol PMS Ex. Strength by Bayer	Canadian DIN 02150506	PMS Relief
MIDOL	Tab, White, Cap Shaped, Film Coated, Blue Ink	Acetaminophen 500 mg, Caffeine 60 mg, Pyrilamine Maleate 15 mg	Midol Ex. Strength by Bayer	Canadian DIN 02236972	PMS Relief
MIDOL	Tab, White, Cap Shaped	Acetaminophen 325 mg, Caffeine 60 mg, Pyrilamine Maleate 15 mg	Midol Teen Complete by Bayer	Canadian DIN 02273454	PMS Relief
MIDOL	Cap, White	Aspirin 500 mg, Caffeine 32 mg	Midol by Bayer	Canadian	Analgesic
MIDOLMIDOL	Cap, White, Midol/Midol	Aspirin 500 mg, Cinnamedrine 5.5 mg, Caffeine 32.4 mg	Midol by Bayer	Canadian	PMS Relief
MIDRIN	Cap, Red, Pink Print	Acetaminophen 325 mg, Dichloralphenazone 100 mg, Isometheptene Mucate 65 mg	Midrin by Women First HealthCare	64248-0120	Analgesic; C IV

ID FRONT <> BACK	DESCRIPTION FRONT <> BACK	INGREDIENT & STRENGTH	BRAND (or Generic Equiv.) by FIRM	NDC#	CLASS; SCH.
MIGRALAM	Cap	Acetaminophen 325 mg, Caffeine 100 mg, Isometheptene Mucate (1:1) 65 mg	Migralam by Sovereign	58716-0039	Analgesic; C IV
MILES <> 512	Tab, Film Coated	Ciprofloxacin HCl 250 mg	Cipro by Quality Care	60346-0433	Antibiotic
MILES <> 513	Tab, Film Coated	Ciprofloxacin HCl 500 mg	Cipro by Nat Pharmpak	55154-4801	Antibiotic
MILES093	Tab, White, Bullet Shaped	Clotrimazole 100 mg	Mycelex G Vaginal by Miles		Antifungal
MILES095	Tab, White, Round, Miles over 095	Clotrimazole 10 mg	by Med Pro	53978-3040	Antifungal
MILES095	Tab, White, Round, Miles over 095	Clotrimazole 10 mg	by Bayer	00026-3095	Antifungal
MILES097	Tab, White, Bullet Shaped	Clotrimazole 500 mg	Mycelex G Vaginal by Miles		Antifungal
MILES121	Tab, White, Round	Dehydrocholic Acid 250 mg	Decholin by Miles		Gastrointestinal
MILES132	Tab, White, Round, Gray Specks	Diethylstilbestrol Diphosphate 50 mg	Stilphostrol by Miles		Hormone
MILES20	Tab, Grayish Pink, Round	Nifedipine 20 mg	Adalat PA by Miles		Antihypertensive
MILES30 <> 884	Tab, Pink	Nifedipine 30 mg	Adalat CC by Direct Dispensing	57866-6719	Antihypertensive
MILES30 <> 884	Tab, Film Coated	Nifedipine 30 mg	by Caremark	00339-5976	Antihypertensive
MILES411	Tab, White, Round	Aluminum Sulfate, Calcium Acetate	Domeboro by Miles		Gastrointestinal
MILES514	Tab, Yellow, Oblong, Film Coated	Ciprofloxacin HCl 750 mg	Cipro by Miles		Antibiotic
MILES521	Tab, White, Oblong	Praziquantel 600 mg	Biltricide by Miles		Antihelmintic
MILES60 <> 885	Tab, Film Coated	Nifedipine 60 mg	Adalat CC by Pharm Util	60491-0010	Antihypertensive
MILES721	Tab, Yellow, Round, Chewable	Niclosamide 500 mg	Niclocide by Miles		Antihelmintic
MILES855	Cap	Nimodipine 30 mg	by Med Pro	53978-2054	Antihypertensive
MILES855	Cap, Ivory	Nimodipine 30 mg	Nimotop by Miles		Antihypertensive
MILES90886	Tab, Brown, Round, Ex Release	Nifedipine 90 mg	Adalat CC by Miles		Antihypertensive
MILES951	Tab, Green, Round	Lithium Carbonate 300 mg	Eskalith by Miles		Antipsychotic
MILESDT	Tab, Grayish Pink, Round	Nifedipine 10 mg	Adalat FT by Miles		Antihypertensive
MINI <> HR225	Tab, White, Round, HR 225/Mini	Ephedrine HCl 25 mg, Guaifenesin 200 mg	Mini Two-Way Action by BDI		Cold Remedy
MINIHR60	Tab, White, Round, Mini/HR60	Pseudoephedrine 60 mg	Mini Pseudo by BDI		Decongestant
MINIPRESSPFIZER431	Cap, White	Prazosin HCl 1 mg	Minipress by Pfizer	00069-4310	Antihypertensive
MINIPRESSPFIZER437	Cap, White & Pink	Prazosin HCl 2 mg	Minipress by Pfizer	00069-4370	Antihypertensive
MINIPRESSPFIZER438	Cap, Blue & White	Prazosin HCl 5 mg	Minipress by Pfizer	00069-4380	Antihypertensive
MINISLIM	Cap, Clear & Red, Red & White Beads	Phenylpropanolamine 75 mg	Mini Slims by BDI		Decongestant; Appetite Suppressant
MINITHIN	Cap, Red Brown	Ephedrine group alkaloids 25 mg, Kola Nut Extract 100 mg	Mini Thin 25/50 by BDI		Dietary Supplement
MINIZIDEPFIZER430	Cap, Blue-Green	Prazosin HCl 1 mg, Polythiazide 0.5 mg	Minizide by Pfizer	00069-4300	Antihypertensive; Diuretic
MINIZIDEPFIZER432	Cap, Blue-Green & Pink	Prazosin HCl 2 mg, Polythiazide 0.5 mg	Minizide by Pfizer	00069-4320	Antihypertensive; Diuretic
MINIZIDEPFIZER436	Cap, Blue-Green & Blue	Prazosin HCl 5 mg, Polythiazide 0.5 mg	Minizide by Pfizer	00069-4360	Antihypertensive
MINOCYCLINE-100DAN5695	Cap, Dark Grey & Yellow, Black Print, Minocycline over 100 over DAN over 5695	Minocycline HCl 100 mg	Minocin by Watson	00591-5695	Antibiotic
MINOCYCLINE-100DAN5695	Cap, Dark Grey & Yellow, Black Print, Minocycline over 100 over DAN over 5695	Minocycline HCl 100 mg	Minocin by Schein	00364-2498	Antibiotic
MINOCYCLINE-100DAN5695	Cap, Dark Grey & Yellow, Black Print, Minocycline over 100 over DAN over 5695	Minocycline HCl 100 mg	Minocin by Danbury	61955-2498	Antibiotic
MINOCYCLINE-50DAN5694	Cap, Light Yellow, Black Print, Minocycline over 50 over DAN over 5694	Minocycline HCl 50 mg	Minocin by Watson	00591-5694	Antibiotic
MINOCYCLINE-50DAN5694	Cap, Light Yellow, Black Print, Minocycline over 50 over DAN over 5694	Minocycline HCl 50 mg	Minocin by Schein	00364-2497	Antibiotic
MINOCYCLINE-50DAN5694	Cap, Light Yellow, Black Print, Minocycline over 50 over DAN over 5694	Minocycline HCl 50 mg	Minocin by Danbury	61955-2497	Antibiotic

ID FRONT <> BACK	DESCRIPTION FRONT <> BACK	INGREDIENT & STRENGTH	BRAND (or Generic Equiv.) by FIRM	NDC#	CLASS; SCH.
MINOXIDIL10 <> PAR257	Tab, White, Round, Scored, Minoxidil over 10 <> par over 257	Minoxidil 10 mg	Loniten by Physician Total Care	54868-3467	Antihypertensive
MINOXIDIL10 <> PAR257	Tab, White, Round, Scored, Minoxidil over 10 <> par over 257	Minoxidil 10 mg	Loniten by Par	49884-0257	Antihypertensive
MINOXIDIL10 <> PAR257	Tab, White, Round, Scored, Minoxidil over 10 <> par over 257	Minoxidil 10 mg	Loniten by URL Mutual	00677-1162	Antihypertensive
MINOXIDIL10 <> PAR257	Tab, White, Round, Scored, Minoxidil over 10 <> par over 257	Minoxidil 10 mg	Loniten by Qualitest	00603-4688	Antihypertensive
MINOXIDIL10 <> PAR257	Tab, White, Round, Scored, Minoxidil over 10 <> par over 257	Minoxidil 10 mg	Loniten by Moore	00839-7342	Antihypertensive
MINOXIDIL212 <> PAR256	Tab, White, Round, Scored, Minoxidil over 2 1/2 <> par over 256	Minoxidil 2.5 mg	Loniten by Par	49884-0256	Antihypertensive
MINOXIDIL212 <> PAR256	Tab, White, Round, Scored, Minoxidil over 2 1/2 <> par over 256	Minoxidil 2.5 mg	Loniten by Qualitest	00603-4687	Antihypertensive
MINOXIDIL212 <> PAR256	Tab, White, Round, Scored, Minoxidil over 2 1/2 <> par over 256	Minoxidil 2.5 mg	Loniten by Ivax	00182-1602	Antihypertensive
MINTEZOL <> MSD907	Tab, White, Round, Chewable	Thiabendazole 500 mg	Mintezol by Merck	00006-0907	Anthelmintic
MISO100 <> APO	Tab, White, Round	Misoprostol 100 mcg	Cytotec by Apotex	Canadian DIN 02244022	Gastrointestinal
MISO200 <> APO	Tab, White, Hexagonal	Misoprostol 200 mcg	Cytotec by Apotex	Canadian DIN 02244023	Gastrointestinal
MISSION <> MPC610	Tab, Light Yellow, Oval	Potassium Citrate 1080 mg	Urocit K by Mission	00178-0610	Electrolytes
MITSUBISHI	Tab, White, Round, Mitsubishi Logo	3,4-Methylenedioxymethamphetamine (MDMA)	Ecstasy by Illegal		Euphoric; Illicit
MJ	Tab, White, Rectangle, Scored	Buspirone HCl 5 mg	Buspar by Thrift Drug	59198-0369	Antianxiety
MJ	Tab, White, Rectangle, Scored	Buspirone HCl 10 mg	Buspar by Caremark	00339-4106	Antianxiety
MJ	Tab, White, Square, Scored	Buspirone HCl 10 mg	Buspar by Va Cmop	65243-0016	Antianxiety
MJ	Tab, White, Rectangle, Scored, Logo	Buspirone HCl 10 mg	Buspar by Thrift Drug	59198-0370	Antianxiety
MJ <> 468	Tab, Chewable	Ascorbic Acid 60 mg, Cholecalciferol 400, Cyanocobalamin 4.5 mcg, Folic Acid 0.3 mg, Niacin 13.5 mg, Niacinamide, Pyridoxine HCl, Riboflavin Phosphate Sodium, Sodium Fluoride, Thiamine Mononitrate, Vitamin A Acetate, Vitamin E 15 Units	Poly Vi Flor by BMS	00087-0468	Vitamin
MJ <> 474	Tab, Orange, Pink & Purple, Pillow Shaped, Chewable	Ascorbic Acid 60 mg, Cyanocobalamin 4.5 mcg, Fluoride Ion 1 mg, Folic Acid 0.3 mg, Niacin 13.5 mg, Pyridoxine HCl 1.05 mg, Riboflavin 1.2 mg, Thiamine 1.05 mg, Vitamin A 2500 Units, Vitamin D 400 Units, Vitamin E 15 Units	Poly Vi Flor by BMS	00087-0474	Vitamin
MJ <> 476	Tab, Pillow Shaped, Chewable	Ascorbic Acid 60 mg, Copper 1 mg, Cyanocobalamin 4.5 mcg, Fluoride Ion 1 mg, Folic Acid 0.3 mg, Iron 12 mg, Niacin 13.5 mg, Pyridoxine HCl 1.05 mg, Riboflavin 1.2 mg, Thiamine 1.05 mg, Vitamin A 2500 Units, Vitamin D 400 Units, Vitamin E 15 Units, Zinc 10 mg	Poly Vi Flor Iron by BMS	00087-0476	Vitamin
MJ <> 477	Tab, Orange, Pink & Purple, Pillow Shaped, Chewable	Ascorbic Acid 60 mg, Cholecalciferol 400 Units, Sodium Fluoride, Vitamin A Acetate 2500 Units	Tri Vi Flor by BMS	00087-0477	Vitamin
MJ <> 482	Tab, Pillow Shaped, Chewable	Ascorbic Acid 60 mg, Copper 1 mg, Cyanocobalamin 4.5 mcg, Fluoride Ion 0.5 mg, Folic Acid 0.3 mg, Iron 12 mg, Niacin 13.5 mg, Pyridoxine HCl 1.05 mg, Riboflavin 1.2 mg, Thiamine 1.05 mg, Vitamin A 2500 Units, Vitamin D 400 Units, Vitamin E 15 Units, Zinc 10 mg	Poly Vi Flor Iron by BMS	00087-0482	Vitamin
MJ <> 487	Tab, Orange, Pink & Purple, Chewable	Cyanocobalamin 4.5 mcg, Folic Acid 0.3 mg, Niacinamide, Pyridoxine HCl 1.05 mg, Riboflavin 1.2 mg, Sodium Ascorbate, Sodium Fluoride, Thiamine Mononitrate, Vitamin A Acetate, Vitamin D 400 Units, Vitamin E Acetate	Poly Vi Flor by BMS	00087-0487	Vitamin

ID FRONT <> BACK	DESCRIPTION FRONT <> BACK	INGREDIENT & STRENGTH	BRAND (or Generic Equiv.) by FIRM	NDC#	CLASS; SCH.
MJ <> 488	Tab, Pillow Shaped, Chewable	Cupric Oxide, Cyanocobalamin 4.5 mcg, Ferrous Fumarate, Folic Acid 0.3 mg, Niacinamide, Pyridoxine HCl 1.05 mg, Riboflavin 1.2 mg, Sodium Ascorbate, Sodium Fluoride, Thiamine Mononitrate, Vitamin A Acetate, Vitamin D 400 Units, Vitamin E Acetate, Zinc Oxide	Poly Vi Flor Iron by BMS	00087-0488	Vitamin
MJ <> 583	Tab, Peach, Round	Ethinyl Estradiol 0.035 mg, Norethindrone 0.4 mg	Ovcon 35 21 by Heartland	61392-0814	Oral Contraceptive
MJ <> 583	Tab, Peach, Round	Ethinyl Estradiol 0.035 mg, Norethindrone 0.4 mg	Ovcon 35 21 by Heartland	61392-0818	Oral Contraceptive
MJ <> 583	Tab, Peach, Round	Ethinyl Estradiol 0.035 mg, Norethindrone 0.4 mg	Ovcon 35 21 by BMS	00087-0583	Oral Contraceptive
MJ <> 583	Tab, Peach, Round	Ethinyl Estradiol 0.035 mg, Norethindrone 0.4 mg	Ovcon 35 21 by Physician Total Care	54868-0509	Oral Contraceptive
MJ <> 583	Tab, Peach, Round	Ethinyl Estradiol 0.035 mg, Norethindrone 0.4 mg	Ovcon 35 21 by Warner Chilcott	00430-0583	Oral Contraceptive
MJ <> 584	Tab, Round, Yellow	Ethinyl Estradiol 0.05 mg, Norethindrone 1 mg	Ovcon 50 28 by Warner Chilcott	00430-0585	Oral Contraceptive
MJ <> 584	Tab, Round, Yellow	Ethinyl Estradiol 0.05 mg, Norethindrone 1 mg	Ovcon 50 28 by BMS	15548-0579	Oral Contraceptive
MJ <> 584	Tab, Round, Yellow	Ethinyl Estradiol 0.05 mg, Norethindrone 1 mg	Ovcon 50 28 by BMS	00087-0579	Oral Contraceptive
MJ <> 584	Tab, Round, Yellow	Ethinyl Estradiol 0.05 mg, Norethindrone 1 mg	Ovcon 50 28 by Physician Total Care	54868-3772	Oral Contraceptive
MJ <> 702	Tab, White, Coated, Speckled	Ascorbic Acid 80 mg, Biotin 0.03 mg, Calcium 200 mg, Copper 3 mg, Cyanocobalamin 2.5 mcg, Folic Acid 1 mg, Iron 54 mg, Magnesium 100 mg, Niacin 17 mg, Pantothenic Acid 7 mg, Pyridoxine HCl 4 mg, Riboflavin 1.6 mg, Thiamine 1.5 mg, Vitamin A 4000 Units, Vitamin D 400 Units, Vitamin E 15 Units, Zinc 25 mg	Natalins Tablets Rx by BMS	00087-0702	Vitamin
MJ <> 755	Tab	Estradiol 1 mg	by Quality Care	60346-0375	Hormone
MJ <> 756	Tab, Blue, Round, Scored	Estradiol 2 mg	Estrace by Rx Pak	65084-0187	Hormone
MJ <> 850	Tab, Green, Cap Shaped	Inert	Ovcon 50 28 by BMS	00087-0579	Oral Contraceptive; Placebo
MJ <> 850	Tab, Green, Cap Shaped	Inert	Ovcon 50 28 by Physician Total Care	54868-3772	Oral Contraceptive; Placebo
MJ <> 850	Tab, Green, Cap Shaped	Inert	Ovcon 50 28 by Warner Chilcott	00430-0585	Oral Contraceptive; Placebo
MJ <> BUSPAR5MG	Tab, White, Rectangle, Scored, MJ Logo <> Buspar 5 mg	Buspirone HCl 5 mg	Buspar by Caremark	00339-4110	Antianxiety
MJ021	Tab, White, Round, Scored	Estradiol 0.5 mg	Estrace by BMS	00087-0021	Hormone
MJ021	Tab, White, Round, Flat-Faced, Bevel-Edged, Compressed	Estradiol-17ß (micronized) 0.5 mg	Estrace by Shire BioChem	Canadian DIN 02225190	Hormone
MJ10 <> BUSPAR	Tab, White, Barrel Shaped, Scored	Buspirone HCl 15 mg	Buspar by PDRX	55289-0556	Antianxiety
MJ10 <> BUSPAR	Tab, White, Barrel Shaped, Scored	Buspirone HCl 10 mg	Buspar by Drug Distr	52985-0156	Antianxiety
MJ10 <> BUSPAR	Tab, White, Barrel Shaped, Scored	Buspirone HCl 10 mg	Buspar by Amerisource	62584-0819	Antianxiety
MJ10 <> BUSPAR	Tab, White, Barrel Shaped, Scored	Buspirone HCl 10 mg	Buspar by Nat Pharmpak	55154-2010	Antianxiety
MJ10 <> BUSPAR	Tab, White, Barrel Shaped, Scored	Buspirone HCl 10 mg	Buspar by Med Pro	53978-3024	Antianxiety
MJ10 <> BUSPAR	Tab, White, Barrel Shaped, Scored	Buspirone HCl 10 mg	Buspar by BMS	15548-0819	Antianxiety
MJ10 <> BUSPAR	Tab, White, Barrel Shaped, Scored	Buspirone HCl 10 mg	Buspar by Rightpak	65240-0618	Antianxiety
MJ10 <> BUSPAR	Tab, White, Barrel Shaped, Scored	Buspirone HCl 10 mg	Buspar by BMS	00087-0819	Antianxiety
MJ10 <> BUSPAR	Tab, White, Barrel Shaped, Scored	Buspirone HCl 10 mg	Buspar by Heartland	61392-0602	Antianxiety
MJ10 <> BUSPAR	Tab, White, Barrel Shaped, Scored	Buspirone HCl 10 mg	Buspar by Caremark	00339-4109	Antianxiety
MJ10 <> BUSPAR	Tab, White, Barrel Shaped, Scored	Buspirone HCl 10 mg	Buspar by Pharmedix	53002-1017	Antianxiety
MJ10 <> BUSPAR	Tab, White, Hexagonal	Buspirone HCl 10 mg	Buspar by CVS	00894-5215	Antianxiety
MJ1202M		Fosinopril Sodium 40 mg	Monopril by BMS		Antihypertensive
MJ158 <> M	Tab, White, Diamond Shaped, MJ over 158	Fosinopril Sodium 10 mg	Monopril by Allscripts		Antihypertensive
MJ158 <> M	Tab, White, Diamond Shaped, MJ over 158	Fosinopril Sodium 10 mg	Monopril by Mead Johnson		Antihypertensive
MJ5 <> BUSPAR	Tab, White, Barrel Shaped, Scored	Buspirone HCl 5 mg	Buspar by Heartland	61392-0601	Antianxiety
MJ5 <> BUSPAR	Tab, White, Barrel Shaped, Scored	Buspirone HCl 5 mg	Buspar by BMS	00087-0818	Antianxiety
MJ5 <> BUSPAR	Tab, White, Barrel Shaped, Scored	Buspirone HCl 5 mg	Buspar by Nat Pharmpak	55154-2008	Antianxiety
MJ5 <> BUSPAR	Tab, White, Barrel Shaped, Scored	Buspirone HCl 5 mg	Buspar by BMS	15548-0818	Antianxiety
MJ5 <> BUSPAR	Tab, White, Barrel Shaped, Scored	Buspirone HCl 5 mg	Buspar by Rightpak	65240-0617	Antianxiety

ID FRONT <> BACK	DESCRIPTION FRONT <> BACK	INGREDIENT & STRENGTH	BRAND (or Generic Equiv.) by FIRM	NDC#	CLASS; SCH.
MJ5 <> BUSPAR	Tab, White, Barrel Shaped, Scored	Buspirone HCl 5 mg	Buspar by Direct Dispensing	57866-0902	Antianxiety
MJ5 <> BUSPAR	Tab, White, Barrel Shaped, Scored	Buspirone HCl 5 mg	Buspar by Med Pro	53978-2044	Antianxiety
MJ5 <> BUSPAR	Tab, White, Barrel Shaped, Scored	Buspirone HCl 5 mg	Buspar by Drug Distr	52985-0155	Antianxiety
MJ5 <> BUSPAR	Tab, White, Barrel Shaped, Scored	Buspirone HCl 5 mg	Buspar by Amerisource	62584-0818	Antianxiety
MJ503 <> 50	Tab, White w/ Blue Flecks, Round, MJ over 503	Cyclophosphamide 50 mg	Cytoxan by BMS	Canadian DIN 00344885	Antineoplastic
MJ503 <> 50	Tab, White w/ Blue Flecks, Round, MJ over 503	Cyclophosphamide 50 mg	Cytoxan by Mead Johnson	00015-0503	Antineoplastic
MJ504 <> 25	Tab, White w/ Blue Flecks, Round, MJ over 504	Cyclophosphamide 25 mg	Cytoxan by Mead Johnson	00015-0504	Antineoplastic
MJ504 <> 25	Tab, White w/ Blue Flecks, Round, MJ over 504	Cyclophosphamide 25 mg	Cytoxan by BMS	Canadian DIN 00344877	Antineoplastic
MJ543 <> 10	Tab, White, Round	Isoxsuprine HCl 10 mg	Vasodilan by BMS	00087-0543	Vasodilator
MJ544 <> 20	Tab, White, Round, Scored	Isoxsuprine HCl 20 mg	Vasodilan by BMS	00087-0544	Vasodilator
MJ595	Tab, Light Blue, Round, Scored, MJ over 595	Megestrol Acetate 20 mg	Megace by Mead Johnson	00015-0595	Hormone
MJ596	Tab, Blue, Round	Megestrol Acetate 40 mg	Megace by Mead Johnson	00015-0596	Hormone
MJ609 <> M	Tab, White, Cap Shaped, MJ over 609	Fosinopril Sodium 20 mg	by Allscripts		Antihypertensive
MJ755	Tab, Lavender, Round, Scored	Estradiol 1 mg	Estrace by Nat Pharmpak	55154-2013	Hormone
MJ755	Tab, Lavender, Round, Scored	Estradiol 1 mg	Estrace by BMS	00087-0755	Hormone
MJ755	Tab, Lavender, Round, Flat-Faced, Bevel-Edged, Compressed	Estradiol-17ß (micronized) 1 mg	Estrace by Shire BioChem	Canadian DIN 02148587	Hormone
MJ756	Tab, Turquoise, Round, Scored	Estradiol 2 mg	Estrace by BMS	00087-0756	Hormone
MJ756	Tab, Turquoise, Round, Scored	Estradiol 2 mg	Estrace by BMS	15548-0756	Hormone
MJ756	Tab, Turquoise, Round, Scored	Estradiol 2 mg	Estrace by Nat Pharmpak	55154-2012	Hormone
MJ756	Tab, Turquoise, Round, Flat-Faced, Bevel-Edged, Compressed	Estradiol-17ß (micronized) 2 mg	Estrace by Shire BioChem	Canadian DIN 02148595	Hormone
MJ778 <> 505050	Tab, Orange, Rectangular, Scored	Trazodone HCl 150 mg	Desyrel by Pharm Util	60491-0912	Antidepressant
MJ778 <> 505050	Tab, Orange, Rectangular, Scored	Trazodone HCl 150 mg	Desyrel by Physician Total Care	54868-2549	Antidepressant
MJ778 <> 505050	Tab, Orange, Rectangular, Scored	Trazodone HCl 150 mg	Desyrel by BMS	00087-0778	Antidepressant
MJ778 <> 505050	Tab, Orange, Rectangular, Scored	Trazodone HCl 150 mg	Desyrel by Amerisource	62584-0778	Antidepressant
MJ778 <> 505050	Tab, Orange, Rectangular, Scored	Trazodone HCl 150 mg	Desyrel by Leiner	59606-0631	Antidepressant
MJ778 <> 505050	Tab, Orange, Rectangular, Scored	Trazodone HCl 150 mg	Desyrel by Nat Pharmpak	55154-2011	Antidepressant
MJ778 <> 505050	Tab, Orange, Rectangular, Scored	Trazodone HCl 150 mg	Desyrel by Rx Pak	65084-0221	Antidepressant
MJ778 <> 505050	Tab, Orange, Rectangular, Scored	Trazodone HCl 150 mg	Desyrel by Apothecon	59772-3171	Antidepressant
MJ784	Cap, Red & White	Cefadroxil Monohydrate 500 mg	Duricef by BMS		Antibiotic
MJ785	Tab, White, Oval	Cefadroxil 1 g	Duricef by BMS		Antibiotic
MJ796 <> 100100100	Tab, Yellow, Scored	Trazodone HCl 300 mg	Desyrel by BMS	00087-0796	Antidepressant
MJ822 <> 555	Tab, White, Rectangular, Scored	Buspirone HCl 15 mg	Buspar by Direct Dispensing	57866-0904	Antianxiety
MJ822 <> 555	Tab, White, Rectangular, Scored	Buspirone HCl 15 mg	Buspar by BMS	00087-0822	Antianxiety
MJ822 <> 555	Tab, White, Rectangular, Scored	Buspirone HCl 15 mg	Buspar by Caremark	00339-4105	Antianxiety
MJ822 <> 555	Tab, White, Rectangular, Scored	Buspirone HCl 15 mg	Buspar by BMS	15548-0822	Antianxiety
MJ822 <> 555	Tab, White, Rectangular, Scored	Buspirone HCl 15 mg	Buspar by Wal Mart	49035-0188	Antianxiety
MJ822 <> 555	Tab, White, Rectangular, Scored	Buspirone HCl 15 mg	Buspar by Murfreesboro	51129-1375	Antianxiety
MJ824 <> 101010	Tab, Pink, Scored, MJ Logo	Buspirone HCl 30 mg	Buspar by BMS	00087-0824	Antianxiety
ML <> 324	Tab, Round, Pink, Film Coated	Folic Acid 2.2 mg, Pyridoxine 25 mg, Cyanocobalamin 500 mcg	Folcaps by Midlothian	68308-0324	Vitamin
ML <> 326	Tab, Round, Pink, Film Coated	Folic Acid 2.2 mg, Vitamin B-6 25 mg, Vitamin B-12 1 mg	FaBB by Midlothian	68308-0326	Vitamin; Supplement
ML <> 516	Tab, Round, Pink, Film Coated	Folic Acid 2.5 mg, Pyridoxine 25 mg, Cyanocobalamin 1 mg	Foltx by Midlothian	68308-0516	Vitamin
ML <> 780	Tab, Round, Peach	Folic Acid 2.5 mg, Vitamin B-12 2 mg, Vitamin B-6 25 mg	Folamin by Midlothian	68308-0780	Vitamin; Supplement
ML15	Tab, Light Yellow, Round, Cobalt Logo <> ML over 15	Meloxicam 15 mg	Mobicox by Cobalt	Canadian DIN 02250020	NSAID
ML19	Tab, White to Off-White, Round, M over L19	Lovastatin 10 mg	Mevacor by Mylan	00378-6510	Antihyperlipidemic
ML19	Tab, White to Off-White, Round, M over L19	Lovastatin 10 mg	Mevacor by UDL	51079-0974	Antihyperlipidemic

ID FRONT <> BACK	DESCRIPTION FRONT <> BACK	INGREDIENT & STRENGTH	BRAND (or Generic Equiv.) by FIRM	NDC#	CLASS; SCH.
ML20	Tab, Yellow, Round, M over L20	Lovastatin 20 mg	Mevacor by Mylan	00378-6520	Antihyperlipidemic
ML20	Tab, Yellow, Round, M over L20	Lovastatin 20 mg	Mevacor by UDL	51079-0975 Discontinued	Antihyperlipidemic
ML21	Tab, Pink, Round, M over L21	Lovastatin 40 mg	Mevacor by Mylan	00378-6540	Antihyperlipidemic
ML21	Tab, Pink, Round, M over L21	Lovastatin 40 mg	Mevacor by UDL	51079-0976 Discontinued	Antihyperlipidemic
ML23	Tab, Peach, Round, Scored, M over L23	Lisinopril 5 mg	Zestril by Mylan	00378-2073	Antihypertensive
ML23	Tab, Peach, Round, Scored	Lisinopril 5 mg	Zestril by UDL	51079-0981 Discontinued	Antihypertensive
ML52	Tab, White to Off-White, Round, Scored	Lamotrigine 100 mg	Lamictal by UDL	51079-0499	Anticonvulsant
ML526	Tab, Blue, Rounded Triangle, Chewable	Diphenhydramine 25 mg, Phenylephrine Tannate 10 mg	D-Tann by Midlothian	68308-0526	Cold Remedy
ML53	Tab, White, Round	Lamotrigine 150 mg	Lamictal by Mylan	00378-4253	Anticonvulsant
ML53	Tab, White, Round	Lamotrigine 150 mg	Lamictal by UDL	51079-0865	Anticonvulsant
ML54	Tab, Blue, Round	Lamotrigine 200 mg	Lamictal by UDL	51079-0866	Anticonvulsant
ML54	Tab, Blue, Round	Lamotrigine 200 mg	Lamictal by Mylan	00378-4254	Anticonvulsant
ML75	Tab, Light Yellow, Round, Convex, Bevelled-Edged, ML over 7.5	Meloxicam 7.5 mg	Mobicox by Cobalt	Canadain DIN 02250012	NSAID
MLA05250	Cap, Blue & White, Opaque, ML-A05 250	Cefaclor 250 mg	Ceclor by Caremark	00339-6150	Antibiotic
MLA06500	Cap, Blue & Gray, Opaque, ML-A06 500	Cefaclor 500 mg	by Caremark	00339-6151	Antibiotic
MLA07	Cap, Green & White	Cephalexin 250 mg	by Southwood	58016-0138	Antibiotic
MLA07	Cap, Green & White	Cephalexin 250 mg	Keflex by Dava	67253-0300	Antibiotic
MLA07250	Cap, Green and White	Cephalexin 250 mg	Keflex by Dava	67253-0104	Antibiotic
MLA08	Cap, Green	Cephalexin 500 mg	Keflex by Dava	67253-0301	Antibiotic
MLA08	Cap, Green	Cephalexin 500 mg	by Southwood	58016-0139	Antibiotic
MLA08500	Cap, Dark Green and Light Green	Cephalexin 500 mg	Keflex by Dava	67253-	Antibiotic
MLP16 <> 1MG	Tab, White, Oblong, Scored	Doxazosin Mesylate 1 mg	Cardura by Dava	67253-0380	Antihypertensive
MLP17 <> 2MG	Tab, Yellow, Oval, Scored	Doxazosin Mesylate 2 mg	Cardura by Dava	67253-0381	Antihypertensive
MLP18 <> 4MG	Tab, Orange, Oblong, Scored	Doxazosin Mesylate 4 mg	Cardura by Dava	67253-0382	Antihypertensive
MLP19 <> 8MG	Tab, Green, Oval	Doxazosin Mesylate 8 mg	Cardura by Dava	67253-0383	Antihypertensive
MLX123	Tab, White, Round, Scored, MLX / 123	Acetaminophen 325 mg	Tylenol by Marlex	10135-0123	Analgesic
MLX125	Tab, White, Round	Acetaminophen 500 mg	Tylenol by Marlex	10135-0152	Analgesic
MLX152	Tab, White, Round	Acetaminophen 500 mg	Tylenol by Marlex	10135-0152	Analgesic
MM	Tab, White to Off-White, Round, Scored, Cobalt Logo <> M / M	Metformin HCl 500 mg	Glucophage by Cobalt	Canadian DIN 02257726	Antidiabetic
MM35	Cap, Light Green	Acetaminophen 300 mg, Phenyltoloxamine Citrate 20 mg, Salicylamide 200 mg	Durabac by Marnel	00682-1444	Analgesic
MM35	Cap	Acetaminophen 300 mg, Phenyltoloxamine Citrate 20 mg, Salicylamide 200 mg	Durabac by Seatrace	00551-1444	Analgesic
MMCNEIL <> NO1	Tab, White, Cap-Shaped	Acetaminophen 300 mg, Caffeine 15 mg, Codeine Phosphate 8 mg	TYLENOL No. 1 by Janssen-Ortho	Canadian DIN 02181061	Analgesic; C III
MMDC	Tab, White, Round	Metformin HCl 500 mg	Glucophage by Marion	Canadian	Antidiabetic
MMDC	Tab, White, Round, Scored	Metoclopramide 10 mg	Reglan by Aventis	Canadian	Gastrointestinal
MMDC30	Tab, Green, MMDC/30	Diltiazem HCl 30 mg	Cardizem by Aventis	Canadian	Antihypertensive
MMDC60	Tab, Yellow, MMDC/60	Diltiazem HCl 60 mg	Cardizem by Aventis	Canadian	Antihypertensive
MMDC850	Tab, White, Oval, MMDC/850	Metformin HCl 850 mg	Glucophage by Marion	Canadian	Antidiabetic
MMS830	Cap, Clear & Orange	Diazoxide 50 mg	Proglycem by MMS		Antihypoglycemic
MMSPBA	Cap, Clear & Orange	Diazoxide 50 mg	Proglycem by MMS		Antihypoglycemic
MN3	Tab, Blue, Round	Paroxetine 30 mg	Paxil by Mylan	00378-7003	Antidepressant
MN4	Tab, Blue, Round	Paroxetine 40 mg	Paxil by Mylan	00378-7004	Antidepressant

ID FRONT <> BACK	DESCRIPTION FRONT <> BACK	INGREDIENT & STRENGTH	BRAND (or Generic Equiv.) by FIRM	NDC#	CLASS; SCH.
MO <> W	Tab, White, Round	Levonorgestrel 150 µg, Ethinyl Estradiol 30 µg	Min-Ovral 21 by Wyeth Canada	Canadian DIN 02042320	Oral Contraceptive
MO <> W	Tab, White, Round	Levonorgestrel 150 µg, Ethinyl Estradiol 30 µg.	Min-Ovral 28 by Wyeth Canada	Canadian DIN 02042339	Oral Contraceptive
MO10	Tab, Peach, Round, Film Coated, Extended Release	Oxybutynin Chloride 10 mg	Ditropan XL by Mylan	00378-6610	Urinary Tract
MO10	Tab, Peach, Round, Film Coated, Extended Release	Oxybutynin Chloride 10 mg	Ditropan XL by UDL	51079-0723 Discontinued	Urinary Tract
MO100	Tab, Purple, Round, Grape Odor	Ibuprofen 100 mg	Children's Motrin Junior Strength by McNeil Consum	Canadian DIN 02247344	NSAIDS
MO17	Tab, Grey, Round, Extended Release	Oxybutynin Chloride 15 mg	Ditropan XL by Mylan	00378-6015	Urinary Tract
MO315 <> MOVA	Tab, White, Oval, MO3 1.5 <> Mova	Glyburide 1.5 mg	Glynase by Watson	52544-0558	Antidiabetic
MO315 <> MOVA	Tab, White, Oval, Scored, MO31.5 <> Mova	Glyburide 1.5 mg	Glynase PresTab by Mova	55370-0146	Antidiabetic
MO315 <> Z	Tab, White, Oval, Scored	Glyburide 1.5 mg	DiaBeta by Zoetica	64909-0101	Antidiabetic
MO430 <> MOVA	Tab, Blue, Oval, Scored, MO43.0 <> Mova	Glyburide 3 mg	Glynase PresTab by Mova	55370-0147	Antidiabetic
MO430 <> MOVA	Tab, Blue, Oval, MO4 3.0 <> Mova	Glyburide 3 mg	Glynase by Watson	52544-0559	Antidiabetic
MO430 <> MOVA	Tab, MO4 3.0	Glyburide 3 mg	by Caremark	00339-5910	Antidiabetic
MO430 <> Z	Tab, Blue, Oval, Scored	Glyburide 3 mg	DiaBeta by Zoetica	64909-0102	Antidiabetic
MO5	Tab, Grey, Round, Extended Release	Oxybutynin Chloride 5 mg	Ditropan XL by Mylan	00378-6605	Urinary Tract
MO50	Tab, Round, Purple, Grape Odor	Ibuprofen 50 mg	Children's Motrin by McNeil Consumer Healthcare	Canadian DIN 02247343	NSAID
MO50	Tab, Orange, Round, Orange Odor	Ibuprofen 50 mg	Children's Motrin by McNeil Consumer Healthcare	Canadian DIN 02247343	NSAIDS
MO52 <> MO52	Tab, Pink, Round, Scored	Sulfamethoxazole 400 mg, Trimethoprim 80 mg	Septra by King	60793-0899	Antibiotic
MO53 <> MO53	Tab, Pink, Oval, Scored	Sulfamethoxazole 800 mg, Trimethoprim 160 mg	Septra DS by King	60793-0900	Antibiotic
MO645 <> MOVA	Tab, MO6 4.5	Glyburide 4.725 mg	by Mova	55370-0149	Antidiabetic
MO760 <> MOVA	Tab, Light Yellow, Oval, MO7 6.0 <> Mova	Glyburide 6 mg	Glynase by Watson	52544-0560	Antidiabetic
MO760 <> MOVA	Tab, Light Yellow, Oval, Scored, MO76.0 <> Mova	Glyburide 6 mg	Glynase PresTab by Mova	55370-0506	Antidiabetic
MO760 <> Z	Tab, Yellow, Oval, Scored	Glyburide 6 mg	DiaBeta by Zoetica	64909-0105	Antidiabetic
MOBAN10	Tab, Purple, Round, Moban over 10	Molindone HCl 10 mg	Moban by Endo	63481-0073	Antipsychotic
MOBAN10 <> DUPONT	Tab, Lavender, Round, Moban over 10	Molindone HCl 10 mg	Moban by BMS	00056-0073	Antipsychotic
MOBAN10 <> GATE	Tab, Lavender, Round, Moban over 10	Molindone HCl 10 mg	Moban by Gate	57844-0915	Antipsychotic
MOBAN100	Tab, Tan, Round, Scored	Molindone HCl 100 mg	Moban by Endo	63481-0077	Antipsychotic
MOBAN100	Tab, Tan, Round, Scored	Molindone HCl 100 mg	Moban by BMS	00056-0077	Antipsychotic
MOBAN100 <> GATE	Tab, Tan, Round, Scored	Molindone HCl 100 mg	Moban by Gate	57844-0918	Antipsychotic
MOBAN25	Tab, Green, Round, Scored	Molindone HCl 25 mg	Moban by Endo	63481-0074	Antipsychotic
MOBAN25	Tab, Green, Round, Scored	Molindone HCl 25 mg	Moban by BMS	00056-0074	Antipsychotic
MOBAN25 <> GATE	Tab, Green, Round, Scored	Molindone HCl 25 mg	Moban by Gate	57844-0916	Antipsychotic
MOBAN5	Tab, Orange, Round	Molindone HCl 5 mg	Moban by BMS	00056-0072	Antipsychotic
MOBAN5	Tab, Orange, Round	Molindone HCl 5 mg	Moban by Endo	63481-0072	Antipsychotic
MOBAN5 <> GATE	Tab, Orange, Round	Molindone HCl 5 mg	Moban by Gate	57844-0914	Antipsychotic
MOBAN50	Tab, Blue, Round, Scored	Molindone HCl 50 mg	Moban by BMS	00056-0076	Antipsychotic
MOBAN50	Tab, Blue, Round, Scored	Molindone HCl 50 mg	Moban by Endo	63481-0076	Antipsychotic
MOBAN50 <> GATE	Tab, Blue, Round, Scored	Molindone HCl 50 mg	Moban by Gate	57844-0917	Antipsychotic
MOC150	Tab, Yellow, MOC/150	Moclobemide 150 mg	by AltiMed	Canadian DIN 02218410	Antidepressant
MOC300	Tab, White to Yellowish-White, Oval, Film Coated, Scored	Moclobemide 300 mg	by AltiMed	Canadian DIN 02218429	Antidepressant
MOD100 <> APO	Tab, White, Round	Modafinil 100 mg	Alertec by Apotex	Canadian DIN 02285398	Stimulant; C IV
MOGADON10	Tab, White, Round, Scored	Nitrazepam 10 mg	Mogadon by Valeant	Canadian DIN 00511536	Sedative; Hypnotic; C IV

ID FRONT <> BACK	DESCRIPTION FRONT <> BACK	INGREDIENT & STRENGTH	BRAND (or Generic Equiv.) by FIRM	NDC#	CLASS; SCH.
MOGADON5	Tab, White, Round, Scored	Nitrazepam 5 mg	Mogadon by Valeant	Canadian DIN 00511528	Sedative; Hypnotic; C IV
MOLE	Cap, Black	Caffeine 200 mg	Molie by BDI		Stimulant
MOLE	Cap, White	Caffeine 200 mg	by B & M Labs		Stimulant
MONOPRIL10 <> BMS	Tab, White, Diamond Shaped, Monopril over 10	Fosinopril Sodium 10 mg	Monopril by Caremark	00339-5745	Antihypertensive
MONOPRIL10 <> BMS	Tab, White, Diamond Shaped, Monopril over 10	Fosinopril Sodium 10 mg	Monopril by BMS	00087-0158	Antihypertensive
MONOPRIL10 <> BMS	Tab, White, Diamond Shaped, Monopril over 10	Fosinopril Sodium 10 mg	Monopril by Va Cmop	65243-0092	Antihypertensive
MONOPRIL10 <> BMS	Tab, White, Diamond Shaped, Monopril over 10	Fosinopril Sodium 10 mg	Monopril by Allscripts		Antihypertensive
MONOPRIL10 <> BMS	Tab, White, Diamond Shaped, Monopril over 10	Fosinopril Sodium 10 mg	Monopril by Direct Dispensing	57866-3800	Antihypertensive
MONOPRIL10 <> BMS	Tab, White, Diamond Shaped, Monopril over 10	Fosinopril Sodium 10 mg	Monopril by BMS	Canadian DIN 01907107	Antihypertensive
MONOPRIL20 <> BMS	Tab, White, Oblong, Monopril over 20	Fosinopril Sodium 20 mg	Monopril by Direct Dispensing	57866-3803	Antihypertensive
MONOPRIL20 <> BMS	Tab, White, Oblong, Monopril over 20	Fosinopril Sodium 20 mg	Monopril by Va Cmop	65243-0093	Antihypertensive
MONOPRIL20 <> BMS	Tab, White, Oblong, Monopril over 20	Fosinopril Sodium 20 mg	Monopril by Allscripts		Antihypertensive
MONOPRIL20 <> BMS	Tab, White, Oblong, Monopril over 20	Fosinopril Sodium 20 mg	Monopril by BMS	00087-0609	Antihypertensive
MONOPRIL20 <> BMS	Tab, White, Oblong, Monopril over 20	Fosinopril Sodium 20 mg	Monopril by BMS	15548-0609	Antihypertensive
MONOPRIL20 <> BMS	Tab, White, Oblong, Monopril over 20	Fosinopril Sodium 20 mg	Monopril by JB	51111-0471	Antihypertensive
MONOPRIL20 <> BMS	Tab, White, Oblong, Monopril over 20	Fosinopril Sodium 20 mg	Monopril by BMS	Canadian DIN 01907115	Antihypertensive
MONOPRIL40 <> BMS	Tab, White, Hexagonal, Monopril over 40	Fosinopril Sodium 40 mg	Monopril by Va Cmop	65243-0094	Antihypertensive
MONOPRIL40 <> BMS	Tab, White, Hexagonal, Monopril over 40	Fosinopril Sodium 40 mg	Monopril by BMS	00087-1202	Antihypertensive
MONOPRIL40 <> BMS	Tab, White, Hexagonal, Monopril over 40	Fosinopril Sodium 40 mg	Monopril by BMS	15548-0202	Antihypertensive
MOSSR <> 30	Tab, Blue, Round, M.O.S.-SR/30	Morphine HCl 30 mg	M.O.S.-S.R. by ICN	Canadian DIN 00776181	Analgesic; C II
MOSSR <> 60	Tab, Red, Round, M.O.S.-SR/60	Morphine HCl 60 mg	M.O.S.-S.R. by ICN	Canadian DIN 00776203	Analgesic; C II
MOTRIN100	Tab, Light Orange, Round, Scored, Chewable	Ibuprofen 100 mg	Motrin by McNeil	50580-0431	NSAID
MOTRIN100	Tab, Light Orange, Round, Scored, Chewable	Ibuprofen 100 mg	Motrin by McNeil	Canadian DIN 02243179	NSAID
MOTRIN300MG	Tab, White, Round, Film Coated	Ibuprofen 300 mg	Motrin by McNeil	Canadian DIN 00327794	NSAID
MOTRIN400	Tab, White, Round, Motrin over 400	Ibuprofen 400 mg	Motrin by Allscripts		NSAID
MOTRIN400	Tab, White, Round, Motrin over 400	Ibuprofen 400 mg	Motrin by Murfreesboro	51129-1511	NSAID
MOTRIN400	Tab, White, Round, Motrin over 400	Ibuprofen 400 mg	Motrin by Thrift Drug	59198-0071	NSAID
MOTRIN400	Tab, White, Round, Motrin over 400	Ibuprofen 400 mg	Motrin by DRX	55045-2422	NSAID
MOTRIN400	Tab, White, Round, Motrin over 400	Ibuprofen 400 mg	Motrin by Nat Pharmpak	55154-3906	NSAID
MOTRIN400	Tab, White, Round, Motrin over 400	Ibuprofen 400 mg	Motrin by Amerisource	62584-0385	NSAID
MOTRIN400	Tab, White, Round, Motrin over 400	Ibuprofen 400 mg	Motrin by Compumed	00403-1377	NSAID
MOTRIN400	Tab, Orange, Black Print, Round, Film Coated, Motrin over 400 mg	Ibuprofen 400 mg	Motrin by Pharmacia	Canadian	NSAID
MOTRIN400MG	Tab, Orange, Black Print, Round, Film Coated, Motrin over 400 mg	Ibuprofen 400 mg	Motrin by McNeil	Canadian DIN 00364142	NSAID
MOTRIN400MG	Tab, White, Round	Ibuprofen 400 mg	Motrin by Pharmacia	00009-7385	NSAID
MOTRIN50	Tab, Light Orange, Round, Scored, Chewable	Ibuprofen 50 mg	Motrin by McNeil	Canadian DIN 02243178	NSAID
MOTRIN50	Tab, Chewable	Ibuprofen 50 mg	Motrin by McNeil	50580-0361	NSAID
MOTRIN600	Tab, White, Oblong, Motrin over 600	Ibuprofen 600 mg	Motrin by Rightpak	65240-0695	NSAID
MOTRIN600	Tab, White, Oblong, Motrin over 600	Ibuprofen 600 mg	Motrin by Thrift Drug	59198-0072	NSAID
MOTRIN600	Tab, White, Oblong, Motrin over 600	Ibuprofen 600 mg	Motrin by Amerisource	62584-0386	NSAID
MOTRIN600	Tab, White, Oblong, Motrin over 600	Ibuprofen 600 mg	Motrin by Murfreesboro	51129-1510	NSAID

ID FRONT <> BACK	DESCRIPTION FRONT <> BACK	INGREDIENT & STRENGTH	BRAND (or Generic Equiv.) by FIRM	NDC#	CLASS; SCH.
MOTRIN600	Tab, White, Oblong, Motrin over 600	Ibuprofen 600 mg	Motrin by Kaiser	00179-1277	NSAID
MOTRIN600MG	Tab, Peach, Black Print, Oval, Film Coated, Motrin over 600 mg	Ibuprofen 600 mg	Motrin by Kaiser	00179-1100	NSAID
MOTRIN600MG	Tab, Peach, Black Print, Oval, Film Coated, Motrin over 600 mg	Ibuprofen 600 mg	Motrin by Med Pro	53978-5006	NSAID
MOTRIN600MG	Tab, Peach, Black Print, Oval, Film Coated, Motrin over 600 mg	Ibuprofen 600 mg	Motrin by Nat Pharmpak	55154-3907	NSAID
MOTRIN600MG	Tab, Peach, Black Print, Oval, Film Coated, Motrin over 600 mg	Ibuprofen 600 mg	Motrin by McNeil	Canadian DIN 00484911	NSAID
MOTRIN600MG	Tab, Peach, Black Print, Oval, Film Coated, Motrin over 600 mg	Ibuprofen 600 mg	Motrin by Pharmacia	Canadian	NSAID
MOTRIN600MG	Tab, White, Cap Shaped	Ibuprofen 600 mg	Motrin by Pharmacia	00009-7386	NSAID
MOTRIN800	Tab, White, Oblong, Motrin over 800	Ibuprofen 800 mg	Motrin by Kaiser	00179-1142	NSAID
MOTRIN800	Tab, White, Oblong, Motrin over 800	Ibuprofen 800 mg	Motrin by Rightpak	65240-0696	NSAID
MOTRIN800	Tab, White, Oblong, Motrin over 800	Ibuprofen 800 mg	Motrin by Thrift Drug	59198-0073	NSAID
MOTRIN800	Tab, White, Oblong, Motrin over 800	Ibuprofen 800 mg	Motrin by Nat Pharmpak	55154-3908	NSAID
MOTRIN800	Tab, White, Oblong, Motrin over 800	Ibuprofen 800 mg	Motrin by Smiths Food & Drug	58341-0060	NSAID
MOTRIN800	Tab, White, Oblong, Motrin over 800	Ibuprofen 800 mg	Motrin by Amerisource	62584-0387	NSAID
MOTRIN800	Tab, White, Oblong, Motrin over 800	Ibuprofen 800 mg	Motrin by Murfreesboro	51129-1509	NSAID
MOTRIN800	Tab, White, Oblong, Motrin over 800	Ibuprofen 800 mg	Motrin by Med Pro	53978-0118	NSAID
MOTRIN800MG	Tab, White, Cap Shaped	Ibuprofen 800 mg	Motrin by Pharmacia	00009-7387	NSAID
MOTRINIB	Cap, Orange & White	Ibuprofen 200 mg	Motrin by McNeil	Canadian DIN 01983873	NSAID
MOTRINIB	Tab, White, Round, Film Coated	Ibuprofen 200 mg	Motrin by McNeil	Canadian DIN 02186934	NSAID
MOTRINIB	Tab, White, Round, Film Coated	Ibuprofen 200 mg	Motrin by McNeil	Canadian DIN 02187124	NSAID
MOTRINIB	Cap, Orange & White	Ibuprofen 200 mg	Motrin by McNeil	Canadian	NSAID
MOVA <> 100M10	Tab, White, Cap Shaped	Captopril 100 mg	Capoten by Mova	55370-0145	Antihypertensive
MOVA <> 250M25	Tab	Naproxen 250 mg	by Caremark	00339-5870	NSAID
MOVA <> 250M25	Tab, Rose, Round	Naproxen 250 mg	Naprosyn by Mova	55370-0139	NSAID
MOVA <> 300M30	Tab, White, Round	Cimetidine HCl 300 mg	Tagamet by Mova	55370-0135	Gastrointestinal
MOVA <> 375M37	Tab, White, Cap Shaped	Naproxen 375 mg	Naprosyn by Mova	55370-0140	NSAID
MOVA <> 375M37	Tab, White, Cap Shaped	Naproxen 375 mg	by Caremark	00339-5872	NSAID
MOVA <> 400M40	Tab, White, Cap Shaped, Scored	Cimetidine HCl 400 mg	Tagamet by Mova	55370-0136	Gastrointestinal
MOVA <> 400M40	Tab, Coated, Mova <> 400/M40	Cimetidine HCl 400 mg	Tagamet by Rosemont	00832-0103	Gastrointestinal
MOVA <> 500M50	Tab, Rose, Cap Shaped	Naproxen 500 mg	Naprosyn by Compumed	00403-1442	NSAID
MOVA <> 500M50	Tab, Rose, Cap Shaped	Naproxen 500 mg	Naprosyn by Mova	55370-0141	NSAID
MOVA <> 500M50	Tab, Rose, Cap Shaped	Naproxen 500 mg	Naprosyn by Caremark	00339-5874	NSAID
MOVA <> 500M50	Tab, Rose, Cap Shaped	Naproxen 500 mg	Naprosyn by JLM	63369-0560	NSAID
MOVA <> 50MO	Tab, Debossed	Captopril 50 mg	Capoten by Mova		Antihypertensive
MOVA <> 50MO5	Tab, White, Cap Shaped	Captopril 50 mg	Capoten by Mova	55370-0144	Antihypertensive
MOVA <> 800M80	Tab, White, Cap Shaped, Scored	Cimetidine HCl 800 mg	Tagamet by Mova	55370-0137	Gastrointestinal
MOVA <> M01	Tab, White, Oval, Scored	Captopril 12.5 mg	Capoten by Mova	55370-0164	Antihypertensive
MOVA <> M01	Tab, Mova <> MO1	Captopril 12.5 mg	Capoten by Caremark	00339-6121	Antihypertensive
MOVA <> MO315	Tab, White, Oval, Scored, Mova <> MO31.5	Glyburide 1.5 mg	Glynase PresTab by Mova	55370-0146	Antidiabetic
MOVA <> MO315	Tab, White, Oval, MO3 1.5 <> Mova	Glyburide 1.5 mg	Glynase by Watson	52544-0558	Antidiabetic
MOVA <> MO430	Tab, MO4 3.0	Glyburide 3 mg	by Caremark	00339-5910	Antidiabetic
MOVA <> MO430	Tab, Blue, Oval, Scored, Mova <> MO43.0	Glyburide 3 mg	Glynase PresTab by Mova	55370-0147	Antidiabetic
MOVA <> MO645	Tab, MO6 4.5	Glyburide 4.725 mg	by Mova	55370-0149	Antidiabetic

653

ID FRONT <> BACK	DESCRIPTION FRONT <> BACK	INGREDIENT & STRENGTH	BRAND (or Generic Equiv.) by FIRM	NDC#	CLASS; SCH.
MOVA <> MO760	Tab, Light Yellow, Oval, Scored, Mova <> MO76.0	Glyburide 6 mg	Glynase PresTab by Mova	55370-0506	Antidiabetic
MOVA25	Tab	Captopril 25 mg	Capoten by Caremark	00339-6122	Antihypertensive
MOVA25	Tab, White, Round	Captopril 25 mg	Capoten by Mova	55370-0142	Antihypertensive
MOVA50M05	Tab	Captopril 50 mg	Capoten by Caremark	00339-6123	Antihypertensive
MOXY <> 5	Tab, White, Round, M-OXY	Oxycodone HCl 5 mg	by Pharmafab	62542-0258	Analgesic; C II
MOXY <> 5	Tab, White, Round, Scored, M-OXY <> 5	Oxycodone HCl 5 mg	Roxicodone/Percolone by Mallinckrodt		Analgesic; C II
MP	Tab	Albuterol Sulfate 2 mg	Proventil by Patient First	57575-0018	Antiasthmatic
MP	Tab, Orange, Oblong, M/P	Guaifenesin 400 mg, Pseudoephedrine HCl 60 mg, Dextromethorphan 20 mg	Anatuss DM by Merz		Cold Remedy
MP	Tab, Sugar Coated	Hydroxyzine HCl 25 mg	by Patient First	57575-0064	Antianxiety; Antihistamine
MP	Tab, Film Coated	Doxycycline Hyclate 100 mg	by Pharmedix	53002-0271	Antibiotic
MP <> 0331	Tab, Dark Red, Cap Shaped, Film Coated	Calcium Carbonate 312 mg, Cyanocobalamin 3 mcg, Ferric Polysaccharide Complex, Folic Acid 1 mg, Niacinamide 10 mg, Pyridoxine HCl 2 mg, Riboflavin 3 mg, Sodium Ascorbate, Thiamine Mononitrate 3 mg, Vitamin A 4000 Units, Vitamin D 400 Units	Nu Iron V by Merz	00259-0331	Vitamin; Mineral
MP <> 112	Tab, Yellow, Round	Sulindac 150 mg	by St. Mary's Med	60760-0415	NSAID
MP <> 52	Tab, White, Round, Scored	Prednisone 10 mg	by Allscripts		Steroid
MP <> 52	Tab, White, Round, Scored	Prednisone 10 mg	by Allscripts		Steroid
MP <> 53	Tab, Peach, Round, Scored	Prednisone 20 mg	by Allscripts		Steroid
MP <> 66	Tab, Off White, Ex Release	Quinidine Gluconate 324 mg	by Quality Care	60346-0555	Antiarrhythmic
MP384	Cap, Brown, Oval	Vitamin E 100 IU, Vitamin C 120, Beta-Carotene 25 mg	Antiox by RP Scherer		Vitamin
MP10	Tab, Pink, Round, Film Coated	Amitriptyline HCl 10 mg	Elavil by Major	00904-0200	Antidepressant
MP10	Tab, Pink, Round, Film Coated	Amitriptyline HCl 10 mg	Elavil by URL Mutual	00677-0475	Antidepressant
MP10	Tab, Pink, Round, Film Coated	Amitriptyline HCl 10 mg	Elavil by Mutual	53489-0104	Antidepressant
MP105	Cap, Light Blue, Black Print, Opaque, MUTUAL over 105	Doxycycline Hyclate 100 mg	Vibramycin by Major	00904-0428	Antibiotic
MP108	Tab, White, Round, Scored	Quinidine Sulfate 200 mg	Quinora by URL Mutual	00677-0122	Antiarrhythmic
MP108	Tab, White, Round, Scored	Quinidine Sulfate 200 mg	Quinora by Mutual	53489-0461	Antiarrhythmic
MP11	Tab, Film Coated	Dipyridamole 25 mg	by Mutual	53489-0115	Antiplatelet
MP111 <> 2	Tab	Acetaminophen 300 mg, Codeine Phosphate 15 mg	Tylenol w/ Codeine by Pharmedix	53002-0122	Analgesic; C III
MP111 <> 2	Tab	Acetaminophen 300 mg, Codeine Phosphate 15 mg	Tylenol w/ Codeine by URL Mutual	00677-0611	Analgesic; C III
MP1112	Tab, MP111 over 2	Acetaminophen 300 mg, Codeine Phosphate 15 mg	Tylenol w/ Codeine by Mutual	53489-0159	Analgesic; C III
MP1112	Tab, White, Round, MP 111 over 2	Acetaminophen 300 mg, Codeine Phosphate 15 mg	Tylenol w/ Codeine by Amerisource	62584-0058	Analgesic; C III
MP112	Tab, Yellow, Round, Film Coated, MP over 112	Sulindac 150 mg	Clinoril by Southwood	58016-0743	NSAID
MP112	Tab, Yellow, Round, Film Coated, MP over 112	Sulindac 150 mg	Clinoril by Rx Dispensing	61807-0036	NSAID
MP112	Tab, Yellow, Round, Film Coated, MP over 112	Sulindac 150 mg	Clinoril by URL Mutual	00677-1173	NSAID
MP112	Tab, Yellow, Round, Film Coated, MP over 112	Sulindac 150 mg	Clinoril by Qualitest	00603-5872	NSAID
MP112	Tab, Yellow, Round, Film Coated, MP over 112	Sulindac 150 mg	Clinoril by Mutual	53489-0478	NSAID
MP112	Tab, Yellow, Round, Film Coated, MP over 112	Sulindac 150 mg	Clinoril by Direct Dispensing	57866-4621	NSAID
MP114	Tab, White, Round, Scored, Film Coated	Trazodone HCl 100 mg	Desyrel by Mutual	53489-0511	Antidepressant
MP114	Tab, White, Round, Scored, Film Coated	Trazodone HCl 100 mg	Desyrel by PDRX	55289-0223	Antidepressant
MP114	Tab, White, Round, Scored, Film Coated	Trazodone HCl 100 mg	Desyrel by Med Pro	53978-0563	Antidepressant
MP114	Tab, White, Round, Scored, Film Coated	Trazodone HCl 100 mg	Desyrel by URL Mutual	00677-1134	Antidepressant
MP114	Tab, White, Round, Scored, Film Coated	Trazodone HCl 100 mg	Desyrel by Teva	00480-0318	Antidepressant
MP114	Tab, White, Round, Scored, Film Coated	Trazodone HCl 100 mg	Desyrel by Major	00904-5220	Antidepressant
MP116	Tab, Yellow, Round, Scored	Sulindac 200 mg	Clinoril by Major	00904-3379	NSAID
MP116	Tab, Yellow, Round, Scored	Sulindac 200 mg	Clinoril by URL Mutual	00677-1174	NSAID
MP116	Tab, Yellow, Round, Scored	Sulindac 200 mg	Clinoril by Qualitest	00603-5873	NSAID
MP116	Tab, Yellow, Round, Scored	Sulindac 200 mg	Clinoril by Mutual	53489-0479	NSAID
MP116	Tab, Yellow, Round, Scored	Sulindac 200 mg	Clinoril by Direct Dispensing	57866-4622	NSAID
MP116	Tab, Yellow, Round, Scored	Sulindac 200 mg	Clinoril by Southwood	58016-0294	NSAID

ID FRONT <> BACK	DESCRIPTION FRONT <> BACK	INGREDIENT & STRENGTH	BRAND (or Generic Equiv.) by FIRM	NDC#	CLASS; SCH.
MP116	Tab, Yellow, Round, Scored	Sulindac 200 mg	Clinoril by Ivax	00182-1706	NSAID
MP118	Tab, White, Round, Scored, Film Coated	Trazodone HCl 50 mg	Desyrel by URL Mutual	00677-1133	Antidepressant
MP118	Tab, White, Round, Scored, Film Coated	Trazodone HCl 50 mg	Desyrel by Mutual	53489-0510	Antidepressant
MP118	Tab, White, Round, Scored, Film Coated	Trazodone HCl 50 mg	Desyrel by Teva	00480-0294	Antidepressant
MP118	Tab, White, Round, Scored, Film Coated	Trazodone HCl 50 mg	Desyrel by Martec	52555-0727	Antidepressant
MP118	Tab, White, Round, Scored, Film Coated	Trazodone HCl 50 mg	Desyrel by Major	00904-5219	Antidepressant
MP12	Tab, Yellow, Round, Film Coated	Thioridazine HCl 10 mg	Mellaril by Taro	52549-4030	Antipsychotic
MP12	Tab, Yellow, Round, Film Coated	Thioridazine HCl 10 mg	Mellaril by Mutual	53489-0148	Antipsychotic
MP12	Tab, Yellow, Round, Film Coated	Thioridazine HCl 10 mg	Mellaril by Qualitest	00603-5992	Antipsychotic
MP12	Tab, Yellow, Round, Film Coated	Thioridazine HCl 10 mg	Mellaril by URL Mutual	00677-0823	Antipsychotic
MP12	Tab, Yellow, Round, Film Coated	Thioridazine HCl 10 mg	Mellaril by Major	00904-5240	Antipsychotic
MP122 <> 3	Tab	Acetaminophen 300 mg, Codeine Phosphate 30 mg	Tylenol w/ Codeine by URL Mutual	00677-0612	Analgesic; C III
MP1223	Tab, MP 122 over 3	Acetaminophen 300 mg, Codeine Phosphate 30 mg	Tylenol w/ Codeine by Mutual	53489-0160	Analgesic; C III
MP124	Tab, White, Round, Scored	Quinidine Sulfate 300 mg	Quinora by URL Mutual	00677-1209	Antiarrhythmic
MP124	Tab, White, Round, Scored	Quinidine Sulfate 300 mg	Quinora by Qualitest	00603-5595	Antiarrhythmic
MP124	Tab, White, Round, Scored	Quinidine Sulfate 300 mg	Quinora by Mutual	53489-0460	Antiarrhythmic
MP127 <> 4	Tab	Acetaminophen 300 mg, Codeine Phosphate 60 mg	Tylenol w/ Codeine by URL Mutual	00677-0632	Analgesic; C III
MP1274	Tab, MP 127 over 4	Acetaminophen 300 mg, Codeine Phosphate 60 mg	Tylenol w/ Codeine by Mutual	53489-0161	Analgesic; C III
MP1274	Tab, White, Round, MP 127 over 4	Acetaminophen 300 mg, Codeine Phosphate 60 mg	Tylenol w/ Codeine by Amerisource	62584-0065	Analgesic; C III
MP13	Tab, Purple, Round, Film Coated	Hydroxyzine HCl 50 mg	Atarax by Mutual	53489-0128	Antianxiety; Antihistamine
MP13	Tab, Purple, Round, Film Coated	Hydroxyzine HCl 50 mg	Atarax by Watson	00591-5565	Antianxiety; Antihistamine
MP13	Tab, Purple, Round, Film Coated	Hydroxyzine HCl 50 mg	Atarax by URL Mutual	00677-0606	Antianxiety; Antihistamine
MP13	Tab, Purple, Round, Film Coated	Hydroxyzine HCl 50 mg	Atarax by Murfreesboro	51129-1474	Antianxiety; Antihistamine
MP135	Tab, White, Round	Acetaminophen 325 mg	Tylenol by Mutual		Analgesic
MP14	Tab, Yellow, Round, Film Coated	Thioridazine HCl 25 mg	Mellaril by Mutual	53489-0149	Antipsychotic
MP14	Tab, Yellow, Round, Film Coated	Thioridazine HCl 25 mg	Mellaril by Taro	52549-4031	Antipsychotic
MP14	Tab, Yellow, Round, Film Coated	Thioridazine HCl 25 mg	Mellaril by Major	00904-5241	Antipsychotic
MP14	Tab, Yellow, Round, Film Coated	Thioridazine HCl 25 mg	Mellaril by URL Mutual	00677-0824	Antipsychotic
MP141	Tab	Acetazolamide 250 mg	Diamox by Mutual	53489-0167	Antiglaucoma Agent
MP142	Tab	Benztropine Mesylate 2 mg	Cogentin by Mutual	53489-0184	Antiparkinson
MP142	Tab	Benztropine Mesylate 2 mg	Cogentin by URL Mutual	00677-0995	Antiparkinson
MP146	Tab, White, Round, Scored	Atenolol 50 mg	Tenormin by Qualitest	00603-2371	Antihypertensive
MP146	Tab, White, Round, Scored	Atenolol 50 mg	Tenormin by URL Mutual	00677-1478	Antihypertensive
MP146	Tab, White, Round, Scored	Atenolol 50 mg	Tenormin by Mutual	53489-0529	Antihypertensive
MP146	Tab, White, Round, Scored	Atenolol 50 mg	Tenormin by Darby Group	66467-3330	Antihypertensive
MP147	Tab, White, Round	Atenolol 100 mg	Tenormin by Mutual	53489-0530	Antihypertensive
MP147	Tab, White, Round	Atenolol 100 mg	Tenormin by Talbert	44514-0885	Antihypertensive
MP147	Tab, White, Round	Atenolol 100 mg	Tenormin by Qualitest	00603-2372	Antihypertensive
MP147	Tab, White, Round	Atenolol 100 mg	Tenormin by URL Mutual	00677-1479	Antihypertensive
MP148	Tab, White, Round	Metoclopramide HCl 5 mg	Reglan by Major	00904-1069	Gastrointestinal
MP148	Tab, White, Round	Metoclopramide HCl 5 mg	Reglan by Mutual	53489-0384	Gastrointestinal
MP15	Tab, Film Coated	Dipyridamole 50 mg	by Mutual	53489-0116	Antiplatelet
MP151	Tab, White, Beveled Bisect	Prednisone 5 mg	by Apotheca	12634-0184	Steroid
MP152	Tab, White, Round	Atenolol 100 mg, Chlorthalidone 25 mg	Tenoretic by Ivax	00182-1943	Antihypertensive; Diuretic
MP152	Tab, White, Round	Atenolol 100 mg, Chlorthalidone 25 mg	Tenoretic by PDRX	55289-0988	Antihypertensive; Diuretic
MP152	Tab, White, Round	Atenolol 100 mg, Chlorthalidone 25 mg	Tenoretic by URL Mutual	00677-1481	Antihypertensive; Diuretic
MP152	Tab, White, Round	Atenolol 100 mg, Chlorthalidone 25 mg	Tenoretic by Mutual	53489-0532	Antihypertensive; Diuretic
MP153	Tab, White, Round, Scored	Atenolol 50 mg, Chlorthalidone 25 mg	Tenoretic by PDRX	55289-0993	Antihypertensive; Diuretic
MP153	Tab, White, Round, Scored	Atenolol 50 mg, Chlorthalidone 25 mg	Tenoretic by Ivax	00182-1942	Antihypertensive; Diuretic
MP153	Tab, White, Round, Scored	Atenolol 50 mg, Chlorthalidone 25 mg	Tenoretic by Sandoz	00781-1315	Antihypertensive; Diuretic

ID FRONT <> BACK	DESCRIPTION FRONT <> BACK	INGREDIENT & STRENGTH	BRAND (or Generic Equiv.) by FIRM	NDC#	CLASS; SCH.
MP153	Tab, White, Round, Scored	Atenolol 50 mg, Chlorthalidone 25 mg	Tenoretic by URL Mutual	00677-1480	Antihypertensive; Diuretic
MP153	Tab, White, Round, Scored	Atenolol 50 mg, Chlorthalidone 25 mg	Tenoretic by Mutual	53489-0531	Antihypertensive; Diuretic
MP153	Tab, White, Round, Scored	Atenolol 50 mg, Chlorthalidone 25 mg	Tenoretic by Murfreesboro	51129-1328	Antihypertensive; Diuretic
MP153	Tab, White, Round, Scored	Atenolol 50 mg, Chlorthalidone 25 mg	Tenoretic by Major	00904-7881	Antihypertensive; Diuretic
MP155	Tab	Quinine Sulfate 260 mg	by Mutual	53489-0462	Antimalarial
MP160	Tab, Yellow, Round, Film Coated	Thioridazine 100 mg	Mellaril by Mutual	53489-0500	Antipsychotic
MP160	Tab, Yellow, Round, Film Coated	Thioridazine 100 mg	Mellaril by URL Mutual	00677-0832	Antipsychotic
MP160	Tab, Yellow, Round, Film Coated	Thioridazine 100 mg	Mellaril by Qualitest	00603-5995	Antipsychotic
MP160	Tab, Yellow, Round, Film Coated	Thioridazine 100 mg	Mellaril by Major	00904-5243	Antipsychotic
MP167	Tab, Film Coated	Fenoprofen Calcium 600 mg	by Mutual	53489-0287	NSAID
MP168 <> 25255050	Tab, White, Round, Scored, 2525 over 5050	Trazodone HCl 150 mg	Desyrel by Teva	00480-0319	Antidepressant
MP168 <> 25255050	Tab, White, Round, Scored, 2525 over 5050	Trazodone HCl 150 mg	Desyrel by Major	00904-5221	Antidepressant
MP168 <> 25255050	Tab, White, Round, Scored, 2525 over 5050	Trazodone HCl 150 mg	Desyrel by Schein	00364-2300	Antidepressant
MP168 <> 25255050	Tab, White, Round, Scored, 2525 over 5050	Trazodone HCl 150 mg	Desyrel by Watson	00591-2300	Antidepressant
MP168 <> 25255050	Tab, White, Round, Scored, 2525 over 5050	Trazodone HCl 150 mg	Desyrel by Mutual	53489-0517	Antidepressant
MP17	Tab, Yellow, Round, Film Coated	Thioridazine 50 mg	Mellaril by Mutual	53489-0150	Antipsychotic
MP17	Tab, Yellow, Round, Film Coated	Thioridazine 50 mg	Mellaril by URL Mutual	00677-0825	Antipsychotic
MP17	Tab, Yellow, Round, Film Coated	Thioridazine 50 mg	Mellaril by Qualitest	00603-5994	Antipsychotic
MP17	Tab, Yellow, Round, Film Coated	Thioridazine 50 mg	Mellaril by Major	00904-5242	Antipsychotic
MP174	Tab, Yellow, Round, Film Coated	Salsalate 500 mg	Disalcid by Mutual	53489-0465	NSAID
MP174	Tab, Yellow, Round, Film Coated	Salsalate 500 mg	Disalcid by Kaiser	00179-1220	NSAID
MP177	Tab, Yellow, Cap Shaped, Film Coated	Salsalate 750 mg	Disalcid by URL Mutual	00677-1024	NSAID
MP177	Tab, Yellow, Cap Shaped, Film Coated	Salsalate 750 mg	Disalcid by Kaiser	00179-1229	NSAID
MP177	Tab, Yellow, Cap Shaped, Film Coated	Salsalate 750 mg	Disalcid by Mutual	53489-0466	NSAID
MP177	Tab, Yellow, Cap Shaped, Film Coated	Salsalate 750 mg	Disalcid by Pharmedix	53002-0488	NSAID
MP177	Tab, Yellow, Cap Shaped, Film Coated	Salsalate 750 mg	Disalcid by Med Pro	53978-0399	NSAID
MP177	Tab, Yellow, Cap Shaped, Film Coated	Salsalate 750 mg	Disalcid by Kaiser	62224-0559	NSAID
MP177	Tab, Yellow, Cap Shaped, Film Coated	Salsalate 750 mg	Disalcid by Golden State	60429-0207	NSAID
MP178	Tab, White, Debossed	Pindolol 5 mg	by Mutual	53489-0430	Antihypertensive
MP178	Tab, Debossed	Pindolol 5 mg	by Major	00904-7893	Antihypertensive
MP178	Tab	Pindolol 5 mg	by Qualitest	00603-5220	Antihypertensive
MP178 <> MP178	Tab	Pindolol 5 mg	by URL Mutual	00677-1457	Antihypertensive
MP18	Tab, Film Coated	Dipyridamole 75 mg	by Mutual	53489-0117	Antiplatelet
MP183	Tab, White	Pindolol 10 mg	by Mutual	53489-0431	Antihypertensive
MP183	Tab, Debossed	Pindolol 10 mg	by Major	00904-7894	Antihypertensive
MP183 <> MP183	Tab	Pindolol 10 mg	by URL Mutual	00677-1458	Antihypertensive
MP184	Tab, Orange, Cap Shaped, Scored, Film Coated	Metoprolol Tartrate 50 mg	Lopressor by Major	00904-7772	Antihypertensive
MP184	Tab, Orange, Cap Shaped, Scored, Film Coated	Metoprolol Tartrate 50 mg	Lopressor by Mutual	53489-0366	Antihypertensive
MP185	Tab, Yellow, Cap Shaped, Scored, Film Coated	Metoprolol Tartrate 100 mg	Lopressor by Murfreesboro	51129-1109	Antihypertensive
MP185	Tab, Yellow, Cap Shaped, Scored, Film Coated	Metoprolol Tartrate 100 mg	Lopressor by URL Mutual	00677-1483	Antihypertensive
MP185	Tab, Yellow, Cap Shaped, Scored, Film Coated	Metoprolol Tartrate 100 mg	Lopressor by Major	00904-7773	Antihypertensive
MP185	Tab, Yellow, Cap Shaped, Scored, Film Coated	Metoprolol Tartrate 100 mg	Lopressor by PDRX	55289-0093	Antihypertensive
MP185	Tab, Yellow, Cap Shaped, Scored, Film Coated	Metoprolol Tartrate 100 mg	Lopressor by Mutual	53489-0367	Antihypertensive
MP20	Tab, White, Round, MP over 20	Dihydro-Alpha-Ergocryptine Mesylate 0.222 mg, Dihydro-Beta-Ergocryptine Mesylate 0.111 mg, Dihydroergocornine Mesylate 0.333 mg, Dihydroergocristine Mesylate 0.333 mg	Ergoloid Mesylates by Direct Dispensing	57866-0303	Ergot Alkaloids
MP20	Tab, White, Round, MP over 20	Dihydro-Alpha-Ergocryptine Mesylate 0.222 mg, Dihydro-Beta-Ergocryptine Mesylate 0.111 mg, Dihydroergocornine Mesylate 0.333 mg, Dihydroergocristine Mesylate 0.333 mg	Ergoloid Mesylates by Mutual	53489-0281	Ergot Alkaloids

ID FRONT <> BACK	DESCRIPTION FRONT <> BACK	INGREDIENT & STRENGTH	BRAND (or Generic Equiv.) by FIRM	NDC#	CLASS; SCH.
MP20	Tab, White, Round, MP over 20	Dihydro-Alpha-Ergocryptine Mesylate 0.222 mg, Dihydro-Beta-Ergocryptine Mesylate 0.111 mg, Dihydroergocornine Mesylate 0.333 mg, Dihydroergocristine Mesylate 0.333 mg	Ergoloid Mesylates by Ivax	00182-1518	Ergot Alkaloids
MP20	Tab, White, Round, MP over 20	Dihydro-Alpha-Ergocryptine Mesylate 0.222 mg, Dihydro-Beta-Ergocryptine Mesylate 0.111 mg, Dihydroergocornine Mesylate 0.333 mg, Dihydroergocristine Mesylate 0.333 mg	Ergoloid Mesylates by Qualitest	00603-3527	Ergot Alkaloids
MP20	Tab, White, Round, MP over 20	Dihydro-Alpha-Ergocryptine Mesylate 0.222 mg, Dihydro-Beta-Ergocryptine Mesylate 0.111 mg, Dihydroergocornine Mesylate 0.333 mg, Dihydroergocristine Mesylate 0.333 mg	Ergoloid Mesylates by URL Mutual	00677-0782	Ergot Alkaloids
MP20	Tab, White, Round, MP over 20	Dihydro-Alpha-Ergocryptine Mesylate 0.222 mg, Dihydro-Beta-Ergocryptine Mesylate 0.111 mg, Dihydroergocornine Mesylate 0.333 mg, Dihydroergocristine Mesylate 0.333 mg	Ergoloid Mesylates by UDL	51079-0110	Ergot Alkaloids
MP20	Tab, White, Round, MP over 20	Dihydro-Alpha-Ergocryptine Mesylate 0.222 mg, Dihydro-Beta-Ergocryptine Mesylate 0.111 mg, Dihydroergocornine Mesylate 0.333 mg, Dihydroergocristine Mesylate 0.333 mg	Ergoloid Mesylates by Major	00904-0336	Ergot Alkaloids
MP22	Tab, Film Coated	Hydralazine HCl 10 mg	by Mutual	53489-0123	Antihypertensive
MP25	Tab, Green, Round, Film Coated	Amitriptyline HCl 25 mg	Elavil by Kaiser	62224-7117	Antidepressant
MP25	Tab, Green, Round, Film Coated	Amitriptyline HCl 25 mg	Elavil by URL Mutual	00677-0476	Antidepressant
MP25	Tab, Green, Round, Film Coated	Amitriptyline HCl 25 mg	Elavil by Kaiser	00179-0042	Antidepressant
MP25	Tab, Green, Round, Film Coated	Amitriptyline HCl 25 mg	Elavil by Mutual	53489-0105	Antidepressant
MP25	Tab, Green, Round, Film Coated	Amitriptyline HCl 25 mg	Elavil by Major	00904-0201	Antidepressant
MP26	Tab, Brown, Round, Film Coated	Amitriptyline HCl 50 mg	Elavil by Major	00904-0202	Antidepressant
MP26	Tab, Brown, Round, Film Coated	Amitriptyline HCl 50 mg	Elavil by Mutual	53489-0106	Antidepressant
MP26	Tab, Brown, Round, Film Coated	Amitriptyline HCl 50 mg	Elavil by URL Mutual	00677-0477	Antidepressant
MP26	Tab, Brown, Round, Film Coated	Amitriptyline HCl 50 mg	Elavil by Kaiser	62224-7220	Antidepressant
MP27	Tab, Purple, Round, Film Coated	Amitriptyline HCl 75 mg	Elavil by URL Mutual	00677-0478	Antidepressant
MP27	Tab, Purple, Round, Film Coated	Amitriptyline HCl 75 mg	Elavil by Mutual	53489-0107	Antidepressant
MP27	Tab, Purple, Round, Film Coated	Amitriptyline HCl 75 mg	Elavil by Major	00904-0203	Antidepressant
MP271	Tab, White, Round, Scored, Film Coated	Labetalol HCl 200 mg	Normodyne by URL Mutual	00677-1702	Antihypertensive
MP271	Tab, White, Round, Scored, Film Coated	Labetalol HCl 200 mg	Normodyne by Murfreesboro	51129-1609	Antihypertensive
MP271	Tab, White, Round, Scored, Film Coated	Labetalol HCl 200 mg	Normodyne by Mutual	53489-0355	Antihypertensive
MP272	Tab, Blue, Round, Film Coated	Labetalol HCl 300 mg	Normodyne by Mutual	53489-0356	Antihypertensive
MP272	Tab, Blue, Round, Film Coated	Labetalol HCl 300 mg	Normodyne by Murfreesboro	51129-1611	Antihypertensive
MP272	Tab, Blue, Round, Film Coated	Labetalol HCl 300 mg	Normodyne by URL Mutual	00677-1703	Antihypertensive
MP273	Tab, White with Blue Specks, Oval, Scored	Phentermine 37.5 mg	Adipex-P by Mutual	53489-0406	Anorexiant; C IV
MP277	Tab, Beige, Round, Scored, Film Coated	Labetalol HCl 100 mg	Normodyne by Murfreesboro	51129-1608	Antihypertensive
MP277	Tab, Beige, Round, Scored, Film Coated	Labetalol HCl 100 mg	Normodyne by Mutual	53489-0354	Antihypertensive
MP28	Tab, Orange, Round, Film Coated	Amitriptyline HCl 100 mg	Elavil by URL Mutual	00677-0568	Antidepressant
MP28	Tab, Orange, Round, Film Coated	Amitriptyline HCl 100 mg	Elavil by Mutual	53489-0108	Antidepressant
MP29	Tab, Peach, Cap Shaped, Film Coated	Amitriptyline HCl 150 mg	Elavil by URL Mutual	00677-0645	Antidepressant
MP29	Tab, Peach, Cap Shaped, Film Coated	Amitriptyline HCl 150 mg	Elavil by Mutual	53489-0109	Antidepressant
MP3	Tab, Lavender, Round, Film Coated	Hydroxyzine HCl 10 mg	Atarax by Mutual		Antianxiety; Antihistamine
MP3	Tab, Lavender, Round, Film Coated	Hydroxyzine HCl 10 mg	by Allscripts		Antianxiety; Antihistamine
MP3	Tab, Lavender, Round, Film Coated	Hydroxyzine HCl 10 mg	by Pharmedix	53002-0390	Antianxiety; Antihistamine
MP3	Tab, Lavender, Round, Film Coated	Hydroxyzine HCl 10 mg	by URL Mutual	00677-0604	Antianxiety; Antihistamine
MP3	Tab, White, Round, Extended Release	Paroxetine HCl 12.5 mg	Paxil CR by Mylan	00378-2003	Antidepressant

ID FRONT <> BACK	DESCRIPTION FRONT <> BACK	INGREDIENT & STRENGTH	BRAND (or Generic Equiv.) by FIRM	NDC#	CLASS; SCH.
MP30	Tab	Chlorthalidone 25 mg	by Mutual	53489-0111	Diuretic
MP303	Tab, White, Oval, Scored, Film Coated	Spironolactone 100 mg	Aldactone by URL Mutual	00677-1708	Diuretic
MP303	Tab, White, Oval, Scored, Film Coated	Spironolactone 100 mg	Aldactone by Sidmak		Diuretic
MP303	Tab, White, Oval, Scored, Film Coated	Spironolactone 100 mg	Aldactone by Mutual	53489-0329	Diuretic
MP303	Tab, White, Round	Spironolactone 100 mg	Aldactone by Qualitest	00603-5766	Diuretic
MP35	Tab, White, Round	Spironolactone 25 mg	Aldactone by Allscripts		Diuretic
MP35	Tab, White, Round	Spironolactone 25 mg	Aldactone by Mutual	53489-0143	Diuretic
MP35	Tab, White, Round	Spironolactone 25 mg	Aldactone by Pharmedix	53002-0472	Diuretic
MP36	Tab	Metoclopramide 10 mg	Reglan by Mutual	53489-0385	Gastrointestinal
MP37	Tab, Light Orange, Round, Film Coated	Doxycycline Hyclate 100 mg	Vibra-Tabs by URL Mutual	00677-0799	Antibiotic
MP37	Tab, Light Orange, Round, Film Coated	Doxycycline Hyclate 100 mg	Vibra-Tabs by Qualitest	00603-3482	Antibiotic
MP37	Tab, Light Orange, Round, Film Coated	Doxycycline Hyclate 100 mg	Vibra-Tabs by Dept Health	53808-0041	Antibiotic
MP37	Tab, Light Orange, Round, Film Coated	Doxycycline Hyclate 100 mg	Vibra-Tabs by H J Harkins Co	52959-0474	Antibiotic
MP37	Tab, Light Orange, Round, Film Coated	Doxycycline Hyclate 100 mg	Vibra-Tabs by Major	00904-0430	Antibiotic
MP37	Tab, Light Orange, Round, Film Coated	Doxycycline Hyclate 100 mg	Vibra-Tabs by Mutual	53489-0120	Antibiotic
MP37	Tab, Light Orange, Round, Film Coated	Doxycycline Hyclate 100 mg	Vibra-Tabs by Golden State	60429-0069	Antibiotic
MP37	Tab, Light Orange, Round, Film Coated	Doxycycline Hyclate 100 mg	Vibra-Tabs by Darby Group	66467-0340	Antibiotic
MP37	Tab, Light Orange, Round, Film Coated	Doxycycline Hyclate 100 mg	Vibra-Tabs by Allscripts		Antibiotic
MP39	Tab, White, Round, Scored	Lorazepam 1 mg	Ativan by URL Mutual	00677-1057	Antianxiety; C IV
MP39	Tab, White	Lorazepam 1 mg	Ativan by Major	00904-1501	Antianxiety; C IV
MP39	Tab, White, Round, Scored	Lorazepam 1 mg	Ativan by Mutual	53489-0358	Antianxiety; C IV
MP392	Tab, White, Cap Shaped, Scored	Acetaminophen 650 mg, Butalbital 50 mg	Promacet by Merz	00259-0392	Analgesic
MP392	Tab, White, Cap Shaped, Scored	Acetaminophen 650 mg, Butalbital 50 mg	Promacet by Mikart	46672-0164	Analgesic
MP4	Tab, Yellow, Round, Film Coated	Imipramine HCl 10 mg	Tofranil by URL Mutual	00677-0421	Antidepressant
MP4	Tab, Yellow, Round, Film Coated	Imipramine HCl 10 mg	Tofranil by Qualitest	00603-4043	Antidepressant
MP4	Tab, Yellow, Round, Film Coated	Imipramine HCl 10 mg	Tofranil by Mutual	53489-0330	Antidepressant
MP4	Tab, Purple, Round, Extended Release	Paroxetine HCl 25 mg	Paxil CR by Mylan	00378-2004	Antidepressant
MP40	Tab, Buff, Round, MP over 40	Hydrochlorothiazide 25 mg, Spironolactone 25 mg	by Allscripts		Diuretic; Antihypertensive
MP40	Tab, Buff, Round	Hydrochlorothiazide 25 mg, Spironolactone 25 mg	by Ivax	00182-1158	Diuretic; Antihypertensive
MP40	Tab, Buff, Round	Hydrochlorothiazide 25 mg, Spironolactone 25 mg	by Sandoz	00781-1149	Diuretic; Antihypertensive
MP40	Tab, Buff, Round	Hydrochlorothiazide 25 mg, Spironolactone 25 mg	by URL Mutual	00677-0624	Diuretic; Antihypertensive
MP40	Tab, Buff, Round	Hydrochlorothiazide 25 mg, Spironolactone 25 mg	Aldactazide by Mutual	53489-0144	Diuretic; Antihypertensive
MP423	Tab, Cap Shaped, Scored	Guaifenesin 600 mg	Robitussin by Mutual	53489-0423	Expectorant
MP424	Tab, White, Oval, Scored	Guaifenesin 600 mg, Pseudoephedrine HCl 120 mg	Entex PSE by Mutual	53489-0424	Cold Remedy
MP424	Tab, White, Oval, Scored	Guaifenesin 600 mg, Pseudoephedrine HCl 120 mg	Entex PSE by URL Mutual	00677-1476	Cold Remedy
MP425	Tab, Blue, Cap Shaped, Scored	Guaifenesin 600 mg, Pseudoephedrine HCl 60 mg	Deconsal II by Mutual	53489-0425	Cold Remedy
MP425	Tab, Blue, Cap Shaped, Scored	Guaifenesin 600 mg, Pseudoephedrine HCl 60 mg	Deconsal II by URL Mutual	00677-1487	Cold Remedy
MP43	Tab	Chlorthalidone 50 mg	by Mutual	53489-0112	Diuretic
MP44	Tab	Benztropine Mesylate 1 mg	Cogentin by URL Mutual	00677-0993	Antiparkinson
MP44	Tab	Benztropine Mesylate 1 mg	Cogentin by Mutual	53489-0183	Antiparkinson
MP441	Tab, Green, Round, Scored	Mixed Amphetamine Salts 5 mg: Amphetamine Aspartate 1.25 mg, Amphetamine Sulfate 1.25 mg, Dextroamphetamine Saccharate 1.25 mg, Dextroamphetamine Sulfate 1.25 mg	Adderall by Mutual	53489-0564	Stimulant; C II
MP442	Tab, Green, Oval, Scored	Mixed Amphetamine Salts 7.5 mg: Amphetamine Aspartate 1.875 mg, Amphetamine Sulfate 1.875 mg, Dextroamphetamine Saccharate 1.875 mg, Dextroamphetamine Sulfate 1.875 mg	Adderall by Mutual	53489-0565	Stimulant; C II
MP443	Tab, Green, Round, Scored	Mixed Amphetamine Salts 10 mg: Amphetamine Aspartate 2.5 mg, Amphetamine Sulfate 2.5 mg, Dextroamphetamine Saccharate 2.5 mg, Dextroamphetamine Sulfate 2.5 mg	Adderall by Mutual	53489-0566	Stimulant; C II

ID FRONT <> BACK	DESCRIPTION FRONT <> BACK	INGREDIENT & STRENGTH	BRAND (or Generic Equiv.) by FIRM	NDC#	CLASS; SCH.
MP444	Tab, Yellow, Round, Scored	Mixed Amphetamine Salts 12.5 mg: Amphetamine Aspartate 3.125 mg, Amphetamine Sulfate 3.125 mg, Dextroamphetamine Saccharate 3.125 mg, Dextroamphetamine Sulfate 3.125 mg	Adderall by Mutual	53489-0567	Stimulant; C II
MP445	Tab, Yellow, Oval, Scored	Mixed Amphetamine Salts 15 mg: Amphetamine Aspartate 3.75 mg, Amphetamine Sulfate 3.75 mg, Dextroamphetamine Saccharate 3.75 mg, Dextroamphetamine Sulfate 3.75 mg	Adderall by Mutual	53489-0568	Stimulant; C II
MP446	Tab, Yellow, Round, Scored	Mixed Amphetamine Salts 20 mg: Amphetamine Aspartate 5 mg, Amphetamine Sulfate 5 mg, Dextroamphetamine Saccharate 5 mg, Dextroamphetamine Sulfate 5 mg	Adderall by Mutual	53489-0569	Stimulant; C II
MP447	Tab, Yellow, Round, Scored	Mixed Amphetamine Salts 30 mg: Amphetamine Aspartate 7.5 mg, Amphetamine Sulfate 7.5 mg, Dextroamphetamine Saccharate 7.5 mg, Dextroamphetamine Sulfate 7.5 mg	Adderall by Mutual	53489-0570	Stimulant; C II
MP45	Tab, White, Round	Metronidazole 250 mg	Flagyl by Pharmedix	53002-0221	Antibiotic
MP45	Tab, White, Round	Metronidazole 250 mg	Flagyl by Mutual	53489-0135	Antibiotic
MP46	Tab, White, Cap Shaped	Metronidazole 500 mg	Flagyl by Pharmedix	53002-0247	Antibiotic
MP46	Tab, White, Cap Shaped	Metronidazole 500 mg	Flagyl by Mutual	53489-0136	Antibiotic
MP47	Tab, White, Round, Scored	Albuterol Sulfate 2 mg	Proventil by URL Mutual	00677-1359	Antiasthmatic
MP47	Tab, White, Round, Scored	Albuterol Sulfate 2 mg	Proventil by Major	00904-2876	Antiasthmatic
MP47	Tab, White, Round, Scored	Albuterol Sulfate 2 mg	Proventil by PDRX	55289-0363	Antiasthmatic
MP47	Tab, White, Round, Scored	Albuterol Sulfate 2 mg	Proventil by Mutual	53489-0176	Antiasthmatic
MP50	Tab, Off-White, Round, Scored	Tolmetin Sodium 200 mg	Tolectin by URL Mutual	00677-1425	NSAID
MP50	Tab, Off-White, Round, Scored	Tolmetin Sodium 200 mg	Tolectin by Mutual	53489-0506	NSAID
MP500	Tab, White to Off-White, Round, Scored	Ketoconazole 200 mg	Nizoral by Mutual	53489-0554	Antifungal
MP500	Tab, White to Off-White, Round, Scored	Ketoconazole 200 mg	Nizoral by Murfreesboro		Antifungal
MP51	Tab, White, Round, Scored	Prednisone 5 mg	Deltasone by URL Mutual	00677-0117	Steroid
MP51	Tab, White, Round, Scored	Prednisone 5 mg	Deltasone by Qualitest	00603-4235	Steroid
MP51	Tab, White, Round, Scored	Prednisone 5 mg	Deltasone by Major	00904-2157	Steroid
MP51	Tab, White, Round, Scored	Prednisone 5 mg	Deltasone by Qualitest	00603-5025	Steroid
MP51	Tab, White, Round, Scored	Prednisone 5 mg	Deltasone by PDRX	55289-0438	Steroid
MP51	Tab, White, Round, Scored	Prednisone 5 mg	Deltasone by Rx Dispensing	61807-0044	Steroid
MP51	Tab, White, Round, Scored	Prednisone 5 mg	Deltasone by Qualitest	00603-3459	Steroid
MP51	Tab, White, Round, Scored	Prednisone 5 mg	Deltasone by H J Harkins Co	52959-0220	Steroid
MP51	Tab, White, Round, Scored	Prednisone 5 mg	Deltasone by Mutual	53489-0138	Steroid
MP51	Tab, White, Round, Scored	Prednisone 5 mg	Deltasone by Pharmedix	53002-0352	Steroid
MP51	Tab, White, Round, Scored	Prednisone 5 mg	Deltasone by Darby Group	66467-4324	Steroid
MP51	Tab, White, Round, Scored	Prednisone 5 mg	Deltasone by Qualitest	00603-5332	Steroid
MP51	Tab, White, Round, Scored	Prednisone 5 mg	Deltasone by UDL	51079-0032 Discontinued	Steroid
MP511	Tab, White, Round, Scored, Film Coated	Propafenone HCl 150 mg	Rythmol by Mutual	53489-0551	Antiarrhythmic
MP511	Tab, White, Round, Scored, Film Coated	Propafenone HCl 150 mg	Rythmol by UDL	51079-0996	Antiarrhythmic
MP512	Tab, White, Round, Scored, Film Coated	Propafenone HCl 225 mg	Rythmol by Mutual	53489-0552	Antiarrhythmic
MP513	Tab, White, Round, Scored, Film Coated	Propafenone HCl 300 mg	Rythmol by Mutual	53489-0553	Antiarrhythmic
MP514	Tab, Blue, Cap Shaped	Sotalol 80 mg	Betapace by URL	00677-1709	Antiarrhythmic
MP52	Tab, White, Round, Scored	Prednisone 10 mg	Deltasone by Major	00904-2141	Steroid
MP52	Tab, White, Round, Scored	Prednisone 10 mg	Deltasone by URL Mutual	00677-0698	Steroid
MP52	Tab, White, Round, Scored	Prednisone 10 mg	Deltasone by Darby Group	66467-4325	Steroid
MP52	Tab, White, Round, Scored	Prednisone 10 mg	Deltasone by Mutual	53489-0139	Steroid
MP52	Tab, White, Round, Scored	Prednisone 10 mg	Deltasone by Qualitest	00603-5333	Steroid
MP52	Tab, White, Round, Scored	Prednisone 10 mg	Deltasone by Pharmedix	53002-0309	Steroid
MP52	Tab, White, Round, Scored	Prednisone 10 mg	Deltasone by H J Harkins Co	52959-0126	Steroid

ID FRONT <> BACK	DESCRIPTION FRONT <> BACK	INGREDIENT & STRENGTH	BRAND (or Generic Equiv.) by FIRM	NDC#	CLASS; SCH.
MP52	Tab, White, Round, Scored	Prednisone 10 mg	Deltasone by UDL	51079-0033 Discontinued	Steroid
MP53	Tab, Peach, Round, Scored	Prednisone 20 mg	Deltasone by Major	00904-2140	Steroid
MP53	Tab, Peach, Round, Scored	Prednisone 20 mg	Deltasone by URL Mutual	00677-0427	Steroid
MP53	Tab, Peach, Round, Scored	Prednisone 20 mg	Deltasone by Qualitest	00603-3763	Steroid
MP53	Tab, Peach, Round, Scored	Prednisone 20 mg	Deltasone by Mutual	53489-0140	Steroid
MP53	Tab, Peach, Round, Scored	Prednisone 20 mg	Deltasone by Rx Dispensing	61807-0067	Steroid
MP53	Tab, Peach, Round, Scored	Prednisone 20 mg	Deltasone by St. Mary's Med	60760-0002	Steroid
MP53	Tab, Peach, Round, Scored	Prednisone 20 mg	Deltasone by PDRX	55289-0352	Steroid
MP53	Tab, Peach, Round, Scored	Prednisone 20 mg	Deltasone by Direct Dispensing	57866-4326	Steroid
MP53	Tab, Peach, Round, Scored	Prednisone 20 mg	Deltasone by UDL	51079-0022 Discontinued	Steroid
MP53 <> 1332	Tab, Peach, Round, Scored	Prednisone 20 mg	Deltasone by Southwood	58016-0217	Steroid
MP532	Tab, Light Orange, Round	Lovastatin 10 mg	Mevacor by Mutual	53489-0607	Antihyperlipidemic
MP533	Tab, Light Blue, Round	Lovastatin 20 mg	Mevacor by Mutual	53489-0608	Antihyperlipidemic
MP534	Tab, Light Green, Round	Lovastatin 40 mg	Mevacor by Mutual	53489-0609	Antihyperlipidemic
MP542	Tab, White, Round, Scored, Film Coated	Spironolactone 50 mg	Aldactone by Pliva	53489-0550	Diuretic
MP542	Tab, White, Round, Scored, Film Coated	Spironolactone 50 mg	Aldactone by Mutual	53489-0328	Diuretic
MP55	Tab	Hydralazine HCl 50 mg	by Mutual	53489-0125	Antihypertensive
MP55	Tab	Hydralazine HCl 50 mg	by Kaiser	00179-0345	Antihypertensive
MP556	Tab, Yellow, Round	Meloxicam 7.5mg	Mobic by Mutual	53489-0620	NSAID
MP557	Tab, Yellow, Round	Meloxicam 15mg	Mobic by Mutual	53489-0621	NSAID
MP573	Tab, White, Round	Doxycycline Hyclate 20 mg	Periostat by Mutual	53489-0550	Antibiotic
MP577	Tab, White, Round	Cyclobenzaprine HCl 10 mg	Flexeril by Mutual	53489-0591	Muscle Relaxant
MP58	Tab, White, Round, MP over 58	Carisoprodol 350 mg	Soma by Major	00904-0355	Muscle Relaxant
MP58	Tab, White, Round, MP over 58	Carisoprodol 350 mg	Soma by Rx Dispensing	61807-0047	Muscle Relaxant
MP58	Tab, White, Round, MP over 58	Carisoprodol 350 mg	Soma by Darby Group	66467-3435	Muscle Relaxant
MP58	Tab, White, Round, MP over 58	Carisoprodol 350 mg	Soma by Direct Dispensing	57866-3435	Muscle Relaxant
MP58	Tab, White, Round, MP over 58	Carisoprodol 350 mg	Soma by PDRX	55289-0049	Muscle Relaxant
MP58	Tab, White, Round, MP over 58	Carisoprodol 350 mg	Soma by Kaiser	62224-7333	Muscle Relaxant
MP58	Tab, White, Round, MP over 58	Carisoprodol 350 mg	Soma by Kaiser	00179-0171	Muscle Relaxant
MP58	Tab, White, Round, MP over 58	Carisoprodol 350 mg	Soma by H J Harkins Co	52959-0026	Muscle Relaxant
MP58	Tab, White, Round, MP over 58	Carisoprodol 350 mg	Soma by Pharmedix	53002-0356	Muscle Relaxant
MP58	Tab, White, Round, MP over 58	Carisoprodol 350 mg	Soma by Mutual	53489-0110	Muscle Relaxant
MP58	Tab, White, Round, MP over 58	Carisoprodol 350 mg	Soma by URL Mutual	00677-0589	Muscle Relaxant
MP58	Tab, White, Round, MP over 58	Carisoprodol 350 mg	Soma by Qualitest	00603-2582	Muscle Relaxant
MP58	Tab, White, Round, MP over 58	Carisoprodol 350 mg	Soma by Urgent Care Center	50716-0202	Muscle Relaxant
MP58	Tab, White, Round, MP over 58	Carisoprodol 350 mg	Soma by UDL	51079-0055	Muscle Relaxant
MP58	Tab, White, Round, MP over 58	Carisoprodol 350 mg	Soma by Ivax	00182-1079	Muscle Relaxant
MP6	Tab, White, Round	Lorazepam 0.5 mg	Ativan by Mutual	53489-0357	Antianxiety; C IV
MP6	Tab, White	Lorazepam 0.5 mg	Ativan by Major	00904-1500	Antianxiety; C IV
MP6	Tab, White, Round	Lorazepam 0.5 mg	Ativan by URL Mutual	00677-1056	Antianxiety; C IV
MP64	Tab	Hydralazine HCl 25 mg	by Mutual	53489-0124	Antihypertensive
MP64	Tab	Hydralazine HCl 25 mg	by Pharmedix	53002-0429	Antihypertensive
MP64	Tab	Hydralazine HCl 25 mg	by URL Mutual	00677-0447	Antihypertensive
MP64	Tab	Hydralazine HCl 25 mg	by Kaiser	00179-0344	Antihypertensive
MP65	Tab, White, Scored	Acetazolamide 125 mg	Diamox by Mutual	53489-0166	Antiglaucoma Agent
MP65	Tab, White, Scored	Acetazolamide 125 mg	Diamox by URL Mutual	00677-1248	Antiglaucoma Agent
MP657	Tab, Yellow, Round	Clonidine HCl 0.1 mg	Catapres by Mutual	53489-0215	Antihypertensive
MP658	Tab, Yellow, Round	Clonidine HCl 0.2 mg	Catapres by Mutual	53489-0216	Antihypertensive

ID FRONT <> BACK	DESCRIPTION FRONT <> BACK	INGREDIENT & STRENGTH	BRAND (or Generic Equiv.) by FIRM	NDC#	CLASS; SCH.
MP659	Tab, Green, Round	Clonidine HCl 0.3 mg	Catapres by Mutual	53489-0217	Antihypertensive
MP66	Tab, White to Off White, Round, Ex Release, MP over 66	Quinidine Gluconate 324 mg	Quinaglute by Qualitest	00603-5598	Antiarrhythmic
MP66	Tab, White to Off White, Round, Ex Release, MP over 66	Quinidine Gluconate 324 mg	Quinaglute by URL Mutual	00677-0675	Antiarrhythmic
MP66	Tab, White to Off White, Round, Ex Release, MP over 66	Quinidine Gluconate 324 mg	Quinaglute by Ivax	00182-1382	Antiarrhythmic
MP66	Tab, White to Off White, Round, Ex Release, MP over 66	Quinidine Gluconate 324 mg	Quinaglute by UDL	51079-0027	Antiarrhythmic
MP66	Tab, White to Off White, Round, Ex Release, MP over 66	Quinidine Gluconate 324 mg	Quinaglute by Mutual	53489-0141	Antiarrhythmic
MP68	Tab	Tolazamide 100 mg	by Mutual	53489-0151	Antidiabetic
MP69	Tab, Film Coated	Verapamil HCl 80 mg	by Mutual	53489-0154	Antihypertensive
MP7	Tab, Purple, Round, Film Coated	Hydroxyzine HCl 25 mg	Atarax by Mutual	53489-0127	Antianxiety; Antihistamine
MP7	Tab, Purple, Round, Film Coated	Hydroxyzine HCl 25 mg	Atarax by Pharmedix	53002-0320	Antianxiety; Antihistamine
MP7	Tab, Purple, Round, Film Coated	Hydroxyzine HCl 25 mg	Atarax by URL Mutual	00677-0605	Antianxiety; Antihistamine
MP70	Tab	Tolazamide 250 mg	by Mutual	53489-0152	Antidiabetic
MP71	Tab, White, Round, Scored	Allopurinol 100 mg	Zyloprim by Major	00904-2613	Antigout
MP71	Tab, White, Round, Scored	Allopurinol 100 mg	Zyloprim by Mutual	53489-0156	Antigout
MP71	Tab, White, Round, Scored	Allopurinol 100 mg	Zyloprim by URL Mutual	00677-0870	Antigout
MP71	Tab, White, Round, Scored	Allopurinol 100 mg	Zyloprim by Qualitest	00603-2117	Antigout
MP711	Tab, Red, Round, Scored, Film Coated	Bisoprolol Fumarate 5 mg	Zebeta by Mutual	53489-0555	Antihypertensive
MP712	Tab, White, Round, Film Coated	Bisoprolol Fumarate 10 mg	Zebeta by Mutual	53489-0556	Antihypertensive
MP717	Tab, White, Round, Film Coated	Tramadol HCl 50 mg	Ultram by Mutual	53489-0499	Analgesic
MP72	Tab	Tolazamide 500 mg	by Mutual	53489-0153	Antidiabetic
MP727	Tab, Yellow, Round	Folic Acid 1 mg	Folic Acid by Mutual	53489-0580	Vitamin
MP737	Tab, White, Round, Scored	Primidone 50 mg	Mysoline by Mutual	53489-0602	Anticonvulsant
MP738	Tab, Yellow, Round, Scored	Primidone 250 mg	Mysoline by Mutual	53489-0603	Anticonvulsant
MP74	Tab	Chlorzoxazone 500 mg	by URL Mutual	00677-1221	Muscle Relaxant
MP74	Tab	Chlorzoxazone 500 mg	by Mutual	53489-0193	Muscle Relaxant
MP751	Tab, White, Round, Film Coated	Metformin HCl 500 mg	Glucophage by Major	00904-5601	Antidiabetic
MP751	Tab, White, Round, Film Coated	Metformin HCl 500 mg	Glucophage by Mutual	53489-0467	Antidiabetic
MP752	Tab, White, Round, Film Coated	Metformin HCl 850 mg	Glucophage by Major	00904-5602	Antidiabetic
MP752	Tab, White, Round, Film Coated	Metformin HCl 850 mg	Glucophage by Mutual	53489-0468	Antidiabetic
MP753	Tab, White, Oval, Film Coated	Metformin HCl 1000 mg	Glucophage by Mutual	53489-0469	Antidiabetic
MP753	Tab, White, Oval, Film Coated	Metformin HCl 1000 mg	Glucophage by Major	00904-5603	Antidiabetic
MP76	Tab, Film Coated	Verapamil HCl 120 mg	by Mutual	53489-0155	Antihypertensive
MP77	Tab, White, Round	Ibuprofen 200 mg	Motrin by Mutual		NSAID
MP771	Tab, Light Green, Round, Film Coated, ER	Felodipine 2.5 mg	Plendil ER by Mutual	53489-0368	Antihypertensive
MP772	Tab, Light Orange, Round, Film Coated, ER	Felodipine 5 mg	Plendil ER by Mutual	53489-0369	Antihypertensive
MP773	Tab, Brown, Film Coated, ER	Felodipine 10 mg	Plendil ER by Mutual	53489-0370	Antihypertensive
MP79	Tab, Green, Round, Film Coated	Imipramine HCl 50 mg	Tofranil by Qualitest	00603-4045	Antidepressant
MP79	Tab, Green, Round, Film Coated	Imipramine HCl 50 mg	Tofranil by Mutual	53489-0332	Antidepressant
MP79	Tab, Green, Round, Film Coated	Imipramine HCl 50 mg	Tofranil by Allscripts		Antidepressant
MP79	Tab, Green, Round, Film Coated	Imipramine HCl 50 mg	Tofranil by URL Mutual	00677-0423	Antidepressant
MP8	Tab, Brown, Round, Film Coated	Imipramine HCl 25 mg	Tofranil by URL Mutual	00677-0422	Antidepressant
MP8	Tab, Brown, Round, Film Coated	Imipramine HCl 25 mg	Tofranil by Allscripts		Antidepressant
MP8	Tab, Brown, Round, Film Coated	Imipramine HCl 25 mg	Tofranil by Mutual	53489-0331	Antidepressant
MP80	Tab, Orange, Round, Scored	Allopurinol 300 mg	Zyloprim by Golden State	60429-0014	Antigout
MP80	Tab, Orange, Round, Scored	Allopurinol 300 mg	Zyloprim by Qualitest	00603-2118	Antigout
MP80	Tab, Orange, Round, Scored	Allopurinol 300 mg	Zyloprim by URL Mutual	00677-0871	Antigout
MP80	Tab, Orange, Round, Scored	Allopurinol 300 mg	Zyloprim by Kaiser	00179-1212	Antigout
MP80	Tab, Orange, Round, Scored	Allopurinol 300 mg	Zyloprim by Mutual	53489-0157	Antigout
MP80	Tab, Orange, Round, Scored	Allopurinol 300 mg	Zyloprim by Major	00904-2614	Antigout

ID FRONT <> BACK	DESCRIPTION FRONT <> BACK	INGREDIENT & STRENGTH	BRAND (or Generic Equiv.) by FIRM	NDC#	CLASS; SCH.
MP80	Tab, Orange, Round, Scored	Allopurinol 300 mg	Zyloprim by Pharmedix	53002-0482	Antigout
MP81	Tab, White, Round, Scored	Sulfamethoxazole 400 mg, Trimethoprim 80 mg	Bactrim by Southwood	58016-0171	Antibiotic
MP81	Tab, White, Round, Scored	Sulfamethoxazole 400 mg, Trimethoprim 80 mg	Bactrim by Ivax	00182-1478	Antibiotic
MP81	Tab, White, Round, Scored	Sulfamethoxazole 400 mg, Trimethoprim 80 mg	Bactrim by ESI Lederle	59911-5859	Antibiotic
MP81	Tab, White, Round, Scored	Sulfamethoxazole 400 mg, Trimethoprim 80 mg	Bactrim by Murfreesboro	51129-1438	Antibiotic
MP81	Tab, White, Round, Scored	Sulfamethoxazole 400 mg, Trimethoprim 80 mg	Bactrim by Major	00904-2726	Antibiotic
MP81	Tab, White, Round, Scored	Sulfamethoxazole 400 mg, Trimethoprim 80 mg	Bactrim by URL Mutual	00677-0783	Antibiotic
MP81	Tab, White, Round, Scored	Sulfamethoxazole 400 mg, Trimethoprim 80 mg	Bactrim by Mutual	53489-0145	Antibiotic
MP81	Tab, White, Round, Scored	Sulfamethoxazole 400 mg, Trimethoprim 80 mg	Bactrim by Kaiser	00179-0371	Antibiotic
MP81	Tab, White, Round, Scored	Sulfamethoxazole 400 mg, Trimethoprim 80 mg	Bactrim by Darby Group	66467-4692	Antibiotic
MP83	Tab, Brown, Round, Film Coated	Nystatin 500,000 Units	Mycostatin by Major	00904-0672	Antifungal
MP83	Tab, Brown, Round, Film Coated	Nystatin 500,000 Units	Mycostatin by Murfreesboro	51129-1360	Antifungal
MP83	Tab, Brown, Round, Film Coated	Nystatin 500,000 Units	Mycostatin by URL Mutual	00677-0613	Antifungal
MP83	Tab, Brown, Round, Film Coated	Nystatin 500,000 Units	Mycostatin by Mutual	53489-0400	Antifungal
MP84	Tab, White, Round, Scored	Minoxidil 2.5 mg	Loniten by Mutual	53489-0386	Antihypertensive
MP85	Tab, White, Oval, Scored	Sulfamethoxazole 800 mg, Trimethoprim 160 mg	Bactrim DS by West-Ward	00143-1625	Antibiotic
MP85	Tab, White, Oval, Scored	Sulfamethoxazole 800 mg, Trimethoprim 160 mg	Bactrim DS by Mutual	53489-0146	Antibiotic
MP85	Tab, White, Oval, Scored	Sulfamethoxazole 800 mg, Trimethoprim 160 mg	Bactrim DS by Apotheca	12634-0177	Antibiotic
MP85	Tab, White, Oval, Scored	Sulfamethoxazole 800 mg, Trimethoprim 160 mg	Bactrim DS by St. Mary's Med	60760-0076	Antibiotic
MP85	Tab, White, Oval, Scored	Sulfamethoxazole 800 mg, Trimethoprim 160 mg	Bactrim DS by ESI Lederle	59911-5860	Antibiotic
MP85	Tab, White, Oval, Scored	Sulfamethoxazole 800 mg, Trimethoprim 160 mg	Bactrim DS by Golden State	60429-0170	Antibiotic
MP85	Tab, White, Oval, Scored	Sulfamethoxazole 800 mg, Trimethoprim 160 mg	Bactrim DS by Qualitest	00603-5779	Antibiotic
MP85	Tab, White, Oval, Scored	Sulfamethoxazole 800 mg, Trimethoprim 160 mg	Bactrim DS by URL Mutual	00677-0784	Antibiotic
MP85	Tab, White, Oval, Scored	Sulfamethoxazole 800 mg, Trimethoprim 160 mg	Bactrim DS by UDL	51079-0128	Antibiotic
MP85	Tab, White, Oval, Scored	Sulfamethoxazole 800 mg, Trimethoprim 160 mg	Bactrim DS by Pharmedix	53002-0210	Antibiotic
MP85	Tab, White, Oval, Scored	Sulfamethoxazole 800 mg, Trimethoprim 160 mg	Bactrim DS by Major	00904-2725	Antibiotic
MP85	Tab, White, Oval, Scored	Sulfamethoxazole 800 mg, Trimethoprim 160 mg	Bactrim DS by Amneal	65162-0313	Antibiotic
MP88	Tab, White, Round, Scored	Albuterol Sulfate 4 mg	Proventil by Mutual	53489-0177	Antiasthmatic
MP88	Tab, White, Round, Scored	Albuterol Sulfate 4 mg	Proventil by URL Mutual	00677-1360	Antiasthmatic
MP88	Tab, White, Round, Scored	Albuterol Sulfate 4 mg	Proventil by Major	00904-2877	Antiasthmatic
MP89	Tab, White, Round, Scored	Minoxidil 10 mg	Loniten by Mutual	53489-0387	Antihypertensive
MP9	Tab, White, Round	Atenolol 25 mg	Tenormin by Mutual	53489-0536	Antihypertensive
MP9	Tab, White, Round	Atenolol 25 mg	Tenormin by URL Mutual	00677-1633	Antihypertensive
MP91	Tab, Yellow, Round, Scored	Sulfasalazine 500 mg	by Murfreesboro	51129-1408	Gastrointestinal
MP91	Tab, Yellow, Round, Scored	Sulfasalazine 500 mg	by Darby Group	66467-4617	Gastrointestinal
MP91	Tab, Yellow, Round, Scored	Sulfasalazine 500 mg	by Ivax	00182-1016	Gastrointestinal
MP91	Tab, Yellow, Round, Scored	Sulfasalazine 500 mg	by Mutual	53489-0147	Gastrointestinal
MP91	Tab, Yellow, Round, Scored	Sulfasalazine 500 mg	by URL Mutual	00677-0483	Gastrointestinal
MP91	Tab, Yellow, Round, Scored	Sulfasalazine 500 mg	by Qualitest	00603-5802	Gastrointestinal
MP93	Tab	Quinidine Sulfate 100 mg	by Mutual	53489-0459	Antiarrhythmic
MP94	Tab, White, Round	Ibuprofen 300 mg	Motrin by Mutual		NSAID
MP95	Tab, Film Coated	Ibuprofen 400 mg	Motrin by West-Ward	00143-1300	NSAID
MP95	Tab, Film Coated	Ibuprofen 400 mg	Motrin by URL Mutual	00677-1031	NSAID
MP96	Tab, White, Round, Scored	Lorazepam 2 mg	Ativan by Mutual	53489-0359	Antianxiety; C IV
MP96	Tab, White, Round, Scored	Lorazepam 2 mg	Ativan by URL Mutual	00677-1058	Antianxiety; C IV
MP98	Tab, Film Coated	Ibuprofen 600 mg	Motrin by West-Ward	00143-1302	NSAID
MP98	Tab, Film Coated	Ibuprofen 600 mg	Motrin by URL Mutual	00677-1032	NSAID
MP98	Tab, Film Coated	Ibuprofen 600 mg	Motrin by St. Mary's Med	60760-0119	NSAID
MP99	Tab, Film Coated	Ibuprofen 800 mg	Motrin by West-Ward	00143-1304	NSAID
MP99 <> 800	Tab, Film Coated	Ibuprofen 800 mg	Motrin by URL Mutual	00677-1119	NSAID

ID FRONT <> BACK	DESCRIPTION FRONT <> BACK	INGREDIENT & STRENGTH	BRAND (or Generic Equiv.) by FIRM by Allscripts	NDC#	CLASS; SCH.
MPALTACE5MG	Cap, Red, Gelatin	Ramipril 5 mg			Antihypertensive
MPC	Tab, Red, Rectangular, Film Coated	Ferrous Fumarate 90 mg	Ferrous Fumarate by Mission	00178-0085	Supplement
MPC <> 500	Tab, White, Round	Acetohydroxamic Acid 250 mg	Lithostat by Mission	00178-0500	Urinary Tract
MPC <> CALCET	Tab, Yellow, Rectangular, Film Coated	Vitamin D 200 IU, Calcium 300 mg	Calcet by Mission	00178-0251	Vitamin; Supplement
MPC <> CITRACAL	Tab, White, Barrel Shaped, Film Coated	Calcium Citrate 200 mg	Citracal by Mission	00178-0800	Vitamin; Supplement
MPC <> CITRACAL	Tab, White, Barrel Shaped, Film Coated	Calcium Citrate 200 mg	Citracal by Mission	Canadian DIN 02150220	Vitamin; Supplement
MPC100	Tab, Yellow, Cap Shaped, Scored	Chlorpheniramine Maleate 4 mg, Hydrocodone Bitartrate 5 mg, Pseudoephedrine HCl 60 mg	Tussend by Monarch	61570-0011	Cold Remedy; C III
MPC188 <> ANEXSIA	Tab, White, Cap Shaped, Scored	Acetaminophen 650 mg, Hydrocodone Bitartrate 7.5 mg	Lorcet Plus by Med Pro	53978-3309	Analgesic; C III
MPC188 <> ANEXSIA	Tab, White, Cap Shaped, Scored	Acetaminophen 650 mg, Hydrocodone Bitartrate 7.5 mg	Lorcet Plus by Nat Pharmpak	55154-7101	Analgesic; C III
MPC188 <> ANEXSIA	Tab, White, Cap Shaped, Scored	Acetaminophen 650 mg, Hydrocodone Bitartrate 7.5 mg	Lorcet Plus by King	60793-0843	Analgesic; C III
MPC207 <> ANEXSIA	Tab, White, Round, Scored	Acetaminophen 500 mg, Hydrocodone Bitartrate 5 mg	Vicodin by King	60793-0842	Analgesic; C III
MPC600	Tab, Light Yellow, Round, Ex Release	Potassium Citrate 540 mg	Urocit K by Mission	Canadian DIN 01914022	Electrolytes
MPC600	Tab, Light Yellow, Round, Ex Release	Potassium Citrate 540 mg	Urocit K by Mission	00178-0600	Electrolytes
MPC610 <> MISSION	Tab, Light Yellow, Oval	Potassium Citrate 1080 mg	Urocit K by Mission	00178-0610	Electrolytes
MPC7	Tab, Coated	Calcium Ascorbate, Calcium Carbonate, Precipitated, Cupric Oxide, Cyanocobalamin 8 mcg, Ferrous Fumarate, Folic Acid 1 mg, Niacinamide, Potassium Iodide, Pyridoxine HCl, Riboflavin 2 mg, Thiamine Mononitrate, Vitamin A Acetate, Vitamin D 400 Units, Zinc Sulfate	Mission Prenatal Rx by Mission	00178-0007 Discontinued	Vitamin; Mineral
MPC900	Tab, Round, White, Sugar Coated	Tiopronin 100 mg	Thiola by Mission	00178-0900	Urinary Tract
MPELDERCAPS	Cap, Red	Ascorbic Acid 200 mg, Calcium Pantothenate 10 mg, Cholecalciferol 400 Units, Folic Acid 1 mg, Magnesium Sulfate, Manganese Sulfate, Niacinamide 25 mg, Pyridoxine HCl 2 mg, Riboflavin 5 mg, Thiamine Mononitrate 10 mg, Vitamin A 4000 Units, Alpha-tocopherol 25 Units, Zinc Sulfate	Eldercaps by Merz	00259-0393	Vitamin
MPELDERCAPS	Cap, Red	Ascorbic Acid 200 mg, Calcium Pantothenate 10 mg, Cholecalciferol 400 Units, Folic Acid 1 mg, Magnesium Sulfate, Manganese Sulfate, Niacinamide 25 mg, Pyridoxine HCl 2 mg, Riboflavin 5 mg, Thiamine Mononitrate 10 mg, Vitamin A 4000 Units, Vitamin E 25 Units, Zinc Sulfate	Eldercaps by Anabolic	00722-6386	Vitamin
MPELDERCAPS	Tab, Red, Oblong	Multivitamin With Folic Acid 1 mg	Eldercaps by Merz		Vitamin
MR	Tab, White, Oblong, M/R	Guaifenesin 200 mg	Aquabid by Merz		Expectorant
MR	Tab	Acetaminophen 325 mg, Dextromethorphan HBr 15 mg, Guaifenesin 100 mg, Phenylpropanolamine HCl 25 mg	Anatuss by Merz	00259-2244	Cold Remedy
MR <> 0379	Tab, Off-White, Film Coated	Guaifenesin 400 mg, Pseudoephedrine HCl 120 mg	Sudafed Sinus by Merz	00259-0379	Cold Remedy
MR <> GEIGY	Tab, White w/ Red Specks, Round, Scored	Carbamazepine 100 mg	Tegretol by Novartis	Canadian DIN 00369810	Anticonvulsant
MR <> P	Tab, White with Red Specks, Scored, P <> M/R	Carbamazepine 100 mg	Tegretol by Pharmascience	Canadian DIN 02231542	Anticonvulsant
MR0382	Tab, Orange, M/R 0382	Guaifenesin 400 mg, Dextromethorphan 20 mg, Pseudoephedrine HCl 60 mg	Robitussin by Vintage		Cold Remedy
MR1278	Tab, White, Oblong, Scored	Butalbital 50 mg, Acetaminophen 650 mg	Sedapap by Merz	00259-1278	Analgesic
MR15 <> G	Tab, Round, Yellow, Scored, Film Coated	Mirtazapine 15 mg	Remeron by Par	49884-0655	Antidepressant
MR30 <> G	Tab, Round, Buff, Scored, Film Coated	Mirtazapine 30 mg	Remeron by Par	49884-0656	Antidepressant
MR45 <> G	Tab, White, Round, Film Coated	Mirtazapine 45 mg	Remeron by Par	49884-0873	Antidepressant
MRK <> 266	Tab, Light Pink, Cap Shaped	Rizatriptan Benzoate 5 mg	Maxalt by Merck	00006-0266	Antimigraine
MRK <> 936	Tab, White, Oval	Alendronate Sodium 10 mg	Fosamax by Merck	00006-0936	Antiosteoporosis
MRK <> 936	Tab, White, Oval	Alendronate Sodium 10 mg	Fosamax by Merck Frosst	Canadian DIN 02201011	Antiosteoporosis

ID FRONT <> BACK	DESCRIPTION FRONT <> BACK	INGREDIENT & STRENGTH	BRAND (or Generic Equiv.) by FIRM	NDC#	CLASS; SCH.
MRK <> 951	Tab, Light Green, Tear Drop Shaped, Film Coated	Losartan Potassium 25 mg	Cozaar by Merck Frosst	Canadian DIN 02182815	Antihypertensive
MRK <> 951	Tab, Light Green, Tear Drop Shaped, Film Coated	Losartan Potassium 25 mg	Cozaar by Nat Pharmpak	55154-5009	Antihypertensive
MRK <> 960	Tab, Dark Green, Teardrop Shaped, Film Coated	Losartan Potassium 100 mg	Cozaar by Merck Frosst	Canadian DIN 02182882	Antihypertensive
MRK110 <> VIOXX	Tab, Yellow, Round	Rofecoxib 25 mg	Vioxx by Allscripts	Discontinued	NSAID
MRK110 <> VIOXX	Tab, Yellow, Round	Rofecoxib 25 mg	Vioxx by RX Pak	65084-0201	NSAID
MRK110 <> VIOXX	Tab, Yellow, Round	Rofecoxib 25 mg	Vioxx by Merck	00006-0110 Discontinued	NSAID
MRK114 <> VIOXX	Tab, Orange, Round	Rofecoxib 50 mg	Vioxx by Merck	00006-0114 Discontinued	NSAID
MRK117 <> SINGULAIR	Tab, Beige, Square, Film Coated	Montelukast Sodium 10 mg	Singulair by Murfreesboro	51129-1398	Antiasthmatic
MRK117 <> SINGULAIR	Tab, Beige, Square, Film Coated	Montelukast Sodium 10 mg	Singulair by Merck	00006-0117	Antiasthmatic
MRK212 <> FOSAMAX	Tab, White, Triangular	Alendronate Sodium 40 mg	Fosamax by Merck Frosst	Canadian DIN 02201038	Antiosteoporosis
MRK212 <> FOSAMAX	Tab, White, Triangular	Alendronate Sodium 40 mg	Fosamax by Merck	00006-0212	Antiosteoporosis
MRK267 <> MAXALT	Tab, Light Pink, Cap Shaped	Rizatriptan Benzoate 10 mg	Maxalt by Merck	00006-0267	Antimigraine
MRK275 <> SINGULAIR	Tab, Pink, Round, Chewable	Montelukast Sodium 5 mg	Singulair by Merck	00006-0275	Antiasthmatic
MRK275 <> SINGULAIR	Tab, Pink, Round, Chewable	Montelukast Sodium 5 mg	Singulair by Neuman	64579-0348	Antiasthmatic
MRK71 <> PROPECIA	Tab, Tan, Octagonal, Film Coated	Finasteride 1 mg	Propecia by Southwood	58016-0329	Antiandrogen
MRK71 <> PROPECIA1	Tab, Tan, Octagonal, Film Coated	Finasteride 1 mg	Propecia by Physician Total Care	54868-4120	Antiandrogen
MRK711 <> SINGULAIR	Tab, Pink, Oval, Chewable	Montelukast Sodium 4 mg	Singulair by Merck	00006-0711	Antiasthmatic
MRK717 <> HYZAAR	Tab, Yellow, Teardrop Shaped, Film Coated	Hydrochlorothiazide 12.5 mg, Losartan Potassium 50 mg	Hyzaar by Merck Frosst	Canadian DIN 02230047	Diuretic; Antihypertensive
MRK717 <> HYZAAR	Tab, Yellow, Teardrop Shaped, Film Coated	Hydrochlorothiazide 12.5 mg, Losartan Potassium 50 mg	Hyzaar by Nat Pharmpak	55154-3011	Diuretic; Antihypertensive
MRK717 <> HYZAAR	Tab, Yellow, Teardrop Shaped, Film Coated	Hydrochlorothiazide 12.5 mg, Losartan Potassium 50 mg	Hyzaar by Merck	00006-0717	Diuretic; Antihypertensive
MRK74 <> VIOXX	Tab, Off-White, Round	Rofecoxib 12.5 mg	Vioxx by DRX	55045-2720 Discontinued	NSAID
MRK74 <> VIOXX	Tab, Off-White, Round	Rofecoxib 12.5 mg	Vioxx by Allscripts	Discontinued	NSAID
MRK74 <> VIOXX	Tab, Off-White, Round	Rofecoxib 12.5 mg	Vioxx by Physician Total Care	54868-4148	NSAID
MRK74 <> VIOXX	Tab, Off-White, Round	Rofecoxib 12.5 mg	Vioxx by RX Pak	65084-0199	NSAID
MRK74 <> VIOXX	Tab, Off-White, Round	Rofecoxib 12.5 mg	Vioxx by Merck	00006-0074 Discontinued	NSAID
MRK747 <> HYZAAR	Tab, Light Yellow, Teardrop Shaped	Hydrochlorothiazide 25 mg, Losartan Potassium 100 mg	Hyzaar by Merck Frosst	Canadian DIN 02241007	Diuretic; Antihypertensive
MRK747 <> HYZAAR	Tab, Light Yellow, Teardrop Shaped	Hydrochlorothiazide 25 mg, Losartan Potassium 100 mg	Hyzaar by Merck	00006-0747	Diuretic; Antihypertensive
MRK925	Tab, White, Round, MRK over 925 <> Bone Logo	Alendronate Sodium 5 mg	Fosamax by Murfreesboro	51129-1356	Antiosteoporosis
MRK925	Tab, White, Round, MRK over 925 <> Bone Logo	Alendronate Sodium 5 mg	Fosamax by Merck	00006-0925	Antiosteoporosis
MRK925	Tab, White, Round, MRK over 925 <> Bone Logo	Alendronate Sodium 5 mg	Fosamax by Merck Frosst	Canadian DIN 02233055	Antiosteoporosis
MRK936 <> FOSAMAX	Tab, White, Round, Bone Logo on both sides	Alendronate Sodium 10 mg	Fosamax by Physician Total Care	54868-3857	Antiosteoporosis
MRK936 <> FOSAMAX	Tab, White, Round, Bone Logo on both sides	Alendronate Sodium 10 mg	Fosamax by Heartland	61392-0854	Antiosteoporosis
MRK936 <> FOSAMAX	Tab, White, Round, Bone Logo on both sides	Alendronate Sodium 10 mg	Fosamax by MSD	Canadian	Antiosteoporosis
MRK952 <> COZAAR	Tab, Green, Teardrop Shaped, Film Coated	Losartan Potassium 50 mg	Cozaar by Physician Total Care	54868-3726	Antihypertensive
MRK952 <> COZAAR	Tab, Green, Teardrop Shaped, Film Coated	Losartan Potassium 50 mg	Cozaar by Merck Frosst	Canadian DIN 02182874	Antihypertensive
MRK952 <> COZAAR	Tab, Green, Teardrop Shaped, Film Coated	Losartan Potassium 50 mg	Cozaar by Nat Pharmpak	55154-5016	Antihypertensive
MS1	Tab, Light Green, Round, Scored, M / S1	Sertraline HCl 25 mg	Zoloft by Mylan	00378-4186	Antidepressant

ID FRONT <> BACK	DESCRIPTION FRONT <> BACK	INGREDIENT & STRENGTH	BRAND (or Generic Equiv.) by FIRM	NDC#	CLASS; SCH.
MS1	Tab, Light Green, Scored, M over S1	Sertraline HCl 25 mg	Zoloft by UDL	51079-0762	Antidepressant
MS2	Tab, Light Green, Scored, M over S2	Sertraline HCl 50 mg	Zoloft by UDL	51079-0763	Antidepressant
MS2	Tab, Light Green, Round, Scored, M / S2	Sertraline HCl 50 mg	Zoloft by Mylan	00378-4187	Antidepressant
MS23	Tab, Light Peach, Round, Scored	Sotalol HCl 80 mg	Betapace by Mylan	00378-0305	Antiarrhythmic
MS24	Tab, Light Peach, Round, Scored	Sotalol HCl 120 mg	Betapace by Mylan	00378-0310	Antiarrhythmic
MS25	Tab, Light Peach, Round, Scored	Sotalol HCl 160 mg	Betapace by Mylan	00378-0314	Antiarrhythmic
MS3	Tab, Light Green, Oval, Scored, M / S3	Sertraline HCl 100 mg	Zoloft by Mylan	00378-4188	Antidepressant
MS3	Tab, Light Green, Scored, M over S3	Sertraline HCl 100 mg	Zoloft by UDL	51079-0764	Antidepressant
MS958	Tab, White, Round	Aspirin 325 mg	Aspirin by Medtech		Analgesic
MSAP	Tab, White, Oblong	Aspirin 500 mg	Aspirin by Medtech		Analgesic
MSD	Cap, Blue & White	Indomethacin 25 mg	Indocin by MSD	Canadian	NSAID
MSD	Cap, Opaque Blue & White	Indomethacin 50 mg	Indocin by MSD	Canadian	NSAID
MSD	Tab, White	Ethacrynic Acid 50 mg	by MSD	Canadian	Diuretic
MSD	Tab	Phytonadione 5 mg	Mephyton by H J Harkins Co	52959-0424	Vitamin
MSD <> 15	Tab, White, Round	Lisinopril 2.5 mg	Prinivil by Merck	00006-0015	Antihypertensive
MSD <> 173	Tab, Green, Squared Cap Shape	Enalapril Maleate 5 mg, Hydrochlorothiazide 12.5 mg	Vaseretic by Merck-Frosst	Canadian DIN 02242826	Antihypertensive; Diuretic
MSD <> 173	Tab, Green, Squared Cap Shape	Enalapril Maleate 5 mg, Hydrochlorothiazide 12.5 mg	Vaseretic by Biovail	64455-0145	Antihypertensive; Diuretic
MSD <> 173	Tab, Green, Squared Cap Shape	Enalapril Maleate 5 mg, Hydrochlorothiazide 12.5 mg	Vaseretic by Merck	00006-0173	Antihypertensive; Diuretic
MSD <> 266	Tab, Pale Pink, Cap-Shaped	Rizatriptan 5 mg	Maxalt by Merck Frosst	Canadian DIN 02240520	Antimigraine
MSD <> 32	Tab, White, Round	Ivermectin 3 mg	Stromectol by Merck	00006-0032	Antihelmintic
MSD <> 32	Tab, White, Round	Ivermectin 3 mg	Stromectol by Murfreesboro	51129-1590	Antihelmintic
MSD102	Tab, Beige, Discoid	Amitriptyline HCl 75 mg	Elavil by MSD	Canadian	Antidepressant
MSD105	Tab, Peach	Hydrochlorothiazide 50 mg	Hydrodiuril by MSD	Canadian	Diuretic; Antihypertensive
MSD105 <> HYDRODIURIL	Tab, Peach, Round, Scored, MSD on Left, 105 on Right	Hydrochlorothiazide 50 mg	Hydrodiuril by Merck	00006-0105	Diuretic; Antihypertensive
MSD106 <> PRINIVIL	Tab, Yellow, Oval	Lisinopril 10 mg	Prinivil by Med Pro	53978-3015	Antihypertensive
MSD106 <> PRINIVIL	Tab, Yellow, Oval	Lisinopril 10 mg	Prinivil by PDRX	55289-0929	Antihypertensive
MSD106 <> PRINIVIL	Tab, Yellow, Oval	Lisinopril 10 mg	Prinivil by DRX	55045-2292	Antihypertensive
MSD106 <> PRINIVIL	Tab, Yellow, Oval	Lisinopril 10 mg	Prinivil by Nat Pharmpak	55154-5015	Antihypertensive
MSD106 <> PRINIVIL	Tab, Yellow, Oval	Lisinopril 10 mg	Prinivil by Merck	00006-0106	Antihypertensive
MSD106 <> PRINIVIL	Tab, Yellow, Oval	Lisinopril 10 mg	Prinivil by Amerisource	62584-0925	Antihypertensive
MSD106 <> PRINIVIL	Tab, Yellow, Oval	Lisinopril 10 mg	Prinivil by Pharmacy Care	65070-0012	Antihypertensive
MSD106 <> PRINIVIL	Tab, Yellow, Oval	Lisinopril 10 mg	Prinivil by Merck Frosst	Canadian DIN 00839396	Antihypertensive
MSD117 <> SINGULAIR	Tab, Beige, Rounded Square, Film Coated	Montelukast Sodium 10 mg	Singulair by Merck-Frosst	Canadian DIN 02238217	Antiasthmatic
MSD126	Tab, White, Discoid	Cortisone Acetate 5 mg	Cortisone Tablets by MSD	Canadian Discontinued	Steroid
MSD135 <> ALDOMET	Tab, Yellow, Round	Methyldopa 125 mg	Aldomet by Merck	00006-0135	Antihypertensive
MSD136 <> BLOCADREN	Tab, White, Round, Scored, MSD over 136	Timolol Maleate 10 mg	Blocadren by Merck	00006-0136	Antihypertensive
MSD139	Tab, White, Round, Scored	Ivermectin 6 mg	Stromectol by Merck	00006-0139	Antihelmintic
MSD139	Tab, White, Round, Scored	Ivermectin 6 mg	Stromectol by Merck Sharp & Dohme	52888-8107	Antihelmintic
MSD139	Tab, White, Round, Scored	Ivermectin 6 mg	Stromectol by Merck Sharp & Dohme	52888-0139	Antihelmintic
MSD14	Tab, White, Oval	Enalapril Maleate 2.5 mg	Vasotec by Merck	00006-0014	Antihypertensive
MSD14	Tab, White, Oval	Enalapril Maleate 2.5 mg	Vasotec by Caremark	00339-5413	Antihypertensive
MSD14	Tab, White, Oval	Enalapril Maleate 2.5 mg	Vasotec by Med Pro	53978-1122	Antihypertensive
MSD14	Tab, White, Oval	Enalapril Maleate 2.5 mg	Vasotec by H J Harkins Co	52959-0507	Antihypertensive
MSD14	Tab, White, Oval	Enalapril Maleate 2.5 mg	Vasotec by Nat Pharmpak	55154-5008	Antihypertensive

ID FRONT <> BACK	DESCRIPTION FRONT <> BACK	INGREDIENT & STRENGTH	BRAND (or Generic Equiv.) by FIRM	NDC#	CLASS; SCH.
MSD14	Tab, White, Oval	Enalapril Maleate 2.5 mg	Vasotec by Southwood	58016-0882	Antihypertensive
MSD14	Tab, White, Oval	Enalapril Maleate 2.5 mg	Vasotec by Amerisource	62584-0482	Antihypertensive
MSD14	Tab, White, Oval	Enalapril Maleate 2.5 mg	Vasotec by Biovail	64455-0140	Antihypertensive
MSD14	Tab, White, Oval	Enalapril Maleate 2.5 mg	Vasotec by Merck-Frosst	Canadian DIN 00851795	Antihypertensive
MSD140	Tab, Yellow, Hexagon-Shaped	Lisinopril 20 mg, Hydrochlorothiazide 12.5 mg	Prinzide by Merck Frosst	Canadian DIN 00884413	Antihypertensive; Diuretic
MSD140 <> PRINZIDE	Tab, Yellow, Flower Shaped	Lisinopril 20 mg, HCTZ 12.5 mg	Prinzide by MSD	Canadian	Antihypertensive; Diuretic
MSD140 <> PRINZIDE	Tab, Yellow, Flower Shaped	Lisinopril 20 mg, HCTZ 12.5 mg	Prinzide by Merck	00006-0140	Antihypertensive; Diuretic
MSD142 <> PRINZIDE	Tab, Peach, Flower Shaped	Lisinopril 20 mg, HCTZ 25 mg	Prinzide by MSD	Canadian DIN 00884421	Antihypertensive; Diuretic
MSD142 <> PRINZIDE	Tab, Peach, Flower Shaped	Lisinopril 20 mg, HCTZ 25 mg	Prinzide by Merck	00006-0142	Antihypertensive; Diuretic
MSD145 <> PRINZIDE	Tab, Light Blue, Hexagonal	Lisinopril 10 mg, HCTZ 12.5 mg	Prinzide by MSD	Canadian	Antihypertensive; Diuretic
MSD145 <> PRINZIDE	Tab, Light Blue, Hexagonal	Lisinopril 10 mg, HCTZ 12.5 mg	Prinzide by Merck	00006-0145	Antihypertensive; Diuretic
MSD145 <> PRINZIDE	Tab, Light Blue, Hexagonal	Lisinopril 10 mg, HCTZ 12.5 mg	Prinzide by Murfreesboro	51129-1397	Antihypertensive; Diuretic
MSD19 <> PRINIVIL	Tab, White, Oval, Scored	Lisinopril 5 mg	Prinivil by Pharmacy Care	65070-0014	Antihypertensive
MSD19 <> PRINIVIL	Tab, White, Oval, Scored	Lisinopril 5 mg	Prinivil by Merck	00006-0019	Antihypertensive
MSD19 <> PRINIVIL	Tab, White, Oval, Scored	Lisinopril 5 mg	Prinivil by Nat Pharmpak	55154-5006	Antihypertensive
MSD19 <> PRINIVIL	Tab, White, Oval, Scored	Lisinopril 5 mg	Prinivil by Merck Frosst	Canadian DIN 00839388	Antihypertensive
MSD207 <> PRINIVIL	Tab, Peach, Oval	Lisinopril 20 mg	Prinivil by Merck Frosst	Canadian DIN 00839418	Antihypertensive
MSD207 <> PRINIVIL	Tab, Peach, Oval	Lisinopril 20 mg	Prinivil by Med Pro	53978-3017	Antihypertensive
MSD207 <> PRINIVIL	Tab, Peach, Oval	Lisinopril 20 mg	Prinivil by Merck	00006-0207	Antihypertensive
MSD207 <> PRINIVIL	Tab, Peach, Oval	Lisinopril 20 mg	Prinivil by Pharmacy Care	65070-0013	Antihypertensive
MSD207 <> PRINIVIL	Tab, Peach, Oval	Lisinopril 20 mg	Prinivil by Nat Pharmpak	55154-5011	Antihypertensive
MSD21 <> COGENTIN	Tab, White, Round	Benztropine Mesylate 0.5 mg	Cogentin by Merck	00006-0021	Antiparkinson
MSD214 <> DIURIL	Tab, White, Round, Scored, MSD over 214	Chlorothiazide 250 mg	Diuril by Merck	00006-0214	Diuretic; Antihypertensive
MSD219	Tab, White, Discoid	Cortisone Acetate 25 mg	Cortisone Tablets by MSD	Canadian Discontinued	Steroid
MSD219 <> CORTONE	Tab	Cortisone Acetate 25 mg	by Merck	00006-0219	Steroid
MSD23	Tab, Blue, Discoid	Amitriptyline HCl 10 mg	Elavil by MSD	Canadian	Antidepressant
MSD237 <> PRINIVIL	Tab, Rose Red, Shield Shaped, MSD over 237	Lisinopril 40 mg	Prinivil by Merck	00006-0237	Antihypertensive
MSD25INDOCIN	Cap, Light Blue & White, MSD25 over Indocin	Indomethacin 25 mg	Indocin by Merck	00006-0025	NSAID
MSD26 <> VIVACTIL	Tab, Orange, Oval, Film Coated, MSD over 26	Protriptyline HCl 5 mg	Vivactil by Merck	00006-0026	Antidepressant
MSD267 <> MAXALT	Tab, Pale Pink, Cap-Shaped	Rizatriptan 10 mg	Maxalt by Merck Frosst	Canadian DIN 02240521	Antimigraine
MSD275 <> SINGULAIR	Tab, Pink, Round, Chewable	Montelukast Sodium 5 mg	Singulair by Merck-Frosst	Canadian DIN 02238216	Antiasthmatic
MSD401 <> ALDOMET	Tab, Yellow, Round, Film Coated	Methyldopa 250 mg	Aldomet by Merck	00006-0401	Antihypertensive
MSD401 <> ALDOMET	Tab, Yellow, Round, Film	Methyldopa 250 mg	Aldomet by Neuman	64579-0017	Antihypertensive
MSD403 <> URECHOLINE	Tab, White	Bethanechol Chloride 5 mg	Urecholine by Merck	00006-0403	Urinary Tract
MSD405 <> DIUPRES	Tab	Chlorothiazide 500 mg, Reserpine 0.125 mg	Diupres by Merck	00006-0405	Diuretic; Antihypertensive
MSD41	Tab, White, Pentagonal	Dexamethasone 0.5 mg	Decadron by MSD	Canadian Discontinued	Steroid
MSD41 <> DECADRON	Tab, Yellow, Pentagonal	Dexamethasone 0.5 mg	Decadron by Merck	00006-0041	Steroid
MSD410	Tab, Peach	Hydrochlorothiazide 100 mg	Hydrodiuril by MSD	Canadian	Diuretic; Antihypertensive
MSD42	Tab, Peach	Hydrochlorothiazide 25 mg	Hydrodiuril by MSD	Canadian	Diuretic; Antihypertensive
MSD42 <> HYDRODIURIL	Tab, Peach, Round, Scored	Hydrochlorothiazide 25 mg	Hydrodiuril by Merck	00006-0042	Diuretic; Antihypertensive
MSD423	Tab, Salmon, Biconvex	Hydrochlorothiazide 15 mg, Methyldopa 250 mg	Aldoril 15 by MSD	Canadian	Diuretic; Antihypertensive

ID FRONT <> BACK	DESCRIPTION FRONT <> BACK	INGREDIENT & STRENGTH	BRAND (or Generic Equiv.) by FIRM	NDC#	CLASS; SCH.
MSD423 <> ALDORIL	Tab, Salmon, Round, Film Coated	Hydrochlorothiazide 15 mg, Methyldopa 250 mg	Aldoril 15 by Merck	00006-0423	Diuretic; Antihypertensive
MSD43 <> MEPHYTON	Tab, Yellow, Round, Scored	Vitamin K 5 mg	by PDRX	55289-0793	Vitamin
MSD43 <> MEPHYTON	Tab, Yellow, Round, Scored	Vitamin K 5 mg	Mephyton by Merck	00006-0043	Vitamin
MSD430	Tab, Orange, Discoid	Amitriptyline HCl 75 mg	Elavil by MSD	Canadian	Antidepressant
MSD432 <> DIURIL	Tab, White, Round	Chlorothiazide 500 mg	Diuril by Merck	00006-0432	Diuretic; Antihypertensive
MSD437 <> BLOCADREN	Tab, Light Blue, Cap Shaped	Timolol Maleate 20 mg	Blocadren by Merck	00006-0437	Antihypertensive
MSD45	Tab, Yellow, Discoid	Amitriptyline HCl 25 mg	Elavil by MSD	Canadian	Antidepressant
MSD456	Tab, White, Biconvex	Hydrochlorothiazide 25 mg, Methyldopa 250 mg	Aldoril 25 by MSD	Canadian	Diuretic; Antihypertensive
MSD456 <> ALDORIL	Tab, White, Round, Film Coated	Hydrochlorothiazide 15 mg, Methyldopa 250 mg	Aldoril by Merck	00006-0456	Diuretic; Antihypertensive
MSD47 <> VIVACTIL	Tab, Yellow, Oval, Film Coated	Protriptyline HCl 10 mg	by MSD	Canadian	Antidepressant
MSD47 <> VIVACTIL	Tab, Yellow, Oval, Film Coated	Protriptyline HCl 10 mg	Vivactil by Merck	00006-0047	Antidepressant
MSD49 <> DARANIDE	Tab, Yellow, Round	Dichlorphenamide 50 mg	Daranide by Merck	Discontinued	Carbonic Anhydrase Inhibitor
MSD501	Tab, White, Round	Probenecid 500 mg	Benemid by MSD	Canadian Discontinued	Antigout
MSD50INDOCIN	Cap, Blue & White	Indomethacin 50 mg	Indocin by Merck	00006-0050	NSAID
MSD516 <> ALDOMET	Tab, Yellow, Round, Film Coated	Methyldopa 500 mg	Aldomet by Merck	00006-0516	Antihypertensive
MSD59 <> BLOCADREN	Tab, Light Blue, Round	Timolol Maleate 5 mg	Blocadren by Merck	00006-0059	Antihypertensive
MSD60	Tab, White, Discoid	Benztropine Mesylate 2 mg	Cogentin by MSD	Canadian	Antiparkinson
MSD60 <> COGENTIN	Tab, White, Round	Benztropine Mesylate 2 mg	Cogentin by Merck	00006-0060	Antiparkinson
MSD602CUPRIMINE	Cap, Ivory	Penicillamine 250 mg	Cuprimine by Merck	00006-0602	Chelating Agent
MSD602CUPRIMINE	Cap, Ivory	Penicillamine 250 mg	by MSD	Canadian	Chelating Agent
MSD612	Tab, Coated	Chlorothiazide 150 mg, Methyldopa 250 mg	Aldoclor 150 by Merck	00006-0612	Diuretic; Antihypertensive
MSD619 <> HYDROCORTONE	Tab, White, Oval, Scored	Hydrocortisone 10 mg	Hydrocortone by Merck	00006-0619	Steroid
MSD62	Tab, White, Round, Scored	Cyproheptadine HCl 4 mg	Periactin by Johnson & Johnson	Canadian DIN 00016454	Antihistamine
MSD62 <> PERIACTIN	Tab, White, Round	Cyproheptadine HCl 4 mg	Periactin by Merck	00006-0062	Antihistamine
MSD63 <> DECADRON	Tab, Bluish-Green, Pentagon Shaped	Dexamethasone 0.75 mg	Decadron by Merck	00006-0063	Steroid
MSD634 <> ALDOCLOR	Tab, Green, Oval, Film Coated	Chlorothiazide 250 mg, Methyldopa 250 mg	Aldoclor by Merck	00006-0634	Diuretic; Antihypertensive
MSD635 <> COGENTIN	Tab, White, Oval	Benztropine Mesylate 1 mg	Cogentin by Merck	00006-0635	Antiparkinson
MSD65 <> EDECRIN	Tab, White, Cap Shaped, Scored	Ethacrynic Acid 25 mg	Edecrin by Merck	00006-0065	Diuretic
MSD661SYPRINE	Cap, Light Brown	Trientine HCl 250 mg	Syprine by Merck	00006-0661	Chelating Agent
MSD67 <> TIMOLIDE	Tab, Light Blue, Hexagonal	Timolol Maleate 10 mg, Hydrochlorothiazide 25 mg	Timolide by Merck	00006-0067	Antihypertensive; Diuretic
MSD672	Cap	Penicillamine 125 mg	by DRX	55045-2486	Chelating Agent
MSD672	Cap, Gray & Yellow	Penicillamine 125 mg	by MSD	Canadian	Chelating Agent
MSD672CUPRIMINE	Cap, Gray & Ivory	Penicillamine 125 mg	Cuprimine by Merck	00006-0672	Chelating Agent
MSD675 <> DOLOBID	Tab, Peach, Cap Shaped, Film Coated	Diflunisal 250 mg	Dolobid by Frosst	Canadian	NSAID
MSD675 <> DOLOBID	Tab, Peach, Cap Shaped, Film Coated	Diflunisal 250 mg	Dolobid by Merck	00006-0675	NSAID
MSD690DEMSER	Cap, Blue, Two-Tone	Metyrosine 250 mg	Demser by Merck	00006-0690	Antipheochromocytoma
MSD693	Cap, Clear & Opaque	Indomethacin 75 mg	Indocin SR by MSD	Canadian	NSAID
MSD693INDOCINSR	Cap, Blue & Clear	Indomethacin 75 mg	Indocin SR by Merck	00006-0693	NSAID
MSD694 <> ALDORIL	Tab, Salmon, Round	Hydrochlorothiazide 30 mg, Methyldopa 500 mg	Aldoril by Merck	00006-0694	Diuretic; Antihypertensive
MSD697 <> DOLOBID	Tab, Orange, Cap Shaped	Diflunisal 500 mg	Dolobid by Merck	00006-0697	NSAID
MSD697 <> DOLOBID	Tab, Orange, Cap Shaped	Diflunisal 500 mg	Dolobid by Allscripts		NSAID
MSD705 <> NOROXIN	Tab, Dark Pink, Oval, Film Coated, MSD over 705	Norfloxacin 400 mg	Noroxin by MSD	Canadian	Antibiotic
MSD705 <> NOROXIN	Tab, Dark Pink, Oval, Film Coated, MSD over 705	Norfloxacin 400 mg	Noroxin by Quality Care	60346-0563	Antibiotic
MSD705 <> NOROXIN	Tab, Dark Pink, Oval, Film Coated, MSD over 705	Norfloxacin 400 mg	Noroxin by DRX	55045-2419	Antibiotic
MSD705 <> NOROXIN	Tab, Dark Pink, Oval, Film Coated, MSD over 705	Norfloxacin 400 mg	Noroxin by Roberts	54092-0097	Antibiotic
MSD705 <> NOROXIN	Tab, Dark Pink, Oval, Film Coated, MSD over 705	Norfloxacin 400 mg	Noroxin by Merck	00006-0705	Antibiotic

ID FRONT <> BACK	DESCRIPTION FRONT <> BACK	INGREDIENT & STRENGTH	BRAND (or Generic Equiv.) by FIRM	NDC#	CLASS; SCH.
MSD705 <> NOROXIN	Tab, Dark Pink, Oval, Film Coated, MSD over 705	Norfloxacin 400 mg	Noroxin by Allscripts		Antibiotic
MSD707 <> TONOCARD	Tab, Yellow, Oval, Scored, Film Coated	Tocainide HCl 400 mg	Tonocard by Merck	00006-0707	Antiarrhythmic
MSD707 <> TONOCARD	Tab, Yellow, Oval, Scored, Film Coated	Tocainide HCl 400 mg	Tonocard by Teva	00480-0089	Antiarrhythmic
MSD709 <> TONOCARD	Tab, Yellow, Oblong, Scored, Film Coated	Tocainide HCl 600 mg	Tonocard by Teva	00480-0090	Antiarrhythmic
MSD709 <> TONOCARD	Tab, Yellow, Oblong, Scored, Film Coated	Tocainide HCl 600 mg	Tonocard by Merck	00006-0709	Antiarrhythmic
MSD711 <> SINGULAIR	Tab, Pink, Oval, Chewable	Montelukast Sodium 4 mg	Singulair by Merck-Frosst	Canadian DIN 02243602	Antiasthmatic
MSD712	Tab, White, Triangle Shaped, Scored	Enalapril Maleate 5 mg	Vasotec by Biovail	64455-0141	Antihypertensive
MSD712	Tab, White, Triangle Shaped, Scored	Enalapril Maleate 5 mg	Vasotec by Merck-Frosst	Canadian DIN 00708879	Antihypertensive
MSD712	Tab, White, Triangle Shaped, Scored	Enalapril Maleate 5 mg	Vasotec by PDRX	55289-0622	Antihypertensive
MSD712	Tab, White, Triangle Shaped, Scored	Enalapril Maleate 5 mg	Vasotec by Southwood	58016-0572	Antihypertensive
MSD712	Tab, White, Triangle Shaped, Scored	Enalapril Maleate 5 mg	Vasotec by Amerisource	62584-0483	Antihypertensive
MSD712	Tab, White, Triangle Shaped, Scored	Enalapril Maleate 5 mg	Vasotec by Merck	00006-0712	Antihypertensive
MSD712	Tab, White, Triangle Shaped, Scored	Enalapril Maleate 5 mg	Vasotec by Med Pro	53978-0176	Antihypertensive
MSD712	Tab, White, Triangle Shaped, Scored	Enalapril Maleate 5 mg	Vasotec by DRX	55045-2319	Antihypertensive
MSD712	Tab, White, Triangle Shaped, Scored	Enalapril Maleate 5 mg	Vasotec by H J Harkins Co	52959-0531	Antihypertensive
MSD712	Tab, White, Triangle Shaped, Scored	Enalapril Maleate 5 mg	Vasotec by Pharmedix	53002-1021	Antihypertensive
MSD712	Tab, White, Triangle Shaped, Scored	Enalapril Maleate 5 mg	Vasotec by Nat Pharmpak	55154-5001	Antihypertensive
MSD713	Tab, Salmon, Triangle Shaped, Scored	Enalapril Maleate 10 mg	Vasotec by Merck	00006-0713	Antihypertensive
MSD713	Tab, Salmon, Triangle Shaped, Scored	Enalapril Maleate 10 mg	Vasotec by H J Harkins Co	52959-0505	Antihypertensive
MSD713	Tab, Salmon, Triangle Shaped, Scored	Enalapril Maleate 10 mg	Vasotec by Nat Pharmpak	55154-5003	Antihypertensive
MSD713	Tab, Salmon, Triangle Shaped, Scored	Enalapril Maleate 10 mg	Vasotec by Med Pro	53978-3013	Antihypertensive
MSD713	Tab, Salmon, Triangle Shaped, Scored	Enalapril Maleate 10 mg	Vasotec by Amerisource	62584-0484	Antihypertensive
MSD713	Tab, Salmon, Triangle Shaped, Scored	Enalapril Maleate 10 mg	Vasotec by Southwood	58016-0569	Antihypertensive
MSD713	Tab, Salmon, Triangle Shaped, Scored	Enalapril Maleate 10 mg	Vasotec by Merck-Frosst	Canadian DIN 00670901	Antihypertensive
MSD713	Tab, Salmon, Triangle Shaped, Scored	Enalapril Maleate 10 mg	Vasotec by Biovail	64455-0142	Antihypertensive
MSD714	Tab, Peach, Triangle Shaped, Scored	Enalapril Maleate 20 mg	Vasotec by Biovail	64455-0143	Antihypertensive
MSD714	Tab, Peach, Triangle Shaped, Scored	Enalapril Maleate 20 mg	Vasotec by Merck-Frosst	Canadian DIN 00670928	Antihypertensive
MSD714	Tab, Peach, Triangle Shaped, Scored	Enalapril Maleate 20 mg	Vasotec by DRX	55045-2364	Antihypertensive
MSD714	Tab, Peach, Triangle Shaped, Scored	Enalapril Maleate 20 mg	Vasotec by Nat Pharmpak	55154-5013	Antihypertensive
MSD714	Tab, Peach, Triangle Shaped, Scored	Enalapril Maleate 20 mg	Vasotec by Med Pro	53978-3016	Antihypertensive
MSD714	Tab, Peach, Triangle Shaped, Scored	Enalapril Maleate 20 mg	Vasotec by Merck	00006-0714	Antihypertensive
MSD714	Tab, Peach, Triangle Shaped, Scored	Enalapril Maleate 20 mg	Vasotec by Caremark	00339-5415	Antihypertensive
MSD714	Tab, Peach, Triangle Shaped, Scored	Enalapril Maleate 20 mg	Vasotec by Southwood	58016-0571	Antihypertensive
MSD72 <> PROSCAR	Tab, Blue, Apple Shaped, Film Coated	Finasteride 5 mg	Proscar by Integrity	64731-0754	Antiandrogen
MSD72 <> PROSCAR	Tab, Blue, Apple Shaped, Film Coated	Finasteride 5 mg	Proscar by Merck-Frosst	Canadian DIN 02010909	Antiandrogen
MSD72 <> PROSCAR	Tab, Blue, Apple Shaped, Film Coated	Finasteride 5 mg	Proscar by Physician Total Care	54868-2719	Antiandrogen
MSD72 <> PROSCAR	Tab, Blue, Apple Shaped, Film Coated	Finasteride 5 mg	Proscar by Merck	00006-0072	Antiandrogen
MSD720	Tab, Rust, Squared Cap Shape, Scored	Enalapril Maleate 10 mg, Hydrochlorothiazide 25 mg	Vaseretic by Merck-Frosst	Canadian DIN 00657298	Antihypertensive; Diuretic
MSD720 <> VASERETIC	Tab, Rust, Squared Cap Shape	Enalapril Maleate 10 mg, Hydrochlorothiazide 25 mg	Vaseretic by Biovail	64455-0146	Antihypertensive; Diuretic
MSD720 <> VASERETIC	Tab, Rust, Squared Cap Shape	Enalapril Maleate 10 mg, Hydrochlorothiazide 25 mg	Vaseretic by Merck	00006-0720	Antihypertensive; Diuretic
MSD726 <> ZOCOR5	Tab, Buff, Oval, Film Coated	Simvastatin 5 mg	Zocor by Merck-Frosst	Canadian DIN 00884324	Antihyperlipidemic
MSD726 <> ZOCOR5	Tab, Buff, Shield Shaped, Film Coated, MSD over 726	Simvastatin 5 mg	Zocor by Merck	00006-0726	Antihyperlipidemic
MSD730 <> MEVACOR	Tab, Peach, Octagonal, MSD over 730	Lovastatin 10 mg	Mevacor by Kaiser	00179-1209	Antihyperlipidemic

ID FRONT <> BACK	DESCRIPTION FRONT <> BACK	INGREDIENT & STRENGTH	BRAND (or Generic Equiv.) by FIRM	NDC#	CLASS; SCH.
MSD730 <> MEVACOR	Tab, Peach, Octagonal, MSD over 730	Lovastatin 10 mg	Mevacor by Nat Pharmpak	55154-3618	Antihyperlipidemic
MSD730 <> MEVACOR	Tab, Peach, Octagonal, MSD over 730	Lovastatin 10 mg	Mevacor by Merck	00006-0730	Antihyperlipidemic
MSD731 <> MEVACOR	Tab, Blue, Octagonal, MSD over 731	Lovastatin 20 mg	Mevacor by Va Cmop	65243-0045	Antihyperlipidemic
MSD731 <> MEVACOR	Tab, Blue, Octagonal, MSD over 731	Lovastatin 20 mg	Mevacor by Allscripts		Antihyperlipidemic
MSD731 <> MEVACOR	Tab, Blue, Octagonal, MSD over 731	Lovastatin 20 mg	Mevacor by Nat Pharmpak	55154-5004	Antihyperlipidemic
MSD731 <> MEVACOR	Tab, Blue, Octagonal, MSD over 731	Lovastatin 20 mg	Mevacor by Merck	00006-0731	Antihyperlipidemic
MSD731 <> MEVACOR	Tab, Blue, Octagonal, MSD over 731	Lovastatin 20 mg	Mevacor by Pharmedix	53002-0570	Antihyperlipidemic
MSD731 <> MEVACOR	Tab, Blue, Octagonal, MSD over 731	Lovastatin 20 mg	Mevacor by Amerisource	62584-0426	Antihyperlipidemic
MSD731 <> MEVACOR	Tab, Blue, Octagonal, MSD over 731	Lovastatin 20 mg	Mevacor by PDRX	55289-0400	Antihyperlipidemic
MSD731 <> MEVACOR	Tab, Blue, Octagonal, MSD over 731	Lovastatin 20 mg	Mevacor by Merck Frosst	Canadian DIN 00795860	Antihyperlipidemic
MSD732 <> MEVACOR	Tab, Light Green, Octagonal, MSD over 732	Lovastatin 40 mg	Mevacor by Merck Frosst	Canadian DIN 00795852	Antihyperlipidemic
MSD732 <> MEVACOR	Tab, Light Green, Octagonal, MSD over 732	Lovastatin 40 mg	Mevacor by PDRX	55289-0548	Antihyperlipidemic
MSD732 <> MEVACOR	Tab, Light Green, Octagonal, MSD over 732	Lovastatin 40 mg	Mevacor by Merck	00006-0732	Antihyperlipidemic
MSD735	Tab, Peach, Oval, Film Coated, MSD over 735	Simvastatin 10 mg	Zocor by Merck-Frosst	Canadian DIN 00884332	Antihyperlipidemic
MSD735	Tab, Peach, Shield Shaped, Film Coated, MSD over 735	Simvastatin 10 mg	Zocor by Southwood	58016-0364	Antihyperlipidemic
MSD735	Tab, Peach, Shield Shaped, Film Coated, MSD over 735	Simvastatin 10 mg	Zocor by Va Cmop	65243-0064	Antihyperlipidemic
MSD735	Tab, Peach, Shield Shaped, Film Coated, MSD over 735	Simvastatin 10 mg	Zocor by Merck	00006-0735	Antihyperlipidemic
MSD735	Tab, Peach, Shield Shaped, Film Coated, MSD over 735	Simvastatin 10 mg	Zocor by Caremark	00339-5795	Antihyperlipidemic
MSD735	Tab, Peach, Shield Shaped, Film Coated, MSD over 735	Simvastatin 10 mg	Zocor by Med Pro	53978-3069	Antihyperlipidemic
MSD735	Tab, Peach, Shield Shaped, Film Coated, MSD over 735	Simvastatin 10 mg	Zocor by Nat Pharmpak	55154-5012	Antihyperlipidemic
MSD735	Tab, Peach, Shield Shaped, Film Coated, MSD over 735	Simvastatin 10 mg	Zocor by DRX	55045-2316	Antihyperlipidemic
MSD740	Tab, Tan, Shield Shaped, Film Coated, MSD over 740	Simvastatin 20 mg	Zocor by Southwood	58016-0385	Antihyperlipidemic
MSD740	Tab, Tan, Shield Shaped, Film Coated, MSD over 740	Simvastatin 20 mg	Zocor by Va Cmop	65243-0065	Antihyperlipidemic
MSD740	Tab, Tan, Shield Shaped, Film Coated, MSD over 740	Simvastatin 20 mg	Zocor by Med Pro	53978-3370	Antihyperlipidemic
MSD740	Tab, Tan, Shield Shaped, Film Coated, MSD over 740	Simvastatin 20 mg	Zocor by Merck	00006-0740	Antihyperlipidemic
MSD740	Tab, Tan, Shield Shaped, Film Coated, MSD over 740	Simvastatin 20 mg	Zocor by Physician Total Care	54868-3104	Antihyperlipidemic
MSD740	Tab, Tan, Oval, Film Coated, MSD over 740	Simvastatin 20 mg	Zocor by Merck-Frosst	Canadian DIN 00884340	Antihyperlipidemic
MSD749	Tab, Brick Red, Oval, Film Coated, MSD over 749	Simvastatin 40 mg	Zocor by Merck-Frosst	Canadian DIN 00884359	Antihyperlipidemic
MSD749	Tab, Peach to Light Red, Shield Shaped, Film Coated, MSD over 749	Simvastatin 40 mg	Zocor by Va Cmop	65243-0082	Antihyperlipidemic
MSD749	Tab, Peach to Light Red, Shield Shaped, Film Coated, MSD over 749	Simvastatin 40 mg	Zocor by Merck	00006-0749	Antihyperlipidemic
MSD749	Tab, Peach to Light Red, Shield Shaped, Film Coated, MSD over 749	Simvastatin 40 mg	Zocor by Caremark	00339-5798	Antihyperlipidemic
MSD749	Tab, Peach to Light Red, Shield Shaped, Film Coated, MSD over 749	Simvastatin 40 mg	Zocor by Kaiser	00179-1331	Antihyperlipidemic
MSD90 <> EDECRIN	Tab, Green, Cap Shaped, Scored	Ethacrynic Acid 50 mg	Edecrin by Merck	00006-0090	Diuretic
MSD907 <> MINTEZOL	Tab, White, Round, Chewable	Thiabendazole 500 mg	Mintezol by Merck	00006-0907	Antihelmintic
MSD917 <> M	Tab, Peach, Diamond Shaped, Scored	Amiloride HCl 5 mg, Hydrochlorothiazide 50 mg	Moduretic by Merck	00006-0917	Antihypertensive; Diuretic
MSD92	Tab, Yellow, Diamond	Amiloride HCl 5 mg	Midamor by MSD	Canadian	Diuretic
MSD92 <> MIDAMOR	Tab, Yellow, Diamond Shaped	Amiloride HCl 5 mg	Midamor by Merck	00006-0092	Diuretic
MSD921	Tab, Orange, Triangular	Amitriptyline 25 mg, Perphenazine 2 mg	Triavil by MSD	Canadian	Antidepressant; Antipsychotic
MSD931	Tab, Yellow, D-Shaped, Film	Cyclobenzaprine HCl 10 mg	Flexeril by DJ Pharma	64455-0014	Muscle Relaxant
MSD931 <> FLEXERIL	Tab, Butterscotch Yellow, D-Shaped, Film Coated	Cyclobenzaprine HCl 10 mg	Flexeril by Merck	00006-0931	Muscle Relaxant

ID FRONT <> BACK	DESCRIPTION FRONT <> BACK	INGREDIENT & STRENGTH	BRAND (or Generic Equiv.) by FIRM	NDC#	CLASS; SCH.
MSD931 <> FLEXERIL	Tab, Butterscotch Yellow, D-Shaped, Film Coated	Cyclobenzaprine HCl 10 mg	Flexeril by Allscripts		Muscle Relaxant
MSD931 <> FLEXERIL	Tab, Butterscotch Yellow, D-Shaped, Film Coated	Cyclobenzaprine HCl 10 mg	Flexeril by Nat Pharmpak	55154-5007	Muscle Relaxant
MSD931 <> FLEXERIL	Tab, Butterscotch Yellow, D-Shaped, Film Coated	Cyclobenzaprine HCl 10 mg	Flexeril by Allscripts		Muscle Relaxant
MSD935 <> ALDORIL	Tab, White, Oval, Film Coated	Hydrochlorothiazide 50 mg, Methyldopa 500 mg	Aldoril by Merck	00006-0935	Diuretic; Antihypertensive
MSD941 <> CLINORIL	Tab, Bright Yellow, Hexagonal	Sulindac 200 mg	Clinoril by Merck	00006-0941	NSAID
MSD942 <> CLINORIL	Tab, Bright Yellow, Hexagonal	Sulindac 200 mg	Clinoril by Merck	00006-0942	NSAID
MSD942 <> CLINORIL	Tab, Bright Yellow, Hexagonal	Sulindac 200 mg	Clinoril by Merck	62904-0942	NSAID
MSD942 <> CLINORIL	Tab, Bright Yellow, Hexagonal	Sulindac 200 mg	Clinoril by Merck	62904-0941	NSAID
MSD963	Tab, Beige, Square, Film Coated	Famotidine 20 mg	Pepcid by Merck Frosst	Canadian DIN 00710121	Gastrointestinal
MSD963 <> PEPCID	Tab, Beige, U-Shaped, MSD over 963, Film Coated	Famotidine 20 mg	Pepcid by Allscripts		Gastrointestinal
MSD963 <> PEPCID	Tab, Beige, U-Shaped, Film Coated	Famotidine 20 mg	by PDRX	55289-0162	Gastrointestinal
MSD963 <> PEPCID	Tab, Beige, U-Shaped, Film Coated	Famotidine 20 mg	Pepcid by H J Harkins Co	52959-0465	Gastrointestinal
MSD963 <> PEPCID	Tab, Beige, U-Shaped, Film Coated	Famotidine 20 mg	by Med Pro	53978-0518	Gastrointestinal
MSD963 <> PEPCID	Tab, Beige, U-Shaped, Film Coated	Famotidine 20 mg	by Amerisource	62584-0440	Gastrointestinal
MSD963 <> PEPCID	Tab, Beige, U-Shaped, Film Coated	Famotidine 20 mg	Pepcid by Merck	00006-0963	Gastrointestinal
MSD963 <> PEPCID	Tab, Beige, U-Shaped, Film Coated	Famotidine 20 mg	by Nat Pharmpak	55154-5005	Gastrointestinal
MSD964	Tab, Dark Reddish Brown, Square, Film Coated	Famotidine 40 mg	Pepcid by Merck Frosst	Canadian DIN 00710113	Gastrointestinal
MSD964 <> PEPCID	Tab, Dark Reddish Brown, U-Shaped, Film Coated	Famotidine 40 mg	Pepcid by Merck	00006-0964	Gastrointestinal
MSD964 <> PEPCID	Tab, Dark Reddish Brown, U-Shaped, Film Coated	Famotidine 40 mg	by PDRX	55289-0146	Gastrointestinal
MSD97	Tab, White, Pentagonal	Dexamethasone 4 mg	Decadron by MSD	Canadian Discontinued	Steroid
MSD97 <> DECADRON	Tab, Blue-Green, Pentagonal	Dexamethasone 4 mg	Decadron by Merck	00006-0097	Steroid
MSM	Tab, White, Oval	Magnesium Salicylate 580 mg	MD Mentom by Medtech		Analgesic
MSM	Tab, White, Football	Magnesium Salicylate 467 mg	Momentum by Whitehall Robins		Analgesic
MSTSM500	Cap, Green	Acetaminophen 500 mg, Pseudoephedrine HCl 30 mg	Tylenol Sinus Ex Strength by McNeil	Canadian DIN 00663980	Cold Remedy
MT11	Tab, White, Round, Film Coated	Topiramate 25 mg	Topamax by UDL	51079-0726	Anticonvulsant
MT12	Tab, White, Round, Film Coated	Topiramate 50 mg	Topamax by UDL	51079-0727	Anticonvulsant
MT13	Tab, White, Round, Film Coated	Topiramate 100 mg	Topamax by UDL	51079-0728	Anticonvulsant
MT20ULTRASE	Cap, Gray & Yellow	Amylase 65,000 Units, Lipase 20,000 Units, Protease 65,000 Units	Ultrase MT 20 by Eurand	57298-0052	Gastrointestinal
MTP10 <> APO	Tab, Pale Green, Round, Scored	Methylphenidate HCl 10 mg	Ritalin by Apotex	Canadian DIN 02249324	Stimulant; C II
MTP20 <> APO	Tab, Yellow, Round, Scored	Methylphenidate HCl 20 mg	Ritalin by Apotex	Canadian DIN 02249332	Stimulant; C II
MTP5 <> APO	Tab, Peach, Round	Methylphenidate HCl 5 mg	Ritalin by Apotex	Canadian DIN 02273950	Stimulant; C II
MU11	Tab, Light Green, Round, ER	Bupropion HCl 100 mg	Wellbutrin SR by Mylan	00378-3411	Antidepressant
MU11	Tab, Light Green, Round, ER	Bupropion HCl 100 mg	Wellbutrin SR by UDL	51079-0391	Antidepressant
MU12	Tab, Light Green, Round, ER	Bupropion HCl 150 mg	Wellbutrin SR by UDL	51079-0392	Antidepressant
MU12	Tab, Light Green, Round, ER	Bupropion HCl 150 mg	Wellbutrin SR by Mylan	00378-3412	Antidepressant
MU13	Tab, Light Green, Round, ER	Bupropion HCl 200 mg	Wellbutrin SR by Mylan	00378-3413	Antidepressant
MUCOFEN	Tab, White, Elliptical, Scored, Ex Release	Guaifenesin 1000 mg	Muco-Fen by Ivax Labs	59310-0118	Cold Remedy
MUCOFEN	Tab, White, Oval, Scored, Ex Release	Guaifenesin 800 mg	Muco-Fen 800 by Ivax Labs	59310-0109	Expectorant
MUCOFEN	Tab, White, Oval, Scored, Ex Release	Guaifenesin 800 mg	Muco-Fen 800 by Eli Lilly		Expectorant
MUCOFEN800DM	Tab, White, Oval, Scored, Mucofen over 800 DM	Guaifenesin 800 mg, Dextromethorphan Hydrobromide 60 mg	by Med Pro	53978-3360	Cold Remedy
MUCOFENDM	Tab, White, Oval, Scored, Ex Release	Guaifenesin 600 mg, Dextromethorphan HBr 30 mg	by Pfab	62542-0726	Cold Remedy
MUCOFENDM	Tab, White, Oval, Scored, Ex Release	Dextromethorphan HBr 30 mg, Guaifenesin 600 mg	Mucofen DM by Anabolic	00722-6355	Cold Remedy

ID FRONT <> BACK	DESCRIPTION FRONT <> BACK	INGREDIENT & STRENGTH	BRAND (or Generic Equiv.) by FIRM	NDC#	CLASS; SCH.
MUCOFENDM	Tab, White, Oval, Scored, Ex Release	Dextromethorphan HBr 30 mg, Guaifenesin 600 mg	Muco Fen DM by Ivax Labs	59310-0108	Cold Remedy
MUCOFENDM	Tab, White, Elliptical, Scored, Ex Release	Dextromethorphan 60 mg, Guaifenesin 1000 mg	Muco-Fen DM by Ivax Labs	59310-0119	Cold Remedy
MUCOFENLA	Tab, White, Oval, Scored, Ex Release	Guaifenesin 600 mg	Robitussin by Anabolic	00722-6249	Expectorant
MUCOFENLA	Tab, White, Oval, Scored, Ex Release	Guaifenesin 600 mg	Robitussin by Pfab	62542-0706	Expectorant
MURO1212BROMFED	Cap, Light Green, Ex Release, MURO 12-120 <>	Brompheniramine Maleate 12 mg, Pseudoephedrine HCl 120 mg	by Thrift Drug	59198-0190	Cold Remedy
MURO1212BROMFED	Cap, Muro 12-120 <> Bromfed	Brompheniramine Maleate 6 mg, Pseudoephedrine HCl 60 mg	Bromfed by Muro	00451-4000	Cold Remedy
MURO40060	Tab, Purple, Muro 400/60	Pseudoephedrine HCl 60 mg, Guaifenesin 400 mg	Guaitab by Central		Cold Remedy
MURO4060	Tab	Brompheniramine Maleate 4 mg, Pseudoephedrine HCl 60 mg	by PDRX	55289-0807	Cold Remedy
MURO4060	Tab	Brompheniramine Maleate 6 mg, Pseudoephedrine HCl 60 mg	Bromfed by Muro		Cold Remedy
MURO660BROMFEDPD	Cap, Muro 6-60 <> Bromfed-PD	Brompheniramine Maleate 6 mg, Pseudoephedrine HCl 60 mg	by Nat Pharmpak	55154-4301	Cold Remedy
MURO660BROMFEDPD	Cap, Muro 6-60 <> Bromfed-PD	Brompheniramine Maleate 6 mg, Pseudoephedrine HCl 60 mg	Bromfed PD by Muro	00451-4001	Cold Remedy
MURO660BROMFEDPD	Cap, Dark Green, Ex Release, Muro 6-60 <> Bromfed-PD	Brompheniramine Maleate 6 mg, Pseudoephedrine HCl 60 mg	Bromfed PD by Thrift Drug	59198-0189	Cold Remedy
MUTUAL100	Cap, Light Blue & White, Black Print, Opaque, MUTUAL over 100	Doxycycline Hyclate 50 mg	Vibramycin by Allscripts		Antibiotic
MUTUAL100	Cap, Light Blue & White, Black Print, Opaque, MUTUAL over 100	Doxycycline Hyclate 50 mg	Vibramycin by Qualitest	00603-3480	Antibiotic
MUTUAL100	Cap, Light Blue & White, Black Print, Opaque, MUTUAL over 100	Doxycycline Hyclate 50 mg	Vibramycin by URL Mutual	00677-0598	Antibiotic
MUTUAL100	Cap, Light Blue & White, Black Print, Opaque, MUTUAL over 100	Doxycycline Hyclate 50 mg	Vibramycin by Mutual	53489-0118	Antibiotic
MUTUAL100	Cap, Light Blue & White, Black Print, Opaque, MUTUAL over 100	Doxycycline Hyclate 50 mg	Vibramycin by DRX	55045-2731	Antibiotic
MUTUAL100	Cap, Light Blue & White, Black Print, Opaque, MUTUAL over 100	Doxycycline Hyclate 50 mg	Vibramycin by Major	00904-0427	Antibiotic
MUTUAL101	Cap	Indomethacin 25 mg	Indocin by Pharmedix	53002-0305	NSAID
MUTUAL101	Cap	Indomethacin 25 mg	Indocin by Mutual	53489-0133	NSAID
MUTUAL101	Cap	Indomethacin 25 mg	Indocin by URL Mutual	00677-0872	NSAID
MUTUAL102	Cap, Clear	Quinine Sulfate 324 mg	Quinine Sulfate by Mutual	53489-0221	Antimalarial
MUTUAL102	Cap, Clear	Quinine Sulfate 324 mg	Quinine Sulfate by URL Mutual	00677-1647	Antimalarial
MUTUAL102	Cap, Clear	Quinine Sulfate 324 mg	Quinine Sulfate by Allscripts		Antimalarial
MUTUAL103	Cap, Clear & Pink	Diphenhydramine HCl 25 mg	by URL Mutual	00677-0063	Antihistamine
MUTUAL103	Cap, Clear & Pink	Diphenhydramine HCl 25 mg	by Pharmedix	53002-0314	Antihistamine
MUTUAL103	Cap, Clear & Pink	Diphenhydramine HCl 25 mg	by Allscripts		Antihistamine
MUTUAL103	Cap, Clear & Pink	Diphenhydramine HCl 100 mg	by Mutual	53489-0113	Antihistamine
MUTUAL103	Cap, Clear & Pink	Diphenhydramine HCl 100 mg	by Direct Dispensing	57866-3594	Antihistamine
MUTUAL105	Cap, Light Blue, Black Print, Opaque, MUTUAL over 105	Doxycycline Hyclate 100 mg	Vibramycin by Allscripts		Antibiotic
MUTUAL105	Cap, Light Blue, Black Print, Opaque, MUTUAL over 105	Doxycycline Hyclate 100 mg	Vibramycin by Darby Group	66467-0230	Antibiotic
MUTUAL105	Cap, Light Blue, Black Print, Opaque, MUTUAL over 105	Doxycycline Hyclate 100 mg	Vibramycin by St. Mary's Med	60760-0562	Antibiotic
MUTUAL105	Cap, Light Blue, Black Print, Opaque, MUTUAL over 105	Doxycycline Hyclate 100 mg	Vibramycin by Direct Dispensing	57866-0341	Antibiotic
MUTUAL105	Cap, Light Blue, Black Print, Opaque, MUTUAL over 105	Doxycycline Hyclate 100 mg	Vibramycin by Mutual	53489-0119	Antibiotic
MUTUAL105	Cap, Light Blue, Black Print, Opaque, MUTUAL over 105	Doxycycline Hyclate 100 mg	Vibramycin by URL Mutual	00677-0562	Antibiotic
MUTUAL105	Cap, Light Blue, Black Print, Opaque, MUTUAL over 105	Doxycycline Hyclate 100 mg	Vibramycin by H J Harkins Co	52959-0055	Antibiotic
MUTUAL105	Cap, Light Blue, Black Print, Opaque, MUTUAL over 105	Doxycycline Hyclate 100 mg	Vibramycin by Qualitest	00603-3481	Antibiotic
MUTUAL106	Cap	Indomethacin 50 mg	Indocin by Pharmedix	53002-0350	NSAID
MUTUAL106	Cap	Indomethacin 50 mg	Indocin by Mutual	53489-0134	NSAID
MUTUAL106	Cap	Indomethacin 50 mg	Indocin by Talbert	44514-0453	NSAID
MUTUAL106	Cap	Indomethacin 50 mg	Indocin by URL Mutual	00677-0873	NSAID
MUTUAL106	Cap	Indomethacin 50 mg	Indocin by Mutual		NSAID
MUTUAL107	Cap	Diphenhydramine HCl 50 mg	by URL Mutual	00677-0064	Antihistamine

ID FRONT <> BACK	DESCRIPTION FRONT <> BACK	INGREDIENT & STRENGTH	BRAND (or Generic Equiv.) by FIRM	NDC#	CLASS; SCH.
MUTUAL107	Cap	Diphenhydramine HCl 50 mg	by Pharmedix	53002-0331	Antihistamine
MUTUAL107	Cap, Pink	Diphenhydramine HCl 50 mg	by Mutual	53489-0114	Antihistamine
MUTUAL107	Cap	Diphenhydramine HCl 50 mg	by Allscripts		Antihistamine
MUTUAL165	Cap	Piroxicam 10 mg	Feldene by URL Mutual	00677-1430	NSAID
MUTUAL166	Cap	Piroxicam 20 mg	Feldene by URL Mutual	00677-1431	NSAID
MUTUAL179	Cap	Tolmetin Sodium 400 mg	by Mutual	53489-0507	NSAID
MUTUAL179	Cap	Tolmetin Sodium 400 mg	by Allscripts		NSAID
MUTUAL179	Cap, Yellow, Opaque	Tolmetin Sodium 400 mg	by URL Mutual	00677-1424	NSAID
MUTUAL274	Cap, Blue, Mutual over 400	Phentermine HCl 30 mg	Phentermine by Mutual	53489-0433	Anorexiant; C IV
MUTUAL400	Cap	Trimethobenzamide HCl 250 mg	by Mutual	53489-0293	Antiemetic
MUTUAL400	Cap, Mutual over 400	Trimethobenzamide HCl 250 mg	by URL Mutual	00677-1383	Antiemetic
MUTUAL400	Cap, Swedish Orange, Opaque	Trimethobenzamide HCl 250 mg	by Qualitest	00603-6256	Antiemetic
MUTUAL401	Cap, Yellow	Trimethobenzamide HCl 300 mg	Tigan by Mutual	53489-0376	Antiemetic
MUTUAL603	Cap, Dark Grey and Light Grey, Opaque	Zonisamide 25 mg	Zonegran by Mutual	53489-0617	Anticonvulsant
MUTUAL604	Cap, Red and Light Grey, Opaque	Zonisamide 50 mg	Zonegran by Mutual	53489-0618	Anticonvulsant
MUTUAL605	Cap, Yellow	Zonisamide 100 mg	Zonegran by Mutual	53489-0619	Anticonvulsant
MUTUAL681	Cap, Biege	Gabapentin 300 mg	Neurontin by Mutual	00677-1936	Anticonvulsant
MUTUAL682	Cap, White	Gabapentin 400 mg	Neurontin by Mutual	00677-1937	Anticonvulsant
MUTUAL688	Cap, Brown, Scored	Pancrelipase 4500I Units	by Mutual	53489-0320	Gastrointestinal
MUTUAL688	Cap, Light Brown	Lipase 4500 Units, Amylase 20,000 Units, Protease 25,000 Units	Pancrelipase by URL Mutual	00677-1653	Gastrointestinal
MUTUAL689	Cap, Light Orange	Lipase 10,000 Units, Protease 37,500 Units, Amylase 33,200 Units	Pancrelipase by URL Mutual	00677-1654	Gastrointestinal
MUTUAL689	Cap, Orange, Enteric Coated	Pancrelipase 10,000I Units	by Mutual	53489-0321	Gastrointestinal
MUTUAL690	Cap, Orange, Enteric Coated	Pancrelipase 16,000I Units	by Mutual	53489-0322	Gastrointestinal
MUTUAL691	Tab, Yellow, Round, Scored	Lipase 20,000 Units, Protease 75,000 Units, Amylase 66,400 Units	Microspheres by URL Mutual	00677-1656	Gastrointestinal
MUTUAL691	Tab, Yellow, Round, Scored	Lipase 20,000 Units, Protease 75,000 Units, Amylase 66,400 Units	Microspheres by Mutual	53489-0323	Gastrointestinal
MV4	Tab, Yellow, Round, Scored	Venlafaxine 75 mg	Effexor by Mylan	00378-4884	Antidepressant
MV4	Tab, Yellow, Round, Scored	Venlafaxine 75 mg	Effexor by UDL	51079-0482	Antidepressant
MV5	Tab, Yellow, Round, Scored	Venlafaxine 100 mg	Effexor by Mylan	00378-4885	Antidepressant
MVC150 <> PFIZER	Tab, Blue, Oval, Film Coated	Maraviroc 150 mg	Celsentri by Pfizer	Canadian DIN 02299844	Antiviral
MVC150 <> PFIZER	Tab, Blue, Oval, Film Coated	Maraviroc 150 mg	Selzentry by Pfizer	00069-0807	Antiviral
MVC300 <> PFIZER	Tab, Blue, Oval, Film Coated	Maraviroc 300 mg	Selzentry by Pfizer	00069-0808	Antiviral
MVC300 <> PFIZER	Tab, Blue, Oval, Film Coated	Maraviroc 300 mg	Celsentri by Pfizer	Canadian DIN 02299852	Antiviral
MX <> 511	Tab, Yellow, Round, Scored	Methotrexate 2.5 mg	Rheumatrex by Lederle	00005-5874	Antineoplastic
MX <> 511	Tab, Yellow, Round, Scored	Methotrexate Sodium 2.5 mg	Rheumatrex by ESI Lederle	59911-5874	Antineoplastic
MX225	Tab, White, Cap Shaped, Scored	Guaifenesin 500 mg, Pseudoephedrine HCl 120 mg	Sudafed Sinus by Sovereign	58716-0669	Cold Remedy
MX225	Tab, White, Cap Shaped, Scored	Guaifenesin 500 mg, Pseudoephedrine HCl 120 mg	Nasatab LA by ECR	00095-0225	Cold Remedy
MX31	Tab, Pink, Round	Citalopram 10 mg	Celexa by Mylan	00378-6231	Antidepressant
MX32	Tab, Salmon, Round, Scored	Citalopram 20 mg	Celexa by Mylan	00378-6232	Antidepressant
MX72	Tab, Light Yellow, Round, Scored	Trazodone HCl 100 mg	Desyrel by Mylan	00378-3472	Antidepressant
MYCELEX10	Tab, White, Round	Clotrimazole 10 mg	Mycelex by Alza	17314-9400	Antifungal
MYCELEX10	Tab, White, Round	Clotrimazole 10 mg	by Med Pro	53978-3040	Antifungal
MYCELEX10	Tab, White, Round	Clotrimazole 10 mg	by Eckerd	19458-0858	Antifungal
MYCOBUTIN-PHARMACIA&UPJOHN	Cap, Red, White Print, Opaque, Mycobutin over Pharmacia & Upjohn	Rifabutin 150 mg	Mycobutin by Pharmacia	00013-5301	Antibiotic
MYCOBUTIN-PHARMACIA&UPJOHN	Cap, Red, White Print, Opaque, Mycobutin over Pharmacia & Upjohn	Rifabutin 150 mg	Mycobutin by Pharmacia	Canadian DIN 02063786	Antibiotic
MYKROX <> 12	Tab, White, Round, Mykrox <> 1/2	Metolazone 0.5 mg	Mykrox by Medeva	53014-0847	Diuretic
MYLAN <> 1155	Tab, White, Cap Shaped, Film Coated	Acetaminophen 650 mg, Propoxyphene Napsylate 100 mg	Darvocet-N 100 by Mylan		Analgesic; C IV

ID FRONT <> BACK	DESCRIPTION FRONT <> BACK	INGREDIENT & STRENGTH	BRAND (or Generic Equiv.) by FIRM	NDC#	CLASS; SCH.
MYLAN <> 1155	Tab, White, Cap Shaped, Film Coated	Acetaminophen 650 mg, Propoxyphene Napsylate 100 mg	Darvocet-N 100 by UDL	51079-0934 Discontinued	Analgesic; C IV
MYLAN <> 130	Tab, Orange, Cap Shaped, Film Coated	Acetaminophen 650 mg, Propoxyphene HCl 65 mg	Wygesic by Qualitest	00603-5463	Analgesic; C IV
MYLAN <> 130	Tab, Orange, Cap Shaped, Film Coated	Acetaminophen 650 mg, Propoxyphene HCl 65 mg	Wygesic by Mylan	00378-0130	Analgesic; C IV
MYLAN <> 130	Tab, Orange, Cap Shaped, Film Coated	Acetaminophen 650 mg, Propoxyphene HCl 65 mg	Wygesic by UDL	51079-0741	Analgesic; C IV
MYLAN <> 155	Tab, Pink, Oblong, Film Coated	Acetaminophen 650 mg, Propoxyphene Napsylate 100 mg	Darvocet-N 100 by Med Pro	53978-5013	Analgesic; C IV
MYLAN <> 155	Tab, Pink, Oblong, Film Coated	Acetaminophen 650 mg, Propoxyphene Napsylate 100 mg	Darvocet-N 100 by UDL	51079-0322 Discontinued	Analgesic; C IV
MYLAN <> 155	Tab, Pink, Oblong, Film Coated	Acetaminophen 650 mg, Propoxyphene Napsylate 100 mg	Darvocet-N 100 by Mylan	00378-0155	Analgesic; C IV
MYLAN <> 155	Tab, Pink, Oblong, Film Coated	Acetaminophen 650 mg, Propoxyphene Napsylate 100 mg	Darvocet-N 100 by Vangard	00615-0455	Analgesic; C IV
MYLAN <> 155	Tab, Pink, Oblong, Film Coated	Acetaminophen 650 mg, Propoxyphene Napsylate 100 mg	Darvocet-N 100 by Qualitest	00603-5466	Analgesic; C IV
MYLAN <> 211	Tab, Green, Coated	Amitriptyline 12.5 mg, Chlordiazepoxide 5 mg	Limbitrol by Mylan	00378-0211	Antianxiety; C IV
MYLAN <> 237	Tab, White, Oval, Film Coated	Etodolac 400 mg	Lodine by Mylan	00378-0237	NSAID
MYLAN <> 237	Tab, White, Oval, Film Coated	Etodolac 400 mg	Lodine by Allscripts		NSAID
MYLAN <> 237	Tab, White, Oval, Film Coated	Etodolac 400 mg	Lodine by Aventis	64734-0002	NSAID
MYLAN <> 242	Tab, Pink, Oval, Film Coated	Etodolac 500 mg	Lodine by Mylan	00378-1242	NSAID
MYLAN <> 242	Tab, Pink, Oval, Film Coated	Etodolac 500 mg	Lodine by Heartland	61392-0912	NSAID
MYLAN <> 244	Tab, Blue, Oval, Film Coated, Ex Release	Verapamil HCl 120 mg	Isoptin SR by Murfreesboro	51129-1298	Antihypertensive
MYLAN <> 244	Tab, Blue, Oval, Film Coated, Ex Release	Verapamil HCl 120 mg	Isoptin SR by UDL	51079-0894	Antihypertensive
MYLAN <> 244	Tab, Blue, Oval, Film Coated, Ex Release	Verapamil HCl 120 mg	Isoptin SR by Mylan	00378-1120	Antihypertensive
MYLAN <> 245	Tab, Green, Oval, Scored	Bumetanide 0.5 mg	Bumex by Caraco	57664-0317	Diuretic
MYLAN <> 245	Tab, Light Green	Bumetanide 0.5 mg	Bumex by Hoffmann La Roche	00004-0290	Diuretic
MYLAN <> 245	Tab, Green, Oval, Scored	Bumetanide 0.5 mg	Bumex by Heartland	61392-0048	Diuretic
MYLAN <> 245	Tab, Light Green, Scored	Bumetanide 0.5 mg	Bumex by Mylan	00378-0245	Diuretic
MYLAN <> 277	Tab, White, Coated	Amitriptyline 25 mg, Chlordiazepoxide 10 mg	Limbitrol DS by Mylan	00378-0277	Antianxiety; C IV
MYLAN <> 302	Tab, White	Acyclovir 800 mg	Zovirax by Mylan	00378-0302	Antiviral
MYLAN <> 323	Tab, Orange, Cap Shaped	Ciprofloxacin 500 mg	Cipro by Mylan	00378-1323	Antibiotic
MYLAN <> 323	Tab, Orange, Cap Shaped	Ciprofloxacin 500 mg	Cipro by UDL	51079-0403	Antibiotic
MYLAN <> 324	Tab, Orange, Cap Shaped	Ciprofloxacin 750 mg	Cipro by Mylan	00378-1324	Antibiotic
MYLAN <> 324	Tab, Orange, Cap Shaped	Ciprofloxacin 750 mg	Cipro by UDL	51079-0234 Discontinued	Antibiotic
MYLAN <> 330	Tab, White, Round	Amitriptyline 10 mg, Perphenazine 2 mg	Triavil by Direct Dispensing	57866-3077	Antidepressant; Antipsychotic
MYLAN <> 330	Tab, White, Round	Amitriptyline 10 mg, Perphenazine 2 mg	Triavil by Mylan	00378-0330	Antidepressant; Antipsychotic
MYLAN <> 357	Tab, Lavender, Cap Shaped, Film Coated, Ex Release	Pentoxifylline 400 mg	Trental by UDL	51079-0889 Discontinued	Anticoagulant
MYLAN <> 357	Tab, Lavender, Cap Shaped, Film Coated, Ex Release	Pentoxifylline 400 mg	Trental by Mylan	00378-0357	Anticoagulant
MYLAN <> 370	Tab, Yellow, Scored	Bumetanide 1 mg	Bumex by Mylan	00378-0370	Diuretic
MYLAN <> 3725	Tab, Beveled Edge, 37 to Left, 25 to Right of Score	Hydrochlorothiazide 25 mg, Triamterene 37.5 mg	Maxzide 25 by Mylan	00378-3725	Diuretic; Antihypertensive
MYLAN <> 377	Tab, White, Round	Naproxen 250 mg	Naprosyn by H J Harkins Co	52959-0190	NSAID
MYLAN <> 377	Tab, White, Round	Naproxen 250 mg	Naprosyn by UDL	51079-0793 Discontinued	NSAID
MYLAN <> 377	Tab, White, Round	Naproxen 250 mg	Naprosyn by Dixon Shane	17236-0076	NSAID
MYLAN <> 377	Tab, White, Round	Naproxen 250 mg	Naprosyn by Novartis	17088-0014	NSAID
MYLAN <> 377	Tab, White, Round	Naproxen 250 mg	Naprosyn by Mylan	00378-0377	NSAID
MYLAN <> 377	Tab, White, Round	Naproxen 250 mg	Naprosyn by Kaiser	00179-1186	NSAID
MYLAN <> 401	Tab, Beveled Edge, Coated	Ibuprofen 400 mg	Motrin by Mylan	00378-0401	NSAID
MYLAN <> 417	Tab, Peach, Oval, Scored	Bumetanide 2 mg	Bumex by Caraco	57664-0367	Diuretic
MYLAN <> 417	Tab, Peach, Scored	Bumetanide 2 mg	Bumex by Mylan	00378-0417	Diuretic

ID FRONT <> BACK	DESCRIPTION FRONT <> BACK	INGREDIENT & STRENGTH	BRAND (or Generic Equiv.) by FIRM	NDC#	CLASS; SCH.
MYLAN <> 417	Tab, Peach, Scored	Bumetanide 2 mg	Bumex by Capellon	64543-	Diuretic
MYLAN <> 421	Tab, Beige, Cap Shaped, Film Coated	Methyldopa 500 mg	Aldomet by Mylan	00378-0421	Antihypertensive
MYLAN <> 421	Tab, Beige, Cap Shaped, Film Coated	Methyldopa 500 mg	Aldomet by UDL	51079-0201	Antihypertensive
MYLAN <> 427	Tab, Yellowish Orange, Round	Sulindac 150 mg	Clinoril by UDL	51079-0666 Discontinued	NSAID
MYLAN <> 427	Tab, Yellowish Orange, Round	Sulindac 150 mg	Clinoril by Mylan	00378-0427	NSAID
MYLAN <> 442	Tab, Purple, Round, Film Coated	Perphenazine 2 mg, Amitriptyline HCl 25 mg	Triavil by Pharmafab	62542-0914	Antidepressant; Antipsychotic
MYLAN <> 442	Tab, Purple, Round, Film Coated	Amitriptyline 25 mg, Perphenazine 2 mg	Triavil by Mylan	00378-0442	Antidepressant; Antipsychotic
MYLAN <> 451	Tab, White, Cap Shaped	Naproxen 500 mg	Naprosyn by UDL	51079-0795	NSAID
MYLAN <> 451	Tab, White, Cap Shaped	Naproxen 500 mg	Naprosyn by Murfreesboro	51129-1314	NSAID
MYLAN <> 451	Tab, White, Cap Shaped	Naproxen 500 mg	Naprosyn by Kaiser	00179-1188	NSAID
MYLAN <> 451	Tab, White, Cap Shaped	Naproxen 500 mg	Naprosyn by OHM	51660-0701	NSAID
MYLAN <> 451	Tab, White, Cap Shaped	Naproxen 500 mg	Naprosyn by Mylan	00378-0451	NSAID
MYLAN <> 451	Tab, White, Cap Shaped	Naproxen 500 mg	Naprosyn by St. Mary's Med	60760-0451	NSAID
MYLAN <> 451	Tab, White, Cap Shaped	Naproxen 500 mg	Naprosyn by Kaiser	62224-2119	NSAID
MYLAN <> 451	Tab, White, Cap Shaped	Naproxen 500 mg	Naprosyn by Dixon Shane	17236-0078	NSAID
MYLAN <> 451	Tab, White, Cap Shaped	Naproxen 500 mg	Naprosyn by Talbert	44514-0651	NSAID
MYLAN <> 457	Tab	Lorazepam 1 mg	Ativan by Vangard	00615-0451	Antianxiety; C IV
MYLAN <> 507	Tab, Green, Beveled Edge, Coated	Hydrochlorothiazide 15 mg, Methyldopa 250 mg	Aldoril by Mylan	00378-0507	Diuretic; Antihypertensive
MYLAN <> 517	Tab, White, Film Coated, Scored	Gemfibrozil 600 mg	by Mylan	00378-0517	Antihyperlipidemic
MYLAN <> 521	Tab, Coated	Acetaminophen 650 mg, Propoxyphene Napsylate 100 mg	Darvocet-N 100 by H J Harkins Co	00378-0521	Analgesic; C IV
MYLAN <> 555	Tab, White, Cap Shaped	Naproxen 375 mg	Naprosyn by H J Harkins Co	52959-0191	NSAID
MYLAN <> 555	Tab, White, Cap Shaped	Naproxen 375 mg	Naprosyn by Mylan	00378-0555	NSAID
MYLAN <> 555	Tab, White, Cap Shaped	Naproxen 375 mg	Naprosyn by Kaiser	00179-1187	NSAID
MYLAN <> 555	Tab, White, Cap Shaped	Naproxen 375 mg	Naprosyn by UDL	51079-0794	NSAID
MYLAN <> 555	Tab, White, Cap Shaped	Naproxen 375 mg	Naprosyn by Dixon Shane	17236-0077	NSAID
MYLAN <> 555	Tab, White, Cap Shaped	Naproxen 375 mg	Naprosyn by Kaiser	62224-4552	NSAID
MYLAN <> 555	Tab, White, Cap Shaped	Naproxen 375 mg	Naprosyn by Novartis	61615-0016	NSAID
MYLAN <> 574	Tab, Orange, Round, Film Coated	Amitriptyline 25 mg, Perphenazine 4 mg	Triavil by Mylan	00378-0574	Antidepressant; Antipsychotic
MYLAN <> 601	Tab, Beveled Edge, Coated	Ibuprofen 600 mg	Motrin by Mylan	00378-0601	NSAID
MYLAN <> 611	Tab, Beige, Round, Film Coated	Methyldopa 250 mg	Aldomet by UDL	51079-0200	Antihypertensive
MYLAN <> 611	Tab, Beige, Round, Film Coated	Methyldopa 250 mg	Aldomet by Mylan	00378-0611	Antihypertensive
MYLAN <> 611	Tab, Beige, Round, Film Coated	Methyldopa 250 mg	Aldomet by Murfreesboro	51129-1293	Antihypertensive
MYLAN <> 711	Tab, Green, Beveled Edge, Coated	Hydrochlorothiazide 25 mg, Methyldopa 250 mg	Aldoril by Mylan	00378-0711	Diuretic; Antihypertensive
MYLAN <> 727	Tab, Blue, Round, Film Coated	Amitriptyline 10 mg, Perphenazine 4 mg	Triavil by Mylan	00378-0042	Antidepressant; Antipsychotic
MYLAN <> 73	Tab, Purple, Round, Coated	Amitriptyline 50 mg, Perphenazine 4 mg	Triavil by Mylan	00378-0073	Antidepressant; Antipsychotic
MYLAN <> 733	Tab, Film Coated	Naproxen 550 mg	by Allscripts		NSAID
MYLAN <> 801	Tab, Beveled Edge, Coated	Ibuprofen 800 mg	Motrin by Mylan	00378-0801	NSAID
MYLAN <> 88	Tab, Purple, Oval, Ex Release	Carbidopa 25 mg, Levodopa 100 mg	Sinemet CR by UDL	51079-0978 Discontinued	Antiparkinson
MYLAN <> 88	Tab, Purple, Oval, Ex Release	Carbidopa 25 mg, Levodopa 100 mg	Sinemet CR by Mylan	00378-0088	Antiparkinson
MYLAN <> 94	Tab, Purple, Oval, Scored, Ex Release, Mylan <> 9/4	Carbidopa 50 mg, Levodopa 200 mg	Sinemet CR by Mylan	00378-0094	Antiparkinson
MYLAN <> 94	Tab, Purple, Oval, Scored, Ex Release, Mylan <> 9/4	Carbidopa 50 mg, Levodopa 200 mg	Sinemet CR by UDL	51079-0923 Discontinued	Antiparkinson
MYLAN <> G11	Tab, White, Oval	Glimepiride 1 mg	Amaryl by Mylan	00378-4011	Antidiabetic

ID FRONT <> BACK	DESCRIPTION FRONT <> BACK	INGREDIENT & STRENGTH	BRAND (or Generic Equiv.) by FIRM	NDC#	CLASS; SCH.
MYLAN <> G12	Tab, Light Green, Oval	Glimepiride 2 mg	Amaryl by Mylan	00378-4012	Antidiabetic
MYLAN <> G12	Tab, Light Yellow, Oval, Scored, G/12	Glimepiride 2 mg	Amaryl by UDL	51079-0425	Antidiabetic
MYLAN <> G13	Tab, Peach, Oval, Scored, G/13	Glimepiride 4 mg	Amaryl by UDL	51079-0426	Antidiabetic
MYLAN <> G13	Tab, Light Pink, Oval	Glimepiride 4 mg	Amaryl by Mylan	00378-4013	Antidiabetic
MYLAN <> TH1	Tab, Green, Scored, Beveled Edge, TH/1	Hydrochlorothiazide 25 mg, Triamterene 37.5 mg	Maxzide 25 by Mylan	00378-1352	Diuretic; Antihypertensive
MYLAN <> TH1	Tab, Green, Scored, Beveled Edge, TH/1	Hydrochlorothiazide 25 mg, Triamterene 37.5 mg	Maxzide 25 by Mylan	55160-0126	Diuretic; Antihypertensive
MYLAN <> TH2	Tab, Yellow, Round, Scored, TH over 2	Hydrochlorothiazide 50 mg, Triamterene 75 mg	Maxzide by Mylan	00378-1355	Diuretic; Antihypertensive
MYLAN <> TH2	Tab, Yellow, Round, Scored, TH over 2	Hydrochlorothiazide 50 mg, Triamterene 75 mg	Maxzide by UDL	51079-0433	Diuretic; Antihypertensive
MYLAN <> TH2	Tab, Yellow, Round, Scored, TH over 2	Hydrochlorothiazide 50 mg, Triamterene 75 mg	Maxzide by Mylan	55160-0127	Diuretic; Antihypertensive
MYLAN1001	Cap, Caramel & Powder Blue, Black Print, Mylan over 1001	Thiothixene 1 mg	Navane by Mylan	00378-1001	Antipsychotic
MYLAN1001	Cap, Caramel & Powder Blue, Black Print, Mylan over 1001	Thiothixene 1 mg	Navane by Med Pro	53978-2003	Antipsychotic
MYLAN1001	Cap, Caramel & Powder Blue, Black Print, Mylan over 1001	Thiothixene 1 mg	Navane by Dixon Shane	17236-0465	Antipsychotic
MYLAN1001	Cap, Caramel & Powder Blue, Black Print, Mylan over 1001	Thiothixene 1 mg	Navane by UDL	51079-0586 Discontinued	Antipsychotic
MYLAN101	Cap, Medium Orange & Yellow, Black Print, Mylan over 101	Tetracycline HCl 500 mg	by Urgent Care Center	50716-0782	Antibiotic
MYLAN101	Cap, Medium Orange & Yellow, Black Print, Mylan over 101	Tetracycline HCl 250 mg	by Mylan	00378-0101	Antibiotic
MYLAN1010	Cap, Dark Green & Olive, Black Print, Mylan over 1010	Piroxicam 10 mg	Feldene by UDL	51079-0742	NSAID
MYLAN1010	Cap, Dark Green & Olive, Black Print, Mylan over 1010	Piroxicam 10 mg	Feldene by H J Harkins Co	52959-0398	NSAID
MYLAN1010	Cap, Dark Green & Olive, Black Print, Mylan over 1010	Piroxicam 10 mg	Feldene by Mylan	55160-0128	NSAID
MYLAN1010	Cap, Dark Green & Olive, Black Print, Mylan over 1010	Piroxicam 10 mg	Feldene by Mylan	00378-1010	NSAID
MYLAN102	Cap, Black & Yellow, White Print, Mylan over 102	Tetracycline HCl 500 mg	by Mylan	00378-0102	Antibiotic
MYLAN1020	Cap, Green & Ivory, Black Print, Mylan over 1020	Nicardipine HCl 20 mg	Cardene by Murfreesboro	51129-1372	Antihypertensive
MYLAN1020	Cap, Green & Ivory, Black Print, Mylan over 1020	Nicardipine HCl 20 mg	Cardene by Mylan	00378-1020	Antihypertensive
MYLAN1049	Cap, Buff, Black Print, Mylan over 1049	Doxepin HCl 10 mg	Sinequan by Major	00904-1260	Antidepressant
MYLAN1049	Cap, Buff, Black Print, Mylan over 1049	Doxepin HCl 10 mg	Sinequan by UDL	51079-0436	Antidepressant
MYLAN1049	Cap, Buff, Black Print, Mylan over 1049	Doxepin HCl 10 mg	Sinequan by Mylan	00378-1049	Antidepressant
MYLAN1049	Cap, Buff, Black Print, Mylan over 1049	Doxepin HCl 10 mg	Sinequan by Pharmedix	53002-0489	Antidepressant
MYLAN106 <> 250	Tab, Film Coated, Mylan over 106 <> 250	Erythromycin Stearate 250 mg	by Diversified Healthcare	55887-0994	Antibiotic
MYLAN106 <> 250	Tab, Yellow, Film Coated, Mylan over 106 <> 250	Erythromycin Stearate 250 mg	by Mylan	00378-0106	Antibiotic
MYLAN106 <> 250	Tab, Film Coated, Mylan over 106 <> 250	Erythromycin Stearate 250 mg	by Rx Dispensing	61807-0013	Antibiotic
MYLAN107 <> 500	Tab, Coated	Erythromycin Stearate 500 mg	by Direct Dispensing	57866-0265	Antibiotic
MYLAN107 <> 500	Tab, Film Coated, Mylan over 107 <> 500	Erythromycin Stearate 500 mg	by St. Mary's Med	60760-0107	Antibiotic
MYLAN107 <> 500	Tab, Film Coated, Mylan over 107 <> 500	Erythromycin Stearate 500 mg	by DRX	55045-1113	Antibiotic
MYLAN107 <> 500	Tab, Film Coated	Erythromycin Stearate 500 mg	by Med Pro	53978-0026	Antibiotic
MYLAN107 <> 500	Tab, Coated	Erythromycin Stearate 500 mg	by PDRX	55289-0705	Antibiotic
MYLAN107 <> 500	Tab, Yellow, Film Coated, Mylan over 107 <> 500	Erythromycin Stearate 500 mg	by Mylan	00378-0107	Antibiotic
MYLAN107 <> 500	Tab, Film Coated, Mylan over 107 <> 500	Erythromycin Stearate 500 mg	by Rx Dispensing	61807-0015	Antibiotic
MYLAN1101	Cap, Dark Green & Light Brown, Mylan over 1101	Prazosin HCl 1 mg	Minipress by Pharmedix	53002-0499	Antihypertensive
MYLAN1101	Cap, Dark Green & Light Brown, Mylan over 1101	Prazosin HCl 1 mg	Minipress by Med Pro	53978-5045	Antihypertensive
MYLAN1101	Cap, Dark Green & Light Brown, Mylan over 1101	Prazosin HCl 1 mg	Minipress by Mylan	00378-1101	Antihypertensive
MYLAN1101	Cap, Dark Green & Light Brown, Mylan over 1101	Prazosin HCl 1 mg	Minipress by UDL	51079-0630	Antihypertensive
MYLAN1101	Cap, Dark Green & Light Brown, Mylan over 1101	Prazosin HCl 1 mg	Minipress by Mylan	00378-1101	Antihypertensive
MYLAN1101	Cap, Dark Green & Light Brown, Mylan over 1101	Prazosin HCl 1 mg	Minipress by Kaiser	62224-0119	Antihypertensive
MYLAN111250	Tab, White, Oval, Mylan 111/250	Penicillin V Potassium 250 mg	V-Cillin K by Mylan		Antibiotic
MYLAN112500	Tab, White, Round, Mylan 112/500	Penicillin V Potassium 500 mg	V-Cillin K by Mylan		Antibiotic
MYLAN115	Cap	Ampicillin 250 mg	Principen by Med Pro	53978-5018	Antibiotic
MYLAN115	Cap, Scarlet, Mylan over 115	Ampicillin 250 mg	Principen by Mylan	00378-0115	Antibiotic
MYLAN116	Cap, Scarlet, Mylan over 116	Ampicillin 500 mg	Principen by Mylan	00378-0116	Antibiotic
MYLAN116	Cap	Ampicillin 500 mg	Principen by Apotheca	12634-0168	Antibiotic
MYLAN1200	Cap, Orange, Black Print, Mylan over 1200	Acebutolol HCl 200 mg	Sectral by Mylan	00378-1200	Antihypertensive

ID FRONT <> BACK	DESCRIPTION FRONT <> BACK	INGREDIENT & STRENGTH	BRAND (or Generic Equiv.) by FIRM	NDC#	CLASS; SCH.
MYLAN121	Tab, White, Round	Penicillin G Potassium 250,000 Units	Pentids by Mylan		Antibiotic
MYLAN122	Tab, White, Round	Penicillin G Potassium 400,000 Units	Pentids by Mylan		Antibiotic
MYLAN129	Cap, Pink, Black Print, Mylan over 129	Propoxyphene HCl 65 mg	by Mylan	00378-0129	Analgesic; C IV
MYLAN129	Cap, Pink, Black Print, Mylan over 129	Propoxyphene HCl 65 mg	by Ranbaxy	63304-0701	Analgesic; C IV
MYLAN129	Cap, Pink, Black Print, Mylan over 129	Propoxyphene HCl 65 mg	by Qualitest	00603-5460	Analgesic; C IV
MYLAN130	Tab, Coated,	Acetaminophen 650 mg, Propoxyphene HCl 65 mg	Wygesic by Med Pro	53978-2020	Analgesic; C IV
MYLAN130	Tab, Coated	Acetaminophen 650 mg, Propoxyphene HCl 65 mg	Wygesic by Allscripts		Analgesic; C IV
MYLAN130	Tab, Coated	Acetaminophen 650 mg, Propoxyphene HCl 65 mg	Wygesic by Heartland	61392-0148	Analgesic; C IV
MYLAN131	Cap, Gray & Red, Mylan over 131	Aspirin 389 mg, Caffeine 32.4 mg, Propoxyphene HCl 65 mg	Propoxyphene Compound 65 by Mylan	00378-0131	Analgesic; C IV
MYLAN1400	Cap, Orange, Black Print, Mylan over 1400	Acebutolol HCl 400 mg	Sectral by ABG	60999-0900	Antihypertensive
MYLAN1400	Cap, Orange, Black Print, Mylan over 1400	Acebutolol HCl 400 mg	Sectral by Caremark	00339-6092	Antihypertensive
MYLAN1400	Cap, Orange, Black Print, Mylan over 1400	Acebutolol HCl 400 mg	Sectral by Mylan	00378-1400	Antihypertensive
MYLAN1401	Tab, White, Beveled Edge, Coated, Mylan over 1401 in Black Ink	Ibuprofen 400 mg	Motrin by Mylan	00378-1401	NSAID
MYLAN141	Tab, Ivory, Round	Hydrochlorothiazide 25 mg, Spironolactone 25 mg	Aldactazide by Mylan		Diuretic; Antihypertensive
MYLAN1410	Cap, Orange, Opaque, Mylan over 1410	Nortriptyline HCl 10 mg	Pamelor by Mylan	00378-1410	Antidepressant
MYLAN1410	Cap, Orange, Opaque, Mylan over 1410	Nortriptyline HCl 10 mg	Pamelor by Dixon Shane	17236-0003	Antidepressant
MYLAN1410	Cap, Orange, Opaque, Mylan over 1410	Nortriptyline HCl 10 mg	Pamelor by UDL	51079-0803 Discontinued	Antidepressant
MYLAN143	Cap, Light Green, Black Print, Mylan over 143	Indomethacin 25 mg	Indocin by Mylan	00378-0143	NSAID
MYLAN143	Cap, Light Green, Black Print, Mylan over 143	Indomethacin 25 mg	Indocin by UDL	51079-0190 Discontinued	NSAID
MYLAN1430	Cap, Bluish-Green & Yellow, Black Print, Mylan over 1430	Nicardipine HCl 30 mg	Cardene by Mylan	00378-1430	Antihypertensive
MYLAN145	Cap, Aqua Blue & White, Black Print, Mylan over 145	Doxycycline Hyclate 50 mg	Vibramycin by Mylan	00378-0145	Antibiotic
MYLAN146 <> 25	Tab, White, Round, Scored, Mylan over 146	Spironolactone 25 mg	Aldactone by Qualitest	00603-5766	Diuretic
MYLAN146 <> 25	Tab, White, Round, Scored, Mylan over 146	Spironolactone 25 mg	Aldactone by Sidmak		Diuretic
MYLAN146 <> 25	Tab, White, Round, Scored, Mylan over 146	Spironolactone 25 mg	Aldactone by Heartland	61392-0083	Diuretic
MYLAN146 <> 25	Tab, White, Round, Scored, Mylan over 146	Spironolactone 25 mg	Aldactone by UDL	51079-0103	Diuretic
MYLAN146 <> 25	Tab, White, Round, Scored, Mylan over 146	Spironolactone 25 mg	Aldactone by Pharmedix	53002-0472	Diuretic
MYLAN146 <> 25	Tab, White, Round, Scored, Mylan over 146	Spironolactone 25 mg	Aldactone by Nat Pharmpak	55154-5517	Diuretic
MYLAN146 <> 25	Tab, White, Round, Scored, Mylan over 146	Spironolactone 25 mg	Aldactone by Mylan	00378-2146	Diuretic
MYLAN146 <> 25	Tab, White, Round, Scored, Mylan over 146	Spironolactone 25 mg	Aldactone by Vangard	00615-1535	Diuretic
MYLAN147	Cap, Light Green, Black Print, Mylan over 147	Indomethacin 50 mg	Indocin by Mylan	00378-0147	NSAID
MYLAN147	Cap, Light Green, Black Print, Mylan over 147	Indomethacin 50 mg	Indocin by UDL	51079-0191	NSAID
MYLAN147	Cap, Light Green, Black Print, Mylan over 147	Indomethacin 50 mg	Indocin by St. Mary's Med	60760-0147	NSAID
MYLAN148	Cap, Aqua Blue, Mylan over 148	Doxycycline Hyclate 100 mg	Vibramycin by UDL	51079-0522	Antibiotic
MYLAN148	Cap, Aqua Blue	Doxycycline Hyclate 100 mg	Vibramycin by Mylan	00378-0148	Antibiotic
MYLAN148	Tab, Blue, Oblong	Doxycycline Hyclate 100 mg	Vibramycin by Family Health	65149-0554	Antibiotic
MYLAN148	Cap, Aqua Blue	Doxycycline Hyclate 100 mg	Vibramycin by Diversified Healthcare	55887-0979	Antibiotic
MYLAN150250	Tab, White, Round, Mylan 150/250	Chlorothiazide 250 mg	Diuril by Mylan		Diuretic; Antihypertensive
MYLAN152	Tab, White, Round, Scored, Mylan over 152	Clonidine HCl 0.1 mg	Catapres by Nat Pharmpak	55154-5561	Antihypertensive
MYLAN152	Tab, White, Round, Scored, Mylan over 152	Clonidine HCl 0.1 mg	Catapres by Prepackage Specialists	58864-0110	Antihypertensive
MYLAN152	Tab, White, Round, Scored, Mylan over 152	Clonidine HCl 0.1 mg	Catapres by Kaiser	62224-7551	Antihypertensive
MYLAN152	Tab, White, Round, Scored, Mylan over 152	Clonidine HCl 0.1 mg	Catapres by PDRX	55289-0073	Antihypertensive
MYLAN152	Tab, White, Round, Scored, Mylan over 152	Clonidine HCl 0.1 mg	Catapres by Southwood	58016-0518	Antihypertensive
MYLAN152	Tab, White, Round, Scored, Mylan over 152	Clonidine HCl 0.1 mg	Catapres by Med Pro	53978-0936	Antihypertensive
MYLAN152	Tab, White, Round, Scored, Mylan over 152	Clonidine HCl 0.1 mg	Catapres by Mylan	00378-0152	Antihypertensive
MYLAN152	Tab, White, Round, Scored, Mylan over 152	Clonidine HCl 0.1 mg	Catapres by Pharmedix	53002-0414	Antihypertensive
MYLAN152	Tab, White, Round, Scored, Mylan over 152	Clonidine HCl 0.1 mg	Catapres by Southwood	58016-0517	Antihypertensive

ID FRONT <> BACK	DESCRIPTION FRONT <> BACK	INGREDIENT & STRENGTH	BRAND (or Generic Equiv.) by FIRM	NDC#	CLASS; SCH.
MYLAN152	Tab, White, Round, Scored, Mylan over 152	Clonidine HCl 0.1 mg	Catapres by UDL	51079-0299	Antihypertensive
MYLAN156 <> 500	Tab, Yellow, Oblong, Film Coated	Probenecid 500 mg	Benemid by Mylan	00378-0156	Antigout
MYLAN156 <> 500	Tab, Yellow, Oblong, Film Coated	Probenecid 500 mg	Benemid by Med Pro	53978-0014	Antigout
MYLAN1560	Cap, Lavender and White, MYLAN over 1560	Extended Phenytoin Sodium 100 mg	Dilantin Kapseals by Mylan	00378-1560	Anticonvulsant
MYLAN1560	Cap, Lavender and White, MYLAN over 1560	Extended Phenytoin Sodium 100 mg	Dilantin Kapseals by UDL	51079-0905 Discontinued	Anticonvulsant
MYLAN1570	Cap, Light Lavender, Mylan over 1570	Terazosin HCl 10 mg	Hytrin by Mylan	00378-1570	Antihypertensive
MYLAN1570	Cap, Light Lavender, Mylan over 1570	Terazosin HCl 10 mg	Hytrin by UDL	51079-0939 Discontinued	Antihypertensive
MYLAN159	Cap, Maroon & White	Disopyramide Phosphate 100 mg	Norpace by Mylan		Antiarrhythmic
MYLAN1601	Tab, White, Beveled Edge, Coated, Mylan over 1601 in Black Ink	Ibuprofen 600 mg	Motrin by Mylan	00378-1601	NSAID
MYLAN161	Cap, Maroon	Disopyramide Phosphate 150 mg	Norpace by Mylan		Antiarrhythmic
MYLAN1610	Cap, Blue, Black Print, Mylan over 1610	Dicyclomine HCl 10 mg	Bentyl by UDL	51079-0118	Gastrointestinal
MYLAN1610	Cap, Blue, Black Print, Mylan over 1610	Dicyclomine HCl 10 mg	Bentyl by Mylan	00378-1610	Gastrointestinal
MYLAN162	Tab, White, Round, Scored, Mylan over 162	Chlorothiazide 500 mg	Diuril by Mylan	00378-0162	Diuretic
MYLAN162	Tab, White, Round, Scored, Mylan over 162	Chlorothiazide 500 mg	Diuril by Med Pro	53978-0020	Diuretic; Antihypertensive
MYLAN162	Tab, White, Round, Scored, Mylan over 162	Chlorothiazide 500 mg	Diuril by UDL	51079-0061	Diuretic; Antihypertensive
MYLAN1650	Cap, Light Brown, Mylan over 1650 in Black Ink	Nitrofurantoin 50 mg	Macrodantin by Mylan	00378-1650	Antibiotic
MYLAN1650	Cap, Light Brown, Opaque, Mylan over 1650	Nitrofurantoin 50 mg	Macrodantin by UDL	51079-0584	Antibiotic
MYLAN167 <> 100	Tab, Beige, Film Coated, Mylan over 167 <> 100	Doxycycline Hyclate 100 mg	by Mylan	00378-0167	Antibiotic
MYLAN167 <> 100	Tab, Beige, Round, Film Coated, Mylan over 167 <> 100	Doxycycline Hyclate 100 mg	Vibra-Tabs by UDL	51079-0554	Antibiotic
MYLAN1700	Cap, Gray, Opaque, Mylan over 1700	Nitrofurantoin 100 mg	Macrodantin by UDL	51079-0585	Antibiotic
MYLAN1700	Cap, Gray, Mylan over 1700 in Black Ink	Nitrofurantoin 100 mg	Macrodantin by Mylan	00378-1700	Antibiotic
MYLAN1730	Cap, Peach and White, Opaque	Ursodiol 300 mg	Actigall by UDL	51079-0383	Gastrointestinal
MYLAN175	Tab, Orange, Round	Chlorothiazide 250 mg, Reserpine 0.125 mg	Diupres by Mylan		Diuretic; Antihypertensive
MYLAN176	Tab, Orange, Round	Chlorothiazide 500 mg, Reserpine 0.125 mg	Diupres by Mylan		Diuretic; Antihypertensive
MYLAN1801	Tab, White, Beveled Edge, Coated, Mylan over 1801 in Black Ink	Ibuprofen 800 mg	Motrin by Mylan	00378-1801	NSAID
MYLAN182 <> 10	Tab, Orange, Round, Scored, Mylan over 182	Propranolol HCl 10 mg	Inderal by UDL	51079-0277 Discontinued	Antihypertensive
MYLAN182 <> 10	Tab, Orange, Round, Scored, Mylan over 182	Propranolol HCl 10 mg	Inderal by Mylan	00378-0182	Antihypertensive
MYLAN183 <> 20	Tab, Blue, Round, Scored, Mylan over 183	Propranolol HCl 20 mg	Inderal by UDL	51079-0278	Antihypertensive
MYLAN183 <> 20	Tab, Blue, Round, Scored, Mylan over 183	Propranolol HCl 20 mg	Inderal by Mylan	00378-0183	Antihypertensive
MYLAN184 <> 40	Tab, Green, Round, Scored, Mylan over 184	Propranolol HCl 40 mg	Inderal by UDL	51079-0279	Antihypertensive
MYLAN184 <> 40	Tab, Green, Round, Scored, Mylan over 184	Propranolol HCl 40 mg	Inderal by Mylan	00378-0184	Antihypertensive
MYLAN185 <> 80	Tab, Yellow, Round, Scored, Mylan over 185	Propranolol HCl 80 mg	Inderal by UDL	51079-0280	Antihypertensive
MYLAN185 <> 80	Tab, Yellow, Round, Scored, Mylan over 185	Propranolol HCl 80 mg	Inderal by Mylan	00378-0185	Antihypertensive
MYLAN186	Tab, White, Round, Scored, Mylan over 186	Clonidine HCl 0.2 mg	Catapres by Kaiser	62224-7555	Antihypertensive
MYLAN186	Tab, White, Round, Scored, Mylan over 186	Clonidine HCl 0.2 mg	Catapres by Prepackage Specialists	58864-0111	Antihypertensive
MYLAN186	Tab, White, Round, Scored, Mylan over 186	Clonidine HCl 0.2 mg	Catapres by Nat Pharmpak	55154-5562	Antihypertensive
MYLAN186	Tab, White, Round, Scored, Mylan over 186	Clonidine HCl 0.2 mg	Catapres by DHHS Prog	11819-0112	Antihypertensive
MYLAN186	Tab, White, Round, Scored, Mylan over 186	Clonidine HCl 0.2 mg	Catapres by Med Pro	53978-0816	Antihypertensive
MYLAN186	Tab, White, Round, Scored, Mylan over 186	Clonidine HCl 0.2 mg	Catapres by Nat Pharmpak	55154-5229	Antihypertensive
MYLAN186	Tab, White, Round, Scored, Mylan over 186	Clonidine HCl 0.2 mg	Catapres by Vangard	00615-2573	Antihypertensive
MYLAN186	Tab, White, Round, Scored, Mylan over 186	Clonidine HCl 0.2 mg	Catapres by Mylan	00378-0186	Antihypertensive
MYLAN186	Tab, White, Round, Scored, Mylan over 186	Clonidine HCl 0.2 mg	Catapres by UDL	51079-0300	Antihypertensive
MYLAN186	Tab, White, Round, Scored, Mylan over 186	Clonidine HCl 0.2 mg	Catapres by Amerisource	62584-0339	Antihypertensive

ID FRONT <> BACK	DESCRIPTION FRONT <> BACK	INGREDIENT & STRENGTH	BRAND (or Generic Equiv.) by FIRM	NDC#	CLASS; SCH.
MYLAN195250	Tab, White, Round, Mylan 195/250	Penicillin V Potassium 250 mg	V-Cillin K by Mylan	51079-0202 Discontinued	Antibiotic
MYLAN197 <> 100	Tab, Green, Round, Scored, Mylan over 197	Chlorpropamide 100 mg	Diabinese by UDL	00378-0197	Antidiabetic
MYLAN197 <> 100	Tab, Green, Round, Scored, Mylan over 197	Chlorpropamide 100 mg	Diabinese by Mylan		Antidiabetic
MYLAN198500	Tab, White, Oval, Mylan 198/500	Penicillin V Potassium 500 mg	V-Cillin K by Mylan		Antibiotic
MYLAN199	Tab, White, Round, Scored, Mylan over 199	Clonidine HCl 0.3 mg	Catapres by UDL	51079-0301	Antihypertensive
MYLAN199	Tab, White, Round, Scored, Mylan over 199	Clonidine HCl 0.3 mg	Catapres by Nat Pharmpak	55154-5570	Antihypertensive
MYLAN199	Tab, White, Round, Scored, Mylan over 199	Clonidine HCl 0.3 mg	Catapres by Mylan	00378-0199	Antihypertensive
MYLAN2002	Cap, Caramel & Yellow, Mylan over 2002	Thiothixene 2 mg	Navane by UDL	51079-0587	Antipsychotic
MYLAN2002	Cap, Caramel & Yellow, Mylan over 2002	Thiothixene 2 mg	Navane by Dixon Shane	17236-0466	Antipsychotic
MYLAN2002	Cap, Caramel & Yellow, Mylan over 2002	Thiothixene 2 mg	Navane by Med Pro	53978-2000	Antipsychotic
MYLAN2002	Cap, Caramel & Yellow, Mylan over 2002	Thiothixene 2 mg	Navane by Mylan	00378-2002	Antipsychotic
MYLAN2020	Cap, Green	Piroxicam 20 mg	Feldene by Va Cmop	65243-0057	NSAID
MYLAN2020	Cap, Green, Opaque, Mylan over 2020	Piroxicam 20 mg	Feldene by Mylan	00378-2020	NSAID
MYLAN2020	Cap, Green, Opaque, Mylan over 2020	Piroxicam 20 mg	Feldene by Compumed	00403-0880	NSAID
MYLAN2020	Cap, Green, Opaque, Mylan over 2020	Piroxicam 20 mg	Feldene by UDL	51079-0743 Discontinued	NSAID
MYLAN204	Cap, Buff & Caramel, Mylan over 204	Amoxicillin 250 mg	Amoxil by Pharmedix	53002-0208	Antibiotic
MYLAN204	Cap, Buff & Caramel, Mylan over 204	Amoxicillin 250 mg	Amoxil by Mylan	00378-0204	Antibiotic
MYLAN205	Cap, Buff, Mylan over 205	Amoxicillin 500 mg	Amoxil by Mylan	00378-0205	Antibiotic
MYLAN205	Cap, Buff, Mylan over 205	Amoxicillin 500 mg	Amoxil by Pharmedix	53002-0216	Antibiotic
MYLAN20820	Tab, White, Round, Mylan 208/20	Furosemide 20 mg	Lasix by Mylan		Diuretic
MYLAN210 <> 250	Tab, Green, Round, Scored, Mylan over 210	Chlorpropamide 250 mg	Diabinese by UDL	51079-0203 Discontinued	Antidiabetic
MYLAN210 <> 250	Tab, Green, Round, Scored, Mylan over 210	Chlorpropamide 250 mg	Diabinese by Mylan	00378-0210	Antidiabetic
MYLAN210 <> 250	Tab, Green, Round, Scored, Mylan over 210	Chlorpropamide 250 mg	Diabinese by Physician Total Care	54868-0036	Antidiabetic
MYLAN2100	Cap, Light Brown, Black Print, Mylan over 2100	Loperamide 2 mg	Imodium by Vangard	00615-0362	Antidiarrheal
MYLAN2100	Cap, Light Brown, Black Print, Mylan over 2100	Loperamide 2 mg	Imodium by Mylan	00378-2100	Antidiarrheal
MYLAN2100	Cap, Light Brown, Black Print, Mylan over 2100	Loperamide 2 mg	Imodium by Compumed	00403-1046	Antidiarrheal
MYLAN2100	Cap, Light Brown, Black Print, Mylan over 2100	Loperamide 2 mg	Imodium by Mylan	55160-0137	Antidiarrheal
MYLAN2100	Cap, Light Brown, Black Print, Mylan over 2100	Loperamide 2 mg	Imodium by UDL	51079-0690	Antidiarrheal
MYLAN211	Tab, Green, Round, Coated	Amitriptyline 12.5 mg, Chlordiazepoxide 5 mg	Limbitrol by Physician Total Care	54868-2206	Antianxiety; C IV
MYLAN21350	Tab, Green, Round, Mylan 213/50	Chlorthalidone 50 mg	Hygroton by Mylan		Diuretic
MYLAN214	Tab, Orange, Round, Scored, Mylan over 214	Haloperidol 2 mg	Haldol by Mylan	00378-0214	Antipsychotic
MYLAN214	Tab, Orange, Round, Scored, Mylan over 214	Haloperidol 2 mg	Haldol by Heartland	61392-0269	Antipsychotic
MYLAN214	Tab, Orange, Round, Scored, Mylan over 214	Haloperidol 2 mg	Haldol by UDL	51079-0735	Antipsychotic
MYLAN2150	Cap, Coral, Mylan over 2150 in Black Ink	Meclofenamate Sodium 50 mg	Meclomen by Med Pro	53978-2015	NSAID
MYLAN2150	Cap, Coral, Mylan over 2150 in Black Ink	Meclofenamate Sodium 50 mg	Meclomen by Qualitest	00603-4344	NSAID
MYLAN2150	Cap, Coral, Mylan over 2150 in Black Ink	Meclofenamate Sodium 50 mg	Meclomen by Mylan	00378-2150	NSAID
MYLAN216 <> 40	Tab, White, Round, Scored, Mylan over 216	Furosemide 40 mg	Lasix by Murfreesboro	51129-1389	Diuretic
MYLAN216 <> 40	Tab, White, Round, Scored, Mylan over 216	Furosemide 40 mg	Lasix by Kaiser	62224-1222	Diuretic
MYLAN216 <> 40	Tab, White, Round, Scored, Mylan over 216	Furosemide 40 mg	Lasix by Heartland	61392-0253	Diuretic
MYLAN216 <> 40	Tab, White, Round, Scored, Mylan over 216	Furosemide 40 mg	Lasix by Mylan	00378-0216	Diuretic
MYLAN216 <> 40	Tab, White, Round, Scored, Mylan over 216	Furosemide 40 mg	Lasix by UDL	51079-0073 Discontinued	Diuretic
MYLAN217 <> 250	Tab, White, Mylan over 217	Tolazamide 250 mg	Tolinase by Mylan	00378-0217	Antidiabetic
MYLAN2200	Cap, Purple, Black Print, Mylan over 2200	Acyclovir 200 mg	Zovirax by Mylan	00378-2200	Antiviral
MYLAN2200	Cap, Purple, Black Print, Mylan over 2200	Acyclovir 200 mg	Zovirax by Allscripts		Antiviral
MYLAN2200	Cap, Purple, Black Print, Mylan over 2200	Acyclovir 200 mg	Zovirax by Amerisource	62584-0694	Antiviral

ID FRONT <> BACK	DESCRIPTION FRONT <> BACK	INGREDIENT & STRENGTH	BRAND (or Generic Equiv.) by FIRM	NDC#	CLASS; SCH.
MYLAN2200	Cap, Purple, Black Print, Mylan over 2200	Acyclovir 200 mg	Zovirax by Physician Total Care	54868-3996	Antiviral
MYLAN2200	Cap, Purple, Black Print, Mylan over 2200	Acyclovir 200 mg	Zovirax by Direct Dispensing	57866-6950	Antiviral
MYLAN22225	Tab, Yellow, Round, Mylan 222/25	Chlorthalidone 25 mg	Hygroton by Mylan		Diuretic
MYLAN2252	Cap, Light Blue & Aqua Blue, Opaque	Selegiline HCl 5 mg	Eldepryl by UDL	51079-0137	Antiparkinson
MYLAN2252	Cap, Light Blue & Aqua Blue, Opaque	Selegiline HCl 5 mg	Eldepryl by Mylan	00378-2252	Antiparkinson
MYLAN2260	Cap, Light Lavender & Yellow, Opaque, Mylan over 2260	Terazosin HCl 1 mg	Hytrin by Mylan	00378-2260	Antihypertensive
MYLAN2260	Cap, Light Lavender & Yellow, Opaque, Mylan over 2260	Terazosin HCl 1 mg	Hytrin by UDL	51079-0936	Antihypertensive
MYLAN2264	Cap, Black & Light Lavender, Opaque, Mylan over 2264	Terazosin HCl 2 mg	Hytrin by UDL	51079-0937	Antihypertensive
MYLAN2264	Cap, Black & Light Lavender, Opaque, Mylan over 2264	Terazosin HCl 2 mg	Hytrin by Mylan	00378-2264	Antihypertensive
MYLAN2268	Cap, Gray & Light Lavender, Opaque, Mylan over 2268	Terazosin HCl 5 mg	Hytrin by Mylan	00378-2268	Antihypertensive
MYLAN2268	Cap, Gray & Light Lavender, Opaque, Mylan over 2268	Terazosin HCl 5 mg	Hytrin by UDL	51079-0938	Antihypertensive
MYLAN2302	Cap, Brown & Light Brown, White Print, Mylan over 2302	Prazosin HCl 2 mg	Minipress by Pharmedix	53002-0453	Antihypertensive
MYLAN2302	Cap, Brown & Light Brown, White Print, Mylan over 2302	Prazosin HCl 2 mg	Minipress by Mylan	00378-2302	Antihypertensive
MYLAN2302	Cap, Brown & Light Brown, White Print, Mylan over 2302	Prazosin HCl 2 mg	Minipress by Caremark	00339-6020	Antihypertensive
MYLAN2302	Cap, Brown & Light Brown, White Print, Mylan over 2302	Prazosin HCl 2 mg	Minipress by Kaiser	62224-0115	Antihypertensive
MYLAN2302	Cap, Brown & Light Brown, White Print, Mylan over 2302	Prazosin HCl 2 mg	Minipress by Actavis		Antihypertensive
MYLAN2302	Cap, Brown & Light Brown, White Print, Mylan over 2302	Prazosin HCl 2 mg	Minipress by UDL	51079-0631	Antihypertensive
MYLAN232 <> 80	Tab, White, Round, Scored, Mylan over 232	Furosemide 80 mg	Lasix by Mylan	00378-0232	Diuretic
MYLAN232 <> 80	Tab, White, Round, Scored, Mylan over 232	Furosemide 80 mg	Lasix by UDL	51079-0527	Diuretic
MYLAN232 <> 80	Tab, White, Round, Scored, Mylan over 232	Furosemide 80 mg	Lasix by Heartland	61392-0254	Diuretic
MYLAN2325	Cap, Orange & Swedish Orange, Imprint in White Ink	Nortriptyline HCl 25 mg	Pamelor by Medirex	57480-0824	Antidepressant
MYLAN2325	Cap, Orange & Swedish Orange, Imprint in White Ink	Nortriptyline HCl 25 mg	Pamelor by Mylan	00378-2325	Antidepressant
MYLAN2325	Cap, Orange & Swedish Orange, Imprint in White Ink	Nortriptyline HCl 25 mg	Pamelor by UDL	51079-0804	Antidepressant
MYLAN2325	Cap, Orange & Swedish Orange, Imprint in White Ink	Nortriptyline HCl 25 mg	Pamelor by Dixon Shane	Discontinued	Antidepressant
MYLAN2325	Cap, Orange & Swedish Orange, Imprint in White Ink	Nortriptyline HCl 25 mg	by UDL	17236-0005	Antidepressant
MYLAN2500	Cap, Blue, Opaque	Tamsulosin HCl 0.4 mg		51079-0294	Antiadrenergic
MYLAN251	Tab, Beveled Edge, Coated, Mylan over 251	Trazodone HCl 50 mg	Desyrel by Mylan	00378-0251	Antidepressant
MYLAN252	Tab, Beveled Edge, Coated, Mylan over 252	Trazodone HCl 100 mg	Desyrel by Mylan	00378-0252	Antidepressant
MYLAN2537	Cap, Green & Yellow, Black Print, Mylan over 2537	Hydrochlorothiazide 25 mg, Triamterene 37.5 mg	Dyazide by Teva	00480-0734	Diuretic; Antihypertensive
MYLAN2537	Cap, Green & Yellow, Black Print, Mylan over 2537	Hydrochlorothiazide 25 mg, Triamterene 37.5 mg	Dyazide by UDL	51079-0935	Diuretic; Antihypertensive
MYLAN2537	Cap, Green & Yellow, Black Print, Mylan over 2537	Hydrochlorothiazide 25 mg, Triamterene 37.5 mg	Dyazide by Mylan	00378-2537	Diuretic; Antihypertensive
MYLAN257	Tab, Orange, Round, Scored, Mylan over 257	Haloperidol 1 mg	Haldol by Mylan	00378-0257	Antipsychotic
MYLAN257	Tab, Orange, Round, Scored, Mylan over 257	Haloperidol 1 mg	Haldol by Heartland	61392-0266	Antipsychotic
MYLAN257	Tab, Orange, Round, Scored, Mylan over 257	Haloperidol 1 mg	Haldol by UDL	51079-0734	Antipsychotic
MYLAN271	Tab, White, Round, Scored, Mylan over 271	Diazepam 2 mg	Valium by Mylan	00378-0271	Antianxiety; C IV
MYLAN271	Tab, White, Round, Scored, Mylan over 271	Diazepam 2 mg	Valium by Allscripts		Antianxiety; C IV
MYLAN271	Tab, White, Round, Scored, Mylan over 271	Diazepam 2 mg	Valium by UDL	51079-0284	Antianxiety; C IV
				Discontinued	
MYLAN3000	Cap, Coral & White, Black Print, Mylan over 3000	Meclofenamate Sodium 100 mg	Meclomen by Qualitest	00603-4345	NSAID
MYLAN3000	Cap, Coral & White, Black Print, Mylan over 3000	Meclofenamate Sodium 100 mg	Meclomen by Mylan	00378-3000	NSAID
MYLAN3000	Cap, Coral & White, Black Print, Mylan over 3000	Meclofenamate Sodium 100 mg	Meclomen by Pharmedix	53002-0400	NSAID
MYLAN3005	Cap, Caramel & White, Black Print, Mylan over 3005	Thiothixene 5 mg	Navane by UDL	51079-0588	Antipsychotic
MYLAN3005	Cap, Caramel & White, Black Print, Mylan over 3005	Thiothixene 5 mg	Navane by Dixon Shane	17236-0467	Antipsychotic
MYLAN3005	Cap, Caramel & White, Black Print, Mylan over 3005	Thiothixene 5 mg	Navane by Mylan	00378-3005	Antipsychotic
MYLAN3025	Cap, Red & Light Orange, Black Print, Mylan over 3025	Clomipramine HCl 25 mg	Anafranil by Mylan	00378-3025	OCD
MYLAN3050	Cap, Flesh & Yellow, Mylan over 3050	Clomipramine HCl 50 mg	Anafranil by Mylan	00378-3050	OCD
MYLAN3075	Cap, Flesh & Swedish Orange, Mylan over 3075	Clomipramine HCl 75 mg	Anafranil by Mylan	00378-3075	OCD
MYLAN3125	Cap, Ivory & Yellow, Black Print, Mylan over 3125	Doxepin HCl 25 mg	Sinequan by H J Harkins Co	52959-0280	Antidepressant
MYLAN3125	Cap, Ivory & Yellow, Black Print, Mylan over 3125	Doxepin HCl 25 mg	Sinequan by Mylan	00378-3125	Antidepressant
MYLAN3125	Cap, Ivory & Yellow, Black Print, Mylan over 3125	Doxepin HCl 25 mg	Sinequan by Allscripts		Antidepressant

ID FRONT <> BACK	DESCRIPTION FRONT <> BACK	INGREDIENT & STRENGTH	BRAND (or Generic Equiv.) by FIRM	NDC#	CLASS; SCH.
MYLAN3125	Cap, Ivory & Yellow, Black Print, Mylan over 3125	Doxepin HCl 25 mg	Sinequan by UDL	51079-0437	Antidepressant
MYLAN3125	Cap, Ivory & Yellow, Black Print, Mylan over 3125	Doxepin HCl 25 mg	Sinequan by Pharmedix	53002-0490	Antidepressant
MYLAN3125	Cap, Ivory & Yellow, Black Print, Mylan over 3125	Doxepin HCl 25 mg	Sinequan by Major	00904-1261	Antidepressant
MYLAN3205	Cap, Light Blue & Light Brown, White Print, Mylan over 3205	Prazosin HCl 5 mg	Minipress by Mylan	00378-3205	Antihypertensive
MYLAN3205	Cap, Light Blue & Light Brown, White Print, Mylan over 3205	Prazosin HCl 5 mg	Minipress by UDL	51079-0632	Antihypertensive
MYLAN3205	Cap, Light Blue & Light Brown, White Print, Mylan over 3205	Prazosin HCl 5 mg	Minipress by Kaiser	62224-0111	Antihypertensive
MYLAN3205	Cap, Light Blue & Light Brown, White Print, Mylan over 3205	Prazosin HCl 5 mg	Minipress by Caremark	00339-6069	Antihypertensive
MYLAN321	Tab, Peach, Round	Haloperidol 5 mg	Haldol by Mylan	00378-0327	Antipsychotic
MYLAN3250	Cap, Orange & Yellow, Opaque, Mylan over 3250	Nortriptyline HCl 50 mg	Pamelor by Dixon Shane	17236-0006	Antidepressant
MYLAN3250	Cap, Orange & Yellow, Opaque, Mylan over 3250	Nortriptyline HCl 50 mg	Pamelor by Mylan	00378-3250	Antidepressant
MYLAN3250	Cap, Orange & Yellow, Opaque, Mylan over 3250	Nortriptyline HCl 50 mg	Pamelor by UDL	51079-0805 Discontinued	Antidepressant
MYLAN327	Tab, Orange, Round, Scored, Mylan over 327	Haloperidol 5 mg	Haldol by UDL	51079-0736	Antipsychotic
MYLAN327	Tab, Orange, Round, Scored, Mylan over 327	Haloperidol 5 mg	Haldol by Heartland	61392-0272	Antipsychotic
MYLAN327	Tab, Orange, Round, Scored, Mylan over 327	Haloperidol 5 mg	Haldol by Murfreesboro	51129-1244	Antipsychotic
MYLAN327	Tab, Orange, Round, Scored, Mylan over 327	Haloperidol 5 mg	Haldol by Mylan	00378-0327	Antipsychotic
MYLAN327	Tab, Orange, Round, Scored, Mylan over 327	Haloperidol 5 mg	Haldol by Vangard	00615-2597	Antipsychotic
MYLAN334	Tab, Light Green, Round, Scored, Mylan over 334	Haloperidol 10 mg	Haldol by UDL	51079-0431	Antipsychotic
MYLAN3422	Cap, Grey and Light Orange, Black Print	Nitrofurantoin 100 mg	Macrobid by Mylan	00378-3422	Antibiotic
MYLAN3422	Cap, Grey and Light Orange, Black Print	Nitrofurantoin 100 mg	Macrobid by UDL	51079-0348	Antibiotic
MYLAN345	Tab, Orange, Round, Scored, Mylan over 345	Diazepam 5 mg	Valium by Mylan	00378-0345	Antianxiety; C IV
MYLAN345	Tab, Orange, Round, Scored, Mylan over 345	Diazepam 5 mg	Valium by H J Harkins Co	52959-0047	Antianxiety; C IV
MYLAN345	Tab, Orange, Round, Scored, Mylan over 345	Diazepam 5 mg	Valium by DRX	55045-2666	Antianxiety; C IV
MYLAN345	Tab, Orange, Round, Scored, Mylan over 345	Diazepam 5 mg	Valium by UDL	51079-0285 Discontinued	Antianxiety; C IV
MYLAN347	Tab, White, Round, Scored, Mylan over 347	Hydrochlorothiazide 25 mg, Propranolol HCl 80 mg	Inderide by Mylan	00378-0347	Diuretic; Antihypertensive
MYLAN351	Tab, Orange, Round, Mylan over 351, Scored	Haloperidol 0.5 mg	Haldol by Mylan	00378-0351	Antipsychotic
MYLAN351	Tab, Orange, Round, Mylan over 351, Scored	Haloperidol 0.5 mg	Haldol by Heartland	61392-0263	Antipsychotic
MYLAN351	Tab, Orange, Round, Mylan over 351, Scored	Haloperidol 0.5 mg	Haldol by UDL	51079-0733	Antipsychotic
MYLAN370	Tab	Bumetanide 1 mg	Bumex by Hoffmann La Roche	00004-0291	Diuretic
MYLAN370	Tab	Bumetanide 1 mg	Bumex by Caremark	00339-6030	Diuretic
MYLAN370	Tab, Mylan/370	Bumetanide 1 mg	Bumex by Heartland	61392-0049	Diuretic
MYLAN377	Tab, Green, Round, Scored	Diazepam 10 mg	by Allscripts		Antianxiety; C IV
MYLAN4010	Cap, Orange, Black Print, Mylan over 4010	Temazepam 15 mg	Restoril by Mylan	00378-4010	Sedative/Hypnotic; C IV
MYLAN4010	Cap, Orange, Black Print, Mylan over 4010	Temazepam 15 mg	Restoril by St. Mary's Med	60760-0607	Sedative/Hypnotic; C IV
MYLAN4010	Cap, Orange, Black Print, Mylan over 4010	Temazepam 15 mg	Restoril by Nat Pharmpak	55154-5591	Sedative/Hypnotic; C IV
MYLAN4010	Cap, Orange, Black Print, Mylan over 4010	Temazepam 15 mg	Restoril by Direct Dispensing	57866-4628	Sedative/Hypnotic; C IV
MYLAN4010	Cap, Orange, Black Print, Mylan over 4010	Temazepam 15 mg	Restoril by UDL	51079-0418	Sedative/Hypnotic; C IV
MYLAN4010	Cap, Orange, Black Print, Mylan over 4010	Temazepam 15 mg	Restoril by Vangard	00615-0470	Sedative/Hypnotic; C IV
MYLAN4070	Cap, Light Celery	Ketoprofen 50 mg	Orudis by Mylan	00378-4070	NSAID
MYLAN41	Tab, Mylan over 41	Hydrochlorothiazide 25 mg, Spironolactone 25 mg	by Mylan		Diuretic; Antihypertensive
MYLAN415	Tab, White, Round	Atropine Sulfate 0.025 mg, Diphenoxylate HCl 2.5 mg	Lomotil by Mylan	00378-0141	Antidiarrheal; C V
MYLAN417	Tab, Mylan/417	Bumetanide 2 mg	Bumex by Heartland	61392-0050	Diuretic
MYLAN417	Cap	Bumetanide 2 mg	Bumex by Caremark	00339-6031	Diuretic
MYLAN4175	Cap, Brown & Orange, Opaque, White Print	Nortriptyline HCl 75 mg	Pamelor by Mylan	00378-4175	Antidepressant
MYLAN4175	Cap, Brown & Orange, Opaque, White Print	Nortriptyline HCl 75 mg	Pamelor by Medirex	57480-0826	Antidepressant
MYLAN4175	Cap, Brown & Orange, Opaque, White Print	Nortriptyline HCl 75 mg	Pamelor by Dixon Shane	17236-0007	Antidepressant
MYLAN4210	Cap, White Opaque, Flesh Opaque	Fluoxetine HCl 10 mg	Prozac by Mylan	51079-0997	Antidepressant
MYLAN4220	Cap, Light Turquoise & Flesh, Opaque, Mylan over 4220	Fluoxetine HCl 20 mg	Prozac by Mylan	00378-4220	Antidepressant
MYLAN4220	Cap, Light Turquoise & Flesh, Opaque, Mylan over 4220	Fluoxetine HCl 20 mg	Prozac by UDL	51079-0971	Antidepressant

ID FRONT <> BACK	DESCRIPTION FRONT <> BACK	INGREDIENT & STRENGTH	BRAND (or Generic Equiv.) by FIRM	NDC#	CLASS; SCH.
MYLAN4250	Cap, Yellow, Black Print, Mylan over 4250	Doxepin HCl 50 mg	Sinequan by Mylan	00378-4250	Antidepressant
MYLAN4250	Cap, Yellow, Black Print, Mylan over 4250	Doxepin HCl 50 mg	Sinequan by UDL	51079-0438	Antidepressant
MYLAN4250	Cap, Yellow, Black Print, Mylan over 4250	Doxepin HCl 50 mg	Sinequan by Major	00904-1262	Antidepressant
MYLAN4350	Cap, White Opaque Body, Light Blue Opaque Cap	Fluoxetine 40 mg	Prozac by Mylan	00378-4350	Antidepressant
MYLAN4415	Cap, Powder Blue & White, Opaque, Mylan over 4415	Flurazepam HCl 15 mg	Dalmane by Mylan	00378-4415	Hypnotic; C IV
MYLAN4415	Cap, Powder Blue & White, Opaque, Mylan over 4415	Flurazepam HCl 15 mg	Dalmane by Southwood	58016-0811	Hypnotic; C IV
MYLAN4415	Cap, Powder Blue & White, Opaque, Mylan over 4415	Flurazepam HCl 15 mg	Dalmane by UDL	51079-0302 Discontinued	Hypnotic; C IV
MYLAN4430	Cap, Powder Blue, Opaque, Mylan over 4430	Flurazepam HCl 30 mg	Dalmane by Southwood	58016-0812	Hypnotic; C IV
MYLAN4430	Cap, Powder Blue, Opaque, Mylan over 4430	Flurazepam HCl 30 mg	Dalmane by UDL	51079-0303	Hypnotic; C IV
MYLAN4430	Cap, Powder Blue, Opaque, Mylan over 4430	Flurazepam HCl 30 mg	Dalmane by Mylan	00378-4430	Hypnotic; C IV
MYLAN451	Tab	Naproxen 500 mg	Naprosyn by Med Pro	53978-2083	NSAID
MYLAN457	Tab, White, Round, Scored, Mylan over 457	Lorazepam 1 mg	Ativan by Mylan	00378-0457	Antianxiety; C IV
MYLAN457	Tab, White, Round, Scored, Mylan over 457	Lorazepam 1 mg	Ativan by Caremark	00339-4020	Antianxiety; C IV
MYLAN457	Tab, White, Round, Scored, Mylan over 457	Lorazepam 1 mg	Ativan by UDL	51079-0386 Discontinued	Antianxiety; C IV
MYLAN457	Tab, White, Round, Scored, Mylan over 457	Lorazepam 1 mg	Ativan by Murfreesboro	51129-1401	Antianxiety; C IV
MYLAN457	Tab, White, Round, Scored, Mylan over 457	Lorazepam 1 mg	Ativan by Nat Pharmpak	55154-2418	Antianxiety; C IV
MYLAN457	Tab, White, Round, Scored, Mylan over 457	Lorazepam 1 mg	Ativan by Nat Pharmpak	55154-1609	Antianxiety; C IV
MYLAN457	Tab, White, Round, Scored, Mylan over 457	Lorazepam 1 mg	Ativan by PDRX	55289-0487	Antianxiety; C IV
MYLAN457	Tab, White, Round, Scored, Mylan over 457	Lorazepam 1 mg	Ativan by Nat Pharmpak	55154-0250	Antianxiety; C IV
MYLAN4700	Tab, Mylan over 4700	Gemfibrozil 300 mg	Lopid by Mylan	00378-4700	Antihyperlipidemic
MYLAN477	Tab, Green, Round, Scored, Mylan over 477	Diazepam 10 mg	Valium by Mylan	00378-0477	Antianxiety; C IV
MYLAN477	Tab, Green, Round, Scored, Mylan over 477	Diazepam 10 mg	Valium by Pharmacy Serv Ctr	00855-3243	Antianxiety; C IV
MYLAN477	Tab, Green, Round, Scored, Mylan over 477	Diazepam 10 mg	Valium by UDL	51079-0286 Discontinued	Antianxiety; C IV
MYLAN5010	Cap, Caramel & Peach, Mylan over 5010	Thiothixene 10 mg	Navane by Mylan	00378-5010	Antipsychotic
MYLAN5010	Cap, Caramel & Peach, Mylan over 5010	Thiothixene 10 mg	Navane by Med Pro	53978-2002	Antipsychotic
MYLAN5010	Cap, Caramel & Peach, Mylan over 5010	Thiothixene 10 mg	Navane by Dixon Shane	17236-0468	Antipsychotic
MYLAN5010	Cap, Caramel & Peach, Mylan over 5010	Thiothixene 10 mg	Navane by UDL	51079-0589	Antipsychotic
MYLAN5050	Cap, Yellow, Black Print, Mylan over 5050	Temazepam 30 mg	Restoril by H J Harkins Co	52959-0459	Sedative/Hypnotic; C IV
MYLAN5050	Cap, Yellow, Black Print, Mylan over 5050	Temazepam 30 mg	Restoril by Direct Dispensing	57866-4629	Sedative/Hypnotic; C IV
MYLAN5050	Cap, Yellow, Black Print, Mylan over 5050	Temazepam 30 mg	Restoril by Mylan	00378-5050	Sedative/Hypnotic; C IV
MYLAN5050	Cap, Yellow, Black Print, Mylan over 5050	Temazepam 30 mg	Restoril by Vangard	00615-0471	Sedative/Hypnotic; C IV
MYLAN5050	Cap, Yellow, Black Print, Mylan over 5050	Temazepam 30 mg	Restoril by St. Mary's Med	60760-0618	Sedative/Hypnotic; C IV
MYLAN5050	Cap, Yellow, Black Print, Mylan over 5050	Temazepam 30 mg	Restoril by UDL	51079-0419 Discontinued	Sedative/Hypnotic; C IV
MYLAN512	Tab, White, Round, Scored, Film Coated, Mylan over 512	Verapamil HCl 80 mg	Isoptin by UDL	51079-0682 Discontinued	Antihypertensive
MYLAN512	Tab, White, Round, Scored, Film Coated, Mylan over 512	Verapamil HCl 80 mg	Isoptin by Thrift Drug	59198-0317	Antihypertensive
MYLAN512	Tab, White, Round, Scored, Film Coated, Mylan over 512	Verapamil HCl 80 mg	Isoptin by Mylan	00378-0512	Antihypertensive
MYLAN5150	Cap, Light & Dark Purple, White Print, Mylan over 5150	Nizatidine 150 mg	Axid by Mylan	00378-5150	Gastrointestinal
MYLAN5150	Cap, Light & Dark Purple, White Print, Mylan over 5150	Nizatidine 150 mg	Axid by UDL	51079-0990 Discontinued	Gastrointestinal
MYLAN517	Tab, White, Oval	Gemfibrozil 600 mg	Lopid by Mylan		Antihyperlipidemic
MYLAN5200	Cap, Blue, Black Print, Mylan over 5200	Tolmetin Sodium 400 mg	Tolectin DS by Mylan	00378-5200	NSAID
MYLAN5211	Cap, Green	Omeprazole 10 mg	Prilosec by Mylan	00378-5211	Gastrointestinal
MYLAN5220	Cap, Flesh & Pink, Opaque, Mylan over 5220	Diltiazem HCl 120 mg	Dilacor XR by Mylan	00378-5220	Antihypertensive
MYLAN5220	Cap, Flesh & Pink, Opaque, Mylan over 5220	Diltiazem HCl 120 mg	Dilacor XR by UDL	51079-0947	Antihypertensive
MYLAN5280	Cap, Flesh & Purple, Opaque, Mylan over 5280	Diltiazem HCl 180 mg	Dilacor XR by UDL	51079-0948	Antihypertensive

ID FRONT <> BACK	DESCRIPTION FRONT <> BACK	INGREDIENT & STRENGTH	BRAND (or Generic Equiv.) by FIRM	NDC#	CLASS; SCH.
MYLAN5280	Cap, Flesh & Purple, Opaque, Mylan over 5280	Diltiazem HCl 180 mg	Dilacor XR by Mylan	00378-5280	Antihypertensive
MYLAN5280	Cap, Flesh & Purple, Opaque, Mylan over 5280	Diltiazem HCl 180 mg	Dilacor XR by Murfreesboro	51129-1681	Antihypertensive
MYLAN5280	Cap, Flesh & Purple, Opaque, Mylan over 5280	Diltiazem HCl 180 mg	Dilacor XR by Physician Total Care	54868-4186	Antihypertensive
MYLAN5300	Cap, Dark Purple, White Print, Mylan over 5300	Nizatidine 300 mg	Axid by Mylan	00378-5300	Gastrointestinal
MYLAN531	Tab, Yellowish Orange, Round, Scored, Mylan over 531	Sulindac 200 mg	Clinoril by Mylan	00378-0531	NSAID
MYLAN531	Tab, Yellowish Orange, Round, Scored, Mylan over 531	Sulindac 200 mg	Clinoril by UDL	51079-0667	NSAID
MYLAN5340	Cap, Blue & Flesh, Black Print, Mylan over 5340	Diltiazem HCl 240 mg	Dilacor XR by Egis	48581-6122	Antihypertensive
MYLAN5340	Cap, Blue & Flesh, Black Print, Mylan over 5340	Diltiazem HCl 240 mg	Dilacor XR by UDL	51079-0949	Antihypertensive
MYLAN5340	Cap, Blue & Flesh, Black Print, Mylan over 5340	Diltiazem HCl 240 mg	Dilacor XR by Mylan	00378-5340	Antihypertensive
MYLAN5340	Cap, Blue & Flesh, Black Print, Mylan over 5340	Diltiazem HCl 240 mg	Dilacor XR by Physician Total Care	54868-4184	Antihypertensive
MYLAN5375	Cap, Bluish-Green, Black Print, Mylan over 5375	Doxepin HCl 75 mg	Sinequan by Mylan	00378-5375	Antidepressant
MYLAN5375	Cap, Bluish-Green, Black Print, Mylan over 5375	Doxepin HCl 75 mg	Sinequan by Major	00904-1263	Antidepressant
MYLAN5375	Cap, Bluish-Green, Black Print, Mylan over 5375	Doxepin HCl 75 mg	Sinequan by PDRX	55289-0258	Antidepressant
MYLAN5375	Cap, Bluish-Green, Black Print, Mylan over 5375	Doxepin HCl 75 mg	Sinequan by UDL	51079-0645	Antidepressant
				Discontinued	
MYLAN5410	Cap, Blue, Opaque	Fluoxetine 10 mg	Sarafem by Mylan	00378-5410	Antidepressant
MYLAN5420	Cap, Pink, Opaque	Fluoxetine 20 mg	Sarafem by Mylan	00378-5420	Antidepressant
MYLAN551	Tab, White, Round, Scored, Mylan over 551	Tolazamide 500 mg	Tolinase by Mylan	00378-0551	Antidiabetic
MYLAN574	Tab, Film Coated	Amitriptyline 25 mg, Perphenazine 4 mg	Triavil by PDRX	55289-0185	Antidepressant; Antipsychotic
MYLAN5750	Cap, Bluish-Green, Black Print, Mylan over 5750	Ketoprofen 75 mg	Orudis by Murfreesboro	51129-1382	NSAID
MYLAN5750	Cap, Bluish-Green, Black Print, Mylan over 5750	Ketoprofen 75 mg	Orudis by Mylan	00378-5750	NSAID
MYLAN5750	Cap, Bluish-Green, Black Print, Mylan over 5750	Ketoprofen 75 mg	Orudis by Direct Dispensing	57866-4639	NSAID
MYLAN6025	Cap, Dark Blue & White, Coated, Mylan over 6025	Cephalexin 250 mg	by Mylan	00378-6025	Antibiotic
MYLAN6050	Cap, Dark Blue & Light Blue, Black Print, Mylan over 6050	Cephalexin 500 mg	by Mylan	00378-6050	Antibiotic
MYLAN6060	Cap, Pink & White, Opaque, Mylan over 6060	Diltiazem HCl 60 mg	Cardizem SR by Mylan	00378-6060	Antihypertensive
MYLAN6060	Cap, Pink & White, Opaque, Mylan over 6060	Diltiazem HCl 60 mg	Cardizem SR by UDL	51079-0924	Antihypertensive
MYLAN6060	Cap, Pink & White, Opaque, Mylan over 6060	Diltiazem HCl 60 mg	Cardizem SR by Egis	48581-6121	Antihypertensive
MYLAN6090	Cap, Pink & White, Mylan over 6090	Diltiazem HCl 90 mg	Cardizem SR by Mylan	00378-6090	Antihypertensive
MYLAN6090	Cap, Pink & White, Mylan over 6090	Diltiazem HCl 90 mg	Cardizem SR by UDL	51079-0925	Antihypertensive
MYLAN6090	Cap, Pink & White, Mylan over 6090	Diltiazem HCl 90 mg	Cardizem SR by Murfreesboro	51129-1365	Antihypertensive
MYLAN611	Tab, Film Coated	Methyldopa 250 mg	by Heartland	61392-0184	Antihypertensive
MYLAN6120	Cap, Pink, Opaque, Mylan over 6120	Diltiazem HCl 120 mg	Cardizem SR by Mylan	00378-6120	Antihypertensive
MYLAN6120	Cap, Pink, Opaque, Mylan over 6120	Diltiazem HCl 120 mg	Cardizem SR by UDL	51079-0926	Antihypertensive
MYLAN6150	Cap, Green and Light Green	Omeprazole 20 mg	Prilosec by Mylan	00378-6150	Gastrointestinal
MYLAN6150	Cap, Dark Green and Blue-Green	Omeprazole 20 mg	Prilosec by Mylan	51079-0007	Gastrointestinal
MYLAN6160	Cap, Violet and Pink, Black Ink, Ex Release	Propranolol HCl 60 mg	Inderal LA by Mylan	00378-6160	Antihypertensive
MYLAN6180	Cap, Orange and Pink, Black Ink, Ex Release	Propranolol HCl 80 mg	Inderal LA by Mylan	00378-6180	Antihypertensive
MYLAN62	Tab	Glipizide 10 mg	by Med Pro	53978-2014	Antidiabetic
MYLAN6201	Cap, Pink, White, Opaque	Verapamil HCl Extended Release 100 mg	Verelan PM by Mylan	00378-6201	Antihypertensive
MYLAN6202	Cap, Orange Opaque Body, Pink Opaque Cap	Verapamil HCl Extended Release 200 mg	Verelan PM by Mylan	00378-6202	Antihypertensive
MYLAN6203	Cap, Pink, Opaque	Verapamil HCl Extended Release 300 mg	Verelan PM by Mylan	00378-6203	Antihypertensive
MYLAN6220	Cap, Violet, Black Ink, Ex Release	Propranolol HCl 120 mg	Inderal LA by Mylan	00378-6220	Antihypertensive
MYLAN6260	Cap, Pink, Black Ink, Ex Release	Propranolol HCl 160 mg	Inderal LA by Mylan	00378-6260	Antihypertensive
MYLAN6320	Cap, Bluish Green & White, Opaque, Ex Release, Mylan over 6320	Verapamil HCl 120 mg	Verelan by UDL	51079-0917	Antihypertensive
MYLAN6320	Cap, Bluish Green & White, Opaque, Ex Release, Mylan over 6320	Verapamil HCl 120 mg	Verelan by Mylan	00378-6320	Antihypertensive
MYLAN6380	Cap, Bluish Green & Light Green, Opaque, Ex Release, Mylan over 6380	Verapamil HCl 180 mg	Verelan by Mylan	00378-6380	Antihypertensive

ID FRONT <> BACK	DESCRIPTION FRONT <> BACK	INGREDIENT & STRENGTH	BRAND (or Generic Equiv.) by FIRM	NDC#	CLASS; SCH.
MYLAN6380	Cap, Bluish Green & Light Green, Opaque, Ex Release, Mylan over 6380	Verapamil HCl 180 mg	Verelan by UDL	51079-0918 Discontinued	Antihypertensive
MYLAN6410	Cap, Light Green & White, Black Print, Mylan over 6410	Doxepin HCl 100 mg	Sinequan by Major	00904-1264	Antidepressant
MYLAN6410	Cap, Light Green & White, Black Print, Mylan over 6410	Doxepin HCl 100 mg	Sinequan by Mylan	00378-6410	Antidepressant
MYLAN6410	Cap, Light Green & White, Black Print, Mylan over 6410	Doxepin HCl 100 mg	Sinequan by UDL	51079-0651	Antidepressant
MYLAN6440	Cap, Bluish Green, Opaque, Ex Release	Verapamil HCl 240 mg	Verelan by UDL	51079-0919	Antihypertensive
MYLAN6440	Cap, Bluish Green, Opaque, Ex Release	Verapamil HCl 240 mg	Verelan by Mylan	00378-6440	Antihypertensive
MYLAN6725	Cap, Purple and Light Blue	Zonisamide 25 mg	Zonegran by Mylan	00378-6725	Anticonvulsant
MYLAN6726	Cap, Purple and White	Zonisamide 50 mg	Zonegran by Mylan	00378-6726	Anticonvulsant
MYLAN6727	Cap, Purple and Light Turquoise	Zonisamide 100 mg	Zonegran by Mylan	00378-6727	Anticonvulsant
MYLAN6727	Cap, Violet and Blue, Opaque	Zonisamide 100 mg	Zonegran by UDL	51079-0768	Anticonvulsant
MYLAN6750	Cap, Peach, Opaque	Balsalazide Disodium 750 mg	Colazal by Mylan	00378-6750	Gastrointestinal
MYLAN6868	Cap, Grey and Red, Opaque, Black Ink	Anagrelide HCl 0.5 mg	Agrylin by Mylan	00378-6868	Antiplatelet
MYLAN6869	Cap, Grey and Greenish-Blue, Black Ink	Anagrelide HCl 1 mg	Agrylin by Mylan	00378-6869	Antiplatelet
MYLAN7005	Tab, Olive, Opaque, Hard Gel, MYLAN over 7005	Loxapine 5 mg	Loxitane by Mylan	00378-7005	Antipsychotic
MYLAN7010	Cap, Olive & Yellow, Opaque, MYLAN over 7010	Loxapine 10 mg	Loxitane by Mylan	00378-7010	Antipsychotic
MYLAN7010	Cap, Olive & Yellow, Opaque, MYLAN over 7010	Loxapine 10 mg	Loxitane by UDL	51079-0901	Antipsychotic
MYLAN7025	Cap, Olive & Light Green, Opaque, MYLAN over 7025	Loxapine 25 mg	Loxitane by UDL	51079-0902	Antipsychotic
MYLAN7025	Cap, Olive & Light Green, Opaque, MYLAN over 7025	Loxapine 25 mg	Loxitane by Mylan	00378-7025	Antipsychotic
MYLAN7050	Cap, Olive & Light Blue, Opaque, Hard Gel, MYLAN over 7050	Loxapine 50 mg	Loxitane by Mylan	00378-7050	Antipsychotic
MYLAN7050	Cap, Olive & Light Blue, Opaque, Hard Gel, MYLAN over 7050	Loxapine 50 mg	Loxitane by UDL	51079-0903	Antipsychotic
MYLAN7065	Cap, Mauve, Opaque, Black Ink	Propoxyphene HCl 65 mg	Darvon Pulvules by Mylan	00378-7065	Analgesic; C IV
MYLAN7096	Cap, Ivory and Tan, Black Ink	Bromocriptine 5 mg	Parlodel by Mylan	00378-7096	Antiparkinson
MYLAN7200	Cap, Brown, Mylan over 7200	Etodolac 200 mg	Lodine by Mylan	00378-7200	NSAID
MYLAN7200	Cap, Brown, Mylan over 7200	Etodolac 200 mg	Lodine by Murfreesboro	51129-1274	NSAID
MYLAN7233	Cap, Light Brown, White Print, Mylan over 7233	Etodolac 300 mg	Lodine by H J Harkins Co	52959-0483	NSAID
MYLAN7233	Cap, Light Brown, White Print, Mylan over 7233	Etodolac 300 mg	Lodine by Allscripts		NSAID
MYLAN7233	Cap, Light Brown, White Print, Mylan over 7233	Etodolac 300 mg	Lodine by Mylan	00378-7233	NSAID
MYLAN7233	Cap, Light Brown, White Print, Mylan over 7233	Etodolac 300 mg	Lodine by DRX	55045-2592	NSAID
MYLAN7250	Cap, Mylan 7250	Cefaclor 250 mg	Ceclor by Qualitest	00603-2586	Antibiotic
MYLAN7250	Cap	Cefaclor 250 mg	Ceclor by Mylan	00378-7250	Antibiotic
MYLAN7250	Cap, Pink & White	Cefaclor 250 mg	Ceclor by Mylan		Antibiotic
MYLAN73	Tab, Coated	Amitriptyline 50 mg, Perphenazine 4 mg	Triavil by Med Pro	53978-2010	Antidepressant; Antipsychotic
MYLAN731	Tab, White, Round, Scored, Mylan over 731	Hydrochlorothiazide 25 mg, Propranolol HCl 40 mg	Inderide by Mylan	00378-0731	Diuretic; Antihypertensive
MYLAN7500	Cap, Gray & Pink, Black Print, Mylan over 7500	Cefaclor 500 mg	Ceclor CD by Mylan	00378-7500	Antibiotic
MYLAN7500	Cap, Gray & Pink, Black Print, Mylan over 7500	Cefaclor 500 mg	by Qualitest	00603-2587	Antibiotic
MYLAN7500	Cap, Gray & Pink, Black Print, Mylan over 7500	Cefaclor 500 mg	by Mylan		Antibiotic
MYLAN7500	Cap, Gray & Pink, Black Print, Mylan over 7500	Cefaclor 500 mg	Ceclor CD by Compumed	00403-0038	Antibiotic
MYLAN772	Tab, White, Round, Scored, Film Coated, Mylan over 772	Verapamil HCl 120 mg	Isoptin by Mylan	00378-0772	Antihypertensive
MYLAN772	Tab, White, Round, Scored, Film Coated, Mylan over 772	Verapamil HCl 120 mg	Isoptin by UDL	51079-0683 Discontinued	Antihypertensive
MYLAN777	Tab, White, Round, Scored, Mylan over 777	Lorazepam 2 mg	Ativan by Compumed	00403-0012	Antianxiety; C IV
MYLAN777	Tab, White, Round, Scored, Mylan over 777	Lorazepam 2 mg	Ativan by Vangard	00615-0452	Antianxiety; C IV
MYLAN777	Tab, White, Round, Scored, Mylan over 777	Lorazepam 2 mg	Ativan by Nat Pharmpak	55154-0913	Antianxiety; C IV
MYLAN777	Tab, White, Round, Scored, Mylan over 777	Lorazepam 2 mg	Ativan by Caremark	00339-4022	Antianxiety; C IV
MYLAN777	Tab, White, Round, Scored, Mylan over 777	Lorazepam 2 mg	Ativan by Mylan	00378-0777	Antianxiety; C IV

ID FRONT <> BACK	DESCRIPTION FRONT <> BACK	INGREDIENT & STRENGTH	BRAND (or Generic Equiv.) by FIRM	NDC#	CLASS; SCH.
MYLAN777	Tab, White, Round, Scored, Mylan over 777	Lorazepam 2 mg	Ativan by UDL	51079-0387 Discontinued	Antianxiety; C IV
MYLAN8030	Cap, Pink, Opaque	Lansoprazole 30 mg	Prevacid by UDL	51079-0121	Gastrointestinal
MYLAN810	Cap, White, Mylan over 810	Hydrochlorothiazide 12.5 mg	Microzide by Mylan	00378-0810	Diuretic; Antihypertensive
MYLAN810	Cap, White, Mylan over 810	Hydrochlorothiazide 12.5 mg	Microzide by UDL	51079-0776	Diuretic; Antihypertensive
MYLAN8200	Cap, Teal and Gray, Exended Release	Ketoprofen 200 mg	Oruvail by Mylan	00378-8200	NSAID
MYLANA	Tab, White, Round, Scored, Mylan over A	Alprazolam 0.25 mg	Xanax by UDL	51079-0788	Antianxiety; C IV
MYLANA	Tab, White, Round, Scored, Mylan over A	Alprazolam 0.25 mg	Xanax by Kaiser	00179-1183	Antianxiety; C IV
MYLANA	Tab, White, Round, Scored, Mylan over A	Alprazolam 0.25 mg	Xanax by Mylan	00378-4001	Antianxiety; C IV
MYLANA	Tab, White, Round, Scored, Mylan over A	Alprazolam 0.25 mg	Xanax by Apotheca	12634-0533	Antianxiety; C IV
MYLANA1	Tab, Blue, Round, Scored, Mylan over A1	Alprazolam 1 mg	Xanax by Mylan	00378-4005	Antianxiety; C IV
MYLANA1	Tab, Blue, Round, Scored, Mylan over A1	Alprazolam 1 mg	Xanax by UDL	51079-0790	Antianxiety; C IV
MYLANA1	Tab, Blue, Round, Scored, Mylan over A1	Alprazolam 1 mg	Xanax by Kaiser	00179-1185	Antianxiety; C IV
MYLANA1	Tab, Blue, Round, Scored, Mylan over A1	Alprazolam 1 mg	Xanax by Compumed	00403-4578	Antianxiety; C IV
MYLANA1	Tab, Blue, Round, Scored, Mylan over A1	Alprazolam 1 mg	Xanax by PDRX	55289-0920	Antianxiety; C IV
MYLANA3	Tab, Peach, Round, Scored, Mylan over A3	Alprazolam 0.5 mg	Xanax by UDL	51079-0789	Antianxiety; C IV
MYLANA3	Tab, Peach, Round, Scored, Mylan over A3	Alprazolam 0.5 mg	Xanax by Apotheca	12634-0525	Antianxiety; C IV
MYLANA3	Tab, Peach, Round, Scored, Mylan over A3	Alprazolam 0.5 mg	Xanax by Murfreesboro	51129-1200	Antianxiety; C IV
MYLANA3	Tab, Peach, Round, Scored, Mylan over A3	Alprazolam 0.5 mg	Xanax by Mylan	00378-4003	Antianxiety; C IV
MYLANA3	Tab, Peach, Round, Scored, Mylan over A3	Alprazolam 0.5 mg	Xanax by Kaiser	00179-1184	Antianxiety; C IV
MYLANA3	Tab, Peach, Round, Scored, Mylan over A3	Alprazolam 0.5 mg	Xanax by PDRX	55289-0945	Antianxiety; C IV
MYLANA4	Tab, White, Round, Mylan over A4	Alprazolam 2 mg	Xanax by Mylan	00378-4007	Antianxiety; C IV
MYLANCYSTA50	Cap, Cysta over 50	Cysteamine Bitartrate 50 mg	Cystagon by Mylan	00378-9040	Nephropathic Cystimosis
MYLANCYSTAGON150	Cap, Cystagon over 150	Cysteamine Bitartrate 150 mg	Cystagon by Mylan	00378-9045	Nephropathic Cystimosis
MYLANCYSTAGON150	Cap, White	Cysteamine Bitartrate 150 mg	Cystagon by Mylan		Urinary Tract
MYLANCYSTAGON50	Cap, White	Cysteamine Bitartrate 50 mg	Cystagon by Mylan		Urinary Tract
MYLANG1	Tab, White, Round, Scored, Mylan over G1	Glipizide 5 mg	Glucotrol by Med Pro	53978-2013	Antidiabetic
MYLANG1	Tab, White, Round, Scored, Mylan over G1	Glipizide 5 mg	Glucotrol by UDL	51079-0810	Antidiabetic
MYLANG1	Tab, White, Round, Scored, Mylan over G1	Glipizide 5 mg	Glucotrol by Nat Pharmpak	55154-5224	Antidiabetic
MYLANG1	Tab, White, Round, Scored, Mylan over G1	Glipizide 5 mg	Glucotrol by Dixon Shane	17236-0441	Antidiabetic
MYLANG1	Tab, White, Round, Scored, Mylan over G1	Glipizide 5 mg	Glucotrol by Compumed	00403-0920	Antidiabetic
MYLANG1	Tab, White, Round, Scored, Mylan over G1	Glipizide 5 mg	Glucotrol by Mylan	00378-1105	Antidiabetic
MYLANG1	Tab, White, Round, Scored, Mylan over G1	Glipizide 5 mg	Glucotrol by Mylan	55160-0122	Antidiabetic
MYLANG1	Tab, White, Round, Scored, Mylan over G1	Glipizide 5 mg	Glucotrol by Heartland	61392-0063	Antidiabetic
MYLANG1	Tab, White, Round, Scored, Mylan over G1	Glipizide 5 mg	Glucotrol by Kaiser	00179-1207	Antidiabetic
MYLANG1	Tab, White, Round, Scored, Mylan over G1	Glipizide 10 mg	Glucotrol by UDL	51079-0811	Antidiabetic
MYLANG2	Tab, White, Round, Scored, Mylan over G2	Glipizide 10 mg	Glucotrol by Dixon Shane	17236-0442	Antidiabetic
MYLANG2	Tab, White, Round, Scored, Mylan over G2	Glipizide 10 mg	Glucotrol by Mylan	00378-1110	Antidiabetic
MYLANG2	Tab, White, Round, Scored, Mylan over G2	Glipizide 10 mg	Glucotrol by Kaiser	00179-1316	Antidiabetic
MYLANG2	Tab, White, Round, Scored, Mylan over G2	Glipizide 10 mg	Glucotrol by Kaiser	00179-1208	Antidiabetic
MYLANG2	Tab, White, Round, Scored, Mylan over G2	Glipizide 10 mg	Glucotrol by Heartland	61392-0064	Antidiabetic
MYLANTM1	Tab, Green, Round	Hydrochlorothiazide 25 mg, Triamterene 37.5 mg	Maxzide 25 by Mylan		Diuretic; Antihypertensive
MYLANTM2	Tab, Yellow, Round	Hydrochlorothiazide 50 mg, Triamterene 75 mg	Maxzide by Mylan		Diuretic; Antihypertensive
MYLERAN <> K2A	Tab, White, Film Coated	Busulfan 2 mg	Myleran by GSK	00173-0713	Antineoplastic
MYLERAN <> K2A	Tab, White, Film Coated	Busulfan 2 mg	Myleran by DSM	63552-0713	Antineoplastic
MYLERAN K2A	Tab, White, Biconvex	Busulfan 2 mg	by GSK	Canadian	Antineoplastic
MYOGESIC	Tab, Green	Magnesium Salicylate 600 mg, Phenyltoloxamine Citrate 25 mg	Myogesic by A J Bart	49326-0182	Analgesic
MYSOLINE250	Tab, Yellow, Square, Scored	Primidone 250 mg	Mysoline by Rightpak	65240-0697	Anticonvulsant
MYSOLINE250	Tab	Primidone 250 mg	Mysoline by Leiner	59606-0697	Anticonvulsant

ID FRONT <> BACK	DESCRIPTION FRONT <> BACK	INGREDIENT & STRENGTH	BRAND (or Generic Equiv.) by FIRM	NDC#	CLASS; SCH.
MYSOLINE250 <> M	Tab	Primidone 250 mg	by Thrift Drug	59198-0181	Anticonvulsant
MYSOLINE250 <> M	Tab	Primidone 250 mg	by Murfreesboro	51129-1168	Anticonvulsant
MYSOLINE250 <> M	Tab	Primidone 250 mg	Mysoline by Wal Mart	49035-0169	Anticonvulsant
MZ1	Tab, Lavender, Round, Film-Coated, M over Z1	Zolpidem 5 mg	Ambien by UDL	51079-0724	Sedative/Hypnotic; C IV
MZ1	Tab, Lavender, Round, Film-Coated, M over Z1	Zolpidem 5 mg	Ambien by Mylan	00378-5305	Sedative/Hypnotic; C IV
MZ2	Tab, Lavender, Round, Film-Coated, M over Z2	Zolpidem 10 mg	Ambien by Mylan	00378-5310	Sedative/Hypnotic; C IV
MZ2	Tab, Lavender, Round, Film-Coated, M over Z2	Zolpidem 10 mg	Ambien by UDL	51079-0725	Sedative/Hypnotic; C IV
MZ50 <> APO	Tab, White, Round, Biconvex	Methazolamide 50 mg	Neptazane by Apotex	Canadian DIN 02245882	Antiglaucoma Agent
N	Tab, Orange, Round, Enteric Coated	Aspirin 325 mg	Aspirin by Neil Labs	60242-0115	Analgesic
N	Tab, White, Round, Enteric Coated	Aspirin 325 mg	Aspirin by Neil Labs	60242-0116	Analgesic
N	Tab, Yellow, Round, Enteric Coated	Aspirin 81 mg	Aspirin by Neil Labs	60242-0118	Analgesic
N	Tab, White, Round, Enteric Coated	Aspirin 81 mg	Aspirin by Neil Labs	60242-0119	Analgesic
N	Tab, White, Oval	Carvedilol 3.125 mg	Coreg by Novopharm	Canadian DIN 02246529	Antihypertensive
N	Tab, Cream, Round	Spironolactone 100 mg	Novo Spiroton by Novopharm	Canadian	Diuretic
N	Tab, White, Oval, Scored	Cimetidine HCl 800 mg	Tagamet by Novopharm	43806-0305	Gastrointestinal
N	Tab, Blue	Diphenhydramine HCl 50 mg	Nytol by GSK	Canadian DIN 00583332	Antihistamine
N	Tab, White	Diphenhydramine HCl 25 mg	Nytol by GSK	Canadian DIN 00450839	Antihistamine
N	Tab, White, Round	Aspirin 325 mg	Aspirin by PG		Analgesic
N	Tab, Red, Oblong	Divalproex Sodium 125 mg	Epival by Novopharm	Canadian DIN 02239701	Anticonvulsant
N	Tab, Beige, Oblong	Divalproex Sodium 250 mg	Epival by Novopharm	Canadian DIN 02239702	Anticonvulsant
N	Tab, Lavender, Oblong	Divalproex Sodium 500 mg	Epival by Novopharm	Canadian DIN 02239703	Anticonvulsant
N	Tab, White, Round, Scored	Gliclazide 80 mg	Diamicron by Novopharm	Canadian DIN 02238103	Antidiabetic
N	Tab, Orange, Oval	Aspirin 650 mg	Entrophen by Novopharm	Canadian DIN 00229296	Analgesic
N	Tab, White, Round, Scored	Selegiline HCl 5 mg	Eldepryl by Novopharm	Canadian DIN 02068087	Antiparkinson
N	Tab, Pink, Oval, Coated, Scripted "N" <> "fleur-de-lis" Symbol	L-Methylfolate 1 mg, Elemental Iron 29 mg, Vitamin C 80 mg, Vitamin D3 400 IU, Vitamin E 30 IU, Vitamin B1 3 mg, Vitamin B2 3.4 mg, Vitamin B3 20 mg, Vitamin B5 7 mg, Vitamin B6 2.6 mg, Vitamin B9 400 mcg, Vitamin B12 500 mcg, Biotin 30 mcg, Copper 2 mg, Zinc 15 mg, Calcium 200 mg, Magnesium 40 mg	Neevo by PAMLAB	00525-2010	Vitamin; Supplement
N	Tab, Reddish Brown, Round, Biconvex, Beveled-Edged, Enteric, Film-Coated	Aspirin 325 mg	Novasen by Novopharm	Canadian DIN 00216666	Muscle Relaxant
N	Cap, Black, "n" logo made of two white outlined shapes	Vitamin C 100 mg, Folate 1 mg, Niacin 20 mg, Thiamine 1.5 mg, Riboflavin 1.7 mg, Vitamin B6 10 mg, Vitamin B12 6 mcg, Pantothenic Acid 5 mg, Biotin 150 mcg	Nephrocaps by Fleming	00256-0185	Supplement
N <> 05	Tab, White, Round, N <> 0.5	Lorazepam 0.5 mg	Ativan by Novopharm	Canadian DIN 00711101	Antianxiety; C IV
N <> 1	Tab, Yellow, Round, Scored, Large N	Haloperidol 1 mg	Haldol by Novopharm	Canadian DIN 00363677	Antipsychotic
N <> 1	Tab, White, Round	Terazosin HCl 1 mg	Hytrin by Novopharm	Canadian DIN 02230805	Antihypertensive

ID FRONT <> BACK	DESCRIPTION FRONT <> BACK	INGREDIENT & STRENGTH	BRAND (or Generic Equiv.) by FIRM	NDC#	CLASS; SCH.
N <> 10	Tab, Green, Round	Terazosin HCl 10 mg	Hytrin by Novopharm	Canadian DIN 02230808	Antihypertensive
N <> 10	Tab, Blue, Round	Amitriptyline HCl 10 mg	Elavil by Novopharm	Canadian DIN 00037400	Antidepressant
N <> 10	Tab, Light Blue, Round, Scored, Large N	Haloperidol 10 mg	Haldol by Novopharm	Canadian DIN 00713449	Antipsychotic
N <> 10	Tab, Yellow, Cap Shaped	Paroxetine HCl 10 mg	Paxil by Novopharm	Canadian DIN 02248556	Antidepressant
N <> 10	Tab, Dark Orange, Round, Large N	Imipramine 10 mg	Tofranil by Novopharm	Canadian DIN 00021504	Antidepressant
N <> 10	Tab, Pink, Rounded Square	Pravastatin Sodium 10 mg	Pravachol by Novopharm	Canadian DIN 02247008	Antihyperlipidemic
N <> 10	Tab, Pink, Shield Shaped	Simvastatin 10 mg	Zocor by Novopharm	Canadian DIN 02250152	Antihyperlipidemic
N <> 10	Tab, White, Round, Black Ink	Ketorolac Tromethamine 10 mg	Toradol by Novopharm	Canadian DIN 02230201	NSAID
N <> 10	Tab, White, Round, Film-Coated	Leflunomide 10 mg	Arava by Novopharm	Canadian DIN 02261251	Antiarthritic
N <> 10	Tab, White, Round, Scored, N/N	Medroxyprogesterone Acetate 10 mg	Provera by Novopharm	Canadian DIN 02221306	Hormone
N <> 10	Tab, White, Diamond Shaped, Scored, 1 / 0	Fosinopril Sodium 10 mg	Monopril by Novopharm	Canadian DIN 02247802	Antihypertensive
N <> 10	Tab, White, Oval	Alendronate Sodium 10 mg	Fosamax by Novopharm	Canadian DIN 02247373	Antiosteoporosis
N <> 10	Tab, White, Oval, Squared Ends, Scored, N <> 1/0	Buspirone HCl	Buspar by Novopharm	Canadian DIN 02231492	Antianxiety
N <> 100	Tab, White, Round, Scored	Chlorpromazine HCl 100 mg	Largactil by Novopharm	Canadian DIN 00232831	Antipsychotic; Antiemetic
N <> 100	Tab, Pink, Shield Shaped	Fluconazole 100 mg	Diflucan by Novopharm	Canadian DIN 02236979	Antifungal
N <> 100	Tab, White, Round	Misoprostol 100 mcg	Cytotec by Novopharm	Canadian DIN 02240754	Gastrointestinal
N <> 100	Tab, Orange, Round	Topiramate 100 mg	Topamax by Novopharm	Canadian DIN 02248861	Anticonvulsant
N <> 100	Tab, Pink, Triangle Shaped	Sumatriptan 100 mg	Imitrex by Novopharm	Canadian DIN 02239367	Antimigraine
N <> 100	Tab, Grey, Round	Morphine Sulfate 100 mg	MS Contin by Novopharm	Canadian DIN 02302799	Analgesic; N
N <> 10025	Tab, White, Round, Scored	Atenolol 100 mg, Chlorthalidone 25 mg	Tenoretic by Novopharm	Canadian DIN 02302926	Antihypertensive
N <> 100MG	Tab, Diamond-Shaped, Yellow, Scored	Azathioprine 100 mg	Azasan by Salix	65649-0241	Immunosuppressant
N <> 100MG	Tab, Light Yellow, Diamond Shaped	Azathioprine 100 mg	Azasan by AAI Pharma	66591-0241	Immunosuppressant
N <> 125	Tab, White, Oval, N <> 12.5	Carvedilol 12.5 mg	Coreg by Novopharm	Canadian DIN 02246531	Antihypertensive
N <> 15	Tab, Off-White, Round, Scored, N <> 1/5	Meloxicam 15 mg	Mobicox by Novopharm	Canadian DIN 02258323	NSAID
N <> 15	Tab, White, Round	Codeine Phosphate 15 mg	by AltiMed	Canadian DIN 00779458	Analgesic; C II
N <> 150	Tab, Lavender, Round Sustained Release	Bupropion HCl 150 mg	Wellbutrin SR by Novopharm	Canadian DIN 02260239	Antidepressant
N <> 150	Tab, White, Round	Ranitidine HCl 150 mg	Zantac by Novopharm	Canadian DIN 00828564	Gastrointestinal

ID FRONT <> BACK	DESCRIPTION FRONT <> BACK	INGREDIENT & STRENGTH	BRAND (or Generic Equiv.) by FIRM	NDC#	CLASS; SCH.
N <> 150	Tab, Yellow, Hexagonal	Sulindac 150 mg	Clinoril by Novopharm	Canadian DIN 00745588	NSAID
N <> 15034	Tab, White, Oval, Scored, 1.5 034	Glyburide 1.5 mg	Glynase by Teva	00093-8034	Antidiabetic
N <> 16	Tab, White, Round, Biconvex, Bevelled-Edge, Scored	Betahistine Dihydrochloride 16 mg	Novo-Betahistine by Novopharm	Canadian DIN 02280191	Antivertigo
N <> 2	Tab, Pink, Round, Scored, Large N	Haloperidol 2 mg	Haldol by Novopharm	Canadian DIN 00363669	Antipsychotic
N <> 2	Tab, Peach, Round	Terazosin HCl 2 mg	Hytrin by Novopharm	Canadian DIN 02230806	Antihypertensive
N <> 20	Tab, Dark Pink, Round, Scored, Large N	Haloperidol 20 mg	Haldol by Novopharm	Canadian DIN 00768820	Antipsychotic
N <> 20	Tab, Pink, Oval, Scored, N <> 2/0	Paroxetine HCl 20 mg	Paxil by Novopharm	Canadian DIN 02248557	Antidepressant
N <> 20	Tab, Cream, Rounded Square	Pravastatin Sodium 20 mg	Pravachol by Novopharm	Canadian DIN 02247009	Antihyperlipidemic
N <> 20	Tab, Blue, Hexagonal, Scored, N <> 2/0	Propranolol HCl 20 mg	Inderal by Novopharm	Canadian DIN 00740675	Antihypertensive
N <> 20	Tab, Light Orange, Shield Shaped	Simvastatin 20 mg	Zocor by Novopharm	Canadian DIN 02250160	Antihyperlipidemic
N <> 20	Tab, White, Shield Shaped	Leflunomide 20 mg	Arava by Novopharm	Canadian DIN 02261278	Antiarthritic
N <> 20	Tab, White, Oblong	Fosinopril Sodium 20 mg	Monopril by Novopharm	Canadian DIN 02247803	Antihypertensive
N <> 20	Tab, Orange, Round, Scored, Film Coated	Isosorbide Dinitrate 20 mg, Hydralazine HCl 37.5 mg	BiDil by NitroMed	12948-0001	Antianginal; Antihypertensive
N <> 20	Tab, White to Off-White, Oval, Scored, Film-Coated tablet	Citalopram 20 mg	Novo-Citalopram by Novopharm	Canadian DIN 02251558	Antidepressant
N <> 200	Tab, Blue, Shield-Shaped, Compressed	Acyclovir 200 mg	Zovirax by Novopharm	Canadian DIN 02285959	Antiviral
N <> 200	Tab, Off-White, Oval	Ofloxacin 200 mg	Floxin by Novopharm	Canadian DIN 02243474	Antibiotic
N <> 200	Tab, Yellow, Cap Shaped	Ibuprofen 200 mg	Motrin by Novopharm	Canadian DIN 00629324	NSAID
N <> 200	Tab, Pink, Round	Topiramate 200 mg	Topamax by Novopharm	Canadian DIN 02248862	Anticonvulsant
N <> 200	Tab, Yellow, Hexagonal	Sulindac 200 mg	Clinoril by Novopharm	Canadian DIN 00745596	NSAID
N <> 24	Tab, White, Round, Biconvex, Bevelled-Edge, Scored	Betahistine Dihydrochloride 24 mg	Novo-Betahistine by Novopharm	Canadian DIN 02280205	Antivertigo
N <> 25	Tab, White, Round	Topiramate 25 mg	Topamax by Novopharm	Canadian DIN 02248860	Anticonvulsant
N <> 25	Tab, Yellow, Round, Scored, N <> 2/5	Spironolactone 25 mg	Aldactone by Novopharm	Canadian DIN 00613215	Diuretic
N <> 25	Tab, Yellow, Round	Amitriptyline HCl 25 mg	Elavil by Novopharm	Canadian DIN 00037419	Antidepressant
N <> 25	Tab, Dark Orange, Round, Large N	Imipramine 25 mg	Tofranil by Novopharm	Canadian DIN 00021512	Antidepressant
N <> 25	Tab, Dark Pink, Round, N <> 2.5	Indapamide 2.5 mg	Lozide by Novopharm	Canadian DIN 02231184	Diuretic
N <> 25	Tab, White, Oval	Carvedilol 25 mg	Coreg by Novopharm	Canadian DIN 02246532	Antihypertensive

ID FRONT <> BACK	DESCRIPTION FRONT <> BACK	INGREDIENT & STRENGTH	BRAND (or Generic Equiv.) by FIRM	NDC#	CLASS; SCH.
N <> 25	Tab, White, Round, Scored, N <> 2 / 5	Chlorpromazine HCl 25 mg	Largactil by Novopharm	Canadian DIN 00232823	Antipsychotic; Antiemetic
N <> 25	Tab, Blue, Round, N/25	Hydralazine HCl 25 mg	Apresoline by Novopharm	Canadian DIN 00759473	Antihypertensive
N <> 250	Tab, Peach, Oblong	Diflunisal 250 mg	Dolobid by Novopharm	Canadian DIN 02048493	NSAID
N <> 250	Tab, Dark Pink, Oval	Azithromycin 250 mg	Zithromax by Novopharm	Canadian DIN 02267845	Antibiotic
N <> 250	Tab, Pink, Oblong	Levofloxacin 250 mg	Levaquin by Novopharm	Canadian DIN 02248262	Antibiotic
N <> 25MG	Tab, Light Yellow, Oval	Azathioprine 25 mg	Azasan by AAI Pharma	66591-0211	Immunosuppressant
N <> 3	Tab, White, Round	Nitroglycerin 0.3 mg	Nitrostat by Parke Davis	Canadian DIN 00037613	Vasodilator
N <> 3	Tab, White, Round	Nitroglycerin 0.3 mg	Nitrostat by Parke Davis	00071-0417	Vasodilator
N <> 30	Tab, Orange, Oval, Scored, N <> 3 / 0	Mirtazapine 30 mg	Remeron by Novopharm	Canadian DIN 02259354	Antidepressant
N <> 30	Tab, Blue, Oval, N <> 3/0	Paroxetine HCl 30 mg	Paxil by Novopharm	Canadian DIN 02248558	Antidepressant
N <> 300	Tab, White, Cap Shaped	Ranitidine HCl 300 mg	Zantac by Novopharm	Canadian DIN 00828556	Gastrointestinal
N <> 300	Tab, White, Oval	Ofloxacin 300 mg	Floxin by Novopharm	Canadian DIN 02243475	Antibiotic
N <> 3035	Tab, Pale Blue, Oval, Scored	Glyburide 3 mg	Glynase by Teva	0093-8035 Discontinued	Antidiabetic
N <> 375	Tab, White, Cap Shaped	Naproxen Sodium 375 mg	Naprelan by Victory	68453-0375	NSAID
N <> 375	Tab, White, Cap Shaped	Naproxen Sodium 375 mg	Naprelan by Elan	00086-0090	NSAID
N <> 4	Tab, White, Round	Nitroglycerin 0.4 mg	Nitrostat by Parke Davis	00071-0418	Vasodilator
N <> 40	Tab, White to Off-White, Oval, Scored, Film-Coated	Citalopram 40 mg	Novo-Citalopram by Novopharm	Canadian DIN 02251566	Antidepressant
N <> 40	Tab, Green, Octagonal	Lovastatin 40 mg	Mevacor by Novopharm	Canadian DIN 02246543	Antihyperlipidemic
N <> 40	Tab, Pink, Shield Shaped	Simvastatin 40 mg	Zocor by Novopharm	Canadian DIN 02250179	Antihyperlipidemic
N <> 40	Tab, Green, Rounded Square	Pravastatin Sodium 40 mg	Pravachol by Novopharm	Canadian DIN 02247010	Antihyperlipidemic
N <> 400	Tab, Gold, Oval	Ofloxacin 400 mg	Floxin by Novopharm	Canadian DIN 02243476	Antibiotic
N <> 400	Tab, Pink, Shield-Shaped, Compressed tablet	Acyclovir 400 mg	Zovirax by Novopharm	Canadian DIN 02285967	Antiviral
N <> 5	Tab, White, Round	Alendronate Sodium 5 mg	Fosamax by Novopharm	Canadian DIN 02248251	Antiosteoporosis
N <> 5	Tab, Light Yellow, Shield Shaped	Simvastatin 5 mg	Zocor by Novopharm	Canadian DIN 02250144	Antihyperlipidemic
N <> 5	Tab, Brown, Round	Terazosin HCl 5 mg	Hytrin by Novopharm	Canadian DIN 02230807	Antihypertensive
N <> 5	Tab, White, Round	Zopiclone 5 mg	Imovane by Novopharm	Canadian DIN 02251450	Hypnotic
N <> 50	Tab, Light Pink, Round	Amitriptyline HCl 50 mg	Elavil by Novopharm	Canadian DIN 00037427	Antidepressant
N <> 50	Tab, Dark Orange, Round, Large N	Imipramine 50 mg	Tofranil by Novopharm	Canadian DIN 00021520	Antidepressant

ID FRONT <> BACK	DESCRIPTION FRONT <> BACK	INGREDIENT & STRENGTH	BRAND (or Generic Equiv.) by FIRM	NDC#	CLASS; SCH.
N <> 50	Tab, Yellow, Cap Shaped, Scored, N <> 5/0	Azathioprine 50 mg	Imuran by Novopharm	Canadian DIN 02236819	Immunosuppressant
N <> 50	Tab, White, Round, N <> 5/0	Cyproterone Acetate 50 mg	Androcur by Novopharm	Canadian DIN 02232872	Antiandrogen
N <> 50	Tab, White, Round, Scored, N <> 5/0	Chlorpromazine HCl 50 mg	Largactil by Novopharm	Canadian	Antipsychotic; Antiemetic
N <> 50	Tab, White, Round, Scored, N <> 5/0	Fluvoxamine Maleate 50 mg	Luvox by Novopharm	Canadian DIN 02239953	OCD
N <> 50	Tab, Reddish Brown, Round, Biconvex, Film-Coated	Diclofenac Potassium 50 mg	Novo-Difenac-K by Novopharm	Canadian DIN 02239355	NSAID
N <> 50	Tab, Pink, Round, N/50	Hydralazine HCl 50 mg	Apresoline by Novopharm	Canadian DIN 00759481	Antihypertensive
N <> 500	Tab, White, Cap Shaped	Naproxen Sodium 500 mg	Naprelan by Victory	68453-0850	NSAID
N <> 500	Tab, Orange, Oblong	Diflunisal 500 mg	Dolobid by Novopharm	Canadian DIN 02048507	NSAID
N <> 500	Tab, Light Pink, Oblong	Levofloxacin 500 mg	Levaquin by Novopharm	Canadian DIN 02248263	Antibiotic
N <> 500	Tab, White, Cap Shaped	Naproxen Sodium 500 mg	Naprelan by Elan	00086-0091	NSAID
N <> 5025	Tab, White, Round, Scored	Atenolol 50 mg, Chlorthalidone 25 mg	Tenoretic by Novopharm	Canadian DIN 02302918	Antihypertensive
N <> 50MG	Tab, Light Yellow, Oblong	Azathioprine 50 mg	Azasan by AAI Pharma	66591-0221	Immunosuppressant
N <> 6	Tab, White, Round	Nitroglycerin 0.6 mg	Nitrostat by Parke Davis	00037621	Vasodilator
N <> 6	Tab, White, Round	Nitroglycerin 0.6 mg	Nitrostat by Parke Davis	00071-0419	Vasodilator
N <> 60	Tab, Orange, Round	Morphine Sulfate 60 mg	MS Contin by Novopharm	Canadian DIN 02302780	Analgesic; N
N <> 600	Tab, White, Oval, Black Ink	Gabapentin 600 mg	Neurontin by Novopharm	Canadian DIN 02248457	Antiepileptic
N <> 6036	Tab, Dark Blue, Oval, Scored	Glyburide 6 mg	Glynase by Teva	00093-8036	Antidiabetic
N <> 625	Tab, White, Oval, N <> 6.25	Carvedilol 6.25 mg	Coreg by Novopharm	Canadian DIN 02246530	Antihypertensive
N <> 70	Tab, White, Oval	Alendronate Sodium 70 mg	Fosamax by Novopharm	Canadian DIN 02261715	Antiosteoporosis
N <> 75	Tab, Off-White, Round, N <> 7.5	Meloxicam 7.5 mg	Mobicox by Novopharm	Canadian DIN 02258315	NSAID
N <> 75MG	Tab, Triangle-Shaped, Yellow, Scored	Azathioprine 75 mg	Azasan by Salix	65649-0231	Immunosuppressant
N <> 75MG	Tab, Light Yellow, Triangle Shaped	Azathioprine 75 mg	Azasan by AAI Pharma	66591-0231	Immunosuppressant
N <> 80	Tab, Pink, Cap Shaped	Simvastatin 80 mg	Zocor by Novopharm	Canadian DIN 02250187	Antihyperlipidemic
N <> 80	Tab, Light Blue, Cap Shaped, Scored, N <> 8/0	Sotalol HCl 80 mg	Sotacor by Novopharm	Canadian DIN 02231181	Antiarrhythmic
N <> 800	Tab, White, Oval, Black Ink	Gabapentin 800 mg	Neurontin by Novopharm	Canadian DIN 02247346	Antiepileptic
N <> 850	Tab, White, Oval	Metformin HCl 850 mg	Glucophage by Novopharm	Canadian DIN 02230475	Antidiabetic
N <> N2	Tab, White, Square	Methazolamide 25 mg	Neptazane by Lederle	00005-4565	Antiglaucoma Agent
N <> SR100	Tab, Pink, Round, N <> SR / 100, Sustained Release	Diclofenac Potassium 100 mg	Voltaren by Novopharm	Canadian DIN 02048698	NSAID
N <> SR75	Tab, Light Pink, Triangle, N <> SR / 75, Sustained Release	Diclofenac Potassium 75 mg	Voltaren by Novopharm	Canadian DIN 02158582	NSAID
N <> WARFARIN1	Tab, Dark Pink, Round, Scored	Warfarin 1 mg	Coumadin by Novopharm	Canadian DIN 02265273	Anticoagulant

ID FRONT <> BACK	DESCRIPTION FRONT <> BACK	INGREDIENT & STRENGTH	BRAND (or Generic Equiv.) by FIRM	NDC#	CLASS; SCH.
N <> WARFARIN2	Tab, Lavender, Round, Scored	Warfarin 2 mg	Coumadin by Novopharm	Canadian DIN 02265281	Anticoagulant
N <> WARFARIN212	Tab, Light Green, Round, Scored, 2 1/2	Warfarin 2.5 mg	Coumadin by Novopharm	Canadian DIN 02265303	Anticoagulant
N <> WARFARIN3	Tab, Light Brown, Round, Scored	Warfarin 3 mg	Coumadin by Novopharm	Canadian DIN 02265311	Anticoagulant
N <> WARFARIN4	Tab, Blue, Round, Scored	Warfarin 4 mg	Coumadin by Novopharm	Canadian DIN 02265338	Anticoagulant
N <> WARFARIN5	Tab, Tan, Round, Scored	Warfarin 5 mg	Coumadin by Novopharm	Canadian DIN 02265346	Anticoagulant
N004	Tab, White, Round	Hydroxyzine HCl 25 mg	Atarax by Northstar RX	16714-0082	Antianxiety; Antihistamine
N007	Tab, Orange, Round, Scored	Propranolol HCl 10 mg	Inderal by Northstar RX	16714-0021	Antihypertensive
N008	Tab, Blue, Round, Scored	Propranolol HCl 20 mg	Inderal by Northstar RX	16714-0022	Antihypertensive
N009	Tab, Yellow, Round, Scored	Propranolol HCl 80 mg	Inderal by Northstar RX	16714-0025	Antihypertensive
N01 <> LU	Tab, Yellow, Cap Shaped, Film Coated	Pravastatin Sodium 10 mg	Pravachol by Lupin	68180-0485	Antihyperlipidemic
N010	Tan, Green, Round, Scored	Propranolol HCl 40 mg	Inderal by Northstar RX	16714-0023	Antihypertensive
N011	Tan, Pink, Round, Scored	Propranolol HCl 60 mg	Inderal by Northstar RX	16714-0024	Antihypertensive
N012	Tab, White, Round	Atenolol 25 mg	Tenormin by Northstar RX	16714-0031	Antihypertensive
N013	Tab, White, Round	Atenolol 50 mg	Tenormin by Northstar RX	16714-0032	Antihypertensive
N014	Tab, White, Round	Atenolol 100 mg	Tenormin by Northstar RX	16714-0033	Antihypertensive
N0172MG	Tab, Green, Oblong, N 017/2 mg	Loperamide 2 mg	Imodium by Novopharm		Antidiarrheal
N019750	Cap, White and Yellow, Black Ink, N/0197 50	Nitrofurantoin 50 mg	Macrodantin by Novopharm	Canadian DIN 02231015	Antibiotic
N02 <> LU	Tab, Yellow, Cap Shaped, Film Coated	Pravastatin Sodium 20 mg	Pravachol by Lupin	68180-0486	Antihyperlipidemic
N020	Tab, White, Round, Scored	Allopurinol 100 mg	Zyloprim by Northstar RX	16714-0041	Antigout
N0202	Cap, Opaque White, N over 020 <> 2	Loperamide 2 mg	Imodium by Mylan	00378-3260	Antidiarrheal
N0202	Cap, N over 020	Loperamide 2 mg	Imodium by Major	00904-7617	Antidiarrheal
N0202	Cap	Loperamide 2 mg	Imodium by Medirex	57480-0830	Antidiarrheal
N0202	Cap	Loperamide 2 mg	Imodium by Heartland	61392-0336	Antidiarrheal
N0202	Cap, N over 020 <> 2	Loperamide 2 mg	Imodium by Amerisource	62584-0768	Antidiarrheal
N0202	Cap	Loperamide 2 mg	Imodium by DHHS Prog	11819-0036	Antidiarrheal
N021	Tab, Orange, Round, Scored	Allopurinol 300 mg	Zyloprim by Northstar RX	16714-0042	Antigout
N022	Tab, Green, Oval	Metoclopramide HCl 5 mg	Reglan by Northstar RX	16714-0061	Gastrointestinal
N02705	Tab, Orange, Oval, Scored, N 027/0.5	Clonazepam 0.5 mg	by Teva	55953-0027 Discontinued	Sedative; C IV
N02810	Tab, Blue, Oval, Scored, N 028/1.0	Clonazepam 1 mg	by Teva	55953-0028	Sedative; C IV
N02920	Tab, White, Oval, Scored, N 029/2.0	Clonazepam 2 mg	by Teva	55953-0029	Sedative; C IV
N03 <> LU	Tab, Yellow, Cap Shaped, Film Coated	Pravastatin Sodium 40 mg	Pravachol by Lupin	68180-0487	Antihyperlipidemic
N03125	Cap, Bright Yellow & Deep Orange, N over 031 <> 25	Clomipramine HCl 25 mg	by Teva	55953-0031 Discontinued	OCD
N03250	Cap, Bright Yellow & Turquoise, N over 032 <> 50	Clomipramine HCl 50 mg	by Teva	55953-0032 Discontinued	OCD
N03375	Cap, Bright Yellow, N over 033 <> 75	Clomipramine HCl 75 mg	by Teva	55953-0033 Discontinued	OCD
N039 <> 50	Tab, N over 039 <> 50	Atenolol 50 mg	Tenormin by Medirex	57480-0446	Antihypertensive
N039 <> 50	Tab, White, Round, N over 039 <> 50	Atenolol 50 mg	Tenormin by Teva	55953-0039	Antihypertensive
N039 <> 50	Tab, White, Round, Scored	Atenolol 50 mg	Tenormin by Novopharm	62528-0039	Antihypertensive
N039 <> 50	Tab, N over 039 <> 50	Atenolol 50 mg	Tenormin by Apotheca	12634-0436	Antihypertensive

ID FRONT <> BACK	DESCRIPTION FRONT <> BACK	INGREDIENT & STRENGTH	BRAND (or Generic Equiv.) by FIRM	NDC#	CLASS; SCH.
N039 <> 50	Tab, N over 039 <> 50	Atenolol 50 mg	Tenormin by DRX	55045-1860	Antihypertensive
N03950	Tab	Atenolol 50 mg	Tenormin by Med Pro	53978-1199	Antihypertensive
N03950	Tab	Atenolol 50 mg	Tenormin by Qualitest	00603-2371	Antihypertensive
N04 <> LU	Tab, Yellow, Oval, Film Coated	Pravastatin Sodium 80 mg	Pravachol by Lupin	68180-0488	Antihyperlipidemic
N084250	Cap, Swedish Orange and Gray, N over 084 and 250 <> N over 084 250	Cephalexin 250 mg	by St. Mary's Med	60760-0008	Antibiotic
N084250	Cap, Swedish Orange and Gray, N over 084 and 250 <> N over 084 250	Cephalexin 250 mg	by URL Mutual	00677-1158	Antibiotic
N084250	Cap, Swedish Orange and Gray, N over 084 and 250 <> N over 084 250	Cephalexin 250 mg	by H J Harkins Co	52959-0030	Antibiotic
N084250	Cap, Swedish Orange and Gray, N over 084 and 250 <> N over 084 250	Cephalexin 250 mg	by Apotheca	12634-0433	Antibiotic
N084250	Cap, Swedish Orange and Gray, N over 084 and 250 <> N over 084 250	Cephalexin 250 mg	by Quality Care	60346-0441	Antibiotic
N084250	Cap, Swedish Orange and Gray, N over 084 and 250 <> N over 084 250	Cephalexin 250 mg	by Rx Dispensing	61807-0005	Antibiotic
N084250	Cap, Swedish Orange and Gray, N over 084 and 250 <> N over 084 250	Cephalexin 250 mg	by Teva	55953-0084 Discontinued	Antibiotic
N0885	Tab, White, Round, N088/5	Pindolol 5 mg	Visken by Novopharm	43806-0088	Antihypertensive
N0885	Tab	Pindolol 5 mg	by Med Pro	53978-2046	Antihypertensive
N093 <> 10	Tab, White, Round, Scored, N over 093 <> 10	Pindolol 10 mg	by Med Pro	53978-2025	Antihypertensive
N09310	Tab, White, Round, N093/10	Pindolol 10 mg	Visken by Novopharm	43806-0093	Antihypertensive
N1	Tab, White, N/1	Acetaminophen 300 mg, Caffeine 15 mg, Codeine Phosphate 8 mg	Novo Gesic C8 by Novopharm	Canadian	Analgesic; C III
N1	Tab, White, Oblong, Scored	Lorazepam 1 mg	Ativan by Novopharm	Canadian DIN 00637742	Antianxiety; C IV
N1 <> LL	Tab, White, Round, Scored	Methazolamide 50 mg	Neptazane by Lederle	00005-4570	Antiglaucoma Agent
N1 <> M	Tab, Blue, Capsule Shaped	Paroxetine 10 mg	Paxil by Mylan	00378-7001	Antidepressant
N10	Tab, Blue, Round, Scored	Diazepam 10 mg	Valium by Novopharm	Canadian DIN 00272450	Antianxiety; C IV
N10	Tab, Cream, Round, N/10	Maprotiline 10 mg	Ludiomil by Novopharm	Canadian Discontinued	Antidepressant
N10	Tab, Yellow, Round, Scored, N/10	Hydralazine HCl 10 mg	Apresoline by Novopharm	Canadian DIN 00759465	Antihypertensive
N10	Tab, White, Round	Domperidone Maleate 10 mg	Motilium by Novopharm	Canadian DIN 02157195	Gastrointestinal
N10	Tab, Light Orange, Scored, N/10	Propranolol HCl 10 mg	Inderal by Novopharm	Canadian DIN 00496480	Antihypertensive
N10	Tab, White to Off-White, Round, Biconvex, Film-Coated, N over 10	Domperidone 10 mg	Novo-Domperidone by Novopharm	Canadian DIN 02157195	Gastrointestinal
N10	Tab, White, Round, N/10	Tamoxifen Citrate 10 mg	Nolvadex by Novopharm	Canadian DIN 00851965	Antiestrogen
N10 <> M	Tab, Green, Round	Ropinirole HCl 1 mg	Requip by Mylan	00378-5501	Antiparkinson
N100	Tab, White, Round, N/100	Sulfinpyrazone 100 mg	Novo Pyrazone by Novopharm	Canadian	Uricosuric
N100	Cap, Yellow, N/100	Nitrofurantoin 100 mg	Macrodantin by Novopharm	Canadian DIN 02231016	Antibiotic
N100	Cap, Orange, Black Ink	Sertraline HCl 100 mg	Zoloft by Novopharm	Canadian DIN 02240481	Antidepressant
N100	Cap, White, Blue Ink	Gabapentin 100 mg	Neurontin by Novopharm	Canadian DIN 02244513	Antiepileptic
N100	Cap, Red and Orange	Mexiletine HCl 100 mg	Mexitil by Novopharm	Canadian DIN 02230359	Antiarrhythmic

ID FRONT <> BACK	DESCRIPTION FRONT <> BACK	INGREDIENT & STRENGTH	BRAND (or Generic Equiv.) by FIRM	NDC#	CLASS; SCH.
N100	Tab, Blue, Oval, N/100	Flurbiprofen 100 mg	Ansaid by Novopharm	Canadian DIN 02100517	NSAID
N100	Tab, White, Round, Scored, N/100	Metoprolol Tartrate 100 mg	Lopressor by Novopharm	Canadian DIN 00842656	Antihypertensive
N100	Tab, Light Blue, Oblong, Scored, N/100	Metoprolol Tartrate 100 mg	Lopressor by Novopharm	Canadian DIN 00648043	Antihypertensive
N100	Tab, White, Round	Acebutolol HCl 100 mg	Monitan by Novopharm	Canadian DIN 02204517	Antihypertensive
N11	Tab, White to Off-White, Round, Film Coated	Methyldopa 250 mg	Aldomet by Teva	00093-2932	Antihypertensive
N11 <> LL	Tab, White, Round	Naproxen 250 mg	Naprosyn by Lederle	00005-3300	NSAID
N110	Tab, White, Barrel, N/110	Buspirone HCl 10 mg	Buspar by Novopharm	Canadian	Antianxiety
N114500	Cap, Orange	Cephalexin 500 mg	by Caremark	00339-6168	Antibiotic
N114500	Cap, N over 114 <> 500	Cephalexin 500 mg	by Apotheca	12634-0434	Antibiotic
N114500	Cap, Orange, N over 114 <> 500	Cephalexin 500 mg	by Teva	55953-0114	Antibiotic
N114500	Cap, N over 114 <> 500	Cephalexin 500 mg	by H J Harkins Co	52959-0031	Antibiotic
N114500	Tab, Coated	Cephalexin	by Med Pro	53978-5021	Antibiotic
N120	Cap, Light Blue, Black Print	Diltiazem HCl 120 mg	Cardizem by Novopharm	Canadian DIN 02242538	Antihypertensive
N125	Cap, Pink	Amoxicillin 250 mg	Amoxil by Southwood	58016-0103	Antibiotic
N125 <> 2	Tab, White, N over 125 <> 2	Alprazolam 2 mg	Xanax by Teva	55953-8125	Antianxiety; C IV
N126 <> 025	Tab, White, Round, Scored, N over 126 <> 0.25	Alprazolam 0.25 mg	Xanax by Teva	55953-8131	Antianxiety; C IV
N126 <> 025	Tab, N over 126 <> 0.25	Alprazolam 0.25 mg	Xanax by PDRX	55289-0962	Antianxiety; C IV
N126 <> 025	Tab, N over 126 <> 0.25	Alprazolam 0.25 mg	Xanax by Medirex	57480-0520	Antianxiety; C IV
N127 <> 05	Tab, N over 127 <> 0.5	Alprazolam 0.5 mg	Xanax by Medirex	57480-0521	Antianxiety; C IV
N127 <> 05	Tab, N over 127 <> 0.5	Alprazolam 0.5 mg	Xanax by Moore	00839-7852	Antianxiety; C IV
N127 <> 05	Tab, Orange, Round, Scored, N over 127 <> 0.5	Alprazolam 0.5 mg	Xanax by Teva	55953-8127	Antianxiety; C IV
N131 <> 10	Tab, N over 131 <> 1.0	Alprazolam 1 mg	Xanax by Medirex	57480-0522	Antianxiety; C IV
N131 <> 10	Tab, Blue, Round, Scored, N over 131 <> 1.0	Alprazolam 1 mg	Xanax by Teva	55953-0131	Antianxiety; C IV
N132 <> 125	Tab, White, Oval, Scored, N score 132 <> 12.5	Captopril 12.5 mg	Capoten by Major		Antihypertensive
N132 <> 125	Tab, White, Oval, Scored, N score 132 <> 12.5	Captopril 12.5 mg	Capoten by Medirex	57480-0838	Antihypertensive
N132 <> 125	Tab, White, Oval, Scored, N score 132 <> 12.5	Captopril 12.5 mg	Capoten by Teva	55953-0132	Antihypertensive
N132 <> 125	Tab, White, Oval, Scored, N score 132 <> 12.5	Captopril 12.5 mg	Capoten by Teva	00093-8132 Discontinued	Antihypertensive
N133	Tab, White, Round, Scored, N over 133	Captopril 25 mg	Capoten by Teva	00093-8133 Discontinued	Antihypertensive
N133	Tab, White, Round, Scored, N over 133	Captopril 25 mg	Capoten by Teva	55953-0133 Discontinued	Antihypertensive
N133	Tab, Quadrisected, N over 133	Captopril 25 mg	Capoten by Medirex	57480-0839	Antihypertensive
N133	Tab, N over 133	Captopril 25 mg	Capoten by Moore	00839-7995	Antihypertensive
N134 <> 50	Tab, White, Oblong, Scored, N score 134 <> 50	Captopril 50 mg	Capoten by Moore	00839-7996	Antihypertensive
N134 <> 50	Tab, White, Oblong, Scored, N score 134 <> 50	Captopril 50 mg	Capoten by Major		Antihypertensive
N134 <> 50	Tab, White, Oblong, Scored, N score 134 <> 50	Captopril 50 mg	Capoten by Caremark	00339-5916	Antihypertensive
N134 <> 50	Tab, White, Oblong, Scored, N score 134 <> 50	Captopril 50 mg	Capoten by Medirex	57480-0840	Antihypertensive
N134 <> 50	Tab, White, Oblong, Scored, N score 134 <> 50	Captopril 50 mg	Capoten by Teva Pharmaceuticals	00093-8134 Discontinued	Antihypertensive
N135 <> 100	Tab, White, Oblong, Scored, N over 135 <> 100	Captopril 100 mg	Capoten by Teva	55953-0135 Discontinued	Antihypertensive
N135 <> 100	Tab, White, Oblong, Scored, N over 135 <> 100	Captopril 100 mg	Capoten by Teva	00093-8135	Antihypertensive
N135 <> 100	Tab, Scored, N over 135 <> 100	Captopril 100 mg	Capoten by Medirex	57480-0841	Antihypertensive
N135 <> 100	Tab, N over 135 <> 100	Captopril 100 mg	Capoten by Major	00904-5048	Antihypertensive

ID FRONT <> BACK	DESCRIPTION FRONT <> BACK	INGREDIENT & STRENGTH	BRAND (or Generic Equiv.) by FIRM	NDC#	CLASS; SCH.
N144500L	Cap	Cephalexin 500 mg	by URL Mutual	0677-1159	Antibiotic
N15	Tab, White	Codeine Phosphate 15 mg	by Rougier	Canadian	Analgesic; C II
N15	Cap, Red and Tan	Temazepam 15 mg	Restoril by Novopharm	Canadian DIN 02230095	Sedative/Hypnotic; C IV
N150	Cap, Red and Purple, White Print	Clindamycin HCl 150 mg	Dalacin C by Novopharm	Canadian DIN 02241709	Antibiotic
N150	Cap, White, Black Print	Fluconazole 150 mg	Diflucan by Novopharm	Canadian DIN 02243645	Antifungal
N150	Cap, Dark Orange, Ex Release	Venlafaxine HCl 150 mg	Novo-Venlafaxine XR by Novopharm	Canadian DIN 02275058	Antidepressant
N160	Tab, White, Oval, Scored, N/160	Trimethoprim 160 mg, Sulfamethoxazole 800 mg	Bactrim by Novopharm	Canadian DIN 00510645	Antibiotic
N17 <> LL	Tab, White, Oblong	Naproxen 375 mg	Naprosyn by Lederle	00005-3301	NSAID
N17 <> LL	Tab, White, Oblong	Naproxen 375 mg	Naprosyn by Physician Total Care	54868-2965	NSAID
N17110	Cap, Brown, White Print, N over 171	Nifedipine 10 mg	Procardia by Teva	00093-8171	Antihypertensive
N17110	Cap, Brown, White Print, N over 171	Nifedipine 10 mg	Procardia by Moore	00839-7564	Antihypertensive
N17110	Cap, Brown, White Print, N over 171	Nifedipine 10 mg	Procardia by Teva	55953-0171	Antihypertensive
N17110	Cap, Brown, White Print, N over 171	Nifedipine 10 mg	Procardia by PDRX	55289-0907	Antihypertensive
N17110	Cap, Brown, White Print, N over 171	Nifedipine 10 mg	Procardia by Warrick	59930-1618	Antihypertensive
N179 <> 5	Tab, N over 179	Selegiline HCl 5 mg	by Warrick	59930-1537	Antiparkinson
N179 <> 5	Tab, White, Round, N over 179 <> 5	Selegiline HCl 5 mg	by Teva	55953-0179	Antiparkinson
N179 <> 5	Tab	Selegiline HCl 5 mg	by Major	00904-5206	Antiparkinson
N180	Cap, Light Blue and Dark Blue, Black Print	Diltiazem HCl 180 mg	Cardizem by Novopharm	Canadian DIN 02242539	Antihypertensive
N181 <> 200	Tab, Coated	Cimetidine HCl 200 mg	Tagamet by URL Mutual	00677-1527	Gastrointestinal
N181 <> 200	Tab, Coated	Cimetidine HCl 200 mg	Tagamet by Brightstone	62939-2111	Gastrointestinal
N181 <> 200	Tab, Film Coated, Engraved	Cimetidine HCl 200 mg	Tagamet by Darby Group	66467-3480	Gastrointestinal
N181 <> 200	Tab, Green, Oval, Film Coated	Cimetidine HCl 200 mg	Tagamet by Teva	00093-8181	Gastrointestinal
N181200	Tab, Film Coated	Cimetidine HCl 200 mg	Tagamet by Sandoz	Discontinued	Gastrointestinal
N192 <> 300	Tab, Green, Oval, Film Coated	Cimetidine HCl 300 mg	Tagamet by Dixon Shane	17236-0171	Gastrointestinal
N192 <> 300	Tab, Film Coated	Cimetidine HCl 300 mg	Tagamet by DRX	55045-2272	Gastrointestinal
N192 <> 300	Tab, Coated, N/192	Cimetidine HCl 300 mg	Tagamet by Brightstone	62939-2121	Gastrointestinal
N192 <> 300	Tab, Green, Oval, Film Coated	Cimetidine HCl 300 mg	Tagamet by Nat Pharmpak	55154-9303	Gastrointestinal
N192 <> 300	Tab, Dark Green, Oval, Film Coated	Cimetidine HCl 300 mg	Tagamet by Teva	00093-8192	Gastrointestinal
N192 <> 300	Tab, Coated	Cimetidine HCl 300 mg	Tagamet by URL Mutual	00677-1528	Gastrointestinal
N192 <> 300	Tab, Film Coated	Cimetidine HCl 300 mg	Tagamet by Warrick	59930-1801	Gastrointestinal
N192 <> 300	Tab, Film Coated	Cimetidine HCl 300 mg	Tagamet by Medirex	57480-0813	Gastrointestinal
N192300	Tab, Film Coated	Cimetidine HCl 300 mg	Tagamet by Sandoz	00781-1448	Gastrointestinal
N2	Tab, White, N/2	Acetaminophen 300 mg, Caffeine 15 mg, Codeine Phosphate 15 mg	Novo Gesic C15 by Novopharm	Canadian	Analgesic; C III
N2	Cap, White	Loperamide 2 mg	Imodium by Moore	00839-7623	Antidiarrheal
N2	Cap, White	Loperamide 2 mg	Imodium by Mova	55370-0169	Antidiarrheal
N2	Cap, White	Loperamide 2 mg	Imodium by Teva	55953-0020	Antidiarrheal
N2	Tab, White, Round, Scored	Diazepam 2 mg	Valium by Novopharm	Canadian DIN 00272434	Antianxiety; C IV
N2	Tab, Orange, Hexagonal, N2 <> Sword Logo	Buprenorphine 2 mg, Naloxone 0.5 mg	Suboxone by Reckitt Benckiser	12496-1283	Detoxification Agent; C III
N2	Tab, Pink, Round	Salbutamol Sulfate 2 mg	Novo Salmol by Novopharm	Canadian	Antiasthmatic
N2	Tab, White, Oval	Lorazepam 2 mg	Ativan by Novopharm	Canadian DIN 00637750	Antianxiety; C IV

ID FRONT <> BACK	DESCRIPTION FRONT <> BACK	INGREDIENT & STRENGTH	BRAND (or Generic Equiv.) by FIRM	NDC#	CLASS; SCH.
N2 <> M	Tab, Blue, Capsule Shaped	Paroxetine 20 mg	Paxil by Mylan	00378-7002	Antidepressant
N2 <> N	Tab, White, Square	Methazolamide 25 mg	Neptazane by Lederle	00005-4565	Antiglaucoma Agent
N20	Tab, Yellow, Oval, N/20	Tenoxicam 20 mg	Mobiflex by Roche	Canadian	NSAID
N20	Cap	Piroxicam 20 mg	Feldene by Rx Dispensing	61807-0039	NSAID
N20	Tab, White, Round, Scored, N/20	Tamoxifen Citrate 20 mg	Nolvadex by Novopharm	Canadian DIN 00851973	Antiestrogen
N20	Tab, White, Round, Scored	Furosemide 20 mg	Lasix by Novopharm	Canadian DIN 00337730	Diuretic
N20 <> M	Tab, Peach, Round	Ropinirole HCl 2 mg	Requip by Mylan	00378-5502	Antiparkinson
N200	Tab, White, Hexagonal, Scored, N/200	Misoprostol 200 mcg	Cytotec by Novopharm	Canadian DIN 02240755	Gastrointestinal
N200	Cap, Blue, Opaque	Acyclovir 200 mg	Zovirax by Teva	55953-8940	Antiviral
N200	Cap, Blue, Convex	Acyclovir 200 mg	Zovirax by Amerisource	62584-0707	Antiviral
N200	Cap, Red	Mexiletine HCl 200 mg	Mexitil by Novopharm	Canadian DIN 02230360	Antiarrhythmic
N200	Cap, Orange, Black Print	Fenofibrate 200 mg	Lipidil Micro by Novopharm	Canadian DIN 02243552	Antihyperlipidemic
N204 <> 400	Tab, Green, Oval, Scored, Film Coated, Scored, N over 204	Cimetidine HCl 400 mg	Tagamet by Medirex	57480-0814	Gastrointestinal
N204 <> 400	Tab, Dark Green, Oval, Scored, Film Coated, N over 204	Cimetidine HCl 400 mg	Tagamet by Teva	00093-8204 Discontinued	Gastrointestinal
N204 <> 400	Tab, Green, Oval, Scored, Film Coated, Scored, N over 204	Cimetidine HCl 400 mg	Tagamet by Rx Dispensing	61807-0066	Gastrointestinal
N204 <> 400	Tab, Green, Oval, Scored, Film Coated, Scored, N over 204	Cimetidine HCl 400 mg	Tagamet by Warrick	59930-1802	Gastrointestinal
N204 <> 400	Tab, Green, Oval, Scored, Film Coated, Scored, N over 204	Cimetidine HCl 400 mg	Tagamet by Brightstone	62939-2131	Gastrointestinal
N204 <> 400	Tab, Green, Oval, Scored, Film Coated, Scored, N over 204	Cimetidine HCl 400 mg	Tagamet by Sandoz	00781-1449	Gastrointestinal
N204 <> 400	Tab, Green, Oval, Scored, Film Coated, Scored, N over 204	Cimetidine HCl 400 mg	Tagamet by URL Mutual	00677-1529	Gastrointestinal
N204 <> 400	Tab, Green, Oval, Scored, Film Coated, Scored, N over 204	Cimetidine HCl 400 mg	Tagamet by Compumed	00403-1005	Gastrointestinal
N21	Tab, White, Round	Nitrazepam 5 mg	by ICN	Canadian	Sedative; Hypnotic; C IV
N21 <> W	Tab, Light Buff, N/21	Nalidixic Acid 250 mg	Neggram by Sanofi	00024-1321	Antibiotic
N214 <> 200	Tab, Pink, Oval, Scored	Amiodarone 200 mg	Cordarone by Teva	55953-0214 Discontinued	Antiarrhythmic
N214 <> 200	Tab, Pink, Oval, N 214/200	Amiodarone 200 mg	Cordarone by Novopharm	43806-0214	Antiarrhythmic
N22	Tab, White, Round	Nitrazepam 10 mg	by ICN	Canadian	Sedative; Hypnotic; C IV
N22 <> M	Tab, Pink, Round	Nisoldipine ER 20 mg	Sular by Mylan	00378-2222	Antihypertensive
N22 <> W	Tab, Light Buff, N/22	Nalidixic Acid 500 mg	Neggram by Sanofi	00024-1322	Antibiotic
N22W	Cap, Yellow, N/22/W	Nalidixic Acid 500 mg	by Sanofi	Canadian	Antibiotic
N23 <> M	Tab, Pink, Round	Nisoldipine ER 30 mg	Sular by Mylan	00378-2223	Antihypertensive
N23 <> W	Tab, Light Buff, N/23	Nalidixic Acid 1 g	Neggram by Sanofi	00024-1323	Antibiotic
N235 <> 800	Tab, Coated, N/235	Cimetidine HCl 800 mg	Tagamet by Brightstone	62939-2141	Gastrointestinal
N235 <> 800	Tab, Film Coated, Scored	Cimetidine HCl 800 mg	Tagamet by Warrick	59930-1803	Gastrointestinal
N235 <> 800	Tab, Coated	Cimetidine HCl 800 mg	Tagamet by URL Mutual	00677-1530	Gastrointestinal
N235800	Tab, Coated	Cimetidine HCl 800 mg	Tagamet by Ivax	00182-1986	Gastrointestinal
N24 <> M	Tab, Orange, Round	Nisoldipine ER 40 mg	Sular by Mylan	00378-2224	Antihypertensive
N240	Cap, Dark Blue, Black Print	Diltiazem HCl 240 mg	Cardizem by Novopharm	Canadian DIN 02242540	Antihypertensive
N24067	Cap, Pink, N <> 240 on cap, 67 on body	Fenofibrate 67 mg	Lofibra by Gate	57844-0322	Antihyperlipidemic
N25	Tab, Pink, Round, N/250	Trimipramine Maleate 25 mg	Novo Tripramine by Novopharm	Canadian	Antidepressant
N25	Tab, Orange, Round	Dipyridamole 25 mg	Novo Dipiradol by Novopharm	Canadian	Antiplatelet
N25	Tab, Orange, Round, N/25	Maprotiline 25 mg	Ludiomil by Novopharm	Canadian DIN 02158612	Antidepressant
N25	Tab, Orange, Round, Coated, N / 25	Diclofenac 25 mg	Voltaren by Novopharm	Canadian DIN 00808539	NSAID

ID FRONT <> BACK	DESCRIPTION FRONT <> BACK	INGREDIENT & STRENGTH	BRAND (or Generic Equiv.) by FIRM	NDC#	CLASS; SCH.
N25	Cap, Yellow, Black Ink	Sertraline HCl 25 mg	Zoloft by Novopharm	Canadian DIN 02240485	Antidepressant
N25 <> M	Tab, White, Round	Ropinirole HCl 0.25 mg	Requip by Mylan	00378-5525	Antiparkinson
N250	Tab, White, Oval, Scored	Chlorpropamide 250 mg	Diabinese by Novopharm	Canadian DIN 00021350	Antidiabetic
N250	Tab, White, N/250	Metronidazole 250 mg	Novo Nidazol by Novopharm	Canadian	Antibiotic
N250	Cap, Gray	Cephalexin 500 mg	by Southwood	58016-0139	Antibiotic
N250	Cap, Gray	Cephalexin 250 mg	by Southwood	58016-0138	Antibiotic
N250	Tab, White, Oval	Ticlopidine HCl 250 mg	Ticlid by Novopharm	Canadian DIN 02236848	Anticoagulant
N250	Cap, Purple and White, N / 250	Cefaclor 250 mg	Ceclor by Novopharm	Canadian DIN 02231691	Antibiotic
N250	Tab, Orange, Oblong, Scored	Cephalexin 250 mg	Keflex by Novopharm	Canadian DIN 00583413	Antibiotic
N251500	Cap, Bright Orange & Gray, Opaque, N over 251 <> 500	Cefaclor 500 mg	Ceclor by UDL	51079-0618	Antibiotic
N251500	Cap, Bright Orange & Gray, Opaque, N over 251 <> 500	Cefaclor 500 mg	by Qualitest	00603-2587	Antibiotic
N251500	Cap, Bright Orange & Gray, Opaque, N over 251 <> 500	Cefaclor 500 mg	by Warrick	59930-1536	Antibiotic
N251500	Cap, Bright Orange & Gray, Opaque, N over 251 <> 500	Cefaclor 500 mg	by Teva	55953-0251 Discontinued	Antibiotic
N251500	Cap, Bright Orange & Gray, Opaque, N over 251 <> 500	Cefaclor 500 mg	Ceclor CD by Major	00904-5205	Antibiotic
N253250	Cap, Bright Orange & White, Opaque, N over 253 <> 250	Cefaclor 250 mg	Ceclor by Major	00904-5204	Antibiotic
N253250	Cap, Bright Orange & White, Opaque, N over 253 <> 250	Cefaclor 250 mg	Ceclor by H J Harkins Co	52959-0367	Antibiotic
N253250	Cap, Bright Orange & White, Opaque, N over 253 <> 250	Cefaclor 250 mg	Ceclor by UDL	51079-0617	Antibiotic
N253250	Cap, Bright Orange & White, Opaque, N over 253 <> 250	Cefaclor 250 mg	Ceclor by Teva	55953-0253 Discontinued	Antibiotic
N253250	Cap, Bright Orange & White, Opaque, N over 253 <> 250	Cefaclor 250 mg	Ceclor by Qualitest	00603-2586	Antibiotic
N3	Tab, White, Round, N/3	Acetaminophen 300 mg, Caffeine 15 mg, Codeine Phosphate 30 mg	Novo Gesic C30 by Novopharm	Canadian	Analgesic; C III
N30	Tab, White	Codeine Phosphate 30 mg	Codeine by Rougier	Canadian	Analgesic; C II
N30	Cap, Red and Blue	Temazepam 30 mg	Restoril by Novopharm	Canadian DIN 02230102	Sedative/Hypnotic; C IV
N30 <> M	Tab, Purple, Round	Ropinirole HCl 3 mg	Requip by Mylan	00378-5503	Antiparkinson
N300	Cap, Yellow, Black Ink	Gabapentin 300 mg	Neurontin by Novopharm	Canadian DIN 02244514	Antiepileptic
N300	Cap, Red and White, Black	Gemfibrozil 300 mg	Lopid by Novopharm	Canadian DIN 02241704	Antihyperlipidemic
N300	Cap, Dark Blue and Grey, Black Print	Diltiazem HCl 300 mg	Cardizem by Novopharm	Canadian DIN 02242541	Antihypertensive
N300	Cap, Light Blue, White Print	Clindamycin HCl 300 mg	Dalacin C by Novopharm	Canadian DIN 02241710	Antibiotic
N305 <> 800	Tab, White, Oval, Scored, 800 <> N score 305	Cimetidine HCl 800 mg	Tagamet by Teva	00093-8305 Discontinued	Gastrointestinal
N325	Tab, White, Round	Aspirin 325 mg	Aspirin by P&G		Analgesic
N3325	Tab, White, Round, N 133/25	Captopril 25 mg	Capoten by Novopharm	43806-0133	Antihypertensive
N342 <> 125	Tab, White, Round, Scored, N over 342 <> 1.25	Glyburide 1.25 mg	Micronase by Brightstone	62939-3211	Antidiabetic
N342 <> 125	Tab, N 342 <> 1.25	Glyburide 1.25 mg	by Warrick	59930-1592	Antidiabetic
N342 <> 125	Tab, White, Round, Scored, N over 342 <> 1.25	Glyburide 1.25 mg	Micronase by Teva	55953-0342	Antidiabetic
N342 <> 125	Tab, White, Round, Scored, N over 342 <> 1.25	Glyburide 1.25 mg	Micronase by Major	00904-5075	Antidiabetic
N342 <> 125	Tab, White, Round, Scored, N over 342 <> 1.25	Glyburide 1.25 mg	Micronase by Ivax	00182-2645	Antidiabetic
N342 <> 125	Tab, White, Round, Scored, N over 342 <> 1.25	Glyburide 1.25 mg	Micronase by Moore	00839-8039	Antidiabetic
N342 <> 125	Tab, White, Round, Scored, N over 342 <> 1.25	Glyburide 1.25 mg	Micronase by Qualitest	00603-3762	Antidiabetic

ID FRONT <> BACK	DESCRIPTION FRONT <> BACK	INGREDIENT & STRENGTH	BRAND (or Generic Equiv.) by FIRM	NDC#	CLASS; SCH.
N342 <> 125	Tab, White, Round, Scored, N over 342 <> 1.25	Glyburide 1.25 mg	Micronase by Teva	00093-8342	Antidiabetic
N343 <> 25	Tab, Peach, Round, Scored, N over 343 <> 2.5	Glyburide 2.5 mg	Micronase by Teva	00093-8343	Antidiabetic
N343 <> 25	Tab, Peach, Round, Scored, N over 343 <> 2.5	Glyburide 2.5 mg	Micronase by Medirex	57480-0408	Antidiabetic
N343 <> 25	Tab, Peach, Round, Scored, N over 343 <> 2.5	Glyburide 2.5 mg	Micronase by UDL	51079-0872 Discontinued	Antidiabetic
N343 <> 25	Tab, Peach, Round, Scored, N over 343 <> 2.5	Glyburide 2.5 mg	Micronase by Major	00904-5076	Antidiabetic
N343 <> 25	Tab, Peach, Round, Scored, N over 343 <> 2.5	Glyburide 2.5 mg	Micronase by Moore	00839-8040	Antidiabetic
N343 <> 25	Tab, Peach, Round, Scored, N over 343 <> 2.5	Glyburide 2.5 mg	Micronase by Heartland	61392-0709	Antidiabetic
N343 <> 25	Tab, Peach, Round, Scored, N over 343 <> 2.5	Glyburide 2.5 mg	Micronase by Brightstone	62939-3221	Antidiabetic
N343 <> 25	Tab, Peach, Round, Scored, N over 343 <> 2.5	Glyburide 2.5 mg	Micronase by Murfreesboro	51129-1405	Antidiabetic
N343 <> 25	Tab, Peach, Round, Scored, N over 343 <> 2.5	Glyburide 2.5 mg	Micronase by Kaiser	62224-1331	Antidiabetic
N343 <> 25	Tab, Peach, Round, Scored, N over 343 <> 2.5	Glyburide 2.5 mg	Micronase by Warrick	59930-1622	Antidiabetic
N343 <> 25	Tab, Peach, Round, Scored, N over 343 <> 2.5	Glyburide 2.5 mg	Micronase by Teva	55953-0343	Antidiabetic
N344 <> 5	Tab, Light Green, Round, Scored, N over 344	Glyburide 5 mg	Micronase by Teva	55953-0344	Antidiabetic
N344 <> 5	Tab, Light Green, Round, Scored, N over 344	Glyburide 5 mg	Micronase by Novopharm	62528-0344	Antidiabetic
N344 <> 5	Tab, Light Green, Round, Scored, N over 344	Glyburide 5 mg	Micronase by PDRX	55289-0892	Antidiabetic
N344 <> 5	Tab, Light Green, Round, Scored, N over 344	Glyburide 5 mg	Micronase by Medirex	57480-0409	Antidiabetic
N344 <> 5	Tab, Light Green, Round, Scored, N over 344	Glyburide 5 mg	Micronase by Warrick	59930-1639	Antidiabetic
N344 <> 5	Tab, Light Green, Round, Scored, N over 344	Glyburide 5 mg	Micronase by Murfreesboro	51129-1288	Antidiabetic
N344 <> 5	Tab, Light Green, Round, Scored, N over 344	Glyburide 5 mg	Micronase by Brightstone	62939-3231	Antidiabetic
N344 <> 5	Tab, Light Green, Round, Scored, N over 344	Glyburide 5 mg	Micronase by Kaiser	00179-1205	Antidiabetic
N344 <> 5	Tab, Light Green, Round, Scored, N over 344	Glyburide 5 mg	Micronase by Qualitest	00603-3764	Antidiabetic
N344 <> 5	Tab, Light Green, Round, Scored, N over 344	Glyburide 5 mg	Micronase by Moore	00839-8041	Antidiabetic
N344 <> 5	Tab, Light Green, Round, Scored, N over 344	Glyburide 5 mg	Micronase by Major	00904-5077	Antidiabetic
N344 <> 5	Tab, Light Green, Round, Scored, N over 344	Glyburide 5 mg	Micronase by UDL	51079-0873	Antidiabetic
N344 <> 5	Tab, Light Green, Round, Scored, N over 344	Glyburide 5 mg	Micronase by Talbert	44514-0385	Antidiabetic
N344 <> 5	Tab, Light Green, Round, Scored, N over 344	Glyburide 5 mg	Micronase by Teva	00093-8344	Antidiabetic
N375	Cap, Grey and Peach, Ex Release	Venlafaxine HCl 37.5 mg	Novo-Venlafaxine XR by Novopharm	Canadian DIN 02275023	Antidepressant
N382	Cap	Clofibrate 500 mg	Atromid-S by Qualitest	00603-2932	Antihyperlipidemic
N392 <> 500	Tab, White, Round	Etodolac 500 mg	Lodine by Teva	55953-0392	NSAID
N393400	Tab, Orange, Round, N 393/400	Etodolac 400 mg	Lodine by Teva	55953-0393 Discontinued	NSAID
N397300	Cap, Opaque & Red, Gray Print, Three Bands, Hard Gel, N397 over 300	Etodolac 300 mg	Lodine by Heartland	61392-0885	NSAID
N397300	Cap, Opaque & Red, Gray Print, Three Bands, Hard Gel, N397 over 300	Etodolac 300 mg	Lodine by Teva	00093-8397	NSAID
N399200	Cap, Opaque & Red, Hard Gel, N 399 over 200 in Gray Ink, 2 Dark Red Bands	Etodolac 200 mg	Lodine by Heartland	61392-0904	NSAID
N399200	Cap, Opaque & Red, Hard Gel, N 399 over 200 in Gray Ink	Etodolac 200 mg	Lodine by Heartland	61392-0903	NSAID
N4	Tab, Pink, Round	Salbutamol Sulfate 4 mg	Novo Salmol by Novopharm	Canadian	Antiasthmatic
N40	Tab, Light Green, Scored, N/40	Propranolol HCl 40 mg	Inderal by Novopharm	Canadian DIN 00496499	Antihypertensive
N40 <> M	Tab, Grey, Round	Ropinirole HCl 4 mg	Requip by Mylan	00378-5504	Antiparkinson
N400	Tab, Dark Orange, Round, N / 400	Ibuprofen 400 mg	Motrin by Novopharm	Canadian DIN 00629340	NSAID
N400	Cap, Orange, Blue Ink	Gabapentin 400 mg	Neurontin by Novopharm	Canadian DIN 02244515	Antiepileptic
N401 <> 100	Tab, White, Round	Atenolol 100 mg	Tenormin by Novopharm	62528-0401	Antihypertensive
N401 <> 100	Tab, White, Round	Atenolol 100 mg	Tenormin by Allscripts		Antihypertensive

ID FRONT <> BACK	DESCRIPTION FRONT <> BACK	INGREDIENT & STRENGTH	BRAND (or Generic Equiv.) by FIRM	NDC#	CLASS; SCH.
N401 <> 100	Tab, White, Round, N over 401 <> 100	Atenolol 100 mg	Tenormin by Teva	55953-0401	Antihypertensive
N401 <> 100	Tab, N over 401 <> 100	Atenolol 100 mg	Tenormin by Medirex	57480-0447	Antihypertensive
N401100	Tab, N over 401 100	Atenolol 100 mg	Tenormin by Qualitest	00603-2372	Antihypertensive
N411134	Cap, Light Blue, N <> 411 on cap, 134 on body	Fenofibrate 134 mg	Lofibra by Gate	57844-0323	Antihyperlipidemic
N412200	Cap, Orange, N <> 412 on cap, 200 on body	Fenofibrate 200 mg	Lofibra by Gate	57844-0324	Antihyperlipidemic
N42025	Cap, Light Green, N420 / 25	Indomethacin 25 mg	Indocin by Allscripts		NSAID
N42025	Cap, Light Green, N420 / 25	Indomethacin 25 mg	Indocin by Murfreesboro	51129-1549	NSAID
N42025	Cap, Light Green, N420 / 25	Indomethacin 25 mg	Indocin by Novopharm	43806-0420	NSAID
N42025	Cap, Light Green, N420 / 25	Indomethacin 25 mg	Indocin by Apotheca	12634-0455	NSAID
N43950	Cap, Green, N 439-50	Indomethacin 50 mg	Indocin by Novopharm	43806-0439	NSAID
N463	Tab, White, Round, N/463	Methyldopa 125 mg	Aldomet by Novopharm		Antihypertensive
N471	Tab, White, Round, N/471	Methyldopa 250 mg	Aldomet by Novopharm		Antihypertensive
N480 <> 2	Tab, White, Round, Scored, N over 480 <> 2	Albuterol Sulfate 2 mg	Proventil by Amerisource	62584-0821	Antiasthmatic
N480 <> 2	Tab, White, Round, Scored, N over 480 <> 2	Albuterol Sulfate 2 mg	Proventil by Apotheca	12634-0090	Antiasthmatic
N480 <> 2	Tab, White, Round, Scored, N over 480 <> 2	Albuterol Sulfate 2 mg	Proventil by Qualitest	00603-2093	Antiasthmatic
N480 <> 2	Tab, White, Round, Scored, N over 480 <> 2	Albuterol Sulfate 2 mg	Proventil by Teva	55953-0480	Antiasthmatic
N480 <> 2	Tab, White, Round, Scored, N over 480 <> 2	Albuterol Sulfate 2 mg	Proventil by Heartland	61392-0567	Antiasthmatic
N480 <> 2	Tab, White, Round, Scored, N over 480 <> 2	Albuterol Sulfate 2 mg	Proventil by Anabolic	00722-6436	Antiasthmatic
N480 <> 2	Tab, White, Round, Scored, N over 480 <> 2	Albuterol Sulfate 2 mg	Proventil by Warner Chilcott	00047-0956	Antiasthmatic
N498	Tab, White, Round, N/498	Methyldopa 500 mg	Aldomet by Novopharm		Antihypertensive
N499 <> 4	Tab, White, Round, Scored, N over 499 <> 4	Albuterol Sulfate 4 mg	Proventil by Allscripts		Antiasthmatic
N499 <> 4	Tab, White, Round, Scored, N over 499 <> 4	Albuterol Sulfate 4 mg	Proventil by DRX	55045-2283	Antiasthmatic
N499 <> 4	Tab, White, Round, Scored, N over 499 <> 4	Albuterol Sulfate 4 mg	Proventil by Qualitest	00603-2094	Antiasthmatic
N499 <> 4	Tab, White, Round, Scored, N over 499 <> 4	Albuterol Sulfate 4 mg	Proventil by Heartland	61392-0570	Antiasthmatic
N499 <> 4	Tab, White, Round, Scored, N over 499 <> 4	Albuterol Sulfate 4 mg	Proventil by Teva	55953-0499 Discontinued	Antiasthmatic
N499 <> 4	Tab, White, Round, Scored, N over 499 <> 4	Albuterol Sulfate 4 mg	Proventil by Medirex	57480-0423	Antiasthmatic
N499 <> 4	Tab, White, Round, Scored, N over 499 <> 4	Albuterol Sulfate 4 mg	Proventil by Anabolic	00722-6437	Antiasthmatic
N5	Tab, White, Round, N/.5	Lorazepam 0.5 mg	Ativan by Novopharm	Canadian	Antianxiety; C IV
N5	Cap, Gray & Red, N/5	Flunarizine HCl 5 mg	by Novopharm	Canadian	Entry Blocker
N5	Cap, Tan	Nifedipine 5 mg	Novo Nifedin by Novopharm	Canadian Discontinued	Antihypertensive
N5	Tab, Yellow, Round, Scored	Diazepam 5 mg	Valium by Novopharm	Canadian DIN 00272442	Antianxiety; C IV
N5	Tab, White, Round, Scored, N / 5	Prednisone 5 mg	Deltasone by Novopharm	Canadian DIN 00021695	Steroid
N5	Tab, Green, Round, Scored, N/5	Haloperidol 5 mg	Haldol by Novopharm	Canadian DIN	Antipsychotic
N5 <> M	Tab, Yellow, Round	Ropinirole HCl 0.5 mg	Requip by Mylan	00378-5550	Antiparkinson
N50	Cap, White & Yellow	Nitrofurantoin 50 mg	by Novopharm	Canadian	Antibiotic
N 50	Tab, Brown, Round	Dipyridamole 50 mg	Novo Dipiradol by Novopharm	Canadian Discontinued	Antiplatelet
N50	Tab, White, Oval, N/50	Flurbiprofen 50 mg	Ansaid by Novopharm	Canadian DIN 02100509	NSAID
N50	Tab, Orange, Round, N/50	Maprotiline 50 mg	Ludiomil by Novopharm	Canadian DIN 02158620	Antidepressant
N50	Tab, White, Round, Scored, N/50	Metoprolol Tartrate 50 mg	Lopressor by Novopharm	Canadian DIN 00842648	Antihypertensive
N50	Tab, Pink, Cap Shaped, Scored, N/50	Metoprolol Tartrate 50 mg	Lopressor by Novopharm	Canadian DIN 00648035	Antihypertensive

ID FRONT <> BACK	DESCRIPTION FRONT <> BACK	INGREDIENT & STRENGTH	BRAND (or Generic Equiv.) by FIRM	NDC#	CLASS; SCH.
N50	Cap, Yellow and White, Black Ink	Sertraline HCl 50 mg	Zoloft by Novopharm	Canadian DIN 02240484	Antidepressant
N50	Tab, Dark Orange, Round, Coated, N / 50	Diclofenac 50 mg	Voltaren by Novopharm	Canadian DIN 00808547	NSAID
N50	Tab, Red, Round, Coated	Diclofenac Potassium 50 mg	Voltaren by Novopharm	Canadian DIN 02239355	NSAID
N50 <> M	Tab, Blue, Round	Ropinirole HCl 5 mg	Requip by Mylan	00378-5505	Antiparkinson
N500	Cap, Orange	Cephalexin 500 mg	by DRX	55045-2787	Antibiotic
N500	Cap	Cephalexin 500 mg	by Rx Dispensing	61807-0006	Antibiotic
N500	Cap, Brown	Amoxicillin 500 mg	Amoxil by Nat Pharmpak	55154-1750	Antibiotic
N500	Tab, Orange, Oblong, novo/500	Cephalexin 500 mg	Keflex by Novopharm	Canadian DIN 00583421	Antibiotic
N500	Cap, Purple and Grey, N / 500	Cefaclor 500 mg	Ceclor by Novopharm	Canadian DIN 02231693	Antibiotic
N500	Cap, Red and White, Black Print, N / 500	Cefadroxil 500 mg	Duricef by Novopharm	Canadian DIN 02235134	Antibiotic
N500	Tab, Yellow, Cap Shaped	Naproxen 500 mg	Novo-Naprox by Novopharm	Canadian DIN 00589861	NSAID
N517 <> 250	Tab, Yellow, Oval	Naproxen 250 mg	Naprosyn by OHM	51660-0714	NSAID
N517 <> 250	Tab, Peach & Yellow, N over 517	Naproxen 250 mg	Naprosyn by Teva	55953-0517	NSAID
				Discontinued	
N517 <> 520	Tab, Film Coated	Naproxen 550 mg	Naprosyn by URL Mutual	00677-1514	NSAID
N518 <> 375	Tab, N over 518	Naproxen 375 mg	Naprosyn by Medirex	57480-0834	NSAID
N518 <> 375	Tab, Pink, N over 518	Naproxen 375 mg	Naprosyn by Teva	55953-0518	NSAID
N52 <> M	Tab, White, Round, Scored, M <> N / 52	Nefazodone HCl 100 mg	Serzone by Mylan	00378-2052	Antidepressant
N520 <> 500	Tab, Yellow, Oval	Naproxen 500 mg	Naprosyn by JLM	63369-0071	NSAID
N520 <> 500	Tab, Light Yellow, Oval, N over 520 <> 500	Naproxen 500 mg	Naprosyn by Teva	55953-0520	NSAID
				Discontinued	
N520 <> 500	Tab, N over 520	Naproxen 500 mg	Naprosyn by Medirex	57480-0835	NSAID
N524 <> 5	Tab, White, Oval, Scored	Glipizide 5 mg	by Novopharm	43806-0524	Antidiabetic
N525 <> 10	Tab, White, Oval, Scored	Glipizide 10 mg	by Novopharm	43806-0525	Antidiabetic
N53 <> M	Tab, White, Round, Scored, M <> N / 53	Nefazodone HCl 150 mg	Serzone by Mylan	00378-2053	Antidepressant
N531 <> 275	Tab, White, Round, Film Coated, N over 531	Naproxen 275 mg	Naprosyn by Moore	00839-7889	NSAID
N531 <> 275	Tab, White, Round, Film Coated, N over 531	Naproxen 275 mg	Naprosyn by Major	00904-5040	NSAID
N531 <> 275	Tab, White, Round, Film Coated, N over 531	Naproxen 275 mg	Naprosyn by Teva	55953-0531	NSAID
				Discontinued	
N533 <> 550	Tab, White, Oval, Film Coated, N over 533	Naproxen 550 mg	Naprosyn by Moore	00839-7890	NSAID
N533 <> 550	Tab, White, Oval, Film Coated, N over 533	Naproxen 550 mg	Naprosyn by Major	00904-5041	NSAID
N533 <> 550	Tab, White, Oval, Film Coated, N over 533	Naproxen 550 mg	Naprosyn by Teva	55953-0533	NSAID
N54 <> M	Tab, White, Round, M <> N / 54	Nefazodone HCl 200 mg	Serzone by Mylan	00378-2054	Antidepressant
N544 <> 150	Tab, White, Round, Film Coated, N over 544	Ranitidine HCl 150 mg	Zantac by RX Pak	65084-0165	Gastrointestinal
N544 <> 150	Tab, White, Round, Film Coated, N over 544	Ranitidine HCl 150 mg	Zantac by RX Pak	65084-0180	Gastrointestinal
N544 <> 150	Tab, White, Round, Film Coated, N over 544	Ranitidine HCl 150 mg	Zantac by Murfreesboro	51129-1197	Gastrointestinal
N544 <> 150	Tab, White, Round, Film Coated, N over 544	Ranitidine HCl 150 mg	Zantac by Pharmacy Care	65070-0053	Gastrointestinal
N544 <> 150	Tab, White, Round, Film Coated, N over 544	Ranitidine HCl 150 mg	Zantac by UDL	51079-0879	Gastrointestinal
N544 <> 150	Tab, White, Round, Film Coated, N over 544	Ranitidine HCl 150 mg	Zantac by Teva	55953-0544	Gastrointestinal
N544 <> 150	Tab, White, Round, Film Coated, N over 544	Ranitidine HCl 150 mg	Zantac by RX Pak	65084-0177	Gastrointestinal
N544 <> 150	Tab, White, Round, Film Coated, N over 544	Ranitidine HCl 150 mg	Zantac by Med Pro	53978-2075	Gastrointestinal
N544 <> 150	Tab, White, Round, Film Coated, N over 544	Ranitidine HCl 150 mg	Zantac by Nat Pharmpak	55154-5581	Gastrointestinal
N544 <> 150	Tab, White, Round, Film Coated, N over 544	Ranitidine HCl 150 mg	Zantac by Teva	00093-8544	Gastrointestinal
				Discontinued	

ID FRONT <> BACK	DESCRIPTION FRONT <> BACK	INGREDIENT & STRENGTH	BRAND (or Generic Equiv.) by FIRM	NDC#	CLASS; SCH.
N547 <> 300	Tab, White, Cap Shaped, Film Coated, N over 547	Ranitidine HCl 300 mg	Zantac by Teva	00093-8547 Discontinued	Gastrointestinal
N547 <> 300	Tab, White, Cap Shaped, Film Coated, N over 547	Ranitidine HCl 300 mg	Zantac by UDL	51079-0880	Gastrointestinal
N547 <> 300	Tab, White, Cap Shaped, Film Coated, N over 547	Ranitidine HCl 300 mg	Zantac by Teva	55953-0547	Gastrointestinal
N548 <> 150	Tab, Peach, Round, N over 548	Fluconazole 150 mg	Diflucan by Teva	00093-7204 Discontinued	Antifungal
N55 <> M	Tab, White, Round, M <> N / 55	Nefazodone HCl 250 mg	Serzone by Mylan	00378-2055	Antidepressant
N550 <> 50	Tab, Peach, Round, N over 550	Fluconazole 50 mg	Diflucan by Teva	00093-0237 Discontinued	Antifungal
N551 <> 100	Tab, Peach, Round, N over 551	Fluconazole 100 mg	Diflucan by Teva	00093-7203 Discontinued	Antifungal
N552 <> 200	Tab, Peach, Round, N over 552	Fluconazole 200 mg	Diflucan by Teva	00093-7205 Discontinued	Antifungal
N557 <> 100	Tab, Blue, Round, Film Coated	Flurbiprofen 100 mg	Ansaid by Invamed	52189-0392	NSAID
N573 <> 50	Tab, Film Coated	Flurbiprofen 50 mg	Ansaid by Moore	00839-8003	NSAID
N573 <> 50	Tab, Film Coated	Flurbiprofen 50 mg	Ansaid by Warrick	59930-1771	NSAID
N57350	Tab, White, Round, N 573/50	Flurbiprofen 50 mg	Ansaid by Novopharm	43806-0573	NSAID
N577 <> 100	Tab, Film Coated	Flurbiprofen 100 mg	Ansaid by Moore	00839-8004	NSAID
N577 <> 100	Tab, Film Coated	Flurbiprofen 100 mg	Ansaid by Qualitest	00603-3700	NSAID
N577 <> 100	Tab, Film Coated	Flurbiprofen 100 mg	Ansaid by Warrick	59930-1772	NSAID
N577100	Tab, Deep Blue, Round, N 577/100	Flurbiprofen 100 mg	Ansaid by Novopharm	43806-0577	NSAID
N590 <> 1	Tab, White to Off-White, Round, Scored, N over 590	Doxazosin Mesylate 1 mg	Cardura by Teva	00093-8120	Antihypertensive
N593 <> 2	Tab, White to Off-White, Cap Shaped, Scored	Doxazosin Mesylate 2 mg	Cardura by Teva	00093-8121	Antihypertensive
N596 <> 4	Tab, White to Off-White, Diamond Shaped, Scored, N over 596	Doxazosin Mesylate 4 mg	Cardura by Teva	00093-8122	Antihypertensive
N598 <> 8	Tab, White to Off-White, Round, Scored, N over 598	Doxazosin Mesylate 8 mg	Cardura by Teva	00093-8123	Antihypertensive
N61710	Cap, Gray & Dark Green, N617/10	Piroxicam 10 mg	Feldene by Teva	55953-0617	NSAID
N61710	Cap, Gray & Dark Green, N617/10	Piroxicam 10 mg	Feldene by Moore	00839-7773	NSAID
N61710	Cap, Gray & Dark Green, N617/10	Piroxicam 10 mg	Feldene by Heartland	61392-0398	NSAID
N634	Tab, Green, Round, N/634	Hydrochlorothiazide 15 mg, Methyldopa 250 mg	Aldoril by Novopharm		Diuretic; Antihypertensive
N635	Tab, Green, Round, N/635	Hydrochlorothiazide 30 mg, Methyldopa 500 mg	Aldoril by Novopharm		Diuretic; Antihypertensive
N64020	Cap, Dark Green, N640/20	Piroxicam 20 mg	Feldene by Teva	55953-0640	NSAID
N64020	Cap, Dark Green	Piroxicam 20 mg	Feldene by Heartland	61392-0401	NSAID
N64020	Cap	Piroxicam 20 mg	Feldene by Med Pro	53978-1255	NSAID
N64020	Cap	Piroxicam 20 mg	Feldene by Moore	00839-7774	NSAID
N642	Tab, White, Round, N/642	Hydrochlorothiazide 25 mg, Methyldopa 250 mg	Aldoril by Novopharm		Diuretic; Antihypertensive
N643	Tab, White, Round, N/643	Hydrochlorothiazide 50 mg, Methyldopa 500 mg	Aldoril by Novopharm		Diuretic; Antihypertensive
N67	Cap, Yellow, Black Print	Fenofibrate 67 mg	Lipidil Micro by Novopharm	Canadian DIN 02243551	Antihyperlipidemic
N716500	Cap, Buff, Opaque, N over 716	Amoxicillin 500 mg	Amoxil by Teva	00093-8716	Antibiotic
N716500	Cap, Buff, Opaque, N over 716	Amoxicillin 500 mg	Amoxil by Teva	55953-0716 Discontinued	Antibiotic
N716500	Cap	Amoxicillin 500 mg	Amoxil by Dept Health	53808-0040	Antibiotic
N716500	Cap, Buff, Opaque, N over 716 <> 500	Amoxicillin 500 mg	Amoxil by Novopharm	43806-0716	Antibiotic
N716500	Cap	Amoxicillin 500 mg	Amoxil by Casa DeAmigos	62138-0601	Antibiotic
N716500	Cap	Amoxicillin 500 mg	Amoxil by Med Pro	53978-5003	Antibiotic
N716500	Cap	Amoxicillin 500 mg	Amoxil by Qualitest	00603-2267	Antibiotic
N716500	Cap, Buff	Amoxicillin 500 mg	Amoxil by Rx Dispensing	61807-0002	Antibiotic
N716500	Cap, N over 716	Amoxicillin 500 mg	Amoxil by St. Mary's Med	60760-0716	Antibiotic

ID FRONT <> BACK	DESCRIPTION FRONT <> BACK	INGREDIENT & STRENGTH	BRAND (or Generic Equiv.) by FIRM	NDC#	CLASS; SCH.
N724250	Cap, Buff & Caramel, N over 724 <> 250	Amoxicillin 250 mg	Amoxil by Apotheca	12634-0185	Antibiotic
N724250	Cap, Buff & Caramel, N over 724 <> 250	Amoxicillin 250 mg	Amoxil by Dept Health	53808-0039	Antibiotic
N724250	Cap, Buff & Caramel, N over 724 <> 250	Amoxicillin 250 mg	Amoxil by Novopharm	43806-0724	Antibiotic
N724250	Cap, Buff & Caramel, N over 724 <> 250	Amoxicillin 250 mg	Amoxil by Qualitest	00603-2266	Antibiotic
N724250	Cap, Buff & Caramel, N over 724 <> 250	Amoxicillin 250 mg	Amoxil by Teva	55953-0724 Discontinued	Antibiotic
N727 <> 50	Tab, Film Coated, N 727	Metoprolol Tartrate 50 mg	Lopressor by Brightstone	62939-2211	Antihypertensive
N727 <> 50	Tab, White, Cap Shaped, Film Coated, Engraved N 727	Metoprolol Tartrate 50 mg	Lopressor by Teva	55953-0727 Discontinued	Antihypertensive
N727 <> 50	Tab, Film Coated	Metoprolol Tartrate 50 mg	Lopressor by Medirex	57480-0802	Antihypertensive
N727 <> 50	Tab, White, Oblong, Scored, Film, N 727	Metoprolol Tartrate 50 mg	Lopressor by Neuman	64579-0095	Antihypertensive
N727 <> 50	Tab, White, Oblong, Scored	Metoprolol Tartrate 50 mg	Lopressor by Va Cmop	65243-0048	Antihypertensive
N727 <> 50	Tab, White, Oblong, Scored	Metoprolol Tartrate 100 mg	Lopressor by Va Cmop	65243-0091	Antihypertensive
N734	Tab, Film Coated, N 734	Metoprolol Tartrate 100 mg	Lopressor by Brightstone	62939-2221	Antihypertensive
N734 <> 100	Tab, Film Coated	Metoprolol Tartrate 100 mg	Lopressor by Medirex	57480-0803	Antihypertensive
N734 <> 100	Tab, White, Oblong, Scored, Film, N 734	Metoprolol Tartrate 100 mg	Lopressor by Neuman	64579-0079	Antihypertensive
N734 <> 100	Tab, White, Cap Shaped, Film Coated, Engraved	Metoprolol Tartrate 100 mg	Lopressor by Teva	55953-0734 Discontinued	Antihypertensive
N734 <> 100	Tab, Film Coated	Metoprolol Tartrate 100 mg	Lopressor by Direct Dispensing	57866-6579	Antihypertensive
N735 <> 50	Tab, Dark Orange, Round, Film Coated	Diclofenac Sodium 50 mg	by Allscripts		NSAID
N73550	Tab, Orange, Round, N 735/50	Diclofenac Sodium 50 mg	by Teva	55953-0735 Discontinued	NSAID
N737 <> 75	Tab, White, Round, Film Coated	Diclofenac Sodium 75 mg	by Allscripts		NSAID
N737 <> 75	Tab, Delayed Release	Diclofenac Sodium 75 mg	by Rx Dispensing	61807-0088	NSAID
N737 <> 75	Tab, Delayed Release, N over 737	Diclofenac Sodium 75 mg	by Warrick	59930-1642	NSAID
N737 <> 75	Tab, White, Round	Diclofenac Sodium 75 mg	by Teva	55953-0737 Discontinued	NSAID
N737 <> 75	Tab, N over 737 <> 75	Diclofenac Sodium 75 mg	by DRX	55045-2247	NSAID
N737 <> 75	Tab, N over 737 <> 75	Diclofenac Sodium 75 mg	by H J Harkins Co	52959-0423	NSAID
N739150	Cap, Light Orange & Tan, N over 739	Mexiletine 150 mg	Mexitil by Physician Total Care	54868-3776	Antiarrhythmic
N739150	Cap, Light Orange & Tan, N over 739	Mexiletine 150 mg	Mexitil by Warrick	59930-1685	Antiarrhythmic
N739150	Cap, Light Orange & Tan, N over 739	Mexiletine 150 mg	Mexitil by Neuman	64579-0186	Antiarrhythmic
N739150	Cap, Light Orange & Tan, N over 739	Mexiletine 150 mg	Mexitil by Brightstone	62939-2312	Antiarrhythmic
N739150	Cap, Light Orange & Tan, N over 739	Mexiletine 150 mg	Mexitil by Teva	55953-0739	Antiarrhythmic
N739150	Cap, Light Orange & Tan, N over 739	Mexiletine 150 mg	Mexitil by Medirex	57480-0836	Antiarrhythmic
N739150	Cap, Light Orange & Tan, N over 739	Mexiletine 150 mg	Mexitil by Teva	00093-8739	Antiarrhythmic
N740200	Cap, Light Orange, N over 740	Mexiletine 200 mg	Mexitil by Teva	00093-8740	Antiarrhythmic
N740200	Cap, Light Orange, N over 740	Mexiletine 200 mg	Mexitil by Medirex	57480-0837	Antiarrhythmic
N740200	Cap, Light Orange, N over 740	Mexiletine 200 mg	Mexitil by Neuman	55953-0740	Antiarrhythmic
N740200	Cap, Light Orange, N over 740	Mexiletine 150 mg	Mexitil by Teva	59930-1686	Antiarrhythmic
N740200	Cap, Light Orange, N over 740	Mexiletine 200 mg	Mexitil by Warrick	62939-2322	Antiarrhythmic
N741250	Cap, Light Orange & Dark Green, N over 741	Mexiletine 250 mg	Mexitil by Teva	55953-0741	Antiarrhythmic
N741250	Cap, Light Orange & Dark Green, N over 741	Mexiletine 250 mg	Mexitil by Brightstone	62939-2332	Antiarrhythmic
N741250	Cap, Light Orange & Dark Green, N over 741	Mexiletine 250 mg	Mexitil by Warrick	59930-1687	Antiarrhythmic
N741250	Cap, Light Orange & Dark Green, N over 741	Mexiletine 250 mg	Mexitil by Teva	00093-8741	Antiarrhythmic
N747 <> 125	Tab, Cherry & Rose, Chewable, N over 747 <> 25	Amoxicillin 155 mg	Amoxil by Teva	55953-0747	Antibiotic
N747 <> 125	Tab, Chewable	Amoxicillin 155 mg	Amoxil by Warrick	59930-1573	Antibiotic
N 75	Tab, Orange, Round	Dipyridamole 75 mg	Novo Dipiradol by Novopharm	Canadian Discontinued	Antiplatelet

ID FRONT <> BACK	DESCRIPTION FRONT <> BACK	INGREDIENT & STRENGTH	BRAND (or Generic Equiv.) by FIRM	NDC#	CLASS; SCH.
N75	Tab, Red, Round, Scored, N/75	Maprotiline 75 mg	Ludiomil by Novopharm	Canadian DIN 02158639	Antidepressant
N75	Cap, Peach, Ex Release	Venlafaxine HCl 75 mg	Novo-Venlafaxine XR by Novopharm	Canadian DIN 02275031	Antidepressant
N751 <> 250	Tab, Pink, Round, Scored, Chewable, 250 <> N over 751	Amoxicillin 250 mg	Amoxil by Teva	55953-0751 Discontinued	Antibiotic
N751 <> 250	Tab, Pink, Round, Scored, Chewable, 250 <> N over 751	Amoxicillin 250 mg	Amoxil by Warrick	59930-1611	Antibiotic
N77 <> LL	Tab, White, Oblong	Naproxen 500 mg	Naprosyn by St. Mary's Med	60760-0452	NSAID
N77 <> LL	Tab, White, Oblong	Naproxen 500 mg	Naprosyn by Lederle	00005-3302	NSAID
N8	Tab, Orange, Hexagonal, N8 <> Sword Logo	Buprenorphine 8 mg, Naloxone 2 mg	Suboxone by Reckitt Benckiser	12496-1306	Detoxification Agent; C III
N80	Tab, Yellow, Cap Shaped, Scored	Furosemide 80 mg	Lasix by Novopharm	Canadian DIN 00765953	Diuretic
N80	Tab, Yellow, Scored, N/80	Propranolol HCl 80 mg	Inderal by Novopharm	Canadian DIN 00496502	Antihypertensive
N80	Tab, White, Round, Scored, N/80	Trimethoprim 80 mg, Sulfamethoxazole 400 mg	Bactrim by Novopharm	Canadian DIN 00510637	Antibiotic
N815400	Cap, Red, Opaque, N over 815	Tolmetin Sodium 400 mg	Tolectin DS by Qualitest	00603-6130	NSAID
N815400	Cap, Red, Opaque, N over 815	Tolmetin Sodium 400 mg	Tolectin DS by URL Mutual	00677-1424	NSAID
N815400	Cap, Red, Opaque, N over 815	Tolmetin Sodium 400 mg	Tolectin DS by Teva	00093-8815 Discontinued	NSAID
N827 <> 200	Tab, Yellow, Round, Scored, Debossed, N over 827	Ketoconazole 200 mg	Nizoral by Murfreesboro	51129-1591	Antifungal
N827200	Tab, Light Peach, Round, N827/200	Ketoconazole 200 mg	Nizoral by Teva	55953-0827 Discontinued	Antifungal
N837 <> 25	Tab, Film Coated, N837 <> 2.5	Indapamide 2.5 mg	Lozol by Teva	55953-0837	Diuretic
N853 <> 125	Tab, Light Yellow, Film Coated, N853 <> 1.25	Indapamide 1.25 mg	Lozol by Teva	55953-0853	Diuretic
N853 <> 125	Tab, Light Yellow, Film Coated, N853 <> 1.25	Indapamide 1.25 mg	Lozol by Novopharm	43806-0853	Diuretic
N894150	Cap, Light Tan & White, Opaque	Nizatidine 150 mg	Axid by Teva	00093-1065	Gastrointestinal
N899300	Cap, Light Tan, Opaque	Nizatidine 300 mg	Axid by Teva	00093-1066	Gastrointestinal
N940200	Cap, Blue, Opaque, N over 940	Acyclovir 200 mg	Zovirax by Teva	00093-8940	Antiviral
N940200	Cap, Blue, Opaque, N 940 over 200	Acyclovir 200 mg	Zovirax by Teva	55953-0940	Antiviral
N940200	Cap, Blue, Opaque, N over 940	Acyclovir 200 mg	Zovirax by Warrick	59930-1538	Antiviral
N940200	Cap, Blue, Opaque, N over 940	Acyclovir 200 mg	Zovirax by Physician Total Care	54868-3996	Antiviral
N940200	Cap, Blue, Opaque, N over 940	Acyclovir 200 mg	Zovirax by Murfreesboro	51129-1359	Antiviral
N940200	Cap, Blue, Opaque, N over 940	Acyclovir 200 mg	Zovirax by Major	00904-5231	Antiviral
N940200	Cap, Blue, Opaque, N over 940	Acyclovir 200 mg	Zovirax by Novopharm	43806-0940	Antiviral
N940200	Cap, Blue, Opaque, N over 940	Acyclovir 200 mg	Zovirax by UDL	51079-0876 Discontinued	Antiviral
N943 <> 400	Tab, Blue, Cap Shaped	Acyclovir 400 mg	Zovirax by Teva	55953-0943	Antiviral
N943 <> 400	Tab, Blue, Cap Shaped	Acyclovir 400 mg	Zovirax by Amerisource	62584-0437	Antiviral
N943 <> 400	Tab, Blue, Cap Shaped	Acyclovir 400 mg	Zovirax by Warrick	59930-1576	Antiviral
N943 <> 400	Tab, Blue, Cap Shaped	Acyclovir 400 mg	Zovirax by Major	00904-5232	Antiviral
N943 <> 400	Tab, Blue, Cap Shaped	Acyclovir 400 mg	Zovirax by UDL	51079-0877 Discontinued	Antiviral
N947 <> 800	Tab, White, Cap Shaped	Acyclovir 800 mg	Zovirax by Teva	00093-8943	Antiviral
N947 <> 800	Tab, White, Cap Shaped	Acyclovir 800 mg	Zovirax by Teva	00093-8947	Antiviral
N947 <> 800	Tab, White, Cap Shaped	Acyclovir 800 mg	Zovirax by Warrick	59930-1584	Antiviral
N947 <> 800	Tab, White, Cap Shaped	Acyclovir 800 mg	Zovirax by Teva	55953-0947	Antiviral
N947 <> 800	Tab, White, Cap Shaped	Acyclovir 800 mg	Zovirax by Amerisource	62584-0429	Antiviral
N947 <> 800	Tab, White, Cap Shaped	Acyclovir 800 mg	Zovirax by UDL	51079-0878 Discontinued	Antiviral

ID FRONT <> BACK	DESCRIPTION FRONT <> BACK	INGREDIENT & STRENGTH	BRAND (or Generic Equiv.) by FIRM	NDC#	CLASS; SCH.
N958 <> 25	Tab, Pale Yellow, Oval, Scored, N/958	Clozapine 25 mg	Clozaril by Teva	00093-0275 Discontinued	Antipsychotic
N958 <> 25	Tab, Pale Yellow, Oval, Scored, N/958	Clozapine 25 mg	Clozaril by Par	49884-0088	Antipsychotic
N9615	Tab, White, Round, N 961-5	Timolol Maleate 5 mg	Blocadren by Novopharm		Antihypertensive
N969 <> 100	Tab, Pale Yellow, Oval, Scored, N/969	Clozapine 100 mg	Clozaril by Par	49884-0089	Antipsychotic
N969 <> 100	Tab, Pale Yellow, Oval, Scored, N/969	Clozapine 100 mg	Clozaril by Teva	00093-0276 Discontinued	Antipsychotic
N97210	Tab, White, Round, N 972-10	Timolol Maleate 10 mg	Blocadren by Novopharm		Antihypertensive
N98420	Tab, White, Round, N 984-20	Timolol Maleate 20 mg	Blocadren by Novopharm		Antihypertensive
NA	Tab, Pink, Round, Abbott Logo	Pargyline HCl 10 mg	Eutonyl by Abbott		Antihypertensive
NALDECON <> BLN1	Tab, White, Red Specks, BL over N1	Chlorpheniramine Maleate 5 mg, Phenylephrine HCl 10 mg, Phenylpropanolamine HCl 40 mg, Phenyltoloxamine Citrate 15 mg	Naldecon by Mead Johnson	00015-5600 Discontinued	Cold Remedy
NALEXJRBLANSETT33	Cap, Green & White Print	Guaifenesin 300 mg, Pseudoephedrine HCl 60 mg	Sudafed Sinus by Sovereign	58716-0006	Cold Remedy
NALFONDISTAH77	Cap	Fenoprofen Calcium 300 mg	Nalfon by Physician Total Care	54868-0856	NSAID
NALFONDISTAH77	Cap	Fenoprofen Calcium 300 mg	Nalfon by Dista Prod	00777-0877	NSAID
NAPROSYN <> 250	Tab	Naproxen 250 mg	Naprosyn by H J Harkins Co	52959-0110	NSAID
NAPROSYN <> 375	Tab, Peach, Oblong	Naproxen 375 mg	Naprosyn by Allscripts		NSAID
NAPROSYN <> 375	Tab, Peach, Oblong	Naproxen 375 mg	Naprosyn by H J Harkins Co	52959-0192	NSAID
NAPROSYN <> 375	Tab, Peach, Oblong	Naproxen 375 mg	Naprosyn by Rightpak	65240-0700	NSAID
NAPROSYN <> 375	Tab, Peach, Oblong	Naproxen 375 mg	Naprosyn by Thrift Drug	59198-0238	NSAID
NAPROSYN <> 375	Tab, Peach, Oblong	Naproxen 375 mg	Naprosyn by Amerisource	62584-0273	NSAID
NAPROSYN <> 375	Tab, Peach, Oblong	Naproxen 375 mg	Naprosyn by Nat Pharmpak	55154-3803	NSAID
NAPROSYN <> 375	Tab, Peach, Oblong	Naproxen 375 mg	Naprosyn by Syntex	18393-0273	NSAID
NAPROSYN <> 500	Tab, Yellow, Round, Scored	Naproxen 500 mg	Naprosyn by H J Harkins Co	52959-0516	NSAID
NAPROSYN <> 500	Tab, Yellow, Round, Scored	Naproxen 500 mg	Naprosyn by Rightpak	65240-0701	NSAID
NAPROSYN <> 500	Tab, Yellow, Round, Scored	Naproxen 500 mg	Naprosyn by Allscripts		NSAID
NAPROSYN <> 500	Tab, Yellow, Round, Scored	Naproxen 500 mg	Naprosyn by Novopharm	43806-0139	NSAID
NAPROSYN <> 500	Tab, Yellow, Round, Scored	Naproxen 500 mg	Naprosyn by Syntex	18393-0277	NSAID
NAPROSYN <> 500	Tab, Yellow, Round, Scored	Naproxen 500 mg	Naprosyn by Thrift Drug	59198-0239	NSAID
NAPROSYN <> 500	Tab, Yellow, Round, Scored	Naproxen 500 mg	Naprosyn by Nat Pharmpak	55154-3804	NSAID
NAPROSYN <> 500	Tab, Yellow, Round, Scored	Naproxen 500 mg	Naprosyn by H J Harkins Co	52959-0111	NSAID
NAPROSYN250 <> ROCHE	Tab, Yellow, Round	Naproxen 250 mg	Naprosyn by Thrift Drug	59198-0237	NSAID
NAPROSYN250 <> ROCHE	Tab, Yellow, Round	Naproxen 250 mg	Naprosyn by Amerisource	62584-0272	NSAID
NAPROSYN250 <> ROCHE	Tab, Yellow, Round	Naproxen 250 mg	Naprosyn by Syntex	18393-0272	NSAID
NAPROSYN250 <> ROCHE	Tab, Yellow, Round	Naproxen 250 mg	Naprosyn by Allscripts		NSAID
NAPROSYN250 <> ROCHE	Tab, Yellow, Round	Naproxen 250 mg	Naprosyn by Hoffmann La Roche	00004-6312	NSAID
NAPROSYN250 <> ROCHE	Tab	Naproxen 250 mg	Naprosyn by Quality Care	60346-0092	NSAID
NAPROSYN500 SYNTEX	Tab	Naproxen 500 mg	Naprosyn by Pharmedix	53002-0311	NSAID
NAPROXEN <> 375	Tab	Naproxen 375 mg	Naprosyn by Quality Care	60346-0817	NSAID
NAPROXEN250 <> SYNTEX	Tab	Naproxen 250 mg	Naprosyn by Pharmedix	53002-0324	NSAID
NAPROXEN375	Tab	Naproxen 375 mg	Naprosyn by Pharmedix	53002-0310	NSAID
NASABID <> SR	Tab, Nasabid <> S/R	Guaifenesin 600 mg, Pseudoephedrine HCl 90 mg	Nasabid Sr by Anabolic	00722-6356	Cold Remedy

ID FRONT <> BACK	DESCRIPTION FRONT <> BACK	INGREDIENT & STRENGTH	BRAND (or Generic Equiv.) by FIRM	NDC#	CLASS; SCH.
NASABID <> SR	Tab, Yellow, Oval, Scored	Guaifenesin 600 mg, Pseudoephedrine HCl 90 mg	Nasabid Sr by Jones	52604-0600	Cold Remedy
NASUTRA	Cap, White, Red Print, Chinese Letter Symbol	Proprietary Blend 300 mg: Cynomorium stem (cynomorium songaricum), Bai Zhu atractylodes rhizome (atractylodes macrocephala), Lycium fruit (lycium barbarum), Epimedium leaf (epimedium sagittatum), Cassia bark (cinnamomum aromaticum), Rehmannia root (rehmannia glutinosa), Fo-Ti stem (polygonum multiflorum), Schisandra fruit (schisandra chinensis), Asian Ginseng root (panax ginseng), Chinese Amomum fruit (amomum villosum)	Nasutra by Nasutra LLC		Supplement
NATAFORT	Tab, Film Coated	Ascorbic Acid 120 mg, Cholecalciferol 400 Units, Cyanocobalamin 12 mcg, Folic Acid 1 mg, Iron 60 mg, Niacinamide 20 mg, Pyridoxine HCl 10 mg, Riboflavin 3 mg, Thiamine Mononitrate 2 mg, Vitamin A 1000 Units, Vitamin E 11 Units	Natafort by Amide	52152-0176	Vitamin
NATURALMINI	Tab, White, Film Coated, Natural/Mini	Ephedra Alkaloids 12.5 mg, Kola Nut Extract 80 mg 50%	Mini Natural by BDI		Supplement
NATURETIN10 <> PPP618	Tab	Bendroflumethiazide 10 mg	Naturetin by BMS	00003-0618	Diuretic; Antihypertensive
NATURETIN5 <> PPP606	Tab, Green, Round, PPP over 606	Bendroflumethiazide 5 mg	Naturetin by BMS	00003-0606	Diuretic; Antihypertensive
NAVANEROERIG571	Cap, Orange & Yellow, Black Print, ROERIG over 571	Thiothixene 1 mg	Navane by Roerig	00049-5710	Antipsychotic
NAVANEROERIG572	Cap, Bluish Green & Yellow, Black Print, ROERIG over 572	Thiothixene 2 mg	Navane by Roerig	00049-5720	Antipsychotic
NAVANEROERIG573	Cap, Orange & White, Black Print, ROERIG over 573	Thiothixene 5 mg	Navane by Roerig	00049-5730	Antipsychotic
NAVANEROERIG574	Cap, Bluish Green & White, Black Print, ROERIG over 574	Thiothixene 10 mg	Navane by Roerig	00049-5740	Antipsychotic
NAVANEROERIG577	Cap, Blue & Green, Black Print, ROERIG over 577	Thiothixene 20 mg	Navane by Roerig	00049-5770	Antipsychotic
NAXEN	Tab, Yellow, Oblong	Naproxen 500 mg	by BW Inc	Canadian	NSAID
NAXEN250	Tab, Yellow, Round, Naxen/250	Naproxen 250 mg	by AltiMed	Canadian DIN 00615315	NSAID
NAXEN375	Tab, Pink, Oval, Naxen/375	Naproxen 375 mg	by AltiMed	Canadian DIN 00615323	NSAID
NAXEN500	Tab, Yellow, Oblong, Naxen/500	Naproxen 500 mg	by AltiMed	Canadian DIN 00615331	NSAID
NB	Tab, Apricot, Round, Abbott Logo	Pargyline HCl 25 mg	Eutonyl by Abbott		Antihypertensive
NC	Tab, White, Round	Juglans Regia (walnut) 6x, Candida Albicans (yeast) 12x, 30x, 60x, 200x, Echinacea Angustifolia (cone flower) 12x, Ledum Palustre (wild rosemary) 12x, Carbo Vegetabilis (vegetable carbon) 30x, Cistus canadensis (frost weed) 30x	Nature's Cure Acne for Females by Nature's Cure		Homeopathic
NC	Tab, White, Round	Calendula Officinalis (marigold) 6x, Hydrastis Canadensis (golden seal) 6x, Echinacea Angustifolia (cone flower) 12x, Sarsaparilla (wild licorice) 12x, Black Cohosh (Cimicifuga racemosa) 30x	Nature's Cure Acne for Males by Nature's Cure		Homeopathic
NC	Tab, White, Round	Juglans Regia (walnut) 6x, Echinacea Angustifolia (cone flower) 6x, Poison Ivy (Rhus toxicodendron) 12x, Antimonious Sulfide (Antimonium Crudum) 12x, Calcium Silica (Calcarea silicata) 12x	Nature's Cure Acne Unisex by Nature's Cure		Homeopathic
NC <> CG	Tab, Yellow, Round, Scored	Artemether 20 mg, Lumefantrine 120 mg	Coartem by Novartis International AG	00078-0568	Antimalarial
ND	Tab, Orange, Round, Abbott Logo	Imipramine HCl 10 mg	Tofranil by Abbott		Antidepressant
NDESEF	Cap, Yellow, ND ES/EF	D-Pseudoephedrine 30 mg, Acetaminophen 500 mg	by Whitehall Robins	Canadian	Analgesic
NE	Tab, Yellow, Round, Abbott Logo	Imipramine HCl 25 mg	Tofranil by Abbott		Antidepressant
NE	Tab, Blue	Phenylpropanolamine HCl 75 mg, Guaifenesin 600 mg	Aquatab D by AstraZeneca	Canadian	Cold Remedy
NE <> 406	Tab, White, Cap Shaped, Scored	Etidronate Disodium 400 mg	Didronel by Pharm Util	60491-0802	Calcium Metabolism
NE <> 406	Tab, White, Cap Shaped, Scored	Etidronate Disodium 400 mg	Didronel by Norwich		Calcium Metabolism
NE <> 406	Tab, White, Cap Shaped, Scored	Etidronate Disodium 400 mg	Didronel by Procter and Gamble	00149-0406	Calcium Metabolism
NE1	Tab, White, Cap Shaped, Scored, Obtained in a kit containing NE2	Etidronate Disodium 400 mg	Didrocal by Proctor & Gambel	Canadian DIN 02177017	Calcium Metabolism

ID FRONT <> BACK	DESCRIPTION FRONT <> BACK	INGREDIENT & STRENGTH	BRAND (or Generic Equiv.) by FIRM	NDC#	CLASS; SCH.
NE10G	Cap, Mustard, Opaque, NE 10/G	Nifedipine 10 mg	by Genpharm	Canadian	Antihypertensive
NE2	Tab, Blue, Cap Shaped, Film Coated, NE2 <> NE2, Obtained in a kit containing NE1	Calcium Carbonate 500 mg	Os-Cal by Proctor & Gamble	Canadian DIN 02176017	Vitamin; Mineral
NE2	Tab, Blue, Cap Shaped, Film Coated, NE2 <> NE2	Calcium Carbonate 500 mg	Os-Cal by Procter and Gamble	00149-0475	Vitamin; Mineral
NE2 <> NE2	Tab, Blue, Oval, Film-Coated	Calcium Carbonate 1250 mg	Actonel with Calcium by Proc & Gamble	Canadian	Bisphosphonate
NE560	Tab, Green, Oblong	Esterified Estrogen 1.25 mg, Methyltestosterone 2.5 mg	Estratest by Econolab		Hormone
NE570	Tab, Green, Oblong	Esterified Estrogen 0.625 mg, Methyltestosterone 1.25 mg	Estratest by Econolab		Hormone
NEEVODHA	Cap, Blue, Soft Gel	L-Methylfolate 1 mg, Calcium 75 mg, Elemental Iron 27 mg, Vitamin C 40 mg, Vitamin E 30 IU, Vitamin B6 25 mg, Vitamin B9 400 mcg, Vitamin B12 1 mg, Docosahexaenoic Acid 250 mg	Neevo DHA by PAMLAB	00525-2030	Vitamin; Supplement
NEORAL100MG	Cap, Bluish Gray, Oblong, Red Print, Neoral over 100 mg	Cyclosporine 100 mg	Neoral by Novartis	00078-0248	Immunosuppressant
NEORAL100MG	Cap, Neoral over 100 mg	Cyclosporine 100 mg	by Nat Pharmpak	55154-3419	Immunosuppressant
NEORAL25MG	Cap, Bluish Gray, Red Print, Oval, Neoral over 25 mg	Cyclosporine 25 mg	by Nat Pharmpak	55154-3418	Immunosuppressant
NEORAL25MG	Cap, Bluish Gray, Red Print, Oval, Neoral over 25 mg	Cyclosporine 25 mg	by Drug Distr	52985-0230	Immunosuppressant
NEORAL25MG	Cap, Bluish Gray, Red Print, Oval, Neoral over 25 mg	Cyclosporine 25 mg	Sandimmun Neoral B63 by RP Scherer	11014-1197	Immunosuppressant
NEORAL25MG	Cap, Bluish Gray, Red Print, Oval, Neoral over 25 mg	Cyclosporine 25 mg	Neoral by Novartis	00078-0246	Immunosuppressant
NEURONTIN100MGPD	Cap, White, Blue Print, Hard Gel, Neurontin over 100 mg over PD Logo	Gabapentin 100 mg	Neurontin by Parke Davis	00071-0803	Anticonvulsant
NEURONTIN100MGPD	Cap, White, Blue Print, Hard Gel, Neurontin over 100 mg over PD Logo	Gabapentin 100 mg	Neurontin by Nat Pharmpak	55154-2414	Anticonvulsant
NEURONTIN100MGPD	Cap, White, Blue Print, Hard Gel, Neurontin over 100 mg over PD Logo	Gabapentin 100 mg	Neurontin by Johnson & Johnson	59604-0301	Anticonvulsant
NEURONTIN100MGPD	Cap, White, Blue Print, Hard Gel, Neurontin over 100 mg over PD Logo	Gabapentin 100 mg	Neurontin by Parke Davis	Canadian DIN 02084260	Anticonvulsant
NEURONTIN100MGPD	Cap, White, Blue Print, Hard Gel, Neurontin over 100 mg over PD Logo	Gabapentin 100 mg	Neurontin by H J Harkins Co	52959-0506	Anticonvulsant
NEURONTIN100MGPD	Cap, White, Blue Print, Hard Gel, Neurontin over 100 mg over PD Logo	Gabapentin 100 mg	Neurontin by Amerisource	62584-0083	Anticonvulsant
NEURONTIN300MGPD	Cap, Yellow, Blue Print, Hard Gel, Neurontin over 300 mg over PD Logo	Gabapentin 300 mg	Neurontin by Johnson & Johnson	59604-0302	Anticonvulsant
NEURONTIN300MGPD	Cap, Yellow, Blue Print, Hard Gel, Neurontin over 300 mg over PD Logo	Gabapentin 300 mg	Neurontin by Heartland	61392-0716	Anticonvulsant
NEURONTIN300MGPD	Cap, Yellow, Blue Print, Hard Gel, Neurontin over 300 mg over PD Logo	Gabapentin 300 mg	Neurontin by Amerisource	62584-0085	Anticonvulsant
NEURONTIN300MGPD	Cap, Yellow, Blue Print, Hard Gel, Neurontin over 300 mg over PD Logo	Gabapentin 300 mg	Neurontin by H J Harkins Co	52959-0434	Anticonvulsant
NEURONTIN300MGPD	Cap, Yellow, Blue Print, Hard Gel, Neurontin over 300 mg over PD Logo	Gabapentin 300 mg	Neurontin by Parke Davis	Canadian DIN 02084279	Anticonvulsant
NEURONTIN300MGPD	Cap, Yellow, Blue Print, Hard Gel, Neurontin over 300 mg over PD Logo	Gabapentin 300 mg	Neurontin by JB	51111-0498	Anticonvulsant
NEURONTIN300MGPD	Cap, Yellow, Blue Print, Hard Gel, Neurontin over 300 mg over PD Logo	Gabapentin 300 mg	Neurontin by Parke Davis	00071-0805	Anticonvulsant
NEURONTIN300MGPD	Cap, Yellow, Blue Print, Hard Gel, Neurontin over 300 mg over PD Logo	Gabapentin 300 mg	Neurontin by Caremark	00339-6101	Anticonvulsant
NEURONTIN300MGPD	Cap, Yellow, Blue Print, Hard Gel, Neurontin over 300 mg over PD Logo	Gabapentin 300 mg	Neurontin by Nat Pharmpak	55154-2415	Anticonvulsant
NEURONTIN300MGPD	Cap, Yellow, Blue Print, Hard Gel, Neurontin over 300 mg over PD Logo	Gabapentin 300 mg	Neurontin by Med Pro	53978-3020	Anticonvulsant
NEURONTIN300MGPD	Cap, Yellow, Blue Print, Hard Gel, Neurontin over 300 mg over PD Logo	Gabapentin 300 mg	Neurontin by Pharm Pkg Ctr	54383-0080	Anticonvulsant

ID FRONT <> BACK	DESCRIPTION FRONT <> BACK	INGREDIENT & STRENGTH	BRAND (or Generic Equiv.) by FIRM	NDC#	CLASS; SCH.
NEURONTIN300MGPD	Cap, Yellow, Blue Print, Hard Gel, Neurontin over 300 mg over PD Logo	Gabapentin 300 mg	Neurontin by Physician Total Care	54868-3768	Anticonvulsant
NEURONTIN400MGPD	Cap, Orange, Blue Print, Hard Gel, Neurontin over 400 mg over PD Logo	Gabapentin 400 mg	Neurontin by DRX	55045-2545	Anticonvulsant
NEURONTIN400MGPD	Cap, Orange, Blue Print, Hard Gel, Neurontin over 400 mg over PD Logo	Gabapentin 400 mg	Neurontin by Amerisource	62584-0086	Anticonvulsant
NEURONTIN400MGPD	Cap, Orange, Blue Print, Hard Gel, Neurontin over 400 mg over PD Logo	Gabapentin 400 mg	Neurontin by Nat Pharmpak	55154-2417	Anticonvulsant
NEURONTIN400MGPD	Cap, Orange, Blue Print, Hard Gel, Neurontin over 400 mg over PD Logo	Gabapentin 400 mg	Neurontin by Parke Davis	Canadian DIN 02084287	Anticonvulsant
NEURONTIN400MGPD	Cap, Orange, Blue Print, Hard Gel, Neurontin over 400 mg over PD Logo	Gabapentin 400 mg	Neurontin by Kaiser	00179-1280	Anticonvulsant
NEURONTIN400MGPD	Cap, Orange, Blue Print, Hard Gel, Neurontin over 400 mg over PD Logo	Gabapentin 400 mg	Neurontin by Parke Davis	00071-0806	Anticonvulsant
NEURONTIN600	Tab, White, Black Print, Oval, Film Coated, Neurontin over 600	Gabapentin 600 mg	Neurontin by Parke Davis	Canadian DIN 02239717	Anticonvulsant
NEURONTIN600	Tab, White, Black Print, Oval, Film Coated, Neurontin over 600	Gabapentin 600 mg	Neurontin by Parke Davis	00071-0416	Anticonvulsant
NEURONTIN800	Tab, White, Orange Print, Oval, Film Coated, Neurontin over 800	Gabapentin 800 mg	Neurontin by Parke Davis	Canadian DIN 02239718	Anticonvulsant
NEURONTIN800	Tab, White, Orange Print, Oval, Film Coated, Neurontin over 800	Gabapentin 800 mg	Neurontin by Parke Davis	00071-0426	Anticonvulsant
NEXIUM20MG	Cap, Purple, Opaque, Hard Gel, Delayed Release, 2 Yellow Bands	Esomeprazole 20 mg	Nexium by AstraZeneca	00186-5020	Proton Pump Inhibitor
NEXIUM20MG	Cap, Purple, Opaque, Hard Gel, Delayed Release, 2 Yellow Bands	Esomeprazole 20 mg	Nexium by AstraZeneca	00186-5022	Proton Pump Inhibitor
NEXIUM40MG	Cap, Purple, Opaque, Hard Gel, Delayed Release, 3 Yellow Bands	Esomeprazole 40 mg	Nexium by AstraZeneca	00186-5042	Proton Pump Inhibitor
NEXIUM40MG	Cap, Purple, Opaque, Hard Gel, Delayed Release, 3 Yellow Bands	Esomeprazole 40 mg	Nexium by AstraZeneca	00186-5040	Proton Pump Inhibitor
NF	Tab, Green, Abbott Logo	Hexocyclium Methylsulfate 25 mg	Tral by Abbott		Antispasmodic
NHAHNA	Cap, HN-A	Terazosin HCl 10 mg	Hytrin by RP Scherer	11014-1034	Antihypertensive
NICHE	Cap, Yellow	Magnesium L-lactate Dihydrate 84 mg	Mag-Tab SR by Niche	59016-0420	Mineral
NIFED2030	Cap, Nifed./20-30	Nifedipine 20 mg	by RP Scherer	11014-0873	Antihypertensive
NIFEDIPINE100364	Cap	Nifedipine 10 mg	by Nat Pharmpak	55154-5206	Antihypertensive
NIFEDIPINE100364	Cap, 10-0364	Nifedipine 10 mg	by Schein	00364-2376	Antihypertensive
NIFEDIPINE100364	Cap	Nifedipine 10 mg	by Schein	00364-2376	Antihypertensive
NIFEDIPINE200364	Cap, Orange, Black Print, Nifedipine over 20-0364	Nifedipine 20 mg	by Amerisource	62584-0802	Antihypertensive
NIFEDIPINE200364	Cap, Orange, Black Print, Nifedipine over 20-0364	Nifedipine 20 mg	by Schein	00364-2377	Antihypertensive
NIFEDIPINE200364	Cap, Orange, Black Print, Nifedipine over 20-0364	Nifedipine 20 mg	by Amerisource	62584-0803	Antihypertensive
NIFEDIPINE200364	Cap, Orange, Black Print, Nifedipine over 20-0364	Nifedipine 20 mg	by Allscripts		Antihypertensive
NIFEDIPINEP10	Cap, Yellow, Opaque, Soft Gel	Nifedipine 10 mg	by Pharmascience	Canadian DIN 5760658982	Antihypertensive
NIKE	Tab, White, Round, Nike Swoosh, Scored	3,4-Methylenedioxymethamphetamine (MDMA) 92 mg	Ecstasy by Illegal		Euphoric; Illicit
NIKESWOOSH	Tab, White, Round, Nike Swoosh, Scored	3,4-Methylenedioxymethamphetamine (MDMA) 92 mg	Ecstasy by Illegal		Euphoric; Illicit
NIMOTOP	Cap, Ivory, Soft Gel	Nimodipine 30 mg	Nimotop by Bayer	00026-2855	Antihypertensive
NIMOTOP	Cap, Ivory, Soft Gel	Nimodipine 30 mg	Nimotop by Par	49884-0632	Antihypertensive
NIMOTOP	Cap, Ivory, Soft Gel	Nimodipine 30 mg	Nimotop by Par	49884-0643	Antihypertensive
NIMOTOP	Cap, Ivory, Soft Gel	Nimodipine 30 mg	Nimotop by RP Scherer	11014-0781	Antihypertensive

ID FRONT <> BACK	DESCRIPTION FRONT <> BACK	INGREDIENT & STRENGTH	BRAND (or Generic Equiv.) by FIRM	NDC#	CLASS; SCH.
NIMOTOP	Cap, Ivory, Soft Gel	Nimodipine 30 mg	Nimotop by Bayer	Canadian DIN 02155923	Antihypertensive
NIT10 <> APO	Tab, Round, White	Nitrazepam 10 mg	Apo Nitrazepam by Apotex	Canadian DIN 02245231	Sedative; Hypnotic; C IV
NIT5 <> APO	Tab, Round, White	Nitrazepam 5 mg	Apo Nitrazepam by Apotex	Canadian DIN 02245230	Sedative; Hypnotic; C IV
NITROFURANTOIN-MACRO	Cap, Yellow	Nitrofurantoin Macrocrystal Ca 100 mg	by Schein	00364-2557	Antibiotic
NITROFURANTOIN-MACRO	Cap, White	Nitrofurantoin Macrocrystal Ca 25 mg	by Schein	00364-2555	Antibiotic
NITROFURANTOIN-MACRO	Cap, White & Yellow	Nitrofurantoin Macrocrystal Ca 50 mg	by Schein	00364-2556	Antibiotic
NITROGLYN25MG	Cap, ER	Nitroglycerin 2.5 mg	Nitroglyn by Kenwood	00482-1025	Vasodilator
NITROGLYN65MG	Cap, ER	Nitroglycerin 6.5 mg	Nitroglyn by Kenwood	00482-1065	Vasodilator
NITROGLYN9MG	Cap, ER, White Beads	Nitroglycerin 9 mg	Nitroglyn by Kenwood	00482-1090	Vasodilator
NIZORAL <> JANSSEN	Tab, White, Scored	Ketoconazole 200 mg	Nizoral by H J Harkins Co	52959-0197	Antifungal
NIZORAL <> JANSSEN	Tab, White, Scored	Ketoconazole 200 mg	Nizoral by Janssen	50458-0220	Antifungal
NIZORAL <> JANSSEN	Tab, White, Scored	Ketoconazole 200 mg	Nizoral by Johnson & Johnson	59604-0220	Antifungal
NIZORAL <> JANSSEN	Tab, White, Scored	Ketoconazole 200 mg	Nizoral by Direct Dispensing	57866-6570	Antifungal
NIZORAL <> JANSSEN	Tab, White, Scored	Ketoconazole 200 mg	Nizoral by Pharm Util	60491-0454	Antifungal
NK	Tab, Purple, Oval, Abb. Logo	Pargyline HCl 25 mg, Methyclothiazide 5 mg	Eutron by Abbott		Antihypertensive; Diuretic
NL	Tab, Peach, Oval, Abb. Logo	Imipramine HCl 50 mg	Tofranil by Abbott		Antidepressant
NL101	Tab, White, Round	Acetaminophen 325 mg	Tylenol by Neil Labs	60242-0101	Analgesic
NL102	Tab, White, Round	Acetaminophen 500 mg	Tylenol Ex Strength by Neil Labs	60242-0102	Analgesic
NL104	Tab, Blue, Cap Shaped	Acetaminophen 500 mg, Diphenhydramine HCl 25 mg	Tylenol PM by Neil Labs	60242-0104	Cold Remedy
NL105	Tab, White, Cap Shaped	Acetaminophen 500 mg	Tylenol Ex Strength by Neil Labs	60242-0105	Analgesic
NL150	Tab, Yellow, Round, Scored	Bisacodyl 5 mg	Dulcolax by Neil Labs	60242-0150	Gastrointestinal
NL151	Tab, Pink, Round, Scored	Bisacodyl 5 mg	Dulcolax by Neil Labs	60242-0151	Gastrointestinal
NL175	Tab, Off-White, Oblong	Polycarbophil 625 mg	Fibercon by Qualitest	00603-0181	Gastrointestinal
NL175	Tab, White, Cap Shaped, Film Coated	Calcium Polycarbophil	Fibercon by Neil Labs	60242-0175	Gastrointestinal
NL200	Tab, Pink, Oval, Film Coated	Diphenhydramine HCl 25 mg	Benadryl by Neil Labs	60242-0200	Antihistamine
NL201	Cap, Pink & Clear	Diphenhydramine HCl 25 mg	Benadryl by Neil Labs	60242-0201	Antihistamine
NL202	Cap, Pink	Diphenhydramine HCl 50 mg	Benadryl by Neil Labs	60242-0202	Antihistamine
NL275	Tab, White, Long	Guaifenesin 400 mg	Humibid E by URL	00677-1929	Cold Remedy
NL325	Tab, White, Round	Ibuprofen 200 mg	Motrin by Neil Labs	60242-0325	NSAID
NL326	Tab, White, Cap Shaped, Film Coated	Ibuprofen 200 mg	Motrin by Neil Labs	60242-0326	NSAID
NL327	Tab, Brown, Round, Film Coated	Ibuprofen 200 mg	Motrin by Neil Labs	60242-0327	NSAID
NL328	Tab, Brown, Cap Shaped, Film Coated	Ibuprofen 200 mg	Motrin by Neil Labs	60242-0328	NSAID
NL575	Tab, Green, Round	Senna Concentrate 8.6 mg	Senokot by Neil Labs	60242-0575	Laxative
NL703	Tab, White, Cap Shaped	Guaifenesin 800 mg, Pseudoephedrine HCl 80 mg	by Neil Labs		Cold Remedy
NL715	Tab, White, Oval	Guaifenesin 1200 mg, Pseudoephedrine 90 mg	Dynax by URL	00677-1850	Cold Remedy
NL716	Tab, White, Cap Shaped, Scored	Chlorpheniramine Maleate 12 mg, Pseudoephedrine HCl 120 mg	Deconamine by Neil Labs	60242-0716	Cold Remedy
NL718	Tab, White, Cap Shaped, Scored	Pseudoephedrine HCl 90 mg, Guaifenesin 800 mg	Profen Forte by Neil Labs	60242-0718	Cold Remedy
NL719	Tab, White, Cap Shaped, Scored	Pseudoephedrine HCl 90 mg, Guaifenesin 800 mg, Dextromethorphan HBr 60 mg	Profen Forte DM by Neil Labs	60242-0719	Cold Remedy
NL734	Tab, White, Oblong	Guaifenesin 795 mg, Pseudoephedrine 85 mg	Panmist LA by Neil Labs	60242-0101	Cold Remedy
NM11	Tab, White, Round, Coated	Ferrous Sulfate 65 mg	Iron by Nature Made		Vitamin
NMA	Tab, Yellow, Oval, Film Coated, Ex Release, Abbott Logo (a)	Potassium Chloride 750 mg	K-Tab ER by Abbott		Electrolytes

ID FRONT <> BACK	DESCRIPTION FRONT <> BACK	INGREDIENT & STRENGTH	BRAND (or Generic Equiv.) by FIRM	NDC#	CLASS; SCH.
NMI	Cap, Peach, Scored, Film Coated	Ascorbic Acid 50 mg, Calcium Carbonate, Cholecalciferol, Cupric Sulfate, Ferrous Fumarate, Folic Acid 1 mg, Magnesium Oxide, Pyridoxine HCl 2 mg, Tocopheryl Acetate, Zinc Sulfate	Prenatal Vitamin by Thrift Drug	59198-0340	Vitamin
NMI	Tab, Coated	Ascorbic Acid 50 mg, Calcium Carbonate, Cholecalciferol, Cupric Sulfate, Ferrous Fumarate, Folic Acid 1 mg, Magnesium Oxide, Pyridoxine HCl 2 mg, Tocopheryl Acetate, Zinc Sulfate	Prenatal Vitamin by Northampton Med	58436-0071	Vitamin
NMI	Cap, Peach, Scored, Film Coated	Ascorbic Acid 50 mg, Calcium Carbonate, Cholecalciferol, Cupric Sulfate, Ferrous Fumarate, Folic Acid 1 mg, Magnesium Oxide, Pyridoxine HCl 2 mg, Tocopheryl Acetate, Zinc Sulfate	Prenatal Vitamin by Physician Total Care	54868-3787	Vitamin
NN <> 05	Tab, Orange, Round, Scored, N / N <> 0.5	Clonazepam 0.5 mg	Rivotril by Novopharm	Canadian DIN 02239024	Anticonvulsant
NN <> 1	Tab, Yellow, Oval, Scored, N / N <> 1	Cilazapril 1 mg	Inhibace by Novopharm	Canadian DIN 02266350	Antihypertensive
NN <> 1	Tab, White, Round, Scored, N / N	Doxazosin Mesylate 1 mg	Cardura by Novopharm	Canadian DIN 02242728	Antihypertensive
NN <> 1	Tab, White, Round, Scored, N/N	Ketotifen Fumarate 1 mg	Zaditen by Novopharm	Canadian DIN 02230730	Antiasthmatic
NN <> 100	Tab, Peach, Shield Shaped, Scored, N/N <> 100	Lamotrigine 100 mg	Lamictal by Novopharm	Canadian DIN 02248233	Antiepileptic
NN <> 100	Tab, Orange, Oval, Scored, N/N	Moclobemide 100 mg	Manerix by Novopharm	Canadian DIN 02239746	Antidepressant
NN <> 100	Tab, White, Oval, Scored, N / N <> 100	Fluvoxamine Maleate 100 mg	Luvox by Novopharm	Canadian DIN 02239954	OCD
NN <> 100	Tab, Light Yellow, Round, Scored, N/N <> 100	Spironolactone 100 mg	Aldactone by Novopharm	Canadian DIN 00613223	Diuretic
NN <> 100	Tab, White, Round, Scored, N/N <> 100	Theophylline Anhydrous 100 mg	Theo-Dur by Novopharm	Canadian DIN 02230085	Antiasthmatic
NN <> 100	Tab, White to Off-White, Oval, Film-Coated	Fluvoxamine Maleate 100 mg	Novo-Fluvoxamine by Novopharm	Canadian DIN 02239954	OCD
NN <> 125	Tab, White, Cap Shaped, Scored, N/N <> 12.5	Captopril 12.5 mg	Capoten by Novopharm	Canadian DIN 01942964	Antihypertensive
NN <> 150	Tab, Tan, Oval, Scored, N/N	Moclobemide 150 mg	Manerix by Novopharm	Canadian DIN 02239747	Antidepressant
NN <> 150	Tab, White, Shield Shaped, Scored, N/N <> 150	Lamotrigine 150 mg	Lamictal by Novopharm	Canadian DIN 02248234	Antiepileptic
NN <> 160	Tab, Light Blue, Cap Shaped, Scored, N/N <> 160	Sotalol HCl 160 mg	Sotacor by Novopharm	Canadian DIN 02231182	Antiarrhythmic
NN <> 2	Tab, White, Oblong, Scored, N / N	Doxazosin Mesylate 2 mg	Cardura by Novopharm	Canadian DIN 02242729	Antihypertensive
NN <> 2	Tab, White, Round, Scored, N / N <> 2	Clonazepam 2 mg	Rivotril by Novopharm	Canadian DIN 02239025	Anticonvulsant
NN <> 20	Tab, White, Oval, Scored, N / N <> 20	Citalopram 20 mg	Celexa by Novopharm	Canadian DIN 02251558	Antidepressant
NN <> 20	Tab, Blue, Octagonal, 20 <> N/N	Lovastatin 20 mg	Mevacor by Novopharm	Canadian DIN 02246542	Antihyperlipidemic
NN <> 200	Tab, White, Round, Scored, N/N <> 200	Ketoconazole 200 mg	Nizoral by Novopharm	Canadian DIN 02231061	Antifungal
NN <> 200	Tab, Pink, Round, Scored, N / N <> 200	Amiodarone HCl 200 mg	Cordarone by Novopharm	Canadian DIN 02239835	Antiarrhythmic
NN <> 200	Tab, Red, Cap Shaped, N/N	Morphine Sulfate 200 mg	MS Contin by Novopharm	Canadian DIN 02302802	Analgesic; N

ID FRONT <> BACK	DESCRIPTION FRONT <> BACK	INGREDIENT & STRENGTH	BRAND (or Generic Equiv.) by FIRM	NDC#	CLASS; SCH.
NN <> 25	Tab, White, Round, N/N <> 25	Atenolol 25 mg	Tenormin by Novopharm	Canadian DIN 02266660	Antihypertensive
NN <> 25	Tab, Pink, Oval, Scored, N / N <> 2.5	Cilazapril 2.5 mg	Inhibace by Novopharm	Canadian DIN 02266369	Antihypertensive
NN <> 25	Tab, Peach, Round, Scored, N/N	Medroxyprogesterone Acetate 2.5 mg	Provera by Novopharm	Canadian DIN 02221284	Hormone
NN <> 25	Tab, White, Shield Shaped, Scored, N/N <> 25	Lamotrigine 25 mg	Lamictal by Novopharm	Canadian DIN 02248232	Antiepileptic
NN <> 250	Tab, Off-White, Round, Scored, N / N	Flutamide 250 mg	Euflex by Novopharm	Canadian DIN 02230089	Antiandrogen
NN <> 250	Tab, White, Round, Scored, N/N <> 250	Terbinafine HCl 250 mg	Lamisil by Novopharm	Canadian DIN 02240346	Antifungal
NN <> 300	Tab, White, Cap Shaped, Scored, N/N <> 300	Theophylline Anhydrous 300 mg	Theo-Dur by Novopharm	Canadian DIN 02230087	Antiasthmatic
NN <> 300	Tab, White, Oval, Scored, N/N	Moclobemide 300 mg	Manerix by Novopharm	Canadian DIN 02239748	Antidepressant
NN <> 4	Tab, White, Diamond-Shaped, Scored, N / N	Doxazosin Mesylate 4 mg	Cardura by Novopharm	Canadian DIN 02247730	Antihypertensive
NN <> 40	Tab, White, Oval, Scored, N / N <> 40	Citalopram 40 mg	Celexa by Novopharm	Canadian DIN 02251566	Antidepressant
NN <> 5	Tab, Orange, Oval, Scored, N / N <> 5	Cilazapril 5 mg	Inhibace by Novopharm	Canadian DIN 02266377	Antihypertensive
NN <> 5	Tab, White, Oblong, Scored, N/N	Glyburide 5 mg	DiaBeta by Novopharm	Canadian DIN 01913689	Antidiabetic
NN <> 5	Tab, Blue, Round, Scored, N/N	Medroxyprogesterone Acetate 5 mg	Provera by Novopharm	Canadian DIN 02221292	Hormone
NN <> 5	Tab, Blue, Round, N/N/5	Oxybutynin Chloride 5 mg	Ditropan by Novopharm	Canadian DIN 02230394	Urinary Tract
NN <> 550	Tab, Pink, Diamond Shaped, N/N <> 5 over 50	Amiloride HCl 5 mg, Hydrochlorothiazide 50 mg	Moduret by Novopharm	Canadian DIN 01937219	Antihypertensive; Diuretic
N|N <> 7.5	Tab, Blue, Oval, N/N <> 7.5	Zopiclone 7.5 mg	Imovane by Novopharm	Canadian DIN 02251469	Hypnotic
NN <> 800	Tab, Blue, Elongated, Scored, Compressed tablet	Acyclovir 800 mg	Zovirax by Novopharm	Canadian DIN 02285975	Antiviral
NN <> 875	Tab, White, Oblong, Scored, N / N <> 875	Amoxicillin 875 mg, Clavulanate Potassium 125 mg	Clavulin by Novopharm	Canadian DIN 02248138	Antibiotic
NN <> C10	Tab, White, Round, Scored, N / N <> C10	Clobazam 10 mg	Frisium by Novopharm	Canadian DIN 02238334	Anticonvulsant
NN <> C50	Tab, White, Round, Biconvex, Film-Coated	Chlorpromazine 50 mg	Largactil by Novopharm	Canadian DIN 00232807	Antipsychotic; Antiemetic
NN2	Tab, White, Square	Methazolamide 25 mg	Neptazane by Lederle		Antiglaucoma Agent
NO	Tab, White, Oval, Coated, Scored, Cobalt Logo <> N / O	Norfloxacin 400 mg	Noroxin by Cobalt	Canadian DIN 02269627	Antibiotic
NO1 <> MMCNEIL	Tab, White, Cap-Shaped	Acetaminophen 300 mg, Caffeine 15 mg, Codeine Phosphate 8 mg	TYLENOL No. 1 by Janssen-Ortho	Canadian DIN 02181061	Analgesic; C III
NO1FORTEMCNEIL	Cap, White, Film Coated, No. 1 Forte <> McNeil	Acetaminophen 500 mg, Caffeine 15 mg, Codeine Phosphate 8 mg	Tylenol No. 1 Forte by McNeil	Canadian DIN 02181088	Analgesic; C III
NO1MCNEIL	Cap, White, Film Coated, No. 1 <> McNeil	Acetaminophen 300 mg, Caffeine 15 mg, Codeine Phosphate 8 mg	Tylenol w/ Codeine by McNeil	Canadian DIN 02181061	Analgesic; C III
NODOZ	Tab, White, Round, Scored	Caffeine 200 mg	NoDoz by BMS		Stimulant
NOLVADEX10	Tab, White, Round	Tamoxifen Citrate 15.2 mg	Nolvadex by Zeneca	Canadian	Antiestrogen
NOLVADEX600	Tab, White, Round, NOLVADEX600 <> CAMEO	Tamoxifen Citrate 10 mg	Nolvadex by AstraZeneca	00310-0600	Antiestrogen

ID FRONT <> BACK	DESCRIPTION FRONT <> BACK	INGREDIENT & STRENGTH	BRAND (or Generic Equiv.) by FIRM	NDC#	CLASS; SCH.
NOLVADEX604	Tab, White, Round, NOLVADEX, NOLVADEX604 <> CAMEO	Tamoxifen Citrate 20 mg	Nolvadex by AstraZeneca	00310-0604	Antiestrogen
NOLVADEXD	Tab, White to Off-White, Octagonal, Film Coated	Tamoxifen 20 mg	Nolvadex-D by AstraZeneca	Canadian DIN 02048485	Antineoplastic
NORCO539	Tab, Yellow, Oblong, Scored	Acetaminophen 325 mg, Hydrocodone Bitartrate 10 mg	Norco 10/325 by Physician Total Care	54868-4034	Analgesic; C III
NORCO539	Tab, Yellow, Oblong, Scored	Acetaminophen 325 mg, Hydrocodone Bitartrate 10 mg	Norco 10/325 by Watson	52544-0539	Analgesic; C III
NORCO539	Tab, Yellow, Oblong, Scored	Acetaminophen 325 mg, Hydrocodone Bitartrate 10 mg	Norco 10/325 by Murfreesboro	51129-1425	Analgesic; C III
NORCO539	Tab, Yellow, Oblong, Scored	Acetaminophen 325 mg, Hydrocodone Bitartrate 10 mg	Norco 10/325 by Nat Pharmpak	55154-1150	Analgesic; C III
NORCO539	Tab, Yellow, Oblong, Scored	Acetaminophen 325 mg, Hydrocodone Bitartrate 10 mg	Norco 10/325 by Eckerd	19458-0916	Analgesic; C III
NORCO729	Tab, Light Orange, Cap Shaped, Scored	Acetaminophen 325 mg, Hydrocodone Bitartrate 7.5 mg	Norco by Watson	52544-0729	Analgesic; C III
NORGESIC <> 3M	Tab, White & Yellow, Round	Aspirin 385 mg, Caffeine 30 mg, Orphenadrine Citrate 25 mg	Norgesic by 3M	00089-0231 Discontinued	Analgesic; Muscle Relaxant
NORGESICFORTE	Tab, White, Oblong, Scored	Orphenadrine Citrate 50 mg, Caffeine 60 mg, Aspirin 770 mg	Norgesic Forte by Rightpak	65240-0704	Muscle Relaxant
NORGESICFORTE <> 3M	Tab, White & Yellow, Oblong	Orphenadrine Citrate 50 mg, Caffeine 60 mg, Aspirin 770 mg	by Med Pro	53978-3384	Muscle Relaxant
NORGESICFORTE <> 3M	Tab	Aspirin 770 mg, Caffeine 60 mg, Orphenadrine Citrate 50 mg	Norgesic Forte by CVS	00894-6767	Analgesic
NORGESICFORTE <> 3M	Tab, Green & White	Aspirin 770 mg, Caffeine 60 mg, Orphenadrine Citrate 50 mg	Norgesic Forte by CVS	51316-0050	Analgesic
NORGESICFORTE <> 3M	Tab, Light Green, Layered, Norgesic over Forte <> 3M	Aspirin 770 mg, Caffeine 60 mg, Orphenadrine Citrate 50 mg	Norgesic Forte by Amerisource	62584-0233	Analgesic
NORGESICFORTE <> 3M	Tab, Light Green, White & Yellow	Aspirin 770 mg, Caffeine 60 mg, Orphenadrine Citrate 50 mg	Norgesic Forte by Allscripts		Analgesic
NORGESICFORTE <> 3M	Tab, Light Green & White & Yellow, Layered	Aspirin 770 mg, Caffeine 60 mg, Orphenadrine Citrate 50 mg	Norgesic Forte by Thrift Drug	59198-0158	Analgesic
NORGESICFORTE <> 3M	Tab, Green & White, Cap Shaped, Scored	Aspirin 770 mg, Caffeine 60 mg, Orphenadrine Citrate 50 mg	Norgesic Forte by 3M	00089-0233 Discontinued	Analgesic
NORGESICFORTE <> 3M	Tab, Green & White	Aspirin 770 mg, Caffeine 60 mg, Orphenadrine Citrate 50 mg	Norgesic Forte by Nat Pharmpak	55154-2905	Analgesic
NORGESICFORTE <> RIKER	Tab, Green	Aspirin 770 mg, Caffeine 60 mg, Orphenadrine Citrate 50 mg	Norgesic Forte by Pharmedix	53002-0376	Analgesic
NORINYLSYNTEX	Tab, White, Circular, Norinyl/Syntex	Norethindrone 1 mg, Mestranol 0.05 mg	by Novartis	Canadian	Oral Contraceptive
NORMODYNE <> SCHERING438	Tab, Blue, Round	Labetalol HCl 300 mg	Normodyne by Rx Pak	65084-0230	Antihypertensive
NORMODYNE <> SCHERING7	Tab, Film Coated	Labetalol HCl 200 mg	Normodyne by Pharmedix	53002-1046	Antihypertensive
NORMODYNE <> SCHERING752	Tab, Film Coated	Labetalol HCl 200 mg	Normodyne by Med Pro	53978-0697	Antihypertensive
NORMODYNE100 <> SCHERING244	Tab, Brown, Round, Scored	Labetalol HCl 100 mg	Normodyne by Rite Aid	11822-5260	Antihypertensive
NORMODYNE100 <> SCHERING244	Tab, Brown, Round, Scored	Labetalol HCl 100 mg	Normodyne by Nat Pharmpak	55154-3511	Antihypertensive
NORMODYNE100 <> SCHERING244	Tab, Brown, Round, Scored	Labetalol HCl 100 mg	Normodyne by Amerisource	62584-0244	Antihypertensive
NORMODYNE100 <> SCHERING244	Tab, Brown, Round, Scored	Labetalol HCl 100 mg	Normodyne by Pharm Util	60491-0458	Antihypertensive
NORMODYNE100 <> SCHERING244	Tab, Brown, Round, Scored	Labetalol HCl 100 mg	Normodyne by Thrift Drug	59198-0080	Antihypertensive
NORMODYNE100 <> SCHERING244	Tab, Brown, Round, Scored	Labetalol HCl 100 mg	Normodyne by Caremark	00339-5265	Antihypertensive
NORMODYNE100 <> SCHERING244	Tab, Brown, Round, Scored	Labetalol HCl 100 mg	Normodyne by Schering	00085-0244	Antihypertensive
NORMODYNE100 <> SCHERING244	Tab, Brown, Round, Scored	Labetalol HCl 100 mg	Normodyne by Rightpak	65240-0705	Antihypertensive
NORMODYNE100 <> SCHERING244	Tab, Brown, Round, Scored	Labetalol HCl 100 mg	Normodyne by Murfreesboro	51129-1618	Antihypertensive
NORMODYNE100 <> SCHERING244	Tab, Brown, Round, Scored	Labetalol HCl 100 mg	Normodyne by Caremark	00339-5265	Antihypertensive

ID FRONT <> BACK	DESCRIPTION FRONT <> BACK	INGREDIENT & STRENGTH	BRAND (or Generic Equiv.) by FIRM	NDC#	CLASS; SCH.
NORMODYNE200 <> SCHERING752	Tab, White, Round, Film Coated	Labetalol HCl 200 mg	Normodyne by Schering	00085-0752	Antihypertensive
NORMODYNE200 <> SCHERING752	Tab, Film Coated	Labetalol HCl 200 mg	Normodyne by Rite Aid	11822-5234	Antihypertensive
NORMODYNE200 <> SCHERING752	Tab, Film Coated	Labetalol HCl 200 mg	Normodyne by Nat Pharmpak	55154-3506	Antihypertensive
NORMODYNE300 <> SCHERING438	Tab, Blue, Round, Film, Schering 438 <> 300 Normodyne	Labetalol HCl 300 mg	Normodyne by Schering	00085-0438	Antihypertensive
NORMODYNE300 <> SCHERING438	Tab, Blue, Round, Film, Schering 438 <> 300 Normodyne	Labetalol HCl 300 mg	Normodyne by Leiner	59606-0670	Antihypertensive
NOROXIN <> MSD705	Tab, Dark Pink, Oval, Film Coated, MSD over 705	Norfloxacin 400 mg	by MSD	Canadian	Antibiotic
NOROXIN <> MSD705	Tab, Dark Pink, Oval, Film Coated, MSD over 705	Norfloxacin 400 mg	Noroxin by Merck	00006-0705	Antibiotic
NOROXIN <> MSD705	Tab, Dark Pink, Oval, Film Coated, MSD over 705	Norfloxacin 400 mg	by Allscripts		Antibiotic
NOROXIN <> MSD705	Tab, Dark Pink, Oval, Film Coated, MSD over 705	Norfloxacin 400 mg	Noroxin by Roberts	54092-0097	Antibiotic
NOROXIN <> MSD705	Tab, Dark Pink, Oval, Film Coated, MSD over 705	Norfloxacin 400 mg	by Quality Care	60346-0563	Antibiotic
NOROXIN <> MSD705	Tab, Dark Pink, Oval, Film Coated, MSD over 705	Norfloxacin 400 mg	by DRX	55045-2419	Antibiotic
NORPACECR100MG- SEARLE2732	Cap, Light Green & White, Black Print, Norpace CR over 100 mg over Searle over 2732	Disopyramide Phosphate 100 mg	Norpace CR by Thrift Drug	59198-0164	Antiarrhythmic
NORPACECR100MG- SEARLE2732	Cap, Light Green & White, Black Print, Norpace CR over 100 mg over Searle over 2732	Disopyramide Phosphate 100 mg	Norpace CR by Leiner	59606-0709	Antiarrhythmic
NORPACECR100MG- SEARLE2732	Cap, Light Green & White, Black Print, Norpace CR over 100 mg over Searle over 2732	Disopyramide Phosphate 100 mg	Norpace CR by Searle	00025-2732	Antiarrhythmic
NORPACECR100MG- SEARLE2732	Cap, Light Green & White, Black Print, Norpace CR over 100 mg over Searle over 2732	Disopyramide Phosphate 100 mg	Norpace CR by Amerisource	62584-0732	Antiarrhythmic
NORPACECR100MG- SEARLE2732	Cap, Light Green & White, Black Print, Norpace CR over 100 mg over Searle over 2732	Disopyramide Phosphate 100 mg	Norpace CR by Rightpak	65240-0709	Antiarrhythmic
NORPACECR100MG- SEARLE2732	Cap, Light Green & White, Black Print, Norpace CR over 100 mg over Searle over 2732	Disopyramide Phosphate 100 mg	Norpace CR by Nat Pharmpak	55154-3609	Antiarrhythmic
NORPACECR100MG- SEARLE2732	Cap, Light Green & White, Black Print, Norpace CR over 100 mg over Searle over 2732	Disopyramide Phosphate 100 mg	Norpace CR by GSK	51947-8310	Antiarrhythmic
NORPACECR150MG- SEARLE2742	Cap, Brown & Light Green, White Print, Norpace CR over 150 mg over Searle over 2742	Disopyramide Phosphate 150 mg	Norpace CR by Golden State	60429-0703	Antiarrhythmic
NORPACECR150MG- SEARLE2742	Cap, Brown & Light Green, White Print, Norpace CR over 150 mg over Searle over 2742	Disopyramide Phosphate 150 mg	Norpace CR by Nat Pharmpak	55154-3610	Antiarrhythmic
NORPACECR150MG- SEARLE2742	Cap, Brown & Light Green, White Print, Norpace CR over 150 mg over Searle over 2742	Disopyramide Phosphate 150 mg	Norpace CR by Amerisource	62584-0742	Antiarrhythmic
NORPACECR150MG- SEARLE2742	Cap, Brown & Light Green, White Print, Norpace CR over 150 mg over Searle over 2742	Disopyramide Phosphate 150 mg	Norpace CR by Searle	00014-2742	Antiarrhythmic
NORPACECR150MG- SEARLE2742	Cap, Brown & Light Green, White Print, Norpace CR over 150 mg over Searle over 2742	Disopyramide Phosphate 150 mg	Norpace CR by Searle	00025-2742	Antiarrhythmic
NORPACECR150MG- SEARLE2742	Cap, Brown & Light Green, White Print, Norpace CR over 150 mg over Searle over 2742	Disopyramide Phosphate 150 mg	Norpace CR by Thrift Drug	59198-0085	Antiarrhythmic
NORPACECR150MG- SEARLE2742	Cap, Brown & Light Green, White Print, Norpace CR over 150 mg over Searle over 2742	Disopyramide Phosphate 150 mg	Norpace CR by Leiner	59606-0710	Antiarrhythmic
NORPRAMIN100	Tab, Peach, Round	Desipramine HCl 100 mg	Norpramin by Marion	Canadian	Antidepressant
NORPRAMIN100	Tab, Peach, Round	Desipramine HCl 100 mg	Norpramin by Merrell	00068-0020	Antidepressant
NORPRAMIN150	Tab, White, Round	Desipramine HCl 150 mg	Norpramin by Merrell	00068-0021	Antidepressant
NORPRAMIN25	Tab, Yellow, Round	Desipramine HCl 25 mg	Norpramin by Marion	Canadian	Antidepressant
NORPRAMIN25	Tab, Yellow, Round	Desipramine HCl 25 mg	Norpramin by Merrell	00068-0011	Antidepressant
NORPRAMIN50	Tab, Green, Round	Desipramine HCl 50 mg	Norpramin by Merrell	00068-0015	Antidepressant
NORPRAMIN50	Tab, Green, Round	Desipramine HCl 50 mg	Norpramin by Marion	Canadian	Antidepressant

ID FRONT <> BACK	DESCRIPTION FRONT <> BACK	INGREDIENT & STRENGTH	BRAND (or Generic Equiv.) by FIRM	NDC#	CLASS; SCH.
NORPRAMIN75	Tab, Orange, Round	Desipramine HCl 75 mg	Norpramin by Merrell	00068-0019	Antidepressant
NORPRAMIN75	Tab, Orange, Round	Desipramine HCl 75 mg	Norpramin by Marion	Canadian	Antidepressant
NORPROLAC <> 150	Tab, White, Round, Flat Bevelled Edge	Quinagolide 0.150 mg	Norprolac by Ferring	Canadian DIN 02223775	Antihyperprolactinaemia
NORPROLAC <> 25	Tab, Light Pink with Pigment Spots, Circular, Flat, Bevelled Edge	Quinagolide 0.025 mg	Norprolac by Ferring	Canadian DIN 02223740	Antihyperprolactinaemia
NORPROLAC <> 50	Tab, Pale Blue with Pigment Spots, Round, Flat Bevelled Edge	Quinagolide 0.050 mg	Norprolac by Ferring	Canadian DIN 02223759	Antihyperprolactinaemia
NORPROLAC <> 75	Tab, White, Round, Flat Bevelled Edge	Quinagolide 0.075 mg	Norprolac by Ferring	Canadian DIN 02223767	Antihyperprolactinaemia
NORTRIPTYLINE10250	Cap, Green & White	Nortriptyline HCl 10 mg	Pamelor by H J Harkins Co	52959-0358	Antidepressant
NORTRIPTYLINE10CP-250	Cap	Nortriptyline HCl 10 mg	Pamelor by Creighton	50752-0250	Antidepressant
NORTRIPTYLINE25251	Cap, Green & White	Nortriptyline HCl 25 mg	Pamelor by H J Harkins Co	52959-0359	Antidepressant
NORTRIPTYLINE25251-CP	Cap, Black & White Print	Nortriptyline HCl 25 mg	Pamelor by Rx Dispensing	61807-0142	Antidepressant
NORTRIPTYLINEDAN-10MG	Cap, Blue & White, Black Print, Nortriptyline over DAN over 10 mg	Nortriptyline HCl 10 mg	Pamelor by PDRX	55289-0405	Antidepressant
NORTRIPTYLINEDAN-10MG	Cap, Blue & White, Black Print, Nortriptyline over DAN over 10 mg	Nortriptyline HCl 10 mg	Pamelor by Watson	00591-5786	Antidepressant
NORTRIPTYLINEDAN-10MG	Cap, Blue & White, Black Print, Nortriptyline over DAN over 10 mg	Nortriptyline HCl 10 mg	Pamelor by Heartland	61392-0361	Antidepressant
NORTRIPTYLINEDAN-10MG	Cap, Blue & White, Black Print, Nortriptyline over DAN over 10 mg	Nortriptyline HCl 10 mg	Pamelor by Danbury	61955-2508	Antidepressant
NORTRIPTYLINEDAN-10MG	Cap, Blue & White, Black Print, Nortriptyline over DAN over 10 mg	Nortriptyline HCl 10 mg	Pamelor by Schein	00364-2508	Antidepressant
NORTRIPTYLINEDAN-25MG	Cap, Green & White, Black Print, Nortriptyline over DAN over 25 mg	Nortriptyline HCl 25 mg	Pamelor by Schein	00364-2509	Antidepressant
NORTRIPTYLINEDAN-25MG	Cap, Green & White, Black Print, Nortriptyline over DAN over 25 mg	Nortriptyline HCl 25 mg	Pamelor by Danbury	61955-2509	Antidepressant
NORTRIPTYLINEDAN-25MG	Cap, Green & White, Black Print, Nortriptyline over DAN over 25 mg	Nortriptyline HCl 25 mg	Pamelor by Watson	00591-5787	Antidepressant
NORTRIPTYLINEDAN-25MG	Cap, Green & White, Black Print, Nortriptyline over DAN over 25 mg	Nortriptyline HCl 25 mg	Pamelor by Nat Pharmpak	55154-5220	Antidepressant
NORTRIPTYLINEDAN-25MG	Cap, Green & White, Black Print, Nortriptyline over DAN over 25 mg	Nortriptyline HCl 25 mg	Pamelor by Heartland	61392-0364	Antidepressant
NORTRIPTYLINEDAN-50MG	Cap, White, Black Print, Nortriptyline over DAN over 50 mg	Nortriptyline HCl 50 mg	Pamelor by Watson	00591-5788	Antidepressant
NORTRIPTYLINEDAN-50MG	Cap, White, Black Print, Nortriptyline over DAN over 50 mg	Nortriptyline HCl 50 mg	Pamelor by Heartland	61392-0367	Antidepressant
NORTRIPTYLINEDAN-50MG	Cap, White, Black Print, Nortriptyline over DAN over 50 mg	Nortriptyline HCl 50 mg	Pamelor by Heartland	61392-0367	Antidepressant
NORTRIPTYLINEDAN-50MG	Cap, White, Black Print, Nortriptyline over DAN over 50 mg	Nortriptyline HCl 50 mg	Pamelor by Danbury	61955-2510	Antidepressant
NORTRIPTYLINEDAN-50MG	Cap, White, Black Print, Nortriptyline over DAN over 50 mg	Nortriptyline HCl 50 mg	Pamelor by Danbury	61955-2510	Antidepressant
NORTRIPTYLINEDAN-50MG	Cap, White, Black Print, Nortriptyline over DAN over 50 mg	Nortriptyline HCl 50 mg	Pamelor by PDRX	55289-0386	Antidepressant
NORTRIPTYLINEDAN-50MG	Cap, White, Black Print, Nortriptyline over DAN over 50 mg	Nortriptyline HCl 50 mg	Pamelor by Schein	00364-2510	Antidepressant

ID FRONT <> BACK	DESCRIPTION FRONT <> BACK	INGREDIENT & STRENGTH	BRAND (or Generic Equiv.) by FIRM	NDC#	CLASS; SCH.
NORTRIPTYLINEDAN-75MG	Cap, Dark Green, Nortriptyline over DAN over 75 mg	Nortriptyline HCl 75 mg	Pamelor by Schein	00364-2511	Antidepressant
NORTRIPTYLINEDAN-75MG	Cap, Dark Green, Nortriptyline over DAN over 75 mg	Nortriptyline HCl 75 mg	Pamelor by Danbury	61955-2511	Antidepressant
NORTRIPTYLINEDAN-75MG	Cap, Dark Green, Nortriptyline over DAN over 75 mg	Nortriptyline HCl 75 mg	Pamelor by Heartland	61392-0370	Antidepressant
NORTRIPTYLINEDAN-75MG	Cap, Dark Green, Nortriptyline over DAN over 75 mg	Nortriptyline HCl 75 mg	Pamelor by Watson	00591-5789	Antidepressant
NORTRIPTYLINEINV75	Cap, Green	Nortriptyline HCl 75 mg	Pamelor by Invamed	52189-0331	Antidepressant
NORTRIPTYLINEINV75	Cap, Green	Nortriptyline HCl 75 mg	Pamelor by Apothecon	62269-0331	Antidepressant
NORVASC <> 25	Tab, White, Diamond Shaped, Norvasc <> 2.5	Amlodipine Besylate 2.5 mg	Norvasc by Murfreesboro	51129-1260	Antihypertensive
NORVASC <> 25	Tab, White, Diamond Shaped, Norvasc <> 2.5	Amlodipine Besylate 2.5 mg	Norvasc by Physician Total Care	54868-3853	Antihypertensive
NORVASC <> 25	Tab, White, Diamond Shaped, Norvasc <> 2.5	Amlodipine Besylate 2.5 mg	Norvasc by DRX	55045-2377	Antihypertensive
NORVASC <> 25	Tab, White, Diamond Shaped, Norvasc <> 2.5	Amlodipine Besylate 2.5 mg	Norvasc by Pfizer	00069-1520	Antihypertensive
NORVASC10	Tab, White, Round, Norvasc over 10	Amlodipine Besylate 10 mg	Norvasc by Va Cmop	65243-0009	Antihypertensive
NORVASC10	Tab, White, Round, Norvasc over 10	Amlodipine Besylate 10 mg	Norvasc by PDRX	55289-0549	Antihypertensive
NORVASC10	Tab, White, Round, Norvasc over 10	Amlodipine Besylate 10 mg	Norvasc by Direct Dispensing	57866-6626	Antihypertensive
NORVASC10	Tab, White, Round, Norvasc over 10	Amlodipine Besylate 10 mg	Norvasc by Pfizer	00069-1540	Antihypertensive
NORVASC10	Tab, White, Round, Norvasc over 10	Amlodipine Besylate 10 mg	Norvasc by Nat Pharmpak	55154-2710	Antihypertensive
NORVASC10	Tab, White, Round, Norvasc over 10	Amlodipine Besylate 10 mg	Norvasc by Med Pro	53978-3073	Antihypertensive
NORVASC10	Tab, White, Round, Norvasc over 10	Amlodipine Besylate 10 mg	Norvasc by Allscripts		Antihypertensive
NORVASC10	Tab, White, Round, Norvasc over 10	Amlodipine Besylate 10 mg	Norvasc by DRX	55045-2305	Antihypertensive
NORVASC10	Tab, White, Round, Norvasc over 10	Amlodipine Besylate 10 mg	Norvasc by Physician Total Care	54868-3464	Antihypertensive
NORVASC10	Tab, White, Round, Norvasc over 10	Amlodipine Besylate 10 mg	Norvasc by Amerisource	62584-0540	Antihypertensive
NORVASC5	Tab, White, Octagonal, Norvasc over 5	Amlodipine Besylate 5 mg	Norvasc by Amerisource	62584-0530	Antihypertensive
NORVASC5	Tab, White, Octagonal, Norvasc over 5	Amlodipine Besylate 5 mg	Norvasc by Heartland	61392-0711	Antihypertensive
NORVASC5	Tab, White, Octagonal, Norvasc over 5	Amlodipine Besylate 5 mg	Norvasc by Direct Dispensing	57866-6625	Antihypertensive
NORVASC5	Tab, White, Octagonal, Norvasc over 5	Amlodipine Besylate 5 mg	Norvasc by Va Cmop	65243-0008	Antihypertensive
NORVASC5	Tab, White, Octagonal, Norvasc over 5	Amlodipine Besylate 5 mg	Norvasc by Rightpac	65240-0794	Antihypertensive
NORVASC5	Tab, White, Octagonal, Norvasc over 5	Amlodipine Besylate 5 mg	Norvasc by Pfizer	00069-1530	Antihypertensive
NORVASC5	Tab, White, Octagonal, Norvasc over 5	Amlodipine Besylate 5 mg	Norvasc by B F Ascher	00225-0570	Antihypertensive
NORVASC5	Tab, White, Octagonal, Norvasc over 5	Amlodipine Besylate 5 mg	Norvasc by Wal Mart	49035-0185	Antihypertensive
NORVASC5	Tab, White, Octagonal, Norvasc over 5	Amlodipine Besylate 5 mg	Norvasc by Med Pro	53978-2045	Antihypertensive
NORVASC5	Tab, White, Octagonal, Norvasc over 5	Amlodipine Besylate 5 mg	Norvasc by PDRX	55289-0103	Antihypertensive
NORVASC5	Tab, White, Octagonal, Norvasc over 5	Amlodipine Besylate 5 mg	Norvasc by Repack Co of America	55306-1530	Antihypertensive
NORVASC5	Tab, White, Octagonal, Norvasc over 5	Amlodipine Besylate 5 mg	Norvasc by Nat Pharmpak	55154-2708	Antihypertensive
NORVASC5	Tab, White, Octagonal, Norvasc over 5	Amlodipine Besylate 5 mg	Norvasc by Drug Distr	52985-0229	Antihypertensive
NORVASC5	Tab, White, Octagonal, Norvasc over 5	Amlodipine Besylate 5 mg	Norvasc by Compumed	00403-0933	Antihypertensive
NORVASC5	Tab, White, Octagonal, Norvasc over 5	Amlodipine Besylate 5 mg	Norvasc by CVS	00894-6780	Antihypertensive
NOVAFEDA	Cap, Orange & Red, Ex Release	Pseudoephedrine 120 mg, Chlorpheniramine Maleate 8 mg	Novafed A by Merrell	00068-0106 Discontinued	Cold Remedy
NOVALDEXD	Tab, White, Octagonal	Tamoxifen Citrate 30.4 mg	Nolvadex by Zeneca	Canadian	Antiestrogen
NOVO	Tab, Rose, Oval	Amoxicillin 125 mg	Amoxil by Novopharm	Canadian	Antibiotic
NOVO	Tab, White, Round	Carbamazepine 200 mg	Tegretol by Novopharm	Canadian	Anticonvulsant
NOVO	Tab, White, Round, Scored	Metformin HCl 500 mg	Glucophage by Novopharm	Canadian DIN 02045710	Antidiabetic
NOVO	Tab, White, Oblong	Sucralfate 1 g	Sulcrate by Novopharm	Canadian DIN 02045702	Gastrointestinal
NOVO	Tab, Orange, Round, Scored	Penicillin V Potassium 300 mg	Pen-Vee K by Novopharm	Canadian DIN 00021202	Antibiotic

ID FRONT <> BACK	DESCRIPTION FRONT <> BACK	INGREDIENT & STRENGTH	BRAND (or Generic Equiv.) by FIRM	NDC#	CLASS; SCH.
NOVO <> 01	Tab, White, Round, No/Vo <> 0.1	Clonidine HCl 0.1 mg	Catapres by Novopharm	Canadian DIN 02046121	Antihypertensive
NOVO <> 02	Tab, Orange, Round, No/Vo <> 0.2	Clonidine HCl 0.2 mg	Catapres by Novopharm	Canadian DIN 02046148	Antihypertensive
NOVO <> 025	Tab, White, Oval, no/vo <> 0.25	Alprazolam 0.25 mg	Xanax by Novopharm	Canadian DIN 01913484	Antianxiety; C IV
NOVO <> 05	Tab, Peach, Oval, no/vo <> 0.5	Alprazolam 0.5 mg	Xanax by Novopharm	Canadian DIN 01913492	Antianxiety; C IV
NOVO <> 1	Tab, Peach, Oblong, NO/VO <> 1	Prazosin HCl 1 mg	Minipress by Novopharm	Canadian DIN 01934198	Antihypertensive
NOVO <> 10	Tab, Light Blue, Round, NO/VO <> 10	Timolol Maleate 10 mg	Blocadren by Novopharm	Canadian DIN 01947818	Antihypertensive
NOVO <> 10	Tab, Yellow, Shield-Shaped	Cyclobenzaprine HCl 10 mg	Flexeril by Novopharm	Canadian DIN 02080052	Muscle Relaxant
NOVO <> 100	Tab, Orange, Round	Doxycycline Hyclate 100 mg	Vibramycin by Novopharm	Canadian DIN 02158574	Antibiotic
NOVO <> 100	Tab, White, Round, Scored	Trazodone HCl 100 mg	Desyrel by Novopharm	Canadian DIN 02144271	Antidepressant
NOVO <> 100	Tab, White, Round, Scored no/vo <> 100	Atenolol 100 mg	Tenormin by Novopharm	Canadian DIN 01912054	Antihypertensive
NOVO <> 100	Tab, White, Oval, novo/100	Captopril 100 mg	Capoten by Novopharm	Canadian DIN 01942999	Antihypertensive
NOVO <> 10010	Tab, Blue, Oval, Scored	Levodopa 100 mg, Carbidopa 10 mg	Sinemet by Novopharm	Canadian DIN 02244494	Antiparkinson
NOVO <> 10025	Tab, Yellow, Oval, Scored	Levodopa 100 mg, Carbidopa 25 mg	Sinemet by Novopharm	Canadian DIN 02244495	Antiparkinson
NOVO <> 125	Tab, Pink, Oval, Scored, NO / VO, Chewable	Amoxicillin 125 mg	Amoxil by Novopharm	Canadian DIN 02036347	Antibiotic
NOVO <> 2	Tab, White, Round, Scored	Prazosin HCl 2 mg	Minipress by Novopharm	Canadian DIN 01934201	Antihypertensive
NOVO <> 20	Tab, Light Blue, Oblong, NO/VO <> 20	Timolol Maleate 20 mg	Blocadren by Novopharm	Canadian DIN 01947826	Antihypertensive
NOVO <> 20	Tab, Beige, D-Shaped, Novo/20	Famotidine 20 mg	Pepcid by Novopharm	Canadian DIN 02022133	Gastrointestinal
NOVO <> 200	Tab, White, Oval	Acebutolol HCl 200 mg	Monitan by Novopharm	Canadian DIN 02204525	Antihypertensive
NOVO <> 240	Tab, Off White, Cap Shaped, Scored, NO/VO <> 2/40, Sustained Release	Verapamil HCl 240 mg	Isoptin SR by Novopharm	Canadian DIN 002211920	Antihypertensive
NOVO <> 25	Tab, White, Round, Scored, no/vo <> 2.5	Glyburide 2.5 mg	DiaBeta by Novopharm	Canadian DIN 01913670	Antidiabetic
NOVO <> 250	Tab, Pink, Oval, Scored, NO / VO, Chewable	Amoxicillin 250 mg	Amoxil by Novopharm	Canadian DIN 02036355	Antibiotic
NOVO <> 250	Tab, White, Round, Film-Coated	Ciprofloxacin Hydrochloride 250 mg	Novo-Ciprofloxacin by Novopharm	Canadian DIN 02161737	Antibiotic
NOVO <> 25025	Tab, Light Blue, Oval, Scored	Levodopa 250 mg, Carbidopa 25 mg	Sinemet by Novopharm	Canadian DIN 02244496	Antiparkinson
NOVO <> 2525	Tab, Light Peach, Round, Scored, NOVO <> 25/25	Hydrochlorothiazide 25 mg, Spironolactone 25 mg	Aldactazide by Novopharm	Canadian DIN 00613231	Diuretic; Antihypertensive
NOVO <> 2550	Tab, Light Orange, Round, Scored, 25/50	Hydrochlorothiazide 25 mg, Triamterene 50 mg	Dyazide by Novopharm	Canadian DIN 00532657	Diuretic; Antihypertensive
NOVO <> 3	Tab, Pink, Round	Bromazepam 3 mg	Lectopam by Novopharm	Canadian DIN 02230584	Sedative; C IV

ID FRONT <> BACK	DESCRIPTION FRONT <> BACK	INGREDIENT & STRENGTH	BRAND (or Generic Equiv.) by FIRM	NDC#	CLASS; SCH.
NOVO <> 30	Tab, Green, Round	Diltiazem HCl 30 mg	Cardizem by Novopharm	Canadian DIN 00862924	Antihypertensive
NOVO <> 325	Tab, White, Oblong	Acetaminophen 325 mg	Tylenol by Novopharm	Canadian DIN 00389218	Analgesic
NOVO <> 40	Tab, Brown & Orange, D-Shaped, novo/40	Famotidine 40 mg	Pepcid by Novopharm	Canadian DIN 02022141	Gastrointestinal
NOVO <> 400	Tab, Green, Oval	Cimetidine 400 mg	Tagamet by Novopharm	Canadian DIN 00603678	Gastrointestinal
NOVO <> 400	Tab, White, Oval	Acebutolol HCl 400 mg	Monitan by Novopharm	Canadian DIN 02204533	Antihypertensive
NOVO <> 5	Tab, White, Round, Scored, NO/VO <> 5	Timolol Maleate 5 mg	Blocadren by Novopharm	Canadian DIN 01947796	Antihypertensive
NOVO <> 5	Tab, White, Diamond, Scored, NO/VO <> 5	Prazosin HCl 5 mg	Minipress by Novopharm	Canadian DIN 01934228	Antihypertensive
NOVO <> 50	Tab, Light Orange, Round, Scored	Trazodone HCl 50 mg	Desyrel by Novopharm	Canadian DIN 02144263	Antidepressant
NOVO <> 50	Tab, Peach, Round, Scored, 50 below Score	Hydrochlorothiazide 50 mg	HydroDiuril by Novopharm	Canadian DIN 00021482	Diuretic; Antihypertensive
NOVO <> 50	Tab, White, Oval, Scored	Captopril 50 mg	Capoten by Novopharm	Canadian DIN 01942980	Antihypertensive
NOVO <> 500	Tab, White, Cap-Shaped, Film-Coated	Ciprofloxacin 500 mg	Novo-Ciprofloxacin by Novopharm	Canadian DIN 02161745	Antibiotic
NOVO <> 5050	Tab, Light Peach, Round, Scored, NOVO <> 50/50	Hydrochlorothiazide 50 mg, Spironolactone 50 mg	Aldactazide by Novopharm	Canadian DIN 00657182	Diuretic; Antihypertensive
NOVO <> 505050	Tab, Light Orange, Rectangular, NOVO <> 50/50/50	Trazodone HCl 150 mg	Desyrel by Novopharm	Canadian DIN 02144298	Antidepressant
NOVO <> 6	Tab, Green, Round	Bromazepam 6 mg	Lectopam by Novopharm	Canadian DIN 02230585	Sedative; C IV
NOVO <> 600	Tab, White, Oval	Gemfibrozil 600 mg	Lopid by Novopharm	Canadian DIN 02142074	Antihyperlipidemic
NOVO <> 600	Tab, Light Orange, Oval	Ibuprofen 600 mg	Motrin by Novopharm	Canadian DIN 00629359	NSAID
NOVO <> 600	Tab, Green, Oval	Cimetidine 600 mg	Tagamet by Novopharm	Canadian DIN 00603686	Gastrointestinal
NOVO <> 750	Tab, White, Cap-Shaped, Film Coated	Ciprofloxacin 750 mg	Novo-Ciprofloxacin by Novopharm	Canadian DIN 02161753	Antibiotic
NOVO <> 800	Tab, Green, Oval	Cimetidine 800 mg	Tagamet by Novopharm	Canadian DIN 00663727	Gastrointestinal
NOVO <> C500	Tab, White, Oblong	Acetaminophen 500 mg	Tylenol by Novopharm	Canadian DIN 00482323	Analgesic
NOVO <> C500	Tab, White, Cap-Shaped, Compressed	Acetaminophen 500 mg	Novo-Gesic by Novopharm	Canadian DIN 00482323	Analgesic
NOVO0125	Tab, Violet, Oval, Novo/0.125	Triazolam 0.125 mg	by Novopharm	Canadian	Sedative/Hypnotic; C IV
NOVO025	Tab, Powder Blue, Oval, Novo/0.25	Triazolam 0.25 mg	Halcion by Novopharm	Canadian	Sedative/Hypnotic; C IV
NOVO10	Cap, Tan	Nifedipine 10 mg	Novo Nifedin by Novopharm	Canadian	Antihypertensive
NOVO10	Tab, White, Round, Scored	Isosorbide Dinitrate 10 mg	Isordil by Novopharm	Canadian DIN 00458686	Antianginal
NOVO10	Tab, White, Round, Novo/10	Medroxyprogesterone Acetate 10 mg	by Novopharm	Canadian	Hormone
NOVO10	Tab, Cream, Round, Novo/10	Maprotiline HCl 10 mg	Novo Maprotiline by Novopharm	Canadian	Antidepressant
NOVO10	Tab, White, Oval, novo/10	Baclofen 10 mg	Lioresal by Novopharm	Canadian	Muscle Relaxant
NOVO10	Tab, Light Yellow, Triangle, Novo/10	Clomipramine HCl 10 mg	by Novopharm	Canadian	OCD
NOVO10	Tab, Blue, Round, Novo/10	Desipramine HCl 10 mg	by Novopharm	Canadian	Antidepressant

ID FRONT <> BACK	DESCRIPTION FRONT <> BACK	INGREDIENT & STRENGTH	BRAND (or Generic Equiv.) by FIRM	NDC#	CLASS; SCH.
NOVO10	Cap, Gray & Green, novo/10	Fluoxetine HCl 10 mg	Prozac by Novopharm	Canadian DIN 02216582	Antidepressant
NOVO10	Tab, White, Round, Scored	Pindolol 10 mg	Novo Pindol by Novopharm	Canadian DIN 00869015	Antihypertensive
NOVO10	Cap, Blue & Maroon	Piroxicam 10 mg	Feldene by Novopharm	Canadian DIN 00695718	NSAID
NOVO100	Cap, Blue & White, Novo/100	Zidovudine 100 mg	Retrovir by Novopharm	Canadian Discontinued	Antiviral
NOVO100	Tab, Pink, Round, Novo/100	Trimipramine Maleate 100 mg	Novo Trimipramine100 by Novopharm	Canadian	Antidepressant
NOVO100	Tab, White, Round, Novo/100	Theophylline Anhydrous 100 mg	Theophylline Anhydrous 100 mg by Novopharm	Canadian	Antiasthmatic
NOVO100	Tab, White, Round, Scored, NOVO/100	Allopurinol 100 mg	Zyloprim by Novopharm	Canadian DIN 00364282	Antigout
NOVO100	Tab, Blue, Oval, novo/100	Flurbiprofen 100 mg	Novo Flurprofen by Novopharm	Canadian	NSAID
NOVO100	Tab, Blue, Oblong	Metoprolol Tartrate 100 mg	Lopressor by Novopharm	Canadian	Antihypertensive
NOVO100	Cap, Orange & Scarlet, Novo/100	Mexiletine HCl 100 mg	Mexiletine HCl 100 mg by Novopharm	Canadian	Antiarrhythmic
NOVO100	Tab, Yellow, Round, Novo/100	Ketoprofen 100 mg	Orudis by Novopharm	Canadian	NSAID
NOVO100	Cap, Orange & Purple, Novo/100	Minocycline HCl 100 mg	Minocin by Novopharm	Canadian DIN 02108151	Antibiotic
NOVO100	Cap, Blue	Doxycycline Hyclate 100 mg	Vibramycin by Novopharm	Canadian DIN 00725250	Antibiotic
NOVO100	Cap, Blue & Pink, Novo/100	Doxepin HCl 100 mg	Sinequan by Novopharm	Canadian DIN 01913468	Antidepressant
NOVO100	Cap, Red, White Print, Clear	Docusate Sodium 100 mg	Colace by Novopharm	Canadian DIN 00842044	Laxative
NOVO120	Tab, White, Round	Verapamil HCl 120 mg	Novo Veramil by Novopharm	Canadian	Antihypertensive
NOVO125	Tab, White, Oblong, novo/12.5	Captopril 12.5 mg	Capoten by Novopharm	Canadian	Antihypertensive
NOVO125	Tab, Green, Oval	Naproxen 125 mg	Novo Naprox by Novopharm	Canadian	NSAID
NOVO125	Tab, Yellow, Round, Novo/125	Methyldopa 125 mg	Methyldopa 125 mg by Novopharm	Canadian	Antihypertensive
NOVO15	Cap, Flesh & Maroon, Novo/15	Temazepam 15 mg	Restoril by Novopharm	Canadian	Sedative/Hypnotic; C IV
NOVO15	Tab, White, Round, Scored	Pindolol 15 mg	Visken by Novopharm	Canadian DIN 00869023	Antihypertensive
NOVO15	Cap, Grey, NOVO 15	Clorazepate Dipotassium 15 mg	Tranxene by Novopharm	Canadian DIN 00628212	Antianxiety; C IV
NOVO150	Cap, Pink, Novo/150	Doxepin HCl 150 mg	Sinequan by Novopharm	Canadian DIN 01913476	Antidepressant
NOVO 180	Cap, Blue	Doxycycline Hyclate 100 mg	Novo Doxylin by Novopharm	Canadian	Antibiotic
NOVO20	Tab, White, Oblong, novo/20	Baclofen 20 mg	Lioresal by Novartis	Canadian	Muscle Relaxant
NOVO20	Cap, Green & Ivory, novo/20	Fluoxetine HCl 20 mg	Prozac by Novopharm	Canadian DIN 02216590	Antidepressant
NOVO20	Cap, Red	Piroxicam 20 mg	Feldene by Novopharm	Canadian DIN 00695696	NSAID
NOVO200	Tab, White, Round, Scored, NOVO/200	Allopurinol 200 mg	Zyloprim by Novopharm	Canadian DIN 00565342	Antigout
NOVO200	Tab, Green, Round, Scored, NOVO / 200	Cimetidine 200 mg	Tagamet by Novopharm	Canadian DIN 00582409	Gastrointestinal
NOVO200	Tab, White, Round	Sulfinpyrazone 200 mg	Novo Pyrazone by Novopharm	Canadian	Uricosuric
NOVO200	Cap, Scarlet, Novo/200	Mexiletine HCl 200 mg	Mexiletine HCl 200 mg	Canadian	Antiarrhythmic
NOVO200	Tab, White, Oval, Scored, Novo/200	Theophylline Anhydrous 200 mg	Theo-Dur by Novopharm	Canadian DIN 02230086	Antiasthmatic
NOVO200	Tab, White, Round, Deep Score, Novo/200	Tiaprofenic Acid 200 mg	Surgam by Novopharm	Canadian DIN 02179679	NSAID

ID FRONT <> BACK	DESCRIPTION FRONT <> BACK	INGREDIENT & STRENGTH	BRAND (or Generic Equiv.) by FIRM	NDC#	CLASS; SCH.
NOVO240	Cap, Red, White Print, Clear	Docusate Calcium 240 mg	Surfak by Novopharm	Canadian DIN 02020084	Laxative
NOVO25	Tab, Cream, Round, Novo/25	Spironolactone 25 mg	Novo Spiroton by Novopharm	Canadian	Diuretic
NOVO25	Tab, Orange, Round, Novo/25	Maprotiline HCl 25 mg	Novo Maprotiline by Novopharm	Canadian	Antidepressant
NOVO25	Tab, Peach, Round, Novo/2.5	Medroxyprogesterone Acetate 2.5 mg	by Novopharm	Canadian	Hormone
NOVO25	Tab, Yellow, Round, Novo/25	Desipramine HCl 25 mg	by Novopharm	Canadian	Antidepressant
NOVO25	Cap, Blue & Pink	Doxepin HCl 25 mg	Sinequan by Novopharm	Canadian DIN 01913425	Antidepressant
NOVO25	Cap, Blue and White, Opaque	Indomethacin 25 mg	Indocin by Novopharm	Canadian DIN 00337420	NSAID
NOVO25	Tab, Square, Scored, Novo / 25	Captopril 25 mg	Capoten by Novopharm	Canadian DIN 01942972	Antihypertensive
NOVO250	Cap, Orange & Yellow	Tetracycline HCl 250 mg	Novo Tetra by Novopharm	Canadian	Antibiotic
NOVO250	Tab, Yellow, Round, Novo/250	Methyldopa 250 mg	by Novopharm	Canadian	Antihypertensive
NOVO250	Tab, Yellow, Oval	Naproxen 250 mg	Novo Naprox by Novopharm	Canadian	NSAID
NOVO250	Tab, Light Yellow, Round, novo/250	Flutamide 250 mg	by Novopharm	Canadian	Antiandrogen
NOVO 250	Cap, Clear & Orange	Erythromycin 250 mg	Novo Rythro Enca by Novopharm	Canadian	Antibiotic
NOVO250	Tab, Peach, Oblong, Novo/250	Diflunisal 250 mg	Novo Diflunisal by Novopharm	Canadian	NSAID
NOVO250	Cap, Orange, novo/250	Cephalexin 250 mg	Keflex by Novopharm	Canadian DIN 00342084	Antibiotic
NOVO250	Cap, Black & Red, White Print	Ampicillin 250 mg	Principen by Novopharm	Canadian DIN 00020877	Antibiotic
NOVO250	Cap, Orange and Brown	Cloxacillin Sodium 250 mg	Orbenin by Novopharm	Canadian DIN 00337765	Antibiotic
NOVO250	Cap, Yellow and Red	Amoxicillin 250 mg	Amoxil by Novopharm	Canadian DIN 00406724	Antibiotic
NOVO250	Cap, Red Cap, Yellow Body, Hard Gel	Amoxicillin 250 mg	Novamoxin by Novopharm	Canadian DIN 00406724	Antibiotic
NOVO275	Tab, Blue, Oblong	Naproxen 275 mg	Novo Naprox Sod by Novopharm	Canadian	NSAID
NOVO288	Tab, White, Round, Film Coated, NOVO288 <> Apis Bull	Estradiol 1 mg, Norethindrone Acetate 0.5 mg	Activella by Novo Nordisk	00169-5174	Hormone
NOVO288	Tab, White, Round, Film Coated, NOVO288 <> Apis Bull	Estradiol 1 mg, Norethindrone Acetate 0.5 mg	Activella by Pharmacia	00009-5174	Hormone
NOVO291 <> APIS	Tab, White, Round, Film Coated	Estradiol 0.5 mg, Norethindrone Acetate 0.1 mg	Activelle LD by Novo Nordisk	Canadian DIN 02309009	Estrogenic and Progestin Hormones
NOVO2MG	Tab, Light Green, Oblong, Novo/2 mg	Loperamide 2 mg	Imodium by Novopharm	Canadian	Antidiarrheal
NOVO30	Tab, White, Round, Scored	Isosorbide Dinitrate 30 mg	Isordil by Novopharm	Canadian DIN 00458694	Antianginal
NOVO30	Cap, Blue & Maroon, Novo/30	Temazepam 30 mg	Restoril by Novopharm	Canadian	Sedative/Hypnotic; C IV
NOVO300	Tab, White, Round, Deep Score, Novo/300	Tiaprofenic Acid 300 mg	Surgam by Novopharm	Canadian DIN 02179687	NSAID
NOVO300	Tab, White, Oblong, Novo/300	Theophylline Anhydrous 300 mg	by Novopharm	Canadian	Antiasthmatic
NOVO300	Tab, Orange, Round, Scored, NOVO/300	Allopurinol 300 mg	Zyloprim by Novopharm	Canadian DIN 00363693	Antigout
NOVO300	Tab, Green, Round, Scored, NOVO / 300	Cimetidine 300 mg	Tagamet by Novopharm	Canadian DIN 00582417	Gastrointestinal
NOVO375	Cap, Cream and Grey, NOVO 3.75	Clorazepate Dipotassium 3.75 mg	Tranxene by Novopharm	Canadian DIN 00628190	Antianxiety; C IV
NOVO375	Tab, Peach, Oblong	Naproxen 375 mg	Novo Naprox by Novopharm	Canadian	NSAID
NOVO4	Tab, Yellow, Round, Scored	Chlorpheniramine Maleate 4 mg	Chlor-Tripolon by Novopharm	Canadian DIN 00021288	Antihistamine
NOVO40	Tab, White, Round, Novo/40	Nadolol 40 mg	Novo Nadolol by Novopharm	Canadian	Antihypertensive

ID FRONT <> BACK	DESCRIPTION FRONT <> BACK	INGREDIENT & STRENGTH	BRAND (or Generic Equiv.) by FIRM	NDC#	CLASS; SCH.
NOVO40	Tab, Light Orange, Round, Scored	Furosemide 40 mg	Lasix by Novopharm	Canadian DIN 00337749	Diuretic
NOVO400	Cap, Opaque & Orange, Novo/400	Tolmetin Sodium 400 mg	Novo Tripramine by Novopharm	Canadian	NSAID
NOVO5	Tab, Blue, Round, Novo/5	Medroxyprogesterone Acetate 5 mg	by Novopharm	Canadian	Hormone
NOVO5	Tab, White, Oblong, Novo/5	Glyburide 5 mg	Novo Glyburide by Novopharm	Canadian DIN 01913689	Antidiabetic
NOVO5	Tab, White, Round, Scored	Pindolol 5 mg	Visken by Novopharm	Canadian DIN 00869007	Antihypertensive
NOVO50	Tab, Pink, Round, Novo/50	Trimipramine Maleate 50 mg	Novo Tripramine by Novopharm	Canadian	Antidepressant
NOVO50	Tab, White, Round, Scored, NOVO / 50	Prednisone 50 mg	Deltasone by Novopharm	Canadian DIN 00232378	Steroid
NOVO50	Tab, White, Oval, novo/50	Flurbiprofen 50 mg	Novo Flurprofen by Novopharm	Canadian	NSAID
NOVO50	Tab, Orange, Round, Novo/50	Maprotiline HCl 50 mg	Novo Maprotiline by Novopharm	Canadian	Antidepressant
NOVO50	Tab, Yellow, Round, Novo/50	Ketoprofen 50 mg	Orudis by Novopharm	Canadian	NSAID
NOVO50	Tab, Pink, Oblong	Metoprolol Tartrate 50 mg	Lopressor by Novopharm	Canadian	Antihypertensive
NOVO50	Tab, Green, Round, Novo/50	Desipramine HCl 50 mg	by Novopharm	Canadian	Antidepressant
NOVO50	Cap, Pink, Novo50	Doxepin HCl 50 mg	Novo Doxepin by Novopharm	Canadian DIN 01913433	Antidepressant
NOVO50	Tab, White, novo/50	Atenolol 50 mg	Tenormin by Novopharm	Canadian DIN 01912062	Antihypertensive
NOVO50	Cap, Orange, Novo/50	Minocycline HCl 50 mg	Minocin by Novopharm	Canadian DIN 02108143	Antibiotic
NOVO50	Cap, Blue & White, Opaque	Indomethacin 50 mg	Indocin by Novopharm	Canadian DIN 00337439	NSAID
NOVO500	Tab, Yellow, Oval	Naproxen 500 mg	Novo Naprox by Novopharm	Canadian	NSAID
NOVO500	Tab, Yellow, Round, Novo/500	Methyldopa 500 mg	by Novopharm	Canadian	Antihypertensive
NOVO500	Tab, Orange, Oblong, Novo/500	Diflunisal 500 mg	Novo Diflunisal by Novopharm	Canadian	NSAID
NOVO500	Cap, Black & Red, White Print	Ampicillin 500 mg	Principen by Novopharm	Canadian DIN 00020885	Antibiotic
NOVO500	Cap, Orange and Brown	Cloxacillin Sodium 500 mg	Orbenin by Novopharm	Canadian DIN 00337773	Antibiotic
NOVO500	Cap, Yellow and Red	Amoxicillin 500 mg	Amoxil by Novopharm	Canadian DIN 00406716	Antibiotic
NOVO500	Cap, Orange and Grey, novo/500	Cephalexin 500 mg	Keflex by Novopharm	Canadian DIN 00342114	Antibiotic
NOVO500	Cap, Red Cap, Yellow Body, Hard Gel	Amoxicillin 500 mg	Novamoxin by Novopharm	Canadian DIN 00406716	Antibiotic
NOVO50MG	Cap, Pink	Doxepin HCl 50 mg	Novo Doxepin by Novopharm	Canadian	Antidepressant
NOVO60	Tab, Yellow, Round, Novo/60	Diltiazem HCl 60 mg	Cardizem by Novopharm	Canadian DIN 00862932	Antihypertensive
NOVO75	Tab, Orange & Red, Round, Novo/75	Maprotiline HCl 75 mg	Novo Maprotiline by Novopharm	Canadian	Antidepressant
NOVO75	Cap, Pink	Doxepin HCl 75 mg	Sinequan by Novopharm	Canadian DIN 01913441	Antidepressant
NOVO75	Tab, Orange, Round, Novo/75	Desipramine HCl 75 mg	by Novopharm	Canadian	Antidepressant
NOVO75	Cap, Red and Grey, NOVO 7.5	Clorazepate Dipotassium 7.5 mg	Tranxene by Novopharm	Canadian DIN 00628204	Antianxiety; C IV
NOVO80	Tab, Yellow, Round	Verapamil HCl 80 mg	Novo Verapamil by Novopharm	Canadian	Antihypertensive
NOVO80	Tab, Light Blue, Oblong, Novo/80	Sotalol HCl 80 mg	by Novopharm	Canadian	Antiarrhythmic
NOVO80	Tab, White, Round, Novo/80	Nadolol 80 mg	Novo Nadolol by Novopharm	Canadian	Antihypertensive

ID FRONT <> BACK	DESCRIPTION FRONT <> BACK	INGREDIENT & STRENGTH	BRAND (or Generic Equiv.) by FIRM	NDC#	CLASS; SCH.
NP	Tab, White, Football Shaped, Film Coated	Ascorbic Acid 60 mg, Biotin 300 mcg, Pantothenic Acid 10 mg, Cobalamin 6 mcg, Folic Acid 1 mg, Niacin 20 mg, Pyridoxine HCl 10 mg, Riboflavin 1.7 mg, Thiamine Mononitrate 1.5 mg, Zinc 12.5 mg	Nephplex Rx by Nephro-Tech	59528-0317	Vitamin
NP	Tab, N-P	Ascorbic Acid 60 mg, Biotin 300 mcg, Calcium Pantothenate, Cyanocobalamin 6 mcg, Folic Acid 1 mg, Niacinamide 20 mg, Pyridoxine HCl 10 mg, Riboflavin 1.7 mg, Thiamine Mononitrate 1.5 mg	Nephplex Rx by Anabolic	00722-6396	Vitamin
NP	Tab, Orange, Football Shaped, Film Coated	Vitamin Combination	RenaPlex by Nephro-Tech	59528-0810	Vitamin; Supplement
NP2	Tab, White, Cap Shaped, Scored, Coated	Clonidine 0.17 mg	Clonidine ER by Tris Pharma	27808-0030	Antihypertensive
NP4	Tab, Yellow, Cap Shaped, Scored, Coated	Clonidine 0.26 mg	Clonidine ER by Tris Pharma	27808-0031	Antihypertensive
NPL430	Tab, White, Round	Chlorpheniramine Maleate 4 mg, Pseudoephedrine HCl 60 mg	Deconamine by Nutripharm		Cold Remedy
NPL510	Tab, White	Carbinoxamine Maleate 4 mg, Pseudoephedrine HCl 60 mg	Carbiset by Nutripharm	Discontinued	Cold Remedy
NPL51081424	Cap, White, NPL 51081/424	Isometheptene Mucate 65 mg, Dichloralphenazone 100 mg, Acetaminophen 325 mg	Isocom by Nutripharm		Analgesic; C IV
NPL512	Tab, White	Carbinoxamine Maleate 8 mg, Pseudoephedrine HCl 120 mg	Carbiset-TR by Nutripharm	Discontinued	Cold Remedy
NPREC250	Tab, White, Round, Enteric Coated	Naproxen 250 mg	Naprosyn by Roche	Canadian DIN 02162792	NSAID
NPREC375	Tab, White, Oval, Enteric Coated	Naproxen 375 mg	Naprosyn by Roche	Canadian DIN 02162415	NSAID
NPREC500	Tab, White, Oblong, Enteric Coated	Naproxen 500 mg	Naprosyn by Roche	Canadian DIN 02162423	NSAID
NPRLE250	Tab, Yellow, Round, Scored	Naproxen 250 mg	Naprosyn by Roche	Canadian	NSAID
NPRLE250	Tab, Yellow, Round, Scored	Naproxen 250 mg	Naprosyn by Hoffmann La Roche	00004-6313	NSAID
NPRLE375	Tab, Pink, Oval	Naproxen 375 mg	Naprosyn by Hoffmann La Roche	00004-6314	NSAID
NPRLE375	Tab, Pink, Oval, Biconvex	Naproxen 375 mg	Prevacid NaraPAC by Tap	00300-1545	NSAID
NPRLE375	Tab, Pink, Oval	Naproxen 375 mg	Naprosyn by Roche	Canadian	NSAID
NPRLE500	Tab, Yellow, Cap Shaped	Naproxen 500 mg	Naprosyn by Roche	Canadian	NSAID
NPRLE500	Tab, Yellow, Cap Shaped, Scored	Naproxen 500 mg	Prevacid NaraPAC by Tap	00300-1546	NSAID
NPRLE500	Tab, Yellow, Cap Shaped	Naproxen 500 mg	Naprosyn by Hoffmann La Roche	00004-6316	NSAID
NPRSR750	Tab, Peach, Oval, SR	Naproxen 750 mg	Naprosyn by Roche	Canadian DIN 02162466	NSAID
NPS275	Tab, Blue, Oval, Film Coated, NPS-275	Naproxen 275 mg	Anaprox by Roche	Canadian DIN 02162725	NSAID
NPS275	Tab, Light Blue, Oval	Naproxen 275 mg	Anaprox by Hoffmann La Roche	00004-6202	NSAID
NPS550	Tab, Dark Blue, Oblong, Scored	Naproxen 550 mg	Anaprox by Hoffmann La Roche	00004-6203	NSAID
NPS550	Tab, Dark Blue, Oblong, Film Coated	Naproxen 550 mg	Anaprox DS by Roche	Canadian DIN 02162717	NSAID
NR <> CIBA	Tab, Tan, Round	Ferrous Sulfate (Dried) 160 mg	Slow FE by Novartis	00067-0125	Supplement
NRP1020MG	Cap, Ivory	Lisdexamfetamine Dimesylate 20 mg	Vyvanse by New River	59417-0102	Stimulant; C II
NRP1030MG	Cap, White and Orange	Lisdexamfetamine Dimesylate 30 mg	Vyvanse by New River	59417-0103	Stimulant; C II
NRP1040MG	Cap, Blue Green and White	Lisdexamfetamine Dimesylate 40 mg	Vyvanse by New River	59417-0104	Stimulant; C II
NRP1050MG	Cap, White and Blue	Lisdexamfetamine Dimesylate 50 mg	Vyvanse by New River	59417-0105	Stimulant; C II
NRP1060MG	Cap, Aqua Blue	Lisdexamfetamine Dimesylate 60 mg	Vyvanse by New River	59417-0106	Stimulant; C II
NRP1070MG	Cap, Blue and Orange	Lisdexamfetamine Dimesylate 70 mg	Vyvanse by New River	59417-0107	Stimulant; C II
NRV10 <> PFIZER	Tab, White, Octagonal	Amlodipine 10 mg	Norvasc by Pfizer	Canadian DIN 00878936	Antihypertensive
NRV10PFIZER	Tab, White, Octagonal, NRV 10/Pfizer	Amlodipine Besylate 10 mg	Norvasc by Pfizer	Canadian	Antihypertensive
NRV5 <> PFIZER	Tab, White, Octagonal, Scored	Amlodipine 5 mg	Norvasc by Pfizer	Canadian DIN 00878928	Antihypertensive
NRV5PFIZER	Tab, White, Octagonal	Amlodipine Besylate 5 mg	Norvasc by Pfizer	Canadian	Antihypertensive

ID FRONT <> BACK	DESCRIPTION FRONT <> BACK	INGREDIENT & STRENGTH	BRAND (or Generic Equiv.) by FIRM	NDC#	CLASS; SCH.
NRX	Tab, Light Blue, Oval, Film Coated	Beta Carotene 4000 IU, Vitamin D 400 IU, dl-Alpha Tocopheryl Acetate 30 IU, Ascorbic Acid 120 mg, Folic Acid 1 mg, Thiamine Mononitrate 3 mg, Riboflavin 3 mg, Niacinamide 20 mg, Pyridoxine HCl 3 mg, Cyanocobalamin 8 mcg, Biotin 30 mcg, Pantothenic Acid 7 mg, Calcium Carbonate 200 mg, Potassium Iodide 150 mcg, Zinc 15 mg, Magnesium 100 mg, Iron 29 mg, Copper 3 mg	Nestabs RX by Fielding	00421-1317	Vitamin
NSR25 <> PFIZER	Tab, Yellow, Diamond Shaped, Film Coated	Eplerenone 25 mg	Inspra by Searle	00025-1710	Antihypertensive
NSR50 <> PFIZER	Tab, Yellow, Diamond Shaped, Film Coated	Eplerenone 50 mg	Inspra by Searle	00025-1720	Antihypertensive
NT	Tab, White, Cap Shaped, Film Coated, Scored, N/T	Ascorbic Acid 40 mg, Biotin 300 mcg, Cobalamin 6 mcg, Docusate Sodium 75 mg, Ferrous Fumarate 200 mg, Folic Acid 1 mg, Niacin 20 mg, Pantothenic Acid 10 mg, Pyridoxine HCl 10 mg, Riboflavin 1.7 mg, Thiamine Mononitrate 1.5 mg	Nephron Fa by Nephro-Tech	59528-4456	Vitamin
NT	Tab, Pink, Black Print, Oval	Ascorbic Acid 40 mg, Biotin 300 mcg, Cyanocobalamin 6 mcg, Docusate Sodium 75 mg, Ferrous Fumarate 200 mg, Folic Acid 1 mg, Niacinamide 20 mg, Pantothenic Acid 10 mg, Pyridoxine HCl 10 mg, Riboflavin 1.7 mg, Thiamine Mononitrate 1.5 mg	Nephron Fa by Anabolic	00722-6392	Vitamin
NT <> HYL	Tab, White, Oblong	Calcarea Phosphorica 3X, Ferrum Phosphorica 3X, Kali Phosphoricum 3X, Natrum Phosphoricum 3X, Magnesia Phosphoricum 3X	Hyland's Nerve Tonic by Hyland's	54973-1129	Homeopathic
NT10MG709	Cap, Yellow and White, Opaque	Nortriptyline HCl 10 mg	Aventyl by Pharmascience	Canadian DIN 02177692	Antidepressant
NT112 <> JMI	Tab, NT over 1 1/2	Thyroid 97.2 mg	Nature Thyroid by Jones	52604-3304	Thyroid Hormone
NT112 <> JMI	Tab, NT over 1 1/2	Thyroid 97.2 mg	Nature Thyroid by JMI Canton	00252-3304	Thyroid Hormone
NT12 <> JMI	Tab, NT over 1/2	Thyroid 32.4 mg	Nature Thyroid by JMI Canton	00252-3299	Thyroid Hormone
NT12 <> JMI	Tab, NT over 1/2	Thyroid 32.4 mg	Nature Thyroid by Jones	52604-3299	Thyroid Hormone
NT16	Tab, White, Elliptical, Film Coated, Scored, NT / 16	Gabapentin 600 mg	Neurontin by Parke Davis	00071-0513	Anticonvulsant
NT25MG710	Cap, Yellow and White, Opaque	Nortriptyline HCl 25 mg	Aventyl by Pharmascience	Canadian DIN 02177706	Antidepressant
NT26	Tab, White, Elliptical, Film Coated, Scored, NT / 26	Gabapentin 800 mg	Neurontin by Parke Davis	00071-0401	Anticonvulsant
NT3 <> JMI	Tab	Thyroid 3 g	Nature Thyroid by Jones	52604-3312	Thyroid Hormone
NTR <> DUPONT	Tab, White w/ Orange Specks, Round, Scored	Naltrexone HCl 50 mg	by BMS	00056-0079	Opioid Antagonist
NTR <> DUPONT	Tab, White w/ Orange Specks, Round, Scored	Naltrexone HCl 50 mg	Revia by Dupont	Canadian	Opioid Antagonist
NU <> 05	Tab, White, Round, NU <> 0.5	Lorazepam 0.5 mg	Ativan by Nu Pharm	00865672	Antianxiety; C IV
NU <> 10	Tab, White, Round, Film Coated	Domperidone 10 mg	by Nu Pharm	Canadian DIN 02231477	Gastrointestinal
NU <> 10	Tab, Grayish-Pink, Round, Film Coated	Nifedipine 10 mg	by Nu Pharm	Canadian DIN 02212102	Antihypertensive
NU <> 100	Tab, White, Oval, Film Coated	Fluvoxamine Maleate 100 mg	Luvox by Nu Pharm	Canadian DIN 02231193	OCD
NU <> 10010	Tab, Blue, Oval, Scored, NU <> 100 over 10	Carbidopa 10 mg, Levodopa 100 mg	by Nu Pharm	Canadian DIN 02182831	Antiparkinson
NU <> 125	Tab, White, Cap Shaped, Scored, NU <> 12.5	Captopril 12.5 mg	Capoten by Nu Pharm	Canadian DIN 01913824	Antihypertensive
NU <> 20	Tab, Grayish-Pink, Round, Film Coated	Nifedipine 20 mg	by Nu Pharm	Canadian DIN 02200937	Antihypertensive
NU <> 250	Tab, White, Oval	Ticlopidine HCl 250 mg	by Nu Pharm	Canadian DIN 02237560	Anticoagulant
NU <> 25025	Tab, Blue, Oval, Scored, NU <> 250 over 25	Carbidopa 25 mg, Levodopa 250 mg	by Nu Pharm	Canadian DIN 02182831	Antiparkinson
NU <> 400	Tab, Pink, Cap Shaped	Pentoxifylline 400 mg	Trental by Nu Pharm	Canadian DIN 02230401	Anticoagulant

ID FRONT <> BACK	DESCRIPTION FRONT <> BACK	INGREDIENT & STRENGTH	BRAND (or Generic Equiv.) by FIRM	NDC#	CLASS; SCH.
NU <> 50	Tab, White, Round, Film Coated	Fluvoxamine Maleate 50 mg	Luvox by Nu Pharm	Canadian DIN 02231192	OCD
NU <> 850	Tab, White, Cap Shaped	Metformin HCl 850 mg	by Nu Pharm	Canadian DIN 02229517	Antidiabetic
NU <> AP	Tab, Round, White, AP <> nu, Chewable	Hyoscyamine Sulfate 0.125 mg	NuLev Chewable Melt by Alaven Pharmaceutical	68220-0118	Gastrointestinal
NU <> BU10	Tab, White, Rectangular, Scored	Buspirone HCl 10 mg	Buspar by Nu Pharm	Canadian DIN 02207672	Antianxiety
NU <> D500	Tab, Orange, Cap Shaped, Film Coated	Diflunisal 500 mg	by Nu Pharm	Canadian DIN 02058413	NSAID
NU <> LOX10	Tab, Green, Round, Film Coated, Scored, NU <> Lox over 10	Loxapine Succinate 10 mg	by Nu Pharm	Canadian DIN 02237535	Antipsychotic
NU <> LOX25	Tab, Pink, Round, Film Coated, Scored, NU <> Lox over 25	Loxapine Succinate 25 mg	by Nu Pharm	Canadian DIN 02237535	Antipsychotic
NU <> LOX5	Tab, Yellow, Round, Film Coated, Scored, NU <> Lox over 5	Loxapine Succinate 5 mg	by Nu Pharm	Canadian DIN 02237534	Antipsychotic
NU <> LOX50	Tab, White, Round, Film Coated, Scored, NU <> Lox over 50	Loxapine Succinate 50 mg	by Nu Pharm	Canadian DIN 02237536	Antipsychotic
NU <> T1	Tab, White, Round	Terazosin HCl 1 mg	by Nu Pharm	Canadian DIN 02233047	Antihypertensive
NU <> T10	Tab, Blue, Round	Terazosin HCl 10 mg	Hytrin by Nu Pharm	Canadian DIN 02233050	Antihypertensive
NU <> T2	Tab, Orange, Round	Terazosin HCl 2 mg	Hytrin by Nu Pharm	Canadian DIN 02233048	Antihypertensive
NU <> T5	Tab, Tan, Round	Terazosin HCl 5 mg	Hytrin by Nu Pharm	Canadian DIN 02233049	Antihypertensive
NU01	Tab, White, Round, NU/0.1	Clonidine HCl 0.1 mg	Nu Clonidine by Nu Pharm	Canadian	Antihypertensive
NU01	Tab, White, Round, Scored, NU over 0.1	Clonidine HCl 0.1 mg	by Nu Pharm	Canadian DIN 01913786	Antihypertensive
NU02	Tab, Orange, Round, Scored, NU over 0.2	Clonidine HCl 0.2 mg	by Nu Pharm	Canadian DIN 01913220	Antihypertensive
NU02	Tab, Orange, Round, N NU/0.2	Clonidine HCl 0.2 mg	Nu Clonidine by Nu Pharm	Canadian	Antihypertensive
NU05	Tab, Peach, Oval, Scored, NU over 0.5	Alprazolam 0.5 mg	Xanax by Nu Pharm	Canadian DIN 01913247	Antianxiety; C IV
NU1	Tab, White, Cap Shaped, Scored, NU over 1	Lorazepam 1 mg	Ativan by Nu Pharm	Canadian DIN 00865680	Antianxiety; C IV
NU1	Tab, Peach, Cap Shaped, Scored	Prazosin HCl 1 mg	Nu Prazo by Nu Pharm	Canadian DIN 01913794	Antihypertensive
NU10	Tab, Peachish Orange, Round, Film Coated, NU over 10	Prochlorperazine 10 mg	Nu Prochlor by Nu Pharm	Canadian DIN 01964402	Antiemetic
NU10	Cap, Blue & Maroon, Gelatin	Piroxicam 10 mg	Feldene by Nu Pharm	Canadian DIN 00865761	NSAID
NU10	Tab, Orange, Round, NU/10	Propranolol HCl 10 mg	Inderal by Nu Pharm	Canadian	Antihypertensive
NU10	Cap, White & Yellow, Opaque, Gelatin	Nortriptyline HCl 10 mg	by Nu Pharm	Canadian DIN 02231139	Antidepressant
NU10	Cap, Dark Yellow, Gelatin	Nifedipine 10 mg	Nu Nifed by Nu Pharm	Canadian DIN 00865591	Antihypertensive
NU10	Tab, White, Round, Scored, NU over 10	Pindolol 10 mg	Nu Pindol by Nu Pharm	Canadian DIN 00886009	Antihypertensive
NU10	Tab, Light Blue, Round, Scored, NU over 10	Timolol Maleate 10 mg	Nu Timolol by Nu Pharm	Canadian DIN 02044617	Antihypertensive

ID FRONT <> BACK	DESCRIPTION FRONT <> BACK	INGREDIENT & STRENGTH	BRAND (or Generic Equiv.) by FIRM	NDC#	CLASS; SCH.
NU10	Tab, White, Round, Film Coated, NU over 10	Ketorolac Tromethamine 10 mg	Toradol by Nu Pharm	Canadian DIN 02237910	NSAID
NU10	Cap, Gray & Light Green, Opaque, Gelatin	Fluoxetine HCl 10 mg	Prozac by Nu Pharm	Canadian DIN 02192756	Antidepressant
NU10	Tab, Yellow, Round, Scored, NU over 10	Hydralazine HCl 10 mg	by Nu Pharm	Canadian DIN 01913204	Antihypertensive
NU10	Tab, White to Off-White, Oval, Scored	Baclofen 10 mg	Lioresal by Nu Pharm	Canadian DIN 02136090	Muscle Relaxant
NU10	Tab, Yellow, D-Shaped, Film Coated, NU over 10	Cyclobenzaprine HCl 10 mg	by Nu Pharm	Canadian DIN 002171848	Muscle Relaxant
NU100	Tab, White, Oval, Scored	Captopril 100 mg	Capoten by Nu Pharm	Canadian DIN 01913859	Antihypertensive
NU100	Tab, White, Round, Scored, NU over 100	Atenolol 100 mg	Tenormin by Nu Pharm	Canadian DIN 00886122	Antihypertensive
NU100	Tab, White, Round, Film Coated, Scored, NU over 100	Acebutolol HCl 100 mg	Sectral by Nu Pharm	Canadian DIN 02165546	Antihypertensive
NU100	Tab, Blue, Oval, Film Coated, NU over 100	Flurbiprofen 100 mg	by Nu Pharm	Canadian DIN 02020688	NSAID
NU100	Tab, Light Orange, Round, Film Coated, NU over 100	Doxycycline Hyclate 100 mg	by Nu Pharm	Canadian DIN 02044676	Antibiotic
NU100	Cap, Blue, Opaque, Gelatin	Doxycycline Hyclate 100 mg	by Nu Pharm	Canadian DIN 02044668	Antibiotic
NU100	Cap, White, Opaque, Gelatin	Fenofibrate 100 mg	by Nu Pharm	Canadian DIN 02223600	Antihyperlipidemic
NU100	Tab, Blue, Oval	Flurbiprofen 100 mg	by Nu Pharm	Canadian	NSAID
NU100	Tab, Orange, Oval, Film Coated, Scored, NU over 100	Moclobemide 100 mg	by Nu Pharm	Canadian DIN 02237111	Antidepressant
NU100	Tab, White, Round, Scored, NU over 100	Sulfinpyrazone 100 mg	Nu Sulfinpyrazone by Nu Pharm	Canadian DIN 02045680	Uricosuric
NU100	Tab, Pink, Round, NU/100	Trimipramine Maleate 100 mg	by Nu Pharm	Canadian	Antidepressant
NU120	Tab, White, Round, Film Coated, NU over 120	Verapamil HCl 120 mg	by Nu Pharm	Canadian DIN 00886041	Antihypertensive
NU120	Tab, Rose, Round, NU/120	Propranolol HCl 120 mg	Inderal LA by Nu Pharm	Canadian	Antihypertensive
NU120	Cap, Light Turquoise, Opaque, Gelatin	Diltiazem HCl 120 mg	Cardizem by Nu Pharm	Canadian DIN 02231052	Antihypertensive
NU125	Tab, Green, Oval, NU-125	Naproxen 125 mg	Nu Naprox by Nu Pharm	Canadian	NSAID
NU125	Tab, Yellow, Round, NU/125	Methyldopa 125 mg	by Nu Pharm	Canadian	Antihypertensive
NU15	Tab, White, Round, Scored, NU over 15	Pindolol 15 mg	Nu Pindol by Nu Pharm	Canadian DIN 00886130	Antihypertensive
NU15	Cap, Maroon & Pink, Opaque, Gelatin	Temazepam 15 mg	Restoril by Nu Pharm	Canadian DIN 02223570	Sedative/Hypnotic; C IV
NU150	Tab, White, Round, Film Coated, NU over 150	Ranitidine HCl 150 mg	Nu Ranit by Nu Pharm	Canadian DIN 00865737	Gastrointestinal
NU150	Tab, Dark Yellow, Hexagonal, Scored, NU over 150	Sulindac 150 mg	by Nu Pharm	Canadian DIN 02042576	NSAID
NU150	Tab, Pale Yellow, Oval, Film Coated, Scored, NU over 150	Moclobemide 150 mg	by Nu Pharm	Canadian DIN 02237112	Antidepressant
NU150 <> 50252550	Tab, Pale Orange, Rectangular, Scored, NU-150 <> 50 over 25 over 25 over 50	Trazodone HCl 150 mg	Desyrel by Nu Pharm	Canadian DIN 02165406	Antidepressant
NU160	Tab, Blue, Cap Shaped, NU-160	Sotalol 160 mg	by Nu Pharm	Canadian DIN 02163772	Antiarrhythmic

ID FRONT <> BACK	DESCRIPTION FRONT <> BACK	INGREDIENT & STRENGTH	BRAND (or Generic Equiv.) by FIRM	NDC#	CLASS; SCH.
NU160	Tab, White, Oval, Scored	Megestrol Acetate 160 mg	by Nu Pharm	Canadian DIN 02185423	Hormone
NU180	Cap, Light Blue & Turquoise, Opaque, Gelatin	Diltiazem HCl 180 mg	Cardizem by Nu Pharm	Canadian DIN 02231053	Antihypertensive
NU1G	Tab, White, Cap Shaped, Scored, NU-1g	Sucralfate 1 g	by Nu Pharm	Canadian DIN 02134829	Gastrointestinal
NU2	Tab, White, Round, Scored, NU over 2	Prazosin HCl 2 mg	Nu Prazo by Nu Pharm	Canadian DIN 01913808	Antihypertensive
NU2	Tab, White, Oval, Scored	Lorazepam 2 mg	Ativan by Nu Pharm	Canadian DIN 00865699	Antianxiety; C IV
NU20	Tab, Beige, D-Shaped, Film Coated, NU over 20	Famotidine 20 mg	by Nu Pharm	Canadian DIN 02024195	Gastrointestinal
NU20	Cap, Green & Ivory, Opaque, Gelatin	Fluoxetine HCl 20 mg	by Nu Pharm	Canadian DIN 02192764	Antidepressant
NU20	Tab, White to Off-White, Oval, Scored	Baclofen 20 mg	Lioresal by Nu Pharm	Canadian DIN 02136104	Muscle Relaxant
NU20	Cap, Maroon, Gelatin	Piroxicam 20 mg	Feldene by Nu Pharm	Canadian DIN 00865788	NSAID
NU20	Tab, Blue, Hexagonal, Scored, NU over 20	Propranolol HCl 20 mg	Inderal by Nu Pharm	Canadian DIN 02044692	Antihypertensive
NU20	Tab, Light Blue, Oblong, NU/20	Timolol Maleate 20 mg	Nu Timolol by Nu Pharm	Canadian	Antihypertensive
NU200	Tab, White, Round, Scored, NU over 200	Sulfinpyrazone 200 mg	Nu Sulfinpyrazone by Nu Pharm	Canadian DIN 02045699	Uricosuric
NU200	Tab, Dark Yellow, Hexagonal, Scored, NU over 200	Sulindac 200 mg	by Nu Pharm	Canadian DIN 02042584	NSAID
NU200	Tab, White, Oval, Film Coated, Scored	Acebutolol HCl 200 mg	Sectral by Nu Pharm	Canadian DIN 02165554	Antihypertensive
NU200	Tab, Blue, Round, NU over 200	Acyclovir 200 mg	Zovirax by Nu Pharm	Canadian DIN 02197405	Antiviral
NU200	Tab, Pale Green, Round, Film Coated, NU over 200	Cimetidine HCl 200 mg	Tagamet by Nu Pharm	Canadian DIN 00865796	Gastrointestinal
NU200	Tab, White, Round, Scored	Carbamazepine 200 mg	Tegretol by Taro	Canadian DIN 02042568	Anticonvulsant
NU240	Cap, Light Blue, Opaque, Gelatin	Diltiazem HCl 240 mg	Cardizem by Nu Pharm	Canadian DIN 02231054	Antihypertensive
NU25	Tab, White, Square, Quadrisected, NU over 25	Captopril 25 mg	Capoten by Nu Pharm	Canadian DIN 02197405	Antihypertensive
NU25	Tab, White, Oval, Scored, NU over .25	Alprazolam 0.25 mg	Xanax by Nu Pharm	Canadian DIN 01913239	Antianxiety; C IV
NU25	Tab, White, Round, Scored, NU over 2.5	Glyburide 2.5 mg	by Nu Pharm	Canadian DIN 02020734	Antidiabetic
NU25	Tab, Yellow, Barrel Shaped, Scored, NU over 2.5	Enalapril Maleate 2.5 mg	Vasotec by Nu Pharm	Canadian DIN 02239498	Antihypertensive
NU25	Cap, Blue & White, Opaque, Gelatin	Indomethacin 25 mg	Indocin by Nu Pharm	Canadian DIN 00865850	NSAID
NU25	Cap, White & Yellow, Opaque, Gelatin	Nortriptyline HCl 25 mg	by Nu Pharm	Canadian DIN 02223147	Antidepressant
NU250	Cap, Orange & Yellow, Opaque, Gelatin	Tetracycline HCl 250 mg	Nu Tetra by Nu Pharm	Canadian DIN 00717606	Antibiotic
NU250	Cap, Blue & Yellow, Opaque, Gelatin	Mefenamic Acid 250 mg	Ponstel by Nu Pharm	Canadian DIN 02229569	NSAID

ID FRONT <> BACK	DESCRIPTION FRONT <> BACK	INGREDIENT & STRENGTH	BRAND (or Generic Equiv.) by FIRM	NDC#	CLASS; SCH.
NU250	Tab, Yellow, Round, Film Coated	Methyldopa 250 mg	by Nu Pharm	Canadian DIN 00717509	Antihypertensive
NU250	Tab, Yellow, Oval, NU-250	Naproxen 250 mg	Nu Naprox by Nu Pharm	Canadian DIN 08865648	NSAID
NU250	Tab, Bright Pink, Round, Film Coated, NU over 250	Erythromycin 250 mg	by Nu Pharm	Canadian DIN 02051850	Antibiotic
NU250	Cap, Gold & Red, Opaque, Gelatin	Amoxicillin 250 mg	Amoxil by Nu Pharm	Canadian DIN 00865567	Antibiotic
NU250	Cap, Black & Red, Opaque, Gelatin	Ampicillin 250 mg	Principen by Nu Pharm	Canadian DIN 00717657	Antibiotic
NU250	Tab, Orange, Oblong, NU-250	Diflunisal 250 mg	by Nu Pharm	Canadian	NSAID
NU250	Cap, Black & Orange, Gelatin	Cloxacillin Sodium 250 mg	Nu Cloxi by Nu Pharm	Canadian DIN 00717584	Antibiotic
NU250	Tab, Orange, Cap Shaped, Film Coated, NU-250	Cephalexin 250 mg	Nu Cephalex by Nu Pharm	Canadian DIN 00865877	Antibiotic
NU250	Cap, Purple & White, Opaque, Gelatin	Cefaclor 250 mg	Ceclor by Nu Pharm	Canadian DIN 02231432	Antibiotic
NU30	Tab, Light Green, Round, Film Coated, NU over 30	Diltiazem HCl 30 mg	Cardizem by Nu Pharm	Canadian DIN 00886068	Antihypertensive
NU30	Cap, Light Blue & Maroon, Opaque, Gelatin	Temazepam 30 mg	Restoril by Nu Pharm	Canadian DIN 02223589	Sedative/Hypnotic; C IV
NU300	Tab, White, Round, Film Coated, Scored, NU over 300	Tiaprofenic Acid 300 mg	by Nu Pharm	Canadian DIN 02146886	NSAID
NU300	Tab, Orange, Round, Film Coated, NU over 300	Penicillin V Potassium 300 mg	by Nu Pharm	Canadian DIN 00717568	Antibiotic
NU300	Tab, Pale Green, Round, Film Coated, NU over 300	Cimetidine HCl 300 mg	Tagamet by Nu Pharm	Canadian DIN 00865818	Gastrointestinal
NU300	Cap, Maroon & White, Opaque, Gelatin	Gemfibrozil 300 mg	by Nu Pharm	Canadian DIN 02058456	Antihyperlipidemic
NU300	Tab, White, Round, Film Coated, NU over 300	Ibuprofen 300 mg	Motrin by Nu Pharm	Canadian DIN 02020696	NSAID
NU300	Tab, White, Cap Shaped, Film Coated	Ranitidine 300 mg	Nu Ranit by Nu Pharm	Canadian DIN 00865745	Gastrointestinal
NU375	Tab, Peach, Cap Shaped, Scored	Naproxen 375 mg	Nu Naprox by Nu Pharm	Canadian DIN 00865656	NSAID
NU40	Tab, Light Blue, Round, Scored, NU over 40	Megestrol Acetate 40 mg	by Nu Pharm	Canadian DIN 02185415	Hormone
NU40	Tab, Light Brown, D-Shaped, Film Coated, NU over 40	Famotidine 40 mg	by Nu Pharm	Canadian DIN 02024209	Gastrointestinal
NU40	Tab, Green, Round, NU/40	Propranolol HCl 40 mg	Inderal by Nu Pharm	Canadian	Antihypertensive
NU400	Tab, Orange, Round, Film Coated, NU over 400	Ibuprofen 400 mg	Motrin by Nu Pharm	Canadian DIN 02020718	NSAID
NU400	Tab, Pale Green, Oblong, Film Coated, NU-400	Cimetidine HCl 400 mg	Tagamet by Nu Pharm	Canadian DIN 00865826	Gastrointestinal
NU400	Tab, Pink, Round, NU over 400	Acyclovir 400 mg	Zovirax by Nu Pharm	Canadian DIN 02197413	Antiviral
NU400	Tab, White, Cap Shaped, Film Coated, Scored	Acebutolol HCl 200 mg	Sectral by Nu Pharm	Canadian DIN 02165562	Antihypertensive
NU40080	Tab, White, Round, Scored, NU over 400-80	Sulfamethoxazole 400 mg, Trimethoprim 80 mg	Nu Cotrimix by Nu Pharm	Canadian DIN 00865753	Antibiotic

ID FRONT <> BACK	DESCRIPTION FRONT <> BACK	INGREDIENT & STRENGTH	BRAND (or Generic Equiv.) by FIRM	NDC#	CLASS; SCH.
NU5	Tab, White, Round, Scored, NU over 5	Pindolol 5 mg	Nu-Pindol by Nu Pharm	Canadian DIN 00886149	Antihypertensive
NU5	Tab, White, Diamond Shaped, Scored, NU over 5	Prazosin HCl 5 mg	Nu Prazo by Nu Pharm	Canadian DIN 01913816	Antihypertensive
NU5	Tab, Peachish Orange, Round, Film Coated, NU over 5	Prochlorperazine Maleate 5 mg	Nu Prochlor by Nu Pharm	Canadian DIN 01964399	Antiemetic
NU5	Tab, Blue, Round, Scored, NU over 5	Oxybutynin Chloride 5 mg	by Nu Pharm	Canadian DIN 02158590	Urinary Tract
NU5	Tab, White, Cap Shaped, Scored	Glyburide 5 mg	by Nu Pharm	Canadian DIN 02020742	Antidiabetic
NU50	Tab, White, Oval, Film Coated, NU over 50	Flurbiprofen 50 mg	by Nu Pharm	Canadian DIN 02020661	NSAID
NU50	Cap, Blue & White, Opaque, Gelatin	Indomethacin 50 mg	Indocin by Nu Pharm	Canadian DIN 00865869	NSAID
NU50	Cap, Green & Ivory, NU-50	Ketoprofen 50 mg	Orudis by Nu Pharm	Canadian	NSAID
NU50	Tab, White, Round, Scored, NU over 50	Atenolol 50 mg	Tenormin by Nu Pharm	Canadian DIN 00886114	Antihypertensive
NU50	Tab, White, Oval, Scored, NU-50	Captopril 50 mg	Capoten by Nu Pharm	Canadian DIN 01913840	Antihypertensive
NU50	Tab, Pink, Round, NU/50	Trimipramine Maleate 50 mg	by Nu Pharm	Canadian	Antidepressant
NU500	Tab, Orange, Cap Shaped, Film Coated, Scored, NU-500	Cephalexin 500 mg	Nu Cephalex by Nu Pharm	Canadian DIN 00865885	Antibiotic
NU500	Cap, Gray & Purple, Opaque, Gelatin	Cefaclor 500 mg	by Nu Pharm	Canadian DIN 02231433	Antibiotic
NU 500	Tab, Orange, Oblong	Diflunisal 500 mg	by Nu Pharm	Canadian	NSAID
NU500	Cap, Black & Orange, Gelatin	Cloxacillin Sodium 500 mg	Nu Cloxi by Nu Pharm	Canadian DIN 00717592	Antibiotic
NU500	Cap, Black & Red, Opaque, Gelatin	Ampicillin 500 mg	Principen by Nu Pharm	Canadian DIN 00717673	Antibiotic
NU500	Cap, Gold & Red, Opaque, Gelatin	Amoxicillin 500 mg	Amoxil by Nu Pharm	Canadian DIN 00865575	Antibiotic
NU500	Tab, Yellow, Round, Film Coated	Methyldopa 500 mg	by Nu Pharm	Canadian DIN 00717576	Antihypertensive
NU500	Tab, Yellow, Cap Shaped, Scored	Naproxen 500 mg	Nu Naprox by Nu Pharm	Canadian DIN 00865664	NSAID
NU550	Tab, Peach, Diamond Shaped, Scored, NU above Score, 5/50 below Score	Amiloride HCl 5 mg, Hydrochlorothiazide 50 mg	Moduretic by Nu Pharm	Canadian DIN 00886106	Antihypertensive; Diuretic
NU60	Tab, Yellow, Round, Film Coated, Scored, NU over 60	Diltiazem HCl 60 mg	Cardizem by Nu Pharm	Canadian DIN 00886076	Antihypertensive
NU600	Tab, Pale Green, Oblong, Film Coated, NU-600	Cimetidine HCl 600 mg	Tagamet by Nu Pharm	Canadian DIN 00865834	Gastrointestinal
NU600	Tab, White, Oval, Film Coated, NU-600	Gemfibrozil 600 mg	by Nu Pharm	Canadian DIN 02058464	Antihyperlipidemic
NU600	Tab, Light Orange, Oval, Film Coated, NU-600	Ibuprofen 600 mg	Motrin by Nu Pharm	Canadian DIN 02020726	NSAID
NU75	Tab, Light Pink, Triangular, Film Coated, NU over 75	Diclofenac Sodium 75 mg	by Nu Pharm	Canadian DIN 02228203	NSAID
NU75	Tab, Blue, Oval, Film Coated, Scored, NU 7.5	Zopiclone 7.5 mg	Nu-Zopiclone by Nu Pharm	Canadian DIN 02228270	Hypnotic
NU80	Tab, Blue, Cap Shaped, NU-80	Sotalol 80 mg	by Nu Pharm	Canadian DIN 02200996	Antiarrhythmic

ID FRONT <> BACK	DESCRIPTION FRONT <> BACK	INGREDIENT & STRENGTH	BRAND (or Generic Equiv.) by FIRM	NDC#	CLASS; SCH.
NU80	Tab, Yellow, Round, Film Coated, NU over 80	Verapamil HCl 80 mg	by Nu Pharm	Canadian DIN 00886033	Antihypertensive
NU80	Tab, Yellow, Round, NU/80	Propranolol HCl 80 mg	Inderal by Nu Pharm	Canadian	Antihypertensive
NU800	Tab, Blue, Oval, Scored	Acyclovir 800 mg	Zovirax by Nu Pharm	Canadian DIN 02197421	Antiviral
NUB15	Tab, White, Round, Scored, NU over B-1.5	Bromazepam 1.5 mg	Lectopam by Nu Pharm	Canadian DIN 02171856	Sedative; C IV
NUB3	Tab, Pink, Round, Scored, NU over B-3	Bromazepam 3 mg	Lectopam by Nu Pharm	Canadian DIN 02171864	Sedative; C IV
NUB6	Tab, Green, Round, Scored, NU over B-6	Bromazepam 6 mg	Lectopam by Nu Pharm	Canadian DIN 02171872	Sedative; C IV
NUC05	Tab, Orange, Round, Scored, NU over C-0.5	Clonazepam 0.5 mg	by Nu Pharm	Canadian DIN 02173344	Sedative; C IV
NUC2	Tab, White, Round, Scored, NU over C-2	Clonazepam 2 mg	by Nu Pharm	Canadian DIN 02173352	Sedative; C IV
NUDS	Tab, White, Cap Shaped, Scored, NU-DS	Sulfamethoxazole 800 mg, Trimethoprim 160 mg	Nu Cotrimix by Nu Pharm	Canadian DIN 00865729	Antibiotic
NUE10	Tab, White, Barrel Shaped, Scored, NU over E10	Enalapril Maleate 10 mg	Vasotec by Nu Pharm	Canadian DIN 02239500	Antihypertensive
NUE25	Tab, Dark Pink, Barrel Shaped, Scored, NU over E25	Enalapril Maleate 20 mg	Vasotec by Nu Pharm	Canadian DIN 02239501	Antihypertensive
NUE5	Tab, White, Barrel Shaped, Scored, NU over E5	Enalapril Maleate 5 mg	Vasotec by Nu Pharm	Canadian DIN 02239599	Antihypertensive
NUIRON1500291	Tab, Red & White, Oblong	Elemental Iron 150 mg	Nu Iron 150 by Merz		Mineral
NUM10	Tab, White, Round, NU over M10	Metoclopramide HCl 10 mg	Reglan by Nu Pharm	Canadian DIN 02143283	Gastrointestinal
NUM5	Tab, White, Square, NU over M5	Metoclopramide HCl 5 mg	Reglan by Nu Pharm	Canadian DIN 02143275	Gastrointestinal
NUM500	Tab, White, Round, Scored, NU over M500	Metformin HCl 500 mg	by Nu Pharm	Canadian DIN 02162822	Antidiabetic
NUMARK <> 1039	Tab, Soluble, Numark <> 10/39	Chlorpheniramine Maleate 4 mg, Phenylephrine HCl 10 mg, Phenylpropanolamine HCl 50 mg, Pyrilamine Maleate 25 mg	by Mikart	46672-0021	Cold Remedy
NUMARK <> 1039	Tab, Soluble	Chlorpheniramine Maleate 4 mg, Phenylephrine 10 mg, Phenylpropanolamine 50 mg, Pyrilamine Maleate 25 mg	Histalet Forte by Numark	55499-1039	Cold Remedy
NUMARK <> 1091	Tab, Orange, Oblong, Scored	Hydrocodone Bitartrate 5 mg, Pseudoephedrine HCl 60 mg	P V Tussin by Numark	55499-1091	Analgesic; C III
NUMARK <> 1091	Tab, Orange, Oblong, Scored	Hydrocodone Bitartrate 5 mg, Pseudoephedrine HCl 60 mg	by Mikart	46672-0133	Analgesic; C III
NUMARK1050	Tab	Guaifenesin 400 mg, Pseudoephedrine HCl 120 mg	Sudafed Sinus by Mikart	46672-0162	Cold Remedy
NUMARK1050	Tab	Guaifenesin 400 mg, Pseudoephedrine HCl 120 mg	Sudafed Sinus by Numark	55499-1050	Cold Remedy
NUMARK1082	Cap, Coated	Phendimetrazine Tartrate 105 mg	Melfiat-105 by Numark	55499-1082	Anorexiant; C III
NUT	Tab, Light Orange, Round, Scored, NU over T	Triamterene 50 mg, Hydrochlorothiazide 25 mg	by Nu Pharm	Canadian DIN 00865532	Diuretic; Antihypertensive
NUT100	Tab, White to Off-White, Round, Scored, NU over T100	Trazodone HCl 100 mg	Desyrel by Nu Pharm	Canadian DIN 02165392	Antidepressant
NUT5	Tab, White, Round, Scored, NU over T5	Timolol Maleate 5 mg	Nu Timolol by Nu Pharm	Canadian DIN 02044609	Antihypertensive
NUT50	Tab, Pale Orange, Round, Scored, NU over T50	Trazodone HCl 50 mg	Desyrel by Nu Pharm	Canadian DIN 02165384	Antidepressant
NVN	Cap, Orange, Oval Shaped	Valproic Acid 125 mg	Stavzor by Banner Pharma	68968-3125	Manic Episode Treatment
NVN1	Cap, Orange, Oval Shaped	Valproic Acid 250 mg	Stavzor by Banner Pharma	68968-3250	Manic Episode Treatment
NVN2	Cap, Orange, Oval Shaped	Valproic Acid 500 mg	Stavzor by Banner Pharma	68968-3500	Manic Episode Treatment
NVR <> 5	Tab, White to Light Yellow, Oblong	Everolimus 5 mg	Afinitor by Novartis	00078-0566	Cancer Therapy

ID FRONT <> BACK	DESCRIPTION FRONT <> BACK	INGREDIENT & STRENGTH	BRAND (or Generic Equiv.) by FIRM	NDC#	CLASS; SCH.
NVR <> C	Tab, White to Yellowish, Round, Marbled	Everolimus 0.25 mg	Zortress by Novartis Consumer Health, Inc.	00078-0417	Immunosuppressant
NVR <> CH	Tab, White to Yellowish, Round, Marbled	Everolimus 0.5 mg	Zortress by Novartis Consumer Health, Inc.	00078-0414	Immunosuppressant
NVR <> CL	Tab, White to Yellowish, Round, Marbled	Everolimus 0.75 mg	Zortress by Novartis Consumer Health, Inc.	00078-0415	Immunosuppressant
NVR <> CLL	Tab, Pale Yellow, Oval, Film Coated	Aliskiren 150 mg, HCTZ 25 mg	Tekturna HCT by Novartis	00078-0522	Antihypertensive; Diuretic
NVR <> CSF	Tab, Dark Yellow, Oval, Film Coated	Amlodipine 5 mg, Valsartan 320 mg	Exforge by Novartis	00078-0490	Antihypertensive
NVR <> CTI	Tab, Yellow, Oval	Hydrochlorothiazide 25 mg, Valsartan 320 mg	Diovan HCT by Novartis	00078-0472	Antihypertensive; Diuretic
NVR <> CVI	Tab, Violet and White, Oval, Film Coated	Aliskiren 300 mg, HCTZ 12.5 mg	Tekturna HCT by Novartis	00078-0523	Antihypertensive; Diuretic
NVR <> CVV	Tab, Light Yellow, Oval, Film Coated	Aliskiren 300 mg, HCTZ 25 mg	Tekturna HCT by Novartis	00078-0524	Antihypertensive; Diuretic
NVR <> DL	Tab, White, Round	Tegaserod Maleate 2 mg	Zelnorm by Novartis	00078-0355	Gastrointestinal
NVR <> DO	Tab, Yellow, Oval	Valsartan 40 mg	Diovan by Novartis	Canadian DIN 02270528	Antihypertensive
NVR <> DO	Tab, Yellow, Oval	Valsartan 40 mg	Diovan by Novartis	00078-0423	Antihypertensive
NVR <> DV	Tab, Pale Red, Round	Valsartan 80 mg	Diovan by Novartis	Canadian DIN 02244781	Antihypertensive
NVR <> DV	Tab, Pale Red, Almond Shaped	Valsartan 80 mg	Diovan by Novartis	00078-0358	Antihypertensive
NVR <> DX	Tab, Greyish Orange, Almond Shaped	Valsartan 160 mg	Diovan by Novartis	00078-0359	Antihypertensive
NVR <> DX	Tab, Greyish Orange, Oblong	Valsartan 160 mg	Diovan by Novartis	Canadian DIN 02244782	Antihypertensive
NVR <> DXL	Tab, Dark Greyish Violet, Almond Shaped	Valsartan 320 mg	Diovan by Novartis	00078-0360	Antihypertensive
NVR <> ECE	Tab, Light Yellow, Oval, Film Coated	Amlodipine 5 mg, Valsartan 160 mg	Exforge by Novartis	00078-0488	Antihypertensive
NVR <> EH	Tab, White, Round	Tegaserod Maleate 6 mg	Zelnorm by Novartis	Canadian DIN 02245566	Gastrointestinal
NVR <> EH	Tab, White, Round	Tegaserod Maleate 6 mg	Zelnorm by Novartis	00078-0426	Gastrointestinal
NVR <> EH	Tab, White, Round	Tegaserod Maleate 6 mg	Zelnorm by Novartis	00078-0356	Gastrointestinal
NVR <> HDU	Tab, Light Red, Oval, Film-Coated	Aliskiren 150 mg, Valsartan 160 mg	Valturna by Novartis Consumer Health, Inc.	00078-0572	Antihypertensive
NVR <> HIL	Tab, Pink, Oval	Hydrochlorothiazide 12.5 mg, Valsartan 320 mg	Diovan HCT by Novartis	00078-0471	Diuretic; Antihypertensive
NVR <> HXH	Tab, Brownish Orange, Oval	Hydrochlorothiazide 25 mg, Valsartan 160 mg	Diovan HCT by Novartis	Canadian DIN 02246955	Antihypertensive
NVR <> HXH	Tab, Brownish Orange, Oval	Hydrochlorothiazide 25 mg, Valsartan 160 mg	Diovan HCT by Novartis	00078-0383	Diuretic; Antihypertensive
NVR <> IL	Tab, Light Pink, Round	Aliskiren 150 mg	Tekturna by Novartis	00078-0485	Antihypertensive
NVR <> IL	Tab, Light Pink, Round	Aliskiren 150 mg	Rasilez by Novartis	Canadian DIN 02302063	Antihypertensive
NVR <> IU	Tab, Light Red, Oval	Aliskiren 300 mg	Rasilez by Novartis	Canadian DIN 02302071	Antihypertensive
NVR <> IU	Tab, Light Red, Oval	Aliskiren 300 mg	Tekturna by Novartis	00078-0486	Antihypertensive
NVR <> J125	Tab, Off-White, Round, Tablet for Oral Suspension	Deferasirox 125 mg	Exjade by Novartis	Canadian DIN 02287420	Chelating Agent
NVR <> J125	Tab, Off-White, Round, Tablet for Oral Suspension	Deferasirox 125 mg	Exjade by Novartis	00078-0468	Chelating Agent
NVR <> J250	Tab, Off-White, Round, Tablet for Oral Suspension	Deferasirox 250 mg	Exjade by Novartis	00078-0469	Chelating Agent
NVR <> J250	Tab, Off-White, Round, Tablet for Oral Suspension	Deferasirox 250 mg	Exjade by Novartis	Canadian DIN 02287439	Chelating Agent
NVR <> J500	Tab, Off-White, Round, Tablet for Oral Suspension	Deferasirox 500 mg	Exjade by Novartis	Canadian DIN 02287447	Chelating Agent
NVR <> J500	Tab, Off-White, Round, Tablet for Oral Suspension	Deferasirox 500 mg	Exjade by Novartis	00078-0470	Chelating Agent
NVR <> LCI	Tab, White, Oval, Film Coated	Aliskiren 150 mg, HCTZ 12.5 mg	Tekturna HCT by Novartis	00078-0521	Antihypertensive; Diuretic
NVR <> LUF	Tab, Dark Yellow, Oval, Film Coated	Amlodipine 10 mg, Valsartan 320 mg	Exforge by Novartis	00078-0491	Antihypertensive
NVR <> OB	Tab, Red, Oval, Film Coated	Lumiracoxib 100 mg	Prexige by Novartis	Canadian DIN 02288036 Discontinued	NSAID
NVR <> SA	Tab, Dark Yellow to Brownish-Orange, Round, Film Coated, Scored	Imatinib 100 mg	Gleevec by Novartis	Canadian DIN 02253275	Antineoplastic

ID FRONT <> BACK	DESCRIPTION FRONT <> BACK	INGREDIENT & STRENGTH	BRAND (or Generic Equiv.) by FIRM	NDC#	CLASS; SCH.
NVR <> SA	Tab, Dark Yellow to Brownish-Orange, Round, Film Coated, Scored	Imatinib 100 mg	Gleevec by Novartis	00078-0401	Antineoplastic
NVR <> SL	Tab, Dark Yellow to Brownish-Orange, Oval, Film Coated	Imatinib 400 mg	Gleevec by Novartis	00078-0402	Antineoplastic
NVR <> SNB	Tab, Light Brown, Oval, Film-Coated	Aliskiren 300 mg, Valsartan 320 mg	Valturna by Novartis Consumer Health, Inc.	00078-0574	Antihypertensive
NVR <> UHE	Tab, White to Light Yellow, Oblong	Everolimus 10 mg	Afinitor by Novartis	00078-0567	Cancer Therapy
NVR <> UIC	Tab, Light Yellow, Oval, Film Coated	Amlodipine 10 mg, Valsartan 160 mg	Exforge by Novartis	00078-0489	Antihypertensive
NVRD10	Cap, Light Caramel, Extended Release	Dexmethylphenidate HCl 10 mg	Focalin XR by Novartis	00078-0431	Stimulant; C II
NVRD15	Cap, Green, Extended Release	Dexmethylphenidate HCl 15 mg	Focalin XR by Novartis	00078-0493	Stimulant; C II
NVRD20	Cap, White, Extended Release	Dexmethylphenidate HCl 20 mg	Focalin XR by Novartis	00078-0432	Stimulant; C II
NVRD5	Cap, Light Blue, Extended Release	Dexmethylphenidate HCl 5 mg	Focalin XR by Novartis	00078-0430	Stimulant; C II
NVRR10	Cap, White and Light Brown	Methylphenidate HCl 10 mg	Ritalin LA by Novartis	00078-0424	Stimulant; C II
NVRR20.	Cap, White	Methylphenidate HCl 20 mg	Ritalin LA by Novartis	00078-0370	Stimulant; C II
NVRR30	Cap, Yellow	Methylphenidate HCl 30 mg	Ritalin LA by Novartis	00078-0371	Stimulant; C II
NVRR40	Cap, Light Brown	Methylphenidate HCl 40 mg	Ritalin LA by Novartis	00078-0372	Stimulant; C II
NVRSI	Cap, Orange to Grayish Orange, Red Print	Imatinib 100 mg	Gleevec by Novartis	00078-0373	Antineoplastic
NVRTKI	Cap, Light Yellow, Opaque, Red Imprint	Nilotinib 200 mg	Tasigna by Novartis	00078-0526	Cancer Treatment
NVRTKI	Cap, Light Yellow, Opaque, Hard Gelatin, Filled with Yellowish Powder	Nilotinib 200 mg	Tasigna by Novartis	Canadian DIN 02315874	Leukemia Cancer Treatment
NYQ	Cap, Green, Oval, Liquid Filled, NyQ	Acetaminophen 500 mg, Dextromethorphan HBr 15 mg, Doxylamine succinate 6.25 mg, Pseudoephedrine HCl 30 mg	NyQuil by P & G Health	23900-0008	Cold Remedy
NYQUIL	Cap, Green, Oval, Liquid Filled, NyQuil	Acetaminophen 500 mg, Dextromethorphan HBr 15 mg, Doxylamine succinate 6.25 mg, Pseudoephedrine HCl 30 mg	NyQuil by P & G Health	37000-0539	Cold Remedy
NYTOL	Cap, Blue	Diphenhydramine HCl 50 mg	by Block Drug	Canadian	Antihistamine
NZ150G	Cap, Yellow, Hard Gel	Nizatidine 150 mg	Axid by Par	49884-0766	Gastrointestinal
NZ300G	Cap, Light Brown, Hard Gel	Nizatidine 300 mg	Axid by Par	49884-0767	Gastrointestinal
O1C	Tab, White, Round, O1C <> Boehringer Ingelheim tower	Clonidine HCl 0.1 mg	Catapres by Boehringer Ingelheim Canada	Canadian DIN 00259527	Antihypertensive
O2C	Tab, Orange, Round, O2C <> Boehringer Ingelheim tower	Clonidine HCl 0.2 mg	Catapres by Boehringer Ingelheim Canada	Canadian DIN 00291889	Antihypertensive
O2C <> SEPTRADS	Tab	Sulfamethoxazole 800 mg, Trimethoprim 160 mg	Septra DS by Leiner	59606-0733	Antibiotic
O4	Tab, White, Round, Orally Disintegrating	Ondansetron 4 mg	Zofran ODT by Sandoz	00781-5265	Antiemetic
O8	Tab, White, Round, Orally Disintegrating	Ondansetron 8 mg	Zofran ODT by Sandoz	00781-5266	Antiemetic
OB <> NVR	Tab, Red, Oval, Film Coated	Lumiracoxib 100 mg	Prexige by Novartis	Canadian DIN 02288036 Discontinued	NSAID
OC <> 10	Tab, White, Round, Film Coated	Oxycodone HCl 10 mg	OxyContin by Purdue	59011-0100	Analgesic; C II
OC <> 15	Tab, Grey, Round, CR	Oxycodone HCl 15 mg	OxyContin by Purdue	59011-0815	Analgesic; C II
OC <> 160	Tab, Blue, Cap Shaped, Film Coated	Oxycodone HCl 160 mg	OxyContin by Purdue	59011-0109	Analgesic; C II
OC <> 20	Tab, Pink, Round, Film Coated	Oxycodone HCl 20 mg	OxyContin by Purdue	59011-0103	Analgesic; C II
OC <> 30	Tab, Round, Brown, CR	Oxycodone HCl 30 mg	OxyContin by Purdue	59011-0830	Analgesic; C II
OC <> 40	Tab, Yellow, Round, Film Coated	Oxycodone HCl 40 mg	OxyContin by Purdue	59011-0105	Analgesic; C II
OC <> 60	Tab, Red, Round, CR	Oxycodone HCl 60 mg	OxyContin by Purdue	59011-0860	Analgesic; C II
OC <> 80	Tab, Green, Round, Film Coated	Oxycodone HCl 80 mg	OxyContin by Purdue	59011-0107	Analgesic; C II
OCL55CINOBAC250MG	Cap, Green & Orange	Cinoxacin 250 mg	Cinobac by Eli Lilly	00002-3055	Antibiotic
OCL55CINOBAC250MG	Cap, Green & Orange	Cinoxacin 250 mg	Cinobac by Eli Lilly	00002-0055	Antibiotic
OCL55CINOBAC250MG	Cap, Green & Orange	Cinoxacin 250 mg	Cinobac by Oclassen	55515-0055	Antibiotic
OCL56CINOBAC500MG	Cap, Green & Orange	Cinoxacin 500 mg	Cinobac by Eli Lilly	00002-0056	Antibiotic
OCL56CINOBAC500MG	Cap, Green & Orange	Cinoxacin 500 mg	Cinobac by Compumed	00403-2041	Antibiotic
OCL56CINOBAC500MG	Cap, Green & Orange	Cinoxacin 500 mg	Cinobac by Oclassen	55515-0056	Antibiotic
OCTK0	Tab, White, Round, Scored, Coated	Acetaminophen 325 mg	Tylenol by Sandoz		Analgesic

ID FRONT <> BACK	DESCRIPTION FRONT <> BACK	INGREDIENT & STRENGTH	BRAND (or Generic Equiv.) by FIRM	NDC#	CLASS; SCH.
OCTK10	Tab, White, Round, Coated	Acetaminophen 500 mg	Tylenol Ex Strength by Sandoz		Analgesic
OCTK48	Tab, White, Film Coated	Aspirin 325 mg	Aspirin by Sandoz		Analgesic
OCUVITE	Tab, Peach, Film Coated, Scored	Vitamin C, Lutein, L-glutathione, Zinc Oxide, Magnesium, Beta Carotene, Copper	Ocuvite by Bausch and Lomb	24208-3876	Vitamin; Supplement
OCUVITELUTEIN	Cap, Yellow, Ocuvite on Cap and Lutein on Body, Black Ink	Vitamin C 60 mg, Vitamin E 30 IU, Lutein 6 mg, Zinc 15 mg, Copper 2 mg	Ocuvite Lutein by Bausch and Lomb	24208-4031	Vitamin; Supplement
ODYSSEY <> 750	Tab, Off-White, Oval	Nystatin Vaginal 10,000 Units	Mycostatin by Odyssey	65473-0705	Antifungal
OGT918100	Cap, White, Hard Gel, Black Ink, OGT918 on cap 100 on body	Miglustat 100 mg	Zavesca by Actelion	Canadian DIN 02250519	Substrate Reduction Therapy
OHM <> 078	Tab, Orange, Round	Acetaminophen 325 mg, Phenyltoloxamine Citrate 30 mg	Percogesic by Ivax	00182-1413 Discontinued	Analgesic
OHM010	Tab, White, Round, Scored, OHM over 010	Acetaminophen 325 mg	Tylenol by OHM		Analgesic
OHM011	Tab, White, Round	Acetaminophen 500 mg	Tylenol Ex Strength by OHM		Analgesic
OHM021	Tab, White, Round	Aspirin 325 mg	Aspirin by OHM		Analgesic
OHM045	Tab, White & Yellow, Round	Acetaminophen, Chlorpheniramine, Phenylephrine	Dristan Adv. Formula by OHM		Cold Remedy
OHM055	Tab, White, Round	Acetaminophen 250 mg, Aspirin 250 mg, Caffeine 65 mg	Excedrin Migraine by Reese	10956-0739	Analgesic
OHM076	Tab, White, Round, OHM/076	Pseudoephedrine 60 mg	Sudafed by OHM		Decongestant
OHM078	Tab, Peach, Round	Acetaminophen 325 mg, Phenyltoloxamine 30 mg	Percogesic by OHM		Analgesic
OHM117	Tab, Brown & Green, Round, OHM/117	Senna Concentrate 217 mg	Senokot by OHM		Gastrointestinal
OHM135	Tab, Yellow, Round	Genacol 325 mg	Comtrex by OHM		Cold Remedy
OHM311	Tab, White, Oblong	Acetaminophen 500 mg	Tylenol Ex Strength by OHM		Analgesic
OIRPF5MG	Cap, Beige & Orange	Oxycodone HCl 5 mg	OxyIR by Purdue	59011-0201	Analgesic; C II
OIRPF5MG	Cap, Beige & Orange	Oxycodone HCl 5 mg	OxyIR by PF	48692-0006	Analgesic; C II
OJF547	Cap, Brown & White	Acetaminophen 325 mg, Butalbital 50 mg, Codeine 30 mg	Bancap w/ Codeine by Forest	00456-0547	Analgesic; C III
OL459743	Cap, OL4/59743	Acetaminophen 325 mg, Butalbital 50 mg, Caffeine 40 mg	Fioricet by Qualitest	00603-2546	Analgesic
OM <> 100	Tab, Orange, Round	Tapentadol Hydrochloride 100 mg	Tapentadol Hydrochloride by Janssen-Ortho	50458-0840	Analgesic; C II
OM <> 180	Tab, White, Round, O-M 180	Ethinyl Estradiol 0.025 mg, Norgestimate 0.180 mg	Ortho Tri-Cyclen Lo by Ortho-McNeil	00062-1251	Oral Contraceptive
OM <> 215	Tab, Light Blue, Round, O-M 215	Ethinyl Estradiol 0.025 mg, Norgestimate 0.215 mg	Ortho Tri-Cyclen Lo by Ortho-McNeil	00062-1251	Oral Contraceptive
OM <> 250	Tab, Dark Blue, Round, O-M 250	Ethinyl Estradiol 0.025 mg, Norgestimate 0.250 mg	Ortho Tri-Cyclen Lo by Ortho-McNeil	00062-1251	Oral Contraceptive
OM <> 50	Tab, Yellow, Round	Tapentadol Hydrochloride 50 mg	Tapentadol Hydrochloride by Janssen-Ortho	50458-0820	Analgesic; C II
OM <> 650	Tab, Yellow, Cap Shaped	Acetaminophen 325 mg, Tramadol HCl 37.5 mg	Ultracet by Ortho-McNeil	00045-0650	Analgesic
OM <> 650	Tab, Light Yellow, Capsule-Shaped, Coated, O-M	Tramadol HCl 37.5 mg, Acetaminophen 325 mg	Tramacet by Ivax	00172-6359	Analgesic
OM <> 75	Tab, Yellow-Orange, Round	Tapentadol Hydrochloride 75 mg	Tapentadol Hydrochloride by Janssen-Ortho	50458-0830	Analgesic; C II
OM <> P	Tab, Dark Green, Round, O-M P	Inert	Ortho Tri-Cyclen Lo by Ortho-McNeil	00062-1251	Oral Contraceptive; Placebo
OME10	Cap, Beige, OME10 on cap and OME10 on body	Omeprazole 10 mg	Prilosec by LEK		Gastrointestinal
OME20	Cap, White, OME20 on cap and OME20 on body	Omeprazole 20 mg	Prilosec by LEK	66685-0422	Gastrointestinal
OMNICEF300MGA	Cap, Lavender & Turquoise, Omnicef 300 mg Abbott Logo (a)	Cefdinir 300 mg	Omnicef by Parke Davis	00071-0067	Antibiotic
OMNICEF300MGA	Cap, Lavender & Turquoise, Omnicef 300 mg Abbott Logo (a)	Cefdinir 300 mg	Omnicef by Abbott	00074-3769	Antibiotic
OMNICEFPD	Cap, Lavender & Turquoise, Omnicef/PD	Cefdinir 300 mg	Omnicef by Eli Lilly		Antibiotic
OND4 <> APO	Tab, Yellow, Oval, Film Coated	Ondansetron HCl 4 mg	Zofran by Apotex	Canadian DIN 02288184	Antiemetic
OND8 <> APO	Tab, Yellow, Oval, Film Coated	Ondansetron HCl 8 mg	Zofran by Apotex	Canadian DIN 02288192	Antiemetic
OP697	Tab, White, Round	Bethanechol Chloride 5 mg	Urecholine by Odyssey	65473-0697	Urinary Tract
OP700	Tab, Yellow, Round	Bethanechol Chloride 50 mg	Urecholine by Odyssey	65473-0700	Urinary Tract
OP701	Tab, Orange, Oval, Film Coated	Protriptyline HCl 5 mg	Vivactil by Odyssey	65473-0701	Antidepressant
OP702	Tab, Yellow, Oval, Film Coated	Protriptyline HCl 10 mg	Vivactil by Odyssey	65473-0702	Antidepressant

ID FRONT <> BACK	DESCRIPTION FRONT <> BACK	INGREDIENT & STRENGTH	BRAND (or Generic Equiv.) by FIRM	NDC#	CLASS; SCH.
OP703	Tab, White, Round	Bethanechol Chloride 10 mg	Urecholine by Odyssey	65473-0703	Urinary Tract
OP704	Tab, Yellow, Round	Bethanechol Chloride 25 mg	Urecholine by Odyssey	65473-0704	Urinary Tract
OP706	Tab, White, Round	Disulfiram 250 mg	Antabuse by Odyssey	65473-0703	Antialcoholism
OP718	Cap, Blue and Yellow, Opaque	Trimipramine Maleate 25 mg	Surmontil by Odyssey	65473-0718	Antidepressant
OP719	Cap, Blue and Orange, Opaque	Trimipramine Maleate 50 mg	Surmontil by Odyssey	65473-0719	Antidepressant
OP720	Cap, Blue and White, Opaque	Trimipramine Maleate 100 mg	Surmontil by Odyssey	65473-0720	Antidepressant
OPPOSINGCS	Tab, White, Round, Opposing C's	Medroxyprogesterone Acetate 2.5 mg	Cycrin by ESI Lederle		Hormone
OPPOSINGCS <> CYCRIN	Tab, Opposing C's <> Cycrin	Medroxyprogesterone Acetate 10 mg	by Kaiser	62224-4331	Hormone
OR606	Tab, Peach, Round	Ranitidine 75 mg	Zantac by Ranbaxy		Gastrointestinal
OR607	Tab, Light Pink, Round, OR <> 607	Ranitidine HCl 75 mg	by Schein		Gastrointestinal
ORAP1	Tab, White, Oval, Scored	Pimozide 1 mg	Orap by Teva	00093-0151 Discontinued	Antipsychotic
ORAP1	Tab, White, Oval, Scored	Pimozide 1 mg	Orap by Gate	57844-0151	Antipsychotic
ORAP2 <> LEMMON	Tab, White, Oval, Scored, Orap/2 <> Lemmon	Pimozide 2 mg	Orap by Teva	00093-0187 Discontinued	Antipsychotic
ORAP2 <> LEMMON	Tab, White, Oval, Scored, Orap/2 <> Lemmon	Pimozide 2 mg	Orap by Gate	57844-0187	Antipsychotic
ORETIC <> A	Tab, White, Round, Scored, Abbott Logo (a)	Hydrochlorothiazide 25 mg	Hydrodiuril by Abbott	00074-6978 Discontinued	Diuretic; Antihypertensive
ORETIC <> A	Tab, White, Round, Scored, Abbott Logo (a)	Hydrochlorothiazide 50 mg	Oretic by Abbott	00074-6985 Discontinued	Diuretic; Antihypertensive
ORETIC <> A	Tab, White, Round, Scored, Abbott Logo (a)	Hydrochlorothiazide 50 mg	Oretic by Kaiser	00179-0352	Diuretic; Antihypertensive
ORETIC <> A	Tab, White, Round, Scored, Abbott Logo (a)	Hydrochlorothiazide 25 mg	Hydrodiuril by Kaiser	00179-0347	Diuretic; Antihypertensive
OREXIS	Cap, Blue, Black Ink	Tribulus Terrestris, Epimedium, Yohimbe extract, Muira Puama, Panax Ginseng, Catuaba bark extract, Damiana (turnera aphrodisiaca)	Orexis by Urban Nutrition Inc		Supplement
OREXISPERVALID-USOBDURO	Cap, Blue, OREXIS (pervalidus obduro)	Tribulus Terrestris, Epimedium, Yohimbe Extract, Muira Puama, Panax Ginseng, Catuaba Bark Extract, Damiana (turnera aphrodisiaca)	Orexis by Urban Nutrition Inc		Supplement
ORFENAGESIC	Tab	Acetaminophen 500 mg, Orphenadrine Citrate 50 mg	Orfenagesic by Lex	49523-2313	Analgesic
ORG <> ORG	Tab, Green	Ethinyl Estradiol 0.035 mg, Norethindrone 1 mg	Jenest-28 by Ortho-McNeil	00062-1790	Oral Contraceptive
ORG07 <> ORG07	Tab, White	Ethinyl Estradiol 0.035 mg, Norethindrone 0.5 mg	Jenest-28 by Ortho-McNeil	00062-1790	Oral Contraceptive
ORG14 <> ORG14	Tab, Peach	Ethinyl Estradiol 0.035 mg, Norethindrone 1 mg	Jenest-28 by Ortho-McNeil	00062-1790	Oral Contraceptive
ORG472	Cap, Off-White, Black Print	Calcifediol, Anhydrous 20 mcg	Sec Calderol by RP Scherer	11014-0763	Vitamin; Mineral
ORG472	Cap, Off-White, Black Print	Calcifediol, Anhydrous 20 mcg	by Organon	00052-0472	Vitamin; Mineral
ORG474	Cap	Calcifediol, Anhydrous 50 mcg	Calderol by RP Scherer	11014-0836	Vitamin; Mineral
ORGANON	Cap, Clear, Gelatin w/ Dark Blue Print, Organon Logo	Amylase 30,000 USP, Lipase 8000 USP, Protease 30,000 USP	Cotazym by Organon	Canadian DIN 00263818	Gastrointestinal
ORGANON <> K2H	Tab, Green, Round, "2" set below K & H	Inert	Linessa 28 by Organon	Canadian DIN 02257238	Oral Contraceptive
ORGANON <> KH2	Tab, Green, Film Coated, KH over 2 <> Organon	Inert	Cesia by Prasco	66993-0615	Oral Contraceptive; Placebo
ORGANON <> KH2	Tab, Green, Round	Inert	Cyclessa by Organon	00052-0283	Oral Contraceptive; Placebo
ORGANON <> KH2	Tab, KH over 2	Desogestrel 0.15 mg, Ethinyl Estradiol 0.03 mg	Desogen by Organon	60889-0261	Oral Contraceptive
ORGANON <> KH2	Tab, Film Coated, Organon <> K H over 2	Inert	Mircette by NV Organon	12860-0281	Oral Contraceptive; Placebo
ORGANON <> KH2	Tab, Film Coated, KH over 2 <> Organon	Inert	Desogen by Organon	00052-0261	Oral Contraceptive; Placebo
ORGANON <> KH2	Tab, Green, Film Coated, KH over 2 <> Organon	Inert	Mircette by Organon	00052-0281	Oral Contraceptive; Placebo

ID FRONT <> BACK	DESCRIPTION FRONT <> BACK	INGREDIENT & STRENGTH	BRAND (or Generic Equiv.) by FIRM	NDC#	CLASS; SCH.
ORGANON <> KH2	Tab, Green, Round	Inert	Marvelon 28 by Organon	Canadian DIN 02042479	Oral Contraceptive; Placebo
ORGANON <> KS2	Tab, Yellow, Film Coated, Organon <> K S over 2	Ethinyl Estradiol 0.01 mg	Mircette by Organon	00052-0281	Oral Contraceptive
ORGANON <> KS2	Tab, Film Coated, Organon <> K S over 2	Ethinyl Estradiol 0.01 mg	Mircette by NV Organon	12860-0281	Oral Contraceptive
ORGANON <> T0R	Tab, Light Yellow, Round, Coated, "0" set below T & R	Desogestrel 0.100 mg, Ethinyl Estradiol 0.025 mg	Linessa 21 by Organon	Canadian DIN 02272903	Oral Contraceptive
ORGANON <> T0R	Tab, Light Yellow, Round, Coated, "0" set below T & R	Desogestrel 0.100 mg, Ethinyl Estradiol 0.025 mg	Linessa 28 by Organon	Canadian DIN 02257238	Oral Contraceptive
ORGANON <> T1R	Tab, Red, Round, Coated, "1" set below T & R	Desogestrel 0.150 mg, Ethinyl Estradiol 0.025 mg	Linessa 28 by Organon	Canadian DIN 02257238	Oral Contraceptive
ORGANON <> T1R	Tab, Red, Round, Coated, "1" set below T & R	Desogestrel 0.150 mg, Ethinyl Estradiol 0.025 mg	Linessa 21 by Organon	Canadian DIN 02272903	Oral Contraceptive
ORGANON <> T6R	Tab, Orange, Round, Coated, "6" set below T & R	Desogestrel 0.125 mg, Ethinyl Estradiol 0.025 mg	Linessa 28 by Organon	Canadian DIN 02257238	Oral Contraceptive
ORGANON <> T6R	Tab, Orange, Round, Coated, "6" set below T & R	Desogestrel 0.125 mg, Ethinyl Estradiol 0.025 mg	Linessa 21 by Organon	Canadian DIN 02272903	Oral Contraceptive
ORGANON <> TR0	Tab, Light Yellow, Round	Desogestrel 0.100 mg, Ethinyl Estradiol 0.025 mg	Cyclessa by Organon	00052-0283	Oral Contraceptive
ORGANON <> TR0	Tab, Light Yellow, Round	Desogestrel 0.100 mg, Ethinyl Estradiol 0.025 mg	Cesia by Prasco	66993-0615	Oral Contraceptive
ORGANON <> TR1	Tab, Red, Round	Desogestrel 0.150 mg, Ethinyl Estradiol 0.025 mg	Cesia by Prasco	66993-0615	Oral Contraceptive
ORGANON <> TR1	Tab, Red, Round	Desogestrel 0.150 mg, Ethinyl Estradiol 0.025 mg	Cyclessa by Organon	00052-0283	Oral Contraceptive
ORGANON <> TR4	Tab, White, Film Coated, Organon <> T R over 4	Desogestrel 0.15 mg, Ethinyl Estradiol 0.02 mg	Mircette by NV Organon	12860-0281	Oral Contraceptive
ORGANON <> TR4	Tab, White, Film Coated, Organon <> T R over 4	Desogestrel 0.15 mg, Ethinyl Estradiol 0.02 mg	Mircette by Organon	00052-0281	Oral Contraceptive
ORGANON <> TR5	Tab, White, Round	Desogestrel 0.15 mg, Ethinyl Estradiol 0.03 mg	Marvelon 21 by Organon	Canadian DIN 02042487	Oral Contraceptive
ORGANON <> TR5	Tab, White, Round	Desogestrel 0.15 mg, Ethinyl Estradiol 0.03 mg	Marvelon 28 by Organon	Canadian DIN 02042479	Oral Contraceptive
ORGANON <> TR5	Tab, White, Round, TR over 5	Desogestrel 0.15 mg, Ethinyl Estradiol 0.03 mg	Desogen by Organon	60889-0261	Oral Contraceptive
ORGANON <> TR5	Tab, White, Round	Desogestrel 0.15 mg, Ethinyl Estradiol 0.03 mg	Desogen by Organon	00052-0261	Oral Contraceptive
ORGANON <> TR6	Tab, Orange, Round	Desogestrel 0.125 mg, Ethinyl Estradiol 0.025 mg	Cyclessa by Organon	00052-0283	Oral Contraceptive
ORGANON <> TR6	Tab, Orange, Round	Desogestrel 0.125 mg, Ethinyl Estradiol 0.025 mg	Cesia by Prasco	66993-0615	Oral Contraceptive
ORGANON <> TZ3	Tab, Yellow, Oval, Scored, Film Coated	Mirtazapine 15 mg	Remeron by Neuman	64579-0390	Antidepressant
ORGANON <> TZ3	Tab, Yellow, Oval, Scored, Film Coated	Mirtazapine 15 mg	Remeron by Organon	00052-0105	Antidepressant
ORGANON <> TZ3	Tab, Yellow, Oval, Scored, Film Coated	Mirtazapine 15 mg	Remeron by NV Organon	12860-0105	Antidepressant
ORGANON <> TZ5	Tab, Red-Brown, Oval, Scored, Film Coated	Mirtazapine 30 mg	Remeron by Organon	00052-0107	Antidepressant
ORGANON <> TZ5	Tab, Red-Brown, Oval, Scored, Film Coated	Mirtazapine 30 mg	Remeron by NV Organon	12860-0107	Antidepressant
ORGANON <> TZ5	Tab, Red-Brown, Oval, Scored, Film Coated	Mirtazapine 30 mg	Remeron by Organon	Canadian DIN 02243910	Antidepressant
ORGANON <> TZ5	Tab, Red Brown, Oval, Scored, Film Coated	Mirtazapine 30 mg	Remeron by Schering-Plough	Canadian DIN 02243910	Antidepressant
ORGANON <> TZ7	Tab, White, Oval, Film Coated	Mirtazapine 45 mg	Remeron by Organon	00052-0109	Antidepressant
ORGANON <> TZ7	Tab, White, Oval, Film Coated	Mirtazapine 45 mg	Remeron by Nv Organon	12860-0109	Antidepressant
ORGANON381	Cap, Green, White Print, Organon in circle	Amylase 30,000 Units, Lipase 8000 Units, Protease 30,000 Units	Viokase by Physician Total Care	54868-3793	Gastrointestinal
ORGANON381	Cap, Green, White Print, Organon in circle	Amylase 30,000 Units, Lipase 8000 Units, Protease 30,000 Units	Cotazyme by Organon	00052-0381	Gastrointestinal
ORGANON388	Cap, Clear, Black Print, Organon in circle	Amylase 20,000 Units, Lipase 5000 Units, Protease 20,000 Units	Cotazyme-S by Organon	00052-0388	Gastrointestinal
ORGANON393	Cap, Clear & Green	Lipase, Protease, Amylase	Zymase by Organon		Gastrointestinal
ORGANON542	Tab, White, Round	Ergotamine Tartrate 1 mg, Caffeine 100 mg	Wigraine by Organon		Antimigraine
ORGANON790	Tab, Peach, Round	Dexamethasone 1.5 mg	Hexadrol by Organon		Steroid
ORGANON791	Tab, White, Round	Dexamethasone 0.75 mg	Hexadrol by Organon		Steroid
ORGANON792	Tab, Yellow, Round	Dexamethasone 0.5 mg	Hexadrol by Organon		Steroid

ID FRONT <> BACK	DESCRIPTION FRONT <> BACK	INGREDIENT & STRENGTH	BRAND (or Generic Equiv.) by FIRM	NDC#	CLASS; SCH.
ORGANON798	Tab, Green, Round	Dexamethasone 4 mg	Hexadrol by Organon		Steroid
ORGANONKH2	Tab, Green, Round	Inert	Desogen 28 by Organon		Oral Contraceptive; Placebo
ORGDV3	Cap, Orange, Oval, Soft Gel	Testosterone Undecanoate 40 mg	Andriol by Schering-Plough	Canadian DIN 00782327	Hormone; C III
ORINASE500	Tab	Tolbutamide 500 mg	by Watson	00591-5508	Antidiabetic
ORLISTAT60	Cap, Light Blue with Dark Blue Band and Imprint	Orlistat 60 mg	Alli by GSK Consumer		Lipase Inhibitor
ORNADESB	Cap, Natural & Red, Ornade/SB	Chlorpheniramine Maleate 12 mg, Phenylpropanolamine 75 mg	Ornade by SKB	00007-4421	Cold Remedy
ORNEX	Tab, Blue, Oblong, Cap Shaped	Pseudoephedrine HCl 30 mg, Acetaminophen 325 mg	Ornex by B F Ascher	00225-0590	Cold Remedy
ORNEXMAX	Tab, White, Oblong, Cap Shaped	Pseudoephedrine HCl 30 mg, Acetaminophen 500 mg	Ornex-Max by B F Ascher	00225-0600	Cold Remedy
ORTHO	Tab, Green, Round	Inert	Ortho-Novum 1/50 28 by Ortho-McNeil	00062-1332	Oral Contraceptive; Placebo
ORTHO	Tab, Green, Round	Inert	Ortho Tri-Cyclen by Ortho-McNeil	00062-1903	Oral Contraceptive; Placebo
ORTHO	Tab, Green, Round	Inert	Ortho Cyclen by Ortho-McNeil	00062-1901	Oral Contraceptive; Placebo
ORTHO	Tab, Green, Round	Inert	Ortho-Novum 1/35 by Ortho-McNeil	00062-1761	Oral Contraceptive; Placebo
ORTHO	Tab, Green, Round	Inert	Modicon by Ortho-McNeil	00062-1714	Oral Contraceptive; Placebo
ORTHO	Tab, Green, Round	Inert	Ortho-Novum 10/11 by Ortho-McNeil	00062-1771	Oral Contraceptive; Placebo
ORTHO	Tab, Green, Round	Inert	Ortho-Novum 7/7/7 28 by Ortho-McNeil	00062-1781	Oral Contraceptive; Placebo
ORTHO	Tab	Ethinyl Estradiol 0.035 mg, Norgestimate 0.25 mg	by Physician Total Care	54868-2606	Oral Contraceptive
ORTHO <> 150	Tab	Ethinyl Estradiol 0.035 mg, Norgestimate 0.215 mg, Norgestimate 0.18 mg, Norgestimate 0.25 mg	Ortho Tri-Cyclen 28 by Dept Health	53808-0043	Oral Contraceptive
ORTHO <> 150	Tab	Mestranol 0.05 mg, Norethindrone 1 mg	Ortho Novum 1 Plus 50 by Dept Health	53808-0030	Oral Contraceptive
ORTHO <> 35	Tab	Ethinyl Estradiol 0.035 mg, Norethindrone 0.5 mg, Norethindrone 1 mg, Norethindrone 0.75 mg	Ortho Novum 777 by Dept Health	53808-0032	Oral Contraceptive
ORTHO <> D150	Tab, Orange	Desogestrel 0.15 mg, Ethinyl Estradiol 0.03 mg	Ortho-Cept 28 by Ortho-McNeil	00062-1796	Oral Contraceptive
ORTHO <> D150	Tab, Peach, Round	Desogestrel 0.15 mg, Ethinyl Estradiol 0.03 mg	Ortho-Cept 21 by Ortho-McNeil	00062-1795	Oral Contraceptive
ORTHO035	Tab, Green, Round	Norethindrone 0.35 mg	Micronor by Janssen-Ortho	Canadian DIN 00037605	Hormone
ORTHO035	Tab, Green, Round	Norethindrone 0.35 mg	Micronor by Ortho-McNeil	00062-1411	Hormone
ORTHO1	Tab, White, Round	Norethindrone 1 mg, Mestranol 0.08 mg	Ortho Novum by Ortho-McNeil		Oral Contraceptive
ORTHO135	Tab, Peach, Round	Ethinyl Estradiol 0.035 mg, Norethindrone 1 mg	Ortho-Novum 10/11 by Ortho-McNeil	00062-1771	Oral Contraceptive
ORTHO135	Tab, Peach, Round	Ethinyl Estradiol 0.035 mg, Norethindrone 1 mg	Ortho-Novum 1/35 by Ortho-McNeil	00062-1761	Oral Contraceptive
ORTHO135	Tab, Peach, Round	Ethinyl Estradiol 0.035 mg, Norethindrone 1 mg	Ortho-Novum 7/7/7 28 by Ortho-McNeil	00062-1781	Oral Contraceptive
ORTHO150	Tab, Yellow	Norethindrone 1 mg, Mestranol 50 mcg	Ortho-Novum by Ortho-McNeil	Canadian	Oral Contraceptive
ORTHO150 <>	Tab, Pale Yellow, Round	Mestranol 0.05 mg, Norethindrone 1 mg	Ortho Novum 21 by Ortho-McNeil	00062-1331	Oral Contraceptive
ORTHO150 <> ORTHO150	Tab, Pale Yellow, Round	Mestranol 0.05 mg, Norethindrone 1 mg	Ortho-Novum 1/50-28 by Ortho-McNeil	00062-1332	Oral Contraceptive
ORTHO1570	Tab, White, Oblong	Metronidazole 250 mg	Protostat by Ortho-McNeil	00062-1570	Antibiotic
ORTHO1571	Tab, White, Oblong	Metronidazole 500 mg	Protostat by Ortho-McNeil	00062-1571	Antibiotic
ORTHO180	Tab, White, Round	Ethinyl Estradiol 0.035 mg, Norgestimate 0.180 mg	Ortho Tri-Cyclen 28 by Ortho-McNeil	00062-1903	Oral Contraceptive
ORTHO1800	Tab, Lavender	Estropipate 1.5 mg	Ortho EST by Ortho-McNeil	00062-1800	Hormone
ORTHO1801	Tab	Estropipate 0.75 mg	Ortho EST by Ortho-McNeil	00062-1801	Hormone
ORTHO2	Tab, White, Round	Norethindrone 2 mg, Mestranol 0.1 mg	Ortho Novum by Ortho-McNeil		Oral Contraceptive

ID FRONT <> BACK	DESCRIPTION FRONT <> BACK	INGREDIENT & STRENGTH	BRAND (or Generic Equiv.) by FIRM	NDC#	CLASS; SCH.
ORTHO211	Tab, White, Round, Scored	Griseofulvin, Microsize 250 mg	Fulvicin P/G by Ortho-McNeil	00062-0211	Antifungal
ORTHO214	Tab, White, Round, Scored	Griseofulvin, Microsize 500 mg	Fulvicin-U/F by Ortho-McNeil	00062-0214	Antifungal
ORTHO215	Tab, Light Blue, Round	Ethinyl Estradiol 0.035 mg, Norgestimate 0.215 mg	Ortho Tri-Cyclen 28 by Ortho-McNeil	00062-1903	Oral Contraceptive
ORTHO250	Tab, Blue, Round	Ethinyl Estradiol 0.035 mg, Norgestimate 0.250 mg	Ortho Tri-Cyclen 28 by Ortho-McNeil	00062-1903	Oral Contraceptive
ORTHO250	Tab, Blue, Round	Norgestimate 0.25 mg, Ethinyl Estradiol 0.035 mg	Ortho Cyclen by Ortho-McNeil	00062-1901	Oral Contraceptive
ORTHO535	Tab, White, Round	Ethinyl Estradiol 0.035 mg, Norethindrone 0.5 mg	Ortho-Novum 10/11 by Ortho-McNeil	00062-1771	Oral Contraceptive
ORTHO535	Tab, White, Round	Ethinyl Estradiol 0.035 mg, Norethindrone 0.5 mg	Modicon by Ortho-McNeil	00062-1714	Oral Contraceptive
ORTHO535	Tab, White	Norethindrone 0.75 mg, Ethinyl Estradiol 0.035 mg	by Kaiser	00179-1298	Oral Contraceptive
ORTHO535	Tab, White, Round	Ethinyl Estradiol 0.035 mg, Norethindrone 0.5 mg	Ortho-Novum 7/7/7 28 by Ortho-McNeil	00062-1781	Oral Contraceptive
ORTHO735	Tab, Peach	Norethindrone 0.75 mg, Ethinyl Estradiol 35 mcg	by Janssen	Canadian	Oral Contraceptive
ORTHO75	Tab, Light Peach, Round	Ethinyl Estradiol 0.035 mg, Norethindrone 0.75 mg	Ortho-Novum 7/7/7 28 by Ortho-McNeil	00062-1781	Oral Contraceptive
ORTHOP	Tab, Green, Round	Inert	Ortho-Cept 28 by Ortho-McNeil	00062-1796	Oral Contraceptive; Placebo
ORTHOP	Tab, Green, Round	Inert	Ortho-Cept 28 by Janssen-Ortho	Canadian DIN 02042533	Oral Contraceptive; Placebo
ORTHOPD150	Tab, Orange, Ortho/p D 150	Desogestrel 0.15 mg, Ethinyl Estradiol 0.03 mg	by Janssen	Canadian	Oral Contraceptive
ORUDIS50	Cap, Green & Ivory	Ketoprofen 50 mg	Orudis by RPR	Canadian	NSAID
ORUDISSR200	Tab, White, Round	Ketoprofen 200 mg	Orudis by RPR	Canadian	NSAID
ORUVAIL100	Cap, Pink & Dark Green, Blue Print, 2 Blue Bands	Ketoprofen 100 mg	Orudis by Wyeth	00008-0821	NSAID
ORUVAIL150	Cap, Pink & Light Green, Blue Print, 2 Blue Bands	Ketoprofen 150 mg	Orudis by May & Baker Pharma	Canadian	NSAID
ORUVAIL150	Cap, Pink & Light Green, Blue Print, 2 Blue Bands	Ketoprofen 150 mg	Orudis by Wyeth	00008-0822	NSAID
ORUVAIL200	Cap, Pink & White, Blue Print, 2 Blue Bands	Ketoprofen 200 mg	Orudis by May & Baker Pharma	Canadian	NSAID
ORUVAIL200	Cap, Pink & White, Blue Print, 2 Blue Bands	Ketoprofen 200 mg	Orudis by Wyeth	00008-0690	NSAID
ORUVAIL200	Cap, Pink & White, Blue Print, 2 Blue Bands	Ketoprofen 200 mg	Orudis by DRX	55045-2118	NSAID
ORUVAIL200	Cap, Pink & White, Blue Print, 2 Blue Bands	Ketoprofen 200 mg	Orudis by Murfreesboro	51129-1597	NSAID
OS301	Tab, White, Round	Venlafaxine Hydrochloride 37.5 mg	Venlafaxine Hydrochloride by Upstate Pharma	65580-0301	Antidepressant
OS302	Tab, White, Round	Venlafaxine Hydrochloride 75 mg	Venlafaxine Hydrochloride by Upstate Pharma	65580-0302	Antidepressant
OS303	Tab, White, Round	Venlafaxine Hydrochloride 150 mg	Venlafaxine Hydrochloride by Upstate Pharma	65580-0303	Antidepressant
OS304	Tab, White, Round	Venlafaxine Hydrochloride 225 mg	Venlafaxine Hydrochloride by Upstate Pharma	65580-0304	Antidepressant
OSCAL	Tab, White, Round, OS-CAL	Elemental Calcium 750 mg	OS-CAL by Wyeth	Canadian	Mineral
OSCAL	Tab, Green, Oblong, OS-CAL	Elemental Calcium 500 mg	OS-CAL by Wyeth	Canadian DIN 02042991	Mineral
OSCALD	Tab, Pale Grey, Cap-Shaped	Calcium Carbonate 1250	Os-Cal D by Wyeth	Canadian DIN 02043025	Mineral
OTSUKA15	Tab, Blue, Triangular	Tolvaptan 15mg	Samsca by Otsuka	59148-0020	Diuretic
OTSUKA30	Tab, Blue, Round	Tolvaptan 30 mg	Samsca by Otsuka	59148-0021	Diuretic
OV <> 12	Tab, White	Methamphetamine HCl 5 mg	Desoxyn by Ovation	67386-0102	Stimulant; C II
OV <> 61	Tab, White, Scored	Ethotoin 250 mg	Peganone by Ovation	67386-0601	Anticonvulsant
OV111 <> 500MG	Tab, White, Oval, Film-Coated, Scored	Vigabatrin 500 mg	Sabril by Lundbeck	67386-0111	Anticonvulsant
OV31 <> T	Tab, Blue, \/ Shaped, Scored	Clorazepate Dipotassium 3.75 mg	Tranxene by Ovation	67386-0301	Antianxiety; C IV
OV32 <> T	Tab, Peach, \/ Shaped, Scored	Clorazepate Dipotassium 7.5 mg	Tranxene by Ovation	67386-0302	Antianxiety; C IV
OV33 <> T	Tab, Lavender, \/ Shaped, Scored	Clorazepate Dipotassium 15 mg	Tranxene by Ovation	67386-0303	Antianxiety; C IV
OV44	Tab, Blue	Clorazepate Dipotassium 11.25 mg	Tranxene SD by Ovation	67386-0404	Antianxiety; C IV
OV45	Tab, Tan	Clorazepate Dipotassium 22.5 mg	Tranxene SD by Ovation	67386-0405	Antianxiety; C IV
OVOL160	Tab, White, Round, Ovol-160	Simethicone 160 mg	Ovol by Horner	Canadian	Antiflatulent
OW	Tab, Pink, Round	Phenolphthalein	Correctol by Barre		Gastrointestinal

ID FRONT <> BACK	DESCRIPTION FRONT <> BACK	INGREDIENT & STRENGTH	BRAND (or Generic Equiv.) by FIRM	NDC#	CLASS; SCH.
OX <> 10	Tab, White, Oval, Scored	Oxandrolone 10 mg	Oxandrin by Watson	00591-3545	Steroid; C III
OX <> 1111	Tab, White, Oval, Scored	Oxandrolone 2.5 mg	Oxandrin by Watson	00591-3544	Steroid; C III
OX15 <> APO	Tab, Yellow, Round, Scored	Oxazepam 15 mg	Serax by Apotex	Canadian DIN 00402745	Sedative/Hypnotic; C IV
OXA600 <> APO	Tab, White to Off-White, Cap Shaped, Scored, Film Coated	Oxaprozin 600 mg	Daypro by Apotex	Canadian DIN 02243661	NSAID
OXA600 <> APO	Tab, White to Off-White, Cap Shaped, Scored, Film Coated	Oxaprozin 600 mg	Daypro by Apotex	60505-0176	NSAID
OXC150 <> APO	Tab, Yellow, Oval, Film Coated, Scored	Oxcarbazepine 150 mg	Trileptal by Apotex	Canadian DIN 02284294	Anticonvulsant
OXC300 <> APO	Tab, Yellow, Oval, Film Coated, Scored	Oxcarbazepine 300 mg	Trileptal by Apotex	Canadian DIN 02284308	Anticonvulsant
OXC6 <> TARO	Tab, Off White, Oval	Oxcarbazepine 600 mg	Trileptal by Taro	51672-4107	Anticonvulsant
OXC600 <> APO	Tab, Yellow, Oval, Film Coated, Scored	Oxcarbazepine 600 mg	Trileptal by Apotex	Canadian DIN 02284316	Anticonvulsant
OXY5 <> P	Tab, Blue, Round, Scored, P Logo <> OXY / 5	Oxybutynin Chloride 5 mg	Ditropan by Pharmascience	Canadian DIN 02240550	Urinary Tract
OXYIR <> 10	Tab, White, Cap-Shaped, Scored	Oxycodone HCl 10 mg.	Oxy IR by Purdue Pharma	Canadian DIN 02240131	Analgesic
OXYIR <> 20	Tab, White, Oval, Scored	Oxycodone HCl 20 mg	Oxy IR by Purdue Pharma	Canadian DIN 02240132	Analgesic
OXYIR <> 5	Tab, White, Round, Scored, Biconvex	Oxycodone HCl 5 mg	Oxy IR by Purdue Pharma	Canadian DIN 02231934	Analgesic
OZ10	Tab, White, Round, Blue Print	Olanzapine 10 mg	Zyprexa by Pharmascience	Canadian DIN 02303175	Antipsychotic
OZ15	Tab, White, Oval	Olanzapine 15 mg	Zyprexa by Pharmascience	Canadian DIN 02303183	Antipsychotic
OZ25	Tab, White, Round, Blue Print, OZ 2.5	Olanzapine 2.5 mg	Zyprexa by Pharmascience	Canadian DIN 02303116	Antipsychotic
OZ5	Tab, White, Round, Blue Print	Olanzapine 5 mg	Zyprexa by Pharmascience	Canadian DIN 02303159	Antipsychotic
OZ75	Tab, White, Round, Blue Print, OZ 7.5	Olanzapine 7.5 mg	Zyprexa by Pharmascience	Canadian DIN 02303167	Antipsychotic
P	Tab, Green, Round	Inert	Tri-Cyclen LO 28 by Janssen-Ortho	Canadian DIN 02258587	Oral Contraceptive; Placebo
P	Cap, Green, Soft Gel, P inside Triangle	Pseudoephedrine HCl 30 mg, Doxylamine Succinate 6.25 mg, Acetaminophen 250 mg, Dextromethorphan HBr 10 mg	Nite Time Liquid Capsules by Perrigo	00113-0193	Cold Remedy
P	Tab, Peach, Elliptical, P over Score	Omeprazole Magnesium 20.6 mg	OTC Prilosec by Procter and Gamble	37000-0455	Gastrointestinal
P	Tab, Pink, Round, Chewable	Famotidine 10 mg, Calcium Carbonate 800 mg, Magnesium Hydroxide 165 mg	by McNeil	Canadian DIN 02243053	Gastrointestinal
P	Tab, White, Round	Docusate Sodium 100 mg	Phillips Liqui Gels by Group Health	58087-0019	Laxative
P	Tab, Orange, Round	Sennosides 8.6 mg, Docusate Sodium 50 mg	Senokot-S by Purdue	00034-1210	Gastrointestinal
P	Tab, Blue, Round, Film Coated, P in a diamond	Desipramine HCl 10 mg	Norpramin by Pharmascience	Canadian DIN 01946250	Antidepressant
P	Tab, White, Scored	Captopril 12.5 mg	Capoten by Pharmascience	Canadian DIN 02230203	Antihypertensive
P	Tab, White to Off-White, Round, Scored	Selegiline HCl 5 mg	by Pharmascience	Canadian DIN 02238102	Antiparkinson
P	Tab, Peach, Round	Hydrochlorothiazide 12.5 mg	PMS-Hydrocholorothiazide by Pharmascience	Canadian DIN 02274086	Diuretic
P	Tab, White, Oval, Film Coated	Carvedilol 3.125 mg	Coreg by Pharmascience	Canadian DIN 02245914	Antihypertensive

ID FRONT <> BACK	DESCRIPTION FRONT <> BACK	INGREDIENT & STRENGTH	BRAND (or Generic Equiv.) by FIRM	NDC#	CLASS; SCH.
P	Tab, Yellow, Oval, Scored	Isosorbide Mononitrate 60 mg	Imdur by Pharmascience	Canadian DIN 02301288	Antianginal
P	Tab, Yellow, Round, Scored, "P" inside circle	Ephedrine HCl 12.5 mg, Guaifenesin 200 mg	Primatene by Wyeth	00573-2952	Antiasthmatic
P <> 011	Tab, Orange, Round, Enteric Coated, P inside Triangle	Aspirin 325 mg	Ecotrin by Qualitest	00603-0167	Analgesic
P <> 05	Tab, White, Round	Lorazepam 0.5 mg	Ativan by Pharmascience	Canadian DIN 00728187	Antianxiety; C IV
P <> 1	Tab, Blue, Round, Scored	Methadone Hydrochloride 1 mg	Metadol by Pharmascience	Canadian DIN 02247698	Analgesic
P <> 1	Tab, White, Round	Terazosin HCl 1 mg	Hytrin by Pharmascience	Canadian DIN 02243518	Antihypertensive
P <> 10	Tab, Blue, Round	Terazosin HCl 10 mg	Hytrin by Pharmascience	Canadian DIN 02243521	Antihypertensive
P <> 10	Tab, Peach, Round, Scored	Bethanechol Chloride 10 mg	Urecholine by Pharmascience	Canadian DIN 00759171	Urinary Tract
P <> 10	Tab, Pale Green, Round, Scored	Methadone Hydrochloride 10 mg	Metadol by Pharmascience	Canadian DIN 02247700	Analgesic
P <> 10	Tab, White, Round, Film Coated	Bisoprolol Fumarate 10 mg	Zym-Bisoprolol by Zymcan Pharm	Canadian DIN 02321572	Antihypertensive
P <> 10	Tab, White, Round	Leflunomide 10 mg	ARAVA by Pharmascience	Canadian DIN 02288265	Antiarthritic
P <> 10	Tab, White, Round	Bisoprolol Fumarate 10 mg	Monocor by Pharmascience	Canadian DIN 02302640	Antihypertensive
P <> 10	Tab, Yellow, Oval, Scored, P Logo <> 1 / 0	Paroxetine HCl 10 mg	Paxil by Pharmascience	Canadian DIN 02247750	Antidepressant
P <> 10	Tab, Light Pink, Shield Shaped	Simvastatin 10 mg	Zocor by Pharmascience	Canadian DIN 02269260	Antihyperlipidemic
P <> 100	Tab, Pink, Round, Pharmascience Logo	Amiodarone 100 mg	Cordarone by Pharmascience	Canadian DIN 02292173	Antiarrhythmic
P <> 100	Tab, Yellow, Round	Topiramate 100 mg	Topamax by Pharmascience	Canadian DIN 02263009	Anticonvulsant
P <> 100	Tab, Light Pink, Trapezoidal	Fluconazole 100 mg	Diflucan by Pharmascience	Canadian DIN 02245644	Antifungal
P <> 10CL	Tab, White, Round, Scored, P <> 10/CL	Clobazam 10 mg	Frisium by Pharmascience	Canadian DIN 02244474	Anticonvulsant
P <> 11	Tab, Dye Free, Round, Chewable, 1.1	Sodium Fluoride 1.1 mg	Pharmaflur 1.1 by Pharmics	00813-0065	Element
P <> 125	Tab, White, Oval, Film Coated, P <> 12.5	Carvedilol 12.5 mg	Coreg by Pharmascience	Canadian DIN 02245916	Antihypertensive
P <> 125	Tab, White, Round	Famciclovir 125 mg	Famvir by Pharmascience	Canadian DIN 02278081	Antiviral
P <> 15	Tab, Yellow, Oval, Scored	Mirtazapine 15 mg	Remeron by Pharmascience	Canadian DIN 02273942	Antidepressant
P <> 15M	Tab, White, Round, Scored	Meloxicam 15 mg	Mobicox by Pharmascience	Canadian DIN 02248268	NSAID
P <> 15MG	Tab, Green, Round, Sustained Release	Morphine Sulfate 15 mg	MS Contin by Pharmascience	Canadian DIN 02245284	Analgesic
P <> 2	Tab, Orange, Round	Terazosin HCl 2 mg	Hytrin by Pharmascience	Canadian DIN 02243519	Antihypertensive
P <> 20	Tab, Pink, Oval, Scored, P Logo <> 2 / 0	Paroxetine HCl 20 mg	Paxil by Pharmascience	Canadian DIN 02247751	Antidepressant
P <> 20	Tab, Beige, Shield Shaped	Simvastatin 20 mg	Zocor by Pharmascience	Canadian DIN 02269279	Antihyperlipidemic

ID FRONT <> BACK	DESCRIPTION FRONT <> BACK	INGREDIENT & STRENGTH	BRAND (or Generic Equiv.) by FIRM	NDC#	CLASS; SCH.
P <> 20	Tab, White, Triangle Shaped	Leflunomide 20 mg	ARAVA by Pharmascience	Canadian DIN 02288273	Antiarthritic
P <> 200	Tab, White, Round, Pharmascience Logo	Bezafibrate 200 mg	Bezalip by Pharmascience	Canadian DIN 02240331	Antihyperlipidemic
P <> 200	Tab, Salmon, Round	Topiramate 200 mg	Topamax by Pharmascience	Canadian DIN 02263017	Anticonvulsant
P <> 22	Tab, White, Round, Chewable, 2.2	Sodium Fluoride 2.21 mg	Pharmaflur by Pharmics	00813-0066	Element
P <> 25	Tab, White, Oval, Film Coated	Carvedilol 25 mg	Coreg by Pharmascience	Canadian DIN 02245917	Antihypertensive
P <> 25	Tab, White, Round	Topiramate 25 mg	Topamax by Pharmascience	Canadian DIN 02262991	Anticonvulsant
P <> 25	Tab, Yellow, Round	Diclofenac Sodium 25 mg	Voltaren by Pharmascience	Canadian DIN 02231502	NSAID
P <> 25	Tab, Yellow, Round	Methotrimeprazine Maleate 25 mg	Nozinan by Pharmascience	Canadian DIN 02232904	Antipsychotic
P <> 25	Tab, Pink, Round, Scored	Loxapine Succinate 25 mg	Loxapac by Pharmascience	Canadian DIN 02230839	Antipsychotic
P <> 25	Tab, White, Round, P logo <> 2.5	Oxybutynin Chloride 2.5 mg	Ditropan by Pharmascience	Canadian DIN 02240549	Urinary Tract
P <> 25	Tab, White to Off White, Caplet Shaped, Scored	Methadone HCl 25 mg	Metadol by Pharmascience	Canadian DIN 02247701	Analgesic
P <> 250	Tab, Red, Oblong	Azithromycin 250 mg	Zithromax by Pharmascience	Canadian DIN 02261634	Antibiotic
P <> 250	Tab, White, Round	Famciclovir 250 mg	Famvir by Pharmascience	Canadian DIN 02278103	Antiviral
P <> 250	Tab, White, Oval	Ursodiol 250 mg	Urso by Pharmascience	Canadian DIN 02273497	Gastrointestinal
P <> 30	Tab, Blue, Oval, P Logo	Paroxetine HCl 30 mg	Paxil by Pharmascience	Canadian DIN 02247752	Antidepressant
P <> 30	Tab, Brown, Oval, Scored	Mirtazapine 30 mg	Remeron by Pharmascience	Canadian DIN 02248762	Antidepressant
P <> 30MG	Tab, Violet, Round, Sustained Release	Morphine Sulfate 30 mg	MS Contin by Pharmascience	Canadian DIN 02245285	Analgesic
P <> 4	Tab, Yellow, Oval, P logo <> 4	Ondansetron HCl 4 mg	Zofran by Pharmascience	Canadian DIN 02258188	Antiemetic
P <> 40	Tab, Green, Oblong, P logo	Paroxetine HCl 40 mg	Paxil by Pharmascience	Canadian DIN 02293749	Antidepressant
P <> 40	Tab, Brick Red, Shield Shaped	Simvastatin 40 mg	Zocor by Pharmascience	Canadian DIN 02269287	Antihyperlipidemic
P <> 425	Tab, White, Round, Scored	Atropine Sulfate 0.0194 mg, Scopolamine HBr 0.0065 mg, Hyoscyamine HBr 0.1037 mg, Phenobarbital 16.2 mg	Donnatal by PBM	66213-0425	Gastrointestinal; C IV
P <> 5	Tab, Brown, Round	Terazosin HCl 5 mg	Hytrin by Pharmascience	Canadian DIN 02243520	Antihypertensive
P <> 5	Tab, White, Shield Shaped	Simvastatin 5 mg	Zocor by Pharmascience	Canadian DIN 02269252	Antihyperlipidemic
P <> 5	Tab, Yellow, Round	Methotrimeprazine Maleate 5 mg	Nozinan by Pharmascience	Canadian DIN 02232903	Antipsychotic
P <> 5	Tab, Peach, Round, Scored	Methadone Hydrochloride 5 mg	Metadol by Pharmascience	Canadian DIN 02247699	Analgesic
P <> 50	Tab, Yellow, Round	Methotrimeprazine Maleate 50 mg	Nozinan by Pharmascience	Canadian DIN 02232905	Antipsychotic

ID FRONT <> BACK	DESCRIPTION FRONT <> BACK	INGREDIENT & STRENGTH	BRAND (or Generic Equiv.) by FIRM	NDC#	CLASS; SCH.
P <> 50	Tab, Pink, Trapezoid Shaped	Fluconazole 50 mg	Diflucan by Pharmascience	Canadian DIN 02245643	Antifungal
P <> 50	Tab, Light Brown, Round	Diclofenac Sodium 50 mg	Voltaren by Pharmascience	Canadian DIN 02231503	NSAID
P <> 500	Tab, White, Oval	Famciclovir 500 mg	Famvir by Pharmascience	Canadian DIN 02278111	Antiviral
P <> 50K	Tab, Orange, Round, White Print, Coated	Diclofenac Sodium 50 mg	Voltaren Rapide by Pharmascience	Canadian DIN 02239753	NSAID
P <> 55	Tab, Pink, Round, Scored, P <> 5 / 5	Bisoprolol Fumarate 5 mg	Monocor by Pharmascience	Canadian DIN 02247573	Antihypertensive
P <> 55	Tab, Salmon Pink, Round, Film Coated	Bisoprolol Fumarate 5 mg	Zym-Bisoprolol by Zymcan Pharm	Canadian DIN 02321556	Antihypertensive
P <> 600	Tab, White, Oblong	Azithromycin 600 mg	by Pharmascience	Canadian DIN 02261642	Antibiotic
P <> 60MG	Tab, Orange, Round, Sustained Release	Morphine Sulfate 60 mg	MS Contin by Pharmascience	Canadian DIN 02245286	Analgesic
P <> 625	Tab, White, Oval, Film Coated, P <> 6.25	Carvedilol 6.25 mg	Coreg by Pharmascience	Canadian DIN 02245915	Antihypertensive
P <> 70	Tab, White, Oval, P logo	Alendronate Sodium 70 mg	Fosamax by Pharmascience	Canadian DIN 02284006	Antiosteoporosis
P <> 75M	Tab, White, Round, Scored, 7.5 / M	Meloxicam 7.5 mg	Mobicox by Pharmascience	Canadian DIN 02248267	NSAID
P <> 75Z	Tab, Blue, Oval, Scored, Z 7.5	Zopiclone 7.5 mg	Imovane by Pharmascience	Canadian DIN 02240606	Hypnotic
P <> 8	Tab, Yellow, Oval, P logo <> 8	Ondansetron HCl 8 mg	Zofran by Pharmascience	Canadian DIN 02258196	Antiemetic
P <> 80	Tab, Pink, Cap Shaped	Simvastatin 80 mg	Zocor by Pharmascience	Canadian DIN 02269295	Antihyperlipidemic
P <> 850	Tab, White, Cap Shaped, Film Coated	Metformin HCl 850 mg	Glucophage by Pharmascience	Canadian DIN 02242589	Antidiabetic
P <> A25	Tab, White, Round	Atenolol 25 mg	Tenormin by Pharmascience	Canadian DIN 02246581	Antihypertensive
P <> BIC50	Tab, White, Round	Bicalutamide 50 mg	Casodex by Pharmascience	Canadian DIN 02275589	Antineoplastic
P <> DOXA	Tab, White, Lozenge-Shaped	Doxazosin Mesylate 4 mg	Cardura by Pharmascience	Canadian DIN 02244529	Antihypertensive
P <> DOXA1	Tab, White, Round	Doxazosin Mesylate 1 mg	Cardura by Pharmascience	Canadian DIN 02244527	Antihypertensive
P <> G600	Tab, White, Elliptical	Gabapentin 600 mg	Neurontin by Pharmascience	Canadian DIN 02255898	Anticonvulsant
P <> G800	Tab, White, Elliptical	Gabapentin 800 mg	Neurontin by Pharmascience	Canadian DIN 02255901	Anticonvulsant
P <> IN25	Tab, Pink, Round	Indapamide 2.5 mg	Lozide by Pharmascience	Canadian DIN 02239620	Antihypertensive; Diuretic
P <> KETOTIFEN	Tab, White, Round, Scored	Ketotifen Fumarate 1 mg	by Pharmascience	Canadian DIN 5760616809	Antiasthmatic
P <> L10	Tab, Green, Round, Scored	Loxapine Succinate 10 mg	Loxapac by Pharmascience	Canadian DIN 02230838	Antipsychotic
P <> L25	Tab, Blue, Round, Scored, L / 2.5	Loxapine Succinate 2.5 mg	Loxapac by Pharmascience	Canadian DIN 02242868	Antipsychotic
P <> L25	Tab, White, Oblong, Scored	Metoprolol Tartrate 25 mg	Lopressor by Pharmascience	Canadian DIN 02248855	Antihypertensive

ID FRONT <> BACK	DESCRIPTION FRONT <> BACK	INGREDIENT & STRENGTH	BRAND (or Generic Equiv.) by FIRM	NDC#	CLASS; SCH.
P <> L5	Tab, Yellow, Round, Scored	Loxapine Succinate 5 mg	Loxapac by Pharmascience	Canadian DIN 02230837	Antipsychotic
P <> L50	Tab, White, Round, Scored	Loxapine Succinate 50 mg	Loxapac by Pharmascience	Canadian DIN 02230840	Antipsychotic
P <> LOVA20	Tab, Blue, Octagonal, Scored	Lovastatin 20 mg	Mevacor by Pharmascience	Canadian DIN 02246013	Antihyperlipidemic
P <> LOVA40	Tab, Green, Octagonal	Lovastatin 40 mg	Mevacor by Pharmascience	Canadian DIN 02246014	Antihyperlipidemic
P <> M10	Tab, White, Round, Scored	Metoclopramide HCl 10 mg	Maxeran by Pharmascience	Canadian DIN 02230432	Gastrointestinal
P <> M5	Tab, White, Square	Metoclopramide HCl 5 mg	Maxeran by Pharmascience	Canadian DIN 02230431	Gastrointestinal
P <> MET500	Tab, White, Round, Scored, Film Coated	Metformin HCl 500 mg	Glucophage by Pharmascience	Canadian DIN 02223562	Antidiabetic
P <> MR	Tab, White with Red Specks, Scored, P <> M/R	Carbamazepine 100 mg	Tegretol by Pharmascience	Canadian DIN 02231542	Anticonvulsant
P <> OM	Tab, Dark Green, Round, O-M P	Inert	Ortho Tri-Cyclen Lo by Ortho-McNeil	00062-1251	Oral Contraceptive; Placebo
P <> OXY5	Tab, Blue, Round, Scored, P <> OXY over 5	Oxybutynin Chloride 5 mg	by Pharmascience	Canadian DIN 02240550	Anticholinergic
P <> P10	Tab, Dark Pink, Rectangular	Pravastatin Sodium 10 mg	Pravachol by Pharmascience	Canadian DIN 02247655	Antihyperlipidemic
P <> P20	Tab, Yellow, Rectangular, P logo <> P 20	Pravastatin Sodium 20 mg	Pravachol by Pharmascience	Canadian DIN 02247656	Antihyperlipidemic
P <> P40	Tab, Green, Rectangular, P logo <> P 40	Pravastatin Sodium 40 mg	Pravachol by Pharmascience	Canadian DIN 02247657	Antihyperlipidemic
P <> PF	Tab, Off-White, Round, Flat-Faced, Scored	Aminophylline USP 225 mg	Phyllocontin by Purdue Pharma	Canadian DIN 02014270	Vasodilator
P <> PF	Tab, Off-White, Square, Scored	Aminophylline USP 350 mg	Phyllocontin 350 by Purdue Pharma	Canadian DIN 02014289	Vasodilator
P <> PF	Tab, White, Round	Aminophylline 225 mg	Aminophylline by Purdue	Canadian	Antiasthmatic
P <> PINDOLOL5	Tab, White, Round, Scored	Pindolol 5 mg	by Pharmascience	Canadian DIN 5760615365	Antihypertensive
P <> PRAVACHOL10	Tab, Pink, Rectangular, Pravachol 10 <> P Logo	Pravastatin Sodium 10 mg	Pravachol by Nat Pharmpak	55154-0606	Antihyperlipidemic
P <> PRAVACHOL10	Tab, Pink, Rectangular, Pravachol 10 <> P Logo	Pravastatin Sodium 10 mg	Pravachol by PDRX	55289-0104	Antihyperlipidemic
P <> PRAVACHOL10	Tab, Pink, Rectangular, Pravachol 10 <> P Logo	Pravastatin Sodium 10 mg	Pravachol by BMS	Canadian DIN 00893749	Antihyperlipidemic
P <> PRAVACHOL10	Tab, Pink, Rounded Square, P Logo <> Pravachol over 10	Pravastatin Sodium 10 mg	Pravachol by BMS	00003-5154	Antihyperlipidemic
P <> PRAVACHOL20	Tab, Yellow, Rectangular, Pravachol over 20	Pravastatin Sodium 20 mg	Pravachol by BMS	00003-0178	Antihyperlipidemic
P <> PRAVACHOL20	Tab, Yellow, Rectangular, Pravachol over 20	Pravastatin Sodium 20 mg	Pravachol by BMS	Canadian	Antihyperlipidemic
P <> PRAVACHOL20	Tab, Yellow, Rounded Square, P Logo <> Pravachol over 20	Pravastatin Sodium 20 mg	Pravachol by Nat Pharmpak	55154-0608	Antihyperlipidemic
P <> PRAVACHOL20	Tab, Yellow, Rounded Square, P Logo <> Pravachol over 20	Pravastatin Sodium 20 mg	Pravachol by BMS	12783-0178	Antihyperlipidemic
P <> PRAVACHOL20	Tab, Yellow, Rounded Square, P Logo <> Pravachol over 20	Pravastatin Sodium 20 mg	Pravachol by BMS	00003-5178	Antihyperlipidemic
P <> PRAVACHOL20	Tab, Yellow, Rounded Square, P Logo <> Pravachol over 20	Pravastatin Sodium 20 mg	Pravachol by BMS	Canadian DIN 00893757	Antihyperlipidemic
P <> PRAVACHOL20	Tab, Yellow, Rounded Rectangular	Pravastatin Sodium 20 mg	Pravigard PAC by BMS	00003-5168 00003-5169	Antihyperlipidemic
P <> PRAVACHOL40	Tab, Green, Rounded Rectangular	Pravastatin Sodium 40 mg	Pravigard PAC by BMS	00003-5173 00003-5174	Antihyperlipidemic
P <> PRAVACHOL40	Tab, Green, Rounded Square, P Logo <> Pravachol over 40	Pravastatin Sodium 40 mg	Pravachol by BMS	00003-5194	Antihyperlipidemic
P <> PRAVACHOL40	Tab, Green, Rounded Square, P Logo <> Pravachol over 40	Pravastatin Sodium 40 mg	Pravachol by Caremark	00339-5746	Antihyperlipidemic

ID FRONT <> BACK	DESCRIPTION FRONT <> BACK	INGREDIENT & STRENGTH	BRAND (or Generic Equiv.) by FIRM	NDC#	CLASS; SCH.
P <> PRAVACHOL40	Tab, Green, Rounded Square, P Logo <> Pravachol over 40	Pravastatin Sodium 40 mg	Pravachol by BMS	Canadian DIN 02222051	Antihyperlipidemic
P <> PRAVACHOL40	Tab, Green, Rounded Square, Pravachol over 40 <> P Logo	Pravastatin Sodium 40 mg	Pravachol by BMS	15548-0194	Antihyperlipidemic
P <> PROPECIA	Tab, Tan, Octagonal, Film Coated, Stylized P	Finasteride 1 mg	Propecia by Merck-Frosst	Canadian DIN 02238213	Antiandrogen
P <> PROPECIA	Tab, Tan, Octagonal, Film Coated, Stylized P	Finasteride 1 mg	Propecia by Merck	00006-0071	Antiandrogen
P <> PU	Tab, White with Red Specks, Oval, Scored, P <> P/U	Carbamazepine 200 mg	Tegretol by Pharmascience	Canadian DIN 02231540	Anticonvulsant
P <> R50	Tab, Purepac Logo <> R/50	Lorazepam 1 mg	Ativan by Kaiser	00179-1093	Antianxiety; C IV
P <> S100	Tab, Pink, Diamond Shaped	Sumatriptan Succinate 100 mg	Imitrex by Pharmascience	Canadian DIN 02256444	Antimigraine
P <> S25	Tab, White, Round	Sumatriptan Succinate 25 mg	Imitrex by Pharmascience	Canadian DIN 02256428	Antimigraine
P <> S50	Tab, White, Diamond Shaped	Sumatriptan Succinate 50 mg	Imitrex by Pharmascience	Canadian DIN 02256436	Antimigraine
P <> SEARLE	Tab	Ethinyl Estradiol 35 mcg, Ethynodiol Diacetate 1 mg	Demulen 1 35 28 by Pharm Util	60491-0181	Oral Contraceptive
P <> SEARLE	Tab	Ethinyl Estradiol 50 mcg, Ethynodiol Diacetate 1 mg	by Physician Total Care	54868-3790	Oral Contraceptive
P <> SEARLE	Tab	Ethinyl Estradiol 50 mcg, Ethynodiol Diacetate 1 mg	Demulen 1 50 28 by Pharm Util	60491-0183	Oral Contraceptive
P <> SEARLE	Tab, White, Round, Placebo	Inert	Demulen 1/35-28 by Searle	00025-0151	Oral Contraceptive; Placebo
P <> SEARLE	Tab	Ethinyl Estradiol 35 mcg, Ethynodiol Diacetate 1 mg	by Physician Total Care	54868-0404	Oral Contraceptive
P <> SEARLE	Tab, Blue, Round	Ethinyl Estradiol 35 mcg, Ethynodiol Diacetate 1 mg	Demulen Compack by Rx Pak	65084-0219	Oral Contraceptive
P <> SEARLE	Tab, Orange, Round	Inert	Synphasic 28 day by Pfizer	Canadian DIN 02187116	Oral Contraceptive; Placebo
P <> SEARLE	Tab, Orange, Round	Inert	Select 1/35 28 day by Pfizer	Canadian DIN 02199297	Oral Contraceptive; Placebo
P <> SEARLE	Tab, Orange, Round	Inert	Demulen 30 28 day by Pfizer	Canadian DIN 0047152	Oral Contraceptive; Placebo
P <> SEARLE	Tab, Orange, Round	Inert	Brevicon .5/35 28 day by Pfizer	Canadian DIN 02187094	Oral Contraceptive; Placebo
P <> SEARLE	Tab, Orange, Round	Inert	Brevicon 1/35 28 day by Pfizer	Canadian DIN 02189062	Oral Contraceptive; Placebo
P <> SEARLE	Tab, Orange, Round	Inert	Demulen 1/50-28 by Searle	00025-0071	Oral Contraceptive; Placebo
P <> SR100	Tab, Pink, Round, Sustained Release	Diclofenac Sodium 100 mg	Voltaren S.R. by Pharmascience	Canadian DIN 02231505	NSAID
P <> SR240	Tab, Light Green, Oblong, Scored	Verapamil HCl 240 mg	Isoptin by Pharmascience	Canadian DIN 02237791	Antihypertensive
P <> SR75	Tab, Pink, Triangle, Sustained Release	Diclofenac Sodium 75 mg	Voltaren S.R. by Pharmascience	Canadian DIN 02231504	NSAID
P <> SUCRALFATE	Tab, White, Oblong, Scored	Sucralfate 1 g	Carafate by Pharmascience	Canadian DIN 02238209	Gastrointestinal
P <> T1	Tab, White, Oblong	Tryptophan 1 g	Tryptan by Pharmascience	Canadian DIN 02230202	Antidepressant
P <> T5	Tab, White, Oblong	Tryptophan 500 mg	Tryptan by Pharmascience	Canadian DIN 02240445	Antidepressant
P <> TRYPTOPHAN500	Tab, White, Cap Shaped, Film Coated	Tryptophan 500 mg	by Pharmascience	Canadian DIN 5760601029	Antidepressant
P <> US144	Tab, White, Round, P <> U-S over 144	Amiodarone HCl 100 mg	Pacerone by Upsher Smith	00245-0144	Antiarrhythmic
P <> WATSON	Tab, Green, Round	Inert	TriNessa by Watson	52544-0935	Oral Contraceptive; Placebo

ID FRONT <> BACK	DESCRIPTION FRONT <> BACK	INGREDIENT & STRENGTH	BRAND (or Generic Equiv.) by FIRM	NDC#	CLASS; SCH.
P <> WATSON	Tab, Green, Round	Inert	Ortho-Cept by Watson	52544-0954	Oral Contraceptive; Placebo
P <> WATSON	Tab, Green, Round	Inert	Necon 7/7/7 by Watson	52544-0936	Oral Contraceptive; Placebo
P <> WATSON	Tab, Green, Round	Inert	Mononessa by Watson	52544-0526	Oral Contraceptive; Placebo
P <> WATSON	Tab, White, Round	Inert	Zovia 1/35 by DRX	55045-2722	Oral Contraceptive; Placebo
P <> WATSON	Tab, White, Round	Inert	Zovia 1/35 by PDRX	55289-0381	Oral Contraceptive; Placebo
P <> WATSON	Tab, White, Round	Inert	Zovia 1/35 by Watson		Oral Contraceptive; Placebo
P <> Z5	Tab, White, Round	Zopiclone 5 mg	Imovane by Pharmascience	Canadian DIN 02243426	Hypnotic
P0	Tab, Red, Round	Pseudoephedrine 30 mg	Sudafed by PFI		Decongestant
P001	Tab, Pink, Cap Shaped, Sugar Coated, P-001	Vitamin A 3000 IU, Vitamin C 120 mg, Vitamin D-3 400 IU, Vitamin E 30 IU, Vitamin B-1 3 mg, Vitamin B-2 3.5 mg, Niacin 20 mg, Vitamin B-6 30 mg, Folic Acid 1 mg, Vitamin B-12 12 mcg, Biotin 30 mcg, Pantothenic Acid 8 mg, Calcium Carbonate 150 mg, Iron 27 mg, Magnesium 75 mg, Zinc 15 mg, Copper 2.5 mg	Natelle by Pharmelle	66663-0317	Vitamin
P001 <> 3	Tab, Purepac Logo	Acetaminophen 300 mg, Codeine Phosphate 30 mg	Tylenol w/ Codeine by Talbert	44514-0223	Analgesic; C III
P0013	Tab, Purepac Logo 001/3	Acetaminophen 300 mg, Codeine Phosphate 30 mg	Tylenol w/ Codeine by Golden State	60429-0500	Analgesic; C III
P0013	Tab, Purepac Logo P 001/3	Acetaminophen 300 mg, Codeine Phosphate 30 mg	Tylenol w/ Codeine by St. Mary's Med	60760-0001	Analgesic; C III
P002	Tab, Blue, Round, Sugar Coated, P-002	Methenamine 81.0 mg, Sodium Biphosphate 40.8 mg, Phenyl Salicylate 32.4 mg, Methylene Blue 10.8 mg, Hyoscyamine Sulfate 0.12 mg	Urelle by Pharmelle	66663-0219	Urinary Antiseptic
P0034	Tab, P003/4 Purepac Logo	Acetaminophen 300 mg, Codeine Phosphate 60 mg	Tylenol w/ Codeine by Actavis		Analgesic; C III
P004	Tab, Light Pink, Cap Shaped, Sugar Coated, P-004	Vitamin A 2700 IU, Vitamin C 120 mg, Vitamin D-3 400 IU, Vitamin E 20 IU, Vitamin B-1 3 mg, Vitamin B-2 3.5 mg, Niacin 20 mg, Vitamin B-6 30 mg, Folic Acid 1 mg, Vitamin B-12 12 mcg, Biotin 30 mcg, Pantothenic Acid 8 mg, Calcium 100 mg, Iron 25 mg, Magnesium 50 mg, Zinc 15 mg, Selenium 50 mcg, Copper 2 mg, Choline Bitartrate 55 mg	Natelle-EZ by Pharmelle	66663-0668	Vitamin
P005	Tab, Light Pink, Cap Shaped, Sugar Coated, P-005	Vitamin A 3000 IU, Vitamin C 120 mg, Vitamin D-3 400 IU, Vitamin E 30 IU, Vitamin B-1 3 mg, Vitamin B-2 3.5 mg, Niacin 20 mg, Vitamin B-6 50 mg, Folic Acid 1 mg, Vitamin B-12 12 mcg, Biotin 30 mcg, Pantothenic Acid 8 mg, Iron 29 mg, Magnesium 75 mg, Zinc 15 mg	Natelle Prefer by Pharmelle	66663-0330	Vitamin
P012	Tab, White, Round, Triangle over P/012	Acetaminophen 325 mg	Tylenol by Advance		Analgesic
P014	Tab, White, Oblong, Lower Case "p" inside inverted triangle	Acetaminophen 500 mg	Tylenol by Advance		Analgesic
P0140	Cap, Gelatin, P in a Triangle	Ergocalciferol 1.25 mg	Vitamin D by Consolidated Midland Corp.	00223-1971	Vitamin
P0140	Cap, Gelatin Coated, P in a Triangle	Ergocalciferol 1.25 mg	Vitamin D by Superior	00144-0639	Vitamin
P0140	Cap, Gelatin, P in a Triangle	Ergocalciferol 1.25 mg	Vitamin D by URL Mutual	00677-0765	Vitamin
P0140	Cap, Gelatin, P in a Triangle 0140	Ergocalciferol 1.25 mg	Vitamin D by Major	00904-0291	Vitamin
P0140	Cap, Gelatin, P in a Triangle	Ergocalciferol 1.25 mg	Vitamin D by Banner Pharma	10888-0140	Vitamin
P02	Tab, Light Yellow to Off White, Diamond Shaped, Scored	Mercaptopurine 50 mg	Purinethol by Par	49884-0922	Antineoplastic
P021	Cap, Purepac Logo 21	Flurazepam HCl 15 mg	by Actavis		Hypnotic; C IV
P022	Cap, Purepac Logo 022	Flurazepam HCl 30 mg	by Actavis		Hypnotic; C IV
P026	Tab, Light Peach, Cushion, P/026	Phenyltoloxamine 325 mg	by Advance		Decongestant
P084	Tab, Yellow, Pentagonal Shaped, Scored	Dexamethasone 0.5 mg	Decadron by Pharmascience	Canadian DIN 01964976	Steroid
P086	Tab, White, Pentagonal, Scored	Dexamethasone 2 mg	Decadron by Pharmascience	Canadian DIN 02279363	Steroid

ID FRONT <> BACK	DESCRIPTION FRONT <> BACK	INGREDIENT & STRENGTH	BRAND (or Generic Equiv.) by FIRM	NDC#	CLASS; SCH.
P087	Cap, White, with Red Bands	Diphenhydramine HCl 25 mg	by Quality Care	60346-0589	Antihistamine
P1	Tab, Brown, Round	Ibuprofen 200 mg	Motrin by PFI		NSAID
P1	Tab, Brown, Round	Ibuprofen 200 mg	Advil by Qualitest	00603-0216	NSAID
P1	Tab, Orange, Oval, Scored	Cilazapril 1 mg	Inhibace by Pharmascience	Canadian DIN 02280442	Antihypertensive
P1	Tab, White, Oblong, Scored	Lorazepam 1 mg	Ativan by Pharmascience	Canadian DIN 00728195	Antianxiety; C IV
P1 <> G	Tab, White, Round, Film Coated	Paroxetine HCl 10 mg	Paxil by Watson	62037-0845	Antidepressant
P1 <> M	Tab, Maroon, Round, Film Coated	Prochlorperazine 5 mg	Compazine by Mylan	00378-5105	Antiemetic
P1 <> M	Tab, Maroon, Round, Film Coated	Prochlorperazine 5 mg	Compazine by UDL	51079-0541 Discontinued	Antiemetic
P1 <> WATSON	Tab, Orange, Round	Inert	Leena by Watson	52544-0219	Oral Contraceptive; Placebo
P1 <> WATSON	Tab, Orange, Round	Inert	Lutera by Watson	52544-0949	Oral Contraceptive; Placebo
P1 <> WATSON	Tab, Orange, Round	Inert	Levora by Watson	52544-0279	Oral Contraceptive; Placebo
P1 <> WATSON	Tab, Orange, Round	Inert	Lo-Ogestrel by Watson	52544-0847	Oral Contraceptive; Placebo
P1 <> WATSON	Tab, Orange, Round	Inert	Tri-Norinyl by Watson	52544-0274	Oral Contraceptive; Placebo
P1 <> WATSON	Tab, Orange, Round	Inert	Quasense by Watson	52544-0966	Oral Contraceptive; Placebo
P10	Tab, White to Off-White, Round, Film-Coated, P over 10	Domperidone 10 mg	Motilium by Pharmascience	Canadian DIN 02236466	Gastrointestinal
P10	Tab, Round, White Scored, P/10	Diazepam 10 mg	Valium by Pharmascience	Canadian DIN 02247492	Antianxiety; C IV
P10	Cap, Red & Beige, Oval, P inside Triangle	Docusate Sodium 100 mg	Colace by Perrigo	00113-0486	Laxative
P10	Tab, Yellow, Round	Meclizine HCl 25 mg	by PFI		Antiemetic
P10	Tab, White, Round, Scored	Medroxyprogesterone Acetate 10 mg	Provera by Pharmascience	Canadian DIN 02246629	Hormone
P10	Tab, Rust Red, Triangular, Scored	Enalapril Maleate 10 mg	Vasotec by Pharmascience	Canadian DIN 02300095	Antihypertensive
P10	Tab, Orange, Round, Scored, P / 10	Propranolol HCl 10 mg	Inderal by Heritage	23155-0110	Antihypertensive
P10	Tab, Pink, Round, Film Coated	Omeprazole 10 mg	PMS-Omeprazole by Pharmascience	Canadian DIN 02310252	Gastrointestinal
P10	Cap, Red and White, Oval, Soft Gel	Docusate Sodium 100 mg	Colace by PL Developments		Laxative
P10 <> G	Tab, White, Round	Pindolol 10 mg	by URL Mutual	00677-1458	Antihypertensive
P10 <> G	Tab, White, Round	Pindolol 10 mg	by Genpharm	55567-0016	Antihypertensive
P10 <> G	Tab, White, Round	Pindolol 10 mg	by Par	49884-0443	Antihypertensive
P10 <> JANSSEN	Tab, White, Round, Scored, Janssen <> P/10	Cisapride 10 mg	by PDRX	55289-0105	Gastrointestinal
P10 <> JANSSEN	Tab, White, Round, Scored, Janssen <> P/10	Cisapride 10 mg	by Nat Pharmpak	55154-1402	Gastrointestinal
P10 <> JANSSEN	Tab, White, Round, Scored, Janssen <> P/10	Cisapride 10 mg	by Pharm Pkg Ctr	54383-0077	Gastrointestinal
P10 <> JANSSEN	Tab, White, Round, Scored, Janssen <> P/10	Cisapride 10 mg	Propulsid by Johnson & Johnson	59604-0430	Gastrointestinal
P10 <> JANSSEN	Tab, White, Round, Scored, Janssen <> P/10	Cisapride 10 mg	by Allscripts		Gastrointestinal
P10 <> P	Tab, Dark Pink, Rectangular	Pravastatin Sodium 10 mg	Pravachol by Pharmascience	Canadian DIN 02247655	Antihyperlipidemic
P100	Cap, Orange & Purple, Opaque, Hard Gel	Minocycline HCl 100 mg	Minocin by Pharmascience	Canadian DIN 5760692391	Antibiotic

ID FRONT <> BACK	DESCRIPTION FRONT <> BACK	INGREDIENT & STRENGTH	BRAND (or Generic Equiv.) by FIRM	NDC#	CLASS; SCH.
P100	Tab, Peach, Shield-Shaped	Lamotrigine 100 mg	Lamictal by Pharmascience	Canadian DIN 02246898	Antiepileptic
P100	Tab, White to Off-White, Oblong, Scored, Film Coated	Fluvoxamine Maleate 100 mg	Luvox by Pharmascience	Canadian DIN 02240683	OCD
P100	Cap, Blue, Opaque	Doxycycline Hyclate 100 mg	Vibramycin by Pharmascience	Canadian DIN 02289539	Antibiotic
P100 <> ATENOLOL	Tab, White, Round, Scored	Atenolol 100 mg	Tenormin by Pharmascience	Canadian DIN 02237601	Antihypertensive
P1015 <> APO	Tab, White, Round	Pioglitazone 15 mg	Actos by Apotex	Canadian DIN 02302942	Antidiabetic
P1030 <> APO	Tab, White, Round	Pioglitazone 30 mg	Actos by Apotex	Canadian DIN 02302950	Antidiabetic
P1045 <> APO	Tab, White, Round	Pioglitazone 45 mg	Actos by Apotex	Canadian DIN 02302977	Antidiabetic
P10G	Tab, White, Round, P10/G	Pindolol 10 mg	Gen Pindolol by Genpharm	Canadian	Antihypertensive
P10JANSSEN	Tab, Beige & White, Circular, P/10/Janssen	Cisapride 10 mg	Propulsid by Janssen	Canadian	Gastrointestinal
P10NIFEDIPINE	Cap, Yellow, Opaque, Soft Gel	Nifedipine 10 mg	by Pharmascience	Canadian DIN 5760658982	Antihypertensive
P10P10	Cap, Grey & Green, Hard Gel, Trade Dress Lic'd	Fluoxetine HCl 10 mg	Prozac by Pharmascience	Canadian DIN 02177579	Antidepressant
P110	Tab, Light Green, Round, Scored, Film Coated, P 1/10	Loxapine 10 mg	by Pharmascience	Canadian DIN 576060 8387	Antipsychotic
P111	Tab, White, Oblong	Acetaminophen 500 mg	Tylenol Ex Strength by PFI		Analgesic
P112	Tab, White, Oblong	Acetaminophen 325 mg, Pseudoephedrine HCl 30 mg, Dextromethorphan HBr 15 mg	by PFI		Cold Remedy
P114	Tab, Yellow, Round	Caffeine 200 mg	by PFI		Stimulant
P115	Tab, Yellow, Round	Acetaminophen 325 mg, Pseudoephedrine HCl 30 mg, Chlorpheniramine 2 mg, Dextromethorphan HBr 15 mg	by PFI		Cold Remedy
P11P11 <> BIBI	Tab, White, Round, Scored	Pramipexole DiHCl 1.5 mg	Mirapex by Boehringer Ingelheim Canada	Canadian DIN 02237147	Antiparkinson
P12	Tab, Blue, Round	Pseudoephedrine 30 mg, Chlorpheniramine 2 mg	by PFI		Cold Remedy
P121	Tab, White, Round	Acetaminophen 500 mg	Tylenol Ex Strength by PFI		Analgesic
P122	Tab, Green, Oblong	Loperamide 2 mg	Imodium by PFI		Antidiarrheal
P125	Tab, Green, Oblong	Pseudoephedrine 30 mg, Diphenhydramine 12.5 mg, Acetaminophen 500 mg	by PFI		Cold Remedy
P125	Tab, Yellow, Round, Scored	Digoxin 0.125 mg	Lanoxin by Pharmascience	Canadian DIN 02245427	Cardiac Agent
P13	Tab, Orange, Round, Enteric Coated	Aspirin 500 mg	Aspirin by PFI		Analgesic
P133	Tab, Reddish Brown, Film Coated, Purepac Logo 133	Amitriptyline HCl 50 mg	Elavil by Actavis		Antidepressant
P14	Tab, Blue, Round	Phenylpropanolamine 25 mg, Brompheniramine 4 mg	by PFI		Cold Remedy
P141	Cap, Yellow	Acetaminophen 500 mg, Pseudoephedrine HCl 30 mg, Chlorpheniramine Maleate 2 mg	by PFI		Cold Remedy
P142	Tab, Orange, Ellipse	Acetaminophen 500 mg, Pseudoephedrine 30 mg	Sudafed Sinus by PFI		Cold Remedy
P144	Tab, Purple, Round, Chewable	Acetaminophen 160 mg	Children's Tylenol by PFI		Analgesic
P147	Tab, Blue, Round	Acetaminophen 500 mg, Pseudoephedrine HCl 30 mg	Sudafed Sinus by PFI		Cold Remedy
P147	Tab, Orange, Oblong	Pseudoephedrine HCl 60 mg, Acetaminophen 500 mg	by PFI		Cold Remedy
P15	Tab, White, Round, P-15	Phenobarbital 15 mg	Phenobarbital by Eon		Sedative/Hypnotic; C IV
P15	Tab, Yellow, Round, Scored, Film Coated, P 1/5	Loxapine 5 mg	by Pharmascience	Canadian DIN 5760603377	Antipsychotic

For updated data, go to www.IdentADrug.com

ID FRONT <> BACK	DESCRIPTION FRONT <> BACK	INGREDIENT & STRENGTH	BRAND (or Generic Equiv.) by FIRM	NDC#	CLASS; SCH.
P15	Tab, White, Round, Chewable	Acetaminophen 80 mg	Children's Tylenol by PFI		Analgesic
P150	Tab, Off-White, Shield-Shaped, Scored	Lamotrigine 150 mg	Lamictal by Pharmascience	Canadian DIN 02246899	Antiepileptic
P150	Tab, Yellow, Oval, Scored, Film Coated	Moclobemide 150 mg	by Pharmascience	Canadian DIN 02243218	Antidepressant
P150	Tab, White, Round, Film Coated	Ranitidine HCl 150 mg	Zantac by Pharmascience	Canadian DIN 02242453	Antihistamine
P150	Cap, Dark Orange	Venlafaxine HCl 150 mg	Effexor XR by Pharmascience	Canadian DIN 02278561	Antidepressant
P150MG	Cap, White	Fluconazole 150 mg	Diflucan by Pharmascience	Canadian DIN 02282348	Antifungal
P151	Tab, Pink, Round	Acetaminophen 325 mg, Pseudoephedrine HCl 30 mg	by PFI		Cold Remedy
P15G	Tab, White, Round, P-15/G	Pindolol 15 mg	Gen Pindolol by Genpharm	Canadian	Antihypertensive
P171	Cap, Yellow	Acetaminophen 650 mg, Pseudoephedrine HCl 60 mg, Dextromethorphan HBr 30 mg	Tylenol Cold Ex Strength by PFI		Cold Remedy
P172	Cap, Blue	Acetaminophen 650 mg, Pseudoephedrine HCl 60 mg, Diphenhydramine HCl 50 mg	Contac Night Allergy Relief by PFI		Cold Remedy
P174	Tab, Yellow, Cap Shaped	Acetaminophen 325 mg, Pseudoephedrine HCl 30 mg, Chlorpheniramine 2 mg, Dextromethorphan HBr 15 mg	Multi-Symptom Cold Relief by PFI		Cold Remedy
P177	Tab, White, Oval	Diphenhydramine HCl 25 mg, Pseudoephedrine HCl 60 mg	by PFI		Antihistamine
P19	Tab, Orange, Round, Enteric Coated	Aspirin 325 mg	Aspirin by PFI		Analgesic
P2	Tab, White, Round	Ibuprofen 200 mg	Motrin by PFI		NSAID
P2	Tab, White, Round, Scored, P/2	Diazepam 2 mg	Valium by Pharmascience	Canadian DIN 02247490	Antianxiety; C IV
P2	Tab, White, Oval, Scored	Lorazepam 2 mg	Ativan by Pharmascience	Canadian DIN 00728209	Antianxiety; C IV
P2 <> DOXA	Tab, White, Oblong, Scored	Doxazosin Mesylate 2 mg	Cardura by Pharmascience	Canadian DIN 02244528	Antihypertensive
P2 <> G	Tab, White, Round, Film Coated	Paroxetine HCl 20 mg	Paxil by Watson	62037-0846	Antidepressant
P2 <> M	Tab, Maroon, Round, Film Coated	Prochlorperazine 10 mg	Compazine by Mylan	00378-5110	Antiemetic
P2 <> M	Tab, Maroon, Round, Film Coated	Prochlorperazine 10 mg	Compazine by UDL	51079-0542 Discontinued	Antiemetic
P20	Tab, White, Round, P-20	Pseudoephedrine 60 mg	Sudafed by Circa		Decongestant
P20	Cap, Amber, Oval, Clear	Docusate Sodium 250 mg	Colace by URL	00677-0192	Laxative
P20	Cap, Orange, Oval, Clear	Docusate Sodium 250 mg	Colace by Major	00904-7891	Laxative
P20	Cap, Red, Oval, P inside inverted Triangle	Docusate Sodium 250 mg	Colace by Paddock	00574-0102	Laxative
P20	Tab, Yellow, Brown Print, Oval	Pantoprazole Sodium 20 mg	Protonix by Wyeth	00008-0843	Gastrointestinal
P20	Tab, White, Round	Acetaminophen 325 mg, Phenylpropanolamine HCl 12.5 mg, Chlorpheniramine Maleate 2 mg	by PFI		Cold Remedy
P20	Tab, Yellow, Brown Print, Oval	Pantoprazole Sodium 20 mg	Protonix by BYK Canada	Canadian DIN 02241804	Gastrointestinal
P20	Tab, Rust Red, Triangular, Scored	Enalapril Maleate 20 mg	Vasotec by Pharmascience	Canadian DIN 02300109	Antihypertensive
P20	Tab, Yellow, Brown Print, Oval	Pantoprazole Sodium 20 mg	Protonix by Ranbaxy	Canadian DIN 02305038	Gastrointestinal
P20	Tab, Blue, Round, Scored, P / 20	Propranolol HCl 20 mg	Inderal by Heritage	23155-0111	Antihypertensive
P20	Tab, Red Brown, Round, Film Coated	Omeprazole 20 mg	PMS-Omeprazole by Pharmascience	Canadian DIN 02310260	Gastrointestinal
P20	Tab, Yellow, Oval, Enteric Coated	Pantoprazole Sodium 20 mg	Pantoprazole by Pro Doc Limitee	Canadian DIN 02318687	Gastrointestinal

ID FRONT <> BACK	DESCRIPTION FRONT <> BACK	INGREDIENT & STRENGTH	BRAND (or Generic Equiv.) by FIRM	NDC#	CLASS; SCH.
P20 <> APO	Tab, Yellow, Oval, Coated	Pantoprazole Sodium 20 mg	Pantoloc by Apotex	Canadian DIN 02292912	Gastrointestinal
P20 <> JANSSEN	Tab, Blue, Oval, P/20 <> Janssen	Cisapride 20 mg	Propulsid by Caremark	00339-6024	Gastrointestinal
P20 <> JANSSEN	Tab, Blue, Oval, P/20 <> Janssen	Cisapride 20 mg	Propulsid by Janssen	50458-0440	Gastrointestinal
P20 <> JANSSEN	Tab, Blue, Oval, P/20 <> Janssen	Cisapride 20 mg	Propulsid by Johnson & Johnson	59604-0440	Gastrointestinal
P20 <> P	Tab, Yellow, Rectangular, P logo <> P 20	Pravastatin Sodium 20 mg	Pravachol by Pharmascience	Canadian DIN 02247656	Antihyperlipidemic
P200	Tab, Pink, Round, Scored	Amiodarone 200 mg	Cordarone by Pharmascience	Canadian DIN 02242472	Antiarrhythmic
P200 <> US0147	Tab, Pink, Round, Scored, U-S over 0147	Amiodarone 200 mg	Cordarone by Pharmascience	Canadian DIN 576063613	Antiarrhythmic
P200 <> US0147	Tab, Pink, Round, Scored, U-S over 0147	Amiodarone HCl 200 mg	Pacerone by Apotheca	12634-0543	Antiarrhythmic
P200 <> US0147	Tab, Pink, Round, Scored, U-S over 0147	Amiodarone 200 mg	Cordarone by Thrift Drug	59198-0362	Antiarrhythmic
P200 <> US0147	Tab, Pink, Round, Scored, U-S over 0147	Amiodarone 200 mg	Cordarone by Upsher Smith	00245-0147	Antiarrhythmic
P203	Tab, Purepac Logo 20/3	Acetaminophen 300 mg, Codeine Phosphate 30 mg	Tylenol w/ Codeine by McNeil	52021-0020	Analgesic; C III
P207	Tab, White, Oblong, Scored	Sucralfate 1000 mg	Carafate by PFI	10916-0429	Gastrointestinal
P20P20	Cap, Yellow and Green, Hard Gel	Fluoxetine HCl 20 mg	Prozac by Pharmascience	Canadian DIN 02177587	Antidepressant
P21	Tab, Blue, Round	Diphenhydramine HCl 25 mg	by PFI		Antihistamine
P21	Tab, Green, Round, P-21	Imipramine HCl 50 mg	Tofranil by Eon		Antidepressant
P210	Tab, Yellow, Oblong	Phenylpropanolamine HCl 75 mg	by PFI		Decongestant; Appetite Suppressant
P211	Tab, Green, Oblong	Acetaminophen 500 mg, Pseudoephedrine 30 mg	Sudafed Sinus by PFI		Cold Remedy
P2120	Cap, White, Soft Gel, P in an Inverted Triangle 2120	Valproic Acid 250 mg	Depakene by Teva	00480-0757	Anticonvulsant
P2120	Cap, Gelatin Coated, P Inside of Upside Down Triangle	Valproic Acid 250 mg	Depakene by URL Mutual	00677-1079	Anticonvulsant
P2120	Cap, Gelatin Coated, P Inside of Upside Down Triangle	Valproic Acid 250 mg	Depakene by Moore	00839-7180	Anticonvulsant
P2120	Cap, Gelatin Coated, P Inside of Upside Down Triangle	Valproic Acid 250 mg	Depakene by Banner Pharma	10888-2120	Anticonvulsant
P2120	Cap, Gelatin Coated	Valproic Acid 250 mg	Depakene by Qualitest	00603-6334	Anticonvulsant
P214	Tab, P 21/4	Acetaminophen 300 mg, Codeine Phosphate 60 mg	Tylenol w/ Codeine by McNeil	52021-0021	Analgesic; C III
P214	Tab, Orange, Oblong	Acetaminophen 325 mg, Pseudoephedrine HCl 30 mg, Dextromethorphan HBr 10 mg	by PFI		Cold Remedy
P218	Tab, Yellow, Oblong	Triprolidine 2.5 mg, Pseudoephedrine 60 mg	Actifed by PFI		Cold Remedy
P219	Tab, Blue, Oblong	Pseudoephedrine HCl 60 mg, Diphenhydramine HCl 25 mg	by PFI		Cold Remedy
P221	Tab, Orange, Round	Acetaminophen 500 mg, Pseudoephedrine 30 mg	Sudafed Sinus by PFI		Cold Remedy
P224	Tab, Blue, Oblong	Acetaminophen 500 mg, Phenylpropanolamine HCl 12.5 mg, Brompheniramine 2 mg	by PFI		Cold Remedy
P225	Tab, White, Oblong	Magnesium Salicylate 467 mg	by PFI		Analgesic
P225	Tab, Green, Oblong	Magnesium Salicylate 500 mg	by PFI		Analgesic
P227	Tab, Yellow, Oblong	Phenylpropanolamine 25 mg, Chlorpheniramine 4 mg	by PFI		Cold Remedy
P23	Tab, White, Round	Aspirin 400 mg, Caffeine 32 mg	Anacin by PFI		Analgesic
P241	Tab, Yellow, Oblong	Pseudoephedrine HCl 30 mg, Acetaminophen 500 mg	by PFI		Cold Remedy
P243	Tab, White, Oblong	Acetaminophen 500 mg, Pamabrom 25 mg, Pyrilamine 15 mg	Midol by PFI		PMS Relief
P25	Tab, White, Round	Dimenhydrinate 50 mg	Dramamine by PFI		Antiemetic
P25	Tab, Peach, Round, P-25	Hydrochlorothiazide 25 mg	Hydrodiuril by Eon		Diuretic; Antihypertensive
P25	Tab, White to Off-White, Shield-Shaped, Scored	Lamotrigine 25 mg	Lamictal by Pharmascience	Canadian DIN 02246897	Antiepileptic
P25	Tab, White, Oval, Scored, P 2.5	Enalapril Maleate 2.5 mg	Vasotec by Pharmascience	Canadian DIN 02300079	Antihypertensive

ID FRONT <> BACK	DESCRIPTION FRONT <> BACK	INGREDIENT & STRENGTH	BRAND (or Generic Equiv.) by FIRM	NDC#	CLASS; SCH.
P25	Tab, Orange, Oval, Scored, P 2.5	Cilazapril 2.5 mg	Inhibace by Pharmascience	Canadian DIN 02280450	Antihypertensive
P25	Tab, Peach, Round, P 2.5	Medroxyprogesterone Acetate 2.5 mg	Provera by Pharmascience	Canadian DIN 02246627	Hormone
P250	Cap, Red and Yellow, Opaque	Amoxicillin 250 mg	Amoxil by Pharmascience	Canadian DIN 02230243	Antibiotic
P250	Cap, Blue & Yellow, Opaque, Hard Gel	Mefenamic Acid 250 mg	Ponstel by Pharmascience	Canadian DIN 02231208	NSAID
P250	Tab, White, Round, Scored	Digoxin 0.25 mg	Lanoxin by Pharmascience	Canadian DIN 02245428	Cardiac Agent
P250 <> FLUTAMIDE	Tab, Pale Yellow, Round, Scored	Flutamide 250 mg	by Pharmascience	Canadian DIN 02230104	Antiandrogen
P250 <> TERBINAFINE	Tab, White, Round, Scored	Terbinafine HCl 250 mg	Lamisil by Pharmascience	Canadian DIN 02240807	Antifungal
P252	Tab, Yellow, Round	Acetaminophen 325 mg, Pseudoephedrine HCl 30 mg, Chlorpheniramine 2 mg, Dextromethorphan HBr 10 mg	by PFI		Cold Remedy
P253	Tab, Yellow, Oblong	Acetaminophen 325 mg, Pseudoephedrine HCl 30 mg, Chlorpheniramine 2 mg, Dextromethorphan HBr 10 mg	by PFI		Cold Remedy
P254	Cap, Purple	Ibuprofen 200 mg	Motrin by PFI		NSAID
P254	Cap, Brown & Ivory	Ibuprofen 200 mg	Motrin by Pharma Formulations		NSAID
P255	Tab, White, Ellipse	Pseudoephedrine 30 mg, Acetaminophen 500 mg, Diphenhydramine 12.5 mg	by PFI		Cold Remedy
P262	Tab, Buff, Round	Phenolphthalein 90 mg	by PFI		Gastrointestinal
P27	Tab, Purepac Logo	Propranolol HCl 10 mg	Inderal by Golden State	60429-0227	Antihypertensive
P29	Tab, Purepac Logo	Propranolol HCl 20 mg	Inderal by Golden State	60429-0164	Antihypertensive
P291	Tab, Off White to Light Yellow, Diamond Shaped	Amiloride HCl 5 mg	Midamor by Paddock	00574-0116	Diuretic
P2M	Tab, Maroon, Round, P2/M	Prochlorperazine 10 mg	Compazine by Mylan		Antiemetic
P2MG <> LOPERAMIDE	Tab, Green, Cap Shaped, Scored, P/2 mg	Loperamide 2 mg	Imodium by Pharmascience	Canadian DIN 02228351	Antidiarrheal
P3	Tab, White, Oblong	Acetaminophen 160 mg	Children's Tylenol by PFI		Analgesic
P3 <> G	Tab, White, Round, Film Coated	Paroxetine HCl 30 mg	Paxil by Andrx	62037-0847	Antidepressant
P30	Cap, Dark Red, Oval, Soft Gel, P inside Triangle	Docusate Sodium 100 mg, Casanthranol 31.5 mg	Peri-Colace by Perrigo	00113-0495	Laxative
P30	Tab, White, Round, P-30	Phenobarbital 30 mg	by Eon		Sedative/Hypnotic; C IV
P30	Tab, Tan, Oblong, Brown Specks	Calcium Polycarbophil 625 mg	Fiberlax by PFI		Vitamin; Mineral
P300	Cap, Green & Ivory	Acetaminophen 325 mg, Chlorpheniramine 2 mg, Pseudoephedrine HCl 30 mg	by PFI		Cold Remedy
P300	Tab, Ivory and Green, Cap Shaped	Acetaminophen 500 mg, Chlorpheniramine 2 mg, Pseudoephedrine HCl	Duadacin by Kenwood	00482-0730	Cold Remedy
P300	Tab, White, Cap Shaped, Film Coated	Ranitidine HCl 300 mg	Zantac by Pharmascience	Canadian DIN 02242454	Antihistamine
P300	Tab, White, Oval, Scored, Film Coated	Moclobemide 300 mg	by Pharmascience	Canadian DIN 02243219	Antidepressant
P300	Cap, Maroon and White	Gemfibrozil 300 mg	Lopid by Pharmascience	Canadian DIN 02239951	Antihyperlipidemic
P300 <> TIAPROFENIC	Tab, White, Round, Scored	Tiaprofenic 300 mg	Surgam by Pharmascience	Canadian DIN 02230828	NSAID
P300 <> US0140	Tab, Peach, Round, Scored, P subscript 300 <> U-S over 0140	Amiodarone HCl 300 mg	Pacerone by Upsher Smith	00245-0140	Antiarrhythmic
P301	Cap, Green & White	Acetaminophen 500 mg, Pseudoephedrine 30 mg	Sudafed Sinus by PFI		Cold Remedy
P31	Tab, Coated, Purepac Logo	Amitriptyline HCl 10 mg	Elavil by Quality Care	60346-0354	Antidepressant

ID FRONT <> BACK	DESCRIPTION FRONT <> BACK	INGREDIENT & STRENGTH	BRAND (or Generic Equiv.) by FIRM	NDC#	CLASS; SCH.
P316	Cap, Red & White	Acetaminophen 500 mg	Tylenol Ex Strength by PFI		Analgesic
P32	Tab, Coated, Purepac Logo 32	Amitriptyline HCl 25 mg	Elavil by Actavis		Antidepressant
P32	Tab, Orange, Round, Chewable	Aspirin 81 mg	Aspirin by PFI		Analgesic
P32	Tab, White, Round, P-32	Reserpine 0.1 mg	Serpasil by Eon		Antihypertensive
P325	Tab, Blue, Oblong	Acetaminophen 500 mg, Diphenhydramine HCl 25 mg	Tylenol PM by PFI		Cold Remedy
P325	Tab, White, Round, Scored	Acetaminophen 325 mg	Tylenol by Pharmascience	Canadian DIN 00891177	Analgesic
P33	Tab, White, Round	Diphenhydramine HCl 25 mg	Benedryl by PFI		Antihistamine
P33 <> LL	Tab, White, Round, Scored, P over 33	Propylthiouracil 50 mg	Propylthiouracil by Lederle	00005-4609	Antithyroid
P33 <> LL	Tab, White, Round, Scored, P over 33	Propylthiouracil 50 mg	Propylthiouracil by Physician Total Care	54868-1752	Antithyroid
P334	Tab, Blue, Round	Acetaminophen 500 mg, Diphenhydramine HCl 25 mg	Tylenol PM by PFI		Cold Remedy
P337	Tab, White, Oblong	Acetaminophen 500 mg, Pseudoephedrine HCl 30 mg, Chlorpheniramine Maleate 2 mg	by PFI		Cold Remedy
P34	Tab, Pink, Round	Acetaminophen 325 mg, Pseudoephedrine HCl 30 mg, Chlorpheniramine Maleate 2 mg	by PFI		Cold Remedy
P345	Tab, Aqua & Ivory, Oblong	Calcium Carbonate 311 mg, Magnesium Carbonate 232 mg			Vitamin; Mineral
P346	Cap, Orange & Red	Acetaminophen 325 mg, Pseudoephedrine HCl 30 mg, Dextromethorphan HBr 15 mg	by PFI		Cold Remedy
P349	Cap, Blue	Acetaminophen 500 mg, Diphenhydramine HCl 25 mg	Tylenol PM by PFI		Cold Remedy
P35	Tab, White, Round, Scored	Clonazepam 2 mg	by Pharmacy Serv Ctr	00855-0762	Sedative; C IV
P35	Tab, Red, Round	Pseudoephedrine 30 mg	Sudafed by Circa		Decongestant
P350 <> PF	Tab, White, Square	Aminophylline 350 mg	Aminophylline by Purdue	Canadian	Antiasthmatic
P36	Tab, White, Round, Scored, P over 36	Pyrazinamide 500 mg	Riftar by Dava	67253-0660	Antibiotic
P36 <> LL	Tab, White, Round, Scored, P over 36	Pyrazinamide 500 mg	by Amerisource	62584-0848	Antibiotic
P36 <> LL	Tab, White, Round, Scored, P over 36	Pyrazinamide 500 mg	by PDRX	55289-0283	Antibiotic
P36 <> LL	Tab, White, Round, Scored, P over 36	Pyrazinamide 500 mg	Pyrazinamide by UDL	51079-0691	Antibiotic
P36 <> LL	Tab, White, Round, Scored, P over 36	Pyrazinamide 500 mg	by Lederle	00005-5093	Antibiotic
P375	Cap, Grey and Peach, P 37.5	Venlafaxine HCl 37.5 mg	Effexor XR by Pharmascience	Canadian DIN 02278545	Antidepressant
P384	Tab, Purple, Round	Acetaminophen 80 mg, Chlorpheniramine Maleate 0.5 mg, Pseudoephedrine HCl 7.5 mg, Dextromethorphan 3.75 mg	Children's Tylenol Cold Plus Cough by PFI		Cold Remedy
P3900	Cap, Gelatin, P in a Triangle	Guaifenesin 90 mg, Theophylline 150 mg	Bronchial by Banner Pharma	10888-3900	Antiasthmatic
P4	Tab, White, Round	Pseudoephedrine 30 mg, Chlorpheniramine 4 mg	by PFI		Cold Remedy
P4 <> G	Tab, White, Round, Film Coated	Paroxetine HCl 40 mg	Paxil by Andrx	62037-0848	Antidepressant
P40	Tab, White, Round, P over 40	Furosemide 40 mg	Lasix by Pharmascience	Canadian DIN 02247494	Diuretic
P40	Tab, Yellow, Oval, Enteric Coated	Pantoprazole Sodium 40 mg	Pantoloc by BYK Canada	Canadian DIN 02229453	Gastrointestinal
P40	Tab, Green, Round, Scored, P / 40	Propranolol HCl 40 mg	Inderal by Heritage	23155-0112	Antihypertensive
P40	Tab, Yellow, Oval, Enteric Coated	Pantoprazole Sodium 40 mg	Pantoloc by Ranbaxy	Canadian DIN 02305046	Gastrointestinal
P40	Tab, Yellow, Oval, Enteric Coated	Pantoprazole Sodium 40 mg	Pantoprazole by Pro Doc Limitee	Canadian DIN 02318695	Gastrointestinal
P40 <> APO	Tab, Yellow, Oval, Coated	Pantoprazole Sodium 40 mg	Pantoloc by Apotex	Canadian DIN 02292920	Gastrointestinal
P40 <> P	Tab, Green, Rectangular, P logo <> P 40	Pravastatin Sodium 40 mg	Pravachol by Pharmascience	Canadian DIN 02247657	Antihyperlipidemic
P400	Tab, White, Oval, Scored	Norfloxacin 400 mg	Noroxin by Pharmascience	Canadian DIN 02246596	Antibiotic

ID FRONT <> BACK	DESCRIPTION FRONT <> BACK	INGREDIENT & STRENGTH	BRAND (or Generic Equiv.) by FIRM	NDC#	CLASS: SCH.
P400 <> 0145	Tab, Light Yellow, Oval, Scored	Amiodarone 400 mg	Cordarone by Upsher Smith	00245-0145	Antiarrhythmic
P406	Cap, Hard Gelatin, Purepac Logo	Tetracycline HCl 500 mg	by Quality Care	60346-0435	Antibiotic
P41	Tab, White, Round	Acetaminophen 325 mg	Tylenol by PFI		Analgesic
P411	Tab, Pink, Oval	Diphenhydramine HCl 25 mg	by PFI		Antihistamine
P412	Tab, White, Round	Aspirin 250 mg, Acetaminophen 250 mg, Caffeine 65 mg	by PFI		Analgesic
P416	Tab, Blue, Round	Phenolphthalein 135 mg	by PFI		Gastrointestinal
P419	Cap, Clear & Red	Acetaminophen 650 mg, Pseudoephedrine HCl 30 mg, Dextromethorphan HBr 15 mg	Tylenol Cold Ex Strength by PFI		Cold Remedy
P42	Tab, White, Oblong	Ibuprofen 200 mg	Motrin by PFI		NSAID
P42	Tab, White, Oblong	Ibuprofen 200 mg	Motrin IB by Qualitest	00603-0217	NSAID
P420	Cap, Beige	Acetaminophen 500 mg, Pseudoephedrine HCl 30 mg, Chlorpheniramine Maleate 2 mg	by PFI		Cold Remedy
P421	Tab, Green, Round, Film Coated	Phenobarbital 48.6 mg, Hyoscyamine Sulfate 0.3111 mg, Atropine Sulfate 0.0582 mg, Scopolamine Hydrobromide 0.0195 mg	Donnatal Extentabs by PBM	66213-0421	Gastrointestinal; C IV
P422	Tab, White, Round	Acetaminophen 500 mg, Pseudoephedrine HCl 30 mg, Chlorpheniramine Maleate 2 mg	Tylenol Allergy by PFI		Cold Remedy
P43	Tab, Brown, Oblong	Ibuprofen 200 mg	Motrin by PFI		NSAID
P431	Tab, Blue, Oblong	Acetaminophen 500 mg, Pseudoephedrine HCl 30 mg, Chlorpheniramine Maleate 2 mg	by PFI		Cold Remedy
P434	Tab, Blue, Round	Naproxen 200 mg	by PFI		NSAID
P434	Tab, Light Blue, Round	Naproxen 220 mg	Aleve by Ivax	00182-1097 Discontinued	NSAID
P44	Tab, Blue, Round	Diphenhydramine HCl 50 mg	by PFI		Antihistamine
P44 <> LL	Tab, Gray, Round, Scored	Propranolol HCl 10 mg	Inderal by Lederle	00005-3109	Antihypertensive
P440	Tab, White, Oblong	Acetaminophen 500 mg, Pamabrom 25 mg, Pyrilamine 15 mg	Midol by PFI		PMS Relief
P441	Tab, Orange, Oblong	Pseudoephedrine HCl 30 mg, Acetaminophen 500 mg	by PFI		Cold Remedy
P445	Tab, Blue, Oblong	Naproxen 200 mg	by PFI		NSAID
P452	Tab, Pink, Round, Chewable	Acetaminophen 80 mg, Dextromethorphan HBr 2.5 mg, Pseudoephedrine HCl 7.5 mg	Tylenol Cold by PFI		Cold Remedy
P454	Tab, Blue, Oblong	Acetaminophen 500 mg, Phenylpropanolamine HCl 12.5 mg, Chlorpheniramine 2 mg, DM 15 mg	by PFI		Cold Remedy
P457	Tab, Maroon, Round	Acetaminophen 500 mg, Diphenhydramine HCl 50 mg	Tylenol PM by PFI		Cold Remedy
P458	Tab, Blue, Round	Acetaminophen 500 mg, Diphenhydramine HCl 38 mg	Tylenol PM by PFI		Cold Remedy
P459	Tab, Purple, Round	Diphenhydramine HCl 12.5 mg	Benadryl by PFI		Antihistamine
P460	Tab, Yellow, Oblong	Acetaminophen 500 mg, Diphenhydramine HCl 12.5 mg	by PFI		Cold Remedy
P4600	Cap, P in a Triangle	Benzonatate 100 mg	Tessalon by URL Mutual	00677-1472	Antitussive
P4600	Cap, Gelatin, P Inside of Triangle	Benzonatate 100 mg	Tessalon by Qualitest	00603-2426	Antitussive
P4600	Cap, Gelatin, P in a Triangle 4600	Benzonatate 100 mg	Tessalon by Murfreesboro	51129-1148	Antitussive
P4600	Cap, Gelatin, P in a Triangle 4600	Benzonatate 100 mg	Tessalon by Kaiser	00179-1256	Antitussive
P4600	Cap, Gelatin, P in a Triangle	Benzonatate 100 mg	Tessalon by Warner Chilcott	00047-0048	Antitussive
P4600	Cap, Gelatin Coated, P in a Triangle 4600	Benzonatate 100 mg	Tessalon by PDRX	55289-0175	Antitussive
P4600	Cap, Gelatin, P in a Triangle	Benzonatate 100 mg	Tessalon by Banner Pharma	10888-4600	Antitussive
P467	Tab, White, Round	Acetaminophen 500 mg, Pseudoephedrine HCl 30 mg, Chlorpheniramine Maleate 2 mg	by PFI		Cold Remedy
P47	Tab, Purple, Round, Chewable	Acetaminophen 80 mg	Children's Tylenol by PFI		Analgesic
P484	Tab, White, Round	Acetaminophen 250 mg, Aspirin 250 mg, Caffeine 65 mg	Excedrin Migraine by PFI		Analgesic

ID FRONT <> BACK	DESCRIPTION FRONT <> BACK	INGREDIENT & STRENGTH	BRAND (or Generic Equiv.) by FIRM	NDC#	CLASS; SCH.
P485	Tab, Yellow, Round	Bisacodyl 5 mg	Dulcolax by PFI	00113-0389	Gastrointestinal
P4900	Cap, Orange, Soft Gel, P inside Triangle	Dextromethorphan 10 mg, Pseudoephedrine 30 mg	Sudafed Cold/Flu by Perrigo	Canadian DIN 02247491	Cold Remedy
P5	Tab, White, Round, Scored, P/5	Diazepam 5 mg	Valium by Pharmascience	Canadian DIN 02246628	Antianxiety; C IV
P5	Tab, White, Round, Scored	Medroxyprogesterone Acetate 5 mg	Provera by Pharmascience	Canadian DIN 02300087	Hormone
P5	Tab, White, Triangular, Scored	Enalapril Maleate 5 mg	Vasotec by Pharmascience	Canadian DIN 02280469	Antihypertensive
P5	Tab, Maroon, Oval, Scored	Cilazapril 5 mg	Inhibace by Pharmascience	49884-0442	Antihypertensive
P5 <> G	Tab	Pindolol 5 mg	by Par	00677-1457	Antihypertensive
P5 <> G	Tab	Pindolol 5 mg	by URL Mutual	55567-0015	Antihypertensive
P5 <> G	Tab	Pindolol 5 mg	by Genpharm	Canadian DIN 5760692381	Antihypertensive
P50	Cap, Orange, Opaque, Hard Gel	Minocycline HCl 50 mg	Minocin by Pharmascience		Antibiotic
P50	Tab, Pink, Round	Diphenhydramine HCl 25 mg	by PFI		Antihistamine
P50 <> ATENOLOL	Tab, White, Round, Scored	Atenolol 50 mg	Tenormin by Pharmascience	Canadian DIN 02237600	Antihypertensive
P500	Cap, Purepac Logo	Prazosin HCl 1 mg	by Actavis	60429-0159	Antihypertensive
P500	Cap, Purepac Logo	Prazosin HCl	by Golden State	Canadian DIN 02230244	Antihypertensive
P500	Cap, Red and Yellow, Opaque	Amoxicillin 500 mg	Amoxil by Pharmascience	50111-0790	Antibiotic
P500	Tab, Pink, Cap Shaped, Film Coated	Acetaminophen 500 mg, Propoxyphene Napsylate 100 mg	Darvocet by Pliva	Canadian DIN 00892505	Analgesic; C IV
P500	Tab, White, Round, Scored	Acetaminophen 500 mg	Tylenol Ex Strength by Pharmascience	60429-0160	Analgesic
P501	Cap, Purepac Logo	Prazosin HCl	by Golden State	60429-0161	Antihypertensive
P502	Cap, Purepac Logo	Prazosin HCl	by Golden State	51079-0019	Antihypertensive
P51	Cap, Clear Bright Orange, Oval, Soft Gel	Docusate Sodium 100 mg	Colace by UDL	Discontinued	Laxative
P51	Cap, Clear Bright Orange, Oval, Soft Gel	Docusate Sodium 100 mg	Colace by Qualitest	00603-0146	Laxative
P51	Cap, Clear Bright Orange, Oval, Soft Gel	Docusate Sodium 100 mg	Colace by Major	00904-7889	Laxative
P51	Cap, Clear Bright Orange, Oval, Soft Gel	Docusate Sodium 100 mg	Colace by Major	00904-2244	Laxative
P51	Cap, Clear Bright Orange, Oval, Soft Gel	Docusate Sodium 100 mg	Colace by Paddock	00574-0101	Laxative
P51	Cap, Clear Bright Orange, Oval, Soft Gel	Docusate Sodium 100 mg	Colace by Ivax	00182-0287 Discontinued	Laxative
P51	Cap, Clear Bright Orange, Oval, Soft Gel	Docusate Sodium 100 mg	Colace by Amneal	65162-0614	Laxative
P51	Cap, Clear Bright Orange, Oval, Soft Gel	Docusate Sodium 100 mg	Colace by Ivax	00182-1417 Discontinued	Laxative
P511	Tab, White & Yellow, Round	Acetaminophen 325 mg, Phenylephrine HCl 5 mg, Chlorpheniramine Maleate 2 mg	by PFI		Cold Remedy
P5124	Cap, White & Blue, Opaque, Hard Gel, P over 5124	Fluoxetine HCl 10 mg	Prozac by Actavis	00228-2702	Antidepressant
P5125	Cap, White & Violet, Opaque, Hard Gel, P over 5125	Fluoxetine HCl 20 mg	Prozac by Actavis	00228-2703	Antidepressant
P513	Tab, Pink, Round	Calcium Carbonate 400 mg	Os-Cal by PFI		Vitamin; Mineral
P514	Tab, Orange, Round, Chewable	Pseudoephedrine HCl 15 mg	by PFI		Decongestant
P515	Tab, Yellow, Oblong	Guaifenesin 200 mg, Pseudoephedrine 30 mg, Acetaminophen 325 mg, Dextromethorphan 15 mg	by PFI		Cold Remedy
P516	Tab, Orange, Round	Calcium Carbonate 400 mg	Os-Cal by PFI		Vitamin; Mineral
P52	Tab, White, Oblong	Acetaminophen 500 mg, Calcium Carbonate 250 mg	by PFI		Analgesic
P537	Tab, Ivory & Orange, Oblong	Acetaminophen 500 mg	Tylenol Ex Strength by PFI		Analgesic

ID FRONT <> BACK	DESCRIPTION FRONT <> BACK	INGREDIENT & STRENGTH	BRAND (or Generic Equiv.) by FIRM	NDC#	CLASS; SCH.
P542	Tab, Blue, Round	Naproxen 220 mg	by Par	60346-0875 Discontinued	NSAID
P547	Tab, Film Coated	Naproxen 275 mg	by Quality Care	53002-0252	NSAID
P553	Cap	Erythromycin 250 mg	by Pharmedix	00182-1398	Antibiotic
P553	Cap	Erythromycin 250 mg	by Ivax	44514-0515	Antibiotic
P555	Tab, Embossed, Film Coated	Metoprolol Tartrate 100 mg	Lopressor by Talbert	51079-0071 Discontinued	Antihypertensive
P58	Cap, Red, Soft Gel, Translucent, P inside Triangle	Docusate Calcium 240 mg	Surfak by UDL	00904-7892	Laxative
P58	Cap, Red, Soft Gel, Translucent, P inside Triangle	Docusate Calcium 240 mg	Surfak by Major	00603-0306	Laxative
P58	Cap, Red, Soft Gel, Translucent, P inside Triangle	Docusate Calcium 240 mg	Surfak by Qualitest	00182-8221	Laxative
P58	Cap, Red, Soft Gel, Translucent, P inside Triangle	Docusate Calcium 240 mg	Surfak by Ivax	00182-1302 Discontinued	Laxative
P593	Tab, White, Cap Shaped	Acetaminophen 500 mg, Pamabrom 25 mg	PMS Formula by PFI		PMS Relief
P5NIFEDIPINE	Cap, Yellow, Opaque, Soft Gel	Nifedipine 5 mg	by Pharmascience	Canadian DIN 5760658972	Antihypertensive
P6	Tab, White, Round	Cimetidine HCl 100 mg	Tagamet HB by PFI		Gastrointestinal
P60	Tab, Pink, Round, Scored, P / 60	Propranolol HCl 60 mg	Inderal by Heritage	23155-0113	Antihypertensive
P62	Cap, Red	Docusate Sodium 250 mg	Colace by Paddock		Laxative
P64	Tab, Pink, Round, Chewable	Acetaminophen 80 mg	Children's Tylenol by PFI		Analgesic
P67	Tab, White, Oval	Cimetidine HCl 200 mg	Tagamet by PFI		Gastrointestinal
P7	Tab, Yellow, Round	Chlorpheniramine Maleate 4 mg	Chlor-Trimeton by PFI		Antihistamine
P71	Cap, Green, Soft Gel	Guaifenesin 200 mg, Pseudoephedrine 30 mg	Sudafed Sinus by Perrigo	00113-0537	Cold Remedy
P72	Cap Red, Soft Gel, P inside Triangle	Pseudoephedrine 30 mg, Dextromethorphan 10 mg, Guaifenesin 200 mg	by Perrigo	00113-0226	Cold Remedy
P73	Tab, Yellow, Round, Enteric Coated	Aspirin 81 mg	Aspirin by PFI		Analgesic
P74	Cap, Green, Soft Gel, P Inside Triangle 74	Pseudoephedrine HCl 30 mg, Doxylamine Succinate 6.25 mg, Acetaminophen 250 mg, Dextromethorphan HBr 10 mg	Nite Time Liquid Capsules by Perrigo	00113-0193	Cold Remedy
P75	Tab, Light Pink, Round	Ranitidine 75 mg	Zantac by Dr. Reddy's	55111-0131	Gastrointestinal
P75	Tab, Green, Oval	Magnesium Salicylate 325 mg	by PFI		Analgesic
P75	Cap, Peach	Venlafaxine HCl 75 mg	Effexor XR by Pharmascience	Canadian DIN 02278553	Antidepressant
P77	Tab, White, Round	Aspirin 325 mg	Aspirin by PFI		Analgesic
P77 <> 511	Tab, White, Oblong, Ex Release	Pentoxifylline 400 mg	Trental by ESI Lederle	59911-3290	Anticoagulant
P771	Tab, White, Round, P over 771	Atropine Sulfate 0.025 mg, Diphenoxylate HCl 2.5 mg	Lomotil by Par	49884-0771	Antidiarrheal; C V
P7P7 <> BIBI	Tab, White, Oval, Scored	Pramipexole DiHCl 0.25 mg	Mirapex by Boehringer Ingelheim Canada	Canadian DIN 02237145	Antiparkinson
P8	Tab, White, Round	Triprolidine 2.5 mg, Pseudoephedrine 60 mg	Actifed by PFI		Cold Remedy
P80	Tab, Yellow, Round, Scored, P / 80	Propranolol HCl 80 mg	Inderal by Heritage	23155-0114	Antihypertensive
P80	Tab, White, Round	Gliclazide 80 mg	Diamicron by Pharmascience	Canadian DIN 02294400	Antidiabetic
P8040	Cap, Red	Amantadine HCl 100 mg	Symmetrel by Pharmascience	Canadian DIN 01990403	Antiviral
P8P8 <> BIBI	Tab, White, Oval, Scored	Pramipexole DiHCl 0.5 mg	Mirapex by Boehringer Ingelheim Canada	Canadian DIN 02241594	Antiparkinson
P9	Tab, Brown, Round, P-9	Imipramine HCl 25 mg	Tofranil by Eon		Antidepressant
P912	Tab, Pink, Round	Docusate Sodium 100 mg, Phenolphthalein 65 mg	Correctol by PFI		Laxative

ID FRONT <> BACK	DESCRIPTION FRONT <> BACK	INGREDIENT & STRENGTH	BRAND (or Generic Equiv.) by FIRM	NDC#	CLASS; SCH.
P9523	Tab, White, Round	Phenobarbital 16 mg	Solfoton by Poythress		Sedative/Hypnotic; C IV
P97 <> W	Tab, Pink, Black Print, Round, Film Coated	Primaquine Phosphate 26.3 mg	Primaquine by Sanofi	00024-1596	Antimalarial
P97 <> W	Tab, Pink, Black Print, Round, Film Coated	Primaquine Phosphate 26.3 mg	by Bayer	00280-1596	Antimalarial
P97 <> W	Tab, Pink, Black Print, Round, Film Coated	Primaquine Phosphate 26.3 mg	Primaquine by Sanofi	Canadian	Antimalarial
P9P9 <> BIBI	Tab, White, Round, Scored	Pramipexole DiHCl 1 mg	Mirapex by Boehringer Ingelheim Canada	Canadian DIN 02237146	Antiparkinson
PA <> 307	Tab, White, Round, Film Coated	Hydroxyzine HCl 10 mg	Atarax by Pliva	50111-0307	Antianxiety; Antihistamine
PA <> 307	Tab, White, Round, Film Coated	Hydroxyzine HCl 10 mg	Atarax by UDL	51079-0413	Antianxiety; Antihistamine
PA <> 308	Tab, White, Round, Sugar Coated	Hydroxyzine HCl 25 mg	Atarax by Pliva	50111-0308	Antianxiety; Antihistamine
PA <> 309	Tab, White, Round, Sugar Coated	Hydroxyzine HCl 50 mg	Atarax by Pliva	50111-0309	Antianxiety; Antihistamine
PA <> 546	Tab, White, Round, Enteric Coated	Diclofenac Sodium 50 mg	Voltaren by Pliva	50111-0546	NSAID
PA <> 547	Tab, White, Round, Enteric Coated	Diclofenac Sodium 75 mg	Voltaren by Pliva	50111-0547	NSAID
PA <> 608	Tab, White, Round, Film Coated	Ketorolac Tromethamine 10 mg	Toradol by Pliva	50111-0608	NSAID
PA09	Cap, Off-White, Oval, Soft Gel	Cyclosporine 25 mg	Neoral by Pliva	50111-0909	Immunosuppressant
PA1000	Cap, Orange & Clear, Oval, Soft Gel	Ethosuximide 250 mg	Zarontin by Pliva	50111-0901	Anticonvulsant
PA140	Cap, Green, Oval, Softgel	Vitamin D 50,000 IU	Drisdol by Pliva	50111-0990	Vitamin
PA20	Cap, Off-White, Oblong, Soft Gel	Cyclosporine 100 mg	Neoral by Pliva	50111-0920	Immunosuppressant
PA2120	Cap, White, Oblong, Soft Gel	Valproic Acid 250 mg	Depakene by Pliva	50111-0852	Anticonvulsant
PA46	Cap, Yellow, White Print, Soft Gel	Benzonatate 100 mg	Tessalon by Pliva	50111-0851	Antitussive
PA550	Tab, White, Black Print, Round, Film Coated	Cimetidine HCl 300 mg	Tagamet by Pliva	50111-0550	Gastrointestinal
PA551	Tab, White, Black Print, Cap Shaped, Scored, Film Coated, PA over 551	Cimetidine HCl 400 mg	Tagamet by Pliva	50111-0551	Gastrointestinal
PA552	Tab, White, Black Print, Cap Shaped, Scored, Film Coated, PA over 552	Cimetidine HCl 800 mg	Tagamet by Pliva	50111-0552	Gastrointestinal
PA614	Tab, Light Green, Cap Shaped, Film Coated	Naproxen 375 mg	Naprosyn by Pliva	50111-0614	NSAID
PA615	Tab, Green, Cap Shaped, Film Coated	Naproxen 500 mg	Naprosyn by Pliva	50111-0615	NSAID
PA675	Tab, Pale Pink, Round	Fluconazole 50 mg	Diflucan by Pliva	50111-0675	Antifungal
PA915	Tab, White, Round, Scored	Torsemide 5 mg	Demadex by Pliva	50111-0915	Diuretic
PA916	Tab, White, Round, Scored	Torsemide 10 mg	Demadex by Pliva	50111-0916	Diuretic
PA917	Tab, White, Round	Torsemide 20 mg	Demadex by Pliva	50111-0917	Diuretic
PA918	Tab, White, Round, Scored	Torsemide 100 mg	Demadex by Pliva	50111-0918	Diuretic
PAC20	Tab, White	Famotidine 20 mg	Pepcid AC Max Strength by Merck	71683-0855	Gastrointestinal
PAD0107	Tab, White, Round, Lozenge	Clotrimazole 10 mg	Mycelex Troches by Paddock	00574-0107	Antifungal
PAD0115	Tab, White, Round, Film Coated	Flavoxate HCl 100 mg	Urispas by Paddock	00574-0115	Antispasmodic
PAD0116	Tab, Round, Film Coated, Scored	Benzphetamine HCl 50 mg	Didrex by Paddock	00574-0116	Sympathomimetic; C III
PAD112	Tab, Dark Beige, Round, Film Coated, Scored	Moexipril HCl 15 mg	Univasc by Paddock	00574-0112	Antihypertensive
PAL	Tab, Beige, Round, PAL <> Heart outline	Folic Acid 2.5 mg, Pyridoxine HCl 25 mg, Cyanocobalamin 2 mg	Foltx by Pamlab	00525-0906	Vitamin
PAL <> 032	Tab, Purple, Oval, Scored	Acetaminophen 712.8 mg, Caffeine 60 mg, Dihydrocodeine Bitartrate 32 mg	Panlor SS by Mikart	46672-0141	Analgesic; C III
PAL <> 032	Tab, Purple, Oval, Scored	Acetaminophen 712.8 mg, Caffeine 60 mg, Dihydrocodeine Bitartrate 32 mg	Panlor SS by Pamlab	00525-0032	Analgesic; C III
PAL <> 0754	Tab, Green, Oblong, Scored	Pseudoephedrine HCl 45 mg, Guaifenesin 600 mg, Dextromethorphan HBr 30 mg	Panmist DM by Sovereign	58716-0687	Cold Remedy
PAL <> 0754	Tab, Green, Oblong, Scored	Pseudoephedrine HCl 45 mg, Guaifenesin 600 mg, Dextromethorphan HBr 30 mg	Panmist DM by Pamlab	00525-0754 Discontinued	Cold Remedy
PAL <> 0759	Tab, Green, Cap Shaped, Scored	Pseudoephedrine HCl 48 mg, Guaifenesin 595 mg, Dextromethorphan HBr 32 mg	Panmist DM by Pamlab	00525-0759 Discontinued	Cold Remedy
PAL <> 0768	Tab, White, Cap Shaped	Pseudoephedrine HCl 48 mg, Guaifenesin 595 mg	Panmist Jr. by Pamlab	00525-0768 Discontinued	Cold Remedy
PAL <> 0775	Tab	Guaifenesin 600 mg, Pseudoephedrine HCl 90 mg	Panmist LA by Pamlab	00525-0775 Discontinued	Cold Remedy

ID FRONT <> BACK	DESCRIPTION FRONT <> BACK	INGREDIENT & STRENGTH	BRAND (or Generic Equiv.) by FIRM	NDC#	CLASS; SCH.
PAL <> 0775	Tab	Guaifenesin 600 mg, Pseudoephedrine HCl 90 mg	Panmist LA by Sovereign	58716-0658 Discontinued	Cold Remedy
PAL <> 0780	Tab, White w/ Green Specks	Chlorpheniramine Maleate 8 mg, Methscopolamine Nitrate 2.5 mg, Phenylpropanolamine HCl 75 mg	Pannaz by Murfreesboro	51129-1429 Discontinued	Cold Remedy
PAL <> 0780	Tab, White w/ Green Specks	Chlorpheniramine Maleate 8 mg, Methscopolamine Nitrate 2.5 mg, Phenylpropanolamine HCl 75 mg	Pannaz by Anabolic	00722-6337 Discontinued	Cold Remedy
PAL <> 0780	Tab, White w/ Green Specks	Chlorpheniramine Maleate 8 mg, Methscopolamine Nitrate 2.5 mg, Phenylpropanolamine HCl 75 mg	Pannaz by Pamlab	00525-0780 Discontinued	Cold Remedy
PAL <> 0788	Tab, White w/ Green Specks, Scored	Pseudoephedrine HCl 90 mg, Chlorpheniramine HCl 8 mg, Methscopolamine 2.5 mg	Rescon by Pamlab	00525-0788 Discontinued	Cold Remedy
PAL <> 0792	Tab, White with Red Spots, Cap Shaped, PAL <> 07/92	Pseudoephedrine HCl 85 mg, Guaifenesin 795 mg	Panmist LA by Pamlab	00525-0792 Discontinued	Cold Remedy
PAL <> 10	Tab, Light Yellow, Round, Coated, PAL <> 1.0	L-methylfolate (Metafolin) 1.0 mg	Zervalx by PAMLAB	00525-1010	Supplement
PAL <> 2	Tab, Peach, Round	Folic Acid 2.5 mg, Pyridoxine HCl 25 mg, Cyanocobalamin 1 mg	Foltx by Pamlab	00525-0855 Discontinued	Vitamin
PAL <> 4	Tab, White, Round, Scored	Carbinoxamine Maleate 4 mg	Palgic by PamLab	00525-6748	Cold Remedy
PAL <> 5	Tab, Yellow, Round	Folacin 5 mg, Niacinamide 20 mg, Cobalamin 1 mg, Pantothenic Acid 10 mg, Pyridoxine HCl 50 mg, D-Biotin 300 mcg, Thiamine HCl 1.5 mg, Vitamin C 60 mg, Riboflavin 1.5 mg	Diatx by PamLab	00525-0316	Vitamin
PAL <> 5FE	Tab, Red, Round, PAL <> 5Fe	Iron 100 mg, Vitamin C 60 mg, D-biotin 0.3 mg, Pantothenic Acid (B5) 10 mg, Niacinamide (B3) 20 mg, Riboflavin (B2) 1.5 mg, Thiamine HCl (B1) 1.5 mg, Pyridoxine HCl (B6) 50 mg, Cyanocobalamin (B12) 1 mg, Folacin 5 mg	Diatx Fe by PamLab	00525-0503	Dietary Supplement
PAL <> 600	Tab, Blue, Oval, Coated	L-methylfolate (Metafolin) 5.6 mg, Methylcobalamin 2 mg, N-acetylcysteine 600 mg	Cerefolin NAC by PamLab	00525-0510	Vitamin; Supplement
PAL <> 6121	Tab, White, Oblong, Scored	Carbinoxamine Maleate 8 mg, Pseudoephedrine HCl 80 mg	Palgic D by PamLab	00525-6121	Cold Remedy
PAL <> 6131	Tab, White, Cap Shaped, Scored	Carbinoxamine Maleate 8 mg, Pseudoephedrine HCl 80 mg	Palgic D by PamLab	00525-6131	Cold Remedy
PAL <> 75	Tab, Blue, Round, Coated, PAL <> 7.5	L-methylfolate (Metafolin) 7.5 mg	Deplin by PamLab	00525-0410	Supplement
PAL <> 762	Tab, White, Oval, Scored	Pseudoephedrine HCl 45 mg, Guaifenesin 600 mg	Panmist JR by Sovereign	58716-0680 Discontinued	Cold Remedy
PAL <> 762	Tab, White, Oval, Scored	Pseudoephedrine HCl 45 mg, Guaifenesin 600 mg	Panmist JR by Pamlab	00525-0762 Discontinued	Cold Remedy
PAL <> 88	Tab, Light Green, Oblong, Scored	Pseudoephedrine HCl 90 mg, Carbinoxamine Maleate 8 mg, Methscopolamine Nitrate 2.5 mg	Pannaz by PamLab	00525-0880	Cold Remedy
PAL <> JUL42	Tab, White, Scored	Pseudoephedrine HCl 85 mg, Guaifenesin 795 mg	Panmist LA by Sovereign	58716-0692	Cold Remedy
PAL <> M	Tab, Purple, Round, Coated	L-methylfolate Calcium (Metafolin) 3 mg, Pyridoxal-5'-Phosphate 35 mg, Methylcobalamin 2 mg	Metanx by PAMLAB, LLC.	00525-8019	Supplement
PAL <> M5	Tab, Blue, Round, Coated	L-methylfolate 5.635 mg, Riboflavin 5 mg, Pyridoxine 50 mg, Cyanocobalamin 1 mg	Cerefolin by Pamlab	00525-0503	Vitamin; Supplement
PAL0016	Cap, Red, White Print	Acetaminophen 356.4 mg, Caffeine 30 mg, Dihydrocodeine Bitartrate 16 mg	Panlor DC by Mikart	46672-0267	Analgesic; C III
PAL0016	Cap, Red, White Print	Acetaminophen 356.4 mg, Caffeine 30 mg, Dihydrocodeine Bitartrate 16 mg	Panlor DC by PAMLAB, LLC.	00525-0016 Discontinued	Analgesic; C III
PAL0305	Cap, Green & Orange	Dyphylline 200 mg, Guaifenesin 100 mg	Panfil G by Pamlab	00525-0305	Antiasthmatic; Expectorant
PAL0305	Cap, Green & Orange	Dyphylline 200 mg, Guaifenesin 100 mg	Panfil G by Mikart	46672-0202	Antiasthmatic; Expectorant
PAL3	Tab, White, Cap Shaped, Extended Release	Paliperidone 3 mg	Invega by Janssen	Canadian DIN 02300273	Antipsychotic
PAL6	Tab, Beige, Cap Shaped, Extended Release	Paliperidone 6 mg	Invega by Janssen	Canadian DIN 02300281	Antipsychotic
PAL9	Tab, Pink, Cap Shaped, Extended Release	Paliperidone 9 mg	Invega by Janssen	Canadian DIN 02300303	Antipsychotic

ID FRONT <> BACK	DESCRIPTION FRONT <> BACK	INGREDIENT & STRENGTH	BRAND (or Generic Equiv.) by FIRM	NDC#	CLASS; SCH.
PALAFER	Cap, Scarlet, White Ink	Ferrous Fumarate 300 mg	Palafer by GSK	Canadian DIN 01923420	Supplement
PALAFERCF	Cap, Pink and Scarlet, White Ink	Ferrous Fumarate 300 mg, Ascorbic Acid 200 mg, Folic Acid 0.5 mg	Palafer CF by GSK	Canadian DIN 01923455	Supplement
PALI3	Tab, White, Cap Shaped, Extended Release	Paliperidone 3 mg	Invega by Janssen	50458-0550	Antipsychotic
PALI6	Tab, Beige, Cap Shaped, Extended Release	Paliperidone 6 mg	Invega by Janssen	50458-0551	Antipsychotic
PALI9	Tab, Pink, Cap Shaped, Extended Release	Paliperidone 9 mg	Invega by Janssen	50458-0552	Antipsychotic
PAMELORSSANDOZ-10MG	Cap, White & Orange, "S" inside Triangle, a Logo Pamelor 10 mg	Nortriptyline HCl 10 mg	Pamelor by Mallinckrodt	00406-9910	Antidepressant
PAMELORSSANDOZ-25MG	Cap, White & Orange, a Logo, Pamelor, "S" inside Triangle, SANDOZ, 25 mg	Nortriptyline HCl 25 mg	Pamelor by Mallinckrodt	00406-9911	Antidepressant
PAMELORSSANDOZ-50MG	Cap, White, "S" inside Triangle, a Logo Pamelor 50 mg	Nortriptyline HCl 50 mg	Pamelor by Mallinckrodt	00406-9912	Antidepressant
PAMELORSSANDOZ-75MG	Cap, Orange, "S" inside Triangle, a Logo Pamelor 75 mg	Nortriptyline HCl 75 mg	Pamelor by Mallinckrodt	00078-0079	Antidepressant
PAMELORSSANDOZ-75MG	Cap, Orange, "S" inside Triangle, a Logo Pamelor 75 mg	Nortriptyline HCl 75 mg	Pamelor by Mallinckrodt	00406-9913	Antidepressant
PAMINE	Tab, White, Round	Methscopolamine Bromide 2.5 mg	Pamine by Kenwood	00482-0061	Gastrointestinal
PAMINE5	Tab, White, Oval	Methscopolamine Bromide 5 mg	Pamine Forte by Kenwood	00482-0062	Gastrointestinal
PAMPRIN	Cap, Yellow/Red	Pamabrom 25 mg, Pyrilamine Maleate 15 mg, Acetaminophen 500 mg	Pamprin ES by Chattem	Canadian	PMS Relief
PAMPRIN	Cap, White	Acetaminophen 500 mg, Pamabrom 25 mg, Pyrilamine Maleate 15 mg	Pamprin by Chattem	Canadian DIN 00718130	PMS Relief
PAMPRINPMS	Cap, White	Acetaminophen 500 mg, Pamabrom 25 mg, Pyrilamine Maleate 15 mg	Pamprin by Chattem	Canadian DIN 02240359	PMS Relief
PAN2000	Cap, White, PAN/2000	Amylase 20,000 Units, Lipase 4500 Units, Protease 25,000 Units	Pancrease by Jones		Gastrointestinal
PAN2001	Cap, Delayed Release, PAN/2001	Pancreatin 195.73 mg	Pancrelipase by JMI Canton	00252-2001	Gastrointestinal
PAN2001	Cap, Delayed Release, PAN/2001	Pancreatin 195.73 mg	Pancrelipase by Jones	52604-2001	Gastrointestinal
PANCREASEMCNEIL	Cap, Clear & White, Red Print, Pancrease over McNeil	Amylase 20,000 Units, Lipase 4500 Units, Protease 25,000 Units	Pancrease by Janssen-Ortho	Canadian DIN 02242374	Gastrointestinal
PANCREASEMCNEIL	Cap, Clear & White, Red Print, Pancrease over McNeil	Amylase 20,000 Units, Lipase 4500 Units, Protease 25,000 Units	Pancrease by Prestige	58056-0350	Gastrointestinal
PANCREASEMCNEIL	Cap, Clear & White, Red Print, Pancrease over McNeil	Amylase 20,000 Units, Lipase 4500 Units, Protease 25,000 Units	Pancrease by Leiner	59606-0714	Gastrointestinal
PANCREASEMCNEIL	Cap, Clear & White, Red Print, Pancrease over McNeil	Amylase 20,000 Units, Lipase 4500 Units, Protease 25,000 Units	Pancrease by McNeil	00045-0095	Gastrointestinal
PANCREASEMCNEIL	Cap, Clear & White, Red Print, Pancrease over McNeil	Amylase 20,000 Units, Lipase 4500 Units, Protease 25,000 Units	Pancrease by McNeil	52021-0095	Gastrointestinal
PANCREASEMT10-MCNEIL	Cap, Clear & Brown, Black Print, Pancrease over MT 10 over McNeil	Amylase 30,000 Units, Lipase 10,000 Units, Protease 30,000 Units	Pancrease Mt 10 by Murfreesboro	51129-9416	Gastrointestinal
PANCREASEMT10-MCNEIL	Cap, Clear & Brown, Black Print, Pancrease over MT 10 over McNeil	Amylase 30,000 Units, Lipase 10,000 Units, Protease 30,000 Units	Pancrease Mt 10 by McNeil	00045-0342	Gastrointestinal
PANCREASEMT10-MCNEIL	Cap, Clear & Brown, Black Print, Pancrease over MT 10 over McNeil	Amylase 30,000 Units, Lipase 10,000 Units, Protease 30,000 Units	Pancrease Mt 10 by McNeil	52021-0342	Gastrointestinal
PANCREASEMT10-MCNEIL	Cap, Clear & Brown, Black Print, Pancrease over MT 10 over McNeil	Amylase 30,000 Units, Lipase 10,000 Units, Protease 30,000 Units	Pancrease Mt 10 by Janssen-Ortho	Canadian DIN 00789437	Gastrointestinal
PANCREASEMT16-MCNEIL	Cap, Clear & Salmon, Black Print, Pancrease over MT 16 over McNeil	Amylase 48,000 Units, Lipase 16,000 Units, Protease 48,000 Units	Pancrease Mt 16 by Janssen-Ortho	Canadian DIN 00789429	Gastrointestinal
PANCREASEMT16-MCNEIL	Cap, Clear & Salmon, Black Print, Pancrease over MT 16 over McNeil	Amylase 48,000 Units, Lipase 16,000 Units, Protease 48,000 Units	Pancrease Mt 16 by McNeil	52021-0343	Gastrointestinal
PANCREASEMT16-MCNEIL	Cap, Clear & Salmon, Black Print, Pancrease over MT 16 over McNeil	Amylase 48,000 Units, Lipase 16,000 Units, Protease 48,000 Units	Pancrease Mt 16 by McNeil	00045-0343	Gastrointestinal
PANCREASEMT16-MCNEIL	Cap, Clear & Salmon, Black Print, Pancrease over MT 16 over McNeil	Amylase 48,000 Units, Lipase 16,000 Units, Protease 48,000 Units	Pancrease Mt 16 by Murfreesboro	51129-1171	Gastrointestinal
PANCREASEMT20-MCNEIL	Cap, White, Opaque	Amylase 56,000 Units, Lipase 20,000 Units, Protease 44,000 Units	Pancrease Mt 20 by Murfreesboro	51129-2530	Gastrointestinal

ID FRONT <> BACK	DESCRIPTION FRONT <> BACK	INGREDIENT & STRENGTH	BRAND (or Generic Equiv.) by FIRM	NDC# Canadian DIN	CLASS; SCH.
PANCREASEMT4MCNEIL	Cap, Clear and Yellow, Black Print, Pancrease over MT 4 over McNeil	Lipase 16,000 Units, Amylase 48,000 Units, Protease 48,000 Units	Pancrease Mt 4 by Janssen-Ortho	00789445	Gastrointestinal
PANCRECARBMS16DCI	Cap, Clear, Hard Gel, Blue Ink	Lipase 16,000 Units, Amylase 52,000 Units, Protease 52,000 Units	Pancrecarb Ms-16 by Digestive Care	59767-0003	Gastrointestinal
PANCRECARBMS4DCI	Cap, Blue Ink, Delayed Release	Amylase 25,000 Units, Lipase 4000 Units, Protease 25,000 Units	Pancrecarb Ms-4 by Digestive Care	59767-0002	Gastrointestinal
PANCRECARBMS8DCI	Cap, Delayed Release	Amylase 40,000 Units, Lipase 8000 Units, Protease 45,000 Units	Pancrecarb Ms-8 by Digestive Care	59767-0001	Gastrointestinal
PAR <> 012	Tab, Coated	Hydroxyzine HCl 10 mg	by Par	49884-0012	Antianxiety; Antihistamine
PAR <> 013	Tab, Coated	Hydroxyzine HCl 25 mg	by Par	49884-0013	Antianxiety; Antihistamine
PAR <> 014	Tab, Coated	Hydroxyzine HCl 50 mg	Atarax by Par	49884-0014	Antianxiety; Antihistamine
PAR <> 015	Tab, Layered	Meclizine HCl 50 mg	by Par	49884-0015	Antiemetic
PAR <> 016	Tab	Chlorzoxazone 250 mg	by Par	49884-0016	Muscle Relaxant
PAR <> 034	Tab, Blue & White, Oval	Meclizine HCl 12.5 mg	Antivert by Ivax	00182-0871	Antiemetic
PAR <> 034	Tab, Blue & White, Oval	Meclizine HCl 12.5 mg	Antivert by Schein	00364-0411	Antiemetic
PAR <> 034	Tab, Blue & White, Oval	Meclizine HCl 12.5 mg	Antivert by Vangard	00615-1553	Antiemetic
PAR <> 034	Tab, Blue & White, Oval	Meclizine HCl 12.5 mg	Antivert by Par	49884-0034	Antiemetic
PAR <> 034	Tab, Blue & White, Oval	Meclizine HCl 12.5 mg	Antivert by PDRX	55289-0982	Antiemetic
PAR <> 034	Tab, Blue & White, Oval	Meclizine HCl 12.5 mg	Antivert by Amerisource	62584-0772	Antiemetic
PAR <> 034	Tab, Blue & White, Oval	Meclizine HCl 12.5 mg	Antivert by URL Mutual	00677-0418	Antiemetic
PAR <> 034	Tab, Blue & White, Oval	Meclizine HCl 12.5 mg	Antivert by Major	00904-2384	Antiemetic
PAR <> 034	Tab, Blue & White, Oval	Meclizine HCl 12.5 mg	Antivert by Qualitest	00603-4319	Antiemetic
PAR <> 034	Tab, Blue & White, Oval	Meclizine HCl 12.5 mg	Antivert by UDL	51079-0089	Antiemetic
PAR <> 035	Tab, Yellow & White, Oval, Scored	Meclizine HCl 25 mg	Antivert by UDL	51079-0090	Antiemetic
PAR <> 035	Tab, Yellow & White, Oval, Scored	Meclizine HCl 25 mg	Antivert by Ivax	00182-0872	Antiemetic
PAR <> 035	Tab, Yellow & White, Oval, Scored	Meclizine HCl 25 mg	Antivert by Schein	00364-0412	Antiemetic
PAR <> 035	Tab, Yellow & White, Oval, Scored	Meclizine HCl 25 mg	Antivert by Par	49884-0035	Antiemetic
PAR <> 035	Tab, Yellow & White, Oval, Scored	Meclizine HCl 25 mg	Antivert by Pharmedix	53002-0351	Antiemetic
PAR <> 035	Tab, Yellow & White, Oval, Scored	Meclizine HCl 25 mg	Antivert by Amerisource	62584-0774	Antiemetic
PAR <> 035	Tab, Yellow & White, Oval, Scored	Meclizine HCl 25 mg	Antivert by Vangard	00615-1554	Antiemetic
PAR <> 035	Tab, Yellow & White, Oval, Scored	Meclizine HCl 25 mg	Antivert by Qualitest	00603-4320	Antiemetic
PAR <> 035	Tab, Yellow & White, Oval, Scored	Meclizine HCl 25 mg	Antivert by URL Mutual	00677-0419	Antiemetic
PAR <> 061	Tab, Film Coated	Fluphenazine HCl 1 mg	by Schein	00364-2265	Antipsychotic
PAR <> 061	Tab, Film Coated	Fluphenazine HCl 1 mg	by Qualitest	00603-3666	Antipsychotic
PAR <> 062	Tab, Coated	Fluphenazine HCl 2.5 mg	by Schein	00364-2266	Antipsychotic
PAR <> 062	Tab, Coated	Fluphenazine HCl 2.5 mg	by Qualitest	00603-3667	Antipsychotic
PAR <> 064	Tab, Film Coated	Fluphenazine HCl 10 mg	by Qualitest	00603-3669	Antipsychotic
PAR <> 064	Tab, Film Coated	Fluphenazine HCl 10 mg	by Schein	00364-2268	Antipsychotic
PAR <> 091	Tab, Yellow, Round, Film Coated	Doxycycline 50 mg	Monoclox by Par	49884-0091	Antibiotic
PAR <> 092	Tab, Light Orange, Round, Film Coated	Doxycycline 75 mg	Monoclox by Par	49884-0092	Antibiotic
PAR <> 093	Tab, Yellow, Round, Film Coated	Doxycycline 100 mg	Monoclox by Par	49884-0093	Antibiotic
PAR <> 114	Tab, Coated, Debossed	Metronidazole 500 mg	by Par		Antibiotic
PAR <> 187	Tab, Film Coated	Hydrochlorothiazide 25 mg, Methyldopa 250 mg	by Par	49884-0187	Diuretic; Antihypertensive
PAR <> 188	Tab, Coated	Hydrochlorothiazide 30 mg, Methyldopa 500 mg	by Par	49884-0188	Diuretic; Antihypertensive
PAR <> 225	Tab	Haloperidol 2 mg	Haldol by Ivax	00182-1264	Antipsychotic
PAR <> 236	Tab, Peach, Round, Scored, Film Coated	Doxycycline 150 mg	Monoclox by Par	49884-0236	Antibiotic
PAR <> 246	Tab, Lavender	Aspirin 325 mg, Carisoprodol 200 mg	Soma Compound by Schein	00364-2524	Analgesic; Muscle Relaxant
PAR <> 265	Tab, Coated	Amitriptyline 12.5 mg, Chlordiazepoxide 5 mg	Limbitrol by Par	49884-0265	Antianxiety; C IV
PAR <> 266	Tab, Coated	Amitriptyline 25 mg, Chlordiazepoxide 10 mg	Limbitrol DS by Par	49884-0266	Antianxiety; C IV
PAR <> 468	Tab, Elongated Shape, Film Coated	Ibuprofen 600 mg	Motrin by Par		NSAID
PAR <> 469	Tab, Film Coated	Ibuprofen 400 mg	Motrin by Par		NSAID

ID FRONT <> BACK	DESCRIPTION FRONT <> BACK	INGREDIENT & STRENGTH	BRAND (or Generic Equiv.) by FIRM	NDC#	CLASS; SCH.
PAR <> 511	Tab, White, Cap Shaped, Coated	Minocycline 50 mg	Dynacin by Par	49884-0511	Antibiotic
PAR <> 512	Tab, White, Cap Shaped, Coated	Minocycline 75 mg	Dynacin by Par	49884-0512	Antibiotic
PAR <> 513	Tab, White, Cap Shaped, Coated	Minocycline 100 mg	Dynacin by Par	49884-0513	Antibiotic
PAR <> 54	Tab, Yellow, Triangle	Imipramine HCl 10 mg	Tofranil by Murfreesboro	51129-1534	Antidepressant
PAR <> 54	Tab, Yellow, Triangular, Sugar Coated	Imipramine HCl 10 mg	Tofranil by Allscripts		Antidepressant
PAR <> 55	Tab, Brown, Black Print, Round, Sugar Coated	Imipramine HCl 25 mg	Tofranil by Amerisource	62584-0750	Antidepressant
PAR <> 55	Tab, Brown, Black Print, Round, Sugar Coated	Imipramine HCl 25 mg	Tofranil by Par	49884-0055	Antidepressant
PAR <> 55	Tab, Brown, Black Print, Round, Sugar Coated	Imipramine HCl 25 mg	Tofranil by Ivax	00182-0827	Antidepressant
PAR <> 55	Tab, Brown, Black Print, Round, Sugar Coated	Imipramine HCl 25 mg	Tofranil by URL Mutual	00677-0422	Antidepressant
PAR <> 556	Tab, White, Oval	Lisinopril 2.5 mg	Zestril by Par	49884-0556	Antihypertensive
PAR <> 557	Tab, White, Cap Shaped	Lisinopril 5 mg	Zestril by Par	49884-0557	Antihypertensive
PAR <> 558	Tab, White, Round	Lisinopril 10 mg	Zestril by Par	49884-0558	Antihypertensive
PAR <> 559	Tab, White, Round	Lisinopril 20 mg	Zestril by Par	49884-0559	Antihypertensive
PAR <> 56	Tab, Green, Round, Sugar Coated	Imipramine HCl 50 mg	Tofranil by Par	49884-0056	Antidepressant
PAR <> 56	Tab, Black Print, Sugar Coated	Imipramine HCl 50 mg	Tofranil by Amerisource	62584-0751	Antidepressant
PAR <> 560	Tab, White to Off-White, Round	Lisinopril 40 mg	Zestril by Par	49884-0560	Antihypertensive
PAR <> 635	Tab, White, Round	Lisinopril 30 mg	Zestril by Par	49884-0635	Antihypertensive
PAR <> 850	Tab, Off-White to Yellow, Round	Meloxicam 7.5 mg	Mobic by Par	49884-0850	NSAID
PAR <> 851	Tab, Off-White to Yellow, Oval	Meloxicam 15 mg	Mobic by Par	49884-0851	NSAID
PAR <> 961	Tab, Blue, Round, Film Coated	Chlordiazepoxide 5 mg, Amitriptyline HCl 12.5 mg	Limbitrol by Par	49884-0961	Antidepressant; Antianxiety
PAR009	Tab, Blue, Round, Scored, par over 009	Isosorbide Dinitrate 30 mg	Isordil by Par	49884-0009	Antianginal
PAR018	Cap, Blue & White	Doxycycline Hyclate 50 mg	Vibramycin by Par		Antibiotic
PAR019	Cap, Blue, Par/019	Doxycycline Hyclate 100 mg	Vibramycin by Par		Antibiotic
PAR020	Tab, White, Round, Scored, par over 020	Isosorbide Dinitrate 5 mg	Isordil by Par	49884-0020	Antianginal
PAR021	Tab, White, Round, Scored, par over 021	Isosorbide Dinitrate 10 mg	Isordil by Par	49884-0021	Antianginal
PAR022	Tab, Green, Round, Scored, par over 022	Isosorbide Dinitrate 20 mg	Isordil by Par	49884-0022	Antianginal
PAR022	Tab, Green, Round, Scored, par over 022	Isosorbide Dinitrate 20 mg	Isordil by UDL	51079-0085	Antianginal
PAR025	Tab, Green, Round	Isosorbide Dinitrate Sustained Action 40 mg	Isordil by Par		Antianginal
PAR027	Tab, Peach, Round, par over 027	Hydralazine HCl 25 mg	Apresoline by Par	49884-0027	Antihypertensive
PAR028	Tab, Peach, Round, par over 028	Hydralazine HCl 50 mg	Apresoline by Par	49884-0028	Antihypertensive
PAR029	Tab, Light Pink, Round	Hydralazine HCl 10 mg	Apresoline by Par	49884-0029	Antihypertensive
PAR030	Tab, White/Blue-Green Speckles, Par/030	Phenylpropanolamine HCl 40 mg, Phenylephrine HCl 10 mg, Phentoloxamine 15 mg, Chlorpheniramine 5 mg	Naldecon by Par		Cold Remedy
PAR036	Tab	Methocarbamol 500 mg	Robaxin by Par	49884-0036	Muscle Relaxant
PAR037	Tab	Methocarbamol 750 mg	Robaxin by Par	49884-0037	Muscle Relaxant
PAR038	Tab	Trichlormethiazide 2 mg	by Par	49884-0038	Diuretic; Antihypertensive
PAR039	Tab	Trichlormethiazide 4 mg	Naquival by Par	49884-0039	Diuretic; Antihypertensive
PAR043	Tab, White, Round, Scored, par over 043	Cyproheptadine HCl 4 mg	Periactin by Par	49884-0043	Antihistamine
PAR053	Tab, Orange, Oblong	B Complex, Folic Acid	Berocca by Par		Vitamin
PAR06	Tab, White, Oval	Dexchlorpheniramine Maleate 6 mg	Polaramine by Par		Antihistamine
PAR061	Tab, White, Round, Film Coated	Fluphenazine HCl 1 mg	Prolixin by Par	49884-0061	Antipsychotic
PAR062	Tab, Blue, Round, Film Coated	Fluphenazine HCl 2.5 mg	Prolixin by Par	49884-0062	Antipsychotic
PAR064	Tab, Orange, Round, Film Coated	Fluphenazine HCl 10 mg	Prolixin by Par	49884-0064	Antipsychotic
PAR066	Tab, Round	Doxylamine Succinate 25 mg	Unisom by Par		Sleep Aid
PAR067	Cap	Indomethacin 25 mg	Indocin by Par	49884-0067	NSAID
PAR068	Cap	Indomethacin 50 mg	Indocin by Par	49884-0068	NSAID
PAR069	Cap, Green, Par/069	Hydroxyzine Pamoate 25 mg	Vistaril by Par		Antianxiety; Antihistamine

ID FRONT <> BACK	DESCRIPTION FRONT <> BACK	INGREDIENT & STRENGTH	BRAND (or Generic Equiv.) by FIRM	NDC#	CLASS; SCH.
PAR070	Cap, White & Green, Par/070	Hydroxyzine Pamoate 50 mg	Vistaril by Par		Antianxiety; Antihistamine
PAR071	Cap, Gray & Green, Par/071	Hydroxyzine Pamoate 100 mg	Vistaril by Par		Antianxiety; Antihistamine
PAR076	Tab, Pink, Round, Film Coated, par over 076	Fluphenazine HCl 5 mg	Prolixin by Par	49884-0076	Antipsychotic
PAR077	Tab	Chlorpropamide 100 mg	by Par	49884-0077	Antidiabetic
PAR078	Tab	Chlorpropamide 250 mg	by Par	49884-0078	Antidiabetic
PAR083	Tab, Orange, Pentagonal, Scored	Dexamethasone 0.25 mg	Decadron by Par	49884-0083	Steroid
PAR084	Tab, Yellow, Pentagonal, Scored	Dexamethasone 0.5 mg	Decadron by Par	49884-0084	Steroid
PAR085	Tab, Blue, Pentagonal, Scored	Dexamethasone 0.75 mg	Decadron by Par	49884-0085	Steroid
PAR085	Tab, Blue, Pentagonal, Scored	Dexamethasone 0.75 mg	Decadron by Pharmascience	Canadian DIN 01964968	Steroid
PAR086	Tab, Pink, Pentagonal, Scored	Dexamethasone 1.5 mg	Decadron by Par	49884-0086	Steroid
PAR087	Tab, White, Pentagonal, Scored	Dexamethasone 4 mg	Decadron by Par	49884-0087	Steroid
PAR087	Tab, White, Pentagonal, Scored	Dexamethasone 4 mg	Decadron by Pharmascience	Canadian DIN 01964070	Steroid
PAR095	Tab	Metronidazole 250 mg	by Par	49884-0095	Antibiotic
PAR095	Tab, White, Round	Metronidazole 250 mg	Metronidazole by Neuman	64579-0106	Antibiotic
PAR101	Tab, Orange, Round, Par/101	Thioridazine 100 mg	Mellaril by Par		Antipsychotic
PAR102	Tab, Orange, Round	Thioridazine 150 mg	Mellaril by Par		Antipsychotic
PAR103	Tab, Orange, Round	Thioridazine 200 mg	Mellaril by Par		Antipsychotic
PAR104	Tab, White, Round, Scored, par over 104	Allopurinol 100 mg	Zyloprim by Med Pro	53978-5000	Antigout
PAR104	Tab, White, Round, Scored, par over 104	Allopurinol 100 mg	Zoloprim by Ivax	00182-1481	Antigout
PAR105	Tab, Orange, Round, Scored, par over 105	Allopurinol 300 mg	Zyloprim by Med Pro	53978-5001	Antigout
PAR105	Tab, Orange, Round, Scored, par over 105	Allopurinol 300 mg	Zoloprim by Ivax	00182-1482	Antigout
PAR106	Tab	Propranolol HCl 10 mg	Inderal by Par	49884-0106	Antihypertensive
PAR107	Tab	Propranolol HCl 20 mg	Inderal by Par	49884-0107	Antihypertensive
PAR108	Tab	Propranolol HCl 40 mg	Inderal by Par	49884-0108	Antihypertensive
PAR109	Tab	Propranolol HCl 80 mg	Inderal by Par	49884-0109	Antihypertensive
PAR110	Tab	Clonidine HCl 0.1 mg	by Quality Care	60346-0786	Antihypertensive
PAR111	Tab, Yellow, Round, Par/111	Clonidine HCl 0.2 mg	Catapres by Par		Antihypertensive
PAR112	Tab, Blue, Round, Par/112	Clonidine HCl 0.3 mg	Catapres by Ivax	00182-1252	Antihypertensive
PAR113	Tab	Chlorthalidone 15 mg, Clonidine HCl 0.1 mg	by Par	49884-0113	Diuretic; Antihypertensive
PAR114	Tab	Metronidazole 500 mg	by Dept Health	53808-0053	Antibiotic
PAR114	Tab	Metronidazole 500 mg	by Par	49884-0114	Antibiotic
PAR115	Tab	Chlorthalidone 15 mg, Clonidine HCl 0.2 mg	by Par	49884-0115	Diuretic; Antihypertensive
PAR116	Tab	Chlorthalidone 15 mg, Clonidine HCl 0.3 mg	by Ivax	00182-1277	Diuretic; Antihypertensive
PAR116	Tab	Chlorthalidone 15 mg, Clonidine HCl 0.3 mg	by Par	49884-0116	Diuretic; Antihypertensive
PAR117	Tab, Yellow, Round, par over 117	Amiloride HCl 5 mg	Midamor by Qualitest	00603-2187	Diuretic
PAR117	Tab, Yellow, Round, par over 117	Amiloride HCl 5 mg	Midamor by Par	49884-0117	Diuretic
PAR117	Tab, Yellow, Round, par over 117	Amiloride HCl 5 mg	Midamor by Ivax	00182-1828	Diuretic
PAR118	Tab, Peach, Round, Par/118	Propantheline Bromide 15 mg	Pro-Banthine by Par		Gastrointestinal
PAR119	Tab, Film Coated	Nystatin 500,000 Units	by Qualitest	00603-4830	Antifungal
PAR119	Tab, Film Coated	Nystatin 500,000 Units	by Ivax	00182-1369	Antifungal
PAR119	Tab, Film Coated	Nystatin 500,000 Units	by Par	49884-0119	Antifungal
PAR119	Tab, Film Coated	Nystatin 500,000 Units	by Allscripts		Antifungal
PAR121	Tab, Peach, Round, par over 121	Hydralazine HCl 100 mg	Apresoline by Par	49884-0121	Antihypertensive
PAR122	Tab	Tolazamide 100 mg	by Par	49884-0122	Antidiabetic
PAR123	Tab	Tolazamide 250 mg	by Par	49884-0123	Antidiabetic
PAR124	Tab	Tolazamide 500 mg	by Par	49884-0124	Antidiabetic

ID FRONT <> BACK	DESCRIPTION FRONT <> BACK	INGREDIENT & STRENGTH	BRAND (or Generic Equiv.) by FIRM	NDC#	CLASS; SCH.
PAR125	Cap	Valproic Acid 250 mg	Depakene by Par	49884-0125	Anticonvulsant
PAR127	Tab, Pink, Round, Par/127	Propranolol HCl 60 mg	Inderal by Par		Antihypertensive
PAR128	Tab	Amiloride HCl 5 mg, Hydrochlorothiazide 50 mg	Moduretic by Par	49884-0128	Antihypertensive; Diuretic
PAR129	Tab, Green, Pentagonal, Scored	Dexamethasone 6 mg	Decadron by Par	49884-0129	Steroid
PAR130	Tab, Coated	Metronidazole 250 mg	by Par	49884-0229	Antibiotic
PAR131	Tab, Coated	Metronidazole 500 mg	by Par	49884-0230	Antibiotic
PAR132	Tab, White, Round, Par/132	Metoclopramide HCl 10 mg	Reglan by Par		Gastrointestinal
PAR133	Tab, Pink, Round, Par/133	Amitriptyline HCl 10 mg	Elavil by Par		Antidepressant
PAR134	Tab, Green, Round, Par/134	Amitriptyline HCl 25 mg	Elavil by Par		Antidepressant
PAR135	Tab, Brown, Round, Par/135	Amitriptyline HCl 50 mg	Elavil by Par		Antidepressant
PAR136	Tab, Purple, Round, Par/136	Amitriptyline HCl 75 mg	Elavil by Par		Antidepressant
PAR137	Tab, Orange, Round, Par/137	Amitriptyline HCl 100 mg	Elavil by Par		Antidepressant
PAR138	Tab, Peach, Round	Amitriptyline HCl 150 mg	Elavil by Par		Antidepressant
PAR139	Tab	Sulfamethoxazole 400 mg, Trimethoprim 80 mg	by Par	49884-0139	Antibiotic
PAR140	Tab	Sulfamethoxazole 800 mg, Trimethoprim 160 mg	by Par	49884-0140	Antibiotic
PAR143	Cap, White, Opaque	Hydralazine 25 mg, Hydrochlorothiazide 25 mg	Apresazide by Par	49884-0143	Antihypertensive; Diuretic
PAR144	Cap, White & Black, Opaque	Hydralazine 50 mg, Hydrochlorothiazide 50 mg	Apresazide by Par	49884-0144	Antihypertensive; Diuretic
PAR145	Cap, Light Blue, Opaque	Hydralazine 100 mg, Hydrochlorothiazide 50 mg	Apresazide by Par	49884-0145	Antihypertensive; Diuretic
PAR147	Tab	Hydroflumethiazide 50 mg	Diucardin by Par	49884-0147	Diuretic; Antihypertensive
PAR148	Tab, Coated	Hydroflumethiazide 50 mg, Reserpine 0.125 mg	by Par	49884-0148	Diuretic; Antihypertensive
PAR150	Tab, Coated	Methyldopa 125 mg	by Par	49884-0150	Antihypertensive
PAR151	Tab, Coated	Methyldopa 250 mg	by Par	49884-0151	Antihypertensive
PAR152	Tab, Coated	Methyldopa 500 mg	by Par	49884-0152	Antihypertensive
PAR153	Tab	Disulfiram 250 mg	Antabuse by Par	49884-0153	Antialcoholism
PAR154	Tab	Disulfiram 500 mg	Antabuse by Par	49884-0154	Antialcoholism
PAR158	Tab	Methylprednisolone 16 mg	by Par	49884-0158	Steroid
PAR159	Tab	Methylprednisolone 24 mg	by Par	49884-0159	Steroid
PAR160	Tab	Methylprednisolone 32 mg	by Par	49884-0160	Steroid
PAR161	Tab, Film Coated	Fluphenazine HCl 1 mg	by Amerisource	62584-0698	Antipsychotic
PAR161300	Tab, White, Round, Par/161 300	Ibuprofen 300 mg	Motrin by Par		NSAID
PAR162 <> 400	Tab, White, Round, Film Coated, Par over 162 <> 400	Ibuprofen 400 mg	Motrin by UDL	51079-0281 Discontinued	NSAID
PAR162 <> 400	Tab, Film Coated	Ibuprofen 400 mg	Motrin by Ivax	00172-4018	NSAID
PAR162 <> 400	Tab, White, Round	Ibuprofen 400 mg	Motrin by Murfreesboro	51129-1524	NSAID
PAR162 <> 400	Tab, Film Coated, Debossed	Ibuprofen 400 mg	Motrin by Amerisource	62584-0746	NSAID
PAR162 <> 400	Tab, Film Coated, Par over 162 <> 400	Ibuprofen 400 mg	Motrin by Par	49884-0162	NSAID
PAR162 <> 400	Tab, Film Coated	Ibuprofen 400 mg	Motrin by PDRX	55289-0590	NSAID
PAR162 <> 400	Tab, Film Coated	Ibuprofen 400 mg	Motrin by Par		NSAID
PAR162 <> 400	Tab, Coated	Ibuprofen 400 mg	Motrin by Rx Dispensing	61807-0027	NSAID
PAR163 <> 600	Tab, Film Coated	Ibuprofen 600 mg	Motrin by Ivax	00172-3646	NSAID
PAR163 <> 600	Tab, Film Coated	Ibuprofen 600 mg	Motrin by Pharmedix	53002-0301	NSAID
PAR163 <> 600	Tab, Film Coated	Ibuprofen 600 mg	Motrin by Med Pro	53978-5006	NSAID
PAR163 <> 600	Tab, Film Coated	Ibuprofen 600 mg	Motrin by Par	49884-0163	NSAID
PAR164	Tab, White, Round, Scored, par over 164	Benztropine Mesylate 0.5 mg	Cogentin by Major	00904-1055	Antiparkinson
PAR164	Tab, White, Round, Scored, par over 164	Benztropine Mesylate 0.5 mg	Cogentin by Par	49884-0164	Antiparkinson
PAR164	Tab, White, Round, Scored, par over 164	Benztropine Mesylate 0.5 mg	Cogentin by Ivax	00182-1299 Discontinued	Antiparkinson
PAR165	Tab, White, Oval, Scored, par over 165	Benztropine Mesylate 1 mg	Cogentin by Major	00904-1056	Antiparkinson

ID FRONT <> BACK	DESCRIPTION FRONT <> BACK	INGREDIENT & STRENGTH	BRAND (or Generic Equiv.) by FIRM	NDC#	CLASS; SCH.
PAR165	Tab, White, Oval, Scored, par over 165	Benztropine Mesylate 1 mg	Cogentin by Par	49884-0165	Antiparkinson
PAR165	Tab, White, Oval, Scored, par over 165	Benztropine Mesylate 1 mg	Cogentin by Ivax	00182-1700 Discontinued	Antiparkinson
PAR166	Tab, White, Round, Scored, par over 166	Benztropine Mesylate 2 mg	Cogentin by Major	00904-1057	Antiparkinson
PAR166	Tab, White, Round, Scored, par over 166	Benztropine Mesylate 2 mg	Cogentin by Par	49884-0166	Antiparkinson
PAR166	Tab, White, Round, Scored, par over 166	Benztropine Mesylate 2 mg	Cogentin by Ivax	00182-1701 Discontinued	Antiparkinson
PAR170	Tab	Sulfinpyrazone 100 mg	by Par	49884-0170	Uricosuric
PAR171	Cap	Sulfinpyrazone 200 mg	by Par	49884-0171	Uricosuric
PAR176	Tab, Green/Orange, Round, Par/176	Aspirin 325 mg, Meprobamate 200 mg	Equagesic by Par		Sedative/Hypnotic; C IV
PAR177	Tab	Methylclothiazide 2.5 mg	by Par	49884-0177	Diuretic; Antihypertensive
PAR178	Tab	Methylclothiazide 5 mg	by Par	49884-0178	Diuretic; Antihypertensive
PAR181	Tab, Blue, Round, Par/181	Amitriptyline 10 mg, Perphenazine 2 mg	Triavil by Par		Antidepressant; Antipsychotic
PAR182	Tab, Orange, Round, Par/182	Amitriptyline 25 mg, Perphenazine 2 mg	Triavil by Par		Antidepressant; Antipsychotic
PAR183	Tab, Salmon, Round, Par/183	Amitriptyline 10 mg, Perphenazine 4 mg	Triavil by Par		Antidepressant; Antipsychotic
PAR184	Tab, Yellow, Round, Par/184	Amitriptyline 25 mg, Perphenazine 4 mg	Triavil by Par		Antidepressant; Antipsychotic
PAR185	Tab, Orange, Round, Par/185	Amitriptyline 50 mg, Perphenazine 4 mg	Triavil by Par		Antidepressant; Antipsychotic
PAR186	Tab, Film Coated	Hydrochlorothiazide 15 mg, Methyldopa 250 mg	by Ivax	00182-1830	Diuretic; Antihypertensive
PAR186	Tab, Film Coated	Hydrochlorothiazide 15 mg, Methyldopa 250 mg	by Par	49884-0186	Diuretic; Antihypertensive
PAR189	Tab, Coated	Hydrochlorothiazide 50 mg, Methyldopa 500 mg	by Par	49884-0189	Diuretic; Antihypertensive
PAR190 <> DIAZEPAM2	Tab	Diazepam 2 mg	by Par	49884-0190	Antianxiety; C IV
PAR191 <> DIAZEPAM5	Tab	Diazepam 5 mg	by Par	49884-0191	Antianxiety; C IV
PAR192 <> DIAZEPAM10	Tab	Diazepam 10 mg	by Par	49884-0192	Antianxiety; C IV
PAR193	Cap, Powder Blue	Flurazepam HCl 15 mg	by Amerisource	62584-0705	Hypnotic; C IV
PAR193	Cap	Flurazepam HCl 15 mg	by Par	49884-0193	Hypnotic; C IV
PAR193	Cap	Flurazepam HCl 15 mg	by Qualitest	00603-3691	Hypnotic; C IV
PAR194	Cap	Flurazepam HCl 30 mg	by Par	49884-0194	Hypnotic; C IV
PAR194	Cap	Flurazepam HCl 30 mg	by Qualitest	00603-3692	Hypnotic; C IV
PAR200 <> 682	Tab, White, Cap Shaped	Ofloxacin 200 mg	Floxin by Par	49884-0682	Antibiotic
PAR202	Tab, Beige, Round, Par/202	Methyldopa 250 mg, Chlorothiazide 150 mg	Aldoclor 150 by Par		Antihypertensive; Diuretic
PAR203	Tab, Green, Round, Par/203	Methyldopa 250 mg, Chlorothiazide 250 mg	Aldoclor 250 by Par		Antihypertensive; Diuretic
PAR206	Tab, White, Round, Par/206	Lorazepam 0.5 mg	Ativan by Par		Antianxiety; C IV
PAR207	Tab, White, Round, Par/207	Lorazepam 1 mg	Ativan by Par		Antianxiety; C IV
PAR208	Tab, White, Round, Par/208	Lorazepam 2 mg	Ativan by Par		Antianxiety; C IV
PAR213	Tab, White & Green, Round, Par/213	Orphenadrine 25 mg, Aspirin 325 mg, Caffeine 30 mg	Orphengesic by Par		Muscle Relaxant
PAR214	Tab, White & Green, Oblong, Par/214	Orphenadrine 50 mg, Aspirin 770 mg, Caffeine 60 mg	Orphengesic Forte by Par		Muscle Relaxant
PAR216	Tab, Film Coated	Ibuprofen 800 mg	Motrin by Med Pro	53978-5007	NSAID
PAR216 <> 800	Tab, Film Coated, Par over 216 <> 800	Ibuprofen 800 mg	Motrin by PDRX	55289-0140	NSAID
PAR216 <> 800	Tab, Coated, Par over 216 <> 800	Ibuprofen 800 mg	Motrin by Baker Cummins	63171-1297	NSAID
PAR216 <> 800	Tab, White, Cap Shaped, Film-Coated, Par over 216 <> 800	Ibuprofen 800 mg	Motrin by UDL	51079-0596 Discontinued	NSAID
PAR216 <> 800	Tab, Coated, Par over 216 <> 800	Ibuprofen 800 mg	Motrin by Nat Pharmpak	55154-5565	NSAID
PAR216 <> 800	Tab, Coated	Ibuprofen 800 mg	Motrin by Par	49884-0216	NSAID
PAR217	Cap, Ivory, Black Print, par over 217	Doxepin HCl 10 mg	Sinequan by Par	49884-0217	Antidepressant

ID FRONT <> BACK	DESCRIPTION FRONT <> BACK	INGREDIENT & STRENGTH	BRAND (or Generic Equiv.) by FIRM	NDC#	CLASS; SCH.
PAR218	Cap, White & Ivory, Black Print, par over 218	Doxepin HCl 25 mg	Sinequan by Par	49884-0218	Antidepressant
PAR219	Cap, Ivory, Black Print, par over 219	Doxepin HCl 50 mg	Sinequan by Par	49884-0219	Antidepressant
PAR220	Cap, Green, Black Print, par over 220	Doxepin HCl 75 mg	Sinequan by Par	49884-0220	Antidepressant
PAR221	Cap, White & Green, Black Print, par over 221	Doxepin HCl 100 mg	Sinequan by Par	49884-0221	Antidepressant
PAR222	Cap, White & Blue, Black Print, par over 222	Doxepin HCl 150 mg	Sinequan by Par	49884-0222	Antidepressant
PAR223	Tab, White, Round, Scored, par over 223	Haloperidol 0.5 mg	Haldol by Par	49884-0223	Antipsychotic
PAR224	Tab	Haloperidol 1 mg	Haldol by Par	49884-0224	Antipsychotic
PAR225	Tab, Pink, Round	Haloperidol 2 mg	Haldol by Par	49884-0225	Antipsychotic
PAR226	Tab, Green, Round	Haloperidol 5 mg	Haldol by Par	49884-0226	Antipsychotic
PAR227	Tab, Light Blue, Round, Scored, par over 227	Haloperidol 10 mg	Haldol by Par	49884-0227	Antipsychotic
PAR228	Tab, Salmon, Round, Par/228	Haloperidol 20 mg	Haldol by Par		Antipsychotic
PAR237	Tab	Leucovorin Calcium	Wellcovorin by Par	49884-0237	Antineoplastic
PAR238	Tab	Leucovorin Calcium	Wellcovorin by Par	49884-0238	Antineoplastic
PAR239	Tab	Propranolol HCl 90 mg	Inderal by Par	49884-0239	Antihypertensive
PAR240	Cap	Temazepam 15 mg	Restoril by Par	49884-0240	Sedative/Hypnotic; C IV
PAR240	Cap, Opaque	Temazepam 15 mg	Restoril by Amerisource	62584-0860	Sedative/Hypnotic; C IV
PAR240	Cap	Temazepam 15 mg	Restoril by Qualitest	00603-5895	Sedative/Hypnotic; C IV
PAR241	Cap, White	Temazepam 30 mg	Restoril by Southwood	58016-0831	Sedative/Hypnotic; C IV
PAR241	Cap	Temazepam 30 mg	Restoril by Amerisource	62584-0862	Sedative/Hypnotic; C IV
PAR241	Cap	Temazepam 30 mg	Restoril by Major	00904-2811	Sedative/Hypnotic; C IV
PAR241	Cap	Temazepam 30 mg	Restoril by Qualitest	00603-5896	Sedative/Hypnotic; C IV
PAR241	Cap	Temazepam 30 mg	Restoril by Par	49884-0241	Sedative/Hypnotic; C IV
PAR246	Tab, White & Light Lavender, Round	Aspirin 325 mg, Carisoprodol 200 mg	Soma Compound by Par	49884-0246	Analgesic; Muscle Relaxant
PAR247	Tab, Coated	Salsalate 500 mg	by Par	49884-0247	NSAID
PAR248	Tab, Coated	Salsalate 750 mg	by Par	49884-0248	NSAID
PAR249	Tab	Aspirin 325 mg, Methocarbamol 400 mg	Robaxisal by Qualitest	00603-4489	Analgesic; Muscle Relaxant
PAR249	Tab	Aspirin 325 mg, Methocarbamol 400 mg	Robaxisal by Allscripts		Analgesic; Muscle Relaxant
PAR249	Tab	Aspirin 325 mg, Methocarbamol 400 mg	Robaxisal by Par	49884-0249	Analgesic; Muscle Relaxant
PAR249	Tab	Aspirin 325 mg, Methocarbamol 400 mg	Robaxisal by Major	00904-0227	Analgesic; Muscle Relaxant
PAR249	Tab	Aspirin 325 mg, Methocarbamol 400 mg	Robaxisal by DRX	55045-2551	Analgesic; Muscle Relaxant
PAR25	Tab, White, Round, Par/25	Dipyridamole 25 mg	Persantine by Par		Antiplatelet
PAR250	Cap, Gray & Orange, Par/250	Cephalexin 250 mg	Keflex by Par		Antibiotic
PAR256 <> MINOXIDIL212	Tab, White, Round, Scored, par over 256 <> Minoxidil over 2 1/2	Minoxidil 2.5 mg	Loniten by Par	49884-0256	Antihypertensive
PAR256 <> MINOXIDIL212	Tab, White, Round, Scored, par over 256 <> Minoxidil over 2 1/2	Minoxidil 2.5 mg	Loniten by Ivax	00182-1602	Antihypertensive
PAR256 <> MINOXIDIL212	Tab, White, Round, Scored, par over 256 <> Minoxidil over 2 1/2	Minoxidil 2.5 mg	Loniten by Qualitest	00603-4687	Antihypertensive
PAR257 <> MINOXIDIL10	Tab, White, Round, Scored, par over 257 <> Minoxidil over 10	Minoxidil 10 mg	Loniten by Physician Total Care	54868-3467	Antihypertensive
PAR257 <> MINOXIDIL10	Tab, White, Round, Scored, par over 257 <> Minoxidil over 10	Minoxidil 10 mg	Loniten by URL Mutual	00677-1162	Antihypertensive
PAR257 <> MINOXIDIL10	Tab, White, Round, Scored, par over 257 <> Minoxidil over 10	Minoxidil 10 mg	Loniten by Moore	00839-7342	Antihypertensive

ID FRONT <> BACK	DESCRIPTION FRONT <> BACK	INGREDIENT & STRENGTH	BRAND (or Generic Equiv.) by FIRM	NDC#	CLASS; SCH.
PAR257 <> MINOXIDIL10	Tab, White, Round, Scored, par over 257 <> Minoxidil over 10	Minoxidil 10 mg	Loniten by Qualitest	00603-4688	Antihypertensive
PAR257 <> MINOXIDIL10	Tab, White, Round, Scored, par over 257 <> Minoxidil over 10	Minoxidil 10 mg	Loniten by Par	49884-0257	Antihypertensive
PAR258	Tab, White, Round, Scored	Metaproterenol Sulfate 10 mg	Alupent by Par	49884-0258	Antiasthmatic
PAR258	Tab, White, Round, Scored	Metaproterenol Sulfate 10 mg	Alupent by Pharm Pkg Ctr	54383-0090	Antiasthmatic
PAR259	Tab, White, Round, Scored, par over 259	Metaproterenol Sulfate 20 mg	Alupent by Par	49884-0259	Antiasthmatic
PAR263	Cap, Maroon & Pink, Par/263	Meclofenamate Sodium 50 mg	Meclomen by Par		NSAID
PAR264	Cap, Maroon & White, Par/264	Meclofenamate Sodium 100 mg	Meclomen by Par		NSAID
PAR279	Tab	Hydrochlorothiazide 50 mg, Triamterene 75 mg	by Par		Diuretic; Antihypertensive
PAR282	Cap, White and Aqua, Opaque, Controlled Release	Propranolol HCl 60 mg	Inderal by Par	49884-0282	Antihypertensive
PAR286	Tab, Coated	Fenoprofen Calcium	by Par	49884-0286	NSAID
PAR287	Cap	Fenoprofen Calcium	by Par	49884-0287	NSAID
PAR288	Cap	Fenoprofen Calcium	by Par	49884-0288	NSAID
PAR289	Tab, White, Round, Scored, par over 289	Megestrol Acetate 20 mg	Megace by Murfreesboro	51129-1305	Hormone
PAR289	Tab, White, Round, Scored, par over 289	Megestrol Acetate 20 mg	Megace by Qualitest	00603-4391	Hormone
PAR289	Tab, White, Round, Scored, par over 289	Megestrol Acetate 20 mg	Megace by Amerisource	62584-0777	Hormone
PAR289	Tab, White, Round, Scored, par over 289	Megestrol Acetate 20 mg	Megace by Schein	00364-2235	Hormone
PAR289	Tab, White, Round, Scored, par over 289	Megestrol Acetate 20 mg	Megace by Par	49884-0289	Hormone
PAR289	Tab, White, Round, Scored, par over 289	Megestrol Acetate 20 mg	Megace by Ivax	00182-1863	Hormone
PAR290	Tab, White, Round, Scored, par over 290	Megestrol Acetate 40 mg	Megace by URL Mutual	00677-1206	Hormone
PAR290	Tab, White, Round, Scored, par over 290	Megestrol Acetate 40 mg	Megace by Par	49884-0290	Hormone
PAR290	Tab, White, Round, Scored, par over 290	Megestrol Acetate 40 mg	Megace by Amerisource	62584-0779	Hormone
PAR290	Tab, White, Round, Scored, par over 290	Megestrol Acetate 40 mg	Megace by Vangard	00615-3570	Hormone
PAR290	Tab, White, Round, Scored, par over 290	Megestrol Acetate 40 mg	Megace by Schein	00364-2234	Hormone
PAR290	Tab, White, Round, Scored, par over 290	Megestrol Acetate 40 mg	Megace by Med Pro	53978-3010	Hormone
PAR290	Tab, White, Round, Scored, par over 290	Megestrol Acetate 40 mg	Megace by Major	00904-3571	Hormone
PAR290	Tab, White, Round, Scored, par over 290	Megestrol Acetate 40 mg	Megace by Ivax	00182-1864	Hormone
				Discontinued	
PAR300 <> 683	Tab, White, Cap Shaped	Ofloxacin 300 mg	Floxin by Par	49884-0683	Antibiotic
PAR304	Tab, Peach, Round	Divalproex sodium 250 mg	Depakote by Par		Anticonvulsant
PAR305	Tab, Lavender, Round	Divalproex sodium 500 mg	Depakote by Par		Anticonvulsant
PAR328	Cap, Aqua Blue, Opaque, Controlled Release	Propranolol HCl 80 mg	Inderal by Par	49884-0328	Antihypertensive
PAR329	Cap, Aqua Blue, Opaque, Controlled Release	Propranolol HCl 120 mg	Inderal by Par	49884-0329	Antihypertensive
PAR330	Cap, Blue, Opaque, Controlled Release	Propranolol HCl 160 mg	Inderal by Par	49884-0330	Antihypertensive
PAR4	Tab, Yellow, Oval, Par/4	Dexchlorpheniramine Maleate 4 mg	Polaramine Repetabs by Par		Antihistamine
PAR400 <> 684	Tab, White, Cap Shaped	Ofloxacin 400 mg	Floxin by Par	49884-0684	Antibiotic
PAR412	Tab, Film Coated	Metoprolol Tartrate 50 mg	Lopressor by Par	49884-0412	Antihypertensive
PAR413	Tab, Blue, Round, Scored, Film	Metoprolol Tartrate 100 mg	Lopressor by Neuman	64579-0059	Antihypertensive
PAR413	Tab, Coated	Metoprolol Tartrate 100 mg	Lopressor by Par	49884-0413	Antihypertensive
PAR444	Tab, Scored	Captopril 12.5 mg	Capoten by Par	49884-0444	Antihypertensive
PAR445	Tab	Captopril 25 mg	Capoten by Par	49884-0445	Antihypertensive
PAR446	Tab	Captopril 50 mg	Capoten by Par	49884-0446	Antihypertensive
PAR447	Tab	Captopril 100 mg	Capoten by Par	49884-0447	Antihypertensive
PAR467	Tab, White, Black Print, Oblong, Film Coated, par over 467	Ibuprofen 400 mg	Motrin by Dixon Shane	17236-0568	NSAID
PAR468	Tab, White, Oblong, Film Coated	Ibuprofen 600 mg	Motrin by Dixon Shane	17236-0569	NSAID
PAR468	Tab, Printed in Black, Film Coated	Ibuprofen 600 mg	Motrin by Amerisource	62584-0747	NSAID
PAR468	Tab, Film Coated	Ibuprofen 600 mg	Motrin by Prepackage Specialists	58864-0286	NSAID

ID FRONT <> BACK	DESCRIPTION FRONT <> BACK	INGREDIENT & STRENGTH	BRAND (or Generic Equiv.) by FIRM	NDC#	CLASS; SCH.
PAR468	Tab, Film Coated	Ibuprofen 600 mg	Motrin by Par		NSAID
PAR469	Tab, Printed in Black, Film Coated	Ibuprofen 800 mg	Motrin by Amerisource	62584-0748	NSAID
PAR469	Tab, White, Oblong, Film Coated	Ibuprofen 800 mg	Motrin by Dixon Shane	17236-0570	NSAID
PAR472	Tab, Green & White, Round	Orphenadrine Citrate 25 mg, Aspirin 385 mg, Caffeine 30 mg	Norgesic by Par	49884-0472	Muscle Relaxant
PAR473	Tab, Green & White, Cap Shaped, Scored	Orphenadrine Citrate 50 mg, Aspirin 770 mg, Caffeine 60 mg	Norgesic Forte by Par	49884-0473	Muscle Relaxant
PAR50	Tab, White, Round, Par/50	Dipyridamole 50 mg	Persantine by Par		Antiplatelet
PAR500	Cap, Orange, Par/500	Cephalexin 500 mg	Keflex by Par		Antibiotic
PAR54	Tab, Yellow, Triangular, Sugar Coated	Imipramine HCl 10 mg	Tofranil by Par	49884-0054	Antidepressant
PAR544	Tab, Peach to Light Brown, Round, par over 544	Ranitidine HCl 150 mg	Zantac by Par	49884-0544	Gastrointestinal
PAR544	Tab, Peach to Light Brown, Round, par over 544	Ranitidine HCl 150 mg	Zantac by RX Pak	65084-0175	Gastrointestinal
PAR545	Tab, Peach to Light Brown, Oval, par next to 545	Ranitidine HCl 300 mg	Zantac by RX Pak	65084-0176	Gastrointestinal
PAR545	Tab, Peach to Light Brown, Oval, par next to 545	Ranitidine HCl 300 mg	Zantac by Par	49884-0545	Gastrointestinal
PAR6	Tab, White, Oval, Par/6	Dexchlorpheniramine Maleate 6 mg	Polaramine Repetabs by Par		Antihistamine
PAR651 <> 5	Tab, White, Round, Scored	Torsemide 5 mg	Demadex by Par	49884-0651	Diuretic
PAR652 <> 10	Tab, White, Round, Scored	Torsemide 10 mg	Demadex by Par	49884-0652	Diuretic
PAR653 <> 20	Tab, White, Round, Scored	Torsemide 20 mg	Demadex by Par	49884-0653	Diuretic
PAR654 <> 100	Tab, White, Round, Scored	Torsemide 100 mg	Demadex by Par	49884-0654	Diuretic
PAR701	Tab, Off-White, Round	Clomiphene Citrate 50 mg	Soma by Par	49884-0701	Infertility
PAR701	Tab, Off White, Round	Clomiphene Citrate 50 mg	Clomid by Par	49884-0701	Fertility
PAR707 <> 5	Tab, Peach, Oval, Scored	Buspirone HCl 5 mg	Buspar by Par	49884-0707	Antianxiety
PAR708 <> 10	Tab, Peach, Oval, Scored	Buspirone HCl 10 mg	Buspar by Par	49884-0708	Antianxiety
PAR721 <> 555	Tab, Peach, Rectangular, Scored, 5-5-5	Buspirone HCl 15 mg	Buspar by Par	49884-0721	Antianxiety
PAR725 <> 75	Tab, Off-White, Oval, Scored, 7.5	Buspirone HCl 7.5 mg	Buspar by Par	49884-0725	Antianxiety
PAR726	Cap, Buff & White, Brown Print, Opaque	Doxycycline Monohydrate 50 mg	Monodox by Par	49884-0726	Antibiotic
PAR727	Cap, Brown & White, Brown Print, Opaque	Doxycycline Monohydrate 100 mg	Monodox by Par	49884-0727	Antibiotic
PAR75	Tab, White, Round, Par/75	Dipyridamole 75 mg	Persantine by Par		Antiplatelet
PAR845	Tab, Pink, Rectangular, Speckled, Scored	Glimepiride 1 mg	Amaryl by Par	49884-0845	Antidiabetic
PAR846	Tab, Green, Rectangular, Scored, par / 846	Glimepiride 2 mg	Amaryl by Par	49884-0846	Antidiabetic
PAR847	Tab, Blue, Rectangular, Scored, par / 847	Glimepiride 4 mg	Amaryl by Par	49884-0847	Antidiabetic
PAR867	Cap, Cream, Oblong, Softgel	Dronabinol 2.5 mg	Marinol by Par	49884-0868	Antiemetic
PAR868	Cap, Brown, Opaque, Oblong, Softgel	Dronabinol 5 mg	Marinol by Par	49884-0868	Antiemetic
PAR869	Cap, Orange, Oblong, Softgel	Dronabinol 10 mg	Marinol by Par	49884-0869	Antiemetic
PAR876	Tab, White, Oval, Scored, Film Coated	Paroxetine HCl 10 mg	Paxil by Par	49884-0876	Antidepressant
PAR877	Tab, White, Oval, Scored, Film Coated	Paroxetine HCl 20 mg	Paxil by Par	49884-0877	Antidepressant
PAR878	Tab, White, Oval, Film Coated	Paroxetine HCl 30 mg	Paxil by Par	49884-0878	Antidepressant
PAR879	Tab, White, Oval, Film Coated	Paroxetine HCl 40 mg	Paxil by Par	49884-0879	Antidepressant
PAR96	Tab, Orange, Round, Par/96	Thioridazine 10 mg	Mellaril by Par		Antipsychotic
PAR962	Tab, White, Round, Film Coated	Chlordiazepoxide 10 mg, Amitriptyline HCl 25 mg	Limbitrol DS by Par	49884-0962	Antidepressant; Antianxiety
PAR97	Tab, Orange, Round, Par/97	Thioridazine 15 mg	Mellaril by Par		Antipsychotic
PAR98	Tab, Orange, Round, Par/98	Thioridazine 25 mg	Mellaril by Par		Antipsychotic
PAR99	Tab, Orange, Round, Par/99	Thioridazine 50 mg	Mellaril by Par		Antipsychotic
PARAFLEX	Tab, Peach, Cap Shaped	Chlorzoxazone 250 mg	Para-Flex by McNeil	00045-0317	Muscle Relaxant
PARAFONFORTEC8M	Tab, Pink/White, Round	Acetaminophen 300 mg, Chlorzoxazone 250 mg, Codeine Phosphate 8 mg	Parafon Forte C8 by Johnson & Johnson	Canadian	Analgesic; C III
PARAFONFORTEDSC <> MCNEIL	Tab, Light Green, Cap Shaped, Scored	Chlorzoxazone 500 mg	Parafon Forte DSC by Nat Pharmpak	55154-1907	Muscle Relaxant
PARAFONFORTEDSC <> MCNEIL	Tab, Light Green, Cap Shaped, Scored	Chlorzoxazone 500 mg	Parafon Forte DSC by McNeil	00045-0325	Muscle Relaxant

ID FRONT <> BACK	DESCRIPTION FRONT <> BACK	INGREDIENT & STRENGTH	BRAND (or Generic Equiv.) by FIRM	NDC#	CLASS; SCH.
PARAFONFORTEDSC <> MCNEIL	Tab, Light Green, Cap Shaped, Scored	Chlorzoxazone 500 mg	Parafon Forte DSC by Allscripts		Muscle Relaxant
PARAFONFORTEDSC <> MCNEIL	Tab, Light Green, Cap Shaped, Scored	Chlorzoxazone 500 mg	Parafon Forte DSC by Compumed	00403-0261	Muscle Relaxant
PARAFONFORTEDSC <> MCNEIL	Tab, Light Green, Cap Shaped, Scored	Chlorzoxazone 500 mg	Parafon Forte DSC by Rightpac	65240-0715	Muscle Relaxant
PARAFONFORTEDSC <> MCNEIL	Tab, Light Green, Cap Shaped, Scored	Chlorzoxazone 500 mg	Parafon Forte DSC by Thrift Drug	59198-0089	Muscle Relaxant
PARAONFORTEC8M	Tab, Pink/White, Round, Paraon Forte C8/M	Chlorzoxazone 250 mg, Acetaminophen 300 mg, Codeine Phosphate 8 mg	Parafon Forte C8 by McNeil	Canadian	Muscle Relaxant; C III
PARKEDAVIS	Cap, Green & Pink, ParkeDavis	Caffeine 100 mg, Diphenhydramine HCl 25 mg, Ergotamine 1 mg	Ergodryl by Pfizer	Canadian DIN 00156086	Antimigraine
PARKEDAVIS	Cap, Orange & Yellow	Methsuximide 300 mg	Celontin by Pfizer	Canadian DIN 00022802	Anticonvulsant
PARKEDAVIS	Cap, Aqua Blue & Ivory, Opaque	Mefenamic Acid 250 mg	Ponstel by Pfizer	Canadian DIN 00155225	NSAID
PARKEDAVIS	Cap, Clear & Yellow, Opaque	Erythromycin 333 mg	Eryc by Parke Davis	Canadian DIN 00873454	Antibiotic
PARKEDAVIS <> LOPID600MG	Tab, White, Ellipsoid, Film Coated	Gemfibrozil 600 mg	Lopid by Parke Davis	Canadian DIN 00659606	Antihyperlipidemic
PARKEDAVISPD100	Cap, Orange & White, Parke-Davis P-D 100	Phenytoin Sodium 100 mg	Dilantin by Parke Davis	Canadian DIN 00022780	Anticonvulsant
PARKEDAVISPD30	Cap, Pink & White, Parke-Davis P-D 30	Phenytoin Sodium 30 mg	Dilantin by Parke Davis	Canadian DIN 00022772	Anticonvulsant
PARLODEL	Tab, White, Oval, Scored	Bromocriptine 2.5 mg	Parlodel by Novartis	Canadian DIN 00371033	Antiparkinson
PARLODEL212	Tab, White, Round, Scored, Parlodel over 2 1/2	Bromocriptine 2.5 mg	Parlodel by Pharm Util	60491-0497	Antiparkinson
PARLODEL212	Tab, White, Round, Scored, Parlodel over 2 1/2	Bromocriptine 2.5 mg	Parlodel by Novartis	00078-0017	Antiparkinson
PARLODEL5MGS	Cap, Brown & White, Red Print, Parlodel over 5 mg, S in Triangle	Bromocriptine 5 mg	Parlodel by Sandoz	Canadian DIN 00566643	Antiparkinson
PARLODEL5MGS	Cap, Brown & White, Red Print, Parlodel over 5 mg, S in Triangle	Bromocriptine 5 mg	Parlodel by Pharm Util	60491-0499	Antiparkinson
PARLODEL5MGS	Cap, Brown & White, Red Print, Parlodel over 5 mg, S in Triangle	Bromocriptine 5 mg	Parlodel by Novartis	00078-0102	Antiparkinson
PARNATESB	Tab, Pink, Round, Parnate/SB	Tranylcypromine 10 mg	Parnate by SKB	00007-4471	Antidepressant
PARNATESB	Tab, Pink, Round, Parnate/SB	Tranylcypromine 10 mg	Parnate by GSK	Canadian DIN 01919598	Antidepressant
PARNATESKF	Tab, Red, Black Print, Round	Tranylcypromine 10 mg	Parnate by SKB	Canadian	Antidepressant
PARNATESR	Tab, Red, Round, Film Coated	Tranylcypromine Sulfate 10 mg	Parnate by Teva	00480-0149	Antidepressant
PATC10	Tab, Yellow, Pentagonal	Cyclobenzaprine HCl 10 mg	Flexeril by Patriot	10147-0740	Muscle Relaxant
PATC5	Tab, Orange, Pentagonal	Cyclobenzaprine HCl 5 mg	Flexeril by Patriot	10147-0790	Muscle Relaxant
PAXIL <> 10	Tab, Yellow, Oblong, Film Coated	Paroxetine HCl 10 mg	Paxil by GSK	Canadian DIN 02027887	Antidepressant
PAXIL <> 10	Tab, Yellow, Oblong, Film Coated	Paroxetine HCl 10 mg	by Med Pro	53978-2059	Antidepressant
PAXIL <> 10	Tab, Yellow, Oblong, Film Coated	Paroxetine HCl 10 mg	Paxil by SB	59742-3210	Antidepressant
PAXIL <> 10	Tab, Yellow, Oblong, Film Coated	Paroxetine HCl 10 mg	Paxil by SKB	00029-3210	Antidepressant
PAXIL <> 10	Tab, Yellow, Oblong, Film Coated	Paroxetine HCl 10 mg	Paxil by Pharmacy Care	65070-0144	Antidepressant
PAXIL <> 20	Tab, Pink, Oblong, Film Coated	Paroxetine HCl 20 mg	Paxil by SKB	00029-3211	Antidepressant
PAXIL <> 20	Tab, Pink, Oblong, Film Coated	Paroxetine HCl 20 mg	by Kaiser	00179-1182	Antidepressant
PAXIL <> 20	Tab, Pink, Oblong, Film Coated	Paroxetine HCl 20 mg	by Nat Pharmpak	55154-4504	Antidepressant
PAXIL <> 20	Tab, Pink, Oblong, Film Coated	Paroxetine HCl 20 mg	by Allscripts		Antidepressant
PAXIL <> 20	Tab, Pink, Oblong, Film Coated	Paroxetine HCl 20 mg	Paxil by H J Harkins Co	52959-0360	Antidepressant

ID FRONT <> BACK	DESCRIPTION FRONT <> BACK	INGREDIENT & STRENGTH	BRAND (or Generic Equiv.) by FIRM	NDC#	CLASS; SCH.
PAXIL <> 20	Tab, Pink, Oblong, Film Coated	Paroxetine HCl 20 mg	by Kaiser	62224-2340	Antidepressant
PAXIL <> 20	Tab, Pink, Oblong, Film Coated	Paroxetine HCl 20 mg	by Amerisource	62584-0211	Antidepressant
PAXIL <> 20	Tab, Pink, Oblong, Film Coated	Paroxetine HCl 20 mg	Paxil by SB	59742-3211	Antidepressant
PAXIL <> 20	Tab, Pink, Oblong, Film Coated	Paroxetine HCl 20 mg	Paxil by GSK	Canadian DIN 01940481	Antidepressant
PAXIL <> 30	Tab, Blue, Oblong, Film Coated	Paroxetine HCl 30 mg	Paxil by GSK	Canadian DIN 01940473	Antidepressant
PAXIL <> 30	Tab, Blue, Oblong, Film Coated	Paroxetine HCl 30 mg	Paxil by SKB	00029-3212	Antidepressant
PAXIL <> 30	Tab, Blue, Oblong, Film Coated	Paroxetine HCl 30 mg	by Physician Total Care	54868-3526	Antidepressant
PAXIL <> 30	Tab, Blue, Oblong, Film Coated	Paroxetine HCl 30 mg	Paxil by SB	59742-3212	Antidepressant
PAXIL <> 40	Tab, Light Green, Oblong, Film Coated	Paroxetine HCl 40 mg	Paxil by SKB	00029-3213	Antidepressant
PAXIL <> 40	Tab, Light Green, Oblong, Film Coated	Paroxetine HCl 40 mg	Paxil by SB	59742-3213	Antidepressant
PAXIL20MG	Tab, Pink, Oval, Paxil/20 mg	Paroxetine HCl 20 mg	Paxil by SKB	Canadian	Antidepressant
PAXIL30MG	Tab, Blue, Oval, Paxil 30 mg	Paroxetine HCl 30 mg	Paxil by SKB	Canadian	Antidepressant
PAXILCR <> 125	Tab, Yellow, Round, Film Coated, Paxil over CR <> 12.5	Paroxetine HCl 12.5 mg	Paxil CR by GSK	Canadian DIN 02248503	Antidepressant
PAXILCR <> 125	Tab, Yellow, Round, Film Coated, Paxil over CR <> 12.5	Paroxetine HCl 12.5 mg	Paxil CR by GSK	00029-3206	Antidepressant
PAXILCR <> 25	Tab, Pink, Round, Film Coated, Paxil CR 25	Paroxetine HCl 25 mg	Paxil CR by GSK	Canadian DIN 02248504	Antidepressant
PAXILCR <> 25	Tab, Pink, Round, Film Coated, Paxil CR 25	Paroxetine HCl 25 mg	Paxil CR by SKB	00029-3207	Antidepressant
PAXILCR <> 375	Tab, Blue, Round, Film Coated, Paxil over CR <> 37.5	Paroxetine HCl 37.5 mg	Paxil CR by SKB	00029-3208	Antidepressant
PBCT5MG	Cap, Beige	Bromocriptine 5 mg	Parlodel by Pharmascience	Canadian DIN 5760669492	Antiparkinson
PBM540	Cap, Red, Opaque	Folic Acid 1 mg, Vitamin B6 12.5 mg, Vitamin B12 500 mcg, Omega-3 Acids 500 mg, Docosahexaenoic Acid (DHA) 350 mg, Eicosapentaenoic Acid (EPA) 35 mg	Animi-3 by PBM	66213-0540	Supplement
PCH <> MEGESTROL40	Tab, White, Scored	Megestrol Acetate 40 mg	by Pharmachemie	57527-0513	Hormone
PCH <> MEGESTROL40	Tab, White, Scored, PCH <> Megestrol over 40	Megestrol Acetate 40 mg	by Teva	00093-5138 Discontinued	Hormone
PCHRES25	Tab, Yellow & White, Round, PCH/RES/25	Leucovorin 25 mg	Wellcovorin by AstraZeneca		Antineoplastic
PCHRES5	Tab, Yellow & White, Round, PCH/RES/5	Leucovorin Calcium 5 mg	Wellcovorin by AstraZeneca		Antineoplastic
PD	Tab, Tan	Thyroid Hormone 30 mg	Thyroid by Parke Davis	Canadian	Thyroid Hormone
PD	Tab, Tan	Thyroid Hormone 125 mg	Thyroid by Pfizer	Canadian DIN 00023965	Thyroid Hormone
PD	Tab, Tan	Thyroid Hormone 30 mg	Thyroid by Pfizer	Canadian DIN 00023949	Thyroid Hormone
PD	Tab, Tan	Thyroid Hormone 60 mg	Thyroid by Pfizer	Canadian DIN 00023957	Thyroid Hormone
PD	Tab, Salmon	Norethindrone Acetate 5 mg	by Parke Davis	Canadian	Hormone
PD <> 144	Tab, White, D-Shaped	Norethindrone Acetate 1 mg, Ethinyl Estradiol 5 mcg	Femhrt by Parke Davis	00071-0144	Oral Contraceptive
PD <> 144	Tab, White, D-Shaped	Norethindrone Acetate 1 mg, Ethinyl Estradiol 5 mcg	Femhrt by Pfizer	Canadian DIN 02242531	Oral Contraceptive
PD001	Tab, Green, Round, P-D 001	Pentaerythritol Tetranitrate 20 mg	Peritrate by Parke Davis		Antianginal
PD004	Tab, Green, Round, P-D 004	Pentaerythritol Tetranitrate SA 80 mg	Peritrate SA by Parke Davis		Antianginal
PD007	Tab, Yellow, Triangular, Scored, Chewable, P-D 007	Phenytoin 50 mg	Dilantin Infatabs by Parke Davis	00071-0007	Anticonvulsant
PD007	Tab, Yellow, Triangular, Scored, Chewable, P-D 007	Phenytoin 50 mg	Dilantin Infatabs by Nat Pharmpak	55154-2416	Anticonvulsant
PD008	Tab, Coral, Round, P-D 008	Pentaerythritol Tetranitrate 40 mg	Peritrate by Parke Davis		Antianginal
PD013	Tab, Green, Round, P-D 013	Pentaerythritol Tetranitrate 10 mg	Peritrate by Parke Davis		Antianginal
PD070	Tab, White, Round, P-D 070	Propranolol HCl 10 mg	Inderal by Parke Davis		Antihypertensive

ID FRONT <> BACK	DESCRIPTION FRONT <> BACK	INGREDIENT & STRENGTH	BRAND (or Generic Equiv.) by FIRM	NDC#	CLASS; SCH.
PD071	Tab, White, Round, P-D 071	Propranolol HCl 20 mg	Inderal by Parke Davis		Antihypertensive
PD072	Tab, White, Round, P-D 072	Propranolol HCl 40 mg	Inderal by Parke Davis		Antihypertensive
PD073	Tab, White, Round, P-D 073	Propranolol HCl 60 mg	Inderal by Parke Davis		Antihypertensive
PD074	Tab, White, Round, P-D 074	Propranolol HCl 80 mg	Inderal by Parke Davis		Antihypertensive
PD111	Tab, Orange, Round, P-D 111	Ergotamine Tartrate 2 mg	Ergostat SL by Parke Davis		Antimigraine
PD121	Tab, Blue, Round, P-D 121	Chlorthalidone 50 mg	Hygroton by Parke Davis		Diuretic
PD123	Tab, Orange, Round, P-D 123	Chlorthalidone 25 mg	Hygroton by Parke Davis		Diuretic
PD1412	Tab, White, Oval, P-D 141/2	Diazepam 2 mg	Valium by Parke Davis		Antianxiety; C IV
PD1425	Tab, White, Triangular, P-D 142/5	Diazepam 5 mg	Valium by Parke Davis		Antianxiety; C IV
PD14310	Tab, White, Round, P-D 143/10	Diazepam 10 mg	Valium by Parke Davis		Antianxiety; C IV
PD15	Tab, Pink	Phenobarbital 15 mg	Phenobarbital by Parke Davis	Canadian	Sedative/Hypnotic; C IV
PD155 <> 10	Tab, White, Oval, Film Coated	Atorvastatin Calcium 10 mg	Lipitor by Parke Davis	Canadian DIN 02230711	Antihyperlipidemic
PD155 <> 10	Tab, White, Oval, Film Coated	Atorvastatin Calcium 10 mg	Lipitor by Pharm Util	60491-0803	Antihyperlipidemic
PD155 <> 10	Tab, White, Oval, Film Coated	Atorvastatin Calcium 10 mg	Lipitor by Parke Davis	00071-0155	Antihyperlipidemic
PD155 <> 10	Tab, White, Oval, Film Coated	Atorvastatin Calcium 10 mg	Lipitor by Goedecke	53869-0155	Antihyperlipidemic
PD156 <> 20	Tab, White, Oval, Film Coated	Atorvastatin Calcium 20 mg	Lipitor by Pharm Util	60491-0804	Antihyperlipidemic
PD156 <> 20	Tab, White, Oval, Film Coated	Atorvastatin Calcium 20 mg	Lipitor by Physician Total Care	54868-3946	Antihyperlipidemic
PD156 <> 20	Tab, White, Oval, Film Coated	Atorvastatin Calcium 20 mg	Lipitor by Parke Davis	00071-0156	Antihyperlipidemic
PD156 <> 20	Tab, White, Oval, Film Coated	Atorvastatin Calcium 20 mg	Lipitor by Goedecke	53869-0156	Antihyperlipidemic
PD156 <> 20	Tab, White, Oval, Film Coated	Atorvastatin Calcium 20 mg	Lipitor by Parke Davis	Canadian DIN 02230713	Antihyperlipidemic
PD157 <> 40	Tab, White, Oval, Film Coated	Atorvastatin Calcium 40 mg	Lipitor by Parke Davis	Canadian DIN 02230714	Antihyperlipidemic
PD157 <> 40	Tab, White, Oval, Film Coated	Atorvastatin Calcium 40 mg	Lipitor by Murfreesboro	51129-1424	Antihyperlipidemic
PD157 <> 40	Tab, White, Oval, Film Coated	Atorvastatin Calcium 40 mg	Lipitor by Physician Total Care	54868-4229	Antihyperlipidemic
PD157 <> 40	Tab, White, Oval, Film Coated	Atorvastatin Calcium 40 mg	Lipitor by Parke Davis	00071-0157	Antihyperlipidemic
PD157 <> 40	Tab, White, Oval, Film Coated	Atorvastatin Calcium 40 mg	Lipitor by Goedecke	53869-0157	Antihyperlipidemic
PD158 <> 80	Tab, White, Oval, Film Coated	Atorvastatin Calcium 80 mg	Lipitor by Parke Davis	00071-0158	Antihyperlipidemic
PD158 <> 80	Tab, White, Oval, Film Coated	Atorvastatin Calcium 80 mg	Lipitor by Parke Davis	Canadian DIN 02243097	Antihyperlipidemic
PD166	Tab, Brown, Oval, P-D 166	Methenamine Mandelate 500 mg	Mandelamine by Parke Davis		Antibiotic; Urinary Tract
PD167	Tab, Purple, Oval, P-D 167	Methenamine Mandelate 1000 mg	Mandelamine by Parke Davis		Antibiotic; Urinary Tract
PD177	Tab, Pink, Oval, P-D 177	Phenylpropanolamine HCl 100 mg, Phenyltoloxamine 66 mg, Acetaminophen 600 mg	Sinubid by Parke Davis		Cold Remedy
PD180	Tab, Maroon, Round, Sugar Coated	Phenazopyridine HCl 100 mg	Pyridium by Parke Davis		Urinary Analgesic
PD180	Tab, Maroon, Round, Sugar Coated	Phenazopyridine HCl 100 mg	Pyridium by Able	53265 Discontinued	Urinary Analgesic
PD181	Tab, Maroon, Round, Sugar Coated	Phenazopyridine HCl 200 mg	Pyridium by Able	53265 Discontinued	Urinary Analgesic
PD181	Tab, Maroon, Round, Sugar Coated	Phenazopyridine HCl 200 mg	Pyridium by Parke Davis	Canadian DIN 00476722	Urinary Analgesic
PD182	Tab, Maroon, Square, P-D 182	Phenazopyridine HCl 150 mg, Hyoscyamine HBr 0.3 mg, Butabarbital 15 mg	Pyridium Plus by Parke Davis		Urinary Analgesic
PD200	Tab, Salmon, Round, P-D 200	Oxtriphylline 200 mg, Guaifenesin 100 mg	Brondecon by Parke Davis		Antiasthmatic
PD202	Tab, Green, Oval, P-D 202	Procainamide HCl SR 250 mg	Procan SR by Parke Davis		Antiarrhythmic
PD204	Tab, Yellow, Oval, P-D 204	Procainamide HCl SR 500 mg	Procan SR by Parke Davis		Antiarrhythmic
PD205	Tab, Orange, Black Print, Oblong, Scored	Procainamide HCl SR 750 mg	Procan SR by Parke Davis	00071-0205	Antiarrhythmic

ID FRONT <> BACK	DESCRIPTION FRONT <> BACK	INGREDIENT & STRENGTH	BRAND (or Generic Equiv.) by FIRM	NDC#	CLASS; SCH.
PD207	Tab, Red, Oblong, Scored	Procainamide HCl SR 1000 mg	Procan SR by Parke Davis	00071-0207	Antiarrhythmic
PD210	Tab, Red, Round, P-D 210	Oxtriphylline 100 mg	Choledyl by Parke Davis		Antiasthmatic
PD211	Tab, Yellow, Round, P-D 211	Oxtriphylline 200 mg	Choledyl by Parke Davis		Antiasthmatic
PD214	Tab, Elliptical-Shaped, Film Coated, P-D 214	Oxtriphylline 400 mg	Choledyl SA by Parke Davis		Antiasthmatic
PD220	Tab, Pink, Triangular, Scored, Film Coated	Hydrochlorothiazide 12.5 mg, Quinapril 20 mg	Accuretic by Parke Davis	00071-0214	Diuretic; Antihypertensive
PD220	Tab, Pink, Triangular, Scored, Film Coated	Hydrochlorothiazide 12.5 mg, Quinapril 20 mg	Accuretic by Parke Davis	Canadian DIN 02237368	Diuretic; Antihypertensive
PD221	Tab, Elliptical-Shaped, Film Coated, P-D 221	Oxtriphylline 600 mg	Choledyl SA by Parke Davis	00071-0221	Antiasthmatic
PD222	Tab, Pink, Oval, Scored, Film Coated	Hydrochlorothiazide 12.5 mg, Quinapril 10 mg	Accuretic by Parke Davis	Canadian DIN 02237367	Diuretic; Antihypertensive
PD222	Tab, Pink, Oval, Scored, Film Coated	Hydrochlorothiazide 12.5 mg, Quinapril 10 mg	Accuretic by Parke Davis	00071-0222	Diuretic; Antihypertensive
PD223	Tab, Pink, Round, Film Coated	Hydrochlorothiazide 25 mg, Quinapril 20 mg	Accuretic by Parke Davis	00071-0223	Diuretic; Antihypertensive
PD223	Tab, Pink, Round, Film Coated	Hydrochlorothiazide 25 mg, Quinapril 20 mg	Accuretic by Parke Davis	Canadian DIN 02237369	Diuretic; Antihypertensive
PD230	Tab, White, Round	Phenobarbital 8 mg, Theophylline 130 mg, Ephedrine 24 mg	Tedral by Parke Davis		Antiasthmatic; C IV
PD231	Tab, Coral & White, Round, P-D 231	Theophylline Anhydrous 180 mg, Ephedrine 48 mg, Phenobarbital SA 25 mg	Tedral SA by Parke Davis		Antiasthmatic; C IV
PD237	Cap, Transparent Orange, White Print, Soft Gel, PD over 237	Ethosuximide 250 mg	Zarontin by Parke Davis	00071-0237	Anticonvulsant
PD237	Cap, Transparent Orange, White Print, Soft Gel, PD over 237	Ethosuximide 250 mg	Zarontin by RP Scherer	11014-0121	Anticonvulsant
PD251	Tab, Gray, Round, P-D 251	Thyroglobulin 32 mg	Proloid by Parke Davis		Thyroid Hormone
PD252	Tab, Gray, Round, P-D 252	Thyroglobulin 65 mg	Proloid by Parke Davis		Thyroid Hormone
PD253	Tab, Gray, Round, P-D 253	Thyroglobulin 100 mg	Proloid by Parke Davis		Thyroid Hormone
PD254	Tab, Gray, Round, P-D 254	Thyroglobulin 200 mg	Proloid by Parke Davis		Thyroid Hormone
PD257	Tab, Gray, Round, P-D 257	Thyroglobulin 130 mg	Proloid by Parke Davis		Thyroid Hormone
PD260	Tab, Peach, Square, P-D 260	Liotrix	Euthroid 1/2 by Parke Davis		Thyroid Hormone
PD261	Tab, Tan, Square, P-D 261	Liotrix	Euthroid 1 by Parke Davis		Thyroid Hormone
PD262	Tab, Lavender, Square, P-D 262	Liotrix	Euthroid 2 by Parke Davis		Thyroid Hormone
PD263	Tab, Gray, Square, P-D 263	Liotrix	Euthroid 3 by Parke Davis		Thyroid Hormone
PD270	Tab, Orange, Brown Print, Round, Sugar Coated, PD over 270	Phenelzine Sulfate 15 mg	Nardil by Parke Davis	00071-0270	Antidepressant
PD271	Tab, Dark Yellow, Round, P-D 271	Amitriptyline HCl 100 mg	Elavil by Parke Davis		Antidepressant
PD272	Tab, Tan, Round, P-D 272	Amitriptyline HCl 10 mg	Elavil by Parke Davis		Antidepressant
PD273	Tab, Coral, Round, P-D 273	Amitriptyline HCl 25 mg	Elavil by Parke Davis		Antidepressant
PD274	Tab, Blue & Purple, Round, P-D 274	Amitriptyline HCl 50 mg	Elavil by Parke Davis		Antidepressant
PD275	Tab, Green, Round, P-D 275	Amitriptyline HCl 75 mg	Elavil by Parke Davis		Antidepressant
PD276	Tab, Blue, Round, P-D 276	Prazepam 10 mg	Centrax by Parke Davis		Sedative/Hypnotic; C IV
PD278	Tab, Orange, Oval, P-D 278	Amitriptyline HCl 150 mg	Elavil by Parke Davis		Antidepressant
PD282	Tab, Yellow, Oblong, P-D 282	Prenatal Vitamin Combination	Natafort Filmseals by Parke Davis		Vitamin
PD30	Tab, Yellow	Phenobarbital 30 mg	by Parke Davis	Canadian	Sedative; Hypnotic; C IV
PD320	Tab, White, Round, P-D 320	Ethopropazine 10 mg	Parsidol by Parke Davis		Antiparkinson
PD321	Tab, White, Round, P-D 321	Ethopropazine 50 mg	Parsidol by Parke Davis		Antiparkinson
PD337	Cap, Blue, P-D 337	Vitamin Combination	Eldec by Parke Davis		Vitamin
PD352 <> 200	Tab, Light Yellow, Oval, Film Coated	Troglitazone 200 mg	by Murfreesboro	51129-1286	Antidiabetic
PD352 <> 200	Tab, Light Yellow, Oval, Film Coated	Troglitazone 200 mg	Rezulin by Parke Davis	00071-0352	Antidiabetic
PD353 <> 400	Tab, Tan, Oval, Film Coated	Troglitazone 400 mg	Rezulin by Parke Davis	00071-0353	Antidiabetic

ID FRONT <> BACK	DESCRIPTION FRONT <> BACK	INGREDIENT & STRENGTH	BRAND (or Generic Equiv.) by FIRM	NDC#	CLASS; SCH.
PD353 <> 400	Tab, Tan, Oval, Film Coated	Troglitazone 400 mg	Rezulin by Teva	00480-0756	Antidiabetic
PD357 <> 300	Tab, White, Oval, Film Coated	Troglitazone 300 mg	by Murfreesboro	51129-1423	Antidiabetic
PD357 <> 300	Tab, White, Oval, Film Coated	Troglitazone 300 mg	Rezulin by Parke Davis	00071-0357	Antidiabetic
PD362	Cap, White w/ Orange Band, Black Print, Ex Release, PD over 362	Phenytoin Sodium 100 mg	Dilantin by Pharmedix	53002-0415	Anticonvulsant
PD362	Cap, White w/ Orange Band, Black Print, Ex Release, PD over 362	Phenytoin Sodium 100 mg	by Med Pro	53978-0298	Anticonvulsant
PD362	Cap, White w/ Orange Band, Black Print, Ex Release, PD over 362	Phenytoin Sodium 100 mg	by Nat Pharmpak	55154-2404	Anticonvulsant
PD362	Cap, White w/ Orange Band, Black Print, Ex Release, PD over 362	Phenytoin Sodium 100 mg	by Kaiser	00179-0222	Anticonvulsant
PD365	Cap, Clear w/ Pink Band, Black Print, Ex Release, PD over 365	Phenytoin Sodium 30 mg	Dilantin by Parke Davis	00071-0365	Anticonvulsant
PD373	Cap, Pink with White Band, P-D 373	Diphenhydramine HCl 50 mg	Benadryl by Parke Davis	00071-0373	Antihistamine
PD375	Cap, White/Red Band, P-D 375	Phenytoin Sodium 100 mg, Phenobarbital 16 mg	Dilantin with PB by Parke Davis		Anticonvulsant; C IV
PD379	Cap, White with Gray Band, PD over 379	Chloramphenicol 250 mg	Chloromycetin by Parke Davis	00071-0379	Antibiotic
PD389	Cap, P-D 389	Bromodiphenhydramine 25 mg	Ambodryl by Parke Davis		Antihistamine
PD390	Cap, Pink & Blue	Vitamin, Mineral Combination	Natabec by Parke Davis		Vitamin
PD393	Cap, Orange, P-D 393	Phensuximide 500 mg	Milontin by Parke Davis		Anticonvulsant
PD402	Cap, Blue & Gray, P-D 402	Ampicillin 250 mg	Principen by Parke Davis		Antibiotic
PD404	Cap, Blue & Gray, P-D 404	Ampicillin 500 mg	Principen by Parke Davis		Antibiotic
PD407	Cap, Red & White, P-D 407	Tetracycline HCl 250 mg	Achromycin V by Parke Davis		Antibiotic
PD425	Tab, White, Square	Norethindrone Acetate 1 mg, Ethinyl Estradiol 30 mcg	Estrostep Fe by Parke Davis	00071-0928	Oral Contraceptive
PD427	Tab, White, Triangular	Norethindrone Acetate 1 mg, Ethinyl Estradiol 20 mcg	Estrostep Fe by Parke Davis	00071-0928	Oral Contraceptive
PD437	Tab, Blue, Round, P-D 437	Quinestrol 100 mcg	Estrovis by Parke Davis		Hormone
PD440	Tab, White, Oval, P-D 440	Furosemide 20 mg	Lasix by Watson		Diuretic
PD441	Tab, White, Round, P-D 441	Furosemide 40 mg	Lasix by Parke Davis		Diuretic
PD442	Tab, White, Round, P-D 442	Furosemide 80 mg	Lasix by Parke Davis		Diuretic
PD443	Tab, Pink, Round, P-D 443	Clonidine HCl 0.1 mg	Catapres by Parke Davis		Antihypertensive
PD444	Tab, White, Round, P-D 444	Clonidine HCl 0.2 mg	Catapres by Parke Davis		Antihypertensive
PD445	Tab, White, Round, P-D 445	Clonidine HCl 0.3 mg	Catapres by Parke Davis		Antihypertensive
PD471	Cap, P-D 471	Diphenhydramine HCl 25 mg	Benadryl by Parke Davis	00071-0471	Antihistamine
PD490	Tab, Rose, Elliptical, Delayed Release	Aspirin 975 mg	Aspirin by Parke Davis		Analgesic
PD525300MG	Cap, Yellow w/ Orange Band, P-D 525	Methsuximide 300 mg	Celontin by Parke Davis	00071-0525	Anticonvulsant
PD527 <> 5	Tab, Brown, Oval, Scored, Film Coated	Quinapril HCl 5 mg	Accupril by PDRX	55289-0552	Antihypertensive
PD527 <> 5	Tab, Brown, Oval, Scored, Film Coated	Quinapril HCl 5 mg	Accupril by Pharm Util	60491-0001	Antihypertensive
PD527 <> 5	Tab, Brown, Oval, Scored, Film Coated	Quinapril HCl 5 mg	Accupril by Parke Davis	00071-0527	Antihypertensive
PD527 <> 5	Tab, Brown, Oval, Scored, Film Coated	Quinapril HCl 5 mg	Accupril by Parke Davis	Canadian DIN 01947664	Antihypertensive
PD529	Cap, Black & Yellow, Opaque	Paromomycin Sulfate 250 mg	Humatin by Pfizer	Canadian DIN 02078759	Antibiotic
PD529	Cap, Black & Yellow, Opaque	Paromomycin Sulfate 250 mg	Humatin by Parke Davis	00071-0529	Antibiotic
PD529	Cap, Black & Yellow, Opaque	Paromomycin Sulfate 250 mg	Humatin by Monarch	61570-0529	Antibiotic
PD530 <> 10	Tab, Brown, Triangular, Film Coated	Quinapril HCl 10 mg	Accupril by RX Pak	65084-0124	Antihypertensive
PD530 <> 10	Tab, Brown, Triangular, Film Coated	Quinapril HCl 10 mg	Accupril by Direct Dispensing	57866-4420	Antihypertensive
PD530 <> 10	Tab, Brown, Triangular, Film Coated	Quinapril HCl 10 mg	Accupril by PDRX	55289-0553	Antihypertensive

ID FRONT <> BACK	DESCRIPTION FRONT <> BACK	INGREDIENT & STRENGTH	BRAND (or Generic Equiv.) by FIRM	NDC#	CLASS; SCH.
PD530 <> 10	Tab, Brown, Triangular, Film Coated	Quinapril HCl 10 mg	Accupril by Parke Davis	Canadian DIN 01947672	Antihypertensive
PD530 <> 10	Tab, Brown, Triangular, Film Coated	Quinapril HCl 10 mg	Accupril by Parke Davis	00071-0530	Antihypertensive
PD531	Cap, White/Black Band, P-D 531	Phenytoin Sodium 100 mg, Phenobarbital 32 mg	Dilantin with PB by Parke Davis		Anticonvulsant; C IV
PD532 <> 20	Tab, Brown, Round, Film Coated, PD over 532	Quinapril HCl 20 mg	Accupril by Parke Davis	00071-0532	Antihypertensive
PD532 <> 20	Tab, Brown, Round, Film Coated, PD over 532	Quinapril HCl 20 mg	Accupril by PDRX	55289-0554	Antihypertensive
PD532 <> 20	Tab, Brown, Round, Film Coated, PD over 532	Quinapril HCl 20 mg	Accupril by Parke Davis	Canadian DIN 01947680	Antihypertensive
PD534	Cap, Pink & Purple, P-D 534	Prenatal Vitamin Combination, Fluoride	Natabec Fluoride by Parke Davis		Vitamin
PD535 <> 40	Tab, Brown, Oval, Film Coated	Quinapril HCl 40 mg	Accupril by Parke Davis	Canadian DIN 01947699	Antihypertensive
PD535 <> 40	Tab, Brown, Oval, Film Coated	Quinapril HCl 40 mg	Accupril by Parke Davis	00071-0535	Antihypertensive
PD535 <> 40	Tab, Brown, Oval, Film Coated	Quinapril HCl 40 mg	Accupril by PDRX	55289-0555	Antihypertensive
PD537150MG	Cap, Yellow, P-D 537 150 mg	Methsuximide 150 mg	Celontin by Parke Davis	00071-0537	Anticonvulsant
PD540PONSTEL	Cap, Yellow with Blue Band, P-D 540	Mefenamic Acid 250 mg	Ponstel by Parke Davis	00071-0540	NSAID
PD541	Cap, Pink & White	Vitamin, Mineral Combination	Natabec FA by Parke Davis		Vitamin
PD544	Cap, Blue & Yellow	Vitamin, Mineral Combination	Geriplex-FS by Parke Davis		Vitamin
PD547	Cap, Blue & White Band, P-D 547	Prenatal Vitamin Combination	Natabec RX by Parke Davis		Vitamin
PD552	Cap, Celery	Prazepam 5 mg	Centrax by Parke Davis		Sedative/Hypnotic; C IV
PD553	Cap, Aqua	Prazepam 10 mg	Centrax by Parke Davis		Sedative/Hypnotic; C IV
PD554	Cap, Ivory	Prazepam 20 mg	Centrax by Parke Davis		Sedative/Hypnotic; C IV
PD555	Tab, White, Round	Norethindrone Acetate 1 mg, Ethinyl Estradiol 35 mcg	Estrostep Fe by Parke Davis	00071-0928	Oral Contraceptive
PD557	Tab, White, Round, P-D 557	Verapamil 80 mg	Isoptin by Parke Davis		Antihypertensive
PD573	Tab, White, Round, P-D 573	Verapamil 120 mg	Isoptin by Parke Davis		Antihypertensive
PD60	Tab, Light Green	Phenobarbital 60 mg	by Parke Davis	Canadian	Sedative/Hypnotic; C IV
PD607	Tab, White, Round, P-D 607	Phenobarbital 60 mg	by Parke Davis		Sedative/Hypnotic; C IV
PD618	Tab, White, Round, P-D 618	Placebo	Placebo by Parke Davis		Placebo
PD622	Tab, Brown, Round, P-D 622	Ferrous Fumarate 75 mg	Estrostep Fe by Parke Davis	00071-0928	Oral Contraceptive; Placebo
PD622	Tab, Brown, Round, P-D 622	Ferrous Fumarate 75 mg	Loestrin Fe by Parke Davis	00071-0917	Oral Contraceptive; Placebo
PD634	Tab, White, Round, P-D 634	Acetaminophen 300 mg, Codeine Phosphate 15 mg	Tylenol w/ Codeine by Parke Davis		Analgesic; C III
PD635	Tab, White, Round, P-D 635	Acetaminophen 300 mg, Codeine Phosphate 30 mg	Tylenol w/ Codeine by Parke Davis		Analgesic; C III
PD637	Tab, White, Round, P-D 637	Acetaminophen 300 mg, Codeine Phosphate 60 mg	Tylenol w/ Codeine by Parke Davis		Analgesic; C III
PD638	Tab, Brown, Oval, P-D 638	Vitamin Combination	Tabron by Parke Davis		Vitamin
PD648	Tab, White, Oval, P-D 648	Penicillin V Potassium 250 mg	V-Cillin K by Parke Davis		Antibiotic
PD663	Cap, Orange, Clear, Delayed Release	Erythromycin 125 mg	Eryc by Parke Davis		Antibiotic
PD669LOPID	Cap, Maroon and White, Hard Gel	Gemfibrozil 300 mg	Lopid by Parke Davis	Canadian DIN 00599026	Antihyperlipidemic
PD672	Tab, Yellow, Round, P-D 672	Erythromycin Stearate 250 mg	Erythrocin by Parke Davis		Antibiotic
PD673	Tab, White, Oval, P-D 673	Penicillin V Potassium 500 mg	V-Cillin K by Parke Davis		Antibiotic
PD692	Cap, P-D 692	Propoxyphene 65 mg	Darvon by Parke Davis		Analgesic; C IV
PD696ERYC	Cap, Clear & Orange	Erythromycin 250 mg	by Murfreesboro	51129-1422	Antibiotic
PD696ERYC	Cap, P-D 696	Erythromycin 250 mg	Eryc by Parke Davis	00071-0696	Antibiotic

ID FRONT <> BACK	DESCRIPTION FRONT <> BACK	INGREDIENT & STRENGTH	BRAND (or Generic Equiv.) by FIRM	NDC# Canadian DIN	CLASS; SCH.
PD696ERYC	Cap, Clear & Orange, Opaque	Erythromycin 250 mg	Eryc by Parke Davis	0607142	Antibiotic
PD696ERYC	Cap, P-D 696	Erythromycin 250 mg	by Allscripts		Antibiotic
PD697	Cap, Orange & White, P-D 697	Tetracycline HCl 500 mg	Achromycin V by Parke Davis		Antibiotic
PD698	Tab, White, Round, P-D 698	Phenobarbital 100 mg	Phenobarbital by Parke Davis		Sedative/Hypnotic; C IV
PD699	Tab, White, Round, P-D 699	Phenobarbital 15 mg	Phenobarbital by Parke Davis		Sedative/Hypnotic; C IV
PD700	Tab, White, Round, P-D 700	Phenobarbital 30 mg	by Parke Davis		Sedative/Hypnotic; C IV
PD702	Tab, White, Round, P-D 702	Hydrochlorothiazide 25 mg	Hydrodiuril by Parke Davis		Diuretic; Antihypertensive
PD710	Tab, White, Round, P-D 710	Hydrochlorothiazide 50 mg	Hydrodiuril by Parke Davis		Diuretic; Antihypertensive
PD712	Tab, White, Round, P-D 712	Hydrochlorothiazide 25 mg, Spironolactone 25 mg	Aldactazide by Parke Davis		Diuretic; Antihypertensive
PD713	Tab, White, Round, P-D 713	Spironolactone 25 mg	Aldactone by Parke Davis		Diuretic
PD725	Tab, White, Round, P-D 725	Aspirin 325 mg, Codeine Phosphate 15 mg	Aspirin w/ Codeine by Parke Davis		Analgesic; C III
PD726	Tab, White, Round, P-D 726	Aspirin 325 mg, Codeine Phosphate 30 mg	Aspirin w/ Codeine by Parke Davis		Analgesic; C III
PD727	Tab, White, Round, P-D 727	Aspirin 325 mg, Codeine Phosphate 60 mg	Aspirin w/ Codeine by Parke Davis		Analgesic; C III
PD730	Cap, Pink & Red, P-D 730	Amoxicillin 250 mg	Amoxil by Parke Davis		Antibiotic
PD731	Cap, Pink & Red, P-D 731	Amoxicillin 500 mg	Amoxil by Parke Davis		Antibiotic
PD737 <> LOPID	Tab, White, Blue Print, Oval, Scored, Film Coated, P-D 737	Gemfibrozil 600 mg	Lopid by Parke Davis	00071-0737	Antihyperlipidemic
PD813	Tab, Orange, Round, P-D 813	Doxycycline Hyclate 100 mg	Vibra-Tab by Parke Davis		Antibiotic
PD829	Cap, Aqua & Cream, P-D 829	Doxycycline Hyclate 50 mg	Vibramycin by Parke Davis		Antibiotic
PD830	Cap, Aqua, P-D 830	Doxycycline Hyclate 100 mg	Vibramycin by Parke Davis		Antibiotic
PD849	Tab, White, Round, P-D 849	Quinidine Sulfate 200 mg	Quinidine by Parke Davis		Antiarrhythmic
PD850	Tab, White, Round, P-D 850	Quinidine Gluconate 330 mg	Duraquin by Parke Davis		Antiarrhythmic
PD865	Tab, Blue, Round, P-D 865	Methyldopa 250 mg	Aldomet by Parke Davis		Antihypertensive
PD866	Tab, Blue, Round, P-D 866	Methyldopa 500 mg	Aldomet by Parke Davis		Antihypertensive
PD882	Tab, White, Round, P-D 882	Norethindrone 5 mg	Norlutin by Parke Davis		Oral Contraceptive
PD887	Cap, Blue & Aqua, P-D 887	Indomethacin 25 mg	Indocin by Parke Davis		NSAID
PD888	Cap, Blue & Aqua, P-D 888	Indomethacin 50 mg	Indocin by Parke Davis		NSAID
PD901	Tab, Pink, Round, P-D 901	Norethindrone Acetate 2.5 mg, Ethinyl Estradiol 50 mcg	Norlestrin by Parke Davis		Oral Contraceptive
PD904	Tab, Yellow, Round, P-D 904	Norethindrone Acetate 1 mg, Ethinyl Estradiol 50 mcg	Norlestrin by Parke Davis		Oral Contraceptive
PD915	Tab, White, Round, P-D 915	Norethindrone Acetate 1 mg, Ethinyl Estradiol 20 mcg	Loestrin 21 by Parke Davis	00071-0915	Oral Contraceptive
PD916	Tab, Green, Round, P-D 916	Norethindrone Acetate 1.5 mg, Ethinyl Estradiol 30 mcg	Loestrin 21 by Parke Davis	00071-0916	Oral Contraceptive
PD917	Tab, Green, Round, P-D 917	Ethinyl Estradiol 30 mcg, Norethindrone Acetate 1.5 mg	Loestrin Fe by Parke Davis	00071-0917	Oral Contraceptive
PD918	Tab, Pink, Round, P-D 918	Norethindrone Acetate 5 mg	Norlutate by Parke Davis		Hormone
PD919	Tab, Yellow, Oval, P-D 919	Erythromycin Stearate 500 mg	Erythrocin by Parke Davis		Antibiotic
PDNEURONTINR300MG	Cap, PD <> Neurontin R/300 mg	Gabapentin 300 mg	by Caremark	00339-6101	Anticonvulsant
PE	Tab, Red, Round	Phenylephrine HCl 10 mg	Sudafed PE by Pfizer		Decongestant
PE220	Tab, Light Yellow, Cap Shaped, Film Coated	Vitamin E 150 IU, Vitamin E 2.5 mg, Vitamin E 9 mg, Selenium 20.0 mcg, Lycopene Complex 5 mg, Zinc 15 mg, Folic Acid 2 mg, Cyanocobalamin 500 mcg, Pyridoxine HCL 25 mg	Udamin by ProEthic	66869-0220	Supplement
PE424	Tab, White, Oval Scored	Chlorpheniramine Maleate 8 mg, Methscopolamine Nitrate 1.25 mg, Pseudoephedrine HCl 60 mg	Durahist by ProEthic Labs	66869-0424	Cold Remedy
PE425	Tab, White, Oval Scored	Chlorpheniramine Maleate 8 mg, Methscopolamine Nitrate 1.25 mg, Phenylephrine HCl 20 mg	Durahist PE by ProEthic Labs	66869-0425	Cold Remedy

ID FRONT <> BACK	DESCRIPTION FRONT <> BACK	INGREDIENT & STRENGTH	BRAND (or Generic Equiv.) by FIRM	NDC#	CLASS; SCH.
PE614	Tab, White, Oval, Scored	Guaifenesin 1200 mg, Phenylephrine HCl 40 mg, Dextromethorphan HBr 20 mg	Duraphen DM by ProEthic Labs	66869-0614	Cold Remedy
PE715	Tab, White, Dye-Free, Scored, PE-715	Guaifenesin 800 mg, Phenylephrine HCl 20 mg, Dextromethorphan HBr 20 mg	Duraphen II DM by ProEthic	66869-0715	Cold Remedy
PE723	Tab, White, Oval, Scored	Acetaminophen 500 mg, Dextromethorphan HBr 20 mg, Guaifenesin 200 mg, Pseudoephedrine HCl 60 mg	DuraFlu by ProEthic Labs	66869-0723	Cold Remedy
PE8 <> APO	Tab, Green, Round	Perindopril Erbumine 8 mg	Coversyl by Apotex	Canadian DIN 02289296	Antihypertensive
PE805	Tab, White, Dye-Free, Scored, PE-805	Guaifenesin 1200 mg, Phenylephrine HCl 30 mg, Dextromethorphan HBr 30 mg	Duraphen Forte by ProEthic	66869-0805	Cold Remedy
PE820	Tab, White, Cap Shaped, Film Coated	Saw Palmetto 320 mg, Vitamin E 75 IU, Vitamin E 12.5 mg, Vitamin E 4.5 mg, Selenium 100 mcg, Lycopene Complex 2.5mg, Zinc 7.5 mg, Folic Acid 1 mg, Cyanocobalamin 25.0 mcg, Pyridoxine 12.5 mg	Udamin SP by ProEthic	66869-0820	Supplement
PE822	Tab, White, Cap Shaped, Scored	Guaifenesin 800 mg, Phenylephrine HCl 25 mg	Duraphen II by ProEthic Labs	66869-0822	Cold Remedy
PE826	Cap, Red and White	Acetaminophen 325 mg, Salicylamide 250 mg, Phenyltoloxamine Citrate 20 mg, Caffeine 50 mg	Durabac by ProEthic Labs	66869-0826	Analgesic
PEC101	Tab, Scored	Ascorbic Acid 100 mg, Biotin 0.03 mg, Calcium Carbonate, Precipitated, Calcium Pantothenate, Cholecalciferol, Chromium 0.025 mg, Cupric Oxide, Cyanocobalamin 0.012 mg, Ferrous Fumarate, Folic Acid 1 mg, Magnesium Oxide, Manganese Sulfate Monohydrate, Niacinamide 20 mg, Potassium Iodide, Pyridoxine HCl 10 mg, Riboflavin 3.4 mg, Sodium Molybdate, Thiamine Mononitrate, Vitamin A Acetate 5000 Units, Zinc Oxide	Pecos Prenatal No 101 by Anabolic	00722-6266	Vitamin
PEC101	Tab, Scored	Ascorbic Acid 100 mg, Biotin, D- 30 mcg, Calcium 250 mg, Calcium Pantothenate 10 mg, Cholecalciferol 400 Units, Chromium 25 mcg, Copper 2 mg, Cyanocobalamin 12 mcg, Folic Acid 1 mg, Iodine 150 mcg, Iron 60 mg, Magnesium 25 mg, Manganese 5 mg, Molybdenum 25 mcg, Niacin 20 mg, Pyridoxine HCl 10 mg, Riboflavin 3.4 mg, Thiamine HCl 3 mg, Vitamin A 5000 Units, Vitamin E 30 Units, Zinc 25 mg	Prenatal M by Mutual	53489-0300	Vitamin
PEC101	Tab, Scored	Ascorbic Acid 100 mg, Biotin, D- 30 mcg, Calcium 250 mg, Calcium Pantothenate 10 mg, Cholecalciferol 400 Units, Chromium 25 mcg, Copper 2 mg, Cyanocobalamin 12 mcg, Folic Acid 1 mg, Iodine 150 mcg, Iron 60 mg, Magnesium 25 mg, Manganese 5 mg, Molybdenum 25 mcg, Niacin 20 mg, Pyridoxine HCl 10 mg, Riboflavin 3.4 mg, Thiamine HCl 3 mg, Vitamin A 5000 Units, Vitamin E 30 Units, Zinc 25 mg	Materna Type by Contract	10267-1371	Vitamin
PEC102	Tab, Scored	Ascorbic Acid 120 mg, Calcium 250 mg, Copper 2 mg, Cyanocobalamin 12 mcg, Docusate Sodium 50 mg, Folic Acid 1 mg, Iodine 0.15 mg, Iron 90 mg, Niacinamide 20 mg, Pyridoxine HCl 20 mg, Riboflavin 3.4 mg, Thiamine HCl 3 mg, Vitamin A 4000 Units, Vitamin D 400 Units, Vitamin E 30 Units, Zinc 25 mg	Maternal Plus 90 by Ivax	00182-4387	Vitamin
PEC102	Tab, Film Coated, Scored	Ascorbic Acid 120 mg, Calcium 250 mg, Copper 2 mg, Cyanocobalamin 12 mcg, Docusate Sodium 50 mg, Folic Acid 1 mg, Iodine 0.15 mg, Iron 90 mg, Niacinamide 20 mg, Pyridoxine HCl 20 mg, Riboflavin 3.4 mg, Thiamine HCl 3 mg, Vitamin A 4000 Units, Vitamin D 400 Units, Vitamin E 30 Units, Zinc 25 mg	Prenatal 90 by Mutual	53489-0301	Vitamin
PEC102	Tab, Film Coated, Scored	Ascorbic Acid 120 mg, Calcium 250 mg, Copper 2 mg, Cyanocobalamin 12 mcg, Docusate Sodium 50 mg, Folic Acid 1 mg, Iodine 0.15 mg, Iron 90 mg, Niacinamide 20 mg, Pyridoxine HCl 20 mg, Riboflavin 3.4 mg, Thiamine HCl 3 mg, Vitamin A 4000 Units, Vitamin D 400 Units, Vitamin E 30 Units, Zinc 25 mg	Prenate 90 by Lini	58215-0307 Discontinued	Vitamin

ID FRONT <> BACK	DESCRIPTION FRONT <> BACK	INGREDIENT & STRENGTH	BRAND (or Generic Equiv.) by FIRM	NDC#	CLASS; SCH.
PEC103	Tab, Coated	Ascorbic Acid 120 mg, Calcium 250 mg, Cholecalciferol 400 Units, Copper 2 mg, Cyanocobalamin 12 mcg, Docusate Sodium 50 mg, Folic Acid 1 mg, Iodine 150 mcg, Iron 90 mg, Niacinamide 20 mg, Pyridoxine HCl 20 mg, Riboflavin 3.4 mg, Thiamine HCl 3 mg, Vitamin A 4000 Units, Vitamin E 30 Units, Zinc 25 mg	Maternity 90 Prenatal Vit & Min by Qualitest	00603-5355	Vitamin
PEC104	Tab	Ascorbic Acid 70 mg, Calcium 200 mg, Cyanocobalamin 2.2 mcg, Folic Acid 1 mg, Iodine 175 mcg, Iron 65 mg, Magnesium 100 mg, Niacin 17 mg, Pyridoxine HCl 2.2 mg, Riboflavin 1.6 mg, Selenium 65 mcg, Thiamine Mononitrate 1.5 mg, Vitamin A 4000 Units, Vitamin D 400 Units, Vitamin E 10 Units, Zinc 15 mg	Z+ Prenatal by Qualitest	00603-6476	Vitamin
PEC105	Cap, Orange & Brown	Polysaccharide Iron Complex	Niferex-150 by Pecos	00677-1597	Vitamin
PEC105	Cap, Brown Cap, Orange Body	Polysaccharide Iron 150 Complex	Niferex 150 by URL Mutual	58215-0323	Vitamin
PEC106	Cap, ER	Pheniramine Maleate 8 mg, Phenylpropanolamine HCl 25 mg, Phenyltoloxamine Citrate 8 mg, Pyrilamine Maleate 8 mg	Multihistamine D Ped by Lini	Discontinued	Cold Remedy
PEC106	Cap, ER	Pheniramine Maleate 8 mg, Phenylpropanolamine HCl 25 mg, Phenyltoloxamine Citrate 8 mg, Pyrilamine Maleate 8 mg	Multihist D Ped by Mutual	53489-0267	Cold Remedy
PEC108	Tab	Guaifenesin 600 mg, Phenylpropanolamine HCl 75 mg	Entex LA by Pecos	59879-0108	Cold Remedy
PEC108	Tab	Guaifenesin 600 mg, Phenylpropanolamine HCl 75 mg	Entex LA by Moore	00839-8018	Cold Remedy
PEC108	Tab	Guaifenesin 600 mg, Phenylpropanolamine HCl 75 mg	Entex LA by Ivax	00182-2626	Cold Remedy
PEC108	Tab	Guaifenesin 600 mg, Phenylpropanolamine HCl 75 mg	Entex LA by Lini	58215-0321 Discontinued	Cold Remedy
PEC109	Cap, Clear, ER	Hyoscyamine Sulfate 0.375 mg	Levsin by Qualitest	00603-4004	Gastrointestinal
PEC110	Tab, Sugar Coated	Atropine Sulfate 0.0582 mg, Hyoscyamine Sulfate 0.3111 mg, Phenobarbital 48.6 mg, Scopolamine 0.0195 mg	Donnatal by Pecos	59879-0110	Gastrointestinal; C IV
PEC110	Tab, Sugar Coated	Atropine Sulfate 0.0582 mg, Hyoscyamine Sulfate 0.3111 mg, Phenobarbital 48.6 mg, Scopolamine 0.0195 mg	Donnatal by Moore	00839-7974	Gastrointestinal; C IV
PEC110	Tab	Atropine Sulfate 0.0582 mg, Hyoscyamine Sulfate 0.311 mg, Phenobarbital 48.6 mg, Scopolamine 0.0195 mg	Donnatal by Physician Total Care	54868-3622	Gastrointestinal; C IV
PEC110	Tab, Sugar Coated	Atropine Sulfate 0.0582 mg, Hyoscyamine Sulfate 0.3111 mg, Phenobarbital 48.6 mg, Scopolamine 0.0195 mg	Donnatal by Lini	58215-0303 Discontinued	Gastrointestinal; C IV
PEC111	Cap, Maroon, Opaque, Ex Release	Chlorpheniramine Maleate 12 mg, Phenylpropanolamine 75 mg	Ornade by Lini	58215-0329 Discontinued	Cold Remedy
PEC111	Cap, Maroon, Opaque, Ex Release	Chlorpheniramine Maleate 12 mg, Phenylpropanolamine 75 mg	Ornade by Circa	71114-4209	Cold Remedy
PEC111	Cap, Gray, Pink & White Beads	Chlorpheniramine Maleate 12 mg, Phenylpropanolamine 75 mg	Ornade by Mutual	53489-0302	Cold Remedy
PEC111	Cap, Maroon, Opaque, Ex Release	Chlorpheniramine Maleate 12 mg, Phenylpropanolamine 75 mg	Ornade by Pecos	59879-0111	Cold Remedy
PEC111	Cap	Chlorpheniramine Maleate 12 mg, Phenylpropanolamine 75 mg	Ornade by Qualitest	00603-4862	Cold Remedy
PEC111	Cap, Red	Chlorpheniramine Maleate 12 mg, Phenylpropanolamine 75 mg	Ornade by Breckenridge	51991-0150	Cold Remedy
PEC112	Tab, Film Coated	Guaifenesin 600 mg, Pseudoephedrine HCl 120 mg	by URL Mutual	00677-1476	Cold Remedy
PEC112	Tab, Film Coated	Guaifenesin 600 mg, Pseudoephedrine HCl 120 mg	Entex PSE by Lini	58215-0310 Discontinued	Cold Remedy
PEC112	Tab, Film Coated	Guaifenesin 600 mg, Pseudoephedrine HCl 120 mg	Guaifed PSE by Pecos	59879-0112	Cold Remedy
PEC114	Tab, Ex Release, PEC 114	Hyoscyamine Sulfate 0.375 mg	Levsin by URL Mutual	00677-1611	Gastrointestinal
PEC114	Tab, Ex Release, PEC 114	Hyoscyamine Sulfate 0.375 mg	Levsin by Mutual	53489-0241	Gastrointestinal
PEC114	Tab, Ex Release, PEC 114	Hyoscyamine Sulfate 0.375 mg	Levsin by Lini	58215-0331 Discontinued	Gastrointestinal
PEC114	Tab, Ex Release, PEC 114	Hyoscyamine Sulfate 0.375 mg	Levsin by Pecos	59879-0114	Gastrointestinal
PEC114	Tab, Ex Release, PEC/114	Hyoscyamine Sulfate 0.375 mg	Levsin by Sovereign	58716-0679	Gastrointestinal
PEC115	Cap	Trimethobenzamide HCl 250 mg	by URL Mutual	00677-1383	Antiemetic
PEC115	Cap	Trimethobenzamide HCl 250 mg	by Qualitest	00603-6256	Antiemetic
PEC115	Cap	Trimethobenzamide HCl 250 mg	by Pecos	59879-0115	Antiemetic

ID FRONT <> BACK	DESCRIPTION FRONT <> BACK	INGREDIENT & STRENGTH	BRAND (or Generic Equiv.) by FIRM	NDC#	CLASS; SCH.
PEC115	Cap	Trimethobenzamide HCl 250 mg	by Lini	58215-0320 Discontinued	Antiemetic
PEC116	Tab, Dark Blue	Guaifenesin 600 mg, Pseudoephedrine HCl 60 mg	by URL Mutual	00677-1487	Cold Remedy
PEC116	Tab, Dark Blue	Guaifenesin 600 mg, Pseudoephedrine HCl 60 mg	Decongest II by Lini	58215-0318 Discontinued	Cold Remedy
PEC116	Tab, Dark Blue	Guaifenesin 600 mg, Pseudoephedrine HCl 60 mg	Decongest II by Pecos	59879-0116	Cold Remedy
PEC117	Cap, ER, PEC 117	Pheniramine Maleate 16 mg, Phenylpropanolamine HCl 50 mg, Phenyltoloxamine Citrate 16 mg, Pyrilamine Maleate 16 mg	Multihist D by Mutual	53489-0266	Cold Remedy
PEC117	Cap, ER, PEC 117	Pheniramine Maleate 16 mg, Phenylpropanolamine HCl 50 mg, Phenyltoloxamine Citrate 16 mg, Pyrilamine Maleate 16 mg	Poly D by Qualitest	00603-5230	Cold Remedy
PEC117	Cap, ER	Pheniramine Maleate 16 mg, Phenylpropanolamine HCl 50 mg, Phenyltoloxamine Citrate 16 mg, Pyrilamine Maleate 16 mg	Multihistamine D by Lini	58215-0317 Discontinued	Cold Remedy
PEC118	Cap, Burgundy	Vitamin, Iron	Chromagen by Pecos		Vitamin
PEC121	Tab, Bluish Green	Belladonna Alkaloids 0.2 mg, Ergotamine Tartrate 0.6 mg, Phenobarbital 40 mg	Bellaphen S by Pecos	59879-0121	Gastrointestinal; C IV
PEC121	Tab, Bluish Green	Belladonna Alkaloids 0.2 mg, Ergotamine Tartrate 0.6 mg, Phenobarbital 40 mg	Bellamine S by Mutual	53489-0232	Gastrointestinal; C IV
PEC121	Tab, Bluish Green	Belladonna Alkaloids 0.2 mg, Ergotamine Tartrate 0.6 mg, Phenobarbital 40 mg	Phenarbal S by Lini	58215-0304 Discontinued	Gastrointestinal; C IV
PEC122	Cap, Clear & Orange, Opaque	Amylase 48,000 Units, Lipase 16,000 Units, Protease 48,000 Units	Pancrelipase 16,000 by Pecos	59879-0122	Gastrointestinal
PEC122	Cap, Clear & Orange, Opaque	Amylase 48,000 Units, Lipase 16,000 Units, Protease 48,000 Units	Pancrelipase 16000 by Lini	58215-0300 Discontinued	Gastrointestinal
PEC122	Cap, Orange Clear & Orange Opaque	Amylase 48,000 Units, Lipase 16,000 Units, Protease 48,000 Units	Pancrelipase 16000 by Mutual	53489-0247	Gastrointestinal
PEC122	Cap, Clear & Orange, Opaque	Amylase 48,000 Units, Lipase 16,000 Units, Protease 48,000 Units	Pancrelipase 16000 by URL Mutual	00677-1543	Gastrointestinal
PEC122	Cap, Orange & Clear	Pancrelipase 16,000 U	Pancrease MT 16 by Pecos		Gastrointestinal
PEC123	Tab, White, Oval	Prenatal Vitamin	Prenate Ultra by Pecos		Vitamin
PEC126	Cap, White & Opaque	Pancron 20	Creon-20 by Pecos		Gastrointestinal
PEC126	Cap	Amylase 66,400 Units, Lipase 20,000 Units, Protease 75,000 Units	Pancrelipase 20000 by Lini	58215-0332 Discontinued	Gastrointestinal
PEC126	Cap, Delayed Release	Amylase 66,400 Units, Lipase 20,000 Units, Protease 75,000 Units	Pancron 20 by Pecos	59879-0126	Gastrointestinal
PEC126	Cap,	Amylase 66,400 Units, Lipase 20,000 Units, Protease 75,000 Units	Pancrelipase 20000 by URL Mutual	00677-1631	Gastrointestinal
PEC126	Cap	Amylase 66,400 Units, Lipase 20,000 Units, Protease 75,000 Units	Pancrelipase 20000 by Mutual	53489-0303	Gastrointestinal
PEC128	Tab, Film Coated	Ascorbic Acid 120 mg, Biotin 30 mcg, Calcium 200 mg, Chromium 25 mcg, Copper 2 mg, Cyanocobalamin 12 mcg, Folic Acid 1 mg, Iodine 150 mcg, Iron 27 mg, Magnesium 25 mg, Manganese 5 mg, Molybdenum 25 mcg, Niacinamide 20 mg, Pantothenic Acid 10 mg, Pyridoxine HCl 10 mg, Riboflavin 3.4 mg, Selenium 20 mcg, Thiamine HCl 3 mg, Vitamin A 5000 Units, Vitamin D 400 Units, Vitamin E 30 Units, Zinc 25 mg	Prenatal M New Form by Pecos	59879-0128	Vitamin
PEC301	Tab, PEC 301	Hyoscyamine Sulfate 0.125 mg	Levsin by Mutual	53489-0239	Gastrointestinal
PEC301	Tab, PEC/301	Hyoscyamine Sulfate 0.125 mg	Levsin by Sovereign	58716-0651	Gastrointestinal
PEC505	Cap	Amylase 33,200 Units, Lipase 10,000 Units, Protease 37,500 Units	Pancrelipase 10000 by URL Mutual	00677-1576	Gastrointestinal
PEC505	Cap	Amylase 33,200 Units, Lipase 10,000 Units, Protease 37,500 Units	Pancreatin 10 by Moore	00839-8016	Gastrointestinal
PEC505	Cap	Amylase 33,200 Units, Lipase 10,000 Units, Protease 37,500 Units	Pancrelipase 10000 by Lini	58215-0322 Discontinued	Gastrointestinal
PEC505	Cap	Amylase 33,200 Units, Lipase 10,000 Units, Protease 37,500 Units	Pancron 10 Pancreatin by Pecos	59879-0505	Gastrointestinal
PEC505	Cap	Amylase 33,200 Units, Lipase 10,000 Units, Protease 37,500 Units	Pancrelipase 10000 by Mutual	53489-0246	Gastrointestinal
PEC506	Cap, ER	Pheniramine Maleate 8 mg, Phenylpropanolamine HCl 25 mg, Phenyltoloxamine Citrate 8 mg, Pyrilamine Maleate 8 mg	Uni Multihist D Ped by URL Mutual	00677-1575	Cold Remedy
PEC512	Tab, Film Coated	Codeine Phosphate 10 mg, Guaifenesin 300 mg	by Anabolic	00722-6373	Cold Remedy; C III
PEC512	Tab	Codeine Phosphate 10 mg, Guaifenesin 300 mg	by Pecos	59879-0512	Cold Remedy; C III

ID FRONT <> BACK	DESCRIPTION FRONT <> BACK	INGREDIENT & STRENGTH	BRAND (or Generic Equiv.) by FIRM	NDC#	CLASS; SCH.
PENGLOBE	Tab, White/Yellow, Pen/Globe	Bacampicillin HCl 371 mg	Penglobe by AstraZeneca	Canadian	Antibiotic
PENGLOBE	Tab, White/Yellow, Pen/Globe	Bacampicillin HCl 742 mg	Penglobe by AstraZeneca	Canadian	Antibiotic
PENTASA <> 500MG	Tab, Speckled Beige, Round, Flat, Beveled Edges	5-ASA 500 mg	Pentasa by Ferring	Canadian DIN 02099683	Gastrointestinal
PENTASA250MG2010	Cap, Green & Blue, Black Print, Starburst Logo	Mesalamine 250 mg	Pentasa by Shire	54092-0189	Gastrointestinal
PENTASA250MG2010	Cap, Green & Blue, Black Print, Starburst Logo	Mesalamine 250 mg	Pentasa by Aventis	Canadian	Gastrointestinal
PENTASA250MG2010	Cap, Green & Blue, Black Print, Starburst Logo	Mesalamine 250 mg	Pentasa by Nat Pharmpak	55154-2216	Gastrointestinal
PENTASA500	Tab, Gray/Light Brown, Pentasa/500	Mesalamine 500 mg	Pentasa by Aventis	Canadian	Gastrointestinal
PENTASA500	Tab, Gray/Light Brown, Pentasa/500	Mesalamine 500 mg	Pentasa by Marion	Canadian	Gastrointestinal
PENTASA500	Cap, Blue, Controlled Release, PENTASA500 / Starburst Logo	Mesalamine 500 mg	Pentasa by Shire	54092-0191	Gastrointestinal
PENTOX <> 672	Tab, White, Oblong, Film Coated	Pentoxifylline 400 mg	Trental by Teva	38245-0672 Discontinued	Anticoagulant
PENTOX <> 672	Tab, White, Oblong, Film Coated	Pentoxifylline 400 mg	Trental by Pharmafab	62542-0761	Anticoagulant
PENTOX <> 672	Tab, White, Oblong, Film Coated	Pentoxifylline 400 mg	Trental by Blue Ridge	59273-0018	Anticoagulant
PENTOX <> 672	Tab, White, Oblong, Film Coated	Pentoxifylline 400 mg	Trental by Merrell	00068-0672	Anticoagulant
PENTOX <> 672	Tab, White, Oblong, Film Coated	Pentoxifylline 400 mg	Trental by Pharmafab	62542-0781	Anticoagulant
PENVEE300	Tab, Orange, Round, PEN VEE/300	Penicillin V 300 mg	Pen-Vee by Wyeth	Canadian	Antibiotic
PEPCID <> MSD963	Tab, Beige, U-Shaped, Film Coated	Famotidine 20 mg	Pepcid by PDRX	55289-0162	Gastrointestinal
PEPCID <> MSD963	Tab, Beige, U-Shaped, Film Coated	Famotidine 20 mg	Pepcid by Nat Pharmpak	55154-5005	Gastrointestinal
PEPCID <> MSD963	Tab, Beige, U-Shaped, MSD over 963, Film Coated	Famotidine 20 mg	Pepcid by Allscripts		Gastrointestinal
PEPCID <> MSD963	Tab, Beige, U-Shaped, Film Coated	Famotidine 20 mg	Pepcid by H J Harkins Co	52959-0465	Gastrointestinal
PEPCID <> MSD963	Tab, Beige, U-Shaped, Film Coated	Famotidine 20 mg	Pepcid by Med Pro	53978-0518	Gastrointestinal
PEPCID <> MSD963	Tab, Beige, U-Shaped, Film Coated	Famotidine 20 mg	Pepcid by Merck	00006-0963	Gastrointestinal
PEPCID <> MSD963	Tab, Beige, U-Shaped, Film Coated	Famotidine 20 mg	Pepcid by Amerisource	62584-0440	Gastrointestinal
PEPCID <> MSD964	Tab, Dark Reddish Brown, U-Shaped, Film Coated	Famotidine 40 mg	Pepcid by PDRX	55289-0146	Gastrointestinal
PEPCID <> MSD964	Tab, Dark Reddish Brown, U-Shaped, Film Coated	Famotidine 40 mg	Pepcid by Merck	00006-0964	Gastrointestinal
PEPCIDAC	Tab, Pink, Square, Film Coated	Famotidine 10 mg	Pepcid AC by Johnson & Johnson	Canadian DIN 02185938	Gastrointestinal
PEPCIDAC	Tab, Pink, Round, Chewable	Famotidine 10 mg	Pepcid AC by Johnson & Johnson	Canadian DIN 02185911	Gastrointestinal
PERCOCET	Tab, White to Off-White, Scored	Oxycodone HCl 5 mg, Acetaminophen 325 mg	Percocet by BMS	Canadian DIN 01916475	Analgesic
PERCOCET <> 10	Tab, Yellow, Oval	Oxycodone HCl 10 mg, Acetaminophen 650 mg	Percocet by Endo	63481-0622	Analgesic; C II
PERCOCET <> 10	Tab, Yellow, Oval	Acetaminophen 650 mg, Oxycodone HCl 10 mg	Percocet by BMS	00056-0622	Analgesic; C II
PERCOCET <> 10	Tab, Yellow, Oval	Acetaminophen 650 mg, Oxycodone HCl 10 mg	Percocet by West Pharm	52967-0280	Analgesic; C II
PERCOCET <> 10325	Tab, Yellow, Oval, 10-325 <> PERCOCET	Oxycodone HCl 10 mg, Acetaminophen 325 mg	Percocet by Endo	63481-0629	Analgesic; C II
PERCOCET <> 25	Tab, Pink, Oval, Percocet <> 2.5	Oxycodone HCl 2.5 mg, Acetaminophen 325 mg	Percocet by Endo	63481-0627	Analgesic; C II
PERCOCET <> 25	Tab, Pink, Oval, Percocet <> 2.5	Oxycodone HCl 2.5 mg, Acetaminophen 325 mg	Percocet by West Pharm	52967-0278	Analgesic; C II
PERCOCET <> 75	Tab, Peach, Cap Shaped, Percocet <> 7.5	Oxycodone HCl 7.5 mg, Acetaminophen 500 mg	Percocet by Endo	63481-0621	Analgesic; C II
PERCOCET <> 75	Tab, Peach, Cap Shaped, Percocet <> 7.5	Oxycodone HCl 7.5 mg, Acetaminophen 500 mg	Percocet by West Pharm	52967-0279	Analgesic; C II
PERCOCET <> 75325	Tab, Peach, Cap Shaped, Percocet <> 7.5 / 325	Oxycodone HCl 7.5 mg, Acetaminophen 325 mg	Percocet by Endo	63481-0628	Analgesic; C II
PERCOCET <> DUPONT	Tab	Acetaminophen 325 mg, Oxycodone HCl 5 mg	Percocet by BMS	00590-0127	Analgesic; C II
PERCOCET5	Tab, Blue, Round, Scored	Oxycodone HCl 5 mg, Acetaminophen 325 mg	Percocet by Endo	63481-0623	Analgesic; C II
PERCOCET5	Tab, Blue, Round, Scored	Oxycodone HCl 5 mg, Acetaminophen 325 mg	Percocet by Physician Total Care	54868-0510	Analgesic; C II
PERCOCETDEMI	Tab, Blue, Scored, Percocet-Demi	Oxycodone HCl 2.5 mg, Acetaminophen 325 mg	Percocet by BMS	Canadian DIN 01916491	Analgesic; C II
PERCOCETDUPONT	Tab, White, Percocet/Dupont	Oxycodone HCl 5 mg, Acetaminophen 325 mg	Percocet by Dupont	Canadian	Analgesic; C II
PERCODAN	Tab, Yellow, Round, Scored	Aspirin 325 mg, Oxycodone HCl 4.5 mg	Percodan by Endo	63481-0135	Analgesic; C II
PERCODAN	Tab, Yellow, Round, Scored	Aspirin 325 mg, Oxycodone HCl 4.5 mg	Percodan by BMS	00590-0135	Analgesic; C II

ID FRONT <> BACK	DESCRIPTION FRONT <> BACK	INGREDIENT & STRENGTH	BRAND (or Generic Equiv.) by FIRM	NDC#	CLASS; SCH.
PERCODAN	Tab, Yellow, Round, Scored	Aspirin 325 mg, Oxycodone HCl 5 mg	Percodan by BMS	Canadian DIN 01916572	Analgesic
PERCODANDEMI	Tab, Pink, Percodan-Demi	Oxycodone 2.5 mg, Aspirin 325 mg	Percodan by Dupont	Canadian	Analgesic; C II
PERCODANDEMI	Tab, White, Round, Scored	Aspirin 325 mg, Oxycodone HCl 2.25 mg	Percodan by Endo	63481-0166	Analgesic; C II
PERCODANDEMI <> DUPONT	Tab, Percodan-Demi <> Dupont	Aspirin 325 mg, Oxycodone HCl 2.25 mg	Percodan by BMS	00590-0166	Analgesic; C II
PERCODANDUPONT	Tab, Yellow, Percodan/Dupont	Oxycodone 5 mg, Aspirin 325 mg	Percodan by Dupont	Canadian	Analgesic; C II
PERCODENDUPONT	Tab, Yellow, Percodan/Dupont	Oxycodone HCl 5 mg, Acetaminophen 325 mg	Percocet by Dupont	Canadian	Analgesic; C II
PERGOSEC	Tab, Orange, Round	Acetaminophen 325 mg, Phenyltoloxamine 30 mg	Pergogesic by Medtech		Analgesic
PERIACTIN <> MSD62	Tab	Cyproheptadine HCl 4 mg	Periactin by Merck	00006-0062	Antihistamine
PERIOSTAT20MG	Cap, White, Opaque	Doxycycline Hyclate 20 mg	Periostat by H J Harkins Co	52959-0446	Antibiotic
PERRIGO0P8	Tab, White, Round, Scored	Prednisone 5 mg	Prednisone by Perrigo	10768-7733	Steroid
PERRIGO3N3	Tab, White, Round, Scored	Prednisone 10 mg	Prednisone by Perrigo	10768-7283	Steroid
PERRIGO4X7	Tab, Peach, Round, Scored	Prednisone 20 mg	Prednisone by Perrigo	10768-7085	Steroid
PF	Tab, Yellow, Black Print, Enteric Coated	Bisacodyl 5 mg	Gentlax by Purdue	00034-4410	Laxative
PF <> 10	Tab, White, Round, Film-Coated	Morphine Sulfate Pentahydrate 10 mg	MS IR by Purdue Pharma	Canadian DIN 02014211	Analgesic
PF <> 100	Tab, Gray, Round	Morphine Sulfate 100 mg	MS Contin by Purdue	59011-0263	Analgesic; C II
PF <> 100MG	Tab, Grey, Round, Sustained-Release, Film-Coated, Biconvex	Morphine Sulfate 100 mg	MS Contin by Purdue Pharma	Canadian DIN 02014319	Analgesic
PF <> 100MG	Tab, Grey, Round, Sustained-Release, Film-Coated, Biconvex	Morphine Sulfate 100 mg	MS Contin by Pharmascience	Canadian DIN 02245287	Analgesic
PF <> 15MG	Tab, Green, Round, Sustained-Release, Film-Coated, Biconvex tablet	Morphine Sulfate 15 mg	MS IR by Purdue Pharma	Canadian DIN 02015439	Analgesic
PF <> 20	Tab, White, Cap-Shaped, Film-Coated,	Morphine Sulfate Pentahydrate 20 mg	MS IR by Purdue Pharma	Canadian DIN 02014238	Analgesic
PF <> 200MG	Tab, Red, Cap-Shaped, Scored, Film-Coated, Sustained-Release	Morphine Sulfate 200 mg	MS Contin by Purdue	Canadian DIN 02014327	Analgesic
PF <> 200MG	Tab, Red, Cap-Shaped, Scored, Film-Coated, Sustained-Release	Morphine Sulfate 200 mg	MS Contin by Pharmascience	Canadian DIN 02245288	Analgesic
PF <> 30	Tab, White, Cap-Shaped, Film-Coated	Morphine Sulfate Pentahydrate 30 mg	MS IR by Purdue Pharma	Canadian DIN 02014254	Analgesic
PF <> 30MG	Tab, Violet, Round, Sustained-Release, Film-Coated, Biconvex	Morphine Sulfate 30 mg	MS Contin by Purdue Pharma	Canadian DIN 02014297	Analgesic
PF <> 5	Tab, White, Round, Film-Coated	Morphine Sulfate Pentahydrate 5 mg	MS IR by Purdue Pharma	Canadian DIN 02014203	Analgesic
PF <> 60MG	Tab, Orange, Round, Sustained-Release, Film-Coated, Biconvex tablet	Morphine Sulfate 60 mg	MS Contin by Purdue Pharma	Canadian DIN 02014300	Analgesic
PF <> C275	Tab, Round, White, Scored	Quinidine Polygalacturonate 275 mg	Cardioquin by Purdue	00034-5470 Discontinued	Antiarrhythmic
PF <> CC100	Tab, Yellow, Round, Scored, Film-Coated tablet	Codeine Monohydrate 53 mg, Codeine Sulfate Trihydrate 62.7 mg	Codeine Contin by Purdue Pharma	Canadian DIN 02163748	Analgesic
PF <> CC150	Tab, Red, Round, Scored, Film-Coated	Codeine Monohydrate 79.5 mg, Codeine Sulfate Trihydrate 94.1 mg	Codeine Contin by Purdue Pharma	Canadian DIN 02163780	Analgesic
PF <> CC200	Tab, Orange, Cap-Shaped, Scored, Film-Coated	Codeine Monohydrate 106 mg, Codeine Sulfate Trihydrate 125.4 mg	Codeine Contin by Purdue Pharma	Canadian DIN 02163799	Analgesic
PF <> CC50	Tab, Blue, Round, Film-Coated	Codeine Monohydrate 26.5 mg, Codeine Sulfate Trihydrate 31.35 mg	Codeine Contin by Purdue Pharma	Canadian DIN 02230302	Analgesic
PF <> M15	Tab, Blue, Round	Morphine Sulfate 15 mg	MS Contin by Purdue	59011-0260	Analgesic; C II
PF <> M200	Tab, Green, Cap Shaped, Ex Release	Morphine Sulfate 200 mg	Ms Contin by Purdue	59011-0264	Analgesic; C II
PF <> M30	Tab, Lavender, Round	Morphine Sulfate 30 mg	MS Contin by Purdue	59011-0261	Analgesic; C II

ID FRONT <> BACK	DESCRIPTION FRONT <> BACK	INGREDIENT & STRENGTH	BRAND (or Generic Equiv.) by FIRM	NDC#	CLASS; SCH.
PF <> M60	Tab, Orange, Round	Morphine Sulfate 60 mg	MS Contin by Purdue	59011-0262	Analgesic; C II
PF <> MI15	Tab, White, Round, Scored	Morphine Sulfate 15 mg	MSIR by Purdue	00034-0518	Analgesic; C II
PF <> MI30	Tab, White, Cap Shaped, Scored	Morphine Sulfate 30 mg	MSIR by Purdue	00034-0519	Analgesic; C II
PF <> T1000	Tab, Red, Scored, Film Coated	Choline Magnesium Trisalicylate 1000 mg	Trilisate by Purdue	00034-0510	NSAID
PF <> T500	Tab, Pink, Oblong, Partially Scored, Film Coated	Choline Magnesium Trisalicylate 500 mg	Trilisate by Purdue	00034-0500	NSAID
PF <> T750	Tab, White, Oblong, Partially Scored, Film Coated	Choline Magnesium Trisalicylate 750 mg	Trilisate by Purdue	00034-0505	NSAID
PF <> U200	Tab, White, Round, Scored, U over 200	Theophylline Anhydrous 200 mg	T-Phyl by Purdue	00034-7102	Antiasthmatic
PF <> U400	Tab, White, Round, Scored, U over 400	Theophylline Anhydrous 400 mg	Uniphyl by Purdue	00034-7004	Antiasthmatic
PF <> U600	Tab, White, Rectangular, Scored, U over 600	Theophylline Anhydrous 600 mg	Uniphyl by Purdue	00034-7006	Antiasthmatic
PF1	Tab, Ex Release, PF/1	Atropine Sulfate 0.04 mg, Chlorpheniramine Maleate 8 mg, Hyoscyamine Sulfate 0.19 mg, Phenylephrine 25 mg, Phenylpropanolamine 50 mg, Scopolamine 0.01 mg	Atrohist Plus by Pharmafab	62542-0001	Cold Remedy
PF12MGHYDRO-MORPHCONTIN	Cap, Orange	Hydromorphone HCl 12 mg	Hydromorph Contin by Purdue	Canadian DIN 02125366	Analgesic; C II
PF24MGHYDRO-MORPHCONTIN	Cap, Gray	Hydromorphone HCl 24 mg	Hydromorph Contin by Purdue	Canadian DIN 02125382	Analgesic; C II
PF30MGHYDRO-MORPHCONTIN	Cap, Red	Hydromorphone HCl 30 mg	Hydromorph Contin by Purdue	Canadian DIN 02125390	Analgesic; C II
PF3MGHYDRO-MORPHCONTIN	Cap, Green	Hydromorphone HCl 3 mg	Hydromorph Contin by Purdue	Canadian DIN 02125323	Analgesic; C II
PF5MGOIR	Cap, Beige & Orange	Oxycodone HCl 5 mg	OxyIR by Purdue	59011-0201	Analgesic; C II
PF5MGOIR	Cap, Beige & Orange	Oxycodone HCl 5 mg	OxyIR by PF	48692-0006	Analgesic; C II
PF6MGHYDRO-MORPHCONTIN	Cap, Pink	Hydromorphone HCl 6 mg	Hydromorph Contin by Purdue	Canadian DIN 02125331	Analgesic; C II
PFE	Tab, Red, Oblong, Film Coated, P-Fe	Iron 106 mg	Ferretts by Pharmics	00813-0012	Mineral
PFENOMICRO	Cap, Orange	Fenofibrate 200 mg	Lipidil Micro by Pharmascience	Canadian DIN 02273551	Antihyperlipidemic
PFI440	Cap, ER, PFI 440	Pheniramine Maleate 16 mg, Phenylpropanolamine HCl 50 mg, Phenyltoloxamine Citrate 16 mg, Pyrilamine Maleate 16 mg	Poly D Sr by Pharmafab	62542-0440	Cold Remedy
PFIZER	Tab, White, Diamond, Scored	Prazosin HCl 5 mg	Minipress by Pfizer	Canadian DIN 00560979	Antihypertensive
PFIZER	Tab, White, Round, Scored	Prazosin HCl 2 mg	Minipress by Pfizer	Canadian DIN 00560960	Antihypertensive
PFIZER	Tab, Orange, Scored	Prazosin HCl 1 mg	Minipress by Pfizer	Canadian DIN 00560952	Antihypertensive
PFIZER	Cap, Flesh, Pfizer Logo	Doxepin HCl 10 mg	Sinequan by Pfizer	Canadian DIN 00024325	Antidepressant
PFIZER	Cap, Blue & Flesh, Pfizer Logo	Doxepin HCl 100 mg	Sinequan by Pfizer	Canadian DIN 00326925	Antidepressant
PFIZER	Cap, Blue & Pink, Pfizer Logo	Doxepin HCl 25 mg	Sinequan by Pfizer	Canadian DIN 00024333	Antidepressant
PFIZER	Cap, Flesh & Pink, Pfizer Logo	Doxepin HCl 50 mg	Sinequan by Pfizer	Canadian DIN 00024341	Antidepressant
PFIZER	Cap, Pink & Scarlet, Pfizer Logo	Doxepin HCl 75 mg	Sinequan by Pfizer	Canadian DIN 00400750	Antidepressant
PFIZER	Cap, Orange & White, Gelatin, Pfizer Logo	Thiothixene 5 mg	by Erfa	Canadian DIN 00024449	Antipsychotic
PFIZER	Cap, White, Gelatin, Pfizer Logo	Thiothixene 2 mg	by Erfa	Canadian DIN 00024430	Antipsychotic
PFIZER	Cap, Orange, Gelatin, Pfizer Logo	Thiothixene 10 mg	by Erfa	Canadian DIN 00024457	Antipsychotic

ID FRONT <> BACK	DESCRIPTION FRONT <> BACK	INGREDIENT & STRENGTH	BRAND (or Generic Equiv.) by FIRM	NDC#	CLASS; SCH.
PFIZER	Tab, White, Round, Scored, Chewable	Meclizine HCl 25 mg	Bonamine by Pfizer	Canadian DIN 00220442	Antiemetic
PFIZER	Tab, White, Round, Oval	Chlorpropamide 250 mg	Diabinese by Pfizer	Canadian	Antidiabetic
PFIZER	Tab, Yellow, Oval	Chlorpropamide 100 mg	Diabinese by Pfizer	Canadian	Antidiabetic
PFIZER <> 306	Tab, Pink, Cap Shaped, Film Coated	Azithromycin 250 mg	Zithromax by Pfizer	Canadian DIN 02212021	Antibiotic
PFIZER <> 306	Tab, Pink, Cap Shaped, Film Coated	Azithromycin 250 mg	Zithromax by Physician Total Care	54868-4183	Antibiotic
PFIZER <> 306	Tab, Pink, Cap Shaped, Film Coated	Azithromycin 250 mg	Zithromax by Pfizer	00069-3060	Antibiotic
PFIZER <> 306	Tab, Pink, Cap Shaped, Film Coated	Azithromycin 250 mg	Zithromax by Allscripts		Antibiotic
PFIZER <> 308	Tab, White, Oval, Film Coated	Azithromycin 600 mg	Zithromax by Pfizer	00069-3080	Antibiotic
PFIZER <> 308	Tab, White, Oval, Film Coated	Azithromycin 600 mg	Zithromax by Pfizer	Canadian DIN 02231143	Antibiotic
PFIZER <> 378	Tab, Blue, Round, Film Coated	Trovafloxacin Mesylate 100 mg	Trovan by Roerig	00049-3780	Antibiotic
PFIZER <> 378	Tab, Blue, Round, Film Coated	Trovafloxacin Mesylate 100 mg	Trovan by Pfizer	Canadian DIN 02239191	Antibiotic
PFIZER <> 379	Tab, Blue, Oval, Film Coated	Trovafloxacin Mesylate 200 mg	Trovan by Pfizer	Canadian DIN 02239192	Antibiotic
PFIZER <> 379	Tab, Blue, Oval, Film Coated	Trovafloxacin Mesylate 200 mg	Trovan by Roerig	00049-3790	Antibiotic
PFIZER <> 551	Tab, Rounded Rectangular, Film Coated	Cetirizine HCl 10 mg		54868-3876	Antihistamine
PFIZER <> 551	Tab, Rounded Rectangular, Film Coated	Cetirizine HCl 10 mg	by Physician Total Care		Antihistamine
PFIZER <> 551	Tab, Rounded Rectangular, Film Coated	Cetirizine HCl 10 mg	by PDRX	55289-0108	Antihistamine
PFIZER <> 551	Tab, Rounded Rectangular, Film Coated	Cetirizine HCl 10 mg	by Caremark	00339-6097	Antihistamine
PFIZER <> CDT051	Tab, White, Oval	Amlodipine Besylate 5 mg, Atorvastatin Calcium 10 mg	Caduet by Pfizer	Canadian DIN 02273233	Antihypertensive; Antihyperlipidemic
PFIZER <> CDT051	Tab, White, Oval	Amlodipine Besylate 5 mg, Atorvastatin Calcium 10 mg	Caduet by Pfizer	00069-2150	Antihypertensive; Antihyperlipidemic
PFIZER <> CDT052	Tab, White, Oval	Amlodipine Besylate 5 mg, Atorvastatin Calcium 20 mg	Caduet by Pfizer	00069-2170	Antihypertensive; Antihyperlipidemic
PFIZER <> CDT052	Tab, White, Oval	Amlodipine Besylate 5 mg, Atorvastatin Calcium 20 mg	Caduet by Pfizer	Canadian DIN 02273241	Antihypertensive; Antihyperlipidemic
PFIZER <> CDT054	Tab, White, Oval	Amlodipine Besylate 5 mg, Atorvastatin Calcium 40 mg	Caduet by Pfizer	00069-2190	Antihypertensive; Antihyperlipidemic
PFIZER <> CDT058	Tab, White, Oval	Amlodipine Besylate 5 mg, Atorvastatin Calcium 80 mg	Caduet by Pfizer	00069-2260	Antihypertensive; Antihyperlipidemic
PFIZER <> CDT058	Tab, White, Oval	Amlodipine Besylate 5 mg, Atorvastatin Calcium 80 mg	Caduet by Pfizer	Canadian DIN 02273276	Antihypertensive; Antihyperlipidemic
PFIZER <> CDT101	Tab, Blue, Oval	Amlodipine Besylate 10 mg, Atorvastatin Calcium 10 mg	Caduet by Pfizer	Canadian DIN 02273284	Antihypertensive; Antihyperlipidemic
PFIZER <> CDT101	Tab, Blue, Oval	Amlodipine Besylate 10 mg, Atorvastatin Calcium 10 mg	Caduet by Pfizer	00069-2160	Antihypertensive; Antihyperlipidemic
PFIZER <> CDT102	Tab, Blue, Oval	Amlodipine Besylate 10 mg, Atorvastatin Calcium 20 mg	Caduet by Pfizer	00069-2180	Antihypertensive; Antihyperlipidemic
PFIZER <> CDT102	Tab, Blue, Oval	Amlodipine Besylate 10 mg, Atorvastatin Calcium 20 mg	Caduet by Pfizer	Canadian DIN 02273292	Antihypertensive; Antihyperlipidemic
PFIZER <> CDT104	Tab, Blue, Oval	Amlodipine Besylate 10 mg, Atorvastatin Calcium 40 mg	Caduet by Pfizer	Canadian DIN 02273306	Antihypertensive; Antihyperlipidemic
PFIZER <> CDT104	Tab, Blue, Oval	Amlodipine Besylate 10 mg, Atorvastatin Calcium 40 mg	Caduet by Pfizer	00069-2250	Antihypertensive; Antihyperlipidemic
PFIZER <> CDT108	Tab, Blue, Oval	Amlodipine Besylate 10 mg, Atorvastatin Calcium 80 mg	Caduet by Pfizer	00069-2270	Antihypertensive; Antihyperlipidemic

ID FRONT <> BACK	DESCRIPTION FRONT <> BACK	INGREDIENT & STRENGTH	BRAND (or Generic Equiv.) by FIRM	NDC#	CLASS; SCH.
PFIZER <> CDT108	Tab, Blue, Oval	Amlodipine Besylate 10 mg, Atorvastatin Calcium 80 mg	Caduet by Pfizer	Canadian DIN 02273314	Antihypertensive; Antihyperlipidemic
PFIZER <> CDT251	Tab, White, Oval	Amlodipine Besylate 2.5 mg, Atorvastatin Calcium 10 mg	Caduet by Pfizer	00069-2960	Antihypertensive; Antihyperlipidemic
PFIZER <> CDT252	Tab, White, Oval	Amlodipine Besylate 2.5 mg, Atorvastatin Calcium 20 mg	Caduet by Pfizer	00069-2970	Antihypertensive; Antihyperlipidemic
PFIZER <> CDT254	Tab, White, Oval	Amlodipine Besylate 2.5 mg, Atorvastatin Calcium 40 mg	Caduet by Pfizer	00069-2980	Antihypertensive; Antihyperlipidemic
PFIZER <> CHX05	Tab, White to Off-White, Film Coated, CHX 0.5	Varenicline 0.5 mg	Champix by Pfizer	Canadian DIN 02291177	Smoking Cessation
PFIZER <> CHX05	Tab, White to Off-White, Film Coated, CHX 0.5	Varenicline 0.5 mg	Chantix by Pfizer	00069-0468	Smoking Cessation
PFIZER <> CHX05	Tab, White to Off-White, Film Coated, CHX 0.5	Varenicline 0.5 mg	Chantix by Pfizer	00069-0471; 00069-0469	Smoking Cessation
PFIZER <> CHX10	Tab, Light Blue, Cap Shaped, Film Coated, CHX 1.0	Varenicline 1 mg	Chantix by Pfizer	00069-0469; 00069-0471	Smoking Cessation
PFIZER <> CHX10	Tab, Light Blue, Cap Shaped, Film Coated, CHX 1.0	Varenicline 1 mg	Champix by Pfizer	Canadian DIN 02291185	Smoking Cessation
PFIZER <> DIFLUCAN100	Tab, Pink, Trapezoid	Fluconazole 100 mg	Diflucan by Pfizer	Canadian DIN 00891819	Antifungal
PFIZER <> DIFLUCAN50	Tab, Pink, Trapezoid	Fluconazole 50 mg	Diflucan by Pfizer	Canadian DIN 00891800	Antifungal
PFIZER <> MVC150	Tab, Blue, Oval, Film Coated	Maraviroc 150 mg	Selzentry by Pfizer	00069-0807	Antiviral
PFIZER <> MVC150	Tab, Blue, Oval, Film Coated	Maraviroc 150 mg	Celsentri by Pfizer	Canadian DIN 02299844	Antiviral
PFIZER <> MVC300	Tab, Blue, Oval, Film Coated	Maraviroc 300 mg	Celsentri by Pfizer	Canadian DIN 02299852	Antiviral
PFIZER <> MVC300	Tab, Blue, Oval, Film Coated	Maraviroc 300 mg	Selzentry by Pfizer	00069-0808	Antiviral
PFIZER <> NRV10	Tab, White, Octagonal	Amlodipine 10 mg	Norvasc by Pfizer	Canadian DIN 00878936	Antihypertensive
PFIZER <> NRV5	Tab, White, Octagonal, Scored	Amlodipine 5 mg	Norvasc by Pfizer	Canadian DIN 00878928	Antihypertensive
PFIZER <> NSR25	Tab, Yellow, Diamond Shaped, Film Coated	Eplerenone 25 mg	Inspra by Searle	00025-1710	Antihypertensive
PFIZER <> NSR50	Tab, Yellow, Diamond Shaped, Film Coated	Eplerenone 50 mg	Inspra by Searle	00025-1720	Antihypertensive
Pfizer <> PFIZER	Cap, Blue, Hard Gelatin	Doxycycline Hyclate 100 mg	Vibramycin by Pfizer	Canadian DIN 00024368	Antibiotic
PFIZER <> REP20	Tab, Orange, Round, Film Coated	Eletriptan HBr 20 mg	Relpax by Pfizer	Canadian DIN 02256290	Antimigraine
PFIZER <> REP20	Tab, Orange, Round, Film Coated	Eletriptan HBr 20 mg	Relpax by Roerig	00049-2330	Antimigraine
PFIZER <> REP40	Tab, Orange, Round, Film Coated	Eletriptan HBr 40 mg	Relpax by Roerig	00049-2340	Antimigraine
PFIZER <> REP40	Tab, Orange, Round, Film Coated	Eletriptan HBr 40 mg	Relpax by Pfizer	Canadian DIN 02256304	Antimigraine
PFIZER <> TVN100	Tab, Blue, Round	Trovafloxacin 100 mg	Trovan by Pfizer	Canadian DIN 02239191	Antibiotic
PFIZER <> TVN200	Tab, Blue, Oval	Trovafloxacin 200 mg	Trovan by Pfizer	Canadian DIN 02239192	Antibiotic
PFIZER <> VGR100	Tab, Blue, Diamond Shaped, Film Coated	Sildenafil Citrate 100 mg	Viagra by Compumed	00403-1989	Impotence Agent
PFIZER <> VGR100	Tab, Blue, Diamond Shaped, Film Coated	Sildenafil Citrate 100 mg	Viagra by Southwood	58016-0371	Impotence Agent
PFIZER <> VGR100	Tab, Blue, Diamond Shaped, Film Coated	Sildenafil Citrate 100 mg	Viagra by Pfizer	Canadian DIN 02239768	Impotence Agent
PFIZER <> VGR100	Tab, Blue, Diamond Shaped, Film Coated	Sildenafil Citrate 100 mg	Viagra by Pfizer	00069-4220	Impotence Agent
PFIZER <> VGR100	Tab, Blue, Diamond Shaped, Film Coated	Sildenafil Citrate 100 mg	Viagra by Allscripts		Impotence Agent

ID FRONT <> BACK	DESCRIPTION FRONT <> BACK	INGREDIENT & STRENGTH	BRAND (or Generic Equiv.) by FIRM	NDC#	CLASS; SCH.
PFIZER <> VGR25	Tab, Blue, Diamond Shaped, Film Coated	Sildenafil Citrate 25 mg	Viagra by Pfizer	Canadian DIN 02239766	Impotence Agent
PFIZER <> VGR25	Tab, Blue, Diamond Shaped, Film Coated	Sildenafil Citrate 25 mg	Viagra by Pfizer	00069-4200	Impotence Agent
PFIZER <> VGR50	Tab, Blue, Diamond Shaped, Film Coated	Sildenafil Citrate 50 mg	Viagra by Allscripts		Impotence Agent
PFIZER <> VGR50	Tab, Blue, Diamond Shaped, Film Coated	Sildenafil Citrate 50 mg	Viagra by Pfizer	00069-4210	Impotence Agent
PFIZER <> VGR50	Tab, Blue, Diamond Shaped, Film Coated	Sildenafil Citrate 50 mg	Viagra by Pfizer	Canadian DIN 02239767	Impotence Agent
PFIZER <> VGR50	Tab, Blue, Diamond Shaped, Film Coated	Sildenafil Citrate 50 mg	Viagra by Compumed	00403-1947	Impotence Agent
PFIZER <> VGR50	Tab, Blue, Diamond Shaped, Film Coated	Sildenafil Citrate 50 mg	Viagra by Southwood	58016-0355	Impotence Agent
PFIZER <> VOR200	Tab, White, Cap Shaped, Film Coated	Voriconazole 200 mg	Vfend by Pfizer	00049-3180	Antifungal
PFIZER <> VOR50	Tab, White, Round, Film Coated	Voriconazole 50 mg	Vfend by Pfizer	00049-3170	Antifungal
PFIZER <> ZTM500	Tab, Pink, Cap Shaped, Film Coated	Azithromycin 500 mg	Zithromax by Pfizer	00069-3070	Antibiotic
PFIZER092	Cap, Yellow & Green	Oxytetracycline 250 mg, Sulfamethizole 250 mg, Phenazopyridine 50 mg	Urobiotic by Pfizer	00049-0920	Antibiotic
PFIZER099 <> VIBRATAB	Tab, Orange, Film Coated	Doxycycline Hyclate 100 mg	Vibra-Tabs by Pfizer	Canadian DIN 00578452	Antibiotic
PFIZER099 <> VIBRATABS	Tab, Salmon, Round, Film Coated	Doxycycline Hyclate 100 mg	Vibra by Pfizer	00069-0990	Antibiotic
PFIZER375	Tab, White, Round, Scored	Polythiazide 1 mg	Renese by Pfizer	00069-3750	Diuretic; Antihypertensive
PFIZER376	Tab, Yellow, Round, Scored	Polythiazide 2 mg	Renese by Pfizer	00069-3760	Diuretic; Antihypertensive
PFIZER377	Tab, White, Round, Scored	Polythiazide 4 mg	Renese by Pfizer	00069-3770	Diuretic; Antihypertensive
PFIZER393	Tab, Blue, D-Shaped, Scored	Chlorpropamide 100 mg	Diabinese by Pfizer	00069-3930	Antidiabetic
PFIZER394	Tab, Blue, D-Shaped, Scored	Chlorpropamide 250 mg	Diabinese by Pfizer	00663-3940	Antidiabetic
PFIZER394	Tab, Blue, D-Shaped, Scored	Chlorpropamide 250 mg	Diabinese by Pfizer	00069-3940	Antidiabetic
PFIZER396	Cap, Blue & White, Black Print, Pfizer over 396	Ziprasidone HCl 20 mg	Geodon by Roerig	00049-3960	Antipsychotic
PFIZER397	Cap, Blue, Black Print, Pfizer over 397	Ziprasidone HCl 40 mg	Geodon by Roerig	00049-3970	Antipsychotic
PFIZER398	Cap, White, Black Print, Pfizer over 398	Ziprasidone HCl 60 mg	Geodon by Roerig	00049-3980	Antipsychotic
PFIZER399	Cap, Blue & White, Black Print, Pfizer over 399	Ziprasidone HCl 80 mg	Geodon by Roerig	00049-3990	Antipsychotic
PFIZER411	Tab, White, Diamond Shaped, Scored, Pfizer over 411	Glipizide 5 mg	Glucotrol by Pharmedix	53002-0446	Antidiabetic
PFIZER411	Tab, White, Diamond Shaped, Scored, Pfizer over 411	Glipizide 5 mg	Glucotrol by Amerisource	62584-0110	Antidiabetic
PFIZER411	Tab, White, Diamond Shaped, Scored, Pfizer over 411	Glipizide 5 mg	Glucotrol by Rightpak	65240-0651	Antidiabetic
PFIZER411	Tab, White, Diamond Shaped, Scored, Pfizer over 411	Glipizide 5 mg	Glucotrol by Roerig	00049-4110	Antidiabetic
PFIZER411	Tab, White, Diamond Shaped, Scored, Pfizer over 411	Glipizide 5 mg	Glucotrol by Kaiser	00179-1296	Antidiabetic
PFIZER411	Tab, White, Diamond Shaped, Scored, Pfizer over 411	Glipizide 5 mg	Glucotrol by Nat Pharmpak	55154-3213	Antidiabetic
PFIZER412	Tab, White, Diamond Shaped, Scored, Pfizer over 412	Glipizide 10 mg	Glucotrol by Med Pro	53978-0183	Antidiabetic
PFIZER412	Tab, White, Diamond Shaped, Scored, Pfizer over 412	Glipizide 10 mg	Glucotrol by Med Pro	53978-0183	Antidiabetic
PFIZER412	Tab, White, Diamond Shaped, Scored, Pfizer over 412	Glipizide 10 mg	Glucotrol by Rightpak	65240-0652	Antidiabetic
PFIZER412	Tab, White, Diamond Shaped, Scored, Pfizer over 412	Glipizide 10 mg	Glucotrol by Roerig	00049-4120	Antidiabetic
PFIZER412	Tab, White, Diamond Shaped, Scored, Pfizer over 412	Glipizide 10 mg	Glucotrol by Kaiser	00179-1299	Antidiabetic
PFIZER412	Tab, White, Diamond Shaped, Scored, Pfizer over 412	Glipizide 10 mg	Glucotrol by Amerisource	62584-0120	Antidiabetic
PFIZER412	Tab, White, Diamond Shaped, Scored, Pfizer over 412	Glipizide 10 mg	Glucotrol by Nat Pharmpak	55154-3212	Antidiabetic
PFIZER441	Tab, Yellow, Oval	Rescinnamine 0.25 mg	Moderil by Pfizer		Antihypertensive
PFIZER442	Tab, Salmon, Oval	Rescinnamine 0.5 mg	Moderil by Pfizer		Antihypertensive
PFIZER446	Tab, Blue, Round	Polythiazide 2 mg, Reserpine 0.25 mg	Renese R by Pfizer		Diuretic; Antihypertensive
PFIZER641	Cap, Green & Yellow	Oxamniquine 250 mg	Vansil by Pfizer		Antihelmintic
PFIZERDIFLUCAN150MG	Cap, White, Gelatin	Fluconazole 150 mg	Diflucan by Pfizer	Canadian DIN 02141442	Antifungal
PFIZERLITHANE150MG	Cap, Ivory, Gelatin	Lithium Carbonate 150 mg	Eskalith by Pfizer	Canadian DIN 02013231	Antipsychotic

ID FRONT <> BACK	DESCRIPTION FRONT <> BACK	INGREDIENT & STRENGTH	BRAND (or Generic Equiv.) by FIRM	NDC#	CLASS; SCH.
PFIZERLITHANE300MG	Cap, Green & Ivory, Gelatin	Lithium Carbonate 300 mg	Eskalith by Pfizer	Canadian DIN 00406775	Antipsychotic
PFIZERPGN100	Cap, Orange, Hard Gel, Black Ink	Pregabalin 100 mg	Lyrica by Pfizer	00071-1015	Anticonvulsant; C V
PFIZERPGN150	Cap, White, Hard Gel, Black Ink	Pregabalin 150 mg	Lyrica by Pfizer	00071-1016	Anticonvulsant; C V
PFIZERPGN150	Cap, White, Hard Gel, Black Ink	Pregabalin 150 mg	Lyrica by Pfizer	Canadian DIN 02268450	Anticonvulsant, Analgesic Agent
PFIZERPGN200	Cap, Light Orange, Hard Gel, Black Ink	Pregabalin 200 mg	Lyrica by Pfizer	00071-1017	Anticonvulsant; C V
PFIZERPGN225	Cap, White and Light Orange, Hard Gel, Black Ink	Pregabalin 225 mg	Lyrica by Pfizer	00071-1019	Anticonvulsant; C V
PFIZERPGN25	Cap, White, Hard Gel, Black Ink	Pregabalin 25 mg	Lyrica by Pfizer	00071-1012	Anticonvulsant; C V
PFIZERPGN25	Cap, White, Hard Gel, Black Ink	Pregabalin 25 mg	Lyrica by Pfizer	Canadian DIN 02268418	Anticonvulsant, Analgesic Agent
PFIZERPGN300	Cap, White and Orange, Hard Gel, Black Ink	Pregabalin 300 mg	Lyrica by Pfizer	Canadian DIN 02268485	Anticonvulsant, Analgesic Agent
PFIZERPGN300	Cap, White and Orange, Hard Gel, Black Ink	Pregabalin 300 mg	Lyrica by Pfizer	00071-1018	Anticonvulsant; C V
PFIZERPGN50	Cap, White, Hard Gel, Black Ink	Pregabalin 50 mg	Lyrica by Pfizer	00071-1013	Anticonvulsant; C V
PFIZERPGN50	Cap, White, Hard Gel, Black Ink	Pregabalin 50 mg	Lyrica by Pfizer	Canadian DIN 02268426	Anticonvulsant, Analgesic Agent
PFIZERPGN75	Cap, White and Orange, Hard Gel, Black Ink	Pregabalin 75 mg	Lyrica by Pfizer	Canadian DIN 02268434	Anticonvulsant, Analgesic Agent
PFIZERPGN75	Cap, White and Orange, Hard Gel, Black Ink	Pregabalin 75 mg	Lyrica by Pfizer	00071-1014	Anticonvulsant; C V
PFIZERSTN125MG	Cap, Orange, Hard Gel, PFIZER on Cap, and STN 12.5 mg on Body	Sunitinib Maleate 12.5 mg	Sutent by Pfizer	00069-0550	Cancer Treatment
PFIZERSTN125MG	Cap, Orange, Hard Gel, PFIZER on Cap, and STN 12.5 mg on Body	Sunitinib Maleate 12.5 mg	Sutent by Pfizer	Canadian DIN 02280795	Cancer Treatment
PFIZERSTN25MG	Cap, Caramel and Orange, Hard Gel	Sunitinib Maleate 25 mg	Sutent by Pfizer	00069-0770	Cancer Treatment
PFIZERSTN25MG	Cap, Caramel and Orange, Hard Gel, Pfizer on Cap, and STN 25 mg on Body	Sunitinib Maleate 25 mg	Sutent by Pfizer	Canadian DIN 02280809	Cancer Treatment
PFIZERSTN50MG	Cap, Caramel, Hard Gel	Sunitinib Maleate 50 mg	Sutent by Pfizer	00069-0980	Cancer Treatment
PFIZERSTN50MG	Cap, Caramel, Hard Gel, Pfizer on Cap, and STN 50 mg on Body	Sunitinib Maleate 50 mg	Sutent by Pfizer	Canadian DIN 02280817	Cancer Treatment
PFIZERZOLOFT100MG	Cap, Orange	Sertraline 100 mg	Zoloft by Pfizer	Canadian DIN 01962779	Antidepressant
PFIZERZOLOFT25MG	Cap, Yellow	Sertraline 25 mg	Zoloft by Pfizer	Canadian DIN 02132702	Antidepressant
PFIZERZOLOFT50MG	Cap, White & Yellow	Sertraline 50 mg	Zoloft by Pfizer	Canadian DIN 01962816	Antidepressant
PFIZERZOLOFT50MG	Cap, White and Yellow, Oblong, Pfizer on Cap, Zoloft 50 mg on Body	Sertraline HCl 50 mg	Zoloft by Pfizer	Canadian DIN 01962817	Antidepressant
PFM15	Tab, White, Round	Morphine Sulfate 15 mg	MS Contin by PF		Analgesic; C II
PFMI15	Tab, White, Round, PF/MI 15	Morphine Sulfate 15 mg	MS Contin by Purdue		Analgesic; C II
PFMI30	Tab, White, Oblong, PF/MI 30	Morphine Sulfate 30 mg	MS Contin by Purdue		Analgesic; C II
PFMISR15THISENDUP	Cap, White & Blue, Opaque	Morphine Sulfate 15 mg	MSIR by Purdue	00034-1025	Analgesic; C II
PFMISR30THISENDUP	Cap, Lavender & Gray, Opaque	Morphine Sulfate 30 mg	MSIR by Purdue	00034-1026	Analgesic; C II
PFNZ	Tab, Yellow, Round	Thiethylperazine Maleate 10 mg	Norzine by PF		Antiemetic
PFT750	Tab, Film Coated	Choline Magnesium Trisalicylate 750 mg	by Med Pro	53978-1306	NSAID
PG <> 15	Tab, White, Round	Pioglitazone HCl 15 mg	Actos by Pharmascience	Canadian DIN 02303124	Antihyperglycemic
PG <> 30	Tab, White, Round	Pioglitazone HCl 30 mg	Actos by Pharmascience	Canadian DIN 02303132	Antihyperglycemic
P&G <> 402	Tab, White, Rectangular	Etidronate Disodium 200 mg	Didronel by Procter and Gamble	00149-0405	Calcium Metabolism

ID FRONT <> BACK	DESCRIPTION FRONT <> BACK	INGREDIENT & STRENGTH	BRAND (or Generic Equiv.) by FIRM	NDC#	CLASS; SCH.
P&G <> 402	Tab, White, Rectangular	Etidronate Disodium 200 mg	Didronel by Pharm Util	60491-0801	Calcium Metabolism
P&G <> 402	Tab, White, Rectangular	Etidronate Disodium 200 mg	Didronel by DRX	55045-2326	Calcium Metabolism
P&G <> 402	Tab, White, Rectangular	Etidronate Disodium 200 mg	Didronel by Proc & Gamble	Canadian DIN 01997629	Calcium Metabolism
PG <> 45	Tab, White, Round	Pioglitazone HCl 45 mg	Actos by Pharmascience	Canadian DIN 02303140	Antihyperglycemic
PG10	Tab, White, Round, Chewable	Metronidazole 250 mg	Helidac Therapy Kit by Prometheus	65483-0495	Antibiotic
PG11	Tab, White, Round, Chewable	Bismuth Subsalicylate 262.4 mg	Helidac Therapy Kit by Prometheus	65483-0495	Antibiotic
PG12	Cap, Pink	Tetracycline HCl 500 mg	Helidac Therapy Kit by Prometheus	65483-0495	Antibiotic
PG12	Cap, Pink	Tetracycline HCl 500 mg	Sumycin by Proc & Gamble		Antibiotic
PG402	Tab, White, Rectangular, P & G 402	Etidronate Disodium 200 mg	Didronel by Norwich		Calcium Metabolism
PG800	Tab, Red Brown, Capsule Shaped	Mesalamine 800 mg	Asacol HD by Procter and Gamble	00149-0783	Gastrointestinal
PGABAPENTIN100MG	Cap, White, Opaque, Hard Gel	Gabapentin 100 mg	by Pharmascience	Canadian DIN 5760603608	Anticonvulsant
PGABAPENTIN300MG	Cap, Yellow, Opaque, Hard Gel	Gabapentin 300 mg	by Pharmascience	Canadian DIN 5760603606	Anticonvulsant
PGABAPENTIN400MG	Cap, Orange, Opaque, Hard Gel	Gabapentin 400 mg	by Pharmascience	Canadian DIN 5760603604	Anticonvulsant
PH <> 023	Tab, Yellow, Round, Enteric Coated	Aspirin 81 mg	Aspirin by Pharbest	16103-0356	Analgesic
PH012	Tab, Yellow, Round	Chlorpheniramine Maleate 4 mg	Pharbechlor by Pharbest	16103-0346	Antihistamine
PH013	Cap, Pink	Diphenhydramine HCl 50 mg	Pharbedryl by Pharbest	16103-0347	Antihistamine
PH014	Cap, Pink and White	Diphenhydramine HCl 25 mg	Pharbedryl by Pharbest	16103-0348	Antihistamine
PH016	Tab, White, Cap Shaped	Acetaminophen 500 mg	Pharbetol Extra Strength by Pharbest	16103-0350	Analgesic
PH019	Tab, Light Blue, Cap Shaped	Acetaminophen 500 mg, Diphenhydramine 25 mg	Pharbetol PM by Pharbest	16103-0352	Analgesic; Sleep Aid
PH020	Tab, White, Round	Acetaminophen 325 mg	Pharbetol by Pharbest	16103-0353	Analgesic
PH023	Tab, Light Yellow, Round, Enteric Coated	Aspirin 81 mg	Aspirin by Pharbest	16103-0356	Analgesic
PH024	Tab, Orange, Round, Enteric Coated	Aspirin 325 mg	Aspirin by Pharbest	16103-0357	Analgesic
PH033	Tab, White, Round	Aspirin 325 mg	Aspirin by Pharbest	16103-0365	Analgesic
PH034	Tab, Orange and White, Mottled, Round, Chewable	Aspirin 81 mg	Aspirin by Pharbest	16103-0366	Analgesic
PH044	Tab, White, Round	Acetaminophen 500 mg	Pharbetol by Pharbest	16103-0376	Analgesic
PHA <> 1710	Tab, Yellow, Diamond Shaped, Film Coated	Eplerenone 25 mg	Inspra by Pharmacia		Antihypertensive
PHA <> 1720	Tab, Pink, Diamond Shaped, Film Coated	Eplerenone 50 mg	Inspra by Pharmacia		Antihypertensive
PHA <> 1730	Tab, Red, Diamond Shaped, Film Coated	Eplerenone 100 mg	Inspra by Searle	00025-1730	Antihypertensive
PHARMACIA&UPJOHN-EMCYT140MG	Cap, White, Opaque	Estramustine Phosphate Sodium 140 mg	Emcyt by Pfizer	Canadian DIN 02063794	Antineoplastic
PHARMACIA&UPJOHN-EMCYT140MG	Cap, White, Opaque	Estramustine Phosphate Sodium 140 mg	Emcyt by Pharmacia	00013-0132	Antineoplastic
PHARMICS	Tab, Off-White, Oblong, Chewable	Ascorbic Acid 60 mg, Cyanocobalamin 4.5 mcg, Folic Acid 0.3 mg, Niacinamide 13.5 mg, Pyridoxine HCl 1.05 mg, Riboflavin 1.2 mg, Sodium Fluoride 2.21 mg, Thiamine Mononitrate 1.05 mg, Vitamin A Acetate 2500 Units, Vitamin D 400 Units, Vitamin E Acetate 15 Units	Soluvite C T by Pharmics	00813-0078	Vitamin
PHARMICS	Tab, Pink, Oblong, Film Coated	Ascorbic Acid 120 mg, Calcium Carbonate, Precipitated, Calcium Pantothenate, Cupric Oxide, Cyanocobalamin 12 mcg, Ergocalciferol 400 Units, Ferrous Fumarate, Folic Acid 1 mg, Magnesium 100 mg, Niacinamide 20 mg, Potassium Iodide, Pyridoxine HCl 12 mg, Riboflavin 3.4 mg, Thiamine Mononitrate, Vitamin A Acetate, Vitamin E 30 Units, Zinc Oxide	Par F by Pharmics	00813-0076	Vitamin

ID FRONT <> BACK	DESCRIPTION FRONT <> BACK	INGREDIENT & STRENGTH	BRAND (or Generic Equiv.) by FIRM	NDC#	CLASS; SCH.
PHARMICS	Tab, White, Dye-Free, Oblong, Film Coated	Ascorbic Acid 90 mg, Calcium Carbonate 200 mg, Copper 2 mg, Cyanocobalamin 12 mcg, Ergocalciferol 400 Units, Ferrous Fumarate 66 mg, Folic Acid 1 mg, Iodine 150 mcg, Magnesium Oxide 100 mg, Niacinamide 20 mg, Pyridoxine HCl 4 mg, Riboflavin 3 mg, Sodium Fluoride 1.1 mg, Thiamine HCl 3 mg, Vitamin A 5000 Units, Vitamin D 400 Units, Vitamin E 30 Units, Zinc 15 mg	O Cal F A by Pharmics	00813-0038	Vitamin
PHARMICS	Tab, Yellow, Oblong, Film Coated	Ascorbic Acid 300 mg, Lemon Bioflavonoid Complex 200 mg, Riboflavin 10 mg, Thiamine HCl 25 mg, Calcium Pantothenate 10 mg, Niacinamide 50 mg	B-Scorbic by Pharmics	00813-0070	Vitamin
PHARMICS	Tab, White, Oblong, Film Coated	Vitamin A 2500 Units, Vitamin D 400 Units, Vitamin E 30 Units, Vitamin C 70 mg, Folic Acid 1 mg, Thiamin 1.5 mg, Riboflavin 1.6 mg, Niacinamide 17 mg, Vitamin B6 12 mg, Vitamin B12 12 mcg, Calcium Carbonate 200 mg, Magnesium 100 mg, Iron 15 mg, Iodine 150 mcg, Copper 2 mg, Zinc 15 mg	O-Cal Prenatal by Pharmics	00813-0202	Vitamin
PHARMICS <> 0025	Tab, 00 over 25	Acetaminophen 500 mg, Hydrocodone Bitartrate 5 mg	Vicodin by Quality Care	60346-0442	Analgesic; C III
PHE	Tab, Green and White, Bilayered, Cap Shaped, Scored, Star Logo PHE	Phenylephrine HCl 40 mg, Chlorpheniramine Maleate 8 mg, Methscopolamine Nitrate 2.5 mg	Rescon Mx by Capellon	64543-0090	Cold Remedy
PHI	Tab, Yellow, Round, Scored	Acetaminophen 375 mg, Caffeine 15 mg, Codeine Phosphate 15 mg	by Frosst	Canadian	Analgesic; C III
PHI292	Tab, Peach, Round, Scored, PHI over 292	Acetaminophen 375 mg, Caffeine 15 mg, Codeine Phosphate 30 mg	by Frosst	Canadian	Analgesic; C III
PHILLIPSPHILLIPS	Tab, White, Round, Phillips/Phillips	Magnesium Hydroxide 311 mg	Phillips by Bayer	Canadian	Mineral Supplement
PHOSCHOL	Cap, Amber	Soybean Lecithin	Phoschol by American Lecithin		
PHOSLO667	Cap, Blue & White	Calcium Acetate 667 mg	PhosLo by Braintree	52268-0210	Vitamin; Mineral
PHPH	Tab, Green, Round	pHos-pHaid 250 mg	pHos-pHaid by Guardian		Urinary Tract
PHPH	Tab, Blue, Round	pHos-pHaid 500 mg	pHos-pHaid by Guardian		Urinary Tract
PHPH	Tab, Orange, Round	pHos-pHaid 500 mg	pHos-pHaid by Guardian		Urinary Tract
PI	Tab, Red, Round, Scored	Ferrous Fumarate 150 mg, Ascorbic Acid 500 mg, Cyanocobalamin 60 mcg, Intrinsic Factor, Concentrate 75 mg, Folic Acid 1 mg, Vitamin E 30 Units, Docusate Sodium 50 mg	Genhemat by Pharmakon	55422-0220	Mineral
PIM2	Tab, White, Round, Scored, PIM / 2	Pimozide 2 mg	ORAP by Pharmascience	Canadian DIN 00313815	Antipsychotic
PIM2 <> APO	Tab, White, Round, Scored	Pimozide 2 mg	ORAP by Apotex	Canadian DIN 02245432	Antipsychotic
PIM4	Tab, Green, Round, Scored, PIM / 4	Pimozide 4 mg	ORAP by Pharmascience	Canadian DIN 00313823	Antipsychotic
PIM4 <> APO	Tab, Green, Round, Scored	Pimozide 4 mg	Apo Pimozide by Apotex	Canadian DIN 02245433	Antipsychotic
PINDOLOL10 <> PP	Tab, White, Round, Scored	Pindolol 10 mg	Visken by Pharmascience	Canadian DIN 02231537	Antihypertensive
PINDOLOL15 <> PP	Tab, White, Round, Scored	Pindolol 15 mg	Visken by Pharmascience	Canadian DIN 02231539	Antihypertensive
PINDOLOL5 <> PP	Tab, White, Round, Scored	Pindolol 5 mg	Visken by Pharmascience	Canadian DIN 5760615365	Antihypertensive
PINDOLOL5 <> PP	Tab, White, Round, Scored	Pindolol 5 mg	Visken by Pharmascience	Canadian DIN 02231536	Antihypertensive
PIR <> 2	Tab, White, Round, Scored	Hydromorphone Hydrochloride 2 mg.	Hydromorph IR by Purdue Pharma	Canadian DIN 02245703	Analgesic
PIR <> 4	Tab, White, Cap-Shaped, Scored	Hydromorphone hydrochloride 4 mg.	Hydromorph IR by Purdue Pharma	Canadian DIN 02245704	Analgesic
PIR <> 8	Tab, White, Scored	Hydromorphone Hydrochloride 8 mg	Hydromorph IR by Purdue Pharma	Canadian DIN 02245705	Analgesic

ID FRONT <> BACK	DESCRIPTION FRONT <> BACK	INGREDIENT & STRENGTH	BRAND (or Generic Equiv.) by FIRM	NDC#	CLASS; SCH.
PIROXICAM10P	Cap, Blue & Maroon, Hard Gel	Piroxicam 10 mg	Feldene by Pharmascience	Canadian DIN 5760636242	NSAID
PIROXICAM20P	Cap, Maroon, Hard Gel	Piroxicam 20 mg	Feldene by Pharmascience	Canadian DIN 5760636232	NSAID
PL <> 250	Tab, Pink, Round, Film Coated, Scored	Tinidazole 250 mg	Tindamax by Presutti Labs	66378-0250 Discontinued	Antibiotic
PL <> 500	Tab, Pink, Cap Shaped, Film Coated, Scored	Tinidazole 500 mg	Tindamax by Presutti Labs	66378-0500 Discontinued	Antibiotic
PL <> C20	Tab, Mottled Pink, Round	Amoxicillin 200 mg, Clavulanate Potassium 20 mg	Augmentin by Ivax	00172-7401	Antibiotic
PL500	Tab, White, Oval, Film Coated	Amoxicillin 500 mg, Clavulanic Acid 125 mg	Augmentin by Par	49884-0298	Antibiotic
PL500125	Tab, White, Oval, Film Coated	Amoxicillin 500 mg, Clavulanate Potassium 125 mg	Augmentin by Ivax	00172-7403	Antibiotic
PL875	Tab, White, Cap Shaped, Scored	Amoxicillin 875 mg, Clavulanate Potassium 125 mg	Augmentin by Ivax	00172-7404	Antibiotic
PL875	Tab, White, Capsule Shaped, Scored	Amoxicillin 875 mg, Clavulanic Acid 125 mg	Augmentin by Par	49884-0299	Antibiotic
PLACIDYL500	Cap, Red, Placidyl over 500	Ethchlorvynol 500 mg	Placidyl by Abbott	00074-6685 Discontinued	Hypnotic; C IV
PLACIDYL750	Cap, Green, Placidyl over 750	Ethchlorvynol 750 mg	Placidyl by Abbott	00074-6630 Discontinued	Hypnotic; C IV
PLAIN <> GG250	Tab, Ex Release	Quinidine Gluconate 324 mg	by Golden State	60429-0167	Antiarrhythmic
PLAIN <> GG288	Tab, Coated	Cyclobenzaprine HCl 10 mg	by Golden State	60429-0052	Muscle Relaxant
PLAIN <> GG60	Tab, Scored	Allopurinol 300 mg	Zyloprim by Golden State	60429-0014	Antigout
PLAQUENIL	Tab, White, Black Print, Peanut Shaped	Hydroxychloroquine Sulfate 200 mg	Plaquenil by Pharmedix	53002-0485	Antimalarial
PLAQUENIL	Tab, White, Black Print, Peanut Shaped	Hydroxychloroquine Sulfate 200 mg	Plaquenil by Sanofi	Canadian	Antimalarial
PLAQUENIL	Tab, White, Black Print, Peanut Shaped	Hydroxychloroquine Sulfate 200 mg	Plaquenil by Sanofi	00024-1562	Antimalarial
PLAT8	Cap, Pink	Amoxicillin 875 mg	Amoxil by Ivax	00172-7411	Antibiotic
PLC <> 40	Tab, Mottled Pink, Round	Amoxicillin 400 mg, Clavulanate Potassium 20 mg	Augmentin by Ivax	00172-7402	Antibiotic
PLCAP500	Cap, Royal Blue, Pink, Opaque	Amoxicillin 500 mg	Amoxil by Ivax	00172-7414	Antibiotic
PLCT4	Tab, Pink, Round, Chewable	Amoxicillin 400 mg	Amoxil by Ivax	00172-7416	Antibiotic
PLENDIL <> 450	Tab, Sage Green, Round, Ex Release	Felodipine 2.5 mg	Plendil by AstraZeneca	00186-0450	Antihypertensive
PLENDIL <> 451	Tab, Light Red-Brown, Round, Ex Release	Felodipine 5 mg	Plendil by AstraZeneca	00186-0451	Antihypertensive
PLENDIL <> 452	Tab, Red-Brown, Round, Ex Release	Felodipine 10 mg	Plendil by AstraZeneca	00186-0452	Antihypertensive
PLETAL100	Tab, White, Round, PLETAL over 100	Cilostazol 100 mg	Pletal by Otsuka	59148-0002	Antiplatelet
PLETAL100	Tab, White, Round, PLETAL over 100	Cilostazol 100 mg	Pletal by Compumed	00403-0803	Antiplatelet
PLETAL50	Tab, White, Triangular, PLETAL over 50	Cilostazol 50 mg	Pletal by Otsuka	59148-0003	Antiplatelet
PLETAL50	Tab, White, Triangular, PLETAL over 50	Cilostazol 50 mg	Pletal by Compumed	00403-0994	Antiplatelet
PLIVA <> 563	Tab, Yellow, Round, Film Coated	Cyclobenzaprine HCl 10 mg	Flexeril by Pliva	50111-0563	Muscle Relaxant
PLIVA <> 563	Tab, Yellow, Round, Film Coated	Cyclobenzaprine HCl 10 mg	Flexeril by Teva	00093-1919	Muscle Relaxant
PLIVA <> 609	Tab, Yellow, Black Print, Cap Shaped, Film Coated, Ex Release	Pentoxifylline 400 mg	Trental by Pliva	50111-0609	Anticoagulant
PLIVA <> 675	Tab, Pale Pink, Round	Fluconazole 50 mg	Diflucan by Par	49884-0935	Antifungal
PLIVA <> 787	Tab, White, Oval, Film Coated	Azithromycin 250 mg	Zithromax by Pliva	50111-0787 Discontinued	Antibiotic
PLIVA <> 788	Tab, Blue, Cap Shaped, Film Coated	Azithromycin 500 mg	Zithromax by Pliva	50111-0788	Antibiotic
PLIVA <> 789	Tab, White, Cap Shaped, Film Coated	Azithromycin 600 mg	Zithromax by Pliva	50111-0789	Antibiotic
PLIVA <> 930	Tab, Light Green, Round, Scored, Film Coated	Sertraline HCl 25 mg	Zoloft by Pliva	50111-0930	Antidepressant
PLIVA <> 931	Tab, Light Blue, Round, Scored, Film Coated	Sertraline HCl 50 mg	Zoloft by Pliva	50111-0931	Antidepressant
PLIVA <> 932	Tab, Light Yellow, Round, Scored, Film Coated	Sertraline HCl 100 mg	Zoloft by Pliva	50111-0932	Antidepressant
PLIVA314	Tab, White, Round, Scored	Cyproheptadine HCl 4 mg	Periactin by Pliva	50111-0314 Discontinued	Antihistamine
PLIVA323	Tab, White, Round, Scored, PLIVA over 323	Bethanechol Chloride 5 mg	Urecholine by Pliva	50111-0323	Urinary Tract
PLIVA324	Tab, White, Round, Scored, PLIVA over 324	Bethanechol Chloride 10 mg	Urecholine by Pliva	50111-0324	Urinary Tract
PLIVA325	Tab, Yellow, Round, Scored	Bethanechol Chloride 25 mg	Urecholine by Pliva	50111-0325	Urinary Tract

ID FRONT <> BACK	DESCRIPTION FRONT <> BACK	INGREDIENT & STRENGTH	BRAND (or Generic Equiv.) by FIRM	NDC#	CLASS; SCH.
PLIVA326	Tab, Yellow, Round, Scored	Bethanechol Chloride 50 mg	Urecholine by Pliva	50111-0326	Urinary Tract
PLIVA327	Tab, Orange, Round	Hydralazine HCl 25 mg	Apresoline by Pliva	50111-0327	Antihypertensive
PLIVA327	Tab, Orange, Round	Hydralazine HCl 25 mg	Apresoline by UDL	51079-0075	Antihypertensive
PLIVA328	Tab, Orange, Round	Hydralazine HCl 50 mg	Apresoline by Pliva	50111-0328	Antihypertensive
PLIVA328	Tab, Orange, Round	Hydralazine HCl 50 mg	Apresoline by UDL	51079-0076	Antihypertensive
				Discontinued	
PLIVA333	Tab, White, Round	Metronidazole 250 mg	Flagyl by Pliva	50111-0333	Antibiotic
PLIVA333	Tab, White, Round	Metronidazole 250 mg	Flagyl by Amneal	65162-0303	Antibiotic
PLIVA334	Tab, White, Oblong	Metronidazole 500 mg	Flagyl by Pliva	50111-0334	Antibiotic
PLIVA334	Tab, White, Oblong	Metronidazole 500 mg	Flagyl by Amneal	65162-0304	Antibiotic
PLIVA362	Tab, Light Orange, Round	Chlorthalidone 25 mg	Hygroton by Major	00904-1349	Diuretic
PLIVA362	Tab, Light Orange, Round	Chlorthalidone 25 mg	Hygroton by Pliva	50111-0362	Diuretic
PLIVA362	Tab, Light Orange, Round	Chlorthalidone 25 mg	Hygroton by Qualitest	00603-2860	Diuretic
PLIVA362	Tab, Light Orange, Round	Chlorthalidone 25 mg	Hygroton by Ivax	00182-1434	Diuretic
PLIVA363	Tab, Light Blue, Round	Chlorthalidone 50 mg	Hygroton by Pliva	50111-0363	Diuretic
				Discontinued	
PLIVA364	Tab, White, Round, Scored	Chlorthalidone 100 mg	Hygroton by Pliva	50111-0364	Diuretic
PLIVA372	Tab, Blue, Round, Scored	Chlorpropamide 100 mg	Diabinese by Pliva	50111-0372	Antidiabetic
PLIVA373	Tab, Blue, Round, Scored	Chlorpropamide 250 mg	Diabinese by Pliva	50111-0373	Antidiabetic
PLIVA375MG	Cap, Light Green, Opaque	Metronidazole 375 mg	Flagyl by Pliva	50111-0884	Antibiotic
PLIVA390	Tab, Yellow, Round, Film Coated	Salsalate 500 mg	Disalcid by Pliva	50111-0390	NSAID
PLIVA390	Tab, Yellow, Round, Film Coated	Salsalate 500 mg	Disalcid by Ivax	00182-1802	NSAID
				Discontinued	
PLIVA391	Tab, Yellow, Cap Shaped, Scored, Film Coated	Salsalate 750 mg	Disalcid by Ivax	00182-1803	NSAID
				Discontinued	
PLIVA391	Tab, Yellow, Oblong, Scored, Pliva over 391	Salsalate 750 mg	Disalcid by Pliva	50111-0391	NSAID
PLIVA395	Tab, White, Round, Scored	Benztropine Mesylate 2 mg	Cogentin by Pliva	50111-0395	Antiparkinson
PLIVA397	Tab, Orange, Round	Hydralazine HCl 100 mg	Apresoline by Pliva	50111-0397	Antihypertensive
PLIVA398	Tab, Orange, Round	Hydralazine HCl 10 mg	Apresoline by Pliva	50111-0398	Antihypertensive
PLIVA398	Tab, Orange, Round	Hydralazine HCl 10 mg	Apresoline by UDL	51079-0074	Antihypertensive
PLIVA430	Tab, Light Green, Round	Metoclopramide HCl 5 mg	Reglan by Ivax	00182-1898	Gastrointestinal
PLIVA430	Tab, White, Round, Scored	Metoclopramide HCl 10 mg	Reglan by Pliva	50111-0430	Gastrointestinal
PLIVA430	Tab, White, Round, Scored, PLIVA over 433	Metoclopramide HCl 10 mg	Reglan by Ivax	00182-1789	Gastrointestinal
PLIVA433	Tab, White, Round, Scored	Trazodone HCl 50 mg	Desyrel by Pliva	50111-0433	Antidepressant
PLIVA434	Tab, White, Round, Scored	Trazodone HCl 100 mg	Desyrel by Pliva	50111-0434	Antidepressant
PLIVA441 <> 505050	Tab, White, Trapezoidal, Scored	Trazodone HCl 150 mg	Desyrel by Pliva	50111-0441	Antidepressant
PLIVA456	Tab, White to Light Blue, Round, Scored	Oxybutynin Chloride 5 mg	Ditropan by Pliva	50111-0456	Urinary Tract
PLIVA456	Tab, White to Light Blue, Round, Scored	Oxybutynin Chloride 5 mg	Ditropan by Amneal	65162-0210	Urinary Tract
PLIVA459	Tab, White, Cap Shaped, Scored, Ex Release	Theophylline Anhydrous 300 mg	Theo-Dur by Pliva	50111-0459	Antiasthmatic
PLIVA467	Tab, Orange, Round, Scored	Propranolol HCl 10 mg	Inderal by Ivax	00182-1812	Antihypertensive
PLIVA467	Tab, Orange, Round, Scored	Propranolol HCl 10 mg	Inderal by Pliva	50111-0467	Antihypertensive
PLIVA468	Tab, Blue, Round, Scored	Propranolol HCl 20 mg	Inderal by Ivax	50111-0468	Antihypertensive
PLIVA468	Tab, Blue, Round, Scored	Propranolol HCl 20 mg	Inderal by Ivax	00182-1813	Antihypertensive
PLIVA469	Tab, Green, Round, Scored	Propranolol HCl 40 mg	Inderal by Ivax	00182-1814	Antihypertensive
PLIVA469	Tab, Green, Round, Scored	Propranolol HCl 40 mg	Inderal by Pliva	50111-0469	Antihypertensive
PLIVA470	Tab, Pink, Round, Scored	Propranolol HCl 60 mg	Inderal by Pliva	50111-0470	Antihypertensive
PLIVA471	Tab, Yellow, Round, Scored	Propranolol HCl 80 mg	Inderal by Pliva	50111-0471	Antihypertensive
PLIVA471	Tab, Yellow, Round	Propranolol HCl 80 mg	Inderal by Ivax	00182-1815	Antihypertensive
PLIVA473	Tab, White, Round, Scored	Hydrochlorothiazide 25 mg, Propranolol HCl 40 mg	Inderide by Pliva	50111-0473	Diuretic; Antihypertensive
PLIVA474	Tab, White, Round, Scored	Hydrochlorothiazide 25 mg, Propranolol HCl 80 mg	Inderide by Pliva	50111-0474	Diuretic; Antihypertensive

ID FRONT <> BACK	DESCRIPTION FRONT <> BACK	INGREDIENT & STRENGTH	BRAND (or Generic Equiv.) by FIRM	NDC#	CLASS; SCH.
PLIVA482	Tab, White, Oval, Scored	Theophylline Anhydrous 200 mg	Theo-Dur by Pliva	50111-0482	Antiasthmatic
PLIVA483	Tab, White, Round, Scored, Ex Release	Theophylline Anhydrous 100 mg	Theo-Dur by Pliva	50111-0483	Antiasthmatic
PLIVA505	Tab, Yellow, Rectangular, Scored	Hydrochlorothiazide 50 mg, Triamterene 75 mg	Maxzide by Pliva	50111-0505	Diuretic; Antihypertensive
PLIVA517	Tab, Light Green, Round	Metoclopramide HCl 5 mg	Reglan by Pliva	50111-0517	Gastrointestinal
PLIVA518	Tab, White, Cap Shaped, Ex Release, Scored	Theophylline Anhydrous 450 mg	Theo-Dur by Pliva	50111-0518	Antiasthmatic
PLIVA528	Tab, Yellow, Cap Shaped, Scored, Film Coated	Choline Magnesium Trisalicylate 500 mg	Trilisate by Pliva	50111-0528	NSAID
PLIVA529	Tab, Blue, Cap Shaped, Scored, Film Coated	Choline Magnesium Trisalicylate 750 mg	Trilisate by Pliva	50111-0529	NSAID
PLIVA530	Tab, Pink, Cap Shaped, Scored, Film Coated	Choline Magnesium Trisalicylate 1000 mg	Trilisate by Pliva	50111-0530	NSAID
PLIVA534	Tab, Orange, Rectangular, Scored	Hydrochlorothiazide 25 mg, Triamterene 37.5 mg	Maxzide 25 by Pliva	50111-0534	Diuretic; Antihypertensive
PLIVA616	Tab, White, Oval, Film Coated	Tramadol 50 mg	Ultram by Pliva	50111-0616	Analgesic
PLIVA621	Tab, White, Round, Scored	Ketoconazole 200 mg	Nizoral by Pliva	50111-0621	Antifungal
PLIVA647	Cap, White w/ Green Band, Opaque	Fluoxetine HCl 10 mg	Prozac by Pliva	50111-0647	Antidepressant
PLIVA647	Cap, White, Opaque	Fluoxetine 10 mg	Prozac by Teva	50111-0647	Antidepressant
PLIVA648	Cap, White w/ Green Band on Cap Only, Opaque	Fluoxetine HCl 20 mg	Prozac by Pliva	50111-0648	Antidepressant
PLIVA648	Cap, White, Opaque	Fluoxetine 20 mg	Prozac by Teva	50111-0648	Antidepressant
PLIVA651	Tab, White, Round, Scored	Doxazosin Mesylate 1 mg	Cardura by Pliva	50111-0651	Antihypertensive
PLIVA652	Tab, Yellow, Round, Scored	Doxazosin Mesylate 2 mg	Cardura by Pliva	50111-0652	Antihypertensive
PLIVA653	Tab, Orange, Round, Scored	Doxazosin Mesylate 4 mg	Cardura by Pliva	50111-0653	Antihypertensive
PLIVA654	Tab, Green, Round, Scored	Doxazosin Mesylate 8 mg	Cardura by Pliva	50111-0654	Antihypertensive
PLIVA676	Tab, Pale Pink, Round	Fluconazole 100 mg	Diflucan by Pliva	50111-0676	Antifungal
PLIVA677	Tab, Pale Pink, Round	Fluconazole 150 mg	Diflucan by Pliva	50111-0677	Antifungal
PLIVA678	Tab, Pale Pink, Round	Fluconazole 200 mg	Diflucan by Pliva	50111-0678	Antifungal
PLIVA708	Tab, White, Round, Scored, Film Coated	Propafenone HCl 150 mg	Rythmol by Pliva	50111-0708	Antiarrhythmic
PLIVA709	Tab, White, Round, Scored, Film Coated	Propafenone HCl 225 mg	Rythmol by Pliva	50111-0709	Antiarrhythmic
PLIVA710	Tab, White, Round, Film Coated, Scored	Propafenone HCl 300 mg	Rythmol by Pliva	50111-0710	Antiarrhythmic
PLOND <> 4	Tab, White, Oval	Ondansetron 4 mg	Zofran by Sandoz	00781-5257	Antiemetic
PLOND <> 8	Tab, White, Oval	Ondansetron 8 mg	Zofran by Sandoz	00781-5258	Antiemetic
PLUS <> CITRACAL	Tab, White, Modified Rectangle, Film Coated	Calcium Citrate, Vitamin D, Magnesium	Citracal Plus by Mission	00178-0825	Vitamin; Supplement
PLUS3	Tab, Yellow, Oval, Heart Shape <> PLUS3	Vitamin Combination	StuartNatal 3 by Integrity	64731-0814	Vitamin
PLZID <> 300	Tab, White, Round, Film-Coated	Zidovudine 300 mg	Retrovir by Teva	00093-5530 Discontinued	Antiviral
PM	Tab, Light Blue, Round	Acetaminophen 500 mg, Diphenhydramine 38 mg	Excedrin PM by Novartis Consumer Health, Inc.	00067-2053	Analgesic; Sleep Aid
PM <> L437	Tab, Light Blue, Cap Shaped	Acetaminophen 500 mg, Diphenhydramine HCl 25 mg	Tylenol PM by Major Pharmaceuticals	00904-7651	Analgesic; Sleep Aid
PM <> L437	Tab, Light Blue, Cap Shaped	Acetaminophen 500 mg, Diphenhydramine HCl 25 mg	Tylenol PM by Perrigo	00113-0437	Analgesic; Sleep Aid
PM <> L465	Tab, Blue, Round	Acetaminophen 500 mg, Diphenhydramine HCl 25 mg	Tylenol PM by Perrigo	00113-0465	Analgesic; Sleep Aid
PM200	Cap, Ex Release	Chlorpheniramine Maleate 8 mg, Pseudoephedrine HCl 120 mg	by Pharma Medica	62441-0200	Cold Remedy
PM200	Cap, Clear	Chlorpheniramine Maleate 8 mg, Pseudoephedrine HCl 120 mg	by Compumed	00403-0010	Cold Remedy
PM200	Cap, Clear	Chlorpheniramine Maleate 8 mg, Pseudoephedrine HCl 120 mg	by Kaiser	62224-0448	Cold Remedy
PM200PM200	Cap, Black Print	Chlorpheniramine Maleate 8 mg, Pseudoephedrine HCl 120 mg	by Kaiser	00179-0376	Cold Remedy
PM300	Tab, White, Oblong, Scored	Guaifenesin 400 mg	GFN IR by PharmaFab	62542-0689	Cold Remedy
PMS	Tab, White, Round, Scored	Tiaprofenic Acid 200 mg	by Pharmascience	Canadian DIN 5760608272	NSAID
PMS	Tab, Yellow, Round, Scored	Salicylazosulfapyridine 500 mg	by Pharmascience	Canadian	Gastrointestinal
PMS	Tab, White, Round, Scored	Nylidrin HCl 6 mg	by Pharmascience	Canadian DIN 5760609752	Vasodilator
PMS	Tab, White, Round	Zinc Sulfate 220 mg	Orazinc by Pharmascience	Canadian	Mineral
PMS	Tab, Orange, Round, Scored	Procyclidine HCl 2.5 mg	by Pharmascience	Canadian	Antiparkinson
PMS	Tab, White, Round	Acetaminophen 325 mg	Tylenol by Pharmascience	Canadian	Analgesic
PMS	Tab, White, Round	Acetaminophen 500 mg	Tylenol Ex Strength by Pharmascience	Canadian	Analgesic

For updated data, go to www.IdentADrug.com

ID FRONT <> BACK	DESCRIPTION FRONT <> BACK	INGREDIENT & STRENGTH	BRAND (or Generic Equiv.) by FIRM	NDC#	CLASS; SCH.
PMS	Tab, Pink, Round, Film Coated	Amitriptyline 2 mg, Perphenazine 25 mg	Elavil Plus by Pharmascience	Canadian DIN 00590495	Antidepressant; Antipsychotic
PMS	Tab, Red	Amitriptyline 4 mg, Perphenazine 25 mg	Triavil by Pharmascience	Canadian	Antidepressant; Antipsychotic
PMS	Tab, White, Round	Isoniazid 50 mg	Laniazid by Pharmascience	Canadian	Antimycobacterial
PMS	Tab, White	Magnesium Gluconate 500 mg	by Pharmascience	Canadian DIN 5760651262	Mineral
PMS	Tab, White, Round	Metoclopramide 5 mg	Reglan by Pharmascience	Canadian	Gastrointestinal
PMS	Tab, White, Round	Metoclopramide 10 mg	Reglan by Pharmascience	Canadian	Gastrointestinal
PMS	Tab, Pink	Fluphenazine HCl 1 mg	by Pharmascience	Canadian	Antipsychotic
PMS	Tab, Yellow, Round	Flutamide 250 mg	by Pharmascience	Canadian	Antiandrogen
PMS	Tab, Dark Pink	Fluphenazine HCl 2 mg	by Pharmascience	Canadian	Antipsychotic
PMS	Tab, White, Round, Film Coated	Fluphenazine HCl 5 mg	Moditen by Pharmascience	Canadian DIN 00726354	Antipsychotic
PMS	Tab, White, Round, Scored	Isoniazid 100 mg	Laniazid by Pharmascience	Canadian DIN 00577790	Antimycobacterial
PMS	Tab, White, Round, Scored	Isoniazid 300 mg	Laniazid by Pharmascience	Canadian	Antimycobacterial
PMS	Tab, Orange, Round, Scored	Propranolol HCl 10 mg	Inderal by Pharmascience	Canadian DIN 00582255	Antihypertensive
PMS	Tab, White, Round, Scored	Pyrazinamide 500 mg	Tebrazid by Pharmascience	Canadian DIN 00618810	Antibiotic
PMS	Tab, Light Green, Round, Scored	Propranolol HCl 40 mg	Inderal by Pharmascience	Canadian DIN 00582263	Antihypertensive
PMS	Tab, Yellow, Round, Scored	Propranolol HCl 80 mg	Inderal by Pharmascience	Canadian DIN 00582271	Antihypertensive
PMS	Tab, Dark Yellow, Round, Scored	Sulfasalazine 500 mg	Salazopyrin by Pharmascience	Canadian DIN 00598461	Gastrointestinal
PMS <> 1	Tab, Pale Green, Round, Scored	Hydromorphone HCl 1 mg	by Pharmascience	Canadian DIN 00885444	Analgesic; C II
PMS <> 111	Tab, Yellow, D Shaped, Film Coated	Cyclobenzaprine HCl 10 mg	Flexeril by Pharmascience	Canadian DIN 02212048	Muscle Relaxant
PMS <> 121	Tab, Orange, Round, Scored	Procyclidine HCl 2.5 mg	Kemadrin by Pharmascience	Canadian DIN 00649392	Antiparkinson
PMS <> 123	Tab, Orange, Round, Scored	Procyclidine HCl 2.5 mg	by Pharmascience	Canadian DIN 5760693922	Antiparkinson
PMS <> 2	Tab, Pale Orange, Round, Scored	Hydromorphone HCl 2 mg	by Pharmascience	Canadian DIN 00885436	Analgesic; C II
PMS <> 305	Tab, White, Round, Scored	Procyclidine HCl 5 mg	Kemadrin by Pharmascience	Canadian DIN 00587354	Antiparkinson
PMS <> 4	Tab, Yellow, Round, Scored	Hydromorphone HCl 4 mg	by Pharmascience	Canadian DIN 00885401	Analgesic; C II
PMS <> 403	Tab, Pink, Round	Sennosides 12 mg	Senokot by Pharmascience	Canadian DIN 00896403	Laxative
PMS <> 411	Tab, White, Round	Sennosides 8.6 mg	Senokot by Pharmascience	Canadian DIN 00896411	Laxative
PMS <> 8	Tab, White, Round, Scored	Hydromorphone HCl 8 mg	Dilaudid by Pharmascience	Canadian DIN 00885428	Analgesic; C II
PMS <> B5	Tab, White, Round, Scored	Buspirone HCl 5 mg	Buspar by Pharmascience	Canadian DIN 5760609410	Antianxiety
PMS <> IN125	Tab, Orange, Round, Coated, IN 12.5	Indapamide 1.25 mg	Lozide by Pharmascience	Canadian DIN 02239619	Diuretic

ID FRONT <> BACK	DESCRIPTION FRONT <> BACK	INGREDIENT & STRENGTH	BRAND (or Generic Equiv.) by FIRM	NDC#	CLASS; SCH.
PMS05 <> CLONAZEPAM	Tab, Orange, Round, Scored, pms over 0.5	Clonazepam 0.5 mg	Rivotril by Pharmascience	Canadian DIN 02048701	Sedative; C IV
PMS05 <> CLONAZEPAM	Tab, Orange, Round, Scored, pms over 0.5	Clonazepam 0.5 mg	Rivotril by Pharmascience	Canadian DIN 02207818	Sedative; C IV
PMS1	Tab, Salmon, Round, x/PMS-1	Benztropine Mesylate 1 mg	Cogentin by Pharmascience	Canadian DIN 00706531	Antiparkinson
PMS10	Tab, Blue, Round, PMS-10	Desipramine HCl 10 mg	by Pharmascience	Canadian	Antidepressant
PMS10	Tab, Peach, Round, Scored, PMS over 10	Prochlorperazine 10 mg	Stemetil by Pharmascience	Canadian DIN 00753637	Antiemetic
PMS10 <> 110	Tab, Blue, Round, Scored	Methylphenidate HCl 10 mg	Ritalin by Pharmascience	Canadian DIN 00584991	Stimulant; C II
PMS10 <> BACLOFEN	Tab, White, Oval, Scored	Baclofen 10 mg	Lioresal by Pharmascience	Canadian DIN 02063735	Muscle Relaxant
PMS10 <> CLONAZEPAM	Tab, Pink, Round, pms 1.0	Clonazepam 1 mg	Rivotril by Pharmascience	Canadian DIN 02048728	Sedative; C IV
PMS100	Tab, Yellow, Round, Logo pms/100	Ketoprofen 100 mg	Orudis by Pharmascience	Canadian	NSAID
PMS100	Cap, Orange, Soft Gel	Docusate Sodium 100 mg	Colace by Pharmascience	Canadian DIN 01994344	Laxative
PMS100 <> METOPL	Tab, Pale Blue, Cap Shaped, Scored, Film Coated	Metoprolol Succinate 100 mg	Toprol XL by Pharmascience	Canadian DIN 02230804	Antihypertensive
PMS100 <> TRAZODONE	Tab, White, Round, Scored	Trazodone HCl 100 mg	Desyrel by Pharmascience	Canadian DIN 01937235	Antidepressant
PMS10110	Tab, Blue/Green, Round, pms/10 110	Methylphenidate HCl 10 mg	Ritalin by Pharmascience	Canadian	Stimulant; C II
PMS10MG <> BUSPIRONE	Tab, White, Cap Shaped, Scored	Buspirone HCl 10 mg	Buspar by Pharmascience	Canadian DIN 02230942	Antianxiety
PMS150LITH	Cap, Orange and Yellow	Lithium Carbonate 150 mg	Carbolith by Pharmascience	Canadian DIN 02216132	Antipsychotic
PMS150MGLITH	Cap, Yellow & Orange, Hard Gel	Lithium Carbonate 150 mg	Eskalith by Pharmascience	Canadian DIN 5760661324	Antipsychotic
PMS160 <> SOTALOL	Tab, Pale Blue, Oblong, Scored	Sotalol HCl 160 mg	Sotacor by Pharmascience	Canadian DIN 02238327	Antiarrhythmic
PMS191	Cap, Pink, Hard Gel	Diphenhydramine HCl 25 mg	by Pharmascience	Canadian DIN 5760676834	Antihistamine
PMS192	Cap, Clear & Pink, Hard Gel	Diphenhydramine HCl 50 mg	by Pharmascience	Canadian DIN 5760676914	Antihistamine
PMS2	Tab, White, Round, Scored	Benztropine 2 mg	Cogentin by Pharmascience	Canadian DIN 00587265	Antiparkinson
PMS20 <> 123	Tab, Yellow, Round, Scored	Methylphenidate HCl 20 mg	Ritalin by Pharmascience	Canadian DIN 00585009	Stimulant; C II
PMS20 <> BACLOFEN	Tab, White, Cap Shaped, Scored	Baclofen 20 mg	Lioresal by Pharmascience	Canadian DIN 02063743	Muscle Relaxant
PMS20 <> CLONAZEPAM	Tab, White, Round, Scored, pms over 2.0	Clonazepam 2 mg	Rivotril by Pharmascience	Canadian DIN 02048736	Sedative; C IV
PMS200	Cap, Orange, Soft Gel	Docusate Sodium 200 mg	Colace by Pharmascience	Canadian DIN 02029529	Laxative
PMS240	Cap, Red, Soft Gel	Docusate Calcium 240 mg	Surfak by Pharmascience	Canadian DIN 00664553	Laxative
PMS25	Tab, Yellow, Round, Film Coated	Desipramine HCl 25 mg	Norpramin by Pharmascience	Canadian DIN 01946269	Antidepressant
PMS250	Cap, Orange	Valproic Acid 250 mg	Depakene by Pharmascience	Canadian DIN 02230768	Anticonvulsant

ID FRONT <> BACK	DESCRIPTION FRONT <> BACK	INGREDIENT & STRENGTH	BRAND (or Generic Equiv.) by FIRM	NDC#	CLASS; SCH.
PMS25PMS	Tab, White, Round, Scored, PMS over 25 over PMS	Bethanechol Chloride 25 mg	Urecholine by Pharmascience	Canadian DIN 00739162	Urinary Tract
PMS300LITH	Cap, Flesh and White	Lithium Carbonate 300 mg	Carbolith by Pharmascience	Canadian DIN 02216140	Antipsychotic
PMS300MGLITH	Cap, White & Flesh, Hard Gel	Lithium Carbonate 300 mg	Eskalith by Pharmascience	Canadian DIN 5760661404	Antipsychotic
PMS403	Tab, Pink, PMS/403	Sennosides 12 mg	by Pharmascience	Canadian	Gastrointestinal
PMS411	Tab, Gray, PMS/411	Sennosides 8.6 mg	by Pharmascience	Canadian	Gastrointestinal
PMS488	Tab, Yellow, Oval, PMS/488	Salicylazosulfapyridine 500 mg	by Pharmascience	Canadian	Gastrointestinal
PMS5	Tab, Peach, Round, Scored, PMS over 5	Prochlorperazine 5 mg	by Pharmascience	Canadian DIN 00753661	Antiemetic
PMS5 <> 130	Tab, Orange, Round, Scored	Methylphenidate HCl 5 mg	by Pharmascience	Canadian DIN 02234749	Stimulant; C II
PMS50	Tab, Green, Round, Film Coated	Desipramine HCl 50 mg	Norpramin by Pharmascience	Canadian DIN 01946277	Antidepressant
PMS50	Tab, Logo pms/50	Ketoprofen 50 mg	Orudis by Pharmascience	Canadian	NSAID
PMS50 <> METOPL	Tab, Pink, Oblong, Scored	Metoprolol Tartrate 50 mg	Lopressor by Pharmascience	Canadian DIN 02230803	Antihypertensive
PMS50 <> TRAZADONE	Tab, Orange, Round, Scored	Trazodone HCl 50 mg	Desyrel by Pharmascience	Canadian DIN 01937227	Antidepressant
PMS50 <> TRAZADONE	Tab, Orange, Round, Scored	Trazodone HCl 50 mg	Desyrel by Pharmascience	Canadian DIN 6952369419	Antidepressant
PMS500MG	Cap, Blue & Green, Opaque	Trikacide 500 mg	by Pharmascience	Canadian DIN 5760631374	Antibacterial
PMS500MG	Cap, Blue and Turquoise, Opaque	Metronidazole 500 mg	Flagyl by Pharmascience	Canadian DIN 00783137	Antifungal
PMS50PMS	Tab, Beige, Round, Scored, PMS over 50 over PMS	Bethanechol Chloride 50 mg	Urecholine by Pharmascience	Canadian DIN 00759198	Urinary Tract
PMS600LITH	Cap, Aqua and White	Lithium Carbonate 600 mg	Carbolith by Pharmascience	Canadian DIN 02216159	Antipsychotic
PMS75	Tab, Orange, Round, Film Coated	Desipramine HCl 75 mg	Norpramin by Pharmascience	Canadian DIN 01946242	Antidepressant
PMS75 <> TRAZADONE	Tab, Salmon	Trazodone HCl 75 mg	Desyrel by Pharmascience	Canadian DIN 02237339	Antidepressant
PMS80 <> SOTALOL	Tab, Pale Blue, Oblong, Scored	Sotalol HCl 80 mg	Sotacor by Pharmascience	Canadian DIN 02238326	Antiarrhythmic
PMSB5	Tab, White, Round, pms/B/5	Buspirone HCl 5 mg	Buspar by Pharmascience	Canadian	Antianxiety
PMSF250	Cap, Orange	Valproic Acid 250 mg	Depakene by Pharmascience	Canadian	Anticonvulsant
PMSKETOPROFEN50	Cap, Ivory & Dark Green	Ketoprofen 50 mg	Orudis by Pharmascience	Canadian DIN 02150808	NSAID
PMSTRAZODONE125	Tab, Pink, Round, pms/Trazodone/12.5	Trazodone HCl 12.5 mg	Desyrel by Pharmascience	Canadian	Antidepressant
PMSTRAZODONE25	Tab, Blue, Round, pms/Trazodone/25	Trazodone HCl 25 mg	Desyrel by Pharmascience	Canadian	Antidepressant
PMSYOHIMBINE	Tab, Pink, Round, PMS/Yohimbine	Yohimbine HCl 6 mg	by Pharmascience	Canadian	Impotence Agent
PN	Tab, White, Oval, Film Coated	Elemental Iron 90 mg, Biotin 30 mcg, Pantothenic acid 6 mg, Calcium 200 mg, Copper 2 mg, Zinc 15 mg, Folate 1 mg, L-methylfolate (as Metafolin) 600 mcg, Folic acid 400 mcg, Vitamin D3 400 IU, Vitamin E 10 IU, Vitamin C 120 mg, Vitamin B1 3 mg, Vitamin B2 3.4 mg, Vitamin B6 20 mg, Vitamin B12 12 mcg, Niacinamide 20 mg, Magnesium 30 mg, Docusate Sodium 50 mg	OptiNate by Horizon	59630-0412	Prenatal Vitamin

ID FRONT <> BACK	DESCRIPTION FRONT <> BACK	INGREDIENT & STRENGTH	BRAND (or Generic Equiv.) by FIRM	NDC#	CLASS; SCH.
PN	Tab, White, Oval, Film Coated	Elemental Iron 90 mg, Biotin 30 mcg, Pantothenic acid 6 mg, Calcium 200 mg, Copper 2 mg, Zinc 15 mg, Folate 1 mg, L-methylfolate (as Metafolin) 600 mcg, Folic acid 400 mcg, Vitamin D3 400 IU, Vitamin E 10 IU, Vitamin C 120 mg, Vitamin B1 3 mg, Vitamin B2 3.4 mg, Vitamin B6 20 mg, Vitamin B12 12 mcg, Niacinamide 20 mg, Magnesium 30 mg, Docusate Sodium 50 mg	Prenate Elite by Horizon	59630-0411	Prenatal Vitamin
PN	Tab, White, Oval, Film-Coated	Vitamin A 2500 IU, Vitamin C 80 mg, Vitamin D3 400 IU, Vitamin E 10 IU, Thiamin (Vitamin B1) 3 mg, Riboflavin (Vitamin B2) 3.4 mg, Niacinamide 20 mg, Vitamin B6 20 mg, Folate 1 mg, (L-methylfolate calcium 676 mcg (as Metafolin) molar equivalent to 600 mcg of Folic Acid) (Folic acid, USP 400 mcg), Vitamin B12 12 mcg, Biotin 300 mcg, Pantothenic acid 6 mg, Calcium Carbonate 120 mg, Iron (ferrous fumarate) 27 mg, Iodine 150 mcg, Magnesium 30 mg, Zinc 15 mg, Copper 2 mg	Prenate Elite by Shionogi	59630-0416	Prenatal Vitamin
PN <> CIBA	Tab, Pale Yellow, Round, Scored	Methylphenidate HCl 20 mg	Ritalin by Novartis	Canadian DIN 00005614	Stimulant; C II
PN <> SANOFI	Tab, Coated	Ascorbic Acid 120 mg, Calcium Citrate 200 mg, Cholecalciferol 400 Units, Cupric Oxide 2 mg, Cyanocobalamin 12 mcg, Docusate Sodium 50 mg, Folic Acid 1 mg, Iron Pentacarbonyl 90 mg, Niacinamide 20 mg, Potassium Iodide 150 mcg, Pyridoxine HCl 20 mg, Riboflavin 3.4 mg, Thiamine HCl 3 mg, Vitamin A 2700 Units, Vitamin E 30 Units, Zinc Oxide 25 mg	Prenate Ultra by Sanofi	00024-1730	Vitamin
PN90 <> BOCK	Tab, PN/90	Ascorbic Acid 120 mg, Calcium 250 mg, Cholecalciferol 10 mcg, Copper 2 mg, Cyanocobalamin 12 mcg, Docusate Sodium 50 mg, Folic Acid 1 mg, Iodine 150 mcg, Iron 90 mg, Niacinamide 20 mg, Pyridoxine HCl 20 mg, Riboflavin 3.4 mg, Thiamine Mononitrate 3 mg, Vitamin A Acetate 1.2 mg, Vitamin E Acetate 30 mg, Zinc 25 mg	by Physician Total Care	54868-2703	Vitamin
PNAXEN250S	Tab, Yellow, Round	Naproxen 250 mg	by AltiMed	Canadian	NSAID
PNAXEN375S	Tab, Pink, Oval	Naproxen 375 mg	by AltiMed	Canadian	NSAID
PNAXEN500S	Tab, Yellow, Oblong	Naproxen 500 mg	by AltiMed	Canadian	NSAID
POLY0101	Tab, Poly over 0101, Ex Release	Chlorpheniramine Maleate 4 mg, Phenylephrine HCl 10 mg, Phenylpropanolamine HCl 50 mg, Pyrilamine Maleate 25 mg	Poly Hist Forte by Pharmafab	62542-0903	Cold Remedy
POLY500 <> FLEXTRADS	Tab, Orange & Red, Oblong, Scored, Poly500<>Flextra-DS	Acetaminophen 500 mg	Tylenol Ex Strength by ABG	60999-0901	Analgesic
POLVENT <> 675	Tab, Poly-Vent <> 6 over 75	Guaifenesin 600 mg, Phenylpropanolamine HCl 75 mg	Entex LA by Poly	50991-0408	Cold Remedy
POLVENT <> 675	Tab, 6 over 75, Ex Release	Guaifenesin 600 mg, Phenylpropanolamine HCl 75 mg	Entex LA by Pharmafab	62542-0780	Cold Remedy
POT10	Tab, White, Oval, Film Coated	Paroxetine Mesylate 10 mg	Pexeva by Synthon	63672-2010	Antidepressant
POT20	Tab, Dark Orange, Oval, Film Coated, Scored	Paroxetine Mesylate 20 mg	Pexeva by Synthon	63672-2020	Antidepressant
POT30	Tab, Yellow, Oval, Film Coated	Paroxetine Mesylate 30 mg	Pexeva by Synthon	63672-2030	Antidepressant
POT40	Tab, Rose, Oval, Film Coated	Paroxetine Mesylate 40 mg	Pexeva by Synthon	63672-2040	Antidepressant
POTABA51	Cap, White	Potassium Aminobenzoate 500 mg	Potaba by Glenwood LLC	00516-0051	Dermatologic
POTABA54	Tab, Off-White, Round	Potassium Aminobenzoate 500 mg	Potaba by Glenwood LLC	00516-0054	Dermatologic
PP	Tab, White, P/P	Proguanil 100 mg	Paludrine by Wyeth	Canadian	Antimalarial
PP	Tab, Beige-Orange, Oval, Scored	Carbamazepine 200 mg	Tegretol by Pharmascience	Canadian DIN 02231543	Anticonvulsant
PP <> 673	Tab, White to Off-White, Oval	Cabergoline 0.5 mg	Dostinex by Par	49884-0673	Antiparkinson
PP <> AA	Tab, White, Oval, Scored, P logo / P logo <> A / A	Pramipexole DiHCl 0.25 mg	Mirapex by Pharmascience	Canadian DIN 02290111	Antiparkinson
PP <> BB	Tab, White, Oval, Scored, P logo / P logo <> B / B	Pramipexole DiHCl 0.5 mg	Mirapex by Pharmascience	Canadian DIN 02290138	Antiparkinson
PP <> CAPTOPRIL100	Tab, White, Oval	Captopril 100 mg	Capoten by Pharmascience	Canadian DIN 02230206	Antihypertensive

ID FRONT <> BACK	DESCRIPTION FRONT <> BACK	INGREDIENT & STRENGTH	BRAND (or Generic Equiv.) by FIRM	NDC#	CLASS; SCH.
PP <> CAPTOPRIL50	Tab, White, Oval, Scored	Captopril 50 mg	Capoten by Pharmascience	Canadian DIN 02230205	Antihypertensive
PP <> CC	Tab, White, Round, Scored, P logo / P logo <> C / C	Pramipexole DiHCl 1 mg	Mirapex by Pharmascience	Canadian DIN 02290146	Antiparkinson
PP <> DD	Tab, White, Round, Scored, P logo / P logo <> D / D	Pramipexole DiHCl 1.5 mg	Mirapex by Pharmascience	Canadian DIN 02290154	Antiparkinson
PP <> ENE	Tab, Brown-Orange, Scored	Carbamazepine 400 mg	Tegretol by Pharmascience	Canadian DIN 02231544	Anticonvulsant
PP <> PINDOLOL10	Tab, White, Round, Scored	Pindolol 10 mg	Visken by Pharmascience	Canadian DIN 02231537	Antihypertensive
PP <> PINDOLOL15	Tab, White, Round, Scored	Pindolol 15 mg	Visken by Pharmascience	Canadian DIN 02231539	Antihypertensive
PP <> PINDOLOL5	Tab, White, Round, Scored	Pindolol 5 mg	Visken by Pharmascience	Canadian DIN 02231536	Antihypertensive
PP040	Tab, White, Round, PP-040	Furosemide 40 mg	Lasix by Eon		Diuretic
PP052	Tab	Diazepam 5 mg	by Pharmedix	53002-0334	Antianxiety; C IV
PP071	Tab, Blue, Round, PP-071	Chlorthalidone 50 mg	Hygroton by Eon		Diuretic
PP073	Tab, White, Round, PP/073	Chlorthalidone 100 mg	Hygroton by Eon		Diuretic
PP081	Tab, Yellow, Round, PP-081	Folic Acid 1 mg	Folvite by Eon		Vitamin
PP100	Tab, White, Round, Beveled Edge	Tramadol Hydrochloride 100 mg	Ryzolt by Purdue Pharma	59011-0334	Analgesic
PP111	Tab, White, Round, PP-111	Sulfamethoxazole 400 mg, Trimethoprim 80 mg	Bactrim by Eon		Antibiotic
PP112	Tab, Eon Logo	Sulfamethoxazole 800 mg, Trimethoprim 160 mg	Trimeth Sulfa DS by Pharmedix		Antibiotic
PP12	Tab, Red, Round, PP-12	Ferrous Sulfate 325 mg	Feosol by Eon	53002-0210	Mineral
PP1217	Cap, Green & Yellow, PP-1217	Nitroglycerin 9 mg	Nitrobid by Eon		Vasodilator
PP1235	Cap, ER, Eon Logo	Nitroglycerin 6.5 mg	by URL Mutual	00677-0486	Vasodilator
PP125	Tab, White, Oval, PP-125	Methylprednisolone 4 mg	Medrol by Eon		Steroid
PP13	Tab, Green, Round, PP-13	Ferrous Sulfate 325 mg	Feosol by Eon		Mineral
PP1303	Cap, Clear	Quinine Sulfate 325 mg	by Eon		Antimalarial
PP1304	Cap	Chlorpheniramine Maleate 8 mg, Pseudoephedrine HCl 120 mg	Pseudo Chlor by Sandoz		Cold Remedy
PP134	Tab, White, Round, PP-134	Reserpine 0.25 mg	Serpasil by Eon	00781-2915	Antihypertensive
PP14	Tab, Yellow, Round	Chlorpheniramine Maleate 4 mg	Chlor-Trimeton by Eon		Antihistamine
PP16	Tab, White, Round, PP-16	Triprolidine 2.5 mg, Pseudoephedrine 60 mg	Actifed by Eon		Cold Remedy
PP17	Tab, White, Round, PP-17	Baclofen 10 mg	Lioresal by Eon		Muscle Relaxant
PP18	Tab, White, Round, PP-18	Baclofen 20 mg	Lioresal by Eon		Muscle Relaxant
PP200	Tab, White, Round, Beveled Edge	Tramadol Hydrochloride 200 mg	Ryzolt by Purdue Pharma	59011-0335	Analgesic
PP2007	Cap, Brown & Clear	Papaverine HCl 150 mg	Pavabid by Pioneer		Vasodilator
PP212	Tab, Blue, Round, PP-212	Butabarbital 30 mg	Butisol Sodium by Eon		Sedative/Hypnotic; C III
PP220	Tab, Blue, Round, PP-220	Urinary Antiseptic #2	Atrosept by Eon		Urinary Tract
PP226	Tab, Green, Round, PP-226	Chlorzoxazone 250 mg, Acetaminophen 300 mg	Parafon Forte by Eon		Muscle Relaxant
PP250	Cap, Blue & Yellow, PP-250	Mefenamic Acid 250 mg	Ponstel by Eon		NSAID
PP256	Cap, Blue & Clear, PP-256	Chlorpheniramine Maleate 12 mg, Phenylpropanolamine 75 mg	Ornade by Eon		Cold Remedy
PP257	Tab, Yellow, Oblong, PP-257	Prenatal Vitamin	by Eon		Vitamin
PP259	Tab, Yellow, Oblong	Prenatal Vitamin	Stuartnatal 1+1 by Eon		Vitamin
PP29	Tab, Purepac Logo	Propranolol HCl 20 mg	Inderal by Pharmedix	53002-0360	Antihypertensive
PP29	Tab, White, Round, PP-29	Desipramine HCl 10 mg	Norpramin by Eon		Antidepressant

ID FRONT <> BACK	DESCRIPTION FRONT <> BACK	INGREDIENT & STRENGTH	BRAND (or Generic Equiv.) by FIRM	NDC#	CLASS; SCH.
PP3	Tab, White, Round, PP-3	Dipyridamole 25 mg	Persantine by Eon		Antiplatelet
PP300	Tab, White, Round, Beveled Edge	Tramadol Hydrochloride 300 mg	Ryzolt by Purdue Pharma	59011-0336	Analgesic
PP3001	Tab, White with Red Specks, Round	Phenylpropanolamine HCl 40 mg, Phenylephrine HCl 10 mg, Phentoloxamine 15 mg, Chlorpheniramine 5 mg	Naldecon by Pioneer		Cold Remedy
PP3008	Tab, Blue, Round	Brompheniramine Maleate 12 mg, Phenylephrine HCl 15 mg, Phenylpropanolamine HCl 15 mg	Dimetapp by Pioneer		Cold Remedy
PP333	Tab, White/Green, Round, PP-333	Aspirin 325 mg, Meprobamate 200 mg	Equagesic by Eon		Sedative/Hypnotic; C IV
PP345	Cap, Clear & White	Phenylpropanolamine HCl 75 mg, Caramiphen Edisylate 40 mg	Tuss-Ornade by Eon		Cold Remedy
PP3602	Tab, White, Round, PP-360 & 2	Acetaminophen 300 mg, Codeine Phosphate 15 mg	Tylenol w/ Codeine by Eon		Analgesic; C III
PP3653	Tab, White, Round, PP-365 & 3	Acetaminophen 300 mg, Codeine Phosphate 30 mg	Tylenol w/ Codeine by Eon		Analgesic; C III
PP3704	Tab, White, Round, PP-370 & 4	Acetaminophen 300 mg, Codeine Phosphate 60 mg	Tylenol w/ Codeine by Eon		Analgesic; C III
PP4001	Cap, Blue	Cyclandelate 200 mg	Cyclospasmol by Pioneer		Vasodilator
PP4002	Cap, Blue & Red	Cyclandelate 400 mg	Cyclospasmol by Pioneer		Vasodilator
PP4005	Cap, Green	Indomethacin 25 mg	Indocin by Pioneer		NSAID
PP4006	Cap, Green	Indomethacin 50 mg	Indocin by Pioneer		NSAID
PP4008	Cap, Pink	Diphenhydramine HCl 50 mg	Benadryl by Pioneer		Antihistamine
PP4009	Cap, Green	Chlordiazepoxide 5 mg, Clidinium Bromide 2.5 mg	Librax by Pioneer		Gastrointestinal
PP4010	Cap, Green & Yellow	Chlordiazepoxide 5 mg	Librium by Pioneer		Antianxiety; C IV
PP4011	Cap, Black & Green	Chlordiazepoxide 10 mg	Librium by Pioneer		Antianxiety; C IV
PP4012	Cap, Green & White	Chlordiazepoxide 25 mg	Librium by Pioneer		Antianxiety; C IV
PP4013	Cap, Clear & Pink	Diphenhydramine HCl 25 mg	Benadryl by Pioneer		Antihistamine
PP4017	Cap, Blue	Dicyclomine HCl 10 mg	Bentyl by Pioneer		Gastrointestinal
PP497	Tab, White, Round, PP-497	Atropine Sulfate 0.025 mg, Diphenoxylate HCl 2.5 mg	Lomotil by Eon		Antidiarrheal; C V
PP50	Tab, PP/50	Hydrochlorothiazide 50 mg	Aquazide H by JMI Canton	00252-9783	Diuretic; Antihypertensive
PP50	Tab, PP/50	Hydrochlorothiazide 50 mg	Aquazide by Jones	52604-9783	Diuretic; Antihypertensive
PP5000	Cap	Phentermine HCl 30 mg	by Sandoz	00781-2415	Anorexiant; C IV
PP5023	Tab, Yellow, Oblong	Vitamin Combination	Strovite by Pioneer		Vitamin
PP511	Tab, White, Round, PP-511	Quinidine Sulfate 200 mg	Quinidine Sulfate by Eon		Antiarrhythmic
PP512	Tab, White, Round, PP-512	Quinidine Sulfate 300 mg	Quinidine Sulfate by Eon		Antiarrhythmic
PP5156	Cap, Brown & Clear, PP-5156	Papaverine HCl 150 mg	Pavabid by Eon		Vasodilator
PP5174	Cap, ER, Eon Logo	Nitroglycerin 2.5 mg	by URL Mutual		Vasodilator
PP5254	Cap, Brown & Clear, PP-5254	Phendimetrazine Tartrate TR 105 mg	by Eon	00677-0485	Anorexiant; C III
PP53	Tab, Pink, Oblong, PP-53	Prenatal Vitamin, Folic Acid	by Eon		Vitamin
PP53010	Tab, White, Round, PP-530 & 10	Isoxsuprine HCl 10 mg	Vasodilan by Eon		Vasodilator
PP53120	Tab, White, Round, PP-531 & 20	Isoxsuprine HCl 20 mg	Vasodilan by Eon		Vasodilator
PP535	Tab, White, Round, PP-535	Tolbutamide 500 mg	Orinase by Eon		Antidiabetic
PP5380	Cap, Red & Maroon	Multivitamin, Mineral	Trinsicon by Eon		Vitamin
PP54	Tab, Yellow, Round, PP-54	Hydrochlorothiazide 50 mg, Triamterene 75 mg	Maxzide by Eon		Diuretic; Antihypertensive
PP551	Tab, White, Round, PP-551	Metronidazole 250 mg	Flagyl by Eon		Antibiotic
PP5511	Cap, Clear & Green, PP-5511	Chlorpheniramine Maleate SR 8 mg	Teldrin by Eon		Antihistamine
PP5512	Cap, Clear & Green, PP-5512	Chlorpheniramine Maleate SR 12 mg	Teldrin by Eon		Antihistamine
PP555	Tab, Eon Logo	Metronidazole 500 mg	by Pharmedix	53002-0247	Antibiotic

ID FRONT <> BACK	DESCRIPTION FRONT <> BACK	INGREDIENT & STRENGTH	BRAND (or Generic Equiv.) by FIRM	NDC#	CLASS; SCH.
PP5730	Cap, Blue & Clear, PP-5730	Phendimetrazine Tartrate 35 mg	by Eon		Anorexiant; C III
PP5740	Cap, Orange/Clear, PP-5740	Phendimetrazine Tartrate 35 mg	by Eon		Anorexiant; C III
PP58	Tab, Yellow, Round, PP-58	Hydroxyzine HCl 50 mg	Atarax by Eon		Antianxiety; Antihistamine
PP585	Tab, White, Round	Methocarbamol 500 mg	Robaxin by Eon		Muscle Relaxant
PP587	Tab, White, Oblong	Methocarbamol 750 mg	Robaxin by Eon		Muscle Relaxant
PP59	Tab, Green, Round, PP-59	Hydroxyzine HCl 25 mg	Atarax by Eon		Antianxiety; Antihistamine
PP60	Tab, Orange, Round, PP-60	Hydroxyzine HCl 10 mg	Atarax by Eon		Antianxiety; Antihistamine
PP6001	Tab, Blue, Round	Ephedrine 25 mg, Hydroxyzine 10 mg, Theophylline 130 mg	Marax by Pioneer		Antiasthmatic
PP6004	Tab, Yellow, Round	Folic Acid 1 mg	Folvite by Pioneer		Vitamin
PP6007	Tab, White, Round	Diazepam 2 mg	Valium by Pioneer		Antianxiety; C IV
PP6008	Tab, Yellow, Round	Diazepam 5 mg	Valium by Pioneer		Antianxiety; C IV
PP6009	Tab, Blue, Round	Diazepam 10 mg	Valium by Pioneer		Antianxiety; C IV
PP6012	Tab, Peach, Round	Chlorzoxazone 250 mg	Parafon by Pioneer		Muscle Relaxant
PP6013	Tab, Blue, Round	Dicyclomine HCl 20 mg	Bentyl by Pioneer		Gastrointestinal
PP6015	Tab, White, Round	Cyproheptadine HCl 4 mg	Periactin by Pioneer		Antihistamine
PP6017	Tab, Green, Round	Acetaminophen 300 mg, Chlorzoxazone 250 mg	Parafon Forte by Pioneer		Muscle Relaxant
PP6018	Tab, White, Round	Carisoprodol 350 mg	Soma by Pioneer		Muscle Relaxant
PP6026	Tab, Yellow, Round	Chlorpheniramine Maleate 4 mg	Chlor-Trimeton by Pioneer		Antihistamine
PP6031	Tab, Orange, Round	Brompheniramine Maleate 4 mg	Dimetane by Pioneer		Antihistamine
PP6036	Tab, White, Round	Methocarbamol 500 mg	Robaxin by Pioneer		Muscle Relaxant
PP6038	Tab, White, Oblong	Methocarbamol 750 mg	Robaxin by Pioneer		Muscle Relaxant
PP6048	Tab, Green, Oblong	Chlorzoxazone 500 mg	Parafon DSC by Pioneer		Muscle Relaxant
PP605	Cap, Green & Yellow, PP-605	Chlordiazepoxide 5 mg	Librium by Eon		Antianxiety; C IV
PP6062	Tab, Peach, Round	Chlorthalidone 25 mg	Hygroton by Pioneer		Diuretic
PP6063	Tab, Blue, Round	Chlorthalidone 50 mg	Hygroton by Pioneer		Diuretic
PP610	Cap, Black & Green, PP-610	Chlordiazepoxide 10 mg	Librium by Eon		Antianxiety; C IV
PP613	Cap, Green & Green, PP-613	Hydroxyzine Pamoate 25 mg	Vistaril by Eon		Antianxiety; Antihistamine
PP615	Cap, Green & White, PP-615	Hydroxyzine Pamoate 50 mg	Vistaril by Eon		Antianxiety; Antihistamine
PP617	Cap, White, PP-617	Chlordiazepoxide 5 mg, Clidinium Bromide 2.5 mg	Librax by Eon		Gastrointestinal
PP625	Cap, Green & White, PP-625	Chlordiazepoxide 25 mg	Librium by Eon		Antianxiety; C IV
PP6265	Cap, Black & Orange, PP-6265	Phendimetrazine Tartrate 35 mg	by Eon		Anorexiant; C III
PP630	Cap, Pink, PP-630	Propoxyphene 65 mg	Darvon by Eon		Analgesic; C IV
PP635	Cap, Red/Black, PP-635	Phentermine HCl 30 mg	by Eon		Anorexiant; C IV
PP640	Cap, Black, PP-640	Phentermine HCl 30 mg	Phentermine HCl by Eon		Anorexiant; C IV
PP647	Cap, Yellow/Yellow, PP-647	Phentermine 30 mg	Ionamin by Eon		Anorexiant; C IV
PP648	Cap, Clear & Pink	Diphenhydramine HCl 25 mg	Benadryl by Eon		Antihistamine
PP649	Cap, Pink	Diphenhydramine HCl 50 mg	Benadryl by Eon		Antihistamine
PP670	Cap, Yellow/Orange, PP-670	Tetracycline HCl 250 mg	Achromycin V by Eon		Antibiotic
PP671	Cap, Black & Yellow, PP-671	Tetracycline HCl 500 mg	Achromycin V by Eon		Antibiotic
PP686	Cap, Red/Gray, PP-686	Aspirin 389 mg, Caffeine 32.4 mg, Propoxyphene 65 mg	Darvon Compound 65 by Eon		Analgesic; C IV

ID FRONT <> BACK	DESCRIPTION FRONT <> BACK	INGREDIENT & STRENGTH	BRAND (or Generic Equiv.) by FIRM	NDC#	CLASS; SCH.
PP698	Cap, Blue & White, PP-698	Doxycycline Hyclate 50 mg	Vibramycin by Eon		Antibiotic
PP699	Cap, Blue, PP-699	Doxycycline Hyclate 100 mg	Vibramycin by Eon		Antibiotic
PP711	Tab, Green, Round	Salsalate 500 mg	Disalcid by Eon		NSAID
PP712	Tab, Green, Oblong	Salsalate 750 mg	Disalcid by Eon		NSAID
PP713	Tab, Green/White, Round, PP-713	Orphenadrine 25 mg, Aspirin 385 mg, Caffeine 60 mg	Norgesic by Eon		Muscle Relaxant
PP714	Tab, Green/White, Round, PP-714	Orphenadrine 50 mg, Aspirin 770 mg, Caffeine 60 mg	Norgesic Forte by Eon		Muscle Relaxant
PP716	Tab, White, Round, PP-716	Meprobamate 200 mg	Equanil by Eon		Sedative/Hypnotic; C IV
PP717	Tab, White, Round, PP-717	Meprobamate 400 mg	Equanil by Eon		Sedative/Hypnotic; C IV
PP717	Tab, Film Coated	Salsalate 750 mg	by Pharmedix	53002-0488	NSAID
PP718	Cap, Green & Opaque, PP-718	Indomethacin 25 mg	Indocin by Eon		NSAID
PP719	Cap, Green & Opaque, PP-719	Indomethacin 50 mg	Indocin by Eon		NSAID
PP720	Cap, Green & Clear, PP-720	Indomethacin 75 mg	Indocin SR by Eon		NSAID
PP721	Tab, Blue, Round	Desipramine HCl 50 mg	Norpramin by Eon		Antidepressant
PP722	Tab, Blue, Round, PP-722	Desipramine HCl 75 mg	Norpramin by Eon		Antidepressant
PP723	Tab, White, Round, PP-723	Carisoprodol 350 mg	Soma by Eon		Muscle Relaxant
PP725	Cap, Rust, PP-725	Meclofenamate Sodium 50 mg	Meclomen by Eon		NSAID
PP726	Cap, Rust/White, PP-726	Meclofenamate Sodium 100 mg	Meclomen by Eon		NSAID
PP736	Tab, Blue, Round, PP-736	Desipramine HCl 100 mg	Norpramin by Eon		Antidepressant
PP737	Cap, Green & Pink, PP-737	Cephradine 250 mg	Anspor by Eon		Antibiotic
PP738	Cap, Green, PP-738	Cephradine 500 mg	Anspor by Eon		Antibiotic
PP739	Cap, Yellow & White	Trimipramine Maleate 25 mg	Surmontil by Eon		Antidepressant
PP740	Cap, Orange & White	Trimipramine Maleate 50 mg	Surmontil by Eon		Antidepressant
PP741	Cap, White, PP-741	Trimipramine Maleate 100 mg	Surmontil by Eon		Antidepressant
PP743	Cap, Green & Clear	Niacin SR 250 mg	Nicobid by Eon		Vitamin
PP745	Tab	Guaifenesin 400 mg, Phenylpropanolamine HCl 75 mg	Entex LA by Pharmedix by Eon	53002-0323	Cold Remedy
PP75	Tab, Pink/White/Blue, Oblong, PP-75	Phendimetrazine Tartrate 35 mg			Anorexiant; C III
PP750	Tab, Brown, Round, PP/750	Nystatin Oral 500,000 Units	Mycostatin by Eon		Antifungal
PP7512	Tab, White, Round, PP-7531 2	Aspirin 325 mg, Codeine Phosphate 15 mg	Aspirin w/ Codeine by Eon		Analgesic; C III
PP7523	Tab, White, Round, PP-7531 3	Aspirin 325 mg, Codeine Phosphate 30 mg	Aspirin w/ Codeine by Eon		Analgesic; C III
PP7534	Tab, White, Round, PP-7531 4	Aspirin 325 mg, Codeine Phosphate 60 mg	Aspirin w/ Codeine by Eon		Analgesic; C III
PP754	Cap, Flesh	Clindamycin HCl 75 mg	Cleocin HCl by Eon		Antibiotic
PP755	Cap, Flesh & Lavender	Clindamycin HCl 150 mg	Cleocin HCl by Eon		Antibiotic
PP756	Cap, Red, PP-756	Hydrochlorothiazide 25 mg, Triamterene 50 mg	Dyazide by Eon		Diuretic; Antihypertensive
PP760	Tab, White, Round, PP-760	Desipramine HCl 150 mg	Norpramin by Eon		Antidepressant
PP761	Tab, Yellow, Round	Salsalate 500 mg	Disalcid by Eon		NSAID
PP762	Tab, Yellow, Oblong	Salsalate 750 mg	Disalcid by Eon		NSAID
PP777	Tab, Yellow, Diamond Shaped, PP-777	Nystatin Vaginal 100,000 Units	Mycostatin by Eon		Antifungal
PP8	Tab, Yellow, Round	Imipramine HCl 10 mg	Tofranil by Eon		Antidepressant
PP84	Tab, Orange, Round	Iodinated Glycerol 30 mg	Organidin by Eon		Expectorant
PP856	Tab, Blue, Round	Salsalate 500 mg	Disalcid by Eon		NSAID

ID FRONT <> BACK	DESCRIPTION FRONT <> BACK	INGREDIENT & STRENGTH	BRAND (or Generic Equiv.) by FIRM	NDC#	CLASS; SCH.
PP857	Tab, Blue, Oblong	Salsalate 750 mg	Disalcid by Eon		NSAID
PP882	Cap, PP 882	Phentermine HCl 15 mg	by Quality Care	60346-0133	Anorexiant; C IV
PP968	Cap, Green	Chlordiazepoxide 5 mg, Clidinium Bromide 2.5 mg	Librax by Eon		Gastrointestinal
PP970	Cap, Red & Gray, PP-970	Cephalexin 250 mg	Keflex by Eon		Antibiotic
PP971	Cap, Red, PP-971	Cephalexin 500 mg	Keflex by Eon		Antibiotic
PP988	Tab, White, Round	Quinine Sulfate 260 mg	Quinamm by Eon		Antimalarial
PP995	Tab, Yellow, Oblong	Choline Magnesium Trisalicylate 500 mg	Trilisate by Eon		NSAID
PP996	Tab, Blue, Oblong	Choline Magnesium Trisalicylate 750 mg	Trilisate by Eon		NSAID
PP997	Tab, Pink, Oblong	Choline Magnesium Trisalicylate 1000 mg	Trilisate by Eon		NSAID
PPIROXICAM10	Cap, Blue & Maroon, Hard Gel	Piroxicam 10 mg	Feldene by Pharmascience	Canadian DIN 5760636242	NSAID
PPIROXICAM20	Cap, Maroon, Hard Gel	Piroxicam 20 mg	Feldene by Pharmascience	Canadian DIN 5760636232	NSAID
PPL54	Tab, Yellow, Round	Hydrochlorothiazide 10 mg, Triamterene 75 mg	Maxzide by Eon		Diuretic; Antihypertensive
PPP207 <> CORGARD40	Tab	Nadolol 40 mg	Nadolol by Pharmedix	53002-1018	Antihypertensive
PPP208	Tab, Blue, Oblong	Nadolol 120 mg	Corgard by BMS		Antihypertensive
PPP232	Tab, Blue, Round	Nadolol 20 mg	Corgard by BMS		Antihypertensive
PPP241	Tab, Blue, Round	Nadolol 80 mg	Corgard by BMS		Antihypertensive
PPP246	Tab, Blue, Oblong	Nadolol 160 mg	Corgard by BMS		Antihypertensive
PPP283	Tab, Blue Specks	Bendroflumethiazide 5 mg, Nadolol 40 mg	Corzide by Pharmedix	53002-1038	Diuretic; Antihypertensive
PPP284	Tab, White/Blue Specks, Round	Bendroflumethiazide 5 mg, Nadolol 80 mg	Corzide by BMS		Diuretic; Antihypertensive
PPP431	Tab, Yellow, Black Print, Cap Shaped, Film Coated, PPP over 431	Procainamide HCl 250 mg	Pronestyl by BMS	00003-0431	Antiarrhythmic
PPP434	Tab, Light Orange, Black Print, Cap Shaped, Film Coated, PPP over 434	Procainamide HCl 375 mg	Pronestyl by BMS	00003-0434	Antiarrhythmic
PPP438	Tab, Red, Black Print, Cap Shaped, Film Coated, PPP over 438	Procainamide HCl 500 mg	Pronestyl by BMS	00003-0438	Antiarrhythmic
PPP606 <> NATURETIN5	Tab, Green, Round, PPP over 606	Bendroflumethiazide 5 mg	Naturetin by BMS	00003-0606	Diuretic; Antihypertensive
PPP618 <> NATURETIN10	Tab	Bendroflumethiazide 10 mg	Naturetin by BMS	00003-0618	Diuretic; Antihypertensive
PPP757	Cap, Yellow & Orange, Black Print, PPP over 757	Procainamide HCl 500 mg	Pronestyl by BMS	00003-0757	Antiarrhythmic
PPP758	Cap, Yellow, Black Print, PPP over 758	Procainamide HCl 250 mg	Pronestyl by BMS	00003-0758	Antiarrhythmic
PPP769	Tab, White Print, PPP over 769	Bendroflumethiazide 4 mg, Rauwolfia Serpentina 50 mg	Rauzide by BMS	00003-0769 Discontinued	Antihypertensive; Diuretic
PPP775	Tab, Greenish Yellow, Black Print, Oval, Film Coated, Ex Release, PPP over 775	Procainamide HCl 500 mg	Pronestyl SR by BMS	00003-0775	Antiarrhythmic
PPP784DURICEF500MG	Cap, White & Red, Black Print, PPP over 784 & Duricef over 500 mg	Cefadroxil Monohydrate 500 mg	Duricef by Warner Chilcott	00430-0780	Antibiotic
PPP784DURICEF500MG	Cap, White & Red, Black Print, PPP over 784 & Duricef over 500 mg	Cefadroxil Monohydrate 500 mg	Duricef by BMS	55961-0784	Antibiotic
PPP784DURICEF500MG	Cap, White & Red, Black Print, PPP over 784 & Duricef over 500 mg	Cefadroxil Monohydrate 500 mg	Duricef by Prestige	58056-0348	Antibiotic
PPP784DURICEF500MG	Cap, White & Red, Black Print, PPP over 784 & Duricef over 500 mg	Cefadroxil Monohydrate 500 mg	Duricef by BMS	00087-0784	Antibiotic
PPP784DURICEF500MG	Cap, White & Red, Black Print, PPP over 784 & Duricef over 500 mg	Cefadroxil Monohydrate 500 mg	Duricef by Nat Pharmpak	55154-2009	Antibiotic
PPP784DURICEF500MG	Cap, White & Red, Black Print, PPP over 784 & Duricef over 500 mg	Cefadroxil Monohydrate 500 mg	Duricef by Pharmedix	53002-0284	Antibiotic

ID FRONT <> BACK	DESCRIPTION FRONT <> BACK	INGREDIENT & STRENGTH	BRAND (or Generic Equiv.) by FIRM	NDC#	CLASS; SCH.
PPP784DURICEF500MG	Cap, White & Red, Black Print, PPP over 784 & Duricef over 500 mg	Cefadroxil Monohydrate 500 mg	Duricef by Allscripts		Antibiotic
PPP785	Tab, White to Off-White, Oval, Scored, PPP / 785	Cefadroxil Monohydrate 1 g	Duricef by BMS	55961-0785	Antibiotic
PPP785	Tab, White to Off-White, Oval, Scored, PPP / 785	Cefadroxil Monohydrate 1 g	Duricef by BMS	00087-0785	Antibiotic
PPP785	Tab, White to Off-White, Oval, Scored, PPP / 785	Cefadroxil Monohydrate 1 g	Duricef by Allscripts		Antibiotic
PPP785	Tab, White to Off-White, Oval, Scored, PPP / 785	Cefadroxil Monohydrate 1 g	Duricef by Warner Chilcott	00430-0781	Antibiotic
PPP863	Tab, Film Coated	Fluphenazine HCl 1 mg	Prolixin by BMS	00003-0863	Antipsychotic
PPP864	Tab, Film Coated	Fluphenazine HCl 2.5 mg	Prolixin by BMS	00003-0864	Antipsychotic
PPP877	Tab, Green, Round, Film Coated	Fluphenazine HCl 5 mg	Prolixin by BMS	00003-0877	Antipsychotic
PPP956	Tab, Pink, Round, Film Coated, PPP over 956	Fluphenazine HCl 10 mg	Prolixin by BMS	00003-0956	Antipsychotic
PR1 <> APO	Tab, White, Round, Scored	Pramipexole DiHCl 1 mg	Mirapex by Apotex	Canadian DIN 02292394	Antiparkinson
PR10 <> G	Tab, White, Square	Pravastatin Sodium 10 mg	Pravachol by Mylan	00378-8210	Antihyperlipidemic
PR10 <> G	Tab, Pink, Rounded Rectangular, PR over 10	Pravastatin Sodium 10 mg	Pravachol by Par	49884-0176	Antihyperlipidemic
PR15 <> APO	Tab, White, Round, Scored, APO <> PR / 1.5	Pramipexole DiHCl 1.5 mg	Mirapex by Apotex	Canadian DIN 02292408	Antiparkinson
PR20 <> G	Tab, White, Square	Pravastatin Sodium 20 mg	Pravachol by Mylan	00378-8220	Antihyperlipidemic
PR20 <> G	Tab, Yellow, Rounded Rectangular, PR over 20	Pravastatin Sodium 20 mg	Pravachol by Par	49884-0179	Antihyperlipidemic
PR25 <> APO	Tab, White, Oval, Scored, APO <> PR / .25	Pramipexole DiHCl 0.25 mg	Mirapex by Apotex	Canadian DIN 02292378	Antiparkinson
PR40 <> G	Tab, White, Square	Pravastatin Sodium 40 mg	Pravachol by Mylan	00378-8240	Antihyperlipidemic
PR40 <> G	Tab, Green, Rounded Rectangular, PR over 40	Pravastatin Sodium 40 mg	Pravachol by Par	49884-0180	Antihyperlipidemic
PR5 <> APO	Tab, White, Oval, Scored, APO <> PR / .5	Pramipexole DiHCl 0.50 mg	Mirapex by Apotex	Canadian DIN 02292386	Antiparkinson
PRA10 <> APO	Tab, Light Pink, Round	Pravastatin Sodium 10 mg	Pravachol by Apotex	60505-0168	Antihyperlipidemic
PRA10 <> APO	Tab, Pink to Peach, Rounded Square	Pravastatin Sodium 10 mg	Apo Pravastatin by Apotex	Canadian DIN 02243506	Antihyperlipidemic
PRA20 <> APO	Tab, Yellow, Rounded Square	Pravastatin Sodium 20 mg	Apo Pravastatin by Apotex	Canadian DIN 02243507	Antihyperlipidemic
PRA20 <> APO	Tab, Off-White to Yellow, Round	Pravastatin Sodium 20 mg	Pravachol by Apotex	60505-0169	Antihyperlipidemic
PRA40 <> APO	Tab, Light Green, Round	Pravastatin Sodium 40 mg	Pravachol by Apotex	60505-0170	Antihyperlipidemic
PRA40 <> APO	Tab, Green, Rounded Square	Pravastatin Sodium 40 mg	Apo Pravastatin by Apotex	Canadian DIN 02243508	Antihyperlipidemic
PRASCO <> 315	Tab, White, Oval	Guaifenesin 600 mg, Phenylephrine HCl 40 mg	WellBid-D by Prasco	66993-0315	Cold Remedy
PRASCO <> 316	Tab, Green, Oblong	Guaifenesin 1200 mg, Phenylephrine HCl 40 mg	WellBid-D 1200 by Prasco	66993-0316	Cold Remedy
PRASCO <> 326	Tab, White, Oblong, Scored	Phenylephrine 25 mg, Guaifenesin 900 mg	by Prasco	66993-0326	Cold Remedy
PRASCO <> KH2	Tab, Green, Round, PRASCO <> KH2	Inert	Solia by Prasco	66993-0611	Oral Contraceptive; Placebo
PRASCO <> TR5	Tab, White, Round, PRASCO <> TR / 5	Desogestrel 0.15 mg, Ethinyl Estradiol 30 mcg	Solia by Prasco	66993-0611	Oral Contraceptive
PRASCO008	Tab, White, Triangular	Cilostazol 50 mg	Pletal by Prasco	66993-0008	Antiplatelet
PRASCO009	Tab, White, Round	Cilostazol 100 mg	Pletal by Prasco	66993-0009	Antiplatelet
PRASCO525	Tab, Tan to Brown, Scored	Phenylephrine Tannate 25 mg, Pyrilamine Tannate 60 mg	K-Tan by Prasco	66993-0525	Cold Remedy
PRAVACHOL10 <> P	Tab, Pink, Rectangular, Pravachol over 10 <> P Logo	Pravastatin Sodium 10 mg	Pravachol by BMS	Canadian DIN 00893749	Antihyperlipidemic
PRAVACHOL10 <> P	Tab, Pink, Rectangular, Pravachol over 10 <> P Logo	Pravastatin Sodium 10 mg	Pravachol by BMS	00003-5154	Antihyperlipidemic
PRAVACHOL10 <> P	Tab, Pink, Rectangular, Pravachol over 10 <> P Logo	Pravastatin Sodium 10 mg	Pravachol by PDRX	55289-0104	Antihyperlipidemic
PRAVACHOL10 <> P	Tab, Pink, Rectangular, Pravachol over 10 <> P Logo	Pravastatin Sodium 10 mg	Pravachol by Nat Pharmpak	55154-0606	Antihyperlipidemic
PRAVACHOL20 <> P	Tab, Yellow, Rounded Square, Pravachol over 20 <> P Logo	Pravastatin Sodium 20 mg	Pravachol by BMS	Canadian DIN 00893757	Antihyperlipidemic
PRAVACHOL20 <> P	Tab, Yellow, Rounded Square, Pravachol over 20 <> P Logo	Pravastatin Sodium 20 mg	Pravachol by BMS	00003-5178	Antihyperlipidemic

ID FRONT <> BACK	DESCRIPTION FRONT <> BACK	INGREDIENT & STRENGTH	BRAND (or Generic Equiv.) by FIRM	NDC#	CLASS; SCH.
PRAVACHOL20 <> P	Tab, Yellow, Rounded Square, Pravachol over 20 <> P Logo	Pravastatin Sodium 20 mg	Pravachol by Allscripts	55154-0608	Antihyperlipidemic
PRAVACHOL20 <> P	Tab, Yellow, Rounded Square, Pravachol over 20 <> P Logo	Pravastatin Sodium 20 mg	Pravachol by Nat Pharmpak	55154-0608	Antihyperlipidemic
PRAVACHOL20 <> P	Tab, Yellow, Rounded Square, Pravachol over 20 <> P Logo	Pravastatin Sodium 20 mg	Pravachol by BMS	12783-0178	Antihyperlipidemic
PRAVACHOL20 <> P	Tab, Yellow, Rounded Rectangular	Pravastatin Sodium 20 mg	Pravigard PAC by BMS	00003-5168 00003-5169	Antihyperlipidemic
PRAVACHOL40 <> P	Tab, Green, Rounded Rectangular	Pravastatin Sodium 40 mg	Pravigard PAC by BMS	00003-5173 00003-5174	Antihyperlipidemic
PRAVACHOL40 <> P	Tab, Green, Rounded Square, Pravachol over 40 <> P Logo	Pravastatin Sodium 40 mg	Pravachol by BMS	Canadian DIN 02222051	Antihyperlipidemic
PRAVACHOL40 <> P	Tab, Green, Rounded Square, Pravachol over 40 <> P Logo	Pravastatin Sodium 40 mg	Pravachol by BMS	00003-5194	Antihyperlipidemic
PRAVACHOL40 <> P	Tab, Green, Rounded Square, Pravachol over 40 <> P Logo	Pravastatin Sodium 40 mg	Pravachol by Caremark	00339-5746	Antihyperlipidemic
PRAVACHOL40 <> P	Tab, Green, Rounded Square, Pravachol over 40 <> P Logo	Pravastatin Sodium 40 mg	Pravachol by BMS	15548-0194	Antihyperlipidemic
PRAZOSIN5DAN5693	Cap, Orange, Black Print, Prazosin over 5 over DAN over 5693	Prazosin HCl 5 mg	by Schein	00364-2391	Antihypertensive
PRECOSE <> 25	Tab, White, Round	Acarbose 25 mg	Precose by Bayer	00026-2863	Antidiabetic
PRECOSE100	Tab, White, Round	Acarbose 100 mg	Precose by Bayer	00026-2862	Antidiabetic
PRECOSE50	Tab, White, Round, Precose over 50	Acarbose 50 mg	Precose by Bayer	00026-2861	Antidiabetic
PRECOSE50	Tab, White, Round, Precose over 50	Acarbose 50 mg	Precose by Caremark	00339-6105	Antidiabetic
PRECOSE50	Tab, White, Round, Precose over 50	Acarbose 50 mg	Precose by Physician Total Care	54868-3823	Antidiabetic
PRECOSE50	Tab, White, Round, Precose over 50	Acarbose 50 mg	Precose by Allscripts		Antidiabetic
PREMARIN	Tab, Green, Oval, Sugar-Coated tablet	Conjugated Estrogens CSD 0.3 mg	Premarin by Wyeth Canada	Canadian DIN 02043394	Hormone
PREMARIN	Tab, Maroon, Oval, Sugar-Coated	Conjugated Estrogens CSD 0.625 mg	Premarin by Wyeth Canada	Canadian DIN 02043408	Hormone
PREMARIN	Tab, Pink, Oval, Sugar-Coated	Conjugated Estrogens CSD 0.9 mg	Premarin by Wyeth Canada	Canadian DIN 02043416	Hormone
PREMARIN	Tab, Yellow, Oval, Sugar-Coated	Conjugated Estrogens CSD 1.25 mg	Premarin by Wyeth Canada	Canadian DIN 02043424	Hormone
PREMARIN03	Tab, Dark Green, White Print, Oval, Sugar Coated, Premarin over 0.3	Conjugated Estrogens 0.3 mg	Premarin by Respa	60575-0078	Hormone
PREMARIN03	Tab, Dark Green, White Print, Oval, Sugar Coated, Premarin over 0.3	Conjugated Estrogens 0.3 mg	Premarin by Kaiser	00179-1173	Hormone
PREMARIN03	Tab, Dark Green, White Print, Oval, Sugar Coated, Premarin over 0.3	Conjugated Estrogens 0.3 mg	Premarin by Ayerst	00046-0868	Hormone
PREMARIN03	Tab, Dark Green, White Print, Oval, Sugar Coated, Premarin over 0.3	Conjugated Estrogens 0.3 mg	Premarin by Wyeth	Canadian DIN 02043394	Hormone
PREMARIN045	Tab, Blue, Oval	Conjugated Estrogens 0.45 mg	Premarin by Ayerst	00046-0936	Hormone
PREMARIN0625	Tab, Maroon, White Print, Oval Sugar Coated, Premarin over 0.625	Conjugated Estrogens 0.625 mg	Premarin by Ayerst	00046-3867	Hormone
PREMARIN0625	Tab, Maroon, White Print, Oval Sugar Coated, Premarin over 0.625	Conjugated Estrogens 0.625 mg	Premarin by Wyeth	Canadian	Hormone
PREMARIN0625	Tab, Maroon, White Print, Oval Sugar Coated, Premarin over 0.625	Conjugated Estrogens 0.625 mg	Premarin by DJ Pharma	64455-0006	Hormone
PREMARIN0625	Tab, Maroon, White Print, Oval Sugar Coated, Premarin over 0.625	Conjugated Estrogens 0.625 mg	Premarin by Heartland	61392-0418	Hormone
PREMARIN0625	Tab, Maroon, White Print, Oval Sugar Coated, Premarin over 0.625	Conjugated Estrogens 0.625 mg	Premarin by Thrift Drug	59198-0092	Hormone
PREMARIN0625	Tab, Maroon, White Print, Oval Sugar Coated, Premarin over 0.625	Conjugated Estrogens 0.625 mg	Premarin by Prepackage Specialists	58864-0422	Hormone

ID FRONT <> BACK	DESCRIPTION FRONT <> BACK	INGREDIENT & STRENGTH	BRAND (or Generic Equiv.) by FIRM	NDC#	CLASS; SCH.
PREMARIN0625	Tab, Maroon, White Print, Oval Sugar Coated, Premarin over 0.625	Conjugated Estrogens 0.625 mg	Premarin by Nat Pharmpak	55154-0213	Hormone
PREMARIN0625	Tab, Maroon, White Print, Oval Sugar Coated, Premarin over 0.625	Conjugated Estrogens 0.625 mg	Premarin by H J Harkins Co	52959-0223	Hormone
PREMARIN0625	Tab, Maroon, White Print, Oval Sugar Coated, Premarin over 0.625	Conjugated Estrogens 0.625 mg	Premarin by Ayerst	00046-0867	Hormone
PREMARIN0625	Tab, Maroon, White Print, Oval Sugar Coated, Premarin over 0.625	Conjugated Estrogens 0.625 mg	Premarin by Kaiser	00179-1172	Hormone
PREMARIN0625	Tab, Maroon, White Print, Oval Sugar Coated, Premarin over 0.625	Conjugated Estrogens 0.625 mg	Premarin by Med Pro	53978-0189	Hormone
PREMARIN0625	Tab, Maroon, White Print, Oval Sugar Coated, Premarin over 0.625	Conjugated Estrogens 0.625 mg	Premarin by Talbert	44514-0493	Hormone
PREMARIN0625	Tab, Maroon, White Print, Oval Sugar Coated, Premarin over 0.625	Conjugated Estrogens 0.625 mg	Premarin by Apotheca	12634-0409	Hormone
PREMARIN0625	Tab, Maroon, White Print, Oval Sugar Coated, Premarin over 0.625	Conjugated Estrogens 0.625 mg	Premarin by Rite Aid	11822-5207	Hormone
PREMARIN09	Tab, White, Pink Print, Oval, Sugar Coated, Premarin over 0.9	Conjugated Estrogens 0.9 mg	Premarin by Wyeth	Canadian	Hormone
PREMARIN09	Tab, White, Pink Print, Oval, Sugar Coated, Premarin over 0.9	Conjugated Estrogens 0.9 mg	Premarin by Ayerst	00046-0864	Hormone
PREMARIN125	Tab, Yellow, Black Print, Oval, Sugar Coated, Premarin over 1.25	Conjugated Estrogens 1.25 mg	Premarin by Wyeth	00046-1104	Hormone
PREMARIN125	Tab, Yellow, Black Print, Oval, Sugar Coated, Premarin over 1.25	Conjugated Estrogens 1.25 mg	Premarin by Wyeth	Canadian	Hormone
PREMARIN125	Tab, Yellow, Black Print, Oval, Sugar Coated, Premarin over 1.25	Conjugated Estrogens 1.25 mg	Premarin by Nat Pharmpak	55154-0211	Hormone
PREMARIN125	Tab, Yellow, Black Print, Oval, Sugar Coated, Premarin over 1.25	Conjugated Estrogens 1.25 mg	Premarin by Thrift Drug	59198-0093	Hormone
PREMARIN125	Tab, Yellow, Black Print, Oval, Sugar Coated, Premarin over 1.25	Conjugated Estrogens 1.25 mg	Premarin by Ayerst	00046-0866	Hormone
PREMARIN125	Tab, Yellow, Black Print, Oval, Sugar Coated, Premarin over 1.25	Conjugated Estrogens 1.25 mg	Premarin by Kaiser	00179-1239	Hormone
PREMARIN125	Tab, Yellow, Black Print, Oval, Sugar Coated, Premarin over 1.25	Conjugated Estrogens 1.25 mg	Premarin by Med Pro	53978-0190	Hormone
PREMARIN125	Tab, Yellow, Black Print, Oval, Sugar Coated, Premarin over 1.25	Conjugated Estrogens 1.25 mg	Premarin by Rite Aid	11822-5200	Hormone
PREMARIN25	Tab, Purple, White Print, Oval, Sugar Coated, Premarin over 2.5	Conjugated Estrogens 2.5 mg	Premarin by Thrift Drug	59198-0094	Hormone
PREMARIN25	Tab, Purple, White Print, Oval, Sugar Coated, Premarin over 2.5	Conjugated Estrogens 2.5 mg	Premarin by Prestige	58056-0353	Hormone
PREMARIN25	Tab, Purple, White Print, Oval, Sugar Coated, Premarin over 2.5	Conjugated Estrogens 2.5 mg	Premarin by Nat Pharmpak	55154-0212	Hormone
PREMARIN25	Tab, Purple, White Print, Oval, Sugar Coated, Premarin over 2.5	Conjugated Estrogens 2.5 mg	Premarin by Amerisource	62584-0865	Hormone
PREMARIN25	Tab, Purple, White Print, Oval, Sugar Coated, Premarin over 2.5	Conjugated Estrogens 2.5 mg	Premarin by Ayerst	00046-0865	Hormone
PREMARIN25	Tab, Purple, White Print, Oval, Sugar Coated, Premarin over 2.5	Conjugated Estrogens 2.5 mg	Premarin by Kaiser	00179-1240	Hormone
PREMARIN25	Tab, Purple, White Print, Oval, Sugar Coated, Premarin over 2.5	Conjugated Estrogens 2.5 mg	Premarin by Repack Co of America	55306-0865	Hormone

ID FRONT <> BACK	DESCRIPTION FRONT <> BACK	INGREDIENT & STRENGTH	BRAND (or Generic Equiv.) by FIRM	NDC#	CLASS; SCH.
PREMARIN25	Tab, Purple, White Print, Oval, Sugar Coated, Premarin over 2.5	Conjugated Estrogens 2.5 mg	Premarin by Wyeth	Canadian	Hormone
PREMPRO	Tab, Peach, Black Print, Oval	Conjugated Estrogens 0.625 mg, Medroxyprogesterone Acetate 2.5 mg	Prempro by Wyeth	55045-2561	Hormone
PREMPRO	Tab, Oval, Cream	Conjugated Estrogens 0.3 mg, Medroxyprogesterone Acetate 1.5 mg	Prempro by Wyeth	00046-0938	Hormone
PREMPRO	Tab, Gold, Black Print, Oval	Conjugated Estrogens 0.45 mg, Medroxyprogesterone Acetate 1.5 mg	Prempro by Ayerst	00046-0937	Hormone
PREMPRO	Tab, Peach, Black Print, Oval	Conjugated Estrogens 0.625 mg, Medroxyprogesterone Acetate 2.5 mg	Prempro by Ayerst	00046-0875	Hormone
PRENATE	Tab, Red, White Print, Oval	Iron Pentacarbonyl 90 mg, Calcium Carbonate 200 mg, Cupric Oxide 2 mg, Zinc Oxide 25 mg, Folic Acid 1 mg, Beta-Carotene 2700 Units, Cholecalciferol 400 Units, Tocopherol Acetate 30 Units, Ascorbic Acid 120 mg, Thiamine Mononitrate 3 mg, Riboflavin 3.4 mg	Prenatal Vitamin by Sanofi	00024-1727	Vitamin; Mineral
PRENATEDHA	Cap, Blue-Green, Opaque, Soft Gel	Vitamin C 85 mg, Vitamin D3 200 IU, Vitamin E 10 IU, Vitamin B6 25 mg, Folate 1 mg, (L-methylfolate calcium 676 mcg (as Metafolin) molar equivalent to 600 mcg of Folic Acid) (Folic acid, USP 400 mcg), Vitamin B12 12 mcg, Calcium 140 mg, Iron (ferrous fumarate) 27 mg, Magnesium 45 mg, Docosahexaenoic Acid (DHA) 300 mg	Prenate DHA by Shionogi	59630-0418	Prenatal Vitamin
PREVACID15	Cap, Pink and Green, Opaque, Hard Gel, TAP Logo and PREVACID15	Lansoprazole 15 mg	Prevacid NaraPAC by Tap	00300-1545	Gastrointestinal
PREVACID15	Cap, Pink and Green, Opaque, Hard Gel, TAP Logo and PREVACID15	Lansoprazole 15 mg	Prevacid NaraPAC by Tap	00300-1546	Gastrointestinal
PREVACID15	Cap, Green & Pink, Opaque, Hard Gel, Delayed Release, Tap Logo & Prevacid 15	Lansoprazole 15 mg	Prevacid by Murfreesboro	51129-1147	Gastrointestinal
PREVACID15	Cap, Green & Pink, Opaque, Hard Gel, Delayed Release, Tap Logo & Prevacid 15	Lansoprazole 15 mg	Prevacid by DRX	55045-2740	Gastrointestinal
PREVACID15	Cap, Green & Pink, Opaque, Hard Gel, Delayed Release, Tap Logo & Prevacid 15	Lansoprazole 15 mg	Prevacid by Tap	00300-1541	Gastrointestinal
PREVACID15	Cap, Green & Pink, Opaque, Hard Gel, Delayed Release, Tap Logo & Prevacid 15	Lansoprazole 15 mg	Prevacid by Tap	Canadian DIN 02165503	Gastrointestinal
PREVACID30	Cap, Black & Pink, Opaque, Hard Gel, Tap Logo & Prevacid 30	Lansoprazole 30 mg	Prevpac by Tap	00300-3702	Gastrointestinal
PREVACID30	Cap, Black & Pink, Opaque, Hard Gel, Tap Logo & Prevacid 30	Lansoprazole 30 mg	Prevacid by Tap	00300-3046	Gastrointestinal
PREVACID30	Cap, Black & Pink, Opaque, Hard Gel, Tap Logo & Prevacid 30	Lansoprazole 30 mg	Prevacid by Murfreesboro	51129-1626	Gastrointestinal
PREVACID30	Cap, Black & Pink, Opaque, Hard Gel, Tap Logo & Prevacid 30	Lansoprazole 30 mg	Prevacid by Tap	Canadian DIN 02165511	Gastrointestinal
PRIFTIN <> 150	Tab, Dark Pink, Round, Film Coated	Rifapentine 150 mg	Priftin by Aventis	00088-2100	Antibiotic
PRIFTIN <> 150	Tab, Dark Pink, Round, Film Coated	Rifapentine 150 mg	Priftin by Gruppo Lepetit	12522-8598	Antibiotic
PRIMUS52001	Cap, Turquoise Green	Flavocoxid 250 mg	Limbrel by Primus	68040-0601	Antiosteoporosis
PRINIVIL <> MSD106	Tab, Yellow, Oval	Lisinopril 10 mg	Prinivil by Amerisource	62584-0925	Antihypertensive
PRINIVIL <> MSD106	Tab, Yellow, Oval	Lisinopril 10 mg	Prinivil by Merck Frosst	Canadian DIN 00839396	Antihypertensive
PRINIVIL <> MSD106	Tab, Yellow, Oval	Lisinopril 10 mg	Prinivil by DRX	55045-2292	Antihypertensive
PRINIVIL <> MSD106	Tab, Yellow, Oval	Lisinopril 10 mg	Prinivil by Med Pro	53978-3015	Antihypertensive
PRINIVIL <> MSD106	Tab, Yellow, Oval	Lisinopril 10 mg	Prinivil by PDRX	55289-0929	Antihypertensive
PRINIVIL <> MSD106	Tab, Yellow, Oval	Lisinopril 10 mg	Prinivil by Merck	00006-0106	Antihypertensive
PRINIVIL <> MSD106	Tab, Yellow, Oval	Lisinopril 10 mg	Prinivil by Pharmacy Care	65070-0012	Antihypertensive
PRINIVIL <> MSD106	Tab, Yellow, Oval	Lisinopril 10 mg	Prinivil by Nat Pharmpak	55154-5015	Antihypertensive
PRINIVIL <> MSD19	Tab, White, Oval, Scored	Lisinopril 5 mg	Prinivil by Nat Pharmpak	55154-5006	Antihypertensive
PRINIVIL <> MSD19	Tab, White, Oval, Scored	Lisinopril 5 mg	Prinivil by Merck	00006-0019	Antihypertensive
PRINIVIL <> MSD19	Tab, White, Oval, Scored	Lisinopril 5 mg	Prinivil by Pharmacy Care	65070-0014	Antihypertensive

ID FRONT <> BACK	DESCRIPTION FRONT <> BACK	INGREDIENT & STRENGTH	BRAND (or Generic Equiv.) by FIRM	NDC#	CLASS; SCH.
PRINIVIL <> MSD19	Tab, White, Oval, Scored	Lisinopril 5 mg	Prinivil by Merck Frosst	Canadian DIN 00839388	Antihypertensive
PRINIVIL <> MSD207	Tab, Peach, Oval	Lisinopril 20 mg	Prinivil by Pharmacy Care	65070-0013	Antihypertensive
PRINIVIL <> MSD207	Tab, Peach, Oval	Lisinopril 20 mg	Prinivil by Med Pro	53978-3017	Antihypertensive
PRINIVIL <> MSD207	Tab, Peach, Oval	Lisinopril 20 mg	Prinivil by Nat Pharmpak	55154-5011	Antihypertensive
PRINIVIL <> MSD207	Tab, Peach, Oval	Lisinopril 20 mg	Prinivil by Merck Frosst	Canadian DIN 00839418	Antihypertensive
PRINIVIL <> MSD207	Tab, Peach, Oval	Lisinopril 20 mg	Prinivil by Merck	00006-0207	Antihypertensive
PRINIVIL <> MSD237	Tab, Rose Red, Shield Shaped, MSD over 237	Lisinopril 40 mg	Prinivil by Merck	00006-0237	Antihypertensive
PRINZIDE <> MSD140	Tab, Yellow, Flower Shaped	Lisinopril 20 mg, HCTZ 12.5 mg	Prinzide by Merck	00006-0140	Antihypertensive; Diuretic
PRINZIDE <> MSD140	Tab, Yellow, Flower Shaped	Lisinopril 20 mg, HCTZ 12.5 mg	Prinzide by MSD	Canadian	Antihypertensive; Diuretic
PRINZIDE <> MSD142	Tab, Peach, Flower Shaped	Lisinopril 20 mg, HCTZ 25 mg	Prinzide by Merck	00006-0142	Antihypertensive; Diuretic
PRINZIDE <> MSD142	Tab, Peach, Flower Shaped	Lisinopril 20 mg, HCTZ 25 mg	Prinzide by MSD	Canadian DIN 00884421	Antihypertensive; Diuretic
PRINZIDE <> MSD145	Tab, Light Blue, Hexagonal	Lisinopril 10 mg, HCTZ 12.5 mg	Prinzide by Merck	00006-0145	Antihypertensive; Diuretic
PRINZIDE <> MSD145	Tab, Light Blue, Hexagonal	Lisinopril 10 mg, HCTZ 12.5 mg	Prinzide by MSD	Canadian	Antihypertensive; Diuretic
PRINZIDE <> MSD145	Tab, Light Blue, Hexagonal	Lisinopril 10 mg, HCTZ 12.5 mg	Prinzide by Murfreesboro	51129-1397	Antihypertensive; Diuretic
PROCANBID <> 1000	Tab, Gray, Black Print, Oval, Film Coated, Ex Release	Procainamide HCl 1000 mg	Procanbid by King	61570-0071	Antiarrhythmic
PROCANBID <> 1000	Tab, Gray, Black Print, Oval, Film Coated, Ex Release	Procainamide HCl 1000 mg	Procanbid by Parke Davis	00071-0564	Antiarrhythmic
PROCANBID500	Tab, White, Oval, Film Coated, Ex Release	Procainamide HCl 500 mg	Procanbid by King	61570-0069	Antiarrhythmic
PROCANSR250MG	Tab, Green, Elliptical, Film Coated	Procainamide HCl 250 mg	Procan SR by Parke Davis	Canadian DIN 00638692	Antiarrhythmic
PROCANSR500MG	Tab, Green, Elliptical, Film Coated	Procainamide HCl 500 mg	Procan by Parke Davis	Canadian DIN 00638676	Antiarrhythmic
PROCANSR750MG	Tab, Orange, Elliptical, Film Coated	Procainamide HCl 750 mg	Procan SR by Parke Davis	Canadian DIN 00638684	Antiarrhythmic
PROCARDIA20PFIZER-261	Cap, Orange & Light Brown, Soft Gel	Nifedipine 20 mg	Procardia by Pfizer	00069-2610	Antihypertensive
PROCARDIAPFIZER260	Cap, Orange, Soft Gel	Nifedipine 10 mg	Procardia by Allscripts	00069-2600	Antihypertensive
PROCARDIAPFIZER260	Cap, Orange, Soft Gel	Nifedipine 10 mg	Procardia by Pfizer	11146-0270	Antihypertensive
PROCARDIAXL30	Tab, Pink, Black Print, Round, Film Coated, Ex Release, Procardia XL over 30	Nifedipine 30 mg	Procardia XL by Giant Food	55154-2706	Antihypertensive
PROCARDIAXL30	Tab, Pink, Black Print, Round, Film Coated, Ex Release, Procardia XL over 30	Nifedipine 30 mg	Procardia XL by Nat Pharmpak		Antihypertensive
PROCARDIAXL30	Tab, Pink, Black Print, Round, Film Coated, Ex Release, Procardia XL over 30	Nifedipine 30 mg	Procardia XL by Allscripts	00069-2650	Antihypertensive
PROCARDIAXL30	Tab, Pink, Black Print, Round, Film Coated, Ex Release, Procardia XL over 30	Nifedipine 30 mg	Procardia XL by Pfizer	53002-1054	Antihypertensive
PROCARDIAXL30	Tab, Pink, Black Print, Round, Film Coated, Ex Release, Procardia XL over 30	Nifedipine 30 mg	Procardia XL by Pharmedix	53978-3035	Antihypertensive
PROCARDIAXL30	Tab, Pink, Black Print, Round, Film Coated, Ex Release, Procardia XL over 30	Nifedipine 30 mg	Procardia XL by Med Pro	62584-0650	Antihypertensive
PROCARDIAXL60	Tab, Pink, Black Print, Round, Film Coated, Ex Release, Procardia XL over 60	Nifedipine 60 mg	Procardia XL by Amerisource	62584-0660	Antihypertensive
PROCARDIAXL60	Tab, Pink, Black Print, Round, Film Coated, Ex Release, Procardia XL over 60	Nifedipine 60 mg	Procardia XL by Pfizer	00069-2660	Antihypertensive
PROCARDIAXL60	Tab, Pink, Black Print, Round, Film Coated, Ex Release, Procardia XL over 60	Nifedipine 60 mg	Procardia XL by Allscripts		Antihypertensive

ID FRONT <> BACK	DESCRIPTION FRONT <> BACK	INGREDIENT & STRENGTH	BRAND (or Generic Equiv.) by FIRM	NDC#	CLASS; SCH.
PROCARDIAXL60	Tab, Pink, Black Print, Round, Film Coated, Ex Release, Procardia XL over 60	Nifedipine 60 mg	Procardia XL by Med Pro	53978-3036	Antihypertensive
PROCARDIAXL60	Tab, Pink, Black Print, Round, Film Coated, Ex Release, Procardia XL over 60	Nifedipine 60 mg	Procardia XL by Nat Pharmpak	55154-2707	Antihypertensive
PROCARDIAXL60	Tab, Pink, Black Print, Round, Film Coated, Ex Release, Procardia XL over 60	Nifedipine 60 mg	Procardia XL by Par	49884-0623	Antihypertensive
PROCARDIAXL90	Tab, Pink, Black Print, Round, Film Coated, Ex Release, Procardia XL over 90	Nifedipine 90 mg	Procardia XL by Allscripts		Antihypertensive
PROCARDIAXL90	Tab, Pink, Black Print, Round, Film Coated, Ex Release, Procardia XL over 90	Nifedipine 90 mg	Procardia XL by Pfizer	00069-2670	Antihypertensive
PRODM	Tab, White, Round, Scored	Dextromethorphan HBr 30 mg, Guaifenesin 600 mg, Pseudoephedrine HCl 60 mg	Protuss DM by Horizon	59630-0160	Cold Remedy
PRODM	Tab, White, Round, Scored	Dextromethorphan HBr 30 mg, Guaifenesin 600 mg, Pseudoephedrine HCl 60 mg	Protuss DM by Anabolic	00722-6370	Cold Remedy
PROFENFORTE <> 315	Tab, White, Oval, Scored, Ex Release	Guaifenesin 800 mg, Pseudoephedrine HCl 90 mg	Profen Forte by Ivax Labs	59310-0315	Cold Remedy
PROFENFORTEDM	Tab, White, Oval, Scored, Ex Release	Dextromethorphan HBr 60 mg, Guaifenesin 800 mg, Pseudoephedrine HCl 90 mg	Profen Forte DM by Ivax Labs	59310-0316	Cold Remedy
PROFENII	Tab, White, Oval, Scored, Ex Release	Guaifenesin 800 mg, Pseudoephedrine HCl 45 mg	Profen II by Ivax Labs	59310-0307	Cold Remedy
PROFENIIDM	Tab, White, Oval, Scored, Ex Release	Guaifenesin 600 mg, Phenylpropanolamine HCl 37.5 mg, Dextromethorphan HBr 30 mg	Profen II DM by Med Pro	53978-3329	Cold Remedy
PROFENIIDM	Tab, White, Oval, Scored, Ex Release	Dextromethorphan HBr 30 mg, Guaifenesin 800 mg, Pseudoephedrine HCl 45 mg	Profen II DM by Ivax Labs	59310-0310	Cold Remedy
PROLEXD	Tab, White, Oval, Scored	Phenylephrine HCl 20 mg, Guaifenesin 600 mg	Prolex D by Sovereign	58716-0686	Cold Remedy
PROLEXD	Tab, White, Oval, Scored	Phenylephrine HCl 20 mg, Guaifenesin 600 mg	Prolex D by Blansett	51674-0124	Cold Remedy
PROLEXPD	Tab, Light Blue, Cap Shaped, Scored	Guaifenesin 600 mg, Phenylephrine HCl 10 mg	Prolex PB by Blansett	51674-0126	Cold Remedy
PROLOPRIM09A	Tab, White, Round, Scored, Proloprim over 09A	Trimethoprim 100 mg	Proloprim by BW Inc	Canadian	Antibiotic
PROLOPRIM09A	Tab, White, Round, Scored, Proloprim over 09A	Trimethoprim 100 mg	Proloprim by DSM	63552-0820	Antibiotic
PROLOPRIM09A	Tab, White, Round, Scored, Proloprim over 09A	Trimethoprim 100 mg	Proloprim by King	61570-0057	Antibiotic
PROLOPRIM200	Tab, Yellow, Round, Scored, Proloprim over 200	Trimethoprim 200 mg	Proloprim by DSM	63552-0825	Antibiotic
PROLOPRIM200	Tab, Yellow, Round, Scored, Proloprim over 200	Trimethoprim 200 mg	Proloprim by King	61570-0058	Antibiotic
PROLOPRIMR2C	Tab, Yellow, Round	Trimethoprim 200 mg	Proloprim by BW Inc	Canadian	Antibiotic
PROMACET <> MCR524	Tab, Blue, Oblong, Scored	Butalbital 50 mg, Acetaminophen 650 mg	Promacet by AM Pharms	58605-0524	Analgesic
PROPACET	Tab, White, Oblong, Film Coated	Acetaminophen 650 mg, Propoxyphene Napsylate 100 mg	Darvocet-N 100 by Teva	00093-0590	Analgesic; C IV
PROPACET	Tab, Coated	Acetaminophen 650 mg, Propoxyphene Napsylate 100 mg	Darvocet-N 100 by Patient First	57575-0019	Analgesic; C IV
PROPECIA <> MRK71	Tab, Tan, Octagonal, Film Coated	Finasteride 1 mg	Propecia by Southwood	58016-0329	Antiandrogen
PROPECIA <> P	Tab, Tan, Octagonal, Film Coated, Stylized P	Finasteride 1 mg	Propecia by Merck	00006-0071	Antiandrogen
PROPECIA <> P	Tab, Tan, Octagonal, Film Coated, Stylized P	Finasteride 1 mg	Propecia by Merck-Frosst	Canadian DIN 02238213	Antiandrogen
PROPECIA1 <> MRK71	Tab, Tan, Octagonal, Film Coated	Finasteride 1 mg	Propecia by Physician Total Care	54868-4120	Antiandrogen
PROSCAR <> MSD72	Tab, Blue, Apple Shaped, Film Coated	Finasteride 5 mg	Proscar by Physician Total Care	54868-2719	Antiandrogen
PROSCAR <> MSD72	Tab, Blue, Apple Shaped, Film Coated	Finasteride 5 mg	Proscar by Merck	00006-0072	Antiandrogen
PROSCAR <> MSD72	Tab, Blue, Apple Shaped, Film Coated	Finasteride 5 mg	Proscar by Physician Total Care	54868-2719	Antiandrogen
PROSCAR <> MSD72	Tab, Blue, Apple Shaped, Film Coated	Finasteride 5 mg	Proscar by Merck-Frosst	Canadian DIN 02010909	Antiandrogen
PROSEDDS	Tab, Deep Blue, Round, Sugar Coated, Prosed/DS	Methenamine 81.6 mg, Phenyl Salicylate 36.2 mg, Methylene Blue 10.8 mg, Benzoic Acid 9.0 mg, Atropine Sulfate 0.06 mg, Hyoscyamine Sulfate 0.06 mg	Prosed DS by Star	00076-0108	Antibiotic; Urinary Tract
PROSEDEC	Tab, Dark Blue, Round, Sugar Coated	Methenamine 81.6 mg, Phenyl Salicylate 36.2 mg, Methylene Blue 10.8 mg, Benzoic Acid 9.0 mg, Atropine Sulfate 0.06 mg, Hyoscyamine Sulfate 0.06 mg	Prosed EC by Star Pharm		Urinary Analgesic
PROSTIGMIN15 <> ICN	Tab, White, Round, Scored	Neostigmine Bromide 15 mg	Prostigmin by ICN	Canadian DIN 00869945	Muscle Stimulant

ID FRONT <> BACK	DESCRIPTION FRONT <> BACK	INGREDIENT & STRENGTH	BRAND (or Generic Equiv.) by FIRM	NDC#	CLASS; SCH.
PROTECTPLUSNR58552	Cap, Purple, Softgel	Coenzyme Q10 30 mg, Alpha-Lipoic Acid 40 mg, Vitamin E 400 IU, Beta Carotene 5,000 IU, Vitamin A 5,000 IU, Vitamin C 500 mg, Vitamin D 400 IU, Grape Seed Extract 500 mcg, Superoxide Dismutase 500 mcg, L-Glutathione 30 mg, Vanadium 50 mcg, Chromium 200 mcg, Selenium 100 mcg, Magnesium 200 mg, Zinc, 30 mg, Manganese 5 mg, Copper 1 mg, Calcium 100 mg, Molybdenum 50 mcg, Folic Acid 1 mg, Vitamin B-1 50 mg, Vitamin B-2 50 mg, Vitamin B-3 50 mg, Vitamin B-5 50 mg, Vitamin B-6 50 mg, Vitamin B-12 50 mcg, Biotin 300 mcg, Inositol 50 mg, Choline 50 mg, Lecithin 100 mg	Protect Plus NR by Gil Pharma	58552-0309	Vitamin
PROTONIX	Tab, Yellow, Brown Print, Oval	Pantoprazole Sodium 40 mg	Protonix by Wyeth	00008-0841	Gastrointestinal
PROTONIX	Tab, Yellow, Brown Print, Oval	Pantoprazole Sodium 40 mg	Protonix by BYK Gulden	47234-0001	Gastrointestinal
PROTONIX	Tab, Yellow, Brown Print, Oval	Pantoprazole Sodium 40 mg	Protonix by Wyeth	00008-0607	Gastrointestinal
PROVENTIL <> 4	Tab, Film Coated	Albuterol Sulfate 4 mg	Proventil by Nat Pharmpak	55154-3507	Antiasthmatic
PROVENTIL2 <> 252252	Tab, Off-White, Round, Proventil 2 <> 252 over 252	Albuterol Sulfate 2 mg	Proventil by Schering	00085-0252	Antiasthmatic
PROVENTIL4 <> 573	Tab, White, Round, Scored	Albuterol Sulfate 4 mg	Proventil by Amide	52152-0188	Antiasthmatic
PROVENTIL4 <> 573	Tab, Film Coated	Albuterol Sulfate 4 mg	Proventil by Amerisource	62584-0463	Antiasthmatic
PROVENTIL4 <> 573	Tab, Film Coated	Albuterol Sulfate 4 mg	Proventil by PDRX	55289-0634	Antiasthmatic
PROVENTIL4 <> 573573	Tab, Off-White, Round, Proventil 4 <> 573/573	Albuterol Sulfate 4 mg	Proventil by Schering	00085-0573	Antiasthmatic
PROVERA10	Tab, White, Round, Scored, Provera over 10	Medroxyprogesterone Acetate 10 mg	Provera by Pharmacia	00009-0050	Hormone
PROVERA10	Tab, White, Round, Scored, Provera over 10	Medroxyprogesterone Acetate 10 mg	Provera by Allscripts	51129-9005	Hormone
PROVERA10	Tab, White, Round, Scored, Provera over 10	Medroxyprogesterone Acetate 10 mg	Provera by Murfreesboro	59198-0197	Hormone
PROVERA10	Tab, White, Round, Scored, Provera over 10	Medroxyprogesterone Acetate 10 mg	Provera by Thrift Drug	55154-3913	Hormone
PROVERA10	Tab, White, Round, Scored, Provera over 10	Medroxyprogesterone Acetate 10 mg	Provera by Nat Pharmpak	11822-5269	Hormone
PROVERA10	Tab, White, Round, Scored, Provera over 10	Medroxyprogesterone Acetate 10 mg	Provera by Rite Aid	51129-0064	Hormone
PROVERA25	Tab, Orange, Round, Scored, Provera over 2.5	Medroxyprogesterone Acetate 2.5 mg	Provera by Murfreesboro	00009-0064	Hormone
PROVERA25	Tab, Orange, Round, Scored, Provera over 2.5	Medroxyprogesterone Acetate 2.5 mg	Provera by Pharmacia	59198-0198	Hormone
PROVERA25	Tab, Orange, Round, Scored, Provera over 2.5	Medroxyprogesterone Acetate 2.5 mg	Provera by Thrift Drug	55154-3911	Hormone
PROVERA25	Tab, Orange, Round, Scored, Provera over 2.5	Medroxyprogesterone Acetate 2.5 mg	Provera by Nat Pharmpak	11822-5267	Hormone
PROVERA25	Tab, Orange, Round, Scored, Provera over 2.5	Medroxyprogesterone Acetate 2.5 mg	Provera by Rite Aid	55154-3912	Hormone
PROVERA5	Tab, White, Hexagonal, Scored, Provera over 5	Medroxyprogesterone Acetate 5 mg	Provera by Nat Pharmpak	11822-5268	Hormone
PROVERA5	Tab, White, Hexagonal, Scored, Provera over 5	Medroxyprogesterone Acetate 5 mg	Provera by Rite Aid	59198-0199	Hormone
PROVERA5	Tab, White, Hexagonal, Scored, Provera over 5	Medroxyprogesterone Acetate 5 mg	Provera by Allscripts	00009-0286	Hormone
PROVERA5	Tab, White, Hexagonal, Scored, Provera over 5	Medroxyprogesterone Acetate 5 mg	Provera by Thrift Drug	63459-0101	Hormone
PROVERA5	Tab, White, Hexagonal, Scored, Provera over 5	Medroxyprogesterone Acetate 5 mg	Provera by Pharmacia	64579-0319	Hormone
PROVIGIL <> 100MG	Tab, White, Cap Shaped	Modafinil 100 mg	Provigil by Cephalon	63459-0201	Stimulant; C IV
PROVIGIL <> 100MG	Tab, White, Cap Shaped	Modafinil 100 mg	Provigil by Neuman	64579-0324	Stimulant; C IV
PROVIGIL <> 200MG	Tab, White, Cap Shaped	Modafinil 200 mg	Provigil by Cephalon	00002-4006	Stimulant; C IV
PROVIGIL <> 200MG	Tab, White, Cap Shaped	Modafinil 200 mg	Provigil by Neuman	59885-3513	Stimulant; C IV
PROZAC10	Tab, Green, Oval, Scored	Fluoxetine HCl 10 mg	Prozac by Eli Lilly	00179-1252	Antidepressant
PROZAC10	Tab, Green, Oval, Scored	Fluoxetine HCl 10 mg	Prozac by Int'l Processing	64682-0008	Antidepressant
PROZAC10DISTA3104	Cap	Fluoxetine HCl 10 mg	Prozac by Kaiser	60999-0904	Antidepressant
PS20	Tab, White, Round	Doxycycline 20 mg	Periostat by Collagenex		Antibiotic
PSA	Tab, White, Oblong, Film Coated	Acetaminophen 300 mg, Phenyltoloxamine Citrate 20 mg, Salicylamide 200 mg	Durabac by ABG		Analgesic
PSERTRALINE100MG	Cap, Orange	Sertraline HCl 100 mg	Zoloft by Pharmascience	Canadian DIN 02244840	Antidepressant
PSERTRALINE25MG	Cap, Yellow	Sertraline HCl 25 mg	Zoloft by Pharmascience	Canadian DIN 02244838	Antidepressant
PSERTRALINE50MG	Cap, Yellow and White	Sertraline HCl 50 mg	Zoloft by Pharmascience	Canadian DIN 02244839	Antidepressant

ID FRONT <> BACK	DESCRIPTION FRONT <> BACK	INGREDIENT & STRENGTH	BRAND (or Generic Equiv.) by FIRM	NDC#	CLASS; SCH.
PT <> GLYNASE15	Tab, White, Oval, Scored	Glyburide 1.5 mg	Glynase by Pharmacia	00009-0341	Antidiabetic
PT <> M	Tab, Peach, Round	Tramadol HCl 37.5 mg, Acetaminophen 325 mg	Ultracet by Mylan	00378-8088	Analgesic
PT150	Cap, Clear, P/T <> 150	Chlorpheniramine Maleate 12 mg, Phenylpropanolamine 75 mg	Omade by Kaiser	00179-1136	Cold Remedy
PT150	Cap, Ex Release, P/T-150	Chlorpheniramine Maleate 12 mg, Phenylpropanolamine 75 mg	Omade by Kaiser	62224-2444	Cold Remedy
PT150	Cap, Clear, P/T <> 150	Chlorpheniramine Maleate 12 mg, Phenylpropanolamine 75 mg	Omade by Jones	52604-0405	Cold Remedy
PT20	Tab, White, Elliptical, Scored, PT20 <> Lloyd Logo	Prednisolone 20 mg	PrednisTab by Lloyd		Steroid; Veterinary
PT5	Tab, White, Cap Shaped, Rectangular, PT5 <> Lloyd Logo	Prednisolone 5 mg	PrednisTab by Lloyd		Steroid; Veterinary
PT500	Cap, White	Tryptophan 500 mg	Tryptan by Pharmascience	Canadian DIN 02241023	Antidepressant
PTEMAZEPAM	Cap, Blue, Hard Gel	Temazepam 15 mg	Restoril by Pharmascience	Canadian DIN 5760694554	Sedative/Hypnotic; C IV
PTEMAZEPAM	Cap, Blue, Hard Gel	Temazepam 30 mg	Restoril by Pharmascience	Canadian DIN 5760694564	Sedative/Hypnotic; C IV
PTP710	Tab, PTP/710	Acetaminophen 500 mg, Hydrocodone Bitartrate 10 mg	Lortab by D M Graham	00756-0257	Analgesic; C III
PTP710	Tab, PTP over 710	Acetaminophen 500 mg, Hydrocodone Bitartrate 10 mg	Lortab by Peachtree	62793-0710 Discontinued	Analgesic; C III
PTP775	Tab, PTP over 775	Acetaminophen 650 mg, Hydrocodone Bitartrate 7.5 mg	Lorcet Plus by Peachtree	62793-0775 Discontinued	Analgesic; C III
PTPT <> GLYNASE3	Tab, Blue, Oblong, Scored, Film Coated, Glynase over 3	Glyburide 3 mg	Glynase by Allscripts		Antidiabetic
PTPT <> GLYNASE3	Tab, Blue, Oblong, Scored, Film Coated, Glynase over 3	Glyburide 3 mg	Glynase by Nat Pharmpak	55154-3909	Antidiabetic
PTPT <> GLYNASE3	Tab, Blue, Oblong, Scored, Film Coated, Glynase over 3	Glyburide 3 mg	Glynase by Amerisource	62584-0352	Antidiabetic
PTPT <> GLYNASE3	Tab, Blue, Oblong, Scored, Film Coated, Glynase over 3	Glyburide 3 mg	Glynase by Thrift Drug	59198-0171	Antidiabetic
PTPT <> GLYNASE3	Tab, Blue, Oblong, Scored, Film Coated, Glynase over 3	Glyburide 3 mg	Glynase by Pharmacia	00009-0352	Antidiabetic
PTPT <> GLYNASE3	Tab, Blue, Oblong, Scored, Film Coated, Glynase over 3	Glyburide 3 mg	Glynase by Physician Total Care	54868-3017	Antidiabetic
PTPT <> GLYNASE3	Tab, Blue, Oblong, Scored, Film Coated, Glynase over 3	Glyburide 3 mg	Glynase by Drug Distr	52985-0224	Antidiabetic
PTPT <> GLYNASE3	Tab, Coated, Glynase 3/PT	Glyburide 3 mg	Glynase by Kiel	59063-0111	Antidiabetic
PTPT <> GLYNASE6	Tab, Blue, Oblong, Scored, Film Coated, Glynase over 6	Glyburide 6 mg	Glynase by Kaiser	00179-1332	Antidiabetic
PTPT <> GLYNASE6	Tab, Yellow to Light Green, Oblong, Scored, Glynase over 6	Glyburide 6 mg	Glynase by Repack Co of America	55306-3449	Antidiabetic
PTPT <> GLYNASE6	Tab, Yellow to Light Green, Oblong, Scored, Glynase over 6	Glyburide 6 mg	Glynase by Amerisource	62584-0449	Antidiabetic
PTPT <> GLYNASE6	Tab, Yellow to Light Green, Oblong, Scored, Glynase over 6	Glyburide 6 mg	Glynase by DRX	55045-2338	Antidiabetic
PTPT <> GLYNASE6	Tab, Yellow to Light Green, Oblong, Scored, Glynase over 6	Glyburide 6 mg	Glynase by Compumed	00403-4629	Antidiabetic
PTPT <> GLYNASE6	Tab, Yellow to Light Green, Oblong, Scored, Glynase over 6	Glyburide 6 mg	Glynase by Drug Distr	52985-0225	Antidiabetic
PTPT <> GLYNASE6	Tab, Yellow to Light Green, Oblong, Scored, Glynase over 6	Glyburide 6 mg	Glynase by Leiner	59606-0723	Antidiabetic
PTPT <> GLYNASE6	Tab, Yellow to Light Green, Oblong, Scored, Glynase over 6	Glyburide 6 mg	Glynase by Kaiser	62224-7447	Antidiabetic
PTPT <> GLYNASE6	Tab, Yellow to Light Green, Oblong, Scored, Glynase over 6	Glyburide 6 mg	Glynase by Pharmacia	00009-3449	Antidiabetic
PTPT <> GLYNASE6	Tab, Yellow to Light Green, Oblong, Scored, Glynase over 6	Glyburide 6 mg	Glynase by Physician Total Care	54868-3711	Antidiabetic
PTPT <> GLYNASE6	Tab, Yellow to Light Green, Oblong, Scored, Glynase over 6	Glyburide 6 mg	Glynase by Rightpac	65240-0723	Antidiabetic
PTPT <> GLYNASE6	Tab, Yellow to Light Green, Oblong, Scored, Glynase over 6	Glyburide 6 mg	Glynase by Allscripts		Antidiabetic
PTPT <> GLYNASE6	Tab, Yellow to Light Green, Oblong, Scored, Glynase over 6	Glyburide 6 mg	Glynase by Nat Pharmpak	55154-3917	Antidiabetic
PTPT <> GLYNASE6	Tab, Yellow to Light Green, Oblong, Scored, Glynase over 6	Glyburide 6 mg	Glynase by Thrift Drug	59198-0003	Antidiabetic
PU <> 700	Tab, Off-White, Cap Shaped, Scored	Cabergoline 0.5 mg	Dostinex by Pharmacia	00013-7001	Antiparkinson
PU <> 700	Tab, Off-White, Cap Shaped, Scored	Cabergoline 0.5 mg	Dostinex by Pharmacia	10829-7001	Antiparkinson
PU <> 700	Tab, Off-White, Cap Shaped, Scored	Cabergoline 0.5 mg	Dostinex by Pharmacia	Canadian DIN 02242471	Antiparkinson
PU <> GEIGY	Tab, White w/ Red Specks, Oval, Scored, Chewable	Carbamazepine 200 mg	Tegretol by Novartis	Canadian DIN 00665088	Anticonvulsant
PU <> P	Tab, White with Red Specks, Oval, Scored, P <> P/U	Carbamazepine 200 mg	Tegretol by Pharmascience	Canadian DIN 02231540	Anticonvulsant
PURDUE	Cap, Light Aqua & Blue Green	Dihydrocodeine Bitartrate 16 mg, Acetaminophen 356.4 mg, Caffeine 30 mg	DHC Plus by Purdue	00034-8400	Analgesic; C III

ID FRONT <> BACK	DESCRIPTION FRONT <> BACK	INGREDIENT & STRENGTH	BRAND (or Generic Equiv.) by FIRM	NDC#	CLASS; SCH.
PURDUE200MG	Tab, White, Elliptical, Film Coated, Blue Ink	Cefditoren Pivoxil	Spectracef by Purdue	67781-0181	Antibiotic
PURINETHOL04A	Tab, White to Off-White, Round, Scored	Mercaptopurine 50 mg	Purinethol by Teva	00093-0522	Antineoplastic
PURINETHOL04A	Tab, Light Yellow, Round, Partially Scored, Purinethol over 04A	Mercaptopurine 50 mg	Purinethol by Gate	57844-0522	Antineoplastic
PURINETHOL04A	Tab, Light Yellow, Round, Partially Scored, Purinethol over 04A	Mercaptopurine 50 mg	Purinethol by Novopharm	Canadian DIN 00004723	Antineoplastic
PURINETHOL04A	Tab, Light Yellow, Round, Partially Scored, Purinethol over 04A	Mercaptopurine 50 mg	Purinethol by Wyeth	Canadian	Antineoplastic
PURINETHOL04A	Tab, Light Yellow, Round, Partially Scored, Purinethol over 04A	Mercaptopurine 50 mg	Purinethol by DSM	63552-0807	Antineoplastic
PURINETHOL04A	Tab, Light Yellow, Round, Partially Scored, Purinethol over 04A	Mercaptopurine 50 mg	Purinethol by GSK	00173-0807	Antineoplastic
PV10	Tab, White, Cap Shaped, PV10 <> Logo	Pravastatin Sodium 10 mg	Pravachol by Cobalt	16252-0526	Antihyperlipidemic
PV10	Tab, Pink to Peach, Rectangle-Shaped, PV10 <> Logo	Pravastatin Sodium 10 mg	Pravachol by Cobalt	Canadian DIN 02248182	Antihyperlipidemic
PV20	Tab, Yellow, Rectangle-Shaped, PV20 <> Logo	Pravastatin Sodium 20 mg	Pravachol by Cobalt	Canadian DIN 02248183	Antihyperlipidemic
PV20	Tab, White, Cap Shaped, PV20 <> Logo	Pravastatin Sodium 20 mg	Pravachol by Cobalt	16252-0527	Antihyperlipidemic
PV40	Tab, White, Cap Shaped, PV40 <> Logo	Pravastatin Sodium 40 mg	Pravachol by Cobalt	16252-0528	Antihyperlipidemic
PV40	Tab, Green, Rectangle-Shaped, PV40 <> Logo	Pravastatin Sodium 40 mg	Pravachol by Cobalt	Canadian DIN 02248184	Antihyperlipidemic
PVK250 <> GG949	Tab, Off-White, Round	Penicillin V Potassium 250 mg	Pen Vee K by Sandoz	00781-1205	Antibiotic
PVK500 <> GG950	Tab, Off-White, Oblong	Penicillin V Potassium 500 mg	Pen Vee K by Sandoz	00781-1655	Antibiotic
PX10	Tab, Yellow, Oval, Film-Coated, Scored, Cobalt Logo <> PX 10	Paroxetine HCl 10 mg	Paxil by Cobalt	Canadian DIN 02262746	Antidepressant
PX20	Tab, Pink, Oval, Film-Coated, Scored, Cobalt Logo <> PX / 20	Paroxetine HCl 20 mg	Paxil by Cobalt	Canadian DIN 02262754	Antidepressant
PX30	Tab, Blue, Oval, Film-Coated, Cobalt Logo <> PX 30	Paroxetine HCl 30 mg	Paxil by Cobalt	Canadian DIN 02262762	Antidepressant
PXL12MG	Cap, Cinnamon Colored, P-XL, Extended Release	Hydromorphone HCl 12 mg	Palladone by Purdue	59011-0312 Discontinued	Analgesic; C II
PXL16MG	Cap, Pink, P-XL, Extended Release	Hydromorphone HCl 16 mg	Palladone by Purdue	59011-0313 Discontinued	Analgesic; C II
PXL24MG	Cap, Blue, P-XL, Extended Release	Hydromorphone HCl 24 mg	Palladone by Purdue	59011-0314 Discontinued	Analgesic; C II
PXL32MG	Cap, White, P-XL, Extended Release	Hydromorphone HCl 32 mg	Palladone by Purdue	59011-0315 Discontinued	Analgesic; C II
Q	Tab, White, Oblong	Anhydrous Cholestyramine 800 mg	Questran by Apothecon		Antihyperlipidemic
Q11 <> LL	Tab, White, Round, Scored, Q over 11	Quinidine Sulfate 200 mg	Quinidine Sulfate by UDL	51079-0031	Antiarrhythmic
Q11 <> LL	Tab, White, Round, Scored, Q over 11	Quinidine Sulfate 200 mg	Quinidine Sulfate by Lederle		Antiarrhythmic
Q2542	Cap, White, Opaque, in Black	Acetaminophen 650 mg, Butalbital 50 mg	Phrenilin Forte by American Pharm	00005-3558	Analgesic
Q2542Q2542	Cap, White, Opaque, Q2542/Q2542	Acetaminophen 650 mg, Butalbital 50 mg	Phrenilin Forte by Alza		Analgesic
Q5 <> APO	Tab, Reddish-Brown, Cap Shaped, Scored, Film Coated, Q / 5	Quinapril 5 mg	Accupril by Apotex	60505-0172	Antihypertensive
QD111	Cap, Blue and White, QD over 111	Chlorpheniramine Maleate 12 mg	QDAll AR by Atley	59702-0111	Antihistamine
QD112	Cap, Blue and Yellow, Extended Release	Pseudoephedrine HCl 100 mg, Chlorpheniramine Maleate 12 mg	QDAll by Atley	59702-0112	Cold Remedy
QPL114	Tab, Brown, Round, QPL-114	Nystatin Oral 500,000 Units	Mycostatin by Quantum		Antifungal
QPL115Q	Tab, White, Round	Benztropine Mesylate 2 mg	Cogentin by Quantum		Antiparkinson

ID FRONT <> BACK	DESCRIPTION FRONT <> BACK	INGREDIENT & STRENGTH	BRAND (or Generic Equiv.) by FIRM	NDC#	CLASS; SCH.
QPL116Q	Tab, White, Round, QPL-116 Q	Benztropine Mesylate 0.5 mg	Cogentin by Quantum		Antiparkinson
QPL117Q	Tab, White, Oval, QPL-117 Q	Benztropine Mesylate 1 mg	Cogentin by Quantum		Antiparkinson
QPL154	Tab, Maroon, Round	Phenazopyridine HCl 100 mg	Pyridium by Quantum		Urinary Analgesic
QPL155	Tab, Maroon, Round	Phenazopyridine HCl 200 mg	Pyridium by Quantum		Urinary Analgesic
QPL156Q	Tab, White, Round, QPL/156 Q	Lorazepam 0.5 mg	Ativan by Quantum		Antianxiety; C IV
QPL157Q	Tab, White, Round, QPL/157 Q	Lorazepam 1 mg	Ativan by Quantum		Antianxiety; C IV
QPL158Q	Tab, White, Round, QPL/158 Q	Lorazepam 2 mg	Ativan by Quantum		Antianxiety; C IV
QPL171	Tab, Green/Yellow, Round	Aspirin 325 mg, Meprobamate 200 mg	Equagesic by Quantum		Sedative/Hypnotic; C IV
QPL179	Cap, Blue & Clear, QPL-179	Phentermine Resin Complex	Ionamin by Quantum		Anorexiant; C IV
QPL194Q	Tab, White, Round, QPL-194/Q	Haloperidol 0.5 mg	Haldol by Quantum		Antipsychotic
QPL195Q	Tab, Yellow, Round, QPL-195/Q	Haloperidol 1 mg	Haldol by Quantum		Antipsychotic
QPL196Q	Tab, Lavender, Round, QPL-196/Q	Haloperidol 2 mg	Haldol by Quantum		Antipsychotic
QPL197Q	Tab, Green, Round, QPL-197/Q	Haloperidol 5 mg	Haldol by Quantum		Antipsychotic
QPL207	Cap, Green & Yellow, QPL-207	Oxazepam 30 mg	Serax by Quantum		Sedative/Hypnotic; C IV
QPL208	Cap, Green & White, QPL-208	Oxazepam 15 mg	Serax by Quantum		Sedative/Hypnotic; C IV
QPL209	Cap, Green/Black, QPL-209	Oxazepam 10 mg	Serax by Quantum		Sedative/Hypnotic; C IV
QPL212	Tab, Green/Yellow, Round	Aspirin 325 mg, Meprobamate 200 mg	Equagesic by Quantum		Sedative/Hypnotic; C IV
QPL213Q	Tab, White, Round, QPL/213 Q	Trazodone HCl 50 mg	Desyrel by Quantum		Antidepressant
QPL214Q	Tab, White, Round, QPL/214 Q	Trazodone HCl 100 mg	Desyrel by Quantum		Antidepressant
QPL217Q	Tab, White, Round, QPL/217/Q	Metoclopramide 10 mg	Reglan by Quantum		Gastrointestinal
QPL2181Q	Tab, White, Round, QPL/2/181 Q	Diazepam 2 mg	Valium by Quantum		Antianxiety; C IV
QPL220Q	Tab, Yellow, Round, QPL-220/Q	Hydrochlorothiazide 50 mg, Triamterene 75 mg	Maxzide by Quantum		Diuretic; Antihypertensive
QPL225Q	Tab, Blue, Round, QPL-225 Q	Clorazepate Dipotassium 30.75 mg	Tranxene by Quantum		Antianxiety; C IV
QPL226Q	Tab, Peach, Round, QPL-226 Q	Clorazepate Dipotassium 7.5 mg	Tranxene by Quantum		Antianxiety; C IV
QPL227Q	Tab, Lavender, Round, QPL-227 Q	Clorazepate Dipotassium 15 mg	Tranxene by Quantum		Antianxiety; C IV
QPL236Q	Cap, Flesh & Lavender, QPL-236/Q	Fenoprofen Calcium 200 mg	Nalfon by Quantum		NSAID
QPL237Q	Cap, Flesh & Orange, QPL-237/Q	Fenoprofen Calcium 300 mg	Nalfon by Quantum		NSAID
QPL238Q	Tab, Peach, QPL-238/Q	Fenoprofen Calcium 600 mg	Nalfon by Quantum		NSAID
QPL242Q	Tab, Green/Yellow, Round, QPL242/Q	Aspirin 325 mg, Meprobamate 400 mg	Equagesic by Quantum		Sedative/Hypnotic; C IV
QPL24325	Tab, White, Round, QPL-243/2.5	Minoxidil 2.5 mg	Loniten by Quantum		Antihypertensive
QPL245Q	Tab, White, Round, QPL/245-Q	Oxybutynin Chloride 5 mg	Ditropan by Quantum		Urinary Tract
QPL270Q	Tab, Pink, Round, QPL-270/Q	Metoclopramide HCl 5 mg	Reglan by Quantum		Gastrointestinal
QPL273Q	Tab, Green, Round, QPL-273/Q	Timolol Maleate 5 mg	Blocadren by Quantum		Antihypertensive
QPL274Q	Tab, Green, Round, QPL-274/Q	Timolol Maleate 10 mg	Blocadren by Quantum		Antihypertensive
QPL275Q	Tab, Green, Round, QPL-275/Q	Timolol Maleate 20 mg	Blocadren by Quantum		Antihypertensive
QU10 <> APO	Tab, Reddish-Brown, Cap Shaped, Film Coated	Quinapril 10 mg	Accupril by Apotex	60505-0173	Antihypertensive
QU20 <> APO	Tab, Reddish-Brown, Cap Shaped, Film Coated	Quinapril 20 mg	Accupril by Apotex	60505-0174	Antihypertensive
QU40 <> APO	Tab, Reddish-Brown, Cap Shaped, Film Coated	Quinapril 40 mg	Accupril by Apotex	60505-0175	Antihypertensive
QUANTUM10183	Tab, Blue, Round, Quantum/10/183	Diazepam 10 mg	Valium by Quantum		Antianxiety; C IV
QUANTUM5182	Tab, Yellow, Round, Quantum/5/182	Diazepam 5 mg	Valium by Quantum		Antianxiety; C IV

ID FRONT <> BACK	DESCRIPTION FRONT <> BACK	INGREDIENT & STRENGTH	BRAND (or Generic Equiv.) by FIRM	NDC#	CLASS; SCH.
QUINIDEXAHR	Tab, White, Black Print, Round, Sugar Coated, Ex Release, Quinidex over AHR	Quinidine Sulfate 300 mg	Quinidex Extentabs by Wyeth	Canadian	Antiarrhythmic
QUINIDEXAHR	Tab, White, Black Print, Round, Sugar Coated, Ex Release, Quinidex over AHR	Quinidine Sulfate 300 mg	Quinidex Extentabs by Rightpac	65240-0728	Antiarrhythmic
QUINIDEXAHR	Tab, White, Black Print, Round, Sugar Coated, Ex Release, Quinidex over AHR	Quinidine Sulfate 300 mg	Quinidex Extentabs by A H Robins	00031-6649	Antiarrhythmic
QUINIDEXAHR	Tab, White, Black Print, Round, Sugar Coated, Ex Release, Quinidex over AHR	Quinidine Sulfate 300 mg	Quinidex Extentabs by Leiner	59606-0728	Antiarrhythmic
QUINIDEXAHR	Tab, White, Black Print, Round, Sugar Coated, Ex Release, Quinidex over AHR	Quinidine Sulfate 300 mg	Quinidex Extentabs by Amerisource	62584-0649	Antiarrhythmic
QUINIDEXAHR	Tab, White, Black Print, Round, Sugar Coated, Ex Release, Quinidex over AHR	Quinidine Sulfate 300 mg	Quinidex Extentabs by Thrift Drug	59198-0098	Antiarrhythmic
QUINIDEXAHR	Tab, White, Black Print, Round, Sugar Coated, Ex Release, Quinidex over AHR	Quinidine Sulfate 300 mg	Quinidex Extentabs by Nat Pharmpak	55154-3003	Antiarrhythmic
QUINIDEXAHR	Tab, White, Black Print, Round, Sugar Coated, Ex Release, Quinidex over AHR	Quinidine Sulfate 300 mg	Quinidex Extentabs by RX Pak	65084-0133	Antiarrhythmic
R	Tab, White, Round, Scored	Atropine Sulfate 0.0194 mg, Hyoscyamine Sulfate 0.1037 mg, Phenobarbital 16.2 mg, Scopolamine 0.0065 mg	Donnatal by RX Pak	65084-0123	Gastrointestinal; C IV
R	Tab, White, Round, Scored	Atropine Sulfate 0.0194 mg, Hyoscyamine Sulfate 0.1037 mg, Phenobarbital 16.2 mg, Scopolamine 0.0065 mg	Donnatal by Pharm Pkg Ctr	54383-0076	Gastrointestinal; C IV
R	Tab, White, Round, Scored	Atropine Sulfate 0.0194 mg, Hyoscyamine Sulfate 0.1037 mg, Phenobarbital 16.2 mg, Scopolamine 0.0065 mg	Donnatal by Leiner	59606-0778	Gastrointestinal; C IV
R	Tab, Yellow, Cap-Shaped, Film-Coated, Cobalt Logo <> R	Risperidone 0.25 mg	Risperdal by Cobalt	Canadian DIN 02282585	Antipsychotic
R <> 023	Tab, White, Round	Aspirin 325 mg, Butalbital 50 mg, Caffeine 40 mg	Fiorinal by Actavis	00228-2023	Analgesic; C III
R <> 025	Tab, Tan, Oblong	Risperidone 0.25 mg	Risperdal by Pharmascience	Canadian DIN 02252007	Antipsychotic
R <> 026	Tab, White, Round	Phenobarbital 15 mg	Phenobarbital by Actavis	00228-2026	Sedative/Hypnotic; C IV
R <> 026	Tab, White, Round	Phenobarbital 15 mg	Phenobarbital by UDL	51079-0094 Discontinued	Sedative/Hypnotic; C IV
R <> 026	Tab, White, Round	Phenobarbital 15 mg	Phenobarbital by Heartland	61392-0382	Sedative/Hypnotic; C IV
R <> 026	Tab, White, Round	Phenobarbital 15 mg	Phenobarbital by Vangard	00615-0420	Sedative/Hypnotic; C IV
R <> 027	Tab, White, Round, Scored	Alprazolam 0.25 mg	Xanax by Ivax	00182-0027	Antianxiety; C IV
R <> 027	Tab, White, Round, Scored	Alprazolam 0.25 mg	Xanax by Actavis	00228-2027	Antianxiety; C IV
R <> 027	Tab, White, Round, Scored	Alprazolam 0.25 mg	Xanax by Heartland	61392-0034	Antianxiety; C IV
R <> 028	Tab, White, Round, Scored	Phenobarbital 30 mg	Phenobarbital by Vangard	00615-0421	Sedative/Hypnotic; C IV
R <> 028	Tab, White, Round, Scored	Phenobarbital 30 mg	Phenobarbital by Actavis	00228-2028	Sedative/Hypnotic; C IV
R <> 029	Tab, Peach, Round, Scored	Alprazolam 0.5 mg	Xanax by Heartland	61392-0035	Antianxiety; C IV
R <> 029	Tab, Peach, Round, Scored	Alprazolam 0.5 mg	Xanax by Ivax	00182-0028	Antianxiety; C IV
R <> 029	Tab, Peach, Round, Scored	Alprazolam 0.5 mg	Xanax by Actavis	00228-2029	Antianxiety; C IV
R <> 031	Tab, Blue, Round, Scored	Alprazolam 1 mg	Xanax by Ivax	00182-0029	Antianxiety; C IV
R <> 031	Tab, Blue, Round, Scored	Alprazolam 1 mg	Xanax by Actavis	00228-2031	Antianxiety; C IV
R <> 05	Tab, Brownish Red, Oblong, Scored	Risperidone 0.5 mg	Risperdal by Pharmascience	Canadian DIN 02252015	Antipsychotic
R <> 051	Tab, White, Round, Scored	Diazepam 2 mg	Valium by Actavis	00228-2051	Antianxiety; C IV
R <> 051	Tab, White, Round, Scored	Diazepam 2 mg	Valium by Heartland	61392-0726	Antianxiety; C IV
R <> 052	Tab, Yellow, Round, Scored	Diazepam 5 mg	Valium by Urgent Care Center	50716-0132	Antianxiety; C IV
R <> 052	Tab, Yellow, Round, Scored	Diazepam 5 mg	Valium by Actavis	00228-2052	Antianxiety; C IV
R <> 052	Tab, Yellow, Round, Scored	Diazepam 5 mg	Valium by Talbert	44514-0955	Antianxiety; C IV
R <> 052	Tab, Yellow, Round, Scored	Diazepam 5 mg	Valium by Physician Total Care	54868-0059	Antianxiety; C IV
R <> 052	Tab, Yellow, Round, Scored	Diazepam 5 mg	Valium by Heartland	61392-0831	Antianxiety; C IV

ID FRONT <> BACK	DESCRIPTION FRONT <> BACK	INGREDIENT & STRENGTH	BRAND (or Generic Equiv.) by FIRM	NDC#	CLASS; SCH.
R <> 053	Tab, Blue, Round, Scored	Diazepam 10 mg	Valium by URL Mutual	00677-1050	Antianxiety; C IV
R <> 053	Tab, Blue, Round, Scored	Diazepam 10 mg	Valium by Actavis	00228-2053	Antianxiety; C IV
R <> 053	Tab, Blue, Round, Scored	Diazepam 10 mg	Valium by H J Harkins Co	52959-0306	Antianxiety; C IV
R <> 063	Tab, White, Round, Scored	Lorazepam 2 mg	Ativan by Talbert	44514-0100	Antianxiety; C IV
R <> 063	Tab, White, Round, Scored	Lorazepam 2 mg	Ativan by Nat Pharmpak	55154-0552	Antianxiety; C IV
R <> 063	Tab, White, Round, Scored	Lorazepam 2 mg	Ativan by Compumed	00403-0012	Antianxiety; C IV
R <> 063	Tab, White, Round, Scored	Lorazepam 2 mg	Ativan by Actavis	00228-2063	Antianxiety; C IV
R <> 085	Tab, Pink, Cap Shaped, Coated	Acetaminophen 650 mg, Propoxyphene Napsylate 100 mg	Darvocet-N 100 by Urgent Care Center	50716-0364	Analgesic; C IV
R <> 085	Tab, Pink, Cap Shaped, Coated	Acetaminophen 650 mg, Propoxyphene Napsylate 100 mg	Darvocet-N 100 by Golden State	60429-0518	Analgesic; C IV
R <> 085	Tab, Pink, Cap Shaped, Coated	Acetaminophen 650 mg, Propoxyphene Napsylate 100 mg	Darvocet-N 100 by Heartland	61392-0446	Analgesic; C IV
R <> 085	Tab, Pink, Cap Shaped, Coated	Acetaminophen 650 mg, Propoxyphene Napsylate 100 mg	Darvocet-N 100 by Rugby	00536-4361	Analgesic; C IV
R <> 085	Tab, Pink, Cap Shaped, Film Coated	Acetaminophen 650 mg, Propoxyphene Napsylate 100 mg	Darvocet-N 100 by Actavis	00228-2085	Analgesic; C IV
R <> 125	Tab, White, Oval, Film Coated	Ciprofloxacin 100 mg	Cipro by Dr. Reddy's	55111-0125	Antibiotic
R <> 126	Tab, White, Oval, Film Coated	Ciprofloxacin 250 mg	Cipro by Dr. Reddy's	55111-0126	Antibiotic
R <> 126	Tab, White, Oval, Film Coated	Ciprofloxacin 250 mg	Cipro by Pharmascience	Canadian DIN 02248437	Antibiotic
R <> 127	Tab, White, Oval, Film Coated	Ciprofloxacin 500 mg	Cipro by Pharmascience	Canadian DIN 02248438	Antibiotic
R <> 127	Tab, White, Oval, Film Coated	Ciprofloxacin 500 mg	Cipro by Dr. Reddy's	55111-0127	Antibiotic
R <> 127	Tab, Orange, Round, Scored	Clonidine HCl 0.1 mg	Catapres by Vangard	00615-2572	Antihypertensive
R <> 127	Tab, Orange, Round, Scored	Clonidine HCl 0.1 mg	Catapres by Ivax	00182-1250	Antihypertensive
R <> 127	Tab, Orange, Round, Scored	Clonidine HCl 0.1 mg	Catapres by Apotheca	12634-0465	Antihypertensive
R <> 127	Tab, Orange, Round, Scored	Clonidine HCl 0.1 mg	Catapres by Qualitest	00603-2954	Antihypertensive
R <> 127	Tab, Orange, Round, Scored	Clonidine HCl 0.1 mg	Catapres by Med Pro	53978-0936	Antihypertensive
R <> 127	Tab, Orange, Round, Scored	Clonidine HCl 0.1 mg	Catapres by PDRX	55289-0073	Antihypertensive
R <> 127	Tab, Orange, Round, Scored	Clonidine HCl 0.1 mg	Catapres by Heartland	61392-0513	Antihypertensive
R <> 127	Tab, Orange, Round, Scored	Clonidine HCl 0.1 mg	Catapres by Golden State	60429-0050	Antihypertensive
R <> 128	Tab, Orange, Round, Scored	Clonidine HCl 0.2 mg	Catapres by Golden State	60429-0051	Antihypertensive
R <> 128	Tab, Orange, Round, Scored	Clonidine HCl 0.2 mg	Catapres by Heartland	61392-0516	Antihypertensive
R <> 128	Tab, Orange, Round, Scored	Clonidine HCl 0.2 mg	Catapres by Actavis	00228-2128	Antihypertensive
R <> 128	Tab, Orange, Round, Scored	Clonidine HCl 0.2 mg	Catapres by Qualitest	00603-2955	Antihypertensive
R <> 128	Tab, Orange, Round, Scored	Clonidine HCl 0.2 mg	Catapres by Ivax	00182-1251	Antihypertensive
R <> 128	Tab, Orange, Round, Scored	Clonidine HCl 0.2 mg	Catapres by Major	00904-5657	Antihypertensive
R <> 128	Tab, White, Cap Shaped, Film Coated	Ciprofloxacin 750 mg	Cipro by Pharmascience	Canadian DIN 02248439	Antibiotic
R <> 128	Tab, White, Cap Shaped, Film Coated	Ciprofloxacin 750 mg	Cipro by Dr. Reddy's	55111-0128	Antibiotic
R <> 129	Tab, Orange, Round, Scored	Clonidine HCl 0.3 mg	Catapres by Major	00904-5658	Antihypertensive
R <> 129	Tab, Orange, Round, Scored	Clonidine HCl 0.3 mg	Catapres by Heartland	61392-0519	Antihypertensive
R <> 129	Tab, Orange, Round, Scored	Clonidine HCl 0.3 mg	Catapres by Ivax	00182-1252	Antihypertensive
R <> 129	Tab, Orange, Round, Scored	Clonidine HCl 0.3 mg	Catapres by Qualitest	00603-2956	Antihypertensive
R <> 129	Tab, Orange, Round, Scored	Clonidine HCl 0.3 mg	Catapres by Actavis	00228-2129	Antihypertensive
R <> 143	Tab, White, Round, Scored	Carbamazepine 200 mg	Tegretol by PDRX	55289-0210	Anticonvulsant
R <> 143	Tab, White, Round, Scored	Carbamazepine 200 mg	Tegretol by Vangard	00615-3505	Anticonvulsant
R <> 143	Tab, White, Round, Scored	Carbamazepine 200 mg	Tegretol by Actavis	00228-2143	Anticonvulsant
R <> 143	Tab, White, Round, Scored	Carbamazepine 200 mg	Tegretol by Heartland	61392-0038	Anticonvulsant
R <> 143	Tab, Peach, Oval	Fluconazole 50 mg	Diflucan by Dr. Reddy's	55111-0143	Antifungal
R <> 144	Tab, Peach, Oval	Fluconazole 100 mg	Diflucan by Dr. Reddy's	55111-0144	Antifungal
R <> 145	Tab, Peach, Oval	Fluconazole 150 mg	Diflucan by Dr. Reddy's	55111-0145	Antifungal
R <> 146	Tab, Peach, Oval	Fluconazole 200 mg	Diflucan by Dr. Reddy's	55111-0146	Antifungal
R <> 146	Tab, Peach, Oval	Fluconazole 200 mg	Diflucan by Dr. Reddy's	55111-0146	Antifungal

ID FRONT <> BACK	DESCRIPTION FRONT <> BACK	INGREDIENT & STRENGTH	BRAND (or Generic Equiv.) by FIRM	NDC#	CLASS; SCH.
R <> 153	Tab, White, Round, Film Coated	Ondansetron HCl 4 mg	Zofran by Dr. Reddy's	55111-0153	Antiemetic
R <> 154	Tab, Yellow, Round, Film Coated	Ondansetron HCl 8 mg	Zofran by Dr. Reddy's	55111-0154	Antiemetic
R <> 155	Tab, White, Round, Film Coated	Ondansetron HCl 16 mg	Zofran by Dr. Reddy's	55111-0155	Antiemetic
R <> 156	Tab, Pink, Round, Film Coated	Ondansetron HCl 24 mg	Zofran by Dr. Reddy's	55111-0156	Antiemetic
R <> 160	Tab, Yellow, Cap Shaped	Ofloxacin 200 mg	Floxin by Dr. Reddy's	55111-0160	Antibiotic
R <> 161	Tab, White, Cap Shaped	Ofloxacin 300 mg	Floxin by Dr. Reddy's	55111-0161	Antibiotic
R <> 162	Tab, Yellow, Cap Shaped	Ofloxacin 400 mg	Floxin by Dr. Reddy's	55111-0162	Antibiotic
R <> 172	Tab, Green, Oval	Finasteride 5 mg	Proscar by Dr. Reddy's	55111-0172	Antiandrogen
R <> 183	Tab, Coated	Dipyridamole 50 mg	by Vangard	00615-1573	Antiplatelet
R <> 192	Tab, Pink, Oval	Fexofenadine 30 mg	Allegra by Dr. Reddy's	55111-0192	Antihistamine
R <> 193	Tab, Pink, Oval	Fexofenadine HCl 60 mg	Allegra by Dr. Reddy's	55111-0193	Antihistamine
R <> 194	Tab, Pink, Oval	Fexofenadine HCl 180 mg	Allegra by Dr. Reddy's	55111-0194	Antihistamine
R <> 221	Tab, Peach, Round, Scored	Hydrochlorothiazide 25 mg	Hydrodiuril by H J Harkins Co	52959-0132	Diuretic; Antihypertensive
R <> 221	Tab, Peach, Round, Scored	Hydrochlorothiazide 25 mg	Hydrodiuril by Actavis	00228-2221	Diuretic; Antihypertensive
R <> 221	Tab, Peach, Round, Scored	Hydrochlorothiazide 25 mg	Hydrodiuril by Apotheca	12634-0445	Diuretic; Antihypertensive
R <> 222	Tab, Peach, Round, Scored	Hydrochlorothiazide 50 mg	Hydrodiuril by Actavis	00228-2222	Diuretic; Antihypertensive
R <> 252	Tab, Yellow, Round	Carvedilol 3.125 mg	Coreg by Dr. Reddy's	55111-0252	Antihypertensive
R <> 253	Tab, White, Round	Carvedilol 6.25 mg	Coreg by Dr. Reddy's	55111-0253	Antihypertensive
R <> 254	Tab, White, Round, Film-Coated	Carvedilol 12.5 mg	Coreg by Dr. Reddy's	55111-0254	Antihypertensive
R <> 255	Tab, White, Round	Carvedilol 25 mg	Coreg by Dr. Reddy's	55111-0255	Antihypertensive
R <> 269	Tab, White, Round, Scored	Metoclopramide HCl 10 mg	Reglan by Nat Pharmpak	55154-5510	Gastrointestinal
R <> 269	Tab, White, Round, Scored	Metoclopramide HCl 10 mg	Reglan by Actavis	00228-2269	Gastrointestinal
R <> 269	Tab, White, Round, Scored	Metoclopramide HCl 10 mg	Reglan by UDL	Discontinued	Gastrointestinal
R <> 27	Tab, Orange, Round	Propranolol HCl 10 mg	Inderal by Actavis	00228-2327	Antihypertensive
R <> 321	Tab, Pink, Round	Propranolol HCl 60 mg	Inderal by Actavis	00228-2321	Antihypertensive
R <> 333	Tab, Yellow, Round	Propranolol HCl 80 mg	Inderal by Actavis	00228-2333	Antihypertensive
R <> 337	Tab, Peach, Round	Prednisone 20 mg	by Actavis	00228-2337	Steroid
R <> 338	Tab, White, Round	Prednisone 10 mg	by Actavis	00228-2338	Steroid
R <> 34625	Tab, Film Coated, Royce Logo, <> 346 25	Hydroxyzine HCl 25 mg	by Quality Care	60346-0086	Antianxiety; Antihistamine
R <> 348	Tab, White, Round, Scored	Propylthiouracil 50 mg	Propylthiouracil by Actavis	00228-2348	Antithyroid
R <> 439	Tab, White to Off-White, Round, Clear Film Coated	Trazodone HCl 50 mg	Desyrel by Actavis	00228-2439	Antidepressant
R <> 439	Tab, White to Off-White, Round, Clear Film Coated	Trazodone HCl 50 mg	Desyrel by Heartland	61392-0487	Antidepressant
R <> 439	Tab, White to Off-White, Round, Clear Film Coated	Trazodone HCl 50 mg	Desyrel by Vangard	00615-2578	Antidepressant
R <> 439	Tab, White to Off-White, Round, Clear Film Coated	Trazodone HCl 50 mg	Desyrel by Med Pro	53978-0495	Antidepressant
R <> 441	Tab, White, Round, Coated	Trazodone HCl 100 mg	Desyrel by Nat Pharmpak	55154-1910	Antidepressant
R <> 441	Tab, White, Round, Coated	Trazodone HCl 100 mg	Desyrel by Heartland	61392-0490	Antidepressant
R <> 441	Tab, White to Off-White, Round, Clear Film Coated	Trazodone HCl 100 mg	Desyrel by Vangard	00615-2579	Antidepressant
R <> 441	Tab, White, Round, Scored, Film Coated	Trazodone HCl 100 mg	Desyrel by Actavis	00228-2441	Antidepressant
R <> 473	Tab, White, Round, Scored, Film Coated	Verapamil HCl 80 mg	Verelan by Actavis	00228-2473	Antihypertensive
R <> 473	Tab, White, Round, Scored, Film Coated	Verapamil HCl 80 mg	Verelan by Heartland	61392-0493	Antihypertensive
R <> 475	Tab, White, Round, Scored, Film Coated	Verapamil HCl 120 mg	Verelan by Heartland	61392-0496	Antihypertensive
R <> 475	Tab, White, Round, Scored, Film Coated	Verapamil HCl 120 mg	Verelan by Prepackage Specialists	58864-0530	Antihypertensive
R <> 475	Tab, White, Round, Scored, Film Coated	Verapamil HCl 120 mg	Verelan by PDRX	55289-0481	Antihypertensive
R <> 475	Tab, White, Round, Scored, Film Coated	Verapamil HCl 120 mg	Verelan by Actavis	00228-2475	Antihypertensive
R <> 480	Tab, White, Oval, Film Coated	Tolmetin Sodium 600 mg	by Actavis	00228-2480	NSAID
R <> 480	Tab, White, Oval, Film Coated	Tolmetin Sodium 600 mg	by Ivax	00182-1932	NSAID
R <> 480	Tab, White, Oval, Film Coated	Tolmetin Sodium 600 mg	by Physician Total Care	54868-2421	NSAID
R <> 480	Tab, White, Oval, Film Coated	Tolmetin Sodium 600 mg	by Qualitest	00603-6131	NSAID
R <> 538	Tab, Mottled Dark Blue, Round, Scored	Carbidopa 10 mg, Levodopa 100 mg	Sinemet by Actavis	00228-2538	Antiparkinson
R <> 538	Tab, Mottled Dark Blue, Round, Scored	Carbidopa 10 mg, Levodopa 100 mg	Sinemet by Murfreesboro	51129-1301	Antiparkinson

ID FRONT <> BACK	DESCRIPTION FRONT <> BACK	INGREDIENT & STRENGTH	BRAND (or Generic Equiv.) by FIRM	NDC#	CLASS; SCH.
R <> 538	Tab, Mottled Dark Blue, Round, Scored	Carbidopa 10 mg, Levodopa 100 mg	Sinemet by Qualitest	00603-2568	Antiparkinson
R <> 538	Tab, Mottled Dark Blue, Round, Scored	Carbidopa 10 mg, Levodopa 100 mg	Sinemet by Ivax	00182-1948	Antiparkinson
R <> 538	Tab, Mottled Dark Blue, Round, Scored	Carbidopa 10 mg, Levodopa 100 mg	Sinemet by Heartland	61392-0177	Antiparkinson
R <> 538	Tab, Mottled Dark Blue, Round, Scored	Carbidopa 25 mg, Levodopa 100 mg	Sinemet by Heartland	61392-0180	Antiparkinson
R <> 539	Tab, Mottled Yellow, Round, Scored	Carbidopa 25 mg, Levodopa 100 mg	Sinemet by Med Pro	53978-2078	Antiparkinson
R <> 539	Tab, Mottled Yellow, Round, Scored	Carbidopa 25 mg, Levodopa 100 mg	Sinemet by Qualitest	00603-2569	Antiparkinson
R <> 539	Tab, Mottled Yellow, Round, Scored	Carbidopa 25 mg, Levodopa 100 mg	Sinemet by Actavis	00228-2539	Antiparkinson
R <> 539	Tab, Mottled Yellow, Round, Scored	Carbidopa 25 mg, Levodopa 100 mg	Sinemet by Heartland	61392-0183	Antiparkinson
R <> 540	Tab, Mottled Light Blue, Round, Scored	Carbidopa 25 mg, Levodopa 250 mg	Sinemet by Qualitest	00603-2570	Antiparkinson
R <> 540	Tab, Mottled Light Blue, Round, Scored	Carbidopa 25 mg, Levodopa 250 mg	Sinemet by Murfreesboro	51129-1292	Antiparkinson
R <> 540	Tab, Mottled Light Blue, Round, Scored	Carbidopa 25 mg, Levodopa 250 mg	Sinemet by Actavis	00228-2540	Antiparkinson
R <> 545	Tab, R <> Purepac Logo 545	Diflunisal 250 mg	by Actavis	00228-2545	NSAID
R <> 550	Tab, White, Round, Enteric Coated, Delayed Release	Diclofenac Sodium 50 mg	Voltaren by PDRX	55289-0166	NSAID
R <> 550	Tab, White, Round, Enteric Coated, Delayed Release	Diclofenac Sodium 50 mg	Voltaren by CVS	00894-5841	NSAID
R <> 550	Tab, White, Round, Enteric Coated, Delayed Release	Diclofenac Sodium 50 mg	Voltaren by Actavis	00228-2550	NSAID
R <> 550	Tab, White, Round, Enteric Coated, Delayed Release	Diclofenac Sodium 50 mg	Voltaren by Ivax	00182-2618	NSAID
R <> 551	Tab, White, Round, Enteric Coated, Delayed Release	Diclofenac Sodium 75 mg	Voltaren by DRX	55045-2247	NSAID
R <> 551	Tab, White, Round, Enteric Coated, Delayed Release	Diclofenac Sodium 75 mg	Voltaren by CVS	00894-5846	NSAID
R <> 551	Tab, White, Round, Enteric Coated, Delayed Release	Diclofenac Sodium 75 mg	Voltaren by PDRX	55289-0150	NSAID
R <> 551	Tab, White, Round, Enteric Coated, Delayed Release	Diclofenac Sodium 75 mg	Voltaren by Actavis	00228-2551	NSAID
R <> 551	Tab, White, Round, Enteric Coated, Delayed Release	Diclofenac Sodium 75 mg	Voltaren by Rugby	00536-5738	NSAID
R <> 551	Tab, White, Round, Enteric Coated, Delayed Release	Diclofenac Sodium 75 mg	Voltaren by Ivax	00182-2619	NSAID
R <> 554	Tab, Film Coated	Metoprolol Tartrate 50 mg	Lopressor by Vangard	00615-3552	Antihypertensive
R <> 57	Tab, White, Round, Scored, Coated	Lorazepam 0.5 mg	Ativan by Nat Pharmpak	55154-1116	Antianxiety; C IV
R <> 57	Tab, White, Round, Scored, Coated	Lorazepam 0.5 mg	Ativan by Actavis	00228-2057	Antianxiety; C IV
R <> 57	Tab, White, Round, Scored, Coated	Lorazepam 0.5 mg	Ativan by Kaiser	00179-1174	Antianxiety; C IV
R <> 57	Tab, White, Round, Scored, Coated	Lorazepam 0.5 mg	Ativan by Mylan	55160-0130	Antianxiety; C IV
R <> 571	Tab, White, Round, Film Coated	Indapamide 2.5 mg	Lozol by Caremark	00339-6183	Diuretic
R <> 571	Tab, White, Round, Film Coated	Indapamide 2.5 mg	Lozol by Actavis	00228-2571	Diuretic
R <> 59	Tab, White, Round, Scored	Lorazepam 1 mg	Ativan by Nat Pharmpak	55154-1115	Antianxiety; C IV
R <> 59	Tab, White, Round, Scored	Lorazepam 1 mg	Ativan by Actavis	00228-2059	Antianxiety; C IV
R <> 59	Tab, White, Round, Scored	Lorazepam 1 mg	Ativan by Mylan	55160-0131	Antianxiety; C IV
R <> 59	Tab, White, Round, Scored	Lorazepam 1 mg	Ativan by Golden State	60429-0512	Antianxiety; C IV
R <> 597	Tab, Orange, Round, Film Coated	Indapamide 1.25 mg	Lozol by Caremark	00339-6182	Diuretic
R <> 597	Tab, Orange, Round, Film Coated	Indapamide 1.25 mg	Lozol by Actavis	00228-2597	Diuretic
R <> 606	Tab, White, Round	Acyclovir 400 mg	Zovirax by Golden State	60429-0712	Antiviral
R <> 606	Tab, White, Round	Acyclovir 400 mg	Zovirax by Actavis	00228-2606	Antiviral
R <> 611	Tab, Yellow, Oblong, Coated, Extended Release	Pentoxifylline 400 mg	Trental by Pharmafab	62542-0753	Anticoagulant
R <> 611	Tab, Yellow, Oblong, Coated, Extended Release	Pentoxifylline 400 mg	Trental by Murfreesboro	51129-1100	Anticoagulant
R <> 611	Tab, Yellow, Oblong, Coated, Extended Release	Pentoxifylline 400 mg	Trental by Caremark	00339-5278	Anticoagulant
R <> 611	Tab, Yellow, Oblong, Coated, Extended Release	Pentoxifylline 400 mg	Trental by Actavis	00228-2611	Anticoagulant
R <> 611	Tab, Yellow, Oblong, Coated, Extended Release	Pentoxifylline 400 mg	Trental by Heartland	61392-0833	Anticoagulant
R <> 611	Tab, Yellow, Oblong, Coated, Extended Release	Pentoxifylline 400 mg	Trental by Murfreesboro	51129-1121	Anticoagulant
R <> 611	Tab, Yellow, Oblong, Coated, Extended Release	Pentoxifylline 400 mg	Trental by Pharmacy Care	65070-0030	Anticoagulant
R <> 613	Tab, White, Oval, Film Coated	Ticlopidine HCl 250 mg	Ticlid by Actavis	00228-2613	Anticoagulant
R <> 617	Tab, Yellow, Cap Shaped, Enteric Coated, Delayed Release	Naproxen 375 mg	Naprosyn by Actavis	00228-2617	NSAID
R <> 618	Tab, Yellow, Cap Shaped, Enteric Coated, Delayed Release	Naproxen 500 mg	Naprosyn by Actavis	00228-2618	NSAID
R <> 618	Tab, Yellow, Cap Shaped, Enteric Coated, Delayed Release	Naproxen 500 mg	Naprosyn by Orion	52483-0014	NSAID
R <> 633	Tab, White, Round	Lovastatin 10 mg	Mevacor by Actavis	00228-2633	Antihyperlipidemic
R <> 633	Tab, White, Round	Lovastatin 10 mg	Mevacor by Major	00904-5581	Antihyperlipidemic

ID FRONT <> BACK	DESCRIPTION FRONT <> BACK	INGREDIENT & STRENGTH	BRAND (or Generic Equiv.) by FIRM	NDC#	CLASS; SCH.
R <> 634	Tab, Pink, Round	Lovastatin 20 mg	Mevacor by Major	00904-5582	Antihyperlipidemic
R <> 634	Tab, Pink, Round	Lovastatin 20 mg	Mevacor by Actavis	00228-2634	Antihyperlipidemic
R <> 635	Tab, Yellow, Round	Lovastatin 40 mg	Mevacor by Actavis	00228-2635	Antihyperlipidemic
R <> 635	Tab, Yellow, Round	Lovastatin 40 mg	Mevacor by Major	00904-5583	Antihyperlipidemic
R <> 641	Tab, Beige, Round, Film Coated	Famotidine 40 mg	by Actavis	00228-2641	Gastrointestinal
R <> 650	Tab, Yellow, Cap Shaped, Film Coated	Bisoprolol 2.5 mg, Hydrochlorothiazide 6.25 mg	Ziac by Actavis	00228-2650	Antihypertensive; Diuretic
R <> 651	Tab, Pink, Cap Shaped, Film Coated	Bisoprolol 5 mg, Hydrochlorothiazide 6.25 mg	Ziac by Actavis	00228-2651	Antihypertensive; Diuretic
R <> 652	Tab, White, Cap Shaped, Film Coated	Bisoprolol 10 mg, Hydrochlorothiazide 6.25 mg	Ziac by Actavis	00228-2652	Antihypertensive; Diuretic
R <> 679	Tab, Yellow, Round, Film Coated	Famotidine 20 mg	by Actavis	00228-2679	Gastrointestinal
R <> 7	Tab, Orange, Octagonal, Film Coated	Indapamide 1.25 mg	Lozol by RPR	00075-0700	Diuretic
R <> 7	Tab, Orange, Octagonal, Film Coated	Indapamide 1.25 mg	Lozol by Thrift Drug	59198-0263	Diuretic
R <> 7	Tab, Orange, Octagonal, Film Coated	Indapamide 1.25 mg	Lozol by Amerisource	62584-0700	Diuretic
R <> 7	Tab, Orange, Octagonal, Film Coated	Indapamide 1.25 mg	Lozol by RPR	00801-0700	Diuretic
R <> 704	Tab, Green, Cap Shaped, Film Coated	Fluvoxamine Maleate 25 mg	Luvox by Actavis	00228-2704	OCD
R <> 717	Tab, Yellow, Round, Film Coated, Ex Release	Diclofenac Sodium 100 mg	Voltaren XR by Actavis	00228-2717	NSAID
R <> 743	Tab, White, Round, Enteric Coated	Diclofenac Sodium 50 mg	Voltaren by Actavis	00228-2743	NSAID
R <> 744	Tab, White, Round, Enteric Coated	Diclofenac Sodium 75 mg	Voltaren by Actavis	00228-2744	NSAID
R <> 745	Tab, Yellow, Cap Shaped, Film Coated, Delayed Release	Naproxen 375 mg	Naprosyn by Actavis	00228-2745	NSAID
R <> 746	Tab, Green, Cap Shaped, Film Coated, Delayed Release	Naproxen 500 mg	Naprosyn by Actavis	00228-2746	NSAID
R <> 755	Tab, Beige, Cap Shaped, Film Coated	Citalopram 10 mg	Celexa by Actavis	00228-2755	Antidepressant
R <> 8	Tab, White, Octagonal, Film Coated	Indapamide 2.5 mg	Lozol by Pharm Util	60491-0382	Diuretic
R <> 8	Tab, White, Octagonal, Film Coated	Indapamide 2.5 mg	Lozol by Thrift Drug	59198-0174	Diuretic
R <> 8	Tab, White, Octagonal, Film Coated	Indapamide 2.5 mg	Lozol by RPR	00075-0082	Diuretic
R <> 8	Tab, White, Octagonal, Film Coated	Indapamide 2.5 mg	Lozol by Allscripts		Diuretic
R <> 8	Tab, White, Octagonal, Film Coated	Indapamide 2.5 mg	Lozol by Nat Pharmpak	55154-4011	Diuretic
R <> 8	Tab, White, Octagonal, Film Coated	Indapamide 2.5 mg	Lozol by Drug Distr	52985-0062	Diuretic
R <> 803	Tab, White to Off-White, Round, Film Coated	Spironolactone 25 mg	Aldactone by Purepac	00228-2803	Diuretic
R <> 83	Tab, White to Off-White, Round, Extended Release	Alprazolam 0.5 mg	Xanax XR by Actavis	00228-3083	Antianxiety; C IV
R <> 84	Tab, Yellow, Round, Extended Release	Alprazolam 1 mg	Xanax XR by Actavis	00228-3084	Antianxiety; C IV
R <> 86	Tab, Light Green, Round, Extended Release	Alprazolam 3 mg	Xanax XR by Actavis	00228-3086	Antianxiety; C IV
R <> 87	Tab, Peach, Round, Extended Release	Alprazolam 2 mg	Xanax XR by Actavis	00228-3087	Antianxiety; C IV
R <> M	Tab, White, Round, Film Coated	Risperidone 0.25 mg	Risperdal by UDL	51079-0460	Antipsychotic
R <> M	Tab	Risperidone .25 mg	Risperdal by Mylan	00378-3502	Antipsychotic
R001 <> 3	Tab, White, Round	Acetaminophen 300 mg, Codeine Phosphate 30 mg	Tylenol w/ Codeine by Pharmedix	53002-0101	Analgesic; C III
R001 <> 3	Tab, White, Round	Acetaminophen 300 mg, Codeine Phosphate 30 mg	Tylenol w/ Codeine by Allscripts		Analgesic; C III
R001 <> 3	Tab, White, Round	Acetaminophen 300 mg, Codeine Phosphate 30 mg	Tylenol w/ Codeine by Actavis	00228-2001	Analgesic; C III
R001 <> 3	Tab, White, Round	Acetaminophen 300 mg, Codeine Phosphate 30 mg	Tylenol w/ Codeine by Vangard	00615-0430	Analgesic; C III
R003 <> 4	Tab, White, Round	Acetaminophen 300 mg, Codeine Phosphate 60 mg	Tylenol w/ Codeine by Allscripts		Analgesic; C III
R003 <> 4	Tab, White, Round	Acetaminophen 300 mg, Codeine Phosphate 60 mg	Tylenol w/ Codeine by Actavis	00228-2003	Analgesic; C III
R003 <> 4	Tab	Acetaminophen 300 mg, Codeine Phosphate 60 mg	Tylenol w/ Codeine by Ivax	00182-1338	Analgesic; C III
R012	Cap, Green	Chloral Hydrate 500 mg	Chloral Hydrate by Rondex		Sedative/Hypnotic; C IV
R012	Tab, White, Round	Meprobamate 200 mg	Miltown by Rondex		Sedative/Hypnotic; C IV
R016	Tab, White, Round	Meprobamate 200 mg	Miltown by Actavis		Sedative/Hypnotic; C IV
R018	Tab, White, Round	Meprobamate 400 mg	Miltown by Actavis		Sedative/Hypnotic; C IV
R021	Cap, Blue & White	Flurazepam HCl 15 mg	by Actavis	00228-2021	Hypnotic; C IV
R022	Cap, Blue	Flurazepam HCl 30 mg	by Actavis	00228-2022	Hypnotic; C IV
R028	Tab, R 028	Phenobarbital 30 mg	by Heartland	61392-0391	Sedative/Hypnotic; C IV
R039	Tab, Yellow, Rectangular, Scored	Alprazolam 2 mg	Xanax by Actavis	00228-2039	Antianxiety; C IV

ID FRONT <> BACK	DESCRIPTION FRONT <> BACK	INGREDIENT & STRENGTH	BRAND (or Generic Equiv.) by FIRM	NDC#	CLASS; SCH.
R039	Tab, Yellow, Rectangular, Scored	Alprazolam 2 mg	Xanax by Ivax	00182-0030	Antianxiety; C IV
R05	Tab, Light Coral, Round, R0.5	Risperidone 0.5 mg	Risperdal M-Tab by Janssen-Ortho	Canadian DIN 02247704	Antipsychotic
R05	Tab, Light Coral, Round, R0.5	Risperidone 0.5 mg	Risperdal M-Tab by Janssen	50458-0395	Antipsychotic
R067	Cap, Pink, Opaque	Oxazepam 10 mg	Serax by Actavis	00228-2067	Sedative/Hypnotic; C IV
R067	Cap, Pink, Opaque	Oxazepam 10 mg	Serax by Direct Dispensing	57866-6970	Sedative/Hypnotic; C IV
R067	Cap, Fink, Opaque	Oxazepam 10 mg	Serax by PF	48692-0031	Sedative/Hypnotic; C IV
R069	Cap, Red, Opaque	Oxazepam 15 mg	Serax by Actavis	00228-2069	Sedative/Hypnotic; C IV
R073R073	Cap, Maroon, Opaque	Oxazepam 30 mg	Serax by Actavis	00228-2073	Sedative/Hypnotic; C IV
R076	Cap, Green & White, Opaque	Temazepam 15 mg	Restoril by Ivax	00182-1822	Sedative/Hypnotic; C IV
R076	Cap, Green & White, Opaque	Temazepam 15 mg	Restoril by Actavis	00228-2076	Sedative/Hypnotic; C IV
R077	Cap, White, Opaque	Temazepam 30 mg	Restoril by Actavis	00228-2077	Sedative/Hypnotic; C IV
R077	Cap, White, Opaque	Temazepam 30 mg	Restoril by Ivax	00182-1823	Sedative/Hypnotic; C IV
R077	Cap, White, Opaque	Temazepam 30 mg	Restoril by Direct Dispensing	57866-4629	Sedative/Hypnotic; C IV
R078	Tab, Blue, Round	Clorazepate Dipotassium 30.75 mg	Tranxene by Actavis		Antianxiety; C IV
R081	Tab, Peach, Round	Clorazepate Dipotassium 7.5 mg	Tranxene by Actavis		Antianxiety; C IV
R082	Cap, Pink	Propoxyphene 65 mg	Darvon 65 by Actavis		Analgesic; C IV
R083	Tab, Pink, Round	Clorazepate Dipotassium 15 mg	Tranxene by Actavis		Antianxiety; C IV
R1	Tab, R/1	Chlorpheniramine Tannate 8 mg, Phenylephrine Tannate 25 mg	Ricobid by Teral	51234-0154	Cold Remedy
R1	Tab, Light Coral, Square	Risperidone 1 mg	Risperdal M-Tab by Janssen	50458-0315	Antipsychotic
R1	Tab, Light Coral, Square	Risperidone 1 mg	Risperdal M-Tab by Janssen-Ortho	Canadian DIN 02247705	Antipsychotic
R1	Tab, White to Off-White, Cap-Shaped, Film-Coated, Cobalt Logo <> R1	Risperidone 1 mg	Risperdal by Cobalt	Canadian DIN 02282607	Antipsychotic
R1	Tab, White, Oblong	Risperidone 1 mg	Risperdal by Pharmascience	Canadian DIN 02255023	Antipsychotic
R1 <> JANSSEN	Tab, White	Risperidone 1 mg	Risperdal by Va Cmop	65243-0061	Antipsychotic
R1 <> JANSSEN	Tab, White, Cap Shaped, Scored	Risperidone 1 mg	Risperdal by Janssen	50458-0300	Antipsychotic
R1 <> JANSSEN	Tab, Coated	Risperidone 1 mg	Risperdal by Johnson & Johnson	59604-0300	Antipsychotic
R10	Tab, Black, Round	Charcoal Activated 250 mg	Activated Charcoal Tabs by Requa	10961-0010	Gastrointestinal
R10	Cap, Green and Gray	Fluoxetine 10 mg	Prozac by Cobalt	Canadian DIN 02242177	Antidepressant
R102	Tab, White, Round	Allopurinol 100 mg	Zyloprim by Actavis		Antigout
R103	Tab, Peach, Round	Allopurinol 300 mg	Zyloprim by Actavis		Antigout
R11	Tab, Blue, Round	Verapamil 40 mg	Isoptin by Rugby		Antihypertensive
R11 <> 50	Tab, Pale Yellow, Cap Shaped, Scored, Film Coated	Naltrexone HCl 50 mg	ReVia by Duramed	51285-0011	Opioid Antagonist
R11 <> 50	Tab, Pale Yellow, Cap Shaped, Scored, Film Coated	Naltrexone HCl 50 mg	ReVia by BMS	00056-0011	Opioid Antagonist
R11 <> M	Tab, White, Round, Film-Coated	Risperidone 1 mg	Risperdal by UDL	51079-0462	Antipsychotic
R11 <> M	Tab, White, Round	Risperidone 1 mg	Risperdal by Mylan	00378-3511	Antipsychotic
R1103	Tab, White, Round	Acetaminophen 325 mg	Tylenol by Actavis		Analgesic
R110BI	Cap, Light Blue Opaque Cap, Cream Opaque Body, Filled with Yellow Pellets	Dabigatran Etexilate 110 mg	Pradax by Boehringer Ingelheim	Canadian DIN 02312441	Anticoagulant
R110BISymbol	Cap, Light Blue Opaque Cap, Cream Opaque Body, Filled with Yellow Pellets	Dabigatran Etexilate 110 mg	Pradax by Boehringer Ingelheim Canada	Canadian DIN 02312441	Anticoagulant
R111	Tab, White, Oval	Ibuprofen 800 mg	Motrin by Actavis		NSAID
R113	Tab, White, Round, Coated	Domperidone 10 mg	Motilium by Ranbaxy	Canadian DIN 02268078	Gastrointestinal
R12 <> M	Tab, Beige, Round, Film-Coated	Risperidone 2 mg	Risperdal by UDL	51079-0463	Antipsychotic

ID FRONT <> BACK	DESCRIPTION FRONT <> BACK	INGREDIENT & STRENGTH	BRAND (or Generic Equiv.) by FIRM	NDC#	CLASS; SCH.
R12 <> M	Tab, Pink, Round	Risperidone 2 mg	Risperdal by Mylan	00378-3512	Antipsychotic
R12 <> RBX	Tab, White, Round, Scored, Film Coated	Metformin HCl 500 mg	Glucophage by Ranbaxy	Canadian DIN 02269031	Antidiabetic
R124	Tab, White, Round	Ibuprofen 400 mg	Motrin by Actavis		NSAID
R125	Tab, White, Oval	Ibuprofen 600 mg	Motrin by Actavis		NSAID
R127	Tab, Orange, Round, Scored	Clonidine HCl 0.1 mg	Catapres by Actavis	00228-2127	Antihypertensive
R127	Tab, Orange, Round, Scored	Clonidine HCl 0.1 mg	Catapres by Major	00904-5656	Antihypertensive
R128	Tab, White, Round	Folacin 5 mg, Cobalamin 1 mg, Pyridoxine 50 mg, Thiamine 1.5 mg, Riboflavin 1.5 mg, Niacinamide 20 mg, Pantothenic Acid 10 mg, D-Biotin 300 mcg, Vitamin C 60 mg	DexFol by Rising	64980-0128	Vitamin; Supplement
R13 <> M	Tab, White, Round, Film-Coated	Risperidone 3 mg	Risperdal by UDL	51079-0464	Antipsychotic
R13 <> M	Tab, White, Round	Risperidone 3 mg	Risperdal by Mylan	00378-3513	Antipsychotic
R133	Tab, Coated	Amitriptyline HCl 50 mg	Elavil by Actavis	00228-2133	Antidepressant
R134	Tab, Coated	Amitriptyline HCl 75 mg	Elavil by Actavis	00228-2134	Antidepressant
R135	Tab, Coated	Amitriptyline HCl 100 mg	Elavil by Actavis	00228-2135	Antidepressant
R14 <> M	Tab, Pink, Round	Risperidone 4 mg	Risperdal by Mylan	00378-3514	Antipsychotic
R14 <> M	Tab, Beige, Round, Film-Coated	Risperidone 4 mg	Risperdal by UDL	51079-0465	Antipsychotic
R147	Tab, Blue, Oblong	Prenatal Vitamins	Pramet FA by Ross		Vitamin
R148	Cap, Light Blue and Light Turquoise-Blue	Fluoxetine 20 mg	Prozac by Par	49884-0751	Antidepressant
R1507	Tab, White, Round	Quinine Sulfate 200 mg	by Actavis		Antimalarial
R1511	Tab, White, Round	Quinine Sulfate 325 mg	by Actavis		Antimalarial
R157	Cap, Lavender and Yellow	Omeprazole 10 mg	Prilosec by Dr. Reddy's	55111-0157	Gastrointestinal
R158	Cap, Lavender and Iron Grey	Omeprazole 20 mg	Prilosec by Dr. Reddy's	55111-0158	Gastrointestinal
R159	Cap, Lavender and Yellow	Omeprazole 40 mg	Prilosec by Dr. Reddy's	55111-0159	Gastrointestinal
R161	Tab, Yellow, Round	Chlorthalidone 25 mg	Hygroton by Actavis		Diuretic
R163	Tab, Green, Round	Chlorthalidone 50 mg	Hygroton by Actavis	00228-2161	Diuretic
R176	Tab, Pink, Round	Digitoxin 0.1 mg	Crystodigin by Actavis		Cardiac Agent
R178	Tab, White, Round	Digitoxin 0.2 mg	Crystodigin by Actavis		Cardiac Agent
R179	Tab, White, Oval, Scored	Tizanidine HCl 2 mg	Zanaflex by Dr. Reddy's	55111-0179	Muscle Relaxant
R179	Tab, White, Oval, Scored	Tizanidine HCl 2 mg	Zanaflex by Par	49884-0782	Muscle Relaxant
R180	Tab, White, Oval, Scored	Tizanidine HCl 4 mg	Zanaflex by Par	49884-0783	Muscle Relaxant
R180	Tab, White, Oval, Scored	Tizanidine HCl 4 mg	Zanaflex by Dr. Reddy's	55111-0180	Muscle Relaxant
R185	Tab, White, Round	Dipyridamole 75 mg	Persantine by Actavis		Antiplatelet
R191	Cap, Clear & Pink	Diphenhydramine HCl 25 mg	Benadryl by Actavis	00228-2185	Antihistamine
R191	Cap, Clear & Pink, R/191	Diphenhydramine HCl 25 mg	by Pharmascience	Canadian	Antihistamine
R192	Cap, Pink	Diphenhydramine HCl 50 mg	Benadryl by Actavis		Antihistamine
R192	Cap, Pink, R/192	Diphenhydramine HCl 50 mg	by Pharmascience	Canadian	Antihistamine
R193	Tab, White, Round	Dipyridamole 25 mg	Persantine by Actavis	00228-2193	Antiplatelet
R194	Cap, Aqua & White	Doxycycline Hyclate 50 mg	Vibramycin by Actavis		Antibiotic
R195	Cap, Blue	Doxycycline Hyclate 100 mg	Vibramycin by Actavis	00228-2195	Antibiotic
R2	Tab, Ex Release, R/2	Guaifenesin 600 mg, Phenylephrine HCl 15 mg	Numonyl Sr by Sovereign	58716-0629	Cold Remedy
R2	Tab, Yellow, Round	Isosorbide Dinitrate SL 2.5 mg	Isordil by Rugby		Antianginal
R2	Tab, Light Coral, Round	Risperidone 2 mg	Risperdal M-Tab by Janssen-Ortho	Canadian DIN 02247706	Antipsychotic
R2	Tab, Tan, Cap-Shaped, Film-Coated, Scored, Cobalt Logo <> R / 2	Risperidone 2 mg	Risperdal by Cobalt	Canadian DIN 02282615	Antipsychotic

ID FRONT <> BACK	DESCRIPTION FRONT <> BACK	INGREDIENT & STRENGTH	BRAND (or Generic Equiv.) by FIRM	NDC#	CLASS; SCH.
R2	Tab, Peach, Oblong, Scored	Risperidone 2 mg	Risperdal by Pharmascience	Canadian DIN 02252031	Antipsychotic
R2 <> JANSSEN	Tab, Orange, Cap Shaped	Risperidone 2 mg	Risperdal by Janssen	50458-0320	Antipsychotic
R2 <> JANSSEN	Tab, Coated	Risperidone 2 mg	Risperdal by Johnson & Johnson	59604-0320	Antipsychotic
R20	Cap, Green and Gray	Fluoxetine 20 mg	Prozac by Cobalt	Canadian DIN 02242178	Antidepressant
R20 <> 3	Tab, White, Round	Acetaminophen 300 mg, Codeine Phosphate 30 mg	Tylenol w/ Codeine by Heartland	61392-0714	Analgesic; C III
R20 <> 3	Tab, White, Round	Acetaminophen 300 mg, Codeine Phosphate 30 mg	Tylenol w/ Codeine by Actavis	00228-3020	Analgesic; C III
R204	Tab, Pink, Round	Erythromycin Stearate 250 mg	Erythrocin by Actavis		Antibiotic
R21 <> 4	Tab, White, Round	Acetaminophen 300 mg, Codeine Phosphate 60 mg	Tylenol w/ Codeine by Actavis	00228-3021	Analgesic; C III
R210	Tab, Yellow, Round	Folic Acid 1 mg	Folvite by Actavis		Vitamin
R212	Tab, White, Round	Hydrocortisone 10 mg	Hydrocortone by Actavis		Steroid
R212	Tab, White, Round, R/212	Hydrocortisone 10 mg	Hydrocortone by Rondex		Steroid
R214	Tab, White, Round	Hydrocortisone 20 mg	Hydrocortone by Actavis		Steroid
R214	Tab, White, Round, R 21/4	Acetaminophen 300 mg, Codeine Phosphate 60 mg	Tylenol w/ Codeine by Actavis		Analgesic; C III
R219	Tab, Green, Round	Hydralazine HCl 25 mg	Apresoline by Actavis		Antihypertensive
R22 <> RBX	Tab, White, Oblong, Film Coated	Metformin HCl 850 mg	Glucophage by Ranbaxy	Canadian DIN 02269058	Antidiabetic
R220	Tab, Green, Round	Hydralazine HCl 50 mg	Apresoline by Actavis		Antihypertensive
R227	Tab, Salmon, Round	Hydralazine 25 mg, Hydrochlorothiazide 15 mg, Reserpine 0.1 mg	Ser-Ap-Es by Rondex		Antihypertensive; Diuretic
R247	Tab, White, Round	Methocarbamol 500 mg	Robaxin by Actavis		Muscle Relaxant
R249	Tab, White, Oblong	Methocarbamol 750 mg	Robaxin by Actavis		Muscle Relaxant
R250	Tab, White, Round	Terbinafine 250 mg	Lamisil by Dr. Reddy's	55111-0250	Antifungal
R253	Tab, Beige, Round	Methyldopa 250 mg	Aldomet by Rondex		Antihypertensive
R253	Tab, White, Round	Methyldopa 250 mg	Aldomet by Actavis		Antihypertensive
R255	Tab, White, Round	Methyldopa 500 mg	Aldomet by Actavis		Antihypertensive
R255	Tab, Beige, Oblong	Methyldopa 500 mg	Aldomet by Rondex		Antihypertensive
R2577	Cap, Aqua Blue & Dark Green, Opaque, Ex Release	Diltiazem HCl 180 mg	Cardizem CD by Heartland	61392-0962	Antihypertensive
R2577	Cap, Aqua Blue & Dark Green, Opaque, Ex Release	Diltiazem HCl 180 mg	Cardizem CD by Actavis	00228-2577	Antihypertensive
R2577	Cap, Aqua Blue & Dark Green, Opaque, Ex Release	Diltiazem HCl 180 mg	Cardizem CD by Amerisource	62584-0975	Antihypertensive
R2578	Cap, Dark Green, Opaque, Ex Release	Diltiazem HCl 240 mg	Cardizem CD by Heartland	61392-0963	Antihypertensive
R2578	Cap, Dark Green, Opaque, Ex Release	Diltiazem HCl 240 mg	Cardizem CD by Actavis	00228-2578	Antihypertensive
R2579	Cap, Dark Green & Light Gray, Opaque, Ex Release	Diltiazem HCl 300 mg	Cardizem CD by Actavis	00228-2579	Antihypertensive
R2579	Cap, Dark Green & Light Gray, Opaque, Ex Release	Diltiazem HCl 300 mg	Cardizem CD by Heartland	61392-0964	Antihypertensive
R2588	Cap, Light Gray, Opaque, Ex Release	Diltiazem HCl 120 mg	Cardizem CD by Actavis	00228-2588	Antihypertensive
R2588	Cap, Light Gray, Opaque, Ex Release	Diltiazem HCl 120 mg	Cardizem CD by Heartland	61392-0961	Antihypertensive
R2598	Cap, White	Doxycycline Hyclate 100 mg	by Faulding	50546-0470	Antibiotic
R2598	Cap, Clear & Yellow	Doxycycline Hyclate 100 mg	Doryx by Faulding		Antibiotic
R261	Tab, Tan, Round	Hydrochlorothiazide 15 mg, Methyldopa 250 mg	Aldoril 15 by Actavis		Diuretic; Antihypertensive
R263	Tab, White, Round	Hydrochlorothiazide 25 mg, Methyldopa 250 mg	Aldoril 25 by Actavis		Diuretic; Antihypertensive
R265	Tab, Tan, Oval	Hydrochlorothiazide 30 mg, Methyldopa 500 mg	Aldoril by Actavis		Diuretic; Antihypertensive
R2666	Cap, Light Brown and Yellow, Black ink	Gabapentin 300 mg	Neurontin by Actavis	00228-2666	Anticonvulsant
R267	Tab, White, Oval	Hydrochlorothiazide 50 mg, Methyldopa 500 mg	Aldoril by Actavis		Diuretic; Antihypertensive
R269	Tab, White, Round	Metoclopramide HCl 10 mg	Reglan by Heartland	61392-0558	Gastrointestinal
R27	Tab	Propranolol HCl 10 mg	Inderal by Heartland	61392-0420	Antihypertensive

ID FRONT <> BACK	DESCRIPTION FRONT <> BACK	INGREDIENT & STRENGTH	BRAND (or Generic Equiv.) by FIRM	NDC#	CLASS; SCH.
R27	Tab	Propranolol HCl 10 mg	Inderal by Med Pro	53978-0034	Antihypertensive
R276	Tab, White, Round	Reserpine 0.25 mg	Serpasil by Rondex		Antihypertensive
R2778	Cap, White and Yellow, Opaque, Extended Release	Propranolol 60 mg	Inderal LA by Actavis	00228-2778	Antihypertensive
R2779	Cap, Yellow, Opaque, Extended Release	Propranolol 80 mg	Inderal LA by Actavis	00228-2779	Antihypertensive
R278	Cap, Yellow	Oxytetracycline 250 mg	Terramycin by Rondex		Antibiotic
R2780	Cap, Grey and Yellow, Opaque, Extended Release	Propranolol 120 mg	Inderal LA by Actavis	00228-2780	Antihypertensive
R2781	Cap, Grey, Opaque, Extended Release	Propranolol 160 mg	Inderal LA by Actavis	00228-2781	Antihypertensive
R280	Tab, Yellow, Round	Haloperidol 1 mg	Haldol by Actavis		Antipsychotic
R281	Tab, Pink, Round	Haloperidol 2 mg	Haldol by Actavis		Antipsychotic
R282	Tab, Green, Round	Haloperidol 5 mg	Haldol by Actavis		Antipsychotic
R286	Tab, Aqua, Round	Haloperidol 10 mg	Haldol by Actavis		Antipsychotic
R287	Tab, Salmon, Round	Haloperidol 20 mg	Haldol by Actavis		Antipsychotic
R289	Tab, White, Round	Haloperidol 0.5 mg	Haldol by Actavis		Antipsychotic
R29	Tab	Propranolol HCl 20 mg	Inderal by Actavis	00228-2329	Antihypertensive
R29	Tab	Propranolol HCl 20 mg	Inderal by Med Pro	53978-5014	Antihypertensive
R29	Tab	Propranolol HCl 20 mg	Inderal by Heartland	61392-0423	Antihypertensive
R292	Cap, Brown & Clear	Papaverine HCl SR 150 mg	Pavabid by Actavis		Vasodilator
R296	Tab, White, Round	Penicillin G Potassium 200,000 Units	Pentids by Rondex		Antibiotic
R3	Tab, Light Coral, Round	Risperidone 3 mg	Risperdal M-Tab by Janssen-Ortho	Canadian DIN 02268086	Antipsychotic
R3	Tab, Yellow, Cap-Shaped, Film-Coated, Scored, Cobalt Logo <> R / 3	Risperidone 3 mg	Risperdal by Cobalt	Canadian DIN 02282623	Antipsychotic
R3	Tab, Yellow, Oblong, Scored	Risperidone 3 mg	Risperdal by Pharmascience	Canadian DIN 02252058	Antipsychotic
R3 <> JANSSEN	Tab, Yellow, Cap Shaped	Risperidone 3 mg	Risperdal by Janssen	50458-0330	Antipsychotic
R3 <> JANSSEN	Tab, Coated	Risperidone 3 mg	Risperdal by Johnson & Johnson	59604-0330	Antipsychotic
R31	Tab, Coated	Amitriptyline HCl 10 mg	Elavil by Actavis	00228-2131	Antidepressant
R31	Tab, Coated	Amitriptyline HCl 10 mg	Elavil by Heartland	61392-0143	Antidepressant
R316	Tab, White, Cap Shaped, Scored	Phentermine 37.5 mg	Fastin by Actavis	00228-3016	Anorexiant; C IV
R317	Tab, Yellow, Cap Shaped, Scored	Fenoprofen Calcium 600 mg	by Actavis	00228-2317	NSAID
R317	Tab, Yellow, Cap Shaped, Scored	Fenoprofen Calcium 600 mg	by Pharmedix	53002-0367	NSAID
R32	Tab, Film Coated	Amitriptyline HCl 25 mg	Elavil by Heartland	61392-0140	Antidepressant
R32	Tab, Film Coated	Amitriptyline HCl 25 mg	Elavil by Actavis	00228-2132	Antidepressant
R33	Tab, Pink, Round, Scored	Clonazepam 0.5 mg	Klonopin by Actavis	00228-3003	Sedative; C IV
R33	Tab, Pink, Round, Scored	Clonazepam 0.5 mg	Klonopin by Murfreesboro	51129-1140	Sedative; C IV
R33	Tab, Pink, Round, Scored	Clonazepam 0.5 mg	Klonopin by Med Pro	53978-3300	Sedative; C IV
R33	Tab, Pink, Round, Scored	Clonazepam 0.5 mg	Klonopin by Golden State	60429-0524	Sedative; C IV
R330	Tab, White, Round	Penicillin V Potassium 500 mg	V-Cillin K by Rondex		Antibiotic
R331	Tab, Green, Round	Propranolol HCl 40 mg	Inderal by Actavis	00228-2331	Antihypertensive
R331	Tab, Green, Round	Propranolol HCl 40 mg	Inderal by Prepackage Specialists	58864-0431	Antihypertensive
R331	Tab, Green, Round	Propranolol HCl 40 mg	Inderal by Heartland	61392-0430	Antihypertensive
R336	Tab, White, Round	Prednisone 5 mg	Deltasone by Actavis		Steroid
R34	Tab, Yellow, Round, Scored	Clonazepam 1 mg	Klonopin by Southwood	58016-0186	Sedative; C IV
R34	Tab, Yellow, Round, Scored	Clonazepam 1 mg	Klonopin by Golden State	60429-0525	Sedative; C IV
R34	Tab, Yellow, Round, Scored	Clonazepam 1 mg	Klonopin by DHHS Prog	11819-0028	Sedative; C IV
R34	Tab, Yellow, Round, Scored	Clonazepam 1 mg	Klonopin by Actavis	00228-3004	Sedative; C IV
R346	Cap, Orange	Procainamide HCl 500 mg	Pronestyl by Rondex		Antiarrhythmic

ID FRONT <> BACK	DESCRIPTION FRONT <> BACK	INGREDIENT & STRENGTH	BRAND (or Generic Equiv.) by FIRM	NDC#	CLASS; SCH.
R3487	Cap, Rugby 3487	Chlordiazepoxide 5 mg	Librium by Rugby	00536-3487	Antianxiety; C IV
R3487	Cap, R in a Diamond Shape	Chlordiazepoxide 5 mg	Librium by Chelsea	46193-0944	Antianxiety; C IV
R3488	Cap, Rugby 3488	Chlordiazepoxide 10 mg	Librium by Rugby	00536-3488	Antianxiety; C IV
R3488	Cap, R in a Diamond Shape	Chlordiazepoxide 10 mg	Librium by Chelsea	46193-0945	Antianxiety; C IV
R3489	Cap, R in a Diamond Shape	Chlordiazepoxide 25 mg	Librium by Rugby	00536-3489	Antianxiety; C IV
R3489	Cap	Chlordiazepoxide 25 mg	Librium by Chelsea	46193-0946	Antianxiety; C IV
R35	Tab, White, Round, Scored	Clonazepam 2 mg	Klonopin by Golden State	60429-0526	Sedative; C IV
R35	Tab, White, Round, Scored	Clonazepam 2 mg	Klonopin by Actavis	00228-3005	Sedative; C IV
R356	Tab, White, Round	Quinidine Sulfate 200 mg	Quinaglute by Actavis	00228-2356	Antiarrhythmic
R358	Tab, White, Round, Scored	Hydrochlorothiazide 25 mg, Propranolol HCl 40 mg	Inderide by Actavis	00228-2358	Diuretic; Antihypertensive
R360	Tab, White, Round, Scored	Hydrochlorothiazide 25 mg, Propranolol HCl 80 mg	Inderide by Actavis	00228-2360	Diuretic; Antihypertensive
R368	Tab, Red, Rcund	Rauwolfia Serpentina 50 mg	Raudixin by Actavis		Antihypertensive
R370	Tab, Red, Round	Rauwolfia Serpentina 100 mg	Raudixin by Actavis		Antihypertensive
R3702	Tab, Rugby Logo R 3702	Diethylpropion HCl 25 mg	Tenuate by Rugby	00536-3702	Anorexiant; C III
R374	Tab, White, Round	Reserpine 0.1 mg	Serpasil by Actavis		Antihypertensive
R376	Tab, White, Round	Reserpine 0.25 mg	Serpasil by Actavis		Antihypertensive
R3763	Tab, Rugby Logo R 3763	Atropine Sulfate 0.025 mg, Diphenoxylate HCl 2.5 mg	Lomotil by Rugby	00536-3763	Antidiarrheal; C V
R386	Tab, White, Round	Sulfisoxazole 500 mg	Gantrisin by Actavis		Antibiotic
R3870	Tab, Rugby Logo R 3870	Glutethimide 500 mg	Doriden by Rugby	00536-3870	Hypnotic; C II
R388	Tab, White, Round	Spironolactone 25 mg	Aldactone by Actavis		Diuretic
R390	Tab, White, Round	Hydrochlorothiazide 25 mg, Spironolactone 25 mg	Aldactazide by Actavis		Diuretic; Antihypertensive
R3924	Cap	Butalbital 50 mg, Aspirin 325 mg, Caffeine 40 mg	Fiorinal by Actavis		Analgesic; C III
R397	Cap, Green	Doxepin HCl 75 mg	Sinequan by Actavis		Antidepressant
R398	Cap, Green & White	Doxepin HCl 100 mg	Sinequan by Actavis		Antidepressant
R4	Tab, Ex Release, R-4	Guaifenesin 675 mg	Numobid by Sovereign	58716-0607	Expectorant
R4	Tab, Light Coral, Round	Risperidone 4 mg	Risperdal M-Tab by Janssen-Ortho	Canadian DIN 02268094	Antipsychotic
R4	Tab, Greer, Cap-Shaped, Film-Coated, Scored, Cobalt Logo <> R / 4	Risperidone 4 mg	Risperdal by Cobalt	Canadian DIN 02282631	Antipsychotic
R4	Tab, Green, Oblong, Scored	Risperidone 4 mg	Risperdal by Pharmascience	Canadian DIN 02252066	Antipsychotic
R4 <> JANSSEN	Tab, Green, Cap Shaped	Risperidone 4 mg	Risperdal by Janssen	50458-0350	Antipsychotic
R4 <> JANSSEN	Tab, Coated	Risperidone 4 mg	Risperdal by Johnson & Johnson	59604-0350	Antipsychotic
R400	Cap, White	Doxepin HCl 150 mg	Sinequan by Actavis		Antidepressant
R404	Cap, Orarge & Yellow	Tetracycline HCl 250 mg	Tetracyn by Actavis		Antibiotic
R406	Cap, Black & Yellow	Tetracycline HCl 500 mg	Tetracyn by Actavis		Antibiotic
R409	Cap, Gray & Orange	Cephalexin 250 mg	Keflex by Rondex		Antibiotic
R418	Cap, Orange	Cephalexin 500 mg	Keflex by Rondex		Antibiotic
R4250	Tab, White, Round	Atropine Sulfate, Hyoscyamine Sulfate, Phenobarbital, Scopolamine	Donnatal by A H Robins		Gastrointestinal; C IV
R4264	Tab, Round	Atropine Sulfate, Hyoscyamine Sulfate, Phenobarbital, Scopolamine Hydrobromide	Donnatal #2 by A H Robins		Gastrointestinal; C IV
R4306	Tab, White, Round	Promethazine 25 mg	Phenergan by Richlyn		Antiemetic; Antihistamine
R4322	Tab, White, Round	Propylthiouracil 50 mg	Propylthiouracil by Richlyn		Antithyroid
R4374	Cap	Aspirin 389 mg, Caffeine 32.4 mg, Propoxyphene HCl 65 mg	Propoxyphene Compound 65 by Allscripts		Analgesic; C IV
R4388	Tab, Burgundy, Round	Phenazopyridine HCl 100 mg	Pyridium by Rugby		Urinary Analgesic

ID FRONT <> BACK	DESCRIPTION FRONT <> BACK	INGREDIENT & STRENGTH	BRAND (or Generic Equiv.) by FIRM	NDC#	CLASS; SCH.
R4392	Tab, Burgundy, Round	Phenazopyridine HCl 200 mg	Pyridium by Rugby		Urinary Analgesic
R440	Tab, White, Round	Tolbutamide 500 mg	Orinase by Actavis		Antidiabetic
R4429	Tab, R inside of a Diamond Shape 4429	Quinidine Sulfate 300 mg	by Rugby	00536-4429	Antiarrhythmic
R497	Cap, Yellow, Opaque, Soft Gel	Nifedipine 10 mg	Adalat by Actavis	00228-2497	Antihypertensive
R497	Cap, Yellow, Opaque, Soft Gel	Nifedipine 10 mg	Adalat by Vangard	00615-0360	Antihypertensive
R497	Cap, Yellow, Opaque, Soft Gel	Nifedipine 10 mg	Adalat by Murfreesboro	51129-1133	Antihypertensive
R497	Cap, Yellow, Opaque, Soft Gel	Nifedipine 10 mg	Adalat by Med Pro	53978-1189	Antihypertensive
R497	Cap, Yellow, Opaque, Soft Gel	Nifedipine 10 mg	Adalat by UDL	51079-0664	Antihypertensive
R497	Cap, Yellow, Opaque, Soft Gel	Nifedipine 10 mg	Adalat by Ivax	00182-1547	Antihypertensive
R497	Cap, Yellow, Opaque, Soft Gel	Nifedipine 10 mg	Adalat by Baker Cummins	63171-1547	Antihypertensive
R497	Cap, Yellow, Opaque, Soft Gel	Nifedipine 10 mg	Adalat by Golden State	60429-0138	Antihypertensive
R497	Cap, Yellow, Opaque, Soft Gel	Nifedipine 10 mg	Adalat by Heartland	61392-0356	Antihypertensive
R497	Cap, Yellow, Opaque, Soft Gel	Nifedipine 10 mg	Adalat by PDRX	55289-0907	Antihypertensive
R497	Cap, Yellow, Opaque, Soft Gel	Nifedipine 10 mg	Adalat by RP Scherer	11014-0870	Antihypertensive
R5	Tab, Ex Release, R/5	Dextromethorphan HBr 30 mg, Guaifenesin 675 mg	Numobid Dx by Sovereign	58716-0637	Cold Remedy
R5	Tab, White, Round	Isosorbide Dinitrate SL 5 mg	Isordil by Rugby		Antianginal
R5 <> M	Tab, Beige, Round, Film-Coated	Risperidone 0.5 mg	Risperdal by UDL	51079-0461	Antipsychotic
R5 <> M	Tab, Pink, Round	Risperidone .5 mg	Risperdal by Mylan	00378-3505	Antipsychotic
R50 <> P	Tab, R/50 <> Purepac Logo	Lorazepam 1 mg	Ativan by Kaiser	00179-1093	Antianxiety; C IV
R500	Cap	Prazosin HCl	by Heartland	61392-0115	Antihypertensive
R500	Cap	Prazosin HCl 1 mg	by Qualitest	00603-5286	Antihypertensive
R500	Cap, White	Prazosin HCl	by Actavis	00228-2500	Antihypertensive
R501	Cap, Pink	Prazosin HCl	by Actavis	00228-2501	Antihypertensive
R502	Cap	Prazosin HCl	by Heartland	61392-0118	Antihypertensive
R502	Cap, Blue	Prazosin HCl 5 mg	by Actavis	00228-2502	Antihypertensive
R502	Cap	Prazosin HCl 5 mg	by Qualitest	00603-5288	Antihypertensive
R520	Cap, Orange & White	Tolmetin Sodium 400 mg	by Actavis	00228-2520	NSAID
R521	Tab, White, Round	Naproxen 250 mg	Naprosyn by Actavis		NSAID
R522	Tab, White, Oblong	Naproxen 375 mg	Naprosyn by Actavis		NSAID
R523	Tab, White, Oblong	Naproxen 500 mg	Naprosyn by Actavis		NSAID
R529	Tab, Light Brown, Cap Shaped	Divalproex Sodium 125 mg	Depakote by Dr. Reddy's	55111-0529	Anticonvulsant
R530	Cap, Reddish Brown, Opaque, Soft Gel	Nifedipine 20 mg	Adalat by Actavis	00228-2530	Antihypertensive
R530	Cap, Reddish Brown, Opaque, Soft Gel	Nifedipine 20 mg	Adalat by Vangard	00615-0359	Antihypertensive
R530	Cap, Reddish Brown, Opaque, Soft Gel	Nifedipine 20 mg	Adalat by Ivax	00182-1548	Antihypertensive
R530	Cap, Reddish Brown, Opaque, Soft Gel	Nifedipine 20 mg	Adalat by Baker Cummins	63171-1548	Antihypertensive
R530	Cap, Reddish Brown, Opaque, Soft Gel	Nifedipine 20 mg	Adalat by UDL	51079-0665	Antihypertensive
R530	Cap, Reddish Brown, Opaque, Soft Gel	Nifedipine 20 mg	Adalat by Med Pro	53978-2038	Antihypertensive
R530	Cap, Reddish Brown, Opaque, Soft Gel	Nifedipine 20 mg	Adalat by H J Harkins Co	52959-0488	Antihypertensive
R530	Cap, Reddish Brown, Opaque, Soft Gel	Nifedipine 20 mg	Adalat by Par	49884-0624	Antihypertensive
R530	Cap, Reddish Brown, Opaque, Soft Gel	Nifedipine 20 mg	Adalat by Golden State	60429-0139	Antihypertensive
R530	Cap, Reddish Brown, Opaque, Soft Gel	Nifedipine 20 mg	Adalat by Heartland	61392-0353	Antihypertensive
R530	Tab, Cream, Cap Shaped	Divalproex Sodium 250 mg	Depakote by Dr. Reddy's	55111-0530	Anticonvulsant
R531	Tab, Light Pink, Cap Shaped	Divalproex Sodium 500 mg	Depakote by Dr. Reddy's	55111-0531	Anticonvulsant
R534	Tab, White, Round	Pindolol 5 mg	Visken by Actavis		Antihypertensive
R535	Tab, White, Round	Pindolol 10 mg	Visken by Actavis		Antihypertensive
R546	Tab, Orange, Round	Diflunisal 500 mg	Dolobid by Actavis	00228-2546	NSAID
R547	Tab, White, Oval	Naproxen 275 mg	Anaprox by Actavis		NSAID
R548	Tab, White, Oval	Naproxen 550 mg	Anaprox by Actavis		NSAID

ID FRONT <> BACK	DESCRIPTION FRONT <> BACK	INGREDIENT & STRENGTH	BRAND (or Generic Equiv.) by FIRM	NDC#	CLASS; SCH.
R553	Cap, Clear with White Beads	Erythromycin 250 mg	by Actavis	00228-2553	Antibiotic
R553	Cap	Erythromycin 250 mg	by Qualitest	00603-3548	Antibiotic
R553	Cap, Clear	Erythromycin 250 mg	by Faulding	50546-0350	Antibiotic
R554	Tab, Film Coated	Metoprolol Tartrate 50 mg	Lopressor by Talbert	44514-0514	Antihypertensive
R554	Tab, Film Coated	Metoprolol Tartrate 50 mg	Lopressor by Ivax	00182-1987	Antihypertensive
R555	Tab, Film Coated	Metoprolol Tartrate 100 mg	Lopressor by Ivax	00182-1988	Antihypertensive
R56 <> 3	Tab, White to Off-White, Round	Acetaminophen 300 mg, Codeine Phosphate 30 mg	Tylenol w/ Codeine by Actavis	00228-3056	Analgesic; C III
R5726	Tab, Tan, Oblong	Carbinoxamine Maleate 4 mg, Pseudoephedrine HCl 60 mg	Rondec by Ross	Discontinued	Cold Remedy
R58 <> 4	Tab, White to Off-White, Round	Acetaminophen 300 mg, Codeine Phosphate 60 mg	Tylenol w/ Codeine by Actavis	00228-3058	Analgesic; C III
R59	Tab, White, Round, Scored	Lorazepam 1 mg	Ativan by Actavis	00228-2059	Antianxiety; C IV
R599	Tab, Light Gray, Football Shaped, Film Coated	Etodolac 400 mg	Lodine by Actavis	00228-2599	NSAID
R599	Tab, Light Gray, Football Shaped, Film Coated	Etodolac 400 mg	Lodine by Heartland	61392-0908	NSAID
R599	Tab, Light Gray, Football Shaped, Film Coated	Etodolac 400 mg	Lodine by DRX	55045-2490	NSAID
R60	Tab, Yellow, Round	Phendimetrazine 35 mg	Plegine by Rugby		Anorexiant; C III
R605	Cap, Green, Opaque	Acyclovir 200 mg	Zovirax by Actavis	00228-2605	Antiviral
R605	Cap, Green, Opaque	Acyclovir 200 mg	Zovirax by Golden State	60429-0711	Antiviral
R607	Tab, Green, Oval	Acyclovir 800 mg	Zovirax by Golden State	60429-0713	Antiviral
R607	Tab, Green, Oval	Acyclovir 800 mg	Zovirax by Actavis	00228-2607	Antiviral
R614	Tab, Orange, Cap Shaped, Film Coated	Oxaprozin 600 mg	Daypro by Actavis	00228-2614	NSAID
R620	Tab, Blue, Round, Scored	Isosorbide Mononitrate 20 mg	Ismo by Actavis	00228-2620	Antianginal
R6240	Tab, Ex Release	Carbinoxamine Maleate 8 mg, Pseudoephedrine HCl 120 mg	Rondec TR by Abbott	Discontinued	Cold Remedy
R63	Tab	Clonazepam 0.5 mg	by Pharmacy Serv Ctr	00855-9215	Sedative; C IV
R631	Tab, Blue, Round, Scored	Isosorbide Mononitrate 10 mg	Ismo by Actavis	00228-2631	Antianginal
R632	Tab, White, Football Shaped, Film Coated	Etodolac 500 mg	Lodine by Heartland	61392-0905	NSAID
R632	Tab, White, Football Shaped, Film Coated	Etodolac 500 mg	Lodine by Actavis	00228-2632	NSAID
R636	Tab, Light Green, Cap Shaped, Film Coated, Scored	Gabapentin 600 mg	Neurontin by Actavis	00228-2636	Anticonvulsant
R637	Tab, Light Gray, Cap Shaped, Film Coated, Scored	Gabapentin 800 mg	Neurontin by Actavis	00228-2637	Anticonvulsant
R642	Tab, White, Round, Scored	Doxazosin Mesylate 1 mg	Cardura by Actavis	00228-2642	Antihypertensive
R643	Tab, White, Cap Shaped, Scored	Doxazosin Mesylate 2 mg	Cardura by Actavis	00228-2643	Antihypertensive
R644	Tab, White, Cap Shaped, Scored	Doxazosin Mesylate 4 mg	Cardura by Actavis	00228-2644	Antihypertensive
R645	Tab, White, Round, Scored	Doxazosin Mesylate 8 mg	Cardura by Actavis	00228-2645	Antihypertensive
R655	Tab, Blue, Cap Shaped, Film Coated, Scored	Fluvoxamine Maleate 50 mg	Luvox by Actavis	00228-2655	OCD
R656	Tab, White, Cap Shaped, Film Coated, Scored	Fluvoxamine Maleate 100 mg	Luvox by Actavis	00228-2656	OCD
R657	Tab, White to Off-White, Oval, Film Coated	Metformin HCl 500 mg	Glucophage by Actavis	00228-2657	Antidiabetic
R665	Cap, Light Brown and White, Black ink	Gabapentin 100 mg	Neurontin by Actavis	00228-2665	Anticonvulsant
R666	Cap, Brown and Yellow	Gabapentin 300 mg	Neurontin by Actavis	00228-2666	Anticonvulsant
R667	Cap, Light Brown and Orange, Black ink	Gabapentin 400 mg	Neurontin by Actavis	00228-2667	Anticonvulsant
R671	Tab, Peach, Oval, Film Coated, Ex Release	Etodolac 400 mg	Lodine XL by Actavis	00228-2671	NSAID
R672	Tab, White to Off-White, Oval, Scored, Film Coated	Spironolactone 50 mg	Aldactone by Actavis	00228-2672	Diuretic
R673	Tab, White to Off-White, Round, Scored, Film Coated	Spironolactone 100 mg	Aldactone by Actavis	00228-2673	Diuretic
R7	Tab, Orange, Octagonal	Indapamide 1.25 mg	Lozol by RPR		Diuretic
R70	Tab, White, Round	Dipyridamole 25 mg	Persantine by Rugby		Antiplatelet
R706	Tab, White to Off-White, Round	Lisinopril 10 mg, HCTZ 12.5 mg	Prinzide by Actavis	00228-2706	Antihypertensive; Diuretic
R707	Tab, Yellow, Round	Lisinopril 20 mg, HCTZ 12.5 mg	Prinzide by Actavis	00228-2707	Antihypertensive; Diuretic
R708	Tab, Pink, Round	Lisinopril 20 mg, HCTZ 25 mg	Prinzide by Actavis	00228-2708	Antihypertensive; Diuretic
R708	Tab, Pink, Round	Lisinopril 20 mg, HCTZ 25 mg	Prinzide by Actavis	00228-2708	Antihypertensive; Diuretic
R711	Tab, Beige, Oval, Film Coated, Scored, Ex Release	Isosorbide Mononitrate 60 mg	Imdur by Actavis	00228-2711	Antianginal
R713	Tab, White, Oval, Film Coated, Scored, Ex Release	Isosorbide Mononitrate 30 mg	Imdur by Actavis	00228-2713	Antianginal

ID FRONT <> BACK	DESCRIPTION FRONT <> BACK	INGREDIENT & STRENGTH	BRAND (or Generic Equiv.) by FIRM	NDC#	CLASS; SCH.
R714	Tab, White, Oval, Film Coated	Tramadol HCl 50 mg	Ultram by Actavis	00228-2714	Analgesic
R715	Tab, White to Off-White, Oval, Film Coated	Metformin HCl 850 mg	Glucophage by Actavis	00228-2715	Antidiabetic
R718	Tab, White to Off-White, Oval, Film Coated	Metformin HCl 1000 mg	Glucophage by Actavis	00228-2718	Antidiabetic
R728	Tab, Light Orange, Cap Shaped, Film Coated, Extended Release	Metformin HCl 750 mg	Glucophage XR by Actavis	00228-2728	Antidiabetic
R740	Tab, Light Yellow, Film Coated, Extended Release	Metformin HCl 500 mg	Glucophage XR by Actavis	00228-2740	Antidiabetic
R741	Tab, Yellow, Round, Scored	Tizanidine HCl 4 mg	Zanaflex by Actavis	00228-2741	Muscle Relaxant
R742	Tab, Yellow, Cap Shaped, Scored	Tizanidine HCl 2 mg	Zanaflex by Actavis	00228-2742	Muscle Relaxant
R747	Tab, Yellow, Cap Shaped, Film Coated, Ex Release	Pentoxifylline 400 mg	Trental by Actavis	00228-2747	Anticoagulant
R751	Tab, White to Off-White, Cap Shaped, Film Coated	Glyburide 1.25 mg, Metformin 250 mg	Glucovance by Actavis	00228-2751	Antidiabetic
R752	Tab, Yellow, Cap Shaped, Film Coated	Glyburide 2.5 mg, Metformin 500 mg	Glucovance by Actavis	00228-2752	Antidiabetic
R753	Tab, Blue, Cap Shaped, Film Coated	Glyburide 5 mg, Metformin 500 mg	Glucovance by Actavis	00228-2753	Antidiabetic
R756	Tab, Pink, Cap Shaped, Scored, Film Coated	Citalopram 20 mg	Celexa by Actavis	00228-2756	Antidepressant
R757	Tab, White to Off-White, Cap Shaped, Scored, Film Coated	Citalopram 40 mg	Celexa by Actavis	00228-2757	Antidepressant
R75BI	Cap, Light Blue Opaque Cap, Cream Opaque Body, Filled with Yellow Pellets	Dabigatran Etexilate 75 mg	Pradax by Boehringer Ingelheim	Canadian DIN 02312433	Anticoagulant
R7621	Tab, Maroon, Oval	Multivitamin, Fluoride, Iron	ViDaylin F with Iron by Ross		Vitamin
R7626	Tab, Yellow, Oval	Multivitamin, Fluoride	ViDaylin F by Ross		Vitamin
R8	Tab, White, Octagonal, Film Coated, R over 8	Indapamide 2.5 mg	Lozol by Amerisource	62584-0082	Diuretic
R8	Tab, White, Octagon	Indapamide 2.5 mg	Lozol by Rightpak	65240-0685	Diuretic
RAFTON	Tab, White, Round	Alginic Acid 200 mg, Aluminum Hydroxide 80 mg	Rafton by Ferring	Canadian	Gastrointestinal
RAM017 <> RAM017	Tab	Yohimbine HCl 5.4 mg	Yovital by Kenwood	00482-0017	Impotence Agent
RAM020	Tab, Sugar Coated	Bile Salts 150 mg, Pancreatin 300 mg, Pepsin 250 mg	Digepepsin by Lini	58215-0302 Discontinued	Gastrointestinal
RAMIPRIL10	Cap, Blue and White, Opaque	Ramipril 10 mg	Altace by Pharmascience	Canadian DIN 02255332	Antihypertensive
RAMIPRIL25	Cap, Orange and White, Opaque	Ramipril 2.5 mg	Altace by Pharmascience	Canadian DIN 02255316	Antihypertensive
RAMIPRIL5	Cap, Red and White, Opaque	Ramipril 5 mg	Altace by Pharmascience	Canadian DIN 02255324	Antihypertensive
RAN150 <> APO	Tab, White to Off-White, Round, Film Coated	Ranitidine HCl 150 mg	Zantac by Apotex	60505-0025	Gastrointestinal
RAN300 <> APO	Tab, White to Off-White, Cap Shaped, Film Coated	Ranitidine HCl 300 mg	Zantac by Apotex	60505-0026	Gastrointestinal
RAPAMUNE1MG	Tab, White, Triangular	Sirolimus 1 mg	Rapamune by Wyeth	00008-1031	Immunosuppressant
RAPAMUNE1MG	Tab, White, Triangular	Sirolimus 1 mg	Rapamune by Wyeth Canada	02247111	Immunosuppressant
RAPAMUNE2MG	Tab, Yellow to Beige, Triangular	Sirolimus 2 mg	Rapamune by Wyeth	00008-1032	Immunosuppressant
RAPIDE50 <> VOLTAREN	Tab, Reddish Brown, Round, Sugar Coated	Diclofenac Potassium 50 mg	Voltaren Rapide by Novartis	Canadian DIN 00881635	NSAID
RB	Tab, Grey, Round, Backwards "R", "b"	3,4-Methylenedioxymethamphetamine (MDMA)	Ecstasy by Illegal		Euphoric; Illicit
RB <> 49	Tab, Light Blue, Oval	Glimepiride 2 mg	Amaryl by Ranbaxy	63304-0426 Discontinued	Antidiabetic
RB <> 49	Tab, White, Dumbbell-Shaped, Scored	Glimepiride 2 mg	Amaryl by Ranbaxy	63304-0426	Antidiabetic
RB41	Tab, White, Oval, Film Coated	Cefprozil 250 mg	Cefzil by Ranbaxy	Canadian DIN 02293528	Antibiotic
RB42	Tab, White to Off-White, Oval, Film Coated	Cefprozil 500 mg	Cefzil by Ranbaxy	Canadian DIN 02293536	Antibiotic
RB80	Tab, White, Round	Cetirizine HCl 10 mg	Zyrtec by OHM		Antihistamine
RB81	Tab, Pink, Oblong	Zolpidem Tartrate 5 mg	Ambien by Ranbaxy	63304-0159	Sedative/Hypnotic; C IV
RB82	Tab, White, Oblong	Zolpidem Tartrate 10 mg	Ambien by Ranbaxy	63304-0160	Sedative/Hypnotic; C IV

ID FRONT <> BACK	DESCRIPTION FRONT <> BACK	INGREDIENT & STRENGTH	BRAND (or Generic Equiv.) by FIRM	NDC#	CLASS; SCH.
RBX	Tab, Light Blue, Octagon Shaped, Scored	Lovastatin 20 mg	Mevacor by Ranbaxy	Canadian DIN 02267969	Antihyperlipidemic
RBX	Tab, Mint Green, Octagon Shaped, Film Coated	Lovastatin 40 mg	Mevacor by Ranbaxy	Canadian DIN 02267977	Antihyperlipidemic
RBX <> 312R	Tab, White, Round, Film Coated	Zopiclone 5 mg	Imovane by Ranbaxy	Canadian DIN 02267918	Sedative; Hypnotic
RBX <> 482A	Tab, White, Oval, Film Coated	Carvedilol 3.125 mg	Coreg by Ranbaxy	Canadian DIN 02268027	Antihypertensive
RBX <> 482B	Tab, White, Oval, Film Coated	Carvedilol 6.25 mg	Coreg by Ranbaxy	Canadian DIN 02268035	Antihypertensive
RBX <> 482C	Tab, White, Oval, Film Coated	Carvedilol 12.5 mg	Coreg by Ranbaxy	Canadian DIN 02268043	Antihypertensive
RBX <> 482D	Tab, White, Oval, Film Coated	Carvedilol 25 mg	Coreg by Ranbaxy	Canadian DIN 02268051	Antihypertensive
RBX <> C19	Tab, White, Oblong	Ciprofloxacin 750 mg	Cipro by Ranbaxy	Canadian DIN 02267950	Antibiotic
RBX <> C29	Tab, White, Oblong	Ciprofloxacin 500 mg	Cipro by Ranbaxy	Canadian DIN 02267942	Antibiotic
RBX <> C39	Tab, White, Round, Film Coated	Ciprofloxacin 250 mg	Cipro by Ranbaxy	Canadian DIN 02267934	Antibiotic
RBX <> R12	Tab, White, Round, Scored, Film Coated	Metformin HCl 500 mg	Glucophage by Ranbaxy	Canadian DIN 02269031	Antidiabetic
RBX <> R22	Tab, White, Oblong, Film Coated	Metformin HCl 850 mg	Glucophage by Ranbaxy	Canadian DIN 02269058	Antidiabetic
RBX312	Tab, Blue, Oval, Scored, Film Coated	Zopiclone 7.5 mg	Imovane by Ranbaxy	Canadian DIN 02267926	Sedative; Hypnotic
RBX582A	Tab, White, Oval, Scored, Film Coated	Citalopram 20 mg	Celexa by Ranbaxy	Canadian DIN 02268000	Antidepressant
RBX582B	Tab, White, Oval, Scored, Film Coated	Citalopram 40 mg	Celexa by Ranbaxy	Canadian DIN 02268019	Antidepressant
RBXR14	Tab, White, Round, Scored, Film Coated	Atenolol 50 mg	Tenormin by Ranbaxy	Canadian DIN 02267985	Antihypertensive
RBXR15	Tab, White, Round, Scored, Film Coated	Atenolol 100 mg	Tenormin by Ranbaxy	Canadian DIN 02267993	Antihypertensive
RC	Tab, Purple, Round, RC/+	Diphenhydramine HCl 25 mg, Pseudoephedrine HCl 60 mg, Acetaminophen 500 mg	Cold Control by Reese	10956-0589	Antihistamine
RC22	Tab, Yellow, Cap Shaped, Scored	Penbutolol Sulfate 20 mg	Levatol by Schwarz	Discontinued	Antihypertensive
RC3	Tab, White to Off-White, Round	Fosinopril Sodium 10 mg, Hydrochlorothiazide 12.5 mg	Monopril HCT by Ranbaxy	63304-0403	Antihypertensive; Diuretic
RC4	Tab, White to Off-White, Round, Scored	Fosinopril Sodium 20 mg, Hydrochlorothiazide 12.5 mg	Monopril HCT by Ranbaxy	63304-0404	Antihypertensive; Diuretic
RC80	Tab, Light Yellow, Cap Shaped, Scored, RC / 80, For Suspension	Cephalexin 125 mg	Panixine DisperDose by Ranbaxy	63304-0573	Antibiotic
RC81	Tab, Light Yellow, Cap Shaped, Scored, RC / 81, For Suspension	Cephalexin 250 mg	Panixine DisperDose by Ranbaxy	63304-0574	Antibiotic
RCA	Tab, White, RC/A	Acetaminophen 650 mg	Tylenol by Reese		Analgesic
RCAPP	Cap, Orange, RC/APP	Phenylpropanolamine HCl 25 mg, Acetaminophen 500 mg	Tetra Caps by Reese	10956-0706	Cold Remedy
RCCGUF	Cap, Pink, RCC/GUF	Guaifenesin 200 mg	Aquabid by Reese	10956-0700	Expectorant
RCD	Tab, Yellow, Round, RC/D	Diphenhydramine HCl 50 mg	Sleep-Ettes D by Reese	10956-0601	Antihistamine
RCE	Cap, Orange, RC/E	Guaifenesin 200 mg, Phenylpropanolamine HCl 37.5 mg	Entex LA by Reese	10956-0685	Cold Remedy
RCGGP	Cap, White, RC/GGP	Guaifenesin 400 mg, Pseudoephedrine HCl 60 mg	Sudafed Sinus by Reese	10956-0724	Cold Remedy
RCNS	Tab, Green, Round, RC/NS	Acetaminophen 500 mg, Pseudoephedrine HCl 60 mg, Dexbrompheniramine Maleate 2 mg	Sinadrin Plus by Reese	10956-0636	Cold Remedy

ID FRONT <> BACK	DESCRIPTION FRONT <> BACK	INGREDIENT & STRENGTH	BRAND (or Generic Equiv.) by FIRM	NDC#	CLASS; SCH.
RCP	Cap, Yellow, RC/P	Guaifenesin 200 mg, Dextromethorphan HBr 15 mg	Tussi-Organidan DM NR by Reese	10956-0659	Cold Remedy
RCP	Cap, Yellow, RC/P	Pyrantel Pamoate 180 mg	Reese's Pinworm by Reese	10956-0658	Anthelmintic
RCSS	Tab, Yellow, Round	Acetaminophen 500 mg, Phenylpropanolamine HCl 25 mg, Chlorpheniramine Maleate 4 mg	Sinadrin Max Strength by Reese	10956-0697	Cold Remedy
RCTC	Cap, Yellow, RC/TC	Acetaminophen 500 mg, Phenylpropanolamine HCl 37.5 mg, Pyrilamine Maleate 50 mg, Dextromethorphan HBr 30 mg	Theracaps by Reese	10956-0637	Cold Remedy
RD02	Tab, Yellow, Round	B and C Vitamin Combinations	Nephro-Vite by Watson	54391-0002	Supplement
RD05 <> CALCICHEW	Tab, White, Round, Scored, CALCI-CHEW, Chewable	Calcium Carbonate 1250 mg	Calci-Chew Cherry by Watson	54391-0025	Vitamin; Mineral
RD12	Tab, Yellow, Round	Ascorbic Acid 60 mg, Biotin, D- 300 mcg, Calcium Pantothenate 10 mg, Cyanocobalamin 6 mcg, Folic Acid 1 mg, Niacinamide 20 mg, Pyridoxine HCl 10 mg, Riboflavin 1.7 mg, Thiamine Mononitrate 1.5 mg	Nephro Vite Rx by Watson	52544-0977	Vitamin
RD12	Tab, Film Coated	Acetaminophen 500 mg, Biotin, D- 300 mcg, Calcium Pantothenate 10 mg, Cyanocobalamin 6 mcg, Folic Acid 1 mg, Niacinamide 20 mg, Pyridoxine HCl 10 mg, Riboflavin 1.7 mg, Thiamine Mononitrate 1.5 mg	Nephro Vite Rx by Anabolic	00722-6191	Vitamin
RD12	Tab, Yellow, Round	Ascorbic Acid 60 mg, Biotin, D- 300 mcg, Calcium Pantothenate 10 mg, Cyanocobalamin 6 mcg, Folic Acid 1 mg, Niacinamide 20 mg, Pyridoxine HCl 10 mg, Riboflavin 1.7 mg, Thiamine Mononitrate 1.5 mg	Nephro Vite Rx by R & D	54391-1002	Vitamin
RD13	Tab, Brown, Oval	Ferrous Fumarate 350 mg	Nephro-Fer by Watson	54391-0013	Supplement
RD20180RELIANT	Cap, Gray & White, Ex Release, 80 2 Bands Reliant Logo	Propranolol HCl 80 mg	InnoPran XL by Reliant	65726-0250	Antihypertensive
RD23	Tab, Film Coated	Ascorbic Acid 60 mg, Biotin 0.3 mg, Calcium Pantothenate, Cyanocobalamin 0.006 mg, Ferrous Fumarate, Folic Acid 1 mg, Niacinamide 20 mg, Pyridoxine HCl, Riboflavin 1.7 mg, Thiamine Mononitrate	Nephro Vite Rx Iron by Anabolic	00722-6244	Vitamin
RD23	Tab, Film Coated	Ascorbic Acid 60 mg, Biotin 0.3 mg, Calcium Pantothenate, Cyanocobalamin 0.006 mg, Ferrous Fumarate, Folic Acid 1 mg, Niacinamide 20 mg, Pyridoxine HCl, Riboflavin 1.7 mg, Thiamine Mononitrate	Nephro Vite Fe by R & D	54391-2213	Vitamin
RD25	Tab, White, Round, Chewable	Calcium Carbonate 1250 mg	Calci-Chew Lemon by Watson	54391-0225	Vitamin; Mineral
RD26	Tab, White, Cap Shaped	Calcium Carbonate 1500 mg	Nephro-Calci by Watson	54391-0026	Supplement
RD33	Tab, Film Coated	Ferrous Fumarate 324 mg, Folic Acid 1 mg	Nephro Fer Rx by Anabolic	00722-6262	Mineral
RD33	Tab, Film Coated	Ferrous Fumarate 324 mg, Folic Acid 1 mg	Nephro Fer Rx by R & D	54391-1313	Mineral
RD35 <> CALCICHEW	Tab, White, Round, CALCI-CHEW, Chewable	Calcium Carbonate 1250 mg	Calci-Chew Orange by Watson	54391-0325	Vitamin; Mineral
RD50	Cap, White, Oval	L-Carnitine 250 mg	L-Carnitine by Watson	54391-0050	Supplement
RDY <> 107	Tab, White, Capsule Shaped	Naproxen Sodium 275 mg	Anaprox by Dr. Reddy's	55111-0107	Anti-inflammatory
RDY <> 108	Tab, White, Capsule Shaped, Scored	Naproxen Sodium 550 mg	Anaprox by Dr. Reddy's	55111-0108	Anti-inflammatory
RDY <> 181	Tab, Beige, Cap Shaped, Scored	Levetiracetam 250 mg	Keppra by Dr. Reddy's	55111-0181	Anticonvulsant
RDY <> 182	Tab, Beige, Cap Shaped, Scored, 1 / 82 <> RDY	Levetiracetam 500 mg	Keppra by Dr. Reddy's	55111-0182	Anticonvulsant
RDY <> 183	Tab, Beige, Cap Shaped, Scored	Levetiracetam 750 mg	Keppra by Dr. Reddy's	55111-0183	Anticonvulsant
RDY <> 197	Tab, Brown, Round, Film Coated	Simvastatin 5 mg	Zocor by Dr. Reddy's	55111-0197	Antihyperlipidemic
RDY <> 198	Tab, Brown, Round, Film Coated	Simvastatin 10 mg	Zocor by Dr. Reddy's	55111-0198	Antihyperlipidemic
RDY <> 199	Tab, Brown, Round, Film Coated	Simvastatin 20 mg	Zocor by Dr. Reddy's	55111-0199	Antihyperlipidemic
RDY <> 200	Tab, Brown, Round, Film Coated	Simvastatin 40 mg	Zocor by Dr. Reddy's	55111-0200	Antihyperlipidemic
RDY <> 201	Tab, Yellow, Round	Risperidone 0.25 mg	Risperdal by Dr. Reddy's	55111-0201	Antipsychotic
RDY <> 202	Tab, Pink, Round	Risperidone 0.5 mg	Risperdal by Dr. Reddy's	55111-0202	Antipsychotic
RDY <> 203	Tab, White, Round	Risperidone 1 mg	Risperdal by Dr. Reddy's	55111-0203	Antipsychotic
RDY <> 204	Tab, White, Round	Risperidone 2 mg	Risperdal by Dr. Reddy's	55111-0204	Antipsychotic
RDY <> 205	Tab, White, Round	Risperidone 3 mg	Risperdal by Dr. Reddy's	55111-0205	Antipsychotic
RDY <> 206	Tab, White, Round	Risperidone 4 mg	Risperdal by Dr. Reddy's	55111-0206	Antipsychotic
RDY <> 220	Tab, Light Yellow, Round	Lamotrigine 25 mg	Lamictal by Dr. Reddy's	55111-0220	Anticonvulsant
RDY <> 221	Tab, Light Yellow, Round	Lamotrigine 100 mg	Lamictal by Dr. Reddy's	55111-0221	Anticonvulsant
RDY <> 222	Tab, Light Yellow, Round	Lamotrigine 150 mg	Lamictal by Dr. Reddy's	55111-0222	Anticonvulsant
RDY <> 223	Tab, Light Yellow, Round	Lamotrigine 200 mg	Lamictal by Dr. Reddy's	55111-0223	Anticonvulsant
RDY <> 225	Tab, White, Round	Lamotrigine 5 mg	Lamictal by Dr. Reddy's	55111-0225	Anticonvulsant

ID FRONT <> BACK	DESCRIPTION FRONT <> BACK	INGREDIENT & STRENGTH	BRAND (or Generic Equiv.) by FIRM	NDC#	CLASS; SCH.
RDY <> 226	Tab, White, Cap Shaped	Lamotrigine 25 mg	Lamictal by Dr. Reddy's	55111-0226	Anticonvulsant
RDY <> 229	Tab, White, Round	Pravastatin Sodium 10 mg	Pravachol by Dr. Reddy's	55111-0229	Antihyperlipidemic
RDY <> 230	Tab, White, Round	Pravastatin Sodium 20 mg	Pravachol by Dr. Reddy's	55111-0230	Antihyperlipidemic
RDY <> 231	Tab, White, Round	Pravastatin Sodium 40 mg	Pravachol by Dr. Reddy's	55111-0231	Antihyperlipidemic
RDY <> 233	Tab, Yellow, Oval	Meloxicam 7.5 mg	Mobic by Dr. Reddy's	55111-0233	NSAID
RDY <> 234	Tab, Yellow, Round	Meloxicam 15 mg	Mobic by Dr. Reddy's	55111-0234	NSAID
RDY <> 248	Tab, Beige, Ova, Scored	Levetiracetam 1000 mg	Keppra by Dr. Reddy's	55111-0248	Anticonvulsant
RDY <> 268	Tab, Brown, Round, Film Coated	Simvastatin 80 mg	Zocor by Dr. Reddy's	55111-0268	Antihyperlipidemic
RDY <> 269	Tab, White, Oval	Amlodipine Besylate 2.5 mg	Norvasc by Dr. Reddy's	55111-0269	Antihypertensive
RDY <> 270	Tab, White, Oval	Amlodipine Besylate 5 mg	Norvasc by Dr. Reddy's	55111-0270	Antihypertensive
RDY <> 271	Tab, White, Oval	Amlodipine Besylate 10 mg	Norvasc by Dr. Reddy's	55111-0271	Antihypertensive
RDY <> 274	Tab, White, Oval	Pravastatin 80 mg	Pravachol by Dr. Reddy's	55111-0274	Antihyperlipidemic
RDY <> 320	Tab, Peach, Oval, Scored, 3/20	Glimepiride 1 mg	Amaryl by Dr. Reddy's	55111-0320	Antidiabetic
RDY <> 321	Tab, Green, Oval, Scored, 3/21	Glimepiride 2 mg	Amaryl by Dr. Reddy's	55111-0321	Antidiabetic
RDY <> 322	Tab, Blue, Oval, Scored, 3/22	Glimepiride 4 mg	Amaryl by Dr. Reddy's	55111-0322	Antidiabetic
RDY <> 342	Tab, Brown, Round, Film Coated	Citalopram 10 mg	Celexa by Dr. Reddy's	55111-0342	Antidepressant
RDY <> 343	Tab, Pink, Round	Citalopram 20 mg	Celexa by Dr. Reddy's	55111-0343	Antidepressant
RDY <> 344	Tab, White, Round	Citalopram 40 mg	Celexa by Dr. Reddy's	55111-0344	Antidepressant
RDY <> 422	Tab, White, Oblong, Ex Release	Ciprofloxacin 500 mg	Cipro XR by Dr. Reddy's	55111-0422	Antibiotic
RDY <> 423	Tab, White, Oblong, Ex Release	Ciprofloxacin 1000 mg	Cipro XR by Dr. Reddy's	55111-0423	Antibiotic
RDY <> 429	Tab, White, Round, Film Coated	Metformin HCl 500 mg	Glucophage by Dr. Reddy's	55111-0429	Antidiabetic
RDY <> 430	Tab, White, Cap Shaped, Film Coated	Metformin HCl 850 mg	Glucophage by Dr. Reddy's	55111-0430	Antidiabetic
RDY <> 431	Tab, White, Oval, Film Coated, Scored, RD / Y <> 43 / 1	Metformin HCl 1000 mg	Glucophage by Dr. Reddy's	55111-0431	Antidiabetic
RDY <> 478	Tab, Light Pink, Cap Shaped, Film Coated	Zolpidem Tartrate 5 mg	Ambien by Dr. Reddy's	55111-0478	Sedative/Hypnotic; C IV
RDY <> 479	Tab, White, Cap Shaped, Film Coated	Zolpidem Tartrate 10 mg	Ambien by Dr. Reddy's	55111-0479	Sedative/Hypnotic; C IV
RDY <> 486	Tab, White, Oval	Nabumetone 500 mg	Relafen by Dr. Reddy's	55111-0486	NSAID
RDY <> 487	Tab, White, Oval	Nabumetone 750 mg	Relafen by Dr. Reddy's	55111-0487	NSAID
RDY <> 545	Tab, Peach, Round, Biconvex	Venlafaxine 25 mg	Effexor by Dr. Reddy's	55111-0545	Antidepressant
RDY <> 546	Tab, Peach, Round, Biconvex	Venlafaxine 37.5 mg	Effexor by Dr. Reddy's	55111-0546	Antidepressant
RDY <> 547	Tab, Peach, Round, Biconvex	Venlafaxine 50 mg	Effexor by Dr. Reddy's	55111-0547	Antidepressant
RDY <> 548	Tab, Peach, Round, Biconvex	Venlafaxine 75 mg	Effexor by Dr. Reddy's	55111-0548	Antidepressant
RDY <> 549	Tab, Peach, Round, Flat	Venlafaxine 100 mg	Effexor by Dr. Reddy's	55111-0549	Antidepressant
RDY272	Tab, Blue, Round	Naproxen Sodium 220 mg	Aleve by Dr. Reddy's	55111-0272	NSAID
RDY273	Tab, Blue, Cap Shaped	Naproxen Sodium 220 mg	Aleve by Dr. Reddy's	55111-0273	NSAID
RDY288	Cap, White and Flesh, Opaque	Zonisamide 100 mg	Zonegran by Dr. Reddy's	55111-0288	Anticonvulsant
RDY310	Cap, Pink and Yellow	Nizatidine 150 mg	Axid by Dr. Reddy's	55111-0310	Gastrointestinal
RDY311	Cap, Pink and White	Nizatidine 300 mg	Axid by Dr. Reddy's	55111-0311	Gastrointestinal
RDY343	Tab, Pink, Round, Scored	Citalopram 20 mg	Celexa by Dr. Reddy's	55111-0343	Antidepressant
RDY344	Cap, Orange Cap, White Body	Citalopram 40 mg	Celexa by Dr. Reddy's	55111-0344	Antidepressant
RDY351	Cap, Swedish Orange Cap, White Body	Cetirizine 10 mg	Zyrtec by Dr. Reddy's	55111-0351	Antihistamine
RDY402	Cap, White, Opaque	Zonisamide 25 mg	Zonegran by Dr. Reddy's	55111-0402	Anticonvulsant
RDY403	Cap, White, Opaque	Zonisamide 50 mg	Zonegran by Dr. Reddy's	55111-0403	Anticonvulsant
RDY438	Cap, Yellow Cap, White Body	Ramipril 1.25 mg	Altace by Dr. Reddy's	55111-0438	Antihypertensive
RDY439	Cap, Orange Cap, White Body	Ramipril 2.5 mg	Altace by Dr. Reddy's	55111-0439	Antihypertensive
RDY440	Cap, Swedish Orange Cap, White Body	Ramipril 5 mg	Altace by Dr. Reddy's	55111-0440	Antihypertensive
RDY441	Cap, Light Elue and White Body	Ramipril 10 mg	Altace by Dr. Reddy's	55111-0441	Antihypertensive
RDY532	Cap, Light Elue and White	Divalproex Sodium 125 mg	Depakote Sprinkles by Dr. Reddy's	55111-0532	Anticonvulsant
RE <> 19	Tab, White, Round	Atenolol 25 mg	Tenormin by Ranbaxy	63304-0621	Antihypertensive
RE16	Tab, White, Cap Shaped, Scored, Coated	Sertraline HCl 25 mg	Zoloft by Ranbaxy	63304-0164	Antidepressant
RE20	Tab, White, Round, Scored	Atenolol 50 mg	Tenormin by Ranbaxy	63304-0622	Antihypertensive

ID FRONT <> BACK	DESCRIPTION FRONT <> BACK	INGREDIENT & STRENGTH	BRAND (or Generic Equiv.) by FIRM	NDC#	CLASS; SCH.
RE22	Tab, White to Off-White, Round	Furosemide 20 mg	Lasix by Ranbaxy	63304-0624	Diuretic
RE23	Tab, White to Off-White, Round	Furosemide 40 mg	Lasix by Ranbaxy	63304-0625	Diuretic
RE24	Tab, White to Off-White, Round	Furosemide 80 mg	Lasix by Ranbaxy	63304-0626	Diuretic
RE25	Tab, Pink to Peach, Rounded Rectangle Shaped	Pravastatin 10 mg	Ran-Pravastatin by Ranbaxy	Canadian DIN 02284421	Antihyperlipidemic
RE26	Tab, Yellow, Rounded Rectangle Shaped	Pravastatin 20 mg	Ran-Pravastatin by Ranbaxy	Canadian DIN 02284448	Antihyperlipidemic
RE27	Tab, Green, Rounded Rectangle Shaped	Pravastatin 40 mg	Ran-Pravastatin by Ranbaxy	Canadian DIN 02284456	Antihyperlipidemic
RE75	Tab, Pink, Round, Scored	Metoprolol Tartrate 50 mg	Lopressor by Ranbaxy	63304-0580	Antihypertensive
RE76	Tab, White, Round	Metoprolol Tartrate 100 mg	Lopressor by Ranbaxy	63304-0581	Antihypertensive
REBETOL200MG	Cap, White, Opaque, Rebetol 200MG <> Schering Logo	Ribavirin 200 mg	Rebetol by Schering	00085-1327	Antiviral
REBETOL200MG	Cap, White, Opaque, Rebetol 200MG <> Schering Logo	Ribavirin 200 mg	Rebetol by Schering	00085-1351	Antiviral
REBETOL200MG	Cap, White, Opaque, Rebetol 200MG <> Schering Logo	Ribavirin 200 mg	Rebetol by Schering	00085-1385	Antiviral
REBETOL200MG	Cap, White, Opaque, Rebetol 200MG <> Schering Logo	Ribavirin 200 mg	Rebetol by Schering	00085-1194	Antiviral
REDKAT	Cap, Red, Black Ink, RED KAT and Cat Head Outline	RED KAT Formula 750 mg: Lauroyl Macrogol-32 Glycerides, Propylene Glycol Monocaprylate, BIOTEST Nano-Dispersed Gel Eurycoma Longifolia extract, Sclaremax (proprietary sclareolide)	Red Kat by BioTest Labs	53922-1194	Supplement
REGLAN <> AHR10	Tab, White, Cap Shaped, Scored	Metoclopramide HCl 10 mg	Reglan by Nat Pharmpak	55154-3004	Gastrointestinal
REGLAN <> AHR10	Tab, White, Cap Shaped, Scored	Metoclopramide HCl 10 mg	Reglan by Thrift Drug	59198-0099	Gastrointestinal
REGLAN <> AHR10	Tab, White, Cap Shaped, Scored	Metoclopramide HCl 10 mg	Reglan by Wal Mart	49035-0157	Gastrointestinal
REGLAN <> AP10	Tab, White, Cap Shaped, Scored	Metoclopramide 10 mg	Reglan by Alaven Pharmaceutical	68220-0151	Gastrointestinal
REGLAN <> SP10	Tab, White, Cap Shaped, Scored	Metoclopramide 10 mg	Reglan by Schwarz	00091-6701	Gastrointestinal
REGLAN5 <> AP	Tab, Green, Elliptical-Shaped	Metoclopramide 5 mg	Reglan by Alaven Pharmaceutical	68220-0150	Gastrointestinal
REGLAN5 <> SP	Tab, Green, Oval	Metoclopramide 5 mg	Reglan by Schwarz	00091-6705	Gastrointestinal
REL900	Cap , Clear filled with Light Yellow Liquid, Soft Gel	Omega-3-Acid Ethyl Esters 1 g	Lovaza by Reliant	65726-0424	Antihyperlipidemic
REL900	Cap, Clear filled with Light Yellow Liquid, Soft Gel	Omega-3-Acid Ethyl Esters 1 g	Lovaza by Abbott	00074-5792	Antihyperlipidemic
RELAFEN <> 500	Tab, White, Oblong, Film Coated	Nabumetone 500 mg	Relafen by SKB	00029-4851	NSAID
RELAFEN <> 500	Tab, White, Oblong, Film Coated	Nabumetone 500 mg	by Eli Lilly	Canadian	NSAID
RELAFEN <> 500	Tab, White, Oblong, Film Coated	Nabumetone 500 mg	Relafen by SKB	Canadian	NSAID
RELAFEN <> 500	Tab, White, Oblong, Film Coated	Nabumetone 500 mg	Relafen by H J Harkins Co	52959-0227	NSAID
RELAFEN <> 500	Tab, White, Oblong, Film Coated	Nabumetone 500 mg	by Allscripts		NSAID
RELAFEN <> 750	Tab, Beige, Oblong, Film Coated	Nabumetone 750 mg	by Nat Pharmpak	55154-4505	NSAID
RELAFEN <> 750	Tab, Beige, Oblong, Film Coated	Nabumetone 750 mg	Relafen by Rx Dispensing	61807-0051	NSAID
RELAFEN <> 750	Tab, Beige, Oblong, Film Coated	Nabumetone 750 mg	by PDRX	55289-0015	NSAID
RELAFEN <> 750	Tab, Beige, Oblong, Film Coated	Nabumetone 750 mg	Relafen by SB	59742-4851	NSAID
RELAFEN <> 750	Tab, Beige, Oblong, Film Coated	Nabumetone 750 mg	by Amerisource	62584-0851	NSAID
RELAFEN <> 750	Tab, Beige, Oblong, Film Coated	Nabumetone 750 mg	Relafen by SKB	00029-4852	NSAID
RELAFEN <> 750	Tab, Beige, Oblong, Film Coated	Nabumetone 750 mg	Relafen by SB	59742-4852	NSAID
RELAFEN <> 750	Tab, Beige, Oblong, Film Coated	Nabumetone 750 mg	by DRX	55045-2440	NSAID
RELAFEN <> 750	Tab, Beige, Oblong, Film Coated	Nabumetone 750 mg	Relafen by H J Harkins Co	52959-0373	NSAID
RELAFEN <> 750	Tab, Beige, Oblong, Film Coated	Nabumetone 750 mg	Relafen by Rx Dispensing	61807-0059	NSAID
RELAFEN <> 750	Tab, Beige, Oblong, Film Coated	Nabumetone 750 mg	Relafen by Allscripts		NSAID
RELAGESIC <> IEL650	Tab, White, Oblong, Scored	Phenyltoloxamine Citrate 50 mg, Acetaminophen 650 mg	Relagesic by Int'l Ethical Labs	11584-0476	Cold Remedy
RELIANT225	Cap, White, Opaque, Hard Gel, Reliant Logo "Reliant 225"	Propafenone HCl 225 mg	Rythmol SR by Reliant	65726-0261	Antiarrhythmic
RELIANT325	Cap, White, Opaque, Hard Gel, Reliant Logo "Reliant 325", Red Band	Propafenone HCl 325 mg	Rythmol SR by Reliant Pharmaceuticals	65726-0262	Antiarrhythmic
RELIANT425	Cap, White, Opaque, Hard Gel, Reliant Logo "Reliant 425", Three Bands	Propafenone HCl 425 mg	Rythmol SR by Abbott	65726-0263	Antiarrhythmic

ID FRONT <> BACK	DESCRIPTION FRONT <> BACK	INGREDIENT & STRENGTH	BRAND (or Generic Equiv.) by FIRM	NDC#	CLASS; SCH.
RENAGEL400	Tab, Off-White with Black Print, Oval, Film Coated	Sevelamer HCl 400 mg	Renagel by Genzyme	58468-0020	Phosphate Binder
RENAGEL800	Tab, Off-White with Black Print, Oval, Film Coated	Sevelamer HCl 800 mg	Renagel by Genzyme	58468-0021	Phosphate Binder
RENVELA800	Tab, White, Oval, Film Coated	Sevelamer Carbonate 800 mg	Renvela by Genzyme	Canadian DIN 02256290	Phosphate Binder
REP20 <> PFIZER	Tab, Orange, Round, Film Coated	Eletriptan HBr 20 mg	Relpax by Pfizer		Antimigraine
REP20 <> PFIZER	Tab, Orange, Round, Film Coated	Eletriptan HBr 20 mg	Relpax by Roerig	00049-2330	Antimigraine
REP40 <> PFIZER	Tab, Orange, Round, Film Coated	Eletriptan HBr 40 mg	Relpax by Roerig	00049-2340	Antimigraine
REP40 <> PFIZER	Tab, Orange, Round, Film Coated	Eletriptan HBr 40 mg	Relpax by Pfizer	Canadian DIN 02256304	Antimigraine
REQUA	Cap, Pink	Activated Charcoal 250 mg	Charcocaps by Requa	10961-0030	Gastrointestinal
RESCON	Cap, Printed in White, Ex Release	Chlorpheniramine Maleate 12 mg, Pseudoephedrine HCl 120 mg	Deconamine SR by Sovereign	58716-0023	Cold Remedy
RESCON	Tab, Green	Chlorpheniramine Maleate 8 mg, Methscopolamine Nitrate 2.5 mg, Pseudoephedrine HCl 120 mg	Rescon-Mx by Sovereign	58716-0674	Cold Remedy
RESCON	Tab, Green	Chlorpheniramine Maleate 8 mg, Methscopolamine Nitrate 2.5 mg, Pseudoephedrine HCl 120 mg	Rescon-Mx by ION	11808-0088 Discontinued	Cold Remedy
RESCON	Tab, White, Oblong, Scored, Res/Con	Chlorpheniramine Maleate 8 mg, Methscopolamine Nitrate 2.5 mg, Pseudoephedrine HCl 120 mg	by Compumed	00403-0002	Cold Remedy
RESCON	Tab, Purple and Yellow, Cap Shaped, Scored, Bilayered	Phenylephrine HCl 40 mg SR, Chlorpheniramine Maleate 12 mg SR, Methscopolamine Nitrate 2 mg IR	Rescon by Capellon	64543-0095	Cold Remedy
RESCON	Tab, Green	Pseudoephedrine HCl 120 mg, Chlorpheniramine Maleate 8 mg, Methscopolamine Nitrate 2.5 mg	Rescon-Mx by Capellon	64543-0089	Cold Remedy
RESCONED	Cap, Green & Clear, Black Ink	Pseudoephedrine HCl 120 mg, Chlorpheniramine Maleate 8 mg	Rescon ED by RX Pak	65084-0112	Cold Remedy
RESCONED	Cap, Ex Release, Rescon ED	Chlorpheniramine Maleate 8 mg, Pseudoephedrine HCl 120 mg	Rescon ED by Sovereign	58716-0021	Cold Remedy
RESCONJR	Tab, Yellow and White, Bilayered, Cap Shaped, Scored	Chlorpheniramine Maleate 4 mg, Pseudoephedrine HCl 60 mg	Rescon Jr by Sovereign	58716-0022	Cold Remedy
RESCONJR	Tab, Yellow and White, Bilayered, Cap Shaped, Scored	Chlorpheniramine Maleate 4 mg, Phenylephrine HCl 20 mg	Rescon Jr by Capellon	64543-0085	Cold Remedy
RESPA733	Tab, White, Oblong, Scored	Dextromethorphan HBr 30 mg, Guaifenesin 600 mg, Pseudoephedrine HCl 37.5 mg	by DRX	55045-2649	Cold Remedy
RESPA733	Tab, White, Oblong, Scored, Respa over 733	Guaifenesin 600 mg, Phenylpropanolamine HCl 37.5 mg, Dextromethorphan HBr 30 mg	by Med Pro	53978-3328	Cold Remedy
RESPA78	Tab, White, Oblong, Scored	Guaifenesin 600 mg, Dextromethorphan HBr 28 mg	Humibid-DM by Med Pro		Cold Remedy
RESPA78	Tab, White, Oblong, Scored	Dextromethorphan HBr 28 mg, Guaifenesin 600 mg	by DRX	55045-2617	Cold Remedy
RESPA786	Tab, Embossed, Ex Release, Respa over 786	Guaifenesin 600 mg	Robitussin by Pharmafab	62542-0702	Expectorant
RESPA786	Tab, Respa786	Guaifenesin 600 mg	Robitussin by Anabolic	00722-6334	Expectorant
RESPA787	Tab, Ex Release	Guaifenesin 600 mg, Pseudoephedrine HCl 60 mg	Respa 1st by Respa	60575-0108	Cold Remedy
RESPA787	Tab, Ex Release, Respa over 787	Guaifenesin 600 mg, Pseudoephedrine HCl 60 mg	Respa 1st by Pharmafab	62542-0742	Cold Remedy
RESPA787	Tab	Guaifenesin 600 mg, Pseudoephedrine HCl 60 mg	Respa 1st by Anabolic	00722-6350	Cold Remedy
RESPA788	Tab, Ex Release, Respa788	Dextromethorphan 30 mg, Guaifenesin 600 mg	Respa-DM by Respa	60575-0123	Cold Remedy
RESPA788	Tab, Ex Release, Respa788	Dextromethorphan 30 mg, Guaifenesin 600 mg	Respa-DM by Pharmafab	62542-0721	Cold Remedy
RESPA788	Tab, Respa788	Dextromethorphan 30 mg, Guaifenesin 600 mg	Respa-DM by Anabolic	00722-6349	Cold Remedy
RESPA789	Cap, Ex Release	Brompheniramine Maleate 6 mg, Pseudoephedrine HCl 60 mg	Respahist by Pharmafab	62542-0102	Cold Remedy
RESPA790	Tab Ex Release	Belladonna Alkaloids 0.24 mg, Chlorpheniramine Maleate 8 mg, Phenylephrine HCl 25 mg, Phenylpropanolamine HCl 50 mg	Respa ARM by Respa	60575-0790	Cold Remedy
RESPA790	Tab	Belladonna Alkaloids 0.24 mg, Chlorpheniramine Maleate 8 mg, Phenylephrine HCl 25 mg, Phenylpropanolamine HCl 50 mg	Respa ARM by Anabolic	00722-6371	Cold Remedy
RESPA87	Tab, White, Oblong, Scored	Guaifenesin 600 mg, Pseudoephedrine HCl 58 mg	by Med Pro	53978-3357	Cold Remedy
RESPA87	Tab, White, Oblong, Scored	Guaifenesin 600 mg, Pseudoephedrine HCl 58 mg	by Med Pro	53978-3347	Cold Remedy
RESTORIL15MG-FORSLEEPM	Cap, Pink & Maroon, M inside Square	Temazepam 15 mg	Restoril by Med Pro	53978-3080	Sedative/Hypnotic; C IV
RESTORIL15MG-FORSLEEPM	Cap, Pink & Maroon, M inside Square	Temazepam 15 mg	Restoril by Mallinckrodt	00406-9916	Sedative/Hypnotic; C IV

ID FRONT <> BACK	DESCRIPTION FRONT <> BACK	INGREDIENT & STRENGTH	BRAND (or Generic Equiv.) by FIRM	NDC#	CLASS; SCH.
RESTORIL225MG-FORSLEEPM	Cap, Blue, 22.5 mg, M inside Square	Temazepam 22.5 mg	Restoril by Mallinckrodt	00406-9914	Sedative/Hypnotic; C IV
RESTORIL30MG-FORSLEEP	Cap, Blue & Maroon	Temazepam 30 mg	Restoril by Med Pro	53978-3081	Sedative/Hypnotic; C IV
RESTORIL30MG-FORSLEEPM	Cap, Blue & Maroon, M inside Square	Temazepam 30 mg	Restoril by Mallinckrodt	00406-9917	Sedative/Hypnotic; C IV
RESTORIL75MG-FORSLEEPM	Cap, Pink & Blue, M inside Square	Temazepam 7.5 mg	Restoril by Mallinckrodt	00406-9915	Sedative/Hypnotic; C IV
RETE	Tab, Blue, Round	Caffeine 65 mg, Potassium Salicylate 75 mg, Salicylamide 3.0 mg	Trim-Elim by Reese	10956-0647	Diuretic
REV10MG	Cap, Blue/Green and Pale Yellow, Opaque	Lenalidomide 10 mg	Revlimid by Celgene	59572-0410	Immunomodulator
REV10MG	Cap, Blue Green Opaque, Pale Yellow Opaque	Lenalidomide 10 mg	Revlimid by Celgene	Canadian DIN 02304902	Antineoplastic and Immunomodulator
REV15MG	Cap, Powder Blue Opaque, White Opaque	Lenalidomide 15 mg	Revlimid by Celgene	Canadian DIN 02317699	Antineoplastic and Immunomodulator
REV15MG	Cap, Powder Blue and White, Opaque	Lenalidomide 15 mg	Revlimid by Celgene	59572-0415	Immunomodulator
REV25MG	Cap, White, Opaque	Lenalidomide 25 mg	Revlimid by Celgene	Canadian DIN 02317710	Antineoplastic and Immunomodulator
REV25MG	Cap, White, Opaque	Lenalidomide 25 mg	Revlimid by Celgene	59572-0425	Immunomodulator
REV5MG	Cap, White, Opaque	Lenalidomide 5 mg	Revlimid by Celgene	59572-0405	Immunomodulator
REV5MG	Cap, White, Opaque	Lenalidomide 5 mg	Revlimid by Celgene	Canadian DIN 02304899	Antineoplastic and Immunomodulator
REVIA <> 177	Tab, Pale Yellow, Cap Shaped, Scored	Naltrexone 50 mg	Revia by Apotex	Canadian DIN 02213826	Opioid Antagonist
RF11	Tab, White, Oval	Metoclopramide 10 mg	Reglan by Ranbaxy	63304-0846	Gastrointestinal
RF26	Cap, Teal, Hard Gel	Hydrochlorothiazide 12.5 mg	by Heritage	23155-0140	Diuretic; Antihypertensive
RG <> 770	Tab, White to Off-White, Triangular-Shaped, Film-Coated	Finasteride 5 mg	Proscar by Barr	00555-0770 Discontinued	Antiandrogen
RG <> F100	Tab, White to Off-White, Rectangular, Rounded	Fluconazole 100 mg	Diflucan by Barr	00555-0772	Antifungal
RG <> F150	Tab, White to Off-White, Rectangular, Rounded	Fluconazole 150 mg	Diflucan by Barr	00555-0773	Antifungal
RG <> F200	Tab, White to Off-White, Rectangular, Rounded	Fluconazole 200 mg	Diflucan by Barr	00555-0774	Antifungal
RG <> F50	Tab, White to Off-White, Round, Film-Coated	Fluconazole 50 mg	Diflucan by Barr	00555-0771	Antifungal
RG <> L		Bicalutamide 50 mg	Casodex by Cobalt	Canadian DIN 02274337	Antiandrogen
RGPBM	Cap	Acetaminophen 300 mg, Phenyltoloxamine Citrate 20 mg, Salicylamide 200 mg	by Pharmakon	55422-0411	Analgesic
RGPBM	Cap	Acetaminophen 300 mg, Phenyltoloxamine Citrate 20 mg, Salicylamide 200 mg	by Seatrace	00551-0411	Analgesic
RH	Tab, Pink, Round	Trimipramine 12.5 mg	Rhotrimine by Rhodiapharm	Canadian	Antidepressant
RH100RHOTRAL	Tab, White, Shield, RH/100-Rhotral	Acebutolol HCl 100 mg	Sectral by Rhodiapharm	Canadian	Antihypertensive
RH200RHOTRAL	Tab, Blue, Shield, RH/200-Rhotral	Acebutolol HCl 200 mg	Sectral by Rhodiapharm	Canadian	Antihypertensive
RH400RHOTRAL	Tab, White, Shield, RH/400-Rhotral	Acebutolol HCl 400 mg	Rhotral by Rhodiapharm	Canadian	Antihypertensive
RHO05	Tab, Orange, Round, RHO/0.5	Clonazepam 0.5 mg	Rho-Clonazepam by Rhoxal Pharma	Canadian	Sedative
RHO1	Tab, Green, Round, RHO/1	Clonazepam 1 mg	Rho-Clonazepam by Rhoxal Pharma	Canadian	Sedative
RHO10	Tab, White, Round, RHO/10	Nitrazepam 10 mg	Rho-Nitrazepam by Rhoxal Pharma	Canadian	Sedative/Hypnotic; C IV
RHO160	Tab, Light Blue, Oblong, RHO-160	Sotalol HCl 160 mg	Rho-Sotalol by Rhoxal Pharma	Canadian	Antiarrhythmic
RHO2	Tab, White, Round, RHO/2	Clonazepam 2 mg	Rho-Clonazepam by Rhoxal Pharma	Canadian	Sedative
RHO2	Tab, Green, Oblong, RHO-2	Loperamide 2 mg	Imodium by Rhoxal Pharma	Canadian	Antidiarrheal
RHO5	Tab, White, Round, RHO/5	Nitrazepam 5 mg	Rho-Nitrazepam by Rhoxal Pharma	Canadian	Sedative/Hypnotic; C IV
RHO500	Tab, White, Round, RHO/500	Metformin HCl 500 mg	Glucophage by Rhoxal Pharma	Canadian	Antidiabetic
RHO80	Tab, Light Blue, Oblong, RHO-80	Sotalol HCl 80 mg	Rho-Sotalol by Rhoxal Pharma	Canadian	Antiarrhythmic

ID FRONT <> BACK	DESCRIPTION FRONT <> BACK	INGREDIENT & STRENGTH	BRAND (or Generic Equiv.) by FIRM	NDC#	CLASS: SCH.
RHODOX10	Cap, Pink & Red, RHO/DOX 10	Doxepin HCl 10 mg	Rho Doxepin by Rhodiapharm	Canadian	Antidepressant
RHODOX25	Cap, Blue & Pink, RHO/DOX 25	Doxepin HCl 25 mg	Rho Doxepin by Rhodiapharm	Canadian	Antidepressant
RHODOX 50	Cap, Pink/Salmon, RHO/DOX 50	Doxepin HCl 50 mg	Rho Doxepin by Rhodiapharm	Canadian	Antidepressant
RHODXY100	Cap, Blue & Opaque, RHO/DXY 100	Doxycycline Hyclate 100 mg	Rho Doxycin by Rhodiapharm	Canadian	Antibiotic
RHODXY100	Tab, Orange, RHO/DXY 200	Doxycycline Hyclate 100 mg	Rho Doxycin Tabs by Rhodiapharm	Canadian	Antibiotic
RHOPIR10	Cap, Maroon/Blue, RHO/PIR 10	Piroxicam 10 mg	Feldene by Rhodiapharm	Canadian	NSAID
RHOPIR20	Cap, Maroon/Opaque, RHO/PIR 20	Piroxicam 20 mg	Feldene by Rhodiapharm	Canadian	NSAID
RHOPRA1	Cap, Orange, RHO/PRA 1	Prazosin HCl 1 mg	Rho Prazosin by Rhodiapharm	Canadian	Antihypertensive
RHOPRA2	Tab, White, Round, RHO/PRA 2	Prazosin HCl 2 mg	Rho Prazosin by Rhodiapharm	Canadian	Antihypertensive
RHOPRA5	Tab, White, Diamond, RHO/PRA 5	Prazosin HCl 5 mg	Rho Prazosin by Rhodiapharm	Canadian	Antihypertensive
RHOVAIL150MG	Cap, Pink & White, Rhovail/150 mg	Ketoprofen 150 mg	Orudis by Rho-Pharm	Canadian	NSAID
RHOVAIL200MG	Cap, Pink & Elue, Rhovail/200 mg	Ketoprofen 200 mg	Orudis by Rho-Pharm	Canadian	NSAID
RHRHODISSR200	Tab, White, Round, RH-Rhodis SR 200	Ketoprofen 200 mg	Orudis by Rhodiapharm	Canadian	NSAID
RHRHRHOVANE	Tab, Blue, Oval, RH/RH-Rhovane	Zopiclone 7.5 mg	Rhovane by Rhodiapharm	Canadian	Hypnotic
RI1 <> APO	Tab, White, Cap Shaped, Scored	Risperidone 1 mg	Risperdal by Apotex	Canadian DIN 02282135	Antipsychotic
RI2 <> APO	Tab, Peach, Cap Shaped, Scored	Risperidone 2 mg	Risperdal by Apotex	Canadian DIN 02282143	Antipsychotic
RI25 <> APO	Tab, Yellowish-Orange, Cap Shaped, APO <> RI .25	Risperidone 0.25 mg	Risperdal by Apotex	Canadian DIN 02282119	Antipsychotic
RI3 <> APO	Tab, Yellow, Cap Shaped, Scored	Risperidone 3 mg	Risperdal by Apotex	Canadian DIN 02282151	Antipsychotic
RI4 <> APO	Tab, Green, Cap Shaped, Scored	Risperidone 4 mg	Risperdal by Apotex	Canadian DIN 02282178	Antipsychotic
RI5 <> APO	Tab, Reddish-Brown, Cap Shaped, Scored, APO <> RI .5	Risperidone 0.50 mg	Risperdal by Apotex	Canadian DIN 02282127	Antipsychotic
RIB200 <> ROCHE	Tab, Pink, Oval, Film Coated	Ribavirin 200 mg	Pegasys RBV by Roche	Canadian DIN 02253410	Antiviral
RIB200 <> ROCHE	Tab, Pink, Oval, Film Coated	Ribavirin 200 mg	Copegus by Hoffmann La Roche	00004-0086	Antiviral
RIBA200RIBA200	Cap, White, Opaque	Ribavirin 200 mg	Ribasphere by Par	49884-0856	Antiviral
RIDAURA	Cap, Red ard White	Auranofin 3 mg	Ridaura by Connetics	63032-0011	Antiarthritic
RIDAURA	Cap, Red and White	Auranofin 3 mg	Ridaura by SKB	Canadian	Antiarthritic
RIFADIN150	Cap, Red, Hard Gel	Rifampin 150 mg	Rifadin by Merrell	00068-0510	Antibiotic
RIFADIN150	Cap, Red, Hard Gel	Rifampin 150 mg	Rifadin by H J Harkins Co	52959-0461	Antibiotic
RIFADIN150	Cap, Red, Hard Gel	Rifampin 150 mg	Rifadin by Dept Health	53808-0011	Antibiotic
RIFADIN300	Cap, Red, Hard Gel, Rifadin over 300	Rifampin 300 mg	Rifadin by Merrell	00068-0508	Antibiotic
RIFADIN300	Cap, Red, Hard Gel, Rifadin over 300	Rifampin 300 mg	Rifadin by Dept Health	53808-0012	Antibiotic
RIFAMATE	Cap, Red, Opaque, Hard Gel	Rifampin 300 mg, Isoniazid 150 mg	Rifamate by Merrell	00068-0509	Antibiotic
RIFAMPIN150VP015	Cap, Red, Opaque, White Print	Rifampin 150 mg	Rifadin by Versapharm	61748-0015	Antibiotic
RIFAMPIN300VP018	Cap, Red, Opaque, White Print	Rifampin 300 mg	Rifadin by Versapharm	61748-0018	Antibiotic
RIFATER	Tab, Light Eeige, Black Print, Round, Sugar Coated	Isoniazid 50 mg, Pyrazinamide 300 mg, Rifampin 120 mg	Rifater by Aventis	00088-0576	Antimycobacterial
RIFATER	Tab, Light Beige, Black Print, Round, Sugar Coated	Isoniazid 50 mg, Pyrazinamide 300 mg, Rifampin 120 mg	Rifater by Gruppo Lepetit	12522-8576	Antimycobacterial
RIKER <> NORGESICFORTE	Tab, Green	Aspirin 770 mg, Caffeine 60 mg, Orphenadrine Citrate 50 mg	Norgesic Forte by Pharmedix	53002-0376	Analgesic
RIKER125PLUS	Tab, White, Round, Riker/125 Plus	Theophylline Anhydrous 125 mg, Guaifenesin 100 mg	Theolair-Plus by Riker		Antiasthmatic
RIKER161	Tab, Green, Round, Riker/161	Orphenadrine HCl 50 mg	Disipal by 3M		Muscle Relaxant
RIKER250PLUS	Cap, White, Riker/250 Plus	Theophylline Anhydrous 250 mg, Guaifenesin 200 mg	Theolair-Plus by 3M		Antiasthmatic
RIKER265	Tab, Browr, Round, Riker/265	Rauwolfia Serpentina 2 mg	Rauwloid by 3M		Antihypertensive
RIOPANPLUS	Tab, White, Round	Magaldrate 480 mg	Riopan by Whitehall Robins	Canadian	Gastrointestinal

ID FRONT <> BACK	DESCRIPTION FRONT <> BACK	INGREDIENT & STRENGTH	BRAND (or Generic Equiv.) by FIRM	NDC#	CLASS; SCH.
RIS025 <> JANSSEN	Tab, Yellow, Round	Risperidone 0.25 mg	Risperdal by Janssen	62579-0301	Antipsychotic
RIS025 <> JANSSEN	Tab, Dark Yellow, Cap Shaped, Ris 0.25	Risperidone 0.25 mg	Risperdal by Janssen	50458-0301	Antipsychotic
RIS025 <> JANSSEN	Tab, Dark Yellow, Cap Shaped, Ris 0.25	Risperidone 0.25 mg	Risperdal by Janssen-Ortho	Canadian DIN 02240551	Antipsychotic
RIS05 <> JANSSEN	Tab, Red-Brown, Cap Shaped, Ris 0.5	Risperidone 0.5 mg	Risperdal by Janssen-Ortho	Canadian DIN 02240552	Antipsychotic
RIS05 <> JANSSEN	Tab, Red-Brown, Cap Shaped, Ris 0.5	Risperidone 0.5 mg	Risperdal by Janssen	50458-0302	Antipsychotic
RIS05 <> JANSSEN	Tab, Red, Janssen <> RIS 0.5	Risperidone 0.5 mg	Risperdal by RX Pak	65084-0197	Antipsychotic
RIS1	Tab, White, Cap Shaped	Risperidone 1 mg	Risperdal by Janssen-Ortho	Canadian DIN 02025280	Antipsychotic
RIS102	Tab, Dark Green, Cap Shaped	Multiple Vitamins and Minerals	Vita S Forte by Rising	64980-0102	Vitamin
RIS107	Tab, Blue, Cap Shaped	Prenatal Vitamins, Ferrous Fumarate 65 mg, FA 1 mg	Natafolic-PN by Rising	64980-0107	Vitamin
RIS108	Tab, White, Cap Shaped, Scored	Dextromethorphan 60 mg, Guaifenesin 1200 mg	Entab-DM by Rising	64980-0108	Cold Remedy
RIS110	Tab, White, Oval, RIS / 110	Niacinamide 750 mg, Zinc 25 mg, Folic Acid 0.5 mg	Niafol by Rising	64980-0110	Dermatologic
RIS118	Tab, Green, Cap Shaped	Multiple Vitamins and Minerals	Nutrifac ZX by Rising	64980-0118	Vitamin
RIS121	Tab, White, Oval	Vitamin Combination	Nu-Natal Advanced by Rising	64980-0125	Vitamin; Supplement
RIS1JANSSEN	Tab, White, Oblong, Ris 1/Janssen	Risperidone 1 mg	Risperdal by Janssen	Canadian	Antipsychotic
RIS2	Tab, Orange, Oblong, Scored	Risperidone 2 mg	Risperdal by Janssen-Ortho	Canadian DIN 02025299	Antipsychotic
RIS3	Tab, Yellow, Oblong, Scored	Risperidone 3 mg	Risperdal by Janssen-Ortho	Canadian DIN 02025302	Antipsychotic
RIS4	Tab, Green, Oblong, Scored	Risperidone 4 mg	Risperdal by Janssen-Ortho	Canadian DIN 02025310	Antipsychotic
RIVA	Tab, Green, Film-Coated	Calcium Carbonate 1250 mg, Vitamin D 125 IU	Calcite D by Riva	Canadian DIN 00688770	Vitamin; Mineral
RIVA	Tab, Yellow, Film-Coated	Calcium Carbonate 1250 mg	Calcite by Riva	Canadian DIN 00646474	Vitamin; Mineral
RIVOTRIL05ROCHE	Tab, Orange, Cylindrical, Rivotril/0.5/Roche	Clonazepam 0.5 mg	Rivotril by Roche	Canadian	Sedative; C IV
RL	Cap	Dronabinol 5 mg	Marinol by Banner Pharma	10888-1039	Antiemetic; C III
RL	Cap	Dronabinol 2.5 mg	Marinol by Banner Pharma	10888-1037	Antiemetic; C III
RL	Cap	Dronabinol 5 mg	Marinol by Banner Pharma	10888-1038	Antiemetic; C III
RL	Cap, White	Dronabinol 2.5 mg	Marinol by Sanofi	Canadian	Antiemetic; C III
RL	Cap, White, Gelatin, Round	Dronabinol 2.5 mg	Marinol by Roxane	00054-2601	Antiemetic; C III
RL	Cap, Brown	Dronabinol 5 mg	Marinol by Sanofi	Canadian	Antiemetic; C III
RL	Cap, Dark Brown, Gelatin, Round	Dronabinol 5 mg	Marinol by Roxane	00054-2602	Antiemetic; C III
RL	Cap, Dark Brown	Dronabinol 5 mg	Marinol by Unimed	00051-0022	Antiemetic; Antivertigo; C III
RL	Cap, White	Dronabinol 2.5 mg	Marinol by Unimed	00051-0021	Antiemetic; Antivertigo; C III
RL	Cap, Orange	Dronabinol 10 mg	Marinol by Unimed	00051-0023	Antiemetic; Antivertigo; C III
RL	Cap, Orange	Dronabinol 10 mg	Marinol by Sanofi	Canadian	Antiemetic; C III
RL	Cap, Orange, Gelatin, Round	Dronabinol 10 mg	Marinol by Roxane	00054-2603	Antiemetic; C III
RO26	Tab, White, Round	Phenobarbital 15 mg	Phenobarbital by Rondex		Sedative/Hypnotic; C IV
RO28	Tab, White, Round	Phenobarbital 30 mg	by Rondex		Sedative/Hypnotic; C IV
ROA10	Cap, Oval, Reddish-Violet, Opaque, Soft Gel, ROA/10	Isotretinoin 10 mg	Accutane by Roche	Canadian DIN 00582344	Dermatologic
ROA40	Cap, Oval, Yellow, Opaque, Soft Gel, ROA/40	Isotretinoin 40 mg	Accutane by Roche	Canadian DIN 00582352	Dermatologic
ROBAXIN500 <> SP	Tab, Light Orange, Round, Scored, Film Coated	Methocarbamol 500 mg	Robaxin by Schwarz	00091-7429	Muscle Relaxant

ID FRONT <> BACK	DESCRIPTION FRONT <> BACK	INGREDIENT & STRENGTH	BRAND (or Generic Equiv.) by FIRM	NDC#	CLASS; SCH.
ROBAXIN750 <> AHR	Tab, Orange, Film Coated	Methocarbamol 750 mg	Robaxin by Schwarz	00031-7449	Muscle Relaxant
ROBAXIN750 <> AHR	Tab, Film Coated, Robaxin over 750	Methocarbamol 750 mg	Robaxin by Amerisource	62584-0450	Muscle Relaxant
ROBAXIN750 <> AHR	Tab, Film Coated	Methocarbamol 750 mg	Robaxin by Leiner	59606-0730	Muscle Relaxant
ROBAXIN750 <> AHR	Tab, Film Coated, Robaxin-750	Methocarbamol 750 mg	Robaxin by Thrift Drug	59198-0182	Muscle Relaxant
ROBAXIN750 <> SP	Tab, Orange, Cap Shaped, Film Coated	Methocarbamol 750 mg	Robaxin by Schwarz	00091-7449	Muscle Relaxant
ROBAXINAHR	Tab, Orange, Round, Scored, Film Coated	Methocarbamol 500 mg	Robaxin by Nat Pharmpak	55154-9001	Muscle Relaxant
ROBAXINAHR	Tab, Light Orange, Film Coated	Methocarbamol 500 mg	Robaxin by Schwarz	00031-7429	Muscle Relaxant
ROBAXINAHR	Tab, Orange, Round	Methocarbamol 750 mg	Robaxin by Rightpac	65240-0730	Muscle Relaxant
ROBAXISALAHR	Tab, Pink & White, Round, Scored	Aspirin 325 mg, Methocarbamol 400 mg	Robaxisal by A H Robins	00031-7469	Analgesic; Muscle Relaxant
ROBERTS <> ETHMOZINE200	Tab, Light Green, Oval, Film Coated	Moricizine HCl 200 mg	Ethmozine by Roberts	54092-0046	Antiarrhythmic
ROBERTS <> ETHMOZINE250	Tab, Light Orange, Oval, Film Coated	Moricizine HCl 250 mg	Ethmozine by Roberts	54092-0047	Antiarrhythmic
ROBERTS <> ETHMOZINE300	Tab, Light Blue, Oval, Film Coated	Moricizine HCl 300 mg	Ethmozine by Roberts	54092-0048	Antiarrhythmic
ROBERTS067	Cap, Yellow	Guaifenesin 91.44 mg, Theophylline 152.4 mg	Quibron by King	00087-0516	Antiasthmatic
ROBERTS067	Cap, Yellow	Guaifenesin 91.44 mg, Theophylline 152.4 mg	Quibron by RP Scherer	11014-0543	Antiasthmatic
ROBERTS068	Cap, Yellow	Guaifenesin 183 mg, Theophylline 305 mg	Quibron by King	00087-0515	Antiasthmatic
ROBERTS068	Cap, Yellow	Guaifenesin 183 mg, Theophylline 305 mg	Quibron by RP Scherer	11014-0730	Antiasthmatic
ROBERTS101 <> 10	Tab, Orange, Round, Flat, Beveled, Bisected	Bethanechol Chloride 10 mg	Duvoid by Shire BioChem	Canadian DIN 01947958	Urinary Tract
ROBERTS102 <> 25	Tab, White, Round, Flat, Beveled, Bisected	Bethanechol Chloride 25 mg	Duvoid by Shire BioChem	Canadian DIN 01947931	Urinary Tract
ROBERTS103 <> 50	Tab, Tan, Round, Flat, Beveled, Bisected	Bethanechol Chloride 50 mg	Duvoid by Shire BioChem	Canadian DIN 01947923	Urinary Tract
ROBERTS103 <> 50	Tab	Bethanechol Chloride 50 mg	Urecholine by Pharm Util	60491-0221	Urinary Tract
ROBERTS130	Tab	Furazolidone 100 mg	Furoxone by Roberts	54092-0130	Antibiotic
ROBERTS135-CHLORAFEDHS	Cap, White, Beads, Black Print	Chlorpheniramine Maleate 4 mg, Pseudoephedrine HCl 60 mg	Chlorafed by Roberts		Cold Remedy
ROBERTS136-CHLORAFED	Cap, Black Print, White Beads	Chlorpheniramine Maleate 8 mg, Pseudoephedrine HCl 120 mg	Chlorafed by Roberts		Cold Remedy
ROBERTS138DOLACET	Cap	Acetaminophen 500 mg, Hydrocodone Bitartrate 5 mg	Vicodin by Mikart	46672-0247	Analgesic; C III
ROBERTS151	Cap, White Beads, Black Print	Guaifenesin 300 mg, Pseudoephedrine HCl 60 mg	Sudafed Sinus by Roberts		Cold Remedy
ROBERTS186TIGAN	Cap	Trimethobenzamide HCl 100 mg	Tigan by Roberts	54092-0186	Antiemetic
ROBERTS187TIGAN	Cap, Roberts 187	Trimethobenzamide HCl 250 mg	Tigan by King	60793-0885	Antiemetic
ROBERTSCOMHISTLA	Cap	Chlorpheniramine Maleate 4 mg, Phenylephrine HCl 20 mg, Phenyltoloxamine Citrate 50 mg	Comhist LA by Roberts	54092-0065	Cold Remedy
ROBITAB8217	Tab, White, Round	Penicillin VK 250 mg	Robicillin by A H Robins		Antibiotic
ROBITAB8227	Tab, White, Round	Penicillin VK 500 mg	Robicillin by A H Robins		Antibiotic
ROCALTROL025ROCHE	Cap, Light Orange, Black Print, Oval, Rocaltrol over 0.25 Roche	Calcitriol 0.25 mcg	Rocaltrol by Hoffmann La Roche	00004-0143	Vitamin; Mineral
ROCALTROL05ROCHE	Cap, Dark Orange, Black Print, Oblong, Rocaltrol over 0.5 Roche	Calcitriol 0.5 mcg	Rocaltrol by Hoffmann La Roche	00004-0144	Vitamin; Mineral
ROCALTROL05ROCHE	Cap, Dark Orange, Black Print, Oblong, Rocaltrol over 0.5 Roche	Calcitriol 0.5 mcg	Rocaltrol by Pharm Util	60491-0562	Vitamin; Mineral
ROCHE	Cap, White	Clodronate Disodium 400 mg	Ostac by Roche	Canadian	Bisphosphonate
ROCHE	Cap, Blue & Pale Pink, ROCHE ROCHE	Levodopa 100 mg, Benseazide 25 mg	Prolopa by Roche	Canadian DIN 00386464	Antiparkinson
ROCHE	Tab, White, Cylindrical	Mefloquine HCl 250 mg	Lariam by Roche	Canadian	Antiprotozoal

ID FRONT <> BACK	DESCRIPTION FRONT <> BACK	INGREDIENT & STRENGTH	BRAND (or Generic Equiv.) by FIRM	NDC#	CLASS; SCH.
ROCHE	Tab, Yellowish-Buff, Round	Tetrabenazine 25 mg	Nitoman by Roche	Canadian	Dyskinesia Agent
ROCHE	Tab, Yellow, Oblong	Tenoxicam 20 mg	Mobiflex by Roche	Canadian	NSAID
ROCHE	Tab, White, Round	Sulfamethoxazole 400 mg, Trimethoprim 80 mg	Bactrim by Roche	Canadian Discontinued	Antibiotic
ROCHE	Tab, White	Sulfadoxine 500 mg	by Roche	Canadian	Antimalarial
ROCHE	Tab, White	Pyramethamine 25 mg, Sulfadoxine 500 mg	Fansidar by Roche	Canadian	Antimalarial
ROCHE	Cap, Light Grey and Blue, ROCHE ROCHE	Levodopa 50 mg, Benseazide 12.5 mg	Prolopa by Roche	Canadian DIN 00522597	Antiparkinson
ROCHE	Cap, Blue and Caramel, ROCHE ROCHE	Levodopa 200 mg, Benseazide 50 mg	Prolopa by Roche	Canadian DIN 00386472	Antiparkinson
ROCHE <> 10VALIUM	Tab, Blue, Round, Scored	Diazepam 10 mg	Valium by Roche	00140-0006	Antianxiety; C IV
ROCHE <> 12KLONOPIN	Tab, Orange, Round, Scored, 1/2 Klonopin, K perforation	Clonazepam 0.5 mg	Klonopin by Hoffmann La Roche	00004-0068	Sedative; C IV
ROCHE <> 1KLONOPIN	Tab, Blue, Round, K perforation	Clonazepam 1 mg	Klonopin by Hoffmann La Roche	00004-0058	Sedative; C IV
ROCHE <> 274	Tab, Light Blue, Film Coated	Naproxen 275 mg	Naprosyn by Syntex	18393-0274	NSAID
ROCHE <> 274	Tab, Light Blue, Oval, Film Coated	Naproxen 275 mg	Naprosyn by Allscripts		NSAID
ROCHE <> 2KLONOPIN	Tab, White, Round, K perforation	Clonazepam 2 mg	Klonopin by Hoffmann La Roche	00004-0098	Sedative; C IV
ROCHE <> 2VALIUM	Tab, White, Round, Scored	Diazepam 2 mg	Valium by Roche	00140-0004	Antianxiety; C IV
ROCHE <> 5VALIUM	Tab, Yellow, Round, Scored	Diazepam 5 mg	Valium by PDRX	55289-0117	Antianxiety; C IV
ROCHE <> 5VALIUM	Tab, Yellow, Round, Scored	Diazepam 5 mg	Valium by Caremark	00339-4073	Antianxiety; C IV
ROCHE <> 5VALIUM	Tab, Yellow, Round, Scored	Diazepam 5 mg	Valium by Roche	00140-0005	Antianxiety; C IV
ROCHE <> ANAPROX	Tab, Film Coated	Naproxen 275 mg	Naprosyn by H J Harkins Co	52959-0015	NSAID
ROCHE <> ANAPROXDS	Tab, Blue, Oblong	Naproxen 550 mg	Naprosyn by Rightpak	65240-0603	NSAID
ROCHE <> ANAPROXDS	Tab, Blue, Oblong	Naproxen 550 mg	Naprosyn by Med Pro	53978-3369	NSAID
ROCHE <> ANAPROXDS	Tab, Film Coated	Naproxen 550 mg	Naprosyn by Allscripts		NSAID
ROCHE <> ANAPROXDS	Tab, Dark Blue, Film Coated, Anaprox DS	Naproxen 550 mg	Naprosyn by Syntex	18393-0276	NSAID
ROCHE <> ANAPROXDS	Tab, Dark Blue, Film Coated, Anaprox DS	Naproxen 550 mg	Naprosyn by H J Harkins Co	52959-0016	NSAID
ROCHE <> ANAPROXDS	Tab, Dark Blue, Debossed <> Anaprox DS, Film Coated	Naproxen 550 mg	Naprosyn by Thrift Drug	59198-0244	NSAID
ROCHE <> ANAPROXDS	Tab, Film Coated, Anaprox DS	Naproxen 550 mg	Naprosyn by Nat Pharmpak	55154-3805	NSAID
ROCHE <> BACTRIMDS	Tab, White, Oblong, Bactrim-DS	Sulfamethoxazole 800 mg, Trimethoprim 160 mg	Bactrim DS by Thrift Drug	59198-0258	Antibiotic
ROCHE <> BACTRIMDS	Tab, White, Oblong, Bactrim-DS	Sulfamethoxazole 800 mg, Trimethoprim 160 mg	Bactrim DS by Nat Pharmpak	55154-3101	Antibiotic
ROCHE <> BACTRIMDS	Tab, White, Oblong, Bactrim-DS	Sulfamethoxazole 800 mg, Trimethoprim 160 mg	Bactrim DS by Amerisource	62584-0117	Antibiotic
ROCHE <> BACTRIMDS	Tab, White, Oblong, Bactrim-DS	Sulfamethoxazole 800 mg, Trimethoprim 160 mg	Bactrim DS by Hoffmann La Roche	00004-0117	Antibiotic
ROCHE <> BACTRIMDS	Tab, White, Oblong, Bactrim-DS	Sulfamethoxazole 800 mg, Trimethoprim 160 mg	Bactrim DS by DRX	55045-2291	Antibiotic
ROCHE <> BUMEX05	Tab, Green, Oval, Bumex over 0.5	Bumetanide 0.5 mg	Bumex by Thrift Drug	59198-0257	Diuretic
ROCHE <> BUMEX05	Tab, Green, Oval, Bumex over 0.5	Bumetanide 0.5 mg	Bumex by Nat Pharmpak	55154-3103	Diuretic
ROCHE <> BUMEX05	Tab, Green, Oval, Bumex over 0.5	Bumetanide 0.5 mg	Bumex by Amerisource	62584-0125	Diuretic
ROCHE <> BUMEX05	Tab, Green, Oval, Bumex over 0.5	Bumetanide 0.5 mg	Bumex by Med Pro	53978-3386	Diuretic
ROCHE <> BUMEX05	Tab, Green, Oval, Bumex over 0.5	Bumetanide 0.5 mg	Bumex by Rightpak	65240-0698	Diuretic
ROCHE <> BUMEX05	Tab, Green, Oval, Bumex over 0.5	Bumetanide 0.5 mg	Bumex by Hoffmann La Roche	00004-0125	Diuretic
ROCHE <> BUMEX1	Tab, Yellow, Oval, Bumex over 1	Bumetanide 1 mg	Bumex by Thrift Drug	59198-0256	Diuretic
ROCHE <> BUMEX1	Tab, Yellow, Oval, Bumex over 1	Bumetanide 1 mg	Bumex by Nat Pharmpak	55154-3104	Diuretic
ROCHE <> BUMEX1	Tab, Yellow, Oval, Bumex over 1	Bumetanide 1 mg	Bumex by Med Pro	53978-0241	Diuretic
ROCHE <> BUMEX1	Tab, Yellow, Oval, Bumex over 1	Bumetanide 1 mg	Bumex by Physician Total Care	54868-1293	Diuretic
ROCHE <> BUMEX1	Tab, Yellow, Oval, Bumex over 1	Bumetanide 1 mg	Bumex by Hoffmann La Roche	00004-0121	Diuretic
ROCHE <> BUMEX1	Tab, Yellow, Oval, Bumex over 1	Bumetanide 1 mg	Bumex by Rightpak	65240-0610	Diuretic
ROCHE <> BUMEX1	Tab, Yellow, Oval, Bumex over 1	Bumetanide 1 mg	Bumex by Amerisource	62584-0121	Diuretic
ROCHE <> BUMEX2	Tab, Peach, Oval, Bumex over 2	Bumetanide 2 mg	Bumex by Caraco	57664-0219	Diuretic
ROCHE <> BUMEX2	Tab, Peach, Oval, Bumex over 2	Bumetanide 2 mg	Bumex by Thrift Drug	59198-0101	Diuretic
ROCHE <> BUMEX2	Tab, Peach, Oval, Bumex over 2	Bumetanide 2 mg	Bumex by Nat Pharmpak	55154-3105	Diuretic
ROCHE <> BUMEX2	Tab, Peach, Oval, Bumex over 2	Bumetanide 2 mg	Bumex by Leiner	59606-0716	Diuretic

ID FRONT <> BACK	DESCRIPTION FRONT <> BACK	INGREDIENT & STRENGTH	BRAND (or Generic Equiv.) by FIRM	NDC#	CLASS; SCH.
ROCHE <> BUMEX2	Tab, Peach, Oval, Bumex over 2	Bumetanide 2 mg	Bumex by Hoffmann La Roche	00004-0162	Diuretic
ROCHE <> BUMEX2	Tab, Peach, Oval, Bumex over 2	Bumetanide 2 mg	Bumex by Amerisource	62584-0162	Diuretic
ROCHE <> BUMEX2	Tab, Peach, Oval, Bumex over 2	Bumetanide 2 mg	Bumex by Drug Distr	52985-0222	Diuretic
ROCHE <> BUMEX2	Tab, Peach, Oval, Bumex over 2	Bumetanide 2 mg	Bumex by Med Pro	53978-2035	Diuretic
ROCHE <> CELLCEPT500	Tab, Lavender, Black Print, Cap Shaped, Film Coated, Cellcept over 500	Mycophenolate Mofetil 500 mg	Cellcept by Syntex	18393-0923	Immunosuppressant
ROCHE <> CELLCEPT500	Tab, Lavender, Black Print, Cap Shaped, Film Coated, Cellcept over 500	Mycophenolate Mofetil 500 mg	Cellcept by Hoffmann La Roche	00004-0260	Immunosuppressant
ROCHE <> CELLCEPT500	Tab, Lavender, Black Print, Cap Shaped, Film Coated, Cellcept over 500	Mycophenolate Mofetil 500 mg	CellCept by Roche	Canadian DIN 02237484	Immunosuppressant
ROCHE <> HIVID0375	Tab, Beige, Black Print, Oval, Film Coated, Hivid over 0.375	Zalcitabine 0.375 mg	Hivid by Roche	Canadian	Antiviral
ROCHE <> HIVID0375	Tab, Beige, Black Print, Oval, Film Coated, Hivid over 0.375	Zalcitabine 0.375 mg	Hivid by Pharm Util	60491-0296	Antiviral
ROCHE <> HIVID0375	Tab, Beige, Black Print, Oval, Film Coated, Hivid over 0.375	Zalcitabine 0.375 mg	Hivid by Hoffmann La Roche	00004-0220	Antiviral
ROCHE <> HIVID0750	Tab, Beige, Black Print, Oval, Film Coated, Hivid over 0.750	Zalcitabine 0.75 mg	Hivid by Pharm Util	60491-0297	Antiviral
ROCHE <> HIVID0750	Tab, Beige, Black Print, Oval, Film Coated, Hivid over 0.750	Zalcitabine 0.750 mg	Hivid by Hoffmann La Roche	00004-0221	Antiviral
ROCHE <> LARIAM250	Tab, White, Round, Scored	Mefloquine HCl 250 mg	Lariam by PDRX	55289-0780	Antiprotozoal
ROCHE <> LARIAM250	Tab, White, Round, Scored	Mefloquine HCl 250 mg	Lariam by DRX	55045-2459	Antiprotozoal
ROCHE <> LARIAM250	Tab, White, Round, Scored	Mefloquine HCl 250 mg	Lariam by Hoffmann La Roche	00004-0172	Antiprotozoal
ROCHE <> LARODOPA100	Tab, Pink, Oval, Scored	Levodopa 100 mg	Larodopa by Hoffmann La Roche	00004-0072	Antiparkinson
ROCHE <> LARODOPA250	Tab, Pink, Round, Scored	Levodopa 250 mg	Larodopa by Hoffmann La Roche	00004-0057	Antiparkinson
ROCHE <> NAPROSYN250	Tab, Yellow, Round	Naproxen 250 mg	Naprosyn by Hoffmann La Roche	00004-6312	NSAID
ROCHE <> NAPROSYN250	Tab, Yellow, Round	Naproxen 250 mg	Naprosyn by Syntex	18393-0272	NSAID
ROCHE <> NAPROSYN250	Tab, Yellow, Round	Naproxen 250 mg	Naprosyn by Allscripts		NSAID
ROCHE <> NAPROSYN250	Tab, Yellow, Round	Naproxen 250 mg	Naprosyn by Amerisource	62584-0272	NSAID
ROCHE <> NAPROSYN250	Tab, Yellow, Round	Naproxen 250 mg	Naprosyn by Thrift Drug	59198-0237	NSAID
ROCHE <> RIB200	Tab, Pink, Oval, Film Coated	Ribavirin 200 mg	Copegus by Hoffmann La Roche	00004-0086	Antiviral
ROCHE <> RIB200	Tab, Pink, Oval, Film Coated	Ribavirin 200 mg	Pegasys RBV by Roche	Canadian DIN 02253410	Antiviral
ROCHE <> TASMAR100	Tab, Beige, Black Print, Hexagonal, Film Coated, TASMAR over 100	Tolcapone 100 mg	Tasmar by Teva	00480-0100	Antiparkinson
ROCHE <> TASMAR100	Tab, Beige, Black Print, Hexagonal, Film Coated, TASMAR over 100	Tolcapone 100 mg	Tasmar by Hoffmann La Roche	00004-5920	Antiparkinson
ROCHE <> TASMAR200	Tab, Reddish Brown, Hexagonal, Film Coated	Tolcapone 200 mg	Tasmar by Hoffmann La Roche	00004-5921	Antiparkinson
ROCHE0245	Cap, Green & Light Brown, White Print, Roche over 0245	Saquinavir Mesylate 200 mg	Invirase by Physician Total Care	54868-3699	Antiviral
ROCHE0245	Cap, Green & Light Brown, White Print, Roche over 0245	Saquinavir Mesylate 200 mg	Invirase by Pharm Util	60491-0336	Antiviral
ROCHE0245	Cap, Green & Light Brown, White Print, Roche over 0245	Saquinavir Mesylate 200 mg	Invirase by Hoffmann La Roche	00004-0245	Antiviral
ROCHE0245	Cap, Green & Light Brown, White Print, Roche over 0245	Saquinavir Mesylate 200 mg	Invirase by Roche	Canadian DIN 02216965	Antiviral
ROCHE0245	Cap, Green & Light Brown, White Print, Roche over 0245	Saquinavir Mesylate 200 mg	Invirase by 3M	Canadian	Antiviral
ROCHE0246	Cap, Beige, Red Print, Opaque, Soft Gel	Saquinavir 200 mg	Fortovase by Roche	Canadian DIN 02239083	Antiviral
ROCHE0246	Cap, Beige, Red Print, Opaque, Soft Gel	Saquinavir 200 mg	Fortovase by Hoffmann La Roche	00004-0246	Antiviral
ROCHE05	Tab, Pale Orange, Cylindrical, Scored, Roche/0.5	Clonazepam 0.5 mg	Rivotril by Roche	Canadian DIN 00382825	Sedative; C IV

ID FRONT <> BACK	DESCRIPTION FRONT <> BACK	INGREDIENT & STRENGTH	BRAND (or Generic Equiv.) by FIRM	NDC#	CLASS; SCH.
ROCHE1	Tab, Yellow, Oval	Cilazapril 1 mg	Inhibace by Roche	Canadian	Antihypertensive
ROCHE10	Tab, Light Blue, Cylindrical, Roche/10	Diazepam 10 mg	Valium Roche by Roche	Canadian	Antianxiety; C IV
ROCHE100	Tab, Orange, Roche/100	Moclobemide 100 mg	Manerix by Roche	Canadian	Antidepressant
ROCHE100	Tab, Light Yellow, Hexagonal	Tolcapone 100 mg	Tasmar by Roche	Canadian	Antiparkinson
ROCHE15	Tab, White, Cylindrical, Scored, Roche 1.5	Bromazepam 1.5 mg	Lectopam by Roche	Canadian	Sedative; C IV
ROCHE150	Tab, Yellow, Biconvex, Scored, Film Coated, Roche/150	Moclobemide 150 mg	Manerix by Roche	Canadian DIN 00899356	Antidepressant
ROCHE2	Tab, White, Cylindrical, Scored, Roche/2	Clonazepam 2 mg	Rivotril by Roche	Canadian DIN 00382841	Sedative; C IV
ROCHE2	Tab, White, Round, Double Scored	Flunitrazepam 2 mg	Rohypnol by Hoffmann La Roche	Foreign	Sedative; Illicit in USA
ROCHE200	Tab, Brown/Orange, Hexagonal	Tolcapone 200 mg	Tasmar by Roche	Canadian	Antiparkinson
ROCHE25	Tab, Pink, Oval, Tannish-Brown, Roche 2.5	Cilazapril 2.5 mg	Inhibace by Roche	Canadian	Antihypertensive
ROCHE3	Tab, Pink, Cylindrical, Scored, Roche/3	Bromazepam 3 mg	Lectopam by Roche	Canadian DIN 00518123	Sedative; C IV
ROCHE300	Tab, White, Biconvex, Scored, Film Coated, Roche/300	Moclobemide 300 mg	Manerix by Roche	Canadian DIN 02166747	Antidepressant
ROCHE 5	Tab, Red & Brown, Oval	Cilazapril 5 mg	Inhibace by Roche	Canadian	Antihypertensive
ROCHE5	Tab, Pale Yellow, Cylindrical, Scored	Diazepam 5 mg	Valium Roche by Roche	Canadian DIN 00013285	Antianxiety; C IV
ROCHE6	Tab, Yellowish Green, Cylindrical, Scored, Roche/6	Bromazepam 6 mg	Lectopam by Roche	Canadian DIN 00518131	Sedative; C IV
ROCHE75MG	Cap, Grey & Light Yellow, Hard Gel	Oseltamivir Phosphate 75 mg	Tamiflu by Roche	Canadian DIN 02241472	Antiviral
ROCHE75MG	Cap, Grey & Light Yellow, Hard Gel	Oseltamivir Phosphate 75 mg	Tamiflu by Hoffmann La Roche	00004-0800	Antiviral
ROCHE800160	Tab, White, Oval, Roche 800 + 160	Sulfamethoxazole 800 mg, Trimethoprim 160 mg	Bactrim DS by Roche	Canadian Discontinued	Antibiotic
ROCHECLIBRAX	Cap, Green, Roche/C/Librax	Chlordiazepoxide 5 mg, Clidinium Bromide 2.5 mg	Librax by Roche	Canadian	Gastrointestinal
ROCHECPROLOPA	Cap, Blue & Flesh, Roche/C/Prolopa	Levodopa 100 mg, Benserazide 25 mg	Prolopa by Roche	Canadian	Antiparkinson
ROCHECPROLOPA	Cap, Light Gray/Blue, Roche/C/Prolopa	Levodopa 50 mg, Benserazide 12.5 mg	Prolopa by Roche	Canadian	Antiparkinson
ROCHEHEXAGON	Tab, White, Cylindrical, Roche/Hexagon	Mefloquine HCl 250 mg	Lariam by Roche	Canadian	Antiprotozoal
ROCHEHEXAGON	Tab, White, Roche/Hexagon	Pyrimethamine 25 mg, Sulfadoxine 500 mg	Fansidar by Roche	Canadian	Antimalarial
ROCHEMARPLAN	Tab, Peach, Round, Scored	Isocarboxazid 10 mg	Marplan by Roche	00004-0032	Antidepressant
ROCHEROCHE	Cap, Brown & White	Acitretin 10 mg	Soriatane by Roche	Canadian DIN 02070847	Dermatologic
ROCHEROCHE	Cap, Brown & Yellow	Acitretin 25 mg	Soriatane by Roche	Canadian DIN 02070863	Dermatologic
ROCHESQV500	Tab, Light Orange, Oval, Film Coated	Saquinavir Mesylate 500 mg	Invirase by Roche	00004-0244	Antiviral
ROCHEXENICAL120	Cap, Turquoise, Hard Gel	Orlistat 120 mg	Xenical by Roche	Canadian DIN 02240325	Lipase Inhibitor
ROERIG <> 143	Tab, Yellow, Cap Shaped, Film Coated	Carbenicillin Indanyl Sodium 382 mg	Geocillin by Roerig	00049-1430	Antibiotic
ROERIG <> DIFLUCAN100	Tab, Pink, Trapezoidal, Diflucan over 100	Fluconazole 100 mg	Diflucan by Roerig	00049-3420	Antifungal
ROERIG <> DIFLUCAN100	Tab, Pink, Trapezoidal, Diflucan over 100	Fluconazole 100 mg	Diflucan by Allscripts		Antifungal
ROERIG <> DIFLUCAN100	Tab, Pink, Trapezoidal, Diflucan over 100	Fluconazole 100 mg	Diflucan by Med Pro	53978-3012	Antifungal
ROERIG <> DIFLUCAN100	Tab, Pink, Trapezoidal, Diflucan over 100	Fluconazole 100 mg	Diflucan by Nat Pharmpak	55154-3214	Antifungal
ROERIG <> DIFLUCAN100	Tab, Pink, Trapezoidal, Diflucan over 100	Fluconazole 100 mg	Diflucan by Amerisource	62584-0362	Antifungal

ID FRONT <> BACK	DESCRIPTION FRONT <> BACK	INGREDIENT & STRENGTH	BRAND (or Generic Equiv.) by FIRM	NDC#	CLASS: SCH.
ROERIG <> DIFLUCAN150	Tab, Pink, Oval, Diflucan over 150	Fluconazole 150 mg	Diflucan by Roerig	00049-3500	Antifungal
ROERIG <> DIFLUCAN200	Tab, Pink, Trapezoidal, Diflucan over 200	Fluconazole 200 mg	Diflucan by Med Pro	53978-3105	Antifungal
ROERIG <> DIFLUCAN200	Tab, Pink, Trapezoidal, Diflucan over 200	Fluconazole 200 mg	Diflucan by Allscripts		Antifungal
ROERIG <> DIFLUCAN200	Tab, Pink, Trapezoidal, Diflucan over 200	Fluconazole 200 mg	Diflucan by Roerig	00049-3430	Antifungal
ROERIG <> DIFLUCAN200	Tab, Pink, Trapezoidal, Diflucan over 200	Fluconazole 200 mg	Diflucan by Nat Pharmpak	55154-3215	Antifungal
ROERIG <> DIFLUCAN200	Tab, Pink, Trapezoidal, Diflucan over 200	Fluconazole 200 mg	Diflucan by Amerisource	62584-0363	Antifungal
ROERIG <> DIFLUCAN50	Tab, Pink, Trapezoidal, Diflucan over 50	Fluconazole 50 mg	Diflucan by Roerig	00049-3410	Antifungal
ROERIG <> DIFLUGAN50	Tab, Pink, Trapezoidal, Diflucan over 50	Fluconazole 50 mg	Diflucan by Pharm Util	60491-0194	Antifungal
ROERIG159TAO	Cap, White	Troleandomycin 250 mg	Tao by Roerig	00049-1590	Antibiotic
ROERIG254 <> MARAX	Tab	Ephedrine 25 mg, Hydroxyzine 10 mg, Theophylline 130 mg	Marax by Roerig	00049-2540	Antiasthmatic
RONDEX278	Cap, Yellow	Oxytetracycline 250 mg	Terramycin by Rondex		Antibiotic
ROSETTE	Tab, White, Round	Pamabrom 25 mg, Pyrilamine Maleate 12.5 mg, Acetaminophen 325 mg	Pamprin by Chattem	Canadian	Menstrual Symptom Relief
ROUGIER	Tab, Pink, Round, Scored, Rougier Logo	Yohimbine HCl 6 mg	by Rougier Pharma	Canadian DIN 00843512 Discontinued	Impotence Agent
ROUGIER	Cap, Yellow, Opaque, Gelatin, Rougier Logo	Diphenhydramine HCl 50 mg		Canadian DIN 02153165	Antihistamine
ROWELL7720	Tab, White, Round	Chenodiol 250 mg	Chenix by RR		Cholelitholytic
ROYCE <> 377200	Tab, Coated, Royce Logo <> 377,200 and a Partial Score	Hydroxychloroquine Sulfate 200 mg	by Ivax	00182-2609	Antimalarial
RP <> 51	Tab, Yellow, Round, Scored	Dextroamphetamine Sulfate 5 mg	Dexedrine by Shire	58521-0451	Stimulant; C II
RP <> 52	Tab, Yellow, Round, Scored	Dextroamphetamine Sulfate 10 mg	Dexedrine by Shire	58521-0452	Stimulant; C II
RP069	Tab, Ivory, Round, RP Monarch Logo 069	Theophylline Anhydrous 300 mg	Quibron T by King	00087-0512	Antiasthmatic
RP070	Tab, White, Round, Ex Release, RP Monarch Logo 070	Theophylline Anhydrous 300 mg	Quibron T Sr by King	00087-0519	Antiasthmatic
RP10	Cap, Blue and White, Cobalt Logo RP 10	Ramipril 10 mg	Altace by Cobalt	16252-0573	Antihypertensive
RP10	Cap, Blue and White, Cobalt Logo RP 10	Ramipril 10 mg	Altace by Cobalt	Canadian DIN 02295512	Antihypertensive
RP102	Tab, Green, Round	Calcium Carbonate 750 mg	Tums by Raritan Pharma		Antacid
RP125	Cap, White and Yellow, Opaque	Ramipril 1.25 mg	Altace by Cobalt	Canadian DIN 02295482	Antihypertensive
RP125	Tab, Pink, Cap Shaped	Bismuth Subsalicylate 262 mg	Pepto Bismol by CVS		Gastrointestinal
RP25	Cap, Orange and White, Cobalt Logo RP 2.5	Ramipril 2.5 mg	Altace by Cobalt	Canadian DIN 02295490	Antihypertensive
RP25	Cap, Orange and White, Cobalt Logo RP 2.5	Ramipril 2.5 mg	Altace by Cobalt	16252-0571	Antihypertensive
RP5	Cap, Red and White, Cobalt Logo RP 5	Ramipril 5 mg	Altace by Cobalt	16252-0572	Antihypertensive
RP5	Cap, Red and White, Cobalt Logo RP 5	Ramipril 5 mg	Altace by Cobalt	Canadian DIN 02295504	Antihypertensive
RP5455	Tab, Pink, Round	Methamphetamine HCl 5 mg	Desoxyn by Richwood		Stimulant; C II
RP5456	Tab, Pink, Round	Methamphetamine HCl 10 mg	Desoxyn by Richwood		Stimulant; C II
RP57	Tab, Pink, Round	Phendimetrazine Tartrate 35 mg	X-Trozine by Richwood		Anorexiant; C III
RP57	Tab, Blue, Round	Phendimetrazine Tartrate 35 mg	X-Trozine by Richwood		Anorexiant; C III
RP57	Tab, Green, Round	Phendimetrazine Tartrate 35 mg	X-Trozine by Richwood		Anorexiant; C III

ID FRONT <> BACK	DESCRIPTION FRONT <> BACK	INGREDIENT & STRENGTH	BRAND (or Generic Equiv.) by FIRM	NDC#	CLASS; SCH.
RP57	Tab, Yellow, Round	Phendimetrazine Tartrate 35 mg	X-Trozine by Richwood		Anorexiant; C III
RP600	Tab	Guaifenesin 600 mg	Robitussin by Seatrace	00551-0189	Expectorant
RPC <> 073	Tab, Sugar Coated	Propantheline Bromide 7.5 mg	Pro Banthine by Roberts	54092-0073	Gastrointestinal
RPC <> 074	Tab, Sugar Coated	Propantheline Bromide 15 mg	Pro Banthine by Roberts	54092-0074	Gastrointestinal
RPC <> 73	Tab, White, Round	Propantheline Bromide 7.5 mg	by Compumed	00403-5167	Gastrointestinal
RPC052	Cap, Clear & Red, White Print, Oval, Soft Gel	Docusate Sodium 50 mg	Colace by Purdue	67618-0050	Laxative
RPC053	Cap, Beige & Pink, Black Print, Oval, Opaque, Soft Gel	Docusate Sodium 100 mg	Colace by Purdue	67618-0100	Laxative
RPC054	Tab, Red, Round	Sennoside 8.6 mg, Docusate Sodium 50 mg	Peri-Colace by Purdue	67618-0106	Laxative
RPC055	Tab, RPC over 055	Hydroflumethiazide 50 mg	Diucardin by Roberts	54092-0055	Diuretic; Antihypertensive
RPC056	Tab, RPC over 056	Hydroflumethiazide 50 mg, Reserpine 0.125 mg	Salutensin by Roberts	54092-0056	Diuretic; Antihypertensive
RPC057	Tab, Pale Yellow, RPC over 05	Hydroflumethiazide 25 mg, Reserpine 0.125 mg	Salutensin-Demi by Mead Johnson	00015-5455	Antihypertensive; Diuretic
RPC059	Tab, White, Scored	Fludrocortisone Acetate 0.1 mg	Florinef by Shire BioChem	Canadian DIN 02086026	Steriod
RPC066 <> COMHIST	Tab	Chlorpheniramine Maleate 2 mg, Phenylephrine HCl 10 mg, Phenyltoloxamine Citrate 25 mg	Comhist by Roberts	54092-0066	Cold Remedy
RPC10 <> 007	Tab, Blue, Round, Scored, RPC over 10	Midodrine HCl 10 mg	ProAmatine by Roberts	54092-0007	Antihypotensive
RPC152	Tab, Ex Release, RPC/152	Guaifenesin 600 mg	Robitussin by Sovereign	58716-0602	Expectorant
RPC25 <> 003	Tab, White, Round, Scored, RPC over 2.5	Midodrine HCl 2.5 mg	ProAmatine by Nycomed	57585-0103	Antihypotensive
RPC25 <> 003	Tab, White, Round, Scored, RPC over 2.5	Midodrine HCl 2.5 mg	ProAmatine by Roberts	54092-0003	Antihypotensive
RPC25 <> 003	Tab, White, Round, Scored, RPC over 2.5	Midodrine HCl 2.5 mg	Amatine by Shire	Canadian DIN 01934392	Antihypotensive
RPC5 <> 004	Tab, Orange, Round, Scored, RPC over 5	Midodrine HCl 5 mg	Amatine by Shire	Canadian DIN 01934406	Antihypotensive
RPC5 <> 004	Tab, Orange, Round, Scored, RPC over 5	Midodrine HCl 5 mg	ProAmatine by Roberts	54092-0004	Antihypotensive
RPC5 <> 004	Tab, Orange, Round, Scored, RPC over 5	Midodrine HCl 5 mg	ProAmatine by Nycomed	57585-0104	Antihypotensive
RPC50 <> 004	Tab, Orange, Round, Scored, RPC over 5.0 <> 004	Midodrine HCl 5 mg	ProAmatine by Shire	54092-0004	Antihypotensive
RPC62	Cap, Brown & Clear	Phendimetrazine Tartrate 105 mg	by Physician Total Care	54868-1336	Anorexiant; C III
RPC62	Cap, Clear with White Beads, Ex Release, RPC/62 <> Clear with White Beads	Phendimetrazine Tartrate 105 mg	Adipost by Jones	52604-0470	Anorexiant; C III
RPC62	Cap	Phendimetrazine Tartrate 105 mg	X Trozine LA by Shire	58521-0105	Anorexiant; C III
RPC62	Cap, ER	Phendimetrazine Tartrate 105 mg	by DRX	55045-2453	Anorexiant; C III
RPC62	Cap, Brown & Clear	Phendimetrazine Tartrate 105 mg	by Compumed	00403-0016	Anorexiant; C III
RPC62	Cap, ER	Phendimetrazine Tartrate 105 mg	X Trozine LA by Shire	58521-0105	Anorexiant; C III
RPC63	Cap, Red & White	Phendimetrazine Tartrate 35 mg	X-Trozine by Richwood		Anorexiant; C III
RPC63	Cap, Black & Orange	Phendimetrazine Tartrate 35 mg	X-Trozine by Richwood		Anorexiant; C III
RPC63	Cap, Black	Phendimetrazine Tartrate 35 mg	X-Trozine by Richwood		Anorexiant; C III
RPC69	Cap, Yellow	Phentermine HCl 30 mg	Oby Trim by Eon	00185-2061 Discontinued	Anorexiant; C IV
RPC69	Cap, Yellow	Phentermine HCl 30 mg	Oby Trim by Allscripts	54569-3248 Discontinued	Anorexiant; C IV
RPC69	Cap, Yellow	Phentermine HCl 30 mg	Oby Trim by Quality Care	62682-7042 Discontinued	Anorexiant; C IV
RPHM12	Tab, White, Round, Film Coated	Metformin 500 mg	Ratio-Metformin by Ratiopharm	Canadian DIN 02242974	Antidiabetic
RPL1050	Tab, White/Green Specks, Round	Pseudoephedrine HCl 120 mg, Guaifenesin 400 mg	Histalet X by RR		Cold Remedy
RPL1082	Cap, Orange/Clear	Phendimetrazine Tartrate 105 mg	Melfiat-105 by RR		Anorexiant; C III
RPR <> 20R	Tab	Chlorthalidone 50 mg	Hygroton by RPR	00075-0020 Discontinued	Diuretic
RPR <> 20R	Tab	Chlorthalidone 50 mg	Hygroton by RPR	00801-0020	Diuretic

ID FRONT <> BACK	DESCRIPTION FRONT <> BACK	INGREDIENT & STRENGTH	BRAND (or Generic Equiv.) by FIRM	NDC#	CLASS; SCH.
RPR <> 22R	Tab	Chlorthalidone 25 mg	Hygroton by RPR	00801-0022	Diuretic
RPR <> 22R	Tab	Chlorthalidone 25 mg	Hygroton by RPR	00075-0022 Discontinued	Diuretic
RPR <> 351	Tab, White, Round	Theophylline Anhydrous 100 mg	Slo Phyllin by RPR		Antiasthmatic
RPR <> 352	Tab, White, Round	Theophylline Anhydrous 200 mg	Slo Phyllin by RPR		Antiasthmatic
RPR <> 5100	Tab, Light Blue, Oblong, Film Coated	Enoxacin 200 mg	Penetrex by RPR	00801-5100	Antibiotic
RPR <> 5100	Tab, Light Blue, Oblong, Film Coated	Enoxacin 200 mg	Penetrex by RPR	00075-5100 Discontinued	Antibiotic
RPR <> 5140	Tab, Dark Blue, Oblong, Film Coated	Enoxacin 400 mg	Penetrex by RPR	00075-5140 Discontinued	Antibiotic
RPR <> 5140	Tab, Dark Blue, Oblong, Film Coated	Enoxacin 400 mg	Penetrex by RPR	00801-5140	Antibiotic
RPR <> DDAVP01	Tab, White, Oblong, Scored, RPR Logo <> DDAVP0.1	Desmopressin Acetate 0.1 mg	DDAVP by Aventis	00075-0016	Antidiuretic
RPR <> DDAVP02	Tab, White, Round, Scored, RPR Logo <> DDAVP over 0.2	Desmopressin Acetate 0.2 mg	DDAVP by Aventis	00075-0026	Antidiuretic
RPR <> DDAVP02	Tab, White, Round, Scored, RPR Logo <> DDAVP over 0.2	Desmopressin Acetate 0.2 mg	DDAVP by Promex Med	62301-0030	Antidiuretic
RPR <> IMOVANE5	Tab, White, Round	Zopiclone 5 mg	Imovane 5 by ICN	Canadian DIN 02216167	Hypnotic
RPR <> SECTRAL100	Tab, White to Off White, Shield Shaped, Film Coated	Acebutolol HCl 100 mg	Sectral by Sanofi-Aventis	Canadian DIN 01926543	Antihypertensive
RPR <> SECTRAL200	Tab, Blue, Shield Shaped, Film Coated	Acebutolol HCl 200 mg	Sectral by Sanofi-Aventis	Canadian DIN 01926551	Antihypertensive
RPR <> SECTRAL400	Tab, White to Off White, Shield Shaped, Film Coated	Acebutolol HCl 400 mg	Sectral by Sanofi-Aventis	Canadian DIN 01926578	Antihypertensive
RPR0251180MG	Cap	Diltiazem HCl 180 mg	Dilacor XR by RPR		Antihypertensive
RPR0252240MG	Cap	Diltiazem HCl 240 mg	Dilacor XR by RPR		Antihypertensive
RPR201	Tab, White, Round, Film Coated	Sparfloxacin 200 mg	Zagam by RPR		Antibiotic
RPR202	Tab, White, Oblong, Film Coated, RPR over 202	Riluzole 50 mg	Rilutek by RPR	00075-7700	Amyotrophic Lateral Sclerosis Agent
RPR202	Tab, White, Capsule Shaped, Film Coated	Riluzole 50 mg	Rilutek by Sanofi-Aventis	Canadian DIN 02242763	Antiglutamate
RPR21	Tab, White, Round	Chlorthalidone 100 mg	Hygroton by RPR		Diuretic
RPRDILACORXR120MG	Cap, Gold & White, Black Print, Ex Release, RPR over Dilacor XR over 120 mg	Diltiazem HCl 120 mg	Dilacor XR by Amerisource	62584-0250	Antihypertensive
RPRDILACORXR120MG	Cap, Gold & White, Black Print, Ex Release, RPR over Dilacor XR over 120 mg	Diltiazem HCl 120 mg	Dilacor XR by Watson	00075-0250	Antihypertensive
RPRDILACORXR120MG	Cap, Gold & White, Black Print, Ex Release, RPR over Dilacor XR over 120 mg	Diltiazem HCl 120 mg	Dilacor XR by Drug Distr	52985-0223	Antihypertensive
RPRDILACORXR120MG	Cap, Gold & White, Black Print, Ex Release, RPR over Dilacor XR over 120 mg	Diltiazem HCl 120 mg	Dilacor XR by Nat Pharmpak	55154-4020	Antihypertensive
RPRDILACORXR120MG	Cap, Gold & White, Black Print, Ex Release, RPR over Dilacor XR over 120 mg	Diltiazem HCl 120 mg	Dilacor XR by Leiner	59606-0776	Antihypertensive
RPRDILACORXR120MG	Cap, Gold & White, Black Print, Ex Release, RPR over Dilacor XR over 120 mg	Diltiazem HCl 120 mg	Dilacor XR by Thrift Drug	59198-0259	Antihypertensive
RPRDILACORXR180MG	Cap, Orange & White, Black Print, Ex Release, RPR over Dilacor XR over 180 mg	Diltiazem HCl 180 mg	Dilacor XR by Leiner	59606-0736	Antihypertensive
RPRDILACORXR180MG	Cap, Orange & White, Black Print, Ex Release, RPR over Dilacor XR over 180 mg	Diltiazem HCl 180 mg	Dilacor XR by Thrift Drug	59198-0260	Antihypertensive
RPRDILACORXR180MG	Cap, Orange & White, Black Print, Ex Release, RPR over Dilacor XR over 180 mg	Diltiazem HCl 180 mg	Dilacor XR by Watson	00075-0251	Antihypertensive
RPRDILACORXR180MG	Cap, Orange & White, Black Print, Ex Release, RPR over Dilacor XR over 180 mg	Diltiazem HCl 180 mg	Dilacor XR by Amerisource	62584-0251	Antihypertensive

ID FRONT <> BACK	DESCRIPTION FRONT <> BACK	INGREDIENT & STRENGTH	BRAND (or Generic Equiv.) by FIRM	NDC#	CLASS; SCH.
RPRDILACORXR180MG	Cap, Orange & White, Black Print, Ex Release, RPR over Dilacor XR over 180 mg	Diltiazem HCl 180 mg	Dilacor XR by Nat Pharmpak	55154-4021	Antihypertensive
RPRDILACORXR240MG	Cap, Brown & White, Black Print, Ex Release, RPR over Dilacor XR over 240 mg over Black Lines	Diltiazem HCl 240 mg	Dilacor XR by Thrift Drug	59198-0261	Antihypertensive
RPRDILACORXR240MG	Cap, Brown & White, Black Print, Ex Release, RPR over Dilacor XR over 240 mg over Black Lines	Diltiazem HCl 240 mg	Dilacor XR by Caremark	00339-5903	Antihypertensive
RPRDILACORXR240MG	Cap, Brown & White, Black Print, Ex Release, RPR over Dilacor XR over 240 mg over Black Lines	Diltiazem HCl 240 mg	Dilacor XR by Nat Pharmpak	55154-4022	Antihypertensive
RPRDILACORXR240MG	Cap, Brown & White, Black Print, Ex Release, RPR over Dilacor XR over 240 mg over Black Lines	Diltiazem HCl 240 mg	Dilacor XR by Amerisource	62584-0252	Antihypertensive
RPRDILACORXR240MG	Cap, Brown & White, Black Print, Ex Release, RPR over Dilacor XR over 240 mg over Black Lines	Diltiazem HCl 240 mg	Dilacor XR by Leiner	59606-0639	Antihypertensive
RPRH20	Tab, Aqua, Square	Chlorthalidone 50 mg	Hygroton by RPR		Diuretic
RPRH22	Tab, Peach, Square	Chlorthalidone 25 mg	Hygroton by RPR		Diuretic
RPRSLOBID	Tab, White, Oval, In Red RPR <> SLO-BID	Theophylline Anhydrous 50 mg	Slo-Bid by Takeda		Antiasthmatic
RPRSLOBID100MG	Cap, White, Red Print, Opaque, Slo-Bid over 100 mg	Theophylline Anhydrous 100 mg	Slo-Bid by RPR	00075-0100 Discontinued	Antiasthmatic
RPRSLOBID100MG	Cap, White, Red Print, Opaque, Slo-Bid over 100 mg	Theophylline Anhydrous 100 mg	Slo-Bid by RPR	Canadian	Antiasthmatic
RPRSLOBID125MG	Cap, White, Hard Gel, Ex Release, RPR Logo <> SLO-BID 125 MG	Theophylline Anhydrous 125 mg	Slo-Bid by RPR	00075-1125 Discontinued	Antiasthmatic
RPRSLOBID125MG	Cap, White, Hard Gel, Ex Release, RPR Logo <> SLO-BID 125 MG	Theophylline Anhydrous 125 mg	Slo-Bid by Murfreesboro	51129-1668	Antiasthmatic
RPRSLOBID200MG	Cap, Off-White, Red Print, Slo-bid over 200 mg	Theophylline Anhydrous 200 mg	Slo-Bid by RPR	Canadian	Antiasthmatic
RPRSLOBID200MG	Cap, Off-White, Red Print, Slo-bid over 200 mg	Theophylline Anhydrous 200 mg	Slo-Bid by RPR	00075-0200 Discontinued	Antiasthmatic
RPRSLOBID300MG	Cap, White, Red Print, Opaque, RPR over Slo-Bid over 300 mg	Theophylline Anhydrous 300 mg	Slo-Bid by RPR	Canadian	Antiasthmatic
RPRSLOBID300MG	Cap, White, Red Print, Opaque, RPR over Slo-Bid over 300 mg	Theophylline Anhydrous 300 mg	Slo-Bid by RPR	00075-0300 Discontinued	Antiasthmatic
RPRSLOBID300MG	Cap, White, Red Print, Opaque, RPR over Slo-Bid over 300 mg	Theophylline Anhydrous 300 mg	Slo-Bid by Talbert	44514-0904	Antiasthmatic
RPRSLOBID50MG	Cap, White, Red Print, Ex Release, Slo-Bid over 50 mg	Theophylline Anhydrous 50 mg	Slo-Bid by RPR	00075-0057 Discontinued	Antiasthmatic
RPRSLOBID50MG	Cap, White, Red Print, Ex Release, Slo-Bid over 50 mg	Theophylline Anhydrous 50 mg	Slo-Bid by RPR	Canadian	Antiasthmatic
RPRSLOBID75MG	Cap, Ex Release, Slo-Bid 75 MG	Theophylline Anhydrous 75 mg	Slo-Bid by RPR	00075-1075 Discontinued	Antiasthmatic
RR	Tab, White, Round	Calcium Sulfate, Belladonna, Potassium Bromide	Acne Relief Tab by Herbal Harvest		Supplement
RR	Tab, Brownish-Red, Cap-Shaped, Film-Coated, Scored, Cobalt Logo <> R / R	Risperidone 0.5 mg	Risperdal by Cobalt	Canadian DIN 02282593	Antipsychotic
RR0840	Cap, Yellow, RR-0840	Acetaminophen 325 mg, Codeine Phosphate 16 mg, Phenylephrine 10 mg, Chlorpheniramine 2 mg	Colrex by RR		Analgesic; C III
RR1	Tab, Pink, Round	Prednisone 1 mg	Orasone 1 by RR		Steroid
RR10	Tab, Blue, Round	Prednisone 10 mg	Orasone 10 by RR		Steroid
RR1007	Tab, White, Round	Medroxyprogesterone Acetate 10 mg	Curretab by RR		Hormone
RR1014	Tab, Blue, Round	Esterified Estrogen 0.3 mg	Estratab by RR		Hormone
RR1022	Tab, Yellow, Round	Esterified Estrogen 0.625 mg	Estratab by RR		Hormone
RR1023	Tab, Green, Oblong	Esterified Estrogen 0.625 mg, Methyltestosterone 2.5 mg	Estratest by RR		Hormone
RR1024	Tab, Red, Round	Esterified Estrogen 1.25 mg	Estratab by RR		Hormone

ID FRONT <> BACK	DESCRIPTION FRONT <> BACK	INGREDIENT & STRENGTH	BRAND (or Generic Equiv.) by FIRM	NDC#	CLASS; SCH.
RR1025	Tab, Pink, Round	Esterified Estrogen 2.5 mg	Estratab by RR		Hormone
RR1026	Tab, Green, Oblong	Esterified Estrogen 1.25 mg, Methyltestosterone 2.5 mg	Estratest by RR		Hormone
RR1039	Tab, White with Blue Specks, Oblong	Chlorpheniramine Maleate 4 mg, Phenylephrine 10 mg, Phenylpropanolamine 50 mg, Pyrilamine Maleate 25 mg	Histalet Forte by RR		Cold Remedy
RR1088	Tab, Brown, Rectangular	Hydrocodone Bitartrate 5 mg, Phenindamine 25 mg, Guaifenesin 200 mg	P-V-Tussin by RR		Analgesic; C III
RR1132	Tab, Yellow, Round	Hydralazine 25 mg, Reserpine 0.1 mg, Hydrochlorothiazide 15 mg	Unipres by RR		Antihypertensive; Diuretic
RR1146	Tab, Blue, Oblong	Prenatal Vitamin	Zenate by RR		Vitamin
RR1216	Cap, Brown	Vitamin Combination	Vio-Bec by RR		Vitamin
RR1218	Tab, Brown, Oblong	Vitamin Combination	Vio-Bec Forte by RR		Vitamin
RR1611	Tab, Peach, Oval	Vitamin, Mineral Combination	Norlac RX by RR		Vitamin
RR20	Tab, Yellow, Round	Prednisone 20 mg	Orasone 20 by RR		Steroid
RR3205	Tab, Yellow, Round	Dexamethasone 0.5 mg	Decadron by RR		Steroid
RR3210	Tab, Green, Round	Dexamethasone 0.75 mg	Decadron by RR		Steroid
RR3215	Tab, Pink, Round	Dexamethasone 1.5 mg	Decadron by RR		Steroid
RR3220	Tab, White, Round	Dexamethasone 4 mg	Decadron by RR		Steroid
RR40	Cap, Red	Amantadine HCl 100 mg	Symmetrel by Reid-Rowell		Antiviral
RR4020	Cap, Clear	Quinidine Sulfate 300 mg	Cin-Quin by RR		Antiarrhythmic
RR4024	Tab, White, Round	Quinidine Sulfate 100 mg	Cin-Quin by RR		Antiarrhythmic
RR4028	Tab, White, Round	Quinidine Sulfate 200 mg	Cin-Quin by RR		Antiarrhythmic
RR4032	Tab, White, Round	Quinidine Sulfate 300 mg	Cin-Quin by RR		Antiarrhythmic
RR4120	Cap, Orange, Oval	Valproic Acid 250 mg	Depakene by Reid-Rowell		Anticonvulsant
RR4140	Cap, Red, Oval	Amantadine HCl 100 mg	Symmetrel by Reid-Rowell		Antiviral
RR5	Tab, White, Round	Prednisone 5 mg	Orasone 5 by RR		Steroid
RR50	Tab, White, Round	Prednisone 50 mg	Orasone 50 by RR		Steroid
RR586	Tab, Green, Octagonal	Fluoxymesterone 10 mg	Halotestin by RR		Steroid; C III
RR7025	Tab, Red, Round	Meclizine HCl 20 mg	Ru-Vert M by RR		Antiemetic
RR7512	Cap, Peach	Lithium Carbonate 300 mg	Eskalith by RR		Antipsychotic
RR7516	Tab, White, Round	Lithium Carbonate 300 mg	Eskalith by RR		Antipsychotic
RS <> 301	Tab, White, Round	Atropine Sulfate 0.025 mg, Diphenoxylate HCl 2.5 mg	Lomotil by Corepharma	64720-0301	Antidiarrheal; C V
RS <> 301	Tab, White, Round	Atropine Sulfate 0.025 mg, Diphenoxylate HCl 2.5 mg	Lomotil by Amneal	65162-0301	Antidiarrheal; C V
RSN <> 150MG	Tab, Blue, Oval, Film Coated	Risedronate Sodium 150 mg	Actonel by Procter and Gamble	00149-0478	Bisphosphonate
RSN <> 30MG	Tab, White, Oval, Film Coated	Risedronate Sodium 30 mg	Actonel by Proc & Gamble	Canadian DIN 02239146	Bisphosphonate
RSN <> 30MG	Tab, White, Oval, Film Coated	Risedronate Sodium 30 mg	Actonel by Procter and Gamble	00149-0470	Bisphosphonate
RSN <> 35MG	Tab, Light Orange, Oval, Film-Coated	Risedronate Sodium 5 mg	Actonel Plus Calcium by Proc and Gamble	Canadian DIN 02279657	Bisphosphonate
RSN <> 35MG	Tab, Orange, Oval, Film Coated	Risedronate Sodium 35 mg	Actonel by Proc & Gamble	Canadian DIN 02246896	Bisphosphonate
RSN <> 35MG	Tab, Orange, Oval, Film Coated	Risedronate Sodium 35 mg	Actonel by Procter and Gamble	00149-0472	Bisphosphonate
RSN <> 5 MG	Tab, Yellow, Oval, Film Coated	Anhydrous Risedronate Sodium 5 mg	Actonel by Proc & Gamble	Canadian DIN 02242518	Bisphosphonate
RSN <> 5MG	Tab, Yellow, Oval, Film Coated	Risedronate Sodium 5 mg	Actonel by Proc & Gamble	Canadian DIN 02242531	Bisphosphonate
RSN <> 5MG	Tab, Yellow, Oval, Film Coated	Risedronate Sodium 5 mg	Actonel by Procter and Gamble	00149-0471	Bisphosphonate

ID FRONT <> BACK	DESCRIPTION FRONT <> BACK	INGREDIENT & STRENGTH	BRAND (or Generic Equiv.) by FIRM	NDC#	CLASS; SCH.
RSN <> 75MG	Tab, Pink, Oval, Film Coated	Risedronate Sodium 75 mg	Actonel by Procter and Gamble	00149-0477	Bisphosphonate
RSTLNE	Tab, Black with Yellow line, Coated	Acetazamorphazine 3.5 mg	Trydox by EST Pharma	99508-0048	Pain Reliever
RSTSM325	Cap, Green	Acetaminophen 325 mg, Pseudoephedrine HCl 30 mg	Regular Tylenol Sinus by McNeil	Canadian DIN 00778400	Cold Remedy
RTSN400	Cap, Brown and Orange	Tamsulosin HCl 0.4 mg	Flomax by Ranbaxy	Canadian DIN 02294885	Antiadrenergic
RUFEN400	Tab, Magenta, Round	Ibuprofen 400 mg	Motrin by Boots		NSAID
RUFEN6	Tab, White, Elongated	Ibuprofen 600 mg	Motrin by Boots		NSAID
RUFEN8	Tab, White, Elongated	Ibuprofen 800 mg	Motrin by Boots		NSAID
RUGBY	Tab, White, Round	Aspirin 325 mg	Aspirin by Rugby	00536-3300 Discontinued	Analgesic
RUGBY0070	Cap	Amoxicillin 250 mg	Amoxil by Rugby	00536-0070 Discontinued	Antibiotic
RUGBY0080	Cap, Cream	Amoxicillin 500 mg	Amoxil by Rugby	00536-0080 Discontinued	Antibiotic
RUGBY0120	Cap, Gray & Red	Cephalexin 250 mg	Keflex by Rugby	00536-0120 Discontinued	Antibiotic
RUGBY0130	Cap, Red	Cephalexin 500 mg	Keflex by Rugby	00536-0130 Discontinued	Antibiotic
RUGBY0230	Cap, Blue	Doxycycline Hyclate 100 mg	Vibramycin by Rugby	00536-0230 Discontinued	Antibiotic
RUGBY0250	Tab, Pink, Round	Erythromycin Stearate 250 mg	Erythrocin by Rugby	00536-0250 Discontinued	Antibiotic
RUGBY0265	Tab, Pink, Oval	Erythromycin Stearate 500 mg	Erythrocin by Rugby	00536-0265 Discontinued	Antibiotic
RUGBY0280	Cap, Aqua & White	Doxycycline Hyclate 50 mg	Vibramycin by Rugby	00536-0280 Discontinued	Antibiotic
RUGBY0340	Tab, Buff	Doxycycline Hyclate 100 mg	Vibra-Tab by Rugby	00536-0340 Discontinued	Antibiotic
RUGBY0390	Tab, Buff	Doxycycline Hyclate 50 mg	Vibra-Tab by Rugby	00536-0390 Discontinued	Antibiotic
RUGBY10	Tab, White, Round	Isoxsuprine HCl 10 mg	Vasodilan by Rugby	Discontinued	Vasodilator
RUGBY1003027	Tab, White, Round, Rugby 100/3027	Allopurinol 100 mg	Zyloprim by Rugby	Discontinued	Antigout
RUGBY1820	Cap, Orange & Yellow, Black Print, Rugby over 1820	Tetracycline HCl 250 mg	Achromycin V by Rugby	00536-1820 Discontinued	Antibiotic
RUGBY1830	Cap, Black & Yellow	Tetracycline HCl 250 mg	Achromycin V by Rugby	00536-1830 Discontinued	Antibiotic
RUGBY1870	Cap, Black & Yellow	Tetracycline HCl 500 mg	Achromycin V by Rugby	00536-1870 Discontinued	Antibiotic
RUGBY20	Tab, White, Round	Isoxsuprine HCl 20 mg	Vasodilan by Rugby	Discontinued	Vasodilator
RUGBY212	Tab, White, Round	Terfenadine 60 mg	Seldane by Rugby	Discontinued	Antihistamine
RUGBY23228	Tab, White, Round, Rugby 2/3228	Acetaminophen 300 mg, Codeine Phosphate 15 mg	Tylenol w/ Codeine by Rugby	Discontinued	Analgesic; C III
RUGBY3003028	Tab, Peach, Round, Rugby 300/3028	Allopurinol 300 mg	Zyloprim by Rugby	Discontinued	Antigout
RUGBY3007	Tab, White, Round, Rugby Logo 3007	Acetazolamide 250 mg	Diamox by Rugby	00536-3007	Antiglaucoma Agent
RUGBY3018	Tab, White, Round	Triprolidine 2.5 mg, Pseudoephedrine 60 mg	Actifed by Rugby	00536-3018 Discontinued	Cold Remedy
RUGBY3044	Tab, Yellow, Round	Amiloride HCl 5 mg, Hydrochlorothiazide 50 mg	Moduretic by Rugby	00536-3044 Discontinued	Antihypertensive; Diuretic

ID FRONT <> BACK	DESCRIPTION FRONT <> BACK	INGREDIENT & STRENGTH	BRAND (or Generic Equiv.) by FIRM	NDC#	CLASS; SCH.
RUGBY3046	Tab, White, Round	Aminophylline 100 mg	Aminophylline by Rugby	00536-3046 Discontinued	Antiasthmatic
RUGBY3060	Tab, White, Round	Aminophylline 200 mg	Aminophylline by Rugby	00536-3060 Discontinued	Antiasthmatic
RUGBY3071	Tab, Pink, Black Print, Round	Amitriptyline HCl 10 mg	Elavil by Rugby	00536-3071 Discontinued	Antidepressant
RUGBY3072	Tab, Green, Black Print, Round	Amitriptyline HCl 25 mg	Elavil by Rugby	00536-3072 Discontinued	Antidepressant
RUGBY3073	Tab, Brown, Round	Amitriptyline HCl 50 mg	Elavil by Rugby	00536-3073 Discontinued	Antidepressant
RUGBY3074	Tab, Purple, Black Print, Round	Amitriptyline HCl 75 mg	Elavil by Rugby	00536-3074 Discontinued	Antidepressant
RUGBY3075	Tab, Orange, Black Print, Round	Amitriptyline HCl 100 mg	Elavil by Rugby	00536-3075 Discontinued	Antidepressant
RUGBY3076	Tab, Peach, Round	Amitriptyline HCl 150 mg	Elavil by Rugby	00536-3076 Discontinued	Antidepressant
RUGBY3077	Tab, Blue, Round	Amitriptyline 10 mg, Perphenazine 2 mg	Triavil by Rugby	00536-3077 Discontinued	Antidepressant; Antipsychotic
RUGBY3078	Tab, Salmon, Round	Amitriptyline 10 mg, Perphenazine 4 mg	Triavil by Rugby	00536-3078 Discontinued	Antidepressant; Antipsychotic
RUGBY3082	Tab, Orange, Round	Amitriptyline 25 mg, Perphenazine 2 mg	Triavil by Rugby	00536-3082 Discontinued	Antidepressant; Antipsychotic
RUGBY3083	Tab, Yellow, Round	Amitriptyline 25 mg, Perphenazine 4 mg	Triavil by Rugby	00536-3083 Discontinued	Antidepressant; Antipsychotic
RUGBY3084	Tab, Orange, Round	Amitriptyline 50 mg, Perphenazine 4 mg	Triavil by Rugby	00536-3084 Discontinued	Antidepressant; Antipsychotic
RUGBY3109	Tab	Clomiphene Citrate 50 mg	by Rugby	00536-3109 Discontinued	Infertility
RUGBY3218	Tab, White, Oblong	Acetaminophen 500 mg	Tylenol Ex Strength by Rugby	00536-3218 Discontinued	Analgesic
RUGBY3222	Tab, White, Rugby Logo 3222	Acetaminophen 325 mg	Tylenol by Rugby	00536-3222 Discontinued	Analgesic
RUGBY3231	Tab, Rugby Logo 3231	Acetaminophen 500 mg	Tylenol Ex Strength by Rugby	00536-3231 Discontinued	Analgesic
RUGBY3235	Tab, White, Round	Alprazolam 0.25 mg	Xanax by Rugby	00536-3235 Discontinued	Antianxiety; C IV
RUGBY3236	Tab, Orange, Round	Alprazolam 0.5 mg	Xanax by Rugby	00536-3236 Discontinued	Antianxiety; C IV
RUGBY3237	Tab, Blue, Round	Alprazolam 1 mg	Xanax by Rugby	00536-3237 Discontinued	Antianxiety; C IV
RUGBY3279	Tab	Hydralazine 25 mg, Hydrochlorothiazide 15 mg	Apresoline-Esidrix by Rugby	00536-3279 Discontinued	Antihypertensive; Diuretic
RUGBY33227	Tab, White, Round, Rugby 3/3227	Acetaminophen 300 mg, Codeine Phosphate 30 mg	Tylenol w/ Codeine by Rugby	00536-3325 Discontinued	Analgesic; C III
RUGBY3325	Tab, White, Round	Atenolol 25 mg	Tenormin by Rugby	00536-3325 Discontinued	Antihypertensive
RUGBY3329	Tab, White, Round	Aspirin 325 mg, Codeine Phosphate 60 mg	Aspirin w/ Codeine by Rugby	00536-3329 Discontinued	Analgesic; C III
RUGBY3360	Tab	Belladonna, Phenobarbital	by Rugby	00536-3360 Discontinued	Gastrointestinal; C IV
RUGBY3364	Tab	Bethanechol Chloride 5 mg	Urecholine by Rugby	00536-3364 Discontinued	Urinary Tract

ID FRONT <> BACK	DESCRIPTION FRONT <> BACK	INGREDIENT & STRENGTH	BRAND (or Generic Equiv.) by FIRM	NDC#	CLASS; SCH.
RUGBY3365	Tab, White, Round	Bethanechol Chloride 10 mg	Urecholine by Rugby	00536-3365 Discontinued	Urinary Tract
RUGBY3367	Cap, Blue, White Print, Rugby over 3367	Dicyclomine HCl 10 mg	by Chelsea	46193-0105	Gastrointestinal
RUGBY3367	Cap, Blue, White Print, Rugby over 3367	Dicyclomine HCl 10 mg	by Rugby	53002-0329 Discontinued	Gastrointestinal
RUGBY3367	Cap, Blue, White Print, Rugby over 3367	Dicyclomine HCl 10 mg	by Rugby	00536-3367 Discontinued	Gastrointestinal
RUGBY3367	Cap, Blue, White Print, Rugby over 3367	Dicyclomine HCl 10 mg	by Caremark	00339-6054	Gastrointestinal
RUGBY3369	Tab, Light Yellow, Round, Scored	Bethanechol Chloride 25 mg	Urecholine by Rugby	00536-3369 Discontinued	Urinary Tract
RUGBY3370	Tab, White, Round	Benztropine Mesylate 0.5 mg	Cogentin by Rugby	00536-3370 Discontinued	Antiparkinson
RUGBY3371	Tab, White, Round	Benztropine Mesylate 1 mg	Cogentin by Rugby	00536-3371 Discontinued	Antiparkinson
RUGBY3372	Tab	Benztropine Mesylate 2 mg	Cogentin by Rugby	00536-3372 Discontinued	Antiparkinson
RUGBY3377	Tab	Dicyclomine HCl 20 mg	by Heartland	61392-0041 Discontinued	Gastrointestinal
RUGBY3377	Tab	Dicyclomine HCl 20 mg	by DRX	55045-1467 Discontinued	Gastrointestinal
RUGBY3377	Tab	Dicyclomine HCl 20 mg	by Pharmedix	53002-0345 Discontinued	Gastrointestinal
RUGBY3377	Tab	Dicyclomine HCl 20 mg	by Chelsea	46193-0115	Gastrointestinal
RUGBY3377	Tab	Dicyclomine HCl 20 mg	by Rugby	00536-3377 Discontinued	Gastrointestinal
RUGBY3377	Tab	Dicyclomine HCl 20 mg	by Allscripts	Discontinued	Gastrointestinal
RUGBY3377	Tab	Dicyclomine HCl 20 mg	by Kaiser	62224-9222 Discontinued	Gastrointestinal
RUGBY3406	Cap	Clorazepate Dipotassium 3.75 mg	Tranxene by Rugby	00536-3406 Discontinued	Antianxiety; C IV
RUGBY3407	Cap	Clorazepate Dipotassium 7.5 mg	Tranxene by Rugby	00536-3407 Discontinued	Antianxiety; C IV
RUGBY3408	Cap	Clorazepate Dipotassium 15 mg	Tranxene by Rugby	00536-3408 Discontinued	Antianxiety; C IV
RUGBY3415	Tab, White	Carbamazepine 200 mg	Tegretol by Rosemont	00536-3415 Discontinued	Anticonvulsant
RUGBY3420	Cap, Blue & Clear	Pseudoephedrine 120 mg, Chlorpheniramine Maleate 8 mg	Novafed A by Rugby	00536-3420 Discontinued	Cold Remedy
RUGBY3435	Tab	Carisoprodol 350 mg	by Rugby	00536-3435 Discontinued	Muscle Relaxant
RUGBY3435	Tab	Carisoprodol 350 mg	by Chelsea	46193-0500	Muscle Relaxant
RUGBY3444	Tab, White, Oblong, Scored	Chlorzoxazone 500 mg	by Chelsea	46193-0809	Muscle Relaxant
RUGBY3444	Tab, White, Oblong, Scored	Chlorzoxazone 500 mg	by Rugby	00536-3444 Discontinued	Muscle Relaxant
RUGBY3450	Tab	Chlorzoxazone 250 mg, Acetaminophen 300 mg	Parafon Forte by Rugby	00536-3450 Discontinued	Muscle Relaxant
RUGBY3455	Tab, Butterscotch Yellow, Round	Chlorpromazine HCl 25 mg	Thorazine by Rugby	00536-3455 Discontinued	Antipsychotic
RUGBY3456	Tab, Butterscotch Yellow, Round	Chlorpromazine HCl 50 mg	Thorazine by Rugby	00536-3456 Discontinued	Antipsychotic

ID FRONT <> BACK	DESCRIPTION FRONT <> BACK	INGREDIENT & STRENGTH	BRAND (or Generic Equiv.) by FIRM	NDC#	CLASS; SCH.
RUGBY3457	Tab, Butterscotch Yellow, Round	Chlorpromazine HCl 100 mg	Thorazine by Rugby	00536-3457 Discontinued	Antipsychotic
RUGBY3458	Tab, Butterscotch Yellow, Round	Chlorpromazine HCl 200 mg	Thorazine by Rugby	00536-3458 Discontinued	Antipsychotic
RUGBY3460	Tab, White, Round	Chlorothiazide 250 mg	Diuril by Rugby	00536-3460 Discontinued	Diuretic; Antihypertensive
RUGBY3461	Tab, White, Round	Chlorothiazide 500 mg	Diuril by Rugby	00536-3461 Discontinued	Diuretic; Antihypertensive
RUGBY3462	Tab, Blue, Round	Chlorpropamide 100 mg	Diabinese by Rugby	00536-3462 Discontinued	Antidiabetic
RUGBY3465	Tab, Blue, Round	Chlorpropamide 250 mg	Diabinese by Rugby	00536-3465 Discontinued	Antidiabetic
RUGBY3466	Cap, Yellow	Clofibrate 500 mg	Atromid-S by Rugby	00536-3466 Discontinued	Antihyperlipidemic
RUGBY3468	Tab, Blue, Round	Chlorthalidone 50 mg	Hygroton by Rugby	00536-3468 Discontinued	Diuretic
RUGBY3469	Tab, White, Round	Chlorthalidone 100 mg	Hygroton by Rugby	00536-3469 Discontinued	Diuretic
RUGBY3471	Tab	Captopril 12.5 mg	Capoten by Rugby	00536-3471 Discontinued	Antihypertensive
RUGBY3471	Tab	Captopril 12.5 mg	Capoten by Chelsea	46193-0552	Antihypertensive
RUGBY3472	Tab	Captopril 25 mg	Capoten by Rugby	00536-3472 Discontinued	Antihypertensive
RUGBY3472	Tab	Captopril 25 mg	Capoten by Chelsea	46193-0553	Antihypertensive
RUGBY3473	Tab	Captopril 50 mg	Capoten by Rugby	00536-3473 Discontinued	Antihypertensive
RUGBY3473	Tab	Captopril 50 mg	Capoten by Chelsea	46193-0554	Antihypertensive
RUGBY3474	Tab	Captopril 100 mg	Capoten by Chelsea	46193-0555	Antihypertensive
RUGBY3474	Tab	Captopril 100 mg	Capoten by Rugby	00536-3474 Discontinued	Antihypertensive
RUGBY3475	Tab, White, Round	Dimenhydrinate 50 mg	Dramamine by Rugby	00536-3475 Discontinued	Antiemetic
RUGBY3477	Cap, Green	Chloral Hydrate 500 mg	Chloral Hydrate by Rugby	00536-3477 Discontinued	Sedative/Hypnotic; C IV
RUGBY3485	Tab, Yellow	Chlorthalidone 25 mg	Hygroton by Rugby	00536-3485 Discontinued	Diuretic
RUGBY3490	Cap	Chlordiazepoxide 5 mg, Clidinium Bromide 2.5 mg	Librax by Rugby	00536-3490 Discontinued	Gastrointestinal
RUGBY3494	Tab, White, Round, Rugby Logo 3494	Colchicine 0.6 mg	by West-Ward	00536-3494	Antigout
RUGBY3496	Tab, White, Round, Rugby Logo 3496	Conjugated Estrogens 0.3 mg	Premarin by Rugby	00536-3496 Discontinued	Hormone
RUGBY3497	Tab, White, Round, Rugby Logo 3497	Conjugated Estrogens 0.625 mg	Premarin by Rugby	00536-3497 Discontinued	Hormone
RUGBY3498	Tab, White, Round, Rugby Logo 3498	Conjugated Estrogens 1.25 mg	Premarin by Rugby	00536-3498 Discontinued	Hormone
RUGBY3501	Tab, White, Round, Rugby Logo 3501	Conjugated Estrogens 2.5 mg	Premarin by Rugby	00536-3501 Discontinued	Hormone
RUGBY3515	Tab, White, Round, Scored	Cyproheptadine HCl 4 mg	Periactin by Rugby	00536-3515 Discontinued	Antihistamine
RUGBY3516	Tab, White, Round	Conjugated Estrogens 0.625 mg	Premarin by Rugby	00536-3516 Discontinued	Hormone

ID FRONT <> BACK	DESCRIPTION FRONT <> BACK	INGREDIENT & STRENGTH	BRAND (or Generic Equiv.) by FIRM	NDC#	CLASS; SCH.
RUGBY3517	Tab, White, Round, Rugby Logo 3517	Conjugated Estrogens 0.3 mg	Premarin by Rugby	00536-3517	Hormone
RUGBY3522	Tab, White, Round	Conjugated Estrogens 1.25 mg	Premarin by Rugby	00536-3522 Discontinued	Hormone
RUGBY3523	Tab, Orange, Round	Clonidine HCl 0.1 mg	Catapres by Rugby	00536-3523 Discontinued	Antihypertensive
RUGBY3524	Tab, Orange, Round	Clonidine HCl 0.2 mg	Catapres by Rugby	00536-3524 Discontinued	Antihypertensive
RUGBY3526	Tab, Orange, Round	Clonidine HCl 0.3 mg	Catapres by Rugby	00536-3526 Discontinued	Antihypertensive
RUGBY3528	Tab, White, Round	Conjugated Estrogens 2.5 mg	Premarin by Rugby	00536-3528 Discontinued	Hormone
RUGBY3529	Cap, Red & Blue	Cyclandelate 400 mg	Cyclospasmol by Rugby	00536-3529 Discontinued	Vasodilator
RUGBY3530	Tab	Cortisone Acetate 25 mg	by Rugby	00536-3530 Discontinued	Steroid
RUGBY3531	Cap, Blue	Cyclandelate 200 mg	Cyclospasmol by Rugby	00536-3531 Discontinued	Vasodilator
RUGBY3571	Tab, White, Round	Dipyridamole 50 mg	Persantine by Rugby	00536-3571 Discontinued	Antiplatelet
RUGBY3572	Tab, White, Round	Dipyridamole 75 mg	Persantine by Rugby	00536-3572 Discontinued	Antiplatelet
RUGBY3583	Tab	Dexamethasone 0.75 mg	Decadron by Rugby	00536-3583 Discontinued	Steroid
RUGBY3591	Tab, White, Round	Diazepam 2 mg	Valium by Rugby	00536-3591 Discontinued	Antianxiety; C IV
RUGBY3592	Tab, Yellow, Round	Diazepam 5 mg	Valium by Rugby	00536-3592 Discontinued	Antianxiety; C IV
RUGBY3593	Tab, Blue, Round	Diazepam 10 mg	Valium by Rugby	00536-3593 Discontinued	Antianxiety; C IV
RUGBY3595	Cap, Blue	Disopyramide Phosphate 100 mg	Norpace by Rugby	00536-3595 Discontinued	Antiarrhythmic
RUGBY3596	Cap, Scarlet	Disopyramide Phosphate 150 mg	Norpace by Rugby	00536-3596 Discontinued	Antiarrhythmic
RUGBY3597	Tab, Purple, Oblong	Diphenhydramine HCl 25 mg	Benadryl by Rugby	00536-3597 Discontinued	Antihistamine
RUGBY3728	Cap, Orange	Doxepin HCl 25 mg	Sinequan by Rugby	00536-3728 Discontinued	Antidepressant
RUGBY3729	Cap, Black & White	Doxepin HCl 50 mg	Sinequan by Rugby	00536-3729 Discontinued	Antidepressant
RUGBY3730	Cap, Yellow	Doxepin HCl 100 mg	Sinequan by Rugby	00536-3730 Discontinued	Antidepressant
RUGBY3736	Cap, Yellow	Doxepin HCl 10 mg	Sinequan by Rugby	00536-3736 Discontinued	Antidepressant
RUGBY3737	Cap, Green	Doxepin HCl 75 mg	Sinequan by Rugby	00536-3737 Discontinued	Antidepressant
RUGBY3738	Cap, Blue & White	Doxepin HCl 150 mg	Sinequan by Rugby	00536-3738 Discontinued	Antidepressant
RUGBY3745	Tab, White, Round	Dimenhydrinate 50 mg	Dramamine by Rugby	00536-3745 Discontinued	Antiemetic
RUGBY3758	Cap, Pink & White	Diphenhydramine 25 mg	Benadryl by Rugby	00536-3758 Discontinued	Antihistamine
RUGBY3762	Cap	Diphenhydramine HCl 50 mg	by Rugby	00536-3762 Discontinued	Antihistamine

ID FRONT <> BACK	DESCRIPTION FRONT <> BACK	INGREDIENT & STRENGTH	BRAND (or Generic Equiv.) by FIRM	NDC#	CLASS; SCH.
RUGBY3764	Cap, White	Prompt Phenytoin Sodium 100 mg	by Rugby	00536-3764 Discontinued	Anticonvulsant
RUGBY3767	Tab, White, Round	Disulfiram 250 mg	Antabuse by Rugby	00536-3767 Discontinued	Antialcoholism
RUGBY3768	Tab, White, Round	Disulfiram 500 mg	Antabuse by Rugby	00536-3768 Discontinued	Antialcoholism
RUGBY3770	Tab, Blue & Green	Trichlormethiazide 4 mg	Metahydrin by Rugby	00536-3770 Discontinued	Diuretic; Antihypertensive
RUGBY3778	Cap	Ephedrine Sulfate 50 mg	by Rugby	00536-3778 Discontinued	Antiasthmatic
RUGBY3780	Cap	Ephedrine Sulfate 25 mg	by Rugby	00536-3780 Discontinued	Antiasthmatic
RUGBY3795	Cap, Blue & White	Flurazepam HCl 15 mg	Dalmane by Rugby	00536-3795 Discontinued	Hypnotic; C IV
RUGBY3796	Cap	Flurazepam HCl 30 mg	by Rugby	00536-3796 Discontinued	Hypnotic; C IV
RUGBY3798	Tab, Salmon & Blue-Green, Round	Aspirin 325 mg, Meprobamate 400 mg	Equagesic by Rugby	00536-3798 Discontinued	Sedative/Hypnotic; C IV
RUGBY3804	Cap	Vitamin Combination	Trinsicon by Rugby	00536-3804 Discontinued	Vitamin
RUGBY3813	Tab, White, Oval	Fenoprofen Calcium 600 mg	Nalfon by Rugby	00536-3813 Discontinued	NSAID
RUGBY3824	Tab, Green, Round	Ferrous Gluconate 5 g	Fergon by Rugby	00536-3824 Discontinued	Mineral
RUGBY3835	Tab, White	Furosemide 80 mg	Lasix by Rugby	00536-3835 Discontinued	Diuretic
RUGBY3840	Tab	Furosemide 20 mg	by Rugby	00536-3840 Discontinued	Diuretic
RUGBY3841	Tab	Furosemide 40 mg	by Rugby	00536-3841 Discontinued	Diuretic
RUGBY3845	Tab, Yellow, Round, Scored, Rugby over 3845	Folic Acid 1 mg	by Rugby	00536-3845 Discontinued	Vitamin
RUGBY3854	Tab, Light Orange, Film Coated, Scored	Gemfibrozil 600 mg	by Rugby	00536-3854 Discontinued	Antihyperlipidemic
RUGBY3854	Tab, Light Orange, Film Coated, Scored	Gemfibrozil 600 mg	by Chelsea	46193-0537	Antihyperlipidemic
RUGBY3856	Tab, White, Round	Ergoloid Mesylate 1 mg	Hydergine by Rugby	00536-3856 Discontinued	Ergot Alkaloids
RUGBY3857	Tab, White, Round	Ergoloid Mesylate 1 mg	Hydergine by Rugby	00536-3857 Discontinued	Ergot Alkaloids
RUGBY3859	Tab, White, Round	Ergoloid Mesylate 0.5 mg	Hydergine by Rugby	00536-3859 Discontinued	Ergot Alkaloids
RUGBY3871	Tab	Guaifenesin 400 mg, Phenylpropanolamine HCl 75 mg	Entex LA by Rugby	00536-3871 Discontinued	Cold Remedy
RUGBY3874	Tab, Lavender	Hydroxyzine HCl 10 mg	Atarax by Rugby	00536-3874 Discontinued	Antianxiety; Antihistamine
RUGBY3875	Tab, Lavender, Round	Hydroxyzine HCl 25 mg	Atarax by Rugby	00536-3875 Discontinued	Antianxiety; Antihistamine
RUGBY3876	Tab, Purple, Round	Hydroxyzine HCl 50 mg	Atarax by Rugby	00536-3876 Discontinued	Antianxiety; Antihistamine
RUGBY3882	Tab, Peach, Round	Hydroflumethiazide 50 mg	Diucardin by Rugby	00536-3882 Discontinued	Diuretic; Antihypertensive
RUGBY3893	Cap, Dark Green & Light Green	Hydroxyzine Pamoate 25 mg	Vistaril by Chelsea	46193-0619	Antianxiety; Antihistamine
RUGBY3894	Cap, Dark Green	Hydroxyzine Pamoate 50 mg	Vistaril by Chelsea	46193-0623	Antianxiety; Antihistamine

ID FRONT <> BACK	DESCRIPTION FRONT <> BACK	INGREDIENT & STRENGTH	BRAND (or Generic Equiv.) by FIRM	NDC#	CLASS; SCH.
RUGBY3894	Cap, Dark Green	Hydroxyzine Pamoate 50 mg	Vistaril by Rugby	00536-3894 Discontinued	Antianxiety; Antihistamine
RUGBY3894	Cap, Green & White, Opaque	Hydroxyzine Pamoate 50 mg	by Murfreesboro	51129-1487 Discontinued	Antianxiety; Antihistamine
RUGBY3895	Cap, Green & Gray	Hydroxyzine Pamoate 100 mg	Vistaril by Rugby	00536-3895 Discontinued	Antianxiety; Antihistamine
RUGBY3906	Tab, White	Ephedrine 24 mg, Phenobarbital 8 mg, Theophylline 130 mg	Tedral by Rugby	00536-3906 Discontinued	Antiasthmatic; C IV
RUGBY3914	Tab	Acetaminophen 500 mg, Hydrocodone Bitartrate 5 mg	Lortab by Rugby	00536-3914 Discontinued	Analgesic; C III
RUGBY3915	Tab, Green, Round	Hydrochlorothiazide 25 mg, Reserpine 0.125 mg	Hydropres by Rugby	00536-3915 Discontinued	Diuretic; Antihypertensive
RUGBY3916	Tab, Green, Round	Hydrochlorothiazide 50 mg, Reserpine 0.125 mg	Hydropres by Rugby	00536-3916 Discontinued	Diuretic; Antihypertensive
RUGBY3918	Tab	Hyoscyamine Sulfate 0.125 mg	Levsin by Rugby	00536-3918 Discontinued	Gastrointestinal
RUGBY3918	Tab, 39/18	Hyoscyamine Sulfate 0.125 mg	Levsin by Anabolic	00722-6286	Gastrointestinal
RUGBY3919	Tab, White, Round, Scored	Hydrochlorothiazide 50 mg	by Rugby	00536-3919 Discontinued	Diuretic; Antihypertensive
RUGBY3920	Tab, Rugby/3920	Atropine Sulfate 0.0194 mg, Hyoscyamine Sulfate 0.1037 mg, Phenobarbital 16.2 mg, Scopolamine 0.0065 mg	Donnatal by Rugby	00536-3920 Discontinued	Gastrointestinal; C IV
RUGBY3920	Tab, Rugby/3920	Atropine Sulfate 0.0194 mg, Hyoscyamine Sulfate 0.1037 mg, Phenobarbital 16.2 mg, Scopolamine 0.0065 mg	Donnatal by JMI Canton	00252-6793	Gastrointestinal; C IV
RUGBY3921	Tab, Yellow, Round	Hydrochlorothiazide 50 mg	Hydrodiuril by Rugby	00536-3921 Discontinued	Diuretic; Antihypertensive
RUGBY3922	Tab	Hydrochlorothiazide 25 mg	Hydrodiuril by Heartland		Diuretic; Antihypertensive
RUGBY3922	Tab, White, Round, Scored	Hydrochlorothiazide 25 mg	Hydrodiuril by Rugby	00536-3922 Discontinued	Diuretic; Antihypertensive
RUGBY3923	Tab, Peach, Round	Hydrochlorothiazide 100 mg	Hydrodiuril by Rugby	00536-3923 Discontinued	Diuretic; Antihypertensive
RUGBY3927	Tab, Green, Round, Scored	Isosorbide Dinitrate 20 mg	Isordil by Rugby	00536-3927 Discontinued	Antianginal
RUGBY3929	Tab, Yellow, Black Print, Round	Imipramine HCl 10 mg	Tofranil by Rugby	00536-3929 Discontinued	Antidepressant
RUGBY3930	Tab, Orange	Imipramine HCl 25 mg	Tofranil by Rugby	00536-3930 Discontinued	Antidepressant
RUGBY3931	Tab, Green, Black Print, Round	Imipramine HCl 50 mg	Tofranil by Rugby	00536-3931 Discontinued	Antidepressant
RUGBY3933	Cap, White, Round, Rugby Logo R 3933	Butalbital 50 mg, Aspirin 325 mg, Caffeine 40 mg	Fiorinal by Rugby	00536-3933 Discontinued	Analgesic; C III
RUGBY3934	Tab	Ibuprofen 200 mg	Motrin by Rugby	00536-3934 Discontinued	NSAID
RUGBY3935	Tab, White, Round	Isoxsuprine HCl 10 mg	Vasodilan by Rugby	00536-3935 Discontinued	Vasodilator
RUGBY3936	Tab, White, Round	Isoxsuprine HCl 20 mg	Vasodilan by Rugby	00536-3936 Discontinued	Vasodilator
RUGBY3937	Tab	Aspirin 325 mg, Butalbital 50 mg, Caffeine 40 mg	Fiorinal by Rugby	00536-3937 Discontinued	Analgesic; C III
RUGBY3938	Tab, Blue-Green, Round, Scored	Isosorbide Dinitrate Oral 30 mg	Isordil by Rugby	00536-3938 Discontinued	Antianginal

ID FRONT <> BACK	DESCRIPTION FRONT <> BACK	INGREDIENT & STRENGTH	BRAND (or Generic Equiv.) by FIRM	NDC#	CLASS; SCH.
RUGBY3940	Tab	Isosorbide Dinitrate TR 40 mg	Isordil by Rugby	00536-3940 Discontinued	Antianginal
RUGBY3941	Tab, White, Round	Isoniazid 300 mg	INH by Rugby	00536-3941 Discontinued	Antimycobacterial
RUGBY3943	Tab, White, Round, Scored	Isosorbide Dinitrate Oral 10 mg	Isordil by Rugby	00536-3943 Discontinued	Antianginal
RUGBY3946	Tab, Pink, Round	Isosorbide Dinitrate Oral 5 mg	Isordil by Rugby	00536-3946 Discontinued	Antianginal
RUGBY3947	Tab, Orange, Round	Levothyroxine Sodium 25 mcg	Synthroid by Rugby	00536-3947 Discontinued	Thyroid Hormone
RUGBY3948	Tab, White, Round	Isoniazid 100 mg	Laniazid by Rugby	00536-3948 Discontinued	Antimycobacterial
RUGBY3950	Tab, White, Round	Isosorbide Dinitrate SL 10 mg	Isordil by Rugby	00536-3950 Discontinued	Antianginal
RUGBY3950	Tab, Pink, Round	Levothyroxine Sodium 50 mcg	Synthroid by Rugby	00536-3950 Discontinued	Thyroid Hormone
RUGBY3951	Tab, Round	Levothyroxine Sodium 75 mcg	Synthroid by Rugby	00536-3951 Discontinued	Thyroid Hormone
RUGBY3952	Tab, Yellow, Round, Scored	Levothyroxine Sodium 0.1 mg	Synthroid by Rugby	00536-3952 Discontinued	Thyroid Hormone
RUGBY3953	Tab, Blue, Round	Levothyroxine Sodium 0.15 mg	Synthroid by Rugby	00536-3953 Discontinued	Thyroid Hormone
RUGBY3954	Tab, Round	Levothyroxine Sodium 0.2 mg	Synthroid by Rugby	00536-3954 Discontinued	Thyroid Hormone
RUGBY3956	Cap	Lithium Carbonate 300 mg	Eskalith by Rugby	00536-3956 Discontinued	Antipsychotic
RUGBY3957	Cap	Prochlorperazine Maleate 10 mg, Isopropamide Iodide 5 mg	Combid by Rugby	00536-3957 Discontinued	Gastrointestinal
RUGBY3958	Tab, Green, Round	Levothyroxine Sodium 0.3 mg	Synthroid by Rugby	00536-3958 Discontinued	Thyroid Hormone
RUGBY3961	Tab, White, Round	Lorazepam 2 mg	Ativan by Watson	00536-3961 Discontinued	Antianxiety; C IV
RUGBY3963	Tab, Beige, Round	Levothyroxine Sodium 125 mcg	Synthroid by Rugby	00536-3963 Discontinued	Thyroid Hormone
RUGBY3976	Tab	Ibuprofen 300 mg	Motrin by Rugby	00536-3976 Discontinued	NSAID
RUGBY3977	Tab, White, Round	Ibuprofen 400 mg	Motrin by Rugby	00536-3977 Discontinued	NSAID
RUGBY3978	Tab, White, Oval	Ibuprofen 600 mg	Motrin by Rugby	00536-3978 Discontinued	NSAID
RUGBY3979	Tab	Ibuprofen 800 mg	Motrin by Rugby	00536-3979 Discontinued	NSAID
RUGBY3980	Cap, Purple & White	Indomethacin 75 mg	Indocin SR by Rugby	00536-3980 Discontinued	NSAID
RUGBY3981	Cap, Green	Indomethacin 25 mg	Indocin by Rugby	00536-3981 Discontinued	NSAID
RUGBY3982	Cap, Green	Indomethacin 50 mg	Indocin by Rugby	00536-3982 Discontinued	NSAID
RUGBY3985	Tab, White	Meclizine HCl 12.5 mg	Antivert by Rugby	00536-3985 Discontinued	Antiemetic
RUGBY3986	Tab, Blue & White, Multilayer	Meclizine HCl 12.5 mg	by Rugby	00536-3986 Discontinued	Antiemetic

ID FRONT <> BACK	DESCRIPTION FRONT <> BACK	INGREDIENT & STRENGTH	BRAND (or Generic Equiv.) by FIRM	NDC#	CLASS; SCH.
RUGBY3988	Tab, Yellow & White, Multilayer	Meclizine HCl 25 mg	by Chelsea	46193-0149	Antiemetic
RUGBY3988	Tab, Yellow & White	Meclizine HCl 25 mg	by Rugby	00536-3988 Discontinued	Antiemetic
RUGBY3990	Tab	Meclizine HCl 25 mg Chewable	Antivert by Rugby	00536-3990 Discontinued	Antiemetic
RUGBY3995	Tab, White, Round	Medroxyprogesterone Acetate 10 mg	Provera by Rugby	00536-3995 Discontinued	Hormone
RUGBY3996	Tab	Hydrochlorothiazide 15 mg, Methyldopa 250 mg	Aldoril by Rugby	00536-3996 Discontinued	Diuretic; Antihypertensive
RUGBY3997	Tab	Hydrochlorothiazide 25 mg, Methyldopa 250 mg	Aldoril by Rugby	00536-3997 Discontinued	Diuretic; Antihypertensive
RUGBY4002	Cap, Yellow	Meclofenamate Sodium 50 mg	Meclomen by Rugby	00536-4002 Discontinued	NSAID
RUGBY4003	Cap, Beige & Yellow	Meclofenamate Sodium 100 mg	Meclomen by Rugby	00536-4003 Discontinued	NSAID
RUGBY4005	Tab, White, Round	Meprobamate 200 mg	Equanil by Rugby	00536-4005 Discontinued	Sedative/Hypnotic; C IV
RUGBY4006	Tab, White, Round	Meprobamate 400 mg	Equanil by Rugby	00536-4006 Discontinued	Sedative/Hypnotic; C IV
RUGBY4010	Tab, White, Round	Methyldopa 250 mg	Aldomet by Rugby	00536-4010 Discontinued	Antihypertensive
RUGBY4011	Tab, White, Round	Methyldopa 500 mg	Aldomet by Rugby	00536-4011 Discontinued	Antihypertensive
RUGBY4012	Tab, White, Round	Methyldopa 125 mg	Aldomet by Rugby	00536-4012 Discontinued	Antihypertensive
RUGBY4012	Tab, Film Coated	Etodolac 400 mg	by Rugby	00536-4012 Discontinued	NSAID
RUGBY4012	Tab, Film Coated	Etodolac 400 mg	by Chelsea	46193-0584	NSAID
RUGBY4018	Tab, White, Round	Metronidazole 250 mg	Flagyl by Rugby	00536-4018 Discontinued	Antibiotic
RUGBY4019	Tab, White, Oval	Metronidazole 500 mg	Flagyl by Rugby	00536-4019 Discontinued	Antibiotic
RUGBY4020	Tab, Peach, Round	Methyldopa 125 mg	Aldomet by Rugby	00536-4020 Discontinued	Antihypertensive
RUGBY4021	Tab, Peach, Round	Methyldopa 250 mg	Aldomet by Rugby	00536-4021 Discontinued	Antihypertensive
RUGBY4023	Tab, Peach, Round	Methyldopa 500 mg	Aldomet by Rugby	00536-4023 Discontinued	Antihypertensive
RUGBY4025	Tab, Yellow, Round	Methyclothiazide 5 mg	Enduron by Rugby	00536-4025 Discontinued	Diuretic; Antihypertensive
RUGBY4025	Tab	Methyclothiazide 5 mg	by Chelsea	46193-0525	Diuretic; Antihypertensive
RUGBY4026	Tab	Methocarbamol 500 mg	Robaxin by Rugby	00536-4026 Discontinued	Muscle Relaxant
RUGBY4026	Tab	Methocarbamol 500 mg	Robaxin by Chelsea	46193-0120	Muscle Relaxant
RUGBY4027	Tab	Methocarbamol 750 mg	Robaxin by Chelsea	46193-0121	Muscle Relaxant
RUGBY4027	Tab	Methocarbamol 750 mg	Robaxin by Rugby	00536-4027 Discontinued	Muscle Relaxant
RUGBY4028	Tab	Aspirin 325 mg, Methocarbamol 500 mg	Robaxisal by Rugby	00536-4028 Discontinued	Analgesic; Muscle Relaxant
RUGBY4036	Tab, White, Oval	Methylprednisolone 4 mg	Medrol by Rugby	00536-4036 Discontinued	Steroid
RUGBY4036	Tab	Methylprednisolone 4 mg	by Chelsea	46193-0604	Steroid

ID FRONT <> BACK	DESCRIPTION FRONT <> BACK	INGREDIENT & STRENGTH	BRAND (or Generic Equiv.) by FIRM	NDC#	CLASS; SCH.
RUGBY4040	Tab, Peach, Round	Methylclothiazide 2.5 mg	Enduron by Rugby	00536-4040 Discontinued	Diuretic; Antihypertensive
RUGBY4041	Tab, Pink, Orange, Round	Methylclothiazide 5 mg	Enduron by Rugby	00536-4041 Discontinued	Diuretic; Antihypertensive
RUGBY4042	Tab, White, Round	Metoclopramide HCl 10 mg	Reglan by Watson	00536-4042 Discontinued	Gastrointestinal
RUGBY4043	Tab, White, Round	Minoxidil 10 mg	Loniten by Rugby	00536-4043 Discontinued	Antihypertensive
RUGBY4052	Tab	Methyldopa 250 mg, Chlorothiazide 150 mg	Aldochlor by Rugby	00536-4052 Discontinued	Antihypertensive; Diuretic
RUGBY4053	Tab	Methyldopa 250 mg, Chlorothiazide 250 mg	Aldochlor by Rugby	00536-4053 Discontinued	Antihypertensive; Diuretic
RUGBY4081	Tab	Nitrofurantoin 50 mg	Furadantin by Rugby	00536-4081 Discontinued	Antibiotic
RUGBY4082	Tab	Nitrofurantoin 100 mg	Furadantin by Rugby	00536-4082 Discontinued	Antibiotic
RUGBY4083	Cap, Lavender & Clear	Nitroglycerin SR 2.5 mg	Nitrobid by Rugby	00536-4083 Discontinued	Vasodilator
RUGBY4084	Cap, Brown and Orange, ER	Nitroglycerin 6.5 mg	by Rugby	00536-4084 Discontinued	Vasodilator
RUGBY4090	Cap, Green and Clear, ER	Nitroglycerin 9 mg	by Rugby	00536-4090 Discontinued	Vasodilator
RUGBY4091	Tab, Off-White	Nystatin Vaginal 100,000 Units	Mycostatin by Rugby	00536-4091 Discontinued	Antifungal
RUGBY4094	Tab, Brown, Round	Nystatin 500,000 Units	Mycostatin by Lemmon	00536-4094 Discontinued	Antifungal
RUGBY4114	Cap, Pink & Clear	Oxazepam 10 mg	Serax by Rugby	00536-4114 Discontinued	Sedative/Hypnotic; C IV
RUGBY4115	Cap, White	Oxazepam 15 mg	Serax by Rugby	00536-4115 Discontinued	Sedative/Hypnotic; C IV
RUGBY4116	Cap, Clear	Oxazepam 30 mg	Serax by Rugby	00536-4116 Discontinued	Sedative/Hypnotic; C IV
RUGBY4124	Cap, Brown & Clear	Papaverine HCl TD 150 mg	Pavabid by Rugby	00536-4124 Discontinued	Vasodilator
RUGBY4130	Tab	Pentaerythritol Tetranitrate 10 mg	Peritrate by Rugby	00536-4130 Discontinued	Antianginal
RUGBY4131	Tab, Round	Perphenazine 2 mg	Trilafon by Rugby	00536-4131 Discontinued	Antipsychotic
RUGBY4132	Tab, Round	Perphenazine 4 mg	Trilafon by Rugby	00536-4132 Discontinued	Antipsychotic
RUGBY4133	Tab, Round	Perphenazine 8 mg	Trilafon by Rugby	00536-4133 Discontinued	Antipsychotic
RUGBY4134	Tab, Round	Perphenazine 16 mg	Trilafon by Rugby	00536-4134 Discontinued	Antipsychotic
RUGBY4138	Tab	Pentaerythritol Tetranitrate 20 mg	Peritrate by Rugby	00536-4138 Discontinued	Antianginal
RUGBY4147	Tab, White, Round	Perphenazine 8 mg	Trilafon by Rugby	00536-4147 Discontinued	Antipsychotic
RUGBY4148	Tab	Leucovorin 5 mg	Wellcovorin by Rugby	00536-4148 Discontinued	Antineoplastic
RUGBY4149	Tab	Leucovorin 25 mg	Wellcovorin by Rugby	00536-4149 Discontinued	Antineoplastic

ID FRONT <> BACK	DESCRIPTION FRONT <> BACK	INGREDIENT & STRENGTH	BRAND (or Generic Equiv.) by FIRM	NDC#	CLASS; SCH.
RUGBY4160	Tab, Yellow	Phendimetrazine Tartrate 35 mg	Plegine by Rugby	00536-4160 Discontinued	Anorexiant; C III
RUGBY4161	Tab, Gray	Phendimetrazine Tartrate 35 mg	Plegine by Rugby	00536-4161 Discontinued	Anorexiant; C III
RUGBY4162	Tab, Pink	Phendimetrazine Tartrate 35 mg	Plegine by Rugby	00536-4162 Discontinued	Anorexiant; C III
RUGBY4167	Tab, White	Phendimetrazine Tartrate 35 mg	Plegine by Rugby	00536-4167 Discontinued	Anorexiant; C III
RUGBY4224	Tab	Phenobarbital 20 mg	by West-Ward		Sedative/Hypnotic; C IV
RUGBY4234	Tab, Blue, Round	Ergotamine Tartrate 0.6 mg, Phenobarbital 40 mg, Belladonna 0.2	Bellergal-S by Rugby	00536-4234 Discontinued	Antispasmodic; C IV
RUGBY4235	Cap, Blue & Clear	Phentermine 30 mg	Fastin by Rugby	00536-4235 Discontinued	Anorexiant; C IV
RUGBY4288	Tab, Green	Phentermine HCl 8 mg	by Rugby	00536-4288 Discontinued	Anorexiant; C IV
RUGBY4290	Tab	Phenylpropanolamine 25 mg	Dexatrim by Rugby	00536-4290 Discontinued	Decongestant; Appetite Suppressant
RUGBY4295	Cap	Piroxicam 20 mg	Feldene by Rugby	00536-4295 Discontinued	NSAID
RUGBY4298	Tab, Orange, Round, Film Coated	Phenylbutazone 100 mg	Butazolidin by Rugby	00536-4298 Discontinued	Anti-Inflammatory
RUGBY4299	Tab, Red, Film Coated	Phenylbutazone 100 mg	Butazolidin by Rugby	00536-4299 Discontinued	Anti-Inflammatory
RUGBY4305	Cap, Orange & Cream	Phenylbutazone 100 mg	Butazolidin by Rugby	00536-4305 Discontinued	Anti-Inflammatory
RUGBY4307	Tab, Chewable	Ascorbic Acid 60 mg, Cyanocobalamin 4.5 mcg, Folic Acid 0.3 mg, Niacinamide, Pyridoxine HCl 1.05 mg, Riboflavin 1.2 mg, Sodium Fluoride, Thiamine Mononitrate, Vitamin A Acetate, Vitamin D 400 Units, Vitamin E Acetate	Poly-Vitamin by Rugby	00536-4307 Discontinued	Vitamin
RUGBY4308	Tab, Chewable	Ascorbic Acid 60 mg, Cupric Oxide, Cyanocobalamin 4.5 mcg, Ferrous Fumarate, Folic Acid 0.3 mg, Niacinamide, Pyridoxine HCl 1.05 mg, Riboflavin 1.2 mg, Sodium Fluoride, Thiamine HCl 1.05 mg, Vitamin A Acetate 2500 Units, Vitamin D 400 Units, Zinc Oxide	Poly-Vitamin by Rugby	00536-4308 Discontinued	Vitamin
RUGBY4309	Tab, Orange, Round	Propranolol HCl 10 mg	Inderal by Rugby	00536-4309 Discontinued	Antihypertensive
RUGBY4312	Tab, Chewable	Ascorbic Acid 60 mg, Cyanocobalamin 4.5 mcg, Fluoride Ion 0.5 mg, Folic Acid 0.3 mg, Niacin 13.5 mg, Pyridoxine HCl 1.05 mg, Riboflavin 1.2 mg, Thiamine Mononitrate 1.05 mg, Vitamin A 2500 Units, Vitamin D 400 Units, Vitamin E 15 Units	Poly-Vitamin by Rugby	00536-4312 Discontinued	Vitamin
RUGBY4313	Tab, Blue, Round	Propranolol HCl 20 mg	Inderal by Rugby	00536-4313 Discontinued	Antihypertensive
RUGBY4314	Tab, Green, Round	Propranolol HCl 40 mg	Inderal by Rugby	00536-4314 Discontinued	Antihypertensive
RUGBY4315	Tab, Pink, Round	Propranolol HCl 60 mg	Inderal by Rugby	00536-4315 Discontinued	Antihypertensive
RUGBY4316	Tab, Yellow, Round	Propranolol HCl 80 mg	Inderal by Rugby	00536-4316 Discontinued	Antihypertensive
RUGBY43215	Tab, White, Round, Rugby 4/3215	Acetaminophen 300 mg, Codeine Phosphate 60 mg	Tylenol w/ Codeine by Rugby	00536-4321 Discontinued	Analgesic; C III
RUGBY4322	Tab, Round	Potassium Chloride 600 mg (8 mEq)	Slow K by Rugby	00536-4322 Discontinued	Electrolytes

ID FRONT <> BACK	DESCRIPTION FRONT <> BACK	INGREDIENT & STRENGTH	BRAND (or Generic Equiv.) by FIRM	NDC#	CLASS; SCH.
RUGBY4324	Tab	Prednisone 5 mg	by Rugby	00536-4324 Discontinued	Steroid
RUGBY4324	Tab	Prednisone 5 mg	by Chelsea	46193-0102	Steroid
RUGBY4325	Tab	Prednisone 10 mg	by Chelsea	46193-0676	Steroid
RUGBY4325	Tab	Prednisone 10 mg	by Rugby	00536-4325 Discontinued	Steroid
RUGBY4326	Tab	Prednisone 20 mg	by Chelsea	46193-0647	Steroid
RUGBY4326	Tab	Prednisone 20 mg	by Rugby	00536-4326 Discontinued	Steroid
RUGBY4328	Tab	Prednisone 50 mg	by Rugby	00536-4328 Discontinued	Steroid
RUGBY4328	Tab, White, Scored	Prednisone 50 mg	by Rugby	00536-4328 Discontinued	Steroid
RUGBY4335	Tab	Prenatal, Folic Acid, Iron Improved	by Rugby	00536-4335 Discontinued	Vitamin
RUGBY4339	Tab, Yellow	Prenatal, Folic Acid, Iron Plus	Prenatal Plus by Rugby	00536-4339 Discontinued	Vitamin
RUGBY4340	Tab, White	Prednisolone 5 mg	by Rugby	00536-4340 Discontinued	Steroid
RUGBY4346	Tab, Salmon	Prednisolone 5 mg	by Rugby	00536-4346 Discontinued	Steroid
RUGBY4352	Tab, Green	Prednisolone 5 mg	by Rugby	00536-4352 Discontinued	Steroid
RUGBY4360	Tab, Pink, Round	Acetaminophen 325 mg, Propoxyphene Napsylate 50 mg	Darvocet-N 50 by Rugby	00536-4360 Discontinued	Analgesic; C IV
RUGBY4361	Tab, Pink, Oblong	Acetaminophen 650 mg, Propoxyphene Napsylate 100 mg	Darvocet-N 100 by Rugby	00536-4361 Discontinued	Analgesic; C IV
RUGBY4365	Tab	Colchicine 0.5 mg, Probenecid 500 mg	ColBenemid by Rugby	00536-4365 Discontinued	Antigout
RUGBY4366	Tab	Probenecid 500 mg	Benemid by Rugby	00536-4366 Discontinued	Antigout
RUGBY4367	Cap, Yellow	Procainamide HCl 250 mg	Pronestyl by Rugby	00536-4367 Discontinued	Antiarrhythmic
RUGBY4368	Cap, Orange & Yellow	Procainamide HCl 500 mg	Pronestyl by Rugby	00536-4368 Discontinued	Antiarrhythmic
RUGBY4369	Tab	Promethazine 50 mg	Phenergan by Rugby	00536-4369 Discontinued	Antiemetic; Antihistamine
RUGBY4374	Cap, Red & Gray	Aspirin 389 mg, Caffeine 32.4 mg, Propoxyphene 65 mg	Darvon Compound 65 by Rugby	00536-4374 Discontinued	Analgesic; C IV
RUGBY4377	Cap, Orange & White	Procainamide HCl 375 mg	Pronestyl by Rugby	00536-4377 Discontinued	Antiarrhythmic
RUGBY4378	Tab	Promethazine 12.5 mg	Phenergan by Rugby	00536-4378 Discontinued	Antiemetic; Antihistamine
RUGBY4379	Tab	Promethazine 25 mg	Phenergan by Rugby	00536-4379 Discontinued	Antiemetic; Antihistamine
RUGBY4380	Tab	Levothyroxine Sodium 0.15 mg	Synthroid by Rugby	00536-4380 Discontinued	Thyroid Hormone
RUGBY4381	Tab, White, Round	Levothyroxine Sodium 0.2 mg	Synthroid by Rugby	00536-4381 Discontinued	Thyroid Hormone
RUGBY4382	Cap, Pink	Propoxyphene 65 mg	Darvon by Lemmon		Analgesic; C IV

ID FRONT <> BACK	DESCRIPTION FRONT <> BACK	INGREDIENT & STRENGTH	BRAND (or Generic Equiv.) by FIRM	NDC#	CLASS; SCH.
RUGBY4384	Tab	Propylthiouracil 50 mg	by Rugby	00536-4384	Antithyroid
RUGBY4387	Tab	Acetaminophen 650 mg, Propoxyphene HCl 65 mg	Wygesic by Rugby	00536-4387 Discontinued	Analgesic; C IV
RUGBY4390	Tab	Pseudoephedrine 60 mg	Sudafed by Rugby	00536-4390 Discontinued	Decongestant
RUGBY4391	Tab	Pseudoephedrine 30 mg	Sudafed by Rugby	00536-4391 Discontinued	Decongestant
RUGBY4399	Tab, Round	Pseudoephedrine 60 mg	Sudafed by Rugby	00536-4399 Discontinued	Decongestant
RUGBY4402	Tab, White, Round	Hydrochlorothiazide 25 mg, Propranolol HCl 40 mg	Inderide by Rugby	00536-4402 Discontinued	Diuretic; Antihypertensive
RUGBY4403	Tab, White, Round	Hydrochlorothiazide 25 mg, Propranolol HCl 80 mg	Inderide by Rugby	00536-4403 Discontinued	Diuretic; Antihypertensive
RUGBY4411	Cap	Pyrilamine 25 mg	by Rugby	00536-4411 Discontinued	Antihistamine
RUGBY4426	Tab, White, Round	Quinine Sulfate 260 mg	Quinamm by Rugby	00536-4426 Discontinued	Antimalarial
RUGBY4429	Tab, White, Round	Quinidine Sulfate 300 mg	Quinidine Sulfate by Rugby	00536-4429 Discontinued	Antiarrhythmic
RUGBY4432	Tab	Quinidine Sulfate 200 mg	by Rugby	00536-4432 Discontinued	Antiarrhythmic
RUGBY4432	Tab	Quinidine Sulfate 200 mg	Quinidine Sulfate by Rugby	00536-4432 Discontinued	Antiarrhythmic
RUGBY4433	Cap	Quinine Sulfate 325 mg	by Rugby	00536-4433 Discontinued	Antimalarial
RUGBY4434	Tab, White, Round	Quinidine Gluconate SR 324 mg	Quinaglute by Rugby	00536-4434 Discontinued	Antiarrhythmic
RUGBY4447	Tab, Green, Cap Shaped	Guaifenesin 600 mg	Robitussin by Rugby	00536-4447 Discontinued	Expectorant
RUGBY4454	Tab	Reserpine 0.1 mg	Serpasil by Rugby	00536-4454 Discontinued	Antihypertensive
RUGBY4455	Tab, Film Coated	Ranitidine HCl 168 mg	by Rugby	00536-4455 Discontinued	Gastrointestinal
RUGBY4455	Tab, Film Coated	Ranitidine HCl 168 mg	by Chelsea	46193-0575 Discontinued	Gastrointestinal
RUGBY4456	Tab, Film Coated	Ranitidine HCl 336 mg	by Rugby	00536-4456 Discontinued	Gastrointestinal
RUGBY4456	Tab, Film Coated	Ranitidine HCl 336 mg	by Chelsea	46193-0576 Discontinued	Gastrointestinal
RUGBY4458	Tab, White, Round	Reserpine 0.25 mg	Serpasil by Rugby	00536-4458 Discontinued	Antihypertensive
RUGBY4494	Tab, White, Round	Nylidrin 6 mg	Arlidin by Rugby	00536-4494 Discontinued	Vasodilator
RUGBY4495	Tab, White, Round	Nylidrin 12 mg	Arlidin by Rugby	00536-4495 Discontinued	Vasodilator
RUGBY4515	Cap, Yellow	Thiothixene 2 mg	Navane by Rugby	00536-4515 Discontinued	Antipsychotic
RUGBY4516	Cap, Orange	Thiothixene 5 mg	Navane by Rugby	00536-4516 Discontinued	Antipsychotic

ID FRONT <> BACK	DESCRIPTION FRONT <> BACK	INGREDIENT & STRENGTH	BRAND (or Generic Equiv.) by FIRM	NDC#	CLASS; SCH.
RUGBY4517	Cap, Orange & Blue	Thiothixene 10 mg	Navane by Rugby	00536-4517 Discontinued	Antipsychotic
RUGBY4522	Tab	Salsalate 500 mg	Disalcid by Able	Discontinued	NSAID
RUGBY4523	Tab	Salsalate 750 mg	Disalcid by Able	Discontinued	NSAID
RUGBY4547	Tab, Pink, Round	Sodium Fluoride 2.2 mg	Luride by Copley		Element
RUGBY4548	Tab	Sodium Fluoride Chewable 1.1 mg	Luride by Rugby	00536-4548 Discontinued	Element
RUGBY4563	Cap, Buff, Rugby Logo 4563	Doxepin HCl 10 mg	Sinequan by Rugby	00536-4563 Discontinued	Antidepressant
RUGBY4564	Cap, Ivory & White, Rugby Logo 4564	Doxepin HCl 25 mg	Sinequan by Rugby	00536-4564 Discontinued	Antidepressant
RUGBY4565	Cap, Yellow, Rugby Logo 4565	Doxepin HCl 50 mg	Sinequan by Rugby	00536-4565 Discontinued	Antidepressant
RUGBY4566	Cap, Green & White, Rugby Logo 4566	Doxepin HCl 100 mg	Sinequan by Rugby	00536-4566 Discontinued	Antidepressant
RUGBY4575	Tab, White, Round	Spironolactone 25 mg	Aldactone by Rugby	00536-4575 Discontinued	Diuretic
RUGBY4576	Tab, White, Round	Hydrochlorothiazide 25 mg, Spironolactone 25 mg	Aldactazide by Rugby	00536-4576 Discontinued	Diuretic; Antihypertensive
RUGBY4604	Tab, White, Ova	Ibuprofen 400 mg	Motrin by Rugby	00536-4604 Discontinued	NSAID
RUGBY4605	Tab, White, Oval	Ibuprofen 600 mg	Motrin by Rugby	00536-4605 Discontinued	NSAID
RUGBY4606	Tab, White, Oval	Ibuprofen 800 mg	Motrin by Rugby	00536-4606 Discontinued	NSAID
RUGBY4617	Tab	Sulfasalazine 500 mg	by Allscripts	Discontinued	Gastrointestinal
RUGBY4617	Tab, Partial Score	Sulfasalazine 500 mg	by Rugby	00536-4617	Gastrointestinal
RUGBY4617	Tab, Mustard	Sulfasalazine 500 mg	by Rugby	00536-4617	Gastrointestinal
RUGBY4617	Tab, Mustard	Sulfasalazine 500 mg	by Chelsea	46193-0166	Gastrointestinal
RUGBY4618	Tab, White, Round	Sulfisoxazole 500 mg	Gantrisin by Rugby	00536-4618 Discontinued	Antibiotic
RUGBY4628	Cap	Temazepam 15 mg	Restoril by Rugby	Discontinued	Sedative/Hypnotic; C IV
RUGBY4629	Cap	Temazepam 30 mg	Restoril by Rugby	Discontinued	Sedative/Hypnotic; C IV
RUGBY4640	Tab, Orange, Round	Thioridazine 15 mg	Mellaril by Rugby	00536-4640 Discontinued	Antipsychotic
RUGBY4641	Tab, Orange, Round	Thioridazine 10 mg	Mellaril by Rugby	00536-4641 Discontinued	Antipsychotic
RUGBY4642	Tab, Orange, Round	Thioridazine 25 mg	Mellaril by Rugby	00536-4642 Discontinued	Antipsychotic
RUGBY4643	Tab, Orange, Round	Thioridazine 50 mg	Mellaril by Rugby	00536-4643 Discontinued	Antipsychotic
RUGBY4644	Tab, Orange, Round	Thioridazine 100 mg	Mellaril by Rugby	00536-4644 Discontinued	Antipsychotic
RUGBY4648	Tab, White, Round	Phenobarbital 8 mg, Theophylline 130 mg, Ephedrine (Azpan) 24 mg	Tedral by Rugby	00536-4648 Discontinued	Antiasthmatic; C IV
RUGBY4649	Tab	Thioridazine 200 mg	by Rugby	00536-4649 Discontinued	Antipsychotic
RUGBY4657	Cap	Theophylline Anhydrous CR 300 mg	by Rugby	00536-4657 Discontinued	Antiasthmatic

ID FRONT <> BACK	DESCRIPTION FRONT <> BACK	INGREDIENT & STRENGTH	BRAND (or Generic Equiv.) by FIRM	NDC#	CLASS; SCH.
RUGBY4668	Tab, White, Round	Tolbutamide 500 mg	Orinase by Rugby	00536-4668 Discontinued	Antidiabetic
RUGBY4687	Tab, Peach, Round	Trazodone HCl 50 mg	Desyrel by Rugby	00536-4687 Discontinued	Antidepressant
RUGBY4688	Tab, White, Round	Trazodone HCl 100 mg	Desyrel by Rugby	00536-4688 Discontinued	Antidepressant
RUGBY4692	Tab, White, Round	Sulfamethoxazole 400 mg, Trimethoprim 80 mg	Bactrim by Rugby	00536-4692 Discontinued	Antibiotic
RUGBY4693	Tab, White, Oval	Sulfamethoxazole 800 mg, Trimethoprim 160 mg	Bactrim DS by Rugby	00536-4693 Discontinued	Antibiotic
RUGBY4694	Tab	Thyroid 30 mg	by Rugby	00536-4694 Discontinued	Thyroid Hormone
RUGBY4698	Tab	Thyroid 30 mg	by Rugby	00536-4698 Discontinued	Thyroid Hormone
RUGBY4702	Tab	Thyroid 60 mg	by Rugby	00536-4702 Discontinued	Thyroid Hormone
RUGBY4706	Tab	Thyroid 60 mg	by Rugby	00536-4706 Discontinued	Thyroid Hormone
RUGBY4710	Tab	Thyroid 125 mg	by Rugby	00536-4710 Discontinued	Thyroid Hormone
RUGBY4714	Tab	Thyroid 125 mg	by Rugby	00536-4714 Discontinued	Thyroid Hormone
RUGBY4717	Tab	Triamcinolone 4 mg	Aristocort by Rugby	00536-4717 Discontinued	Steroid
RUGBY4720	Tab, Round	Hydralazine 25 mg, Hydrochlorothiazide 15 mg, Reserpine 0.1 mg	Ser-Ap-Es by Rugby	00536-4720 Discontinued	Antihypertensive; Diuretic
RUGBY4721	Tab, White, Round	Hydralazine 25 mg, Hydrochlorothiazide 15 mg, Reserpine 0.1 mg	Ser-Ap-Es by Rugby	00536-4721 Discontinued	Antihypertensive; Diuretic
RUGBY4725	Tab	Phenylpropanolamine HCl 40 mg, Phenylephrine HCl 10 mg, Phentoloxamine 15 mg, Chlorpheniramine 5 mg	Naldecon by Rugby	00536-4725 Discontinued	Cold Remedy
RUGBY4729	Tab	Chlorpheniramine Tannate 8 mg, Phenylephrine Tannate 25 mg, Pyrilamine Tannate 25 mg	Tri Tannate by Rugby	00536-4729 Discontinued	Cold Remedy
RUGBY4736	Tab	Tripelennamine HCl 50 mg	PBZ by Rugby	00536-4736 Discontinued	Antihistamine
RUGBY4737	Tab, Chewable	Ascorbic Acid 30 mg, Sodium Ascorbate 33 mg, Sodium Fluoride, Vitamin A Acetate, Vitamin D 400 Units	Tri Vitamins by Rugby	00536-4737 Discontinued	Vitamin
RUGBY4738	Tab	Tolazamide 100 mg	Tolinase by Rugby	00536-4738 Discontinued	Antidiabetic
RUGBY4739	Tab	Tolazamide 250 mg	Tolinase by Rugby	00536-4739 Discontinued	Antidiabetic
RUGBY4744	Tab	Tolazamide 500 mg	Tolinase by Rugby	00536-4744 Discontinued	Antidiabetic
RUGBY4759	Tab	Therapeutic Vitamins	Berocca by Amide	00536-4759 Discontinued	Vitamin
RUGBY4812	Tab, Aqua, Round	Verapamil HCl 80 mg	Calan by Rugby	00536-4812 Discontinued	Antihypertensive
RUGBY4813	Tab, Blue, Round	Verapamil HCl 120 mg	Calan by Rugby	00536-4813 Discontinued	Antihypertensive
RUGBY4840	Tab, Film Coated	Cyclobenzaprine HCl 10 mg	by Rugby	00536-4840 Discontinued	Muscle Relaxant
RUGBY4840	Tab, White, Round, Rugby Logo 4840	Cyclobenzaprine HCl 10 mg	Flexeril by Rugby	00536-4840 Discontinued	Muscle Relaxant

ID FRONT <> BACK	DESCRIPTION FRONT <> BACK	INGREDIENT & STRENGTH	BRAND (or Generic Equiv.) by FIRM	NDC#	CLASS; SCH.
RUGBY4841	Tab, Film Coated	Naproxen 275 mg	by Chelsea	46193-0530	NSAID
RUGBY4841	Tab, Film Coated	Naproxen 275 mg	by Rugby	00536-4841 Discontinued	NSAID
RUGBY4842	Tab	Naproxen 250 mg	by Chelsea	46193-0527	NSAID
RUGBY4842	Tab	Naproxen 250 mg	by Rugby	00536-4842 Discontinued	NSAID
RUGBY4843	Tab	Naproxen 375 mg	by Rugby	00536-4843	NSAID
RUGBY4843	Tab	Naproxen 375 mg	by Rugby	00536-4843 Discontinued	NSAID
RUGBY4843	Tab	Naproxen 375 mg	by Chelsea	46193-0528	NSAID
RUGBY4844	Tab	Naproxen 500 mg	by Rugby	00536-4844 Discontinued	NSAID
RUGBY4844	Tab	Naproxen 500 mg	by Chelsea	46193-0529	NSAID
RUGBY4848	Tab, Film Coated	Naproxen 550 mg	by Rugby	00536-4848 Discontinued	NSAID
RUGBY4848	Tab, Film Coated	Naproxen 550 mg	by Chelsea	46193-0531	NSAID
RUGBY4861	Tab	Desipramine HCl 25 mg	Norpramin by Rugby	00536-4861 Discontinued	Antidepressant
RUGBY4862	Tab	Desipramine HCl 50 mg	Norpramin by Rugby	00536-4862 Discontinued	Antidepressant
RUGBY4863	Tab	Desipramine HCl 75 mg	Norpramin by Rugby	00536-4863 Discontinued	Antidepressant
RUGBY4864	Tab	Desipramine HCl 100 mg	Norpramin by Rugby	00536-4864 Discontinued	Antidepressant
RUGBY4881	Tab, Yellow, Round, Rugby over 4881	Desipramine HCl 25 mg	by DRX	55045-2278 Discontinued	Antidepressant
RUGBY4881	Tab, Yellow, Round, Rugby over 4881	Desipramine HCl 25 mg	Norpramin by Rugby	52544-0808	Antidepressant
RUGBY4881	Tab, Yellow, Round, Rugby over 4881	Desipramine HCl 25 mg	by Blue Ridge	59273-0009	Antidepressant
RUGBY4882	Tab, Green	Desipramine HCl 50 mg	by Blue Ridge	59273-0010	Antidepressant
RUGBY4882	Tab, Coated	Desipramine HCl 50 mg	by Rugby	00536-4882 Discontinued	Antidepressant
RUGBY4882	Tab, Green, Rugby over 4882	Desipramine HCl 50 mg	by DRX	55045-2352 Discontinued	Antidepressant
RUGBY4883	Tab, Orange, Round	Desipramine HCl 75 mg	Norpramin by Rugby	00536-4883 Discontinued	Antidepressant
RUGBY4884	Tab, Peach, Round, Rugby/4884	Desipramine HCl 50 mg	by DRX	55045-2548 Discontinued	Antidepressant
RUGBY4884	Tab, Peach	Desipramine HCl 100 mg	by Blue Ridge	59273-0012	Antidepressant
RUGBY4884	Tab, Coated	Desipramine HCl 100 mg	by Rugby	00536-4884 Discontinued	Antidepressant
RUGBY4884	Tab, Peach, Round	Desipramine HCl 100 mg	Norpramin by Rugby	51544-0545 Discontinued	Antidepressant
RUGBY4884	Tab, Peach, Rugby over 4884	Desipramine HCl 100 mg	by DRX	55045-2569 Discontinued	Antidepressant
RUGBY4903	Tab, Tan Round	Chlorpromazine HCl 10 mg	Thorazine by Rosemont		Antipsychotic
RUGBY4903	Tab, Butterscotch Yellow, Round	Chlorpromazine HCl 10 mg	Thorazine by Rugby	00536-4903 Discontinued	Antipsychotic
RUGBY4906	Tab, Butterscotch Yellow, Round	Chlorpromazine HCl 25 mg	Thorazine by Rugby	00536-4906 Discontinued	Antipsychotic
RUGBY4906	Tab, Tar, Round	Chlorpromazine HCl 25 mg	Thorazine by Rosemont		Antipsychotic

ID FRONT <> BACK	DESCRIPTION FRONT <> BACK	INGREDIENT & STRENGTH	BRAND (or Generic Equiv.) by FIRM	NDC#	CLASS; SCH.
RUGBY4909	Tab	Hydralazine 25 mg, Hydrochlorothiazide 15 mg, Reserpine 0.1 mg	Serapes by Rugby	00536-4909 Discontinued	Antihypertensive; Diuretic
RUGBY4915	Tab, White, Round	Chlorpromazine HCl 50 mg	Thorazine by Rugby	00536-4915 Discontinued	Antipsychotic
RUGBY4916	Tab, Tan, Round	Chlorpromazine HCl 100 mg	Thorazine by Rosemont	00536-4916 Discontinued	Antipsychotic
RUGBY4916	Tab, Butterscotch Yellow, Round	Chlorpromazine HCl 100 mg	Thorazine by Rugby	00536-4916 Discontinued	Antipsychotic
RUGBY4918	Tab, Butterscotch Yellow, Round	Chlorpromazine HCl 200 mg	Thorazine by Rugby	00536-4918 Discontinued	Antipsychotic
RUGBY4918	Tab, Tan, Round	Chlorpromazine HCl 200 mg	Thorazine by Rosemont		Antipsychotic
RUGBY4926	Cap, Red	Hydrochlorothiazide 25 mg, Triamterene 50 mg	Dyazide by Rugby	00536-4926 Discontinued	Diuretic; Antihypertensive
RUGBY4930	Cap, White	Hydrochlorothiazide 25 mg, Triamterene 50 mg	Dyazide by Rugby	00536-4930 Discontinued	Diuretic; Antihypertensive
RUGBY4931	Tab, White, Round	Verapamil HCl 80 mg	by Rugby	00536-4931 Discontinued	Antihypertensive
RUGBY4932	Tab, White, Round	Verapamil HCl 120 mg	by Rugby	00536-4932 Discontinued	Antihypertensive
RUGBY4939	Cap, Clear & Lavender w/ White Beads	Indomethacin 75 mg	Indocin SR by Rugby	00536-4939 Discontinued	NSAID
RUGBY4939	Cap, Clear & Lavender w/ White Beads	Indomethacin 75 mg	Indocin SR by Inwood	00258-3607 Discontinued	NSAID
RUGBY4940	Tab, Blue, Round	Clorazepate Dipotassium 3.75 mg	Tranxene by Watson		Antianxiety; C IV
RUGBY4941	Tab, Beige, Round	Clorazepate Dipotassium 7.5 mg	Tranxene by Watson		Antianxiety; C IV
RUGBY4942	Tab, Pink, Round	Clorazepate Dipotassium 15 mg	Tranxene by Watson		Antianxiety; C IV
RUGBY4948	Tab, Round	Desipramine HCl 25 mg	Norpramin by Rugby	00536-4948 Discontinued	Antidepressant
RUGBY4949	Tab, Round	Desipramine HCl 50 mg	Norpramin by Rugby	00536-4949 Discontinued	Antidepressant
RUGBY4950	Tab, White	Theophylline Anhydrous CR 100 mg	Theo-Dur by Rugby	00536-4950 Discontinued	Antiasthmatic
RUGBY4951	Cap, Yellow	Thiothixene 1 mg	Navane by Rugby		Antipsychotic
RUGBY4952	Cap, Green	Thiothixene 2 mg	Navane by Rugby		Antipsychotic
RUGBY4956	Tab, Yellow, Round	Hydrochlorothiazide 50 mg, Triamterene 75 mg	Maxzide by Watson		Diuretic; Antihypertensive
RUGBY4957	Tab, Round	Desipramine HCl 75 mg	Norpramin by Rugby	00536-4957 Discontinued	Antidepressant
RUGBY4958	Tab, Round	Desipramine HCl 100 mg	Norpramin by Rugby	00536-4958 Discontinued	Antidepressant
RUGBY4959	Tab	Baclofen 10 mg	Lioresal by Chelsea	46193-0869	Muscle Relaxant
RUGBY4960	Tab	Baclofen 20 mg	Lioresal by Rugby	00536-4960 Discontinued	Muscle Relaxant
RUGBY4960	Tab	Baclofen 20 mg	Lioresal by Chelsea	46193-0870	Muscle Relaxant
RUGBY4963	Cap	Danazol 200 mg	Danocrine by Rugby	00536-4963 Discontinued	Steroid
RUGBY4989	Tab, White, Round	Yohimbine HCl 5.4 mg	Yocon by Rugby	00536-4989 Discontinued	Impotence Agent
RUGBY4989	Tab, White, Round	Yohimbine HCl 5.4 mg	by Rugby	00536-4989 Discontinued	Impotence Agent
RUGBY4996	Tab, White	Theophylline Anhydrous CR 100 mg	Theo-Dur by Rugby	00536-4996 Discontinued	Antiasthmatic

ID FRONT <> BACK	DESCRIPTION FRONT <> BACK	INGREDIENT & STRENGTH	BRAND (or Generic Equiv.) by FIRM	NDC#	CLASS; SCH.
RUGBY4997	Tab, White	Theophylline Anhydrous CR 200 mg	Theo-Dur by Rugby	00536-4997 Discontinued	Antiasthmatic
RUGBY4998	Tab, White	Theophylline Anhydrous CR 300 mg	Theo-Dur by Rugby	00536-4998 Discontinued	Antiasthmatic
RUGBY5506	Tab, Beige, Round	Levothyroxine Sodium 0.125 mg	Synthroid by Rugby	00536-5506 Discontinued	Thyroid Hormone
RUGBY5535	Tab, Coated	Guaifenesin 600 mg, Pseudoephedrine HCl 120 mg	Guaitex PSE by Rugby	00536-5535 Discontinued	Cold Remedy
RUGBY5573	Cap	Nicardipine HCl 20 mg	by Chelsea	46193-0559	Antihypertensive
RUGBY5574	Cap	Nicardipine HCl 30 mg	by Chelsea	46193-0560	Antihypertensive
RUGBY5574	Cap	Nicardipine HCl 30 mg	by Chelsea	46193-0560	Antihypertensive
RUGBY5575	Tab, Blue & Green	Hyoscyamine Sulfate 0.125 mg	Levsin by Rugby	00536-5575 Discontinued	Gastrointestinal
RUGBY5595	Tab, White, Round	Clorazepate Dipotassium 15 mg	Tranxene by Rugby	00536-5595 Discontinued	Antianxiety; C IV
RUGBY5661	Tab, White, Round	Cimetidine HCl 200 mg	Tagamet by Rugby	00536-5661 Discontinued	Gastrointestinal
RUGBY5663	Tab, Film Coated	Cimetidine HCl 400 mg	Tagamet by Rugby	00536-5663 Discontinued	Gastrointestinal
RUGBY5670	Tab, White, Round	Oxycodone HCl 5 mg, Acetaminophen 325 mg	Percocet by Rugby	00536-5670 Discontinued	Analgesic; C II
RUGBY5673	Tab, White, Oblong	Diethylpropion HCl 75 mg	by BMS	00590-0623	Anorexiant; C IV
RUGBY5673	Tab, White, Cap Shaped	Diethylpropion HCl 75 mg	by Allscripts	Discontinued	Anorexiant; C IV
RUGBY5673	Tab, White, Oblong	Diethylpropion HCl 75 mg	by BMS	00056-0668	Anorexiant; C IV
RUGBY5673	Tab	Diethylpropion HCl 75 mg	by Rugby	00536-5673 Discontinued	Anorexiant; C IV
RUGBY5673	Tab, White, Oblong	Diethylpropion HCl 75 mg	by Blue Ridge	59273-0008	Anorexiant; C IV
RUGBY5683	Tab, Yellow	Prenatal, Beta Carotene	Prenatal Plus by Rugby	00536-5683 Discontinued	Vitamin
RUGBY5721	Tab, Film Coated	Ketorolac Tromethamine 10 mg	Toradol by Rugby	00536-5721 Discontinued	NSAID
RUGBY5721	Tab, White, Round	Ketorolac Tromethamine 10 mg	Toradol by Murfreesboro	51129-1605 Discontinued	NSAID
RUGBY5721	Tab, Film Coated	Ketorolac Tromethamine 10 mg	Toradol by Chelsea	46193-0564	NSAID
RUGBY5725	Cap, White and Light Blue, Opaque	Acyclovir 200 mg	Zovirax by Chelsea	46193-0569	Antiviral
RUGBY5725	Cap, White and Light Blue, Opaque	Acyclovir 200 mg	Zovirax by Rugby	00536-5725 Discontinued	Antiviral
RUGBY5925	Tab, Rugby over 5925	Diethylpropion HCl 25 mg	by Rugby	00536-5925 Discontinued	Anorexiant; C IV
RUGBY5925	Tab, White, Round	Diethylpropion HCl 25 mg	by BMS	00056-0669	Anorexiant; C IV
RUGBY5925	Tab, White, Round	Diethylpropion HCl 25 mg	by BMS	00056-0675	Anorexiant; C IV
RUGBY5925	Tab, Rugby over 5525	Diethylpropion HCl 25 mg	by Merrell	00068-5925	Anorexiant; C IV
RUGBY5925	Tab, White, Round	Diethylpropion HCl 25 mg	by Blue Ridge	59273-0007	Anorexiant; C IV
RUGBY5925	Tab, White, Round	Diethylpropion HCl 25 mg	by Allscripts	Discontinued	Anorexiant; C IV
RUGBY5926	Tab, Orange, Round	Ranitidine HCl 75 mg	Zantac by Rugby	00536-5926 Discontinued	Gastrointestinal
RUSS316	Cap, Orange & Black	Vitamin, Mineral Combination	Vicon Forte by Eon		Vitamin
RUSS500	Tab, Pink, Oblong	Aspirin 500 mg, Hydrocodone Bitartrate 5 mg	Lortab ASA by Russ		Analgesic; C III
RUSS901	Tab, White & Pink Specks, Oblong	Acetaminophen 500 mg, Hydrocodone Bitartrate 2.5 mg	Lortab by Russ		Analgesic; C III
RUSS902	Tab, White & Blue Specks, Oblong	Acetaminophen 500 mg, Hydrocodone Bitartrate 5 mg	Lortab-5 by Russ		Analgesic; C III

ID FRONT <> BACK	DESCRIPTION FRONT <> BACK	INGREDIENT & STRENGTH	BRAND (or Generic Equiv.) by FIRM	NDC#	CLASS; SCH.
RUSS903	Tab, White & Green Specks, Oblong	Acetaminophen 500 mg, Hydrocodone Bitartrate 7.5 mg	Lortab by Russ		Analgesic; C III
RUSS906	Tab, White & Green Specks, Oblong	Acetaminophen 500 mg, Hydrocodone Bitartrate 7.5 mg	Lortab by Russ		Analgesic; C III
RVT20	Tab, White, Round, Film Coated	Sildenafil Citrate 20 mg	Revatio by Pfizer	00069-4190	Antihypertensive
RVT20 <> PFIZER	Tab, White, Round, Film-Coated	Sildenafil Citrate equivalent to 20 mg of Sildenafil	Revatio by Pfizer	Canadian DIN 02279401	Antihypertensive
RW2	Tab, Orange, Round	Hydromorphone HCl 2 mg	Dilaudid by Richwood		Analgesic; C II
RW4	Tab, Yellow, Round	Hydromorphone HCl 4 mg	Dilaudid by Richwood		Analgesic; C II
RW81	Tab, White, Round	Aspirin 81 mg	Aspirin by Richwood		Analgesic
RX <> 11	Tab, White, Oblong, Scored, R / X <> 1 / 1	Fosinopril 10 mg	Monopril by Ranbaxy	63304-0775	Antihypertensive
RX165	Tab, White, Oblong, Scored	Sertraline HCl 50 mg	Zoloft by Ranbaxy	63304-0165	Antidepressant
RX166	Tab, White, Cap Shaped, Scored, Coated	Sertraline HCl 100 mg	Zoloft by Ranbaxy	63304-0166	Antidepressant
RX167	Tab, White, Cap Shaped, Scored, Coated	Sertraline HCl 150 mg	Zoloft by Ranbaxy	63304-0167	Antidepressant
RX168	Tab, White, Cap Shaped, Scored, Coated	Sertraline HCl 200 mg	Zoloft by Ranbaxy	63304-0168	Antidepressant
RX496	Tab, White, Oblong, Scored, RX / 496	Hydrocodone Bitartrate 7.5 mg, Acetaminophen 750 mg	Vicodin by Ranbaxy	63304-0496	Analgesic; C III
RX498	Tab, White, Round, Scored	Acetaminophen 500 mg, Hydrocodone Bitartrate 10 mg	Vicodin by Ranbaxy	63304-0498	Analgesic; C III
RX5	Tab, Light Pink, Round	Lisinopril 2.5 mg	Prinivil by Ranbaxy	63304-0531	Antihypertensive
RX504	Tab, White, Oval	Acyclovir 400 mg	Zovirax by Ranbaxy	63304-0504	Antiviral
RX505	Tab, White, Oval	Acyclovir 800 mg	Zovirax by Ranbaxy	63304-0505	Antiviral
RX509	Tab, White, Cap Shaped, Film Coated	Amoxicillin 875 mg, Clavulanate Potassium 125 mg	Augmentin by Ranbaxy	63304-0509	Antibiotic
RX509	Tab, White, Cap Shaped, Film Coated, Scored	Amoxicillin 875 mg, Clavulanate Potassium 125 mg	Augmentin by UDL	51079-0267 Discontinued	Antibiotic
RX512	Tab, White, Oblong, Scored, Film Coated	Cefadroxil 1 g	Duricef by Ranbaxy	63304-0512	Antibiotic
RX512	Tab, White, Oblong, Scored, Film Coated	Cefadroxil 1 g	Duricef by Barr	00555-0512	Antibiotic
RX514	Tab, Pink, Round, Chewable	Amoxicillin 125 mg	Amoxil by Ranbaxy	63304-0514	Antibiotic
RX515	Tab, Pink, Round, Chewable	Amoxicillin 250 mg	Amoxil by Ranbaxy	63304-0515	Antibiotic
RX518	Cap, Black and Yellow, Opaque, Hard Gelatin	Nitrofurantoin (Macrocrystals) 100 mg	Macrobid by Ranbaxy	63304-0518	Antibiotic
RX520	Tab, White, Cap-Shaped, Film Coated	Cefpodoxime Proxetil 100 mg	Vantin by Ranbaxy	63304-0520	Antibiotic
RX521	Tab, White, Oblong, Black Print	Cefpodoxime Proxetil 200 mg	Vantin by Ranbaxy	63304-0521	Antibiotic
RX522	Tab, Yellow, Round, Scored	Enalapril Maleate 2.5 mg	Vasotec by Ranbaxy	63304-0522	Antihypertensive
RX523	Tab, White, Round, Scored	Enalapril Maleate 5 mg	Vasotec by Ranbaxy	63304-0523	Antihypertensive
RX523	Tab, White, Round, Scored	Enalapril Maleate 5 mg	Vasotec by Major	00904-5502	Antihypertensive
RX524	Tab, Reddish Brown, Round	Enalapril Maleate 10 mg	Vasotec by Ranbaxy	63304-0524	Antihypertensive
RX525	Tab, Orange, Round	Enalapril Maleate 20 mg	Vasotec by Ranbaxy	63304-0525	Antihypertensive
RX525	Tab, Orange, Round	Enalapril Maleate 20 mg	Vasotec by Major	00904-5611	Antihypertensive
RX526	Tab, White, Round	Loratadine 10 mg	Claritin by UDL	51079-0132	Antihistamine
RX532	Tab, Light Pink, Round, Scored	Lisinopril 5 mg	Prinivil by Ranbaxy	63304-0532	Antihypertensive
RX532	Tab, Light Pink, Round, Scored	Lisinopril 5 mg	Zestril by Ranbaxy	Canadian DIN 02294230	Antihypertensive
RX533	Tab, Light Pink, Round	Lisinopril 10 mg	Zestril by Ranbaxy	Canadian DIN 02294249	Antihypertensive
RX533	Tab, Light Pink, Round	Lisinopril 10 mg	Prinivil by Ranbaxy	63304-0533	Antihypertensive
RX534	Tab, Light Brown, Round	Lisinopril 20 mg	Prinivil by Ranbaxy	63304-0534	Antihypertensive
RX534	Tab, Light Brown, Round	Lisinopril 20 mg	Zestril by Ranbaxy	Canadian DIN 02294257	Antihypertensive
RX535	Tab, Light Yellow, Round	Lisinopril 40 mg	Prinivil by Ranbaxy	63304-0535	Antihypertensive
RX536	Tab, Blue, Round	Lisinopril 10 mg, HCTZ 12.5 mg	Prinzide by Ranbaxy	63304-0536	Antihypertensive; Diuretic
RX537	Tab, Yellow, Round	Lisinopril 20 mg, HCTZ 12.5 mg	Prinzide by Ranbaxy	63304-0537	Antihypertensive; Diuretic
RX538	Tab, Light Peach, Round	Lisinopril 20 mg, HCTZ 25 mg	Prinzide by Ranbaxy	63304-0538	Antihypertensive; Diuretic

ID FRONT <> BACK	DESCRIPTION FRONT <> BACK	INGREDIENT & STRENGTH	BRAND (or Generic Equiv.) by FIRM	NDC#	CLASS; SCH.
RX549	Tab, White to Off-White, Round, Film Coated	Quinapril HCl 10 mg	Accupril by Teva	00093-5457 Discontinued	Antihypertensive
RX550	Tab, White to Off-White, Round, Film Coated	Quinapril HCl 20 mg	Accupril by Teva	00093-5458 Discontinued	Antihypertensive
RX551	Tab, White to Off-White, Round, Film Coated	Quinapril HCl 40 mg	Accupril by Teva	00093-5459 Discontinued	Antihypertensive
RX552	Tab, Blue, Round, Scored, RX / 552	Clorazepate Dipotassium 3.75 mg	Tranxene by Ranbaxy	63304-0552	Antianxiety; C IV
RX553	Tab, Peach, Round, Scored, RX / 553	Clorazepate Dipotassium 7.5 mg	Tranxene by Ranbaxy	63304-0553	Antianxiety; C IV
RX554	Tab, Red, Round, Scored, RX / 554	Clorazepate Dipotassium 15 mg	Tranxene by Ranbaxy	63304-0554	Antianxiety; C IV
RX561 <> 4	Tab, White, Round	Acetaminophen 300 mg, Codeine Phosphate 60 mg	Tylenol w/ Codeine by Ranbaxy	63304-0561	Analgesic; C III
RX562 <> 3	Tab, White, Round	Acetaminophen 300 mg, Codeine Phosphate 30 mg	Tylenol w/ Codeine by Ranbaxy	63304-0562	Analgesic; C III
RX565	Tab, Light Pink, Mottled, Round, Tab for Oral Suspension	Amoxicillin 200 mg	DisperMox by Ranbaxy	63304-0565	Antibiotic
RX567	Tab, Light Pink, Mottled, Round, Tab for Oral Suspension	Amoxicillin 400 mg	DisperMox by Ranbaxy	63304-0567	Antibiotic
RX597	Tab, Light Gold	Pravastatin Sodium 40 mg	Pravachol by Ranbaxy	63304-0597	Antihyperlipidemic
RX598	Tab, Yellow, Oblong	Pravastatin Sodium 80 mg	Pravachol by Ranbaxy	63304-0598	Antihyperlipidemic
RX6	Tab, Peach, Round, Film-Coated	Simvastatin 5 mg	Zocor by Ranbaxy	63304-0789	Antihyperlipidemic
RX6	Tab, Peach, Round	Simvastatin 5 mg	Zocor by Blu	24658-0210	Antihyperlipidemic
RX627	Cap, White, Opaque, Black Ink	Gabapentin 100 mg	Neurontin by Ranbaxy	63304-0627	Anticonvulsant
RX628	Cap, Ivory, Opaque, Black Ink	Gabapentin 300 mg	Neurontin by Ranbaxy	63304-0628	Anticonvulsant
RX629	Cap, Orange, Opaque, Black Ink	Gabapentin 400 mg	Neurontin by Ranbaxy	63304-0629	Anticonvulsant
RX632	Cap, Green and Orange, Opaque	Fluoxetine 40 mg	Prozac by Ranbaxy	63304-0632	Antidepressant
RX636	Cap, Green, Opaque, Black Ink	Ganciclovir Sodium 250 mg	Cytovene by Ranbaxy	63304-0636	Antiviral
RX637	Cap, Ivory Yellow and Green, Opaque, Black Ink	Ganciclovir Sodium 500 mg	Cytovene by Ranbaxy	63304-0637	Antiviral
RX652	Cap, White, Opaque	Acyclovir 200 mg	Zovirax by Ranbaxy	63304-0652	Antiviral
RX654	Cap, Yellow, Opaque	Amoxicillin 250 mg	Amoxil by Ranbaxy	63304-0654	Antibiotic
RX654	Cap, Yellow, Opaque	Amoxicillin 250 mg	Amoxil by UDL	51079-0600 Discontinued	Antibiotic
RX655	Cap, Maroon & Yellow, Opaque	Amoxicillin 500 mg	Amoxil by Ranbaxy	63304-0655	Antibiotic
RX655	Cap, Maroon & Yellow, Opaque	Amoxicillin 500 mg	Amoxil by Ranbaxy	63304-0655	Antibiotic
RX656	Cap, Green & White, Opaque	Cephalexin 250 mg	Keflex by Ranbaxy	63304-0656	Antibiotic
RX657	Cap, Dark Green & Light Green, Opaque	Cephalexin 500 mg	Keflex by Ranbaxy	63304-0657	Antibiotic
RX657	Cap, Dark Green and Light Green	Cephalexin 500 mg	Keflex by UDL	51079-0605 Discontinued	Antibiotic
RX658	Cap, Blue and Gray	Cefaclor 250 mg	Ceclor by Ranbaxy	63304-0658	Antibiotic
RX659	Cap, Blue Green	Cefaclor 500 mg	Ceclor CD by Ranbaxy	63304-0659	Antibiotic
RX675	Cap, Imprint in Edible Black Ink	Cephalexin 250 mg	Keflex by Ranbaxy	63304-0675	Antibiotic
RX676	Cap, Dark Green & Light Green	Cephalexin 500 mg	Keflex by Ranbaxy	63304-0676	Antibiotic
RX677	Cap, Imprint in Edible Black Ink	Propoxyphene HCl 65 mg	by Ranbaxy	63304-0677	Analgesic; C IV
RX678	Cap, Imprint in Edible Black Ink	Aspirin 389 mg, Caffeine 32.4 mg, Propoxyphene HCl 65 mg	Propoxyphene Compound 65 by Ranbaxy	63304-0678	Analgesic; C IV
RX679	Cap, Orange	Secobarbital Sodium 100 mg	by Ranbaxy	63304-0679	Sedative/Hypnotic; C II
RX680	Cap, Blue & Orange	Amobarbital Sodium 50 mg, Secobarbital 50 mg	Tuinal by Ranbaxy	63304-0680	Sedative/Hypnotic; C II
RX681	Cap, Yellow and White, Opaque	Fenoprofen Calcium 200 mg	Nalfon by Pedinol	00884-6600	NSAID
RX682	Cap, Yellow, Opaque	Fenoprofen Calcium 300 mg	Nalfon by Pedinol	00884-6700	NSAID
RX692	Cap, Blue & Light Green, Opaque	Clindamycin HCl 150 mg	Cleocin HCl by Ranbaxy	63304-0692	Antibiotic
RX693	Cap, Blue, Opaque	Clindamycin HCl 300 mg	Cleocin HCl by Ranbaxy	63304-0693	Antibiotic
RX694	Cap, White, Opaque	Minocycline HCl 50 mg	Minocin by Ranbaxy	63304-0694	Antibiotic
RX695	Cap, Gray, Opaque	Minocycline HCl 75 mg	Minocin by Ranbaxy	63304-0695	Antibiotic
RX696	Cap, Gray & White, Opaque	Minocycline HCl 100 mg	Minocin by Ranbaxy	63304-0696	Antibiotic
RX7	Tab, White, Round, RX over 7	Lorazepam 0.5 mg	Ativan by Ranbaxy	63304-0772	Antianxiety; C IV
RX701	Tab, Yellow, Oval, Film Coated	Etodolac 400 mg	by Ranbaxy	63304-0701	NSAID

ID FRONT <> BACK	DESCRIPTION FRONT <> BACK	INGREDIENT & STRENGTH	BRAND (or Generic Equiv.) by FIRM	NDC#	CLASS; SCH.
RX709	Tab, White to Off-White	Ciprofloxacin 250 mg	Cipro by Ranbaxy	63304-0709	Antibiotic
RX709	Tab, White to Off-White	Ciprofloxacin 250 mg	Cipro by UDL	51079-0218	Antibiotic
RX710	Tab, White, Oblong	Ciprofloxacin 500 mg	Cipro by Ranbaxy	63304-0710	Antibiotic
RX710	Tab, White, Oblong	Ciprofloxacin 500 mg	Cipro by UDL	51079-0233	Antibiotic
				Discontinued	
RX711	Tab	Ciprofloxacin 750 mg	Cipro by Ranbaxy	63304-0711	Antibiotic
RX713	Tab, White, Oval, Film Coated	Amoxicillin 500 mg, Clavulanate Potassium 125 mg	Augmentin by Ranbaxy	63304-0713	Antibiotic
RX713	Tab, White, Oval, Film Coated	Amoxicillin 500 mg, Clavulanate Potassium 125 mg	Augmentin by UDL	51079-0265	Antibiotic
				Discontinued	
RX714	Tab, Blue, Oval, Film Coated	Etodolac 500 mg	by Ranbaxy	63304-0714	NSAID
RX715	Tab, White, Oval	Ofloxacin 300 mg	Floxin by Ranbaxy	63304-0715	Antibiotic
RX716	Tab, White, Oblong, Film Coated	Ofloxacin 200 mg	Floxin by Ranbaxy	63304-0716	Antibiotic
RX717	Tab, White, Oval	Ofloxacin 400 mg	Floxin by Ranbaxy	63304-0717	Antibiotic
RX724	Tab, White, Oblong	Pseudoephedrine 240 mg, Loratadine 10 mg	Claritin D 24 hour by OHM Labs	51660-0724	Decongestant; Antihistamine
RX725	Tab, Light Yellow, Cap Shaped, Film Coated	Clarithromycin 250 mg	Biaxin by Ranbaxy	63304-0725	Antibiotic
RX726	Tab, Light Yellow, Cap Shaped, Film Coated	Clarithromycin 500 mg	Biaxin by Ranbaxy	63304-0726	Antibiotic
RX736	Tab, Light Yellow, Round, Film Coated	Benazepril HCl 5 mg	Lotensin by Ranbaxy	63304-0736	Antihypertensive
RX737	Tab, Dark Yellow	Benazepril HCl 10 mg	Lotensin by Ranbaxy	63304-0737	Antihypertension
RX738	Tab, Light Pink, Round, Film Coated	Benazepril HCl 20 mg	Lotensin by Ranbaxy	63304-0738	Antihypertensive
RX739	Tab, Pink	Benazepril HCl 40 mg	Lotensin by Ranbaxy	63304-0739	Antihypertensive
RX741	Tab, White	Phenobarbital 15 mg	Phenobarbital by Ranbaxy	63304-0741	Sedative/Hypnotic; C IV
RX742	Tab, White, Round	Phenobarbital 30 mg	by Ranbaxy	63304-0742	Sedative/Hypnotic; C IV
RX743	Tab, White, Round, Scored	Phenobarbital 60 mg	by Ranbaxy	63304-0743	Sedative/Hypnotic; C IV
RX744	Tab, White	Phenobarbital 100 mg	Phenobarbital by Ranbaxy	63304-0744	Sedative/Hypnotic; C IV
RX745	Tab, White	Morphine Sulfate 10 mg	MS Contin by Ranbaxy	63304-0706	Analgesic; C II
RX746	Tab, White	Morphine Sulfate 15 mg	MS Contin by Ranbaxy	63304-0707	Analgesic; C II
RX747	Tab, White	Morphine Sulfate 30 mg	MS Contin by Ranbaxy	63304-0708	Analgesic; C II
RX748	Tab, White, Round	Codeine Phosphate 30 mg	Codeine by Ranbaxy	63304-0748	Analgesic; C II
RX749	Tab, White, Round	Codeine Phosphate 60 mg	Codeine by Ranbaxy	63304-0749	Analgesic; C II
RX751	Tab, Blue, Cap Shaped	Cefuroxime Axetil 250 mg	Ceftin by Ranbaxy	63304-0751	Antibiotic
RX751	Tab, Blue, Cap Shaped	Cefuroxime Axetil 250 mg	Ceftin by UDL	51079-0016	Antibiotic
				Discontinued	
RX752	Tab, Blue, Cap Shaped	Cefuroxime Axetil 500 mg	Ceftin by Ranbaxy	63304-0752	Antibiotic
RX752	Tab, Blue, Cap Shaped	Cefuroxime Axetil 500 mg	Ceftin by UDL	51079-0017	Antibiotic
				Discontinued	
RX756	Tab, Yellow, Round, Film Coated	Ranitidine 150 mg	by Ranbaxy	63304-0756	Gastrointestinal
RX757	Tab, Yellow, Oblong	Ranitidine 300 mg	by Ranbaxy	63304-0757	Gastrointestinal
RX760	Tab, Light Pink, Mottled, Round, Chewable	Amoxicillin 200 mg	DisperMox by Ranbaxy	63304-0760	Antibiotic
RX761	Tab, Light Pink, Mottled, Round, Chewable	Amoxicillin 400 mg	DisperMox by Ranbaxy	63304-0761	Antibiotic
RX762	Tab, Pink, Cap Shaped, Film Coated, Scored	Amoxicillin 500 mg	DisperMox by Ranbaxy	63304-0762	Antibiotic
RX763	Tab, Pink, Cap Shaped, Film Coated, Scored	Amoxicillin 875 mg	DisperMox by Ranbaxy	63304-0763	Antibiotic
RX770	Tab, White, Round, Film Coated	Ranitidine 150 mg	by Ranbaxy	63304-0770	Gastrointestinal
RX771	Tab, White, Oblong	Ranitidine 300 mg	by Ranbaxy	63304-0771	Gastrointestinal
RX773	Tab, White, Round	Lorazepam 1 mg	Ativan by Ranbaxy	63304-0773	Antianxiety; C IV
RX774	Tab, White, Round	Lorazepam 2 mg	Ativan by Ranbaxy	63304-0774	Antianxiety; C IV
RX776	Tab, White to Off-White, Round	Fosinopril Sodium 20 mg	Monopril by Ranbaxy	63304-0776	Antihypertensive
RX777	Tab, White, Round	Fosinopril Sodium 40 mg	Monopril by Ranbaxy	63304-0777	Antihypertensive
RX790	Tab, Peach, Round, Film-Coated	Simvastatin 10 mg	Zocor by Ranbaxy	63304-0790	Antihyperlipidemic
RX790	Tab, Peach, Round	Simvastatin 10 mg	Zocor by Blu	24658-0211	Antihyperlipidemic

ID FRONT <> BACK	DESCRIPTION FRONT <> BACK	INGREDIENT & STRENGTH	BRAND (or Generic Equiv.) by FIRM	NDC#	CLASS; SCH.
RX791	Tab, Tan, Round, Film-Coated	Simvastatin 20 mg	Zocor by Ranbaxy	63304-0791	Antihyperlipidemic
RX791	Tab, Tan, Round	Simvastatin 20 mg	Zocor by Blu	24658-0212	Antihyperlipidemic
RX792	Tab, Brick Red, Round, Film-Coated	Simvastatin 40 mg	Zocor by Ranbaxy	63304-0792	Antihyperlipidemic
RX792	Tab, Brick Red, Round	Simvastatin 40 mg	Zocor by Blu	24658-0213	Antihyperlipidemic
RX793	Tab, Brick Red, Round, Film-Coated	Simvastatin 80 mg	Zocor by Ranbaxy	63304-0793	Antihyperlipidemic
RX793	Tab, Brick Red, Round	Simvastatin 80 mg	Zocor by Blu	24658-0210	Antihyperlipidemic
RX794	Tab, White to Off-White, Round	Flecainide Acetate 50 mg	Tambocor by Ranbaxy	63304-0794	Antiarrhythmic
RX795	Tab, White to Off-White, Round, Scored	Flecainide Acetate 100 mg	Tambocor by Ranbaxy	63304-0795	Antiarrhythmic
RX796	Tab, White to Off-White, Oval, Scored	Flecainide Acetate 150 mg	Tambocor by Ranbaxy	63304-0796	Antiarrhythmic
RX803	Tab, Pink, Round	Fluconazole 50 mg	Diflucan by Ranbaxy	63304-0803	Antifungal
RX804	Tab, Pink, Round	Fluconazole 100 mg	Diflucan by Ranbaxy	63304-0804	Antifungal
RX804	Tab, Pink, Round	Fluconazole 100 mg	Diflucan by UDL	51079-0259 Discontinued	Antifungal
RX805	Tab, Pink, Round	Fluconazole 150 mg	Diflucan by Ranbaxy	63304-0805	Antifungal
RX806	Tab, Pink, Round	Fluconazole 200 mg	Diflucan by Ranbaxy	63304-0806	Antifungal
RX806	Tab, Pink, Round	Fluconazole 200 mg	Diflucan by UDL	51079-0260 Discontinued	Antifungal
RX860	Tab, White, Oblong, Extended Release	Metformin HCl 500 mg	Glucophage by Ranbaxy	63304-0860	Antidiabetic
RX900	Tab, White, Oblong	Fenofibrate 54 mg	TriCor by Ranbaxy	63304-0900	Antihyperlipidemic
RX901	Tab, White, Oblong	Fenofibrate 160 mg	TriCor by Ranbaxy	63304-0901	Antihyperlipidemic
RX920	Tab, White, Oval	Zidovudine 300 mg	Retrovir by Ranbaxy	63304-0920	Antiviral
RYNA1708	Tab, Blue, Oval, Scored	Phenylephrine 25 mg, Pyrilamine 60 mg, Pseudoephedrine Sulfate 120 mg, Guaifenesin 200 mg	Ryna-12X by MedPointe	00037-1708	Cold Remedy
RYNATAN711	Tab, Red, Black Print, Sugar Coated, Rynatan over 711	Azatadine Maleate 1 mg, Pseudoephedrine Sulfate 120 mg	Rynatan by Wallace	00037-0711	Cold Remedy
RYNEZE	Tab, Blue, Cap Shaped, Scored	Chlorpheniramine Maleate 8 mg, Methscopolamine Nitrate 2.5 mg	Ryneze by Stewart Jackson	45985-0659	Cold Remedy
RYR	Tab, White, Circular, RY R/Roussel Logo	Disopyramide Phosphate 250 mg	Norpace CR by Aventis	Canadian	Antiarrhythmic
S	Tab, White, Round, Scored	Clomiphene Citrate 50 mg	Serophene by Serono	Canadian	Infertility
S	Tab, Dark Green, Light Yellow & Orange, Speckled, Scored, S in Triangle	Belladonna 0.2 mg, Ergotamine 0.6 mg, Phenobarbital 40 mg	Bellergal by Novartis	Canadian DIN 00176141	Gastrointestinal; C III
S	Tab, White, Round	Acetaminophen 325 mg, Codeine Phosphate 8 mg, Doxylamine Succinate 5 mg	Mersyndol by Marion	Canadian	Analgesic; C IV
S	Tab, Brown, Round	Sennosides 8.6 mg	Senokot by Purdue	00034-1200	Gastrointestinal
S	Cap, Off-White	Ergoloid Mesylate 1 mg	Hydergine by RP Scherer	11014-0775	Ergot Alkaloids
S	Tab, Brownish-Yellow, Round, Biconvex, Coated, Black Ink, Capital "S"	Trospium Chloride 20 mg	Sanctura by Odyssey	65473-0980	Antispasmodic; Urinary Tract
S	Tab, Brownish-Yellow, Round, Biconvex, Coated, Black Ink, Capital "S"	Trospium Chloride 20 mg	Sanctura by Odyssey	67979-0631	Antispasmodic; Urinary Tract
S	Cap, Bluish-Green, Opaque, White Ink, Shire Logo, Extended Release	Carbamazepine 100 mg	Carbatrol by Shire	54092-0171	Anticonvulsant
S	Cap, Light Gray and Bluish-Green, Opaque, White Ink, Shire Logo, Extended Release	Carbamazepine 200 mg	Carbatrol by Shire	54092-0172	Anticonvulsant
S	Cap, Black and Bluish-Green, Opaque, White Ink, Shire Logo, Extended Release	Carbamazepine 300 mg	Carbatrol by Shire	54092-0173	Anticonvulsant
S	Tab, White, Round, Scored	Clomiphene Citrate 50 mg	by Serono	Canadian DIN 00893722	Hormone
S	Tab, Light Brown, Round	Standardized Sennosides 8.6 mg	Senokot by Purdue Pharma	Canadian DIN 00026158	Gastrointestinal
S	Tab, Round, Orange, Film-Coated	Indapamide Hemihydrate 1.25 mg	Lozide by Servier	Canadian DIN 02179709	Diuretic; Antihypertensive
S <> 100	Tab, Orange, Round, Film Coated	Pinaverium Bromide 100 mg	Dicetel by Solvay	Canadian DIN 02230684	Gastrointestinal
S <> 100	Tab, White, Triangle Shaped	Sumatriptan 100 mg	Imitrex by Dr. Reddy's	55111-0737	Antimigraine

ID FRONT <> BACK	DESCRIPTION FRONT <> BACK	INGREDIENT & STRENGTH	BRAND (or Generic Equiv.) by FIRM	NDC#	CLASS; SCH.
S <> 197	Tab, White Round	Inert	Seasonale by Duramed	51285-0058	Oral Contraceptive; Placebo
S <> 25	Tab, White, Triangle Shaped	Sumatriptan 25 mg	Imitrex by Dr. Reddy's	55111-0738	Antimigraine
S <> 256	Tab, White to Off-White, Round	Betahistine DiHCl 8 mg	by Solvay	Canadian DIN 02240601	Antivertigo
S <> 267267	Tab, White to Off-White, Round, Scored	Betahistine Dihydrochloride 16 mg	Serc by Solvay	Canadian DIN 02243878	Antivertigo
S <> 289289	Tab, White to Off-White, Round, Scored	Betahistine Dihydrochloride 24 mg	Serc by Solvay	Canadian DIN 02247998	Antivertigo
S <> 291291	Tab, White, Round, Scored, Film Coated	Fluvoxamine Maleate 50 mg	Luvox by Solvay	Canadian DIN 01919342	OCD
S <> 313313	Tab, White, Oval, Scored, Film Coated	Fluvoxamine Maleate 100 mg	Luvox by Solvay	Canadian DIN 01919369	OCD
S <> 420	Tab, White, Round	Atenolol 25 mg	Tenormin by Dava	67253-0420	Antihypertensive
S <> 422	Tab, White, Round	Atenolol 100 mg	Tenormin by Dava	67253-0422	Antihypertensive
S <> 5	Tab, White, Shield Shaped	Selegiline 5 mg	Eldepryl by Watson	52544-0136	Antiparkinson
S <> 50	Tab, Orange, Round, Film Coated, S over Triangle <> 50	Pinaverium Bromide 50 mg	Dicetel by Solvay	Canadian DIN 01950592	Gastrointestinal
S <> 50	Tab, White, Triangle Shaped	Sumatriptan 50 mg	Imitrex by Dr. Reddy's	55111-0736	Antimigraine
S <> 62	Tab, Pink, Round, Film-Coated	Ethinyl Estradiol 0.03 mg, Levonorgestrel 0.15 mg	Seasonale by Duramed	51285-0058	Oral Contraceptive
S <> 741	Tab, White to Off-White, Oval	Gemfibrozil 600 mg	Lopid by Dava	67253-0741	Antihyperlipidemic
S <> 770	Tab, Green, Oval, Scored	Isosorbide Dinitrate 5 mg	Isordil by Zeneca	00310-0770	Antianginal
S <> 773	Tab	Isosorbide Dinitrate 30 mg	Isordil by Zeneca	00310-0773	Antianginal
S <> 774	Tab, Light Blue, Oval, Scored	Isosorbide Dinitrate 40 mg	Isordil by Zeneca	00310-0774	Antianginal
S <> 780	Tab, Yellow, Oval, Scored	Isosorbide Dinitrate 10 mg	Isordil by Zeneca	00310-0780	Antianginal
S <> 782	Tab, Light Green, Black Print, Round, Film Coated, S in Triangle <> 78-2	Thioridazine 10 mg	Mellaril by Novartis	00078-0002	Antipsychotic
S <> 788	Tab, Pink, Black Print, Round, Film Coated, 78-8 <> S in Triangle	Thioridazine 15 mg	Mellaril by Novartis	00078-0008	Antipsychotic
S <> 810	Tab, Green, Round, Scored, Chewable	Isosorbide Dinitrate 5 mg	Isordil by Zeneca	00310-0810	Antianginal
S <> 815	Tab, Chewable	Isosorbide Dinitrate 10 mg	Isordil by Zeneca	00310-0815	Antianginal
S <> 820	Tab	Isosorbide Dinitrate 20 mg	Isordil by Nat Pharmpak	55154-4402	Antianginal
S <> 820	Tab, Blue, Oval, Scored	Isosorbide Dinitrate 20 mg	Isordil by Zeneca	00310-0820	Antianginal
S <> 853	Tab	Isosorbide Dinitrate 2.5 mg	Isordil by Zeneca	00310-0853	Antianginal
S <> 8667	Tab, Pink, Oblong, Scored	Metaxalone 800 mg	Skelaxin by King	60793-0136	Muscle Relaxant
S <> 8667	Tab, Pink, Oblong, Scored	Metaxalone 800 mg	Skelaxin by Elan	59075-0068	Muscle Relaxant
S <> FIORINAL	Tab, White, Round, Fiorinal <> S in a Triangle	Butalbital 50 mg, Caffeine 40 mg, Aspirin 330 mg	Fiorinal by Novartis	Canadian DIN 00275328	Analgesic; C III
S <> HYDERGINE	Tab, White, Round	Ergoloid Mesylate 1 mg	Hydergine by Novartis	61615-0102	Ergot Alkaloids
S <> MELLARIL100	Tab, Light Yellow, Black Print, Round, Film Coated, S in Triangle <> Mellaril over 100	Thioridazine 100 mg	Mellaril by Novartis	00078-0005	Antipsychotic
S <> MELLARIL150	Tab, Yellow, Black Print, Round, Film Coated, Mellaril over 150 <> S in Triangle	Thioridazine 150 mg	Mellaril by Novartis	00078-0006	Antipsychotic
S <> MELLARIL200	Tab, Purple, Black Print, Round, Film Coated, S in Triangle <> Mellaril over 200	Thioridazine 200 mg	Mellaril by Novartis	00078-0007	Antipsychotic
S <> MELLARIL25	Tab, Brown, Black Print, Round, Film Coated, S in Triangle <> Mellaril over 25	Thioridazine 25 mg	Mellaril by Novartis	00078-0003	Antipsychotic
S <> MELLARIL50	Tab, White, Black Print, Round, Film Coated, S in Triangle <> Mellaril over 50	Thioridazine 50 mg	Mellaril by Novartis	00078-0004	Antipsychotic
S <> S80	Tab, White, Oblong	Sotalol HCl 80 mg	Betapace by Genpharm	55567-0057	Antiarrhythmic

ID FRONT <> BACK	DESCRIPTION FRONT <> BACK	INGREDIENT & STRENGTH	BRAND (or Generic Equiv.) by FIRM	NDC#	CLASS; SCH.
S0260	Cap, Gelatin	Ascorbic Acid 250 mg, Cyanocobalamin 10 mcg, Ferrous Fumarate 200 mg, Zinc Sulfate 25 mg	Chromagen by RP Scherer	11014-1173	Vitamin
S0262	Cap, Gelatin	Ascorbic Acid 60 mg, Cyanocobalamin 10 mcg, Ferrous Fumarate 460 mg, Folic Acid 1 mg	Chromagen by RP Scherer	11014-1176	Vitamin
S063	Cap, White, Black Print, Opaque, Shire Logo	Anagrelide HCl 0.5 mg	Agrylin by Shire	54092-0063	Antiplatelet
S063	Cap, White, Black Print, Opaque, Shire Logo	Anagrelide HCl 0.5 mg	Agrylin by Shire	Canadian DIN 02236859	Antiplatelet
S064	Cap, Gray, Black Print, Opaque, Shire Logo	Anagrelide HCl 1 mg	Agrylin by Shire	54092-0064	Antiplatelet
S1 <> GPI	Tab, White with Green Specks	Acetaminophen 325 mg, Phenylephrine HCl 5 mg, Chlorpheniramine Maleate 2 mg	Super Cold Tabs by Reese	10956-0771	Cold Remedy
S100 <> P	Tab, Pink, Diamond Shaped	Sumatriptan Succinate 100 mg	Imitrex by Pharmascience	Canadian DIN 02256444	Antimigraine
S100MG	Cap, Bluish-Gray, S in a Triangle	Cyclosporine 100 mg	Neoral by Novartis	Canadian DIN 02150670	Immunosuppressant
S103	Tab, Brown, Round, S-103		Duravent by Dura		Cold Remedy
S10MG	Cap, Yellowish-White, Oval, S in a Triangle	Cyclosporine 10 mg	Neoral by Novartis	Canadian DIN 02237671	Immunosuppressant
S11	Tab, White, Round	Selegiline 5 mg	Eldepryl by Dava	67253-0701	Antiparkinson
S11 <> LL	Tab, White, Round	Selegiline 5 mg	Eldepryl by ESI Lederle	59911-3254	Antiparkinson
S111	Cap, Purple	Methenamine 118 mg, Sodium Phosphate Monobasic 40.8 mg, Phenyl Salicylate 36 mg, Methylene Blue 10 mg, Hyoscyamine Sulfate 0.12 mg	Uribel by Mission	00076-0111	Urinary Tract
S1124	Tab, Pink, Round, Scored, S over 1124	Dyphylline 200 mg, Guaifenesin 200 mg	Dilor-G by Savage	00281-1124	Antiasthmatic; Expectorant
S120 <> G	Tab, White, Cap Shaped, Scored	Sotalol HCl 120 mg	Betapace by Par	49884-0583	Antiarrhythmic
S120 <> G	Tab, White, Oblong	Sotalol HCl 120 mg	by Genpharm	55567-0076	Antiarrhythmic
S120 <> G	Tab, White, Cap Shaped, Scored, S/120	Sotalol HCl 120 mg	Betapace by Genpharm	15330-0209	Antiarrhythmic
S145	Tab, White, Oblong	Amoxicillin 875 mg	Amoxil by Dava	67253-0145	Antibiotic
S15WYETH317	Tab, Yellow, Pentagonal, S15/Wyeth 317	Oxazepam 15 mg	Serax by Wyeth		Sedative/Hypnotic; C IV
S16 <> LL	Tab	Sulindac 150 mg	by Lederle	00005-3550	NSAID
S16 <> LL	Tab	Sulindac 150 mg	by Caremark	00339-5696	NSAID
S160 <> G	Tab, White, Oblong	Sotalol HCl 160 mg	by Genpharm	55567-0058	Antiarrhythmic
S160 <> G	Tab, White, Cap Shaped, Scored	Sotalol HCl 160 mg	Betapace by Par	49884-0584	Antiarrhythmic
S160 <> G	Tab, White, Cap Shaped, Scored, S/160	Sotalol HCl 160 mg	Betapace by Genpharm	15330-0210	Antiarrhythmic
S17 <> LL	Tab	Sulindac 200 mg	by Quality Care	60346-0686	NSAID
S190	Tab, Light Blue, Round, Film-Coated	Eszopiclone 1 mg	Lunesta by Sepracor	63402-0190	Hypnotic; C IV
S191	Tab, White, Round, Film-Coated	Eszopiclone 2 mg	Lunesta by Sepracor	63402-0191	Hypnotic; C IV
S193	Tab, Dark Blue, Round, Film Coated	Eszopiclone 3 mg	Lunesta by Sepracor	63402-0193	Hypnotic; C IV
S20	Tab, White, Oval	Penicillin VK 250 mg	V-Cillin K by Dava	67253-0200	Antibiotic
S20LESCOL	Cap, Brown & Yellow, Red & White Print, S in Triangle over 20 over Lescol	Fluvastatin Sodium 20 mg	Lescol by Novartis	Canadian DIN 02061562	Antihyperlipidemic
S20LESCOL	Cap, Brown & Yellow, Red & White Print, S in Triangle over 20 over Lescol	Fluvastatin Sodium 20 mg	Lescol by Pharm Util	60491-0355	Antihyperlipidemic
S20LESCOL	Cap, Brown & Yellow, Red & White Print, S in Triangle over 20 over Lescol	Fluvastatin Sodium 20 mg	Lescol by Amerisource	62584-0176	Antihyperlipidemic
S20LESCOL	Cap, Brown & Yellow, Red & White Print, S in Triangle over 20 over Lescol	Fluvastatin Sodium 20 mg	Lescol by Novartis	00078-0176	Antihyperlipidemic
S20LESCOL	Cap, Brown & Yellow, Red & White Print, S in Triangle over 20 over Lescol	Fluvastatin Sodium 20 mg	Lescol by Allscripts		Antihyperlipidemic
S21	Tab, White, Oval	Penicillin V Potassium 500 mg	Pen*Vee K by Dava	67253-0201	Antibiotic

ID FRONT <> BACK	DESCRIPTION FRONT <> BACK	INGREDIENT & STRENGTH	BRAND (or Generic Equiv.) by FIRM	NDC#	CLASS; SCH.
S240 <> G	Tab, White, Cap Shaped, Scored	Sotalol 240 mg	Betapace by Par	49884-0585	Antiarrhythmic
S240 <> G	Tab, White, Oblong	Sotalol HCl 240 mg	Betapace by Genpharm	55567-0059	Antiarrhythmic
S25 <> P	Tab, White, Round	Sumatriptan Succinate 25 mg	Imitrex by Pharmascience	Canadian DIN 02256428	Antimigraine
S25DYNACIRC	Cap, White, Red Print, S in Triangle over 2.5 over DynaCirc	Isradipine 2.5 mg	by Novartis	00078-0226	Antihypertensive
S25DYNACIRC	Cap, White, Red Print, S in Triangle over 2.5 over DynaCirc	Isradipine 2.5 mg	by Caremark	00339-5719	Antihypertensive
S25MG	Cap, Blue-Gray, Oval, S in a Triangle	Cyclosporine 25 mg	Neoral by Novartis	Canadian DIN 02150689	Immunosuppressant
S263	Tab, Light Blue, Round, Scored	Clonidine HCl 0.1 mg	Catapres by Dava	67253-0263	Antihypertensive
S264	Tab, Light Yellow, Round, Scored	Clonidine HCl 0.2 mg	Catapres by Dava	67253-0264	Antihypertensive
S265	Tab, Light Green, Round, Scored	Clonidine HCl 0.3 mg	Catapres by Dava	67253-0265	Antihypertensive
S4051000	Tab, White to Off-White, Round	Elemental Lanthanum 1000 mg	Fosrenol by Shire	54092-0254	Phosphate Binder
S4051000MG	Tab, White to Off-White, Round, Flat with Beveled Edge, Chewable	Elemental Lanthanum 1000 mg	Fosrenol by Shire BioChem	Canadian DIN 02287188	Phosphate Binder
S405250MG	Tab, White to Off-White, Round, Biconvex	Lanthanum Carbonate 250 mg	Fosrenol by Shire	54092-0247	Phosphate Binder
S405250MG	Tab, White to Off-White, Round, Flat with Beveled Edge, Chewable	Elemental Lanthanum 250 mg	Fosrenol by Shire BioChem	Canadian DIN 02287145	Phosphate Binder
S405500	Tab, White to Off-White, Round, Convex	Lanthanum Carbonate 500 mg	Fosrenol by Shire	54092-0252	Phosphate Binder
S405500MG	Tab, White to Off-White, Round, Flat with Beveled Edge, Chewable	Elemental Lanthanum 500 mg	Fosrenol by Shire BioChem	Canadian DIN 02287153	Phosphate Binder
S405750	Tab, White to Off-White, Round	Elemental Lanthanum 750 mg	Fosrenol by Shire	54092-0253	Phosphate Binder
S405750MG	Tab, White to Off-White, Round, Flat with Beveled Edge, Chewable	Elemental Lanthanum 750 mg	Fosrenol by Shire BioChem	Canadian DIN 02287161	Phosphate Binder
S40LESCOL	Cap, Brown & Gold, White & Red Print, S in Triangle over 40 over Lescol	Fluvastatin Sodium 40 mg	Lescol by Allscripts		Antihyperlipidemic
S40LESCOL	Cap, Brown & Gold, White & Red Print, S in Triangle over 40 over Lescol	Fluvastatin Sodium 40 mg	Lescol by DRX	55045-2369	Antihyperlipidemic
S40LESCOL	Cap, Brown & Gold, White & Red Print, S in Triangle over 40 over Lescol	Fluvastatin Sodium 40 mg	Lescol by Pharm Util	60491-0356	Antihyperlipidemic
S40LESCOL	Cap, Brown & Gold, White & Red Print, S in Triangle over 40 over Lescol	Fluvastatin Sodium 40 mg	Lescol by Novartis	00078-0234	Antihyperlipidemic
S40LESCOL	Cap, Brown & Gold, White & Red Print, S in Triangle over 40 over Lescol	Fluvastatin Sodium 40 mg	Lescol by Novartis	Canadian DIN 02061570	Antihyperlipidemic
S40S	Cap, Brown & Yellow, Lescol Logo 40	Fluvastatin Sodium 40 mg	Lescol by Inwood		Antihyperlipidemic
S4131	Tab, Ivory colored, Modified Rectangle-Shaped, Scored	Pergolide Mesylate 0.05 mg	Permax by Shire BioChem	Canadian DIN 02123320 Discontinued	Antiparkinson
S4133	Tab, Green, Modified Rectangle-Shaped, Scored	Pergolide Mesylate 0.25 mg	Permax by Shire BioChem	Canadian DIN 02123339 Discontinued	Antiparkinson
S4135	Tab, Pink, Modified Rectangle-Shaped, Scored	Pergolide Mesylate 1 mg	Permax by Shire BioChem	Canadian DIN 02123347 Discontinued	Antiparkinson
S4140	Cap	Amantadine HCl 100 mg	Symmetrel by Pharmedix	53002-0375	Antiviral
S4140	Cap	Amantadine HCl 100 mg	Symmetrel by URL Mutual	00677-1452	Antiviral
S4140	Cap, Gelatin	Amantadine HCl 100 mg	Symmetrel by Qualitest	00603-2163	Antiviral
S4140	Cap, Dark Red	Amantadine HCl 100 mg	Symmetrel by RP Scherer	11014-0813	Antiviral
S421	Tab, White, Round, Scored, S / 421	Atenolol 50 mg	Tenormin by Dava	67253-0421	Antihypertensive
S476	Tab, Reddish Brown, Elliptical, Film Coated	Mesalamine 1.2 g	Lialda by Shire	54092-0476	Gastrointestinal
S48920MG	Cap, Ivory	Lisdexamfetamine Dimesylate 20 mg	Vyvanse by New River	59417-0102	Stimulant; C II
S48930MG	Cap, White and Orange	Lisdexamfetamine Dimesylate 30 mg	Vyvanse by New River	59417-0103	Stimulant; C II

ID FRONT <> BACK	DESCRIPTION FRONT <> BACK	INGREDIENT & STRENGTH	BRAND (or Generic Equiv.) by FIRM	NDC#	CLASS; SCH.
S48940MG	Cap, Blue Green and White	Lisdexamfetamine Dimesylate 40 mg	Vyvanse by New River	59417-0104	Stimulant; C II
S48950MG	Cap, White and Blue	Lisdexamfetamine Dimesylate 50 mg	Vyvanse by New River	59417-0105	Stimulant; C II
S48960MG	Cap, Aqua Blue	Lisdexamfetamine Dimesylate 60 mg	Vyvanse by New River	59417-0106	Stimulant; C II
S48970MG	Cap, Blue and Orange	Lisdexamfetamine Dimesylate 70 mg	Vyvanse by New River	59417-0107	Stimulant; C II
S5	Tab, White, Round	Selegiline HCl 5 mg	by Apotex	Canadian DIN 02230641	Antiparkinson
S50 <> P	Tab, White, Diamond Shaped	Sumatriptan Succinate 50 mg	Imitrex by Pharmascience	Canadian DIN 02256436	Antimigraine
S50MG	Cap, Yellowish-White, Oval, S in a Triangle	Cyclosporine 50 mg	Neoral by Novartis	Canadian DIN 02150662	Immunosuppressant
S540	Tab, White, Round	Furosemide 20 mg	Lasix by Dava	67253-0540	Diuretic
S541	Tab, White, Round, Scored	Furosemide 40 mg	Lasix by Dava	67253-0541	Diuretic
S542	Tab, White, Round, Scored	Furosemide 80 mg	Lasix by Dava	67253-0542	Diuretic
S547	Tab, Aqua, Clover-Shaped	Trichlormethiazide 4 mg	Naqua by Schering	00085-0547	Diuretic; Antihypertensive
S5DYNACIRC	Cap, Pink, Red Print, S in Triangle over 5 over DynaCirc	Isradipine 5 mg	by Novartis	00078-0227	Antihypertensive
S5E <> G	Tab, White, Round	Selegiline HCl 5 mg	by Par	49884-0610	Antiparkinson
S700	Cap, White, Red Ink	Selegiline HCl 5 mg	Eldepryl by Dava	67253-0700	Antiparkinson
S760	Tab, Pink, Round	Isosorbide Dinitrate SL 5 mg	Isordil by Zeneca		Antianginal
S761	Tab, Yellow, Round	Isosorbide Dinitrate SL 10 mg	Isordil by Zeneca		Antianginal
S770	Tab, Green, Oval	Isosorbide Dinitrate Oral 5 mg	Isordil by Zeneca		Antianginal
S7720	Tab, White, Round	Chenodiol 250 mg	Chenix by Solvay		Cholelitholytic
S78240	Cap, Pink, Gelatin, 78/240, S inside Triangle	Cyclosporine 25 mg	Sandimmune by Nat Pharmpak	55154-3415	Immunosuppressant
S78240	Cap, Pink, Gelatin, 78/240, S inside Triangle	Cyclosporine 25 mg	Sandimmune by Novartis	00078-0240	Immunosuppressant
S78241	Cap, Dusty Rose, Gelatin, 78/241, S inside Triangle	Cyclosporine 100 mg	Sandimmune by Novartis	00078-0241	Immunosuppressant
S7830	Tab, White, Round, S 78-30	Belladonna Alkaloids 0.25 mg	Bellafoline by Sandoz		Gastrointestinal
S7836	Tab, Green, Round, S 78-36	Ergotamine Tartrate 1 mg, Caffeine 100 mg, Bellafoline 0.125 mg, Pentobarbital 30 mg	Cafergot by Sandoz		Antimigraine; C IV
S788	Tab, Rose, Round, S 78-8	Thioridazine 15 mg	Mellaril by Sandoz		Antipsychotic
S80 <> G	Tab, White, Cap Shaped, Scored	Sotalol HCl 80 mg	Betapace by Par	49884-0582	Antiarrhythmic
S80 <> G	Tab, White, Cap Shaped, Scored, S/80	Sotalol HCl 80 mg	Betapace by Genpharm by Genpharm	15330-0208	Antiarrhythmic
S80 <> S	Tab, White, Oblong	Sotalol HCl 80 mg		55567-0057	Antiarrhythmic
S820	Tab, Peach, Round	Hydrochlorothiazide 25 mg	Hydrodiuril by Dava	67253-0820	Diuretic; Antihypertensive
S821	Tab, Peach, Round, Scored	Hydrochlorothiazide 50 mg	Hydrodiuril by Dava	67253-0821	Diuretic; Antihypertensive
S822	Tab, Pink, Clover-Shaped	Trichlormethiazide 2 mg	Naqua by Schering		Diuretic; Antihypertensive
S880	Tab, Yellow, Round	Isosorbide Dinitrate SR Oral 40 mg	Isordil by Zeneca		Antianginal
S900	Tab, White, Oval, Scored	Alprazolam 0.25 mg	Xanax by Dava	67253-0900	Antianxiety; C IV
S901	Tab, Yellow, Oval, Scored	Alprazolam 0.5 mg	Xanax by Dava	67253-0901	Antianxiety; C IV
S902	Tab, Green, Oval, Scored	Alprazolam 1 mg	Xanax by Dava	67253-0902	Antianxiety; C IV
S903	Tab, Green, Rectangle, Double Scored	Alprazolam 2 mg	Xanax by Dava	67253-0903	Antianxiety; C IV
SA <> NVR	Tab, Dark Yellow to Brownish-Orange, Round, Film Coated, Scored	Imatinib 100 mg	Gleevec by Novartis	Canadian DIN 02253275	Antineoplastic
SA <> NVR	Tab, Dark Yellow to Brownish-Orange, Round, Film Coated, Scored	Imatinib 100 mg	Gleevec by Novartis	00078-0401	Antineoplastic
SA100	Tab, Pink, Triangle-Shaped, Cobalt Logo <> SA over 100	Sumatriptan Succinate 100 mg	Imitrex DF by Cobalt	Canadian DIN 02257904	Antimigraine
SA25	Tab, White to Off-White, Round, Cobalt Logo <> SA over 25	Sumatriptan Succinate 25 mg	Imitrex DF by Cobalt	Canadian DIN 02257882	Antimigraine
SA50	Tab, White to Off-White, Triangle-Shaped, Cobalt Logo <> SA over 50	Sumatriptan Succinate 50 mg	Imitrex DF by Cobalt	Canadian DIN 02257890	Antimigraine

ID FRONT <> BACK	DESCRIPTION FRONT <> BACK	INGREDIENT & STRENGTH	BRAND (or Generic Equiv.) by FIRM	NDC#	CLASS; SCH.
SABRIL	Tab, White, Oval	Vigabatrin 500 mg	Sabril by Marion	Canadian	Anticonvulsant
SAHG	Tab, Pink, Clover-Shaped	Trichlormethiazide 2 mg	Naqua by Schering		Diuretic; Antihypertensive
SAHH	Tab, Aqua, Clover-Shaped	Trichlormethiazide 4 mg	Naqua by Schering	00085-0547	Diuretic; Antihypertensive
SAL <> 5	Tab, White, Round, Film Coated	Pilocarpine HCl 5 mg	Salagen by MGI	58063-0705	Cholinergic Agonist
SAL <> 5	Tab, White, Round, Biconvex, Film-Coated	Pilocarpine HCl 5 mg	Salagen by Pfizer	Canadian DIN 02216345	Cholinergic Agonist
SAL <> 75	Tab, Blue, Round, Biconvex, Coated, SAL <> 7.5	Pilocarpine HCl 7.5 mg	Salagen by MGI	58063-0775	Cholinergic Agonist
SAL5	Tab, White, Round, Film Coated, SAL-5	Pilocarpine HCl 5 mg	Salagen by Actavis	00228-2801	Cholinergic Agonist
SAL5	Tab, White, Round, SAL/5	Pilocarpine HCl 5 mg	by Pharmacia	Canadian	Cholinergic Agonist
SAMPLE <> 4	Tab, Film Coated	Ondansetron HCl 4 mg	Zofran by GSK		Antiemetic
SAMPLE <> 8	Tab	Ondansetron HCl 8 mg	Zofran by GSK		Antiemetic
SAMPLE <> ZOFRAN	Tab	Ondansetron HCl 8 mg	Zofran by GSK		Antiemetic
SAMPLE <> ZOFRAN	Tab, Film Coated	Ondansetron HCl 4 mg	Zofran by GSK		Antiemetic
SAN60	Cap, White and Orange Opaque, Extended Release	Trospium Chloride 60 mg	Sanctura XR by Esprit	15456-0981	Antispasmodic; Urinary Tract
SAN60	Cap, White and Orange Opaque, Extended Release	Trospium Chloride 60 mg	Sanctura XR by Allergan	Canadian DIN 02339706	Antispasmodic; Urinary Tract
SANDOZ	Tab, White, Round, Scored	Pizotifen 1 mg	Sandomigran DS by Sandoz	Canadian DIN 00511552	Antimigraine
SANDOZ	Tab, Green/Yellow, Circular, SAN/DOZ	Methysergide Maleate 2 mg	Sansert by Sandoz	Canadian	Antimigraine
SANDOZ	Tab, Red	Mesoridazine Besylate 10 mg	Serentil by Sandoz	Canadian	Antipsychotic
SANDOZ	Tab, Coated	Methylergonovine Maleate 0.2 mg	Methergine by Apotheca	12634-0179	Ergot Alkaloids
SANDOZ <> 25	Tab, Red, Round, Sugar Coated	Mesoridazine Besylate 25 mg	Serentil by Novartis	Canadian DIN 00027456	Antipsychotic
SANDOZ <> 7854	Tab, Orchid, Coated, 78-54 in Black Ink	Methylergonovine Maleate 0.2 mg	Methergine by Allscripts		Ergot Alkaloids
SANDOZ <> 7854	Tab, Orchid, Coated, 78-54 in Black Ink	Methylergonovine Maleate 0.2 mg	Methergine by Novartis	00078-0054	Ergot Alkaloids
SANDOZ <> 7854	Tab, Orchid, Coated, 78-54 in Black Ink	Methylergonovine Maleate 0.2 mg	Methergine by PDRX	55289-0708	Ergot Alkaloids
SANDOZ <> 7854	Tab, Orchid, Coated, 78-54 in Black Ink	Methylergonovine Maleate 0.2 mg	Methergine by Kaiser	00179-0432	Ergot Alkaloids
SANDOZ <> 7858	Tab, Yellow, Black Print, Round, Film Coated, 78-58	Methysergide Maleate 2 mg	Sansert by Novartis	00078-0058	Antimigraine
SANDOZ <> BC	Tab, Ivory, Round, Sugar Coated	Pizotifen 0.5 mg	Sandomigran by Novartis	Canadian DIN 00329320	Antimigraine
SANDOZ <> VJ	Tab, White, Round	Ergoloid Mesylate 1 mg	Hydergine by Novartis	Canadian DIN 00176176	Ergot Alkaloids
SANDOZ10	Tab, Red, Round, Sandoz/10	Mesoridazine Besylate 10 mg	Serentil by Novartis	Canadian	Antipsychotic
SANDOZ10MG	Cap, Yellow-Orange & White, Pamelor Logo <> Sandoz 10 mg	Nortriptyline HCl 10 mg	by Allscripts		Antidepressant
SANDOZ50	Tab, Red, Round, Sandoz/50	Mesoridazine Besylate 50 mg	Serentil by Novartis	Canadian	Antipsychotic
SANDOZ50MG	Cap	Cyclosporine 50 mg	Sandimmun Neoral B17 by RP Scherer	11014-1196	Immunosuppressant
SANDOZ571	Cap, White, Gold Band	Amlodipine 2.5 mg, Benazepril 10 mg	Lotrel by Sandoz	00781-2271	Antihypertensive
SANDOZ572	Cap, Light Brown, White Band	Amlodipine 5 mg, Benazepril 10 mg	Lotrel by Sandoz	00781-2272	Antihypertensive
SANDOZ573	Cap, Pink, White Band	Amlodipine 5 mg, Benazepril 20 mg	Lotrel by Sandoz	00781-2273	Antihypertensive
SANDOZ574	Cap, Purple, White Band	Amlodipine 10 mg, Benazepril 20 mg	Lotrel by Sandoz	00781-2274	Antihypertensive
SANDO663	Cap, Blue	Cefdinir 300 mg	Omnicef by Sandoz	00781-2176	Antibiotic
SANDOZ78107FC	Cap, Sandoz 78-107 <> Sandoz Logo F-C	Aspirin 325 mg, Butalbital 50 mg, Caffeine 40 mg, Codeine Phosphate 30 mg	Fiorinal w/ Codeine by Allscripts		Analgesic; C III
SANDOZ78107SFC	Cap, Sandoz 78-107 <> S in Triangle F-C	Aspirin 325 mg, Butalbital 50 mg, Caffeine 40 mg, Codeine Phosphate 30 mg	Fiorinal w/ Codeine by Physician Total Care	54868-0530	Analgesic; C III
SANDOZ7858	Tab, Yellow, Round, Sandoz 78-58	Methysergide Maleate 2 mg	Sansert by Sandoz		Antimigraine
SANDOZ7866	Tab, White, Round, Sandoz 78-66	Mazindol 2 mg	Sanorex by Sandoz		Anorexiant; C IV
SANDOZME100	Tab, Blue/Green, Circular, SAN/DOZ/MEL100	Thioridazine 100 mg	Mellaril by Sandoz	Canadian	Antipsychotic

ID FRONT <> BACK	DESCRIPTION FRONT <> BACK	INGREDIENT & STRENGTH	BRAND (or Generic Equiv.) by FIRM	NDC#	CLASS; SCH.
SANDOZMEL10	Tab, Light Green, Circular, SAN/DOZ/MEL/10	Thioridazine 10 mg	Mellaril by Sandoz	Canadian	Antipsychotic
SANDOZMEL25	Tab, Light Brown, Circular, SAN/DOZ/MEL/25	Thioridazine 25 mg	Mellaril by Sandoz	Canadian	Antipsychotic
SANDOZMEL50	Tab, White, Circular, SAN/DOZ/MEL/50	Thioridazine 50 mg	Mellaril by Sandoz	Canadian	Antipsychotic
SANDOZRESTORIL15	Cap, Flesh & Maroon, Gelatin	Temazepam 15 mg	Restoril by Sandoz	Canadian DIN 00604453	Sedative/Hypnotic; C IV
SANDOZRESTORIL15	Cap, Flesh & Maroon, Gelatin	Temazepam 15 mg	Restoril by Cobalt	Canadian DIN 02244814	Sedative/Hypnotic; C IV
SANDOZRESTORIL30	Cap, Blue & Maroon, Gelatin	Temazepam 30 mg	Restoril by Sandoz	Canadian DIN 00604461	Sedative/Hypnotic; C IV
SANDZO <> 7854	Tab, Purple, Round	Methylergonovine Maleate 0.2 mg	Methergine by Novartis	61615-0107	Ergot Alkaloids
SANKYO <> C12	Tab, Yellow, Round, Film Coated	Olmesartan Medoxomil 5 mg	Benicar by Sankyo	65597-0101	Antihypertensive
SANKYO <> C14	Tab, White, Round, Film Coated	Olmesartan Medoxomil 20 mg	Benicar by Sankyo	65597-0103	Antihypertensive
SANKYO <> C15	Tab, White, Oval, Film Coated	Olmesartan Medoxomil 40 mg	Benicar by Sankyo	65597-0104	Antihypertensive
SANKYO <> C22	Tab, Reddish-Yellow, Round, Film Coated	Hydrochlorothiazide 12.5 mg, Olmesartan Medoxomil 20 mg	Benicar HCT by Sankyo	65597-0105	Antihypertensive; Diuretic
SANKYO <> C23	Tab, Reddish-Yellow, Oval, Film Coated	Hydrochlorothiazide 12.5 mg, Olmesartan Medoxomil 40 mg	Benicar HCT by Sankyo	65597-0106	Antihypertensive; Diuretic
SANKYO <> C25	Tab, Pink, Oval, Film Coated	Hydrochlorothiazide 25 mg, Olmesartan Medoxomil 40 mg	Benicar HCT by Sankyo	65597-0107	Antihypertensive; Diuretic
SANKYOC01	Tab, Off White, Black Print, Cap Shaped, Film Coated, SANKYO over C01	Colesevelam HCl 625 mg	WelChol by Sankyo	65597-0701	Bile Acid Resin
SANOFI <> PN	Tab, Coated	Ascorbic Acid 120 mg, Calcium Citrate 200 mg, Cholecalciferol 400 Units, Cupric Oxide 2 mg, Cyanocobalamin 12 mcg, Docusate Sodium 50 mg, Folic Acid 1 mg, Iron Pentacarbonyl 90 mg, Niacinamide 20 mg, Potassium Iodide 150 mcg, Pyridoxine HCl 20 mg, Riboflavin 3.4 mg, Thiamine HCl 3 mg, Vitamin A 2700 Units, Vitamin E 30 Units, Zinc Oxide 25 mg	Prenate Ultra by Sanofi	00024-1730	Vitamin
SANOFI <> ZLA	Tab, Orange, Oval, Film Coated, Z / LA	Guaifenesin 600 mg, Pseudoephedrine HCl 120 mg	Zephrex, LA by Sanofi	00024-2627	Cold Remedy
SANOREX	Tab	Mazindol 1 mg	by Allscripts		Anorexiant; C IV
SANOREX <> 7871	Tab, White, Elliptical, Sanorex <> 78-71	Mazindol 1 mg	by Allscripts		Anorexiant; C IV
SANOREX <> JC	Tab, Peach, Round, Scored	Mazindol 2 mg	Sanorex by Novartis	Canadian DIN 00285544	Anorexiant; C IV
SANTHERALOGO <> 150	Tab, Orange, Round, Film Coated	Idebenone 150 mg	Catena by Santhera Pharm	Canadian DIN 02314150	Neuromuscular
SB <> 2	Tab, Pink, Pentagonal, Film Coated	Rosiglitazone Maleate 2 mg	Avandia by SKB	00029-3158	Antidiabetic
SB <> 2	Tab, Pink, Pentagonal, Film Coated	Rosiglitazone Maleate 2 mg	Avandia by GSK	Canadian DIN 02241112	Antidiabetic
SB <> 39	Tab, White, Oval, Film Coated	Carvedilol 3.125 mg	Coreg by SKB	59742-4139	Antihypertensive
SB <> 39	Tab, White, Oval, Film Coated	Carvedilol 3.125 mg	Coreg by SKB	00007-4139	Antihypertensive
SB <> 39	Tab, White, Oval, Film Coated	Carvedilol 3.125 mg	Coreg by Murfreesboro	51129-1126	Antihypertensive
SB <> 4	Tab, Orange, Pentagonal, Film Coated	Rosiglitazone Maleate 4 mg	Avandia by GSK	Canadian DIN 02241113	Antidiabetic
SB <> 4	Tab, Orange, Pentagonal, Film Coated	Rosiglitazone Maleate 4 mg	Avandia by SKB	00029-3159	Antidiabetic
SB <> 4890	Tab, White, Pentagonal, Film Coated	Ropinirole HCl 0.25 mg	Requip by GSK	Canadian DIN 02232565	Antiparkinson
SB <> 4890	Tab, White, Pentagonal, Film Coated	Ropinirole HCl 0.25 mg	Requip by RX Pak	65084-0202	Antiparkinson
SB <> 4890	Tab, White, Pentagonal, Film Coated	Ropinirole HCl 0.25 mg	Requip by SKB	00007-4890	Antiparkinson
SB <> 4890	Tab, White, Pentagonal, Film Coated	Ropinirole HCl 0.25 mg	Requip by SKB	60351-4890	Antiparkinson
SB <> 4891	Tab, Yellow, Pentagonal, Film Coated	Ropinirole HCl 0.5 mg	Requip by SKB	00007-4891	Antiparkinson
SB <> 4891	Tab, Yellow, Pentagonal, Film Coated	Ropinirole HCl 0.5 mg	Requip by SKB	60351-4891	Antiparkinson
SB <> 4892	Tab, Green, Pentagonal, Film Coated	Ropinirole HCl 1 mg	Requip by SKB	00007-4892	Antiparkinson
SB <> 4892	Tab, Green, Pentagonal, Film Coated	Ropinirole HCl 1 mg	Requip by SKB	60351-4892	Antiparkinson
SB <> 4892	Tab, Green, Pentagonal, Film Coated	Ropinirole HCl 1 mg	Requip by RX Pak	65084-0203	Antiparkinson

ID FRONT <> BACK	DESCRIPTION FRONT <> BACK	INGREDIENT & STRENGTH	BRAND (or Generic Equiv.) by FIRM	NDC#	CLASS; SCH.
SB <> 4892	Tab, Green, Pentagonal, Film Coated	Ropinirole HCl 1 mg	Requip by GSK	Canadian DIN 02232567	Antiparkinson
SB <> 4893	Tab, Light Pink, Pentagonal, Film Coated	Ropinirole HCl 2 mg	Requip by GSK	Canadian DIN 02232568	Antiparkinson
SB <> 4893	Tab, Light Pink, Pentagonal, Film Coated	Ropinirole HCl 2 mg	Requip by SKB	60351-4893	Antiparkinson
SB <> 4893	Tab, Light Pink, Pentagonal, Film Coated	Ropinirole HCl 2 mg	Requip by SKB	00007-4893	Antiparkinson
SB <> 4894	Tab, Blue, Pentagonal, Film Coated	Ropinirole HCl 5 mg	Requip by SKB	00007-4894	Antiparkinson
SB <> 4894	Tab, Blue, Pentagonal, Film Coated	Ropinirole HCl 5 mg	Requip by SKB	60351-4894	Antiparkinson
SB <> 4894	Tab, Blue, Pentagonal, Film Coated	Ropinirole HCl 5 mg	Requip by GSK	Canadian DIN 02232569	Antiparkinson
SB <> 4895	Tab, Purple, Pentagonal	Ropinirole HCl 3 mg	Requip by SKB	00007-4895	Antiparkinson
SB <> 4896	Tab, Brown, Pentagonal	Ropinirole HCl 4 mg	Requip by SKB	00007-4896	Antiparkinson
SB <> 8	Tab, Reddish Brown, Pentagonal	Rosiglitazone Maleate 8 mg	Avandia by SKB	00029-3160	Antidiabetic
SB <> 8	Tab, Reddish Brown, Pentagonal, Film Coated	Rosiglitazone Maleate 8 mg	Avandia by GSK	Canadian DIN 02241114	Antidiabetic
SB10MG334610MG	Cap, Black/Natural, SB 10mg/3346 10mg	Prochlorperazine 15 mg	Compazine Spansule by SKB		Antiemetic
SB4140	Tab, White, Oval, Film Coated	Carvedilol 6.25 mg	Coreg by SB	59742-4140	Antihypertensive
SB4140	Tab, White, Oval, Film Coated	Carvedilol 6.25 mg	Coreg by SKB	Canadian	Antihypertensive
SB4140	Tab, White, Oval, Film Coated	Carvedilol 6.25 mg	Coreg by SKB	00007-4140	Antihypertensive
SB4141	Tab, White, Oval, Film Coated	Carvedilol 12.5 mg	Coreg by SB	59742-4141	Antihypertensive
SB4141	Tab, White, Oval, Film Coated	Carvedilol 12.5 mg	Coreg by SKB	Canadian	Antihypertensive
SB4141	Tab, White, Oval, Film Coated	Carvedilol 12.5 mg	Coreg by SKB	00007-4141	Antihypertensive
SB4142	Tab, White, Oval, Film Coated	Carvedilol 25 mg	Coreg by SB	59742-4142	Antihypertensive
SB4142	Tab, White, Oval, Film Coated	Carvedilol 25 mg	Coreg by SKB	Canadian	Antihypertensive
SB4142	Tab, White, Oval, Film Coated	Carvedilol 25 mg	Coreg by SKB	00007-4142	Antihypertensive
SB4896	Tab, Brown, Pentagon, Beveled, Film, SB over 4896	Ropinirole HCl 4 mg	Requip by RX Pak	65084-0205	Antiparkinson
SB4896	Tab, Brown, Pentagon, Beveled, Film, SB over 4896	Ropinirole HCl 4 mg	Requip by RX Pak	65084-0204	Antiparkinson
SB5043	Tab, White, Oval, Film Coated, SB5043 <> SB5043	Eprosartan 300 mg	Teveten by Solvay	Canadian DIN 02240431	Antihypertensive
SB5044	Tab, Pink, Oval, Film Coated, SB5044 <> SB5044	Eprosartan 400 mg	Teveten by Solvay	Canadian DIN 02240432	Antihypertensive
SB5500	Tab, White, Round, Raised Pentagon Imprint, SB/5500	Albendazole 200 mg	Albenza by SKB	00007-5500	Antihelmintic
SB5MG35125MG	Cap, Brown & Clear	Dextroamphetamine Sulfate 5 mg	Dexedrine by SKB	00007-3512	Stimulant; C II
SC <> A	Tab, Light Violet, Oval, Film Coated, Abbott Logo (a)	Verapamil HCl 120 mg	Isoptin SR by Abbott	00074-1149	Antihypertensive
SCHEIN0765400	Tab, White, Black Print, Oblong, Film Coated, Schein over 0765/400	Ibuprofen 400 mg	Motrin by Nat Pharmpak	55154-5214	NSAID
SCHEIN0765400	Tab, White, Black Print, Oblong, Film Coated, Schein over 0765/400	Ibuprofen 400 mg	Motrin by Med Pro	53978-5005	NSAID
SCHEIN0765400	Tab, White, Black Print, Oblong, Film Coated, Schein over 0765/400	Ibuprofen 400 mg	Motrin by Schein	00364-0765	NSAID
SCHEIN0765400	Tab, White, Black Print, Oblong, Film Coated, Schein over 0765/400	Ibuprofen 400 mg	Motrin by Murfreesboro	51129-1512	NSAID
SCHEIN0766600	Tab, White, Black Print, Oblong, Film Coated, Schein over 0766/600	Ibuprofen 600 mg	Motrin by Talbert	44514-0636	NSAID
SCHEIN0766600	Tab, White, Black Print, Oblong, Film Coated, Schein over 0766/600	Ibuprofen 600 mg	Motrin by Nat Pharmpak	55154-5207	NSAID
SCHEIN0766600	Tab, White, Black Print, Oblong, Film Coated, Schein over 0766/600	Ibuprofen 600 mg	Motrin by Murfreesboro	51129-1514	NSAID
SCHEIN0766600	Tab, White, Black Print, Oblong, Film Coated, Schein over 0766/600	Ibuprofen 600 mg	Motrin by Schein	00364-0766	NSAID
SCHEIN20	Cap, Schein over 20	Nifedipine 10 mg	by RP Scherer	11014-0955	Antihypertensive

ID FRONT <> BACK	DESCRIPTION FRONT <> BACK	INGREDIENT & STRENGTH	BRAND (or Generic Equiv.) by FIRM	NDC#	CLASS; SCH.
SCHEIN213780	Tab, White, Black Print, Oblong, Film Coated, Schein over 2137/800	Ibuprofen 800 mg	Motrin by Talbert	44514-0637	NSAID
SCHEIN213780	Tab, White, Black Print, Oblong, Film Coated, Schein over 2137/800	Ibuprofen 800 mg	Motrin by Heartland	61392-0528	NSAID
SCHEIN213780	Tab, White, Black Print, Oblong, Film Coated, Schein over 2137/800	Ibuprofen 800 mg	Motrin by Nat Pharmpak	55154-5233	NSAID
SCHEIN213780	Tab, White, Black Print, Oblong, Film Coated, Schein over 2137/800	Ibuprofen 800 mg	Motrin by Murfreesboro	51129-1531	NSAID
SCHEIN213780	Tab, White, Black Print, Oblong, Film Coated, Schein over 2137/800	Ibuprofen 800 mg	Motrin by Med Pro	53978-5007	NSAID
SCHEIN213780	Tab, White, Black Print, Oblong, Film Coated, Schein over 2137/800	Ibuprofen 800 mg	Motrin by Schein	00364-2137	NSAID
SCHERING	Tab, Blue, Round	Betamethasone 1 mg	Celestone by Schering	Canadian Discontinued	Steroid
SCHERING	Tab, White, Round, Scored, Schering Logo	Azatadine Maleate 1 mg	Optimine by Schering	Canadian DIN 00355666	Antihistamine
SCHERING <> 080	Tab, Yellow, Round, Scored, "Schering" over a Logo <> / 080	Chlorpheniramine 4 mg	Chlor-Trimeton by Schering-Plough	00085-0080	Antihistamine
SCHERING <> 100NORMODYNE	Tab, Light Brown, Film Coated	Labetalol HCl 100 mg	Normodyne by Pharm Util	60491-0458	Antihypertensive
SCHERING <> 228	Tab, White, Round, Score, Schering Logo	Griseofulvin, Ultramicrosize 125 mg	Fulvicin P/G by Schering	00085-0228	Antifungal
SCHERING <> 496	Tab, White, Round, Scored	Griseofulvin, Microsize 500 mg	Fulvicin U/F by Schering	00085-0496	Antifungal
SCHERING <> 795	Tab, Pink, Oval, Scored	Anisindione 50 mg	Miradon by Schering	00085-0795	Anticoagulant
SCHERING <> 948	Tab, White, Mortar and Pestle to Right of Schering	Griseofulvin, Microsize 250 mg	Fulvicin P/G by Schering	00085-0948	Antifungal
SCHERING <> A	Tab, Orange, Round, Film Coated	Amitriptyline HCl 10 mg, Perphenazine 4 mg	Etrafon-A by Pharmascience	Canadian DIN 00176958	Antidepressant; Antipsychotic
SCHERING244 <> NORMODYNE100	Tab, Light Brown, Film Coated	Labetalol HCl 100 mg	Normodyne by Pharm Util	60491-0458	Antihypertensive
SCHERING244 <> NORMODYNE100	Tab, Brown, Round, Scored	Labetalol HCl 100 mg	Normodyne by Nat Pharmpak	55154-3511	Antihypertensive
SCHERING244 <> NORMODYNE100	Tab, Brown, Round, Scored	Labetalol HCl 100 mg	Normodyne by Amerisource	62584-0244	Antihypertensive
SCHERING244 <> NORMODYNE100	Tab, Brown, Round, Scored	Labetalol HCl 100 mg	Normodyne by Thrift Drug	59198-0080	Antihypertensive
SCHERING244 <> NORMODYNE100	Tab, Brown, Round, Scored	Labetalol HCl 100 mg	Normodyne by Rite Aid	11822-5260	Antihypertensive
SCHERING244 <> NORMODYNE100	Tab, Brown, Round, Scored	Labetalol HCl 100 mg	Normodyne by Murfreesboro	51129-1618	Antihypertensive
SCHERING244 <> NORMODYNE100	Tab, Brown, Round, Scored	Labetalol HCl 100 mg	Normodyne by Rightpak	65240-0705	Antihypertensive
SCHERING244 <> NORMODYNE100	Tab, Brown, Round, Scored	Labetalol HCl 100 mg	Normodyne by Caremark	00339-5265	Antihypertensive
SCHERING244 <> NORMODYNE100	Tab, Brown, Round, Scored	Labetalol HCl 100 mg	Normodyne by Schering	00085-0244	Antihypertensive
SCHERING396	Tab, White, Bullet Shaped	Clotrimazole 500 mg	Gyne Lotrimin by Schering		Antifungal
SCHERING438	Tab, Blue, Round	Labetalol HCl 300 mg	Normodyne by Schering		Antihypertensive
SCHERING438 <> 300	Tab, Blue, Round	Labetalol HCl 300 mg	Normodyne by Rightpak	65240-0670	Antihypertensive
SCHERING438 <> 300NORMODYNE	Tab, Blue, Round, Film, Schering 438 <> 300 Normodyne	Labetalol HCl 300 mg	Normodyne by Murfreesboro	51129-1607	Antihypertensive
SCHERING438 <> 300NORMODYNE	Tab, Blue, Round, Film, Schering 438 <> 300 Normodyne	Labetalol HCl 300 mg	Normodyne by Murfreesboro	51129-1606	Antihypertensive

ID FRONT <> BACK	DESCRIPTION FRONT <> BACK	INGREDIENT & STRENGTH	BRAND (or Generic Equiv.) by FIRM	NDC#	CLASS; SCH.
SCHERING438 <> 300NORMODYNE	Tab, Blue, Round, Film, Schering 438 <> 300 Normodyne	Labetalol HCl 300 mg	Normodyne by Thrift Drug	59198-0082	Antihypertensive
SCHERING438 <> NORMODYNE	Tab, Blue, Round, Film, Schering 438 <> 300 Normodyne	Labetalol HCl 300 mg	Normodyne by Rx Pak	65084-0230	Antihypertensive
SCHERING438 <> NORMODYNE300	Tab, Blue, Round, Film, Schering 438 <> 300 Normodyne	Labetalol HCl 300 mg	Normodyne by Leiner	59606-0670	Antihypertensive
SCHERING438 <> NORMODYNE300	Tab, Blue, Round, Film, Schering 438 <> 300 Normodyne	Labetalol HCl 300 mg	Normodyne by Schering	00085-0438	Antihypertensive
SCHERING525	Cap, Lt. Brown & Dark Brown, Black Print, Schering over 525	Flutamide 125 mg	Eulexin by Schering	00085-0525	Antiandrogen
SCHERING525	Cap, Lt. Brown & Dark Brown, Black Print, Schering over 525	Flutamide 125 mg	Eulexin by Eckerd	19458-0919	Antiandrogen
SCHERING7 <> NORMODYNE	Tab, Film Coated	Labetalol HCl 200 mg	Normodyne by Pharmedix	53002-1046	Antihypertensive
SCHERING703	Tab, Sugar Coated	Azatadine Maleate 1 mg, Pseudoephedrine Sulfate 120 mg	Trinalin by Pharmedix	53002-0413	Cold Remedy
SCHERING752	Tab, White, Round	Labetalol HCl 200 mg	Normodyne by Schering		Antihypertensive
SCHERING752 <> 200	Tab, White, Round, Scored	Labetalol HCl 200 mg	Normodyne by Rightpak	65240-0706	Antihypertensive
SCHERING752 <> 200NORMODYNE	Tab, Film Coated, Schering 752 <> 200 Normodyne	Labetalol HCl 200 mg	Normodyne by Thrift Drug	59198-0081	Antihypertensive
SCHERING752 <> 200NORMODYNE	Tab, White, Round, Scored, Film Coated, Schering 752 <> 200 Normodyne	Labetalol HCl 200 mg	Normodyne by Murfreesboro	51129-1617	Antihypertensive
SCHERING752 <> NORMODYNE	Tab, Film Coated, Schering 752	Labetalol HCl 200 mg	Normodyne by Med Pro	53978-0697	Antihypertensive
SCHERING752 <> NORMODYNE 200	Tab, Film Coated, Schering 438 <> Normodyne 300	Labetalol HCl 200 mg	Normodyne by Schering	53922-0752	Antihypertensive
SCHERING752 <> NORMODYNE 200	Tab, White, Round, Film Coated	Labetalol HCl 200 mg	Normodyne by Schering	00085-0752	Antihypertensive
SCHERING752 <> NORMODYNE200	Tab, Film Coated	Labetalol HCl 200 mg	Normodyne by Amerisource	62584-0752	Antihypertensive
SCHERING752 <> NORMODYNE200	Tab, Film Coated, Schering 752 <> Normodyne 200	Labetalol HCl 200 mg	Normodyne by Nat Pharmpak	55154-3506	Antihypertensive
SCHERING752 <> NORMODYNE200	Tab, Film Coated	Labetalol HCl 200 mg	Normodyne by Rite Aid	11822-5234	Antihypertensive
SCHERINGGROOVE	Tab, Blue, Round, Schering/Groove	Betamethasone 0.5 mg	Celestone by Schering	Canadian Discontinued	Steroid
SCHERINGLOGO	Tab, Orange, Round, Schering Logo	Chlorpheniramine Maleate 12 mg	Chlor-Trimeton by Schering	Canadian Discontinued	Antihistamine
SCHWARZ <> 531	Tab, White, Round, Scored	Hyoscyamine Sulfate 0.125 mg	Levsin by Prestige	58056-0351	Gastrointestinal
SCHWARZ <> 531	Tab, White, Round, Scored	Hyoscyamine Sulfate 0.125 mg	Levsin by Thrift Drug	59198-0287	Gastrointestinal
SCHWARZ <> 531	Tab, White, Round, Scored	Hyoscyamine Sulfate 0.125 mg	Levsin by Schwarz	00091-3531	Gastrointestinal
SCHWARZ <> 532	Tab, White, Octagonal, Scored, Sublingual	Hyoscyamine Sulfate 0.125 mg	Levsin by Schwarz	00091-3532	Gastrointestinal
SCHWARZ <> 532	Tab, White, Octagonal, Scored, Sublingual	Hyoscyamine Sulfate 0.125 mg	Levsin by Med Pro	53978-3372	Gastrointestinal
SCHWARZ <> 532	Tab, White, Octagonal, Scored, Sublingual	Hyoscyamine Sulfate 0.125 mg	Levsin by Nat Pharmpak	55154-0952	Gastrointestinal
SCHWARZ <> 532	Tab, White, Octagonal, Scored, Sublingual	Hyoscyamine Sulfate 0.125 mg	Levsin by Prestige	58056-0352	Gastrointestinal
SCHWARZ <> 532	Tab, White, Octagonal, Scored, Sublingual	Hyoscyamine Sulfate 0.125 mg	Levsin by Amerisource	62584-0007	Gastrointestinal
SCHWARZ <> 532	Tab, White, Octagonal, Scored, Sublingual	Hyoscyamine Sulfate 0.125 mg	Levsin by Physician Total Care	54868-1767	Gastrointestinal
SCHWARZ <> 532	Tab, White, Octagonal, Scored, Sublingual	Hyoscyamine Sulfate 0.125 mg	Levsin by Murfreesboro	51129-1489	Gastrointestinal
SCHWARZ <> 532	Tab, White, Octagonal, Scored, Sublingual	Hyoscyamine Sulfate 0.125 mg	Levsin by Thrift Drug	59198-0173	Gastrointestinal
SCHWARZ <> 534	Tab, Pink	Hyoscyamine Sulfate 0.125 mg, Phenobarbital 15 mg	Levsin Phenobarb by Schwarz	00091-3534	Gastrointestinal; C IV
SCHWARZ053	Cap, White & Yellow	Pseudoephedrine HCl 65 mg, Chlorpheniramine 10 mg	Fedahist Gyrocaps by Schwarz		Cold Remedy
SCHWARZ055	Cap, Clear	Pseudoephedrine HCl 120 mg, Chlorpheniramine 8 mg	Fedahist Timecaps by Schwarz		Cold Remedy
SCHWARZ0920	Cap, Clear & Pink, Black Print, Opaque	Isosorbide Dinitrate 40 mg	Dilatrate-SR by Schwarz	00091-0920	Antianginal

ID FRONT <> BACK	DESCRIPTION FRONT <> BACK	INGREDIENT & STRENGTH	BRAND (or Generic Equiv.) by FIRM	NDC#	CLASS; SCH.
SCHWARZ2489-VERELAN180MG	Cap, Gray & Yellow, Schwarz over 2489, Verelan over 180 mg	Verapamil HCl 180 mg	Verelan by Schwarz	00091-2489	Antihypertensive
SCHWARZ2490-VERELAN120MG	Cap, Yellow, Black Print, Schwarz over 2490, Verelan over 120 mg	Verapamil HCl 120 mg	Verelan by Schwarz	00091-2490	Antihypertensive
SCHWARZ2491-VERELAN240MG	Cap, Blue & Yellow, Black Print, Schwarz over 2491, Verelan over 240 mg	Verapamil HCl 240 mg	Verelan by Schwarz	00091-2491	Antihypertensive
SCHWARZ2495-VERELAN360MG	Cap, Purple & Yellow, Schwarz over 2495, Verelan over 360 mg	Verapamil HCl 360 mg	Verelan by Schwarz	00091-2495	Antihypertensive
SCHWARZ4085100MG	Cap, Purple & White, Opaque, Hard Gel, Ex Release	Verapamil HCl 100 mg	Verelan PM by Teva	00480-0832	Antihypertensive
SCHWARZ4085100MG	Cap, Purple & White, Opaque, Hard Gel, Ex Release	Verapamil HCl 100 mg	Verelan PM by Schwarz	00091-4085	Antihypertensive
SCHWARZ4086200MG	Cap, Purple, Opaque, Hard Gel, Ex Release	Verapamil HCl 200 mg	Verelan PM by Teva	00480-0833	Antihypertensive
SCHWARZ4086200MG	Cap, Purple, Opaque, Hard Gel, Ex Release	Verapamil HCl 200 mg	Verelan PM by Schwarz	00091-4086	Antihypertensive
SCHWARZ4087300MG	Cap, Purple, Opaque, Hard Gel, Ex Release	Verapamil HCl 300 mg	Verelan PM by Teva	00480-0834	Antihypertensive
SCHWARZ4087300MG	Cap, Purple, Opaque, Hard Gel, Ex Release	Verapamil HCl 300 mg	Verelan PM by Schwarz	00091-4087	Antihypertensive
SCHWARZ4122	Cap, White & Yellow, Red Print	Amylase 15000 Units, Lipase 1200 Units, Protease 15000 Units	Ku-Zyme by Schwarz	00091-4122	Gastrointestinal
SCHWARZ4175	Cap, Green & White, Opaque	Amylase 30,000 USP, Lipase 2,400 USP, Protease 30,000 USP	Kutrase by Schwarz	00091-4175	Gastrointestinal
SCHWARZ475	Cap, Green & White, Opaque	Amylase 30 mg, Cellulase 2 mg, Hyoscyamine Sulfate 0.0625 mg, Lipase 1200 Units, Phenyltoloxamine Citrate 15 mg, Protease 6 mg	Kutrase by Schwarz	00091-3475 Discontinued	Gastrointestinal
SCHWARZ505	Cap, Orange & White, Opaque	Lactase Enzyme 250 mg	Lactrase by Schwarz	00091-3505	Gastrointestinal
SCHWARZ505	Cap, Orange & White, Opaque	Lactase Enzyme 250 mg	Lactrase by Schwarz		Gastrointestinal
SCHWARZ522	Cap, Yellow & White, Red Print	Amylase 30 mg, Cellulase 2 mg, Lipase 1200 Units, Protease 30,000 Units	Ku-Zyme by Schwarz	00091-3522 Discontinued	Gastrointestinal
SCHWARZ525	Cap, White, Red Print	Amylase 30,000 Units, Lipase 8000 Units, Protease 30,000 Units	Ku-Zyme HP by Schwarz	00091-3525	Gastrointestinal
SCHWARZ537	Cap, Brown & White, Schwarz 537, Extended Release	Hyoscyamine Sulfate 0.375 mg	Levsinex Timecaps by Nat Pharmpak	55154-0950	Gastrointestinal
SCHWARZ537	Cap, Brown & White, Schwarz 537, Extended Release	Hyoscyamine Sulfate 0.375 mg	Levsinex Timecaps by Med Pro	53978-3399	Gastrointestinal
SCHWARZ537	Cap, Brown & White, Schwarz 537, Extended Release	Hyoscyamine Sulfate 0.375 mg	Levsinex Timecaps by Schwarz	00091-3537	Gastrointestinal
SCHWARZ537	Cap, Brown & White, Schwarz 537, Extended Release	Hyoscyamine Sulfate 0.375 mg	Levsinex Timecaps by Schwarz		Gastrointestinal
SCHWARZ537	Cap, Brown & White, Schwarz 537, Extended Release	Hyoscyamine Sulfate 0.375 mg	Levsinex Timecaps by CVS	51316-0251	Gastrointestinal
SCHWARZ537	Cap, Brown & White, Schwarz 537, Extended Release	Hyoscyamine Sulfate 0.375 mg	Levsinex Timecaps by Thrift Drug	59198-0288	Gastrointestinal
SCHWARZ537	Cap, Brown & White, Schwarz 537, Extended Release	Hyoscyamine Sulfate 0.375 mg	Levsinex Timecaps by Amerisource	62584-0010	Gastrointestinal
SCHWARZ537	Cap, Brown & White, Schwarz 537, Extended Release	Hyoscyamine Sulfate 0.375 mg	Levsinex Timecaps by Eckerd	19458-0836	Gastrointestinal
SCHWARZ610 <> 10	Tab, White, Round, Scored	Isosorbide Mononitrate 10 mg	Monoket by Schwarz	00091-3610	Antianginal
SCHWARZ620 <> 20	Tab, White, Round, Scored	Isosorbide Mononitrate 20 mg	Monoket by Schwarz	00091-3620	Antianginal
SCHWARZ620 <> 20	Tab, White, Round, Scored	Isosorbide Mononitrate 20 mg	Monoket by Heartland	61392-0630	Antianginal
SCORED <> C	Tab	Conjugated Estrogens 0.625 mg, Medroxyprogesterone Acetate 2.5 mg	Prempro by Pharm Util	60491-0904	Hormone
SCS <> 1530	Tab	Ethinyl Estradiol 0.03 mg, Levonorgestrel 0.15 mg	Levora by Patheon	63285-0100	Oral Contraceptive
SCS <> 1530	Tab, White, Round	Ethinyl Estradiol 0.03 mg, Levonorgestrel 0.15 mg	by SCS Pharms	00905-0279	Oral Contraceptive
SCS12530	Tab, Pink, Round, SCS 125/30	Levonorgestrel 0.125 mg, Ethinyl Estradiol 0.03 mg	Trivora by Watson		Oral Contraceptive
SCS1530	Tab, Round, SCS/15/30	Ethinyl Estradiol 0.03 mg, Levonorgestrel 0.15 mg	Levora by Watson		Oral Contraceptive
SCS221	Tab, Round	Norethindrone 1 mg, Ethinyl Estradiol 35 mcg	Norethin 1/35E by Searle		Oral Contraceptive
SCS431	Tab, Round	Norethindrone 1 mg, Mestranol 50 mcg	Norethin 1/50M by Searle		Oral Contraceptive
SCS5030	Tab, Round, SCS 50/30	Levonorgestrel 0.05 mg, Ethinyl Estradiol 0.03 mg	Trivora by Watson		Oral Contraceptive
SCS5752	Cap	Piroxicam 10 mg	Feldene by SCS Pharms	00905-5752	NSAID
SCS5762	Cap	Piroxicam 20 mg	Feldene by SCS Pharms	00905-5762	NSAID
SCS7540	Tab, Round, SCS 75/40	Levonorgestrel 0.075 mg, Ethinyl Estradiol 0.04 mg	Trivora by Watson		Oral Contraceptive
SCSP	Tab, Peach, Round	Placebo	Placebo by Watson		Placebo
SCSP	Tab, Round, SCS/P	Placebo	Placebo by Watson		Placebo
SDA1201	Tab, White, Cap Shaped	Guaifenesin 1200 mg, Pseudoephedrine 120 mg	Robitussin by Major	00904-5543	Cold Remedy

ID FRONT <> BACK	DESCRIPTION FRONT <> BACK	INGREDIENT & STRENGTH	BRAND (or Generic Equiv.) by FIRM	NDC#	CLASS; SCH.
SE25 <> APO	Tab, Light Green, Oval, Scored, Film Coated, SE / 25	Sertraline HCl 25 mg	Zoloft by Apotex	60505-0180	Antidepressant
SE5 <> G	Tab, White, Round, SE over 5	Selegiline HCl 5 mg	by Draxis	Canadian	Antiparkinson
SE5 <> G	Tab, White, Round, SE over 5	Selegiline HCl 5 mg	Selegiline HCl by Schein		Antiparkinson
SE50 <> APO	Tab, Bluish Purple, Oval, Scored, Film Coated, SE / 50	Sertraline HCl 50 mg	Zoloft by Apotex	60505-0181	Antidepressant
SEARLE	Tab, Peach, Round	Inert	Demulen 30 28 by Pharmacia	Canadian DIN 00471526	Oral Contraceptive; Placebo
SEARLE	Tab, Blue, Round	Placebo	Placebo by Searle		Placebo
SEARLE <> 1	Tab	Mestranol 0.05 mg, Norethindrone 1 mg	Norinyl 1 50 21 Day by Searle	00025-0263	Oral Contraceptive
SEARLE <> 1451	Tab, White, Round	Misoprostol 100 mcg	Cytotec by Searle	00025-1451	Gastrointestinal
SEARLE <> 1451	Tab, White, Round	Misoprostol 100 mcg	Cytotec by H J Harkins Co	52959-0353	Gastrointestinal
SEARLE <> 151	Tab, White, Round	Ethinyl Estradiol 35 mcg, Ethynodiol Diacetate 1 mg	Demulen 1/35 by Nat Pharmpak	55154-3612	Oral Contraceptive
SEARLE <> 151	Tab, White, Round	Ethinyl Estradiol 35 mcg, Ethynodiol Diacetate 1 mg	Demulen 1/35 by Rx Pak	65084-0219	Oral Contraceptive
SEARLE <> 151	Tab, White, Round	Ethinyl Estradiol 35 mcg, Ethynodiol Diacetate 1 mg	Demulen 1/35 by Physician Total Care	54868-0404	Oral Contraceptive
SEARLE <> 151	Tab, White, Round	Ethinyl Estradiol 35 mcg, Ethynodiol Diacetate 1 mg	Demulen 1/35 by Pharm Util	60491-0181	Oral Contraceptive
SEARLE <> 151	Tab, White, Round	Ethinyl Estradiol 35 mcg, Ethynodiol Diacetate 1 mg	Demulen 1/35 by Searle	00025-0151	Oral Contraceptive
SEARLE <> 6	Tab	Ethinyl Estradiol 0.035 mg, Norethindrone 0.5 mg, Norethindrone 1 mg	Tri Norinyl 21 Day by Searle	00025-0272	Oral Contraceptive
SEARLE <> 6	Tab, Searle <> Underlined 6	Ethinyl Estradiol 0.035 mg, Norethindrone 0.5 mg	Brevicon 21 Day by Searle	00025-0252	Oral Contraceptive
SEARLE <> 61	Tab, White, Round	Atropine Sulfate 0.025 mg, Diphenoxylate HCl 2.5 mg	Lomotil by Nat Pharmpak	55154-3614	Antidiarrheal; C V
SEARLE <> 61	Tab, White, Round	Atropine Sulfate 0.025 mg, Diphenoxylate HCl 2.5 mg	Lomotil by Searle	00014-0061	Antidiarrheal; C V
SEARLE <> 61	Tab, White, Round	Atropine Sulfate 0.025 mg, Diphenoxylate HCl 2.5 mg	Lomotil by St. Mary's Med	60760-0061	Antidiarrheal; C V
SEARLE <> 61	Tab, White, Round	Atropine Sulfate 0.025 mg, Diphenoxylate HCl 2.5 mg	Lomotil by Amerisource	62584-0027	Antidiarrheal; C V
SEARLE <> 61	Tab, White, Round	Atropine Sulfate 0.025 mg, Diphenoxylate HCl 2.5 mg	Lomotil by Searle	00025-0061	Antidiarrheal; C V
SEARLE <> 61	Tab, White, Round	Atropine Sulfate 0.025 mg, Diphenoxylate HCl 2.5 mg	Lomotil by Med Pro	53978-3088	Antidiarrheal; C V
SEARLE <> 61	Tab, White, Round	Diphenoxylate HCl 2.5 mg	Lomotil by Searle	Canadian DIN 00036323	Antidiarrheal; C V
SEARLE <> 7	Tab, Yellowish Green	Ethinyl Estradiol 0.035 mg, Norethindrone 0.5 mg, Norethindrone 1 mg	Tri Norinyl 21 Day by Searle	00025-0272	Oral Contraceptive
SEARLE <> 7	Tab, Yellowish Green	Ethinyl Estradiol 0.035 mg, Norethindrone 1 mg	Norinyl 1 35 21 Day by Searle	00025-0257	Oral Contraceptive
SEARLE <> 71	Tab, White, Round	Ethinyl Estradiol 50 mcg, Ethynodiol Diacetate 1 mg	Demulen 1/50 by Pharm Util	60491-0183	Oral Contraceptive
SEARLE <> 71	Tab, White, Round	Ethinyl Estradiol 50 mcg, Ethynodiol Diacetate 1 mg	Demulen 1/50 by Searle	00025-0071	Oral Contraceptive
SEARLE <> 71	Tab, White, Round	Ethinyl Estradiol 50 mcg, Ethynodiol Diacetate 1 mg	Demulen 1/50 by Physician Total Care	54868-3790	Oral Contraceptive
SEARLE <> ALDACTONE	Tab, Film Coated	Spironolactone 25 mg	by Nat Pharmpak	55154-3602	Diuretic
SEARLE <> BX	Tab, White, Round	Norethindrone 1 mg, Ethinyl Estradiol 0.035 mg	Select 1/35 21 day by Pfizer	Canadian DIN 02197502	Oral Contraceptive
SEARLE <> BX	Tab, White, Round	Norethindrone 1 mg, Ethinyl Estradiol 0.035 mg	Select 1/35 28 day by Pfizer	Canadian DIN 02199297	Oral Contraceptive
SEARLE <> BX	Tab, White, Round	Norethindrone 1 mg, Ethinyl Estradiol 0.035 mg	Brevicon 1/35 28 day by Pfizer	Canadian DIN 02189062	Oral Contraceptive
SEARLE <> BX	Tab, White, Round	Norethindrone 1 mg, Ethinyl Estradiol 0.035 mg	Brevicon 1/35 21 day by Pfizer	Canadian DIN 02189054	Oral Contraceptive
SEARLE <> BX	Tab, White, Round	Norethindrone 1 mg, Ethinyl Estradiol 0.035 mg	Synphasic 21 day by Pfizer	Canadian DIN 02187108	Oral Contraceptive
SEARLE <> BX	Tab, Blue, Round	Norethindrone 0.5 mg, Ethinyl Estradiol 0.035 mg	Synphasic 28 day by Pfizer	Canadian DIN 02187116	Oral Contraceptive
SEARLE <> BX	Tab, Blue, Round	Norethindrone 0.5 mg, Ethinyl Estradiol 0.035 mg	Brevicon .5/35 28 day by Pfizer	Canadian DIN 02187094	Oral Contraceptive
SEARLE <> BX	Tab, Blue, Round	Norethindrone 0.5 mg, Ethinyl Estradiol 0.035 mg	Brevicon .5/35 21 day by Pfizer	Canadian DIN 02187086	Oral Contraceptive
SEARLE <> BX	Tab, White, Round	Norethindrone 1 mg, Ethinyl Estradiol 0.035 mg	Synphasic 28 day by Pfizer	Canadian DIN 02187116	Oral Contraceptive

ID FRONT <> BACK	DESCRIPTION FRONT <> BACK	INGREDIENT & STRENGTH	BRAND (or Generic Equiv.) by FIRM	NDC#	CLASS; SCH.
SEARLE <> BX	Tab, Blue, Round	Norethindrone 0.5 mg, Ethinyl Estradiol 0.035 mg	Synphasic 21 day by Pfizer	Canadian DIN 02187108	Oral Contraceptive
SEARLE <> CYTOTEC	Tab, White to Off-White, Round	Misoprostol 100 mcg	by Pharmacia	Canadian DIN 00813966 Discontinued	Gastrointestinal
SEARLE <> P	Tab	Ethinyl Estradiol 50 mcg, Ethynodiol Diacetate 1 mg	by Physician Total Care	54868-3790	Oral Contraceptive
SEARLE <> P	Tab	Ethinyl Estradiol 50 mcg, Ethynodiol Diacetate 1 mg	Demulen 1 50 28 by Pharm Util	60491-0183	Oral Contraceptive
SEARLE <> P	Tab	Ethinyl Estradiol 35 mcg, Ethynodiol Diacetate 1 mg	Demulen 1/35 by Physician Total Care	54868-0404	Oral Contraceptive
SEARLE <> P	Tab, Blue, Round, Placebo	Inert	Demulen 1/35 by Searle	00025-0151	Oral Contraceptive; Placebo
SEARLE <> P	Tab, Blue, Round	Ethinyl Estradiol 35 mcg, Ethynodiol Diacetate 1 mg	Demulen 1/35 by Rx Pak	65084-0219	Oral Contraceptive
SEARLE <> P	Tab	Ethinyl Estradiol 35 mcg, Ethynodiol Diacetate 1 mg	Demulen 1 35 28 by Pharm Util	60491-0181	Oral Contraceptive
SEARLE <> P	Tab, Orange, Round	Inert	Brevicon 1/35 28 day by Pfizer	Canadian DIN 02189062	Oral Contraceptive; Placebo
SEARLE <> P	Tab, Orange, Round	Inert	Synphasic 28 day by Pharmacia	Canadian DIN 02187116	Oral Contraceptive; Placebo
SEARLE <> P	Tab, Orange, Round	Inert	Select 1/35 28 day by Pfizer	Canadian DIN 02199297	Oral Contraceptive; Placebo
SEARLE <> P	Tab, Orange, Round	Inert	Demulen by Pfizer	Canadian DIN 0047152	Oral Contraceptive; Placebo
SEARLE <> P	Tab, Orange, Round	Inert	Brevicon .5/35 28 day by Pfizer	Canadian DIN 02187094	Oral Contraceptive; Placebo
SEARLE <> P	Tab, Orange, Round	Inert	Demulen 1/50-28 by Searle	00025-0071	Oral Contraceptive; Placebo
SEARLE1001 <> ALDACTONE25	Tab, Light Yellow, Round, Film Coated	Spironolactone 25 mg	Aldactone by Pfizer	Canadian DIN 00028606	Diuretic
SEARLE1001 <> ALDACTONE25	Tab, Light Yellow, Round, Film Coated	Spironolactone 25 mg	Aldactone by Rx Pak	65084-0106	Diuretic
SEARLE1001 <> ALDACTONE25	Tab, Light Yellow, Round, Film Coated	Spironolactone 25 mg	Aldactone by Thrift Drug	59198-0001	Diuretic
SEARLE1001 <> ALDACTONE25	Tab, Light Yellow, Round, Film Coated	Spironolactone 25 mg	Aldactone by Caremark	00339-5531	Diuretic
SEARLE1001 <> ALDACTONE25	Tab, Light Yellow, Round, Film Coated	Spironolactone 25 mg	Aldactone by DRX	55045-2716	Diuretic
SEARLE1001 <> ALDACTONE25	Tab, Light Yellow, Round, Film Coated	Spironolactone 25 mg	Aldactone by Searle	00025-1001	Diuretic
SEARLE1001 <> ALDACTONE25	Tab, Light Yellow, Round, Film Coated	Spironolactone 25 mg	Aldactone by Rightpak	65240-0601	Diuretic
SEARLE1001 <> ALDACTONE25	Tab, Light Yellow, Round, Film Coated	Spironolactone 25 mg	Aldactone by Amerisource	62584-0001	Diuretic
SEARLE101	Tab, Brown, Round	Norethynodrel 10 mg, Mestranol 75 mcg	Enovid by Searle		Oral Contraceptive
SEARLE1011 <> ALDACTAZIDE25	Tab, Tan, Round, Film Coated	Hydrochlorothiazide 25 mg, Spironolactone 25 mg	Aldactazide by Rightpak	65240-0600	Diuretic; Antihypertensive
SEARLE1011 <> ALDACTAZIDE25	Tab, Tan, Round, Film Coated	Hydrochlorothiazide 25 mg, Spironolactone 25 mg	Aldactazide by Med Pro	53978-3382	Diuretic; Antihypertensive
SEARLE1011 <> ALDACTAZIDE25	Tab, Tan, Round, Film Coated	Hydrochlorothiazide 25 mg, Spironolactone 25 mg	Aldactazide by Pfizer	Canadian DIN 00180408	Diuretic; Antihypertensive
SEARLE1011 <> ALDACTAZIDE25	Tab, Tan, Round, Film Coated	Hydrochlorothiazide 25 mg, Spironolactone 25 mg	Aldactazide by Searle	00025-1011	Diuretic; Antihypertensive
SEARLE1011 <> ALDACTAZIDE25	Tab, Tan, Round, Film Coated	Hydrochlorothiazide 25 mg, Spironolactone 25 mg	Aldactazide by Nat Pharmpak	55154-3601	Diuretic; Antihypertensive

ID FRONT <> BACK	DESCRIPTION FRONT <> BACK	INGREDIENT & STRENGTH	BRAND (or Generic Equiv.) by FIRM	NDC#	CLASS; SCH.
SEARLE1011 <> ALDACTAZIDE25	Tab, Tan, Round, Film Coated	Hydrochlorothiazide 25 mg, Spironolactone 25 mg	Aldactazide by Murfreesboro	51129-1377	Diuretic; Antihypertensive
SEARLE1011 <> ALDACTAZIDE25	Tab, Tan, Round, Film Coated	Hydrochlorothiazide 25 mg, Spironolactone 25 mg	Aldactazide by Thrift Drug	59198-0170	Diuretic; Antihypertensive
SEARLE1011 <> ALDACTAZIDE25	Tab, Tan, Round, Film Coated	Hydrochlorothiazide 25 mg, Spironolactone 25 mg	Aldactazide by Amerisource	62584-0011	Diuretic; Antihypertensive
SEARLE1021 <> ALDACTAZIDE50	Tab, Tan, Oblong, Film Coated	Hydrochlorothiazide 50 mg, Spironolactone 50 mg	Aldactazide by Searle	00025-1021	Diuretic; Antihypertensive
SEARLE1021 <> ALDACTAZIDE50	Tab, Tan, Oblong, Film Coated	Hydrochlorothiazide 50 mg, Spironolactone 50 mg	Aldactazide by Pfizer	Canadian DIN 00594377	Diuretic; Antihypertensive
SEARLE1031 <> ALDACTONE100	Tab, Peach, Round, Scored, Film Coated	Spironolactone 100 mg	Aldactone by Pfizer	Canadian DIN 00285455	Diuretic
SEARLE1031 <> ALDACTONE100	Tab, Peach, Round, Scored, Film Coated	Spironolactone 100 mg	Aldactone by Sidmak		Diuretic
SEARLE1031 <> ALDACTONE100	Tab, Peach, Round, Scored, Film Coated	Spironolactone 100 mg	Aldactone by Searle	00025-1031	Diuretic
SEARLE1041 <> ALDACTONE50	Tab, Light Orange, Oval, Film Coated	Spironolactone 50 mg	Aldactone by Searle	00025-1041	Diuretic
SEARLE1231	Tab, White, Round	Aminophylline 100 mg	Aminophylline by Searle		Antiasthmatic
SEARLE1251	Tab, White, Oval	Aminophylline 200 mg	Aminophylline by Searle		Antiasthmatic
SEARLE131	Tab, Peach, Round	Norethynodrel 2.5 mg, Mestranol 0.1 mg	Enovid-E by Searle		Oral Contraceptive
SEARLE1391	Tab, Blue, Cap Shaped, Film Coated	Oxaprozin 600 mg	Daypro by Searle	00025-5500	NSAID
SEARLE1401	Tab, White, Oval	Oxandrolone 2.5 mg	Anavar by Searle		Steroid; C III
SEARLE1411 <> AAAA50	Tab, White to Off-White, Round, Film Coated, A's around 50	Diclofenac Sodium 50 mg, Misoprostol 200 mcg	Arthrotec 50 by Searle	00025-1411	NSAID
SEARLE1411 <> AAAA50	Tab, White to Off-White, Round, Film Coated, A's around 50	Diclofenac Sodium 50 mg, Misoprostol 200 mcg	Arthrotec 50 by Searle	00014-1411	NSAID
SEARLE1411 <> AAAA50	Tab, White to Off-White, Round, Film Coated, A's around 50	Diclofenac Sodium 50 mg, Misoprostol 200 mcg	Arthrotec 50 by Searle	51227-6169	NSAID
SEARLE1411 <> AAAA50	Tab, White to Off-White, Round, Film Coated, A's around 50	Diclofenac Sodium 50 mg, Misoprostol 200 mcg	Arthrotec 50 by Pfizer	Canadian DIN 01917056	NSAID
SEARLE1421 <> AAAA75	Tab, White to Off-White, Round, A's around 75	Diclofenac Sodium 75 mg, Misoprostol 200 mcg	Arthrotec 75 by Pfizer	Canadian DIN 02229837	NSAID
SEARLE1421 <> AAAA75	Tab, White to Off-White, Round, A's around 75	Diclofenac Sodium 75 mg, Misoprostol 200 mcg	Arthrotec 75 by Searle	51227-6179	NSAID
SEARLE1421 <> AAAA75	Tab, White to Off-White, Round, A's around 75	Diclofenac Sodium 75 mg, Misoprostol 200 mcg	Arthrotec 75 by Searle	Canadian	NSAID
SEARLE1421 <> AAAA75	Tab, White to Off-White, Round, A's around 75	Diclofenac Sodium 75 mg, Misoprostol 200 mcg	Arthrotec 75 by Searle	00025-1421	NSAID
SEARLE1421 <> AAAA75	Tab, White to Off-White, Round, A's around 75	Diclofenac Sodium 75 mg, Misoprostol 200 mcg	Arthrotec 75 by Searle	00014-1421	NSAID
SEARLE1461	Tab, White, Hexagonal, Scored, Searle over 1461	Misoprostol 200 mcg	Cytotec by Searle	00025-1461	Gastrointestinal
SEARLE1461	Tab, White, Hexagonal, Scored, Searle over 1461	Misoprostol 200 mcg	Cytotec by H J Harkins Co	52959-0354	Gastrointestinal
SEARLE1461	Tab, White, Hexagonal, Scored, Searle over 1461	Misoprostol 200 mcg	Cytotec by Nat Pharmpak	55154-3613	Gastrointestinal
SEARLE1461	Tab, White, Hexagonal, Scored, Searle over 1461	Misoprostol 200 mcg	Cytotec by Pharmacia	Canadian DIN 00632600 Discontinued	Gastrointestinal
SEARLE1461	Tab, White, Hexagonal, Scored, Searle over 1461	Misoprostol 200 mcg	Cytotec by Apotheca	12634-0502	Gastrointestinal
SEARLE1461	Tab, White, Hexagonal, Scored, Searle over 1461	Misoprostol 200 mcg	Cytotec by Neuman	64579-0314	Gastrointestinal
SEARLE1501	Tab, Peach, Round	Methantheline Bromide 50 mg	Banthine by Searle		Gastrointestinal
SEARLE1701	Tab, White, Round	Dimenhydrinate 50 mg	Dramamine by Searle		Antiemetic
SEARLE1831 <> FLAGYL250	Tab, Blue, Round, Film Coated	Metronidazole 250 mg	Flagyl by Thrift Drug	59198-0311	Antibiotic
SEARLE1831 <> FLAGYL250	Tab, Blue, Round, Film Coated	Metronidazole 250 mg	Flagyl by Amerisource	62584-0831	Antibiotic

ID FRONT <> BACK	DESCRIPTION FRONT <> BACK	INGREDIENT & STRENGTH	BRAND (or Generic Equiv.) by FIRM	NDC#	CLASS; SCH.
SEARLE1831 <> FLAGYL250	Tab, Blue, Round, Film Coated	Metronidazole 250 mg	Flagyl by Searle	00025-1831	Antibiotic
SEARLE1831 <> FLAGYL250	Tab, Blue, Round, Film Coated	Metronidazole 250 mg	Flagyl by Neuman	64579-0102	Antibiotic
SEARLE1961 <> FLAGYLER	Tab, Blue, Oval, Film Coated	Metronidazole 750 mg	Flagyl by Mova	55370-0562	Antibiotic
SEARLE1961 <> FLAGYLER	Tab, Blue, Oval, Film Coated, Ex Release	Metronidazole 750 mg	Flagyl by Searle	00025-1961	Antibiotic
SEARLE201	Tab, White, Round	Hydrochlorothiazide 25 mg, Spironolactone 25 mg	Aldactazide by Searle		Diuretic; Antihypertensive
SEARLE2011	Tab, Blue, Round, Film Coated	Verapamil HCl 180 mg	Verelan by Pharmacia	Canadian DIN 02231676	Antihypertensive
SEARLE2021	Tab, White, Round, Film Coated	Verapamil HCl 240 mg	by Pharmacia	Canadian DIN 02231677	Antihypertensive
SEARLE205	Tab, White to Off-White, Round	Spironolactone 25 mg	Aldactone by Searle	Canadian DIN 00028606	Diuretic
SEARLE210	Tab, White to Off-White, Round	Spironolactone 100 mg	Aldactone by Searle	Canadian DIN 00285455	Diuretic
SEARLE221	Tab, White, Round	Norethindrone 1 mg, Ethinyl Estradiol 35 mcg	Norethin 1/35 by Searle		Oral Contraceptive
SEARLE244	Tab, White, Round	Hydrochlorothiazide 50 mg, Spironolactone 50 mg	Aldactazide by Searle		Diuretic; Antihypertensive
SEARLE2752- NORPACE100MG	Cap, Orange & White, Black Print, Searle over 2752 over Norpace over 100 mg	Disopyramide Phosphate 100 mg	Norpace by Rightpak	65240-0707	Antiarrhythmic
SEARLE2752- NORPACE100MG	Cap, Orange & White, Black Print, Searle over 2752 over Norpace over 100 mg	Disopyramide Phosphate 100 mg	Norpace by Thrift Drug	59198-0083	Antiarrhythmic
SEARLE2752- NORPACE100MG	Cap, Orange & White, Black Print, Searle over 2752 over Norpace over 100 mg	Disopyramide Phosphate 100 mg	Norpace by Nat Pharmpak	55154-3607	Antiarrhythmic
SEARLE2752- NORPACE100MG	Cap, Orange & White, Black Print, Searle over 2752 over Norpace over 100 mg	Disopyramide Phosphate 100 mg	Norpace by Searle	00025-2752	Antiarrhythmic
SEARLE2752- NORPACE100MG	Cap, Orange & White, Black Print, Searle over 2752 over Norpace over 100 mg	Disopyramide Phosphate 100 mg	Norpace by Amerisource	62584-0753	Antiarrhythmic
SEARLE2752- NORPACE100MG	Cap, Orange & White, Black Print, Searle over 2752 over Norpace over 100 mg	Disopyramide Phosphate 100 mg	Norpace by Leiner	59606-0707	Antiarrhythmic
SEARLE2762- NORPACE150MG	Cap, Brown & Orange, White Print, Searle over 2762 over Norpace over 150 mg	Disopyramide Phosphate 150 mg	Norpace by Amerisource	62584-0762	Antiarrhythmic
SEARLE2762- NORPACE150MG	Cap, Brown & Orange, White Print, Searle over 2762 over Norpace over 150 mg	Disopyramide Phosphate 150 mg	Norpace by Searle	00025-2762	Antiarrhythmic
SEARLE2762- NORPACE150MG	Cap, Brown & Orange, White Print, Searle over 2762 over Norpace over 150 mg	Disopyramide Phosphate 150 mg	Norpace by Nat Pharmpak	55154-3608	Antiarrhythmic
SEARLE2762- NORPACE150MG	Cap, Brown & Orange, White Print, Searle over 2762 over Norpace over 150 mg	Disopyramide Phosphate 150 mg	Norpace by Thrift Drug	59198-0084	Antiarrhythmic
SEARLE2762- NORPACE150MG	Cap, Brown & Orange, White Print, Searle over 2762 over Norpace over 150 mg	Disopyramide Phosphate 150 mg	Norpace by Leiner	59606-0708	Antiarrhythmic
SEARLE2762- NORPACE150MG	Cap, Brown & Orange, White Print, Searle over 2762 over Norpace over 150 mg	Disopyramide Phosphate 150 mg	Norpace by Rightpak	65240-0710	Antiarrhythmic
SEARLE2762- NORPACE150MG	Cap, Brown & Orange, White Print, Searle over 2762 over Norpace over 150 mg	Disopyramide Phosphate 150 mg	Norpace by Rightpak	65240-0708	Antiarrhythmic
SEARLE401	Tab, White, Pentagonal	Ethynodiol Diacetate 1 mg, Mestranol 0.1 mg	Ovulen by Searle		Oral Contraceptive
SEARLE431	Tab, White, Round	Norethindrone 1 mg, Mestranol 50 mcg	Norethin 1/50 by Searle		Oral Contraceptive
SEARLE501	Tab, Rose, Round	Metolazone 2.5 mg	Diulo by Searle		Diuretic
SEARLE51	Tab, Tan, Round	Norethynodrel 5 mg, Mestranol 75 mcg	Enovid 5mg by Searle		Oral Contraceptive

ID FRONT <> BACK	DESCRIPTION FRONT <> BACK	INGREDIENT & STRENGTH	BRAND (or Generic Equiv.) by FIRM	NDC#	CLASS; SCH.
SEARLE511	Tab, Blue, Round	Metolazone 5 mg	Diulo by Searle		Diuretic
SEARLE521	Tab, Yellow, Round	Metolazone 10 mg	Diulo by Searle		Diuretic
SEARLE531	Tab, Yellow, Round	Chlorthalidone 25 mg	Hygroton by Searle		Diuretic
SEARLE541	Tab, Green, Round	Chlorthalidone 50 mg	Hygroton by Searle		Diuretic
SEARLE571	Tab, White, Round	Furosemide 20 mg	Lasix by Searle		Diuretic
SEARLE581	Tab, White, Round	Furosemide 40 mg	Lasix by Searle		Diuretic
SEARLE601	Tab, Peach, Round	Propantheline Bromide 15 mg	Pro-Banthine by Searle		Gastrointestinal
SEARLE611	Tab, White, Round	Propantheline Bromide 7.5 mg	Pro-Banthine by Searle		Gastrointestinal
SEARLE71	Tab, White, Round, Searle/71	Ethynodiol Diacetate 1 mg	by Searle	Canadian	Oral Contraceptive
SEARLE831	Tab, White, Round	Haloperidol 0.5 mg	Haldol by Searle		Antipsychotic
SEARLE841	Tab, White, Round	Haloperidol 1 mg	Haldol by Searle		Antipsychotic
SEARLE851	Tab, White, Round	Haloperidol 2 mg	Haldol by Searle		Antipsychotic
SEARLE861	Tab, White, Round	Haloperidol 5 mg	Haldol by Searle		Antipsychotic
SEARLE871	Tab, White, Round	Haloperidol 10 mg	Haldol by Searle		Antipsychotic
SEARLE881	Tab, White, Round	Haloperidol 20 mg	Haldol by Searle		Antipsychotic
SEARLE930	Tab, White, Round, Film Coated	Ethynodiol Diacetate 2 mg, Ethinyl Estradiol 0.03 mg	Demulen 30 21 by Pharmacia	Canadian DIN 00469327	Oral Contraceptive
SEARLE930	Tab, White, Round, Film Coated	Ethynodiol Diacetate 2 mg, Ethinyl Estradiol 0.03 mg	Demulen 30 28 by Pharmacia	Canadian DIN 00471526	Oral Contraceptive
SEARLECYOTEC	Tab, White, Round, Searle/Cyotec	Misoprostol 100 mcg	Cyotec by Searle	Canadian	Gastrointestinal
SEATRACE	Cap, Blue Print	Acetaminophen 500 mg, Hydrocodone Bitartrate 5 mg	Vicodin by Seatrace	00551-0180	Analgesic; C III
SEATRACELOBAC0176	Cap, Egg Shell, Seatrace <> Lobac-0176	Acetaminophen 300 mg, Phenyltoloxamine Citrate 20 mg, Salicylamide 200 mg	Durabac by Seatrace	00551-0176	Analgesic
SEATRACETENAKE	Cap, Green Print	Acetaminophen 325 mg, Butalbital 50 mg, Caffeine 40 mg	Fioricet by Seatrace	00551-0181	Analgesic
SECTRAL100	Tab, White, Shield	Acebutolol HCl 100 mg	Sectral by RPR		Antihypertensive
SECTRAL100 <> RPR	Tab, White to Off White, Shield Shaped, Film Coated	Acebutolol HCl 100 mg	Sectral by Sanofi-Aventis	Canadian DIN 01926543	Antihypertensive
SECTRAL200	Tab, Blue, Shield	Acebutolol HCl 200 mg	Sectral by RPR	Canadian	Antihypertensive
SECTRAL200 <> RPR	Tab, Blue, Shield Shaped, Film Coated	Acebutolol HCl 200 mg	Sectral by Sanofi-Aventis	Canadian DIN 01926551	Antihypertensive
SECTRAL400	Tab, White, Shield	Acebutolol HCl 400 mg	Sectral by RPR	Canadian	Antihypertensive
SECTRAL400	Tab, White, Shield, Rorer Logo	Acebutolol HCl 400 mg	Sectral by RPR	Canadian	Antihypertensive
SECTRAL400 <> RPR	Tab, White to Off White, Shield Shaped, Film Coated	Acebutolol HCl 400 mg	Sectral by Sanofi-Aventis	Canadian DIN 01926578	Antihypertensive
SELDANE	Tab, White, Round	Terfenadine 60 mg	by Pharmedix	53002-0409	Antihistamine
SELDANE	Tab, White, Round	Terfenadine 60 mg	by Merrell	00068-0723	Antihistamine
SELDANED	Tab, Seldane over D, Ex Release	Pseudoephedrine HCl 120 mg, Terfenadine 60 mg	by Quality Care	60346-0664	Cold Remedy
SEMPREXDMEDEVA	Cap, SEMPREX-D in White Ink	Acrivastine 8 mg, Pseudoephedrine HCl 60 mg	Semprex D by DSM	63552-0404	Cold Remedy
SEPTRADS	Tab, Pink, Oval	Sulfamethoxazole 800 mg, Trimethoprim 160 mg	Septra DS by King		Antibiotic
SEPTRADS02C	Tab, Pink, Oval, Scored	Sulfamethoxazole 800 mg, Trimethoprim 160 mg	by Thrift Drug	59198-0322	Antibiotic
SEPTRADS02C	Tab, Septra DS 02C	Sulfamethoxazole 800 mg, Trimethoprim 160 mg	by Thrift Drug	59198-0212	Antibiotic
SEPTRADS02C	Tab, Septra DS 02C	Sulfamethoxazole 800 mg, Trimethoprim 160 mg	Septra DS by Pharm Util	60491-0581	Antibiotic
SEPTRADS02C	Tab, Septra DS over 02C	Sulfamethoxazole 800 mg, Trimethoprim 160 mg	by Amerisource	62584-0853	Antibiotic
SEPTRADS02C	Tab	Sulfamethoxazole 800 mg, Trimethoprim 160 mg	Septra DS by DSM	63552-0853	Antibiotic
SEPTRADS02C	Tab, Oval	Sulfamethoxazole 800 mg, Trimethoprim 160 mg	by GSK	Canadian	Antibiotic
SEPTRAY2B	Tab, Septra Y2B	Sulfamethoxazole 400 mg, Trimethoprim 80 mg	Septra by DSM	63552-0852	Antibiotic
SEPTRAY2B	Tab, Round	Trimethoprim 80 mg, Sulfamethoxazole 400 mg	by GSK	Canadian	Antibiotic

ID FRONT <> BACK	DESCRIPTION FRONT <> BACK	INGREDIENT & STRENGTH	BRAND (or Generic Equiv.) by FIRM	NDC#	CLASS; SCH.
SEPTRAY2B	Tab, Pink, Round	Sulfamethoxazole 400 mg, Trimethoprim 80 mg	Septra by King		Antibiotic
SER100 <> APO	Tab, Yellow, Oval, Scored, Film Coated, SER / 100	Sertraline HCl 100 mg	Zoloft by Apotex	60505-0182	Antidepressant
SERAX	Tab, Light Yellow	Oxazepam 10 mg	Serax by Wyeth	Canadian	Sedative/Hypnotic; C IV
SERAX30	Tab, Peach, Serax/30	Oxazepam 30 mg	by Wyeth	Canadian	Sedative/Hypnotic; C IV
SERAX51SERAX10	Cap, Pink & White	Oxazepam 10 mg	Serax by Wyeth	52903-0051	Sedative/Hypnotic; C IV
SEROQUEL <> 300	Tab, White, Cap Shaped, Film Coated	Quetiapine Fumarate 300 mg	Seroquel by AstraZeneca	Canadian DIN 02244107	Antipsychotic
SEROQUEL <> 300	Tab, White, Cap Shaped, Film Coated	Quetiapine Fumarate 300 mg	Seroquel by AstraZeneca	00310-0274	Antipsychotic
SEROQUEL <> 400	Tab, Yellow, Cap Shaped, Film Coated	Quetiapine Fumarate 400 mg	Seroquel by AstraZeneca	00310-0279	Antipsychotic
SEROQUEL100	Tab, Yellow, Round, Film Coated	Quetiapine Fumarate 100 mg	Seroquel by Direct Dispensing	57866-1032	Antipsychotic
SEROQUEL100	Tab, Yellow, Round, Film Coated	Quetiapine Fumarate 100 mg	Seroquel by AstraZeneca	00310-0271	Antipsychotic
SEROQUEL100	Tab, Yellow, Round, Film Coated	Quetiapine Fumarate 100 mg	Seroquel by AstraZeneca	Canadian DIN 02236952	Antipsychotic
SEROQUEL200	Tab, White, Round, Film Coated	Quetiapine Fumarate 200 mg	Seroquel by AstraZeneca	00310-0272	Antipsychotic
SEROQUEL200	Tab, White, Round, Film Coated	Quetiapine Fumarate 200 mg	Seroquel by AstraZeneca	Canadian DIN 02236953	Antipsychotic
SEROQUEL25	Tab, Peach, Round, Film Coated	Quetiapine Fumarate 25 mg	Seroquel by Murfreesboro	51129-1559	Antipsychotic
SEROQUEL25	Tab, Peach, Round, Film Coated	Quetiapine Fumarate 25 mg	Seroquel by AstraZeneca	00310-0275	Antipsychotic
SEROQUEL25	Tab, Peach, Round, Film Coated	Quetiapine Fumarate 25 mg	Seroquel by RX Pak	65084-0115	Antipsychotic
SEROQUEL25	Tab, Peach, Round, Film Coated	Quetiapine Fumarate 25 mg	Seroquel by RX Pak	65084-0113	Antipsychotic
SEROQUEL25	Tab, Peach, Round, Film Coated	Quetiapine Fumarate 25 mg	Seroquel by AstraZeneca	Canadian DIN 02236951	Antipsychotic
SEROQUEL50	Tab, White, Round, Film Coated	Quetiapine Fumarate 50 mg	Seroquel by AstraZeneca	00310-0278	Antipsychotic
SFC3512	Cap, Maroon, SFC-3512	Docusate Calcium 60 mg, Phenolphthalein 65 mg	Doxidan by Chase	Canadian	Laxative
SFCSANDOZ78107	Cap, S in Triangle F-C <> Sandoz 78-107	Aspirin 325 mg, Butalbital 50 mg, Caffeine 40 mg, Codeine Phosphate 30 mg	Fiorinal w/ Codeine by Physician Total Care	54868-0530	Analgesic; C III
SFCSANDOZ78107	Cap, Blue & Yellow, S in Triangle, F-C Sandoz 78-107	Aspirin 325 mg, Butalbital 50 mg, Caffeine 40 mg, Codeine 30 mg	Fiorinal #3 by Novartis	00078-0107	Analgesic; C III
SGP0535	Tab, White, Round, SGP 0.5/35	Genora 0.5 mg	Modicon by Searle		Oral Contraceptive
SGP135	Tab, Blue, Round, SGP 1/35	Genora	Ortho Novum by Searle		Oral Contraceptive
SGP150	Tap, White, Round, SGP 1/50	Genora	Ortho Novum by Searle		Oral Contraceptive
SHIRE38110MG	Cap, Blue, Ex Release	Mixed Amphetamine Salts 10 mg: Amphetamine Aspartate 2.5 mg, Amphetamine Sulfate 2.5 mg, Dextroamphetamine Saccharate 2.5 mg, Dextroamphetamine Sulfate 2.5 mg	Adderall XR by Shire	54092-0383	Stimulant; C II
SHIRE38120MG	Cap, Orange, Ex Release	Mixed Amphetamine Salts 20 mg: Amphetamine Aspartate 5 mg, Amphetamine Sulfate 5 mg, Dextroamphetamine Saccharate 5 mg, Dextroamphetamine Sulfate 5 mg	Adderall XR by Shire	54092-0387	Stimulant; C II
SHIRE38130MG	Cap, Natural & Orange, Ex Release	Mixed Amphetamine Salts 30 mg: Amphetamine Aspartate 7.5 mg, Amphetamine Sulfate 7.5 mg, Dextroamphetamine Saccharate 7.5 mg, Dextroamphetamine Sulfate 7.5 mg	Adderall XR by Shire	54092-0391	Stimulant; C II
SHIRECARBATROL-200MG	Cap, Grey and Green, White Print, SHIRE on cap, CARBATROL200MG on body	Carbamazepine 200 mg	Carbatrol ER by Shire	58521-0172	Anticonvulsant
SHIRECARBATROL-300MG	Cap, Black and Green, White Print, SHIRE on cap, CARBATROL300MG on body	Carbamazepine 300 mg	Carbatrol SR by Shire	58521-0173	Anticonvulsant
SHNKETOPROFENER-200	Cap, Ex Release, Ketoprofen ER 200 MG	Ketoprofen 200 mg	Orudis by Schein	00364-2667	NSAID
SHNKETOPROFENER-200	Cap, ER, Ketoprofen ER 200 MG	Ketoprofen 200 mg	Orudis by Watson	00591-8847	NSAID
SHNKETOPROFENER-200	Cap, Ex Release, Ketoprofen ER 200 MG	Ketoprofen 200 mg	Orudis by Elan	56125-0102	NSAID
SIDMAK <> 375	Tab, Off-White, Oval	Nystatin 100,000 Units	Mycostatin by Qualitest	00603-4831	Antifungal
SIDMAK <> 375	Tab, Off-White, Oval	Nystatin 100,000 Units	Mycostatin by Pliva	50111-0375	Antifungal

ID FRONT <> BACK	DESCRIPTION FRONT <> BACK	INGREDIENT & STRENGTH	BRAND (or Generic Equiv.) by FIRM	NDC#	CLASS; SCH.
SILVER	Tab, Grey, Oval, Scored	Vitamin A 3500 IU, Vitamin C 60 mg, Vitamin D 400 IU, Vitamin E 45 IU, Vitamin K 10 mcg, Thiamin 1.5 mg, Riboflavin 1.7 mg, Niacin 20 mg, Vitamin B6 3 mg, Folic Acid 400 mcg, Vitamin B12 25 mcg, Biotin 30 mcg, Pantothenic Acid 10 mg, Calcium 200 mg, Phosphorus 48 mg, Iodine 150 mcg, Magnesium 100 mg, Zinc 15 mcg, Selenium 20 mcg, Copper 2 mg, Manganese 2 mg, Chromium 150 mcg, Molybdenum 75 mcg, Nickel 5 mcg, Silicon 2 mg, Potassium 80 mg, Boron 150 mcg, Chloride 72 mg, Vanadium 10 mcg, Lutein 250 mcg, Lycopene 300 mcg	Centrum Silver by Wyeth		Vitamin
SINA6301		Phenylephrine 25 mg, Guaifenesin 200 mg	Sina-12X by MedPointe	00037-6301	Cold Remedy
SINEMET <> 647	Tab, Purple, Cap Shaped, Scored	Carbidopa 10 mg, Levodopa 100 mg	Sinemet by BMS	Canadian DIN 00355658	Antiparkinson
SINEMET <> 647	Tab, Dark Blue, Oval, Scored	Carbidopa 10 mg, Levodopa 100 mg	Sinemet by BMS	00056-0647	Antiparkinson
SINEMET <> 650	Tab, Yellow, Oval, Scored	Carbidopa 25 mg, Levodopa 100 mg	Sinemet by BMS	00056-0650	Antiparkinson
SINEMET <> 650	Tab, Yellow, Oval, Scored	Carbidopa 25 mg, Levodopa 100 mg	Sinemet by BMS	Canadian DIN 00513997	Antiparkinson
SINEMET <> 654	Tab, Light Blue, Oval, Scored	Carbidopa 25 mg, Levodopa 250 mg	Sinemet by BMS	Canadian DIN 00328219	Antiparkinson
SINEMET <> 654	Tab, Light Blue, Oval, Scored	Carbidopa 25 mg, Levodopa 250 mg	Sinemet by BMS	00056-0654	Antiparkinson
SINEMET10010	Tab, Blue, Oval, Sinemet/100/10	Levodopa 100 mg, Carbidopa 10 mg	Sinemet by Dupont	Canadian	Antiparkinson
SINEMETCR <> 521	Tab, Peach, Oval, Scored, Sustained Release, SINEMET over CR	Carbidopa 50 mg, Levodopa 200 mg	Sinemet CR by BMS	00056-0521	Antiparkinson
SINEMETCR <> 521	Tab, Peach, Oval, Scored, Sustained Release, SINEMET over CR	Carbidopa 50 mg, Levodopa 200 mg	Sinemet CR by BMS	Canadian DIN 00870935	Antiparkinson
SINEMETCR <> 601	Tab, Pink, Oval, Sustained Release, SINEMET over CR	Carbidopa 25 mg, Levodopa 100 mg	Sinemet CR by BMS	Canadian DIN 02028786	Antiparkinson
SINEMETCR <> 601	Tab, Pink, Oval, Sustained Release, SINEMET over CR	Carbidopa 25 mg, Levodopa 100 mg	Sinemet CR by BMS	00056-0601	Antiparkinson
SINEQUANROERIG534	Cap, Pink & Red	Doxepin HCl 10 mg	Sinequan by Roerig	00049-5340	Antidepressant
SINEQUANROERIG535	Cap, Blue & Pink	Doxepin HCl 25 mg	Sinequan by Nat Pharmpak	55154-3209	Antidepressant
SINEQUANROERIG535	Cap, Blue & Pink	Doxepin HCl 25 mg	Sinequan by Rightpac	65240-0734	Antidepressant
SINEQUANROERIG535	Cap, Blue & Pink	Doxepin HCl 25 mg	Sinequan by Roerig	00049-5350	Antidepressant
SINEQUANROERIG536	Cap, Pink & White	Doxepin HCl 50 mg	Sinequan by Rightpac	65240-0735	Antidepressant
SINEQUANROERIG536	Cap, Pink & White	Doxepin HCl 50 mg	Sinequan by Roerig	00049-5360	Antidepressant
SINEQUANROERIG536	Cap, Pink & White	Doxepin HCl 50 mg	Sinequan by Nat Pharmpak	55154-3210	Antidepressant
SINEQUANROERIG537	Cap, Blue	Doxepin HCl 75 mg	Sinequan by Roerig	00049-5370	Antidepressant
SINEQUANROERIG538	Cap, Blue & White	Doxepin HCl 100 mg	Sinequan by Roerig	00049-5380	Antidepressant
SINEQUANROERIG539	Cap, White	Doxepin HCl 75 mg	Sinequan by Roerig	00049-5390	Antidepressant
SINGULAIR <> MRK117	Tab, Beige, Square, Film Coated	Montelukast Sodium 10 mg	Singulair by Murfreesboro	51129-1398	Antiasthmatic
SINGULAIR <> MRK117	Tab, Beige, Square, Film Coated	Montelukast Sodium 10 mg	Singulair by Merck	00006-0117	Antiasthmatic
SINGULAIR <> MRK275	Tab, Pink, Round, Chewable	Montelukast Sodium 5 mg	Singulair by Neuman	64579-0348	Antiasthmatic
SINGULAIR <> MRK275	Tab, Pink, Round, Chewable	Montelukast Sodium 5 mg	Singulair by Merck	00006-0275	Antiasthmatic
SINGULAIR <> MRK711	Tab, Pink, Oval, Chewable	Montelukast Sodium 4 mg	Singulair by Merck	00006-0711	Antiasthmatic
SINGULAIR <> MSD117	Tab, Beige, Rounded Square, Film Coated	Montelukast Sodium 10 mg	Singulair by Merck-Frosst	Canadian DIN 02238217	Antiasthmatic
SINGULAIR <> MSD275	Tab, Pink, Round, Chewable	Montelukast Sodium 5 mg	Singulair by Merck-Frosst	Canadian DIN 02238216	Antiasthmatic
SINGULAIR <> MSD711	Tab, Pink, Oval, Chewable	Montelukast Sodium 4 mg	Singulair by Merck-Frosst	Canadian DIN 02243602	Antiasthmatic
SINUPAN	Cap, Ex Release	Guaifenesin 200 mg, Phenylephrine HCl 40 mg	by Sovereign	58716-0013	Cold Remedy
SINUTAB	Cap, Orange	Acetaminophen 325 mg	Sinutab by Warner Wellcome	Canadian	Analgesic
SINUTAB	Cap, Yellow	Acetaminophen 500 mg	Sinutab by Warner Wellcome	Canadian	Analgesic
SINUTAB	Cap, Orange	Acetaminophen 500 mg	Sinutab by Warner Wellcome	Canadian	Analgesic

ID FRONT <> BACK	DESCRIPTION FRONT <> BACK	INGREDIENT & STRENGTH	BRAND (or Generic Equiv.) by FIRM	NDC#	CLASS: SCH.
SJ <> GEIGY	Tab, Peach, Round	Desipramine HCl 50 mg	Norpramin by Geigy		Antidepressant
SJ630	Cap, Blue Print, S-J 630	Acetaminophen 500 mg, Hydrocodone Bitartrate 5 mg	Vicodin by Stewart Jackson	45985-0630 Discontinued	Analgesic; C III
SJ631	Tab, Pink Specks	Guaifenesin 600 mg	Robitussin by Anabolic	00722-6348	Expectorant
SJ631	Tab	Guaifenesin 800 mg	Bidex by Stewart Jackson	45985-0637	Expectorant
SJ631	Tab	Guaifenesin 800 mg	by Mikart	46672-0167	Expectorant
SJ638	Tab, White, Oblong, Scored	Guaifenesin 800 mg, Dextromethorphan Hydrobromide 300 mg	Bidex DM by Stewart-Jackson	45985-0638	Cold Remedy
SJ638	Tab, White, Oblong, Scored	Guaifenesin 800 mg, Dextromethorphan Hydrobromide 300 mg	Bidex DM by Pfab	62542-0916	Cold Remedy
SJ641	Tab, White, Oval, Scored	Guaifenesin 800 mg, Pseudoephedrine HCl 60 mg, Dextromethorphan Hydrobromide 30 mg	Medent DM by Pfab	62542-0775	Cold Remedy
SJ641	Tab, White, Oblong	Guaifenesin 800 mg, Pseudoephedrine HCl 60 mg, Dextromethorphan Hydrobromide 30 mg	Medent DM by Stewart-Jackson	45985-0641	Cold Remedy
SJ642	Tab, White, Oval, Scored	Guaifenesin 800 mg, Pseudoephedrine HCl 60 mg	Medent LD by Pfab	62542-0754	Cold Remedy
SJ642	Tab, White, Oblong	Guaifenesin 800 mg, Pseudoephedrine HCl 60 mg	Medent LD by Stewart-Jackson	45985-0642	Cold Remedy
SJ645	Tab, White, Oblong, Scored	Guaifenesin 1000 mg	Bidex by Stewart-Jackson	45985-0645	Cold Remedy
SJ646	Cap, Blue	Hyoscyamine 0.12 mg, Methenamine 120 mg, Methylene Blue 10 mg, Phenyl Salicylate 36 mg, Sodium Phosphate Monobasic 40.8 mg	UTA by Stewart-Jackson	45985-0646	Urinary Tract
SJ647	Tab, White, Oblong	Dyphylline 200 mg, Guaifenesin 300 mg	Difil-G by Stewart Jackson	45985-0647	Antiasthmatic; Expectorant
SJGEIGY	Tab, Peach, Round, SJ/Geigy	Desipramine HCl 50 mg	Pertofrane by Geigy	Canadian	Antidepressant
SK <> AA	Tab, Light Pink, Oval, Scored, Film Coated, double Abbott Logo (aa)	Verapamil HCl 180 mg	Isoptin SR by Abbott	00074-1486	Antihypertensive
SKF	Tab, Peach, Round	Triamterene 50 mg, Hydrochlorothiazide 25 mg	by SKB	Canadian	Diuretic; Antihypertensive
SKF	Tab, Coated	Prochlorperazine 8.1 mg	Compazine by Patient First	57575-0099	Antiemetic
SKF <> C66	Tab, Yellow-Green, Coated	Prochlorperazine Maleate 8.1 mg	by Allscripts		Antiemetic
SKF <> C67	Tab, Yellow-Green, Coated	Prochlorperazine Maleate 16.2 mg	by Quality Care	60346-0860	Antiemetic
SKF <> E19	Tab, Orange, Triangular	Dextroamphetamine Sulfate 5 mg	Dexedrine by Abbott	00074-3241	Stimulant; C II
SKF1	Tab, Yellow, Round	Isopropamide Iodide 5 mg, Trifluoperazine HCl 1 mg	Stelabid by SKB		Antipsychotic
SKF1	Tab, Blue, Round	Trifluoperazine HCl 1 mg	Stelazine by SKB	00108-4903	Antipsychotic
SKF1	Tab, Blue, Round, SKF/1	Trifluoperazine 1 mg	Stelazine by SKB	Canadian	Antipsychotic
SKF10	Tab, Blue, Round, SKF/10	Trifluoperazine 10 mg	Stelazine by SKB	Canadian	Antipsychotic
SKF2	Tab, Blue, Round, SKF/2	Trifluoperazine 2 mg	Stelazine by SKB	Canadian	Antipsychotic
SKF2	Tab, Blue, Round	Trifluoperazine HCl 2 mg	Stelazine by SKB	00108-4904	Antipsychotic
SKF200	Tab, Green, Round	Cimetidine HCl 200 mg	Tagamet by SKB		Gastrointestinal
SKF25	Tab, Yellow, Round	Diphenidol HCl 25 mg	Vontrol by SKB		Antiemetic
SKF300	Tab, Green, Round, SK & F/300	Cimetidine HCl 300 mg	Tagamet by Frosst	Canadian	Gastrointestinal
SKF300TAGAMENT	Tab, Green, Round, SK & F/300/Tagament	Cimetidine HCl 300 mg	Tagamet by SKB	Canadian	Gastrointestinal
SKF400	Tab, Green, Ovoid, SK & F/400	Cimetidine HCl 400 mg	Tagamet by Frosst	Canadian	Gastrointestinal
SKF400TAGAMENT	Tab, Green, Ovoid, SK & F/400/Tagament	Cimetidine HCl 400 mg	Tagamet by SKB	Canadian	Gastrointestinal
SKF5	Tab, Blue, Round, SKF/5	Trifluoperazine 5 mg	Stelazine by SKB	Canadian	Antipsychotic
SKF5	Tab, Blue, Round	Trifluoperazine HCl 5 mg	Stelazine by SKB		Antipsychotic
SKF600	Tab, Green, Ovoid SK & F/600	Cimetidine HCl 600 mg	Tagamet by Frosst	Canadian	Gastrointestinal
SKF600TAGAMENT	Tab, Green, Ovoid, SK & F/600/Tagament	Cimetidine HCl 600 mg	Tagamet by SKB	Canadian	Gastrointestinal
SKFC44	Cap, Clear Black with Beads, Ex Release, SKF over C44	Prochlorperazine Maleate 16.2 mg	by Quality Care	60346-0434	Antiemetic
SKFC46	Cap, Black/Natural	Prochlorperazine 15 mg	Compazine Spansule by SKB		Antiemetic
SKFC47	Cap, Black/Natural	Prochlorperazine 30 mg	Compazine Spansule by SKB		Antiemetic
SKFC66	Tab, Yellow w/ Black Print, Round, Film Coated, SKF over C66	Prochlorperazine 5 mg	Compazine by SKB	00007-3366	Antiemetic

ID FRONT <> BACK	DESCRIPTION FRONT <> BACK	INGREDIENT & STRENGTH	BRAND (or Generic Equiv.) by FIRM	NDC#	CLASS; SCH.
SKFC66	Tab, Yellow w/ Black Print, Round, Film Coated, SKF over C66	Prochlorperazine Maleate 5 mg	by PDRX	55289-0113	Antiemetic
SKFC67	Tab, Yellow w/ Black Print, Round, Film Coated, SKF over C67	Prochlorperazine 10 mg	Compazine by SKB	00007-3367	Antiemetic
SKFC67	Tab, Yellow w/ Black Print, Round, Film Coated, SKF over C67	Prochlorperazine Maleate 10 mg	by Nat Pharmpak	55154-4502	Antiemetic
SKFC67	Tab, Yellow w/ Black Print, Round, Film Coated, SKF over C67	Prochlorperazine 10 mg	Compazine by Ranbaxy Labs	54907-5120	Antiemetic
SKFC69	Tab, Yellow, Round	Prochlorperazine 25 mg	Compazine by SKB		Antiemetic
SKFD11	Tab, Yellow, Round	Triamterene 50 mg	Dyrenium by SKB	Canadian	Diuretic
SKFD14	Tab, White, Round	Liothyronine Sodium 5 mcg	Cytomel by SKB	Canadian	Thyroid Hormone
SKFD16	Tab, White, Round, Scored, SKF over D16	Liothyronine Sodium 25 mcg	Cytomel by SKB	Canadian	Thyroid Hormone
SKFD16	Tab, White, Round, Scored, SKF over D16	Liothyronine Sodium 25 mcg	Cytomel by SKB	00007-3416	Thyroid Hormone
SKFD62	Tab, Pink, Round	Isopropamide Iodide 5 mg	Darbid by SKB		Antipsychotic
SKFE12	Cap, Brown & Natural	Dextroamphetamine Sulfate 5 mg	Dexedrine by SKB		Stimulant; C II
SKFE12	Cap	Dextroamphetamine Sulfate 5 mg	Dexedrine by Physician Total Care	54868-3402	Stimulant; C II
SKFE13	Cap, Brown & Natural	Dextroamphetamine Sulfate 10 mg	Dexedrine by SKB		Stimulant; C II
SKFE13	Cap, Brown	Dextroamphetamine Sulfate 10 mg	Dexedrine by SKB	Canadian	Stimulant; C II
SKFE14	Cap, Brown	Dextroamphetamine Sulfate 15 mg	Dexedrine by SKB	Canadian	Stimulant; C II
SKFE14	Cap, Brown & Natural	Dextroamphetamine Sulfate 15 mg	Dexedrine by SKB		Stimulant; C II
SKFE19	Tab, Orange, Shield-Shaped	Dextroamphetamine Sulfate 5 mg	Dexedrine by SKB	00007-3519	Stimulant; C II
SKFE19	Tab, Orange, Shield-Shaped	Dextroamphetamine Sulfate 5 mg	Dexedrine by GSK	Canadian DIN 01924516	Stimulant; C II
SKFE33	Cap, Red w/ White Print, SKF over E33	Phenoxybenzamine HCl 10 mg	Dibenzyline by SKB		Antihypertensive
SKFE93	Tab, Peach, Round, SKF/E93	Hydrochlorothiazide 25 mg, Triamterene 50 mg	Maxzide 25 by SKB		Diuretic; Antihypertensive
SKFH10	Tab, Yellow, Round	Triamterene 100 mg	Dyrenium by SKB	Canadian	Diuretic
SKFH10	Cap, Red, SKF/H10	Triamterene 100 mg	Dyrenium by SKB		Diuretic
SKFH10	Tab, Yellow, Round, SKF/H10	Triamterene 100 mg	Dyrenium by SKB		Diuretic
SKFH11	Cap, Red, SKF/H11	Triamterene 50 mg	Dyrenium by SKB		Diuretic
SKFH11	Tab, Yellow, Round, SKF/H11	Triamterene 50 mg	Dyrenium by SKB		Diuretic
SKFH11	Tab, Yellow, Round	Triamterene 50 mg	Dyrenium by SKB	Canadian	Diuretic
SKFJ09	Tab, Gray, Round	Lithium Carbonate 300 mg	Eskalith by SKB		Antipsychotic
SKFJ10	Tab, Yellow, Round, Scored, SKF over J10	Lithium Carbonate 450 mg	Eskalith by SKB	00007-4010	Antipsychotic
SKFN30	Cap, Blue & Clear, SKF/N30	Chlorpheniramine Maleate 8 mg, Phenylpropanolamine 75 mg	Ornade by SKB		Cold Remedy
SKFN31	Cap, Orange & Clear, SKF/N31	Chlorpheniramine Maleate 12 mg, Phenylpropanolamine 75 mg	Ornade by SKB		Cold Remedy
SKFP90	Tab, Yellow, Round	Isopropamide Iodide 5 mg, Trifluoperazine 1 mg	Stelabid No 1 by SKB		Antipsychotic
SKFP90	Tab, Yellow, Round	Isopropamide Iodide 5 mg	Stelabid No 1 by SKB		Antipsychotic
SKFP90	Tab, Maize, Round	Isopropamide Iodide 5 mg, Trifluoperazine 1 mg	Stelabid by SKB	Canadian	Antipsychotic
SKFP91	Tab, Maize, Round	Isopropamide Iodide 5 mg, Trifluoperazine 2 mg	Stelabid by SKB	Canadian	Antipsychotic
SKFP91	Tab, Yellow, Round	Isopropamide Iodide 5 mg, Trifluoperazine HCl 2 mg	Stelabid No 2 by SKB		Antipsychotic
SKFP92	Tab, Yellow, Round	Isopropamide Iodide 7.5 mg, Trifluoperazine HCl 2 mg	Stelabid Forte by SKB		Antipsychotic
SKFP92	Tab, Maize, Round	Isopropamide Iodide 7.5 mg, Trifluoperazine 2 mg	Stelabid by SKB	Canadian	Antipsychotic
SKFP93	Tab, Yellow, Round	Isopropamide Iodide 10 mg, Trifluoperazine HCl 2 mg	Stelabid Ultra by SKB		Antipsychotic
SKFS03	Tab, Blue, Round	Trifluoperazine HCl 1 mg	Stelazine by SKB	00108-4903	Antipsychotic
SKFS04	Tab, Blue, Round	Trifluoperazine HCl 2 mg	Stelazine by SKB	00108-4904	Antipsychotic

ID FRONT <> BACK	DESCRIPTION FRONT <> BACK	INGREDIENT & STRENGTH	BRAND (or Generic Equiv.) by FIRM	NDC#	CLASS; SCH.
SKFS06	Tab, Blue, Round	Trifluoperazine HCl 5 mg	Stelazine by SKB	00108-4906	Antipsychotic
SKFS07	Tab, Blue, Round	Trifluoperazine HCl 10 mg	Stelazine by SKB	00108-4907	Antipsychotic
SKFT12	Tab, Green, Round	Cimetidine HCl 200 mg	Tagamet by SKB		Gastrointestinal
SKFT13	Tab, Green, Round	Cimetidine HCl 300 mg	Tagamet by SKB		Gastrointestinal
SKFT25	Tab, Orange, Round	Diphenidol HCl 25 mg	Vontrol by SKB		Antiemetic
SKFT63	Cap, Orange & Clear	Chlorpromazine HCl 30 mg	Thorazine Spansule by SKB	00007-5063	Antipsychotic
SKFT64	Cap, Orange & Clear	Chlorpromazine HCl 75 mg	Thorazine Spansule by SKB	00007-5064	Antipsychotic
SKFT66	Cap, Orange & Clear, Black Print, SKF over T66	Chlorpromazine HCl 150 mg	Thorazine Spansule by SKB	00007-5066	Antipsychotic
SKFT67	Cap, Orange & Clear	Chlorpromazine HCl 200 mg	Thorazine Spansule by SKB		Antipsychotic
SKFT69	Tab, Orange, Round	Chlorpromazine HCl 300 mg	Thorazine Spansule by SKB		Antipsychotic
SKFT73	Tab, Orange, Black Print, Round, SKF over T73	Chlorpromazine HCl 10 mg	Thorazine by SKB	00007-5073	Antipsychotic
SKFT74	Tab, Orange, Black Print, Round, SKF over T74	Chlorpromazine HCl 25 mg	Thorazine by SKB	00007-5074	Antipsychotic
SKFT76	Tab, Orange, Black Print, Round, SKF over T76	Chlorpromazine HCl 50 mg	Thorazine by SKB	00007-5076	Antipsychotic
SKFT77	Tab, Orange, Black Print, Round, SKF over T77	Chlorpromazine HCl 100 mg	Thorazine by SKB	00007-5077	Antipsychotic
SKFT79	Tab, Orange, Round	Chlorpromazine HCl 200 mg	Thorazine by SKB	00007-5079	Antipsychotic
SKFV36	Cap, White	Phenylpropanolamine 50 mg, Caramiphen 20 mg, Chlorpheniramine 8 mg	Tuss-Ornade by SKB	Canadian	Cold Remedy
SKFX42	Tab, Yellow, Round	Diphenidol HCl 25 mg	Vontrol by SKB		Antiemetic
SKY	Tab, Blue, Mottled, Round	3,4-Methylenedioxymethamphetamine (MDMA)	Ecstasy by Illegal		Euphoric; Illicit
SKY	Tab, Red, Mottled, Round	3,4-Methylenedioxymethamphetamine (MDMA)	Ecstasy by Illegal		Euphoric; Illicit
SL	Cap, Light Blue, Film Coated	Diphenhydramine HCl 25 mg	Simply Sleep by McNeil	Canadian DIN 02239548	Antihistamine
SL	Tab, Film Coated	Guaifenesin 400 mg, Phenylpropanolamine HCl 75 mg	Entex LA by Patient First	57575-0090	Cold Remedy
SL <> 07	Tab, White, Round, Sugar Coated	Hydroxyzine HCl 10 mg	Atarax by Kaiser	00179-0294	Antianxiety; Antihistamine
SL <> 07	Tab, White, Round, Sugar Coated	Hydroxyzine HCl 10 mg	Atarax by Murfreesboro	51129-1475	Antianxiety; Antihistamine
SL <> 07	Tab, White, Round, Sugar Coated	Hydroxyzine HCl 10 mg	Atarax by Sidmak	Discontinued	Antianxiety; Antihistamine
SL <> 07	Tab, White, Round, Sugar Coated	Hydroxyzine HCl 10 mg	Atarax by Murfreesboro	51129-1478	Antianxiety; Antihistamine
SL <> 07	Tab, White, Round, Sugar Coated	Hydroxyzine HCl 10 mg	Atarax by Qualitest	00603-3970	Antianxiety; Antihistamine
SL <> 07	Tab, White, Round, Sugar Coated	Hydroxyzine HCl 10 mg	Atarax by Talbert	44514-0418	Antianxiety; Antihistamine
SL <> 07	Tab, White, Round, Film Coated	Hydroxyzine HCl 10 mg	Atarax by Mutual	53489-0126	Antianxiety; Antihistamine
SL <> 08	Tab, White, Black Print, Round, Sugar Coated	Hydroxyzine HCl 25 mg	Atarax by Ivax	00182-1493	Antianxiety; Antihistamine
SL <> 08	Tab, White, Black Print, Round, Sugar Coated	Hydroxyzine HCl 25 mg	Atarax by Caremark	00339-6009	Antianxiety; Antihistamine
SL <> 08	Tab, White, Black Print, Round, Sugar Coated	Hydroxyzine HCl 25 mg	Atarax by Pharmedix	53002-0320	Antianxiety; Antihistamine
SL <> 08	Tab, White, Black Print, Round, Sugar Coated	Hydroxyzine HCl 25 mg	Atarax by H J Harkins Co	52959-0074	Antianxiety; Antihistamine
SL <> 08	Tab, White, Black Print, Round, Sugar Coated	Hydroxyzine HCl 25 mg	Atarax by Physician Total Care	54868-0063	Antianxiety; Antihistamine
SL <> 08	Tab, White, Black Print, Round, Sugar Coated	Hydroxyzine HCl 25 mg	Atarax by Richmond	54738-0308	Antianxiety; Antihistamine
SL <> 08	Tab, White, Black Print, Round, Sugar Coated	Hydroxyzine HCl 25 mg	Atarax by Murfreesboro	51129-1481	Antianxiety; Antihistamine
SL <> 08	Tab, White, Black Print, Round, Sugar Coated	Hydroxyzine HCl 25 mg	Atarax by Med Pro	53978-3066	Antianxiety; Antihistamine
SL <> 08	Tab, White, Black Print, Round, Sugar Coated	Hydroxyzine HCl 25 mg	Atarax by Amerisource	62584-0743	Antianxiety; Antihistamine
SL <> 08	Tab, White, Black Print, Round, Sugar Coated	Hydroxyzine HCl 25 mg	Atarax by Darby Group	66467-4568	Antianxiety; Antihistamine
SL <> 08	Tab, White, Black Print, Round, Sugar Coated	Hydroxyzine HCl 25 mg	Atarax by Baker Cummins	63171-1493	Antianxiety; Antihistamine
SL <> 08	Tab, White, Black Print, Round, Sugar Coated	Hydroxyzine HCl 25 mg	Atarax by Kaiser	00179-0295	Antianxiety; Antihistamine
SL <> 08	Tab, White, Black Print, Round, Sugar Coated	Hydroxyzine HCl 25 mg	Atarax by Rx Dispensing	61807-0032	Antianxiety; Antihistamine
SL <> 08	Tab, White, Black Print, Round, Sugar Coated	Hydroxyzine HCl 25 mg	Atarax by Talbert	44514-0419	Antianxiety; Antihistamine
SL <> 08	Tab, White, Black Print, Round, Sugar Coated	Hydroxyzine HCl 25 mg	Atarax by Moore	00839-7438	Antianxiety; Antihistamine
SL <> 08	Tab, White, Black Print, Round, Sugar Coated	Hydroxyzine HCl 25 mg	Atarax by Sandoz	00781-1334	Antianxiety; Antihistamine
SL <> 08	Tab, White, Black Print, Round, Sugar Coated	Hydroxyzine HCl 25 mg	Atarax by Qualitest	00603-3971	Antianxiety; Antihistamine
SL <> 08	Tab, White, Black Print, Round, Sugar Coated	Hydroxyzine HCl 25 mg	Atarax by Major	00904-0358	Antianxiety; Antihistamine
SL <> 08	Tab, White, Black Print, Round, Sugar Coated	Hydroxyzine HCl 25 mg	Atarax by Apotheca	12634-0474	Antianxiety; Antihistamine

ID FRONT <> BACK	DESCRIPTION FRONT <> BACK	INGREDIENT & STRENGTH	BRAND (or Generic Equiv.) by FIRM	NDC#	CLASS; SCH.
SL <> 11	Tab, Sugar Coated	Dipyridamole 25 mg	Persantine by Pliva	50111-0311	Antiplatelet
SL <> 309	Tab, White, Black Print, Round, Sugar Coated	Hydroxyzine HCl 50 mg	Atarax by Darby Group	66467-4569	Antianxiety; Antihistamine
SL <> 309	Tab, White, Black Print, Round, Sugar Coated	Hydroxyzine HCl 50 mg	Atarax by Direct Dispensing	57866-3876	Antianxiety; Antihistamine
SL <> 309	Tab, White, Black Print, Round, Sugar Coated	Hydroxyzine HCl 50 mg	Atarax by Baker Cummins	63171-1494	Antianxiety; Antihistamine
SL <> 309	Tab, White, Black Print, Round, Sugar Coated	Hydroxyzine HCl 50 mg	Atarax by Sidmak		Antianxiety; Antihistamine
SL <> 309	Tab, White, Black Print, Round, Sugar Coated	Hydroxyzine HCl 50 mg	Atarax by Ivax	00182-1494	Antianxiety; Antihistamine
SL <> 309	Tab, White, Black Print, Round, Sugar Coated	Hydroxyzine HCl 50 mg	Atarax by Richmond	54738-0309	Antianxiety; Antihistamine
SL <> 309	Tab, White, Black Print, Round, Sugar Coated	Hydroxyzine HCl 50 mg	Atarax by Qualitest	00603-3972	Antianxiety; Antihistamine
SL <> 309	Tab, White, Black Print, Round, Sugar Coated	Hydroxyzine HCl 50 mg	Atarax by Murfreesboro	51129-1473	Antianxiety; Antihistamine
SL <> 309	Tab, White, Black Print, Round, Sugar Coated	Hydroxyzine HCl 50 mg	Atarax by Major	00904-0359	Antianxiety; Antihistamine
SL <> 309	Tab, White, Black Print, Round, Sugar Coated	Hydroxyzine HCl 50 mg	Atarax by Sandoz	00781-1336	Antianxiety; Antihistamine
SL <> 309	Tab, White, Black Print, Round, Sugar Coated	Hydroxyzine HCl 50 mg	Atarax by Moore	00839-7439	Antianxiety; Antihistamine
SL <> 312	Tab, Sugar Coated	Dipyridamole 50 mg	by Pliva	50111-0312	Antiplatelet
SL <> 313	Tab, Sugar Coated	Dipyridamole 75 mg	by Pliva	50111-0313	Antiplatelet
SL <> 36	Tab, Light Yellow, Round, Sugar Coated	Desipramine HCl 25 mg	Norpramin by Pliva	50111-0436	Antidepressant
SL <> 36	Tab, Light Yellow, Sugar Coated	Desipramine HCl 25 mg	by Schein	00364-2209	Antidepressant
SL <> 368	Tab, Brown, Black Print, Round	Amitriptyline HCl 50 mg	Elavil by Pliva	50111-0368	Antidepressant
SL <> 368	Tab, Brown, Black Print, Round	Amitriptyline HCl 50 mg	Elavil by H J Harkins Co	52959-0514	Antidepressant
SL <> 368	Tab, Brown, Black Print, Round	Amitriptyline HCl 50 mg	Elavil by Qualitest	00603-2214	Antidepressant
SL <> 368	Tab, Brown, Black Print, Round	Amitriptyline HCl 50 mg	Elavil by Ivax	00182-1020	Antidepressant
SL <> 368	Tab, Brown, Black Print, Round	Amitriptyline HCl 50 mg	Elavil by Apothecon	59772-8554	Antidepressant
SL <> 368	Tab, Brown, Black Print, Round	Amitriptyline HCl 50 mg	Elavil by Nat Pharmpak	55154-5809	Antidepressant
SL <> 368	Tab, Brown, Black Print, Round	Amitriptyline HCl 50 mg	Elavil by Baker Cummins	63171-1020	Antidepressant
SL <> 368	Tab, Brown, Black Print, Round	Amitriptyline HCl 50 mg	Elavil by Amerisource	62584-0308	Antidepressant
SL <> 370	Tab, Orange, Round	Amitriptyline HCl 100 mg	Elavil by Ivax	00182-1063	Antidepressant
SL <> 387	Tab, Film Coated	Ibuprofen 400 mg	Motrin by Pliva	50111-0387	NSAID
SL <> 388	Tab, Film Coated	Ibuprofen 600 mg	Motrin by Pliva	50111-0388	NSAID
SL <> 400	Tab, Dark Yellow to Brownish-Orange, Oval, Film Coated, Scored	Imatinib 400 mg	Gleevec by Novartis	Canadian DIN 02253283	Antineoplastic
SL <> 400	Tab, Dark Yellow to Brownish-Orange, Oval, Film Coated, Scored	Imatinib 400 mg	Gleevec by Novartis	00078-0438	Antineoplastic
SL <> 437	Tab, Light Green, Black Print, Round, Sugar Coated	Desipramine HCl 50 mg	by Warner Chilcott	00047-0595	Antidepressant
SL <> 437	Tab, Light Green, Black Print, Round, Sugar Coated	Desipramine HCl 50 mg	by Schein	00364-2210	Antidepressant
SL <> 437	Tab, Light Green, Black Print, Round, Sugar Coated	Desipramine HCl 50 mg	by Ivax	00182-1333	Antidepressant
SL <> 437	Tab, Light Green, Black Print, Round, Sugar Coated	Desipramine HCl 50 mg	by Med Pro	53978-2077	Antidepressant
SL <> 437	Tab, Light Green, Black Print, Round, Sugar Coated	Desipramine HCl 50 mg	Norpramin by Pliva	50111-0437	Antidepressant
SL <> 437	Tab, Light Green, Black Print, Round, Sugar Coated	Desipramine HCl 50 mg	by DRX	55045-1909	Antidepressant
SL <> 437	Tab, Light Green, Black Print, Round, Sugar Coated	Desipramine HCl 50 mg	by Moore	00839-7552	Antidepressant
SL <> 437	Tab, Light Green, Black Print, Round, Sugar Coated	Desipramine HCl 50 mg	by Qualitest	00603-3167	Antidepressant
SL <> 437	Tab, Light Green, Black Print, Round, Sugar Coated	Desipramine HCl 50 mg	by URL Mutual	00677-1199	Antidepressant
SL <> 437	Tab, Light Green, Black Print, Round, Sugar Coated	Desipramine HCl 50 mg	by Richmond	54738-0437	Antidepressant
SL <> 437	Tab, Light Green, Black Print, Round, Sugar Coated	Desipramine HCl 75 mg	by Schein	00364-2243	Antidepressant
SL <> 438	Tab, Light Orange, Sugar Coated	Desipramine HCl 75 mg	Norpramin by Pliva	50111-0438	Antidepressant
SL <> 438	Tab, Light Orange, Round, Sugar Coated	Desipramine HCl 75 mg	Motrin by Pliva		Antidepressant
SL <> 451	Tab, Film Coated, Debossed	Ibuprofen 800 mg		50111-0451	NSAID
SL <> 471	Tab, Yellow, Round, Scored	Propranolol HCl 80 mg	Inderal by Ivax	00182-1815	Antihypertensive
SL <> 557	Tab, Debossed	Naproxen 500 mg	Naprosyn by Pliva	50111-0557	NSAID
SL <> 563	Tab, Yellow, Round, Film Coated	Cyclobenzaprine HCl 10 mg	Flexeril by URL Mutual	00677-1429	Muscle Relaxant
SL <> 563	Tab, Yellow, Round, Film Coated	Cyclobenzaprine HCl 10 mg	Flexeril by Qualitest	00603-3077	Muscle Relaxant
SL <> 563	Tab, Yellow, Round, Film Coated	Cyclobenzaprine HCl 10 mg	Flexeril by Warner Chilcott		Muscle Relaxant
SL <> 563	Tab, Yellow, Round, Film Coated	Cyclobenzaprine HCl 10 mg	Flexeril by Sidmak	00047-0057	Muscle Relaxant

ID FRONT <> BACK	DESCRIPTION FRONT <> BACK	INGREDIENT & STRENGTH	BRAND (or Generic Equiv.) by FIRM	NDC#	CLASS; SCH.
SL <> 604	Tab, Green, Oblong, Scored, Film Coated	Guaifenesin 600 mg, Pseudoephedrine HCl 120 mg	Entex PSE by Pliva	Discontinued 50111-0604	Cold Remedy
SL <> 608	Tab, White, Round, Film Coated	Ketorolac Tromethamine 10 mg	Toradol by Sidmak		NSAID
SL <> 616	Tab, White	Tramadol HCl 50 mg	Ultram by Sidmak		Analgesic
SL <> 66	Tab, Pink, Round, Film Coated	Amitriptyline HCl 10 mg	Elavil by Pliva	50111-0366	Antidepressant
SL <> 66	Tab, Pink, Round, Film Coated	Amitriptyline HCl 10 mg	Elavil by Vangard	00615-0828	Antidepressant
SL <> 67	Tab, Green, Black Print, Round, Film Coated	Amitriptyline HCl 25 mg	Elavil by Rx Dispensing	61807-0129	Antidepressant
SL <> 67	Tab, Green, Black Print, Round, Film Coated	Amitriptyline HCl 25 mg	Elavil by Apotheca	12634-0401	Antidepressant
SL <> 67	Tab, Green, Black Print, Round, Film Coated	Amitriptyline HCl 25 mg	Elavil by Major		Antidepressant
SL <> 67	Tab, Green, Black Print, Round, Film Coated	Amitriptyline HCl 25 mg	Elavil by Allscripts		Antidepressant
SL <> 67	Tab, Green, Black Print, Round, Film Coated	Amitriptyline HCl 25 mg	Elavil by Pliva	50111-0367	Antidepressant
SL <> 67	Tab, Green, Black Print, Round, Film Coated	Amitriptyline HCl 25 mg	Elavil by Med Pro	53978-0023	Antidepressant
SL <> 67	Tab, Green, Black Print, Round, Film Coated	Amitriptyline HCl 25 mg	Elavil by H J Harkins Co	52959-0348	Antidepressant
SL <> 67	Tab, Green, Black Print, Round, Film Coated	Amitriptyline HCl 25 mg	Elavil by St. Mary's Med	60760-0367	Antidepressant
SL <> 67	Tab, Green, Black Print, Round, Film Coated	Amitriptyline HCl 25 mg	Elavil by Amerisource	62584-0614	Antidepressant
SL <> 67	Tab, Green, Black Print, Round, Film Coated	Amitriptyline HCl 25 mg	Elavil by Nat Pharmpak	55154-5814	Antidepressant
SL <> 67	Tab, Green, Black Print, Round, Film Coated	Amitriptyline HCl 25 mg	Elavil by Apothecon	59772-2593	Antidepressant
SL <> 67	Tab, Green, Black Print, Round, Film Coated	Amitriptyline HCl 25 mg	Elavil by Baker Cummins	63171-1019	Antidepressant
SL <> 67	Tab, Green, Black Print, Round, Film Coated	Amitriptyline HCl 25 mg	Elavil by Vangard	00615-0829	Antidepressant
SL <> 67	Tab, Green, Black Print, Round, Film Coated	Amitriptyline HCl 25 mg	Elavil by Qualitest	00603-2213	Antidepressant
SL <> 67	Tab, Green, Black Print, Round, Film Coated	Amitriptyline HCl 25 mg	Elavil by Ivax	00182-1019	Antidepressant
SL <> 67	Tab, Green, Black Print, Round, Film Coated	Amitriptyline HCl 25 mg	Elavil by Kaiser	00179-1275	Antidepressant
SL <> NVR	Tab, Dark Yellow to Brownish-Orange, Oval, Film Coated	Imatinib 400 mg	Gleevec by Novartis	00078-0402	Antineoplastic
SL07	Tab, Sugar Coated	Hydroxyzine HCl 10 mg	by Moore	00839-7437	Antianxiety; Antihistamine
SL07	Tab, Sugar Coated	Hydroxyzine HCl 10 mg	by Major	00904-0357	Antianxiety; Antihistamine
SL07	Tab, Sugar Coated, SL/07	Hydroxyzine HCl 10 mg	by URL Mutual	00677-0604	Antianxiety; Antihistamine
SL07	Tab, Sugar Coated	Hydroxyzine HCl 10 mg	by Sandoz	00781-1332	Antianxiety; Antihistamine
SL07	Tab, Sugar Coated, SL/07	Hydroxyzine HCl 10 mg	by St. Mary's Med	60760-0307	Antianxiety; Antihistamine
SL07	Tab, Sugar Coated, SL/07	Hydroxyzine HCl 10 mg	by Richmond	54738-0317	Antianxiety; Antihistamine
SL07	Tab, Sugar Coated, SL/07	Hydroxyzine HCl 10 mg	by H J Harkins Co	52959-0481	Antianxiety; Antihistamine
SL07	Tab, Film Coated, Sidmak	Hydroxyzine HCl 10 mg	by Pharmedix	53002-0390	Antianxiety; Antihistamine
SL07	Tab, White, Round, SL/07	Hydroxyzine HCl 10 mg	by Murfreesboro	51129-1479	Antianxiety; Antihistamine
SL07	Tab, Sugar Coated	Hydroxyzine HCl 10 mg	by Darby Group	66467-4567	Antianxiety; Antihistamine
SL07	Tab, White, Round	Hydroxyzine HCl 10 mg	by Direct Dispensing	57866-3875	Antianxiety; Antihistamine
SL07	Tab, Sugar Coated, SL over 07	Hydroxyzine HCl 10 mg	by Baker Cummins	63171-1492	Antianxiety; Antihistamine
SL07	Tab, Sugar Coated	Hydroxyzine HCl 10 mg	by Ivax	00182-1492	Antianxiety; Antihistamine
SL07	Tab, Purple or White, Round	Hydroxyzine HCl 10 mg	by Allscripts		Antianxiety; Antihistamine
SL100	Tab, White, Cap Shaped, Scored, SL / 100 <> Logo	Sertraline HCl 100 mg	Zoloft by Cobalt	16252-0535	Antidepressant
SL100	Cap, Orange, Opaque, Black Ink, Cobalt Logo	Sertraline HCl 100 mg	Zoloft by Cobalt	Canadian DIN 02287412	Antidepressant
SL11	Tab, Film Coated, SL over 11	Dipyridamole 25 mg	by Sidmak		Antiplatelet
SL125	Tab, Mint Green, Round, Scored	Hyoscyamine Sulfate 0.125 mg	Levsin by Murfreesboro	51129-1491	Gastrointestinal
SL125	Tab, Mint Green, Round, Scored	Hyoscyamine Sulfate 0.125 mg	Levsin by Sovereign	58716-0670	Gastrointestinal
SL125	Tab, Mint Green, Round, Scored	Hyoscyamine Sulfate 0.125 mg	Symax SL by Capellon	64543-0111	Gastrointestinal
SL236	Tab, Red, Round	Pseudoephedrine 30 mg	Sudafed by Sidmak		Decongestant
SL25	Cap, Yellow, Opaque, Black Ink, Cobalt Logo	Sertraline HCl 25 mg	Zoloft by Cobalt	Canadian DIN 02287390	Antidepressant
SL25	Tab, White, Cap Shaped, Scored, SL / 25 <> Logo	Sertraline HCl 25 mg	Zoloft by Cobalt	16252-0533	Antidepressant
SL301	Cap, Lavender & Clear	Nitroglycerin TD 2.5 mg	Nitrobid by Sidmak		Vasodilator

ID FRONT <> BACK	DESCRIPTION FRONT <> BACK	INGREDIENT & STRENGTH	BRAND (or Generic Equiv.) by FIRM	NDC#	CLASS; SCH.
SL302	Cap, Blue & Clear	Nitroglycerin TD 6.5 mg	Nitrobid by Sidmak		Vasodilator
SL303	Cap, Green & Yellow	Nitroglycerin TD 9 mg	Nitrobid by Sidmak		Vasodilator
SL314	Tab, White, Round, Scored, SL over 314	Cyproheptadine HCl 4 mg	Periactin by Direct Dispensing	57866-3515	Antihistamine
SL314	Tab, White, Round, Scored, SL over 314	Cyproheptadine HCl 4 mg	Periactin by Major	00904-1145	Antihistamine
SL314	Tab, White, Round, Scored, SL over 314	Cyproheptadine HCl 4 mg	Periactin by Heartland	61392-0209	Antihistamine
SL314	Tab, White, Round, Scored, SL over 314	Cyproheptadine HCl 4 mg	Periactin by Amerisource	62584-0355	Antihistamine
SL314	Tab, White, Round, Scored, SL over 314	Cyproheptadine HCl 4 mg	Periactin by Sidmak		Antihistamine
SL314	Tab, White, Round, Scored, SL over 314	Cyproheptadine HCl 4 mg	Periactin by Moore	00839-7866	Antihistamine
SL314	Tab, White, Round, Scored, SL over 314	Cyproheptadine HCl 4 mg	Periactin by Qualitest	00603-3098	Antihistamine
SL318	Cap, ER	Papaverine HCl 150 mg	by URL Mutual	00677-0171	Vasodilator
SL318	Cap, White Beads, Ex Release	Papaverine HCl 150 mg	by Pliva	50111-0318	Vasodilator
SL32	Tab	Bethanechol Chloride 5 mg	Urecholine by Qualitest		Urinary Tract
SL320	Tab, White, Round, Orange Specks, Chewable	Florvite	Poly-Vi-Flor by Sidmak	00603-2455	Mineral
SL32110	Tab, White, Round	Isoxsuprine HCl 10 mg	Vasodilan by Sidmak		Vasodilator
SL32220	Tab, White, Round	Isoxsuprine HCl 20 mg	Vasodilan by Sidmak		Vasodilator
SL323	Tab, SL over 323	Bethanechol Chloride 5 mg	Urecholine by UDL	51079-0053	Urinary Tract
SL324	Tab, SL over 324	Bethanechol Chloride 10 mg	Urecholine by UDL	51079-0054	Urinary Tract
SL324	Tab	Bethanechol Chloride 10 mg	Urecholine by Med Pro	53978-3072	Urinary Tract
SL324	Tab	Bethanechol Chloride 10 mg	Urecholine by Sidmak		Urinary Tract
SL324	Tab	Bethanechol Chloride 10 mg	Urecholine by Major	00904-0591	Urinary Tract
SL324	Tab	Bethanechol Chloride 10 mg	Urecholine by URL Mutual	00677-0506	Urinary Tract
SL324	Tab	Bethanechol Chloride 10 mg	Urecholine by Qualitest	00603-2456	Urinary Tract
SL325	Tab, Yellow, Round, Scored, SL/325	Bethanechol Chloride 25 mg	Urecholine by UDL	51079-0123	Urinary Tract
SL325	Tab, Yellow, Round, Scored, SL/325	Bethanechol Chloride 25 mg	Urecholine by URL Mutual	00677-0507	Urinary Tract
SL325	Tab, Yellow, Round, Scored, SL/325	Bethanechol Chloride 25 mg	Urecholine by Qualitest	00603-2457	Urinary Tract
SL325	Tab, Yellow, Round, Scored, SL/325	Bethanechol Chloride 25 mg	Urecholine by Bryant	63629-0387	Urinary Tract
SL325	Tab, Yellow, Round, Scored, SL/325	Bethanechol Chloride 25 mg	Urecholine by Major	00904-0592	Urinary Tract
SL326	Tab	Bethanechol Chloride 50 mg	Urecholine by URL Mutual	00677-0940	Urinary Tract
SL326	Tab, SL over 326	Bethanechol Chloride 50 mg	Urecholine by Qualitest	00603-2458	Urinary Tract
SL326	Tab, SL over 326	Bethanechol Chloride 50 mg	Urecholine by UDL	51079-0056	Urinary Tract
SL327	Tab, Orange, Round, SL over 327	Hydralazine HCl 25 mg	Apresoline by Ivax	00182-0554	Antihypertensive
SL327	Tab, Orange, Round, SL over 327	Hydralazine HCl 25 mg	Apresoline by Baker Cummins	63171-0554	Antihypertensive
SL327	Tab, Orange, Round, SL over 327	Hydralazine HCl 25 mg	Apresoline by Kaiser	00179-1290	Antihypertensive
SL327	Tab, Orange, Round, SL over 327	Hydralazine HCl 25 mg	Apresoline by Major	00904-5170	Antihypertensive
SL327	Tab, Orange, Round, SL over 327	Hydralazine HCl 25 mg	Apresoline by Sidmak		Antihypertensive
SL327	Tab, Orange, Round, SL over 327	Hydralazine HCl 25 mg	Apresoline by Med Pro	53978-3051	Antihypertensive
SL327	Tab, Orange, Round, SL over 327	Hydralazine HCl 25 mg	Apresoline by Richmond	54738-0327	Antihypertensive
SL327	Tab, Orange, Round, SL over 327	Hydralazine HCl 25 mg	Apresoline by Qualitest	00603-3831	Antihypertensive
SL327	Tab, Orange, Round, SL over 327	Hydralazine HCl 25 mg	Apresoline by Heartland	61392-0043	Antihypertensive
SL327	Tab, Orange, Round, SL over 327	Hydralazine HCl 25 mg	Apresoline by Nat Pharmpak	55154-5821	Antihypertensive
SL328	Tab, Orange, Round, SL over 328	Hydralazine HCl 50 mg	Apresoline by Nat Pharmpak	55154-5818	Antihypertensive
SL328	Tab, Orange, Round, SL over 328	Hydralazine HCl 50 mg	Apresoline by Monarch	61570-0022	Antihypertensive
SL328	Tab, Orange, Round, SL over 328	Hydralazine HCl 50 mg	Apresoline by Med Pro	53978-3001	Antihypertensive
SL328	Tab, Orange, Round, SL over 328	Hydralazine HCl 50 mg	Apresoline by Sidmak		Antihypertensive
SL328	Tab, Orange, Round, SL over 328	Hydralazine HCl 50 mg	Apresoline by Richmond	54738-0328	Antihypertensive
SL328	Tab, Orange, Round, SL over 328	Hydralazine HCl 50 mg	Apresoline by Kaiser	00179-1274	Antihypertensive
SL328	Tab, Orange, Round	Hydralazine HCl 50 mg	Apresoline by Ivax	00182-0555	Antihypertensive
SL328	Tab, Orange, Round, SL over 328	Hydralazine HCl 50 mg	Apresoline by Qualitest	00603-3832	Antihypertensive

ID FRONT <> BACK	DESCRIPTION FRONT <> BACK	INGREDIENT & STRENGTH	BRAND (or Generic Equiv.) by FIRM	NDC#	CLASS; SCH.
SL328	Tab, Orange, Round, SL over 328	Hydralazine HCl 50 mg	Apresoline by Moore	00839-1363	Antihypertensive
SL329	Cap, Orange	Cyclandelate 200 mg	Cyclospasmol by Sidmak		Vasodilator
SL330	Cap, Green & White	Cyclandelate 400 mg	Cyclospasmol by Sidmak		Vasodilator
SL331	Tab, White, Round	Disulfiram 250 mg	Antabuse by Qualitest	00603-3431	Antialcoholism
SL331	Tab, White, Round	Disulfiram 250 mg	Antabuse by Sandoz	00781-1060	Antialcoholism
SL331	Tab, White, Round	Disulfiram 250 mg	Antabuse by Pliva	50111-0331	Antialcoholism
SL331	Tab, White, Round	Disulfiram 250 mg	Antabuse by Major	00904-1180	Antialcoholism
SL331	Tab, White, Round	Disulfiram 250 mg	Antabuse by DRX	55045-2423	Antialcoholism
SL332	Tab, White, Round, Scored	Disulfiram 500 mg	Antabuse by Ivax	00182-0533	Antialcoholism
SL332	Tab, White, Round, Scored	Disulfiram 500 mg	Antabuse by Pliva	50111-0332	Antialcoholism
SL333	Tab, White, Round	Metronidazole 250 mg	Flagyl by Baker Cummins	63171-1330	Antibiotic
SL333	Tab, White, Round	Metronidazole 250 mg	Flagyl by Darby Group	66467-4032	Antibiotic
SL333	Tab, White, Round	Metronidazole 250 mg	Flagyl by Apotheca	12634-0165	Antibiotic
SL333	Tab, White, Round	Metronidazole 250 mg	Flagyl by Diversified Healthcare	55887-0978	Antibiotic
SL333	Tab, White, Round	Metronidazole 250 mg	Flagyl by Physician Total Care	54868-0108	Antibiotic
SL333	Tab, White, Round	Metronidazole 250 mg	Flagyl by Sidmak		Antibiotic
SL333	Tab, White, Round	Metronidazole 250 mg	Flagyl by Med Pro	53978-0215	Antibiotic
SL333	Tab, White, Round	Metronidazole 250 mg	Flagyl by Moore	00839-6415	Antibiotic
SL333	Tab, White, Round	Metronidazole 250 mg	Flagyl by Rx Dispensing	61807-0023	Antibiotic
SL333	Tab, White, Round	Metronidazole 250 mg	Flagyl by St. Mary's Med	60760-0333	Antibiotic
SL333	Tab, White, Round	Metronidazole 250 mg	Flagyl by Major	00904-1453	Antibiotic
SL333	Tab, White, Round	Metronidazole 250 mg	Flagyl by Qualitest	00603-4640	Antibiotic
SL333	Tab, White, Round	Metronidazole 250 mg	Flagyl by URL Mutual	00677-0690	Antibiotic
SL333	Tab, White, Round	Metronidazole 250 mg	Flagyl by Southwood	58016-0129	Antibiotic
SL334	Tab, White, Oblong	Metronidazole 500 mg	Flagyl by Baker Cummins	63171-1517	Antibiotic
SL334	Tab, White, Oblong	Metronidazole 500 mg	Flagyl by Dixon Shane	17236-0304	Antibiotic
SL334	Tab, White, Oblong	Metronidazole 500 mg	Flagyl by Apotheca	12634-0172	Antibiotic
SL334	Tab, White, Oblong	Metronidazole 500 mg	Flagyl by Moore	00839-6620	Antibiotic
SL334	Tab, White, Oblong	Metronidazole 500 mg	Flagyl by URL Mutual	00677-0816	Antibiotic
SL334	Tab, White, Oblong	Metronidazole 500 mg	Flagyl by Qualitest	00603-4641	Antibiotic
SL334	Tab, White, Oblong	Metronidazole 500 mg	Flagyl by Rx Dispensing	61807-0024	Antibiotic
SL334	Tab, White, Oblong	Metronidazole 500 mg	Flagyl by Med Pro	53978-3056	Antibiotic
SL334	Tab, White, Oblong	Metronidazole 500 mg	Flagyl by Sidmak		Antibiotic
SL334	Tab, White, Oblong	Metronidazole 500 mg	Flagyl by St. Mary's Med	60760-0641	Antibiotic
SL334	Tab, White, Oblong	Metronidazole 500 mg	Flagyl by H J Harkins Co	52959-0102	Antibiotic
SL334	Tab, White, Oblong	Metronidazole 500 mg	Flagyl by Dept Health	53808-0053	Antibiotic
SL335	Cap, Blue & Clear	Ethaverine HCl 100 mg			Vasodilator
SL337	Tab, White, Round	Nylidrin 6 mg	Arlidin by Sidmak		Vasodilator
SL338	Tab, White, Round	Nylidrin 12 mg	Arlidin by Sidmak		Vasodilator
SL339	Tab, Oval, Blue, Film Coated	Procainamide HCl 250 mg	by Pliva	50111-0339	Antiarrhythmic
SL340	Tab, ER	Procainamide HCl 500 mg	by Pliva	50111-0340	Antiarrhythmic
SL340	Tab	Metoclopramide HCl 10 mg	Reglan by URL Mutual	00677-1039	Gastrointestinal
SL341	Tab	Sulfamethoxazole 400 mg, Trimethoprim 80 mg	by Major	00904-2726	Antibiotic
SL341	Tab	Sulfamethoxazole 400 mg, Trimethoprim 80 mg	by Sandoz	00781-1062	Antibiotic
SL341	Tab	Sulfamethoxazole 400 mg, Trimethoprim 80 mg	by Qualitest	00603-5778	Antibiotic
SL341	Tab	Sulfamethoxazole 400 mg, Trimethoprim 80 mg	by Moore	00839-6487	Antibiotic
SL341	Tab, SL over 341	Sulfamethoxazole 400 mg, Trimethoprim 80 mg	by Amerisource	62584-0856	Antibiotic
SL341	Tab	Sulfamethoxazole 400 mg, Trimethoprim 80 mg	SMZ TMP by Casa DeAmigos	62138-7383	Antibiotic

ID FRONT <> BACK	DESCRIPTION FRONT <> BACK	INGREDIENT & STRENGTH	BRAND (or Generic Equiv.) by FIRM	NDC#	CLASS; SCH.
SL341	Tab, SL/341	Sulfamethoxazole 400 mg, Trimethoprim 80 mg	by Pliva	50111-0341	Antibiotic
SL342	Tab, SL/342	Sulfamethoxazole 800 mg, Trimethoprim 160 mg	by Amerisource	62584-0857	Antibiotic
SL342	Tab, Sidmak	Sulfamethoxazole 800 mg, Trimethoprim 160 mg	by Apotheca	12634-0177	Antibiotic
SL342	Tab	Sulfamethoxazole 800 mg, Trimethoprim 160 mg	by Qualitest	00603-5779	Antibiotic
SL342	Tab	Sulfamethoxazole 800 mg, Trimethoprim 160 mg	by Talbert	44514-0826	Antibiotic
SL342	Tab, SL/342	Sulfamethoxazole 800 mg, Trimethoprim 160 mg	by Major	00904-2725	Antibiotic
SL342	Tab, Sidmak	Sulfamethoxazole 800 mg, Trimethoprim 160 mg	Trimeth Sulfa DS by Pharmedix	53002-0210	Antibiotic
SL342	Tab	Sulfamethoxazole 800 mg, Trimethoprim 160 mg	by Pliva	50111-0342	Antibiotic
SL342	Tab	Sulfamethoxazole 800 mg, Trimethoprim 160 mg	by Urgent Care Center		Antibiotic
SL343	Tab, Peach, Oval	Papaverine HCl HP 300 mg	Pavabid HP by Sidmak	50716-0163	Vasodilator
SL346	Tab, White, Round	Isosorbide Dinitrate SL 10 mg	Isordil by Sidmak		Antianginal
SL347	Tab, Pink, Round	Isosorbide Dinitrate 5 mg	Isordil by Sidmak		Antianginal
SL348	Tab, White, Round	Isosorbide Dinitrate 10 mg	Isordil by Sidmak		Antianginal
SL348	Tab, Sugar Coated	Desipramine HCl 75 mg	by Ivax	00182-1335	Antidepressant
SL349	Tab, Green, Round	Isosorbide Dinitrate 20 mg	Isordil by Sidmak		Antianginal
SL350	Tab, Blue, Round	Isosorbide Dinitrate 30 mg	Isordil by Sidmak		Antianginal
SL351	Tab, Yellow, Round	Isosorbide Dinitrate SR 40 mg	Isordil by Sidmak		Antianginal
SL353	Tab, Blue & White, Oval, Layered, SL/353	Meclizine HCl 12.5 mg	Antivert by Qualitest	00603-4319	Antiemetic
SL353	Tab, Blue & White, Oval, Layered, SL/353	Meclizine HCl 12.5 mg	Antivert by URL Mutual	00677-0418	Antiemetic
SL353	Tab, Blue & White, Oval, Layered, SL/353	Meclizine HCl 12.5 mg	Antivert by Baker Cummins	63171-0871	Antiemetic
SL353	Tab, Blue & White, Oval, Layered, SL/353	Meclizine HCl 12.5 mg	Antivert by Heartland	61392-0338	Antiemetic
SL353	Tab, Blue & White, Oval, Layered, SL/353	Meclizine HCl 12.5 mg	Antivert by Ivax	00182-0871	Antiemetic
SL353	Tab, Blue & White, Oval, Layered, SL/353	Meclizine HCl 12.5 mg	Antivert by Pliva	50111-0353	Antiemetic
SL354	Tab, White & Yellow, Oval, Scored, SL over 354	Meclizine HCl 25 mg	by Qualitest	00603-4320	Antiemetic
SL354	Tab, White & Yellow, Oval, Scored, SL over 354	Meclizine HCl 25 mg	by URL Mutual	00677-0419	Antiemetic
SL354	Tab, White & Yellow, Oval, Scored, SL over 354	Meclizine HCl 25 mg	by Major	00904-5363	Antiemetic
SL354	Tab, White & Yellow, Oval, Scored, SL over 354	Meclizine HCl 25 mg	by H J Harkins Co	52959-0033	Antiemetic
SL354	Tab, White & Yellow, Oval, Scored, SL over 354	Meclizine HCl 25 mg	Antivert by Pliva	50111-0354	Antiemetic
SL354	Tab, White & Yellow, Oval, Scored, SL over 354	Meclizine HCl 25 mg	by Pharmedix	53002-0351	Antiemetic
SL354	Tab, White & Yellow, Oval, Scored, SL over 354	Meclizine HCl 25 mg	by Heartland	61392-0339	Antiemetic
SL354	Tab, White & Yellow, Oval, Scored, SL over 354	Meclizine HCl 25 mg	by Ivax	00182-0872	Antiemetic
SL354 <> SL354	Tab, Yellow & White, Oval, Scored	Meclizine HCl 25 mg	by Nat Pharmpak	55154-5559	Antiemetic
SL355	Tab, Chewable	Meclizine HCl 25 mg	by Pliva	50111-0355	Antiemetic
SL359	Tab, Pink, Oval	Dexchlorpheniramine Maleate 2 mg	Polaramine by Sidmak		Antihistamine
SL36	Tab, Sugar Coated	Desipramine HCl 25 mg	by Warner Chilcott	00047-0594	Antidepressant
SL36	Tab, Sugar Coated	Desipramine HCl 25 mg	by Richmond	54738-0436	Antidepressant
SL36	Tab, Sugar Coated	Desipramine HCl 25 mg	by Qualitest	00603-3166	Antidepressant
SL36	Tab, Sugar Coated	Desipramine HCl 25 mg	by URL Mutual	00677-1198	Antidepressant
SL36	Tab, Sugar Coated	Desipramine HCl 25 mg	by Amerisource	62584-0661	Antidepressant
SL36	Tab, Yellow, Oval	Ethaverine HCl 100 mg	Ethatab by Sidmak		Vasodilator
SL363	Tab, Light Blue, Round, Scored, SL over 363	Chlorthalidone 50 mg	Hygroton by Ivax	00182-1435	Diuretic
SL363	Tab, Light Blue, Round, Scored, SL over 363	Chlorthalidone 50 mg	Hygroton by Qualitest	00603-2861	Diuretic
SL363	Tab, Light Blue, Round, Scored, SL over 363	Chlorthalidone 50 mg	Hygroton by Major	00904-1350	Diuretic
SL364	Tab, White, Round, Scored	Chlorthalidone 100 mg	Hygroton by Major	00904-1351	Diuretic
SL364	Tab, White, Round, Scored	Chlorthalidone 100 mg	Hygroton by Qualitest	00603-2862	Diuretic
SL369	Tab, Purple, Black Print, Round, Film Coated, SL over 369	Amitriptyline HCl 50 mg	Elavil by Major		Antidepressant
SL369	Tab, Purple, Black Print, Round, Film Coated, SL over 369	Amitriptyline HCl 75 mg	Elavil by Baker Cummins	63171-1021	Antidepressant
SL369	Tab, Purple, Black Print, Round, Film Coated, SL over 369	Amitriptyline HCl 75 mg	Elavil by Parmed	00349-1043	Antidepressant

ID FRONT <> BACK	DESCRIPTION FRONT <> BACK	INGREDIENT & STRENGTH	BRAND (or Generic Equiv.) by FIRM	NDC#	CLASS; SCH.
SL369	Tab, Purple, Black Print, Round, Film Coated, SL over 369	Amitriptyline HCl 75 mg	Elavil by Pliva	50111-0369	Antidepressant
SL369	Tab, Purple, Black Print, Round, Film Coated, SL over 369	Amitriptyline HCl 75 mg	Elavil by H J Harkins Co	52959-0284	Antidepressant
SL369	Tab, Purple, Black Print, Round, Film Coated, SL over 369	Amitriptyline HCl 75 mg	Elavil by Ivax	00182-1021	Antidepressant
SL369	Tab, Purple, Black Print, Round, Film Coated, SL over 369	Amitriptyline HCl 75 mg	Elavil by Compumed	00403-0792	Antidepressant
SL370	Tab, Film Coated, SL/370	Amitriptyline HCl 100 mg	Elavil by Major	00904-0204	Antidepressant
SL370	Tab, Film Coated, SL/370	Amitriptyline HCl 100 mg	Elavil by Qualitest	00603-2216	Antidepressant
SL370	Tab, Orange, Round, Film Coated	Amitriptyline HCl 100 mg	Elavil by Pliva	50111-0370	Antidepressant
SL371	Tab, Light Peach, Oval, Film Coated	Amitriptyline HCl 150 mg	Elavil by Pliva	50111-0371	Antidepressant
SL371	Tab, Film Coated	Amitriptyline HCl 150 mg	Elavil by Major	00904-0205	Antidepressant
SL371	Tab, Film Coated, SL/371	Amitriptyline HCl 150 mg	Elavil by Qualitest	00603-2217	Antidepressant
SL371	Tab, Film Coated	Amitriptyline HCl 150 mg	Elavil by Moore	00839-6401	Antidepressant
SL371	Tab, Film Coated	Amitriptyline HCl 150 mg	Elavil by Ivax	00182-1486	Antidepressant
SL372	Tab, Blue, Round, Scored, SL over 372	Chlorpropamide 100 mg	Diabinese by Major	00904-0225	Antidiabetic
SL372	Tab, Blue, Round, Scored, SL over 372	Chlorpropamide 100 mg	Diabinese by Moore	00839-7011	Antidiabetic
SL372	Tab, Blue, Round, Scored, SL over 372	Chlorpropamide 100 mg	Diabinese by Ivax	00182-1851	Antidiabetic
SL372	Tab, Blue, Round, Scored, SL over 372	Chlorpropamide 100 mg	Diabinese by Qualitest	00603-2835	Antidiabetic
SL372	Tab, Blue, Round, Scored, SL over 372	Chlorpropamide 100 mg	Diabinese by Compumed		Antidiabetic
SL373	Tab, Blue, Round, Scored, SL over 373	Chlorpropamide 250 mg	Diabinese by Qualitest	00603-2836	Antidiabetic
SL373	Tab, Blue, Round, Scored, SL over 373	Chlorpropamide 250 mg	Diabinese by Pharmedix	53002-0347	Antidiabetic
SL373	Tab, Blue, Round, Scored, SL over 373	Chlorpropamide 250 mg	Diabinese by Moore	00839-7012	Antidiabetic
SL373	Tab, Blue, Round, Scored, SL over 373	Chlorpropamide 250 mg	Diabinese by Compumed		Antidiabetic
SL373	Tab, Blue, Round, Scored, SL over 373	Chlorpropamide 250 mg	Diabinese by Ivax	00182-1852	Antidiabetic
SL375	Tab, Green, Oblong, Scored	Hyoscyamine Sulfate 0.375 mg	Levsin by Murfreesboro	51129-1492	Gastrointestinal
SL375	Tab	Nystatin 100,000 Units	by Ivax	00182-0981	Antifungal
SL375	Tab	Nystatin 100,000 Units	by URL Mutual	00677-1165	Antifungal
SL375	Tab, Green, Oblong, Scored	Hyoscyamine Sulfate 0.375 mg	Symax SR by Capellon	64543-0112	Gastrointestinal
SL377	Cap, Lemon Yellow & Teal Blue, Coated	Doxycycline Hyclate 125 mg	by Pliva		Antibiotic
SL381	Tab, Blue with Blue Specks, Round	Phenylpropanolamine HCl 40 mg, Phenylephrine HCl 10 mg, Phentoloxamine 15 mg, Chlorpheniramine 5 mg	Naldecon by Sidmak	50111-0377	Cold Remedy
SL383	Tab, White, Round	Dextrobrompheniramine Maleate 6 mg, Pseudoephedrine Sulfate 120 mg	Drixoral by Sidmak		Cold Remedy
SL384	Tab, Pink, Round	Isosorbide Dinitrate SR 20 mg	Isordil by Sidmak		Antianginal
SL385	Tab, Blue, Oval, Scored	Guaifenesin 400 mg, Phenylpropanolamine HCl 75 mg	Entex LA by Talbert	44514-0348	Cold Remedy
SL385	Tab, Blue, Oval, Scored	Guaifenesin 400 mg, Phenylpropanolamine HCl 75 mg	Entex LA by Pliva	50111-0385	Cold Remedy
SL385	Tab, Blue, Oval, Scored	Guaifenesin 400 mg, Phenylpropanolamine HCl 75 mg	Entex LA by Sandoz	00781-1503	Cold Remedy
SL385	Tab, Blue, Oval, Scored	Guaifenesin 400 mg, Phenylpropanolamine HCl 75 mg	Entex LA by Ivax	00172-4370	Cold Remedy
SL385	Tab, Blue, Oval, Scored	Guaifenesin 400 mg, Phenylpropanolamine HCl 75 mg	Entex LA by URL Mutual	00677-1026	Cold Remedy
SL387	Tab, Coated, Sidmak	Ibuprofen 400 mg	Motrin by Pharmedix	53002-0337	NSAID
SL388	Tab, Film Coated, Sidmak	Ibuprofen 600 mg	Motrin by Pharmedix	53002-0301	NSAID
SL390	Tab, Yellow, Round, Film Coated	Salsalate 500 mg	Disalcid by Richmond	54738-0306	NSAID
SL390	Tab, Yellow, Round, Film Coated	Salsalate 500 mg	Disalcid by PDRX	55289-0275	NSAID
SL390	Tab, Yellow, Round, Film Coated	Salsalate 500 mg	Disalcid by Major	00904-1250	NSAID
SL391	Tab, Yellow, Cap Shaped, Scored, Film Coated	Salsalate 750 mg	Disalcid by Major	00904-1251	NSAID
SL391	Tab, Yellow, Cap Shaped, Scored, Film Coated	Salsalate 750 mg	Disalcid by RX Pak	65084-0217	NSAID
SL391	Tab, Yellow, Cap Shaped, Scored, Film Coated	Salsalate 750 mg	Disalcid by RX Pak	65084-0218	NSAID
SL391	Tab, Yellow, Cap Shaped, Scored, Film Coated	Salsalate 750 mg	Disalcid by Med Pro	53978-0399	NSAID
SL391	Tab, Yellow, Cap Shaped, Scored, Film Coated	Salsalate 750 mg	Disalcid by DRX	55045-1935	NSAID
SL391	Tab, Yellow, Cap Shaped, Scored, Film Coated	Salsalate 750 mg	Disalcid by Compumed	00403-0088	NSAID
SL391	Tab, Yellow, Cap Shaped, Scored, Film Coated	Salsalate 750 mg	Disalcid by Apotheca	12634-0463	NSAID
SL391	Tab, Yellow, Cap Shaped, Scored, Film Coated	Salsalate 750 mg	Disalcid by Moore	00839-7168	NSAID

ID FRONT <> BACK	DESCRIPTION FRONT <> BACK	INGREDIENT & STRENGTH	BRAND (or Generic Equiv.) by FIRM	NDC#	CLASS; SCH.
SL391	Tab, Yellow, Cap Shaped, Scored, Film Coated	Salsalate 750 mg	Disalcid by Apotheca	12634-0431	NSAID
SL393	Tab, White, Round, Scored	Benztropine Mesylate 0.5 mg	Cogentin by Sidmak	Discontinued	Antiparkinson
SL393	Tab, White, Round, Scored	Benztropine Mesylate 0.5 mg	Cogentin by Qualitest	00603-2430	Antiparkinson
SL394	Tab, White, Oval, Scored	Benztropine Mesylate 1 mg	Cogentin by Qualitest	00603-2431	Antiparkinson
SL395	Tab, White, Round, Scored, SL over 395	Benztropine Mesylate 2 mg	Cogentin by Qualitest	00603-2432	Antiparkinson
SL396	Tab, Peach, Oval	Procainamide HCl SR 750 mg	Procan SR by Sidmak		Antiarrhythmic
SL397	Tab, Orange, Round, SL over 397	Hydralazine HCl 100 mg	Apresoline by Qualitest	00603-3833	Antihypertensive
SL397	Tab, Orange, Round, SL over 397	Hydralazine HCl 100 mg	Apresoline by Ivax	00182-1553	Antihypertensive
SL398	Tab, Orange, Round, SL over 398	Hydralazine HCl 10 mg	Apresoline by Ivax	00182-0905	Antihypertensive
SL398	Tab, Orange, Round, SL over 398	Hydralazine HCl 10 mg	Apresoline by Qualitest	00603-3830	Antihypertensive
SL398	Tab, Orange, Round, SL over 398	Hydralazine HCl 10 mg	Apresoline by Richmond	54738-0398	Antihypertensive
SL398	Tab, Orange, Round, SL over 398	Hydralazine HCl 10 mg	Apresoline by Sidmak		Antihypertensive
SL398	Tab, Orange, Round, SL over 398	Hydralazine HCl 10 mg	Apresoline by Monarch		Antihypertensive
SL398	Tab, Orange, Round, SL over 398	Hydralazine HCl 10 mg	Apresoline by Nat Pharmpak	55154-5827	Antihypertensive
SL398	Tab, Orange, Round, SL over 398	Hydralazine HCl 10 mg	Apresoline by Baker Cummins	63171-0905	Antihypertensive
SL398	Tab, Orange, Round, SL over 398	Hydralazine HCl 10 mg	Apresoline by Major	00904-5169	Antihypertensive
SL404	Cap, White	Phenytoin Sodium 100 mg	Dilantin by Sidmak		Anticonvulsant
SL406	Cap, Green, Black Print, SL over 406	Indomethacin 25 mg	Indocin by Pliva	50111-0406	NSAID
SL406	Cap, Green, Black Print, SL over 406	Indomethacin 25 mg	Indocin by Richmond	54738-0406	NSAID
SL406	Cap, Green, Black Print, SL over 406	Indomethacin 25 mg	Indocin by H J Harkins Co	52959-0080	NSAID
SL406	Cap, Green, Black Print, SL over 406	Indomethacin 25 mg	Indocin by URL Mutual	00677-0872	NSAID
SL406	Cap, Green, Black Print, SL over 406	Indomethacin 25 mg	Indocin by Qualitest	00603-4067	NSAID
SL406	Cap, Green, Black Print, SL over 406	Indomethacin 25 mg	Indocin by Murfreesboro	51129-1552	NSAID
SL407	Cap	Indomethacin 50 mg	Indocin by Richmond	54738-0407	NSAID
SL407	Cap, Green, Gelatin	Indomethacin 50 mg	Indocin by Pliva	50111-0407	NSAID
SL407	Cap, SL 407 <> Sidmak	Indomethacin 50 mg	Indocin by Qualitest	00603-4068	NSAID
SL407	Cap, SL 407 <> Sidmak	Indomethacin 50 mg	Indocin by URL Mutual	00677-0873	NSAID
SL410	Tab	Carbamazepine 200 mg	Tegretol by Pliva	50111-0410	Anticonvulsant
SL415	Tab	Griseofulvin, Ultramicrosize 165 mg	Fulvicin P/G by Pliva	50111-0415	Antifungal
SL416	Tab	Griseofulvin, Ultramicrosize 330 mg	Fulvicin P/G by Pliva	50111-0416	Antifungal
SL425	Tab, Pink, Oblong, Enteric Coated	Aspirin 975 mg	Aspirin by Sidmak		Analgesic
SL427	Cap, Orange & Beige, Oblong	Guaifenesin 200 mg, Phenylephrine HCl 5 mg, Phenylpropanolamine HCl 45 mg	Entex by Sidmak		Cold Remedy
SL430	Tab, White, Round, Scored, SL over 430	Metoclopramide HCl 10 mg	Reglan by Sidmak		Gastrointestinal
SL430	Tab, White, Round, Scored, SL over 430	Metoclopramide HCl 10 mg	Reglan by Neuman	64579-0048	Gastrointestinal
SL430	Tab, White, Round, Scored, SL over 430	Metoclopramide HCl 10 mg	Reglan by Qualitest	00603-4617	Gastrointestinal
SL430	Tab, White, Round, Scored, SL over 430	Metoclopramide HCl 10 mg	Reglan by Major	00904-1070	Gastrointestinal
SL430	Tab, White, Round, Scored, SL over 430	Metoclopramide HCl 10 mg	Reglan by Richmond	54738-0430	Gastrointestinal
SL433	Tab, White, Round, Scored, SL over 433	Trazodone HCl 50 mg	Desyrel by Kaiser	00179-1118	Antidepressant
SL433	Tab, White, Round, Scored, SL over 433	Trazodone HCl 50 mg	Desyrel by Direct Dispensing	57866-4715	Antidepressant
SL433	Tab, White, Round, Scored, SL over 433	Trazodone HCl 50 mg	Desyrel by Warner Chilcott	00047-0577	Antidepressant
SL433	Tab, White, Round, Scored, SL over 433	Trazodone HCl 50 mg	Desyrel by Qualitest	00603-6144	Antidepressant
SL433	Tab, White, Round, Scored, SL over 433	Trazodone HCl 50 mg	Desyrel by Baker Cummins	63171-1259	Antidepressant
SL433	Tab, White, Round, Scored, SL over 433	Trazodone HCl 50 mg	Desyrel by Rx Dispensing	61807-0143	Antidepressant
SL433	Tab, White, Round, Scored, SL over 433	Trazodone HCl 50 mg	Desyrel by Kaiser	62224-0555	Antidepressant
SL433	Tab, White, Round, Scored, SL over 433	Trazodone HCl 50 mg	Desyrel by Moore	00839-7251	Antidepressant
SL433	Tab, White, Round, Scored, SL over 433	Trazodone HCl 50 mg	Desyrel by H J Harkins Co	52959-0378	Antidepressant
SL433	Tab, White, Round, Scored, SL over 433	Trazodone HCl 50 mg	Desyrel by DRX	55045-1715	Antidepressant
SL433	Tab, White, Round, Scored, SL over 433	Trazodone HCl 50 mg	Desyrel by Ivax	00182-1259	Antidepressant

ID FRONT <> BACK	DESCRIPTION FRONT <> BACK	INGREDIENT & STRENGTH	BRAND (or Generic Equiv.) by FIRM	NDC#	CLASS; SCH.
SL433	Tab, White, Round, Scored, SL over 433	Trazodone HCl 50 mg	Desyrel by Major	00904-3990	Antidepressant
SL434	Tab, White, Round, Scored, SL over 434	Trazodone HCl 100 mg	Desyrel by Qualitest	00603-6145	Antidepressant
SL434	Tab, White, Round, Scored	Trazodone HCl 100 mg	Desyrel by Major	00904-3991	Antidepressant
SL434	Tab, White, Round, Scored, SL over 434	Trazodone HCl 100 mg	Desyrel by Amerisource	62584-0883	Antidepressant
SL434	Tab, White, Round, Scored, SL over 434	Trazodone HCl 100 mg	Desyrel by Baker Cummins	63171-1260	Antidepressant
SL434	Tab, White, Round, Scored, SL over 434	Trazodone HCl 100 mg	Desyrel by Teva	00480-0280	Antidepressant
SL434	Tab, White, Round, Scored, SL over 434	Trazodone HCl 100 mg	Desyrel by Warner Chilcott	00047-0578	Antidepressant
SL434	Tab, White, Round, Scored, SL over 434	Trazodone HCl 100 mg	Desyrel by Teva	00480-0293	Antidepressant
SL434	Tab, White, Round, Scored, SL over 434	Trazodone HCl 100 mg	Desyrel by Ivax	00182-1260	Antidepressant
SL434	Tab, White, Round, Scored, SL over 434	Trazodone HCl 100 mg	Desyrel by Southwood	58016-0862	Antidepressant
SL436	Tab, Sugar Coated	Desipramine HCl 25 mg	Norpramin by Ivax	00182-1332	Antidepressant
SL438	Tab, Sugar Coated	Desipramine HCl 75 mg	Norpramin by Warner Chilcott	00047-0596	Antidepressant
SL438	Tab, Sugar Coated	Desipramine HCl 75 mg	Norpramin by Qualitest	00603-3168	Antidepressant
SL438	Tab, Sugar Coated	Desipramine HCl 75 mg	Norpramin by Moore	00839-7553	Antidepressant
SL439	Tab, Peach, Round, Sugar Coated	Desipramine HCl 100 mg	Norpramin by Pliva	50111-0439	Antidepressant
SL440	Tab, White, Round, Sugar Coated	Desipramine HCl 150 mg	Norpramin by Pliva	50111-0440	Antidepressant
SL441 <> 50100	Tab, White, Trapezoid, Scored, SL 441<> 50/100	Trazodone HCl 150 mg	Desyrel by Teva	00480-0154	Antidepressant
SL441 <> 50100	Tab, White, Trapezoid, Scored, SL 441<> 50/100	Trazodone HCl 150 mg	Desyrel by Heartland	61392-0179	Antidepressant
SL441 <> 50100	Tab, White, Trapezoid, Scored, SL 441<> 50/100	Trazodone HCl 150 mg	Desyrel by Physician Total Care	54868-1959	Antidepressant
SL441 <> 505050	Tab, White, Trapezoidal, Scored, SL441 <> 50 50 50	Trazodone HCl 150 mg	Desyrel by Sandoz	00781-1826	Antidepressant
SL441 <> 505050	Tab, White, Trapezoidal, Scored, SL441 <> 50 50 50	Trazodone HCl 150 mg	Desyrel by Warner Chilcott	00047-0716	Antidepressant
SL441 <> 505050	Tab, White, Trapezoidal, Scored, SL441 <> 50 50 50	Trazodone HCl 150 mg	Desyrel by Ivax	00182-1298	Antidepressant
SL441 <> 505050	Tab, White, Trapezoidal, Scored, SL441 <> 50 50 50	Trazodone HCl 150 mg	Desyrel by Parmed	00349-8824	Antidepressant
SL441 <> 505050	Tab, White, Trapezoidal, Scored, SL441 <> 50 50 50	Trazodone HCl 150 mg	Desyrel by Qualitest	00603-6146	Antidepressant
SL441 <> 505050	Tab, White, Trapezoidal, Scored, SL441 <> 50 50 50	Trazodone HCl 150 mg	Desyrel by URL Mutual	00677-1302	Antidepressant
SL441 <> 505050	Tab, White, Trapezoidal, Scored, SL441 <> 50 50 50	Trazodone HCl 150 mg	Desyrel by Major	00904-3992	Antidepressant
SL441 <> 505050	Tab, White, Trapezoidal, Scored, SL441 <> 50 50 50	Trazodone HCl 150 mg	Desyrel by Moore	00839-7507	Antidepressant
SL4415010OTRPZ	Tab, White, Trapezoidal, Scored, Compressed, SL 441 50/100 TRPZ	Trazodone HCl 150 mg	Desyrel by Sandoz	00781-1826	Antidepressant
SL451	Tab, White, Oblong	Ibuprofen 800 mg	Motrin by Sidmak		NSAID
SL454	Cap, Red	Ethchlorvynol 500 mg	Placidyl by Rosemont		Hypnotic; C IV
SL455	Cap, Green	Ethchlorvynol 750 mg	Placidyl by Rosemont		Hypnotic; C IV
SL456	Tab, Pale Blue, Round, Scored, SL over 456	Oxybutynin Chloride 5 mg	Ditropan by Sidmak	00182-1289 Discontinued	Urinary Tract
SL456	Tab, Pale Blue, Round, Scored, SL over 456	Oxybutynin Chloride 5 mg	Ditropan by Ivax		Urinary Tract
SL456	Tab, Pale Blue, Round, Scored, SL over 456	Oxybutynin Chloride 5 mg	Ditropan by Richmond	54738-0456	Urinary Tract
SL456	Tab, Pale Blue, Round, Scored, SL over 456	Oxybutynin Chloride 5 mg	Ditropan by Nat Pharmpak	55154-5537	Urinary Tract
SL456	Tab, Pale Blue, Round, Scored, SL over 456	Oxybutynin Chloride 5 mg	Ditropan by Baker Cummins	63171-1289	Urinary Tract
SL456	Tab, Pale Blue, Round, Scored, SL over 456	Oxybutynin Chloride 5 mg	Ditropan by Heartland	61392-0138	Urinary Tract
SL456	Tab, Pale Blue, Round, Scored, SL over 456	Oxybutynin Chloride 5 mg	Ditropan by Amerisource	62584-0815	Urinary Tract
SL456	Tab, Pale Blue, Round, Scored, SL over 456	Oxybutynin Chloride 5 mg	Ditropan by URL Mutual	00677-1255	Urinary Tract
SL456	Tab, Pale Blue, Round, Scored, SL over 456	Oxybutynin Chloride 5 mg	Ditropan by Vangard	00615-3512	Urinary Tract
SL456	Tab, Pale Blue, Round, Scored, SL over 456	Oxybutynin Chloride 5 mg	Ditropan by Qualitest	00603-4975	Urinary Tract
SL456	Tab, Pale Blue, Round, Scored, SL over 456	Oxybutynin Chloride 5 mg	Ditropan by Major	00904-2821	Urinary Tract
SL458	Tab, White, Oblong	Theophylline Anhydrous 300 mg	Theo-Dur by Sidmak	Discontinued	Antiasthmatic
SL459	Tab, White, Cap Shaped, Scored, Ex Release	Theophylline Anhydrous 300 mg	Theo-Dur by URL Mutual	00677-0817	Antiasthmatic
SL459	Tab, White, Cap Shaped, Scored, Ex Release	Theophylline Anhydrous 300 mg	Theo-Dur by Qualitest	00603-5946	Antiasthmatic
SL459	Tab, White, Cap Shaped, Scored, Ex Release	Theophylline Anhydrous 300 mg	Theo-Dur by Pharmedix	53002-0335	Antiasthmatic
SL459	Tab, White, Cap Shaped, Scored, Ex Release	Theophylline Anhydrous 300 mg	Theo-Dur by Warner Chilcott	00047-0592	Antiasthmatic

ID FRONT <> BACK	DESCRIPTION FRONT <> BACK	INGREDIENT & STRENGTH	BRAND (or Generic Equiv.) by FIRM	NDC#	CLASS; SCH.
SL459	Tab, White, Cap Shaped, Scored, Ex Release	Theophylline Anhydrous 300 mg	Theo-Dur by Dey LP	49502-0433	Antiasthmatic
SL459	Tab, White, Cap Shaped, Scored, Ex Release	Theophylline Anhydrous 300 mg	Theo-Dur by Heartland	61392-0017	Antiasthmatic
SL459	Tab, White, Cap Shaped, Scored, Ex Release	Theophylline Anhydrous 300 mg	Theo-Dur by Sandoz	00781-1005	Antiasthmatic
SL459	Tab, White, Cap Shaped, Scored, Ex Release	Theophylline Anhydrous 300 mg	Theo-Dur by Med Pro	53978-0320	Antiasthmatic
SL460	Tab, Green, Round	Clonidine HCl 0.1 mg	Catapres by Sidmak		Antihypertensive
SL461	Tab, Yellow, Round	Clonidine HCl 0.2 mg	Catapres by Sidmak		Antihypertensive
SL462	Tab, Blue, Round	Clonidine HCl 0.3 mg	Catapres by Sidmak		Antihypertensive
SL463	Tab, Pink, Round	Clonidine HCl 0.1 mg, Chlorthalidone 15 mg	Combipres by Sidmak		Antihypertensive; Diuretic
SL464	Tab, Blue, Round	Clonidine HCl 0.2 mg, Chlorthalidone 15 mg	Combipres by Sidmak		Antihypertensive; Diuretic
SL465	Tab, White, Round	Clonidine HCl 0.3 mg, Chlorthalidone 15 mg	Combipres by Sidmak		Antihypertensive; Diuretic
SL467	Tab, Orange, Round, Scored, SL over 467	Propranolol HCl 10 mg	Inderal by Qualitest	00603-5489	Antihypertensive
SL467	Tab, Orange, Round, Scored, SL over 467	Propranolol HCl 10 mg	Inderal by Vangard	00615-2561	Antihypertensive
SL467	Tab, Orange, Round, Scored, SL over 467	Propranolol HCl 10 mg	Inderal by Sandoz	00781-1344	Antihypertensive
SL467	Tab, Orange, Round, Scored, SL over 467	Propranolol HCl 10 mg	Inderal by Med Pro	53978-0034	Antihypertensive
SL467	Tab, Orange, Round, Scored, SL over 467	Propranolol HCl 10 mg	Inderal by Kaiser	62224-0224	Antihypertensive
SL467	Tab, Orange, Round, Scored, SL over 467	Propranolol HCl 10 mg	Inderal by Major	00904-0411	Antihypertensive
SL467	Tab, Orange, Round, Scored, SL over 467	Propranolol HCl 10 mg	Inderal by Baker Cummins	63171-1812	Antihypertensive
SL467	Tab, Orange, Round, Scored, SL over 467	Propranolol HCl 10 mg	Inderal by Richmond	54738-0467	Antihypertensive
SL467	Tab, Orange, Round, Scored, SL over 467	Propranolol HCl 10 mg	Inderal by Kaiser	00179-1088	Antihypertensive
SL467	Tab, Orange, Round, Scored, SL over 467	Propranolol HCl 10 mg	Inderal by Warner Chilcott	00047-0070	Antihypertensive
SL468	Tab, Blue, Round, Scored, SL over 468	Propranolol HCl 20 mg	Inderal by Baker Cummins	63171-1813	Antihypertensive
SL468	Tab, Blue, Round, Scored, SL over 468	Propranolol HCl 20 mg	Inderal by PDRX	55289-0233	Antihypertensive
SL468	Tab, Blue, Round, Scored, SL over 468	Propranolol HCl 20 mg	Inderal by Med Pro	53978-5014	Antihypertensive
SL468	Tab, Blue, Round, Scored, SL over 468	Propranolol HCl 20 mg	Inderal by Richmond	54738-0468	Antihypertensive
SL468	Tab, Blue, Round, Scored, SL over 468	Propranolol HCl 20 mg	Inderal by H J Harkins Co	52959-0212	Antihypertensive
SL468	Tab, Blue, Round, Scored, SL over 468	Propranolol HCl 20 mg	Inderal by Kaiser	00179-1089	Antihypertensive
SL468	Tab, Blue, Round, Scored, SL over 468	Propranolol HCl 20 mg	Inderal by Qualitest	00603-5490	Antihypertensive
SL468	Tab, Blue, Round, Scored, SL over 468	Propranolol HCl 20 mg	Inderal by Major	00904-0412	Antihypertensive
SL468	Tab, Blue, Round, Scored, SL over 468	Propranolol HCl 20 mg	Inderal by Kaiser	00179-1090	Antihypertensive
SL468	Tab, Blue, Round, Scored, SL over 468	Propranolol HCl 20 mg	Inderal by Kaiser	62224-0222	Antihypertensive
SL468	Tab, Blue, Round, Scored, SL over 468	Propranolol HCl 20 mg	Inderal by Sandoz	00781-1354	Antihypertensive
SL468	Tab, Blue, Round, Scored, SL over 468	Propranolol HCl 20 mg	Inderal by Warner Chilcott	00047-0071	Antihypertensive
SL469	Tab, Green, Round, Scored, SL over 469	Propranolol HCl 40 mg	Inderal by Warner Chilcott	00047-0072	Antihypertensive
SL469	Tab, Green, Round, Scored, SL over 469	Propranolol HCl 40 mg	Inderal by Baker Cummins	63171-1814	Antihypertensive
SL469	Tab, Green, Round, Scored, SL over 469	Propranolol HCl 40 mg	Inderal by Major	00904-0414	Antihypertensive
SL469	Tab, Green, Round, Scored, SL over 469	Propranolol HCl 40 mg	Inderal by Qualitest	00603-5491	Antihypertensive
SL469	Tab, Green, Round, Scored, SL over 469	Propranolol HCl 40 mg	Inderal by Sandoz	00781-1364	Antihypertensive
SL469	Tab, Green, Round, Scored, SL over 469	Propranolol HCl 40 mg	Inderal by Richmond	54738-0469	Antihypertensive
SL469	Tab, Green, Round, Scored, SL over 469	Propranolol HCl 40 mg	Inderal by Kaiser	62224-0339	Antihypertensive
SL470	Tab, Pink, Round, Scored, SL over 470	Propranolol HCl 60 mg	Inderal by Warner Chilcott	00047-0073	Antihypertensive
SL470	Tab, Pink, Round, Scored, SL over 470	Propranolol HCl 60 mg	Inderal by Richmond	54738-0470	Antihypertensive
SL470	Tab, Pink, Round, Scored, SL over 470	Propranolol HCl 60 mg	Inderal by Sidmak		Antihypertensive
SL470	Tab, Pink, Round, Scored, SL over 470	Propranolol HCl 60 mg	Inderal by Sandoz	00781-1374	Antihypertensive
SL470	Tab, Pink, Round, Scored, SL over 470	Propranolol HCl 60 mg	Inderal by Moore	00839-7117	Antihypertensive
SL470	Tab, Pink, Round, Scored, SL over 470	Propranolol HCl 60 mg	Inderal by Qualitest	00603-5492	Antihypertensive
SL471	Tab, Yellow, Round, Scored, SL over 471	Propranolol HCl 80 mg	Inderal by Baker Cummins	63171-1815	Antihypertensive
SL471	Tab, Yellow, Round, Scored, SL over 471	Propranolol HCl 80 mg	Inderal by Warner Chilcott	00047-0074	Antihypertensive
SL471	Tab, Yellow, Round, Scored, SL over 471	Propranolol HCl 80 mg	Inderal by Qualitest	00603-5493	Antihypertensive

ID FRONT <> BACK	DESCRIPTION FRONT <> BACK	INGREDIENT & STRENGTH	BRAND (or Generic Equiv.) by FIRM	NDC#	CLASS; SCH.
SL471	Tab, Yellow, Round, Scored, SL over 471	Propranolol HCl 80 mg	Inderal by Richmond	54738-0471	Antihypertensive
SL471	Tab, Yellow, Round, Scored, SL over 471	Propranolol HCl 80 mg	Inderal by Kaiser	00179-1091	Antihypertensive
SL471	Tab, Yellow, Round, Scored, SL over 471	Propranolol HCl 80 mg	Inderal by Sandoz	00781-1384	Antihypertensive
SL471	Tab, Yellow, Round, Scored, SL over 471	Propranolol HCl 80 mg	Inderal by Sidmak		Antihypertensive
SL471	Tab, Yellow, Round, Scored, SL over 471	Propranolol HCl 80 mg	Inderal by Kaiser	62224-0335	Antihypertensive
SL472	Tab	Propranolol HCl 90 mg	Inderal by Pliva	50111-0472	Antihypertensive
SL473	Tab, White, Round, Scored	Hydrochlorothiazide 25 mg, Propranolol HCl 40 mg	Inderide by Qualitest	00603-5503	Diuretic; Antihypertensive
SL474	Tab, White, Round, Scored	Hydrochlorothiazide 25 mg, Propranolol HCl 80 mg	Inderide by Ivax	00182-1834	Diuretic; Antihypertensive
SL474	Tab, White, Round, Scored	Hydrochlorothiazide 25 mg, Propranolol HCl 80 mg	Inderide by Qualitest	00603-5504	Diuretic; Antihypertensive
SL475	Tab, Film Coated	Methyldopa 125 mg	by Pliva	50111-0475	Antihypertensive
SL476	Tab, Film Coated	Methyldopa 250 mg	by Pliva	50111-0476	Antihypertensive
SL477	Tab, Film Coated	Methyldopa 500 mg	by Pliva	50111-0477	Antihypertensive
SL478	Tab, Brown, Round	Hydrochlorothiazide 15 mg, Methyldopa 250 mg	Aldoril by Sidmak		Diuretic; Antihypertensive
SL479	Tab, White, Round	Hydrochlorothiazide 25 mg, Methyldopa 250 mg	Aldoril by Sidmak		Diuretic; Antihypertensive
SL480	Tab, Brown, Oval	Hydrochlorothiazide 30 mg, Methyldopa 500 mg	Aldoril by Sidmak		Diuretic; Antihypertensive
SL481	Tab, White, Oval	Hydrochlorothiazide 50 mg, Methyldopa 500 mg	Aldoril by Sidmak		Diuretic; Antihypertensive
SL482	Tab, White, Oval, Scored, Ex Release	Theophylline Anhydrous 200 mg	Theo-Dur by Warner Chilcott	00047-0659	Antiasthmatic
SL482	Tab, White, Oval, Scored, Ex Release	Theophylline Anhydrous 200 mg	Theo-Dur by Heartland	61392-0016	Antiasthmatic
SL482	Tab, White, Oval, Scored, Ex Release	Theophylline Anhydrous 200 mg	Theo-Dur by Dey LP	49502-0432	Antiasthmatic
SL482	Tab, White, Oval, Scored, Ex Release	Theophylline Anhydrous 200 mg	Theo-Dur by Sandoz	00781-1004	Antiasthmatic
SL482	Tab, White, Oval, Scored, Ex Release	Theophylline Anhydrous 200 mg	Theo-Dur by Physician Total Care	54868-0028	Antiasthmatic
SL482	Tab, White, Oval, Scored, Ex Release	Theophylline Anhydrous 200 mg	Theo-Dur by Pharmedix	53002-0330	Antiasthmatic
SL482	Tab, White, Oval, Scored, Ex Release	Theophylline Anhydrous 200 mg	Theo-Dur by URL Mutual	00677-0846	Antiasthmatic
SL483	Tab, White, Round, Scored, Ex Release	Theophylline Anhydrous 100 mg	Theo-Dur by Sandoz	00781-1003	Antiasthmatic
SL483	Tab, White, Round, Scored, Ex Release	Theophylline Anhydrous 100 mg	Theo-Dur by Dey LP	49502-0431	Antiasthmatic
SL483	Tab, White, Round, Scored, Ex Release	Theophylline Anhydrous 100 mg	Theo-Dur by Warner Chilcott	00047-0657	Antiasthmatic
SL483	Tab, White, Round, Scored, Ex Release	Theophylline Anhydrous 100 mg	Theo-Dur by Qualitest	00603-5944	Antiasthmatic
SL484	Tab, Yellow, Round	Sulindac 150 mg	Clinoril by Sidmak		NSAID
SL485	Tab, Yellow, Round	Sulindac 200 mg	Clinoril by Sidmak		NSAID
SL486	Tab, Film Coated	Verapamil HCl 80 mg	by Qualitest	00603-6357	Antihypertensive
SL486	Tab, White, Round, Film Coated, Scored	Verapamil HCl 80 mg	Isoptin by Sidmak	Discontinued	Antihypertensive
SL486	Tab, Film Coated	Verapamil HCl 80 mg	by Warner Chilcott	00047-0328	Antihypertensive
SL487	Tab, White, Round, Film Coated, Scored	Verapamil HCl 120 mg	Isoptin by Sidmak	Discontinued	Antihypertensive
SL487	Tab, Film Coated	Verapamil HCl 120 mg	Verelan by Qualitest	00603-6358	Antihypertensive
SL487	Tab, Film Coated	Verapamil HCl 120 mg	by Warner Chilcott	00047-0329	Antihypertensive
SL488	Tab, Green, Oblong	Verapamil SR 240 mg	Isoptin SR by Sidmak	Discontinued	Antihypertensive
SL491	Tab, White, Round, Scored	Albuterol Sulfate 2 mg	Proventil by Pliva	50111-0491	Antiasthmatic
SL491	Tab	Albuterol Sulfate 2 mg	Proventil by Sandoz	00781-1671	Antiasthmatic
SL492	Tab, White, Round, Scored	Albuterol Sulfate 4 mg	Proventil by Pliva	50111-0492	Antiasthmatic
SL493	Tab, White, Oval, Controlled Release	Aspirin 800 mg	Aspirin by Sidmak		Analgesic
SL497	Tab, Yellow, Oblong	Fenoprofen Calcium 600 mg	Nalfon by Sidmak		NSAID
SL50	Tab, White and Yellow, Cap Shaped, Scored, SL / 50 <> Logo	Sertraline HCl 50 mg	Zoloft by Cobalt	16252-0534	Antidepressant
SL50	Cap, Yellow and White, Opaque, Black Ink, Cobalt Logo	Sertraline HCl 50 mg	Zoloft by Cobalt	Canadian DIN 02287404	Antidepressant
SL505	Tab, Yellow, Rectangular, Scored	Hydrochlorothiazide 50 mg, Triamterene 75 mg	Maxzide by Richmond	54738-0127	Diuretic; Antihypertensive
SL505	Tab, Yellow, Rectangular, Scored	Hydrochlorothiazide 50 mg, Triamterene 75 mg	Maxzide by Qualitest	00603-6182	Diuretic; Antihypertensive
SL506	Tab	Atenolol 50 mg	Tenormin by Pliva	50111-0506	Antihypertensive

ID FRONT <> BACK	DESCRIPTION FRONT <> BACK	INGREDIENT & STRENGTH	BRAND (or Generic Equiv.) by FIRM	NDC#	CLASS; SCH.
SL507	Tab	Atenolol 100 mg	Tenormin by Pliva	50111-0507	Antihypertensive
SL508	Tab	Atenolol 50 mg, Chlorthalidone 25 mg	Tenoretic by Pliva	50111-0508	Antihypertensive; Diuretic
SL509	Tab	Atenolol 100 mg, Chlorthalidone 25 mg	Tenoretic by Pliva	50111-0509	Antihypertensive; Diuretic
SL514	Tab, Blue & Yellow, Round	Meclizine HCl 50 mg	Antivert by Sidmak		Antiemetic
SL515	Tab, Sugar Coated, SL/515	Hydroxyzine HCl 100 mg	Atarax by Pliva	50111-0515	Antianxiety; Antihistamine
SL516	Tab, Film Coated, Debossed	Verapamil HCl 40 mg	by Qualitest	00603-6356	Antihypertensive
SL516	Tab, White, Round, Film Coated, Scored	Verapamil HCl 40 mg	Isoptin by Sidmak	Discontinued	Antihypertensive
SL517	Tab, Light Green, Round, SL over 517	Metoclopramide HCl 5 mg	Reglan by Moore	00839-7530	Gastrointestinal
SL517	Tab, Light Green, Round, SL over 517	Metoclopramide HCl 5 mg	Reglan by Sidmak		Gastrointestinal
SL517	Tab, Light Green, Round, SL over 517	Metoclopramide HCl 5 mg	Reglan by Sidmak	51285-0585	Gastrointestinal
SL517	Tab, Light Green, Round, SL over 517	Metoclopramide HCl 5 mg	Reglan by Richmond	54738-0517	Gastrointestinal
SL517	Tab, Light Green, Round, SL over 517	Metoclopramide HCl 5 mg	Reglan by Qualitest	00603-4616	Gastrointestinal
SL517	Tab, Light Green, Round, SL over 517	Metoclopramide HCl 5 mg	Reglan by Ivax	00182-1898	Gastrointestinal
SL517	Tab, Light Green, Round, SL over 517	Metoclopramide HCl 5 mg	Reglan by URL Mutual	00677-1323	Gastrointestinal
SL518	Tab, White, Cap Shaped, Ex Release, Scored	Theophylline Anhydrous 450 mg	Theo-Dur by Warner Chilcott	00047-0593	Antiasthmatic
SL518	Tab, White, Cap Shaped, Ex Release, Scored	Theophylline Anhydrous 450 mg	Theo-Dur by Ivax	00182-1941	Antiasthmatic
SL518	Tab, White, Cap Shaped, Ex Release, Scored	Theophylline Anhydrous 450 mg	Theo-Dur by Qualitest	00603-5747	Antiasthmatic
SL520	Tab, Orange, Oblong	Chlorpheniramine 8 mg, Phenylephrine 25 mg, Pyrilamine 25 mg	Rynatan by Sidmak		Cold Remedy
SL521	Tab, Pink, Oblong	Carbetapentane Tannate 60 mg, Chlorpheniramine Tannate 5 mg, Ephedrine Tannate 10 mg, Phenylephrine Tannate 10 mg	Rynatuss by Sidmak		Cold Remedy
SL522	Tab, Green, Oval, Film Coated, Scored	Guaifenesin 400 mg, Phenylpropanolamine HCl 75 mg	Entex LA by Ivax	50111-0522	Cold Remedy
SL523	Tab, Orange, Round, Film Coated, SL over 523	Protriptyline HCl 5 mg	by Ivax	00182-2643	Antidepressant
SL523	Tab, Orange, Round, Film Coated, SL over 523	Protriptyline HCl 5 mg	by Qualitest	00603-5531	Antidepressant
SL523	Tab, Orange, Round, Film Coated, SL over 523	Protriptyline HCl 5 mg	by Pliva	50111-0523	Antidepressant
SL524	Tab, Orange, Round, Film Coated, SL over 524	Protriptyline HCl 10 mg	by Ivax	00182-2644	Antidepressant
SL524	Tab, Orange, Round, Film Coated, SL over 524	Protriptyline HCl 10 mg	by Qualitest	00603-5532	Antidepressant
SL524	Tab, Orange, Round, Film Coated, SL over 524	Protriptyline HCl 10 mg	Vivactil by Pliva	50111-0524	Antidepressant
SL528	Tab, Yellow, Cap Shaped, Scored, Film Coated	Choline Magnesium Trisalicylate 500 mg	Trilisate by Sandoz	00781-1637	NSAID
SL528	Tab, Yellow, Cap Shaped, Scored, Film Coated	Choline Magnesium Trisalicylate 500 mg	Trilisate by Compumed	00403-0532	NSAID
SL528	Tab, Yellow, Cap Shaped, Scored, Film Coated	Choline Magnesium Trisalicylate 500 mg	Trilisate by Compumed	00403-0318	NSAID
SL528	Tab, Yellow, Cap Shaped, Scored, Film Coated	Choline Magnesium Trisalicylate 500 mg	Trilisate by URL Mutual	00677-1390	NSAID
SL528	Tab, Yellow, Cap Shaped, Scored, Film Coated	Choline Magnesium Trisalicylate 500 mg	Trilisate by Sidmak	Discontinued	NSAID
SL528	Tab, Yellow, Cap Shaped, Scored, Film Coated	Choline Magnesium Trisalicylate 500 mg	Trilisate by Kaiser	00179-1218	NSAID
SL528	Tab, Yellow, Cap Shaped, Scored, Film Coated	Choline Magnesium Trisalicylate 500 mg	Trilisate by Compumed	00403-0759	NSAID
SL529	Tab, Blue, Cap Shaped, Scored, Film Coated	Choline Magnesium Trisalicylate 750 mg	Trilisate by Sandoz	00781-1638	NSAID
SL529	Tab, Blue, Cap Shaped, Scored, Film Coated	Choline Magnesium Trisalicylate 750 mg	Trilisate by PDRX	55289-0282	NSAID
SL529	Tab, Blue, Cap Shaped, Scored, Film Coated	Choline Magnesium Trisalicylate 750 mg	Trilisate by Kaiser	00179-1219	NSAID
SL529	Tab, Blue, Cap Shaped, Scored, Film Coated	Choline Magnesium Trisalicylate 750 mg	Trilisate by Medirex	57480-0402	NSAID
SL529	Tab, Blue, Cap Shaped, Scored, Film Coated	Choline Magnesium Trisalicylate 750 mg	Trilisate by Heartland	61392-0181	NSAID
SL529	Tab, Blue, Cap Shaped, Scored, Film Coated	Choline Magnesium Trisalicylate 750 mg	Trilisate by URL Mutual	00677-1391	NSAID
SL529	Tab, Blue, Cap Shaped, Scored, Film Coated	Choline Magnesium Trisalicylate 750 mg	Trilisate by Sidmak	Discontinued	NSAID
SL530	Tab, Pink, Cap Shaped, Scored, Film Coated	Choline Magnesium Trisalicylate 1000 mg	Trilisate by Ivax	00182-2604	NSAID
SL530	Tab, Pink, Cap Shaped, Scored, Film Coated	Choline Magnesium Trisalicylate 1000 mg	Trilisate by Moore	00839-7619	NSAID
SL530	Tab, Pink, Cap Shaped, Scored, Film Coated	Choline Magnesium Trisalicylate 1000 mg	Trilisate by Sidmak	Discontinued	NSAID
SL534	Tab, Orange, Rectangular, Scored	Hydrochlorothiazide 25 mg, Triamterene 37.5 mg	Maxzide 25 by Ivax	00182-1903	Diuretic; Antihypertensive
SL534	Tab, Orange, Rectangular, Scored	Hydrochlorothiazide 25 mg, Triamterene 37.5 mg	Maxzide 25 by Richmond	54738-0117	Diuretic; Antihypertensive
SL534	Tab, Orange, Rectangular, Scored	Hydrochlorothiazide 25 mg, Triamterene 37.5 mg	Maxzide 25 by Major	00904-5281	Diuretic; Antihypertensive
SL534	Tab, Orange, Rectangular, Scored	Hydrochlorothiazide 25 mg, Triamterene 37.5 mg	Maxzide 25 by Sidmak		Diuretic; Antihypertensive
SL534	Tab, Orange, Rectangular, Scored	Hydrochlorothiazide 25 mg, Triamterene 37.5 mg	Maxzide 25 by Qualitest	00603-6180	Diuretic; Antihypertensive

ID FRONT <> BACK	DESCRIPTION FRONT <> BACK	INGREDIENT & STRENGTH	BRAND (or Generic Equiv.) by FIRM	NDC#	CLASS; SCH.
SL535	Tab, White, Oblong, Scored	Guaifenesin 600 mg	Robitussin by Eli Lilly	00110-4415	Expectorant
SL535	Tab, White, Oblong, Scored	Guaifenesin 600 mg	Robitussin by Pliva	50111-0535	Expectorant
SL535	Tab, White, Oblong, Scored	Guaifenesin 600 mg	Robitussin by Physician Total Care	54868-1778	Expectorant
SL549	Tab, Film Coated	Cimetidine HCl 200 mg	Tagamet by Pliva	50111-0549	Gastrointestinal
SL550	Tab, White, Black Print, Round, Film Coated, SL over 550	Cimetidine HCl 300 mg	Tagamet by ESI Lederle	59911-5550	Gastrointestinal
SL550	Tab, White, Black Print, Round, Film Coated, SL over 550	Cimetidine HCl 300 mg	Tagamet by Compumed	00403-1068	Gastrointestinal
SL550	Tab, White, Black Print, Round, Film Coated, SL over 550	Cimetidine HCl 300 mg	Tagamet by Sidmak		Gastrointestinal
SL551	Tab, White, Black Print, Cap Shaped, Scored, Film Coated, SL over 551	Cimetidine HCl 400 mg	Tagamet by Va Cmop	65243-0021	Gastrointestinal
SL551	Tab, White, Black Print, Cap Shaped, Scored, Film Coated, SL over 551	Cimetidine HCl 400 mg	Tagamet by ESI Lederle	59911-5551	Gastrointestinal
SL551	Tab, White, Black Print, Cap Shaped, Scored, Film Coated, SL over 551	Cimetidine HCl 400 mg	Tagamet by Dixon Shane	17236-0447	Gastrointestinal
SL551	Tab, White, Black Print, Cap Shaped, Scored, Film Coated, SL over 551	Cimetidine HCl 400 mg	Tagamet by Compumed	00403-1083	Gastrointestinal
SL552	Tab, White, Black Print, Cap Shaped, Scored, Film Coated, SL over 552	Cimetidine HCl 800 mg	Tagamet by Richmond	54738-0114	Gastrointestinal
SL552	Tab, White, Black Print, Cap Shaped, Scored, Film Coated, SL over 552	Cimetidine HCl 800 mg	Tagamet by ESI Lederle	59911-5552	Gastrointestinal
SL552	Tab, White, Black Print, Cap Shaped, Scored, Film Coated, SL over 552	Cimetidine HCl 800 mg	Tagamet by Compumed	00403-1091	Gastrointestinal
SL553	Tab	Atenolol 25 mg	Tenormin by Pliva	50111-0553	Antihypertensive
SL555	Tab	Naproxen 250 mg	Naprosyn by Pliva	50111-0555	NSAID
SL556	Tab	Naproxen 375 mg	Naprosyn by Pliva	50111-0556	NSAID
SL558	Tab, Film Coated	Naproxen 275 mg	Naprosyn by Pliva	50111-0558	NSAID
SL559	Tab, Film Coated	Naproxen 550 mg	Naprosyn by Pliva	50111-0559	NSAID
SL584	Tab	Glipizide 5 mg	by Pliva	50111-0584	Antidiabetic
SL585	Tab	Glipizide 10 mg	by Pliva	50111-0585	Antidiabetic
SL605	Tab, Coated, SL over 605	Flurbiprofen 50 mg	by Pliva	50111-0605	NSAID
SL606	Tab, Coated	Flurbiprofen 100 mg	by Pliva	50111-0606	NSAID
SL609	Tab, Yellow, Black Print, Cap Shaped, Film Coated, Ex Release	Pentoxifylline 400 mg	Trental by Pharmfab	62542-0743	Anticoagulant
SL614	Tab, Green, Oblong, Film Coated	Naproxen 375 mg	Naprosyn by Novopharm	43806-0397	NSAID
SL615	Tab, Green, Oblong, Film Coated	Naproxen 500 mg	Naprosyn by Novopharm	43806-0399	NSAID
SL621	Tab, White, Round, Scored	Ketoconazole 200 mg	Nizoral by Murfreesboro	51129-1595	Antifungal
SL648	Cap, White w/ Green Band on Cap Only, Opaque	Fluoxetine HCl 20 mg	Prozac by Sidmak		Antidepressant
SL66	Tab, Film Coated, SL/66	Amitriptyline HCl 10 mg	Elavil by Qualitest	00603-2212	Antidepressant
SL66	Tab, Film Coated	Amitriptyline HCl 10 mg	Elavil by H J Harkins Co	52959-0008	Antidepressant
SL66	Tab, Film Coated, SL/66	Amitriptyline HCl 10 mg	Elavil by Major		Antidepressant
SL66	Tab, Round, Film Coated	Amitriptyline HCl 10 mg	Elavil by Apothecon	59772-2592	Antidepressant
SL66	Tab, Pink, Round, Film Coated	Amitriptyline HCl 10 mg	Elavil by Ivax	00182-1018	Antidepressant
SL66 <> SL66	Tab, Coated	Amitriptyline HCl 10 mg	Elavil by Heartland	61392-0143	Antidepressant
SLFKJ10	Tab, Film Coated	Lithium Carbonate 450 mg	Eskalith by Physician Total Care	54868-2557	Antipsychotic
SLOWK	Tab, Light Orange, Round, Sugar Coated	Potassium Chloride 600 mg	Slow-K by Ciba	Canadian DIN 00074225	Electrolytes
SLOWMAG	Tab, White, Blue Print, Round, Enteric Coated	Elemental Magnesium 64 mg, Elemental Calcium 106 mg	Slow Mag by Purdue	67618-0107	Vitamin; Mineral
SLVSLV <> ACN2	Tab, White, Oblong, Scored	Perindopril Erbumine 2 mg	Aceon by Solvay	00032-1101	Antihypertensive
SLVSLV <> ACN4	Tab, Pink, Oblong, Scored	Perindopril Erbumine 4 mg	Aceon by RPR	00801-1102	Antihypertensive
SLVSLV <> ACN4	Tab, Pink, Oblong	Perindopril Erbumine 4 mg	Aceon by Solvay	00032-1102	Antihypertensive
SLVSLV <> ACN8	Tab, Orange, Oblong, Scored, SLV Score SLV<>ACN 8	Perindopril Erbumine 8 mg	Aceon by Pharmafab	62542-0790	Antihypertensive

ID FRONT <> BACK	DESCRIPTION FRONT <> BACK	INGREDIENT & STRENGTH	BRAND (or Generic Equiv.) by FIRM	NDC#	CLASS; SCH.
SLVSLV <> ACN8	Tab, Orange, Oblong, Scored, SLV Score SLV<>ACN 8	Perindopril Erbumine 8 mg	Aceon by RPR	00801-1103	Antihypertensive
SLVSLV <> ACN8	Tab, Orange, Oblong, Scored, SLV Score SLV<>ACN 8	Perindopril Erbumine 8 mg	Aceon by Solvay	00032-1103	Antihypertensive
SLX <> 102	Tab, White to Off-White, Oval, Scored	Sodium phosphate (Monobasic, monohydrate) 1.102 g, Sodium Phosphate (Dibasic, Anhydrous) 0.398 g	OsmoPrep by Salix	65649-0701	Gastrointestinal
SMP <> I	Tab, Coated	Sumatriptan Succinate 25 mg	Imitrex by GSK	00173-0460	Antimigraine
SMS	Cap	Acetaminophen 250 mg, Dextromethorphan HBr 10 mg, Guaifenesin 100 mg, Pseudoephedrine HCl 30 mg	Tylenol Cold by Warner Wellcome	Canadian	Cold Remedy
SNB <> NVR	Tab, Light Brown, Oval, Film-Coated	Aliskiren 300 mg, Valsartan 320 mg	Valturna by Novartis Consumer Health, Inc.	00078-0574	Antihypertensive
SOLI3NT	Tab, Tan, Round, Soli/3NT	Thyroid 194.4 mg	Nature Thyroid by Jones		Thyroid Hormone
SOLINT3	Tab, Soli/NT3	Thyroid 3 g	Parloid Thyroid Rn3 by JMI Canton	00252-3312	Thyroid Hormone
SOLVAY <> 1022	Tab, Sugar Coated	Esterified Estrogens 0.625 mg	by Apotheca	12634-0509	Hormone
SOLVAY <> 1472	Tab, Coated	Ascorbic Acid 70 mg, Calcium 200 mg, Cyanocobalamin 2.2 mcg, Folic Acid 1 mg, Iodine 175 mcg, Iron 65 mg, Magnesium 100 mg, Niacin 17 mg, Pyridoxine HCl 2.2 mg, Riboflavin 1.6 mg, Thiamine Mononitrate 1.5 mg, Vitamin A 3000 Units, Vitamin D 400 Units, Vitamin E 10 Units, Zinc 15 mg	Zenate by Leiner	59606-0497	Vitamin
SOLVAY <> 1472	Tab, Coated	Ascorbic Acid 70 mg, Calcium 200 mg, Cyanocobalamin 2.2 mcg, Folic Acid 1 mg, Iodine 175 mcg, Iron 65 mg, Magnesium 100 mg, Niacin 17 mg, Pyridoxine HCl 2.2 mg, Riboflavin 1.6 mg, Thiamine Mononitrate 1.5 mg, Vitamin A 3000 Units, Vitamin D 400 Units, Vitamin E 10 Units, Zinc 15 mg	Zenate by Solvay	00032-1472	Vitamin
SOLVAY <> 5044	Tab, Pink, Oval	Eprosartan 400 mg	Teveten by Solvay	Canadian DIN 02240432	Antihypertensive
SOLVAY <> 5044	Tab, Pink, Oval	Eprosartan 400 mg	Teveten by Biovail	64455-0130	Antihypertensive
SOLVAY <> 5046	Tab, White, Cap Shaped	Eprosartan 600 mg	Teveten by Biovail	64455-0131	Antihypertensive
SOLVAY <> 5046	Tab, White, Cap Shaped	Eprosartan 600 mg	Teveten by Solvay	Canadian DIN 02243942	Antihypertensive
SOLVAY <> 5046	Tab, White, Oblong	Eprosartan 600 mg	Teveten by Halsey		Antihypertensive
SOLVAY <> 5147	Tab, Butterscotch, Cap Shaped, Film Coated	Eprosartan 600 mg, Hydrochlorothiazide 12.5 mg	Teveten HCT by Solvay	Canadian DIN 02253631	Antihypertensive; Diuretic
SOLVAY <> 5147	Tab, Butterscotch, Cap Shaped, Film Coated	Eprosartan 600 mg, Hydrochlorothiazide 12.5 mg	Teveten HCT by Biovail	64455-0132	Antihypertensive; Diuretic
SOLVAY <> 5150	Tab, Brick Red, Cap Shaped, Film Coated	Eprosartan 600 mg, Hydrochlorothiazide 25 mg	Teveten HCT by Biovail	64455-0133	Antihypertensive; Diuretic
SOLVAY0840	Cap, Yellow	Acetaminophen 325 mg, Codeine Phosphate 16 mg, Phenylephrine 10 mg, Chlorpheniramine 2 mg	Colrex by Solvay		Analgesic; C III
SOLVAY1007	Tab	Medroxyprogesterone Acetate 10 mg	Curretab by Solvay	00032-1007	Hormone
SOLVAY1014	Tab, Blue, Black Print, Round, Sugar Coated, Solvay over 1014	Esterified Estrogens 0.3 mg	by Heartland	61392-0318	Hormone
SOLVAY1014	Tab, Blue, Black Print, Round, Sugar Coated, Solvay over 1014	Esterified Estrogens 0.3 mg	by Solvay	00032-1014	Hormone
SOLVAY1022	Tab, Yellow, Black Print, Round, Sugar Coated, Solvay over 1022	Esterified Estrogens 0.625 mg	by Amerisource	62584-0022	Hormone
SOLVAY1022	Tab, Yellow, Black Print, Round, Sugar Coated, Solvay over 1022	Esterified Estrogens 0.625 mg	by Solvay	00032-1022	Hormone
SOLVAY1023	Tab, Light Green, Cap Shaped, Sugar Coated	Esterified Estrogens 0.625 mg, Methyltestosterone 1.25 mg	Estratab HS by Solvay	00032-1023	Hormone
SOLVAY1023	Tab, Light Green, Cap Shaped, Sugar Coated	Esterified Estrogens 0.625 mg, Methyltestosterone 1.25 mg	by Physician Total Care	54868-3564	Hormone
SOLVAY1024	Tab, Red, Round	Esterified Estrogens 1.25 mg	Estratab by Solvay	00032-1024	Hormone
SOLVAY1025	Tab, Sugar Coated	Esterified Estrogens 2.5 mg	Estratab by Solvay	00032-1025	Hormone
SOLVAY1026	Tab, Dark Green, Cap Shaped, Sugar Coated	Esterified Estrogens 1.25 mg, Methyltestosterone 2.5 mg	by Nat Pharmpak	55154-6501	Hormone
SOLVAY1026	Tab, Dark Green, Cap Shaped, Sugar Coated	Esterified Estrogens 1.25 mg, Methyltestosterone 2.5 mg	Estratest by Solvay	00032-1026	Hormone
SOLVAY1026	Tab, Dark Green, Cap Shaped, Sugar Coated	Esterified Estrogens 1.25 mg, Methyltestosterone 2.5 mg	by Physician Total Care	54868-3565	Hormone

ID FRONT <> BACK	DESCRIPTION FRONT <> BACK	INGREDIENT & STRENGTH	BRAND (or Generic Equiv.) by FIRM	NDC#	CLASS; SCH.
SOLVAY1039	Tab, White & Blue Specks, Oblong	Chlorpheniramine Maleate 4 mg, Phenylephrine 10 mg, Phenylpropanolamine 50 mg, Pyrilamine Maleate 25 mg	Histalet Forte by Solvay		Cold Remedy
SOLVAY1050	Tab, White & Green Specks, Round	Pseudoephedrine HCl 120 mg, Guaifenesin 400 mg	Histalet X by Solvay		Cold Remedy
SOLVAY1082	Cap, Orange & Clear	Phendimetrazine Tartrate 105 mg	Melfiat-105 by Solvay		Anorexiant; C III
SOLVAY1088	Tab, Peach, Oblong	Hydrocodone Bitartrate 5 mg, Phenindamine 25 mg, Guaifenesin 200 mg	P-V-Tussin by Solvay		Analgesic; C III
SOLVAY1091	Tab, Peach, Oblong	Hydrocodone Bitartrate 5 mg, Pseudoephedrine HCl 60 mg	P-V-Tussin by Solvay		Analgesic; C III
SOLVAY1132	Tab, Yellow, Round	Hydralazine 25 mg, Reserpine 0.1 mg, Hydrochlorothiazide 15 mg	Unipres by Solvay		Antihypertensive; Diuretic
SOLVAY1146	Tab, Blue, Oblong	Prenatal Vitamin	Zenate by Solvay		Vitamin
SOLVAY1200	Cap, Brown & Clear	Pancreatin, Lipase, Protease, Amylase	Creon by Solvay		Gastrointestinal
SOLVAY1205	Cap, Red and Blue	Amylase 16,600 Units, Lipase 5000 Units, Protease 18,750 Units	Creon-5 by Solvay	Canadian DIN 02239007	Gastrointestinal
SOLVAY1205	Cap, Red and Blue	Amylase 16,600 Units, Lipase 5000 Units, Protease 18,750 Units	Creon-5 by Solvay	00032-1205	Gastrointestinal
SOLVAY1210	Cap, Brown & Clear, White Print, Solvay over 1210	Lipase 10,000 Units, Protease 37,500 Units, Amylase 33,200 Units	by Murfreesboro	51129-1671	Gastrointestinal
SOLVAY1210	Cap, Brown & Clear, White Print, Solvay over 1210	Amylase 33,200 Units, Lipase 10,000 Units, Protease 37,500 Units	Creon-10 by Solvay	00032-1210	Gastrointestinal
SOLVAY1210	Cap, Brown & Clear, White Print, Solvay over 1210	Amylase 33,200 Units, Lipase 10,000 Units, Protease 37,500 Units	Creon-10 by Solvay	Canadian DIN 02200104	Gastrointestinal
SOLVAY1216	Cap, Brown	Vitamin Combination	Vio-Bec by Solvay		Vitamin
SOLVAY1220	Cap, Brown & Clear, White Print, Solvay over 1220	Amylase 66,400 Units, Lipase 20,000 Units, Protease 75,000 Units	Creon-20 by Solvay	00032-1220	Gastrointestinal
SOLVAY1220	Cap, Brown & Clear, White Print, Solvay over 1220	Lipase 20,000 Units, Protease 75,000 Units, Amylase 66,400 Units	by Physician Total Care	54868-3475	Gastrointestinal
SOLVAY1220	Cap, Brown & Clear, White Print, Solvay over 1220	Amylase 66,400 Units, Lipase 20,000 Units, Protease 75,000 Units	Creon-20 by Solvay	Canadian DIN 02239008	Gastrointestinal
SOLVAY1225	Cap, Orange & Yellow	Pancreatin, Lipase, Protease, Amylase	Creon-25 by Solvay		Gastrointestinal
SOLVAY1611	Tab, Peach, Oval	Vitamin, Mineral Combination	Norlac RX by Solvay		Vitamin
SOLVAY2808	Tab	Prednisone 1 mg	Orasone by Solvay	00032-2808	Steroid
SOLVAY2810	Tab	Prednisone 5 mg	Orasone by Solvay	00032-2810	Steroid
SOLVAY2812	Tab	Prednisone 10 mg	Orasone by Solvay	00032-2812	Steroid
SOLVAY2814	Tab	Prednisone 20 mg	Orasone by Solvay	00032-2814	Steroid
SOLVAY2816	Tab, Coated	Prednisone 50 mg	Orasone by Solvay	00032-2816	Steroid
SOLVAY3205	Tab	Dexamethasone 0.5 mg	Dexone by Solvay	00032-3205	Steroid
SOLVAY3210	Tab	Dexamethasone 0.75 mg	Dexone by Solvay	00032-3210	Steroid
SOLVAY3215	Tab	Dexamethasone 1.5 mg	Dexone by Solvay	00032-3215	Steroid
SOLVAY3220	Tab	Dexamethasone 4 mg	Dexone by Solvay	00032-3220	Steroid
SOLVAY4020	Cap, Clear	Quinidine Sulfate 300 mg	Cin-Quin by Solvay		Antiarrhythmic
SOLVAY4028	Tab, White, Round	Quinidine Sulfate 200 mg	Cin-Quin by Solvay		Antiarrhythmic
SOLVAY4032	Tab, White, Round	Quinidine Sulfate 300 mg	Cin-Quin by Solvay		Antiarrhythmic
SOLVAY4120	Cap, Orange, Oval	Valproic Acid 250 mg	Depakene by Solvay		Anticonvulsant
SOLVAY4202	Tab, Film Coated	Fluvoxamine Maleate 25 mg	Luvox by Solvay	00032-4202	OCD
SOLVAY4205	Tab, Yellow, Oval, Scored, Film Coated, Solvay over 4205	Fluvoxamine Maleate 50 mg	Luvox by Heartland	61392-0849	OCD
SOLVAY4205	Tab, Yellow, Oval, Scored, Film Coated, Solvay over 4205	Fluvoxamine Maleate 50 mg	Luvox by Solvay	00032-4205	OCD
SOLVAY4205	Tab, Yellow, Oval, Scored, Film Coated, Solvay over 4205	Fluvoxamine Maleate 50 mg	Luvox by Pharm Util	60491-0810	OCD
SOLVAY4210	Tab, Brown, Oval, Scored, Film Coated, Solvay over 4210	Fluvoxamine Maleate 100 mg	Luvox by Solvay	00032-4210	OCD
SOLVAY4210	Tab, Brown, Oval, Scored, Film Coated, Solvay over 4210	Fluvoxamine Maleate 100 mg	Luvox by Pharm Util	60491-0811	OCD
SOLVAY4492	Tab, Light Red, Round, Film Coated, Solvay over 4492	Lithium Carbonate 300 mg	Lithobid by Solvay	00032-4492	Antipsychotic
SOLVAY7512	Cap, Light Pink to Peach, Red Print	Lithium Carbonate 300 mg	Eskalith by Solvay		Antipsychotic
SOLVAY7516	Tab, White, Round, Scored, Solvay over 7516	Lithium Carbonate 300 mg	Eskalith by Solvay	00032-7516	Antipsychotic
SOMA <> 37WALLACE2001	Tab, White, Round	Carisoprodol 350 mg	Soma by Nat Pharmpak	55154-4102	Muscle Relaxant

ID FRONT <> BACK	DESCRIPTION FRONT <> BACK	INGREDIENT & STRENGTH	BRAND (or Generic Equiv.) by FIRM	NDC#	CLASS; SCH.
SOMA <> 37WALLACE2001	Tab, White, Round	Carisoprodol 350 mg	Soma by Wallace	00037-2001	Muscle Relaxant
SOMA <> 37WALLACE2001	Tab, White, Round	Carisoprodol 350 mg	Soma by Caremark	00339-6143	Muscle Relaxant
SOMA <> 37WALLACE2001	Tab, White, Round	Carisoprodol 350 mg	Soma by Rightpac	65240-0738	Muscle Relaxant
SOMA <> 37WALLACE2001	Tab, White, Round	Carisoprodol 350 mg	Soma by Thrift Drug	59198-0361	Muscle Relaxant
SOMA <> 37WALLACE2001	Tab, White, Round	Carisoprodol 350 mg	Soma by Quality Care	60346-0149	Muscle Relaxant
SOMAC <> WALLACE2103	Tab, Yellow & Light Orange, Round	Aspirin 325 mg, Carisoprodol 200 mg	Soma Compound by Wallace	00037-2103	Analgesic; Muscle Relaxant
SOMACC <> WALLACE2403	Tab, White & Yellow, Oval	Aspirin 325 mg, Carisoprodol 200 mg, Codeine Phosphate 16 mg	Soma Compound w/ Codeine by Wallace	00037-2403	Analgesic; C III
SOMACC <> WALLACE2403	Tab, White & Yellow, Oval	Aspirin 325 mg, Carisoprodol 200 mg, Codeine Phosphate 16 mg	Soma Compound w/ Codeine by Pharmedix	53002-0124	Analgesic; C III
SORIATANE10MG	Cap, Brown and White	Acitretin 10 mg	Soriatane by Connetics	63032-0090	Dermatologic
SORIATANE10ROCHE	Cap, Brown & White, Black Print, Soriatane over 10 Roche	Acitretin 10 mg	Soriatane by Hoffmann La Roche	00004-0288	Dermatologic
SORIATANE10ROCHE	Cap, Brown & White, Black Print, Soriatane over 10 Roche	Acitretin 10 mg	Soriatane by Amerisource	62584-0075	Dermatologic
SORIATANE10ROCHE	Cap, Brown & White, Black Print, Soriatane over 10 Roche	Acitretin 10 mg	Soriatane by Hoffmann La Roche	00004-0213	Dermatologic
SORIATANE25MG	Cap, Brown and Yellow	Acitretin 25 mg	Soriatane by Connetics	63032-0091	Dermatologic
SORIATANE25ROCHE	Cap, Brown & Yellow, Black Print, Soriatane over 25 Roche	Acitretin 25 mg	Soriatane by Hoffmann La Roche	00004-0289	Dermatologic
SORIATANE25ROCHE	Cap, Brown & Yellow, Black Print, Soriatane over 25 Roche	Acitretin 25 mg	Soriatane by Amerisource	62584-0096	Dermatologic
SORIATANE25ROCHE	Cap, Brown & Yellow, Black Print, Soriatane over 25 Roche	Acitretin 25 mg	Soriatane by Hoffmann La Roche	00004-0214	Dermatologic
SOT120 <> APO	Tab, White to Off-White, Cap Shaped, APO <> SOT over 120	Sotalol HCl 120 mg	Betapace by Apotex	60505-0159	Antiarrhythmic
SOT160 <> APO	Tab, White to Off-White, Cap Shaped, APO <> SOT over 160	Sotalol HCl 160 mg	Betapace by Apotex	60505-0081	Antiarrhythmic
SOT240 <> APO	Tab, White to Off-White, Cap Shaped, APO <> SOT over 240	Sotalol HCl 240 mg	Betapace by Apotex	60505-0082	Antiarrhythmic
SOT80 <> APO	Tab, White to Off-White, Cap Shaped, APO <> SOT over 80	Sotalol HCl 80 mg	Betapace by Apotex	60505-0080	Antiarrhythmic
SOTACORBL160	Tab, Light Blue, Oblong, Sotacor/BL/160	Sotalol 160 mg	Sotacor by BMS	Canadian	Antiarrhythmic
SOTACORBL240	Tab, Light Blue, Oblong, Sotacor/BL/240	Sotalol 240 mg	Sotacor by BMS	Canadian	Antiarrhythmic
SOTACORBL80	Tab, Light Blue, Oblong, Sotacor/BL/80	Sotalol 80 mg	Sotacor by BMS	Canadian	Antiarrhythmic
SOTALOL <> PMS160	Tab, Pale Blue, Oblong, Scored	Sotalol HCl 160 mg	Sotacor by Pharmascience	Canadian DIN 02238327	Antiarrhythmic
SOTALOL <> PMS80	Tab, Pale Blue, Oblong, Scored	Sotalol HCl 80 mg	Sotacor by Pharmascience	Canadian DIN 02238326	Antiarrhythmic
SP <> 03	Tab, Yellow, Round	Aspirin 81 mg	Aspirin by Amneal	65162-0241	Analgesic
SP <> 100	Tab, Dark Yellow, Oval, Film Coated	Lacosamide 100 mg	Vimpat by Schwarz	00091-2478	Antiepileptic
SP <> 150	Tab, Salmon, Oval, Film Coated	Lacosamide 150 mg	Vimpat by Schwarz	00091-2479	Antiepileptic
SP <> 200	Tab, Blue, Oval, Film Coated	Lacosamide 200 mg	Vimpat by Schwarz	00091-2480	Antiepileptic
SP <> 3	Tab, Blue, Oval	Doxepin 3 mg	Silenor by Somaxon	42847-0103	Sedative/Hypnotic
SP <> 50	Tab, Pink, Oval, Film Coated	Lacosamide 50 mg	Vimpat by Schwarz	00091-2477	Antiepileptic
SP <> 500	Tab, Light Orange, Round, Scored, Film Coated	Methocarbamol 500 mg	Robaxin by Schwarz		Muscle Relaxant
SP <> 6	Tab, Green, Oval	Doxepin 6 mg	Silenor by Somaxon	42847-0106	Sedative/Hypnotic
SP <> 712	Tab, Yellow, Oval, Scored, Film Coated	Moexipril HCl 7.5 mg, Hydrochlorothiazide 12.5 mg	Uniretic by Schwarz	00091-3712	Antihypertensive; Diuretic
SP <> 720	Tab, White, Oval, Scored, Film Coated	Moexipril HCl 15 mg, Hydrochlorothiazide 12.5 mg	Uniretic by Schwarz	00091-3720	Antihypertensive; Diuretic
SP <> 725	Tab, Yellow, Oval, Scored, Film Coated	Moexipril HCl 15 mg, HCTZ 25 mg	Uniretic by Schwarz	51217-3725	Antihypertensive; Diuretic
SP <> 725	Tab, Yellow, Oval, Scored, Film Coated	Moexipril HCl 15 mg, Hydrochlorothiazide 25 mg	Uniretic by Schwarz	00091-3725	Antihypertensive; Diuretic
SP <> 750	Tab, Orange, Cap Shaped, Film Coated	Methocarbamol 750 mg	Robaxin by Schwarz		Muscle Relaxant
SP <> REGLAN5	Tab, Green, Oval	Metoclopramide 5 mg	Reglan by Schwarz	00091-6705	Gastrointestinal
SP <> ROBAXIN500	Tab, Light Orange, Round, Scored, Film Coated	Methocarbamol 500 mg	Robaxin by Schwarz	00091-7429	Muscle Relaxant

ID FRONT <> BACK	DESCRIPTION FRONT <> BACK	INGREDIENT & STRENGTH	BRAND (or Generic Equiv.) by FIRM	NDC#	CLASS; SCH.
SP <> ROBAXIN750	Tab, Orange, Cap Shaped, Film Coated	Methocarbamol 750 mg	Robaxin by Schwarz	00091-7449	Muscle Relaxant
SP006	Tab, Green, Hexagonal	Acetaminophen 300 mg, Chlorzoxazone 250 mg	Parafon Forte by Superpharm		Muscle Relaxant
SP01	Tab, White, Round	Furosemide 40 mg	Lasix by Superpharm		Diuretic
SP02	Tab, White, Oval	Furosemide 20 mg	Lasix by Superpharm		Diuretic
SP062	Tab, White, Round	Acetaminophen 300 mg, Codeine Phosphate 60 mg	Tylenol w/ Codeine by Superpharm		Analgesic; C III
SP063	Tab, White, Round	Acetaminophen 300 mg, Codeine Phosphate 30 mg	Tylenol w/ Codeine by Superpharm		Analgesic; C III
SP091	Tab, White, Round	Allopurinol 100 mg	Zyloprim by Superpharm		Antigout
SP092	Tab, Peach, Round	Allopurinol 300 mg	Zyloprim by Superpharm		Antigout
SP094	Tab, White, Round	Chlorpropamide 100 mg	Diabinese by Superpharm		Antidiabetic
SP095	Tab, White, Round	Chlorpropamide 250 mg	Diabinese by Superpharm		Antidiabetic
SP10 <> REGLAN	Tab, White, Cap Shaped, Scored	Metoclopramide 10 mg	Reglan by Schwarz	00091-6701	Gastrointestinal
SP100	Tab, Yellow, Round	Doxycycline Hyclate 100 mg	Vibramycin by Superpharm		Antibiotic
SP101	Cap, Blue & White	Doxycycline Hyclate 50 mg	Vibramycin by Superpharm		Antibiotic
SP102	Cap, Blue	Doxycycline Hyclate 100 mg	Vibramycin by Superpharm		Antibiotic
SP103	Tab, Peach, Round	Hydralazine 10 mg	Apresoline by Superpharm		Antihypertensive
SP104	Tab, Peach, Round	Hydralazine 25 mg	Apresoline by Superpharm		Antihypertensive
SP105	Tab, Peach, Round	Hydralazine 50 mg	Apresoline by Superpharm		Antihypertensive
SP106	Tab, Lavender, Round	Hydroxyzine HCl 10 mg	Atarax by Superpharm		Antianxiety; Antihistamine
SP107	Tab, Violet, Round	Hydroxyzine HCl 25 mg	Atarax by Superpharm		Antianxiety; Antihistamine
SP108	Tab, Purple, Round	Hydroxyzine HCl 50 mg	Atarax by Superpharm		Antianxiety; Antihistamine
SP109	Cap, Orange & Yellow	Tetracycline HCl 250 mg	Achromycin V by Superpharm		Antibiotic
SP110	Cap, Black & Yellow	Tetracycline HCl 500 mg	Achromycin V by Superpharm		Antibiotic
SP111	Tab, White, Round, Orally Disintegrating	Hyoscyamine Sulfate 0.125 mg	NuLev by Superpharm		Gastrointestinal
SP111	Tab, White, Round, Orally Disintegrating	Hyoscyamine Sulfate 0.125 mg	NuLev by Schwarz	00091-3111	Gastrointestinal
SP112	Tab, Pink, Round	Amitriptyline HCl 10 mg	Elavil by Superpharm		Antidepressant
SP113	Tab, Green, Round	Amitriptyline HCl 25 mg	Elavil by Superpharm		Antidepressant
SP114	Tab, Brown, Round	Amitriptyline HCl 50 mg	Elavil by Superpharm		Antidepressant
SP115	Tab, Purple, Round	Amitriptyline HCl 75 mg	Elavil by Superpharm		Antidepressant
SP116	Tab, Orange, Round	Amitriptyline HCl 100 mg	Elavil by Superpharm		Antidepressant
SP118	Cap, Dark Green & Light Green	Hydroxyzine Pamoate 25 mg	Vistaril by Sidmak		Antianxiety; Antihistamine
SP119	Cap, Dark Green & White	Hydroxyzine Pamoate 50 mg	Vistaril by Superpharm		Antianxiety; Antihistamine
SP120	Cap, Dark Green & Gray	Hydroxyzine Pamoate 100 mg	Vistaril by Superpharm		Antianxiety; Antihistamine
SP121	Tab, Salmon, Round	Prednisolone 5 mg	by Superpharm		Steroid
SP122	Tab, White, Round	Prednisone 5 mg	Deltasone by Superpharm		Steroid
SP123	Tab, White, Round	Prednisone 10 mg	Deltasone by Superpharm		Steroid
SP124	Tab, Peach, Round	Prednisone 20 mg	Deltasone by Superpharm		Steroid
SP126	Cap, Green & Yellow	Chlordiazepoxide 5 mg	Librium by Superpharm		Antianxiety; C IV
SP127	Cap, Black & Green	Chlordiazepoxide 10 mg	Librium by Superpharm		Antianxiety; C IV
SP128	Cap, Green & White	Chlordiazepoxide 25 mg	Librium by Superpharm		Antianxiety; C IV
SP129	Tab, Peach, Round	Hydrochlorothiazide 25 mg	Hydrodiuril by Superpharm		Diuretic; Antihypertensive
SP130	Tab, Peach, Round	Hydrochlorothiazide 50 mg	Hydrodiuril by Superpharm		Diuretic; Antihypertensive

ID FRONT <> BACK	DESCRIPTION FRONT <> BACK	INGREDIENT & STRENGTH	BRAND (or Generic Equiv.) by FIRM	NDC#	CLASS; SCH.
SP131	Tab, Peach, Round	Hydrochlorothiazide 100 mg	Hydrodiuril by Superpharm		Diuretic; Antihypertensive
SP132	Tab, White, Round	Quinidine Sulfate 200 mg	by Superpharm		Antiarrhythmic
SP136	Tab, Orange, Round	Thioridazine 10 mg	Mellaril by Superpharm		Antipsychotic
SP137	Tab, Orange, Round	Thioridazine 25 mg	Mellaril by Superpharm		Antipsychotic
SP138	Tab, Orange, Round	Thioridazine 50 mg	Mellaril by Superpharm		Antipsychotic
SP14	Tab, White, Round	Diazepam 2 mg	Valium by Superpharm		Antianxiety; C IV
SP140	Tab, White, Round	Quinidine Gluconate SR 324 mg	Quinaglute by Superpharm		Antiarrhythmic
SP141	Tab, White, Round	Atropine Sulfate 0.025 mg, Diphenoxylate HCl 2.5 mg	Lomotil by Superpharm		Antidiarrheal; C V
SP142	Cap, Clear & Pink	Diphenhydramine HCl 25 mg	Benadryl by Superpharm		Antihistamine
SP143	Cap, Pink	Diphenhydramine HCl 50 mg	Benadryl by Superpharm		Antihistamine
SP144	Tab, Blue & White, Oval	Meclizine HCl 12.5 mg	Antivert by Superpharm		Antiemetic
SP145	Tab, Yellow & White, Oval	Meclizine HCl 25 mg	Antivert by Superpharm		Antiemetic
SP146	Tab, White, Round	Sulfamethoxazole 400 mg, Trimethoprim 80 mg	Septra by Superpharm		Antibiotic
SP147	Tab, White, White	Sulfamethoxazole 800 mg, Trimethoprim DS 160 mg	Septra DS by Superpharm		Antibiotic
SP148	Tab, Yellow, Round	Sulfasalazine 500 mg	Azulfidine by Superpharm		Gastrointestinal
SP15	Tab, Yellow, Round	Diazepam 5 mg	Valium by Superpharm		Antianxiety; C IV
SP15 <> 715	Tab, Salmon, Round, Scored, Film Coated	Moexipril HCl 15 mg	Univasc by Schwarz	00091-3715	Antihypertensive
SP152	Cap, Green	Indomethacin 25 mg	Indocin by Superpharm		NSAID
SP153	Cap, Green	Indomethacin 50 mg	Indocin by Superpharm		NSAID
SP154	Tab, White, Round	Hydrochlorothiazide 25 mg, Spironolactone 25 mg	Aldactazide by Superpharm		Diuretic; Antihypertensive
SP16	Tab, Blue, Round	Diazepam 10 mg	Valium by Superpharm		Antianxiety; C IV
SP161	Tab, White, Round	Metoclopramide 10 mg	Reglan by Superpharm		Gastrointestinal
SP164	Cap, Blue & Scarlet	Disopyramide Phosphate 100 mg	Norpace by Superpharm		Antiarrhythmic
SP165	Cap, Buff & Scarlet	Disopyramide Phosphate 150 mg	Norpace by Superpharm		Antiarrhythmic
SP166	Tab, White, Round	Spironolactone 25 mg	Aldactone by Superpharm		Diuretic
SP170	Tab, White, Round	Ibuprofen 400 mg	Motrin by Superpharm		NSAID
SP171	Tab, White, Oval	Ibuprofen 600 mg	Motrin by Superpharm		NSAID
SP175	Tab, Pink, Oblong	Acetaminophen 650 mg, Propoxyphene Napsylate 100 mg	Darvocet-N 100 by Superpharm		Analgesic; C IV
SP181	Tab, White, Round	Lorazepam 0.5 mg	Ativan by Superpharm		Antianxiety; C IV
SP182	Tab, White, Round	Lorazepam 1 mg	Ativan by Superpharm		Antianxiety; C IV
SP183	Tab, White, Round	Lorazepam 2 mg	Ativan by Superpharm		Antianxiety; C IV
SP184	Cap, Blue & White	Flurazepam HCl 15 mg	Dalmane by Superpharm		Hypnotic; C IV
SP185	Cap, Blue	Flurazepam HCl 30 mg	Dalmane by Superpharm		Hypnotic; C IV
SP189	Tab, Orange, Round	Propranolol HCl 10 mg	Inderal by Superpharm		Antihypertensive
SP190	Tab, Blue, Round	Propranolol HCl 20 mg	Inderal by Superpharm		Antihypertensive
SP191	Tab, Green, Round	Propranolol HCl 40 mg	Inderal by Superpharm		Antihypertensive
SP192	Tab, Yellow, Round	Propranolol HCl 80 mg	Inderal by Superpharm		Antihypertensive
SP20	Tab, White, Round	Pseudoephedrine 60 mg	Sudafed by Superpharm		Decongestant
SP200MG	Cap, White, Opaque, Blue Ink	Ribavirin 200 mg	Pegetron by Schering	Canadian	Antiviral
SP2055 <> GUAIMAXD	Tab, White to Off-White, Cap Shaped, Scored	Guaifenesin 600 mg, Pseudoephedrine HCl 120 mg	Guaimax-D by Schwarz	00131-2055	Cold Remedy
SP2104 <> 5005	Tab, White, Oval, Scored	Acetaminophen 500 mg, Hydrocodone Bitartrate 5 mg	Co-Gesic by Schwarz	00131-2104	Analgesic; C III

ID FRONT <> BACK	DESCRIPTION FRONT <> BACK	INGREDIENT & STRENGTH	BRAND (or Generic Equiv.) by FIRM	NDC#	CLASS; SCH.
SP2164 <> 750MG	Tab, Pink, Oval, Scored, Film Coated	Salsalate 750 mg	Mono-Gesic by Schwarz	00131-2164	NSAID
SP22	Tab, Yellow, Cap Shaped, Scored	Penbutolol Sulfate 20 mg	Levatol by Schwarz	00091-4500	Antihypertensive
SP2200	Tab, Brown, Round, Film Coated	Polysaccharide Iron Complex 50 mg	Niferex Tablets by Ther-RX	00131-2200	Vitamin
SP2209 <> 13105	Tab, Blue, Oval, Film Coated	Calcium Carbonate 125 mg, Cyanocobalamin 3 mcg, Vitamin D 400 Units, Polysaccharide Iron Complex 60 mg, Folic Acid 1 mg, Niacinamide 10 mg, Pyridoxine HCl 1.64 mg, Riboflavin 3 mg, Sodium Ascorbate 50 mg, Thiamine Mononitrate 2.43 mg, Vitamin A 4000 Units, Zinc Sulfate 18 mg	Niferex PN by Schwarz	00131-2209	Vitamin; Mineral
SP23	Tab, Peach, Round	Chlorthalidone 25 mg	Hygroton by Superpharm		Diuretic
SP2309 <> 10	Tab, White, Cap Shaped, Film Coated, Scored	Ascorbic Acid, Calcium Carbonate, Cupric Oxide, Cyanocobalamin 12 mcg, Vitamin D, Polysaccharide Iron Complex, Folic Acid 1 mg, Magnesium Oxide, Niacinamide 20 mg, Potassium Iodide, Pyridoxine HCl, Riboflavin 3.4 mg, Thiamine Mononitrate, Vitamin A, Vitamin E Acetate, Zinc Sulfate	Niferex PN Forte by Ther-Rx	00131-2309	Vitamin
SP24	Tab, Blue, Round	Chlorthalidone 50 mg	Hygroton by Superpharm		Diuretic
SP26	Tab, White, Round	Methocarbamol 500 mg	Robaxin by Superpharm		Muscle Relaxant
SP27	Tab, White, Oblong	Methocarbamol 750 mg	Robaxin by Superpharm		Muscle Relaxant
SP321 <> 025	Tab, Yellow, Round, Scored, Orally Disintegrating, 0.25	Alprazolam 0.25 mg	Niravam by Schwarz	00091-3321	Antianxiety; C IV
SP322 <> 05	Tab, Yellow, Round, Scored, Orally Disintegrating, 05	Alprazolam 0.5 mg	Niravam by Schwarz	00091-3322	Antianxiety; C IV
SP323 <> 1	Tab, White, Round, Scored, Orally Disintegrating	Alprazolam 1 mg	Niravam by Schwarz	00091-3323	Antianxiety; C IV
SP324 <> 2	Tab, White, Round, Scored, Orally Disintegrating	Alprazolam 2 mg	Niravam by Schwarz	00091-3324	Antianxiety; C IV
SP341 <> 10100	Tab, Blue, Round, Scored, 10/100 <> SP over 341, Orally Disintegrating	Carbidopa 10 mg, Levodopa 100 mg	Parcopa by Schwarz	00091-3341	Antiparkinson
SP342 <> 25100	Tab, Yellow, Round, Scored, 25/100 <> SP over 342, Orally Disintegrating	Carbidopa 25 mg, Levodopa 100 mg	Parcopa by Schwarz	00091-3342	Antiparkinson
SP343 <> 25250	Tab, Blue, Round, Scored, 25/250 <> SP over 343, Orally Disintegrating	Carbidopa 25 mg, Levodopa 250 mg	Parcopa by Schwarz	00091-3343	Antiparkinson
SP351 <> 10	Tab, White, Round, Orally Disintegrating, SP above Score, 351 below	Baclofen 10 mg	Kemstro by Schwarz	00091-3351	Muscle Relaxant
SP352 <> 20	Tab, White, Round, Orally Disintegrating, SP above Score, 352 below	Baclofen 20 mg	Kemstro by Schwarz	00091-3352	Muscle Relaxant
SP38	Cap, Green	Hydralazine 25 mg, Hydrochlorothiazide 25 mg	Apresazide by Superpharm		Antihypertensive; Diuretic
SP39	Cap, Dark Green & Light Green	Hydralazine 50 mg, Hydrochlorothiazide 50 mg	Apresazide by Superpharm		Antihypertensive; Diuretic
SP41	Tab, White, Round	Cyproheptadine HCl 4 mg	Periactin by Superpharm		Antihistamine
SP4220	Cap, Clear & Orange, Opaque	Polysaccharide-Iron Complex 150 mg	Niferex-150 by Ther-Rx	00131-4220	Vitamin
SP43	Tab, White, Round	Dipyridamole 25 mg	Persantine by Superpharm		Antiplatelet
SP431	Tab, White, Round, Film Coated, Ex Release, Schering Logo over 431	Albuterol Sulfate 4 mg	Proventil by Amerisource	62584-0895	Antiasthmatic
SP431	Tab, White, Round, Film Coated, Ex Release, Schering Logo over 431	Albuterol Sulfate 4 mg	Proventil by Schering	00085-0431	Antiasthmatic
SP4330	Cap, Clear & Red, White Print, Opaque	Cyanocobalamin 25 mcg, Polysaccharide-Iron Complex 150 mg, Folic Acid 1 mg	Niferex-150 Forte by Ther-Rx	00131-4330	Vitamin
SP4330	Cap, Clear & Red, White Print, Opaque	Cyanocobalamin 25 mcg, Polysaccharide-Iron Complex 150 mg, Folic Acid 1 mg	Niferex-150 Forte by Physician Total Care	54868-2600	Vitamin
SP44	Tab, White, Round	Dipyridamole 50 mg	Persantine by Superpharm		Antiplatelet
SP45	Tab, White, Round	Dipyridamole 75 mg	Persantine by Superpharm		Antiplatelet
SP49	Tab, White, Round	Triprolidine 2.5 mg, Pseudoephedrine 60 mg	Actifed by Superpharm		Cold Remedy
SP52	Tab, Pink, Round	Isosorbide Dinitrate 5 mg	Isordil by Superpharm		Antianginal
SP53	Tab, White, Round	Isosorbide Dinitrate 10 mg	Isordil by Superpharm		Antianginal
SP538	Tab, Orange, Cap Shaped, Scored, Ex Release	Hyoscyamine Sulfate 0.375 mg	Levbid by Amerisource	62584-0019	Gastrointestinal

ID FRONT <> BACK	DESCRIPTION FRONT <> BACK	INGREDIENT & STRENGTH	BRAND (or Generic Equiv.) by FIRM	NDC#	CLASS; SCH.
SP538	Tab, Orange, Cap Shaped, Scored, Ex Release	Hyoscyamine Sulfate 0.375 mg	Levbid by Murfreesboro	51129-1490	Gastrointestinal
SP538	Tab, Light Orange, Cap Shaped, Scored, Ex Release	Hyoscyamine Sulfate 0.375 mg	Levbid by Eckerd	19458-0850	Gastrointestinal
SP538	Tab, Orange, Cap Shaped, Scored, Ex Release	Hyoscyamine Sulfate 0.375 mg	Levbid by Caremark	00339-5930	Gastrointestinal
SP538	Tab, Light Orange, Cap Shaped, Scored, Ex Release	Hyoscyamine Sulfate 0.375 mg	Levbid by Schwarz	00091-3538	Gastrointestinal
SP538	Tab, Orange, Cap Shaped, Scored, Ex Release	Hyoscyamine Sulfate 0.375 mg	Levbid by Nat Pharmpak	55154-0951	Gastrointestinal
SP538	Tab, Orange, Cap Shaped, Scored, Ex Release	Hyoscyamine Sulfate 0.375 mg	Levbid by Thrift Drug	59198-0321	Gastrointestinal
SP54	Tab, Green, Round	Isosorbide Dinitrate 20 mg	Isordil by Superpharm		Antianginal
SP57	Tab, White, Round	Tolazamide 250 mg	Tolinase by Superpharm		Antidiabetic
SP58	Tab, White, Round	Tolazamide 500 mg	Tolinase by Superpharm		Antidiabetic
SP62	Tab, White, Round	Acetaminophen 300 mg, Codeine Phosphate 60 mg	Tylenol w/ Codeine by Superpharm		Analgesic; C III
SP63	Tab, White, Round	Acetaminophen 300 mg, Codeine Phosphate 30 mg	Tylenol w/ Codeine by Superpharm		Analgesic; C III
SP64	Tab, White, Round	Acetaminophen 300 mg, Codeine Phosphate 15 mg	Tylenol w/ Codeine by Superpharm		Analgesic; C III
SP74	Cap, Clear & Green	Chlordiazepoxide 5 mg, Clidinium Bromide 2.5 mg	Librax by Superpharm		Gastrointestinal
SP75 <> 707	Tab, Pink, Round, Scored, Film Coated, SP 7.5	Moexipril HCl 7.5 mg	Univasc by Schwarz	00091-3707	Antihypertensive
SP78	Tab, White, Round	Ergoloid Mesylate 1 mg	Hygergine by Superpharm		Ergot Alkaloids
SP84	Tab, White, Round	Quinine Sulfate 260 mg	Quinamm by Superpharm		Antimalarial
SP89	Tab, White, Oval	Ergoloid Mesylate 1 mg	Hydergine by Superpharm		Ergot Alkaloids
SP90	Tab, White, Round	Ergoloid Mesylate 0.5 mg	Hydergine by Superpharm		Ergot Alkaloids
SP96	Tab, White, Round	Metronidazole 250 mg	Flagyl by Superpharm		Antibiotic
SP97	Tab, White, Round	Metronidazole 500 mg	Flagyl by Superpharm		Antibiotic
SP98	Tab, White, Round	Chlorthalidone 100 mg	Hygroton by Superpharm		Diuretic
SPD417SPD417100MG	Cap, Yellow and Bluish-Green, Opaque, White Ink, Shire Logo SPD417 100 mg, Extended Release	Carbamazepine 100 mg	Equetro by Shire	54092-0419	Anticonvulsant
SPD417SPD417200MG	Cap, Yellow and Blue, Opaque, White Ink, Shire Logo SPD417 200 mg, Extended Release	Carbamazepine 200 mg	Equetro by Shire	54092-0421	Anticonvulsant
SPD417SPD417300MG	Cap, Yellow and Blue, Opaque, White Ink, Shire Logo SPD417 300 mg, Extended Release	Carbamazepine 300 mg	Equetro by Shire	54092-0423	Anticonvulsant
SPI	Cap, Oval, Orange, Soft Gel	Lubiprostone 24 mcg	Amitiza by Sucampo	64764-0240	Gastrointestinal
SPI	Cap, Oval, Pink, Soft Gel	Lubiprostone 8 mcg	Amitiza by Sucampo	64764-0080	Gastrointestinal
SPIA5	Tab, White, Oblong	Acetaminophen 500 mg	Tylenol by Amneal	65162-0607	Analgesic
SPIKE	Tab, Yellow, Oval	SPIKE Formula 400 mg: T-MAX (Biotest proprietary thiamine di(2-methylpropionate) disulfide), Caffeine	Spike by BioTest Labs	Discontinued	Supplement
SPSP <> EUFLEX	Tab, Yellow, Round, Scored, SP logo	Flutamide 250 mg	Euflex by Schering	Canadian DIN 00637726	Antiandrogen
SQUARE	Tab, Off-White, Round, Debossed Modified Square, Orally Disintegrating	Rizatriptan Benzoate 10 mg	Maxalt-MLT by Merck	00006-3801	Antimigraine
SQUARE	Tab, White to Off-White, Round, Rapidly Disintegrating Peppermint Flavor	Rizatriptan 10 mg	Maxalt RPD 10 mg by Merck Frosst	Canadian DIN 02240519	Antimigraine
SQUIBB <> 138	Tab, White, Round, Scored	Sulfamethoxazole 400 mg, Trimethoprim 80 mg	by Mutual	53489-0145	Antibiotic
SQUIBB <> 138	Tab, White, Round, Scored	Sulfamethoxazole 400 mg, Trimethoprim 80 mg	SMZ TMP 400/80 by Apothecon	59772-0139	Antibiotic
SQUIBB <> 171	Tab, White, Oval Shaped, Scored	Sulfamethoxazole 800 mg, Trimethoprim 160 mg	SMZ TMP 800/160 by Apothecon	59772-0174	Antibiotic
SQUIBB <> 171	Tab, White, Oval Shaped, Scored	Sulfamethoxazole 800 mg, Trimethoprim 160 mg	by Mutual	53489-0146	Antibiotic
SQUIBB113	Cap, Blue & Orange, Squibb over 113	Cephradine 250 mg	Velosef by BMS	00003-0113	Antibiotic
SQUIBB113	Cap, Blue & Orange, Squibb over 113	Cephradine 250 mg	Velosef by BMS	55961-0113	Antibiotic
SQUIBB114	Cap, Blue, White Print, Squibb over 114	Cephradine 500 mg	Velosef by BMS	55961-0114	Antibiotic
SQUIBB114	Cap, Blue, White Print, Squibb over 114	Cephradine 500 mg	Velosef by BMS	00003-0114	Antibiotic

ID FRONT <> BACK	DESCRIPTION FRONT <> BACK	INGREDIENT & STRENGTH	BRAND (or Generic Equiv.) by FIRM	NDC#	CLASS; SCH.
SQUIBB138	Tab, White, Round	Sulfamethoxazole, Trimethoprim	Septra by BMS	00003-0138 Discontinued	Antibiotic
SQUIBB158M	Tab, White, Diamond	Fosinopril Sodium 10 mg	Monopril by BMS		Antihypertensive
SQUIBB160	Tab	Erythromycin Stearate 250 mg	Ethril by BMS		Antibiotic
SQUIBB161	Tab	Erythromycin Stearate 500 mg	Ethril by BMS		Antibiotic
SQUIBB164	Tab	Penicillin G Potassium 125 mg	Pentids by BMS		Antibiotic
SQUIBB165	Tab	Penicillin G Potassium 250 mg	Pentids 400 by BMS		Antibiotic
SQUIBB168	Tab	Penicillin G Potassium 500 mg	Pentids 800 by BMS		Antibiotic
SQUIBB171	Tab, White, Oval	Sulfamethoxazole, Trimethoprim	Septra by BMS	00003-0171 Discontinued	Antibiotic
SQUIBB178 <> 20	Tab, White, Round, Squibb over 178 <> 20	Pravastatin Sodium 20 mg	Pravachol by BMS	00003-0178	Antihyperlipidemic
SQUIBB178 <> 20	Tab, White, Round, Squibb over 178 <> 20	Pravastatin Sodium 20 mg	Pravachol by BMS	Canadian	Antihyperlipidemic
SQUIBB181	Cap, Red & Gray, Black Print, Squibb over 181	Cephalexin 250 mg	Keflex by Med Pro	53978-5020	Antibiotic
SQUIBB181	Cap, Red & Gray, Black Print, Squibb over 181	Cephalexin 250 mg	Keflex by BMS	00003-0749 Discontinued	Antibiotic
SQUIBB181	Cap, Red & Gray, Black Print, Squibb over 181	Cephalexin 250 mg	Keflex by BMS		Antibiotic
SQUIBB193	Tab	Amitriptyline 10 mg, Perphenazine 2 mg	Triavil by BMS	55961-0749	Antidepressant; Antipsychotic
SQUIBB19440	Tab, White, Round, Squibb 194/40	Pravastatin Sodium 40 mg	Pravachol by BMS		Antihyperlipidemic
SQUIBB195	Tab	Tolazamide 100 mg	Tolinase by BMS		Antidiabetic
SQUIBB202	Cap	Dicloxacillin Sodium 250 mg	Dynapen by BMS		Antibiotic
SQUIBB203	Cap	Dicloxacillin Sodium 500 mg	Dynapen by BMS		Antibiotic
SQUIBB207	Tab, Blue, Round	Nadolol 40 mg	Corgard by Princeton		Antihypertensive
SQUIBB208	Tab, Blue, Oblong	Nadolol 120 mg	Corgard by Princeton		Antihypertensive
SQUIBB211	Cap	Cloxacillin Sodium 250 mg	Tegopen by BMS		Antibiotic
SQUIBB212	Cap	Cloxacillin Sodium 500 mg	Tegopen by BMS		Antibiotic
SQUIBB230	Cap, Green	Amoxicillin 250 mg	Amoxil by BMS		Antibiotic
SQUIBB231	Cap, Green & Light Green	Amoxicillin 500 mg	Amoxil by BMS		Antibiotic
SQUIBB232	Tab, Blue, Round	Nadolol 20 mg	Corgard by Princeton		Antihypertensive
SQUIBB239	Cap, Red, Black Print, Squibb over 239	Cephalexin 500 mg	Keflex by BMS	55961-0874 Discontinued	Antibiotic
SQUIBB239	Cap, Red, Black Print, Squibb over 239	Cephalexin 500 mg	Keflex by BMS	00003-0874 Discontinued	Antibiotic
SQUIBB239	Cap, Red, Black Print, Squibb over 239	Cephalexin 500 mg	Keflex by Med Pro	53978-5021 Discontinued	Antibiotic
SQUIBB241	Tab, Blue, Round	Nadolol 80 mg	Corgard by Princeton		Antihypertensive
SQUIBB246	Tab, Blue, Oblong	Nadolol 160 mg	Corgard by Princeton		Antihypertensive
SQUIBB259	Tab	Amitriptyline 25 mg, Perphenazine 2 mg	Triavil by BMS		Antidepressant; Antipsychotic
SQUIBB267	Tab	Amitriptyline 10 mg, Perphenazine 4 mg	Triavil by BMS		Antidepressant; Antipsychotic
SQUIBB271	Tab	Amitriptyline 25 mg, Perphenazine 4 mg	Triavil by BMS		Antidepressant; Antipsychotic
SQUIBB277	Tab	Tolazamide 250 mg	Tolinase by BMS		Antidiabetic
SQUIBB279	Tab	Isosorbide Dinitrate SA 40 mg	Isordil by BMS		Antianginal

ID FRONT <> BACK	DESCRIPTION FRONT <> BACK	INGREDIENT & STRENGTH	BRAND (or Generic Equiv.) by FIRM	NDC#	CLASS; SCH.
SQUIBB283	Tab, White & Blue Specks, Round	Bendroflumethiazide 5 mg, Nadolol 40 mg	Corzide by Princeton		Diuretic; Antihypertensive
SQUIBB284	Tab, White & Blue Specks, Round	Bendroflumethiazide 5 mg, Nadolol 80 mg	Corzide by Princeton		Diuretic; Antihypertensive
SQUIBB286	Tab	Quinidine Gluconate 324 mg	Quinaglute by BMS		Antiarrhythmic
SQUIBB288	Tab, Round	Allopurinol 300 mg	Zyloprim by BMS		Antigout
SQUIBB429	Tab, White, Round, Scored, Squibb over 429	Fludrocortisone Acetate 0.1 mg	Florinef Acetate by Integrity	64731-0947	Steroid
SQUIBB429	Tab, White, Round, Scored, Squibb over 429	Fludrocortisone Acetate 0.1 mg	Florinef Acetate by King	00003-0429	Steroid
SQUIBB431	Tab, Yellow, Oblong	Procainamide HCl 250 mg	Pronestyl by Princeton		Antiarrhythmic
SQUIBB434	Tab, Gold, Oblong	Procainamide HCl 375 mg	Pronestyl by Princeton		Antiarrhythmic
SQUIBB438	Tab, Orange, Oblong	Procainamide HCl 500 mg	Pronestyl by Princeton		Antiarrhythmic
SQUIBB450	Tab, White, Oblong	Captopril 12.5 mg	Capoten by BMS		Antihypertensive
SQUIBB452	Tab	Captopril 25 mg	Capoten by Pharmedix	53002-0431	Antihypertensive
SQUIBB455	Cap, Squibb over 455	Ipodate Sodium 500 mg	by Banner Pharma	10888-1051	Diagnostic
SQUIBB457	Tab, Beige, Oval	Nystatin 100,000 Units	Mycostatin Vaginal by BMS		Antifungal
SQUIBB482	Tab, White, Oval	Captopril 50 mg	Capoten by BMS		Antihypertensive
SQUIBB485	Tab, White, Oval	Captopril 100 mg	Capoten by BMS		Antihypertensive
SQUIBB512	Tab	Triamcinolone 4 mg	Kenacort by BMS		Steroid
SQUIBB518	Tab	Triamcinolone 8 mg	Kenacort by BMS		Steroid
SQUIBB535	Tab, Pink, Cap Shaped, Black Print, Squibb over 535	Retinol 0.42 mg, Vitamin D 0.67 mg, Thiamine Mononitrate 3.3 mg, Riboflavin 3.3 mg, Pyridoxine HCl 3.3 mg, Niacinamide 33.3 mg, Calcium Pantothenate 11.7 mg, Vitamin E 5 mg, Copper 0.67 mg, Magnesium Carbonate 41.7 mg, Iron 66.7 mg, Cyanocobalamin 50 mcg, Folic Acid 0.33 mg, Vitamin C 100 mg	Theragran Hematinic by BMS	00003-0535	Vitamin; Mineral
SQUIBB537	Tab, White, Round	Niacin 500 mg	Niacin by BMS	00003-0537	Vitamin
SQUIBB573	Tab	Fluoxymesterone 5 mg	Ora-Testryl by BMS		Steroid; C III
SQUIBB580	Tab, Light Yellow to Light Brown, Film Coated	Nystatin 500,000 Units	Mycostatin by BMS	00003-0580	Antifungal
SQUIBB603	Tab, Pink, Black Print, Oval, Squibb over 603	Tetracycline HCl 500 mg	Sumycin 500 by Par	00003-0603	Antibiotic
SQUIBB606	Tab, Green, Round	Bendroflumethiazide 5 mg	Naturetin by Princeton		Diuretic; Antihypertensive
SQUIBB611	Tab, White, Round	Niacin 50 mg	Niacin by BMS	00003-0611 Discontinued	Vitamin
SQUIBB612	Tab, White, Round	Niacin 100 mg	Niacin by BMS	00003-0612 Discontinued	Vitamin
SQUIBB618	Tab, Peach, Round	Bendroflumethiazide 10 mg	Naturetin by Princeton		Diuretic; Antihypertensive
SQUIBB622	Cap	Meclofenamate Sodium 50 mg	Meclomen by BMS		NSAID
SQUIBB623	Cap	Chloral Hydrate 250 mg	Chloral Hydrate by BMS		Sedative/Hypnotic; C IV
SQUIBB626	Cap	Chloral Hydrate 500 mg	Chloral Hydrate by BMS		Sedative/Hypnotic; C IV
SQUIBB629	Cap	Meclofenamate Sodium 100 mg	Meclomen by BMS		NSAID
SQUIBB637	Tab	Isoniazid 100 mg	Laniazid by BMS		Antimycobacterial
SQUIBB647	Cap, White	Doxycycline Hyclate 50 mg	Vibramycin by BMS		Antibiotic
SQUIBB648	Tab, White, Oblong	Penicillin V Potassium 500 mg	Veetids by BMS		Antibiotic
SQUIBB655	Cap	Tetracycline HCl 250 mg	Sumycin 250 by Golden State	60429-0208 Discontinued	Antibiotic
SQUIBB655	Cap	Tetracycline HCl 250 mg	Sumycin 250 by Par	00003-0655 Discontinued	Antibiotic
SQUIBB655	Cap	Tetracycline HCl 250 mg	Sumycin 250 by Prepackage Specialists	58864-0493	Antibiotic

ID FRONT <> BACK	DESCRIPTION FRONT <> BACK	INGREDIENT & STRENGTH	BRAND (or Generic Equiv.) by FIRM	NDC#	CLASS; SCH.
SQUIBB655	Cap	Tetracycline HCl 250 mg	Sumycin 250 by Med Pro	53978-5048 Discontinued	Antibiotic
SQUIBB663	Tab, Light Pink	Tetracycline HCl 250 mg	Sumycin 250 by Par		Antibiotic
SQUIBB674	Cap	Doxycycline Hyclate 50 mg	Vibramycin by BMS	00003-0663	Antibiotic
SQUIBB684	Tab, Peach, Oblong	Penicillin V Potassium 250 mg	Veetids by BMS		Antibiotic
SQUIBB713	Tab, Red, Round	Rauwolfia Serpentina 50 mg	Raudixin by Princeton		Antihypertensive
SQUIBB723	Cap	Phenytoin 100 mg	by BMS		Anticonvulsant
SQUIBB726	Tab	Procainamide HCl SR 250 mg	Pronestyl by BMS		Antiarrhythmic
SQUIBB738	Cap	Temazepam 15 mg	Restoril by BMS		Sedative/Hypnotic; C IV
SQUIBB742	Tab	Procainamide HCl SR 500 mg	Pronestyl by BMS		Antiarrhythmic
SQUIBB747	Cap	Temazepam 30 mg	Restoril by BMS		Sedative/Hypnotic; C IV
SQUIBB749	Cap	Cephalexin 250 mg	Keflex by BMS		Antibiotic
SQUIBB756	Cap, White & Orange	Procainamide HCl 375 mg	Pronestyl by Princeton		Antiarrhythmic
SQUIBB757	Cap, Yellow & Orange	Procainamide HCl 500 mg	Pronestyl by Princeton		Antiarrhythmic
SQUIBB758	Cap, Yellow & Orange	Procainamide HCl 250 mg	Pronestyl by Princeton		Antiarrhythmic
SQUIBB763	Cap	Tetracycline HCl 500 mg	Sumycin 500 by Par	00003-0763 Discontinued	Antibiotic
SQUIBB763	Cap	Tetracycline HCl 500 mg	Sumycin 500 by Golden State		Antibiotic
SQUIBB769	Tab, Green, Round	Bendroflumethiazide 4 mg, Rauwolfia Serpentina 50 mg	Rauzide by Princeton	60429-0209	Antihypertensive, Diuretic
SQUIBB775	Tab, Yellow, Oval	Procainamide HCl SR 500 mg	Pronestyl-SR by Princeton		Antiarrhythmic
SQUIBB776	Tab, Red, Round	Rauwolfia Serpentina 100 mg	Raudixin by Princeton		Antihypertensive
SQUIBB777	Tab	Procainamide HCl SR 750 mg	Pronestyl by Princeton		Antiarrhythmic
SQUIBB779	Cap	Tetracycline 250 mg, Amphotericin B 50 mg	Mysteclin-F by BMS		Antibiotic
SQUIBB788	Tab, Round	Allopurinol 300 mg	Zyloprim by BMS		Antigout
SQUIBB812	Tab, Tan, Round	Doxycycline Hyclate 100 mg	Vibramycin by BMS		Antibiotic
SQUIBB830	Cap, Pink & Green	Hydroxyurea 500 mg	Hydrea by BMS		Antineoplastic
SQUIBB834	Tab	Multivitamin, Iron, Biotin	Theragran Stress by BMS		Vitamin
SQUIBB842	Tab	Multivitamin	Theragran by BMS		Vitamin
SQUIBB845	Tab, Round	Allopurinol 100 mg	Zyloprim by BMS		Antigout
SQUIBB849	Tab	Multivitamin, Minerals	Theragran M by BMS		Vitamin
SQUIBB863	Tab, Pink, Round	Fluphenazine HCl 1 mg	Prolixin by BMS		Antipsychotic
SQUIBB864	Tab, Yellow, Round	Fluphenazine HCl 2.5 mg	Prolixin by Princeton		Antipsychotic
SQUIBB874	Cap	Cephalexin 500 mg	Keflex by BMS		Antibiotic
SQUIBB877	Tab, Green, Round	Fluphenazine HCl 5 mg	Prolixin by Princeton		Antipsychotic
SQUIBB940	Cap, White	Doxycycline Hyclate 100 mg	Vibramycin by BMS		Antibiotic
SQUIBB956	Tab, Dark Pink, Round	Fluphenazine HCl 10 mg	Prolixin by Princeton		Antipsychotic
SQUIBB971	Cap, Gray	Ampicillin 250 mg	Principen by BMS		Antibiotic
SQUIBB974	Cap, Dark Gray & Gray	Ampicillin 500 mg	Principen by BMS		Antibiotic
SQUIBBUNILOG181	Cap, Swedish Orange, Squibb and Unilog 181, Swedish	Cephalexin	by BMS		Antibiotic
SQUIBBW028	Cap	Cloxacillin Sodium 250 mg	by Apothecon	59772-6028	Antibiotic
SQUIBBW038	Cap, Orange, Opaque, Squibb/W 038	Cloxacillin Sodium 500 mg	Tegopen by BMS		Antibiotic
SQUIBBW048	Cap, Blue	Dicloxacillin Sodium 250 mg	by DRX	55045-2727	Antibiotic

ID FRONT <> BACK	DESCRIPTION FRONT <> BACK	INGREDIENT & STRENGTH	BRAND (or Generic Equiv.) by FIRM	NDC#	CLASS; SCH.
SQUIBBW048	Cap, Blue, Black Print, Squibb over W048	Dicloxacillin Sodium 250 mg	Pathocil by Apothecon	59772-6048	Antibiotic
SQUIBBW048	Cap	Dicloxacillin Sodium 250 mg	by Golden State	60429-0059	Antibiotic
SQUIBBW058	Cap, Blue, Black Print, Squibb over W058	Dicloxacillin Sodium 500 mg	Pathocil by Apothecon	59772-6058	Antibiotic
SR <> NASABID	Tab, S/R <> Nasabid	Guaifenesin 600 mg, Pseudoephedrine HCl 90 mg	Nasabid Sr by Anabolic	00722-6356	Cold Remedy
SR <> NASABID	Tab, Yellow, Oval, Scored	Guaifenesin 600 mg, Pseudoephedrine HCl 90 mg	Nasabid Sr by Jones	52604-0600	Cold Remedy
SR089	Cap, Opaque Peach and Clear	Brompheniramine Maleate 10 mg, Pseudoephedrine HCl 120 mg	Histex SR by Pharmafab	62542-0125	Cold Remedy
SR089	Cap, Opaque Peach and Clear	Brompheniramine Maleate 10 mg, Pseudoephedrine HCl 120 mg	Histex SR by Teamm	67336-0089	Cold Remedy
SR100	Tab, Pink, Round, SR/100	Diclofenac Sodium 100 mg	Novo Difenac by Novopharm	Canadian	NSAID
SR100 <> N	Tab, Pink, Round, N <> SR / 100, Sustained Release	Diclofenac Potassium 100 mg	Voltaren by Novopharm	Canadian DIN 02048698	NSAID
SR100 <> P	Tab, Pink, Round, Sustained Release	Diclofenac Sodium 100 mg	Voltaren S.R. by Pharmascience	Canadian DIN 02231505	NSAID
SR100NOVO	Tab, White, Round, SR/100/Novo	Diclofenac Sodium 100 mg	Novo Difenac by Novopharm	Canadian	NSAID
SR120 <> CALAN	Tab, Light Violet, Oval, Film Coated	Verapamil HCl 120 mg	Calan SR by Searle	00025-1901	Antihypertensive
SR180 <> 7711	Tab, Film Coated	Verapamil 180 mg	Calan SR by Qualitest	06603-6359	Antihypertensive
SR180 <> CALAN	Tab, Light Pink, Oval, Scored, Film Coated	Verapamil HCl 180 mg	Calan SR by Nat Pharmpak	55154-3616	Antihypertensive
SR180 <> CALAN	Tab, Light Pink, Oval, Scored, Film Coated	Verapamil HCl 180 mg	Calan SR by Searle	00025-1911	Antihypertensive
SR180 <> KNOLL	Tab, Pink, Oval, Scored	Verapamil HCl 180 mg	Isoptin SR by Abbott	Canadian DIN 01934317	Antihypertensive
SR180 <> Z4286	Tab, Film Coated	Verapamil HCl 180 mg	Calan SR by Major	00904-7956	Antihypertensive
SR180 <> Z4286	Tab, Film Coated	Verapamil HCl 180 mg	Calan SR by Warner Chilcott	00047-0472	Antihypertensive
SR180 <> Z4286	Tab, Film Coated	Verapamil 180 mg	Calan SR by Qualitest	06603-6359	Antihypertensive
SR20 <> APO	Tab, White, Round, SR	Methylphenidate HCl 20 mg	Ritalin SR by Apotex	Canadian DIN 02266687	Stimulant; C II
SR200	Tab, White, Round	Theophylline Anhydrous 200 mg	Theolair SR by 3M	Canadian	Antiasthmatic
SR200	Tab, Yellow, Cap Shaped, Film Coated, Extended Release	Quetiapine Fumarate 200 mg	Seroquel XR by AstraZeneca	00310-0282	Antipsychotic
SR200 <> 3M	Tab, Ex Release	Theophylline Anhydrous 200 mg	Theolair SR by Urgent Care Center	50716-0505	Antiasthmatic
SR200 <> 3M	Tab, White, Round, Scored	Theophylline Anhydrous 200 mg	Theolair SR by 3M	00089-0341	Antiasthmatic
SR240 <> 7722	Tab, Film Coated	Verapamil HCl 240 mg	Calan SR by URL Mutual	00677-1453	Antihypertensive
SR240 <> 7722	Tab, Film Coated	Verapamil HCl 240 mg	Calan SR by Qualitest	06603-6360	Antihypertensive
SR240 <> 7722	Tab, Off White, Film Coated	Verapamil HCl 240 mg	Calan SR by DRX	55045-2321	Antihypertensive
SR240 <> CALAN	Tab, Light Green, Oblong, Scored, Film Coated	Verapamil HCl 240 mg	Calan SR by Med Pro	53978-0588	Antihypertensive
SR240 <> CALAN	Tab, Light Green, Oblong, Scored, Film Coated	Verapamil HCl 240 mg	Calan SR by Nat Pharmpak	55154-3615	Antihypertensive
SR240 <> CALAN	Tab, Light Green, Oblong, Scored, Film Coated	Verapamil HCl 240 mg	Calan SR by Rx Pak	65084-0141	Antihypertensive
SR240 <> CALAN	Tab, Light Green, Oblong, Scored, Film Coated	Verapamil HCl 240 mg	Calan SR by Searle	00014-1891	Antihypertensive
SR240 <> CALAN	Tab, Light Green, Oblong, Scored, Film Coated	Verapamil HCl 240 mg	Calan SR by Searle	00025-1891	Antihypertensive
SR240 <> CALAN	Tab, Light Green, Oblong, Scored, Film Coated	Verapamil HCl 240 mg	Calan SR by Teva	00480-0788	Antihypertensive
SR240 <> P	Tab, Light Green, Oblong, Scored	Verapamil HCl 240 mg	Isoptin by Pharmascience	Canadian DIN 02237791	Antihypertensive
SR240 <> Z4280	Tab, Film Coated	Verapamil HCl 240 mg	Calan SR by Warner Chilcott	00047-0474	Antihypertensive
SR240 <> Z4280	Tab, Film Coated	Verapamil HCl 240 mg	Calan SR by Med Pro	53978-2029	Antihypertensive
SR240 <> Z4280	Tab, Film Coated	Verapamil HCl 240 mg	Calan SR by Qualitest	06603-6360	Antihypertensive
SR240 <> Z4280	Tab, Film Coated	Verapamil HCl 240 mg	Calan SR by Major	00904-7957	Antihypertensive
SR240 <> Z4280	Tab, Film Coated	Verapamil HCl 240 mg	Calan SR by Moore	00839-7670	Antihypertensive
SR250 <> 3M	Tab, White, Round, Scored, SR over 250	Theophylline Anhydrous 250 mg	Theolair by 3M	Canadian	Antiasthmatic
SR250 <> 3M	Tab, White, Round, Scored, SR over 250	Theophylline Anhydrous 250 mg	Theolair SR by 3M	00089-0345	Antiasthmatic
SR300	Tab, White, Oval	Theophylline Anhydrous 300 mg	Theolair by 3M	Canadian	Antiasthmatic
SR300	Tab, Pale Yellow, Cap Shaped, Film Coated, Extended Release	Quetiapine Fumarate 300 mg	Seroquel XR by AstraZeneca	00310-0283	Antipsychotic
SR300 <> 3M	Tab, White, Oval, Scored	Theophylline Anhydrous 300 mg	Theolair SR by 3M	00089-0343	Antiasthmatic

ID FRONT <> BACK	DESCRIPTION FRONT <> BACK	INGREDIENT & STRENGTH	BRAND (or Generic Equiv.) by FIRM	NDC#	CLASS: SCH.
SR400	Tab, White, Cap Shaped, Film Coated, Extended Release	Quetiapine Fumarate 400 mg	Seroquel XR by AstraZeneca	00310-0284	Antipsychotic
SR500 <> 3M	Tab, White, Oblong, Scored	Theophylline Anhydrous 500 mg	Theolair by 3M	Canadian	Antiasthmatic
SR500 <> 3M	Tab, White, Oblong, Scored	Theophylline Anhydrous 500 mg	Theolair SR by 3M	00089-0347	Antiasthmatic
SR672	Tab, Ex Release	Hyoscyamine Sulfate 0.375 mg	Levsin by Sovereign	58716-0672	Gastrointestinal
SR672	Tab, Ex Release	Hyoscyamine Sulfate 0.375 mg	Levsin by ION	11808-0112 Discontinued	Gastrointestinal
SR75	Tab, Pink, Triangular, SR75	Diclofenac Sodium 75 mg	Novo Difenac by Novopharm	Canadian	NSAID
SR75 <> N	Tab, Light Pink, Triangle, N <> SR / 75, Sustained Release	Diclofenac Potassium 75 mg	Voltaren by Novopharm	Canadian DIN 02158582	NSAID
SR75 <> P	Tab, Pink, Triangle, Sustained Release	Diclofenac Sodium 75 mg	Voltaren S.R. by Pharmascience	Canadian DIN 02231504	NSAID
SR75 <> VOLTAREN	Tab, Light Pink, Triangular, Film Coated	Diclofenac Sodium 75 mg	Voltaren SR by Novartis	Canadian DIN 00782459	NSAID
SR75NOVO	Tab, White, Triangular, SR75/Novo	Diclofenac Sodium 75 mg	by Novopharm	Canadian	NSAID
SR80 <> DESPECSR	Tab, White, Scored	Pseudoephedrine HCl 800 mg, Guaifenesin 120 mg	Despec SR by Int'l Ethical Labs	11584-0442	Cold Remedy
SRM100 <> APO	Tab, Orange, Round, SR	Metoprolol Tartrate 100 mg	Lopresor SR by Apotex	Canadian DIN 02285169	Antihypertensive
SRM200 <> APO	Tab, Light Yellow, Round, SR	Metoprolol Tartrate 200 mg	Lopresor SR by Apotex	Canadian DIN 02285177	Antihypertensive
SRNASABID	Tab, Yellow, Oval, SR/Nasabid	Guaifenesin 600 mg, Pseudoephedrine HCl 60 mg	Nasabid SR by Jones		Cold Remedy
SS	Tab, Lavender, Oval, Scored	Acetaminophen 712.8 mg, Caffeine 60 mg, Dihydrocodeine Bitartrate 32mg	Zerlor by PamLab	18011-0032	Analgesic; C III
SS	Tab, Orange, Round, S/S	Sennosides 8.6 mg, Docusate Sodium 50 mg	Senokot-S by Purdue	Canadian	Gastrointestinal
S/S	Tab, Orange, Round, Film-Coated	Standardized Sennosides 8.6 mg, Docusate Sodium 50 mg	Senokot S by Purdue Pharma	Canadian DIN 00026123	Gastrointestinal
SS121	Tab, White, Round	Tiopronin 100 mg	Thiola by Mission		Urinary Tract
SSANDOZ7852	Tab, White, Round	Mephenytoin 100 mg	Mesantoin by Sandoz		Anticonvulsant
ST <> AA	Tab, Light Green, Cap Shaped, Scored, Film Coated, double Abbott Logo (aa)	Verapamil HCl 240 mg	Isoptin SR by Abbott	00074-1625	Antihypertensive
ST2243850	Cap, Purple and Yellow, ST-2	Proprietary Blend 198 mg (Kola Nut, 3 mg caffeine group alkaloids, Yerba Mate, Cassia Mimosoides Extract, White Willow Bark), Caffeine 200 mg, Tri-GuggLyptoid3 Complex 25 mg (Green Tea, < 1 mg caffeine group alkaloids, Guggulsterone, Gymmema)	Stacker-2 by NVE		Supplement
ST3243850	Cap, Blue & Pink, ST-3 <> 224 3850	Ephedra, White Willow Bark, Grapefruit, Kola Nut, Chitosan	Stacker 3 by NVE		Supplement
ST3EF2243850	Cap, Grey and Purple, ST-3EF <> 224 / 3850	Proprietary Blend 225 mg: (Kola Nut, Caffeine Group Alkaloids 4 mg, Cactus Extract 12:1, White Willow Bark, Grapefruit Extract, Chitosan), Caffeine 250 mg, Tri-Guarcinia3 Complex 25 mg (Green Tea, Caffeine Group Alkaloids, Guarana, Garcinia)	Stacker III by NVE		Supplement
ST3XPLC	Cap, Purple and Pink, White Ink	Proprietary Blend 195 mg: Yohimbine Alkaloids, Yerba Mate, Camellia Sinensis, Capsaicin; Caffeine 200 mg	Stacker 3 XPLC by NVE		Supplement
STAGESIC	Cap, Blue Ink	Acetaminophen 500 mg, Hydrocodone Bitartrate 5 mg	Vicodin by Huckaby	58407-0091	Analgesic; C III
STAHIST	Tab, STA/Hist	Atropine Sulfate 40 mcg, Chlorpheniramine Maleate 8 mg, Hyoscyamine Sulfate 190 mcg, Phenylephrine HCl 25 mg, Phenylpropanolamine HCl 50 mg, Scopolamine Hydrobromide 10 mcg	Stahist by Anabolic	00722-6243	Cold Remedy
STARDUST	Tab, White, Round, Star Symbol	3,4-Methylenedioxymethamphetamine (MDMA)	Ecstasy by Illegal		Euphoric; Illicit
STARLIX <> 120	Tab, Yellow, Oval	Nateglinide 120 mg	Starlix by Novartis	00078-0352	Antidiabetic
STARLIX <> 120	Tab, Yellow, Oval	Nateglinide 120 mg	Starlix by Novartis	Canadian DIN 02245439	Antidiabetic
STARLIX <> 180	Tab, Red, Oval, Film-Coated	Nateglinide 180 mg	Starlix by Novartis	Canadian DIN 02245440	Antidiabetic

Copyright © 2010 Ident-A-Drug (209) 472-2240 • May not be reproduced without permission • For updated data, go to www.IdentADrug.com

ID FRONT <> BACK	DESCRIPTION FRONT <> BACK	INGREDIENT & STRENGTH	BRAND (or Generic Equiv.) by FIRM	NDC#	CLASS; SCH.
STARLIX <> 60	Tab, Pink, Round	Nateglinide 60 mg	Starlix by Novartis	Canadian DIN 02245438	Antidiabetic
STARLIX <> 60	Tab, Pink, Round	Nateglinide 60 mg	Starlix by Novartis	00078-0351	Antidiabetic
STASON <> 1011	Tab, 10/11	Captopril 12.5 mg	Capoten by Stason	60763-1011	Antihypertensive
STASON <> 1012	Tab, Off-White, Diamond Shaped, Scored	Captopril 25 mg	Capoten by Stason	60763-1012	Antihypertensive
STASON <> 1013	Tab, White, Diamond Shaped, Stason <> 10/13	Captopril 50 mg	Capoten by Duramed	51285-0957	Antihypertensive
STASON <> 1013	Tab, White, Diamond, Scored	Captopril 50 mg	Capoten by Stason	60763-1013	Antihypertensive
STASON <> 1014	Tab, Oblong, Scored	Captopril 100 mg	Capoten by Stason	60763-1014	Antihypertensive
STASON <> 10X12	Tab, White, Diamond Shaped	Captopril 25 mg	Capoten by Duramed	51285-0956	Antihypertensive
STASON1020	Tab, Off-White, Round, Stason-1020	Selegiline 5 mg	Eldepryl by Stason	51285-0020	Antiparkinson
STDS911	Tab, White, Oval, S/T DS 911	Sulfamethoxazole 800 mg, Trimethoprim 160 mg	Septra DS by Lemmon		Antibiotic
STIEFELMINOCIN100	Cap, Orange and Purple, Opaque, White Ink	Minocycline HCl 100 mg	Minocin by Stiefel Canada Inc.	Canadian DIN 02173506	Antibiotic
STIEFELMINOCIN50	Cap, Orange, Opaque, White and Black Ink	Minocycline HCl 50 mg	Minocin by Stiefel Canada Inc.	Canadian DIN 02173514	Antibiotic
STJ	Tab, Round, Black Print, Peach, Enteric Coated	Aspirin 81 mg	Aspirin by McNeil		Analgesic
STSS <> 910	Tab, White, ST/SS, Round	Sulfamethoxazole 400 mg, Trimethoprim 80 mg	by Teva	Discontinued	Antibiotic
STUART021	Tab, Yellow, Oblong	Multivitamin, Multimineral combination	Stuartnatal 1+1 by Zeneca		Vitamin
STUART071	Tab, Pink, Oblong	Multivitamin, Multimineral combination	Stuart Prenatal by Zeneca		Vitamin
STUART380	Cap, Brown	Docusate Potassium 240 mg	Kasof by Zeneca		Laxative
STUART41	Tab, Film Coated	Amitriptyline HCl 50 mg	Elavil by Leiner	59606-0638	Antidepressant
STUART41	Tab, Film Coated	Amitriptyline HCl 50 mg	Elavil by Prestige	58056-0292	Antidepressant
STUART45	Tab, Film Coated	Amitriptyline HCl 25 mg	Elavil by Prestige	58056-0291	Antidepressant
STUART450	Tab, White, Round	Simethicone 40 mg	Mylicon by Zeneca		Antiflatulent
STUART455	Tab, Pink, Round	Simethicone 125 mg	Mylicon by Zeneca		Antiflatulent
STUART470	Cap, Pink	Docusate Potassium 100 mg	Dialose by Zeneca		Laxative
STUART475	Cap, Yellow	Docusate Potassium 100 mg, Casanthranol 30 mg	Dialose Plus by Zeneca		Laxative
STUART620	Tab, White & Yellow, Round	Aluminum 200 mg, Magnesium Hydroxide 200 mg, Simethicone 20 mg	Mylanta by Zeneca		Gastrointestinal
STUART650	Tab, Brown & Yellow, Round	Chewable Hematinic	Ferancee by Zeneca		Vitamin
STUART651	Tab, Green & White, Round	Aluminum 400 mg, Magnesium Hydroxide 400 mg, Simethicone 40 mg	Mylanta II by Zeneca		Gastrointestinal
STUART710	Tab, Orange, Round	Fluoride, Multivitamins	Mulvidren-F by Zeneca		Vitamin; Mineral
STUART858	Tab, Pink, Round	Simethicone 80 mg	Mylicon by Zeneca		Antiflatulent
STUART864	Tab, Yellow, Round	Buclizine HCl 50 mg	Bucladin-S Softab by Zeneca		Antiemetic
SU	Tab, Red, Round, Coated	Pseudoephedrine HCl 30 mg	Sudafed by Pfizer	00501-2850	Cold Remedy
SU24	Tab, White, Round, SU-24	Pseudoephedrine HCl 240 mg	Sudafed 24 Hr by Pfizer	00501-2790	Decongestant
SUCRALFATE <> P	Tab, White, Oblong, Scored	Sucralfate 1 g	Carafate by Pharmascience	Canadian DIN 02238209	Gastrointestinal
SUDAFED12HOUR	Cap, White	Pseudoephedrine 120 mg	Sudafed by Warner Wellcome	Canadian	Decongestant
SUDAFEDA7C	Cap, White, Sudafed/A7C	Acetaminophen 50 mg, Pseudoephedrine 60 mg,	Sudafed by Warner Wellcome	Canadian	Decongestant
SUDAFEDS7A	Tab, White, Biconvex	Pseudoephedrine 60 mg	Sudafed by Warner Wellcome	Canadian	Decongestant
SUDAFEDSINUS	Cap, Blue, Clear	Pseudoephedrine HCl 30 mg, Guaifenesin 200 mg	Sudafed Non-Drying Sinus by Pfizer	00501-2206	Cold Remedy
SUDAL60 <> AP	Tab, White, Cap Shaped, Scored	Guaifenesin 500 mg, Pseudoephedrine HCl 60 mg	Sudafed Sinus by Atley	59702-0060	Cold Remedy
SUDAL60 <> AP	Tab, White, Cap Shaped, Scored	Guaifenesin 500 mg, Pseudoephedrine HCl 60 mg	Sudafed Sinus by Anabolic	00722-6395	Cold Remedy
SUDAL60 <> AP	Tab, White, Cap Shaped, Scored	Guaifenesin 500 mg, Pseudoephedrine HCl 60 mg	Sudafed Sinus by Martec		Cold Remedy
SUDALDM <> AP	Tab, White, Oblong, Scored, Sudal DM <> A over P	Guaifenesin 500 mg, Dextromethorphan HBr 30 mg	Sudal DM by Martec		Cold Remedy
SUDALDM <> AP	Tab, White, Cap Shaped, Scored	Guaifenesin 500 mg, Dextromethorphan HBr 30 mg	Sudal DM by Atley	59702-0305	Cold Remedy

ID FRONT <> BACK	DESCRIPTION FRONT <> BACK	INGREDIENT & STRENGTH	BRAND (or Generic Equiv.) by FIRM	NDC#	CLASS; SCH.
SUDALSR <> AP	Tab, White, Cap Shaped, Scored	Pseudoephedrine HCl 50 mg, Guaifenesin 1200 mg	Cephadyn by Atley	59702-0050	Cold Remedy
SULCRATE <> HMR	Tab, White, Cap Shape	Sucralfate 1 g	Sulcrate by Axcan	Canadian DIN 02100622	Gastrointestinal
SULCRATEMMDC	Tab, White, Oblong, Sulcrate/MMDC	Sucralfate 1 g	by Aventis	Canadian	Gastrointestinal
SULFAMETHOXAZO <> TRIMETHOPRIM160	Tab	Sulfamethoxazole 800 mg, Trimethoprim 160 mg	by Moore	00839-6406	Antibiotic
SUM100 <> APO	Tab, Pink, Triangle Shaped	Sumatriptan Succinate 100 mg	Imitrex DF by Apotex	Canadian DIN 02268396	Antimigraine
SUM50 <> APO	Tab, White, Triangle Shaped	Sumatriptan Succinate 50 mg	Imitrex DF by Apotex	Canadian DIN 02268388	Antimigraine
SUPE <> WL89	Tab, Orange, Cap Shaped	Acetaminophen 325 mg, Dextromethorphan HBr 10 mg, Guaifenesin 100 mg, Phenylephrine HCl 5 mg	Sudafed PE Cold and Cough by Pfizer	00501-2909	Cold Remedy
SUPERMINI	Tab, Dark Brown, Round	Ephedra 250 mg	Super Mini by BDI	Discontinued	Supplement
SUPRAX <> LL200	Tab, White, Rectangular, Scored	Cefixime 200 mg	Suprax by Lederle	00005-3899	Antibiotic
SUPRAX <> LL400	Tab, White, Rectangular, Scored	Cefixime 400 mg	Suprax by PDRX	55289-0954	Antibiotic
SUPRAX <> LL400	Tab, White, Rectangular, Scored	Cefixime 400 mg	Suprax by Lederle	00005-3897	Antibiotic
SUPRAX <> LL400	Tab, White, Rectangular, Scored	Cefixime 400 mg	Suprax by Dept Health	53808-0062	Antibiotic
SUPRAX <> LL400	Tab, White, Rectangular, Scored	Cefixime 400 mg	Suprax by Physician Total Care	54868-1383	Antibiotic
SUPROPD	Cap, Orange & Opaque, Supro/PD	Gabapentin 400 mg	Neurontin by Parke Davis	Canadian	Anticonvulsant
SUPROPD	Cap, Opaque, Supro/PD	Gabapentin 100 mg	Neurontin by Parke Davis	Canadian	Anticonvulsant
SUPROPD	Cap, Yellow & Opaque, Supro/PD	Gabapentin 300 mg	Neurontin by Parke Davis	Canadian	Anticonvulsant
SURGAM200	Tab, White, Biconvex, Surgam/200	Tiaprofenic 200 mg	Surgam by Aventis	Canadian	NSAID
SURGAM300	Tab, White, Biconvex, Surgam/300	Tiaprofenic 300 mg	Surgam by Aventis	Canadian	NSAID
SURGAMSR	Cap, Pink & Maroon	Tiaprofenic 300 mg	Surgam by Aventis	Canadian	NSAID
SUSTIVA	Tab, Yellow, Cap Shaped, Film Coated	Efavirenz 600 mg	Sustiva by BMS	Canadian DIN 02246045	Antiviral
SUSTIVA	Tab, Yellow, Cap Shaped, Film Coated	Efavirenz 600 mg	Sustiva by BMS	00056-0510	Antiviral
SUSTIVA100MG	Cap, White	Efavirenz 100 mg	Sustiva by BMS	Canadian DIN 02239887	Antiviral
SUSTIVA100MG	Cap, White	Efavirenz 100 mg	Sustiva by BMS	00056-0473	Antiviral
SUSTIVA200MG	Cap, Gold	Efavirenz 200 mg	Sustiva by BMS	00056-0474	Antiviral
SUSTIVA200MG	Cap, Gold	Efavirenz 200 mg	Sustiva by BMS	Canadian DIN 02239888	Antiviral
SUSTIVA50MG	Cap, Gold & White	Efavirenz 50 mg	Sustiva by BMS	Canadian DIN 02239886	Antiviral
SUSTIVA50MG	Cap, Gold & White	Efavirenz 50 mg	Sustiva by BMS	00056-0470	Antiviral
SV	Cap, Peach	Progesterone 100 mg	Prometrium by West Pharm	52967-0290	Hormone
SV	Cap, Peach, Round	Progesterone 100 mg	Prometrium by Solvay	00032-1708	Hormone
SV	Cap, Cap Gelatin Coated	Progesterone 100 mg	Prometrium by RP Scherer	11014-0856	Hormone
SV	Cap, Peach	Progesterone 100 mg	Prometrium by Schering	00085-0869	Hormone
SV10	Tab, Pink, Round, SV10 <> Logo	Simvastatin 10 mg	Zocor by Cobalt	16252-0506	Antihyperlipidemic
SV10	Tab, Pink, Shield-Shaped, Cobalt Logo <> SV 10	Simvastatin 10 mg	Zocor by Cobalt	Canadian DIN 02248104	Antihyperlipidemic
SV2	Cap, Yellow	Progesterone 200 mg	Prometrium by RP Scherer	11014-1147	Hormone
SV2	Cap, Yellow	Progesterone 200 mg	Prometrium by Solvay	00032-1711	Hormone
SV20	Tab, Tan, Shield-Shaped, Cobalt Logo <> SV 20	Simvastatin 20 mg	Zocor by Cobalt	Canadian DIN 02248105	Antihyperlipidemic
SV20	Tab, Tan, Round, SV20 <> Logo	Simvastatin 20 mg	Zocor by Cobalt	16252-0507	Antihyperlipidemic
SV40	Tab, Pink, Round, SV40 <> Logo	Simvastatin 40 mg	Zocor by Cobalt	16252-0508	Antihyperlipidemic
SV40	Tab, Dark Pink, Shield-Shaped, Cobalt Logo <> SV 40	Simvastatin 40 mg	Zocor by Cobalt	Canadian DIN 02248106	Antihyperlipidemic

ID FRONT <> BACK	DESCRIPTION FRONT <> BACK	INGREDIENT & STRENGTH	BRAND (or Generic Equiv.) by FIRM	NDC#	CLASS; SCH.
SV5	Tab, Cream, Shield-Shaped, Cobalt Logo <> SV 5	Simvastatin 5 mg	Zocor by Cobalt	Canadian DIN 02248103	Antihyperlipidemic
SV5	Tab, Cream, Round, SV5 <> Logo	Simvastatin 5 mg	Zocor by Cobalt	16252-0505	Antihyperlipidemic
SV80	Tab, Pink, Cap Shaped, SV80 <> Logo	Simvastatin 80 mg	Zocor by Cobalt	16252-0509	Antihyperlipidemic
SV80	Tab, Pink, Cap-Shaped, Cobalt Logo <> SV 80	Simvastatin 80 mg	Zocor by Cobalt	Canadian DIN 02248107	Antihyperlipidemic
SW <> 200	Tab	Tiludronate Disodium 240 mg	Skelid by Sanofi Winthrop	53360-1800	Bisphosphonate
SW <> 200	Tab	Tiludronate Disodium 240 mg	Skelid by Sanofi	00024-1800	Bisphosphonate
SX	Tab, Pink, Round, Biconvex	Rifaximin 200 mg	Xifaxan by Salix	65649-0301	Antibiotic
SYC160	Tab, Light Blue, Oblong	Sotalol HCl 160 mg	Betapace by AltiMed	Canadian DIN 02084236	Antiarrhythmic
SYC80	Tab, Light Blue, Oblong	Sotalol HCl 80 mg	by AltiMed	Canadian DIN 02084228	Antiarrhythmic
SYCAMSYCAM	Tab, Peach, Diamond, Syc/AM/Syc-AM	Hydrochlorothiazide 50 mg, Amiloride 5 mg	by MSD	Canadian DIN 02174596	Diuretic; Antihypertensive
SYCB	Tab, White, Oval	Bromocriptine 2.5 mg	Parlodel by SynCare	Canadian	Antiparkinson
SYCB5MG	Cap, Caramel & White	Bromocriptine 5 mg	Parlodel by SynCare	Canadian	Antiparkinson
SYCBMZ15	Tab, White, Cylindrical, Syc-BMZ/1.5	Bromazepam 1.5 mg	Lectopam by AltiMed	Discontinued	Sedative; C IV
SYCBMZ3	Tab, Pink, Cylindrical, Syc-BMZ/3	Bromazepam 3 mg	Lectopam by AltiMed	Canadian	Sedative; C IV
SYCBMZ6	Tab, Green, Cylindrical, Syc-BMZ/6	Bromazepam 6 mg	Lectopam by AltiMed	Discontinued	Sedative; C IV
SYCC125	Tab, White, Oblong, Syc/C12.5	Captopril 12.5 mg	Capoten by SynCare	Canadian	Antihypertensive
SYCC25	Tab, White, Square, Syc/C25	Captopril 25 mg	Capoten by SynCare	Canadian	Antihypertensive
SYCCL05	Tab, Pale Peach, Cylindrical, Syc-CL 0.5	Clonazepam 0.5 mg	by AltiMed	Canadian DIN 02103656	Sedative; C IV
SYCCL05	Tab, Orange, Cylindrical, Syc-CL 0.5	Clonazepam 0.5 mg	by AltiMed	Canadian	Sedative; C IV
SYCCL2	Tab, White, Cylindrical, Syc-CL 2	Clonazepam 2 mg	by AltiMed	Canadian DIN 02103737	Sedative; C IV
SYCCY10	Tab, Yellow, D-Shaped, Syc/CY 10	Cyclobenzaprine HCl 10 mg	by AltiMed	Canadian DIN 02174618	Muscle Relaxant
SYCCYU10	Tab, White, Syc/CYu10	LL Aminocaproic Acid, A10 Aminocaproic Acid	by BMS	Discontinued Canadian	Hemostatic
SYCD30	Tab, Green, Syc-D30	Diltiazem HCl 30 mg	Cardizem by AltiMed	Canadian DIN 00088524	Antihypertensive
SYCD60	Tab, Yellow, Syc-D60	Diltiazem HCl 60 mg	Cardizem by AltiMed	Discontinued Canadian DIN 00088532	Antihypertensive
SYCN160	Tab, Blue, Oblong, Syc/N160	Nadolol 160 mg	by AltiMed	Discontinued Canadian	Antihypertensive
SYCN40	Tab, White, Round, Scored	Nadolol 40 mg	by AltiMed	Canadian DIN 00851663	Antihypertensive
SYCN40	Tab, Off-White, Round, Syc/N40	Nadolol 40 mg	by AltiMed	Canadian	Antihypertensive
SYCN80	Tab, White, Round, Syc/N80	Nadolol 80 mg	by AltiMed	Canadian	Antihypertensive
SYCT100	Tab, White, Round, Syc/T100	Trazodone HCl 100 mg	Desyrel by AltiMed	Canadian DIN 02053195	Antidepressant
SYCT50	Tab, Orange, Round, Syc/T50	Trazodone HCl 50 mg	Desyrel by AltiMed	Canadian DIN 02053187	Antidepressant
SYCT50	Tab, Orange, Round, Syc/T50	Trazodone HCl 50 mg	Desyrel by AltiMed	Canadian	Antidepressant

ID FRONT <> BACK	DESCRIPTION FRONT <> BACK	INGREDIENT & STRENGTH	BRAND (or Generic Equiv.) by FIRM	NDC#	CLASS; SCH.
SYCT75	Tab, Orange, Rectangular, Syc-T/75	Trazodone HCl 150 mg	Desyrel by AltiMed	Canadian DIN 02053209	Antidepressant
SYCTCP <> 250	Tab, White, Oval, Film Coated, Syc-TCP <> 250	Ticlopidine HCl 250 mg	by AltiMed	Canadian DIN 02194422	Anticoagulant
SYMAX <> DUOTAB	Tab, Purple and White, Cap-Shaped, Bilayered	Hyoscyamine Sulfate 0.125 mg IR, Hyoscyamine Sulfate 0.250 mg ER	Symax DuoTab by Capellon	64543-0118	Gastrointestinal
SYMAX <> FASTAB	Tab, Light Blue, Round	Hyoscyamine Sulfate 0.125 mg	Symax FasTab by Capellon	64543-0114	Gastrointestinal
SYMMETREL	Cap, Red, Softgel	Amantadine HCl 100 mg	Symmetrel by BMS	Canadian DIN 01914006	Antiviral
SYMMETREL	Tab, Light Orange, Triangular	Amantadine HCl 100 mg	Symmetrel by Endo	63481-0108	Antiviral
SYMMETREL	Tab, Light Orange, Triangular	Amantadine HCl 100 mg	Symmetrel by BMS	00056-0108	Antiviral
SYMMETREL- DUPONTPHARMA	Cap	Amantadine HCl 100 mg	Symmetrel by BMS	00056-0315	Antiviral
SYNCAREM2MIN50MG	Cap, Orange, SynCare M2/Min 50 mg	Minocycline HCl 50 mg	Minocin by AltiMed	Canadian	Antibiotic
SYNCAREM4MIN100MG	Cap, Orange & Purple, SynCare M4/Min 100 mg	Minocycline HCl 100 mg	Minocin by AltiMed	Canadian	Antibiotic
SYNCARESYC100	Tab, White, Oval, SynCare/Syc/100	Captopril 100 mg	Capoten by SynCare	Canadian	Antihypertensive
SYNCARESYC50	Tab, White, Oval, SynCare/Syc/50	Captopril 50 mg	Capoten by SynCare	Canadian	Antihypertensive
SYNCARESYCC100	Tab, White, Oval, Syncare/Syc/C100	Captopril 100 mg	Capoten by AltiMed	Canadian DIN 00851655	Antihypertensive
SYNCARESYCC50	Tab, White, Oval, SynCare/Syc/C50	Captopril 50 mg	Capoten by AltiMed	Canadian DIN 00851647	Antihypertensive
SYNCARESYCN160	Tab, Blue, Oblong, SynCare/Syc/N160	Nadolol 160 mg	by AltiMed	Canadian DIN 00851698	Antihypertensive
SYNCARESYCN80	Tab, Off-White, Round, SynCare/Syc/N80	Nadolol 80 mg	by AltiMed	Canadian DIN 00851671	Antihypertensive
SYNFLEX	Tab, Blue, Oval	Naproxen 275 mg	by AltiMed	Canadian DIN 00675369	NSAID
SYNFLEX DS	Tab, Blue, Oval	Naproxen 550 mg	by AltiMed	Canadian DIN 01900897	NSAID
SYNTEC	Tab, Blue, Round	Norethindrone 0.5 mg, Ethinyl Estradiol 35 mcg	Brevicon by Searle	Canadian	Oral Contraceptive
SYNTEX	Tab, Film Coated	Naproxen 275 mg	by Amerisource	62584-0274	NSAID
SYNTEX	Tab, Peach, Oblong	Naproxen 375 mg	Naprosyn by Roche	Canadian	NSAID
SYNTEX	Tab, Yellow, Oblong	Naproxen 500 mg	Naprosyn by Roche	Canadian	NSAID
SYNTEX <> 274	Tab, Film Coated	Naproxen 275 mg	by Allscripts		NSAID
SYNTEX <> ANAPROXDS	Tab, Anaprox DS, Film Coated	Naproxen 550 mg	by Quality Care	60346-0035 Discontinued	NSAID
SYNTEX <> NAPROXEN250	Tab	Naproxen 250 mg	by Pharmedix	53002-0324	NSAID
SYNTEX <> TORADOL	Tab, Red Print, Film Coated	Ketorolac Tromethamine 10 mg	Toradol by Quality Care	60346-0446	NSAID
SYNTEX1	Tab, White, Round	Mestranol 0.05 mg, Norethindrone 1 mg	Norinyl by Syntex		Oral Contraceptive
SYNTEX1110	Tab, Blue, Round	Norethindrone 0.5 mg, Ethinyl Estradiol 0.035 mg	Brevicon by Syntex		Oral Contraceptive
SYNTEX111	Tab, Green, Round	Norethindrone 1 mg, Ethinyl Estradiol 0.035 mg	Norinyl by Syntex		Oral Contraceptive
SYNTEX2440-CARDENESR30MG	Cap	Nicardipine HCl 30 mg	by Physician Total Care	54868-3817	Antihypertensive
SYNTEX272	Tab, Yellow, Round	Naproxen 250 mg	Naprosyn by Syntex		NSAID
SYNTEX273	Tab, Peach, Oblong	Naproxen 375 mg	Naprosyn by Syntex		NSAID
SYNTEX277	Tab, Yellow, Oblong	Naproxen 500 mg	Naprosyn by Syntex		NSAID
SYNTEX2902	Tab, White, Round	Oxymetholone 50 mg	Anadrol-50 by Syntex		Steroid; C III
SYNTEX3	Tab, Yellow, Round	Norethindrone 1 mg, Mestranol 0.08 mg	Norinyl by Syntex		Oral Contraceptive

ID FRONT <> BACK	DESCRIPTION FRONT <> BACK	INGREDIENT & STRENGTH	BRAND (or Generic Equiv.) by FIRM	NDC#	CLASS; SCH.
SYNTEX50	Tab, White, Round	Oxymetholone 50 mg	Anapolon by Syntex		Steroid; C III
SYNTEX50	Tab, White, Syntex/50	Oxymethelone 50 mg	Syntex by Roche	Canadian	Steroid; C III
SYNTEXBX	Tab, Blue, Circular, Syntex/BX	Norethindrone 0.5 mg, Ethinyl Estradiol 0.035 mg	by Searle	Canadian	Oral Contraceptive
SYNTHO <> 230	Tab, Light Blue, Cap Shaped, Film Coated	Esterified Estrogens 0.625 mg, Methyltestosterone 1.25 mg	Syntest H.S. by Breckenridge	66756-0230	Hormone
SYNTHO <> 230	Tab, Light Blue, Cap Shaped, Film Coated	Esterified Estrogens 0.625 mg, Methyltestosterone 1.25 mg	Syntest H.S. by Breckenridge	51991-0078	Hormone
SYNTHO <> 231	Tab, Light Green, Cap Shaped, Film Coated	Esterified Estrogens 1.25 mg, Methyltestosterone 2.5 mg	Syntest D.S. by Breckenridge	51991-0079	Hormone
SYNTHO <> 231	Tab, Light Green, Cap Shaped, Film Coated	Esterified Estrogens 1.25 mg, Methyltestosterone 2.5 mg	Syntest D.S. by Breckenridge	66756-0231	Hormone
SYNTHROID <> 100	Tab, Yellow, Round, Scored	Levothyroxine Sodium 100 mcg	Synthroid by Abbott	00074-6624	Thyroid Hormone
SYNTHROID <> 112	Tab, Pink, Round, Scored	Levothyroxine Sodium 112 mcg	Synthroid by Abbott	00074-9296	Thyroid Hormone
SYNTHROID <> 125	Tab, Brown, Round, Scored	Levothyroxine Sodium 125 mcg	Synthroid by Abbott	00074-7068	Thyroid Hormone
SYNTHROID <> 137	Tab, Turquoise-Blue, Round, Scored	Levothyroxine Sodium 137 mcg	Synthroid by Abbott	00074-3727	Thyroid Hormone
SYNTHROID <> 150	Tab, Blue, Round, Scored	Levothyroxine Sodium 150 mcg	Synthroid by Abbott	00074-7069	Thyroid Hormone
SYNTHROID <> 175	Tab, Purple, Round, Scored	Levothyroxine Sodium 175 mcg	Synthroid by Abbott	00074-7070	Thyroid Hormone
SYNTHROID <> 200	Tab, Pink, Round, Scored	Levothyroxine Sodium 200 mcg	Synthroid by Abbott	00074-7148	Thyroid Hormone
SYNTHROID <> 25	Tab, Orange, Round, Scored	Levothyroxine Sodium 25 mcg	Synthroid by Abbott	00074-4341	Thyroid Hormone
SYNTHROID <> 300	Tab, Green, Round, Scored	Levothyroxine Sodium 300 mcg	Synthroid by Abbott	00074-7149	Thyroid Hormone
SYNTHROID <> 50	Tab, White, Round, Scored	Levothyroxine Sodium 50 mcg	Synthroid by Abbott	00074-4552	Thyroid Hormone
SYNTHROID <> 75	Tab, Violet, Round, Scored	Levothyroxine Sodium 75 mcg	Synthroid by Abbott	00074-5182	Thyroid Hormone
SYNTHROID <> 88	Tab, Green, Round, Scored	Levothyroxine Sodium 88 mcg	Synthroid by Abbott	00074-6594	Thyroid Hormone
SZ <> 104	Tab, Round, Peach, Chewable	Cetirizine HCl 5 mg	Zyrtec by Sandoz	00781-5283	Antihistamine
SZ <> 106	Tab, Round, Peach, Chewable	Cetirizine HCl 10 mg	Zyrtec by Sandoz	00781-5284	Antihistamine
SZ <> 116	Tab, White, Oblong	Carvedilol 12.5 mg	Coreg by Sandoz	00781-5223	Antihypertensive
SZ <> 117	Tab, White, Oval	Carvedilol 25 mg	Coreg by Sandoz	00781-5224	Antihypertensive
SZ <> 327	Tab, Grayish Lavender, Oblong, Film Coated	Mycophenolate Mofetil 500 mg	CellCept by Sandoz	00781-5175	Immunosuppressant
SZ <> 61	Tab, White, Oval	Carvedilol 3.125 mg	Coreg by Sandoz	00781-5221	Antihypertensive
SZ <> 62	Tab, White, Oval	Carvedilol 6.25 mg	Coreg by Sandoz	00781-5222	Antihypertensive
SZ <> 780	Tab, White, Round, Sustained Release	Methylphenidate HCl 20 mg	Ritalin SR by Sandoz	00781-5754	Stimulant; C II
SZ <> 789	Tab, Pale Bluish Green, Round	Methylphenidate HC 10 mg	Ritalin by Sandoz	00781-5749	Stimulant; C II
SZ <> 789	Tab, Pale Bluish Green, Round	Methylphenidate HC 10 mg	Ritalin by Sandoz	00781-5749	Stimulant; C II
SZ <> 790	Tab, Light Yellow, Round	Methylphenidate HCl 20 mg	Ritalin by Sandoz	00781-5753	Stimulant; C II
SZ <> 905	Tab, Off White, Round, Film Coated	Cetirizine HCl 5 mg	Zyrtec by Sandoz	00781-1683	Antihistamine
SZ <> 906	Tab, Off White, Round, Film Coated	Cetirizine HCl 10 mg	Zyrtec by Sandoz	00781-1684	Antihistamine
SZ <> 996	Tab, Yellow, Round	Simvastatin 5 mg	Zocor by Sandoz	00781-5070	Antihyperlipidemic
SZ <> 997	Tab, Round, Light Pink	Simvastatin 10 mg	Zocor by Sandoz	00781-5071	Antihyperlipidemic
SZ286	Tab, White, Oval, Scored	Sulfamethoxazole 800 mg, Trimethoprim 160 mg	Bactrim/Septra by Sandoz	00185-0112	Antibiotic
SZ306	Tab, Dark Pink, Oblong	Simvastatin 80 mg	Zocor by Sandoz	00781-5074	Antihyperlipidemic
SZ465	Tab, White, Round, Scored	Nadolol 20 mg	Corgard by Sandoz	00781-1181	Antihypertensive
SZ466	Tab, White, Round, Scored	Nadolol 40 mg	Corgard by Sandoz	00781-1182	Antihypertensive
SZ467	Tab, White, Round, Scored	Nadolol 80 mg	Corgard by Sandoz	00781-1183	Antihypertensive
SZ912	Tab, Yellow, Round, Film Coated	Cetirizine 5 mg, Pseudoephedrine 120 mg	Zyrtec-D by Sandoz	00781-5285	Antihistamine; Decongestant
SZ998	Tab, Brown, Round	Simvastatin 20 mg	Zocor by Sandoz	00781-5072	Antihyperlipidemic
SZ999	Tab, Dark Pink, Round	Simvastatin 40 mg	Zocor by Sandoz	00781-5073	Antihyperlipidemic
T	Tab, Red, Round, Raised T Imprint	Aspirin 325 mg	Aspirin by Time Caps	49483-0060	Analgesic
T	Tab, Orange, Round, Enteric Coated, Raised T	Aspirin 325 mg	Ecotrin by Time Caps	49483-0052	Analgesic
T	Tab, Orange, Round	Aspirin 325 mg	Aspirin by Paddock	00574-0002	Analgesic
				Discontinued	
T	Tab, Orange, Round, Raised T	Aspirin 325 mg	Ecotrin by Rugby	00536-3313	Analgesic
T	Tab, Orange, Round	Potassium Bicarbonate 2500 mg	Efferv Potassium by Major	00904-2720	Electrolytes
T	Cap, Yellow, Round, Soft Gel	Benzonatate 100 mg	Tessalon by Major	00904-7737	Antitussive

ID FRONT <> BACK	DESCRIPTION FRONT <> BACK	INGREDIENT & STRENGTH	BRAND (or Generic Equiv.) by FIRM	NDC#	CLASS; SCH.
T	Tab, Effervescent	Potassium Bicarbonate 2500 mg	K Efferv Potassium by Qualitest	00603-4170	Electrolytes
T	Tab, Lime Green, Round, Effervescent	Potassium Bicarbonate 2500 mg	Efferv Potassium by Bajamar	44184-0024 Discontinued	Electrolytes
T	Tab, Orange, Round	Potassium Bicarbonate 2500 mg	Efferv Potassium by Tower	50201-2400	Electrolytes
T	Tab, Green, Round	Potassium Bicarbonate 2500 mg	Efferv Potassium by Tower	50201-2401	Electrolytes
T	Tab, Orange, Round	Potassium Bicarbonate 2500 mg	Efferv Potassium by Watson	00591-6035	Electrolytes
T	Tab, Red, Round, Raised T	Aspirin 325 mg	Aspirin by Rugby	00536-3318	Analgesic
T	Tab, Orange, Round	Iodinated Glycerol 30 mg	Organidin by Trinity		Expectorant
T	Tab, Orange, Round, Effervescent	Potassium Bicarbonate 2500 mg	Efferv Potassium by Bajamar	44184-0016 Canadian	Electrolytes
T	Tab, Lavender, Round	Acetaminophen 80 mg	Children's Tylenol by Mead Johnson	Canadian	Analgesic
T	Cap, Yellow, Round, Soft Gel	Benzonatate 100 mg	Tessalon by RP Scherer	11014-0732	Antitussive
T	Cap, Yellow, Round, Soft Gel	Benzonatate 100 mg	Tessalon by Ivax	00182-1080	Antitussive
T	Cap, Yellow, Round, Soft Gel	Benzonatate 100 mg	Tessalon by Forest	00456-0688	Antitussive
T	Tab, Orange, Round	Aspirin 325 mg	Aspirin by Sandoz	00781-1603	Analgesic
T	Tab, Red, Round, Raised T Imprint	Aspirin 325 mg	Aspirin by Ivax	00182-1415 Discontinued	Analgesic
T	Tab, Orange, Round, Raised T	Aspirin 325 mg	Ecotrin by Ivax	00182-0448 Discontinued	Analgesic
T	Tab, White to Off-White, Round, Scored	Terbinafine HCl 250 mg	Lamisil by Cobalt	Canadian DIN 02254727	Antifungal
T <> 061	Tab, Pink, Oblong, Line under 061	Diphenhydramine HCl 25 mg	Benadryl by Time Caps	49483-0061	Antihistamine
T <> 100MG	Tab, White, Yellow Imprint, Round, Film Coated, Ex Release	Carbamazepine 100 mg	Tegretol by Caremark	00339-6131	Anticonvulsant
T <> 100MG	Tab, White, Yellow Imprint, Round, Film Coated, Ex Release	Carbamazepine 100 mg	Tegretol by Novartis	00083-0061	Anticonvulsant
T <> 107	Tab, White, Round	Atenolol 25 mg	Tenormin by AstraZeneca	00310-0107	Antihypertensive
T <> 109	Tab	Carbamazepine 200 mg	Tegretol by Baker Cummins	63171-1233	Anticonvulsant
T <> 200MG	Tab, White, Pink Imprint, Round, Film Coated, Ex Release	Carbamazepine XR 200 mg	Tegretol XR by Novartis	00083-0062	Anticonvulsant
T <> 250	Tab, Pink, Round, Scored	Tinidazole 250 mg	Tindamax by BioComp	44523-0042	Antibiotic
T <> 35	Tab, Yellow, Round, Scored, 3 / 5, Stylized T	Phendimetrazine Tartrate 35 mg	Bontril by Mikart	46672-0138	Anorexiant; C III
T <> 400MG	Tab, Brown, Round, Film Coated, Ex Release	Carbamazepine 400 mg	Tegretol by Physician Total Care	54868-3862	Anticonvulsant
T <> 400MG	Tab, Brown, Round, Film Coated, Ex Release	Carbamazepine XR 400 mg	Tegretol XR by Novartis	00083-0060	Anticonvulsant
T <> 50	Tab, Light Yellow, Round	Topiramate 50 mg	Topamax by Pharmascience	Canadian DIN 02312085	Anticonvulsant
T <> ATL	Tab, Blue, _/ Shaped, Scored, Abbott Logo (aTL <> T)	Clorazepate Dipotassium 3.75 mg	Tranxene T-Tab by Ovation		Antianxiety; C IV
T <> ATM	Tab, Peach, _/ Shaped, Scored, Abbott Logo (aTM <> T)	Clorazepate Dipotassium 7.5 mg	Tranxene T-Tab by Med Pro	53978-3079	Antianxiety; C IV
T <> ATN	Tab, Lavender, _/ Shaped, Scored, Abbott Logo (aTN <> T)	Clorazepate Dipotassium 15 mg	Tranxene T-Tab by Ovation		Antianxiety; C IV
T <> OV31	Tab, Blue, _/ Shaped, Scored	Clorazepate Dipotassium 3.75 mg	Tranxene by Ovation	67386-0301	Antianxiety; C IV
T <> OV32	Tab, Peach, _/ Shaped, Scored	Clorazepate Dipotassium 7.5 mg	Tranxene by Ovation	67386-0302	Antianxiety; C IV
T <> OV33	Tab, Lavender, _/ Shaped, Scored	Clorazepate Dipotassium 15 mg	Tranxene by Ovation	67386-0303	Antianxiety; C IV
T013	Tab, White, Round, Scored, T over 013	Hyoscyamine Sulfate 0.125 mg	Levsin by Murfreesboro	51129-1498	Gastrointestinal
T024	Tab, White, Round, Scored, T over 024	Colchicine 0.6 mg	by Dixon Shane	17236-0635	Antigout
T024	Tab	Colchicine 0.6 mg	by Major	00904-2047	Antigout
T024	Tab, Yellow, Round	Colchicine 0.6 mg	by Qualitest	00603-3052	Antigout
T024	Tab, White, Round	Colchicine 0.6 mg	by DRX	55045-2420	Antigout
T03	Tab, Greenish White	Hyoscyamine Sulfate 0.125 mg	Levsin by Ivax	00182-2603	Gastrointestinal
T03	Tab, Green, Round, Scored, T over 03	Hyoscyamine Sulfate 0.125 mg	Levsin by Murfreesboro	51129-1499	Gastrointestinal
T03	Tab, Pale Blue, Round	Hyoscyamine Sulfate 0.125 mg	Levsin by Trinity		Gastrointestinal
T04	Tab, Light Blue, T/04	Hyoscyamine Sulfate 0.15 mg	Levsin by Shire	58521-0295	Gastrointestinal
T04	Tab, Blue, Round, Scored	Hyoscyamine Sulfate 0.15 mg	Levsin by Murfreesboro	51129-1497	Gastrointestinal
T04	Tab, Blue, Round	Meperidine HCl 50 mg	Cytospaz by Trinity		Analgesic; C II

ID FRONT <> BACK	DESCRIPTION FRONT <> BACK	INGREDIENT & STRENGTH	BRAND (or Generic Equiv.) by FIRM	NDC#	CLASS; SCH.
T05	Tab, White, Round	Yohimbine HCl 5.4 mg	Yocon by Trinity		Impotence Agent
T0R <> ORGANON	Tab, Light Yellow, Round, Coated, "0" set below T & R	Desogestrel 0.100 mg, Ethinyl Estradiol 0.025 mg	Linessa 28 by Organon	Canadian DIN 02257238	Oral Contraceptive
T0R <> ORGANON	Tab, Light Yellow, Round, Coated, "0" set below T & R	Desogestrel 0.100 mg, Ethinyl Estradiol 0.025 mg	Linessa 21 by Organon	Canadian DIN 02272903	Oral Contraceptive
T1 <> APO	Tab, White, Round	Terazosin HCl 1 mg	Terazosin by Apotex	Canadian DIN 02234502	Antihypertensive
T1 <> LL	Tab, Dark Red, Coated	Ascorbic Acid 600 mg, Cobalamin Concentrate 25 mcg, Docusate Sodium 50 mg, Ferrous Fumarate 350 mg, Folic Acid 1 mg, Intrinsic Factor 75 mg, Tocopheryl Succinate 30 Units	Trihemic 600 by Lederle	00005-4590	Vitamin
T1 <> NU	Tab, White, Round	Terazosin HCl 1 mg	by Nu Pharm	Canadian DIN 02233047	Antihypertensive
T1 <> P	Tab, White, Oblong	Tryptophan 1 g	Tryptan by Pharmascience	Canadian DIN 02230202	Antidepressant
T10	Tab, White, Round, T/10	Tamoxifen Citrate 10 mg	Nolvadex by RPR	Canadian	Antiestrogen
T10	Tab, Pink, Round	Enalapril Maleate 10 mg	Vasotec by Taro	51672-4039	Antihypertensive
T10	Tab, Aqua, Round	Haloperidol 10 mg	Haldol by Technilab	Canadian	Antipsychotic
T10	Tab, Aquamarine, Round, Scored	Haloperidol 10 mg	Haldol by AltiMed	Canadian DIN 00728306	Antipsychotic
T10 <> APO	Tab, Blue, Round	Terazosin HCl 10 mg	Hytrin by Apotex	Canadian DIN 02234505	Antihypertensive
T10 <> NU	Tab, Blue, Round	Terazosin HCl 10 mg	Hytrin by Nu Pharm	Canadian DIN 02233050	Antihypertensive
T100	Tab, White, Round, Biconvex, Film Coated, Gray Print	Erlotinib 100 mg	Tarceva by Genentech	50242-0063	Chemotherapy Agent
T1000 <> PF	Tab, Red, Scored, Film Coated	Choline Magnesium Trisalicylate 1000 mg	Trilisate by Purdue	00034-0510	NSAID
T109	Tab, White, Round, Scored, T over 109	Carbamazepine 200 mg	Tegretol by Physician Total Care	54868-0147	Anticonvulsant
T109	Tab, White, Round, Scored, T over 109	Carbamazepine 200 mg	Tegretol by Med Pro	53978-1070	Anticonvulsant
T109	Tab, White, Round, Scored, T over 109	Carbamazepine 200 mg	Tegretol by UDL	51079-0385 Discontinued	Anticonvulsant
T109	Tab, White, Round, Scored, T over 109	Carbamazepine 200 mg	Tegretol by Teva	00093-0109	Anticonvulsant
T109	Tab, White, Round, Scored, T over 109	Carbamazepine 200 mg	Tegretol by Caremark	00339-5941	Anticonvulsant
T11	Tab, White, Round, T-11	Carbamazepine 200 mg	Tegretol by Taro	52549-4005	Anticonvulsant
T121	Tab, Blue, Round	Atropine Sulfate, Benzoic Acid, Hyoscyamine Sulfate, Methenamine, Phenyl Salicylate	Urised by Trinity		Urinary Tract
T127	Tab, White, Round	Phenylephrine HCl 10 mg, Chlorpheniramine Maleate 4 mg	Cold-Time PE by Time Caps		Cold Remedy
T129	Tab, Blue, Oblong	Diphenhydramine HCl 25 mg	Sleepy-Time by Time Caps	49483-0127	Antihistamine; Sleep Aid
T142	Tab, Burgundy, Round	Phenazopyridine HCl 200 mg	Pyridium by Trinity	49483-0129	Urinary Analgesic
T147	Tab, Burgundy, Round	Phenazopyridine HCl 200 mg	Pyridium by Trinity		Urinary Analgesic
T150	Tab, White, Round, Biconvex, Film Coated, Maroon Print	Erlotinib 150 mg	Tarceva by Genentech	50242-0064	Chemotherapy Agent
T150	Tab, White, Oval, Film-Coated	Tramadol HCl 150 mg	Zytram XL by Purdue Pharma	Canadian DIN 02286424	Analgesic
T17	Tab, White, Oval	Aspirin 800 mg	Aspirin by Interpharm		Analgesic
T1R <> ORGANON	Tab, Red, Round, Coated, "1" set below T & R	Desogestrel 0.150 mg, Ethinyl Estradiol 0.025 mg	Linessa 21 by Organon	Canadian DIN 02272903	Oral Contraceptive
T1R <> ORGANON	Tab, Red, Round, Coated, "1" set below T & R	Desogestrel 0.150 mg, Ethinyl Estradiol 0.025 mg	Linessa 28 by Organon	Canadian DIN 02257238	Oral Contraceptive
T2	Tab, Yellow, Round, Scored	Enalapril Maleate 2.5 mg	Vasotec by Taro	51672-4037	Antihypertensive
T2	Tab, Pink, Round	Haloperidol 2 mg	Haldol by Technilab	Canadian	Antipsychotic
T2	Tab, Pink, Round, Scored	Haloperidol 2 mg	Haldol by AltiMed	Canadian DIN 00728292	Antipsychotic

ID FRONT <> BACK	DESCRIPTION FRONT <> BACK	INGREDIENT & STRENGTH	BRAND (or Generic Equiv.) by FIRM	NDC#	CLASS; SCH.
T2 <> APO	Tab, Orange, Round	Terazosin HCl 2 mg	Hytrin by Apotex	Canadian DIN 02234503	Antihypertensive
T2 <> NU	Tab, Orange, Round	Terazosin HCl 2 mg	Hytrin by Nu Pharm	Canadian DIN 02233048	Antihypertensive
T20	Tab, White, Round, T/20	Tamoxifen Citrate 20 mg	Nolvadex by RPR	Canadian	Antiestrogen
T20	Tab, Orange, Round	Enalapril Maleate 20 mg	Vasotec by Taro	51672-4040	Antihypertensive
T200	Tab, White, Oval, Film-Coated	Tramadol HCl 200 mg	Zytram XL by Purdue Pharma	Canadian DIN 02286432	Analgesic
T234	Tab, Red, Round	Phenylephrine HCl 10 mg	Pseudo-Time PE by Time Caps	49483-0234	Decongestant
T25	Tab, White, Round, Biconvex, Film Coated, Orange Print	Erlotinib 25 mg	Tarceva by Genentech	50242-0062	Chemotherapy Agent
T250 <> G	Tab, White to Off-White, Oval, Film Coated	Ticlopidine HCl 250 mg	Ticlid by Par	49884-0599	Anticoagulant
T27	Tab, White with Pink Speckles, Oval, Scored	Carbamazepine 200 mg	Tegretol by Taro	Canadian DIN 02244404	Anticonvulsant
T27 <> WINTHROP	Tab	Aspirin 325 mg, Pentazocine HCl	Talwin Compound by Searle	00966-1927	Analgesic; C IV
T27 <> WINTHROP	Tab	Aspirin 325 mg, Pentazocine HCl	Talwin Compound by Sanofi	00024-1927	Analgesic; C IV
T3	Tab, Orange, Cap Shaped	Enalapril Maleate 10 mg, Hydrochlorothiazide 25 mg	Vaseretic by Taro	51672-4046	Antihypertensive; Diuretic
T3 <> M	Tab, White, Round, Film Coated	Trifluoperazine HCl 1 mg	Stelazine by UDL	51079-0572	Antipsychotic
T3 <> M	Tab, White, Film Coated, Beveled Edge	Trifluoperazine HCl 1 mg	Stelazine by Mylan	00378-2401	Antipsychotic
T300	Tab, White, Oval, Film-Coated	Tramadol HCl 300 mg	Zytram XL by Purdue Pharma	Canadian DIN 02286440	Analgesic
T31	Tab, Pink, Oblong, Flat, Scored	Warfarin Sodium 1 mg	by Thrift Drug	59198-0351	Anticoagulant
T31	Tab, Pink, Oblong, Scored	Warfarin Sodium 1 mg	by Ivax	00182-2671	Anticoagulant
T31 <> W	Tab, T and 31, Coated	Iopanoic Acid 500 mg	Telepaque by Nycomed	00407-1931	Diagnostic
T32	Tab, Pink, Round	Amobarbital 100 mg	Amytal by Eli Lilly		Sedative/Hypnotic; C II
T32	Tab, Purple, Oblong, Flat, Scored	Warfarin Sodium 2 mg	by Thrift Drug	59198-0352	Anticoagulant
T32	Tab, Purple, Oblong, Scored	Warfarin Sodium 2 mg	by Ivax	00182-2672	Anticoagulant
T33	Tab, Green, Oblong, Scored	Warfarin Sodium 2.5 mg	by Ivax	00182-2673	Anticoagulant
T33	Tab, Green, Oblong, Flat, Scored	Warfarin Sodium 2.5 mg	by Thrift Drug	59198-0353	Anticoagulant
T34	Tab, Blue, Oblong, Scored	Warfarin Sodium 4 mg	by Ivax	00182-2675	Anticoagulant
T34	Tab, Blue, Oblong, Flat, Scored	Warfarin Sodium 4 mg	by Thrift Drug	59198-0357	Anticoagulant
T35	Tab, Peach, Oblong, Flat, Scored	Warfarin Sodium 5 mg	Warfarin Sodium by Torpharm	62318-0018	Anticoagulant
T35	Tab, Peach, Oblong, Scored	Warfarin Sodium 5 mg	by Ivax	00182-2676	Anticoagulant
T35	Tab, White, Round	Calcium Carbonate 10 g	Os-Cal by Eli Lilly		Vitamin; Mineral
T36	Tab, Yellow, Oblong, Flat, Scored	Warfarin Sodium 7.5 mg	Warfarin Sodium by Torpharm	62318-0020	Anticoagulant
T36	Tab, Yellow, Oblong, Scored	Warfarin Sodium 7.5 mg	by Ivax	00182-2678	Anticoagulant
T37	Tab, White, Oblong, Flat, Scored	Warfarin Sodium 10 mg	Warfarin Sodium by Torpharm	62318-0021	Anticoagulant
T37	Tab, White, Oblong, Scored	Warfarin Sodium 10 mg	by Ivax	00182-2679	Anticoagulant
T37	Tab, Orange, Round	Amobarbital 50 mg	Amytal by Eli Lilly		Sedative/Hypnotic; C II
T37 <> WINTHROP	Tab, Pale Blue, Cap Shaped, Scored	Pentazocine HCl 25 mg, Acetaminophen 650 mg	Talacen by Sanofi	00024-1937	Analgesic; C IV
T38	Tab, Tan, Oblong, Flat, Scored	Warfarin Sodium 3 mg	by Thrift Drug	59198-0354	Anticoagulant
T38	Tab, Tan, Oblong, Scored	Warfarin Sodium 3 mg	by Ivax	00182-2674	Anticoagulant
T39	Tab, Yellow, Oblong, Flat, Scored	Warfarin Sodium 6 mg	Warfarin Sodium by Torpharm	62318-0019	Anticoagulant
T39	Tab, Green, Oblong, Scored	Warfarin Sodium 6 mg	by Ivax	00182-2677	Anticoagulant
T4	Tab, Ivory, Cap Shaped	Enalapril Maleate 5 mg, Hydrochlorothiazide 12.5 mg	Vaseretic by Taro	51672-4045	Antihypertensive; Diuretic
T4 <> 100	Tab, Yellow, Cap Shaped, Scored	Levothyroxine Sodium 100 mcg	Levothroid by Forest	00456-1323	Thyroid Hormone
T4 <> 112	Tab, Rose, Cap Shaped	Levothyroxine Sodium 112 mcg	Levothroid by Forest	00456-1330	Thyroid Hormone
T4 <> 125	Tab, Brown, Cap Shaped	Levothyroxine Sodium 125 mcg	Levothroid by Forest	00456-1324	Thyroid Hormone
T4 <> 137	Tab, Cap Shaped, Dark Blue, Scored	Levothyroxine Sodium 137 mcg	Levothroid by Forest	00456-1331	Thyroid Hormone
T4 <> 150	Tab, Blue, Cap Shaped, Scored	Levothyroxine Sodium 150 mcg	Levothroid by Forest	00456-1325	Thyroid Hormone
T4 <> 175	Tab, Lilac, Cap Shaped	Levothyroxine Sodium 175 mcg	Levothroid by Forest	00456-1326	Thyroid Hormone

ID FRONT <> BACK	DESCRIPTION FRONT <> BACK	INGREDIENT & STRENGTH	BRAND (or Generic Equiv.) by FIRM	NDC#	CLASS; SCH.
T4 <> 200	Tab, Pink, Cap Shaped	Levothyroxine Sodium 200 mcg	Levothroid by Forest	00456-1327	Thyroid Hormone
T4 <> 25	Tab, Orange, Cap Shaped	Levothyroxine Sodium 25 mcg	Levothroid by Forest	00456-1320	Thyroid Hormone
T4 <> 300	Tab, Green, Cap Shaped	Levothyroxine Sodium 300 mcg	Levothroid by Forest	00456-1328	Thyroid Hormone
T4 <> 50	Tab, White, Cap Shaped	Levothyroxine Sodium 50 mcg	Levothroid by Forest	00456-1321	Thyroid Hormone
T4 <> 75	Tab, Violet, Cap Shaped	Levothyroxine Sodium 75 mcg	Levothroid by Forest	00456-1322	Thyroid Hormone
T4 <> 88	Tab, Mint Green, Cap Shaped	Levothyroxine Sodium 88 mcg	Levothroid by Forest	00456-1329	Thyroid Hormone
T4 <> M	Tab, White, Round, Film Coated	Trifluoperazine HCl 2 mg	Stelazine by Mylan	00378-2402	Antipsychotic
T4 <> M	Tab, White, Round, Film Coated	Trifluoperazine HCl 2 mg	Stelazine by UDL	51079-0573	Antipsychotic
T4 <> M	Tab, White, Round, Film Coated	Trifluoperazine HCl 2 mg	Stelazine by Dixon Shane	17236-0293	Antipsychotic
T400	Tab, Pink, Round, Film Coated, Extended Release	Etodolac 400 mg	Lodine XL by Taro	51672-4051	NSAID
T400	Tab, White, Oval, Film-Coated	Tramadol HCl 400 mg	Zytram XL by Purdue Pharma	Canadian DIN 02286459	Analgesic
T41	Tab, Burgundy, Round	Phenazopyridine HCl 100 mg	Pyridium by Trinity		Urinary Analgesic
T41 <> M	Tab, White, Oblong, Scored, M <> T / 41	Trandolapril 1 mg	Mavik by Mylan	00378-3241	Antihypertensive
T42 <> M	Tab, White, Round	Trandolapril 2 mg	Mavik by Mylan	00378-3242	Antihypertensive
T43 <> M	Tab, Peach, Round	Trandolapril 4 mg	Mavik by Mylan	00378-3243	Antihypertensive
T45	Tab, Purple, Round, Scored	Clorazepate Dipotassium 3.75 mg	Tranxene by Taro	51672-4042	Antianxiety; C IV
T46	Tab, Orange, Round, Scored	Clorazepate Dipotassium 7.5 mg	Tranxene by Taro	51672-4043	Antianxiety; C IV
T46	Tab, White, Round	Sulfapyridine 500 mg	by Eli Lilly		Dermatitis Herpetiformis Suppressant
T47	Tab, Pink, Round, Scored	Clorazepate Dipotassium 15 mg	Tranxene by Taro	51672-4044	Antianxiety; C IV
T5	Tab, Green, Round	Haloperidol 5 mg	Haldol by Technilab	Canadian	Antipsychotic
T5	Tab, Green, Round, Scored	Haloperidol 5 mg	Haldol by AltiMed	Canadian DIN 00647969	Antipsychotic
T5	Tab, Yellow, Round, Scored	Enalapril Maleate 5 mg	Vasotec by Taro	51672-4038	Antihypertensive
T5 <> APO	Tab, White to Off-White, Cap Shaped, Scored, APO <> T / 5	Torsemide 5 mg	Demadex by Apotex	60505-0232	Diuretic
T5 <> APO	Tab, Tan, Round	Terazosin HCl 5 mg	Hytrin by Apotex	Canadian DIN 02234504	Antihypertensive
T5 <> M	Tab, Purple, Round, Film Coated	Trifluoperazine HCl 5 mg	Stelazine by UDL	51079-0574	Antipsychotic
T5 <> M	Tab, Purple, Round, Film Coated	Trifluoperazine HCl 5 mg	Stelazine by Dixon Shane	17236-0296	Antipsychotic
T5 <> M	Tab, Purple, Round, Film Coated	Trifluoperazine HCl 5 mg	Stelazine by Mylan	00378-2405	Antipsychotic
T5 <> NU	Tab, Tan, Round	Terazosin HCl 5 mg	Hytrin by Nu Pharm	Canadian DIN 02233049	Antihypertensive
T5 <> P	Tab, White, Oblong	Tryptophan 500 mg	Tryptan by Pharmascience	Canadian DIN 02240445	Antidepressant
T500	Tab, Green, Oblong, Extended Release	Etodolac 500 mg	Lodine XL by Taro	51672-4052	NSAID
T500 <> PF	Tab, Pink, Partially Scored, Film Coated	Choline Magnesium Trisalicylate 500 mg	Trilisate by Purdue	00034-0500	NSAID
T51 <> W	Tab, T 51	Naloxone HCl 0.5 mg, Pentazocine HCl 50 mg	Talwin Nx by Sanofi	00024-1951	Analgesic; C IV
T51 <> W	Tab, T 51	Naloxone HCl 0.5 mg, Pentazocine HCl 50 mg	Talwin Nx by Searle	00966-1951	Analgesic; C IV
T51 <> W	Tab, Yellow, Oblong, Scored	Naloxone HCl 50 mg	by Novartis	17088-0005	Opioid Antagonist
T52	Tab, White, Round, Scored	Acetazolamide 125 mg	Diamox by Taro	51672-4022	Antiglaucoma Agent
T53	Tab, White, Round, Scored	Acetazolamide 250 mg	Diamox by Taro	51672-4023	Antiglaucoma Agent
T54	Tab, White, Round	Sulfadiazine 500 mg	by Eli Lilly		Antibiotic
T55.	Tab, White, Round	Papaverine HCl 100 mg	by Eli Lilly		Vasodilator
T56	Tab, Yellow, Round	Amobarbital 30 mg	Amytal by Eli Lilly		Sedative/Hypnotic; C II
T57	Tab, White, Round, Scored	Atropine Sulfate 0.04 mg, Chlorpheniramine Maleate 8 mg, Hyoscyamine Sulfate 0.19 mg, Phenylephrine 25 mg, Phenylpropanolamine 50 mg, Scopolamine 0.01 mg	Atrohist Plus by URL Mutual	00677-1418	Cold Remedy

ID FRONT <> BACK	DESCRIPTION FRONT <> BACK	INGREDIENT & STRENGTH	BRAND (or Generic Equiv.) by FIRM	NDC#	CLASS; SCH.
T57	Tab, White, Round, Scored	Atropine Sulfate 40 mcg, Chlorpheniramine Maleate 8 mg, Hyoscyamine Sulfate 190 mcg, Phenylephrine HCl 25 mg, Phenylpropanolamine HCl 50 mg, Scopolamine Hydrobromide 10 mcg	Pro Tuss by Anabolic	00722-6073	Cold Remedy
T57	Tab, White, Round, Scored	Ketoconazole 200 mg	Nizoral by Murfreesboro	51129-1593	Antifungal
T57	Tab, White, Round, Scored	Ketoconazole 200 mg	Nizoral by Taro	51672-4026	Antifungal
T6 <> M	Tab, Purple, Round, Film Coated	Trifluoperazine HCl 10 mg	Stelazine by Mylan	00378-2410	Antipsychotic
T6 <> M	Tab, Purple, Round, Film Coated	Trifluoperazine HCl 10 mg	Stelazine by Dixon Shane	17236-0334	Antipsychotic
T6 <> M	Tab, Purple, Round, Film Coated	Trifluoperazine HCl 10 mg	Stelazine by UDL	51079-0575	Antipsychotic
T600	Tab, Grey, Oval, Extended Release	Etodolac 600 mg	Lodine XL by Taro	51672-4053	NSAID
T62	Tab, Tan, Oval	Polycarbophil 625 mg	Fiber Tab by Major	00904-2500	Gastrointestinal
T62	Tab, Tan, Oval	Polycarbophil 625 mg	FiberCon by Time Caps	49483-0062	Gastrointestinal
T66	Tab	Carbinoxamine Maleate 8 mg, Pseudoephedrine HCl 120 mg	Carbodec by Rugby	00536-4453 Discontinued	Cold Remedy
T67	Tab, Purple, Oval, Scored, Film Coated, T-67	Carbinoxamine Maleate 8 mg, Pseudoephedrine HCl 120 mg	Andec TR by Anabolic	00722-6077 Discontinued	Cold Remedy
T6R <> ORGANON	Tab, Orange, Round, Coated, "6" set below T & R	Desogestrel 0.125 mg, Ethinyl Estradiol 0.025 mg	Linessa 28 by Organon	Canadian DIN 02257238	Oral Contraceptive
T6R <> ORGANON	Tab, Orange, Round, Coated, "6" set below T & R	Desogestrel 0.125 mg, Ethinyl Estradiol 0.025 mg	Linessa 21 by Organon	Canadian DIN 02272903	Oral Contraceptive
T7 <> M	Tab, White, Round, Film Coated	Tramadol HCl 50 mg	Ultram by Mylan	00378-4151	Analgesic
T7 <> M	Tab, White, Round, Film Coated	Tramadol HCl 50 mg	Ultram by UDL	51079-0991 Discontinued	Analgesic
T73	Tab, White, Round	Papaverine HCl 200 mg	P 200 by Eli Lilly		Vasodilator
T750 <> PF	Tab, White, Oblong, Partially Scored, Film Coated	Choline Magnesium Trisalicylate 750 mg	Trilisate by Purdue	00034-0505	NSAID
T77	Tab, Coated, T-77	Carbinoxamine Maleate 4 mg, Pseudoephedrine HCl 60 mg	Cardec by Ivax	00182-1199 Discontinued	Cold Remedy
T77	Tab, Coated, T-77	Carbinoxamine Maleate 4 mg, Pseudoephedrine HCl 60 mg	Andec by Anabolic	00722-6082 Discontinued	Cold Remedy
T88	Tab, Peach, Oval, Film Coated	Etodolac 400 mg	Lodine by Taro	51672-4018	NSAID
T92	Tab, White, Film Coated, Round	Ciprofloxacin HCl 250 mg	Cipro by Taro	Canadian DIN 02266962	Antibiotic
T93	Tab, White, Round	Isoniazid 100 mg	Laniazid by Eli Lilly		Antimycobacterial
T95	Tab, White, Film Coated, Oblong	Ciprofloxacin HCl 500 mg	Cipro by Taro	Canadian DIN 02266970	Antibiotic
T95	Tab, White, Round	Sulfamerazine 167 mg, Sulfamethazine 167 mg	Neotrizine by Eli Lilly		Antibiotic
T96	Tab, White, Round	Neomycin Sulfate 500 mg	by Eli Lilly		Antibiotic
T99	Tab, Yellow, Round	Paramethasone Acetate 1 mg	Haldrone by Eli Lilly		Steroid
TA	Tab, Pink, Round	Metronidazole 250 mg	Flagyl by McNeil	50580-0827	Antibiotic
TA	Tab, Pink, Round, Chewable	Acetaminophen 80 mg, Diphenhydramine HCl 6.25 mg, Pseudoephedrine HCl 7.5 mg	Children's Tylenol Allergy by McNeil	Canadian DIN 02240560	Cold Remedy
TA <> A	Tab, Yellow, Oblong, Abbott Logo (a)	Fenofibrate 54 mg	TriCor by Abbott	00074-4009	Antihyperlipidemic
TA <> DP406	Tab, White, Sustained-Release	Pseudoephedrine HCl 45 mg, Brompheniramine Maleate 6 mg	Touro Allergy by Dartmouth	58869-0406	Cold Remedy
TAGAMET <> 300SKF	Tab, Film Coated	Cimetidine HCl 300 mg	Tagamet by Pharmedix	53002-0328	Gastrointestinal
TAGAMET200	Tab, White, Diamond Shaped, Convex Diamond shape between TAGAMET and 200	Cimetidine HCl 200 mg	Tagamet HB by SKB		Gastrointestinal
TAGAMET300SB	Tab, Light Green, Film Coated	Cimetidine HCl 300 mg	Tagamet by Quality Care	60346-0001	Gastrointestinal
TAGAMET300SB	Tab, Light Green, Round, Tagamet/300/SB	Cimetidine HCl 300 mg	Tagamet by SKB	00108-5013	Gastrointestinal
TAGAMET300SB	Tab, Light Green, Film Coated, Tagamet-SB-300	Cimetidine HCl 300 mg	Tagamet by Kaiser	00179-0156	Gastrointestinal
TAGAMET300SB	Tab, Film Coated	Cimetidine HCl 300 mg	Tagamet by H J Harkins Co	52959-0270	Gastrointestinal
TAGAMET400SB	Tab, Film Coated, Tagamet/400/SB	Cimetidine HCl 400 mg	Tagamet by Kaiser	00179-1108	Gastrointestinal

ID FRONT <> BACK	DESCRIPTION FRONT <> BACK	INGREDIENT & STRENGTH	BRAND (or Generic Equiv.) by FIRM	NDC#	CLASS; SCH.
TAGAMET400SB	Tab, Light Green, Round, Tagamet/400/SB	Cimetidine HCl 400 mg	Tagamet by SKB	00108-5026	Gastrointestinal
TAGAMET400SB	Tab, Light Green, Film Coated	Cimetidine HCl 400 mg	Tagamet by Quality Care	60346-0706	Gastrointestinal
TAGAMET800SB	Tab, Light Green, Round, Tagamet/800/SB	Cimetidine HCl 800 mg	Tagamet by SKB	00108-5027	Gastrointestinal
TAGAMETSB400	Tab, Film Coated	Cimetidine HCl 400 mg	Tagamet by Allscripts		Gastrointestinal
TAKRAM8	Tab, Pale Orangish Yellow, Round, Film-Coated, TAK RAM-8	Ramelteon 8 mg	Rozerem by Takeda	64764-0805	Melatonin Receptor Agonist
TAM10 <> APO	Tab, White, Round	Tamoxifen Citrate 10 mg	Nolvadex by Apotex	Canadian DIN 00812404	Antiestrogen
TAM20 <> APO	Tab, White, Hexagonal, Scored	Tamoxifen Citrate 20 mg	Nolvadex by Apotex	Canadian DIN 00812390	Antiestrogen
TAP <> 40	Tab, Green, Round	Febuxostat 40 mg	Uloric by Takeda	64764-0918	Antigout
TAP200MG	Tab, White, Blue Print, Oval, Film Coated	Cefditoren Pivoxil 200 mg	Spectracef by Tap	00300-7535	Antibiotic
TAP30	Cap, Blue and Gray, Opaque, Extended Release	Dexlansoprazole 30 mg	Kapidex by Takeda	64764-0905	Gastrointestinal
TAP60	Cap, Blue, Opaque, Extended Release	Dexlansoprazole 60 mg	Kapidex by Takeda	64764-0915	Gastrointestinal
TARCEVA100	Tab, White to Yellowish, Round, Tarceva 100 and Logo	Erlotinib 100 mg	Tarceva by Hoffmann-La Roche	Canadian DIN 02269015	Chemotherapy Agent
TARCEVA150	Tab, White to Yellowish, Round, Tarceva 150 and Logo	Erlotinib 150 mg	Tarceva by Hoffmann-La Roche	Canadian DIN 02269023	Chemotherapy Agent
TARCEVA25	Tab, White to Yellowish, Round, Tarceva 25 and Logo	Erlotinib 25 mg	Tarceva by Hoffmann-La Roche	Canadian DIN 02269007	Chemotherapy Agent
TARGRETIN	Cap, White, Soft Gel	Bexarotene 75 mg	Targretin by Ligand	64365-0502	Antineoplastic - Retinoid
TARGRETIN	Cap, White, Soft Gel	Bexarotene 75 mg	Targretin by RP Scherer	11014-1263	Antineoplastic - Retinoid
TARKA <> 182	Tab, Pink, Oval, Film Coated	Trandolapril 2 mg, Verapamil 180 mg	Tarka by Abbott	00044-5921	Antihypertensive
TARKA <> 241	Tab, White, Oval, Film Coated	Trandolapril 1 mg, Verapamil 240 mg	Tarka by Abbott	00044-5912	Antihypertensive
TARKA <> 242	Tab, Gold, Oval, Film Coated	Trandolapril 2 mg, Verapamil 240 mg	Tarka by Abbott	00044-5922	Antihypertensive
TARKA <> 244	Tab, Reddish Brown, Oval, Film Coated	Trandolapril 4 mg, Verapamil 240 mg	Tarka by Abbott	00044-5942	Antihypertensive
TARO <> 10	Tab, Peach, Shield-Shaped, Film-Coated	Simvastatin 10 mg	Zocor by Taro	Canadian DIN 02265885	Antihyperlipidemic
TARO <> 20	Tab, Tan, Shield-Shaped, Film-Coated	Simvastatin 20 mg	Zocor by Taro	Canadian DIN 02265893	Antihyperlipidemic
TARO <> 40	Tab, Brick Red, Shield-Shaped, Film-Coated	Simvastatin 40 mg	Zocor by Taro	Canadian DIN 02265907	Antihyperlipidemic
TARO <> 89	Tab, Blue, Oval, Film Coated	Etodolac 500 mg	Lodine by Taro	51672-4036	NSAID
TARO <> FL100	Tab, Pink, Rectangular	Fluconazole 100 mg	Diflucan by Taro	Canadian DIN 02249308	Antifungal
TARO <> FL100	Tab, Pink, Rectangular	Fluconazole 100 mg	Diflucan by Taro	51672-4065	Antifungal
TARO <> FL150	Tab, Pink, Rectangular	Fluconazole 150 mg	Diflucan by Taro	51672-4066	Antifungal
TARO <> FL200	Tab, Pink, Rectangular	Fluconazole 200 mg	Diflucan by Taro	51672-4067	Antifungal
TARO <> FL50	Tab, Pink, Rectangular	Fluconazole 50 mg	Diflucan by Taro	51672-4064	Antifungal
TARO <> FL50	Tab, Pink, Rectangular	Fluconazole 50 mg	Diflucan by Taro	Canadian DIN 02249294	Antifungal
TARO <> LMT100	Tab, Peach, Round	Lamotrigine 100 mg	Lamictal by Taro	51672-4131	Anticonvulsant
TARO <> LMT150	Tab, Off White, Round	Lamotrigine 150 mg	Lamictal by Taro	51672-4132	Anticonvulsant
TARO <> LMT200	Tab, Light Blue, Round	Lamotrigine 200 mg	Lamictal by Taro	51672-4133	Anticonvulsant
TARO <> OXC6	Tab, Off White, Oval	Oxcarbazepine 600 mg	Trileptal by Taro	51672-4107	Anticonvulsant
TARO <> WARFARIN1	Tab, Pink, Round, Scored	Warfarin Sodium 1 mg	Coumadin by Taro	Canadian DIN 02242680	Anticoagulant
TARO <> WARFARIN10	Tab, White, Round, Scored	Warfarin Sodium 10 mg	Coumadin by Taro	Canadian DIN 02242687	Anticoagulant
TARO <> WARFARIN2	Tab, Purple, Round, Scored	Warfarin Sodium 2 mg	Coumadin by Taro	Canadian DIN 02242681	Anticoagulant

ID FRONT <> BACK	DESCRIPTION FRONT <> BACK	INGREDIENT & STRENGTH	BRAND (or Generic Equiv.) by FIRM	NDC#	CLASS; SCH.
TARO <> WARFARIN212	Tab, Turquoise, Round, Scored, WARFARIN 2 1/2	Warfarin Sodium 2.5 mg	Coumadin by Taro	Canadian DIN 02242682	Anticoagulant
TARO <> WARFARIN3	Tab, Light Pink, Round, Scored	Warfarin Sodium 3 mg	Coumadin by Taro	Canadian DIN 02242683	Anticoagulant
TARO <> WARFARIN4	Tab, Blue, Round, Scored	Warfarin Sodium 4 mg	Coumadin by Taro	Canadian DIN 02242684	Anticoagulant
TARO <> WARFARIN5	Tab, Light Pink, Round, Scored	Warfarin Sodium 5 mg	Coumadin by Taro	Canadian DIN 02242685	Anticoagulant
TARO <> WARFARIN6	Tab, Green, Round, Scored	Warfarin Sodium 6 mg	Coumadin by Taro	Canadian DIN 02242686	Anticoagulant
TARO <> WARFARIN712	Tab, Yellow, Round, Scored, 7 1/2	Warfarin Sodium 7.5 mg	Coumadin by Taro	Canadian DIN 02242697	Anticoagulant
TARO100MG <> LMT25	Tab, White, Round	Lamotrigine 25 mg	Lamictal by Taro	51672-4131	Anticonvulsant
TARO11	Tab, White, Round, Scored	Carbamazepine 200 mg	Tegretol by Taro	51672-4005	Anticonvulsant
TARO11	Tab, White, Round, Taro over 11	Carbamazepine 200 mg	Tegretol by Taro	51672-4005	Anticonvulsant
TARO11	Tab, White, Round, Scored	Carbamazepine 200 mg	Tegretol by Teva	00093-1233	Anticonvulsant
TARO16	Tab, White w/ Pink Specks, Round, Scored, Chewable	Carbamazepine 100 mg	Tegretol by Taro	51672-4041	Anticonvulsant
TARO16	Tab, White w/ Pink Specks, Round, Scored, Chewable	Carbamazepine 100 mg	Tegretol by Taro	Canadian DIN 02244403	Anticonvulsant
TARO56	Tab, Peach, Round, Scored, TARO over 56	Amiodarone 200 mg	Cordarone by Taro	51672-4025	Antiarrhythmic
TARO59	Tab, Light Yellow, Round, Scored	Amiodarone 400 mg	Cordarone by Taro	51672-4057	Antiarrhythmic
TARONTP10	Cap, Light Green, Opaque	Nortriptyline HCl 10 mg	Pamelor by Taro	51672-4001	Antidepressant
TARONTP25	Cap, Ivory, Opaque	Nortriptyline HCl 25 mg	Pamelor by Taro	51672-4002	Antidepressant
TARONTP50	Cap, Dark Green and White, Opaque	Nortriptyline HCl 50 mg	Pamelor by Taro	51672-4003	Antidepressant
TARONTP75	Cap, Dark Green, Opaque	Nortriptyline HCl 75 mg	Pamelor by Taro	51672-4004	Antidepressant
TAROPHN100	Cap, Orange, Opaque, Hard Gelatin	Phenytoin Sodium 100 mg	Dilantin Kapseals by Taro	51672-4111	Anticonvulsant
TAS500	Cap, Yellow, Film Coated	Acetaminophen 500 mg, Chlorpheniramine Maleate 2 mg, Pseudoephedrine HCl 30 mg	Extra Strength Tylenol Allergy Sinus by McNeil	Canadian DIN 01933728	Cold Remedy
TASMAR100 <> ROCHE	Tab, Beige, Black Print, Hexagonal, Film Coated, TASMAR over 100	Tolcapone 100 mg	Tasmar by Hoffmann La Roche	00004-5920	Antiparkinson
TASMAR100 <> ROCHE	Tab, Beige, Black Print, Hexagonal, Film Coated, TASMAR over 100	Tolcapone 100 mg	Tasmar by Teva	00480-0100	Antiparkinson
TASMAR100 <> V	Tab, Beige, Hexagonal, Film Coated, Black Ink	Tolcapone 100 mg	Tasmar by ICN	00187-0938	Antiparkinson
TASMAR200 <> ROCHE	Tab, Reddish Brown, Hexagonal, Film Coated	Tolcapone 200 mg	Tasmar by Hoffmann La Roche	00004-5921	Antiparkinson
TASMAR200 <> V	Tab, Reddish Brown, Hexagonal, Film Coated, Black Ink	Tolcapone 200 mg	Tasmar by ICN	00187-0939	Antiparkinson
TAVIST	Cap, White & Red, Gel Caps	Acetaminophen 500 mg, Pseudoephedrine 30 mg	Sudafed Sinus by Perrigo	00113-0075	Cold Remedy
TAVISTD	Tab	Clemastine Fumarate 1.34 mg, Phenylpropanolamine 75 mg	Tavist D by Pharmedix	53002-0371	Cold Remedy
TC	Tab, White, Round, Abbott Logo	Methamphetamine HCl 2.5 mg	Desoxyn by Abbott	Discontinued	Stimulant; C II
TC <> 15	Tab, Green, Oval	Morphine Sulfate 15 mg ER	Ratio-Morphine by Ratiopharm	Canadian DIN 02244790	Analgesic; C II
TC <> A	Tab, White, Oblong, Abbott Logo (a)	Fenofibrate 160 mg	TriCor by Abbott	00074-4013	Antihyperlipidemic
TCL001	Tab, Orange, Round, Enteric Coated	Aspirin 325 mg	Aspirin by Time Caps	49483-0001	Analgesic
TCL002	Tab, Red, Round, Enteric Coated	Aspirin 650 mg	Ecotrin by Time Caps	49483-0002	Analgesic
TCL002	Tab, Red, Round, Enteric Coated	Aspirin 650 mg	Ecotrin by Rugby	00536-3326	Analgesic
TCL002	Tab, Red, Round, Enteric Coated	Aspirin 650 mg	Ecotrin by Ivax	00182-0449 Discontinued	Analgesic
TCL003	Tab, Yellowish Orange, Black Print, Round, TCL over 003	Bisacodyl 5 mg	Dulcolax by Paddock	00574-0004	Gastrointestinal
TCL003	Tab, Yellowish Orange, Black Print, Round, TCL over 003	Bisacodyl 5 mg	Dulcolax by Time Caps	49483-0003	Gastrointestinal
TCL003	Tab, Yellowish Orange, Black Print, Round, TCL over 003	Bisacodyl 5 mg	Dulcolax by Able	Discontinued	Gastrointestinal

ID FRONT <> BACK	DESCRIPTION FRONT <> BACK	INGREDIENT & STRENGTH	BRAND (or Generic Equiv.) by FIRM	NDC#	CLASS; SCH.
TCL003	Tab, Yellowish Orange, Black Print, Round, TCL over 003	Bisacodyl 5 mg	Dulcolax by Ivax	00182-1992 Discontinued	Gastrointestinal
TCL005	Tab, Orange, Round	Aspirin 500 mg	Ecotrin Maximum Strength by Time Caps	49483-0005	Analgesic
TCL005	Tab, Orange, Round	Aspirin 500 mg	Aspirin by Perrigo	00113-0511	Analgesic
TCL011	Tab, White, Round	Aspirin 325 mg	Bayer by Time Caps	49483-0011	Analgesic
TCL011	Tab, White, Round	Aspirin 325 mg	Aspirin by Rugby	00536-3305	Analgesic
TCL016	Tab, Red, Round	Pseudoephedrine 30 mg	Sudafed by Time Caps	49483-0016	Decongestant
TCL016	Tab, Red, Round	Pseudoephedrine 30 mg	Sudafed by Rugby	00536-4391	Decongestant
TCL019	Cap, Brown and Clear, Black Ink, Ex Release	Papaverine HCl 150 mg	Pavabid by Time Caps	49483-0019	Vasodilator
TCL019	Cap, Brown and Clear, Black Ink, Ex Release	Papaverine HCl 150 mg	Pavabid by Qualitest	00603-5043	Vasodilator
TCL019	Cap, Brown and Clear, Black Ink, Ex Release	Papaverine HCl 150 mg	Pavabid by UDL	51079-0010	Vasodilator
TCL019	Cap, Brown and Clear, Black Ink, Ex Release	Papaverine HCl 150 mg	Pavabid by Schein	00364-0181	Vasodilator
TCL021	Tab, Tan, Round	Thyroid 30 mg	by Time Caps	49483-0021	Thyroid Hormone
TCL022	Tab, Tan, Round	Thyroid 65 mg	Thyroid by Time Caps	49483-0022	Thyroid Hormone
TCL022	Tab, Tan, Round	Thyroid 65 mg	Thyroid by Major	00904-0761	Thyroid Hormone
TCL023	Tab, Tan, Round	Thyroid 130 mg	Thyroid by Major	00904-0762	Thyroid Hormone
TCL023	Tab, Tan, Round	Thyroid 130 mg	Thyroid by Time Caps	49483-0023	Thyroid Hormone
TCL025	Tab, Yellow, Round	Aspirin 81 mg	Aspirin by Time Caps	00113-0937	Analgesic
TCL025	Tab, Yellow, Round	Aspirin 81 mg	Aspirin by Perrigo	00113-0535	Analgesic
TCL027	Tab, Red, Round, TCL/027	Ferrous Sulfate 324 mg	Feosol by Time Caps	49483-0027	Mineral
TCL028	Cap, Banded	Phenylpropanolamine HCl 4 mg, Chlorphen Mal (Time Rel) 75 mg	Aler-Releaf by Reese	10956-0703	Cold Remedy
TCL031	Tab, Green, Cap Shaped	Ferrous Fumarate 150 mg, Docusate Sodium 100 mg	Ferro-Sequels by Time Caps	49483-0031	Supplement
TCL032	Tab, Red, Round, Enteric Coated, Raised T	Aspirin 325 mg	Aspirin by Time Caps	49483-0032	Analgesic
TCL036	Cap, Black Print	Chlorpheniramine Maleate 4 mg, Phenylephrine HCl 20 mg, Phenyltoloxamine Citrate 50 mg	Com Time by Time Caps	49483-0036	Cold Remedy
TCL036	Cap	Chlorpheniramine Maleate 4 mg, Phenylephrine HCl 20 mg, Phenyltoloxamine Citrate 50 mg	Q Hist LA by Qualitest	00603-5537	Cold Remedy
TCL038	Tab, Tan, Round	Thyroid 195 mg	Thyroid by Major	00904-0763	Thyroid Hormone
TCL038	Tab, Tan, Round	Thyroid 195 mg	Thyroid by Time Caps	49483-0038	Thyroid Hormone
TCL039	Tab, Blue, White Print, Round, Sugar Coated, TCL over 039	Brompheniramine Maleate 12 mg, Phenylephrine HCl 15 mg, Phenylpropanolamine HCl 15 mg	Dime Time by Time Caps	49483-0039	Cold Remedy
TCL041	Cap, Green, Clear	Chlorpheniramine Maleate 8.8 mg	Teldrin by Qualitest	00603-2784	Antihistamine
TCL041	Cap, Blue-Green and Clear, White Print	Chlorpheniramine Maleate 8 mg	Teldrin by Time Caps	49483-0041	Antihistamine
TCL043	Cap, Blue-Green and Clear, Black Print	Chlorpheniramine Maleate 12 mg	Teldrin by Time Caps	49483-0043	Antihistamine
TCL050	Cap, White	Guaifenesin 250 mg, Pseudoephedrine HCl 120 mg	Sudafed Sinus by Time Caps	49483-0050	Cold Remedy
TCL050	Cap, White	Guaifenesin 250 mg, Pseudoephedrine HCl 120 mg	Sudafed Sinus by Ivax	00182-2601	Cold Remedy
TCL050	Cap, White	Guaifenesin 250 mg, Pseudoephedrine HCl 120 mg	Sudafed Sinus by Qualitest	00603-3776	Cold Remedy
TCL051	Cap, Blue & Clear	Guaifenesin 300 mg, Pseudoephedrine HCl 60 mg	Sudafed Sinus by Qualitest	00603-3777	Cold Remedy
TCL051	Cap, Blue & Clear	Guaifenesin 300 mg, Pseudoephedrine HCl 60 mg	Sudafed Sinus by Time Caps	49483-0051	Cold Remedy
TCL051	Cap, Blue, Opaque	Guaifenesin 300 mg, Pseudoephedrine HCl 60 mg	Sudafed Sinus by Ivax	00182-2602	Cold Remedy
TCL057	Tab, Pink, Round	Bisacodyl 5 mg	Correctol by Time Cap Labs	49483-0057	Laxative
TCL079	Tab, White, Round, Sugar Coated	Sennosides 15 mg	Ex-Lax by Time Caps	49483-0079	Gastrointestinal
TCL080	Tab, Tan to Brown, Mottled	Sennosides 8.6 mg	Senokot by Time Caps	49483-0080	Gastrointestinal
TCL081	Tab, Orange, Round	Sennosides 8.6 mg, Docusate Sodium 50 mg	Senokot-S by Time Caps	49483-0081	Gastrointestinal
TCL081 <> CL220	Tab, Orange, Round	Sennosides 8.6 mg, Docusate Sodium 50 mg	Senokot-S by Ivax	00182-1113	Gastrointestinal
TCL083	Tab, Blue, Round, Sugar Coated	Sennosides 25 mg	Ex-Lax Maximum Strength by Time Caps	49483-0083	Gastrointestinal
TCL086	Tab, Tan, Round	Meclizine HCl 25 mg	Dramamine by Time Caps	49483-0086	Antiemetic
TCL088	Cap, Red and Clear, Black Ink	Phenylpropanolamine 75 mg	Veterinary by Time Caps	49483-0228	Decongestant; Appetite Suppressant (Veterinary)
TCL090	Tab, White, Round	Triprolidine 2.5 mg, Pseudoephedrine 60 mg	Actifed by Time Caps	49483-0090	Cold Remedy

ID FRONT <> BACK	DESCRIPTION FRONT <> BACK	INGREDIENT & STRENGTH	BRAND (or Generic Equiv.) by FIRM	NDC#	CLASS; SCH.
TCL090	Tab, White, Round	Triprolidine 2.5 mg, Pseudoephedrine 60 mg	Actifed by Rugby	00536-3421	Cold Remedy
TCL093	Tab, Off-White, Round	Iron 50 mg	Slow Fe by Rugby	00536-3478	Vitamin
TCL093	Tab, Off-White, Round	Iron 50 mg	Slow Fe by Time Caps	49483-0077	Vitamin
TCL097	Tab, Red, Round	Sennosides 8.6 mg, Docusate 50 mg	Senokot-S by Time Caps		Laxative
TCL108	Tab, Pink, Round, Mottled, Chewable	Bismuth Subsalicylate 262 mg	Pepto-Bismol by Time Caps	49483-0108	Gastrointestinal
TCL121	Tab, Pink, Round, Mottled	Bismuth Subsalicylate 262 mg	Pepto-Bismol by Time Caps	49483-0121	Gastrointestinal
TCL1221	Cap, Lavender & Clear, in Black Ink, Ex Release	Nitroglycerin 2.5 mg	Nitro-Bid by Qualitest	00603-4782	Vasodilator
TCL1221	Cap, Lavender & Clear, in Black Ink, Ex Release	Nitroglycerin 2.5 mg	Nitro-Bid by Major	00904-0643	Vasodilator
TCL1221	Cap, Lavender & Clear, in Black Ink, Ex Release	Nitroglycerin 2.5 mg	Nitro-Bid by Time Caps	49483-0221	Vasodilator
TCL1221	Cap, Lavender & Clear, in Black Ink, Ex Release	Nitroglycerin 2.5 mg	Nitro-Bid by URL Mutual	00677-0485	Vasodilator
TCL1221	Cap, Lavender & Clear, in Black Ink, Ex Release	Nitroglycerin 2.5 mg	Nitro-Bid by Schein	00364-0174	Vasodilator
TCL1222	Cap, Yellow and Dark Blue, White Ink, Ex Release	Nitroglycerin 6.5 mg	Nitro-Bid by URL Mutual	00677-0486	Vasodilator
TCL1222	Cap, Yellow and Dark Blue, White Ink, Ex Release	Nitroglycerin 6.5 mg	Nitro-Bid by Qualitest	00603-4783	Vasodilator
TCL1222	Cap, Yellow and Dark Blue, White Ink, Ex Release	Nitroglycerin 6.5 mg	Nitro-Bid by Time Caps	49483-0222	Vasodilator
TCL1222	Cap, Yellow and Dark Blue, White Ink, Ex Release	Nitroglycerin 6.5 mg	Nitro-Bid by Schein	00364-0432	Vasodilator
TCL1223	Cap, Green & Yellow, Ex Release	Nitroglycerin 9 mg	Nitro-Bid by Baker Cummins	63171-1670	Vasodilator
TCL1223	Cap, Green & Yellow, Ex Release	Nitroglycerin 9 mg	Nitro-Bid by URL Mutual	00677-0967	Vasodilator
TCL1223	Cap, Green & Yellow, Ex Release	Nitroglycerin 9 mg	Nitro-Bid by Time Caps	49483-0223	Vasodilator
TCL1223	Cap, Green & Yellow, Ex Release	Nitroglycerin 9 mg	Nitro-Bid by Qualitest	00603-4784	Vasodilator
TCL1223	Cap, Green & Yellow, Ex Release	Nitroglycerin 9 mg	Nitro-Bid by Ivax	00182-1670 Discontinued	Vasodilator
TCL1223	Cap, Green & Yellow, Ex Release	Nitroglycerin 9 mg	Nitro-Bid by Schein	00364-0664	Vasodilator
TCL124	Tab, Blue, Oval	Phenylephrine HCl 10 mg, Diphenhydramine HCl 25 mg	Allergy-Time PE by Time Caps	49483-0124	Cold Remedy
TCL134	Tab, Tan, Round	Sennosides 17.2 mg	Senna-Time Ex Strength by Time Caps	49483-0134	Gastrointestinal
TCL224	Tab, White, Cap Shaped, Enteric Coated	Aspirin 975 mg	Easprin by Time Caps	49483-0224	Analgesic
TCL272	Tab, White, Round	Guaifenesin 400 mg	Mucinex by Time Cap Labs	49483-0272	Cold Remedy
TCL280	Tab, White, Oval, Scored	Guaifenesin 400 mg, Dextromethorphan HBr 20 mg	Mucinex DM by Time Cap Labs	49483-0280	Cold Remedy
TCLO50	Cap	Guaifenesin 250 mg, Pseudoephedrine HCl 120 mg	Sudafed Sinus by Ivax	00182-2601	Cold Remedy
TCLO51	Cap	Guaifenesin 300 mg, Pseudoephedrine HCl 60 mg	Sudafed Sinus by Ivax	00182-2602	Cold Remedy
TCM325	Cap, Yellow	Acetaminophen 325 mg, Chlorpheniramine Maleate 2 mg, Pseudoephedrine HCl 30 mg, Dextromethorphan HBr 15 mg	Alka Seltzer Plus Liquid Gels by McNeil	Canadian	Cold Remedy
TCM500	Cap, Yellow, Film Coated	Acetaminophen 500 mg, Chlorpheniramine Maleate 2 mg, Pseudoephedrine HCl 30 mg, Dextromethorphan Hydrobromide 15 mg	Tylenol Cold Ex Strength by McNeil	Canadian DIN 00743275	Cold Remedy
TCMDM <> 160	Tab, Purple, Round	Acetaminophen 160 mg, Chlorpheniramine maleate 1 mg, Pseudoephedrine 15 mg, Dextromethorphan HBr 7.5 mg	Tylenol Junior Strength Cold and Cough by McNeil C	Canadian DIN 00890677	Cold Remedy
TCMND325	Cap, Yellow, Film Coated	Acetaminophen 325 mg, Pseudoephedrine HCl 30 mg, Dextromethorphan HBr 15 mg	Regular Tylenol Daytime by McNeil	Canadian DIN 00743283	Cold Remedy
TCMND500	Cap, Yellow, Film Coated	Acetaminophen 500 mg, Pseudoephedrine HCl 30 mg, Dextromethorphan HBr 15 mg	Tylenol Flu Daytime Ex Strength by McNeil	Canadian DIN 00743267	Cold Remedy
TD <> A	Tab	Levothyroxine 19 mcg, Liothyronine 4.5 mcg	Armour Thyroid by Amerisource	62584-0457	Thyroid Hormone
TD <> CG	Tab, Pale Grey-Green, Oval, Scored, Film Coated	Oxcarbazepine 150 mg	Trileptal by Novartis	Canadian DIN 02242067	Anticonvulsant
TD <> CG	Tab, Pale Grey-Green, Oval, Scored, Film Coated	Oxcarbazepine 150 mg	Trileptal by Novartis	00078-0456	Anticonvulsant
TE	Tab, Tan, Round, Convex, Debossed with a Mortar and Pestle	Levothyroxine 38 mcg, Liothyronine 9 mcg	Armour Thyroid by Murfreesboro	51129-1637	Thyroid Hormone
TE <> A	Tab, White, Round, Abbott Logo (a)	Methamphetamine HCl 5 mg	Desoxyn by Abbott	00074-3377	Stimulant; C II
TEC	Tab, White, Oval, Scored	Metformin HCl 850 mg	Glucophage by AltiMed	Canadian DIN 02242931	Antidiabetic
TEC	Cap, Red, Gelatin	Docusate Calcium 240 mg	by AltiMed	Canadian DIN 00809055	Laxative

ID FRONT <> BACK	DESCRIPTION FRONT <> BACK	INGREDIENT & STRENGTH	BRAND (or Generic Equiv.) by FIRM	NDC#	CLASS; SCH.
TEC	Tab, White, Round	Acetaminophen 330 mg, Butalbital 50 mg, Caffeine 40 mg	by AltiMed	Canadian DIN 00608211	Analgesic
TEC	Cap, Orange & White, Scored	Acetaminophen 325 mg, Codeine Phosphate 15 mg, Methocarbamol 400 mg	by AltiMed	Canadian DIN 01966367	Analgesic; C III
TEC	Tab, White, Round, Scored	Acetaminophen 325 mg, Oxycodone HCl 5 mg	Percocet by AltiMed	Canadian DIN 00608165	Analgesic; C II
TEC	Tab, Yellow, Scored	Acetaminophen 325 mg, Oxycodone HCl 5 mg	Percocet by AltiMed	Canadian DIN 00608157	Analgesic; C II
TEC	Cap, Light Green & White, Scored	Acetaminophen 325 mg, Methocarbamol 400 mg	by AltiMed	Canadian DIN 02230521	Muscle Relaxant
TEC	Cap, Pink & White, Scored	Acetaminophen 325 mg, Methocarbamol 400 mg	by AltiMed	Canadian DIN 00868868	Muscle Relaxant
TEC	Cap, Light Blue & White, Scored	Acetaminophen 325 mg, Codeine Phosphate 8 mg, Methocarbamol 400 mg	by AltiMed	Canadian DIN 02236872	Analgesic; C III
TEC	Cap, Yellow & White, Scored	Acetaminophen 325 mg, Codeine Phosphate 8 mg, Methocarbamol 400 mg	by AltiMed	Canadian DIN 01941895	Analgesic; C III
TEC	Cap, Peach & White, Scored	Acetaminophen 325 mg, Codeine Phosphate 30 mg, Methocarbamol 400 mg	by AltiMed	Canadian DIN 01966375	Analgesic; C III
TEC	Tab, Pink, Round	Chlorzoxazone 250 mg, Acetaminophen 300 mg, Codeine Phosphate 8 mg	Acetazone Forte C8 by Rougier Pharma	Canadian DIN 00834319	Muscle Relaxant; C III
TEC	Tab, Green, Round	Chlorzoxazone 250 mg, Acetaminophen 300 mg	Acetazone Forte by Rougier Pharma	Canadian DIN 00834300	Muscle Relaxant
TEC	Tab, Pink, Round, Film Coated	Nystatin 500,000 Units	by AltiMed	Canadian DIN 02194198	Antifungal
TEC	Tab, Yellowish, Oval	Nystatin 100,000 Units	by AltiMed	Canadian DIN 02194171	Antifungal
TEC	Cap, Green and White, Oblong, Film-Coated	Methocarbamol 400 mg, Acetaminophen 325 mg.	Methoxacet by Rougier Pharma	Canadian DIN 02230521	Analgesic
TEC	Cap, Light Blue and White	Methocarbamol 400 mg, Acetaminophen 325 mg, Codeine Phosphate 8 mg	Methoxacet-C 1/8 by Rougier Pharma	Canadian DIN 02236872	Muscle Relaxant
TEC	Tab, Green and White, Oval, Double Layer	Methocarbamol 400 mg, Acetaminophen 500 mg	Methoxacet Extra Strength by Rougier Pharma	Canadian DIN 02242960	Muscle Relaxant
TEC	Cap, Pink and White, Oblong	Methocarbamol 400 mg, ASA 325 mg	Methoxisal by Rougier Pharma	Canadian DIN 00868868	Muscle Relaxant
TEC	Cap, Yellow and White, Oblong	Methocarbamol 400 mg, ASA 325 mg, Codeine Phosphate 8 mg.	Methoxisal-C 1/8 by Rougier Pharma	Canadian DIN 01941895	Muscle Relaxant
TEC	Cap, Orange and White, Oblong	Methocarbamol 400 mg, ASA 325 mg, Codeine Phosphate 16.2 mg	Methoxisal-C 1/4 by Rougier Pharma	Canadian DIN 01966367	Muscle Relaxant
TEC	Cap, Peach and White, Oblong	Methocarbamol 400 mg, ASA 325 mg, Codeine Phosphate 32.4 mg	Methoxisal-C 1/2 by Rougier Pharma	Canadian DIN 01966375	Muscle Relaxant
TEC	Cap, Pink and White, Oblong	Methocarbamol 400 mg, ASA 500 mg	Methoxisal Extra Strength by Rougier Pharma	Canadian DIN 02242978	Muscle Relaxant
TEC	Cap, Red, Gelatin	Docusate Calcium 100 mg	Ratio Docusate by AltiMed	Canadian DIN 00870196	Laxative
TEC <> 10	Tab, Yellow, Pentagonal, Film Coated	Cyclobenzaprine HCl 10 mg	by AltiMed	Canadian DIN 02236506 Discontinued	Muscle Relaxant
TEC <> 203A	Tab, White to Off-White, Round, Scored	Doxazosin Mesylate 1 mg	Cardura by Ratiopharm	Canadian DIN 02243215 Discontinued	Antihypertensive

ID FRONT <> BACK	DESCRIPTION FRONT <> BACK	INGREDIENT & STRENGTH	BRAND (or Generic Equiv.) by FIRM	NDC#	CLASS; SCH.
TEC <> 203B	Tab, White to Off-White, Rectangular, Scored	Doxazosin Mesylate 2 mg	Cardura by AltiMed	Canadian DIN 02243216 Discontinued	Antihypertensive
TEC <> 79B	Tab, Brown, D-Shaped, Film Coated, Scored	Famotidine 40 mg	by AltiMed	Canadian DIN 02242328	Gastrointestinal
TEC <> 79B	Tab, Beige, D-Shaped, Film Coated, Scored	Famotidine 20 mg	by AltiMed	Canadian DIN 02242327	Gastrointestinal
TEC05	Tab, White, Round, TEC 0.5	Haloperidol 0.5 mg	Haldol by Technilab	Canadian	Antipsychotic
TEC050	Tab, White, Pentagonal, Scored, TEC 0.50	Dexamethasone 0.50 mg	by AltiMed	Canadian DIN 02240684	Steroid
TEC075	Tab, White, Pentagonal, Scored, TEC 0.75	Dexamethasone 0.75 mg	by AltiMed	Canadian DIN 02240685	Steroid
TEC1	Cap, White	Acetaminophen 300 mg, Caffeine 15 mg, Codeine Phosphate 8 mg	Lenoltec 1 by Technilab	Canadian	Analgesic; C III
TEC1	Tab, White, Round	Acetaminophen 300 mg, Caffeine 15 mg, Codeine Phosphate 8 mg	Lenoltec 1 by Technilab	Canadian	Analgesic; C III
TEC 1	Tab, Yellow, Round	Haloperidol 1 mg	Haldol by Technilab	Canadian	Antipsychotic
TEC100	Cap, Blue, Opaque, Gelatin w/ Light Yellow Powder	Doxycycline Hyclate 100 mg	by AltiMed	Canadian DIN 02093103 Discontinued	Antibiotic
TEC102A	Tab, White, Cap Shaped, Scored	Baclofen 10 mg	Lioresal by AltiMed	Canadian DIN 02236507	Muscle Relaxant
TEC102B	Tab, White, Cap Shaped, Scored	Baclofen 20 mg	Lioresal by AltiMed	Canadian DIN 02236508	Muscle Relaxant
TEC137A	Cap, Green & Grey	Fluoxetine HCl 10 mg	Prozac by AltiMed	Canadian DIN 02241371	Antidepressant
TEC137B	Cap, Green & Ivory	Fluoxetine HCl 20 mg	by AltiMed	Canadian DIN 02241374	Antidepressant
TEC145	Tab, White, Round, Scored	Metformin HCl 500 mg	Glucophage by AltiMed	Canadian DIN 02242974	Antidiabetic
TEC15	Tab, White, Round	Codeine Phosphate 15 mg	by AltiMed	Canadian DIN 00593435	Analgesic; C II
TEC173A	Cap, White & Yellow, Opaque w/ White Powder	Nortriptyline HCl 10 mg	by AltiMed	Canadian DIN 02240789	Antidepressant
TEC173B	Cap, White & Yellow, Opaque w/ White Powder	Nortriptyline HCl 25 mg	by AltiMed	Canadian DIN 02240790	Antidepressant
TEC177X	Tab, Blue, Scored	Sotalol HCl 80 mg	by AltiMed	Canadian DIN 02238415	Antiarrhythmic
TEC177Y	Tab, Blue, Scored	Sotalol HCl 160 mg	by AltiMed	Canadian DIN 02238416	Antiarrhythmic
TEC185A	Cap, Maroon & Peach, Gelatin	Temazepam 15 mg	Restoril by AltiMed	Canadian DIN 02243023	Sedative/Hypnotic; C IV
TEC185B	Cap, Maroon & Peach, Gelatin	Temazepam 30 mg	Restoril by AltiMed	Canadian DIN 02243024	Sedative/Hypnotic; C IV
TEC186B	Tab, White, Square, Quadrisected	Captopril 25 mg	Capoten by AltiMed	Canadian DIN 02237862	Antihypertensive
TEC186C	Tab, White, Oval, Scored	Captopril 50 mg	Capoten by AltiMed	Canadian DIN 02237863	Antihypertensive
TEC186D	Tab, White, Oval, Scored	Captopril 100 mg	Capoten by AltiMed	Canadian DIN 02237864	Antihypertensive
TEC2	Tab, White, Round	Acetaminophen 300 mg, Caffeine 15 mg, Codeine Phosphate 15 mg	Lenoltec 2 by Technilab	Canadian	Analgesic; C III
TEC203C	Tab, White to Off-White, Diamond Shaped, Scored	Doxazosin Mesylate 4 mg	Cardura by AltiMed	Canadian DIN 02243217	Antihypertensive

ID FRONT <> BACK	DESCRIPTION FRONT <> BACK	INGREDIENT & STRENGTH	BRAND (or Generic Equiv.) by FIRM	NDC#	CLASS; SCH.
TEC250	Cap, Orange w/ Yellowish Liquid	Valproic Acid 250 mg	Depakene by AltiMed	Canadian DIN 02217414	Anticonvulsant
TEC3	Tab, White, Round	Acetaminophen 300 mg, Caffeine 15 mg, Codeine Phosphate 30 mg	Lenoltec 3 by Technilab	Canadian	Analgesic; C III
TEC30	Tab, White, Round, Scored	Codeine Phosphate 30 mg	Codeine by AltiMed	Canadian DIN 00593451	Analgesic; C II
TEC39	Tab, White, Round, Coated	Domperidone 10 mg	by AltiMed	Canadian DIN 02230473	Gastrointestinal
TEC4	Tab, White, Pentagonal, Scored	Dexamethasone 4 mg	by AltiMed	Canadian DIN 02240687	Steroid
TEC4	Tab, White, Round	Acetaminophen 300 mg, Codeine Phosphate 60 mg	Tylenol w/ Codeine by Technilab	Canadian	Analgesic; C III
TEC90	Tab, White to Brownish-White, Oval, Scored	Buspirone HCl 10 mg	Buspar by AltiMed	Canadian DIN 02237858	Antianxiety
TECNALC12TECHNILAB	Cap, Blue & Light Blue, Tecnal C 1/2: Technilab	Acetaminophen 330 mg, Butalbital 50 mg, Caffeine 40 mg, Codeine Phosphate 30 mg	by AltiMed	Canadian DIN 00608181	Analgesic; C III
TECNALC14TECHNILAB	Cap, Light Blue & White, Opaque, Tecnal C 1/4: Technilab	Acetaminophen 330 mg, Butalbital 50 mg, Caffeine 40 mg, Codeine Phosphate 15 mg	by AltiMed	Canadian DIN 00608203	Analgesic; C III
TECNALTECHNILAB	Cap, Light Blue & Violet, Tecnal:Technilab	Acetaminophen 330 mg, Butalbital 50 mg, Caffeine 40 mg	Tecnal by Technilab	Canadian DIN 00608238	Analgesic
TECZEM5180	Tab, Film Coated, Teczem 5/180	Diltiazem Malate 180 mg, Enalapril Maleate 5 mg	Teczem by Merck	00006-0764	Antihypertensive
TEGRETOL <> 2727	Tab, Pink, Cap Shaped, Scored	Carbamazepine 200 mg	Tegretol by Novartis	00083-0027	Anticonvulsant
TEGRETOL <> 2727	Tab, Pink, Cap Shaped, Scored	Carbamazepine 200 mg	Tegretol by Nat Pharmpak	55154-1012	Anticonvulsant
TEGRETOL <> 5252	Tab, White w/ Pink Specks, Round, Scored, 52 over 52, Chewable	Carbamazepine 100 mg	Tegretol by Neuman	64579-0325	Anticonvulsant
TEGRETOL <> 5252	Tab, White w/ Pink Specks, Round, Scored, 52 over 52, Chewable	Carbamazepine 100 mg	Tegretol by Novartis	00083-0052	Anticonvulsant
TEGRETOL <> 5252	Tab, White w/ Pink Specks, Round, Scored, 52 over 52, Chewable	Carbamazepine 100 mg	Tegretol by Allscripts		Anticonvulsant
TEGRETOL <> 5252	Tab, White w/ Pink Specks, Round, Scored, 52 over 52, Chewable	Carbamazepine 100 mg	Tegretol by Basel	58887-0052	Anticonvulsant
TEGRETOL <> 5252	Tab, White w/ Pink Specks, Round, Scored, 52 over 52, Chewable	Carbamazepine 100 mg	Tegretol by Nat Pharmpak	55154-1011	Anticonvulsant
TEMAZEPAM15MG	Cap, Aqua & White, Red Print	Temazepam 15 mg	Restoril by PDRX	55289-0196	Sedative/Hypnotic; C IV
TEMAZEPAM15MG272	Cap, in Red Ink, 272 Creighton Logo	Temazepam 15 mg	Restoril by Kaiser	00179-1106	Sedative/Hypnotic; C IV
TEMAZEPAM15MG272CP	Cap	Temazepam 15 mg	Restoril by Creighton	50752-0272	Sedative/Hypnotic; C IV
TEMAZEPAM30MG273CP	Cap	Temazepam 30 mg	Restoril by Creighton	50752-0273	Sedative/Hypnotic; C IV
TEMAZEPAM75MG271CP	Cap, Pink & White, Red Print, Temazepam over 7.5 mg over 271 over cp	Temazepam 7.5 mg	Restoril by Sandoz	00781-2209	Sedative/Hypnotic; C IV
TEMAZEPAM75MG271CP	Cap, Pink & White, Red Print, Temazepam over 7.5 mg over 271 over cp	Temazepam 7.5 mg	Restoril by Mallinckrodt	00406-9960	Sedative/Hypnotic; C IV
TEMAZEPAMP	Cap, Blue, Hard Gel	Temazepam 30 mg	Restoril by Pharmascience	Canadian DIN 5760694564	Sedative/Hypnotic; C IV
TEMAZEPAMP	Cap, Blue, Hard Gel	Temazepam 15 mg	Restoril by Pharmascience	Canadian DIN 5760694554	Sedative/Hypnotic; C IV
TEMODAL100MG	Cap, White, Opaque, Blue Ink	Temozolomide 100 mg	Temodal by Schering	Canadian DIN 02241095	Antineoplastic
TEMODAL20MG	Cap, White, Opaque, Brown Ink	Temozolomide 20 mg	Temodal by Schering	Canadian DIN 02241094	Antineoplastic
TEMODAL250MG	Cap, White, Opaque, Black Ink	Temozolomide 250 mg	Temodal by Schering	Canadian DIN 02241096	Antineoplastic
TEMODAL5MG	Cap, White, Opaque, Green Ink	Temozolomide 5 mg	Temodal by Schering	Canadian DIN 02241093	Antineoplastic

ID FRONT <> BACK	DESCRIPTION FRONT <> BACK	INGREDIENT & STRENGTH	BRAND (or Generic Equiv.) by FIRM	NDC#	CLASS; SCH.
TEMOZOLOMIDE100MG	Cap, White, Blue Ink	Temozolomide 100 mg	Temodar by Schering	00085-1259	Chemotherapy Agent
TEMOZOLOMIDE20MG	Cap, White, Red Ink	Temozolomide 20 mg	Temodar by Schering	00085-1244	Chemotherapy Agent
TEMOZOLOMIDE250MG	Cap, White, Black Ink	Temozolomide 250 mg	Temodar by Schering	00085-1252	Chemotherapy Agent
TEMOZOLOMIDE5MG	Cap, White	Temozolomide 5 mg	Temodar by Schering	00085-1248	Chemotherapy Agent
TEMPRA	Tab, Light Purple, Round	Acetaminophen 80 mg	Children's Tylenol by Mead Johnson	Canadian	Analgesic
TEMPRA160	Tab, Purple, Tempra/160	Acetaminophen 160 mg	Children's Tylenol by Sanofi	Canadian	Analgesic
TEMPRA160	Tab, Purple, Rectangular	Acetaminophen 160 mg	Children's Tylenol by Mead Johnson	Canadian	Analgesic
TEMPRA80	Tab, Purple, Tempra/80	Acetaminophen 80 mg	Children's Tylenol by Mead Johnson	Canadian	Analgesic
TENAKESEATRACE	Cap, Green Print	Acetaminophen 325 mg, Butalbital 50 mg, Caffeine 40 mg	Fioricet by Seatrace	00551-0181	Analgesic
TENCON <> 029	Tab, White, Cap Shaped	Acetaminophen 650 mg, Butalbital 50 mg	Tencon by Int'l Ethical Labs	11584-0029	Analgesic
TENEX <> 1AHR	Tab, Light Pink, Diamond Shaped, AHR imprinted inside 1	Guanfacine HCl 1 mg	Tenex by Pharmedix	53002-1045	Antihypertensive
TENEX <> 1AHR	Tab, Light Pink, Diamond Shaped, AHR imprinted inside 1	Guanfacine HCl 1 mg	Tenex by A H Robins	00031-8901	Antihypertensive
TENEX <> 1AHR	Tab, Light Pink, Diamond Shaped, AHR imprinted inside 1	Guanfacine HCl 1 mg	Tenex by Nat Pharmpak	55154-3008	Antihypertensive
TENEX <> 1AHR	Tab, Light Pink, Diamond Shaped, AHR imprinted inside 1	Guanfacine HCl 1 mg	Tenex by Leiner	59606-0748	Antihypertensive
TENEX <> 1AHR	Tab, Light Pink, Diamond Shaped, AHR imprinted inside 1	Guanfacine HCl 1 mg	Tenex by Rightpac	65240-0748	Antihypertensive
TENEX <> 1AHR	Tab, Light Pink, Diamond Shaped, AHR imprinted inside 1	Guanfacine HCl 1 mg	Tenex by Amerisource	62584-0901	Antihypertensive
TENEX <> 2AHR	Tab, Yellow, Diamond Shaped, 2 over AHR	Guanfacine HCl 2 mg	Tenex by Rightpac	65240-0748	Antihypertensive
TENOLIN100	Tab, White, Biconvex	Atenolol 100 mg	Tenormin by Technilab	Canadian	Antihypertensive
TENOLIN50	Tab, White, Biconvex	Atenolol 50 mg	Tenormin by Technilab	Canadian	Antihypertensive
TENORETIC <> 115	Tab, White, Round	Atenolol 50 mg, Chlorthalidone 25 mg	Tenoretic by AstraZeneca	00310-0115	Antihypertensive; Diuretic
TENORETIC <> 117	Tab, White, Round	Atenolol 100 mg, Chlorthalidone 25 mg	Tenoretic by AstraZeneca	00310-0117	Antihypertensive; Diuretic
TENORMIN	Tab, White to Off-White, Bioconvex, Film Coated, Scored	Atenolol 100 mg	Tenormin by AstraZeneca	Canadian DIN 02039540	Antihypertensive
TENORMIN <> 101	Tab, White, Round	Atenolol 100 mg	Tenormin by AstraZeneca	00310-0101	Antihypertensive
TENORMIN <> 105	Tab, White, Round, Scored	Atenolol 50 mg	Tenormin by AstraZeneca	00310-0105	Antihypertensive
TENORMIN50	Tab, White, Biconvex, Film Coated, Scored	Atenolol 50 mg	Tenormin by AstraZeneca	Canadian DIN 02039532	Antihypertensive
TENUATE25	Tab, White, Round	Diethylpropion HCl 25 mg	Tenuate by Merrell	00068-0697	Anorexiant; C IV
TENUATE75	Tab, White, Cap Shaped	Diethylpropion HCl 75 mg	Tenuate by Merrell	00068-0698	Anorexiant; C IV
TEQUIN200 <> BMS	Tab, White, Almond Shaped, Film Coated	Gatifloxacin 200 mg	Tequin by Mead Johnson	00015-1117 Discontinued	Antibiotic
TEQUIN200 <> BMS	Tab, White, Almond Shaped, Film Coated	Gatifloxacin 200 mg	Tequin by BMS	12783-0117 Discontinued	Antibiotic
TEQUIN400 <> BMS	Tab, White, Biconvex, Film Coated	Gatifloxacin 400 mg	Tequin by Mead Johnson	00015-1177 Discontinued	Antibiotic
TEQUIN400 <> BMS	Tab, White, Biconvex, Film Coated	Gatifloxacin 400 mg	Tequin by BMS	12783-0177 Discontinued	Antibiotic
TER250 <> APO	Tab, White, Round, Scored	Terbinafine HCl 250 mg	Lamisil by Apotex	Canadian DIN 02239893	Antifungal
TERBINAFINE <> P250	Tab, White, Round, Scored	Terbinafine HCl 250 mg	Lamisil by Pharmascience	Canadian DIN 02240807	Antifungal
TERF60	Tab, White, Round, Terf/60	Terfenadine 60 mg	Novo Terfenadine by Novopharm	Canadian	Antihistamine
TETE <> CGCG	Tab, Yellow, Oval, Scored, Film Coated	Oxcarbazepine 300 mg	Trileptal by Novartis	00078-0337	Anticonvulsant
TETE <> CGCG	Tab, Yellow, Oval, Scored, Film Coated	Oxcarbazepine 300 mg	Trileptal by Novartis	Canadian DIN 02242068	Anticonvulsant
TEVA <> 5715	Tab, White to Off-White, Cap Shaped, Chewable	Lamotrigine 5 mg	Lamictal by Teva	00093-5715 Discontinued	Anticonvulsant
TEVA <> 5716	Tab, White, Elliptical, Chewable, 57 over 16	Lamotrigine 25 mg	Lamictal by Teva	00093-5716 Discontinued	Anticonvulsant
TEVA <> 7202	Tab, Light Green, Round	Pravastatin Sodium 40 mg	Pravachol by Teva Pharmaceuticals	00093-7202	Antihyperlipidemic
TEVA <> 74	Tab, White to Off-White, Film Coated, Round	Zolpidem Tartrate 10 mg	Ambien by Teva Pharmaceuticals	00093-0074	Sedative/Hypnotic; C IV

ID FRONT <> BACK	DESCRIPTION FRONT <> BACK	INGREDIENT & STRENGTH	BRAND (or Generic Equiv.) by FIRM	NDC#	CLASS; SCH.
TEVA <> A10	Tab, White to Off White, Round, Film Coated	Anastrozole 1 mg	Arimidex by Teva Pharmaceuticals	00093-7536	Antineoplastic
TEVA081010MG	Cap, Orange & White, Black Print	Nortriptyline HCl 10 mg	Pamelor by Teva Pharmaceuticals	00093-0810	Antidepressant
TEVA081125MG	Cap, Orange & White, Black Print	Nortriptyline HCl 25 mg	Pamelor by Teva Pharmaceuticals	00093-0811	Antidepressant
TEVA081250MG	Cap, White, Black Print	Nortriptyline HCl 50 mg	Pamelor by Teva Pharmaceuticals	00093-0812	Antidepressant
TEVA081375MG	Cap, Orange, Black Print	Nortriptyline HCl 75 mg	Pamelor by Teva Pharmaceuticals	00093-0813	Antidepressant
TF	Tab, Abb. Logo	Metharbital 100 mg	Gemonil by Abbott		Sedative
TF <> A	Tab, Tan, Round	Levothyroxine Sodium 76 mcg, Liothyronine 18 mcg	Armour Thyroid by Amerisource	62584-0461	Thyroid Hormone
TFTF <> CGCG	Tab, Light Pink, Oval, Scored, Film Coated	Oxcarbazepine 600 mg	Trileptal by Novartis	Canadian DIN 02242069	Anticonvulsant
TFTG <> CGCG	Tab, Light Pink, Oval, Scored, Film Coated	Oxcarbazepine 600 mg	Trileptal by Novartis	00078-0457	Anticonvulsant
TH <> A	Tab, White, Round, Scored, Abbott Logo (a)	Pemoline 18.75 mg	Cylert by Abbott	00074-6025 Discontinued	Stimulant; C IV
TH1 <> MYLAN	Tab, Green, Scored, Beveled Edge, TH/1	Hydrochlorothiazide 25 mg, Triamterene 37.5 mg	Maxzide by Mylan	55160-0126	Diuretic; Antihypertensive
TH1 <> MYLAN	Tab, Green, Scored, Beveled Edge, TH/1	Hydrochlorothiazide 25 mg, Triamterene 37.5 mg	Maxzide by Mylan	00378-1352	Diuretic; Antihypertensive
TH2 <> MYLAN	Tab, Yellow, Round, Scored, TH over 2	Hydrochlorothiazide 50 mg, Triamterene 75 mg	Maxzide by UDL	51079-0433	Diuretic; Antihypertensive
TH2 <> MYLAN	Tab, Yellow, Round, Scored, TH over 2	Hydrochlorothiazide 50 mg, Triamterene 75 mg	Maxzide by Mylan	00378-1355	Diuretic; Antihypertensive
TH2 <> MYLAN	Tab, Yellow, Round, Scored, TH over 2	Hydrochlorothiazide 50 mg, Triamterene 75 mg	Maxzide by Mylan	55160-0127	Diuretic; Antihypertensive
THCA09	Tab, White, Round, THC over A09	Ephedrine 12.5 mg, Guaifenesin 200 mg	by Halsey		Cold Remedy
THCP07	Tab, White, Round	Ephedrine 20 mg, Guaifenesin 100 mg	by Hammer		Cold Remedy
THE100 <> APO	Tab, White, Round, The/100	Theophylline Anhydrous 100 mg	Theo LA by Apotex	Canadian DIN 00692689	Antiasthmatic
THE200 <> APO	Tab, White, Oval	Theophylline Anhydrous 200 mg	Theo LA by Apotex	Canadian DIN 00692697	Antiasthmatic
THE300	Tab, White, Oblong	Theophylline Anhydrous 300 mg	Theo LA by Apotex	Canadian	Antiasthmatic
THE300 <> APO	Tab, White, Cap Shaped, Scored	Theophylline 300 mg	Theo-DUR by Apotex	Canadian DIN 00692700	Muscle Relaxant
THEO24100MGUCB2832	Cap, Yellowish Orange & Clear, Ex Release	Theophylline Anhydrous 100 mg	Theo-24 by UCB	50474-0100	Antiasthmatic
THEO24200MGUCB2842	Cap, Reddish Orange & Clear, Ex Release	Theophylline Anhydrous 300 mg	Theo-24 by UCB	50474-0200	Antiasthmatic
THEO24200MGUCB2842	Cap, Reddish Orange & Clear, Ex Release	Theophylline Anhydrous 200 mg	Theo-24 by Taro	52549-4028	Antiasthmatic
THEO24200MGUCB2842	Cap, Reddish Orange & Clear, Ex Release	Theophylline Anhydrous 200 mg	Theo-24 by DRX	55045-2354	Antiasthmatic
THEO24300MGUCB2852	Cap, Clear & Red, Ex Release	Theophylline Anhydrous 300 mg	Theo-24 by Taro	52549-4029	Antiasthmatic
THEO24300MGUCB2852	Cap, Clear & Red, Ex Release	Theophylline Anhydrous 300 mg	Theo-24 by Taro	52549-4026	Antiasthmatic
THEO24300MGUCB2852	Cap, Clear & Red, Ex Release	Theophylline Anhydrous 300 mg	Theo-24 by UCB	50474-0300	Antiasthmatic
THEO24400MGUCB2902	Cap, Pink & Clear, Ex Release	Theophylline Anhydrous 400 mg	Theo-24 by UCB	50474-0400	Antiasthmatic
THEODUR100	Tab, White, Round, Scored, Theodur over 100	Theophylline Anhydrous 100 mg	Theo-Dur by Thrift Drug	59198-0235	Antiasthmatic
THEODUR100	Tab, White, Round, Scored, Theodur over 100	Theophylline Anhydrous 300 mg	Theo-Dur by Amerisource	62584-0487	Antiasthmatic
THEODUR100	Tab, White, Round, Scored, Theodur over 100	Theophylline Anhydrous 100 mg	Theo-Dur by Schering	00085-0487	Antiasthmatic
THEODUR200	Tab, White, Oval, Scored, THEO-DUR over 200	Theophylline Anhydrous 200 mg	Theo-Dur by Rightpac	65240-0750	Antiasthmatic
THEODUR200	Tab, White, Oval, Scored, THEO-DUR over 200	Theophylline Anhydrous 200 mg	Theo-Dur by Schering	00085-0933	Antiasthmatic
THEODUR200	Tab, White, Oval, Scored, THEO-DUR over 200	Theophylline Anhydrous 200 mg	Theo-Dur by AstraZeneca	Canadian	Antiasthmatic
THEODUR200	Tab, White, Oval, Scored, THEO-DUR over 200	Theophylline Anhydrous 200 mg	Theo-Dur by Thrift Drug	59198-0108	Antiasthmatic
THEODUR200	Tab, White, Oval, Scored, THEO-DUR over 200	Theophylline Anhydrous 200 mg	Theo-Dur by Amerisource	62584-0933	Antiasthmatic
THEODUR200	Tab, White, Oval, Scored, THEO-DUR over 200	Theophylline Anhydrous 200 mg	Theo-Dur by CVS	51316-0018	Antiasthmatic
THEODUR200	Tab, White, Oval, Scored, THEO-DUR over 200	Theophylline Anhydrous 200 mg	Theo-Dur by Nat Pharmpak	55154-1502	Antiasthmatic
THEODUR200	Tab, White, Oval, Scored, THEO-DUR over 200	Theophylline Anhydrous 200 mg	Theo-Dur by Kaiser	00179-1047	Antiasthmatic
THEODUR300	Tab, White, Oblong, Scored, THEO-DUR over 300	Theophylline Anhydrous 300 mg	Theo-Dur by Rightpac	65240-0751	Antiasthmatic
THEODUR300	Tab, White, Oblong, Scored, THEO-DUR over 300	Theophylline Anhydrous 300 mg	Theo-Dur by Taro	52549-4027	Antiasthmatic
THEODUR300	Tab, White, Oblong, Scored, THEO-DUR over 300	Theophylline Anhydrous 300 mg	Theo-Dur by Amerisource	62584-0584	Antiasthmatic
THEODUR300	Tab, White, Oblong, Scored, THEO-DUR over 300	Theophylline Anhydrous 300 mg	Theo-Dur by Thrift Drug	59198-0109	Antiasthmatic
THEODUR300	Tab, White, Oblong, Scored, THEO-DUR over 300	Theophylline Anhydrous 300 mg	Theo-Dur by Rite Aid	11822-5278	Antiasthmatic

ID FRONT <> BACK	DESCRIPTION FRONT <> BACK	INGREDIENT & STRENGTH	BRAND (or Generic Equiv.) by FIRM	NDC#	CLASS; SCH.
THEODUR300	Tab, White, Oblong, Scored, THEO-DUR over 300	Theophylline Anhydrous 300 mg	Theo-Dur by Pharmedix	53002-0575	Antiasthmatic
THEODUR300	Tab, White, Oblong, Scored, THEO-DUR over 300	Theophylline Anhydrous 300 mg	Theo-Dur by Nat Pharmpak	55154-1503	Antiasthmatic
THEODUR300	Tab, White, Oblong, Scored, THEO-DUR over 300	Theophylline Anhydrous 300 mg	Theo-Dur by Kaiser	00179-0365	Antiasthmatic
THEODUR300	Tab, White, Oblong, Scored, THEO-DUR over 300	Theophylline Anhydrous 300 mg	Theo-Dur by Caremark	00339-5395	Antiasthmatic
THEODUR300	Tab, White, Oblong, Scored, THEO-DUR over 300	Theophylline Anhydrous 300 mg	Theo-Dur by AstraZeneca	Canadian	Antiasthmatic
THEODUR300	Tab, White, Oblong, Scored, THEO-DUR over 300	Theophylline Anhydrous 300 mg	Theo-Dur by Schering	00085-0584	Antiasthmatic
THEODUR450	Tab, Off White, Cap Shaped, Scored, THEO-DUR over 450	Theophylline Anhydrous 450 mg	Theo-Dur by Schering	00085-0806	Antiasthmatic
THEODUR450	Tab, Off White, Cap Shaped, Scored, THEO-DUR over 450	Theophylline Anhydrous 450 mg	Theo-Dur by AstraZeneca	Canadian	Antiasthmatic
THEODUR450	Tab, Off White, Cap Shaped, Scored, THEO-DUR over 450	Theophylline Anhydrous 450 mg	Theo-Dur by Pharmedix	53002-1042	Antiasthmatic
THEODUR75	Tab	Theophylline Anhydrous 75 mg	Theo-Dur by Pharmedix	53002-1058	Antiasthmatic
THEOLAIR250 <> 3M	Tab, White, Cap Shaped, Scored	Theophylline Anhydrous 250 mg	Theo-Dur by 3M	00089-0344	Antiasthmatic
THEOPHYLLINE200	Tab, Debossed, Ex Release	Theophylline Anhydrous 200 mg	Theo-Dur by Repack Co of America	55306-1660	Antiasthmatic
THEOPHYLLINE300	Tab, Theophylline/300 Debossed, Ex Release	Theophylline Anhydrous 300 mg	Theo-Dur by Quality Care	60346-0596	Antiasthmatic
THEOPHYLLINE-XR1ARCOLA	Cap, White, Ex Release	Theophylline Anhydrous 100 mg	Theo-Dur by RPR	00801-2340	Antiasthmatic
THEOPHYLLINE-XR1ARCOLA	Cap, White, Ex Release	Theophylline Anhydrous 125 mg	Theo-Dur by Murfreesboro	51129-1670	Antiasthmatic
THEOPHYLLINE-XR1ARCOLA	Cap, White, Ex Release	Theophylline Anhydrous 125 mg	Theo-Dur by RPR	00801-2341	Antiasthmatic
THEOPHYLLINE-XR1ARCOLA	Cap, White, Ex Release	Theophylline Anhydrous 200 mg	Theo-Dur by Arcola	00070-2342 Discontinued	Antiasthmatic
THEOPHYLLINE-XR2ARCOLA	Cap, White, Ex Release	Theophylline Anhydrous 200 mg	Theo-Dur by RPR	00801-2342	Antiasthmatic
THEOPHYLLINE-XR2ARCOLA	Cap, White, Ex Release	Theophylline Anhydrous 300 mg	Theo-Dur by RPR	00801-2343	Antiasthmatic
THEOPHYLLINE-XR3ARCOLA	Cap, White, Ex Release	Theophylline Anhydrous 300 mg	Theo-Dur by Arcola	00070-2343 Discontinued	Antiasthmatic
THEOPHYLLINE-XR3ARCOLA	Cap, White, Ex Release	Theophylline Anhydrous 200 mg	Theo-Dur by DRX	55045-2279	Antiasthmatic
THEOPHYLLINE-XRARCOLA	Cap, White, Ex Release	Theophylline Anhydrous 125 mg	Theo-Dur by Arcola	00070-2341 Discontinued	Antiasthmatic
THEOPHYLLINE-XRARCOLA	Cap, White, Ex Release	Theophylline Anhydrous 100 mg	Theo-Dur by Arcola	00070-2340 Discontinued	Antiasthmatic
THERRX	Cap, White, Pink Print, Soft Gel	Omega-3 Fatty Acids 150 mg, Linoleic Acid 25 mg, Linolenic Acid 25 mg, Calcium Carbonate 150 mg, Vitamin D3 170 IU, Vitamin E 30 IU	PrimaCare by KV Pharma	64011-0015	Vitamin; Mineral
THERRX <> 014	Tab, Yellow, Diamond Shaped, Film Coated	Ascorbic Acid 60 mg, Calcium Carbonate 200 mg, Iron 30 mg, Vitamin E 30 IU, Thiamine Mononitrate 3 mg, Riboflavin 3.4 mg, Niacinamide 20 mg, Pyridoxine HCl 50 mg, Folic Acid 1 mg, Magnesium Oxide 100 mg, Cyanocobalamin 12 mcg, Zinc Oxide 15 mg, Cupric Oxide 2 mg, Folic Acid 1 mg	Precare Conceive by Ther Rx	64011-0014	Vitamin; Mineral
THERRX <> 019	Tab, Blue, Oval, Film Coated	Calcium 200 mg, Folic Acid 1 mg, Vitamin B6 75 mg, Vitamin B12 12 mcg	PremesisRx by KV Pharma	64011-0019	Vitamin; Mineral
THERRX <> 025	Tab, Peach, Cap Shaped, Scored, Film Coated	Ascorbic Acid 50 mg, Calcium Carbonate 250 mg, Cyanocobalamin 12 mcg, Cholecalciferol 6 mcg, Thiamine Mononitrate 3 mg, Riboflavin 3.4 mg, Niacinamide 20 mg, Pyridoxine HCl 20 mg, Folic Acid 1 mg, Magnesium Oxide 50 mg, Zinc Sulfate 15 mg, Cupric Sulfate 2 mg	Precare Prenatal by Ther Rx	64011-0025	Vitamin
THERRX <> 118	Tab, Peach, Cap Shaped, Film Coated	Folic Acid 1 mg, Vitamin B1 3 mg, Vitamin B2 3.4 mg, Vitamin B3 20 mg, Vitamin B6 50 mg, Vitamin B12 12 mcg, Vitamin C 50 mg, Vitamin D3 6 mcg, Vitamin E 3.5 IU, Calcium Carbonate 250 mg, Copper 2 mg, Iron 40 mg, Magnesium 50 mg, Zinc 15 mg	PreCare by KV Pharma	64011-0118	Vitamin; Mineral

ID FRONT <> BACK	DESCRIPTION FRONT <> BACK	INGREDIENT & STRENGTH	BRAND (or Generic Equiv.) by FIRM	NDC#	CLASS; SCH.
THERRX <> 119	Tab, White, Pink Print, Oval, Film Coated	Biotin 35 mcg, Folic Acid 1 mg, Vitamin B1 3 mg, Vitamin B2 3.4 mg, Vitamin B3 20 mg, Vitamin B6 10 mg, Vitamin B12 12 mcg, Vitamin C 100 mg, Vitamin D3 230 IU, Vitamin K 90 mcg, Pantothenic Acid 7 mg, Calcium Carbonate 250 mg, Chromium 45 mcg, Copper 1.3 mg, Iron 30 mg, Molybdenum 50 mcg, Selenium 75 mcg, Zinc 11 mg	PrimaCare by KV Pharma	64011-0015	Vitamin; Mineral
THERRX <> 147	Tab, Oval, Light Pink, Film-Coated, Scored	Calcium 400 mg, Vitamin D3 200 IU, Vitamin C 25 mg, Folic Acid 2 mg, Vitamin B6 25 mg	Encora AM by Ther-Rx	64011-0166	Supplement
THERRX <> 161	Tab, Oval, Purple, Film-Coated, Scored	Calcium 600 mg, Vitamin D3 600 IU, Vitamin C 25 mg, Folic Acid 0.5 mg, Vitamin B6 12.5 mg	Encora PM by Ther-Rx	64011-0166	Supplement
THERRX <> 195	Tab, Peach, Cap Shaped, Film Coated	Vitamin C 50 mg, Vitamin D3 6 mcg, Vitamin E 3.5 IU, Vitamin B1 3 mg, Vitamin B2 3.4 mg, Vitamin B3 20 mg, Vitamin B6 50 mg, Folic Acid 1 mg, Vitamin B12 12 mcg, Calcium 250 mg, Iron 30 mg, Magnesium 25 mg, Zinc 15 mg, Copper 2 mg, Docusate Sodium 50 mg, Succinic Acid 35 mg	PreCare Premier by Ther-Rx	64011-0195	Supplement
THERRX <> 197	Tab, Maroon, Cap Shaped, Film Coated, Ther-Rx <> 197	Iron 151 mg (Iron Sumalate 50 mg) (Iron Fumarate 101 mg), Succinic Acid 50 mg, Vitamin C 60.8 mg (Ascorbic Acid 60 mg) (Threonic Acid 0.8 mg), Folic Acid 1 mg, Vitamin B12 10 mcg	Chromagen Forte by Ther-Rx	64011-0197	Supplement
THERRX <> 198	Tab, Maroon, Cap Shaped, Film Coated, Ther-Rx <> 198	Iron 70 mg, Succinic Acid 75 mg, Vitamin C 152 mg (Ascorbic Acid 150 mg) (Threonic Acid 2 mg), Vitamin B12 10 mcg, Desiccated Stomach Substance 50 mg	Chromagen by Ther-Rx	64011-0198	Supplement
THERRX <> 199	Tab, Green, Cap Shaped, Film Coated, Ther-Rx <> 199	Iron 70 mg, Succinic Acid 75 mg, Vitamin C 152 mg (Ascorbic Acid 150 mg) (Threonic Acid 2 mg), Folic Acid 1 mg, Vitamin B12 10 mcg	Chromagen FA by Ther-Rx	64011-0199	Supplement
THERRX <> 201	Tab, Red, Scored, Film-Coated	Iron Sumalate 70 mg, Iron Ferrous Fumarate 81 mg, Succinic Acid 150 mg, Vitamin C 140 mg, Vitamin C (Ascorbic Acid 60 mg) (Threonic Acid 0.8 mg), Folic Acid 1 mg, Vitamin B12 10 mcg	Repliva 21/7 by Ther-Rx	64011-0207	Supplement
THERRX <> 206	Tab, Purple, Scored, Film-Coated	Succinic Acid 150 mg	Repliva 21/7 by Ther-Rx	64011-0207	Supplement
THERRX148	Cap, Pink, Soft Gel	Essential Fatty Acids (Omega-3) 650 mg, Linoleic Acid 10 mg, Vitamin E 50 IU	Encora AM and PM by Ther-Rx	64011-0166	Supplement
THERRX200	Cap, Purple, Ther-Rx 200	Omega-3 Fatty Acids 300 mg, Linoleic Acid 30 mg, Linolenic Acid 30 mg, Vitamin C 25 mg, Vitamin D3 170 IU, Vitamin E 30 IU, Folic Acid 1 mg, Vitamin B6 25 mg, Calcium 150 mg, Iron 27 mg (Elemental Carbonyl Iron 20 mg, Sumalate Iron 7 mg)	PrimaCare ONE by Ther-Rx	64011-0200	Prenatal Vitamin
THISENDUP DEPAKOTESPRINKLE-125MG	Cap, Blue & White, Black Print, THIS END UP on blue, DEPAKOTE over SPRINKLE over 125 mg on white	Divalproex Sodium 125 mg	Depakote by Abbott	00074-6114	Anticonvulsant
THUMBSUP	Tab, White, Round, Thumbs Up Logo	3,4-Methylenedioxymethamphetamine (MDMA)	Ecstasy by Illegal		Euphoric; Illicit
THX <> 024	Tab, Orange, Oval, Film Coated, Chewable	Calcium 250 mg, Copper 2 mg, Folic Acid 1 mg, Iron 40 mg, Magnesium 50 mg, Vitamin B6 2 mg, Vitamin C 50 mg, Vitamin D3 6 mcg, Vitamin E 3.5 IU, Zinc 15 mg	Precare Prenatal by Ther Rx	64011-0024	Vitamin; Mineral
THX0135	Cap, Red, Clear	Elemental Iron 150 mg, Vitamin C 50 mg	Niferex 150 by Ther-Rx	64011-0135	Vitamin
THX0136	Cap, Red, Clear	Ferrochel (elemental iron) 80 mg, Polysaccharide iron 70 mg, Vitamin C 60 mg, Threonic acid 0.8 mg, Folic Acid 1 mg, Vitamin B12 25 mcg	Niferex 150 Forte by Ther-Rx	64011-0136	Vitamin
THX164	Cap, Red and Clear, Brown Powder	Iron Sumalate 50 mg, Polysaccharide Iron 100 mg, Succinic Acid 50 mg, Vitamin C 60 mg, Threonic acid 0.8 mg, Folic Acid 1 mg, Vitamin B12 25 mcg	Niferex-150 Forte by Ther-Rx	64011-0164	Vitamin
TI	Tab, White, Scored	Tizanidine HCl 4 mg	Zanaflex by Genpharm	15330-0248	Muscle Relaxant
TI <> A	Tab, Orange, Round, Scored, Abbott Logo (a)	Pemoline 37.5 mg	Cylert by Abbott	00074-6057 Discontinued	Stimulant; C IV
TI <> G	Tab, White, Scored	Tizanidine HCl 2 mg	Zanaflex by Genpharm	15330-0247	Muscle Relaxant
TI01	Cap, Light Green, TI01 <> Boehringer Ingelheim Logo, Cap contains powder for inhalation	Tiotropium 18 mcg	Spiriva by Boehringer Ingelheim	00597-0075	Antiasthmatic
TIAFEN200	Tab, White	Tiaprofenic Acid 200 mg	Albert Tiafen by Aventis	Canadian Discontinued	NSAID

For updated data, go to www.IdentADrug.com

ID FRONT <> BACK	DESCRIPTION FRONT <> BACK	INGREDIENT & STRENGTH	BRAND (or Generic Equiv.) by FIRM	NDC#	CLASS; SCH.
TIAFEN200	Tab, White	Tiaprofenic Acid 200 mg	Tiafen by AltiMed	Canadian DIN 01924613	NSAID
TIAFEN300	Tab, White	Tiaprofenic Acid 300 mg	Tiafen by AltiMed	Canadian DIN 01924621	NSAID
TIAFEN300	Tab, White	Tiaprofenic Acid 300 mg	Albert Tiafen by Aventis	Canadian Discontinued	NSAID
TIAMATE120	Tab	Diltiazem Malate 120 mg	Tiamate by Merck	00006-0760	Antihypertensive
TIAMATE180	Tab	Diltiazem Malate 180 mg	Tiamate by Merck	00006-0762	Antihypertensive
TIAMATE240	Tab	Diltiazem Malate 240 mg	Tiamate by Merck	00006-0763	Antihypertensive
TIAPROFENIC <> P300	Tab, White, Round, Scored	Tiaprofenic 300 mg	Surgam by Pharmascience	Canadian DIN 02230828	NSAID
TIAZAC120	Cap, Purple, Ex Release	Diltiazem HCl 120 mg	Tiazac by Biovail	55542-0001	Antihypertensive
TIAZAC120	Cap, Purple, Ex Release	Diltiazem HCl 120 mg	Tiazac by Wal Mart	49035-0160	Antihypertensive
TIAZAC120	Cap, Purple, Ex Release	Diltiazem HCl 120 mg	Tiazac by Physician Total Care	54868-3774	Antihypertensive
TIAZAC120	Cap, Purple, Ex Release	Diltiazem HCl 120 mg	Tiazac by Forest	00456-2612	Antihypertensive
TIAZAC120	Cap, Purple, Ex Release	Diltiazem HCl 120 mg	Tiazac by Rx Pak	65084-0227	Antihypertensive
TIAZAC120	Cap, Purple, Ex Release	Diltiazem HCl 120 mg	Tiazac by Eckerd	19458-0860	Antihypertensive
TIAZAC120	Cap, Purple, Ex Release	Diltiazem HCl 120 mg	Tiazac by Biovail	62660-0001	Antihypertensive
TIAZAC180	Cap, White & Blue-Green, Ex Release	Diltiazem HCl 180 mg	Tiazac by Biovail	55542-0002	Antihypertensive
TIAZAC180	Cap, White & Blue-Green, Ex Release	Diltiazem HCl 180 mg	Tiazac by Physician Total Care	54868-3956	Antihypertensive
TIAZAC180	Cap, White & Blue-Green, Ex Release	Diltiazem HCl 180 mg	Tiazac by Rx Pak	65084-0226	Antihypertensive
TIAZAC180	Cap, White & Blue-Green, Ex Release	Diltiazem HCl 180 mg	Tiazac by Wal Mart	49035-0161	Antihypertensive
TIAZAC180	Cap, White & Blue-Green, Ex Release	Diltiazem HCl 180 mg	Tiazac by CVS	51316-0244	Antihypertensive
TIAZAC180	Cap, White & Blue-Green, Ex Release	Diltiazem HCl 180 mg	Tiazac by Biovail	62660-0002	Antihypertensive
TIAZAC180	Cap, White & Blue-Green, Ex Release	Diltiazem HCl 180 mg	Tiazac by Forest	00456-2613	Antihypertensive
TIAZAC180	Cap, White & Blue-Green, Ex Release	Diltiazem HCl 180 mg	Tiazac by Thrift Drug	59198-0350	Antihypertensive
TIAZAC180	Cap, White & Blue-Green, Ex Release	Diltiazem HCl 180 mg	Tiazac by Eckerd	19458-0861	Antihypertensive
TIAZAC240	Cap, Blue-Green & Purple, Ex Release	Diltiazem HCl 240 mg	Tiazac by Biovail	55542-0003	Antihypertensive
TIAZAC240	Cap, Blue-Green & Purple, Ex Release	Diltiazem HCl 240 mg	Tiazac by Biovail	62660-0003	Antihypertensive
TIAZAC240	Cap, Blue-Green & Purple, Ex Release	Diltiazem HCl 240 mg	Tiazac by Rx Pak	65084-0228	Antihypertensive
TIAZAC240	Cap, Blue-Green & Purple, Ex Release	Diltiazem HCl 240 mg	Tiazac by Wal Mart	49035-0162	Antihypertensive
TIAZAC240	Cap, Blue-Green & Purple, Ex Release	Diltiazem HCl 240 mg	Tiazac by CVS	51316-0243	Antihypertensive
TIAZAC240	Cap, Blue-Green & Purple, Ex Release	Diltiazem HCl 240 mg	Tiazac by Forest	00456-2614	Antihypertensive
TIAZAC240	Cap, Blue-Green & Purple, Ex Release	Diltiazem HCl 240 mg	Tiazac by Egis	48581-6124	Antihypertensive
TIAZAC240	Cap, Blue-Green & Purple, Ex Release	Diltiazem HCl 240 mg	Tiazac by Eckerd	19458-0862	Antihypertensive
TIAZAC300	Cap, Purple & White	Diltiazem HCl 300 mg	Tiazac by Astellas	61276-0607	Antihypertensive
TIAZAC300	Cap, Purple & White	Diltiazem HCl 300 mg	Tiazac by Biovail	55542-0004	Antihypertensive
TIAZAC300	Cap, Purple & White	Diltiazem HCl 300 mg	Tiazac by Biovail	62660-0004	Antihypertensive
TIAZAC300	Cap, Purple & White	Diltiazem HCl 300 mg	Tiazac by Wal Mart	49035-0163	Antihypertensive
TIAZAC300	Cap, Purple & White	Diltiazem HCl 300 mg	Tiazac by Thrift Drug	59198-0323	Antihypertensive
TIAZAC300	Cap, Purple & White	Diltiazem HCl 300 mg	Tiazac by Rx Pak	65084-0134	Antihypertensive
TIAZAC300	Cap, Purple & White	Diltiazem HCl 300 mg	Tiazac by Forest	00456-2615	Antihypertensive
TIAZAC300	Cap, Purple & White	Diltiazem HCl 300 mg	Tiazac by Nat Pharmpak	55154-4607	Antihypertensive
TIAZAC300	Cap, Purple & White	Diltiazem HCl 300 mg	Tiazac by Eckerd	19458-0863	Antihypertensive
TIAZAC360	Cap, Blue-Green, Ex Release	Diltiazem HCl 360 mg	Tiazac by Biovail	55542-0005	Antihypertensive
TIAZAC360	Cap, Blue-Green, Ex Release	Diltiazem HCl 360 mg	Tiazac by Biovail	62660-0005	Antihypertensive
TIAZAC360	Cap, Blue-Green, Ex Release	Diltiazem HCl 360 mg	Tiazac by Forest	00456-2616	Antihypertensive
TIAZAC360	Cap, Blue-Green, Ex Release	Diltiazem HCl 360 mg	Tiazac by Wal Mart	49035-0164	Antihypertensive
TIAZAC360	Cap, Blue-Green, Ex Release	Diltiazem HCl 360 mg	Tiazac by Eckerd	19458-0864	Antihypertensive
TIAZAC360	Cap, Blue-Green, Ex Release	Diltiazem HCl 360 mg	Tiazac by Nat Pharmpak	55154-4608	Antihypertensive

ID FRONT <> BACK	DESCRIPTION FRONT <> BACK	INGREDIENT & STRENGTH	BRAND (or Generic Equiv.) by FIRM	NDC#	CLASS; SCH.
TIAZAC420	Cap, White, Ex Release	Diltiazem HCl 420 mg	Tiazac by Forest	00456-2617	Antihypertensive
TICLID <> 250	Tab, White, Blue Print, Oval, Film Coated	Ticlopidine HCl 250 mg	Ticlid by Roche	Canadian DIN 02162776 Discontinued	Anticoagulant
TICLID <> 250	Tab, White, Blue Print, Oval, Film Coated	Ticlopidine HCl 250 mg	Ticlid by Hoffmann La Roche	00004-0018	Anticoagulant
TICLID <> 250	Tab, White, Blue Print, Oval, Film Coated	Ticlopidine HCl 250 mg	Ticlid by Syntex	18393-0431	Anticoagulant
TICLID <> 250	Tab, White, Blue Print, Oval, Film Coated	Ticlopidine HCl 250 mg	Ticlid by Wal Mart	49035-0165	Anticoagulant
TICLID <> 250	Tab, White, Blue Print, Oval, Film Coated	Ticlopidine HCl 250 mg	Ticlid by Physician Total Care	54868-3783	Anticoagulant
TICLID <> 250	Tab, White, Blue Print, Oval, Film Coated	Ticlopidine HCl 250 mg	Ticlid by Med Pro	53978-3027	Anticoagulant
TIGAN	Cap	Trimethobenzamide HCl 100 mg	Tigan by King	60793-0857	Antiemetic
TIGAN	Cap, Blue & White	Trimethobenzamide HCl 100 mg	by Murfreesboro	51129-1432	Antiemetic
TIGAN100MG	Cap, Blue & White	Trimethobenzamide HCl 100 mg	Tigan by Roberts	54092-0186	Antiemetic
TIGAN250MG	Cap, Blue, White Print, Tigan over 250 mg	Trimethobenzamide HCl 250 mg	by Thrift Drug	59198-0273	Antiemetic
TIGAN250MG	Cap, Blue, White Print, Tigan over 250 mg	Trimethobenzamide HCl 250 mg	Tigan by Roberts	54092-0187	Antiemetic
TIGAN250MG	Cap, Blue, White Print, Tigan over 250 mg	Trimethobenzamide HCl 250 mg	by SKB	00029-4083	Antiemetic
TIGANM079	Cap, Dark Blue, White Ink	Trimethobenzamide HCl 300 mg	Tigan by Monarch	61570-0079	Antiemetic
TIGANM187	Cap, Blue, Opaque	Trimethobenzamide HCl 250 mg	Tigan by Monarch	61570-0187	Antiemetic
TIGANM187	Cap, Blue, Opaque	Trimethobenzamide HCl 250 mg	Tigan by Roberts	54092-0186	Antiemetic
TIGANROBERTS187	Cap	Trimethobenzamide HCl 250 mg	Tigan by King	60793-0885	Antiemetic
TIMEHISTMCR	Cap, Clear, Time-Hist MCR	Chlorpheniramine Maleate 8 mg, Pseudoephedrine HCl 120 mg	by Compumed	00403-0010	Cold Remedy
TIMEHISTMCR	Cap, Time Hist Printed in Red, Ex Release	Chlorpheniramine Maleate 8 mg, Pseudoephedrine HCl 120 mg	Time Hist by Sovereign	58716-0016	Cold Remedy
TIMOLIDE <> MSD67	Tab, Light Blue, Hexagonal	Timolol Maleate 10 mg, Hydrochlorothiazide 25 mg	Timolide by Merck	00006-0067	Antihypertensive; Diuretic
TISH <> 3618	Tab, Beige, Oblong	Polycarbophil 500 mg	Fibercon by Rugby		Laxative
TISH <> 3712	Tab, Green, Triangular	Ferrous Sulfate 324 mg	Feosol by ADH Health Products		Mineral
TISH <> 8962	Tab, Beige, Oblong	Polycarbophil 500 mg	FiberCon by Rugby	00536-4306	Laxative
TISH8441	Tab, Yellow & White, Round	Aluminum Hydroxide 200 mg, Magnesium Hydroxide 200 mg, Simethicone 20 mg	Mylanta by Rugby	00536-3035	Antacid
TJ	Tab, Logo TJ	Levothyroxine 57 mcg, Liothyronine 13.5 mcg	Armour Thyroid by Allscripts		Thyroid Hormone
TJ <> A	Tab, Tan, Round, Scored, Abbott Logo (a)	Pemoline 75 mg	Cylert by Abbott	00074-6073 Discontinued	Stimulant; C IV
TK <> A	Tab, Orange, Square, Scored, Chewable, Abbott Logo (a)	Pemoline 37.5 mg	Cylert Chewable by Abbott	00074-6088 Discontinued	Stimulant; C IV
TKN125PFIZER	Cap, Light Orange & White	Dofetilide 125 mcg	Tikosyn by Pfizer	00069-5800	Antiarrhythmic
TKN250PFIZER	Cap, Peach	Dofetilide 250 mcg	Tikosyn by Pfizer	00069-5810	Antiarrhythmic
TKN500PFIZER	Cap, Peach & White	Dofetilide 500 mcg	Tikosyn by Pfizer	00069-5820	Antiarrhythmic
TL001	Tab, White, Oval, Scored	Methylprednisolone 4 mg	Medrol by Par	49884-0490	Steroid
TL001	Tab, White, Oval, Scored	Methylprednisolone 4 mg	Medrol by Neuman	64579-0042	Steroid
TL001	Tab, White, Oval, Scored	Methylprednisolone 4 mg	Medrol by Trigen	59746-0001	Steroid
TL001	Tab, White, Oval, Scored	Methylprednisolone 4 mg	Medrol by Lannett	00527-1296	Steroid
TL001	Tab, White, Oval, Scored	Methylprednisolone 4 mg	Medrol by Ranbaxy	63304-0591	Steroid
TL001	Tab, White, Oval, Scored	Methylprednisolone 4 mg	Medrol by Prasco	66993-0840	Steroid
TL001	Tab, White, Oval, Scored	Methylprednisolone 4 mg	Medrol by Major	00904-2175	Steroid
TL001	Tab, White, Oval, Scored	Methylprednisolone 4 mg	Medrol by Dava	67253-0360	Steroid
TL002	Tab, White, Scored	Methylprednisolone 8 mg	Medrol by Prasco	66993-0842	Steroid
TL012	Tab, Yellow, Round	Folic Acid 1 mg	Folvite by Dava	67253-0981	Vitamin
TL113	Tab, Yellow, Round, Scored, Film Coated	Prochlorperazine 5 mg	Compazine by Prasco	66993-0805	Antiemetic
TL113	Tab, Yellow, Round, Scored, Film Coated	Prochlorperazine 5 mg	Compazine by Ranbaxy	63304-0590	Antiemetic
TL113	Tab, Yellow, Round, Scored, Film Coated	Prochlorperazine 5 mg	Compazine by Par	49884-0549	Antiemetic
TL115	Tab, Yellow, Round, Scored, Film Coated	Prochlorperazine 10 mg	Compazine by Par	49884-0550	Antiemetic
TL115	Tab, Yellow, Round, Scored, Film Coated	Prochlorperazine 10 mg	Compazine by Prasco	66993-0810	Antiemetic

ID FRONT <> BACK	DESCRIPTION FRONT <> BACK	INGREDIENT & STRENGTH	BRAND (or Generic Equiv.) by FIRM	NDC#	CLASS; SCH.
TL115	Tab, Yellow, Round, Scored, Film Coated	Prochlorperazine 10 mg	Compazine by Ranbaxy	63304-0589	Antiemetic
TL171	Tab, White, Round	Prednisone 1 mg	Deltasone by Cadista	59746-0171	Steroid
TL177	Tab, Yellow, Round	Cyclobenzaprine HCl 10 mg	Flexeril by Trigen	59746-0177	Muscle Relaxant
TL211	Tab, Orange, Round	Cyclobenzaprine HCl 5 mg	Flexeril by Jubilant		Muscle Relaxant
TL382	Cap, Blue and White	Hydrochlorothiazide 12.5 mg	Hydrodiuril by Cadista	59746-0382	Antihypertensive
TL383	Cap, Gray, Opaque, Black Ink	Terazosin 1 mg	Hytrin by Trigen	59746-0383	Antihypertensive
TL384	Cap, Ivory, Opaque, Black Ink	Terazosin 2 mg	Hytrin by Trigen	59746-0384	Antihypertensive
TL385	Cap, Orange, Opaque, Black Ink	Terazosin 5 mg	Hytrin by Trigen	59746-0385	Antihypertensive
TL386	Cap, Light Green, Opaque, Black Ink	Terazosin 10 mg	Hytrin by Trigen	59746-0386	Antihypertensive
TL50 <> G	Tab, White, Film Coated	Tramadol HCl 50 mg	Ultram by Par	49884-0742	Analgesic
TLC037	Cap, Blue & Clear w/ Blue & White Beads, Ex Release	Phenylpropanolamine 75 mg	Mini Thin Diet Aid by BDI		Decongestant; Appetite Suppressant
TLC1221	Cap, Pink & Clear, Ex Release	Nitroglycerin 2.5 mg	Nitrobid by Ivax	00182-0702 Discontinued	Vasodilator
TLC1222	Cap, Yellow & Blue, Ex Release	Nitroglycerin 6.5 mg	Nitrobid by Ivax	00182-0703 Discontinued	Vasodilator
TM <> 250	Tab, Pink, Round, Film Coated	Tinidazole 250 mg	Tindamax by Mission	00178-8250	Antibiotic
TM <> 500	Tab, Pink, Oval, Film Coated	Tinidazole 500 mg	Tindamax by Mission	00178-8500	Antibiotic
TMB100 <> APO	Tab, White, Round, Scored	Trimebutine Maleate 100 mg	Modulon by Apotex	Canadian DIN 02245663	Motility Regulator
TMB200 <> APO	Tab, White, Round, Scored	Trimebutine Maleate 100 mg	Modulon by Apotex	Canadian DIN 02245664	Motility Regulator
TMC <> 150	Tab, White, Oval, Film Coated	Darunavir 150 mg	Prezista by Tibotec	59676-0564	Antiviral
TMC <> 400	Tab, Light Orange, Oval, Film Coated	Darunavir 400 mg	Prezista by Tibotec	59676-0561	Antiviral
TMC <> 400mg	Tab, Light Orange, Oval, Film Coated	Darunavir 400 mg	Prezista by Janssen-Ortho	Canadian DIN 02324016	Antiviral
TMC <> 600	Tab, Orange, Oval, Film Coated	Darunavir 600 mg	Prezista by Tibotec	59676-0562	Antiviral
TMC <> 600mg	Tab, Orange, Oval, Film Coated	Darunavir 600 mg	Prezista by Janssen-Ortho	Canadian DIN 02324024	Antiviral
TMC <> 75	Tab, White, Cap Shaped, Film Coated	Darunavir 75 mg	Prezista by Tibotec	59676-0563	Antiviral
TMC114 <> 300	Tab, Orange, Oval, Film-Coated	Darunavir 300 mg	Prezista by Tibotec	59676-0560 Discontinued	Antiviral
TMC114 <> 300MG	Tab, Orange, Oval, Film-Coated	Darunavir 300 mg	Prezista by Janssen-Ortho	Canadian DIN 02284057	Antiviral
TMC125 <> 100	Tab, White to Off-White, Oval	Etravirine 100 mg	Intelence by Tibotec	59676-0570	Antiviral
TN1	Tab, White, Round, Scored, Cobalt Logo <> TN / 1	Trandolapril 1 mg	Mavik by Cobalt	16252-0541	Antihypertensive
TN10G	Tab, White, Biconvex, TN 10/G	Tamoxifen Citrate 10 mg	Nolvadex by Genpharm	Canadian	Antiestrogen
TN120	Tab, White, Round	Sodium Bicarbonate 10 g	by Watson	00536-4544	Antacid
TN2	Tab, White, Round, Cobalt Logo <> TN2	Trandolapril 2 mg	Mavik by Cobalt	16252-0542	Antihypertensive
TN20G	Tab, White, Octagonal, TN-20/G	Tamoxifen Citrate 20 mg	Nolvadex by Genpharm	Canadian	Antiestrogen
TN4	Tab, White, Round, Cobalt Logo <> TN4	Trandolapril 4 mg	Mavik by Cobalt	16252-0543	Antihypertensive
TO	Tab, White, Round	Tolterodine 1 mg	Detrol by Pharmacia	10829-4541	Urinary Tract
TO	Tab, White, Round	Tolterodine 1 mg	Detrol by Pharmacia	00009-4541	Urinary Tract
TO	Tab, White, Round	Tolterodine 1 mg	Detrol by Pharmacia	Canadian DIN 02239064	Urinary Tract
TO10 <> APO	Tab, White to Off-White, Cap Shaped, Scored, APO <> TO / 10	Torsemide 10 mg	Demadex by Apotex	60505-0233	Diuretic
TO20 <> APO	Tab, White to Off-White, Cap Shaped, Scored, APO <> TO / 20	Torsemide 20 mg	Demadex by Apotex	60505-0234	Diuretic
TO60	Tab, White, Round	Toremifene Citrate 60 mg	Fareston by Schering	00085-1126	Antiestrogen

ID FRONT <> BACK	DESCRIPTION FRONT <> BACK	INGREDIENT & STRENGTH	BRAND (or Generic Equiv.) by FIRM	NDC#	CLASS; SCH.
TO60	Tab, White, Round	Toremifene Citrate 60 mg	Fareston by Roberts	54092-0170	Antiestrogen
TOA1	Tab, White, Cylindrical, T/O/A1	Glyburide 2.5 mg	by Boehringer Mannheim	Canadian	Antidiabetic
TOFRANILPM100MGM	Cap, Yellow & Orange, Black Print, M inside square	Imipramine Pamoate 100 mg	Tofranil PM by Mallinckrodt	00406-9924	Antidepressant
TOFRANILPM125MGM	Cap, Coral & Ivory, Black Print, M inside square	Imipramine Pamoate 125 mg	Tofranil PM by Mallinckrodt	00406-9925	Antidepressant
TOFRANILPM150MGM	Cap, Coral, Black Print	Imipramine Pamoate 150 mg	Tofranil PM by Mallinckrodt	00406-9926	Antidepressant
TOFRANILPM75MGM	Cap, Coral, Black Print, M inside square	Imipramine Pamoate 75 mg	Tofranil PM by Mallinckrodt	00406-9923	Antidepressant
TOLECTIN200 <> MCNEIL	Tab, White, Round, Scored, Tolectin over 200	Tolmetin Sodium 200 mg	Tolectin by McNeil	Canadian	NSAID
TOLECTIN200 <> MCNEIL	Tab, White, Round, Scored, Tolectin over 200	Tolmetin Sodium 200 mg	Tolectin by McNeil	00045-0412	NSAID
TOLECTIN600MCNEIL	Tab, Orange, Black Print, Oval, Film Coated, Tolectin over 600 over McNeil	Tolmetin Sodium 400 mg	Tolectin by McNeil	Canadian	NSAID
TOLECTIN600MCNEIL	Tab, Orange, Black Print, Oval, Film Coated, Tolectin over 600 over McNeil	Tolmetin Sodium 738 mg	by Pharmedix	53002-0597	NSAID
TOLECTIN600MCNEIL	Tab, Orange, Black Print, Oval, Film Coated, Tolectin over 600 over McNeil	Tolmetin Sodium 738 mg	by Amerisource	62584-0416	NSAID
TOLECTIN600MCNEIL	Tab, Orange, Black Print, Oval, Film Coated, Tolectin over 600 over McNeil	Tolmetin Sodium 600 mg	Tolectin by McNeil	00045-0416	NSAID
TOLECTINDSMCNEIL	Cap, Orange, Gray Print	Tolmetin Sodium 492 mg	Tolectin Ds by Amerisource	62584-0414	NSAID
TOLECTINDSMCNEIL	Cap, Orange, Gray Print	Tolmetin Sodium 492 mg	Tolectin Ds by McNeil	00045-0414	NSAID
TOLECTINDSMCNEIL	Cap, Orange, Gray Print	Tolmetin Sodium 492 mg	Tolectin Ds by Pharmedix	53002-0318	NSAID
TOLECTINDSMCNEIL	Cap, Orange, Gray Print	Tolmetin Sodium 492 mg	Tolectin Ds by Thrift Drug	59198-0127	NSAID
TOLINASE100	Tab, White, Round, Scored, Tolinase over 100	Tolazamide 100 mg	Tolinase by Pharmacia	00009-0070	Antidiabetic
TOLINASE250	Tab, White, Half Oval, Scored	Tolazamide 250 mg	Tolinase by Pharmacia	00009-0114	Antidiabetic
TOLINASE500	Tab, White, Half Oval, Scored	Tolazamide 500 mg	Tolinase by Pharmacia	00009-0477	Antidiabetic
TOLMENTIN600	Tab, Film Coated	Tolmetin Sodium 738 mg	by Major	00904-5149	NSAID
TOLMETIN200	Tab	Sodium 18 mg, Tolmetin Sodium 245 mg	by McNeil	52021-0846	NSAID
TOLMETIN200	Tab, White, Round	Sodium 18 mg, Tolmetin Sodium 245 mg	by Duramed	51285-0846	NSAID
TOLMETIN400	Cap, Orange, Parallel Bands	Sodium 36 mg, Tolmetin Sodium 490 mg	by Duramed	51285-0847	NSAID
TOLMETIN400	Cap, Parallel Bands	Sodium 36 mg, Tolmetin Sodium 490 mg	by McNeil	52021-0847	NSAID
TOLMETIN400	Cap	Tolmetin Sodium 492 mg	by Quality Care	60346-0615	NSAID
TOLMETIN400	Cap	Tolmetin Sodium 492 mg	Tolectin by Quality Care	60346-0615	NSAID
TOLMETIN600	Tab, Orange, Coated, Football Shaped	Sodium 54 mg, Tolmetin Sodium 735 mg	by Duramed	51285-0848	NSAID
TOLMETIN600	Tab, Coated	Sodium 54 mg, Tolmetin Sodium 735 mg	by McNeil	52021-0848	NSAID
TONOCARD <> 707	Tab, Yellow, Oval, Scored, Film Coated	Tocainide HCl 400 mg	Tonocard by AstraZeneca	00186-0707	Antiarrhythmic
TONOCARD <> 709	Tab, Yellow, Oblong, Scored, Film Coated	Tocainide HCl 600 mg	Tonocard by AstraZeneca	00186-0709	Antiarrhythmic
TONOCARD <> MSD707	Tab, Yellow, Oval, Scored, Film Coated	Tocainide HCl 400 mg	Tonocard by Merck	00006-0707	Antiarrhythmic
TONOCARD <> MSD707	Tab, Yellow, Oval, Scored, Film Coated	Tocainide HCl 400 mg	Tonocard by Teva	00480-0089	Antiarrhythmic
TONOCARD <> MSD709	Tab, Yellow, Oblong, Scored, Film Coated	Tocainide HCl 600 mg	Tonocard by Teva	00480-0090	Antiarrhythmic
TONOCARD <> MSD709	Tab, Yellow, Oblong, Scored, Film Coated	Tocainide HCl 600 mg	Tonocard by Merck	00006-0709	Antiarrhythmic
TOP <> 100	Tab, Yellow to Light Brown, Round, Film Coated	Topiramate 100 mg	Topamax by Janssen-Ortho	Canadian DIN 02230894	Anticonvulsant
TOP <> 200	Tab, Salmon, Round, Film Coated	Topiramate 200 mg	Topamax by Janssen-Ortho	Canadian DIN 02230896	Anticonvulsant
TOP <> 25	Tab, White, Round, Film Coated	Topiramate 25 mg	Topamax by Ortho-McNeil	00062-0639	Anticonvulsant
TOP <> 25	Tab, White, Round, Film Coated	Topiramate 25 mg	Topamax by Janssen-Ortho	Canadian DIN 02230893	Anticonvulsant
TOP <> 25	Tab, White, Round, Film Coated	Topiramate 25 mg	Topamax by McNeil	00045-0639	Anticonvulsant
TOP <> 25	Tab, White, Round, Film Coated	Topiramate 25 mg	Topamax by McNeil	52021-0639	Anticonvulsant
TOP15MG	Cap, White & Clear, Opaque	Topiramate 15 mg	Topamax Sprinkles by McNeil	00045-0647	Anticonvulsant
TOP15MG	Cap, White & Clear, Opaque	Topiramate 15 mg	Topamax by Janssen-Ortho	Canadian DIN 02239907	Anticonvulsant

ID FRONT <> BACK	DESCRIPTION FRONT <> BACK	INGREDIENT & STRENGTH	BRAND (or Generic Equiv.) by FIRM	NDC#	CLASS; SCH.
TOP25MG	Cap, White & Clear, Opaque	Topiramate 25 mg	Topamax by Janssen-Ortho	Canadian DIN 02239908	Anticonvulsant
TOP25MG	Cap, White & Clear, Opaque	Topiramate 25 mg	Topamax Sprinkles by McNeil	00045-0645	Anticonvulsant
TOP25MG	Cap, White & Clear, Opaque	Topiramate 25 mg	Topamax Sprinkles by Teva	00480-0109	Anticonvulsant
TOPAMAX <> 100	Tab, Yellow to Light Brown, Round, Film Coated	Topiramate 100 mg	Topamax by McNeil	52021-0641	Anticonvulsant
TOPAMAX <> 100	Tab, Yellow to Light Brown, Round, Film Coated	Topiramate 100 mg	Topamax by Ortho-McNeil	00062-0641	Anticonvulsant
TOPAMAX <> 100	Tab, Yellow to Light Brown, Round, Film Coated	Topiramate 100 mg	Topamax by McNeil	00045-0641	Anticonvulsant
TOPAMAX <> 200	Tab, Salmon, Round, Film Coated	Topiramate 200 mg	Topamax by McNeil	52021-0642	Anticonvulsant
TOPAMAX <> 200	Tab, Salmon, Round, Film Coated	Topiramate 200 mg	Topamax by Ortho-McNeil	00062-0642	Anticonvulsant
TOPAMAX <> 200	Tab, Salmon, Round, Film Coated	Topiramate 200 mg	Topamax by McNeil	00045-0642	Anticonvulsant
TOPAMAX <> 50	Tab, Light Yellow, Round, Coated	Topiramate 50 mg	Topamax by Ortho-McNeil	00045-0640	Anticonvulsant
TOR100 <> APO	Tab, White to Off-White, Cap Shaped, Scored, APO <> TOR / 100	Torsemide 100 mg	Demadex by Apotex	60505-0235	Diuretic
TOUROAH	Cap, Orange & White, Touro A & H	Pseudoephedrine HCl 60 mg, Brompheniramine Maleate 6 mg	Touro A&H by Dartmouth	58869-0301 Discontinued	Cold Remedy
TOUROALLERGY	Cap, Orange & White, Ex Release	Brompheniramine Maleate 5.75 mg, Pseudoephedrine HCl 60 mg	Touro Allergy by Dartmouth	58869-0401	Cold Remedy
TOUROALLERGY	Cap, Orange & Clear, Ex Release	Brompheniramine Maleate 5.75 mg, Pseudoephedrine HCl 60 mg	Touro Allergy by Pharmafab	62542-0106	Cold Remedy
TOUROCC <> DP	Tab, White, Cap Shaped, Scored	Guaifenesin 575 mg, Pseudoephedrine HCl 60 mg, Dextromethorphan HBr 30 mg	by Pfab	62542-0770	Cold Remedy
TOUROCC <> DP	Tab, White, Cap Shaped, Scored	Guaifenesin 575 mg, Pseudoephedrine HCl 60 mg, Dextromethorphan HBr 30 mg	Touro CC by Dartmouth	58869-0441	Cold Remedy
TOUROCCLD <> DP445	Tab, Scored	Dextromethorphan 30 mg, Pseudoephedrine 25 mg, Guaifenesin 575 mg	Touro CC-LD by Dartmouth	58869-0445	Cold Remedy
TOURODM <> DP311	Tab, Light Blue, Cap Shaped, Scored	Dextromethorphan HBr 30 mg, Guaifenesin 575 mg	Touro DM by Dartmouth	58869-0411	Cold Remedy
TOURODM <> DP311	Tab, Light Blue, Scored	Dextromethorphan HBr 30 mg, Guaifenesin 575 mg	Touro DM by Anabolic	00722-6297	Cold Remedy
TOUROEX <> DP321	Tab, White, Ex Release	Guaifenesin 575 mg	Robitussin by Dartmouth	58869-0421 Discontinued	Expectorant
TOUROHC <> DP581	Tab, White, Cap Shaped, Scored	Hydrocodone Bitartrate 5 mg, Guaifenesin 575 mg	Touro HC by Dartmouth	58869-0581	Cold Remedy; C III
TOUROLA <> DP436	Tab, White, Cap Shaped	Pseudoephedrine HCl 120 mg, Guaifenesin 500 mg	Touro LA by Dartmouth	58869-0536 Discontinued	Cold Remedy
TOUROLA <> DP636	Tab, White, Oblong	Guaifenesin 525 mg, Pseudoephedrine HCl 120 mg	Sudafed Sinus by Dartmouth	58869-0636	Cold Remedy
TOUROLALD <> DP635	Tab, Scored	Pseudoephedrine 50 mg, Guaifenesin 525 mg	Touro LA-LD by Dartmouth	58869-0635	Cold Remedy
TP <> 10300	Tab, White, Oblong, Scored, TP <> 10 / 300	Hydrocodone 10 mg, Acetaminophen 300 mg	Xodol by Teamm	67336-0911	Analgesic; C III
TP <> JC	Tab, Light Yellow, Cap Shaped, Film Coated, J-C <> T/P	Tramadol HCl 37.5 mg, Acetaminophen 325 mg	Tramacet by Janssen-Ortho	Canadian DIN 02264846	Analgesic
TP100 <> APO	Tab, Mustard, Round	Topiramate 100 mg	Topamax by Apotex	Canadian DIN 02279630	Anticonvulsant
TP189 <> 375	Tab, White, Oval	Naproxen 375 mg	Naprosyn by Major	00904-5590	NSAID
TP190 <> 500	Tab, White, Oval	Naproxen 500 mg	Naprosyn by Major	00904-5591	NSAID
TP200 <> APO	Tab, Pink, Round	Topiramate 200 mg	Topamax by Apotex	Canadian DIN 02279649	Anticonvulsant
TP25 <> APO	Tab, White, Round	Topiramate 25 mg	Topamax by Apotex	Canadian DIN 02279614	Anticonvulsant
TP305	Tab, White, Round	Colchicine 0.6 mg	by Towne Paulsen		Antigout
TP352	Cap, Pink	Zinc Sulfate 220 mg	Orazinc by Towne Paulsen		Mineral
TP403	Tab, Peach, Round	Hydrochlorothiazide 100 mg	Hydrodiuril by Towne Paulsen		Diuretic; Antihypertensive
TP404	Tab, Peach, Round	Hydrochlorothiazide 25 mg	Hydrodiuril by Towne Paulsen		Diuretic; Antihypertensive
TP405	Tab, Peach, Round	Hydrochlorothiazide 50 mg	Hydrodiuril by Towne Paulsen		Diuretic; Antihypertensive
TP4214	Tab, White, Round, TP421/4	Aspirin 325 mg, Codeine Phosphate 60 mg	Aspirin w/ Codeine by Towne Paulsen		Analgesic; C III
TP4243	Tab, White, Round	Aspirin 325 mg, Codeine Phosphate 30 mg	Aspirin w/ Codeine by Towne Paulsen		Analgesic; C III

ID FRONT <> BACK	DESCRIPTION FRONT <> BACK	INGREDIENT & STRENGTH	BRAND (or Generic Equiv.) by FIRM	NDC#	CLASS; SCH.
TP4653	Tab, White, Round, TP 465/3	Acetaminophen 300 mg, Codeine Phosphate 30 mg	Tylenol w/ Codeine by Towne Paulsen		Analgesic; C III
TP4664	Tab, White, Round, TP 466-4	Acetaminophen 300 mg, Codeine Phosphate 60 mg	Tylenol w/ Codeine by Towne Paulsen		Analgesic; C III
TP520	Tab, White, Round	Meprobamate 400 mg	Miltown by Towne Paulsen		Sedative/Hypnotic; C IV
TP522	Tab, White, Round	Meprobamate 200 mg	Miltown by Towne Paulsen		Sedative/Hypnotic; C IV
TP601	Tab, White, Round	Colchicine 0.5 mg	by Towne Paulsen		Antigout
TP604	Tab, White, Round	Cortisone Acetate 25 mg	Cortone by Towne Paulsen		Steroid
TP606	Tab, White, Round	Hydrocortisone 20 mg	Cortef by Towne Paulsen		Steroid
TP608	Tab, White, Round	Hydrocortisone 10 mg	by Towne Paulsen		Steroid
TP758	Tab, White, Round, TP-758	Acetaminophen 325 mg	Tylenol by Rosemont		Analgesic
TP783	Tab, Bluish Green, Round	Butabarbital 30 mg	Butisol Sodium by Towne Paulsen		Sedative/Hypnotic; C III
TP816	Tab, Yellow, Round	Chlorpheniramine Maleate 4 mg	Chlor-Trimeton by Towne Paulsen		Antihistamine
TP827	Cap, Pink	Diphenhydramine HCl 50 mg	Benadryl by Towne Paulsen		Antihistamine
TP833	Cap, Pink & White	Diphenhydramine HCl 25 mg	Benadryl by Towne Paulsen		Antihistamine
TP865	Tab, Yellow, Round	Isoniazid 100 mg	Laniazid by Towne Paulsen		Antimycobacterial
TP873	Tab, Yellow, Round	Folic Acid 1 mg	Folvite by Rosemont		Vitamin
TP900	Tab, White, Octagonal	Quinidine Sulfate 200 mg	Quinidine Sulfate by Towne Paulsen		Antiarrhythmic
TP913	Tab, White, Round	Prednisone 10 mg	Deltasone by Towne Paulsen		Steroid
TP922	Tab, Orange, Round	Prednisone 5 mg	Deltasone by Towne Paulsen		Steroid
TP924	Tab, White, Round	Prednisone 5 mg	Deltasone by Towne Paulsen		Steroid
TP925	Tab, Peach, Round	Prednisone 20 mg	Deltasone by Towne Paulsen		Steroid
TP926	Tab, Peach, Round	Prednisone 2.5 mg	Deltasone by Towne Paulsen		Steroid
TPV250	Cap, Pink, Oblong, Black Ink, Soft Gel	Tipranavir 250 mg	Aptivus by Boehringer Ingelheim	00597-0003	Antiviral
TPV250	Cap, Pink, Oblong, Black Ink, Soft Gel	Tipranavir 250 mg	Aptivus by Boehringer Ingelheim	Canadian DIN 02273322	Antiviral
TR0 <> ORGANON	Tab, Light Yellow, Round	Desogestrel 0.100 mg, Ethinyl Estradiol 0.025 mg	Cesia by Prasco	66993-0615	Oral Contraceptive
TR0 <> ORGANON	Tab, Light Yellow, Round	Desogestrel 0.100 mg, Ethinyl Estradiol 0.025 mg	Cyclessa by Organon	00052-0283	Oral Contraceptive
TR012	Tab, Pale Yellow, Round, Scored	Folic Acid 1 mg	Folic Acid by Dava	67253-0981	Vitamin
TR1 <> ORGANON	Tab, Red, Round	Desogestrel 0.150 mg, Ethinyl Estradiol 0.025 mg	Cyclessa by Organon	00052-0283	Oral Contraceptive
TR1 <> ORGANON	Tab, Red, Round	Desogestrel 0.150 mg, Ethinyl Estradiol 0.025 mg	Cesia by Prasco	66993-0615	Oral Contraceptive
TR100 <> 3M	Tab, White, Round, Scored, TR over 100	Flecainide Acetate 100 mg	Tambocor by 3M	00089-0307	Antiarrhythmic
TR125 <> G	Tab, White, Oval	Triazolam 0.125 mg	Halcion by Genpharm	15330-0249	Sedative/Hypnotic; C IV
TR125 <> G	Tab, White, Oval	Triazolam 0.125 mg	Halcion by Qualitest	00603-6186	Sedative/Hypnotic; C IV
TR125 <> G	Tab, White, Oval	Triazolam 0.125 mg	Halcion by Par	49884-0453	Sedative/Hypnotic; C IV
TR150 <> 3M	Tab, White, Oval, Scored	Flecainide Acetate 150 mg	Tambocor by Integrity	64731-0945	Antiarrhythmic
TR150 <> 3M	Tab, White, Oval, Scored	Flecainide Acetate 150 mg	Tambocor by 3M	00089-0314	Antiarrhythmic
TR250 <> G	Tab, Pale Yellow, Oval	Triazolam 0.25 mg	Halcion by Par	49884-0454	Sedative/Hypnotic; C IV
TR250 <> G	Tab, Pale Yellow, Oval	Triazolam 0.25 mg	Halcion by Qualitest	00603-6187	Sedative/Hypnotic; C IV
TR250 <> G	Tab, Pale Yellow, Oval	Triazolam 0.25 mg	Halcion by Genpharm	15330-0250	Sedative/Hypnotic; C IV
TR4 <> ORGANON	Tab, White, Film Coated, Organon <> T R over 4	Desogestrel 0.15 mg, Ethinyl Estradiol 0.02 mg	Mircette by Organon	00052-0281	Oral Contraceptive
TR4 <> ORGANON	Tab, Film Coated, T R over 4 <> Organon	Desogestrel 0.15 mg, Ethinyl Estradiol 0.02 mg	Mircette by NV Organon	12860-0281	Oral Contraceptive
TR5 <> ORGANON	Tab, White, Round	Desogestrel 0.15 mg, Ethinyl Estradiol 0.03 mg	Marvelon 28 by Organon	Canadian DIN 02042479	Oral Contraceptive
TR5 <> ORGANON	Tab, White, Round	Desogestrel 0.15 mg, Ethinyl Estradiol 0.03 mg	Desogen by Organon	00052-0261	Oral Contraceptive
TR5 <> ORGANON	Tab, White, Round	Desogestrel 0.15 mg, Ethinyl Estradiol 0.03 mg	Desogen by Organon	60889-0261	Oral Contraceptive

ID FRONT <> BACK	DESCRIPTION FRONT <> BACK	INGREDIENT & STRENGTH	BRAND (or Generic Equiv.) by FIRM	NDC#	CLASS; SCH.
TR5 <> ORGANON	Tab, White, Round	Desogestrel 0.15 mg, Ethinyl Estradiol 0.03 mg	Marvelon 21 by Organon	Canadian DIN 02042487	Oral Contraceptive
TR5 <> PRASCO	Tab, White, Round, PRASCO <> TR / 5	Desogestrel 0.15 mg, Ethinyl Estradiol 30 mcg	Solia by Prasco	66993-0611	Oral Contraceptive
TR50 <> 3M	Tab, White, Round, TR over 50	Flecainide Acetate 50 mg	by Murfreesboro	51129-1378	Antiarrhythmic
TR50 <> 3M	Tab, White, Round, TR over 50	Flecainide Acetate 50 mg	Tambocor by 3M	00089-0305	Antiarrhythmic
TR50 <> APO	Tab, White to Off-White, Oblong	Tramadol HCl 50 mg	Ultram by Major	00904-5556	Analgesic
TR50 <> APO	Tab, White to Off-White, Oblong	Tramadol HCl 50 mg	Ultram by Apotex	60505-0171	Analgesic
TR6 <> ORGANON	Tab, Orange, Round	Desogestrel 0.125 mg, Ethinyl Estradiol 0.025 mg	Cesia by Prasco	66993-0615	Oral Contraceptive
TR6 <> ORGANON	Tab, Orange, Round	Desogestrel 0.125 mg, Ethinyl Estradiol 0.025 mg	Cyclessa by Organon	00052-0283	Oral Contraceptive
TRANDATE100	Tab, Light Orange, Round, Scored	Labetalol HCl 100 mg	Trandate by Amerisource	62584-0346	Antihypertensive
TRANDATE100	Tab, Light Orange, Round, Scored	Labetalol HCl 100 mg	Trandate by Rightpac	65240-0754	Antihypertensive
TRANDATE100	Tab, Light Orange, Round, Scored	Labetalol HCl 100 mg	Trandate by GSK	00173-0346	Antihypertensive
TRANDATE100	Tab, Light Orange, Round, Scored	Labetalol HCl 100 mg	Trandate by Nat Pharmpak	55154-1100	Antihypertensive
TRANDATE100	Tab, Light Orange, Round, Scored	Labetalol HCl 100 mg	Trandate by Leiner	59606-0754	Antihypertensive
TRANDATE100	Tab, Light Orange, Round, Scored	Labetalol HCl 100 mg	Trandate by Thrift Drug	59198-0284	Antihypertensive
TRANDATE100	Tab, Light Orange, Round, Scored	Labetalol HCl 100 mg	Trandate by Murfreesboro	51129-1615	Antihypertensive
TRANDATE100	Tab, Light Orange, Round, Scored	Labetalol HCl 100 mg	Trandate by Drug Distr	52985-0219	Antihypertensive
TRANDATE100	Tab, Light Orange, Round, Scored	Labetalol HCl 100 mg	Trandate by Roberts	Canadian	Antihypertensive
TRANDATE100	Tab, Light Orange, Round, Scored	Labetalol HCl 100 mg	Trandate by Med Pro	53978-3374	Antihypertensive
TRANDATE100	Tab, Light Orange, Round, Scored	Labetalol HCl 100 mg	Trandate by Faro Pharms	60976-0346	Antihypertensive
TRANDATE100 <> RP	Tab, Orange, Capsule-Shaped, Film-Coate	Labetalol HCl 100 mg	Trandate by Shire BioChem	Canadian DIN 02106272	Antihypertensive
TRANDATE200	Tab, White, Oblong	Labetalol HCl 200 mg	Trandate by Roberts	Canadian	Antihypertensive
TRANDATE200	Tab, White, Round	Labetalol HCl 200 mg	Trandate by GSK	00173-0347	Antihypertensive
TRANDATE200	Tab, White, Round, Scored	Labetalol HCl 200 mg	Trandate by Rightpac	65240-0755	Antihypertensive
TRANDATE200	Tab, White, Round, Scored	Labetalol HCl 200 mg	Trandate by Med Pro	53978-3388	Antihypertensive
TRANDATE200	Tab, Film Coated	Labetalol HCl 200 mg	Trandate by Amerisource	62584-0347	Antihypertensive
TRANDATE200	Tab, Film Coated	Labetalol HCl 200 mg	Trandate by Nat Pharmpak	55154-1101	Antihypertensive
TRANDATE200	Tab, Film Coated	Labetalol HCl 200 mg	Trandate by Thrift Drug	59198-0285	Antihypertensive
TRANDATE200	Tab, Film Coated	Labetalol HCl 200 mg	Trandate by Leiner	59606-0755	Antihypertensive
TRANDATE200	Tab, Film Coated	Labetalol HCl 200 mg	Trandate by GSK	00173-0347	Antihypertensive
TRANDATE200	Tab, White, Round, Scored, Film Coated	Labetalol HCl 200 mg	Trandate by Murfreesboro	51129-1616	Antihypertensive
TRANDATE200 <> RP	Tab, White, Cap-Shaped, Film-Coated	Labetalol HCl 200 mg	Trandate by Shire BioChem	Canadian DIN 02106280	Antihypertensive
TRANDATE300	Tab, Peach, Round, Film Coated, Scored	Labetalol HCl 300 mg	Trandate by Neuman	64579-0386	Antihypertensive
TRANDATE300	Tab, Peach, Round	Labetalol HCl 300 mg	Trandate by GSK	00173-0348	Antihypertensive
TRANDATE300	Tab, Peach, Round, Scored	Labetalol HCl 300 mg	Trandate by Rightpac	65240-0770	Antihypertensive
TRANDATE300	Tab, Film Coated	Labetalol HCl 300 mg	Trandate by GSK	00173-0348	Antihypertensive
TRANDATE300	Tab, Film Coated	Labetalol HCl 300 mg	Trandate by GSK	51947-3332	Antihypertensive
TRANDATE300	Tab, Film Coated	Labetalol HCl 300 mg	Trandate by Leiner	59606-0770	Antihypertensive
TRANDATE300	Tab, Film Coated	Labetalol HCl 300 mg	Trandate by Thrift Drug	59198-0286	Antihypertensive
TRAZADONE <> PMS50	Tab, Orange, Round, Scored	Trazodone HCl 50 mg	Desyrel by Pharmascience	Canadian DIN 01937227	Antidepressant
TRAZADONE <> PMS75	Tab, Salmon	Trazodone HCl 75 mg		Canadian DIN 02237339	Antidepressant
TRAZODONE <> PMS100	Tab, White, Round, Scored	Trazodone HCl 100 mg	Desyrel by Pharmascience	Canadian DIN 01937235	Antidepressant
TRAZODONE <> PMS50	Tab, Orange, Round, Scored	Trazodone HCl 50 mg	Desyrel by Pharmascience	Canadian DIN 6952369419	Antidepressant
TRENTAL <> HOECHST	Tab, Pink, Oblong, Film Coated	Pentoxifylline 400 mg	Trental by Merrell	00068-0780	Anticoagulant

ID FRONT <> BACK	DESCRIPTION FRONT <> BACK	INGREDIENT & STRENGTH	BRAND (or Generic Equiv.) by FIRM	NDC#	CLASS; SCH.
TRENTAL <> HOECHST	Tab, Pink, Oblong, Film Coated	Pentoxifylline 400 mg	Trental by Aventis	00039-0078	Anticoagulant
TRENTAL <> HOECHST	Tab, Pink, Oblong, Film Coated	Pentoxifylline 400 mg	Trental by Amerisource	62584-0078	Anticoagulant
TRENTAL <> HOECHST	Tab, Pink, Oblong, Film Coated	Pentoxifylline 400 mg	Trental by Med Pro	53978-0374	Anticoagulant
TRENTAL <> HOECHST	Tab, Pink, Oblong, Film Coated	Pentoxifylline 400 mg	Trental by DRX	55045-2327	Anticoagulant
TRENTAL <> HOECHST	Tab, Pink, Oblong, Film Coated	Pentoxifylline 400 mg	Trental by Nat Pharmpak	55154-1205	Anticoagulant
TRENTAL <> HOECHST	Tab, Pink, Oblong, Film Coated	Pentoxifylline 400 mg	Trental by Pharmedix	53002-1040	Anticoagulant
TREXAN <> DUPONT	Tab, White w/ Brown Specks, Round, Scored	Naltrexone HCl 50 mg	Trexan by BMS	00056-0080	Opioid Antagonist
TRI100 <> APO	Tab, White, Round, Scored, TRI / 100	Trimethoprim 100 mg	Apo Trimethoprim by Apotex	Canadian DIN 02243116	Antibiotic
TRI200 <> APO	Tab, Yellow, Round, Scored, TRI / 200	Trimethoprim 200 mg	Apo Trimethoprim by Apotex	Canadian DIN 02243117	Antibiotic
TRIADUAD305	Cap, White, Opaque, Green Ink	Butalbital 50 mg, Acetaminophen 325 mg, Caffeine 40 mg	Triad by Forest	00785-2305	Analgesic
TRIANAL	Cap, Blue	Butalbital 50 mg, Caffeine 40 mg, Aspirin 330 mg	by Trianon	Canadian	Analgesic; C III
TRIANAL	Tab, White	Butalbital 50 mg, Caffeine 40 mg, Aspirin 330 mg	by Trianon	Canadian	Analgesic; C III
TRIANALC12	Cap, Blue, Trianal C 1/2	Butalbital 50 mg, Caffeine 40 mg, Aspirin 330 mg	by Trianon	Canadian	Analgesic; C III
TRIANALC14	Cap, Blue, Trianal C 1/4	Butalbital 50 mg, Caffeine 40 mg, Aspirin 330 mg	by Trianon	Canadian	Analgesic; C III
TRIANGLE	Tab, Off-White, Round, Debossed Modified Triangle, Orally Disintegrating	Rizatriptan Benzoate 5 mg	Maxalt-MLT by Merck	00006-3800	Antimigraine
TRIANGLE	Tab, White to Off-White, Round, Rapidly Disintegrating, Peppermint Flavor	Rizatriptan 5 mg	Maxalt RPD 5 mg by Merck Frosst	Canadian DIN 02240518	Antimigraine
TRIANGLE150	Tab, White, Round	Propafenone HCl 150 mg	Rythmol by Knoll		Antiarrhythmic
TRIANGLE225	Tab, White, Round	Propafenone HCl 225 mg	Rythmol by Knoll		Antiarrhythmic
TRIANGLE300	Tab, White, Round	Propafenone HCl 300 mg	Rythmol by Knoll		Antiarrhythmic
TRIANGLES	Tab, White, Round, Three Triangles in a circle	3,4-Methylenedioxymethamphetamine (MDMA)	Ecstasy by Illegal		Euphoric; Illicit
TRIATEC30	Tab, Salmon, Round, Scored	Acetaminophen 300 mg, Codeine Phosphate 30 mg	Triatec 30 by Trianon	Canadian DIN	Analgesic
TRIBEX	Cap, Blue, Oval	Tribex Full-Spectrum Active Extracts 2000 mg: Tribulus Terrestris, Avena Sativa	Tribex by BioTest Labs	00789828	Supplement
TRIMETHOPRIM160 <> SULFAMETHOXAZO	Tab	Sulfamethoxazole 800 mg, Trimethoprim 160 mg	by Moore	00839-6406	Antibiotic
TRINALIN703	Tab, Red, Black Print, Round, Sugar Coated	Azatadine Maleate 1 mg, Pseudoephedrine Sulfate 120 mg	by Schering	00085-0703	Cold Remedy
TRINALIN703	Tab, Red, Black Print, Round, Sugar Coated	Azatadine Maleate 1 mg, Pseudoephedrine Sulfate 120 mg	by Caremark	00339-5411	Cold Remedy
TRINITY <> 60030	Tab, Film Coated, Scored	Dextromethorphan HBr 30 mg, Guaifenesin 600 mg	by URL Mutual	00677-1486	Cold Remedy
TRITEC	Tab, Blue, Octagonal, Stomach Logo	Ranitidine Bismuth Citrate 400 mg	Tritec by GSK	00173-0488	Gastrointestinal
TRM5MG	Tab, White, Round, TRM/5 mg	Trihexyphenidyl HCl 2 mg	by Pharmascience	Canadian	Antiparkinson
TROCHE <> TORADOL	Tab, White, Round, Film Coated	Ketorolac Tromethamine 10 mg	Toradol by Syntex	18393-0435	NSAID
TROCHE <> TORADOL	Tab, White, Round, Film Coated	Ketorolac Tromethamine 10 mg	Toradol by Hoffmann La Roche	00004-0273	NSAID
TROCHE <> TORADOL	Tab, White, Round, Film Coated	Ketorolac Tromethamine 10 mg	Toradol by H J Harkins Co	52959-0224	NSAID
TROCHE <> TORADOL	Tab, White, Round, Film Coated	Ketorolac Tromethamine 10 mg	Toradol by Murfreesboro	51129-1151	NSAID
TRYPTAN <> 250MG	Tab, White, Oval, Film Coated	L-Tryptophan 250 mg	Tryptan by Valeant	Canadian DIN 02239326	Supplement
TRYPTAN <> 500MG	Tab, White, Oval, Film Coated	L-Tryptophan 500 mg	Tryptan by Valeant	Canadian DIN 02029456	Supplement
TRYPTAN <> 500MG	Tab, White, Oval, Film Coated	L-Tryptophan 500 mg	by AltiMed	Canadian DIN 02240333	Supplement
TRYPTAN <> 750MG	Tab, White, Oval, Film Coated	L-Tryptophan 750 mg	Tryptan by Valeant	Canadian DIN 02239327	Supplement
TRYPTAN1G	Tab, White, Oval, Film Coated	L-Tryptophan 1 g	Tryptan by Valeant	Canadian DIN 00654531	Supplement

ID FRONT <> BACK	DESCRIPTION FRONT <> BACK	INGREDIENT & STRENGTH	BRAND (or Generic Equiv.) by FIRM	NDC#	CLASS; SCH.
TRYPTOPHAN500 <> P	Tab, White, Cap Shaped, Film Coated	Tryptophan 500 mg	by Pharmascience	Canadian DIN 5760601029	Antidepressant
TS	Tab, Red, Round, Chewable	Acetaminophen 80 mg, Pseudoephedrine HCl 7.5 mg	Children's Tylenol Sinus by McNeil	Canadian DIN 02240419	Cold Remedy
TSH9199	Tab, White, Oblong	Lactase 3000 Fcc Units	Lactaid by Rugby	00536-7811	Gastrointestinal
TT	Tab, Pink, Oblong	Acetaminophen 650 mg, Chlorpheniramine 4 mg, Pseudoephedrine HCl 60 mg	Singlet by Trinity		Cold Remedy
TT <> 207	Tab	Guaifenesin 600 mg, Pseudoephedrine HCl 60 mg	by URL Mutual	00677-1487	Cold Remedy
TT10110	Tab, White, Round, TT/101 10	Isoxsuprine HCl 10 mg	Vasodilan by Trinity		Vasodilator
TT10220	Tab, White, Round, TT/102 20	Isoxsuprine HCl 20 mg	Vasodilan by Trinity		Vasodilator
TT177	Tab, Yellow, Oblong, T/T 177	Guaifenesin 600 mg, Pseudoephedrine HCl 120 mg	Entex PSE by Trinity		Cold Remedy
TT207	Tab	Guaifenesin 600 mg, Pseudoephedrine HCl 60 mg	by Major	00904-5150	Cold Remedy
TT60075	Tab, White, Oblong, TT 600/75	Guaifenesin 600 mg, Phenylpropanolamine 75 mg	Duravent by Trinity		Cold Remedy
TTC <> G600	Tab	Guaifenesin 600 mg	Robitussin by URL Mutual	00677-1475	Expectorant
TTC40075	Tab, Blue, Oblong, TTC 400/75	Guaifenesin 400 mg, Phenylpropanolamine HCl 75 mg	Entex LA by Trinity		Cold Remedy
TTG200	Tab, Pink, Round, TT/G200	Guaifenesin 200 mg	Aquabid by Trinity		Expectorant
TTORADOL <> TROCHE	Tab, White, Round, Film Coated	Ketorolac Tromethamine 10 mg	Toradol by Syntex	18393-0435	NSAID
TTORADOL <> TROCHE	Tab, White, Round, Film Coated	Ketorolac Tromethamine 10 mg	Toradol by Murfreesboro	51129-1151	NSAID
TTORADOL <> TROCHE	Tab, White, Round, Film Coated	Ketorolac Tromethamine 10 mg	Toradol by Hoffmann La Roche	00004-0273	NSAID
TTORADOL <> TROCHE	Tab, White, Round, Film Coated	Ketorolac Tromethamine 10 mg	Toradol by H J Harkins Co	52959-0224	NSAID
TTS500	Tab, Blue, Round	Salsalate 500 mg	Disalcid by Trinity		NSAID
TTS750	Tab, Blue, Oblong	Salsalate 750 mg	Disalcid by Trinity		NSAID
TUMS	Tab, Purple, Round	Calcium Carbonate 1000 mg	Os-Cal by Caremark	00339-5423	Vitamin; Mineral
TUMSSD	Tab, Multi-Colored, Round, Chewable	Calcium Carbonate 750 mg	Tums by GSK		Antacid
TUSSIGON <> DP082	Tab, Blue, Round, Scored, dp/082	Homatropine Methylbromide 1.5 mg, Hydrocodone Bitartrate 5 mg	Tussigon by JMI Daniels	00689-0082	Cold Remedy; C III
TVN100 <> PFIZER	Tab, Blue, Round	Trovafloxacin 100 mg	Trovan by Pfizer	Canadian DIN 02239191	Antibiotic
TVN200 <> PFIZER	Tab, Blue, Oval	Trovafloxacin 200 mg	Trovan by Pfizer	Canadian DIN 02239192	Antibiotic
TX	Tab, Blue, Round, TX over Abbott Logo	Clorazepate Dipotassium 11.25 mg	Tranxene-SD by Ovation		Antianxiety; C IV
TY	Tab, Tan, Round, TY over Abbott Logo	Clorazepate Dipotassium 22.5 mg	Tranxene-SD by Ovation		Antianxiety; C IV
TY <> 160	Tab, Pink or Purple, Round, Scored, Chewable	Acetaminophen 160 mg	Children's Tylenol by McNeil	Canadian DIN 02241361	Analgesic
TY <> 160	Tab, Pink, Round, Scored, Chewable	Acetaminophen 160 mg	Junior Tylenol Meltaways by McNeil	50580-0513	Analgesic
TY <> 160	Tab, Purple, Round, Scored, Chewable	Acetaminophen 160 mg	Junior Tylenol Meltaways by McNeil	50580-0514	Analgesic
TY500	Cap, Red, Dark Gray and Blue, Black Print, Rapid Release	Acetaminophen 500 mg	Tylenol Ex Strength Rapid Release Gels by McNeil	50580-0488	Analgesic
TY500	Tab, Red and Grey and Blue, Capsule-Shaped Gel-Coated	Acetaminophen 500 mg	Tylenol Ex Strength Rapid Release Gels by McNeil C	Canadian DIN 00863270	Analgesic
TY80	Tab, Pink, Round, Chewable	Acetaminophen 80 mg	Children's Tylenol Meltaways by McNeil	50580-0519	Analgesic
TY80	Tab, Purple, Round, Chewable	Acetaminophen 80 mg	Children's Tylenol Meltaways by McNeil	50580-0518	Analgesic
TY80	Tab, Dark Pink, Round, Chewable	Acetaminophen 80 mg	Children's Tylenol Meltaways by McNeil	50580-0516	Analgesic
TY80	Tab, Pink or Purple, Round, Chewable	Acetaminophen 80 mg	Children's Tylenol by McNeil	Canadian DIN 02238295	Analgesic
TYC1078	Tab, White, Cap-Shaped	Acetaminophen 325 mg, Dextromethorphan 10 mg, Phenylephrine 5 mg	Regular Strength Tylenol Cold Daytime by McNeil Co	Canadian DIN 02275627	Cold Remedy
TYC1080	Tab, Light Green, Cap-Shaped	Acetaminophen 325 mg, Phenylephrine 5 mg	Tylenol Regular Strength Sinus Daytime by McNeil C	Canadian DIN 02275708	Analgesic

ID FRONT <> BACK	DESCRIPTION FRONT <> BACK	INGREDIENT & STRENGTH	BRAND (or Generic Equiv.) by FIRM	NDC#	CLASS; SCH.
TYC365	Tab, Light Blue, Cap-Shaped	Acetaminophen 500 mg, Diphenhydramine HCl 25 mg	Tylenol Cold Nighttime by McNeil		Cold Relief
TYCNT	Cap, Dark Blue, Grey Band, TY C-NT	Acetaminophen 325 mg, Phenylephrine HCl 5 mg, Dextromethorphan HBr 10 mg, Chlorpheniramine Maleate 2 mg	Tylenol Cold Multi-Symptom Nighttime by McNeil	Canadian DIN 02017377	Cold Remedy
TYCOF500	Cap, Red, Film Coated	Acetaminophen 500 mg, Dextromethorphan HBr 15 mg	Tylenol Cough Ex Strength by McNeil		Cold Remedy
TYLCODEINE3 <> MCNEIL	Tab, TYL over Codeine 3	Acetaminophen 300 mg, Codeine Phosphate 30 mg	Tylenol w/ Codeine by McNeil	Canadian DIN 02017377	Analgesic; C III
TYLENOL <> 325	Tab, White, Round, Scored	Acetaminophen 325 mg	Tylenol by McNeil	Canadian DIN 00559393	Analgesic
TYLENOL <> 325	Tab, White, Round	Acetaminophen 325 mg	Tylenol by McNeil Consumer Healthcare	Canadian DIN 00559393	Analgesic
TYLENOL <> 500	Tab, White, Round	Acetaminophen 500 mg	Tylenol Ex Strength by McNeil	Canadian DIN 00559407	Analgesic
TYLENOL <> 80	Tab, Pink or Purple, Round, Scored, Chewable	Acetaminophen 80 mg	Children's Tylenol by McNeil	Canadian DIN 02229539	Analgesic
TYLENOL160	Tab, Pink or Purple, Round, Scored, Chewable	Acetaminophen 160 mg	Children's Tylenol by McNeil	Canadian DIN 01967819	Analgesic
TYLENOL325	Cap, White, Film Coated, Scored	Acetaminophen 325 mg	Tylenol by McNeil	Canadian DIN 00723894	Analgesic
TYLENOL3CODEINE <> MCNEIL	Tab, Round, White	Acetaminophen 300 mg, Codeine Phosphate 30 mg	Tylenol w/ Codeine by McNeil	00045-0513	Analgesic; C III
TYLENOL4CODEINE <> MCNEIL	Tab, Round, White	Acetaminophen 300 mg, Codeine Phosphate 60 mg	Tylenol w/ Codeine by McNeil	00045-0515	Analgesic; C III
TYLENOL500	Tab, White, Cap Shaped, Film Coated, Red Print	Acetaminophen 500 mg	Tylenol Ex Strength by McNeil	50580-0449	Analgesic
TYLENOL500	Tab, White, Cap Shaped, Film Coated, Red Print	Acetaminophen 500 mg	Tylenol Ex Strength by McNeil	Canadian DIN 00723908	Analgesic
TYLENOL500	Tab, Red & Yellow, Cap Shaped, Film Coated	Acetaminophen 500 mg	Tylenol Ex Strength by McNeil	Canadian DIN 00863270	Analgesic
TYLENOL500	Tab, Red, Round, Sweet-Coated	Acetaminophen 500 mg	Tylenol Extra Strength Tab 500mg by McNeil Consumer	Canadian DIN 00559407	Analgesic
TYLENOLALLERGY	Tab, Light Yellow, Round, Coated, Mint Odor	Acetaminophen 500 mg, Phenylephrine 5 mg, Chlorpheniramine maleate 2 mg	Tylenol Extra Strength Allergy by McNeil Consumer	Canadian DIN 02276054	Analgesic
TYLENOLAS	Cap, Light Blue, Film Coated, Tylenol A/S	Acetaminophen 500 mg, Pseudoephedrine HCl 30 mg, Diphenhydramine HCl 25 mg	Tylenol PM Ex Strength by McNeil	Canadian DIN 02237483	Cold Remedy
TYLENOLCODEINE2 <> MCNEIL	Tab	Acetaminophen 300 mg, Codeine Phosphate 15 mg	Tylenol w/ Codeine by Murfreesboro	51129-1393	Analgesic; C III
TYLENOLCODEINE2 <> MCNEIL	Tab	Acetaminophen 300 mg, Codeine Phosphate 15 mg	Tylenol w/ Codeine by McNeil	00045-0511	Analgesic; C III
TYLENOLCODEINE3 <> MCNEIL	Tab	Acetaminophen 300 mg, Codeine Phosphate 30 mg	Tylenol w/ Codeine by Med Pro	53978-3087	Analgesic; C III
TYLENOLCODEINE3 <> MCNEIL	Tab	Acetaminophen 300 mg, Codeine Phosphate 30 mg	Tylenol w/ Codeine by Allscripts		Analgesic; C III
TYLENOLCODEINE4 <> MCNEIL	Tab	Acetaminophen 300 mg, Codeine Phosphate 60 mg	Tylenol w/ Codeine by Med Pro	53978-3094	Analgesic; C III
TYLENOLCODEINE4 <> MCNEIL	Tab, White, Round	Codeine Phosphate 60 mg, Acetaminophen 300 mg	by Nat Pharmpak	55154-1916	Analgesic; C III
TYLENOLCOLD <> 80	Tab, Pink or Orange, Round, Scored, Chewable	Acetaminophen 80 mg, Chlorpheniramine Maleate 0.5 mg, Pseudoephedrine HCl 7.5 mg	Children's Tylenol Cold by McNeil	Canadian DIN 00743224	Cold Remedy
TYLENOLCOLDDM <> 80	Tab, Pink or Purple, Round, Chewable	Acetaminophen 80 mg, Chlorpheniramine Maleate 0.5 mg, Pseudoephedrine HCl 7.5 mg, Dextromethorphan 3.75 mg	Children's Tylenol Cold Plus Cough by McNeil	Canadian DIN 00870455	Cold Remedy
TYLENOLER	Tab, White, Cap Shaped	Acetaminophen 650 mg	Tylenol Arthritis Pain by McNeil		Analgesic

ID FRONT <> BACK	DESCRIPTION FRONT <> BACK	INGREDIENT & STRENGTH	BRAND (or Generic Equiv.) by FIRM	NDC#	CLASS; SCH.
TYLENOLER	Tab, White, Elongated, Extended Release	Acetaminophen 650 mg	Tylenol Arthritis Pain by McNeil Consumer Healthca	Canadian DIN 02238885	Analgesic
TYLENOLER	Tab, White, Elongated, Extended Release	Acetaminophen 650 mg	Tylenol 8 Hour by McNeil Consumer Healthcare	Canadian DIN 02246060	Analgesic
TYLENOLFLU	Cap, Dark Red & White, Film Coated	Acetaminophen 500 mg, Pseudoephedrine HCl 30 mg, Dextromethorphan HBr 15 mg	Tylenol Flu Daytime Ex Strength by McNeil	Canadian DIN 02241526	Cold Remedy
TYLENOLFLUDT	Tab, Yellow, Round, Coated, Tylenol over Flu DT	Acetaminophen 500 mg, Dextromethorphan 10 mg, Phenylephrine 5 mg	Tylenol Flu Extra Strength Daytime by McNeil Consumer Healthcare	Canadian DIN 02275996	Cold Remedy
TYLENOLFLUNT	Cap, Blue & White, Film Coated	Acetaminophen 500 mg, Diphenhydramine HCl 25 mg, Pseudoephedrine HCl 30 mg	Tylenol PM Ex Strength by McNeil	Canadian DIN 02167670	Cold Remedy
TYLENOLPM	Tab, Light Blue, Cap Shaped	Acetaminophen 500 mg, Diphenhydramine 25 mg	Tylenol PM by McNeil	50580-0482	Cold Remedy
TYLENOLPM	Tab, Blue and White, Cap Shaped, Gel Coated	Acetaminophen 500 mg, Diphenhydramine 25 mg	Tylenol PM by McNeil	50580-0182	Cold Remedy
TYLENOLPM	Tab, Blue and White, Round, Gel Coated	Acetaminophen 500 mg, Diphenhydramine 25 mg	Tylenol PM by McNeil	50580-0176	Cold Remedy
TYLENOLSINUSDT	Tab, Light Green, Round, Coated, Mint Odor	Acetaminophen 500 mg, Phenylephrine 5 mg	Tylenol Extra Strength Sinus Daytime by McNeil Consumer Healthcare	Canadian DIN 02276003	Analgesic
TYLENOLSINUSNT	Cap, Teal, Film Coated	Acetaminophen 500 mg, Pseudoephedrine HCl 30 mg, Doxylamine Succinate 6.25 mg	Ex Strength Tylenol Sinus Nighttime by McNeil Consumer Healthcare	Canadian DIN 02240302	Cold Remedy
TYLENOLULTRA	Tab, Red, Round, Sweet-Coated	Acetaminophen 500 mg, Caffeine 65 mg	Tylenol Ultra Relief by McNeil Consumer Healthcare	Canadian DIN 02254468	Analgesic
TYLOXMCNEIL	Cap, Red, Black Print	Acetaminophen 500 mg, Oxycodone HCl 5 mg	Tylox by McNeil	00045-0526	Analgesic; C II
TYME500	Cap, Peach, Film Coated	Acetaminophen 500 mg, Pamabrom 25 mg, Pyrilamine Maleate 15 mg	Midol Ex Strength by McNeil	Canadian DIN 02231239	PMS Relief
TZ	Tab, Mauve, Oval	Triazolam 0.125 mg	Gen Triazolam by Genpharm	Canadian	Sedative/Hypnotic; C IV
TZ	Tab, Blue, Oval	Triazolam 0.25 mg	Gen Triazolam by Genpharm	Canadian	Sedative/Hypnotic; C IV
TZ1	Tab, Round, White, Orally Disintegrating, TZ over 1	Mirtazapine 15 mg	Remeron RD by Organon	Canadian DIN 02248542	Antidepressant
TZ1	Tab, Round, White, Orally Disintegrating, TZ over 1	Mirtazapine 15 mg	Remeron SolTab by Prasco	66993-0709	Antidepressant
TZ1	Tab, Round, White, Orally Disintegrating, TZ over 1	Mirtazapine 15 mg	Remeron SolTab by Organon	00052-0106	Antidepressant
TZ1	Tab, White, Round, Flat, Orally Disintegrating	Mirtazapine 15 mg	Remeron RD by Schering-Plough	Canadian DIN 02248542	Antidepressant
TZ15	Cap, Maroon and Tan, Hard Gel	Temazepam 15 mg	CO Temazepam by Cobalt	Canadian DIN 02244814	Sedative/Hypnotic; C IV
TZ2	Tab, Round, White, Orally Disintegrating, TZ over 2	Mirtazapine 30 mg	Remeron RD by Organon	Canadian DIN 02248543	Antidepressant
TZ2	Tab, Round, White, Orally Disintegrating, TZ over 2	Mirtazapine 30 mg	Remeron SolTab by Organon	00052-0108	Antidepressant
TZ2	Tab, Round, White, Orally Disintegrating, TZ over 2	Mirtazapine 30 mg	Remeron SolTab by Prasco	66993-0711	Antidepressant
TZ2	Tab, White, Round, Flat, Orally Disintegrating	Mirtazapine 30 mg	Remeron RD by Schering-Plough	Canadian DIN 02248543	Antidepressant
TZ3 <> ORGANON	Tab, Yellow, Oval, Scored, Film Coated	Mirtazapine 15 mg	Remeron by Organon	00052-0105	Antidepressant
TZ3 <> ORGANON	Tab, Yellow, Oval, Scored, Film Coated	Mirtazapine 15 mg	Remeron by Neuman	64579-0390	Antidepressant
TZ3 <> ORGANON	Tab, Yellow, Oval, Scored, Film Coated	Mirtazapine 15 mg	Remeron by NV Organon	12860-0105	Antidepressant
TZ30	Cap, Blue & Maroon, Gelatin	Temazepam 30 mg	Restoril by Cobalt	Canadian DIN 02244815	Sedative/Hypnotic; C IV
TZ4	Tab, Round, White, Orally Disintegrating, TZ over 4	Mirtazapine 45 mg	Remeron RD by Organon	Canadian DIN 02248544	Antidepressant
TZ4	Tab, Round, White, Orally Disintegrating, TZ over 4	Mirtazapine 45 mg	Remeron SolTab by Prasco	66993-0712	Antidepressant
TZ4	Tab, Round, White, Orally Disintegrating, TZ over 4	Mirtazapine 45 mg	Remeron SolTab by Organon	00052-0110	Antidepressant
TZ4	Tab, White, Round, Flat, Orally Disintegrating	Mirtazapine 45 mg	Remeron RD by Schering-Plough	Canadian DIN 02248544	Antidepressant
TZ5	Tab, Red Brown, Oval, Scored, Film Coated	Mirtazapine 30 mg	Remeron by Schering-Plough	Canadian DIN 02243910	Antidepressant

ID FRONT <> BACK	DESCRIPTION FRONT <> BACK	INGREDIENT & STRENGTH	BRAND (or Generic Equiv.) by FIRM	NDC#	CLASS; SCH.
TZ5 <> ORGANON	Tab, Red-Brown, Oval, Scored, Film Coated	Mirtazapine 30 mg	Remeron by Organon	00052-0107	Antidepressant
TZ5 <> ORGANON	Tab, Red-Brown, Oval, Scored, Film Coated	Mirtazapine 30 mg	Remeron by NV Organon	12860-0107	Antidepressant
TZ5 <> ORGANON	Tab, Red-Brown, Oval, Scored, Film Coated	Mirtazapine 30 mg	Remeron by Organon	Canadian DIN 02243910	Antidepressant
TZ7 <> ORGANON	Tab, White, Oval, Film Coated	Mirtazapine 45 mg	Remeron by Organon	00052-0109	Antidepressant
TZ7 <> ORGANON	Tab, White, Oval, Film Coated	Mirtazapine 45 mg	Remeron by Nv Organon	12860-0109	Antidepressant
TZD100832	Tab, White, Round	Trazodone HCl 100 mg	Desyrel by Rosemont		Antidepressant
TZD50832	Tab, White, Round	Trazodone HCl 50 mg	Desyrel by Rosemont		Antidepressant
U	Tab, Light Yellow, Oblong, Film Coated	Colestipol HCl 1 g	Colestid by Pharmacia	00009-0450	Bile Acid Resin
U	Tab, White	Prednisone 50 mg	Deltasone by Upjohn	Canadian	Steroid
U	Tab, Light Yellow, Oblong, Film Coated	Colestipol HCl 1 g	Colestid by Pfizer	Canadian DIN 02132680	Bile Acid Resin
U <> 10	Tab, Yellow, Round, Film Coated	Oxybutynin Chloride 10 mg	Uromax by Purdue Pharma	Canadian DIN 02273578	Antispasmodic
U <> 15	Tab, Pink, Oval, Film Coated	Oxybutynin Chloride 15 mg	Uromax by Purdue Pharma	Canadian DIN 02273586	Antispasmodic
U <> 2	Tab, White, Round	Pramipexole DiHCl 0.125 mg	Mirapex by Boehringer Ingelheim	00597-0083	Antiparkinson
U <> 2	Tab, White, Round	Pramipexole DiHCl 0.125 mg	Mirapex by Pharmacia	00009-0002	Antiparkinson
U <> 2	Tab, White, Round	Pramipexole DiHCl 0.125 mg	Mirapex by Promex Med	62301-0026	Antiparkinson
U <> 76	Tab, White, Rectangular	Dinoprostone 0.5 mg	by Pharmacia	00400688	Labor Inducer
U01	Tab, Orange, Round	Paramethasone Acetate 2 mg	Haldrone by Eli Lilly		Steroid
U03	Tab, White, Cap Shaped	Acetohexamide 250 mg	Dymelor by Eli Lilly		Antidiabetic
U05	Tab, Pink, Square, Chewable	Erythromycin Estolate 125 mg	Ilosone by Eli Lilly		Antibiotic
U07	Tab, Yellow, Oblong	Acetohexamide 500 mg	Dymelor by Eli Lilly		Antidiabetic
U09	Tab, Blue, Oblong	Cyclothiazide 2 mg	Anhydron by Eli Lilly		Diuretic; Antihypertensive
U121	Tab, White, Round	Minoxidil 2.5 mg	Loniten by Upjohn	Canadian	Antihypertensive
U121 <> 212	Tab, White, Half Oval, Scored, U/121 <> 2 1/2	Minoxidil 2.5 mg	Loniten by Upjohn		Antihypertensive
U121 <> 212	Tab, White, Half Oval, Scored, U/121 <> 2 1/2	Minoxidil 2.5 mg	Loniten by Pharmacia	Canadian DIN 0514497	Antihypertensive
U121 <> 212	Tab, White, Half Oval, Scored, U/121 <> 2 1/2	Minoxidil 2.5 mg	Loniten by Pharmacia	00009-0121	Antihypertensive
U137	Tab, White, Round	Minoxidil 10 mg	Loniten by Upjohn	Canadian	Antihypertensive
U137 <> 10	Tab, White, Round, Scored	Minoxidil 10 mg	Loniten by Pharmacia	Canadian DIN 00514500	Antihypertensive
U2	Tab, White, Round	Pramipexole DiHCl 0.125 mg	Mirapex by Upjohn		Antiparkinson
U200 <> PF	Tab, White, Round, Scored, U over 200	Theophylline Anhydrous 200 mg	T-Phyl by Purdue	00034-7102	Antiasthmatic
U23	Tab, White, Round	Isoniazid 300 mg	Laniazid by Eli Lilly		Antimycobacterial
U25	Tab, Pink, Square, Chewable	Erythromycin Estolate 250 mg	Ilosone by Eli Lilly		Antibiotic
U26	Tab, Salmon, Oblong	Erythromycin Estolate 500 mg	Ilosone by Eli Lilly		Antibiotic
U286	Tab, Blue, Round, Scored	Medroxyprogesterone Acetate 5 mg	Provera by Upjohn	Canadian DIN 00030937	Hormone
U29	Tab, Green, Round	Reserpine 0.25 mg	Sandril by Eli Lilly		Antihypertensive
U3617	Tab, Light Orange, Oval	Cefpodoxime Proxetil 100 mg	Vantin by Pharmacia	00009-3617	Antibiotic
U3617	Tab, Orange, Oval	Cefpodoxime Proxetil 100 mg	Vantin by Allscripts		Antibiotic
U3618	Tab, Red, Oval, Film Coated, U over 3618	Cefpodoxime Proxetil 200 mg	Vantin by Pharmacia	59267-3618	Antibiotic
U3618	Tab, Red, Oval, Film Coated, U over 3618	Cefpodoxime Proxetil 200 mg	Vantin by Pharmacia	00009-3618	Antibiotic
U3618	Tab, Red, Oval, Film Coated, U over 3618	Cefpodoxime Proxetil 200 mg	Vantin by PDRX	55289-0390	Antibiotic

ID FRONT <> BACK	DESCRIPTION FRONT <> BACK	INGREDIENT & STRENGTH	BRAND (or Generic Equiv.) by FIRM	NDC#	CLASS; SCH.
U3761	Tab	Delavirdine Mesylate 100 mg	Rescriptor by Agouron	63010-0020	Antiviral
U3761	Tab, White, Cap Shaped, Film Coated	Delavirdine Mesylate 100 mg	Rescriptor by Pfizer	Canadian DIN 2238348	Antiviral
U3772	Tab, Yellow, Oval, Scored	Estropipate 0.75 mg	Ogen by Apotheca	12634-0512	Hormone
U3772	Tab, Yellow, Oval, Scored	Estropipate 0.75 mg	Ogen by Eckerd	19458-0873	Hormone
U3772	Tab, Yellow, Oval, Scored	Estropipate 0.75 mg	Ogen by Abbott	60692-3943	Hormone
U3772	Tab, Yellow, Oval, Scored	Estropipate 0.75 mg	Ogen by Pharmacia	Canadian	Hormone
U3772	Tab, Yellow, Oval, Scored	Estropipate 0.75 mg	Ogen by Pharmacia	Canadian DIN 02089793	Hormone
U3772	Tab, Yellow, Oval, Scored	Estropipate 0.75 mg	Ogen by Wal Mart	49035-0175	Hormone
U3772	Tab, Yellow, Oval, Scored	Estropipate 0.75 mg	Ogen by Pharmacia	00009-3772	Hormone
U3773	Tab, Peach, Oval, Scored	Estropipate 1.5 mg	Ogen by Pharmacia	Canadian	Hormone
U3773	Tab, Peach, Oval, Scored	Estropipate 1.5 mg	Ogen by Heartland	61392-0492	Hormone
U3773	Tab, Peach, Oval, Scored	Estropipate 1.5 mg	Ogen by Pharmacia	Canadian DIN 02089769	Hormone
U3773	Tab, Peach, Oval, Scored	Estropipate 1.5 mg	Ogen by Abbott	60692-3946	Hormone
U3773	Tab, Peach, Oval, Scored	Estropipate 1.5 mg	Ogen by Pharmacia	00009-3773	Hormone
U3773	Tab, Peach, Oval, Scored	Estropipate 1.5 mg	Ogen by Wal Mart	49035-0174	Hormone
U3773	Tab, Peach, Oval, Scored	Estropipate 1.5 mg	Ogen by Eckerd	19458-0874	Hormone
U3773	Tab, Peach, Oval, Scored	Estropipate 1.5 mg	Ogen by Heartland	61392-0500	Hormone
U3774	Tab, Blue, Oval, Scored	Estropipate 3 mg	Ogen by Pharmacia	Canadian DIN 02089777	Hormone
U3774	Tab, Blue, Oval, Scored	Estropipate 3 mg	Ogen by Abbott	60692-3951	Hormone
U3774	Tab, Blue, Oval, Scored	Estropipate 3 mg	Ogen by Wal Mart	49035-0173	Hormone
U3774	Tab, Blue, Oval, Scored	Estropipate 3 mg	Ogen by Pharmacia	Canadian	Hormone
U3774	Tab, Blue, Oval, Scored	Estropipate 3 mg	Ogen by Eckerd	19458-0875	Hormone
U3774	Tab, Blue, Oval, Scored	Estropipate 3 mg	Ogen by Pharmacia	00009-3774	Hormone
U400 <> PF	Tab, White, Round, Flat-Faced, Scored, U over 400	Theophylline 400 mg	Uniphyl by Purdue Pharma	Canadian DIN 02014165	Antiasthmatic
U400 <> PF	Tab, White, Round, Scored, U over 400	Theophylline Anhydrous 400 mg	Uniphyl by Purdue	00034-7004	Antiasthmatic
U467	Tab, White, Round, Scored	Medroxyprogesterone Acetate 100 mg	Provera by Upjohn	Canadian DIN 0030945	Hormone
U4AZYLOPRIM	Tab, White, Round, U4A/Zyloprim	Allopurinol 100 mg	Zyloprim by GSK	Canadian	Antigout
U53	Tab, Peach, Square, Chewable	Methadone HCl 40 mg	Dolophine by Eli Lilly		Analgesic; C II
U56	Tab, Yellow, Round	Folic Acid 1 mg	Folvite by Eli Lilly		Vitamin
U60	Tab, Green, Oblong	Cephalexin 1 g	Keflex by Eli Lilly		Antibiotic
U600 <> PF	Tab, White, Rectangular, Scored, U over 600	Theophylline Anhydrous 600 mg	Uniphyl by Purdue	00034-7006	Antiasthmatic
U600 <> PF	Tab, White, Cap-Shaped, Concave-Faced, Scored	Theophylline 600 mg	Uniphyl by Purdue Pharma	Canadian DIN 02014181	Antiasthmatic
U64	Tab, Orange, Round, Scored	Medroxyprogesterone Acetate 2.5 mg	Provera by Upjohn	Canadian DIN 00708917	Hormone
U76	Tab, White, Rectangular, U/76	Dinoprostone 0.5 mg	by Pharmacia	Canadian	Labor Inducer
UAD <> 204	Tab, White, Oblong	Guaifenesin 300 mg, Phenylephrine HCl 20 mg	Endal by Mikart	46672-0145	Cold Remedy
UAD <> 204	Tab, White, Oblong	Guaifenesin 300 mg, Phenylephrine HCl 20 mg	Endal by Forest	00785-2204	Cold Remedy
UAD <> 204	Tab, White, Oblong	Guaifenesin 300 mg, Phenylephrine HCl 20 mg	Endal by Physician Total Care	54868-4094	Cold Remedy
UAD <> 400	Tab, White, Scored	Guaifenesin 400 mg, Pseudoephedrine HCl 120 mg	Sudafed Sinus by Forest	00785-6301	Cold Remedy
UAD <> 6350	Tab, Light Blue, Cap Shaped, Scored	Acetaminophen 650 mg, Hydrocodone Bitartrate 10 mg	Lorcet by Southwood	58016-0232	Analgesic; C III
UAD <> 6350	Tab, Light Blue, Cap Shaped, Scored	Acetaminophen 650 mg, Hydrocodone Bitartrate 10 mg	Lorcet by Forest	00785-6350	Analgesic; C III
UAD <> 6350	Tab, Light Blue, Cap Shaped, Scored	Acetaminophen 650 mg, Hydrocodone Bitartrate 10 mg	Lorcet by Med Pro	53978-2068	Analgesic; C III
UAD <> 6350	Tab, Light Blue, Cap Shaped, Scored	Acetaminophen 650 mg, Hydrocodone Bitartrate 10 mg	Lorcet by DRX	55045-2122	Analgesic; C III

ID FRONT <> BACK	DESCRIPTION FRONT <> BACK	INGREDIENT & STRENGTH	BRAND (or Generic Equiv.) by FIRM	NDC#	CLASS; SCH.
UAD <> 6350	Tab, Light Blue, Cap Shaped, Scored	Acetaminophen 650 mg, Hydrocodone Bitartrate 10 mg	Lorcet by Mikart	46672-0103	Analgesic; C III
UAD <> 6350	Tab, Light Blue, Cap Shaped, Scored	Acetaminophen 650 mg, Hydrocodone Bitartrate 10 mg	Lorcet by Nat Pharmpak	55154-7301	Analgesic; C III
UAD <> 6350	Tab, Light Blue, Cap Shaped, Scored	Acetaminophen 650 mg, Hydrocodone Bitartrate 10 mg	Lorcet by Amerisource	62584-0021	Analgesic; C III
UAD111	Tab, Orange, UAD/111	Propoxyphene HCl 65 mg, Acetaminophen 650 mg	E-Lor by Forest	00785-1117	Analgesic; C IV
UAD111	Tab, Orange, UAD/111	Propoxyphene HCl 65 mg, Acetaminophen 650 mg	by Forest	00785-1117	Analgesic; C IV
UAD1120	Cap, Maroon, Opaque	Acetaminophen 500 mg, Hydrocodone Bitartrate 5 mg	Lorcet by Forest		Analgesic; C III
UAD202	Tab, Yellow, UAD/202	Acetaminophen 325 mg, Hydrocodone Bitartrate 2.5 mg	Lortab by Forest	00785-1120	Analgesic; C III
UAD207	Tab, Red, UAD/207	Acetaminophen 325 mg, Hydrocodone Bitartrate 7.5 mg	Anexsia by Forest		Analgesic; C III
UAD210	Tab, Burgundy, UAD/210	Acetaminophen 325 mg, Hydrocodone Bitartrate 10 mg	Norco by Forest		Analgesic; C III
UAD2404	Cap, Blue	Dimenhydrinate 50 mg	Vertab by Forest	00785-2404	Antiemetic
UAD308	Tab, Peach, UAD/308	Acetaminophen 150 mg, Aspirin 180 mg, Hydrocodone 5 mg	by Forest		Analgesic; C III
UAD309	Tab, Purple, UAD/309	Acetaminophen 150 mg, Aspirin 180 mg, Hydrocodone 7.5 mg	by Forest		Analgesic; C III
UAD310	Tab, Red, UAD/310	Acetaminophen 150 mg, Aspirin 180 mg, Hydrocodone 10 mg	by Forest		Analgesic; C III
UAD505	Cap, Red, UAD/505	Acetaminophen 325 mg, Hydrocodone Bitartrate 5 mg	Anexsia by Forest		Analgesic; C III
UADCEZINS811	Cap, Yellow	Vitamin A, D, E, Ascorbic Acid	Cezin-S by Forest	00785-4811	Vitamin
UADENDAFED206	Cap, Blue & Clear	Pseudoephedrine HCl 120 mg, Brompheniramine Maleate 12 mg	Endafed by Forest	00785-2206	Cold Remedy
UC5337 <> A625	Tab, Green, Round, Scored	Pergolide Mesylate 0.25 mg	Epermax by Pharmacy Care	65070-0513	Antiparkinson
UC5364	Tab, Coated	Dirithromycin 250 mg	Dynabac by Sanofi	00024-0490	Antibiotic
UC5364	Tab, Delayed Release	Dirithromycin 250 mg	Dynabac by Promex Med	62301-0012	Antibiotic
UC5364 <> DYNABAC	Tab, White, Oval, Coated	Dirithromycin 250 mg	Dynabac by Eli Lilly	00002-0490	Antibiotic
UC5391	Tab, Blue, Ex Release	Cefaclor 375 mg	Ceclor CD by Dura	51479-0036	Antibiotic
UC5392	Tab, Blue, Ex Release	Cefaclor 500 mg	Ceclor CD by Dura	51479-0035	Antibiotic
UC5392	Tab, Blue, Ex Release	Cefaclor 500 mg	Ceclor CD by Promex Med	62301-0028	Antibiotic
UC5395	Tab, Dark Green, Elliptical	Cephalexin 500 mg	Keftab by Dura		Antibiotic
UC5966RX681	Cap, White & Ocher	Fenoprofen Calcium 200 mg	Nalfon by Ranbaxy	63004-0681	NSAID
UC5967RX682	Cap, Yellow & Ocher	Fenoprofen Calcium 300 mg	Nalfon by Ranbaxy	63004-0682	NSAID
UCB <> 250	Tab, Blue, Oblong, Scored, Film Coated	Levetiracetam 250 mg	Keppra by UCB	50474-0591	Anticonvulsant
UCB <> 500	Tab, Yellow, Oblong, Scored, Film Coated	Levetiracetam 500 mg	Keppra by UCB	50474-0592	Anticonvulsant
UCB <> 612	Tab, White, Oval, Scored, Film Coated	Guaifenesin 600 mg, Pseudoephedrine 120 mg	Duratuss by Mikart	46672-0126	Cold Remedy
UCB <> 612	Tab, White, Oval, Scored, Film Coated	Guaifenesin 600 mg, Pseudoephedrine HCl 120 mg	Duratuss by UCB	50474-0612	Cold Remedy
UCB <> 612	Tab, White, Oval, Scored, Film Coated	Guaifenesin 600 mg, Pseudoephedrine HCl 120 mg	Duratuss by Nat Pharmpak	55154-7203	Cold Remedy
UCB <> 612	Tab, White, Oval, Scored, Film Coated	Guaifenesin 600 mg, Pseudoephedrine 120 mg	Duratuss by Physician Total Care	54868-3943	Cold Remedy
UCB <> 750	Tab, Orange, Oblong, Scored, Film Coated	Levetiracetam 750 mg	Keppra by UCB	50474-0593	Anticonvulsant
UCB <> 901	Tab, White, Cap Shaped, Scored	Acetaminophen 500 mg, Hydrocodone Bitartrate 2.5 mg	Lortab by UCB	50474-0925	Analgesic; C III
UCB <> 902	Tab, White, Cap Shaped, Scored	Acetaminophen 500 mg, Hydrocodone Bitartrate 5 mg	Lortab by Murfreesboro	51129-1434	Analgesic; C III
UCB <> 902	Tab, White, Cap Shaped, Scored	Acetaminophen 500 mg, Hydrocodone Bitartrate 7.5 mg	Lortab by H J Harkins Co	52959-0185	Analgesic; C III
UCB <> 902	Tab, White, Cap Shaped, Scored	Acetaminophen 500 mg, Hydrocodone Bitartrate 5 mg	Lortab by Nat Pharmpak	55154-7204	Analgesic; C III
UCB <> 902	Tab, White, Cap Shaped, Scored	Acetaminophen 500 mg, Hydrocodone Bitartrate 5 mg	Lortab by UCB	50474-0902	Analgesic; C III
UCB <> 902	Tab, White, Cap Shaped, Scored	Acetaminophen 500 mg, Hydrocodone Bitartrate 5 mg	Lortab by Allscripts		Analgesic; C III
UCB <> 903	Tab, White, Cap Shaped, Scored	Acetaminophen 500 mg, Hydrocodone Bitartrate 7.5 mg	Lortab by UCB	50474-0907	Analgesic; C III
UCB <> 903	Tab, White, Cap Shaped, Scored	Acetaminophen 500 mg, Hydrocodone Bitartrate 7.5 mg	Lortab by Med Pro	53978-2069	Analgesic; C III
UCB <> 903	Tab, White, Cap Shaped, Scored	Acetaminophen 500 mg, Hydrocodone Bitartrate 7.5 mg	Lortab by H J Harkins Co	52959-0186	Analgesic; C III
UCB <> 903	Tab, White, Cap Shaped, Scored	Acetaminophen 500 mg, Hydrocodone Bitartrate 7.5 mg	Lortab by Amerisource	62584-0907	Analgesic; C III
UCB <> 903	Tab, White, Cap Shaped, Scored	Acetaminophen 500 mg, Hydrocodone Bitartrate 7.5 mg	Lortab by Allscripts		Analgesic; C III
UCB <> 903	Tab, White, Pink, Cap Shaped, Scored	Acetaminophen 500 mg, Hydrocodone Bitartrate 7.5 mg	Lortab by Nat Pharmpak	55154-7201	Analgesic; C III
UCB <> 910	Tab, Pink, Cap Shaped, Scored	Acetaminophen 500 mg, Hydrocodone Bitartrate 10 mg	Lortab by UCB	50474-0910	Analgesic; C III
UCB <> 910	Tab, Pink, Cap Shaped, Scored	Acetaminophen 500 mg, Hydrocodone Bitartrate 10 mg	Lortab by D M Graham	00756-0249	Analgesic; C III
UCB <> 910	Tab, Pink, Cap Shaped, Scored	Acetaminophen 500 mg, Hydrocodone Bitartrate 10 mg	Lortab by Amerisource	62584-0016	Analgesic; C III

ID FRONT <> BACK	DESCRIPTION FRONT <> BACK	INGREDIENT & STRENGTH	BRAND (or Generic Equiv.) by FIRM	NDC#	CLASS; SCH.
UCB <> 910	Tab, Pink, Cap Shaped, Scored	Acetaminophen 500 mg, Hydrocodone Bitartrate 10 mg	Lortab by H J Harkins Co	52959-0453	Analgesic; C III
UCB <> 910	Tab, Pink, Cap Shaped, Scored	Acetaminophen 500 mg, Hydrocodone Bitartrate 10 mg	Lortab by Nat Pharmpak	55154-7202	Analgesic; C III
UCB <> 935	Tab, White, Oblong, Scored, with Orange Specks	Acetaminophen 325 mg, Hydrocodone Bitartrate 5 mg	by Murfreesboro	51129-1452	Analgesic; C III
UCB1000	Tab, White, Oblong, Film Coated	Levetiracetam 1000 mg	Keppra by Lundbeck	50474-0597	Anticonvulsant
UCB250	Tab, Blue, Oblong, Scored, Film Coated	Levetiracetam 250 mg	Keppra by UCB	50474-0591	Anticonvulsant
UCB250	Tab, Blue, Oblong, Film-Coated	Levetiracetam 250 mg	Keppra by Lundbeck	Canadian DIN 02247027	Anticonvulsant
UCB315	Cap, Black & Orange	Niacinamide 25 mg, Vitamin A 8000 Units, Magnesium Sulfate 70 mg, Zinc Sulfate 80 mg, Ascorbic Acid 150 mg, Vitamin E 50 Units, Thiamine Mononitrate 10 mg, Calcium Pantothenate 10 mg, Riboflavin 5 mg, Manganese Chloride 4 mg, Pyridoxine HCl 2 mg, Folic Acid 1 mg	Vicon Forte by Rx Pak	65084-0211	Vitamin
UCB316	Cap, Black & Orange	Ascorbic Acid 150 mg, Calcium Pantothenate 10 mg, Cyanocobalamin 10 mcg, Folic Acid 1 mg, Magnesium Sulfate 70 mg, Manganese Chloride 4 mg, Niacinamide 25 mg, Pyridoxine HCl 2 mg, Riboflavin 5 mg, Thiamine Mononitrate 10 mg, Vitamin A 8000 Units, Vitamin E 50 Units, Zinc Sulfate 80 mg	Vicon Forte by Rightpac	65240-0780	Vitamin
UCB316	Cap, Black & Orange	Ascorbic Acid 150 mg, Calcium Pantothenate 10 mg, Cyanocobalamin 10 mcg, Folic Acid 1 mg, Magnesium Sulfate 70 mg, Manganese Chloride 4 mg, Niacinamide 25 mg, Pyridoxine HCl 2 mg, Riboflavin 5 mg, Thiamine Mononitrate 10 mg, Vitamin A 8000 Units, Vitamin E 50 Units, Zinc Sulfate 80 mg	Vicon Forte by D M Graham	00756-0235	Vitamin
UCB316	Cap, Black & Orange	Ascorbic Acid 150 mg, Calcium Pantothenate 10 mg, Cyanocobalamin 10 mcg, Folic Acid 1 mg, Magnesium Sulfate 70 mg, Manganese Chloride 4 mg, Niacinamide 25 mg, Pyridoxine HCl 2 mg, Riboflavin 5 mg, Thiamine Mononitrate 10 mg, Vitamin A 8000 Units, Vitamin E 50 Units, Zinc Sulfate 80 mg	Vicon Forte by UCB	50474-0316	Vitamin
UCB316	Cap, Black & Orange	Ascorbic Acid 150 mg, Calcium Pantothenate 10 mg, Cyanocobalamin 10 mcg, Folic Acid 1 mg, Magnesium Sulfate 70 mg, Manganese Chloride 4 mg, Niacinamide 25 mg, Pyridoxine HCl 2 mg, Riboflavin 5 mg, Thiamine Mononitrate 10 mg, Vitamin A 8000 Units, Vitamin E 50 Units, Zinc Sulfate 80 mg	by Eckerd	19458-0847	Vitamin
UCB364	Cap, Dark Pink & Dark Red	Ascorbic Acid 75 mg, Cyanocobalamin 15 mcg, Ferrous Fumarate 110 mg, Folic Acid 0.5 mg, Liver w/ Stomach 240 mg	Trinsicon by UCB	50474-0364	Vitamin
UCB500	Tab, Yellow, Oblong, Scored, Film Coated	Levetiracetam 500 mg	Keppra by UCB	50474-0592	Anticonvulsant
UCB500	Tab, Yellow, Oblong, Film-Coated	Levetiracetam 500 mg	Keppra by Lundbeck	Canadian DIN 0224702	Anticonvulsant
UCB500XR	Tab, White, Oblong, Film Coated	Levetiracetam 500 mg	Keppra XR by UCB	50474-0598	Antiepileptic
UCB57910MG	Cap, Green and White, Extended Release	Methylphenidate HCl 10 mg	Metadate CD by UCB	53014-0579	Stimulant; C II
UCB58020MG	Cap, Blue and White, Extended Release	Methylphenidate HCl 20 mg	Metadate CD by UCB	53014-0580	Stimulant; C II
UCB58130MG	Cap, Reddish Brown and White, Extended Release	Methylphenidate HCl 30 mg	Metadate CD by UCB	53014-0581	Stimulant; C II
UCB58240MG	Cap, Yellow and White, Extended Release	Methylphenidate HCl 40 mg	Metadate CD by UCB	53014-0582	Stimulant; C II
UCB58350MG	Cap, Purple and White, Extended Release	Methylphenidate HCl 50 mg	Metadate CD by UCB	53014-0583	Stimulant; C II
UCB58460MG	Cap, White, Extended Release	Methylphenidate HCl 60 mg	Metadate CD by UCB	53014-0584	Stimulant; C II
UCB620	Tab, White, Oblong, Scored, Film Coated	Guaifenesin 1200 mg	Robitussin by Eckerd	19458-0869	Expectorant
UCB620	Tab, White, Oblong, Scored, Film Coated	Guaifenesin 1200 mg	Robitussin by UCB	50474-0650	Expectorant
UCB620	Tab, White, Oblong, Scored, Film Coated	Guaifenesin 1200 mg	Robitussin by Mikart	46672-0163	Expectorant
UCB620	Tab, White, Oblong, Scored, Film Coated	Guaifenesin 1200 mg	Robitussin by Nat Pharmpak	55154-7205	Expectorant
UCB620	Tab, White, Oblong, Scored, Film Coated	Guaifenesin 1200 mg	Robitussin by Thrift Drug	59198-0329	Expectorant
UCB620	Tab, White, Oblong, Scored, Film Coated	Guaifenesin 1200 mg	Robitussin by Rx Pak	65084-0224	Expectorant
UCB620	Tab, White, Oblong, Scored, Film Coated	Guaifenesin 1200 mg	Robitussin by Eli Lilly	00110-0895	Expectorant
UCB640	Tab, White, Cap Shaped, Scored, Film Coated	Guaifenesin 1200 mg, Pseudoephedrine HCl 120 mg	Aquabid D by UCB	50474-0650	Cold Remedy

ID FRONT <> BACK	DESCRIPTION FRONT <> BACK	INGREDIENT & STRENGTH	BRAND (or Generic Equiv.) by FIRM	NDC#	CLASS; SCH.
UCB750	Tab, Orange, Oblong, Scored, Film Coated	Levetiracetam 750 mg	Keppra by UCB	50474-0593	Anticonvulsant
UCB750	Tab, Orange, Oblong, Film-Coated	Levetiracetam 750 mg	Keppra by Lundbeck	Canadian DIN 02247029	Anticonvulsant
UCB750XR	Tab, White, Oblong, Film Coated	Levetiracetam 750 mg	Keppra XR by UCB	50474-0599	Antiepileptic
UCBUCB	Cap, Orange & Yellow w/ Blue Band	Ascorbic Acid 300 mg, Magnesium 6.4 mg, Niacin 95 mg, Pantothenic Acid 22 mg, Pyridoxine 4 mg, Riboflavin 10 mg, Vitamin B1 17.9 mg, Zinc 15.9 mg	Vicon-C by UCB	50474-0273	Vitamin
UCBUCB	Cap, Orange w/ Blue Band	Alpha-tocopherol 45 Units, Ascorbic Acid 480 mg, Retinol 5000 Units, Zinc 17 mg	Vi-Zac by UCB	50474-0292	Vitamin
UCBUCB	Cap, Red & Light Yellow w/ Blue Band	Alpha-tocopherol 45 Units, Ascorbic Acid 140 mg, Magnesium 5 mg, Manganese 1 mg, Niacin 24 mg, Pantothenic Acid 11 mg, Pyridoxine 1.5 mg, Retinol 3400 Units, Riboflavin 4.6 mg, Thiamine 9.3 mg, Zinc 10 mg	Vicon Plus by UCB	50474-0305	Vitamin
UCY500	Tab, Beige, Oval	Sodium Phenylbutyrate 500 mg	Buphenyl by Pharmaceutics Int'l	61916-0496	Antihyperammonemic
UCY500	Tab, Beige, Oval	Sodium Phenylbutyrate 500 mg	Buphenyl by Ucyclyd	62592-0496	Antihyperammonemic
UDANL5347	Tab, White, Round, U:DAN L.5347	Minoxidil 10 mg	Loniten by Danbury		Antihypertensive
UG604	Tab, Purple, Cap-Shaped, Scored	Carbetapentane Tannate 60 mg, Chlorpheniramine Tannate 5 mg	Tussi-12 by URL	00677-1825	Cold Remedy
UHE <> NVR	Tab, White to Light Yellow, Oblong	Everolimus 10 mg	Afinitor by Novartis	00078-0567	Cancer Therapy
UIC <> NVR	Tab, Light Yellow, Oval, Film Coated	Amlodipine 10 mg, Valsartan 160 mg	Exforge by Novartis	00078-0489	Antihypertensive
ULTRADOL200MG	Cap, Light Gray w/ Two Red Bands	Etodolac 200 mg	Ultradol by Proc & Gamble	Canadian DIN 02142023	NSAID
ULTRADOL300MG	Cap, Light Gray w/ Red Bands	Etodolac 300 mg	Ultradol by Proc & Gamble	Canadian DIN 02142031	NSAID
ULTRAM <> 0659	Tab, White, Oblong	Tramadol HCl 50 mg	Ultram by Ortho-McNeil	00045-0659	Analgesic
ULTRASE	Cap, White	Lipase 4,500 Units, Amylase 20,000 Units, Protease 25,000 Units	Ultrase by Scandipharm	58914-0045	Gastrointestinal
ULTRASEMS4	Cap, White, Opaque	Lipase 4500 Units, Amylase 20,000 Units, Protease 25,000 Units	Ultrase by Axcan	Canadian DIN 02203324	Gastrointestinal
ULTRASEMT12	Cap, White & Yellow	Lipase 12,000 Units, Amylase 39,000 Units, Protease 39,000 Units	Ultrase MT12 by Axcan	Canadian DIN 02045834	Gastrointestinal
ULTRASEMT12	Cap, White & Yellow	Lipase 12,000 Units, Amylase 39,000 Units, Protease 39,000 Units	Ultrase MT by Scandipharm	58914-0002	Gastrointestinal
ULTRASEMT18	Cap, White & Gray	Lipase 18,000 Units, Amylase 58,500 Units, Protease 58,500 Units	Ultrase MT by Scandipharm	58914-0018	Gastrointestinal
ULTRASEMT20	Cap, Gray & Yellow, Oblong	Lipase 20,000 Units, Amylase 65,000 Units, Protease 65,000 Units	Ultrace MT 20 by Scandipharm	58914-0004	Gastrointestinal
ULTRASEMT20	Cap, Gray & Yellow, Oblong	Lipase 20,000 Units, Amylase 65,000 Units, Protease 65,000 Units	Ultrase MT20 by Axcan	Canadian DIN 02045869	Gastrointestinal
ULTRASEMT20	Cap, Gray & Yellow	Amylase 65,000 Units, Lipase 20,000 Units, Protease 65,000 Units	Ultrase MT 20 by Eurand	57298-0052	Gastrointestinal
UM	Cap, White	Dronabinol 2.5 mg	Marinol by Unimed	00051-0021	Antiemetic; Antivertigo; C III
UM	Cap, Dark Brown	Dronabinol 5 mg	Marinol by Unimed	00051-0022	Antiemetic; Antivertigo; C III
UM	Cap, Orange	Dronabinol 10 mg	Marinol by Unimed	00051-0023	Antiemetic; Antivertigo; C III
UM	Cap, White	Dronabinol 2.5 mg	Marinol by Solvay	Canadian DIN 00611190	Antiemetic; Antivertigo; C III
UM	Cap, Dark Brown	Dronabinol 5 mg	Marinol by Solvay	Canadian DIN 00611204	Antiemetic; Antivertigo; C III
UM	Cap, Orange	Dronabinol 10 mg	Marinol by Solvay	Canadian DIN 00611212	Antiemetic; Antivertigo; C III
UNIGEN601	Tab, Purple, Oblong, Scored	Carbetapentane Tannate 60 mg, Chlorpheniramine Tannate 5 mg, Ephedrine Tannate 10 mg, Phenylephrine Tannate 10 mg	Quadratuss by Unigen	62305-0601	Cold Remedy
UNIGEN601	Tab, Pink, Oblong, Scored	Carbetapentane Tannate 60 mg, Chlorpheniramine Tannate 5 mg, Ephedrine Tannate 10 mg, Phenylephrine Tannate 10 mg	Ry Tuss by Cypress	60258-0271	Cold Remedy

ID FRONT <> BACK	DESCRIPTION FRONT <> BACK	INGREDIENT & STRENGTH	BRAND (or Generic Equiv.) by FIRM	NDC#	CLASS; SCH.
UNIMED	Tab, Mottled Pink, Round, Scored	Betahistine DiHCl 4 mg	by Solvay	Canadian DIN 02222035	Antivertigo
UPJOHN	Cap, Light Blue	Lincomycin HCl 500 mg	by Pharmacia	Canadian	Antibiotic
UPJOHN	Tab, Green, Round, Scored	Fluoxymesterone 5 mg	Halotestin by Upjohn	Canadian DIN 00030902	Steroid; C III
UPJOHN10	Tab, Violet	Triazolam 0.125 mg	by Pharmacia	Canadian	Sedative/Hypnotic; C IV
UPJOHN15	Tab, White, Round, Scored, Upjohn over 15	Cortisone Acetate 5 mg	by Pharmacia	00009-0015 Discontinued	Steroid
UPJOHN17	Tab, Powder Blue, Scored	Triazolam 0.25 mg	Halcion by Pharmacia	Canadian DIN 00443158	Sedative/Hypnotic; C IV
UPJOHN18	Tab, Yellow, Round	Benzphetamine HCl 25 mg	Didrex by Upjohn		Sympathomimetic; C III
UPJOHN225	Cap, Lavender & Maroon, Gelatin	Clindamycin HCl 150 mg	Dalacin C by Pharmacia	Canadian DIN 00030570	Antibiotic
UPJOHN23	Tab, White, Scored	Cortisone Acetate 10 mg	Cortone Acetate by Pharmacia	00009-0023	Steroid
UPJOHN29	Tab, White, Scored	Alprazolam 0.25 mg	Xanax by Upjohn	Canadian DIN 00548359	Antianxiety; C IV
UPJOHN29	Tab, White, Single Score	Alprazolam 0.25 mg	Xanax by Pfizer	Canadian DIN 00548359	Antianxiety
UPJOHN34	Tab, White, Scored	Cortisone Acetate 25 mg	Cortone Acetate by Pharmacia	00009-0034	Steroid
UPJOHN395	Cap, Light Blue, Gelatin	Clindamycin HCl 300 mg	Dalacin C by Pharmacia	Canadian DIN 02182866	Antibiotic
UPJOHN45	Tab, White	Prednisone 5 mg	Deltasone by Upjohn	Canadian	Steroid
UPJOHN50	Tab, White, Round, Scored	Medroxyprogesterone Acetate 10 mg	Provera by Upjohn	Canadian DIN 00729973	Hormone
UPJOHN55	Tab, Peach, Scored	Alprazolam 0.5 mg	Xanax by Upjohn	Canadian DIN 00548367	Antianxiety; C IV
UPJOHN55	Tab, Peach, Single Score	Alprazolam 0.5 mg.	Xanax by Pfizer	Canadian DIN 00548367	Antianxiety
UPJOHN56	Tab, White, Elliptical, Scored	Methylprednisolone 4 mg	by Upjohn	Canadian DIN 00030988	Steroid
UPJOHN90	Tab, Lavender, Scored	Alprazolam 1 mg	Xanax by Upjohn	Canadian DIN 00723770	Antianxiety; C IV
UPJOHN90	Tab, Lavender, Single Score	Alprazolam 1 mg.	Xanax by Pfizer	Canadian DIN 00723770	Antianxiety
UPJOHN949	Cap, Yellow & Blue	Uracil Mustard 1 mg	by Upjohn		Antineoplastic
UR500	Tab, White, Oval	Ursodiol 500 mg	Urso DS by Pharmascience	Canadian DIN 02273500	Gastrointestinal
URECHOLINE <> MSD403	Tab, White	Bethanechol Chloride 5 mg	Urecholine by Merck	00006-0403	Urinary Tract
URECHOLINE <> MSD412	Tab, Pink	Bethanechol Chloride 10 mg	Urecholine by Merck	00006-0412	Urinary Tract
URECHOLINE <> MSD457	Tab, Yellow	Bethanechol Chloride 25 mg	Urecholine by Merck	00006-0457	Urinary Tract
URECHOLINE <> MSD460	Tab, Yellow	Bethanechol Chloride 50 mg	Urecholine by Merck	00006-0460	Urinary Tract
URETRONDS	Tab, Sugar Coated, Uretron D/S	Hyoscyamine Sulfate 0.12 mg, Methenamine 81.6 mg, Methylene Blue 10.8 mg, Phenyl Salicylate 36.2 mg, Sodium Phosphate, Monobasic 40.8 mg	Uretron DS by A G Marin	12539-0144	Gastrointestinal
URETRONDS	Tab, Purple, Round, Uretron D/S	Phenyl Phosphate 36.2 mg, Methylene Blue 10.8 mg, Methenamine 81.6, Hyoscyamine Sulfate 0.12 mg	Uretron DS by Physician Total Care		Urinary Tract
UREX <> 3M	Tab, White, Cap Shaped, Scored	Methenamine Hippurate 1 g	Urex by 3M	00089-0371	Antibiotic; Urinary Tract
UREX <> VP	Tab, White, Oblong, Scored	Methenamine Hippurate 1 g	Urex by Virco Pharms	65199-1201	Antibiotic; Urinary Tract
URIMAX	Tab, Round, Magenta, Film Coated, Black Ink	Methenamine 81.60 mg, Sodium Biphosphate 40.80 mg, Phenyl Salicylate 36.20 mg, Methylene Blue 10.80 mg, Hyoscyamine Sulfate 0.12 mg	Urimax by Xanodyne	64731-0860	Urinary Tract

ID FRONT <> BACK	DESCRIPTION FRONT <> BACK	INGREDIENT & STRENGTH	BRAND (or Generic Equiv.) by FIRM	NDC#	CLASS; SCH.
URISPAS	Tab, White, Round, Film Coated	Flavoxate HCl 100 mg	Urispas by Alza	17314-9220	Antispasmodic
URISPASSKF	Tab, White, Round, Film Coated, URISPAS over SKF	Flavoxate HCl 100 mg	by SKB	00007-5290	Antispasmodic
URISPASSKF	Tab, White, Round, Film Coated, URISPAS over SKF	Flavoxate HCl 100 mg	Urispas by Integrity		Antispasmodic
URL401	Cap, White, Opaque	Mefenamic Acid 250 mg	Ponstel by URL Mutual	00677-1934	NSAID
UROKPNEUTRAL	Tab, Light Peach, Cap Shaped, Film Coated, Debossed, URO-KP-Neutral	Phosphorous 250 mg, Potassium 49.4 mg, Sodium 250.5 mg	Uro-KP-Neutral by Star	00076-0109	Supplement
UROLENEBLUE	Tab, Dark Blue	Methylene Blue 65 mg	Urolene Blue by Star	00076-0501	Analgesic
URS785	Tab, White, Elliptical, Film Coated	Ursodiol 250 mg	Urso by Global	55963-0785	Gastrointestinal
URS785	Tab, White	Ursodeoxycholic Acid 250 mg	Urso by Schwarz		Gastrointestinal
URS785	Tab, White, Elliptical, Film Coated	Ursodiol 250 mg	Urso by Axcan	58914-0785	Gastrointestinal
URS785	Tab, White, Elliptical, Film Coated	Ursodiol 250 mg	Urso by Axcan	Canadian DIN 02238984	Gastrointestinal
URS790	Tab, White, Elliptical, Film Coated	Ursodiol 500 mg	Urso DS by Axcan	Canadian DIN 02245894	Gastrointestinal
URS790	Tab, White, Elliptical, Film Coated	Ursodiol 500 mg	Urso Forte by Axcan	58914-0790	Gastrointestinal
URSODIOL300MG-COPLEY380	Cap, Red & White	Ursodiol 300 mg	Urso by Teva	38245-0380	Gastrointestinal
US	Cap, Maroon, Black Print	Ferrous Fumarate 324 mg, Sodium Ascorbate 200 mg, Thiamine Mononitrate 10 mg, Riboflavin 6 mg, Pyridoxine HCl 5 mg, Cyanocobalamin Concentrate 15 mcg, Folic Acid 1 mg, Nicotinamide 30 mg, Calcium Pantothenate 10 mg, Zinc Sulfate 18.2 mg, Magnesium Sulfate 6.9 mg, Manganese Sulfate 1.3 mg, Copper Sulfate 0.8 mg	Hemocyte Plus by US Pharma	52747-0800	Vitamin/Mineral
US	Tab, Maroon, Round	Ferrous Fumarate, Folic Acid	Hemocyte-F by US Pharma	52747-0306	Mineral
US	Tab, Red, Round	Ferrous Fumarate 324 mg	Hemocyte by US Pharma	52747-0307	Mineral
US	Tab, Peach, Football Shaped	Vitamin E di-Alpha Tocopheryl Acetate 100 IU, Vitamin C Ascorbic Acid 300 mg, Vitamin B-12 Cyanocobalamin Concentrate 25 mcg, Vitamin B-1 Thiamine 25 mg, Niacinamide 100 mg, Vitamin B-6 Pyridoxine 10 mg, Calcium Pantothenate 25 mg, Zinc 18 mg, Magnesium 7 mg, Manganese 13 mg, Copper (as Cupric Sulfate) 8 mg, Folic Acid 4 mg 52747-0305 Discontinued	Mediplex- Ultra by US Pharma	52747-0305 Discontinued	Vitamin
US	Cap, White, Green Print	Acetaminophen 325 mg, Butalbital 50 mg, Caffeine 40 mg	Fioricet by US Pharma	52747-0600	Analgesic
US	Cap, Yellow & White, Black Print	Acetaminophen 325 mg, Chlorpheniramine Maleate 4 mg, Phenylpropanolamine HCl 25 mg, Phenyltoloxamine Citrate 25 mg	Norel Plus by US Pharma	52747-0128 Discontinued	Cold Remedy
US <> 016	Tab, Yellow, Oval, Film Coated	Folic Acid 2.2 mg, Vitamin B-6 25 mg, Vitamin B-12 500 mcg	Folgard Rx by Upsher Smith	00245-0183	Vitamin
US <> 016	Tab, Yellow, Oval, Film Coated	Folic Acid 2.2 mg, Vitamin B-6 25 mg, Vitamin B-12 500 mcg	Folgard Rx by Upsher Smith	00245-0016	Vitamin
US <> 017	Tab, Green, Round, Film Coated	Folic Acid 800 mcg, Vitamin B 115 mcg, Vitamin B-6 10 mg	Folgard by Upsher Smith	00245-0017	Vitamin
US <> 750	Tab, Blue, Oblong	Salsalate 750 mg	Salsitab by Upsher Smith	00228-2769	NSAID
US <> A	Tab, White, Round	Amiodarone 200 mg	Cordarone by Heartland	61392-0935	Antiarrhythmic
US0140 <> P300	Tab, Peach, Round, Scored, P subscript 300 <> U-S over 0140	Amiodarone HCl 300 mg	Pacerone by Upsher Smith	00245-0140	Antiarrhythmic
US0147 <> P200	Tab, Pink, Round, Scored, U-S over 0147	Amiodarone 200 mg	Cordarone by Pharmascience	Canadian DIN 5760603613	Antiarrhythmic
US0147 <> P200	Tab, Pink, Round, Scored, U-S over 0147	Amiodarone 200 mg	Cordarone by Thrift Drug	59198-0362	Antiarrhythmic
US0147 <> P200	Tab, Pink, Round, Scored, U-S over 0147	Amiodarone 200 mg	Cordarone by Upsher Smith	00245-0147	Antiarrhythmic
US0147 <> P200	Tab, Pink, Round, Scored, U-S over 0147	Amiodarone HCl 200 mg	Pacerone by Apotheca	12634-0549	Antiarrhythmic
US027	Tab, Light Pink, Cap Shaped, Film Coated, U-S 027, Extended Release	Pentoxifylline 400 mg	Trental by Upsher-Smith	00228-2769	Anticoagulant
US027	Tab, Pink, Oblong, Film Coated, Ex Release	Pentoxifylline 400 mg	Trental by Zoetica	64909-0001	Anticoagulant
US027	Tab, Pink, Oblong, Film Coated, Ex Release	Pentoxifylline 400 mg	Trental by Upsher Smith	00245-0027	Anticoagulant
US027	Tab, Pink, Oblong, Film Coated, Ex Release	Pentoxifylline 400 mg	Trental by Pharmafab	62542-0751	Anticoagulant

ID FRONT <> BACK	DESCRIPTION FRONT <> BACK	INGREDIENT & STRENGTH	BRAND (or Generic Equiv.) by FIRM	NDC#	CLASS; SCH.
US10	Tab, White, Oblong, Ex Release	Potassium Chloride 10 mEq	K-Dur by Teva	00093-5310 Discontinued	Electrolytes
US10 <> 213	Tab, Purple, Round, Scored, US over 10 <> 213	Midodrine HCl 10 mg	Orvaten by Upsher Smith	00245-0213	Antihypertensive
US12 <> 80	Tab, White, Cap Shaped	Sotalol HCl 80 mg	Sorine by Upsher Smith	00245-0012	Antiarrhythmic
US13 <> 120	Tab, White, Cap Shaped	Sotalol HCl 120 mg	Sorine by Upsher Smith	00245-0013	Antiarrhythmic
US14 <> 160	Tab, White, Cap Shaped	Sotalol HCl 160 mg	Sorine by Upsher Smith	00245-0014	Antiarrhythmic
US144 <> P	Tab, White, Round, P <> U-S over 144	Amiodarone HCl 100 mg	Pacerone by Upsher Smith	00245-0144	Antiarrhythmic
US15 <> 240	Tab, White, Cap Shaped	Sotalol HCl 240 mg	Sorine by Upsher Smith	00245-0015	Antiarrhythmic
US180	Tab, Rose, Cap Shaped, Enteric-Coated, Delayed Release	Divalproex Sodium 125 mg	Depakote by Upsher Smith	00245-0180	Anticonvulsant
US181	Tab, Peach, Cap Shaped, Enteric-Coated, Delayed Release	Divalproex Sodium 250 mg	Depakote by Upsher-Smith	00245-0181	Anticonvulsant
US182	Tab, Pink, Cap Shaped, Enteric-Coated, Delayed Release	Divalproex Sodium 500 mg	Depakote by Upsher Smith	00245-0182	Anticonvulsant
US20	Tab, White, Oblong, Scored	Potassium Chloride 20 mEq ER	K-Dur by Qualitest	00603-5244	Electrolytes
US20	Tab, White, Oblong, Scored, Ex Release	Potassium Chloride 20 mEq ER	K-Dur by Teva	00093-5311 Discontinued	Electrolytes
US200 <> A	Tab, White, Round, Scored, U-S over 200	Amiodarone 200 mg	Cordarone by Sandoz	00781-1203	Antiarrhythmic
US200 <> A	Tab, White, Round, Scored, U-S over 200	Amiodarone 200 mg	Cordarone by Upsher Smith	00245-1480	Antiarrhythmic
US25 <> 211	Tab, White, Round, Scored, US over 2.5 <> 211	Midodrine HCl 2.5 mg	Orvaten by Upsher Smith	00245-0211	Antihypertensive
US411	Tab, Green Mottled, Ex Release	Nitroglycerin 2.6 mg	Nitrong by RPR		Vasodilator
US412	Tab, Orange Mottled, Ex Release	Nitroglycerin 6.5 mg	Nitrong by RPR		Vasodilator
US5 <> 212	Tab, Pink, Round, Scored, US over 5 <> 212	Midodrine HCl 5 mg	Orvaten by Upsher Smith	00245-0212	Antihypertensive
US500	Tab, Blue, Round	Salsalate 500 mg	Salsitab by Upsher Smith		NSAID
US67 <> 500	Tab, White, Oval, Scored, US over 67	Niacin 500 mg	Niacor by Upsher Smith	00245-0067	Vitamin
USANA	Tab, White, Cap Shaped	Calcium 200 mg, Magnesium 100 mg, Silicon 2.25 mg, Vitamin D3 100 Units	Active Calcium Plus by Usana	Canadian DIN 02245629	Vitamin; Mineral
USB001	Cap, Clear	Altretamine 50 mg	Hexalen by MGI	58063-0001	Antineoplastic
USB001HEXALEN50MG	Cap, Clear	Altretamine 50 mg	Hexalen by US Bioscience	58178-0001	Antineoplastic
USB001HEXALEN50MG	Cap	Altretamine 50 mg	Hexalen by AAI Pharma	27280-0001	Antineoplastic
USCENOGEN	Cap, Pink & Blue, Black Print	Ferrous Fumarate 324 mg, Sodium Ascorbate 200 mg, Thiamine Mononitrate 10 mg, Riboflavin 6 mg, Pyridoxine HCl 5 mg, Cyanocobalamin Concentrate 15 mcg, Folic Acid 1 mg, Nicotinamide 30 mg, Calcium Pantothenate 10 mg, Manganese Sulfate 1.3 mg, Copper Sulfate 0.8 mg	Cenogen Ultra by US Pharma	52747-0140	Vitamin/Mineral
USE <> 411	Tab, Scored, US over E	Nitroglycerin 2.6 mg	Nitrong by RPR	00075-0221	Vasodilator
USE <> 412	Tab, Scored, Film Coated, US over E	Nitroglycerin 6.5 mg	Nitrong by RPR	00075-0274	Vasodilator
USL <> 070	Tab, Yellow, Round	Potassium Citrate 5 mEq	Potassium Citrate by Upsher-Smith	00245-0070	Electrolytes
USL <> 071	Tab, Yellow, Oval	Potassium Citrate 10 mEq	Potassium Citrate by Upsher-Smith	00245-0071	Electrolytes
USL10	Tab, White, Round, Slow Release	Potassium Chloride 750 mg	K-Tab by Sandoz	00781-1526	Electrolytes
USL10	Tab, White, Round, Slow Release	Potassium Chloride 750 mg	K-Tab by Ivax	00182-1840	Electrolytes
USL10	Tab, White, Round, Slow Release	Potassium Chloride 750 mg	K-Tab by Upsher Smith	00245-0041	Electrolytes
USL10	Tab, White, Round	Potassium Chloride 10 mEq	K-Tab by Qualitest	00603-5241	Electrolytes
USL8	Tab, Dark Blue, Round, Film Coated	Potassium Chloride 600 mg	K-Tab by Upsher Smith	00245-0040	Electrolytes
USL8	Tab, Orange, Round, Film Coated, Copley over 225	Potassium Citrate 600 mg	Slow-K by Sandoz	00781-1516	Electrolytes
USL8	Tab, Dark Blue, Round, Film Coated	Potassium Chloride 600 mg	K-Tab by Ivax	00182-1839	Electrolytes
USL8	Tab, Dark Blue, Round, Film Coated	Potassium Chloride 600 mg	K-Tab by Qualitest	00603-5237	Electrolytes
USL80	Cap, Pink, Black Print, USL over 80	Zinc Sulfate 220 mg	Orazinc by Upsher Smith	00245-0080	Mineral
USV2835	Cap, Black & Clear	Nicotinic Acid Time Release 125 mg	Nicobid by RPR		Vitamin
USV2840	Cap, Green & Clear	Nicotinic Acid Time Release 250 mg	Nicobid by RPR		Vitamin
USV2841	Cap, Blue & White	Nicotinic Acid Time Release 500 mg	Nicobid by RPR		Vitamin
USVHK	Tab, Orange, Round, USV Logo HK	Levothyroxine Sodium 25 mcg	Levothroid by USV		Thyroid Hormone

ID FRONT <> BACK	DESCRIPTION FRONT <> BACK	INGREDIENT & STRENGTH	BRAND (or Generic Equiv.) by FIRM	NDC#	CLASS; SCH.
UU <> 201	Tab, White, Cap Shaped, Scored	Acetaminophen 650 mg, Hydrocodone Bitartrate 7.5 mg	Lorcet Plus by Amerisource	62584-0028	Analgesic; C III
UU <> 201	Tab, White, Cap Shaped, Scored	Acetaminophen 650 mg, Hydrocodone Bitartrate 7.5 mg	Lorcet Plus by Nat Pharmpak	55154-7302	Analgesic; C III
UU <> 201	Tab, White, Cap Shaped, Scored	Acetaminophen 650 mg, Hydrocodone Bitartrate 7.5 mg	Lorcet Plus by Med Pro	53978-2071	Analgesic; C III
UU <> 201	Tab, White, Cap Shaped, Scored	Acetaminophen 650 mg, Hydrocodone Bitartrate 7.5 mg	Lorcet Plus by Forest	00785-1122	Analgesic; C III
UU <> 201	Tab, White, Cap Shaped, Scored	Acetaminophen 650 mg, Hydrocodone Bitartrate 7.5 mg	Lorcet Plus by Murfreesboro	51129-0053	Analgesic; C III
UU <> 201	Tab, White, Cap Shaped, Scored	Acetaminophen 650 mg, Hydrocodone Bitartrate 7.5 mg	Lorcet Plus by Mikart	46672-0025	Analgesic; C III
UU <> 3737	Tab, White, Round, Scored	Pramipexole DiHCl 1.5 mg	Mirapex by Pharmacia	00009-0037	Antiparkinson
UU <> 3737	Tab, White, Round, Scored	Pramipexole DiHCl 1.5 mg	Mirapex by Boehringer Ingelheim	00597-0091	Antiparkinson
UU <> 44	Tab, White, Oval, Scored	Pramipexole DiHCl 0.25 mg	Mirapex by Boehringer Ingelheim	00597-0084	Antiparkinson
UU <> 44	Tab, White, Oval, Scored	Pramipexole DiHCl 0.25 mg	Mirapex by Pharmacia	00009-0004	Antiparkinson
UU <> 66	Tab, White, Round, Scored	Pramipexole DiHCl 1 mg	Mirapex by Boehringer Ingelheim	00009-0006	Antiparkinson
UU <> 66	Tab, White, Round, Scored	Pramipexole DiHCl 1 mg	Mirapex by Boehringer Ingelheim	00597-0090	Antiparkinson
UU <> 88	Tab, White, Oval, Scored	Pramipexole DiHCl 0.5 mg	Mirapex by Boehringer Ingelheim	00597-0085	Antiparkinson
UU <> 88	Tab, White, Oval, Scored	Pramipexole DiHCl 0.5 mg	Mirapex by Pharmacia	00009-0008	Antiparkinson
UU33	Tab, White, Oval	Pramipexole DiHCl 1.25 mg	Mirapex by Pharmacia		Antiparkinson
V	Tab, Pale Yellow, Orally Disintegrating, Stylized "V"	Selegiline HCl 1.25 mg	Zelapar by Valeant	00187-0453	Antiparkinson
V	Tab, White, Round, Sublingual, Roman Numeral V	Zolpidem 5 mg	Edluar by Orexo AB	42447-0112	Sedative/Hypnotic; C IV
V <> 2090	Tab, White, Oblong	Alprazolam 2 mg	Xanax by Qualitest	00603-2130	Antianxiety; C IV
V <> 2102	Tab, Yellow, Round	Amitriptyline HCl 25 mg	Elavil by Vintage	00603-2213	Antidepressant
V <> 2106	Tab, Blue, Oblong	Amitriptyline HCl 150 mg	Elavil by Vintage		Antidepressant
V <> 2265	Tab, Off-White, Oval, Scored	Baclofen 10 mg	Lioresal by Vintage	00254-2265	Muscle Relaxant
V <> 2265	Tab, Off-White, Oval, Scored	Baclofen 10 mg	Lioresal by Qualitest	00603-2406	Muscle Relaxant
V <> 2266	Tab, Off-White, Cap Shaped, Scored	Baclofen 20 mg	Lioresal by Qualitest	00603-2407	Muscle Relaxant
V <> 2266	Tab, Off-White, Cap Shaped, Scored	Baclofen 20 mg	Lioresal by Vintage	00254-2266	Muscle Relaxant
V <> 2325	Tab, White, Round, Scored	Benztropine Mesylate 0.5 mg	Cogentin by Qualitest	00603-2433	Antiparkinson
V <> 2325	Tab, White, Round, Scored	Benztropine Mesylate 0.5 mg	Cogentin by UDL	51079-0404	Antiparkinson
V <> 2326	Tab, White, Oval, Scored	Benztropine Mesylate 1 mg	Cogentin by UDL	51079-0406	Antiparkinson
V <> 2326	Tab, White, Oval, Scored	Benztropine Mesylate 1 mg	Cogentin by Qualitest	00603-2434	Antiparkinson
V <> 2327	Tab, White, Round, Scored	Benztropine Mesylate 2 mg	Cogentin by Qualitest	00603-2435	Antiparkinson
V <> 2327	Tab, White, Round, Scored	Benztropine Mesylate 2 mg	Cogentin by UDL	51079-0407	Antiparkinson
V <> 2355	Tab, White, Round, Scripted V	Acetaminophen 325 mg, Butalbital 50 mg, Caffeine 40 mg	Fioricet by Qualitest	00603-2546	Analgesic
V <> 2357	Tab, White, Oblong	Acetaminophen 500, Butalbital 50 mg, Caffeine 40 mg	Esgic Plus by Vintage	00254-2357	Analgesic
V <> 2357	Tab, White, Oblong	Acetaminophen 500, Butalbital 50 mg, Caffeine 40 mg	Esgic Plus by Qualitest	00603-2545	Analgesic
V <> 2530	Tab, Yellow, Round, Scored	Clonazepam 0.5 mg	Klonopin by Vintage	00254-2530	Sedative; C IV
V <> 2531	Tab, Light Blue, Round	Clonazepam 1 mg	Klonopin by Vintage	00254-2531	Sedative; C IV
V <> 2532	Tab, White, Round	Clonazepam 2 mg	Klonopin by Vintage	00254-2532	Sedative; C IV
V <> 2541	Tab, Light Tan, Oval, Scored	Clonidine HCl 0.1 mg	Catapres by Vintage	00254-2541	Antihypertensive
V <> 2542	Tab, Orange, Oval, Scored	Clonidine HCl 0.2 mg	Catapres by Vintage	00254-2542	Antihypertensive
V <> 2543	Tab, Peach, Oval, Scored	Clonidine HCl 0.3 mg	Catapres by Vintage	00254-2543	Antihypertensive
V <> 2577	Tab, Yellow, Round	Colchicine 0.6 mg	by Vintage	00254-2577	Antigout
V <> 2631	Tab, Orange, Round	Cyclobenzaprine HCl 5 mg	Flexeril by Qualitest	00603-3078	Muscle Relaxant
V <> 2632	Tab, Yellow, Round	Cyclobenzaprine HCl 10 mg	Flexeril by Qualitest	00603-3079	Muscle Relaxant
V <> 2682	Tab, White, Round, Scored	Diazepam 2 mg	Valium by Vintage	00254-2682	Antianxiety; C IV
V <> 2683	Tab, Yellow, Round, Scored	Diazepam 5 mg	Valium by Vintage	00254-2683	Antianxiety; C IV
V <> 2684	Tab, Blue, Round, Scored	Diazepam 10 mg	Valium by Vintage	00254-2684	Antianxiety; C IV
V <> 2722	Tab, White, Oblong	Guaifenesin 1200 mg, Pseudoephedrine 120 mg	Entex PSE by Qualitest	00603-3504	Cold Remedy
V <> 3169	Tab, White, Oval	Furosemide 20 mg	Lasix by Vintage	00254-3169	Diuretic
V <> 3180	Tab, White, Round	Glycopyrrolate 1 mg	Robinul by UDL	51079-0700	Gastrointestinal
V <> 3186	Tab, Coated	Codeine Phosphate 10 mg, Guaifenesin 300 mg	by Vintage	00254-3186	Cold Remedy; C III
V <> 3186	Tab, Red, Oblong	Guaifenesin 300 mg, Codeine Phosphate 10 mg	Robitussin by Qualitest	00603-3781	Analgesic; C III

ID FRONT <> BACK	DESCRIPTION FRONT <> BACK	INGREDIENT & STRENGTH	BRAND (or Generic Equiv.) by FIRM	NDC#	CLASS; SCH.
V <> 3190	Tab, Yellow, Cap Shaped	Guaifenesin 600 mg, Pseudoephedrine 120 mg	Entex PSE by Qualitest	00603-3767	Cold Remedy
V <> 3585	Tab, White, Film-Coated, Round	Hydrocodone Bitartrate 7.5 mg, Ibuprofen 200 mg	Vicoprofen by Vintage	00254-3585	Analgesic; C III
V <> 3586	Tab, Purple, Film-Coated, Oval, Scored	Hydrocodone Bitartrate 10 mg, Ibuprofen 200 mg	Vicoprofen by Vintage	00254-3586	Analgesic; C III
V <> 3591	Tab, White, Red Specks, Cap Shaped, Scored, 35/91 V	Acetaminophen 500 mg, Hydrocodone Bitartrate 2.5 mg	Lortab by Vintage	00254-3591	Analgesic; C III
V <> 3592	Tab, White, Oblong, Scored, 35/92	Acetaminophen 500 mg, Hydrocodone Bitartrate 5 mg	Vicodin by UDL	51079-0780	Analgesic; C III
V <> 3592	Tab, White, Oblong, Scored, 35/92	Acetaminophen 500 mg, Hydrocodone Bitartrate 5 mg	Vicodin by Pharmedix	53002-0119	Analgesic; C III
V <> 3592	Tab, White, Oblong, Scored, 35/92	Acetaminophen 500 mg, Hydrocodone Bitartrate 5 mg	by Vangard	00615-0400	Analgesic; C III
V <> 3592	Tab, White, Oblong, Scored, 35/92	Acetaminophen 500 mg, Hydrocodone Bitartrate 5 mg	Vicodin by Kaiser	00179-1026	Analgesic; C III
V <> 3592	Tab, White, Cap Shaped, Scored	Acetaminophen 500 mg, Hydrocodone Bitartrate 5 mg	Vicodin by Vintage	00254-3592	Analgesic; C III
V <> 3594	Tab, White w/ Green Specks, Oblong, V <> 35 over 94	Acetaminophen 500 mg, Hydrocodone Bitartrate 7.5 mg	Lortab by Ivax	00182-0691	Analgesic; C III
V <> 3594	Tab, White w/ Green Specks, Oblong, V <> 35 over 94	Acetaminophen 500 mg, Hydrocodone Bitartrate 7.5 mg	Lortab by Qualitest	00603-3882	Analgesic; C III
V <> 3594	Tab, White w/ Green Specks, Oblong, V <> 35 over 94	Acetaminophen 500 mg, Hydrocodone Bitartrate 7.5 mg	Lortab by UDL	51079-0781 Discontinued	Analgesic; C III
V <> 3594	Tab, White w/ Green Specks, Cap Shaped, Scored, V <> 35 over 94	Acetaminophen 500 mg, Hydrocodone Bitartrate 7.5 mg	Lortab by Vintage	00254-3594	Analgesic; C III
V <> 3595	Tab, White, Cap Shaped, Scored	Acetaminophen 650 mg, Hydrocodone Bitartrate 7.5 mg	Lorcet Plus by Vintage	00254-3595	Analgesic; C III
V <> 3596	Tab, White, Cap Shaped, Scored	Acetaminophen 750 mg, Hydrocodone Bitartrate 7.5 mg	Vicodin ES by Vintage	00603-3596	Analgesic; C III
V <> 3596	Tab, White, Oblong	Acetaminophen 750 mg, Hydrocodone Bitartrate 7.5 mg	Vicodin ES by Qualitest	00603-3883	Analgesic; C III
V <> 3596	Tab, White, Oblong	Acetaminophen 750 mg, Hydrocodone Bitartrate 7.5 mg	Vicodin ES by Ivax	00182-0681	Analgesic; C III
V <> 3597	Tab, Light Blue, Cap Shaped, 35/97 V	Acetaminophen 650 mg, Hydrocodone Bitartrate 10 mg	Lorcet by Vintage	00254-3597	Analgesic; C III
V <> 3597	Tab, Light Blue, 35/97 V	Acetaminophen 650 mg, Hydrocodone Bitartrate 10 mg	Lorcet by Qualitest	00603-3885	Analgesic; C III
V <> 3598	Tab, White, Oblong, Scored	Acetaminophen 660 mg, Hydrocodone Bitartrate 10 mg	Lorcet by Vintage	00254-3598	Analgesic; C III
V <> 3598	Tab, Pink, Oval	Acetaminophen 500 mg, Hydrocodone Bitartrate 10 mg	Lortab by Qualitest	00603-3888	Analgesic; C III
V <> 3600	Tab, Pink, Cap Shaped	Hydrocodone Bitartrate 10 mg, Acetaminophen 500 mg	Lortab by Vintage	00254-3600	Analgesic; C III
V <> 3600	Tab, Pink, Cap Shaped	Acetaminophen 500 mg, Hydrocodone Bitartrate 10 mg	Lortab by UDL	51079-0254	Analgesic; C III
V <> 3601	Tab, Yellow, Oblong	Acetaminophen 325 mg, Hydrocodone Bitartrate 10 mg	Norco by UDL	51079-0779	Analgesic; C III
V <> 3601	Tab, Yellow, Oblong	Acetaminophen 325 mg, Hydrocodone Bitartrate 10 mg	Norco by Vintage	00254-3601	Analgesic; C III
V <> 3604	Tab, White with Orange Specks, Oblong	Hydrocodone Bitartrate 5 mg, Acetaminophen 325 mg	Norco by UDL	51079-0777	Analgesic; C III
V <> 3604	Tab, White with Orange Specks, Oblong	Hydrocodone Bitartrate 5 mg, Acetaminophen 325 mg	Norco by Vintage	00254-3604	Analgesic; C III
V <> 3605	Tab, Light Orange, Oval, Scored	Hydrocodone Bitartrate 7.5 mg, Acetaminophen 325 mg	Norco by UDL	51079-0778	Analgesic; C III
V <> 3615	Tab, Orange, Round	Hydroxyzine HCl 10 mg	Atarax by Vintage	00254-3615	Antianxiety; Antihistamine
V <> 3616	Tab, Green, Round	Hydroxyzine HCl 25 mg	Atarax by Vintage	00254-3616	Antianxiety; Antihistamine
V <> 3616	Tab, Green, Round	Hydroxyzine HCl 25 mg	Atarax by Qualitest	00603-3968	Antianxiety; Antihistamine
V <> 3617	Tab, Light Orange, Round	Hydroxyzine HCl 50 mg	Atarax by Vintage	00254-3617	Antianxiety; Antihistamine
V <> 3913	Tab, Bluish Purple, Round, Scored	Levothyroxine Sodium 0.075 mg	Synthroid by Allscripts		Thyroid Hormone
V <> 4	Tab, Green, Round, Ex Release	Albuterol Sulfate 4 mg	Vospire ER by Dava	68774-0600	Antiasthmatic
V <> 4	Tab, Green, Round, Ex Release	Albuterol Sulfate 4 mg	Vospire ER by Odyssey	65473-0754	Antiasthmatic
V <> 4140	Tab, Double Layered	Meclizine HCl 12.5 mg	by Qualitest	00603-4319	Antiemetic
V <> 4212	Tab, White, Oblong	Methocarbamol 750 mg	Robaxin by Qualitest	00603-4486	Muscle Relaxant
V <> 4234	Tab, White, Oval	Metoclopramide 5 mg	Reglan by Qualitest	00603-4614	Gastrointestinal
V <> 4235	Tab, White, Oval	Metoclopramide 10 mg	Reglan by Qualitest	00603-4615	Gastrointestinal
V <> 4810	Tab, White, Round, Scored	Oxycodone HCl 5 mg	OxyContin by Qualitest	00603-4990	Analgesic; C II
V <> 4811	Tab, Light Green, Round, Scored	Oxycodone HCl 15 mg	OxyContin by Qualitest	00603-4991	Analgesic; C II
V <> 4811	Tab, Light Green, Round, Scored	Oxycodone HCl 15 mg	Roxicodone by Vintage	00254-4811	Analgesic; C II
V <> 4812	Tab, Light Blue, Round, Scored	Oxycodone HCl 30 mg	Roxicodone by Vintage	00254-4812	Analgesic; C II
V <> 4812	Tab, Light Blue, Round, Scored	Oxycodone HCl 30 mg	OxyContin by Qualitest	00603-4992	Analgesic; C II
V <> 5030	Tab, Light Blue with Dark Blue Specks	Phentermine 37.5 mg	Adipex-P by Vintage	00254-5030	Anorexiant; C IV
V <> 5030	Tab, Light Blue with Dark Blue Specks	Phentermine 37.5 mg	Adipex-P by Qualitest	00603-5192	Anorexiant; C IV
V <> 5051	Tab, Blue, Oblong	Guaifenesin 400 mg, Phenylpropanolamine HCl 75 mg	Entex LA by Vintage		Cold Remedy
V <> 5053	Tab, V <> 50/53	Guaifenesin 600 mg, Phenylpropanolamine HCl 75 mg	Entex LA by Vintage	00254-5053	Cold Remedy

ID, FRONT <> BACK	DESCRIPTION FRONT <> BACK	INGREDIENT & STRENGTH	BRAND (or Generic Equiv.) by FIRM	NDC#	CLASS; SCH.
V <> 5053	Tab	Guaifenesin 600 mg, Phenylpropanolamine HCl 75 mg	Entex LA by Qualitest	00603-3778	Cold Remedy
V <> 5084	Tab, White, Round, Scored	Prednisone 1 mg	Deltasone by Vintage	00254-5084	Steroid
V <> 5085	Tab, White, Round, Scored	Prednisone 2.5 mg	Deltasone by Vintage	00254-5085	Steroid
V <> 5092	Tab, Peach, Round, Scored	Prednisone 20 mg	Deltasone by Vintage	00254-5092	Steroid
V <> 5093	Tab, White, Round, Scored	Prednisone 10 mg	Deltasone by Qualitest	00603-5338	Steroid
V <> 5093	Tab, White, Round, Scored	Prednisone 10 mg	Deltasone by Vintage	00254-5093	Steroid
V <> 5094	Tab, White, Round, Scored	Prednisone 5 mg	Deltasone by Qualitest	00603-5337	Steroid
V <> 5094	Tab, White, Round, Scored	Prednisone 5 mg	Deltasone by Vintage	00254-5094	Steroid
V <> 5124	Tab, White, Round, Scored, Film Coated	Propafenone HCl 150 mg	Rythmol by Vintage	00254-5124	Antiarrhythmic
V <> 5125	Tab, White, Round, Scored, Film Coated	Propafenone HCl 225 mg	Rythmol by Vintage	00254-5125	Antiarrhythmic
V <> 5126	Tab, White, Round, Scored, Film Coated	Propafenone HCl 300 mg	Rythmol by Vintage	00254-5126	Antiarrhythmic
V <> 5130	Tab, White, Round, Scored	Primidone 50 mg	Mysoline by Vintage	00254-5130	Anticonvulsant
V <> 5136	Tab, Pink, Round	Promethazine HCl 50 mg	Phenergan by Vintage	00254-5136	Antiemetic; Antihistamine
V <> 5137	Tab, White, Round, Scored	Promethazine HCl 25 mg	Phenergan by Vintage	00254-5137	Antiemetic; Antihistamine
V <> 5138	Tab, Orange, Round, Scored	Promethazine HCl 12.5 mg	Phenergan by Vintage	00254-5138	Antiemetic; Antihistamine
V <> 5401	Tab, White, Round, Scored	Quinine Sulfate 260 mg	Quinamm by Qualitest	00603-5618	Antimalarial
V <> 5812	Tab, Turquoise, Coated, Scored, 58 to Left 12 to Right over V	Salsalate 750 mg	Disalcid by Quality Care	60346-0034	NSAID
V <> 5812	Tab, Turquoise, Coated, Scored, 58 to Left 12 to Right over V	Salsalate 750 mg	Disalcid by Vintage	00254-5812	NSAID
V <> 5812	Tab, Turquoise, Coated, Scored, 58 to Left 12 to Right over V	Salsalate 750 mg	Disalcid by Quality Care	60346-0034	NSAID
V <> 5812	Tab, Turquoise, Coated, Scored, 58 to Left 12 to Right over V	Salsalate 750 mg	Disalcid by Vintage	00254-5812	NSAID
V <> 5812	Tab, Turquoise, Coated, Scored, 58 to Left 12 to Right over V	Salsalate 750 mg	Disalcid by Qualitest	00603-5755	NSAID
V <> 5875	Tab, Light Blue, Oval	Sotalol 80 mg	Betapace by Vintage	00254-5875	Antiarrhythmic
V <> 5876	Tab, Light Blue, Oval	Sotalol 120 mg	Betapace by Vintage	00254-5876	Antiarrhythmic
V <> 5876	Tab, Blue, Oval	Sotalol HCl 120 mg	Betapace by Qualitest	00603-5770	Antiarrhythmic
V <> 5877	Tab, Light Blue, Oval	Sotalol 160 mg	Betapace by Vintage	00254-5877	Antiarrhythmic
V <> 5878	Tab, Light Blue, Oval	Sotalol 240 mg	Betapace by Vintage	00254-5878	Antiarrhythmic
V <> 5880	Tab, White, Round, Film-Coated	Spironolactone 25 mg	Aldactone by Vintage	00254-5880	Diuretic
V <> 5881	Tab, White, Oval, Scored, Film-Coated	Spironolactone 50 mg	Aldactone by Vintage	00254-5881	Diuretic
V <> 5882	Tab, White, Round, Scored, Film-Coated	Spironolactone 100 mg	Aldactone by Vintage	00254-5882	Diuretic
V <> 5897	Tab, White to Off-White, Round, Scored	Sulfamethoxazole 400 mg, Trimethoprim 80 mg	Bactrim by Vintage	00254-5897	Antibiotic
V <> 5898	Tab, White to Off-White, Oval, Scored	Sulfamethoxazole 800 mg, Trimethoprim 160 mg	Bactrim DS by Vintage	00254-5898	Antibiotic
V <> 5905	Tab, Gold, Oval, Enteric Coated	Sulfasalazine EC 500 mg	Sulfazine by Vintage	00254-5905	Gastrointestinal
V <> 5905	Tab, Gold, Oval, Enteric Coated	Sulfasalazine EC 500 mg	Sulfazine by Qualitest	00603-5803	Gastrointestinal
V <> 6211	Tab, Yellow, Oval, Scored, 62 over 11	Guaifenesin 600 mg, Pseudoephedrine HCl 120 mg	Entex PSE by Quality Care	60346-0933	Cold Remedy
V <> 6211	Tab, Yellow, Oval, Scored, 62 over 11	Guaifenesin 600 mg, Pseudoephedrine HCl 120 mg	by Ivax	00182-1740	Cold Remedy
V <> 625	Tab, White, Oval-Shaped, Clear Film-Coated	Nelfinavir Mesylate 625 mg	Viracept by Pfizer	Canadian DIN 0224876	Antiviral
V <> 625	Tab, White, Oval, Film Coated	Nelfinavir Mesylate 625 mg	Viracept by Agouron	63010-0027	Antiviral
V <> 8	Tab, White, Round, Ex Release	Albuterol Sulfate 8 mg	Vospire ER by Dava	68774-0601	Antiasthmatic
V <> 8	Tab, White, Round, Ex Release	Albuterol Sulfate 8 mg	Vospire ER by Odyssey	65473-0758	Antiasthmatic
V <> TASMAR100	Tab, Beige, Hexagonal, Film Coated, Black Ink	Tolcapone 100 mg	Tasmar by ICN	00187-0938	Antiparkinson
V <> TASMAR200	Tab, Reddish Brown, Hexagonal, Film Coated, Black Ink	Tolcapone 200 mg	Tasmar by ICN	00187-0939	Antiparkinson
V <> VISKEN5	Tab, White, Heart Shaped	Pindolol 5 mg	Visken by Prepackage Specialists	58864-0488	Antihypertensive
V <> VISKEN5	Tab, White, Heart Shaped	Pindolol 5 mg	by Novartis	00078-0111	Antihypertensive
V1 <> M	Tab, Yellow, Round, Scored	Venlafaxine 25 mg	Effexor by Mylan	00378-4881	Antidepressant

ID FRONT <> BACK	DESCRIPTION FRONT <> BACK	INGREDIENT & STRENGTH	BRAND (or Generic Equiv.) by FIRM	NDC#	CLASS; SCH.
V16 <> 9116	Tab, Tan, Oval, '16' in superscript	Amylase 60,000 Units, Protease 60,000 Units, Lipase 16,000 Units	Viokase by Axcan	58914-0116	Gastrointestinal
V16 <> 9116	Tab, Tan, Oval, '16' in superscript	Amylase 60,000 Units, Protease 60,000 Units, Lipase 16,000 Units	Viokase by Axcan	Canadian DIN 02241933	Gastrointestinal
V2 <> M	Tab, Yellow, Round, Scored	Venlafaxine 37.5 mg	Effexor by Mylan	00378-4882	Antidepressant
V2 <> M	Tab, Yellow, Round, Scored	Venlafaxine 37.5 mg	Effexor by UDL	51079-0480	Antidepressant
V2063	Tab, White, Round	Acetaminophen 300 mg, Codeine Phosphate 15 mg	Tylenol w/ Codeine by Qualitest	00603-2337	Analgesic; C III
V2063 <> 2	Tab, White, V-Scored, Round	Acetaminophen 300 mg, Codeine Phosphate 15 mg	Tylenol w/ Codeine by Vintage	00254-2063	Analgesic; C III
V2065	Tab, White, Round	Acetaminophen 300 mg, Codeine Phosphate 60 mg	Tylenol w/ Codeine by Qualitest	00603-2339	Analgesic; C III
V2065	Tab, V-Scored	Acetaminophen 300 mg, Codeine Phosphate 60 mg	Tylenol w/ Codeine by Vintage	00254-2065	Analgesic; C III
V2721	Tab, White, Oblong	Guaifenesin 1200 mg	Duratuss G by Qualitest	00603-3503	Expectorant
V2732	Cap, Light Green	Chlordiazepoxide 5 mg, Clidinium Bromide 2.5 mg	Librax by Qualitest	00603-2714	Gastrointestinal
V2732	Cap	Chlordiazepoxide 5 mg, Clidinium Bromide 2.5 mg	Librax by Quality Care	60346-0780	Gastrointestinal
V3 <> M	Tab, Yellow, Round, Scored	Venlafaxine 50 mg	Effexor by Mylan	00378-4883	Antidepressant
V3109	Cap, Light Blue and Grey, Opaque	Codeine Phosphate 30 mg, Butalbital 50 mg, Caffeine 40 mg, Acetaminophen 325 mg	Fioricet w/ Codeine by Vintage	00254-3109	Analgesic; C III
V3566	Cap, Teal, Opaque	Hydrochlorothiazide 12.5 mg	Hydrodiuril by Vintage	00254-3566	Diuretic; Antihypertensive
V3566	Cap, Teal, Opaque	Hydrochlorothiazide 12.5 mg	Hydrodiuril by Qualitest	00603-3855	Diuretic; Antihypertensive
V3592	Tab, White, Oblong	Acetaminophen 500 mg, Hydrocodone Bitartrate 5 mg	Vicodin by Ivax	00172-5643	Analgesic; C III
V3592	Tab, White, Oblong	Acetaminophen 500 mg, Hydrocodone Bitartrate 5 mg	Vicodin by Qualitest	00603-3881	Analgesic; C III
V3595	Tab, White, Oblong	Acetaminophen 650 mg, Hydrocodone Bitartrate 7.5 mg	Lorcet Plus by Ivax	00182-0692	Analgesic; C III
V3595	Tab, White, Oblong	Acetaminophen 650 mg, Hydrocodone Bitartrate 7.5 mg	Lorcet Plus by Qualitest	00603-3884	Analgesic; C III
V3598	Tab, White, Oval	Acetaminophen 660 mg, Hydrocodone Bitartrate 10 mg	Vicodin HP by Qualitest	00603-3886	Analgesic; C III
V3601	Tab, Yellow, Oblong	Acetaminophen 325 mg, Hydrocodone Bitartrate 10 mg	Norco by Qualitest	00603-3887	Analgesic; C III
V3611	Tab	Hydromorphone HCl 2 mg	by Qualitest	00603-3925	Analgesic; C II
V3612	Tab, White, Round	Hydromorphone HCl 4 mg	by Qualitest	00603-3926	Analgesic; C II
V3911	Tab	Levothyroxine Sodium 25 mcg	by Qualitest	00603-4192	Thyroid Hormone
V3912	Tab	Levothyroxine Sodium 50 mcg	by Qualitest	00603-4193	Thyroid Hormone
V3912	Tab, White, Round	Levothyroxine Sodium 50 mcg	Synthroid by Vintage		Thyroid Hormone
V3913	Tab	Levothyroxine Sodium 75 mcg	Synthroid by Qualitest	00603-4194	Thyroid Hormone
V3914	Tab	Levothyroxine Sodium 100 mcg	by Qualitest	00603-4195	Thyroid Hormone
V3915	Tab	Levothyroxine Sodium 150 mcg	by Qualitest	00603-4196	Thyroid Hormone
V3915	Tab	Levothyroxine Sodium 150 mcg	by Vintage	00254-3915	Thyroid Hormone
V3916	Tab	Levothyroxine Sodium 200 mcg	by Qualitest	00603-4197	Thyroid Hormone
V3917	Tab	Levothyroxine Sodium 300 mcg	by Qualitest	00603-4198	Thyroid Hormone
V4130	Tab, Coated	Ascorbic Acid 100 mg, Biotin 30 mcg, Calcium 250 mg, Cholecalciferol 400 Units, Chromium 25 mcg, Copper 2 mg, Cyanocobalamin 12 mcg, Folic Acid 1 mg, Iron 60 mg, Magnesium 25 mg, Manganese 5 mg, Molybdenum 25 mcg, Niacinamide 20 mg, Pantothenic Acid 10 mg, Potassium Iodide 150 mcg, Pyridoxine HCl 10 mg, Riboflavin 3.4 mg, Thiamine Mononitrate 3 mg, Vitamin A 5000 Units, Vitamin E Acetate 30 Units, Zinc 25 mg	Maternity by Qualitest	00603-4304	Vitamin
V4206	Cap, Red	Meperidine 50 mg, Promethazine 25 mg	Mepergan by Wyeth		Analgesic; C II
V4206	Cap	Meperidine HCl 50 mg, Promethazine HCl 25 mg	Meprozine by Vintage	00254-4206	Analgesic; C II
V4206	Cap, Red	Meperidine HCl 50 mg, Promethazine HCl 25 mg	Meprozine by Qualitest	00603-4424	Analgesic; C II
V4216	Tab, White, Oval	Methylprednisolone 4 mg	by Ivax	00182-1050	Steroid
V4740	Tab, Salmon, Round	Guaifenesin 200 mg	Organidin NR by Qualitest	00603-4886	Expectorant
V4839	Tab, White, Round	Oxycodone HCl 5 mg, Acetaminophen 325 mg	Percocet by Vintage		Analgesic; C II
V4929	Tab, White, Round	Pemoline 18.75 mg	Cylert by Qualitest	00603-5055 Discontinued	Stimulant; C IV

ID FRONT <> BACK	DESCRIPTION FRONT <> BACK	INGREDIENT & STRENGTH	BRAND (or Generic Equiv.) by FIRM	NDC#	CLASS; SCH.
V4930	Tab, Orange, Round	Pemoline 37.5 mg	Cylert by Qualitest	00603-5056 Discontinued	Stimulant; C IV
V4931	Tab, Tan, Round	Pemoline 75 mg	Cylert by Qualitest	00603-5057 Discontinued	Stimulant; C IV
V4943	Tab, Gray	Perphenazine 16 mg	Trilafon by Qualitest	00603-5093	Antipsychotic
V4971	Tab, Maroon, Round	Phenazopyridine HCl 100 mg	Pyridium by Qualitest	00603-5141	Urinary Analgesic
V4971	Tab, Coated	Phenazopyridine HCl 100 mg	by Vintage	00254-4971	Urinary Analgesic
V4972	Tab, Sugar Coated	Phenazopyridine HCl 200 mg	by Vintage	00254-4972	Urinary Analgesic
V4972	Tab, Maroon, Round, Sugar Coated	Phenazopyridine HCl 200 mg	Pyridium by Qualitest	00603-5142	Urinary Analgesic
V5013	Tab	Phenobarbital 64.8 mg	by Ivax	00182-0590	Sedative/Hypnotic; C IV
V5013	Tab, Bisected V	Phenobarbital 64.8 mg	by Vintage	00254-5013	Sedative/Hypnotic; C IV
V5013	Tab, White, Round	Phenobarbital 64.8 mg	by Qualitest	00603-5167	Sedative/Hypnotic; C IV
V5014	Tab, Bisected V	Phenobarbital 100 mg	Phenobarbital by Vintage	00254-5014	Sedative/Hypnotic; C IV
V5014	Tab, White, Round	Phenobarbital 100 mg	Phenobarbital by Qualitest	00603-5168	Sedative/Hypnotic; C IV
V5051	Tab, Film Coated, V-Scored	Guaifenesin 400 mg, Phenylpropanolamine HCl 75 mg	Entex LA by Vintage	00254-5051	Cold Remedy
V5051	Tab	Guaifenesin 400 mg, Phenylpropanolamine HCl 75 mg	Entex LA by Qualitest	00603-5214	Cold Remedy
V5052	Tab, Film Coated	Guaifenesin 400 mg, Phenylpropanolamine HCl 75 mg	Entex LA by Qualitest	00603-5215	Cold Remedy
V5097	Tab, Coated	Ascorbic Acid 80 mg, Beta-Carotene, Biotin 0.03 mg, Calcium Carbonate, Cholecalciferol 400 Units, Cupric Oxide, Cyanocobalamin 2.5 mcg, Ferrous Fumarate, Folic Acid 1 mg, Magnesium Oxide, Niacinamide 17 mg, Pantothenic Acid 7 mg, Pyridoxine HCl 4 mg, Riboflavin 1.6 mg, Thiamine Mononitrate 1.5 mg, Vitamin A Acetate, Vitamin E Acetate 15 mg, Zinc Oxide	Prenatal Rx by Qualitest	00603-5359	Vitamin
V5098	Tab, Coated	Ascorbic Acid 120 mg, Calcium 250 mg, Cholecalciferol 400 Units, Copper 2 mg, Cyanocobalamin 12 mcg, Docusate Sodium 50 mg, Folic Acid 1 mg, Iodine 150 mcg, Iron 90 mg, Niacinamide 20 mg, Pyridoxine HCl 20 mg, Riboflavin 3.4 mg, Thiamine HCl 3 mg, Vitamin A 4000 Units, Vitamin E 30 Units, Zinc 25 mg	Maternity 90 Prenatal Vit & Min by Qualitest	00603-5355	Vitamin
V5099	Tab, Coated	Ascorbic Acid 80 mg, Calcium Carbonate, Precipitated, Cholecalciferol 400 Units, Cyanocobalamin 12 mcg, Ferrous Fumarate, Folic Acid 1 mg, Magnesium Oxide, Niacinamide 20 mg, Potassium Iodide, Pyridoxine HCl 10 mg, Riboflavin 3 mg, Thiamine Mononitrate 3 mg, Vitamin A Palmitate 5000 Units, Vitamin E Acetate 30 mg, Zinc Oxide	Z Plus Prenatal by Qualitest	00603-6475	Vitamin
V5100	Tab, Coated	Ascorbic Acid 120 mg, Calcium Sulfate, Cupric Oxide, Cyanocobalamin 12 mcg, Ferrous Fumarate, Folic Acid 1 mg, Niacin 20 mg, Pyridoxine HCl 10 mg, Riboflavin 3 mg, Thiamine HCl 1.5 mg, Vitamin A 4000 Units, Vitamin D 400 Units, Vitamin E 11 mg, Zinc Oxide	Prenatal 1 Plus Iron by Qualitest	00603-5357	Vitamin
V5101	Tab, Yellow	Prenatal Vitamin	Prenatal Improved by Vintage		Vitamin
V5114	Tab, Pink, Cap Shaped	Propoxyphene Napsylate 100 mg, Acetaminophen 650 mg	Darvocet by Vintage	00254-5114	Analgesic; C IV
V5131	Tab, Yellow, Round, Scored, 51 / 31	Primidone 250 mg	Mysoline by Qualitest	00603-5372	Anticonvulsant
V5311	Tab, Green, Oblong, Film Coated	Dextromethorphan HBr 30 mg, Guaifenesin 600 mg	Q-Bid DM by Qualitest	00603-5542	Cold Remedy
V5312	Tab, Green, Oblong, Scored	Guaifenesin 600 mg	Robitussin by Mason	11845-0975	Expectorant
V5312	Tab	Guaifenesin 600 mg	Robitussin by Qualitest	00603-5543	Expectorant
V5811	Tab, Aqua, Round, Film Coated	Salsalate 500 mg	Disalcid by Qualitest	00603-5754	NSAID
V5935	Tab, White, Coated	Choline Magnesium Trisalicylate 500 mg	Tricosal by Qualitest	00603-6215	NSAID
V5936	Tab, White, Coated	Choline Magnesium Trisalicylate 986.835 mg	Tricosal by Qualitest	00603-6216	NSAID
V5937	Tab, Pink, Cap Shaped, Film Coated	Choline Magnesium Trisalicylate 1000 mg	Tricosal by Qualitest	00603-6217	NSAID
V5972	Tab, White, Round	Trihexyphenidyl HCl 5 mg	Artane by Qualitest	00603-6241	Antiparkinson
V60	Tab, Orange, Round	Bisacodyl 5 mg	Dulcolax by Qualitest	00603-2481	Gastrointestinal
V60	Tab, Orange, Round	Bisacodyl 5 mg	Dulcolax by Vintage		Gastrointestinal
V6211	Tab, Film Coated	Guaifenesin 600 mg, Pseudoephedrine HCl 120 mg	Guaifen PSE by Vintage	00254-6211	Cold Remedy

ID FRONT <> BACK	DESCRIPTION FRONT <> BACK	INGREDIENT & STRENGTH	BRAND (or Generic Equiv.) by FIRM	NDC#	CLASS; SCH.
V6211	Tab, Film Coated	Guaifenesin 600 mg, Pseudoephedrine HCl 120 mg	Quaifen PSE by Qualitest	00603-5668	Cold Remedy
V6377	Tab, White, Round	Yohimbine HCl 5.4 mg	Yocon by Qualitest	00603-6430	Impotence Agent
V6377	Tab	Yohimbine HCl 5.4 mg	by Vintage	00254-6377	Impotence Agent
VA250	Cap, Orange	Valproic Acid 250 mg	Depakene by Genpharm	Canadian	Anticonvulsant
VAD <> 6330	Tab, Blue, Oblong, Scored	Acetaminophen 650 mg, Hydrocodone Bitartrate 10 mg	Lorcet by H J Harkins Co	52959-0403	Analgesic; C III
VAL500 <> APO	Tab, Blue, Cap Shaped, Film Coated	Valacyclovir 500 mg	Valtrex by Apotex	Canadian DIN 02295822	Antiviral
VALPROIC25003	Cap, Yellow, Soft Gel	Valproic Acid 250 mg	Depakene by Ivax	00182-1754 Discontinued	Anticonvulsant
VALPROIC2500364	Cap, Off-White, Black Print, VALPROIC over 250-0364	Valproic Acid 250 mg	Depakene by Schein	00364-0822	Anticonvulsant
VALPROIC2500364	Cap, Off-White, Black Print, VALPROIC over 250-0364	Valproic Acid 250 mg	Depakene by RP Scherer	11014-0879	Anticonvulsant
VALPROIC2500364	Cap, Off-White, Black Print, Soft Gel, VALPROIC over 250-0364	Valproic Acid 250 mg	Depakene by UDL	51079-0298	Anticonvulsant
VALPROIC2500364	Cap, Off-White, Black Print, VALPROIC over 250-0364	Valproic Acid 250 mg	Depakene by Vangard	00615-1325	Anticonvulsant
VALPROIC2500364	Cap, Off-White, Black Print, Soft Gel, VALPROIC over 250-0364	Valproic Acid 250 mg	Depakene by Watson	00591-4012	Anticonvulsant
VALTREX1GRAM	Tab, Blue, Cap Shaped, Film Coated	Valacyclovir HCl 1 g	Valtrex by DSM	63552-0565	Antiviral
VALTREX1GRAM	Tab, Blue, Cap Shaped, Film Coated	Valacyclovir HCl 1 g	Valtrex by GSK	00173-0565	Antiviral
VALTREX500MG	Tab, Blue, Cap Shaped, Film Coated	Valacyclovir HCl 500 mg	Valtrex by GSK	Canadian DIN 02219492	Antiviral
VALTREX500MG	Tab, Blue, Cap Shaped, Film Coated	Valacyclovir HCl 500 mg	Valtrex by DSM	63552-0933	Antiviral
VALTREX500MG	Tab, Blue, Cap Shaped, Film Coated	Valacyclovir HCl 500 mg	Valtrex by Promex Med	62301-0040	Antiviral
VALTREX500MG	Tab, Blue, Cap Shaped, Film Coated	Valacyclovir HCl 500 mg	Valtrex by GSK	00173-0933	Antiviral
VALTREX500MG	Tab, Blue, Cap Shaped, Film Coated	Valacyclovir HCl 500 mg	Valtrex by Physician Total Care	54868-3804	Antiviral
VALTREX500MG	Tab, Blue, Cap Shaped, Film Coated	Valacyclovir HCl 500 mg	Valtrex by Allscripts		Antiviral
VALTREX500MG	Tab, Blue, Cap Shaped, Film Coated	Valacyclovir HCl 500 mg	Valtrex by PDRX	55289-0926	Antiviral
VASCOR200	Tab, Blue, Film Coated, Scored	Bepridil HCl 200 mg	Vascor by McNeil	52021-0682	Antianginal
VASCOR200	Tab, Light Blue, Film Coated, Scored	Bepridil HCl 200 mg	Vascor by McNeil	00045-0682	Antianginal
VASCOR300	Tab, Blue, Film Coated	Bepridil HCl 300 mg	Vascor by McNeil	00045-0683	Antianginal
VASCOR300	Tab, Coated	Bepridil HCl 300 mg	Vascor by McNeil	52021-0683	Antianginal
VASCOR400	Tab, Dark Blue, Film Coated	Bepridil HCl 400 mg	Vascor by McNeil	00045-0684	Antianginal
VASERETIC <> MSD720	Tab, Rust, Squared Cap Shape	Enalapril Maleate 10 mg, Hydrochlorothiazide 25 mg	Vaseretic by Merck	00006-0720	Antihypertensive; Diuretic
VASERETIC <> MSD720	Tab, Rust, Squared Cap Shape	Enalapril Maleate 10 mg, Hydrochlorothiazide 25 mg	Vaseretic by Biovail	64455-0146	Antihypertensive; Diuretic
VASOTEC <> 712	Tab	Enalapril Maleate 5 mg	Vasotec by Med Pro	53978-0176	Antihypertensive
VC500	Tab, Blue, Oblong	Valacyclovir HCl 500 mg	Valtrex by Pharmascience	Canadian DIN 02298457	Antiviral
VC5364 <> DYNABAC	Tab, Delayed Release	Dirithromycin 250 mg	by Quality Care	60346-0601	Antibiotic
VCILLINK250LILL	Tab, V-Cillin K 250, Lilly	Penicillin V Potassium 250 mg	V-Cillin K by Eli Lilly	00002-0329	Antibiotic
VCILLINK500LILL	Tab, V-Cillin K 500, Lilly	Penicillin V Potassium 500 mg	V-Cillin K by Eli Lilly	00002-0346	Antibiotic
VECTRIN100MG	Cap	Minocycline HCl 100 mg	Vectrin by Parke Davis	00071-0688	Antibiotic
VECTRIN100MG	Cap	Minocycline HCl 100 mg	Vectrin by Warner Chilcott	00047-0688	Antibiotic
VECTRIN50MG	Cap	Minocycline HCl 50 mg	Vectrin by Warner Chilcott	00047-0687	Antibiotic
VECTRIN50MG	Cap	Minocycline HCl 50 mg	Vectrin by Parke Davis	00071-0687	Antibiotic
VENTOLIN2 <> GLAXOGLAXO	Tab, Ventolin over 2, Glaxo over Glaxo	Albuterol Sulfate 2 mg	Ventolin by GSK	00173-0341	Antiasthmatic
VENTOLIN200GLAXO	Cap, Light Blue, Ventolin 200/Glaxo	Albuterol Sulfate 2 mg	Ventolin by GSK		Antiasthmatic
VENTOLIN4 <> GLAXOGLAXO	Tab, Ventolin over 4, Glaxo over Glaxo	Albuterol Sulfate 4 mg	Ventolin by GSK	00173-0342	Antiasthmatic
VERMOX <> JANSSEN	Tab, Chewable	Mebendazole 100 mg	Vermox by Janssen	50458-0110	Antihelmintic
VERMOX <> JANSSEN	Tab, Chewable	Mebendazole 100 mg	Vermox C by Johnson & Johnson	59604-0110	Antihelmintic

Copyright © 2010 Ident-A-Drug (209) 472-2240 • May not be reproduced without permission •

For updated data, go to www.IdentADrug.com

ID FRONT <> BACK	DESCRIPTION FRONT <> BACK	INGREDIENT & STRENGTH	BRAND (or Generic Equiv.) by FIRM	NDC#	CLASS; SCH.
VERMOX <> JANSSEN	Tab, Pink, Round	Mebendazole 100 mg	Vermox by H J Harkins Co	52959-0160	Antihelmintic
VERSACAP2AMPM	Cap, White to Off White Beads, 2-AM over PM, Ex Release	Guaifenesin 300 mg, Pseudoephedrine HCl 60 mg	Sudafed Sinus by Pharmafab	62542-0403	Cold Remedy
VERSACAPS2AMPM	Cap, Versacap/2-AM/PM	Guaifenesin 300 mg, Pseudoephedrine HCl 60 mg	Sudafed Sinus by Seatrace	00551-0173	Cold Remedy
VESANOID10ROCHE	Cap, Orange & Red	Tretinoin 10 mg	Vesanoid by Hoffmann La Roche	00004-0250	Retinoid
VESANOID10ROCHE	Cap, Orange & Red	Tretinoin 10 mg	Vesanoid by Teva	00480-0537	Retinoid
VGC <> 450	Tab, Pink, Oval, Film Coated	Valganciclovir HCl 450 mg	Valcyte by Roche	Canadian DIN 02245777	Antiviral
VGC <> 450	Tab, Pink, Oval, Film Coated	Valganciclovir HCl 450 mg	Valcyte by Hoffmann La Roche	00004-0038	Antiviral
VGR100 <> PFIZER	Tab, Blue, Diamond Shaped, Film Coated	Sildenafil Citrate 100 mg	Viagra by Allscripts	Canadian DIN 02239766	Impotence Agent
VGR100 <> PFIZER	Tab, Blue, Diamond Shaped, Film Coated	Sildenafil Citrate 100 mg	Viagra by Compumed	00403-1989	Impotence Agent
VGR100 <> PFIZER	Tab, Blue, Diamond Shaped, Film Coated	Sildenafil Citrate 100 mg	Viagra by Southwood	58016-0371	Impotence Agent
VGR100 <> PFIZER	Tab, Blue, Diamond Shaped, Film Coated	Sildenafil Citrate 100 mg	Viagra by Pfizer	00069-4220	Impotence Agent
VGR100 <> PFIZER	Tab, Blue, Diamond Shaped, Film Coated	Sildenafil Citrate 100 mg	Viagra by Pfizer	Canadian DIN 02239768	Impotence Agent
VGR25 <> PFIZER	Tab, Blue, Diamond Shaped, Film Coated	Sildenafil Citrate 25 mg	Viagra by Pfizer	Canadian DIN 02239766	Impotence Agent
VGR25 <> PFIZER	Tab, Blue, Diamond Shaped, Film Coated	Sildenafil Citrate 25 mg	Viagra by Pfizer	00069-4200	Impotence Agent
VGR50 <> PFIZER	Tab, Blue, Diamond Shaped, Film Coated	Sildenafil Citrate 50 mg	Viagra by Southwood	58016-0355	Impotence Agent
VGR50 <> PFIZER	Tab, Blue, Diamond Shaped, Film Coated	Sildenafil Citrate 50 mg	Viagra by Pfizer	00069-4210	Impotence Agent
VGR50 <> PFIZER	Tab, Blue, Diamond Shaped, Film Coated	Sildenafil Citrate 50 mg	Viagra by Compumed	00403-1947	Impotence Agent
VGR50 <> PFIZER	Tab, Blue, Diamond Shaped, Film Coated	Sildenafil Citrate 50 mg	Viagra by Pfizer	Canadian DIN 02239767	Impotence Agent
VIBRAPFIZER094	Cap, White & Light Blue	Doxycycline Hyclate 50 mg	Vibramycin by Pfizer	00069-0940	Antibiotic
VIBRAPFIZER095	Cap, Light Blue	Doxycycline Hyclate 100 mg	Vibramycin by Pfizer	00069-0950	Antibiotic
VIBRATABS <> PFIZER099	Tab, Salmon, Round, Film Coated	Doxycycline Hyclate 100 mg	Vibra by Pfizer	00069-0990	Antibiotic
VICODIN	Tab, White, Cap Shaped, Scored	Acetaminophen 500 mg, Hydrocodone Bitartrate 5 mg	Vicodin by Abbott	00074-1949	Analgesic; C III
VICODIN	Tab, White, Cap Shaped, Scored	Acetaminophen 500 mg, Hydrocodone Bitartrate 5 mg	Vicodin by DRX	55045-2464	Analgesic; C III
VICODIN	Tab, White, Cap Shaped, Scored	Acetaminophen 500 mg, Hydrocodone Bitartrate 5 mg	Vicodin by PDRX	55289-0116	Analgesic; C III
VICODIN	Tab, White, Cap Shaped, Scored	Acetaminophen 500 mg, Hydrocodone Bitartrate 5 mg	Vicodin by Caremark	00339-4072	Analgesic; C III
VICODIN	Tab, White, Cap Shaped, Scored	Acetaminophen 500 mg, Hydrocodone Bitartrate 5 mg	Vicodin by Allscripts		Analgesic; C III
VICODIN	Tab, White, Cap Shaped, Scored	Acetaminophen 500 mg, Hydrocodone Bitartrate 5 mg	Vicodin by Abbott	00044-0727	Analgesic; C III
VICODIN	Tab, White, Cap Shaped, Scored	Acetaminophen 500 mg, Hydrocodone Bitartrate 5 mg	Vicodin by Amerisource	62584-0023	Analgesic; C III
VICODIN	Tab, White, Cap Shaped, Scored	Acetaminophen 500 mg, Hydrocodone Bitartrate 5 mg	Vicodin by Nat Pharmpak	55154-1603	Analgesic; C III
VICODIN	Tab, White, Cap Shaped, Scored	Acetaminophen 500 mg, Hydrocodone Bitartrate 5 mg	Vicodin by Med Pro	53978-3093	Analgesic; C III
VICODINES	Tab, White, Oval, Scored	Acetaminophen 750 mg, Hydrocodone Bitartrate 7.5 mg	Vicodin ES by Abbott	00044-0728	Analgesic; C III
VICODINES	Tab, White, Oval, Scored	Acetaminophen 750 mg, Hydrocodone Bitartrate 7.5 mg	Vicodin ES by Amerisource	62584-0025	Analgesic; C III
VICODINES	Tab, White, Oval, Scored	Acetaminophen 750 mg, Hydrocodone Bitartrate 7.5 mg	Vicodin ES by Amerisource	62584-0039	Analgesic; C III
VICODINES	Tab, White, Oval, Scored	Acetaminophen 750 mg, Hydrocodone Bitartrate 7.5 mg	Vicodin ES by Nat Pharmpak	55154-1604	Analgesic; C III
VICODINES	Tab	Acetaminophen 750 mg, Hydrocodone Bitartrate 7.5 mg	Vicodin ES by Med Pro	53978-1104	Analgesic; C III
VICODINES	Tab, White, Oval, Scored	Acetaminophen 750 mg, Hydrocodone Bitartrate 7.5 mg	Vicodin ES by Abbott	00074-1973	Analgesic; C III
VICODINHP	Tab, White, Oval, Scored	Acetaminophen 660 mg, Hydrocodone Bitartrate 10 mg	Vicodin HP by Abbott	00074-2274	Analgesic; C III
VICODINHP	Tab, White, Oval, Scored	Acetaminophen 660 mg, Hydrocodone Bitartrate 10 mg	Vicodin HP by Nat Pharmpak	55154-1607	Analgesic; C III
VICODINHP	Tab, White, Oval, Scored	Acetaminophen 660 mg, Hydrocodone Bitartrate 10 mg	Vicodin HP by Eckerd	19458-0872	Analgesic; C III
VICODINHP	Tab, White, Oval, Scored	Acetaminophen 660 mg, Hydrocodone Bitartrate 10 mg	Vicodin HP by Abbott	00044-0725	Analgesic; C III
VIDEX <> 100	Tab, Off-White to Light Orange/Yellow, Round, Chewable	Didanosine 100 mg	Videx by BMS	00087-6652	Antiviral
VIDEX <> 100	Tab, Off-White to Light Orange/Yellow, Round, Chewable	Didanosine 100 mg	Videx by BMS	Canadian DIN 01940546	Antiviral
VIDEX <> 150	Tab, Off-White to Light Orange/Yellow, Round, Chewable	Didanosine 150 mg	Videx by BMS	Canadian DIN 01940554	Antiviral

ID FRONT <> BACK	DESCRIPTION FRONT <> BACK	INGREDIENT & STRENGTH	BRAND (or Generic Equiv.) by FIRM	NDC#	CLASS; SCH.
VIDEX <> 150	Tab, Off-White to Light Orange/Yellow, Round, Chewable	Didanosine 150 mg	Videx by BMS	00087-6653	Antiviral
VIDEX <> 200	Tab, Off-White to Light Orange/Yellow, Round, Chewable	Didanosine 200 mg	Videx by BMS	00087-6665	Antiviral
VIDEX <> 25	Tab, Off-White to Light Orange/Yellow, Round, Chewable	Didanosine 25 mg	Videx by BMS	00087-6650	Antiviral
VIDEX <> 25	Tab, Off-White to Light Orange/Yellow, Round, Chewable	Didanosine 25 mg	Videx by BMS	Canadian DIN 01940511	Antiviral
VIDEX <> 50	Tab, Off-White to Light Orange/Yellow, Round, Chewable	Didanosine 50 mg	Videx by BMS	00087-6651	Antiviral
VIDEX100	Tab, Off-White to Light Orange/Yellow, Round, Chewable	Didanosine 100 mg	Videx by BMS	Canadian	Antiviral
VIDEX150	Tab, Off-White to Light Orange/Yellow, Round, Chewable	Didanosine 150 mg	Videx by BMS	Canadian	Antiviral
VIDEXBL	Tab, White, Round, Videx/BL	Didanosine 25 mg	Videx by BMS	Canadian	Antiviral
VIDEXBL	Tab, White, Round, Videx/BL	Didanosine 50 mg	Videx by BMS	Canadian	Antiviral
VIOKASE <> 9111	Tab, Tan, Round	Amylase 30,000 Units, Protease 30,000 Units, Lipase 8,000 Units	Viokase by Axcan	Canadian DIN 02230019	Gastrointestinal
VIOKASEAHR <> 9111	Tab, Light Brown & White, Round, Viokase over AHR	Amylase 30,000 Units, Lipase 8000 Units, Protease 30,000 Units	Viokase by A H Robins	58914-0111	Gastrointestinal
VIOKASEAHR <> 9111	Tab, Light Brown & White, Round, Viokase over AHR	Amylase 30,000 Units, Lipase 8000 Units, Protease 30,000 Units	Viokase by Eckerd	00031-0111	Gastrointestinal
VIOKASEAHR <> 9111	Tab, Light Brown & White, Round, Viokase over AHR	Amylase 30,000 Units, Lipase 8000 Units, Protease 30,000 Units	Viokase by Paddock	19458-0871	Gastrointestinal
VIOKASEAHR <> 9111	Tab, Light Brown & White, Round, Viokase over AHR	Amylase 30,000 Units, Lipase 8000 Units, Protease 30,000 Units	Viokase by BMS	00574-9111	Gastrointestinal
VIOXX <> MRK110	Tab, Yellow, Round	Rofecoxib 25 mg	Vioxx by Allscripts	Discontinued	NSAID
VIOXX <> MRK110	Tab, Yellow, Round	Rofecoxib 25 mg	Vioxx by Merck	00006-0110 Discontinued	NSAID
VIOXX <> MRK110	Tab, Yellow, Round	Rofecoxib 25 mg	Vioxx by RX Pak	65084-0201 Discontinued	NSAID
VIOXX <> MRK114	Tab, Orange, Round	Rofecoxib 50 mg	Vioxx by Merck	00006-0114 Discontinued	NSAID
VIOXX <> MRK74	Tab, Off-White, Round	Rofecoxib 12.5 mg	Vioxx by RX Pak	65084-0199 Discontinued	NSAID
VIOXX <> MRK74	Tab, Off-White, Round	Rofecoxib 12.5 mg	Vioxx by Merck	00006-0074 Discontinued	NSAID
VIOXX <> MRK74	Tab, Off-White, Round	Rofecoxib 12.5 mg	Vioxx by DRX	55045-2720 Discontinued	NSAID
VIOXX <> MRK74	Tab, Off-White, Round	Rofecoxib 12.5 mg	Vioxx by Physician Total Care	54868-4148	NSAID
VIOXX <> MRK74	Tab, Off-White, Round	Rofecoxib 12.5 mg	Vioxx by Allscripts	Discontinued	NSAID
VIRACEPT <> 250MG	Tab, Light Blue, Capsule-Shaped, Clear Film-Coated	Nelfinavir Mesylate 250 mg	Viracept by Pfizer	Canadian DIN 02238617	Antiviral
VIRACEPT <> 250MG	Tab, Light Blue, Oblong	Nelfinavir Mesylate 250 mg	Viracept by Mova	55370-0560	Antiviral
VIRACEPT <> 250MG	Tab, Light Blue, Oblong	Nelfinavir Mesylate 250 mg	Viracept by Circa	71114-4206	Antiviral
VIRACEPT <> 250MG	Tab, Light Blue, Oblong	Nelfinavir Mesylate 250 mg	Viracept by Patheon	63285-0010	Antiviral
VIRACEPT <> 250MG	Tab, Light Blue, Oblong	Nelfinavir Mesylate 250 mg	Viracept by Agouron	63010-0010	Antiviral
VIRAVAN	Tab, Brown Mottled, Round, Scored	Phenylephrine Tannate 25 mg, Pyrilamine Tannate 30 mg	Viravan-T by Kiel	66346-0032	Cold Remedy
VIRAVANDM	Tab, Brown Mottled, Oval, Scored	Phenylephrine Tannate 25 mg, Pyrilamine Tannate 30 mg, Dextromethorphan Tannate 25 mg	Viravan DM by Kiel	66346-0142	Cold Remedy
VIRILON10MG	Cap, Black, Opaque	Methyltestosterone 10 mg	Virilon by Star	00076-0301	Hormone; C III
VISKAZIDES <> 10251025	Tab, Peach, Round, Scored, Viskazide S in a Triangle <> 10/25 10/25	Hydrochlorothiazide 25 mg, Pindolol 10 mg	Viskazide by Novartis	Canadian DIN 00568627	Diuretic; Antihypertensive
VISKAZIDES <> 10501050	Tab, Orange, Round, Scored, Viskazide S in a Triangle <> 10/50 10/50	Hydrochlorothiazide 50 mg, Pindolol 10 mg	Viskazide by Novartis	Canadian DIN 00568635	Diuretic; Antihypertensive
VISKEN10	Tab, White, Round, Scored	Pindolol 10 mg	Visken by Novartis	Canadian DIN 00443174	Antihypertensive
VISKEN10	Tab, White, Round, Scored	Pindolol 10 mg	Visken by Novartis	Canadian DIN 00443174	Antihypertensive
VISKEN10 <> V	Tab, White, Round	Pindolol 10 mg	Visken by Prepackage Specialists	58864-0489	Antihypertensive

ID FRONT <> BACK	DESCRIPTION FRONT <> BACK	INGREDIENT & STRENGTH	BRAND (or Generic Equiv.) by FIRM	NDC#	CLASS; SCH.
VISKEN15 <> JU	Tab, White, Round, Scored	Pindolol 15 mg	Visken by Novartis	Canadian DIN 00417289	Antihypertensive
VISKEN5 <> LB	Tab, White, Round, Scored	Pindolol 5 mg	Visken by Novartis	Canadian DIN 00417270	Antihypertensive
VISKEN5 <> V	Tab, White, Heart Shaped	Pindolol 5 mg	Visken by Prepackage Specialists	58864-0488	Antihypertensive
VISKEN5 <> V	Tab, White, Heart Shaped	Pindolol 5 mg	by Novartis	58864-0488	Antihypertensive
VISTA065 <> 20	Tab, White, Round, Scored	Isoxsuprine HCl 20 mg	Vasodilan by Vista	61970-0066	Vasodilator
VISTA065 <> 20	Tab, Film Coated, Embossed	Isoxsuprine HCl 20 mg	Vasodilan by Vista	61970-0065	Vasodilator
VISTARILPFIZER541	Cap, Light Green & Dark Green	Hydroxyzine Pamoate 25 mg	Vistaril by Pfizer	00069-5410	Antianxiety; Antihistamine
VISTARILPFIZER542	Cap, Green & White	Hydroxyzine Pamoate 50 mg	Vistaril by Pfizer	00069-5420	Antianxiety; Antihistamine
VISTARILPFIZER543	Cap, Green & Gray	Hydroxyzine Pamoate 100 mg	Vistaril by Pfizer	00069-5430	Antianxiety; Antihistamine
VIVACTIL <> MSD26	Tab, Orange, Oval, Film Coated, MSD over 26	Protriptyline HCl 5 mg	Vivactil by Merck	00006-0026	Antidepressant
VIVACTIL <> MSD47	Tab, Yellow, Oval, Film Coated	Protriptyline HCl 10 mg	Vivactil by MSD	Canadian	Antidepressant
VIVACTIL <> MSD47	Tab, Yellow, Oval, Film Coated	Protriptyline HCl 10 mg	Vivactil by Merck	00006-0047	Antidepressant
VJ <> SANDOZ	Tab, White, Round	Ergoloid Mesylate 1 mg	Hydergine by Novartis	Canadian DIN 00176176	Ergot Alkaloids
VM	Tab, White, Round, Scored	Methimazole 5 mg	Tapazole by URL	0677-1945	Antithyroid
VM	Tab, White, Round	Methimazole 5 mg	Methimazole by URL Mutual	0677-1945	Antithyroid
VOLMAX <> 4	Tab, Powder Blue, Dark Blue Print, Hexagonal, Ex Release	Albuterol Sulfate 4 mg	Volmax by Med Pro	53978-2026	Antiasthmatic
VOLMAX <> 4	Tab, Powder Blue, Dark Blue Print, Hexagonal, Ex Release	Albuterol Sulfate 4 mg	Volmax by Anabolic	00722-6429	Antiasthmatic
VOLMAX <> 4	Tab, Powder Blue, Dark Blue Print, Hexagonal, Ex Release	Albuterol Sulfate 4 mg	Volmax by Muro	00451-0398	Antiasthmatic
VOLMAX <> 4	Tab, Powder Blue, Dark Blue Print, Hexagonal, Ex Release	Albuterol Sulfate 4 mg	Volmax by CVS	51316-0240	Antiasthmatic
VOLMAX <> 4	Tab, Powder Blue, Dark Blue Print, Hexagonal, Ex Release	Albuterol Sulfate 4 mg	Volmax by Nat Pharmpak	55154-4304	Antiasthmatic
VOLMAX <> 4	Tab, Powder Blue, Dark Blue Print, Hexagonal, Ex Release	Albuterol Sulfate 4 mg	Volmax by Eckerd	19458-0848	Antiasthmatic
VOLMAX <> 4	Tab, Powder Blue, Dark Blue Print, Hexagonal, Ex Release	Albuterol Sulfate 4 mg	Volmax by Wal Mart	49035-0159	Antiasthmatic
VOLMAX <> 4	Tab, Powder Blue, Dark Blue Print, Hexagonal, Ex Release	Albuterol Sulfate 4 mg	Volmax by McNeil	00045-1039	Antiasthmatic
VOLMAX <> 8	Tab, White, Hexagonal, 8 in Dark Blue	Albuterol Sulfate 8 mg	Volmax by Thrift Drug	59198-0355	Antiasthmatic
VOLMAX <> 8	Tab, White, Hexagonal, 8 in Dark Blue	Albuterol Sulfate 8 mg	Volmax by Eckerd	19458-0849	Antiasthmatic
VOLMAX <> 8	Tab, White, Hexagonal, 8 in Dark Blue	Albuterol Sulfate 8 mg	Volmax by Amerisource	62584-0873	Antiasthmatic
VOLMAX <> 8	Tab, White, Hexagonal, 8 in Dark Blue	Albuterol Sulfate 8 mg	Volmax by Amerisource	62584-0874	Antiasthmatic
VOLMAX <> 8	Tab, White, Hexagonal, 8 in Dark Blue	Albuterol Sulfate 8 mg	Volmax by Muro	00451-0399	Antiasthmatic
VOLTAREN <> 25	Tab, Yellow, Round, Enteric Coated	Diclofenac Sodium 25 mg	Voltaren by Novartis	Canadian DIN 00514004	NSAID
VOLTAREN <> 50	Tab, Light Brown, Round, Enteric Coated	Diclofenac Sodium 50 mg	Voltaren by Novartis	Canadian DIN 00514012	NSAID
VOLTAREN <> RAPIDE50	Tab, Reddish Brown, Round, Sugar Coated	Diclofenac Potassium 50 mg	Voltaren Rapide by Novartis	Canadian DIN 00881635	NSAID
VOLTAREN <> SR75	Tab, Light Pink, Triangular, Film Coated	Diclofenac Sodium 75 mg	Voltaren SR by Novartis	Canadian DIN 00782459	NSAID
VOLTAREN25	Tab, Yellow, Triangular	Diclofenac Sodium 25 mg	Voltaren by Novartis	00028-0258	NSAID
VOLTAREN50	Tab, Light Brown, Black Print, Triangular, Voltaren over 50	Diclofenac Potassium 50 mg	Cataflam by Rx Dispensing	61807-0084	NSAID
VOLTAREN50	Tab, Light Brown, Black Print, Triangular, Voltaren over 50	Diclofenac Potassium 50 mg	by Novartis	61615-0109	NSAID
VOLTAREN50	Tab, Light Brown, Black Print, Triangular, Voltaren over 50	Diclofenac Sodium 50 mg	Voltaren by Pharm Util	60491-0705	NSAID
VOLTAREN50	Tab, Light Brown, Black Print, Triangular, Voltaren over 50	Diclofenac Sodium 50 mg	by DRX	55045-2691	NSAID
VOLTAREN50	Tab, Light Brown, Black Print, Triangular, Voltaren over 50	Diclofenac Sodium 50 mg	by Nat Pharmpak	55154-1008	NSAID
VOLTAREN50	Tab, Light Brown, Black Print, Triangular, Voltaren over 50	Diclofenac Sodium 50 mg	by Med Pro	53978-1059	NSAID
VOLTAREN50	Tab, Light Brown, Black Print, Triangular, Voltaren over 50	Diclofenac Sodium 50 mg	Voltaren by Novartis	00028-0262	NSAID
VOLTAREN50	Tab, Light Brown, Black Print, Triangular, Voltaren over 50	Diclofenac Sodium 50 mg	by Pharmedix	53002-0537	NSAID
VOLTAREN50	Tab, Light Brown, Black Print, Triangular, Voltaren over 50	Diclofenac Sodium 50 mg	by Allscripts		NSAID
VOLTAREN75	Tab, Light Pink, Black Print, Triangular, Voltaren over 75	Diclofenac Sodium 75 mg	by Med Pro	53978-1049	NSAID

ID FRONT <> BACK	DESCRIPTION FRONT <> BACK	INGREDIENT & STRENGTH	BRAND (or Generic Equiv.) by FIRM	NDC#	CLASS; SCH.
VOLTAREN75	Tab, Light Pink, Black Print, Triangular, Voltaren over 75	Diclofenac Sodium 75 mg	by Pharmedix	53002-0536	NSAID
VOLTAREN75	Tab, Light Pink, Black Print, Triangular, Voltaren over 75	Diclofenac Sodium 75 mg	by Allscripts		NSAID
VOLTAREN75	Tab, Light Pink, Black Print, Triangular, Voltaren over 75	Diclofenac Sodium 75 mg	by Nat Pharmpak	55154-1007	NSAID
VOLTAREN75	Tab, Light Pink, Black Print, Triangular, Voltaren over 75	Diclofenac Sodium 75 mg	Voltaren by Rx Pak	65084-0119	NSAID
VOLTAREN75	Tab, Light Pink, Black Print, Triangular, Voltaren over 75	Diclofenac Sodium 75 mg	Voltaren by Rx Dispensing	61807-0049	NSAID
VOLTAREN75	Tab, Light Pink, Black Print, Triangular, Voltaren over 75	Diclofenac Sodium 75 mg	Voltaren by Novartis	00028-0264	NSAID
VOLTARENSR <> 100	Tab, Light Pink, Round, Coated, Voltaren-XR	Diclofenac Sodium 100 mg	Voltaren XR by Novartis	Canadian DIN 00590827	NSAID
VOLTARENXR <> 100	Tab, Light Pink, Round, Coated, Voltaren-XR	Diclofenac Sodium 100 mg	Voltaren XR by Novartis	17088-0205	NSAID
VOLTARENXR <> 100	Tab, Light Pink, Round, Coated, Voltaren-XR	Diclofenac Sodium 100 mg	Voltaren XR by Novartis	00028-0205	NSAID
VOLTARENXR <> 100	Tab, Light Pink, Round, Coated, Voltaren-XR	Diclofenac Sodium 100 mg	Voltaren XR by Caremark	00339-6091	NSAID
VOLTARENXR <> 100	Tab, Light Pink, Round, Coated, Voltaren-XR	Diclofenac Sodium 100 mg	Voltaren XR by H J Harkins Co	52959-0472	NSAID
VOO31	Tab	Acetaminophen 500 mg	Tylenol Ex Strength by Diversified Healthcare	55887-0945	Analgesic
VOR200 <> PFIZER	Tab, White, Cap Shaped, Film Coated	Voriconazole 200 mg	Vfend by Pfizer	00049-3180	Antifungal
VOR50 <> PFIZER	Tab, White, Round, Film Coated	Voriconazole 50 mg	Vfend by Pfizer	00049-3170	Antifungal
VOR50 <> PFIZER	Tab, White, Round, Film-Coated	Voriconazole 50 mg	Vfend by Pfizer	Canadian DIN 02256460	Antifungal
VOR50 <> PFIZER	Tab, White, Cap-shaped, Film-Coated	Voriconazole 200 mg	Vfend by Pfizer	Canadian DIN 02256479	Antifungal
VP	Tab, White, Round, Convex, Film, VP over the Knoll Triangle	Hydrocodone Bitartrate 7.5 mg, Ibuprofen 200 mg	Vicoprofen by Murfreesboro	51129-1457	Analgesic; C III
VP	Tab, White, Round, Convex, Film, Knoll Triangle	Hydrocodone Bitartrate 7.5 mg, Ibuprofen 200 mg	Vicoprofen by Murfreesboro	51129-1459	Analgesic; C III
VP	Tab, White, Round, Convex, Film, VP over the Knoll Triangle	Hydrocodone Bitartrate 7.5 mg, Ibuprofen 200 mg	Vicoprofen by Murfreesboro	51129-1458	Analgesic; C III
VP	Tab, White, Round, Convex, Film, Knoll Triangle	Hydrocodone Bitartrate 7.5 mg, Ibuprofen 200 mg	Vicoprofen by Murfreesboro	51129-1456	Analgesic; C III
VP	Tab, White, Round, Convex, Film, VP over the Knoll Triangle	Hydrocodone Bitartrate 7.5 mg, Ibuprofen 200 mg	Vicoprofen by Physician Total Care	54868-4035	Analgesic; C III
VP	Tab, White, Round, Convex, Film, VP over the Knoll Triangle	Hydrocodone Bitartrate 7.5 mg, Ibuprofen 200 mg	Vicoprofen by Southwood	58016-0442	Analgesic; C III
VP	Tab, White, Round, Convex, Film, VP over Knoll Triangle	Hydrocodone Bitartrate 7.5 mg, Ibuprofen 200 mg	Vicoprofen by Murfreesboro	51129-1463	Analgesic; C III
VP <> 11	Tab, White, Round, Scored	Ethambutol HCl 100 mg	Myambutol by Versapharm	61748-0011	Antituberculosis
VP <> 11	Tab, White, Round, Film Coated	Ethambutol HCl 100 mg	by West-Ward	00143-9100	Antituberculosis
VP <> 14	Tab, White, Round, Scored	Ethambutol HCl 400 mg	Myambutol by Versapharm	61748-0014	Antituberculosis
VP <> 14	Tab, White, Round, Film Coated, Scored	Ethambutol HCl 400 mg	by West-Ward	00143-9101	Antituberculosis
VP <> UREX	Tab, White, Oblong, Scored	Methenamine Hippurate 1 g	Urex by Virco Pharms	65199-1201	Antibiotic; Urinary Tract
VP012	Tab, White, Round, Scored, VP over 012	Pyrazinamide 500 mg	Pyrazinamide by Versapharm	61748-0012	Antibiotic
VP045	Tab, White, Round, Scored	Aminocaproic Acid 500 mg	Amicar by Versa Pharm	61748-0045	Hemostatic
VP120	Tab, White, Oval	Sulfamethoxazole 800 mg, Trimethoprim 160 mg	Septra by Midland Pharms	15686-0102	Antibiotic
VPA	Tab, White, Round, Film Coated, VP over Abbott Logo (a)	Hydrocodone Bitartrate 7.5 mg, Ibuprofen 200 mg	Vicoprofen by Abbott	00044-0723	Analgesic; C III
VPA	Tab, White, Round, Film Coated, VP over Abbott Logo (a)	Hydrocodone Bitartrate 7.5 mg, Ibuprofen 200 mg	Vicoprofen by Abbott	00074-2277	Analgesic; C III
VSR120 <> APO	Tab, White, Round, Film Coated	Verapamil HCl 120 mg	Apo Verapamil by Apotex	Canadian DIN 02246893	Antihypertensive
VSR180 <> APO	Tab, Pink, Oval, Scored	Verapamil HCl 180	Apo Verapamil by Apotex	Canadian DIN 02246894	Antihypertensive
VSR240 <> APO	Tab, Off-White, Cap Shaped, Scored, Film Coated	Verapamil HCl 240 mg	Apo Verapamil by Apotex	Canadian DIN 02246895	Antihypertensive
VT1052	Cap, Brown & Clear, VT-1052	Theophylline Anhydrous SR 260 mg	by Eon		Antiasthmatic
VT5720	Cap, Red & Clear, VT-5720	Phendimetrazine Tartrate 35 mg	by Eon		Anorexiant; C III
VT76	Tab, Yellow, Round	Phendimetrazine Tartrate 35 mg	Plegine by Eon		Anorexiant; C III
VT77	Tab, Pink, Oblong, VT-77	Phendimetrazine Tartrate 35 mg	by Eon		Anorexiant; C III
VW	Tab, Orange, Round, V on top of W, intersecting	3,4-Methylenedioxymethamphetamine (MDMA)	Ecstasy by Illegal		Euphoric; Illicit

ID FRONT <> BACK	DESCRIPTION FRONT <> BACK	INGREDIENT & STRENGTH	BRAND (or Generic Equiv.) by FIRM	NDC#	CLASS; SCH.
VXR150	Cap, Dark Orange, Opaque, Extended Release	Venlafaxine 150 mg	Effexor XR by Cobalt	Canadian DIN 02304333	Antidepressant
VXR375	Tab, Peach and Grey, Opaque, Extended Release	Venlafaxine 37.5 mg	Effexor XR by Cobalt	Canadian DIN 02304317	Antidepressant
VXR75	Cap, Peach, Opaque, Extended Release	Venlafaxine 75 mg	Effexor XR by Cobalt	Canadian DIN 02304325	Antidepressant
W	Tab, Maroon, Round	Phenazopyridine HCl 95 mg	by Able	Discontinued	Urinary Analgesic
W	Tab, Green, Round	Inert	Alesse 28 by Wyeth	Canadian DIN 02236975	Oral Contraceptive; Placebo
W	Cap, Brown & Gray, Opaque	Dihydrotachysterol 170 mg	Hytakerol by RP Scherer	11014-0300	Vitamin
W	Cap, Yellow	Danazol 100 mg	Cyclomen by Sanofi	Canadian	Steroid
W	Cap, Orange	Danazol 200 mg	Cyclomen by Sanofi	Canadian	Steroid
W	Cap, Orange & White	Danazol 50 mg	Cyclomen by Sanofi	Canadian	Steroid
W	Cap, Brown	Dihydrotachysterol 0.125 mg	Hytakerol by Sanofi	Canadian	Vitamin
W	Cap, Brown, Soft Gel	Dihydrotachysterol 0.125 mg	Hytakerol by Sanofi	00024-0792	Vitamin
W	Tab, White, Round, Scored	Chloroquine Diphosphate 250 mg	Aralen by Sanofi	Canadian DIN 02017539	Antimalarial
W	Tab, White, Round	Floctafenine 200 mg	Idarac by Sanofi	Canadian	Anti-Inflammatory
W	Tab, White, Round	Floctafenine 400 mg	Idarac by Sanofi	Canadian	Anti-Inflammatory
W	Tab	Lead 12 X	Scleron by Weleda	00164-1193	Homeopathic
W	Tab	Lead 12 X	Scleron by Weleda	55946-0396	Homeopathic
W	Tab, Pink, Round	Ethinyl Estradiol 20 mg, Levonorgestrel 100 mg	Alesse 21 by Wyeth	Canadian DIN 02236974	Oral Contraceptive
W	Tab, Pink, Round	Ethinyl Estradiol 20 mg, Levonorgestrel 100 mg	Alesse 28 by Wyeth	Canadian DIN 02236975	Oral Contraceptive
W <> 05	Tab, Pale Green, Round, W <> 0.5, Sublingual	Lorazepam 0.5 mg	Ativan by Wyeth	Canadian DIN 02041456	Antianxiety; C IV
W <> 05	Tab, White, Round, W/0.5	Lorazepam 0.5 mg	Ativan by Wyeth	Canadian DIN 02041413	Antianxiety; C IV
W <> 1	Tab, White, Round, Sublingual	Lorazepam 1 mg	Ativan by Wyeth	Canadian DIN 02041464	Antianxiety; C IV
W <> 1117	Tab, Yellow, Round, Film-Coated	Levonorgestrel 90 mcg, Ethinyl Estradiol 20 mcg	Lybrel by Wyeth	00008-1117	Oral Contraceptive
W <> 1605	Tab, Branded in Blue, Sugar Coated	Perphenazine 8 mg	by Schein	00364-2625	Antipsychotic
W <> 171	Tab, Green, Hexagon Shaped	Ropinirole HCl 1 mg	Requip by Wockhardt	64679-0171	Antiparkinson
W <> 2	Tab, Blue, Round, Sublingual	Lorazepam 2 mg	Ativan by Wyeth	Canadian DIN 02041472	Antianxiety; C IV
W <> 25	Tab, Yellow, Round	Isosorbide Dinitrate 2.5 mg	Isordil by Wyeth	00008-4139	Antianginal
W <> 4117	Tab, Orange, Film Coated	Ethionamide 250 mg	Trecator by Wyeth	00008-4117	Antituberculosis
W <> 5	Tab, Pink, Round	Isosorbide Dinitrate 5 mg	Isordil by Wyeth	00008-4126	Antianginal
W <> 56	Tab, Yellow, Oval	Sertraline HCl 100 mg	Zoloft by West-Ward	00143-9580	Antidepressant
W <> 724	Tab, White, Oval, Film Coated, Extended Release	Divalproex Sodium 250 mg	Depakote by Wockhardt	64679-0724	Anticonvulsant
W <> 743	Tab, White, Round	Terbinafine HCl 250 mg	Lamisil by Wockhardt	64679-0743	Antifungal
W <> 82	Tab, White, Round	Primidone 50 mg	Mysoline by West-Ward	00143-1482	Anticonvulsant
W <> 82	Tab, White, Round	Primidone 50 mg	Mysoline by Blu	24658-0150	Anticonvulsant
W <> 902	Tab, Film Coated	Naproxen 550 mg	Naprelan by Quality Care	62682-2001 Discontinued	NSAID
W <> 902	Tab, Film Coated	Naproxen 550 mg	by Physician Total Care	54868-3973	NSAID
W <> 902	Tab, White, Oblong	Naproxen 550 mg	by PDRX	55289-0304	NSAID
W <> 902	Tab, Film Coated	Naproxen 550 mg	by Caremark	00339-6102	NSAID
W <> 912	Tab, Pink, Round, Scored	Levonorgestrel 0.1 mg, Ethinyl Estradiol 0.02 mg	Alesse 28 by Wyeth	00008-2576	Oral Contraceptive
W <> 912	Tab, Pink, Round, Scored	Levonorgestrel 0.1 mg, Ethinyl Estradiol 0.02 mg	Alesse 21 by Wyeth	00008-0912	Oral Contraceptive

ID FRONT <> BACK	DESCRIPTION FRONT <> BACK	INGREDIENT & STRENGTH	BRAND (or Generic Equiv.) by FIRM	NDC#	CLASS; SCH.
W <> A77	Tab, Bright Pink, Black Print, Film Coated	Chloroquine Phosphate 500 mg	Aralen Phosphate by Bayer	00280-0084	Antimalarial
W <> A77	Tab, Bright Pink, Black Print, Film Coated	Chloroquine Phosphate 500 mg	Aralen Phosphate by Sanofi	00024-0084	Antimalarial
W <> A77	Tab, Bright Pink, Black Print, Film Coated	Chloroquine Phosphate 500 mg	Aralen Phosphate by Allscripts		Antimalarial
W <> D35	Tab, D35	Meperidine 50 mg	Demerol by Sanofi	00280-0335	Analgesic; C II
W <> D35	Tab, D35, Tab Coated	Meperidine 50 mg	Demerol by Bayer	00280-0335	Analgesic; C II
W <> D37	Tab, D37, Tab Coated	Meperidine 100 mg	Demerol by Bayer	00280-0337	Analgesic; C II
W <> D37	Tab, D37	Meperidine 100 mg	Demerol by Sanofi	00024-0337	Analgesic; C II
W <> M87	Tab, Coated, W <> M/87	Ambenonium Chloride 10 mg	Mytelase by Bayer	00280-1287	Myasthenia Gravis
W <> M87	Tab, W <> M/87	Ambenonium Chloride 10 mg	Mytelase by Sanofi	00024-1287	Myasthenia Gravis
W <> MERRELL547	Tab, White, Round, Merrell over 547	Quinine Sulfate 260 mg	Quinamm by Merrell	00068-0547	Antimalarial
W <> N21	Tab, Light Buff, N/21	Nalidixic Acid 250 mg	Neggram by Sanofi	00024-1321	Antibiotic
W <> N22	Tab, Light Buff, N/22	Nalidixic Acid 500 mg	Neggram by Sanofi	00024-1322	Antibiotic
W <> N23	Tab, Light Buff, N/23	Nalidixic Acid 1 g	Neggram by Sanofi	00024-1323	Antibiotic
W <> P97	Tab, Pink, Black Print, Round, Film Coated	Primaquine Phosphate 26.3 mg	Primaquine by Sanofi	Canadian	Antimalarial
W <> P97	Tab, Pink, Black Print, Round, Film Coated	Primaquine Phosphate 26.3 mg	by Bayer	00280-1596	Antimalarial
W <> P97	Tab, Pink, Black Print, Round, Film Coated	Primaquine Phosphate 26.3 mg	by Sanofi	00024-1596	Antimalarial
W <> T31	Tab, T and 31, Tab Coated	Iopanoic Acid 500 mg	Telepaque by Nycomed	00407-1931	Diagnostic
W <> T51	Tab, T 51	Naloxone HCl 0.5 mg, Pentazocine HCl 50 mg	Talwin Nx by Sanofi	00024-1951	Analgesic; C IV
W <> T51	Tab, T 51	Naloxone HCl 0.5 mg, Pentazocine HCl 50 mg	Talwin Nx by Searle	00966-1951	Analgesic; C IV
W01	Tab, White, Round	Leflunomide 10 mg	Arava by Prasco	66993-0160	Antiarthritic
W02	Tab, Light Yellow, Triangular	Leflunomide 20 mg	Arava by Prasco	66993-0161	Antiarthritic
W028SQUIBB	Cap	Cloxacillin Sodium 250 mg	by Apothecon	59772-6028	Antibiotic
W03	Tab, Pink, Oblong, Notched Sides	Glimepiride 1 mg	Amaryl by Prasco	66993-0162	Antidiabetic
W03	Tab, Green, Oblong, Notched Sides	Glimepiride 2 mg	Amaryl by Prasco	66993-0163	Antidiabetic
W03	Tab, Blue, Oblong, Notched Sides	Glimepiride 4 mg	Amaryl by Prasco	66993-0164	Antidiabetic
W038	Cap, Orange, White Ink	Cloxacillin Sodium 500 mg	by Apothecon	59772-6038	Antibiotic
W04	Tab, White, Round	Ondansetron HCl 4 mg	Zofran by West-Ward	00143-2422	Antiemetic
W048SQUIBB	Cap	Dicloxacillin Sodium 250 mg	by Golden State	60429-0059	Antibiotic
W06255	Tab, Blue, Black Print, Oval, W over 0.625/5	Conjugated Estrogens 0.625 mg, Medroxyprogesterone Acetate 2.5 mg	Prempro by Ayerst	00046-0975	Hormone
W1	Tab, Yellow, Round	Isosorbide Dinitrate 2.5 mg	Isordil by Qualitest	00603-4122	Antianginal
W1	Tab, Yellow, Round	Isosorbide Dinitrate 2.5 mg	Isordil by West-Ward	00143-1765	Antianginal
W1 <> ICN	Tab, White, Round	Prednisone 1 mg	Winpred by ICN	Canadian DIN 00271373	Steroid
W100	Tab, Reddish-Orange, Square Pyramid Shaped, W / 100	Desvenlafaxine 100 mg	Pristiq by Wyeth	00008-1222	Antidepressant
W100	Tab, Reddish Orange, Square Pyramid	Desvenlafaxine 100 mg	Pristiq by Wyeth Canada	Canadian DIN 02321106	Antidepressant
W100 <> 705	Tab, Peach, Shield Shaped, Scored, W over 100	Venlafaxine 100 mg	Effexor by Wyeth	00008-0705	Antidepressant
W1502	Tab, White, Cap Shaped, Scored, Extended Release	Isosorbide Mononitrate 30 mg	Imdur by Warrick	59930-3094	Antianginal
W152200MG	Cap, White, Opaque	Ribavirin 200 mg	Rebetol by Warrick	59930-1523	Antiviral
W154	Tab, White, Hexagon Shaped	Ropinirole HCl 0.25 mg	Requip by Wockhardt	64679-0154	Antiparkinson
W1549	Tab, White, Cap Shaped, Ex Release	Isosorbide Mononitrate 60 mg	Imdur by Warrick	59930-3144	Antianginal
W155	Tab, Yellow, Hexagon Shaped	Ropinirole HCl 0.5 mg	Requip by Wockhardt	64679-0155	Antiparkinson
W1587	Tab, White, Cap Shaped, Extended Release	Isosorbide Mononitrate 120 mg	Imdur by Warrick	59930-3605	Antianginal
W1600	Tab, Gray, Round, Sugar Coated	Perphenazine 2 mg	by Warrick	59930-1600	Antipsychotic
W1600	Tab, Gray, Round, Sugar Coated	Perphenazine 2 mg	by Martec	52555-0569	Antipsychotic
W1603	Tab, Gray, Round, Sugar Coated	Perphenazine 4 mg	by Martec	52555-0570	Antipsychotic
W1603	Tab, Gray, Round, Sugar Coated	Perphenazine 4 mg	by Warrick	59930-1603	Antipsychotic
W1605	Tab, Gray, Sugar Coated	Perphenazine 8 mg	Trilafon by Warrick		Antipsychotic
W1605	Tab, Gray, Sugar Coated	Perphenazine 8 mg	by Qualitest		Antipsychotic

ID FRONT <> BACK	DESCRIPTION FRONT <> BACK	INGREDIENT & STRENGTH	BRAND (or Generic Equiv.) by FIRM	NDC#	CLASS; SCH.
W1606	Tab, Gray, Sugar Coated	Perphenazine 8 mg	by Martec	52555-0571	Antipsychotic
W1610	Tab, Gray, Sugar Coated	Perphenazine 16 mg	by Martec	52555-0572	Antipsychotic
W16WYETH92	Tab, White, Pentagonal, W16/Wyeth 92	Guanabenz Acetate 16 mg	Wytensin by Wyeth		Antihypertensive
W1714	Tab, White, Oblong, Scored	Potassium Chloride 20 mEq	K-Dur by Warrick	59930-1714	Electrolytes
W1715	Tab, White, Oblong	Potassium Chloride 10 mEq	K-Dur by Warrick	59930-1715	Electrolytes
W172	Tab, Pale Yellowish Pink, Hexagon Shaped	Ropinirole HCl 2 mg	Requip by Wockhardt	64679-0172	Antiparkinson
W174	Tab, Purple, Hexagon Shaped	Ropinirole HCl 3 mg	Requip by Wockhardt	64679-0174	Antiparkinson
W175	Tab, Brown, Hexagon Shaped	Ropinirole HCl 4 mg	Requip by Wockhardt	64679-0175	Antiparkinson
W177	Tab, Blue, Hexagon Shaped	Ropinirole HCl 5 mg	Requip by Wockhardt	64679-0177	Antiparkinson
W2 <> GPI	Tab, Light Brown, Round	Sennosides 8.6 mg	Senokot by Amneal	65162-0440	Gastrointestinal
W200	Tab, Orange, Round, W/200	Peripheral Vasodilator 200 mg	Cyclospasmol by Wyeth	Canadian	Vasodilator
W200	Tab, Orange, Round	Cyclandelate 200 mg	by Wyeth	Canadian	Vasodilator
W209	Tab, White, Round	Terbinafine HCl 250 mg	Lamisil by Wockhardt	64679-0209	Antifungal
W2183	Tab, Purple, Round	Atropine Sulfate, Benzoic Acid, Hyoscyamine Sulfate, Methenamine, Phenyl Salicylate	Urised by Webcon		Urinary Tract
W2183	Tab, Purple, Round	Phenyl Salicylate 18.1 mg, Methylene Blue 5.4 mg, Atropine Sulfate 0.03 mg, Benzoic Acid 4.5 mg, Hyoscyamine 0.03 mg, Methenamine 40.8 mg	Urised by Polymedica	61451-2183	Urinary Tract
W2225	Tab, Light Blue, Round	Hyoscyamine Sulfate 0.15 mg	Cystospaz by Polymedica	61451-2225	Gastrointestinal
W2225	Tab	Hyoscyamine Sulfate 0.15 mg	Levsin by Pegasus	55246-0956	Gastrointestinal
W2260	Cap, Light Blue	Hyoscyamine Sulfate 0.375 mg	Levsin by Polymedica	61451-2260 Discontinued	Gastrointestinal
W23	Tab, White, W/23	D-Norgestrel 250 mcg, Ethinyl Estradiol 50 mcg	Ovral by Wyeth	Canadian DIN 02043033	Oral Contraceptive
W23	Tab, White, W/23	Norgestrel 250 mcg	Orval 21 by Wyeth	Canadian DIN 02043033	Oral Contraceptive
W25 <> 701	Tab, Peach, Shield Shaped, Scored, W over 25	Venlafaxine 25 mg	Effexor by Wyeth	00008-0701	Antidepressant
W3	Tab, White, Round	Isosorbide Dinitrate 5 mg	Isordil by Qualitest	00603-4123	Antianginal
W3	Tab, White, Round	Isosorbide Dinitrate 5 mg	Isordil by URL Mutual	00677-0409	Antianginal
W3	Tab, White, Round	Isosorbide Dinitrate 5 mg	Isordil by West-Ward	00143-1767	Antianginal
W300	Tab	Furosemide 20 mg	by Qualitest	00603-3736	Diuretic
W302	Tab	Furosemide 80 mg	by Qualitest	00603-3738	Diuretic
W332	Tab, Cap Shaped	Ascorbic Acid 500 mg, Biotin 0.15 mg, Calcium Pantothenate, Chromic Nitrate, Cupric Oxide, Cyanocobalamin 50 mcg, Ferrous Fumarate, Folic Acid 0.8 mg, Magnesium Oxide, Manganese Dioxide, Niacinamide, Pyridoxine HCl 25 mg, Riboflavin 20 mg, Thiamine Mononitrate, Vitamin A Acetate, Vitamin E Acetate, Zinc Oxide	Vitalize Plus by West-Ward	00143-2332	Vitamin
W363	Tab, Blue, Round	Clorazepate Dipotassium 3.75 mg	by Qualitest	00603-3004	Antianxiety; C IV
W365	Tab, Peach, Round	Clorazepate Dipotassium 7.5 mg	by Qualitest	00603-3005	Antianxiety; C IV
W365	Tab, White, Round	Clorazepate Dipotassium 15 mg	by Qualitest	00603-3006	Antianxiety; C IV
W369	Cap	Loxapine Succinate	by Qualitest	00603-4268	Antipsychotic
W371	Cap	Loxapine Succinate	by Qualitest	00603-4270	Antipsychotic
W373	Tab, Film Coated	Maprotiline HCl 25 mg	by Qualitest	00603-4294	Antidepressant
W375 <> 781	Tab, Peach, Shield Shaped, Scored, W over 37.5	Venlafaxine 37.5 mg	Effexor by Wyeth	00008-0781	Antidepressant
W375 <> 781	Tab, Peach, Shield Shaped, Scored, W over 37.5	Venlafaxine 37.5 mg	Effexor by Caremark	00339-6035	Antidepressant
W379	Tab	Amoxapine 25 mg	Asendin by Qualitest	00603-2240	Antidepressant
W380	Tab, Salmon	Amoxapine 50 mg	Asendin by Qualitest	00603-2241	Antidepressant
W381	Tab	Amoxapine 100 mg	Asendin by Qualitest	00603-2242	Antidepressant
W382	Tab	Amoxapine 150 mg	Asendin by Qualitest	00603-2243	Antidepressant
W4	Tab, White, Round, Scored	Trihexyphenidyl HCl 2 mg	Artane by West-Ward	00143-1764	Antiparkinson
W4 <> WYETH73	Tab, Coated, W 4 <> Wyeth 73	Guanabenz Acetate 4 mg	Wytensin by Wyeth	00008-0073	Antihypertensive

ID FRONT <> BACK	DESCRIPTION FRONT <> BACK	INGREDIENT & STRENGTH	BRAND (or Generic Equiv.) by FIRM	NDC#	CLASS; SCH.
W40	Tab, Yellow, Round, Scored	Digoxin 125 mcg	Lanoxin by UDL	51079-0847	Cardiac Agent
W400	Tab, Film Coated	Ibuprofen 400 mg	Motrin by Quality Care	60346-0430	NSAID
W404	Tab, Film Coated, Debossed	Verapamil HCl 40 mg	by Qualitest	00603-6356	Antihypertensive
W414	Tab	Estropipate 0.75 mg	by Qualitest	00603-3559	Hormone
W415	Tab	Estropipate 1.5 mg	by Qualitest	00603-3560	Hormone
W416	Tab	Estropipate 3 mg	by Qualitest	00603-3561	Hormone
W421	Tab, White to Off White, Triangle Shaped	Amlodipine Besylate 2.5 mg	Norvasc by Wockhardt	64679-0421	Antihypertensive
W422	Tab, White to Off White, Cap Shaped	Amlodipine Besylate 5 mg	Norvasc by Wockhardt	64679-0422	Antihypertensive
W423	Tab, White to Off White, Round	Amlodipine Besylate 10 mg	Norvasc by Wockhardt	64679-0423	Antihypertensive
W424	Tab	Hydrochlorothiazide 25 mg, Triamterene 37.5 mg	by Qualitest	00603-6180	Diuretic; Antihypertensive
W425	Cap	Aspirin 325 mg, Butalbital 50 mg, Caffeine 40 mg, Codeine Phosphate 30 mg	Fiorinal w/ Codeine by Qualitest	00603-2549	Analgesic; C III
W431	Tab, White, Round	Lorazepam 0.5 mg	Ativan by Watson		Antianxiety; C IV
W451	Tab	Guanabenz Acetate	by Qualitest	00603-3779	Antihypertensive
W452	Tab	Guanabenz Acetate	by Qualitest	00603-3780	Antihypertensive
W454	Tab, Film Coated	Gemfibrozil 600 mg	by Qualitest	00603-3750	Antihyperlipidemic
W460	Tab	Glipizide 5 mg	by Qualitest	00603-3755	Antidiabetic
W462	Tab	Metoprolol Tartrate 50 mg	Lopressor by Qualitest	00603-4627	Antihypertensive
W480	Tab, White, Round	Propylthiouracil 50 mg	by Rondex		Antithyroid
W49	Tab, Pink, Round	Aluminum 180 mg, Magnesium Hydroxide 160 mg	Wingel by Sanofi		Gastrointestinal
W50	Tab, Light Pink, Square Pyramid Shaped, W / 50	Desvenlafaxine 50 mg	Pristiq by Wyeth	00008-1211	Antidepressant
W50	Tab, Light Pink, Square Pyramid	Desvenlafaxine 50 mg	Pristiq by Wyeth Canada	Canadian DIN 02321092	Antidepressant
W50 <> 703	Tab, Peach, Shield Shaped, Scored, W over 50	Venlafaxine 50 mg	Effexor by Wyeth	00008-0703	Antidepressant
W53	Tab, W over 53	Stanozolol 2 mg	Winstrol by Searle	00966-2253 Discontinued	Anabolic Steroid; C III
W53	Tab, W over 53	Stanozolol 2 mg	Winstrol by Sanofi	00024-2253 Discontinued	Anabolic Steroid; C III
W553	Tab, Yellow, Cap Shaped, Film Coated	Risperidone 0.25 mg	Risperdal by Wockhardt	64679-0553	Antipsychotic
W554	Tab, Brown, Cap Shaped, Film Coated	Risperidone 0.5 mg	Risperdal by Wockhardt	64679-0554	Antipsychotic
W555	Tab, White, Cap Shaped, Film Coated	Risperidone 1 mg	Risperdal by Wockhardt	64679-0555	Antipsychotic
W557	Tab, Orange, Cap Shaped, Film Coated	Risperidone 2 mg	Risperdal by Wockhardt	64679-0557	Antipsychotic
W57	Tab, Light Blue	Sertraline 50 mg	Zoloft by West-Ward	00143-9581	Antidepressant
W571	Tab, Yellow, Cap Shaped, Film Coated	Risperidone 3 mg	Risperdal by Wockhardt	64679-0571	Antipsychotic
W572	Tab, Green, Cap Shaped, Film Coated	Risperidone 4 mg	Risperdal by Wockhardt	64679-0572	Antipsychotic
W587 <> 120	Tab, White, Oval, Scored	Isosorbide Mononitrate 120 mg	Imdur by Warrick	59930-1587	Antianginal
W587 <> 120	Tab, White, Oval, Scored	Isosorbide Mononitrate 120 mg	Imdur by Murfreesboro	51129-1569	Antianginal
W587 <> 120	Tab, White, Oval, Ex Release, W-587	Isosorbide Mononitrate 120 mg	Imdur by Murfreesboro	51129-1581	Antianginal
W6255	Tab, Light Blue, Black Print, Oval, W0.625/5	Conjugated Estrogens 0.625 mg, Medroxyprogesterone Acetate 5 mg	Prempro by Ayerst	00046-0975	Hormone
W641	Tab, Brown, Round	Ethinyl Estradiol 0.03 mg, Levonorgestrel 0.05 mg	Triphasil by Wyeth	00008-2536	Oral Contraceptive
W641	Tab, Brown, Round	Ethinyl Estradiol 0.03 mg, Levonorgestrel 0.05 mg	Triphasil by Wyeth	00008-0641	Oral Contraceptive
W641	Tab, Brown, Round	Ethinyl Estradiol 0.03 mg, Levonorgestrel 0.05 mg	Triphasil by Dept Health	53808-0060	Oral Contraceptive
W641	Tab, Brown, Round	Ethinyl Estradiol 0.04 mg, Levonorgestrel 0.075 mg	Triphasil by Physician Total Care	54868-0518	Oral Contraceptive
W642	Tab, White, Round	Ethinyl Estradiol 0.04 mg, Levonorgestrel 0.075 mg	Triphasil by Physician Total Care	54868-0518	Oral Contraceptive
W642	Tab, White, Round	Ethinyl Estradiol 0.04 mg, Levonorgestrel 0.075 mg	Triphasil by Dept Health	53808-0060	Oral Contraceptive
W642	Tab, White, Round	Ethinyl Estradiol 0.04 mg, Levonorgestrel 0.075 mg	Triphasil by Wyeth	00008-0642	Oral Contraceptive
W642	Tab, White, Round	Ethinyl Estradiol 0.03 mg, Levonorgestrel 0.125 mg	Triphasil by Wyeth	00008-2536	Oral Contraceptive
W643	Tab, Yellow, Round	Ethinyl Estradiol 0.03 mg, Levonorgestrel 0.125 mg	Triphasil by Wyeth	00008-2536	Oral Contraceptive
W643	Tab, Yellow, Round	Ethinyl Estradiol 0.03 mg, Levonorgestrel 0.125 mg	Triphasil by Wyeth	00008-0643	Oral Contraceptive
W643	Tab, Yellow, Round	Ethinyl Estradiol 0.03 mg, Levonorgestrel 0.125 mg	Triphasil by Dept Health	53808-0060	Oral Contraceptive

ID FRONT <> BACK	DESCRIPTION FRONT <> BACK	INGREDIENT & STRENGTH	BRAND (or Generic Equiv.) by FIRM	NDC#	CLASS; SCH.
W643	Tab, Yellow, Round	Ethinyl Estradiol 0.03 mg, Levonorgestrel 0.125 mg	Triphasil by Physician Total Care	54868-0518	Oral Contraceptive
W650	Tab, Green, Round	Inert	by Physician Total Care	54868-0518	Oral Contraceptive; Placebo
W650	Tab, Green, Round	Inert	Triphasil 28 by Dept Health	53808-0060	Oral Contraceptive; Placebo
W650	Tab, Green, Round	Inert	Alesse 28 by Wyeth	00008-2576	Oral Contraceptive; Placebo
W650	Tab, Light Green, Round	Inert	Triphasil 28 by Wyeth	00008-0650	Oral Contraceptive; Placebo
W650	Tab, Light Green, Round	Inert	Triphasil 28 by Wyeth	00008-2536	Oral Contraceptive; Placebo
W7	Tab, White, Round, Scored, W-7	Captopril 12.5 mg	Capoten by Major	00904-5045	Antihypertensive
W7	Tab, White, Round, Scored	Captopril 12.5 mg	Capoten by ESI Lederle	59911-5832	Antihypertensive
W7	Tab, White, Round, Scored	Captopril 12.5 mg	Capoten by West-Ward	00143-1171	Antihypertensive
W712	Tab, White, Cap Shaped, Film Coated	Cefprozil 250 mg	Cefzil by Wockhardt	64679-0712	Antibiotic
W713	Tab, White, Cap Shaped, Film Coated	Cefprozil 500 mg	Cefzil by Wockhardt	64679-0713	Antibiotic
W714	Tab, Pink, Cap Shaped, Film Coated	Zolpidem Tartrate 5 mg	Ambien by Wockhardt	64679-0714	Sedative/Hypnotic; C IV
W715	Tab, White, Cap Shaped, Film Coated	Zolpidem Tartrate 10 mg	Ambien by Wockhardt	64679-0715	Sedative/Hypnotic; C IV
W718	Tab, White, Oval, Scored, Watson Logo on one end, 718 on other	Buspirone HCl 15 mg	BuSpar by Watson	00591-0718	Antianxiety
W719	Cap, Pink, Extended Release	Phenytoin Sodium 30 mg	Dilantin by Wockhardt	64679-0719	Anticonvulsant
W720	Cap, Orange, Extended Release	Phenytoin Sodium 100 mg	Dilantin by Wockhardt	64679-0720	Anticonvulsant
W720	Cap, Orange, Extended Release	Phenytoin Sodium 100 mg	Dilantin by Wockhardt	64679-0720	Anticonvulsant
W725	Tab, Dark Grey, Oval, Film Coated, Extended Release	Divalproex Sodium 500 mg	Depakote by Wockhardt	64679-0725	Anticonvulsant
W7300	Tab, Pink, Round, Chewable	Methdilazine HCl 3.6 mg	Tacaryl by Westwood		Antihistamine
W7400	Tab, Peach, Round	Methdilazine HCl 8 mg	Tacaryl by Westwood		Antihistamine
W741	Tab, White, Six Sided, Film Coated	Ranitidine 150 mg	Zantac by Wockhardt	64679-0906	Gastrointestinal
W741	Tab, Orange, Six Sided, Coated	Ranitidine 150 mg	Zantac by Major Pharmaceuticals	00904-5832	Gastrointestinal
W75 <> 704	Tab, Peach, Shield Shaped, Scored, W over 75	Venlafaxine 75 mg	Effexor by Wyeth	00008-0704	Antidepressant
W75 <> 704	Tab, Peach, Shield Shaped, Scored, W over 75	Venlafaxine 75 mg	Effexor by Caremark	00339-6034	Antidepressant
W752	Tab, Blue, Cap Shaped, Film Coated, Scored	Sertraline HCl 50 mg	Zoloft by Wockhardt	64679-0752	Antidepressant
W753	Tab, Yellow, Cap Shaped, Film Coated, Scored	Sertraline HCl 100 mg	Zoloft by Wockhardt	64679-0753	Antidepressant
W8WYETH74	Tab, Gray, Pentagonal, W8/Wyeth 74	Guanabenz Acetate 8 mg	Wytensin by Wyeth		Antihypertensive
W901	Cap, Film Coated	Naproxen 375 mg	Naprelan by Wyeth	00008-0901	NSAID
W902	Cap, Film Coated	Naproxen 550 mg	Naprelan by Wyeth	00008-0902	NSAID
W902	Tab, White, Round, Scored, W over 902	Captopril 12.5 mg	Capoten by Wockhardt	64679-0902	Antihypertensive
W903	Tab, White, Round, Scored, W over 903	Captopril 25 mg	Capoten by Wockhardt	64679-0903	Antihypertensive
W904	Tab, White, Round, Scored, W over 904	Captopril 50 mg	Capoten by Wockhardt	64679-0904	Antihypertensive
W905	Tab, White, Round, Scored, W over 905	Captopril 100 mg	Capoten by Wockhardt	64679-0905	Antihypertensive
W906	Tab, White, Hexagonal, Film Coated, W over 906	Ranitidine HCl 150 mg	Zantac by Wockhardt Americas	64679-0906	Gastrointestinal
W906	Tab, White, Hexagonal, Film Coated, W over 906	Ranitidine HCl 150 mg	Zantac by Pliva	50111-0899	Gastrointestinal
W906	Tab, White, Hexagonal, Film Coated, W over 906	Ranitidine HCl 150 mg	Zantac by Ranbaxy	63304-0838	Gastrointestinal
W906	Tab, White, Hexagonal, Film Coated, W over 906	Ranitidine HCl 150 mg	Zantac by Amneal	65162-0258	Gastrointestinal
W907	Tab, White, Hexagonal, Film Coated, W over 907	Ranitidine HCl 300 mg	Zantac by Ranbaxy	63304-0839	Gastrointestinal
W907	Tab, White, Hexagonal, Film Coated, W over 907	Ranitidine HCl 300 mg	Zantac by Pliva	50111-0900	Gastrointestinal
W907	Tab, White, Hexagonal, Film Coated, W over 907	Ranitidine HCl 300 mg	Zantac by Wockhardt Americas	64679-0906	Gastrointestinal
W907	Tab, White to Off-White, Cap Shaped, Film Coated	Ranitidine HCl 300 mg	Zantac by Ivax	00172-4358	Gastrointestinal
W907	Tab, White, Hexagonal, Film Coated, W over 907	Ranitidine HCl 300 mg	Zantac by Amneal	65162-0260	Gastrointestinal
W920	Tab, White, Round, Film Coated	Cefuroxime Axetil 125 mg	Ceftin by Wockhardt	64679-0920	Antibiotic
W921	Tab, White, Round, Film Coated	Cefuroxime Axetil 250 mg	Ceftin by Wockhardt	64679-0921	Antibiotic

ID FRONT <> BACK	DESCRIPTION FRONT <> BACK	INGREDIENT & STRENGTH	BRAND (or Generic Equiv.) by FIRM	NDC#	CLASS; SCH.
W921 <> BMS	Tab	Metoprolol Tartrate 50 mg	Lopressor by Apothecon	59772-3692	Antihypertensive
W922	Tab, White, Round, Film Coated	Cefuroxime Axetil 500 mg	Ceftin by Wockhardt	64679-0922	Antibiotic
W923	Tab, White, Round, Scored, W over 923	Enalapril Maleate 2.5 mg	Vasotec by Wockhardt	64679-0923	Antihypertensive
W923	Tab, White, Round	Enalapril Maleate 2.5 mg	Vasotec by Ivax	00172-4195 Discontinued	Antihypertensive
W923	Tab, White, Round, Scored, W over 923	Enalapril Maleate 2.5 mg	Vasotec by Major	00904-5609	Antihypertensive
W923	Tab, White, Round, Scored, W over 923	Enalapril Maleate 2.5 mg	Vasotec by Pliva	50111-0891	Antihypertensive
W923	Tab, White, Round, Scored, W over 923	Enalapril Maleate 2.5 mg	Vasotec by Ranbaxy	63304-0834	Antihypertensive
W924	Tab, White, Round, Scored, W over 924	Enalapril Maleate 5 mg	Vasotec by Ranbaxy	63304-0835	Antihypertensive
W924	Tab, White, Round, Scored, W over 924	Enalapril Maleate 5 mg	Vasotec by Pliva	50111-0892	Antihypertensive
W924	Tab, White, Round, Scored, W over 924	Enalapril Maleate 5 mg	Vasotec by Ivax	00172-4196 Discontinued	Antihypertensive
W924	Tab, White, Round, Scored, W over 924	Enalapril Maleate 5 mg	Vasotec by Wockhardt	64679-0924	Antihypertensive
W925	Tab, Pink, Round, W over 925	Enalapril Maleate 10 mg	Vasotec by Wockhardt	64679-0925	Antihypertensive
W925	Tab, Pink, Round	Enalapril Maleate 10 mg	Vasotec by Ivax	00172-4197 Discontinued	Antihypertensive
W925	Tab, Pink, Round, W over 925	Enalapril Maleate 10 mg	Vasotec by Major	00904-5610	Antihypertensive
W925	Tab, Pink, Round, W over 925	Enalapril Maleate 10 mg	Vasotec by Ranbaxy	63304-0836	Antihypertensive
W925	Tab, Pink, Round, W over 925	Enalapril Maleate 10 mg	Vasotec by Pliva	50111-0893	Antihypertensive
W926	Tab, Pink to Light Beige, Round, W over 926	Enalapril Maleate 20 mg	Vasotec by Pliva	50111-0894	Antihypertensive
W926	Tab, Pink to Light Beige, Round, W over 926	Enalapril Maleate 20 mg	Vasotec by Ranbaxy	63304-0837	Antihypertensive
W926	Tab, Pink to Light Beige, Round, W over 926	Enalapril Maleate 20 mg	Vasotec by Ivax	00172-4198 Discontinued	Antihypertensive
W926	Tab, Pink to Light Beige, Round, W over 926	Enalapril Maleate 20 mg	Vasotec by Wockhardt	64679-0926	Antihypertensive
W927	Tab, White to Off White, Round	Lisinopril 2.5 mg	Zestril by Wockhardt	64679-0927	Antihypertensive
W928	Tab, White to Off White, Round, Scored	Lisinopril 5 mg	Zestril by Wockhardt	64679-0928	Antihypertensive
W929	Tab, White to Off White, Round	Lisinopril 10 mg	Zestril by Wockhardt	64679-0929	Antihypertensive
W933 <> BMS	Tab	Metoprolol Tartrate 100 mg	Lopressor by Apothecon	59772-3693	Antihypertensive
W936	Tab, Beige, Barrel Shaped, Film Coated, W over 936	Famotidine 20 mg	Pepcid by Wockhardt	64679-0936	Gastrointestinal
W937	Tab, White, Barrel Shaped, Film Coated, W over 937	Famotidine 40 mg	Pepcid by Wockhardt	64679-0937	Gastrointestinal
W941	Tab, Light yellow, Round	Lisinopril 20 mg	Zestril by Wockhardt	64679-0941	Antihypertensive
W942	Tab, Light Brown, Round	Lisinopril 40 mg	Zestril by Wockhardt	64679-0942	Antihypertensive
W945	Cap, White, Opaque	Zonisamide 25 mg	Zonegran by Wockhardt	64679-0945	Anticonvulsant
W946	Cap, White and Grey, Opaque	Zonisamide 50 mg	Zonegran by Wockhardt	64679-0946	Anticonvulsant
W949	Tab, White, Oval, Film Coated	Clarithromycin 500 mg	Biaxin by Wockhardt	64679-0949	Antibiotic
W953	Tab, Light Red, Round	Lisinopril 30 mg	Zestril by Wockhardt	64679-0953	Antihypertensive
W954	Tab, White, Oval, Film Coated	Clarithromycin 250 mg	Biaxin by Wockhardt	64679-0954	Antibiotic
W961	Tab, White, Oval	Azithromycin 250 mg	Zithromax by Wockhardt	64679-0961	Antibiotic
W962	Tab, White, Oval	Azithromycin 600 mg	Zithromax by Wockhardt	64679-0962	Antibiotic
W964	Tab, White, Oval	Azithromycin 500 mg	Zithromax by Wockhardt	64679-0964	Antibiotic
W965	Tab, White, Oval, Scored	Bethanechol Chloride 5 mg	Urecholine by Wockhardt	64679-0965	Urinary Tract
W965	Tab, White, Oval, Scored	Bethanechol Chloride 5 mg	Urecholine by Ranbaxy	63304-0993	Urinary Tract
W966	Tab, Pink, Oval	Bethanechol 10 mg	Urecholine by Ranbaxy	63304-0994	Urinary Tract
W966	Tab, Pink, Oval	Bethanechol Chloride 10 mg	Urecholine by Wockhardt	64679-0966	Urinary Tract
W967	Tab, Light Yellow, Oval, Scored	Bethanechol Chloride 25 mg	Urecholine by Wockhardt	64679-0967	Urinary Tract
W967	Tab, Light Yellow, Oval, Scored	Bethanechol Chloride 25 mg	Urecholine by Ranbaxy	63304-0995	Urinary Tract
W968	Tab, Yellow, Oval, Scored	Bethanechol Chloride 50 mg	Urecholine by Wockhardt	64679-0968	Urinary Tract
W968	Tab, Yellow, Oval, Scored	Bethanechol Chloride 50 mg	Urecholine by Ranbaxy	63304-0996	Urinary Tract
W973	Tab, White, Round, Delayed Release	Divalproex Sodium 125 mg	Depakote by Wockhardt	64679-0973	Anticonvulsant
W974	Tab, White, Oval, Delayed Release	Divalproex Sodium 250 mg	Depakote by Wockhardt	64679-0974	Anticonvulsant

ID FRONT <> BACK	DESCRIPTION FRONT <> BACK	INGREDIENT & STRENGTH	BRAND (or Generic Equiv.) by FIRM	NDC#	CLASS; SCH.
W975	Tab, White, Oval, Delayed Release	Divalproex Sodium 500 mg	Depakote by Wockhardt	64679-0975	Anticonvulsant
W990	Cap, White and Orange, Opaque	Zonisamide 100 mg	Zonegran by Wockhardt	64679-0990	Anticonvulsant
WA79	Tab, Orange, Round	Chloroquine Phosphate 500 mg, Primaquine Phosphate 79 mg	Aralen / Primaquine by Sanofi		Antimalarial
WA82	Tab, Yellow, Round	Quinacrine HCl 100 mg	Atabrine by Sanofi		Antimalarial
WALLACE <> 0430	Tab, Yellow, Cap Shaped, Scored	Felbamate 400 mg	Felbatol by Wallace	00037-0430	Anticonvulsant
WALLACE <> 0431	Tab, Peach, Cap Shaped, Scored	Felbamate 600 mg	Felbatol by Wallace	00037-0431	Anticonvulsant
WALLACE <> 0431	Tab, Peach, Oblong, Scored	Felbamate 600 mg	Felbatol by Hoffmann La Roche	00004-6200	Anticonvulsant
WALLACE <> 371001	Tab, White, Round, Scored, Wallace <> 37-1001	Meprobamate 400 mg	Miltown by Wallace	00037-1001	Sedative/Hypnotic; C IV
WALLACE <> 371101	Tab, White, Round, Sugar Coated, Wallace 37-1101	Meprobamate 200 mg	Miltown by Wallace	00037-1101	Sedative/Hypnotic; C IV
WALLACE <> 374401	Tab, White, Oval, Scored, 37 over 4401	Penicillamine 250 mg	Depen Titratable by Wallace	00037-4401	Chelating Agent
WALLACE0430	Tab, Yellow, Oval	Felbamate 400 mg	Felbatol by Wallace		Anticonvulsant
WALLACE0640	Tab, Mauve, Cap Shaped, Scored	Carbetapentane Tannate 60 mg, Chlorpheniramine Tannate 5 mg, Phenylephrine Tannate 10 mg	Tussi-12 by Wallace	00037-0640	Cold Remedy
WALLACE0640	Tab, Purple, Oblong, Scored	Carbetapentane Tannate 60 mg, Chlorpheniramine Tannate 5 mg, Phenylephrine Tannate 10 mg	by Allscripts		Cold Remedy
WALLACE0692	Tab, Pink, Cap Shaped, Scored	Carbetapentane 60 mg, Pyrilamine 40 mg, Phenylephrine 10 mg	Tussi by MedPointe	00037-0692	Cold Remedy
WALLACE153	Tab, Peach, Rectangular	Methyclothiazide 5 mg	Aquatensen by Wallace	00037-0153	Diuretic; Antihypertensive
WALLACE2103 <> SOMAC	Tab, Yellow & Light Orange, Round, Wallace 2103 <> Soma C	Aspirin 325 mg, Carisoprodol 200 mg	Soma Compound by Wallace	00037-2103	Analgesic; Muscle Relaxant
WALLACE24 <> SOMACC	Tab	Aspirin 325 mg, Carisoprodol 200 mg, Codeine Phosphate 16 mg	Soma Compound w/ Codeine by Pharmedix	53002-0124	Analgesic; C III
WALLACE2403 <> SOMACC	Tab, White & Yellow, Oval	Aspirin 325 mg, Carisoprodol 200 mg, Codeine Phosphate 16 mg	Soma Compound w/ Codeine by Wallace	00037-2403	Analgesic; C III
WALLACE272	Tab, White, Round	Cryptenamine 2 mg, Methyclothiazide 2.5 mg	Diutensen by Wallace		Antihypertensive; Diuretic
WALLACE274	Tab, Pink & White, Round	Methyclothiazide 2.5 mg, Reserpine 0.1 mg	Diutensen-R by Wallace	00037-0274	Diuretic; Antihypertensive
WALLACE3001	Tab, Pink, Round	Meprobamate 400 mg, Benactyzine HCl 1 mg	Deprol by Wallace		Sedative/Hypnotic; C IV
WALLACE301	Tab, White, Round, Scored	Atropine Sulfate 0.025 mg, Hyoscyamine Sulfate 0.1286 mg, Phenobarbital 16 mg, Scopolamine Hydrobromide 0.0074 mg	Barbidonna by Wallace	00037-0301	Gastrointestinal; C IV
WALLACE311	Tab, Light Brown, Round, Scored	Atropine Sulfate 0.025 mg, Hyoscyamine Sulfate 0.1286 mg, Phenobarbital 32 mg, Scopolamine Hydrobromide 0.0074 mg	Barbidonna No. 2 by Wallace	00037-0311	Gastrointestinal; C IV
WALLACE370120	Tab, Orange & White, Cap Shaped, Wallace 37-0120	Aspirin 325 mg, Meprobamate 200 mg	Micrainin by Wallace	00037-0120	Analgesic; C IV
WALLACE371001	Tab, White, Round	Meprobamate 400 mg	Miltown by Wallace	00037-1001	Sedative/Hypnotic; C IV
WALLACE371101	Tab, White, Round	Meprobamate 200 mg	Miltown by Wallace	00037-1101	Sedative/Hypnotic; C IV
WALLACE371601 <> 600	Tab, Wallace over 37-1601	Meprobamate 600 mg	Miltown by Wallace	00037-1601	Sedative/Hypnotic; C IV
WALLACE472	Tab, White, Round	Potassium Iodide 130 mg	Thyro-Block by Wallace	00037-0472	Antithyroid
WALLACE521	Tab, White, Rectangular, Scored	Dyphylline 200 mg	Lufyllin by Wallace	00037-0521	Antiasthmatic
WALLACE541	Tab, Light Yellow, Round, Scored	Dyphylline 200 mg, Guaifenesin 200 mg	Lufyllin-GG by Wallace	00037-0541	Antiasthmatic; Expectorant
WALLACE561	Tab, Pink, Round, Scored	Dyphylline 100 mg, Ephedrine HCl 16 mg, Guaifenesin 200 mg, Phenobarbital 16 mg	Lufyllin-EPG by Wallace	00037-0561	Antiasthmatic; Antiasthmatic; Expectorant; C IV
WALLACE713	Tab	Chlorpheniramine 8 mg, Phenylephrine 25 mg, Pyrilamine 25 mg	Rynatan by Leiner	59606-0732	Cold Remedy
WALLACE713	Tab, Buff	Chlorpheniramine Tannate 8 mg, Phenylephrine Tannate 25 mg, Pyrilamine Tannate 25 mg	by Amerisource	62584-0713	Cold Remedy
WALLACE713	Tab	Chlorpheniramine Tannate 8 mg, Phenylephrine 25 mg, Pyrilamine 25 mg	Rynatan by Wallace	00037-0713	Cold Remedy
WALLACE713	Tab	Chlorpheniramine Tannate 8 mg, Phenylephrine Tannate 25 mg, Pyrilamine Tannate 25 mg	by Nat Pharmpak	55154-4105	Cold Remedy
WALLACE713	Tab	Chlorpheniramine Tannate 8 mg, Phenylephrine Tannate 25 mg, Pyrilamine Tannate 25 mg	by Caremark	00339-5495	Cold Remedy
WALLACE717	Tab, Mauve, Cap Shaped, Scored	Carbetapentane Tannate 60 mg, Chlorpheniramine Tannate 5 mg, Ephedrine Tannate 10 mg, Phenylephrine Tannate 10 mg	Rynatuss by Wallace	00037-0717	Cold Remedy

ID FRONT <> BACK	DESCRIPTION FRONT <> BACK	INGREDIENT & STRENGTH	BRAND (or Generic Equiv.) by FIRM	NDC#	CLASS; SCH.
WALLACE731	Tab, White, Cap Shaped, Scored	Dyphylline 400 mg	Lufyllin-400 by Wallace	00037-0731	Antiasthmatic
WAR1	Tab, Pink, Oval, Scored	Warfarin Sodium 1 mg	Coumadin by Zydus	68382-0052	Anticoagulant
WAR1	Tab, Pink, Oval	Warfarin Sodium 1 mg	Coumadin by Mallinckrodt	00406-2052	Anticoagulant
WAR1 <> APO	Tab, Pink, Round, Scored, WAR / 1	Warfarin Sodium 1 mg	Apo Warfarin by Apotex	Canadian DIN 02242924	Anticoagulant
WAR10	Tab, White to Off-White, Oval, Scored	Warfarin Sodium 10 mg	Coumadin by Zydus	68382-0059	Anticoagulant
WAR10	Tab, Off White, Oval	Warfarin Sodium 10 mg	Coumadin by Mallinckrodt	00406-2059	Anticoagulant
WAR10 <> APO	Tab, White, Round, Scored, WAR / 10	Warfarin Sodium 10 mg	Apo Warfarin by Apotex	Canadian DIN 02242929	Anticoagulant
WAR2	Tab, Lavender, Oval, Scored	Warfarin Sodium 2 mg	Coumadin by Zydus	68382-0053	Anticoagulant
WAR2	Tab, Lavender, Oval	Warfarin Sodium 2 mg	Coumadin by Mallinckrodt	00406-2053	Anticoagulant
WAR2 <> APO	Tab, Lavender, Round, Scored, WAR / 2	Warfarin Sodium 2 mg	Apo Warfarin by Apotex	Canadian DIN 02242925	Anticoagulant
WAR212	Tab, Green, Oval, Scored, 2 1/2	Warfarin Sodium 2.5 mg	Coumadin by Zydus	68382-0064	Anticoagulant
WAR212	Tab, Green, Oval	Warfarin Sodium 2.5 mg	Coumadin by Mallinckrodt	00406-2064	Anticoagulant
WAR25 <> APO	Tab, Green, Round, Scored, WAR / 2.5	Warfarin Sodium 2.5 mg	Apo Warfarin by Apotex	Canadian DIN 02242926	Anticoagulant
WAR3	Tab, Tan, Oval, Scored	Warfarin Sodium 3 mg	Coumadin by Zydus	68382-0054	Anticoagulant
WAR3	Tab, Tan, Oval	Warfarin Sodium 3 mg	Coumadin by Mallinckrodt	00406-2054	Anticoagulant
WAR3 <> APO	Tab, Tan, Round, Scored, WAR / 3	Warfarin Sodium 3 mg	Apo Warfarin by Apotex	Canadian DIN 02245618	Anticoagulant
WAR4	Tab, Blue, Oval, Scored	Warfarin Sodium 4 mg	Coumadin by Zydus	68382-0055	Anticoagulant
WAR4	Tab, Blue, Oval	Warfarin Sodium 4 mg	Coumadin by Mallinckrodt	00406-2055	Anticoagulant
WAR4 <> APO	Tab, Blue, Round, Scored, WAR / 4	Warfarin Sodium 4 mg	Apo Warfarin by Apotex	Canadian DIN 02242927	Anticoagulant
WAR5	Tab, Peach, Oval, Scored	Warfarin Sodium 5 mg	Coumadin by Zydus	68382-0056	Anticoagulant
WAR5	Tab, Peach, Oval	Warfarin Sodium 5 mg	Coumadin by Mallinckrodt	00406-2056	Anticoagulant
WAR5 <> APO	Tab, Round, Peach, Scored, WAR / 5	Warfarin Sodium 5 mg	Apo Warfarin by Apotex	Canadian DIN 02242928	Anticoagulant
WAR6	Tab, Teal, Oval, Scored	Warfarin Sodium 6 mg	Coumadin by Zydus	68382-0057	Anticoagulant
WAR6	Tab, Teal, Oval	Warfarin Sodium 6 mg	Coumadin by Mallinckrodt	00406-2057	Anticoagulant
WAR712	Tab, Yellow, Oval, Scored, 7 1/2	Warfarin Sodium 7.5 mg	Coumadin by Zydus	68382-0058	Anticoagulant
WAR712	Tab, Yellow, Oval	Warfarin Sodium 7.5 mg	Coumadin by Mallinckrodt	00406-2058	Anticoagulant
WARFARIN1 <> N	Tab, Dark Pink, Round, Scored	Warfarin 1 mg	Coumadin by Novopharm	Canadian DIN 02265273	Anticoagulant
WARFARIN1 <> TARO	Tab, Pink, Round, Scored	Warfarin Sodium 1 mg	Coumadin by Taro	Canadian DIN 02242680	Anticoagulant
WARFARIN10 <> TARO	Tab, White, Round, Scored	Warfarin Sodium 10 mg	Coumadin by Taro	Canadian DIN 02242687	Anticoagulant
WARFARIN2 <> N	Tab, Lavender, Round, Scored	Warfarin 2 mg	Coumadin by Novopharm	Canadian DIN 02265281	Anticoagulant
WARFARIN2 <> TARO	Tab, Purple, Round, Scored	Warfarin Sodium 2 mg	Coumadin by Taro	Canadian DIN 02242681	Anticoagulant
WARFARIN212 <> N	Tab, Light Green, Round, Scored, 2 1/2	Warfarin 2.5 mg	Coumadin by Novopharm	Canadian DIN 02265303	Anticoagulant
WARFARIN212 <> TARO	Tab, Turquoise, Round, Scored, WARFARIN 2 1/2	Warfarin Sodium 2.5 mg	Coumadin by Taro	Canadian DIN 02242682	Anticoagulant
WARFARIN3 <> N	Tab, Light Brown, Round, Scored	Warfarin 3 mg	Coumadin by Novopharm	Canadian DIN 02265311	Anticoagulant
WARFARIN3 <> TARO	Tab, Light Pink, Round, Scored	Warfarin Sodium 3 mg	Coumadin by Taro	Canadian DIN 02242683	Anticoagulant

ID FRONT <> BACK	DESCRIPTION FRONT <> BACK	INGREDIENT & STRENGTH	BRAND (or Generic Equiv.) by FIRM	NDC#	CLASS; SCH.
WARFARIN4 <> N	Tab, Blue, Round, Scored	Warfarin 4 mg	Coumadin by Novopharm	Canadian DIN 02265338	Anticoagulant
WARFARIN4 <> TARO	Tab, Blue, Round, Scored	Warfarin Sodium 4 mg	Coumadin by Taro	Canadian DIN 02242684	Anticoagulant
WARFARIN5 <> N	Tab, Tan, Round, Scored	Warfarin 5 mg	Coumadin by Novopharm	Canadian DIN 02265346	Anticoagulant
WARFARIN5 <> TARO	Tab, Light Pink, Round, Scored	Warfarin Sodium 5 mg	Coumadin by Taro	Canadian DIN 02242685	Anticoagulant
WARFARIN6 <> TARO	Tab, Green, Round, Scored	Warfarin Sodium 6 mg	Coumadin by Taro	Canadian DIN 02242686	Anticoagulant
WARFARIN712 <> TARO	Tab, Yellow, Round, Scored, 7 1/2	Warfarin Sodium 7.5 mg	Coumadin by Taro	Canadian DIN 02242697	Anticoagulant
WARFARINTARO <> 1	Tab, Light Pink, Cap Shaped	Warfarin Sodium 1 mg	Coumadin by Taro	51672-4027	Anticoagulant
WARFARINTARO <> 10	Tab, White, Cap Shaped	Warfarin Sodium 10 mg	Coumadin by Taro	51672-4035	Anticoagulant
WARFARINTARO <> 2	Tab, Lavender, Cap Shaped	Warfarin Sodium 2 mg	Coumadin by Taro	51672-4028	Anticoagulant
WARFARINTARO <> 212	Tab, Green, Cap Shaped, 2 1/2	Warfarin Sodium 2.5 mg	Coumadin by Taro	51672-4029	Anticoagulant
WARFARINTARO <> 3	Tab, Tan, Cap Shaped	Warfarin Sodium 3 mg	Coumadin by Taro	51672-4030	Anticoagulant
WARFARINTARO <> 4	Tab, Blue, Cap Shaped	Warfarin Sodium 4 mg	Coumadin by Taro	51672-4031	Anticoagulant
WARFARINTARO <> 5	Tab, Peach, Cap Shaped	Warfarin Sodium 5 mg	Coumadin by Taro	51672-4032	Anticoagulant
WARFARINTARO <> 6	Tab, Teal, Cap Shaped	Warfarin Sodium 6 mg	Coumadin by Taro	51672-4033	Anticoagulant
WARFARINTARO <> 712	Tab, Yellow, Cap Shaped, 7 1/2	Warfarin Sodium 7.5 mg	Coumadin by Taro	51672-4034	Anticoagulant
WARRICK <> 1520	Tab, White, Round, Scored	Albuterol Sulfate 2 mg	Proventil by Allscripts		Antiasthmatic
WARRICK <> 1520	Tab, White, Round, Scored	Albuterol Sulfate 2 mg	Proventil by Southwood	58016-0473	Antiasthmatic
WARRICK1520	Tab, White, Round	Albuterol Sulfate 2 mg	Proventil by Warrick		Antiasthmatic
WARRICK1530	Tab, White, Round	Albuterol Sulfate 4 mg	Proventil by Warrick		Antiasthmatic
WARRICK1620	Tab, White, Round, Scored, Ultramicrosize	Griseofulvin, Ultramicrosize 125 mg	Fulvicin P/G by Martec	52555-0583	Antifungal
WARRICK1620	Tab, White, Round	Griseofulvin, Ultramicrosize 125 mg	Fulvicin P/G by Warrick		Antifungal
WARRICK1621	Tab, White, Round, Scored, Ultramicrosize	Griseofulvin, Ultramicrosize 250 mg	Fulvicin P/G by Martec	52555-0584	Antifungal
WARRICK1624	Tab, Off-White, Oval, Scored, Ultramicrosize	Griseofulvin, Ultramicrosize 330 mg	Fulvicin P/G by Martec	52555-0585	Antifungal
WARRICK1624	Tab, Off-White, Oval	Griseofulvin, Ultramicrosize 330 mg	Fulvicin P/G by Warrick		Antifungal
WARRICK16421	Tab, White, Round	Griseofulvin, Ultramicrosize 250 mg	Fulvicin P/G by Warrick		Antifungal
WARRICK1648	Tab, White, Round	Griseofulvin 250 mg	Fulvicin P/G by Warrick	59930-1648	Antifungal
WARRICK1649	Tab, White, Round	Griseofulvin 500 mg	Fulvicin P/G by Warrick	59930-1649	Antifungal
WARRICK1653 <> 300	Tab, Blue, Round	Labetalol 300 mg	Normodyne by Warrick		Antihypertensive
WARRICK1670	Tab, Ex Release	Theophylline Anhydrous 300 mg	by Repack Co of America	55306-1670	Antiasthmatic
WATSON	Tab	Furosemide 40 mg	by URL Mutual	00677-0659	Diuretic
WATSON	Tab, Peach, Round	Desipramine HCl 100 mg	by Blue Ridge	59273-0012	Antidepressant
WATSON	Tab, Peach, Round	Desipramine HCl 25 mg	by Blue Ridge	59273-0009	Antidepressant
WATSON	Tab, Peach, Round	Desipramine HCl 50 mg	by Blue Ridge	59273-0010	Antidepressant
WATSON <> 12530	Tab, Pink, Round	Ethinyl Estradiol 0.03 mg, Levonorgestrel 0.125 mg	Trivora-28 by Watson	52544-0291	Oral Contraceptive
WATSON <> 12530	Tab, Pink, Round	Ethinyl Estradiol 0.03 mg, Levonorgestrel 0.125 mg	Trivora-28 by Murfreesboro	51129-1632	Oral Contraceptive
WATSON <> 1530	Tab, White, Round	Ethinyl Estradiol 0.03 mg, Levonorgestrel 0.15 mg	Levora by Watson	52544-0279	Oral Contraceptive
WATSON <> 235	Tab, Yellow	Norethindrone 0.35 mg	Aygestin by Watson	52544-0235	Hormone
WATSON <> 24005	Tab, White, Round, Scored, 240 over 0.5	Lorazepam 0.5 mg	Ativan by Watson	00591-0240	Antianxiety; C IV
WATSON <> 24005	Tab, White, Round, Scored, 240 over 0.5	Lorazepam 0.5 mg	Ativan by Watson	52544-0240	Antianxiety; C IV
WATSON <> 2411	Tab, White, Round, Scored, 241 over 1	Lorazepam 1 mg	Ativan by Watson	52544-0241	Antianxiety; C IV
WATSON <> 2411	Tab, White, Round, Scored, 241 over 1	Lorazepam 1 mg	Ativan by Watson	00591-0241	Antianxiety; C IV
WATSON <> 2422	Tab, White, Round, Scored, 242 over 2	Lorazepam 2 mg	Ativan by Watson	52544-0242	Antianxiety; C IV
WATSON <> 2422	Tab, White, Round, Scored, 242 over 2	Lorazepam 2 mg	Ativan by Watson	00591-0242	Antianxiety; C IV

ID FRONT <> BACK	DESCRIPTION FRONT <> BACK	INGREDIENT & STRENGTH	BRAND (or Generic Equiv.), by FIRM	NDC#	CLASS; SCH.
WATSON <> 243	Tab, Light Blue, Round	Norethindrone 0.5 mg, Ethinyl Estradiol 0.035 mg	Leena by Watson	52544-0219	Oral Contraceptive
WATSON <> 244	Tab, Yellowish Green, Round	Norethindrone 1 mg, Ethinyl Estradiol 0.035 mg	Leena by Watson	52544-0219	Oral Contraceptive
WATSON <> 254	Tab, Blue, Round	Norethindrone 0.5 mg, Ethinyl Estradiol 0.035 mg	Tri-Norinyl by Watson	52544-0274	Oral Contraceptive
WATSON <> 254	Tab, Blue, Round	Norethindrone 0.5 mg, Ethinyl Estradiol 0.035 mg	Brevicon by Watson	52544-0254	Oral Contraceptive
WATSON <> 25650	Tab, Light Aqua, Cap Shaped, Watson <> 25/650	Pentazocine HCl 25 mg, Acetaminophen 650 mg	Talacen by Watson	52544-0396	Analgesic; C IV
WATSON <> 259	Tab, Yellowish Green, Round	Norethindrone 1 mg, Ethinyl Estradiol 0.035 mg	Norinyl 1+35 28 by Watson	52544-0259	Oral Contraceptive
WATSON <> 259	Tab, Yellowish Green, Round	Norethindrone 1 mg, Ethinyl Estradiol 0.035 mg	Tri-Norinyl by Watson	52544-0274	Oral Contraceptive
WATSON <> 265	Tab, White, Round	Norethindrone 1 mg, Mestranol 0.05 mg	Norinyl 1+50 28 by Watson	52544-0265	Oral Contraceptive
WATSON <> 301	Tab, White, Round	Furosemide 40 mg	Lasix by Allscripts		Diuretic
WATSON <> 311	Tab	Furosemide 20 mg	Lasix by DRX	55045-1553	Diuretic
WATSON <> 311	Tab	Furosemide 20 mg	Lasix by Major	00904-1580	Diuretic
WATSON <> 311	Tab	Furosemide 20 mg	Lasix by Watson	52544-0311	Diuretic
WATSON <> 311	Tab	Furosemide 20 mg	Lasix by Golden State	60429-0078	Diuretic
WATSON <> 311	Tab	Furosemide 20 mg	Lasix by Macnary	55982-0010	Diuretic
WATSON <> 3202	Tab, White, Orange Specks, Cap Shaped, Bisected	Hydrocodone 5 mg, Acetaminophen 325 mg	Norco by Watson	00591-3202	Analgesic; C III
WATSON <> 3256	Tab, White, Round	Cyclobenzaprine HCl 5 mg	Flexeril by Watson	00591-3256	Muscle Relaxant
WATSON <> 33205	Tab, White, Round, Scored	Lorazepam 0.5 mg	Ativan by Murfreesboro		Antianxiety; C IV
WATSON <> 33310	Tab, Watson <> 333 1.0	Lorazepam 1 mg	Ativan by Watson	51129-1410	Antianxiety; C IV
WATSON <> 3369	Tab, White, Round, Scored	Butalbital 50 mg, Acetaminophen 325 mg, Caffeine 40 mg	Fioricet by Watson	00591-3369 Discontinued	Analgesic
WATSON <> 3436	Tab, White, Oval	Furosemide 20 mg	Lasix by Watson	00591-3436	Diuretic
WATSON <> 3494	Tab, White, Cap Shaped, Scored, 34 / 94	Oxycodone 5 mg, Ibuprofen 400 mg	Combunox by Watson	00591-3494	Analgesic; NSAID; C II
WATSON <> 3955005	Tab, Green, Cap Shaped, Scored, 50 0.5	Naloxone HCl 0.5 mg, Pentazocine HCl 50 mg	Talwin NX by Watson	00591-0395	Analgesic; C IV
WATSON <> 3955005	Tab, Green, Cap Shaped, Scored	Pentazocine HCl 50 mg, Naloxone HCl 0.5 mg	Talwin by Watson	52544-0395	Analgesic; C IV
WATSON <> 39625650	Tab, Light Aqua, Cap Shaped, Scored	Pentazocine HCl 25 mg, Acetaminophen 650 mg	Talacen by Watson	00591-0396	Analgesic; C IV
WATSON <> 405	Tab, White, Round	Lisinopril 2.5 mg	Prinivil by Watson	00591-0405	Antihypertensive
WATSON <> 406	Tab, White, Cap Shaped	Lisinopril 5 mg	Prinivil by Watson	00591-0406	Antihypertensive
WATSON <> 418	Tab, White, Round, Film Coated	Cyclobenzaprine HCl 10 mg	Flexeril by Watson	52544-0418	Muscle Relaxant
WATSON <> 418	Tab, White, Round, Film Coated	Cyclobenzaprine HCl 10 mg	Flexeril by Apotheca	12634-0528	Muscle Relaxant
WATSON <> 418	Tab, White, Round, Film Coated	Cyclobenzaprine HCl 10 mg	Flexeril by DHHS Prog	11819-0069	Muscle Relaxant
WATSON <> 418	Tab, White, Round, Film Coated	Cyclobenzaprine HCl 10 mg	Flexeril by Prepackage Specialists	58864-0128	Muscle Relaxant
WATSON <> 454	Tab, Orange, Oblong	Gemfibrozil 600 mg	Lopid by Watson	00591-0454	Antihyperlipidemic
WATSON <> 466	Tab, White, Round	Tramadol HCl 50 mg	Ultram by Watson	00591-0466	Analgesic
WATSON <> 5030	Tab, Blue, Round	Ethinyl Estradiol 0.03 mg, Levonorgestrel 0.05 mg	Trivora-28 by Watson	52544-0291	Oral Contraceptive
WATSON <> 5030	Tab, Blue, Round	Ethinyl Estradiol 0.03 mg, Levonorgestrel 0.05 mg	Trivora-28 by Murfreesboro	51129-1631	Oral Contraceptive
WATSON <> 507	Tab, Light Yellow, Round	Ethinyl Estradiol 0.035 mg, Norethindrone 0.5 mg	Necon 0.5 35 21 by Watson	52544-0507	Oral Contraceptive
WATSON <> 507	Tab, Light Yellow, Round	Ethinyl Estradiol 0.035 mg, Norethindrone 0.5 mg	Necon 0.5 35 21 by Watson	52544-0507	Oral Contraceptive
WATSON <> 507	Tab, Light Yellow, Round	Ethinyl Estradiol 0.035 mg, Norethindrone 0.5 mg	Necon 0.5 35 28 by Watson	52544-0550	Oral Contraceptive
WATSON <> 507	Tab, Light Yellow, Round	Ethinyl Estradiol 0.035 mg, Norethindrone 0.5 mg	Necon 1 10/11-21 by Watson	52544-0553	Oral Contraceptive
WATSON <> 507	Tab, Light Yellow, Round	Ethinyl Estradiol 0.035 mg, Norethindrone 0.5 mg	Necon 1 10/11-28 by Watson	52544-0554	Oral Contraceptive
WATSON <> 508	Tab, Dark Yellow, Round	Ethinyl Estradiol 0.035 mg, Norethindrone 1 mg	Necon 1 10/11-28 by Watson	52544-0554	Oral Contraceptive
WATSON <> 508	Tab, Dark Yellow, Round	Ethinyl Estradiol 0.035 mg, Norethindrone 1 mg	Necon 1 10/11-21 by Watson	52544-0553	Oral Contraceptive
WATSON <> 508	Tab, Dark Yellow, Round	Ethinyl Estradiol 0.035 mg, Norethindrone 1 mg	Necon 1 35 21 by Watson	52544-0508	Oral Contraceptive
WATSON <> 508	Tab, Dark Yellow, Round	Ethinyl Estradiol 0.035 mg, Norethindrone 1 mg	Necon 1 35 28 by Watson	52544-0552	Oral Contraceptive
WATSON <> 510	Tab, Light Blue, Round	Norethindrone 1 mg, Mestranol 0.05 mg	Necon 1 50 21 by Watson	52544-0510	Oral Contraceptive
WATSON <> 510	Tab, Light Blue, Round	Norethindrone 1 mg, Mestranol 0.05 mg	Necon 1 50 28 by Watson	52544-0556	Oral Contraceptive
WATSON <> 510	Tab, Light Blue, Round	Norethindrone 1 mg, Mestranol 0.05 mg	Necon 1 50 21 by PDRX	55289-0379	Oral Contraceptive
WATSON <> 510	Tab, Light Blue, Round	Norethindrone 1 mg, Mestranol 0.05 mg	Necon 1 50 21 by DRX	55045-2722	Oral Contraceptive
WATSON <> 524	Tab, White, Round	Norgestimate 0.180 mg, Ethinyl Estradiol 0.035 mg	TriNessa by Watson	52544-0935	Oral Contraceptive
WATSON <> 525	Tab, Light Blue, Round	Norgestimate 0.215 mg, Ethinyl Estradiol 0.035 mg	TriNessa by Watson	52544-0935	Oral Contraceptive

ID FRONT <> BACK	DESCRIPTION FRONT <> BACK	INGREDIENT & STRENGTH	BRAND (or Generic Equiv.) by FIRM	NDC#	CLASS; SCH.
WATSON <> 526	Tab, Blue, Round	Norgestimate 0.250 mg, Ethinyl Estradiol 0.035 mg	TriNessa by Watson	52544-0935	Oral Contraceptive
WATSON <> 526	Tab, Blue, Round	Norgestimate 0.250 mg, Ethinyl Estradiol 0.035 mg	Mononessa by Watson	52544-0526	Oral Contraceptive
WATSON <> 657	Tab, White, Oval, Scored	Buspirone HCl 5 mg	BuSpar by Watson	00591-0657	Antianxiety
WATSON <> 658	Tab, White, Oval, Scored	Buspirone HCl 10 mg	BuSpar by Watson	00591-0658	Antianxiety
WATSON <> 667400	Tab, Watson <> 667 over 400	Etodolac 400 mg	Lodine by Major	00904-5246	NSAID
WATSON <> 667400	Tab, Watson <> 667 over 400	Etodolac 400 mg	Lodine by Watson	52544-0667	NSAID
WATSON <> 667400	Tab, Watson <> 667 over 400	Etodolac 400 mg	Lodine by Qualitest	00603-3570	NSAID
WATSON <> 682025	Tab, White, Oval, Scored, Watson <> 682 0.25	Alprazolam 0.25 mg	Xanax by Allscripts		Antianxiety; C IV
WATSON <> 68305	Tab, Peach, Oval, Scored	Alprazolam 0.5 mg	Xanax by Allscripts		Antianxiety; C IV
WATSON <> 68410	Tab, Blue, Oval, Scored, Watson <> 684-1.0	Alprazolam 1 mg	Xanax by Allscripts		Antianxiety; C IV
WATSON <> 685550	Tab, Peach, Round, 685 over 5-50	Amiloride HCl 5 mg, Hydrochlorothiazide 50 mg	Moduretic by Major	00904-2114	Antihypertensive; Diuretic
WATSON <> 685550	Tab, Peach, Round, 685 over 5-50	Amiloride HCl 5 mg, Hydrochlorothiazide 50 mg	Moduretic by Qualitest	00603-2188	Antihypertensive; Diuretic
WATSON <> 685550	Tab, Peach, Round, 685 over 5-50	Amiloride HCl 5 mg, Hydrochlorothiazide 50 mg	Moduretic by Watson	52544-0685	Antihypertensive; Diuretic
WATSON <> 68610	Tab, White, Oval, Scored, 686 over 10	Baclofen 10 mg	Lioresal by Watson	52544-0686	Muscle Relaxant
WATSON <> 68610	Tab, White, Oval, Scored, 686 over 10	Baclofen 10 mg	Lioresal by Major	00904-5216	Muscle Relaxant
WATSON <> 68610	Tab, White, Oval, Scored, 686 over 10	Baclofen 10 mg	Lioresal by Moore	00839-7472	Muscle Relaxant
WATSON <> 68610	Tab, White, Oval, Scored, 686 over 10	Baclofen 10 mg	Lioresal by DRX	55045-2724	Muscle Relaxant
WATSON <> 68610	Tab, White, Oval, Scored, 686 over 10	Baclofen 10 mg	Lioresal by Supremus	62114-0120	Muscle Relaxant
WATSON <> 68610	Tab, White, Oval, Scored, 686 over 10	Baclofen 10 mg	Lioresal by Murfreesboro	51129-1409	Muscle Relaxant
WATSON <> 68720	Tab, White, Oval, Scored, 687/20 <> Watson	Baclofen 20 mg	Lioresal by Supremus	62114-0122	Muscle Relaxant
WATSON <> 68720	Tab, White, Oval, Scored, 687/20 <> Watson	Baclofen 20 mg	Lioresal by Watson	52544-0687	Muscle Relaxant
WATSON <> 68720	Tab, White, Oval, Scored, 687/20 <> Watson	Baclofen 20 mg	Lioresal by Major		Muscle Relaxant
WATSON <> 688125	Tab, White, Oblong, Scored, 688 12.5	Captopril 12.5 mg	Capoten by Qualitest	00603-2555	Antihypertensive
WATSON <> 688125	Tab, White, Oblong, Scored, 688 12.5	Captopril 12.5 mg	Capoten by Watson	52544-0688	Antihypertensive
WATSON <> 688125	Tab, White, Oblong, Scored, 688 12.5	Captopril 12.5 mg	Capoten by Major		Antihypertensive
WATSON <> 68925	Tab	Captopril 25 mg	Capoten by Qualitest	00603-2556	Antihypertensive
WATSON <> 68925	Tab	Captopril 25 mg	Capoten by Watson	52544-0689	Antihypertensive
WATSON <> 69050	Tab	Captopril 50 mg	Capoten by Major		Antihypertensive
WATSON <> 69050	Tab, Football Shaped	Captopril 50 mg	Capoten by Watson	52544-0690	Antihypertensive
WATSON <> 69050	Tab	Captopril 50 mg	Capoten by Qualitest	00603-2557	Antihypertensive
WATSON <> 691	Tab	Captopril 100 mg	Capoten by Major	00904-5048	Antihypertensive
WATSON <> 691100	Tab	Captopril 100 mg	Capoten by Watson	52544-0691	Antihypertensive
WATSON <> 693500	Tab, Green, Cap Shaped, Scored	Chlorzoxazone 500 mg	by Watson	52544-0693	Muscle Relaxant
WATSON <> 693500	Tab	Chlorzoxazone 500 mg	by Martec	52555-0263	Muscle Relaxant
WATSON <> 693500	Tab, Green, Cap Shaped, Scored	Chlorzoxazone 500 mg	by Major	00904-0302	Muscle Relaxant
WATSON <> 693500	Tab, Green, Cap Shaped, Scored	Chlorzoxazone 500 mg	by Allscripts		Muscle Relaxant
WATSON <> 698200	Tab, White, Oval, Scored	Hydroxychloroquine Sulfate 200 mg	Plaquenil by Watson	00591-0698	Antimalarial
WATSON <> 698200	Tab, White, Oval, Scored	Hydroxychloroquine Sulfate 200 mg	Plaquenil by Moore	00839-7963	Antimalarial
WATSON <> 698200	Tab, White, Oval, Scored	Hydroxychloroquine Sulfate 200 mg	Plaquenil by Major	00904-5107	Antimalarial
WATSON <> 698200	Tab, White, Oval, Scored	Hydroxychloroquine Sulfate 200 mg	Plaquenil by Qualitest	00603-3944	Antimalarial
WATSON <> 69910	Tab, Orange, Round, Film Coated	Hydroxyzine HCl 10 mg	Atarax by Watson	52544-0699	Antianxiety; Antihistamine
WATSON <> 70025	Tab, Green, Round, Film Coated	Hydroxyzine HCl 25 mg	Atarax by Watson	52544-0700	Antianxiety; Antihistamine
WATSON <> 70450	Tab, Yellow, Round, Film Coated	Hydroxyzine HCl 50 mg	Atarax by Watson	52544-0704	Antianxiety; Antihistamine
WATSON <> 706210	Tab, Blue, Round	Perphenazine 2 mg, Amitriptyline HCl 10 mg	Etrafon by Watson	52544-0706	Antipsychotic; Antidepressant
WATSON <> 707225	Tab, Orange, Round	Amitriptyline 25 mg, Perphenazine 2 mg	Triavil by Major	00904-1825	Antidepressant; Antipsychotic

ID FRONT <> BACK	DESCRIPTION FRONT <> BACK	INGREDIENT & STRENGTH	BRAND (or Generic Equiv.) by FIRM	NDC#	CLASS; SCH.
WATSON <> 707225	Tab, Orange, Round	Amitriptyline 25 mg, Perphenazine 2 mg	Triavil by Watson	52544-0707	Antidepressant; Antipsychotic
WATSON <> 708410	Tab, Beige, Round	Perphenazine 4 mg, Amitriptyline HCl 10 mg	Etrafon by Watson	52544-0708	Antipsychotic; Antidepressant
WATSON <> 709425	Tab, Yellow, Round	Perphenazine 4 mg, Amitriptyline HCl 25 mg	Etrafon by Watson	52544-0709	Antipsychotic; Antidepressant
WATSON <> 7105	Tab, Watson <> 710 over 5	Pindolol 5 mg	Visken by Qualitest	00603-5220	Antihypertensive
WATSON <> 7105	Tab, Watson <> 710 over 5	Pindolol 5 mg	Visken by Major	00904-7893	Antihypertensive
WATSON <> 7105	Tab, Watson <> 710 over 5	Pindolol 5 mg	Visken by Moore	00839-7761	Antihypertensive
WATSON <> 7105	Tab, White, Round	Pindolol 5 mg	Visken by Watson	52544-0710	Antihypertensive
WATSON <> 71110	Tab, White, Round	Pindolol 10 mg	Visken by Watson	52544-0711	Antihypertensive
WATSON <> 71465650	Tab, Orange, Cap Shaped, Film Coated, 71465 over 650	Acetaminophen 650 mg, Propoxyphene HCl 65 mg	Wygesic by Watson	00591-0714	Analgesic; C IV
WATSON <> 71465650	Tab, Orange, Cap Shaped, Film Coated, 71465 over 650	Acetaminophen 650 mg, Propoxyphene HCl 65 mg	Wygesic by Qualitest	00603-5463	Analgesic; C IV
WATSON <> 715260	Tab, White, Round, 715 over 260	Quinine Sulfate 260 mg	Quinamm by RX Pak	65084-0143	Antimalarial
WATSON <> 715260	Tab, White, Round, 715 over 260	Quinine Sulfate 260 mg	Quinamm by Watson	00591-0715	Antimalarial
WATSON <> 71754	Tab, Watson <> 717 over 5.4	Yohimbine HCl 5.4 mg	by Watson	52544-0717	Impotence Agent
WATSON <> 72650	Tab, White, Round, 726 over 50	Meperidine 50 mg	Demerol by Watson	00591-0726	Analgesic; C II
WATSON <> 72650	Tab, White, Round, 726 over 50	Meperidine 50 mg	Demerol by Watson	52544-0726	Analgesic; C II
WATSON <> 727100	Tab, White, Round, 727 over 100	Meperidine 100 mg	Demerol by Watson	00591-0727	Analgesic; C II
WATSON <> 727100	Tab, White, Round, 727 over 100	Meperidine 100 mg	Demerol by Watson	52544-0727	Analgesic; C II
WATSON <> 728500	Tab, Blue, Oblong, Film Coated	Etodolac 500 mg	by Watson	52544-0728	NSAID
WATSON <> 7441	Tab, White, Diamond Shaped, Scored	Estazolam 1 mg	Prosom by Watson	00591-0744	Sedative/Hypnotic; C IV
WATSON <> 7452	Tab, Pink, Diamond Shaped, Scored, 745 on left of Score, 2 on right	Estazolam 2 mg	Prosom by Watson	00591-0745	Sedative/Hypnotic; C IV
WATSON <> 7540	Tab, White, Round	Ethinyl Estradiol 0.04 mg, Levonorgestrel 0.075 mg	Trivora-28 by Watson	52544-0291	Oral Contraceptive
WATSON <> 7540	Tab, White, Round	Ethinyl Estradiol 0.04 mg, Levonorgestrel 0.075 mg	Trivora-28 by Murfreesboro	51129-1633	Oral Contraceptive
WATSON <> 7711875	Tab, White, Round, Scored, Watson <> 771 over 18.75	Pemoline 18.75 mg	by Watson	52544-0771	Stimulant; C IV
WATSON <> 772375	Tab, Peach, Round, Scored, Watson <> 772 over 37.5	Pemoline 37.5 mg	by Watson	52544-0772	Stimulant; C IV
WATSON <> 7731875	Tab, Yellow, Round, Scored, Watson <> 773 over 18.75	Pemoline 75 mg	by Watson	52544-0773	Stimulant; C IV
WATSON <> 774	Tab, White, Round, Scored	Oxycodone HCl 5 mg	Percolone by Watson	52544-0774	Analgesic; C II
WATSON <> 784	Tab, White, Round	Carisoprodol 350 mg	Soma by Watson	52544-0784	Muscle Relaxant
WATSON <> 803	Tab, Yellow & White, Oval	Meclizine HCl 25 mg	Antivert by Watson	52544-0803	Antiemetic
WATSON <> 804	Tab, White, Round	Meprobamate 200 mg	Equanil by Watson	52544-0804	Sedative/Hypnotic; C IV
WATSON <> 805	Tab, White, Round	Meprobamate 400 mg	Equanil by Watson	52544-0805	Sedative/Hypnotic; C IV
WATSON <> 808	Tab, Yellow, Round	Desipramine HCl 25 mg	Norpramin by Watson	52544-0808	Antidepressant
WATSON <> 809	Tab, Green, Round	Desipramine HCl 50 mg	Norpramin by Watson	52544-0809	Antidepressant
WATSON <> 831	Tab, White, Round	Prednisone 10 mg	Merticorten by Watson	00591-0831	Steroid
WATSON <> 83675	Tab, Peach, Triangular, Scored, WATSON written down middle <> 836 / 7.5	Clorazepate Dipotassium 7.5 mg	Tranxene by Watson	52544-0836	Antianxiety; C IV
WATSON <> 83715	Tab, Purple, Triangular, Scored	Clorazepate Dipotassium 15 mg	Tranxene by Watson	52544-0837	Antianxiety; C IV
WATSON <> 847	Tab, White, Round	Norgestrel 0.3 mg, Ethinyl Estradiol 0.03 mg	Lo-Ogestrel by Watson	52544-0847	Oral Contraceptive
WATSON <> 848	Tab, White, Round	Norgestrel 0.5 mg, Ethinyl Estradiol 0.05 mg	Ogestrel by Watson	52544-0848	Oral Contraceptive
WATSON <> 892	Tab, Lime Green, Round	Norethindrone 0.35 mg	Jolivette by Watson	52544-0892	Oral Contraceptive
WATSON <> 913	Tab, White w/ Orange Specks, Cap Shaped, Scored	Acetaminophen 325 mg, Hydrocodone Bitartrate 5 mg	Norco by Watson	52544-0913	Analgesic; C III
WATSON <> 949	Tab, White, Round	Levonorgestrel 0.1 mg, Ethinyl Estradiol 0.02 mg	Lutera by Watson	52544-0949	Oral Contraceptive
WATSON <> 954	Tab, White, Round	Desogestrel 0.15 mg, Ethinyl Estradiol 0.03 mg	Ortho-Cept by Watson	52544-0954	Oral Contraceptive
WATSON <> 966	Tab, White, Round	Levonorgestrel 0.15 mg, Ethinyl Estradiol 0.03 mg	Quasense by Watson	52544-0966	Oral Contraceptive
WATSON <> P	Tab, Green, Round	Inert	Ortho-Cept by Watson	52544-0954	Oral Contraceptive; Placebo

ID FRONT <> BACK	DESCRIPTION FRONT <> BACK	INGREDIENT & STRENGTH	BRAND (or Generic Equiv.) by FIRM	NDC#	CLASS; SCH.
WATSON <> P	Tab, Green, Round	Inert	Necon 7/7/7 by Watson	52544-0936	Oral Contraceptive; Placebo
WATSON <> P	Tab, Green, Round	Inert	Mononessa by Watson	52544-0526	Oral Contraceptive; Placebo
WATSON <> P	Tab, Green, Round	Inert	TriNessa by Watson	52544-0935	Oral Contraceptive; Placebo
WATSON <> P	Tab, White, Round	Inert	Zovia 1/35 by PDRX	55289-0381	Oral Contraceptive; Placebo
WATSON <> P	Tab, White, Round	Inert	Zovia 1/35 by DRX	55045-2722	Oral Contraceptive; Placebo
WATSON <> P	Tab, White, Round	Inert	Zovia 1/35 by Watson	52544-0935	Oral Contraceptive; Placebo
WATSON <> P1	Tab, Orange, Round	Inert	Leena by Watson	52544-0219	Oral Contraceptive; Placebo
WATSON <> P1	Tab, Orange, Round	Inert	Tri-Norinyl by Watson	52544-0274	Oral Contraceptive; Placebo
WATSON <> P1	Tab, Orange, Round	Inert	Lutera by Watson	52544-0949	Oral Contraceptive; Placebo
WATSON <> P1	Tab, Orange, Round	Inert	Levora by Watson	52544-0279	Oral Contraceptive; Placebo
WATSON <> P1	Tab, Orange, Round	Inert	Lo-Ogestrel by Watson	52544-0847	Oral Contraceptive; Placebo
WATSON <> P1	Tab, Orange, Round	Inert	Quasense by Watson	52544-0966	Oral Contraceptive; Placebo
WATSON137	Cap, Aqua Blue & Light Blue	Selegiline 5 mg	Eldepryl by Watson	52544-0137	Antiparkinson
WATSON213	Tab, Blue, Round	Estropipate 3 mg	Ogen by Watson		Hormone
WATSON235	Tab, Yellow, Round, Watson/235	Norethindrone 0.35 mg	Nor-QD by Watson	52544-0235	Hormone
WATSON300	Tab, White, Round, Watson over 300	Furosemide 20 mg	Lasix by Schein	00378-0568	Diuretic
WATSON300	Tab, White, Round, Watson over 300	Furosemide 20 mg	Lasix by Kaiser	62224-1220	Diuretic
WATSON300	Tab, White, Round, Watson over 300	Furosemide 20 mg	Lasix by Golden State	60429-0078	Diuretic
WATSON300	Tab, White, Round, Watson over 300	Furosemide 20 mg	Lasix by Amerisource	62584-0709	Diuretic
WATSON300	Tab, White, Round, Watson over 300	Furosemide 20 mg	Lasix by Allscripts		Diuretic
WATSON300	Tab, White, Round, Watson over 300	Furosemide 20 mg	Lasix by Major	00904-1480	Diuretic
WATSON300	Tab, White, Round, Watson over 300	Furosemide 20 mg	Lasix by Watson	52544-0300	Diuretic
WATSON300	Tab, White, Round, Watson over 300	Furosemide 20 mg	Lasix by Kaiser	00179-0380	Diuretic
WATSON301	Tab, White, Round, Scored	Furosemide 40 mg	Lasix by Golden State	60429-0079	Diuretic
WATSON301	Tab, White, Round, Scored	Furosemide 40 mg	Lasix by Kaiser	62224-1222	Diuretic
WATSON301	Tab, White, Round, Scored	Furosemide 40 mg	Lasix by Macnary	55982-0011	Diuretic
WATSON301	Tab, White, Round, Scored	Furosemide 40 mg	Lasix by Amerisource	62584-0710	Diuretic
WATSON301	Tab, White, Round, Scored	Furosemide 40 mg	Lasix by Major	00904-1481	Diuretic
WATSON301	Tab, White, Round, Scored	Furosemide 40 mg	Lasix by Watson	52544-0301	Diuretic
WATSON301	Tab, White, Round, Scored	Furosemide 40 mg	Lasix by JB	51111-0479	Diuretic
WATSON301	Tab, White, Round, Scored	Furosemide 40 mg	Lasix by Kaiser	00179-0381	Diuretic
WATSON301	Tab, White, Round, Scored	Furosemide 80 mg	Lasix by Ivax	00182-1736	Diuretic
WATSON302	Tab, White, Round, Scored	Furosemide 80 mg	Lasix by Physician Total Care	54868-2180	Diuretic
WATSON302	Tab, White, Round, Scored	Furosemide 80 mg	Lasix by Watson	52544-0302	Diuretic
WATSON302	Tab, White, Round, Scored	Furosemide 80 mg	Lasix by URL Mutual	00677-0976	Diuretic
WATSON302	Tab, White, Round, Scored	Furosemide 80 mg	Lasix by Moore	00839-6777	Diuretic
WATSON302	Tab, White, Round, Scored	Furosemide 80 mg	Lasix by Major	00904-1482	Diuretic
WATSON302	Tab, White, Round, Scored	Furosemide 80 mg	Lasix by Murfreesboro	51129-1161	Diuretic
WATSON302	Tab, White, Round, Scored	Furosemide 80 mg	Lasix by Kaiser	00179-0382	Diuretic
WATSON302	Tab, White, Round, Scored	Furosemide 80 mg	Lasix by Amerisource	62584-0711	Diuretic

ID FRONT <> BACK	DESCRIPTION FRONT <> BACK	INGREDIENT & STRENGTH	BRAND (or Generic Equiv.) by FIRM	NDC#	CLASS; SCH.
WATSON303	Cap	Indomethacin 25 mg	Indocin by Warner Chilcott	00047-0887	NSAID
WATSON304	Cap	Indomethacin 50 mg	Indocin by Warner Chilcott	00047-0888	NSAID
WATSON305	Tab, White, Round, Scored	Propranolol HCl 10 mg	Inderal by Amerisource	62584-0842	Antihypertensive
WATSON305	Tab, White, Round, Scored	Propranolol HCl 10 mg	Inderal by Watson	52544-0305	Antihypertensive
WATSON306	Tab, White, Round, Scored	Propranolol HCl 20 mg	Inderal by Watson	52544-0306	Antihypertensive
WATSON306	Tab, White, Round, Scored	Propranolol HCl 20 mg	Inderal by Amerisource	62584-0843	Antihypertensive
WATSON307	Tab, White, Round, Scored	Propranolol HCl 40 mg	Inderal by Amerisource	62584-0844	Antihypertensive
WATSON307	Tab, White, Round, Scored	Propranolol HCl 40 mg	Inderal by Apotheca	12634-0472	Antihypertensive
WATSON308	Tab, White, Round, Scored	Propranolol HCl 80 mg	Inderal by Nat Pharmpak	55154-5538	Antihypertensive
WATSON308	Tab, White, Round, Scored	Propranolol HCl 80 mg	Inderal by Major	00904-0418	Antihypertensive
WATSON308	Tab, White, Round, Scored	Propranolol HCl 80 mg	Inderal by Amerisource	62584-0845	Antihypertensive
WATSON308	Tab, White, Round, Scored	Propranolol HCl 80 mg	Inderal by Watson	52544-0308	Antihypertensive
WATSON30950	Cap, Green & Yellow, Watson 309/50	Doxycycline Monohydrate 50 mg	Monodox by Watson	52544-0309	Antibiotic
WATSON310100	Cap, Green	Doxycycline Monohydrate 100 mg	Monodox by Watson	52544-0310	Antibiotic
WATSON312	Tab, White	Metoclopramide 10 mg	Reglan by Watson	52544-0312	Gastrointestinal
WATSON312	Tab, White	Metoclopramide 10 mg	Reglan by Nat Pharmpak	55154-5804	Gastrointestinal
WATSON3159	Cap, White, Opaque	Ursodiol 300 mg	Actigall by Watson	00591-3159	Gastrointestinal
WATSON3191	Tab, White, Round, Scored	Pyridostigmine Bromide 60 mg	Mestinon by Watson	00591-3191	Muscle Stimulant
WATSON3203	Tab, Light Orange, Cap Shaped, Scored	Hydrocodone 7.5 mg, Acetaminophen 325 mg	Norco by Watson	00591-3203	Analgesic; C III
WATSON3219	Cap, Yellow and Green, Red Imprint	Butalbital 50 mg, Aspirin 325 mg, Caffeine 40 mg	Fiorinal by Watson	00591-3219	Analgesic; C II
WATSON3220	Cap, White and Dark Blue, White and Pink Imprint	Butalbital 50 mg, Acetaminophen 325 mg, Caffeine 40 mg, Codeine Phosphate 30 mg	Fioricet by Watson	00591-3220	Analgesic
WATSON3228	Tab, Yellow, Cap Shaped, Scored	Hydrocodone 10 mg, Acetaminophen 750 mg	Maxidone by Watson	00591-3228	Analgesic; C III
WATSON3250	Cap, Yellow and Black	Nitrofurantoin 100 mg	Macrobid by Watson	00591-3250	Antibiotic
WATSON3253	Cap, Yellow and White	Nitrofurantoin Macrocrystals 50 mg	Macrodantin by Watson	00591-3253	Antibiotic
WATSON3254	Cap, Yellow	Nitrofurantoin Macrocrystals 100 mg	Macrodantin by Watson	00591-3254	Antibiotic
WATSON332	Tab, White	Lorazepam 0.5 mg	Ativan by Ivax	00182-1806	Antianxiety; C IV
WATSON332	Tab, White	Lorazepam 0.5 mg	Ativan by Qualitest	00603-4243	Antianxiety; C IV
WATSON332	Tab, White	Lorazepam 0.5 mg	Ativan by Watson	52544-0332	Antianxiety; C IV
WATSON333	Tab, White	Lorazepam 1 mg	Ativan by Nat Pharmpak	55154-0550	Antianxiety; C IV
WATSON333	Tab, White	Lorazepam 1 mg	Ativan by Amerisource	62584-0770	Antianxiety; C IV
WATSON333	Tab, White	Lorazepam 1 mg	Ativan by PDRX	55289-0487	Antianxiety; C IV
WATSON333	Tab, White	Lorazepam 1 mg	Ativan by Watson	52544-0333	Antianxiety; C IV
WATSON333	Tab, White	Lorazepam 1 mg	Ativan by Med Pro	53978-5008	Antianxiety; C IV
WATSON333	Tab, White	Lorazepam 1 mg	Ativan by URL Mutual	00677-1057	Antianxiety; C IV
WATSON333	Tab, White	Lorazepam 1 mg	Ativan by Qualitest	00603-4244	Antianxiety; C IV
WATSON334	Tab, White, Round, Scored	Lorazepam 2 mg	Ativan by Major	00904-1502	Antianxiety; C IV
WATSON334	Tab, White, Round, Scored	Lorazepam 2 mg	Ativan by Compumed	00403-0012	Antianxiety; C IV
WATSON334	Tab, White, Round, Scored	Lorazepam 2 mg	Ativan by PDRX	55289-0594	Antianxiety; C IV
WATSON334	Tab, White, Round, Scored	Lorazepam 2 mg	Ativan by Ivax	00182-1808	Antianxiety; C IV
WATSON334	Tab, White, Round, Scored	Lorazepam 2 mg	Ativan by Watson	52544-0334	Antianxiety; C IV
WATSON334	Tab, White, Round, Scored	Lorazepam 2 mg	Ativan by Amerisource	62584-0771	Antianxiety; C IV
WATSON334	Tab, White, Round, Scored	Lorazepam 2 mg	Ativan by Nat Pharmpak	55154-0914	Antianxiety; C IV
WATSON335	Tab, White, Oval	Acyclovir 400 mg	Zovirax by Watson	00591-0335	Antiviral
WATSON336	Tab, White, Oval	Acyclovir 800 mg	Zovirax by Watson	00591-0336	Antiviral
WATSON338	Tab, White, Round, Delayed Release	Diclofenac Sodium 50 mg	Voltaren by Watson	52544-0338	NSAID
WATSON338	Tab, White, Round, Delayed Release	Diclofenac Sodium 50 mg	Voltaren by Watson	00591-0338	NSAID
WATSON343	Tab, White, Round, Scored	Verapamil HCl 80 mg	Verelan by Thrift Drug	59198-0251	Antihypertensive
WATSON343	Tab, White, Round, Scored	Verapamil HCl 80 mg	Verelan by Watson	00591-0343	Antihypertensive
WATSON343	Tab, White, Round, Scored	Verapamil HCl 80 mg	Verelan by Ivax	00182-1300	Antihypertensive

ID FRONT <> BACK	DESCRIPTION FRONT <> BACK	INGREDIENT & STRENGTH	BRAND (or Generic Equiv.) by FIRM	NDC#	CLASS; SCH.
WATSON343	Tab, White, Round, Scored	Verapamil HCl 80 mg	Verelan by Kaiser	62224-8558	Antihypertensive
WATSON343	Tab, White, Round, Scored	Verapamil HCl 80 mg	Verelan by Major	00904-2920	Antihypertensive
WATSON343	Tab, Film Coated, Debossed	Verapamil HCl 80 mg	Verelan by URL Mutual	00677-1130	Antihypertensive
WATSON3437	Tab, White, Round, Scored	Furosemide 40 mg	Lasix by Watson	00591-3437	Diuretic
WATSON3438	Tab, White, Round, Scored	Furosemide 80 mg	Lasix by Watson	00591-3438	Diuretic
WATSON344	Tab, White, Round, Scored	Verapamil HCl 80 mg	Verelan by Caremark	00339-6174	Antihypertensive
WATSON344	Tab, White, Round, Scored	Verapamil HCl 80 mg	Verelan by Med Pro	53978-7001	Antihypertensive
WATSON344	Tab, White, Round, Scored	Verapamil HCl 80 mg	Verelan by Watson	00591-0344	Antihypertensive
WATSON345	Tab, White, Round, Scored	Verapamil HCl 120 mg	Verelan by Major	00904-2924	Antihypertensive
WATSON345	Tab, White, Round, Scored	Verapamil HCl 120 mg	Verelan by Ivax	00182-1301	Antihypertensive
WATSON345	Tab, White, Round, Scored	Verapamil HCl 120 mg	Verelan by Watson	00591-0345	Antihypertensive
WATSON346	Tab, Peach, Round, Scored	Verapamil HCl 120 mg	Verelan by Watson	00591-0346	Antihypertensive
WATSON347125MG	Cap, Teal & White, Opaque, Watson 347/12.5	Hydrochlorothiazide 12.5 mg	Microzide by Watson	00591-0347	Diuretic; Antihypertensive
WATSON348	Tab, Yellow to Light Green, Round, Scored, Watson over 348	Hydrochlorothiazide 50 mg, Triamterene 75 mg	Maxzide by Apotheca	12634-0270	Diuretic; Antihypertensive
WATSON348	Tab, Yellow to Light Green, Round, Scored, Watson over 348	Hydrochlorothiazide 50 mg, Triamterene 75 mg	Maxzide by Moore	00839-7422	Diuretic; Antihypertensive
WATSON348	Tab, Yellow to Light Green, Round, Scored, Watson over 348	Hydrochlorothiazide 50 mg, Triamterene 75 mg	Maxzide by Watson	52544-0348	Diuretic; Antihypertensive
WATSON348	Tab, Yellow to Light Green, Round, Scored, Watson over 348	Hydrochlorothiazide 50 mg, Triamterene 75 mg	Maxzide by Par	49884-0017	Diuretic; Antihypertensive
WATSON348	Tab, Yellow to Light Green, Round, Scored, Watson over 348	Hydrochlorothiazide 50 mg, Triamterene 75 mg	Maxzide by Murfreesboro	51129-1420	Diuretic; Antihypertensive
WATSON348	Tab, Yellow to Light Green, Round, Scored, Watson over 348	Hydrochlorothiazide 50 mg, Triamterene 75 mg	Maxzide by Ivax	00182-1872	Diuretic; Antihypertensive
WATSON348	Tab, Yellow to Light Green, Round, Scored, Watson over 348	Hydrochlorothiazide 50 mg, Triamterene 75 mg	Maxzide by Baker Cummins	63171-1872	Diuretic; Antihypertensive
WATSON348	Tab, Yellow to Light Green, Round, Scored, Watson over 348	Hydrochlorothiazide 50 mg, Triamterene 75 mg	Maxzide by Warner Chilcott	00047-0833	Diuretic; Antihypertensive
WATSON348	Tab, Yellow to Light Green, Round, Scored, Watson over 348	Hydrochlorothiazide 50 mg, Triamterene 75 mg	Maxzide by Martec	52555-0974	Diuretic; Antihypertensive
WATSON348	Tab, Yellow to Light Green, Round, Scored, Watson over 348	Hydrochlorothiazide 50 mg, Triamterene 75 mg	Maxzide by Watson	00591-0348	Diuretic; Antihypertensive
WATSON349	Tab, White, Cap Shaped, Scored, Watson over 349	Acetaminophen 500 mg, Hydrocodone Bitartrate 5 mg	Vicodin by Murfreesboro	51129-1448	Analgesic; C III
WATSON349	Tab, White, Cap Shaped, Scored, Watson over 349	Acetaminophen 500 mg, Hydrocodone Bitartrate 5 mg	Vicodin by Murfreesboro	51129-1439	Analgesic; C III
WATSON349	Tab, White, Cap Shaped, Scored, Watson over 349	Acetaminophen 500 mg, Hydrocodone Bitartrate 5 mg	Vicodin by Pharmedix	53002-0119	Analgesic; C III
WATSON349	Tab, White, Cap Shaped, Scored, Watson over 349	Acetaminophen 500 mg, Hydrocodone Bitartrate 5 mg	Vicodin by Talbert	44514-0413	Analgesic; C III
WATSON349	Tab, White, Cap Shaped, Scored, Watson over 349	Acetaminophen 500 mg, Hydrocodone Bitartrate 5 mg	Vicodin by Major	00904-3440	Analgesic; C III
WATSON349	Tab, White, Cap Shaped, Scored, Watson over 349	Acetaminophen 500 mg, Hydrocodone Bitartrate 5 mg	Vicodin by Moore	00839-7176	Analgesic; C III
WATSON349	Tab, White, Cap Shaped, Scored, Watson over 349	Acetaminophen 500 mg, Hydrocodone Bitartrate 5 mg	Vicodin by Apotheca	12634-0514	Analgesic; C III
WATSON349	Tab, White, Cap Shaped, Scored, Watson over 349	Acetaminophen 500 mg, Hydrocodone Bitartrate 5 mg	Vicodin by Warner Chilcott	00047-0448	Analgesic; C III
WATSON349	Tab, White, Cap Shaped, Scored, Watson over 349	Acetaminophen 500 mg, Hydrocodone Bitartrate 5 mg	Vicodin by PDRX	55289-0137	Analgesic; C III
WATSON349	Tab, White, Cap Shaped, Scored, Watson over 349	Acetaminophen 500 mg, Hydrocodone Bitartrate 5 mg	Vicodin by URL Mutual	00677-1184	Analgesic; C III
WATSON349	Tab, White, Cap Shaped, Scored, Watson over 349	Acetaminophen 500 mg, Hydrocodone Bitartrate 5 mg	Vicodin by Sandoz	00781-1606	Analgesic; C III
WATSON349	Tab, White, Cap Shaped, Scored, Watson over 349	Acetaminophen 500 mg, Hydrocodone Bitartrate 5 mg	Vicodin by Amerisource	62584-0738	Analgesic; C III
WATSON349	Tab, White, Cap Shaped, Scored, Watson over 349	Acetaminophen 500 mg, Hydrocodone Bitartrate 5 mg	Vicodin by Nat Pharmpak	55154-5549	Analgesic; C III
WATSON349	Tab, White, Cap Shaped, Scored, Watson over 349	Acetaminophen 500 mg, Hydrocodone Bitartrate 5 mg	Vicodin by UDL	51079-0420 Discontinued	Analgesic; C III
WATSON349	Tab, White, Cap Shaped, Scored, Watson over 349	Acetaminophen 500 mg, Hydrocodone Bitartrate 5 mg	Vicodin by Watson	00591-0349	Analgesic; C III
WATSON3497	Cap, Pink and White, Opaque, Hard Gelatin	Galantamine Hydrobromide 16 mg	Galantamine Hydrobromide by Watson	00591-3497	Acetylcholinesterase Inhibitor

ID FRONT <> BACK	DESCRIPTION FRONT <> BACK	INGREDIENT & STRENGTH	BRAND (or Generic Equiv.) by FIRM	NDC#	CLASS; SCH.
WATSON352	Tab, Pink, Round	Propranolol HCl 60 mg	Inderal by Watson	52544-0352	Antihypertensive
WATSON353	Tab, Lavender, Round	Propranolol HCl 90 mg	Inderal by Watson	52544-0353	Antihypertensive
WATSON357	Tab, White, Round	Hydrochlorothiazide 15 mg, Methyldopa 250 mg	Aldoril 15 by Watson	52544-0357	Diuretic; Antihypertensive
WATSON358	Tab, White, Round	Hydrochlorothiazide 25 mg, Methyldopa 250 mg	Aldoril 25 by Watson	52544-0358	Diuretic; Antihypertensive
WATSON359	Tab, White, Round	Hydrochlorothiazide 30 mg, Methyldopa 500 mg	Aldoril by Watson	52544-0359	Diuretic; Antihypertensive
WATSON360	Tab, White, Round	Hydrochlorothiazide 50 mg, Methyldopa 500 mg	Aldoril by Watson	52544-0360	Diuretic; Antihypertensive
WATSON363 <> 375	Tab, Blue, Round, Scored, 3.75 <> Watson 363	Clorazepate Dipotassium 3.75 mg	Tranxene by Major	00904-3970	Antianxiety; C IV
WATSON363 <> 375	Tab, Blue, Round, Scored, 3.75 <> Watson 363	Clorazepate Dipotassium 3.75 mg	Tranxene by Watson	52544-0363	Antianxiety; C IV
WATSON363 <> 375	Tab, Blue, Round, Scored, 3.75 <> Watson 363	Clorazepate Dipotassium 3.75 mg	Tranxene by Ivax	00182-0009	Antianxiety; C IV
WATSON363 <> 375	Tab, Blue, Round, Scored, 3.75 <> Watson 363	Clorazepate Dipotassium 3.75 mg	Tranxene by Watson	00591-0363	Antianxiety; C IV
WATSON364 <> 75	Tab, Light Beige, Round, Scored, 7.5	Clorazepate Dipotassium 7.5 mg	Tranxene by Ivax	00182-0010	Antianxiety; C IV
WATSON364 <> 75	Tab, Light Beige, Round, Scored, 7.5	Clorazepate Dipotassium 7.5 mg	Tranxene by Watson	00591-0364	Antianxiety; C IV
WATSON364 <> 75	Tab, Light Beige, Round, Scored, 7.5	Clorazepate Dipotassium 7.5 mg	Tranxene by Major	00904-5160	Antianxiety; C IV
WATSON365 <> 15	Tab, Pink, Round, Scored	Clorazepate Dipotassium 15 mg	Tranxene by Ivax	00182-0014	Antianxiety; C IV
WATSON365 <> 15	Tab, Pink, Round, Scored	Clorazepate Dipotassium 15 mg	Tranxene by Watson	00591-0365	Antianxiety; C IV
WATSON365 <> 15	Tab, Pink, Round, Scored	Clorazepate Dipotassium 15 mg	Tranxene by Major	00904-5159	Antianxiety; C IV
WATSON366	Tab	Fenoprofen Calcium 600 mg	by Pharmedix	53002-0367	NSAID
WATSON366	Tab, Coated	Fenoprofen Calcium 600 mg	by Physician Total Care	54868-0775	NSAID
WATSON366	Tab	Fenoprofen Calcium 600 mg	by Watson	52544-0366	NSAID
WATSON367	Cap, White & Yellow	Fenoprofen Calcium 200 mg	Nalfon by Watson	52544-0367	NSAID
WATSON368	Cap, Yellow	Fenoprofen Calcium 300 mg	Nalfon by Watson	52544-0368	NSAID
WATSON3695MG	Cap, White, Black Print, Opaque, Watson over 369	Loxapine 5 mg	Loxitane by UDL	51079-0900	Antipsychotic
WATSON3695MG	Cap, White, Black Print, Opaque, Watson over 369	Loxapine 5 mg	Loxitane by Nat Pharmpak	55154-4605	Antipsychotic
WATSON3695MG	Cap, White, Black Print, Opaque, Watson over 369	Loxapine 5 mg	Loxitane by Sandoz	00781-2710	Antipsychotic
WATSON3695MG	Cap, White, Black Print, Opaque, Watson over 369	Loxapine 5 mg	Loxitane by Major	00904-2310	Antipsychotic
WATSON3695MG	Cap, White, Black Print, Opaque, Watson over 369	Loxapine 5 mg	Loxitane by Nat Pharmpak	55154-4611	Antipsychotic
WATSON3695MG	Cap, White, Black Print, Opaque, Watson over 369	Loxapine 5 mg	Loxitane by Ivax	00182-1305	Antipsychotic
WATSON3695MG	Cap, White, Black Print, Opaque, Watson over 369	Loxapine 5 mg	Loxitane by UDL	51079-0677	Antipsychotic
WATSON3695MG	Cap, White, Black Print, Opaque, Watson over 369	Loxapine 5 mg	Loxitane by Moore	00839-7495	Antipsychotic
WATSON3695MG	Cap, White, Black Print, Opaque, Watson over 369	Loxapine 5 mg	Loxitane by Dixon Shane	17236-0698	Antipsychotic
WATSON3695MG	Cap, White, Black Print, Opaque, Watson over 369	Loxapine 5 mg	Loxitane by Watson	00591-0369	Antipsychotic
WATSON3695MG	Cap, White, Black Print, Opaque, Watson over 369	Loxapine 5 mg	Loxitane by Watson	00591-0370	Antipsychotic
WATSON37010MG	Cap, White & Yellow, Opaque, Watson over 370	Loxapine 10 mg	Loxitane by Ivax	00182-1306	Antipsychotic
WATSON37010MG	Cap, White & Yellow, Opaque, Watson over 370	Loxapine 10 mg	Loxitane by Physician Total Care	54868-2327	Antipsychotic
WATSON37010MG	Cap, White & Yellow, Opaque, Watson over 370	Loxapine 10 mg	Loxitane by UDL	51079-0678	Antipsychotic
WATSON37010MG	Cap, White & Yellow, Opaque, Watson over 370	Loxapine 10 mg	Loxitane by Sandoz	00781-2711	Antipsychotic
WATSON37010MG	Cap, White & Yellow, Opaque, Watson over 370	Loxapine 10 mg	Loxitane by Qualitest	00603-4269	Antipsychotic
WATSON37010MG	Cap, White & Yellow, Opaque, Watson over 370	Loxapine 10 mg	Loxitane by Nat Pharmpak	55154-4606	Antipsychotic
WATSON37010MG	Cap, White & Yellow, Opaque, Watson over 370	Loxapine 10 mg	Loxitane by Dixon Shane	17236-0694	Antipsychotic
WATSON37010MG	Cap, White & Yellow, Opaque, Watson over 370	Loxapine 10 mg	Loxitane by Major	00904-2311	Antipsychotic
WATSON37010MG	Cap, White & Yellow, Opaque, Watson over 370	Loxapine 10 mg	Loxitane by Moore	00839-7496	Antipsychotic
WATSON37125MG	Cap, Green & White, Opaque, Watson over 371	Loxapine 25 mg	Loxitane by Dixon Shane	17236-0695	Antipsychotic
WATSON37125MG	Cap, Green & White, Opaque, Watson over 371	Loxapine 25 mg	Loxitane by Nat Pharmpak	55154-4609	Antipsychotic
WATSON37125MG	Cap, Green & White, Opaque, Watson over 371	Loxapine 25 mg	Loxitane by Major	00904-2312	Antipsychotic
WATSON37125MG	Cap, Green & White, Opaque, Watson over 371	Loxapine 25 mg	Loxitane by Sandoz	00781-2712	Antipsychotic
WATSON37125MG	Cap, Green & White, Opaque, Watson over 371	Loxapine 25 mg	Loxitane by Moore	00839-7497	Antipsychotic
WATSON37125MG	Cap, Green & White, Opaque, Watson over 371	Loxapine 25 mg	Loxitane by URL Mutual	00677-1320	Antipsychotic
WATSON37125MG	Cap, Green & White, Opaque, Watson over 371	Loxapine 25 mg	Loxitane by UDL	51079-0679	Antipsychotic
WATSON37125MG	Cap, Green & White, Opaque, Watson over 371	Loxapine 25 mg	Loxitane by Physician Total Care	54868-2478	Antipsychotic
WATSON37125MG	Cap, Green & White, Opaque, Watson over 371	Loxapine 25 mg	Loxitane by Ivax	00182-1307	Antipsychotic

ID FRONT <> BACK	DESCRIPTION FRONT <> BACK	INGREDIENT & STRENGTH	BRAND (or Generic Equiv.) by FIRM	NDC#	CLASS; SCH.
WATSON37125MG	Cap, Green & White, Opaque, Watson over 371	Loxapine 25 mg	Loxitane by Watson	00591-0371	Antipsychotic
WATSON37250MG	Cap, White & Blue, Opaque, Hard Gel, Watson over 372	Loxapine 50 mg	Loxitane by Ivax	00182-1308	Antipsychotic
WATSON37250MG	Cap, White & Blue, Opaque, Hard Gel, Watson over 372	Loxapine 50 mg	Loxitane by Nat Pharmpak	55154-4610	Antipsychotic
WATSON37250MG	Cap, White & Blue, Opaque, Hard Gel, Watson over 372	Loxapine 50 mg	Loxitane by UDL	51079-0680	Antipsychotic
WATSON37250MG	Cap, White & Blue, Opaque, Hard Gel, Watson over 372	Loxapine 50 mg	Loxitane by Physician Total Care	54868-2479	Antipsychotic
WATSON37250MG	Cap, White & Blue, Opaque, Hard Gel, Watson over 372	Loxapine 50 mg	Loxitane by Major	00904-2313	Antipsychotic
WATSON37250MG	Cap, White & Blue, Opaque, Hard Gel, Watson over 372	Loxapine 50 mg	Loxitane by Moore	00839-7498	Antipsychotic
WATSON37250MG	Cap, White & Blue, Opaque, Hard Gel, Watson over 372	Loxapine 50 mg	Loxitane by URL Mutual	00677-1321	Antipsychotic
WATSON37250MG	Cap, White & Blue, Opaque, Hard Gel, Watson over 372	Loxapine 50 mg	Loxitane by Sandoz	00781-2713	Antipsychotic
WATSON37250MG	Cap, White & Blue, Opaque, Hard Gel, Watson over 372	Loxapine 50 mg	Loxitane by Dixon Shane	17236-0696	Antipsychotic
WATSON37250MG	Cap, White & Blue, Opaque, Hard Gel, Watson over 372	Loxapine 50 mg	Loxitane by Murfreesboro	51129-1351	Antipsychotic
WATSON37250MG	Cap, White & Blue, Opaque, Hard Gel, Watson over 372	Loxapine 50 mg	Loxitane by Watson	00591-0372	Antipsychotic
WATSON373	Tab, Film Coated	Maprotiline HCl 25 mg	by Watson	52544-0373	Antidepressant
WATSON373	Tab, Film Coated	Maprotiline HCl 25 mg	by Ivax	00182-1882	Antidepressant
WATSON373	Tab, Film Coated	Maprotiline HCl 25 mg	by Medirex	57480-0493	Antidepressant
WATSON373	Tab, Film Coated	Maprotiline HCl 25 mg	by Sandoz	00781-1631	Antidepressant
WATSON374	Tab, Film Coated	Maprotiline HCl 50 mg	by Watson	52544-0374	Antidepressant
WATSON374	Tab, Film Coated	Maprotiline HCl 50 mg	by Ivax	00182-1883	Antidepressant
WATSON374	Tab, Film Coated	Maprotiline HCl 50 mg	by Sandoz	00781-1632	Antidepressant
WATSON374	Tab, Film Coated	Maprotiline HCl 50 mg	by Medirex	57480-0494	Antidepressant
WATSON375	Tab, White, Oval	Maprotiline 75 mg	Ludiomil by Watson	52544-0375	Antidepressant
WATSON379	Tab, White, Round, Scored	Amoxapine 25 mg	Asendin by Watson	52544-0379	Antidepressant
WATSON379	Tab, White, Round, Scored	Amoxapine 25 mg	Asendin by Medirex	57480-0480	Antidepressant
WATSON379	Tab, White, Round, Scored	Amoxapine 25 mg	Asendin by Dixon Shane	17236-0888	Antidepressant
WATSON380	Tab	Amoxapine 50 mg	Asendin by Medirex	57480-0481	Antidepressant
WATSON380	Tab, Pink, Round, Scored	Amoxapine 50 mg	Asendin by Watson	52544-0380	Antidepressant
WATSON380	Tab, Salmon	Amoxapine 50 mg	Asendin by URL Mutual	00677-1378	Antidepressant
WATSON380	Tab, Salmon	Amoxapine 50 mg	Asendin by Major	00904-3995	Antidepressant
WATSON380	Tab, Orange, Round, Scored	Amoxapine 50 mg	Asendin by Dixon Shane	17236-0889	Antidepressant
WATSON381	Tab, Blue, Round, Scored	Amoxapine 100 mg	Asendin by Dixon Shane	17236-0890	Antidepressant
WATSON381	Tab	Amoxapine 100 mg	Asendin by Ivax	00182-1045	Antidepressant
WATSON381	Tab	Amoxapine 100 mg	Asendin by URL Mutual	00677-1379	Antidepressant
WATSON381	Tab, Blue, Round, Scored	Amoxapine 100 mg	Asendin by Watson	52544-0380	Antidepressant
WATSON382	Tab, Peach, Round, Scored	Amoxapine 150 mg	Asendin by Watson	00591-0381	Antidepressant
WATSON382	Tab, Peach, Round, Scored	Amoxapine 150 mg	Asendin by Watson	00591-0382	Antidepressant
WATSON382	Tab, Peach, Round, Scored	Amoxapine 150 mg	Asendin by Dixon Shane	17236-0891	Antidepressant
WATSON383	Tab, Light Pink, Round	Ethinyl Estradiol 35 mcg, Ethynodiol Diacetate 1 mg	Zovia 1/35 by Watson	52544-0383	Oral Contraceptive
WATSON384	Tab, Pink, Round	Ethinyl Estradiol 50 mcg, Ethynodiol Diacetate 1 mg	Zovia 1/50 by Watson	52544-0384	Oral Contraceptive
WATSON385	Tab, White, Cap Shaped, Scored	Acetaminophen 500 mg, Hydrocodone Bitartrate 7.5 mg	Lortab by Sandoz Pharms	00781-1513	Analgesic; C III
WATSON385	Tab, White, Cap Shaped, Scored	Acetaminophen 500 mg, Hydrocodone Bitartrate 7.5 mg	Lortab by Southwood	58016-0195	Analgesic; C III
WATSON385	Tab, White, Cap Shaped, Scored	Acetaminophen 500 mg, Hydrocodone Bitartrate 7.5 mg	Lortab by Heartland	61392-0729	Analgesic; C III
WATSON385	Tab, White, Cap Shaped, Scored	Acetaminophen 500 mg, Hydrocodone Bitartrate 7.5 mg	Lortab by Direct Dispensing	57866-3915	Analgesic; C III
WATSON385	Tab, White, Cap Shaped, Scored	Acetaminophen 500 mg, Hydrocodone Bitartrate 7.5 mg	Lortab by PDRX	55289-0268	Analgesic; C III
WATSON385	Tab, White, Cap Shaped, Scored	Acetaminophen 500 mg, Hydrocodone Bitartrate 7.5 mg	Lortab by Major	00904-7631	Analgesic; C III
WATSON385	Tab, White, Cap Shaped, Scored	Acetaminophen 500 mg, Hydrocodone Bitartrate 7.5 mg	Lortab by Moore	00839-7781	Analgesic; C III
WATSON385	Tab, White, Cap Shaped, Scored	Acetaminophen 500 mg, Hydrocodone Bitartrate 7.5 mg	Lortab by Qualitest	00603-3882	Analgesic; C III
WATSON385	Tab, White, Cap Shaped, Scored	Acetaminophen 500 mg, Hydrocodone Bitartrate 7.5 mg	Lortab by Warner Chilcott	00047-0319	Analgesic; C III
WATSON385	Tab, White, Cap Shaped, Scored	Acetaminophen 500 mg, Hydrocodone Bitartrate 7.5 mg	Lortab by Watson	52544-0385	Analgesic; C III
WATSON385	Tab, White, Cap Shaped, Scored	Acetaminophen 500 mg, Hydrocodone Bitartrate 7.5 mg	Lortab by Watson	00591-0385	Analgesic; C III
WATSON385	Cap, White	Hydrocodone 7.5 mg, Acetaminophen 500 mg	Lortab by Watson	00591-0385	Analgesic; C III
WATSON387	Tab, White, Oblong, Scored, Watson over 387	Acetaminophen 750 mg, Hydrocodone Bitartrate 7.5 mg	Vicodin ES by Watson	00591-0387	Analgesic; C III

ID FRONT <> BACK	DESCRIPTION FRONT <> BACK	INGREDIENT & STRENGTH	BRAND (or Generic Equiv.) by FIRM	NDC#	CLASS; SCH.
WATSON387	Tab, White, Oblong, Scored, Watson over 387	Acetaminophen 750 mg, Hydrocodone Bitartrate 7.5 mg	Vicodin ES by Watson	52544-0387	Analgesic; C III
WATSON387	Tab, White, Oblong, Scored, Watson over 387	Acetaminophen 750 mg, Hydrocodone Bitartrate 7.5 mg	Vicodin ES by Warner Chilcott	00047-0486	Analgesic; C III
WATSON387	Tab, White, Oblong, Scored, Watson over 387	Acetaminophen 750 mg, Hydrocodone Bitartrate 7.5 mg	Vicodin ES by URL Mutual	00677-1504	Analgesic; C III
WATSON387	Tab, White, Oblong, Scored, Watson over 387	Acetaminophen 750 mg, Hydrocodone Bitartrate 7.5 mg	Vicodin ES by Qualitest	00603-3883	Analgesic; C III
WATSON387	Tab, White, Oblong, Scored, Watson over 387	Acetaminophen 750 mg, Hydrocodone Bitartrate 7.5 mg	Vicodin ES by Schein	00364-2505	Analgesic; C III
WATSON387	Tab, White, Oblong, Scored, Watson over 387	Acetaminophen 750 mg, Hydrocodone Bitartrate 7.5 mg	Vicodin ES by Sandoz	00781-1532	Analgesic; C III
WATSON387	Tab, White, Cap Shaped, Scored	Acetaminophen 750 mg, Hydrocodone Bitartrate 7.5 mg	Vicodin ES by PDRX	55289-0360	Analgesic; C III
WATSON387	Tab, White, Oblong, Scored, Watson over 387	Acetaminophen 750 mg, Hydrocodone Bitartrate 7.5 mg	Vicodin ES by Major	00904-7632	Analgesic; C III
WATSON387	Tab, White, Oblong, Scored, Watson over 387	Acetaminophen 750 mg, Hydrocodone Bitartrate 7.5 mg	Vicodin ES by Moore	00839-7728	Analgesic; C III
WATSON387	Tab, White, Oblong, Scored, Watson over 387	Acetaminophen 750 mg, Hydrocodone Bitartrate 7.5 mg	Vicodin ES by Southwood	58016-0758	Analgesic; C III
WATSON387	Tab, White, Oblong, Scored, Watson over 387	Acetaminophen 750 mg, Hydrocodone Bitartrate 7.5 mg	Vicodin ES by Murfreesboro	51129-1440	Analgesic; C III
WATSON388	Tab, White, Oblong, Scored	Acetaminophen 500 mg, Hydrocodone Bitartrate 2.5 mg	Lortab by Watson	52544-0388	Analgesic; C III
WATSON388	Tab, White, Oblong, Scored	Acetaminophen 500 mg, Hydrocodone Bitartrate 2.5 mg	Lortab by Warner Chilcott	00047-0318	Analgesic; C III
WATSON388	Tab, White, Oblong, Scored	Acetaminophen 500 mg, Hydrocodone Bitartrate 2.5 mg	Lortab by Watson	00591-0388	Analgesic; C III
WATSON403	Tab, Peach, Round	Verapamil HCl 40 mg	Isoptin by Watson	52544-0403	Antihypertensive
WATSON404	Tab, Light Peach, Round	Verapamil HCl 40 mg	Isoptin by Watson	00591-0404	Antihypertensive
WATSON404	Tab, Light Peach, Round	Verapamil HCl 40 mg	Isoptin by Ivax	00182-1601	Antihypertensive
WATSON404	Tab, Light Peach, Round	Verapamil HCl 40 mg	Isoptin by Moore	00839-7921	Antihypertensive
WATSON404	Tab, Light Peach, Round	Verapamil HCl 40 mg	Isoptin by Major	00904-7799	Antihypertensive
WATSON404	Tab, Light Peach, Round	Verapamil HCl 40 mg	Isoptin by Watson	52544-0404	Antihypertensive
WATSON407	Tab, Blue, Round	Lisinopril 10 mg	Prinivil by Watson	00591-0407	Antihypertensive
WATSON408	Tab, Yellow, Round	Lisinopril 20 mg	Prinivil by Watson	00591-0408	Antihypertensive
WATSON409	Tab, Yellow, Round	Lisinopril 40 mg	Prinivil by Watson	00591-0409	Antihypertensive
WATSON41050MG	Cap, White and Ivory, Opaque	Doxycycline Monohydrate 50 mg	Monodox by Watson	00591-0410	Antibiotic
WATSON41100MG	Cap, Ivory and Brown, Opaque	Doxycycline Monohydrate 100 mg	Monodox by Watson	00591-0411	Antibiotic
WATSON414	Tab, Yellow, Round, Scored	Estropipate 0.75 mg	Ogen by Ivax	00182-1976	Hormone
WATSON414	Tab, Yellow, Round, Scored	Estropipate 0.75 mg	Ogen by Watson	52544-0414	Hormone
WATSON414	Tab, Yellow, Round, Scored	Estropipate 0.75 mg	Ogen by Watson	00591-0414	Hormone
WATSON415	Tab, Peach, Round, Scored	Estropipate 1.5 mg	Ogen by Watson	00591-0415	Hormone
WATSON416	Tab, Blue, Round, Scored	Estropipate 3 mg	Ogen by Watson	52544-0416	Hormone
WATSON416	Tab, Blue, Round, Scored	Estropipate 3 mg	Ogen by Watson	00591-0416	Hormone
WATSON417	Tab, Green, Round	Estropipate 6 mg	Ogen by Watson	52544-0417	Hormone
WATSON418	Tab, Coated	Cyclobenzaprine HCl 10 mg	by Med Pro	53978-1035	Muscle Relaxant
WATSON424	Tab, Light Green, Round, Scored	Hydrochlorothiazide 25 mg, Triamterene 37.5 mg	Maxzide 25 by Watson	52544-0424	Diuretic; Antihypertensive
WATSON424	Tab, Light Green, Round, Scored	Hydrochlorothiazide 25 mg, Triamterene 37.5 mg	Maxzide 25 by Major	00904-7873	Diuretic; Antihypertensive
WATSON424	Tab, Light Green, Round, Scored	Hydrochlorothiazide 25 mg, Triamterene 37.5 mg	Maxzide 25 by Ivax	00182-1903	Diuretic; Antihypertensive
WATSON424	Tab, Light Green, Round, Scored	Hydrochlorothiazide 25 mg, Triamterene 37.5 mg	Maxzide 25 by Watson	00591-0424	Diuretic; Antihypertensive
WATSON424	Tab, Light Green, Round, Scored	Hydrochlorothiazide 25 mg, Triamterene 37.5 mg	Maxzide 25 by Teva	00480-0670	Diuretic; Antihypertensive
WATSON425	Cap, Yellow & Blue	Aspirin 325 mg, Butalbital 50 mg, Caffeine 40 mg, Codeine Phosphate 30 mg	Fiorinal w/ Codeine by Watson	00591-0425	Analgesic; C III
WATSON425	Cap, Yellow & Blue	Aspirin 325 mg, Butalbital 50 mg, Caffeine 40 mg, Codeine Phosphate 30 mg	Fiorinal w/ Codeine by Physician Total Care	54868-1037	Analgesic; C III
WATSON425	Cap, Yellow & Blue	Aspirin 325 mg, Butalbital 50 mg, Caffeine 50 mg, Codeine Phosphate 30 mg	Fiorinal w/ Codeine by Caremark	00339-5120	Analgesic; C III
WATSON425	Cap, Yellow & Blue	Aspirin 325 mg, Butalbital 50 mg, Caffeine 40 mg, Codeine Phosphate 30 mg	Fiorinal w/ Codeine by Moore	00839-6689	Analgesic; C III
WATSON425	Cap, Yellow & Blue	Aspirin 325 mg, Butalbital 50 mg, Caffeine 40 mg, Codeine Phosphate 30 mg	Fiorinal w/ Codeine by Major		
WATSON425	Cap, Yellow & Blue	Aspirin 325 mg, Butalbital 50 mg, Caffeine 40 mg, Codeine Phosphate 30 mg	Fiorinal w/ Codeine by Watson	52544-0425	Analgesic; C III
WATSON425	Cap, Yellow & Blue	Aspirin 325 mg, Butalbital 50 mg, Caffeine 40 mg, Codeine Phosphate 30 mg	Fiorinal w/ Codeine by Ivax	00182-0036	Analgesic; C III
WATSON430	Tab, Blue, Round	Carbidopa 10 mg, Levodopa 100 mg	Sinemet by Watson	52544-0430	Antiparkinson
WATSON431	Tab, Tan, Round	Carbidopa 25 mg, Levodopa 100 mg	Sinemet by Watson	52544-0431	Antiparkinson
WATSON432	Tab, Blue, Round	Carbidopa 25 mg, Levodopa 250 mg	Sinemet by Watson	52544-0432	Antiparkinson
WATSON437	Cap, Gray & Red	Acebutolol HCl 200 mg	Sectral by Watson	52544-0437	Antihypertensive
WATSON437	Cap	Acebutolol HCl 200 mg	Sectral by Major	00904-5138	Antihypertensive

ID FRONT <> BACK	DESCRIPTION FRONT <> BACK	INGREDIENT & STRENGTH	BRAND (or Generic Equiv.) by FIRM	NDC#	CLASS; SCH.
WATSON437	Cap	Acebutolol HCl 200 mg	Sectral by Qualitest	00603-2046	Antihypertensive
WATSON437	Cap	Acebutolol HCl 200 mg	Sectral by Ivax	00182-2629	Antihypertensive
WATSON438	Cap	Acebutolol HCl 400 mg	Sectral by Major	00904-5139	Antihypertensive
WATSON438	Cap	Acebutolol HCl 400 mg	Sectral by Ivax	00182-2630	Antihypertensive
WATSON438	Cap	Acebutolol HCl 400 mg	Sectral by Qualitest	00603-2047	Antihypertensive
WATSON438	Cap, Green & Maroon	Acebutolol HCl 400 mg	Sectral by Watson	52544-0438	Antihypertensive
WATSON444	Tab, Pink, Round, WATSON over 444	Guanfacine HCl 1 mg	Tenex by Watson	52544-0444	Antihypertensive
WATSON444	Tab, Pink, Round, WATSON over 444	Guanfacine HCl 1 mg	Tenex by Warner Chilcott	00047-0312	Antihypertensive
WATSON444	Tab, Pink, Round, WATSON over 444	Guanfacine HCl 1 mg	Tenex by Ivax	00182-2641	Antihypertensive
WATSON444	Tab, Pink, Round, WATSON over 444	Guanfacine HCl 1 mg	Tenex by Moore	00839-8046	Antihypertensive
WATSON444	Tab, Pink, Round, WATSON over 444	Guanfacine HCl 1 mg	Tenex by Sandoz	00781-1366	Antihypertensive
WATSON444	Tab, Pink, Round, WATSON over 444	Guanfacine HCl 1 mg	Tenex by Caremark	00339-6089	Antihypertensive
WATSON444	Tab, Pink, Round, WATSON over 444	Guanfacine HCl 1 mg	Tenex by Qualitest	00603-3774	Antihypertensive
WATSON444	Tab, Pink, Round, WATSON over 444	Guanfacine HCl 1 mg	Tenex by Med Pro	53978-3365	Antihypertensive
WATSON444	Tab, Pink, Round, WATSON over 444	Guanfacine HCl 1 mg	Tenex by Major	00904-5133	Antihypertensive
WATSON444	Tab, Pink, Round, WATSON over 444	Guanfacine HCl 1 mg	Tenex by Watson	00591-0444	Antihypertensive
WATSON451	Tab	Guanabenz Acetate	by Warner Chilcott	00047-0560	Antihypertensive
WATSON451	Tab, Orange, Round	Guanabenz Acetate 4 mg	Wytensin by Watson	52544-0451	Antihypertensive
WATSON452	Tab, Grey, Round	Guanabenz Acetate 8 mg	Wytensin by Watson	52544-0452	Antihypertensive
WATSON452	Tab	Guanabenz Acetate	by Warner Chilcott	00047-0561	Antihypertensive
WATSON453	Tab, Peach, Round	Guanfacine HCl 2 mg	Tenex by Warner Chilcott	00047-0313	Antihypertensive
WATSON453	Tab, Peach, Round	Guanfacine HCl 2 mg	Tenex by Caremark	00339-6090	Antihypertensive
WATSON453	Tab, Peach, Round	Guanfacine HCl 2 mg	Tenex by Sandoz	00781-1373	Antihypertensive
WATSON453	Tab, Peach, Round	Guanfacine HCl 2 mg	Tenex by Major	00904-5134	Antihypertensive
WATSON453	Tab, Peach, Round	Guanfacine HCl 2 mg	Tenex by Qualitest	00603-3775	Antihypertensive
WATSON453	Tab, Peach, Round	Guanfacine HCl 2 mg	Tenex by Moore	00839-8047	Antihypertensive
WATSON453	Tab, Peach, Round	Guanfacine HCl 2 mg	Tenex by Ivax	00182-2642	Antihypertensive
WATSON453	Tab, Peach, Round	Guanfacine HCl 2 mg	Tenex by Watson	52544-0453	Antihypertensive
WATSON453	Tab, Peach, Round	Guanfacine HCl 2 mg	Tenex by Watson	00591-0453	Antihypertensive
WATSON460	Tab, White, Round, Scored	Glipizide 5 mg	Glucotrol by PDRX	55289-0806	Antidiabetic
WATSON460	Tab, White, Round, Scored	Glipizide 5 mg	Glucotrol by Warner Chilcott	00047-0463	Antidiabetic
WATSON460	Tab, White, Round, Scored	Glipizide 5 mg	Glucotrol by Watson	52544-0460	Antidiabetic
WATSON460	Tab, White, Round, Scored	Glipizide 5 mg	Glucotrol by Kaiser	00179-1300	Antidiabetic
WATSON460	Tab, White, Round, Scored	Glipizide 5 mg	Glucotrol by Moore	00839-7939	Antidiabetic
WATSON460	Tab, White, Round, Scored	Glipizide 5 mg	Glucotrol by Compumed	00403-0920	Antidiabetic
WATSON460	Tab, White, Round, Scored	Glipizide 5 mg	Glucotrol by URL Mutual	00677-1544	Antidiabetic
WATSON460	Tab, White, Round, Scored	Glipizide 5 mg	Glucotrol by Watson	00591-0460	Antidiabetic
WATSON461	Tab, White, Round, Scored	Glipizide 10 mg	Glucotrol by URL Mutual	00677-1545	Antidiabetic
WATSON461	Tab, White, Round, Scored	Glipizide 10 mg	Glucotrol by Qualitest	00603-3756	Antidiabetic
WATSON461	Tab, White, Round, Scored	Glipizide 10 mg	Glucotrol by Watson	52544-0461	Antidiabetic
WATSON461	Tab, White, Round, Scored	Glipizide 10 mg	Glucotrol by Kaiser	00179-1315	Antidiabetic
WATSON461	Tab, White, Round, Scored	Glipizide 10 mg	Glucotrol by Schein	00364-2605	Antidiabetic
WATSON461	Tab, White, Round, Scored	Glipizide 10 mg	Glucotrol by Moore	00839-7940	Antidiabetic
WATSON461	Tab, White, Round, Scored	Glipizide 10 mg	Glucotrol by Warner Chilcott	00047-0464	Antidiabetic
WATSON461	Tab, White, Round, Scored	Glipizide 10 mg	Glucotrol by PDRX	55289-0976	Antidiabetic
WATSON461	Tab, White, Round, Scored	Glipizide 10 mg	Glucotrol by Watson	00591-0461	Antidiabetic
WATSON462	Tab, Pink, Round, Scored	Metoprolol Tartrate 50 mg	Lopressor by Watson	00591-0462	Antihypertensive
WATSON462	Tab, Pink, Round, Scored	Metoprolol Tartrate 50 mg	Lopressor by Watson	52544-0462	Antihypertensive
WATSON462	Tab, Pink, Round, Scored	Metoprolol Tartrate 50 mg	Lopressor by Major	00904-5110	Antihypertensive
WATSON463	Tab, Blue, Round, Scored	Metoprolol Tartrate 100 mg	Lopressor by Major	00904-5111	Antihypertensive

ID FRONT <> BACK	DESCRIPTION FRONT <> BACK	INGREDIENT & STRENGTH	BRAND (or Generic Equiv.) by FIRM	NDC#	CLASS; SCH.
WATSON463	Tab, Blue, Round, Scored	Metoprolol Tartrate 100 mg	Lopressor by Watson	52544-0463	Antihypertensive
WATSON463	Tab, Blue, Round, Scored	Metoprolol Tartrate 100 mg	Lopressor by Watson	00591-0463	Antihypertensive
WATSON485	Tab, White, Round	Acetaminophen 325 mg, Butalbital 50 mg, Caffeine 40 mg	Fioricet by Watson	52544-0485	Analgesic
WATSON487	Tab, Gray, Round, Scored	Estradiol 1 mg	Estrace by Major	00904-5178	Hormone
WATSON487	Tab, Gray, Round, Scored	Estradiol 1 mg	Estrace by Sandoz	00781-1898	Hormone
WATSON487	Tab, Gray, Round, Scored	Estradiol 1 mg	Estrace by Ivax	00182-2649	Hormone
WATSON487	Tab, Gray, Round, Scored	Estradiol 1 mg	Estrace by Qualitest	00603-3557	Hormone
WATSON487	Tab, Gray, Round, Scored	Estradiol 1 mg	Estrace by Moore	00839-8077	Hormone
WATSON487	Tab, Gray, Round, Scored	Estradiol 1 mg	Estrace by Watson	52544-0487	Hormone
WATSON487	Tab, Gray, Round, Scored	Estradiol 1 mg	Estrace by Heartland	61392-0024	Hormone
WATSON487	Tab, Gray, Round, Scored	Estradiol 1 mg	Estrace by Haines	59564-0121	Hormone
WATSON487	Tab, Grey, Round, Scored	Estradiol 1 mg	Estrace by Watson	00591-0487	Hormone
WATSON488	Tab, Light Green, Round, Scored	Estradiol 2 mg	Estrace by Major	00904-5179	Hormone
WATSON488	Tab, Light Green, Round, Scored	Estradiol 2 mg	Estrace by Qualitest	00603-3558	Hormone
WATSON488	Tab, Light Green, Round, Scored	Estradiol 2 mg	Estrace by Moore	00839-8078	Hormone
WATSON488	Tab, Light Green, Round, Scored	Estradiol 2 mg	Estrace by Sandoz	00781-1899	Hormone
WATSON488	Tab, Light Green, Round, Scored	Estradiol 2 mg	Estrace by Ivax	00182-2650	Hormone
WATSON488	Tab, Light Green, Round, Scored	Estradiol 2 mg	Estrace by Watson	52544-0488	Hormone
WATSON49150MG	Cap, Light Brown, Watson 491 150 mg	Mexiletine 150 mg	Mexitil by Watson	00591-0491	Antiarrhythmic
WATSON49200MG	Cap, Brown, Opaque, Watson 492 200 mg	Mexiletine 200 mg	Mexitil by Watson	00591-0492	Antiarrhythmic
WATSON49250MG	Cap, Brown & Light Green, Opaque, Watson 493 250 mg	Mexiletine 250 mg	Mexitil by Watson	00591-0493	Antiarrhythmic
WATSON498100MG	Cap, Blue, 100MG on Cap and WATSON498 on body	Doxycycline Hyclate 100 mg	Vibramycin by Watson	52544-0498	Antibiotic
WATSON499	Tab, Beige, Round, Film Coated, 499 below WATSON	Doxycycline Hyclate 100 mg	Vibra Tabs by Watson	52544-0499	Antibiotic
WATSON502	Tab, Pink, Cap Shaped, Scored	Acetaminophen 650 mg, Hydrocodone Bitartrate 7.5 mg	Lorcet Plus by Murfreesboro	51129-1690	Analgesic; C III
WATSON502	Tab, Pink, Cap Shaped, Scored	Acetaminophen 650 mg, Hydrocodone Bitartrate 7.5 mg	Lorcet Plus by Compumed	00403-5196	Analgesic; C III
WATSON502	Tab, Pink, Cap Shaped, Scored	Acetaminophen 650 mg, Hydrocodone Bitartrate 7.5 mg	Lorcet Plus by Direct Dispensing	57866-5507	Analgesic; C III
WATSON502	Tab, Pink, Cap Shaped, Scored	Acetaminophen 650 mg, Hydrocodone Bitartrate 7.5 mg	Lorcet Plus by Sandoz	00781-1523	Analgesic; C III
WATSON502	Tab, Pink, Cap Shaped, Scored	Acetaminophen 650 mg, Hydrocodone Bitartrate 7.5 mg	Lorcet Plus by Major	00904-5158	Analgesic; C III
WATSON502	Tab, Pink, Cap Shaped, Scored	Acetaminophen 650 mg, Hydrocodone Bitartrate 7.5 mg	Lorcet Plus by Warner Chilcott	00047-0355	Analgesic; C III
WATSON502	Tab, Pink, Cap Shaped, Scored	Acetaminophen 650 mg, Hydrocodone Bitartrate 7.5 mg	Lorcet Plus by Watson	52544-0502	Analgesic; C III
WATSON502	Tab, Pink, Cap Shaped, Scored	Acetaminophen 650 mg, Hydrocodone Bitartrate 7.5 mg	Lorcet Plus by Watson	00591-0502	Analgesic; C III
WATSON503	Tab, Light Green, Cap Shaped, Scored	Acetaminophen 650 mg, Hydrocodone Bitartrate 10 mg	Lorcet by Major	00904-5288	Analgesic; C III
WATSON503	Tab, Light Green, Cap Shaped, Scored	Acetaminophen 650 mg, Hydrocodone Bitartrate 10 mg	Lorcet by Physician Total Care	54868-3729	Analgesic; C III
WATSON503	Tab, Light Green, Cap Shaped, Scored	Acetaminophen 650 mg, Hydrocodone Bitartrate 10 mg	Lorcet by Amerisource	62584-0068	Analgesic; C III
WATSON503	Tab, Light Green, Cap Shaped, Scored	Acetaminophen 650 mg, Hydrocodone Bitartrate 10 mg	Lorcet by Amerisource	62584-0072	Analgesic; C III
WATSON503	Tab, Light Green, Cap Shaped, Scored	Acetaminophen 650 mg, Hydrocodone Bitartrate 10 mg	Lorcet by Sandoz	00781-1524	Analgesic; C III
WATSON503	Tab, Light Green, Cap Shaped, Scored	Acetaminophen 650 mg, Hydrocodone Bitartrate 10 mg	Lorcet by Warner Chilcott	00047-0164	Analgesic; C III
WATSON503	Tab, Light Green, Cap Shaped, Scored	Acetaminophen 650 mg, Hydrocodone Bitartrate 10 mg	Lorcet by Ivax	00182-0034	Analgesic; C III
WATSON503	Tab, Light Green, Cap Shaped, Scored	Acetaminophen 650 mg, Hydrocodone Bitartrate 10 mg	Lorcet by Watson	52544-0503	Analgesic; C III
WATSON503	Tab, Light Green, Cap Shaped, Scored	Acetaminophen 650 mg, Hydrocodone Bitartrate 10 mg	Lorcet by Southwood	58016-0239	Analgesic; C III
WATSON503	Tab, Light Green, Cap Shaped, Scored	Acetaminophen 650 mg, Hydrocodone Bitartrate 10 mg	Lorcet by Compumed	00403-5306	Analgesic; C III
WATSON503	Tab, Light Green, Cap Shaped, Scored	Acetaminophen 650 mg, Hydrocodone Bitartrate 10 mg	Lorcet by Watson	00591-0503	Analgesic; C III
WATSON504	Tab, White, Round	Indapamide 2.5 mg	Lozol by Watson	52544-0504	Diuretic
WATSON527	Tab, Film Coated, Debossed	Indapamide 1.25 mg	Lozol by Physician Total Care	54868-3885	Diuretic
WATSON527	Tab, Orange, Round	Indapamide 1.25 mg	Lozol by Watson	52544-0527	Diuretic
WATSON527	Tab	Estradiol 0.5 mg	by Moore	00839-8076	Hormone
WATSON528	Tab, White, Round, Scored	Estradiol 0.5 mg	Estrace by Qualitest	00603-3556	Hormone
WATSON528	Tab, White, Round, Scored	Estradiol 0.5 mg	Estrace by Watson	52544-0528	Hormone
WATSON528	Tab, White, Round, Scored	Estradiol 0.5 mg	Estrace by Major	00904-5177	Hormone
WATSON528	Tab, White, Round, Scored	Estradiol 0.5 mg	Estrace by Ivax	00182-2648	Hormone

ID FRONT <> BACK	DESCRIPTION FRONT <> BACK	INGREDIENT & STRENGTH	BRAND (or Generic Equiv.) by FIRM	NDC#	CLASS; SCH.
WATSON528	Tab, White, Round, Scored	Estradiol 0.5 mg	Estrace by Sandoz	00781-1897	Hormone
WATSON528	Tab, White, Round, Scored	Estradiol 0.5 mg	Estrace by Watson	00591-0528	Hormone
WATSON540	Tab, Blue, Cap Shaped, Scored	Acetaminophen 500 mg, Hydrocodone Bitartrate 10 mg	Lortab by Southwood	58016-0229	Analgesic; C III
WATSON540	Tab, Blue, Cap Shaped, Scored	Acetaminophen 500 mg, Hydrocodone Bitartrate 10 mg	Lortab by St. Mary's Med	60760-0540	Analgesic; C III
WATSON540	Tab, Blue, Cap Shaped, Scored	Acetaminophen 500 mg, Hydrocodone Bitartrate 10 mg	Lortab by Watson	52544-0540	Analgesic; C III
WATSON540	Tab, Blue, Cap Shaped, Scored	Acetaminophen 500 mg, Hydrocodone Bitartrate 10 mg	Lortab by Murfreesboro	51129-1104	Analgesic; C III
WATSON540	Tab, Blue, Cap Shaped, Scored	Acetaminophen 500 mg, Hydrocodone Bitartrate 10 mg	Lortab by Watson	00591-0540	Analgesic; C III
WATSON544	Tab, Orange, Round	Desipramine HCl 75 mg	Norpramin by Watson	00591-0544	Antidepressant
WATSON544	Tab, Orange, Round	Desipramine HCl 75 mg	Norpramin by Watson	52544-0544	Antidepressant
WATSON545	Tab, Peach, Black Print, Round, Film Coated, Watson over 545	Desipramine HCl 100 mg	Norpramin by DRX	55045-2308	Antidepressant
WATSON545	Tab, Peach, Black Print, Round, Film Coated, Watson over 545	Desipramine HCl 100 mg	Norpramin by DRX	55045-2576	Antidepressant
WATSON545	Tab, Peach, Black Print, Round, Film Coated, Watson over 545	Desipramine HCl 100 mg	Norpramin by Watson	52544-0545	Antidepressant
WATSON545	Tab, Peach, Black Print, Round, Film Coated, Watson over 545	Desipramine HCl 100 mg	Norpramin by Blue Ridge	59273-0012	Antidepressant
WATSON545	Tab, Peach, Black Print, Round, Film Coated, Watson over 545	Desipramine HCl 100 mg	Norpramin by Watson	00591-0545	Antidepressant
WATSON575	Tab, White, Round, Scored	Trihexyphenidyl HCl 2 mg	Artane by Watson	52544-0575	Antiparkinson
WATSON576	Tab, White, Round, Scored	Trihexyphenidyl HCl 5 mg	Artane by Watson	52544-0576	Antiparkinson
WATSON576	Tab, White, Round, Scored	Trihexyphenidyl HCl 5 mg	Artane by Teva	00480-0755	Antiparkinson
WATSON582	Tab, White, Round, Film Coated, Scored	Propafenone HCl 150 mg	Rythmol by Watson	00591-0582	Antiarrhythmic
WATSON583	Tab, White, Round, Film Coated, Scored	Propafenone HCl 225 mg	Rythmol by Watson	00591-0583	Antiarrhythmic
WATSON585	Tab, Brown, Round, Film Coated	Diclofenac Potassium 50 mg	by Watson	52544-0585	NSAID
WATSON59425MG	Cap, Blue, Black Print, WATSON over 594	Clomipramine HCl 25 mg	Anafranil by Watson	52544-0594	OCD
WATSON59950MG	Cap, Yellow, Black Print, WATSON over 595	Clomipramine HCl 50 mg	Anafranil by Andrx	62022-0088	OCD
WATSON59950MG	Cap, Yellow, Black Print, WATSON over 595	Clomipramine HCl 50 mg	Anafranil by Watson	52544-0595	OCD
WATSON59675MG	Cap, Green, Black Print, WATSON over 596	Clomipramine HCl 75 mg	Anafranil by Watson	52544-0596	OCD
WATSON605	Tab, Beige, Round, Scored, Film Coated	Labetalol HCl 100 mg	Trandate by Watson	00591-0605	Antihypertensive
WATSON606	Tab, White, Round, Scored, Film Coated	Labetalol HCl 200 mg	Trandate by Watson	00591-0606	Antihypertensive
WATSON607	Tab, Blue, Round	Labetalol HCl 300 mg	Trandate by Watson	00591-0607	Antihypertensive
WATSON613	Tab, Blue, Oblong, Scored	Acetaminophen 500 mg, Butalbital 50 mg, Caffeine 40 mg	Esgic Plus by Watson	52544-0613	Analgesic
WATSON617	Tab, Gray, Round, Ex Release	Morphine Sulfate 100 mg	MS Contin by Watson	00591-0617	Analgesic; C II
WATSON629	Tab, White, Round	Norethindrone 0.35 mg	Nora-BE by Watson	52544-0629	Oral Contraceptive
WATSON630	Tab, White, Round	Norethindrone Acetate 1 mg, Ethinyl Estradiol 20 mcg	Microgestin by Watson	52544-0950	Oral Contraceptive
WATSON630	Tab, White, Round	Norethindrone Acetate 1 mg, Ethinyl Estradiol 20 mcg	Microgestin FE by Watson	52544-0630	Oral Contraceptive
WATSON631	Tab, Green, Round	Norethindrone Acetate 1.5 mg, Ethinyl Estradiol 30 mcg	Microgestin FE by Watson	52544-0631	Oral Contraceptive
WATSON631	Tab, Green, Round	Norethindrone Acetate 1.5 mg, Ethinyl Estradiol 30 mcg	Microgestin by Watson	52544-0951	Oral Contraceptive
WATSON632	Tab, Brown, Round	Inert	Microgestin FE by Watson	52544-0630	Oral Contraceptive; Placebo
WATSON632	Tab, Brown, Round	Inert	Microgestin FE by Watson	52544-0631	Oral Contraceptive; Placebo
WATSON637	Tab, Red, Oblong, Film Coated	Pentoxifylline 400 mg	Trental by Andrx	62037-0951	Anticoagulant
WATSON637	Tab, Red, Oblong, Film Coated, Scored	Pentoxifylline 400 mg	Trental by Watson	52544-0637	Anticoagulant
WATSON639	Tab, White to Off-White, Round, Scored	Doxazosin Mesylate 1 mg	Cardura by Watson	52544-0639	Antihypertensive
WATSON640	Tab, Light Orange, Round, Scored	Doxazosin Mesylate 2 mg	Cardura by Watson	52544-0640	Antihypertensive
WATSON641	Tab, Light Orange, Round, Scored	Doxazosin Mesylate 4 mg	Cardura by Watson	52544-0641	Antihypertensive
WATSON642	Tab, Green, Round, Scored	Doxazosin Mesylate 8 mg	Cardura by Watson	52544-0642	Antihypertensive
WATSON654	Tab, Light Blue, Oval	Sotalol 80 mg	Betapace by Watson	52544-0654	Antiarrhythmic

ID FRONT <> BACK	DESCRIPTION FRONT <> BACK	INGREDIENT & STRENGTH	BRAND (or Generic Equiv.) by FIRM	NDC#	CLASS; SCH.
WATSON655	Tab, Light Blue, Oval	Sotalol 160 mg	Betapace by Watson	52544-0655	Antiarrhythmic
WATSON656	Tab, Light Blue, Oval	Sotalol 240 mg	Betapace by Watson	52544-0665	Antiarrhythmic
WATSON665	Tab, Light Blue, Oval	Sotalol HCl 120 mg	Betapace by Watson	52544-0665	Antiarrhythmic
WATSON667400	Tab, Yellow, Oblong, Watson 667/400	Etodolac 400 mg	Lodine by Watson	52544-0667	NSAID
WATSON668	Tab, White to Off-White, Round, Scored	Enalapril Maleate 2.5 mg	Vasotec by Watson	00591-0668	Antihypertensive
WATSON669	Tab, White to Off-White, Round, Scored	Enalapril Maleate 5 mg	Vasotec by Watson	00591-0669	Antihypertensive
WATSON670	Tab, White w/ Pink Specks, Round	Enalapril Maleate 10 mg	Vasotec by Watson	00591-0670	Antihypertensive
WATSON671	Tab, Peach w/ White Specks, Round	Enalapril Maleate 20 mg	Vasotec by Watson	00591-0671	Antihypertensive
WATSON682	Tab, White, Oval	Alprazolam 0.25 mg	Xanax by Watson	52544-0682	Antianxiety; C IV
WATSON683	Tab, Peach, Oval	Alprazolam 0.5 mg	Xanax by Watson	52544-0683	Antianxiety; C IV
WATSON684	Tab, Blue, Oval	Alprazolam 1 mg	Xanax by Watson	52544-0684	Antianxiety; C IV
WATSON685	Tab, Peach, Round	Amiloride HCl 5 mg, Hydrochlorothiazide 50 mg	Moduretic by Watson	52544-0685	Antihypertensive; Diuretic
WATSON686	Tab, White, Oval	Baclofen 10 mg	Lioresal by Watson	52544-0686	Muscle Relaxant
WATSON687	Tab, White, Oval	Baclofen 20 mg	Lioresal by Watson	52544-0687	Muscle Relaxant
WATSON688	Tab, White, Oblong	Captopril 12.5 mg	Capoten by Watson	52544-0688	Antihypertensive
WATSON689	Tab, White, Round	Captopril 25 mg	Capoten by Watson	52544-0689	Antihypertensive
WATSON690	Tab, White, Oval	Captopril 50 mg	Capoten by Watson	52544-0690	Antihypertensive
WATSON692	Tab, White, Round	Carisoprodol 350 mg	Soma by Watson	52544-0692	Muscle Relaxant
WATSON693	Tab, Green, Oblong	Chlorzoxazone 500 mg	Parafon by Watson	52544-0693	Muscle Relaxant
WATSON69410	Tab, Dark Yellow, Round, Watson/694/10	Cyclobenzaprine HCl 10 mg	by Watson	52544-0694	Muscle Relaxant
WATSON69510MG	Cap	Doxepin HCl 10 mg	Sinequan by Watson	52544-0695	Antidepressant
WATSON69625MG	Cap, Blue, Opaque	Doxepin HCl 25 mg	Sinequan by H J Harkins Co	52959-0351	Antidepressant
WATSON69750MG	Cap, Pink, Opaque	Doxepin HCl 50 mg	Sinequan by H J Harkins Co	52959-0361	Antidepressant
WATSON69750MG	Cap, Pink, Opaque	Doxepin HCl 50 mg	Sinequan by Watson	52544-0697	Antidepressant
WATSON710	Tab, White, Round	Pindolol 5 mg	Visken by Watson	52544-0710	Antihypertensive
WATSON711	Tab, White, Round	Pindolol 10 mg	Visken by Watson	52544-0711	Antihypertensive
WATSON71210MG	Cap, Light Blue & White	Piroxicam 10 mg	Feldene by Watson	52544-0712	NSAID
WATSON71320MG	Cap, Filled with Off White to Yellow Powder	Piroxicam 20 mg	Feldene by Watson	52544-0713	NSAID
WATSON716325MG	Cap, White, Opaque	Quinine Sulfate 325 mg	Quinamm by RX Pak	65084-0137	Antimalarial
WATSON716325MG	Cap, White, Opaque	Quinine Sulfate 325 mg	Quinamm by Watson	52544-0716	Antimalarial
WATSON716325MG	Cap, White, Opaque	Quinine Sulfate 325 mg	Quinamm by Golden State	60429-0242	Antimalarial
WATSON716325MG	Cap, White, Opaque	Quinine Sulfate 325 mg	Quinamm by Watson	00591-0716	Antimalarial
WATSON717	Tab, White, Round	Yohimbine HCl 5.4 mg	Yocon by Watson	52544-0717	Impotence Agent
WATSON735200MG	Cap, Light Gray & Brown	Etodolac 200 mg	Lodine by Watson	00591-0735	NSAID
WATSON736300MG	Cap, Light Gray & Orange	Etodolac 300 mg	Lodine by Watson	00591-0736	NSAID
WATSON7375500MG	Cap, White & Red, Opaque, Watson 737 5-500 mg	Oxycodone 5 mg, Acetaminophen 500 mg	Percocet by Watson	00591-0737	Analgesic; C II
WATSON7375500MG	Cap, Red & White, Opaque, 5-500 <> Watson 737	Oxycodone 5 mg, Acetaminophen 500 mg	Tylox by Watson	00591-0737	Analgesic; C II
WATSON746	Tab, Yellow, Round, Scored	Clonazepam 0.5 mg	Klonopin by Watson	00591-0746	Sedative; C IV
WATSON746	Tab, Yellow, Round, Scored	Clonazepam 0.5 mg	Klonopin by Watson	52544-0746	Sedative; C IV
WATSON747	Tab, Aqua, Round, Scored	Clonazepam 1 mg	Klonopin by Watson	00591-0747	Sedative; C IV
WATSON747	Tab, Aqua, Round, Scored	Clonazepam 1 mg	Klonopin by Watson	52544-0747	Sedative; C IV
WATSON748	Tab, White, Round, Scored	Clonazepam 2 mg	Klonopin by Watson	00591-0748	Sedative; C IV
WATSON748	Tab, White, Round, Scored	Clonazepam 2 mg	Klonopin by Watson	52544-0748	Sedative; C IV
WATSON749	Tab, White, Round, Scored	Oxycodone 5 mg, Acetaminophen 325 mg	Percocet by Watson	00591-0749	Analgesic; C II
WATSON760	Tab, Beige, Round	Ranitidine 150 mg	Zantac by Watson	00591-0760	Gastrointestinal
WATSON761	Tab, Beige, Cap Shaped	Ranitidine 300 mg	Zantac by Watson	00591-0761	Gastrointestinal
WATSON775	Tab, Blue, Round, Scored	Diltiazem HCl 30 mg	Cardizem by Blue Ridge	59273-0002	Antihypertensive
WATSON775	Tab, Blue, Round, Scored	Diltiazem HCl 30 mg	Cardizem by Watson	00591-0775	Antihypertensive
WATSON776	Tab, White, Round, Scored	Diltiazem HCl 60 mg	Cardizem by Blue Ridge	59273-0003	Antihypertensive
WATSON776	Tab, White, Round, Scored	Diltiazem HCl 60 mg	Cardizem by Watson	52544-0776	Antihypertensive

ID FRONT <> BACK	DESCRIPTION FRONT <> BACK	INGREDIENT & STRENGTH	BRAND (or Generic Equiv.) by FIRM	NDC#	CLASS; SCH.
WATSON777	Tab, Blue, Oblong, Scored	Diltiazem HCl 90 mg	Cardizem by Endo		Antihypertensive
WATSON777	Tab, Blue, Oblong, Scored	Diltiazem HCl 90 mg	Cardizem by Watson	00591-0777	Antihypertensive
WATSON777	Tab, Blue, Oblong, Scored	Diltiazem HCl 120 mg	Cardizem by Blue Ridge	59273-0005	Antihypertensive
WATSON778	Tab, White, Oblong, Scored	Diltiazem HCl 120 mg	Cardizem by Excellium		Antihypertensive
WATSON778	Tab, White, Oblong, Scored	Diltiazem HCl 120 mg	Cardizem by Watson	00591-0778	Antihypertensive
WATSON779	Tab, Blue, Round, Scored	Oxybutynin Chloride 5 mg	Ditropan by Watson	00591-0779	Urinary Tract
WATSON780	Tab, Light Blue, Oblong, Scored, Watson over 780	Sucralfate 1 g	Carafate by SKB	00135-0181	Gastrointestinal
WATSON780	Tab, Light Blue, Oblong, Scored, Watson over 780	Sucralfate 1 g	Carafate by Blue Ridge	59273-0001	Gastrointestinal
WATSON780	Tab, Light Blue, Oblong, Scored, Watson over 780	Sucralfate 1 g	Carafate by Watson	00591-0780	Gastrointestinal
WATSON781	Tab, Off-White, Round	Clomiphene Citrate 50 mg	Serophene by Watson	00591-0781	Infertility
WATSON782	Tab, White, Oblong	Diethylpropion HCl 75 mg	Tenuate by Blue Ridge	59273-0008	Anorexiant; C IV
WATSON782	Tab, White, Oblong	Diethylpropion HCl 75 mg	Tenuate by BMS	00590-0627	Anorexiant; C IV
WATSON782	Tab, White, Cap Shaped, Ex Release	Diethylpropion HCl 75 mg	Tenuate by Watson	00591-0782	Anorexiant; C IV
WATSON783	Tab, White, Round	Diethylpropion HCl 25 mg	Tenuate by Blue Ridge	59273-0007	Anorexiant; C IV
WATSON783	Tab, White, Round	Diethylpropion HCl 25 mg	Tenuate by BMS	00056-0698	Anorexiant; C IV
WATSON783	Tab, White, Round	Diethylpropion HCl 25 mg	Tenuate by Watson	00591-0783	Anorexiant; C IV
WATSON785MG	Cap, Green & Yellow, Opaque	Chlordiazepoxide 5 mg	Librium by Watson	52544-0785	Antianxiety; C IV
WATSON785MG	Cap, Green & Yellow, Opaque	Chlordiazepoxide 5 mg	Librium by CCA	61543-0017	Antianxiety; C IV
WATSON785MG	Cap, Green & Yellow, Opaque	Chlordiazepoxide 5 mg	Librium by Blue Ridge	59273-0045	Antianxiety; C IV
WATSON785MG	Cap, Green & Yellow, Opaque	Chlordiazepoxide 5 mg	Librium by Watson	00591-0785	Antianxiety; C IV
WATSON78610MG	Cap, Black & Green, Opaque	Chlordiazepoxide 10 mg	Librium by Watson	52544-0786	Antianxiety; C IV
WATSON78610MG	Cap, Black & Green, Opaque	Chlordiazepoxide 10 mg	Librium by Watson	00591-0786	Antianxiety; C IV
WATSON78725MG	Cap, Green & White, Opaque	Chlordiazepoxide 25 mg	Librium by Watson	52544-0787	Antianxiety; C IV
WATSON78725MG	Cap, Green & White, Opaque	Chlordiazepoxide 25 mg	Librium by Watson	00591-0787	Antianxiety; C IV
WATSON790	Tab, White, Oval, Scored	Methylprednisolone 4 mg	Medrol by Watson	00591-0790	Steroid
WATSON791	Tab, White to Off-White, Cap Shaped	Naproxen 500 mg	Naprosyn by Watson	00591-0791	NSAID
WATSON791	Tab, White to Off-White, Cap Shaped	Naproxen 500 mg	Naprosyn by Blue Ridge	59273-0039	NSAID
WATSON792	Tab, White, Oval	Naproxen 275 mg	Naprosyn by Blue Ridge	59273-0040	NSAID
WATSON792	Tab, White, Oval	Naproxen 275 mg	Naprosyn by Watson	00591-0792	NSAID
WATSON792	Tab, White, Oval	Naproxen 275 mg	Naprosyn by Watson	52544-0792	NSAID
WATSON793	Tab, Green, Oval	Naproxen 550 mg	Naprosyn by Watson	52544-0793	NSAID
WATSON793	Tab, Green, Oval	Naproxen 550 mg	Naprosyn by Watson	00591-0793	NSAID
WATSON79410MG	Cap, Blue, White Print, Watson over 794	Dicyclomine HCl 10 mg	Bentyl by Watson	00591-0794	Gastrointestinal
WATSON795	Tab, Blue, Round, Watson over 795	Dicyclomine HCl 20 mg	Bentyl by Watson	00591-0795	Gastrointestinal
WATSON796	Tab, Yellow, Round, Scored	Sulfasalazine 500 mg	Azulfidine by Watson	00591-0796	Gastrointestinal
WATSON797	Tab, White, Round	Prednisone 50 mg	Merticorten by Watson	52544-0797	Steroid
WATSON80025MG	Cap, Green	Hydroxyzine Pamoate 25 mg	Vistaril by Watson	00591-0800	Antianxiety; Antihistamine
WATSON80150MG	Cap, Green & White	Hydroxyzine Pamoate 50 mg	Vistaril by Watson	00591-0801	Antianxiety; Antihistamine
WATSON80150MG	Cap, Green & White	Hydroxyzine Pamoate 50 mg	Vistaril by Murfreesboro	51129-1486	Antianxiety; Antihistamine
WATSON80150MG	Cap, Green & White	Hydroxyzine Pamoate 50 mg	Vistaril by Blue Ridge	59273-0044	Antianxiety; Antihistamine
WATSON802	Tab, Blue & White, Oval	Meclizine HCl 12.5 mg	Antivert by Watson	52544-0802	Antiemetic
WATSON803	Tab, Yellow and White, Oval	Meclizine 25 mg	Antivert by Watson	00591-0803	Antiemetic
WATSON806	Tab, White, Round, Scored	Methocarbamol 500 mg	Robaxin by Watson	52544-0806	Muscle Relaxant
WATSON807	Tab, White, Cap Shaped, Scored	Methocarbamol 750 mg	Robaxin by Watson	52544-0807	Muscle Relaxant
WATSON808	Tab, Yellow, Round, Watson over 808	Desipramine HCl 25 mg	Norpramin by Blue Ridge	59273-0009	Antidepressant
WATSON808	Tab, Yellow, Round, Watson over 808	Desipramine HCl 25 mg	Norpramin by DRX	55045-2339	Antidepressant
WATSON808	Tab, Yellow, Round, Watson over 808	Desipramine HCl 25 mg	Norpramin by Watson	00591-0808	Antidepressant
WATSON809	Tab, Green, Round, Watson over 809	Desipramine HCl 50 mg	Norpramin by Watson	00591-0809	Antidepressant
WATSON809	Tab, Green, Round, Watson over 809	Desipramine HCl 50 mg	Norpramin by Blue Ridge	59273-0010	Antidepressant
WATSON809	Tab, Green, Round, Watson over 809	Desipramine HCl 50 mg	Norpramin by DRX	55045-2565	Antidepressant

ID FRONT <> BACK	DESCRIPTION FRONT <> BACK	INGREDIENT & STRENGTH	BRAND (or Generic Equiv.) by FIRM	NDC#	CLASS; SCH.
WATSON819	Cap, Green, Oblong	Indomethacin 50 mg	Indocin by Watson	52544-0819	NSAID
WATSON820	Tab, Yellow, Round, Scored	Oxycodone 4.5 mg, Oxycodone Terephthalate 0.38 mg, Aspirin 325 mg	Percodan by Watson	00591-0820	Analgesic; C II
WATSON821	Tab, White, Round	Naproxen 250 mg	Naprosyn by Watson	00591-0821	NSAID
WATSON822	Tab, Grey, Cap Shaped	Naproxen 375 mg	Naprosyn by Watson	00591-0822	NSAID
WATSON824	Tab, White, Cap Shaped, Scored	Oxycodone 7.5 mg, Acetaminophen 500 mg	Percocet by Watson	00591-0824	Analgesic; C II
WATSON824	Tab, White, Cap Shaped, Scored	Oxycodone 7.5 mg, Acetaminophen 500 mg	Percocet by Watson	52544-0824	Analgesic; C II
WATSON825	Tab, White, Cap Shaped, Scored	Oxycodone 10 mg, Acetaminophen 650 mg	Percocet by Watson	00591-0825	Analgesic; C II
WATSON825	Tab, White, Cap Shaped, Scored	Oxycodone 10 mg, Acetaminophen 650 mg	Percocet by Watson	52544-0825	Analgesic; C II
WATSON82610MG	Cap, Light Green, Opaque, Hard Gel	Fluoxetine HCl 10 mg	Prozac by Watson	00591-0826	Antidepressant
WATSON82720MG	Cap, Light Green & White, Opaque, Hard Gel	Fluoxetine HCl 20 mg	Prozac by Watson	00591-0827	Antidepressant
WATSON830	Tab, White, Round	Prednisone 5 mg	Deltasone by Watson	00591-0830	Steroid
WATSON832	Tab, White, Round	Prednisone 20 mg	Deltasone by Watson	00591-0832	Steroid
WATSON835	Tab, Blue, Triangular, Scored	Clorazepate Dipotassium 3.75 mg	Tranxene by Watson	00591-0835	Antianxiety; C IV
WATSON841	Tab, Yellow, Round	Bisoprolol 2.5 mg, Hydrochlorothiazide 6.25 mg	Ziac by Watson	00591-0841	Antihypertensive; Diuretic
WATSON842	Tab, Pink, Round	Bisoprolol 5 mg, Hydrochlorothiazide 6.25 mg	Ziac by Watson	52544-0842	Antihypertensive; Diuretic
WATSON842	Tab, Pink, Round	Bisoprolol 5 mg, Hydrochlorothiazide 6.25 mg	Ziac by Watson	00591-0842	Antihypertensive; Diuretic
WATSON843	Tab, White, Round	Bisoprolol 10 mg, Hydrochlorothiazide 6.25 mg	Ziac by Watson	52544-0843	Antihypertensive; Diuretic
WATSON843	Tab, White, Round	Bisoprolol 10 mg, Hydrochlorothiazide 6.25 mg	Ziac by Watson	00591-0843	Antihypertensive; Diuretic
WATSON850	Tab, White, Round, Scored	Acetaminophen 300 mg, Codeine Phosphate 15 mg	Tylenol w/ Codeine by Watson	52544-0850	Analgesic; C III
WATSON851	Tab, White, Round, Scored	Acetaminophen 300 mg, Codeine Phosphate 30 mg	Tylenol w/ Codeine by Watson	52544-0851	Analgesic; C III
WATSON852	Tab, White, Round, Scored	Acetaminophen 300 mg, Codeine Phosphate 60 mg	Tylenol w/ Codeine by Watson	52544-0852	Analgesic; C III
WATSON853	Tab, Yellow, Cap Shaped, Scored	Acetaminophen 325 mg, Hydrocodone Bitartrate 10 mg	Norco by Watson	00591-0853	Analgesic; C III
WATSON854	Tab, Light Blue, Oval	Sotalol HCl 80 mg	Betapace by Watson	00591-0654	Antiarrhythmic
WATSON860	Tab, Pink, Round	Hydrochlorothiazide 12.5 mg, Lisinopril 10 mg	Lisinopril/HCTZ by Watson	00591-0860	Diuretic; Antihypertensive
WATSON861	Tab, Blue, Round	Hydrochlorothiazide 12.5 mg, Lisinopril 20 mg	Lisinopril/HCTZ by Watson	00591-0861	Diuretic; Antihypertensive
WATSON862	Tab, Pink, Round	Hydrochlorothiazide 25 mg, Lisinopril 20 mg	Lisinopril/HCTZ by Watson	00591-0862	Diuretic; Antihypertensive
WATSON885	Tab, Yellow, Round	Lisinopril HCl 30 mg	Prinivil by Watson	00591-0885	Antihypertensive
WATSON932	Tab, White, Round	Acetaminophen 325 mg, Oxycodone 10 mg	Percocet by Watson	00591-0932	Analgesic; C II
WATSON933	Tab, White, Round	Acetaminophen 325 mg, Oxycodone 7.5 mg	Percocet by Watson	00591-0933	Analgesic; C II
WATSON937	Tab, Light Peach, Round	Norethindrone 0.5 mg, Ethinyl Estradiol 0.035 mg	Necon 7/7/7 by Watson	52544-0936	Oral Contraceptive
WATSON938	Tab, Light Peach, Round	Norethindrone 0.75 mg, Ethinyl Estradiol 0.035 mg	Necon 7/7/7 by Watson	52544-0936	Oral Contraceptive
WATSON939	Tab, Peach, Round	Norethindrone 1 mg, Ethinyl Estradiol 0.035 mg	Necon 7/7/7 by Watson	52544-0936	Oral Contraceptive
WATSONACYCLOVIR200	Cap, Light Blue and Aqua, Black Ink	Acyclovir 200 mg	Zovirax by Watson	00591-2692	Antiviral
WATSONDILACOR120	Cap, Gold & White, Watson/Dilacor/120	Diltiazem HCl 120 mg	Dilacor XR by Watson		Antihypertensive
WATSONDILACOR180	Cap, Gold & White, Watson/Dilacor/180	Diltiazem HCl 180 mg	Dilacor XR by Watson		Antihypertensive
WATSONDILACOR240	Cap, Gold & White, Watson/Dilacor/240	Diltiazem HCl 240 mg	Dilacor XR by Watson		Antihypertensive
WATSONLOXITANE10MG	Cap, Yellow & Dark Green, Loxitane over 10 mg	Loxapine 10 mg	Loxitane by Watson	52544-0495	Antipsychotic
WATSONLOXITANE25MG	Cap, Dark Green & Light Green, Loxitane over 25 mg	Loxapine 25 mg	Loxitane by Watson	52544-0496	Antipsychotic
WATSONLOXITANE50MG	Cap, Blue & Dark Green, Loxitane over 50 mg	Loxapine 50 mg	Loxitane by Watson	52544-0497	Antipsychotic
WATSONLOXITANE5MG	Cap, Green, Opaque, Loxitane over 5 mg	Loxapine 5 mg	Loxitane by Watson	52544-0494	Antipsychotic
WB34	Cap, Tan & Cream	Tyropanoate 750 mg	Bilopaque by Sanofi		Diagnostic
WBS	Tab, Blue & White, Round, Schering Logo WBS	Dexbrompheniramine Maleate 2 mg, Pseudoephedrine Sulfate 60 mg	Disophrol by Schering		Cold Remedy
WC <> 084	Tab, White, Blue Print, Oval, Partially Scored, Film Coated	Gemfibrozil 600 mg	by Pliva	50111-0857	Antihyperlipidemic
WC <> 084	Tab, White, Blue Print, Oval, Partially Scored, Film Coated	Gemfibrozil 600 mg	by Kaiser	62224-1226	Antihyperlipidemic
WC <> 084	Tab, White, Blue Print, Oval, Partially Scored, Film Coated	Gemfibrozil 600 mg	by Moore	00839-7787	Antihyperlipidemic
WC <> 084	Tab, White, Blue Print, Oval, Partially Scored, Film Coated	Gemfibrozil 600 mg	by Kaiser	00179-1171	Antihyperlipidemic
WC <> 084	Tab, White, Blue Print, Oval, Partially Scored, Film Coated	Gemfibrozil 600 mg	by Warner Chilcott	00047-0084	Antihyperlipidemic
WC <> 084	Tab, White, Blue Print, Oval, Partially Scored, Film Coated	Gemfibrozil 600 mg	by Allscripts		Antihyperlipidemic
WC <> 084	Tab, White, Blue Print, Oval, Partially Scored, Film Coated	Gemfibrozil 600 mg	by Med Pro	53978-2033	Antihyperlipidemic

ID FRONT <> BACK	DESCRIPTION FRONT <> BACK	INGREDIENT & STRENGTH	BRAND (or Generic Equiv.) by FIRM	NDC#	CLASS; SCH.
WC <> 176	Tab, White, Cap Shaped, Scored, Ex Release	Isosorbide Mononitrate 60 mg	Imdur by Warner Chilcott	00047-0176	Antianginal
WC <> 227	Tab, Round	Vitamin A 1000 Units, Cholecalciferol 400 Units, Vitamin E 11 Units, Ascorbic Acid 120 mg, Folic Acid 1 mg, Thiamine Mononitrate 2 mg, Riboflavin 3 mg, Niacinamide 20 mg, Cyanocobalamin 12 mcg, Pyridoxine HCl 10 mg, Iron 29 mg	Natachew by Amide	52152-0210	Vitamin
WC <> 227	Tab, Light Buff, Round	Vitamin A 1000 Units, Cholecalciferol 400 Units, Vitamin E 11 Units, Ascorbic Acid 120 mg, Folic Acid 1 mg, Thiamine Mononitrate 2 mg, Riboflavin 3 mg, Niacinamide 20 mg, Cyanocobalamin 12 mcg, Pyridoxine HCl 10 mg, Iron 29 mg	Natachew by Warner Chilcott	00430-0227	Vitamin
WC <> 481	Tab, Green, Cap Shaped, W / C	Inert	Ovcon 35 by Warner Chilcott	00430-0582	Oral Contraceptive; Placebo
WC <> 530	Tab, White, Round	Norethindrone Acetate 1 mg, Ethinyl Estradiol 20 mcg	Loestrin 24 Fe by Warner Chilcott	00430-0530	Oral Contraceptive
WC <> 581	Tab, White, Round, Scored, W / C	Ethinyl Estradiol 0.035 mg, Norethindrone 0.4 mg	Ovcon 35 by Warner Chilcott	00430-0582	Oral Contraceptive
WC <> 72012	Tab, White to Off-White, Oval, Scored	Estradiol 0.5 mg	Estrace by Warner Chilcott	00430-0720	Hormone
WC <> 7211	Tab, Light purple, Oval, Scored	Estradiol 1 mg	Estrace by Warner Chilcott	00430-0721	Hormone
WC <> 7222	Tab, Green, Oval, Scored	Estradiol 2 mg	Estrace by Warner Chilcott	00430-0722	Hormone
WC014	Tab, White, Round	Hydrochlorothiazide 25 mg, Propranolol HCl 40 mg	Inderide by WC		Diuretic; Antihypertensive
WC015	Tab, White, Round	Hydrochlorothiazide 25 mg, Propranolol HCl 80 mg	Inderide by WC		Diuretic; Antihypertensive
WC030	Tab, Green, Round	Hydrochlorothiazide 15 mg, Methyldopa 250 mg	Aldoril by WC		Diuretic; Antihypertensive
WC031	Tab, White, Oblong	Hydrochlorothiazide 25 mg, Methyldopa 250 mg	Aldoril by WC		Diuretic; Antihypertensive
WC032	Tab, Maroon	Hydrochlorothiazide 30 mg, Methyldopa 500 mg	Aldoril by WC		Diuretic; Antihypertensive
WC033	Tab, Gray	Hydrochlorothiazide 50 mg, Methyldopa 500 mg	Aldoril by WC		Diuretic; Antihypertensive
WC038	Tab, Off-White, Chewable	Amoxicillin 250 mg	Amoxil by WC		Antibiotic
WC048	Cap, Yellow	Benzonatate 100 mg	Tessalon by WC		Antitussive
WC049	Tab, White, Round	Butalbital 50 mg, Aspirin 325 mg, Caffeine 40 mg	Fiorinal by WC		Analgesic; C III
WC057	Tab, White, Round	Cyclobenzaprine HCl 10 mg	Flexeril by WC		Muscle Relaxant
WC070	Tab, Orange, Round	Propranolol HCl 10 mg	Inderal by WC		Antihypertensive
WC071	Tab, Blue, Round	Propranolol HCl 20 mg	Inderal by WC		Antihypertensive
WC072	Tab, Green, Round	Propranolol HCl 40 mg	Inderal by WC		Antihypertensive
WC073	Tab, Pink, Round	Propranolol HCl 60 mg	Inderal by WC		Antihypertensive
WC074	Tab, Yellow, Round	Propranolol HCl 80 mg	Inderal by WC		Antihypertensive
WC077	Tab, Peach, Oval	Fenoprofen Calcium 600 mg	Nalfon by WC		NSAID
WC078	Cap, Yellow	Nifedipine 10 mg	Procardia by WC		Antihypertensive
WC079	Cap, Orange, Red & Brown	Nifedipine 20 mg	Procardia by WC		Antihypertensive
WC081	Cap, Yellow	Fenoprofen Calcium 300 mg	Nalfon by WC		NSAID
WC121	Tab, Blue, Round	Chlorthalidone 50 mg	Hygroton by WC		Diuretic
WC123	Tab, Orange, Round	Chlorthalidone 25 mg	Hygroton by WC		Diuretic
WC124	Tab, Yellow, Round	Estropipate 0.75 mg	Ogen by WC		Hormone
WC126	Tab, Peach, Round	Estropipate 1.5 mg	Ogen by WC		Hormone
WC128	Tab, Blue, Round	Estropipate 3 mg	Ogen by WC		Hormone
WC141	Tab, White, Oval	Diazepam 2 mg	Valium by WC		Antianxiety; C IV
WC142	Tab, White, Triangular	Diazepam 5 mg	Valium by WC		Antianxiety; C IV
WC143	Tab, White, Round	Diazepam 10 mg	Valium by WC		Antianxiety; C IV
WC180	Tab, Maroon, Round, Coated	Phenazopyridine HCl 100 mg	Pyridium by Warner Chilcott	00430-0180	Urinary Analgesic

ID FRONT <> BACK	DESCRIPTION FRONT <> BACK	INGREDIENT & STRENGTH	BRAND (or Generic Equiv.) by FIRM	NDC#	CLASS; SCH.
WC180	Tab, Maroon, Round, Coated	Phenazopyridine HCl 100 mg	Pyridium by Warner Chilcott	00430-0180	Urinary Analgesic
WC180	Tab, Maroon, Round, Coated	Phenazopyridine HCl 100 mg	Pyridium by Murfreesboro	51129-1346	Urinary Analgesic
WC181	Tab, Maroon, Round, Coated	Phenazopyridine HCl 200 mg	Pyridium by Pharmafab	62542-0919	Urinary Analgesic
WC181	Tab, Maroon, Round, Coated	Phenazopyridine HCl 200 mg	Pyridium by Physician Total Care	54868-0878	Urinary Analgesic
WC181	Tab, Maroon, Round, Coated	Phenazopyridine HCl 200 mg	Pyridium by Warner Chilcott	00430-0181	Urinary Analgesic
WC182	Tab, Maroon, Oval, Coated	Phenazopyridine HCl 150 mg, Hyoscyamine HBr 0.3 mg, Butabarbital 15 mg	Pyridium Plus by Warner Chilcott	00430-0182	Urinary Analgesic
WC196	Cap, Clear & White	Theophylline Anhydrous CR 100 mg	Slo-Bid by WC		Antiasthmatic
WC197	Cap, Clear	Theophylline Anhydrous CR 125 mg	Slo-Bid by WC		Antiasthmatic
WC198	Cap, Clear & White	Theophylline Anhydrous CR 200 mg	Slo-Bid by WC		Antiasthmatic
WC199	Cap, Clear & White	Theophylline Anhydrous CR 300 mg	Slo-Bid by WC		Antiasthmatic
WC214	Tab, Pink, Oblong, Ex Release	Oxtriphylline 400 mg	Choledyl SA by Warner Chilcott	00430-0214	Antiasthmatic
WC214	Tab, Film Coated	Oxtriphylline 400 mg	Choledyl SA by Warner Chilcott	00430-0214	Antiasthmatic
WC221	Tab, Tan, Oblong, Ex Release	Oxtriphylline 600 mg	Choledyl SA by Warner Chilcott	00430-0221	Antiasthmatic
WC221	Tab, Film Coated	Oxtriphylline 600 mg	Choledyl SA by Warner Chilcott	00430-0221	Antiasthmatic
WC242	Tab, Pink, Round, Chewable	Carbamazepine 100 mg	Tegretol by WC		Anticonvulsant
WC243	Tab, White	Carbamazepine 200 mg	Tegretol by WC		Anticonvulsant
WC271	Tab, Mustard, Round	Amitriptyline HCl 100 mg	Elavil by WC		Antidepressant
WC272	Tab, Tan, Round, W-C 272	Amitriptyline HCl 10 mg	Elavil by WC		Antidepressant
WC273	Tab, Coral, Round, W-C 273	Amitriptyline HCl 25 mg	Elavil by WC		Antidepressant
WC274	Tab, Blue, Round, W-C274	Amitriptyline HCl 50 mg	Elavil by WC		Antidepressant
WC275	Tab, Green, Round, W-C 275	Amitriptyline HCl 75 mg	Elavil by WC		Antidepressant
WC278	Tab, Orange, Round	Amitriptyline HCl 150 mg	Elavil by WC		Antidepressant
WC314	Tab, White, Round	Amoxapine 25 mg	Asendin by WC		Antidepressant
WC315	Tab, Salmon, Round	Amoxapine 50 mg	Asendin by WC		Antidepressant
WC316	Tab, Salmon, Round	Amoxapine 100 mg	Asendin by WC		Antidepressant
WC317	Tab, Peach, Round	Amoxapine 150 mg	Asendin by WC		Antidepressant
WC318	Tab, White, Oblong	Acetaminophen 500 mg, Hydrocodone Bitartrate 2.5 mg	Lortab by WC		Analgesic; C III
WC319	Tab, White, Oblong	Acetaminophen 500 mg, Hydrocodone Bitartrate 5 mg	Vicodin by WC		Analgesic; C III
WC323	Tab, White, Round	Methyldopa 250 mg	Aldomet by WC		Antihypertensive
WC324	Tab, White, Round	Methyldopa 500 mg	Aldomet by WC		Antihypertensive
WC328	Tab, White, Round	Verapamil HCl 80 mg	Isoptin, Calan by WC		Antihypertensive
WC329	Tab, White, Round	Verapamil HCl 120 mg	Isoptin, Calan by WC		Antihypertensive
WC334	Tab, Orange, Round	Levothyroxine Sodium 0.25 mg	Synthroid by WC		Thyroid Hormone
WC336	Tab, White, Round	Levothyroxine Sodium 0.5 mg	Synthroid by WC		Thyroid Hormone
WC338	Tab, Violet, Round	Levothyroxine Sodium 0.075 mg	Synthroid by WC		Thyroid Hormone
WC341	Tab, Yellow, Round	Levothyroxine Sodium 0.1 mg	Synthroid by WC		Thyroid Hormone
WC343	Tab, Brown, Round	Levothyroxine Sodium 0.125 mg	Synthroid by WC		Thyroid Hormone
WC344	Tab, Blue, Round	Levothyroxine Sodium 0.15 mg	Synthroid by WC		Thyroid Hormone
WC347	Tab, Pink, Round	Levothyroxine Sodium 0.2 mg	Synthroid by WC		Thyroid Hormone
WC348	Tab, Green, Round	Levothyroxine Sodium 0.3 mg	Synthroid by WC		Thyroid Hormone
WC389	Tab, Cream, Round, WC389 <> Logo	Estradiol 0.45 mg	Femtrace by Warner Chilcott	00430-0389	Hormone
WC390	Tab, White, Round, WC390 <> Logo	Estradiol 0.9 mg	Femtrace by Warner Chilcott	00430-0390	Hormone
WC391	Tab, Yellow, Round, WC391 <> Logo	Estradiol 1.8 mg	Femtrace by Warner Chilcott	00430-0391	Hormone

ID FRONT <> BACK	DESCRIPTION FRONT <> BACK	INGREDIENT & STRENGTH	BRAND (or Generic Equiv.) by FIRM	NDC#	CLASS; SCH.
WC402	Cap, Blue & Gray, Black Print, WC over 402	Ampicillin 250 mg	Polycillin by Dava	67253-0180	Antibiotic
WC402	Cap, Blue & Gray, Black Print, WC over 402	Ampicillin 250 mg	Principen by Warner Chilcott	00047-0402	Antibiotic
WC402	Cap, Blue & Gray, Black Print, WC over 402	Ampicillin 250 mg	Principen by Clonmell	55190-0402	Antibiotic
WC402	Cap, Blue & Gray, Black Print, WC over 402	Ampicillin 250 mg	Principen by Pharmedix	53002-0230	Antibiotic
WC402	Cap, Blue & Gray, Black Print, WC over 402	Ampicillin 250 mg	Principen by Mova	55370-0880	Antibiotic
WC404	Cap, Blue & Gray, Black Print, WC over 404	Ampicillin 500 mg	Principen by Mova	55370-0881	Antibiotic
WC404	Cap, Blue & Gray, Black Print, WC over 404	Ampicillin 500 mg	Principen by Clonmell	55190-0404	Antibiotic
WC404	Cap, Blue & Gray, Black Print, WC over 404	Ampicillin 500 mg	Principen by Pharmedix	53002-0231	Antibiotic
WC404	Cap, Blue & Gray, Black Print, WC over 404	Ampicillin 500 mg	Polycillin by Dava	67253-0181	Antibiotic
WC407	Cap, Red & Beige, Black Print, WC over 407	Tetracycline HCl 250 mg	by Warner Chilcott	00047-0407	Antibiotic
WC420	Tab, White, Round	Quinine Sulfate 325 mg	by WC		Antimalarial
WC431	Tab, White, Round	Lorazepam 0.5 mg	Ativan by WC		Antianxiety; C IV
WC432	Tab, White, Round	Lorazepam 1 mg	Ativan by WC		Antianxiety; C IV
WC433	Tab, White, Round	Lorazepam 2 mg	Ativan by WC		Antianxiety; C IV
WC440	Tab, White, Oval	Furosemide 20 mg	Lasix by WC		Diuretic
WC441	Tab, White, Round	Furosemide 40 mg	Lasix by WC		Diuretic
WC442	Tab, White, Round	Furosemide 80 mg	Lasix by WC		Diuretic
WC443	Tab, Pink, Round	Clonidine HCl 0.1 mg	Catapres by WC		Antihypertensive
WC444	Tab, White, Round	Clonidine HCl 0.2 mg	Catapres by WC		Antihypertensive
WC445	Tab, White, Round	Clonidine HCl 0.3 mg	Catapres by WC		Antihypertensive
WC448	Tab, White, Oblong	Acetaminophen 500 mg, Hydrocodone Bitartrate 5 mg	Vicodin by WC		Analgesic; C III
WC451	Tab, Blue, Round	Clorazepate Dipotassium 30.75 mg	Tranxene by WC		Antianxiety; C IV
WC452	Tab, Beige, Round	Clorazepate Dipotassium 7.5 mg	Tranxene by WC		Antianxiety; C IV
WC453	Tab, Pink, Round	Clorazepate Dipotassium 15 mg	Tranxene by WC		Antianxiety; C IV
WC463	Tab, White, Round	Glipizide 5 mg	Glucotrol by WC		Antidiabetic
WC464	Tab, White, Round	Glipizide 10 mg	Glucotrol by WC		Antidiabetic
WC472	Tab, White, Oval	Verapamil HCl SR 180 mg	Calan by WC		Antihypertensive
WC474	Tab, White, Oval	Verapamil HCl SR 240 mg	Calan by WC		Antihypertensive
WC486	Tab, White, Oblong	Acetaminophen 750 mg, Hydrocodone Bitartrate 7.5 mg	Vicodin ES by WC		Analgesic; C III
WC508	Tab, Green, Oval	Cimetidine HCl 800 mg	Tagamet by WC		Gastrointestinal
WC515	Tab, White, Round	Allopurinol 100 mg	Zyloprim by WC		Antigout
WC516	Tab, White, Elongated	Ibuprofen 400 mg	Motrin by WC		NSAID
WC517	Tab, Peach, Round	Allopurinol 300 mg	Zyloprim by WC		Antigout
WC528	Cap, Blue	Ketoprofen 50 mg	Orudis by WC		NSAID
WC538	Cap, Blue & Yellow	Cefadroxil Monohydrate 500 mg	Duricef by WC		Antibiotic
WC548	Tab, White, Round	Cephalexin 250 mg	Keflex by WC		Antibiotic
WC549	Tab, White, Round	Cephalexin 500 mg	Keflex by WC		Antibiotic
WC551	Tab, Yellow, Round	Oxazepam 15 mg	Serax by WC		Sedative/Hypnotic; C IV
WC557	Tab, White, Round	Verapamil 80 mg	Isoptin by WC		Antihypertensive
WC558	Cap, Purple & Yellow, Ex Release	Disopyramide Phosphate 100 mg	Norpace CR by WC		Antiarrhythmic
WC560	Tab, Orange, Round	Guanabenz Acetate 4 mg	Wytensin by WC		Antihypertensive
WC561	Tab, Gray, Round	Guanabenz Acetate 8 mg	Wytensin by WC		Antihypertensive

ID FRONT <> BACK	DESCRIPTION FRONT <> BACK	INGREDIENT & STRENGTH	BRAND (or Generic Equiv.) by FIRM	NDC#	CLASS; SCH.
WC566	Cap, Blue & White	Ketoprofen 75 mg	Orudis by WC		NSAID
WC573	Tab, White, Round	Verapamil 120 mg	Isoptin by WC		Antihypertensive
WC575	Cap, Orange & Clear	Danazol 200 mg	Danocrine by WC		Steroid
WC577	Tab, White, Round	Trazodone HCl 50 mg	Desyrel by WC		Antidepressant
WC578	Tab, White, Round	Trazodone HCl 100 mg	Desyrel by WC		Antidepressant
WC592	Tab, White, Round	Theophylline Anhydrous CR 300 mg	Theo-Dur by WC		Antiasthmatic
WC593	Tab, White, Oval	Theophylline Anhydrous CR 450 mg	Theo-Dur by WC		Antiasthmatic
WC594	Tab, Yellow, Round	Desipramine HCl 25 mg	Norpramin by WC		Antidepressant
WC594	Tab, Green, Round	Desipramine HCl 25 mg	Norpramin by WC		Antidepressant
WC595	Tab, Green, Round	Desipramine HCl 50 mg	Norpramin by WC		Antidepressant
WC596	Tab, Orange, Round	Desipramine HCl 75 mg	Norpramin by WC		Antidepressant
WC606	Tab, White, Round, WC over 606	Aspirin 325 mg	Aspirin by Warner Chilcott by WC	00047-0606	Analgesic
WC607	Tab, White, Round	Phenobarbital 60 mg			Sedative/Hypnotic; C IV
WC611	Tab, White, Round	Baclofen 10 mg	Lioresal by WC		Muscle Relaxant
WC612	Tab, White, Round	Baclofen 20 mg	Lioresal by WC		Muscle Relaxant
WC615	Cap, Olive Green & Brown, White Print, WC over 615	Minocycline HCl 50 mg	Minocin by Warner Chilcott	00047-0615	Antibiotic
WC615	Cap, Olive Green & Brown, White Print, WC over 615	Minocycline HCl 50 mg	Minocin by Parke Davis	00071-0615	Antibiotic
WC615	Cap, Olive Green & Brown, White Print, WC over 615	Minocycline HCl 50 mg	Minocin by Pharmedix	53002-0288	Antibiotic
WC616	Cap, Green & White, Black Print, WC over 616	Minocycline HCl 100 mg	Minocin by Parke Davis	00071-0616	Antibiotic
WC616	Cap, Green & White, Black Print, WC over 616	Minocycline HCl 100 mg	Minocin by Warner Chilcott	00047-0616	Antibiotic
WC617	Tab, White, Round	Quinidine Gluconate 324 mg	Quinaglute by WC		Antiarrhythmic
WC621	Cap, White	Loxapine 5 mg	Loxitane by WC		Antipsychotic
WC630	Tab, White, Round	Pindolol 5 mg	Visken by WC		Antihypertensive
WC631	Tab, White, Round	Pindolol 10 mg	Visken by WC		Antihypertensive
WC632	Cap, Yellow & White	Loxapine 10 mg	Loxitane by WC		Antipsychotic
WC634	Tab, White, Round, W-C 634	Acetaminophen 300 mg, Codeine Phosphate 15 mg	Tylenol w/ Codeine by WC		Analgesic; C III
WC635	Tab, White, Round, W-C 635	Acetaminophen 300 mg, Codeine Phosphate 30 mg	Tylenol w/ Codeine by WC		Analgesic; C III
WC637	Tab, White, Round, W-C 637	Acetaminophen 300 mg, Codeine Phosphate 60 mg	Tylenol w/ Codeine by WC		Analgesic; C III
WC640	Tab, White, Round	Acetaminophen 325 mg	Tylenol by WC		Analgesic
WC648	Tab, White, Oval	Penicillin V Potassium	by Clonmell	55190-0648	Antibiotic
WC648	Tab, White, Oval	Penicillin V Potassium	by Urgent Care Center	50716-0648	Antibiotic
WC648	Tab, White, Oval	Penicillin V Potassium	by Pharmedix	53002-0201	Antibiotic
WC650	Cap, Green & White	Loxapine 25 mg	Loxitane by WC		Antipsychotic
WC651	Cap, Blue & White	Loxapine 50 mg	Loxitane by WC		Antipsychotic
WC657	Tab, White, Round	Theophylline Anhydrous CR 100 mg	Theo-Dur by WC		Antiasthmatic
WC659	Tab, White, Oval	Theophylline Anhydrous CR 200 mg	Theo-Dur by WC		Antiasthmatic
WC665	Cap, Natural	Oxazepam 15 mg	Serax by WC		Sedative/Hypnotic; C IV
WC667	Cap, Orange & White	Oxazepam 30 mg	Serax by WC		Sedative/Hypnotic; C IV
WC672	Tab, Yellow, Round	Erythromycin Stearate 250 mg	Erythrocin by WC		Antibiotic
WC673	Tab, White, Oval	Penicillin V Potassium 500 mg	V-Cillin K by WC		Antibiotic
WC690	Cap, Blue & White	Oxazepam 10 mg	Serax by WC		Sedative/Hypnotic; C IV
WC696ERYC	Cap, Clear & Orange	Erythromycin 250 mg	Eryc Delayed Release by Halsey	00904-5394	Antibiotic

ID FRONT <> BACK	DESCRIPTION FRONT <> BACK	INGREDIENT & STRENGTH	BRAND (or Generic Equiv.) by FIRM	NDC#	CLASS; SCH.
WC697	Cap	Tetracycline HCl 500 mg	by Pharmedix	53002-0217	Antibiotic
WC698	Tab, White, Round	Phenobarbital 100 mg	Phenobarbital by WC		Sedative/Hypnotic; C IV
WC699	Tab, White, Round	Phenobarbital 15 mg	Phenobarbital by WC		Sedative/Hypnotic; C IV
WC700	Tab, White, Round	Phenobarbital 30 mg	by WC		Sedative/Hypnotic; C IV
WC702	Tab, White, Round	Hydrochlorothiazide 25 mg	Hydrodiuril by WC		Diuretic; Antihypertensive
WC710	Tab, White, Round	Hydrochlorothiazide 50 mg	Hydrodiuril by WC		Diuretic; Antihypertensive
WC712	Tab, White, Round	Hydrochlorothiazide 25 mg, Spironolactone 25 mg	Aldactazide by WC		Diuretic; Antihypertensive
WC713	Tab, White, Round	Spironolactone 25 mg	Aldactone by WC		Diuretic
WC716	Tab, White	Trazodone HCl 150 mg	Desyrel by WC		Antidepressant
WC720	Cap, Orange & Purple, Controlled Release	Disopyramide Phosphate 150 mg	Norpace CR by WC		Antiarrhythmic
WC724	Tab, White, Oblong	Timolol Maleate 20 mg	Blocadren by WC		Antihypertensive
WC725	Tab, White, Round	Aspirin 325 mg, Codeine Phosphate 15 mg	Aspirin w/ Codeine by WC		Analgesic; C III
WC726	Tab, White, Round	Aspirin 325 mg, Codeine Phosphate 30 mg	Aspirin w/ Codeine by WC		Analgesic; C III
WC727	Tab, White, Round	Aspirin 325 mg, Codeine Phosphate 60 mg	Aspirin w/ Codeine by WC		Analgesic; C III
WC728	Tab, White, Round	Timolol Maleate 10 mg	Blocadren by WC		Antihypertensive
WC729	Tab, White, Round	Timolol Maleate 5 mg	Blocadren by WC		Antihypertensive
WC730	Cap, Orange & Peach	Amoxicillin 250 mg	Amoxil by Dava	67253-0140	Antibiotic
WC730	Cap, Orange & Peach	Amoxicillin 250 mg	Amoxil by Clonmell	55190-0730	Antibiotic
WC730	Cap, Orange & Peach	Amoxicillin 250 mg	Amoxil by Mova	55370-0884	Antibiotic
WC730	Cap, Orange & Peach	Amoxicillin 250 mg	Amoxil by H J Harkins Co	52959-0011	Antibiotic
WC730	Cap, Orange & Peach	Amoxicillin 250 mg	Amoxil by Compumed	00403-0254	Antibiotic
WC730	Cap, Orange & Peach	Amoxicillin 250 mg	Amoxil by Pharmedix	53002-0208	Antibiotic
WC731	Cap, Red and Pink	Amoxicillin 500 mg	Amoxil by Pharmedix	53002-0216	Antibiotic
WC731	Cap, Red and Pink	Amoxicillin 500 mg	Amoxil by Compumed	00403-0260	Antibiotic
WC731	Cap, Red and Pink	Amoxicillin 500 mg	Amoxil by H J Harkins Co	52959-0020	Antibiotic
WC731	Cap, Red and Pink	Amoxicillin 500 mg	Amoxil by Apotheca	12634-0182	Antibiotic
WC731	Cap, Red and Pink	Amoxicillin 500 mg	Amoxil by Mova	55370-0885	Antibiotic
WC731	Cap, Red and Pink	Amoxicillin 500 mg	Amoxil by Clonmell	55190-0731	Antibiotic
WC731	Cap, Red and Pink	Amoxicillin 500 mg	Amoxil by Dava	67253-0141	Antibiotic
WC759	Tab, White, Round	Acetaminophen 500 mg	Tylenol Ex Strength by WC		Analgesic
WC765	Tab, Green, Oval	Cimetidine HCl 400 mg	Tagamet by WC		Gastrointestinal
WC768	Tab, Green, Oval	Cimetidine HCl 300 mg	Tagamet by WC		Gastrointestinal
WC773	Tab, Yellow, Round, Scored, WC over 773	Sulindac 150 mg	by Warner Chilcott	00047-0773	NSAID
WC773	Tab, Yellow, Round, Scored, WC over 773	Sulindac 150 mg	by Kaiser	00179-1144	NSAID
WC773	Tab, Yellow, Round, Scored, WC over 773	Sulindac 150 mg	by Parke Davis	00071-0773	NSAID
WC773	Tab, Yellow, Round, Scored, WC over 773	Sulindac 150 mg	by Ivax	00182-1705	NSAID
WC773	Tab, Yellow, Round, Scored, WC over 773	Sulindac 150 mg	by Kaiser	62224-8119	NSAID
WC774	Tab, Yellow, Oval, Scored	Sulindac 200 mg	by Kaiser	62224-8117	NSAID
WC774	Tab, Yellow, Oval, Scored	Sulindac 200 mg	by Warner Chilcott	00047-0774	NSAID
WC774	Tab, Yellow, Oval, Scored	Sulindac 200 mg	by Kaiser	00179-1145	NSAID
WC774	Tab, Yellow, Oval, Scored	Sulindac 200 mg	by Parke Davis	00071-0774	NSAID
WC784	Tab, Yellow, Round, Ex Release	Potassium Chloride 10 mEq	K-Tab by WC		Electrolytes
WC785	Tab, Blue, Round	Alprazolam 1 mg	Xanax by WC		Antianxiety; C IV
WC786	Tab, White, Round	Alprazolam 0.5 mg	Xanax by WC		Antianxiety; C IV
WC787	Tab, Orange, Round	Alprazolam 0.25 mg	Xanax by WC		Antianxiety; C IV

ID FRONT <> BACK	DESCRIPTION FRONT <> BACK	INGREDIENT & STRENGTH	BRAND (or Generic Equiv.) by FIRM	NDC#	CLASS; SCH.
WC788	Cap, Pink & Yellow	Nitrofurantoin 50 mg	Macrodantin by WC		Antibiotic
WC789	Cap, Pink	Nitrofurantoin 100 mg	Macrodantin by WC		Antibiotic
WC790	Tab, Peach, Round	Maprotiline 25 mg	Ludiomil by WC		Antidepressant
WC791	Tab, Peach, Round	Maprotiline 50 mg	Ludiomil by WC		Antidepressant
WC795	Tab, White, Round	Maprotiline 75 mg	Ludiomil by WC		Antidepressant
WC796	Tab, White, Round	Fluphenazine HCl 1 mg	Prolixin by WC		Antipsychotic
WC797	Tab, Beige, Round	Fluphenazine HCl 2.5 mg	Prolixin by WC		Antipsychotic
WC798	Tab, Blue, Round	Fluphenazine HCl 5 mg	Prolixin by WC		Antipsychotic
WC799	Tab, Red, Round	Fluphenazine HCl 10 mg	Prolixin by WC		Antipsychotic
WC808	Cap, Green & Pink	Cephradine 250 mg	Velosef by WC		Antibiotic
WC809	Cap, Green, & Green	Cephradine 500 mg	Velosef by WC		Antibiotic
WC813	Tab, Beige, Round	Doxycycline Hyclate 100 mg	Vibra-Tab by WC		Antibiotic
WC829	Cap, Blue & White	Doxycycline Hyclate 50 mg	Vibramycin by WC		Antibiotic
WC830	Cap, Blue	Doxycycline Hyclate 100 mg	Vibramycin by WC		Antibiotic
WC832	Tab, Yellow, W-C 832	Amiloride HCl 5 mg, Hydrochlorothiazide 50 mg	Moduretic by WC		Antihypertensive; Diuretic
WC833	Tab, Yellow, Round	Hydrochlorothiazide 50 mg, Triamterene 75 mg	Maxzide by Watson		Diuretic; Antihypertensive
WC834	Cap, Red	Hydrochlorothiazide 25 mg, Triamterene 50 mg	Dyazide by WC		Diuretic; Antihypertensive
WC843	Cap, Ivory & Opaque	Prazosin HCl 1 mg	Minipress by WC		Antihypertensive
WC844	Cap, Pink & Opaque	Prazosin HCl 2 mg	Minipress by WC		Antihypertensive
WC845	Cap, Blue & Opaque	Prazosin HCl 5 mg	Minipress by WC		Antihypertensive
WC849	Tab, White, Round	Quinidine Sulfate 200 mg	Quinidine by WC		Antiarrhythmic
WC850	Tab, White, Round	Quinidine Gluconate 330 mg	Duraquin by WC		Antiarrhythmic
WC853	Cap, Red, W-C 853	Amantadine HCl 100 mg	Symmetrel by WC		Antiviral
WC865	Tab, Blue, Round	Methyldopa 250 mg	Aldomet by WC		Antihypertensive
WC866	Tab, Blue, Round	Methyldopa 500 mg	Aldomet by WC		Antihypertensive
WC868	Cap, Green	Hydralazine 25 mg, Hydrochlorothiazide 25 mg	Apresazide by WC		Antihypertensive; Diuretic
WC871	Cap, Green	Hydralazine 50 mg, Hydrochlorothiazide 50 mg	Apresazide by WC		Antihypertensive; Diuretic
WC872	Tab, Green, Round	Fluoxymesterone 10 mg	Halotestin by WC		Steroid; C III
WC874	Tab, White, Round	Medroxyprogesterone 10 mg	Provera by WC		Hormone
WC875	Cap, Clear & Lavender w/ White Beads	Indomethacin 75 mg	Indocin SR by Inwood	00258-3607	NSAID
WC875	Cap, Lavender & Clear	Indomethacin 75 mg	Indocin SR by WC		NSAID
WC878	Tab, White, Round	Metoclopramide 10 mg	Reglan by Watson		Gastrointestinal
WC887	Cap, Blue & Aqua	Indomethacin 25 mg	Indocin by WC		NSAID
WC888	Cap, Blue & Aqua	Indomethacin 50 mg	Indocin by WC		NSAID
WC914	Tab, White, Elongated	Ibuprofen 800 mg	Motrin by WC		NSAID
WC919	Tab, Yellow, Oval	Erythromycin Stearate 500 mg	Erythrocin by WC		Antibiotic
WC922	Tab, White, Elongated	Ibuprofen 600 mg	Motrin by WC		NSAID
WC926	Tab, Yellow, Round	Norethindrone 0.5 mg, Ethinyl Estradiol 35 mcg	Nelova 0.5/35 E by WC		Oral Contraceptive
WC927	Tab, Yellow, Round	Norethindrone 1 mg, Ethinyl Estradiol 35 mcg	Nelova 1/35 by WC		Oral Contraceptive
WC929	Tab, Yellow, Round	Norethindrone 0.5 mg, Ethinyl Estradiol 35 mcg	Nelova 0.5/35 E by WC		Oral Contraceptive

ID FRONT <> BACK	DESCRIPTION FRONT <> BACK	INGREDIENT & STRENGTH	BRAND (or Generic Equiv.) by FIRM	NDC#	CLASS; SCH.
WC930	Tab, Yellow, Round	Norethindrone 1 mg, Ethinyl Estradiol 35 mcg	Nelova 1/35 by WC		Oral Contraceptive
WC938	Cap, Gray & Orange	Cephalexin 250 mg	Keflex by WC		Antibiotic
WC939	Cap, Orange	Cephalexin 500 mg	Keflex by WC		Antibiotic
WC940	Tab, Beige, Oblong	Chlorpheniramine 8 mg, Phenylephrine 25 mg, Pyrilamine 25 mg	Rynatan by WC		Cold Remedy
WC941	Tab, White, Round	Norethindrone 0.5 mg, Ethinyl Estradiol 35 mcg	Nelova 0.5/35 E by WC		Oral Contraceptive
WC942	Tab, Blue, Round	Norethindrone 1 mg, Mestranol 50 mcg	Nelova 1/50M by WC		Oral Contraceptive
WC944	Tab, Yellow, Round	Norethindrone 10 mg, Mestranol 11 mg	Nelova 10/11 by WC		Oral Contraceptive
WC945	Cap, Green	Dicloxacillin Sodium 250 mg	Dynapen by WC		Antibiotic
WC946	Cap, Green	Dicloxacillin Sodium 500 mg	Dynapen by WC		Antibiotic
WC947	Tab, Yellow, Round	Norethindrone 10 mg, Mestranol 11 mg	Nelova 10/11 by WC		Oral Contraceptive
WC949	Cap, Green & Red	Cloxacillin Sodium 250 mg	Tegopen by WC		Antibiotic
WC950	Cap, Green & Red	Cloxacillin Sodium 500 mg	Tegopen by WC		Antibiotic
WC951	Tab, Peach, Round	Potassium Chloride ER 8 mEq	Slow K by WC		Electrolytes
WC951	Tab, Blue, Round	Potassium Chloride ER 8 mEq	Slow K by WC		Electrolytes
WC954	Tab, Pink, Round	Metoprolol Tartrate 50 mg	Lopressor by WC		Antihypertensive
WC954	Tab, White, Oblong	Metoprolol Tartrate 50 mg	Lopressor by WC		Antihypertensive
WC955	Tab, Blue, Round	Metoprolol Tartrate 100 mg	Lopressor by WC		Antihypertensive
WC955	Tab, White, Oblong	Metoprolol Tartrate 100 mg	Lopressor by WC		Antihypertensive
WC956	Tab, White, Round	Albuterol Sulfate 2 mg	Proventil by WC		Antiasthmatic
WC957	Tab, White, Round	Albuterol Sulfate 4 mg	Proventil by WC		Antiasthmatic
WC966	Tab, Orange, Round	Thioridazine 10 mg	Mellaril by WC		Antipsychotic
WC967	Tab, Orange, Round	Thioridazine 25 mg	Mellaril by WC		Antipsychotic
WC968	Tab, Orange, Round	Thioridazine 50 mg	Mellaril by WC		Antipsychotic
WC969	Tab, Orange, Round	Thioridazine 100 mg	Mellaril by WC		Antipsychotic
WC970	Cap	Thiothixene 1 mg	Navane by WC		Antipsychotic
WC971	Cap, Caramel & Yellow	Thiothixene 2 mg	Navane by WC		Antipsychotic
WC972	Cap, Caramel & White	Thiothixene 5 mg	Navane by WC		Antipsychotic
WC973	Tab, White, Round	Placebo	Placebo by WC		Placebo
WC975	Cap, Caramel & Peach	Thiothixene 10 mg	Navane by WC		Antipsychotic
WC977	Cap, Green & White	Temazepam 15 mg	Restoril by WC		Sedative/Hypnotic; C IV
WC978	Cap, White	Temazepam 30 mg	Restoril by WC		Sedative/Hypnotic; C IV
WC979	Tab, Orange, Oblong	Acetaminophen 650 mg, Propoxyphene HCl 65 mg	Wygesic by WC		Analgesic; C IV
WC980	Tab, Pink	Acetaminophen 650 mg, Propoxyphene Napsylate 100 mg	Darvocet-N 100 by WC		Analgesic; C IV
WC981	Tab, Orange, Round	Haloperidol 0.5 mg	Haldol by WC		Antipsychotic
WC982	Tab, Orange, Round	Haloperidol 1 mg	Haldol by WC		Antipsychotic
WC983	Tab, Orange, Round	Haloperidol 2 mg	Haldol by WC		Antipsychotic
WC984	Tab, Orange, Round	Haloperidol 5 mg	Haldol by WC		Antipsychotic
WC985	Tab, Yellow, Round	Clonidine HCl 0.1 mg, Chlorthalidone 15 mg	Combipres by WC		Antihypertensive; Diuretic
WC986	Tab, Yellow, Round	Clonidine HCl 0.2 mg, Chlorthalidone 15 mg	Combipres by WC		Antihypertensive; Diuretic
WC987	Tab, Yellow, Round	Clonidine HCl 0.3 mg, Chlorthalidone 15 mg	Combipres by WC		Antihypertensive; Diuretic

ID FRONT <> BACK	DESCRIPTION FRONT <> BACK	INGREDIENT & STRENGTH	BRAND (or Generic Equiv.) by FIRM	NDC#	CLASS; SCH.
WC988	Cap, Blue & White	Flurazepam HCl 15 mg	Dalmane by WC		Hypnotic; C IV
WC988	Cap, Peach & Orange	Flurazepam HCl 15 mg	Dalmane by WC		Hypnotic; C IV
WC989	Cap, Blue	Flurazepam HCl 30 mg	Dalmane by WC		Hypnotic; C IV
WC989	Cap, Peach & Red	Flurazepam HCl 30 mg	Dalmane by WC		Hypnotic; C IV
WD03	Cap, Orange & White	Danazol 50 mg	Danocrine by Sanofi	00024-0303	Steroid
WD04	Cap, Yellow	Danazol 100 mg	Danocrine by Sanofi	00024-0304	Steroid
WD05	Cap, Orange	Danazol 200 mg	Danocrine by Sanofi	00024-0305	Steroid
WD35	Tab, White, Round	Meperidine 50 mg	Demerol by Sanofi		Analgesic; C II
WD35	Tab, White, W/D/35	Meperidine 50 mg	Demerol by Sanofi	Canadian	Analgesic; C II
WD37	Tab, White, Round, W/D37	Meperidine 100 mg	Demerol by Sanofi		Analgesic; C II
WD92	Cap, Green, White Print, Soft Gel, W in circle	Ergocalciferol 1.25 mg	Drisdol by RP Scherer	11014-0890	Vitamin
WD92	Cap, Green, White Print, Soft Gel, W in circle	Ergocalciferol 1.25 mg	Drisdol by Sanofi	00024-0392	Vitamin
WD92	Cap, Green, White Print, Soft Gel, W in circle	Ergocalciferol 1.25 mg	Drisdol by Bayer	00280-0392	Vitamin
WDILACORXR120MG	Cap, Peach & Pink	Diltiazem HCl 120 mg	Dilacor XR by Rx Pak	65084-0241	Antihypertensive
WDILACORXR120MG	Cap, Yellow & White, Watson Logo	Diltiazem HCl 120 mg	Dilacor XR by Excellium		Antihypertensive
WDR	Tab, Orange, Oval, Schering Logo WDR	Fluphenazine HCl 2.5 mg	Permitil by Schering	00085-0442	Antipsychotic
WE01	Tab, WE/01, Ex Release	Guaifenesin 600 mg, Phenylpropanolamine HCl 75 mg	Entex LA by Sovereign	58716-0631	Cold Remedy
WE02	Tab, WE/02, Ex Release	Chlorpheniramine Maleate 8 mg, Methscopolamine Nitrate 2.5 mg, Phenylephrine HCl 20 mg	Omnihist LA by Sovereign	58716-0620	Cold Remedy
WE03	Tab, WE/03, Chewable	Chlorpheniramine Maleate 2 mg, Methscopolamine Nitrate 1.25 mg, Phenylephrine HCl 10 mg	AH Chew by Sovereign	58716-0619	Cold Remedy
WE04	Cap, Ex Release	Brompheniramine Maleate 6 mg, Pseudoephedrine HCl 60 mg	Ultrabrom PD by Sovereign by Kiel	58716-0026	Cold Remedy
WE05	Tab, WE/05, Ex Release	Guaifenesin 600 mg, Pseudoephedrine HCl 60 mg	D Feda II by Sovereign	59063-0110	Cold Remedy
WE05	Tab, WE/05, Ex Release	Guaifenesin 600 mg, Pseudoephedrine HCl 60 mg	D Feda II by Sovereign	58716-0625	Cold Remedy
WE05	Tab, WE/05, Ex Release	Guaifenesin 600 mg, Pseudoephedrine HCl 60 mg	D Feda II by WE	59196-0005	Cold Remedy
WE06	Cap, Ex Release	Brompheniramine Maleate 12 mg, Pseudoephedrine HCl 120 mg	Ultrabrom by Sovereign	58716-0025	Cold Remedy
WE07	Tab, Scored, Chewable	Phenylephrine HCl 10 mg	AH Chew D by WE	59196-0007	Decongestant
WE07	Tab, Chewable	Phenylephrine HCl 10 mg	AH Chew D by Nadin	14836-0007	Decongestant
WE35	Tab, Green, Oblong, Scored	Phenylephrine HCl 15 mg, Guaifenesin 600 mg	Sinuvent PE by We Pharma	59196-0035	Cold Remedy
WEFFEXORXR150	Cap, Dark Orange, Pink Print, W over Effexor XR over 150	Venlafaxine 150 mg	Effexor XR by Wyeth	52903-0836	Antidepressant
WEFFEXORXR150	Cap, Dark Orange, Pink Print, W over Effexor XR over 150	Venlafaxine 150 mg	Effexor ER by Murfreesboro	51129-1677	Antidepressant
WEFFEXORXR150	Cap, Dark Orange, Pink Print, W over Effexor XR over 150	Venlafaxine 150 mg	Effexor ER by Ayerst	00046-0836	Antidepressant
WEFFEXORXR150	Cap, Dark Orange, Pink Print, W over Effexor XR over 150	Venlafaxine 150 mg	Effexor XR by Wyeth	00008-0836	Antidepressant
WEFFEXORXR150	Cap, Dark Orange, Hard Gelatin, W over Effexor XR on Cap, 150 on Body	Venlafaxine 150 mg	Effexor XR by Wyeth Canada	Canadian DIN 02237282	Antidepressant
WEFFEXORXR375	Cap, Gray & Peach, Orange Print, W over Effexor XR over 37.5	Venlafaxine 37.5 mg	Effexor XR by Ayerst	00046-0837	Antidepressant
WEFFEXORXR375	Cap, Gray & Peach, Orange Print, W over Effexor XR over 37.5	Venlafaxine 37.5 mg	Effexor XR by Wyeth	52903-0837	Antidepressant
WEFFEXORXR375	Cap, Gray & Peach, Orange Print, W over Effexor XR over 37.5	Venlafaxine 37.5 mg	Effexor ER by Murfreesboro	51129-1678	Antidepressant
WEFFEXORXR375	Cap, Gray & Peach, Orange Print, W over Effexor XR over 37.5	Venlafaxine 37.5 mg	Effexor XR by Wyeth	00008-0837	Antidepressant
WEFFEXORXR375	Cap, Gray Cap, Peach Body, W over Effexor XR over 37.5	Venlafaxine 37.5 mg	Effexor by Wyeth Canada	Canadian DIN 02237279	Antidepressant
WEFFEXORXR75	Cap, Peach, Orange Print, W over Effexor XR over 75	Venlafaxine 75 mg	Effexor XR by Wyeth	52903-0833	Antidepressant
WEFFEXORXR75	Cap, Peach, Orange Print, W over Effexor XR over 75	Venlafaxine 75 mg	Effexor XR by Wyeth	00008-0833	Antidepressant
WEFFEXORXR75	Cap, Peach, Orange Print, W over Effexor XR over 75	Venlafaxine 75 mg	Effexor XR by Ayerst	00046-0833	Antidepressant

ID FRONT <> BACK	DESCRIPTION FRONT <> BACK	INGREDIENT & STRENGTH	BRAND (or Generic Equiv.) by FIRM	NDC#	CLASS; SCH.
WEFFEXORXR75	Cap, Peach, Hard Gelatin, W over Effexor XR on Cap, 75 Body	Venlafaxine 75 mg	Effexor XR by Wyeth Canada	Canadian DIN 02237280	Antidepressant
WELLBUTRIN100	Tab, Dark Pink, Round, Film Coated	Bupropion HCl 100 mg	Wellbutrin by Allscripts		Antidepressant
WELLBUTRIN100	Tab, Dark Pink, Round, Film Coated	Bupropion HCl 100 mg	Wellbutrin by DSM	63552-0178	Antidepressant
WELLBUTRIN75	Tab, Orange, Round, Film Coated	Bupropion HCl 75 mg	Wellbutrin by DSM	63552-0177	Antidepressant
WELLBUTRIN75	Tab, Orange, Round, Film Coated	Bupropion HCl 75 mg	Wellbutrin by GSK	00173-0177	Antidepressant
WELLBUTRINSR100	Tab, Blue, Round, Wellbutrin SR 100, Film Coated	Bupropion HCl 100 mg	Wellbutrin SR by GSK	Canadian	Antidepressant
WELLBUTRINSR100	Tab, Blue, Round, Wellbutrin SR 100, Film Coated	Bupropion HCl 100 mg	Wellbutrin SR by GSK	00173-0947	Antidepressant
WELLBUTRINSR100	Tab, Blue, Round, Wellbutrin SR 100, Film Coated	Bupropion HCl 100 mg	Wellbutrin SR by DSM	63552-0947	Antidepressant
WELLBUTRINSR100	Tab, Blue, Round, Wellbutrin SR 100, Film Coated	Bupropion HCl 100 mg	Wellbutrin SR by Biovail	Canadian DIN 02237824	Antidepressant
WELLBUTRINSR150	Tab, Purple, Round, Wellbutrin SR 150, Film Coated	Bupropion HCl 150 mg	Wellbutrin SR by Biovail	Canadian DIN 02237825	Antidepressant
WELLBUTRINSR150	Tab, Purple, Round, Wellbutrin SR 150, Film Coated	Bupropion HCl 150 mg	Wellbutrin SR by Allscripts		Antidepressant
WELLBUTRINSR150	Tab, Purple, Round, Wellbutrin SR 150, Film Coated	Bupropion HCl 150 mg	Wellbutrin SR by Caremark	00339-4032	Antidepressant
WELLBUTRINSR150	Tab, Purple, Round, Wellbutrin SR 150, Film Coated	Bupropion HCl 150 mg	Wellbutrin SR by Physician Total Care	54868-3984	Antidepressant
WELLBUTRINSR150	Tab, Purple, Round, Wellbutrin SR 150, Film Coated	Bupropion HCl 150 mg	Wellbutrin SR by GSK	Canadian	Antidepressant
WELLBUTRINSR150	Tab, Purple, Round, Wellbutrin SR 150, Film Coated	Bupropion HCl 150 mg	Wellbutrin SR by DSM	63552-0135	Antidepressant
WELLBUTRINSR150	Tab, Purple, Round, Wellbutrin SR 150, Film Coated	Bupropion HCl 150 mg	Wellbutrin SR by Direct Dispensing	57866-0901	Antidepressant
WELLBUTRINSR150	Tab, Purple, Round, Wellbutrin SR 150, Film Coated	Bupropion HCl 150 mg	Wellbutrin SR by GSK	00173-0135	Antidepressant
WELLBUTRINSR200	Tab, Light Pink, Round, Film Coated	Bupropion HCl 200 mg	Wellbutrin SR by GSK	00173-0722	Antidepressant
WELLBUTRINXL150	Tab, Off-White, Round	Bupropion HCl 150 mg	Wellbutrin XL by GSK	00173-0730	Antidepressant
WELLBUTRINXL300	Tab, Off-White, Round	Bupropion HCl 300 mg	Wellbutrin XL by GSK	00173-0731	Antidepressant
WELLCOMEP4B	Tab, White, Round	Triprolidine 4 mg, Pseudoephedrine 60 mg, Codeine Phosphate 20 mg	CoActifed by GSK	Canadian DIN 00068608	Cold Remedy, C III
WELLCOMEU3B	Tab, Greenish-Yellow, Round, Scored	Thioguanine 40 mg	Tabloid by DSM	63552-0880	Antineoplastic
WELLCOMEU3B	Tab, Greenish-Yellow, Round, Scored	Thioguanine 40 mg	Tabloid by GSK	00173-0880	Antineoplastic
WELLCOMEU3B	Tab, Greenish-Yellow, Round, Scored	Thioguanine 40 mg	Lanvis by GSK	Canadian DIN 00282081	Antineoplastic
WELLCOMEX2F	Cap, White	Acetaminophen 500 mg, Dextromethorphan 30 mg, Pseudoephedrine 60 mg	Sudafed by Warner Wellcome	Canadian	Decongestant
WELLCOMEY9C100	Cap, White w/ Blue Band, Black Print, Unicorn Logo over Wellcome over Y9C over 100	Zidovudine 100 mg	Retrovir by GSK	00173-0108	Antiviral
WELLCOMEY9C100	Cap, White w/ Blue Band, Black Print, Unicorn Logo over Wellcome over Y9C over 100	Zidovudine 100 mg	Retrovir by Med Pro	53978-2098	Antiviral
WELLCOMEY9C100	Cap, White w/ Blue Band, Black Print, Unicorn Logo over Wellcome over Y9C over 100	Zidovudine 100 mg	Retrovir by Amerisource	62584-0464	Antiviral
WELLCOMEY9C100	Cap, White w/ Blue Band, Black Print, Unicorn Logo over Wellcome over Y9C over 100	Zidovudine 100 mg	Retrovir by Prepackage Specialists	58864-0462	Antiviral
WELLCOMEY9C100	Cap, White w/ Blue Band, Black Print, Unicorn Logo over Wellcome over Y9C over 100	Zidovudine 100 mg	Retrovir by Pharm Util	60491-0561	Antiviral
WELLCOMEY9C100	Cap, White w/ Blue Band, Black Print, Unicorn Logo over Wellcome over Y9C over 100	Zidovudine 100 mg	Retrovir by DSM	63552-0108	Antiviral
WELLCOMEY9C100	Cap, White w/ Blue Band, Black Print, Unicorn Logo over Wellcome over Y9C over 100	Zidovudine 100 mg	Retrovir by GSK	Canadian DIN 01902660	Antiviral
WELLCOMEZOVIRAX200	Cap, Blue, Black Print, Unicorn Logo over Wellcome over Zovirax over 200	Acyclovir 200 mg	Zovirax by Prepackage Specialists	58864-0563	Antiviral
WELLCOMEZOVIRAX200	Cap, Blue, Black Print, Unicorn Logo over Wellcome over Zovirax over 200	Acyclovir 200 mg	Zovirax by Nat Pharmpak	55154-0706	Antiviral
WELLCOMEZOVIRAX200	Cap, Blue, Black Print, Unicorn Logo over Wellcome over Zovirax over 200	Acyclovir 200 mg	Zovirax by DSM	63552-0991	Antiviral

ID FRONT <> BACK	DESCRIPTION FRONT <> BACK	INGREDIENT & STRENGTH	BRAND (or Generic Equiv.) by FIRM	NDC#	CLASS; SCH.
WELLCOMEZOVIRAX200	Cap, Blue, Black Print, Unicorn Logo over Wellcome over Zovirax over 200	Acyclovir 200 mg	Zovirax by Amerisource	62584-0494	Antiviral
WELLCOMEZOVIRAX200	Cap, Blue, Black Print, Unicorn Logo over Wellcome over Zovirax over 200	Acyclovir 200 mg	Zovirax by GSK	00173-0991	Antiviral
WELLCOMEZOVIRAX200	Cap, Blue, Black Print, Unicorn Logo over Wellcome over Zovirax over 200	Acyclovir 200 mg	Zovirax by Allscripts		Antiviral
WELLCOMEZOVIRAX200	Cap, Blue, Black Print, Unicorn Logo over Wellcome over Zovirax over 200	Acyclovir 200 mg	Zovirax by Apotheca	12634-0180	Antiviral
WELLCOMEZOVIRAX200	Cap, Blue, Black Print, Unicorn Logo over Wellcome over Zovirax over 200	Acyclovir 200 mg	Zovirax by Pharmedix	53002-0245	Antiviral
WESTWARD	Tab, White, Round	Metoclopramide 10 mg	Reglan by West-Ward		Gastrointestinal
WESTWARD <> 260	Tab, White, Round, Scored	Isoniazid 100 mg	Laniazid by Versapharm	61748-0016	Antimycobacterial
WESTWARD <> 260	Tab, White, Round, Scored	Isoniazid 100 mg	Laniazid by Amerisource	62584-0759	Antimycobacterial
WESTWARD <> 260	Tab, White, Round, Scored	Isoniazid 100 mg	Laniazid by West-Ward	00143-1260	Antimycobacterial
WESTWARD <> 260	Tab, White, Round, Scored	Isoniazid 100 mg	Laniazid by Amneal	65162-0180	Antimycobacterial
WESTWARD <> 473	Tab	Prednisone 10 mg	by West-Ward		Steroid
WESTWARD <> 785	Tab	Aspirin 325 mg, Butalbital 50 mg, Caffeine 40 mg	Fiorinal by Schein	00364-0677	Analgesic; C III
FLURAZEPAM15	Tab, Blue & White, Oblong	Flurazepam HCl 15 mg	by Southwood	58016-0811	Hypnotic; C IV
FLURAZEPAM30	Tab, Blue, Oblong	Flurazepam HCl 30 mg	by Southwood	58016-0812	Hypnotic; C IV
WESTWARD004	Tab, White, Round	Acetaminophen 300 mg, Codeine Phosphate 30 mg	Tylenol w/ Codeine by West-Ward		Analgesic; C III
WESTWARD005	Tab, White, Round	Acetaminophen 300 mg, Codeine Phosphate 60 mg	Tylenol w/ Codeine by West-Ward		Analgesic; C III
WESTWARD010	Tab, White, Round	Allopurinol 100 mg	Zyloprim by West-Ward		Antigout
WESTWARD013	Tab, Orange, Round	Allopurinol 300 mg	Zyloprim by West-Ward		Antigout
WESTWARD020	Tab, White, Round	Aminophylline 100 mg	Aminophylline by Schein	00364-0004	Antiasthmatic
WESTWARD020	Tab, White, Round	Aminophylline 100 mg	Aminophylline by West-Ward	00143-1020	Antiasthmatic
WESTWARD020	Tab, White, Round	Aminophylline 100 mg	Aminophylline by URL Mutual	00677-0003	Antiasthmatic
WESTWARD020	Tab, White, Round	Aminophylline 100 mg	Aminophylline by Watson	00591-7904	Antiasthmatic
WESTWARD025	Tab, White, Round, Scored	Aminophylline 200 mg	Aminophylline by Watson	00591-7905	Antiasthmatic
WESTWARD025	Tab, White, Round	Aminophylline 200 mg	Aminophylline by West-Ward	00143-1025	Antiasthmatic
WESTWARD025	Tab, White, Round	Aminophylline 200 mg	Aminophylline by URL Mutual	00677-0007	Antiasthmatic
WESTWARD025	Tab, White, Round	Aminophylline 200 mg	Aminophylline by Schein	00364-0005	Antiasthmatic
WESTWARD045	Tab, Pink, Round, West-ward 045	Amitriptyline HCl 10 mg	Elavil by West-Ward		Antidepressant
WESTWARD046	Tab, Green, Round, West-ward 046	Amitriptyline HCl 25 mg	Elavil by West-Ward		Antidepressant
WESTWARD047	Tab, Brown, Round, West-ward 047	Amitriptyline HCl 50 mg	Elavil by West-Ward		Antidepressant
WESTWARD048	Tab, Purple, Round, West-ward 048	Amitriptyline HCl 75 mg	Elavil by West-Ward		Antidepressant
WESTWARD049	Tab, Orange, Round, West-ward 049	Amitriptyline HCl 100 mg	Elavil by West-Ward		Antidepressant
WESTWARD050	Tab, Peach, Round, West-ward 050	Amitriptyline HCl 150 mg	Elavil by West-Ward		Antidepressant
WESTWARD060	Tab, White, Round, West-ward 060	Ascorbic Acid 500 mg	by West-Ward		Vitamin
WESTWARD074	Tab, Blue, Round, West-ward 074	Brompheniramine, Phenylpropanolamine	Bro-Phen Time Release by West-Ward		Antihistamine
WESTWARD087	Tab, Butterscotch Yellow, Round, West-ward 087	Chlorpromazine HCl 100 mg	Thorazine by West-Ward		Antipsychotic
WESTWARD090	Cap, Green & Yellow, West-ward 090	Chlordiazepoxide 5 mg	Librium by West-Ward		Antianxiety; C IV
WESTWARD090	Tab, Butterscotch Yellow, Round, West-ward 090	Chlorpromazine HCl 200 mg	Thorazine by West-Ward		Antipsychotic
WESTWARD093	Cap, Black & Green, West-ward 093	Chlordiazepoxide 10 mg	Librium by West-Ward		Antianxiety; C IV
WESTWARD095	Cap, Green & White, West-ward 095	Chlordiazepoxide 25 mg	Librium by West-Ward		Antianxiety; C IV

ID FRONT <> BACK	DESCRIPTION FRONT <> BACK	INGREDIENT & STRENGTH	BRAND (or Generic Equiv.) by FIRM	NDC#	CLASS; SCH.
WESTWARD107	Tab, White, Round, West-ward 107	Dipyridamole 25 mg	Persantine by West-Ward		Antiplatelet
WESTWARD109	Tab, White, Round, West-ward 109	Dipyridamole 50 mg	Persantine by West-Ward		Antiplatelet
WESTWARD110	Cap, Green, Oval, West-ward 110	Chloral Hydrate 500 mg	Chloral Hydrate by West-Ward		Sedative/Hypnotic; C IV
WESTWARD111	Tab, White, Round, West-ward 111	Dipyridamole 75 mg	Persantine by West-Ward		Antiplatelet
WESTWARD136	Cap, Clear & Pink, West-ward 136	Diphenhydramine HCl 25 mg	Benadryl by West-Ward		Antihistamine
WESTWARD137	Cap, Pink, West-ward 137	Diphenhydramine HCl 50 mg	Benadryl by West-Ward		Antihistamine
WESTWARD140	Tab, White, Round, Scored	Atropine Sulfate 0.0194 mg, Hyoscyamine Sulfate 0.1037 mg, Phenobarbital 16.2 mg, Scopolamine 0.0065 mg	Donnatal by URL Mutual	00677-0074	Gastrointestinal; C IV
WESTWARD140	Tab, White, Round, Scored	Atropine Sulfate 0.0194 mg, Hyoscyamine Sulfate 0.1037 mg, Phenobarbital 16.2 mg, Scopolamine 0.0065 mg	Donnatal by West-Ward	00143-1140	Gastrointestinal; C IV
WESTWARD140	Tab, White, Round, Scored	Atropine Sulfate 0.0194 mg, Hyoscyamine Sulfate 0.1037 mg, Phenobarbital 16.2 mg, Scopolamine 0.0065 mg	Donnatal by Kaiser	00179-1276	Gastrointestinal; C IV
WESTWARD140	Tab, White, Round, Scored	Atropine Sulfate 0.0194 mg, Hyoscyamine Sulfate 0.1037 mg, Phenobarbital 16.2 mg, Scopolamine 0.0065 mg	Donnatal by Kaiser	00179-0027	Gastrointestinal; C IV
WESTWARD140	Tab, White, Round, Scored	Atropine Sulfate 0.0194 mg, Hyoscyamine Sulfate 0.1037 mg, Phenobarbital 16.2 mg, Scopolamine 0.0065 mg	Donnatal by H J Harkins Co	52959-0023	Gastrointestinal; C IV
WESTWARD143	Tab, White, Round	Benztropine Mesylate 1 mg	Cogentin by West-Ward		Antiparkinson
WESTWARD144	Tab, White, Round	Benztropine Mesylate 2 mg	Cogentin by West-Ward		Antiparkinson
WESTWARD147	Tab, Rust, Round	Imipramine HCl 25 mg	Tofranil by West-Ward		Antidepressant
WESTWARD15	Cap	Flurazepam HCl 15 mg	by Sandoz	00781-2806	Hypnotic; C IV
WESTWARD150	Tab, Green, Round	Imipramine HCl 50 mg	Tofranil by West-Ward		Antidepressant
WESTWARD153	Tab, White, Round	Methyldopa 250 mg	Aldomet by West-Ward		Antihypertensive
WESTWARD155	Tab, White, Oblong	Methyldopa 500 mg	Aldomet by West-Ward		Antihypertensive
WESTWARD155	Tab, Lavender, Round	Butabarbital 15 mg	Butisol Sodium by West-Ward		Sedative/Hypnotic; C III
WESTWARD157	Tab, Lavender, Round	Butabarbital 30 mg	Butisol Sodium by West-Ward		Sedative/Hypnotic; C III
WESTWARD178	Tab, White, Round	Acetaminophen 325 mg, Propoxyphene Napsylate 50 mg	Darvocet-N 50 by West-Ward		Analgesic; C IV
WESTWARD179	Tab, White, Oblong	Acetaminophen 650 mg, Propoxyphene Napsylate 100 mg	Darvocet-N 100 by West-Ward		Analgesic; C IV
WESTWARD181	Tab, White, Round, West-ward 181	Carbamazepine 200 mg	Tegretol by West-Ward		Anticonvulsant
WESTWARD183	Tab, Blue, Round, West-ward 183	Chlorpropamide 100 mg	Diabinese by West-Ward		Antidiabetic
WESTWARD185	Tab, Blue, Round, West-ward 185	Chlorpropamide 250 mg	Diabinese by West-Ward		Antidiabetic
WESTWARD186	Tab, Yellow, Round, West-ward 186	Clonidine HCl 0.1 mg	Catapres by West-Ward		Antihypertensive
WESTWARD187	Tab, White, Round, West-ward 187	Clonidine HCl 0.2 mg	Catapres by West-Ward		Antihypertensive
WESTWARD195	Tab, White, Round, Scored, West-Ward 195	Chloroquine Phosphate 250 mg	Aralen Phosphate by West-Ward	00143-1195	Antimalarial
WESTWARD195	Tab, White, Round	Chloroquine Phosphate 250 mg	Aralen by Global	00115-7056	Antimalarial
WESTWARD200	Tab, Yellow, Round, West-ward 200	Chlorpheniramine Maleate 4 mg	Chlor-Trimeton by West-Ward		Antihistamine
WESTWARD201	Tab, White, Round	Colchicine 0.6 mg	by Ivax	00182-1648	Antigout
WESTWARD201	Tab, White, Round	Colchicine 0.6 mg	by Dixon Shane		Antigout
WESTWARD201	Tab, White, Round	Colchicine 0.6 mg	by Allscripts	54569-0236	Antigout
WESTWARD201	Tab, White, Round	Colchicine 0.6 mg	by URL Mutual	00677-0040	Antigout
WESTWARD201	Tab, White, Round	Colchicine 0.6 mg	by Ivax	00182-0174	Antigout
WESTWARD201	Tab, White, Round	Colchicine 0.6 mg	by West-Ward	00143-1201	Antigout
WESTWARD201	Tab, White, Round	Colchicine 0.6 mg	by Caremark	00339-5450	Antigout
WESTWARD202	Tab, White, Round, Scored	Cortisone Acetate 25 mg	Cortone by DJ Pharma	64455-0008	Steroid
WESTWARD202	Tab, White, Round, Scored	Cortisone Acetate 25 mg	Cortone by Qualitest	00603-3062	Steroid
WESTWARD202	Tab, White, Round, Scored	Cortisone Acetate 25 mg	Cortone by URL Mutual	00677-0046	Steroid

ID FRONT <> BACK	DESCRIPTION FRONT <> BACK	INGREDIENT & STRENGTH	BRAND (or Generic Equiv.) by FIRM	NDC#	CLASS; SCH.
WESTWARD202	Tab, White, Round, Scored	Cortisone Acetate 25 mg	Cortone by West-Ward	00143-1202	Steroid
WESTWARD202	Tab, White, Round, Scored	Cortisone Acetate 25 mg	Cortone by Major	00904-2043	Steroid
WESTWARD205	Tab, Butterscotch Yellow, Round, West-ward 205	Chlorpromazine HCl 25 mg	Thorazine by West-Ward		Antipsychotic
WESTWARD207	Tab, Butterscotch Yellow, Round, West-ward 207	Chlorpromazine HCl 50 mg	Thorazine by West-Ward		Antipsychotic
WESTWARD209	Tab, White, Round, Scored	Chlorothiazide 250 mg	Diuril by Ivax	00182-0790	Diuretic; Antihypertensive
WESTWARD209	Tab, White, Round, Scored	Chlorothiazide 250 mg	Diuril by West-Ward	00143-1209	Diuretic; Antihypertensive
WESTWARD210	Tab, White, Round, Scored	Chlorothiazide 500 mg	Diuril by Physician Total Care	54868-0672	Diuretic; Antihypertensive
WESTWARD210	Tab, White, Round, Scored	Chlorothiazide 500 mg	Diuril by West-Ward	00143-1210	Diuretic; Antihypertensive
WESTWARD217	Tab, Pink, Round	Chlorothiazide 250 mg, Reserpine 0.125 mg	Diupres by West-Ward		Diuretic; Antihypertensive
WESTWARD218	Tab, Pink, Round	Chlorothiazide 500 mg, Reserpine 0.125 mg	Diupres by West-Ward		Diuretic; Antihypertensive
WESTWARD220	Tab, White, Round, West-ward 220	Diazepam 2 mg	Valium by West-Ward		Antianxiety; C IV
WESTWARD222	Tab, Yellow, Round, West-ward 222	Diazepam 5 mg	Valium by West-Ward		Antianxiety; C IV
WESTWARD225	Tab, Blue, Round, West-ward 225	Diazepam 10 mg	Valium by West-Ward		Antianxiety; C IV
WESTWARD227	Cap, White	Prazosin HCl 1 mg	Minipress by West-Ward		Antihypertensive
WESTWARD228	Cap, Pink	Prazosin HCl 2 mg	Minipress by West-Ward		Antihypertensive
WESTWARD229	Cap, Blue	Prazosin HCl 5 mg	Minipress by West-Ward		Antihypertensive
WESTWARD235	Cap, Pink, Opaque, West-Ward	Propoxyphene 65 mg	Darvon by Qualitest	00603-5459	Analgesic; C IV
WESTWARD235	Cap, Pink, Opaque, West-Ward	Propoxyphene 65 mg	Darvon by West-Ward	00143-3235	Analgesic; C IV
WESTWARD239	Tab, White, Round, West-ward 239	Dimenhydrinate 50 mg	Dramamine by West-Ward		Antiemetic
WESTWARD245	Tab, White, Round, West-ward 245	Atropine Sulfate 0.025 mg, Diphenoxylate HCl 2.5 mg	Lomotil by West-Ward		Antidiarrheal; C V
WESTWARD247	Tab, White, Round, West-ward 247	Ergoloid Mesylate 1 mg	Hydergine by West-Ward		Ergot Alkaloids
WESTWARD248	Tab, Yellow, Round, Scored, West-Ward 248	Folic Acid 1 mg	Folvite by Nat Pharmpak	55154-5502	Vitamin
WESTWARD248	Tab, Yellow, Round, Scored, West-Ward 248	Folic Acid 1 mg	Folvite by UDL	51079-0041	Vitamin
WESTWARD248	Tab, Yellow, Round, Scored, West-Ward 248	Folic Acid 1 mg	Folvite by Med Pro	53978-0913	Vitamin
WESTWARD248	Tab, Yellow, Round, Scored, West-Ward 248	Folic Acid 1 mg	Folvite by Caremark	00339-5564	Vitamin
WESTWARD248	Tab, Yellow, Round, Scored, West-Ward 248	Folic Acid 1 mg	Folvite by URL Mutual	00677-0449	Vitamin
WESTWARD248	Tab, Yellow, Round, Scored, West-Ward 248	Folic Acid 1 mg	Folvite by West-Ward	00143-1248	Vitamin
WESTWARD248	Tab, Yellow, Round, Scored, West-Ward 248	Folic Acid 1 mg	Folvite by Golden State	60429-0212	Vitamin
WESTWARD248	Tab, Yellow, Round, Scored, West-Ward 248	Folic Acid 1 mg	Folvite by Heartland	61392-0244	Vitamin
WESTWARD248	Tab, Yellow, Round, Scored, West-Ward 248	Folic Acid 1 mg	Folvite by Major	00904-0625	Vitamin
WESTWARD248	Tab, Yellow, Round, Scored, West-Ward 248	Folic Acid 1 mg	Folvite by Qualitest	00603-3714	Vitamin
WESTWARD248	Tab, Yellow, Round, Scored, West-Ward 248	Folic Acid 1 mg	Folvite by Deca	68552-0529	Vitamin
WESTWARD248	Tab, Yellow, Round, Scored, West-Ward 248	Folic Acid 1 mg	Folvite by Ivax	00182-0507	Vitamin
WESTWARD248	Tab, Yellow, Round, Scored	Folic Acid 1 mg	Folvite by Blu	Discontinued	Vitamin
WESTWARD248	Tab, Yellow, Round, Scored, West-Ward 248	Folic Acid 1 mg	Folvite by West-Ward	24658-0110	Vitamin
WESTWARD249	Tab, White, Round, West-ward 249	Furosemide 20 mg	Lasix by West-Ward	00093-0507	Diuretic
WESTWARD250	Tab, White, Round, West-ward 250	Furosemide 40 mg	Lasix by West-Ward		Diuretic
WESTWARD253	Tab, White, Round, West-ward 253	Furosemide 80 mg	Lasix by West-Ward		Diuretic
WESTWARD254	Tab, White, Round, Scored, West-Ward 254	Hydrocortisone 20 mg	Hydrocortone by Physician Total Care	54868-1743	Steroid
WESTWARD254	Tab, White, Round, Scored, West-Ward 254	Hydrocortisone 20 mg	Hydrocortone by URL Mutual	00677-0076	Steroid
WESTWARD254	Tab, White, Round, Scored, West-Ward 254	Hydrocortisone 20 mg	Hydrocortone by Murfreesboro	51129-1464	Steroid
WESTWARD254	Tab, White, Round, Scored, West-Ward 254	Hydrocortisone 20 mg	Hydrocortone by West-Ward	00143-1254	Steroid
WESTWARD254	Tab, White, Round, Scored, West-Ward 254	Hydrocortisone 20 mg	Hydrocortone by Major	00904-2674	Steroid
WESTWARD256	Tab, Peach, Round	Hydrochlorothiazide 25 mg	Hydrodiuril by West-Ward		Diuretic; Antihypertensive
WESTWARD257	Tab, Peach, Round	Hydrochlorothiazide 50 mg	Hydrodiuril by West-Ward		Diuretic; Antihypertensive

ID FRONT <> BACK	DESCRIPTION FRONT <> BACK	INGREDIENT & STRENGTH	BRAND (or Generic Equiv.) by FIRM	NDC#	CLASS; SCH.
WESTWARD258	Tab, White, Round	Isoxsuprine HCl 10 mg	Vasodilan by West-Ward		Vasodilator
WESTWARD259	Tab, White, Round	Isoxsuprine HCl 20 mg	Vasodilan by West-Ward		Vasodilator
WESTWARD261	Tab, White, Round, Scored	Isoniazid 300 mg	Laniazid by Amerisource	62584-0760	Antimycobacterial
WESTWARD261	Tab, White, Round, Scored	Isoniazid 300 mg	Laniazid by Golden State	60429-0115	Antimycobacterial
WESTWARD261	Tab, White, Round, Scored	Isoniazid 300 mg	Laniazid by Heartland	61392-0803	Antimycobacterial
WESTWARD261	Tab, White, Round, Scored	Isoniazid 300 mg	Laniazid by Versapharm	61748-0013	Antimycobacterial
WESTWARD261	Tab, White, Round, Scored	Isoniazid 300 mg	Laniazid by West-Ward	00143-1261	Antimycobacterial
WESTWARD261	Tab, White, Round, Scored	Isoniazid 300 mg	Laniazid by Amneal	65162-0182	Antimycobacterial
WESTWARD265	Tab, Green, Round	Hydrochlorothiazide 50 mg, Reserpine 0.125 mg	Hydropres 50 by West-Ward		Diuretic; Antihypertensive
WESTWARD269	Tab, Orange, Round, West-ward 269	Hydralazine HCl 25 mg	Apresoline by West-Ward		Antihypertensive
WESTWARD271	Tab, Orange, Round, West-ward 271	Hydralazine HCl 50 mg	Apresoline by West-Ward		Antihypertensive
WESTWARD272	Tab, White, Round	Lorazepam 0.5 mg	Ativan by West-Ward		Antianxiety; C IV
WESTWARD273	Tab, White, Round	Lorazepam 1 mg	Ativan by West-Ward		Antianxiety; C IV
WESTWARD274	Tab, White, Round	Lorazepam 2 mg	Ativan by West-Ward		Antianxiety; C IV
WESTWARD279	Tab, White, Pink Specks	Chlorpheniramine Maleate 5 mg, Phenylephrine HCl 10 mg, Phenylpropanolamine HCl 40 mg, Phenyltoloxamine Citrate 15 mg	Decongestant by Qualitest	00603-3120	Cold Remedy
WESTWARD285	Tab, White, Oblong	Acetaminophen 500 mg, Hydrocodone Bitartrate 5 mg	Vicodin by West-Ward		Analgesic; C III
WESTWARD285	Cap, Orange	Sulfinpyrazone 200 mg	Anturane by West-Ward		Uricosuric
WESTWARD290	Tab, Round, White, Scored	Methocarbamol 500 mg	Robaxin by Qualitest	00603-4487	Muscle Relaxant
WESTWARD290	Tab, White, Round, Scored	Methocarbamol 500 mg	Robaxin by Compumed	00403-1836	Muscle Relaxant
WESTWARD290	Tab, White, Round, Scored	Methocarbamol 500 mg	Robaxin by H J Harkins Co	52959-0167	Muscle Relaxant
WESTWARD290	Tab, White, Round, Scored	Methocarbamol 500 mg	Robaxin by DRX	55045-1531	Muscle Relaxant
WESTWARD290	Tab, White, Round, Scored	Methocarbamol 500 mg	Robaxin by Amerisource	62584-0780	Muscle Relaxant
WESTWARD290	Tab, White, Round, Scored	Methocarbamol 500 mg	Robaxin by Ivax	00182-0572	Muscle Relaxant
WESTWARD290	Tab, White, Round, Scored	Methocarbamol 500 mg	Robaxin by West-Ward	00143-1290	Muscle Relaxant
WESTWARD290	Tab, White, Round, Scored	Methocarbamol 500 mg	Robaxin by Kaiser	00179-1268	Muscle Relaxant
WESTWARD290	Tab, White, Round, Scored	Methocarbamol 500 mg	Robaxin by Allscripts		Muscle Relaxant
WESTWARD292	Tab, White, Cap Shaped, Scored	Methocarbamol 750 mg	Robaxin by West-Ward	00143-1292	Muscle Relaxant
WESTWARD292	Tab, White, Cap Shaped, Scored	Methocarbamol 750 mg	Robaxin by Pharmedix	53002-0359	Muscle Relaxant
WESTWARD292	Tab, White, Cap Shaped, Scored	Methocarbamol 750 mg	Robaxin by H J Harkins Co	52959-0099	Muscle Relaxant
WESTWARD292	Tab, White, Cap Shaped, Scored	Methocarbamol 750 mg	Robaxin by Amerisource	62584-0781	Muscle Relaxant
WESTWARD292	Tab, White, Cap Shaped, Scored	Methocarbamol 750 mg	Robaxin by Qualitest	00603-4488	Muscle Relaxant
WESTWARD292	Tab, White, Cap Shaped, Scored	Methocarbamol 750 mg	Robaxin by URL Mutual	00677-0431	Muscle Relaxant
WESTWARD292	Tab, White, Cap Shaped, Scored	Methocarbamol 750 mg	Robaxin by Kaiser	00179-1279	Muscle Relaxant
WESTWARD292	Tab, White, Cap Shaped, Scored	Methocarbamol 750 mg	Robaxin by Ivax	00182-0573	Muscle Relaxant
WESTWARD292	Tab, White, Cap Shaped, Scored	Methocarbamol 750 mg	Robaxin by Allscripts		Muscle Relaxant
WESTWARD292	Tab, White, Cap Shaped, Scored	Methocarbamol 750 mg	Robaxin by Southwood	58016-0258	Muscle Relaxant
WESTWARD292	Tab, White, Cap Shaped, Scored	Methocarbamol 750 mg	Robaxin by Bryant	63629-1292	Muscle Relaxant
WESTWARD295	Tab, White, Round	Metronidazole 250 mg	Flagyl by West-Ward		Antibiotic
WESTWARD295	Cap, Orange & Yellow	Tetracycline HCl 250 mg	Tetracyn by West-Ward		Antibiotic
WESTWARD296	Tab, Beige, Round	Thioridazine 10 mg	Mellaril by West-Ward		Antipsychotic
WESTWARD297	Tab, Blue, Round	Thioridazine 15 mg	Mellaril by West-Ward		Antipsychotic
WESTWARD297	Tab, White, Oblong	Metronidazole 500 mg	Flagyl by West-Ward		Antibiotic
WESTWARD298	Tab, Yellow, Round	Thioridazine 25 mg	Mellaril by West-Ward		Antipsychotic
WESTWARD299	Tab, Pink, Round	Thioridazine 50 mg	Mellaril by West-Ward		Antipsychotic

ID FRONT <> BACK	DESCRIPTION FRONT <> BACK	INGREDIENT & STRENGTH	BRAND (or Generic Equiv.) by FIRM	NDC#	CLASS; SCH.
WESTWARD30	Cap	Flurazepam HCl 30 mg	by West-Ward		Hypnotic; C IV
WESTWARD30	Cap	Flurazepam HCl 30 mg	by Sandoz	00781-2807	Hypnotic; C IV
WESTWARD300	Tab, White, Round	Ibuprofen 400 mg	Motrin by West-Ward		NSAID
WESTWARD3000	Cap, Blue & Gray	Acetaminophen 500 mg, Butalbital 50 mg, Caffeine 40 mg, Codeine Phosphate 30 mg	Fioricet w/ Codeine by West-Ward	00143-3000	Analgesic; C III
WESTWARD3000	Cap, Blue & Gray	Acetaminophen 325 mg, Butalbital 50 mg, Caffeine 40 mg, Codeine Phosphate 30 mg	Fioricet w/ Codeine by Ivax	00182-2693	Analgesic; C III
WESTWARD3001	Cap, Pink & Red, White Print, West-Ward 3001	Acetaminophen 500 mg, Butalbital 50 mg, Caffeine 40 mg	Esgic Plus by Caremark	00339-4112	Analgesic
WESTWARD3001	Cap, Pink & Red, White Print, West-Ward 3001	Acetaminophen 500 mg, Butalbital 50 mg, Caffeine 40 mg	Esgic Plus by West-Ward	00143-3001	Analgesic
WESTWARD302	Tab, White, Oblong	Ibuprofen 600 mg	Motrin by West-Ward		NSAID
WESTWARD302	Tab, White, Round	Thioridazine 100 mg	Mellaril by West-Ward		Antipsychotic
WESTWARD303	Tab, Green, Round	Thioridazine 150 mg	Mellaril by West-Ward		Antipsychotic
WESTWARD304	Tab, Orange, Round	Thioridazine 200 mg	Mellaril by West-Ward		Antipsychotic
WESTWARD304	Tab, White, Oblong	Ibuprofen 800 mg	Motrin by West-Ward		NSAID
WESTWARD307	Tab, Lavender, Round	Trifluoperazine HCl 1 mg	Stelazine by West-Ward		Antipsychotic
WESTWARD309	Tab, Lavender, Round	Trifluoperazine HCl 2 mg	Stelazine by West-Ward		Antipsychotic
WESTWARD311	Tab, Lavender, Round	Trifluoperazine HCl 5 mg	Stelazine by West-Ward		Antipsychotic
WESTWARD3126	Cap, Dark Blue	Dicyclomine HCl 10 mg	Bentyl by URL Mutual	00677-0341	Gastrointestinal
WESTWARD3126	Cap, Dark Blue	Dicyclomine HCl 10 mg	Bentyl by Qualitest	00603-3265	Gastrointestinal
WESTWARD3126	Cap, Dark Blue	Dicyclomine HCl 10 mg	Bentyl by West-Ward	00143-3126	Gastrointestinal
WESTWARD3126	Cap, Dark Blue	Dicyclomine HCl 10 mg	Bentyl by Warner Chilcott	00047-0403	Gastrointestinal
WESTWARD3126	Cap, Dark Blue	Dicyclomine HCl 10 mg	Bentyl by Heartland	61392-0182	Gastrointestinal
WESTWARD313	Tab, Lavender, Round	Trifluoperazine HCl 10 mg	Stelazine by West-Ward		Antipsychotic
WESTWARD3141	Cap, Blue & White	Doxycycline Hyclate 50 mg	Vibramycin by Warner Chilcott	00047-0829	Antibiotic
WESTWARD3141	Cap, Blue & White	Doxycycline Hyclate 50 mg	Vibramycin by West-Ward	00143-3141	Antibiotic
WESTWARD3142	Cap, Blue, Opaque	Doxycycline Hyclate 100 mg	Vibramycin by West-Ward	00143-3142	Antibiotic
WESTWARD3142	Cap, Blue, Opaque	Doxycycline Hyclate 100 mg	Vibramycin by West-Ward	00143-9410	Antibiotic
WESTWARD3142	Cap, Blue, Opaque	Doxycycline Hyclate 100 mg	Vibramycin by Comm Action	59214-0839	Antibiotic
WESTWARD3142	Cap, Blue, Opaque	Doxycycline Hyclate 100 mg	Vibramycin by Prepackage Specialists	58864-0190	Antibiotic
WESTWARD3142	Cap, Blue, Opaque	Doxycycline Hyclate 100 mg	Vibramycin by Versapharm	61748-0111	Antibiotic
WESTWARD3142	Cap, Blue, Opaque	Doxycycline Hyclate 100 mg	Vibramycin by Amneal	65162-0527	Antibiotic
WESTWARD3145	Cap, Pink, Black Ink	Ephedrine Sulfate 25 mg	by West-Ward	00143-3145	Antiasthmatic
WESTWARD3188	Cap, White, Black Print	Lithium Carbonate 150 mg	Eskalith by West-Ward	00143-3188	Antipsychotic
WESTWARD3189	Cap, Grey and Yellow, Opaque, West-Ward 3189	Lithium Carbonate 300 mg	Eskalith by UDL	51079-0269	Antipsychotic
WESTWARD3189	Cap, Grey and Yellow, Opaque, West-Ward 3189	Lithium Carbonate 300 mg	Eskalith by West-Ward	00143-3189	Antipsychotic
WESTWARD3189	Cap, Grey and Yellow, Opaque, West-Ward 3189	Lithium Carbonate 300 mg	Eskalith by Ivax	00182-1781 Discontinued	Antipsychotic
WESTWARD320	Cap, Ivory & Fuchsia	Hydroxyzine Pamoate 25 mg	Vistaril by West-Ward		Antianxiety; Antihistamine
WESTWARD3238	Cap, Red, Opaque, White Ink	Isoniazid 150 mg, Rifampin 300 mg	Rifamate by Versapharm	61748-0017	Antibiotic
WESTWARD325	Cap, Green & White	Temazepam 15 mg	Restoril by West-Ward		Sedative/Hypnotic; C IV
WESTWARD325	Cap, Ivory & Red	Hydroxyzine Pamoate 50 mg	Vistaril by West-Ward		Antianxiety; Antihistamine
WESTWARD327	Cap, White	Temazepam 30 mg	Restoril by West-Ward		Sedative/Hypnotic; C IV
WESTWARD329	Cap, Maroon	Hydrochlorothiazide 25 mg, Triamterene 50 mg	Dyazide by West-Ward		Diuretic; Antihypertensive
WESTWARD330	Cap, Ivory & Fuchsia	Hydroxyzine Pamoate 100 mg	Vistaril by West-Ward		Antianxiety; Antihistamine
WESTWARD330	Tab, Yellow, Round	Methyltestosterone 25 mg	by West-Ward		Hormone; C III

ID FRONT <> BACK	DESCRIPTION FRONT <> BACK	INGREDIENT & STRENGTH	BRAND (or Generic Equiv.) by FIRM	NDC#	CLASS; SCH.
WESTWARD332	Tab, Yellow, Oblong	Vitamin B Complex	Berocca Plus by West-Ward		Vitamin
WESTWARD336	Tab, White, Round, West-ward 336	Acetaminophen 325 mg	Tylenol by West-Ward		Analgesic
WESTWARD339	Tab, White, Round, West-ward 339	Acetaminophen 500 mg	Tylenol Ex Strength by West-Ward		Analgesic
WESTWARD346	Tab, White, Round	Naproxen 250 mg	Naprosyn by West-Ward	00143-1346	NSAID
WESTWARD347	Tab, White, Oblong	Naproxen 375 mg	Naprosyn by West-Ward	00143-1347	NSAID
WESTWARD348	Tab, White, Oblong, West-Ward 348	Naproxen 500 mg	Naprosyn by West-Ward	00143-1348	NSAID
WESTWARD367	Cap, Blue & White, West-ward 367	Flurazepam HCl 15 mg	Dalmane by West-Ward		Hypnotic; C IV
WESTWARD370	Cap, Blue, West-ward 370	Flurazepam HCl 30 mg	Dalmane by West-Ward		Hypnotic; C IV
WESTWARD445	Tab, White, Round	Phenobarbital 15 mg	Phenobarbital by West-Ward	00143-1445	Sedative/Hypnotic; C IV
WESTWARD445	Tab, White, Round	Phenobarbital 15 mg	Phenobarbital by URL Mutual	00677-1667	Sedative/Hypnotic; C IV
WESTWARD445	Tab, White, Round	Phenobarbital 15 mg	Phenobarbital by Sandoz	00781-1091	Sedative/Hypnotic; C IV
WESTWARD450	Tab, White, Round, Scored	Phenobarbital 30 mg	Phenobarbital by UDL	51079-0095	Sedative/Hypnotic; C IV
WESTWARD450	Tab, White, Round, Scored	Phenobarbital 30 mg	Phenobarbital by West-Ward	00143-1450	Sedative/Hypnotic; C IV
WESTWARD450	Tab, White, Round, Scored	Phenobarbital 30 mg	Phenobarbital by Sandoz	00781-1110	Sedative/Hypnotic; C IV
WESTWARD450	Tab, White, Round, Scored	Phenobarbital 30 mg	Phenobarbital by URL Mutual	00677-1666	Sedative/Hypnotic; C IV
WESTWARD455	Tab, White, Round	Phenobarbital 60 mg	Phenobarbital by West-Ward		Sedative/Hypnotic; C IV
WESTWARD473	Tab, White, Round, Scored, West-Ward 473	Prednisone 10 mg	Deltasone by Baker Cummins	63171-1334	Steroid
WESTWARD473	Tab, White, Round, Scored, West-Ward 473	Prednisone 10 mg	Deltasone by West-Ward	00143-9412	Steroid
WESTWARD473	Tab, White, Round, Scored, West-Ward 473	Prednisone 10 mg	Deltasone by West-Ward	00143-1473	Steroid
WESTWARD473	Tab, White, Round, Scored, West-Ward 473	Prednisone 10 mg	Deltasone by Qualitest	00603-5333	Steroid
WESTWARD473	Tab, White, Round, Scored, West-Ward 473	Prednisone 10 mg	Deltasone by Sandoz	00781-1500	Steroid
WESTWARD473	Tab, White, Round, Scored, West-Ward 473	Prednisone 10 mg	Deltasone by Ivax	00182-1334	Steroid
WESTWARD473	Tab, White, Round, Scored, West-Ward 473	Prednisone 10 mg		Discontinued	Steroid
WESTWARD475	Tab, White, Round, Scored, West-Ward 475	Prednisone 5 mg	Deltasone by West-Ward	00143-1475	Steroid
WESTWARD475	Tab, White, Round, Scored, West-Ward 475	Prednisone 5 mg	Deltasone by Qualitest	00603-5332	Steroid
WESTWARD475	Tab, White, Round, Scored, West-Ward 475	Prednisone 5 mg	Deltasone by Med Pro	53978-0060	Steroid
WESTWARD475	Tab, White, Round, Scored, West-Ward 475	Prednisone 5 mg	Deltasone by Sandoz	00781-1495	Steroid
WESTWARD475	Tab, White, Round, Scored, West-Ward 475	Prednisone 5 mg	Deltasone by Ivax	00182-0201	Steroid
WESTWARD477	Tab, Peach, Round, Scored, West-Ward 477	Prednisone 20 mg		Discontinued	Steroid
WESTWARD477	Tab, Peach, Round, Scored, West-Ward 477	Prednisone 20 mg	Deltasone by Sandoz	00781-1485	Steroid
WESTWARD477	Tab, Peach, Round, Scored, West-Ward 477	Prednisone 20 mg	Deltasone by URL Mutual	00677-0427	Steroid
WESTWARD477	Tab, Peach, Round, Scored, West-Ward 477	Prednisone 20 mg	Deltasone by Baker Cummins	63171-1086	Steroid
WESTWARD477	Tab, Peach, Round, Scored, West-Ward 477	Prednisone 20 mg	Deltasone by West-Ward	00143-1477	Steroid
WESTWARD477	Tab, Peach, Round, Scored, West-Ward 477	Prednisone 20 mg	Deltasone by West-Ward	00143-9413	Steroid
WESTWARD477	Tab, Peach, Round, Scored, West-Ward 477	Prednisone 20 mg	Deltasone by Qualitest	00603-5334	Steroid
WESTWARD477	Tab, Peach, Round, Scored, West-Ward 477	Prednisone 20 mg	Deltasone by Ivax	00182-1086	Steroid
WESTWARD480	Tab, White, Round, Scored, West-Ward 480	Propylthiouracil 50 mg	Propylthiouracil by DRX		Antithyroid
WESTWARD480	Tab, White, Round, Scored, West-Ward 480	Propylthiouracil 50 mg	Propylthiouracil by West-Ward	55045-2747	Antithyroid
WESTWARD481	Tab, White, Round	Prednisone 50 mg	Deltasone by West-Ward	00143-1480	Steroid
WESTWARD485	Tab, White, Round	Pseudoephedrine HCl 60 mg	by West-Ward	00143-1485	Decongestant
WESTWARD485	Tab, White, Round	Pseudoephedrine HCl 60 mg	by Pharmascience	Canadian	Decongestant
WESTWARD502	Tab, Peach, Round	Propranolol HCl 10 mg	Inderal by West-Ward		Antihypertensive
WESTWARD503	Tab, Blue, Round	Propranolol HCl 20 mg	Inderal by West-Ward		Antihypertensive
WESTWARD504	Tab, Green, Round	Propranolol HCl 40 mg	Inderal by West-Ward		Antihypertensive
WESTWARD505	Tab, Pink, Round	Propranolol HCl 60 mg	Inderal by West-Ward		Antihypertensive
WESTWARD506	Tab, Yellow, Round	Propranolol HCl 80 mg	Inderal by West-Ward		Antihypertensive

ID FRONT <> BACK	DESCRIPTION FRONT <> BACK	INGREDIENT & STRENGTH	BRAND (or Generic Equiv.) by FIRM	NDC#	CLASS; SCH.
WESTWARD508	Tab, White, Round	Quinidine Gluconate 324 mg	Quinaglute by West-Ward		Antiarrhythmic
WESTWARD510	Cap, Clear	Quinidine Sulfate 200 mg	by West-Ward		Antiarrhythmic
WESTWARD530	Tab, White, Round	Reserpine 0.1 mg	Serpasil by West-Ward		Antihypertensive
WESTWARD535	Tab, White, Round	Reserpine 0.25 mg	Serpasil by West-Ward		Antihypertensive
WESTWARD625	Tab, White, Oval	Sulfamethoxazole 800 mg, Trimethoprim 160 mg	Bactrim DS by West-Ward		Antibiotic
WESTWARD680	Tab, White, Round	Sulfinpyrazone 100 mg	Anturane by West-Ward		Uricosuric
WESTWARD683	Tab, White, Round	Sulfisoxazole 500 mg	Gantrisin by West-Ward		Antibiotic
WESTWARD689	Tab, White, Oval	Theophylline Anhydrous CR 200 mg	Theo-Dur by West-Ward		Antiasthmatic
WESTWARD690	Tab, White, Oblong	Theophylline Anhydrous CR 300 mg	Theo-Dur by West-Ward		Antiasthmatic
WESTWARD695	Tab, White, Round	Theophylline Anhydrous 118 mg, Ephedrine 24 mg, Phenobarbital 8 mg	Tedral by West-Ward		Antiasthmatic; C IV
WESTWARD737	Tab, White, Round, West-ward 737	Acetaminophen 325 mg, Butalbital 50 mg, Caffeine 40 mg	Fioricet by Qualitest	00603-2547	Analgesic
WESTWARD737	Tab, White, Round, West-ward 737	Acetaminophen 325 mg, Butalbital 50 mg, Caffeine 40 mg	Fioricet by West-Ward	00143-1737	Analgesic
WESTWARD737	Tab, White, Round, West-ward 737	Acetaminophen 325 mg, Butalbital 50 mg, Caffeine 40 mg	by URL Mutual	00677-1748	Analgesic
WESTWARD750	Tab, Round	Hydrochlorothiazide 50 mg, Triamterene 75 mg	Maxzide by West-Ward		Diuretic; Antihypertensive
WESTWARD769	Tab, White, Round, Scored	Isosorbide Dinitrate 5 mg	Isordil by Major	00904-2150	Antianginal
WESTWARD769	Tab, White, Round, Scored	Isosorbide Dinitrate 5 mg	Isordil by West-Ward	00143-1769	Antianginal
WESTWARD769	Tab, White, Round, Scored	Isosorbide Dinitrate 5 mg	Isordil by Heartland	61392-0311	Antianginal
WESTWARD769	Tab, White, Round, Scored	Isosorbide Dinitrate 5 mg	Isordil by Vangard	00615-1564	Antianginal
WESTWARD769	Tab, White, Round, Scored	Isosorbide Dinitrate 5 mg	Isordil by Qualitest	00603-4116	Antianginal
WESTWARD769	Tab, White, Round, Scored	Isosorbide Dinitrate 5 mg	Isordil by Ivax	00182-0550 Discontinued	Antianginal
WESTWARD771	Tab, White, Round	Isosorbide Dinitrate 10 mg	Isordil by West-Ward	00143-9401	Antianginal
WESTWARD771	Tab, White, Round	Isosorbide Dinitrate 10 mg	Isordil by Qualitest	00603-4117	Antianginal
WESTWARD771	Tab, White, Round	Isosorbide Dinitrate 10 mg	Isordil by Vangard	00615-1560	Antianginal
WESTWARD771	Tab, White, Round	Isosorbide Dinitrate 10 mg	Isordil by Talbert	44514-0465	Antianginal
WESTWARD771	Tab, White, Round	Isosorbide Dinitrate 10 mg	Isordil by PDRX	55289-0667	Antianginal
WESTWARD771	Tab, White, Round	Isosorbide Dinitrate 10 mg	Isordil by Major	00904-2151	Antianginal
WESTWARD772	Tab, Green, Round	Isosorbide Dinitrate 20 mg	Isordil by Major	00904-2154	Antianginal
WESTWARD772	Tab, Green, Round	Isosorbide Dinitrate 20 mg	Isordil by West-Ward	00143-9402	Antianginal
WESTWARD772	Tab, Green, Round	Isosorbide Dinitrate 20 mg	Isordil by Talbert	44514-0477	Antianginal
WESTWARD772	Tab, Green, Round	Isosorbide Dinitrate 20 mg	Isordil by Vangard	00615-1575	Antianginal
WESTWARD772	Tab, Green, Round	Isosorbide Dinitrate 20 mg	Isordil by Qualitest	00603-4118	Antianginal
WESTWARD785	Tab, White, Round	Aspirin 325 mg, Butalbital 50 mg, Caffeine 40 mg	Fiorinal by Med Pro	53978-3164	Analgesic; C III
WESTWARD785	Tab, White, Round	Aspirin 325 mg, Butalbital 50 mg, Caffeine 40 mg	Fiorinal by Talbert	44514-0088	Analgesic; C III
WESTWARD785	Tab, White, Round	Aspirin 325 mg, Butalbital 50 mg, Caffeine 40 mg	Fiorinal by Moore	00839-6733	Analgesic; C III
WESTWARD785	Tab, White, Round	Aspirin 325 mg, Butalbital 50 mg, Caffeine 40 mg	Fiorinal by Sandoz	00781-1435	Analgesic; C III
WESTWARD785	Tab, White, Round	Aspirin 325 mg, Butalbital 50 mg, Caffeine 40 mg	Fiorinal by West-Ward	00143-1785	Analgesic; C III
WESTWARD785	Tab, White, Round	Aspirin 325 mg, Butalbital 50 mg, Caffeine 40 mg	Fiorinal by Kaiser	00179-1042	Analgesic; C III
WESTWARD785	Tab, White, Round	Aspirin 325 mg, Butalbital 50 mg, Caffeine 40 mg	Fiorinal by Major	00904-3892	Analgesic; C III
WESTWARD785	Tab, White, Round, West-Ward	Aspirin 325 mg, Butalbital 50 mg, Caffeine 40 mg	Fiorinal by Qualitest	00603-2548	Analgesic; C III
WESTWARD785	Tab, White, Round	Aspirin 325 mg, Butalbital 50 mg, Caffeine 40 mg	Fiorinal by Ivax	00182-1631 Discontinued	Analgesic; C III
WESTWARD787	Tab, Blue, Round, West-Ward over 787	Acetaminophen 325 mg, Butalbital 50 mg, Caffeine 40 mg	Fioricet by Moore	00839-7831	Analgesic
WESTWARD787	Tab, Blue, Round, West-Ward over 787	Acetaminophen 325 mg, Butalbital 50 mg, Caffeine 40 mg	Fioricet by West-Ward	00143-1787	Analgesic
WESTWARD787	Tab, Blue, Round, West-Ward over 787	Acetaminophen 325 mg, Butalbital 50 mg, Caffeine 40 mg	Fioricet by Teva Pharmaceuticals	00093-0854 Discontinued	Analgesic
WESTWARD787	Tab, Blue, Round, West-Ward over 787	Acetaminophen 325 mg, Butalbital 50 mg, Caffeine 40 mg	Fioricet by Ivax	00182-2659 Discontinued	Analgesic

ID FRONT <> BACK	DESCRIPTION FRONT <> BACK	INGREDIENT & STRENGTH	BRAND (or Generic Equiv.) by FIRM	NDC#	CLASS; SCH.
WESTWARD900	Tab, Round	Triprolidine 2.5 mg, Pseudoephedrine 60 mg	Actifed by West-Ward		Cold Remedy
WESTWARD-FLURAZEPAM15	Cap, Blue & White	Flurazepam HCl 15 mg	Dalmane by Invamed	52189-0375	Hypnotic; C IV
WESTWARD-FLURAZEPAM15	Cap, Black Print	Flurazepam HCl 15 mg	by Kaiser	00179-1098	Hypnotic; C IV
WESTWARD-FLURAZEPAM15	Cap, Blue & White	Flurazepam HCl 15 mg	Dalmane by West-Ward	00143-3367	Hypnotic; C IV
WESTWARD-FLURAZEPAM15	Cap, Blue & White	Flurazepam HCl 15 mg	Dalmane by Invamed	52189-0315	Hypnotic; C IV
WESTWARD-FLURAZEPAM30	Cap, Blue	Flurazepam HCl 30 mg	Dalmane by West-Ward	00143-3370	Hypnotic; C IV
WESTWARD-FLURAZEPAM30	Cap, Black Print	Flurazepam HCl 30 mg	by Kaiser	00179-1099	Hypnotic; C IV
WESTWARD-FLURAZEPAM30	Cap, Blue	Flurazepam HCl 30 mg	Dalmane by Invamed	52189-0383	Hypnotic; C IV
WF1 <> G	Tab, Dark Pink, Round, Scored	Warfarin Sodium 1 mg	Coumadin by Genpharm	15330-0100	Anticoagulant
WF10 <> G	Tab, White, Round, Scored	Warfarin Sodium 10 mg	Coumadin by Genpharm	15330-0108	Anticoagulant
WF2 <> G	Tab, Lavender, Round, Scored	Warfarin Sodium 2 mg	Coumadin by Genpharm	15330-0101	Anticoagulant
WF25 <> G	Tab, Green, Round, Scored, WF / 2.5	Warfarin Sodium 2.5 mg	Coumadin by Genpharm	15330-0102	Anticoagulant
WF3 <> G	Tab, Brown, Round, Scored	Warfarin Sodium 3 mg	Coumadin by Genpharm	15330-0266	Anticoagulant
WF4 <> G	Tab, Blue, Round, Scored	Warfarin Sodium 4 mg	Coumadin by Genpharm	15330-0267	Anticoagulant
WF5 <> G	Tab, Peach, Round, Scored	Warfarin Sodium 5 mg	Coumadin by Genpharm	15330-0268	Anticoagulant
WF6 <> G	Tab, Dark Green, Round, Scored	Warfarin Sodium 6 mg	Coumadin by Genpharm	15330-0106	Anticoagulant
WF75 <> G	Tab, Yellow, Round, Scored, WF / 7.5	Warfarin Sodium 7.5 mg	Coumadin by Genpharm	15330-0107	Anticoagulant
WFF	Tab, Pinkish Purple, Oval, Schering Logo WFF	Fluphenazine HCl 5 mg	Permitil by Schering	00085-0550	Antipsychotic
WFG	Tab, Red, Oval, Schering Logo WFG	Fluphenazine HCl 10 mg	Permitil by Schering	00085-0316	Antipsychotic
WFHC <> BACTRIM	Tab, White, Round, Scored	Sulfamethoxazole 400 mg, Trimethoprim 80 mg	Bactrim by Women First HealthCare	64248-0004	Antibiotic
WFHC <> BACTRIMDS	Tab, White, Oval, Scored	Sulfamethoxazole 800 mg, Trimethoprim 160 mg	Bactrim DS by Women First HealthCare	64248-0117	Antibiotic
WFHC101	Tab, White, Diamond Shaped, Scored	Estropipate 0.75 mg	Ortho EST by Women First HealthCare	64248-0101	Hormone
WFHC101	Tab, White, Diamond, Scored	Estropipate 0.625 mg	by Heartland	61392-0557	Hormone
WFHC102	Tab, Purple, Diamond Shaped, Scored	Estropipate 1.5 mg	Ortho EST by Women First HealthCare	64248-0102	Hormone
WFHC4191	Cap, Blue & Grey	Aspirin 356.4 mg, Caffeine 30 mg, Dihydrocodeine Bitartrate 16 mg	Synalgos DC by Women First HealthCare	64248-0419	Analgesic; C III
WFHC91	Tab, Pink & Yellow, Round, Scored	Aspirin 325 mg, Meprobamate 200 mg	Equagesic by Women First HealthCare	64248-0091	Sedative/Hypnotic; C IV
WHITBY <> 612	Tab, Film Coated	Guaifenesin 600 mg, Pseudoephedrine 120 mg	Duratuss by CVS	51316-0238	Cold Remedy
WHITBY <> 612	Tab, Film Coated	Guaifenesin 600 mg, Pseudoephedrine 120 mg	Duratuss by UCB	50474-0612	Cold Remedy
WHITBY <> 901	Tab, White, Oblong, Pink Specks	Acetaminophen 500 mg, Hydrocodone Bitartrate 2.5 mg	Lortab by Alphapharm		Analgesic; C III
WHITBY <> 902	Tab, White, Blue Specks	Acetaminophen 500 mg, Hydrocodone Bitartrate 5 mg	Vicodin by UCB	50474-0902	Analgesic; C III
WHITBY500	Tab, Pink, Oblong	Acetaminophen 500 mg, Hydrocodone Bitartrate 5 mg	Lortab by UCB		Analgesic; C III
WHITBY901	Tab, White, Pink Specks, Oblong	Acetaminophen 500 mg, Hydrocodone Bitartrate 2.5 mg	Lortab by UCB		Analgesic; C III
WHITBY902	Tab, White, Blue Specks, Whitby/902	Acetaminophen 500 mg, Hydrocodone Bitartrate 5 mg	Vicodin by Allscripts		Analgesic; C III
WHITBY903 <> WHITBY903	Tab, White, Green Specks, Whitby/903	Atropine Sulfate 0.025 mg, Diphenoxylate HCl 2.5 mg	Lomotil by Nat Pharmpak	55154-7201	Antidiarrheal; C V
WHITE <> RELAFEN500	Tab, Film Coated	Nabumetone 500 mg	Relafen by Rx Dispensing	61807-0051	NSAID
WHITEHALLLOGO	Tab, Pink	Aspirin 325 mg, Caffeine 32 mg, Codeine Phosphate 8 mg	Anacin w/ Codeine by Whitehall Robins	Canadian	Analgesic; C III
WHR100	Cap, Clear & White	Theophylline Anhydrous 100 mg	Slo-Bid Gyrocaps by RPR		Antiasthmatic
WHR125	Cap, White	Theophylline Anhydrous 125 mg	Slo-Bid Gyrocaps by RPR		Antiasthmatic
WHR1354	Cap, White	Theophylline Anhydrous 60 mg	Slo phyllin Gyrocaps by Rorer		Antiasthmatic
WHR1355	Cap, Brown	Theophylline Anhydrous 125 mg	Slo phyllin Gyrocaps by Rorer		Antiasthmatic

ID FRONT <> BACK	DESCRIPTION FRONT <> BACK	INGREDIENT & STRENGTH	BRAND (or Generic Equiv.) by FIRM	NDC#	CLASS; SCH.
WHR1356	Cap, Purple	Theophylline Anhydrous 250 mg	Slo phyllin Gyrocaps by Rorer		Antiasthmatic
WHR200	Cap, Clear & White	Theophylline Anhydrous 200 mg	Slo-Bid Gyrocaps by RPR		Antiasthmatic
WHR300	Cap, Clear & White	Theophylline Anhydrous 300 mg	Slo-Bid Gyrocaps by RPR		Antiasthmatic
WHR50MG	Cap, Clear & White	Theophylline Anhydrous 50 mg	Slo-Bid Gyrocaps by RPR		Antiasthmatic
WHR75MG	Cap, Clear & White	Theophylline Anhydrous 75 mg	Slo-Bid Gyrocaps by RPR		Antiasthmatic
WI200	Tab, White, Round, W/I/200	Floctafenine 200 mg	Idarac by Sanofi	Canadian	Anti-Inflammatory
WI400	Tab, White, Round, W/I/400	Floctafenine 400 mg	Idarac by Sanofi	Canadian	Anti-Inflammatory
WINTHROP <> T27	Tab	Aspirin 325 mg, Pentazocine HCl	Talwin Compound by Searle	00966-1927	Analgesic; C IV
WINTHROP <> T27	Tab	Aspirin 325 mg, Pentazocine HCl	Talwin Compound by Sanofi	00024-1927	Analgesic; C IV
WINTHROP <> T37	Tab, Pale Blue, Cap Shaped, Scored	Pentazocine HCl 25 mg, Acetaminophen 650 mg	Talacen by Sanofi	00024-1937	Analgesic; C IV
WINTHROPT37	Tab, Blue, Oblong	Pentazocine HCl 25 mg, Acetaminophen 500 mg	Talacen by Sanofi		Analgesic; C IV
WL	Tab, Pink, Round, Scored	Quinidine Phenylethylbarbiturate 100 mg	by AltiMed	Canadian DIN 00249424	Antiarrhythmic
WL	Tab, Pink, Round	Digitoxin 0.1 mg	by Welcker-Lyster	Canadian	Cardiac Agent
WL	Tab, Yellow, Round, Scored, W.L. Logo	Colchicine 0.6 mg	by AltiMed	Canadian DIN 00287873	Antigout
WL	Tab, Pink, Round, Scored, W.L. Logo	Colchicine 1 mg	by AltiMed	Canadian DIN 00206032	Antigout
WL118	Cap, Yellow, W & L 118	Diphenhydramine 50 mg	Sominex by Weeks & Leo		Sleep Aid
WL25 <> B	Tab, Bright Pink	Diphenhydramine HCl 25 mg	Benadryl by Pfizer	00501-2009	Antihistamine
WL26 <> B	Tab, White	Diphenhydramine HCl 12.5 mg, Pseudoephedrine HCl 30 mg, Acetaminophen 500 mg	Benadryl Allergy-Cold by Pfizer	00501-2006	Cold Remedy
WL26 <> B	Tab, Green, Cap Shaped	Diphenhydramine HCl 12.5 mg, Pseudoephedrine HCl 30 mg, Acetaminophen 500 mg	Benadryl Allergy Sinus Headache by Pfizer	00501-2005	Cold Remedy
WL26 <> B	Tab, Green, Cap Shaped	Diphenhydramine HCl 12.5 mg, Pseudoephedrine HCl 30 mg, Acetaminophen 500 mg	Benadryl Total Allergy by Pfizer	Canadian DIN 02255472	Cold Remedy
WL28 <> B	Tab, Blue, Cap Shaped	Diphenhydramine HCl 25 mg, Pseudoephedrine HCl 30 mg, Acetaminophen 500 mg	Benadryl Total Allergy Ex Strength by Pfizer	Canadian DIN 02250993	Cold Remedy
WL28 <> B	Tab, Blue, Cap Shaped	Diphenhydramine HCl 25 mg, Pseudoephedrine HCl 30 mg, Acetaminophen 500 mg	Benadryl Severe Allergy Sinus Headache by Pfizer	00501-2030	Cold Remedy
WL53	Tab, White, Round	Talbutal 120 mg	Lotusate by Sanofi		Hypnotic; C III
WL89 <> SUPE	Tab, Orange, Cap Shaped	Acetaminophen 325 mg, Dextromethorphan HBr 10 mg, Guaifenesin 100 mg, Phenylephrine HCl 5 mg	Sudafed PE Cold and Cough by Pfizer	00501-2909	Cold Remedy
WM31	Tab, White, Round	Mephobarbital 32 mg	Mebaral by Sanofi		Sedative/Hypnotic; C IV
WM32	Tab, White, Round	Mephobarbital 50 mg	Mebaral by Sanofi		Sedative/Hypnotic; C IV
WM33	Tab, White, Round	Mephobarbital 100 mg	Mebaral by Sanofi		Sedative/Hypnotic; C IV
WM87	Tab, White, Round	Ambenonium 10 mg	Symmetrel by Sanofi		Myasthenia Gravis
WM9060MG	Cap, Black & Pink, W M-90 60 mg	Trilostane 60 mg	Modrastane by Sanofi		Steroid Inhibitor
WM9130MG	Cap, Pink, W M-91 30 mg	Trilostane 30 mg	Modrastane by Sanofi		Steroid Inhibitor
WMO	Tab, White, W/M-O	Levonogestrel 150 mcg, Ethinyl Estradiol 30 mcg	Levora by Wyeth	Canadian	Oral Contraceptive
WMP	Cap, Green	Atropine Sulfate 0.195 mg, Phenobarbital 16 mg	Anthrocol by Poythress		Gastrointestinal; C IV
WMP9525	Cap, Brown & Yellow	Phenobarbital 16 mg	Solfoton by Poythress		Sedative/Hypnotic; C IV
WN21	Tab, Tan, Oblong	Nalidixic Acid 250 mg	NegGram by Sanofi		Antibiotic
WN22	Tab, Tan, Oblong	Nalidixic Acid 500 mg	NegGram by Sanofi		Antibiotic
WN23	Tab, Tan, Oval	Nalidixic Acid 1000 mg	NegGram by Sanofi		Antibiotic

ID FRONT <> BACK	DESCRIPTION FRONT <> BACK	INGREDIENT & STRENGTH	BRAND (or Generic Equiv.) by FIRM	NDC#	CLASS; SCH.
WP101	Tab	Carbinoxamine Maleate 8 mg, Pseudoephedrine HCl 120 mg	Biohist LA by Anabolic	00722-6250 Discontinued	Cold Remedy
WP102	Tab, White, Oval, Scored, Ex Release	Dextromethorphan HBr 30 mg, Guaifenesin 600 mg, Phenylpropanolamine HCl 37.5 mg	Profen II DM by Anabolic	00722-6385	Cold Remedy
WP12	Tab, White, Oval, Scored, Ex Release	Guaifenesin 1200 mg	Robitussin by Anabolic	00722-6412	Expectorant
WP12	Tab, White, Oval, Scored, Ex Release	Guaifenesin 1200 mg	Robitussin by Ivax Labs	59310-0120	Expectorant
WP61	Tab, White, Round	Hydroxychloroquine Sulfate 200 mg	Plaquenil by Sanofi		Antimalarial
WPC004 <> DUVOID10	Tab, White, Round	Bethanechol Chloride 10 mg	Urecholine by Abrika	67767-0144	Urinary Tract
WPC005 <> DUVOID25	Tab, White, Round	Bethanechol Chloride 25 mg	Urecholine by Abrika	67767-0145	Urinary Tract
WPC006 <> DUVOID50	Tab, Tan, Round	Bethanechol Chloride 50 mg	Urecholine by Abrika	67767-0146	Urinary Tract
WPHH <> 170	Tab	Sulindac 150 mg	by Merck Sharp & Dohme	62904-0170	NSAID
WPI <> 1117	Tab, White, Oblong, Scored	Mirtazapine 15 mg	Remeron by Watson	00591-1117	Antidepressant
WPI <> 2713	Tab, Light Peach, Cap Shaped, Film Coated	Metformin HCl 500 mg	Glucophage by Watson	00591-2713	Antidiabetic
WPI <> 2775	Tab, Light Peach, Cap Shaped, Film Coated	Metformin HCl 850 mg	Glucophage by Watson	00591-2775	Antidiabetic
WPI <> 3111	Tab, Mottled White to Off-White, Oval, Extended-Release	Methylphenidate HCl 20 mg	Ritalin by Watson	00591-3111	Stimulant; C II
WPI <> 3176	Tab, White, Round, Film Coated	Citalopram HBr 10 mg	Celexa by Watson	00591-3176	Antidepressant
WPI <> 3238	Tab, Green, Cap Shaped, Film Coated, Scored, 32 / 38	Sertraline HCl 25 mg	Zoloft by Watson	00591-3238	Antidepressant
WPI <> 3239	Tab, Blue, Cap Shaped, Film Coated, Scored, 32 / 39	Sertraline HCl 50 mg	Zoloft by Watson	00591-3239	Antidepressant
WPI <> 3240	Tab, Yellow, Cap Shaped, Film Coated, Scored, 32 / 40	Sertraline HCl 100 mg	Zoloft by Watson	00591-3240	Antidepressant
WPI <> 3366	Tab, Pink, Cap Shaped, Film Coated	Zolpidem Tartrate 5 mg	Ambien by Watson	00591-3366	Sedative/Hypnotic; C IV
WPI <> 3367	Tab, White, Cap Shaped, Film Coated	Zolpidem Tartrate 10 mg	Ambien by Watson	00591-3367	Sedative/Hypnotic; C IV
WPI <> 3416	Tab, White, Cap Shaped, Scored	Butalbital 50 mg, Acetaminophen 325 mg, Caffeine 40 mg	Fioricet by Watson	00591-3416	Analgesic
WPI1118	Tab, Yellow, Oval, Scored, Film Coated	Mirtazapine 30 mg	Remeron by Watson	00591-1118	Antidepressant
WPI1119	Tab, White, Oval, WPI over 1119	Mirtazapine 45 mg	Remeron by Watson	00591-1119	Antidepressant
WPI2137	Tab, White, Oval, Film Coated	Ibuprofen 800 mg	Motrin by Watson	00591-2137	NSAID
WPI3177	Tab, White, Round, Film Coated, Scored, WPI curves across top, 3177 around bottom	Citalopram HBr 20 mg	Celexa by Watson	00591-3177	Antidepressant
WPI3178	Tab, White, Round, Film Coated, Scored, WPI curves across top, 3178 around bottom	Citalopram HBr 40 mg	Celexa by Watson	00591-3178	Antidepressant
WPI3231	Tab, Yellow, Round	Meloxicam 15 mg	Mobic by Watson	00591-3231	NSAID
WPI3331	Tab, White to Off White, Round, Extended Release	Bupropion HCl 150 mg	Wellbutrin XL by Watson	00591-3331	Antidepressant
WPI3332	Tab, Off White, Round, Film Coated, Extended Release	Bupropion HCl 300 mg	Wellbutrin XL by Watson	00591-3332	Antidepressant
WPI3332	Tab, Off-White, Round, Film-Coated, Extended Release	Bupropion HCl 300 mg	Wellbutrin XL by Watson	00591-3332	Antidepressant
WPI338	Tab, White, Round, Delayed Release	Diclofenac Sodium 50 mg	Voltaren by Watson	00591-0338	NSAID
WPI3385	Tab, White, Round, Sustained Release	Bupropion HCl 200 mg	Wellbutrin SR by Watson	00591-3385	Antidepressant
WPI339	Tab, White, Round, Ex Release	Diclofenac Sodium 75 mg	Voltaren by Watson	00591-0339	NSAID
WPI339	Tab, White, Round, Ex Release	Diclofenac Sodium 75 mg	Voltaren by Watson	52544-0339	NSAID
WPI3496	Cap, White, Opaque, Hard Gelatin	Galantamine Hydrobromide 8 mg	GALANTAMINE HYDROBROMIDE by Watson	00591-3496	Acetylcholinesterase Inhibitor
WPI3498	Cap, Pink, Extended Release	Galantamine 24 mg	Razadyne ER by Watson	00591-3498	Antialzheimers
WPI4010	Tab, White, Oval, Film Coated	Ibuprofen 400 mg	Motrin by Watson	00591-4010	NSAID
WPI4011	Tab, White, Oval, Film Coated	Ibuprofen 600 mg	Motrin by Watson	00591-4011	NSAID
WPI839	Tab, White, Round, WPI over 839, SR	Bupropion HCl 150 mg	Wellbutrin SR by Watson	00591-0839	Antidepressant
WPI844	Tab, Orange, Round, Extended Release	Glipizide 5 mg	Glucotrol XL by Watson	00591-0844	Antidiabetic
WPI845	Tab, White, Round, Extended Release	Glipizide 10 mg	Glucotrol XL by Watson	00591-0845	Antidiabetic
WPI858	Tab, White, Round, SR	Bupropion HCl 100 mg	Wellbutrin SR by Watson	00591-0858	Antidepressant
WPI867	Tab, White, Round, Film Coated	Bupropion HCl 150 mg	Zyban SR by Watson	00591-0867	Antidepressant
WPI900	Tab, Light Orange, Round, Black Ink, Extended Release	Glipizide 2.5 mg	Glucotrol XL by Watson	00591-0900	Antidiabetic
WPIMINOCYCLINE75	Cap, White & Yellow	Minocycline HCl 75 mg	Minocin by Watson	00591-3153	Antibiotic
WPIWPI <> 2455	Tab, Light Peach, Cap Shaped, Scored, Film Coated	Metformin HCl 1000 mg	Glucophage by Watson	00591-2455	Antidiabetic

ID FRONT <> BACK	DESCRIPTION FRONT <> BACK	INGREDIENT & STRENGTH	BRAND (or Generic Equiv.) by FIRM	NDC#	CLASS; SCH.
WPN325	Tab, White, Round	Phenylpropanolamine HCl 37.5 mg	Revive by NVE		Decongestant; Appetite Suppressant
WPN375	Tab, White, Round, WPN/37.5	Phenylpropanolamine 37.5 mg	Revive Diet Aid by NVE		Decongestant; Appetite Suppressant
WPPH <> 152	Tab, Yellow, Round, Film Coated	Methyldopa 250 mg	by Endo	60951-0776	Antihypertensive
WPPH <> 153	Tab, White, Round, Film Coated	HCTZ 25 mg, Methyldopa 250 mg	by Endo	60951-0779	Diuretic; Antihypertensive
WPPH <> 153	Tab, White, Round, Film Coated	Hydrochlorothiazide 25 mg, Methyldopa 250 mg	by West Point	59591-0153	Diuretic; Antihypertensive
WPPH <> 153	Tab, White, Round, Film Coated	HCTZ 25 mg, Methyldopa 250 mg	by Merck	00006-0153	Diuretic; Antihypertensive
WPPH <> 154	Tab, Bright Yellow, Hexagonal, Scored	Sulindac 200 mg	by West Point	59591-0154	NSAID
WPPH <> 154	Tab, Bright Yellow, Hexagonal, Scored	Sulindac 200 mg	by Endo	60951-0781	NSAID
WPPH <> 154	Tab, Bright Yellow, Hexagonal, Scored	Sulindac 200 mg	by Merck Sharp & Dohme	62904-0154	NSAID
WPPH <> 156	Tab, Butterscotch Yellow, D-Shaped, Film Coated	Cyclobenzaprine HCl 10 mg	by Med Pro	53978-1035	Muscle Relaxant
WPPH <> 156	Tab, Butterscotch Yellow, D-Shaped, Film Coated	Cyclobenzaprine HCl 10 mg	by Endo	60951-0767	Muscle Relaxant
WPPH <> 156	Tab, Butterscotch Yellow, D-Shaped, Film Coated	Cyclobenzaprine HCl 10 mg	by PDRX	55289-0567	Muscle Relaxant
WPPH <> 156	Tab, Butterscotch Yellow, D-Shaped, Film Coated	Cyclobenzaprine HCl 10 mg	by West Point	59591-0156	Muscle Relaxant
WPPH <> 162	Tab, Peach, Diamond Shaped, Scored	Amiloride HCl 5 mg, Hydrochlorothiazide 50 mg	Moduretic by West Point	59591-0162	Antihypertensive; Diuretic
WPPH <> 162	Tab, Peach, Diamond Shaped, Scored	Amiloride HCl 5 mg, Hydrochlorothiazide 50 mg	Moduretic by Endo	60951-0764	Antihypertensive; Diuretic
WPPH <> 170	Tab, Bright Yellow, Round	Sulindac 150 mg	by West Point	59591-0170	NSAID
WPPH <> 170	Tab, Bright Yellow, Round	Sulindac 150 mg	by Endo	60951-0780	NSAID
WPPH <> 174	Tab, Yellow, Round, Film Coated	Methyldopa 125 mg	Aldomet by Endo	60951-0775	Antihypertensive
WPPH <> 176	Tab, Yellow, Round, Film Coated	Methyldopa 500 mg	by Merck	00006-0176	Antihypertensive
WPPH <> 176	Tab, Yellow, Round, Film Coated	Methyldopa 500 mg	by Endo	60951-0777	Antihypertensive
WPPH <> 179	Tab, Salmon, Round, Film Coated	Hydrochlorothiazide 15 mg, Methyldopa 250 mg	by Endo	60951-0778	Diuretic; Antihypertensive
WPPH <> 179	Tab, Salmon, Round, Film Coated	Hydrochlorothiazide 15 mg, Methyldopa 250 mg	by Merck	00006-0179	Diuretic; Antihypertensive
WPPH <> 192	Tab, Light Blue, Round	Timolol Maleate 5 mg	Blocadren by West Point	59591-0192	Antihypertensive
WPPH <> 192	Tab, Light Blue, Round	Timolol Maleate 5 mg	Blocadren by Endo	60951-0782	Antihypertensive
WPPH <> 194	Tab, Light Blue, Round, Scored	Timolol Maleate 10 mg	by West Point	59591-0194	Antihypertensive
WPPH <> 194	Tab, Light Blue, Round, Scored	Timolol Maleate 10 mg	by Endo	60951-0783	Antihypertensive
WPPH <> 195	Tab, Peach, Cap Shaped, Film Coated	Diflunisal 250 mg	by Endo	60951-0768	NSAID
WPPH <> 196	Tab, Orange, Cap Shaped, Film Coated	Diflunisal 500 mg	by Endo	60951-0769	NSAID
WPPH <> 196	Tab, Orange, Cap Shaped, Film Coated	Diflunisal 500 mg	by Duramed	51285-0503	NSAID
WPPH <> 196	Tab, Orange, Cap Shaped, Film Coated	Diflunisal 500 mg	by H J Harkins Co	52959-0379	NSAID
WPPH <> 240	Tab, White, Round, Scored	Chlorothiazide 250 mg	Diuril by Endo	60951-0765	Diuretic; Antihypertensive
WPPH <> 240	Tab, White, Round, Scored	Chlorothiazide 250 mg	Diuril by Merck	00006-0240	Diuretic; Antihypertensive
WPPH <> 241	Tab, Peach, Round, Scored	Hydrochlorothiazide 25 mg	Hydrodiuril by Endo	60951-0770	Diuretic; Antihypertensive
WPPH <> 241	Tab, Peach, Round, Scored	Hydrochlorothiazide 25 mg	Hydrodiuril by Merck	00006-0241	Diuretic; Antihypertensive
WPPH <> 243	Tab, Peach, Round, Scored	Hydrochlorothiazide 50 mg	by Merck	00006-0243	Diuretic; Antihypertensive
WPPH <> 243	Tab, Peach, Round, Scored	Hydrochlorothiazide 50 mg	by Endo	60951-0771	Diuretic; Antihypertensive
WPPH <> 245	Tab, White, Round, Scored	Chlorothiazide 500 mg	Diuril by Endo	60951-0766	Diuretic; Antihypertensive
WPPH157	Cap, Blue and White Pellets, Ex Release	Indomethacin 75 mg	Indocin SR by West Point	59591-0157	NSAID
WPPH157	Cap, Blue and White Pellets, Ex Release	Indomethacin 75 mg	Indocin SR by Endo	60951-0774	NSAID
WPPH159	Cap, Blue	Indomethacin 50 mg	Indocin by Endo	60951-0773	NSAID
WPPH159	Cap, Blue	Indomethacin 50 mg	Indocin by West Point	59591-0159	NSAID
WPPH159	Cap, Blue	Indomethacin 50 mg	Indocin by Southwood	58016-0236	NSAID
WPPH172	Cap	Indomethacin 25 mg	Indocin by West Point	59591-0172	NSAID
WPPH172	Cap, Blue & White	Indomethacin 25 mg	Indocin by West Point	59591-0172	NSAID
WPPH172	Cap	Indomethacin 25 mg	Indocin by Endo	60951-0772	NSAID
WPPH172	Cap, Blue & White	Indomethacin 25 mg	Indocin by Endo	60951-0772	NSAID
WR	Tab, White, Oblong	Methocarbamol 750 mg	Robaxin by Whitehall Robins	Canadian	Muscle Relaxant
WR	Tab, White, Round, Scored	Methocarbamol 500 mg	Robaxin by Whitehall Robins		Muscle Relaxant

ID FRONT <> BACK	DESCRIPTION FRONT <> BACK	INGREDIENT & STRENGTH	BRAND (or Generic Equiv.) by FIRM	NDC#	CLASS; SCH.
WR	Tab, White, Oblong, Scored	Methocarbamol 750 mg	Robaxin by Whitehall Robins		Muscle Relaxant
WR	Tab, White	Methocarbamol 500 mg	Robaxin by Whitehall Robins	Canadian	Muscle Relaxant
WR	Cap, Green & White	Methocarbamol 400 mg, Acetaminophen 325 mg	Robaxacet by Whitehall Robins	Canadian	Muscle Relaxant
WR	Tab, Green & White	Methocarbamol 400 mg, Acetaminophen 325 mg	Robaxacet by Whitehall Robins	Canadian	Muscle Relaxant
WR	Cap, Green & White, Layers, Scored	Methocarbamol 400 mg, Acetaminophen 325 mg	Robaxacet by Whitehall Robins		Muscle Relaxant
WR	Tab, Green & White, Round, Scored	Methocarbamol 400 mg, Acetaminophen 325 mg	Robaxacet by Whitehall Robins		Muscle Relaxant
WR	Tab, Blue & White, Round	Methocarbamol 400 mg, Acetaminophen 325 mg, Codeine Phosphate 8 mg	Robaxacet by Whitehall Robins	Canadian	Muscle Relaxant; C III
WR	Tab, Blue & White, Blue & White Layers, Round, Scored	Methocarbamol 400 mg, Acetaminophen 325 mg, Codeine Phosphate 8 mg	Robaxacet by Whitehall Robins		Muscle Relaxant; C III
WR;	Cap, White & Pink, White & Pink Layers, Scored, W-R	Aspirin 325 mg, Methocarbamol 400 mg	Robaxisal by Whitehall Robins		Analgesic; Muscle Relaxant
WR;	Tab, White, Pink Layers, Round, Scored, W-R	Aspirin 325 mg, Methocarbamol 400 mg	Robaxisal by Whitehall Robins		Analgesic; Muscle Relaxant
WR;	Tab, White & Yellow, Round, Scored, W-R	Aspirin 325 mg, Methocarbamol 400 mg	Robaxisal by Whitehall Robins		Analgesic; Muscle Relaxant
WR	Tab, Coral & White, Coral & White Layers, Round, Scored, W-R	Aspirin 325 mg, Codeine 32.4 mg, Methocarbamol 400 mg	Robaxisal-C by Whitehall Robins		Muscle Relaxant; C III
WR;	Tab, Orange & White, Round, Scored, W-R	Aspirin 325 mg, Codeine 16.2 mg, Methocarbamol 400 mg	Robaxisal-C by Whitehall Robins		Analgesic; Muscle Relaxant; C III
WR	Tab, Orange & White	Aspirin 325 mg, Codeine 16.2 mg, Methocarbamol 400 mg	Robaxisal-C by Whitehall Robins	Canadian	Muscle Relaxant; C III
WR	Tab, Coral & White	Aspirin 325 mg, Codeine 32.4 mg, Methocarbamol 400 mg	Robaxisal-C by Whitehall Robins	Canadian	Muscle Relaxant; C III
WR	Tab, Yellow & White	Aspirin 325 mg, Codeine 8 mg, Methocarbamol 400 mg	Robaxisal-C by Whitehall Robins	Canadian	Muscle Relaxant; C III
WR	Tab, Peach, W-R	Brompheniramine Maleate 4 mg	Dimetane by Whitehall Robins	Discontinued	Antihistamine
WR	Tab, Peach, Round, Scored, W-R	Brompheniramine Maleate 4 mg, Phenylpropanolamine HCl 5 mg	Dimetapp by Whitehall Robins		Cold Remedy
WR	Tab, Blue, Round, W-R	Brompheniramine Maleate 12 mg, Phenylpropanolamine HCl 15 mg	Dimetapp by Whitehall Robins		Cold Remedy
WRF1 <> 832	Tab, Pink, Round, Scored	Warfarin Sodium 1 mg	Jantoven by Upsher Smith	00832-1211	Anticoagulant
WRF10 <> 832	Tab, White, Round, Scored	Warfarin Sodium 10 mg	Jantoven by Upsher Smith	00832-1219	Anticoagulant
WRF2 <> 832	Tab, Lavender, Round, Scored	Warfarin Sodium 2 mg	Jantoven by Upsher Smith	00832-1212	Anticoagulant
WRF212 <> 832	Tab, Green, Round, Scored, WRF 2 1/2 <> 832	Warfarin Sodium 2.5 mg	Jantoven by Upsher Smith	00832-1213	Anticoagulant
WRF3 <> 832	Tab, Tan, Round, Scored	Warfarin Sodium 3 mg	Jantoven by Upsher Smith	00832-1214	Anticoagulant
WRF4 <> 832	Tab, Blue, Round, Scored	Warfarin Sodium 4 mg	Jantoven by Upsher Smith	00832-1215	Anticoagulant
WRF5 <> 832	Tab, Peach, Round, Scored	Warfarin Sodium 5 mg	Jantoven by Upsher Smith	00832-1216	Anticoagulant
WRF6 <> 832	Tab, Teal, Round, Scored	Warfarin Sodium 6 mg	Jantoven by Upsher Smith	00832-1217	Anticoagulant
WRF712 <> 832	Tab, Yellow, Round, Scored, WRF 7 1/2 <> 832	Warfarin Sodium 7.5 mg	Jantoven by Upsher Smith	00832-1218	Anticoagulant
WRP1	Cap, Mauve, WR/P-1	Multivitamins	Paramettes by Whitehall Robins		Vitamin
WRP2	Cap, Lime, WR/P-2	Multivitamins	Paramettes by Whitehall Robins		Vitamin
WRS1	Tab, Orange, Oval, W-R/S1	Multivitamins	by Whitehall Robins	Canadian	Vitamin
WRS1	Tab, Orange & Red, Oval, W-R/S/1	Vitamin B Complex Vitamins C & E & Iron	Stresstabs by Whitehall Robins		Vitamin
WRS2	Tab, Red, Oval, W-R/S2	Multivitamins	by Whitehall Robins	Canadian	Vitamin
WRS3	Tab, Peach, Oval, W-R/S3	Multivitamins	by Whitehall Robins		Vitamin
WRS3	Tab, Light Apricot, Oval, W-R/S/3	Vitamin B Complex Vitamins C & E Zinc	Stresstabs by Whitehall Robins		Vitamin
WRS4	Tab, Light Orange, Oval, WR/S/4	Vitamin B Complex Vitamins C & E	Stresstabs by Whitehall Robins		Vitamin
WRS4	Tab, Orange, Oval, W-R/S4	Multivitamins	by Whitehall Robins	Canadian	Vitamin
WRU10	Tab, Orange, Oval, WR/U/10	Multimineral Multivitamin	Centrum by Whitehall Robins		Vitamin
WRU12	Tab, Peach, Oval, W-R/U/12	Multimineral Multivitamin	Centrum by Whitehall Robins		Vitamin
WRU23	Tab, Orange, Oval, W-R/U/23	Multimineral Multivitamin	Centrum by Whitehall Robins		Vitamin
WRU7	Tab, Light Peach, Oval, W-R/U/7	18 Multimineral Multivitamin	Centrum by Whitehall Robins		Vitamin

ID FRONT <> BACK	DESCRIPTION FRONT <> BACK	INGREDIENT & STRENGTH	BRAND (or Generic Equiv.) by FIRM	NDC#	CLASS; SCH.
WRWR	Cap, Green & Yellow, WR/WR	Therapeutic B-Complex with Vitamin C	Allbee by Whitehall Robins		Vitamin
WT21	Tab, Peach, W/T/21	Pentazocine HCl 50 mg	Talwin by Sanofi	Canadian	Analgesic; C IV
WT31	Tab, White, Discoid, W/T/31	Iopanoic Acid 500 mg	Telepaque by Sanofi	Canadian	Diagnostic
WT31	Tab, Yellow, Round	Iopanoic Acid 500 mg	Telepaque by Sanofi		Diagnostic
WT4111	Tab, White, Oblong, W-T 4111	Magnesium Salicylate 500 mg	Efficin by Adria		Analgesic
WV22	Tab, Speckled Buff, Oblong	Stanozolol 2 mg	Winstrol-V Chewable by Sanofi	Discontinued	Anabolic Steroid; C III
WW	Tab, Red with Specks	Chlorpheniramine Maleate 5 mg, Phenylephrine HCl 10 mg, Phenylpropanolamine HCl 40 mg, Phenyltoloxamine Citrate 15 mg	De Con by Patient First	57575-0034	Cold Remedy
WW <> 12	Tab, White, Oblong	Ondansetron HCl 8 mg	Zofran by West-Ward	00143-2423	Antiemetic
WW <> 24	Tab, White, Cap Shaped	Ondansetron HCl 24 mg	Zofran by West-Ward	00143-2424	Antiemetic
WW <> 267	Tab, Pink, Round	Lisinopril 10 mg	Zestril by West-Ward	00143-1267	Antihypertensive
WW <> 30	Tab, Pink, Oval, Scored, Extended Release	Isosorbide Mononitrate 30 mg	Imdur by West-Ward	00143-2230	Antianginal
WW <> 484	Tab, White, Round	Primidone 250 mg	Mysoline by Blu	24658-0151	Anticonvulsant
WW <> 60	Tab, Yellow, Oval	Isosorbide Mononitrate 60 mg	Imdur by West-Ward	00143-2260	Antianginal
WW <> 771	Tab, White, Round, Scored	Isosorbide Dinitrate 10 mg	Isordil by Heartland	61392-0305	Antianginal
WW <> 771	Tab, White, Round, Scored	Isosorbide Dinitrate 10 mg	Isordil by West-Ward	00143-1771	Antianginal
WW <> 772	Tab, Green, Round, Scored	Isosorbide Dinitrate 20 mg	Isordil by Heartland	61392-0321	Antianginal
WW <> 772	Tab, Green, Round, Scored	Isosorbide Dinitrate 20 mg	Isordil by West-Ward	00143-1772	Antianginal
WW112	Tab, Orange, Round	Doxycycline Hyclate 100 mg	Vibra-Tabs by West-Ward	00143-2112	Antibiotic
WW115	Tab, White, Oblong, Scored	Acetaminophen 500 mg, Butalbital 50 mg, Caffeine 40 mg	Esgic Plus by URL Mutual	00677-1738	Analgesic
WW115	Tab, White, Oblong, Scored	Acetaminophen 500 mg, Butalbital 50 mg, Caffeine 40 mg	Esgic Plus by West-Ward	00143-1115	Analgesic
WW115	Tab, White, Oblong, Scored	Acetaminophen 500 mg, Butalbital 50 mg, Caffeine 40 mg	Esgic Plus by Ivax	00182-2694	Analgesic
				Discontinued	
WW120	Tab, White, Round, Coated	Ergotamine Tartrate 1 mg, Caffeine 100 mg	Cafergot by West-Ward	00143-2120	Antimigraine
WW125	Tab, Pink, Round, Film Coated	Chloroquine Phosphate 500 mg	Aralen Phosphate by West-Ward	00143-2125	Antimalarial
WW172	Tab, White, Round, Scored	Captopril 25 mg	Capoten by ESI Lederle	59911-5833	Antihypertensive
WW172	Tab, White, Round, Scored	Captopril 25 mg	Capoten by West-Ward	00143-1172	Antihypertensive
WW172	Tab, White, Round, Scored, WW-172	Captopril 25 mg	Capoten by Major	00904-5046	Antihypertensive
WW173	Tab, White, Oblong, Scored, WW-173	Captopril 50 mg	Capoten by Major	00904-5047	Antihypertensive
WW173	Tab, White, Oblong, Scored	Captopril 50 mg	Capoten by West-Ward	00143-1173	Antihypertensive
WW173	Tab, White, Oblong, Scored	Captopril 50 mg	Capoten by ESI Lederle	59911-5834	Antihypertensive
WW174	Tab, White, Oval, Scored	Captopril 100 mg	Capoten by ESI Lederle	59911-5835	Antihypertensive
WW174	Tab, White, Oval, Scored	Captopril 100 mg	Capoten by West-Ward	00143-1174	Antihypertensive
WW176	Tab, White, Round	Carisoprodol 350 mg	Soma by Amerisource	62584-0644	Muscle Relaxant
WW176	Tab, White, Round	Carisoprodol 350 mg	Soma by West-Ward	00143-1176	Muscle Relaxant
WW176	Tab, White, Round	Carisoprodol 350 mg	Soma by Ivax	00182-1079	Muscle Relaxant
WW25	Tab, White, Round, Scored	Prednisone 2.5 mg	Deltasone by West-Ward	00143-1425	Steroid
WW267	Tab, Pink, Round	Lisinopril 10 mg	Zestril by Blu	24658-0242	Antihypertensive
WW268	Tab, Red, Round	Lisinopril 20 mg	Zestril by West-Ward	00143-1268	Antihypertensive
WW268	Tab, Red, Round	Lisinopril 20 mg	Zestril by Blu	24658-0243	Antihypertensive
WW27	Tab, Blue, Round	Dicyclomine HCl 20 mg	Bentyl by Major	00904-0195	Gastrointestinal
WW27	Tab, Blue, Round	Dicyclomine HCl 20 mg	Bentyl by Direct Dispensing	57866-3377	Gastrointestinal
WW27	Tab, Blue, Round	Dicyclomine HCl 20 mg	Bentyl by Mova	55370-0879	Gastrointestinal
WW27	Tab, Blue, Round	Dicyclomine HCl 20 mg	Bentyl by Teva	55953-0667	Gastrointestinal
WW27	Tab, Blue, Round	Dicyclomine HCl 20 mg	Bentyl by Heartland	61392-0041	Gastrointestinal
WW27	Tab, Blue, Round	Dicyclomine HCl 20 mg	Bentyl by Kaiser	62224-9222	Gastrointestinal
WW27	Tab, Blue, Round	Dicyclomine HCl 20 mg	Bentyl by Amerisource	62584-0671	Gastrointestinal
WW27	Tab, Blue, Round	Dicyclomine HCl 20 mg	Bentyl by Moore	00839-8099	Gastrointestinal
WW27	Tab, Blue, Round	Dicyclomine HCl 20 mg	Bentyl by Qualitest	00603-3266	Gastrointestinal

ID FRONT <> BACK	DESCRIPTION FRONT <> BACK	INGREDIENT & STRENGTH	BRAND (or Generic Equiv.) by FIRM	NDC#	CLASS; SCH.
WW27	Tab, Blue, Round	Dicyclomine HCl 20 mg	Bentyl by URL Mutual	00677-0498	Gastrointestinal
WW27	Tab, Blue, Round	Dicyclomine HCl 20 mg	Bentyl by Warner Chilcott	00047-0405	Gastrointestinal
WW27	Tab, Blue, Round	Dicyclomine HCl 20 mg	Bentyl by West-Ward	00143-1227	Gastrointestinal
WW270	Tab, Gold, Round	Lisinopril 40 mg	Zestril by West-Ward	00143-1270	Antihypertensive
WW270	Tab, Golden Yellow, Round	Lisinopril 40 mg	Zestril by Blu	24658-0245	Antihypertensive
WW277	Tab, Light Brown, Scored	Lithium Carbonate 450 mg	Eskalith by West-Ward	00143-1277	Antipsychotic
WW279	Tab, Red Specks	Chlorpheniramine Maleate 5 mg, Phenylephrine HCl 10 mg, Phenylpropanolamine HCl 40 mg, Phenyltoloxamine Citrate 15 mg	by Kaiser	62224-9116	Cold Remedy
WW279	Tab	Chlorpheniramine Maleate 5 mg, Phenylephrine HCl 10 mg, Phenylpropanolamine HCl 40 mg, Phenyltoloxamine Citrate 15 mg	Uni Decon by URL Mutual	00677-0472	Cold Remedy
WW279	Tab, Pink Specks	Chlorpheniramine Maleate 5 mg, Phenylephrine HCl 10 mg, Phenylpropanolamine HCl 40 mg, Phenyltoloxamine Citrate 15 mg	Decongest by Pharmedix	53002-0306	Cold Remedy
WW279	Tab, Red Specks	Chlorpheniramine Maleate 5 mg, Phenylephrine HCl 10 mg, Phenylpropanolamine HCl 40 mg, Phenyltoloxamine Citrate 15 mg	Tri Phen Mine Sr by Ivax	00182-1094	Cold Remedy
WW279	Tab	Chlorpheniramine Maleate 5 mg, Phenylephrine HCl 10 mg, Phenylpropanolamine HCl 40 mg, Phenyltoloxamine Citrate 15 mg	by Kaiser	00179-1217	Cold Remedy
WW279	Tab	Chlorpheniramine Maleate 5 mg, Phenylephrine HCl 10 mg, Phenylpropanolamine HCl 40 mg, Phenyltoloxamine Citrate 15 mg	West-Decon by West-Ward	00143-1279	Cold Remedy
WW280	Tab, Red, Round	Lisinopril 30 mg	Zestril by Blu	24658-0244	Antihypertensive
WW33	Tab, White, Round, Scored, Film Coated	Isosorbide Mononitrate 20 mg	Ismo by West-Ward	00143-1333	Vasodilator
WW40	Tab, Yellow, Round	Digoxin 0.125 mg	Lanoxin by West-Ward	00143-1240	Cardiac Agent
WW41	Tab, White, Round, Scored	Digoxin 250 mcg	Lanoxin by UDL	51079-0848	Cardiac Agent
WW455	Tab, White, Round, WW-455	Phenobarbital 60 mg	Phenobarbital by West-Ward	00143-1455	Sedative/Hypnotic; C IV
WW455	Tab, White, Round, WW-455	Phenobarbital 60 mg	Phenobarbital by Physician Total Care	54868-3997	Sedative/Hypnotic; C IV
WW456	Tab, White, Round	Phenobarbital 90 mg	Phenobarbital by Physician Total Care	54868-3998	Sedative/Hypnotic; C IV
WW456	Tab, White, Round	Phenobarbital 90 mg	Phenobarbital by West-Ward	00143-1456	Sedative/Hypnotic; C IV
WW458	Tab, White, Round, Scored, WW-458	Phenobarbital 100 mg	Phenobarbital by West-Ward	00143-1458	Sedative/Hypnotic; C IV
WW48	Tab, Green, Film Coated, Ex Release	Phenobarbital 48.6 mg, Hyoscyamine Sulfate 0.3111 mg, Atropine Sulfate 0.0582 mg, Scopolamine Hydrobromide 0.0195 mg	Belladonna Phenobarbital by West-Ward	00143-2148	Gastrointestinal; C IV
WW53	Tab, Pink, Round	Stanozolol 2 mg	Winstrol by Sanofi	Discontinued	Anabolic Steroid; C III
WW62	Tab, Blue with White Mottling, Round	Lisinopril 10 mg, HCTZ 12.5 mg	Prinzide by West-Ward	00143-1262	Antihypertensive; Diuretic
WW63	Tab, Yellow with White Mottling, Round	Lisinopril 20 mg, HCTZ 12.5 mg	Prinzide by West-Ward	00143-1263	Antihypertensive; Diuretic
WW64	Tab, Peach, Red & White, Round	Lisinopril 20 mg, HCTZ 25 mg	Prinzide by West-Ward	00143-1264	Antihypertensive; Diuretic
WW65	Tab, White, Oblong	Lisinopril 2.5 mg	Zestril by West-Ward	00143-1265	Antihypertensive
WW65	Tab, White, Oblong	Lisinopril 2.5 mg	Zestril by Blu	24658-0240	Antihypertensive
WW66	Tab, Red, Oblong, Scored	Lisinopril 5 mg	Zestril by West-Ward	00143-1266	Antihypertensive
WW66	Tab, Red, Oblong	Lisinopril 5 mg	Zestril by Blu	24658-0241	Antihypertensive
WW763	Tab, White, Round, Scored	Trihexyphenidyl HCl 5 mg	Artane by West-Ward	00143-1763	Antiparkinson
WW763	Tab, White, Round, Scored	Trihexyphenidyl HCl 5 mg	Artane by URL Mutual	00677-1752	Antiparkinson
WW771	Tab, White, Round	Isosorbide Dinitrate 10 mg	Isordil by Ivax	00182-0514 Discontinued	Antianginal
WW772	Tab, Green, Round	Isosorbide Dinitrate 20 mg	Isordil by Ivax	00182-0868 Discontinued	Antianginal
WW927	Tab, Round, White	Ciprofloxacin 250 mg	Cipro by West-Ward		Antibiotic
WW928	Tab, White, Oblong	Ciprofloxacin HCl 500 mg	Cipro by West-Ward		Antibiotic
WXG <> GS	Tab, Light Brown, Cap Shaped, Film Coated	Ropinirole HCl 4 mg	Requip XL by GSK	00007-4887	Antiparkinson
WXL150	Tab, Off White to Light Yellow, Round, Purple Ink, Extended-Release	Bupropion HCl 150 mg	Wellbutrin XL by Biovail	Canadian DIN 02275090	Antidepressant
WXL300	Tab, Off White to Light Yellow, Round, Gray Ink, Extended-Release	Bupropion HCl 300 mg	Wellbutrin XL by Biovail	Canadian DIN 02275104	Antidepressant

ID FRONT <> BACK	DESCRIPTION FRONT <> BACK	INGREDIENT & STRENGTH	BRAND (or Generic Equiv.) by FIRM	NDC#	CLASS; SCH.
WYETH	Tab, Yellow, Round, Scored	Lorazepam 2 mg	Ativan by Wyeth		Antianxiety; C IV
WYETH	Tab, White, Round, Scored	Lorazepam 1 mg	Ativan by Wyeth		Antianxiety; C IV
WYETH <> 10	Tab, White, Round	Isosorbide Dinitrate 10 mg	Isordil by Wyeth	00008-4161	Antianginal
WYETH <> 19	Tab, Orange, Round, Scored	Promethazine 12.5 mg	Phenergan by Wyeth	00008-0019	Antiemetic; Antihistamine
WYETH <> 227	Tab, Pink, Scored	Promethazine HCl 50 mg	Phenergan by Wyeth	52903-0227	Antiemetic; Antihistamine
WYETH <> 227	Tab, Pink, Round	Promethazine HCl 50 mg	Phenergan by Wyeth	00008-0227	Antiemetic; Antihistamine
WYETH <> 390	Tab, White, Round, Scored	Penicillin V Potassium 500 mg	Pen Vee K by Casa DeAmigos	62138-0390	Antibiotic
WYETH <> 390	Tab, White, Round, Scored	Penicillin V Potassium 500 mg	Pen Vee K by Wyeth	00008-0390	Antibiotic
WYETH <> 4125	Tab, Light Green, Ex Release	Isosorbide Dinitrate 40 mg	Isordil by Wyeth	00008-4125	Antianginal
WYETH <> 56	Tab, White, Round	Ethinyl Estradiol 0.05 mg, Norgestrel 0.5 mg	Ovral by PDRX	55289-0245	Oral Contraceptive
WYETH <> 56	Tab, White, Round	Ethinyl Estradiol 0.05 mg, Norgestrel 0.5 mg	Ovral by Wyeth	00008-0056	Oral Contraceptive
WYETH <> 59	Tab, White, Round, Scored	Penicillin V Potassium	by Med Pro	53978-5042	Antibiotic
WYETH <> 59	Tab, White, Round, Scored	Penicillin V Potassium	by Kaiser	00179-0081	Antibiotic
WYETH <> 59	Tab, White, Round, Scored	Penicillin V Potassium	by Wyeth	00008-0059	Antibiotic
WYETH <> 62	Tab, Yellow, Round	Norgestrel 0.075 mg	Ovrette by Wyeth	00008-0062	Oral Contraceptive
WYETH <> 78	Tab, White, Round	Ethinyl Estradiol 0.03 mg, Norgestrel 0.3 mg	Lo Ovral by PDRX	55289-0246	Oral Contraceptive
WYETH <> 78	Tab, White, Round	Ethinyl Estradiol 0.03 mg, Norgestrel 0.3 mg	Lo Ovral by Dept Health	53808-0028	Oral Contraceptive
WYETH <> 85	Tab, Coated	Acetaminophen 650 mg, Propoxyphene HCl 65 mg	Wygesic by Wyeth	00008-0085	Analgesic; C IV
WYETH1	Tab, White, Round	Meprobamate 400 mg	Equanil by Wyeth	00008-0001	Sedative/Hypnotic; C IV
WYETH2	Tab, White, Pentagonal	Meprobamate 200 mg	Equanil by Wyeth	00008-0002	Sedative/Hypnotic; C IV
WYETH200	Tab, Pink, Round	Promazine 100 mg	Sparine by Wyeth	00008-0200	Antipsychotic
WYETH261	Cap, Maroon, Blue Print, Opaque	Meperidine 50 mg, Promethazine 25 mg	Mepergan Fortis by Wyeth	00008-0261	Analgesic; C II
WYETH261	Cap, Red	Meperidine HCl 50 mg, Promethazine HCl 25 mg	Meprozine by Ayerst	00046-0261	Analgesic; C II
WYETH27	Tab, White, Round, Scored, Wyeth over 27	Promethazine HCl 25 mg	Phenergan by Wyeth	00008-0027	Antiemetic; Antihistamine
WYETH28	Tab, Red, Round	Promazine 50 mg	Sparine by Wyeth	00008-0028	Antipsychotic
WYETH29	Tab, Yellow, Round	Promazine 25 mg	Sparine by Wyeth	00008-0029	Antipsychotic
WYETH309	Cap, Pink & Purple	Ampicillin 500 mg	Principen by Wyeth		Antibiotic
WYETH33	Tab, Yellow, Round	Meprobamate 400 mg	Equanil by Wyeth	00008-0033	Sedative/Hypnotic; C IV
WYETH360	Cap, Purple & White	Dicloxacillin Sodium 250 mg	Pathocil by Wyeth		Antibiotic
WYETH389	Cap, Yellow & Blue	Tetracycline HCl 250 mg	Achromycin V by Wyeth		Antibiotic
WYETH4130	Tab, Orange, Black Print, Round, Sugar Coated	Ethionamide 250 mg	Trecator SC by Wyeth	00008-4130	Antituberculosis
WYETH4132	Cap, Blue & Yellow, Black Print	Trimipramine Maleate 25 mg	Surmontil by Wyeth	00008-4132	Antidepressant
WYETH4133	Cap, Blue & Red, Black Print	Trimipramine Maleate 50 mg	Surmontil by Wyeth	00008-4133	Antidepressant
WYETH4140	Cap, Blue & Clear	Isosorbide Dinitrate SA 40 mg	Isordil by Wyeth	00008-4140	Antianginal
WYETH4152	Tab, Pink, Round, Scored, Wyeth over 4152	Isosorbide Dinitrate 5 mg	Isordil by Wyeth	52903-4152	Antianginal
WYETH4152	Tab, Pink, Round, Scored, Wyeth over 4152	Isosorbide Dinitrate 5 mg	Isordil by Biovail	00008-4152	Antianginal
WYETH4153	Tab, White, Round, Scored, Wyeth over 4153	Isosorbide Dinitrate 10 mg	Isordil by Wyeth	00008-4153	Antianginal
WYETH4153	Tab, White, Round, Scored, Wyeth over 4153	Isosorbide Dinitrate 10 mg	Isordil by Rx Pak	65084-0214	Antianginal
WYETH4153	Tab, White, Round, Scored, Wyeth over 4153	Isosorbide Dinitrate 10 mg	Isordil by Amerisource	62584-0061	Antianginal
WYETH4153	Tab, White, Round, Scored, Wyeth over 4153	Isosorbide Dinitrate 10 mg	Isordil by Thrift Drug	59198-0283	Antianginal
WYETH4154	Tab, Green, Round, Scored, Wyeth over 4154	Isosorbide Dinitrate 20 mg	Isordil by Thrift Drug	59198-0146	Antianginal
WYETH4154	Tab, Green, Round, Scored, Wyeth over 4154	Isosorbide Dinitrate 20 mg	Isordil by Wyeth	00008-4154	Antianginal
WYETH4158	Cap, Blue & Yellow	Trimipramine Maleate 100 mg	Surmontil by Wyeth		Antidepressant
WYETH4159	Tab, Powder Blue, Round, Scored, Wyeth over 4159	Isosorbide Dinitrate 30 mg	Isordil by Wyeth	00008-4159	Antianginal
WYETH4177SECTRAL-200	Cap, Orange & Purple, Black Print, Opaque, WYETH over 4177, SECTRAL over L200	Acebutolol HCl 200 mg	Sectral by Wyeth	52903-4177	Antihypertensive
WYETH4177SECTRAL-200	Cap, Orange & Purple, Black Print, Opaque, WYETH over 4177, SECTRAL over L200	Acebutolol HCl 200 mg	Sectral by Wyeth	00008-4177	Antihypertensive

ID FRONT <> BACK	DESCRIPTION FRONT <> BACK	INGREDIENT & STRENGTH	BRAND (or Generic Equiv.) by FIRM	NDC#	CLASS; SCH.
WYETH4179SECTRAL-400	Cap, Brown & Orange, Black Print, Opaque, WYETH over 4179, SECTRAL over L400	Acebutolol HCl 400 mg	Sectral by Watson	52903-4179	Antihypertensive
WYETH4179SECTRAL-400	Cap, Brown & Orange, Black Print, Opaque, WYETH over 4179, SECTRAL over L400	Acebutolol HCl 400 mg	Sectral by Abbott	60692-3871	Antihypertensive
WYETH4181ORUDIS50	Cap, Dark Green & Light Green, Opaque	Ketoprofen 50 mg	Orudis by Wyeth	00008-4181	NSAID
WYETH4186ORUDIS-25MG	Cap, Green & Red, Opaque	Ketoprofen 25 mg	Orudis by Wyeth	00008-4186	NSAID
WYETH4187ORUDIS75	Cap, Dark Green & White, Opaque	Ketoprofen 75 mg	Orudis by Pharmedix	53002-0531	NSAID
WYETH4187ORUDIS75	Cap, Dark Green & White, Opaque	Ketoprofen 75 mg	Orudis by Nat Pharmpak	55154-4201	NSAID
WYETH4187ORUDIS75	Cap, Dark Green & White, Opaque	Ketoprofen 75 mg	Orudis by Thrift Drug	59198-0087	NSAID
WYETH4187ORUDIS75	Cap, Dark Green & White, Opaque	Ketoprofen 75 mg	Orudis by Amerisource	62584-0187	NSAID
WYETH4187ORUDIS75	Cap, Dark Green & White, Opaque	Ketoprofen 75 mg	Orudis by Wyeth	00008-4187	NSAID
WYETH4188 <> 200	Tab, Pink, Round, Scored, Wyeth over 4188 <> 200 inside C	Amiodarone 200 mg	Cordarone by Wyeth	00008-4188	Antiarrhythmic
WYETH4188 <> C200	Tab, Pink, Round, Scored, Wyeth over 4188 <> 200 inside C	Amiodarone 200 mg	Cordarone by Wyeth	Canadian	Antiarrhythmic
WYETH4188 <> C200	Tab, Pink, Round, Scored, Wyeth over 4188 <> 200 inside C	Amiodarone 200 mg	Cordarone by Amerisource	62584-0345	Antiarrhythmic
WYETH4188 <> C200	Tab, Pink, Round, Scored, Wyeth over 4188 <> 200 inside C	Amiodarone 200 mg	Cordarone by Wyeth	00008-4188	Antiarrhythmic
WYETH4188 <> C200	Tab, Pink, Round, Scored, Wyeth over 4188 <> 200 inside C	Amiodarone 200 mg	Cordarone by Caremark	00339-6082	Antiarrhythmic
WYETH4188 <> C200	Tab, Pink, Round, Scored, Wyeth over 4188 <> 200 inside C	Amiodarone 200 mg	Cordarone by Med Pro	53978-2092	Antiarrhythmic
WYETH4188 <> C200	Tab, Pink, Round, Scored, Wyeth over 4188 <> 200 inside C	Amiodarone 200 mg	Cordarone by Nat Pharmpak	55154-4202	Antiarrhythmic
WYETH4191	Cap	Aspirin 356.4 mg, Caffeine 30 mg, Dihydrocodeine Bitartrate 16 mg	Synalgos DC by Wyeth	00008-4191	Analgesic; C III
WYETH4191	Cap	Aspirin 356.4 mg, Caffeine 30 mg, Dihydrocodeine Bitartrate 16 mg	Synalgos DC by Pharmedix	53002-0118	Analgesic; C III
WYETH4192	Tab, Green, Round, Scored, Wyeth over 4192	Isosorbide Dinitrate 40 mg	Isordil by Wyeth	00008-4192	Antianginal
WYETH434	Tab, Orange & White, Round	Promethazine 6.25 mg, Pseudoephedrine 60 mg	Phenergan D by Wyeth		Cold Remedy
WYETH445	Tab, Pink, Round	Inert	Ovral 28 by Wyeth	00008-0445	Oral Contraceptive; Placebo
WYETH464	Tab, White, Oblong	Nafcillin Sodium 500 mg	Unipen by Wyeth		Antibiotic
WYETH471	Cap, Yellow & Blue	Tetracycline HCl 500 mg	Achromycin V by Wyeth		Antibiotic
WYETH486	Tab, Pink, Round	Inert	Lo/Ovral 28 by Wyeth	00008-0486	Oral Contraceptive; Placebo
WYETH51SERAX10	Cap, Pink & White, Wyeth-51 x3 w/ 10 connected Triangles <> Serax 10 x5	Oxazepam 10 mg	Serax by Wyeth	00008-0051	Sedative/Hypnotic; C IV
WYETH53	Cap, Pink & Purple	Ampicillin 250 mg	Principen by Wyeth		Antibiotic
WYETH56	Tab	Ethinyl Estradiol 0.05 mg, Norgestrel 0.5 mg	Ovral by Apotheca	12634-0480	Oral Contraceptive
WYETH560	Cap, Gray & Green	Amoxicillin 500 mg	Amoxil by Wyeth		Antibiotic
WYETH57	Cap, Green & Yellow	Nafcillin Sodium 250 mg	Unipen by Wyeth		Antibiotic
WYETH576	Tab, Pink, Round	Erythromycin Ethylsuccinate 250 mg	Wyamycin S by Wyeth		Antibiotic
WYETH578	Tab, Pink, Oval	Erythromycin Ethylsuccinate 500 mg	Wyamycin S by Wyeth		Antibiotic
WYETH593	Cap, Purple & White	Dicloxacillin Sodium 500 mg	Pathocil by Wyeth		Antibiotic
WYETH614	Tab, Yellow, Oblong	Cyclacillin 250 mg	Cyclapen-W by Wyeth		Antibiotic
WYETH615	Tab, Yellow, Oblong	Cyclacillin 500 mg	Cyclapen-W by Wyeth		Antibiotic
WYETH64 <> A	Tab, White, Shield Shaped, Scored	Lorazepam 1 mg	Ativan by Med Pro	53978-3086	Antianxiety; C IV
WYETH64 <> A	Tab, White, Shield Shaped, Scored	Lorazepam 1 mg	Ativan by Physician Total Care	54868-1339	Antianxiety; C IV
WYETH64 <> A	Tab, White, Shield Shaped, Scored	Lorazepam 1 mg	Ativan by Wyeth	00008-0064	Antianxiety; C IV
WYETH64 <> A	Tab, White, Shield Shaped, Scored	Lorazepam 1 mg	Ativan by Nat Pharmpak	55154-4204	Antianxiety; C IV
WYETH641	Tab, Brown, Round	Levonorgestrel 0.05 mg, Ethinyl Estradiol 0.03 mg	Triphasil by Wyeth		Oral Contraceptive
WYETH642	Tab, White, Round	Levonorgestrel 0.075 mg, Ethinyl Estradiol 0.04 mg	Triphasil by Wyeth		Oral Contraceptive
WYETH643	Tab, Yellow, Round	Levonorgestrel 0.125 mg, Ethinyl Estradiol 0.03 mg	Triphasil by Wyeth		Oral Contraceptive

ID FRONT <> BACK	DESCRIPTION FRONT <> BACK	INGREDIENT & STRENGTH	BRAND (or Generic Equiv.) by FIRM	NDC#	CLASS; SCH.
WYETH65 <> A2	Tab, White, Pentagonal	Lorazepam 2 mg	Ativan by Wyeth	00008-0065	Antianxiety; C IV
WYETH650	Tab, Blue, Round	Inert	Triphasil 28 by Wyeth		Oral Contraceptive; Placebo
WYETH6SERAX15	Cap, Red & White, Wyeth-6 x3 w/ 10 Connected Triangles	Oxazepam 15 mg	Serax by Wyeth	00008-0006	Sedative/Hypnotic; C IV
WYETH71	Tab, White, Round	Mazindol 1 mg	Mazanor by Wyeth		Anorexiant; C IV
WYETH73 <> W4	Tab, Coated	Guanabenz Acetate 4 mg	Wytensin by Wyeth	00008-0073	Antihypertensive
WYETH75	Tab, Light Orange, Round	Levonorgestrel 0.15 mg, Ethinyl Estradiol 0.03 mg	Nordette by Wyeth	00008-2533	Oral Contraceptive
WYETH78	Tab, White, Round	Ethinyl Estradiol 0.03 mg, Ferrous Fumarate 75 mg, Norgestrel 0.3 mg	Lo/Ovral by Wyeth	52903-2542	Oral Contraceptive
WYETH78	Tab, White, Round	Ethinyl Estradiol 0.03 mg, Norgestrel 0.3 mg	by Physician Total Care	54868-0428	Oral Contraceptive
WYETH78	Tab, White, Round	Ethinyl Estradiol 0.03 mg, Norgestrel 0.3 mg	Lo/Ovral by Wyeth	00008-0078	Oral Contraceptive
WYETH78 <> WYETH486	Tab	Ethinyl Estradiol 0.03 mg, Norgestrel 0.3 mg	Lo Ovral 28 by Pharm Util	60491-0367	Oral Contraceptive
WYETH81 <> A	Tab, White, Pentagonal	Lorazepam 0.5 mg	Ativan by Wyeth	00008-0081	Antianxiety; C IV
WYETH81 <> A	Tab, White, Pentagonal	Lorazepam 0.5 mg	Ativan by Med Pro	53978-3085	Antianxiety; C IV
WYETH91	Tab, Pink/Yellow, Round	Aspirin 325 mg, Meprobamate 200 mg	Equagesic by Wyeth		Sedative/Hypnotic; C IV
X	Tab, Brown, Round	Sennosides 17 mg	Senokot XTRA by Purdue	00034-1201	Gastrointestinal
X	Tab, White, Round, Sublingual, Roman Numeral X	Zolpidem 10 mg	Edluar by Orexo AB	42447-0122	Sedative/Hypnotic; C IV
X	Tab, White, Round, X with Curly Edges	3,4-Methylenedioxymethamphetamine (MDMA)	Ecstasy by Illegal		Euphoric; Illicit
X	Tab, Pink, Triangular	3,4-Methylenedioxymethamphetamine (MDMA)	Ecstasy by Illegal		Euphoric; Illicit
X <> 05	Tab, White, Pentagonal, Ex Release, 0.5 <> X	Alprazolam 0.5 mg	Xanax XR by Pharmacia	00009-0057	Antianxiety; C IV
X <> 05	Tab, White, Pentagonal, Ex Release, X <> 0.5	Alprazolam 0.5 mg	Xanax by Pharmacia	00009-5252	Antianxiety; C IV
X <> 1	Tab, Yellow, Square, Ex Release	Alprazolam 1 mg	Xanax by Pharmacia	00009-5255	Antianxiety; C IV
X <> 1	Tab, Yellow, Square, Ex Release	Alprazolam 1 mg	Xanax XR by Pharmacia	00009-0059	Antianxiety; C IV
X <> 2	Tab, Blue, Round, Ex Release	Alprazolam 2 mg	Xanax XR by Pharmacia	00009-0066	Antianxiety; C IV
X <> 2	Tab, Blue, Round, Ex Release	Alprazolam 2 mg	Xanax by Pharmacia	00009-5257	Antianxiety; C IV
X <> 3	Tab, Green, Triangular, Ex Release	Alprazolam 3 mg	Xanax by Pharmacia		Antianxiety; C IV
X <> 3	Tab, Green, Triangular, Ex Release	Alprazolam 3 mg	Xanax XR by Pharmacia	00009-0068	Antianxiety; C IV
X <> 35	Tab, White, Round, Scored	Phendimetrazine Tartrate 35 mg	Bontril by Mikart	46672-0174	Anorexiant; C III
X <> 35	Tab, White, Round	Phendimetrazine Tartrate 35 mg	by Allscripts		Anorexiant; C III
X <> 7301	Tab, Hourglass Logo, Film Coated	Verapamil HCl 180 mg	Verelan by Heartland	61392-0345	Antihypertensive
X01 <> LU	Tab, Blue, Oblong, Film Coated, Scored	Levetiracetam 250 mg	Keppra by Lupin	68180-0112	Anticonvulsant
X02 <> LU	Tab, Yellow, Oblong, Scored, Film Coated	Levetiracetam 500 mg	Keppra by Lupin	68180-0113	Anticonvulsant
X03 <> LU	Tab, Orange, Oblong, Scored, Film Coated	Levetiracetam 750 mg	Keppra by Lupin	68180-0114	Anticonvulsant
X04 <> LU	Tab, White, Oblong, Scored, Film Coated	Levetiracetam 1 g	Keppra by Lupin	68180-0115	Anticonvulsant
X10	Tab, White and Yellow, Round, Layered	Alfuzosin HCl 10 mg	Uroxatral by Sanofi	00024-4200	Antihypertensive
X592	Cap, Pale Yellow, Black Ink	Diclofenac Potassium 25 mg	Zipsor by Xanodyne	66479-0592	NSAID
X7300	Tab, Ivory, Oblong	Verapamil HCl ER 240 mg	Isoptin, Calan SR by Baker		Antihypertensive
X732 <> DQ	Tab, Green, Scored	Pseudoacline 10 mg	Sudaamox by TRC Chem	99598-9999	Anti-Congestion
X92	Tab, White to Off-White, Oval, Scored, Film Coated	Gabapentin 600 mg	Neurontin by Ranbaxy	63304-0592	Anticonvulsant
X93	Tab, White to Off-White, Oval, Scored, Film Coated	Gabapentin 800 mg	Neurontin by Ranbaxy	63304-0593	Anticonvulsant
XANAX <> 2	Tab, white, Triscored (3 scores)	Alprazolam 2 mg	Xanax TS by Pfizer	Canadian DIN 00813958	Antianxiety
XANAX <> 2	Tab, White, Cap Shaped, Film Coated, Scored	Alprazolam 2 mg	Xanax by Pharmacia	Canadian	Antianxiety; C IV
XANAX <> 2	Tab, White, Cap Shaped, Film Coated, Scored	Alprazolam 2 mg	Xanax by Pharmacia	00009-0094	Antianxiety; C IV
XANAX025	Tab, White, Oval, Scored, Xanax 0.25	Alprazolam 0.25 mg	Xanax by Pharmacia	00009-0029	Antianxiety; C IV
XANAX025	Tab, White, Oval, Scored, Xanax 0.25	Alprazolam 0.25 mg	Xanax by Med Pro	53978-1300	Antianxiety; C IV
XANAX025	Tab, White, Oval, Scored, Xanax 0.25	Alprazolam 0.25 mg	Xanax by Nat Pharmpak	55154-3921	Antianxiety; C IV
XANAX025	Tab, White, Oval, Scored, Xanax 0.25	Alprazolam 0.25 mg	Xanax by Nat Pharmpak	55154-3921	Antianxiety; C IV
XANAX025	Tab, White, Oval, Scored, Xanax 0.25	Alprazolam 0.25 mg	Xanax by Med Pro	53978-3091	Antianxiety; C IV

ID FRONT <> BACK	DESCRIPTION FRONT <> BACK	INGREDIENT & STRENGTH	BRAND (or Generic Equiv.) by FIRM	NDC#	CLASS; SCH.
XANAX025	Tab, White, Oval, Scored, Xanax 0.25	Alprazolam 0.25 mg	Xanax by Amerisource	62584-0035	Antianxiety; C IV
XANAX05	Tab, Peach, Oval, Scored, Xanax 0.5	Alprazolam 0.5 mg	Xanax by Amerisource	62584-0036	Antianxiety; C IV
XANAX05	Tab, Peach, Oval, Scored, Xanax 0.5	Alprazolam 0.5 mg	Xanax by Caremark	00339-4041	Antianxiety; C IV
XANAX05	Tab, Peach, Oval, Scored, Xanax 0.5	Alprazolam 0.5 mg	Xanax by Pharmacia	00009-0055	Antianxiety; C IV
XANAX05	Tab, Peach, Oval, Scored, Xanax 0.5	Alprazolam 0.5 mg	Xanax by Allscripts		Antianxiety; C IV
XANAX05	Tab, Peach, Oval, Scored, Xanax 0.5	Alprazolam 0.5 mg	Xanax by Nat Pharmpak	55154-3919	Antianxiety; C IV
XANAX05	Tab, Peach, Oval, Scored, Xanax 0.5	Alprazolam 0.5 mg	Xanax by Pharmedix	53002-0395	Antianxiety; C IV
XANAX05	Tab, Peach, Oval, Scored, Xanax 0.5	Alprazolam 0.5 mg	Xanax by Med Pro	53978-3090	Antianxiety; C IV
XANAX10	Tab, Lavender, Oval, Scored, Xanax 1.0	Alprazolam 1 mg	Xanax by Amerisource	62584-0037	Antianxiety; C IV
XANAX10	Tab, Lavender, Oval, Scored, Xanax 1.0	Alprazolam 1 mg	Xanax by Pharmacia	00009-0090	Antianxiety; C IV
XANAX10	Tab, Lavender, Oval, Scored, Xanax 1.0	Alprazolam 1 mg	Xanax by Nat Pharmpak	55154-3920	Antianxiety; C IV
XANAX10	Tab, Lavender, Oval, Scored, Xanax 1.0	Alprazolam 1 mg	Xanax by Med Pro	53978-3089	Antianxiety; C IV
XANAX10	Tab, Lavender, Oval, Scored, Xanax 1.0	Alprazolam 1 mg	Xanax by Allscripts		Antianxiety; C IV
XELODA <> 150	Tab, Light Peach, Oblong, Film Coated	Capecitabine 150 mg	Xeloda by Roche	Canadian DIN 02238453	Antineoplastic
XELODA <> 150	Tab, Light Peach, Oblong, Film Coated	Capecitabine 150 mg	Xeloda by Hoffmann La Roche	00004-1101	Antineoplastic
XELODA <> 500	Tab, Peach, Oblong, Film Coated	Capecitabine 500 mg	Xeloda by Hoffmann La Roche	00004-1100	Antineoplastic
XELODA <> 500	Tab, Peach, Oblong, Film Coated	Capecitabine 500 mg	Xeloda by Roche	Canadian DIN 02238454	Antineoplastic
XENICAL120ROCHE	Cap, Dark Blue, Light Blue Print, Hard Gel	Orlistat 120 mg	Xenical by Hoffmann La Roche	00004-0256	Lipase Inhibitor
XENICAL120ROCHE	Cap, Dark Blue, Light Blue Print, Hard Gel	Orlistat 120 mg	Xenical by Southwood	58016-0361	Lipase Inhibitor
XENICAL120ROCHE	Cap, Dark Blue, Light Blue Print, Hard Gel	Orlistat 120 mg	Xenical by Pegasus	55246-0020	Lipase Inhibitor
XENICAL120ROCHE	Cap, Dark Blue, Light Blue Print, Hard Gel	Orlistat 120 mg	Xenical by PDRX	55289-0512	Lipase Inhibitor
XL	Tab, Yellowish-White, Speckled, Round, Scored	Caffeine 100 mg, Ergotamine Tartrate 1 mg	Cafergot by Novartis	Canadian DIN 00176095	Antimigraine
XM	Tab, White, Round	Methimazole 10 mg	Methimazole by URL Mutual	00677-1946	Antithyroid
XP650	Tab, White, Oval	Tranexamic Acid 650 mg	Lysteda by Xanodyne	66479-0650	Antifibrinolytic
XR150	Tab, White, Capsule Shaped	Quetiapine Fumarate 150 mg	Seroquel XR by AstraZeneca	Canadian DIN 02321513	Antipsychotic
XR150	Tab, White, Cap Shaped, Extended Release	Quetiapine Fumarate 150 mg	Seroquel XR by AstraZeneca	00310-0281	Antipsychotic
XR200	Tab, Yellow, Cap Shaped, Extended Release	Quetiapine Fumarate 200 mg	Seroquel XR by AstraZeneca	00310-0282	Antipsychotic
XR200	Tab, Yellow, Cap Shaped, Extended Release	Quetiapine Fumarate 200 mg	Seroquel XR by AstraZeneca	Canadian DIN 02300192	Antipsychotic
XR300	Tab, Pale Yellow, Cap Shaped, Extended Release	Quetiapine Fumarate 300 mg	Seroquel XR by AstraZeneca	00310-0283	Antipsychotic
XR300	Tab, Pale Yellow, Capsule Shaped	Quetiapine Fumarate 300 mg	Seroquel XR by AstraZeneca	Canadian DIN 02300206	Antipsychotic
XR400	Tab, White, Capsule Shaped	Quetiapine Fumarate 400 mg	Seroquel XR by AstraZeneca	Canadian DIN 02300214	Antipsychotic
XR400	Tab, White, Cap Shaped, Film Coated, Extended Release	Quetiapine Fumarate 400 mg	Seroquel XR by AstraZeneca	00310-0284	Antipsychotic
XR50	Tab, Peach, Cap Shaped, Extended Release	Quetiapine Fumarate 50 mg	Seroquel XR by AstraZeneca	00310-0280	Antipsychotic
XR50	Tab, Peach, Cap Shaped, Extended Release	Quetiapine Fumarate 50 mg	Seroquel XR by AstraZeneca	Canadian DIN 02300184	Antipsychotic
XR500 <> APO	Tab, White, Cap Shaped, Extended Release	Metformin HCl 500 mg	Glucophage XR by Apotex	60505-0260	Antidiabetic
Y	Tab, White, Oval, Film Coated, Scored, Y / Y	Levocetirizine 5 mg	Xyzal by UCB	00024-5800	Antihistamine
Y	Tab, Pink, Round	Yohimbine HCl 2 mg	by Pharmascience	Canadian	Impotence Agent
YELLOW780	Tab	Isosorbide Dinitrate 10 mg	Isordil by Pharmedix	53002-1047	Antianginal
YJ2243850	Cap, Yellow with Black Stripes	Caffeine 300 mg, Green Tea Extract, Yerba Mate, Guarana, Capsicum, Kola Nut, Siberian Ginseng	Yellow Jacket by NVE		Supplement
YJ244385	Cap, Black & Yellow, with 3 Black Stripes	Ephedra Extract 300 mg, Colanut, Ginseng	by NVE	Discontinued	Supplement
YOCON53	Tab, White, Round, Scored, YOCON over 53	Yohimbine HCl 5.4 mg	by Nat Pharmpak	55154-6001	Impotence Agent

ID FRONT <> BACK	DESCRIPTION FRONT <> BACK	INGREDIENT & STRENGTH	BRAND (or Generic Equiv.) by FIRM	NDC#	CLASS; SCH.
YOCON53	Tab, White, Round, Scored, YOCON over 53	Yohimbine HCl 5.4 mg	by Thrift Drug	59198-0116	Impotence Agent
YOCON53	Tab, White, Round, Scored, YOCON over 53	Yohimbine HCl 5.4 mg	Yocon by Glenwood LLC	00516-0001	Impotence Agent
YODOXIN92	Tab, Greenish-Yellow, Round	Iodoquinol 210 mg	Yodoxin by Glenwood LLC	00516-0092	Antiprotozoal
YODOXIN93	Tab, Greenish-Yellow, Round	Iodoquinol 650 mg	Yodoxin by Glenwood LLC	00516-0093	Antiprotozoal
YSP173	Tab, White, Round, Film Coated	Zolpidem Tartrate 10 mg	Ambien by Actavis	00228-2889	Sedative/Hypnotic; C IV
YSP174	Tab, White, Round, Film Coated	Zolpidem Tartrate 5 mg	Ambien by Actavis	00228-2888	Sedative/Hypnotic; C IV
YUTOPAR	Tab, Yellow, Round	Ritodrine HCl 10 mg	by BMS	Canadian	Urinary Relaxant
Z	Tab, White, Round, Orally Disintegrating	Zolmitriptan 2.5 mg	Zomig by AstraZeneca	Canadian DIN 02243045	Antimigraine
Z		Zolmitriptan 2.5 mg	Zomig by AstraZeneca	Canadian DIN 02238660	Antimigraine
Z	Tab, White, Round	Zolmitriptan 2.5 mg	Zomig by AstraZeneca	00310-0209	Antimigraine
Z	Cap, Light Yellow, Round, Soft Gel	Benzonatate 100 mg	Tessalon by Zydus	68382-0247	Antitussive
Z	Cap, Light Yellow, Soft Gelatin	Benzonatate 100 mg	Tessalon by Mallinckrodt	00406-2247	Antitussive
Z <> 1	Tab, White to Off-White, Round, Film Coated	Carvedilol 3.125 mg	Coreg by Zydus	68382-0092	Antihypertensive
Z <> 100M	Tab, Yellow, Round, Scored	Levothyroxine Sodium 100 mcg	Levo-T by Zoetica	64909-0109	Thyroid Hormone
Z <> 112M	Tab, Pink, Round, Scored	Levothyroxine Sodium 112 mcg	Levo-T by Zoetica	64909-0116	Thyroid Hormone
Z <> 125M	Tab, Brown, Round, Scored	Levothyroxine Sodium 125 mcg	Levo-T by Zoetica	64909-0110	Thyroid Hormone
Z <> 150	Tab, Rust Colored, Five-Sided	Ranitidine 150 mg	Zantac OTC by Pfizer		Gastrointestinal
Z <> 150M	Tab, Blue, Round, Scored	Levothyroxine Sodium 150 mcg	Levo-T by Zoetica	64909-0117	Thyroid Hormone
Z <> 175M	Tab, Purple, Round, Scored	Levothyroxine Sodium 175 mcg	Levo-T by Zoetica	64909-0111	Thyroid Hormone
Z <> 200M	Tab, Pink, Round, Scored	Levothyroxine Sodium 200 mcg	Levo-T by Zoetica	64909-0119	Thyroid Hormone
Z <> 25M	Tab, Orange, Round, Scored	Levothyroxine Sodium 25 mcg	Levo-T by Zoetica	64909-0106	Thyroid Hormone
Z <> 300M	Tab, Green, Round, Scored	Levothyroxine Sodium 300 mcg	Levo-T by Zoetica	64909-0112	Thyroid Hormone
Z <> 4	Tab, Dark Yellow, Round, Film Coated	Risperidone .25 mg	Risperdal by Zydus	68382-0112	Antipsychotic
Z <> 4107	Tab, White, Round, Uncoated	Naproxen 250 mg	by Novartis	61615-0017	NSAID
Z <> 4226	Tab, Peach, Round	Guanabenz Acetate 4 mg	Wytensin by Ivax	00172-4226	Antihypertensive
Z <> 4227	Tab, Gray, Round	Guanabenz Acetate 8 mg	Wytensin by Ivax	00172-4227	Antihypertensive
Z <> 4259	Tab, White, Round	Indapamide 2.5 mg	Lozol by Qualitest	00603-4061	Diuretic
Z <> 4259	Tab, White, Round	Indapamide 2.5 mg	Lozol by Major	00904-5074	Diuretic
Z <> 4259	Tab, White, Round	Indapamide 2.5 mg	Lozol by Ivax	00172-4259	Diuretic
Z <> 4259		Indapamide 2.5 mg	Lozol by Physician Total Care	54868-3106	Diuretic
Z <> 4259	Tab, White, Round	Indapamide 2.5 mg	Lozol by Ivax	00182-2610	Diuretic
Z <> 4259	Tab, White, Round	Indapamide 2.5 mg	Lozol by Sandoz	Discontinued	Diuretic
Z <> 4259	Tab, White, Round	Indapamide 2.5 mg	Lozol by Qualitest	00781-1051	Diuretic
Z <> 50M	Tab, White, Round, Scored	Levothyroxine Sodium 50 mcg	Levo-T by Zoetica	00603-4161	Diuretic
Z <> 6	Tab, Red, Round, Film Coated	Risperidone 0.5 mg	Risperdal by Zydus	64909-0114	Thyroid Hormone
Z <> 65	Tab, White to Off-White, Round	Atenolol 25 mg	Tenormin by Zydus	68382-0113	Antipsychotic
Z <> 65	Tab, White to Off-White, Round	Atenolol 25 mg	Tenormin by Mallinckrodt	00406-2022	Antihypertensive
Z <> 69	Tab, White to Off-White, Oval, Film-Coated	Metformin HCl 850 mg	Glucophage by Zydus	68382-0029	Antidiabetic
Z <> 69	Tab, White to Off-White, Oval, Film-Coated	Metformin HCl 850 mg	Glucophage by Mallinckrodt	00406-2029	Antidiabetic
Z <> 7	Tab, White to Off-White, Round	Amlodipine Besylate 2.5 mg	Norvasc by Zydus	68382-0121	Antihypertensive
Z <> 70	Tab, White to Off-White, Round, Film-Coated	Metformin HCl 500 mg	Glucophage by Mallinckrodt	00406-2028	Antidiabetic
Z <> 70	Tab, White to Off-White, Round, Film-Coated	Metformin HCl 500 mg	Glucophage by Zydus	68382-0028	Antidiabetic
Z <> 75	Tab, Salmon, Pentagonal	Ranitidine HCl 75 mg	Zantac by Pfizer		Gastrointestinal
Z <> 75M	Tab, Purple, Round, Scored	Levothyroxine Sodium 75 mcg	Synthroid by Zoetica	64909-0107	Thyroid Hormone
Z <> 88M	Tab, Green, Round, Scored	Levothyroxine Sodium 88 mcg	Synthroid by Zoetica	64909-0115	Thyroid Hormone
Z <> M0315	Tab, White, Oval, Scored	Glyburide 1.5 mg	Glycron by Mova	55370-0592	Antidiabetic

ID FRONT <> BACK	DESCRIPTION FRONT <> BACK	INGREDIENT & STRENGTH	BRAND (or Generic Equiv.) by FIRM	NDC#	CLASS; SCH.
Z <> M0430	Tab, Blue, Oval, Scored	Glyburide 3 mg	Glycron by Mova	55370-0594	Antidiabetic
Z <> M0645	Tab, Green, Oval, Scored	Glyburide 4.5 mg	Glycron by Mova	55370-0595	Antidiabetic
Z <> M0760	Tab, Yellow, Oval, Scored	Glyburide 6 mg	Glycron by Mova	55370-0596	Antidiabetic
Z <> MO315	Tab, White, Oval, Scored	Glyburide 1.5 mg	DiaBeta by Zoetica	64909-0101	Antidiabetic
Z <> MO430	Tab, Blue, Oval, Scored	Glyburide 3 mg	DiaBeta by Zoetica	64909-0102	Antidiabetic
Z <> MO760	Tab, Yellow, Oval, Scored	Glyburide 6 mg	DiaBeta by Zoetica	64909-0105	Antidiabetic
Z12	Tab, White to Off White, Round, Chewable, Dispersible	Lamotrigine 25 mg	Lamictal CD by Zydus	68382-0109	Anticonvulsant
Z12916	Tab, Lavender, Round, Z-1 2916	Trifluoperazine HCl 1 mg	Stelazine by Ivax		Antipsychotic
Z13	Tab, White to Off White, Round, Chewable, Dispersible	Lamotrigine 5 mg	Lamictal CD by Zydus	68382-0108	Anticonvulsant
Z200 <> 7111	Tab, Coated	Cimetidine HCl 200 mg	Tagamet by Ivax	00172-7111	Gastrointestinal
Z2047	Tab, White, Round	Colchicine 0.6 mg	Colchicine by Ivax	00172-2047	Antigout
Z2055	Cap, Clear & Pink	Diphenhydramine HCl 25 mg	Benadryl by Ivax		Antihistamine
Z2056	Cap, Pink	Diphenhydramine HCl 50 mg	Benadryl by Ivax	00172-2056	Antihistamine
Z2057	Cap, Natural	Phenytoin Sodium 100 mg	Phenytoin by Ivax	00172-2057	Anticonvulsant
Z2058		Digoxin 0.25 mg	Lanoxin by Ivax	Discontinued	
Z2058	Tab, White, Round			00172-2058	Cardiac Agent
Z2083	Tab, Peach, Round, Scored, Z over 2083	Hydrochlorothiazide 25 mg	Hydrodiuril by Kaiser	62224-1441	Diuretic; Antihypertensive
Z2083	Tab, Peach, Round, Scored, Z over 2083	Hydrochlorothiazide 25 mg	Hydrodiuril by Baker Cummins	63171-0556	Diuretic; Antihypertensive
Z2083	Tab, Peach, Round, Scored, Z over 2083	Hydrochlorothiazide 25 mg	Hydrodiuril by Ivax	00172-2083	Diuretic; Antihypertensive
Z2083	Tab, Peach, Round, Scored, Z over 2083	Hydrochlorothiazide 25 mg	Hydrodiuril by Ivax	00182-0556	Diuretic; Antihypertensive
Z2089		Hydrochlorothiazide 50 mg		Discontinued	
Z2089	Tab, Peach, Round, Scored, Z over 2089	Hydrochlorothiazide 50 mg	Hydrodiuril by Golden State	60429-0213	Diuretic; Antihypertensive
Z2089	Tab, Peach, Round, Scored, Z over 2089	Hydrochlorothiazide 50 mg	Hydrodiuril by Baker Cummins	63171-0557	Diuretic; Antihypertensive
Z2089	Tab, Peach, Round, Scored, Z over 2089	Hydrochlorothiazide 50 mg	Hydrodiuril by Compumed	00403-1026	Diuretic; Antihypertensive
Z2089	Tab, Peach, Round, Scored, Z over 2089	Hydrochlorothiazide 50 mg	Hydrodiuril by Ivax	00172-2089	Diuretic; Antihypertensive
Z2089	Tab, Peach, Round, Scored, Z over 2089	Hydrochlorothiazide 50 mg	Hydrodiuril by DRX	55045-1431	Diuretic; Antihypertensive
Z2089	Tab, Peach, Round, Scored, Z over 2089	Hydrochlorothiazide 50 mg	Hydrodiuril by Pharmedix	53002-0362	Diuretic; Antihypertensive
Z2089	Tab, Peach, Round, Scored, Z over 2089	Hydrochlorothiazide 50 mg	Hydrodiuril by Kaiser	62224-1445	Diuretic; Antihypertensive
Z2089	Tab, Peach, Round, Scored, Z over 2089	Hydrochlorothiazide 50 mg	Hydrodiuril by Ivax	00182-0557	Diuretic; Antihypertensive
Z2130	Cap, Pink & White	Nitrofurantoin 50 mg	Macrodantin by Ivax	Discontinued	Antibiotic
Z2130	Cap, Pink & White	Nitrofurantoin 50 mg	Macrodantin by Ivax	00172-1944	Antibiotic
Z2130	Cap, Pink & White	Nitrofurantoin 50 mg	Macrodantin by Qualitest	00603-4776	Antibiotic
Z2130	Cap, Pink & White	Nitrofurantoin 50 mg	Macrodantin by Ivax	00182-1944	Antibiotic
Z2131		Nitrofurantoin 100 mg		Discontinued	
Z2131	Cap, Pink	Nitrofurantoin 100 mg	Macrodantin by URL Mutual	00677-1225	Antibiotic
Z2131	Cap, Pink	Nitrofurantoin 100 mg	Macrodantin by Qualitest	00603-4777	Antibiotic
Z2131	Cap, Light Pink	Nitrofurantoin 100 mg	Macrodantin by Ivax		Antibiotic
Z2131	Cap, Pink	Nitrofurantoin 100 mg	Macrodantin by Ivax	00182-1945	Antibiotic
Z2168	Tab, Green, Round	Hydrochlorothiazide 50 mg, Reserpine (Hydroserpine #2) 0.125 mg	Hydropres by Ivax	Discontinued	Diuretic; Antihypertensive
Z2168	Tab, Green, Round		Hydropres by Ivax	00172-2168	Diuretic; Antihypertensive
Z2169	Tab, Green, Round	Hydrochlorothiazide 25 mg, Reserpine (Hydroserpine #1) 0.125 mg	Hydropres by Ivax	00172-2169	Diuretic; Antihypertensive
Z2186	Cap, Pink	Propoxyphene HCl 65 mg	Darvon-65 by Ivax	00172-2186	Analgesic; C IV
Z2186	Cap, Pink	Propoxyphene HCl 65 mg	Darvon-65 by Ivax	00182-0698	Analgesic; C IV
Z2190	Tab, Yellow, Oblong	Probenecid 500 mg	Benemid by Ivax	00172-2190	Antigout
Z2190				Discontinued	
Z2190	Tab, Yellow, Oblong	Probenecid 500 mg	Benemid by Qualitest	00603-5381	Antigout
Z2190	Tab, Yellow, Oblong	Probenecid 500 mg	Benemid by Sandoz	00781-1021	Antigout

ID FRONT <> BACK	DESCRIPTION FRONT <> BACK	INGREDIENT & STRENGTH	BRAND (or Generic Equiv.) by FIRM	NDC#	CLASS, SCH.
Z2193	Tab, White, Oblong, Scored	Colchicine 0.5 mg, Probenecid 500 mg	ColBenemid by Ivax	00172-2193 Discontinued	Antigout
Z2193	Tab, White, Oblong, Scored	Colchicine 0.5 mg, Probenecid 500 mg	ColBenemid by Sandoz	00781-1023	Antigout
Z2201	Tab, White, Round	Quinidine Sulfate 200 mg	Quinaglute by Ivax	00172-2201	Antiarrhythmic
Z2218	Tab, White, Round, Scored, Z over 2218	Sulfisoxazole 500 mg	Gantrisin by Ivax	00172-2218 Discontinued	Antibiotic
Z2218	Tab, White, Round, Scored, Z over 2218	Sulfisoxazole 500 mg	Gantrisin by Physician Total Care	54868-1535	Antibiotic
Z2218	Tab, White, Round, Scored, Z over 2218	Sulfisoxazole 500 mg	Gantrisin by DRX	55045-1450	Antibiotic
Z2245 <> G1084	Tab, White, Round	Tolbutamide 500 mg	Orinase by Ivax	00172-2245	Antidiabetic
Z22940	Tab, Lavender, Round, Z-2 2940	Trifluoperazine HCl 2 mg	Stelazine by Ivax	00172-2940	Antipsychotic
Z2335	Tab, White, Round	Hydralazine 25 mg, Hydrochlorothiazide 15 mg, Reserpine 0.1 mg	Ser-Ap-Es by Ivax	00172-2335	Antihypertensive; Diuretic
Z2338	Tab, Orange, Round	Hydralazine HCl 10 mg	Apresoline by Ivax	00172-2338	Antihypertensive
Z2339	Tab, Orange, Round	Hydralazine HCl 25 mg	Apresoline by Ivax	00172-2339	Antihypertensive
Z2345	Cap, Yellow, Black Print	Procainamide HCl 250 mg	Pronestyl by Qualitest	00603-5404	Antiarrhythmic
Z2345	Cap, Yellow, Black Print	Procainamide HCl 250 mg	Pronestyl by Ivax	00172-2345 Discontinued	Antiarrhythmic
Z2346	Cap, Orange & White	Procainamide HCl 375 mg	Pronestyl by Ivax	00182-0925	Antiarrhythmic
Z2346	Cap, Orange & White	Procainamide HCl 375 mg	Pronestyl by Qualitest	00603-5405	Antiarrhythmic
Z2346	Cap, Orange & White	Procainamide HCl 375 mg	Pronestyl by Ivax	00172-2346	Antiarrhythmic
Z2347	Cap, Orange & Yellow, Black Print	Procainamide HCl 500 mg	Pronestyl by Qualitest	00603-5406	Antiarrhythmic
Z2347	Cap, Orange & Yellow, Black Print	Procainamide HCl 500 mg	Pronestyl by Ivax	00182-0521	Antiarrhythmic
Z2347	Cap, Orange & Yellow, Black Print	Procainamide HCl 500 mg	Pronestyl by Ivax	00172-2347	Antiarrhythmic
Z2348	Tab, White, Round	Nylidrin 6 mg	Arlidin by Ivax	00172-2348	Vasodilator
Z2349	Tab, White, Round	Nylidrin 12 mg	Arlidin by Ivax	00172-2349	Vasodilator
Z2350	Tab, Yellow with White, Oval	Meclizine HCl 25 mg	Antivert by Ivax	00172-2350	Antiemetic
Z2359	Cap, Off-White, Black Print	Quinine Sulfate 200 mg	Quinamm by Ivax	00172-2359	Antimalarial
Z2384	Tab, Blue/White, Oval	Meclizine HCl 12.5 mg	Antivert by Ivax	00172-2384	Antiemetic
Z2387	Tab, White, Round	Isoxsuprine HCl 10 mg	Vasodilan by Ivax	00172-2387	Vasodilator
Z2388	Tab, White, Round	Isoxsuprine HCl 20 mg	Vasodilan by Ivax	00172-2388	Vasodilator
Z2407	Cap, Black & Yellow, White Print	Tetracycline HCl 500 mg	Tetrex BID by Baker Cummins	63171-0679	Antibiotic
Z2407	Cap, Black & Yellow, White Print	Tetracycline HCl 500 mg	Tetrex BID by Ivax	00172-2407	Antibiotic
Z2407	Cap, Black & Yellow, White Print	Tetracycline HCl 500 mg	Tetrex BID by Ivax	00182-0679 Discontinued	Antibiotic
Z2416	Cap, Orange & Yellow, Black Print	Tetracycline HCl 250 mg	Tetrex by Kaiser	00179-1020	Antibiotic
Z2416	Cap, Orange & Yellow, Black Print	Tetracycline HCl 250 mg	Tetrex by Ivax	00172-2416	Antibiotic
Z2416	Cap, Orange & Yellow, Black Print	Tetracycline HCl 250 mg	Tetrex by Apotheca	12634-0186	Antibiotic
Z2416	Cap, Orange & Yellow, Black Print	Tetracycline HCl 250 mg	Tetrex by Baker Cummins	63171-0112	Antibiotic
Z2416	Cap, Orange & Yellow, Black Print	Tetracycline HCl 250 mg	Tetrex by Ivax	00182-0112 Discontinued	Antibiotic
Z2430	Cap, Purple & Yellow	Tetracycline HCl 250 mg	Achromycin V by Ivax	00172-2430	Antibiotic
Z2458	Tab, Pink, Round	Erythromycin Stearate 250 mg	Erythrocin by Ivax	00172-2458	Antibiotic
Z2485	Tab, Light Orange, Round, Z-2485	Hydrochlorothiazide 100 mg	Hydrodiuril by Ivax	00172-2485	Diuretic; Antihypertensive
Z2493	Tab, Orange, Round	Hydralazine HCl 50 mg	Apresoline by Ivax	00172-2493	Antihypertensive
Z2507	Tab, Green, Round	Hydroflumethiazide 50 mg, Reserpine 0.125 mg	Salutensin by Ivax	00172-2507	Diuretic; Antihypertensive
Z2813	Tab, Pink & White, Round	Aspirin 325 mg, Methocarbamol 400 mg	Robaxisal by Ivax	00172-2813	Analgesic; Muscle Relaxant
Z2813	Tab, Pink & White, Round	Aspirin 325 mg, Methocarbamol 400 mg	Robaxisal by Ivax	00182-1911	Analgesic; Muscle Relaxant
Z2814	Cap, Orange	Cyclandelate 200 mg	Cyclospasmol by Ivax	00172-2814	Vasodilator

ID FRONT <> BACK	DESCRIPTION FRONT <> BACK	INGREDIENT & STRENGTH	BRAND (or Generic Equiv.) by FIRM	NDC#	CLASS; SCH.
Z2815	Cap, Green & White	Cyclandelate 400 mg	Cyclospasmol by Ivax	00172-2815	Vasodilator
Z2823	Tab, Pink, Oval	Erythromycin Stearate 500 mg	Erythrocin by Ivax	00172-2823	Antibiotic
Z2902	Tab, Blue, Round	Chlorpropamide 250 mg	Diabinese by Ivax	00172-2902	Antidiabetic
Z2903	Tab, White, Round	Spironolactone 25 mg	Aldactone by Ivax	00172-2903	Diuretic
Z2904	Tab, White, Round	Chlorthalidone 100 mg	Hygroton by Ivax	00172-2904	Diuretic
Z2907	Tab, White, Round, Scored, Z over 2907	Furosemide 40 mg	Lasix by Nat Pharmpak	55154-5803	Diuretic
Z2907	Tab, White, Round, Scored, Z over 2907	Furosemide 40 mg	Lasix by Pharmedix	53002-0430	Diuretic
Z2907	Tab, White, Round, Scored, Z over 2907	Furosemide 40 mg	Lasix by DRX	55045-1217	Diuretic
Z2907	Tab, White, Round, Scored, Z over 2907	Furosemide 40 mg	Lasix by Ivax	00172-2907	Antihypertensive; Diuretic
Z2907	Tab, White, Round, Scored, Z over 2907	Furosemide 40 mg	Lasix by Ivax	00182-1161	Diuretic
				Discontinued	
Z2907	Tab, White, Round, Scored, Z over 2907	Furosemide 40 mg	Lasix by Baker Cummins	63171-1161	Diuretic
Z2907	Tab, White, Round, Scored, Z over 2907	Furosemide 40 mg	Lasix by Qualitest	00603-3737	Diuretic
Z2907	Tab, White, Round	Furosemide 40 mg	Lasix by Teva	00172-2907	Antihypertensive/Diuretic
Z2909	Cap, Green & White	Hydroxyzine Pamoate 50 mg	Vistaril by Vangard	00615-0332	Antianxiety; Antihistamine
Z2909	Cap, Green & White	Hydroxyzine Pamoate 50 mg	Vistaril by Medirex	57480-0396	Antianxiety; Antihistamine
Z2909	Cap, Green & White	Hydroxyzine Pamoate 50 mg	Vistaril by Heartland	61392-0010	Antianxiety; Antihistamine
Z2909	Cap, Green & White	Hydroxyzine Pamoate 50 mg	Vistaril by Baker Cummins	63171-1099	Antianxiety; Antihistamine
Z2909	Cap, Green & White	Hydroxyzine Pamoate 50 mg	Vistaril by Schein	00364-0484	Antianxiety; Antihistamine
Z2909	Cap, Green & White	Hydroxyzine Pamoate 50 mg	Vistaril by Moore	00839-6271	Antianxiety; Antihistamine
Z2909	Cap, Green & White	Hydroxyzine Pamoate 50 mg	Vistaril by URL Mutual	00677-0597	Antianxiety; Antihistamine
Z2909	Cap, Green & White	Hydroxyzine Pamoate 50 mg	Vistaril by Sandoz	00781-2254	Antianxiety; Antihistamine
Z2909	Cap, Green & White	Hydroxyzine Pamoate 50 mg	Vistaril by Ivax	00182-1099	Antianxiety; Antihistamine
				Discontinued	
Z2909	Cap, Green & White	Hydroxyzine Pamoate 50 mg	Vistaril by Ivax	00172-2909	Antianxiety; Antihistamine
				Discontinued	
Z2911	Cap, Light Green & Dark Green	Hydroxyzine Pamoate 25 mg	Vistaril by URL Mutual	00677-0596	Antianxiety; Antihistamine
Z2911	Cap, Light Green & Dark Green	Hydroxyzine Pamoate 25 mg	Vistaril by Ivax	00182-1098	Antianxiety; Antihistamine
				Discontinued	
Z2911	Cap, Light Green & Dark Green	Hydroxyzine Pamoate 25 mg	Vistaril by Ivax	00172-2911	Antianxiety; Antihistamine
				Discontinue	
Z2911	Cap, Light Green & Dark Green	Hydroxyzine Pamoate 25 mg	Vistaril by PDRX	55289-0226	Antianxiety; Antihistamine
Z2911	Cap, Light Green & Dark Green	Hydroxyzine Pamoate 25 mg	Vistaril by Medirex	57480-0395	Antianxiety; Antihistamine
Z2911	Cap, Light Green & Dark Green	Hydroxyzine Pamoate 25 mg	Vistaril by Baker Cummins	63171-1098	Antianxiety; Antihistamine
Z2911	Cap, Light Green & Dark Green	Hydroxyzine Pamoate 25 mg	Vistaril by Sandoz	00781-2252	Antianxiety; Antihistamine
Z2911	Cap, Light Green & Dark Green	Hydroxyzine Pamoate 25 mg	Vistaril by Nat Pharmpak	55154-5564	Antianxiety; Antihistamine
Z2929	Tab, White, Round, Scored, Z over 2929	Cyproheptadine HCl 4 mg	Periactin by Baker Cummins	63171-1132	Antihistamine
Z2929	Tab, White, Round, Scored, Z over 2929	Cyproheptadine HCl 4 mg	Periactin by Major	00904-1145	Antihistamine
Z2929	Tab, White, Round, Scored, Z over 2929	Cyproheptadine HCl 4 mg	Periactin by Ivax	00182-1132	Antihistamine
				Discontinued	
Z2929	Tab, White, Round, Scored, Z over 2929	Cyproheptadine HCl 4 mg	Periactin by Ivax	00172-2929	Antihistamine
				Discontinued	
Z2931	Tab, White, Round, Z over 2931	Methyldopa 250 mg	Aldomet by Kaiser	00179-1061	Antihypertensive
Z2931	Tab, White, Round, Z over 2931	Methyldopa 250 mg	Aldomet by Ivax	00182-1732	Antihypertensive
Z2931	Tab, White, Round, Z over 2931	Methyldopa 250 mg	Aldomet by Baker Cummins	63171-1732	Antihypertensive
Z2931	Tab, White, Round, Z over 2931	Methyldopa 250 mg	Aldomet by Qualitest	00603-4536	Antihypertensive
Z2931	Tab, White, Round, Z over 2931	Methyldopa 250 mg	Aldomet by Ivax	00172-2931	Antihypertensive
				Discontinued	
Z2932	Tab, White, Round, Z over 2932	Methyldopa 500 mg	Aldomet by Baker Cummins	63171-1733	Antihypertensive
Z2932	Tab, White, Round, Z over 2932	Methyldopa 500 mg	Aldomet by Ivax	00182-1733	Antihypertensive

ID FRONT <> BACK	DESCRIPTION FRONT <> BACK	INGREDIENT & STRENGTH	BRAND (or Generic Equiv.) by FIRM	NDC#	CLASS; SCH.
Z2932	Tab, White, Round, Z over 2932	Methyldopa 500 mg	Aldomet by Qualitest	00603-4537	Antihypertensive
Z2932	Tab, White, Round, Z over 2932	Methyldopa 500 mg	Aldomet by URL Mutual	00677-0974	Antihypertensive
Z2932	Tab, White, Round, Z over 2932	Methyldopa 500 mg	Aldomet by Kaiser	00179-1062	Antihypertensive
Z2932	Tab, White, Round, Z over 2932	Methyldopa 500 mg	Aldomet by Ivax	00172-2932 Discontinued	Antihypertensive
Z2936	Tab, Blue, Round	Amitriptyline 10 mg, Perphenazine 2 mg	Triavil by Ivax	00172-2936	Antidepressant; Antipsychotic
Z2937	Tab, Orange, Round	Amitriptyline 25 mg, Perphenazine 2 mg	Triavil by Ivax	00172-2937	Antidepressant; Antipsychotic
Z2938	Tab, Salmon, Round	Amitriptyline 10 mg, Perphenazine 4 mg	Triavil by Ivax	00172-2938	Antidepressant; Antipsychotic
Z2939	Tab, Yellow, Round	Amitriptyline 25 mg, Perphenazine 4 mg	Triavil by Ivax	00172-2939	Antidepressant; Antipsychotic
Z2942	Tab, Lavender, Round	Trifluoperazine HCl 10 mg	Stelazine by Ivax	00172-2942	Antipsychotic
Z2950	Cap, Maroon, White Print	Hydrochlorothiazide 25 mg, Triamterene 50 mg	Dyazide by Ivax	00182-1750	Diuretic; Antihypertensive
Z2950	Cap, Maroon, White Print	Hydrochlorothiazide 25 mg, Triamterene 50 mg	Dyazide by Major	00904-5016	Diuretic; Antihypertensive
Z2950	Cap, Maroon, White Print	Hydrochlorothiazide 25 mg, Triamterene 50 mg	Dyazide by Moore	00839-8043	Diuretic; Antihypertensive
Z2950	Cap, Maroon, White Print	Hydrochlorothiazide 25 mg, Triamterene 50 mg	Dyazide by Ivax	00172-2950 Discontinued	Diuretic; Antihypertensive
Z2958	Tab, White, Round	Ergoloid Mesylate 0.5 mg	Hydergine SL by Ivax	00172-2958	Ergot Alkaloids
Z2959	Tab, White, Oval, Sublingual	Ergoloid Mesylate 1 mg	Hydergine SL by Ivax	00172-2959 Discontinued	Ergot Alkaloids
Z2960	Cap, White	Chloramphenicol 250 mg	Chloromycetin by Ivax	00172-2960	Antibiotic
Z2962	Tab, White, Round	Ephedrine 25 mg, Hydroxyzine 10 mg, Theophylline 130 mg	Marax by Ivax	00172-2962	Antiasthmatic
Z2963	Cap, Amethyst/Natural	Nitroglycerin TD 2.5 mg	Nitrobid by Ivax	00172-2963	Vasodilator
Z2964	Cap, Blue & Yellow	Nitroglycerin TD 6.5 mg	Nitrobid by Ivax	00173-2964	Vasodilator
Z2969	Cap	Sulfinpyrazone 200 mg	Anturane by Ivax	00172-2969	Uricosuric
Z2970	Tab, White, Round	Sulfinpyrazone 100 mg	Anturane by Ivax	00172-2970	Uricosuric
Z2971	Tab, White, Round, Z over 2791	Metronidazole 250 mg	Flagyl by Ivax	00182-1330	Antibiotic
Z2971	Tab, White, Round, Z over 2791	Metronidazole 250 mg	Flagyl by Ivax	00172-2971 Discontinued	Antibiotic
Z2971	Tab, White, Round, Z over 2791	Metronidazole 250 mg	Flagyl by Med Pro	53978-0215	Antibiotic
Z2971	Tab, White, Round, Z over 2791	Metronidazole 250 mg	Flagyl by Kaiser	00179-0690	Antibiotic
Z2971	Tab, White, Round, Z over 2791	Metronidazole 250 mg	Flagyl by Pharmedix	53002-0221	Antibiotic
Z2971	Tab, White, Round, Z over 2791	Metronidazole 250 mg	Flagyl by Nat Pharmpak	55154-5509	Antibiotic
Z2971	Tab, White, Round, Z over 2791	Metronidazole 250 mg	Flagyl by Ivax	00182-1330	Antibiotic
Z2971 <> G1330	Tab, White, Round, Z over 2791	Metronidazole 250 mg	Flagyl by Ivax	00172-4291	Antibiotic
Z2974	Tab, Off-White, Round, Z over 2974	Chlorthalidone 25 mg	by Ivax	00172-2974	Diuretic
Z2976	Tab, White, Round	Dipyridamole 50 mg	Persantine by Ivax		Antiplatelet
Z2977	Tab, White, Round	Dipyridamole 75 mg	Persantine by Ivax		Antiplatelet
Z2978	Tab, White, Round, Scored, Z over 2978	Tolazamide 100 mg	Tolinase by Ivax	00172-2978 Discontinued	Antidiabetic
Z2978	Tab, White, Round, Scored, Z over 2978	Tolazamide 100 mg	Tolinase by Qualitest	00603-6096	Antidiabetic
Z2979	Tab, White, Round, Scored, Z over 2979	Tolazamide 250 mg	Tolinase by Apotheca	12634-0490	Antidiabetic
Z2979	Tab, White, Round, Scored, Z over 2979	Tolazamide 250 mg	Tolinase by Ivax	00172-2979 Discontinued	Antidiabetic
Z2980	Tab, White, Round, Scored, Z over 2980	Tolazamide 500 mg	Tolinase by Ivax	00182-1679 Discontinued	Antidiabetic
Z2980	Tab, White, Round, Scored, Z over 2980	Tolazamide 500 mg	Tolinase by Ivax	00172-2980 Discontinued	Antidiabetic

ID FRONT <> BACK	DESCRIPTION FRONT <> BACK	INGREDIENT & STRENGTH	BRAND (or Generic Equiv.) by FIRM	NDC#	CLASS; SCH.
Z2982	Cap, White	Chlordiazepoxide 5 mg, Clidinium Bromide 2.5 mg	Librax by Ivax	00172-2982	Gastrointestinal
Z2984	Cap, Blue & White, Black Print	Doxycycline Hyclate 50 mg	Vibramycin by PDRX	55289-0502	Antibiotic
Z2984	Cap, Blue & White, Black Print	Doxycycline Hyclate 50 mg	Vibramycin by Ivax	00172-2984 Discontinued	Antibiotic
Z2985	Cap, Light Blue, Black Print	Doxycycline Hyclate 100 mg	Vibramycin by Apotheca	12634-0169	Antibiotic
Z2985	Cap, Light Blue, Black Print	Doxycycline Hyclate 100 mg	Vibramycin by Quality Care	60346-0109	Antibiotic
Z2985	Cap, Light Blue, Black Print	Doxycycline Hyclate 100 mg	Vibramycin by Darby Group	66467-0230	Antibiotic
Z2985	Cap, Light Blue, Black Print	Doxycycline Hyclate 100 mg	Vibramycin by Baker Cummins	63171-1035	Antibiotic
Z2985	Cap, Light Blue, Black Print	Doxycycline Hyclate 100 mg	Vibramycin by Ivax	00172-2985 Discontinued	Antibiotic
Z2985	Cap, Light Blue, Black Print	Doxycycline Hyclate 100 mg	Vibramycin by Ivax	00182-1035 Discontinued	Antibiotic
Z2986	Tab, Light Orange	Methylclothiazide 2.5 mg	by Ivax	00172-2986	Diuretic; Antihypertensive
Z2987	Tab, Salmon, Round	Methylclothiazide 5 mg	Enduron by Ivax		Diuretic; Antihypertensive
Z2994	Tab, White, Round	Dipyridamole 25 mg	Persantine by Ivax		Antiplatelet
Z2999	Tab	Chlorthalidone 50 mg	by Ivax	00172-2999	Diuretic
Z3	Tab, White to Off-White, Round	Amlodipine Besylate 5 mg	Norvasc by Zydus	68382-0122	Antihypertensive
Z300 <> 7117	Tab, White, Round, Z over 300	Cimetidine HCl 300 mg	Tagamet by Ivax	00172-7117	Gastrointestinal
Z300 <> 7117	Tab, White, Round, Z over 300	Cimetidine HCl 300 mg	Tagamet by Ivax	00182-1984	Gastrointestinal
Z300 <> 7117	Tab, White to Off White, Round	Cimetidine 300 mg	Tagamet by Teva	00712-7117	Gastrointestinal
Z3001	Tab, White, Round, Z over 3001	Quinine Sulfate 260 mg	Quinamm by Vangard	00615-1579	Antimalarial
Z3001	Tab, White, Round, Z over 3001	Quinine Sulfate 260 mg	Quinamm by Ivax	00172-3001 Discontinued	Antimalarial
Z3007	Tab, White, Oval	Metronidazole 500 mg	Flagyl by Ivax	00172-3007 Discontinued	Antibiotic
Z3007	Tab, White, Oval	Metronidazole 500 mg	Flagyl by Kaiser	00179-1227	Antibiotic
Z3007	Tab, White, Oval	Metronidazole 500 mg	Flagyl by Med Pro	53978-3056	Antibiotic
Z3007	Tab, White, Oval	Metronidazole 500 mg	Flagyl by Pharmedix	53002-0247	Antibiotic
Z3007	Tab, White, Oval	Metronidazole 500 mg	Flagyl by Ivax	00182-1517	Antibiotic
Z3606	Tab, Orange, Round	Thioridazine 10 mg	Mellaril by Ivax		Antipsychotic
Z3607	Tab, Orange, Round	Thioridazine 15 mg	Mellaril by Ivax		Antipsychotic
Z3608	Tab, Orange, Round	Thioridazine 25 mg	Mellaril by Ivax		Antipsychotic
Z3609	Tab, Orange, Round	Thioridazine 50 mg	Mellaril by Ivax		Antipsychotic
Z3610	Tab, White, Round	Thioridazine 100 mg	Mellaril by Ivax		Antipsychotic
Z3614	Tab, Orange, Round	Propranolol HCl 10 mg	Inderal by Ivax		Antihypertensive
Z3615	Tab, Blue, Round	Propranolol HCl 20 mg	Inderal by Ivax		Antihypertensive
Z3616	Tab, Green, Round	Propranolol HCl 40 mg	Inderal by Ivax		Antihypertensive
Z3617	Tab, Yellow, Round	Propranolol HCl 80 mg	Inderal by Ivax		Antihypertensive
Z3626	Tab, Peach, Round, Scored, Z over 3626	Doxycycline Hyclate 100 mg	Vibramycin by Ivax	00172-3626	Antibiotic
Z3626	Tab, Peach, Round, Scored, Z over 3626	Doxycycline Hyclate 100 mg	Vibramycin by Ivax	00182-1535	Antibiotic
Z3626	Tab, Peach, Round, Scored, Z over 3626	Doxycycline Hyclate 100 mg	Vibramycin by Apotheca	12634-0167	Antibiotic
Z3626	Tab, Peach, Round, Scored, Z over 3626	Doxycycline Hyclate 100 mg	Vibramycin by Pharmedix	53002-0271	Antibiotic
Z3626	Tab, Peach, Round, Scored, Z over 3626	Doxycycline Hyclate 100 mg	Vibramycin by Baker Cummins	63171-1535	Antibiotic
Z3626	Tab, Peach, Round, Scored, Z over 3626	Doxycycline Hyclate 100 mg	Vibramycin by Golden State	60429-0069	Antibiotic
Z3626	Tab, Peach, Round, Scored, Z over 3626	Doxycycline Hyclate 100 mg	Vibramycin by Prepackage Specialists	58864-0189	Antibiotic
Z3626	Tab, Peach, Round, Scored, Z over 3626	Doxycycline Hyclate 100 mg	Vibramycin by UDL	51079-0554	Antibiotic
Z3638	Tab, Red, Round	Propranolol HCl 60 mg	Inderal by Ivax		Antihypertensive

ID FRONT <> BACK	DESCRIPTION FRONT <> BACK	INGREDIENT & STRENGTH	BRAND (or Generic Equiv.) by FIRM	NDC#	CLASS; SCH.
Z3643	Cap, Green & Yellow	Nitroglycerin TD 9 mg	Nitrobid by Ivax		Vasodilator
Z3657	Tab, Blue, Round	Chlorpropamide 100 mg	Diabinese by Ivax		Antidiabetic
Z36672	Tab, Gray, Round, Z over 3667 over 2	Perphenazine 2 mg	Trilafon by UDL	51079-0738	Antipsychotic
Z36672	Tab, Gray, Round, Z over 3667 over 2	Perphenazine 2 mg	by Pharmafab	62542-0905	Antipsychotic
Z36672	Tab, Gray, Round, Hourglass Logo over 3667	Perphenazine 2 mg	Trilafon by Ivax	00172-3667 Discontinued	Antipsychotic
Z36684	Tab, Gray, Round, Z over 3668 over 4	Perphenazine 4 mg	by Pharmafab	62542-0910	Antipsychotic
Z36684	Tab, Gray, Round, Hourglass Logo over 3668	Perphenazine 4 mg	Trilafon by Ivax	00172-3668 Discontinued	Antipsychotic
Z36684	Tab, Gray, Round, Z over 3668 over 4	Perphenazine 4 mg	Trilafon by UDL	51079-0739	Antipsychotic
Z36698	Tab, Gray, Round, Z over 3668 over 4	Perphenazine 8 mg	Trilafon by UDL	51079-0740	Antipsychotic
Z36698	Tab, Gray, Round, Z over 3668 over 4	Perphenazine 8 mg	Trilafon by UDL	00182-1867	Antipsychotic
Z36698	Tab, White, Round, Hourglass Logo over 3669	Perphenazine 8 mg	Trilafon by Ivax	00172-3669 Discontinued	Antipsychotic
Z367016	Tab, Gray, Round, Z over 3670 over 16	Perphenazine 16 mg	Trilafon by UDL	51079-0823	Antipsychotic
Z367016	Tab, Gray, Round, Z over 3670 over 16	Perphenazine 16 mg	by Pharmafab	62542-0912	Antipsychotic
Z367016	Tab, Gray, Round, Hourglass Logo over 3670	Perphenazine 16 mg	Trilafon by Ivax	00172-3670 Discontinued	Antipsychotic
Z367016	Tab, Gray, Round, Tab Sugar Coated	Perphenazine 16 mg	Trilafon by Ivax	00182-1868	Antipsychotic
Z367016	Tab, Gray, Round, Z over 3670 over 16	Perphenazine 16 mg	by Physician Total Care	54868-2857	Antipsychotic
Z367016	Tab, Gray, Round, Z over 3670 over 16	Perphenazine 16 mg	by Direct Dispensing	57866-1058	Antipsychotic
Z3671	Tab, Orange, Round	Amitriptyline 50 mg, Perphenazine 4 mg	Triavil by Ivax		Antidepressant; Antipsychotic
Z3747	Tab, White, Round	Phenobarbital 8 mg, Theophylline 130 mg, Ephedrine (Azpan) 24 mg	Tedral by Ivax		Antiasthmatic; C IV
Z3904	Tab, White, Round	Meprobamate 400 mg	Miltown by Ivax		Sedative/Hypnotic; C IV
Z3905	Tab, White, Round	Meprobamate 200 mg	Miltown by Ivax		Sedative/Hypnotic; C IV
Z3915	Tab, White, Round	Acetaminophen 300 mg, Codeine Phosphate 30 mg	Tylenol w/ Codeine by Ivax		Analgesic; C III
Z3916	Tab, White, Round	Acetaminophen 300 mg, Codeine Phosphate 60 mg	Tylenol w/ Codeine by Ivax		Analgesic; C III
Z3925 <> 2	Tab, White, Round, Scored, Z over 3925	Diazepam 2 mg	Valium by Ivax	00182-1755	Antianxiety; C IV
Z3925 <> 2	Tab, White, Round, Scored, Z over 3925	Diazepam 2 mg	Valium by Ivax	00172-3925	Antianxiety; C IV
Z3925 <> 2	Tab, White, Round, Scored, Z over 3925	Diazepam 2 mg	Valium by Kaiser	00179-1085	Antianxiety; C IV
Z3926 <> 5	Tab, Yellow, Round, Scored, Z over 3926	Diazepam 5 mg	Valium by Qualitest	00603-3217	Antianxiety; C IV
Z3926 <> 5	Tab, Yellow, Round, Scored, Z over 3926	Diazepam 5 mg	Valium by Pharmedix	53002-0334	Antianxiety; C IV
Z3926 <> 5	Tab, Yellow, Round, Scored, Z over 3926	Diazepam 5 mg	Valium by Ivax	00172-3926	Antianxiety; C IV
Z3927 <> 10	Tab, Light Blue, Round, Scored, Z over 3927	Diazepam 10 mg	Valium by PDRX	55289-0091	Antianxiety; C IV
Z3927 <> 10	Tab, Light Blue, Round, Scored, Z over 3927	Diazepam 10 mg	Valium by Ivax	00172-3927	Antianxiety; C IV
Z3927 <> 10	Tab, Light Blue, Round, Scored, Z over 3927	Diazepam 10 mg	Valium by Ivax	00182-1757	Antianxiety; C IV
Z3964	Tab, White	Aspirin 325 mg, Codeine Phosphate 30 mg	Aspirin w/ Codeine by Qualitest	00603-2361	Analgesic; C III
Z3981	Tab, Film Coated	Acetaminophen 650 mg, Propoxyphene Napsylate 100 mg	Darvocet-N 100 by Talbert	44514-0750	Analgesic; C IV
Z3981	Tab, Coated	Acetaminophen 650 mg, Propoxyphene Napsylate 100 mg	Darvocet-N 100 by Ivax	00172-3981	Analgesic; C IV
Z3984	Tab, White, Round, Z over 3984	Aspirin 325 mg, Codeine Phosphate 30 mg	Aspirin w/ Codeine by URL Mutual	00677-0647	Analgesic; C III
Z3984	Tab, White, Round, Z over 3984	Aspirin 325 mg, Codeine Phosphate 30 mg	Aspirin w/ Codeine by Qualitest	00603-2361	Analgesic; C III
Z3984	Tab, White, Round, Z over 3984	Aspirin 325 mg, Codeine Phosphate 30 mg	Aspirin w/ Codeine by Pharmedix	53002-0109	Analgesic; C III
Z3984 <> 3	Tab, White, Round, Z over 3984	Aspirin 325 mg, Codeine Phosphate 30 mg	Aspirin w/ Codeine by Ivax	00172-3984 Discontinued	Analgesic; C III
Z3985	Tab, White, Round, Z over 3985	Aspirin 325 mg, Codeine Phosphate 60 mg	Aspirin w/ Codeine by Qualitest	00603-2362	Analgesic; C III
Z3985	Tab, White, Round, Z over 3985	Aspirin 325 mg, Codeine Phosphate 60 mg	Aspirin w/ Codeine by URL Mutual	00677-0676	Analgesic; C III
Z3985 <> 4	Tab, White, Round, Z over 3985	Aspirin 325 mg, Codeine Phosphate 60 mg	Aspirin w/ Codeine by Ivax	00172-3985 Discontinued	Analgesic; C III

ID FRONT <> BACK	DESCRIPTION FRONT <> BACK	INGREDIENT & STRENGTH	BRAND (or Generic Equiv.) by FIRM	NDC#	CLASS; SCH.
Z3996	Tab, White, Round	Butalbital 50 mg, Aspirin 325 mg, Caffeine 40 mg	Fiorinal by Ivax	00172-3996	Analgesic; C III
Z4	Tab, White, Round, Orally Disintegrating	Ondansetron 4 mg	Zofran ODT by GSK	00173-0569	Antiemetic
Z400 <> 7171	Tab, White, Oblong, Scored	Cimetidine HCl 400 mg	Tagamet by Golden State	60429-0047	Gastrointestinal
Z400 <> 7171	Tab, White, Oblong, Scored	Cimetidine HCl 400 mg	Tagamet by Murfreesboro	51129-1336	Gastrointestinal
Z400 <> 7171	Tab, White, Oblong, Scored	Cimetidine HCl 400 mg	Tagamet by Med Pro	53978-2009	Gastrointestinal
Z400 <> 7171	Tab, White, Oblong, Scored	Cimetidine HCl 400 mg	Tagamet by Ivax	00182-1985	Gastrointestinal
Z400 <> 7171	Tab, White to Off White, Capsule Shaped	Cimetidine 400 mg	Tagamet by Teva	00172-7171	Gastrointestinal
Z4029	Cap, Green, Black Print	Indomethacin 25 mg	Indocin by Baker Cummins	63171-1681	NSAID
Z4029	Cap, Green, Black Print	Indomethacin 25 mg	Indocin by Kaiser	00179-1059	NSAID
Z4029	Cap, Green, Black Print	Indomethacin 25 mg	Indocin by Qualitest	00603-4067	NSAID
Z4029	Cap, Green, Black Print	Indomethacin 25 mg	Indocin by Moore	00839-6762	NSAID
Z4029	Cap, Green, Black Print	Indomethacin 25 mg	Indocin by Kaiser	62224-3446	NSAID
Z4029	Cap, Green, Black Print	Indomethacin 25 mg	Indocin by Ivax	00172-4029 Discontinued	NSAID
Z4029	Cap, Green, Black Print	Indomethacin 25 mg	Indocin by Ivax	00182-1681 Discontinued	NSAID
Z4029	Cap, Green, Black Print	Indomethacin 25 mg	Indocin by Med Pro	53978-0039	NSAID
Z4029	Cap, Green, Black Print	Indomethacin 25 mg	Indocin by Mova	55370-0858	NSAID
Z4029	Cap, Green, Black Print	Indomethacin 25 mg	Indocin by Pharmedix	53002-0305	NSAID
Z4029	Cap, Green, Black Print	Indomethacin 25 mg	Indocin by Schein	00364-0691	NSAID
Z4029	Cap, Green	Indomethacin 25 mg	Indocin by Teva	00093-4029	NSAID
Z4030	Cap, Green, Black Print	Indomethacin 50 mg	Indocin by Ivax	00182-1682 Discontinued	NSAID
Z4030	Cap, Green, Black Print	Indomethacin 50 mg	Indocin by Ivax	00172-4030 Discontinued	NSAID
Z4030	Cap, Green, Black Print	Indomethacin 50 mg	Indocin by Mova	55370-0859	NSAID
Z4030	Cap, Green, Black Print	Indomethacin 50 mg	Indocin by Med Pro	53978-5037	NSAID
Z4030	Cap, Green, Black Print	Indomethacin 50 mg	Indocin by Pharmedix	53002-0350	NSAID
Z4030	Cap, Green, Black Print	Indomethacin 50 mg	Indocin by Baker Cummins	63171-1682	NSAID
Z4030	Cap, Green, Black Print	Indomethacin 50 mg	Indocin by Rx Dispensing	61807-0041	NSAID
Z4030	Cap, Green, Black Print	Indomethacin 50 mg	Indocin by PDRX	55289-0663	NSAID
Z4030	Cap, Green, Black Print	Indomethacin 50 mg	Indocin by Kaiser	62224-3557	NSAID
Z4030	Cap, Green, Black Print	Indomethacin 50 mg	Indocin by Qualitest	00603-4068	NSAID
Z4030	Cap, Green, Black Print	Indomethacin 50 mg	Indocin by Moore	00839-6763	NSAID
Z4030	Cap, Green	Indomethacin 50 mg	Indocin by Kaiser	00179-1060	NSAID
Z4030	Cap, Green	Indomethacin 50 mg	Indocin by Teva	00093-4030	NSAID
Z4051	Cap, Blue & Clear	Disopyramide Phosphate 100 mg	Norpace by Ivax	00172-4051	Antiarrhythmic
Z4052	Cap, Blue & Clear	Disopyramide Phosphate 150 mg	Norpace by Ivax	00172-4052	Antiarrhythmic
Z4058	Cap, Clear & White	Cefadroxil Monohydrate 500 mg	Duricef by Ivax	00172-4058 Discontinued	Antibiotic
Z4063	Cap, Maroon	Cephradine 250 mg	Anspor by Ivax	00172-4063	Antibiotic
Z4064	Cap, Pink	Cephradine 500 mg	Anspor by Ivax	00172-4064	Antibiotic
Z4067	Cap, Ivory, Black Print	Prazosin HCl 1 mg	Minipress by Ivax	00172-4067 Discontinued	Antihypertensive
Z4068	Cap, Pink, Black Print	Prazosin HCl 2 mg	Minipress by Ivax	00172-4068 Discontinued	Antihypertensive
Z4069	Cap, Blue, White Print	Prazosin HCl 5 mg	Minipress by Ivax	00172-4069 Discontinued	Antihypertensive
Z4069	Cap, Blue, White Print	Prazosin HCl 5 mg	Minipress by Ivax	00182-1257	Antihypertensive
Z4073	Cap, Gray & Red, Black Print	Cephalexin 250 mg	Keflex by Ivax	00182-1278	Antibiotic

ID FRONT <> BACK	DESCRIPTION FRONT <> BACK	INGREDIENT & STRENGTH	BRAND (or Generic Equiv.) by FIRM	NDC#	CLASS; SCH.
Z4073	Cap, Gray & Red, Black Print	Cephalexin 250 mg	Keflex by Ivax	00172-4073 Discontinued	Antibiotic
Z4074	Cap, Red, Black Print	Cephalexin 500 mg	Keflex by Ivax	00182-1279	Antibiotic
Z4074	Cap, Red, Black Print	Cephalexin 500 mg	Keflex by Quality Care	60346-0055	Antibiotic
Z4074	Cap, Red, Black Print	Cephalexin 500 mg	Keflex by Ivax	00172-4074 Discontinued	Antibiotic
Z4077	Cap, Blue & Red	Piroxicam 10 mg	Feldene by Ivax	00172-4077	NSAID
Z4079	Cap, Red, Opaque	Piroxicam 20 mg	Feldene by Ivax	00182-1934	NSAID
Z4079	Cap, Red	Piroxicam 20 mg	Feldene by Ivax	00172-4079	NSAID
Z4079	Cap, Red, Opaque	Piroxicam 20 mg	Feldene by Promeco SA	64674-0007	NSAID
Z4079	Cap, Goldline	Piroxicam 20 mg	Feldene by H J Harkins Co	52959-0232	NSAID
Z4096 <> 10	Tab, White, Round, Scored, Z over 4096	Baclofen 10 mg	Lioresal by Major	00904-3365	Muscle Relaxant
Z4096 <> 10	Tab, White, Round, Scored, Z over 4096	Baclofen 10 mg	Lioresal by Baker Cummins	63171-1295	Muscle Relaxant
Z4096 <> 10	Tab, White, Round, Scored, Z over 4096	Baclofen 10 mg	Lioresal by Ivax	00172-4096	Muscle Relaxant
Z4096 <> 10	Tab, White, Round, Scored, Z over 4096	Baclofen 10 mg	Lioresal by Ivax	00182-1295	Muscle Relaxant
Z4096 <> 10	Tab, White, Round, Scored, Z over 4096	Baclofen 10 mg	Lioresal by Caremark	00339-5834	Muscle Relaxant
Z4097 <> 20	Tab, White, Round, Scored, Z over 4097	Baclofen 20 mg	Lioresal by Ivax	00172-4097	Muscle Relaxant
Z4097 <> 20	Tab, White, Round, Scored, Z over 4097	Baclofen 20 mg	Lioresal by Baker Cummins	63171-1296	Muscle Relaxant
Z4097 <> 20	Tab, White, Round, Scored, Z over 4097	Baclofen 20 mg	Lioresal by Rx Dispensing	61807-0131	Muscle Relaxant
Z4097 <> 20	Tab, White, Round, Scored, Z over 4097	Baclofen 20 mg	Lioresal by UDL		Muscle Relaxant
Z4097 <> 20	Tab, White, Round, Scored, Z over 4097	Baclofen 20 mg	Lioresal by Med Pro	53978-3167	Muscle Relaxant
Z4097 <> 20	Tab, White, Round, Scored, Z over 4097	Baclofen 20 mg	Lioresal by Ivax	00182-1296	Muscle Relaxant
Z4097 <> 20	Tab, White, Round, Scored, Z over 4097	Baclofen 20 mg	Lioresal by Major	00904-5222	Muscle Relaxant
Z4107	Tab	Naproxen 250 mg	Naprosyn by Ivax	00182-1971	NSAID
Z4108	Tab	Naproxen 375 mg	Naprosyn by Ivax	00182-1972	NSAID
Z4109	Tab	Naproxen 500 mg	Naprosyn by Ivax	00182-1973	NSAID
Z4116275	Tab, White, Oval, Z 4116/275	Naproxen 275 mg	Naprosyn by Ivax	00172-4116	NSAID
Z4141	Tab, Peach, Oblong, Z over 4141	Fenoprofen Calcium 600 mg	Nalfon by Ivax	00182-1902	NSAID
Z4141 <> 600	Tab, Peach, Oblong, Z over 4141	Fenoprofen Calcium 600 mg	Nalfon by Ivax	00172-4141 Discontinued	NSAID
Z4141 <> 600	Tab, Orange, Film Coated, 600 and Zenith Logo	Fenoprofen Calcium 600 mg	Nalfon by Quality Care	60346-0233	NSAID
Z4141600	Tab, Coated	Fenoprofen Calcium 600 mg	Nalfon by Ivax	00182-1902	NSAID
Z4172	Cap, Natural Clear, Black Print	Quinine Sulfate 325 mg	Quinamm by Ivax	00172-4172 Discontinued	Antimalarial
Z4217 <> 5	Tab, White, Round, Z over 4217	Pindolol 5 mg	Visken by Ivax	00172-4217 Discontinued	Antihypertensive
Z4218 <> 10	Tab, White, Round, Z over 4218	Pindolol 10 mg	Visken by Ivax	00172-4218 Discontinued	Antihypertensive
Z4219	Tab, White, Round	Diltiazem HCl 30 mg	Cardizem by Ivax	00172-4219	Antihypertensive
Z4220	Tab, White, Round	Diltiazem HCl 60 mg	Cardizem by Ivax	00172-4220	Antihypertensive
Z4221	Tab, White, Oblong	Diltiazem HCl 90 mg	Cardizem by Ivax	00172-4221	Antihypertensive
Z4222	Tab, White, Oblong	Diltiazem HCl 120 mg	Cardizem by Ivax	00172-4222	Antihypertensive
Z4229	Cap, Red	Hydrochlorothiazide 25 mg, Triamterene 50 mg	Dyazide by Ivax	00172-4229	Diuretic; Antihypertensive
Z4232 <> 05	Tab, Green, Round, Scored, 0.5 <> Z over 4232	Bumetanide 0.5 mg	Bumex by Teva	00093-4232	Diuretic
Z4232 <> 05	Tab, Green, Round, Scored, Z 4232 <> 0.5	Bumetanide 0.5 mg	Bumex by Major	00904-5102	Diuretic
Z4232 <> 05	Tab, Green, Round, Scored, Z 4232 <> 0.5	Bumetanide 0.5 mg	Bumex by Sandoz	00781-1821	Diuretic
Z4232 <> 05	Tab, Green, Round, Scored, Z 4232 <> 0.5	Bumetanide 0.5 mg	Bumex by Vangard	00615-4541	Diuretic
Z4232 <> 05	Tab, Green, Round, Scored, Z 4232 <> 0.5	Bumetanide 0.5 mg	Bumex by Ivax	00182-2615	Diuretic
Z4232 <> 05	Tab, Green, Round, Scored, Z 4232 <> 0.5	Bumetanide 0.5 mg	Bumex by Moore	00839-8011	Diuretic

ID FRONT <> BACK	DESCRIPTION FRONT <> BACK	INGREDIENT & STRENGTH	BRAND (or Generic Equiv.) by FIRM	NDC#	CLASS; SCH.
Z4232 <> 05	Tab, Green, Round, Scored, Z over 4232 <> 0.5	Bumetanide 0.5 mg	Bumex by Ivax	00172-4232 Discontinued	Diuretic
Z4233 <> 1	Tab, Yellow, Round, Scored, Z over 4233	Bumetanide 1 mg	Bumex by Nat Pharmpak	55154-5819	Diuretic
Z4233 <> 1	Tab, Yellow, Round, Scored, Z over 4233	Bumetanide 1 mg	Bumex by Murfreesboro	51129-1337	Diuretic
Z4233 <> 1	Tab, Yellow, Round, Scored, Z over 4233	Bumetanide 1 mg	Bumex by Major	00904-5103	Diuretic
Z4233 <> 1	Tab, Yellow, Round, Scored, Z over 4233	Bumetanide 1 mg	Bumex by Ivax	00172-4233 Discontinued	Diuretic
Z4233 <> 1	Tab, Yellow, Round, Scored, Z over 4233	Bumetanide 1 mg	Bumex by Moore	00839-8012	Diuretic
Z4233 <> 1	Tab, Yellow, Round, Scored, Z over 4233	Bumetanide 1 mg	Bumex by Ivax	00182-2616	Diuretic
Z4233 <> 1	Tab, Yellow, Round, Scored, Z over 4233	Bumetanide 1 mg	Bumex by Sandoz	00781-1822	Diuretic
Z4234 <> 2	Tab, Peach, Round, Scored, Z over 4234	Bumetanide 2 mg	Bumex by Teva	00093-4233	Diuretic
Z4234 <> 2	Tab, Peach, Round, Scored, Z over 4234	Bumetanide 2 mg	Bumex by Teva	00093-4234	Diuretic
Z4234 <> 2	Tab, Peach, Round, Scored, Z over 4234	Bumetanide 2 mg	Bumex by Ivax	00182-2617	Diuretic
Z4234 <> 2	Tab, Peach, Round, Scored, Z over 4234	Bumetanide 2 mg	Bumex by Major	00904-5104	Diuretic
Z4234 <> 2	Tab, Peach, Round, Scored, Z over 4234	Bumetanide 2 mg	Bumex by Ivax	00172-4234	Diuretic
Z4234 <> 2	Tab, Peach, Round, Scored, Z over 4234	Bumetanide 2 mg	Bumex by Murfreesboro	51129-1383	Diuretic
Z4234 <> 2	Tab, Peach, Round, Scored, Z over 4234	Bumetanide 2 mg	Bumex by Sandoz	00781-1823	Diuretic
Z4235 <> 20	Tab, White, Round, Z over 4235	Nadolol 20 mg	Corgard by Ivax	00093-4235	Antihypertensive
Z4235 <> 20	Tab, White, Round, Z over 4235	Nadolol 20 mg	Corgard by Ivax	00182-2632	Antihypertensive
Z4236 <> 40	Tab, White, Round, Z over 4236	Nadolol 40 mg	Corgard by Ivax	00093-4236	Antihypertensive
Z4237 <> 80	Tab, White, Round, Scored, Z over 4237	Nadolol 80 mg	Corgard by Ivax	00093-4237	Antihypertensive
Z4237 <> 80	Tab, White, Round, Scored, Z over 4237	Nadolol 80 mg	Nadolol by Ivax	00182-2634	Antihypertensive
Z4238 <> 120	Tab, White, Cap Shaped	Nadolol 120 mg	Corgard by Ivax	00172-4238 Discontinued	Antihypertensive
Z4239 <> 160	Tab, White, Cap Shaped	Nadolol 160 mg	Corgard by Ivax	00172-4239 Discontinued	Antihypertensive
Z4262 <> 125	Tab, Orange, Round, Z over 4262 <> 1.25	Indapamide 1.25 mg	Lozol by Ivax	00182-8201	Diuretic
Z4262 <> 125	Tab, Orange, Round, Z over 4262 <> 1.25	Indapamide 1.25 mg	Lozol by Ivax	00172-4262 Discontinued	Diuretic
Z4266200	Cap, White, Opaque	Acyclovir 200 mg	Zovirax by Schein	00364-2692	Antiviral
Z4275550	Tab, White, Oval, Z 4275/550	Naproxen 550 mg	Naprosyn by Ivax		NSAID
Z4280 <> SR240	Tab, Film Coated	Verapamil HCl 240 mg	by Major	00904-7957	Antihypertensive
Z4280 <> SR240	Tab, Film Coated	Verapamil HCl 240 mg	by Moore	00839-7670	Antihypertensive
Z4280 <> SR240	Tab, Film Coated	Verapamil HCl 240 mg	by Qualitest	00603-6360	Antihypertensive
Z4280 <> SR240	Tab, Film Coated	Verapamil HCl 240 mg	by Warner Chilcott	00047-0474	Antihypertensive
Z4280 <> SR240	Tab, Film Coated	Verapamil HCl 240 mg	by Med Pro	53978-2029	Antihypertensive
Z4286 <> SR180	Tab, Film Coated	Verapamil HCl 180 mg	Verelan by Major	00904-7956	Antihypertensive
Z4286 <> SR180	Tab, Film Coated	Verapamil HCl 180 mg	Verelan by Warner Chilcott	00047-0472	Antihypertensive
Z4286 <> SR180	Tab, Film Coated	Verapamil 180 mg	by Qualitest	00603-6359	Antihypertensive
Z4361	Tab, White, Oval, Z-4361	Flurbiprofen 50 mg	Ansaid by Ivax	00172-4361	NSAID
Z4362	Tab, Green, Oval, Z-4362	Flurbiprofen 100 mg	Ansaid by Ivax	00182-2621	NSAID
Z4362	Tab, Green, Oval, Z-4362	Flurbiprofen 100 mg	Ansaid by Ivax	00172-4362	NSAID
Z4761CEFACLOR500MG	Cap	Cefaclor 500 mg	Ceclor CD by Ivax	00172-4761	Antibiotic
Z4804	Cap, Blue & White, Black Print	Oxazepam 10 mg	Serax by Ivax	00172-4804	Sedative/Hypnotic; C IV
Z4804	Cap, Blue & White, Black Print	Oxazepam 10 mg	Serax by Qualitest	00603-4950	Sedative/Hypnotic; C IV
Z4805	Cap, White, Black Print	Oxazepam 15 mg	Serax by Ivax	00182-1231	Sedative/Hypnotic; C IV
Z4805	Cap, White, Black Print	Oxazepam 15 mg	Serax by Ivax	00172-4805	Sedative/Hypnotic; C IV
Z4805	Cap, White, Black Print	Oxazepam 15 mg	Serax by UDL	51079-0478	Sedative/Hypnotic; C IV
Z4805	Cap, White, Black Print	Oxazepam 15 mg	Serax by Qualitest	00603-4951	Sedative/Hypnotic; C IV

ID FRONT <> BACK	DESCRIPTION FRONT <> BACK	INGREDIENT & STRENGTH	BRAND (or Generic Equiv.) by FIRM	NDC#	CLASS; SCH.
Z4806	Cap, Orange & White	Oxazepam 30 mg	Serax by UDL	51079-0479	Sedative/Hypnotic; C IV
Z4806	Cap, Orange & White	Oxazepam 30 mg	Serax by Qualitest	00603-4952	Sedative/Hypnotic; C IV
Z4806	Cap, Orange & White	Oxazepam 30 mg	Serax by Ivax	00172-4806	Sedative/Hypnotic; C IV
Z4811	Cap, Red/Gray	Aspirin 389 mg, Caffeine 32.4 mg, Propoxyphene 65 mg	Darvon Compound 65 by Ivax	00172-4811	Analgesic; C IV
Z4835	Tab	Alprazolam 0.25 mg	Xanax by Ivax	00182-0027	Antianxiety; C IV
Z4835025	Tab, White, Round, Z 4835/0.25	Alprazolam 0.25 mg	Xanax by Ivax	00172-4835	Antianxiety; C IV
Z483605	Tab, Peach, Round, Z 4836/0.5	Alprazolam 0.5 mg	Xanax by Ivax	00172-4836	Antianxiety; C IV
Z48371	Tab, Blue, Round, Z 4837/1	Alprazolam 1 mg	Xanax by Ivax	00172-4837/1	Antianxiety; C IV
Z4845ZENITH	Tab, White, Rectangular, Z 4845/Zenith	Alprazolam 2 mg	Xanax by Ivax	00172-4845	Antianxiety; C IV
Z5	Tab, White, Round	Zolmitriptan 5 mg	Zomig by AstraZeneca	00310-0213	Antimigraine
Z5	Tab, White, Round, Cobalt Logo <> Z 5	Zopiclone 5 mg	Imovane by Cobalt	Canadian DIN 02271931	Hypnotic
Z5	Tab, White to Off-White, Round	Amlodipine Besylate 10 mg	Norvasc by Zydus	68382-0123	Antihypertensive
Z5 <> P	Tab, White, Round	Zopiclone 5 mg	Imovane by Pharmascience	Canadian DIN 02243426	Hypnotic
Z50MG2130	Cap, Zenith Logo	Nitrofurantoin 50 mg	by Apotheca	12634-0181	Antibiotic
Z52941	Tab, Lavender, Round, Z-5 2941	Trifluoperazine HCl 5 mg	Stelazine by Ivax	00172-2941	Antipsychotic
Z5600	Tab, White, Round	Lorazepam 0.5 mg	Ativan by Ivax	00172-5600	Antianxiety; C IV
Z5800	Tab, White, Round	Lorazepam 1 mg	Ativan by Ivax	00172-5800	Antianxiety; C IV
Z6000	Tab, White, Round	Lorazepam 2 mg	Ativan by Ivax	00172-6000	Antianxiety; C IV
Z6100	Tab, Lavender, Round	Hydroxyzine HCl 10 mg	Atarax by Ivax	00172-6100	Antianxiety; Antihistamine
Z6200	Tab, Magenta, Round	Hydroxyzine HCl 25 mg	Atarax by Ivax	00172-6200	Antianxiety; Antihistamine
Z6300	Tab, Purple, Round	Hydroxyzine HCl 50 mg	Atarax by Ivax	00172-6300	Antianxiety; Antihistamine
Z66	Tab, White to Off-White, Round, Scored, Z / 66	Atenolol 50 mg	Tenormin by Zydus	68382-0023	Antihypertensive
Z66	Tab, White to Off-White, Round, Scored, Z / 66	Atenolol 50 mg	Tenormin by Mallinckrodt	00406-2023	Antihypertensive
Z67	Tab, White to Off-White, Round	Atenolol 100 mg	Tenormin by Mallinckrodt	00406-2024	Antihypertensive
Z67	Tab, White to Off-White, Round	Atenolol 100 mg	Tenormin by Zydus	68382-0024	Antihypertensive
Z71	Tab, White to Off-White, Oval, Film Coated, Scored	Metformin HCl 1000 mg	Glucophage by Zydus	68382-0030	Antidiabetic
Z71	Tab, White to Off-White, Oval, Film Coated, Scored	Metformin HCl 1000 mg	Glucophage by Mallinckrodt	00406-2030	Antidiabetic
Z75	Tab, Blue, Oval, Scored, Cobalt Logo <> Z / 7.5	Zopiclone 7.5 mg	Imovane by Cobalt	Canadian DIN 02271958	Hypnotic
Z8	Tab, White, Round, Orally Disintegrating	Ondansetron 8 mg	Zofran ODT by GSK	00173-0570	Antiemetic
Z800 <> 7711	Tab, White, Oval, Scored, Z over 800	Cimetidine HCl 800 mg	Tagamet by Ivax	00172-7711	Gastrointestinal
Z800 <> 7711	Tab, White, Oval, Scored, Z over 800	Cimetidine HCl 800 mg	Tagamet by Direct Dispensing	57866-6753	Gastrointestinal
Z800 <> 7711	Tab, White, Oval, Z over 800	Cimetidine HCl 800 mg	Tagamet by Golden State	60429-0048	Gastrointestinal
Z800 <> 7711	Tab, White, Oval, Scored, Z over 800	Cimetidine HCl 800 mg	Tagamet by Ivax	00182-1986	Gastrointestinal
Z800 <> 7711	Tab, White to Off White, Oval Shaped, Scored	Cimetidine 800 mg	Tagamet by Teva	00172-7711	Gastrointestinal
ZA <> 74	Tab, White	Terazosin 1 mg	by AltiMed	Canadian DIN 02218941	Antihypertensive
ZA1200MG	Cap, White, Black Ink, ZA-12 over 200 mg	Ribavirin 200 mg	Rebetol by Mallinckrodt	00406-2260	Antiviral
ZA1200MG	Cap, White, Black Ink, ZA-12 over 200 mg	Ribavirin 200 mg	Rebetol by Zydus	68382-0260	Antiviral
ZA175MG	Cap, White Body, Tan Cap, Hard Gelatin Filled With White to Off White Powder	Bromocriptine Mesylate 5 mg	Parlodel by Zydus	68382-0110	Antiparkinson
ZA19	Tab, White, Oval, Film Coated, Black Ink	Simvastatin 5 mg	Zocor by Zydus	68382-0065	Antihyperlipidemic
ZA19	Tab, White, Oval	Simvastatin 5 mg	Zocor by Mallinckrodt	00406-2065	Antihyperlipidemic
ZA20	Tab, Pink, Oval, Film Coated, Black Ink	Simvastatin 10 mg	Zocor by Zydus	68382-0066	Antihyperlipidemic
ZA20	Tab, Pink, Oval	Simvastatin 10 mg	Zocor by Mallinckrodt	00406-2066	Antihyperlipidemic
ZA21	Tab, Brown, Oval, Film Coated, Black Ink	Simvastatin 20 mg	Zocor by Zydus	68382-0067	Antihyperlipidemic
ZA21	Tab, Brown, Oval	Simvastatin 20 mg	Zocor by Mallinckrodt	00406-2067	Antihyperlipidemic
ZA22	Tab, Pink, Oval, Film Coated, Black Ink	Simvastatin 40 mg	Zocor by Zydus	68382-0068	Antihyperlipidemic

ID FRONT <> BACK	DESCRIPTION FRONT <> BACK	INGREDIENT & STRENGTH	BRAND (or Generic Equiv.) by FIRM	NDC#	CLASS; SCH.
ZA22	Tab, Pink, Oval	Simvastin 40 mg	Zocor by Mallinckrodt	00406-2068	Antihyperlipidemic
ZA23	Tab, White to Off-White, Cap Shaped, Film Coated, Black Ink	Simvastatin 80 mg	Zocor by Zydus	68382-0069	Antihyperlipidemic
ZA23	Tab, White, Capsule Shaped	Simvastin 80 mg	Zocor by Mallinckrodt	00406-2069	Antihyperlipidemic
ZA66125MG	Cap, White Body, Blue Cap, Hard Gelatin, Filled With White to Off White Pellets	Divalproex Sodium 125 mg	Depakote by Zydus	68382-0106	Anticonvulsant
ZADITEN	Tab, White, Round, Scored	Ketotifen Fumarate 1 mg	Zaditen by Novartis	Canadian DIN 00577308	Antiasthmatic
ZANTAC150 <> 427	Tab, Effervescent	Ranitidine HCl 168 mg	Zantac Efferdose by GSK	60937-0427	Gastrointestinal
ZANTAC150 <> 427	Tab, White to Yellow, Round, Effervescent	Ranitidine HCl 150 mg	Zantac Efferdose by GSK	00173-0427	Gastrointestinal
ZANTAC150 <> 427	Tab, White to Yellow, Round, Effervescent	Ranitidine HCl 150 mg	Zantac Efferdose by GSK	00173-0427	Gastrointestinal
ZANTAC150 <> GLAXO	Tab, Peach, Pentagon, Film Coated	Ranitidine HCl 150 mg	Zantac by Amerisource	62584-0488	Gastrointestinal
ZANTAC150 <> GLAXO	Tab, Peach, Pentagon, Film Coated	Ranitidine HCl 150 mg	Zantac by Med Pro	53978-2075	Gastrointestinal
ZANTAC150 <> GLAXO	Tab, Peach, Pentagon, Film Coated	Ranitidine HCl 150 mg	Zantac by Nat Pharmpak	55154-1110	Gastrointestinal
ZANTAC150 <> GLAXO	Tab, Peach, Pentagon, Film Coated	Ranitidine HCl 150 mg	Zantac by Rx Dispensing	61807-0054	Gastrointestinal
ZANTAC150 <> GLAXO	Tab, Peach, Pentagon, Film Coated	Ranitidine HCl 150 mg	Zantac by Nat Pharmpak	55154-1107	Gastrointestinal
ZANTAC150 <> GLAXO	Tab, Peach, Pentagon, Film Coated	Ranitidine HCl 150 mg	Zantac by GSK	00173-0344	Gastrointestinal
ZANTAC150 <> GLAXO	Tab, Peach, Pentagon, Film Coated	Ranitidine HCl 150 mg	Zantac by Pharmedix	53002-0552	Gastrointestinal
ZANTAC150 <> GLAXO	Tab, Peach, Pentagon, Film Coated	Ranitidine HCl 150 mg	Zantac by Kaiser	00179-1079	Gastrointestinal
ZANTAC150 <> GLAXO	Tab, Peach, Pentagon, Film Coated	Ranitidine HCl 150 mg	Zantac by RX Pak	65084-0183	Gastrointestinal
ZANTAC150 <> GLAXO	Tab, White, Round, Glaxo <> Zantac/150	Ranitidine HCl 150 mg	Zantac by GSK	Canadian DIN 02212331	Gastrointestinal
ZANTAC150427	Tab, White, Tab-Yellow, Round, Zantac 150/427	Ranitidine HCl 150 mg	Zantac 150 EFFER by GSK	00173-0422	Gastrointestinal
ZANTAC150GLAXO	Cap, Beige, Zantac 150/Glaxo	Ranitidine HCl 150 mg	Zantac 150 GEL by GSK		Gastrointestinal
ZANTAC150-GLAXOWELLCOME	Cap, Blue Ink, Blue Ink	Ranitidine HCl 150 mg	Zantac Geldose by GSK	00173-0428	Gastrointestinal
ZANT AC150-GLAXOWELLCOME	Cap, Blue Ink, Blue Ink	Ranitidine HCl 150 mg	Zantac Geldose by GSK	00173-0481	Gastrointestinal
ZANTAC300 <> GLAXO	Tab, Film Coated	Ranitidine HCl 300 mg	by Kaiser	00179-1211	Gastrointestinal
ZANTAC300 <> GLAXO	Tab, Yellow, Cap Shaped, Film Coated	Ranitidine HCl 300 mg	Zantac by GSK	00173-0393	Gastrointestinal
ZANTAC300 <> GLAXO	Tab	Ranitidine HCl 336 mg	Zantac by Pharmedix	53002-1028	Gastrointestinal
ZANTAC300 <> GLAXO	Tab	Ranitidine HCl 336 mg	by Allscripts		Gastrointestinal
ZANTAC300 <> GLAXO	Tab, Embossed	Ranitidine HCl 336 mg	by Amerisource	62584-0393	Gastrointestinal
ZANTAC300 <> GLAXO	Tab, White, Oblong, Glaxo <> Zantac 300	Ranitidine HCl 300 mg	Zantac by GSK	Canadian DIN 02212358	Gastrointestinal
ZANTAC300GLAXO	Cap, Beige, Zantac 300/Glaxo	Ranitidine HCl 300 mg	Zantac 300 GEL by Prescript	00247-1311	Gastrointestinal
ZANT AC300-GLAXOWELLCOME	Cap, Blue Ink	Ranitidine HCl 300 mg	Zantac Geldose by GSK	00173-0429	Gastrointestinal
ZANTACC150	Cap, Beige, Zantac-C/150	Ranitidine HCl 168 mg	Zantac by GSK	Canadian	Gastrointestinal
ZANTACC300	Cap, Beige, Zantac-C/300	Ranitidine HCl 300 mg	Zantac by GSK	Canadian	Gastrointestinal
ZAROXOLYN	Tab, Blue	Metolazone 5 mg	Zaroxolyn by RPR	Canadian	Diuretic
ZAROXOLYN <> 10	Tab, Yellow	Metolazone 10 mg	Zaroxolyn by Medeva	53014-0835	Diuretic
ZAROXOLYN <> 212	Tab, Pink, Round	Metolazone 2.5 mg	Zaroxolyn by Compumed	00403-1597	Diuretic
ZAROXOLYN <> 212	Tab, Zaroxolyn <> 2 1/2	Metolazone 2.5 mg	Zaroxolyn by Prestige	58056-0355	Diuretic
ZAROXOLYN <> 212	Tab, Zaroxolyn <> 2 1/2	Metolazone 2.5 mg	Zaroxolyn by Amerisource		Diuretic
ZAROXOLYN <> 212	Tab, Zaroxolyn <> 2 1/2	Metolazone 2.5 mg	Zaroxolyn by Nat Pharmpak	55154-2504	Diuretic
ZAROXOLYN <> 212	Tab, Zaroxolyn <> 2 1/2	Metolazone 2.5 mg	Zaroxolyn by Caremark	00339-5426	Diuretic
ZAROXOLYN <> 212	Tab, Pink, Round, Convex	Metolazone 2.5 mg	Zaroxolyn by Neuman	64579-0053	Diuretic
ZAROXOLYN <> 212	Tab, Pink, Zaroxolyn <> 2 1/2	Metolazone 2.5 mg	Zaroxolyn by Medeva	53014-0975	Diuretic
ZAROXOLYN <> 25	Tab, Zaroxolyn <> 2.5	Metolazone 2.5 mg	Zaroxolyn by Drug Distr	52985-0218	Diuretic
ZAROXOLYN <> 5	Tab, Blue, Round	Metolazone 5 mg	Zaroxolyn by Neuman	64579-0057	Diuretic

ID FRONT <> BACK	DESCRIPTION FRONT <> BACK	INGREDIENT & STRENGTH	BRAND (or Generic Equiv.) by FIRM	NDC#	CLASS; SCH.
ZAROXOLYN <> 5	Tab, Blue, Round	Metolazone 5 mg	Zaroxolyn by Caremark	00339-5428	Diuretic
ZAROXOLYN <> 5	Tab, Blue, Round	Metolazone 5 mg	Zaroxolyn by Medeva	53014-0850	Diuretic
ZAROXOLYN <> 5	Tab, Blue, Round	Metolazone 5 mg	Zaroxolyn by Nat Pharmpak	55154-2505	Diuretic
ZAROXOLYN <> 5	Tab, Blue, Round	Metolazone 5 mg	Zaroxolyn by Prestige	58056-0356	Diuretic
ZAROXOLYN <> 5	Tab, Blue, Round	Metolazone 5 mg	Zaroxolyn by Amerisource	62584-0850	Diuretic
ZAROXOLYN <> 5	Tab, Blue, Round	Metolazone 5 mg	Zaroxolyn by Compumed	00403-1603	Diuretic
ZB <> 74	Tab, Orange	Terazosin HCl 2 mg	Hytrin by AltiMed	Canadian DIN 02218968	Antihypertensive
ZBECAHR	Tab, Green, Elliptical, Zbec/AHR	Therapeutic B-Complex Zinc & Vitamin E	Zbec by Whitehall Robins		Vitamin
ZBN	Tab, White, Round, Film Coated	Leflunomide 10 mg	Arava by Aventis	Canadian DIN 02241888	Antiarthritic
ZBN	Tab, White, Round, Film Coated	Leflunomide 10 mg	Arava by Aventis	00088-2160	Antiarthritic
ZBN	Tab, White, Round, Film Coated	Leflunomide 10 mg	Arava by Aventis	12579-0509	Antiarthritic
ZBO	Tab, Yellow, Triangle, Film Coated	Leflunomide 20 mg	Arava by Aventis	00088-2161	Antiarthritic
ZBO	Tab, Yellow, Triangle, Film Coated	Leflunomide 20 mg	Arava by Aventis	12579-0510	Antiarthritic
ZBO	Tab, Yellow, Triangle, Film Coated	Leflunomide 20 mg	Arava by Aventis	Canadian DIN 02241889	Antiarthritic
ZBP	Tab, White, Round, Film Coated	Leflunomide 100 mg	Arava by Aventis	Canadian DIN 02241890	Antiarthritic
ZBP	Tab, White, Round, Film Coated	Leflunomide 100 mg	Arava by Aventis	00088-2162	Antiarthritic
ZBP	Tab, White, Round, Film Coated	Leflunomide 100 mg	Arava by Aventis	12579-0511	Antiarthritic
ZC <> 74	Tab, Tan	Terazosin 5 mg	by AltiMed	Canadian DIN 02218976	Antihypertensive
ZC01	Tab, White, Scored, Round, "Z C" over "0 1"	Promethazine 12.5 mg	Phenergan by Zydus	68382-0040	Antiemetic; Antihistamine
ZC01	Tab, White, Scored, Round, "Z C" over "0 1"	Promethazine 12.5 mg	Phenergan by Mallinckrodt	00406-2040	Antiemetic; Antihistamine
ZC02	Tab, White, Round, Scored, "Z / C" over "0 / 2"	Promethazine 25 mg	Phenergan by Mallinckrodt	00406-2041	Antiemetic; Antihistamine
ZC02	Tab, White, Round, Scored, "Z / C" over "0 / 2"	Promethazine 25 mg	Phenergan by Zydus	68382-0041	Antiemetic; Antihistamine
ZC02	Tab, White, Round, Scored, "Z / C" over "0 / 2"	Promethazine HCl 25 mg	Phenergan by UDL	51079-0895	Antiemetic; Antihistamine
ZC03	Tab, White, Round, "Z C" over "0 3"	Promethazine 50 mg	Phenergan by Zydus	68382-0042	Antiemetic; Antihistamine
ZC03	Tab, White, Round, "Z C" over "0 3"	Promethazine 50 mg	Phenergan by Mallinckrodt	00406-2042	Antiemetic; Antihistamine
ZC08	Tab, Light Green, Capsule Shaped	Haloperidol 10 mg	Haldol by Mallinckrodt	00406-2080	Antipsychotic
ZC08	Tab, Light Green, Cap Shaped, Scored	Haloperidol 10 mg	Haloperidol by Zydus	68382-0080	Antipsychotic
ZC09	Tab, Pink, Cap Shaped, Scored	Haloperidol 20 mg	Haloperidol by Zydus	68382-0081	Antipsychotic
ZC09	Tab, Coral, Capsule Shaped	Haloperidol 20 mg	Haldol by Mallinckrodt	00406-2081	Antipsychotic
ZC15	Tab, White to Off White, Round	Paroxetine 10 mg	Paxil IR by Mallinckrodt	00406-2097	Antidepressant
ZC15	Tab, White, Round, Scored, Film Coated, ZC / 15	Paroxetine 10mg	Paxil by Zydus	68382-0097	Antidepressant
ZC16	Tab, White, Round, Scored, Film Coated, ZC / 16	Paroxetine 20 mg	Paxil by Zydus	68382-0098	Antidepressant
ZC16	Tab, White to Off White, Round	Paroxetine 20 mg	Paxil IR by Mallinckrodt	00406-2098	Antidepressant
ZC17	Tab, White to Off White, Round	Paroxetine 30 mg	Paxil IR by Mallinckrodt	00406-2099	Antidepressant
ZC17	Tab, White to Off-White, Round, Film Coated	Paroxetine 30 mg	Paxil by Zydus	68382-0099	Antidepressant
ZC18	Tab, White to Off-White, Round, Film Coated	Paroxetine 40 mg	Paxil by Zydus	68382-0100	Antidepressant
ZC18	Tab, White to Off White, Round	Paroxetine 40 mg	Paxil IR by Mallinckrodt	00406-2001	Antidepressant
ZC19	Tab, Pink, Round, Film Coated	Ribavirin 200 mg	Copegus by Mallinckrodt	00406-2046	Antiviral
ZC19	Tab, Pink, Round, Film Coated	Ribavirin 200 mg	Copegus by Zydus	68382-0046	Antiviral
ZC25	Tab, Yellow, Round	Meloxicam 7.5 mg	Mobic by Zydus	68382-0050	NSAID
ZC25	Tab, Yellow, Round	Meloxicam 7.5 mg	Mobic by Mallinckrodt	00406-2050	NSAID
ZC26	Tab, Yellow, Round, ZC over 26	Meloxicam 15 mg	Mobic by Zydus	68382-0051	NSAID
ZC26	Tab, Yellow, Round	Meloxicam 15 mg	Mobic by Mallinckrodt	00406-2051	NSAID
ZC38	Tab, White to Off White, Capsule Shaped	Hydroxychloroquine Sulfate	Plaquenil by Mallinckrodt	00406-2096	00406-2096
ZC38	Tab, White to Off White, Cap Shaped, Film Coated	Hydroxychloroquine Sulfate 200 mg	Plaquenil by Zydus	68382-0096	Antimalarial

ID FRONT <> BACK	DESCRIPTION FRONT <> BACK	INGREDIENT & STRENGTH	BRAND (or Generic Equiv.) by FIRM	NDC#	CLASS; SCH.
ZC40	Tab, White to Off-White, Round, Film Coated	Carvedilol 6.25 mg	Coreg by Zydus	68382-0093	Antihypertensive
ZC41	Tab, White, Round	Carvedilol 12.5 mg	Coreg by Zydus	68382-0094	Antihypertensive
ZC42	Tab, White to Off White, Round, Film Coated	Carvedilol 25 mg	Coreg by Zydus	68382-0095	Antihypertensive
ZC59	Tab, Yellow, Round, Scored	Azathioprine 50 mg	Imuran by Zydus	68382-0003	Immunosuppressant
ZC59	Tab, Yellow, Round	Azathioprine 50 mg	Imuran by Mallinckrodt	00406-2003	Immunosuppressant
ZC64	Tab, Peach, Round, Scored	Venlafaxine HCl 25 mg	Effexor by Zydus	68382-0018	Antidepressant
ZC65	Tab, Peach, Round, Scored	Venlafaxine HCl 37.5 mg	Effexor by Zydus	68382-0019	Antidepressant
ZC66	Tab, Peach, Round, Scored	Venlafaxine HCl 50 mg	Effexor by Zydus	68382-0020	Antidepressant
ZC67	Tab, Peach, Round, Scored	Venlafaxine HCl 75 mg	Effexor by Zydus	68382-0021	Antidepressant
ZC68	Tab, Peach, Round, Scored	Venlafaxine HCl 100 mg	Effexor by Zydus	68382-0101	Antidepressant
ZC75	Tab, White to Off-White, Round, Film Coated	Risperidone 1 mg	Risperdal by Zydus	68382-0114	Antipsychotic
ZC76	Tab, Orange, Round, Film Coated	Risperidone 2 mg	Risperdal by Zydus	68382-0115	Antipsychotic
ZC77	Tab, Yellow, Round, Film Coated	Risperidone 3 mg	Risperdal by Zydus	68382-0116	Antipsychotic
ZC78	Tab, Green, Round, Film Coated	Risperidone 4 mg	Risperdal by Zydus	68382-0117	Antipsychotic
ZC79	Tab, White to Off White, Round	Lamotrigine 25 mg	Lamictal by Zydus	68382-0006	Anticonvulsant
ZC80	Tab, White to Off White, Round	Lamotrigine 100 mg	Lamictal by Zydus	68382-0008	Anticonvulsant
ZC81	Tab, White to Off White, Round	Lamotrigine 150 mg	Lamictal by Zydus	68382-0009	Anticonvulsant
ZC82	Tab, White to Off White, Round	Lamotrigine 200 mg	Lamictal by Zydus	68382-0010	Anticonvulsant
ZD <> 74	Tab, Blue	Terazosin 10 mg	by AltiMed	Canadian DIN 02218984	Antihypertensive
ZD13	Tab, White, Round	Topiramate 200 mg	Topamax by Zydus	68382-0141	Anticonvulsant
ZD14	Tab, White, Round	Topiramate 100 mg	Topamax by Zydus	68382-0140	Anticonvulsant
ZD15	Tab, White, Round	Topiramate 50 mg	Topamax by Zydus	68382-0139	Anticonvulsant
ZD16	Tab, White, Round	Topiramate 25 mg	Topamax by Zydus	68382-0138	Anticonvulsant
ZD4522 <> 40	Tab, Pink, Oval, Coated	Rosuvastatin 40 mg	Crestor by AstraZeneca	Canadian DIN 02247164	Antihyperlipidemic
ZD4522 <> 40	Tab, Pink, Oval, Coated	Rosuvastatin 40 mg	Crestor by AstraZeneca	00310-0754	Antihyperlipidemic
ZD452210	Tab, Pink, Round, Coated	Rosuvastatin 10 mg	Crestor by AstraZeneca	00310-0751	Antihyperlipidemic
ZD452210	Tab, Pink, Round, Coated	Rosuvastatin 10 mg	Crestor by AstraZeneca	Canadian DIN 02247162	Antihyperlipidemic
ZD452220	Tab, Pink, Round, Coated	Rosuvastatin 20 mg	Crestor by AstraZeneca	00310-0752	Antihyperlipidemic
ZD452220	Tab, Pink, Round, Coated	Rosuvastatin 20 mg	Crestor by AstraZeneca	Canadian DIN 02247163	Antihyperlipidemic
ZD45225	Tab, Yellow, Round, Coated	Rosuvastatin 5 mg	Crestor by AstraZeneca	00310-0755	Antihyperlipidemic
ZD45225	Tab, Yellow, Round, Coated	Rosuvastatin 5 mg	Crestor by AstraZeneca	Canadian DIN 02265540	Antihyperlipidemic
ZEE <> HF	Tab, Bright Orange, Round, ZEE <> H/F	Acetaminophen 325 mg, Dextromethorphan 10 mg, Pseudoephedrine 30 mg	Histenol Forte by Zee		Cold Remedy
ZE <> 74	Tab, Film Coated	Erythromycin 500 mg	by Quality Care	60346-0646	Antibiotic
ZE43	Tab, Light Yellow, Round	Dipyridamole 25 mg	Persantine by Zydus	68382-0187	Antiplatelet
ZE43	Tab, Light Yellow, Round, Film Coated	Dipyridamole 25 mg	Persantine by Mallinckrodt	00406-2187	Antiplatelet
ZE4760	Cap, Zenith Logo	Cefaclor 250 mg	Ceclor by Quality Care	60346-0202	Antibiotic
ZE49	Tab, Light Yellow, Round, Film Coated	Dipyridamole 50 mg	Persantine by Mallinckrodt	00406-2188	Antiplatelet
ZE49	Tab, Light Yellow, Round, Film Coated	Dipyridamole 50 mg	Persantine by Zydus	68382-0188	Antiplatelet
ZE50	Tab, Light Yellow, Round, Film-Coated	Dipyridamole 75 mg	Persantine by Zydus	68382-0189	Antiplatelet
ZE50	Tab, Light Yellow, Round, Film Coated	Dipyridamole 75 mg	Persantine by Mallinckrodt	00406-2189	Antiplatelet
ZELODA500	Tab, Peach, Oblong, Zeloda/500	Capecitabine 500 mg	Xeloda by Roche	Canadian	Antineoplastic
ZEN50MG2130	Cap, Zenith Logo	Nitrofurantoin 50 mg	by Quality Care	60346-0616	Antibiotic
ZENECA <> ACCOLATE20	Tab, White to Off-White, Round, Film-Coated	Zafirlukast 20 mg	Accolate by AstraZeneca	Canadian DIN 02236606	Antiasthmatic
ZENECA10 <> 891	Tab, Ex Release	Nisoldipine 10 mg	Sular by Bayer	12527-0891	Antihypertensive

ID FRONT <> BACK	DESCRIPTION FRONT <> BACK	INGREDIENT & STRENGTH	BRAND (or Generic Equiv.) by FIRM	NDC#	CLASS; SCH.
ZENECA10 <> 891	Tab, Oyster, Round, Film Coated, Ex Release	Nisoldipine 10 mg	Sular by AstraZeneca	00310-0891	Antihypertensive
ZENECA20 <> 892	Tab, Dark Yellow, Round	Nisoldipine 20 mg	by Murfreesboro	51129-1278	Antihypertensive
ZENECA20 <> 892	Tab, Dark Yellow, Round, Film Coated, Ex Release	Nisoldipine 20 mg	Sular by AstraZeneca	00310-0892	Antihypertensive
ZENECA20 <> 892	Tab, Dark Yellow, Round	Nisoldipine 20 mg	Sular by Bayer	12527-0892	Antihypertensive
ZENECA30 <> 893	Tab, Mustard, Round, Film Coated, Ex Release	Nisoldipine 30 mg	Sular by AstraZeneca	00310-0893	Antihypertensive
ZENECA30 <> 893	Tab, Mustard Yellow, Zeneca 30 <> 893 Underlined	Nisoldipine 30 mg	by Murfreesboro	51129-1334	Antihypertensive
ZENECA30 <> 893	Tab	Nisoldipine 30 mg	Sular by Bayer	12527-0893	Antihypertensive
ZENECA40 <> 894	Tab, Burnt Orange, Round, Film Coated, Ex Release	Nisoldipine 40 mg	Sular by AstraZeneca	00310-0894	Antihypertensive
ZENECA40 <> 894	Tab	Nisoldipine 40 mg	Sular by Bayer	12527-0894	Antihypertensive
ZENITH100MG2131	Cap, Light Pink, Black Print, Zenith over 100 mg over 2131 over 3 Black Lines	Nitrofurantoin 100 mg	Macrodantin by Direct Dispensing	57866-6590	Antibiotic
ZENITH100MG2131	Cap, Light Pink, Black Print, Zenith over 100 mg over 2131 over 3 Black Lines	Nitrofurantoin 100 mg	Macrodantin by H J Harkins Co	52959-0405	Antibiotic
ZENITH100MG2131	Cap, Light Pink, Black Print, Zenith over 100 mg over 2131 over 3 Black Lines	Nitrofurantoin 100 mg	Macrodantin by Prepackage Specialists	58864-0371	Antibiotic
ZENITH100MG2131	Cap, Light Pink, Black Print, Zenith over 100 mg over 2131 over 3 Black Lines	Nitrofurantoin 100 mg	Macrodantin by Thrift Drug	59198-0243	Antibiotic
ZENITH100MG2131	Cap, Light Pink, Black Print, Zenith over 100 mg over 2131 over 3 Black Lines	Nitrofurantoin 100 mg	Macrodantin by Medirex	57480-0817	Antibiotic
ZENITH100MG2131	Cap, Light Pink, Black Print, Zenith over 100 mg over 2131 over 3 Black Lines	Nitrofurantoin 100 mg	Macrodantin by Teva	00093-2131	Antibiotic
ZENITH200MG4171	Cap, Off-White, Black Print, Zenith over 200 mg over 4171	Quinine Sulfate 200 mg	Quinamm by Ivax	00172-4171 Discontinued	Antimalarial
ZENITH20MG4288	Cap, White, Black Print, Zenith over 20 mg over 4288	Nicardipine HCl 20 mg	Cardene by Ivax	00172-4288	Antihypertensive
ZENITH30MG4289	Cap, Light Blue, Black Print, Zenith over 30 mg over 4289	Nicardipine HCl 30 mg	Cardene by Ivax	00172-4289	Antihypertensive
ZENITH405800	Cap, Zenith Logo	Cefadroxil Monohydrate 500 mg	by Rx Dispensing	61807-0123	Antibiotic
ZENITH4266200	Cap, White, Black Print, Zenith over 4266 over 200	Acyclovir 200 mg	Zovirax by Ivax	00172-4266 Discontinued	Antiviral
ZENITH4266200	Cap, White, Black Print, Zenith over 4266 over 200	Acyclovir 200 mg	Zovirax by Murfreesboro	51129-1252	Antiviral
ZENITH4266200	Cap, White, Black Print, Zenith over 4266 over 200	Acyclovir 200 mg	Zovirax by Ivax	00182-2666 Discontinued	Antiviral
ZENITH4280	Tab, Off-White, Oblong	Verapamil 240 mg	Isoptin, Calan by Ivax		Antihypertensive
ZENITH4286	Tab, Off-White, Oval	Verapamil 180 mg	Isoptin, Calan by Ivax		Antihypertensive
ZENITH4760-CEFACLOR250	Cap	Cefaclor 250 mg	Ceclor by PDRX	55289-0749	Antibiotic
ZENITH500MG	Cap, Yellowish White Powder	Cefadroxil Monohydrate 500 mg	by Physician Total Care	54868-3742	Antibiotic
ZENITH500MG4058	Cap, Clear & White, Red Print, Zenith over 500 mg over 4058	Cefadroxil Monohydrate 500 mg	Duricef by Pharmedix	53002-0229	Antibiotic
ZENITH500MG4058	Cap, Clear & White, Red Print, Zenith over 500 mg over 4058	Cefadroxil Monohydrate 500 mg	Duricef by Caremark	00339-6155	Antibiotic
ZENITH500MG4058	Cap, Clear & White, Red Print, Zenith over 500 mg over 4058	Cefadroxil Monohydrate 500 mg	Duricef by H J Harkins Co	52959-0428	Antibiotic
ZENITH500MG4058	Cap, Clear & White, Red Print, Zenith over 500 mg over 4058	Cefadroxil Monohydrate 500 mg	Duricef by CVS	00894-5133	Antibiotic
ZENITH500MG4058	Cap, Clear & White, Red Print, Zenith over 500 mg over 4058	Cefadroxil Monohydrate 500 mg	Duricef by Ivax	00172-4058 Discontinued	Antibiotic
ZENITH50MG2130	Cap, Light Pink & White, Black Print, Zenith over 50 mg over 2130 over 2 Black Lines	Nitrofurantoin 50 mg	Macrodantin by Compumed	00403-1528	Antibiotic
ZENITH50MG2130	Cap, Light Pink & White, Black Print, Zenith over 50 mg over 2130 over 2 Black Lines	Nitrofurantoin 50 mg	Macrodantin by Caremark	00339-6037	Antibiotic

ID FRONT <> BACK	DESCRIPTION FRONT <> BACK	INGREDIENT & STRENGTH	BRAND (or Generic Equiv.) by FIRM	NDC#	CLASS; SCH.
ZENITH50MG2130	Cap, Light Pink & White, Black Print, Zenith over 50 mg over 2130 over 2 Black Lines	Nitrofurantoin 50 mg	Macrodantin by PDRX	55289-0055	Antibiotic
ZENITH50MG2130	Cap, Light Pink & White, Black Print, Zenith over 50 mg over 2130 over 2 Black Lines	Nitrofurantoin 50 mg	Macrodantin by Thrift Drug	59198-0242	Antibiotic
ZENITH50MG2130	Cap, Light Pink & White, Black Print, Zenith over 50 mg over 2130 over 2 Black Lines	Nitrofurantoin 50 mg	Macrodantin by Medirex	57480-0816	Antibiotic
ZENITH50MG2130	Cap, Light Pink & White, Black Print, Zenith over 50 mg over 2130 over 2 Black Lines	Nitrofurantoin 50 mg	Macrodantin by Teva	00093-2130	Antibiotic
ZER <> 4	Tab, White, Round, Scored	Carbinoxamine Maleate 4 mg	Palgic by Zerxis	18011-0674 Discontinued	Cold Remedy
ZESTORETIC	Tab, White, Round	Hydrochlorothiazide 12.5 mg, Lisinopril 20 mg	Zestoretic by AstraZeneca	Canadian DIN 02045737	Diuretic; Antihypertensive
ZESTORETIC	Tab, Peach, Round	Hydrochlorothiazide 25 mg, Lisinopril 20 mg	Zestoretic by AstraZeneca	Canadian DIN 02045729	Diuretic; Antihypertensive
ZESTORETIC <> 141	Tab, Peach, Round	Hydrochlorothiazide 12.5 mg, Lisinopril 10 mg	Zestoretic by AstraZeneca	00310-0141	Diuretic; Antihypertensive
ZESTORETIC <> 141	Tab, Peach, Round	Hydrochlorothiazide 12.5 mg, Lisinopril 10 mg	Zestoretic by IPR	54921-0141	Diuretic; Antihypertensive
ZESTORETIC <> 142	Tab, White, Round	Hydrochlorothiazide 12.5 mg, Lisinopril 20 mg	Zestoretic by AstraZeneca	00310-0142	Diuretic; Antihypertensive
ZESTORETIC <> 142	Tab, White, Round	Hydrochlorothiazide 12.5 mg, Lisinopril 20 mg	Zestoretic by IPR	54921-0142	Diuretic; Antihypertensive
ZESTORETIC <> 145	Tab, Peach, Round	Hydrochlorothiazide 25 mg, Lisinopril 20 mg	Zestoretic by Zeneca	00310-0145	Diuretic; Antihypertensive
ZESTORETIC <> 145	Tab, Peach, Round	Hydrochlorothiazide 25 mg, Lisinopril 20 mg	Zestoretic by IPR	54921-0145	Diuretic; Antihypertensive
ZESTRIL <> 130	Tab, Pink, Cap Shaped, Scored	Lisinopril 5 mg	Prinivil by Kaiser	00179-1168	Antihypertensive
ZESTRIL <> 130	Tab, Pink, Cap Shaped, Scored	Lisinopril 5 mg	Prinivil by Med Pro	53978-3063	Antihypertensive
ZESTRIL <> 130	Tab, Pink, Cap Shaped, Scored	Lisinopril 5 mg	Zestril by AstraZeneca	00310-0130	Antihypertensive
ZESTRIL10 <> 131	Tab, Pink, Round	Lisinopril 10 mg	Prinivil by Med Pro	53978-1000	Antihypertensive
ZESTRIL10 <> 131	Tab, Pink, Round	Lisinopril 10 mg	Prinivil by Kaiser	00179-1157	Antihypertensive
ZESTRIL10 <> 131	Tab, Pink, Round	Lisinopril 10 mg	Zestril by AstraZeneca	00310-0131	Antihypertensive
ZESTRIL20 <> 132	Tab, Red, Round	Lisinopril 20 mg	Zestril by AstraZeneca	00310-0132	Antihypertensive
ZESTRIL20 <> 132	Tab, Red, Round	Lisinopril 20 mg	Prinivil by Kaiser	00179-1169	Antihypertensive
ZESTRIL20 <> 132	Tab, Red, Round	Lisinopril 20 mg	Prinivil by Med Pro	53978-1017	Antihypertensive
ZESTRIL212 <> 135	Tab, White, Round	Lisinopril 2.5 mg	Zestril by AstraZeneca	00310-0135	Antihypertensive
ZESTRIL30 <> 133	Tab, Red, Round	Lisinopril 30 mg	Zestril by AstraZeneca	00310-0133	Antihypertensive
ZESTRIL40 <> 134	Tab, Yellow, Round	Lisinopril 40 mg	Prinivil by Kaiser	00179-1203	Antihypertensive
ZESTRIL40 <> 134	Tab, Yellow, Round	Lisinopril 40 mg	Zestril by AstraZeneca	00310-0134	Antihypertensive
ZINCATEPADDOCK	Cap, Orange & White, ZINCATE in White Print, PADDOCK in Orange Print	Zinc Sulfate 220 mg	Zincate by Paddock	00574-9167	Mineral
ZITHROMAXPFIZER	Cap, Red, Zithromax/Pfizer	Azithromycin 250 mg	Zithromax by Pfizer	Canadian	Antibiotic
ZL <> 600	Tab, White, Oval, Scored, Film Coated, Abbott Logo ZL	Zileuton 600 mg	by Murfreesboro	51129-1380	Antiasthmatic
ZLA <> SANOFI	Tab, Orange, Oval, Film Coated, Z / LA	Guaifenesin 600 mg, Pseudoephedrine HCl 120 mg	Zephrex LA by Sanofi	00024-2627	Cold Remedy
ZLP <> 10	Tab, Yellow, Round, Film Coated	Zolpidem Tartrate 10 mg	Ambien by Sandoz	00781-5318	Sedative/Hypnotic; C IV
ZLP <> 5	Tab, White, Round, Film Coated	Zolpidem Tartrate 5 mg	Ambien by Sandoz	00781-5317	Sedative/Hypnotic; C IV
ZM <> 10	Tab, White, Round, Film Coated	Zolpidem Tartrate 10 mg	Ambien by Genpharm	15330-0265	Sedative/Hypnotic; C IV
ZM <> 5	Tab, Pink, Round, Film Coated	Zolpidem Tartrate 5 mg	Ambien by Genpharm	15330-0264	Sedative/Hypnotic; C IV
ZM10 <> 5422	Tab, White, Cap-Shaped, Film-Coated	Zolpidem Tartrate 10 mg	Ambien by Prasco	66993-0716	Sedative/Hypnotic; C IV
ZM5 <> 5411	Tab, Pink, Cap-Shaped, Film-Coated	Zolpidem Tartrate 5 mg	Ambien by Prasco	66993-0715	Sedative/Hypnotic; C IV
ZOCOR5 <> MSD726	Tab, Buff, Oval, Film Coated	Simvastatin 5 mg	Zocor by Merck-Frosst	Canadian DIN 0884324	Antihyperlipidemic
ZOCOR5 <> MSD726	Tab, Buff, Shield Shaped, Film Coated, MSD over 726	Simvastatin 5 mg	Zocor by Merck	00006-0726	Antihyperlipidemic
ZOFRAN <> 4	Tab, White, Oval, Film	Ondansetron HCl 4 mg	Zofran by PDRX	55289-0480	Antiemetic
ZOFRAN <> 4	Tab, White, Oval, Film Coated	Ondansetron HCl 4 mg	Zofran by GSK	00173-0446	Antiemetic
ZOFRAN <> 8	Tab, Yellow, Oval, Film Coated	Ondansetron HCl 8 mg	Zofran by GSK	00173-0447	Antiemetic
ZOFRAN <> 8	Tab, Yellow, Oval, Film Coated	Ondansetron HCl 8 mg	Zofran by PDRX	55289-0478	Antiemetic

ID FRONT <> BACK	DESCRIPTION FRONT <> BACK	INGREDIENT & STRENGTH	BRAND (or Generic Equiv.) by FIRM	NDC#	CLASS; SCH.
ZOFRAN <> SAMPLE	Tab, Film Coated	Ondansetron HCl 8 mg	Zofran by GSK		Antiemetic
ZOFRAN <> SAMPLE	Tab	Ondansetron HCl 4 mg	Zofran by GSK		Antiemetic
ZOL5 <> APO	Tab, Pink, Cap Shaped, Film Coated	Zolpidem Tartrate 5 mg	Ambien by Apotex	60505-2604	Sedative/Hypnotic; C IV
ZOLLERTM	Cap, Blue	Supplement Blend 1312 mg (Yerba Mate, Caffeine, Guarana seed, Damiana, Schizonepeta, Green Tea, Piper Nigrum, Tibetan Ginseng, Panax Ginseng, Maca Root, Cocoa Nut, Kola Nut, Thea Sinensis Complex)	Zantrex-3 by Zoller Labs		Supplement
ZOLOFT <> 100MG	Tab, Light Yellow, Cap Shaped, Scored, Film Coated	Sertraline HCl 100 mg	Zoloft by Allscripts		Antidepressant
ZOLOFT <> 100MG	Tab, Light Yellow, Cap Shaped, Scored, Film Coated	Sertraline HCl 100 mg	Zoloft by DRX	55045-2208	Antidepressant
ZOLOFT <> 100MG	Tab, Light Yellow, Cap Shaped, Scored, Film Coated	Sertraline HCl 100 mg	Zoloft by Direct Dispensing	57866-6305	Antidepressant
ZOLOFT <> 100MG	Tab, Light Yellow, Cap Shaped, Scored, Film Coated	Sertraline HCl 100 mg	Zoloft by Amerisource	62584-0910	Antidepressant
ZOLOFT <> 100MG	Tab, Light Yellow, Cap Shaped, Scored, Film Coated	Sertraline HCl 100 mg	Zoloft by Heartland	61392-0939	Antidepressant
ZOLOFT <> 100MG	Tab, Light Yellow, Cap Shaped, Scored, Film Coated	Sertraline HCl 100 mg	Zoloft by Physician Total Care	54868-2637	Antidepressant
ZOLOFT <> 100MG	Tab, Light Yellow, Cap Shaped, Scored, Film Coated	Sertraline HCl 100 mg	Zoloft by Nat Pharmpak	55154-2712	Antidepressant
ZOLOFT <> 100MG	Tab, Light Yellow, Cap Shaped, Scored, Film Coated	Sertraline HCl 100 mg	Zoloft by Va Cmop	65243-0063	Antidepressant
ZOLOFT <> 100MG	Tab, Light Yellow, Cap Shaped, Scored, Film Coated	Sertraline HCl 100 mg	Zoloft by PDRX	55289-0550	Antidepressant
ZOLOFT <> 100MG	Tab, Light Yellow, Cap Shaped, Scored, Film Coated	Sertraline HCl 100 mg	Zoloft by Roerig	00049-4910	Antidepressant
ZOLOFT <> 25MG	Tab, Light Green, Cap Shaped, Scored, Film Coated	Sertraline HCl 25 mg	Zoloft by Murfreesboro	51129-1333	Antidepressant
ZOLOFT <> 25MG	Tab, Light Green, Cap Shaped, Scored, Film Coated	Sertraline HCl 25 mg	Zoloft by Pharmacy Care	65070-0210	Antidepressant
ZOLOFT <> 25MG	Tab, Light Green, Cap Shaped, Scored, Film Coated	Sertraline HCl 25 mg	Zoloft by Direct Dispensing	57866-1057	Antidepressant
ZOLOFT <> 25MG	Tab, Light Green, Cap Shaped, Scored, Film Coated	Sertraline HCl 25 mg	Zoloft by Roerig	00049-4960	Antidepressant
ZOLOFT <> 25MG	Tab, Light Green, Cap Shaped, Scored, Film Coated	Sertraline HCl 25 mg	Zoloft by Nat Pharmpak	55154-2709	Antidepressant
ZOLOFT <> 50MG	Tab, Light Blue, Cap Shaped, Scored, Film Coated	Sertraline HCl 50 mg	Zoloft by Roerig	00049-4900	Antidepressant
ZOLOFT <> 50MG	Tab, Light Blue, Cap Shaped, Scored, Film Coated	Sertraline HCl 50 mg	Zoloft by Pharmacy Care	65070-0035	Antidepressant
ZOLOFT <> 50MG	Tab, Light Blue, Cap Shaped, Scored, Film Coated	Sertraline HCl 50 mg	Zoloft by Southwood	58016-0366	Antidepressant
ZOLOFT <> 50MG	Tab, Light Blue, Cap Shaped, Scored, Film Coated	Sertraline HCl 50 mg	Zoloft by Direct Dispensing	57866-6304	Antidepressant
ZOLOFT <> 50MG	Tab, Light Blue, Cap Shaped, Scored, Film Coated	Sertraline HCl 50 mg	Zoloft by Compumed	00403-4721	Antidepressant
ZOLOFT <> 50MG	Tab, Light Blue, Cap Shaped, Scored, Film Coated	Sertraline HCl 50 mg	Zoloft by Heartland	61392-0629	Antidepressant
ZOLOFT <> 50MG	Tab, Light Blue, Cap Shaped, Scored, Film Coated	Sertraline HCl 50 mg	Zoloft by Med Pro	53978-3019	Antidepressant
ZOLOFT <> 50MG	Tab, Light Blue, Cap Shaped, Scored, Film Coated	Sertraline HCl 50 mg	Zoloft by Amerisource	62584-0900	Antidepressant
ZOMIG25	Tab, Yellow, Round, Scored, Film Coated, Zomig 2.5	Zolmitriptan 2.5 mg	Zomig by AstraZeneca	00310-0210	Antimigraine
ZOMIG5	Tab, Pink, Round, Film Coated	Zolmitriptan 5 mg	Zomig by AstraZeneca	00310-0211	Antimigraine
ZONEGRAN100	Cap, White and Red, Opaque, Hard Gel	Zonisamide 100 mg	Zonegran by Eisai	62856-0680	Anticonvulsant
ZONEGRAN100	Cap, White and Red, Opaque, Hard Gel	Zonisamide 100 mg	Zonegran by Elan	59075-0680 Discontinued	Anticonvulsant
ZONEGRAN25	Cap, White, Opaque, Hard Gel	Zonisamide 25 mg	Zonegran by Elan	59075-0681 Discontinued	Anticonvulsant
ZONEGRAN25	Cap, White, Opaque, Hard Gel	Zonisamide 25 mg	Zonegran by Eisai	62856-0681	Anticonvulsant
ZONEGRAN50	Cap, White and Gray, Opaque, Hard Gel	Zonisamide 50 mg	Zonegran by Eisai	62856-0682	Anticonvulsant
ZONEGRAN50	Cap, White and Gray, Opaque, Hard Gel	Zonisamide 50 mg	Zonegran by Elan	59075-0682 Discontinued	Anticonvulsant
ZOP5 <> APO	Tab, White, Round	Zopiclone 5 mg	Imovane by Apotex	Canadian DIN 02245077	Sedative; Hypnotic
ZOVIRAX	Tab, Blue, Shield Shaped, Triangle Logo	Acyclovir 200 mg	Zovirax by GSK	Canadian DIN 00634506	Antiviral
ZOVIRAX	Tab, Blue, Shield Shaped, Triangle Logo	Acyclovir 400 mg	Zovirax by Murfreesboro	51129-1289	Antiviral
ZOVIRAX	Tab, Blue, Shield Shaped, Triangle Logo	Acyclovir 400 mg	Zovirax by Allscripts		Antiviral
ZOVIRAX	Tab, Blue, Shield Shaped, Triangle Logo	Acyclovir 400 mg	Zovirax by GSK	00173-0949	Antiviral
ZOVIRAX	Tab, Blue, Shield Shaped, Triangle Logo	Acyclovir 400 mg	Zovirax by DRX	55045-2293	Antiviral
ZOVIRAX	Tab, Blue, Shield Shaped, Triangle Logo	Acyclovir 400 mg	Zovirax by DSM	63552-0949	Antiviral

ID FRONT <> BACK	DESCRIPTION FRONT <> BACK	INGREDIENT & STRENGTH	BRAND (or Generic Equiv.) by FIRM	NDC#	CLASS; SCH.
ZOVIRAX400	Tab, Pink, Shield Shaped, Triangle Logo	Acyclovir 400 mg	Zovirax by GSK	Canadian DIN 01911627	Antiviral
ZOVIRAX800	Tab, Blue Gray, Oval, Zovirax over 800	Acyclovir 800 mg	Zovirax by PDRX	55289-0564	Antiviral
ZOVIRAX800	Tab, Blue Gray, Oval, Zovirax over 800	Acyclovir 800 mg	Zovirax by Nat Pharmpak	55154-0708	Antiviral
ZOVIRAX800	Tab, Blue Gray, Oval, Zovirax over 800	Acyclovir 800 mg	Zovirax by DSM	63552-0945	Antiviral
ZOVIRAX800	Tab, Blue Gray, Oval, Scored, Zovirax over 800	Acyclovir 800 mg	Zovirax by GSK	Canadian DIN 01911635	Antiviral
ZOVIRAX800	Tab, Blue Gray, Oval, Zovirax over 800	Acyclovir 800 mg	Zovirax by GSK	00173-0945	Antiviral
ZP01	Tab, Red, Round, Coated	Ibuprofen 200 mg	Ibuprofen by Zara Pharm	56489-0001	NSAID
ZP09	Tab, Blue, Oblong, Scored	Acetaminophen 500 mg	Acetaminophen by Zara Pharm	56489-0009	Analgesic
ZT <> 10	Tab, Blue, Round, White Specks, Orally Disintegrating	Zolpidem Tartrate 10 mg	Tovalt ODT by Biovail	64455-0159	Sedative/Hypnotic; C IV
ZT <> 5	Tab, White, Round, Off-White Specks, Orally Disintegrating	Zolpidem Tartrate 5 mg	Tovalt ODT by Biovail	64455-0158	Sedative/Hypnotic; C IV
ZT10	Tab, Peach, Round, Zt/10	Hydrochlorothiazide 12.5 mg, Lisinopril 10 mg	Zestoretic by AstraZeneca	Canadian DIN 02103729	Diuretic; Antihypertensive
ZTM500 <> PFIZER	Tab, Pink, Cap Shaped, Film Coated	Azithromycin 500 mg	Zithromax by Pfizer	00069-3070	Antibiotic
ZVR100	Cap, Blue, White	Zidovudine 100 mg	Retrovir by Dava	67253-0109	Antiviral
ZYBAN150	Tab, Purple, Round, Film Coated, Sustained Release	Bupropion HCl 150 mg	Zyban by Biovail	Canadian DIN 02238441	Antidepressant
ZYBAN150	Tab, Purple, Round, Film Coated	Bupropion HCl 150 mg	Zyban by GSK	00173-0556	Antidepressant
ZYBAN150	Tab, Purple, Round, Film Coated	Bupropion HCl 150 mg	Zyban by DSM	63552-0556	Antidepressant
ZYBAN150	Tab, Purple, Round, Film Coated	Bupropion HCl 150 mg	Zyban by Murfreesboro	51129-1340	Antidepressant
ZYDONE	Cap, White	Acetaminophen 500 mg, Hydrocodone Bitartrate 5 mg	Zydone by Endo		Analgesic; C III
ZYLOPRIM100	Tab, White, Round, Zyloprim 100 on Raised Hexagon	Allopurinol 100 mg	Zyloprim by GSK	00173-0996	Antigout
ZYLOPRIM100	Tab, White, Round, Zyloprim 100 on Raised Hexagon	Allopurinol 100 mg	Zyloprim by DSM	63552-0996	Antigout
ZYLOPRIM300	Tab, Peach, Round, Zyloprim 300 on raised Hexagon, Scored	Allopurinol 300 mg	Zyloprim by DSM	63552-0998	Antigout
ZYLOPRIM300	Tab, Peach, Round, Zyloprim 200 on raised Hexagon, Scored	Allopurinol 300 mg	Zyloprim by Apotheca	12634-0520	Antigout
ZYLOPRIM300	Tab, Peach, Round, Zyloprim 200 on raised Hexagon, Scored	Allopurinol 300 mg	Zyloprim by GSK	00173-0998	Antigout
ZYLOPRIMC9B	Tab, Peach, Round, Scored	Allopurinol 300 mg	Zyloprim by GSK	Canadian DIN 00294322	Antigout
ZYLOPRIMF9B	Tab, White, Round, Scored	Allopurinol 200 mg	Zyloprim by GSK	Canadian DIN 00506370	Antigout
ZYLOPRIMU4A	Tab, White, Round, Scored	Allopurinol 100 mg	Zyloprim by GSK	Canadian DIN 00004588	Antigout
ZYRTEC <> 10	Tab, White, Rectangular, Film Coated	Cetirizine HCl 10 mg	Zyrtec by Southwood	58016-0367	Antihistamine
ZYRTEC <> 10	Tab, White, Rectangular, Film Coated	Cetirizine HCl 10 mg	Zyrtec by Murfreesboro	51129-1379	Antihistamine
ZYRTEC <> 10	Tab, White, Rectangular, Film Coated	Cetirizine HCl 10 mg	Zyrtec by Pfizer	00069-5510	Antihistamine
ZYRTEC <> 5	Tab, White, Rectangular, Film Coated	Cetirizine HCl 5 mg	Zyrtec by Murfreesboro	51129-1192	Antihistamine
ZYRTEC <> 5	Tab, White, Rectangular, Film Coated	Cetirizine HCl 5 mg	Zyrtec by Pfizer	00069-5500	Antihistamine
ZYRTECC10	Tab, Purple, Round, Chewable	Cetirizine HCl 10 mg	Zyrtec by Pfizer	00069-1450	Antihistamine
ZYRTECC5	Tab, Purple, Round, Chewable	Cetirizine HCl 5 mg	Zyrtec by Pfizer	00069-1440	Antihistamine
ZYRTECD	Tab, White, Round, Ex Release, ZYRTEC-D	Cetirizine HCl 5 mg, Pseudoephedrine HCl 120 mg	Zyrtec-D by Pfizer	00069-1630	Antihistamine; Decongestant
ZYVOX400MG	Tab, White, Cap Shaped, Film Coated	Linezolid 400 mg	Zyvox by Pharmacia	00009-5134	Antibiotic
ZYVOX600MG	Tab, White, Cap Shaped, Film Coated	Linezolid 600 mg	Zyvox by Pharmacia	00009-5135	Antibiotic
ZYVOXAM600MG	Tab, White, Oval, Film-Coated	Linezolid 600 mg	Zyvoxam by Pfizer	Canadian DIN 02243684	Antibacterial

Order Book, Web, or PDA

☐ **Yes, I want to start a new subscription to *Ident-A-Drug Reference*.**

☐ Book . . . . $39 ($56 CAN)
☐ Online Version: 1 year access to IdentADrug.com (single-user price) . . . . $39 ($56 CAN)
☐ PDA Version: Includes Online Version with full featured searches . . . . $39 ($56 CAN)
☐ Combination: Online + PDA Versions . . . . $59 ($76 CAN)

☐ **Yes, I want to EXTEND my existing subscription.**

☐ Book: Send me a new edition of the Book as soon as it's published . . . . $39 ($56 CAN)
☐ Online Version: 1 year access to IdentADrug.com (single-user price) . . . . $39 ($56 CAN)
☐ PDA Version: Includes Online Version with full featured searches . . . . $39 ($56 CAN)
☐ Combination: Online + PDA Version . . . . $59 ($76 CAN)

If you are purchasing an *Ident-A-Drug Reference* <u>book</u>, please add:

Only in California, add 9% sales tax ($3.51 per book) . . . . $ _____
Shipping inside U.S. and Canada . . . . FREE
Shipping outside of North America $24

TOTAL . . . . $ _____

---

* PDA Version for Palm or Pocket PC requires min. 6 MB, or 18 MB for photos (memory card supported).

Name _____ Degree _____ Member # (optional) _____
Address _____
City _____ State/Province _____ Zip/Postal Code _____
Email _____ Phone _____

☐ Payment enclosed (please make check payable to *Ident-A-Drug*).
☐ Charge my VISA, MasterCard, American Express, or Discover Card.
   Card No. _____ Exp. Date _____
☐ Bill me with this Purchase Order # _____

Website users will have an opportunity to agree to the license agreement on the website, or get a full refund.

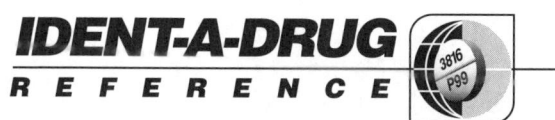

For instant access, order online at IdentADrug.com
Call: (209) 472-2240 • Fax: (209) 472-2249
Email: mail@IdentADrug.com
3120 W. March Lane, PO Box 8190, Stockton, CA 95208

Ident-A-Drug PDA version: access the whole Database wherever you go

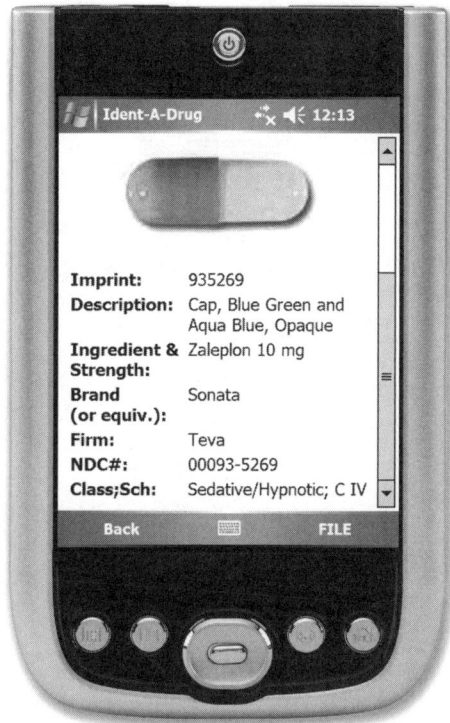

For Palm & Pocket PC

Professionals asked us to put the *Ident-A-Drug Reference* in an easy-to-use handheld format. And we delivered...with a user-friendly version packed with over 39,000 listings, and growing each day.

The handheld version now offers:
- Photos
- Searchable index
- Ingredient and strength listings
- NDC numbers, Canadian DIN, and DEA classifications

(Purchase along with web access and save!)

[X] **YES! I want to purchase the NEW PDA version.**

☐ Handheld version for your PDA (Palm or Pocket PC)*................$39 ($56 CAN)

☐ **SAVE MORE and buy PDA Version plus one year web access** (single-user price)... $59 ($76 CAN)

Name _____ Degree _____ Member # (optional) _____
Address _____
City _____ State/Province _____ Zip/Postal Code _____
Email _____ Phone _____

☐ Payment enclosed (please make check payable to *Ident-A-Drug*).

☐ Charge my VISA, MasterCard, American Express, or Discover Card.
   Card No. _____ Exp. Date _____

☐ Bill me with this Purchase Order # _____

*** PDA Version for Palm or Pocket PC requires min. 6 MB, or 18 MB for photos (memory card supported).**

Website users will have an opportunity to agree to the license agreement on the website, or get a full refund.

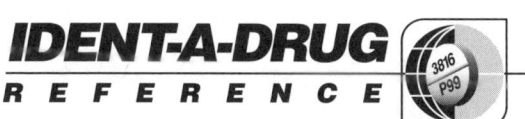

For instant access, order online at IdentADrug.com
Call: (209) 472-2240 • Fax: (209) 472-2249
Email: mail@IdentADrug.com
3120 W. March Lane, PO Box 8190, Stockton, CA 95208

Add access to IdentADrug.com for only $26 and stay current all year!

The *Ident-A-Drug Reference* book was current the day it was printed, but our website is updated each business day with new data.

If you have not yet purchased access to IdentADrug.com, now is a great time to do so. <u>If you already purchased a book, you can add on one year of single-user web access for only $26.</u> You can sign up by phone, mail, fax, or by going to the website.

[X] **YES!** Please give me the reduced price to upgrade my subscription now.*

    * $26 price applies to individuals who have purchased current book and are adding on single-user web access.

- ☐ Add Online Version to my subscription: 1 year access to IdentADrug.com (single-user price) .. $26 ($38 CAN)
- ☐ Book: Send me a new edition of the Book as soon as it's published................ $39 ($56 CAN)
  - In California only, add 9% sales tax ($3.51 per book)
  - If shipping outside of the US or Canada, add $24 postage
- ☐ Give me the PDA Version of *Ident-A-Drug* .... $39 ($56 CAN)

Name _____ Degree _____ Member # (optional) _____

Address _____

City _____ State/Province _____ Zip/Postal Code _____

Email _____ Phone _____

- ☐ Payment enclosed (please make check payable to *Ident-A-Drug*).
- ☐ Charge my VISA, MasterCard, American Express, or Discover Card.
  - Card No. _____ Exp. Date _____
- ☐ Bill me with this Purchase Order # _____

If you have not yet purchased an *Ident-A-Drug Reference* book, you can use the order forms in this book to order the book, Web access, or PDA version in any combination you choose. Or simply call us with your order.

Website users will have an opportunity to agree to the license agreement on the website, or get a full refund.

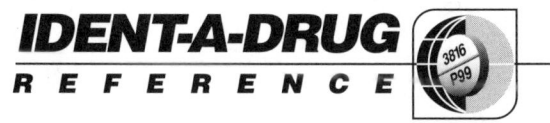

For instant access, order online at IdentADrug.com
Call: (209) 472-2240 ♦ Fax: (209) 472-2249
Email: mail@IdentADrug.com
3120 W. March Lane, PO Box 8190, Stockton, CA 95208

Add access to IdentADrug.com for only $26 and stay current all year!

The *Ident-A-Drug Reference* book was current the day it was printed, but our website is updated each business day with new data.

If you have not yet purchased access to IdentADrug.com, now is a great time to do so. <u>If you already purchased a book, you can add on one year of single-user web access for only $26</u>. You can sign up by phone, mail, fax, or by going to the website.

[X] **YES!** Please give me the reduced price to upgrade my subscription now.*

* $26 price applies to individuals who have purchased current book and are adding on single-user web access.

☐ Add Online Version to my subscription: 1 year access to IdentADrug.com (single-user price) .. $26 ($38 CAN)
☐ Book: Send me a new edition of the Book as soon as it's published. . . . . $39 ($56 CAN)
    In California only, add 9% sales tax ($3.51 per book)
    If shipping outside of the US or Canada, add $24 postage
☐ Give me the PDA Version of *Ident-A-Drug* . . . . $39 ($56 CAN)

Name _____ Degree _____ Member # (optional) _____
Address _____
City _____ State/Province _____ Zip/Postal Code _____
Email _____ Phone _____

☐ Payment enclosed (please make check payable to *Ident-A-Drug*).
☐ Charge my VISA, MasterCard, American Express, or Discover Card.
   Card No. _____ Exp. Date _____
☐ Bill me with this Purchase Order # _____

If you have not yet purchased an *Ident-A-Drug Reference* book, you can use the order forms in this book to order the book, Web access, or PDA version in any combination you choose. Or simply call us with your order.

Website users will have an opportunity to agree to the license agreement on the website, or get a full refund.

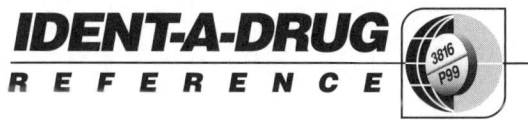

For instant access, order online at IdentADrug.com
Call: (209) 472-2240 ♦ Fax: (209) 472-2249
Email: mail@IdentADrug.com
3120 W. March Lane, PO Box 8190, Stockton, CA 95208